Stroke

Stroke

Pathophysiology, Diagnosis, and Management

SIXTH EDITION

James C. Grotta, MD
Director, Stroke Research
Clinical Innovation and Research Institute;
Director, Mobile Stroke Unit Consortium
Memorial Hermann Hospital-Texas Medical Center
Houston, Texas, USA

Gregory W. Albers, MD
Professor of Neurology and Neurological Sciences
Director, Stanford Stroke Center
Stanford School of Medicine
Stanford, CA, USA

Joseph P. Broderick, MD
Professor, Department of Neurology and Rehabilitation Medicine;
Director, University of Cincinnati Neuroscience Institute
Cincinnati, OH, USA

Scott E. Kasner, MD
Professor, Department of Neurology
Perelman School of Medicine
University of Pennsylvania;
Director, Comprehensive Stroke Center
University of Pennsylvania Health System
Philadelphia, PA, USA

Eng H. Lo, PhD
Professor of Neurology and Radiology
Massachusetts General Hospital
Harvard Medical School
Boston, MA, USA

A. David Mendelow, MB BCh, PhD
William Leech Professor of Neurosurgery
Newcastle University
Consultant Neurosurgeon
Department of Neurosurgery
Royal Victoria Infirmary
Newcastle upon Tyne, UK

Ralph L. Sacco, MD, MS
Professor and Olemberg Chair of Neurology;
Miller Professor of Neurology, Public Health Sciences, Human Genetics, and Neurosurgery;
Executive Director, McKnight Brain Institute;
Chief of Neurology, Jackson Memorial Hospital
Miller School of Medicine
University of Miami
Miami, FL, USA

Lawrence K.S. Wong, MD
Mok Hing Yiu Professor of Medicine
Chief of Neurology
Department of Medicine and Therapeutics
The Chinese University of Hongkong
Prince of Wales Hospital
Shatin, Hong Kong Special Administrative Region
China

ELSEVIER

For additional online content visit www.expertconsult.com

ELSEVIER

First edition 1986
Second edition 1992
Third edition 1998
Fourth edition 2004
Fifth edition 2011
Sixth edition 2016

Notices

Knowledge and best practice in this field are constantly changing. As new research and experience broaden our understanding, changes in research methods, professional practices, or medical treatment may become necessary.

Practitioners and researchers must always rely on their own experience and knowledge in evaluating and using any information, methods, compounds, or experiments described herein. In using such information or methods they should be mindful of their own safety and the safety of others, including parties for whom they have a professional responsibility.

With respect to any drug or pharmaceutical products identified, readers are advised to check the most current information provided (i) on procedures featured or (ii) by the manufacturer of each product to be administered, to verify the recommended dose or formula, the method and duration of administration, and contraindications. It is the responsibility of practitioners, relying on their own experience and knowledge of their patients, to make diagnoses, to determine dosages and the best treatment for each individual patient, and to take all appropriate safety precautions.

To the fullest extent of the law, neither the Publisher nor the authors, contributors, or editors, assume any liability for any injury and/or damage to persons or property as a matter of products liability, negligence or otherwise, or from any use or operation of any methods, products, instructions, or ideas contained in the material herein.

ISBN: 978-0-323-29544-4
INK: 978-0-323-32806-7

Senior Content Strategist: Lotta Kryhl
Senior Content Development Specialist: Nani Clansey
Content Coordinator: Trinity Hutton
Senior Project Manager: Beula Christopher
Design: Christian Bilbow
Illustration Manager: Karen Giacomucci
Illustrator: Angie MacAllister
Marketing Manager: Deborah Davis

Printed in United States of America

Last digit is the print number: 9 8 7 6 5 4 3

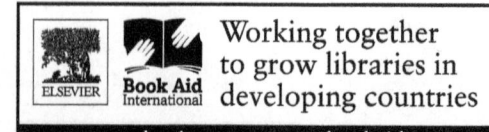

Contents

Foreword to the Sixth Edition

This, the sixth edition of *Stroke*, has passed from the hands of the last of the original four editors to a distinguished and experienced group now numbering eight. The chapter numbers have also increased from the original 61 to 76. The content of these chapters is altered by the very advances the first-edition authors had hoped for.

The few involved in the brief hallway discussion that led to the first edition could not foresee – but certainly hoped for – the expansion in the scope of interest in the field. In 1986 it was still struggling for independence as a justifiable multidisciplinary specialty. Considerable latitude existed for management using experience-based bias, heavy reliance on clinical semiology, and for some an uncertainty of the value of imaging. Few clinicians focused disproportionately on stroke, and most of them were in major centers. Many outside the field still thought of stroke as a bed-occupying distraction lacking therapy, suitable for early discharge. "It's just a stroke" was a common observation.

Contrast that with today, where stroke is the main inpatient service for the clinical neurosciences – for many also including a separate neuro-intensive care unit. Success in very early therapy has changed the attitude of patients toward the disease. Career efforts are made from many disciplines, subspecialty ACGME certification exists, heavy reliance is placed on imaging, emergency management is focused on the very earliest intervention, sophisticated statistical models dictate plans for clinical trials, and we are expected to "Get with the Guidelines".

Along the way semiology has properly given way to pathophysiology as revealed by imaging, biomarkers, and intervention – both physical and medical. While there is an asymptote of treatment effect in sight, a resurgence of interest in semiology is in the offing. Given the current opportunities to understand brain reorganization, ways will eventually be found to ameliorate those syndromes that occur despite the best efforts at their prevention. This emeritus editor sees a bright future ahead.

J. P. Mohr, MD, MS
Daniel Sciarra Professor of Neurology
Department of Neurology
Columbia University
New York, NY, USA

Preface

Welcome to the 6th edition of *Stroke: Pathophysiology, Diagnosis, and Management*. Much has changed in the world of cerebrovascular disease since the first edition edited by Barnett, Mohr, Stein, and Yatsu in 1986. One thing that has remained constant, however, is that this textbook continues to be the most authoritative resource in the field of stroke. Nevertheless, a major milestone with this text has occurred with the baton of editorship being passed from JP Mohr, the sole remaining editor from the first edition, to a new generation of editors to carry the text forward into future decades. Dr Mohr has left an indelible mark on the body of knowledge surrounding many aspects of cerebrovascular disease, including his scholarship and leadership as senior author of *Stroke: Pathophysiology, Diagnosis, and Management*. He will be missed, though the reader will recognize many of his teachings and observations preserved throughout; especially in the section on Clinical Manifestations.

While the basic organization of the text is maintained, and the various sections and many of the chapter titles are the same, there have been some important changes and additions. Within most sections, chapters have been re-ordered into a more logical sequence. The titles of many chapters have been updated to reflect the new information contained in each, and the authorships altered to include clinicians/investigators who are current experts on each topic. Several new chapters have been added, and most importantly, there has been an almost complete change in the cadre of editors.

The editors reflect the "new" generation of senior leadership in the field. The section editor of Pathophysiology has been turned over from Mike Moskowitz to Eng Lo. This was an easy transition since the two have worked together at the same institution for many years, and Dr Lo's expertise in cell signaling and cell death mechanisms reflects the current focus in the understanding of the process of cell injury after stroke. The section contains new chapters on the Neurovascular Unit, and on Mechanisms of Cerebral Hemorrhage. The Epidemiology and Risk Factor section has transitioned from Phil Wolf to Ralph Sacco. Dr Sacco has been a leader in the understanding of ethnic stroke trends based on his work with the Northern Manhattan study and has led the American Heart Association and American Stroke Association as they have focused on stroke risk factors and prevention. Dr Mohr's section on Clinical Manifestations is now edited by Lawrence Wong, a world-class clinical neurologist, who not only understands classical clinical neurology, but also has identified how these may differ in various parts of the world, in particular Asia with its huge burden of stroke.

The section on Specific Conditions and Stroke, also previously edited by Dr Mohr, is now edited by Scott Kasner. Dr Kasner's career as a Vascular Neurologist has paralleled the explosive growth in our ability to diagnose and understand the multifaceted causes and manifestations of stroke, in particular dissections and other vasculopathies. Several new chapters have been added to this section; Stroke Related to Surgery and Other Procedures, Cryptogenic Stroke, and Cerebral Venous Thrombosis. Nowhere has technology advanced faster than in diagnosis, and Greg Albers now assumes editorship of the Diagnostic Studies section from Rüdiger von Kummer. Dr Albers has been a pioneer in the application of brain imaging, in particular MRI to identify, prognosticate and guide treatment of acute stroke, and his innovations reflect the growing integration of imaging into all aspects of stroke management.

James Grotta remains the editor of the section on Medical Therapy which still centers on the appropriate use of tPA – a topic on which he has devoted a substantial part of his productive career. The section now includes a new chapter on Interventions to Improve Recovery after Stroke, reflecting emerging and ongoing research in this area. Exciting new data have been generated in several aspects of Interventional Therapy, and the editorship of that section has passed from Rüdiger von Kummer to Joseph Broderick, who has led one of the major clinical trials in that area. As this text goes to press, recent results and perspectives in the field of endovascular thrombectomy are outlined in Dr Broderick's Introduction to that section. Finally, David Mendelow brings his perspective as a clinical trialist in the surgical management of intracranial hemorrhage to the editorship of the Surgical Therapy section, which he assumes from Marc Mayberg. Under his supervision, the previous 14 chapters in the section have been distilled into eight, all of which have been updated with important information.

The text continues to be developed and guided by experienced and able hands at Elsevier, namely Charlotta Kryhl, Senior Content Strategist, and Nani Clansey, Senior Content Development Specialist.

The 6th edition of *Stroke: Pathophysiology, Diagnosis, and Management* includes an interactive online version housed on www.expertconsult.inkling.com, which can also be downloaded for offline use on phones or tablets.

James C. Grotta, MD
on behalf of the Editors

List of Contributors

Harold P. Adams Jr., MD
Professor
Department of Neurology
University of Iowa
Iowa City, IA, USA

Tarek Y. El Ahmadieh, MD
Neurosurgery Resident
The University of Texas Southwestern Medical Center
Dallas, TX, USA

Gregory W. Albers, MD
Professor of Neurology and Neurological Sciences
Director, Stanford Stroke Center
Stanford School of Medicine
Stanford, CA, USA

Andrei V. Alexandrov, MD, RVT
Semmes-Murphey Professor and Chairman
Department of Neurology
The University of Tennessee Health Science Center
Memphis, TN, USA

Josef Anrather, MD
Associate Professor of Neuroscience
Feil Family Brain and Mind Research Institute
Weill Cornell Medical College
New York, NY, USA

Ken Arai, PhD
The Neuroprotection Research Laboratory
Department of Radioloty and Neurology
Massachusetts General Hospital
Harvard Medical School
Boston, MA, USA

Jaroslaw (Jarek) Aronowski, MD, PhD
Professor and Vice Chair
Department of Neurology
Roy M. and Phyllis Gough Huffington;
Chair in Neurology
Director of Research – Vascular Neurology Program
Houston, TX, USA

Roland N. Auer, MD, PhD, FRCPC
Hôpital Ste-Justine
Département de Pathologie
Université de Montréal
Québec, Canada

Issam A. Awad, MD, MSc, FACS
The John Harper Seeley Professor of Surgery (Neurosurgery) and Neurology
Director of Neurovascular Surgery
University of Chicago Medicine
Chicago, IL, USA

Hakan Ay, MD
Associate Professor
Stroke Service, Department of Neurology
A.A. Martinos Center for Biomedical Imaging, Department of Radiology
Massachusetts General Hospital, Harvard Medical School
Boston, MA, USA

Selva Baltan, MD, PhD
Assistant Staff
Department of Neurosciences
Lerner Research Institute
Cleveland Clinic
Cleveland, OH, USA

Hunt H. Batjer, MD
Lois C.A. and Darwin E. Smith Distinguished Chair in Neurological Surgery
The University of Texas Southwestern Medical Center
Dallas, TX, USA

Oscar R. Benavente, MD, FRCPC
Professor and Director of Stroke Research
Department of Medicine, Division of Neurology
Brain Research Center
University of British Columbia
Vancouver, Canada

Bernard R. Bendok, MD, MSCI
Professor and chair of Neurological Surgery
Department of Neurological Surgery
Mayo Clinic
Phoenix, AZ, USA

Eric M. Bershad, MD
Assistant Professor of Neurology and Space Medicine
Associate Neurology Residency Program Director
Section of Neurocritical Care and Vascular Neurology
Department of Neurology, Baylor College of Medicine
Houston, TX, USA

Leo H. Bonati, MD
Head Intermediate Care Stroke Unit
Department of Neurology
University Hospital Basel
Basel, Switzerland;
Stroke Research Group
UCL Institute of Neurology
Department of Brain Repair and Rehabilitation
The National Hospital for Neurology and Neurosurgery
London, UK

Markus J. Bookland, MD
Associate Professor, Division of Neurosurgery
Connecticut Children's Medical Center
Hartford, CT, USA

Marie-Germaine Bousser, MD
Service de Neurologie
Hôpital Lariboisiére
Université Paris Denis Diderot
Paris, France

John A. Braca III, MD, MMS
Chief Resident, Department of Neurosurgery
Loyola University Medical Center
Maywood, IL, USA

Joseph P. Broderick, MD
Professor, Department of Neurology and Rehabilitation Medicine;
Director, University of Cincinnati Neuroscience Institute
Cincinnati, OH, USA

Martin M. Brown, MD
Professor of Stroke Medicine
Institute of Neurology
University College of London
London, UK

Wendy E. Brown, MD
Department of Neurosciences
Sutter Medical Center Sacramento
Sacramento, CA, USA

John C. M. Brust, MD
Professor of Clinical Neurology
Columbia University College of Physicians and Surgeons
New York Neurological Institute
New York, NY, USA

Cheryl Bushnell, MD, MHS
Associate Professor of Neurology
Director, Wake Forest Baptist Stroke Center
Wake Forest Baptist School of Medicine
Medical Center Boulevard
Winston Salem, NC, USA

Julian Bösel, MD
Department of Neurology
University Heidelberg
Heidelberg, Germany

Patrícia Canhão, MD, PhD
MD, Invited Professor of Neurology
Neurosciences Department, Neurology Service
Hospital de Santa Maria
University of Lisbon
Av. Prof. Egas Moniz
Lisboa, Portugal

Louis R. Caplan, MD
Professor of Neurology
Harvard Medical School
Senior Member
Division of Cerebrovascular Disease
Beth Israel Deaconess Medical Center
Boston, MA, USA

Mar Castellanos, MD, PhD
University Hospital Doctor Josep Trueta
Department of Neurology/Biomedical Research Institute
Girona, Spain

Angel Chamorro, MD
Director, Comprehensive Stroke Center
Hospital Clinic of Barcelona
University of Barcelona and Institut d'Investigacions Biomediques ugust PiSnyer (IIDIBAPS)
Barcelona, Spain

James P. Chandler, MD
Professor of Neurological Surgery
Northwestern Memorial Hospital
Chicago, IL, USA

Jun Chen, MD, PhD
Professor
Department of Neurology
University of Pittsburgh
Pittsburgh, PA, USA

Michael Chopp, PhD
Department of Physics
Oakland University
Rochester, Michigan Neurology Department, Research Division
Henry Ford Hospital
Detroit, MI, USA

Sophocles Chrissobolis, PhD
Vascular Biology and Immunopharmacology Group
Department of Pharmacology
Monash University
Victoria, Australia

Hugues Chabriat, MD
Service de Neurologie
Hôpital Lariboisiére
Université Paris Denis Diderot
INSERM U1161
Paris, France

Steven C. Cramer, MD
Professor
Departments of Neurology, Anatomy and Neurobiology, and Physical Medicine and Rehabilitation
University of California, Irvine
Irvine, CA, USA

Brett L. Cucchiara, MD
Associate Professor of Neurology
Department of Neurology
Comprehensive Stroke Center
University of Pennsylvania Medical Center
Philadelphia, PA, USA

Mark J. Dannenbaum, MD
Assistant Professor
The Vivian L. Smith Department of Neurosurgery
Brigham and Women's Hospital
Harvard Medical School
Boston, MA, USA

Patricia H. Davis, MD
Professor Emeritus
Department of Neurology
University of Iowa
Iowa City, IA, USA

Ted M. Dawson, MD, PhD
Neuroregeneration and Stem Cell Programs
Institute for Cell Engineering
Departments of Neurology, Neuroscience, and Pharmacology and Molecular Sciences
Johns Hopkins University School of Medicine
Baltimore, MD, USA

Valina L. Dawson, PhD
Neuroregeneration and Stem Cell Programs
Institute for Cell Engineering
Departments of Neurology
Solomon H. Snyder Department of Neuroscience and Physiology
Johns Hopkins University School of Medicine
Baltimore, MD, USA

Arthur L. Day, MD
Director of Cerebrovascular Center
Brigham and Women's Hospital
Boston, MA, USA

Gregory J. del Zoppo, MD
Professor of Medicine (in Hematology)
Adjunct Professor of Neurology
University of Washington School of Medicine
Harborview Medical Center
Seattle, WA, USA

Hans-Christoph Diener, MD, PhD
Professor
Department of Neurology and Stroke Center
University Hospital Essen
University Duisburg-Essen
Essen, Germany

Marco R. Di Tullio, MD
Professor of Medicine at CUMC
Associate Director, Cardiovascular Ultrasound Laboratories
Director, Echocardiography Research
Director, CME Cardiology Grand Rounds
Columbia University Medical Center
New York, NY, USA

Bruce H. Dobkin, MD, FRCP
Professor of Neurology
Director, Neurologic Rehabilitation Program
Department of Neurology
Geffen School of Medicine at UCLA
Los Angeles, CA, USA

Imanuel Dzialowski, MD
Senior Physician, Stroke Neurologist
Department of Neurology
Elblandklinikm Meissen Academic Teaching Hospital of Technical University Dresden
Dresden, Germany

Alexis Economos, MD
Post-doctoral Fellow
Harvard Medical School/Partners
Neurology
Brigham and Women's Hospital
Department of Neurology
Boston, MA, USA

Christopher S. Eddleman, MD
Neurosurgeon
Hendrick Medical Center
Abilene, TX, USA

Mitchell S.V. Elkind, MD, MS, FAAN, FAHA
Professor of Neurology and Epidemiology
Fellowships Director, Department of Neurology
Columbia University
New York, NY, USA

Valery L. Feigin, MD, MSc, PhD, FAAN
Professor of Epidemiology and Neurology
National Institute for Stroke and Applied Neurosciences
Faculty of Health and Environmental Studies
AUT University
Auckland, New Zealand

José M. Ferro, MD, PhD
Head of Neurosciences Department
Professor and Chairman of Neurology
Neurosciences Department, Neurology Service
Hospital de Santa Maria
University of Lisbon
Av. Prof. Egas Moniz
Lisboa, Portugal

J. Max Findlay, MD, PhD, FRCSC
Clinical Professor
University of Alberta
Alberta, Canada

Karen L. Furie, MD
Chief of Neurology at Rhode Island
The Miriam and Bradley Hospitals
Chair of Neurology
Warren Alpert Medical School of Brown University
Providence, RI, USA

Matthew R. Fusco, MD
Assistant Professor, Neurological Surgery
Vanderbilt University Medical Center
Nashville, TN, USA

Thalia S. Field, MD, FRCPC
Associate Professor, Department of Medicine, Division of Neurology
Brain Research Center
University of British Columbia
Vancouver, Canada

Sasikhan Geibprasert, MD
Lecturer, Department of Radiology
Ramathibodi Hospital
Mahidol University
Bangkok, Thailand

Anna P. Gensic, MD
Assistant Professor
Department of Emergency Medicine
University of Cincinnati
Cincinnati, OH, USA

Y. Pierre Gobin, MD
Professor of Radiology in Neurology and Neurosurgery
Director, Interventional Neurology
Weill Cornell Medical Center
New York Presbyterian Hospital
New York, NY, USA

Mark P. Goldberg, MD
Professor and Chair
Department of Neurology
University of Texas Southwestern Medical Center
Dallas, TX, USA

Larry B. Goldstein, MD, FAAN, FANA, FAHA
Ruth L. Works Professor and Chairman, Department of Neurology
Co-Director, Kentucky Neuroscience Institute
KY Clinic – University of Kentucky
Lexington, KY, USA

Nicole R. Gonzales, MD
Associate Professor of Neurology
Department of Neurology
University of Texas Medical School-Houston
Houston, TX, USA

Matthew J. Gounis, PhD
Director, New England Center for Stroke Research;
Assistant Professor
Department of Radiology
University of Massachusetts Medical School
Worcester, MA, USA

Steven M. Greenberg, MD, PhD
Professor of Neurology
Harvard Medical School
John J. Conway Endowed Chair
Department of Neurology
Massachusetts General Hospital
Director
Hemorrhagic Stroke Program
Massachusetts General Hospital
Boston, MA, USA

Barbara A. Gregson, PhD
Neurosurgical Trials Director
Newcastle University
Newcastle upon Tyne, UK

James C. Grotta, MD
Director, Stroke Research
Clinical Innovation and Research Institute;
Director, Mobile Stroke Unit Consortium
Memorial Hermann Hospital-Texas Medical Center
Houston, Texas, USA

Jose Gutierrez, MD, MPH
Assistant Professor of Neurology
Department of Neurology
College of Physicians and Surgeons
Columbia University
New York, NY, USA

Werner Hacke, MD, PhD
Chief of the Department
Department of Neurology
University of Heidelberg
Heidelberg, Germany

John M. Hallenbeck, MD
Senior Investigator
Clinical Investigations Section
Stroke Branch, NINDS
Bethesda, MD, USA

Michal Haršány, MD
PhD student
International Clinical Research Center, St. Anne's University Hospital, Brno, Czech Republic
Department of Neurology, St. Anne's University Hospital and Medical Faculty of Masaryk University, Brno, Czech Republic
Comprehensive Stroke Center, Department of Neurology
University of Alabama at Birmingham
Birmingham, AL, USA

Daniel M. Heiferman, MD
Resident Physician
Department of Neurosurgery
Loyola University Medical Center
Maywood, IL, USA

Shunichi Homma, MD
Margaret Milliken Hatch Professor of Medicine
Associate Chief, Cardiology Division
Director, Noninvasive Cardiac Imaging
Columbia University Medical center
New York, NY, USA

George Howard, DrPH, FAHA
Department of Biostatistics
School of Public Health
University of Alabama at Birmingham
Birmingham, AL, USA

Virginia J. Howard, PhD, FAHA, FSCT
Department of Epidemiology
School of Public Health
University of Alabama at Birmingham
Birmingham, AL, USA

Jee-Yeon Hwang, PhD
Associate
Dominick P. Purpura Department of Neuroscience
Albert Einstein College of Medicine
New York, NY, USA

Costantino Iadecola, MD
Anne Parrish Titzell Professor of Neurology and Neuroscience
Director, Feil Family Brain and Mind Research Institute
Weill Cornell Medical College
New York, NY, USA

Reza Jahan, MD
Professor
Division of Interventional Neuroradiology
Department of Radiology
David Geffen School of Medicine at UCLA
Los Angeles, CA, USA

Anne Joutel, MD
INSERM U1161
Faculté de Médecine Villemin
Paris, France

Eric Jüttler, MD, MSc
Assistant Medical Director
Department of Neurology
RKU - University and Rehabilitation Hospitals Ulm
Ulm, Germany

Carlos S. Kase, MD
Professor of Neurology
Boston University School of Medicine
Neurologist-in-Chief and Chair
Department of Neurology
Boston Medical Center
Boston, MA, USA

Scott E. Kasner, MD
Professor, Department of Neurology
Perelman School of Medicine
University of Pennsylvania;
Director, Comprehensive Stroke Center
University of Pennsylvania Health System
Philadelphia, PA, USA

Mira Katan, MD, MS
Oberassistentin
Department of Neurology
University Hospital of Zurich
Zurich, Switzerland

Javed Khader Eliyas, MD
Resident, Section of Neurosurgery
University of Chicago Medicine
Chicago, IL, USA

Muhib Khan, MD
Assistant Professor
Department of Neurology
The Warren Alpert Medical School of Brown University
Providence, RI, USA

Helen Kim, PhD
Associate Professor
Department of Anesthesia and Perioperative Care
Department of Epidemiology and Biostatistics
Institute for Human Genetics
Center for Cerebrovascular Research
University of California
San Francisco, CA, USA

Chelsea S. Kidwell, MD
Professor, Vice Chair of Neurology
Departments of Neurology and Medical Imaging
University of Arizona
Tucson, AZ, USA

Jong S. Kim, MD, PhD
Professor
Department of Neurology
University of Ulsan, Asan Medical Center
Seoul, Korea

Timo Krings, MD, PhD, FRCP
Professor, Departments of Medical Imaging and Surgery
Director, Neuroradiology Program, University of Toronto
Ontorio, Canada

Rita Krishnamurthi, BSc, MApplSc, PhD
National Institute for Stroke and Applied Neurosciences
Faculty of Health and Environmental Studies
AUT University
Auckland, New Zealand

Tobias Kurth, MD, ScD
Research Director
Inserm Research Center for Epidemiology and Biostatistics
University of Bordeaux, Team Neuroepidemiololgy
Bordeaux, France

Catherine Lamy, MD
Praticien Hospitalier
Université Paris Descartes
Service de Neurologie et Unité Neurovasculaire
Hôpital Sainte-Anne
Paris, France

Maarten G. Lansberg, MD, PhD
Associate Professor of Neurology and Neurological Sciences
Stanford Stroke Center
Stanford, CA, USA

Elad I. Levy, MD, MBA
Professor and Chair of Neurosurgery and Professor of Radiology
University at Buffalo, State University of New York
Medical Director of Neuroendovascular Services
Gates Vascular Institute at Kaleida Health
Co-Director, Gates Stroke Center at Kaleida Health
Co-Director, Toshiba Stroke and Vascular Research Center
Buffalo, NY, USA

David S. Liebeskind, MD, FAAN, FAHA, FANA
Professor of Neurology
Director, Neurovascular Imaging Research Core
Director, Outpatient Stroke and Neurovascular Programs
Director, UCLA Cerebral Blood Flow Laboratory
Director, UCLA Vascular Neurology Residency Program
UCLA Department of Neurology
Los Angeles, CA, USA

Eng H. Lo, PhD
Professor of Neurology and Radiology
Massachusetts General Hospital
Harvard Medical School
Boston, MA, USA

Christopher M. Loftus, MD
Treasurer, WFNS
Chair, AANS International Programs
Professor and Chairman, Department of Neurosurgery
Professor of Neurology
Loyola University Stritch School of Medicine
Maywood, IL, USA

Patrick D. Lyden, MD
Chair, Department of Neurology
Cedars-Sinai Medical Center
Los Angeles, CA, USA

Jean-Louis Mas, MD
Professor of Neurology
Department of Neurology
Université Paris Descartes
Hôpital Sainte-Anne
Paris, France

Francesco Massari, MD, PhD
NeuroInterventional Radiology Fellow
Division Neuroimaging and Intervention (NII)
Department of Radiology
University of Massachusetts
Worcester, MA, USA

Jason M. Meckler, MD
Neurologist
Norton Neurology Services
Louisville, KY, USA

A. David Mendelow, MB BCh, PhD
William Leech Professor of Neurosurgery
Newcastle University
Consultant Neurosurgeon
Department of Neurosurgery
Royal Victoria Infirmary
Newcastle upon Tyne, UK

James F. Meschia, MD
Professor of Neurology
Chair, Department of Neurology
Mayo Clinic Florida
Jacksonville, FL, USA

Steven R. Messé, MD
Associate Professor
Department of Neurology
The University of Pennsylvania
Philadelphia, PA, USA

Patrick Mitchel, FRCS, PhD
Consultant and Senior Lecturer Neurosurgery
Royal Victoria Infirmary
University of Newcastle
Newcastle upon Tyne, UK

Lewis B. Morgenstern, MD
Director of the Stroke Program
Professor of Neurology, Epidemiology
Emergency Medicine and Neurosurgery
The University of Michigan Medical School and School of Public Health
Ann Arbor, MI, USA

Maxim Mokin, MD, PhD
Assistant Professor of Neurology and Neurosurgery
Department of Neurosurgery and Brain Repair
University of South Florida
Tampa, FL, USA

Michael A. Moskowitz, MD
Professor of Neurology
Harvard-MIT Division of Health Science and Technology
Boston, MA, USA

Michael T. Mullen, MD, MS
Assistant Professor
Department of Neurology
University of Pennsylvania
School of Medicine
Philadelphia, PA, USA

Maiken Nedergaard, MD, DMSc
Frank P. Smith Professor of Neurosurgery
Department of Neurosurgery
University of Rochester Medical Center
School of Medicine and Dentistry
Rochester, NY, USA

Hermann Neugebauer, MD, MSc
Clinical Fellow
Department of Neurology
RKU – University and Rehabilitation Hospitals Ulm
Ulm, Germany

David W. Newell, MD
Chief of Neurosciences
Swedish Neuroscience Institute
Seattle, WA, USA

Bo Norrving, MD
Professor in Neurology
Department of Clinical Sciences, Neurology
Lund University
Lund, Sweden

Martin O'Donnell, MB, PhD
National University of Ireland Galway
Galway, Ireland

Dimitry Ofengeim, PhD
Research Fellow in Cell Biology (EXT)
Harvard Medical School
Boston, MA, USA

Jun Ogata, MD, PhD
President
Hirakata General Hospital for Developmental Disorders
Osaka, Japan

Christopher S. Ogilvy, MD
Robert G. and A. Jean Ojemann Professor of Surgery
(Neurosurgery)
Director
Endovascular and Operative Neurovascular Surgery
Harvard Medical School
Massachusetts General Hospital
Boston, MA, USA

Arthur M. Pancioli, MD, FACEP
Professor and Chairman
Department of Emergency Medicine
University of Cincinnati, College of Medicine
Cincinnati, OH, USA

Kaushik Parsha, MD
Research Assistant
Department of Neurology
University of Texas
Health Science Center
Houston, TX, USA

Mark W. Parsons, MD, PhD
Director Acute Stroke Services
Department Neurology, John Hunter Hospital;
Senior Staff Neurologist
Department Neurology, John Hunter Hospital;
Professor of Medicine (Neurology), Faculty of Health
University of Newcastle
Newcastle, Australia

Ludmila Pawlikowska, PhD
Associate Professor
Department of Anesthesia and Perioperative Care
Institute for Human Genetics
Center for Cerebrovascular Research
University of California
San Francisco, CA, USA

Adriana Pérez, MS, PhD
Associate Professor
Department of Biostatistics, The University of Texas Health Science Center at Houston
School of Public Health, Austin Regional Campus
Austin, TX, USA

Miguel A. Perez-Pinzon, PhD
Cerebral Vascular Disease Research Laboratories
Department of Neurology and Neuroscience Program
Miller School of Medicine
University of Miami
Miami, FL, USA

William J. Powers, MD
H. Houston Merritt Distinguished Professor and Chair
Department of Neurology
University of North Carolina at Chapel Hill
Chapel Hill, NC, USA

Volker Puetz, MD
Senior Physician, Stroke Neurologist
Department of Neurology
Dresden University Stroke Center
Technical University Dresden
Dresden, Germany

Ajit S. Puri, MD
Assistant Professor of Radiology and Neurosurgery
Co-Director, Division of Neurointerventional Surgery
Director, Neurointerventional Fellowship Program
Department of Radiology
University of Massachusetts Medical Center
Worcester, MA, USA

Bruce R. Ransom, MD, PhD
Magnuson Professor and Chair
Department of Neurology
University of Washington
Seattle, WA, USA

Risto O. Roine, MD, PhD
Professor of Neurology, Chairman
Division of Clinical Neurosciences
Turku University Hospital
University of Turku
Turku, Finland

Tatjana Rundek, MD, PhD, FANA
Professor of Neurology and Public Health Sciences
Vice Chair, Clinical and Translational Research in Neurology
Department of Neurology
University of Miami Miller School of Medicine
Miami, FL, USA

Jonathan J. Russin, MD
Cerebrovascular Fellow
Division of Neurological Surgery
Barrow Neurological Institute
Phoenix, AZ, USA

Ralph L. Sacco, MD, MS
Professor and Olemberg Chair of Neurology;
Miller Professor of Neurology, Public Health Sciences, Human Genetics, and Neurosurgery;
Executive Director, McKnight Brain Institute;
Chief of Neurology, Jackson Memorial Hospital
Miller School of Medicine
University of Miami
Miami, FL, USA

Robert F. Spetzler, MD
Director, Barrow Neurological Institute
J. N. Harber Chairman and Professor of Neurological Surgery
Division of Neurological Surgery
Barrow Neurological Institute
Phoenix, AZ, USA

Ronald J. Sattenberg, MD
Louisville, KY, USA

Jeffrey L. Saver, MD, FAHA, FAAN
Professor of Neurology
David Geffen School of Medicine at UCLA
Director, UCLA Stroke Center
University of California, Los Angeles
Los Angeles, CA, USA

Sean I. Savitz, MD
Frank M. Yatsu Chair in Neurology
Professor of Neurology
Director, Stroke Program
University of Texas Medical School at Houston
Houston, TX, USA

Silvia Schönenberger, MD
Department of Neurology
University Heidelberg
Heidelberg, Germany

Sudha Seshadri, MD
Professor of Neurology
Boston University School of Medicine
Boston, MA, USA

Vijay K. Sharma, MD
Associate Professor
Yong Loo Lin School of Medicine
National University of Singapore;
Senior Consultant
Division of Neurology
University Medicine Cluster, National University Health System
Singapore

Yejie Shi, MD, PhD
Postdoctoral Associate
Department of Neurology
University of Pittsburgh
Pittsburgh, PA, USA

Ashkan Shoamanesh, MD, FRCPC
Assistant Professor of Medicine (Neurology)
Marta and Owen Boris Chair in Stroke Research and Care
Department of Medicine, Division of Neurology
McMaster University
Hamilton, Ontario, Canada

Gerald Silverboard, MD
Pediatric Neurologist
Atlanta Family Neurology
Atlanta, GA, USA

Aneesh B. Singhal, MD
Vice-Chair of Neurology, Quality and Safety
Associate Professor of Neurology, Harvard Medical School
Department of Neurology, Stroke Service
Massachusetts General Hospital
Boston, MA, USA

Christopher G. Sobey, PhD
Professorial Fellow, Vascular Biology and Immunopharmacology Group
Department of Pharmacology
Monash University
Victoria, Australia

Christian Stapf, MD
Tenured Professor of Neurology
Université Paris Diderot - Sorbonne Paris Cité
Department of Neurology
Paris, France

Hua Su, MD
Professor
Department of Anesthesia and Perioperative Care
Center for Cerebrovascular Research
University of California
San Francisco, CA, USA

Jose I. Suarez, MD
Head Vascular Neurology and Neurocritical Care
Professor of Neurology
Baylor College of Medicine
Houston, TX, USA

Marek Sykora, MD, PhD, MSc
Department of Neurology
St. Johns Hospital, Vienna, Austria
Department of Neurology
University Heidelberg
Heidelberg, Germany

Turgut Tatlisumak, MD, PhD
Institute of Neuroscience and Physiology
Sahlgrenska Academy at University of Gothenburg;
Department of Neurology
Sahlgrenska University Hospital
Gothenburg, Sweden

Najib El Tecle, MD, MS
Neurosurgery Resident
Saint Louis University Hospital
Department of Neurosurgery
St. Louis, MO, USA

Karel G. terBrugge, MD, FRCPC
Professor, Departments of Medical Imaging and Surgery
The David Braley and Nancy Gordon Chair in Interventional Neuroradiology
Division Head, Neuroradiology, Toronto Western Hospital
Ontorio, Canada

John W. Thompson, PhD
Cerebral Vascular Disease
Research Laboratories
Department of Neurology and Neuroscience Program
Miller School of Medicine
University of Miami
Miami, FL, USA

Barbara C. Tilley, MS, PhD
Lorne Bain Distinguished Professor in Public Health and Medicine
Director, Department of Biostatistics
The University of Texas Health Science Center at Houston
School of Public Health
Houston, TX, USA

Elisabeth Tournier-Lasserve, MD
Laboratoire de Génétique
Hôpital Lariboisiére
Université Paris Denis Diderot
INSERM 1161
Paris, France

Georgios Tsivgoulis, MD, RVT
Assistant Professor of Neurology
Second Department of Neurology
University of Athens, School of Medicine, "Attikon" University Hospital
Athens, Greece

Marcelo D. Vilela, MD
Staff Neurosurgeon
Mater Dei Hospital
Belo Horizonte MG, Brazil
Affiliated Assistant Professor
Department of Neurological Surgery
University of Washington
Seattle, WA, USA

Rüdiger von Kummer, MD
Senior Professor of Neuroradiology
Department of Neuroradiology
University Hospital
Dresden, Germany

Ajay K. Wakhloo, MD, PhD
Professor of Radiology, Neurology and Surgery
Director, Neuroimaging and Intervention
Director, Clinical Research
New England Center for Stroke Research
University of Massachusetts Medical School
Worcester, MA, USA

Kenneth R. Wagner, PhD
Associate Professor of Neurology
University of Cincinnati College of Medicine
Research Scientist
Veterans Affairs Medical Center
Cincinnati, OH, USA

Steven Warach, MD
Professor and Executive Director
Department of Neurology and Neurotherapeutics
UT Southwestern Medical Center
Austin, TX, USA

Babette B. Weksler, MD
Professor of Medicine
Weill Cornel Medical College
Weill Cornel Cancer Care and Blood Disorders
New York, NY, USA

David Werring, MD
Honorary Consultant Neurologist
The National Hospital for Neurology and Neurosurgery
Department of Neurology
University College London
London, UK

Joshua Z. Willey, MD, MS
Assistant Professor of Neurology
Division of Stroke
Columbia University Medical Center
New York, NY, USA

Max Wintermark, MD
Professor of Radiology
Department of Radiology
Stanford University
Stanford, CA, USA

Philip A. Wolf, MD
Professor of Neurology, Medicine and Epidemiology
Boston University School of Medicine
Boston, MA, USA

Lawrence K.S. Wong, MD
Mok Hing Yiu Professor of Medicine
Chief of Neurology
Department of Medicine and Therapeutics
The Chinese University of Hongkong
Prince of Wales Hospital
Shatin, Hong Kong Special Administrative Region
China

Daniel Woo, MD, MS
Professor of Neurology
Departments of Neurology and Rehabilitation Medicine
University of Cincinnati
Cincinnati, OH, USA

Clinton Wright, MD
Associate Professor of Neurology
Evelyn F. McKnight Brain Institute
Leonard M. Miller School of Medicine, University of Miami
Miami, FL, USA

Guohua Xi, MD
Professor of Neurosurgery
Associate Director, Crosby Neurosurgical Laboratories
R5018 BSRB
University of Michigan
Ann Arbor, MI, USA

Takenori Yamaguchi, MD, PhD
President Emeritus
National Cerebral and Cardiovascular Center
Osaka, Japan

Masahiro Yasaka, MD, PhD
Director
Department of Cerebrovascular Medicine and Neurology
National Hospital Organization
Kyushu Medical Center
Fukuoka, Japan

William L. Young, MD (†)
Professor
Department of Anesthesia and Perioperative Care
Department of Neurological Surgery
Department of Neurology
Center for Cerebrovascular Research
University of California
San Francisco, CA, USA
(†) Deceased

Samer G. Zammar, MD
Post Doctoral Research Fellow
Department of Neurological Surgery
Northwestern Memorial Hospital
Chicago, IL, USA

Darin B. Zahuranec, MD
Assistant Professor of Neurology
The University of Michigan Health System
Ann Arbor, MI, USA

Feng Zhang, MD, PhD
Research Assistant Professor
Department of Neurology
University of Pittsburgh
Pittsburgh, PA, USA

Haiyue Zhang, MD
Department of Neurology
University of Pittsburgh
Pittsburgh, PA, USA

John H. Zhang, MD, PhD
Professor of Neurosurgery, Anesthesiology, Neurology, and Physiology and Pharmacology
Director of Neuroscience Research
Associate Chair and Physiology Graduate Program Coordinator
Loma Linda University School of Medicine
Loma Linda, CA, USA

Zheng Gang Zhang, MD, PhD
Senior Scientist
Department of Neurology
Henry Ford Hospital
Detroit, MI, USA

R. Suzzane Zukin, PhD
F.M. Kirby Professor of Neural Repair and Protection
Director, Neuropsychopharmacology Center
Dominick P. Purpura Department of Neuroscience
Albert Einstein College of Medicine
New York, NY, USA

Richard M. Zweifler, MD
System Chair of Neurology
Ochsner Health System
New Orleans, LA, USA

AHA Evidence-based Classifications

TABLE 1 Applying Classification of Recommendations and Level of Evidence

SIZE OF TREATMENT EFFECT →

ESTIMATE OF CERTAINTY (PRECISION) OF TREATMENT EFFECT ↑

	CLASS I	CLASS IIa	CLASS IIb	CLASS III *No Benefit* or CLASS III *Harm*
	Benefit > > > Risk **Procedure/ Treatment SHOULD be performed/ administered**	***Benefit > > Risk*** ***Additional studies with focused objectives needed*** **IT IS REASONABLE** to perform procedure/ administer treatment	***Benefit ≥ Risk*** ***Additional studies with broad objectives needed; additional registry data would be helpful*** Procedure/Treatment **MAY BE CONSIDERED**	| | **Procedure/ Test** | **Treatment** | | **COR III: No benefit** | **Not Helpful** | **No Proves Benefit** | | **COR III: Harm** | **Excess Cost w/o Benefit or Harmful** | **Harmful to Patients** |
LEVEL A **Multiple populations evaluated*** **Data derived from multiple randomized clinical trials or meta-analyses**	• **Recommendation that procedure or treatment is useful/effective** • **Sufficient evidence from multiple randomized trails or meta-analyses**	• **Recommendation in favor of treatment or procedure being useful/effective** • **Some conflicting evidence from multiple randomized trials or meta-analyses**	• **Recommendation's usefulness/efficacy less well established** • **Greater conflicting evidence from multiple randomized trials or meta-analyses**	• **Recommendation that procedure or treatment is not useful/effective and may be harmful** • **Sufficient evidence from multiple randomized trials or meta-analyses**
LEVEL B **Limited populations evaluated*** **Data derived from a single randomized trial or nonrandomized studies**	• **Recommendation that procedure or treatment is useful/effective** • **Evidence from single randomized trial or nonrandomized studies**	• **Recommendation in favor of treatment or procedure being useful/effective** • **Some conflicting evidence from single randomized trial or nonrandomized studies**	• **Recommendation's usefulness/efficacy less well established** • **Greater conflicting evidence from single randomized trial or nonrandomized studies**	• **Recommendation that procedure or treatment is not useful/effective and may be harmful** • **Evidence from single randomized trial or nonrandomized studies**
LEVEL C **Very limited populations evaluated*** **Only consensus opinion of experts, case studies, or standard of care**	• **Recommendation that procedure or treatment is useful/effective** • **Only expert opinion, case studies, or standard of care**	• **Recommendation in favor of treatment or procedure being useful/effective** • **Only diverging expert opinion, case studies, or standard of care**	• **Recommendation's usefulness/efficacy less well established** • **Only diverging expert opinion, case studies, or standard of care**	• **Recommendation that procedure or treatment is not useful/effective and may be harmful** • **Only expert opinion, case studies, or standard of care**
Suggested phrases for writing recommendations†	should is recommended is indicated is useful/effective/ beneficial	is reasonable can be useful/effective/ beneficial is probably recommended or indicated	may/might be considered may/might be reasonable usefulness/effectiveness is unknown/unclear/ uncertain or not well established	COR III No Benefit: is not recommended is not indicated should not be done is not useful/ beneficial/effective COR III Harm: potentially harmful causes harm associated with excess morbidity/ mortality should not be done
Comparative effectiveness phrases†	treatment/strategy A is recommended/ indicated in preference to treatment B treatment A should be chosen over treatment B	treatment/strategy A is probably recommended/ indicated in preference to treatment B it is reasonable to choose treatment A over treatment B		

(*Reprinted with permission Circulation. 2010;121:1544–1579 ©2010, American Heart Association, Inc.*)

Box: Evidence Classifications

- Size of treatment effect
  - Class I: Benefit >>> Risk. Procedure/treatment **SHOULD** be performed/administered
  - Class IIa: Benefit >> Risk. **IT IS REASONABLE** to perform procedure/administer treatment
  - Class IIb: Benefit ≥ Risk. Procedure/treatment **MAY BE CONSIDERED**
  - Class III: No Benefit/Harm. Procedure/treatment is not useful/ effective and may be harmful
- Certainty of treatment effect
  - Level A: Data derived from multiple randomized clinical trials or meta-analyses.
  - Level B: Data derived from a single randomized trial or nonrandomized studies
  - Level C: Only consensus opinion of experts, case studies, or standard of care

Adapted from Sacco RL, Adams R, Albers G, et al. Guidelines for prevention of stroke in patients with ischemic stroke or transient ischemic attack: a statement for healthcare professionals from the American Heart Association/American Stroke Association Council on Stroke. Stroke 2006;37:577–617.

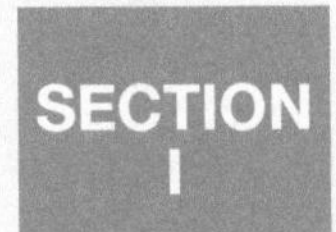

Pathophysiology

Eng H. Lo

Despite impressive advances in the molecular biology of cell death, the development of clinically effective neuroprotectants for the stroke patient remains challenging. An emerging hypothesis now states that a purely intracellular and "neurocentric" focus may not suffice. Stroke is a complex disease and so its pathophysiology comprises multiple signals and mechanisms in multiple cells and systems. The first section in this new edition of *Stroke* surveys the state-of-the-art in the field from this perspective.

At the cellular level, stroke affects mechanisms of hemostasis and perturbs interactions between circulating blood elements, the blood vessel itself, and brain parenchyma. At the functional level, the regulation and dysregulation of hemodynamics and metabolism remains a central event. At the organ level, stroke induces histopathologic reactions in all neural, glial and vascular cells. Hence, this section begins with chapters that define basic principles of vascular biology, cerebral blood flow and metabolism, and the brain tissue response to injury.

Building on this initial survey of key principles, the next few chapters then explore the molecular mechanisms of cell death and survival. Genes and pathways underlying necrosis and programmed cell death are balanced against an expanding family of endogenous neuroprotection and tolerance mediators. Beyond the brain itself, interactions with other organ systems are discussed in terms of crosstalk with neuroinflammatory cascades and immune cells. Stroke recovery is discussed in terms of multi-cellular signals for remodeling in the neurovascular unit, as well as compensatory response in resident and circulating progenitor cells. Because brain compartments are heterogeneous, two chapters are dedicated to assessing the nuances of molecular and cellular phenomena in white matter and hemorrhage. Finally, the section concludes with a chapter that links these molecular, cellular and physiologic principles in stroke to important categories of vascular malformations that contribute to cerebrovascular disease.

Stroke science will continue to advance. Molecular details may be revised and clinical opportunities may evolve. But it is hoped that the basic principles in this section will stand the test of time by providing the mechanistic foundations for stroke pathophysiology and a rational basis for pursuing potential therapeutics and diagnostics.

SECTION I Pathophysiology

1 Vascular Biology and Atherosclerosis of Cerebral Vessels

Sophocles Chrissobolis, Christopher G. Sobey

KEY POINTS

- Cerebral artery tone is substantially modulated under physiological conditions by endothelium-derived nitric oxide, reactive oxygen species, and through hyperpolarization mediated by several types of K^+ channels.
- Cerebral vascular function is very sensitive to endothelial dysfunction that occurs during chronic disease, resulting in impairment of vasodilator mechanisms.
- Oxidative stress and inflammation occur in the cerebral circulation in response to cardiovascular risk factors present during atherosclerosis and chronic hypertension, such as elevated plasma levels of cholesterol and angiotensin II, respectively.

INTRODUCTION

The brain has a limited supply of nutrients, thus normal brain function relies on adequate perfusion by the cerebral circulation for the delivery of oxygen and nutrients, as well as the removal of waste products. It is for this reason that cerebral vascular tone is tightly regulated, and why any alterations in mechanisms that modulate cerebral vessel function can predispose to cerebrovascular disease and stroke. Atherosclerosis is the underlying pathological process for both coronary and cerebral artery disease, which are the two most common forms of cardiovascular disease.[1]

The purpose of this chapter is thus to provide insight into major mechanisms that regulate cerebral artery function, and alterations in these mechanisms in two major clinical conditions which have a significant negative impact on health worldwide – hypertension and atherosclerosis. The scope is mostly limited to discussion of cerebral blood vessels and mechanisms that regulate their tone, either under basal conditions or in response to physiologically relevant agonists.

PHYSIOLOGICAL REGULATION OF CEREBRAL VASCULAR TONE

Numerous mechanisms regulate cerebral artery function. Most of the recent experimental evidence regarding such mechanisms has come from pharmacological studies and the use of genetically modified mice. Major mechanisms include: the release of nitric oxide (NO) from the endothelium to underlying smooth muscle cells (discussed under Nitric Oxide (NO) and Cyclic Guanosine Monophosphate); potassium ion (K^+) channels (see under K^+ Channels), which includes a discussion of the newly described two-pore domain (K_{2P}) channels, rho/rho-kinase activity (see under Rho/rho-kinase); reactive oxygen species (ROS); and the recently described transient receptor potential (TRP) channels.

Cyclic AMP-mediated Mechanisms

Activation of adenylate cyclase and production of cyclic adenosine monophosphate (cAMP) in vascular muscle mediates relaxation of blood vessels in response to a variety of endogenous substances, and represents a major mechanism of vasodilatation in cerebral vessels. Stimuli that activate adenylate cyclase include prostanoids (prostacyclin and prostaglandin E_2), adenosine, calcitonin gene-related peptide (CGRP), vasoactive intestinal peptide, β-adrenergic agonists, pituitary adenylate cyclase activating peptide (PACAP), and adrenomedullin. A recent concept is that increases in intracellular cAMP in vascular muscle produce vasodilatation only in part by a direct effect and, in part, by activation of K^+ channels (see below).

Nitric Oxide (NO) and Cyclic Guanosine Monophosphate

Another major mechanism for maintenance of vascular tone by the endothelium involves production of endothelium-derived NO. In endothelium, NO is synthesized from endothelial nitric oxide synthase (eNOS); it then diffuses to the underlying smooth muscle where it activates soluble guanylate cyclase, which in turn leads to increased intracellular cGMP levels and subsequent relaxation of the smooth muscle.[2] Experimental evidence for modulation of cerebral vascular tone by endothelium-derived NO has been obtained by applying inhibitors of NOS to cerebral blood vessels from several different species, both in vivo and in vitro, and have involved such inhibitors causing vasoconstriction (reviewed extensively in Reference 3).

NO release from the endothelium can also be stimulated in response to receptor (e.g., acetylcholine, bradykinin) or non-receptor-mediated agonists, or in response to shear stress. Endothelium-dependent, NO-mediated cerebral vascular relaxation in response to such agonists is often used to determine the functional integrity of the endothelium. Endothelial dysfunction, manifested as diminished NO bioavailability experimentally by impaired endothelium-dependent vasodilatation, or reduced vasoconstriction in response to a NOS inhibitor, is a common feature of many cerebrovascular-related diseases (discussed in Alterations in Cerebral Vascular Function during Hypertension and Atherosclerosis). Such exogenously applied agonists are often useful in this way experimentally, and they may also be important endogenously. For example, neurovascular coupling in some brain regions is mediated by neuronally released acetylcholine acting on the endothelium to stimulate eNOS.[4]

K^+ Channels

Activity of K^+ channels is a major regulator of smooth muscle cell membrane potential, and as such an important regulator of vascular tone. This is because vessel diameter is in large part dependent on cytosolic Ca^{2+} concentration, which in turn is dependent on membrane potential. There are five major types of K^+ channels known to be expressed in cerebral blood vessels: calcium (Ca^{2+})-activated (K_{Ca}) K^+ channels, ATP-sensitive K^+ (K_{ATP}) channels, voltage-sensitive K^+ (K_V) channels, inwardly rectifying K^+ (K_{IR}) channels, and tandem-pore (TREK-1) channels; and all are regulators of vascular tone. This is supported by the wealth of information using both pharmacological inhibitors and gene-targeted mice to study the regulation of membrane potential and vascular function. Potassium channels are also important mediators of vasodilator responses to several vasodilators that regulate vascular tone, and this will also be discussed.

K_{Ca}-activated K^+ Channels

There are three sub-types of K_{Ca} channels present in the vasculature: large-conductance K_{Ca} (BK_{Ca}) channels; intermediate-conductance (IK_{Ca}) channels, and small-conductance (SK_{Ca}) channels. Most research regarding the functional importance of this channel, especially in cerebral arteries, has centered on the BK_{Ca} channel.

As the name suggests, these channels are activated in response to increases in intracellular Ca^{2+}. Membrane depolarization, myogenic responses (i.e., pressure-induced vasoconstriction, important in development and maintenance of basal vascular tone) and elevations in arterial pressure are associated with elevations in intracellular Ca^{2+} concentration in cells of the vasculature.[5] Thus, an important function of these channels appears to be to act as a negative feedback mechanism during increases in Ca^{2+} to limit vasoconstriction. A major mechanism of elevations in intracellular Ca^{2+} appears to be via Ca^{2+} sparks, which are localized elevations in cytosolic Ca^{2+} due to the opening of ryanodine-sensitive Ca^{2+} release channels in the sarcoplasmic reticulum to K_{Ca} channels located on the plasma membrane.

These channels are important in modulating basal tone of cerebral arteries, as selective inhibition of BK_{Ca} channels with tetraethylammonium ion (TEA) produces vasoconstriction.[5-7] In mice deficient in the β1 subunit of BK_{Ca} channels, increased intracellular Ca^{2+} concentration in response to ryanodine (which at low concentrations depletes Ca^{2+} stores from the sarcoplasmic reticulum so that intracellular Ca^{2+} concentration increases) and cerebral vascular constriction to iberiotoxin (selective inhibitor of BK_{Ca} channels) was reduced, suggesting that Ca^{2+} spark activity modulates myogenic tone through BK_{Ca} channel activation.[8] These channels may be more important in modulation of basal tone in larger cerebral arteries.[5]

Recent evidence of the importance of Ca^{2+} spark activity and BK_{Ca} channels as mediators of vasodilators has emerged, as TEA and iberiotoxin inhibit vasodilator responses in response to vasodilators that activate adenylate cyclase and guanylate cyclase.[9] Acidosis markedly increased Ca^{2+} spark activity and caused dilatation of brain parenchymal arterioles. Dilatation was inhibited by inhibitors of ryanodine receptors (ryanodine) and BK_{Ca} channels (paxilline), as well as in mice lacking the BK_{Ca} channel.[10] Hydrogen sulfide (an important signaling molecule in regulation of vascular tone and blood pressure) also increased Ca^{2+} spark and BK_{Ca} current frequency, as well as causing dilatation in cerebral arterioles – the vasodilatation was inhibited by ryanodine and iberiotoxin, suggesting Ca^{2+} spark activity is important in the response.[11] Intermittent hypoxia increased myogenic tone through loss of hydrogen sulfide activation of K_{Ca} channels.[12] Hypoxia had no effect on Ca^{2+} spark frequency, but reduced K_{Ca} channel activity.[13] Protein expression of $K_{Ca}2.2$, 2.3 and 3.1,[13] as well as α- and β1-subunits of BK_{Ca} channels[14] in cerebral arteries has been reported.

K_{ATP} Channels

K_{ATP} channels are defined by their sensitivity to intracellular ATP, with their activity being inhibited by intracellular ATP.[15] Generally speaking, the intracellular concentration of ATP is normally sufficient that these channels have a low open probability in most vascular smooth muscle cells under normal conditions,[16] and this appears to also be the case in the cerebral circulation, where glibenclamide, a selective inhibitor of K_{ATP} channels, has no effect on cerebral vascular tone.[17] However, K_{ATP} channels appear to be present and functional in cerebral vessels based on direct evidence for their expression (discussed below) and a wealth of evidence reporting glibenclamide-sensitive relaxation of cerebral arteries in response to K_{ATP} channel activators.[15]

Several endogenous substances produce hyperpolarization and relaxation of cerebral vascular muscle that is mediated, either fully or partly, by activation of K_{ATP} channels. These substances include CGRP,[18] norepinephrine (noradrenaline),[19] and increased intracellular concentration of cyclic AMP.[19] The concept that K_{ATP} channels may be activated by increased concentrations of cAMP is supported by evidence that dilatation of the basilar artery in response to forskolin, a direct activator of adenylate cyclase, can be attenuated with glibenclamide.[18,19] In contrast, vasodilators which increase cGMP in cerebral vessels are usually not inhibited by glibenclamide.

Several more recent studies have investigated the expression of K_{ATP} in cerebral vessels. K_{ATP} channels are thought to be a heteromultimeric complex of two subunits – the pore forming inward-rectifying K^+ channel type 6 (i.e., 6.1 or 6.2), and the other is a sulfonylurea receptor (SUR), either SUR1 or SUR2, with the SUR2 gene generating the two splice variants SUR2A and SUR2B.[20] Messenger RNA (mRNA) expression for both the pore-forming subunits ($K_{IR}6.1$ and 6.2) and SUR1, 2A and 2B has been demonstrated in cerebral arteries,[20,21] although another study investigating SUR expression found no expression of SUR1, and reported only SUR2B expression.[22] Protein expression of $K_{IR}6.1$ and 6.2, as well as SUR1 and 2B, was also reported.[21] Cerebral arterioles were found to express $K_{IR}6.1$ and SUR2B,[23] with human cerebral arteries found to express SUR2B.[22]

Acidosis and reductions in intracellular pO_2 are known to produce cerebral vasodilatation. K_{ATP} channels have been shown to be involved in cerebral vasodilatation in response to acidosis,[24,25] as well as in vasodilatation to N-methyl-D-aspartate (NMDA), which may be important in the coupling of cerebral metabolism and blood flow.[26] More direct evidence for a role of K_{ATP} channels in mediating vasodilatation in response to oxygen/glucose deprivation was reported in that vasodilatation was impaired in SUR-deficient compared to wild-type mice.[22] Myogenic tone and vasodilatation in response to hypoxia are not dependent on SUR2 expression,[22] although relaxation to hypoxia is inhibited by glibenclamide,[15,27] suggesting a role for K_{ATP} channels in hypoxia-induced vasodilatation where the K_{ATP} subunit composition does not involve SUR2. Hydrogen sulfide also dilates cerebral arteries, an effect that is inhibited by glibenclamide and in SUR2-deficient mice.[23]

K_V Channels

K_V channels are activated in response to increases in pressure in cerebral arteries and modulate cerebral vascular tone, in that pharmacological inhibition of K_V channels with 4-aminopyridine causes cerebral artery depolarization and constriction.[28,29] K_V channels are also known to mediate cerebral artery dilations, including in response to NO.[28,30] K_V channel subunits are expressed in cerebral vessels (e.g., $K_V1.2$ and 1.5,[31–33] and $K_V2.1$ and 2.2[34,35]) – including in humans.[36] K_V2-mediated current is proposed to underlie K_V-dependent modulation of cerebral artery tone in that inhibition of the K_V2 channel with stromatoxin caused cerebral artery constriction.[35]

K_{IR} Channels

This channel is so named since it conducts K^+ current more readily into than out of the cell over a wide range of membrane potentials. However, at membrane potentials within the physiological range, these channels actually conduct a small outward current. Consequently, when this channel is inhibited with the pharmacological blocker, barium ion (Ba^{2+}), depolarization and constriction of cerebral arteries are observed.[37–43] Furthermore, in mice lacking the $K_{IR}2.1$ subunit – the subunit thought to be important in mediating vascular K_{IR} current – cerebral artery K_{IR} channel currents are absent.[44]

In the cerebral circulation, K^+ is released during neuronal activity and may be siphoned to cerebral vessels directly by astrocytes after neuronal activation.[45] Basal concentration of K^+ in cerebrospinal fluid is ~3 mM, and may increase to between 4 and 7 mM during neuronal activity. In this concentration range (i.e., from 3 to 10 mM), K^+ causes dilatation of cerebral arteries[37,39–41,46,47] and arterioles.[38,42,43,48–55] Moreover, K^+-induced hyperpolarization and vasodilatation in this concentration range is inhibited by Ba^{2+},[37–41,47,52–54,56–58] suggesting K_{IR}-mediated K^+-induced vasodilation may be an important mechanism in coupling of cerebral metabolism and blood flow. Furthermore, cerebral vascular relaxation responses to K^+ are absent in mice lacking the $K_{IR}2.1$ subunit.[44] There have been reports of $K_{IR}2.1$ channel expression in cerebral arteries.[37,57]

K_{2P} Channels

A new family of channels – two pore domain K^+ (K_{2P}) channels – have recently been characterized.[59] These channels require two protein subunits, each contributing two pore domains, to form a functional channel. There are several members of the K_{2P} family expressed in the vasculature, with some reported to be functionally important in the cerebral vasculature. Expression of TREK-1, TREK-2, TASK-1, TWIK-2, TRAAK and THIK-1 has been reported in cerebral arteries, with TREK-1 being the most abundant.[60,61] Protein and mRNA expression of TREK-1 in the basilar artery was associated with vasodilatation induced by polyunsaturated fatty acids (which are important as they improve brain resistance against cerebral ischemia) such as α-linolenic acid in wild-type mice that are absent in mice deficient in TREK-1.[62] Nevertheless, another study reported similar vasodilator responses of the basilar artery to α-linolenic acid in wild-type and TREK-1-deficient mice.[63] Cerebral artery expression of TRAAK was associated with an important role in mediating endothelium-independent vasodilatation.[64]

Rho/rho-kinase

Smooth muscle cell contractility is ultimately governed by the phosphorylation state of myosin light chain (MLC), vascular smooth muscle tone occurring in association with increasing levels of MLC phosphorylation. MLC is phosphorylated by MLC-kinase – a Ca^{2+}-calmodulin-dependent enzyme – and is dephosphorylated by MLC phosphatase (MLCP). MLC phosphorylation and smooth muscle contractility is not always directly proportional to intracellular Ca^{2+} concentration. Other mechanisms can regulate smooth muscle contractility independent of changes in intracellular Ca^{2+} concentration, a phenomenon known as Ca^{2+}-sensitization. Ca^{2+}-sensitization can occur through several pathways, and ultimately results in inhibition of MLCP. One such pathway is the rho/rho-kinase pathway. When rho-kinase is activated, it phosphorylates the myosin binding (i.e., regulatory) subunit of MLCP, and thus inhibits MLCP activity, which ultimately leads to smooth muscle (and thus vascular) contractility.[65,66]

In vascular muscle, rhoA can be activated by stretch. This is important since myogenic tone is characterized by pressure-induced vasoconstriction, making it important for the development of basal vascular tone. The contribution of rho-kinase activity to the cerebral artery myogenic response has been studied over the past decade through the use of Y-27632 and fasudil (HA-1077), pharmacological inhibitors of rho-kinase.[67] For example, Y-27632 relaxes cerebral artery segments following pressure-induced constriction,[68] and pressure-induced cerebral artery constriction is inhibited by Y-27632 and fasudil.[69–71] In vivo, where myogenic tone is present, several studies have reported that Y-27632 and fasudil cause dilatation of cerebral arteries[72–76] and arterioles,[77] thus providing good evidence that the rhoA/rho-kinase pathway is a major mechanism contributing to cerebral vascular tone.

Reactive Oxygen Species (ROS)

ROS are known to influence cerebral vascular tone, and this is reviewed extensively elsewhere.[78] These ROS include the parent molecule superoxide (O_2^-), as well as hydroxyl radical (OH) and hydrogen peroxide (H_2O_2). The closely related reactive nitrogen species (RNS) – peroxynitrite – is also commonly involved in such effects.

Superoxide, a negatively charged anion, can elicit either dilatation[79–82] or constriction[79,83] of cerebral arteries. Superoxide reacts extremely efficiently with NO. As has been discussed, NO is a major regulator of cerebral vascular tone, thus reduced NO bioavailability following increased superoxide levels will likely result in vasoconstriction, with vasoconstriction being reported in response to higher concentrations of superoxide,[79,80] and vasorelaxation at low concentrations.[79]

H_2O_2 is a chemically more stable species than superoxide, and it diffuses much more readily across cell membranes, thus potentially being important as a signaling molecule. Many studies have reported that H_2O_2 acts as a cerebral vasodilator, both in vivo and in vitro,[82,84–91] although vasoconstriction has also been reported.[92]

Peroxynitrite, formed from the rapid chemical reaction of superoxide with NO, can also affect cerebral vascular tone, with both dilatation[93,94] and constriction[94–96] of cerebral arteries reported. Lower concentrations of peroxynitrite appear to cause cerebral vasoconstriction, with higher concentrations typically causing vasodilatation.[94,97]

Transient Receptor Potential (TRP) Channels

TRP channels are a superfamily of cation channels comprising at least 28 members, and are assigned to six subfamilies based on their sequence homology.[98] These are TRPC (classical), TRPV (vanilloid), TRPM (melastatin), TRPA (ankyrin), TRPP (polycystin) and TRPML (mucolipin).[99] One such subfamily – TRPA1 channels – is known to be expressed in cerebral vessels, specifically in endothelium, and mediate endothelium-dependent vasodilatation.[100] The melastatin TRP channel 4 (TRPM 4) is activated by high levels of intracellular Ca^{2+} and is known to be expressed in cerebral arteries.[101] Expression in smooth muscle cells is consistent with a role in the myogenic response, in that myogenic vasoconstriction was attenuated in cerebral arteries administered TRPM4 antisense.[102] Pharmacological inhibition of the TRPM4 channel with

9-phenanthrol was able to cause hyperpolarization and prevent the development and maintenance of myogenic tone, further underlining its importance in maintenance of myogenic tone in the cerebral circulation.[103] Another study also reported cerebral vascular expression of TRPM4 protein, which, once inactivated, results in reduced myogenic vasoconstriction in response to a PKC activator.[104] Myogenic tone in cerebral arteries isolated from hypertensive mice was inhibited by treatment with SKF93635 (a specific inhibitor of TRPC6 channels at the concentration used in that study). SKF93635 was without effect in arteries from aged mice, suggesting TRP channel function is disrupted in cerebral arteries from aged mice.[105] Some TRP channels, such as the TRPV1 channel are chemosensitive. The TRPV1 channel is expressed in the endothelium of cerebral arteries, and the dietary agonist carvacol, which may be cardioprotective, mediates endothelium-dependent cerebral vasodilatation that is inhibited by a pharmacological inhibitor of TRPV1-4 channels.[106] TRPV1, TRPV5 and TRPV6 channels do not appear to be expressed in cerebral arteries.[107]

ALTERATIONS IN CEREBRAL VASCULAR FUNCTION DURING HYPERTENSION AND ATHEROSCLEROSIS

Atherosclerosis

Atherosclerosis is the underlying pathological process for both coronary and cerebral artery disease.[1] Atherosclerosis is thought to be initiated by trapping of lipids in the subendothelial layer, leading to the generation of biologically active oxidized species (i.e., oxidized low-density lipoprotein [LDL]), ultimately leading to recruitment of leukocytes to the artery wall.[108] Oxidative modification of LDL present in the intima by ROS may thus be a key initiating step in atherosclerosis.[109] Endothelial dysfunction is an early step in the development of atherosclerosis, and traditional cardiovascular risk factors (e.g., dyslipidemia, hypertension) are associated with endothelial dysfunction.[110] Furthermore, atherosclerosis is characterized by chronic inflammation of the vasculature, thus these three key processes characteristic of atherosclerosis – oxidative stress, endothelial dysfunction and inflammation – will be discussed here (also summarized in Fig. 1-1), with much of the discussion referring to data from the apolipoprotein E-deficient (ApoE$^{-/-}$) mouse. The ApoE$^{-/-}$ mouse, characterized by high levels of plasma cholesterol due to deletion of the APOE gene (important in cholesterol metabolism), provides a very useful experimental model for understanding the mechanisms of disease initiation.[1]

Cerebral Vascular Oxidative Stress in Models of Atherosclerosis

Some evidence suggests the prevalence of oxidative stress in cerebral vessels during hypercholesterolemia or atherosclerosis. For example, in wild-type mice placed on a high-cholesterol diet for 2 weeks,[111] and ApoE$^{-/-}$ mice on a high-fat diet for 7 weeks,[112] oxidative stress was found to be present in cerebral arteries. The study by Miller et al.[112] went on to suggest that Nox2 oxidase was the source of the oxidative stress, as the oxidative stress present in ApoE$^{-/-}$ mice was abolished in mice deficient in both ApoE and Nox2 (i.e., ApoE$^{-/-}$/Nox2$^{-/y}$).

Cerebral Vascular Endothelial Dysfunction in Models of Atherosclerosis

Several lines of evidence suggest that atherosclerosis is associated with reduced NO bioavailability and endothelial dysfunction. In earlier reports, relaxation responses of the basilar artery to acetylcholine were impaired in hypercholesterolemic vs normal rabbits,[113] although cerebral vascular responses to acetylcholine were reportedly preserved[114,115] or even augmented[116] during atherosclerosis. In atherosclerotic monkeys, contraction of basilar arteries in response to inhibition of soluble guanylate cyclase was reduced compared to that in normal monkeys, suggesting the basal influence of soluble guanylate cyclase on basal tone of cerebral arteries is diminished during atherosclerosis, perhaps reflecting a reduced production/activity of NO during atherosclerosis.[117] Similarly, cerebral artery contractions in response to application of L-NAME (a NOS inhibitor) were reduced in vessels from ApoE$^{-/-}$ compared to normal mice,[112] suggesting reduced NO bioavailability was present during atherosclerosis. Reduced cerebral vascular relaxation to acetylcholine in ApoE$^{-/-}$ versus normal mice further suggests that reduced NO bioavailability is associated with endothelial dysfunction in the cerebral circulation during atherosclerosis.[118,119] Interestingly, consistent with these data, cerebral arteries in rabbits fed a diet high in cholesterol were narrower compared to their control counterparts.[120]

Further experiments were conducted to provide a link between oxidative stress and vascular dysfunction. Impaired NO-dependent responses of cerebral vessels from ApoE$^{-/-}$

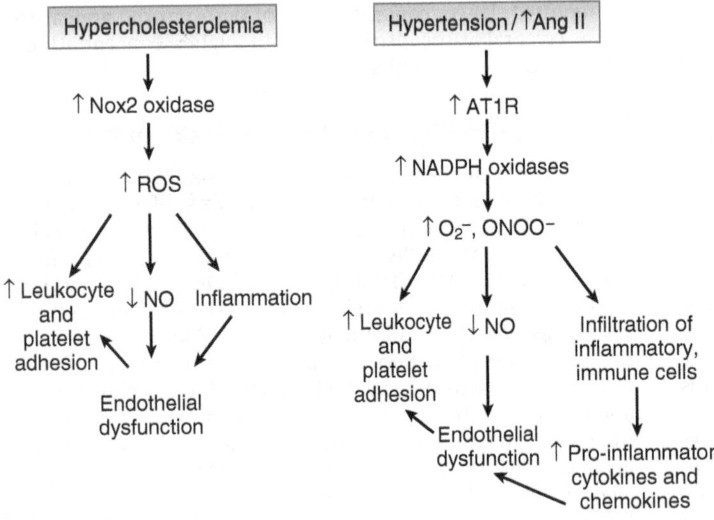

Figure 1-1. Schematic diagram summarizing cerebrovascular effects of hypercholesterolemia, and elevated Ang II and hypertension. Hypercholesterolemia induces oxidative stress, and ultimately inflammation – comprising leukocyte and platelet adhesion, and endothelial dysfunction. These effects are all attenuated in Nox2-deficient mice. Ang II increases leukocyte and platelet adhesion, infiltration of inflammatory/immune cells and causes endothelial dysfunction due to reduced NO bioavailability. These effects are largely inhibited by: AT1 Receptor (AT1R) inhibitors and in AT1R-deficient mice; ROS scavengers and Nox2-deficiency, as well as in lymphocyte-deficiency (RAG$^{-/-}$) mice, implicating AT1R, NADPH oxidase-derived ROS and the adaptive immune system in the detrimental effects of chronic hypertension in the cerebral circulation.

mice were reversed in vessels from ApoE$^{-/-}$ mice treated with a scavenger of ROS (tempol),[112,118] the NADPH oxidase inhibitor apocynin[118] or in ApoE$^{-/-}$/Nox2$^{-/y}$ mice,[112] strongly suggesting that Nox2-derived superoxide is a major mediator of cerebral vascular dysfunction during atherosclerosis. Oxidative stress and endothelial dysfunction is present despite the apparent absence of lesions in cerebral blood vessels.[112,118]

Cerebral Vascular Inflammation in Models of Atherosclerosis

Atherosclerosis is characterized by chronic inflammation of the vasculature. Platelet endothelial cell adhesion molecule-1 (PECAM-1) is involved in the inflammatory process and in leukocyte–endothelial interactions, and its expression is increased in cerebral arterioles of ApoE$^{-/-}$ mice.[121] Leukocyte and platelet adhesion, as well as oxidative stress, were elevated in cerebral vessels of hypercholesterolemic mice – leukocyte and platelet adhesion was prevented by immunoneutralization of P-selectin, and in Nox2-deficient mice, suggesting that P-selectin and Nox2-dependent oxidative stress are important mechanisms in hypercholesterolemia-induced inflammation in the brain.[111] Arginase type 1 expression was also increased in cerebral vessels from ApoE$^{-/-}$ mice,[122] which is relevant since oxidized LDL increases arginase activity and decreases endothelial NO levels, ultimately leading to impaired NO function in the vascular endothelium.[123] Vascular cell adhesion molecule-1 (VCAM-1) expression was not altered in brain microvessels of ApoE$^{-/-}$ mice.[124]

Hypertension

Hypertension profoundly and negatively impacts the cerebral circulation and brain, and is a major risk factor for stroke and a leading cause of cognitive decline and dementia.[125] Hypertension may promote the formation of atherosclerotic plaques in cerebral arteries and arterioles,[125] and there is a wealth of experimental evidence demonstrating detrimental functional consequences of hypertension on the cerebral circulation. Many initial studies focused on the spontaneously hypertensive rat (SHR), where augmented NADPH oxidase-derived superoxide production[88] and impaired endothelium-dependent responses have been reported.[57,73,126–129] What follows is a discussion of more recent data regarding the influence of hypertension on the cerebral circulation – specifically hypertension in response to elevated angiotensin II (Ang II) levels (also summarized in Fig. 1-1). Ang II is of major importance because it is involved in many of the functional and structural changes occurring in the cerebral circulation during chronic hypertension.[2,125]

Oxidative Stress In Hypertension Involving Elevated Ang II

Ang II increases ROS production in the cerebral circulation. Work from Iadecola's group has found that acute intravenous infusion of mice with Ang II increases both blood pressure and ROS production by cerebral blood vessels.[129–133] Increased ROS levels were prevented by treatment with the ROS scavenger MnTBAP.[134] This treatment also reportedly increases 3-nitrotyrosine immunoreactivity (indicative of nitrosative stress) in mouse cerebral vascular endothelial cells, an effect that was prevented by a peroxynitrite scavenger and a NOS inhibitor, and was also absent in Nox2-deficient mice.[131] Thus, these findings suggest that Ang II increases peroxynitrite formation in the cerebral vasculature largely via the reaction of Nox2-oxidase-derived superoxide with NO.

Endothelial Dysfunction in Hypertension Involving Elevated Ang II

Acute intravenous administration of Ang II has been reported to impair NO-dependent increases in cerebral blood flow (CBF),[133,134] an effect that was reversed by MnTBAP and the Ang II type 1 (AT_1) receptor antagonist losartan.[134] Topical application of Ang II to cerebral arterioles in vivo causes impaired NO-dependent responses that can be prevented by the superoxide scavenger, tiron.[135] Similarly, Ang II-induced endothelial dysfunction in cerebral arterioles of ECSOD-deficient mice in vivo was reversed by tempol.[136] In a more chronic model of Ang II-dependent hypertension, Ang II increased blood pressure and caused endothelial dysfunction of the basilar artery. This effect of Ang II was absent in Nox2-deficient mice, and partially attenuated in Nox1-deficient mice, suggesting Ang II-induced endothelial dysfunction is dependent on Nox2-oxidase and, perhaps to some extent, Nox1-oxidase.[137] In spite of these findings, Ang II increases blood pressure in both Nox2- and Nox1-deficient mice, suggesting that the cerebral vascular and pressor actions of Ang II are independent of one another.[137] To further confirm this point, previous studies have reported that systemic administration of a non-pressor dose of Ang II caused endothelial dysfunction in the cerebral circulation.[138,139] Endothelial dysfunction in response to Ang II was reversed by ROS scavengers.[138,139] In a genetic model of hypertension (mice overexpressing human renin and angiotensinogen), endothelial dysfunction of the basilar artery was completely reversed by administration of polyethylene glycol superoxide dismutase (PEG-SOD).[140] Taken together, these data suggest that Ang II causes endothelial dysfunction in the cerebral circulation by activating AT_1 receptors expressed in the vessel wall, leading to an increase in superoxide production, and subsequent oxidative inactivation of NO.

Cerebrovascular Inflammation in Hypertension Involving Elevated Ang II

Hypertension induces inflammation in the cerebral circulation. This includes models in which Ang II is involved. Ang II results in elevated leukocyte and platelet adhesion in cerebral vessels, an effect prevented by the AT1 receptor antagonists, candesartan and losartan, as well as diphenyleneiodonium, an inhibitor of flavoproteins such as NADPH oxidase.[141] In studies performed to extend these findings, Ang II-induced hypertension was associated with a marked increase in leukocyte and platelet adhesion in cerebral vessels which was attenuated in RAG$^{-/-}$ mice (i.e., deficient in T and B lymphocytes), AT1R$^{-/-}$ mice, and by treatment with losartan,[142] suggesting the involvement of immune cells and AT1 receptors in this effect. Leukocyte adhesion in response to Ang II in pial vessels in vivo was also prevented by tempol,[143] further confirming that cerebrovascular inflammation involves ROS production and oxidative stress. Interestingly, although leukocyte and platelet adhesion in cerebral vessels was enhanced in models of Ang II and deoxycorticosterone acetate (DOCA)-salt hypertension, these effects were prevented in the presence of mild hypercholesterolemia, possibly due to the involvement of high-density lipoprotein, suggesting that mild elevations in certain types of cholesterol may be beneficial in the setting of hypertension.[144]

Other models of hypertension have also implicated a role for Ang II in cerebrovascular inflammation. For example, in a DOCA-salt model of hypertension, leukocyte and platelet adhesion was prevented by losartan and in AT1R$^{-/-}$ mice.[145] Furthermore, not only were these effects inhibited by tempol, they were also inhibited by mito-tempol,[145] implicating mitochondria-derived ROS in the cerebrovascular inflammatory response. These anti-inflammatory effects occurred in the absence of any depressor action, suggesting that blood pressure is not necessarily a key mediator of cerebrovascular inflammation where Ang II is involved. In the SHR, increased expression of intracellular adhesion molecule-1 (ICAM-1), as well as increased number of infiltrating and adherent macrophages in brain microvessels, was inhibited by candesartan.[146] Widespread inflammation in many brain regions of the SHR was also inhibited by candesartan,[147] further implicating a role for activation of AT1R by Ang II and demonstrating a beneficial use for AT1R inhibitors in preventing inflammation associated with cerebrovascular disease.

K^+ Channel Function in Chronic Hypertension

Expression of K^+ channels in the cerebral vasculature and the importance of their role in modulating arterial tone, including mediation of vasodilator responses, have been described. The deleterious actions of chronic hypertension in the cerebral vasculature are also well known;[122] it is thus unsurprising that K^+ channel function is altered in association with chronic hypertension.

BK_{Ca} Channels. Basal activity of BK_{Ca} channels may be greater in cerebral arteries during chronic hypertension, in that pharmacological inhibition of these channels (with TEA and iberiotoxin) elicits greater contraction of cerebral arteries from hypertensive vs normotensive rats.[7] Consistent with this, iberiotoxin elicited enhanced contraction of cerebral arterioles from hypertensive vs normotensive rats, an effect associated with enhanced cerebral vascular expression of the K_{Ca} channel α subunit.[148] Inhibition of BK_{Ca} channels with TEA and charybdotoxin caused cerebral vascular contraction in hypertensive but not normotensive rats[149] (Fig. 1-2).

By contrast, in a model of Ang II-dependent hypertension, contraction of cerebral arteries in response to iberiotoxin was reduced in hypertensive vs normotensive rats, and this was associated with reduced coupling efficiency between Ca^{2+} sparks and BK_{Ca} channels, as well as reduced β1 subunit expression, although α subunit expression was unaltered during chronic hypertension.[150] The mechanism may involve calcineurin/NFATc3 signaling, as Ang II-induced reduction in β1 subunit expression was absent in calcineurin/NFATc3-deficient mice. Calcineurin/NFATc3 is also important in the development of Ang II-dependent hypertension.[151] Furthermore, although iberiotoxin caused myogenic constriction in normal mice, in a model of Ang II-dependent hypertension it had no effect on myogenic constriction in cerebral arteries.[105] In a model of diet-induced obesity where blood pressure was elevated, cerebral vascular $BK_{Ca}\beta1$ subunit expression was increased, although myogenic tone was not altered.[14] Thus, functional alterations in K_{Ca} channels appear to be dependent on the model of experimental hypertension studied.

K_{ATP} Channels. To our knowledge, there is little information regarding K_{ATP} channel function in hypertension. Vasodilator responses to the K_{ATP} channel activator aprikalim were significantly impaired in cerebral arteries from hypertensive vs normotensive rats, suggesting impaired K_{ATP} channel function during hypertension[126] (Fig. 1-2). Although SUR2B expression appears to be increased in small cerebral arteries from hypertensive rats compared to their normotensive controls,[152] the functional significance of this finding is unknown.

K_V Channels. Experimental hypertension may be associated with cerebral artery depolarization and increased myogenic response, perhaps indicating impaired K_V channel function (Fig. 1-2). Pharmacological inhibition of K_V channels with correolide and psora-4 constricted cerebral arteries from normotensive rats, but was without effect in cerebral arteries from two models of hypertension, suggesting a reduced contribution of K_V channels to the modulation of basal tone. This was associated with reduced expression of the pore-forming $\alpha_{1.2}$ and $\alpha_{1.5}$ subunits that compose K_V channels in hypertensive vs normotensive rats.[153] This is in agreement with impaired K_V2 channel function of cerebral arteries reported in a model of Ang II-dependent hypertension, in that stromatoxin-induced contraction of cerebral arteries was decreased in arteries from hypertensive vs normotensive rats.[35] In Dahl salt-sensitive rats, K_V channel current density was decreased in cerebral artery myocytes from hypertensive vs normotensive rats.[154] Lower K_V current density was reported in cerebral vascular smooth muscle cells from SHR compared with WKY.[155]

K_{IR} Channels. The first evidence for impaired K_{IR} channel function during chronic hypertension was the finding that Ba^{2+}-sensitive cerebral vascular relaxant responses to K^+ in hypertensive rats were impaired when compared with normotensive controls.[156] A subsequent study reported altered K_{IR} channel function during chronic hypertension, whereby K_{IR} channels were not the predominant mediator of cerebral vasodilator responses to K^+, unlike in normal animals. This was despite responses to K^+ being preserved (or even

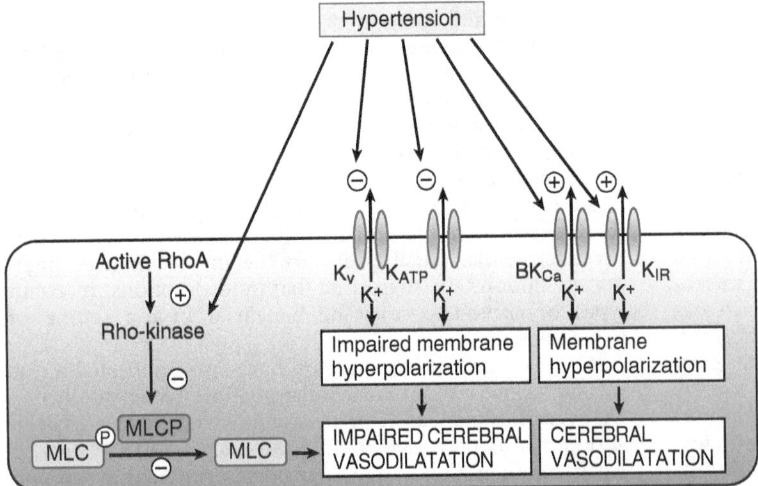

Figure 1-2. Hypertension profoundly influences two major mechanisms modulating cerebral artery tone. Rho-kinase phosphorylates (and inactivates) myosin light chain phosphatase (MLCP), thus leading to enhanced phosphorylation of MLC and increased contractility. Rho-kinase is critically involved in normal maintenance of cerebral vascular tone. During hypertension, rho-kinase activity is increased, leading to further enhanced MLCP phosphorylation and, consequently, enhanced myogenic tone. K^+ channel activity modulates vascular tone. Most studies have investigated the effect of hypertension on BK_{Ca} channel function, with the outcome (i.e., increased or decreased channel function) depending on the model of hypertension studied (see text). Baseline K_V channel function is impaired, as is K_{ATP}-mediated vasodilatation compared with normotensive conditions. Baseline K_{IR} channel function is augmented, whereas K_{IR}-mediated K^+-induced vasodilatation is impaired.

enhanced), $K_{IR}2.1$ expression being preserved, and an enhanced role for K_{IR} channels in modulating arterial tone during chronic hypertension[57] (Fig. 1-2). In the cerebral microvasculature, preserved (or even enhanced) vasorelaxation to K^+ during chronic hypertension was mediated by K_{IR} channels[54] (Fig. 1-2). K_{IR} channel function may thus be preserved in smaller arterioles[54] during chronic hypertension as opposed to impaired function in larger arteries,[57,156] at least in mediating responses to K^+.

Rho-kinase in Hypertension

Enhanced dilator responses of the basilar artery to Y-27632 in models of chronic hypertension suggest an increase in rho-kinase function in hypertension[73,75,76] (Fig. 1-2). Furthermore, pressure-dependent development of myogenic tone of cerebral arteries is inhibited by Y-27632 to a greater extent in hypertensive vs normotensive rats,[157] thus supporting an important role for rho-kinase in increased myogenic tone of cerebral arteries. A recent study demonstrated that acute systemic elevations in endothelin-1 levels impaired cerebral vascular endothelial function, an effect that was reversed by Y-27632.[158] Interestingly, the role of rho-kinase as a key mediator of cerebral vascular dysfunction during chronic hypertension may be dependent on the cause of the hypertension, as Ang II-induced cerebral endothelial dysfunction was not reversed by Y-27632.[158]

CONCLUSION

Experimental evidence for some major mechanisms regulating cerebral vascular function has been presented, together with how many of these mechanisms are altered during hypertension and atherosclerosis – two disease states that predispose to clinical stroke. Consequently, molecular targets that may be of benefit in cerebrovascular disease, and perhaps the prevention and/or treatment of ischemic stroke, are being identified. However, clearly further work is needed to ultimately identify effective therapies as these diseases are currently poorly controlled.

REFERENCES

1. Hansson GK, Hermansson A. The immune system in atherosclerosis. Nat Immunol 2011;12:204–12.
2. Chrissobolis S, Miller AA, Drummond GR, et al. Oxidative stress and endothelial dysfunction in cerebrovascular disease. Front Biosci 2011;16:1733–45.
3. Faraci FM, Heistad DD. Regulation of the cerebral circulation: role of endothelium and potassium channels. Physiol Rev 1998;78:53–97.
4. Zhang F, Xu S, Iadecola C. Role of nitric oxide and acetylcholine in neocortical hyperemia elicited by basal forebrain stimulation: evidence for an involvement of endothelial nitric oxide. Neuroscience 1995;69:1195–204.
5. Faraci FM, Sobey CG. Role of potassium channels in regulation of cerebral vascular tone. J Cereb Blood Flow Metab 1998;18:1047–63.
6. Sobey CG, Faraci FM. Effect of nitric oxide and potassium channel agonists and inhibitors on basilar artery diameter. Am J Physiol Heart Circ Physiol 1997;272:H256–62.
7. Paterno R, Heistad DD, Faraci FM. Functional activity of Ca^{2+}-dependent K+ channels is increased in basilar artery during chronic hypertension. Am J Physiol Heart Circ Physiol 1997;272:H1287–91.
8. Lohn M, Lauterbach B, Haller H, et al. β(1)-Subunit of BK channels regulates arterial wall[Ca(2+)] and diameter in mouse cerebral arteries. J Appl Physiol 2001;91:1350–4.
9. Paterno R, Faraci FM, Heistad DD. Role of Ca^{2+}-dependent K^+ channels in cerebral vasodilatation induced by increases in cyclic GMP and cyclic AMP in the rat. Stroke 1996;27:1603–8.
10. Dabertrand F, Nelson MT, Brayden JE. Acidosis dilates brain parenchymal arterioles by conversion of calcium waves to sparks to activate BK channels. Circ Res 2012;110:285–94.
11. Liang GH, Xi Q, Leffler CW, et al. Hydrogen sulfide activates Ca(2)(+) sparks to induce cerebral arteriole dilatation. J Physiol 2012;590:2709–20.
12. Jackson-Weaver O, Paredes DA, Gonzalez Bosc LV, et al. Intermittent hypoxia in rats increases myogenic tone through loss of hydrogen sulfide activation of large-conductance Ca^{2+}-activated potassium channels. Circ Res 2011;108:1439–47.
13. Zhao G, Adebiyi A, Xi Q, et al. Hypoxia reduces KCa channel activity by inducing Ca^{2+} spark uncoupling in cerebral artery smooth muscle cells. Am J Physiol Cell Physiol 2007;292:C2122–8.
14. Howitt L, Sandow SL, Grayson TH, et al. Differential effects of diet-induced obesity on BKCa β1-subunit expression and function in rat skeletal muscle arterioles and small cerebral arteries. Am J Physiol Heart Circ Physiol 2011;301:H29–40.
15. Kitazono T, Faraci FM, Taguchi H, et al. Role of potassium channels in cerebral blood vessels. Stroke 1995;26:1713–23.
16. Sobey CG. Potassium channel function in vascular disease. Arterioscler Thromb Vasc Biol 2001;21:28–38.
17. Faraci FM, Heistad DD. Role of ATP-sensitive potassium channels in the basilar artery. Am J Physiol Heart Circ Physiol 1993;264:H8–13.
18. Kitazono T, Heistad DD, Faraci FM. Role of ATP-sensitive K+ channels in CGRP-induced dilatation of basilar artery in vivo. Am J Physiol Heart Circ Physiol 1993;265:H581–5.
19. Kitazono T, Faraci FM, Heistad DD. Effect of norepinephrine on rat basilar artery in vivo. Am J Physiol Heart Circ Physiol 1993;264:H178–82.
20. Jansen-Olesen I, Mortensen CH, El-Bariaki N, et al. Characterization of K(ATP)-channels in rat basilar and middle cerebral arteries: studies of vasomotor responses and mRNA expression. Eur J Pharmacol 2005;523:109–18.
21. Ploug KB, Edvinsson L, Olesen J, et al. Pharmacological and molecular comparison of K(ATP) channels in rat basilar and middle cerebral arteries. Eur J Pharmacol 2006;553:254–62.
22. Adebiyi A, McNally EM, Jaggar JH. Vasodilation induced by oxygen/glucose deprivation is attenuated in cerebral arteries of SUR2 null mice. Am J Physiol Heart Circ Physiol 2011;301:H1360–8.
23. Liang GH, Adebiyi A, Leo MD, et al. Hydrogen sulfide dilates cerebral arterioles by activating smooth muscle cell plasma membrane KATP channels. Am J Physiol Heart Circ Physiol 2011;300:H2088–95.
24. Lindauer U, Vogt J, Schuh-Hofer S, et al. Cerebrovascular vasodilation to extraluminal acidosis occurs via combined activation of ATP-sensitive and Ca^{2+}-activated potassium channels. J Cereb Blood Flow Metab 2003;23:1227–38.
25. Rosenblum WI, Wei EP, Kontos HA. Vasodilation of brain surface arterioles by blockade of Na-H+ antiport and its inhibition by inhibitors of KATP channel openers. Brain Res 2004;1005:77–83.
26. Philip S, Armstead WM. NMDA dilates pial arteries by KATP and KCa channel activation. Brain Res Bull 2004;63:127–31.
27. Taguchi H, Heistad DD, Kitazono T, et al. ATP-sensitive K^+ channels mediate dilatation of cerebral arterioles during hypoxia. Circ Res 1994;74:1005–8.
28. Sobey CG, Faraci FM. Inhibitory effect of 4-aminopyridine on responses of the basilar artery to nitric oxide. Br J Pharmacol 1999;126:1437–43.
29. Quan L, Sobey CG. Selective effects of subarachnoid hemorrhage on cerebral vascular responses to 4-aminopyridine in rats. Stroke 2000;31:2460–5.
30. Jarajapu YP, Oomen C, Uteshev VV, et al. Histamine decreases myogenic tone in rat cerebral arteries by H2-receptor-mediated KV channel activation, independent of endothelium and cyclic AMP. Eur J Pharmacol 2006;547:116–24.
31. Albarwani S, Nemetz LT, Madden JA, et al. Voltage-gated K+ channels in rat small cerebral arteries: molecular identity of the functional channels. J Physiol 2003;551:751–63.
32. Cheong A, Dedman AM, Beech DJ. Expression and function of native potassium channel [K(V)α] subunits in terminal arterioles of rabbit. J Physiol 2001;534:691–700.

33. Ishiguro M, Morielli AD, Zvarova K, et al. Oxyhemoglobin-induced suppression of voltage-dependent K+ channels in cerebral arteries by enhanced tyrosine kinase activity. Circ Res 2006;99:1252–60.
34. Jahromi BS, Aihara Y, Ai J, et al. Voltage-gated K+ channel dysfunction in myocytes from a dog model of subarachnoid hemorrhage. J Cereb Blood Flow Metab 2008;28:797–811.
35. Amberg GC, Santana LF. Kv2 channels oppose myogenic constriction of rat cerebral arteries. Am J Physiol Cell Physiol 2006;291:C348–56.
36. Cheong A, Dedman AM, Xu SZ, et al. K(V)α1 channels in murine arterioles: differential cellular expression and regulation of diameter. Am J Physiol Heart Circ Physiol 2001;281: H1057–65.
37. Chrissobolis S, Ziogas J, Chu Y, et al. Role of inwardly rectifying K(+) channels in K(+)-induced cerebral vasodilatation in vivo. Am J Physiol Heart Circ Physiol 2000;279: H2704–12.
38. Horiuchi T, Dietrich HH, Tsugane S, et al. Role of potassium channels in regulation of brain arteriolar tone: comparison of cerebrum versus brain stem. Stroke 2001;32:218–24.
39. Johnson TD, Marrelli SP, Steenberg ML, et al. Inward rectifier potassium channels in the rat middle cerebral artery. Am J Physiol Reg Int Comp Physiol 1998;274:R541–7.
40. Knot HJ, Zimmerman PA, Nelson MT. Extracellular K^+-induced hyperpolarizations and dilatations of rat coronary and cerebral arteries involve inward rectifier K^+ channels. J Physiol 1996;492: 419–30.
41. Prior HM, Webster N, Quinn K, et al. K^+-induced dilation of a small renal artery: no role for inward rectifier K^+ channels. Cardiovasc Res 1998;37:780–90.
42. Sun H, Zhao H, Sharpe GM, et al. Influence of chronic alcohol consumption on inward rectifier potassium channels in cerebral arterioles. Microvasc Res 2008;75:367–72.
43. Weyer GW, Jahromi BS, Aihara Y, et al. Expression and function of inwardly rectifying potassium channels after experimental subarachnoid hemorrhage. J Cereb Blood Flow Metab 2006;26: 382–91.
44. Zaritsky JJ, Eckman DM, Wellman GC, et al. Targeted disruption of Kir2.1 and Kir2.2 genes reveals the essential role of the inwardly rectifying K^+ current in K^+-mediated vasodilation. Circ Res 2000;87:160–6.
45. Filosa JA, Bonev AD, Straub SV, et al. Local potassium signaling couples neuronal activity to vasodilation in the brain. Nat Neurosci 2006;9:1397–403.
46. Fujii K, Heistad DD, Faraci FM. Ionic mechanisms in spontaneous vasomotion of the rat basilar artery *in vivo*. J Physiol 1990;430:389–98.
47. McCarron JG, Halpern W. Potassium dilates rat cerebral arteries by two independent mechanisms. Am J Physiol Heart Circ Physiol 1990;259:H902–8.
48. Busija DW, Chen J. Reversal by increased CSF [H+] and [K+] of phorbol ester-induced arteriolar constriction in piglets. Am J Physiol Heart Circ Physiol 1992;263:H1455–9.
49. Iadecola C, Kraig RP. Focal elevations in neocortical interstitial K+ produced by stimulation of the fastigial nucleus in rat. Brain Res 1991;563:273–7.
50. Kuschinsky W, Wahl M, Bosse O, et al. Perivascular potassium and pH as determinants of local pial arterial diameter in cats. Circ Res 1972;31:240–7.
51. McCulloch J, Edvinsson L, Watt P. Comparison of the effects of potassium and pH on the calibre of cerebral veins and arteries. Pflugers Arch 1982;393:95–8.
52. Nguyen TS, Winn HR, Janigro D. ATP-sensitive potassium channels may participate in the coupling of neuronal activity and cerebrovascular tone. Am J Physiol Heart Circ Physiol 2000;278: H878–85.
53. Paisansathan C, Xu H, Vetri F, et al. Interactions between adenosine and K+ channel-related pathways in the coupling of somatosensory activation and pial arteriolar dilation. Am J Physiol Heart Circ Physiol 2010;299:H2009–17.
54. Nakahata K, Kinoshita H, Tokinaga Y, et al. Vasodilation mediated by inward rectifier K^+ channels in cerebral microvessels of hypertensive and normotensive rats. Anesth Analg 2006;102: 571–6.
55. Jin CZ, Kim HS, Seo EY, et al. Exercise training increases inwardly rectifying K^+ current and augments K^+-mediated vasodilatation in deep femoral artery of rats. Cardiovasc Res 2011;91:142–50.
56. Chrissobolis S, Sobey CG. Inhibitory effects of protein kinase C on inwardly rectifying K^+- and ATP-sensitive K^+ channel-mediated responses of the basilar artery. Stroke 2002;33:1692–7.
57. Chrissobolis S, Ziogas J, Anderson CR, et al. Neuronal NO mediates cerebral vasodilator responses to K^+ in hypertensive rats. Hypertension 2002;39:880–5.
58. Marrelli SP, Johnson TD, Khorovets A, et al. Altered function of inward rectifier potassium channels in cerebrovascular smooth muscle after ischemia/reperfusion. Stroke 1998;29:1469–74.
59. Ketchum KA, Joiner WJ, Sellers AJ, et al. A new family of outwardly rectifying potassium channel proteins with two pore domains in tandem. Nature 1995;376:690–5.
60. Lloyd EE, Marrelli SP, Bryan RM Jr. cGMP does not activate two-pore domain K+ channels in cerebrovascular smooth muscle. Am J Physiol Heart Circ Physiol 2009;296:H1774–80.
61. Bryan RM Jr, You J, Phillips SC, et al. Evidence for two-pore domain potassium channels in rat cerebral arteries. Am J Physiol Heart Circ Physiol 2006;291:H770–80.
62. Blondeau N, Petrault O, Manta S, et al. Polyunsaturated fatty acids are cerebral vasodilators via the TREK-1 potassium channel. Circ Res 2007;101:176–84.
63. Namiranian K, Lloyd EE, Crossland RF, et al. Cerebrovascular responses in mice deficient in the potassium channel, TREK-1. Am J Physiol Regul Integr Comp Physiol 2010;299:R461–9.
64. Parelkar NK, Silswal N, Jansen K, et al. 2,2,2-trichloroethanol activates a nonclassical potassium channel in cerebrovascular smooth muscle and dilates the middle cerebral artery. J Pharmacol Exp Ther 2010;332:803–10.
65. Somlyo AP, Somlyo AV. Signal transduction by G-proteins, rho-kinase and protein phosphatase to smooth muscle and non-muscle myosin II. J Physiol 2000;522(Pt 2):177–85.
66. Somlyo AP, Somlyo AV. Ca^{2+} Sensitivity of smooth muscle and nonmuscle myosin II: modulated by G proteins, kinases, and myosin phosphatase. Physiol Rev 2003;83:1325–58.
67. Chrissobolis S, Sobey CG. Recent evidence for an involvement of rho-kinase in cerebral vascular disease. Stroke 2006;37: 2174–80.
68. Gokina NI, Park KM, McElroy-Yaggy K, et al. Effects of Rho kinase inhibition on cerebral artery myogenic tone and reactivity. J Appl Physiol 2005;98:1940–8.
69. Lagaud G, Gaudreault N, Moore ED, et al. Pressure-dependent myogenic constriction of cerebral arteries occurs independently of voltage-dependent activation. Am J Physiol Heart Circ Physiol 2002;283:H2187–95.
70. Lim M, Choi SK, Cho YE, et al. The role of sphingosine kinase 1/sphingosine-1-phosphate pathway in the myogenic tone of posterior cerebral arteries. PLoS ONE 2012;7:e35177.
71. Kold-Petersen H, Brondum E, Nilsson H, et al. Impaired myogenic tone in isolated cerebral and coronary resistance arteries from the goto-kakizaki rat model of type 2 diabetes. J Vasc Res 2012;49:267–78.
72. Chrissobolis S, Budzyn K, Marley PD, et al. Evidence that estrogen suppresses rho-kinase function in the cerebral circulation in vivo. Stroke 2004;35:2200–5.
73. Chrissobolis S, Sobey CG. Evidence that rho-kinase activity contributes to cerebral vascular tone in vivo and is enhanced during chronic hypertension: comparison with protein kinase C. Circ Res 2001;88:774–9.
74. Erdos B, Snipes JA, Kis B, et al. Vasoconstrictor mechanisms in the cerebral circulation are unaffected by insulin resistance. Am J Physiol Regul Integr Comp Physiol 2004;287:R1456–61.
75. Kitayama J, Kitazono T, Ooboshi H, et al. Long-term effects of benidipine on cerebral vasoreactivity in hypertensive rats. Eur J Pharmacol 2002;438:153–8.
76. Kitazono T, Ago T, Kamouchi M, et al. Increased activity of calcium channels and Rho-associated kinase in the basilar artery during chronic hypertension in vivo. J Hypertens 2002;20: 879–84.
77. Didion SP, Lynch CM, Baumbach GL, et al. Impaired endothelium-dependent responses and enhanced influence of Rho-kinase in cerebral arterioles in type II diabetes. Stroke 2005;36:342–7.

78. Miller AA, Drummond GR, Sobey CG. Reactive oxygen species in the cerebral circulation: are they all bad? Antioxid Redox Signal 2006;8:1113–20.
79. Didion SP, Faraci FM. Effects of NADH and NADPH on superoxide levels and cerebral vascular tone. Am J Physiol Heart Circ Physiol 2002;282:H688–95.
80. Park L, Anrather J, Zhou P, et al. Exogenous NADPH increases cerebral blood flow through NADPH oxidase-dependent and -independent mechanisms. Arterioscler Thromb Vasc Biol 2004; 24:1860–5.
81. Wei EP, Christman CW, Kontos HA, et al. Effects of oxygen radicals on cerebral arterioles. Am J Physiol 1985;248:H157–62.
82. Wei EP, Kontos HA, Beckman JS. Mechanisms of cerebral vasodilation by superoxide, hydrogen peroxide, and peroxynitrite. Am J Physiol 1996;271:H1262–6.
83. Cosentino F, Sill JC, Katusic ZS. Role of superoxide anions in the mediation of endothelium-dependent contractions. Hypertension 1994;23:229–35.
84. Iida Y, Katusic ZS. Mechanisms of cerebral arterial relaxations to hydrogen peroxide. Stroke 2000;31:2224–30.
85. Leffler CW, Busija DW, Armstead WM, et al. H_2O_2 effects on cerebral prostanoids and pial arteriolar diameter in piglets. Am J Physiol 1990;258:H1382–7.
86. Miller AA, Drummond GR, Mast AE, et al. Effect of gender on NADPH-oxidase activity, expression, and function in the cerebral circulation: role of estrogen. Stroke 2007;38:2142–9.
87. Miller AA, Drummond GR, Schmidt HHW, et al. NADPH oxidase activity and function are profoundly greater in cerebral versus systemic arteries. Circ Res 2005;97:1055–62.
88. Paravicini TM, Chrissobolis S, Drummond GR, et al. Increased NADPH-oxidase activity and Nox4 expression during chronic hypertension is associated with enhanced cerebral vasodilatation to NADPH in vivo. Stroke 2004;35:584–9.
89. Sobey CG, Heistad DD, Faraci FM. Mechanisms of bradykinin-induced cerebral vasodilatation in rats. Evidence that reactive oxygen species activate K+ channels. Stroke 1997;28:2290–4.
90. Sobey CG, Heistad DD, Faraci FM. Potassium channels mediate dilatation of cerebral arterioles in response to arachidonate. Am J Physiol 1998;275:H1606–12.
91. You J, Golding EM, Bryan RM Jr. Arachidonic acid metabolites, hydrogen peroxide, and EDHF in cerebral arteries. Am J Physiol Heart Circ Physiol 2005;289:H1077–83.
92. De Silva TM, Broughton BR, Drummond GR, et al. Gender influences cerebral vascular responses to angiotensin II through Nox2-derived reactive oxygen species. Stroke 2009;40:1091–7.
93. Li J, Li W, Altura BT, et al. Peroxynitrite-induced relaxation in isolated canine cerebral arteries and mechanisms of action. Toxicol Appl Pharmacol 2004;196:176–82.
94. Maneen MJ, Hannah R, Vitullo L, et al. Peroxynitrite diminishes myogenic activity and is associated with decreased vascular smooth muscle F-actin in rat posterior cerebral arteries. Stroke 2006;37:894–9.
95. Brzezinska AK, Gebremedhin D, Chilian WM, et al. Peroxynitrite reversibly inhibits Ca^{2+}-activated K^+ channels in rat cerebral artery smooth muscle cells. Am J Physiol Heart Circ Physiol 2000;278:H1883–90.
96. Elliott SJ, Lacey DJ, Chilian WM, et al. Peroxynitrite is a contractile agonist of cerebral artery smooth muscle cells. Am J Physiol 1998;275:H1585–91.
97. Maneen MJ, Cipolla MJ. Peroxynitrite diminishes myogenic tone in cerebral arteries: role of nitrotyrosine and F-actin. Am J Physiol Heart Circ Physiol 2007;292:H1042–50.
98. Earley S. TRPA1 channels in the vasculature. Br J Pharmacol 2012;167:13–22.
99. Earley S. Endothelium-dependent cerebral artery dilation mediated by transient receptor potential and Ca2+-activated K+ channels. J Cardiovasc Pharmacol 2011;57:148–53.
100. Earley S, Gonzales AL, Crnich R. Endothelium-dependent cerebral artery dilation mediated by TRPA1 and Ca2+-Activated K+ channels. Circ Res 2009;104:987–94.
101. Earley S. TRPM4 channels in smooth muscle function. Pflugers Arch 2013;465:1223–31.
102. Earley S, Waldron BJ, Brayden JE. Critical role for transient receptor potential channel TRPM4 in myogenic constriction of cerebral arteries. Circ Res 2004;95:922–9.
103. Gonzales AL, Garcia ZI, Amberg GC, et al. Pharmacological inhibition of TRPM4 hyperpolarizes vascular smooth muscle. Am J Physiol Cell Physiol 2010;299:C1195–202.
104. Crnich R, Amberg GC, Leo MD, et al. Vasoconstriction resulting from dynamic membrane trafficking of TRPM4 in vascular smooth muscle cells. Am J Physiol Cell Physiol 2010;299: C682–94.
105. Toth P, Csiszar A, Tucsek Z, et al. Role of 20-HETE,TRP channels & BKCa in dysregulation of pressure-induced Ca^{2+} signaling and myogenic constriction of cerebral arteries in aged hypertensive mice. Am J Physiol Heart Circ Physiol 2013.
106. Earley S, Gonzales AL, Garcia ZI. A dietary agonist of transient receptor potential cation channel V3 elicits endothelium-dependent vasodilation. Mol Pharmacol 2010;77:612–20.
107. Inoue R, Jensen LJ, Shi J, et al. Transient receptor potential channels in cardiovascular function and disease. Circ Res 2006;99: 119–31.
108. Charo IF, Taub R. Anti-inflammatory therapeutics for the treatment of atherosclerosis. Nat Rev Drug Discov 2011;10: 365–76.
109. Weber C, Noels H. Atherosclerosis: current pathogenesis and therapeutic options. Nat Med 2011;17:1410–22.
110. Sitia S, Tomasoni L, Atzeni F, et al. From endothelial dysfunction to atherosclerosis. Autoimmun Rev 2011;9:830–4.
111. Ishikawa M, Stokes KY, Zhang JH, et al. Cerebral microvascular responses to hypercholesterolemia: roles of NADPH oxidase and P-selectin. Circ Res 2004;94:239–44.
112. Miller AA, De Silva TM, Judkins CP, et al. Augmented superoxide production by Nox2-containing NADPH oxidase causes cerebral artery dysfunction during hypercholesterolemia. Stroke 2010;41: 784–9.
113. Rossitch E Jr, Alexander E 3rd, Black PM, et al. L-arginine normalizes endothelial function in cerebral vessels from hypercholesterolemic rabbits. J Clin Invest 1991;87:1295–9.
114. Simonsen U, Ehrnrooth E, Gerdes LU, et al. Functional properties in vitro of systemic small arteries from rabbits fed a cholesterol-rich diet for 12 weeks. Clin Sci (Lond) 1991;80: 119–29.
115. Kanamaru K, Waga S, Tochio H, et al. The effect of atherosclerosis on endothelium-dependent relaxation in the aorta and intracranial arteries of rabbits. J Neurosurg 1989;70:793–8.
116. Stewart-Lee AL, Burnstock G. Changes in vasoconstrictor and vasodilator responses of the basilar artery during maturation in the Watanabe heritable hyperlipidemic rabbit differ from those in the New Zealand White rabbit. Arterioscler Thromb 1991;11: 1147–55.
117. Didion SP, Heistad DD, Faraci FM. Mechanisms that produce nitric oxide-mediated relaxation of cerebral arteries during atherosclerosis. Stroke 2001;32:761–6.
118. Kitayama J, Faraci FM, Lentz SR, et al. Cerebral vascular dysfunction during hypercholesterolemia. Stroke 2007;38:2136–41.
119. Yamashiro K, Milsom AB, Duchene J, et al. Alterations in nitric oxide and endothelin-1 bioactivity underlie cerebrovascular dysfunction in ApoE-deficient mice. J Cereb Blood Flow Metab 2010;30:1494–503.
120. Schreurs BG, Smith-Bell CA, Lemieux SK. Dietary cholesterol increases ventricular volume and narrows cerebrovascular diameter in a rabbit model of Alzheimer's disease. Neuroscience 2013;254C:61–9.
121. Bengrine A, Da Silveira C, Massy ZA, et al. Cerebral arterioles preparation and PECAM-1 expression in C57BL/6J and $ApoE^{-/-}$ mice. Front Biosci (Landmark Ed) 2011;16:2367–71.
122. Badaut J, Copin JC, Fukuda AM, et al. Increase of arginase activity in old apolipoprotein-E deficient mice under Western diet associated with changes in neurovascular unit. J Neuroinflammation 2012;9:132.
123. Ryoo S, Lemmon CA, Soucy KG, et al. Oxidized low-density lipoprotein-dependent endothelial arginase II activation contributes to impaired nitric oxide signaling. Circ Res 2006;99: 951–60.
124. Bugnicourt JM, Da Silveira C, Bengrine A, et al. Chronic renal failure alters endothelial function in cerebral circulation in mice. Am J Physiol Heart Circ Physiol 2011;301:H1143–52.
125. Iadecola C, Davisson RL. Hypertension and cerebrovascular dysfunction. Cell Metab 2008;7:476–84.

126. Kitazono T, Heistad DD, Faraci FM. ATP-sensitive potassium channels in the basilar artery during chronic hypertension. Hypertension 1993;22:677–81.
127. Kitazono T, Heistad DD, Faraci FM. Enhanced responses of the basilar artery to activation of endothelin-B receptors in stroke-prone spontaneously hypertensive rats. Hypertension 1995;25: 490–4.
128. Mayhan WG. Impairment of endothelium-dependent dilatation of basilar artery during chronic hypertension. Am J Physiol Heart Circ Physiol 1990;259:H1455–62.
129. Sobey CG, Moffatt JD, Cocks TM. Evidence for selective effects of chronic hypertension on cerebral artery vasodilatation to protease-activated receptor-2 activation. Stroke 1999;30:1933–41.
130. Kazama K, Anrather J, Zhou P, et al. Angiotensin II impairs neurovascular coupling in neocortex through NADPH oxidase-derived radicals. Circ Res 2004;95:1019–26.
131. Girouard H, Park L, Anrather J, et al. Cerebrovascular nitrosative stress mediates neurovascular and endothelial dysfunction induced by angiotensin II. Arterioscler Thromb Vasc Biol 2007;27:303–9.
132. Capone C, Faraco G, Anrather J, et al. Cyclooxygenase 1-derived prostaglandin E2 and EP1 receptors are required for the cerebrovascular dysfunction induced by angiotensin II. Hypertension 2010;55:911–17.
133. Capone C, Anrather J, Milner TA, et al. Estrous cycle dependent neurovascular dysfunction induced by angiotensin II in the mouse neocortex. Hypertension 2009;54:302–7.
134. Girouard H, Park L, Anrather J, et al. Angiotensin II attenuates endothelium-dependent responses in the cerebral microcirculation through nox-2-derived radicals. Arterioscler Thromb Vasc Biol 2006;26:826–32.
135. Didion SP, Faraci FM. Angiotensin II produces superoxide-mediated impairment of endothelial function in cerebral arterioles. Stroke 2003;34:2038–42.
136. Kitayama J, Chu Y, Faraci FM, et al. Modulation of dilator responses of cerebral arterioles by extracellular superoxide dismutase. Stroke 2006;37:2802–6.
137. Chrissobolis S, Banfi B, Sobey CG, et al. Role of Nox isoforms in angiotensin II-induced oxidative stress and endothelial dysfunction in brain. J Appl Physiol 2012;113:184–91.
138. Chrissobolis S, Faraci FM. Sex differences in protection against angiotensin II-induced endothelial dysfunction by manganese superoxide dismutase in the cerebral circulation. Hypertension 2010;55:905–10.
139. Capone C, Faraco G, Park L, et al. The cerebrovascular dysfunction induced by slow pressor doses of angiotensin II precedes the development of hypertension. Am J Physiol Heart Circ Physiol 2011;300:H397–407.
140. Faraci FM, Lamping KG, Modrick ML, et al. Cerebral vascular effects of angiotensin II: new insights from genetic models. J Cereb Blood Flow Metab 2006;26:449–55.
141. Ishikawa M, Sekizuka E, Yamaguchi N, et al. Angiotensin II type 1 receptor signaling contributes to platelet-leukocyte-endothelial cell interactions in the cerebral microvasculature. Am J Physiol Heart Circ Physiol 2007;292:H2306–15.
142. Vital SA, Terao S, Nagai M, et al. Mechanisms underlying the cerebral microvascular responses to angiotensin II-induced hypertension. Microcirculation 2010;17:641–9.
143. Zhang M, Mao Y, Ramirez SH, et al. Angiotensin II induced cerebral microvascular inflammation and increased blood-brain barrier permeability via oxidative stress. Neuroscience 2010;171: 852–8.
144. Rodrigues SF, Vital SA, Granger DN. Mild hypercholesterolemia blunts the proinflammatory and prothrombotic effects of hypertension on the cerebral microcirculation. J Cereb Blood Flow Metab 2013;33:483–9.
145. Rodrigues SF, Granger DN. Cerebral microvascular inflammation in DOCA salt-induced hypertension: role of angiotensin II and mitochondrial superoxide. J Cereb Blood Flow Metab 2012;32: 368–75.
146. Ando H, Zhou J, Macova M, et al. Angiotensin II AT1 receptor blockade reverses pathological hypertrophy and inflammation in brain microvessels of spontaneously hypertensive rats. Stroke 2004;35:1726–31.
147. Benicky J, Sanchez-Lemus E, Honda M, et al. Angiotensin II AT1 receptor blockade ameliorates brain inflammation. Neuropsychopharmacology 2011;36:857–70.
148. Liu Y, Hudetz AG, Knaus HG, et al. Increased expression of Ca^{2+}-sensitive K+ channels in the cerebral microcirculation of genetically hypertensive rats: evidence for their protection against cerebral vasospasm. Circ Res 1998;82:729–37.
149. Kamouchi M, Kitazono T, Nagao T, et al. Role of Ca^{2+}-activated K^+ channels in the regulation of basilar arterial tone in spontaneously hypertensive rats. Clin Exp Pharmacol Physiol 2002;29:575–81.
150. Amberg GC, Bonev AD, Rossow CF, et al. Modulation of the molecular composition of large conductance, Ca^{2+} activated K^+ channels in vascular smooth muscle during hypertension. J Clin Invest 2003;112:717–24.
151. Nieves-Cintron M, Amberg GC, Nichols CB, et al. Activation of NFATc3 down-regulates the β1 subunit of large conductance, calcium-activated K+ channels in arterial smooth muscle and contributes to hypertension. J Biol Chem 2007;282:3231–40.
152. Kirsch T, Wellner M, Luft FC, et al. Altered gene expression in cerebral capillaries of stroke-prone spontaneously hypertensive rats. Brain Res 2001;910:106–15.
153. Tobin AA, Joseph BK, Al-Kindi HN, et al. Loss of cerebrovascular Shaker-type K^+ channels: a shared vasodilator defect of genetic and renal hypertensive rats. Am J Physiol Heart Circ Physiol 2009;297:H293–303.
154. Wellman GC, Cartin L, Eckman DM, et al. Membrane depolarization, elevated Ca^{2+} entry, and gene expression in cerebral arteries of hypertensive rats. Am J Physiol Heart Circ Physiol 2001;281:H2559–67.
155. Xie MJ, Zhang LF, Ma J, et al. Functional alterations in cerebrovascular K^+ and Ca^{2+} channels are comparable between simulated microgravity rat and SHR. Am J Physiol Heart Circ Physiol 2005;289:H1265–76.
156. McCarron JG, Halpern W. Impaired potassium-induced dilatation in hypertensive rat cerebral arteries does not reflect altered Na^+, K^+-ATPase dilation. Circ Res 1990;67:1035–9.
157. Jarajapu YP, Knot HJ. Relative contribution of Rho-kinase and PKC to myogenic tone in rat cerebral arteries in hypertension. Am J Physiol Heart Circ Physiol 2005;289:1917–22.
158. Faraco G, Moraga A, Moore J, et al. Circulating endothelin-1 alters critical mechanisms regulating cerebral microcirculation. Hypertension 2013;62:759–66.

2 Mechanisms of Thrombosis and Thrombolysis

Gregory J. del Zoppo

KEY POINTS

- The fundamental processes involved in thrombus formation, thrombus dissolution, and thrombus stability and their relevance to the CNS are described.
- The role(s) of endogenous plasminogen activators (PAs, including tissue-type plasminogen activator, urokinase-type plasminogen activator) in thrombus dissolution are presented, together with considerations of their regulation in vivo. Their relevance to derived therapeutics is emphasized.
- Fibrinolytic agents tested or used as pharmaceuticals including recombinant and purified endogenous PAs and exogenous PAs (including streptokinase, staphylokinase, PAs derived from *Desmodus* species, and novel plasminogen activators) are presented.
- The molecular basis for PA inhibition and modulation of vascular fibrinolysis is made.
- These considerations form a basis for exploration of current information about the impact of PAs and of plasmin generation on CNS vessel and microvessel integrity.
- Exploration of the role(s) of endogenous PAs in CNS development, CNS integrity, and on neuronal function in the CNS is presented, and the potential effects of therapeutic PAs on the CNS.
- The pioneering use of therapeutic plasminogen activation in the acute setting in ischemic/thrombotic stroke, acute cerebral arterial recanalization, and its consequences are described.
- The use of PAs in experimental cerebral ischemia, recanalization and tissue injury reduction, and their limitations and relevance to the clinical setting are discussed.
- The risks of PAs in the acute intervention in ischemic stroke and the quantitative effects on intracerebral hemorrhage are presented. Limitations to the clinical use of fibrinolytic agents in ischemic stroke are considered.

Thrombosis, and thrombus growth, dissolution, and migration are inextricably connected. Thrombus formation involves activation of platelets, activation of the coagulation system, and the processes of fibrin dissolution. The central feature of each of these processes is the generation of thrombin from pro-thrombin. Thrombin, in turn, generates the thrombus fibrin network by the cleavage of circulating fibrinogen. Excess local vascular fibrin deposition can contribute to thrombus growth, while excess fibrin degradation and vascular injury can lead to hemorrhage. Plasmin can degrade fibrin and fibrinogen. Plasminogen activators have been exploited to dissolve clinically significant vascular thrombi acutely, based upon the mechanism that plasminogen is thereby converted to plasmin. Notably, all substances that promote plasmin formation retain the potential to increase the risk of hemorrhage.

The acute use of plasminogen activators (PAs) has been associated with detectable clinical improvement in selected patients with symptoms of focal cerebral ischemia.[1–9] Acute thrombolysis has thus attained pride of place in the treatment of ischemic stroke so far. Currently, recombinant tissue-type plasminogen activator (rt-PA) is licensed in the United States, Japan, Europe, and many other countries for the treatment of ischemic stroke within 3 hours of symptom onset (and up to 4.5 hours in some jurisdictions).[6,9] Early studies and a recent phase III prospective trial suggest that extension of the treatment window is possible with strict limitations to patient selection.[3–5,9] Few studies have correlated the improvement in patient outcome with recanalization of an occluded brain-supplying artery, however.[4]

The development of agents that promote fibrin degradation in the clinical setting stems from observations in the 19th century of the spontaneous liquefaction of clotted blood and the dissolution of fibrin thrombi. A growing understanding of plasma proteolytic digestion of fibrin paralleled enquiry into the mechanisms of streptococcal fibrinolysis. Streptokinase was first employed to dissolve closed space (intrapleural) fibrin clots, but purified preparations were required for lysis of intravascular thrombi. The development of PAs for therapeutic lysis of vascular thrombi has progressed along with insights into the mechanisms of thrombus formation and degradation.

THROMBUS FORMATION

The relative platelet-fibrin composition of a specific thrombus depends on the vascular bed, the local development of fibrin, platelet activation, and regional blood flow or shear stress. Pharmacologic inhibition of the platelet activation/aggregation and coagulation processes can also alter thrombus composition and volume. At arterial flow rates thrombi are predominantly platelet-rich, whereas at lower shear rates characteristic of venous flow, activation of coagulation seems to predominate. It has been suggested that the efficacy of pharmacologic thrombus lysis depends on (i) the relative fibrin content and (ii) the extent of fibrin cross-linking of the thrombus that may reflect thrombus age and thrombus remodeling. The latter may vary with location within a vascular bed (e.g., arterial, capillary, or venular).

Thrombin (factor IIa) is the central player in clot formation (Fig. 2-1). Thrombin, a serine protease, cleaves fibrinogen to generate fibrin, which forms the scaffolding for the growing thrombus. Inter-fibrin strand cross-linking requires active factor XIII, a transglutaminase bound to fibrinogen that is itself activated by thrombin. Factor XIIIa stabilizes the fibrin network (Fig. 2-2).[10,11] Thrombin-mediated fibrin polymerization leads to the generation of fibrin I and fibrin II monomers and to the release of fibrinopeptide A (FPA) and fibrinopeptide B (FPB).

Platelet activation is required for thrombus formation under arterial flow conditions and accompanies thrombin-mediated fibrin formation. Platelet membrane receptors and phospholipids form a workbench for the generation of

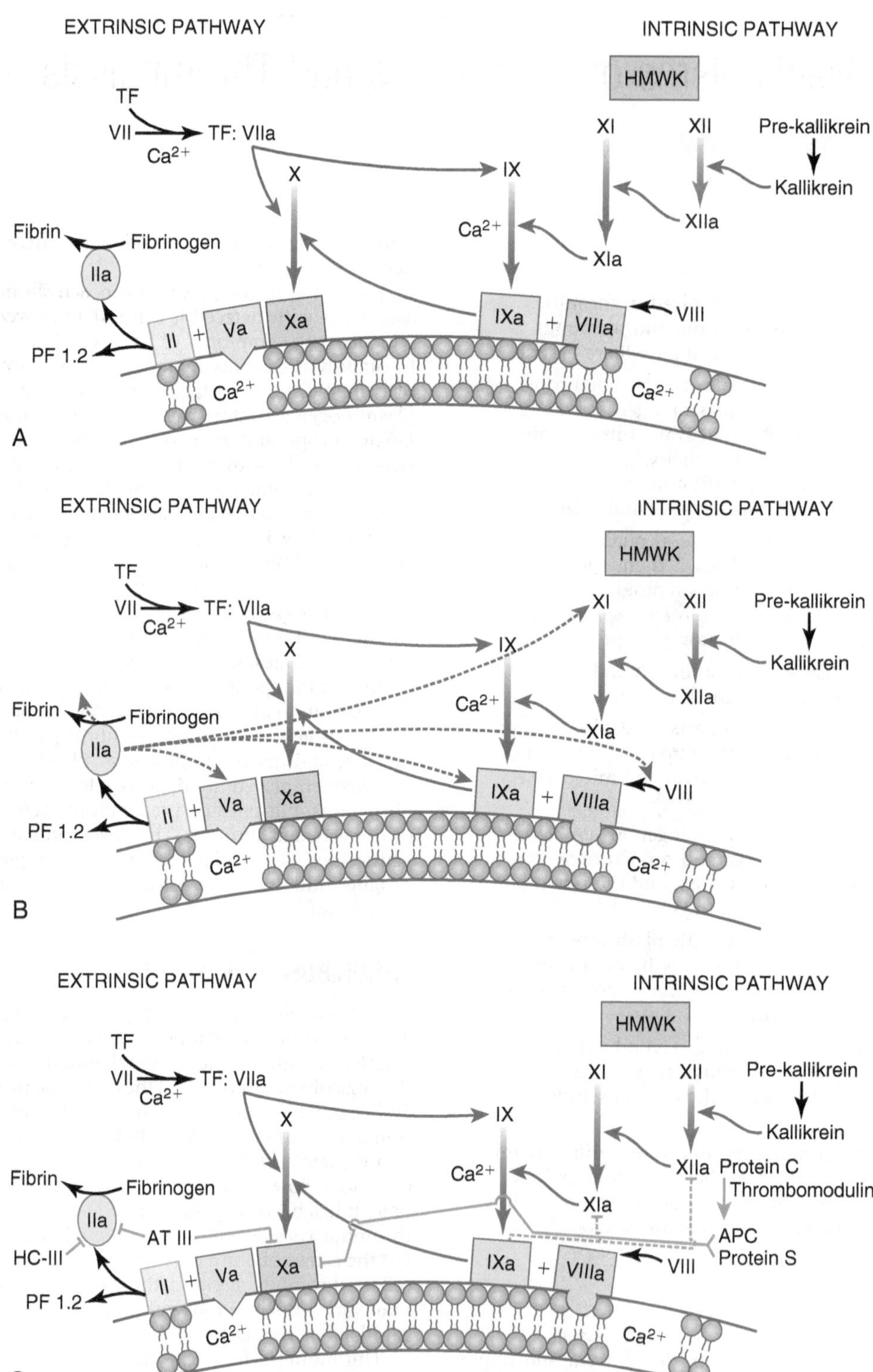

Figure 2-1. Intrinsic and extrinsic coagulation pathways (see text). Phospholipid-containing membranes (e.g., platelets) provide the scaffold for acceleration of coagulation pathway activation. Both intrinsic and extrinsic pathways lead to prothrombin (factor II) activation, with fibrin generation from circulating fibrinogen. The extrinsic pathway initiates coagulation through the interaction of factor VII with tissue factor (TF) in the vascular adventitia, brain perivascular parenchyma, and activated monocytes. The TF:VIIa complex catalyzes activation of factor X and acceleration of thrombin generation. The extrinsic system involves activation of components within the vascular lumen. Initiation of coagulation through this pathway involves pre-kallikrein, kallikrein, high-molecular-weight kininogen (HMWK), and factors XI and XII. A, Thrombin generation. The intrinsic system activates factor X through the "tenase" complex (factors VIIIa and IXa, and Ca^{2+} on phospholipid). Both intrinsic and extrinsic pathways activate prothrombin through the common "prothrombinase" complex (factors Xa and Va, and Ca^{2+}). The platelet surface has receptors for factors Va and VIIIa. Cleavage of prothrombin generates the prothrombin fragment 1.2 (PF 1.2) and thrombin (factor IIa). B, Thrombin has multiple stimulatory positive feedback effects. It catalyzes activation of factors XI and VIII as well as the activities of the tenase and prothrombinase complexes. Thrombin also stimulates activation of platelets and granule secretion via specific thrombin receptors on their surface. C, Coagulation activation is regulated by interleaving inhibitor pathways. The effects of factors Va, Xa, and VIIIa are modulated by the protein C pathway. Activated protein C (APC), generated by the action of the endothelial cell receptor thrombomodulin on protein C, with its cofactor protein S, inhibits the action of factor V. AT-III, antithrombin-III; HC-III, heparin cofactor-III.

thrombin through both the intrinsic and extrinsic coagulation pathways.[12] Platelets promote activation of the early stages of intrinsic coagulation by a process that involves the factor XI receptor and high-molecular-weight kininogen (HMWK) (see Fig. 2-1).[13] Also, factors V and VIII interact with specific platelet membrane phospholipids (receptors) to facilitate the activation of factor X to Xa (the "tenase complex") and the conversion of prothrombin to thrombin (the "prothrombinase complex") on the platelet surface.[14] Platelet-bound thrombin-modified factor V (factor Va) serves as a high-affinity platelet receptor for factor Xa.[15] These mechanisms accelerate the rate of thrombin generation, further catalyzing fibrin formation and the fibrin network.

This process also leads to the conversion of plasminogen to plasmin and to the activation of *endogenous* fibrinolysis. Thrombin provides one direct connection between thrombus formation and plasmin generation, through the localized release of tissue-type plasminogen activator (t-PA) and single chain urokinase (scu-PA) from endothelial cells. Thrombin has been shown in vitro and in vivo to markedly stimulate t-PA release from endothelial stores.[15,16] In one experiment, infusion of factor Xa and phospholipid into non-human primates resulted in a pronounced increase in circulating t-PA activity, suggesting that significant vascular stores of this PA can be released by active components of coagulation. Other vascular and cellular stimuli also augment PA release, thereby pushing the hemostatic balance toward thrombolysis (see below).

The development of arterial or venous thrombi requires loss of the constitutive antithrombotic characteristics of endothelial cells. In addition to both the antithrombotic properties of endothelial cells and the circulating anticoagulants and their cofactors (i.e., activated protein C, protein S), thrombus growth is limited by the *endogenous* thrombolytic system.

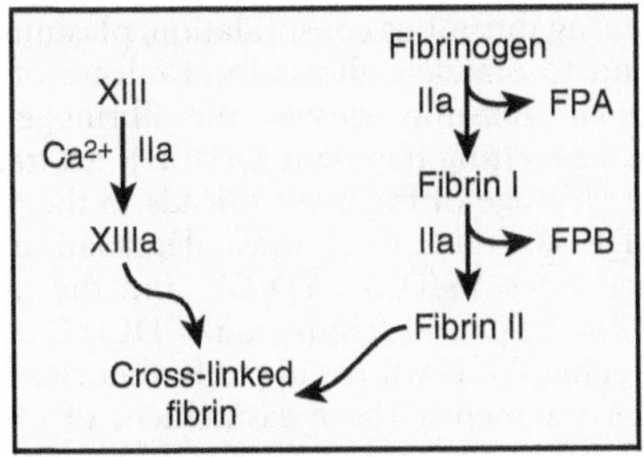

Figure 2-2. Generation of cross-linked fibrin. Fibrinogen is cleaved successively to form fibrin I and fibrin II by thrombin (factor IIa) with the release of fibrinopeptides A and B (FPA and FPB). Thrombin activates factor XIII to the active transglutaminase, which promotes cross-linking of fibrin and stabilization of the growing thrombus.

Thrombus dissolution or remodeling results from the preferential conversion of plasminogen to plasmin on the thrombus surface. There, fibrin binds t-PA in proximity to its substrate (fibrin-bound) plasminogen, thereby accelerating local plasmin formation, in concert with local shear stress.[17] These processes may also promote embolization into the downstream cerebral vasculature. However, little is known about the endogenous generation and secretion of PAs within cerebral vessels.[18] *Exogenous* application of pharmacologic doses of PAs can accelerate conversion plasminogen to plasmin and thereby prevent thrombus formation and promote thrombus dissolution, as discussed later.

FIBRINOLYSIS

Plasmin formation is central to the lysis of vascular thrombi. The endogenous fibrinolytic system comprises plasminogen, scu-PA, urokinase (u-PA), and t-PA, and their inhibitors. Hence, plasmin degrades fibrin (and fibrinogen). Plasminogen, its activators, and their inhibitors contribute to the balance between vascular thrombosis and hemorrhage (Fig. 2-3; Tables 2-1 and 2-2).

Plasmin formation occurs (i) in the plasma, where it can cleave circulating fibrinogen and fibrin into soluble products,[19] and (ii) on reactive surfaces (e.g., thrombi or cells). The fibrin network provides the scaffold for plasminogen activation, whereas various cells, including polymorphonuclear (PMN) leukocytes, platelets, and endothelial cells, express receptors for plasminogen to bind to.[19] Specific cellular receptors concentrate plasminogen and specific activators (e.g., urokinase-type plasminogen activator [u-PA]) on the cell surface, thereby enhancing local plasmin production. Similar receptors on tumor cells (e.g., the urokinase plasminogen activator receptor [u-PAR], which concentrates u-PA) also facilitate dissolution of basement membranes and matrix, promoting metastases. u-PA and u-PAR are both expressed by

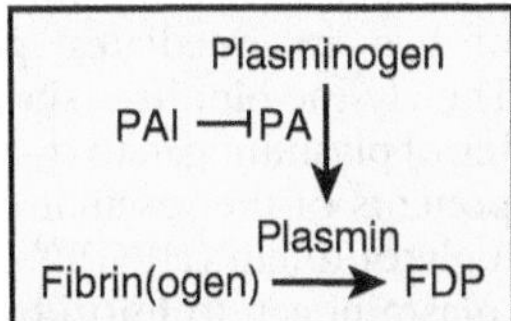

Figure 2-3. Plasminogen activation and fibrin(ogen)olysis. Degradation of fibrinogen and fibrin is catalyzed by plasmin. Plasminogen activators (PAs), including tissue-type PA (t-PA), urokinase-type PA (u-PA), and novel constructs, cleave plasminogen to the active plasmin. Characteristic products of fibrin and fibrinogen degradation (FDP) are generated (see text). PAI, plasminogen activator inhibitor.

TABLE 2-1 Plasminogen Activators

Plasmfinogen Activators	Molecular Weight (kDa)	Chains	Plasma Concentration (mg/dL)	Plasma Concentration Half-Life ($t_{1/2}$)	Substrates
ENDOGENOUS					
Plasminogen	92	2	20	2.2 days	(fibrin)
Tissue-type PA (t-PA)	68 (59)	1→2	5×10^{-4}	5–8 min	fibrin/plasminogen
Single-chain urokinase-type PA (scu-PA)	54 (46)	1→2	$2–20 \times 10^{-4}$	8 min	fibrin/plasmin(ogen)
Urokinase-type PA (u-PA)	54 (46)	2	8×10^{-4}	9–12 min	plasminogen
EXOGENOUS					
Streptokinase	47	1	0	41 and 30 min	plasminogen, fibrin(ogen)
Anisoylated plasminogen-streptokinase activator complex (APSAC)	131	complex	0	70–90 min	fibrin(ogen)
Staphylokinase	16.5		0		plasminogen

TABLE 2-2 Plasminogen Activator Inhibitors

Inhibitor	Molecular Weight (kDa)	Chains	Plasma Concentration ($mgdL^{-1}$)	Plasma Concentration Half-Life($t_{1/2}$)	Inhibitor Substrates
Plasmin Inhibitors					
α_2-antiplasmin	65	1	7	3.3 min	plasmin
α_2-macroglobulin	740	4	250		plasmin (excess)
Plasminogen Activator Inhibitors					
PAI-1	48–52	1	5×10^{-2}	7 min	t-PA, u-PA
PAI-2	47, 70	1	$<5 \times 10^{-4}$	24 h	t-PA, u-PA
PAI-3	50				u-PA, t-PA

PAI, plasminogen activator inhibitor; t-PA, tissue-type plasminogen activator; u-PA, urokinase-type plasminogen activator.

microvessels and neurons in the ischemic bed.[20,21] Plasmin can also cleave various basal lamina and extracellular matrix (ECM) ligands (e.g., laminins, collagen IV, perlecan) found in the basal lamina of microvessels of the central nervous system, and in other organs.[22-24]

Plasminogen

The naturally circulating PAs, single-chain t-PA and single-chain u-PA (scu-PA or pro-UK), catalyze plasmin formation.[25,26] Plasmin derives from the zymogen plasminogen, a glycosylated single-chain 92-kDa serine protease.[27,28] Structurally, plasminogen contains five kringles and a protease domain, two of which (K1 and K5) mediate the binding of plasminogen to fibrin through characteristic lysine-binding sites (Fig. 2-4).[27,29,30] Glu-plasminogen has an NH_2-terminal glutamic acid, and lys-plasminogen, which lacks an 8-kDa peptide, has an NH_2-terminal lysine. Plasmin cleavage of the NH_2-terminal fragment of glu-plasminogen generates lys-plasminogen. Glu-plasminogen has a plasma clearance half-life ($t_{1/2}$) of ~2.2 days, whereas the $t_{1/2}$ of lys-plasminogen is 0.8 days. Both t-PA and u-PA catalyze the conversion of glu-plasminogen to lys-plasmin through either of two intermediates, glu-plasmin or lys-plasminogen.[31] The lysine-binding sites of plasminogen mediate the binding of plasminogen to α_2-antiplasmin, thrombospondin, components of the vascular extracellular matrix, and histidine-rich glycoprotein (HRG).[28] α_2-Antiplasmin prevents binding of plasminogen to fibrin by this mechanism.[31] Partial degradation of the fibrin network enhances the binding of glu-plasminogen to fibrin, promoting further local fibrinolysis.

Plasminogen Activation

Plasminogen activation is tied to activation of the coagulation system and can involve secretion of physiologic PAs ("extrinsic activation"). It has been suggested that kallikrein, factor XIa, and factor XIIa, in the presence of HMWK, can directly activate plasminogen.[31,32] Several lines of evidence suggest that scu-PA activates plasminogen under physiologic conditions. Tissue-type PA, which is secreted from the endothelium and other cellular sources, appears to be the primary PA in the vasculature. Thrombin, generated by either intrinsic or extrinsic coagulation, stimulates secretion of t-PA from endothelial stores.[15,33]

Several serine proteases can convert plasminogen to plasmin by cleaving the arg^{560}–val^{561} bond.[27] Serine proteases have common structural features, including an NH_2-terminal "A" chain with substrate-binding affinity, a COOH-terminal "B" chain with the active site, and intra-chain disulfide bridges. Plasminogen-cleaving serine proteases include the coagulation proteins factor IX, factor X, and prothrombin (factor II), protein C, chymotrypsin and trypsin, various leukocyte elastases, the plasminogen activators u-PA and t-PA, and plasmin itself.[27]

Activation of plasminogen by t-PA is accelerated in a ternary complex with fibrin. In the circulation, plasmin binds rapidly to the inhibitor α_2-antiplasmin and is thereby inactivated. Activation of thrombus-bound plasminogen also protects plasmin from the inhibitors α_2-antiplasmin and α_2-macroglobulin.[27] Here, the lysine-binding sites and the catalytic site of plasmin are occupied by fibrin, thereby blocking its interaction with α_2-antiplasmin.[27] Furthermore, fibrin and fibrin-bound plasminogen render t-PA relatively inaccessible to inhibition by other circulating plasma inhibitors.

Thrombus Dissolution

Fibrinolysis occurs predominantly within the thrombus and at its surface but may be augmented by increased local blood flow.[34,35] During thrombus consolidation, plasminogen bound to fibrin and to platelets allows local release of plasmin. In the *circulation*, plasmin cleaves the fibrinogen Aα chain appendage, generating fragment X (DED), Aα fragments, and Bβ. Further cleavage of fragment X leads to the generation of fragments DE, D, and E. By contrast, degradation of the fibrin network generates YY/DXD, YD/DY, and the unique DD/E (fragment X = DED and fragment Y = DE). Cross-linkage of DD with fragment E is vulnerable to further cleavage, producing D-dimer fragments. The measurement of D-dimer levels has clinical utility, in that the absence of circulating D dimer correlates with the absence of massive thrombosis.[36] Ordinarily, in the setting of focal cerebral ischemia, the thrombus load is small and the meaning of D-dimer elevations uncertain. The generation of the degradation products has two consequences: (i) incorporation of some of these products into the forming thrombus destabilizes the fibrin network and (ii) reduced circulating fibrinogen and the generation of breakdown products of fibrin(ogen) limits the protection from hemorrhage by hemostatic thrombi.

PLASMINOGEN ACTIVATORS

All fibrinolytic agents are obligate plasminogen activators (see Table 2-1). Tissue-type PA, scu-PA, and u-PA are *endogenous* plasminogen activators involved in physiologic fibrinolysis. Recombinant t-PA, scu-PA, and u-PA, as well as streptokinase (SK), acylated plasminogen streptokinase activator complex (APSAC), staphylokinase, PAs from *Desmodus* species, and other newer novel agents in clinical use (e.g., reteplase (r-PA), and tenecteplase (TNK)), are termed *exogenous* plasminogen activators.[34,35] t-PA, scu-PA, and a number of novel agents have relative fibrin and thrombus specificity.[36]

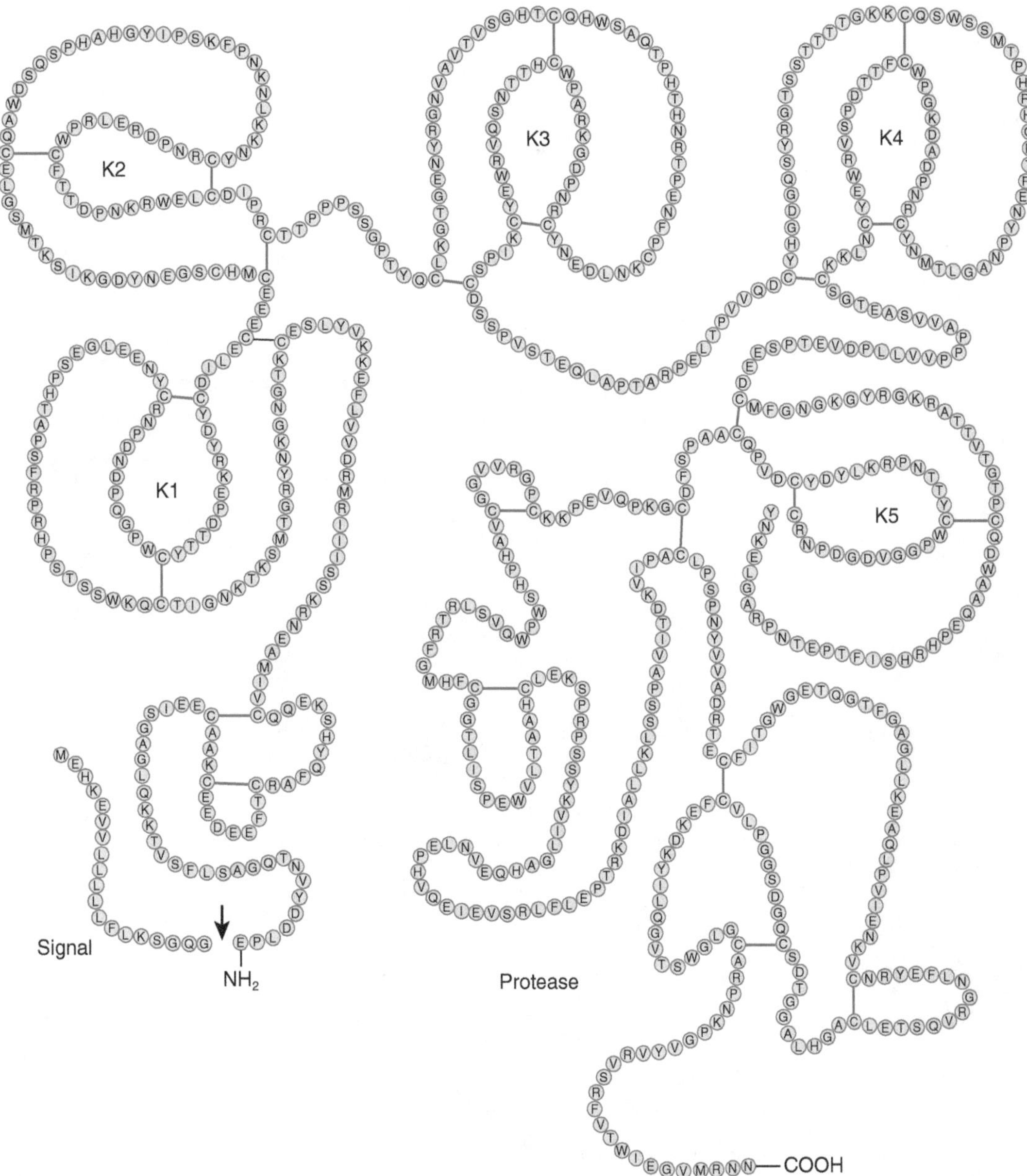

Figure 2-4. The secondary structure of plasminogen.

Endogenous Plasminogen Activators

Tissue-type Plasminogen Activator

Tissue-type PA is a 70-kDa, single-chain glycosylated serine protease that has four distinct domains – a finger (F-) domain, an epidermal growth factor (EGF) domain (residues 50–87), two kringle regions (K1 and K2), and a serine protease domain (Fig. 2-5).[37] The COOH-terminal serine protease domain contains the active site for plasminogen cleavage, and the finger and K2 domains are responsible for fibrin affinity.[37,38] The two kringle domains are homologous to the kringle regions of plasminogen.

The single-chain form is converted to the two-chain form by plasmin cleavage of the arg^{275}–isoleu^{276} bond. Both single-chain and two-chain species are enzymatically active and have relatively fibrin-selective properties. Infusion studies in humans indicate that both single-chain and two-chain t-PA have circulating plasma $t_{1/2}$ values of 3 to 8 minutes, although the biologic $t_{1/2}$ are longer. Tissue-type PA is considered to be fibrin-selective because of its favorable binding constant for fibrin-bound plasminogen and its activation of plasminogen in association with fibrin. Significant inactivation of circulating factors V and VIII does not occur with infused rt-PA, and an anticoagulant state is generally not produced. However, if sufficiently high rt-PA dose-rates are employed, clinically measurable fibrinogenolysis and plasminogen consumption can be produced.

Secretion of t-PA from cultured endothelial cells is stimulated by thrombin,[33,39] activated protein C (APC),[40] histamine,[33] phorbol myristate esterase, and other mediators.[41] Physical exercise and certain vasoactive substances produce measurable increases in circulating t-PA levels, and 1-deamino(8-D-arginine) vasopressin (DDAVP) may produce a 3–4-fold increase in t-PA antigen levels within 60 minutes of parenteral infusion in some patients. Both t-PA and u-PA have been reported to be secreted by endothelial cells, neurons, astrocytes, and microglia in vivo or in vitro.[18,42–47] The reasons for this broad cell expression are not known, however.

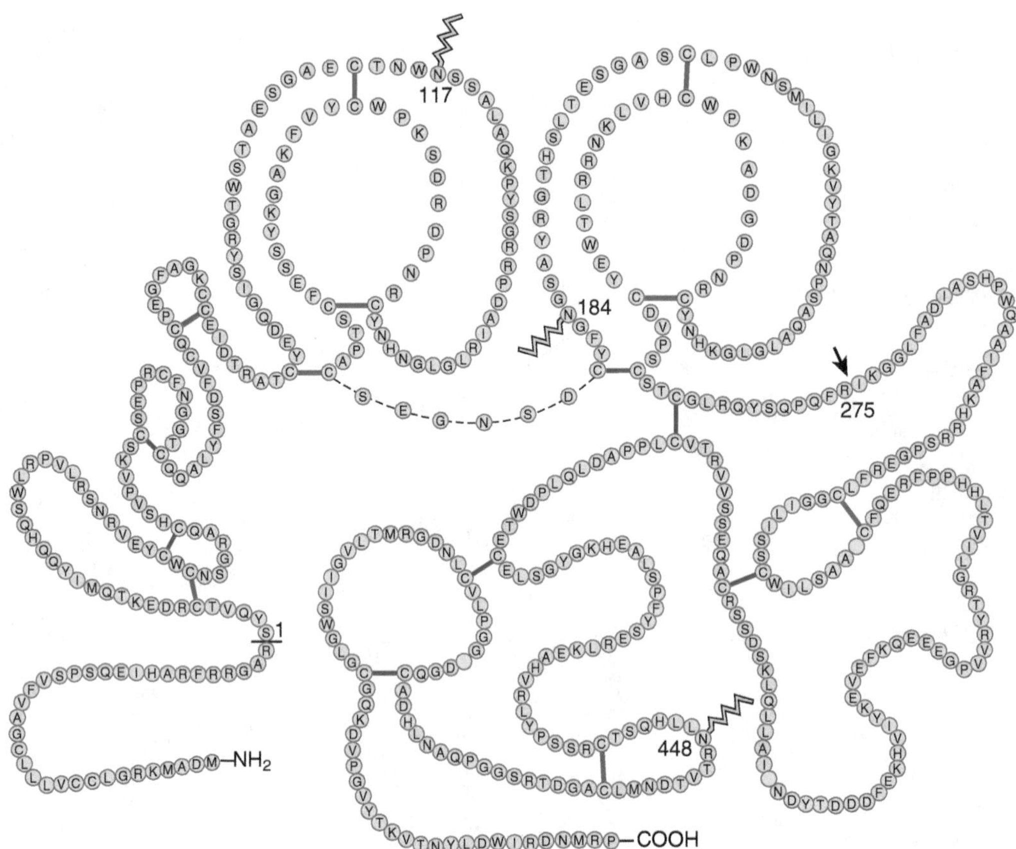

Figure 2-5. The secondary structure of tissue-type plasminogen activator (t-PA). Conversion of single-chain t-PA to two-chain t-PA by plasmin occurs at the arg^{275}-isoleu^{276} bond (arrow).

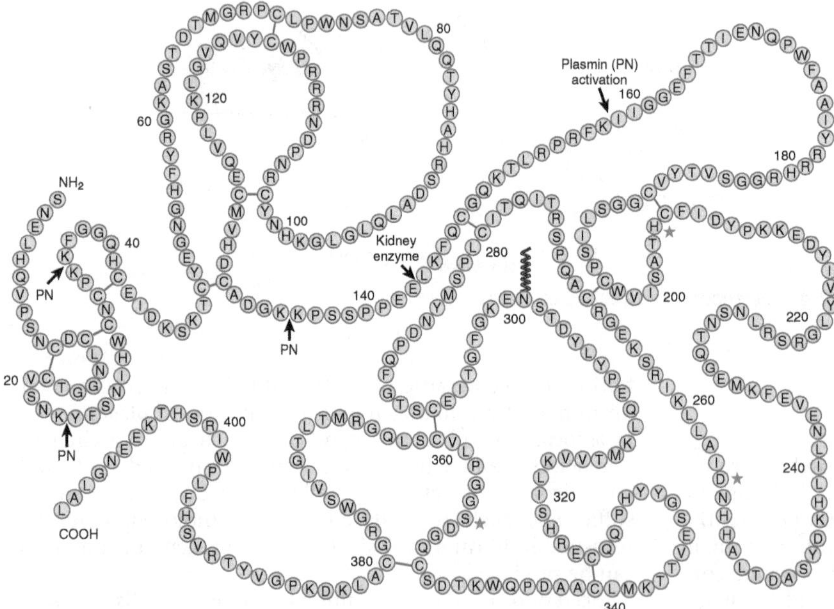

Figure 2-6. The secondary structure of single-chain urokinase-type plasminogen activator (scu-PA; 54 kDa). Activation by plasmin takes place at the 158–159 bond (arrow). The zigzag line represents the glycosylation site.

Urokinase-type Plasminogen Activator (u-PA)

Single-chain u-PA is a 54-kDa glycoprotein synthesized by endothelial and renal cells as well as by certain malignant cells (Fig. 2-6).[19] This single-chain proenzyme of u-PA is unusual in that it has fibrin-selective plasmin-generating activity[48] and also has been synthesized by recombinant techniques.[49]

The relationship of scu-PA to u-PA is complex: cleavage or removal of lys^{158} from scu-PA by plasmin produces 54-kDa, two-chain u-PA. This PA consists of an A-chain (157 residues) and a glycosylated B-chain (253 residues), which are linked by the disulfide bridge between cys^{148} and cys^{279}. Further cleavages at lys^{135} and arg^{156} produce low-molecular-weight (31-kDa) u-PA.[37] Both high- and low-molecular-weight species are enzymatically active.

The 54-kDa urokinase (u-PA) activates plasminogen by first-order kinetics.[34,49] The two forms of u-PA exhibit measurable fibrinolytic and fibrinogenolytic activities in vitro and in vivo, and have plasma $t_{1/2}$ values of 9 to 12 minutes.[50,51] When infused as an *exogenous* therapeutic agent, u-PA leads to plasminogen consumption and inactivation of factors II (prothrombin), V, and VIII. The latter changes constitute the systemic lytic state.

It has been postulated that t-PA is primarily involved in the maintenance of hemostasis through the dissolution of fibrin, whereas u-PA is involved in generating pericellular proteolytic activity by cells expressing the u-PA receptor, which is needed for degradation of the extracellular matrix for migration. The roles of these two PAs in central nervous system cell function are not fully understood.

Exogenous Plasminogen Activators

Streptokinase

Streptokinase (SK) is a 47-kDa, single-chain polypeptide derived from group C β-hemolytic streptococci. The active [SK–plasminogen] complex converts circulating plasminogen directly to plasmin and undergoes further activation to form the [SK–plasmin] complex. The [SK–plasminogen], [SK–plasmin], and plasmin species circulate together.[52] The [SK–plasmin] complex (not bound by the inhibitor α_2-antiplasmin), and free circulating plasmin degrade both fibrinogen and fibrin and inactivate prothrombin, factor V, and factor VIII.

The kinetics of SK elimination are complex. Antistreptococcal antibodies formed from antecedent infections neutralize infused SK and arise maximally by 4 to 7 days after initiation of an SK infusion. Therefore, the doses of SK required to achieve steady-state plasminogen activation must be individualized. Plasminogen depletion through conversion to plasmin and by, as yet, poorly understood clearance mechanisms for the [SK–plasminogen] complex can lead to hypoplasminogenemia. Generation of plasmin is limited at both low and high SK infusion dose-rates because of inadequate plasminogen conversion and depletion of plasminogen, respectively.

APSAC (e.g., Anistreplase) was an artificial activator construct consisting of plasminogen and SK bound non-covalently. Fibrin selectivity relies on the fibrin-attachment properties of the plasminogen kringles. The activity of APSAC depends on the deacylation rate of the acyl-plasminogen component. Hydrolytic activation of the acyl-protected active site of plasminogen allows plasmin formation by SK within the complex in the presence of fibrin. From those observations and on the basis of the terminal $t_{1/2}$ of SK and the $t_{1/2}$ for APSAC deacylation, APSAC has a longer circulation time than streptokinase.[53,54] However, despite these clinically favorable characteristics APSAC has not found a place in the treatment of vascular thrombosis.

Staphylokinase

Staphylokinase (STK) is a 16.5-kDa polypeptide derived from certain strains of *Staphylococcus aureus.*[54–56] STK combines stoichiometrically (1 : 1) with plasminogen to form an irreversible complex that activates free plasminogen. The binding of staphylokinase to plasmin has been worked out in detail.[54,56,57] Recombinant staphylokinase has been prepared from the known gene nucleotide sequence and has been tested in the setting of acute myocardial infarction. STK has been in preliminary testing of ischemic stroke, based upon animal model studies.[58,59]

Plasminogen Activators Derived from *Desmodus rotundus*

Recombinant PAs identical to those derived from the saliva of *Desmodus* species are fibrin-dependent. The α form of *Desmodus* salivary PA (DSPA-α; desmoteplase) and vampire bat salivary plasminogen activator (bat-PA) are more fibrin-dependent than t-PA and may be superior to t-PA in terms of sustained recanalization without fibrinogenolysis.[60,61] The plasma $t_{1/2}$ of DSPA-α is significantly longer than that of rt-PA.[60] A program of studies of desmoteplase as acute treatment for ischemic stroke has so far failed to demonstrate improved outcomes in patients.[62] Significant issues in trial design have been discussed, and a new phase III study is completed.

Novel Plasminogen Activators

Efforts to alter the stability and thrombus selectivity of endogenous PAs have led to a growing list of possible pharmacologic agents. Point and deletion mutations in t-PA and u-PA have provided molecules with unique specificities.[63] For instance, t-PA sequences lacking the K1 and K2 domains possess fibrin specificity, normal specific activity, but reduced inhibition by PA inhibitor-1 (PAI-1).[38] In theory, the increased fibrin selectivity might provide greater thrombolytic effect; however, in studies of the use of this agent in coronary artery thromboses, significant advantages were not evident.

For the clinical target of myocardial ischemia, several t-PA mutants with prolonged $t_{1/2}$ and delayed clearance have been devised that may have benefit when infused as a single bolus.[64,65] Reteplase, a non-glycosylated PA consisting of the K2 and protease domains of t-PA, has a 4.5- to 12.3-fold longer $t_{1/2}$ owing in part to lower affinity for the hepatic cell t-PA receptor.[65,66] It also possesses lower fibrin selectivity. Tenectaplase (TNK-t-PA) differs from t-PA at three mutation sites (T103N, N117Q, and KHRR[296–299]AAAA), which alter two glycosylation sites and increase fibrin selectivity. The changes also result in decreased clearance and prolonged $t_{1/2}$.[67] Another t-PA mutant with greater $t_{1/2}$, lanoteplase (n-PA), derives from deletion of the fibronectin finger and epidermal growth factor domains and mutation of asn^{117} to gln^{117}.[64] In addition to enhanced fibrin selectivity, TNK has relative resistance to inhibition by PAI-1. A t-PA-like construct with moderate fibrin selectivity is monteplase (E6010). This molecule differs from t-PA in the location and organization of disulfide bridges and the complexity of glycosylation. In contrast, the fibrin selectivity and specific activity of pamiteplase (YM866) are nearly identical to those of t-PA, but pamiteplase has a longer $t_{1/2}$.[68,69] These mutants have been developed for bolus infusion application in the setting of myocardial infarction (MI). Application of TNK to clinical ischemic stroke has been formally tested in a small trial,[70] based upon limited experimental studies. A recent report of a non-randomized pilot study indicates the feasibility of testing intravenous TNK treatment within 3 to 6 hours of symptom onset.[71]

What advantage delayed clearance or prolonged $t_{1/2}$ may have in acute application in ischemic stroke is yet to be demonstrated.[72] Dose-adjustment studies in patients with stroke have not been reported. One unproven concern with long $t_{1/2}$ molecules is that they may augment the intercerebral hemorrhage risk in the setting of ischemic stroke.

A similar situation obtains for other novel PA constructs. These have included single-site mutants and variants of rt-PA and recombinant scu-PA, t-PA/scu-PA and t-PA/u-PA chimerae, u-PA/antifibrin monoclonal antibodies, u-PA/antiplatelet monoclonal antibodies, bifunctional antibody conjugates, and scu-PA deletion mutants.[73–75]

REGULATION OF ENDOGENOUS FIBRINOLYSIS

Endogenous fibrinolysis is modulated by several families of inhibitors of plasmin and of the PAs.

In the circulation, α_2-antiplasmin is the primary inhibitor of fibrinolysis, inhibiting plasmin directly. Excess plasmin is inactivated by α_2-macroglobulin. The potential risk of vascular thrombosis then depends on the balance between plasminogen activation and plasmin activity and their respective inhibitors in the circulation.

Thrombospondin interferes with fibrin-associated plasminogen activation by t-PA. Inhibitors of the contact activation system and complement (C1 inhibitor) have an indirect effect on fibrinolysis. Histidine-rich glycoprotein (HRG) is a competitive inhibitor of plasminogen. Generally, though, these physiologic modulators of plasmin activity are overwhelmed by pharmacologic concentrations of PAs.

For streptokinase, APSAC, and staphylokinase, circulating neutralizing antibodies appear, which directly inhibit their activation of plasminogen.

α_2-Antiplasmin and α_2-Macroglobulin

Circulating plasmin generated during fibrinolysis is bound by α_2-antiplasmin in the plasma. The two forms of α_2-antiplasmin are (i) the native form, which binds plasminogen, and (ii) a second form that cannot bind plasminogen.[76] Ordinarily, α_2-antiplasmin is found in either plasminogen-bound or free circulating forms. Fibrin-bound plasmin is protected because of its interaction with fibrin and because α_2-antiplasmin is already occupied. Excess free plasmin is bound by α_2-macroglobulin. α_2-Macroglobulin is a relatively nonspecific inhibitor of fibrinolysis that inactivates plasmin, kallikrein, t-PA, and u-PA.

Inhibitors of Plasminogen Activators and Fibrinolysis

PAIs also reduce the activity of t-PA, scu-PA, and u-PA by direct binding (see Table 2-2).

PAI-1 specifically inhibits both plasma t-PA and u-PA. PAI-1 is derived from both endothelial cell and platelet sources.[77] Several lines of evidence indicate that the K2 domain of t-PA is responsible for the interaction between t-PA and PAI-1, and that this interaction is altered by the presence of fibrin.[78] PAI-1 is also an acute-phase reactant,[79] and deep venous thrombosis, septicemia, and type II diabetes mellitus, for instance, are associated with elevated plasma PAI-1 levels.

PAI-2, which is found in a 70-kDa form and a 47-kDa low-molecular-weight form, has a lower Ki for u-PA and two-chain t-PA. PAI-2 is derived from placental tissue, granulocytes, monocytes/macrophages, and histiocytes.[80] This inhibitor probably plays little role in the physiologic antagonism of t-PA, and is most important in the utero-placental circulation.[81] The kinetics of PA inhibition by PAI-2 differs from those for PAI-1.

PAI-3 is a serine protease inhibitor of u-PA, t-PA, and activated protein C (APC) found in plasma and urine.

Thrombin-activable fibrinolysis inhibitor (TAFI) is an endogenous inhibitor of glu-plasminogen and, therefore, fibrinolysis. TAFI is a precursor of plasma carboxypeptidase B and, when activated by thrombin in the plasma, produces an antifibrinolytic effect.

CLINICAL CONSEQUENCES OF THERAPEUTIC PLASMINOGEN ACTIVATION

Plasminogen activators given at pharmacologic doses significantly alter hemostasis. u-PA, SK, and occasionally t-PA produce systemically detectable fibrin(ogen) degradation, measured by a fall in fibrinogen concentration, and a reduction in circulating plasminogen and α_2-antiplasmin (through binding of the plasmin generated). Both u-PA and SK inactivate factors V and VIII, which contribute to the "systemic lytic state" or "anticoagulant state." Fragments of fibrin(ogen) interfere with fibrin multimerization and contribute to thrombus destabilization, whereas the circulating fragments, hypofibrinogenemia, and factor depletion produce an anticoagulant state that limits thrombus formation and extension. The clinical consequences of u-PA or SK infusion include a progressive decrease or depletion of circulating plasminogen and fibrinogen, prolongation of the aPTT due to significant fibrinogen reduction, and inactivation of factors V and VIII. With repletion of these elements the anticoagulant state may be transient.

Platelet function can also be affected. Clinical studies of rt-PA have demonstrated prolongation of standardized template bleeding times.[82] In experimental systems, infusion of rt-PA produces greater hemorrhage.[83] Furthermore, t-PA is known to cause disaggregation of human platelets through selective proteolysis of inter-platelet fibrin, which is inhibitable by α_2-antiplasmin.[84] Lys-plasminogen and glu-plasminogen can potentiate the platelet disaggregatory effect of rt-PA. It is likely that the risk of intracerebral hemorrhage that attends PA infusion involves disruption of sustained platelet aggregation and lysis of fibrin formed at the site of vascular injury.

LIMITATIONS TO THE CLINICAL USE OF FIBRINOLYTIC AGENTS FOR ISCHEMIC STROKE

The clinical setting in which PAs are used is an important and relevant variable for both the efficacy and the reduction of hemorrhagic risk. Intracerebral hemorrhage is a known risk of the clinical use of PAs. The use of rt-PA in pharmacologic doses in the acute setting of ischemic stroke must conform to the original report,[6] as confirmed subsequently. An abbreviated summary of the strict contraindications to the use of fibrinolytic agents includes: (i) a history of previous intracranial hemorrhage, (ii) septic embolism, (iii) malignant hypertension or sustained diastolic or systolic blood pressure in excess of 180/110, (iv) conditions consistent with ongoing parenchymal hemorrhage (e.g., gastrointestinal source), (v) pregnancy or parturition, (vi) a history of recent trauma or surgery, and (vii) known acquired (e.g., from anticoagulant use) or inherited hemorrhagic diatheses. These contraindications currently apply to the use of rt-PA in selected patients with ischemic stroke less than 3 hours after symptom onset as well as other approved clinical indications for the use of rt-PA, u-PA, or SK. Somewhat different selection criteria were used for the 4.5-hour entry window in a subsequent randomized placebo-controlled study.[9]

PLASMINOGEN ACTIVATORS IN CEREBRAL TISSUE

Although current clinical focus is on the use of PAs as therapeutic agents for vascular reperfusion, cerebral tissue also generates and uses PAs. PA activity has been associated with brain tissue development, vascular remodeling, cell migration, neuron viability, tumor development, and vascular invasion in the central nervous system. However, the pathways involved are still under study.

In normal cerebral tissue, t-PA antigen is expressed by microvessels similar in size to those of the vasa vasorum of the aorta.[17] Expression of PA activity has been reported in non-ischemic tissues of mice, spontaneously hypertensive and

Wistar-Kyoto rats, and primates.[85] Sappino et al. described the localization of t-PA and PN-1 in the adult mouse brain,[86] while u-PA mRNA has been shown to be expressed in the adult brain.[46] Tissue-type PA and u-PA are secreted by endothelial cells, neurons, astrocytes, and microglia in vivo or in vitro.[42–47] u-PA mRNA is expressed in neurons and oligodendrocytes during process outgrowth in the rodent brain.[86] Although t-PA is expressed by neurons in many brain regions, extracellular proteolysis seems confined to specific, discrete brain regions. Studies suggesting that t-PA can mediate neurodegeneration during excitotoxicity or following focal cerebral ischemia in the hippocampus have opened a discussion about whether PAs play roles in cellular viability outside the fibrinolytic system in the circulation.[87]

Plasminogen generation is confined to discrete regions of the CNS.[86] Early during focal ischemia, activators of plasminogen are expressed by microvessels and adjacent neurons (e.g., u-PA),[21] however there is little evidence yet that plasmin activity per se is generated in the ischemic territory. Although, the loss of basal lamina components is compatible with its action,[24] other proteases are generated that can account for this. In addition, evidence of local plasminogen activation has been shown by in situ zymography.[88] Proteolytic fragments of matrix constituents (e.g., laminin) have been associated with enhanced excitotoxicity in the CNS in experimental settings.[89] The roles for t-PA, while not overtly up-regulated in non-human primate ischemia,[21] have been implicated in neuron survival and injury.[90]

Plasminogen Activators and Neuronal Functions

PAs participate in CNS development.[86,91] It is not surprising that as many cells harbor receptors for PAs, the PA system could play distinct roles in CNS development and function. u-PA has been shown to participate in (i) forebrain postnatal development (along with u-PAR), (ii) neuron and axonal growth in the CNS,[91] and (iii) epileptogenesis (along with u-PAR).[92,93] In experimental systems under normoxia t-PA is synthesized by neurons and appears to participate in (i) hippocampal neuron function and responses,[94] (ii) epileptogenesis,[93,95] and (iii) excitotoxic injury of neurons.[45] Microglia appear to require t-PA for proper function in phagocytosis.[96]

Tsirka et al. have demonstrated that deletion of t-PA prevents the excitotoxic generation of neuron injury (in the hippocampus).[45] In contrast, it had been suggested that rt-PA (alteplase) promotes neuron injury during ischemic stroke. Wang et al. reported that injury volumes were significantly smaller in t-PA$^{-/-}$ mice (129/Sv and C57 Bl/6 backgrounds) subject to transient ischemia, compared with wild-type companions.[97] In both strains infusion of human rt-PA at 0.9–1.0 mg/kg increased infarction volumes.[97,98] The increase in injury volume was attributed directly to neuron injury by the ability of rt-PA (alteplase) to potentiate NMDA receptor signaling,[99] evidence of direct proteolytic cleavage of the NR1 subunit of that receptor by rt-PA,[99] or t-PA expression in the hippocampus and amygdala.[95] Concerns have been raised that the proteolytic activity could be associated with the serum in which cells were grown and/or supra-pharmacologic concentrations of human rt-PA used in the mouse preparations. The role(s) and the mechanisms of PA action in individual reports are often difficult to define, in part because the methodologies and the settings of experimental testing have often not been fully described. In another setting, modulation of the NR2B component of the NMDA receptor by rt-PA (alteplase, 100 µg/ml) increased ethanol-withdrawal seizures in mice (C57 Bl/6 background).[95]

Further technical concerns have appeared. Yi et al. have demonstrated that reduction in infarction volume in a MCA occlusion model in the Sprague-Dawley rat occurred when rt-PA (alteplase), the S478A mutant of t-PA, or denatured rt-PA were given by intracerebroventricular injection compared to control.[100] It has also been noted that low-molecular-weight contaminants (potentially L-arginine) in commercial preparations of human rt-PA (alteplase) could cause cell toxicity, and similarly contaminants in plasmin preparations could stimulate neuron Ca^{+2} flux.[101] Those studies suggest that some non-fibrinolytic off-target effects may be responsible for the increased injury observed with high concentrations of human rt-PA in model systems. How these observations relate to ischemic stroke is uncertain.

Many studies have not taken into account the importance of species differences with regard to coagulation system activation. Korninger et al. have demonstrated that for thrombus lysis, non-human systems require a ten-fold higher concentration of human rt-PA than human-relevant thrombus lysis systems ex vivo.[102] Often, with non-thromboembolic models of MCA occlusion, the use of rt-PA has been associated with an increase in infarction volume.

In the non-human primate no change in infarction volume was observed at several doses of rt-PA (alteplase or duteplase).[103] Furthermore, Overgaard et al. had demonstrated significant reduction in infarction volume with rt-PA following ischemia in rodent models.[104–106] In culture, injury to cells occurs consistently at suprapharmacologic concentrations of rt-PA (del Zoppo GJ, Gu Y-H, personal observation; and,[107–109]). Furthermore, there is no clear indication that rt-PA results in a worsening of the injury territories in human stroke patients independent of hemorrhage, who are so treated. Therefore, further investigation of the interactions of the PA system and its substrates within the neurovascular unit is required to understand better the roles of this system.

Plasminogen Activators and Cerebral Microvessel Integrity

A clinically relevant notion proposed is that rt-PA can increase cerebral vascular permeability and the risk of hemorrhage by increasing the vascular matrix degradation. Work has focused on the matrix metalloproteinases (MMPs).

Loss of the basal lamina matrix,[24,110–115] and rapid reorganization of microvessel endothelial cell and astrocyte matrix adhesion receptors occurs during focal ischemia.[24,113,116–118] Heo et al. first described the acute appearance of pro-MMP-2 in ischemic tissue, and the association of pro-MMP-9 with hemorrhagic transformation in the primate.[119] Rosenberg et al. have explored the role(s) that gelatinases play in permeability barrier loss, neuron injury, and the evolution of infarction.[120–123] Within the ECM, collagen IV, laminin, and fibronectin decrease significantly.[24,118]

A plausible explanation for the cerebral vascular ECM changes seen following MCA occlusion is the acute appearance of active matrix-cleaving proteases in the ischemic territory. Four families of matrix-altering enzymes acutely increase following MCA occlusion in the non-human primate: (i) (pro-)MMP-2 and (pro-)MMP-9,[119] and the activation system for pro-MMP-2,[20] (ii) serine proteases, including u-PA,[20] (iii) cathepsin-L,[113] and (iv) heparanase.[24,113] Their individual involvement in brain injury is now certain.[113,115,119,121,124–129] However, no study to date has shown a clear causal relationship; they have been mostly correlational.

In the setting of experimental focal ischemia, it is not known whether the proteases are released in active form and degrade microvessel ECM directly. The inactive gelatinases pro-MMP-2 and pro-MMP-9 are released from vascular endothelium, leukocytes, and other cells during inflammation; pro-MMP-2 is activated by membrane-bound MT1- and

MT3-MMP, plasmin, and other proteases. Considerable experimental work employing focal ischemia models has focused on the active gelatinases.[98,123,130] In the primate MMP-2 antigen is found throughout the ischemic core acutely,[20] but only the inactive pro-MMP-2 form is observed by high-sensitivity zymography.[119] Less than 1% of total MMP-2 in ischemic basal ganglia appears to be active.[119]

It has been suggested that hemorrhage observed with rt-PA use in murine focal cerebral ischemia models is caused by the generation of MMP-9 by rt-PA in the ischemic tissue.[131] Data to support this claim have been developed in murine models,[98,109,132-134] however recently this notion has been countered in another model system.[134] This question is clearly unresolved.

Technical issues confound confirmation of matrix-cleaving activity in tissue derived from ischemia models, including (i) retention of plasma from unperfused brain samples, (ii) the presence of hemorrhage, (iii) activation of samples during extraction, (iv) inconsistencies in assigning molecular masses to active forms, and (v) the absence of sufficient details in the preparation methods to be certain. Species differences in protease expression during focal ischemia between primate (pro-MMP-2) and mouse strains (pro-MMP-9) accentuate this problem.[113,126] Gene deletion studies provide only an indirect impression of the possible impact of specific matrix proteases on evolving ischemic injury,[98,126,127,130,135] and are subject to significant limitations. These include compensatory changes during development, several MMP-9$^{-/-}$ constructs with different phenotypes, failure to identify other protease families, unknown cell sources, and the appearance of similar injury phenoytpes with different gene constructs (e.g., within the PA family, for instance).[136] These concerns argue strongly for identifying the exact enzyme pathways and their cell sources in the CNS during injury.

Plasminogen Activators in Experimental Cerebral Ischemia

Focal cerebral ischemia rapidly increases the endogenous expression of u-PA and PAI-1 within striatal tissue of the primate.[21,119] Endogenous t-PA decreases transiently as it binds PAI-1, but otherwise does not change. u-PA is an indirect activator of pro-MMP-2, which is also generated early following MCA occlusion.[20] It has been postulated that loss of basal lamina integrity contributes to hemorrhagic transformation of the evolving infarction.[24,118] Whether exogenous PAs contribute to the loss in microvessel integrity in this manner is under study.

A limited number of experimental studies have tested the ability of PAs to increase arterial recanalization. Improved clinical (behavioral and/or neurologic) outcomes have been reported in rodent models of focal cerebral ischemia treated with PAs (mostly rt-PA) very soon after thromboembolism. Early infusion of rt-PA in a rabbit multiple-thromboembolism model demonstrated significant improvement in clinical outcome in comparison with untreated controls.[137] The use of rt-PA with putative inhibitors of polymorphonuclear leukocyte adhesion supports this notion, although differences among rt-PA cohorts were observed in various experimental sets. In an acute rt-PA dose-rate study in a nonembolic nonhuman primate stroke model, no significant difference in motor-weighted neurologic outcome was observed, compared with controls.[103] However, another study demonstrated a significant reduction in infarction volume after reperfusion of the MCA territory in a single model.[138]

PLASMINOGEN ACTIVATORS AND RECANALIZATION IN ISCHEMIC STROKE

Experimental and clinical studies indicate that timely restoration of blood flow to the ischemic cerebral parenchyma is required for improved clinical outcome. The substrate and condition requirements of PAs have supported their potential use in cerebrovascular ischemia. Angiographic studies have provided valuable information about the anatomy of the vasculature, the magnitude of thrombus burden, and the success of recanalization with PAs.[3,139-141] u-PA and rt-PA appear to contribute to arterial reperfusion as anticipated by their known activities (Table 2-3).

The frequency of arterial recanalization appears to be greater when the PA is administered by the intra-arterial route than by intravenous delivery (see Table 2-3). That observation

TABLE 2-3 Plasminogen Activators in Acute Ischemic Stroke: Carotid Territory

Study	Year	Agent	Patients (n)	Δ (T-0)[a] (hours)	Recanalization (%)	Total Hemorrhage (%)	Symptomatic Hemorrhage (%)
INTRA-ARTERIAL DELIVERY							
del Zoppo et al.[1]	1988	SK/u-PA	20	<24	90.0	20.0	0.0
Mori et al.[2]	1988	u-PA	22	<7	45.5	18.2	9.1
Matsumoto et al.[150]	1991	u-PA	39	<24	59.0	33.3	–
PROACT[139]	1997	scu-PA/h	26	<6	57.7	42.3	15.4
		C/h	14	<6	14.3	7.1	7.1
Gönner et al.[151]	1998	u-PA	33	<6	58.0	21.2	6.1
PROACT II[142]	1999	scu-PA/h	121	<6	65.7	35.2	10.2
		-/h (IV)	59	<6	18.0	13.0	1.8
INTRAVENOUS DELIVERY							
Yamaguchi[152]	1991	rt-PA	58	<6	43.1	20.7	–
von Kummer and Hacke[153]	1991	rt-PA	32	<6	53.1	37.5	9.4
del Zoppo et al.[3]	1992	rt-PA	93 (104)[b]	<8	34.4	30.8	9.6
Mori et al.[4]	1992	rt-PA	19	<6	47.4	52.6	–
		C	12		16.7	41.7	–
Yamaguchi et al.[5]	1993	rt-PA	47 (51)	<6	21.3	47.1	7.8
		C	46 (47)		4.4	46.8	10.6

[a]Time from symptom onset to treatment.
[b]Intention to treat.
C, control or placebo; h, heparin; rt-PA, recombinant tissue-type plasminogen activator; IV, intravenous; scu-PA, single-chain urokinase-type plasmiogen activator; SK, streptokinase; u-PA, urokinase-type plasminogen activator.

is consistent with the notion that enhanced efficacy may be due to the higher local concentration of the PA at the thrombus surface. However, this has not been shown in the clinical setting.

Only a handful of studies have prospectively compared recanalization rates in PA-treated patients with a matched control group.[4,139,142] In those studies, recanalization was significantly greater in patients receiving the PA for angiographically proven occlusion of the MCA. In a phase II study of recombinant scu-PA (pro-UK), the recanalization frequency was significantly improved by the co-administration of heparin,[139] and was confirmed in a follow-on open phase III study.[142] Many, but not all, subjects in those studies in whom early recanalization was documented experienced clinical improvement. Lack of clinical improvement despite recanalization may be influenced by increased time to reperfusion, poor perfusion, and/or poor collateralization, although this issue is unproven.

Mechanical disruption with either catheter-type devices or ultrasonography has been employed to enhance recanalization in limited clinical series. High ultrasound frequencies have been shown to alter the properties of the fibrin network to increase transport of rt-PA into the structure, increase thrombus penetration,[143] increase rt-PA binding to fibrin,[144] and to increase flow through fibrin gel in in vitro systems. Fibrin disaggregation can also occur. It has been postulated that such high frequencies will also cause injury to the brain parenchyma and to the vessel wall structure.

PLASMINOGEN ACTIVATORS AND CEREBRAL HEMORRHAGE IN ISCHEMIC STROKE

Acute rt-PA administration in ischemic stroke can be complicated by the development of symptomatic parenchymal hemorrhage. A number of randomized studies have documented the increased risk of symptomatic hemorrhagic transformation associated with intravenous infusion of PAs.[6–8] Rates of symptomatic hemorrhage for hemispheric stroke in the cerebral artery territory range from 3.3% to 9.6% in this setting.[3,7–9,139] In addition, the development of symptomatic hemorrhage in rt-PA-treated patients contributed to mortality in properly controlled trials, including the National Institute of Neurological Disorders and Stroke (NINDS) study,[6–8] and ECASS-3.[9] Overall, however, those well-designed trials have shown benefit from the use of systemic rt-PA.

Clinical features that have been associated with higher intracerebral hemorrhage risk in the setting of PA use include advancing age and signs of early infarction on initial cranial computed tomography. Early signs of infarction may reflect otherwise undetectable injury to the matrix of the microvascular bed.[6–8] Increased time to treatment, low body mass (higher relative rt-PA dose), diastolic hypertension, older age, early signs of ischemia, and the use of rt-PA are associated with the risk of intracerebral hemorrhage.[3,145,146] From recent perfusion weighted imaging (PWI) and diffusion weighted imaging (DWI) studies subgroups of patients receiving rt-PA have been identified for whom the risk of hemorrhage is increased.[147,148] This accords with evidence that the depth and duration of focal ischemia is a contributor to the ultimate cerebral hemorrhage risk during exposure to plasminogen activators.[149]

These latter features of focal ischemia also accord with the observation of microvessel matrix degradation in the ischemic territories observed in experimental systems.[23,113,119] The possibility that these processes are augmented by PA exposure (e.g., rt-PA) and interactions with the baseline metabolic environment of the tissue (e.g., hyperglycemia) has not been sufficiently explored.

Both tissue injury and pharmacologic interventions can augment the risk of hemorrhage. Despite the higher risk of hemorrhage associated with rt-PA, a robust clinical benefit results with proper use of this agent.[6] The results of two randomized trials of intra-arterial recombinant scu-PA are consistent with the effect of anticoagulation (heparin) to increase the risk of symptomatic cerebral hemorrhage with scu-PA.[139,142] A significant excess of symptomatic hemorrhages and a significant increase in recanalization rate occurred in patients receiving the higher heparin dose. Nonetheless, there is no evidence so far that the increase in hemorrhage associated with the use of PAs is related to greater recanalization. Early infusion of a PA in selected patients is associated, however, with a decrease in the enhanced hemorrhage risk.[3]

CONCLUSION

Thrombus development and the processes of endogenous thrombus-remodeling and dissolution involve discrete well-understood biochemical pathways. They require the interaction of the vasculature and its lining, platelet activation, and the activation of coagulation. These processes are responsible for thrombotic occlusion of brain-supplying arteries that is a cause of ischemic stroke. Anti-thrombotic agents are derived from naturally occurring endogenous factors or agents that interfere with individual steps in the pathways of thrombosis.

As an example, the pharmacologic use of PAs is based upon the known activities and properties of *endogenous* PAs, and the purification of proteins with PA activity from natural sources. The acute use of PAs for dissolution of cerebral arterial thrombi and recanalization of the occluded artery during ischemic stroke has devolved from a clear understanding of PAs and their actions.

The interactions between PAs and the evolving ischemic cerebral tissue are still incompletely understood. However, it is clear that (i) thrombus dissolution in the CNS can be achieved with PAs, (ii) rt-PA delivered acutely can cause clinical improvement, and (iii) increased intracerebral hemorrhage risk accompanies PA use. Vascular injury is a necessary component of hemorrhage both with ischemic stroke and the use of anti-thrombotic agents, including PAs. Current unknowns regarding the generation of intracerebral hemorrhage include (i) whether the PA (e.g., rt-PA) can cause vascular matrix dissolution, (ii) whether rt-PA can stimulate matrix protease generation, where, and how, (iii) the timing of these events in the clinical setting, and (iv) non-vascular contributors. A growing understanding of non-vascular PA effects covers (i) brain development, (ii) individual cerebral cell activities, and (iii) neuron injury, specifically. Also, work proceeds to understand non-vascular roles of coagulation factors in the CNS. Determinations of outcomes for these studies require the high-quality application of the scientific method, as in the study of the thrombus pathways.

REFERENCES

1. del Zoppo GJ, Ferbert A, Otis S, et al. Local intra-arterial fibrinolytic therapy in acute carotid territory stroke: a pilot study. Stroke 1988;19:307–13.
2. Mori E, Tabuchi M, Yoshida T, et al. Intracarotid urokinase with thromboembolic occlusion of the middle cerebral artery. Stroke 1988;19:802–12.
3. del Zoppo GJ, Poeck K, Pessin MS, et al. Recombinant tissue plasminogen activator in acute thrombotic and embolic stroke. Ann Neurol 1992;32:78–86.
4. Mori E, Yoneda Y, Tabuchi M, et al. Intravenous recombinant tissue plasminogen activator in acute carotid artery territory stroke. Neurology 1992;42:976–82.

5. Yamaguchi T, Hayakawa T, Kikuchi H. Intravenous tissue plasminogen activator ameliorates the outcome of hyperacute embolic stroke. Cerebrovasc Dis 1993;3:269–72.
6. The National Institutes of Neurological Disorders and Stroke rt-PA Stroke Study Group. Tissue plasminogen activator for acute ischemic stroke. N Engl J Med 1995;333:1581–7.
7. Hacke W, Kaste M, Fieschi C, et al. Intravenous thrombolysis with recombinant tissue plasminogen activator for acute hemispheric stroke. The European Cooperative Acute Stroke Study (ECASS). JAMA 1995;274:1017–25.
8. Hacke W, Kaste M, Fieschi C, et al. Randomised double-blind placebo-controlled trial of thrombolytic therapy with intravenous alteplase in acute ischaemic stroke (ECASS II). Second European-Australasian acute Stroke Study Investigators. Lancet 1998;352:1245–51.
9. Hacke W, Kaste M, Bluhmki E, et al. Thrombolysis with alteplase 3 to 4.5 hours after acute ischemic stroke. N Engl J Med 2008;359:1317–29.
10. Davie EW, Fujikawa K, Kisiel W. The coagulation cascade: initiation, maintenance, and regulation. Biochemistry 1991;30: 10363–70.
11. Alkjaersig N, Fletcher AP. Catabolism and excretion of fibrinopeptide A. Blood 1982;60:148–56.
12. Majerus PW, Miletich JP, Kane WP, et al. The formation of thrombin on the platelet surface. In: Mann KG, Taylor FB, editors. The Regulation of Coagulation. New York: Elsevier/North Holland; 1980. p. 215.
13. Kaplan AP. Initiation of the intrinsic coagulation and fibrinolytic pathways of man: The role of surfaces, Hageman factor, prekallikrein, high molecular weight kininogen, and factor XI. Prog Hemost Thromb 1978;4:127–75.
14. Nesheim ME, Hibbard LS, Tracy PB, et al. Participation of factor Va in prothrombinase. In: Mann KG, Tayler FB, editors. The Regulation of Coagulation. New York: Elsevier/North Holland; 1980. p. 145–59.
15. Levin EG, Marzec U, Anderson J, et al. Thrombin stimulates tissue plasminogen activator release from cultured human endothelial cells. J Clin Invest 1984;74:1988–95.
16. van Hinsbergh VW. Regulation of the synthesis and secretion of plasminogen activators by endothelial cells. Haemostasis 1988;18:307–27.
17. Collen D, de Maeyer L. Molecular biology of human plasminogen. I. Physiocochemical properties and microheterogeneity. Thromb Diath Haemorrh 1975;34:396–402.
18. Levin EG, del Zoppo GJ. Localization of tissue plasminogen activator in the endothelium of a limited number of vessels. Am J Pathol 1994;144:855–61.
19. Plow EF, Felez J, Miles LA. Cellular regulation of fibrinolysis. Thromb Haemost 1991;66:132–6.
20. Chang DI, Hosomi N, Lucero J, et al. Activation systems for latent matrix metalloproteinase-2 are upregulated immediately after focal cerebral ischemia. J Cereb Blood Flow Metab 2003;23:1408–19.
21. Hosomi N, Lucero J, Heo JH, et al. Rapid differential endogenous plasminogen activator expression after acute middle cerebral artery occlusion. Stroke 2001;32:1341–8.
22. Whitelock JM, Murdoch AD, Iozzo RV, et al. The degradation of human endothelial cell-derived perlecan and release of bound basic fibroblast growth factor by stromelysin, collagenase, plasmin, and heparanases. J Biol Chem 1996;271: 10079–86.
23. Lijnen HR. Plasmin and matrix metalloproteinases in vascular remodeling. Thromb Haemost 2001;86:324–33.
24. Hamann GF, Okada Y, Fitridge R, et al. Microvascular basal lamina antigens disappear during cerebral ischemia and reperfusion. Stroke 1995;26:2120–6.
25. Bachmann F, Kruithof IE. Tissue plasminogen activator: Chemical and physiological aspects. Semin Thromb Hemost 1984; 10:6–17.
26. Collen D, Lijnen HR. New approaches to thrombolytic therapy. Arteriosclerosis 1984;4:579–85.
27. Bachmann F. Molecular aspects of plasminogen, plasminogen activators and plasmin. In: Bloom AL, Forbes CD, Thomas DP, et al., editors. Haemostasis and Thrombosis. Edinburgh: Churchill Livingstone; 1994. p. 575–613.
28. Peterson LC, Serenson E. Effect of plasminogen and tissue-type plasminogen activator on fibrin gel structure. Fibrinolysis 1990;5:51–9.
29. Tran-Thang C, Kruithof EK, Atkinson J, et al. High-affinity binding sites for human glu-plasminogen unveiled by limited plasmic degradation of human fibrin. Eur J Biochem 1986; 160:559–604.
30. Wallen P, Wiman B. Characterization of human plasminogen. II. Separation and partial characterization of different molecular forms of human plasminogen. Biochim Biophys Acta 1973;257:122–34.
31. Miles LA, Greengard JS, Griffin JH. A comparison of the abilities of plasma kallikrein, Beta-Factor XIIa, Factor XIa and urokinase to activate plasminogen. Thromb Res 1983;29:407–17.
32. Kluft C, Dooijewaard G, Emeis JJ. Role of the contact system in fibrinolysis. Semin Thromb Hemost 1987;13:50–68.
33. Hanss M, Collen D. Secretion of tissue-type plasminogen activator and plasminogen activator inhibitor by cultured human endothelial cells: Modulation by thrombin endotoxin and histamine. J Lab Clin Med 1987;109:97–104.
34. Kakkar VV, Scully MF. Thrombolytic therapy. Br Med Bull 1978;34:191–9.
35. Sharma GVRK, Cella G, Parish AF, et al. Drug therapy: Thrombolytic therapy. N Engl J Med 1982;306:1268–76.
36. Bounameaux H, de Moerloose P, Perrier A, et al. Plasma measurement of D-dimer as diagnostic aid in suspected venous thromboembolism: An overview. Thromb Haemost 1994;71:1–6.
37. Rijken DC. Structure/function relationships of t-PA. In: Kluft C, editor. Tissue Type Plasminogen Activator (t-PA): Physiological and Clinical Aspects, vol. 1. Boca Raton: CRC Press; 1988. p. 101–22.
38. Ehrlich HJ, Bang NW, Little SP, et al. Biological properties of a kringleless tissue plasminogen activator (t-PA) mutant. Fibrinolysis 1987;1:75–81.
39. Gelehrter TD, Sznycer-Laszuk R. Thrombin induction of plasminogen activator-inhibitor in cultured human endothelial cells. J Clin Invest 1986;77:165–9.
40. Sakata Y, Curriden S, Lawrence D, et al. Activated protein C stimulates the fibrinolytic activity of cultured endothelial cells and decreases antiactivator activity. Proc Natl Acad Sci U S A 1985;82:1121–5.
41. Saksela O, Moscatelli D, Rifkin DB. The opposing effects of basic fibroblast growth factor and transforming growth factor beta on the regulation of plasminogen activator activity in capillary endothelial cells and decreases antiactivator activity. J Cell Biol 1987;105:957–63.
42. Pittman RN. Release of plasminogen activator and a calcium-dependent metalloprotease from cultured sympathetic and sensory neurons. Dev Biol 1985;110:91–101.
43. Vincent VA, Lowik CW, Verheijen JH, et al. Role of astrocyte-derived tissue-type plasminogen activator in the regulation of endotoxin-stimulated nitric oxide production by microglial cells. Glia 1998;22:130–7.
44. Toshniwal PK, Firestone SL, Barlow GH, et al. Characterization of astrocyte plasminogen activator. J Neurol Sci 1987; 80:277–87.
45. Tsirka SE, Rogove AD, Bugge TH, et al. An extracellular proteolytic cascade promotes neuronal degeneration in the mouse hippocampus. J Neurosci 1997;17:543–52.
46. Masos T, Miskin R. Localization of urokinase-type plasminogen activator mRNA in the adult mouse brain. Brain Res Mol Brain Res 1996;35:139–48.
47. Nakajima K, Tsuzaki N, Shimojo M, et al. Microglia isolated from rat brain secrete a urokinase-type plasminogen activator. Brain Res 1992;577:285–92.
48. Lijnen HR, Zamarron C, Blaber M, et al. Activation of plasminogen by pro-urokinase. I. Mechanism. J Biol Chem 1986; 261:1253–8.
49. White FW, Barlow GH, Mozen MM. The isolation and characterization of plasminogen activators (urokinase) from human urine. Biochemistry 1966;5:2160–9.
50. Fletcher AP, Alkjaersig N, Sherry S, et al. The development of urokinase as a thrombolytic agent. Maintenance of a sustained thrombolytic state in man by its intravenous infusion. J Lab Clin Med 1965;65:713–31.

51. Stump DC, Mann KH. Mechanisms of thrombus formation and lysis. Ann Emerg Med 1988;17:1138–47.
52. Reddy KN, Marcus B. Mechanisms of activation of human plasminogen by streptokinase. J Biol Chem 1972;246: 1683–91.
53. Standing R, Fears R, Ferres H. The protective effect of acylation on the stability of APSAC (Eminase) in human plasma. Fibrinolysis 1988;2:157.
54. Lijnen HR, de Cock F, Matsuo O, et al. Comparative fibrinolytic and fibrinogenolytic properties of staphylokinase and streptokinase in plasma of different species in vitro. Fibrinolysis 1992;6:33–7.
55. Collen D. Staphylokinase: a potent, uniquely fibrin-selective thrombolytic agent. Nat Med 1998;4(3):279–82.
56. Jespers L, Vanwetswinkel S, Lijnen HR, et al. Structural and functional basis of plasminogen activation by staphylokinase. Thromb Haemost 1999;81(4):479–84.
57. Lijnen HR, Van Hoef B, Matsuo O, et al. On the molecular, interactions between plasminogen- staphylokinase, α_2-antiplasmin and fibrin. Biochim Biophys Acta 1992;1118: 144–8.
58. Vanderschueren S, Van V I, Collen D. Intravenous thrombolysis with recombinant staphylokinase versus tissue-type plasminogen activator in a rabbit embolic stroke model. Stroke 1997;28:1783–8.
59. Nagai N, Vanlinthout I, Collen D. Comparative effects of tissue plasminogen activator, streptokinase, and staphylokinase on cerebral ischemic infarction and pulmonary clot lysis in hamster models. Circulation 1999;100:2541–6.
60. Witt W, Maass B, Baldus B, et al. Coronary thrombosis with Desmodus salivary plasminogen activator in dogs. Fast and persistent recanalization by intravenous bolus administration. Circulation 1994;90:421–6.
61. Bergum PW, Gardell SJ. Vampire bat salivary plasminogen activator exhibits a strict and fastidious requirement for polymeric fibrin as its cofactor, unlike human tissue-type plasminogen activator. A kinetic analysis. J Biol Chem 1992;267:17726–31.
62. Hacke W, Albers G, Al-Rawi Y, et al. The Desmoteplase in Acute Ischemic Stroke Trial (DIAS): a phase II MRI-based 9-hour window acute stroke thrombolysis trial with intravenous desmoteplase. Stroke 2005;36:66–73.
63. Lijnen HR, Collen D. Development of new fibrinolytic agents. In: Bloom AL, Forbes CD, Thomas DP, et al., editors. Haemostasis and Thrombosis. Edinburgh: Churchill-Livingstone; 1994. p. 625–37.
64. Benedict CR, Refino CJ, Keyt BA, et al. New variant of human tissue plasminogen activator (TPA) with enhanced efficacy and lower incidence of bleeding compared with recombinant human TPA. Circulation 1995;92(10):3032–40.
65. Kohnert U, Horsch B, Fischer S. A variant of tissue plasminogen activator (t-PA) comprised of the kringle 2 and the protease domain shows a significant difference in the in vitro rate of plasmin formation as compared to the recombinant human t-PA from transformed Chinese hamster ovary cells. Fibrinolysis 1993;7:365–72.
66. Fischer S, Kohnert U. Major mechanistic differences explain the higher clot lysis potency of reteplase over alteplase: Lack of fibrin binding is an advantage for bolus application of fibrin-specific thrombolytics. Fibrinolysis Proteolysis 1997;11:129–35.
67. Refino CJ, Paoni NF, Keyt BA, et al. A variant of t-PA T103N, KHRR 296-299 AAAA; that, by bolus, has increased potency and decreased systemic activation of plasminogen. Thromb Haemost 1993;70:313–19.
68. Katoh M, Suzuki Y, Miyamoto I, et al. Biochemical and pharmacokinetic properties of YM866, a novel fibrinolytic agent. Thromb Haemost 1991;65:1193.
69. Katoh M, Shimizu Y, Kawauchi Y, et al. Comparison of clearance rate of various tissue plasminogen activator (t-PA) analogues. Thromb Haemost 1989;62:542.
70. Haley EC Jr, Lyden PD, Johnston KC, et al. A pilot dose-escalation safety study of tenecteplase in acute ischemic stroke. Stroke 2005;36:607–12.
71. Parsons MW, Miteff F, Bateman GA, et al. Acute ischemic stroke: imaging-guided tenecteplase treatment in an extended time window. Neurology 2009;72:915–21.
72. Modi NB, Eppler S, Breed J, et al. Pharmacokinetics of a slower clearing tissue plasminogen activator variant, TNK-tPA, in patients with acute myocardial infarction. Thromb Haemost 1998;79(1):134–9.
73. Runge MS, Bode C, Matsueda GR, et al. Antibody-enhanced thrombolysis: Targeting of tissue plasminogen activator *in vivo*. Proc Natl Acad Sci U S A 1987;84:7659–62.
74. Kasper W, Erbel R, Meinertz T, et al. Intracoronary thrombolysis with an acylated streptokinase-plasminogen activator (BRL 26921) in patients with acute myocardial infarction. J Am Coll Cardiol 1984;4:357–63.
75. Pierard L, Jacobs P, Gheysen D, et al. Mutant and chimeric recombinant plasminogen activators. J Biol Chem 1987;262: 11771–8.
76. Kluft C, Los N. Demonstration of two forms of α_2-antiplasmin in plasma by modified crossed immunoelectrophoresis. Thromb Res 1981;21:65–71.
77. Loskutoff DJ, van Mourik JA, Erickson LA, et al. Detection of an unusually stable fibrinolytic inhibitor produced by bovine endothelial cells. Proc Natl Acad Sci U S A 1983;80: 2956–60.
78. Juhan-Vague I, Moerman B, de Cock F, et al. Plasma levels of a specific inhibitor of tissue-type plasminogen activator (and urokinase) in normal and pathological conditions. Thromb Res 1984;33:523–30.
79. Schleuning WD, Medcalf RL, Hession C, et al. Plasminogen activator inhibitor 2: Regulation of gene transcription during phorbol ester-mediated differentiation of U- 937 human histiocytic lymphoma cells. Mol Cell Biol 1987;7:4564–7.
80. Kruithof EK, Tran-Thang C, Gudinchet A, et al. Fibrinolysis in pregnancy: A study of plasminogen activator inhibitors. Blood 1987;69:460–6.
81. Stump DC, Thienpont M, Collen D. Purification and characterization of a novel inhibitor of urokinase from human urine: Quantitation and preliminary characterization in plasma. J Biol Chem 1986;261:12759–66.
82. Agnelli G, Buchanan MR, Fernandez F, et al. A comparison of the thrombolytic and hemorrhagic effects of tissue-type plasminogen activator and streptokinase in rabbits. Circulation 1985;72:178–82.
83. Loscalzo J, Vaughan DB. Tissue plasminogen activator promotes platelet disaggregation in plasma. J Clin Invest 1987;79: 1749–55.
84. Chen LY, Muhta JL. Lys- and glu-plasminogen potentiate the inhibtory effect of recombinant tissue plasminogen activator on human platelet aggregation. Thromb Res 1994;74:555–63.
85. Dent MA, Sumi Y, Morris RJ, et al. Urokinase-type plasminogen activator expression by neurons and oligodendrocytes during process outgrowth in developing rat brain. Eur J Neurosci 1993;5:633–47.
86. Sappino AP, Madani R, Huarte J, et al. Extracellular proteolysis in adult murine brain. J Clin Invest 1993;92:679–85.
87. del Zoppo GJ. t-PA: A neuron buster, too? (Editorial). Nat Med 1998;4:148–50.
88. Sironi L, Maria CA, Bellosta S, et al. Endogenous proteolytic activity in a rat model of spontaneous cerebral stroke. Brain Res 2003;974:184–92.
89. Chen ZL, Yu H, Yu WM, et al. Proteolytic fragments of laminin promote excitotoxic neurodegeneration by up-regulation of the KA1 subunit of the kainate receptor. J Cell Biol 2008;183: 1299–313.
90. Tsirka SE. Tissue plasminogen activator as a modulator of neuronal survival and function. Biochem Soc Trans 2002;30: 222–5.
91. Dent MA, Sumi Y, Morris RJ, et al. Urokinase-type plasminogen activator expression by neurons and oligodendrocytes during process outgrowth in developing rat brain. Eur J Neurosci 1993;5:633–47.
92. Lahtinen L, Huusko N, Myohanen H, et al. Expression of urokinase-type plasminogen activator receptor is increased during epileptogenesis in the rat hippocampus. Neuroscience 2009;163:316–28.
93. Iyer AM, Zurolo E, Boer K, et al. Tissue plasminogen activator and urokinase plasminogen activator in human epileptogenic pathologies. Neuroscience 2010;167:929–45.

94. Carroll PM, Tsirka SE, Richards WG, et al. The mouse tissue plasminogen activator gene 5′ flanking region directs appropriate expression in development and a seizure-enhanced response in the CNS. Development 1994;120:3173–83.
95. Pawlak R, Melchor JP, Matys T, et al. Ethanol-withdrawal seizures are controlled by tissue plasminogen activator via modulation of NR2B-containing NMDA receptors. Proc Natl Acad Sci U S A 2005;102:443–8.
96. Rogove AD, Siao C, Keyt B, et al. Activation of microglia reveals a non-proteolytic cytokine function for tissue plasminogen activator in the central nervous system. J Cell Sci 1999;112(Pt 22):4007–16.
97. Wang YF, Tsirka SE, Strickland S, et al. Tissue plasminogen activator (tPA) increases neuronal damage after focal cerebral ischemia in wild-type and tPA-deficient mice. Nat Med 1998;4:228–31.
98. Tsuji K, Aoki T, Tejima E, et al. Tissue plasminogen activator promotes matrix metalloproteinase-9 upregulation after focal cerebral ischemia. Stroke 2005;36:1954–9.
99. Nicole O, Docagne F, Ali C, et al. The proteolytic activity of tissue-plasminogen activator enhances NMDA receptor-mediated signaling. Nat Med 2001;7:59–64.
100. Yi JS, Kim YH, Koh JY. Infarct reduction in rats following intraventricular administration of either tissue plasminogen activator (tPA) or its non-protease mutant S478A-tPA. Exp Neurol 2004;189:354–60.
101. Samson AL, Nevin ST, Medcalf RL. Low molecular weight contaminants in commercial preparations of plasmin and t-PA activate neurons. J Thromb Haemost 2008;6:2218–20.
102. Korninger C, Collen D. Studies on the specific fibrinolytic effect of human extrinsic (tissue-type) plasminogen activator in human blood and in various animal species *in vitro*. Thromb Haemost 1981;46:561–5.
103. del Zoppo GJ, Copeland BR, Anderchek K, et al. Hemorrhagic transformation following tissue plasminogen activator in experimental cerebral infarction. Stroke 1990;21:596–601.
104. Overgaard K, Sereghy T, Pedersen H, et al. Effect of delayed thrombolysis with rt-PA in a rat embolic stroke model. J Cereb Blood Flow Metab 1994;14:472–7.
105. Overgaard K, Sereghy T, Boysen G, et al. Reduction of infarct volume by thrombolysis with rt-PA in an embolic rat stroke model. Scand J Clin Lab Invest 1993;53:383–93.
106. Rasmussen RS, Overgaard K, Meden P, et al. Thrombolytic and anticoagulation treatment in a rat embolic stroke model. Acta Neurol Scand 2003;108:185–92.
107. Wang X, Lee SR, Arai K, et al. Lipoprotein receptor-mediated induction of matrix metalloproteinase by tissue plasminogen activator. Nat Med 2003;9:1313–17.
108. Suzuki Y, Nagai N, Yamakawa K, et al. Tissue-type plasminogen activator (t-PA) induces stromelysin-1 (MMP-3) in endothelial cells through activation of lipoprotein receptor-related protein. Blood 2009;114:3352–8.
109. Lee SR, Guo SZ, Scannevin RH, et al. Induction of matrix metalloproteinase, cytokines and chemokines in rat cortical astrocytes exposed to plasminogen activators. Neurosci Lett 2007;417:1–5.
110. del Zoppo GJ, Mabuchi T. Cerebral microvessel responses to focal ischemia. J Cereb Blood Flow Metab 2003;23:879–94.
111. Hamann GF, Liebetrau M, Martens H, et al. Microvascular basal lamina injury after experimental focal cerebral ischemia and reperfusion in the rat. J Cereb Blood Flow Metab 2002;22:526–33.
112. Tagaya M, Haring H-P, Stuiver I, et al. Rapid loss of microvascular integrin expression during focal brain ischemia reflects neuron injury. J Cereb Blood Flow Metab 2001;21:835–46.
113. Fukuda S, Fini CA, Mabuchi T, et al. Focal cerebral ischemia induces active proteases that degrade microvascular matrix. Stroke 2004;35:998–1004.
114. Milner R, Hung S, Wang X, et al. Responses of endothelial cell and astrocyte matrix-integrin receptors to ischemia mimic those observed in the neurovascular unit. Stroke 2008;39:191–7.
115. Milner R, Hung S, Wang X, et al. The rapid decrease in astrocyte-associated dystroglycan expression by focal cerebral ischemia is protease-dependent. J Cereb Blood Flow Metab 2008;28:812–23.
116. Galis ZS, Kranzhöfer R, Fenton JWII, et al. Thrombin promotes activation of matrix metalloproteinase-2 produced by cultured vascular smooth muscle cells. Arterioscler Thromb Vasc Biol 1997;17:483–9.
117. Heck LW, Blackburn WD, Irwin MH, et al. Degradation of basement membrane laminin by human neutrophil elastase and cathepsin G. Am J Pathol 1990;136:1267–74.
118. Hamann GF, Okada Y, del Zoppo GJ. Hemorrhagic transformation and microvascular integrity during focal cerebral ischemia/reperfusion. J Cereb Blood Flow Metab 1996;16:1373–8.
119. Heo JH, Lucero J, Abumiya T, et al. Matrix metalloproteinases increase very early during experimental focal cerebral ischemia. J Cereb Blood Flow Metab 1999;19:624–33.
120. Mun-Bryce S, Rosenberg GA. Matrix metalloproteinases in cerebrovascular disease. J Cereb Blood Flow Metab 1998;18:1163–72.
121. Rosenberg GA, Estrada EY, Dencoff JE. Matrix metalloproteinases and TIMPs are associated with blood–brain barrier opening after reperfusion in rat brain. Stroke 1998;29:2189–95.
122. Rosenberg GA, Cunningham LA, Wallace J, et al. Immunohistochemistry of matrix metalloproteinases in reperfusion injury to rat brain: activation of MMP-9 linked to stromelysin-1 and microglia in cell cultures. Brain Res 2001;893:104–12.
123. Yang Y, Estrada EY, Thompson JF, et al. Matrix metalloproteinase-mediated disruption of tight junction proteins in cerebral vessels is reversed by synthetic matrix metalloproteinase inhibitor in focal ischemia in rat. J Cereb Blood Flow Metab 2007;27:697–709.
124. Rosenberg GA, Navratil M. Metalloproteinase inhibition blocks edema in intracerebral hemorrhage in the rat. Neurology 1997;48:921–6.
125. Asahi M, Asahi K, Jung JC, et al. Role for matrix metalloproteinase 9 after focal cerebral ischemia: Effects of gene knockout and enzyme inhibition with BB-94. J Cereb Blood Flow Metab 2000;20:1681–9.
126. Asahi M, Wang X, Mori T, et al. Effects of matrix metalloproteinase-9 gene knock-out on the proteolysis of blood–brain barrier and white matter components after cerebral ischemia. J Neurosci 2001;21:7724–32.
127. Tejima E, Zhao BQ, Tsuji K, et al. Astrocytic induction of matrix metalloproteinase-9 and edema in brain hemorrhage. J Cereb Blood Flow Metab 2007;27:460–8.
128. Montaner J, Alvarez-Sabin J, Molina C, et al. Matrix metalloproteinase expression after human cardioembolic stroke: temporal profile and relation to neurological impairment. Stroke 2001;32:1759–66.
129. Montaner J, Molina CA, Monasterio J, et al. Matrix metalloproteinase-9 pretreatment level predicts intracranial hemorrhagic complications after thrombolysis in human stroke. Circulation 2003;107:598–603.
130. Gidday JM, Gasche YG, Copin JC, et al. Leukocyte-derived matrix metalloproteinase-9 mediates blood–brain barrier breakdown and is proinflammatory after transient focal cerebral ischemia. Am J Physiol Heart Circ Physiol 2005;289:H558–68.
131. Lo E, Wang X, Cuzner M. Extracellular proteolysis in brain injury and inflammation: role for plasminogen activators and matrix metalloproteinases. J Neurosci Res 2002;69:1–9.
132. Wang X, Tsuji K, Lee SR, et al. Mechanisms of hemorrhagic transformation after tissue plasminogen activator reperfusion therapy for ischemic stroke. Stroke 2004;35:2726–30.
133. Ning M, Furie KL, Koroshetz WJ, et al. Association between tPA therapy and raised early matrix metalloproteinase-9 in acute stroke. Neurology 2006;66:1550–5.
134. Foerch C, Rosidi NL, Schlunk F, et al. Intravenous tPA therapy does not worsen acute intracerebral hemorrhage in mice. PLoS ONE 2013;8:e54203.
135. Barber PA, Darby DG, Desmond PM, et al. Prediction of stroke outcome with echoplanar perfusion- and diffusion-weighted MRI. Neurology 1998;51:418–26.
136. del Zoppo GJ. Focal cerebral ischemia and hemostasis: a PAI-1 conundrum. J Thromb Haemost 2005;3:1376–8.
137. Zivin JA, Fisher M, DeGirolami U, et al. Tissue plasminogen activator reduced neurological damage after cerebral embolism. Science 1985;230:1289–92.

138. Young AR, Touzani O, Derlon J-M, et al. Early reperfusion in the anesthetized baboon reduces brain damage following middle cerebral artery occlusion: A quantitative analysis of infarction volume. Stroke 1997;28:632–7.
139. del Zoppo GJ, Higashida RT, Furlan AJ, et al. PROACT: a phase II randomized trial of recombinant pro-urokinase by direct arterial delivery in acute middle cerebral artery stroke. Stroke 1998;29:4–11.
140. Fieschi C, Argentino C, Lenzi GL, et al. Clinical and instrumental evaluation of patients with ischemic stroke within the first six hours. J Neurol Sci 1989;91:311–21.
141. Solis OJ, Roberson GR, Taveras JM, et al. Cerebral angiography in acute cerebral infarction. Rev Interam Radiol 1977;2: 19–25.
142. Furlan AJ, Higashida R, Wechsler L, et al. Intra-arterial prourokinase for acute ischemic stroke. The PROACT II study: a randomized controlled trial. JAMA 1999;282:2003–11.
143. Francis CW, Blinc A, Lee S, et al. Ultrasound accelerates transport of recombinant tissue plasminogen activator into clots. Ultrasound Med Biol 1995;21:419–24.
144. Siddiqi F, Odrljin TM, Fay PJ, et al. Binding of tissue-plasminogen activator to fibrin: effect of ultrasound. Blood 1998;91: 2019–25.
145. The NINDS t-PA Stroke Study Group. Intracerebral hemorrhage after intravenous t-PA therapy for ischemic stroke. Stroke 1997;28:2109–18.
146. Larrue V, von Kummer R, del Zoppo GJ, et al. Hemorrhagic transformation in acute ischemic stroke. Potential contributing factors in the European Cooperative Acute Stroke Study. Stroke 1997;28:957–60.
147. Albers GW, Thijs VN, Wechsler L, et al. Magnetic resonance imaging profiles predict clinical response to early reperfusion: the diffusion and perfusion imaging evaluation for understanding stroke evolution (DEFUSE) study. Ann Neurol 2006; 60:508–17.
148. Singer OC, Humpich MC, Fiehler J, et al. Risk for symptomatic intracerebral hemorrhage after thrombolysis assessed by diffusion-weighted magnetic resonance imaging. Ann Neurol 2008;63:52–60.
149. Ueda T, Hatakeyama T, Kumon Y, et al. Evaluation of risk of hemorrhagic transformation in local intra-arterial thrombolysis in acute ischemic stroke by initial SPECT. Stroke 1994;25: 298–303.
150. Matsumoto K, Satoh K. Topical intraarterial urokinase infusion for acute stroke. In: Hacke W, del Zoppo GJ, Hirschberg M, editors. Thrombolytic Therapy in Acute Ischemic Stroke. Heidelberg, Germany: Springer-Verlag; 1991. p. 207–12.
151. Gönner F, Remonda L, Mattle H, et al. Local intra-arterial thrombolysis in acute ischemic stroke. Stroke 1998;29:1894–900.
152. Yamaguchi T. Intravenous rt-PA in acute embolic stroke. In: Hacke W, del Zoppo GJ, Hirschberg M, editors. Thrombolytic Therapy in Acute Ischemic Stroke. Heidelberg, Germany: Springer-Verlag; 1991. p. 168–74.
153. von Kummer R, Hacke W. Safety and efficacy of intravenous tissue plasminogen activator and heparin in acute middle cerebral artery. Stroke 1992;23:646–52.

3 Cerebral Blood Flow and Metabolism: Regulation and Pathophysiology in Cerebrovascular Disease

William J. Powers

KEY POINTS

- Since storage of substrates for energy metabolism in the brain is minimal, the brain is highly dependent on a continuous supply of oxygen and glucose from the blood for its functional and structural integrity.
- Control of cerebral blood flow (CBF) under conditions of normal cerebral perfusion pressure is determined by the caliber of the resistance vessels, primarily arterioles, which dilate and constrict in response to a variety of stimuli. The metabolic factor controlling CBF in the normal resting brain is cerebral oxygen metabolism. Vasodilation and vasoconstriction maintain the balance between oxygen delivery (CBF x CaO_2) and oxygen metabolism. When there is a primary reduction in the oxygen metabolic rate of brain cells, there is a secondary decline in cerebral blood flow to a comparable degree.
- The responses of the cerebral vasculature to acute changes in arterial pCO_2 represent a notable instance in which the oxidative metabolic control of resting CBF is overridden. Acute decreases in arterial pCO_2 decrease CBF, whereas increases in arterial pCO_2 increase CBF with little or no changes in oxygen metabolism.
- Autoregulation is the physiological compensatory response that insures that changes in cerebral perfusion pressure over a wide range from 70 to 150 mm Hg have little effect on CBF. Chronic hypertension shifts both the lower and upper limits of autoregulation to higher levels.
- The ability of brain cells to survive CBF below 20–25 mL $100g^{-1}$ min^{-1} depends on both the magnitude and duration of the CBF reduction. CBF of 5–10 mL $100g^{-1}$ min^{-1} may be tolerated for a period of less than 1 hour whereas CBF of 10–15 mL $100g^{-1}$ min^{-1} may not produce cell death for 2–3 hours. In addition, the rapidity at which cell death occurs depends on individual properties of the neurons. Some neurons may tolerate the same reduction in CBF for a period of time that is lethal to other cells. White matter is more tolerant than gray matter.
- Pioneering studies performed in experimental animals and humans laid the basis for the current widespread teaching that autoregulation is impaired in acute ischemic stroke. However, more recent data from humans have shown no selective impairment of autoregulation in the peri-infarct region.
- In acute intracerebal hemorrhage, neither is there a zone of ischemia around the hematoma nor is autoregulation impaired.

NORMAL CEREBRAL ENERGY METABOLISM AND HEMODYNAMICS

Introduction

Energy production in the brain relies on metabolism of exogenous compounds with a high-energy content, primarily the oxidation of glucose. Since storage of substrates for energy metabolism in the brain is minimal, the brain is highly dependent on a continuous supply of oxygen and glucose from the blood for its functional and structural integrity.[1]

Cerebral Blood Flow and Other Measurements of Cerebral Perfusion

Cerebral blood flow (CBF) is the volume of blood that flows into a specified amount of brain in a defined time, expressed most commonly as mL $100g^{-1}$ min^{-1} or mL g^{-1} min^{-1} (Figs 3-1A and 3-2). Cerebral blood volume (CBV) is the volume of circulating intravascular blood within a specified amount of brain at a given time, usually expressed as mL $100g^{-1}$ (Figs 3-1B and 3-2). The vascular mean transit time (MTT) is the mean time it takes for intravascular particles to transit through the vasculature within a specified amount of brain (Figs 3-1C and 3-2). These particles may be red blood cells, plasma proteins, iodinated X-ray contrast agents or magnetic resonance imaging (MRI) contrast agents. The vascular MTT will be slightly different for different particles.[2] By the central volume principle vascular MTT = CBV/CBF.[3] Time-to-peak (TTP) and Tmax are two other cerebral perfusion measurements not directly related to CBF or CBV that are commonly used in MRI studies of cerebrovascular disease (Figs 3-1D and 3-2).[4] Both are measurements of the time after intravenous injection it takes for a contrast bolus to reach a region of the brain. TTP is the actual measured time after injection for peak concentration to arrive. Tmax is the arrival time for an idealized bolus corrected for dispersion within the vasculature. Both TTP and Tmax are determined primarily by the length of the circulatory pathway and are prolonged when arterial obstruction forces blood through collateral vessels.

Normal Values of Cerebral Blood Flow and Cerebral Metabolism

Healthy young adults have an average whole-brain CBF of approximately 46 mL $100g^{-1}$ min^{-1}, cerebral metabolic rate of oxygen ($CMRO_2$) of 3.0 mL $100g^{-1}$ min^{-1}(134 µmol $100g^{-1}$ min^{-1}) and cerebral metabolic rate of glucose (CMRglc) of 25 µmol $100g^{-1}$ min^{-1} using the Kety–Schmidt technique.[5–8] Normal whole-brain values obtained by positron emission tomography (PET) are comparable: CBF 48 mL $100g^{-1}$ min^{-1}, $CMRO_2$ 2.8 mL $100g^{-1}$ min^{-1} (125 µmol $100g^{-1}$ min^{-1}) and CMRglc of 22 µmol $100g^{-1}$ min^{-1}. PET measured CBV is 3.7 mL $100g^{-1}$ and vascular MTT is 4.7 seconds (author's data).

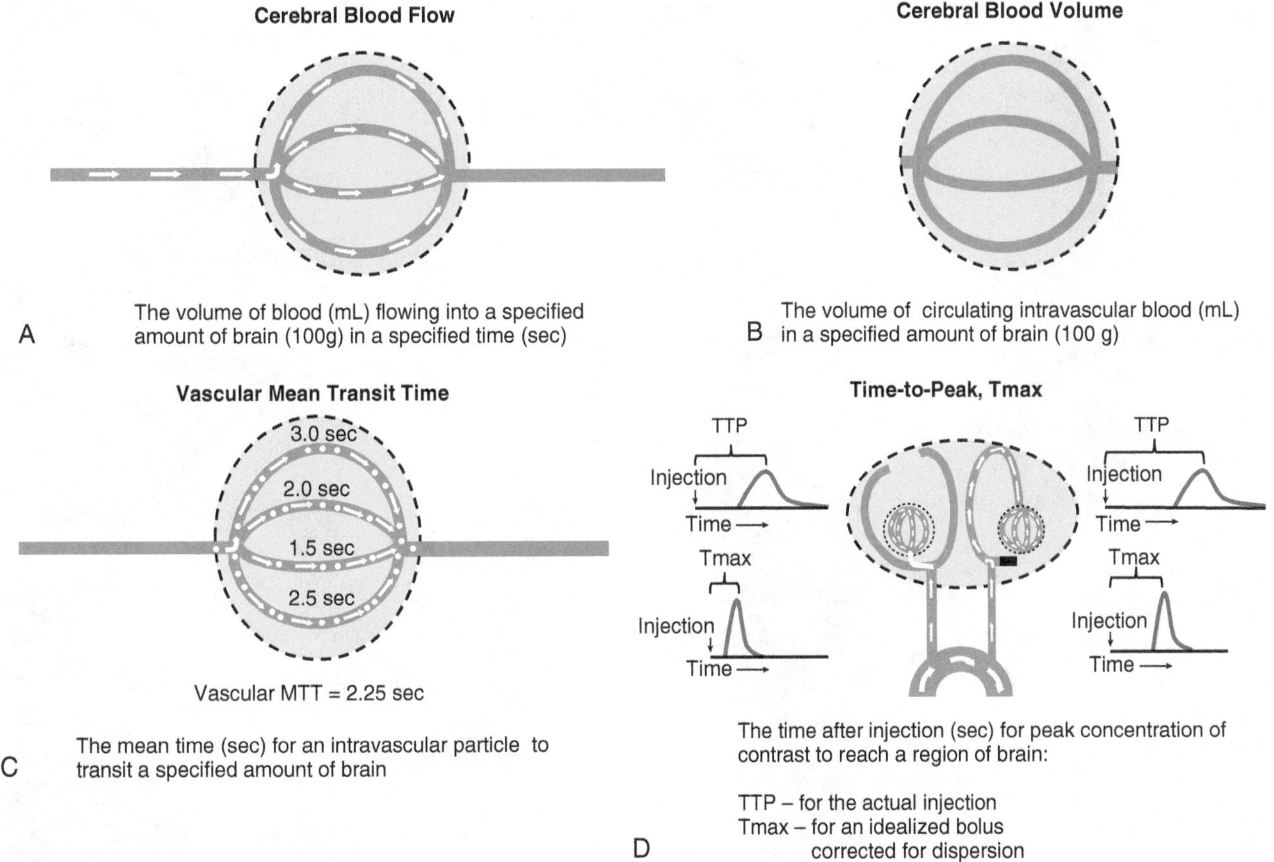

Figure 3-1. Diagrammatic representations of different indices of cerebral perfusion: A, cerebral blood flow; B, cerebral blood volume; C, vascular mean transit time, and D, time-to-peak and Tmax.

In newborn infants, mean whole-brain CBF is much lower, 6– 35 mL $100g^{-1}$ min^{-1}.[9–14] Pre-term infants with subsequently normal development at 6 months of age may have CBF below 10 mL $100g^{-1}$ min^{-1}.[15] Whole-brain $CMRO_2$ in the normal newborn is also very low, often below 1.3 mL $100g^{-1}$ min^{-1}.[9,16] Mean whole-brain CMRglc in the newborn has been reported to be 4 to 19 μmol $100g^{-1}$ min^{-1}.[17–19]

Beyond the neonatal period, average whole-brain CBF, $CMRO_2$ and CMRglc progressively increase, reaching a maximum at 3–10 years with peak CBF 60–140 mL $100g^{-1}$ min^{-1}, peak $CMRO_2$ 4.3–6.2 mL $100g^{-1}$ min^{-1}, and peak CMRglc 49–65 μmol $100g^{-1}$ min^{-1}.[13,20–25] By late adolescence, cerebral flow, oxygen and glucose metabolism decrease to adult levels.[13,20,21,24] Many studies report that CBF declines further from the third decade onward, albeit much more slowly than the decrease in adolescence.[26–29] The changes in $CMRO_2$ and CMRglc with age are less clear, with several studies showing a decrease[26,28,30–32] and others showing no change.[33–35] Studies that have corrected for brain atrophy, show lesser or absent changes in CBF with increasing age.[31,36–38] The author's own data corrected for brain atrophy from 23 normal subjects, ages 23–71 years, show no significant change in CBF or $CMRO_2$, but a small decline in CMRglc.

Control of Cerebral Blood Flow

CBF is regulated by the cerebral perfusion pressure (CPP) and the cerebrovascular resistance (CVR).

$$CBF = \frac{CPP}{CVR}$$

CPP is equal to the difference between arterial and cerebral venous pressures. Cerebral venous pressure is negligible unless there is elevated intracranial pressure (ICP) or venous obstruction. Under constant CPP, changes in CBF must occur as a result of changes in CVR. CVR is determined by blood viscosity, vessel length, and vessel radius. Only vessel radius is amenable to rapid physiological regulation. Thus, the control of CBF under conditions of normal CPP is determined by the caliber of the resistance vessels, primarily arterioles, which dilate and constrict in response to a variety of stimuli.

Relationship of Cerebral Blood Flow and Metabolism

Although it may seem self-contradictory, the term "resting brain" has proven to be a useful concept for understanding the relationship between CBF and metabolism. The brain is considered to be "resting" in awake humans not specifically engaged in any cognitive or behavioral task, often stipulated with eyes closed. In resting brain, CBF in gray matter (80 mL $100g^{-1}$ min^{-1}) is approximately four times higher than in white matter (20 mL $100g^{-1}$ min^{-1}).[39] Regional blood flow is closely matched to the resting metabolic rates of oxygen and glucose, both also higher in gray than in white matter[40–42] (Fig. 3-3). For both oxygen and glucose, the amount delivered to the brain by the arterial blood (CBF x arterial concentration) exceeds the normal metabolic rate. Only approximately one-third of the oxygen and one-tenth of the glucose delivered to the brain by the blood is metabolized.[40,41,43–45] As a consequence of the close regional coupling of resting CBF with both $CMRO_2$ and CMRglc, the fractions extracted by the brain of

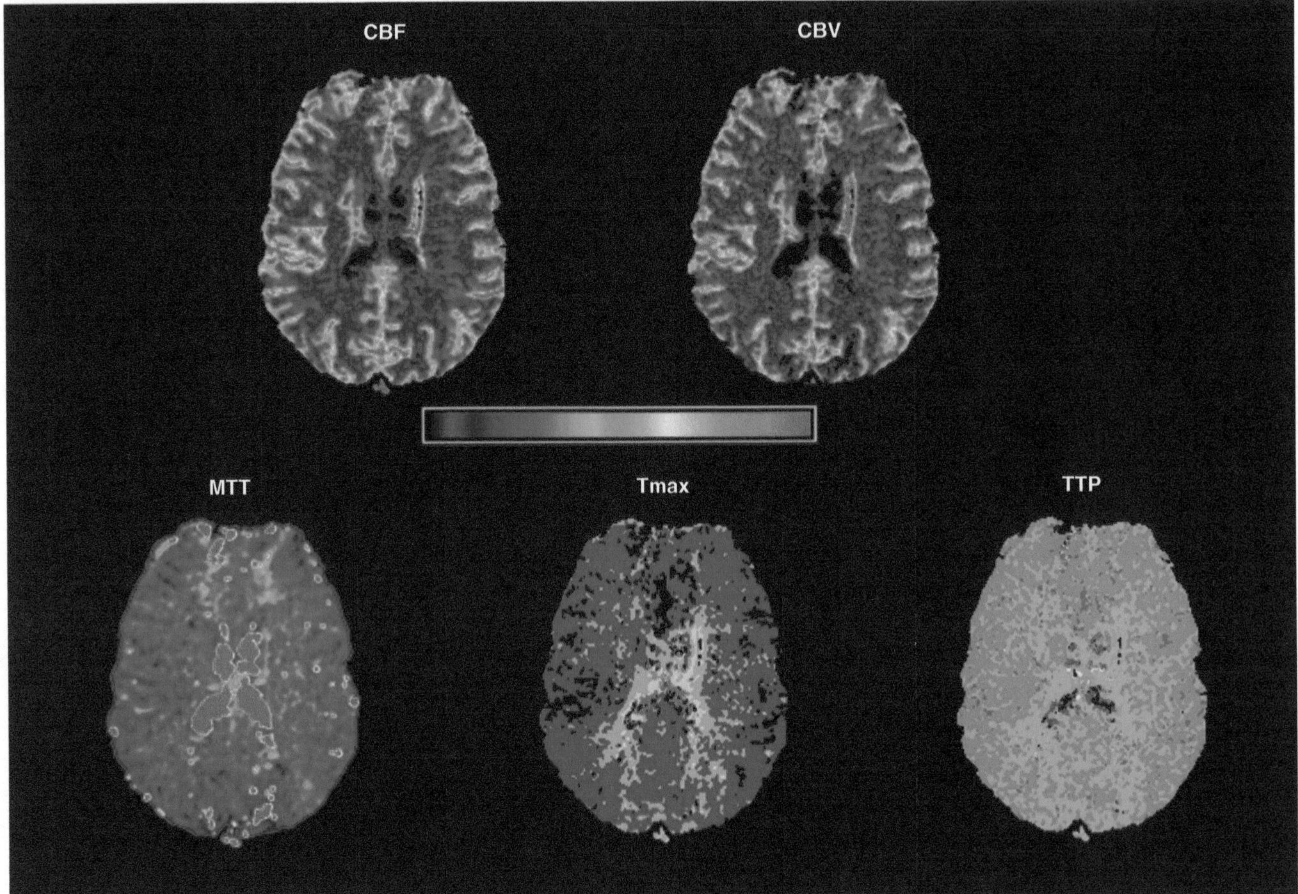

Figure 3-2. Magnetic resonance images from a normal 27-year-old woman depicting cerebral blood flow (CBF), cerebral blood volume (CBV), vascular mean transit time (MTT), Tmax and time-to-peak (TTP). *(Images courtesy of Hongyu An, University of North Carolina.)*

available oxygen (oxygen extraction fraction, OEF) and glucose (glucose extraction fraction, GEF) are strikingly more uniform than either CBF or metabolism (see Fig. 3-3). Similarly, resting CBV is also higher in gray than white matter and closely matched to CBF resulting in a uniform vascular MTT (CBV/CBF) throughout the normal brain (see Fig. 3-2).

There is substantial inter-individual variation in resting whole-brain values of CBF, $CMRO_2$ and CMRglc among normal humans. Normal CBF variation is significantly correlated with normal variations in $CMRO_2$ and arterial oxygen content, but not with normal variations in CMRglc or arterial plasma glucose concentration, thus indicating that the metabolic factor controlling CBF in the normal resting brain is $CMRO_2$ and not CMRglc.[46] When there is a primary reduction in the metabolic rate of brain cells, there is a secondary decline in CBF to a comparable degree with little or no change in OEF. This close coupling of reduced CBF to reduced $CMRO_2$ in the resting brain can be demonstrated experimentally during metabolic depression from hypothermia or barbiturate anesthesia but is also an essential CBF regulatory mechanism than influences CBF in a variety of physiological and pathological conditions[47–51] (Fig. 3-4). Because of the coupling of CBF to $CRMO_2$ in the resting state, it isn't possible to accurately interpret CBF values without knowledge of $CMRO_2$. Low CBF may be due to simply reduced metabolic demand and not an indication of restriction in supply.[50,52]

When simultaneously measured from arterial–jugular venous differences in the human resting brain, the $CMRO_2$ / CMRglc molar ratio is 5.4 rather than 6.0 as would occur with complete oxidation of glucose. A small amount of lactate is produced by glycolysis even under normal conditions of excess oxygen supply.[5,7,53] The $CMRO_2$ /CMRglc molar ratio is not uniform throughout the brain. It is lower in prefrontal cortex, lateral parietal cortex, posterior cingulate/precuneus, lateral temporal gyrus, gyrus rectus, and caudate nuclei and higher in the inferior temporal gyrus and throughout the cerebellum.[54] Compartmentalization of metabolism by cell type between mainly oxidative neurons and mainly glycolytic astrocytes has been proposed with the astrocytes acting to produce and distribute lactate to active neurons.[55]

When brain neurons are engaged in a specific cognitive or behavioral task, both regional CBF and CMRglc increase in the area of increased neuronal activity.[56] Increases in $CMRO_2$, if they occur at all, are much lower.[57,58] As a consequence, the oxygen delivery further outstrips the oxygen demands in these areas causing a decrease in OEF and an increase in the venous oxygen concentration. Metabolism in these areas shifts to non-oxidative glycolysis with increased lactate production even in the face of excess oxygen supply.[59] Blood-oxygen-level-dependent (BOLD) magnetic resonance imaging is sensitive to the changes in blood deoxygenated hemoglobin.[60] Changes in BOLD contrast can be used to detect increases in the venous oxygen concentration that occur with physiologic neuronal activity and the measurement of this signal allows particular brain regions to be implicated in the performance of motor, sensory, language, or cognitive tasks.[61] Examining the intercorrelation of regional BOLD activity over time in the resting brain has revealed multiple networks of brain regions that are tightly coupled. This analysis method, termed resting state functional connectivity, provides insight into intrinsic

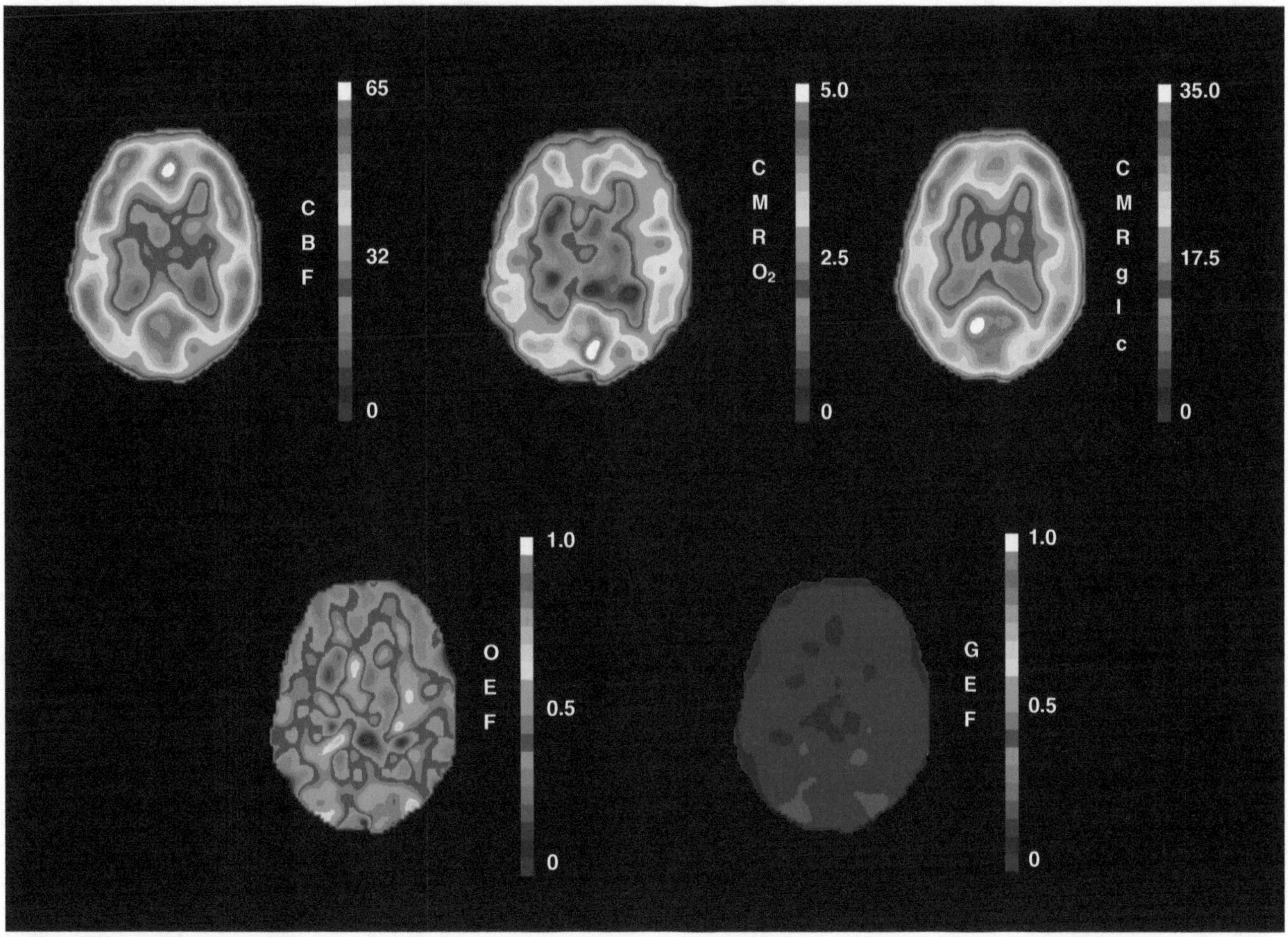

Figure 3-3. Normal positron emission tomography scans of cerebral blood flow (CBF) in mL $100g^{-1} min^{-1}$, cerebral metabolic rate of oxygen ($CMRO_2$) in mL $100g^{-1} min^{-1}$, cerebral metabolic rate of glucose (CMRglc) in μmol $100g^{-1} min^{-1}$, oxygen extraction fraction (OEF) and glucose extraction fraction (GEF).

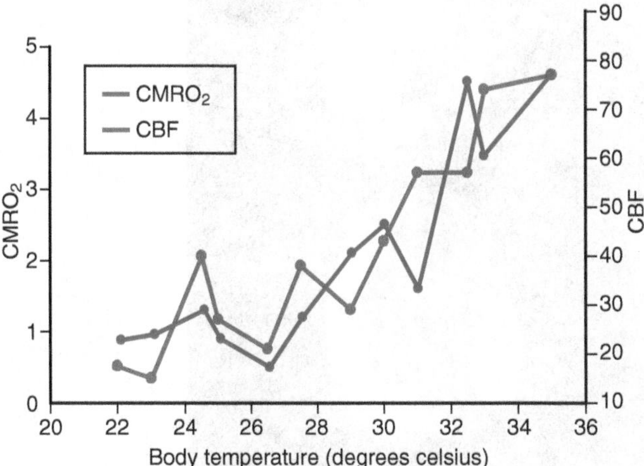

Figure 3-4. Effect of hypothermia on cerebral metabolic rate of oxygen ($CMRO_2$) and cerebral blood flow (CBF) in rhesus macaques. *(Data from Table 3.1 in Bering EAJ, Taren JA, McMurrrey JD, Bernhard WF. Studies on hypothermia in monkeys. II. The effect of hypothermia on the general physiology and cerebral metabolism of monkeys in the hypothermic state,* Surg Gynecol Obstet *102:134–138, 1956.)*

brain function.[62] The mechanism by which increases in neuronal activity cause increases in regional CBF remains unsettled.[63,64]

Response of Cerebral Blood Flow to Changes in Arterial Partial Pressure of Oxygen and Oxygen Content

Because of the sigmoid shape of the hemoglobin-oxygen dissociation curve, a significant reduction in arterial oxygen content (CaO_2) and arterial oxygen delivery (CBF x CaO_2) does not occur until arterial pO_2 falls to about 50–60 mm Hg.[65,66] During arterial hypoxemia, CBF does not increase until arterial pO_2 is reduced below about 30–50 mm Hg,[66,67] indicating that it is primarily CaO_2 and not pO_2 that drives this vasodilatory response. Reductions in CaO_2 due to anemia cause compensatory increases in CBF and increases in CaO_2 with polycythemia are associated with a decrease in CBF.[5,66,68–70] In neither of these cases does cerebral oxygen metabolism change.[66,70] With chronic changes in CaO_2, there is a reciprocal inverse relationship between CaO_2 and CBF throughout the range of oxygen content levels.[69] Acute changes in CaO_2 due to reduction in hemoglobin or pO_2 also produce reciprocal increases in CBF, but less so than do chronic changes.[71,72] These changes are best interpreted as an active cerebrovascular mechanism that produces vasodilation or vasoconstriction to maintain the balance between oxygen delivery (CBF x CaO_2) and $CMRO_2$ at a relatively constant OEF.

Response of Cerebral Blood Flow to Changes in Blood Glucose

In contrast to the clear reciprocal relationship between CBF and CaO_2, alterations in arterial plasma glucose concentration have little effect on CBF. Decreasing blood glucose concentration to 2.3–3 mmol/L in normal subjects has generally been reported to cause no change in CBF.[73–76] More recently, a study with greater measurement precision reported a slight decrease in CBF of 6–8% at a blood glucose concentration of 3.0 mmol/L.[77] More severe reductions in blood glucose down to 1.1–2.2 mmol/L produced a modest but significant increase in CBF.[78–82] This likely does not represent a compensatory mechanism to maintain glucose delivery to the brain. A blood glucose level of 2 mmol/L is well below the level at which brain dysfunction and counter-regulatory hormone response occur.[74] Furthermore, increases in CBF do not increase blood-brain glucose transport.[83,84]

Response of Cerebral Blood Flow to Changes in Arterial pCO_2

The responses of the cerebral vasculature to acute changes in arterial pCO_2 represent a notable instance in which the oxidative metabolic control of resting CBF is overridden. Acute decreases in arterial pCO_2 to approximately 25 mm Hg via hyperventilation produce vasoconstriction and lead to a decrease in CBF of 30–35%, whereas increases in arterial pCO_2 to over 50 mm Hg via CO_2 inhalation cause vasodilation and an increase in CBF of about 75%.[68,85–88] With passive hyperventilation, CBF decreases but there is no reduction in $CMRO_2$,[85,89,90] however, with active hyperventilation, a slight increase in $CMRO_2$ has been reported.[68,85]

The cerebral vasoconstriction with hyperventilation is accompanied by a reduction in CBV[91] (Fig. 3-5). In conditions of increased intracranial pressure, this reduction in the volume of the intracranial contents can be used to temporarily reduce intracranial pressure. However, the cerebrovascular response to hyperventilation attenuates with time such that CBF returns to normal in about 6 hours. If hyperventilation is abruptly ceased after a prolonged period, arterial vasodilation will occur and CBF will rise above baseline levels.[88]

Response of Cerebral Blood Flow to Changes in Blood Viscosity

It is unlikely that viscosity is an independent determinant of CBF under most circumstances. Hematocrit is an important determinant of viscosity and thus viscosity often varies with CaO_2 making it difficult to determine if it has an independent role regulating CBF. In anemic, paraproteinemic subjects in whom reduced CaO_2 is dissociated from changes in viscosity, there is no correlation between viscosity and CBF, but there is a highly significant inverse relationship between CaO_2 and CBF.[92] In normal subjects, reduction of viscosity by plasma exchange without a concomitant change in hemoglobin concentration or CaO_2 does not increase CBF.[93] In these circumstances, any changes in blood viscosity induce compensatory vasodilation or vasoconstriction to maintain CBF and cerebral oxygen delivery. Viscosity may have an effect on CBF in the presence of pre-existing vasodilation. In rats with increased CBF due to hemodilution, hypercapnia, and hypoxia, doubling plasma viscosity reduced CBF by as much as half.[94,95] Thus, the vascular compensatory mechanism to increased

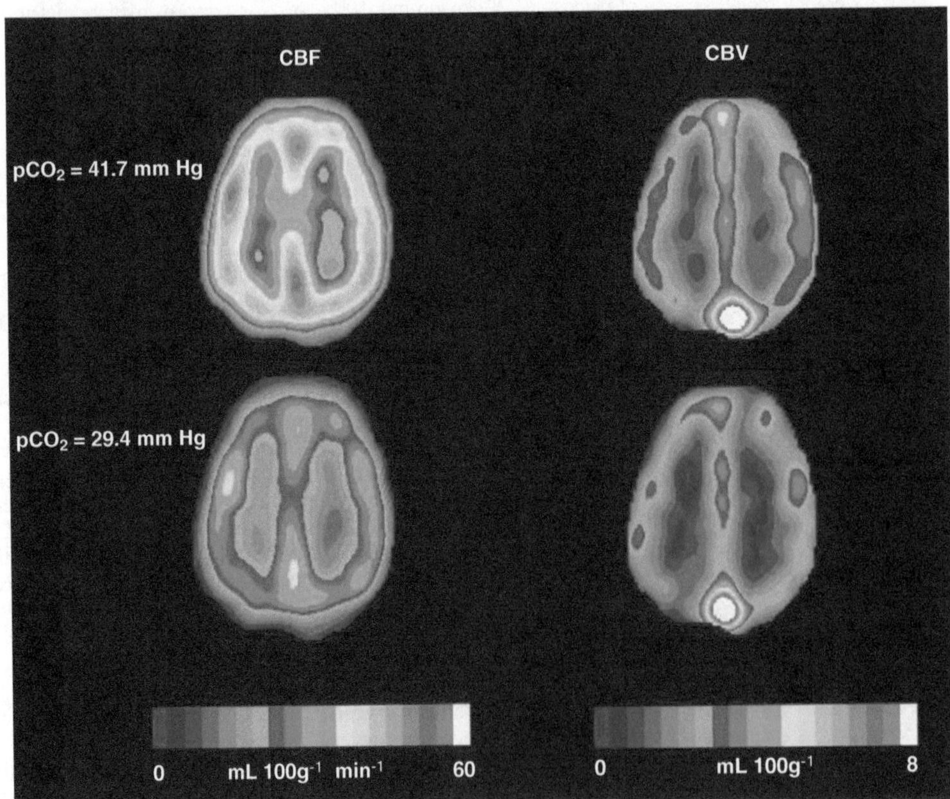

Figure 3-5. Reduction of cerebral blood flow (CBF) and cerebral blood volume (CBV) with hyperventilation in a patient with traumatic brain injury.

viscosity may be exhausted when pre-existing vasodilation impairs the ability of vessels to dilate further and then increases in viscosity can reduce CBF.[95]

Autoregulation of Cerebral Blood Flow to Changes in Cerebral Perfusion Pressure

Changes in CPP over a wide range from 70 to 150 mm Hg have little effect on CBF.[96,97] This compensatory physiological response to maintain CBF in the face of changing CPP is known as autoregulation. Reductions of CPP below the lower autoregulatory limit of 70 mm Hg produce a steep fall in CBF and increases above the upper limit of 150 mm Hg cause a steep rise.[98,99] Chronic hypertension shifts both the lower and upper limits of autoregulation to higher levels. In chronically hypertensive subjects, the lower autoregulatory limit is 100–120 mm Hg[98,100] (Fig. 3-6). This limit is variably and unpredictably affected by chronic antihypertensive drug treatment.[98] Thus, acute reductions in CPP to levels that would cause no change in CBF in normal subjects may precipitate cerebral ischemia in patients with chronic hypertension. It is important to emphasize that cerebral blood vessels autoregulate in response to local CPP not to systemic mean arterial blood pressure (MAP). If intracranial pressure is high, the lower limit of autoregulation will occur at a higher systemic MAP (Fig. 3-6).

This compensatory mechanism of autoregulation is mediated by changes in vessel caliber. When CPP decreases, vasodilation of the small arteries or arterioles reduces CVR. When CPP increases, vasoconstriction of the small arteries or arterioles increases CVR.[101–104] The vasodilation induced by reductions in CPP can be indirectly measured as an increase in CBV.[105] The response of the blood vessels lags about 10 seconds from the change in blood pressure.[104] Investigations into the mechanism of the autoregulatory vascular responses have engendered differences of opinion regarding the importance of myogenic and metabolic factors. Isolated arterioles studied ex vivo demonstrate a marked myogenic response in that reduced transmural pressure causes vasodilation and increased transmural pressure causes vasoconstriction.[106] In vivo, the arterial vasodilatory response to reduced CPP can be reversed by direct local delivery of oxygen to the tissue indicating that the vasodilation is a response to maintain CBF and oxygen delivery.[107] In a living animal model of increased jugular venous pressure in which CPP is reduced in the setting of increased transmural pressure, autoregulation was preserved demonstrating that the metabolic vasodilatory response is dominant over the myogenic vasoconstrictive response in vivo.[108]

These observations of the effect of changes in CPP on CBF were made by changing CPP over minutes, then measuring CBF at the new stable pressure. These responses have recently been termed "static cerebral autoregulation" to differentiate

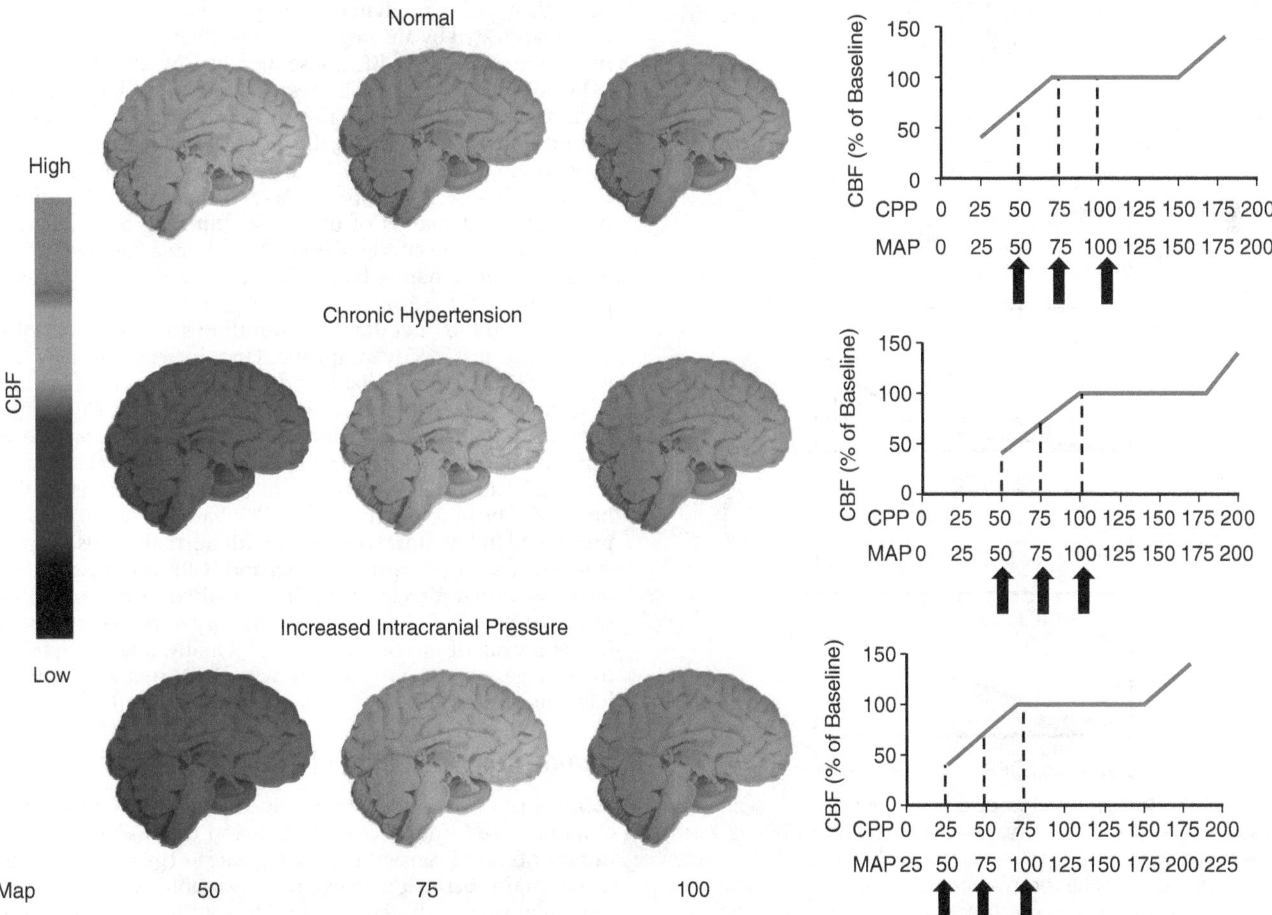

Figure 3-6. Diagrammatic representation of the autoregulation of cerebral blood flow (CBF) at mean arterial pressures (MAP) of 50, 75 and 100 mm Hg in three different conditions. (Top) Normal autoregulation with MAP equal to cerebral perfusion pressure (CPP) (Middle) Chronic hypertension with intact autoregulatory curve shifted upwards and MAP equal to CPP. (Bottom) Increased intracranial pressure of 25 mm Hg with MAP 25 mm Hg higher than CPP.

them from "dynamic cerebral autoregulation" which is based on studies of the dynamic responses of the cerebral vasculature to transient, more rapid fluctuations in CPP or the transfer function analysis of beat-to-beat changes in systemic MAP with spontaneous oscillations in cerebrovascular tone, cortical oxygenation, or intracranial pressure.[109] The physiological basis for dynamic autoregulation is complex and the data are very dependent on the specific measurement techniques and analytic algorithms used.[110-114] Static and dynamic cerebral autoregulation each measure different cerebrovascular functions. Abnormalities of dynamic cerebral autoregulation may be associated with normal or abnormal static autoregulation.[115-117] The clinical relevance of the two measures differs as well. Static autoregulation studies replicate the clinical use of vasoactive drugs to acutely manipulate systemic blood pressure and thus provide some guidance regarding the effect of these therapies on CBF. The clinical relevance of dynamic autoregulation studies rests on the empiric demonstration of a correlation with a clinically relevant outcome.

Compensatory Responses to Reduced Cerebral Blood Flow

As CPP falls below the static lower autoregulatory limit and the maximal vasodilatory capacity of the cerebral circulation has been exceeded, CBF begins to decline and a progressive increase in OEF maintains oxygen metabolism.[52,118] The normal OEF of 30–40% may increase by a factor of two or even more[52] (Fig. 3-7). This compensatory mechanism of increased OEF can adequately maintain cerebral metabolism and normal brain function for long periods of time.[119]

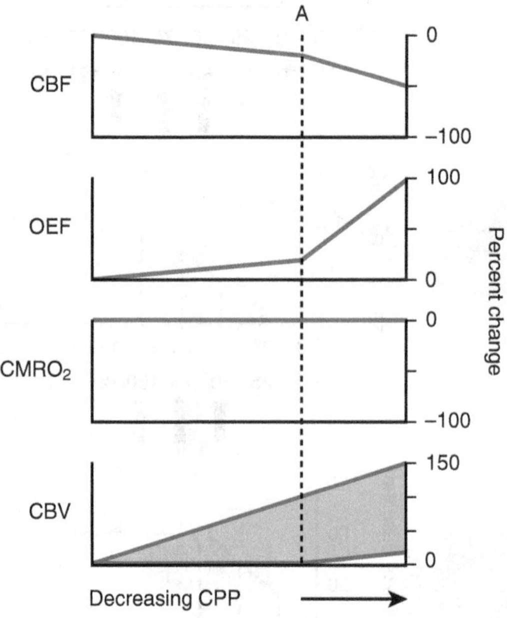

Figure 3-7. Compensatory responses to reduced cerebral perfusion pressure (CPP). As CPP falls, cerebral blood flow (CBF) is initially maintained (with only slight reduction) by arteriolar dilation. When vasodilatory capacity has been exceeded, cerebral autoregulation fails and CBF begins to decrease rapidly (A). A progressive increase in oxygen extraction (OEF) preserves cerebral oxygen metabolism ($CMRO_2$). The response of cerebral blood volume (CBV) to reduced CPP is variable, ranging from a steady rise (of as much as 150%) to only a modest increase beginning at the point of autoregulatory failure.

Response of Cerebral Blood Flow to Multiple Simultaneous Stimuli

Cerebral blood vessels only have a finite capacity to constrict or dilate. Thus, when subjected to multiple simultaneous stimuli, the cerebrovascular response to a single stimulus may be attenuated or lost. For example, when the cerebral blood vessels are already dilated in response to reduced CPP, the normal CBF responses to pCO_2 and increased neuronal activity may be lost.[120,121] Similarly, when already dilated in response to some other stimulus, cerebral blood vessels respond less to vasodilation induced by reduced CPP. As a consequence, the autoregulatory response is attenuated or lost in the setting of pre-existing hypercapnia, anemia, or hypoxemia.[122,123]

HEMODYNAMIC EFFECTS OF ARTERIAL OCCLUSIVE DISEASE

Three-stage Classification System of Cerebral Hemodynamics

Based on the physiological responses of CBF, CBV, and OEF to reductions in CPP, a three-stage sequential classification system has been used to describe the regional cerebral hemodynamic effects of arterial occlusive disease (Figs 3-7 and 3-8).[124] Stage 0 is normal CPP with closely matched flow and metabolism such that OEF is relatively uniform throughout the brain. CBV and vascular MTT are not elevated and the CBF response to vasodilatory stimuli such as hypercapnia is normal. Stage I hemodynamic compromise occurs at decreased CPP manifested by autoregulatory vasodilation of arterioles to maintain a constant CBF. Consequently, CBV and the vascular MTT are increased, the CBF response to vasodilatory stimuli is decreased, but OEF remains uniform. In Stage II hemodynamic failure, CPP is below the autoregulatory capacity. There is increased OEF since CBF has declined with respect to $CMRO_2$. $CMRO_2$ is preserved at a level that reflects the underlying energy demands of the tissue, but may be lower than normal due to the effects of previous ischemic damage.[52,125-127] Stage II hemodynamic failure has also been termed "misery perfusion."[128,129]

Although the three-stage classification scheme is conceptually useful, it is overly simplistic. First, increases in CBV and vascular MTT are not reliable indices of reduced CPP. While it is sometimes possible to measure an increase in CBV that is presumed to be due to autoregulatory vasodilation during experimental reductions in CPP, this is not always evident and a decrease in CBV in response to severe reductions in CPP has even been observed.[105,118,130-133] Vascular MTT may be prolonged in low-flow conditions with normal perfusion pressure, such as hypocapnia.[91,134] Second, CBF responses to different vasodilatory agents may be impaired or normal in the same patient.[135-137] A normal vasodilatory response may occur in the setting of increased CBV.[138,139] Finally, according to the three-stage system, all patients with increased OEF should have increased CBV, but this is not always evident.[140]

Hemodynamic Effects of Arterial Stenosis

Stenosis of the carotid artery produces no intravascular hemodynamic effect until a critical reduction of 60–70% in vessel lumen occurs. Even with this or greater degrees of stenosis, distal brain perfusion pressure is variable and may even remain normal with stenosis exceeding 90%.[141] This is because the downstream hemodynamic effect of carotid artery stenosis depends not only on the degree of stenosis, but also on the adequacy of the collateral circulation. However, the pattern of arteriographic collateral circulation to the MCA distal to an

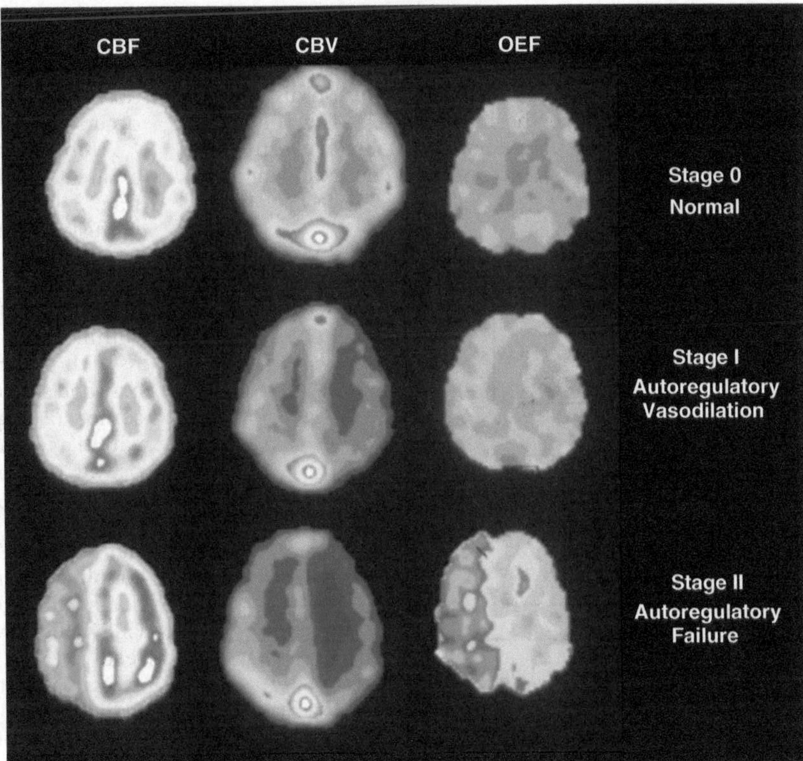

Figure 3-8. Positron emission tomography scans depicting the three-stage classification system of cerebral hemodynamics in three different patients with left carotid occlusion. In all images, the left side of the brain is on the reader's left. Stage 0 shows symmetrical cerebral blood flow (CBF), cerebral blood volume (CBV) and oxygen extraction fraction (OEF). In Stage I, autoregulatory vasodilation in the left hemisphere manifested by increased CBV maintains symmetrical CBF and OEF. In Stage II, autoregulatory vasodilation in the left hemisphere can no longer maintain CBF. Left hemisphere CBF is reduced and OEF is increased.

occluded carotid artery does not consistently differentiate those patients with poor cerebral hemodynamics.[130,142–144] Vascular imaging techniques such as angiography or Doppler ultrasonography can identify the presence of these collateral vessels, but not the adequacy of the blood supply they provide.[143]

Correlation of Cerebral Hemodynamics with Stroke Risk

Several studies have evaluated the prognostic value of measurements of cerebral hemodynamics on stroke risk in symptomatic carotid occlusion or middle cerebral artery stenosis/occlusion. Impaired reactivity to the vasodilating stimuli of acetazolamide or hypercapnia (Stage I hemodynamic compromise) has been an inconsistent predictor of subsequent stroke.[142,145–151] In contrast, Stage II hemodynamic failure, defined as increased OEF, has been consistently shown to be a predictor of subsequent ipsilateral ischemic stroke. The aggregate 2-year risk for ipsilateral ischemic stroke from four studies was 22/71 (31%) for those with increased OEF and 7/200 (3.5%) for those without.[126,130,152,153]

ISCHEMIC STROKE

Changes in Cerebral Blood Flow and Metabolism with Acute Ischemic Stroke

When CPP and CBF decline such that the increase in OEF is no longer adequate to supply the oxygen needs of the brain, a series of functional and biochemical changes occur. The first is a progressive reduction in protein synthesis when CBF falls below 50%. CMRglc increases at CBF of 20–30 mL $100g^{-1}$ min^{-1} and then declines as CBF falls below 20 mL $100g^{-1}$ min^{-1}. At CBF of 15–20 mL $100g^{-1}$ min^{-1}, normal cellular function is disrupted. Neuronal electrical activity is at first impaired and then abolished. Neurological deficits appear. High-energy phosphate levels decline, pH drops and lactate levels rise. With further declines in CBF below 10 mL $100g^{-1}$ min^{-1}, potassium floods out of the cell into the extracellular space. If restoration of blood flow occurs quickly enough, these changes are reversible. If CBF remains below 20–25 mL $100g^{-1}$ min^{-1}, cells may die. The ability of brain cells to survive CBF below 20–25 mL $100g^{-1}$ min^{-1} depends on both the magnitude and duration of the CBF reduction. CBF of 5–10 mL $100g^{-1}$ min^{-1} may be tolerated for a period of less than 1 hour whereas CBF of 10–15 may not produce cell death for 2–3 hours. In addition, the rapidity at which cell death occurs depends not only on the magnitude and duration of the CBF reduction, but also on individual properties of the neurons. Some neurons may tolerate the same reduction in CBF for a period of time that is lethal to other cells. White matter is more tolerant than gray matter.[154–160] In a baboon model of transient MCA occlusion, evidence of reversibility manifested by immediate improvement of hemiparesis was observed in 14/14 with occlusion of less than 1 hour, 8/11 with occlusion of 2–4 hours, 1/3 with occlusion of 8 hours and 1/6 with occlusion of 16–24 hours.[159,161–163]

The evolution of changes in flow and metabolism after acute ischemic stroke has been established from experimental studies of cerebral arterial occlusion in large mammals and by studying patients at different time points after symptom onset (Fig. 3-9). Experimental data from large mammals show an initial reduction in CBF that is most severe in the central perfusion territory of the artery and becomes increasingly less so in more peripheral areas where collateral circulation from other arteries provides additional flow.[164] Accompanying this initial prominent reduction in CBF within 1 hour post-occlusion, there is an increase in OEF. $CMRO_2$ is reduced somewhat initially, but falls further over the subsequent 2–3 hours even though CBF falls only slightly.[165–169] The initially markedly increased OEF progressively decreases. By 24 hours,

CBF in the center of the ischemic region reaches its nadir at less than 20% of baseline values and $CMRO_2$ reaches 25% of baseline values. Also at this time point, increased OEF is seen to develop outside the area of primary perfusion disturbance in the tissue adjacent to the infarct core.[169] The volume of severely hypometabolic tissue remains stable between 1 and 7 hours post-occlusion, but increases by 24 hours and increases even further an average of 17 days after occlusion.[170] The fate of high OEF regions in the core and surrounding regions is variable; some portions may go on to infarct and other portions may survive.[165] An area of selective neuronal necrosis occurs outside the infarction itself.[171]

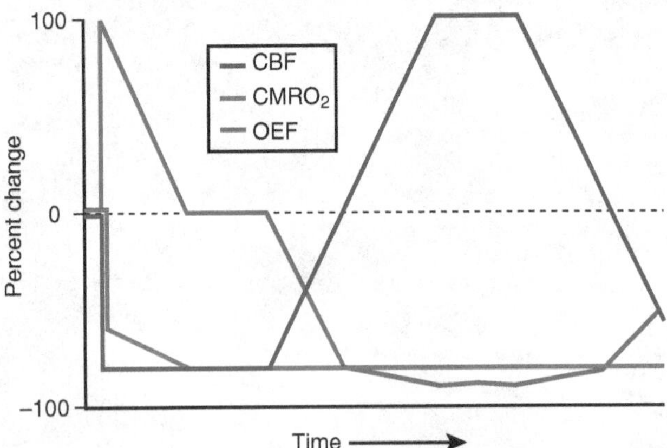

Figure 3-9. Pathophysiological changes in cerebral infarction. At the onset of ischemia, the initial fall in regional cerebral blood flow (CBF) is mirrored by a rise in regional oxygen extraction fraction (OEF). Since the increase in OEF is no longer able to maintain the energy needs of the brain, regional cerebral oxygen metabolism ($CMRO_2$) falls to the level of oxygen delivery. With time, $CMRO_2$ falls further even though there is no further decrease in CBF, resulting in a decrease in OEF. Reperfusion via recanalization of the occluded artery or recruitment of collateral pathways results in an increase in CBF ("luxury perfusion") and a concomitant fall in OEF below baseline with no change in $CMRO_2$. With evolution to the stage of chronic infarction, CBF progressively declines and OEF increases, but often remains below baseline values.

Human data obtained at 2–24 hours after ictus show an area of reduced CBF, reduced $CMRO_2$, and high OEF[172,173] (Fig. 3-10). During the first hours after stroke onset, tissue perfusion is highly dynamic with both reperfusion and new hypoperfusion occurring.[174] In the rim of tissue surrounding the infarct core, areas demonstrating reduced CBF and increased OEF with variable $CMRO_2$ can often be identified within hours after ictus and may persist for up to 16 hours. As with the animal data, the fate of high OEF regions in the core and surrounding regions is variable; some will infarct and some will not.[175,176] Spontaneous reperfusion may take place within a few hours of infarction,[177] but peaks at day 14.[178] This rise in CBF occurs without a concomitant rise in $CMRO_2$; rather, $CMRO_2$ generally falls further. Consequently, a decrease in regional OEF below normal mirrors the rise in CBF. This state, termed "luxury perfusion"[179] indicates that the normal coupling of CBF to oxygen metabolism in the resting brain is deranged. Luxury perfusion may be absolute (Fig. 3-11A) with CBF values greater than normal or luxury perfusion may be relative (Fig. 3-11B) with low or normal CBF that is still in excess of that required to produce a normal OEF for the reduced $CMRO_2$.[180] Luxury perfusion is evident by 48 hours in one-third of patients[181,182] and peaks at 1–2 weeks, paralleling the time course of spontaneous reperfusion.[180] Following this subacute period, CBF progressively declines and OEF normalizes such that the chronic stable infarct demonstrates flow and metabolism that are close to zero with OEF at or below baseline values[183] (Fig. 3-12).

Studies with PET and ^{18}FDG in subacute infarcts have shown that glucose metabolism is not reduced as much as oxygen metabolism.[41,45,173,181] This finding of relatively increased glycolysis in the presence of adequate oxygen delivery has been attributed to glycolytic activity in neutrophils and macrophages.[45]

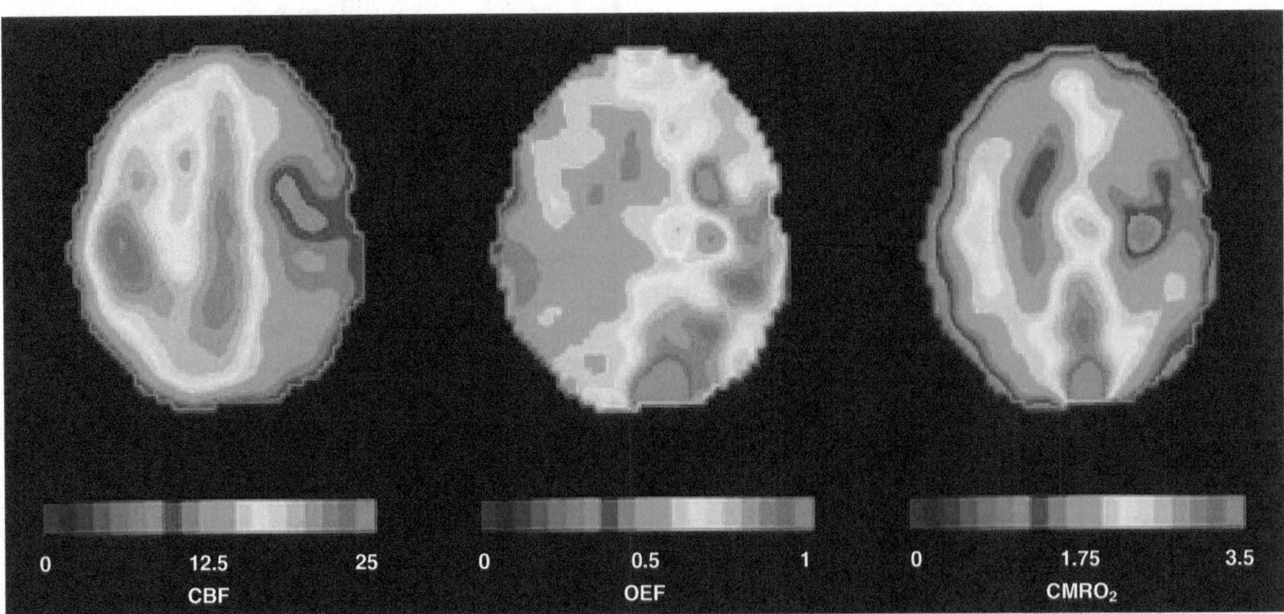

Figure 3-10. Positron emission tomography study in a 54-year-old woman who developed left hemiparesis due to vasospasm 9 days after subarachnoid hemorrhage. In all images, the left side of the brain is on the reader's left. Right hemispheric cerebral blood flow and oxygen metabolism are reduced and oxygen extraction is increased, indicative of ischemia.

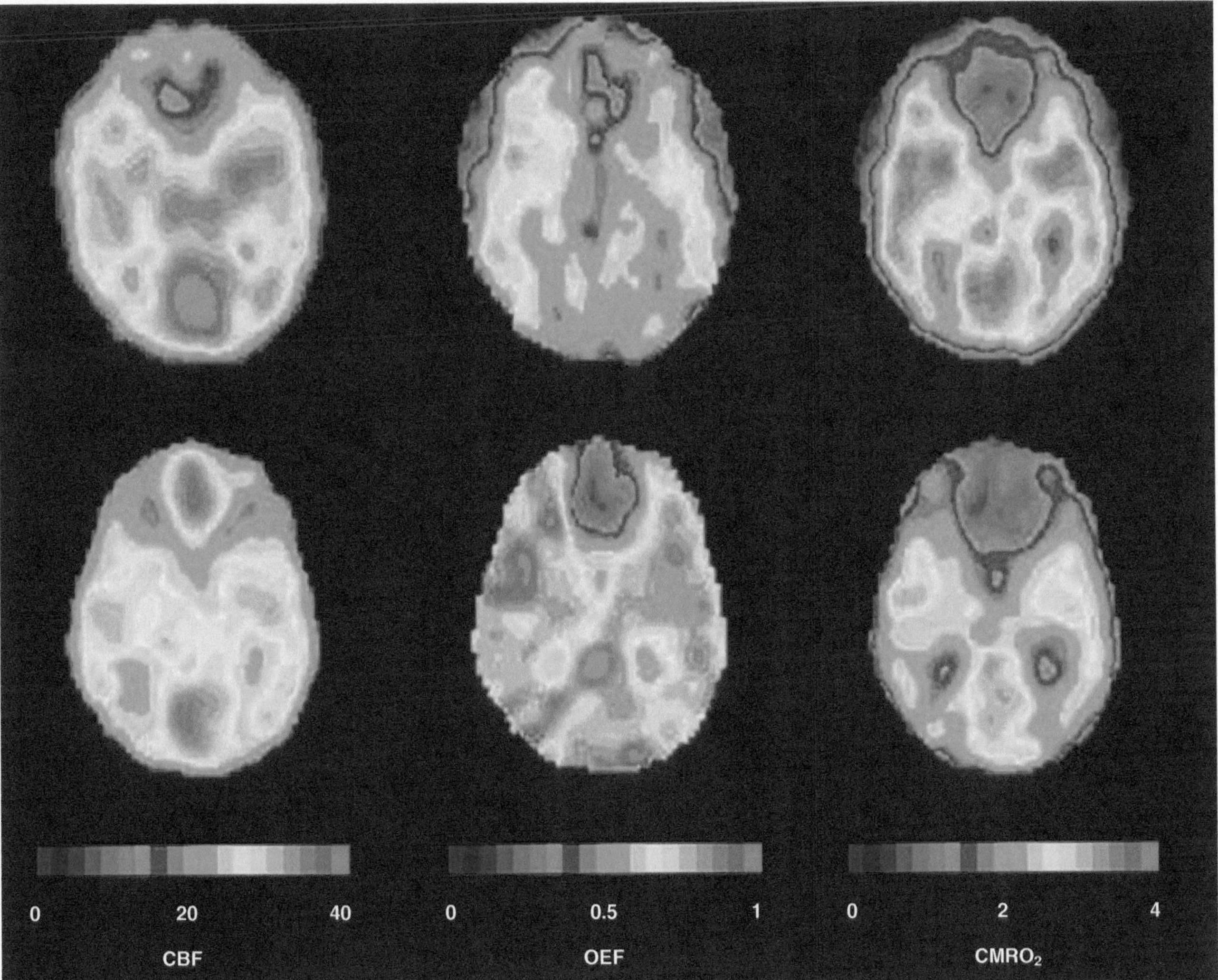

Figure 3-11. Sequential positron emission tomographic studies in a 22-year-old woman with bifrontal infarcts associated with subarachnoid-hemorrhage-induced vasospasm demonstrating luxury perfusion. The first study, performed on day 6 after hemorrhage, reveals *relative* luxury perfusion, with cerebral blood flow (CBF) that is reduced, but that is still in excess of oxygen requirements ($CMRO_2$) such that oxygen extraction fraction (OEF) is reduced (top row). The second study, performed on day 20, shows increased CBF with reduced $CMRO_2$ and OEF, consistent with *absolute* luxury perfusion (bottom row).

Flow-Metabolism Thresholds of Tissue Function and Viability in Acute Ischemic Stroke

In the early hours after cerebral arterial occlusion, the area of the brain with reduced blood flow consists of a mixture of cells that are already irreversibly damaged and destined for death along with some that exhibit abnormal biochemical changes and will go on to die later, but may recover if the biochemical processes leading to cell death are interrupted by pharmacologic treatment or re-establishment of CBF. Irreversibly damaged cells are more common in the central areas with the greatest reduction of blood flow whereas potentially salvageable cells are more common in the periphery. The latter cells have been termed the ischemic penumbra.[184] Identification of the ischemic penumbra by measurements of CBF alone is difficult because of the importance of both magnitude and duration in determining cell death, the different sensitivity of white matter and gray matter, the different sensitivity of different neurons within gray matter and the occurrence of luxury perfusion in dead tissue.[44,176,185] CBF > 20 mL $100g^{-1}$ min^{-1} may indicate the tissue is not at risk, but it may already be dead and undergoing luxury perfusion. CBF 10–20 mL $100g^{-1}$ min^{-1} may indicate tissue that is at risk though salvageable by immediate reperfusion if gray matter, but may be already dead or may not be at risk if white matter. CBF < 10 mL $100g^{-1}$ min^{-} may indicate tissue is at risk but salvageable or already dead. Thus, while CBF measurements are moderately successful at identifying tissue that is in trouble, they cannot reliably differentiate tissue at risk but salvageable from dead tissue. In contrast, measurements of $CMRO_2$ have been shown to be quite reliable for identifying dead tissue within studies, but with some variation across studies. $CMRO_2$ thresholds for irreversible infarction in humans have been reported from 0.87 to 1.7 mL $100g^{-1}$ min^{-1} in different studies.[44,172,186,187] The different threshold values are due to different study methodologies with those at the lower end of the ranges derived from single voxel measurements of both gray and white matter and those at the higher end derived from larger regions primarily in gray matter. The combination of CBF <60% of normal and $CMRO_2$ >40% of normal accurately identifies areas of the brain that will go on to infarct if untreated and live if treated, in these studies treatment being successful

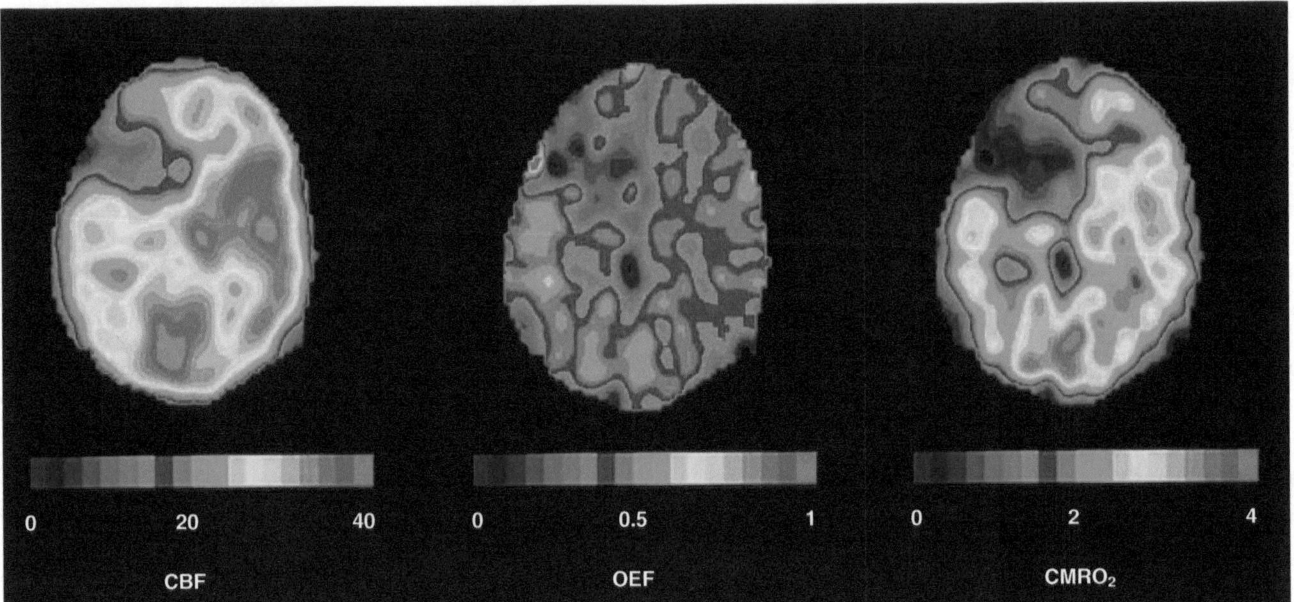

Figure 3-12. Positron emission tomography 5 months after left frontal infarct. In all images, the left side of the brain is on the reader's left. Cerebral blood flow (CBF) and oxygen metabolism ($CMRO_2$) are severely reduced and oxygen extraction (OEF) is below normal in the affected area.

reperfusion.[44,165,170,185,187–189] These data represent a mix from humans and non-human primates with minimal human reperfusion data. Further human reperfusion studies are needed to demonstrate reliability of these criteria for identifying preventable infarction in clinically heterogeneous patient populations. Because tissue regions demonstrating increased OEF represent areas with reduced blood supply relative to oxygen demand but still with metabolically active cells, OEF has received much attention as the factor capable of predicting tissue viability, but it has been shown to be a poor predictor of tissue outcome.[165,176,185,189]

In newborns having subsequent normal neurodevelopmental outcome, values of CBF and $CMRO_2$ that would indicate lethal damage to the adult brain have been observed. CBF as low as 5 mL $100g^{-1}$ min^{-1} and $CMRO_2$ <1.3 mL $100g^{-1}$ min^{-1} (and sometimes virtually absent) have been observed in newborns without evidence of brain injury.[9,15,16,190]

Vasoreactivity and Autoregulation in Ischemic Stroke

Pioneering studies performed in experimental animals and humans laid the basis for the current widespread teaching that autoregulation is impaired in acute ischemic stroke. However, more recent data from humans have forced reconsideration. In baboons immediately after middle cerebral artery occlusion, autoregulation was absent where flow was less than 20%, but partially preserved where flow was greater than 40% of basal flow.[164] Similar results were obtained in spontaneously hypertensive rats with acute experimental focal brain ischemia produced by ipsilateral/middle cerebral artery occlusion. Autoregulation was lost in areas with flow below 30% of pre-occlusion values and partly preserved in ischemic brain tissue with CBF greater than 30%.[96] When baboons were studied 3 years after occlusion of the MCA, autoregulation to decreased MAP was lost in the infarct and impaired in the peri-infarct area, the impairment being progressively less severe further away from the infarct.[191] All of these studies were conducted by altering systemic MAP during persisting arterial occlusion raising the possibility that there is no effect of ischemia on the intrinsic vascular mechanism that regulates autoregulation, but that the changes in CBF were simply a reflection that the CPP downstream from the occlusion was below the lower autoregulatory limit (Fig. 3-13A). Against this interpretation is the demonstration of impaired autoregulation to induced hypertension immediately after transient forebrain ischemia in gerbils suggesting true autoregulatory impairment, at least temporarily (Fig. 3-13D).[192] In monkeys with acute middle cerebral artery occlusion, increased cardiac output induced by intravascular volume expansion in the absence of increased blood pressure increases CBF in ischemic areas of the brain whereas it has no effect on CBF in normal areas of brain.[193]

Early studies in humans, prior to the advent of cerebral imaging modalities such as CT, PET and MRI, used the technique of radioisotope injection into the carotid artery with radioactivity detection by scintillation crystals on the scalp to measure CBF. During the initial days following ischemic stroke, the normal vasodilatory response to increased pCO_2 often disappeared. Other abnormalities such as intracerebral steal (decreased CBF in ischemic areas produced by vasodilation elsewhere), inverse steal (increased CBF in ischemic area due to vasoconstriction elsewhere), and false autoregulation (decreased CBF in ischemic area produced by increased CPP) also occurred. These abnormalities in cerebrovascular control could persist for several weeks and even longer.[194–198] These studies used mostly rapid increases in MAP to study autoregulation and demonstrated focal abnormalities in the affected hemisphere. One study investigated the effect of rapid MAP reductions of 12–67 mm Hg in six subjects without arterial occlusion studied from 1 day to 11 years later and reported non-focal hemispheric deceases in CBF of 9–24% in all.[195] It is not possible to determine whether these changes were in infarcted tissue, the peri-infarct region or non-ischemic tissue This is important clinically because further reductions in CBF in already infarcted tissue have no clinical consequences whereas even slight reductions in CBF in the peri-infarct region could result in the transition from CBF levels barely able to sustain tissue viability to lethal levels (Fig. 3-13).

More recent data from humans with acute ischemic stroke, using tomographic imaging techniques for CBF measurement that have better spatial resolution, have produced different

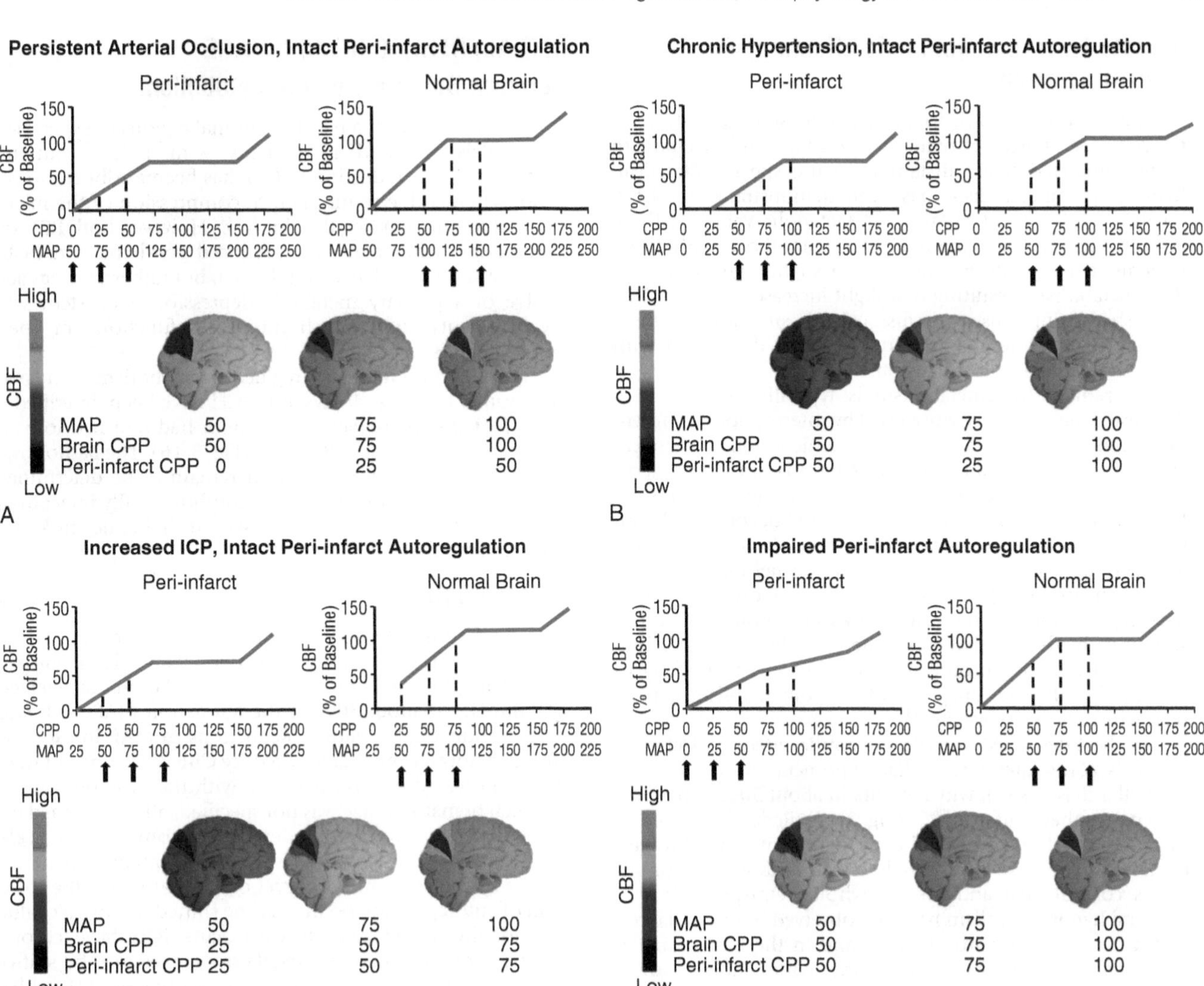

Figure 3-13. Diagrammatic representation of the effect of mean arterial pressures (MAP) of 50, 75 and 100 mm Hg on cerebral blood flow (CBF) in the ischemic penumbra in four different conditions. A, Persistent arterial occlusion with normal autoregulation in the penumbra such that the CPP in the penumbra is 50 mm Hg lower than MAP and CPP in the rest of the brain. B, Chronic hypertension with intact autoregulatory curve shifted upwards in the penumbra without persistent arterial occlusion such that CPP in the penumbra is equal to MAP and CPP in the rest of the brain and MAP equal to CPP. C, Increased intracranial pressure (ICP) of 25 mm Hg with normal autoregulation in the penumbra such that the CPP in the penumbra and rest of brain is 25 mm Hg lower than MAP. D, Impaired autoregulation in the penumbra without persistent arterial occlusion such that CPP in the penumbra is equal to MAP and CPP in the rest of the brain.

results from the earlier studies. In the three studies that replicate best the design of the animal and earlier human studies by using intravenous agents to produce rapid reduction then stabilization of blood pressure, there was no selective impairment of autoregulation in the peri-infarct region to reduced MAP produced by calcium channel blockers in patients studied within 6 hours or 1–11 days after onset.[199–201] In one of these studies, two chronically hypertensive individuals had global reductions of CBF in both hemispheres with MAP reductions consistent with a shift upwards in the whole-brain autoregulatory curve due to chronic hypertension. Two additional studies using oral administration of the angiotensin-converting enzyme inhibitor perindopril or the angiotensin receptor blocker losartan to produce MAP reduction over 6–8 hours also failed to demonstrate impaired autoregulation in patients 2–8 days from onset.[202,203]

Studies of dynamic autoregulation in human ischemic stroke have in general shown that vascular regulation is impaired even after minor strokes and often bilaterally. Studies comparing static and dynamic autoregulation in the same patients found only dynamic impairment. The clinical relevance of these findings is unclear.[117]

At this time it is not possible to reconcile the disparate data regarding autoregulation of CBF to reduction in MAP following acute ischemic stroke. The clinical studies with adequate spatial resolution have not shown selective decreases in CBF with reductions in MAP in the penumbra area, but this does not mean that lowering of systemic MAP cannot produce reductions in CBF. These studies did not address patients with large edematous infarcts causing local increases in ICP or those with persistent large artery occlusion, both of which can lead to apparent ("false") autoregulatory impairment because local CPP is reduced below the lower autoregulatory limit when systemic MAP is still normal (Figs 3-13A and 3-13C). In these circumstances and in patients with chronic hypertension whose lower autoregulatory limit is shifted up, reduction of MAP even within the normal autoregulatory range could lead to reduced CBF (Fig. 3-13B).

Remote Flow and Metabolic Effects of Ischemic Stroke

A common finding in regional metabolic studies of stroke is the presence of areas of reduced blood flow and metabolism in non-infarcted tissue distant from the site of infarction. Remote hypometabolism has been demonstrated for both $CMRO_2$[180,204–206] and CMRglc.[207,208] Metabolic values at these distant sites always remain greater than those within the ischemic core.[207] CBF is reduced to a slightly greater degree than metabolism, resulting in a slight increase in OEF.[209] Distinguished from "misery perfusion," this situation has been interpreted to represent primary metabolic depression with secondary reduction in perfusion.

The remote hypometabolism is typically ascribed to a decrease in neuronal activity caused by interruption of afferent or efferent fiber pathways by the ischemic lesion, a phenomenon often termed *diaschisis*.[204] This term is not strictly accurate though, because diaschisis refers to an acute and reversible functional depression at sites distant from but connected with the site of injury,[210] whereas these remote effects of ischemia are often stable for months[205,211] and may be permanent. Transsynaptic neuronal degeneration has been proposed as an alternate explanation for the remote hypometabolism[206] and is supported by the fact that contralateral $CMRO_2$ often declines between acute and chronic studies,[212] but this is unlikely to account for all cases since remote hypometabolism can be seen within hours of stroke.[213]

The best-described remote metabolic effect of ischemic stroke is contralateral cerebellar hypometabolism ("crossed cerebellar diaschisis"), which occurs in about 50% of patients with hemispheric infarcts[206,213] (Fig. 3-14). Reduction in blood flow and metabolism in the hemisphere contralateral to cerebral infarction have also been described for both the homologous cortical area and for the whole hemisphere.[180,214,215] Cerebral hypometabolism has been observed in the ipsilateral cortex overlying subcortical stroke and in the basal ganglia, thalamus, and distant sites in the cortex after cortical stroke.[207,214,216–219]

The clinical correlate of these remote changes is unclear. Single case reports have suggested an association with focal neurological deficits, including ataxia,[220,221] aphasia,[222–224] neglect,[225] and hemianopia,[214] but larger series of infarcts at various locations have revealed no such relationships.[206,226]

INTRACEREBRAL HEMORRHAGE

Cerebral Blood Flow and Metabolism

CBF is often reduced in peri-hematomal regions in experimental models[227,228] and in patients with ICH,[229] but not always.[230,231] This reduction in CBF has been attributed to cerebral ischemia due to mechanical compression of the microvasculature surrounding the clot.[227,232] However, both PET and MRI studies, while confirming reduced peri-hematomal CBF, have not shown evidence of ischemia, but rather findings suggestive of a primary metabolic depression, consistent with measurements of mitochondrial dysfunction in peri-hematomal tissue[233–235] (Fig. 3-15).

Transient focal increases in glucose metabolism in the peri-hematomal region 2–4 days after ICH have been described in some patients. These were resolving or had returned to baseline on repeat scans at 5–8 days[236] (Fig. 3-16). The pathophysiological basis and clinical import remain to be determined. Remote depression of CMRglc in morphologically intact brain structures in ICH similar to that seen in ischemic stroke has been described as well.[237,238,238]

Autoregulation

Studies of both static and dynamic autoregulation in patients with recent ICH demonstrate that regional and global autoregulation are preserved down to a lower MAP limit that averages 110 mm Hg or about 80% of the admission MAP, with substantial individual variation. Reductions of MAP in excess of 20% or below 84 mm Hg may reduce CBF.[239–241] None of these studies provided data on ICP and, with the exception of one in which hematoma size was not specified, all were carried out on patients with small-to-moderate hematomas. If ICP is elevated due to large hematomas or hydrocephalus, then CPP will be below MAP and the level of MAP at which the lower limit of autoregulation occurs may be shifted to a higher value. Additionally, many patients with acute ICH have chronic hypertension and their autoregulatory curves may be shifted upwards. In both these situations, reductions of MAP within the normal autoregulatory limit could reduce CBF.

ARTERIOVENOUS MALFORMATIONS

Cerebral arteriovenous malformations (AVMs) are high-flow vascular structures lacking capillaries between arteries and

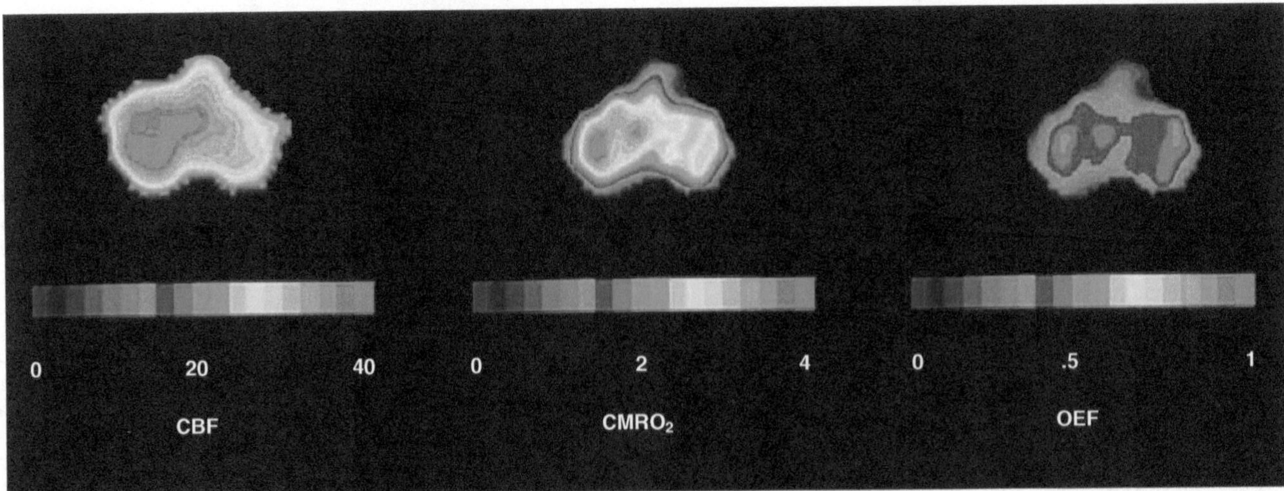

Figure 3-14. Positron emission tomography of the cerebellum 5 months after left frontal infarct demonstrates crossed cerebellar hypometabolism with secondary hypoperfusion. In all images, the left side of the brain is on the reader's left.

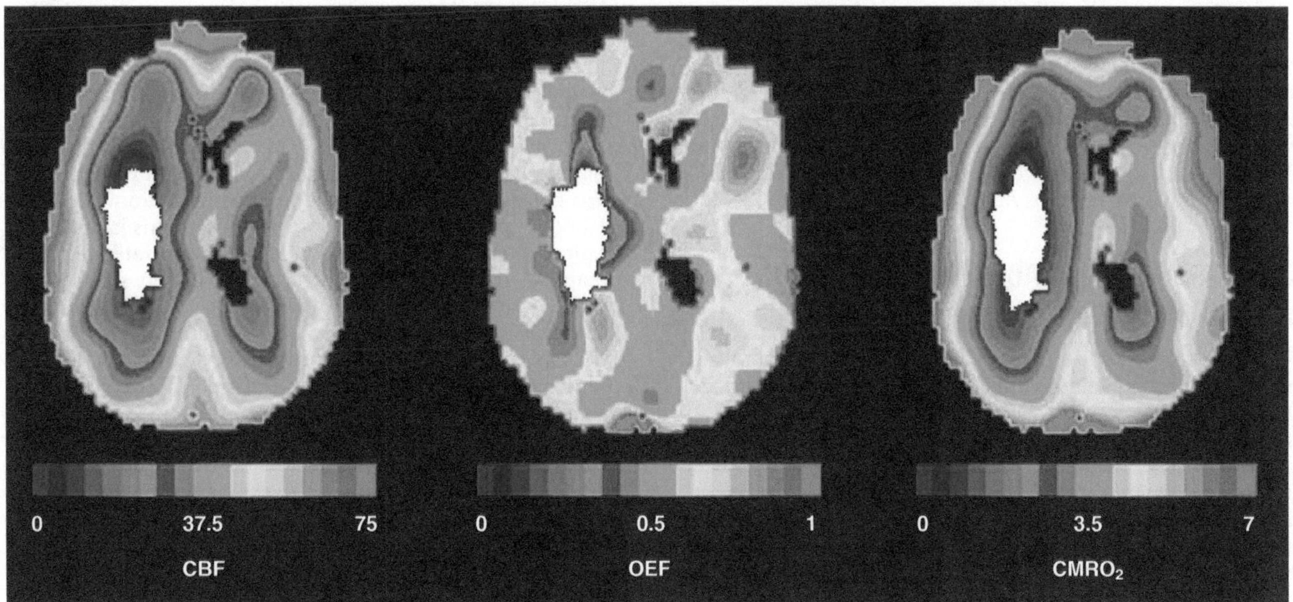

Figure 3-15. Partial volume-corrected positron emission tomographic images of a 44-year-old hypertensive man with a left putaminal hemorrhage studied 21 hours after onset. In all images, the left side of the brain is on the reader's left and the hemorrhage is depicted in white. Perihematomal blood flow, metabolism, and oxygen extraction are all reduced compared to the contralateral hemisphere, suggestive of primary metabolic depression

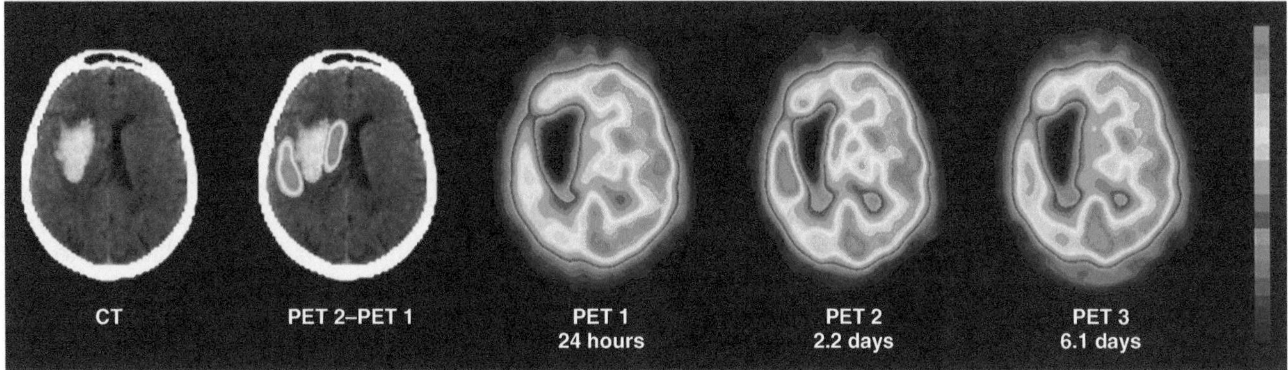

Figure 3-16. Co-registered CT and ^{18}F-fluorodeoxyglucose (FDG) PET images normalized to mean activity in PET 1 from a 77-year-old woman with left putaminal hemorrhage studied 24 hours, 2.2 days, and 6.2 days after onset. In all images, the left side of the brain is on the reader's left. PET 2-PET 1 represents the subtraction image of these two PET studies superimposed on the CT and demonstrates the region of increased glucose metabolism. The color scale is relative, with blue representing the lowest values and red the highest.

veins. Many,[155,242-244] but not all,[245] physiological studies have demonstrated regions of decreased blood flow in the tissue adjacent to the AVM or even far removed in the ipsilateral or contralateral hemisphere. An intracerebral "steal" syndrome, in which blood flow is shunted through the low-resistance AVM and away from other areas of the brain has been postulated to cause both local and distant ischemia.[246] This concept is controversial.[247,248] Support for the "steal" hypothesis has been provided by PET studies that show increased OEF and CBF consistent with ischemia in the peri-lesional area. The increases in OEF in the peri-lesional region were more common in patients with high-flow AVMs, large AVMs and progressive neurological deficits.[249] Similarly, it has been postulated that the occasionally encountered post-treatment complications of edema and hemorrhage are due to a sudden redistribution of previously shunted blood after AVM removal. This *normal perfusion pressure breakthrough* assumes that (1) CPP is reduced below the lower limit of autoregulation by arterial hypotension and venous hypertension in neighboring vascular territories, (2) blood vessels in these territories are maximally dilated such that any decrease in CPP results in ischemia, (3) chronic hypoperfusion results in vasomotor paralysis and impaired autoregulatory capacity, and (4) reversal of reduced CPP after treatment is not matched by a corresponding increase in CVR, leading to hyperemia and sometimes swelling and hemorrhage.[250-254]

Data counter to this theory have emerged, with studies suggesting that autoregulation is intact in tissue adjacent to the AVM both before and after surgery[247,255,256] and that AVM removal may be associated with a decrease in regional CBF.[257] In addition, since the majority of patients with AVMs have feeding artery pressures below the standard lower limit of autoregulation,[258] it would be expected that normalization of these pressures after AVM obliteration would result in a large number of "breakthrough" complications. Such complications are uncommon, however.[259-261] Finally, while there are some reports of impaired vascular reactivity in tissue adjacent to and distant from the AVM,[248,262,263] others indicate that regional vasoreactivity may be preserved.[243,258] In fact, patients who develop hyperemic complications have been shown to exhibit enhanced vasoreactivity to the vasodilatory agent acetazolamide.[243,261,263] As a result, others have postulated that there is an adaptive compensatory shift to the left of the autoregulatory curve in the areas of low CPP surrounding the AVM such that CBF and autoregulation are maintained. Postoperatively, this curve shifts back to the right.[247]

ANEURYSMAL SUBARACHNOID HEMORRHAGE

Cerebral Blood Flow and Metabolism

Interpreting the alterations in CBF and metabolism that follow aneurysmal subarachnoid hemorrhage (SAH) is difficult because of the many different factors that can interact to produce these changes. Chief among these is the occurrence of large artery vasospasm causing ischemia. Vasospasm, defined as segmental or diffuse narrowing of the large arteries at the base of the brain, can be detected angiographically in up to 70% of patients beginning at 4–12 days after aneurysm rupture.[264–266] The time course of angiographic vasospasm is paralleled by a progressive fall in CBF over the first 2 weeks and abnormally low CBF for at least 3 weeks after SAH.[267] Much of the CBF and metabolism data obtained in patients following aneurysmal SAH supports the straightforward pathophysiological sequence of large artery vasospasm causing ischemia which, if severe enough, will cause either reversible ischemic neurological deficits or permanent infarction. Reduced angiographic vessel caliber correlates well with reduced CBF when the CBF study and angiogram are done serially, preferably within 1 hour.[268–273] Not all patients with vasospasm have neurological deficits, but this is to be expected if the spasm does not reduce CBF below 20 mL $100g^{-1}$ min^{-1}.[273] Those regions with CBF falling below the critical level for long enough go on to infarct.[274] Patients with more severe neurological deficits (Hunt and Hess grades III and IV) have a more marked reduction in regional CBF than do patients with a more favorable clinical grade (Hunt and Hess grades I and II). Patients with mean CBF of 41–42 mL 100 g^{-1} min^{-1} achieve better outcomes than those with a mean CBF of 25–33 mL 100 g^{-1} min^{-1}.[275,276]

In contrast to acute ischemic stroke, in which the large artery flow reduction is caused by a single, sudden, well-timed event, large artery vasospasm occurs gradually over a period of days in different vessels at different times to variable degrees and resolves in the same gradual heterogeneous manner. As in the situation of the carotid artery discussed above, no effect of the spasm on downstream flow will occur until there is at least a 70% reduction in diameter and even after this the effect will be dependent on the degree of collateral circulation and the autoregulatory capacity of the distal smaller arteries. At any given time the effect of large artery vasospasm on CBF, CBV, $CMRO_2$, and OEF can correspond to any of the three stages in Figure 13-7 if the resultant reduction in CPP is not severe enough to produce infarction or to any of the time points in Figure 13-9 if CPP was severe enough at some previous time to produce infarction. Regions supplied by vessels not currently in spasm may have suffered ischemic damage when those vessels were previously in spasm with a subsequent permanent reduction in CBF and $CMRO_2$.[274] Thus, a poor correlation between low CBF levels and the presence of hypodense lesions on CT, or the occurrence of new focal deficits in patients evaluated from 1 to 13 days after aneurysm rupture, likely represents the occurrence of subacute infarcts with high flow due to luxury perfusion.[277]

Depression of CBF and $CMRO_2$ has been reported by several investigators with OEF variably described as normal or elevated.[270,274,278–282] While reduced CBF and $CMRO_2$ with elevated OEF is indicative of vasospasm-induced ischemia, reduced metabolism with normal OEF has been interpreted as evidence for non-ischemic primary metabolic depression with vasospasm not causing ischemia but occurring as compensatory vascular constriction in to reduced metabolic demand. Alternatively, reduced metabolism with normal OEF is also consistent with subacute cerebral infarction in which OEF had returned to normal. Consistent with this latter interpretation, some investigators who have demonstrated reduced CBF and $CMRO_2$ with no change in OEF report subsequent cerebral infarction or moderate-to-severe disability in the majority of patients.[280,281] To investigate whether large artery vasospasm is caused by primary metabolic depression without ischemia, Carpenter and colleagues studied a group of patients with vasospasm who did not develop subsequent infarction.[283] CBF was decreased, $CMRO_2$ was normal, and OEF was increased, indicative of ischemia.[283]

Several studies have suggested the presence of smaller vessel spasm as a contributing cause of cerebral ischemia following aneurysmal SAH. Dhar et al. demonstrated regions of reduced CBF below 25 mL $100g^{-1}$ min^{-1} outside the vascular territories of large arteries in spasm.[284] In these territories $CMRO_2$ is depressed and OEF is elevated to the same degree as in low CBF regions within the territory of large arteries in spasm (Michael Diringer, personal communication). These findings suggest that there is primary constriction of smaller arteries as a cause of ischemia. In another PET study, regional CBV was reduced, not elevated, in regions with increased OEF supplied by vessels with angiographic spasm in contrast to a group of patients with carotid occlusion who showed increased CBV in regions with increased OEF. These findings of reduced parenchymal CBV during vasospasm under similar conditions of tissue ischemia that produce increased CBV in patients with carotid occlusion were interpreted as evidence that parenchymal vessels distal to arteries with angiographic spasm following SAH do not demonstrate normal autoregulatory vasodilation.[285]

In addition to the effects of vasospasm-induced ischemia, SAH itself has effects on cerebral metabolism. In a series of patients studied 1 to 4 days after aneurysmal SAH, who had not undergone surgery and who did not have vasospasm, hydrocephalus, or ICH, there was a significant reduction in bihemispheric $CMRO_2$ and CBF with normal OEF.[283] This was interpreted by the authors as indicating that the initial aneurysm rupture produced a primary reduction in metabolism at this stage and the reduction in CBF occurred secondary to reduced metabolic demands. Microdialysis studies have shown both evidence of ischemia and evidence of impaired oxidative metabolism consistent with mitochondrial dysfunction.[286–290]

Additional complicating factors that will also affect CBF and metabolism include increased intracranial pressure, intracerebral hematomas (both discussed above), and injury due to brain retraction. A small PET study before and after right fronto-temporal craniotomies for clipping of ruptured anterior circulation aneurysms showed a 45% reduction in regional $CMRO_2$ and 32% reduction in regional OEF without significant change in CBF in the region of retraction.[291] These changes indicate a primary reduction in metabolism and uncoupling of flow and metabolism (relative luxury perfusion).

Autoregulation

In the absence of ICH, hydrocephalus, infarction, or vasospasm, static cerebral autoregulation of CBF to changes in CPP is probably preserved within the first few days following SAH.[275,292–294] Static autoregulation is defective in the majority of patients with angiographic vasospasm of large arteries following aneurysmal SAH to both decreases[275,292,293,295] and increases[296,297] in MAP, even in those patients with only slight vasospasm (reduction of arterial caliber of 25–50%).[293]

Studies of dynamic autoregulation have described abnormalities in the early period after SAH prior to vasospasm, although they confirm that autoregulation is likely preserved for the first 2–3 days post-ictus except in those with severe initial brain injury. These early abnormalities in dynamic autoregulation are predictive of subsequent neurological deficits.[298]

CONCLUSIONS

The valuable insights into the pathophysiology of cerebrovascular disease provided by measurements of CBF and metabolism provide the basis for current treatments and have been instrumental for the design of clinical trials. Understanding the CBF response to changes in pCO_2 is essential for correctly managing increased intracranial pressure. Knowledge of the interplay between the different effects of ischemia, hypoxemia, hypocarbia, and hypotension on cerebral blood flow is important when dealing with complex clinical situations. Understanding the hemodynamic effects of arterial stenosis or occlusion on the downstream perfusion pressure has been instrumental in designing new trials for treatment.[299] In acute ischemic stroke, CBF and metabolism thresholds for tissue viability have been critical in forming the concept of the "ischemic penumbra" and guiding the design of trials of early intervention.[300] Blood flow and metabolic studies in ICH have documented the integrity of autoregulation and suggested that hematomas exert a primary depression of metabolism rather than inducing ischemia in the surrounding tissue. This fundamental observation has paved the way for clinical trials of acute blood pressure reduction in ICH to try to limit hematoma expansion.[301,301] In aneurysmal SAH, impaired autoregulation during the period of vasospasm is the basis for current therapies to augment CBF.[302] Studies of metabolism that have demonstrated derangements that cannot be attributed to vasospasm-induced ischemia have opened the way for new therapeutic trials.[303] In summary, defining the pathophysiological changes in CBF and metabolism in human cerebrovascular disease has provided and will continue to provide the basic foundation for development and testing of new treatment strategies.

Acknowledgments

This work was supported by the H. Houston Merritt Professorship of Neurology at the University of North Carolina Chapel Hill.

The complete reference list can be found on the companion Expert Consult website at www.expertconsult.inkling.com.

KEY REFERENCES

3. Zierler KL. Equations for measuring blood flow by external monitoring of radioisotopes. Circ Res 1965;16:309–21.
4. Ostergaard L. Principles of cerebral perfusion imaging by bolus tracking. J Magn Reson Imaging 2005;22:710–17.
7. Gottstein U, Bernsmeier A, Sedlmeyer I. Der Kohlenhydratstoffweehsel des menschlichen Gehirns bei Schlafmittelvergiftung. Klin Wschr 1963;41:943–8.
8. Scheinberg P, Stead EA. The cerebral blood flow in male subjects as measured by the nitrous oxide technique: normal values for blood flow, oxygen utilization, glucose utilization and peripheral resistance, with observations on the effect of tilting and anxiety. J Clin Invest 1949;28:1163–71.
9. Altman DI, Perlman JM, Volpe JJ, et al. Cerebral oxygen metabolism in newborns. Pediatrics 1993;92:99–104.
15. Altman DI, Powers WJ, Perlman JM, et al. Cerebral blood flow requirement for brain viability in newborn infants is lower than in adults. Ann Neurol 1988;24:218–26.
17. Powers WJ, Rosenbaum JL, Dence CS, et al. Cerebral glucose transport and metabolism in preterm human infants. J Cereb Blood Flow Metab 1998;18:632–8.
24. Chugani HT, Phelps ME, Mazziotta JC. Positron emission tomography study of human brain functional development. Ann Neurol 1987;22:487–97.
25. Kennedy C, Sokoloff L. An adaptation of the nitrous oxide method to the study of the cerebral circulation in children: normal values for cerebral blood flow and cerebral metabolic rate in childhood. J Clin Invest 1957;36:1130–7.
31. Marchal G, Rioux P, Petit-Taboue MC, et al. Regional cerebral oxygen consumption, blood flow, and blood volume in healthy human aging. Arch Neurol 1992;49:1013–20.
37. Meltzer CC, Cantwell MN, Greer PJ, et al. Does cerebral blood flow decline in healthy aging? A PET study with partial-volume correction. J Nucl Med 2000;41:1842–8.
38. Ibanez V, Pietrini P, Furey ML, et al. Resting state brain glucose metabolism is not reduced in normotensive healthy men during aging, after correction for brain atrophy. Brain Res Bull 2004;63:147–54.
39. McHenry LC Jr, Merory J, Bass E, et al. Xenon-133 inhalation method for regional cerebral blood flow measurements: normal values and test–retest results. Stroke 1978;9:396–9.
40. Lebrun-Grandie P, Baron JC, Soussaline F, et al. Coupling between regional blood flow and oxygen utilization in the normal human brain. A study with positron tomography and oxygen 15. Arch Neurol 1983;40:230–6.
41. Baron JC, Rougemont D, Soussaline F, et al. Local interrelationships of cerebral oxygen consumption and glucose utilization in normal subjects and in ischemic stroke patients: a positron tomography study. J Cereb Blood Flow Metab 1984;4:140–9.
44. Powers WJ, Grubb RL Jr, Darriet D, et al. Cerebral blood flow and cerebral metabolic rate of oxygen requirements for cerebral function and viability in humans. J Cereb Blood Flow Metab 1985;5:600–8.
45. Wise RJ, Rhodes CG, Gibbs JM, et al. Disturbance of oxidative metabolism of glucose in recent human cerebral infarcts. Ann Neurol 1983;14:627–37.
46. Powers WJ, Videen TO, Markham J, et al. Metabolic control of resting hemispheric cerebral blood flow is oxidative, not glycolytic. J Cereb Blood Flow Metab 2011;31:1223–8.
48. Bering EAJ, Taren JA, McMurrey JD, et al. Studies on hypothermia in monkeys. II. The effect of hypothermia on the general physiology and cerebral metabolism of monkeys in the hypothermic state. Surg Gynecol Obstet 1956;102:134–8.
49. Nilsson L, Siesjo BK. The effect of phenobarbitone anaesthesia on blood flow and oxygen consumption in the rat brain. Acta Anaesthesiol Scand Suppl 1975;57:18–24.
50. Diringer MN, Videen TO, Yundt K, et al. Regional cerebrovascular and metabolic effects of hyperventilation after severe traumatic brain injury. J Neurosurg 2002;96:103–8.
51. Frackowiak RS, Pozzilli C, Legg NJ, et al. Regional cerebral oxygen supply and utilization in dementia. A clinical and physiological study with oxygen-15 and positron tomography. Brain 1981;104:753–78.
52. Powers WJ. Cerebral hemodynamics in ischemic cerebrovascular disease. Ann Neurol 1991;29:231–40.
54. Vaishnavi SN, Vlassenko AG, Rundle MM, et al. Regional aerobic glycolysis in the human brain. Proc Natl Acad Sci U S A 2010;107:17757–62.
55. Pellerin L, Magistretti PJ. Sweet sixteen for ANLS. J Cereb Blood Flow Metab 2012;32:1152–66.
56. Sokoloff L. Relationships among local functional activity, energy metabolism, and blood flow in the central nervous system. Fed Proc 1981;40:2311–16.
57. Fox PT, Raichle ME. Focal physiological uncoupling of cerebral blood flow and oxidative metabolism during somatosensory stimulation in human subjects. Proc Natl Acad Sci U S A 1986;83:1140–4.
58. Fox PT, Raichle ME, Mintun MA, et al. Nonoxidative glucose consumption during focal physiologic neural activity. Science 1988;241:462–4.
59. Sappey-Marinier D, Calabrese G, Fein G, et al. Effect of photic stimulation on human visual cortex lactate and phosphates

using ^{1}H and ^{31}P magnetic resonance spectroscopy. J Cereb Blood Flow Metab 1992;12:584–92.
60. Ogawa S, Lee TM, Kay AR, et al. Brain magnetic resonance imaging with contrast dependent on blood oxygenation. Proc Natl Acad Sci 1990;87:9868–72.
61. Kwong K, Belliveau JW, Chesler DA, et al. Dynamic magnetic resonance imaging of human brain activity during primary sensory stimulation. Proc Natl Acad Sci U S A 1992;89:5675–9.
62. van den Heuvel MP, Mandl RC, Kahn RS, et al. Functionally linked resting-state networks reflect the underlying structural connectivity architecture of the human brain. Hum Brain Mapp 2009;30:3127–41.
64. Jensen LJ, Holstein-Rathlou NH. The vascular conducted response in cerebral blood flow regulation. J Cereb Blood Flow Metab 2013;33:649–56.
66. Shimojyo S, Scheinberg P, Kogure K, et al. The effects of graded hypoxia upon transient cerebral blood flow and oxygen consumption. Neurology 1968;18:127–33.
69. Brown MM, Wade JP, Marshall J. Fundamental importance of arterial oxygen content in the regulation of cerebral blood flow in man. Brain 1985;108:81–93.
72. Mintun MA, Lundstrom BN, Snyder AZ, et al. Blood flow and oxygen delivery to human brain during functional activity: theoretical modeling and experimental data. Proc Natl Acad Sci U S A 2001;98:6859–64.
73. Powers WJ, Boyle PJ, Hirsch IB, et al. Unaltered cerebral blood flow during hypoglycemic activation of the sympathochromaffin system in humans. Am J Physiol 1993;265:R883–7.
76. Boyle PJ, Kempers SF, O'Connor AM, et al. Brain glucose uptake and unawareness of hypoglycemia in patients with insulin-dependent diabetes mellitus. N Engl J Med 1995;333:1726–31.
77. Teves D, Videen TO, Cryer PE, et al. Activation of human medial prefrontal cortex during autonomic responses to hypoglycemia. Proc Natl Acad Sci U S A 2004;101:6217–21.
78. Tallroth G, Ryding E, Agardh CD. Regional cerebral blood flow in normal man during insulin-induced hypoglycemia and in the recovery period following glucose infusion. Metabolism 1992;41: 717–21.
85. Kety SS, Schmidt CF. The effects of active and passive hyperventilation on cerebral blood flow, cerebral oxygen consumption, cardiac output, and blood pressure of normal young men. J Clin Invest 1946;25:107–19.
86. Wollman H, Smith TC, Stephen GW, et al. Effects of extremes of respiratory and metabolic alkalosis on cerebral blood flow in man. J Appl Physiol 1968;24:60–5.
88. Raichle ME, Posner JB, Plum F. Cerebral blood flow during and after hyperventilation. Arch Neurol 1970;23:394–403.
89. Alexander SC, Smith TC, Strobel G, et al. Cerebral carbohydrate metabolism of man during respiratory and metabolic alkalosis. J Appl Physiol 1968;24:66–72.
91. Grubb RL Jr, Raichle ME, Eichling JO, et al. The effects of changes in $PaCO_2$ on cerebral blood volume, blood flow, and vascular mean transit time. Stroke 1974;5:630–9.
92. Brown MM, Marshall J. Regulation of cerebral blood flow in response to changes in blood viscosity. Lancet 1985;1:604–9.
94. Tomiyama Y, Brian JE Jr, Todd MM. Plasma viscosity and cerebral blood flow. Am J Physiol Heart Circ Physiol 2000;279: H1949–54.
95. Rebel A, Lenz C, Krieter H, et al. Oxygen delivery at high blood viscosity and decreased arterial oxygen content to brains of conscious rats. Am J Physiol Heart Circ Physiol 2001;280:H2591–7.
96. Dirnagl U, Pulsinelli W. Autoregulation of cerebral blood flow in experimental focal brain ischemia. J Cereb Blood Flow Metab 1990;10:327–36.
98. Strandgaard S. Autoregulation of cerebral blood flow in hypertensive patients. The modifying influence of prolonged antihypertensive treatment on the tolerance to acute, drug-induced hypotension. Circulation 1976;53:720–7.
100. Strandgaard S, Olesen J, Skinhoj E, et al. Autoregulation of brain circulation in severe arterial hypertension. Br Med J 1973; 1:507–10.
102. Symon L, Pasztor E, Dorsch NW, et al. Physiological responses of local areas of the cerebral circulation in experimental primates determined by the method of hydrogen clearance. Stroke 1973;4:632–42.
104. Kontos HA, Wei EP, Navari RM, et al. Responses of cerebral arteries and arterioles to acute hypotension and hypertension. Am J Physiol 1978;234:H371–83.
105. Grubb RL Jr, Phelps ME, Raichle ME, et al. The effects of arterial blood pressure on the regional cerebral blood volume by X-ray fluorescence. Stroke 1973;4:390–9.
106. Paulson OB, Strandgaard S, Edvinsson L. Cerebral autoregulation. Cerebrovasc Brain Metab Rev 1990;2:161–92.
107. Kontos HA, Wei EP, Raper AJ, et al. Role of tissue hypoxia in local regulation of cerebral microcirculation. Am J Physiol 1978; 234:H582–91.
108. McPherson RW, Koehler RC, Traystman RJ. Effect of jugular venous pressure on cerebral autoregulation in dogs. Am J Physiol 1988;255:H1516–24.
109. van Beek AH, Claassen JA, Rikkert MG, et al. Cerebral autoregulation: an overview of current concepts and methodology with special focus on the elderly. J Cereb Blood Flow Metab 2008;28:1071–85.
110. Li Z, Zhang M, Xin Q, et al. Age-related changes in spontaneous oscillations assessed by wavelet transform of cerebral oxygenation and arterial blood pressure signals. J Cereb Blood Flow Metab 2013;33:692–9.
111. Zhang R, Behbehani K, Levine BD. Dynamic pressure-flow relationship of the cerebral circulation during acute increase in arterial pressure. J Physiol 2009;587:2567–77.
112. Tzeng YC, Ainslie PN. Blood pressure regulation IX: cerebral autoregulation under blood pressure challenges. Eur J Appl Physiol 2013;113(11):2869–70.
113. Budohoski KP, Czosnyka M, Smielewski P, et al. Cerebral autoregulation after subarachnoid hemorrhage: comparison of three methods. J Cereb Blood Flow Metab 2013;33:449–56.
114. Tzeng YC, Ainslie PN, Cooke WH, et al. Assessment of cerebral autoregulation: the quandary of quantification. Am J Physiol Heart Circ Physiol 2012;303:H658–71.
115. Dawson SL, Panerai RB, Potter JF. Serial changes in static and dynamic cerebral autoregulation after acute ischaemic stroke. Cerebrovasc Dis 2003;16:69–75.
117. Aries MJ, Elting JW, De Keyser J, et al. Cerebral autoregulation in stroke: a review of transcranial Doppler studies. Stroke 2010;41:2697–704.
118. Schumann P, Touzani O, Young AR, et al. Evaluation of the ratio of cerebral blood flow to cerebral blood volume as an index of local cerebral perfusion pressure. Brain 1998;121:1369–79.
120. Harper AM, Glass HI. Effect of alterations in the arterial carbon dioxide tension on the blood flow through the cerebral cortex at normal and low arterial blood pressures. J Neurol Neurosurg Psychiatry 1965;28:449–52.
121. Powers WJ, Fox PT, Raichle ME. The effect of carotid artery disease on the cerebrovascular response to physiologic stimulation. Neurology 1988;38:1475–8.
122. Maruyama M, Shimoji K, Ichikawa T, et al. The effects of extreme hemodilutions on the autoregulation of cerebral blood flow, electroencephalogram and cerebral metabolic rate of oxygen in the dog. Stroke 1985;16:675–9.
123. Haggendal E, Johansson B. Effect of arterial carbon dioxide tension and oxygen saturation on cerebral blood flow autoregulation in dogs. Acta Physiol Scand 1965;66:27–53.
124. Powers WJ, Press GA, Grubb RL Jr, et al. The effect of hemodynamically significant carotid artery disease on the hemodynamic status of the cerebral circulation. Ann Intern Med 1987;106: 27–34.
127. Kuroda S, Shiga T, Houkin K, et al. Cerebral oxygen metabolism and neuronal integrity in patients with impaired vasoreactivity attributable to occlusive carotid artery disease. Stroke 2006; 37:393–8.
129. Baron JC, Bousser MG, Rey A, et al. Reversal of focal "misery-perfusion syndrome" by extra-intracranial arterial bypass in hemodynamic cerebral ischemia. A case study with 15O positron emission tomography. Stroke 1981;12:454–9.
130. Grubb RL Jr, Derdeyn CP, Fritsch SM, et al. Importance of hemodynamic factors in the prognosis of symptomatic carotid occlusion. JAMA 1998;280:1055–60.
131. Grubb RL Jr, Raichle ME, Phelps ME, et al. Effects of increased intracranial pressure on cerebral blood volume, blood flow, and oxygen utilization in monkeys. J Neurosurg 1975;43:385–98.

132. Ferrari M, Wilson DA, Hanley DF, et al. Effects of graded hypotension on cerebral blood flow, blood volume, and mean transit time in dogs. Am J Physiol 1992;262:H1908–14.
133. Zaharchuk G, Mandeville JB, Bogdanov AA Jr, et al. Cerebrovascular dynamics of autoregulation and hypoperfusion. An MRI study of CBF and changes in total and microvascular cerebral blood volume during hemorrhagic hypotension. Stroke 1999; 30:2197–204.
134. Powers WJ. Is the ratio of cerebral blood volume to cerebral blood flow a reliable indicator of cerebral perfusion pressure. J Cereb Blood Flow Metab 1993;13(Suppl. 1):S325.
140. Derdeyn CP, Videen TO, Yundt KD, et al. Variability of cerebral blood volume and oxygen extraction: stages of cerebral hemodynamic impairment revisited. Brain 2002;125:595–607.
150. Ogasawara K, Ogawa A, Terasaki K, et al. Use of cerebrovascular reactivity in patients with symptomatic major cerebral artery occlusion to predict 5-year outcome: comparison of xenon-133 and iodine-123-IMP single-photon emission computed tomography. J Cereb Blood Flow Metab 2002;22:1142–8.
151. Ogasawara K, Ogawa A, Yoshimoto T. Cerebrovascular reactivity to acetazolamide and outcome in patients with symptomatic internal carotid or middle cerebral artery occlusion: a xenon-133 single-photon emission computed tomography study. Stroke 2002;33:1857–62.
152. Yamauchi H, Fukuyama H, Nagahama Y, et al. Significance of increased oxygen extraction fraction in five-year prognosis of major cerebral arterial occlusive diseases. J Nucl Med 1999;40: 1992–8.
153. Yamauchi H, Higashi T, Kagawa S, et al. Is misery perfusion still a predictor of stroke in symptomatic major cerebral artery disease? Brain 2012;135:2515–16.
154. Heiss WD, Rosner G. Functional recovery of cortical neurons as related to degree and duration of ischemia. Ann Neurol 1983;14:294–301.
156. Hossmann KA. Pathophysiology and therapy of experimental stroke. Cell Mol Neurobiol 2006;26:1057–83.
164. Symon L, Branston NM, Strong AJ. Autoregulation in acute focal ischemia: an experimental study. Stroke 1976;7:547–54.
165. Giffard C, Young AR, Kerrouche N, et al. Outcome of acutely ischemic brain tissue in prolonged middle cerebral artery occlusion: a serial positron emission tomography investigation in the baboon. J Cereb Blood Flow Metab 2004;24:495–508.
167. Sakoh M, Ostergaard L, Rohl L, et al. Relationship between residual cerebral blood flow and oxygen metabolism as predictive of ischemic tissue viability: sequential multitracer positron emission tomography scanning of middle cerebral artery occlusion during the critical first 6 hours after stroke in pigs. J Neurosurg 2000;93:647–57.
168. Pappata S, Fiorelli M, Rommel T, et al. PET study of changes in local brain hemodynamics and oxygen metabolism after unilateral middle cerebral artery occlusion in baboons. J Cereb Blood Flow Metab 1993;13:416–24.
169. Heiss WD, Graf R, Wienhard K, et al. Dynamic penumbra demonstrated by sequential multitracer PET after middle cerebral artery occlusion in cats. J Cereb Blood Flow Metab 1994;14: 892–902.
170. Touzani O, Young AR, Derlon JM, et al. Sequential studies of severely hypometabolic tissue volumes after permanent middle cerebral artery occlusion. A positron emission tomographic investigation in anesthetized baboons. Stroke 1995; 26:2112–19.
171. Giffard C, Landeau B, Kerrouche N, et al. Decreased chronic-stage cortical 11C-flumazenil binding after focal ischemia-reperfusion in baboons: a marker of selective neuronal loss? Stroke 2008;39:991–9.
173. Heiss WD, Huber M, Fink GR, et al. Progressive derangement of periinfarct viable tissue in ischemic stroke. J Cereb Blood Flow Metab 1992;12:193–203.
174. An H, Ford A, Chen Y, et al. Early perfusion instability profoundly impacts tissue outcome in acute ischemic stroke. 2013 International Stroke Conference Oral Abstracts 2013; Abstract 182.
175. Furlan M, Marchal G, Viader F, et al. Spontaneous neurological recovery after stroke and the fate of the ischemic penumbra. Ann Neurol 1996;40:216–26.
176. Shimosegawa E, Hatazawa J, Ibaraki M, et al. Metabolic penumbra of acute brain infarction: a correlation with infarct growth. Ann Neurol 2005;57:495–504.
177. Molina CA, Montaner J, Abilleira S, et al. Timing of spontaneous recanalization and risk of hemorrhagic transformation in acute cardioembolic stroke. Stroke 2001;32:1079–84.
180. Lenzi GL, Frackowiak RS, Jones T. Cerebral oxygen metabolism and blood flow in human cerebral ischemic infarction. J Cereb Blood Flow Metab 1982;2:321–35.
184. Astrup J. Energy-requiring cell functions in the ischemic brain. Their critical supply and possible inhibition in protective therapy. J Neurosurg 1982;56:482–97.
185. Frykholm P, Andersson JL, Valtysson J, et al. A metabolic threshold of irreversible ischemia demonstrated by PET in a middle cerebral artery occlusion-reperfusion primate model. Acta Neurol Scand 2000;102:18–26.
186. Baron JC, Rougemont D, Bousser MG, et al. Local CBF, oxygen extraction fraction (OEF), and $CMRO_2$: Prognostic value in recent supratentorial infarction in humans. J Cereb Blood Flow Metab 1983;3(Suppl. 1):S1–2.
187. Marchal G, Benali K, Iglesias S, et al. Voxel-based mapping of irreversible ischaemic damage with PET in acute stroke. Brain 1999;122:2387–400.
189. Young AR, Sette G, Touzani O, et al. Relationships between high oxygen extraction fraction in the acute stage and final infarction in reversible middle cerebral artery occlusion: an investigation in anesthetized baboons with positron emission tomography. J Cereb Blood Flow Metab 1996;16:1176–88.
190. Rosenbaum JL, Almli CR, Yundt KD, et al. Higher neonatal cerebral blood flow correlates with worse childhood neurologic outcome. Neurology 1997;49:1035–41.
191. Symon L, Crockard HA, Dorsch NW, et al. Local cerebral blood flow and vascular reactivity in a chronic stable stroke in baboons. Stroke 1975;6:482–92.
192. Hosomi N, Mizushige K, Kitadai M, et al. Induced hypertension treatment to improve cerebral ischemic injury after transient forebrain ischemia. Brain Res 1999;835:188–96.
193. Tranmer BI, Keller TS, Kindt GW, et al. Loss of cerebral regulation during cardiac output variations in focal cerebral ischemia. J Neurosurg 1992;77:253–9.
194. Agnoli A, Fieschi C, Bozzao L, et al. Autoregulation of cerebral blood flow. Studies during drug-induced hypertension in normal subjects and in patients with cerebral vascular diseases. Circulation 1968;38:800–12.
195. Paulson OB, Lassen NA, Skinhoj E. Regional cerebral blood flow in apoplexy without arterial occlusion. Neurology 1970;20: 125–38.
196. Paulson OB. Regional cerebral blood flow in apoplexy due to occlusion of the middle cerebral artery. Neurology 1970;20: 63–77.
199. Pozzilli C, Di P V, Pantano P, et al. Influence of nimodipine on cerebral blood flow in human cerebral ischaemia. J Neurol 1989;236:199–202.
200. Vorstrup S, Andersen A, Blegvad N, et al. Calcium antagonist (PY 108-068) treatment may further decrease flow in ischemic areas in acute stroke. J Cereb Blood Flow Metab 1986;6:222–9.
201. Powers WJ, Videen TO, Diringer MN, et al. Autoregulation after ischaemic stroke. J Hypertens 2009;27:2218–22.
202. Nazir FS, Overell JR, Bolster A, et al. Effect of perindopril on cerebral and renal perfusion on normotensives in mild early ischaemic stroke: a randomized controlled trial. Cerebrovasc Dis 2005;19:77–83.
203. Nazir FS, Overell JR, Bolster A, et al. The effect of losartan on global and focal cerebral perfusion and on renal function in hypertensives in mild early ischaemic stroke. J Hypertens 2004;22:989–95.
205. Martin WR, Raichle ME. Cerebellar blood flow and metabolism in cerebral hemisphere infarction. Ann Neurol 1983;14:168–76.
226. Feeney DM, Baron JC. Diaschisis. Stroke 1986;17:817–30.
235. Kim-Han JS, Kopp SJ, Dugan LL, et al. Perihematomal mitochondrial dysfunction after intracerebral hemorrhage. Stroke 2006;37:2457–62.
238. Dal-Bianco P. Positron emission tomography of 2(18F)-fluorodeoxyglucose in cerebral vascular disease: clinicometabolic correlations in patients with nontraumatic spontaneous

intracerebral hematoma and ischemic infarction. In: Meyer JS, Lechner H, Reivich M, et al., editors. Cerebral Vascular Disease 6: Proceedings of the World Federation of Neurology 13th International Salzburg Conference. Amsterdam: Excerpta Medica; 1987. p. 257–62.

239. Powers WJ, Zazulia AR, Videen TO, et al. Autoregulation of cerebral blood flow surrounding acute (6 to 22 hours) intracerebral hemorrhage. Neurology 2001;57:18–24.

240. Gould B, McCourt R, Asdaghi N, et al. Autoregulation of cerebral blood flow is preserved in primary intracerebral hemorrhage. Stroke 2013;44:1726–8.

246. Moftakhar P, Hauptman JS, Malkasian D, et al. Cerebral arteriovenous malformations. Part 2: physiology. Neurosurg Focus 2009;26:E11.

247. Stuer C, Ikeda T, Stoffel M, et al. Norepinephrine and cerebral blood flow regulation in patients with arteriovenous malformations. Neurosurgery 2008;62:1254–60.

248. Fierstra J, Conklin J, Krings T, et al. Impaired peri-nidal cerebrovascular reserve in seizure patients with brain arteriovenous malformations. Brain 2011;134:100–9.

254. Spetzler RF, Wilson CB, Weinstein P, et al. Normal perfusion pressure breakthrough theory. Clin Neurosurg 1978; 25:651–72.

273. Dankbaar JW, Rijsdijk M, van dS I, et al. Relationship between vasospasm, cerebral perfusion, and delayed cerebral ischemia after aneurysmal subarachnoid hemorrhage. Neuroradiology 2009;51:813–19.

274. Powers WJ, Grubb RL Jr, Baker RP, et al. Regional cerebral blood flow and metabolism in reversible ischemia due to vasospasm. Determination by positron emission tomography. J Neurosurg 1985;62:539–46.

284. Dhar R, Scalfani MT, Blackburn S, et al. Relationship between angiographic vasospasm and regional hypoperfusion in aneurysmal subarachnoid hemorrhage. Stroke 2012;43:1788–94.

285. Yundt KD, Grubb RL Jr, Diringer MN, et al. Autoregulatory vasodilation of parenchymal vessels is impaired during cerebral vasospasm. J Cereb Blood Flow Metab 1998;18:419–24.

286. Sakowitz OW, Santos E, Nagel A, et al. Clusters of spreading depolarizations are associated with disturbed cerebral metabolism in patients with aneurysmal subarachnoid hemorrhage. Stroke 2013;44:220–3.

287. Nielsen TH, Olsen NV, Toft P, et al. Cerebral energy metabolism during mitochondrial dysfunction induced by cyanide in piglets. Acta Anaesthesiol Scand 2013;57:793–801.

291. Yundt KD, Grubb RL Jr, Diringer MN, et al. Cerebral hemodynamic and metabolic changes caused by brain retraction after aneurysmal subarachnoid hemorrhage. Neurosurgery 1997; 40:442–50.

298. Budohoski KP, Czosnyka M, Kirkpatrick PJ, et al. Clinical relevance of cerebral autoregulation following subarachnoid haemorrhage. Nat Rev Neurol 2013;9:152–63.

303. Fujii M, Yan J, Rolland WB, et al. Early brain injury, an evolving frontier in subarachnoid hemorrhage research. Transl Stroke Res 2013;4:432–46.

4 Histopathology of Brain Tissue Response to Stroke and Injury

Roland N. Auer

KEY POINTS

- The four kinds of ischemia are transient focal, permanent focal, transient global and permanent global.
- Small vessel disease of arterioles can involve either blockage or breakage, and in hypertension, both can occur simultaneously.
- Large vessel carotid artery pathology is comprised of endothelial ulceration, intramural hemorrhage into carotid plaque and intraluminal thrombosis with detachment and embolization.
- Infarction is a well-demarcated tissue lesion, a pH thresholded pan-necrosis, while selective neuronal loss is a lesser tissue lesion clinically manifest most commonly with memory loss due to bilateral hippocampal neuronal loss after global ischemia.
- Important diseases of the arteriole distinct from hypertension are amyloid angiopathy and CADASIL (cerebral autosomal dominant arteriopathy with subcortical infarcts and leukoencephalopathy).

This chapter illustrates the pathology causing stroke due to large and small vessel disease, as well as heart disease. The pathologic reactions of the brain itself to the ischemic processes are also illustrated and discussed. The repertoire of brain tissue response to ischemia is remarkably limited to two tissue entities: selective neuronal death and infarction. Low blood flow may cause the neurons to selectively die (selective neuronal necrosis), sparing glia and neuropil. The second possibility is that the entire tissue undergoes necrosis (pan-necrosis), termed infarction in the setting of ischemia. All tissue responses to ischemia in the brain and spinal cord are variants of either selective neuronal loss or infarction.

When ischemia affects the entire brain, a much shorter duration of ischemia produces necrosis than in focal ischemia. Cardiac arrest can be tolerated for only a matter of minutes, whereas focal ischemia can be tolerated for much longer durations. This simple fact suggests that trans-synaptic effects must operate, and that they are detrimental in cerebral ischemia. We begin by considering the landscape of possible permutations of the general classes of ischemia.

FOUR BROAD CATEGORIES OF CEREBRAL ISCHEMIA

Lack of blood flow can affect the entire brain (global ischemia) or just a portion of it (focal ischemia). Ischemia can also be permanent, or transient if reperfusion occurs. This gives rise to a natural permutation of four general types of cerebral ischemia (Table 4-1).

In addition to the basic type of ischemia, outcome is determined by basic physiologic parameters such as the degree of reduction in blood flow, the brain temperature and the glucose levels. If blood flow to the entire brain is interrupted, reperfusion is accompanied by damage in remarkably restricted areas. This is termed selective vulnerability, and the principle of selective vulnerability obtains in most neurologic disease, not only stroke and cardiac arrest.

When ischemia is focal, the size and location of the vessel, together with the nature of the occlusion (or leak, in a hemorrhage), determine the outcome of the stroke. The disease is already focal by virtue of a locally occluded vessel, substituting for the principle of selective vulnerability in global ischemia to determine the final neurologic deficit of the patient.

Stroke is aptly named in English, being the most rapidly changing deficit of all neurologic conditions. There are exactly two potential underlying pathologic causes of a stroke: infarct or hemorrhage. This is because only two things can go wrong with a blood vessel: it can block or break.

The fact that vessels can only be blocked or broken in giving rise to brain tissue pathology, has widespread implications for vessels of all sizes. The major named arteries of the brain can occlude, giving rise to large infarcts, or they can rupture, giving rise to fatal hemorrhages. At the level of the arteriole as well as the artery, the principle of blockage vs breakage applies. Lacunes are due to *occlusions* of arterioles, while microhemorrhages are due to *leaking* arterioles.

Some diseases affect brain arterioles in a manner that can produce both hemorrhage and occlusion. The classic example is hypertension, which can break and block arterioles, often simultaneously. In the retina, this blocked-or-broken principle applies as well, where cotton wool spots represent infarcts of the nerve fiber layer, while ophthalmoscopically visible hemorrhages represent leakage of retinal arterioles.

The sudden nature of occlusion or leakage of vessels is the feature that originally gave rise to the term stroke, engendering a rapidly changing clinical deficit that evolves over seconds, to minutes, to hours. There is nothing like it in neurology, with respect to speed of onset.

A slower clinical evolution is unusual and is seen mainly in the entity termed hemodynamic stroke, where progression can occur over hours to days.[1] Hemodynamic stroke results from a cardiac cause that lowers the blood pressure to such an extent that critically low cerebral blood flow levels occur in either an artery that is only partially occluded, or in the watershed zone between two or three major cerebral arteries, leading to infarction. Hemodynamic stroke thus has its origin in the heart, not in a blood vessel of the brain, and comprises the major exception to the above principles of a "blocked or broken" vessel as a cause of the pathology of stroke.

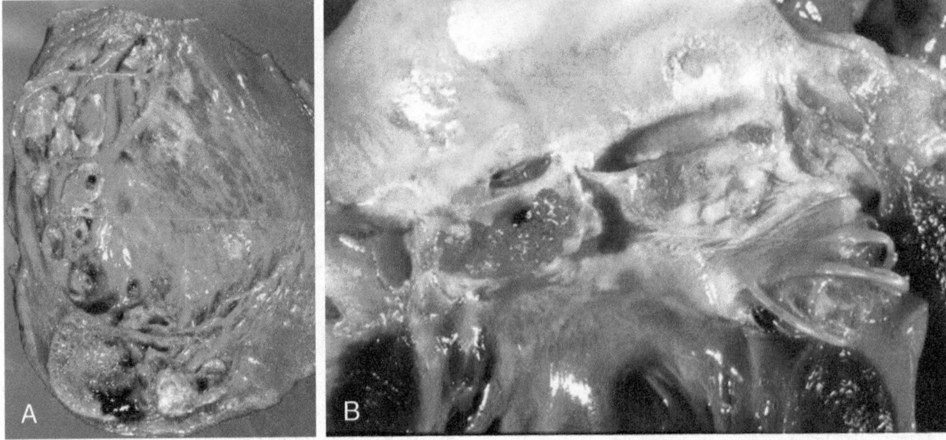

Figure 4-1. Heart causes of stroke include both myocardial and valvular disease. A, Mural clots (white) adhere, and then detach, to ischemic myocardium due to the altered kinetic properties of ischemic heart muscle. B, Non-bacterial thrombotic endocarditis is seen (red) on the aortic valve of a cancer patient. The detached clots embolize to brain in both cases.

TABLE 4-1 The 4 Broad Types of Ischemia

	Focal	Global
Transient	Embolus with reperfusion	Cardiac arrest with reperfusion
Permanent	End-vessel occlusion	Brain death

LARGE VESSEL STROKES

Most large vessel strokes of an ischemic nature arise from causes outside the brain (the carotid arteries or the heart), the most common being atherosclerosis (Chapter 1). Atherosclerosis causes stroke in two major ways, the first being coronary atherosclerosis with consequent heart disease, the second being atherosclerosis of the carotid artery bifurcation. Both the heart (Fig. 4-1) and the carotid (Fig. 4-2) causes of stroke lead to brain infarcts by releasing emboli to the brain. The consequences of cardiac arrest or carotid thrombosis are quite different from the usual stroke. If the heart itself stops, the brain response is that of cardiac arrest encephalopathy, which can take several forms (neocortical, hippocampal, basal ganglia or cerebellar impairment in various combinations). If the carotid artery occludes, this usually results in malignant ischemic hemispheric edema and death. We will first cover the common cardiac and carotid causes of stroke, following the flow of blood and the route emboli actually travel to cause stroke. The brain histopathologic response to these events will follow, in the context of stroke and the related conditions of global ischemia and edema.

Heart Disease and Cerebral Emboli

In ischemic heart disease, poorly contracting or akinetic myocardial segments accumulate mural clot which can dislodge emboli to the brain, from the left ventricle (see Fig. 4-1A). Heart disease need not be ischemic to give rise to embolic brain infarcts: the many forms of valvular disease can also do this, including, e.g., rheumatic endocarditis, non-bacterial thrombotic endocarditis and bacterial endocarditis (see Fig. 4-1B).

Carotid Artery Atherosclerosis

Atherosclerosis is a generalized disease of large and medium-sized arteries that begins in the descending abdominal aorta. Over time, atherosclerosis tends to involve the thoracic aorta and iliac arteries, often affecting the renal arteries. Despite the ascending aorta and aortic arch having greater flow than the distal aorta, they show less atherosclerosis than the descending aorta. Less frequently a source than the carotid artery, the aortic arch and the great vessels which branch from the aortic arch (Chapter 33) can also emboli to the brain.[2]

The atherosclerotic carotid plaque[3] consists of an accumulation of lipid, cholesterol, smooth muscle, fibroblasts, capillaries and hemorrhage.[4] The intramural expansion gives rise to a space-occupying effect of these atheromatous tissue components, and their slow accumulation can lead to occlusion of the carotid artery. But with a smooth overlying endothelium, such slow occlusion is not the usual mechanism of stroke, because collateral circulation can develop when occlusion occurs slowly due to the mass of atheroma building up over years to decades.

The mechanism of stroke in carotid atherosclerosis is not slow, steady occlusion; this allows time for growth of collateral vessels to circumvent the blockage. Instead, carotid atherosclerosis commonly results in a sudden event that breaches the endothelial integrity. The endothelial rent exposes sub-endothelial connective tissue to blood, causing platelet aggregation, and accounting for emboli sent to the brain from a locus of atherosclerosis in the neck.

Two major mechanisms seem to play a role in generating this sudden endothelial breach. One is hemorrhage into the atherosclerotic plaque (see Figs 4-2A,B).[5] The second is ulceration of the plaque (see Figs 4-2C,D). Hemorrhage into the wall occurs too rapidly for endothelial cell cytoplasm to maintain complete integrity of the endothelial lining, resulting in a rent. An ulcer, by definition, involves a more permanent denudation of endothelium. Thus, both of these complications of carotid atherosclerosis breach the integrity of the endothelium, expose sub-endothelial connective tissue, activate clotting systems and release thromboemboli. Endothelial breach explains the therapeutic benefit of aspirin,[6,7] which inhibits platelet aggregation and emboli formed as a result of such carotid disease. Such mural mechanisms are important, as when carotid stenosis is less than 70%, hemodynamic factors poorly account for stroke.

Hemorrhage into the plaque (see Figs 4-2B,D,E) has become increasingly recognized in the pathogenesis of carotid-artery-induced stroke. The suddenness of the hemorrhage means the overlying endothelial cells are torn apart. Any rent in the intercellular junctions of endothelial cells will expose

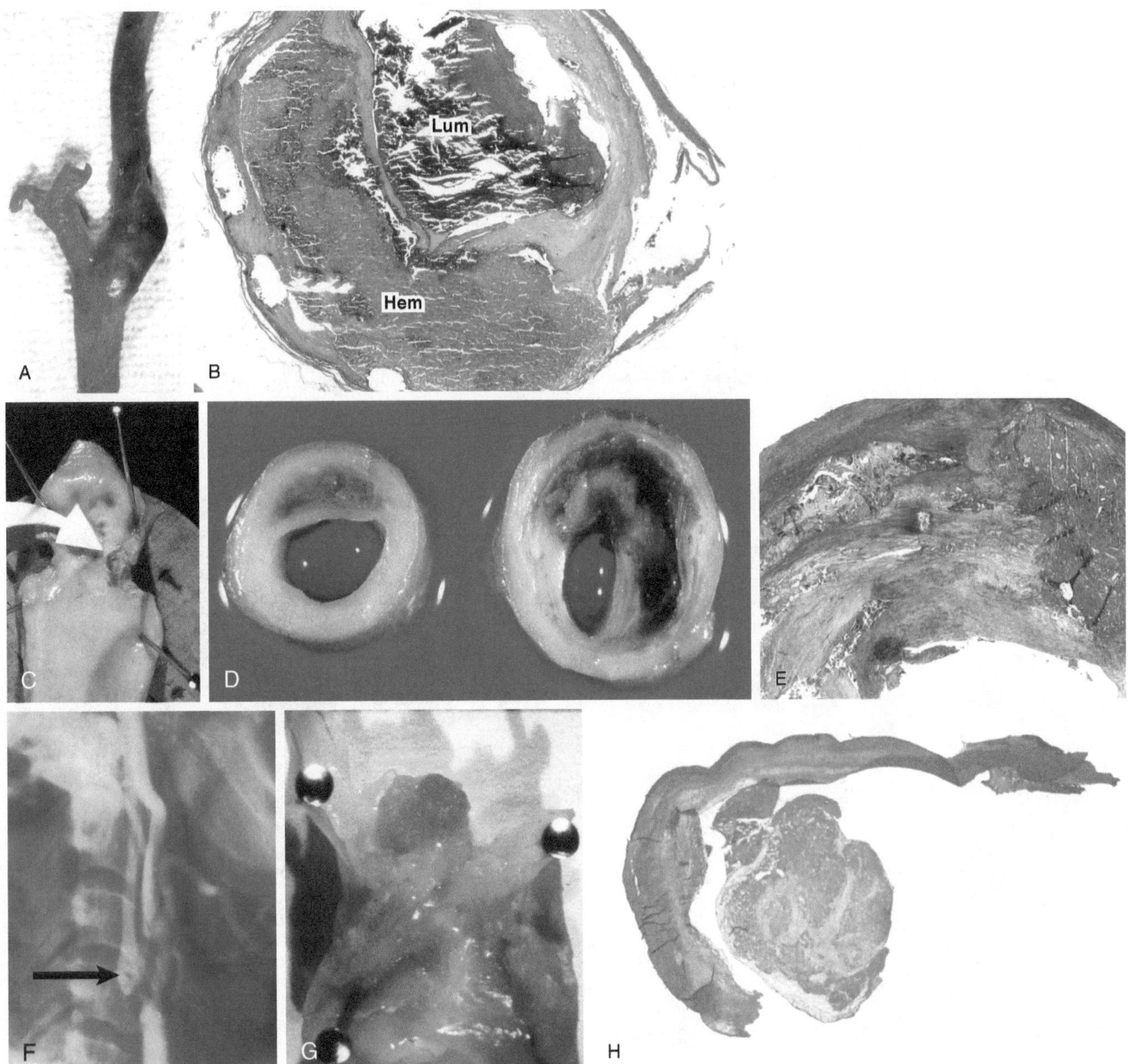

Figure 4-2. Carotid artery causes of stroke. Hemorrhage into atherosclerotic plaque regularly occurs as the plaque enlarges, as seen in an autopsy specimen, where internal carotid artery mural hemorrhage has occurred into a plaque (A) located just above the bifurcation. Section B through an endarterectomy reveals the degree of luminal compression, the lumen (Lum) here equal in size to the intramural hematoma (Hem). An endarterectomy specimen opened and pinned to a cork (C) reveals an ulcer (white arrow) in the right carotid of a 79-year-old man with a right hemisphere infarct. Gross appearance (D) reveals smooth covering of the atheroma on the left, but an ulcer interrupting the normal white appearance of the endothelial and subendothelial connective tissue on the upper aspect of the lumen on the right. A major portion of the atheroma is blood, revealed by a Masson trichrome stain (E) which shows the hemorrhage as violet, admixed with collagen seen as blue. A ball-like thrombus (arrow) seen angiographically (F) prior to endarterectomy, is revealed to be an adherent "red clot" macroscopically (G) and microscopically (H) after endarterectomy.

Continued

sub-endothelial collagen, leading to clot formation. The blood clotting system, especially Hageman factor (XII, initiating the intrinsic coagulation pathway) is very sensitive to collagen connective tissue components located beneath the endothelium. This may lead to clot formation seen in endarterectomy specimens (see Figs 4-2F,G,H) where the clot has not yet detached and embolized to the brain. Intraluminal clot can, if it can persist without detachment and embolization, show a pavement-like growth of endothelium (Fig. 4-2I) over it. Such endothelial overgrowth reduces the chances further, of subsequent detachment, and may eventuate in the clot scarring and becoming incorporated into the carotid artery wall as a healed mural nodule.

Other than blood clot, the pathology of embolic infarction may reveal embolism of atheromatous material itself (see Fig. 4-2J), with fragments of atheroma including cholesterol clefts and giant cells seen lodged in brain vessels (see Fig. 4-2K). Some clots contain calcium (see Fig. 4-2L).[8] When the emboli

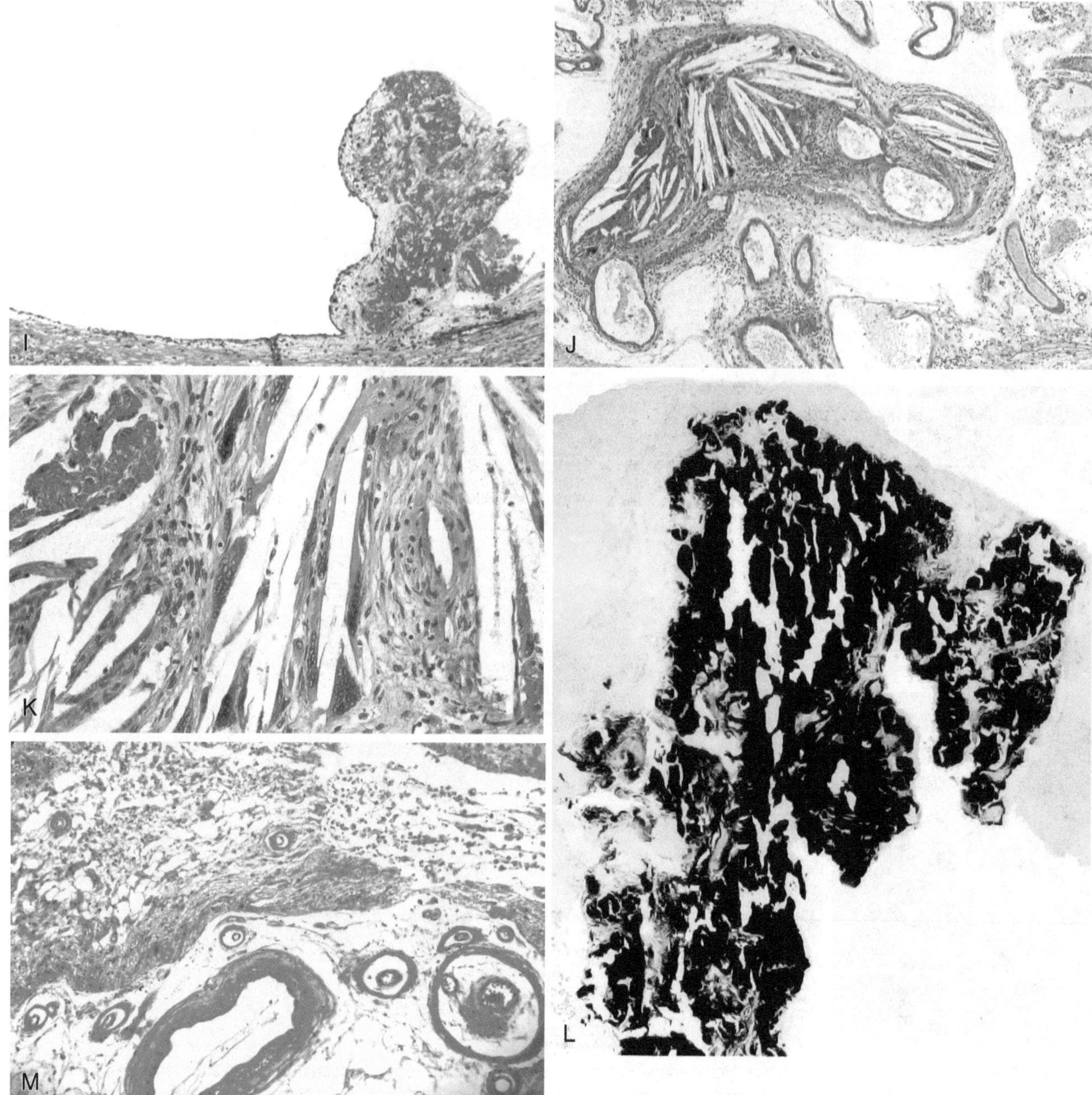

Figure 4-2., cont'd Endothelium overgrows such mural clots (I) over time, converting them to a mural nodule with little residual risk of detachment and embolism. Fragments of the atheroma itself may also detach and embolize, resulting in intravascular contents of embolized cerebral vessels (J) that resemble the wall of a carotid artery, complete with cholesterol clefts, giant cells and hemorrhage (K). Extensive calcium deposits may be present as seen in black on von Kossa stain for calcium in this MERCI-retrieved clot (L), rendering t-PA ineffective in effecting complete dissolution of clot. More commonly though, when clots are composed of pure thrombus, recanalization occurs, leaving telescoped, double lumen, or "lumen within a lumen" vessels (M). Hematoxylin and eosin – B,H,I,J,K,M. Masson trichrome – E. von Kossa stain for calcium – L.

consist of simple clot, there is recanalization leading to a new lumen within the old lumen giving a "lumen-within-a-lumen" appearance of telescoped vessels (see Fig. 4-2M).

Infarction Versus Selective Neuronal Necrosis

Infarction can be defined as ischemic pan-necrosis. By pan-necrosis we mean death of all cellular elements in the brain, including neurons, glia and vascular cells. By selective neuronal necrosis we mean selective death of neurons, sparing glia (oligodendrocytes and astrocytes). The differences in these two fundamentally different ways in which the brain can respond to ischemia are illustrated (Fig. 4-3).

The clinical significance of pan-necrosis and selective neuronal necrosis is quite different. Selective neuronal necrosis leaves the tissue architecture intact, whether in the hippocampus (see Fig. 4-3A) or neocortex (see Fig. 4-3B). Any remaining neurons may still function, including their processes (axons and dendrites), which remain surrounded by glia. Pan-necrosis, in contrast, removes all cellular elements of the brain including glia, leaving a cyst filled with interstitial fluid. Pan-necrosis is the histologic lesion that underlies the

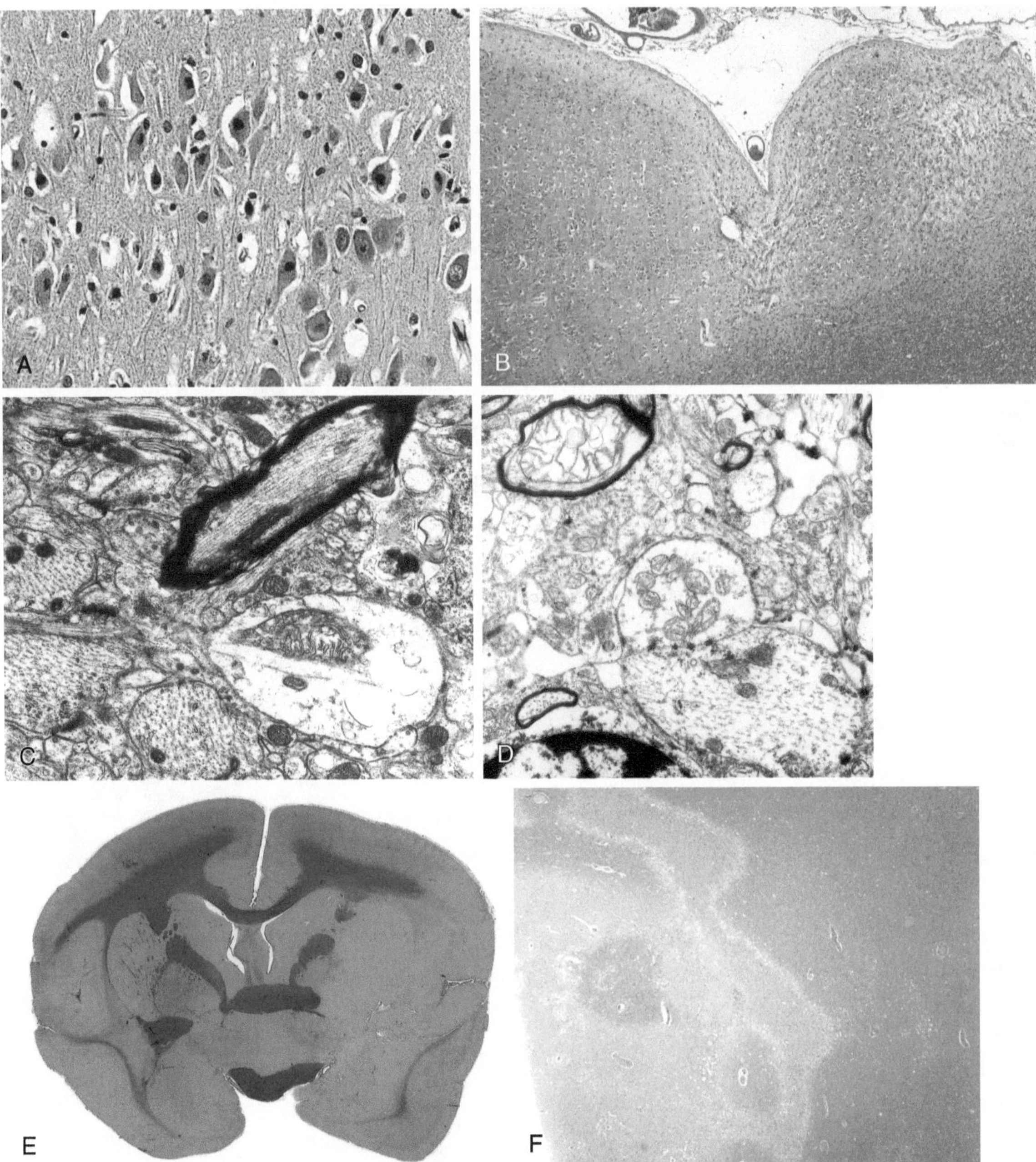

Figure 4-3. Selective neuronal necrosis versus pan-necrosis (infarct). Selective neuronal necrosis is seen here as acidophilic, red neurons in the selectively vulnerable CA1 neurons of the hippocampus (A). In the neocortex, selective neuronal necrosis leaves a glial scar (B) without cyst formation, often termed incomplete infarction. Selective neuronal necrosis shows early dendritic swelling (C), whereas pan-necrosis shows early axonal swelling (D). Pan-necrosis in an MCA infarct shows early demarcation where a line of demarcation is seen to cross gray and white matter indiscriminately as seen experimentally in monkeys (E) and in humans (F).

Continued

permanent clinical deficit of a focal ischemic stroke. Selective neuronal necrosis, in contrast, underlies the memory deficit in cardiac arrest encephalopathy, which requires necrosis of at least 50% of the CA1 pyramidal cells.[9]

The early lesion differs ultrastructurally between selective neuronal necrosis and pan-necrosis. Selective neuronal necrosis shows early dendritic swelling (see Fig. 4-3C), due to the dendritic location of NMDA receptors and other excitatory amino acid receptors, chiefly on neurons. Pan-necrosis shows the inverse lesion ultrastructurally, with axonal swelling, sparing dendrites (see Fig. 4-3D).

The characteristic, early sharp demarcation of an infarct (see Figs 4-3E,F) continues as pan-necrosis becomes cystic (see Fig. 4-3G). Neocortical layer 1 is often spared (see Fig. 4-3H), suggesting a neuroanatomic pattern superimposed upon the initiating vascular pattern that begins the ischemic insult. The old adage that this commonly seen preservation of layer 1 is due to "sparing by CSF" is untenable and must be retired from ischemic pathology descriptions, as the demarcation line of tissue response follows the layer 1–2 junction neuroanatomically, parallel to the pia mater. Furthermore, CSF is not a source of oxygen. The hippocampus may show either selective

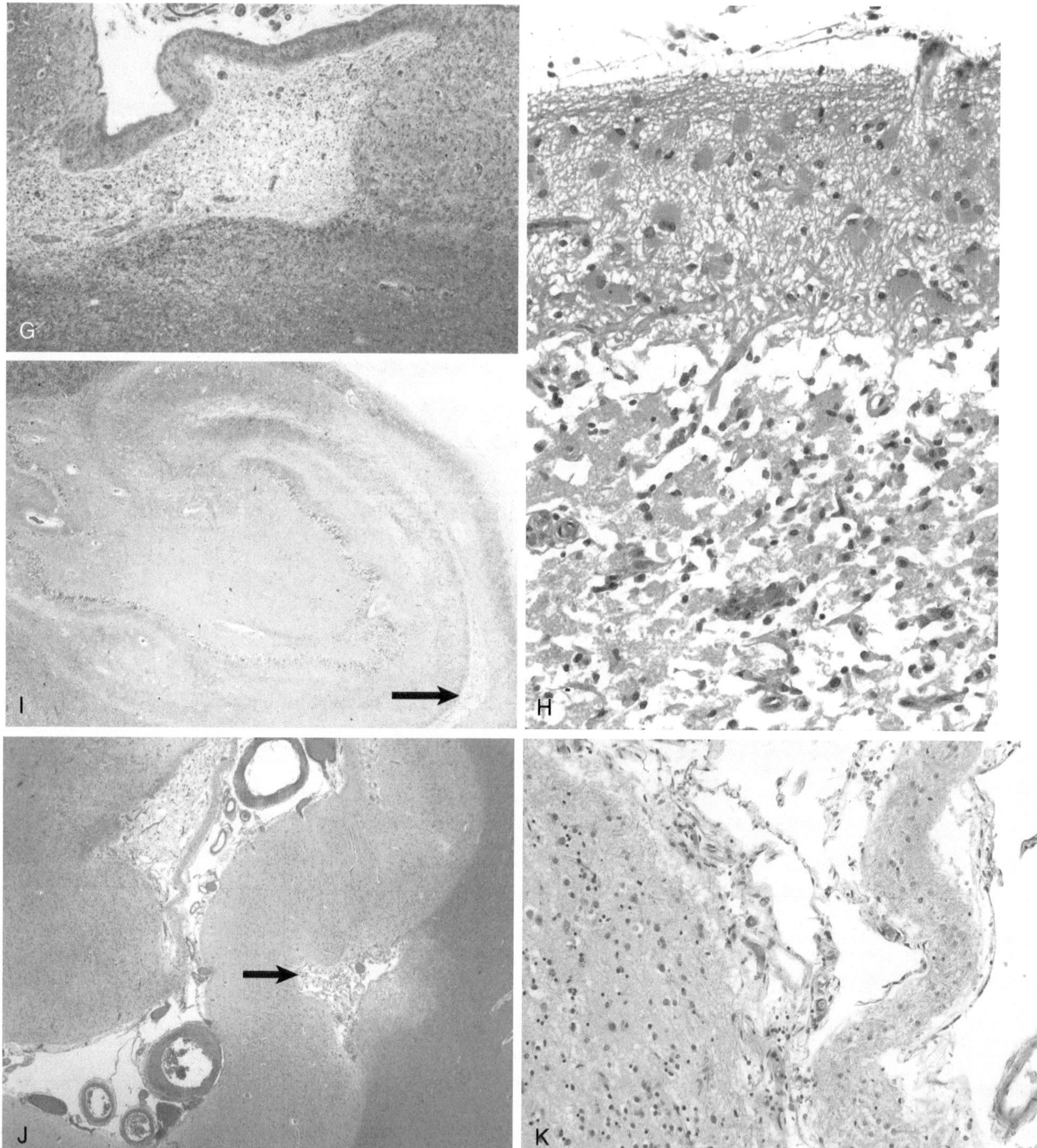

Figure 4-3., cont'd The cysts developing later are filled with brain interstitial fluid, and continue to be sharply outlined (G) often sparing cortical layer one (H). Pan-necrosis may also occur in the hippocampal CA1 stratum pyramidale (I). Surrounding even a small cystic infarct (J, arrow), little selective neuronal necrosis is the rule, and neurons are spared adjacent to the cyst (K, left).

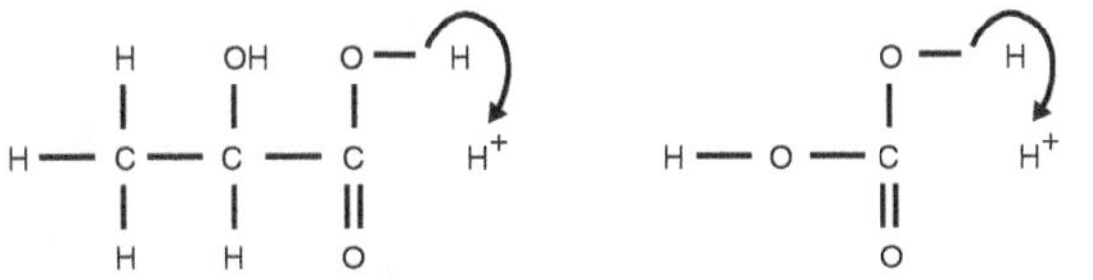

Lactic acid $pK_a = 3.86$ Carbonic acid $pK_a = 6.37$

Figure 4-4. Two acids in brain tissue with different pK_a values, 3.86 and 6.37. Tissue pH changes caused by an acid tend to drift toward the pK_a for that acid due to deprotonation. Carbonic acid has an insufficiently low pK_a to cause pan-necrosis, whereas lactic acidosis causes pan-necrosis in several disease states (see text), including ischemic stroke.

neuronal necrosis (see Fig. 4-3A) or pan-necrosis (see Fig. 4-3I) in the CA1 stratum pyramidale, a selectively vulnerable brain region.

The sharply delimited border of pan-necrosis is an ischemic clue often overlooked, but suggests that a threshold effect is operant in the pathophysiologic mechanism effecting tissue necrosis, likely pH. Acidosis is known to cause tissue necrosis[10,9] and acidosis also leads to a neuron-sparing pan-necrosis in conditions other than ischemia such as Wernicke's encephalopathy and Leigh's disease, both of which produce large amounts of tissue lactate. There exists a threshold of pH in brain tissue below which necrosis occurs, suggested by the experiments of Kraig, where lactic-acid-induced necrosis was pH-dependent, not dependent on the lactate concentration.[10] This would explain the sharp border of infarcts, since the initial fall in CBF is graded in the ischemic penumbra.

Two brain acids[11] are especially relevant to consideration of brain tissue response to acidosis: lactic acid and carbonic acid (Fig. 4-4). Lactic acid has a pK_a of 3.86 and causes tissue necrosis, while carbon dioxide has a tissue pK_a of 6.37, which means lactate deprotonates over 300 times more easily than carbonic acid. By comparison, acetic acid has a pK_a of 4.76, and is thus a weaker acid by almost one log unit, than lactate. At the tissue level, respiratory acidosis does not cause brain necrosis, even when examining the brain by light and electron microscopy in extreme respiratory acidosis.[12,13] Tissue acidosis alone seems to require a $pH \leq 5.3$ to cause necrosis,[10] but in conjunction with other diseases, worsens outcome. Thus, acidosis augments histopathologic damage in cerebral ischemia[14] and even hypoglycemia.[15]

Infarction and selective neuronal necrosis can each occur in any region of the brain. That is to say, all tissue elements may die (infarct) or neurons may die, leaving glia and other cells intact (selective neuronal necrosis), and both can occur anywhere in the brain. The distinction is one of degree of brain damage, not the location of brain damage. The connotation of the location of the brain damage is carried in the term selective vulnerability, not selective neuronal necrosis.

Selective vulnerability occurs in virtually all brain diseases, and implies that certain regions of the brain are more vulnerable than others. And so it is with cerebral ischemia which, in global form, renders the hippocampus selectively vulnerable. Specifically, the CA1 pyramidal neurons of the hippocampus are the first to die in most cases of cardiac arrest encephalopathy. Selective neuronal necrosis occurs in the highly vulnerable CA1 region after global cerebral ischemia is best explained by CA1 dendrites having the highest density of NMDA receptors in the brain,[16] making them most vulnerable to ischemia-induced glutamate release and calcium influx.

The term incomplete infarction has been used in the pathology of ischemic stroke.[17] This is best thought of as selective neuronal necrosis in an area of potential infarction that could have become pan-necrotic with a further reduction in blood supply (see Figs 4-3A,B). Selective GABAergic receptor loss has been shown in such focal areas.[17] A similar selective GABAergic neuron loss has been shown in the telencephalon (specifically in the GABAergic nucleus reticularis thalami[18]) in animal[19] and human[20] global ischemia. That GABAergic transmission is so affected[21] by both focal and global ischemia speaks strongly to a loss of inhibition in ischemia, resulting in a tilt towards an excitatory mechanism leading to the pathology, rather than ischemia simply and directly leading to cell and tissue death.

SMALL VESSEL STROKES

Arterioles are small, unnamed branches resulting from three levels of bifurcation between the larger arteries, and capillaries. They range in size from 40 to 250 µm in diameter. If a vessel is neither blocked nor broken, as in Mönckeberg's medial calcific sclerosis,[22] there is no CNS tissue response because the disease remains intrinsic to the vascular wall (see Figs 4-5A,B). Mural processes that remain within the vessel wall cause no strokes. A vessel which is neither blocked nor broken does not cause parenchymal disease of nervous tissue.

Hypertensive arterioles can be conceived of as going through three stages: hyperplastic arteriolosclerosis, smooth muscle cell death in the tunic media and finally ectasia or occlusion. The first two stages (see Figs 4-5C,D) are pre-ischemic and normal neurons and tissue can be seen around the diseased vessels (see Fig. 4-5D).

When occlusion finally occurs (see Fig. 4-5E) after prolonged hypertension (Chapter 27), the brain tissue response to small vessel disease contrasts with the large infarcts and areas of selective neuronal necrosis seen in disease of the heart and large vessels (see Figs 4-1–4-3). Instead, due to the small size of arterioles, small areas of pan-necrosis termed lacunes characteristically result (see Fig. 4-5F).

Lacunes arise from a different array of diseases than those affecting large vessels, and further give rise to a different localization of tissue response to ischemia within the brain or spinal cord. Hypertensive arteriolosclerosis, amyloid angiopathy and CADASIL (Chapter 41) rank as the top three diseases of arterioles causing stroke, of either ischemic (Chapter 27) or hemorrhagic (Chapter 28) nature and all replace smooth muscle with protein as part of the disease process.[23]

Hypertensive Arteriolosclerosis

Arteriolar smooth muscle cells die in hypertension (see Fig. 4-5C), after an initial proliferative phase (see Fig. 4-5D). The tunica media becomes acellular, replaced by collagen. If too much collagen is laid down inward disease can result in occlusion (see Fig. 4-5E), giving rise to a segment with a disorganized structure[24] lacking tunica intima, media and adventitia. If too little collagen is laid down to prevent pressure dilatation, ectasia and rupture can occur, rarely forming Charcôt-Bouchard aneurysms.[25,26] Thus, hypertensive arteriolosclerosis can lead to both inward and outward disease, in turn leading to the two kinds of stroke, infarcts and hemorrhages. These parallel processes occur in the same vessel over time: occluded arterioles can show no lumen, yet surrounding iron indicating they have shed blood (see Fig. 4-5E).

The early arteriolar change, before medial cells all die, comprises a hyperplasia of smooth muscle cells in reaction to the hypertension. The vessels become longer as well as thicker, giving rise to a tortuous, glomeruloid appearance (see

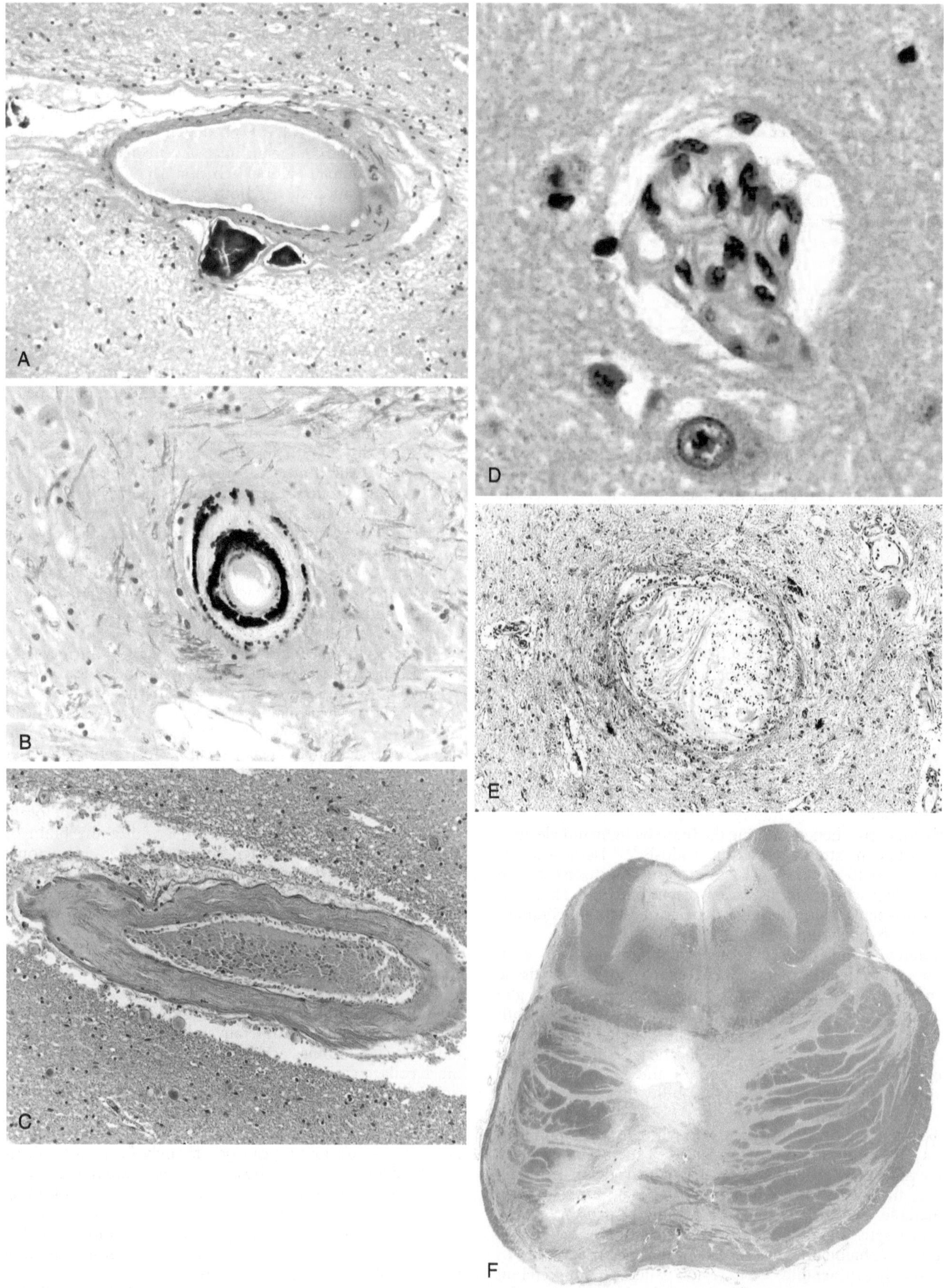

Figure 4-5. Vascular processes that neither break nor block a vessel are asymptomatic. Mönckeberg's medial calcific sclerosis and its variants (A,B) are a prime example. Despite dramatic deposition of calcium, the vessel shows smooth muscle cell nuclei in the tunica media (A), contrasting with the fibrous tunica media (C) that is seen to be acellular. This is preceded by hypertensive arteriolosclerosis, where smooth muscle cells multiply and the vessel at this early stage shows a cellular, tortuous, glomeruloid appearance (D). With continued disease, the arteriole eventually occludes (E), but the dark deposits around the occluded vessel are iron, and show that it has bled as well. Arteriolar occlusion results in lacunes, as seen here in the pons (F), in a location causing ataxia plus hemiparesis.

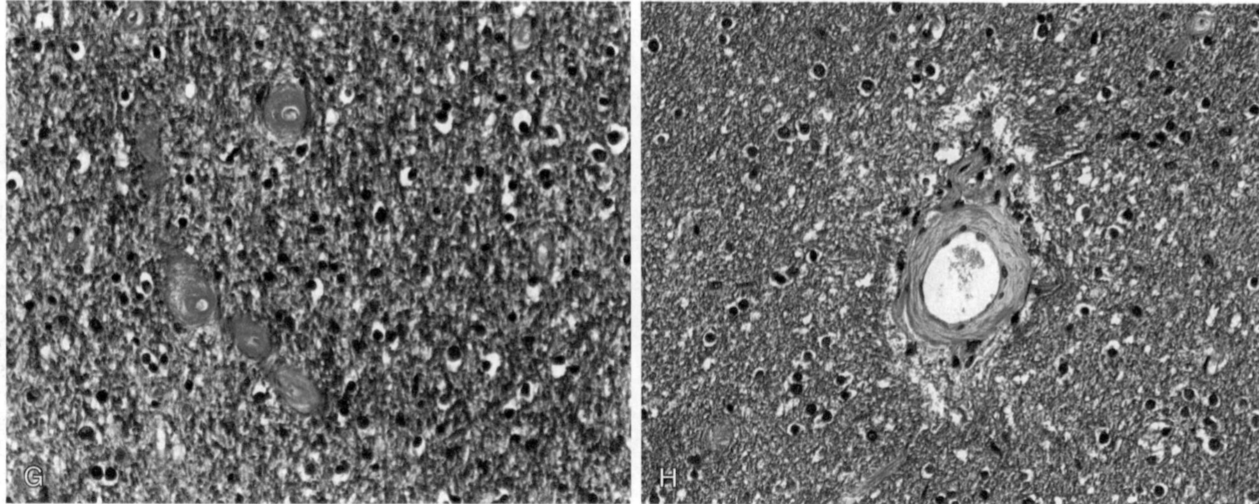

Figure 4-5., cont'd In periventricular white matter, occlusion of small vessels (G) occurs earlier than in larger arterioles (H), as a result of their differing diameters.

Fig. 4-5D) that has been termed arteriolar coils.[25] Similar angioblastic-like nodules of arterioles are found in other organs including the pancreas, kidney and heart of hypertensive patients.[27]

The susceptibility of arterioles to hypertension results from their physiologic role in reducing the blood pressure from arterial levels to pressure levels seen in the capillary bed. Occlusive disease in these small vessels leads to a brain tissue response of formation of small lacunae, rather than large areas of selective neuronal necrosis or pan-necrosis. Lacunes are characteristically seen proximal to arteriolar origins from large vessels and there are three favored locations: basal ganglia, pons (see Fig. 4-5F) and cerebellum, but they can occur elsewhere in the brain and spinal cord. This is quite different from amyloid angiography (Fig. 4-6), where stroke usually occurs distally in the hemisphere, at a distance from the circle of Willis and major cerebral vessels. Hypertensive encephalopathy is covered in detail in Chapter 38.

White Matter Incomplete Infarction

In the posterior hemispheric white matter surrounding the cerebral ventricles, there is often neuroradiologic and pathologic loss of tissue elements seen in elderly patients. Hypertension, intrinsic heart disease or carotid disease[28] may be present and the term "leukoaraiosis" has been applied.[29] These areas, when examined pathologically, show small vessel disease at the arteriolar level (Chapter 27) including arteriolar tortuosities.[30] Subsequently, an occlusive, collagenizing process of arterioles may be seen in the periventricular white matter (see Figs 4-5G,H) that may relate to the white matter change radiologically termed leukoaraiosis, a rarefaction seen around the ventricles.

Of the three branches of arterioles (see Fig. 4-6), it is the smallest which occlude first (see Fig. 4-5H) when collagen is laid down, due to their small diameter. Larger arterioles can be thickened by collagen without occluding.

Diffuse disease in these smallest of vessels gives rise to small infarcts/white matter ischemia, and may contribute to vascular cognitive impairment (Chapter 17).[31,32] The effect of ischemia in the white matter (Chapter 9) causes damage more to myelin than axons, due to axoplasmic flow continuously carrying axoplasm to ischemic areas from non-ischemic zones. A selective demyelination thus represents the early ischemic lesion, but it is the harbinger of the axonal loss that follows with continued or more severe ischemia. The early demyelinative lesion can be thought of as the white matter analog of incomplete infarction of the gray matter. When it eventually gives way to total tissue breakdown involving axons as well, ischemic demyelination can give rise to a radiologic appearance that has been termed leukoaraiosis and Binswanger's disease.[33]

Amyloid Angiopathy

This generally sporadic disease can be conceptualized as a stagnant β-fibrillosis, with impaired egress of amyloid from the brain.[23] This occurs in a complementary distribution to the distribution of hypertensive small vessel disease within the brain. That is to say, the gross pathologic distribution is a negative of the distribution of hypertensive stroke (see Fig. 4-6A), although both give rise to intracranial hemorrhage.[34]

A second major difference from hypertension in this arteriolar disease is the fact that there is less of a tendency for arteriolar occlusion than in hypertension, whereas rupture is a common manifestation of amyloid angiography and hypertension. Amyloid β-fibrils are extremely difficult to remove from the vascular wall after having been produced by secretases in brain parenchyma. The arteriolar rupture is due to the physically brittle nature of a vascular wall whose smooth muscle and elastica have been almost entirely replaced by β-fibril protein. The results of arteriolar death of smooth muscle and mural replacement of mural elastica by other proteins are thus the same, and explain the commonality of hemorrhage (Fig. 4-7A) as a manifestation of both hypertensive and amyloid small vessel brain disease.

The double-stained H & E appearance of arterioles resembles hypertension, in that the vessel wall is replaced by a proteinaceous substance that stains poorly. The replacement of normal tunica media of the arteriole with brittle proteins, results in an arteriole that cannot perform its function of bringing down the blood pressure from that seen in the large

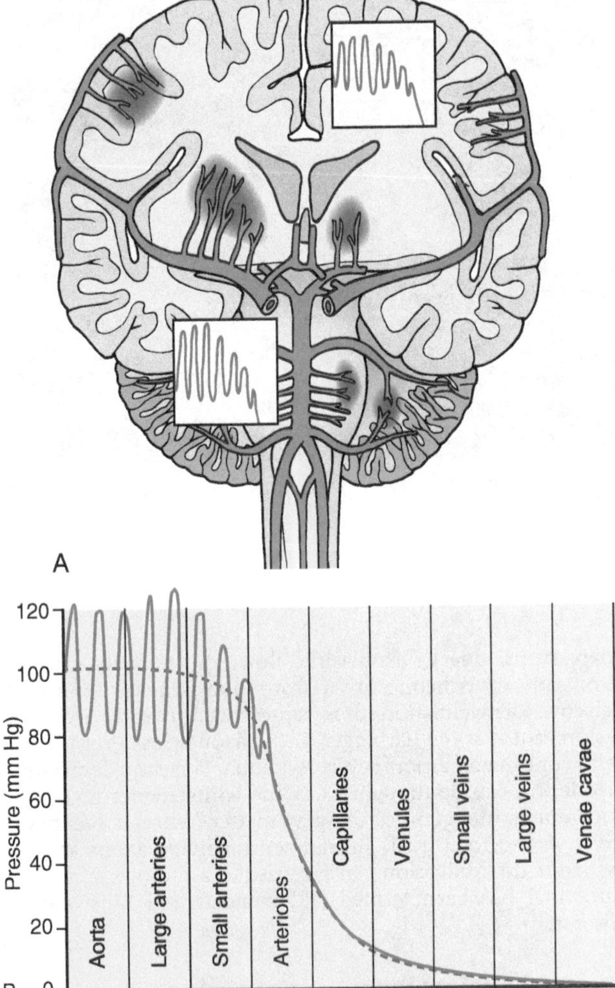

Figure 4-6. Complementary distribution of arteriolar disease due to hypertension and amyloid. Whereas hypertension affects the deep telencephalon and pons/cerebellum, amyloid is deposited further away from the circle of Willis and the vertebrobasilar circulation. The two distributions are inverse negatives of each other (A). Amyloid angiopathy, a stagnant ß-fibrillosis of arteriolar walls, tends to occur far away from the dynamic pressures near the circle of Willis and the vertebrobasilar system (outside dashed line), whereas hypertensive disease predominates near the high-pressure origin of vessels ventral to the brain (inside dashed line). Blood pressure and pulse pressure are both higher at physical locations closer to the brain's ventral vessels (B) and arterioles are located within the circulation where these pressures are reduced. *(Adapted with permission from Qureshi AI, et al. Spontaneous intracerebral hemorrhage.* N Engl J Med *344: 1450–1460, 2001.)*

arteries to the low pressure of the capillary bed (Fig. 4-6B), nor perform the autoregulatory function in regulating CBF.

CADASIL

Cerebral autosomal dominant arteriopathy with subcortical infarcts and leukoencephalopathy (CADASIL) is actually an arteriolopathy that presents as dementia and white matter infarcts, due to a variety of mutations in the notch 3 gene.[35] It can be a very difficult diagnosis to make, clinically, especially with a psychiatric presentation.[36] Detailed coverage is given in Chapter 41. CADASIL gives rise to a leukoencephalopathic picture macroscopically and often few focal lesions on gross brain examination (Fig. 4-7F). Ultrastructurally, it is characterized by accumulation of granular osmiophilic material in the tunica media of arterioles, which eventually kills the smooth muscle cells. CADASIL (together with amyloid angiopathy) can be conceptualized as a protein elimination failure angiopathy.[23]

Arteriolar occlusion in CADASIL gives rise to lacunar infarcts (Fig. 4-7G) characteristically located in the white matter, and ischemic demyelination, discussed above. Small vessels are selectively vulnerable to occlusion (Fig. 4-7H).

In comparing hypertension, amyloid angiopathy and CADASIL, we note that all three arteriolar diseases occlude the smallest vessels most easily, due to their smaller initial diameter. These final arteriolar branches lie just proximal to the capillary circulation. Occlusion of these 40-µm-sized vessels located just proximal to the microcirculation, adds a component of ischemia with each microvascular occlusion, to the respective disease process. All three diseases replace smooth muscle of the tunica media with a protein, chiefly collagen in hypertension,[26] amyloid in cerebral amyloid angiopathy and Notch 3 protein in CADASIL.

TISSUE RESPONSE TO THERAPY OF CEREBRAL ISCHEMIA

In addition to the brain response to ischemia, we briefly consider the tissue response to therapy and reperfusion. An explosion of knowledge in the therapy of cerebral ischemia has occurred recently (see section VI), and influences the final pathology of a stroke. Thrombolysis (Chapter 51) is often successful in salvaging neocortex but not the underlying striatum, due to its end-arterial supply. Although a recent, intense investigative era using small animal models yielded promising pharmacologic agents, these have generally not translated into human use. The most successful therapy presently available is not pharmacotherapy but reperfusion therapy.[37] While it remains obvious that reperfusion is needed to restore ischemic tissue at risk, concerns over injury due to reperfusion have been expressed. While tissue reperfusion injury is accepted and the theoretical basis for possible concerns associated with a toxicity of reperfusion appears sound, there is little evidence that the pathology of an infarct is augmented by reperfusion after transient ischemia. Indeed, it can be experimentally shown that reperfusion, even with high oxygen, seems to reduce, not augment, infarct size.[38] This obtains even if hyperoxemia is limited to the reperfusion period.[39] There is also little evidence from the pathology of human ischemic stroke that early reperfusion should be avoided as a therapeutic maneuver, at whatever blood oxygen levels. Since ischemic brain injury intrinsically involves and has a time course of maturation, it is easy to mistake the natural maturation of the injury process for an exacerbating injury, when in reality, augmentation of infarct size by reperfusion is not actually taking place.

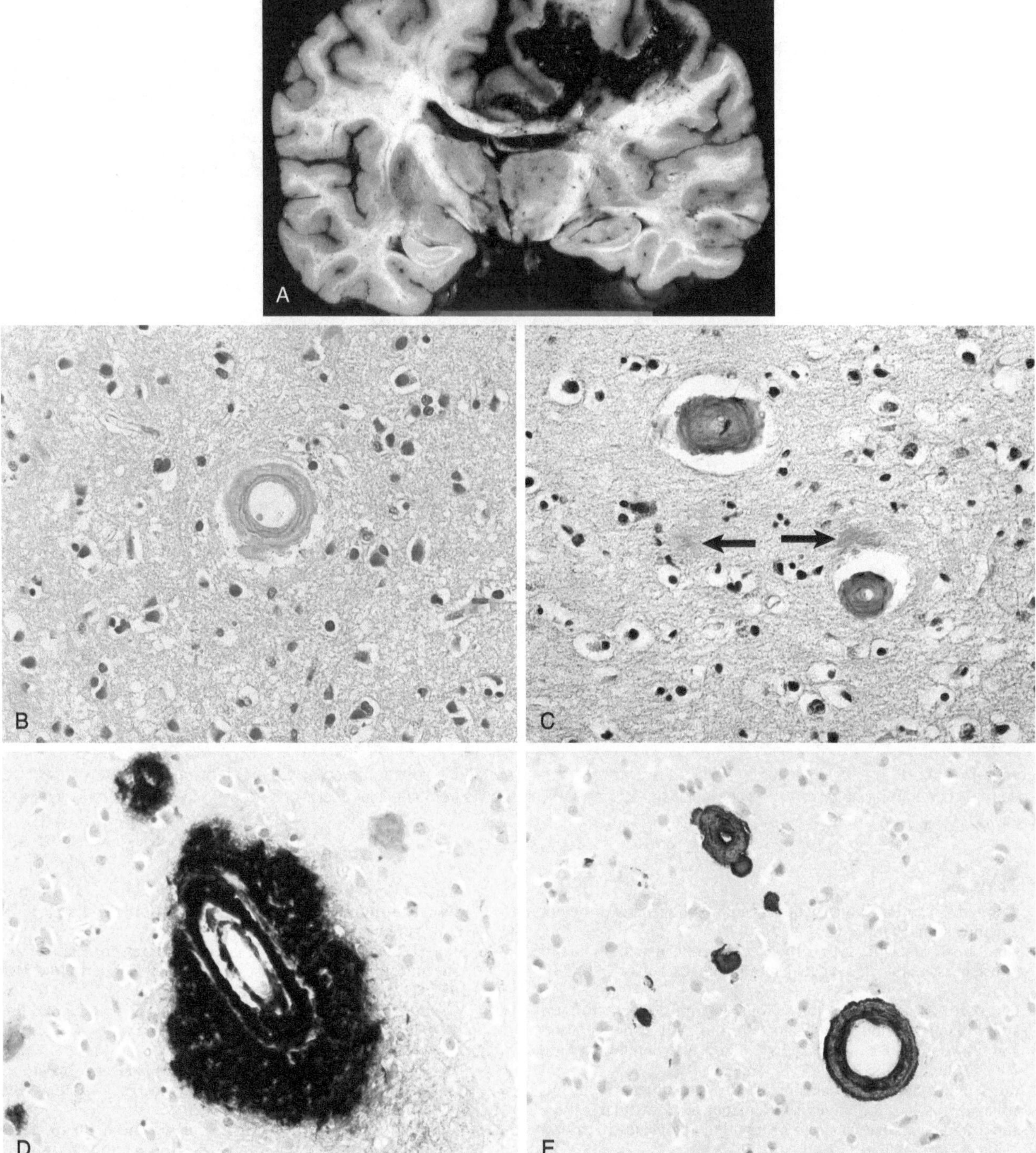

Figure 4-7. Pathology of stroke in amyloidosis and CADASIL. Amyloid gives rise to superficial hemorrhages, far away from the high-pressure arterial circulation supplying the brain, as seen (A) in this 78-year-old woman who suffered a hemiparesis during the night. The vessel microscopically resembles hypertension in being acellular and having the medial smooth muscle cells replaced (B). More sensitive is Congo red (C), which here reveals amyloid in the neuropil (arrows) surrounding the vessels thickened with amyloid. Most sensitive is immunohistochemistry, which reveals massive obstruction of amyloid egress from brain parenchyma into the vessel, resulting in accumulation not only in the vessel, but the surrounding Virchow-Robin space and even the neuropil (D). Mural thickening with amyloid occludes smaller vessels more easily than larger arterioles, due to their smaller diameter (E).

Continued

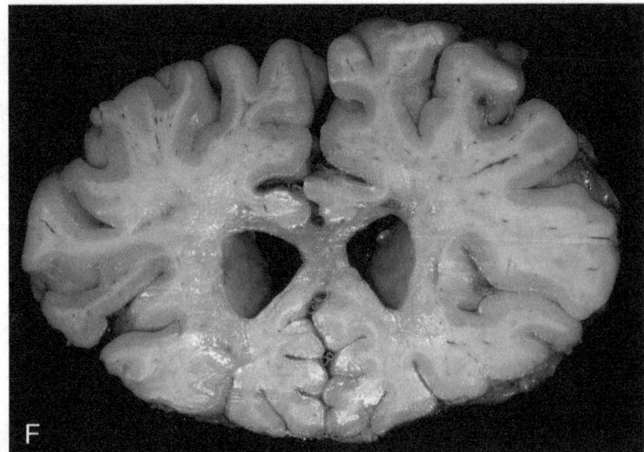

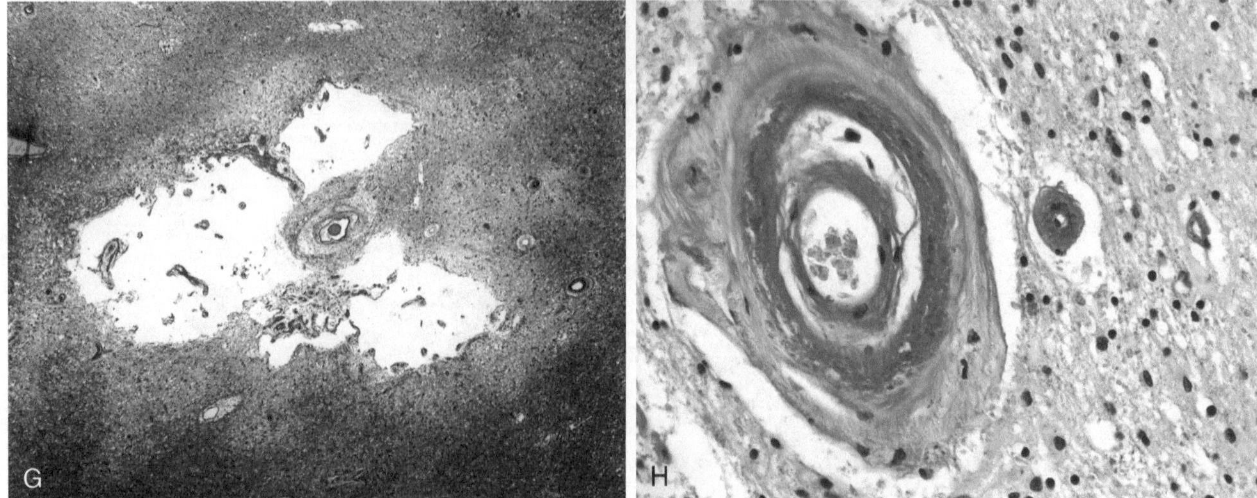

Figure 4-7., cont'd The white matter in CADASIL is diffusely moth-eaten, and is seen to be collapsed and brown in the genu of the corpus callosum (F), due to multiple ischemic lesions including lacunes (G). This results from arteriolar occlusions affecting the smallest branches selectively (H).

REFERENCES

1. Bladin CF, Chambers BR. Frequency and pathogenesis of hemodynamic stroke. Stroke 1994;25:2179–82.
2. Guidoux C, Mazighi M, Lavallée P, et al. Aortic arch atheroma in transient ischemic attack patients old. Atherosclerosis 2013;231: 124–8.
3. European Carotid Plaque Study Group. Reprinted article "Carotid artery plaque composition–relationship to clinical presentation and ultrasound B-mode imaging". Eur J Vasc Endovasc Surg 2011;42(Suppl. 1):S32–8.
4. van Lammeren GW, Pasterkamp G, de Vries JP, et al. Platelets enter atherosclerotic plaque via intraplaque microvascular leakage and intraplaque hemorrhage: a histopathological study in carotid plaques. Atherosclerosis 2012;222:355–9.
5. Hosseini AA, Kandiyil N, Macsweeney ST, et al. Carotid plaque hemorrhage on magnetic resonance imaging strongly predicts recurrent ischemia and stroke. Ann Neurol 2013;73: 774–84.
6. The Canadian Cooperative Study Group. A randomized trial of aspirin and sulfinpyrazone in threatened stroke. N Engl J Med 1978;299:53–9.
7. Wong KS, Chen C, Fu J, et al. CLAIR Study Investigators. Clopidogrel plus aspirin versus aspirin alone for reducing embolisation in patients with acute symptomatic cerebral or carotid artery stenosis (CLAIR study): a randomised, open-label, blinded-endpoint trial. Lancet Neurol 2010;9:489–97.
8. Almekhlafi MA, Hu WY, Hill MD, et al. Calcification and endothelialization of thrombi in acute stroke. Ann Neurol 2008;64: 344–8.
9. Auer RN, Jensen ML, Whishaw IQ. Neurobehavioral deficit due to ischemic brain damage limited to half of the CA1 sector of the hippocampus. J Neurosci 1989;9:1641–7.
10. Kraig RP, Petito CK, Plum F, et al. Hydrogen ions kill brain at concentrations reached in ischemia. J Cereb Blood Flow Metab 1987;7:379–86.
11. Ekholm A, Katsura K, Siesjö BK. Tissue lactate content and tissue PCO_2 in complete brain ischaemia: implications for compartmentation of H+. Neurol Res 1991;13:74–6.
12. Bakay L, Lee JC. The effect of acute hypoxia and hypercapnia on the ultrastructure of the central nervous system. Brain 1968;91:697–709.
13. Paljärvi L, Söderfeldt B, Kalimo H, et al. The brain in extreme respiratory acidosis. A light- and electron-microscopic study in the rat. Acta Neuropathol (Berl) 1982;58:87–94.
14. Kalimo H, Rehncrona S, Söderfeldt H, et al. Brain lactic acidosis and ischemic cell damage. 2. Histopathology. J Cereb Blood Flow Metab 1981;1:313–27.
15. Kristián T, Gidö G, Siesjö BK. The influence of acidosis on hypoglycemic brain damage. J Cereb Blood Flow Metab 1995; 15:78–87.
16. Monaghan DT, Cotman CW. Distribution of N-methyl-D-aspartate-sensitive L-[3H]glutamate-binding sites in rat brain. J Neurosci 1985;5:2909–19.
17. Garcia JH, Lassen NA, Weiller C, et al. Ischemic stroke and incomplete infarction. Stroke 1996;27:761–5.
18. Houser CR, Vaughn JE, Barber RP, et al. GABA neurons are the major cell type of the nucleus reticularis thalami. Brain Res 1980;200:341–54.

19. Smith ML, Auer RN, Siesjö BK. The density and distribution of ischemic brain injury in the rat following 2–10 min of forebrain ischemia. Acta Neuropathol (Berl) 1984;64:319–32.
20. Ross DT, Graham DI. Selective loss and selective sparing of neurons in the thalamic reticular nucleus following human cardiac arrest. J Cereb Blood Flow Metab 1993;13:558–67.
21. Schwartz-Bloom RD, Sah R. gamma-Aminobutyric acid(A) neurotransmission and cerebral ischemia. J Neurochem 2001;77: 353–71.
22. Micheletti RG, Fishbein GA, Currier JS, et al. Mönckeberg sclerosis revisited: a clarification of the histologic definition of Mönckeberg sclerosis. Arch Pathol Lab Med 2008;132:43–7.
23. Carare RO, Hawkes CA, Jeffrey M, et al. Review: cerebral amyloid angiopathy, prion angiopathy, CADASIL and the spectrum of protein elimination failure angiopathies (PEFA) in neurodegenerative disease with a focus on therapy. Neuropathol Appl Neurobiol 2013;39:593–611.
24. Fisher CM. The arterial lesions underlying lacunes. Acta Neuropathol (Berl) 1969;12:1–15.
25. Challa VR, Moody DM, Bell MA. The Charcôt-Bouchard aneurysm controversy: impact of a new histologic technique. J Neuropathol Exp Neurol 1992;51:264–71.
26. Kojima H, Eguchi H, Mizutani T, et al. Three-dimensional analysis of pathological characteristics of a microaneurysm. Clin Neuropathol 2007;26:74–9.
27. Hughson MD, Harley RA, Henninger GR. Cellular arteriolar nodules. Their presence in heart, pancreas, and kidneys of patients with malignant nephrosclerosis. Arch Pathol Lab Med 1982;106: 71–4.
28. Altaf N, Morgan PS, Moody A, et al. Brain white matter hyperintensities are associated with carotid intraplaque hemorrhage. Radiology 2008;248:202–9.
29. Norrving B. Leucoaraiosis and silent subcortical infarcts. Rev Neurol (Paris) 2008;164:801–4.
30. Spangler KM, Challa VR, Moody DM, et al. Arteriolar tortuosity of the white matter in aging and hypertension. A microradiographic study. J Neuropathol Exp Neurol 1994;53:22–6.
31. Manolio TA, Olson J, Longstreth WT. Hypertension and cognitive function: pathophysiologic effects of hypertension on the brain. Curr Hypertens Rep 2003;5:255–61.
32. Pantoni L. Cerebral small vessel disease: from pathogenesis and clinical characteristics to therapeutic challenges. Lancet Neurol 2010;9:689–701.
33. Kelley RE. Ischemic demyelination. Neurol Res 2006;28: 334–40.
34. Sutherland GR, Auer RN. Primary intracerebral hemorrhage. J Clin Neurosci 2006;13:511–17.
35. Kalaria RN, Viitanen M, Kalimo H, et al. The pathogenesis of CADASIL: an update. J Neurol Sci 2004;226:35–9.
36. Valenti R, Poggesi A, Pescini F, et al. Psychiatric disturbances in CADASIL: a brief review. Acta Neurol Scand 2008;118:291–5.
37. Mazighi M, Amarenco P. Reperfusion therapy in acute cerebrovascular syndrome. Curr Opin Neurol 2011;24:59–62.
38. Singhal AB, Wang X, Sumii T, et al. Effects of normobaric hyperoxia in a rat model of focal cerebral ischemia-reperfusion. J Cereb Blood Flow Metab 2002;22:861–8.
39. Flynn EP, Auer RN. Eubaric hyperoxemia and experimental cerebral infarction. Ann Neurol 2002;52:566–72.

5 Molecular and Cellular Mechanisms of Ischemia-Induced Neuronal Death

Haiyue Zhang, Dimitry Ofengeim, Yejie Shi, Feng Zhang, Jee-Yeon Hwang, Jun Chen, R. Suzanne Zukin

KEY POINTS

- Emerging role of RIP1- and RIP3-regulated necroptosis in ischemic cell death.
- Both glutamate excitotoxicity and non-excitotoxic mechanisms trigger ischemic cell death.
- Ca^{2+}: key signal in ischemic neuronal death.
- Epigenetic dysregulation contributes to ischemic cell death.
- Modulation of microglia/macrophage polarization as a new therapy.

Cerebral ischemia is a severe clinical condition in which the blood flow to the brain is insufficient due to a narrowing or occlusion of the arterial blood vessel or low blood flow supply. Cerebral ischemia can be divided into two types, global ischemia and focal ischemia, both of which are detailed below.

GLOBAL ISCHEMIA

Transient global ischemia affects approximately 200,000 Americans annually.[1] It is usually triggered by cardiac arrest, cardiac surgery, profuse bleeding, near-drowning, or carbon monoxide poisoning. In most cases, global ischemia causes selective, delayed neuronal death, which leads to serious cognitive deficits. Hippocampal CA1 neurons are particularly vulnerable. Other neurons that can be damaged include medium aspiny neurons of the striatum, pyramidal neurons in neocortical layers II, V, and VI, and Purkinje neurons of the cerebellum.

FOCAL ISCHEMIA

Focal ischemia in humans is most commonly caused by ischemic stroke due to a vascular occlusion in the cerebral circulation.[1–4] It is the fourth leading cause of death in the US and the primary cause of disabilities in adults. Of the approximately 600,000 new victims each year, nearly 30% die and 20–30% become severely and permanently disabled. Neurological deficits resulting from focal ischemia include paralysis and abnormalities in co-ordination, sensory function, and language ability.

The tissues at risk are at the core or center of the stroke, which contains cells that are highly dependent on blood from the blocked artery but receive essentially no blood, and the penumbra or surrounding region, which contains cells that receive some blood from other arteries.[5] Cells in the core die from several overwhelming causes and probably cannot be salvaged by any treatment short of immediate clot removal. Although the infarct starts in the core, at its maximum it encompasses both the core and penumbra, generally by 6–24 hours after induction of permanent ischemia.[5] The duration of the ischemic episode determines the extent or grade of damage, which is assessed 1–2 days after reperfusion.[6] At 10–20 minutes after induction of focal ischemia, only a few scattered dead neurons are observed in the core. At 1 hour, infarct is observed in the core, and the infarct size is maximal. The mechanisms underlying death of cells in the core are complicated, but they most certainly include glutamate receptor-mediated necrotic cell death (see below).

EXPERIMENTAL MODELS OF GLOBAL AND FOCAL ISCHEMIA

Models of Global Ischemia

Global ischemia can be produced by permanent occlusion of the vertebral arteries and transient occlusion of the common carotid arteries (in rats) or by transient occlusion of the common carotid arteries (in gerbils and mice), followed by reperfusion.[7] The most commonly used models of global ischemia are (1) the four-vessel occlusion (4-VO) model in rats (Fig. 5-1A);[8,9] (2) the two-vessel occlusion (2-VO, also known as temporary bilateral common carotid occlusion or BCCO) model in gerbils[10] or in mice;[11,12] and (3) two-vessel occlusion (2-VO) in combination with hypotension in rats.[7,13] Global ischemia can also be induced in large mammals including monkeys,[14] goats,[15] and pigs.[16] The duration of global ischemia is typically short – in the order of 5–20 minutes. During the ischemic episode, blood flow to the entire brain is immediately reduced to <1% and remains blocked until reperfusion. As a consequence, adenosine triphosphate (ATP) is depleted in cells throughout the brain, but recovers to near-physiologic levels by the time of reperfusion (see below).

Four-VO in rats provides a well-established and widely used model of global ischemia in which neuronal death is largely restricted to pyramidal neurons of the hippocampal CA1 and does not manifest itself until 3 days after insult.[8,9] Briefly, the vertebral arteries of rats are exposed and subjected to permanent electrocauterization. The common carotid arteries are exposed and isolated with a 3-0 silk thread, and the wound is sutured. Twenty-four hours later, the wound is reopened and the common carotid arteries are subjected to temporary occlusion with surgical clasps (4 minutes for sublethal ischemia and 10 minutes for global ischemia). When the carotid arteries are occluded, blood flow is typically reduced to less than 3% of normal in the hippocampus, striatum, and neocortex.[9]

Models of Focal Ischemia

Focal ischemia is the animal model that most closely approximates stroke or cerebral infarction in humans.[17] It is typically performed on rats and mice and is produced experimentally by occlusion of the middle cerebral artery (MCAO). Arterial

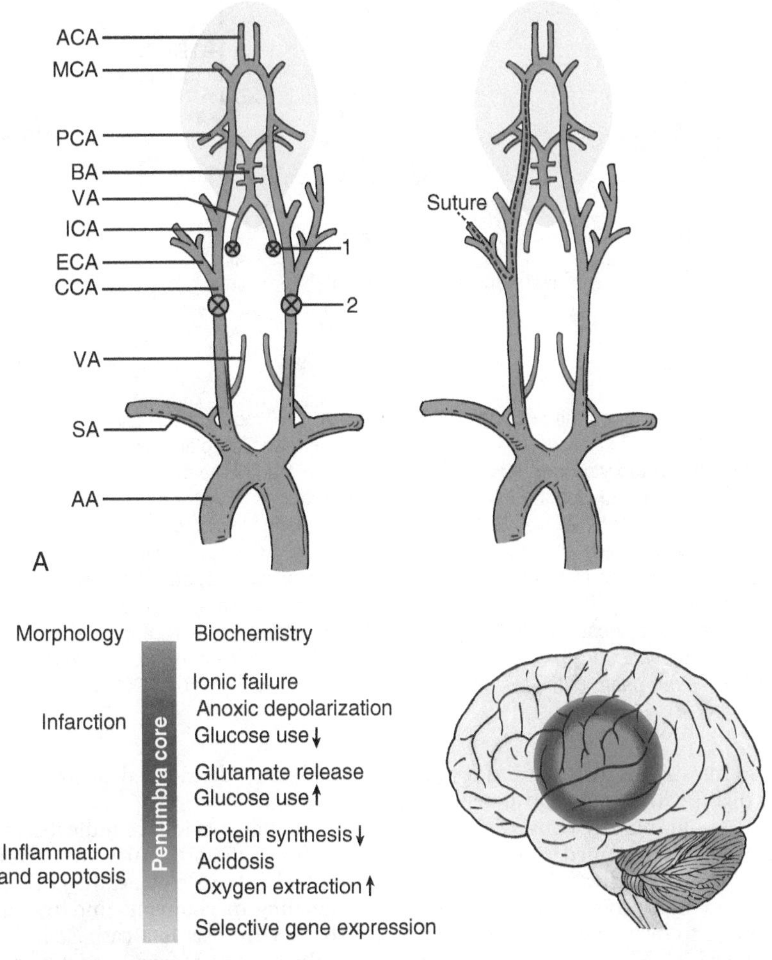

Figure 5-1. Experimental models of global and focal ischemia. A, Diagram of the cerebrovascular anatomy of the rat, illustrating the permanent electrocauterization of the vertebral arteries (1) and the position of the surgical clips in the common carotid arteries (2) in 4-VO model (left) and the intraluminal suture during occlusion in the temporary focal ischemia model (right). AA, Arch of the aorta; ACA, anterior cerebral artery; BA, basilar artery; CCA, common carotid artery; ECA, external carotid artery; ICA, internal carotid artery; MCA, middle cerebral artery; PCA, posterior cerebral artery; SA, subclavian artery; VA, vertebral artery. B, The core and penumbra of ischemia are induced by focal blockade of cerebral arteries. A brain region of low perfusion in which cells have lost their membrane potential terminally ("core") is surrounded by an area in which intermediate perfusion prevails ("penumbra") and cells depolarize intermittently ("peri-infarct depolarization"). Note that from the onset of the focal perfusion deficit, the core and penumbra are dynamic in space and time. Perfusion thresholds exist below which certain biochemical functions are impeded (color-coded scale). *(A, Adapted from Longa EZ, Weinstein PR, Carlson S, et al: Reversible middle cerebral artery occlusion without craniectomy in rats.* Stroke *20:84–91, 1989. B, Reprinted with permission from Dirnagl U, Iadecola C, Moskowitz MA: Pathobiology of ischaemic stroke: an integrated view.* Trends Neurosci *22:391–397, 1999.)*

occlusion can be permanent (i.e., the arterial blockade is maintained throughout the experiment) or temporary (the occlusion is for up to 3 hours, followed by reperfusion) and is either proximal or distal (see below). These procedures induce a necrotic core of cells that are irreversibly damaged and a penumbra of cells that can be revived (Fig. 5-1B).

Proximal MCAO is most commonly induced by ligation of the common carotid and external carotid arteries, followed by insertion of a suture into the internal carotid artery. The coding part of the suture is supposed to be beyond the origin of the posterior communicating artery and past the origin of the MCA.[18] The center of the core is the region in which blood flow is reduced to less than 15% and encompasses the lateral portion of the caudate putamen, and the parietal cortex. The penumbra, the region in which blood flow is reduced to less than 40%, encompasses the remainder of the neocortex, the entorhinal cortex, and medial caudate-putamen. In distal MCAO, blood flow to the basal ganglia is not interrupted and damage is restricted to the neocortex. This type of occlusion can be induced surgically with a clip or thrombotic clots in combination with transient unilateral occlusion of the common carotid arteries.[19,20] The reduction of blood flow in the core and penumbra is similar to that in the proximal model.

Hypoxia/Ischemia

This ischemic model involves transient unilateral occlusion of the common carotid artery in combination with systemic hypoxia, such that oxygen flow to the brain is reduced to 3% in adults or to 8% in neonates.[21,22] After 15–30 minutes of hypoxia, infarct occurs in the cortex, striatum, and hippocampus.

MODALITIES OF ISCHEMIC CELL DEATH

Injurious stimuli such as ischemic insults activate multiple death cascades. There are three main classifications of

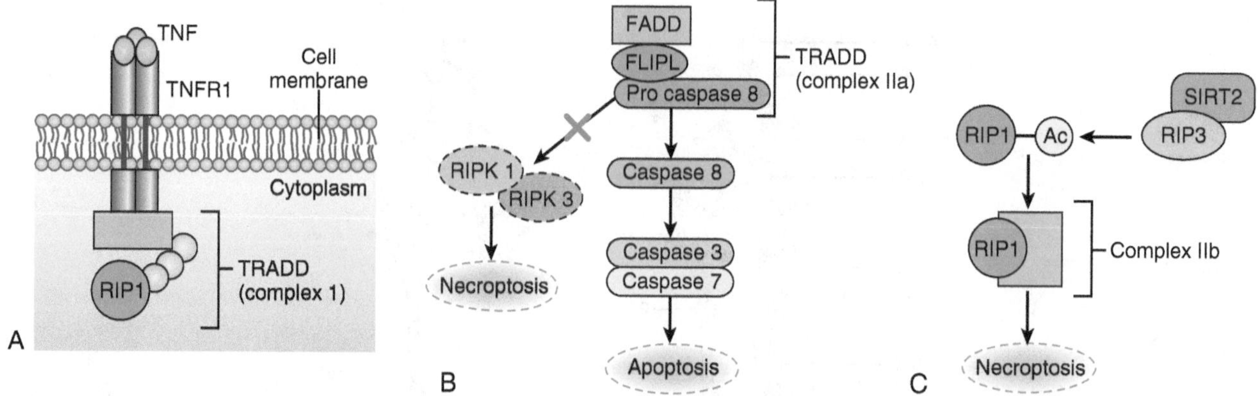

Figure 5-2. Regulation of necroptosis and formation of death complexes. A, TNF receptor-associated death domain (TRADD) is formed upon binding of tumor necrosis factor (TNF) and TNF receptor 1 (TNFR1), which is termed Complex I. The death domain receptors engage intracellular signaling cascades that activate the obligatory serine/threonine kinase RIP1. RIP1 activates the NF-κB signaling pathway to promote cell survival and inflammation. B–C, Complex II, which includes the FAS associated death domain (FADD), RIPK3, FLIPs, and procaspase 8, determines cell apoptosis (Complex IIa) and necroptosis (Complex IIb). B. In Complex IIa, the long isotype of FLIP (FLIPL) and procaspase 8 inactivate RIPK1 and RIPK3 by forming a heterodimeric caspase, thereby preventing necroptosis. Complex IIa also results in apoptosis by activating caspase 8, which mediates the executioner caspases 3 and 7 signaling pathways. C, In Complex IIb, acetylated RIP1 dissociates from Complex I to form an unstable connection between RIP1 and RIP3. The interaction with deacetylase enzyme sirtuin-2 (SIRT2) and RIP3 is required to deacetylate RIP1. Deacetylated RIP1 becomes a prominent part of Complex IIb, directly leading to necroptosis. *(Adapted from Zhou W and Yuan J: Cell biology: Death by deacetylation. Nature 492:194–195, 2012. Vanden Berghe T, Linkermann A, Jouan-Lanhouet S, et al: Regulated necrosis: the expanding network of non-apoptotic cell death pathways.* Nat Rev Mol Cell Biol *15(2):135–147, 2014.)*

mammalian cell death: apoptosis, necrosis, and autophagy, each of which exhibits a distinct histologic and biochemical signature.[23] Apoptosis is an evolutionarily conserved process of cell death by an internally programmed series of events mediated by a dedicated set of gene products.[23-26] Necrosis was traditionally thought to be a non-programmed, accidental form of cell death in response to overwhelming stress that is incompatible with cell survival.[23,25] However, recent evidence indicates that necrosis can also be tightly regulated and that cells such as neurons can die by a form of necrosis, termed necroptosis or regulated necrosis.[27-29] Necroptosis is characterized morphologically by cell swelling and eventual rupture, which releases contents into the surroundings, thus triggering inflammation.[30] The signaling pathways of necroptosis intersect with the regulation of apoptosis.[31] Autophagy is a catabolic process in which cells generate energy and metabolites by digesting their own organelles and macromolecules via the lysosomal pathway.[23,32] It is a tightly regulated process that is essential to embryonic development, tissue homeostasis, and cell survival, helping to maintain a balance between the synthesis, degradation, and subsequent recycling of cellular products.[33] Autophagy is protective in that it allows an energy-deprived cell to survive during starvation by reallocating nutrients from unnecessary processes to more essential activities; however, it also functions in dying cells to mediate cell death.[34] Increasing evidence indicates that inducing autophagy confers neuroprotection against global ischemia;[35] however, a role for autophagy in ischemic injury is largely unknown.[4,30,33]

Necrosis

Necrotic cell death, or necrosis, is morphologically characterized by cell swelling (oncosis) that culminates in the rupture of the plasma membrane, swelling of mitochondria and other organelles, loss of integrity of the plasma membrane, and subsequent loss (disorganized dismantling) of intracellular contents.[30] The nucleus exhibits pyknosis and irregular clumping of the chromatin (peripheral chromatolysis), a pattern that contrasts sharply with the sparse, regularly shaped and uniformly distributed aggregates of chromatin observed in apoptosis.[25]

Emerging evidence indicates that necroptosis, which exhibits both characteristics of necrosis and apoptosis, plays a pivotal role in cell death. Little is known about the precise signaling mechanisms underlying the induction of necroptosis. Necroptosis is a caspase-independent necrotic cell death pathway that is regulated by receptor interacting protein 1 (RIP1) kinase and its downstream mediator RIP3 kinase.[36] Among the proposed necroptosis signaling pathways, the TNF-TNFR1-mediated pathway is the most prominent. Briefly, upon binding of tumor necrosis factor (TNF) and TNF receptor 1 (TNFR1), TNF receptor-associated death domain (TRADD) is formed, which is termed Complex I. Then, the death domain receptors engage intracellular signaling cascades that activate the obligatory serine/threonine kinase known as RIP1.[37] RIP1 activates the nuclear factor (NF)-κB signaling pathway to promote cell survival and inflammation (Fig. 5-2A).[38] The FAS associated death domain (FADD), RIPK3, FLIPs, and procaspase 8 form Complex II, which regulates both apoptosis (Complex IIa) and necroptosis (Complex IIb).[39] In Complex IIa, the long isotype of FLIP ($FLIP_L$) and procaspase 8 inactivate RIPK1 and RIPK3 by forming a heterodimeric caspase, thus preventing necroptosis. Meanwhile, Complex IIa results in apoptosis by activating caspase 8, which mediates the executioner caspases 3 and 7 signaling pathways (Fig. 5-2B).

In Complex IIb, acetylated RIP1 dissociates from Complex I to form an unstable connection between RIP1 and RIP3. However, studies indicate the interaction with deacetylase enzyme sirtuin-2 (SIRT2) and RIP3 is required to deacetylate RIP1. Deacetylated RIP1 becomes a prominent part of Complex IIb, which directly leads to necroptosis (Fig. 5-2C).[38,40] Activated RIP3 can steer TNF-induced apoptosis toward necroptosis or even full-blown necrosis, in part through disruption of energy metabolism, generation of reactive oxygen species (ROS) and nitroxidative stress by nitric acid,[4,41] increases in intracellular Ca^{2+}, activation of Ca^{2+}-dependent, non-caspase proteases such as calpains and cathepsins, activation

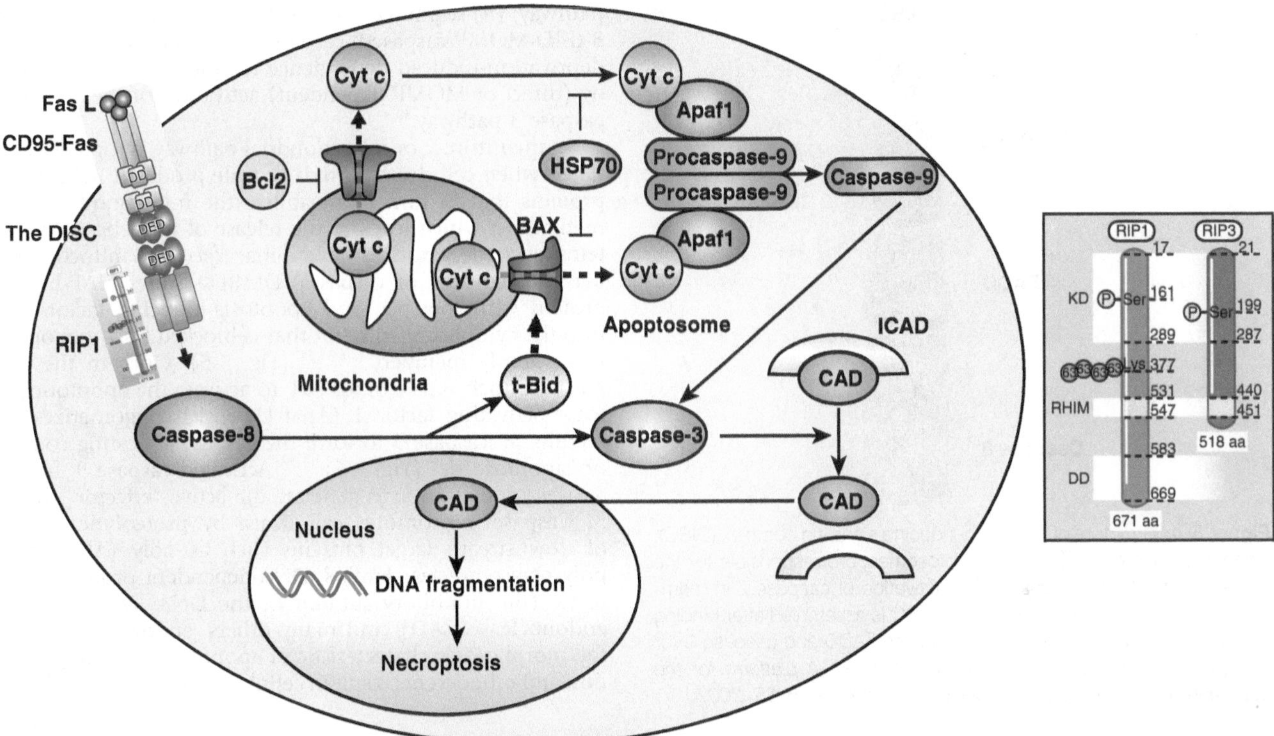

Figure 5-3. The extrinsic or death receptor pathway of caspase activation. In the extrinsic or death receptor-dependent pathway, apoptosis is triggered by stimulation of CD95-Fas, a member of the tumor necrosis factor (TNF) receptor–nerve growth factor superfamily of death domain receptors that includes TNF receptor 1 (TNFR1), CD95-Fas, and the TRAIL receptor. Within seconds of activation, CD95-Fas (receptor for CD95-Fas ligand) forms a cytosolic death-inducing signaling complex (DISC), which recruits procaspase 8. DISC activates procaspase 8 to generate the "instigator" caspase 8. The extrinsic pathway can connect to the intrinsic pathway when caspase 8 cleaves the Bcl-2 family protein Bid to generate truncated tBid, which translocates to the mitochondria where it initiates permeabilization of the outer mitochondrial membrane and the mitochondrial apoptotic pathways. In addition, caspase 8 activates the effector caspases 3, 6, and 7, which promote proteolytic cleavage and destruction of an array of cellular targets, including DNases, paving the way for apoptotic cell death. Arrows indicate the activation of the targets, whereas lines with blunt ends indicate their inactivation. *(Adapted from Vandenabeele P, Declercq W, Van Herreweghe F, et al: The role of the kinases RIP1 and RIP3 in TNF-induced necrosis. Sci Signal 3(115):re4, 2010. Zimmermann KC, Bonzon C, Green DR: The machinery of programmed cell death.* Pharmacol Ther *92:57–70, 2001.)*

of cyclophilin D, opening of the mitochondrial membrane transition pore, and mitochondrial release of poly(adenosine diphosphate [ADP]-ribose)polymerase-1 (PARP-1).[42–44]

In the final stage of necrotic cell death, swollen cells are internalized by a process known as macropinocytosis, in which only parts of the cell are taken up by phagocytes.[27] Necrosis is currently believed to be the predominant form of neuronal death in models of focal ischemia and ischemic stroke in humans.[4] Genetic ablation of cyclophilin D, which abolishes necrotic cell death,[45–47] or pharmacologic inhibition of necrosis by necrostatin 1 (Nec-1), a small-molecule inhibitor of RIP1,[48] affords a significant reduction of infarct volume and improves neurologic outcome in animal models of focal ischemia. These observations implicate RIP1 as a potential therapeutic target in ischemic stroke.

Apoptosis

The Caspase Death Cascade

Caspases are a family of structurally related cysteine proteases and are the executioners of apoptosis.[25] The human genome encodes 13–14 distinct caspases; of these, caspases 2, 3, 6, 7, 8, 9, and 10 predominantly function in cell death, whereas the others are involved in regulating immune responses.[49] Caspases are classified as "initiator caspases" (caspases 2, 8, 9, and 10), which integrate upstream apoptotic stimuli, and "effector caspases" (caspases 3, 6, and 7), which are activated by initiator caspases and cleave an array of diverse cellular targets.

The caspase cascade can be activated by either extrinsic or intrinsic pathways. In the extrinsic or death receptor-dependent pathway, apoptosis is initiated when injurious stimuli such as ischemia lead to activation of CD95-Fas, a member of the TNF receptor–nerve growth factor superfamily of death domain receptors that includes TNFR1, CD95-Fas, and TRAIL receptor[37,50,51] (Fig. 5-3). Within seconds of activation, CD95-Fas (receptor for CD95-Fas ligand) forms a cytosolic DISC (death-inducing signaling complex), known as Complex II, also consisting of the adapter proteins TRADD and FADD, which act via their death domains to bind CD95-Fas and via their death effector domain to recruit procaspase 8 (Fig. 5-4).[37,50–52] DISC may also contain additional cofactors and regulatory proteins such as c-FLIP. DISC catalyzes the cleavage and inactivation of RIP1 and RIP3 and activation of procaspase 8 to generate the "instigator" caspase 8. The extrinsic pathway can connect to the intrinsic pathway when caspase 8 cleaves the Bcl-2 family protein Bid to generate truncated tBid, which translocates to the mitochondria, where it initiates permeabilization of the outer mitochondrial membrane and initiates the mitochondrial pathway of apoptosis. The extrinsic pathway may activate a caspase-dependent cell death execution pathway via one of the following routes: (i) death receptor-mediated and -triggered caspase-8 (or -10)-caspase-3

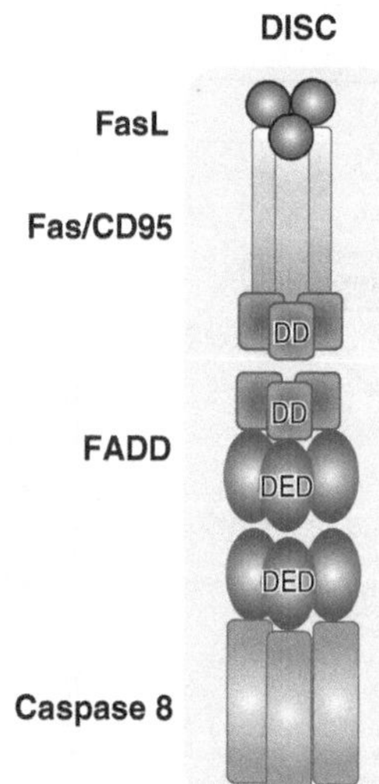

Figure 5-4. Structure of the death-inducing signaling complex (DISC). Adapter protein complexes, or apoptosomes, are responsible for the activation of initiator caspases. The activation of caspase 2 in mammalian cells is mediated by the DISC. DISC is assembled after binding of death ligand to its receptor and contains FADD and caspase 8 (or 10). *(Adapted from Bao Q, Shi Y: Apoptosome: A platform for the activation of initiator caspases.* Cell Death Differ *14:56–65, 2007.)*

pathway; (ii) death receptor-mediated and -triggered caspase-8-tBID-MOMP-caspase-9-caspase-3 pathway; or (iii) ligand deprivation-induced dependence receptor signaling followed by (direct or MOMP-dependent) activation of the caspase-9-caspase-3 pathway.[30]

In the intrinsic or mitochondrial pathway, apoptosis is initiated when cell death stimuli activate prodeath Bcl-2 family proteins that in turn permeabilize the mitochondrial outer membrane, which leads to the release of mitochondrial proteins such as cytochrome *c*, Smac (second mitochondria-derived activator of caspases)/DIABLO (direct IAP-binding protein with low pI), and apoptosis-inducing factor (AIF) into the cytoplasm, an event that is blocked by antiapoptotic Bcl-2 family members[25,26,53,54] (Fig. 5-5). Once in the cytoplasm, cytochrome *c* binds ATP to activate the apoptotic protease activating factor 1 (Apaf-1), which oligomerizes and recruits procaspase 9 to form the caspase-activating complex or "apoptosome" (Fig. 5-6).[55–58] Activated caspase 9, in turn, cleaves procaspase 3 to generate the active "effector" caspase 3. Caspase 3 promotes cell death by proteolytic cleavage of downstream target proteins such as poly (ADP-ribose) polymerase, nuclear lamins, DNA-dependent protein kinase, ICAD (the inhibitory subunit of the DNA ladder-inducing endonuclease CAD), and many others, endowing cells with the morphologic characteristic of apoptosis. DNA fragmentation and other events result in cellular disintegration, followed

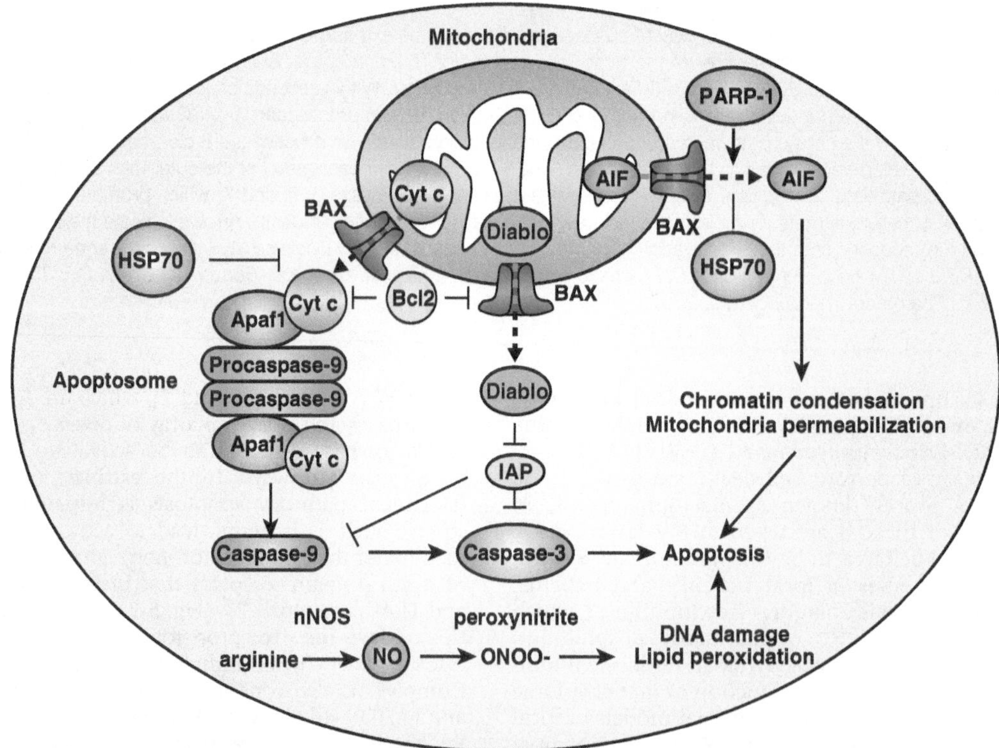

Figure 5-5. The intrinsic or mitochondrial pathway of caspase activation. In the intrinsic or mitochondrial pathway, apoptosis is initiated when injurious stimuli such as ischemia lead to activation of prodeath Bcl-2 family proteins that in turn permeabilize the mitochondrial membrane, leading to the release of mitochondrial proteins such as cytochrome c, second mitochondria-derived activator of caspases (Smac)/direct IAP-binding protein with low pI (DIABLO), and apoptosis inducing factor (AIF) into the cytoplasm, an event that is blocked by antiapoptotic Bcl-2 family members. Once in the cytoplasm, cytochrome c binds ATP to activate the apoptotic protease activating factor 1 (Apaf-1), which oligomerizes and recruits procaspase 9 to form the caspase-activating complex or apoptosome. Activated caspase 9, in turn, cleaves procaspase 3 to generate active caspase 3. Caspase 3 promotes cell death by proteolytic cleavage of downstream target proteins such as poly (ADP-ribose) polymerase, nuclear lamins, DNA-dependent protein kinase, ICAD (the inhibitory subunit of the DNA ladder-inducing endonuclease CAD), and many others, endowing cells with the morphologic characteristic of apoptosis. Mitochondrial permeabilization and DNA fragmentation result in cell death, followed by engulfment by macrophages. Whereas cytochrome c activates Apaf-1, Smac/DIABLO neutralizes the inhibitor of apoptosis proteins (IAPs). Heat shock protein 70 (Hsp70) inhibits apoptosis by preventing the release of cytochrome c and formation of the apoptosome and by inhibiting release of AIF. *(Adapted from Zimmermann KC, Bonzon C, Green DR: The machinery of programmed cell death.* Pharmacol Ther *92:57–70, 2001.)*

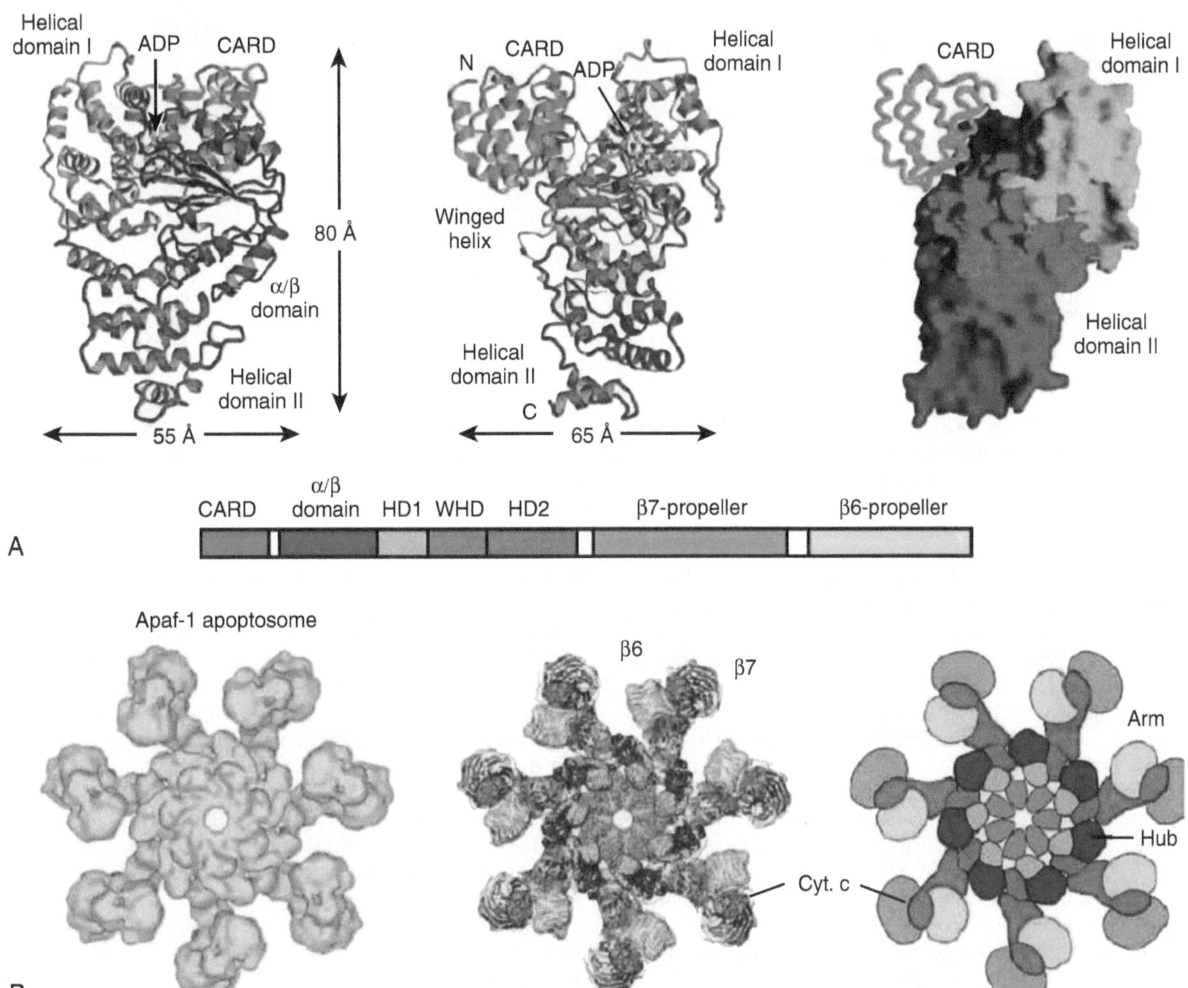

Figure 5-6. Structures of Apaf-1 and the apoptosome. A, Overall structure of the WD40-deleted Apaf-1. The left and middle panels display two perpendicular views of the ribbon diagram of the structure of Apaf-1 (residues 1591, bound to ADP). ADP binds to the hinge region between the α/β-fold and HD1 (right arrow) but is also coordinated by two critical residues from the WHD. The right panel shows the structure in surface representation except for the CARD domain. B, Domain organization in Apaf-1 apoptosome. Left panel shows a top view of the apoptosome. Middle panel shows the proposed domain organization in the apoptosome within semitransparent surfaces. Right panel shows a cartoon model of the apoptosome. Color-coding scheme for the panels is the same as in (A). In the presence of dATP or ATP, cytochrome c and Apaf-1 assemble into an approximately 1.4-MDa complex, termed the apoptosome. The apoptosome is composed of seven molecules of Apaf-1, which bind to cytochrome c in an ATP/dATP-dependent manner. Apaf-1 acts via its CARD domain to form a signaling platform known as the apoptosome. The apoptosome recruits and activates procaspase 9 to generate activated caspase 9. Thus, the apoptosome initiates apoptosis via the intrinsic mitochondrial pathway. *(Reprinted with permission from Bao Q, Shi Y: Apoptosome: A platform for the activation of initiator caspases.* Cell Death Differ *14:56–65, 2007.)*

by engulfment of fragmented cells by surrounding cells.[25,26,53,54] Thus, the apoptosome enables cytochrome *c* to jump-start a caspase cascade of proteolysis independently of ligand-activated death receptors.

Alternative Pathways of Caspase Activation

An additional pathway critical to activation of the initiator caspases, such as caspase 2, is that of DNA damage. DNA damage promotes p53-dependent transcriptional upregulation of p53-induced protein with a death domain (PIDD).[59] In response to injurious stimuli, PIDD forms the PIDDosome death complex, a large (molecular weight >670 kDa) macromolecular signaling platform that recruits and activates procaspase 2 in response to DNA damage and stress (Fig. 5-7).[60] The PIDDosome contains PIDD, the adapter protein RIP-associated Ich-1/Ced-3-homologue protein with a death domain (RAIDD), and procaspase 2. PIDD interacts via its death domain to bind RAIDD and acts via its caspase-recruitment domain (CARD) to recruit procaspase 2.[61] Although the details of caspase 2 activation are not well delineated, the PIDDosome is thought to promote autocleavage of procaspase 2 to generate caspase 2.[62] Upon activation, caspase 2 acts upstream of mitochondria to promote proteolytic cleavage of the BH3-only protein Bid, translocation of Bax to the mitochondria, opening of the mitochondrial permeability transition pore, and release of cytochrome *c*.[52] It is the only caspase that when added to purified mitochondria can directly induce cytochrome *c* release. A 2008 article by the Chan group[63] demonstrates that brief global ischemia promotes

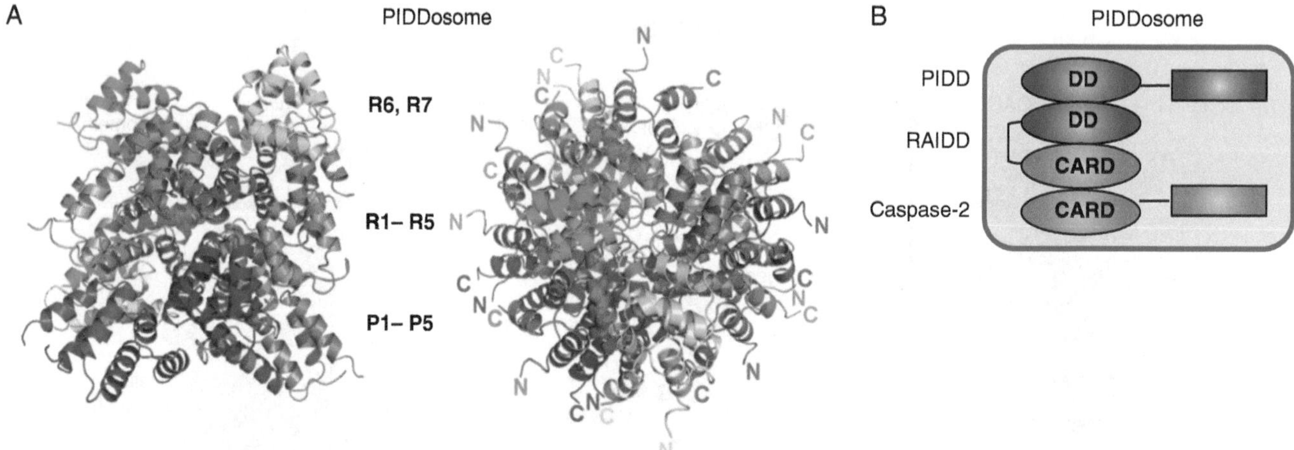

Figure 5-7. Structure of the PIDDosome complex. A, Side view of the complex. The top layer contains two RAIDD DD molecules (green and yellow). The middle layer contains five RAIDD DD molecules (red, purple, orange, magenta, and pink). The bottom layer contains five PIDD DD molecules (different shades of blue). B, Top view of the complex. *(Reprinted with permission from Park HH, Logette E, Raunser S, et al: Death domain assembly mechanism revealed by crystal structure of the oligomeric PIDDosome core complex.* Cell *128:533–546, 2007.)*

expression of a short cleaved fragment of PIDD (PIDD-CC), formation of the PIDDosome, PIDD-dependent activation of procaspase 2, cleavage of Bid, and neuronal death in the hippocampal CA1. These findings implicate the PIDDosome in neuronal death induced by global ischemia.

Recent studies show that PIDD can act as a sensor to determine cell fate, controlling the balance between cell survival and death in response to genotoxic stress.[64,65] PIDD can form a distinct prosurvival complex by binding with kinase RIP1 and the sumoylated form of NF-κB essential modulator (NEMO) to activate cell survival pathway.[64] This complex phosphorylates the inhibitor of NF-κB, IκB, and releases it from NF-κB. Upon activation, NF-κB enters the nucleus, where it promotes transcription of mainly prosurvival genes. In addition, PIDD recruits RAIDD to form PIDDosome and then trigger cell proapoptosis via caspase 2.[66]

The Bcl-2 Family of Proteins

The Bcl-2 proteins are a family of structurally related proteins that serve as central regulators of intrinsic programmed cell death.[53,54,67–70] Bcl-2 family proteins are documented as either antiapoptotic or proapoptotic. Antiapoptotic members are Bcl-xL, Bcl-2, Bcl-w, and Mcl-1; they contain four Bcl-2 homology (BH1-4) domains. They localize to the cytosol and to the mitochondrial and endoplasmic reticulum membrane. Proapoptotic members are further classified as multidomain proteins that contain three BH domains: BH1-3 (Bak and Bax) and the "BH3-only" proteins (Bid, Bad, Bim, Puma, Noxa BIK, BMF, HKR/DP5).[53,67,68] Because they are thought to induce cell death by inhibiting the antiapoptotic family members, BH3-only proteins are divided into two groups: the "inactivators" (e.g., Bad, Noxa) and the "direct activators" (e.g., tBid and, possibly, also Bim and Puma), which bind transiently and activate the multidomain proteins Bax and Bak.[70] When the intracellular concentrations of Bax, Bim, Bad, and Bid exceed that of antiapoptotic Bcl-2 family members, cytochrome *c* and other apoptogenic factors are released from the mitochondria, thus initiating apoptosis.

In the intrinsic pathway, a prevailing view is that under physiologic conditions, prosurvival Bcl-2 family members bind and inhibit the proapoptotic direct-activator BH3-only proteins Bid and Bim and/or they bind and inhibit the multidomain prodeath proteins Bax and Bak.[53,67] The association between the antiapoptotic proteins and the multidomain proapoptotic Bcl-2 proteins prevents the homooligomerization of Bax and Bak, which would otherwise permeabilize the outer mitochondrial membrane. In addition, antiapoptotic Bcl-2 proteins such as Bcl-2 can directly bind the "effectors" Bax and Bak and inhibit channel/pore formation. In response to injurious stimuli, "inactivator" BH3-only proteins such as Bad bind and inhibit the antiapoptotic family members, liberating Bax and Bak and, possibly, "activator" BH3-only proteins Bid and Bim.[71] When unleashed, Bid and Bim trigger homooligomerization of Bak and Bax, which form channels in the outer mitochondrial membrane that permit the escape of apoptogenic proteins such as cytochrome c, Smac/DIABLO, and AIF.[54,67,68]

Until relatively recently, it was thought that permeabilization of the outer mitochondrial membrane and activation of the "effector" caspase 3, was a "point of no return" in the execution of apoptotic cell death of post-ischemic neurons and most other cell types.[72] The importance of early caspase 3 activation to global ischemia-induced neuronal death is underscored by the finding that Z-DEVD-FMK, a selective caspase 3 inhibitor, is neuroprotective if administered at the time of ischemia but not at 24 hours or later.[73] Thus, the apoptotic machinery is engaged early in the post-ischemic period. However, it is now well established that neurons can survive cytochrome *c* release and caspase 3 activation.[74–76] Because of the dual nature of caspase 3,[77] a causal role for caspases or caspase substrates in global ischemia is challenged by the recent consensus that ischemic neurons in adult brain may not die by classical apoptosis.[4,78,79]

Inhibitors of Apoptosis

The IAP proteins are described as a family of proteins that have key roles in inhibiting caspase activation.[80] IAP proteins contain baculoviruses IAP repeat domains that can suppress apoptosis in mammalian cells by directly binding to and inhibiting caspase activities.[80,81] Eight human IAPs have been identified, including XIAP, c-IAP, c-IAP2, and survivin, which, unlike the other IAP family members, lack a C-terminal RING finger (E3 ubiquitin ligase) domain; all exhibit antiapoptotic activity in cell culture. X-chromosome-linked IAP (XIAP) is known as the black sheep of the IAP family for its potent suppression of apoptosis. XIAP binds caspase 3 and caspase 7 reversibly and with high affinity and it suppresses caspase activity, at least in part by masking the caspase active site. The main functional unit in the IAPs is the BIR (or baculoviral IAP repeat) domain, which contains approximately 80 amino acids folded around a zinc atom. Most IAPs have multiple BIR domains, which mediate specialized functions such as binding to caspases. For example, BIR3 and adjacent sequences in XIAP mediate inhibition of activated caspase 9, whereas the linker region between BIR1 and BIR2 selectively targets caspase 3.

IAPs promote neuronal survival not limited to caspase inhibition.[75] The presence of a zinc-binding motif or RING (E3 ubiquitin ligase) domain at the distal end of the carboxy-termini of a subset of IAPs confers protein degradation activity. These IAPs trigger degradation of target proteins via ubiquitin-based proteasomal degradation. IAPs catalyze sequential covalent additions of ubiquitin (a 76-amino-acid moiety) linked to specific lysine residues within target proteins. Then the modified residues form multimeric polyubiquitin chains, which tag the protein and mark it for destruction.

Recent reports indicate that IAPs possess additional functions. For example, c-IAPs and XIAP can act as vital regulators of cell migration and development by linking ubiquitin to substrates as opposed to halting the caspase cascade.[82] In addition, due to the ubiquitin ligase activity of IAP, its roles are reported to range from modulating NF-κB, mitogen-activated protein kinase (MAPK), or IRF signaling pathways to regulating innate immunity and inflammation.[83,84]

Caspase-Independent Programmed Cell Death

Focal and global ischemia is canonically thought to induce apoptotic cell death by activation of caspases. However, an alternative pathway of cell death can occur in animal models of focal and global ischemia even in the presence of caspase inhibitors.[59,85,86] This caspase-independent apoptosis is characterized by effecting permeabilization of the outer mitochondrial membrane and the release of apoptogenic mitochondrial proteins. This pathway deploys the mitochondrial proteins AIF and endonuclease (Endo) G inducing neuronal death rather than forming an apoptosome.[87,88] AIF is a mitochondrial protein essential to oxidative phosphorylation and the integrity of mitochondrial structure.[88] Endo G is a mitochondrial endonuclease that contains a nuclear localization sequence.[88] Thus, in response to injurious stimuli such as ischemia, AIF and Endo G are released from the mitochondria and translocate to the nucleus, where they promote DNA fragmentation and chromatin condensation.

AIF induces cell death by overactivation of PARP-1.[89] PARP-1 is an abundant nuclear enzyme with approximately one molecule per 1000 DNA base pairs.[26,89,90] The obligatory trigger of PARP-1 activation is nicks and breaks in double-stranded DNA, which are recognized by PARP-1 via its DNA binding domain. PARP-1 catalyzes the conversion of β-nicotinamide adenine dinucleotide (NAD+) into nicotinamide and poly(ADP-ribose). Once activated, PARP-1 transfers between 50 and 200 molecules of ADP-ribose to target proteins, which may activate or inhibit their function. Targets of PARP-1 include histones, DNA polymerases, topoisomerases I and II, and PARP-1 itself.[91] In the case of histones, poly-ADP-ribosylation promotes chromatin relaxation.

Overactivation of PARP-1 promotes excessive production of poly(ADP-ribose) and depletion of NAD+, which together induce energy failure and signal the mitochondrial release of AIF (Fig. 5-8).[89-91] Upon release from the mitochondria, AIF is transformed into a powerful cytotoxin that rapidly translocates to the nucleus, where it promotes chromatin condensation and fragmentation. In addition, cytosolic AIF acts on the mitochondria to further compromise the integrity of the outer mitochondrial membrane and initiate the release of cytochrome c, which activates caspase 3. PARP-1 is a critical downstream target of caspase 3. However, caspase activation is apparently not required for PARP-1-dependent cell death, because caspase inhibitors do not afford protection.[90]

PARP-1-dependent cell death exhibits morphologic features that are distinct from those of necrosis, apoptosis, and autophagy. To distinguish it from other forms of cell death, PARP-1-mediated cell death has been termed parthanatos, after the PAR polymer and Thanatos, the Greek personification of death and mortality.[91] The observations that inhibitors of PARP-1 or deletion of the parp-1 gene can protect against the neuronal death associated with cerebral ischemia, myocardial infarction, and inflammatory injury in animal models implicate PARP-1 as an important player in these disorders.[89,90,92] Caspase-independent death can also result from permeabilization of the lysosomal membrane and lysosomal release of cathepsin, which activates Endo G.[93] OGD in primary cultures of hippocampal neurons, an in vitro model of ischemia, promotes translocation of Endo G from the mitochondrion to the nucleus, where it plays a role in neuronal death.[94]

Autophagy

The definition of macroautophagy is forming vacuoles or autophagosomes, which sequester and engulf overly abundant, old, or damaged intracellular organelles and/or portions of the cytoplasm for bulk degradation by lysosomes.[95,96] The last stages of autophagy are marked by the fusion between autophagosomes and lysosomes to form autolysosomes, in which the inner membrane of the autophagosome and its luminal contents are degraded by acidic lysosomal hydrolases. Autophagic cell death is morphologically characterized by the absence of chromatin condensation and by the presence of massive autophagic vacuoles or autophagosomes. Shen and Codogno[97] have introduced three criteria to elucidate autophagic cell death: (i) the cell death pathway is independent of apoptosis; (ii) the increase of autophagic flux is more important than that of autophagic markers; (iii) autophagic cell death can be inhibited by both genetic means and chemical inhibitors.

Recently, an increasing number of studies have shown that there is an interplay between apoptosis and autophagy. The balance between apoptosis and autophagy regulates cell death pathways in many pathophysiological conditions.[98] In regard to ischemia, the cytoprotective effects of autophagy may prevail over its cytotoxic effects. For example, under ischemic preconditioning, a sublethal ischemia-induced autophagic response may provide protection from a subsequent severe brain ischemia.[99,100]

Cell Death Pathways

The canonical hallmarks of induced neuronal death are necrosis and apoptosis (for review, see [4] and [30]). Ultrastructural studies of CA1 neurons undergoing delayed death in rat and gerbil models of global ischemia[101,102] and in humans who die of cardiac arrest[103,104] exhibit morphological features of necrosis (see below) but do not exhibit critical characteristics of apoptosis, such as apoptotic bodies. However, there is strong evidence that apoptosis – as defined as activation of specific cell-signaling events that result in cellular suicide – also occurs during induced neuronal death. Such support comes from molecular studies demonstrating a mitochondrial release of cytochrome *c* and other apoptogenic proteins and activation of the caspase death cascade (see below). Recently, a study has demonstrated that global ischemia can also induce neuronal death via the necroptosis pathway. In the in vitro global ischemia model, OGD elevated the endogenous RIP3 protein level sequentially promoting the assemblage of necrosome

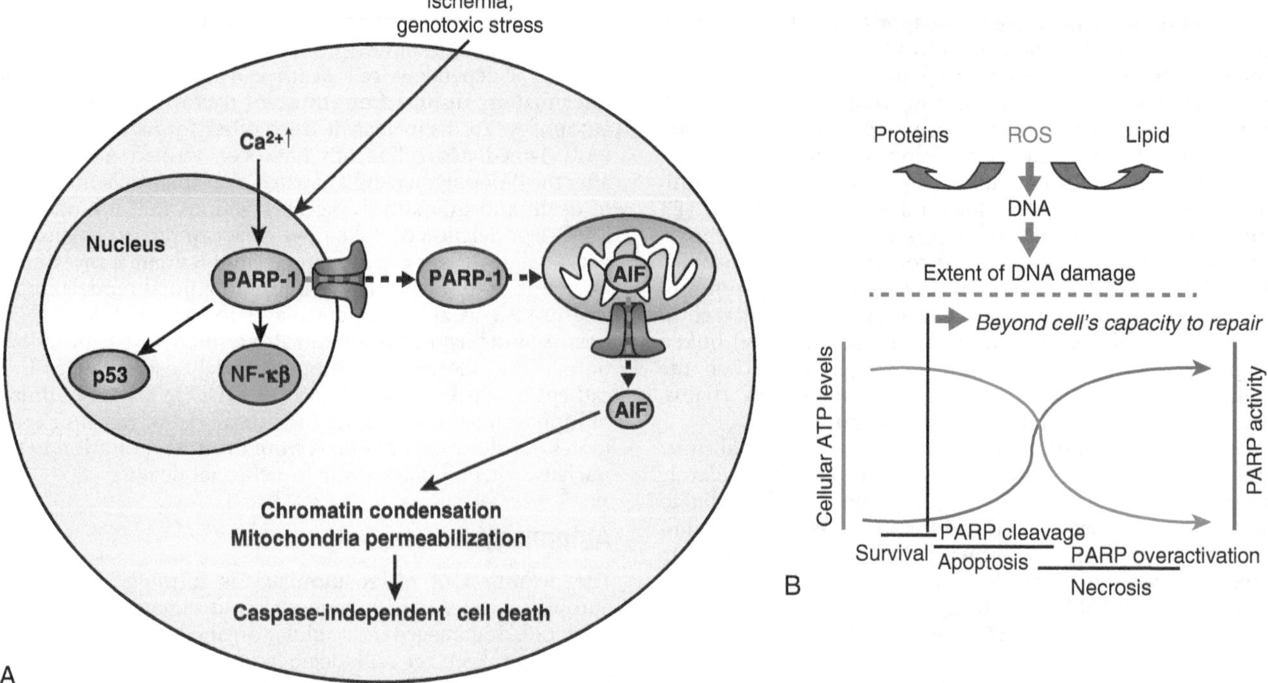

Figure 5-8. PARP-1 mediates a caspase-independent pathway of programmed cell death. A, The role of PARP-1 in apoptotic cell death. Insults to cells such as ischemia and stress can activate PARP-1, which promotes the release of AIF from the mitochondria. AIF can induce chromatin condensation and mitochondrial permeabilization independent of cytochrome c, thus triggering apoptotic cell death. PARP-1 can activate NF-κB, a transcription factor that has a crucial role in the regulation of genes involved in inflammatory responses. PARP-1 also transactivates p53, a transcription factor critical in the execution of apoptosis. On release from the mitochondria, AIF rapidly translocates to the nucleus, where it promotes chromatin condensation and fragmentation. In addition, cytosolic AIF promotes permeabilization of the mitochondria, releasing cytochrome c and other apoptogenic factors into the cytosol. ATP depletion inhibits caspase activation and shifts the balance of death cascades in favor of necrosis. B, A model of PARP-1 overactivation-mediated cytotoxicity. Reactive oxygen species (ROS) such as nitric oxide, $O2^-$, or peroxynitrite are generated during inflammation or ischemia–reperfusion. ROS damages proteins, lipids, and DNA. DNA damage activates PARP-1, a DNA surveillance enzyme, which transforms NAD+ into poly(ADP-ribose) and nicotinamide. Overactivation of PARP-1 promotes excessive production of poly(ADP-ribose) and depletion of NAD+, which together induce energy failure and signal the mitochondrial release of AIF.

complex. That study provides pivotal evidence of the necroptotic neuronal death pathway after global ischemia injury.[105]

Focal ischemia also induces neuronal death with hallmarks of both necrosis and apoptosis.[4,106] Focal ischemia elicits early cell shrinkage and swelling of mitochondria, followed by cell dispersal, and shrinkage of the nucleus without surrounding cytoplasm. The early mitochondrial swelling and loss of integrity of the plasma membrane are key characteristics of necrotic cell death. Recently, evidence in support of apoptotic death in the penumbra has been reported, including DNA fragmentation, activation of death receptors, mitochondrial release of cytochrome c, and activation of the caspase death cascade (see below). Strong evidence in support of necrosis, defined as activation of specific signaling proteins, comes from genetic and pharmacologic studies that show a critical role for RIP1 and cyclophilin D, and from biochemical studies that show a disruption of energy metabolism, generation of ROS and nitroxidative stress by nitric acid, a rise in intracellular Ca^{2+}, activation of non-caspase proteases, activation of cyclophilin-D-dependent mitochondrial outer-membrane permeabilization, and mitochondrial release of AIF (see above).

Both focal and global ischemia trigger caspase activation in neurons destined to die. Global ischemia induces activation of death receptors such as CD95-Fas and TRAIL, effector caspases such as caspases 9 and 3, and DNA fragmentation factor, which promotes fragmentation of DNA.[73,107,108] Focal ischemia leads to delayed neuronal death in the penumbra, with classical features of apoptosis, including CD95-Fas receptor activation,[109] mitochondrial release of cytochrome *c*,[110] activation of caspase 3,[111] and DNA fragmentation.[112-114]

TRIGGERS OF ISCHEMIC CELL DEATH

Glutamate Excitotoxicity

Excitotoxicity refers to the form of cell death by which supraphysiologic levels of excitatory amino acids, such as glutamate, excessively activate excitatory amino acid receptors such as the N-methyl-D-aspartate (NMDA) receptor, leading to cytosolic Ca^{2+} overload and activation of lethal signaling pathways.[78] A half century ago, Lucas and Newhouse observed that glutamate administered to animals in vivo caused death of retinal neurons, indicating that glutamate is toxic.[115] In the glutamate-induced neuronal death, postsynaptic structures such as dendrites and somata were destroyed, whereas axons, presynaptic terminals, and non-neuronal cells survived.[116]

Glutamate is pivotal in the pathogenesis of global and focal ischemia. Raising the extracellular concentration of magnesium markedly reduced the vulnerability of cultured hippocampal neurons to anoxia.[117,118] Moreover, glutamate antagonists have been shown to reduce neuronal injury in in vitro and in vivo models of ischemia.[119,120] Furthermore, over the past 15–20 years, mounting evidence has shown that glutamate antagonists afford neuroprotection in global and focal ischemia. Thus, it is now widely accepted that excitotoxicity plays a critical role in the neuronal death associated with ischemia and other neurologic disorders and diseases.

During an ischemic episode, anoxic depolarization activates voltage-sensitive Ca^{2+} channels, which trigger a massive release of synaptic glutamate.[78] Synaptically released glutamate acts via the ionotropic glutamate receptors, N-methyl-D-aspartate receptors (NMDARs), α-amino-3-hydroxy-5-methyl-4-isoxazole-propionic acid receptors (AMPARs), and kainate receptors to further depolarize the postsynaptic cell. Glutamate also activates metabotropic glutamate receptors (mGluRs).[121-123] Group I mGluRs, mGluR1 and 5, engage the prosurvival ERK/MAPK and phosphatidylinositol 3-kinase (PI3K)/protein kinase B (Akt) signaling pathways. In addition, mGluR1/5 acts via phospholipase C and Ins(1,4,5) P3 to trigger release of Ca^{2+} from intracellular stores. Depletion of Ca^{2+} from the endoplasmic reticulum triggers endoplasmic reticulum stress, which activates apoptosis. The cytosolic Ca^{2+} influx causes cells to further depolarize and become inexcitable. Anoxic depolarization also drives the reverse operation of glutamate transporters in astrocytes, contributing to the rise in extracellular glutamate.[124] During global ischemia, extracellular glutamate increased from approximately 0.6 μM to 1 to 2 μM,[125] whereas in focal ischemia, glutamate rose to 16–30 μM in the core.[126,127] A major consequence of the rise in extracellular glutamate is activation of not only synaptic but also extrasynaptic ionotropic glutamate receptors (AMPARs, NMDAs, and kainate receptors), with consequent influx of toxic Ca^{2+} and shutoff of the CREB-initiated program of cell survival (see below).

NMDARs

NMDARs are glutamate-gated ion channels, which play a pivotal role in the regulation of synaptic function in the brain.[128-131] NMDARs are heteromeric assemblies of NR1, NR2, and NR3 subunits that cotranslationally assemble in the endoplasmic reticulum to form functional channels with differing physiologic and pharmacologic properties. NMDAR-mediated Ca^{2+} influx is essential for synaptogenesis, experience-dependent synaptic remodeling, and long-lasting changes in synaptic efficacy such as long-term potentiation (LTP) and depression (LTD), which are cellular processes widely believed to underlie learning and memory.[132,133] Recent studies indicate that NMDARs not only serve as a trigger of synaptic plasticity but may also contribute to the expression of LTP and LTD.[131] NMDARs mediate the influx of toxic Ca^{2+} in a number of neurologic disorders, insults, and neurodegenerative diseases.[78,131] They are widely accepted as a critical player in both focal and global ischemia-induced neuronal death.

Hypoxia and focal ischemia cause overactivation of NMDARs, excessive Ca^{2+} influx, and excitotoxic cell death (see later). Targets of NMDAR-mediated Ca^{2+} influx include nNOS, JNK signaling, calpains and cathepsins, and Ca^{2+}-dependent transcription factors. Beside the NO signaling pathway, NMDARs can also promote cell death via activation of the JNK.[134] Upon activation, JNK phosphorylates and induces mitochondrial translocation of Bim long (BimL), which leads to MOMP by forming Bax channels.[135] JNK also phosphorylates and activates pyruvate dehydrogenase, which leads to ATP depletion. JNK signaling also contributes to neuronal death as evidenced by several studies in which the inhibition or genetic deletion of JNK has had a neuroprotective effect.[136,137]

Findings by Hardingham et al. reveal that the location of surface NMDARs influences the fate of neurons.[138,139] Whereas synaptic NMDARs activate CREB, extrasynaptic NMDARs elicit CREB shutoff.[128,131] Interestingly, contemporaneous activation of synaptic and extrasynaptic NMDARs by bath-applied NMDA also turns off CREB, which suggests that extrasynaptic NMDARs act via a dominant, cell-death signal to override the CREB-promoting effects of synaptic NMDARs and/or L-type Ca^{2+} channels and protein kinase A (PKA).[131,138] The finding that the synaptic or extrasynaptic location of NMDARs determines cell survival or death after ischemic insults may lead to a broad understanding of potential therapeutic strategies.[140,141]

Recent studies reveal important mechanisms for enhancing NMDA receptor activity and Ca^{2+} influx. Studies using electrophysiology and two-photon laser scanning show that Ca^{2+} permeation through NMDARs is under the control of the cAMP/PKA signaling system.[142] Direct activation of PKA markedly enhances Ca^{2+} influx through NMDARs; direct activation of γ-aminobutyric acid (GABA)B receptors, which negatively couple to cAMP/PKA signaling, strongly inhibits NMDAR-mediated Ca^{2+} signaling in spines in a PKA-dependent manner.[143] An important prediction of these findings is that extracellular signals that modulate cAMP at postsynaptic sites (e.g., norepinephrine, dopamine, and GABA) can bidirectionally regulate Ca^{2+} permeation through synaptic NMDARs. Given the widespread distribution of NMDARs and PKA throughout the CNS, this represents a powerful mechanism for modulating Ca^{2+} signaling in neurons under physiologic and pathologic conditions.

Functional NMDARs are also expressed in glial cells.[144] In oligodendrocytes, NMDARs localize primarily to the processes.[145] Under physiologic conditions, they respond to glutamate released from neighboring neurons; whereas under pathologic conditions such as ischemia, they are overactivated.[146] All glial and neuronal NMDARs are permeable to Ca^{2+}; it is their variable sensitivity to a Mg^{2+} blockade that accounts for their differences in functions. Activation of glial NMDARs in response to ischemia triggers Ca^{2+}-dependent damage of oligodendrocytes.[147] Ca^{2+} influx via glial NMDARs disrupts axoglial junctions and exposed juxtaparanodal K^+ channels, resulting in impaired axonal conduction of neurons.[148] Recent reports document that NMDARs can regulate the migration of oligodendrocyte precursor cells during CNS development by inducing the Tiam1/Rac1 signaling pathway. This further confirms the participation of NMDARs in white matter injury.[149] In addition, astroglial NMDARs are involved in synaptic transmission under physiologic conditions in the cortex.

Ca^{2+}-Permeable AMPARs

AMPARs mediate fast synaptic transmission at excitatory synapses in the CNS. These receptors are tetrameric assemblies of subunits GluR1-4.[150,151] A critical feature of AMPARs lacking the GluR2 subunit is their permeability to Ca^{2+} and Zn^{2+}; the presence of GluR2 in heteromeric AMPARs renders the channel impermeable to Ca^{2+} and Zn^{2+}.[150,151] Under physiologic conditions the principal pyramidal neurons of the hippocampus abundantly express GluR2-containing Ca^{2+}-impermeable AMPARs (see above). Because these cells do not express high levels of Ca^{2+} binding proteins or fast local Ca^{2+} extrusion pumps, the immediate loss of GluR2 would be expected to confer enhanced pathogenicity of endogenous glutamate and vulnerability to neuronal insults.

The dual role of Ca^{2+} permeable AMPARs in both synaptic plasticity and excitotoxicity is widely exhibited in neurologic disorders and diseases.[150,152,153] Accordingly, ischemic insults trigger downregulation of GluR2 mRNA expression and protein abundance in selectively vulnerable CA1 neurons and induce a long-lasting switch in AMPAR phenotype from GluR2-containing to GluR2-lacking (Fig. 5-9).[154-160] In addition to their role in mediating Ca^{2+} entry, GluR2-lacking AMPARs are thought to mediate the late rise in toxic Zn^{2+}.[153]

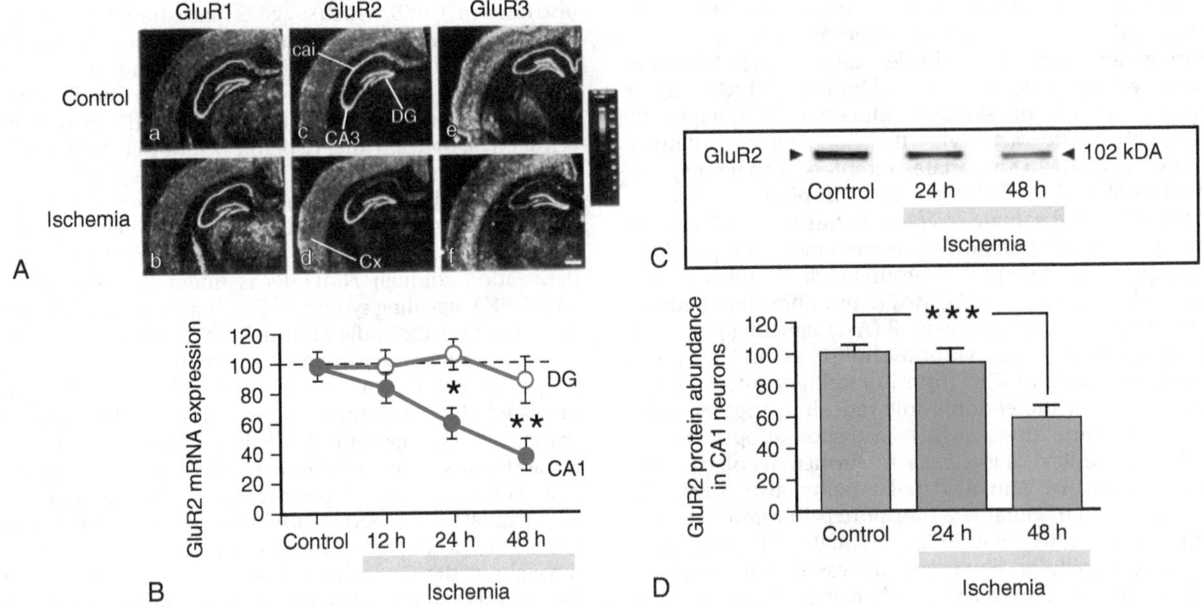

Figure 5-9. Global ischemia suppresses GluR2 mRNA and protein expression in CA1. A, Film autoradiograms of GluR2 mRNA expression, as detected by in-situ hybridization, in the hippocampus of control and experimental rats at 12, 24, and 48 hours after global ischemia. B, Quantitative analysis of GluR2 mRNA expression in the pyramidal cell layer of the CA1 (•) and in the granule cell layer of the dentate gyrus (DG, ○). Global ischemia induced a marked suppression of GluR2 mRNA expression specifically in the pyramidal neurons of the CA1 at 24 hours and was maximal at 48 hours. No changes were detected in the DG or CA3. Mean optical densities are reported after normalization to the corresponding control value for a given region. Statistical significance was assessed by ANOVA followed by Newman-Keuls test (*, $P < 0.05$; **, $P < 0.01$). C, Representative Western blots probed with a monoclonal antibody against a sequence within the N-terminal domain of the GluR2 subunit. D, Relative GluR2 subunit abundance (defined as the ratio of band densities of experimental versus control samples) for protein samples isolated from the CA1 of control and experimental rats at 24 and 48 hours after ischemia. GluR2 abundance was determined from band densities for GluR2 after normalization to the band densities for actin, which served as a loading control. Relative GluR2 subunit abundance was markedly decreased in CA1 at 48 hours. Bars are means ± SEMs. Statistical significance was assessed by means of the Student's unpaired t-test (***, $P < 0.001$). *(A, Adapted from Pellegrini-Giampietro DE, Zukin RS, Bennett MV, et al: Switch in glutamate receptor subunit gene expression in CA1 subfield of hippocampus following global ischemia in rats. Proc Natl Acad Sci U S A 89:10499–10503, 1992. B, Reprinted with permission from Calderone A, Jover T, Noh K-M, et al: Ischemic insults de-repress the gene silencer rest in neurons destined to die.* J Neurosci *23:2112–2121, 2003.)*

AMPAR antagonists protect against global ischemia-induced cell death, even when administered hours after the ischemic insults.[161] Immediate knockdown of GluR2 by antisense oligonucleotides, even in the absence of an ischemic insult, causes death of pyramidal neurons.[159] Overexpression of Ca^{2+}-permeable GluR2 channels in vivo promotes ischemia-induced death of normally resistant CA3 pyramidal cells and dentate gyrus granule cells; overexpression of Ca^{2+}-impermeable GluR2(R) channels protects CA1 neurons against ischemic death.[162] The subunit-specific channel blockers N-naphthylspermine and philanthotoxin, which selectively inhibit GluR2-lacking AMPARs, afford neuroprotection in models of global ischemia.[160,163]

Non-excitotoxic Mechanisms

The pivotal role of NMDARs and AMPARs in the excitotoxicity linked to ischemia is well documented, but other channels are also involved in ischemia-induced neuronal death. Those include the transient receptor potential (TRP) channels and the acid sensing ion channels (ASIC). Both types of channel are discussed below.

TRP Channels

The TRP cation channel superfamily is a group of weakly voltage-sensitive, largely non-selective cation channels that sense and respond to changes in their local environments.[164,165] In the CNS, TRP channels participate in neurite outgrowth, maintain membrane excitability, integrate external signals, and regulate Ca^{2+}-sensitive intracellular signaling. Also, as osmosensors, TRP channels actively regulate homeostasis of body fluids.[164–166] The three major families of TRP genes are the canonical TRPC channels, the melastatin or long TRP (TRPM) channels, and vanilloid TRP (TRPV) V channels. Of these, TRPM2 and 7 are implicated in the cell death resulting from anoxia ROS and stroke.[167]

TRPM7 channels are activated in response to a decrease in extracellular divalent cations, ROS, and extracellular activity, all of which occur in ischemia.[168] Studies have shown that TRPM7 is involved in the excitotoxicity and neuronal death in OGD and MCAO models of ischemia.[168,169] TRP or TRP-like channels are activated by cellular stress and contribute to ischemia-induced membrane depolarization, the accumulation of intracellular Ca^{2+}, and cell swelling.[170] Based on these findings, it has been hypothesized that the neuroprotective effects of hypothermia might be mediated by closure of the temperature-sensitive TRPV3 and TRPV4 channels in response to a lower temperature. Recent studies also provide strong evidence that TRPM2, which has homology to TRPM7, is pivotal in neuronal cell death by downregulating prosurvival signaling pathways.[171] Infarct volume was found to be smaller in TRPM2$^{-/-}$ mice as compared to WT mice following transient MCAO. This result indicated that TRPM2 has a neuroprotective function. Moreover, in vitro, the increased excitability of TRPM2$^{-/-}$ neurons promoted cell survival via prosurvival Akt and ERK cell signaling pathways. Thus, taken together, TRPM2 is a promising therapeutic target for treating ischemic injuries.

Two members of the TRP cation channel (TRPC) family, TRPC3 and 6, protect cerebellar granule neurons against serum-deprivation-induced cell death in cultures and promote the survival of cerebellar granule neurons in rat brain.[172] Although pharmacologic blockade or siRNA to TRPC3 or TRPC6 suppressed a brain-derived neurotrophic-factor (BDNF)-triggered rise in intracellular Ca^{2+}, CREB activation, and neuronal survival, overexpression of TRPC3 or 6 increased CREB-dependent gene transcription and prevented apoptosis in serum-deprived neurons. Increasing evidence exhibits a prosurvival role of TRPC6, including that TRPC6 protect neurons from excitotoxicity by inhibition of NMDAR,[173] inhibition of TRPC6 channels sequentially induced CREB activation which contributed to neuroprotection.[174]

ASIC Channels

ASIC channels also boost Ca^{2+} influx in neuronal injury. ASICs are ligand-gated multimeric channels that belong to the epithelial sodium channel superfamily. They are Na^{+}-selective cation channels sensitive to amiloride, are widely expressed in the CNS, and can be trigged by low pH, membrane stretching, lactate, arachidonic acid, and degraded extracellular Ca^{2+}.[175,176] In mammals there are four genes that encode six ASIC subunit proteins: ASIC1a, ASIC1b, ASIC2a, ASIC2b, ASIC3, and ASIC4. ASICs are abundantly expressed in neurons throughout the brain, including those in the cerebral cortex, cerebellum, hippocampus, amygdala, and olfactory bulb. The ASIC1a subunit is permeable to Ca^{2+}, a major excitotoxic ion, and contributes to acidosis-elicited neuronal injury.[177,178]

Studies by Xiong et al. point to a role for ASIC channels in ischemia-induced acidosis and neuronal death.[179] Acidosis that occurs as a consequence of focal ischemia activates Ca^{2+}-permeable ASICs, which trigger glutamate receptor-independent, Ca^{2+}-dependent, neuronal injury. Whereas cells lacking ASICs are resistant to acid injury, overloading a Ca^{2+}-permeable ASIC1a channel confers enhanced sensitivity to acidosis-induced cell death. Administration of ASIC1a blockers or knockout of the ASIC1a gene in living animals protects the brain from focal-ischemia-induced brain injury and is more potent than glutamate antagonists.[179] Recently, a study revealed that mitochondrial ASIC1a modulate on mitochondrial permeability transition (MPT) pores, which induce oxidative neuronal cell death.[180]

Calcium

Ca^{2+} is a neuronal signaling molecule that is critical to ischemic neuronal death. During the ischemic episode, anoxic depolarization triggers the release of synaptic glutamate. Synaptically released glutamate acts via ionotropic and metabotropic receptors to induce a massive influx of Ca^{2+} from the extracellular space and mobilization of Ca^{2+} from intracellular stores. Depletion of Ca^{2+} from the endoplasmic reticulum initiates endoplasmic reticulum stress, which induces apoptosis (see above). Glutamate induces reverse operation of the Na^{+}/Ca^{2+} exchanger, which exacerbates the buildup of cytosolic Ca^{2+} and elicits a depletion of extracellular Ca^{2+} by more than 90%.[78] Ultimately, the robust rise in cytosolic Ca^{2+} leads to further cell depolarization and the cell then becomes inexcitable. After reperfusion, Ca^{2+} homeostasis is restored; cells appear morphologically normal, exhibit normal intracellular Ca^{2+}, and regain the ability to generate action potentials for 24 to 72 hours after the insult. Ultimately, ambient glutamate elicits a late rise in intracellular Ca^{2+} and Zn^{2+} (see below), and death of CA1 neurons ensues, exhibiting the hallmarks of apoptosis and necrosis.

The robust rise in intracellular Ca^{2+} during the ischemic episode initiates a series of cytoplasmic and nuclear events that impairs cellular activity and profoundly damages the tissue.[78] High cytosolic Ca^{2+} triggers Ca^{2+}-dependent ATPase, which depletes the energy stores of the cell, and interrupts mitochondrial oxidative phosphorylation, leading to cell death.[181] In addition, the influx of intracellular Ca^{2+} activates phospholipases, endonucleases, and non-caspase proteases such as calpains and cathepsins, which perturb cytoskeletal proteins, such as actin and spectrin, extracellular matrix proteins such as laminin, and Ca^{2+}-sensitive transcription factors.[182] Calpains are Ca^{2+}-dependent proteases with papain-like activity and are thought to be key players in the neurodegeneration associated with a number of neurologic disorders and diseases.[78] In addition, high cytosolic concentrations of Ca^{2+} induce excessive activation of nitric oxide synthase, which promotes the generation of free radicals and oxidants. Other targets of calpains include the antiapoptotic Bcl-2 family member Bcl-x_L, which is cleaved to generate its proapoptotic counterpart ΔN-Bcl-x_L[81] (see above), NMDARs and AMPARs, the Na^{+}/Ca^{2+} exchanger NCX, L-type Ca^{2+} channels, sarcoplasmic/endoplasmic reticulum Ca^{2+} ATPases, ryanodine receptors, and Ins (1,4,5)P_3, which regulates the release of Ca^{2+} from intracellular stores.[78]

Zinc

The transition metal Zn^{2+}, like Ca^{2+}, is a neuronal signaling molecule and pivotal player in ischemic cell death.[152,183] In the brain, Zn^{2+} colocalizes with glutamate in presynaptic vesicles at a subset of excitatory synapses. In the hippocampus, Zn^{2+} is uniquely high in mossy fiber tracts, which project to the CA3 (Fig. 5-10).[184] Zn^{2+} is coreleased with glutamate spontaneously and in an activity-dependent manner; it achieves synaptic concentrations of 10–100 μM.[185] Upon release, synaptic Zn^{2+} modulates the activity of a number of postsynaptic receptors. Whereas Zn^{2+} inhibits NMDARs and $GABA_A$ receptors,[186–188] it potentiates AMPARs.[189,190] Zn^{2+} enters neurons via voltage-sensitive Ca^{2+} channels, NMDARs, GluR2-lacking AMPARs, and the Na^{+}/Zn^{2+} antiporter.[150,152,153] Of these, GluR2-lacking AMPARs exhibit the highest permeability to Zn^{2+} but under physiologic conditions they are expressed at low density on distal dendrites of hippocampal pyramidal neurons.[191–193] Within neurons, Zn^{2+} serves as a functionally important component of metalloenzymes and zinc finger-containing transcription factors. Synaptically released Zn^{2+} is thought to be essential for LTP induction at CA3 synapses.[194,195] Accordingly, Zn^{2+} deficiency causes cognitive impairment.[152]

The idea that Zn^{2+}, like glutamate, might be neurotoxic, emerged from findings that perforant path stimulation releases Zn^{2+} and that Zn^{2+} damages postsynaptic target hilar interneurons and CA3 pyramidal cells in vivo[196,197] and in vitro.[198] Exposure of cortical neurons in culture to 300 μM Zn^{2+} for 15 minutes, or to 1 mM Zn^{2+} for 5 minutes, kills virtually all neurons. Moreover, vulnerability to Zn^{2+} is substantially enhanced by concurrent membrane depolarization. Zn^{2+} at high concentrations is a critical mediator of the neuronal injury associated with global ischemia, seizures, traumatic brain injury, and other brain disorders.[150,152,153]

A striking feature of transient global or forebrain ischemia is an early rise in intracellular Ca^{2+} concentrations during the ischemic episode followed by a late rise in intracellular free Zn^{2+} in CA1 neurons at 24–48 hours after ischemia, just prior to the onset of neuronal death (see Fig. 5-10).[161,199] Recent studies reveal a role for Zn^{2+} in the early post-ischemic period.[71,199,200] These studies report proteolytic cleavage of the

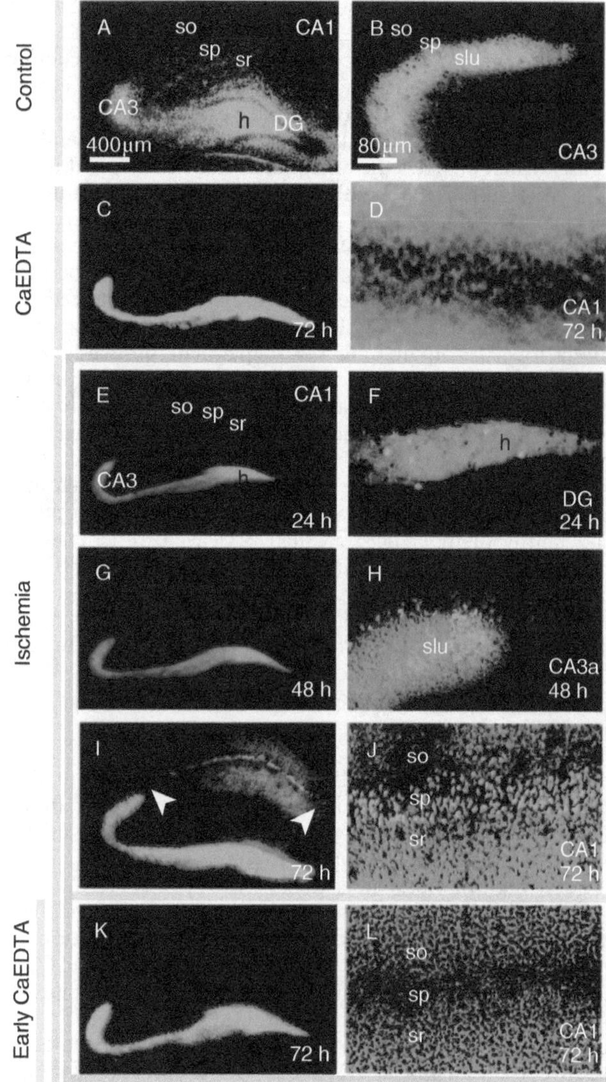

Figure 5-10. Global ischemia elicits a delayed rise in Zn^{2+} levels in selectively vulnerable CA1 neurons. Zn^{2+} fluorescence in TSQ-stained coronal brain sections from sham (A–D) and experimental animals subjected to global ischemia (E-L) or to CaEDTA, followed by global ischemia (K, L). CaEDTA injection at 30 minutes before surgery did not detectably alter the pattern of Zn^{2+} fluorescence in sham-operated control animals, assessed at 72 hours after surgery (C, D). In control hippocampus, TSQ labeling revealed intense fluorescence in the mossy fiber axon terminals of dentate granule neurons in the hilus and stratum lucidum of CA3 (B) and faint fluorescence in the stratum radiatum and stratum oriens of CA1 (A). Global ischemia induced a pronounced increase in Zn^{2+} fluorescence in the cell bodies of scattered hilar neurons, evident at 24 hours after insult (E, F). At 48 hours, Zn^{2+} fluorescence was visible in CA3a pyramidal neurons, extending into the CA1/CA3 transition zone but was not in CA1 (G, F, H). At 72 hours, Zn^{2+} fluorescence was pronounced in cell bodies of CA1 pyramidal neurons (I [arrowheads], J). Injection of CaEDTA 30 minutes before ischemia did not affect the increase in Zn^{2+} in the transition zone but attenuated the late rise in Zn^{2+} fluorescence in the CA1 (K, L). Scale bars: 400 μm in A, C, E, G, I, K; 80 μm in B, D, F, H, J, and L. slu, Stratum lucidum; so, stratum oriens; sp, stratum pyramidale; sr, stratum radiatum. *(Reprinted with permission from Calderone A, Jover T, Mashiko T, et al: Calcium EDTA rescues hippocampal CA1 neurons from global ischemia-induced death.* J Neurosci *24:9903–9913, 2004.)*

antiapoptotic Bcl-2 family protein, Bcl-x_L, to generate its proapoptotic counterpart ΔN-Bcl-x_L as well as the formation of large, Zn^{2+}-dependent channels in the loss of mitochondrial functional integrity in post-ischemic neurons.[71,200] At later times (i.e., 48–72 hours after global ischemia), Zn^{2+} accumulates in degenerating hilar and selectively vulnerable CA1 neurons, concurrent with $p75^{NTR}$ expression and DNA fragmentation.[199,201] Studies with Zn^{2+} indicator dyes show that intracellular concentrations of Zn^{2+} may reach as high as 0.5 μM. Zn^{2+} enters post-ischemic neurons via GluR2-lacking AMPARs[161,199,202] and is released from intracellular stores.[203] Ultimately, Zn^{2+} induces death of CA1 neurons, exhibiting the morphologic features of necrosis. However, if administered before ischemia, the membrane-impermeant metal chelator CaEDTA blocks the rise in Zn^{2+} and protects CA1 neurons. Zn^{2+} exerts its neurotoxic effects via several mechanisms over different timeframes,[157] including potentiation of AMPAR-mediated currents,[189] generation of ROS,[204] and disruption of metabolic enzyme activity,[205] ultimately leading to acute necrosis and apoptosis.[152,157]

MECHANISMS OF ISCHEMIC CELL DEATH

Metabolic Stress

Cells undergoing ischemia exhibit ATP depletion and altered energy dynamics. Neurons and glia consume high amounts of oxygen and glucose and are nearly dependent on oxidative phosphorylation for energy production. When ischemia occurs, obstruction of cerebral blood flow largely limits the delivery of oxygen and glucose, meanwhile impairing the balance of ionic gradients.[181] Anoxic depolarization triggers the release of glutamate, which associates with ionotropic and metabotropic receptors and elevates the concentration of Ca^{2+} in the cytosol while simultaneously reducing it extracellularly.[4,78]

In global ischemia, high cytosolic Ca^{2+} activates Ca^{2+}-ATPase, interrupting mitochondrial oxidative phosphorylation, instantly causing dendrites and cell bodies to swell and undergo necrotic cell death.[25,30,181] ATP drops dramatically in cells throughout the brain but is restored to roughly physiologic levels by reperfusion.[113,206] Low levels of ATP cause neurons to die because of ion pump failure, depolarization, massive release of glutamate, reverse operation of glutamate transporters, swelling of cells (edema), and rupture of the plasma membrane, a canonical necrosis.[181] Because ATP is essential to forming the apoptosome that activates the caspase death cascade, depletion of ATP depletion shifts the balance of death cascades in favor of necrosis.[181] Despite this, global ischemia also activates caspase 3, which catalyzes the cleavage and activation of downstream targets such as PARP-1. Excessive PARP-1 activation depletes the cell of NAD+. NAD+ depletion in mitochondria causes pronounced slowing of glycolysis, electron transport, and ATP formation, resulting in further energy failure and cellular demise.[89-91,181]

Focal ischemia elicits different patterns of metabolic changes in the core and penumbra. Within 1–3 minutes, cells in the core are depleted of ATP and undergo anoxic depolarization. This catalyzes the release of synaptic glutamate.[4,78] Na^+ enters neurons via NMDARs, AMPARs, and other channels permeable to monovalent ions, and K^+ flows out of cells via NMDARs. Water follows passively, driven by the influx of Na^+ and Cl^-, which greatly exceed the efflux of K^+. At the same time, as cells lose energy, the pumps that normally force ions in and out of the cell, which require energy to operate, fail or operate in reverse. These factors result in elevated extracellular K^+ and a reduced extracellular Ca^{2+}. After 2 hours of temporary focal ischemia, the extracellular concentration of K^+ returns to a physiologic level.[4,78]

In contrast, cells in the penumbra face energy reduction but they do not show anoxic depolarization or increases in extracellular K^+.[181] There, low levels of ATP favor necrosis by inducing the reverse operation or failure of ion pumps, swelling of cells, and rupture of the plasma membrane. Meanwhile, ATP depletion inhibits formation of the apoptosome and opposes caspase activation, yet apoptosis ensues in the penumbra. As in global ischemia, activated caspase 3 activates PARP-1, leading to NAD+ depletion and further energy failure.

Mitochondrial Permeabilization

Mitochondria house not only proteins involved in oxidative phosphorylation but also proapoptotic proteins including cytochrome *c*. Under physiologic conditions, cytochrome *c* is localized to the outer compartment of the mitochondria, where it serves as an electron carrier and participates in oxidative phosphorylation. Apoptotic and necrotic stimuli converge when the cytosolic concentration of Ca^{2+} is high, disrupting the integrity of the outer mitochondrial membrane and enabling the release of cytochrome *c* and other apoptogenic factors.[78] Once in the cytoplasm, cytochrome *c* binds dATP to form the apoptosome, a molecular signaling platform that recruits and transactivates procaspase 9 to generate activated caspase 9.

Ischemia triggers high intracellular concentrations of Ca^{2+}, which promote activation of calcineurin, a serine-threonine phosphatase. Calcineurin dephosphorylates Bad, Bad binds Bcl-2 and Bcl-xL and liberates Bak and Bax in mitochondria. Bax and Bak form channels in the mitochondrial membrane that promote permeabilization of the mitochondrial membrane and initiate apoptosis (see above). Growth factors such as BDNF and IGF and other prosurvival factors engage the PI3K/Akt signaling cascade and oppose the actions of pro-death stimuli.[207] Akt phosphorylates Bad, which promotes binding to 14-3-3, which, in turn, sequesters Bad in the cytosol, blocking its proapoptotic actions. A recent study showed that global ischemia triggers the expression and activation of a potent and selective endogenous inhibitor of Akt, carboxyl-terminal modulator protein (CTMP), in vulnerable hippocampal neurons and that CTMP binds to Akt and extinguishes its activity.[208] Although ischemia induces a marked phosphorylation and nuclear translocation of Akt, phosphorylated Akt is not active in post-ischemic neurons, as assessed by kinase assays and phosphorylation of the downstream targets GSK-3β and FOXO-3A. RNA interference-mediated depletion of CTMP in a clinically relevant model of stroke restored Akt activity and rescued hippocampal neurons.[208] More recently, anti-apoptotic activating transcription factor 3 (ATF3) regulated neuronal death together with pro-apoptotic CTMP via ATF3-CTMP signaling cascade, thus indicating a novel therapeutic target for cerebral ischemia.[209]

Nitric Oxide

Nitric oxide (NO) is a small, diffusible signaling molecule that is not released from vesicles and does not act via classic membrane receptors.[210,211] It is synthesized by the neuronal isoform of nitric oxide synthetase (nNOS). At excitatory synapses, nNOS is physically anchored to NMDARs in the postsynaptic membrane via the scaffolding protein, postsynaptic density (PSD) protein-95 (PSD-95)/synapse-associated protein-90 (SAP-90). Activation of NMDARs triggers a rise in postsynaptic Ca^{2+} levels and activation of Ca^{2+}-dependent calmodulin, which rapidly activates nNOS and stimulates production of NO.[210–212]

NO is an important downstream mediator of NMDA-dependent neuronal signaling and synaptic plasticity and NMDA-induced excitotoxicity.[213] Injurious stimuli such as hypoxia and focal ischemia cause overactivation of NMDARs, excessive Ca^{2+} influx, and excitotoxic cell death. Overproduction of NO is a major mediator of excitotoxicity and focal-ischemia-induced neuronal death. The free radical form of NO and the superoxide anion are implicated in the oxidative damage of cellular DNA, lipid peroxidation, and excitotoxic cell death.[212] NO diffuses from the mitochondria and cytoplasm to the nucleus, where it is cleaved to form hydroxyl radicals or singlet oxygen. It reacts with the superoxide anion ($\bullet O2^-$) to form peroxynitrite ($ONOO^-$) (see below). In addition, NO interferes with superoxide dismutase, thereby reducing its antioxidant action, and complexes with non-heme iron within enzymes critical to DNA replication and mitochondrial energy production, thereby inhibiting their activity (see below). Recent evidence indicates that excessive Ca^{2+}-induced generation of NO leads to the formation of S-nitrosylated dynamin-related protein 1, which causes abnormal mitochondrial fragmentation and impairs synaptic function.[213] Studies also have shown that mice that lack nNOS, or are treated with the nNOS inhibitor 7-nitroindazole, are protected against neuronal death in experimental models of stroke.[213,214]

Free Radicals and Lipid Peroxidation

Free radicals, including superoxide anion, hydroxyl radical, singlet oxygen, and radical nitric oxide, are pivotal mediators of neuronal injury. Free radicals perturb the membrane potential by blocking relevant membrane proteins, induce lipid peroxidation, damage DNA, and elicit neuronal death with morphologic features of apoptosis and necrosis.[213–215] NMDAR-mediated Ca^{2+} influx promotes free radical production through the stimulation of NO, which reacts with superoxide free radical ($\bullet O2^-$) to form peroxynitrite, leading to apoptosis.[214,216] In addition to causing DNA damage, ROS such as peroxynitrite oxidize key mitochondrial enzymes such as mitochondrial cytochrome c oxidase, promote the formation of the mitochondrial transition pore and mitochondrial release of AIF, which activates PARP-1, and initiate lipid peroxidation by reaction with unsaturated fatty acids in membranes.[214,215] In addition, ROS activate Ca^{2+}-permeable TRPM7 channels.[167] Peroxynitrite also nitrosylates cysteine residues in target proteins such as NMDARs, thereby impairing synaptic transmission.

NMDAR-mediated Ca^{2+} influx promotes the production of superoxide, which is essential to normal functioning of the cell under physiologic conditions.[213–215] However, overactivation of NMDARs leads to excessive superoxide production and neuronal death. An important source of NMDA-induced superoxide production is the cytoplasmic enzyme NADPH oxidase. NADPH oxidase-2 (NOX2), an isotype of NADPH oxidase, is also a major producer of neuronal superoxide, and thus plays a pivotal role in the outcome of stroke. Studies reviewed by Brennan-Minnella and Won suggest that in addition to an overload of mitochondrial calcium, NMDA receptor-mediated NOX2 signaling is also involved in the production of neuronal superoxide under ischemic insults.[217]

In neurons, free radicals inhibit and damage critical membrane proteins such as Na^+ and Ca^{2+} pumps, creatine kinase, and mitochondrial dehydrogenases. They also promote the oxidation of the Na^+–K^+–ATPase exchanger, rendering it susceptible to calpain-mediated proteolysis.[218] Free radicals damage proteins mainly through the oxidation of side chains and disulfide bonds. Free radicals also damage DNA by causing single- and double-strand breaks, chemically modifying nucleic acid bases, breaking the glycosylic bond between ribose and individual bases, and cross-linking protein to DNA.[219]

Epigenetic Mechanisms and Transcriptional Regulation

Injurious stimuli such as ischemia trigger a number of transcriptional pathways. Transcription factors that are thought to direct programs of changes in gene expression after ischemia include CREB and NF-κB, which direct prosurvival programs, and the forkhead family of transcription factors and REST/NRSF, which direct prodeath pathways in adult neurons.

The Transcription Activator CREB

CREB is a member of the leucine-zipper superfamily of transcription factors. It is triggered in response to external stimuli that activate intracellular signaling cascades that culminate in the phosphorylation of CREB. Upon phosphorylation, CREB forms a functionally active dimer that binds the cis-acting CRE element within the promoters of target genes.[220,221] Immediate-early genes, such as c-fos, Bcl-2, the IAPs, nNOS, and BDNF are important to neuronal survival and are gene targets of CREB.[221] Findings by Hardingham et al.[138] indicate that synaptic and extrasynaptic NMDARs signal through different intracellular signaling cascades (see above). Ca^{2+} influx via synaptic NMDARs promotes the activation of CaMKIV and ERK/MAPK (p42/44) signaling. Upon activation, MAPK phosphorylates and activates the pp90 ribosomal S6 kinases (Rsks), the "synapse to nuclear signal." Rsks then translocate from the synapse to the nucleus, where they regulate gene expression by phosphorylation and activation of transcription factors such as CREB.[131] Rsks act in a coordinated manner to promote robust, sustained phosphorylation of CREB at Ser133 and CREB activation.

Whereas CaMKIV mediates the early phase of Ser133 phosphorylation, the ERK/MAPK pathway mediates late, prolonged phosphorylation of CREB.[220,221] In addition, CaMKIV phosphorylates and activates the coadapter protein, CREB binding protein, at Ser301. On activation, CREB recruits phosphorylated CREB binding protein (CBP) to the promoters of CREB target genes, where it promotes epigenetic modifications and active gene transcription.[222] Considerable evidence indicates that phosphorylation of Ser142 and Ser143 also contributes to CREB activation, but inhibits the interaction of CREB with CBP.[220,221]

Nuclear Factor-κB: A Balance between Neuronal Survival and Death

NF-κB is expressed in almost all mammalian cells. Under physiologic (resting) conditions, NF-κB exists as an inactive form composed of a dimeric form of the transcription factor and its binding partner, IκB.[223] NF-κB is activated in response to a diverse range of external stimuli including the cytokine TNF-α, neurotrophic factors such as nerve growth factor (NGF), neurotransmitters such as glutamate, cell adhesion molecules, and various types of stress. Initiation of NF-κB induces phosphorylation and proteasomal degradation of IκB, which releases active, dimeric NF-κB. Upon activation, NF-κB translocates to the nucleus, where it binds to upstream regulatory elements in κB-responsive genes. These include the Ca^{2+}-binding protein calbindin, cytokines such as TNF-α and interleukin 2κ manganese superoxide dismutase (MnSOD), the antiapoptotic proteins Bcl-xL and Bcl-2, the IAPs, and BDNF.[223] NF-κB also plays an important role in regulating cell survival and synaptic plasticity in neurons. Focal ischemia activates NF-κB and relocalizes it to the nucleus of ischemic neurons, where it binds target genes.[224]

The Pro-Death Transcription Activator FOXO

Forkhead1 (FOXO-3A or FKHRL-1) is a member of the forkhead family of transcription factors (FOXO-3A, FOXO-1, and AFX) and induces expression of proapoptotic target genes.[225-228] In mammals, there are four evolutionarily conserved members of the forkhead family of transcription (FOXO-1, FOXO-3, FOXO-4, and FOXO-6) that are negatively regulated by the PI3K/Akt signaling pathway. Forkhead transcription factors are central to cellular functions such as cell cycle arrest at the G1-S and G2-M checkpoints, detoxification of ROS, repair of damaged DNA, and apoptosis.[225-228] It is thought that these functions of the forkhead family of transcription factors could be related to their ability to promote longevity.

Under physiologic conditions, FOXO-3A resides in the cytosol away from target genes and is thus inactive (Fig. 5-11). The neurotrophins NGF and BDNF and other growth factors such as IGF-I act via the PI3K/protein kinase B (Akt) pathway to promote FOXO-3A phosphorylation.[228] FOXO-3A is a critical target of Akt phosphorylation and inactivation. PI3K promotes neuronal survival by phosphorylation and activation of the serine-threonine kinase Akt. Akt then promotes cell survival by phosphorylation and inactivation of target genes in apoptotic cell death.[228] FOXO-3A is a critical target of Akt phosphorylation and inactivation.[225-228] Phosphorylation of FOXO-3A promotes its binding to the retention factor 14-3-3, which retains FOXO-3A in the cytoplasm, away from target genes such as FasL. Injurious stimuli trigger FOXO-3A dephosphorylation and nuclear translocation. Putative targets of FOXO-3A are the cytokines TNF-α, CD95-Fas ligand, and TRAIL, and their cognate death-domain-containing TNF superfamily of receptors.[50,51] The death cytokines act via the extrinsic or death receptor-mediated pathway to initiate the caspase death cascade. Global ischemia triggers the expression of CD95-Fas ligand, which is implicated in the extrinsic or death-receptor pathway of caspase activation.[50,51] FOXO also regulates oxidative stress-induced neuronal death. For example, the methyltransferase Set9-mediated methylation of FOXO3 at lysine 270 inhibits the transcriptional activity of FOXO3 and thus reduced neuronal cell death.[229]

The Signal Transducer and Activator of Transcription 3 (STAT3)

Signal transducer and activator of transcription 3 (STAT3) is a transcription factor implicated in neuronal function and survival.[230-232] Cytokines, growth factors, and receptor and non-receptor tyrosine kinases activate STAT signaling by phosphorylation of JAK2, a member of the Janus kinase (JAK) family of intracellular non-receptor tyrosine kinases that transduce cytokine-mediated signals, at Tyr1138.[233,234] Upon activation, JAK2 promotes phosphorylation and activation of STAT3.[234] Upon phosphorylation, STAT3 dimerizes and translocates to the nucleus, where it acts by epigenetic remodeling to regulate the transcription of target genes such as MnSOD, ERα, survivin, Bcl-2, and Bcl-xL.[233] MnSOD is a mitochondrial antioxidant enzyme that scavenges free radicals. A recent article[232] indicates that focal ischemia suppresses STAT3 expression and blocks the recruitment of STAT3 to the MnSOD promoter and MnSOD transcription and that downregulation of MnSOD results in overproduction of superoxide anion (•$O2^-$). These findings suggest that STAT3 and its target MnSOD are critical to neuronal survival. Recently, another study demonstrated that IL-32α overexpression could activate anti-inflammation to improve stroke outcome by enhancing STAT3 signaling pathway and perturbing neuroinflammatory cytokines expression and NF-κB initiation.[235]

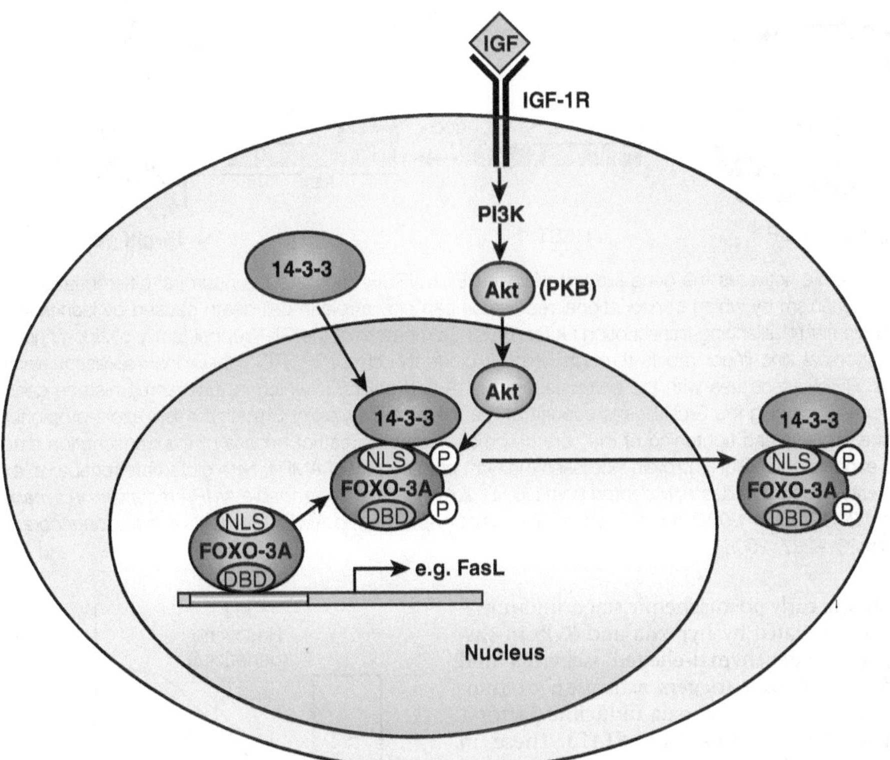

Figure 5-11. Global ischemia activates the forkhead family of transcription factors, implicated in longevity and cell death. Within the nucleus, FOXO-3A triggers apoptosis by transactivation of target genes such as Fas ligand (FasL) and TRAIL. FasL, in turn, activates the cell surface death receptor Fas, which initiates the caspase death cascade via the extrinsic pathway of apoptotic cell death. In the presence of survival factors, the serine/threonine kinase Akt phosphorylates FOXO-3A, leading to its association with 14-3-3 proteins and cytoplasmic retention and sequestration away from nuclear target genes. Ischemia promotes dephosphorylation (activation) of FOXO-3A in CA1, evident at 12 and 24 hours. Estrogen induces phosphorylation (inactivation) of FOXO-3A in control CA1 and attenuates ischemia-induced dephosphorylation of FOXO-3A. *(Adapted from Burgering BM, Kops GJ: Cell cycle and death control: long live forkheads.* Trends Biochem Sci *27:352–360, 2002.)*

The Restrictive Element-1 Silencing Transcription Factor (REST)/Neuron Restrictive Silencing Factor (NRSF)

REST/NRSF is widely expressed during embryogenesis and plays a strategic role in terminal neuronal differentiation.[1,236,237] In pluripotent stem cells and neural progenitors, REST represses a large array of coding and non-coding neuron-specific genes critical to synaptic plasticity and structural remodeling.[238,239] An abundance of REST is modulated via SCF (Skp1-Cul1-F-box protein)/β-TrCP-dependent, ubiquitin proteasomal degradation.[240,241] Disturbance of REST expression during embryogenesis leads to fatal cellular events including apoptosis, aberrant differentiation, and patterning.[236,237]

Epigenetic remodeling is believed to be the profound function of REST genes targeting.[236,237] REST binds the RE1 element of target genes and recruits CoREST and mSin3A, corepressor platforms that, in turn, recruit histone deacetylases (HDACs)-1 and -2. HDACs deacetylate core histone proteins and effect dynamic and reversible gene silencing. REST mediates long-term gene silencing by association with the site-specific histone methyltransferase G9a, which promotes dimethylation of histone 3 at lysine 9 (H3K9me2) via CoREST-dependent and independent mechanisms, and with the site-specific histone demethylase LSD1, which removes methyl groups from H3 at K4 (H3K4). In addition, REST recruits methyl CpG binding protein 2 (MeCP2), a protein that reads epigenetic marks and recruits the machinery that mediates DNA methylation. Whereas histone deacetylation is primarily a mark of dynamic gene repression, cytosine methylation is implicated in long-term gene repression.[242]

In mature neurons REST is quiescent. However, it can be activated in selectively vulnerable hippocampal neurons by insults such as global ischemia[155,243] and epileptic seizures.[244] It accumulates aberrantly in the nucleus of selectively vulnerable striatal neurons in Huntington's disease.[245] Global ischemia triggers a pronounced upregulation of REST mRNA and protein in selectively vulnerable CA1 neurons (Fig. 5-12).[243] Consistent with an induction of REST, core histone proteins over the GluR2 promoter exhibit pronounced deacetylation, which is indicative of reduced GluR2 promoter activity, and GluR2 mRNA and protein expression are suppressed in CA1 neurons.[243] Because the GluR2 subunit governs AMPAR Ca^{2+} permeability and AMPARs are implicated in the excitotoxic death associated with global ischemia, these changes are expected to affect neuronal survival.[150,153] Consistent with this concept, immediate knockdown of the REST gene by antisense administration rescues neurons from ischemic death.[243] These findings suggest a causal relation between REST induction and neuronal death and implicate REST-dependent gene silencing and chromatin remodeling in the transcriptional repression of GluR2 in insulted neurons. Dysregulation of REST and its target genes is also implicated in medulloblastomas, Down's syndrome, Alzheimer's disease, and X-linked mental retardation.[237,246]

Inflammation

Mounting evidence indicates that inflammation exacerbates ischemic injury.[4,247–249] Inflammation signaling plays a fundamental role from the onset of ischemia to the late stage of

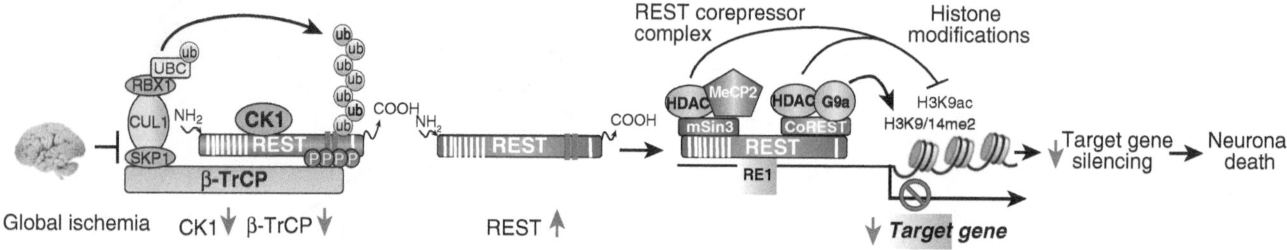

Figure 5-12. Global ischemia activates the gene silencing factor REST/NRSF, implicated in neuronal differentiation and cell death. The model shows the molecular mechanism by which transcriptional repression can play a role in cell death caused by ischemia. Global ischemia induces the neuronal repressor element-1 silencing transcription factor (REST), a member of the Gli-Krüppel family of zinc-finger transcriptional repressors containing nine non-canonical zinc finger motifs through which it binds the cis-acting RE-1 (neuronal repressor element) within the promoter region of target genes. REST associates with the corepressors Sin3A and coREST, which in turn recruit histone deacetylases (HDACs) to the promoters of target genes, including the GluR2 gene subunit of the α-amino-3-hydroxy-5-methyl-4-isoxazole-propionic acid receptor (AMPAR). Deacetylation of histone proteins and tightening of the core chromatin complex restrict access of the transcription machinery required for gene activation. Decreased expression of GluR2 protein increases the Ca^{2+} permeability of AMPA-type glutamate receptors, exacerbating excitotoxicity and increasing the severity of neuronal death. *(Adapted from Liu SJ, Zukin RS: Ca^{2+}-permeable AMPA receptors in synaptic plasticity and neuronal death, Trends Neurosci 30:126–134, 2007. Kwak S, Weiss JH: Calcium-permeable AMPA channels in neurodegenerative disease and ischemia,* Curr Opin Neurobiol *16:281–287, 2006.)*

brain regeneration. In the early post-ischemic stage, inflammatory cellular events are initiated by hypoxia and ROS in vascular, perivascular, and parenchymal-elicited ischemia and reperfusion.[248] Ischemia/hypoxia triggers activation of transcription factors such as NF-κB, hypoxia-inducible factor-1 (HIF-1), interferon regulatory factor-1, and STAT3. These, in turn, orchestrate the expression of an array of proinflammatory target genes such as platelet-activating factor and the cytokines TNF-α and interleukin-1 beta (IL-1β).[4,247,250]

Ischemia/hypoxia triggers the expression of adhesion molecules such as intercellular adhesion molecule-1 (ICAM-1), P-selectins, and E-selectins by endothelial cells on their luminal surface. The adhesion molecules interact with cognate receptors on neutrophils, guiding their migration across the vascular wall and inside the brain parenchyma to the site of injury. Neutrophils are present in large numbers in an ischemic brain by 24–48 hours. Then follows infiltration of lymphocytes, macrophages, and monocytes. Lymphocytes release inflammatory cytokines such as TNF-α, which triggers production of chemokines such as IL-8 and monocyte chemoattractant protein-1, thereby initiating the inflammatory reaction.[4,247] Chemokines rapidly recruit leukocytes (blood-borne inflammatory cells) from the circulation across the endothelial barrier to the site of injury by promoting their adhesion and chemotaxis. Within the brain parenchyma, proinflammatory signals induce the release of cytokines and chemokines from damaged cells. Disruption of the neuronal-microglial connection (CX3CL1, CD200) also contributes to this proinflammatory state. Macrophages appear in large quantity between 1 and 5 days after induction of focal ischemia in the MCAO model; by 5–7 days, they become the predominant cell type in the injured region, where they phagocytose dead cells. The activation of inflammatory cascades and release of cytokines exacerbates neuronal death.[4,247]

An increasing number of studies indicate that microglia/macrophages can transfer from an early "beneficial" M2 phenotype to a late "sick" M1 phenotype when ischemic injuries occur (Fig. 5-13). Thus, traditional therapies for stroke should be updated from simply inhibiting microglia/macrophage toward balancing the polarization of microglia/macrophages.[251] In addition, the in vivo increase of regulatory T cells (Tregs) is believed to be neuroprotective, as it promotes the integrity of the BBB and benefits cellular immune functions.[252,253] This crosstalk between the immune system and ischemic-induced neuronal death illuminates new strategies for stroke therapies, which include as targets Tregs and NK cells.[32,253]

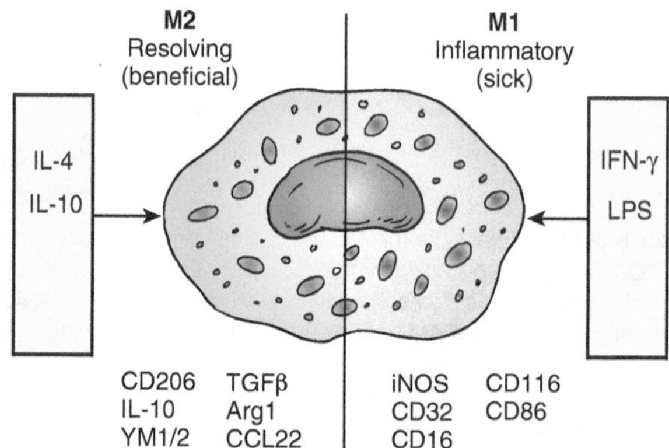

Figure 5-13. Dualistic roles of microglia/macrophages in ischemic injuries. Microglia/macrophages can transfer from an early "beneficial" M2 phenotype to a late "sick" M1 phenotype when ischemic injuries occur. In vitro stimulation with lipopolysaccharide (LPS) and interferon-γ (IFN-γ) promotes the differentiation of "classically activated" M1 microglia/macrophages that typically release destructive proinflammatory mediators. In contrast, interleukin (IL)-4 and IL-10 can trigger a "healthy" M2 phenotype that plays a neuroprotective role. The M1 phenotype markers include iNOS, CD32, CD16, CD116, and CD86; the M2 markers include CD206, IL-10, YM1/2, TGF β, Arg 1, and CCL2. *(Adapted from Bohlson SS, O'conner SD, Hulsebus HJ, et al: Complement, C1q, and C1q-related molecules regulate macrophage polarization. Front Immunol 5:1–7, 2014.)*

Acknowledgments

This work was supported by NIH grants NS 46742 (to R.S.Z.), NS045048, NS062157, and NS089534 (to J.C.), VA grant RX000420 (to J.C), and a Chinese Natural Science Foundation grant (81228008 to J.C). R.S.Z is the F.M. Kirby Endowed Professor in Neural Repair and Protection. J.C. is the R.K. Mellon Endowed Professor in Neurology and Pharmacology.

The complete reference list can be found on the companion Expert Consult website at www.expertconsult.inkling.com. 

KEY REFERENCES

1. Etgen AM, Jover-Mengual T, Zukin RS. Neuroprotective actions of estradiol and novel estrogen analogs in ischemia: translational implications. Front Neuroendocrinol 2011;32:336–52.
2. Liou AKF, Clark RS, Henshall DC, et al. To die or not to die for neurons in ischemia, traumatic brain injury and epilepsy: a

review on the stress-activated signaling pathways and apoptotic pathways. Prog Neurobiol 2003;69:103–42.
3. Lo EH, Dalkara T, Moskowitz MA. Mechanisms, challenges and opportunities in stroke. Nat Rev Neurosci 2003;4:399–415.
4. Moskowitz MA, Lo EH, Iadecola C. The science of stroke: mechanisms in search of treatments. Neuron 2010;67(2):181–98.
5. Garcia JH, Yoshida Y, Chen H, et al. Progression from ischemic injury to infarct following middle cerebral artery occlusion in the rat. Am J Pathol 1993;142:623–35.
6. Memezawa H, Smith ML, Siesjo BK. Penumbral tissues salvaged by reperfusion following middle cerebral artery occlusion in rats. Stroke 1992;23:552–9.
8. Pulsinelli WA, Brierley JB. A new model of bilateral hemispheric ischemia in the unanesthetized rat. Stroke 1979;10:267–72.
9. Pulsinelli WA, Buchan AM. The four-vessel occlusion rat model: method for complete occlusion of vertebral arteries and control of collateral circulation. Stroke 1988;19:913–14.
10. Raghavendra Rao VL, Rao AM, Dogan A, et al. Glial glutamate transporter GLT-1 down-regulation precedes delayed neuronal death in gerbil hippocampus following transient global cerebral ischemia. Neurochem Int 2000;36:531–7.
11. Kitagawa K, Matsumoto M, Yang G, et al. Cerebral ischemia after bilateral carotid artery occlusion and intraluminal suture occlusion in mice: evaluation of the patency of the posterior communicating artery. J Cereb Blood Flow Metab 1998;18(5):570–9.
12. Oguro K, Jover T, Tanaka H, et al. Global ischemia-induced increases in the gap junctional proteins connexin 32 (Cx32) and Cx36 in hippocampus and enhanced vulnerability of Cx32 knock-out mice. J Neurosci 2001;21(19):7534–42.
18. Longa EZ, Weinstein PR, Carlson S, et al. Reversible middle cerebral artery occlusion without craniectomy in rats. Stroke 1989;20(1):84–91.
19. Buchan AM, Xue D, Slivka A. A new model of temporary focal neocortical ischemia in the rat. Stroke 1992;23(2):273–9.
23. Kroemer G, Galluzzi L, Vandenabeele P, et al. Classification of cell death: recommendations of the Nomenclature Committee on Cell Death 2009. Differentiation 2009;16(1):3–11.
24. Green DR. Apoptotic pathways: ten minutes to dead. Cell 2005; 121(5):671–4.
25. Galluzzi L, Blomgren K, Kroemer G. Mitochondrial membrane permeabilization in neuronal injury. Nat Rev Neurosci 2009; 10(7):481–94.
28. Degterev A, Yuan J. Expansion and evolution of cell death programmes. Nat Rev Mol Cell Biol 2008;9(5):378–90.
29. Christofferson DE, Yuan J. Necroptosis as an alternative form of programmed cell death. Curr Opin Cell Biol 2010;22(2):263–8.
30. Galluzzi L, Vitale I, Abrams JM, et al. Molecular definitions of cell death subroutines: recommendations of the Nomenclature Committee on Cell Death 2012. Differentiation 2012;19(1):107–20.
31. Chan JZaFK-M. RIPK3 takes another deadly turn. Science 2014;343:1322.
32. Green DR, Levine B. To be or not to be? How selective autophagy and cell death govern cell fate. Cell 2014;157(1):65–75.
35. Papadakis M, Hadley G, Xilouri M, et al. Tsc1 (hamartin) confers neuroprotection against ischemia by inducing autophagy. Nat Med 2013;19(3):351–7.
36. Ofengeim D, Yuan J. Regulation of RIP1 kinase signalling at the crossroads of inflammation and cell death. Nat Rev Mol Cell Biol 2013;14(11):727–36.
37. Vandenabeele P, Declercq W, Van Herreweghe F, et al. The role of the kinases RIP1 and RIP3 in TNF-induced necrosis. Sci Signal 2010;3(115):re4.
38. Wen Zhou JY. Death by deacetylation. Nature 2012;492:194–5.
39. Vanden Berghe T, Linkermann A, Jouan-Lanhouet S, et al. Regulated necrosis: the expanding network of non-apoptotic cell death pathways. Nat Rev Mol Cell Biol 2014;15(2):135–47.
40. Vanlangenakker N, Vanden Berghe T, Vandenabeele P. Many stimuli pull the necrotic trigger, an overview. Differentiation 2012;19(1):75–86.
41. Cho YS, Challa S, Moquin D, et al. Phosphorylation-driven assembly of the RIP1-RIP3 complex regulates programmed necrosis and virus-induced inflammation. Cell 2009;137(6):1112–23.
42. Galluzzi L, Aaronson SA, Abrams J, et al. Guidelines for the use and interpretation of assays for monitoring cell death in higher eukaryotes. Differentiation 2009;16(8):1093–107.
45. Baines CP, Kaiser RA, Purcell NH, et al. Loss of cyclophilin D reveals a critical role for mitochondrial permeability transition in cell death. Nature 2005;434(7033):658–62.
46. Nakagawa T, Shimizu S, Watanabe T, et al. Cyclophilin D-dependent mitochondrial permeability transition regulates some necrotic but not apoptotic cell death. Nature 2005; 434(7033):652–8.
47. Schneider MD. Cyclophilin D: knocking on death's door. Sci STKE 2005;2005(287):pe26.
48. Degterev A, Hitomi J, Germscheid M, et al. Identification of RIP1 kinase as a specific cellular target of necrostatins. Nat Chem Biol 2008;4(5):313–21.
51. Haase G, Pettmann B, Raoul C, et al. Signaling by death receptors in the nervous system. Curr Opin Neurobiol 2008;18(3):284–91.
52. Bao Q, Shi Y. Apoptosome: a platform for the activation of initiator caspases. Cell Death Differ 2007;14(1):56–65.
53. Youle RJ, Strasser A. The BCL-2 protein family: opposing activities that mediate cell death. Nat Rev Mol Cell Biol 2008;9(1):47–59.
54. Martinou JC, Youle RJ. Mitochondria in apoptosis: Bcl-2 family members and mitochondrial dynamics. Dev Cell 2011;21(1):92–101.
56. Kurokawa M, Kornbluth S. Caspases and kinases in a death grip. Cell 2009;138(5):838–54.
58. Qi S, Pang Y, Hu Q, et al. Crystal structure of the Caenorhabditis elegans apoptosome reveals an octameric assembly of CED-4. Cell 2010;141(3):446–57.
59. Kroemer G, Martin SJ. Caspase-independent cell death. Nat Med 2005;11(7):725–30.
61. Tinel A, Tschopp J. The PIDDosome, a protein complex implicated in activation of caspase-2 in response to genotoxic stress. Science 2004;304(5672):843–6.
62. Janssens S, Tinel A. The PIDDosome, DNA-damage-induced apoptosis and beyond. Differentiation 2012;19(1):13–20.
64. Janssens S, Tinel A, Lippens S, et al. PIDD mediates NF-kappaB activation in response to DNA damage. Cell 2005;123(6):1079–92.
65. McCoy F, Eckard L, Nutt LK. Janus-faced PIDD: a sensor for DNA damage-induced cell death or survival? Mol Cell 2012;47(5):667–8.
66. Ando K, Kernan JL, Liu PH, et al. PIDD death-domain phosphorylation by ATM controls prodeath versus prosurvival PIDDosome signaling. Mol Cell 2012;47(5):681–93.
67. Galonek HL, Hardwick JM. Upgrading the BCL-2 network. Nat Cell Biol 2006;8(12):1317–19.
68. Yip KW, Reed JC. Bcl-2 family proteins and cancer. Oncogene 2008;27(50):6398–406.
69. Hardwick JM, Youle RJ. SnapShot: BCL-2 proteins. Cell 2009; 138(2):404–404.e401.
70. Chipuk JE, Moldoveanu T, Llambi F, et al. The BCL-2 family reunion. Mol Cell 2010;37(3):299–310.
73. Chen J, Nagayama T, Jin K, et al. Induction of caspase-3-like protease may mediate delayed neuronal death in the hippocampus after transient cerebral ischemia. J Neurosci 1998;18(13):4914–28.
76. Garnier P, Ying W, Swanson RA. Ischemic preconditioning by caspase cleavage of poly(ADP-ribose) polymerase-1. J Neurosci 2003;23(22):7967–73.
77. Fan W, Dai Y, Xu H, et al. Caspase-3 modulates regenerative response after stroke. Stem Cells 2014;32(2):473–86.
78. Szydlowska K, Tymianski M. Calcium, ischemia and excitotoxicity. Cell Calcium 2010;47(2):122–9.
80. Gyrd-Hansen M, Meier P. IAPs: from caspase inhibitors to modulators of NF-kappaB, inflammation and cancer. Nat Rev Cancer 2010;10(8):561–74.
82. Kenneth NS, Duckett CS. IAP proteins: regulators of cell migration and development. Curr Opin Cell Biol 2012;24(6):871–5.
83. Estornes Y, Bertrand MJ. IAPs, regulators of innate immunity and inflammation. Semin Cell Dev Biol 2014;S1084-9521(14):00073-1.

84. Beug ST, Cheung HH, LaCasse EC, et al. Modulation of immune signalling by inhibitors of apoptosis. Trends Immunol 2012; 33(11):535–45.
88. Hangen E, Blomgren K, Benit P, et al. Life with or without AIF. Trends Biochem Sci 2010;35(5):278–87.
89. Chiarugi A, Moskowitz MA. Cell biology. PARP-1–a perpetrator of apoptotic cell death? Science 2002;297(5579):200–1.
90. Yu SW, Wang H, Poitras MF, et al. Mediation of poly(ADP-ribose) polymerase-1-dependent cell death by apoptosis-inducing factor. Science 2002;297(5579):259–63.
92. Moroni F, Cozzi A, Chiarugi A, et al. Long-lasting neuroprotection and neurological improvement in stroke models with new, potent and brain permeable inhibitors of poly(ADP-ribose) polymerase. Br J Pharmacol 2012;165(5):1487–500.
93. Boya P, Kroemer G. Lysosomal membrane permeabilization in cell death. Oncogene 2008;27(50):6434–51.
96. Wong E, Cuervo AM. Autophagy gone awry in neurodegenerative diseases. Nat Neurosci 2010;13(7):805–11.
97. Shen H-M, Codogno P. Autophagic cell death: Loch Ness monster or endangered species? Autophagy 2011;7(5):457–65.
98. Marino G, Niso-Santano M, Baehrecke EH, et al. Self-consumption: the interplay of autophagy and apoptosis. Nat Rev Mol Cell Biol 2014;15(2):81–94.
99. Perez-Pinzon MA, Stetler RA, Fiskum G. Novel mitochondrial targets for neuroprotection. J Cereb Blood Flow Metab 2012; 32(7):1362–76.
104. Yamashima T. Implication of cysteine proteases calpain, cathepsin and caspase in ischemic neuronal death of primates. Prog Neurobiol 2000;62(3):273–95.
105. Vieira M, Fernandes J, Carreto L, et al. Ischemic insults induce necroptotic cell death in hippocampal neurons through the up-regulation of endogenous RIP3. Neurobiol Dis 2014;68: 26–36.
107. Ofengeim D, Chen YB, Miyawaki T, et al. N-terminally cleaved Bcl-xL mediates ischemia-induced neuronal death. Nat Neurosci 2012;15(4):574–80.
109. Martin-Villalba A, Herr I, Jeremias I, et al. CD95 ligand (Fas-L/APO-1L) and tumor necrosis factor-related apoptosis-inducing ligand mediate ischemia-induced apoptosis in neurons. J Neurosci 1999;19(10):3809–17.
111. Namura S, Zhu J, Fink K, et al. Activation and cleavage of caspase-3 in apoptosis induced by experimental cerebral ischemia. J Neurosci 1998;18(10):3659–68.
113. Cardell M, Koide T, Wieloch T. Pyruvate dehydrogenase activity in the rat cerebral cortex following cerebral ischemia. J Cereb Blood Flow Metab 1989;9(3):350–7.
115. Lucas DR, Newhouse JP. The toxic effect of sodium L-glutamate on the inner layers of the retina. AMA Arch Ophthalmol 1957; 58(2):193–201.
116. Olney JW, Ho OL. Brain damage in infant mice following oral intake of glutamate, aspartate or cysteine. Nature 1970; 227(5258):609–11.
117. Kass IS, Lipton P. Mechanisms involved in irreversible anoxic damage to the in vitro rat hippocampal slice. J Physiol 1982; 332:459–72.
118. Rothman SM. Synaptic activity mediates death of hypoxic neurons. Science 1983;220(4596):536–7.
119. Rothman SM. The neurotoxicity of excitatory amino acids is produced by passive chloride influx. J Neurosci 1985;5(6): 1483–9.
120. Simon RP, Swan JH, Griffiths T, et al. Blockade of N-methyl-D-aspartate receptors may protect against ischemic damage in the brain. Science 1984;226(4676):850–2.
121. Hermans E, Challiss RA. Structural, signalling and regulatory properties of the group I metabotropic glutamate receptors: prototypic family C G-protein-coupled receptors. Biochem J 2001; 359(Pt 3):465–84.
122. Ronesi JA, Huber KM. Metabotropic glutamate receptors and fragile x mental retardation protein: partners in translational regulation at the synapse. Sci Signal 2008;1(5):pe6.
123. Wang X, Michaelis EK. Selective neuronal vulnerability to oxidative stress in the brain. Front Aging Neurosci 2010;2:12.
125. Meldrum B, Garthwaite J. Excitatory amino acid neurotoxicity and neurodegenerative disease. Trends Pharmacol Sci 1990; 11(9):379–87.
127. Mitani A, Kataoka K. Critical levels of extracellular glutamate mediating gerbil hippocampal delayed neuronal death during hypothermia: brain microdialysis study. Neuroscience 1991; 42(3):661–70.
128. Parsons MP, Raymond LA. Extrasynaptic NMDA receptor involvement in central nervous system disorders. Neuron 2014;82(2): 279–93.
129. Cull-Candy SG, Leszkiewicz DN. Role of distinct NMDA receptor subtypes at central synapses. Sci STKE 2004;2004(255):re16.
131. Lau CG, Zukin RS. NMDA receptor trafficking in synaptic plasticity and neuropsychiatric disorders. Nat Rev Neurosci 2007;8(6): 413–26.
133. Malenka RC, Bear MF. LTP and LTD: an embarrassment of riches. Neuron 2004;44(1):5–21.
136. Coffey ET. Nuclear and cytosolic JNK signalling in neurons. Nat Rev Neurosci 2014;15(5):285–99.
137. Nijboer CH, Bonestroo HJ, Zijlstra J, et al. Mitochondrial JNK phosphorylation as a novel therapeutic target to inhibit neuroinflammation and apoptosis after neonatal ischemic brain damage. Neurobiol Dis 2013;54:432–44.
138. Hardingham GE, Fukunaga Y, Bading H. Extrasynaptic NMDARs oppose synaptic NMDARs by triggering CREB shut-off and cell death pathways. Nat Neurosci 2002;5(5):405–14.
140. Zhang SJ, Buchthal B, Lau D, et al. A signaling cascade of nuclear calcium-CREB-ATF3 activated by synaptic NMDA receptors defines a gene repression module that protects against extrasynaptic NMDA receptor-induced neuronal cell death and ischemic brain damage. J Neurosci 2011;31(13):4978–90.
141. Wroge CM, Hogins J, Eisenman L, et al. Synaptic NMDA receptors mediate hypoxic excitotoxic death. J Neurosci 2012;32(19): 6732–42.
142. Skeberdis VA, Chevaleyre V, Lau CG, et al. Protein kinase A regulates calcium permeability of NMDA receptors. Nat Neurosci 2006;9(4):501–10.
143. Chalifoux JR, Carter AG. GABAB receptors modulate NMDA receptor calcium signals in dendritic spines. Neuron 2010;66(1): 101–13.
145. Salter MG, Fern R. NMDA receptors are expressed in developing oligodendrocyte processes and mediate injury. Nature 2005; 438(7071):1167–71.
146. Karadottir R, Cavelier P, Bergersen LH, et al. NMDA receptors are expressed in oligodendrocytes and activated in ischaemia. Nature 2005;438(7071):1162–6.
147. Micu I, Jiang Q, Coderre E, et al. NMDA receptors mediate calcium accumulation in myelin during chemical ischaemia. Nature 2006;439(7079):988–92.
148. Fu Y, Sun W, Shi Y, et al. Glutamate excitotoxicity inflicts paranodal myelin splitting and retraction. PLoS ONE 2009;4(8):e6705.
149. Xiao L, Hu C, Yang W, et al. NMDA receptor couples Rac1-GEF Tiam1 to direct oligodendrocyte precursor cell migration. Glia 2013;61(12):2078–99.
150. Liu SJ, Zukin RS. Ca^{2+}-permeable AMPA receptors in synaptic plasticity and neuronal death. Trends Neurosci 2007;30(3): 126–34.
151. Isaac JT, Ashby MC, McBain CJ. The role of the GluR2 subunit in AMPA receptor function and synaptic plasticity. Neuron 2007; 54(6):859–71.
152. Sensi SL, Paoletti P, Bush AI, et al. Zinc in the physiology and pathology of the CNS. Nat Rev Neurosci 2009;10(11): 780–91.
154. Pellegrini-Giampietro DE, Zukin RS, Bennett MV, et al. Switch in glutamate receptor subunit gene expression in CA1 subfield of hippocampus following global ischemia in rats. Proc Natl Acad Sci U S A 1992;89(21):10499–503.
156. Opitz T, Grooms SY, Bennett MV, et al. Remodeling of alpha-amino-3-hydroxy-5-methyl-4-isoxazole-propionic acid receptor subunit composition in hippocampal neurons after global ischemia. Proc Natl Acad Sci U S A 2000;97(24):13360–5.
157. Shuttleworth CW, Weiss JH. Zinc: new clues to diverse roles in brain ischemia. Trends Pharmacol Sci 2011;32(8):480–6.
160. Liu S, Lau L, Wei J, et al. Expression of Ca(2+)-permeable AMPA receptor channels primes cell death in transient forebrain ischemia. Neuron 2004;43(1):43–55.
161. Noh KM, Yokota H, Mashiko T, et al. Blockade of calcium-permeable AMPA receptors protects hippocampal neurons

against global ischemia-induced death. Proc Natl Acad Sci U S A 2005;102(34):12230–5.
163. Ying HS, Weishaupt JH, Grabb M, et al. Sublethal oxygen-glucose deprivation alters hippocampal neuronal AMPA receptor expression and vulnerability to kainate-induced death. J Neurosci 1997;17(24):9536–44.
166. Noda M, Sakuta H. Central regulation of body-fluid homeostasis. Trends Neurosci 2013;36(11):661–73.
168. Aarts M, Iihara K, Wei WL, et al. A key role for TRPM7 channels in anoxic neuronal death. Cell 2003;115(7):863–77.
169. Sun HS, Jackson MF, Martin LJ, et al. Suppression of hippocampal TRPM7 protein prevents delayed neuronal death in brain ischemia. Nat Neurosci 2009;12(10):1300–7.
171. Alim I, Teves L, Li R, et al. Modulation of NMDAR subunit expression by TRPM2 channels regulates neuronal vulnerability to ischemic cell death. J Neurosci 2013;33(44):17264–77.
172. Jia Y, Zhou J, Tai Y, et al. TRPC channels promote cerebellar granule neuron survival. Nat Neurosci 2007;10(5):559–67.
174. Lin Y, Zhang JC, Fu J, et al. Hyperforin attenuates brain damage induced by transient middle cerebral artery occlusion (MCAO) in rats via inhibition of TRPC6 channels degradation. J Cereb Blood Flow Metab 2013;33(2):253–62.
176. Immke DC, McCleskey EW. Protons open acid-sensing ion channels by catalyzing relief of Ca2+ blockade. Neuron 2003;37(1): 75–84.
179. Xiong ZG, Zhu XM, Chu XP, et al. Neuroprotection in ischemia: blocking calcium-permeable acid-sensing ion channels. Cell 2004;118(6):687–98.
180. Wang YZ, Zeng WZ, Xiao X, et al. Intracellular ASIC1a regulates mitochondrial permeability transition-dependent neuronal death. Cell Death Differ 2013;20(10):1359–69.
181. Nicotera P, Leist M, Fava E, et al. Energy requirement for caspase activation and neuronal cell death. Brain PatholBrain Pathol 2000;10(2):276–82.
183. Frederickson CJ, Koh JY, Bush AI. The neurobiology of zinc in health and disease. Nat Rev Neurosci 2005;6(6):449–62.
186. Peters S, Koh J, Choi DW. Zinc selectively blocks the action of N-methyl-D-aspartate on cortical neurons. Science 1987; 236(4801):589–93.
187. Westbrook GL, Mayer ML. Micromolar concentrations of Zn^{2+} antagonize NMDA and GABA responses of hippocampal neurons. Nature 1987;328(6131):640–3.
189. Rassendren FA, Lory P, Pin JP, et al. Zinc has opposite effects on NMDA and non-NMDA receptors expressed in Xenopus oocytes. Neuron 1990;4(5):733–40.
195. Li Y, Hough CJ, Frederickson CJ, et al. Induction of mossy fiber -> Ca3 long-term potentiation requires translocation of synaptically released Zn2+. J Neurosci 2001;21(20):8015–25.
196. Sloviter RS. A selective loss of hippocampal mossy fiber Timm stain accompanies granule cell seizure activity induced by perforant path stimulation. Brain Res 1985;330(1):150–3.
198. Weiss JH, Hartley DM, Koh JY, et al. AMPA receptor activation potentiates zinc neurotoxicity. Neuron 1993;10(1):43–9.
200. Bonanni L, Chachar M, Jover-Mengual T, et al. Zinc-dependent multi-conductance channel activity in mitochondria isolated from ischemic brain. J Neurosci 2006;26(25):6851–62.
201. Koh JY, Suh SW, Gwag BJ, et al. The role of zinc in selective neuronal death after transient global cerebral ischemia. Science 1996;272(5264):1013–16.
202. Rosenbaum DM, Degterev A, David J, et al. Necroptosis, a novel form of caspase-independent cell death, contributes to neuronal damage in a retinal ischemia-reperfusion injury model. J Neurosci Res 2010;88(7):1569–76.
206. Pulsinelli WA, Duffy TE. Regional energy balance in rat brain after transient forebrain ischemia. J Neurochem 1983;40(5): 1500–3.
208. Miyawaki T, Ofengeim D, Noh KM, et al. The endogenous inhibitor of Akt, CTMP, is critical to ischemia-induced neuronal death. Nat Neurosci 2009;12(5):618–26.
213. Nakamura T, Lipton SA. Preventing Ca2+-mediated nitrosative stress in neurodegenerative diseases: possible pharmacological strategies. Call Cal 2010;47(2):190–7.
217. Brennan-Minnella AM, Shen Y, El-Benna J, et al. Phosphoinositide 3-kinase couples NMDA receptors to superoxide release in excitotoxic neuronal death. Cell Death Dis 2013;4:e580.
221. Lonze BE, Riccio A, Cohen S, et al. Apoptosis, axonal growth defects, and degeneration of peripheral neurons in mice lacking CREB. Neuron 2002;34(3):371–85.
224. Schneider A, Martin-Villalba A, Weih F, et al. NF-kappaB is activated and promotes cell death in focal cerebral ischemia. Nat Med 1999;5(5):554–9.
227. Hannenhalli S, Kaestner KH. The evolution of Fox genes and their role in development and disease. Nat Rev Genet 2009; 10(4):233–40.
230. Dziennis S, Jia T, Ronnekleiv OK, et al. Role of signal transducer and activator of transcription-3 in estradiol-mediated neuroprotection. J Neurosci 2007;27(27):7268–74.
233. Aaronson DS, Horvath CM. A road map for those who don't know JAK-STAT. Science 2002;296(5573):1653–5.
235. Hwang CJ, Yun HM, Jung YY, et al. Reducing effect of il-32alpha in the development of stroke through blocking of NF-kappaB, but enhancement of STAT3 pathways. Mol Neurobiol 2014; 51(2):648–60.
236. Ballas N, Mandel G. The many faces of REST oversee epigenetic programming of neuronal genes. Curr Opin Neurobiol 2005; 15(5):500–6.
237. Ooi L, Wood IC. Chromatin crosstalk in development and disease: lessons from REST. Nat Rev Genet 2007;8(7):544–54.
240. Westbrook TF, Hu G, Ang XL, et al. SCFbeta-TRCP controls oncogenic transformation and neural differentiation through REST degradation. Nature 2008;452(7185):370–4.
241. Guardavaccaro D, Frescas D, Dorrello NV, et al. Control of chromosome stability by the beta-TrCP-REST-Mad2 axis. Nature 2008;452(7185):365–9.
242. Borrelli E, Nestler EJ, Allis CD, et al. Decoding the epigenetic language of neuronal plasticity. Neuron 2008;60(6):961–74.
245. Zuccato C, Tartari M, Crotti A, et al. Huntingtin interacts with REST/NRSF to modulate the transcription of NRSE-controlled neuronal genes. Nat Genet 2003;35(1):76–83.
246. Pozzi D, Lignani G, Ferrea E, et al. REST/NRSF-mediated intrinsic homeostasis protects neuronal networks from hyperexcitability. EMBO J 2013;32(22):2994–3007.
248. Iadecola C, Anrather J. The immunology of stroke: from mechanisms to translation. Nat Med 2011;17(7):796–808.
249. Hu X, Liou AK, Leak RK, et al. Neurobiology of microglial action in CNS injuries: Receptor-mediated signaling mechanisms and functional roles. Prog Neurobiol 2014;11:56–64.
251. Hu X, Li P, Guo Y, et al. Microglia/macrophage polarization dynamics reveal novel mechanism of injury expansion after focal cerebral ischemia. Stroke 2012;43(11):3063–70.
252. Liesz A, Zhou W, Na SY, et al. Boosting regulatory T cells limits neuroinflammation in permanent cortical stroke. J Neurosci 2013;33(44):17350–62.
253. Li P, Gan Y, Sun BL, et al. Adoptive regulatory T-cell therapy protects against cerebral ischemia. Ann Neurol 2013;74(3): 458–71.

6 Intracellular Signaling: Mediators and Protective Responses

John W. Thompson, Valina L. Dawson, Miguel A. Perez-Pinzon, Ted M. Dawson

KEY POINTS

- Preconditioning of the brain and other organs is an adaptive response to a noxious but non-lethal experience that activates an intracellular reaction rendering the tissue resistant to a subsequent potentially lethal event. Preconditioning consists of an early and a delayed window of protection which are characterized not only by their temporal profiles of protection but also by the mechanisms of activation and the robustness of the neuroprotective response.
- Cross-tolerance is preconditioning that can be activated by diverse insults that increase brain resistance to future injurious events due to a different stressor. The degree of efficacy in cross-tolerance may be somewhat diminished compared to preconditioning to the same stress.
- Preconditioning induces a network response of increased expression of proteins involved in cellular defense, cellular maintenance and regeneration and repair mechanisms.
- Preconditioning induces plasticity and neurogenesis which may allow for the replacement of dying cells and a reshaping of neuronal circuitry to prevent further loss of function.
- Preconditioning and ischemic tolerance are particularly attractive targets for clinical development because all compartments of the nervous system, neurons, glia and endothelial cells, are protected.

The brain is arguably the most complex organ in the body. In the human brain there are billions of neurons that make trillions of connections necessary for normal brain function. Although the brain is only 2% of total body weight it is the most metabolically active organ consuming 25% of total body glucose and oxygen. This high level of energy metabolism generates oxidative stress in an organ that is comprised mostly of lipid and cells that are structurally elaborate with extensive processes. An expectation would be that the cells of the brain would be exquisitely sensitive to stress. However, neurons are terminally differentiated post-mitotic cells with a limited capacity for replacement. Therefore, neurons have evolved powerful adaptive strategies to protect against the high level of oxidative stress produced during normal activity and possess a capacity for repair following injury. These neuroprotective and repair signaling pathways are largely not known, but are an active area of scientific investigation. It is possible that the next generation of therapeutic targets for neuroprotection will be derived from investigations into neuronal survival and repair strategies activated during periods of stress, a process termed preconditioning.

PRECONDITIONING

Preconditioning of the brain and other organs is an adaptive response to a noxious but non-lethal experience that activates an intracellular reaction rendering the tissue resistant to a subsequent potentially lethal event.[1,2] The ability of cells to increase their tolerance to a damaging stress was first described in the heart by Murry et al.[3] and was followed shortly thereafter by studies in the brain by Schurr et al.[4] Since these seminal studies research in laboratories around the world demonstrated the protective effects of preconditioning at the organismal, tissue, and cellular levels and in numerous species. Preconditioning is also observed in nature where certain species of animals appear to exist in a continuous preconditioned state, which allows them to survive in extreme environmental conditions. For example, a few species of turtles such as the freshwater turtles of the genus *Trachemys* and *Chrysemys*[5] and the marine loggerhead turtle *Caretta carreta*,[6] as well as the freshwater fish, *Carassius carassius*,[7] are known to tolerate extended periods of anoxia. In fact tolerance to an extreme or otherwise lethal environment is found ubiquitously in nature with the first published accounts of anoxia tolerance in reptiles being reported by Belkin in the 1960s.[8,9] Metabolic adaptation is also seen in higher euthermic animals such as the Artic ground squirrel, *Spermophilus parryii*, which experiences extreme reductions in cerebral blood perfusion during months of hibernation.[10,11]

Preconditioning is a term applied to the noxious but not lethal event that activates the protective response. The state of enhanced resistance to subsequent lethal events is termed tolerance. The clinical utility of preconditioning is not yet apparent. In the heart, retrospective studies demonstrate that patients that experience angina prior to an acute myocardial infarction have smaller infarct size, a reduction in ventricular dysfunction and arrhythmias, and a better in-hospital outcome following thrombolytic therapy than patients without preinfarction angina.[12,13] Similarly retrospective studies in patients with a history of transient ischemic attack suggests that preconditioning and tolerance occur in human brain as these patients have a more favorable outcome with smaller infarct size, milder clinical impairment and decreased morbidity following stroke.[14–17] Despite a more favorable outcome, patients who experience transient ischemic attack have a tenfold or higher increased risk of stroke[18,19] and these retrospective studies did not assess patients who did not survive their stroke. In addition, doubts have been raised about whether this type of intrinsic protection prevails with age.[20,21] However, these data provide a provocative possibility that the human brain and heart can be preconditioned and experience a state of tolerance. Thus understanding this process may provide new therapies targeted toward patients at risk of stroke and myocardial infarction.

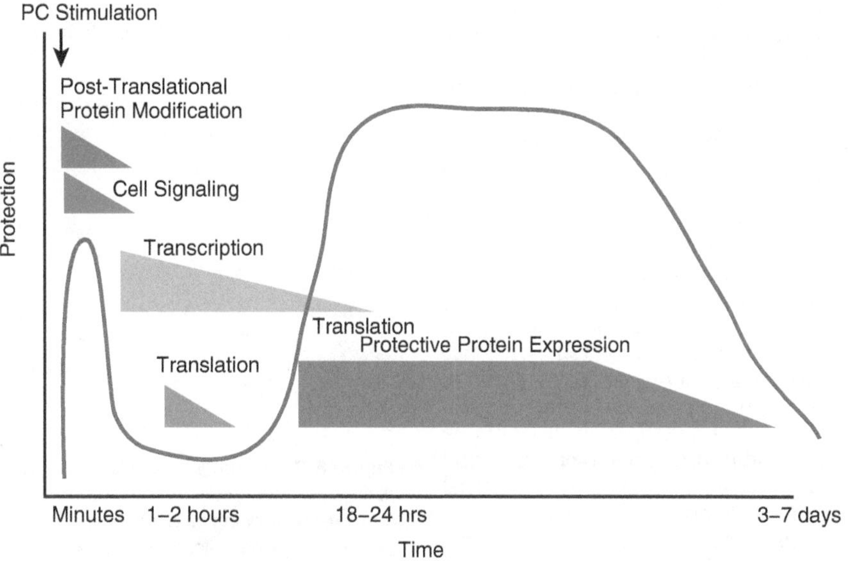

Figure 6-1. A preconditioning stimulation results in an acute transient period of neuroprotection lasting from minutes to 1–2 hours and is due to post-translational protein modifications. Subsequently new gene transcription and protein translation occur, leading the acquisition of neuroprotection that is stable for 24–48 hours, dissipating by 72 hours in most experimental models, although some models have described protection up to 7 days.

WINDOWS OF PRECONDITIONING

Preconditioning consists of early and delayed windows of protection which are characterized not only by their temporal profiles of protection but also by the mechanisms of activation and the robustness of the neuroprotective response (Fig. 6-1). The early or rapid window of protection is activated immediately following the preconditioning stimuli and lasts approximately 1 hour.[22] This rapid onset of protection is mediated by the combination of releasable factors and metabolites, which alter intercellular signaling cascades. The second window of protection is activated 24–48 hours following preconditioning and lasts for at least several days.[23] This delayed window of protection is characterized by an epigenetic reprogramming of the cell, which allows for a more robust and sustained state of tolerance when compared to the early window of protection.[24,25]

The preconditioning response is initiated by various trigger signals that activate receptors and downstream effector pathways leading to both the early and delayed windows of protection. Numerous trigger mechanisms have been described and include neuroactive cytokines,[26] glutamate,[27] adenosine,[28] ATP-sensitive potassium (K^{+}ATP) channels[29] and hypoxia[30] to name a few. Our laboratory and others have shown that both adenosine and post-synaptic NMDA receptors are required for ischemia-triggered preconditioning.[27,31,32] Adenosine is the final product of ATP metabolism and is released following ischemic preconditioning (IPC) where it activates adenosine A1 receptors (A1R).[33] Activation of both NMDA and A1 receptor pathways lead to the activation of the novel protein kinase c family member PKC epsilon (PKCε).[33] PKCε is central to the preconditioning response and is sufficient in and of itself to induce tolerance.[34] Numerous other signaling pathways have also been characterized during the induction of tolerance including AKT,[35] and the MAP kinase signaling cascade, ERK, JNK, and p38.[35–37] The activation of numerous signaling cascades following precondition suggests that there is likely cross-talk between the pro-survival kinase cascades such that tolerance may be the result of the coordination of several signaling pathways that act in concert to target many of the pathophysiological mechanisms leading to cell damage. Numerous reviews are written which provide in-depth overviews of these signaling pathways and their effect on IPC.[38]

INDUCTION OF PRECONDITIONING

As mentioned above, preconditioning can be activated by nearly any stressful stimulus. In cell culture preconditioning can be triggered by a wide variety of stimulations including: adenosine,[28,29] norepinephrine (noradrenaline),[39,40] calcium,[41] bradykinin,[42,43] heat shock,[44,45] mitochondrial uncouplers,[46,47] chemical inhibition of oxidative phosphorylation,[48–50] exposure to excitotoxins,[27,51] cytokines,[26,52] ceramide,[53,54] nitric oxide (NO),[55,56] potassium chloride,[57,58] hypoxia,[30,59] anoxia,[56,60] and oxygen glucose deprivation.[61] Several intracellular signaling pathways mediate preconditioning. The molecular events that mediate tolerance are an active area of investigation. In vivo, preconditioning in the brain can also be experimentally induced by a variety of stimuli. Both global ischemia (occlusion of both common carotid arteries) and focal ischemia (occlusion of the middle cerebral artery) for short durations can activate tolerance within 24 hours.[62,63] Placing animals in a chamber and exposing them to hypoxia for 1–6 hours induces tolerance to either transient or permanent focal ischemia 1–3 days following the hypoxic incident.[64] A small dose of lipopolysaccharide (LPS) injected into the peritoneal cavity is sufficient to induce tolerance within 2–3 days following injection that is sustained for approximately 7 days.[65–69] Inhibition of oxidative phosphorylation by the irreversible inhibitor of succinate dehydrogenase, 3-nitropropionic acid, activates preconditioning in gerbils and rats that develops over 1–4 days, providing protection against transient focal ischemia.[70–72] Exposure to cold or heat can trigger tolerance in experimental animals. Hypothermic (25–32 °C)[73,74] or hyperthermic temperatures (42–43 °C),[75,76] induce tolerance to focal ischemia 24 hours later. However, this preconditioning appears to have a shorter window of opportunity compared to other stressors in which tolerance is sustained from 24 to 72 hours, temperature stress provides protection between 18 and 24 hours, but this protection resolves by 48 hours. Cortical spreading depression of slowly propagating waves of depolarization across the cortex can be triggered experimentally by the application of potassium chloride on the surface of the dura mater or the cortex. Cortical spreading depression induces a prolonged phase of ischemic tolerance that lasts 1–7 days[57,77,78] providing protection against transient and permanent focal ischemia. Surprisingly inhalational anesthetics can chemically precondition the brain in experimental animal models. Isoflurane, sevoflurane, and halothane when given to animals provide protection against permanent or focal ischemia. In the case of isoflurane the protective effects are immediate and last at least 24 hours. This suggests that isoflurane can activate both acute and chronic preconditioning.[79] These observations introduce a significant confound in exploring preconditioning in animal models since all experimental stroke studies are conducted under anesthesia. Since preconditioning can be activated by a diverse set of stressors, the molecular mechanisms initiating and sustaining the protective response are active areas of investigation. It would be simple to understand if preconditioning altered cerebral blood flow in a positive manner. However, measurements of cerebral blood flow showed that tolerance was not accompanied by an improvement of regional tissue perfusion during or after the ischemia that induced tolerance.[63,80] Thus, ischemic tolerance is likely a result of changes in the neurons, glia, and blood vessels of the brain at the cellular level in response to stress.

CROSS-TOLERANCE

Numerous studies indicate that preconditioning can be activated by a wide range of insults, chemical, pharmacological or physical. Virtually any stimulus that can alter brain function appears to have the capacity to increase brain resistance to future injurious events. Furthermore, one stressor that activates preconditioning can induce tolerance towards a different injurious stressor such as LPS inducing tolerance against ischemia. This phenomenon is termed cross-tolerance. The degree of efficacy in cross-tolerance may be somewhat diminished in comparison to ischemic preconditioning inducing ischemic tolerance. Also, the window for the development of tolerance may be altered. For example in many models it takes between 2 and 3 days for maximal tolerance to be realized following injection of LPS rather than 1 day for ischemic tolerance.[81] Since tolerance is observed across organ systems and tolerance can be induced by a wide variety of stressors, it is logical but perhaps simplistic, to presume that these stress signals would converge onto a final common pathway to promote cellular survival. While very attractive this hypothesis does not appear to be valid. A number of genetic analyses of tissue following exposure to different preconditioning stressors show that different gene sets are differentially expressed depending on the nature of the preconditioning stimulus.[81,82] Studies of individual proteins and their involvement in preconditioning and tolerance support this observation as well.[2,81,83] Conceptually, potential mechanisms could include both enhanced cellular defense functions and increased cellular surveillance improving cell maintenance through the stress response. Evidence for both pathways exists. Preconditioning can arise both by post-translational modification of proteins or by expression of new proteins. These newly expressed proteins and enhanced signaling cascades can either strengthen survival mechanisms or may inhibit cell death signaling. Activation of the cell stress response and synthesis of stress proteins will increase the capacity for general cell maintenance allowing for proper cell function. The best known stress response proteins are protein chaperones that unfold damaged or misfolded proteins to facilitate the disposal of these unneeded proteins by the cell. It is not yet known if these two strategies work in concert or independently. However, it is curious that in many experimental model

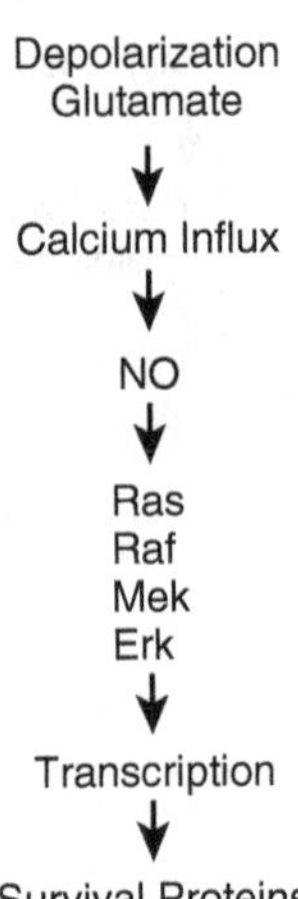

Figure 6-2. Neuronal depolarization leading to glutamate release and glutamate receptor stimulation activates production of nitric oxide (NO) and preconditioning and tolerance through the Ras, Raf, mitogen-activated protein kinase (Mek), extracellular signal-regulated kinase (Erk) signal cascade that triggers gene transcription and production of survival proteins.

systems knockdown or knockout of a single preconditioning molecule is sufficient to block the development of preconditioning and the expression of a single molecule is often sufficient to provide protection. These observations would suggest some sort of a network response to provide protection, even if there is no final common pathway.

CELLULAR DEFENSE

Reactive Oxygen Species

There is strong evidence that reactive oxygen species (ROS) are essential during the preconditioning response. Both in vitro and in vivo, NO generation following glutamate receptor stimulation activates preconditioning and tolerance[84,85] through the Ras, Raf, Mek, Erk signal cascade[85] to trigger gene transcription (Fig. 6-2). Superoxide anion production is also important as increasing levels of superoxide dismutase, the enzyme that degrades superoxide anion, are sufficient to block the development of tolerance in rats.[86] It is not surprising that ROS would be a strong inducer for preconditioning since the primary role of ROS is considered to be involved in is the pathogenesis of brain injury from ischemia. High levels of ROS are generated during both ischemia and reperfusion in all compartments of the brain, neurons, glia, and endothelial cells. Additionally during reperfusion excessive NO generated during ischemia can be converted to peroxynitrite following the reaction with superoxide anion to generate highly toxic reactive nitrogen species. Thus one might expect that a component of the tolerance response would be the increased expression of antioxidant enzymes including the superoxide dismutases, catalase, glutathione peroxidase, and thioredoxin. Both in vitro and in vivo, following ischemic preconditioning and some other stressors, significant induction of the superoxide dismutases, catalase, glutathione peroxidase, thioredoxin has been observed. Although the development of tolerance has not been associated with the increased expression of these enzymes indicating that increased antioxidant capacity can facilitate tolerance, but it is not essential for tolerance.

Mitochondria

Mitochondrial dysfunction following ischemia/reperfusion is a major contributing factor to neuronal cell death. Therefore mitochondrial protection is a primary target of preconditioning mediated tolerance.[87] As mentioned above, mild increases in ROS formation serve as a trigger in inducing preconditioning signaling pathways.[88,89] This mild increase in ROS formation appears to be the result of a temporary opening of the mitochondrial ATP-sensitive potassium channels (mitoK^+_{ATP}). Numerous studies have demonstrated that inhibitors of the mitoK^+_{ATP} block preconditioning neuroprotection whereas mitoK^+_{ATP} agonists induce a preconditioning response.[90,91] For example, use of a mitoK^+_{ATP} channel antagonist, such as 5-hydroxydecanoic acid, blocked IPC-mediated protection in the rat heart[92] whereas the mitoK^+_{ATP} channel agonist, diazoxide, induced a preconditioning response.[93,94] In contrast, excess ROS formation is a major contributing factor to mitochondrial damage following ischemia/reperfusion.[87] Mitochondria are highly sensitive to reactive oxygen and nitrogen species formation (ROS and RNS, respectively), which is generated primarily, but not exclusively, in the mitochondria. ROS and RNS target proteins of the electron transport chain and Krebs cycle, DNA, and mitochondrial specific phospholipid cardiolipin.[95-97] ROS formation also increases sensitivity of the mitochondrial permeability transition pore opening to calcium allowing for the release of apoptogenic factors from the mitochondria.[98] Thus, as would be expected, mitochondria have several defense mechanisms against oxidative stress, such as antioxidant enzymes, that aid in quelling a substantial rise in ROS levels. Therefore, part of preconditioning-induced tolerance stems from the ability of the mitochondria to up-regulate antioxidant defense systems and thereby maintain normal mitochondrial physiology.[99] These antioxidant defense systems include both low-molecular-weight antioxidants, such as glutathione, coenzyme Q, lipoic acid, and ascorbate and antioxidant-related proteins such as manganese superoxide dismutase (SOD2), glutathione peroxidase, peroxiredoxin, glutaredoxin, thioredoxin, glutathione reductase, and thioredoxin reductase.[100-102]

Neurotrophin Support

Known survival-promoting molecules are often observed to be increased during the tolerance phase. Neurotrophins support survival and growth. Molecules that show increased expression include nerve growth factor,[103] brain-derived growth factor,[103,104] basic fibroblast growth factor,[105,106] insulin-like growth factor,[107] epidermal growth factor,[108,109] vascular endothelial growth factor,[64,110,111] and neuregulin.[112] Expression of these proteins provides protection against a variety of neurotoxic insults and thus increased expression following a preconditioning stimulation would reasonably provide resistance to subsequent injury. These growth factors are important in the maintenance and survival of not only neurons, but glia and endothelial cells as well. Furthermore, these growth factors have been implicated in neurogenesis, vascular genesis and remodeling events following ischemic injury and may play a similar role in the development of tolerance.

Survival Kinases

Protein kinases phosphorylate proteins to activate signaling responses. The serine/threonine-specific protein kinase Akt (protein kinase B), when phosphorylated by phosphotidylinositol-3-kinase, is a key mediator of tolerance.[113] This protection appears to occur through Akt phosphorylation and activation of mixed lineage kinase-3. However, the role of Akt in tolerance presented in the literature is mixed. In some model systems phospho-Akt is readily observed and mechanistic investigations can link it to neuronal survival.[114,115] In other studies investigators have not observed a role for

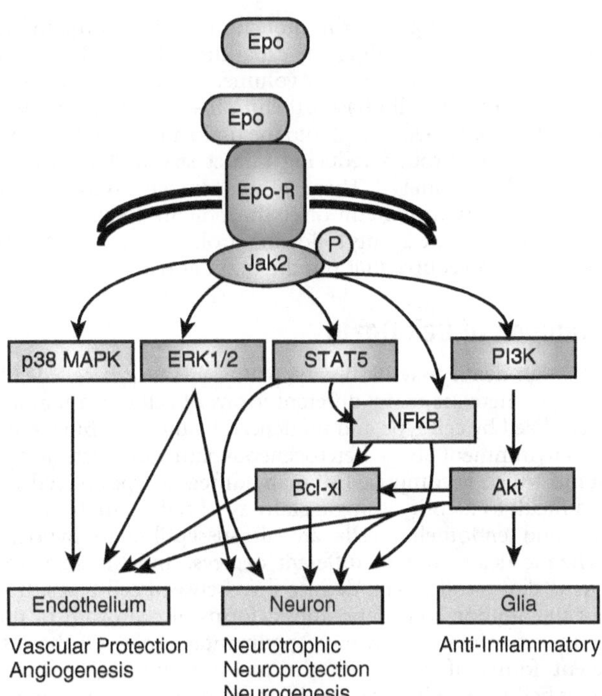

Figure 6-3. During conditions of low oxygen the transcription factor hypoxia-inducible factor is stabilized leading to the expression of erythropoietin (Epo) which binds to its receptor (EpoR) on endothelial cells, neurons and glia. Activation of the EpoR promotes phosphorylation of Janus tyrosine kinase 2 (JAK2) triggering other signaling molecules including the mitogen-activated protein kinase p38 (p38 MAPK), extracellular signal-regulated kinase 1/2 (ERK1/2) signal transducer and activator of transcription 5 (STAT5), and phosphotidylinositol-3-kinase (PI3K). Additionally Akt and nuclear factor-κB (NF-κB) are activated. ERK1/2 are essential for Epo-mediated neuroprotection and angiogenesis. STAT5 may be involved in Epo-mediated NF-κB nuclear translocation but whether this contributes to neuroprotection is not yet clear. Epo-mediated activation of PI3K/Akt phosphorylation, is involved in preventing inflammation, vascular protection and angiogenesis. Through stimulating Bcl-xl, PI3K/Akt mediates Epo-dependent vascular protection and neuroprotection. The translocation of NF-κB to the nucleus triggers events leading to neurogenesis and neuroprotection.

Akt.[116,117] The discrepancy in these observations is likely due to differences in the experimental models used in these studies and reflects the diversity of tolerance pathways. Recently hypoxic preconditioning was shown to involve phosphotidylinositol-3-kinase activation of Akt and subsequent phosphorylation of survivin to promote endothelial cell survival[118] once again suggesting that understanding the role of Akt and its phosphorylation targets such as survivin may provide insight and therapeutic targets for protecting the brain from ischemic insult.

Erythropoietin

Erythropoietin (EPO) is an interesting molecule in the preconditioning and tolerance field (Fig. 6-3). Erythropoietin is a clinically approved glycoprotein hormone that is induced by ischemic preconditioning by activation of (HIF)-1α. Due to the potential clinical utility of erythropoietin rapid progress defined erythropoietin signaling cascades including the Janus kinase-2 pathway, the phosphoinositide-3 kinase,[119] Akt[120,121] pathway, the extracellular signal-regulated kinase (ERK) and signal transducers and activators of transcription (STAT) pathways.[122] In part, the protective actions of erythropoietin are thought to converge on the induction of Bcl-2 proteins to block cell death signaling. In experimental focal ischemia, erythropoietin reduces infarct volume.[120] Erythropoietin was forwarded for a small Phase I/II clinical stroke study and was found to be safe, penetrated into the brain and provided some improvement through reducing infarct size and improving functional outcome.[123] These results are encouraging and suggest that erythropoietin or erythropoietin derivatives may be useful protective agents following stroke or as pre-treatment agents for procedures that put the brain at risk.

Inhibition of Cell Death

Although death may be binary, pathways towards cell death are not. There are many different forms of cell death that are specialized by cell type and influenced by the local biochemical environment. In a heterogeneous structure such as the brain, which is comprised of many different types of cells, it is difficult to identify a single pathway of cell death. Neurons, glia and endothelial cells are all susceptible to hypoxic-ischemic death, but to different degrees, and the signaling events that result in cell demise vary between cell types. It is not uncommon to observe mixed forms of cell death in the brains of animals following experimental stroke. Of the different forms of cell death the major forms in the brain described to date include: extrinsic apoptosis, intrinsic apoptosis, necroptosis, paraptosis, parthanatos, unfolded-protein response (endoplasmic reticulum stress) and autophagy.[124] Apoptosis has been widely studied and defined as occurring through two primary signaling pathways which are termed the extrinsic pathway, which originates through the activation of cell-surface death receptors resulting in the activation of caspase-8 or caspase-10 and the intrinsic pathway, which originates from mitochondrial release of cytochrome c and associated activation of caspase-9. Recently, a less well-characterized intrinsic pathway originating from the endoplasmic reticulum also results in the activation of caspase-9. Caspases are cysteine-aspartyl-specific proteases that are the biochemical hallmark behind apoptosis. Through the action of these proteases the cell is deconstructed and apoptotic bodies are formed. Necroptosis is a form of cell death where features of both apoptosis and necrosis are observed. Paraptosis is a non-apoptotic form of cell death that is programmatic as transcription and translation are required, as are activation of extracellular signal-regulated kinase 2 and ASK-interacting protein-1. Parthanatos is cell death mediated by excess production of poly(ADP-ribose) (PAR) by PAR polymerase-1 (PARP-1). Parthanatos is observed in many tissues throughout the body, including the brain, following hypoxic-ischemic insult. The generation of PAR leads to release of apoptosis inducing factor (AIF) from the mitochondria that enters the nucleus triggering chromosomal degradation, nuclear shrinkage, and cell death. The unfolded-protein response is activated following cellular stress that leads to new protein expression to facilitate the efficiency of the endoplasmic reticulum and proper protein folding. This is a carefully choreographed response to prevent the accumulation of proteins in order to allow time for the elimination of unfolded proteins, and re-establishes cellular homeostasis. However, if the stress cannot be resolved the system becomes overwhelmed and the cell dies. The exact mechanisms of cell death are not yet known but involve in part transcription factor regulation as well as activation of the caspase cascade. Autophagy is subdivided into macroautophagy, microautophagy and chaperone-mediated autophagy and it is a complementary pathway to the ubiquitin-proteasomal system to degrade proteins, protein aggregates, and organelles through the lysosome. It is generally thought that autophagy is a pro-survival response facilitating the clearance of damaged proteins and organelles and recent data show that interfering with autophagy results in neuronal demise while stimulating autophagy can improve survival.[125]

It is no surprise that induction of proteins that oppose these cell death signaling cascades would be part of the expression of tolerance. For the most part, the most studied events are those involved in the apoptotic cascade and most studies describe changes in protein expression, but the relative functional value of altered protein expression is not always apparent. In many cases it is likely that depressing cell death programs is part of a larger response that provides protection, survival and restoration of function. For example, the tumor suppressor transcription factor protein, p53, that can mediate cell death, is suppressed in the tolerant brain.[126] Hippocampal cell cultures preconditioned with the K_{ATP} channel antagonist diazoxide express less p53 and are resistant to apoptosis.[127] Furthermore, overexpression of p53 exacerbates cell death. Taken together, these data point to a role for p53 in regulating the degree of tolerance. Many investigators have explored the role of the Bcl family proteins in preconditioning and tolerance due to their active role in promoting or preventing apoptosis.[128–135] While there is some disparity in findings, most studies indicate that tolerance is associated with a persistent increase in the pro-survival Bcl-2 or Bcl-xl proteins. Less consistent are the observations of the pro-death Bax protein. Intriguingly there are reports that activation of caspase-3, an event most commonly associated with rapid and pronounced cell death, is important for the development of tolerance.[136] Iduna (RNF146), a PAR-dependent ubiquitin E3 ligase is induced by preconditioning and blocks the ability of PAR to release AIF and prevents cell death both in vitro and in vivo.[137] We do not yet know if there is production of proteins that block the other forms of cell death that are observed in ischemic injury. However, it is likely that the ability of preconditioning to reduce ischemic cell death probably involves networks of, as yet unidentified, proteins that have direct and unique cell survival functions. These novel proteins may not function entirely through existing pro-apoptotic or pro-death pathways.

CELLULAR MAINTENANCE

Following a significant stressful event, cells respond by synthesizing a class of proteins called stress proteins. Increased expression of stress proteins can render cells resistant to subsequent potentially injurious stresses.[138] This stress response has been under investigation for several decades and dates back to the acquisition of tolerance to heat shock, resulting in these stress proteins being termed heat-shock proteins (designated Hsp). Heat-shock proteins can be divided into six subfamilies comprised of many members[139] that facilitate the folding of newly synthesized polypeptides into functional proteins. Heat shock proteins also play an important role in maintaining properly folded protein, as well as promoting protein–protein interactions and preventing protein aggregation. These actions are commonly referred to as chaperone functions. Through their interactions with co-chaperones and client proteins both constitutive and inducible Hsp's regulate signal cascades. There are numerous reports on regulated expression of Hsp70 in response to preconditioning, tolerance and cerebral ischemia[140,141] (Fig. 6-4). There exists a large body of published work indicating a prominent role for Hsp70 in adaptive cytoprotection and tolerance and that elevated expression of Hsp70 is neuroprotective. The roles that Hsp70 plays in the development and maintenance of tolerance is not entirely clear and is likely due to the different stresses that trigger Hsp70 expression and the model systems studied.

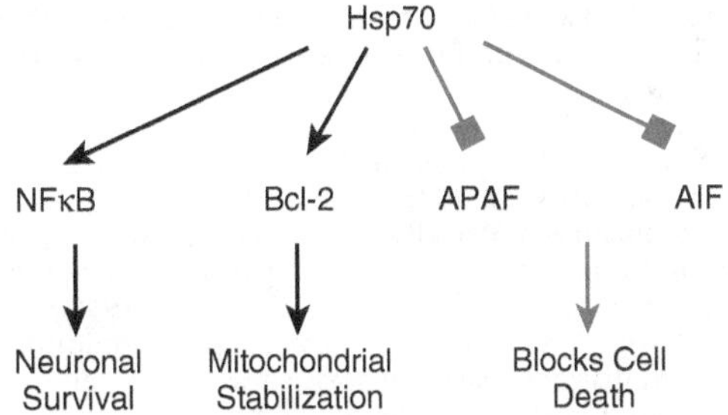

Figure 6-4. Heat shock proteins (Hsp) have been implicated in the development and maintenance of tolerance. Hsp70 expression can be activated early and may facilitate preconditioning induced activation of the transcription factor, nuclear factor κB (NFκB) as well as stabilizing mitochondrial function and actions on Bcl-2. Hsp70 can block cell death signaling by binding to apoptosis protease activating factor-1 (Apaf-1) preventing the development of the apoptosome and by blocking mitochondrial release of AIF and translocation to the nucleus.

Hsp70 expression can be activated early and its increased expression sustained. In the early phase of expression it may facilitate preconditioning-induced activation of the transcription factor, nuclear factor κB (NFκB) that is well described as promoting preconditioning.[38] Hsp70 can also promote cell survival during the tolerance phase through maintenance of mitochondrial physiology. However, the direct actions of Hsp70 on the observed preservation of mitochondrial function are not yet understood. Hsp70 is a regulator of Bcl-2 expression in both normal and injured neurons.[142] Hsp70 can also bind to apoptosis protease activating factor-1 (Apaf-1) preventing the development of the apoptosome and subsequence caspase activation and cell death.[143] Importantly, Hsp70 both prevents mitochondrial release of AIF and sequesters AIF in the cytosol leading to degradation.[144] As AIF is a primary mediator of ischemic injury, preventing its entry to the nucleus could have profound neuroprotective effects. While Hsp70 and family members have been explored in brain ischemia the role of the other Hsp family members in the development of preconditioning and tolerance or in response to ischemic injury is not well studied or developed yet. The strength of the data on Hsp70 as a neuroprotective molecule highlights the importance in understanding protein maintenance as a relevant therapeutic strategy.

REGENERATION AND REPAIR

For over a century it was believed that the mature nervous system was the one organ system that lacked the capacity for renewal and repair. Recently, we have come to appreciate that the brain has a limited capacity to replace and repair neural cells. This process of neurogenesis arises from progenitor or stem cells in specialized regions of the nervous system. The cells of the dentate gyrus and the subventricular zone have been the most intensively studied.[145,146] On-going studies are just defining the role these new cells play and how they integrate into the existing circuitry. From the limited literature currently available it is reasonable to propose that the newborn cells are not just replacing old and damaged cells, but may be important for plasticity required to shape existing neural circuitry in response to experience in learning and memory, mood, and response to injury. Preconditioning produces enough stress to trigger plasticity and a neurogenesis response.[147–149] This neurogenesis corresponds with improved memory scores[149] and may be important in the development of tolerance;[148] however, the latter is difficult to determine with currently available tools to block neurogenesis. While a general focus of current research is to facilitate endogenous neurogenesis to replace cells lost to injury, it is also possible that these newly born cells may play an important role in remodeling the nervous system to resist further injury and loss of function. These possibilities await further scientific investigation.

CLINICAL IMPLICATIONS

With the failure of so many neuroprotective drug trials for the treatment of stroke,[150] investigators are looking for new approaches to develop effective therapies. Preconditioning and ischemic tolerance are particularly attractive phenomena because all compartments of the nervous system, neurons, glia and endothelial cells, appear to be protected. The hope is that understanding the molecular events during preconditioning or those active during tolerance, will provide a window through which we can discover new treatments. Functional and descriptive studies have facilitated the understanding of the initial cellular events that trigger gene transcription and lead to new protein translation resulting in the phenomena of preconditioning and tolerance. Genomic and proteomic experiments have generated large "laundry" lists of putative candidate proteins that may mediate the profound neuroprotection afforded by preconditioning. However, as our knowledge grows it is becoming clear that these events set in motion a complicated network of signaling.

There are several challenges in harnessing preconditioning as a therapeutic tool. One challenge is the observation that the most effective stressors in triggering preconditioning such as ischemia, glutamate, NO and cytokines also play important roles in acute stroke to promote ischemic tissue damage. In order to develop new therapeutic strategies it is important to separate the neuroprotective pathways from the neurotoxic pathways induced by these agents and to functionally identify the molecules that mediate neuroprotection. Another challenge is the possibility that combinatorial therapy will be necessary in order to fully protect the nervous system from ischemic injury since ischemic preconditioning is a complicated network of signaling events. It is possible that a chemical preconditioning drug could be found. The challenge is identifying a compound that will activate the stress response without itself being toxic, as well as having a wide therapeutic window. The other challenge is to identify clinical populations that could measurably benefit from the treatment. Logically these might be scenarios where ischemic injury can occur, such as surgical settings. Coronary artery bypass surgery, while lifesaving, often has adverse effects, such as neurological damage and cognitive impairment from ischemic events. Preconditioning directed therapies might be useful in this setting and other surgical settings. Depending on the treatment there might also be a utility for treating the acute stroke patient during the period of maturation of the stroke. Our understanding of the plasticity of the nervous system is just emerging, harnessing the power of preconditioning and tolerance has promise as a new arena to develop novel therapies to protect the nervous system from ischemic injury.

Acknowledgments

This work was supported by grants from NIH/NIDA DA000266 (T.M.D. & V.L.D.); NIH/NINDS NS67525 (T.M.D.), NS45676 (M.P.P), NS054147 (M.P.P), NS34773 (M.P.P); MDSCRF 2009-MSCRFII-0125-00 Independent Investigator Award (State of Maryland) (V.L.D.); and AHA Postdoctoral award 12POST12090006 (J.W.T). T.M.D. is the Leonard and Madlyn Abramson Professor in Neurodegenerative Diseases.

REFERENCES

1. Nandagopal K, Dawson TM, Dawson VL. Critical role for nitric oxide signaling in cardiac and neuronal ischemic preconditioning and tolerance. J Pharmacol Exp Ther 2001;297:474–8.

2. Obrenovitch TP. Molecular physiology of preconditioning-induced brain tolerance to ischemia. Physiol Rev 2008;88:211–47.
3. Murry CE, Jennings RB, Reimer KA. Preconditioning with ischemia: a delay of lethal cell injury in ischemic myocardium. Circulation 1986;74:1124–36.
4. Schurr A, Reid KH, Tseng MT, et al. Adaptation of adult brain tissue to anoxia and hypoxia in vitro. Brain Res 1986;374: 244–8.
5. Lutz PL, Nilsson GE, Perez-Pinzon MA. Anoxia tolerant animals from a neurobiological perspective. Comp Biochem Physiol B Biochem Mol Biol 1996;113:3–13.
6. Lutz PL, LaManna JC, Adams MR, et al. Cerebral resistance to anoxia in the marine turtle. Respir Physiol 1980;41:241–51.
7. Nilsson GE, Renshaw GM. Hypoxic survival strategies in two fishes: extreme anoxia tolerance in the North European crucian carp and natural hypoxic preconditioning in a coral-reef shark. J Exp Biol 2004;207:3131–9.
8. Belkin DA. Anoxia: tolerance in reptiles. Science 1963;139: 492–3.
9. Belkin DA. Anaerobic brain function: effects of stagnant and anoxic anoxia on persistence of breathing in reptiles. Science 1968;162:1017–18.
10. Dave KR, Christian SL, Perez-Pinzon MA, et al. Neuroprotection: lessons from hibernators. Comp Biochem Physiol B Biochem Mol Biol 2012;162:1–9.
11. Drew KL, Harris MB, LaManna JC, et al. Hypoxia tolerance in mammalian heterotherms. J Exp Biol 2004;207:3155–62.
12. Reiter R, Henry TD, Traverse JH. Preinfarction angina reduces infarct size in ST-elevation myocardial infarction treated with percutaneous coronary intervention. Circ Cardiovasc Interv 2013;6:52–8.
13. Rezkalla SH, Kloner RA. Ischemic preconditioning and preinfarction angina in the clinical arena. Nat Clin Pract Cardiovasc Med 2004;1:96–102.
14. Arboix A, Cabeza N, Garcia-Eroles L, et al. Relevance of transient ischemic attack to early neurological recovery after nonlacunar ischemic stroke. Cerebrovasc Dis 2004;18:304–11.
15. Moncayo J, de Freitas GR, Bogousslavsky J, et al. Do transient ischemic attacks have a neuroprotective effect? Neurology 2000; 54:2089–94.
16. Schaller B. Ischemic preconditioning as induction of ischemic tolerance after transient ischemic attacks in human brain: its clinical relevance. Neurosci Lett 2005;377:206–11.
17. Weih M, Kallenberg K, Bergk A, et al. Attenuated stroke severity after prodromal TIA: a role for ischemic tolerance in the brain? Stroke 1999;30:1851–4.
18. Giles MF, Rothwell PM. Prediction and prevention of stroke after transient ischemic attack in the short and long term. Expert Rev Neurother 2006;6:381–95.
19. Johnston SC, Gress DR, Browner WS, et al. Short-term prognosis after emergency department diagnosis of TIA. JAMA 2000;284: 2901–6.
20. Della-Morte D, Cacciatore F, Salsano E, et al. Age-related reduction of cerebral ischemic preconditioning: myth or reality? Clin Interv Aging 2013;8:1055–61.
21. Abete P, Cacciatore F, Testa G, et al. Ischemic preconditioning in the aging heart: from bench to bedside. Ageing Res Rev 2010;9: 153–62.
22. Perez-Pinzon MA, Xu GP, Dietrich WD, et al. Rapid preconditioning protects rats against ischemic neuronal damage after 3 but not 7 days of reperfusion following global cerebral ischemia. J Cereb Blood Flow Metab 1997;17:175–82.
23. Kato H, Araki T, Kogure K. Preserved neurotransmitter receptor binding following ischemia in preconditioned gerbil brain. Brain Res Bull 1992;29:395–400.
24. Thompson JW, Dave KR, Young JI, et al. Ischemic preconditioning alters the epigenetic profile of the brain from ischemic intolerance to ischemic tolerance. Neurother 2013;10:789–97.
25. Pagliaro P, Gattullo D, Rastaldo R, et al. Ischemic preconditioning: from the first to the second window of protection. Life Sci 2001;69:1–15.
26. Lin HY, Huang CC, Chang KF. Lipopolysaccharide preconditioning reduces neuroinflammation against hypoxic ischemia and provides long-term outcome of neuroprotection in neonatal rat. Pediatr Res 2009;66:254–9.
27. Grabb MC, Choi DW. Ischemic tolerance in murine cortical cell culture: critical role for NMDA receptors. J Neurosci 1999;19: 1657–62.
28. Liu Y, Xiong L, Chen S, et al. Isoflurane tolerance against focal cerebral ischemia is attenuated by adenosine A1 receptor antagonists. Can J Anaesth 2006;53:194–201.
29. Perez-Pinzon MA, Born JG. Rapid preconditioning neuroprotection following anoxia in hippocampal slices: role of the K+ ATP channel and protein kinase C. Neuroscience 1999;89:453–9.
30. Liu J, Ginis I, Spatz M, et al. Hypoxic preconditioning protects cultured neurons against hypoxic stress via TNF-alpha and ceramide. Am J Physiol Cell Physiol 2000;278:C144–53.
31. Raval AP, Dave KR, Mochly-Rosen D, et al. Epsilon PKC is required for the induction of tolerance by ischemic and NMDA-mediated preconditioning in the organotypic hippocampal slice. J Neurosci 2003;23:384–91.
32. Bond A, Lodge D, Hicks CA, et al. NMDA receptor antagonism, but not AMPA receptor antagonism attenuates induced ischaemic tolerance in the gerbil hippocampus. Eur J Pharmacol 1999; 380:91–9.
33. Lange-Asschenfeldt C, Raval AP, Dave KR, et al. Epsilon protein kinase C mediated ischemic tolerance requires activation of the extracellular regulated kinase pathway in the organotypic hippocampal slice. J Cereb Blood Flow Metab 2004;24:636–45.
34. Simkhovich BZ, Przyklenk K, Kloner RA. Role of protein kinase C in ischemic "conditioning": from first evidence to current perspectives. J Cardiovasc Pharmacol Ther 2013;18:525–32.
35. Zhang H, Xue G, Zhang W, et al. Akt and Erk1/2 activate the ornithine decarboxylase/polyamine system in cardioprotective ischemic preconditioning in rats: the role of mitochondrial permeability transition pores. Mol Cell Biochem 2014;390: 133–42.
36. Bi XY, Wang TS, Zhang M, et al. [The up-regulation of p-p38 MAPK during the induction of brain ischemic tolerance induced by intermittent hypobaric hypoxia preconditioning in rats]. Zhongguo Ying Yong Sheng Li Xue Za Zhi 2014;30:97–100.
37. Zhang Y, Li YW, Wang YX, et al. Remifentanil preconditioning alleviating brain damage of cerebral ischemia reperfusion rats by regulating the JNK signal pathway and TNF-alpha/TNFR1 signal pathway. Mol Biol Rep 2013;40:6997–7006.
38. Dirnagl U, Simon RP, Hallenbeck JM. Ischemic tolerance and endogenous neuroprotection. Trends Neurosci 2003;26: 248–54.
39. Bankwala Z, Hale SL, Kloner RA. Alpha-adrenoceptor stimulation with exogenous norepinephrine or release of endogenous catecholamines mimics ischemic preconditioning. Circulation 1994;90:1023–8.
40. Imani A, Faghihi M, Sadr SS, et al. Noradrenaline protects in vivo rat heart against infarction and ventricular arrhythmias via nitric oxide and reactive oxygen species. J Surg Res 2011;169:9–15.
41. Ashraf M, Suleiman J, Ahmad M. Ca^{2+} preconditioning elicits a unique protection against the Ca^{2+} paradox injury in rat heart. Role of adenosine. Fixed. Circ Res 1994;74:360–7.
42. Goto M, Liu Y, Yang XM, et al. Role of bradykinin in protection of ischemic preconditioning in rabbit hearts. Circ Res 1995; 77:611–21.
43. Mechirova E, Danielisova V, Domorakova I, et al. Bradykinin preconditioning affects the number of degenerated neurons and the level of antioxidant enzymes in spinal cord ischemia in rabbits. Acta Histochem 2014;116:252–7.
44. Zhong GQ, Tu RH, Zeng ZY, et al. Novel functional role of heat shock protein 90 in protein kinase C-mediated ischemic postconditioning. J Surg Res 2014;189:198–206.
45. Jiang B, Xiao W, Shi Y, et al. Heat shock pretreatment inhibited the release of Smac/DIABLO from mitochondria and apoptosis induced by hydrogen peroxide in cardiomyocytes and C2C12 myogenic cells. Cell Stress Chaperones 2005;10:252–62.
46. Modriansky M, Gabrielova E. Uncouple my heart: the benefits of inefficiency. J Bioenerg Biomembr 2009;41:133–6.
47. Hoerter J, Gonzalez-Barroso MD, Couplan E, et al. Mitochondrial uncoupling protein 1 expressed in the heart of transgenic mice protects against ischemic-reperfusion damage. Circulation 2004;110:528–33.
48. Riepe MW, Niemi WN, Megow D, et al. Mitochondrial oxidation in rat hippocampus can be preconditioned by selective chemical

inhibition of succinic dehydrogenase. Exp Neurol 1996;138: 15–21.
49. Kasischke K, Ludolph AC, Riepe MW. NMDA-antagonists reverse increased hypoxic tolerance by preceding chemical hypoxia. Neurosci Lett 1996;214:175–8.
50. Hellweg R, von Arnim CA, Buchner M, et al. Neuroprotection and neuronal dysfunction upon repetitive inhibition of oxidative phosphorylation. Exp Neurol 2003;183:346–54.
51. Severino PC, Muller Gdo A, Vandresen-Filho S, et al. Cell signaling in NMDA preconditioning and neuroprotection in convulsions induced by quinolinic acid. Life Sci 2011;89:570–6.
52. Valeur HS, Valen G. Innate immunity and myocardial adaptation to ischemia. Basic Res Cardiol 2009;104:22–32.
53. Bhuiyan MI, Islam MN, Jung SY, et al. Involvement of ceramide in ischemic tolerance induced by preconditioning with sublethal oxygen-glucose deprivation in primary cultured cortical neurons of rats. Biol Pharm Bull 2010;33:11–17.
54. Lecour S, Owira P, Opie LH. Ceramide-induced preconditioning involves reactive oxygen species. Life Sci 2006;78:1702–6.
55. Rakhit RD, Edwards RJ, Marber MS. Nitric oxide, nitrates and ischaemic preconditioning. Cardiovasc Res 1999;43:621–7.
56. Centeno JM, Orti M, Salom JB, et al. Nitric oxide is involved in anoxic preconditioning neuroprotection in rat hippocampal slices. Brain Res 1999;836:62–9.
57. Matsushima K, Hogan MJ, Hakim AM. Cortical spreading depression protects against subsequent focal cerebral ischemia in rats. J Cereb Blood Flow Metab 1996;16:221–6.
58. Gniel HM, Martin RL. Cortical spreading depression-induced preconditioning in mouse neocortex is lamina specific. J Neurophysiol 2013;109:2923–36.
59. Shao G, Lu GW. Hypoxic preconditioning in an autohypoxic animal model. Neurosci Bull 2012;28:316–20.
60. Lushnikova I, Orlovsky M, Dosenko V, et al. Brief anoxia preconditioning and HIF prolyl-hydroxylase inhibition enhances neuronal resistance in organotypic hippocampal slices on model of ischemic damage. Brain Res 2011;1386:175–83.
61. Tauskela JS, Brunette E, Monette R, et al. Preconditioning of cortical neurons by oxygen-glucose deprivation: tolerance induction through abbreviated neurotoxic signaling. Am J Physiol Cell Physiol 2003;285:C899–911.
62. Speetzen LJ, Endres M, Kunz A. Bilateral common carotid artery occlusion as an adequate preconditioning stimulus to induce early ischemic tolerance to focal cerebral ischemia. J Vis Exp 2013;e4387.
63. Matsushima K, Hakim AM. Transient forebrain ischemia protects against subsequent focal cerebral ischemia without changing cerebral perfusion. Stroke 1995;26:1047–52.
64. Bernaudin M, Nedelec AS, Divoux D, et al. Normobaric hypoxia induces tolerance to focal permanent cerebral ischemia in association with an increased expression of hypoxia-inducible factor-1 and its target genes, erythropoietin and VEGF, in the adult mouse brain. J Cereb Blood Flow Metab 2002;22: 393–403.
65. Ahmed SH, He YY, Nassief A, et al. Effects of lipopolysaccharide priming on acute ischemic brain injury. Stroke 2000;31: 193–9.
66. Dawson DA, Furuya K, Gotoh J, et al. Cerebrovascular hemodynamics and ischemic tolerance: lipopolysaccharide-induced resistance to focal cerebral ischemia is not due to changes in severity of the initial ischemic insult, but is associated with preservation of microvascular perfusion. J Cereb Blood Flow Metab 1999;19:616–23.
67. Furuya K, Zhu L, Kawahara N, et al. Differences in infarct evolution between lipopolysaccharide-induced tolerant and nontolerant conditions to focal cerebral ischemia. J Neurosurg 2005;103: 715–23.
68. Tasaki K, Ruetzler CA, Ohtsuki T, et al. Lipopolysaccharide pretreatment induces resistance against subsequent focal cerebral ischemic damage in spontaneously hypertensive rats. Brain Res 1997;748:267–70.
69. Zimmermann C, Ginis I, Furuya K, et al. Lipopolysaccharide-induced ischemic tolerance is associated with increased levels of ceramide in brain and in plasma. Brain Res 2001;895:59–65.
70. Horiguchi T, Kis B, Rajapakse N, et al. Opening of mitochondrial ATP-sensitive potassium channels is a trigger of 3-nitropropionic acid-induced tolerance to transient focal cerebral ischemia in rats. Stroke 2003;34:1015–20.
71. Hoshi A, Nakahara T, Ogata M, et al. The critical threshold of 3-nitropropionic acid-induced ischemic tolerance in the rat. Brain Res 2005;1050:33–9.
72. Wiegand F, Liao W, Busch C, et al. Respiratory chain inhibition induces tolerance to focal cerebral ischemia. J Cereb Blood Flow Metab 1999;19:1229–37.
73. Nishio S, Chen ZF, Yunoki M, et al. Hypothermia-induced ischemic tolerance. Ann N Y Acad Sci 1999;890:26–41.
74. Urrea C, Danton GH, Bramlett HM, et al. The beneficial effect of mild hypothermia in a rat model of repeated thromboembolic insults. Acta Neuropathol 2004;107:413–20.
75. Xu H, Aibiki M, Nagoya J. Neuroprotective effects of hyperthermic preconditioning on infarcted volume after middle cerebral artery occlusion in rats: role of adenosine receptors. Crit Care Med 2002;30:1126–30.
76. Yang YL, Lin MT. Heat shock protein expression protects against cerebral ischemia and monoamine overload in rat heatstroke. Am J Physiol 1999;276:H1961–7.
77. Chazot PL, Lawrence S, Thompson CL. Studies on the subtype selectivity of CP-101,606: evidence for two classes of NR2B-selective NMDA receptor antagonists. Neuropharmacology 2002;42:319–24.
78. Otori T, Greenberg JH, Welsh FA. Cortical spreading depression causes a long-lasting decrease in cerebral blood flow and induces tolerance to permanent focal ischemia in rat brain. J Cereb Blood Flow Metab 2003;23:43–50.
79. Wang L, Traystman RJ, Murphy SJ. Inhalational anesthetics as preconditioning agents in ischemic brain. Curr Opin Pharmacol 2008;8:104–10.
80. Barone FC, White RF, Spera PA, et al. Ischemic preconditioning and brain tolerance: temporal histological and functional outcomes, protein synthesis requirement, and interleukin-1 receptor antagonist and early gene expression. Stroke 1998;29:1937–50, discussion 1950–1.
81. Kirino T. Ischemic tolerance. J Cereb Blood Flow Metab 2002;22: 1283–96.
82. Stenzel-Poore MP, Stevens SL, King JS, et al. Preconditioning reprograms the response to ischemic injury and primes the emergence of unique endogenous neuroprotective phenotypes: a speculative synthesis. Stroke 2007;38:680–5.
83. Shpargel KB, Jalabi W, Jin Y, et al. Preconditioning paradigms and pathways in the brain. Cleve Clin J Med 2008;75(Suppl. 2):S77–82.
84. Gidday JM, Shah AR, Maceren RG, et al. Nitric oxide mediates cerebral ischemic tolerance in a neonatal rat model of hypoxic preconditioning. J Cereb Blood Flow Metab 1999;19: 331–40.
85. Gonzalez-Zulueta M, Feldman AB, Klesse LJ, et al. Requirement for nitric oxide activation of p21(ras)/extracellular regulated kinase in neuronal ischemic preconditioning [In Process Citation]. Proc Natl Acad Sci U S A 2000;97:436–41.
86. Mori T, Muramatsu H, Matsui T, et al. Possible role of the superoxide anion in the development of neuronal tolerance following ischaemic preconditioning in rats. Neuropathol Appl Neurobiol 2000;26:31–40.
87. Silachev DN, Plotnikov EY, Pevzner IB, et al. The mitochondrion as a key regulator of ischaemic tolerance and injury. Heart Lung Circ 2014;23(10):897–904.
88. Kalogeris T, Bao Y, Korthuis RJ. Mitochondrial reactive oxygen species: a double edged sword in ischemia/reperfusion vs preconditioning. Redox Biol 2014;2:702–14.
89. Correia SC, Cardoso S, Santos RX, et al. New insights into the mechanisms of mitochondrial preconditioning-triggered neuroprotection. Curr Pharm Des 2011;17:3381–9.
90. Ghosh S, Standen NB, Galinanes M. Evidence for mitochondrial K ATP channels as effectors of human myocardial preconditioning. Cardiovasc Res 2000;45:934–40.
91. Raval AP, Dave KR, DeFazio RA, et al. epsilonPKC phosphorylates the mitochondrial K(+) (ATP) channel during induction of ischemic preconditioning in the rat hippocampus. Brain Res 2007;1184:345–53.
92. Schultz JE, Qian YZ, Gross GJ, et al. The ischemia-selective KATP channel antagonist, 5-hydroxydecanoate, blocks ischemic

preconditioning in the rat heart. J Mol Cell Cardiol 1997;29: 1055–60.
93. Forbes RA, Steenbergen C, Murphy E. Diazoxide-induced cardioprotection requires signaling through a redox-sensitive mechanism. Circ Res 2001;88:802–9.
94. Carroll R, Gant VA, Yellon DM. Mitochondrial K(ATP) channel opening protects a human atrial-derived cell line by a mechanism involving free radical generation. Cardiovasc Res 2001;51: 691–700.
95. Andreyev AY, Kushnareva YE, Starkov AA. Mitochondrial metabolism of reactive oxygen species. Biochemistry (Mosc) 2005;70: 200–14.
96. Chaturvedi RK, Beal MF. Mitochondrial approaches for neuroprotection. Ann N Y Acad Sci 2008;1147:395–412.
97. Sparvero LJ, Amoscato AA, Kochanek PM, et al. Mass-spectrometry based oxidative lipidomics and lipid imaging: applications in traumatic brain injury. J Neurochem 2010;115: 1322–36.
98. Greco T, Fiskum G. Neuroprotection through stimulation of mitochondrial antioxidant protein expression. J Alzheimers Dis 2010;20(Suppl. 2):S427–37.
99. Thompson JW, Narayanan SV, Perez-Pinzon MA. Redox signaling pathways involved in neuronal ischemic preconditioning. Curr Neuropharmacol 2012;10:354–69.
100. Venditti P, Di Stefano L, Di Meo S. Mitochondrial metabolism of reactive oxygen species. Mitochondrion 2013;13:71–82.
101. Busija DW, Gaspar T, Domoki F, et al. Mitochondrial-mediated suppression of ROS production upon exposure of neurons to lethal stress: mitochondrial targeted preconditioning. Adv Drug Deliv Rev 2008;60:1471–7.
102. Fiskum G, Rosenthal RE, Vereczki V, et al. Protection against ischemic brain injury by inhibition of mitochondrial oxidative stress. J Bioenerg Biomembr 2004;36:347–52.
103. Truettner J, Busto R, Zhao W, et al. Effect of ischemic preconditioning on the expression of putative neuroprotective genes in the rat brain. Brain Res Mol Brain Res 2002;103:106–15.
104. Yanamoto H, Xue JH, Miyamoto S, et al. Spreading depression induces long-lasting brain protection against infarcted lesion development via BDNF gene-dependent mechanism. Brain Res 2004;1019:178–88.
105. Matsushima K, Schmidt-Kastner R, Hogan MJ, et al. Cortical spreading depression activates trophic factor expression in neurons and astrocytes and protects against subsequent focal brain ischemia. Brain Res 1998;807:47–60.
106. Sakaki T, Yamada K, Otsuki H, et al. Brief exposure to hypoxia induces bFGF mRNA and protein and protects rat cortical neurons from prolonged hypoxic stress. Neurosci Res 1995;23:289–96.
107. Wang X, Deng J, Boyle DW, et al. Potential role of IGF-I in hypoxia tolerance using a rat hypoxic-ischemic model: activation of hypoxia-inducible factor 1alpha. Pediatr Res 2004;55: 385–94.
108. Gustavsson M, Wilson MA, Mallard C, et al. Global gene expression in the developing rat brain after hypoxic preconditioning: involvement of apoptotic mechanisms? Pediatr Res 2007;61: 444–50.
109. Mallard C, Hagberg H. Inflammation-induced preconditioning in the immature brain. Semin Fetal Neonatal Med 2007;12: 280–6.
110. Bernaudin M, Tang Y, Reilly M, et al. Brain genomic response following hypoxia and re-oxygenation in the neonatal rat. Identification of genes that might contribute to hypoxia-induced ischemic tolerance. J Biol Chem 2002;277:39728–38.
111. Wick A, Wick W, Waltenberger J, et al. Neuroprotection by hypoxic preconditioning requires sequential activation of vascular endothelial growth factor receptor and Akt. J Neurosci 2002; 22:6401–7.
112. Xu Z, Ford GD, Croslan DR, et al. Neuroprotection by neuregulin-1 following focal stroke is associated with the attenuation of ischemia-induced pro-inflammatory and stress gene expression. Neurobiol Dis 2005;19:461–70.
113. Miao B, Yin XH, Pei DS, et al. Neuroprotective effects of preconditioning ischemia on ischemic brain injury through down-regulating activation of JNK1/2 via N-methyl-D-aspartate receptor-mediated Akt1 activation. J Biol Chem 2005;280: 21693–9.
114. Nakajima T, Iwabuchi S, Miyazaki H, et al. Preconditioning prevents ischemia-induced neuronal death through persistent Akt activation in the penumbra region of the rat brain. J Vet Med Sci 2004;66:521–7.
115. Gao X, Zhang H, Takahashi T, et al. The Akt signaling pathway contributes to postconditioning's protection against stroke; the protection is associated with the MAPK and PKC pathways. J Neurochem 2008;105:943–55.
116. Namura S, Nagata I, Kikuchi H, et al. Serine-threonine protein kinase Akt does not mediate ischemic tolerance after global ischemia in the gerbil. J Cereb Blood Flow Metab 2000;20: 1301–5.
117. Shibata M, Yamawaki T, Sasaki T, et al. Upregulation of Akt phosphorylation at the early stage of middle cerebral artery occlusion in mice. Brain Res 2002;942:1–10.
118. Zhang Y, Park TS, Gidday JM. Hypoxic preconditioning protects human brain endothelium from ischemic apoptosis by Akt-dependent survivin activation. Am J Physiol Heart Circ Physiol 2007;292:H2573–81.
119. Ruscher K, Freyer D, Karsch M, et al. Erythropoietin is a paracrine mediator of ischemic tolerance in the brain: evidence from an in vitro model. J Neurosci 2002;22:10291–301.
120. Siren AL, Fratelli M, Brines M, et al. Erythropoietin prevents neuronal apoptosis after cerebral ischemia and metabolic stress. Proc Natl Acad Sci U S A 2001;98:4044–9.
121. Siren AL, Knerlich F, Poser W, et al. Erythropoietin and erythropoietin receptor in human ischemic/hypoxic brain. Acta Neuropathol 2001;101:271–6.
122. Digicaylioglu M, Lipton SA. Erythropoietin-mediated neuroprotection involves cross-talk between Jak2 and NF-kappaB signalling cascades. Nature 2001;412:641–7.
123. Ehrenreich H, Hasselblatt M, Dembowski C, et al. Erythropoietin therapy for acute stroke is both safe and beneficial. Mol Med 2002;8:495–505.
124. Bredesen DE, Rao RV, Mehlen P. Cell death in the nervous system. Nature 2006;443:796–802.
125. Levine B, Yuan J. Autophagy in cell death: an innocent convict? J Clin Invest 2005;115:2679–88.
126. Tomasevic G, Shamloo M, Israeli D, et al. Activation of p53 and its target genes p21(WAF1/Cip1) and PAG608/Wig-1 in ischemic preconditioning. Brain Res Mol Brain Res 1999;70:304–13.
127. Huang L, Li W, Li B, et al. Activation of ATP-sensitive K channels protects hippocampal CA1 neurons from hypoxia by suppressing p53 expression. Neurosci Lett 2006;398:34–8.
128. Brambrink AM, Schneider A, Noga H, et al. Tolerance-Inducing dose of 3-nitropropionic acid modulates bcl-2 and bax balance in the rat brain: a potential mechanism of chemical preconditioning. J Cereb Blood Flow Metab 2000;20:1425–36.
129. Kato K, Shimazaki K, Kamiya T, et al. Differential effects of sublethal ischemia and chemical preconditioning with 3-nitropropionic acid on protein expression in gerbil hippocampus. Life Sci 2005;77:2867–78.
130. Meller R, Minami M, Cameron JA, et al. CREB-mediated Bcl-2 protein expression after ischemic preconditioning. J Cereb Blood Flow Metab 2005;25:234–46.
131. Rybnikova E, Sitnik N, Gluschenko T, et al. The preconditioning modified neuronal expression of apoptosis-related proteins of Bcl-2 superfamily following severe hypobaric hypoxia in rats. Brain Res 2006;1089:195–202.
132. Shimazaki K, Ishida A, Kawai N. Increase in bcl-2 oncoprotein and the tolerance to ischemia-induced neuronal death in the gerbil hippocampus. Neurosci Res 1994;20:95–9.
133. Shimizu S, Nagayama T, Jin KL, et al. bcl-2 Antisense treatment prevents induction of tolerance to focal ischemia in the rat brain. J Cereb Blood Flow Metab 2001;21:233–43.
134. Wu C, Fujihara H, Yao J, et al. Different expression patterns of Bcl-2, Bcl-xl, and Bax proteins after sublethal forebrain ischemia in C57Black/Crj6 mouse striatum. Stroke 2003;34:1803–8.
135. Wu LY, Ding AS, Zhao T, et al. Involvement of increased stability of mitochondrial membrane potential and overexpression of Bcl-2 in enhanced anoxic tolerance induced by hypoxic preconditioning in cultured hypothalamic neurons. Brain Res 2004;999: 149–54.
136. Miyawaki T, Mashiko T, Ofengeim D, et al. Ischemic preconditioning blocks BAD translocation, Bcl-xL cleavage, and large

channel activity in mitochondria of postischemic hippocampal neurons. Proc Natl Acad Sci U S A 2008;105:4892–7.
137. Andrabi SA, Kang HC, Haince JF, et al. Iduna protects the brain from glutamate excitotoxicity and stroke by interfering with poly(ADP-ribose) polymer-induced cell death. Nat Med 2011;17: 692–9.
138. Jaattela M. Heat shock proteins as cellular lifeguards. Ann Med 1999;31:261–71.
139. Morimoto RI. Proteotoxic stress and inducible chaperone networks in neurodegenerative disease and aging. Genes Dev 2008;22:1427–38.
140. Giffard RG, Han RQ, Emery JF, et al. Regulation of apoptotic and inflammatory cell signaling in cerebral ischemia: the complex roles of heat shock protein 70. Anesthesiology 2008;109: 339–48.
141. Yenari MA, Liu J, Zheng Z, et al. Antiapoptotic and anti-inflammatory mechanisms of heat-shock protein protection. Ann N Y Acad Sci 2005;1053:74–83.
142. Kelly S, Zhang ZJ, Zhao H, et al. Gene transfer of HSP72 protects cornu ammonis 1 region of the hippocampus neurons from global ischemia: influence of Bcl-2. Ann Neurol 2002;52: 160–7.
143. Saleh A, Srinivasula SM, Balkir L, et al. Negative regulation of the Apaf-1 apoptosome by Hsp70. Nat Cell Biol 2000;2: 476–83.
144. Ruchalski K, Mao H, Li Z, et al. Distinct hsp70 domains mediate apoptosis-inducing factor release and nuclear accumulation. J Biol Chem 2006;281:7873–80.
145. Duan X, Kang E, Liu CY, et al. Development of neural stem cell in the adult brain. Curr Opin Neurobiol 2008;18:108–15.
146. Ge S, Sailor KA, Ming GL, et al. Synaptic integration and plasticity of new neurons in the adult hippocampus. J Physiol 2008; 586:3759–65.
147. Lee SH, Kim YJ, Lee KM, et al. Ischemic preconditioning enhances neurogenesis in the subventricular zone. Neuroscience 2007;146:1020–31.
148. Maysami S, Lan JQ, Minami M, et al. Proliferating progenitor cells: a required cellular element for induction of ischemic tolerance in the brain. J Cereb Blood Flow Metab 2008;28:1104–13.
149. Pourie G, Blaise S, Trabalon M, et al. Mild, non-lesioning transient hypoxia in the newborn rat induces delayed brain neurogenesis associated with improved memory scores. Neuroscience 2006;140:1369–79.
150. Ford GA. Clinical pharmacological issues in the development of acute stroke therapies. Br J Pharmacol 2008;153(Suppl. 1): S112–19.

7 The Neurovascular Unit and Responses to Ischemia

Gregory J. del Zoppo, Michael Moskowitz, Maiken Nedergaard

KEY POINTS

- The "neurovascular unit" is a structural and functional concept that seeks to integrate microvessel events with those of the neurons, glia, and brain matrix and serves as a framework for fundamental new findings (e.g., the glymphatic CSF transport network).
- Within each compartment, networks of cells, matrix, and membranes interact and are moderated by supportive cells.
- Coordinated changes in brain vascular and microvascular caliber and in blood flow provide an example of neurovascular coupling, although the precise signaling mechanisms are under study.
- Disease processes (e.g., ischemic stroke, innate immunity and inflammation) negatively impact the functional integrity of the neurovascular unit, and may lead to territorial dysfunction.
- Knowledge of cell–cell and compartment–compartment interactions is incomplete (e.g., precise roles of pericytes in microvessels and microglia and oligodendroglia in the neuropil). A full understanding of the signaling interactions between and among elements of the neurovascular unit may have predictive value.

INTRODUCTION

The central nervous system (CNS) consists of regions of microvessels and neural tissue that interact to maintain homeostasis and neuronal function, prevent entry of substances from the vascular compartment that are toxic to neurons, promote organized neuronal and vascular responses to peripheral stimuli, and limit injury to cerebral regions. It was previously thought of as regions of neurons with cells supporting their nutrition, viability, and function, however, studies of the responses of cerebral tissue to ischemic injury reveal more complex cooperative relationships.

Cells of the CNS can be seen as belonging to at least six interacting networks: (i) neuron networks that relay electrical information; (ii) syncytia of astrocytes that serve both neurons and are a part of microvessels; (iii) the endothelium that covers the microvessel and large vessel interiors; (iv) the extracellular matrix (ECM) that comprises the basal lamina of the vascular tree; (v) pericytes, positioned between the endothelium and astrocyte components of the microvasculature, that form a network within the vascular ECM; and, (vi) a glymphatic cerebrospinal fluid (CSF) transport network.

Control and modulation of regional and local cerebral blood flow (CBF) under conditions of normoxia depend upon neurovascular coupling.[1-3] The proximity of microvessel endothelial cells to the circumferential astrocyte end-feet of capillaries, separated by the thin basal lamina ECM,[2,4] and the support of neurons by astrocytes suggest that communication could be directed from microvessels to the neurons they supply.[5,6] Neuron–microvessel interactions can be described within the context of a *neurovascular unit* that consists of microvessels (endothelial cells, basal lamina ECM, astrocyte end-feet, and pericytes), astrocytes, neurons and their axons, in addition to the supporting cells of the neuropil.[7] This "unit" provides a structural framework for considering bidirectional actions of neurons and their supply microvessels via the intervening astrocytes, and the potential modulation of these actions by other cells (e.g., microglia, oligodendroglia). It also provides a functional framework for considering the elements of the "unit" in their responses to changes in flow, ischemia, inflammatory stimuli, and other processes. These structural and functional relationships are built during the development of the brain tissue as the vasculature matures. Growing insight into these cell and structural relationships sharpens research focus and explains the outcomes and limitations of fundamental and clinical research trials.

ARCHITECTURE OF THE CNS AND THE NEUROVASCULAR UNIT

Although the neuronal network subserves continuous input and output of the cerebral tissue, its functional complexity is supported by an organized vascular supply that contains the individual endothelial, basal lamina ECM, astrocyte, and pericyte networks. Complexity within the vasculature is marked by endothelial cell specialization and variation in basal lamina ECM composition along the vascular axes.[8,9] It is likely that other networks have a similar local specialization.

Structural Relationships: Anatomy of the Cerebral Vasculature

Under normoxic conditions the cerebral vasculature uniquely protects the neuropil from changes in plasma ion concentrations, as well as exposure to plasma substances toxic to neurons and other cells. It preserves neuronal cell function through shifting blood flow to regions of activation on demand, maintains an intravascular anti-thrombotic and anti-inflammatory milieu, and supplies essential nutrients. This protection may be disrupted under conditions of focal or global ischemia, or injury.

The general strategy protecting cortical and deep brain structures from flow obstruction involves interconnection of territories of brain-supplying arteries via pial collateral anastomoses over the cerebral hemispheres and the circle of Willis. Pial and cortical penetrating arteries consist of (i) an endothelial cell layer, (ii) the basal lamina, (iii) layers of smooth muscle cells encased in ECM (myointima), and (iv) an adventitia derived from the leptomeninges.[4] In the cortex and striatum, an extension of the subarachnoid space forms the Virchow-Robins (V-R) space, which surrounds penetrating arterioles until it "disappears" into the *glia limitans*. The abluminal boundary of the *glia limitans* is formed by the astrocyte end-feet. With further arborization of the microvasculature, the *glia limitans* at the capillary level fuses with the thin basal

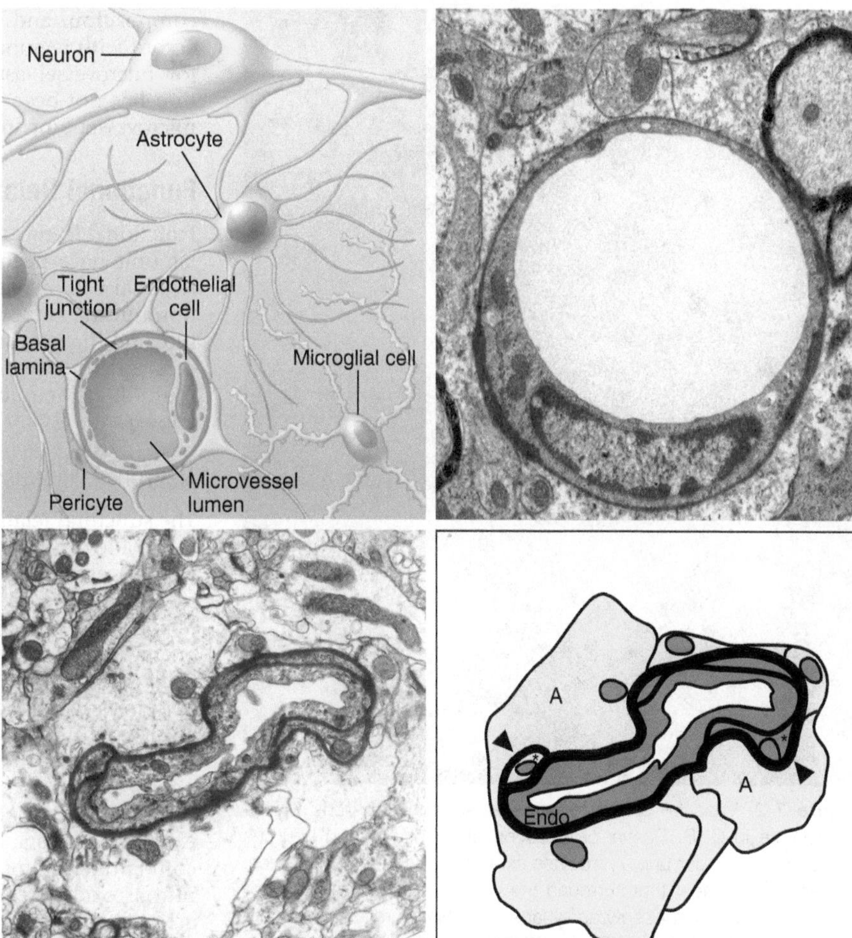

Figure 7-1. Characteristics of cerebral microvessels under normoxic conditions. *Upper left panel,* Depiction of neurovascular unit displaying relationships between neurons and their supply capillaries. (From del Zoppo GJ: Stroke and neurovascular protection. *N Engl J Med* 354:553-555, 2006.) *Upper right panel,* Capillary from rat inferior colliculus. Note endothelial cell, basal lamina matrix, and surrounding astrocyte end-foot. 4.5-5.0 μm diameter. (Courtesy of Dr. C. Willis.) *Lower left panel,* Post-capillary venule from rat cortex. ≈10 μm diameter. (Courtesy of J. H. Heo.) *Lower right panel,* Key to the *lower left panel,* indicating the endothelium (endo), basal lamina matrix *(arrowheads),* astrocyte and astrocyte end-feet (A), and pericytes (*)

lamina. The ECM composition varies depending upon the vessel of interest.[9,10] Astrocytes serve both microvessels and neurons in this setting (Figs 7-1–7-3), and are considered the vascular portion of the *neurovascular unit.* The post-capillary venule network bears close ultrastructural resemblance to the capillaries, except for the presence of a limited myointimal layer.

Also, recent work suggests that the paravascular space plays an important physiological function as a highway for influx of cerebrospinal fluid that subsequently mixes with interstitial fluid as part of the so-called "glymphatic clearance system."[11] The glymphatic fluid system intersects with the V-R space, and affords clearance of CSF and solutes from the CNS.[12]

The neuropil consists of neurons of a variety of subtypes, astrocytes, oligodendroglia, microglia, mast cells, and ECM containing chondroitin sulfate proteoglycans (CSPG) (e.g., CAT-301pg), neurexin, and other proteoglycans.[13] The relative content of these cells and components and their inter-relationships likely depend upon the region of the CNS under consideration.

A unique feature of the cerebral capillary is the permeability barrier, a strategy that prevents contact of the neuropil with the blood and its plasma constituents. The permeability barrier consists of (i) the inter-endothelial cell tight junctions, and limited pinocytosis,[14] (ii) the basal lamina ECM,[15,16] and (iii) adhesion to the intact subtending basal lamina.[6] Developmental interrelationships between the endothelium and astrocytes highlight the close functional association of endothelial cells and astrocytes in cerebral capillaries. Astrocytes and endothelial cells interact to form the intervening basal lamina barrier and the inter-endothelial tight junctions as part of the capillary permeability barrier.[17-21] Elegant xenograft experiments indicate that endothelial cells and astrocyte end-feet are required for the appearance and maintenance of the low-permeability barrier phenotype.[22] Cerebral microvessel endothelial cells display regional functional specialization along the microvascular axis,[8,23] which appear to depend on the interaction of its cellular components.[24,25] It has been postulated that soluble factors generated by astrocytes maintain the endothelial characteristics of the blood–brain barrier, including the tight junctions, transendothelial resistance, and the polarity of glucose-amino acid transport.[22,26]

Two additional barriers include the intact basal lamina and receptor-associated adhesion of the endothelium and astrocyte end-feet to the ECM components. The intact ECM protects the brain parenchyma from hemorrhage.[15,27-31] The basal lamina contains laminins, collagen type IV, fibronectin, and other components, including heparan sulfate proteoglycans (HSPGs; e.g., perlecan), entactin, nidogen, and other minor components.[27,32] Adhesion of both endothelial cells and astrocytes to the subtending basal lamina requires the interaction of cells to their matrix ligands.[27,28] Haring et al. described integrin receptor expression patterns of integrin subunits in normal CNS microvessel subclasses.[28] Their potential roles in microvessel and permeability barrier have been considered recently.[6] Integrin $\alpha_1\beta_1$ on endothelial cells appears in all cerebral microvessels, including cerebral capillaries.[28,30,33,34] Integrins $\alpha_3\beta_1$ and $\alpha_6\beta_1$ are also expressed by cerebral endothelial cells.

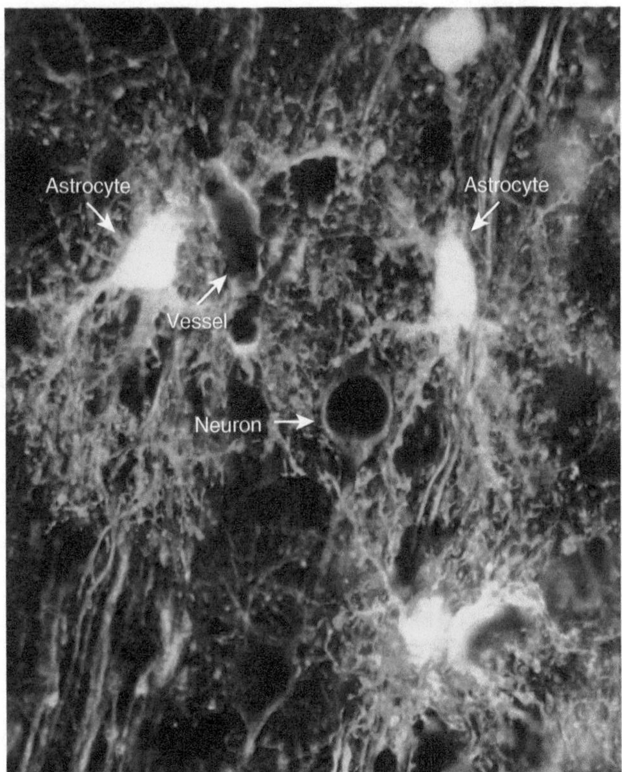

Figure 7-2. Vascular astrocyte end-feet surround all parts of the vasculature in CNS. Spatial organization of astrocytes and neurons in the neurovascular unit. Astrocytes extend two types of processes: (1) vascular end-feet that surround the vessel wall, and (2) fine perisynaptic processes that enwrap synapses. In this figure astrocytes are expressing enhanced green-fluorescent protein (eGFP; yellow), whereas neurons are labeled with antibody to microtubule-associated protein 2 (MAP-2; blue). A small vessel is outlined by eGFP-positive astrocytic end-feet *(From Nedergaard M, Ransom, B, Goldman SA. Trends Neurosci 26: 523–530, 2003.)*

Integrin $\alpha_6\beta_4$ is expressed on astrocyte end-feet around select microvessels, whereas integrin $\alpha_1\beta_1$ is found on their fibers.[29,30] $\alpha\beta$-Dystroglycan, the sole member of a separate family of matrix adhesion receptors, is predominantly expressed by astrocyte end-feet.[35] Adhesion receptor–matrix relationships are perturbed during middle cerebral artery occlusion (MCA:O), which coincide with the detachment of astrocyte end-feet from the basal lamina.[35] Little is known, yet, about the signaling functions of the adhesion receptors expressed in cerebral microvessels. Osada et al. have demonstrated that interference with integrin–matrix adhesion can disrupt permeability and tight junction fidelity,[36] indicating that inter-endothelial cohesion and endothelial-cell–basal-lamina adhesion are connected.

Embedded within the basal lamina matrix of all cerebral microvessels are pericytes. These pluripotential cells become activated and can migrate in response to specific stimuli including focal ischemia and inflammation.[37] Pericytes also have been shown to have properties found in select inflammatory cells.[37,38] A role for pericytes in the formation of the microvessel permeability barrier and its fidelity has been demonstrated.[39] The number of pericytes is sharply decreased during ageing.[40] Pericytes have also been postulated to influence capillary diameter and may contribute to local blood flow regulation, however the mechanisms are uncertain.[41]

Specialization of the microvasculature is implied by differences in endothelial function, basal lamina ECM composition, and adhesion receptor expression which may accord with regional specialization of the neurons. Currently for microvessel–astrocyte–neuron partners, such specialization has not been explored. However, evidence for neuron–microvessel functional relations is known.

Functional Relationships

Functional features supporting the concept of the neurovascular unit have been exposed by (i) physiological studies of regional CBF dynamics, and (ii) inter-neuronal communication hinting at functional pairings between the microvasculature and the neuropil. These may appear to be unidirectional (e.g., neuron $\gg$ microvessel), however they are more likely multi-directional based on the established networks (see above).

Neuron–Microvessel Communication

The structural relationships established during brain development allow neurons to effect changes in flow through the (micro)vasculature. *Neurovascular coupling* has been recognized since the time of Sherrington,[42] and refers to the interrelationship between CBF and neuronal activity that balances energy demand with nutrient supply. The mechanism that achieves coupling between flow and neuronal activity does not appear to involve direct sensing of energy consumption per se, at least under physiological conditions. It depends upon the integrity of the neurovascular unit and cross-talk among neurons, astrocytes, arterioles (vascular smooth muscle), and microvessels via neurotransmitters, astrocyte signaling, and exocrine effectors. Effectors released from neuronal and glial compartments implicated in the vascular response include nitrous oxide (NO), adenosine, H^+, K^+, CO_2, and arachidonic acid metabolites.[1-3] Astrocytes provide one link between neuronal activity and transmitter release (i.e., glutamate) and local CBF changes.[43] In the formulation reviewed below, astrocytes release vasoactive molecules that regulate diameter changes of supply vessels.[44] According to another formulation, axon terminals releasing neurotransmitters approximate vascular smooth muscle cells and may contribute to flow. Currently, the view of neurovascular coupling is incomplete. Alterations in local CBF may reflect (i) astrocyte–smooth muscle endothelial interactions, (ii) neuron–vascular interactions, and/or (iii) other couplings.

Neuron–Astrocyte Communication. Neurovascular coupling supports the communication of neurons with astrocytes. However, interactions between neurons and astrocytes are bidirectional.[45] Synaptic communications employ high-affinity slowly desensitizing receptors, and involve signaling via specific astrocyte receptors (e.g., Eph tyrosine kinases and ephrin).[46] In vivo Ca^{+2} transients within astrocytes are initiated by norepinephrine (noradrenaline) release from activated neurons.[47,48] Neuron–astrocyte metabolic interactions connect glutamate/Na^+ uptake with glucose uptake,[49,50] and degradation of glycogen induced by norepinephrine.[51,52] Furthermore, in vitro studies suggest that the environment of the neuron–astrocyte interactions is pertinent; modulation of neurite outgrowth by astrocytes can depend upon exposure to ECM or ECM products (e.g., laminins).[53] Hence, the proximity of astrocytes with neurons allows intimate cross-talk.

Astrocyte–Endothelial Cell (Vascular) Communication. Changes in CBF can be initiated by central neural activation. Specific pathways of neural-dependent vascular control may vary regionally; however, a general pattern is indicated by control of cortical flow, with three variants: (i) cortical pyramidal glutamatergic neurons when activated by basal forebrain

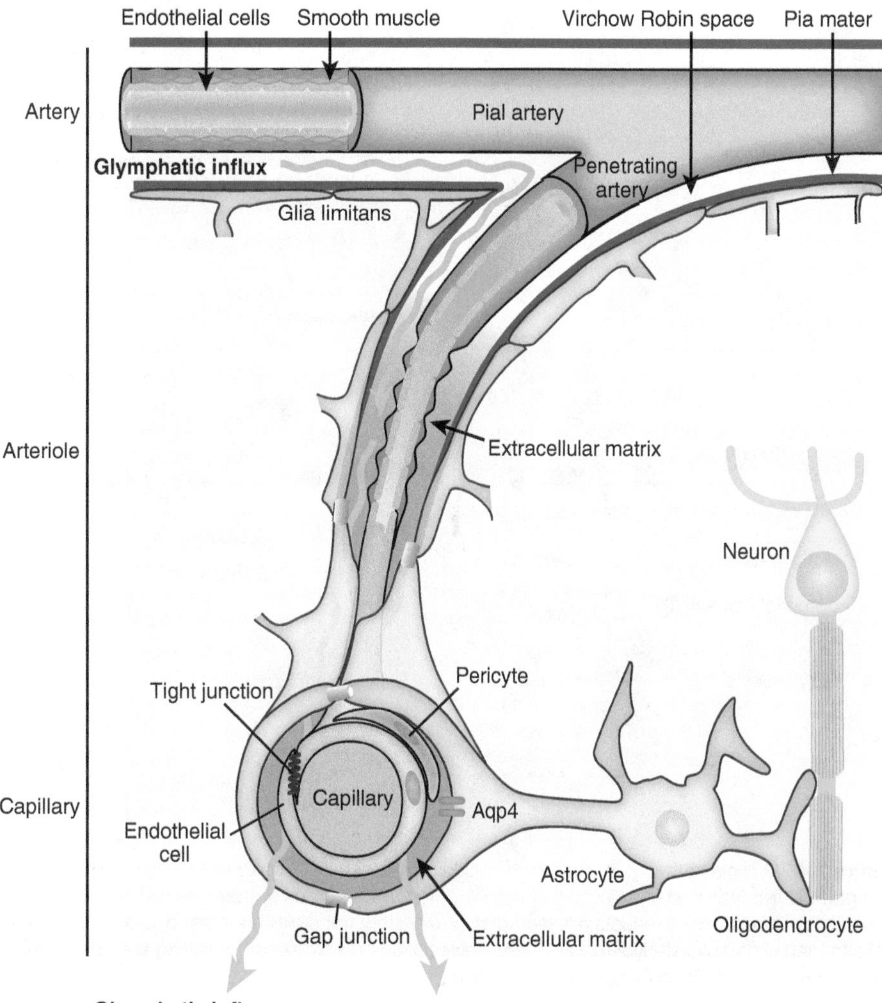

Figure 7-3. A schematic drawing of the vascular tree (pial artery→penetrating artery→arteriole→capillary). The cross-section is at the level of the capillary. Astrocytic vascular end-feet, that are connected by gap junctions and express the aquaporin-4 (AQP4), surround the entire vasculature in CNS. The perivascular space is a donut-shaped tunnel system formed by vascular astrocytic end-feet (outer wall) and the vessel (inner wall). The peri-vascular space around penetrating arteries is also called the Virchow-Robins space. The term "basal lamina" refers to the matrix between the endothelium and the astrocyte end-feet, and is the perivascular space in microvessels. The glymphatic system utilizes the peri-vascular space for rapid influx (arteries) of cerebrospinal fluid (CSF) that flow out along veins. (Prepared by T Takano.)

stimulation contribute to the evoked CBF response.[54] Additionally, acetylcholine released from terminal projections approximates blood vessels and appears to contribute to flow regulation along with GABA interneurons. GABA interneurons have been further implicated whereby firing of single interneurons can modify the caliber of neighboring microvessels.[55] (ii) Similar to basal forebrain stimulation, blood flow regulation following whisker barrel stimulation appears to employ prostanoid synthesis within pyramidal cells as a mediator,[55] or astrocytes as the mediator. (iii) Furthermore, both glutamatergic and GABA receptor blockade can attenuate stimulation of evoked blood flow responses by the locus coeruleus.[56,57] Hence, a complex pattern of blood flow regulation implicates long projecting neurons, pyramidal cells, interneurons and particularly astrocytes in the cross-talk with vascular smooth muscle and possibly the endothelium to regulate CBF. Variations on some of these themes (including the importance of NO[58]) could well mediate the elegant spatial and temporal localization that characterizes neurovascular coupling as suggested by functional neuroimaging.[59]

Astrocyte–Smooth Muscle Communication. Pre-capillary arterioles are instrumental in regional CBF regulation, receiving input from astrocytes, and the microvascular endothelium.[60] In neurovascular coupling, astrocytes interact with smooth muscle; however, the manner in which this occurs is still under study (Fig. 7-4). Astrocytes can regulate Ca^{+2} signaling within vascular smooth muscle cells.[61] In addition, the Strickland group has shown that the ECM features of the astrocyte–smooth muscle cell environment are very important to intercellular communication.[62]

Microvessel–Neuron Communication

In complex (biological) systems feedback loops maintain homeostasis and communication. Although the case for neurovascular coupling is robust, little is known about how the microvasculature could communicate with the dependent neurons beyond variations in nutrient supply. That such communication takes place is suggested by the rapid response of the endothelium, astrocytes, and the intervening matrix to focal ischemia, which accords with the time-frame of alterations in neuron function in the same systems.[63]

Astrocyte–Neuron Communication. In normoxia, astrocytes play dual roles in communication between neurons and the vasculature: end-feet constitute a portion of cerebral microvessels, and astrocytes communicate with neurons directly. The distribution of astrocytes to neurons in mice/rats is 3 : 1, whereas in humans it is 4 : 1.[3] One astrocyte may envelope 4–8 neuron somata and 300–600 dendrites, organized in such a way as to imply a functional association.[64,65] Astrocytes are known to release D-serine, glutamate, ATP, taurine, and cytokines (e.g., TNF-α).[65] ATP can be a source of adenosine. Glutamate released from astrocytes exposed to bradykinin has been shown to stimulate NMDA-receptor-mediated release of Ca^{+2} within the neuron.[66] There is evidence that the signaling within astrocytes and neurons may be reciprocal.[65] This is

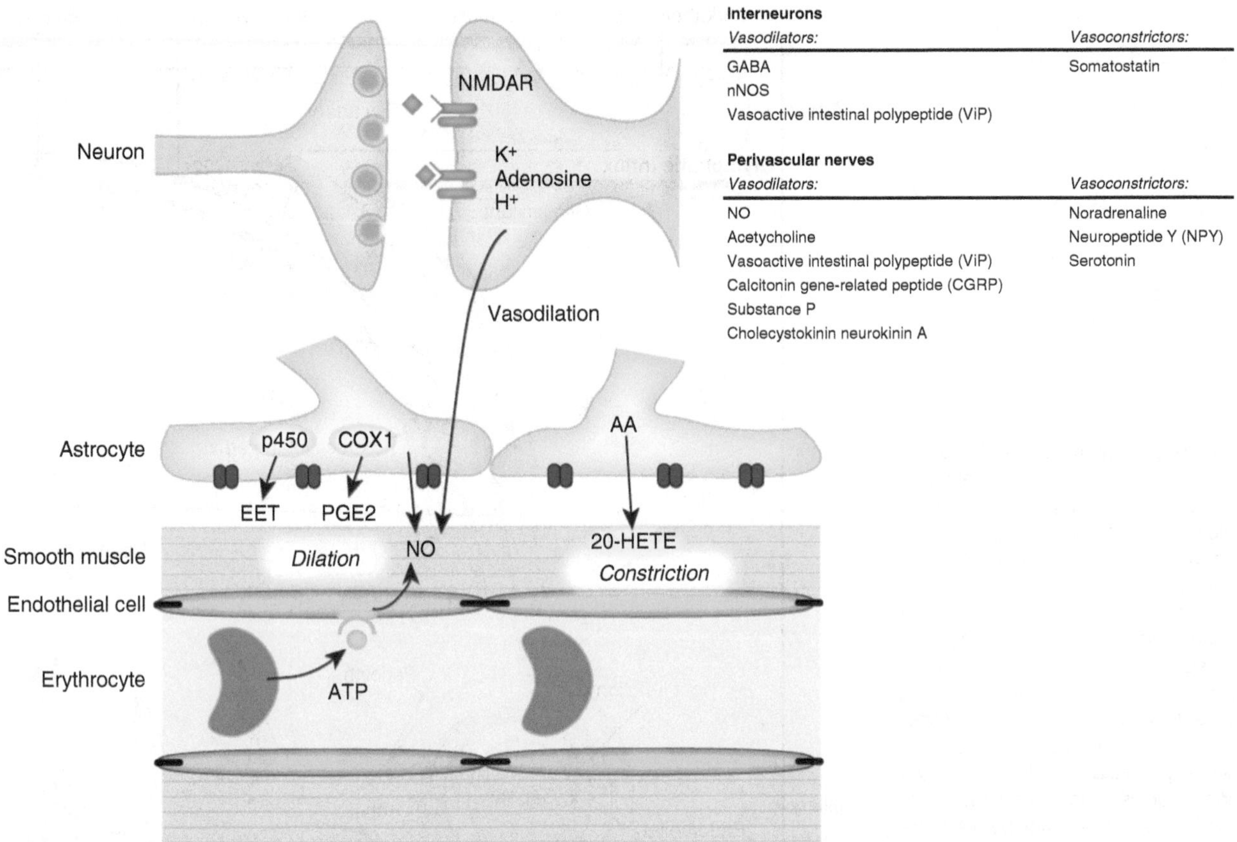

Interneurons	
Vasodilators:	*Vasoconstrictors:*
GABA	Somatostatin
nNOS	
Vasoactive intestinal polypeptide (ViP)	

Perivascular nerves	
Vasodilators:	*Vasoconstrictors:*
NO	Noradrenaline
Acetycholine	Neuropeptide Y (NPY)
Vasoactive intestinal polypeptide (ViP)	Serotonin
Calcitonin gene-related peptide (CGRP)	
Substance P	
Cholecystokinin neurokinin A	

Figure 7-4. Multiple pathways can mediate functional hyperemia. Multiple mechanisms contribute to functional hyperemia. Release of vasoactive compounds from the nerve projections (primarily autonomic nervous system), as well as interneurons can contribute to both arterial dilation and constriction. In addition, products released during excitatory transmission, often byproducts of cellular metabolism, including lactate, adenosine, K^+, can mediate functional hyperemia. Finally, several signaling pathways, including Ca^{2+}-dependent PGE_2 release or receptor-mediated production of nitric oxide (NO) can trigger arterial dilation.

likely to involve intercellular Ca^{+2} transients mediated by ATP release within the astrocyte networks.[67] Clinically, astrocyte–neuron communication can be manifest in plasticity, memory, and perception.[68–70]

Endothelial Cell–Astrocyte Communication. Astrocyte end-feet envelope cerebral capillaries and larger microvessels, thus implying, by their proximity, a potential direct communication with the endothelium. Studies in model systems have confirmed that astrocytes alter the behavior of endothelial cells to increase the fidelity of the blood–brain barrier.[71,72] However, little is yet known about whether, and in what manner, endothelial cells could communicate through astrocyte end-feet to effect glial responses. Several avenues are possible, with most as yet theoretical.

The porosity of the basal lamina ECM is likely to allow bidirectional diffusion of small molecules between the endothelium and the subjacent astrocyte network. For instance, it has been suggested that NO derived from endothelial cells can participate in the maintenance of high glycolytic activity in astrocytes when HIF-1α is activated within astrocytes.[73] In addition, in pre-capillary arterioles NO, from endothelial sources, modulates smooth muscle activation.[60] Because of their participation in cerebral (micro)vascular endothelial cell and astrocyte adhesion to the matrix, β_1 integrins and $\alpha\beta$-dystroglycan, respectively, are known also to participate in signaling events. It is as yet unknown whether trans-matrix communication between endothelium and astrocyte end-feet occurs via these receptors, although this is an attractive hypothesis. In addition, ATP/ADP can be converted to adenosine by ecto-apyrase activity on the endothelial luminal surface, and contributes to the anti-thrombotic milieu.[74,75] Whether ATP/ADP or adenosine generated by the endothelium is used in the abluminal space as a signaling principle with the neuropil, with astrocytes specifically, is unknown.

However, ATP/ADP can activate astrocytes, and initiate Ca^{+2}-dependent signaling within astrocyte networks resulting in the release of PGE2.[44,61] ATP released by astrocytes can be degraded by CD 39 to ADP which could in turn activate endothelial P2Y1 receptors resulting in NO release.[76] Astrocyte end-feet have been regarded as a site of purine signaling, with localization of the $P2Y_2$ and $P2Y_4$ receptors at these sites.[77,78]

Stretch responses are known for endothelium and astrocytes, and the ECM could be a transducer. Mechanotransduction is employed by endothelial cells for signaling in their response to stretching,[79–81] or alterations in ECM (e.g., laminin) behavior.[82,83] Mechanical forces have also been shown to effect astrocyte endothelin and volume responses.[84] Hence, there are theoretical bases for endothelial-astrocyte responses to mechanical events within the microvasculature that might also involve torsion of the basal lamina ECM.

EVIDENCE FOR THE NEUROVASCULAR UNIT

The fundamental relationship that defines the neurovascular unit entails the function of cerebral microvessels to supply nutrients to the neurons and for neurons to regulate flow through their microvascular fields, with astrocytes playing intermediary roles. Potential intercellular interactions have been exposed by responses of the cellular components to specific challenges.

Interactions Suggesting Unit Communication

Both active and passive processes participate in the intercellular interactions that suggest communication within the unit. Under physiologic conditions, individual groups of units do not announce themselves. However, during the acute phase of focal ischemia, and the inflammatory consequences, rather active features of the unit are exposed. With sustained flow cessation alterations in all components of the neurovascular unit are initiated.

Structural Changes During Focal Ischemia. The sine qua non of focal cerebral ischemia is the disturbance of neuron function by threshold loss of local CBF within the microvasculature of the territory-at-risk due to persistent obstruction of supply arteries. Ischemic stroke is a vascular disorder of the CNS. In addition, neuron dysfunction can cause dysfunction of the associated glial and microvascular components of the neurovascular unit, evident by (i) effects on cell viability,[29] (ii) ECM alterations, and (iii) the consequences of spreading depression.

Microvessel (Endothelial–Astrocyte) Communication. During focal cerebral ischemia, a series of metabolic and morphologic alterations occur in the ischemic microvasculature, in concert with responses of the glial and neuron components of the "unit."[85,86] Injury to neurons in the target area reflects both characteristics of the neurons ("selective vulnerability"),[87–89] and the distance of neurons from their neighboring microvessels.[90]

Acute responses of microvessels within the regions of neuron injury occur after the onset of cerebral ischemia: (i) loss of the endothelial cell permeability barrier with subsequent edema development, (ii) loss of the basal lamina ECM, (iii) alterations in microvessel endothelial cell–matrix and astrocyte–matrix adhesion, (iv) loss of microvessel patency (development of focal "no-reflow"), and (v) generation of endothelial cell leukocyte adhesion receptors. These events lead to the extravascular accumulation of fluid as edema, decreased basal lamina integrity, extravasation of blood elements as hemorrhage, and the activation of inflammatory responses.[5,91] Within the ischemic regions those injury events are heterogeneously distributed, and in time (if unchecked) becoming confluent. They negatively affect neuron function.

Capillary permeability barrier function is lost as early as 30 minutes after focal cerebral ischemia. This loss is associated with ultrastructural changes of the endothelium and of astrocytes within the microvasculature.[92,93] In both clinical and experimental settings, edema within the region of injury follows leakage of the vascular permeability barrier.[16,94,95] Loss of selective K^+ channels is associated with the swelling of astrocyte end-feet.[94,96] SUR-1 channels, that facilitate H_2O transit into the injured tissue, are expressed on astrocytes during focal ischemia.[78,97] Swelling of the cellular compartments can contribute to the focal "no-reflow" phenomenon.[98] There is evidence that the loss of the blood–brain barrier and the microvessel ECM results from the actions of bradykinin,[99,100] vascular endothelial growth factor (VEGF),[101–103] thrombin,[100,104] active matrix metalloproteinases (MMPs),[105] cysteine proteases,[32] proteases released by activated leukocytes,[106,107] and other enzyme activities.[108] Blockade of bradykinin receptors has been associated with reduced injury and edema formation,[109] as has blockade of SUR-1 channels.[97]

Garcia et al. demonstrated that capillaries can expand and rupture.[110] In the basal lamina, local decrease in the expression of the major vascular matrix components laminin-1 and laminin-5, collagen IV, and cellular fibronectin follows focal ischemia,[27,111] which is associated with the extravascular accumulation of hemoglobin (hemorrhagic transformation) within the regions of ischemic injury.[111] Note is made that endothelial cell P-selectin and E-selectin and expression of β_1 integrins within the ischemic territory occur only on those microvessels with an intact basal lamina.[112,113]

β_1 integrins are lost from microvessel endothelium, in concert with increased microvessel permeability.[29,30,35,36] Separate studies suggest that β_1 integrins, through their participation in cell matrix adherence, may play a role in preventing transudation and edema formation, in conjunction with other contributors to the intact blood–brain barrier, and might be disturbed during ischemia by action of cytokines locally generated by microglia and astrocytes.[114–116] $\alpha\beta$-Dystroglycan is lost from astrocyte end-feet within the first 2 hours of focal ischemia.[35] This correlates with the detachment of the end-feet from their basal lamina following ischemia onset,[110,117] and alterations in H_2O transit.[118]

All of these events begin within 1–2 hours after the onset of focal ischemia, indicating that microvessel functional integrity and ultrastructure can be rapidly affected. Furthermore, the spatial distribution of altered microvessel adhesion receptor expression is not homogeneous, and coincides with neuron injury.[29,30,101]

Innate Inflammation. The inflammatory responses within the territory-at-risk initiated by focal cerebral ischemia involve all cells of the neurovascular unit. The peripheral inflammatory response is initiated by up-regulation of endothelial cell–PMN leukocyte adhesion receptors in a rapid and orderly way. Transmigration of PMN leukocytes into the ischemic core occurs as early as 1 hour after MCA:O in the non-human primate.[101,119] These observations have been confirmed in rodent models of focal cerebral ischemia, although the details vary, and have been documented in both experimental and patient systems.[120] In anesthetized rodent models IL-1β and TNF-α are generated during early phases of focal ischemia.[121–123]

Endothelial cells, within cerebral capillaries and post-capillary venules, respond to TNF-α and IL-1β by translocation of P-selectin (stored in Weibel-Palade bodies) to the luminal surface, the synthesis of ICAM-1 and its expression on the luminal surface, and the later surface appearance of E-selectin,[112,113] which facilitate firm adhesion of PMN leukocytes to the local endothelium.[124,125] Both cytokines can down-regulate the integrin $\alpha_6\beta_1$ found on endothelial cells.[126] This change parallels the rapid loss in β_1 integrin expression from cerebral microvessels observed in vivo.[30,127]

We and others have hypothesized that these events could contribute to the development of edema during focal ischemia, in addition to recognized changes in the inter-endothelial tight junction proteins (known to occur later).[6,128] Increased permeability by the endothelium leads to exposure of the perivascular tissue factor (TF) to the plasma column of blood, and the abrogation of the anti-thrombotic milieu of the endothelium.[129,130]

Transient occlusion of a brain-supplying artery significantly reduces the patency of the distal microvascular bed, causing the focal "no-reflow" phenomenon.[119,131,132] Intravascular obstruction occurs with the local adherence of PMN leukocytes within the microvasculature, together with activated platelets and fibrin in both capillaries and post-capillary venules of the ischemic bed.[113,119,129]

Astrocytes serve immune function, can potentially present antigens, have phagocytic properties, and generate cytokines

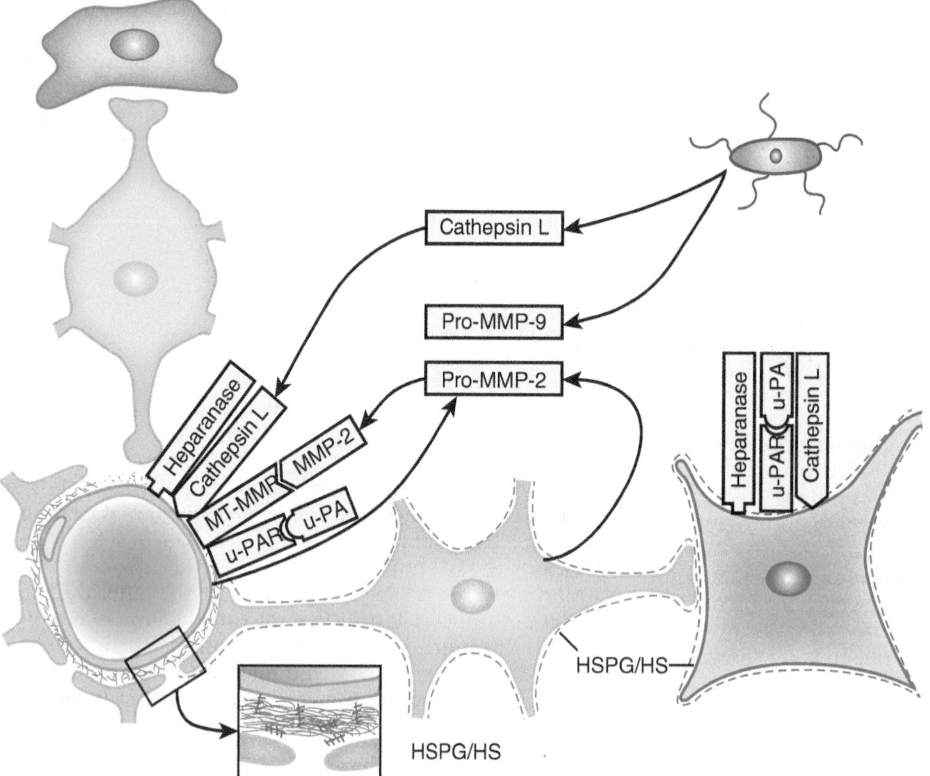

Figure 7-5. Graphic representation of potential consequences to the neurovascular unit of focal ischemia. Coordinate expression of membrane-type matrix metalloproteinases (MT-MMP), pro-MMP-2, u-PA, u-PAR, cathepsin L, and heparanase on microvessels and neurons in the non-human primate basal ganglia. Microglia express pro-MMP-9 and cathepsin L. HSPG = heparan sulfate proteoglycan (perlecan); HS = heparan sulfate side-chains. The hypothesis depicted here states that the alterations of matrix components of the microvasculature and the pericellular matrix during focal ischemia lead to structural and functional alterations within the neurovascular unit. *(From del Zoppo G. Stroke 44: 263–269, 2013.)*

and chemokines in response to a variety of stimuli,[133] including TNF-α and IL-1β. Astrocytes can generate the latent metalloproteinase-2 ((pro-)MMP-2) under a number of conditions. In contrast, circulating PMN leukocytes release pro-MMP-8 and pro-MMP-9, pericytes appear to generate (pro-) MMP-9,[134] and cells of the monocyte/macrophage lineage generate pro-MMP-9. The activation and potential impact of these matrix proteases on the basal laminin and the endothelial permeability is under study.

Significant changes in *basal lamina ECM* integrity and in cell–matrix adhesion receptor expression occur simultaneously with neuron injury, and reflect rapid dynamic changes in response to focal ischemia. Proteases that could process ECM are generated rapidly within the ischemic core under the conditions of focal ischemia in the non-human primate,[32] and belong to four families: the MMPs (e.g., pro-MMP-2 and -9, and their MMP activators), serine proteases (e.g., urokinase plasminogen activator, u-PA), cysteine proteases (e.g., cathepsin L), and heparanase (Fig. 7-5). Members of all four families appear within 1–2 hours after MCA:O in the ischemic core. Degradation products of some matrix proteins have cytokine or chemokine activity. Elastase released upon degranulation of PMN leukocytes can cleave laminin-5 to generate a peptide capable of promoting granulocyte chemotaxis.[135] Similarly, PMN leukocyte released MMP-8 can generate the chemotactic pro-gly-pro-containing peptide from collagen.[136] Cathepsin L-mediated cleavage of perlecan yields the domain V fragment which has pro-angiogenic properties.[137] Degradation of collagen IV, for instance, can generate peptides with anti-angiogenic activities.[138,139] Rosenberg and associates have described a temporal correlation between pro-MMP-9 "activity" and edema formation in rat strains after MCA:O.[140,141] In the primate, increased pro-MMP-9 expression within the ischemic tissue is associated with hemorrhagic transformation.[105,142]

Neuron responses to ischemia include inflammatory responses to cytokines generated acutely. The manner in which IL-1β could mediate neuron injury in the CNS has been the subject of vigorous exploration. For instance, the Dietrich group have shown that a molecular platform consisting of caspase-1, apoptosis-associated speck-like protein containing a caspase-activating recruitment domain (ASC), and nucleotide-binding, leucine-rich repeat, pyrin domain containing 1 (NLRP1) is expressed in neurons, astrocytes, and macrophage/monocytes shortly after focal ischemia onset.[143] Additionally, enzymes with matrix protease activity, generated during ischemia, could promote neuron injury either directly or indirectly.[144]

Microglia participate in the early inflammatory responses of the CNS to focal ischemia. While normally quiescent, these cells have Fc receptors, complement receptors, receptors for a number of cytokines, chemokine receptors, CD40, Fas and Fas ligand.[145] Microglia also generate TNF-α and IL-1β in addition to other cytokines, and are known to regulate T-cell-mediated immune processes.[145] In response to activators, microglia express pro-MMP-9.[146] Mabuchi et al. have detailed the relative appearance and kinetics of microglia and cells of the monocyte/macrophage lineage in the ischemic brain parenchyma.[147]

Located in association with astroglial processes in the vicinity of microvessels at their branch points, and on their luminal aspect,[148,149] *mast cells* associate with astrocytes and matrix substrates (e.g., laminin, fibronectin).[150] Mast cells can release TNF-α and IL-1β.

The *glymphatic clearance network* for CSF may also play roles in innate inflammation, as an extension of the Virchow-Robins space.[151] Perivascular influx of CSF via glymphatic transport may also contribute to edema.[151]

These individual cell responses to cytokines are defined; however, how cells within the neurovascular unit communicate with each other and influence each other under the conditions of ischemia and innate inflammation has not been studied.

Propagating Depolarizations and Neurovascular Unit Dysfunction. Injury and metabolic stress can disturb the

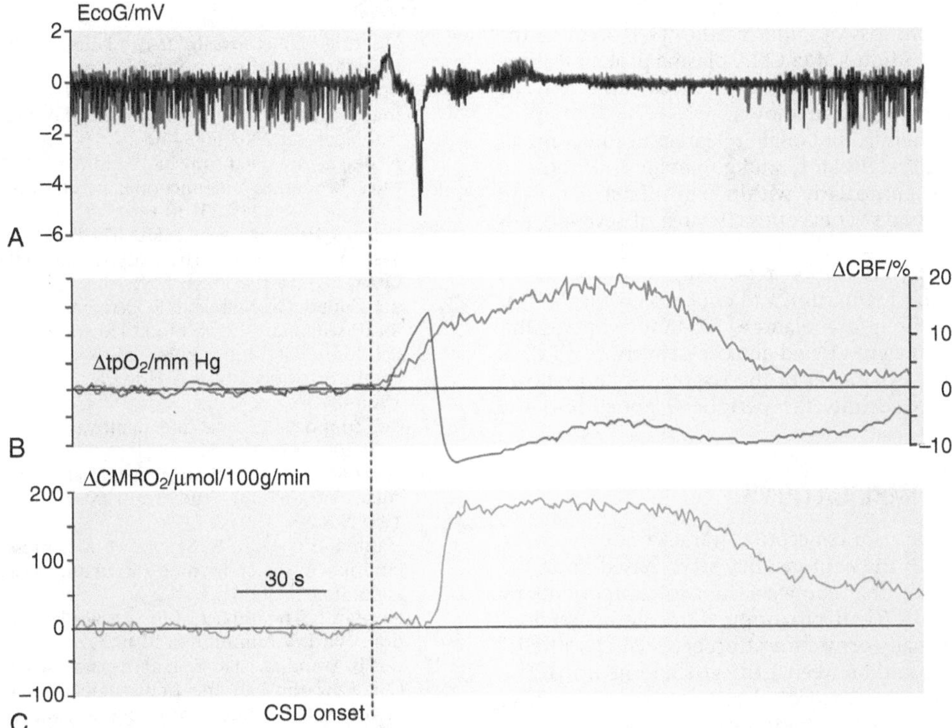

Figure 7-6. CSD – a vascular and bioenergetic stress. A single CSD causes significant perturbations in the neurovascular unit in a healthy rat cortex including disruptions in blood flow, tissue oxygenation and oxygen consumption. Physiological recordings show that following CSD onset (A; vertical broken line), very large increases in blood flow and tissue pO_2 (B) anticipate robust and sustained (hours) metabolic demand for oxygen as measured by the cerebral rate of oxygen metabolism ($CMRO_2$) (C). Following an increase in tissue pO_2, a subsequent decrease (B) reflects the fact that oxygen utilization and metabolism greatly exceed its delivery by large blood flow increases. These mismatches between flow and metabolism are also reflected by indices of impaired mitochondrial redox state and oxidative phosphorylation as well as by relatively long-lasting abnormal vascular responses (see text). Hence, CSD provides an excellent example of integrative gray matter responses that reflect disruptions of the neurovascular unit. tpO_2 = tissue partial pressure of oxygen; eCoG = electrocorticogram; CBF = cerebral blood flow. *(Redrawn from Pilgaard H, Lauritzen M J Cereb Blood Flow Metab 29: 1517–1527; 2009.)*

integrative functioning of the neurovascular unit disrupting neurovascular coupling and, potentially, blood–brain barrier integrity. Alterations within the neuron-vascular networks can generate spreading depolarizations. Spreading depolarization (SD) comprises a continuum of entities.[152] Cortical spreading depression (CSD) is a slowly propagating depolarization of neurons and glia that spreads at a characteristic rate and erupts in otherwise normal tissue. These can explain the migraine aura. Spreading depolarization describes propagating depolarizations that occur in the context of compromised or injured brain and delayed recovery. Anoxic depolarization occurs in the absence of membrane potential recovery, such as in the core of an ischemic lesion.

Propagating depolarizing waves disrupt the neurovascular unit and impose a significant bioenergetic burden on healthy brain. CSD is characterized by collapse of ionic homeostasis, disruption of ionic gradients (Ca^{+2}, Cl^- and Na^+ and H_2O influx with K^+/H^+ efflux), and neurotransmitter release into the extracellular space by neurons.[153]

To support this metabolic demand and to restore the ionic gradients, O_2 and glucose are utilized and delivered to the brain by large transient CBF increases.[154] These increases in flow begin during the direct current (DC) shift and are followed by prolonged oligemia, in part due to impaired vascular responsiveness. Recently, the release of arachidonate during CSD and the synthesis of a vasoconstrictor, 20-hydroxyeicosatetraenoic acid (20-HETE), have been implicated.[155] Synthesis of 20-HETE, however, does not explain the prolonged uncoupling of blood flow to neuronal activity that is characteristic of CSD (Fig. 7-6).[154] Despite the transient rise in flow during CSD, O_2 delivery is insufficient to support the increased tissue energy demand.[156] Moreover, ATP levels decrease along with rising NAD levels in vivo.[156] Glucose utilization surges causing a decrease in brain glucose levels and an increase in lactate which can contribute to mild acidosis.[157,158] To meet this demand, O_2 consumption ($CMRO_2$) increases early and remains elevated for up to 2 hours,[154] well beyond the time needed by Na^+K^+ ATPase activity to restore the ionic gradients.[159] Despite these compensatory adjustments, brain tissue remains O_2-deprived and functionally compromised for 1–2 hours, although the vascular and metabolic changes following CSD are fully reversible in an otherwise healthy brain.[160,161] CSD is accompanied by significant neuronal, but not astrocyte, swelling and a reduction in the extracellular space.[156] Most of these metabolic and blood-flow variables return towards baseline within 2 hours,[154] and both the speed and extent of recovery are determined in part by adequate cerebral perfusion pressure ensuring energy substrate delivery. While cell swelling could negatively impact O_2 diffusion gradients and also blood flow regulated by direct neurovascular connections, the impact of these changes on neurovascular unit function has not been explored. Several excellent reviews on the topic are available.[1,162,163]

CSD can be accompanied by changes in matrix integrity, perhaps by processes involving select MMPs.[164] MMP-9 levels increase ipsilateral to the CSD, reaching a maximum at 24 hours and persisting for at least 48 hours. Gelatinolytic activity is detectable within cortical blood vessels and later within neurons and blood-vessel-rich pia arachnoid by 3 hours. At 3–24 hours, apparent loss of laminin and ZO-1 occur in the ipsilateral cortex. At 3 hours after CSD, plasma protein leakage and brain edema develop, but not in MMP 9 null mice. The source of the MMP remains unknown.

During focal ischemia, glutamate release and ionic imbalances occur:[165–167] extracellular K^+ and glutamate contribute to the genesis of SD, particularly within peri-infarct zones. In animal models, a single SD expands the area of severe hypoperfusion by more than 20%,[168] and the frequency and cumulative duration of DC shifts reportedly correspond to accelerated infarction maturation and core expansion.[169,170] At least part of the tissue injury relates to SD-induced perfusion decreases with insufficient O_2 and glucose delivery.[171,172] It has been proposed that expansion of the regions of "no-reflow" by secondary injury recruits the peripheral zones into the ischemic core.[30,173]

SUMMARY AND IMPLICATIONS

The *neurovascular unit* is a conceptual framework connecting the microvessels with the neurons they serve, based upon the structural relationship that connects the two components by intervening astrocytes. Their proximity within intact cerebral capillaries implies ready communication between endothelial cells and astrocytes, and between astrocytes and neurons. The evidence for neuron ≫ microvessel communication is firm, and microvessel ≫ neuron communication is implied by some modes of signaling already known within microvessels, among astrocytes, between astrocytes and neurons, and across network boundaries. Further evidence comes from the coordinated responses to ischemic injury, as evidenced by CSD, matrix protease release and their cell associations, and the impact of plasma contents on the neuropil when permeability increases.

Among the many implications, the neurovascular unit provides a construct for considering a single element in conjunction with the others. This framework is relevant for understanding the effects of pathophysiologic states (e.g., ischemic stroke) that affect multiple cell compartments and not neurons exclusively, and a reminder that intercellular interactions underlie the ultimate injury and recovery processes. As an example, within the neurovascular unit all individual cell types have immune and/or inflammatory response properties, however the response of the whole unit to a stimulus, and how the elements interact, is not yet understood. This construct may offer significant insights into the difficulties and limitations of achieving clinical neuroprotectant effects with pharmaceutical agents intended to reduce post-stroke CNS injury.

There are many unresolved issues that emerge. Regional differences in composition of the neurovascular unit and routes of communication are likely. Proof of how ischemic processes proceed and how they affect microvessel integrity, neovascularization, and outcome and the roles of neurons in this event after arterial occlusion is still lacking. For instance, in angiogenesis the coordination of VEGF expression and receptor binding among cellular elements of the neurovascular unit is not worked out. Also unresolved are the combined effects of members of the several protease families, the relative specificities of protease family inhibitors, and the impact of active proteases on hemostasis and intravascular cell–matrix interactions.

Offered as a framework for scientific enquiry the *neurovascular unit* is intended to reflect the anatomic and functional relationships that compose the cerebral tissue at rest and targeted by ischemic injury. It is likely to undergo much revision over time.

REFERENCES

1. Iadecola C. Neurovascular regulation in the normal brain and in Alzheimer's disease. Nat Rev Neurosci 2004;5:347–60.
2. Zonta M, Angulo M, Gobbo S, et al. Neuron-to-astrocyte signaling is central to the dynamic control of brain microcirculation. Nat Neurosci 2003;6:43–50.
3. Nedergaard M, Ransom BR, Goldman SA. New roles for astrocytes: Redefining the functional architecture of the brain. Trends Neurosci 2003;26:523–30.
4. Peters A, Palay SL, Webster HD. The Fine Structure of the Nervous System: Neurons and Their Supporting Cells. 3rd ed. New York: Oxford University Press; 1991.
5. del Zoppo GJ, Mabuchi T. Cerebral microvessel responses to focal ischemia. J Cereb Blood Flow Metab 2003;23:879–94.
6. del Zoppo GJ, Milner R. Integrin-matrix interactions in the cerebral microvasculature. Arterioscler Thromb Vasc Biol 2006;26: 1966–75.
7. del Zoppo GJ. Stroke and neurovascular protection. N Engl J Med 2006;354:553–5.
8. Spatz M, Bacic F, McCarron RM, et al. Human cerebromicrovascular endothelium: Studies *in vitro*. J Cereb Blood Flow Metab 1989;9:S393.
9. Hallmann R, Horn N, Selg M, et al. Expression and function of laminins in the embryonic and mature vasculature. Physiol Rev 2005;85:979–1000.
10. Sorokin L. The impact of the extracellular matrix on inflammation. Nat Rev Immunol 2010;10:712–23.
11. Iliff JJ, Wang M, Liao Y, et al. A paravascular pathway facilitates CSF flow through the brain parenchyma and the clearance of interstitial solutes, including amyloid beta. Sci Transl Med 2012;4:147ra111.
12. Iliff JJ, Nedergaard M. Is there a cerebral lymphatic system? Stroke 2013;44:S93–5.
13. Carlson SS, Hockfield S. Central nervous system. In: Comper WD, editor. Extracellular Matrix, Volume 1. Melbourne: Harwood Academic Publishers; 1996. p. 1–23.
14. Hawkins BT, Davis TP. The blood–brain barrier/neurovascular unit in health and disease. Pharmacol Rev 2005;57:173–85.
15. Risau W, Wolburg H. Development of the blood–brain barrier. Trends Neurosci 1990;13:174–8.
16. Risau W, Esser S, Engelhardt B. Differentiation of blood–brain barrier endothelial cells. Pathol Biol (Paris) 1998;46: 171–5.
17. Janzer RC, Raff MC. Astrocytes induce blood–brain barrier properties in endothelial cells. Nature 1987;325:253–7.
18. Webersinke G, Bauer H, Amberger A, et al. Comparison of gene expression of extracellular matrix molecules in brain microvascular endothelial cells and astrocytes. Biochem Biophys Res Commun 1992;189:877–84.
19. Furuse M, Hirase T, Itoh M, et al. Occludin: A novel integral membrane protein localizing at tight junctions. J Cell Biol 1993;123:1777–88.
20. Furuse M, Itoh M, Hirase T, et al. Direct association of occludin with ZO-1 and its possible involvement in the localization of occludin at tight junctions. J Cell Biol 1994;127:1617–26.
21. Furuse M, Sasaki H, Tsukita S. Manner of interaction of heterogeneous claudin species within and between tight junction strands. J Cell Biol 1999;147:891–903.
22. Hurwitz AA, Berman JW, Rashbaum WK, et al. Human fetal astrocytes induce the expression of blood-brain barrier specific proteins by autologous endothelial cells. Brain Res 1993;625: 238–43.
23. Micic D, Swink M, Micic J, et al. The ischemic and postischemic effect on the uptake of neutral amino acids in isolated cerebral capillaries. Experientia 1993;15:625–6.
24. Tran ND, Schreiber SS, Fisher M. Astrocyte regulation of endothelial tissue plasminogen activator in a blood–brain barrier model. J Cereb Blood Flow Metab 1998;18:1316–24.
25. Wang L, Tran ND, Kittaka M, et al. Thrombomodulin expression in bovine brain capillaries. Anticoagulant function of the blood–brain barrier, regional differences, and regulatory mechanisms. Arterioscler Thromb Vasc Biol 1997;17:3139–46.
26. Estrada C, Bready JV, Berliner JA, et al. Astrocyte growth stimulation by a soluble factor produced by cerebral endothelial cells in vitro. J Neuropathol Exp Neurol 1990;49:539–49.

27. Hamann GF, Okada Y, Fitridge R, et al. Microvascular basal lamina antigens disappear during cerebral ischemia and reperfusion. Stroke 1995;26:2120–6.
28. Haring H-P, Akamine P, Habermann R, et al. Distribution of integrin-like immunoreactivity on primate brain microvasculature. J Neuropathol Exp Neurol 1996;55:236–45.
29. Wagner S, Tagaya M, Koziol JA, et al. Rapid disruption of an astrocyte interaction with the extracellular matrix mediated by integrin alpha6beta4 during focal cerebral ischemia/reperfusion. Stroke 1997;28:858–65.
30. Tagaya M, Haring H-P, Stuiver I, et al. Rapid loss of microvascular integrin expression during focal brain ischemia reflects neuron injury. J Cereb Blood Flow Metab 2001;21:835–46.
31. Hamann GF, Liebetrau M, Martens H, et al. Microvascular basal lamina injury after experimental focal cerebral ischemia and reperfusion in the rat. J Cereb Blood Flow Metab 2002;22: 526–33.
32. Fukuda S, Fini CA, Mabuchi T, et al. Focal cerebral ischemia induces active proteases that degrade microvascular matrix. Stroke 2004;35:998–1004.
33. Kramer RH, Cheng Y-F, Clyman R. Human microvascular endothelial cells use β_1 and β_3 integrin receptor complexes to attach to laminin. J Cell Biol 1990;111:1233–43.
34. Paulus W, Baur I, Schuppan D, et al. Characterization of integrin receptors in normal and neoplastic human brain. Am J Pathol 1993;143:154–63.
35. Milner R, Hung S, Wang X, et al. The rapid decrease in astrocyte-associated dystroglycan expression by focal cerebral ischemia is protease-dependent. J Cereb Blood Flow Metab 2008;28: 812–23.
36. Osada T, Gu Y-H, Kanazawa M, et al. Interendothelial claudin-5 expression depends upon cerebral endothelial cell-matrix adhesion by β_1-integrins. J Cereb Blood Flow Metab 2011;31: 1972–85.
37. Dore-Duffy P. Pericytes: Pluripotent cells of the blood brain barrier. Curr Pharm Des 2008;14:1581–93.
38. Balabanov R, Washington R, Wagnerova J, et al. CNS microvascular pericytes express macrophage-like function, cell surface integrin alpha M, and macrophage marker ED-2. Microvasc Res 1996;52:127–42.
39. Daneman R, Zhou L, Kebede AA, et al. Pericytes are required for blood-brain barrier integrity during embryogenesis. Nature 2010;468:562–6.
40. Bell RD, Winkler EA, Sagare AP, et al. Pericytes control key neurovascular functions and neuronal phenotype in the adult brain and during brain aging. Neuron 2010;68:409–27.
41. Hall CN, Reynell C, Gesslein B, et al. Capillary pericytes regulate cerebral blood flow in health and disease. Nature 2014;508: 55–60.
42. Roy CS, Sherrington CS. On the regulation of the blood-supply of the brain. J Physiol 1890;11:85–158.
43. Pellerin L, Magistretti PJ. Neuroenergetics: calling upon astrocytes to satisfy hungry neurons. Neuroscientist 2004;10: 53–62.
44. Takano T, Tian GF, Peng W, et al. Astrocyte-mediated control of cerebral blood flow. Nat Neurosci 2006;9:260–7.
45. Nedergaard M, Verkhratsky A. Artifact versus reality – how astrocytes contribute to synaptic events. Glia 2012;60:1013–23.
46. Murai KK, Pasquale EB. Eph receptors and ephrins in neuron-astrocyte communication at synapses. Glia 2011;59:1567–78.
47. Paukert M, Agarwal A, Cha J, et al. Norepinephrine controls astroglial responsiveness to local circuit activity. Neuron 2014; 82:1263–70.
48. Ding F, O'Donnell J, Thrane AS, et al. alpha1-Adrenergic receptors mediate coordinated Ca^{2+} signaling of cortical astrocytes in awake, behaving mice. Cell Calcium 2013;54:387–94.
49. Schummers J, Yu H, Sur M. Tuned responses of astrocytes and their influence on hemodynamic signals in the visual cortex. Science 2008;320:1638–43.
50. Escartin C, Valette J, Lebon V, et al. Neuron–astrocyte interactions in the regulation of brain energy metabolism: a focus on NMR spectroscopy. J Neurochem 2006;99:393–401.
51. Hutchinson DS, Catus SL, Merlin J, et al. alpha(2)-Adrenoceptors activate noradrenaline-mediated glycogen turnover in chick astrocytes. J Neurochem 2011;117:915–26.
52. Harik SI, Busto R, Martinez E. Norepinephrine regulation of cerebral glycogen utilization during seizures and ischemia. J Neurosci 1982;2:409–14.
53. Costa S, Planchenault T, Charriere-Bertrand C, et al. Astroglial permissivity for neuritic outgrowth in neuron-astrocyte cocultures depends on regulation of laminin bioavailability. Glia 2002;37:105–13.
54. Lecrux C, Toussay X, Kocharyan A, et al. Pyramidal neurons are "neurogenic hubs" in the neurovascular coupling response to whisker stimulation. J Neurosci 2011;31:9836–47.
55. Cauli B, Tong XK, Rancillac A, et al. Cortical GABA interneurons in neurovascular coupling: relays for subcortical vasoactive pathways. J Neurosci 2004;24:8940–9.
56. Bekar LK, Wei HS, Nedergaard M. The locus coeruleus-norepinephrine network optimizes coupling of cerebral blood volume with oxygen demand. J Cereb Blood Flow Metab 2012; 32:2135–45.
57. Toussay X, Basu K, Lacoste B, et al. Locus coeruleus stimulation recruits a broad cortical neuronal network and increases cortical perfusion. J Neurosci 2013;33:3390–401.
58. Duchemin S, Boily M, Sadekova N, et al. The complex contribution of NOS interneurons in the physiology of cerebrovascular regulation. Front Neural Circuits 2012;6:51.
59. Logothetis NK, Pauls J, Augath M, et al. Neurophysiological investigation of the basis of the fMRI signal. Nature 2001;412: 150–7.
60. Koehler RC, Gebremedhin D, Harder DR. Role of astrocytes in cerebrovascular regulation. J Appl Physiol (1985) 2006;100: 307–17.
61. Xi Q, Umstot E, Zhao G, et al. Glutamate regulates Ca^{2+} signals in smooth muscle cells of newborn piglet brain slice arterioles through astrocyte- and heme oxygenase-dependent mechanisms. Am J Physiol Heart Circ Physiol 2010;298:H562–9.
62. Chen ZL, Yao Y, Norris EH, et al. Ablation of astrocytic laminin impairs vascular smooth muscle cell function and leads to hemorrhagic stroke. J Cell Biol 2013;202:381–95.
63. Tagaya M, Liu KF, Copeland B, et al. DNA scission after focal brain ischemia. Temporal differences in two species. Stroke 1997;28:1245–54.
64. Halassa MM, Fellin T, Takano H, et al. Synaptic islands defined by the territory of a single astrocyte. J Neurosci 2007;27:6473–7.
65. Theodosis DT, Poulain DA, Oliet SH. Activity-dependent structural and functional plasticity of astrocyte-neuron interactions. Physiol Rev 2008;88:983–1008.
66. Parpura V, Basarsky TA, Liu F, et al. Glutamate-mediated astrocyte-neuron signalling. Nature 1994;369:744–7.
67. Cotrina ML, Lin JH, Alves-Rodrigues A, et al. Connexins regulate calcium signaling by controlling ATP release. Proc Natl Acad Sci USA 1998;95:15735–40.
68. Sofroniew MV. Astrocyte failure as a cause of CNS dysfunction. Mol Psychiatry 2000;5:230–2.
69. Ben Achour S, Pascual O. Astrocyte-neuron communication: functional consequences. Neurochem Res 2012;37:2464–73.
70. Jo S, Yarishkin O, Hwang YJ, et al. GABA from reactive astrocytes impairs memory in mouse models of Alzheimer's disease. Nat Med 2014;20:886–96.
71. Beck DW, Roberts RL, Olson JJ. Glial cells influence membrane-associated enzyme activity at the blood–brain barrier. Brain Res 1986;381:131–7.
72. Abbruscato TJ, Davis TP. Protein expression of brain endothelial cell E-cadherin after hypoxia/aglycemia: influence of astrocyte contact. Brain Res 1999;842:277–86.
73. Brix B, Mesters JR, Pellerin L, et al. Endothelial cell-derived nitric oxide enhances aerobic glycolysis in astrocytes via HIF-1alpha-mediated target gene activation. J Neurosci 2012;32:9727–35.
74. Marcus AJ, Broekman MJ, Drosopoulos JH, et al. The endothelial cell ecto-ADPase responsible for inhibition of platelet function is CD39. J Clin Invest 1997;99:1351–60.
75. Kawashima Y, Nagasawa T, Ninomiya H. Contribution of ecto-5′-nucleotidase to the inhibition of platelet aggregation by human endothelial cells. Blood 2000;96:2157–62.
76. Albert JL, Boyle JP, Roberts JA, et al. Regulation of brain capillary endothelial cells by P2Y receptors coupled to Ca^{2+}, phospholipase C and mitogen-activated protein kinase. Br J Pharmacol 1997;122:935–41.

77. Lin JH, Takano T, Arcuino G, et al. Purinergic signaling regulates neural progenitor cell expansion and neurogenesis. Dev Biol 2007;302:356–66.
78. Simard M, Arcuino G, Takano T, et al. Signaling at the gliovascular interface. J Neurosci 2003;23:9254–62.
79. Berrout J, Jin M, O'Neil RG. Critical role of TRPP2 and TRPC1 channels in stretch-induced injury of blood–brain barrier endothelial cells. Brain Res 2012;1436:1–12.
80. Zheng W, Christensen LP, Tomanek RJ. Stretch induces upregulation of key tyrosine kinase receptors in microvascular endothelial cells. Am J Physiol Heart Circ Physiol 2004;287:H2739–45.
81. Suresh Babu S, Wojtowicz A, Freichel M, et al. Mechanism of stretch-induced activation of the mechanotransducer zyxin in vascular cells. Sci Signal 2012;5:ra91.
82. Yousif LF, Di RJ, Sorokin L. Laminin isoforms in endothelial and perivascular basement membranes. Cell Adh Migr 2013;7:101–10.
83. Hahn C, Schwartz MA. Mechanotransduction in vascular physiology and atherogenesis. Nat Rev Mol Cell Biol 2009;10:53–62.
84. Hua SZ, Gottlieb PA, Heo J, et al. A mechanosensitive ion channel regulating cell volume. Am J Physiol Cell Physiol 2010;298:C1424–30.
85. Dietrich WD. Neurobiology of stroke. Int Rev Neurobiol 1998;42:55–101.
86. Dirnagl U, Iadecola C, Moskowitz MA. Pathobiology of ischaemic stroke: an integrated view. Trends Neurosci 1999;22:391–7.
87. Francis A, Pulsinelli W. The response of GABAergic and cholinergic neurons to transient cerebral ischemia. Brain Res 1982;243:271–8.
88. Gonzales C, Lin RCS, Chesselet MF. Relative sparing of GABAergic interneurons in the striatum of gerbils with ischemia-induced lesions. Neurosci Lett 1992;135:53–8.
89. Nitsch C, Goping G, Klatzo I. Preservation of GABAergic perikarya and boutons after transient ischemia in the gerbil hippocampal CA1 field. Brain Res 1989;495:243–52.
90. Mabuchi T, Lucero J, Feng A, et al. Focal cerebral ischemia preferentially affects neurons distant from their neighboring microvessels. J Cereb Blood Flow Metab 2005;25:257–66.
91. del Zoppo GJ, Becker KJ, Hallenbeck JM. Inflammation after stroke: Is it harmful? Arch Neurol 2001;58:669–72.
92. Naganuma Y. Changes of the cerebral microvascular structure and endothelium during the course of permanent ischemia. Keio J Med 1990;39:26–31.
93. Okumura Y, Sakaki T, Hiramatsu K, et al. Microvascular changes associated with postischaemic hypoperfusion in rats. Acta Neurochir (Wien) 1997;139:670–6.
94. Chan PH, Chu L. Mechanisms underlying glutamate-induced swelling of astrocytes in primary culture. Acta Neurochir Suppl 1990;51:7–10.
95. Olesen S-P. Rapid increase in blood-brain barrier permeability during severe hypoxia and metabolic inhibition. Brain Res 1986;368:24–9.
96. Bender AS, Norenberg MD. Calcium dependence of hypoosmotically induced potassium release in cultured astrocytes. J Neurosci 1994;14:4237–43.
97. Simard JM, Chen M, Tarasov KV, et al. Newly expressed SUR1-regulated NC(Ca-ATP) channel mediates cerebral edema after ischemic stroke. Nat Med 2006;12:433–40.
98. Ames A, Wright LW, Kowada M, et al. Cerebral ischemia. II. The no-reflow phenomenon. Am J Pathol 1968;52:437–53.
99. Kamiya T, Katayama Y, Kashiwagi F, et al. The role of bradykinin in mediating ischemic brain edema in rats. Stroke 1993;24:571–5.
100. Aschner JL, Lum H, Fletcher PW, et al. Bradykinin- and thrombin-induced increases in endothelial permeability occur independently of phospholipase C but require protein kinease C activation. J Cell Physiol 1997;173:387–96.
101. Abumiya T, Lucero J, Heo JH, et al. Activated microvessels express vascular endothelial growth factor and integrin alpha(v) beta3 during focal cerebral ischemia. J Cereb Blood Flow Metab 1999;19:1038–50.
102. Zhang ZG, Zhang L, Jiang Q, et al. VEGF enhances angiogenesis and promotes blood–brain barrier leakage in the ischemic brain. J Clin Invest 2000;106:829–38.
103. Suarez S, Ballmer-Hofer K. VEGF transiently disrupts gap junctional communciation in endothelial cells. J Cell Sci 2001;114:1229–35.
104. Kubo Y, Suzuki M, Kudo A, et al. Thrombin inhibitor ameliorates secondary damage in rat brain injury: suppression of inflammatory cells and vimentin-positive astrocytes. J Neurotrauma 2000;2:163–72.
105. Heo JH, Lucero J, Abumiya T, et al. Matrix metalloproteinases increase very early during experimental focal cerebral ischemia. J Cereb Blood Flow Metab 1999;19:624–33.
106. Garcia JH, Liu KF, Yoshida Y, et al. Influx of leukocytes and platelets in an evolving brain infarct (Wistar rat). Am J Pathol 1994;144:188–99.
107. Armao D, Kornfeld M, Estrada EY, et al. Neutral proteases and disruption of the blood–brain barrier in rat. Brain Res 1997;767:259–64.
108. Hosomi N, Lucero J, Heo JH, et al. Rapid differential endogenous plasminogen activator expression after acute middle cerebral artery occlusion. Stroke 2001;32:1341–8.
109. Relton JK, Beckey VE, Hanson WL, et al. CP-0597, a selective bradykinin β_2 receptor antagonist, inhibits brain injury in a rat model of reversible middle cerebral artery occlusion. Stroke 1997;28:1430–6.
110. Garcia JH, Lowry SL, Briggs L, et al. Brain capillaries expand and rupture in areas of ischemia and reperfusion. In: Reivich M, Hurtig HI, editors. Cerebrovascular Diseases. 1st ed. New York: Raven Press; 1983. p. 169–82.
111. Hamann GF, Okada Y, del Zoppo GJ. Hemorrhagic transformation and microvascular integrity during focal cerebral ischemia/reperfusion. J Cereb Blood Flow Metab 1996;16:1373–8.
112. Haring H-P, Berg EL, Tsurushita N, et al. E-selectin appears in non-ischemic tissue during experimental focal cerebral ischemia. Stroke 1996;27:1386–92.
113. Okada Y, Copeland BR, Mori E, et al. P-selectin and intercellular adhesion molecule-1 expression after focal brain ischemia and reperfusion. Stroke 1994;25:202–11.
114. Liu T, McDonnell PC, Young PR, et al. Interleukin-1β mRNA expression in ischemic rat cortex. Stroke 1993;24:1746–51.
115. Buttini M, Appel K, Sauter A, et al. Expression of tumor necrosis factor alpha after focal cerebral ischaemia in the rat. Neuroscience 1996;71:1–16.
116. Loddick SA, Rothwell NJ. Neuroprotective effects of human recombinant interleukin-1 receptor antagonist in focal cerebral ischaemia in the rat. J Cereb Blood Flow Metab 1996;16:932–40.
117. Garcia JH, Cox JV, Hudgins WR. Ultrastructure of the microvasculature in experimental cerebral infarction. Arch Neuropathol (Berlin) 1971;18:273–85.
118. Hawkins BT, Gu YH, Izawa Y, et al. Disruption of dystroglycan-laminin interactions modulates water uptake by astrocytes. Brain Res 2013;1503:89–96.
119. del Zoppo GJ, Schmid-Schönbein GW, Mori E, et al. Polymorphonuclear leukocytes occlude capillaries following middle cerebral artery occlusion and reperfusion in baboons. Stroke 1991;22:1276–83.
120. Kalimo H, del Zoppo GJ, Paetau A, et al. Polymorphonuclear neutrophil infiltration into ischemic infarctions: myth or truth? Acta Neuropathol 2013;125:313–16.
121. Siren AL, Heldman E, Doron D, et al. Release of proinflammatory and prothrombotic mediators in the brain and peripheral circulation in spontaneously hypertensive and normotensive Wistar-Kyoto rats. Stroke 1992;23:1643–51.
122. Wang X, Barone FC, Aiyar NV, et al. Increased interleukin-1 receptor and receptor antagonist gene expression after focal stroke. Stroke 1997;28:155–61.
123. Wang X, Yue T-L, Barone FC, et al. Concommitant cortical expression of TNF-α and IL-1β mRNA following transient focal ischemia. Mol Chem Neuropathol 1994;23:103–14.
124. Bevilacqua MP, Stengelin S, Gembrone MA Jr, et al. Endothelial leukocyte adhesion molecule 1: An inducible receptor for neutrophils related to complement regulatory proteins and lectins. Science 1989;243:1162–5.
125. Granger DN, Benoit JN, Suzuki M, et al. Leukocyte adherence to venular endothelium during ischemia- reperfusion. Am J Physiol 1989;257:G683–8.

126. Defilippi P, Silengo L, Tarone G. $\alpha_6\beta_1$ integrin (laminin receptor) is down-regulated by tumor necrosis factor α and interleukin-1 beta in human endothelial cells. J Biol Chem 1992;267: 18303–7.
127. Milner R, Hung S, Wang X, et al. Responses of endothelial cell and astrocyte matrix-integrin receptors to ischemia mimic those observed in the neurovascular unit. Stroke 2008;39:191–7.
128. Yamasaki Y, Suzuki T, Yamaya H, et al. Possible involvement of interleukin-1 brain edema formation. Neurosci Lett 1992;142: 45–7.
129. del Zoppo GJ, Yu JQ, Copeland BR, et al. Tissue factor localization in non-human primate cerebral tissue. Thromb Haemost 1992;68:642–7.
130. Okada Y, Copeland BR, Fitridge R, et al. Fibrin contributes to microvascular obstructions and parenchymal changes during early focal cerebral ischemia and reperfusion. Stroke 1994;25: 1847–53.
131. Little JR, Kerr FWL, Sundt TM Jr. Microcirculatory obstruction in focal cerebral ischemia. Relationship to neuronal alterations. Mayo Clin Proc 1975;50:264–70.
132. Little JR, Kerr FWL, Sundt TM Jr. Microcirculatory obstruction in focal cerebral ischemia: An electron microscopic investigation in monkeys. Stroke 1976;7:25–30.
133. Dong Y, Benveniste EN. Immune function of astrocytes. Glia 2001;36:180–90.
134. Zozulya A, Weidenfeller C, Galla HJ. Pericyte–endothelial cell interaction increases MMP-9 secretion at the blood–brain barrier in vitro. Brain Res 2008;1189:1–11.
135. Mydel P, Shipley JM, Adair-Kirk TL, et al. Neutrophil elastase cleaves laminin-332 (laminin-5) generating peptides that are chemotactic for neutrophils. J Biol Chem 2008;283:9513–22.
136. Lin M, Jackson P, Tester AM, et al. Matrix metalloproteinase-8 facilitates neutrophil migration through the corneal stromal matrix by collagen degradation and production of the chemotactic peptide Pro-Gly-Pro. Am J Pathol 2008;173:144–53.
137. Lee B, Clarke D, Al Ahmad A, et al. Perlecan domain V is neuroprotective and proangiogenic following ischemic stroke in rodents. J Clin Invest 2011;121:3005–23.
138. Mundel TM, Kalluri R. Type IV collagen-derived angiogenesis inhibitors. Microvasc Res 2007;74:85–9.
139. Marneros AG, Olsen BR. The role of collagen-derived proteolytic fragments in angiogenesis. Matrix Biol 2001;20:337–45.
140. Rosenberg GA, Cunningham LA, Wallace J, et al. Immunohistochemistry of matrix metalloproteinases in reperfusion injury to rat brain: activation of MMP-9 linked to stromelysin-1 and microglia in cell cultures. Brain Res 2001;893:104–12.
141. Rosenberg GA, Navratil M. Metalloproteinase inhibition blocks edema in intracerebral hemorrhage in the rat. Neurology 1997; 48:921–6.
142. del Zoppo GJ, Izawa Y, Hawkins BT. Hemostasis and alterations of the central nervous system. Semin Thromb Hemost 2013;39: 856–75.
143. Abulafia DP, de Rivero Vaccari JP, Lozano JD, et al. Inhibition of the inflammasome complex reduces the inflammatory response after thromboembolic stroke in mice. J Cereb Blood Flow Metab 2009;29:534–44.
144. Thornton P, Pinteaux E, Allan SM, et al. Matrix metalloproteinase-9 and urokinase plasminogen activator mediate interleukin-1-induced neurotoxicity. Mol Cell Neurosci 2008;37:135–42.
145. Aloisi F. Immune function of microglia. Glia 2001;36:165–79.
146. del Zoppo GJ, Frankowski H, Gu YH, et al. Microglial cell activation is a source of metalloproteinase generation during hemorrhagic transformation. J Cereb Blood Flow Metab 2012;32: 919–32.
147. Mabuchi T, Kitagawa K, Ohtsuki T, et al. Contribution of microglia/macrophages to expansion of infarction and response of oligodendrocytes after focal cerebral ischemia in rats. Stroke 2000;31:1735–43.
148. Dimitriadou V, Lambracht-Hall M, Reichler J, et al. Histochemical and ultrastructural characteristics of rat brain perivascular mast cells stimulated with compound 48/80 and carbachol. Neuroscience 1990;39:209–24.
149. Goldschmidt RC, Hough LB, Glick SD, et al. Mast cells in rat thalamus: nuclear localization, sex difference and left-right asymmetry. Brain Res 1984;323:209–17.
150. Thompson HL, Thomas L, Metcalfe DD. Murine mast cells attach to and migrate on laminin-, fibronectin-, and matrigel-coated surfaces in response to Fc epsilon RI-mediated signals. Clin Exp Allergy 1993;23:270–5.
151. Thrane AS, Nedergaard M. Drowning stars: Reassessing the role of astrocytes in brain edema. Trends Neurosci 2014;37(11): 620–8.
152. Dreier JP. The role of spreading depression, spreading depolarization and spreading ischemia in neurological disease. Nat Med 2011;17:439–47.
153. Somjen GG. Mechanisms of spreading depression and hypoxic spreading depression-like depolarization. Physiol Rev 2001;81: 1065–96.
154. Piilgaard H, Lauritzen M. Persistent increase in oxygen consumption and impaired neurovascular coupling after spreading depression in rat neocortex. J Cereb Blood Flow Metab 2009;29: 1517–27.
155. Fordsmann JC, Ko RW, Choi HB, et al. Increased 20-HETE synthesis explains reduced cerebral blood flow but not impaired neurovascular coupling after cortical spreading depression in rat cerebral cortex. J Neurosci 2013;33:2562–70.
156. Takano T, Tian GF, Peng W, et al. Cortical spreading depression causes and coincides with tissue hypoxia. Nat Neurosci 2007; 10:754–62.
157. Shinohara M, Dollinger B, Brown G, et al. Cerebral glucose utilization: local changes during and after recovery from spreading cortical depression. Science 1979;203:188–90.
158. Cruz NF, Adachi K, Dienel GA. Rapid efflux of lactate from cerebral cortex during K+-induced spreading cortical depression. J Cereb Blood Flow Metab 1999;19:380–92.
159. Gault LM, Lin CW, LaManna JC, et al. Changes in energy metabolites, cGMP and intracellular pH during cortical spreading depression. Brain Res 1994;641:176–80.
160. Nedergaard M, Hansen AJ. Spreading depression is not associated with neuronal injury in the normal brain. Brain Res 1988; 449:395–8.
161. Florence G, Bonvento G, Charbonne R, et al. Spreading depression reversibly impairs autoregulation of cortical blood flow. Am J Physiol 1994;266:R1136–40.
162. Leithner C, Royl G. The oxygen paradox of neurovascular coupling. J Cereb Blood Flow Metab 2014;34:19–29.
163. Dunn KM, Nelson MT. Neurovascular signaling in the brain and the pathological consequences of hypertension. Am J Physiol Heart Circ Physiol 2014;306:H1–14.
164. Gursoy-Ozdemir Y, Qiu J, Matsuoka N, et al. Cortical spreading depression activates and upregulates MMP-9. J Clin Invest 2004;113:1447–55.
165. Moskowitz MA, Lo EH, Iadecola C. The science of stroke: mechanisms in search of treatments. Neuron 2010;67:181–98.
166. Hossmann KA. Periinfarct depolarizations. Cerebrovasc Brain Metab Rev 1996;8:195–208.
167. Nedergaard M, Astrup J. Infarct rim: effect of hyperglycemia on direct current potential and [14C]2-deoxyglucose phosphorylation. J Cereb Blood Flow Metab 1986;6:607–15.
168. Shin HK, Dunn AK, Jones PB, et al. Vasoconstrictive neurovascular coupling during focal ischemic depolarizations. J Cereb Blood Flow Metab 2006;26:1018–30.
169. Dijkhuizen RM, Beekwilder JP, van der Worp HB, et al. Correlation between tissue depolarizations and damage in focal ischemic rat brain. Brain Res 1999;840:194–205.
170. Mies G, Iijima T, Hossmann KA. Correlation between peri-infarct DC shifts and ischaemic neuronal damage in rat. Neuroreport 1993;4:709–11.
171. Yuzawa I, Sakadzic S, Srinivasan VJ, et al. Cortical spreading depression impairs oxygen delivery and metabolism in mice. J Cereb Blood Flow Metab 2012;32:376–86.
172. Sukhotinsky I, Yaseen MA, Sakadzic S, et al. Perfusion pressure-dependent recovery of cortical spreading depression is independent of tissue oxygenation over a wide physiologic range. J Cereb Blood Flow Metab 2010;30:1168–77.
173. del Zoppo GJ, Sharp FR, Heiss W-D, et al. Heterogeneity in the penumbra. J Cereb Blood Flow Metab 2011;31:1836–51.

8 Mechanisms of Cerebral Hemorrhage

Jaroslaw Aronowski, Kenneth R. Wagner, Guohua Xi, John H. Zhang

KEY POINTS

- The mechanisms triggering brain damage after intracerebral hemorrhage (ICH) are pleiotropic and are, in many respects, distinct from those contributing to ischemic brain injury.
- The toxicity of extravasated blood toward all structural components of the neurovascular unit represents a unique feature of ICH-mediated brain damage.
- Inflammation and oxidative stress appear to play prominent roles in the pathobiology of ICH.
- The secondary injury after ICH develops over days suggesting the presence of a considerably long window for therapeutic intervention.
- Approaches aimed at detoxification of blood-derived noxious components represent a promising target for the treatment of ICH.
- Pre-clinical animal models provide useful guidance on the pathogenesis of ICH. However, better models to assess re-bleeding (hematoma enlargement) are urgently needed.

Intracerebral hemorrhage (ICH) is a devastating form of stroke with a high mortality and poor prognosis, for which no effective therapy is currently available.[1-8] Rapid accumulation of blood within the brain parenchyma causes increased intracranial pressure and initial cell/tissue damage.[9] Since only half of ICH-related deaths occur in the first 2 days after ICH,[10,11] the contributions of toxic hematoma-derived products (e.g., hemolysis products[12-22]), oxidative stress and pro-inflammatory responses to secondary brain injury are clearly important.[23-26] Indeed, as compared to ischemic stroke, ICH may have a long therapeutic time-window. This chapter will outline selected aspects of our current knowledge from experimental models of ICH, regarding cellular mechanisms of injury and experimental approaches to combat ICH-mediated brain injury (Fig. 8-1).

EXPERIMENTAL MODELS OF INTRACEREBRAL HEMORRHAGE

Over past two decades numerous animal models have been developed to study the pathobiology of ICH. However, most experimental studies of ICH have been conducted in two models, i.e., autologous blood infusion or collagenase injection (reviewed in[27-30]). In the blood infusion model, arterial blood is directly infused into a specific brain structure, e.g., basal ganglia in rodents or frontal white matter in pigs. In the collagenase model, the injected bacterial enzyme, collagenase, degrades the basal lamina that surrounds cerebral blood vessels causing them to rupture and bleed.[31] An additional model in swine involves the creation of a cavity in white matter by balloon inflation followed by infusion of blood into the cavity.[32]

All ICH models have their limitations.[30,33] Direct autologous blood infusion does not capture blood vessel rupture that is the basis for bleeding in human ICH. In the collagenase model, the bacterial enzyme induces considerable inflammation and has a significantly different time course, extent and robustness of perihematomal blood–brain barrier (BBB) opening versus ICH in humans or in blood infusion models. Furthermore, collagenase also produces an injury volume that is considerably larger despite similar initial hematoma volumes.[34] In the balloon inflation model, white matter tracts are "torn" and otherwise damaged in a manner different than that which occurs in blood infusion models and in human ICH. Lastly, unfortunately none of these models replicate the blood vessel pathologic changes that may be present with aging, e.g., amyloidosis.[2]

Despite their limitations, and as presented in this chapter, findings from these models (reviewed in[2,5,35,36]) have provided significant new understanding of ICH pathophysiology and pathochemistry. In addition, these models support potential pharmacologic and surgical treatments, including the recent development of a minimally invasive surgical approach using magnetic resonance-guided focused ultrasound.[37] It is noteworthy that findings directly from ICH animal models have provided the basis for several ongoing clinical therapy trials including iron chelation with deferoxamine,[38] pioglitazone for hematoma resolution (SHRINC),[39] and minimally invasive surgery plus thrombolysis for clot evacuation (MISTIE).[40]

MECHANISM OF BRAIN INJURY AFTER INTRACEREBRAL HEMORRHAGE

Inflammatory Responses after Intracerebral Hemorrhage

A considerable body of literature demonstrates the participation of inflammatory cells in the pathophysiologic processes following ICH, including blood-derived leukocytes and macrophages, resident microglia, astrocytes, and mast cells. These cells can aggravate ICH-induced secondary brain injury by releasing a variety of toxic factors, including cytokines, chemokines, free radicals and nitric oxide.[41]

Activated microglia, which are likely the first non-neuronal cells to acutely react to brain injury, are the main locus of cytokine production. Microglia are activated through a variety of different mechanisms, and undergo morphological and functional changes. Microglial cells classified as the activated phenotype (M1) are involved in pro-inflammatory processes following ICH, while the alternative phenotype (M2) may contribute to cell healing and repair. Microglial cells are activated within minutes after the onset of ICH.[1] The activation

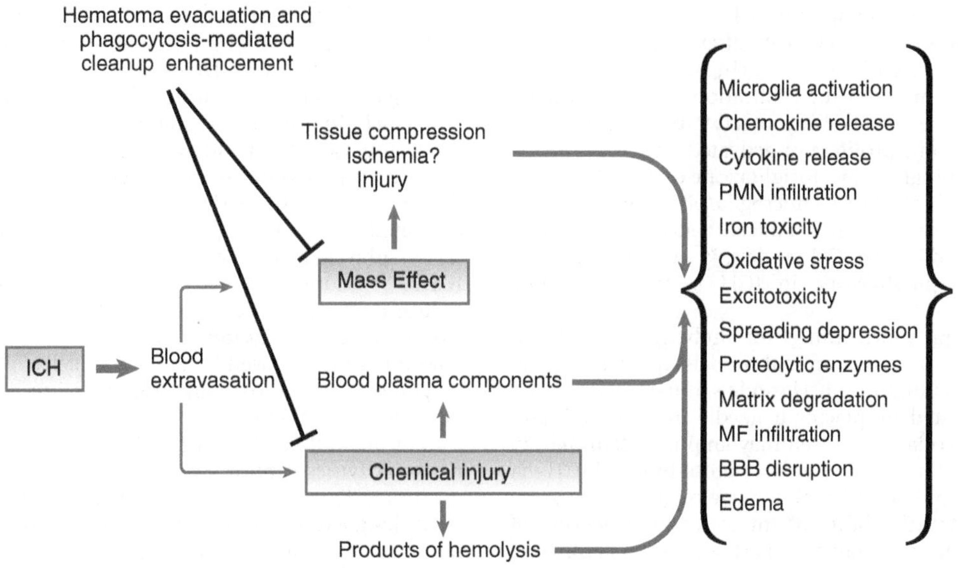

Hematoma evacuation and phagocytosis-mediated cleanup enhancement

Tissue compression ischemia? Injury

Mass Effect

ICH

Blood extravasation

Blood plasma components

Chemical injury

Products of hemolysis

Microglia activation
Chemokine release
Cytokine release
PMN infiltration
Iron toxicity
Oxidative stress
Excitotoxicity
Spreading depression
Proteolytic enzymes
Matrix degradation
MF infiltration
BBB disruption
Edema

Figure 8-1. In response to blood extravasation during ICH, brain tissue is subjected to physical injury associated with the mass effect and potentially to ischemia (in case of large hematomas), and also to chemical injury via toxicity of blood plasma component (e.g., coagulation factors, complement components or immunoglobulins) and product of hemolysis (e.g., hemoglobin, heme or iron). These deleterious events trigger pro-inflammatory responses comprised of activation of microglia, polymorphonuclear (PMN) leukocyte infiltration and entry of blood-borne monocytes. These responses together with the local brain cell death/damage amplify oxidative stress, cause excitotoxicity, ionic imbalance, spreading depression and promote proteolysis-mediated extracellular matrix damage leading to disintegration of neurovascular unit, blood brain damage and deadly edema.

of these cells, particularly the M1 phenotype, results in the production of pro-inflammatory cytokines, including tumor necrosis factors (TNF)-α, interleukin (IL)-1β, IL-6[5] and various chemokines,[42] which triggers neuroinflammation and leukocyte brain infiltration.[25] Several studies have shown that inhibition of microglia activation, for example by minocycline or tuftsin 1–3 fragment, reduces secondary brain injury and improves neurological function in rodents models of ICH.[43,44] Timely clearance of the extravasated hematoma components and damaged tissue debris by activated microglia can reduce local damage from RBC lysis, thereby favoring a nurturing environment and promoting tissue recovery.[19,45]

The roles of other blood-borne inflammatory cells, such as leukocytes and macrophages, have increasingly gained attention in ICH-induced inflammation. In preclinical animal models, neutrophils (polymorphonuclear leukocytes, PMNs) are the earliest leukocyte subtype to infiltrate the hemorrhagic brain, occurring within 4–5 hours after the onset of ICH, and peaking at 3 days after hemorrhage induction.[46–49] PMNs can occlude capillaries, release various proteolytic enzymes, generate NADPH-oxidase- and myeloperoxidase-dependent oxidative stress, which can damage local cells and compromise the BBB.[50–55] Apoptotic cell death of these infiltrating PMNs, without timely removal by phagocytes, may lead to secondary necrosis and further exacerbation of secondary brain injury by stimulating microglia/macrophages to release pro-inflammatory mediators. Recently, Rolland et al. found that fingolimod, an anti-inflammatory drug used as pharmacotherapy for multiple sclerosis, effectively reduced cerebral infiltration of T-lymphocytes, thereby inhibiting local inflammation and improving neurobehavioral and cognitive outcomes following experimental ICH.[56]

Activated astrocytes can secrete inflammatory mediators and increase production of glial fibrillary acidic protein (GFAP), causing so-called reactive gliosis, which can interfere with axonal regeneration. Astrocytes also express and release a variety of matrix metalloproteinases that participate in brain inflammation. Thus, blocking microglia–astrocyte interactions might be a potentially effective strategy to minimize secondary brain damage following ICH.[57] On the other hand, astrocytes may promote neuroprotection by modulating the production of microglial inflammatory mediators.[58,59] Additionally, the inhibition of mast cells has been reported to reduce brain edema and hematoma volume, which was associated with ameliorated neurological deficits following experimental ICH.[60] Hydrogen gas inhalation also diminished brain edema and enhanced BBB preservation by reducing mast cell activation and degranulation in an ICH mouse model.[61]

Accumulating evidence shows that cytokines exacerbate secondary injury after ICH. TNF-α and IL-1β are the two prominent mediators of pro-inflammatory responses in the progression of ICH-induced brain injury.[1,43,62,63] IL-10 and transforming growth factor-β are anti-inflammatory cytokines, which act to eliminate inflammation. Following ICH, perihematomal levels of TNF-α are significantly increased,[23,64,65] which contributes to brain edema and neurological deficits. Clinical evidence is consistent with animal studies, supporting the theory that TNF-α can aggravate ICH-induced brain injury.[66] Similarly, IL-1β has been found to be upregulated after ICH; and increased IL-β expression is associated with severe brain edema and BBB disruption.[43] Inhibition of IL-1β with the receptor antagonist, IL-1Rα, reduces ICH-mediated damage. In addition, IL-6 possesses both pro- and anti-inflammatory properties and may play a significant role in ICH pathophysiology.

Toll-like receptor 4 (TLR4) recruits a specific set of adaptor molecules that interact with the TIR domain, such as MyD88 and TRIF, and subsequently activate a transcription factor, nuclear factor kappa B (NF-κB). The TLR4/NF-κB signaling pathway plays a major role in ICH-induced pathology.[67,68] Heme degradation products lead to production of TNF-α, IL-1β, and IL-6 through activation of the TLR4 pathway. NF-κB is an important transcriptional regulator of pro-inflammatory cytokine production, including TNF-α and IL-1β. Activation of NF-κB occurs in the perihematoma within minutes, lasts for at least 1 week after the onset of ICH,[24,69] and is positively associated with perilesional cell death after ICH in rats. TLR4/NF-κB inhibition, by significantly reducing the perihematomal inflammatory response and the infiltration of the peripheral inflammatory cells, is remarkably protective. In addition, treatment with peroxisome proliferator-activated receptor (PPAR)γ agonists, such as pioglitazone, rosiglitazone or 15d-PGJ_2, promoted phagocytosis of RBCs by microglia/phagocytes, accelerated hematoma resolution and reduced neurological deficits in both in vitro and in vivo ICH models.[19,45] A Phase 2 clinical study evaluating pioglitazone in ICH is currently being carried out.[39]

There are several shortcomings for studying ICH-induced inflammation in our current animal models. In both the collagenase and blood injection ICH models, inflammatory reactions are exacerbated by placing a needle into the animal's brain. Moreover, collagenase itself may amplify inflammatory responses. Focused ultrasound or laser pulse-induced ICH via capillary rupture and endothelial damage might be necessary to improve the translatability of intracerebral injections of collagenase or blood products.[70] Furthermore, establishing animals models of spontaneously occurring ICH, without the injection of foreign agents (such as collagenase), would be a substantial advancement in this field. Since preclinical ICH models are different from the human condition, human histopathologic studies are required to confirm their validity. A better understanding of the inflammation signaling pathways underlying ICH, especially newly identified pathways or molecules should facilitate the identification of therapeutic targets for this malady.

Oxidative Stress after Intracerebral Hemorrhage

Reactive oxygen species (ROS) levels dramatically increase following ICH. High levels of oxidative stress, as measured by protein carbonyl formation, have been found shortly after the intracerebral injection of autologous blood injection in pigs.[71,72] High levels of the ROS marker, ethidium or 4-hydroxynonenal, have been observed in the perihematomal brain region on days 1 and 3 after ICH in the mouse model.[73,74] ROS are produced as a natural byproduct of the oxygen metabolism. Iron and thrombin, released from the hematoma, can generate hydroxyl radicals.[5] One of the ROS sources after ICH is peripheral immune cells, which start invading the brain shortly after the hemorrhage and participate in microglial activation. Subsequently, the activated microglia further enhance the generation of ROS.

Excess generation of ROS is lethal to cells. Hemoglobin degradation products can directly injure DNA by means of oxidative strand breaks.[75] ROS also cause lipid peroxidation, protein oxidation, mitochondrial dysfunction and altered signal transduction, eventually leading to cell death. Beneficial effects of free radical scavengers in preclinical ICH models have been recently demonstrated, including α-phenyl-N-tert-butyl nitrone (PBN), NXY-059 (a derivative of PBN), and edaravone.[1,76–78] In addition, gp91phox KO mice with deleted NADPH oxidase, a key enzyme involved in ROS generation, showed milder damage than wild-type mice in response to ICH.[79] Furthermore, given the potential sources of ROS production following ICH, other efforts targeting pro-oxidant heme or iron such as deferoxamine or porphyrin derivatives have gained increasing promise.[75,80]

In response to heme toxicity and the generation of free radicals, depletion/malfunction of the scavenging antioxidant system may further enhance the oxidative injury of ICH. The pathway involving Kelch-like ECH-associated protein 1 (Keap1) and nuclear factor erythroid 2-related factor 2 (Nrf2) is currently recognized as the central endogenous antioxidant system. Nrf2 expression was significantly increased at 2 hours with a peak at 24 hours following intracerebral blood infusion, while Keap1 was decreased at 8 hours after ICH induction. The downstream antioxidative enzymes regulated by Nrf2, including hemeoxygenase-1 (HO-1), catalase, superoxide dismutase (SOD), glutathione (GSH), thioredoxin (TRX), and glutathione-S-transferase (GST-α1) increased to different degrees during the early stages of ICH.[74,81,82] $Nrf2^{-/-}$ mice exhibited more severe neurologic damage than did wild-type mice subjected to the whole-blood injection model of ICH.[74,81,83] Conversely, Nrf2 inducer sulforaphane exerted to reduce oxidative damage, increased haptoglobin production (to improve hemoglobin elimination), reduced neutrophil amount, and improved behavioral deficits.[74,84]

Drugs with antioxidant properties are promising candidates for ICH therapy. However, conventional antioxidants cannot neutralize ROS formed intracellularly, because the native enzymes cannot cross the membrane of neurons and astrocytes. Thus, different alternatives of enzyme delivery have been designed to improve fusion of enzymes, such as: nanoparticles, PEGylation and lecithinization.[85] More recently, mitochondrial ROS amplified the inflammatory response by triggering NLRP3 inflammasome activation after ICH.[86] Thus, the inhibition of the NLRP3 inflammasome may effectively block the interactions between oxidative stress and inflammation following ICH. The novel free radical neutralizers with clear pharmacokinetics still need to be explored.

Blood Components and Intracerebral-Hemorrhage-induced Injury

As described below, studies have shown that red blood cell (RBC) lysis and coagulation cascade activation are major factors leading to brain edema, BBB disruption, neuronal death and neurological deficits following ICH.

Red Blood Cell Lysis and Hemoglobin Toxicity

RBCs within a clot preserve their normal biconcave configuration for a few days after ICH.[87] Thereafter, they lose their normal shape and start to lyse. RBC lysis appears to begin very early in the brain after hemorrhage. In rodent models of brain hemorrhage, for example, RBCs start to lyse within 24 hours.[88–91] In ICH patients, hemoglobin levels in the CSF increase during the first few days after ictus.[92] However, lysis of RBCs occurs mostly several days after ICH,[18,93,94] which may result from either depletion of intracellular energy reserves or formation of membrane attack complex after activation of the complement system, or both.[95,96] RBC lysis causes edema formation, oxidative stress and neuronal death following ICH.[97,98] A clinical study of edema and ICH indicates that delayed brain edema is related to significant midline shift after ICH in humans.[99] This delayed brain edema (in the second or third weeks after the onset in human) is probably due to hemoglobin and its degradation products.[100] A recent study showed that haptoglobin, an acute response protein and a key hemoglobin neutralizing component, is neuroprotective against ICH-induced brain injury.[101] In addition, carbonic anhydrase-1, one of 14 carbonic anhydrase isozymes, is present at high concentrations in RBCs. Extracellular carbonic anhydrase-1 also contributes to BBB disruption and ICH-induced brain injury.[87,102]

Hemoglobin-induced brain injury results from heme degradation products. Heme is degraded by heme oxygenases in the brain into iron, carbon monoxide and biliverdin.[16] An intracerebral injection of hemoglobin or its degradation products caused brain damage.[103] Studies have shown that heme oxygenase-1 protein levels are increased after brain hemorrhage[90,104] and heme oxygenase inhibitors, tin-mesoporphyrin and zinc protoporphyrin, reduce perihematomal edema, neuronal loss and neurological deficits in ICH animal models.[105–107]

Brain Iron Overload

Iron accumulates in the brain after ICH and results in brain injury.[94,108–110] The release of iron from the degradation of hemoglobin during clot resolution leads to a build up in non-heme brain tissue iron. The high level of non-heme iron remains in the brain for a long time in experimental ICH models and ICH patients.[90] By enhanced Perls' reaction, iron-positive cells are found in the perihematomal zone as early as the first day.[90,111] Studies also have shown that free iron levels in CSF increase significantly on the third day after ICH, and remain high for at least 1 month.[16]

Iron has a key role in brain edema formation following ICH.[94,112] Perihematomal brain edema develops immediately after an ICH and peaks several days later.[112–114] Edema formation following ICH elevates intracranial pressure and may result in herniation.[115] In experimental ICH models, brain edema peaks around the third or fourth days after the hemorrhage, then declines slowly.[98,116–118] In species with significant white matter, perihematomal edema is mainly located within that tissue.[117,119] In humans perihematomal edema develops within 3 hours of symptom onset and peaks between 1 and 3 weeks after the ictus.[99,120,121] Several studies show that the degree of brain edema around the hematoma correlates with poor outcome in patients.[99,115,122] Recent studies have shown that iron chelation with deferoxamine reduces perihematomal brain edema and ICH-induced brain injury in aged rats and pigs (Fig. 8-2).[18,123–125]

Brain iron overload also contributes to neuronal death and brain atrophy after ICH. Clinical and experimental studies have demonstrated that brain atrophy occurs after ICH.[9,126] A recent study demonstrated that brain atrophy developed gradually and peaked between 1 and 2 months after ICH in the rat.[126] Brain atrophy was associated with prolonged neurological deficits. Deferoxamine, an iron chelator, reduced brain atrophy, brain ferritin levels, and improved neurological deficits after rat ICH.[122,124,126] These studies have led to a clinical trial to test use of deferoxamine, an iron chelator, for ICH patients.[127]

Thrombin Formation

Thrombin is a serine protease and an essential component in the coagulation cascade. It is produced immediately in the hematoma after an ICH. Although thrombin formation is essential to stop bleeding, thrombin at high concentrations is neurotoxic. For example, direct intracerebral injection of thrombin causes inflammatory cell infiltration, BBB disruption, brain edema formation and neuronal death.[38,94,128] Thrombin-induced brain injury is partially through activation of its receptors.[128,129] Three protease-activated receptors (PARs), PAR-1, PAR-3 and PAR-4, are thrombin receptors.[130]

To examine whether there is a time window for systemic administration of a thrombin inhibitor could reduce ICH-induced injury, ICH rats were treated with argatroban. The systemic administration of argatroban starting 6 hours after ICH significantly reduced edema but did not increase collagenase-induced hematoma volume.[131]

Thrombin-induced brain injury may be mediated by the complement cascade.[132] Intracerebral infusion of thrombin in rat resulted in a sevenfold increase in complement C9 and deposition of complement C9 on neuronal membranes. Clusterin, an inhibitor of the membrane attack complex formation, was also upregulated by the thrombin and found in neurons. The effects of coagulation cascade on complement activation are not well studied. However, studies suggest that there is a very close relationship between thrombin and

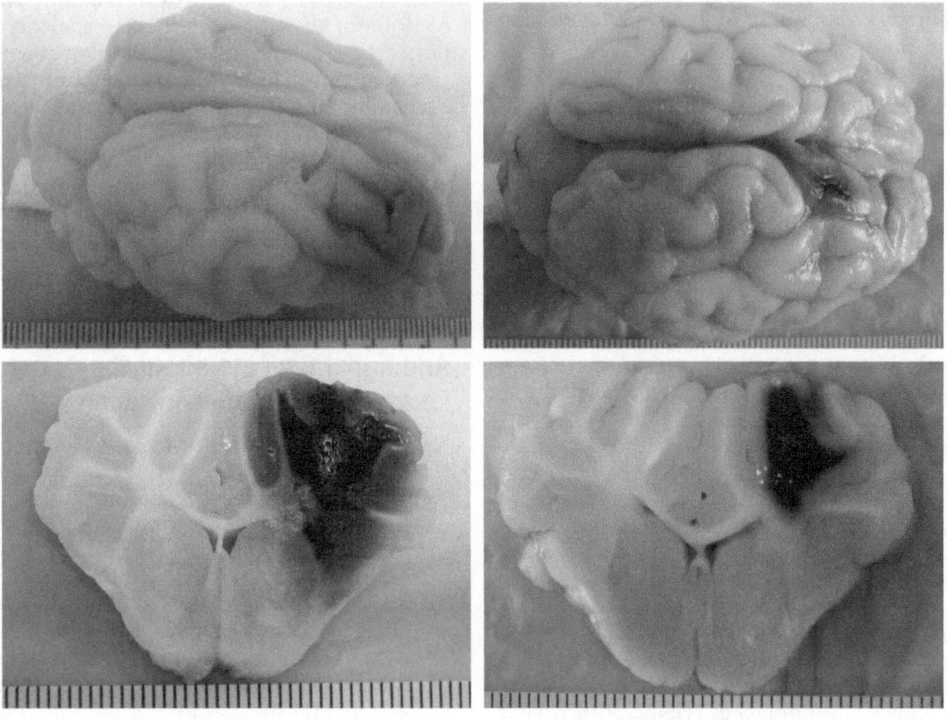

Figure 8-2. Deferoxamine reduces reddish zone around hematoma at day 3 in a pig ICH model. Pigs were treated with deferoxamine (50 mg/kg; administered intramuscularly every 12 hours for 3 days, starting 2 hours post-ICH) or vehicle.

complement. For example, thrombin-cleaved C3a-like fragments are chemotactic for leukocytes and induce enzyme release from neutrophils.[133]

Tumor necrosis factor alpha (TNF-α) is one of the major pro-inflammatory cytokines and it may contribute to brain injury after ICH. TNF-α levels in the brain are increased after intracerebral infusion of thrombin and ICH.[134] ICH-induced brain edema was less in TNF-α knockout mice compared with wild-type mice.[135] In addition, thrombin activates matrix metalloproteinase 2 in endothelial cells.[136]

MECHANISMS OF CELL DEATH AFTER INTRACEREBRAL HEMORRHAGE

Apoptosis

Cell death can be primarily divided into necrosis and apoptosis.[137] Necrosis is a more "chaotic" way of dying, which is characterized by cellular edema and disruption of the plasma membrane, leading to release of cellular components and inflammatory tissue response. Apoptosis is a programmed cellular death that is characterized by morphologic changes such as cell shrinkage, nuclear condensation and scission of chromosomal DNA into internucleosomal fragments and formation of "apoptosis bodies", which can be removed by phagocytic cells.

Using TUNEL staining (to assess DNA fragmentation) and histological evaluation of sections from 12 patients who underwent a blood evacuation procedure after ICH, the abundance of apoptotic cells in the peri-hematoma brain were observed in ten of these patients. Although TUNEL staining is not selective in labeling apoptotic cells, since it may label necrotic and mitotic cells as well, the authors indicated that neither of the TUNEL-positive cells displayed necrotic morphology. In agreement with this human study, the presence of TUNEL-positive cells with appearance of apoptotic morphology, in the peri-hematoma areas of the brain, was also reported in animal models of ICH, suggesting the important role of apoptosis as a pathway contributing to brain cell death after intracerebral hemorrhage.[69,138–140]

It is worth emphasizing that IL-1β is normally translated as a proenzyme (proIL-1β) and requires proteolysis by caspase-1 (interleukin-1 converting enzyme, ICE) to generate the biologically active peptide.[141,142] Therefore, the robust increase in IL-1β levels after ICH[1,143] may represent additional evidence for caspase activation after ICH. IL-1β is one of the most potent activators for NF-κB, which consequently leads to amplification of the inflammatory response regulated by transcriptional activation of several proinflammatory genes including IL-1β itself[144] positioning caspase-1 as a key regulator of ICH-induced inflammation.

It is well documented that release of cytochrome *c* from mitochondria to cytosol activates the proteolytic pathway involving caspase-9 and -3 activation which initiates caspase-activated DNase (CAD) and poly(ADP-ribose) polymerase (PARP), leading to apoptotic cell death.[145–147] Analysis of rat brain at 24 hours post-ICH demonstrated the presence of cells with increased staining intensity for cytosolic cytochrome *c* in the peri-hematoma transition zone.[9] Cytochrome *c*-positive cells were still present at 3 days, but not at 7 days, after ICH, suggesting that mitochondrial damage and cytochrome *c*-mediated caspase activation may play an important role in ICH-induced apoptosis. In agreement with this notion, injection of zVADfmk, a broad-spectrum caspase inhibitor, prior to ICH, significantly reduced the number of TUNEL-positive cells in the ICH-affected hemisphere.[1,138]

In addition to mitochondrial pathways the receptor-mediated pathway of apoptosis through activation of death-inducing ligand/receptor systems such as Fas ligand (FasL)/Fas receptor (FasR) plays a pathological role in cerebrovascular pathologies.[148,149] Increased Fas antigen after ICH was documented,[150,151] suggesting that Fas-mediated death could also play a role in cell death after ICH. This receptor-mediated apoptosis pathway may exist independently from the mitochondrial pathway and lead to PARP cleavage and CAD activation, producing DNA damage and cell death.

Excitotoxicity and Cell Death after Intracerebral Hemorrhage

It is documented that excessive Ca^{++} influx through NMDA- and AMPA-glutamate subtype receptors, in response to prolonged increase of extracellular excitatory amino acids (EAA) or upregulation of these receptors, causes damage to neurons, termed excitotoxicity.[152–154] Glutamate level after ICH was shown to be robustly increased in the perihematoma brain region,[155] suggesting a possible damaging effect. In agreement with this notion, memantine, a non-competitive blocker of NMDA-subtype of glutamate receptor, used at a very high 20 mg/kg dose, was demonstrated to reduce injury, including inflammation and neurological deficit, in the rat ICH model which uses intracerebral injection of bacterial collagenase to induce bleeding.[156] In addition memantine induced the expression of anti-apoptotic mitochondrial protein Bcl-2 and ameliorated ICH-induced caspase-3 activation. Memantine reduced collagenase-induced hematoma volume and inhibited the ICH-induced expression of tPA, uPA and MMP-9, proteases that have been documented to affect vascular integrity and produce hemorrhagic transformation. In another study, MK-801, a different non-competitive NMDA antagonist when used in a pig model of ICH helped to reduce delayed perihematoma edema when used in combination with rt-PA.[157]

The role of EAA in ICH pathogenicity could also be inferred from the studies showing that the glucose hypermetabolism in perihematomal brain could be ameliorated with AMPA- or NMDA-receptor antagonists.[158] Finally, overexcitation as a contributor to ICH-mediated damage could be further supported by the findings that neurological outcome after ICH (induced by collagenase) could be improved with the agonist of γ-aminobutyric acid-A receptor (GABA-A; a major inhibitory neurotransmitter receptor), muscimol.[159] However, inconsistent with the earlier work the NMDA-receptor antagonist, MK-801, did not affect ICH outcome in the same study. One likely explanation for these negative results with MK-801 is that the drug was administered 4 hours after the onset of ICH, in contrast to studies with hypermetabolism that used MK-801 30 minutes prior to ICH.

Additional Caveats about the Apoptosis and Other Forms of Death after Intracerebral Hemorrhage

Autophagy occurs at a low basal level in most cells and is involved in protein and organelle turnover. Amongst other catabolic functions, autophagy has been proposed as one of the forms of programmed cell death[160] that involve formation of autophagosomes and degradation of the cell's own components. The formation of which could have a role in catabolism during starvation. Recently, it was proposed that autophagy takes place after ICH.[161,162] Specifically, conversion of microtubule-associated protein light chain-3 (LC3-I) to its phosphatidylethanolamine conjugate (LC3-II;), cathepsin D expression, and vacuole formation were increased after ICH, and in particular in aged rats, and this process was mimicked by intracerebral infusion of iron and blocked by administration of the iron-chelating agent, deferoxamine. Finally, more recent work with necrostatin-1 (RIPK kinase inhibitor), a compound that selectively inhibits a programmed cell death named regulated necrosis or necroptosis[163] and being stimulated by exposure to damage-associated molecular patterns (DAMPs),[164] was demonstrated to reduce damage after ICH.[165]

BLOOD–BRAIN BARRIER DISRUPTION

The BBB is a physical barrier that maintains a separation between the brain's interstitial compartment and the cerebral circulation.[166] The tight junctions of the cerebral microvessel endothelial cells are the cellular basis of this physical barrier.[167] Clinical studies suggest a pathogenetic association between BBB damage and hemorrhagic stroke through increased levels of matrix metalloproteinases (MMPs) which can cleave structural proteins of the BBB (reviewed in[168]). Following ICH, damage to the BBB through various mechanisms leads to the development of vasogenic brain edema.[35]

Animal studies demonstrate that during the early hours after ICH, Evans blue leakage is absent indicating that the BBB remains intact to large molecules.[35,169] However, by 8–12 hours, BBB permeability is increased.[35,170] Blood clot formation and the components of the clotting cascade, in particular thrombin, importantly contribute to BBB damage and perihematomal edema formation.[120,134,171] In white matter, edema fluid accumulation along fiber tracts can be prominent after ICH and BBB disruption as evidenced by Evans blue staining distant from the hematoma[36] and hyperintensities on T2-weighted imaging.[13] Recent studies suggest that Src kinase signaling is involved in multiple mechanisms of thrombin-induced BBB injury after ICH.[8]

The inflammatory response following ICH (described elsewhere) also contributes to BBB damage following ICH. Circulating neutrophils, a component of this response, rapidly enter the brain after ICH.[25,172,173] Decreasing neutrophil numbers with an anti-polymorphonuclear leukocyte antibody, reduced BBB breakdown and dramatically spared white matter.[25]

MMPs which can modify the extracellular matrix and damage the BBB are also important components in ICH-induced inflammatory responses.[23,174–176] This is seen with MMP gene expression which is generally low, but is upregulated after ICH.[140] Pharmacologic MMP inhibition can reduce edema development, suggesting that MMPs play a role in BBB damage.[1,177] Furthermore, in MMP-9 knockout mice, edema is reduced suggesting that astrocytic MMP-9 can contribute to BBB injury after ICH.[23] Also, hemoglobin generation following red cell lysis after ICH can lead to oxidative stress, MMP upregulation and BBB injury.[178] Minocycline, which can reduce TNF-alpha levels and MMP activity, protects the BBB and reduces edema following ICH.[179] In addition, local hypothermia after ICH markedly down-regulates the pro-inflammatory cytokine, interleukin-1 beta, mRNA expression, and protects the BBB, thereby attenuating vasogenic edema in porcine white matter.[180]

Modifiers of Intracerebral-hemorrhage-induced Injury

Hypertension

Hypertension is a major cause of spontaneous ICH. A recent study showed that moderate chronic hypertension (< 200 mm Hg SBP) did not enlarge the hematoma or exacerbate brain edema after ICH in spontaneously hypertensive rats. However, it did result in increased neuronal death and worse functional outcome, which may be associated with microglia activation and iron toxicity.[181]

Gender

Female animals have a reduced susceptibility to ischemic and hemorrhagic brain injury.[182,183] The greater neuroprotection afforded to females is likely due to the effects of circulating estrogens and progestins.[184] Treatment of male but not female rats with exogenous estrogen reduced ICH-induced brain injury, suggesting that normal circulating levels of estrogen in the female rats are sufficient to induce neuroprotection.[182] Estrogen can reduce hemoglobin- and iron-induced neurotoxicity[185,186] and it is well known that hemoglobin and iron are two major players in the causation of brain damage following ICH.[187] Therefore, estrogen-induced protection after ICH may result from less hemoglobin- and iron-toxicity.

Age

ICH is mostly a disease of the elderly, but current experimental ICH models have primarily used young animals. Age is a significant factor determining brain injury after ICH in animals and humans.[6,188] Experimental data showed that ICH results in more severe brain swelling, white matter injury and neurological deficits in aged animals compared to young animals.[188,189] Severe brain injury in aged animals is associated with enhanced microglial activation. Animal behavioral data also showed that the temporal profiles of recovery in aging and young animals are identical. This result suggests that it is differences in acute injury that cause the greater brain swelling and neurological deficits in aged rats rather than less plasticity.

THERAPEUTIC APPROACHES TARGETING INTRACEREBRAL HEMORRHAGE PATHOGENESIS IN ANIMAL RESEARCH

Surgical Treatment for Intracerebral Hemorrhage

Experimental studies of clot removal surgery in ICH animal models have been relatively limited. Two reports described the use of thrombolytics to liquefy intracerebral clots that are notoriously difficult to aspirate. One study in the 1980s showed that tPA rapidly liquefied clots and induced resorption.[190] A study in the late 1990s in a pig lobar ICH model demonstrated that early (3.5 hours) tPA-induced clot lysis plus aspiration was highly effective in reducing clot and white matter edema volumes by >70% and in preventing BBB opening.[191] In contrast, other experimental studies conducted in a porcine balloon inflation hematoma model have suggested that tPA use for clot lysis and removal enhances delayed edema development.[192] However, it is noteworthy that traumatic injury to white matter produced by balloon inflation is a different insult than the white matter tract dissection that occurs in blood infusion models. Interestingly, a new methodology for hematoma liquification has been recently reported in a swine ICH model in which transcranial MR-guided focused ultrasound (MRgFUS) sonothrombolysis facilitated minimally invasive clot evacuation via craniostomy and an aspiration tube.[37]

Findings in animal models plus results demonstrating that tPA could be used to liquefy hematomas in ICH patients,[193–195] have provided support for the ongoing multicenter Minimally Invasive Surgery plus rt-PA for ICH Evacuation (MISTIE) trial. Hanley and colleagues[40] recently reported that successful hematoma evacuation with a minimally invasive approach after tPA-induced clot lysis, led to significant edema volume reduction. Furthermore, in ICH patients with intraventricular extension of their hematomas, the instillation of rtPA into the ventricles resulted in faster clearance of blood and a reduction in perihematomal edema.[196] At the 2013 International Stroke Meeting, Dr. Hanley presented the trial's 365-day results that

TABLE 8-1

Intervention/target	Proposed mechanism	ICH model	Outcome tested
Porphyrin analogs[110–112]	HO-1 inhibition	Rat and pig AB	Edema, behavior, atrophy
NS-398[204]	COX-2 inhibitor	Rat AB	Edema
Erythropoietin[205–208]	Pleotropic	Rat, Mouse, AB, C	Behavior, tissue loss, inflammation
Sulforaphane/Nrf2[77,84,86,87]	Antioxidative	Rat, mouse, AB, C	Behavior, inflammation
Statins[209–212]	HMG-CoA reductase inhibitor/ Pleiotropic	Rat, AB, C	Behavior, tissue loss, neurogenesis, inflammation
G-CSF[213–215]	Growth factor, Pleotropic	Rat, C	Behavior, edema, inflammation, neurogenesis, astrogliosis
Minocycline[147, 216–219]	Antiinflammatory, Pleiotropic	Rat, mouse, AB, C	Behavior, inflammation, edema, brain tissue loss, BBB integrity
Rosiglitazone, Pioglitazone[5,19,45]	PPARγ agonist	Rat, Mouse, AC	Behavior, edema, hematoma resolution, inflammation
Deferoxamine[94,117,220–223]	Iron chelator	Rat, mouse, piglet,C, AC,	Behavior, edema, inflammation
Memantine[183]	NMDA receptor antagonist	Rat, C	Cell loss, inflammation, behavior
Argatroban[138,224–227]	Thrombin inhibitor	Rat, mouse, AC, C	Edema, inflammation
Citocoline[228]	Cell membranes precursor	Mouse, C	Behavior
Hyperbaric oxygen[229]	Oxygenation, HIF 1α	Rat, AB	Edema
Dexamethasone[230–232]	Glucocorticoid receptor	Rat, C	Behavior, edema, hematoma volume, inflammation
Estrogen[195,233–235]	Estrogen receptor	Rat, AB,	Edema, Behavior
Cell therapy[236–247]	Pleotropic	Rat, mouse, C, AB	Behavior, hematoma volume,
Glycyrrhizin[248]	HMGB1 inhibitor	Rat, C	Edema, behavior, neuronal loss
CP-1[249]	Cathepsin B and L inhibitor	Rat, AB	Behavior, cytoprotection
Hypothermia[250]	Pleotropic	Rat, AB	Behavior, edema, inflammation, oxidative damage
Telmisartan[251]	Angiotensin II receptor (AT1) inhibitor	Rat, C	Edema, hematoma volume, inflammation, cytoprotection
Valproic Acid[252]	Histone deacetylase inhibitor	Rat C	Behavior, neuroprotection markers
PP1[253]	Src kinase inhibitor	Rat, AB	Glucose hypermetabolism, cell death, behavior
Bortezomib[254], PS-519[255]	Proteasome inhibitor	Rat, AB, C	Inflammation, behavior, hematoma volume, edema
15d-Prostaglandin J_2[256]	PPARγ agonist/NF-κB antagonist	Rat, AB	Behavior, oxidative stress
CGS 21680[257]	Adenosine 2A receptor agonist	Rat, C	Inflammation, cell death
NXY-059[258]	Free radical trapping agent	Rat, C	Behavior, inflammation
Xenon[259]	NMDA antagonist, pleotropic	Mouse C	Inflammation, behavior, edema
Gleevec[260]	PDGF receptor antagonist	Mouse, AB	Edema, behavior, BBB

AB: an autologous blood injection model; C: collagenase model.

demonstrated an improving long-term beneficial clinical outcome versus 180 days and a 14% upward shift across all modified Rankin Score levels. Fewer MISTIE-treated subjects were in long-term care facilities and these had shorter hospital stays with significant cost savings (Hanley: Stroke Meeting Website Reference).

These latter results are in contrast to the randomized clinical trials of surgical clot removal without clot thrombolytic treatment (n = 7) that have been conducted for more than 50 years (reviewed in[197]). The largest of these, the Surgical Trial in IntraCerebral Hemorrhage (STICH), was reported in 2005 and demonstrated that surgical and medical management of ICH were equivocal.[198,199] Various reasons for this outcome have been discussed including the late timing of surgery, operative techniques that induced damage and the presence of intraventricular hemorrhage, among others.[197,200,201] Most recently, STICH II, a randomized controlled trial in 601 patients with superficial lobar ICH of early (within 48 hour of ictus), open craniotomy surgery and no IVH versus conservative management demonstrated that surgery might have a small but clinically relevant advantage without increasing death or disability rates at 6 months.[202,203] In summary, clot removal in experimental animals as well as human ICH studies support the conclusion that surgery can improve outcome and that liquefying the hematoma especially facilitates evacuation and reduces perihematomal edema. The comprehensive description of surgical treatments is addressed more thoroughly in Chapter 3.

Pharmacologic and other Experimental Treatment for Intracerebral Hemorrhage

Besides surgical approaches aiming at blood evacuation, numerous experimental pharmacologic or physical (e.g., hypothermia) strategies have been evaluated in animal models of ICH over many years. It appears that in addition to the mechanical damage caused to the brain by tissue displacement with extravasating blood (hematoma), which could theoretically be medically addressed by the hematoma evacuation procedure or by blocking the subsequent hematoma enlargement, neutralization of blood toxicity in the brain parenchyma represents an important and promising target for ICH therapy. As mentioned elsewhere in this chapter, the components damaging brain tissue after ICH include products of hemolysis. Since red blood cell lysis and release of cytotoxic hemoglobin and iron including oxidative stress and inflammation progress over days after the ictus, it is likely that the therapy aiming at neutralization of blood-derived injury may have a longer window of opportunity, as compared to ischemic stroke. Many therapeutic approaches have been evaluated in animal ICH models with many of them showing significant benefit regarding edema or behavioral dysfunction. The following table lists selected experimental approaches targeting various aspects of ICH pathogenesis that have demonstrated beneficial effects in pre-clinical testing (Table 8-1).

CONCLUSION

The most notable conclusion derived from pre-clinical research with ICH is that the pathobiology of ICH is highly complex and in many ways distinct from that of ischemic stroke. These differences primarily pertain to a limited contribution of ischemia (in the majority of cases) and presence of chemical insults associated with toxicity of extravasated blood cells and molecular mediators. Experimental models may also suggest that brain damage after ICH (at least those involving cascades of secondary injury) progresses slower and as such may offer a longer time window for the successful intervention, as compared to ischemic stroke. This extended window may provide therapeutic opportunities for not only surgical and cytoprotective approaches, but also open doors to novel approaches using pre- and post-conditioning paradigms. Finally, it is important to note that, although pre-clinical ICH models have not yet provided ultimate validation of their translational value, it appears that the existing spectrum of models can recapitulate many of ICH-induced pathological events and hopefully serve as meaningful tools to evaluate and develop future therapeutic opportunities.

The complete reference list can be found on the companion Expert Consult website at www.expertconsult.inkling.com.

KEY REFERENCES

1. Aronowski J, Hall CE. New horizons for primary intracerebral hemorrhage treatment: Experience from preclinical studies. Neurol Res 2005;27:268–79.
2. Qureshi AI, Mendelow AD, Hanley DF. Intracerebral haemorrhage. Lancet 2009;373:1632–44.
3. Adeoye O, Broderick JP. Advances in the management of intracerebral hemorrhage. Nat Rev Neurol 2010;6:593–601.
5. Aronowski J, Zhao X. Molecular pathophysiology of cerebral hemorrhage: Secondary brain injury. Stroke 2011;42:1781–6.
6. Keep RF, Hua Y, Xi G. Intracerebral haemorrhage: Mechanisms of injury and therapeutic targets. Lancet Neurol 2012;11:720–31.
8. Xi G, Keep RF, Hoff JT. Mechanisms of brain injury after intracerebral haemorrhage. Lancet Neurol 2006;5:53–63.
9. Felberg RA, Grotta JC, Shirzadi AL, et al. Cell death in experimental intracerebral hemorrhage: The "black hole" model of hemorrhagic damage. Ann Neurol 2002;51:517–24.
11. Broderick J, Connolly S, Feldmann E, et al. Guidelines for the management of spontaneous intracerebral hemorrhage in adults: 2007 update: A guideline from the American Heart Association/American Stroke Association Stroke Council, High Blood Pressure Research Council, and the Quality of Care and Outcomes in Research Interdisciplinary Working Group. Stroke 2007;38:2001–23.
12. Koeppen AH. The history of iron in the brain. J Neurol Sci 1995;134(Suppl.):1–9.
13. Xi G, Wagner KR, Keep RF, et al. Role of blood clot formation on early edema development after experimental intracerebral hemorrhage. Stroke 1998;29:2580–6.
14. Belayev L, Saul I, Curbelo K, et al. Experimental intracerebral hemorrhage in the mouse: Histological, behavioral, and hemodynamic characterization of a double-injection model. Stroke 2003;34:2221–7.
16. Wagner KR, Sharp FR, Ardizzone TD, et al. Heme and iron metabolism: Role in cerebral hemorrhage. J Cereb Blood Flow Metab 2003;23:629–52.
18. Xi G, Fewel ME, Hua Y, et al. Intracerebral hemorrhage: Pathophysiology and therapy. Neurocrit Care 2004;1:5–18.
19. Zhao X, Sun G, Zhang J, et al. Hematoma resolution as a target for intracerebral hemorrhage treatment: Role for peroxisome proliferator-activated receptor gamma in microglia/macrophages. Ann Neurol 2007;61:352–62.
22. Chen-Roetling J, Sinanan J, Regan RF. Effect of iron chelators on methemoglobin and thrombin preconditioning. Transl Stroke Res 2012;3:452–9.
23. Wang J, Dore S. Inflammation after intracerebral hemorrhage. J Cereb Blood Flow Metab 2007;27:894–908.
24. Zhao X, Zhang Y, Strong R, et al. Distinct patterns of intracerebral hemorrhage-induced alterations in NF-kappaB subunit, iNOS, and COX-2 expression. J Neurochem 2007;101: 652–63.
25. Wang J. Preclinical and clinical research on inflammation after intracerebral hemorrhage. Prog Neurobiol 2010;92: 463–77.
27. Andaluz N, Zuccarello M, Wagner KR. Experimental animal models of intracerebral hemorrhage. Neurosurg Clin N Am 2002;13:385–93.
28. James ML, Warner DS, Laskowitz DT. Preclinical models of intracerebral hemorrhage: A translational perspective. Neurocrit Care 2008;9:139–52.
30. MacLellan CL, Paquette R, Colbourne F. A critical appraisal of experimental intracerebral hemorrhage research. J Cereb Blood Flow Metab 2012;32:612–27.
31. Rosenberg GA, Mun-Bryce S, Wesley M, et al. Collagenase-induced intracerebral hemorrhage in rats. Stroke 1990;21:801–7.
33. Adeoye O, Clark JF, Khatri P, et al. Animal models of hemorrhagic stroke: Do current models mirror the human pathologies? Transl Stroke Res 2011;2:17–25.
34. MacLellan CL, Silasi G, Poon CC, et al. Intracerebral hemorrhage models in rat: Comparing collagenase to blood infusion. J Cereb Blood Flow Metab 2008;28:516–25.
36. Wagner KR. White matter injury after experimental intracerebral hemorrhage. In: Baltan S, Carmichael ST, Matute C, et al., editors. White matter injury in stroke and CNS diseases. Springer; 2014 in press.
37. Monteith SJ, Harnof S, Medel R, et al. Minimally invasive treatment of intracerebral hemorrhage with magnetic resonance-guided focused ultrasound. J Neurosurg 2013;118:1035–45.
38. Selim M, Yeatts S, Goldstein JN, et al. Safety and tolerability of deferoxamine mesylate in patients with acute intracerebral hemorrhage. Stroke 2011;42:3067–74.
39. Gonzales NR, Shah J, Sangha N, et al. Design of a prospective, dose-escalation study evaluating the safety of pioglitazone for hematoma resolution in intracerebral hemorrhage (SCHRINC). Int J Stroke 2013;8:388–96.
40. Mould WA, Carhuapoma JR, Muschelli J, et al. Minimally invasive surgery plus recombinant tissue-type plasminogen activator for intracerebral hemorrhage evacuation decreases perihematomal edema. Stroke 2013;44:627–34.
42. Taylor RA, Sansing LH. Microglial responses after ischemic stroke and intracerebral hemorrhage. Clin Dev Immunol 2013;2013: 746068.

43. Wu J, Yang S, Xi G, et al. Microglial activation and brain injury after intracerebral hemorrhage. Acta Neurochir Suppl 2008;105: 59–65.
44. Wang J, Rogove AD, Tsirka AE, et al. Protective role of tuftsin fragment 1-3 in an animal model of intracerebral hemorrhage. Ann Neurol 2003;54:655–64.
45. Zhao X, Grotta J, Gonzales N, et al. Hematoma resolution as a therapeutic target: The role of microglia/macrophages. Stroke 2009;40:S92–4.
46. Del Bigio MR, Yan HJ, Buist R, et al. Experimental intracerebral hemorrhage in rats. Magnetic resonance imaging and histopathological correlates. Stroke 1996;27:2312–19, discussion 2319–20.
48. Wang J, Dore S. Heme oxygenase-1 exacerbates early brain injury after intracerebral haemorrhage. Brain 2007;130: 1643–52.
49. Zhao X, Sun G, Zhang H, et al. Polymorphonuclear neutrophil in brain parenchyma after experimental intracerebral hemorrhage. Trans Stroke Res 2014;5:554–61.
51. Garcia JH, Liu KF, Yoshida Y, et al. Influx of leukocytes and platelets in an evolving brain infarct (wistar rat). Am J Pathol 1994;144:188–99.
52. Hallenbeck JM, Dutka AJ, Tanishima T, et al. Polymorphonuclear leukocyte accumulation in brain regions with low blood flow during the early postischemic period. Stroke 1986;17: 246–53.
54. Sansing LH, Harris TH, Kasner SE, et al. Neutrophil depletion diminishes monocyte infiltration and improves functional outcome after experimental intracerebral hemorrhage. Acta Neurochir Suppl 2011;111:173–8.
56. Rolland WB, Lekic T, Krafft PR, et al. Fingolimod reduces cerebral lymphocyte infiltration in experimental models of rodent intracerebral hemorrhage. Exp Neurol 2013;241:45–55.
57. Wang J, Tsirka SE. Neuroprotection by inhibition of matrix metalloproteinases in a mouse model of intracerebral haemorrhage. Brain 2005;128:1622–33.
59. Brahmachari S, Fung YK, Pahan K. Induction of glial fibrillary acidic protein expression in astrocytes by nitric oxide. J Neurosci 2006;26:4930–9.
60. Lindsberg PJ, Strbian D, Karjalainen-Lindsberg ML. Mast cells as early responders in the regulation of acute blood-brain barrier changes after cerebral ischemia and hemorrhage. J Cereb Blood Flow Metab 2010;30:689–702.
61. Manaenko A, Lekic T, Ma Q, et al. Hydrogen inhalation ameliorated mast cell-mediated brain injury after intracerebral hemorrhage in mice. Crit Care Med 2013;41:1266–75.
62. Mayne M, Ni W, Yan HJ, et al. Antisense oligodeoxynucleotide inhibition of tumor necrosis factor- alpha expression is neuroprotective after intracerebral hemorrhage. Stroke 2001;32: 240–8.
63. Masada T, Hua Y, Xi G, et al. Overexpression of interleukin-1 receptor antagonist reduces brain edema induced by intracerebral hemorrhage and thrombin. Acta Neurochir Suppl 2003;86: 463–7.
65. Hua Y, Wu J, Keep RF, et al. Tumor necrosis factor-alpha increases in the brain after intracerebral hemorrhage and thrombin stimulation. Neurosurgery 2006;58(3):542–50, discussion 542–50.
67. Sansing LH, Harris TH, Welsh FA, et al. Toll-like receptor 4 contributes to poor outcome after intracerebral hemorrhage. Ann Neurol 2011;70:646–56.
69. Hickenbottom SL, Grotta JC, Strong R, et al. Nuclear factor-kappab and cell death after experimental intracerebral hemorrhage in rats. Stroke 1999;30:2472–7, discussion 2477–8.
70. Morgan T, Zuccarello M, Narayan R, et al. Preliminary findings of the minimally-invasive surgery plus rtPA for intracerebral hemorrhage evacuation (MISTIE) clinical trial. Acta Neurochir Suppl 2008;105:147–51.
71. Arima H, Huang Y, Wang JG, et al. Earlier blood pressure-lowering and greater attenuation of hematoma growth in acute intracerebral hemorrhage: Interact pilot phase. Stroke 2012;43: 2236–8.
74. Wagner KR, Packard BA, Hall CL, et al. Protein oxidation and heme oxygenase-1 induction in porcine white matter following intracerebral infusions of whole blood or plasma. Dev Neurosci 2002;24:154–60.
75. Wang J, Tsirka SE. Tuftsin fragment 1-3 is beneficial when delivered after the induction of intracerebral hemorrhage. Stroke 2005;36:613–18.
76. Zhao X, Sun G, Zhang J, et al. Transcription factor nrf2 protects the brain from damage produced by intracerebral hemorrhage. Stroke 2007;38:3280–6.
79. Lyden PD, Shuaib A, Lees KR, et al. Safety and tolerability of NXY-059 for acute intracerebral hemorrhage: The CHANT trial. Stroke 2007;38:2262–9.
80. Nakamura T, Kuroda Y, Yamashita S, et al. Edaravone attenuates brain edema and neurologic deficits in a rat model of acute intracerebral hemorrhage. Stroke 2008;39:463–9.
81. Tang J, Liu J, Zhou C, et al. Role of nadph oxidase in the brain injury of intracerebral hemorrhage. J Neurochem 2005;94: 1342–50.
82. Hatakeyama T, Okauchi M, Hua Y, et al. Deferoxamine reduces neuronal death and hematoma lysis after intracerebral hemorrhage in aged rats. Trans Stroke Res 2013;4.
83. Zhao X, Aronowski J. Nrf2 to pre-condition the brain against injury caused by products of hemolysis after ich. Trans Stroke Res 2013;4:71–5.
84. Shang H, Yang D, Zhang W, et al. Time course of Keap1-Nrf2 pathway expression after experimental intracerebral haemorrhage: Correlation with brain oedema and neurological deficit. Free Radic Res 2013;47:368–75.
85. Wang J, Fields J, Zhao C, et al. Role of nrf2 in protection against intracerebral hemorrhage injury in mice. Free Radic Biol Med 2007;43:408–14.
86. Zhao X, Song S, Sun G, et al. Neuroprotective role of haptoglobin after intracerebral hemorrhage. J Neurosci 2009;29: 15819–27.
88. Ma Q, Chen S, Hu Q, et al. Nlrp3 inflammasome contributes to inflammation after intracerebral hemorrhage. Ann Neurol 2014;75(2):209-19.
91. Koeppen AH, Dickson AC, McEvoy JA. The cellular reactions to experimental intracerebral hemorrhage. J Neurol Sci 1995; 134(Suppl.):102–12.
92. Wu J, Hua Y, Keep RF, et al. Iron and iron-handling proteins in the brain after intracerebral hemorrhage. Stroke 2003;34: 2964–9.
93. Nakamura T, Keep R, Hua Y, et al. Deferoxamine-induced attenuation of brain edema and neurological deficits in a rat model of intracerebral hemorrhage. J Neurosurg 2004;100:672–8.
95. Xi G, Keep RF, Hoff JT. Mechanisms of brain injury after intracerebral hemorrhage. Lancet Neurol 2006;5:53–63.
96. Gu Y, Hua Y, Keep RF, et al. Deferoxamine reduces intracerebral hematoma-induced iron accumulation and neuronal death in piglets. Stroke 2009;40:2241–3.
99. Wu J, Hua Y, Keep RF, et al. Oxidative brain injury from extravasated erythrocytes after intracerebral hemorrhage. Brain Res 2002;953:45–52.
101. Zazulia AR, Diringer MN, Derdeyn CP, et al. Progression of mass effect after intracerebral hemorrhage. Stroke 1999;30:1167–73.
102. Wu G, Xi G, Huang F. Spontaneous intracerebral hemorrhage in humans: Hematoma enlargement, clot lysis, and brain edema. Acta Neurochir Suppl 2006;96:78–80.
103. Gao BB, Clermont A, Rook S, et al. Extracellular carbonic anhydrase mediates hemorrhagic retinal and cerebral vascular permeability through prekallikrein activation. Nat Med 2007;13:181–8.
104. Guo F, Hua Y, Wang J, et al. Inhibition of carbonic anhydrase reduces brain injury after intracerebral hemorrhage. Trans Stroke Res 2012;3:130–7.
107. Wagner KR, Hua Y, de Courten-Myers GM, et al. Tin-mesoporphyrin, a potent heme oxygenase inhibitor, for treatment of intracerebral hemorrhage: In vivo and in vitro studies. Cell Mol Biol 2000;46:597–608.
109. Gong Y, Tian H, Xi G, et al. Systemic zinc protoporphyrin administration reduces intracerebral hemorrhage-induced brain injury. Acta Neurochir (Wien) 2006;96(Suppl.):232–6.
110. Perez de la Ossa N, Sobrino T, Silva Y, et al. Iron-related brain damage in patients with intracerebral hemorrhage. Stroke 2010; 41:810–13.
111. Selim M. Deferoxamine mesylate: A new hope for intracerebral hemorrhage: From bench to clinical trials. Stroke 2009;40: S90–1.

113. Wan S, Hua Y, Keep RF, et al. Deferoxamine reduces CSF free iron levels following intracerebral hemorrhage. Acta Neurochir (Wien) Acta Neurochir Suppl 2006;96:199–202.
114. Xi G, Keep RF, Hoff JT. Pathophysiology of brain edema formation. Neurosurg Clin North Am 2002;13:371–83.
116. Wagner KR, Xi G, Hua Y, et al. Lobar intracerebral hemorrhage model in pigs: Rapid edema development in perihematomal white matter. Stroke 1996;27:490–7.
117. Ropper AH. Lateral displacement of the brain and level of consciousness in patients with an acute hemispheral mass. New Engl J Med 1986;314:953–8.
120. Yang GY, Betz AL, Chenevert TL, et al. Experimental intracerebral hemorrhage: Relationship between brain edema, blood flow, and blood-brain barrier permeability in rats. J Neurosurg 1994; 81:93–102.
121. Garcia JH, Ho KL, Caccamo D. Intracerebral hemorrhage: Pathology of selected topics. In: Kase CS, Caplan LR, editors. Intracerebral hemorrhage. Boston: Butterworths; 1994. p. 45–72.
122. Broderick J, Brott T, Kothari R. Very early edema growth with ich. Stroke 1995;26:184.
125. Okauchi M, Hua Y, Keep RF, et al. Deferoxamine treatment for intracerebral hemorrhage in aged rats: Therapeutic time window and optimal duration. Stroke 2010;41:375–82.
127. Xie Q, Gu Y, Hua Y, et al. Deferoxamine attenuates white matter injury in a piglet intracerebral hemorrhage model. Stroke 2014; 45(1):290-2.
129. Xi G, Reiser G, Keep RF. The role of thrombin and thrombin receptors in ischemic, hemorrhagic and traumatic brain injury: Deleterious or protective? J Neurochem 2003;84:3–9.
131. Xue M, Hollenberg MD, Demchuk A, et al. Relative importance of proteinase-activated receptor-1 versus matrix metalloproteinases in intracerebral hemorrhage-mediated neurotoxicity in mice. Stroke 2009;40:2199–204.
132. Coughlin SR. Thrombin signalling and protease-activated receptors. Nature 2000;407:258–64.
134. Gong Y, Xi G, Keep R, et al. Complement inhibition attenuates brain edema and neurological deficits induced by thrombin. Acta Neurochir (Wien) 2005;95(Suppl.):389–92.
137. Hua Y, Keep R, Hoff J, et al. Brain injury after intracerebral hemorrhage: The role of thrombin and iron. Stroke 2007;38: 759–62.
138. Nguyen M, Arkell J, Jackson CJ. Thrombin rapidly and efficiently activates gelatinase A in human microvascular endothelial cells via a mechanism independent of active MT1 matrix metalloproteinase. Lab Invest 1999;79:467–75.
139. Bonfoco E, Krainc D, Ankarcrona M, et al. Apoptosis and necrosis: Two distinct events induced, respectively, by mild and intense insults with N-methyl-D-aspartate or nitric oxide/superoxide in cortical cell cultures. Proc Natl Acad Sci U S A 1995;92: 7162–6.
140. Matsushita K, Meng W, Wang X, et al. Evidence for apoptosis after intercerebral hemorrhage in rat striatum. J Cereb Blood Flow Metab 2000;20:396–404.
142. Power C, Henry S, Del Bigio MR, et al. Intracerebral hemorrhage induces macrophage activation and matrix metalloproteinases. Ann Neurol 2003;53:731–42.
143. Kuida K, Lippke JA, Ku G, et al. Altered cytokine export and apoptosis in mice deficient in interleukin- 1 beta converting enzyme. Science 1995;267:2000–3.
144. Hara H, Friedlander RM, Gagliardini V, et al. Inhibition of interleukin 1beta converting enzyme family proteases reduces ischemic and excitotoxic neuronal damage. Proc Natl Acad Sci U S A 1997;94:2007–12.
145. Lu A, Tang Y, Ran R, et al. Brain genomics of intracerebral hemorrhage. J Cereb Blood Flow Metab 2006;26:230–52.
150. Rosenbaum DM, Gupta G, D'Amore J, et al. Fas (cd95/apo-1) plays a role in the pathophysiology of focal cerebral ischemia. J Neurosci Res 2000;61:686–92.
154. Choi DW. Calcium and excitotoxic neuronal injury. Ann N Y Acad Sci 1994;747:162–71.
157. Qureshi AI, Ali Z, Suri MF, et al. Extracellular glutamate and other amino acids in experimental intracerebral hemorrhage: An in vivo microdialysis study. Crit Care Med 2003;31:1482–9.
158. Lee ST, Chu K, Jung KH, et al. Memantine reduces hematoma expansion in experimental intracerebral hemorrhage, resulting in functional improvement. J Cereb Blood Flow Metab 2006;26: 536–44.
160. Ardizzone TD, Lu A, Wagner KR, et al. Glutamate receptor blockade attenuates glucose hypermetabolism in perihematomal brain after experimental intracerebral hemorrhage in rat. Stroke 2004;35:2587–91.
163. He Y, Wan S, Hua Y, et al. Autophagy after experimental intracerebral hemorrhage. J Cereb Blood Flow Metab 2008;28: 897–905.
168. Betz AL, Iannotti F, Hoff JT. Brain edema: A classification based on blood-brain barrier integrity. Cerebrovasc Brain Metabol Rev 1989;1:133–54.
170. Florczak-Rzepka M, Grond-Ginsbach C, Montaner J, et al. Matrix metalloproteinases in human spontaneous intracerebral hemorrhage: An update. Cerebrovasc Dis 2012;34:249–62.
171. Yang GY, Betz AL, Hoff JT. The effects of blood or plasma clot on brain edema in the rat with intracerebral hemorrhage. Acta Neurochir Suppl (Wien) 1994;60:555–7.
172. Brown MS, Kornfeld M, Mun-Bryce S, et al. Comparison of magnetic resonance imaging and histology in collagenase-induced hemorrhage in the rat. J Neuroimaging 1995;5:23–33.
173. Liu DZ, Sharp FR. The dual role of src kinases in intracerebral hemorrhage. Acta Neurochir Suppl 2011;111:77–81.
174. Moxon-Emre I, Schlichter LC. Neutrophil depletion reduces blood-brain barrier breakdown, axon injury, and inflammation after intracerebral hemorrhage. J Neuropathol Exp Neurol 2011;70:218–35.
175. Tejima E, Zhao BQ, Tsuji K, et al. Astrocytic induction of matrix metalloproteinase-9 and edema in brain hemorrhage. J Cereb Blood Flow Metab 2007;27:460–8.
176. Wang X, Jung J, Asahi M, et al. Effects of matrix metalloproteinase-9 gene knock-out on morphological and motor outcomes after traumatic brain injury. J Neurosci 2000;20:7037–42.
177. Rosenberg GA. Matrix metalloproteinases in neuroinflammation. Glia 2002;39:279–91.
178. del Zoppo GJ, Milner R, Mabuchi T, et al. Microglial activation and matrix protease generation during focal cerebral ischemia. Stroke 2007;38:646–51.
179. Rosenberg GA, Navratil M. Metalloproteinase inhibition blocks edema in intracerebral hemorrhage in the rat. Neurology 1997;48:921–6.
180. Katsu M, Niizuma K, Yoshioka H, et al. Hemoglobin-induced oxidative stress contributes to matrix metalloproteinase activation and blood-brain barrier dysfunction in vivo. J Cereb Blood Flow Metab 2010;30:1939–50.
181. Wasserman JK, Schlichter LC. Minocycline protects the blood-brain barrier and reduces edema following intracerebral hemorrhage in the rat. Exp Neurol 2007;207:227–37.
182. Wagner KR, Beiler S, Beiler C, et al. Delayed profound local brain hypothermia markedly reduces interleukin-1beta gene expression and vasogenic edema development in a porcine model of intracerebral hemorrhage. Acta Neurochir (Wien) Acta Neurochir Suppl 2006;96:177–82.
183. Wu G, Bao X, Xi G, et al. Brain injury after intracerebral hemorrhage in spontaneously hypertensive rats. J Neurosurg 2011;114: 1805–11.
184. Nakamura T, Hua Y, Keep R, et al. Estrogen therapy for experimental intracerebral hemorrhage. J Neurosurg 2005;103: 97–103.
185. Hurn PD, Macrae IM. Estrogen as a neuroprotectant in stroke. J Cereb Blood Flow Metab 2000;20:631–52.
186. Roof RL, Hall ED. Gender differences in acute CNS trauma and stroke: Neuroprotective effects of estrogen and progesterone. J Neurotrauma 2000;17:367–88.
187. Regan RF, Guo Y. Estrogens attenuate neuronal injury due to hemoglobin, chemical hypoxia, and excitatory amino acids in murine cortical cultures. Brain Res 1997;764:133–40.
188. Culmsee C, Vedder H, Ravati A, et al. Neuroprotection by estrogens in a mouse model of focal cerebral ischemia and in cultured neurons: Evidence for a receptor-independent antioxidative mechanism. J Cereb Blood Flow Metab 1999;19: 1263–9.
189. Gong Y, Hua Y, Keep RF, et al. Intracerebral hemorrhage: Effects of aging on brain edema and neurological deficits. Stroke 2004;35:2571–5.

190. Daverat P, Castel JP, Dartigues JF, et al. Death and functional outcome after spontaneous intracerebral hemorrhage. A prospective study of 166 cases using multivariate analysis. Stroke 1991;22:1–6.
191. Wasserman JK, Schlichter LC. White matter injury in young and aged rats after intracerebral hemorrhage. Exp Neurol 2008;214:266–75.
192. Kaufman HH, Schochet S, Koss W, et al. Efficacy and safety of tissue plasminogen activator. Neurosurgery 1987;20:403–7.
193. Wagner KR, Xi G, Hua Y, et al. Ultra-early clot aspiration after lysis with tissue plasminogen activator in a porcine model of intracerebral hemorrhage: Edema reduction and blood-brain barrier protection. J Neurosurg 1999;90:491–8.
194. Thiex R, Kuker W, Muller HD, et al. The long-term effect of recombinant tissue-plasminogen-activator (rt-PA) on edema formation in a large-animal model of intracerebral hemorrhage. Neurol Res 2003;25:254–62.
195. Lippitz BE, Mayfrank L, Spetzger U, et al. Lysis of basal ganglia haematoma with recombinant tissue plasminogen activator (rtPA) after stereotactic aspiration: Initial results. Acta Neurochir (Wien) 1994;127:157–60.
196. Rohde V, Schaller C, Hassler WE. Intraventricular recombinant tissue plasminogen activator for lysis of intraventricular haemorrhage. J Neurol Neurosurg Psychiatry 1995;58:447–51.
197. Schaller C, Rohde V, Meyer B, et al. Stereotactic puncture and lysis of spontaneous intracerebral hemorrhage using recombinant tissue-plasminogen activator. Neurosurg 1995;36:328–33.
198. Ziai W, Moullaali T, Nekoovaght-Tak S, et al. No exacerbation of perihematomal edema with intraventricular tissue plasminogen activator in patients with spontaneous intraventricular hemorrhage. Neurocrit Care 2013;18:354–61.
199. Vespa PM, Martin N, Zuccarello M, et al. Surgical trials in intracerebral hemorrhage. Stroke 2013;44:S79–82.
200. Mendelow AD, Gregson BA, Fernandes HM, et al. Early surgery versus initial conservative treatment in patients with spontaneous supratentorial intracerebral haematomas in the international surgical trial in intracerebral haemorrhage (STICH): A randomised trial. Lancet 2005;365:387–97.
201. Broderick JP. The STICH trial: What does it tell us and where do we go from here? Stroke 2005;36:1619–20.
202. Mendelow AD, Unterberg A. Surgical treatment of intracerebral haemorrhage. Curr Opin Crit Care 2007;13:169–74.
203. Mendelow AD, Gregson BA, Rowan EN, et al. Early surgery versus initial conservative treatment in patients with spontaneous supratentorial lobar intracerebral haematomas (STICH II): A randomised trial. Lancet 2013;382:397–408.

9 White Matter Pathophysiology

Bruce R. Ransom, Mark P. Goldberg, Ken Arai, Selva Baltan

KEY POINTS

- Most ischemic strokes involve both white matter and gray matter, and 20% of strokes predominantly involve white matter.
- Mechanisms of white matter ischemic injury are less well understood than, and distinctly different from, the mechanisms of gray matter ischemic injury.
- Axons and oligodendrocytes are most vulnerable to ischemic injury in white matter: axons suffer loss of their sodium gradient and accumulate toxic levels of calcium, while oligodendroctyes, and their myelin, suffer non-NMDA-mediated glutamate excitotoxicity.
- Potential therapeutic approaches include modulation of ionic disruptions, suppression of glutamate-mediated damage and recruitment of endogenous repair mechanisms.
- The dream of meaningful stroke neuroprotection can only be realized when the different pathophysiologies of white matter and gray matter injury are both effectively addressed.

Anoxia or ischemia of the mammalian central nervous system (CNS), including the secondary vascular embarrassment that frequently accompanies traumatic brain and spinal cord insults,[1,2] damages both gray and white matter (Fig. 9-1). In fact, 20% of ischemic strokes involve predominantly white matter, as a result of occlusion of small penetrating arteries that supply the deep areas of the cerebral hemispheres (see Chapter 27).[3] Clinically, damage to white matter can result in serious disability, as seen in stroke, spinal cord and traumatic brain injury, some forms of vascular dementia, and hypoglycemia.[2,4,5] The glaring failure of stroke clinical trials testing "neuroprotective" drugs may be due, at least in part, to a lack of benefit on injured white matter. In spite of these facts, how white matter is injured by ischemia has received far less attention than is the case for gray matter. Two reasons are foremost in explanation of this neglect: first, the brain of rodents, which is most often used to study stroke, has very little white matter (far less than the human brain), second, there is a tendency to think that protection of neuron cell bodies alone is sufficient to rescue stroke-imperiled brain tissue.

Great progress has been made in understanding the pathophysiology of anoxic-ischemic white matter injury in the past decade, and the pace of this work is increasing. Models have been developed that allow white matter to be studied independently of gray matter. Basic knowledge about the ionic and molecular events initiated by ischemia in white matter is spawning testable hypotheses for protecting this unique part of the brain during stroke. Most significant, there is a growing awareness about the importance of this topic in achieving the goal of effective, early treatment of ischemic stroke. In this chapter, we review what is currently known about the cellular and molecular events triggered by anoxia or ischemia in white matter and how these events lead to loss of function and irreversible injury.

WHITE MATTER ANATOMY AND PHYSIOLOGY

White matter of the mammalian CNS consists of afferent and efferent axonal tracts that interconnect cortical and neuronal-cell-body-containing nuclear areas of the brain and spinal cord. White matter contains no neuronal cell bodies or synapses. It consists of tightly packed glial cells and myelinated and unmyelinated axons; the presence of myelin lends a white appearance to this tissue. White matter regions vary widely with regard to the ratio of myelinated to unmyelinated axons; for example, all the axons of the optic nerve are myelinated, but only about 30% are myelinated in the corpus callosum.[6,7] The anatomy, physiology and metabolism of myelinated axons are highly specialized and unique compared with those of unmyelinated axons.[8,9] It is not surprising, therefore, that regional differences have been noted in the pathophysiology of white matter injury.[10–12]

Most axons in cerebral white matter provide connections within cortical regions. These connections include short fiber bundles between adjacent cortical regions (U fibers) and longer axons projecting between contralateral hemispheres (callosal fibers) or distinct brain areas (association fibers). Output or input projections to basal ganglia, brainstem, or spinal cord are only a small proportion of total CNS axons. Because most white matter axons connect cortical regions, the massive growth in cortical area from small lissencephalic animals to animals with larger, gyrencephalic brains is associated with a great and disproportionate expansion in white matter volume (Fig. 9-2). White matter constitutes only a small fraction of forebrain volume in rodents (for mice, approximately 10% white matter; total forebrain volume 125 mm^3) but occupies a large proportion of the human brain (approximately 50%; total volume 1,000,000 mm^3) (see Fig. 9-2).[13] This massive, greater than fourfold expansion in the percent volume of brain occupied by white matter means that the human brain has far more white matter at risk during ischemia. It may also help explain why successful therapies in animal models of stroke have not yet proven to be successful in humans.[14]

Although the roles of glial cells in CNS functions continue to evolve,[15,16] it is clear that astrocytes are crucial for ionic homeostasis of brain extracellular space (ECS), glutamate uptake,[17] and synaptogenesis.[16] Astrocytes have a complicated but central role in supporting antioxidant synthesis in the brain.[18] Only astrocytes contain glycogen, and they can provide neurons and axons (and possibly oligodendrocytes) with usable energy substrate in the form of lactate when glucose is restricted.[19] Because astrocytes are natural anaerobes and contain glycogen, they are the only cells in the brain that are able to maintain enough adenosine triphosphate (ATP) to function, at least temporarily, during ischemia.[20,21] Oligodendrocytes provide myelin for CNS axons; conduction

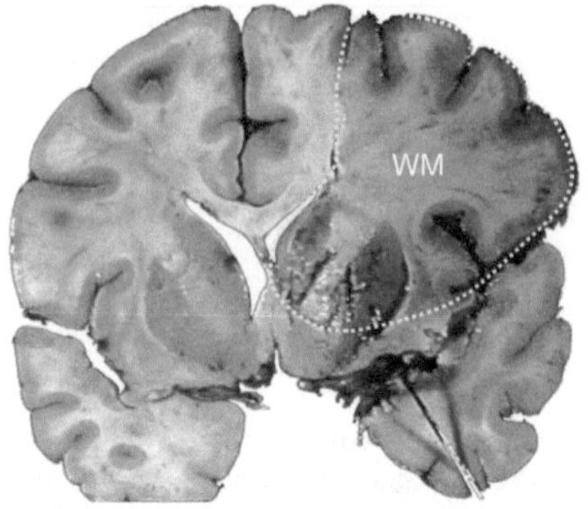

Figure 9-1. Human stroke affects white matter and gray matter. Subacute infarct in vascular distribution of the middle cerebral artery demonstrates damage of a large volume of white matter (WM), including subcortical white matter, centrum semiovale, and internal capsule, as well as gray matter structures such as neocortex and basal ganglia. *(Image provided by Dr. Kevin A. Roth.)*

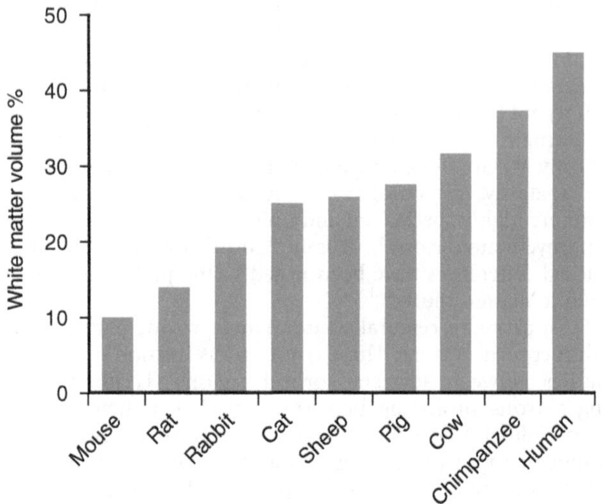

Figure 9-2. The proportion of brain white matter greatly increases as brain size enlarges. Bars show the percentage of cerebral hemisphere volume composed of white matter in several mammals, ranging from mouse to human. *(Data calculated from Zhang K, Sejnowski TJ: A universal scaling law between gray matter and white matter of cerebral cortex.* Proc Natl Sci U S A *97:5621–5626, 2000.)*

fails in myelinated axons with injury to oligodendrocytes or their myelin. Ischemia will, of course, eventually affect all the elements in white matter, leading to axon–glial interactions that are important for understanding how injury occurs. These complex cellular interactions during ischemia or other disruptions in energy metabolism[22] have just begun to be explored in white matter. For example, microglial cells are thought to produce damaging free radical species during ischemia, and astrocytes are the key cell type capable of defending against free radical-mediated injury.[17] Little is known, however, about these topics as they pertain to anoxic-ischemic injury in white matter.

It is essential to understand that an axon's energy metabolism is independent from that of its cell body of origin. Axons extend for great distances from their cell bodies and depend on local production of ATP to maintain ion gradients and sustain energy-consuming functions. This metabolic isolation also means that axons suffer energy deprivation in a manner that is independent of neuron cell bodies. The metabolic rate

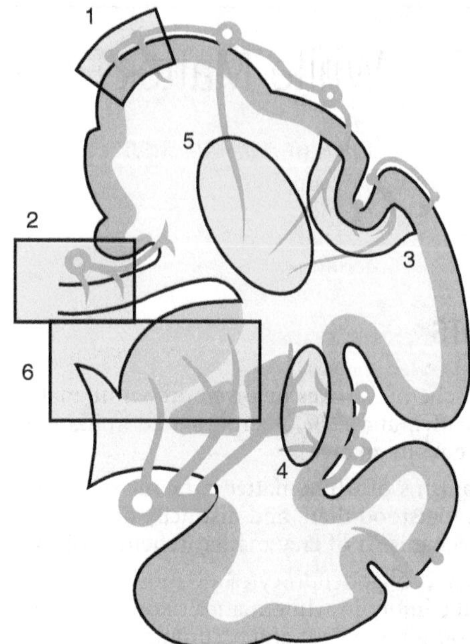

Figure 9-3. Distinct patterns of vascular supply to the supratentorial brain. Regions: *1,* cortex; *2,* corpus callosum; *3,* subcortical U fibers; *4,* external capsule/claustrum/extreme capsule; *5,* centrum semiovale; *6,* basal ganglia and thalamus. Microradiography studies demonstrate much denser capillary beds in gray matter than in white matter structures. The regions of highest vulnerability to anoxic or hypoperfusion damage (cortex, centrum semiovale, basal ganglia, thalamus) are supplied by isolated penetrating arterioles with minimal overlap, whereas more resistant areas (U fibers, external capsule) have interdigitating vessels from two or more arterial supplies. *(Redrawn from Moody DM, Bell MA, Challa VR: Features of the cerebral vascular pattern that predict vulnerability to perfusion or oxygenation deficiency: An anatomic study.* AJNR Am J Neuroradiol *11:431–439, 1990.)*

of white matter is about half that of gray matter on the basis of oxygen consumption.[23] Axons, more than glial cells, are calculated to contribute to this high metabolic rate.[24] The adult mammalian CNS is generally presumed to fail rapidly in the absence of oxygen. There are little actual data on this question, however, because making an animal anoxic without compromising blood supply is challenging. Surprisingly, about 25% of myelinated axons in young adult rodent optic nerve can function anaerobically,[25] but this ability declines and then is lost in older mice.[26] This finding implies that some axons in younger adult white matter could tolerate prolonged periods of pure anoxia without permanent injury.

Because white matter is less metabolically active than gray matter, it requires a lower blood flow (per volume of tissue). The blood flow in cerebral white matter averages 30 mL/100 mg per minute compared with 50 mL/100 mg per minute in gray matter. White matter has a much less dense capillary network than gray matter.[27] Much of the cerebral white matter is perfused by penetrating arterioles that originate from larger pial vessels. Deeper regions of the subcortical white matter are supplied by the striate arteries that arise from the Circle of Willis. The most important of these are the medial striate arteries, which arise directly from the internal carotid artery and supply much of the internal capsule as it courses through the basal ganglia. As white matter tracts descend through the brainstem they are perfused by penetrating arteries from the vertebral and basilar arteries or their circumferential branches.

Different regions of white matter have distinct patterns of vascular supply (Fig. 9-3).[28] For example, in the centrum semiovale, the blood supply consists of long arterioles, which are characteristically terminal vessels with few anastomoses; occlusion of one of these vessels results in an area of ischemia that cannot be rescued by blood flow redistribution because there are no anastomotic connections with neighboring vessels. In contrast, the immediately subcortical association bundles (U fibers), corpus callosum, external capsule-claustrum, and extreme capsule are supplied by interdigitating arterioles derived from two or more pial vessels. Dual vascular supply may account for the relative resistance of these white matter areas to damage after anoxia or hypoperfusion.

MODEL SYSTEMS FOR STUDYING WHITE MATTER ISCHEMIA

Research in white matter anoxia or ischemia requires experimental systems that appropriately model the cell biology and physiology of myelinated axons and glia. Improved understanding of the pathways leading to white matter injury can lead to therapeutic approaches that can be tested in progressively more complex in vitro and in vivo systems and, ultimately, in clinical trials. However, it is important to understand the potential strengths and limitations of each model system and ensure that experiments appropriately examine specific facets of injury and recovery.

Cell Culture

Cell culture models provide the opportunity to examine individual cellular elements of white matter in isolation, separate from the effects of perfusion and vascular supply. Experiments in primary cultures allow assessment of enriched populations of brain cells to effects of energy deprivation, which is typically produced by transient removal of oxygen and glucose. Under these conditions, the relative vulnerabilities of cells, from greatest to least, are approximately as follows: neurons > oligodendrocytes = microglia > endothelial cells > astrocytes.[29–32] Within the oligodendrocyte lineage, immature oligodendrocytes are more vulnerable than slightly more mature cells to energy deprivation.[33] Reasons proposed for the high vulnerability of oligodendrocytes to ischemic damage include their high metabolic demands, poor resistance to oxidative stress, and vulnerability to extracellular glutamate.[34,35]

Cell culture models provide excellent systems for studying the molecular biology, pharmacology, and neurochemistry of ischemic injury, but important limitations must be considered. Most cultured cells are derived from brains of perinatal animals and so may reflect immature phenotypes not found in the adult brain. Relatively few studies of cultured central axons physically isolated from their neuronal cell bodies, as occurs in vivo, have been performed. More importantly, culture models generally exclude the important cell–cell interactions that characterize intact white matter. It is possible to address some of these concerns because systems for isolating axons are well described[36] and oligodendrocytes selectively myelinate axons in coculture.[37] With the use of such a compartmented chamber system, for example, it was possible to determine that ischemic injury to isolated axons (cell bodies in another compartment) is mediated primarily by influx of Ca^{2+} and Na^{+}, but is independent of glutamate receptor activation.[38]

In vitro Tissue Models

Many of the limitations of cell cultures are avoided in models that use immediately isolated, perfused preparations of intact white matter. Considerable progress in understanding white matter injury comes from studies of the isolated rodent optic nerve,[39–44] a CNS white matter tract consisting solely of myelinated axons. Other preparations of CNS white matter regions include isolated spinal cord dorsal column[45] and brain slices, including corpus callosum.[10] These ex vivo white matter tract preparations offer several advantages for studying the mechanisms of white matter injury, including the capacity to quantitatively assess axon function with the use of electrophysiology and perform confocal imaging of cellular components.[42,44] Importantly, each white matter tract offers intact, 3D interactions between glial cells and axons. The use of different white matter tracts facilitates detection of region-specific differences in the mechanisms of white matter injury.[10,44] Although these preparations are not suitable for studies of long-term outcomes after hypoxic or ischemic injury, the axons remain electrically functional for at least several hours in vitro, permitting assessment of short-term recovery. It is imperative to emphasize the importance of studying white matter injury at normal body temperature. Brain slices are commonly studied at several degrees below body temperature because they survive better at these cooler temperatures. Anoxic-ischemic injury of white matter, however, is very sensitive to temperature;[46] the degree of injury decreases markedly with cooling. The real pitfall is that lower temperatures alter injury mechanisms, which can lead to false conclusions.[47]

In vivo Models

Hundreds of studies of focal ischemia in rodent models have been conducted, but the extent of white matter injury has been examined in only a handful (see Pantoni et al.[48] and Dietrich et al.[49–52]). This situation is, in part, due to the very small proportion of cerebral white matter in mice and rats (see Fig. 9-2); the most common outcome measure – infarct volume – is not significantly altered in such models regardless of whether or not white matter is injured. Moreover, middle cerebral artery occlusion (MCAO), the most used model of focal ischemia, consistently spares the corpus callosum, one of the largest white matter tracts in rodents (reviewed by Ginsberg and Busto[53]). Furthermore, a frequently used method of infarct volume assessment in rodent models involves staining with a vital dye, triphenyltetrazolium chloride, which provides little labeling of intact white matter.[54] Careful examination of white matter injury requires special histologic techniques to identify injury of axons, myelin, and glial cells.

Current efforts to injure corpus callosum involve local injections of glutamate analogues,[30,55] demyelinating substances,[56] or vasoconstrictive agents.[57] These models do not mimic ischemia well and can cause confounding tissue injury due to trauma. Primate brain contains about 35% white matter volume and has a middle cerebral artery (MCA) perfusion territory closer to that of human brain. For these reasons, model systems of white matter injury based on the primate are attractive for further development.[58,59] Such studies will likely be necessary in the future to validate promising findings in rodents about white matter ischemic protection before considering human trials.

EFFECTS OF ISCHEMIA ON WHITE MATTER

One can monitor white matter function by electrically evoking a compound action potential (CAP) from constituent axons (Fig. 9-4A). Function (i.e., excitability) of CNS white matter fails rapidly during ischemia at 37 °C.[10,42–44,60,61] In a completely myelinated white matter tract, the mouse optic nerve, the CAP begins to decline within 5–10 minutes of onset of ischemia and virtually disappears after 15–20 minutes (see Fig. 9-4B).[42,44] During reoxygenation after ischemia or anoxia, the CAP partially returns to a new stable level within 1 hour. The speed and magnitude of white matter recovery both

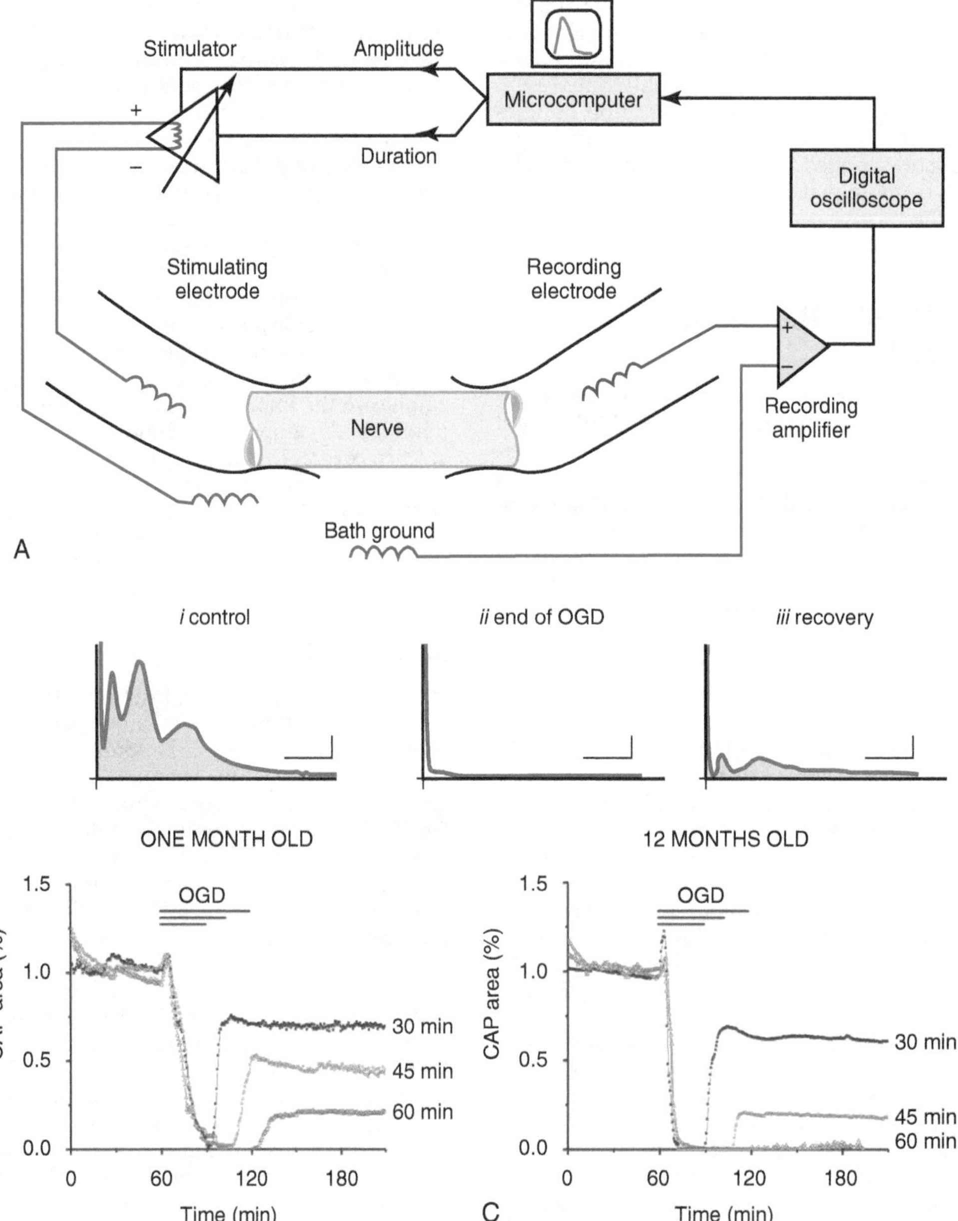

Figure 9-4. Quantifying mouse optic nerve (MON) function before and after ischemia. A, Diagram of recording arrangement. The MON is stimulated with a supramaximal voltage pulse via one suction electrode. The compound action potential (CAP) is recorded from the other end of the nerve with a second suction electrode; signals are amplified, digitized, and transferred to a microcomputer for processing and storage. B, Effects of ischemia on white matter function. The function of the MON was monitored as the area under the CAP (shaded areas). Examples are shown of the CAP before, during, and 60 minutes after ischemia (recovery). Changes in CAP area are shown graphically as percentage of the control CAP integral for young and very mature mice (1 and 12 months old, respectively). Ischemia lasting between 30 and 60 minutes was begun at 60 minutes on the time scale. CAP area rapidly declined, becoming virtually zero after 15–20 minutes of ischemia. After oxygen and glucose were reintroduced, CAP area gradually recovered to a mean of about 25% of control for the 60-minute insult and to a greater extent for shorter periods of ischemia. The extent of final injury was significantly worse in very mature, compared to young, animals for insults lasting 45 or 60 minutes. Calibration marks are 1 ms and 1 mV. *(Modified from Stys PK, et al: Role of extracellular calcium in anoxic injury of mammalian central white matter.* Proc Natl Acad Sci U S A *87:4212–4218, 1990; Baltan S, Besancon EF, Mbow B, et al: White matter vulnerability to ischemic injury increases with age because of enhanced excitotoxicity.* J Neurosci *28:1479–1489, 2008.)*

decrease as the duration of ischemia or anoxia increases. Following 60 minutes of ischemia, however, the mean recovery of function is about 25%.[43,44] This result is interpreted to mean that about 75% of the axons in the tract have been irreversibly injured. Indeed, electron microscopic analysis shows that a majority of axons subjected to 60 minutes of ischemia or anoxia have severe structural changes.[10,62,63] Large axons are more severely affected than small ones. In vitro experiments indicate that white matter recovers better from a given period of insult than gray matter.[60,64] The implication is that the therapeutic window for rescuing white matter from an ischemic insult is longer than that for gray matter. There are regional differences in the pattern of white matter dysfunction due to ischemia.[64] Ischemia causes a monophasic loss of function in both the optic nerve and the corpus callosum, but the pattern of CAP recovery is more complex in the corpus

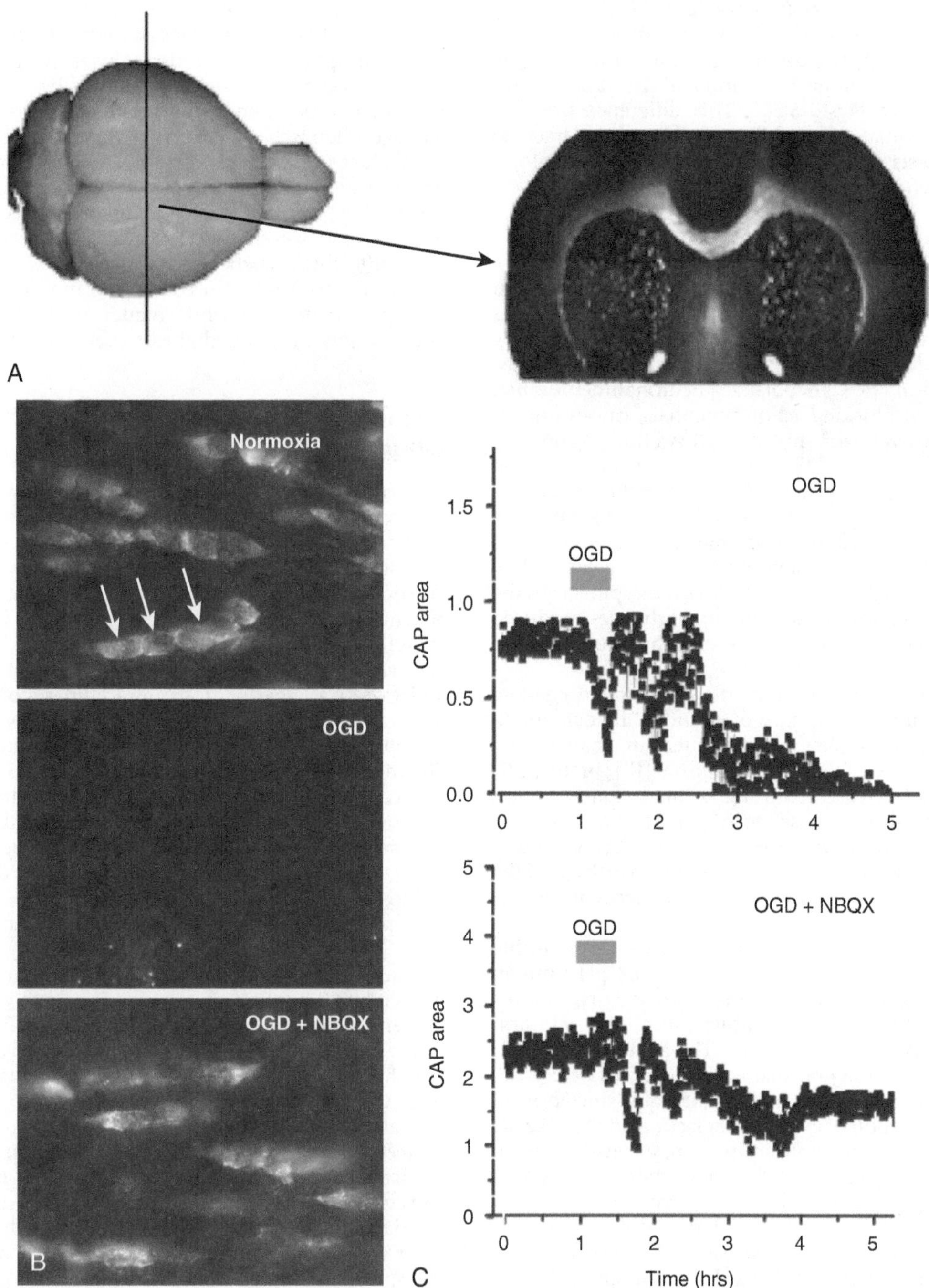

Figure 9-5. Glutamate receptor blockade protects oligodendrocytes and axons in an in vitro model of cerebral white matter injury. A, Acute coronal brain slices, 400 μM in thickness, are derived from adult mice. The slice includes subcortical white matter and intact corpus callosum. B, Immunofluorescence microscopy identifies oligodendrocyte cell bodies in the corpus callosum. Under normoxic perfusion conditions *(top panel),* oligodendrocytes remain intact *(arrows)* for several hours. Oligodendrocytes die within 2 hours after exposure to oxygen and glucose deprivation (OGD) for 30 minutes *(middle panel)* but are preserved in OGD performed with the addition of a glutamate antagonist, NBQX *(bottom panel),* which selectively inhibits the α-amino-3-hydroxy-5-methyl-4-isoxazole-propionic acid (AMPA) and kainate subtypes of glutamate receptors. C, Transient OGD disrupts axonal conduction in white matter, as demonstrated by loss of the stimulus-evoked compound action potential (CAP) recorded across the corpus callosum *(top).* Addition of NBQX preserves the CAP *(bottom)* and prevents disruption of axonal morphology (not shown). These results suggest that glutamate receptor-mediated glial injury may contribute to axon damage under hypoxic-ischemic conditions. *(Modified from Tekkök SB, Goldberg MP: AMPA/kainate receptor activation mediates hypoxic oligodendrocyte death and axonal injury in cerebral white matter.* J Neurosci *21:4237–4248, 2001.)*

callosum (Fig. 9-5).[10] In the optic nerve, recovery of excitability is monophasic and stable after 30–60 minutes of restored glucose and oxygen.[42,44] The corpus callosum, however, recovers excitability in a multiphasic fashion and shows a late progressive decline (see Fig. 9-5C).[10] This difference provides evidence of differential susceptibility of white matter tracts to injury and suggests the possibility that different pathologic mechanisms might operate in different regions.

Derangement of Transmembrane Ion Gradients

Rapid changes in brain extracellular ion concentrations occur with deprivation of oxygen, glucose, or both.[65] These changes reflect the metabolic state of local brain tissue[66] and can have direct effects on neural behavior. Elevated extracellular potassium concentration ($[K^+]_o$) depolarizes neuronal membranes, reducing and then blocking action potentials, causes uncontrolled transmitter release,[67] induces cell swelling,[68] and may affect cerebral blood flow.[69] Elevated $[K^+]_o$ does not, in and of itself, reduce electrogenic glial uptake of the excitotoxin glutamate,[70] as was anticipated.[71] Extracellular acidosis can have direct toxic effects on both neuronal and glial membranes,[72,73] alter ion channel function,[74] and block currents generated by activation of *N*-methyl-D-aspartate (NMDA) receptors.[75] In the case of white matter, the extracellular ionic changes produced by anoxia predispose to other ionic events that are critical for injury (see later).

In white matter, anoxia or ischemia causes rapid changes in the extracellular concentrations of K^+ and H^+ that are qualitatively similar to those seen in gray matter but smaller.[65,76,77] Within 3 or 4 minutes of the onset of anoxia, $[K^+]_o$ in the optic nerve begins to increase, reaching a final concentration of about 15 mM from a baseline of 3 mM. No spreading depression-like event occurs in white matter during anoxia, in contrast to most gray matter areas,[65,78] which partially explains why $[K^+]_o$ increases less in white matter than in gray matter.[77,79]

An acid shift in extracellular pH (pH_o) develops during anoxia and has a maximum value of about 0.3 pH units in standard physiologic solution.[77] After anoxia, pH_o returns slowly to its baseline level and exhibits a secondary acidification phase of unknown significance. The acid shifts in pH_o seen in white matter and gray matter during anoxia are probably the consequence of increased anaerobic metabolism leading to accumulation of extracellular lactic acid.[76,77,80] Lactic acid can exit cells by diffusion, in its undissociated form, or by a direct transport mechanism.[81] In vitro studies suggest that during anoxia, glial cells and neurons contain equivalent amounts of intracellular lactate but that glial cells transport more lactic acid to the ECS.[81] Astrocytes, but not neurons, contain glycogen,[19] which is broken down and anaerobically metabolized to lactate during ischemia. Astrocytes may, therefore, have an important role in producing the acid shift in pH_o seen with anoxia or ischemia.[77] Ischemia causes brain ATP to rapidly decline.[66,82] What is not well publicized is that the ATP decline appears to be significantly slower in white matter than in gray matter.[83] The simple hypothesis for the slower loss of white matter ATP during ischemia is the lower metabolic rate of this tissue compared with gray matter. The implication is that white matter may retain sufficient ATP to prolong the time it can endure ischemia without sustaining irreversible injury. Reduction of ATP causes energy-dependent ion pumps to fail, including the Na^+–K^+ and Ca^{2+}–ATPases, and this failure would affect both axons and glial cells (see later). As a consequence, ions redistribute down their concentration gradients, which leads to membrane depolarization that activates voltage-gated ion channels. Other K^+ channels may be activated and contribute to the increase in $[K^+]_o$, including Ca^{2+}-dependent K^+ channels, ATP-dependent K^+ channels, and Na^+-dependent K^+ channels.[65,84] Anoxia or ischemia causes the volume of the ECS of the rat optic nerve to decrease by as much as 20%,[85] probably because of glial swelling triggered by increases in $[K^+]_o$.[68] In animal experiments, gray matter appears to suffer more damage when ischemia occurs in the presence of higher-than-usual glucose concentrations.[86,87] It is not known whether this observation is also true for white matter. During anoxia, however, white matter is functionally protected by elevated bath glucose,[77] even though it causes a greater extracellular acid shift, which is believed to worsen stroke outcomes.[88] Curiously, in vitro studies, in contrast to in vivo studies, indicate that gray matter and white matter are both protected from anoxic injury by elevated glucose concentrations.[77,89]

The Ca^{2+} Hypothesis and Anoxic-Ischemic White Matter Injury

The calcium hypothesis holds that unregulated increases in intracellular calcium concentration ($[Ca^{2+}]_i$) represent a "final common pathway" for cellular damage.[66,90] This hypothesis appears to be true in the case of white matter ischemic or anoxic injury, but not all the details are yet understood. In general, ischemia causes $[Ca^{2+}]_i$ to increase in axons within minutes of insult onset (see Nikolaeva et al.[64]). Intracellular Ca^{2+} accumulation is the result of Ca^{2+} influx from the ECS and from Ca^{2+} release from intracellular stores. The relative importance of these two mechanisms appears to vary depending on animal age and possibly also on white matter region. The calcium hypothesis probably also applies to white matter glial cells, especially astrocytes and oligodendrocytes, but little is known about this. The collapse of ion gradients leading to increased $[Ca^{2+}]_i$ likely occurs first in oligodendrocytes because astrocyte glycogen supports ATP production during ischemia for 15–20 minutes.

Representative data indicating that extracellular Ca^{2+} ($[Ca^{2+}]_o$) is necessary for white matter injury in young adult animals are shown in Figure 9-6A.[42] White matter is severely injured by 60 minutes of ischemia (i.e., zero glucose and zero oxygen); about 80% of the axons are irreversibly damaged. In contrast, CAP area recovers to 100% of control after 60 minutes of ischemia when the insult is delivered during perfusion with zero $[Ca^{2+}]$ solution (see Fig. 9-6A). This recovery is stable for several hours, which indicates that the tissue is completely protected from an hour of total ischemia in the absence of extracellular Ca^{2+}. In young adult mice this effect is graded, and even modest reductions in $[Ca^{2+}]_o$ (i.e., 2–0.5 mM) during anoxia provide some benefit.[39] Anoxic-ischemic injury in other white matter preparations, specifically corpus callosum and spinal cord dorsal column, also depends on $[Ca^{2+}]_o$.[10,91] In young adult animals, therefore, $[Ca^{2+}]_o$ probably acts as the source for inward flux of Ca^{2+} into a cytoplasmic compartment. This is supported by the observation that $[Ca^{2+}]_o$ falls during anoxia and has a time course that fits well with the development of irreversible injury.[92]

Because white matter axons become dysfunctional during ischemia, on the basis of the loss of the CAP, a damaging increase in intra-axonal $[Ca^{2+}]$ seems likely. Indeed, 60 minutes of anoxia causes striking pathologic alterations within rat optic nerve axons.[62] Large vacuolar spaces appear between axons and their myelin sheaths, axoplasmic mitochondria are swollen and disrupted, and neurofilaments and microtubules disappear from the axoplasm (Fig. 9-7). Strengthening the argument that such changes are due to toxic increases in $[Ca^{2+}]_i$ is the observation that peripheral axons show similar ultrastructural abnormalities after a drug-induced increase in $[Ca^{2+}]_i$.[93] These changes are most prominent in large axons.

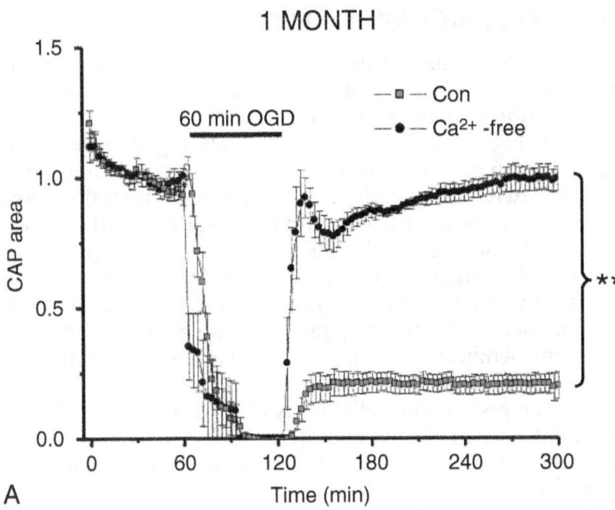

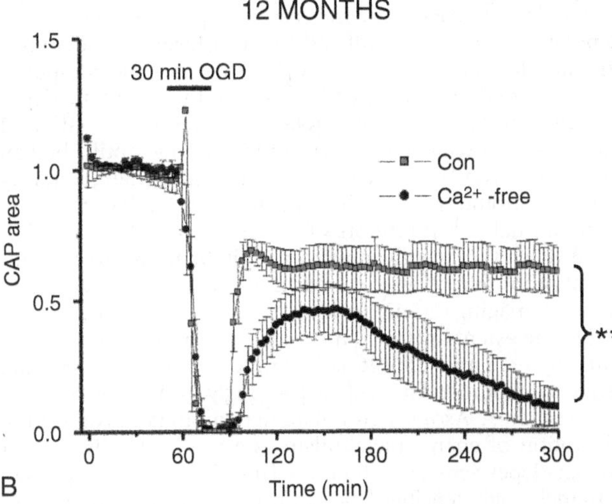

Figure 9-6. Ischemia-induced injury in white matter depends on the presence of extracellular Ca^{2+} in young adult animals but the situation is more complicated in older animals. Mouse optic nerves (MONs) were exposed to oxygen and glucose deprivation (OGD) in normal artificial cerebrospinal fluid (ACSF) (containing 2 mM Ca^{2+}) or in ACSF with no Ca^{2+} (plus 200 μM EGTA). Superfusion conditions were maintained starting 30 minutes before, during, and 30 minutes after OGD. A, Pretreatment with Ca^{2+}-free ACSF offered nearly complete recovery from 60 minutes OGD injury in 1-month-old MONs (95.6 ± 4.3%; n = 6). B, The compound action potential (CAP) area recovery in 12-month-old MONs failed to show improvement over control recovery when OGD was applied in the absence of Ca^{2+}. *(From Tekkök S, Ye Z, Ransom BR: Excitotoxic mechanisms of ischemic injury in myelinated white matter.* J Cereb Blood Flow Metab *27:1540–1552, 2007; and from Baltan S, Besancon EF, Mbow B, et al: White matter vulnerability to ischemic injury increases with age because of enhanced excitotoxicity.* J Neurosci *28:1479–1489, 2008.)*

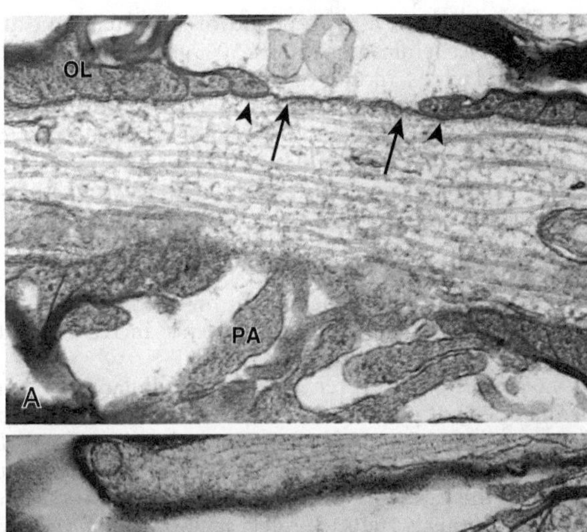

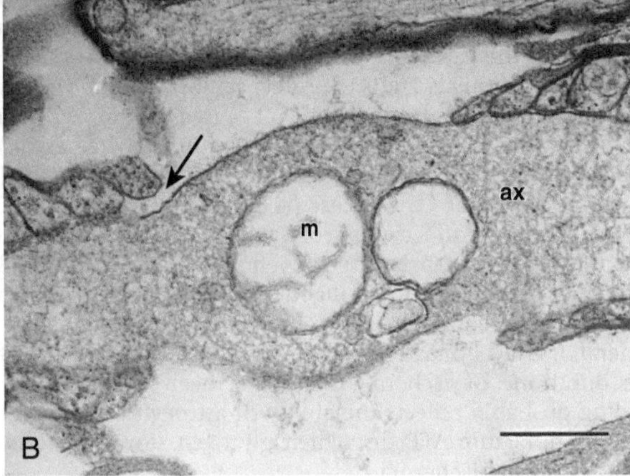

Figure 9-7. Electron micrographs showing ultrastructural changes at nodes of Ranvier in the anoxic optic nerve. A, In the control optic nerve, note the close opposition of terminating oligodendroglial loops *(OL)* to the axon in the paranode *(arrowheads)* and the dense undercoating of the normal axon membrane *(arrows)*. Perinodal astrocyte processes *(PA)* approach the node. The axoplasm contains a dense network of microtubules. B, In the anoxic optic nerve, there is occasional detachment of terminal myelin loops from the axon *(arrow)*. Mitochondria are swollen with distorted cristae *(m)*. There is destruction of microtubules within the axoplasm *(ax)*. A and B, ×40,000; *bar,* 0.5 microns. *(Modified from Waxman SG, Black JA, Stys PK, et al: Ultrastructural concomitants of anoxic injury and early post-anoxic recovery in rat optic nerve.* Brain Res *574:105–119, 1992.)*

Paranodal myelin retracts from the node in some fibers, which is a change that may adversely affect saltatory conduction (see Fig. 9-7B, *arrow*). Although some of the ultrastructural changes seen after 60 minutes of anoxia can partially recover after 60 minutes of reoxygenation, neurofilament and microtubule damage persists. There is a partial restitution in many fibers of the normal relation between axon membrane and paranodal myelin, which might represent the ultrastructural substrate for some of the postanoxic recovery that is measured as a partial return of the CAP (see Fig. 9-4B). We must emphasize, however, that the return of the CAP to a new steady level after anoxia is likely to be a multifactorial process and certainly involves the reestablishment of critical transmembrane ion gradients that are the basis of axonal excitability.[94]

If the nerve is exposed to anoxia in the absence of bath Ca^{2+}, the ultrastructural abnormalities previously described are not seen.[95] The correlation, therefore, between changes in axonal structure and changes in axonal function (i.e., CAP area) is excellent in young animals; in the presence of normal extracellular Ca^{2+}, anoxia disrupts both axonal structure and function, whereas in the absence of extracellular Ca^{2+}, anoxia does not produce long-term disruption of either. These ultrastructural observations were made on young adult mouse optic nerves that suffered anoxia, not ischemia, and while undoubtedly relevant to the pathophysiology of true ischemia, further ultrastructural studies are needed to verify this.

In older adult animals, ischemia is more damaging, and the role of $[Ca^{2+}]_o$ in mediating injury is less certain (see Figs

9-4B and 9-6B).[42] For a given period of ischemia, the extent of irreversible ischemic injury can be 50% greater in 12-month-old compared with 1-month-old mice.[42] In other words, white matter in older animals is intrinsically more susceptible to ischemic injury, completely independent of vascular factors such as vessel patency. In addition, the mechanisms of injury differ between young and old animals (see below). These facts make two emphatic points: (1) animal age is a crucial variable in preclinical studies of stroke pathophysiology, and (2) it is likely that studies on older animals are most relevant in attempting to understand the cellular mechanisms of human ischemic stroke, a disease whose incidence increases greatly with age.

In 12-month-old mice, removal of extracellular Ca^{2+} during ischemia does not protect white matter from irreversible loss of function (see Fig. 9-6B).[42] After the insult in Ca^{2+}-free solution, the CAP makes a partial recovery and then deteriorates slowly over the next 2 hours. In spinal cord dorsal column, Ca^{2+}-free solution also fails to protect against ischemic injury.[96] A number of studies have directly measured axonal $[Ca^{2+}]_i$ and found it to increase with ischemia, even in Ca^{2+}-free extracellular solution.[64,96,97] As suggested by this finding, ischemia also causes intracellular Ca^{2+} release (see below).

Ischemia also affects glial cells and myelin in white matter in a manner that can be Ca^{2+}-dependent.[10,91] In corpus callosum and dorsal column, oligodendrocytes and myelin are severely damaged, according to histopathologic studies.[10,91] In general, the level of astrocyte injury seems relatively minor for the durations of ischemia that have been evaluated. This finding probably reflects the ability of astrocytes to anaerobically manufacture ATP from their glycogen stores for tens of minutes during ischemia.[19,20]

MECHANISMS OF WHITE MATTER INJURY

Ca^{2+} Entry and Intracellular Ca^{2+} Release in Axons during Ischemia

The importance of Ca^{2+} influx in mediating anoxic-ischemic damage in neuron cell bodies[98] and axons[92] is well established, but in the case of white matter, Ca^{2+} influx appears to be a predominant mechanism only in younger animals.[42] As will become clear, however, it is difficult to judge the relative importance of a specific pathologic mechanism when it operates in parallel with other pathologic processes. In gray matter, where synapses abound, the predominant mechanism for Ca^{2+} entry into neurons is through NMDA-type glutamate receptors. White matter has no conventional synapses and appears to be resistant to prolonged application of high concentrations of glutamate[42,99] (but see Li et al.[100]), which would quickly kill neuron cell bodies. However, the story of how white matter is disabled by ischemia has turned out to be more complicated and interesting than anticipated. Some early presumptions about white matter injury, most prominently that glutamate is not involved, have proved incorrect. There are still many unanswered questions about how white matter is injured, and the current model of ischemia-induced white matter injury will undoubtedly require major modifications. At present, there is good evidence that ischemia injures both axons and glial cells in white matter and does so by very different mechanisms. With this in mind, we discuss axon and glial injuries separately. The ionic mechanisms that mediate pathologic increases of $[Ca^{2+}]_i$ in axons during ischemia or anoxia are (1) reverse operation of the Na^+–Ca^{2+} exchanger, a ubiquitous (with the exception of red blood cells) membrane protein that normally operates to extrude cytoplasmic Ca^{2+} in exchange for Na^+ influx, (2) voltage-gated Ca^{2+} channels, and (3) Ca^{2+} release from intracellular stores.

Reversal of Na^+–Ca^{2+} Exchange

The Na^+–Ca^{2+} exchanger does not consume ATP and is driven primarily by the transmembrane Na^+ gradient. The exchanger can function equally well in forward and reverse directions and is a high-capacity, relatively low-affinity transporter of Ca^{2+}.[101] The typical stoichiometry of this process is that three Na^+ ions exchange for each Ca^{2+} ion; this exchange ratio causes the process to be electrogenic and membrane current is generated by its operation.[102] For this reason, the exchanger is also influenced by membrane potential;[103] membrane depolarization favors reverse exchange (i.e., Na^+ efflux and Ca^{2+} influx). The manner in which $[Ca^{2+}]_i$ can be modulated by changes in the transmembrane Na^+ gradient, membrane potential, or both can be calculated.[11] It is important to note that relatively small changes in intracellular $[Na^+]$ ($[Na^+]_i$) or membrane potential can markedly alter $[Ca^{2+}]_i$. Specifically, increases in $[Na^+]_i$ and membrane depolarization lead to large increases in $[Ca^{2+}]_i$.

The hypothesized sequence of events leading to ischemic injury of white matter axons is as follow: (1) Ischemia causes a rapid drop in ATP with an increase in $[K^+]_o$, resulting in axonal depolarization. (2) Na^+ influx through voltage-dependent Na^+ channels leads to an increase in $[Na^+]_i$ because the Na^+ pump function would be impaired.[104,105] (3) Both membrane depolarization and the increase in $[Na^+]_i$ favor reverse operation of the Na^+–Ca^{2+} exchanger, which would continue until a higher, steady-state $[Ca^{2+}]_i$ is reached. Blocking the exchanger during ischemia should improve the outcome - and it does in young adult animals.[11,42] Inhibitors of this transporter (e.g., bepridil or KB-R 7943) markedly improve post-ischemic recovery. Additional proof that reverse operation of the Na^+–Ca^{2+} exchanger causes damaging Ca^{2+} influx into axons, at least during anoxia, is that the extent of $[Ca^{2+}]_o$ drop seen during anoxia is diminished by exchange inhibitors.[92] It follows from the preceding sequence that increases in $[Na^+]_i$ strongly propel reverse Na^+–Ca^{2+} exchange. Axons accumulate net amounts of Na^+ during disruption of energy metabolism as a result of activation of voltage-dependent Na^+ channels (myelinated axons possess extremely high densities [$>10^3/mm^2$] of nodal Na^+ channels).[8] Blocking Na^+ channels with tetrodotoxin (TTX) or removing Na^+ during the insult significantly improves CAP recovery after anoxia.[106] In the optic nerve, entry of Na^+ during anoxia continues throughout the entire period of exposure.[11] Conventional Na^+ channels quickly inactivate with depolarization and would not be available to mediate persistent Na^+ influx. Some Na^+ channels, however, inactivate slowly or not at all.[107] Non-inactivating Na^+ channels are present in optic nerve axons[106] and contribute to the pathologic Na^+ influx that leads to axonal dysfunction in white matter. Curiously, TTX fails to block CAP recovery after ischemia in mouse corpus callosum,[10] perhaps because of differences in the types of Na^+ channels expressed in these two white matter tracts.

Activation of Voltage-Gated Ca^{2+} Channels

Voltage-gated Ca^{2+} channels are known to participate in some models of energy-disruption injury.[108] Calcium channel blockers reduce the extent of this injury, presumably by preventing damaging influx of Ca^{2+} into neurons that are depolarized because of anoxia or ischemia.[108,109] Indeed, L-type Ca^{2+} channels are present on CNS myelinated axons[92] and mediate toxic Ca^{2+} influx during anoxia in CNS white matter.[92,110] Blockers of L-type Ca^{2+} channels applied during anoxia or ischemia improve functional recovery.

Reverse operation of the Na^+–Ca^{2+} exchanger and activation of Ca^{2+} channels may act in parallel to allow entry of Ca^{2+} into axons during anoxia or ischemia. Alternatively, Ca^{2+} influx

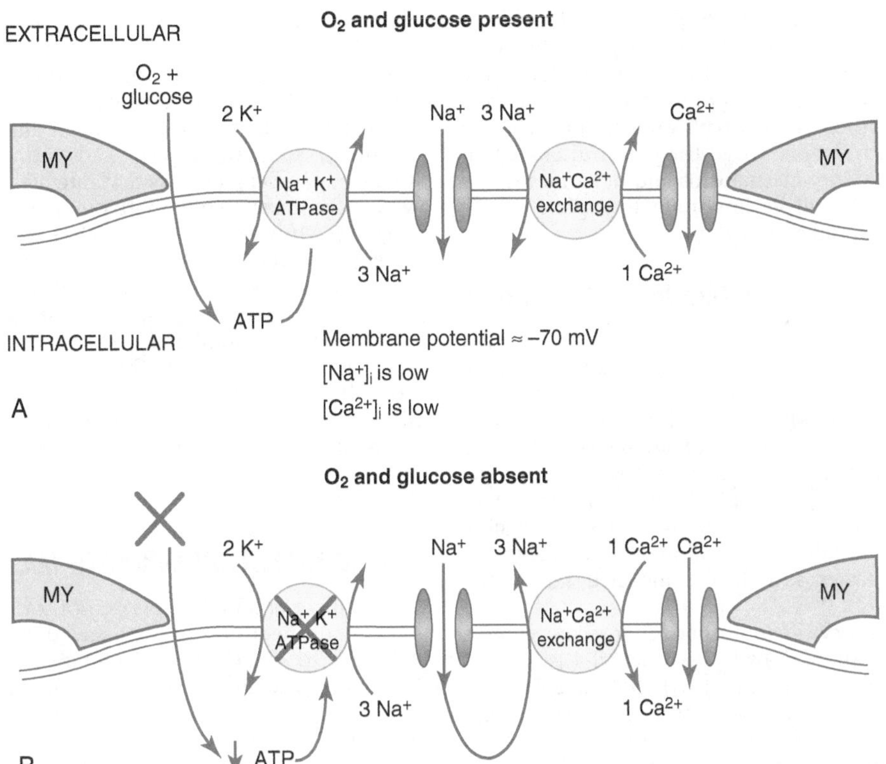

Figure 9-8. Key ionic events that lead to intracellular Ca^{2+} accumulation during ischemia at nodes of Ranvier of central nervous system axons. A, Under normal conditions, sufficient oxygen and glucose are present to generate enough adenosine triphosphate (ATP) to operate the necessary ion pumps for maintaining excitability. If $[Na^+]_i$ increases because of action potentials, this increase is easily compensated by enhanced Na^+ pump activity. The steep Na^+ gradient produced by the Na^+ pump in conjunction with high negative membrane potential drives the high-capacity Na^+–Ca^{2+} exchanger in the forward direction, helping to maintain low $[Ca^{2+}]_i$. There is reason to believe that both the Na^+ pump and the Na^+–Ca^{2+} exchanger might be preferentially located at the nodes because that is where activity-dependent ion fluxes occur in myelinated axons. Voltage-gated Ca^{2+} channels are also present but are not necessary for generation of action potentials. B, In the absence of oxygen and glucose, the generation of ATP is seriously reduced because it is now coming exclusively from glycolysis. The shortfall of ATP causes ion gradients to deteriorate, and the speed of deterioration is augmented by voltage-gated Na^+ channels, some of which are non-inactivating, increasing the workload on the Na^+ pump. As the transmembrane Na^+ gradient falls and the membrane depolarizes, the Na^+–Ca^{2+} exchanger is driven to work in reverse and begins loading the axon with Ca^{2+}. Ca^{2+} also enters the axon by way of voltage-gated Ca^{2+} channels. The ultimate destruction of cellular integrity is probably mediated by Ca^{2+}-activated destructive enzymes, such as proteases and lipases, and the generation of free radicals. *(Modified from Ransom BR, Stys PK, Waxman SG: Anoxic injury of central myelinated axons: Ionic mechanisms and pharmacology. In Waxman SG, editor:* Molecular and cellular approaches to the treatment of brain disease, *New York, 1993, Raven Press, pp 121–151.)*

through Ca^{2+} channels might trigger reverse Na^+–Ca^{2+} exchange. For unclear reasons, higher-than-normal $[Ca^{2+}]_i$ is a necessary precondition for reversal of Na^+–Ca^{2+} exchange.[111] Axonal Ca^{2+} channels, therefore, might act to "kick-start" the phase of Ca^{2+} accumulation mediated by the Na^+–Ca^{2+} exchanger.

A summary diagram of how ischemia leads to Ca^{2+} accumulation in white matter axons is shown in Figure 9-8. In the presence of oxygen and glucose, sufficient ATP is generated to operate the Na^+ pump. The Na^+ pump maintains a low $[Na^+]_i$ and prevents large increases in $[Na^+]_i$ with nerve action potentials.[105] It is also responsible for the axon's high negative resting membrane potential. These two conditions – normal transmembrane Na^+ gradient and negative membrane potential – dictate that the Na^+–Ca^{2+} exchanger operates in the "forward" mode, extruding Ca^{2+} (see Fig. 9-8A). In the absence of oxygen and glucose, ATP drops sharply and the Na^+ pump, which consumes about half of all the energy used in neurons,[104] is no longer able to maintain transmembrane gradients of K^+ and Na^+. Increases in $[Na^+]_i$ secondary to influx through Na^+ channels, some of which are non-inactivating, can no longer be corrected.[105] Myelinated axons may be especially susceptible to this cascade of events because their very high densities of Na^+ channels at nodes of Ranvier would predispose to large focal increases in $[Na^+]_i$. Ca^{2+} channels would be open persistently under these conditions, and the resulting Ca^{2+} influx would lead to elevation of $[Ca^{2+}]_i$. The progressive deterioration of membrane potential and transmembrane Na^+ gradient, along with an increase in $[Ca^{2+}]_i$, causes reverse operation of the Na^+–Ca^{2+} exchanger, leading to a rapid rise in $[Ca^{2+}]_i$[101] (see Fig. 9-8). This summary highlights the ionic disruptions that lead to increased $[Ca^{2+}]_i$ and ultimately to irreversible damage.[90] The downstream events promoted by increased $[Ca^{2+}]_i$ that are the ultimate cause of cell death.[66,112,113] have yet to be defined in white matter. They are likely to include a set of biochemical reactions mediated by enzymes such as proteases and lipases, as well as the generation of free radicals.[114]

Activation of Intracellular Ca^{2+} Release

Axons exposed to ischemia show rapid increases in $[Ca^{2+}]_i$.[64,96] A significant portion of this increase occurs in the absence of $[Ca^{2+}]_o$ and has been linked to Ca^{2+} release from intracellular stores, specifically from axonal endoplasmic reticulum (ER) and possibly also mitochondria.[96,97] The mechanisms of $[Ca^{2+}]_i$ release during ischemia have proved complex. Axon depolarization can lead to activation of L-type Ca^{2+} channels[92] coupled to ryanodine receptors, leading to Ca^{2+} release from axonal ER.[96] Other pathways may also operate, including Ca^{2+} activation of second messenger cascades leading to nitric oxide formation and release of Ca^{2+} from mitochondria.[97] Pharmacologic blockade of these several pathways during ischemia improves functional outcome. Given the powerful effect that age has on ischemic injury mechanisms and outcomes in the rodent optic nerve,[42] it will be important to explore $[Ca^{2+}]_i$ release mechanisms in older animals.

Excitotoxic Pathways Injure Glia in White Matter

Release of endogenous glutamate and activation of neuronal glutamate receptors (*excitotoxicity*) is a major pathway leading to gray matter injury in ischemic stroke. Excitotoxicity was not expected to contribute to white matter injury because white matter lacks synapses and is devoid of the usual excitotoxic targets, neuronal cell bodies, and dendrites; however, this logic proved wrong.[14] During ischemia, glutamate is released in abundance from white matter[44] and mediates irreversible white matter injury, probably by activation of glutamate receptors on oligodendrocytes and their compacted membrane extensions, myelin.

Like neurons, astrocytes and oligodendrocytes express functionally active α-amino-3-hydroxy-5-methyl-4-isoxazole-propionic acid (AMPA) and kainate (KA) glutamate receptor subunits.[115-117] More recently, NMDA-type glutamate receptors were found on white matter oligodendrocytes during development[118-120] and in more mature animals.[42] The physiologic significance of these different glutamate receptors remains to be established. In culture, oligodendrocyte lineage cells are highly vulnerable to glutamate excitotoxicity, and they can be rescued from hypoxic injury by glutamate receptor blockade.[30,33,117,121]

These in vitro studies raised the hypothesis that activation of AMPA/KA receptors contributes to hypoxic-ischemic death of oligodendrocytes in vivo and, in so doing, is a crucial step in white matter injury. However, cultured oligodendrocytes differ from their in vivo counterparts in several important respects, including maturational state, receptor expression, and axonal–glial cellular interactions. Subsequent studies have confirmed a role for glutamate-mediated injury to oligodendrocytes in intact tissue preparations from mature white matter, including corpus callosum slices (see Fig. 9-5),[10] spinal cord white matter,[45] and mouse optic nerve.[42,44] In fact, the more severe ischemic injury seen in older animals is attributable, at least in part, to more intense excitotoxicity related to earlier and more robust glutamate release.[42] Potential nonsynaptic sources for toxic glutamate release within ischemic white matter are axons,[45] astrocytes,[122,123] and oligodendrocytes.[33] While this question remains open, it is our opinion that astrocytes are the more probable source of glutamate. The release is mediated by reverse Na^+-dependent glutamate transport, and astrocytes are the cells with the highest density of these transporters.[42,44]

White matter excitotoxicity is mediated predominately by AMPA/KA-type glutamate receptors, but there is some variability in the subtype that is most important in different white matter regions.[42,124-127] Although NMDA receptors exist on oligodendrocytes, these receptors do not appear to participate in ischemic white matter injury in adult animals (e.g., see Baltan et al.[42]), whereas they may do so during development.[119] White matter injury due to hypoglycemia alone, however, depends heavily on activation of NMDA receptors.[22] In several experimental situations, AMPA/KA receptor blockade has been shown to protect axons as well as glial cells.[10] Axons were not suspected of expressing functional glutamate receptors until recently[97] (see also Brand-Schieber and Werner[128]); still it seems likely that axonal protection associated with glutamate receptor blockade is primarily mediated indirectly, through actions on associated glia.[10] These results support the hypothesis that glial cell injury mediated by glutamate, and axon injury mediated by ion channels, ion exchangers, and intracellular Ca^{2+} release, involves parallel pathways that interact, in currently unknown ways, to enhance white matter vulnerability to energy failure (Fig. 9-9). It is too early to conclude that this scheme applies to white matter everywhere in the brain. In fact, we predict that this will not be the case. It is logical to think that myelinated fibers would be more susceptible than unmyelinated fibers to failure and, perhaps, injury after oligodendrocyte and myelin damage, but this theory has not yet been critically tested. What about the comparative time courses of these parallel pathways? In other words, does one proceed more quickly than the other? Answers to these questions will be important in the development of therapeutic interventions.

AUTOPROTECTION IN WHITE MATTER

Nerve fiber tracts in the CNS do not contain synapses, but they do contain neurotransmitters and their cognate receptors. In addition to glutamate and glutamate receptors (see earlier discussion), white matter contains the neurotransmitters γ-aminobutyric acid (GABA)[129] and adenosine,[83] and their receptors.[130] Although the normal physiologic functions of GABA or adenosine in white matter are not known, both substances appear in extracellular fluid during ischemia.[129,131] Both GABA and adenosine, at very low concentrations, attenuate the severity of anoxia-induced white matter injury and therefore constitute a unique autoprotective system for this tissue.[132,133]

The effect of GABA on the extent of CAP recovery from a standard 60 minute period of anoxia is shown in Figure 9-10.[133] Application of GABA (1 μM) to the optic nerve during anoxia significantly enhances improvement. The beneficial effect of GABA was mediated by GABA-B-type receptors (GABABRs); thus, GABA-induced protection was duplicated by the selective $GABA_B$ agonist baclofen and blocked by the $GABA_B$ antagonist phaclofen. High concentrations of GABA or baclofen did not afford protection, probably because of receptor desensitization.[132] The $GABA_B$ receptor blocker phaclofen significantly worsened outcomes from anoxia. This implied that GABA was being released from endogenous stores and was providing a protective action in the absence of bath application.[132] $GABA_B$ receptors are known to act through G-proteins, and G-protein antagonists blocked the protective effect of GABA against anoxic injury.[132] The second messenger sequence of GABA's action was followed one step further and found to involve protein kinase C (PKC). Direct activation of PKC, in the absence of added GABA, mimicked the action of GABA, which is to say it was significantly protective.[132] Blockade of PKC prevented expression of GABA's protective action.

These findings suggest the following scheme. During ischemia-anoxia in white matter, GABA is released into the ECS, presumably from endogenous stores. The cellular origin of GABA under these conditions has not been determined, but glial cells contain GABA and have the capacity to release it if the ionic gradients that sustain uptake are degraded, as they would be during ischemia.[132] Once released, GABA acts at $GABA_B$ receptors, through a G-protein/PKC pathway, to partially protect the optic nerve from injury. Presumably, protection is a result of PKC phosphorylation of a critical protein within axons, but currently this target is not known. Phosphorylation and downregulation of the Na^+–Ca^{2+} exchanger would be one possibility. Curtailing the conductance of

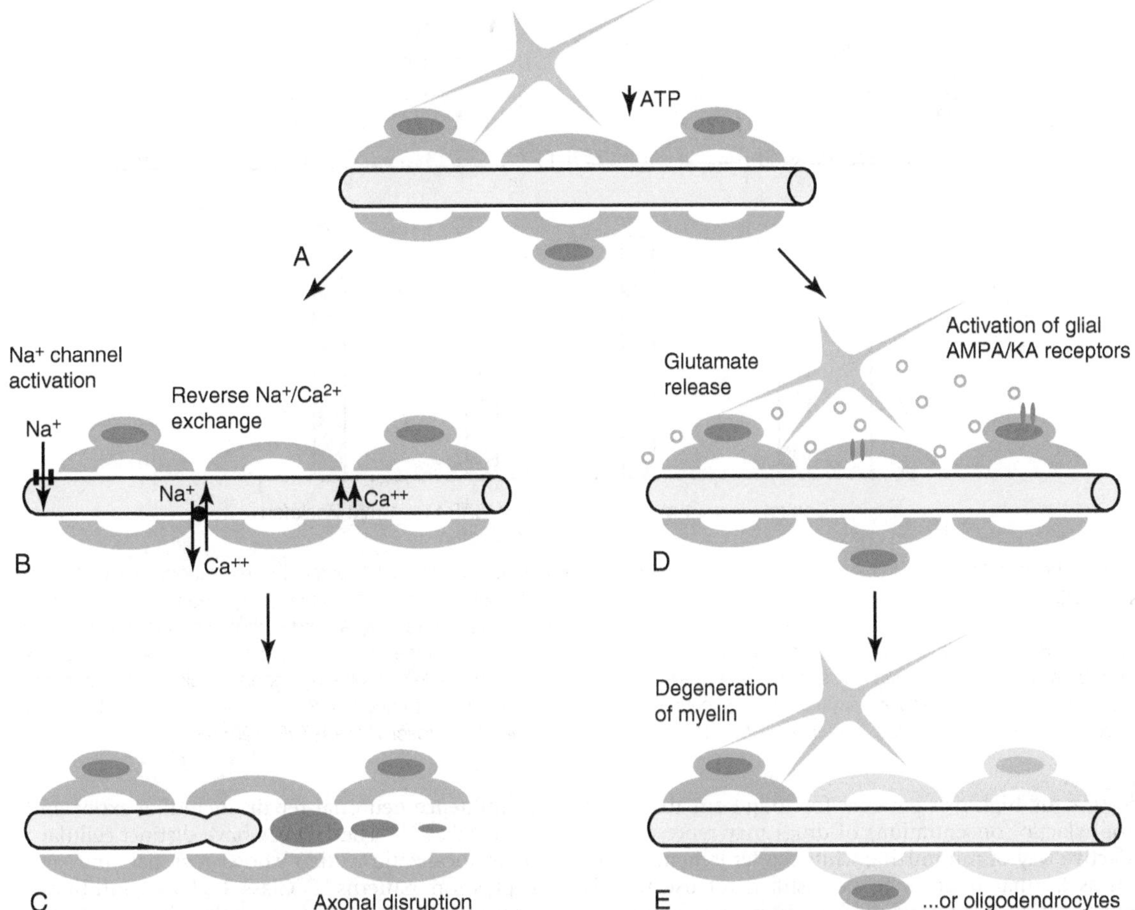

Figure 9-9. Proposed axon and glial injury pathways in hypoxic-ischemic white matter injury. Schematic shows myelinated axon, oligodendrocytes (attached to myelin), and astrocytes *(star-shaped)*. A, Hypoxia, ischemia, or glucose deprivation results in energy depletion and loss of adenosine triphosphate (ATP). B, Failure of Na/K-ATPase and depolarization leads to opening of non-inactivating axon voltage-gated Na^+ channels. Ca^{2+} enters axons by reversal of Na–Ca exchange and activation of voltage-gated Ca^{2+} channels. Action potentials are halted reversibly by loss of ionic gradients. C, Excessive axoplasmic Ca^{2+} levels trigger destructive pathways, leading to degradation of axonal cytoskeleton and organelles, focal axonal swelling, and eventual interruption of axonal integrity. D, Another effect of energy deprivation is release of glutamate into the extracellular space from axons, astrocytes, and/or oligodendrocytes. Glutamate activates ionotropic AMPA/KA (α-amino-3-hydroxy-5-methyl-4-isoxazole-propionic acid/kainate) receptors on glial cells. E, Sustained glutamate receptor activation triggers excitotoxic damage of oligodendrocyte processes (myelin) and death of oligodendrocytes. Myelin damage might result in conduction delay or block. *(From Tekkök SB, Goldberg MP: AMPA/kainate receptor activation mediates hypoxic oligodendrocyte death and axonal injury in cerebral white matter.* J Neurosci *21:4237–4248, 2001.)*

non-inactivating Na^+ channels or voltage-gated Ca^{2+} channels are other possibilities that could serve to lessen the impact of a period of ischemia or anoxia.

Adenosine acts at specific receptors within white matter to reduce the extent of CAP loss associated with anoxic exposure and, in this way, closely mimics the behavior of GABA previously described.[132] In fact, GABA and adenosine act synergistically to protect white matter via the same G-protein/PKC pathway. Both are believed to be released at nanomolar concentrations during anoxia to recruit the "autoprotection" mechanism.[132] The extent to which this novel aspect of the pathophysiology of white matter damage can be pharmacologically manipulated remains to be investigated.

Strategies for Protecting White Matter from Anoxic-Ischemic Injury are Diverse

The clinical importance and the pathophysiologic uniqueness of white matter ischemic injury have never seemed more obvious. The complexity of the injury process in white matter presents many potential strategies for therapeutic intervention. These injury cascades have not been completely explored, especially in older animals, but experiments with isolated white matter have shown that inhibitors of voltage-gated Na^+ channels, voltage-gated Ca^{2+} channels, the Na^+–Ca^{2+} exchanger, $[Ca^{2+}]_i$ release, and AMPA/KA receptors are all protective against anoxic-ischemic injury.[10,42,92,96,106,134] Potentiation of the GABA–adenosine ($GABA_A$) autoprotective system is also protective in isolated white matter.[132,133] These pharmacologic manipulations act to block events that occur relatively early in the injury cascade. For example, the Na^+–Ca^{2+} exchanger inhibitor bepridil is protective because it prevents Ca^{2+} influx during anoxia, eliminating the downstream events that follow from high $[Ca^{2+}]_i$, such as the activation of destructive enzymes. This is advantageous because interrupting the chain of events during the early stages represents the best opportunity for complete arrest of the injury process. The disadvantage of these drugs is that they must be present either before or immediately after the onset of an anoxic-ischemic event if they are to have a significantly protective effect. Therefore,

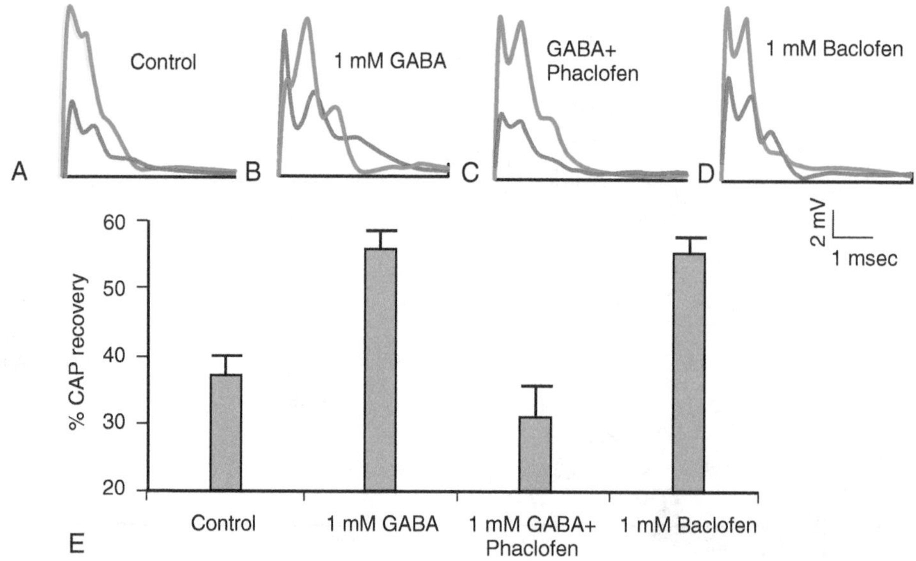

Figure 9-10. The inhibitory neurotransmitter γ-aminobutyric acid (GABA) acts at low concentrations to protect rat optic nerve axons from anoxia-induced damage. Superimposed preanoxic (green) and postanoxic (red) compound action potentials (CAPs) measured under control conditions and in the presence of various agents are shown along with a graphic summary of these results. A, Under control conditions, the mean postanoxic CAP recovery is 36.5 ± 2.9%. B, GABA at 1 mM significantly increased recovery to a mean of 55.7 ± 2.5%. C, The selective $GABA_B$ antagonist phaclofen (500 mM) blocked GABA's protective effect against anoxic injury. D, The selective $GABA_B$ agonist baclofen (1 mM) protected against anoxic injury. E, Summarized results from numerous experiments like those shown in A through D. *(Modified from Fern R, Waxman SG, Ransom BR: Endogenous GABA attenuates CNS white matter dysfunction after anoxia.* J Neurosci *15:699–708, 1995.)*

identification of high-risk patients for long-term treatment with prophylactic concentrations of drugs may represent the most effective way of minimizing white matter ischemic injuries such as lacunar infarcts. To be justified for use in this preemptive way, such drugs would have to be very well tolerated and have few side effects.

The utility of a therapeutic strategy will, therefore, be governed by both its efficacy and the extent to which it is tolerated by patients. Within these constraints, two types of intervention seem most promising. A number of drugs currently in clinical use for other conditions have been shown to protect white matter from anoxic-ischemic injury as a result of blocking Na^+ channels. They include antiarrhythmic drugs such as prajmaline and mexiletine[135,136] and the antiepileptic drugs phenytoin and carbamazepine.[137] Some of these drugs have been shown to protect isolated white matter from injury at concentrations below those in current clinical use. For example, phenytoin improves recovery from a 60-minute period of anoxia by about 80% at 1 μM, a concentration below that found in the cerebrospinal fluid of patients taking phenytoin to treat epilepsy.[137]

Drugs that interfere with GABA uptake and degradation represent a second way of interrupting the injury cascade with minimal side effects. These drugs, which include vigabatrin and gabapentin, have been developed to treat epilepsy and act by increasing the extracellular concentration of GABA.[138] Raising extracellular GABA levels reduces injury in white matter,[132,133] which suggests a secondary use for these drugs in white matter ischemia. The relatively benign side effects of drugs such as gabapentin suggest that long-term treatment in patients at high risk of white matter injury may be possible.

In addition to therapies that involve neurotransmitter and ionic modulation, other approaches are being explored. For example, modulation of epigenetic pathways regulated by histone deacetylases (HDACs) have been tested in white matter ischemia. While alteration of epigenetic mechanisms is generally a slow process, some evidence suggests that meaningful changes can occur within minutes. HDACs appear to influence neuronal repair, including axons and associated glial cells.[139,140] The HDACs have distinct cellular and subcellular localizations that show regional and age-dependent expression patterns.[139] Class I HDAC inhibitors appear to protect white matter from ischemia.[140,141] The mechanisms underlying this protection may include improved glutamate clearance and preservation of mitochondrial structure and function. HDAC inhibitors are already in clinical use to treat cancer patients, and these might have a future role in stroke therapy.[140]

Finally, it is important to consider if endogenous repair mechanisms could be recruited in white matter after ischemic injury. In this regard, oligodendrocyte precursor cells (OPCs) may play an important role. In healthy adult brains, myelin-forming mature oligodendrocytes in white matter can be generated from their precursor cells (i.e., OPCs)[142-146] and may participate in myelin repair after injury.[147,148] When white matter is damaged in stroke or vascular dementia, residual OPCs rapidly proliferate, migrate to fill demyelinated areas,[149,150] and differentiate into mature oligodendrocytes to restore myelin integrity.[150-152] Progenitor cells in the subventricular zone (SVZ) serve as primary precursors for new oligodendrocytes in injured brains. Differentiating cells in this lineage move out of the SVZ into the corpus callosum, neighboring striatum, and fimbria fornix to differentiate into non-myelinated and myelinated oligodendrocytes.[153] The number of OPCs/oligodendrocytes derived from SVZ cells is increased after a demyelinating lesion. Recent studies using mouse models of chronic hypoxic stress demonstrated that activating pro-survival signaling or inhibiting ROS signaling may promote compensatory mechanisms of OPC-into-oligodendrocyte renewal, thus providing a potential method to promote repair after white matter injury.[154,155] Although many translational hurdles remain, drugs that can activate endogenous compensatory mechanisms offer hope for improving function in injured white matter.

The way forward in our quest for practical neuroprotective and/or restorative therapies for white matter ischemia depends on further advances in our fundamental understanding of how these injuries occur acutely and evolve over time.

Acknowledgments

Work in the authors' laboratories has been supported in part by grants from the National Institutes of Health (BRR, SB, MPG, KA), Eastern Paralyzed Veterans Association (BRR), American Heart Association (MPG, SB), and the Juvenile Diabetes Research Foundation (MPG). Selva Baltan has published previously as Selva Tekkök.

REFERENCES

1. Young W. Blood flow, metabolic and neurophysiological mechanisms in spinal cord injury. In: Becker D, Povlishock JT, editors. Central Nervous System Trauma Status Report. Bethesda, MD: NIH, NINCDS; 1985. p. 463.
2. Loizou LA, Kendall BE, Marshall J. Subcortical arteriosclerotic encephalopathy: a clinical and radiological investigation. J Neurol Neurosurg Psychiatry 1981;44:294–304.
3. Fisher CM. Capsular infarcts: the underlying vascular lesions. Arch Neurol 1979;36:65–73.
4. McQuinn BA, O'Leary DH. White matter lucencies on computed tomography, subacute arteriosclerotic encephalopathy (Binswanger's disease), and blood pressure. Stroke 1987;18:900–5.
5. Ma JH, Kim YJ, Yoo WJ, et al. MR imaging of hypoglycemic encephalopathy: lesion distribution and prognosis prediction by diffusion-weighted imaging. Neuroradiology 2009;51:641–9.
6. Foster RE, Connors BW, Waxman SG. Rat optic nerve: electrophysiological, pharmacological and anatomical studies during development. Brain Res 1982;255:371–86.
7. Sturrock RR. Myelination of the mouse corpus callosum. Neuropathol Appl Neurobiol 1980;6:415–20.
8. Waxman SG, Ritchie JM. Organization of ion channels in the myelinated nerve fiber. Science 1985;228:1502–7.
9. Nave KA. Myelination and the trophic support of long axons. Nat Rev Neurosci 2010;11:275–83.
10. Tekkok SB, Goldberg MP. AMPA/Kainate receptor activation mediates hypoxic oligodendrocyte death and axonal injury in cerebral white matter. J Neurosci 2001;21:4237–48.
11. Stys PK, Waxman SG, Ransom BR. Ionic mechanisms of anoxic injury in mammalian CNS white matter: role of Na^+ channels and Na(+)-Ca^{2+} exchanger. J Neurosci 1992;12(2):430–9.
12. Baltan S. Surviving anoxia: a tale of two white matter tracts. Crit Rev Neurobiol 2006;18(1–2):95–103.
13. Zhang K, Sejnowski TJ. A universal scaling law between gray matter and white matter of cerebral cortex. Proc Natl Acad Sci U S A 2000;97(10):5621–6.
14. Ransom BR, Baltan SB. Axons get excited to death. Ann Neurol 2009;65(2):120–1.
15. Ransom B, Behar T, Nedergaard M. New roles for astrocytes (stars at last). Trends Neurosci 2003;26(10):520–2.
16. Barres BA. The mystery and magic of glia: a perspective on their roles in health and disease. Neuron 2008;60(3):430–40.
17. Chen Y, Swanson RA. Astrocytes and brain injury. J Cereb Blood Flow Metab 2003;23(2):137–49.
18. Swanson RA, Ying W, Kauppinen TM. Astrocyte influences on ischemic neuronal death. Curr Mol Med 2004;4(2): 193–205.
19. Wender R, Brown AM, Fern R, et al. Astrocytic glycogen influences axon function and survival during glucose deprivation in central white matter. J Neurosci 2000;20(18):6804–10.
20. Rose CR, Waxman SG, Ransom BR. Effects of glucose deprivation, chemical hypoxia, and simulated ischemia on Na^+ homeostasis in rat spinal cord astrocytes. J Neurosci 1998;18(10): 3554–62.
21. Ransom BR, Fern R. Anoxic-ischemic glial cell injury: Mechanisms and consequences. In: Haddad G, Lister G, editors. Tissue Oxygen Deprivation. New York: Marcel Dekker, Inc.; 1996. p. 617–52.
22. Yang X, Hamner MA, Brown AM, et al. Novel hypoglycemic injury mechanism: N-methyl-D-aspartate receptor-mediated white matter damage. Ann Neurol 2014;75(4):492–507.
23. Nishizaki T, Yamauchi R, Tanimoto M, et al. Effects of temperature on the oxygen consumption in thin slices from different brain regions. Neurosci Lett 1988;86:301–5.
24. Attwell D, Laughlin SB. An energy budget for signaling in the grey matter of the brain. J Cereb Blood Flow Metab 2001;21(10): 1133–45.
25. Tekkok SB, Brown AM, Ransom BR. Axon function persists during anoxia in mammalian white matter. J Cereb Blood Flow Metab 2003;23(11):1340–7.
26. Hamner MA, Moller T, Ransom BR. Anaerobic function of CNS white matter declines with age. J Cereb Blood Flow Metab 2011;31(4):996–1002.
27. Gross PM, Sposito NM, Pettersen SE, et al. Differences in function and structure of the capillary endothelium in gray matter, white matter and a circumventricular organ of rat brain. Blood Vessels 1986;23(6):261–70.
28. Moody DM, Bell MA, Challa VR. Features of the cerebral vascular pattern that predict vulnerability to perfusion or oxygenation deficiency: an anatomic study. AJNR Am J Neuroradiol 1990; 11(3):431–9.
29. Lyons SA, Kettenmann H. Oligodendrocytes and microglia are selectively vulnerable to combined hypoxia and hypoglycemia injury in vitro. J Cereb Blood Flow Metab 1998;18(5):521–30.
30. McDonald JW, Althomsons SP, Hyrc KL, et al. Oligodendrocytes from forebrain are highly vulnerable to AMPA/kainate receptor-mediated excitotoxicity. Nat Med 1998;4(3):291–7.
31. Goldberg MP, Choi DW. Combined oxygen and glucose deprivation in cortical cell culture: calcium-dependent and calcium-independent mechanisms of neuronal injury. J Neurosci 1993; 13(8):3510–24.
32. Xu J, He L, Ahmed SH, et al. Oxygen-glucose deprivation induces inducible nitric oxide synthase and nitrotyrosine expression in cerebral endothelial cells. Stroke 2000;31(7):1744–51.
33. Fern R, Moller T. Rapid ischemic cell death in immature oligodendrocytes: a fatal glutamate release feedback loop. J Neurosci 2000;20(1):34–42.
34. Dewar D, Underhill SM, Goldberg MP. Oligodendrocytes and ischemic brain injury. J Cereb Blood Flow Metab 2003;23(3): 263–74.
35. Oka A, Belliveau MJ, Rosenberg PA, et al. Vulnerability of oligodendroglia to glutamate: pharmacology, mechanisms, and prevention. J Neurosci 1993;13(4):1441–53.
36. Campenot RB. Local control of neurite development by nerve growth factor. Proc Natl Acad Sci U S A 1977;74(10):4516–19.
37. Lubetzki C, Demerens C, Anglade P, et al. Even in culture, oligodendrocytes myelinate solely axons. Proc Natl Acad Sci U S A 1993;90(14):6820–4.
38. Underhill SM, Goldberg MP. Hypoxic injury of isolated axons is independent of ionotropic glutamate receptors. Neurobiol Dis 2007;25(2):284–90.
39. Stys PK, Ransom BR, Waxman SG, et al. Role of extracellular calcium in anoxic injury of mammalian central white matter. Proc Natl Acad Sci U S A 1990;87(11):4212–16.
40. Ransom BR, Waxman SG, Stys PK. Anoxic injury of central myelinated axons: ionic mechanisms and pharmacology. Res Publ Assoc Res Nerv Ment Dis 1993;71:121–51.
41. Stys PK. Anoxic and ischemic injury of myelinated axons in CNS white matter: from mechanistic concepts to therapeutics. J Cereb Blood Flow Metab 1998;18(1):2–25.
42. Baltan S, Besancon EF, Mbow B, et al. White matter vulnerability to ischemic injury increases with age because of enhanced excitotoxicity. J Neurosci 2008;28(6):1479–89.
43. Baltan S, Inman DM, Danilov CA, et al. Metabolic vulnerability disposes retinal ganglion cell axons to dysfunction in a model of glaucomatous degeneration. J Neurosci 2010;30(16):5644–52.
44. Tekkok SB, Ye Z, Ransom BR. Excitotoxic mechanisms of ischemic injury in myelinated white matter. J Cereb Blood Flow Metab 2007;27(9):1540–52.
45. Li S, Mealing GA, Morley P, et al. Novel injury mechanism in anoxia and trauma of spinal cord white matter: glutamate release via reverse Na(+)-dependent glutamate transport. J Neurosci 1999;19(14):RC16.
46. Stys PK, Waxman SG, Ransom BR. Effects of temperature on evoked electrical activity and anoxic injury in CNS white matter. J Cereb Blood Flow Metab 1992;12(6):977–86.
47. Li S, Jiang Q, Stys PK. Important role of reverse Na(+)-Ca(2+) exchange in spinal cord white matter injury at physiological temperature. J Neurophysiol 2000;84(2):1116–19.

48. Pantoni L, Garcia JH, Gutierrez JA. Cerebral white matter is highly vulnerable to ischemia. Stroke 1996;27(9):1641–6, discussion 1647.
49. Dietrich WD, Kraydieh S, Prado R, et al. White matter alterations following thromboembolic stroke: a beta-amyloid precursor protein immunocytochemical study in rats. Acta Neuropathol (Berl) 1998;95(5):524–31.
50. Schabitz WR, Li F, Fisher M. The N-methyl-D-aspartate antagonist CNS 1102 protects cerebral gray and white matter from ischemic injury following temporary focal ischemia in rats. Stroke 2000;31(7):1709–14.
51. Yam PS, Dunn LT, Graham DI, et al. NMDA receptor blockade fails to alter axonal injury in focal cerebral ischemia. J Cereb Blood Flow Metab 2000;20(5):772–9.
52. Imai H, Masayasu H, Dewar D, et al. Ebselen protects both gray and white matter in a rodent model of focal cerebral ischemia. Stroke 2001;32(9):2149–54.
53. Ginsberg MD, Busto R. Rodent models of cerebral ischemia. Stroke 1989;20(12):1627–42.
54. Goldlust EJ, Paczynski RP, He YY, et al. Automated measurement of infarct size with scanned images of triphenyltetrazolium chloride-stained rat brains. Stroke 1996;27(9):1657–62.
55. Leroux P, Hennebert O, Legros H, et al. Role of tissue-plasminogen activator (t-PA) in a mouse model of neonatal white matter lesions: interaction with plasmin inhibitors and anti-inflammatory drugs. Neuroscience 2007;146(2):670–8.
56. Gadea A, Schinelli S, Gallo V. Endothelin-1 regulates astrocyte proliferation and reactive gliosis via a JNK/c-Jun signaling pathway. J Neurosci 2008;28(10):2394–408.
57. Sozmen EG, Kolekar A, Havton LA, et al. A white matter stroke model in the mouse: axonal damage, progenitor responses and MRI correlates. J Neurosci Methods 2009;180(2):261–72.
58. Frykholm P, Andersson JL, Valtysson J, et al. A metabolic threshold of irreversible ischemia demonstrated by PET in a middle cerebral artery occlusion-reperfusion primate model. Acta Neurol Scand 2000;102(1):18–26.
59. Enblad P, Frykholm P, Valtysson J, et al. Middle cerebral artery occlusion and reperfusion in primates monitored by microdialysis and sequential positron emission tomography. Stroke 2001;32(7):1574–80.
60. Fern R, Davis P, Waxman SG, et al. Axon conduction and survival in CNS white matter during energy deprivation: a developmental study. J Neurophysiol 1998;79(1):95–105.
61. Stys PK, Ransom BR, Waxman SG. Compound action potential of nerve recorded by suction electrode: a theoretical and experimental analysis. Brain Res 1991;546(1):18–32.
62. Waxman SG, Black JA, Stys PK, et al. Ultrastructural concomitants of anoxic injury and early post-anoxic recovery in rat optic nerve. Brain Res 1992;574(1–2):105–19.
63. Tekkok SB, Brown AM, Westenbroek R, et al. Transfer of glycogen-derived lactate from astrocytes to axons via specific monocarboxylate transporters supports mouse optic nerve activity. J Neurosci Res 2005;81(5):644–52.
64. Nikolaeva MA, Mukherjee B, Stys PK. Na^+-dependent sources of intra-axonal Ca^{2+} release in rat optic nerve during in vitro chemical ischemia. J Neurosci 2005;25(43):9960–7.
65. Hansen AJ. Effect of anoxia on ion distribution in the brain. Physiol Rev 1985;65(1):101–48.
66. Siesjo BK. Cell damage in the brain: a speculative synthesis. J Cereb Blood Flow Metab 1981;1(2):155–85.
67. Benveniste H, Drejer J, Schousboe A, et al. Elevation of the extracellular concentrations of glutamate and aspartate in rat hippocampus during transient cerebral ischemia monitored by intracerebral microdialysis. J Neurochem 1984;43(5):1369–74.
68. Kimelberg HK, Ransom BR. Physiological and pathological aspects of astrocytic swelling. In: Federoff S, Vernadakis A, editors. Astrocytes. Orlando: Academic Press; 1986. p. 129–66.
69. Paulson OB, Newman EA. Does the release of potassium from astrocyte endfeet regulate cerebral blood flow? Science 1987;237(4817):896–8.
70. Longuemare MC, Rose CR, Farrell K, et al. K(+)-induced reversal of astrocyte glutamate uptake is limited by compensatory changes in intracellular Na. Neuroscience 1999;93(1):285–92.
71. Schwartz EA, Tachibana M. Electrophysiology of glutamate and sodium co-transport in a glial cell of the salamander retina. J Physiol (Lond) 1990;426:43–80.
72. Goldman SA, Pulsinelli WA, Clarke WY, et al. The effects of extracellular acidosis on neurons and glia in vitro. J Cereb Blood Flow Metab 1989;9(4):471–7.
73. Kraig RP, Petito CK, Plum F, et al. Hydrogen ions kill brain at concentrations reached in ischemia. J Cereb Blood Flow Metab 1987;7(4):379–86.
74. Tombaugh GC, Somjen GG. pH modulation of voltage-gated ion channels. In: Kaila K, Ransom BR, editors. pH and Brain Function. New York: Wiley-Liss; 1998. p. 395–416.
75. Traynelis SF. pH Modulation of ligand-gated ion channels. In: Kaila K, Ransom BR, editors. pH and Brain Function. New York: Wiley-Liss; 1998. p. 417–46.
76. Kraig RP, Pulsinelli WA, Plum F. Hydrogen ion buffering during complete brain ischemia. Brain Res 1985;342(2):281–90.
77. Ransom BR, Walz W, Davis PK, et al. Anoxia-induced changes in extracellular K^+ and pH in mammalian central white matter. J Cereb Blood Flow Metab 1992;12(4):593–602.
78. Somjen GG, Aitken PG, Balestrino M, et al. Spreading depression-like depolarization and selective vulnerability of neurons. A brief review. Stroke 1990;21(11 Suppl.):III179–83.
79. Kraig RP, Nicholson C. Extracellular ionic variations during spreading depression. Neuroscience 1978;3(11):1045–59.
80. Kraig RP, Ferreira-Filho CR, Nicholson C. Alkaline and acid transients in cerebellar microenvironment. J Neurophysiol 1983;49(3):831–50.
81. Walz W, Mukerji S. Lactate release from cultured astrocytes and neurons: a comparison. Glia 1988;1(6):366–70.
82. Lowry OH, Passonneau JV, Hasselberger FH, et al. Effect of ischemia on known substrates and cofactors of the glycolytic pathway in brain. J Biol Chem 1964;239:18–30.
83. Dohmen C, Kumura E, Rosner G, et al. Adenosine in relation to calcium homeostasis: comparison between gray and white matter ischemia. J Cereb Blood Flow Metab 2001;21(5):503–10.
84. Haimann C, Bernheim L, Bertrand D, et al. Potassium current activated by intracellular sodium in quail trigeminal ganglion neurons. J Gen Physiol 1990;95(5):961–79.
85. Ransom BR, Yamate CL, Connors BW. Activity-dependent shrinkage of extracellular space in rat optic nerve: a developmental study. J Neurosci 1985;5(2):532–5.
86. Li PA, He QP, Csiszar K, et al. Does long-term glucose infusion reduce brain damage after transient cerebral ischemia? Brain Res 2001;912(2):203–5.
87. Plum F. What causes infarction in ischemic brain? The Robert Wartenberg Lecture. Neurology 1983;33(2):222–33.
88. Siesjo BK, Katsura KI, Kristian T, et al. Molecular mechanisms of acidosis-mediated damage. Acta Neurochir Suppl (Wien) 1996;66:8–14.
89. Schurr A, West CA, Reid KH, et al. Increased glucose improves recovery of neuronal function after cerebral hypoxia in vitro. Brain Res 1987;421(1–2):135–9.
90. Schanne FA, Kane AB, Young EE, et al. Calcium dependence of toxic cell death: a final common pathway. Science 1979;206(4419):700–2.
91. Li S, Stys PK. Mechanisms of ionotropic glutamate receptor-mediated excitotoxicity in isolated spinal cord white matter. J Neurosci 2000;20(3):1190–8.
92. Brown AM, Westenbroek RE, Catterall WA, et al. Axonal L-type Ca^{2+} channels and anoxic injury in rat CNS white matter. J Neurophysiol 2001;85(2):900–11.
93. Schlaepfer WW. Structural alterations of peripheral nerve induced by the calcium ionophore A23187. Brain Res 1977;136(1):1–9.
94. Hodgkin AL. The conduction of the nervous impulse. London: Liverpool University Press; 1964.
95. Waxman SG, Black JA, Ransom BR, et al. Protection of the axonal cytoskeleton in anoxic optic nerve by decreased extracellular calcium. Brain Res 1993;614(1–2):137–45.
96. Ouardouz M, Nikolaeva MA, Coderre E, et al. Depolarization-induced Ca^{2+} release in ischemic spinal cord white matter involves L-type Ca^{2+} channel activation of ryanodine receptors. Neuron 2003;40(1):53–63.

97. Ouardouz M, Coderre E, Basak A, et al. Glutamate receptors on myelinated spinal cord axons: I. GluR6 kainate receptors. Ann Neurol 2009;65(2):151–9.
98. Choi DW. Calcium-mediated neurotoxicity: relationship to specific channel types and role in ischemic damage. Trends Neurosci 1988;11(10):465–9.
99. Ransom BR, Waxman SG, Davis PK. Anoxic injury of CNS white matter: protective effect of ketamine. Neurology 1990;40(9): 1399–403.
100. Li PA, Shuaib A, Miyashita H, et al. Hyperglycemia enhances extracellular glutamate accumulation in rats subjected to forebrain ischemia. Stroke 2000;31(1):183–92.
101. Blaustein MP. Calcium transport and buffering in neurons. Trends Neurosci 1988;11(10):438–43.
102. Lagnado L, Cervetto L, McNaughton PA. Ion transport by the Na-Ca exchange in isolated rod outer segments. Proc Natl Acad Sci U S A 1988;85(12):4548–52.
103. Blaustein MP, Lederer WJ. Sodium/calcium exchange: its physiological implications. Physiol Rev 1999;79(3):763–854.
104. Ames AD, Li YY, Heher EC, et al. Energy metabolism of rabbit retina as related to function: high cost of Na^+ transport. J Neurosci 1992;12(3):840–53.
105. Rose CR, Ransom BR. Regulation of intracellular sodium in cultured rat hippocampal neurones. J Physiol (Lond) 1997; 499(Pt 3):573–87.
106. Stys PK, Sontheimer H, Ransom BR, et al. Noninactivating, tetrodotoxin-sensitive Na^+ conductance in rat optic nerve axons. Proc Natl Acad Sci U S A 1993;90(15):6976–80.
107. Taylor CP. Na^+ currents that fail to inactivate. Trends Neurosci 1993;16(11):455–60.
108. Lipton SA. Calcium channel antagonists in the prevention of neurotoxicity. Adv Pharmacol 1991;22:271–97.
109. Weiss JH, Hartley DM, Koh J, et al. The calcium channel blocker nifedipine attenuates slow excitatory amino acid neurotoxicity. Science 1990;247(4949 Pt 1):1474–7.
110. Fern R, Ransom BR, Waxman SG. Voltage-gated calcium channels in CNS white matter: role in anoxic injury. J Neurophysiol 1995;74(1):369–77.
111. DiPolo R, Beauge L. Regulation of Na^+-Ca^{2+} exchange. An overview. Ann N Y Acad Sci 1991;639:100–11.
112. Flamm ES, Demopoulos HB, Seligman ML, et al. Free radicals in cerebral ischemia. Stroke 1978;9(5):445–7.
113. Nicotera P, McConkey DJ, Dypbukt JM, et al. Ca^{2+}-activated mechanisms in cell killing. Drug Metab Rev 1989;20(2–4): 193–201.
114. Garthwaite G, Goodwin DA, Neale S, et al. Soluble guanylyl cyclase activator YC-1 protects white matter axons from nitric oxide toxicity and metabolic stress, probably through Na(+) channel inhibition. Mol Pharmacol 2002;61(1): 97–104.
115. David JC, Yamada KA, Bagwe MR, et al. AMPA receptor activation is rapidly toxic to cortical astrocytes when desensitization is blocked. J Neurosci 1996;16(1):200–9.
116. Gallo V, Ghiani CA. Glutamate receptors in glia: new cells, new inputs and new functions. Trends Pharmacol Sci 2000;21(7): 252–8.
117. Matute C, Sanchez-Gomez MV, Martinez-Millan L, et al. Glutamate receptor-mediated toxicity in optic nerve oligodendrocytes. Proc Natl Acad Sci U S A 1997;94(16):8830–5.
118. Micu I, Jiang Q, Coderre E, et al. NMDA receptors mediate calcium accumulation in myelin during chemical ischaemia. Nature 2006;439(7079):988–92.
119. Salter MG, Fern R. NMDA receptors are expressed in developing oligodendrocyte processes and mediate injury. Nature 2005; 438(7071):1167–71.
120. Karadottir R, Cavelier P, Bergersen LH, et al. NMDA receptors are expressed in oligodendrocytes and activated in ischaemia. Nature 2005;438(7071):1162–6.
121. Yoshioka A, Hardy M, Younkin DP, et al. Alpha-amino-3-hydroxy-5-methyl-4-isoxazolepropionate (AMPA) receptors mediate excitotoxicity in the oligodendroglial lineage. J Neurochem 1995;64(6):2442–8.
122. Anderson CM, Swanson RA. Astrocyte glutamate transport: review of properties, regulation, and physiological functions [In Process Citation]. Glia 2000;32(1):1–14.
123. Ye ZC, Wyeth MS, Baltan-Tekkok S, et al. Functional hemichannels in astrocytes: a novel mechanism of glutamate release. J Neurosci 2003;23(9):3588–96.
124. Wrathall JR, Choiniere D, Teng YD. Dose-dependent reduction of tissue loss and functional impairment after spinal cord trauma with the AMPA/kainate antagonist NBQX. J Neurosci 1994; 14(11 Pt 1):6598–607.
125. Kanellopoulos GK, Xu XM, Hsu CY, et al. White matter injury in spinal cord ischemia: protection by AMPA/kainate glutamate receptor antagonism. Stroke 2000;31(8):1945–52.
126. Follett PL, Rosenberg PA, Volpe JJ, et al. NBQX attenuates excitotoxic injury in developing white matter. J Neurosci 2000; 20(24):9235–41.
127. McCracken E, Fowler JH, Dewar D, et al. Grey matter and white matter ischemic damage is reduced by the competitive AMPA receptor antagonist, SPD 502. J Cereb Blood Flow Metab 2002; 22(9):1090–7.
128. Brand-Schieber E, Werner P. AMPA/kainate receptors in mouse spinal cord cell-specific display of receptor subunits by oligodendrocytes and astrocytes and at the nodes of Ranvier. Glia 2003;42(1):12–24.
129. Van der Heyden JA, de Kloet ER, Korf J, et al. GABA content of discrete brain nuclei and spinal cord of the rat. J Neurochem 1979;33(4):857–61.
130. Bowery NG, Hudson AL, Price GW. GABAA and GABAB receptor site distribution in the rat central nervous system. Neuroscience 1987;20(2):365–83.
131. Shimada N, Graf R, Rosner G, et al. Ischemia-induced accumulation of extracellular amino acids in cerebral cortex, white matter, and cerebrospinal fluid. J Neurochem 1993;60(1):66–71.
132. Fern R, Waxman SG, Ransom BR. Modulation of anoxic injury in CNS white matter by adenosine and interaction between adenosine and GABA. J Neurophysiol 1994;72(6): 2609–16.
133. Fern R, Waxman SG, Ransom BR. Endogenous GABA attenuates CNS white matter dysfunction following anoxia. J Neurosci 1995;15(1 Pt 2):699–708.
134. Ransom BR, Philbin DM Jr. Anoxia-induced extracellular ionic changes in CNS white matter: the role of glial cells. Can J Physiol Pharmacol 1992;70(Suppl.):S181–9.
135. Stys PK. Protective effects of antiarrhythmic agents against anoxic injury in CNS white matter. J Cereb Blood Flow Metab 1995;15(3):425–32.
136. Stys PK, Lesiuk H. Correlation between electrophysiological effects of mexiletine and ischemic protection in central nervous system white matter. Neuroscience 1996;71(1):27–36.
137. Fern R, Ransom BR, Stys PK, et al. Pharmacological protection of CNS white matter during anoxia: actions of phenytoin, carbamazepine and diazepam. J Pharmacol Exp Ther 1993;266(3): 1549–55.
138. Sayin U, Timmerman W, Westerink BH. The significance of extracellular GABA in the substantia nigra of the rat during seizures and anticonvulsant treatments. Brain Res 1995;669(1):67–72.
139. Baltan S, Bachleda A, Morrison RS, et al. Expression of histone deacetylases in cellular compartments of the mouse brain and the effects of ischemia. Transl Stroke Res 2011;2(3):411–23.
140. Baltan S, Morrison RS, Murphy SP. Novel protective effects of histone deacetylase inhibition on stroke and white matter ischemic injury. Neurother 2013;10(4):798–807.
141. Baltan S, Murphy SP, Danilov CA, et al. Histone deacetylase inhibitors preserve white matter structure and function during ischemia by conserving ATP and reducing excitotoxicity. J Neurosci 2011;31(11):3990–9.
142. Menn B, Garcia-Verdugo JM, Yaschine C, et al. Origin of oligodendrocytes in the subventricular zone of the adult brain. J Neurosci 2006;26(30):7907–18.
143. Blakemore WF. Observations on oligodendrocyte degeneration, the resolution of status spongiosus and remyelination in cuprizone intoxication in mice. J Neurocytol 1972;1(4):413–26.
144. Prineas JW, Connell F. Remyelination in multiple sclerosis. Ann Neurol 1979;5(1):22–31.
145. Kaplan MS, Hinds JW. Gliogenesis of astrocytes and oligodendrocytes in the neocortical grey and white matter of the adult rat: electron microscopic analysis of light radioautographs. J Comp Neurol 1980;193(3):711–27.

146. McCarthy GF, Leblond CP. Radioautographic evidence for slow astrocyte turnover and modest oligodendrocyte production in the corpus callosum of adult mice infused with 3H-thymidine. J Comp Neurol 1988;271(4):589–603.
147. Gensert JM, Goldman JE. Endogenous progenitors remyelinate demyelinated axons in the adult CNS. Neuron 1997;19(1): 197–203.
148. Chari DM, Blakemore WF. Efficient recolonisation of progenitor-depleted areas of the CNS by adult oligodendrocyte progenitor cells. Glia 2002;37(4):307–13.
149. Miyamoto N, Tanaka R, Shimura H, et al. Phosphodiesterase III inhibition promotes differentiation and survival of oligodendrocyte progenitors and enhances regeneration of ischemic white matter lesions in the adult mammalian brain. J Cereb Blood Flow Metab 2010;30(2):299–310.
150. Yong VW. Prospects of repair in multiple sclerosis. J Neurol Sci 2009;277(Suppl. 1):S16–18.
151. Li Q, Brus-Ramer M, Martin JH, et al. Electrical stimulation of the medullary pyramid promotes proliferation and differentiation of oligodendrocyte progenitor cells in the corticospinal tract of the adult rat. Neurosci Lett 2010;479(2):128–33.
152. Zhang J, Kramer EG, Asp L, et al. Promoting myelin repair and return of function in multiple sclerosis. FEBS Lett 2011;585(23): 3813–20.
153. Fancy SP, Zhao C, Franklin RJ. Increased expression of Nkx2.2 and Olig2 identifies reactive oligodendrocyte progenitor cells responding to demyelination in the adult CNS. Mol Cell Neurosci 2004;27(3):247–54.
154. Miyamoto N, Pham LD, Hayakawa K, et al. Age-related decline in oligodendrogenesis retards white matter repair in mice. Stroke 2013;44(9):2573–8.
155. Miyamoto N, Maki T, Pham LD, et al. Oxidative stress interferes with white matter renewal after prolonged cerebral hypoperfusion in mice. Stroke 2013;44(12):3516–21.

10 Inflammation and Immune Response

Josef Anrather, Costantino Iadecola, John Hallenbeck

KEY POINTS

- Inflammation is a predominant feature of clinical and experimental stroke.
- Brain-resident and hematogenous immune cells participate in the inflammatory response.
- Inflammation is deleterious during the acute phase, but may aid repair processes.
- Scavenger receptors and toll-like receptors act as sensors for molecules produced by the ischemic tissue and initiate the inflammatory cascade.
- NF-κB, IRF-1 and C/EBPβ are key transcriptional activators of pro-inflammatory cytokines, adhesion molecules, and enzymes involved in post-ischemic inflammation, while PPARs are the main anti-inflammatory transcription factors.
- Initiation of endogenous neuroprotective programs by local or systemic preconditioning is dependent on the activation of several inflammatory pathways.
- Target-specific immune therapies hold the potential to benefit clinical stroke management.

Ischemic stroke triggers an inflammatory reaction in the affected area, which progresses for days to weeks after the onset of symptoms. There is evidence that selected aspects of such inflammatory processes contribute to the progression of ischemic brain injury, worsen the tissue damage, and exacerbate neurologic deficits. Therefore, interventions aimed at suppressing post-ischemic inflammation offer attractive therapeutic strategies for human stroke, with a potentially wide therapeutic window. On the other hand, inflammation can also have beneficial effects observed in the setting of ischemic tolerance and tissue repair (Fig. 10-1). A large body of work has addressed the inflammatory process in the post-ischemic brain.[1-4] In this chapter, we review the basic cellular and molecular features of post-ischemic inflammation, focusing on recent advances and insights on the potential mechanisms by which such inflammation influences stroke outcome. Furthermore, we examine the role of inflammatory mediators in the mechanisms of ischemic tolerance. Finally, we analyze the potential therapeutic implications of modulators of specific inflammatory targets from the perspective of near-future translational approaches.

CEREBRAL ISCHEMIA, CYTOKINES, AND INFLAMMATION

Cerebral ischemia is associated with infiltration of inflammatory cells into ischemic territory (Fig. 10-2). Histopathologic studies, investigations using biochemical markers of leukocytes, and human studies using radioactive-indium-labeled circulating leukocytes have demonstrated that early accumulation of blood-borne inflammatory cells in the ischemic brain persists for hours and even days after the initial insult.[5-8] The infiltration of hematogenous cells into the ischemic territory is the hallmark of the inflammatory reaction, which parallels activation of brain microglia and astrocytes (see Fig. 10-2).[9] Cytokines are important molecular signals in the inflammatory response to cerebral ischemia. In experimental models of stroke, ischemia induces expression of proinflammatory cytokines, such as tumor necrosis factor (TNF) and interleukin (IL)-6 and IL-1β, in the ischemic brain.[9] Increased production of cytokines has also been reported in patients with ischemic stroke.[7,10-12] Proinflammatory cytokines upregulate the expression of adhesion molecules such as intercellular adhesion molecule-1 (ICAM-1), selectins (especially E-selectin and P-selectin), and integrins on endothelial cells, leukocytes, and platelets.[9] Adhesion receptors mediate the interaction between endothelial cells and leukocytes that results in an initial "rolling" of leukocytes, which in turn leads to adhesion to the endothelium of venules, followed by leukocyte transmigration into the brain parenchyma.[7,13,14] Chemokines, the expression of which is upregulated in the ischemic territory, are believed to promote the infiltration of inflammatory cells toward the injured areas.[15]

Several lines of evidence suggest that post-ischemic inflammation has deleterious effects on the outcome of experimental cerebral ischemia (Tables 10-1–10-4). First, interventions aimed at reducing the number of circulating neutrophils ameliorate ischemic damage in most studies, as indicated by reduction in infarct volume and improvement in functional outcome (see Table 10-1).[16-18] Second, antibodies blocking the action of adhesion molecules reduce the influx of neutrophils and lessen tissue damage (see Table 10-2).[19-24] Third, genetically engineered mice lacking adhesion molecules, such as ICAM-1 and P-selectin, are less susceptible to ischemic damage (see Table 10-2).[25-27] Furthermore, compounds that block the interaction of E-selectin with Sleux – the counterpart adhesion molecule on leukocytes that binds to E-selectin – reduce ischemic brain damage.[22] Fourth, interventions that inactivate cytokines or block cytokine receptors lessen ischemic damage (see Table 10-3).[28-35]

MECHANISMS BY WHICH INFLAMMATION CONTRIBUTES TO ISCHEMIC BRAIN INJURY

The mechanisms by which post-ischemic inflammation contributes to cerebral ischemic damage are not well understood. Although infiltrating immune cells and activated microglia may produce tissue damage by generating reactive oxygen species (ROS) and reactive nitrogen species (RNS),[9,13] microvascular occlusion produced by intravascular neutrophils, lymphocytes, and platelets may also contribute by compromising microvascular flow.[1,3,14,36,37] New data have provided insight into additional mechanisms that may also play a role in the neurotoxicity of inflammation. In experimental models of stroke, TNF and IL-1β have been linked to the associated brain injury.[38-45] Intracerebral injection of TNF exacerbates ischemic injury, whereas anti-TNF monoclonal antibody or soluble TNF receptor (TNFR; TNF-binding protein) treatment reverses the effect.[46] Furthermore, the administration of IL-1 receptor antagonist (IL-1ra), a naturally occurring IL-1 inhibitor, or overexpression of IL-1ra in genetically engineered animals diminishes ischemic injury.[47-51] In addition, studies using IL-1 receptor I (IL-1RI) knockout mice suggest an involvement of this receptor in IL-1-mediated injury in brain trauma, possibly via microglia-macrophage activation as well as expression of cyclooxygenase-2 (COX-2), IL-1, and IL-6.[52] Interferon-γ (IFN-γ) produced after cerebral ischemia is also involved in tissue damage.[37,53] Consistent with a deleterious role of IFN-γ, mice lacking the interferon regulatory factor 1 (IRF1) are less susceptible to focal cerebral ischemia.[54] The mechanisms by which IFN-γ contribute to ischemic injury are multifactorial and include upregulation of adhesion molecules, prothrombotic effects, microglial activation, and formation of NADPH-oxidase-derived ROS.[37,55]

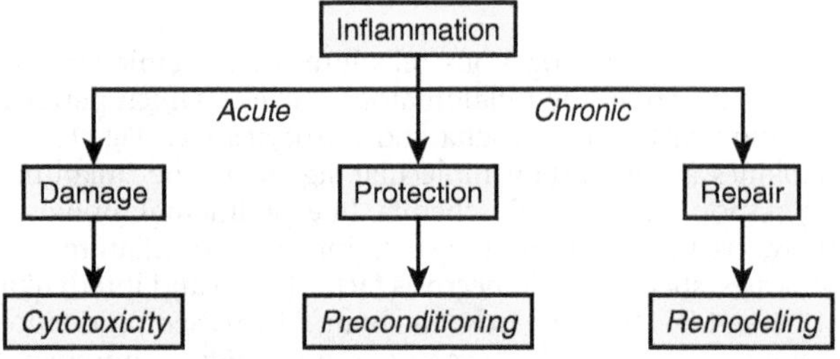

Figure 10-1. Beneficial and deleterious effects of inflammation. Inflammation leads to cytotoxicity in the acute setting but is also essential for brain protection in the setting of ischemic tolerance. Inflammation sets the stage for tissue repair and, as such, is beneficial during the recovery phase after stroke.

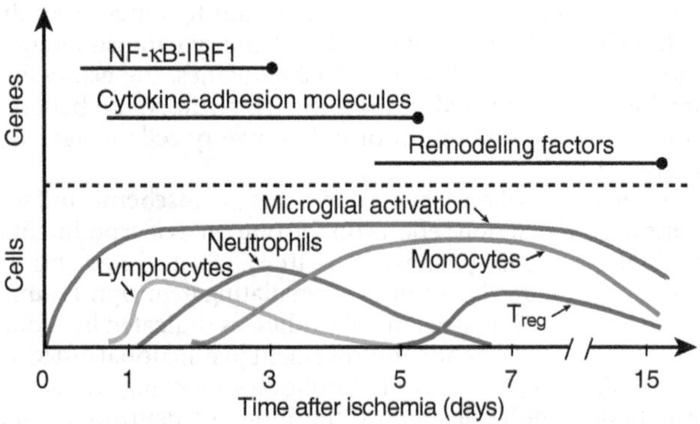

Figure 10-2. Temporal profile of the gene expression and associated cellular events that occur after focal cerebral ischemia in mice. Activation of inflammatory transcription factors leads to expression of cytokines and adhesion molecules. These molecular changes drive the trafficking of leukocytes (neutrophils and lymphocytes) and macrophages across the blood–brain barrier and into the brain. Microglia (i.e., resident brain macrophages) become activated and contribute to the inflammatory reaction. NF-κB, nuclear factor-κB; IRF-1, interferon regulatory factor-1. *(Cell data modified from Schilling M, Besselmann M, Leonhard C, et al. Microglial activation precedes and predominates over macrophage infiltration in transient focal cerebral ischemia: a study in green fluorescent protein transgenic bone marrow chimeric mice.* Exp Neurol *183:25–33, 2003.)*

There are instances in which cytokines ameliorate neuronal injury. For example, TNF can induce protection from subsequent ischemic injury (see section on ischemic preconditioning), and TNF receptor knockout mice have greater sensitivity to brain injury.[56,57] In the case of TNF preconditioning, TNF is presumed to act as a noxious stimulus that activates feedback control mechanisms and confers tolerance to subsequent ischemia by generating cell survival agonists and cell death inhibitors. The response of TNF-receptor-deficient mice is more difficult to explain in light of the TNF inhibition studies just cited. One possible interpretation is that TNFRI/TNFRII-null mice are exposed to long-term deprivation because of TNF homeostatic effects and may have developed compensatory mechanisms that render them different from wild-type mice that experience a sudden block of TNF activity. Such discrepancy may also be due to the specific TNF receptor involved in the process. For example, some studies indicate that different receptor subtypes (e.g., TNFRI and TNFRII) exert opposite roles in TNF-induced neuronal injury and survival.[58,59]

Another member of the TNF receptor superfamily, Fas, has been implicated in ischemic brain damage. Martin-Villalba et al.[60] have reported that infarct volumes in both FasL (Fas ligand) and TNF knockout mice were 54% and 67% smaller,

TABLE 10-1 Effects of Leukocyte Depletion on the Outcome of Experimental Focal Cerebral Ischemia

Intervention	Outcome	Selected Chapter Reference
Mechlorethamine and vinblastine	Improved histologic or functional outcome in models of focal ischemia	Heinel et al.[16]
Antineutrophilic antibodies	Reduction in infarct size or edema in a rat model of focal cerebral ischemia	Matsuo et al.[17]
Neutrophil inhibitory factor	Reduction in infarct size in rats with transient middle cerebral artery occlusion	Jiang et al.[18]
Leukocyte depletion	No effect on brain injury	Hayward et al.[223]

TABLE 10-2 Role of Adhesion Molecules in the Mechanisms of Experimental Focal Cerebral Ischemia

Intervention	Outcome	Selected Chapter Reference
Anti-ICAM-1 antibodies	Reduction in infarct size in rats with transient MCAO	Zhang et al.[19]
ICAM-1-null mice	Reduction in infarct size in transient MCAO	Connolly et al.[27]
Anti-CD18 monoclonal antibodies	Increased reflow in microvessels of different sizes in primates	Mori et al.[20]
Anti-CD11b monoclonal antibody	Reduction in infarct size in rats with transient MCAO	Chen et al.[21]
Mac-1 (CD11b/CD18)	Reduction in infarct size in rats with MCAO	Soriano et al.[26]
CY-1503, analog of sialyl-Lewis (x)	Reduction in infarct size in rats with transient MCAO	Zhang et al.[22]
Synthetic oligopeptide corresponding to the lectin domain of selectins	Reduction in infarct size in rats with MCAO	Morikawa et al.[23]
P-selectin-null mice	Reduction in infarct size with transient MCAO	Connolly et al.[25]
Anti-P-selectin monoclonal antibody	Reduction in infarct size in rats with transient or permanent MCAO	Suzuki et al.[24]

ICAM-1, intercellular adhesion molecule-1; Mac-1, macrophage-1 antigen complex; MCAO, middle cerebral artery occlusion.

TABLE 10-3 Evidence that Cytokines Play a Role in the Mechanisms of Experimental Focal Cerebral Ischemia

Intervention	Outcome	Selected Chapter Reference(s)
TNF-soluble receptor type 1	Reduction in infarct size in rats and mice with permanent MCAO	Dawson et al.[28]
Anti-TNF monoclonal antibody	Reduction in infarct size in rats and mice with MCAO	Yang et al.,[29] Barone et al.[46]
IL-1β administration	Increase in infarct size in rats with transient MCAO	Yamasaki et al.[30]
IL-1 receptor antagonist	Reduction in infarct size in rats with MCAO	Loddick et al.[31]
IL-1 converting enzyme-null mice	Reduction in ICAM-positive vessels in mice with permanent MCAO	Yang et al.[33]
IL-6 administration	Reduction in infarct size in rats with permanent MCAO	Loddick et al.[32]
Anti-IL-8 monoclonal antibody	Reduction in infarct size in rabbits with transient ischemia	Matsumoto et al.[34]
Anti-CINC antibody	Reduction in infarct size in rats with transient MCAO	Yamasaki et al.[35]
IL-1R1-null mice	Suppression of inflammation; reduced microglia activation; reduced IL-1, IL-6, ICAM-1, COX-2 expression	Basu et al.[52]

CINC, cytokine-induced neutrophil chemoattractant; ICAM-1, intercellular adhesion molecule-1; IL, interleukin; MCAO, middle cerebral artery occlusion; TNF, tumor necrosis factor.

TABLE 10-4 Role of Scavenger Receptors and Toll-Like Receptors in the Mechanisms of Experimental Focal Cerebral Ischemia

Intervention	Outcome	Selected Chapter Reference(s)
SCAVENGER RECEPTORS		
CD36-null mice	Reduction in infarct size in transient MCAO	Cho et al.,[144] Kunz et al.,[145] Kim et al.,[224] Abe et al.[225]
RAGE-null mice	Reduction in infarct size in permanent MCAO	Muhammad et al.[131]
TLRs		
TLR2-null mice	Reduction in infarct size in transient MCAO	Tang et al.,[120] Lehnardt et al.,[124] Abe et al.[225]
TLR4-null mice	Reduction in infarct size in transient and permanent MCAO	Tang et al.,[120] Caso et al.[123]

MCAO, middle cerebral artery occlusion; RAGE, receptor for advanced glycation end products; TLR, toll-like receptor.

respectively, than those in controls. Hybrid mice lacking both cytokines showed a 93% reduction in infarct volume, and a combination of antibodies that neutralized FasL and TNF decreased infarct volume by 70%. Ligation of Fas by trimerized FasL leads to recruitment of adapter proteins that form the death-inducing signaling complex (DISC) and, eventually, apoptosis. TNFRI recruits the TNFR-associated death domain protein (TRADD), which can interact with both Fas-associated death domain protein (FADD) and TNFR-associated factor 2 (TRAF2) that can activate nuclear factor-κB (NF-κB). Accordingly, these receptors can activate both pro-inflammatory and apoptotic pathways, which is a feature that may account for the potency of their dual blockade in ischemia.

Immune Cells Participating in Ischemic Injury and Tissue Repair

Microglia, Monocytes/Macrophages, and Dendritic Cells

Post-ischemic inflammation is characterized by the orchestrated recruitment of various blood-borne immune cells and by activation of resident microglia. Because microglia and blood-derived macrophages are not readily distinguishable by morphology or protein expression patterns, most results derived from in vivo studies could either implicate microglia or macrophages or both. Only recently, multi-label flow cytometry of brain immune cells and bone marrow chimeric animals that express discernible markers (fluorescent proteins or CD45 alloantigen) in hematogenous cells have allowed a clear distinction of microglia and blood-derived myeloid cells. A recently developed mouse model, that expresses myeloid-restricted tamoxifen-inducible Cre-recombinase, could be useful to generate microglia-selective gene deletions to further dissect the contribution of brain-resident and hematogenous myeloid cells in stroke.[61] Furthermore, the cellular and functional phenotype of immune cells in the post-ischemic microenvironment is not static but fluent as exemplified by the rapid transformation of microglia after cerebral ischemia. Microglial activation occurs before the appearance of neuronal cell death[62] and this early response is characterized by increased arborisation and exploratory behavior giving way to de-arborisation and amoeboid transformation within the first 24 hours after stroke while the cells remain stationary.[63,64] In a study in GFP+ bone marrow chimeric mice Schilling et al.[65] showed that microglia contributed to increased numbers of macrophage-like cells during the first days after cerebral ischemia while GFP+ blood-borne cells appeared in robust numbers only after day 2. While pro-inflammatory and cytotoxic activities of microglia have been demonstrated in vitro, elimination of proliferating microglia/macrophages by ganciclovir treatment in mice that express HSV1-thymidine kinase in the myeloid lineage increased ischemic injury and reduced expression of the neurotrophic cytokine IGF-1.[66]

Blood monocytes exist as two functionally distinct subpopulations (inflammatory and patrolling) best characterized by the expression of CCR2 and CX3CR1 chemokine receptors, both of which are important for monocyte entry into the ischemic brain,[67,68] and the relative abundance of these subsets in the blood has been linked to clinical stroke outcome.[69,70] Initially, infiltrating monocytes are of the inflammatory subtype while patrolling monocytes are prevalent at later time points.[71] The pathophysiological importance of this finding, however, has yet to be determined. In experimental stroke monocytes/macrophages infiltrate the brain parenchyma 48 hours after ischemia and can persist for several weeks.[65] There is also evidence that inhibition of adhesion molecules involved in lymphocyte and monocyte trafficking, such as the very late activation antigen-4 (VLA-4) or the lymphocyte function antigen-1 (LIF-1), can reduce infarct volumes in stroke models.[72–75] These studies suggest that lymphocytes and monocytes, in addition to neutrophils, participate in post-ischemic brain inflammation.[76] However, the precise role that these cells have remains to be defined. Depending on molecular cues encountered in the post-ischemic brain parenchyma, monocytes/macrophages can undergo classical (M1, pro-inflammatory) or alternative (M2, anti-inflammatory in most settings) activation, thus contributing to the resolution of inflammation.[63,77] Phagocytosis, which is mainly seen in microglia and not macrophages and is tied to MerTK, MFG-E8 and TREM2 expression,[78,79] can contribute to delayed neuronal cell death after ischemia[79,80] and a subset of microglia and infiltrating macrophages express the dendritic cell (DC) marker CD11c and MHC class II molecules.[81] Using chimeric animals that express EYFP under the control of the CD11c promoter in bone-marrow-derived cells, the same study showed that DCs originate from brain-resident myeloid cells early after ischemia, while peripheral immune cells contribute the majority of CD11c/EYFP+ cells 3 days after stroke.[81] Although brain DCs have the capacity to present antigen and induce T cell proliferation in vitro,[82] it remains to be shown whether these cells engage in antigen presentation after brain ischemia.

Neutrophils

Although intravascular adhesion of neutrophils is a relatively early post-ischemic event, parenchymal accumulation is generally observed later, when most of the ischemic damage may have already occurred.[3] In addition, no consistent relationship has been found between the level of leukocyte infiltration and the extent of ischemic damage.[83] These observations raise questions about the role of neutrophils in the mechanisms of ischemic brain injury and suggest that our understanding of the mechanisms and pathophysiologic implications of post-ischemic leukocyte trafficking is rather limited. Neutrophils are among the first hematogenous immune cells found in the brain after experimental stroke peaking at 48–72 hours in most models and declining rapidly afterwards. Although it is not clear whether they enter the brain parenchyma in all circumstances,[84] there is evidence that neutrophils play a part in post-ischemic inflammation by limiting tissue perfusion due to intravascular clogging,[36,85] destabilizing the BBB by releasing MMP9,[86,87] and by generating ROS and NO.[88] However, a cause-and-effect relationship between the extent of neutrophil trafficking and the severity of ischemic damage has not been firmly established.[1,3] Attesting to the complex role of neutrophils in cerebral ischemic injury, a recent study postulates a protective role of neutrophils, that have undergone N2 polarization as characterized by Ym1 (chitinase 3-like 3, Chi3l3) expression, in stroke pathology.[89]

Mast Cells

Mast cells are brain-resident immune cells, located in the perivascular space, that are rich in peptidases and vasoactive molecules. Mast cells are activated early after cerebral ischemia and contribute to the BBB breakdown and brain edema by releasing gelatinase.[90,91]

Lymphocytes

T cells are detrimental in the early phase of ischemia and lymphocyte-deficient mice are protected in models of focal ischemia.[92,93] The mechanism does not involve classical antigen-mediated T cell activation and the cytotoxic activity might be tied to innate T cell functions.[93] Accordingly, IL-17-secreting γδT cells, that do not undergo classical antigen-dependent T cell activation, have been shown to contribute to ischemic injury.[94,95] While effector T lymphocytes may contribute to focal ischemic injury,[37,92] regulatory T cells (Treg) could have a protective effect by downregulating post-ischemic inflammation. Tregs appear in the ischemic tissue after the acute phase and confer neuroprotection by IL-10 secretion, an effect that might be antigen-independent.[53,96,97] Similarly, regulatory B cells (Bregs) confer neuroprotection through an IL-10-dependent mechanism, but do not enter the ischemic brain.[98,99] Recent work that has extended the compass of stroke-related inflammation beyond innate immune mechanisms to include adaptive immunity has been reviewed.[100] Disruption of the blood–brain barrier during acute stroke releases novel central nervous system (CNS) antigens that are normally sequestered in the brain and exposes them to the systemic immune system. Absent activation of the systemic immune system, autoimmune responses to these antigens do not seem to occur. However, cerebral ischemia induces a state of systemic immunodepression that predisposes to post-stroke infections.[101,102] Stroke is frequently complicated by pulmonary or urinary tract infections; under these circumstances, T-effector lymphocytes can become primed to brain antigens and excite a CNS autoimmune response. Activated CD8+ T lymphocytes can secrete cytotoxic and proinflammatory cytokines and can also kill brain cells by direct lysis (e.g., perforin and granzyme) or by inducing apoptosis via the TNF family of receptors (e.g., Fas receptor and FasL).[55]

DANGER SENSORS: SCAVENGER RECEPTORS AND TOLL-LIKE RECEPTORS

In a disorder such as stroke that results from multiple interacting mechanisms,[103–107] therapeutic targets that beneficially affect multiple mechanisms are arguably the most attractive. If the multifactorial progression of ischemic brain injury could be likened to a bad performance by a symphony orchestra, stopping the conductor should be far more effective than stopping the piccolo player. It is interesting in this regard to consider the relationship to ischemic injury of recently identified networks of ligands, receptors, transcription factors, and effector molecules that appear to "conduct" the response to ischemic stress and orchestrate ongoing brain damage. Evolutionarily conserved pattern recognition receptors respond not only to pathogen-associated molecular patterns (PAMPs), but also to endogenous danger signals (termed either alarmins or danger-associated molecular patterns [DAMPs]) that can initiate responses to stresses such as ischemia.[108,109] Such receptor-mediated signaling may provide the first inkling to cells that they are in trouble. Examples of alarmins/DAMPs include cathelicidins,[110] high mobility group box protein 1 (HMGB1),[111] S100/calgranulins,[112] heparan sulfate, hyaluronic acid, cytochrome c, and advanced glycation end products (AGE).[113] Other endogenous ligands that may serve as stress signals are heat shock proteins (HSPs), degraded extracellular matrix components, ROS, denatured proteins, and changes in lipid, carbohydrate, or protein moieties that are expressed on the outer cell membrane of stressed cells.[114] In addition, nucleic acids such as DNA and RNA and their metabolites (i.e., polynucleotides, oligonucleotides, nucleosides, free bases, and uric acid) that are normally sequestered can be released by injured cells and modulate innate immune responses.[115]

Receptors for endogenous stress molecules, which nucleate multiprotein signaling complexes, include toll-like receptor (TLR) and NACHT (domain present in neuronal apoptosis inhibitory protein)-leucine-rich repeat (NLR) receptor families on sentinel cells (macrophages, microglia, dendritic cells).[109,114] TLRs are key receptors of the innate immune system, comprising at least 13 families. On ligand binding, TLRs form homodimers (TLR4/4) or heterodimers (TLR2/6 or TLR2/1) (Fig. 10-3).[116] TLR2 forms functional heterodimers with TLR1 or TLR6[116,117] and recognizes a variety of PAMPs, including triacylated lipopeptides from bacteria, such as peptidoglycan, diacylated lipopeptides such as Pam2CSK4, LPSs from Gram-negative bacteria, fungal zymosan, and mycoplasma lipopeptides.[118] TLR4 predominantly recognizes

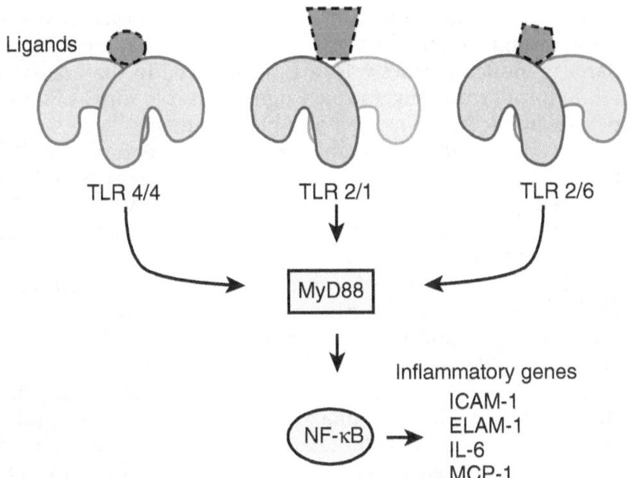

Figure 10-3. Toll-like receptors (TLR) are present as homodimers or heterodimers and, on ligand binding, lead to NF-κB activation through the adapter protein MyD88. NF-κB, nuclear factor-κB; ICAM-1, intercellular adhesion molecule-1; ELAM-1, endothelial-leukocyte adhesion molecule-1; IL-6, interleukin-6; MCP-1, monocyte chemotactic protein-1. *(Modified from Abe T, Shimamura M, Jackman K, et al. Key role of CD36 in Toll-like receptor 2 signaling in cerebral ischemia.* Stroke *41:898–904, 2010.)*

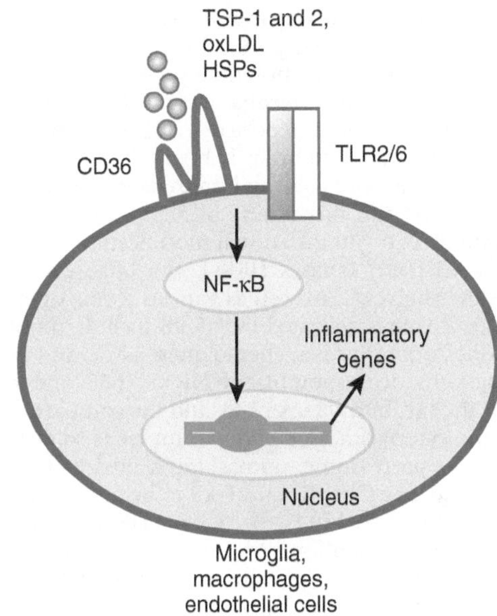

Figure 10-4. The scavenger receptor CD36 is present in microglia, macrophages, and endothelial cells. CD36 can signal independently or as part of a molecular cluster including TLR2/6, which is formed in response to a wide variety of ligands. On ligand binding, CD36 triggers inflammatory signaling through NF-κB activation. TSP-1 and -2, thrombospondin-1 and -2; oxLDL, oxidized low-density lipoprotein; HSPs, heat shock proteins; TLR, toll-like receptor; NF-κB, nuclear factor-κB.

LPS.[119] Activation of TLRs leads to NF-κB activation via the adapter protein MyD88 (see Fig. 10-3).[116] Recent expression studies have demonstrated that cerebral ischemia results in the upregulation of mRNA for TLR2, TLR4, and TLR9, and mice lacking TLR2 or TLR4 exhibit reduced infarct size after focal cerebral ischemic injury (see Table 10-4).[120–125] The expression of IRF-1, iNOS, COX-2, and metalloproteinase-9 is reduced in TLR4-null mouse brains after MCA occlusion,[123] attesting to the key role of TLR4 in postischemic inflammation.

The receptor for advanced glycation end products (RAGE) and acutephase proteins of the pentraxin family (including C-reactive protein) can sense the presence of endogenous danger signals.[109,126] RAGE is a multiligand membrane receptor, and several of the established ligands may activate RAGE in cerebral ischemia. Administration of AGE, a RAGE ligand, increases ischemic injury in a rat model of focal cerebral ischemia.[127] Furthermore, HMGB1 is a well-known RAGE activator released, for example, from activated macrophages, stressed neurons, and necrotic cells after cerebral ischemia.[128–130] A neutralizing anti-HMGB1 antibody and HMGB1 box A, an antagonist of HMGB1 at the receptor RAGE, ameliorates ischemic brain damage.[131] Consistent with a deleterious role of RAGE signaling, RAGE$^{-/-}$ mice have significantly smaller infarcts than controls (see Table 10-4).[131] The roles in brain ischemia of nucleic acid metabolite complexes that may contain both coreceptors and accessory molecules,[132] activate one or more of the inflammasomes through TLRs 7, 8, or 9, and induce both pyroptotic and apoptotic forms of cell death,[133] have received relatively little attention. The Stenzel-Poore lab has clearly linked RNA and DNA metabolite signaling pathways to induction of ischemic tolerance,[134] but fuller understanding of the roles for released endogenous nucleic acid DAMPS in the pathobiology of brain ischemia will come with further study.

Signal transduction from these receptors can lead to the formation of multiprotein complexes that nucleate on a scaffold protein, which characteristically has a region involved in ligand sensing, an oligomerization domain, and a domain involved in recruiting caspases.[135,136] The multiprotein complexes integrate cellular signals, promote activation of initiator caspases (caspase 2, 8, 9, or 10), and initiate signaling cascades that can lead to apoptosis, to inflammation or to cell survival. Examples of these multiprotein complexes include the apoptosome, the inflammasome, the DISC, and the PIDDosome.[137,138]

The class B scavenger receptor CD36 is a surface glycoprotein found in microglia, macrophages, microvascular endothelium, cardiac and skeletal muscle, adipocytes, and platelets.[139] CD36 recognizes a multitude of ligands, including oxidized low-density lipoprotein (LDL), long-chain fatty acids, thrombospondin-1, fibrillar-amyloid (Ab), and the membrane of cells undergoing apoptosis.[139–141] CD36 recognizes pathogen-associated molecular patterns and induces an inflammatory response through activation of NF-κB (Fig. 10-4).[142,143] Focal cerebral ischemia upregulates CD36 in the ischemic brain, and CD36-null mice have smaller infarcts and better neurologic outcomes after focal ischemia.[144] Three of the above complexes – inflammasome, DISC, and PIDDosome – as well as TLR, CD36, and RAGE[113,114,137] activate signal transduction pathways that induce nuclear translocation of a transcription factor, NF-κB, which serves as a critical nexus in the pathways regulating inflammation, cell death, and cell survival. CD36 may well play a key role in focal cerebral ischemia through its augmented NF-κB activation that supports full expression of the cellular and molecular signals driving post-ischemic inflammation.[145]

TRANSCRIPTION FACTORS INVOLVED IN POST-ISCHEMIC INFLAMMATION

The molecular mechanisms that lead to activation of transcription of inflammatory genes in the post-ischemic brain are not fully understood. Gene expression is controlled by transcription factors, DNA-binding proteins that initiate mRNA transcription. Several transcription factors have been studied in the context of post-ischemic inflammation. NF-κB is a multifunctional switch that transactivates the expression of more than 150 target genes, of which some are potentially cytotoxic and others are potentially cytoprotective.[146,147] It functions in the negative feedback control of TNF cytotoxicity,[148,149] and it has been reported to be a key factor in the induction of tolerance to brain ischemia.[150,151] The activity of NF-κB proteins is regulated by hundreds of different stimuli in all cell types, and fine-tuning of NF-κB functional consequences involves posttranslational modification of the inhibitor of NF-κB (IκB) kinases (IKKs), the IκBs, or the NF-κB subunits themselves,[152] as well as various forms of epigenetic regulation.[153] Genes activated by NF-κB include those encoding for adhesion molecules, chemokines, iNOS, and COX-2.[149] In resting cells, two subunits of NF-κB, p65 and p50, are bound to the inhibitory factor IκB, and the complex is sequestered in the cytoplasm. Cell stimulation leads to degradation of IκB in the proteasome, unmasking a nuclear localization signaling sequence that allows NF-κB to be translocated to the nucleus. NF-κB then binds to cognate DNA sequences and activates gene transcription.[154] Ischemia-reperfusion, physical stress, cytokines, and ROS are potent stimuli for NF-κB activation.[149] Cerebral ischemia activates NF-κB.[145,149,155,156] After transient focal ischemia in the rat, greater immunoreactivity of p65 is found in neurons at the periphery of the infarct, in reactive glia, and in inflammatory cells.[157,158] NF-κB activation is observed 6 to 96 hours after ischemia, depending on experimental models and species.[157–159] Immunoreactivity for NF-κB is also observed in glial cells of human infarcts, particularly at the border of the zone between ischemic and non-ischemic areas.[160]

Several studies have investigated the role of NF-κB in ischemic brain injury in vivo.[149] Thus, genetic deletion of the NF-κB subunit p50 reduces ischemic injury.[159,161] Similarly, expression of an NF-κB repressor[162] or deletion of the upstream kinase IKK[163] is neuroprotective. One study in which NF-κB was pharmacologically inhibited with diethyldithiocarbamate (DDTC) suggested a neuroprotective role of NF-κB.[164] However, this study has been questioned because of the lack of specificity of DDTC.[165,166] Currently, the weight of the evidence favors a deleterious role of NF-κB in acute focal ischemic injury. Although NF-κB and other inflammatory mediators may be protective in the setting of ischemic tolerance,[150,167,168] this is not surprising considering the well-established preconditioning effects of injurious stimuli.[169]

IRF-1 is a transcription factor that is thought to coordinate the expression of multiple inflammatory genes, including cytokines, adhesion molecules, iNOS, and COX-2.[170] Data now suggest that IRF-1 is also involved in the mechanisms of cerebral ischemia. In rodents, IRF-1 mRNA is upregulated after permanent MCA occlusion, reaching a peak 3 to 4 days after ischemia.[54,171] Cerebral ischemia increases IRF-1 binding activity, as demonstrated on gel-shift assays.[172] Furthermore, mice lacking IRF-1 have less brain damage and milder neurologic deficits after MCA occlusion.[54] The difference in infarct volume could not be attributed to differences in the reduction of cerebral blood flow produced by MCA occlusion.[54] These findings suggest that IRF-1-dependent gene expression plays a prominent role in the expression of ischemic brain injury. However, the cellular and molecular mechanisms responsible for the protection afforded by IRF-1 deletion remain to be defined.

CCAAT/enhancer binding protein β (C/EBPβ) is a leucine-zipper transcription factor that binds to CCAAT sequences in promoters of eukaryotic genes and regulates cell growth and differentiation.[173] C/EBPβ gene expression is significantly upregulated after MCA occlusion, and C/EBPβ-null mice have significantly smaller infarcts.[174] Also, in C/EBPβ-null mice brain after cerebral ischemia, numbers of ICAM-1-positive capillaries and infiltrated neutrophils and macrophages are reduced.[174] In addition, GeneChip analysis showed that the post-ischemic induction of many inflammatory and neuronal-damage-inducing genes was less pronounced in the brains of C/EBPβ-null mice, suggesting a significant role for C/EBPβ in post-ischemic inflammation and brain damage.[174]

The peroxisome-proliferator-activated receptors (PPARs) are the ligand-activated nuclear proteins, of which at least three subtypes exist (i.e., PPARα, PPARδ, and PPARγ).[175] PPARs regulate gene transcription by binding to conserved DNA sequences termed peroxisome proliferator response elements (PPREs) as heterodimers with the retinoic acid receptor (RXR).[176] Recent studies using animal stroke models suggest that PPARγ activation with thiazolidinediones (TZDs), which are potent PPARγ agonists,[177] is a potent therapeutic option for preventing inflammation and neuronal damage after stroke. TZDs, such as troglitazone, pioglitazone, or rosiglitazone, reduced infarct volume and resulted in a reduction of numbers of microglia/macrophages, myeloperoxidase (MPO) levels and activity, cytokine levels (TNF, IL-6, monocyte chemotactic protein-1 [MCP-1]), and decreased expression of COX-2, IL-1β, and iNOS mRNA or protein in the ischemic brain, which supported the link between anti-inflammatory effects of TZDs acting via PPARγ.[178–181] Treatment with the PPARγ antagonist T0070907 abrogates the protection.[182] Oral administration of the PPARα agonist fenofibrate reduced vascular cell adhesion molecule-1 (VCAM-1) and ICAM-1 expression and cortical infarction after transient MCA occlusion.[183] Furthermore, PPARα antagonist WY14643 decreased oxidative stress, iNOS, and ICAM-1 expression in a model of global ischemia.[184] These observations attest to a protective role of PPAR activation in ischemic injury. Given that PPARγ agonists are in clinical use for the treatment of type 2 diabetes, these agents could also have a therapeutic role in stroke. A recent meta-analysis indicated that the PPARγ agonist rosiglitazone increases the risk of ischemic myocardial events and cardiovascular deaths,[185] but the reliability of these findings has been questioned.[186] However, PPARγ agonists do cause fluid retention and increased incidence of heart failure,[186] which suggests that their potential use in stroke patients needs to be scrutinized further.

INFLAMMATORY MEDIATORS AND ISCHEMIC PRECONDITIONING

As previously discussed, ischemic brain cells produce a large array of mediators that may participate in progression of ischemic brain injury. This is one factor that has complicated efforts to develop clinically effective therapies for stroke. Surprisingly, these inflammatory mediators, under certain conditions, can confer tolerance to cerebral ischemia. Study of the regulation of the endogenous neuroprotection associated with inflammatory mediators may enable investigators to guide the search for effective stroke therapy through the morass of interlaced injury mechanisms.

The earliest observations of tolerance were in the heart and involved preconditioning with brief sublethal ischemia. Preconditioning is the phenomenon whereby a stressful but sublethal stimulus sets in motion a cascade of molecular and biochemical events that renders cells, tissues, or the whole organism tolerant to a future more lethal stimulus. Myocardial ischemia preconditioning in animal models has been studied since the mid-1980s, and later clinical studies suggest that similar preconditioning may be operative in human coronary syndromes.[187–189] Murry et al.[190] were the first to develop a preconditioning paradigm that reduced myocardial infarct size during a subsequent severe ischemia. Later, other groups attempted to replicate the preconditioned responses to ischemia observed in the myocardium in neurologic models.

Kitagawa et al.[191] showed that preconditioning with brief ischemia (2 minutes) protected against a later 5-minute episode of bilateral common carotid artery occlusion in gerbils that otherwise caused damage to pyramidal neurons in the CA1 region of the hippocampus, a region of brain selectively vulnerable to ischemia. Subsequently, many groups have demonstrated that diverse preconditioning strategies can induce tolerance to global or focal brain ischemia, and tolerance has been modeled in cell culture systems to facilitate the study of regulatory mechanisms. As with clinically relevant myocardial preconditioning, there is some clinical evidence for induction of neuroprotection after "preconditioning" that occurs from transient ischemic attacks.[192,193]

Proinflammatory cytokines IL-1 and TNF activate intracellular signaling pathways that mediate stress responses[194] and could, therefore, function in ligand–receptor interactions that induce the tolerant state. IL-1 has been observed to induce tolerance to global brain ischemia with protection of hippocampal CA1 neurons in the gerbil.[195] LPS is a potent stimulus for release of proinflammatory cytokines. Its administration in animal models has been reported to protect against ischemia in both the heart[196–198] and the brain.[199] NO, HSP70, and superoxide dismutase have been implicated in LPS-induced tolerance to brain ischemia.[200,201] A major cytokine elicited by LPS is TNF. Preconditioning with TNF has been reported to confer cytoprotection in an embryonic kidney cell line[202] and has also been reported to reduce injury in isolated perfused rat hearts subjected to ischemia[203] by increasing manganese superoxide dismutase. TNF preconditioning has also been shown to reduce infarct volumes in mice subjected to MCA occlusion[204] and to protect cultured neurons from severe hypoxic stress.[56] Downstream signaling in this pathway involves ceramide and the transcription factor NF-κB.[205] Such studies are moving toward points of intersection for multiple regulatory pathways and have the potential to identify molecular targets that can simultaneously affect multiple mechanisms of ischemic damage.

Important recent work has shown that tolerance to severe ischemia induced by preconditioning fundamentally involves reprogramming of the genetic response to injury.[206] During exposure to severe ischemia, both a high percentage of unique transcripts and widespread, gene-specific repression of gene expression have been found in brain samples that had been preconditioned by sublethal ischemia compared with samples from non-preconditioned brains. Also, the profiles of gene expression during severe ischemia appear to differ depending on the nature of the preconditioning stimulus, as shown for ischemic preconditioning versus LPS preconditioning. These preconditioning-specific phenotypes appear to be adapted to counter the specific cytotoxicity mechanisms of the preconditioning stimulus. This suggests that multiple non-overlapping pathways may subserve tolerance to brain ischemia.[206]

In addition, preconditioning protects cerebral blood vessels from the vasoparalysis induced by cerebral ischemia. Administration of LPS 24 hours before MCA occlusion reduced ischemic brain injury and prevented the dysfunction in cerebrovascular regulation induced by MCA occlusion, as demonstrated by normalization of the increase in cerebral blood flow produced by neural activity, hypercapnia, or the endothelium-dependent vasodilator acetylcholine.[168] These beneficial effects of LPS were not observed in mice lacking iNOS or the NOX2 subunit of the superoxide-producing enzyme NADPH oxidase.[168] LPS increased ROS and the peroxynitrite marker 3-nitrotyrosine in cerebral blood vessels of wild-type mice but not in NOX2 nulls, and the peroxynitrite decomposition catalyst 5,10,15,20-tetrakis(4-sulfonatophenyl)porphyrinato iron (III) counteracted the beneficial effects of LPS, which suggests that the vasoprotective effects of LPS are mediated by peroxynitrite produced by the reaction of iNOS-derived NO with NOX2-derived superoxide.[168] As discussed by Kunz et al.,[168] these findings are of interest because they indicate that peroxynitrite, in addition to its well-known deleterious vascular actions, can also protect cerebral blood vessels from the vascular dysregulation associated with cerebral ischemia.

FROM BENCH TO BEDSIDE

As already discussed, data from animal stroke models provide a strong rationale for therapies directed at limiting the effects of certain components of inflammation in the post-ischemic period. Several clinical trials have used anti-inflammatory approaches to treat ischemic stroke, with mixed results (Table 10-5). A clinical trial using murine antibodies against ICAM-1 has failed to show a benefit in patients with ischemic stroke. This murine monoclonal antibody against ICAM-1 (enlimomab) was evaluated for clinical efficacy in a prospective, randomized, blinded, phase 3 trial in 625 patients presenting within 6 hours after onset of symptoms.[207] Treatment with anti-ICAM-1 antibodies was associated with a higher mortality rate and slightly larger infarct sizes.[208] Fever affected nearly twice as many patients treated with enlimomab as patients receiving placebo. The reasons for the failure of anti-ICAM antibodies to ameliorate ischemic stroke in humans are not entirely clear and have been the subject of extensive debates.[103,209] One likely possibility is that administration of heterologous antibodies leads to immunologic side effects, resulting in the worsening of tissue damage. This scenario is supported by the findings that enlimomab promotes activation of human neutrophils[208] and, in preclinical stroke models, was found to activate complement, induce anti-mouse antibodies, and enhance expression of the adhesion molecules P- and E-selectin as well as ICAM-1.[209,210] Furthermore, sensitization to enlimomab before induction of cerebral ischemia enhances infarct volume.[210] Therefore, future clinical studies testing anti-inflammatory strategies based on heterologous proteins will have to take these factors into consideration to avoid deleterious immune-mediated side effects in patients with stroke.

The HALT stroke trial used humanized anti Mac-1 antibodies (Hu23F2G; LeukoArrest) in patients presenting within 12 hours after onset of symptoms. The trial was stopped after enrolling 400 patients because of lack of improvement of functional outcomes.[211] However, in preclinical studies, Hu23F2G was effective when administered 20 minutes after ischemia[212] and was not tested at the time window used in the clinical trial (12 hours after a stroke).[211] The ASTIN trial tested the recombinant neutrophil inhibitory factor (rNIF), a non-antibody small molecule, in acute stroke with a 6-hour time window. Patients presenting within 3 hours were also treated with tissue plasminogen activator (t-PA) or placebo. The trial was terminated prematurely after enrolling 966 patients because of lack of efficacy.[213] Notwithstanding the limitations of the ICAM-1 and rNIF trials, these clinical observations raise the possibility that modification of leukocyte trafficking by agents like enlimomab and NIF does not offer apparent benefit in human stroke. Therefore, therapeutic approaches based solely on prevention of leukocyte infiltration must be carefully reevaluated before further application in patients with stroke. In particular, clinical trials need to be based on rigorous preclinical studies designed to mimic as closely as possible the conditions of the trial (e.g., dosing, therapeutic window, sexually dimorphic effects, and effective brain concentrations). These efforts will be facilitated by new imaging approaches to monitor treatment effects by examination of the trafficking of inflammatory cells in the postischemic brain.[5] In contrast to these negative results, phase 2 trials with IL-1

TABLE 10-5 Selected Clinical Trials of Anti-Inflammatory Treatments in Ischemic Stroke

Name of Trial	Phase	No. of Patients	Agent(s) Used	Time Window	Primary Endpoint	Effect	Reference
High-dose steroid treatment in cerebral infarction	2a	113	Dexamethasone	<48 h	Death at day 21, TSSS at days 2, 4, 6, 8, 10, 12, 21	No	Norris et al.[226]
EAST (Enlimomab Acute Stroke Trial)	3	625	Enlimomab (murine anti-ICAM-1 antibody)	<6 h	mRS at 90 days	No	Investigators EAST[207]
HALT (Hu23F2G Phase 3 Stroke Trial)	3	400 (stopped)	LeukoArrest (Hu23F2G, humanized anti-Mac-1 antibody)	<12 h	—	No	Becker[227]
ASTIN (Acute Stroke Therapy by Inhibition of Neutrophils)	3	966	rNIF (recombinant neutrophil inhibitory factor), UK-279, 276	<6 h	SSS at 90 days	No	Krams et al.[213]
Study of interleukin-1 receptor antagonist in acute stroke patients	2	34	IL-1ra (interleukin-1 receptor antagonist)	<6 h	Increase in NIHSS score >4 points within 72 h	Improved outcome	Emsley et al.[228]
Minocycline treatment in acute stroke	2	152	Minocycline (inhibitor of microglial activation)	6–24 h	NIHSS at 90 days	Improved outcome	Lampl et al.[229]
ONO-2506 in Acute Ischemic Stroke	2/3	757	Arundic acid (synonym: ONO-2506, MK0724; modulator of astrocytic activation)	<72 h	mRS at 90 days	N/A	Completed
RREACT (Rapid Response with an Astrocyte Modulator for the Treatment of Acute Cortical Stroke)	2	1320	Arundic acid (ONO-2506, MK0724; modulator of astrocytic activation)	<6 h	mRS at 90 days	N/A	Terminated
MINOS (Minocycline to Improve Neurologic Outcome Study)	2	60	Minocycline (inhibitor of microglial activation)	<6 h	Adverse events within 90 days	Safe and well tolerated alone or with rt-PA	Fagan et al.[230]
APCAST (Activated Protein C in Acute Stroke Trial)	2	72	Activated protein C	<6 h	Adverse events (major ICH) at 36–48 h	N/A	Terminated
Enoxaparin and/or minocycline in acute stroke		64	Minocycline + Enoxaparin	<6 h	Indices of salvaged brain tissue	N/A	Terminated

ICAM-1, intercellular adhesion molecule-1; ICH, intracranial hemorrhage; Mac-1, macrophage-1 antigen complex; mRS, modified Rankin Scale; N/A, not available; NIHSS, National Institutes of Health Stroke Scale; SSS, Scandinavian Stroke Scale; TSSS, Toronto Stroke Scoring System.

receptor antagonists or with the broad-spectrum anti-inflammatory agent minocycline have reported improvement in functional outcomes (see Table 10-5). The outcomes of these trials suggest optimism in the quest for an effective treatment for stroke, but the findings need to be confirmed and expanded in larger double-blind trials. A current large double-blind trial with Canakinumab, a human monoclonal antibody that selectively neutralizes IL-1β, will help in this regard.[214]

Immunologic tolerance to antigens found in the brain or on luminal endothelium has found application in preclinical stroke models. Oral tolerance is a well-established model whereby immunologic tolerance is induced to a specific antigen through feeding of that antigen.[215] Orally administered antigen encounters the gut-associated lymphoid tissue (GALT), which forms a well-developed immune network. GALT has evolved to protect the host from ingested pathogens and, perhaps by necessity, has developed the inherent property of preventing the host from reacting to ingested proteins that are innocuous. The nature of the tolerance depends on the schedule and amount of antigen feeding. Clonal deletion of antigen-reactive T cells can occur after a single feeding of very high doses of antigen.[216] Active tolerance with production of regulatory T cells occurs after repetitive feedings of low doses of antigen.[217,218] On antigen restimulation, T cells made tolerant with a low-dose regimen secrete cytokines such as transforming growth factor β1 (TGF-β1) and IL-10, which suppress cell-mediated, or TH1, immune responses.[218] Although activation of these T cells is specific for the tolerance-causing antigen, the immunomodulatory cytokines secreted in response to activation have non-specific effects. Thus, local immunosuppression occurs wherever the tolerance-causing antigen is present. This phenomenon, known as active cellular regulation or bystander suppression, leads to relatively organ-specific immunosuppression.[219] Other forms of mucosal tolerance have also been investigated, specifically the administration of antigen via the nasal or aerosol route. The nasal route appears equal in efficiency to, and in some instances even more effective than, the oral route in suppressing autoimmune diseases in animal models.[220] Controlling inflammation in the brain by inducing oral tolerance to the CNS antigen, myelin basic protein (MBP), has been reported to result in smaller infarcts after MCA occlusion in the rat.[221] Repetitive intranasal administration of E-selectin to induce mucosal tolerance in the spontaneously hypertensive, genetically stroke-prone rat with untreated hypertension has been observed to potently inhibit development of ischemic and hemorrhagic strokes.[222] Translational development of mucosal tolerance to E-selectin is continuing. Assessment of the clinical utility of these approaches will require further testing.

Another approach targets the effector proteins that initiate the cellular changes and damage triggered by post-ischemic inflammation. Cytokines, their receptors and iNOS would be suitable targets. Interventions targeting more broadly inflammatory signaling might be an attractive opportunity. Such signaling elements may include the transcription factors IRF-1 and NF-κB and their activators, including TLRs and scavenger receptors. However, considering the double-edged role of inflammation – destructive in the acute phase and beneficial in the repair phase – modulation of inflammatory signaling has to be carefully timed to the stage of evolution of the damage and tailored to target specific immune cell populations.

CONCLUSIONS

A growing body of evidence suggests that ischemia-induced inflammation might play an important role in various stages of cerebral ischemic injury. The use of anti-inflammatory strategies in ischemic stroke therapy is attractive because they have a wider therapeutic window than the now-predominant approaches based on reperfusion. Studies in animal stroke models indicate that interventions aimed at attenuating the infiltration of leukocytes may have a beneficial effect in ameliorating the progression of ischemic brain damage. However, clinical trials that utilize anti-leukocyte agents have failed to show benefits. Results of preclinical studies have recently revealed a previously unrecognized role for lymphocytes in ischemic brain injury. Therefore, modulation of the trafficking and/or function of specific lymphocyte subtypes might be a powerful new tool for influencing the outcome of ischemic brain injury. New strategies that create tolerance to selected brain antigens also offer the potential of considerable neuroprotection. However, additional translational studies are needed to develop strategies that would be suitable for application in stroke patients. Theoretically, given the multiplicity of the factors controlling post-ischemic inflammation, strategies targeted against upstream regulatory elements that control a wide array of inflammatory pathways, such as transcription factors or immunomodulatory cells, would be preferable to strategies targeting individual effectors of damage. However, because certain aspects of inflammation are needed for tissue repair, silencing specific effectors of damage at a certain time after the unfolding of the ischemic cascade should also be considered. A comprehensive therapeutic approach based on anti-inflammatory strategies will require a more complete understanding of the multifaceted effects of inflammation in the ischemic brain.

Acknowledgments

Supported by grants from the National Institutes of Health (JA: NS081179; CI: NS034179 and NS073666).

The complete reference list can be found on the companion Expert Consult website at www.expertconsult.inkling.com.

KEY REFERENCES

1. Lipton P. Ischemic cell death in brain neurons. Physiol Rev 1999;79:1431–568.
2. Allan SM, Rothwell NJ. Cytokines and acute neurodegeneration. Nat Rev Neurosci 2001;2:734–44.
3. Emerich DF, Dean RL 3rd, Bartus RT. The role of leukocytes following cerebral ischemia: pathogenic variable or bystander reaction to emerging infarct? Exp Neurol 2002;173:168–81.
4. Iadecola C, Anrather J. The immunology of stroke: from mechanisms to translation. Nat Med 2011;17:796–808. PMCID: 3137275.
6. Barone FC, Feuerstein GZ. Inflammatory mediators and stroke: new opportunities for novel therapeutics. J Cereb Blood Flow Metab 1999;19:819–34.
7. Frijns CJ, Kappelle LJ. Inflammatory cell adhesion molecules in ischemic cerebrovascular disease. Stroke 2002;33:2115–22.
8. Ogata J, Yamanishi H, Pantoni L. Neuropathology of ischemic brain injury. Handb Clin Neurol 2009;92:93–116.
9. Wang Q, Tang XN, Yenari MA. The inflammatory response in stroke. J Neuroimmunol 2007;184:53–68. PMCID: 1868538.
13. del Zoppo G, Ginis I, Hallenbeck JM, et al. Inflammation and stroke: putative role for cytokines, adhesion molecules and iNOS in brain response to ischemia. Brain Pathol 2000;10:95–112.
14. Ritter LS, Orozco JA, Coull BM, et al. Leukocyte accumulation and hemodynamic changes in the cerebral microcirculation during early reperfusion after stroke. Stroke 2000;31: 1153–61.
15. Feuerstein GZ, Wang X, Barone FC. The role of cytokines in the neuropathology of stroke and neurotrauma. Neuroimmunomodulation 1998;5:143–59.
16. Heinel LA, Rubin S, Rosenwasser RH, et al. Leukocyte involvement in cerebral infarct generation after ischemia and reperfusion. Brain Res Bull 1994;34:137–41.
17. Matsuo Y, Onodera H, Shiga Y, et al. Correlation between myeloperoxidase-quantified neutrophil accumulation and ischemic brain injury in the rat. Effects of neutrophil depletion. Stroke 1994;25:1469–75.
18. Jiang N, Moyle M, Soule HR, et al. Neutrophil inhibitory factor is neuroprotective after focal ischemia in rats. Ann Neurol 1995;38:935–42.
19. Zhang RL, Chopp M, Li Y, et al. Anti-ICAM-1 antibody reduces ischemic cell damage after transient middle cerebral artery occlusion in the rat. Neurology 1994;44:1747–51.
20. Mori E, del Zoppo GJ, Chambers JD, et al. Inhibition of polymorphonuclear leukocyte adherence suppresses no-reflow after focal cerebral ischemia in baboons. Stroke 1992;23:712–18.
21. Chen H, Chopp M, Zhang RL, et al. Anti-CD11b monoclonal antibody reduces ischemic cell damage after transient focal cerebral ischemia in rat. Ann Neurol 1994;35:458–63.
23. Morikawa E, Zhang SM, Seko Y, et al. Treatment of focal cerebral ischemia with synthetic oligopeptide corresponding to lectin domain of selectin. Stroke 1996;27:951–5, discussion 956.
25. Connolly ES Jr, Winfree CJ, Prestigiacomo CJ, et al. Exacerbation of cerebral injury in mice that express the P-selectin gene: identification of P-selectin blockade as a new target for the treatment of stroke. Circ Res 1997;81:304–10.
26. Soriano SG, Coxon A, Wang YF, et al. Mice deficient in Mac-1 (CD11b/CD18) are less susceptible to cerebral ischemia/reperfusion injury. Stroke 1999;30:134–9.
27. Connolly ES Jr, Winfree CJ, Springer TA, et al. Cerebral protection in homozygous null ICAM-1 mice after middle cerebral artery occlusion. Role of neutrophil adhesion in the pathogenesis of stroke. J Clin Invest 1996;97:209–16. PMCID: 507081.
28. Dawson DA, Martin D, Hallenbeck JM. Inhibition of tumor necrosis factor-alpha reduces focal cerebral ischemic injury in the spontaneously hypertensive rat. Neurosci Lett 1996;218:41–4.
30. Yamasaki Y, Matsuura N, Shozuhara H, et al. Interleukin-1 as a pathogenetic mediator of ischemic brain damage in rats. Stroke 1995;26:676–80, discussion 681.
32. Loddick SA, Turnbull AV, Rothwell NJ. Cerebral interleukin-6 is neuroprotective during permanent focal cerebral ischemia in the rat. J Cereb Blood Flow Metab 1998;18:176–9.
33. Yang GY, Schielke GP, Gong C, et al. Expression of tumor necrosis factor-alpha and intercellular adhesion molecule-1 after focal cerebral ischemia in interleukin-1beta converting enzyme deficient mice. J Cereb Blood Flow Metab 1999;19:1109–17.
34. Matsumoto T, Ikeda K, Mukaida N, et al. Prevention of cerebral edema and infarct in cerebral reperfusion injury by an antibody to interleukin-8. Lab Invest 1997;77:119–25.

35. Yamasaki Y, Matsuo Y, Zagorski J, et al. New therapeutic possibility of blocking cytokine-induced neutrophil chemoattractant on transient ischemic brain damage in rats. Brain Res 1997;759: 103–11.
36. del Zoppo GJ, Schmid-Schonbein GW, Mori E, et al. Polymorphonuclear leukocytes occlude capillaries following middle cerebral artery occlusion and reperfusion in baboons. Stroke 1991; 22:1276–83.
37. Yilmaz G, Arumugam TV, Stokes KY, et al. Role of T lymphocytes and interferon-gamma in ischemic stroke. Circulation 2006;113: 2105–12.
41. Wang X, Yue TL, Barone FC, et al. Concomitant cortical expression of TNF-alpha and IL-1 beta mRNAs follows early response gene expression in transient focal ischemia. Mol Chem Neuropathol 1994;23:103–14.
46. Barone FC, Arvin B, White RF, et al. Tumor necrosis factor-alpha. A mediator of focal ischemic brain injury. Stroke 1997;28: 1233–44.
47. Garcia JH, Liu KF, Relton JK. Interleukin-1 receptor antagonist decreases the number of necrotic neurons in rats with middle cerebral artery occlusion. Am J Pathol 1995;147:1477–86. PMCID: 1869513.
48. Relton JK, Rothwell NJ. Interleukin-1 receptor antagonist inhibits ischaemic and excitotoxic neuronal damage in the rat. Brain Res Bull 1992;29:243–6.
49. Rothwell NJ, Relton JK. Involvement of interleukin-1 and lipocortin-1 in ischaemic brain damage. Cerebrovasc Brain Metab Rev 1993;5:178–98.
50. Martin D, Chinookoswong N, Miller G. The interleukin-1 receptor antagonist (rhIL-1ra) protects against cerebral infarction in a rat model of hypoxia-ischemia. Exp Neurol 1994;130:362–7.
53. Liesz A, Suri-Payer E, Veltkamp C, et al. Regulatory T cells are key cerebroprotective immunomodulators in acute experimental stroke. Nat Med 2009;15:192–9.
54. Iadecola C, Salkowski CA, Zhang F, et al. The transcription factor interferon regulatory factor 1 is expressed after cerebral ischemia and contributes to ischemic brain injury. J Exp Med 1999; 189:719–27. PMCID: 2192924.
57. Bruce AJ, Boling W, Kindy MS, et al. Altered neuronal and microglial responses to excitotoxic and ischemic brain injury in mice lacking TNF receptors. Nat Med 1996;2:788–94.
58. Yang L, Lindholm K, Konishi Y, et al. Target depletion of distinct tumor necrosis factor receptor subtypes reveals hippocampal neuron death and survival through different signal transduction pathways. J Neurosci 2002;22:3025–32.
61. Goldmann T, Wieghofer P, Muller PF, et al. A new type of microglia gene targeting shows TAK1 to be pivotal in CNS autoimmune inflammation. Nat Neurosci 2013;16:1618–26.
62. Rupalla K, Allegrini PR, Sauer D, et al. Time course of microglia activation and apoptosis in various brain regions after permanent focal cerebral ischemia in mice. Acta Neuropathol 1998;96: 172–8.
64. Morrison HW, Filosa JA. A quantitative spatiotemporal analysis of microglia morphology during ischemic stroke and reperfusion. J Neuroinflammation 2013;10:4. PMCID: 3570327.
65. Schilling M, Besselmann M, Leonhard C, et al. Microglial activation precedes and predominates over macrophage infiltration in transient focal cerebral ischemia: a study in green fluorescent protein transgenic bone marrow chimeric mice. Exp Neurol 2003;183:25–33.
66. Lalancette-Hebert M, Gowing G, Simard A, et al. Selective ablation of proliferating microglial cells exacerbates ischemic injury in the brain. J Neurosci 2007;27:2596–605.
69. Kaito M, Araya S, Gondo Y, et al. Relevance of distinct monocyte subsets to clinical course of ischemic stroke patients. PLoS ONE 2013;8:e69409. PMCID: 3732285.
70. Urra X, Villamor N, Amaro S, et al. Monocyte subtypes predict clinical course and prognosis in human stroke. J Cereb Blood Flow Metab 2009;29:994–1002.
71. Gliem M, Mausberg AK, Lee JI, et al. Macrophages prevent hemorrhagic infarct transformation in murine stroke models. Ann Neurol 2012;71:743–52.
72. Becker K, Kindrick D, Relton J, et al. Antibody to the alpha4 integrin decreases infarct size in transient focal cerebral ischemia in rats. Stroke 2001;32:206–11.
73. Relton JK, Sloan KE, Frew EM, et al. Inhibition of alpha4 integrin protects against transient focal cerebral ischemia in normotensive and hypertensive rats. Stroke 2001;32:199–205.
74. Prestigiacomo CJ, Kim SC, Connolly ES Jr, et al. CD18-mediated neutrophil recruitment contributes to the pathogenesis of reperfused but not nonreperfused stroke. Stroke 1999;30:1110–17.
77. Hu X, Li P, Guo Y, et al. Microglia/macrophage polarization dynamics reveal novel mechanism of injury expansion after focal cerebral ischemia. Stroke 2012;43:3063–70.
78. Schilling M, Besselmann M, Muller M, et al. Predominant phagocytic activity of resident microglia over hematogenous macrophages following transient focal cerebral ischemia: an investigation using green fluorescent protein transgenic bone marrow chimeric mice. Exp Neurol 2005;196:290–7.
79. Neher JJ, Emmrich JV, Fricker M, et al. Phagocytosis executes delayed neuronal death after focal brain ischemia. Proc Natl Acad Sci U S A 2013;110:E4098–107. PMCID: 3808587.
81. Felger JC, Abe T, Kaunzner UW, et al. Brain dendritic cells in ischemic stroke: time course, activation state, and origin. Brain Behav Immun 2010;24:724–37. PMCID: 2885548.
83. Ahmed SH, He YY, Nassief A, et al. Effects of lipopolysaccharide priming on acute ischemic brain injury. Stroke 2000;31: 193–9.
84. Enzmann G, Mysiorek C, Gorina R, et al. The neurovascular unit as a selective barrier to polymorphonuclear granulocyte (PMN) infiltration into the brain after ischemic injury. Acta Neuropathol 2013;125:395–412. PMCID: 3578720.
85. Dawson DA, Ruetzler CA, Carlos TM, et al. Polymorphonuclear leukocytes and microcirculatory perfusion in acute stroke in the SHR. Keio J Med 1996;45:248–52, discussion 252–3.
86. Rosell A, Cuadrado E, Ortega-Aznar A, et al. MMP-9-positive neutrophil infiltration is associated to blood-brain barrier breakdown and basal lamina type IV collagen degradation during hemorrhagic transformation after human ischemic stroke. Stroke 2008;39:1121–6.
89. Cuartero MI, Ballesteros I, Moraga A, et al. N2 neutrophils, novel players in brain inflammation after stroke: modulation by the PPARgamma agonist rosiglitazone. Stroke 2013;44:3498–508.
91. Strbian D, Kovanen PT, Karjalainen-Lindsberg ML, et al. An emerging role of mast cells in cerebral ischemia and hemorrhage. Ann Med 2009;41:438–50.
92. Hurn PD, Subramanian S, Parker SM, et al. T- and B-cell-deficient mice with experimental stroke have reduced lesion size and inflammation. J Cereb Blood Flow Metab 2007;27:1798–805. PMCID: 2592689.
93. Kleinschnitz C, Schwab N, Kraft P, et al. Early detrimental T-cell effects in experimental cerebral ischemia are neither related to adaptive immunity nor thrombus formation. Blood 2010;115: 3835–42.
94. Gelderblom M, Weymar A, Bernreuther C, et al. Neutralization of the IL-17 axis diminishes neutrophil invasion and protects from ischemic stroke. Blood 2012;120:3793–802.
95. Shichita T, Sugiyama Y, Ooboshi H, et al. Pivotal role of cerebral interleukin-17-producing gammadeltaT cells in the delayed phase of ischemic brain injury. Nat Med 2009;15:946–50.
97. Planas AM, Chamorro A. Regulatory T cells protect the brain after stroke. Nat Med 2009;15:138–9.
98. Ren X, Akiyoshi K, Dziennis S, et al. Regulatory B cells limit CNS inflammation and neurologic deficits in murine experimental stroke. J Neurosci 2011;31:8556–63. PMCID: 3111929.
100. Becker KJ. Sensitization and tolerization to brain antigens in stroke. Neuroscience 2009;158:1090–7. PMCID: 2684331.
101. Prass K, Meisel C, Hoflich C, et al. Stroke-induced immunodeficiency promotes spontaneous bacterial infections and is mediated by sympathetic activation reversal by poststroke T helper cell type 1-like immunostimulation. J Exp Med 2003;198:725–36. PMCID: 2194193.
103. Moskowitz MA, Lo EH, Iadecola C. The science of stroke: mechanisms in search of treatments. Neuron 2010;67:181–98. PMCID: 2957363.
104. Hallenbeck JM, Frerichs KU. Secondary ischemic neuronal damage may involve multiple factors acting as an aggregate of minor causes. In: Robertson JT, Nowak TS, editors. Frontiers in cerebrovascular disease: Mechanisms, diagnosis, and treatment. Armonk, NY: Futura Publishing Company, Inc; 1998. p. 95–101.

107. Lee YJ, Hallenbeck JM. Insights into cytoprotection from ground squirrel hibernation, a natural model of tolerance to profound brain oligaemia. Biochem Soc Trans 2006;34:1295–8. PMCID: 1850989.
109. Zedler S, Faist E. The impact of endogenous triggers on trauma-associated inflammation. Curr Opin Crit Care 2006;12: 595–601.
111. Kim JB, Sig Choi J, Yu YM, et al. HMGB1, a novel cytokine-like mediator linking acute neuronal death and delayed neuroinflammation in the postischemic brain. J Neurosci 2006;26:6413–21.
114. Akira S, Takeda K, Kaisho T. Toll-like receptors: critical proteins linking innate and acquired immunity. Nat Immunol 2001;2: 675–80.
119. Arumugam TV, Okun E, Tang SC, et al. Toll-like receptors in ischemia-reperfusion injury. Shock 2009;32:4–16.
120. Tang SC, Arumugam TV, Xu X, et al. Pivotal role for neuronal Toll-like receptors in ischemic brain injury and functional deficits. Proc Natl Acad Sci U S A 2007;104:13798–803. PMCID: 1959462.
121. Ziegler G, Harhausen D, Schepers C, et al. TLR2 has a detrimental role in mouse transient focal cerebral ischemia. Biochem Biophys Res Commun 2007;359:574–9.
122. Cao CX, Yang QW, Lv FL, et al. Reduced cerebral ischemia-reperfusion injury in Toll-like receptor 4 deficient mice. Biochem Biophys Res Commun 2007;353:509–14.
123. Caso JR, Pradillo JM, Hurtado O, et al. Toll-like receptor 4 is involved in brain damage and inflammation after experimental stroke. Circulation 2007;115:1599–608.
124. Lehnardt S, Lehmann S, Kaul D, et al. Toll-like receptor 2 mediates CNS injury in focal cerebral ischemia. J Neuroimmunol 2007;190:28–33.
125. Hua F, Ma J, Ha T, et al. Activation of Toll-like receptor 4 signaling contributes to hippocampal neuronal death following global cerebral ischemia/reperfusion. J Neuroimmunol 2007;190:101–11. PMCID: 2453597.
127. Zimmerman GA, Meistrell M 3rd, Bloom O, et al. Neurotoxicity of advanced glycation endproducts during focal stroke and neuroprotective effects of aminoguanidine. Proc Natl Acad Sci U S A 1995;92:3744–8. PMCID: 42038.
129. Scaffidi P, Misteli T, Bianchi ME. Release of chromatin protein HMGB1 by necrotic cells triggers inflammation. Nature 2002;418:191–5.
130. Qiu J, Nishimura M, Wang Y, et al. Early release of HMGB-1 from neurons after the onset of brain ischemia. J Cereb Blood Flow Metab 2008;28:927–38.
131. Muhammad S, Barakat W, Stoyanov S, et al. The HMGB1 receptor RAGE mediates ischemic brain damage. J Neurosci 2008; 28:12023–31.
132. Piccinini AM, Midwood KS. DAMPening inflammation by modulating TLR signalling. Mediators Inflamm 2010;2010:PMCID: 2913853.
133. Sagulenko V, Thygesen SJ, Sester DP, et al. AIM2 and NLRP3 inflammasomes activate both apoptotic and pyroptotic death pathways via ASC. Cell Death Differ 2013;20:1149–60. PMCID: 3741496.
134. Leung PY, Stevens SL, Packard AE, et al. Toll-like receptor 7 preconditioning induces robust neuroprotection against stroke by a novel type I interferon-mediated mechanism. Stroke 2012; 43:1383–9.
135. Martinon F, Tschopp J. Inflammatory caspases and inflammasomes: master switches of inflammation. Cell Death Differ 2007;14:10–22.
139. Silverstein RL, Febbraio M. CD36, a scavenger receptor involved in immunity, metabolism, angiogenesis, and behavior. Sci Signal 2009;2:re3. PMCID: 2811062.
140. Hirano K, Kuwasako T, Nakagawa-Toyama Y, et al. Pathophysiology of human genetic CD36 deficiency. Trends Cardiovasc Med 2003;13:136–41.
142. Stuart LM, Deng J, Silver JM, et al. Response to Staphylococcus aureus requires CD36-mediated phagocytosis triggered by the COOH-terminal cytoplasmic domain. J Cell Biol 2005;170:477–85. PMCID: 2171464.
144. Cho S, Park EM, Febbraio M, et al. The class B scavenger receptor CD36 mediates free radical production and tissue injury in cerebral ischemia. J Neurosci 2005;25:2504–12.
145. Kunz A, Abe T, Hochrainer K, et al. Nuclear factor-kappaB activation and postischemic inflammation are suppressed in CD36-null mice after middle cerebral artery occlusion. J Neurosci 2008;28:1649–58. PMCID: 2588435.
146. Ghosh S, Karin M. Missing pieces in the NF-kappaB puzzle. Cell 2002;109(Suppl.):S81–96.
148. Hallenbeck JM. The many faces of tumor necrosis factor in stroke. Nat Med 2002;8:1363–8.
149. Schwaninger M, Inta I, Herrmann O. NF-kappaB signalling in cerebral ischaemia. Biochem Soc Trans 2006;34:1291–4.
150. Blondeau N, Widmann C, Lazdunski M, et al. Activation of the nuclear factor-kappaB is a key event in brain tolerance. J Neurosci 2001;21:4668–77.
151. Pradillo JM, Romera C, Hurtado O, et al. TNFR1 upregulation mediates tolerance after brain ischemic preconditioning. J Cereb Blood Flow Metab 2005;25:193–203.
152. Perkins ND. Post-translational modifications regulating the activity and function of the nuclear factor kappa B pathway. Oncogene 2006;25:6717–30.
153. Vanden Berghe W, Ndlovu MN, Hoya-Arias R, et al. Keeping up NF-kappaB appearances: epigenetic control of immunity or inflammation-triggered epigenetics. Biochem Pharmacol 2006; 72:1114–31.
156. Carroll JE, Hess DC, Howard EF, et al. Is nuclear factor-kappaB a good treatment target in brain ischemia/reperfusion injury? Neuroreport 2000;11:R1–4.
157. Gabriel C, Justicia C, Camins A, et al. Activation of nuclear factor-kappaB in the rat brain after transient focal ischemia. Brain Res Mol Brain Res 1999;65:61–9.
159. Schneider A, Martin-Villalba A, Weih F, et al. NF-kappaB is activated and promotes cell death in focal cerebral ischemia. Nat Med 1999;5:554–9.
160. Terai K, Matsuo A, McGeer EG, et al. Enhancement of immunoreactivity for NF-kappa B in human cerebral infarctions. Brain Res 1996;739:343–9.
162. Xu L, Zhan Y, Wang Y, et al. Recombinant adenoviral expression of dominant negative IkappaBalpha protects brain from cerebral ischemic injury. Biochem Biophys Res Commun 2002;299: 14–17.
163. Herrmann O, Baumann B, de Lorenzi R, et al. IKK mediates ischemia-induced neuronal death. Nat Med 2005;11:1322–9.
167. Ravati A, Ahlemeyer B, Becker A, et al. Preconditioning-induced neuroprotection is mediated by reactive oxygen species and activation of the transcription factor nuclear factor-kappaB. J Neurochem 2001;78:909–19.
168. Kunz A, Park L, Abe T, et al. Neurovascular protection by ischemic tolerance: role of nitric oxide and reactive oxygen species. J Neurosci 2007;27:7083–93.
169. Gidday JM. Cerebral preconditioning and ischaemic tolerance. Nat Rev Neurosci 2006;7:437–48.
172. Iadecola C, Alexander M, Nogawa S, et al. Inflammation-related genes and ischemic brain injury. In: Krieglstein J, Klumpp S, editors. Pharmacology of cerebral ischemia 2000. Stuttgart: Medpharm Scientific Publishers; 2000. p. 241–51.
173. Yi JH, Park SW, Kapadia R, et al. Role of transcription factors in mediating post-ischemic cerebral inflammation and brain damage. Neurochem Int 2007;50:1014–27. PMCID: 2040388.
176. Berger J, Moller DE. The mechanisms of action of PPARs. Annu Rev Med 2002;53:409–35.
178. Sundararajan S, Gamboa JL, Victor NA, et al. Peroxisome proliferator-activated receptor-gamma ligands reduce inflammation and infarction size in transient focal ischemia. Neuroscience 2005;130:685–96.
179. Luo Y, Yin W, Signore AP, et al. Neuroprotection against focal ischemic brain injury by the peroxisome proliferator-activated receptor-gamma agonist rosiglitazone. J Neurochem 2006; 97:435–48.
180. Zhao Y, Patzer A, Gohlke P, et al. The intracerebral application of the PPARgamma-ligand pioglitazone confers neuroprotection against focal ischaemia in the rat brain. Eur J Neurosci 2005;22: 278–82.
183. Deplanque D, Gele P, Petrault O, et al. Peroxisome proliferator-activated receptor-alpha activation as a mechanism of preventive neuroprotection induced by chronic fenofibrate treatment. J Neurosci 2003;23:6264–71.

185. Nissen SE, Wolski K. Effect of rosiglitazone on the risk of myocardial infarction and death from cardiovascular causes. N Engl J Med 2007;356:2457–71.
188. Noda T, Minatoguchi S, Fujii K, et al. Evidence for the delayed effect in human ischemic preconditioning: prospective multicenter study for preconditioning in acute myocardial infarction. J Am Coll Cardiol 1999;34:1966–74.
189. Marber MS, Baxter GF, Yellon DM. Prodromal angina limits infarct size: a role for ischemic preconditioning. Circulation 1995;92:1061–2.
191. Kitagawa K, Matsumoto M, Tagaya M, et al. 'Ischemic tolerance' phenomenon found in the brain. Brain Res 1990;528:21–4.
192. Weih M, Kallenberg K, Bergk A, et al. Attenuated stroke severity after prodromal TIA: a role for ischemic tolerance in the brain? Stroke 1999;30:1851–4.
193. Moncayo J, de Freitas GR, Bogousslavsky J, et al. Do transient ischemic attacks have a neuroprotective effect? Neurology 2000;54:2089–94.
195. Ohtsuki T, Ruetzler CA, Tasaki K, et al. Interleukin-1 mediates induction of tolerance to global ischemia in gerbil hippocampal CA1 neurons. J Cereb Blood Flow Metab 1996;16:1137–42.
196. Song W, Furman BL, Parratt JR. Delayed protection against ischaemia-induced ventricular arrhythmias and infarct size limitation by the prior administration of *Escherichia coli* endotoxin. Br J Pharmacol 1996;118:2157–63. PMCID: 1909876.
197. Eising GP, Mao L, Schmid-Schonbein GW, et al. Effects of induced tolerance to bacterial lipopolysaccharide on myocardial infarct size in rats. Cardiovasc Res 1996;31:73–81.
199. Tasaki K, Ruetzler CA, Ohtsuki T, et al. Lipopolysaccharide pretreatment induces resistance against subsequent focal cerebral ischemic damage in spontaneously hypertensive rats. Brain Res 1997;748:267–70.
204. Nawashiro H, Tasaki K, Ruetzler CA, et al. TNF-alpha pretreatment induces protective effects against focal cerebral ischemia in mice. J Cereb Blood Flow Metab 1997;17:483–90.
206. Stenzel-Poore MP, Stevens SL, King JS, et al. Preconditioning reprograms the response to ischemic injury and primes the emergence of unique endogenous neuroprotective phenotypes: a speculative synthesis. Stroke 2007;38:680–5.
207. Investigators EAST. Use of anti-ICAM-1 therapy in ischemic stroke: results of the Enlimomab Acute Stroke Trial. Neurology 2001;57:1428–34.
210. Furuya K, Takeda H, Azhar S, et al. Examination of several potential mechanisms for the negative outcome in a clinical stroke trial of enlimomab, a murine anti-human intercellular adhesion molecule-1 antibody: a bedside-to-bench study. Stroke 2001;32:2665–74.
211. Sughrue ME, Mehra A, Connolly ES Jr, et al. Anti-adhesion molecule strategies as potential neuroprotective agents in cerebral ischemia: a critical review of the literature. Inflamm Res 2004;53:497–508.
212. Yenari MA, Kunis D, Sun GH, et al. Hu23F2G, an antibody recognizing the leukocyte CD11/CD18 integrin, reduces injury in a rabbit model of transient focal cerebral ischemia. Exp Neurol 1998;153:223–33.
213. Krams M, Lees KR, Hacke W, et al. Acute Stroke Therapy by Inhibition of Neutrophils (ASTIN): an adaptive dose-response study of UK-279,276 in acute ischemic stroke. Stroke 2003;34:2543–8.
214. Ridker PM, Thuren T, Zalewski A, et al. Interleukin-1beta inhibition and the prevention of recurrent cardiovascular events: rationale and design of the Canakinumab Anti-inflammatory Thrombosis Outcomes Study (CANTOS). Am Heart J 2011;162:597–605.
215. Weiner HL. Oral tolerance: immune mechanisms and treatment of autoimmune diseases. Immunol Today 1997;18:335–43.
216. Chen Y, Inobe J, Marks R, et al. Peripheral deletion of antigen-reactive T cells in oral tolerance. Nature 1995;376:177–80.
218. Chen Y, Kuchroo VK, Inobe J, et al. Regulatory T cell clones induced by oral tolerance: suppression of autoimmune encephalomyelitis. Science 1994;265:1237–40.
219. Faria AM, Weiner HL. Oral tolerance: mechanisms and therapeutic applications. Adv Immunol 1999;73:153–264.
220. Metzler B, Wraith DC. Mucosal tolerance in a murine model of experimental autoimmune encephalomyelitis. Ann N Y Acad Sci 1996;778:228–42.
221. Becker KJ, McCarron RM, Ruetzler C, et al. Immunologic tolerance to myelin basic protein decreases stroke size after transient focal cerebral ischemia. Proc Natl Acad Sci U S A 1997;94:10873–8. PMCID: 23514.
222. Takeda H, Spatz M, Ruetzler C, et al. Induction of mucosal tolerance to E-selectin prevents ischemic and hemorrhagic stroke in spontaneously hypertensive genetically stroke-prone rats. Stroke 2002;33:2156–63.
223. Hayward NJ, Elliott PJ, Sawyer SD, et al. Lack of evidence for neutrophil participation during infarct formation following focal cerebral ischemia in the rat. Exp Neurol 1996;139:188–202.
224. Kim E, Tolhurst AT, Qin LY, et al. CD36/fatty acid translocase, an inflammatory mediator, is involved in hyperlipidemia-induced exacerbation in ischemic brain injury. J Neurosci 2008;28:4661–70. PMCID: 2830708.
225. Abe T, Shimamura M, Jackman K, et al. Key role of CD36 in Toll-like receptor 2 signaling in cerebral ischemia. Stroke 2010;41:898–904. PMCID: 2950279.
226. Norris JW, Hachinski VC. High dose steroid treatment in cerebral infarction. Br Med J (Clin Res Ed) 1986;292:21–3. PMCID: 1338973.
227. Becker KJ. Anti-leukocyte antibodies: LeukArrest (Hu23F2G) and Enlimomab (R6.5) in acute stroke. Curr Med Res Opin 2002;18(Suppl. 2):s18–22.
228. Emsley HC, Smith CJ, Georgiou RF, et al. A randomised phase II study of interleukin-1 receptor antagonist in acute stroke patients. J Neurol Neurosurg Psychiatry 2005;76:1366–72. PMCID: 1739363.
229. Lampl Y, Boaz M, Gilad R, et al. Minocycline treatment in acute stroke: an open-label, evaluator-blinded study. Neurology 2007;69:1404–10.
230. Fagan SC, Waller JL, Nichols FT, et al. Minocycline to improve neurologic outcome in stroke (MINOS): a dose-finding study. Stroke 2010;41:2283–7.

11 Mechanisms of Plasticity, Remodeling and Recovery

Zheng Gang Zhang, Michael Chopp

KEY POINTS

- Neurogenesis, oligodendrogenesis, angiogenesis, astrogliosis and axonal plasticity are major interwoven brain repair processes during stroke recovery.
- Molecules including miRNAs play an important role in mediating these processes.
- Exosomes are mediators of communication among cells and respond to stroke by transferring select RNAs and proteins.
- Cell and pharmacologically based therapies amplify brain repair process, leading to improvement of neurological function.
- New therapies, by targeting miRNAs themselves or by exosomes to deliver target miRNAs, have great potential for promoting brain repair and neurological recovery after stroke.

INTRODUCTION

The ischemic brain has limited repair capacity that leads to some degree of functional recovery. The repair process is multifaceted and involves neurogenesis, angiogenesis, and axonal sprouting and synaptogenesis. Emerging preclinical data indicate that neurorestorative therapies facilitate and amplify these interwoven restorative events and thereby improve functional outcome after stroke. In this chapter, we first review stroke-induced neurogenesis, angiogenesis, and axonal remodeling as well as the coupling of these interacting remodeling events. We restrict discussion to neurogenesis in the ventricular-subventricular zone (V/SVZ) of the lateral ventricle, because stroke primarily induces neuroblasts in the V/SVZ to migrate long distances to the ischemic boundary, where these cells likely contribute to the remodeling of cerebral tissue.[1-5] We then discuss the ways to amplify these events.

Neurogenesis, oligodendrogenesis, angiogenesis, and astrogliosis are major brain repair processes during stroke recovery.[6] Insight into mechanisms that control and coordinate these tightly regulated processes are essential for improving our understanding of developmental and post-stroke brain remodeling and for developing novel strategies to facilitate repair in adult injured brain. Since the last edition, much progress has been made on cellular and molecular mechanisms underlying brain repair after stroke. MicroRNAs (miRNAs), short noncoding RNA molecules of 20 to 25 nucleotides, are involved in physiologic function and in disease processes by controlling the expression of the majority of protein coding genes, mainly at the post-transcriptional level.[7] Circulating miRNAs are transported by exosomes between cells.[8] Recent studies have provided valuable insight into miRNAs and exosomes that regulate brain repair processes after stroke. [9-15] In this chapter, we will review these findings and discuss their potential therapeutic applications to facilitate brain remodeling and neurological recovery post stroke.

NEUROGENESIS IN THE VENTRICULAR-SUBVENTRICULAR ZONE

Neurogenesis in the adult mammalian brain has been investigated and well documented during the last 20 years, although neurogenesis was originally observed in the adult rat brain in the 1960s.[16] In the adult rodent brain, neurogenesis occurs in the SVZ of the lateral ventricle throughout the life of the animal.[1] Neural stem cells have the capacity to undergo unlimited self-renewal and are multipotent, whereas neural progenitor cells exhibit limited self-renewal ability and generate differentiated cell types.[17] During developmental cortical neurogenesis in the rodent, neural stem cells reside in the ventricular zone (VZ) and generate cortical neurons.[18] Radial glial cells located in the VZ and containing radial processes and astroglial properties are neural stem cells, and a subpopulation of radial glia transform into SVZ astrocytes expressing glial fibrillary acidic protein (GFAP) during the early postnatal stage.[1,18] Although earlier studies showed that the VZ is replaced by an ependymal layer while the SVZ shrinks and persists in the adult,[19] new evidence indicates that adult GFAP-positive neural stem cells extend apical processes with a single cilium anchored at the ependymal layer of the ventricular surface to directly contact the cerebrospinal fluid (CSF) and extend their long basal processes to reach blood vessels in the SVZ just beneath the ependymal layer; this localized architecture is referred to as a ventricular-subventricular zone (V/SVZ) niche.[20] GFAP-positive neural stem cells (type B cells) produce neural progenitor cells that are transient amplifying cells (type C cells).[1,21] The neural progenitor cells in turn differentiate into neuroblasts (type A cells) and oligodendrocytes. More than 30,000 neuroblasts are generated daily in the adult rodent V/SVZ.[1,22,23] Neuroblasts generated in the V/SVZ travel via the rostral migratory stream (RMS) to the olfactory bulb, where they differentiate into granule and periglomerular neurons.[1] In the adult human brain, neural stem cells are present in a ribbon of SVZ astrocytes, and a rostral migratory stream is organized around a lateral ventricular extension to the olfactory bulb.[24]

During 2001 and 2002, using 5-bromo-2′-deoxyuridine (BrdU; labels new DNA in the S phase of the cell cycle) and antibodies against β -tubulin III (TuJ1, a marker of immature neurons) and doublecortin (DCX, a marker of neuroblasts), several groups demonstrated that experimental focal cerebral ischemia induces neurogenesis in the ipsilateral SVZ of the adult rodent.[2,25-27] Newly generated neuroblasts in the SVZ migrate to the ischemic boundary where they exhibit neuronal phenotypes.[2,25-27] Since then, many experimental studies have confirmed these findings.[28-30] Patients with stroke also exhibit an increase in neural progenitor cells and neuroblasts in the ipsilateral SVZ, even in patients of advanced age.[31-35] Although cortical neurogenesis has been reported in human stroke, recent studies using genomic and carbon-14 dating approaches fail to demonstrate the presence of neurogenesis in the human neocortex after stroke.[36]

PROLIFERATION AND DIFFERENTIATION OF NEURAL STEM AND PROGENITOR CELLS AFTER STROKE

In a rat model of focal cerebral ischemia, neural progenitor cell proliferation is increased starting 2 days after stroke. The proliferation reaches a maximum between 4 and 7 days after stroke and then decreases to levels observed 2 days after stroke.[37,38] These data indicate that proliferation of neural progenitor cells contributes to stroke-induced neurogenesis. Under physiologic conditions, proliferation of progenitor cells is tightly controlled by cell-cycle kinetics.[39] The proportion of proliferating cells and the length of the cell cycle are two critical parameters of the cytokinetics for neocortical neurogenesis.[39] In the V/SVZ of the adult rat, approximately 15–21% of the neural progenitor cells are actively dividing with a cell cycle ranging from 18 to 21 hours.[37,40] Stroke transiently increases the percentage of dividing V/SVZ neural progenitor cells to 31%.[37] Analysis of cell-cycle phases of actively proliferating V/SVZ neural progenitor cells reveals that the cell-cycle length of these mitotic cells changes dynamically over a period of 2–14 days after stroke.[37,41] The cell-cycle length reduces to 11 hours at 2 days after stroke, which is significantly shorter than the cell-cycle length of 19 hours in non-ischemic V/SVZ cells.[37,41] Reduction of the cell cycle induced by stroke likely results from a decrease of the G1 phase of the cell cycle because the G2, M, and S phases are unchanged. The length of the cell cycle returns to the non-stroke level 14 days after stroke.[37,41] The reduction of the G1 phase is correlated with an increase in the dividing SVZ cell population, whereas an augmentation of the cell population that exits the cell cycle is associated with lengthening of the G1 phase.[37,41] The cells that exit the cell cycle differentiate into neuroblasts.[37,41] Thus, these data suggest that stroke triggers early expansion of the progenitor pool via shortening of the cell-cycle length and a retention of daughter cells within the cell cycle, and the lengthening of G1 leads to exit of daughter cells from the cell cycle and their differentiation into neurons.

The stem cells in the SVZ of the adult rodent constitute approximately 2% of the total population of V/SVZ cells and are relatively quiescent with a cell cycle of approximately 15 days.[17,42] To allow investigation of the effect of stroke on neural stem cells, neural progenitor cells and neuroblasts in the V/SVZ are eliminated by infusion of an antimitotic agent (cytosine-β-D-arabiofuranoside, Ara-C) for 7 days; this infusion does not ablate the relatively quiescent neural stem cells in the SVZ.[3] Seven days after termination of the Ara-C infusion, neural progenitor cells are entirely repopulated in the SVZ after stroke, whereas repopulation of neural progenitor cells in the SVZ takes 14 days in non-ischemic SVZ.[3] These findings suggest that after stroke, neural stem cells accelerate the generation of neural progenitor cells, leading to augmentation of neurogenesis.

Gene profile analysis demonstrates that adult SVZ neural progenitor cells are actively proliferating.[43,44] The neural progenitor cells express many genes that are involved in the biologic processes of cell proliferation and cell cycle, which are not expressed by cells in the cerebral cortex, the hippocampus, and the olfactory bulb.[45] Among these genes are minichromosome maintenance (MCM) genes, cyclin-dependent kinases (CDKs), and CDK inhibitors.[43,46] MCM genes are essential for all dividing cells, and CDK and CDK inhibitors mediate the cell cycle during G1 phase.[43,46–48] Knockout of p21cip and p27kip genes results in increased proliferation of SVZ neural stem and progenitor cells, respectively.[48] Stroke substantially upregulates MCM2 expression and downregulates p27Kip1 in neural progenitor cells.[37,49]

miRNAs complementarily bind to 3′ untranslated regions of target mRNAs to repress their translation and stability.[7] Expression of miRNAs in neural progenitor cells after experimental stroke has been profiled.[50] Stroke down- and up regulated 18 and 21 mature miRNAs, respectively, in SVZ neural progenitor cells compared to non-stroke.[50] Bioinformatics analysis revealed that these stroke-altered miRNAs selectively affect several signaling pathways including transforming growth factor β (TGFβ), Wnt, and Shh signals that are known to regulate neural stem cell function.[50]

The miR17-92 cluster is one of the more robustly upregulated miRNAs in V/SVZ neural progenitor cells after stroke.[50,51] The miR17-92 cluster comprises a cluster of six miRNAs (miR-17, miR-18a, miR-19a, miR-20a, miR-19b-1, and miR-92a-1) on chromosome 13, which is transcribed as a single polycistronic unit.[52] The biological function of the miR-17-92 cluster has been extensively studied in cancer research, but its impact on stroke-induced neurogenesis is just being explored.[12] Overexpression of the miR17-92 cluster in neural progenitor cells enhanced stroke-induced progenitor cell proliferation, whereas attenuation of endogenous members of the miR-17-92 cluster, miR-18a and miR-19a, abolished the neural progenitor cell proliferation increased by stroke. The positive effect of the miR17-92 cluster on neurogenesis is partially attributed to suppression of phosphatase and tensin homolog deleted on chromosome 10 (PTEN), a protein known to negatively regulate embryonic neural stem cell proliferation and survival.[53,54] In the development of mouse neurocortex, the miR17-92 cluster controls neural progenitor cell proliferation by targeting PTEN and the transcription factor Tbr 2.[55,56] Germline deletion of the miR17-92 cluster in patients with Feingold syndrome, an autosomal dominant syndrome, causes microcephaly and skeletal abnormalities.[57] Collectively, these data suggest that the miR17-92 cluster is required for maintaining pools of neural progenitor cells.

The sonic-hedgehog (Shh) pathway is a key signaling pathway in regulating adult neurogenesis and also mediates stroke-induced neurogenesis.[58] Recent studies indicate that the Shh signaling pathway in neural progenitor cells regulates miR17-92 cluster expression by one of the Shh downstream proteins, c-Myc, which binds to the promoter region of the miR17-92 cluster.[59] Stroke enhances the binding of c-Myc to the promoter region of the miR17-92 cluster in neural progenitor cells.[51] In cultured neural progenitor cells, attenuation of endogenous Shh and addition of exogenous Shh down- and up regulate the miR17-92 cluster expression, respectively.[51] Intraventricular administration of exogenous Shh to stroke animals further upregulates the miR17-92 cluster expression in V/SVZ neural progenitor cells, whereas blockage of the Shh pathway suppresses ischemia-upregulated miR17-92 cluster expression and ischemia-increased neural progenitor cell proliferation.[51] Thus, the miR17-92 cluster in neural progenitor cells likely mediates processes of Shh-induced neural progenitor cell proliferation.

miR-124a is abundant in the adult brain.[60] In adult neural progenitor cells, miR-124a regulates neuronal differentiation by targeting SRY-box transcription factor 9 (SOX9).[61] Stroke reduces miR-124a expression in SVZ neural progenitor cells, which induces neural progenitor cell proliferation by targeting Jagged-1 (JAG1), a ligand that activates the Notch receptors.[62] The Notch signaling pathway plays a pivotal role in maintaining the embryonic neural stem cell pool and promotes gliogenesis.[63] Activation of the Notch pathway by stroke increases neural progenitor cell proliferation, whereas blockage of the Notch pathway abolishes stroke-increased progenitor cell proliferation.[64] These data suggest that miR-124a mediates adult neurogenesis either by targeting SOX9 or the Notch signaling pathway under non-ischemic and ischemic conditions.

In addition, stroke downregulates Let-7 and miR-9 in neural progenitor cells[50] and these miRNAs regulate adult neurogenesis by controlling the balance between the proliferation and differentiation of neural stem cells through the TLX nuclear receptor.[65] Wnt/β-catenin signaling represses Let 7 in tumor cells, while miR-92 regulates bone morphogenic protein (BMP) signals.[66,67] Wnt and BMP regulate neurogenesis in the adult brain.[68,69] Stroke changes expression of Wnt and BMP family genes in SVZ neural progenitor cells of the adult rodent.[70,71] Collectively, these data suggest that stroke-altered miRNAs in adult neural progenitor cells are closely associated with signaling pathways known to regulate stroke-induced neurogenesis. Manipulation of selective miRNAs could potentially amplify endogenous neurogenesis after brain injury including stroke.

MIGRATION AND SURVIVAL OF NEUROBLASTS AFTER STROKE

Neuroblasts generated in the ipsilateral V/SVZ migrate to the ischemic boundary.[2-4] Non-invasive MRI measurements show that intracisternal transplantation SVZ cells labeled by ferromagnetic particles selectively migrate into the ischemic boundary.[72] Among many molecules that regulate neuroblast migration, stromal-derived factor-1 α (SDF-1 α), a CXC chemokine, appears to play an important role in mediating neuroblast migration to the ischemic boundary. SDF-1 α secreted by astrocytes and endothelial cells in the ischemic boundary attracts SVZ neuroblasts that express the SDF-1 α receptor, CXCR4.[73,74] Blockage of either SDF-1 α or CXCR4 suppresses neuroblast migration to the ischemic boundary.[75] In addition, vascular endothelial growth factor (VEGF), angiopoietin-1 (Ang1) and matrix metalloproteinases (MMPs) regulate neuroblast migration after stroke.[6] Thus, multiple factors in the ischemic brain may orchestrate neuroblast migration. Neuroblasts generated in the V/SVZ migrate to peri-infarct regions and some of them express phenotypes of mature neurons in young and aged animals.[2,30,76] Stroke-induced neurogenesis persists for at least 6 months.[77] Studies using the patch-clamp technique show that the new neurons in the ischemic boundary have electrophysiologic characteristics of mature neurons, suggesting that neuroblasts mature into resident neurons and integrate into local neuronal circuitry.[78] Although few newly generated neurons survive in the peri-infarct region after stroke, ablation of neuroblasts after stroke substantially impairs brain repair and exacerbates functional recovery.[79] These data suggest that in addition to replacing dead neurons, neuroblasts have functions involving brain repair processes.

OLIGODENDROGENESIS

Oligodendrocytes are derived from non-myelinating oligodendrocyte progenitor cells (OPCs) that comprise 3–9% of the total cell number in the adult CNS.[80] OPCs, are present in the corpus callosum, the striatum, and the cortex and are derived from neural progenitor cells in the V/SVZ.[81] In the adult brain, OPCs continuously differentiate into mature oligodendrocytes to myelinate the previously unmyelinated axons throughout the gray and white matter.[82] Recent studies show that in addition to serving as a source to generate myelinating oligodendrocytes,[83] OPCs act as a surveillance network to detect brain injury, while myelination in adult brain contributes to maintaining axonal integrity, neural plasticity and circuitry function in addition to facilitating saltatory conduction.[84]

Mature oligodendrocytes are vulnerable to stroke, and damage of mature oligodendrocytes leads to loss of myelin and axons.[85] New oligodendrocytes are required to form myelin sheaths for sprouting axons during brain repair processes after stroke, because mature oligodendrocytes do not proliferate in the adult brain and injured oligodendrocytes no longer form new myelin sheets.[81,82] Failure of remyelination of axons after stroke likely leads to axonal degeneration and consequently to cognitive impairment.[86] However, there is a paucity of studies which investigate oligodendrogenesis, including OPC proliferation and differentiation, during brain repair processes after stroke.[87] Using an inducible cre-lox fate mapping strategy in adult neural progenitor cells of transgenic mice, recent studies demonstrate that mature oligodendrocytes differentiate from OPCs originating in white matter and from SVZ neural progenitor cells and are involved in white matter remodeling after stroke.[88-91] For example, during the first 2 weeks of stroke, there is a robust increase in OPCs in ischemic boundary regions of the gray and white matter. Two months later, some of the OPCs in peri-infarct white matter exhibit myelin sheet morphology and express protein components of myelin, cyclic nucleotide 3′-phosphodiesterase (CNPase) and myelin basic protein (MBP).[89,90,92] These data suggest that OPCs in the adult brain contribute to oligodendrogenesis after stroke. Elucidating molecular mechanisms underlying stroke-induced oligodendrogenesis may lead to therapies designed specifically to enhance remyelination.

Oligodendrogenesis is controlled by intrinsic and extrinsic molecules.[81,82] Emerging data indicate that miRNAs are required for maintaining OPCs in the undifferentiated state and for preserving myelin in mature oligodendrocytes.[9] For example, miR-219 and miR-338 are enriched in myelinating oligodendrocytes compared to their levels in OPCs.[93,94] Elevation of miR-219 and miR-338 in OPCs promotes OPC differentiation into mature oligodendrocytes by repressing genes of platelet-derived growth factor receptor α (PDGFRα), Sox6, and Hes5, which are known to inhibit OPC differentiation.[93,94] In addition to differentiation, miRNAs play an important role in OPC survival and proliferation.[93,94] Embryonic deletion of the miR17-92 cluster in OPCs leads to an increase in OPC death and decrease of OPC proliferation, which is likely attributed to inactivation of Akt signals caused by augmentation of PTEN proteins.[95] More importantly, miR-219, miR-338, and the miR-17-92 cluster are enriched in human white matter and expressed in cultured primary human oligodendrocytes.[96] However, the effect of miRNAs on stroke-induced oligodendrogenesis is just beginning to be investigated. Preclinical studies show that stroke considerably downregulates miR-9 and miR-200b in white matter and their levels inversely correlate with the expression of serum response factor (SRF), a transcription factor.[97] Overexpression of miR-9 and miR-200 in cultured rodent OPCs inhibits OPC differentiation by targeting SRF.[97] Additional in vivo experiments focusing on amplification of stroke-induced oligodendrogenesis by modulating miRNA levels are warranted.

ANGIOGENESIS

Vasculogenesis indicates that new vessels are formed by endothelial progenitor cells whereas angiogenesis represents the sprouting of new capillaries from preexisting vessels.[98] Angiogenesis is a multistep process involving endothelial cell proliferation, migration, tube formation, branching, and anastomosis.[99] In the rodent, the cerebral vascular system develops primarily by angiogenesis.[98] The endothelial cells of cerebral capillaries differ functionally and morphologically from those of non-cerebral capillaries.[98] The cerebral endothelial cells are linked by complex tight junctions that form the blood–brain barrier (BBB).[98] The vasculature in the V/SVZ niche forms a planar vascular plexus that extends throughout the entire

SVZ.[100,101] Under physiologic conditions, proliferation of the cerebral endothelial cells ceases and the turnover rate of endothelial cells is approximately 3 years in the adult rodent brain.[102] However, stroke induces angiogenesis in both adult human and rodent brains.[103,104] Angiogenesis is initiated at the border of the infarct areas, and sprouting capillaries develop into new vessels in the ischemic boundary during the first few weeks after the onset of stroke.[105,106] Studies also indicate that angiogenesis in the ischemic boundary lasts for several months.[77] To examine whether newly formed cerebral vessels have function, temporal and spatial profiles of vascular permeability and cerebral blood flow (CBF) in the ischemic brain were analyzed by MRI indices.[107,108] Vascular permeability can be quantified and detected using T1 indices of brain-to-blood transfer constants of extrinsic contrast agents, such as gadolinium DTPA, as well as intrinsic magnetization contrast methods.[107,108] Cerebral blood flow can be measured by perfusion-weighted MRI. Analysis of these MRI indices reveals that the ischemic boundary exhibits transient increase in vascular permeability 2–3 weeks after stroke, which leads to elevation of cerebral blood flow 6 weeks after stroke.[108] Areas with angiogenesis exhibit a remarkable correspondence of elevation of cerebral blood flow.[108] These data demonstrate that stroke induces functional new vessels in the ischemic brain.[108] Analysis of gene expression reveals that stroke up regulates expression of VEGF, its receptor VEGFR2, Ang1 and Ang2 and their receptor, tyrosine kinase with immunoglobulin, and epidermal growth factor homology domains 2 (Tie2) in the ischemic boundary.[103,106,109] Microarray analysis of cerebral endothelial cells isolated from ischemic rat brain demonstrated that stroke robustly alters cerebral endothelial miRNA profiles and many of stroke-changed miRNAs are involved in maintaining cerebral endothelial function and regulating angiogenesis either directly or indirectly[110] (unpublished data). A recent study showed that over expression of miR-15a in endothelial cells reduced stroke-induced angiogenesis and increased infarction in ischemic brain as well as exacerbated neurological deficits in mice.[15] In vitro study showed that miR-15a exerts anti-angiogenic effects on endothelial cells by targeting FGF2 and VEGF.[111] Collectively, these emerging data suggest that miRNAs regulate processes of cerebral angiogenesis after stroke and potentially can be used as therapeutic targets for facilitating stroke-induced angiogenesis during brain repair.

COUPLING OF NEUROGENESIS AND ANGIOGENESIS

Angiogenesis and neurogenesis are coupled.[6] Goldman et al.[112] found that migrating neuroblasts localize to angiogenic vessels within brain parenchyma. Others[100,101] demonstrated that actively proliferating intermediate neural progenitor cells closely localize to the vascular plexus in the V/SVZ niche. Endothelial cells release factors that stimulate the self-renewal of both embryonic and adult neural stem cells.[113] In vivo studies show that under physiologic conditions, cerebral vasculature in the V/SVZ of adult mice secretes factors such as integrin α6β1 that regulate neural stem and progenitor cell biologic function.[100,101] Coupling of angiogenesis and neurogenesis has also been observed in the adult human.[114] An MRI study showed that exercise specifically changes cerebral blood volume (CBV) in the adult human dentate gyrus, where exercise-induced neurogenesis has been demonstrated in the animal.[114] In the ischemic brain, neuroblasts are closely associated with cerebral vessels when neuroblasts migrate to the ischemic boundary.[6] Blockage of stroke-induced angiogenesis with systemic administration of endostatin substantially attenuates migration of neuroblasts newly born in the V/SVZ to the ischemic region.[29] Activated endothelial cells in the angiogenic areas secrete SDF-1 α, MMPs, and Ang1 to attract neuroblasts.[6,115] Blockage of the SDF-1 α /CXCR4, Ang1/Tie2, or MMP signaling suppresses neuroblast migration to the ischemic boundary.[6,75,115,116] To investigate the direct effect of endothelial cells on coupling with neural progenitor cells after stroke, coculture experiments were performed in which cerebral endothelial cells harvested from microvessels in the ischemic boundary were cultured with neural progenitor cells derived from the non-ischemic V/SVZ. The endothelial cells activated by stroke increased neural progenitor cell proliferation by 38% and the neuronal population by 44%,[117] suggesting that activated endothelial cells enhance neurogenesis. Symmetrically, neural progenitor cells isolated from ischemic SVZ promoted in vitro angiogenesis as measured by a capillary tube formation assay.[117] VEGF likely mediates this coupling because blockage of VEGFR2 with VEGFR2 antagonists suppresses coupling of angiogenesis with neurogenesis.[117] These in vitro data are further supported by in vivo gene profile analysis showing that ischemic neural progenitor cells isolated by laser capture microdissection in the SVZ express an array of angiogenic factors, including Ang2, VEGFR2, and fibroblast growth factor.[44] Collectively, these in vitro and in vivo findings indicate that induction of angiogenesis couples to and promotes neurogenesis and migration within the ischemic brain.

THE EFFECT OF CELL- AND PHARMACOLOGICALLY BASED THERAPIES ON ANGIOGENESIS AND NEUROGENESIS

Angiogenesis and neurogenesis in response to stroke are limited during stroke recovery and many newborn neurons die,[2] which may contribute to incomplete functional recovery. Experimental studies show that cell-based and pharmacological therapies targeting amplification of angiogenesis and neurogenesis substantially improve functional recovery after stroke.[6] Among cell-based therapies, treatment of stroke with marrow stromal cells (MSCs) has been the most studied.[6,118] MSC therapy causes an improvement in neurologic function that lasts for at least 12 months when cells are administered days after stroke onset.[118–121] It is unlikely that the therapeutic benefits result from the replacement of cerebral tissue by administration of cells, because only a small fraction of MSCs in the host brain express parenchymal cell phenotypes.[6] We tested the hypothesis that MSCs induce changes within the parenchymal cells that lead to a remodeling of the intact non-infarcted brain, which thereby promotes functional improvement. Intravenous administration of MSCs increased angiogenesis and neurogenesis in the ischemic brain.[118,119] When they were administered to the ischemic rat, human MSCs induced a significant increase in rat VEGF levels in the ischemic brain, indicating that MSCs interact with parenchymal cells.[122] In addition to upregulation of VEGF in astrocytes and cerebral endothelial cells, MSCs induce astrocytes to secrete Ang1.[123] Thus, injected MSCs interact with cerebral parenchymal cells to produce VEGF, leading to angiogenesis, whereas Ang 1 generated by MSC-stimulated astrocytes interacts with the Tie2 receptor in the endothelial cells, promoting the maturation of newly formed vessels primarily in the ischemic boundary zone. This vascular niche not only enhances tissue perfusion but also attracts endogenous neuroblasts originating in the SVZ by the expression of chemotactic molecules such as VEGF, SDF-1 α, and MMP9.[6] Furthermore, treatment of stroke with MSCs stimulates brain parenchymal cells to induce an array of neurotrophic factors, including basic fibroblast growth factor (bFGF) and brain-derived neurotrophic factor (BDNF), which promote neurogenesis and the survival of newly formed neurons.[6,124,125]

Pharmacologic therapies also foster endogenous angiogenesis and neurogenesis and improve functional outcome during stroke recovery. The pharmacological agents are drugs that increase cyclic guanosine monophosphate (cGMP) (phosphodiesterase-5 inhibitors, such as sildenafil and tadalafil), statins, erythropoietin (EPO), granulocyte-colony stimulating factor (G-CSF), niacin extended-release tablets (Niaspan), and minocycline.[126–132] EPO interacts with its receptor, EPOR, to induce angiogenesis and neurogenesis.[133,134,135] Systemic administration of recombinant human EPO (rhEPO) augments angiogenesis and neurogenesis in the ischemic brain.[129,136,137] Cerebral endothelial cells activated by rhEPO secrete active forms of MMP2 and MMP9, which promote neuroblast migration.[138] Application of MMP inhibitors abolishes the endothelially enhanced neuroblast migration.[138] On the other hand, EPO elevates VEGF levels in neural progenitor cells, thereby augmenting in vitro angiogenesis.[138] Blockage of VEGFR2 with a VEGFR2 antagonist or small interfering RNA (siRNA) against VEGFR2 suppresses neural progenitor-cell-increased angiogenesis.[138] These data indicate that MMPs and VEGF likely mediate coupling of EPO-enhanced angiogenesis and neurogenesis. Similar and complementary data demonstrating the coupling of neurogenesis and angiogenesis and functional recovery after stroke have been reported for statins, phosphodiesterase type 5 (PDE5) inhibitors, nitric oxide (NO) donors, granulocyte colony stimulating factor, and agents that increase high-density lipoprotein.[126–132]

Exosomes, small lipid microvesicles (40–100 nm), play an important role in intercellular communication by delivering functional miRNAs.[8,139] For example, delivery of endothelial cell exosomes enriched in miR-143/145 to smooth muscle cells suppresses miR-143/145 target gene expression that are involved in atherosclerotic lesion formation and leads to atheroprotection in the recipient cells.[140] In addition to endothelial cells, neurons, astrocytes and oligodendrocytes release exosomes.[141] Whether these endogenous exosomes regulate intercellular communication in ischemic brain has not been studied. However, recent studies have shown the therapeutic effect of exogenous exosomes on brain remodeling after stroke.[10,11] Treatment of stroke with exosomes derived from MSCs substantially enhances axonal remodeling, angiogenesis and neurogenesis as well as improves neurological outcomes in a rat model of focal cerebral ischemia.[10] In vitro experiments have revealed that delivery of MSC exosomes enriched in miR-133b into cultured neurons promotes neurite outgrowth, which is likely mediated through targeting genes of connective tissue growth factor and RhoA in recipient neurons. These studies suggest that delivery of exogenous exosomes containing enriched cargo miRNAs has a therapeutic effect on brain repair after stroke by mediating their miRNA target genes in host brain. Therapeutic delivery of exosomes for the treatment of stroke and neurological diseases is in its infancy.

THE EFFECT OF CELL- AND PHARMACOLOGICALLY BASED THERAPIES ON AXONAL REMODELING

In addition to angiogenesis and neurogenesis, cell- and pharmacologically based therapies substantially remodel white matter in the ischemic brain.[142–145] Treatment of experimental stroke with MCSs, rhEPO, or sildenafil significantly increases axonal density encapsulating the ischemic lesion.[142–144] Dynamic changes of white matter structure along the ischemic boundary have been imaged in living animals by diffusion tensor imaging (DTI) and fractional anisotropy (FA) measurements.[144] Data from these MRI indices demonstrate that administration of rhEPO or sildenafil augments axonal remodeling and angiogenesis and that both of them are spatially and temporally correlated.[144,145] Administration of MSCs, rhEPO, and thymosin beta 4 (Tβ4) dramatically increases the number of oligodendrocyte progenitor cells in the corpus callosum, the striatum, and the V/SVZ of the ischemic hemisphere and mature oligodendrocytes in the ischemic boundary adjacent to myelinated axons.[142,146] These findings suggest that cell- and pharmacologically based therapies promote generation of oligodendrocyte progenitor cells in the ischemic brain that migrate to target axons, where they extend their processes myelinating the axons.

Astrocytes constitute the largest population of cells in the central nervous system, constituting approximately 90% of human parenchymal cells.[147] Astrocytes are highly responsive to injury, undergoing rapid hyperplasia and hypertrophy.[148] Astrocytes act as physical and biochemical barriers to axonal regeneration by forming glial scars along ischemic lesions and producing axonal growth-inhibitory proteoglycans.[149] Administration of MSCs significantly attenuates the glial scar in the ischemic boundary and reduces expression of inhibitory proteins, such as Nogo.[143,150] Analysis of single-cell astrocytes isolated from the ischemic boundary by laser capture microdissection reveals that administration of MSCs dramatically down regulates neurocan, an axonal growth-inhibitory proteoglycan.[150] Coculture of MSCs with astrocytes also substantially reduces neurocan expression in astrocytes activated by oxygen glucose deprivation.[150] These findings suggest that injected MSCs reduce physical and biochemical barriers of astrocytes, which also contribute to axonal and neurite outgrowth.

CONCLUSION

The brain undergoes dramatic remodeling in response to ischemic stroke, which involves a tapestry of restorative events, including angiogenesis, neurogenesis, oligodendrogenesis, and axonal remodeling. Induction of angiogenesis couples to and promotes neurogenesis. These interacting remodeling events create a microenvironment via the interaction with astrocytes and oligodendrocytes that foster axonal and neurite outgrowth and plasticity within the brain. These sets of interwoven restorative events can be amplified by the restorative cell and pharmacologic therapies that lead to improved functional outcome.

REFERENCES

1. Alvarez-Buylla A, Herrera DG, Wichterle H. The subventricular zone: Source of neuronal precursors for brain repair. Prog Brain Res 2000;127:1–11.
2. Arvidsson A, Collin T, Kirik D, et al. Neuronal replacement from endogenous precursors in the adult brain after stroke. Nat Med 2002;8:963–70.
3. Zhang R, Zhang Z, Wang L, et al. Activated neural stem cells contribute to stroke-induced neurogenesis and neuroblast migration toward the infarct boundary in adult rats. J Cereb Blood Flow Metab 2004;24:441–8.
4. Jin K, Sun Y, Xie L, et al. Directed migration of neuronal precursors into the ischemic cerebral cortex and striatum. Mol Cell Neurosci 2003;24:171–89.
5. Parent JM. Injury-induced neurogenesis in the adult mammalian brain. Neuroscientist 2003;9:261–72.
6. Zhang ZG, Chopp M. Neurorestorative therapies for stroke: Underlying mechanisms and translation to the clinic. Lancet Neurol 2009;8:491–500.
7. Kawahara H, Imai T, Okano H. Micrornas in neural stem cells and neurogenesis. Front Neurosci 2012;6:30.

8. Taylor DD, Gercel-Taylor C. The origin, function, and diagnostic potential of RNA within extracellular vesicles present in human biological fluids. Front Genet 2013;4:142.
9. Zhang R, Chopp M, Zhang ZG. Oligodendrogenesis after cerebral ischemia. Front Cell Neurosci 2013;7:201.
10. Xin H, Li Y, Cui Y, et al. Systemic administration of exosomes released from mesenchymal stromal cells promote functional recovery and neurovascular plasticity after stroke in rats. J Cereb Blood Flow Metab 2013;33:1711–15.
11. Xin H, Li Y, Buller B, et al. Exosome-mediated transfer of miR-133b from multipotent mesenchymal stromal cells to neural cells contributes to neurite outgrowth. Stem Cells 2012;30: 1556–64.
12. Liu XS, Chopp M, Wang XL, et al. MicroRNA-17-92 cluster mediates the proliferation and survival of neural progenitor cells after stroke. J Biol Chem 2013;288:12478–88.
13. Liu XS, Chopp M, Zhang RL, et al. Micrornas in cerebral ischemia-induced neurogenesis. J Neuropathol Exp Neurol 2013;72:718–22.
14. Zhang Y, Ueno Y, Liu XS, et al. The microRNA-17-92 cluster enhances axonal outgrowth in embryonic cortical neurons. J Neurosci 2013;33:6885–94.
15. Yin KJ, Hamblin M, Chen YE. Angiogenesis-regulating microRNAs and ischemic stroke. Curr Vasc Pharmacol 2013. [Epub ahead of print].
16. Altman J. Autoradiographic and histological studies of postnatal neurogenesis. Iv. Cell proliferation and migration in the anterior forebrain, with special reference to persisting neurogenesis in the olfactory bulb. J Comp Neurol 1969;137:433–57.
17. Morshead CM, van der Kooy D. Disguising adult neural stem cells. Curr Opin Neurobiol 2004;14:125–31.
18. Noctor SC, Martinez-Cerdeno V, Ivic L, et al. Cortical neurons arise in symmetric and asymmetric division zones and migrate through specific phases. Nat Neurosci 2004;7:136–44.
19. Morshead CM, Craig CG, van der Kooy D. In vivo clonal analyses reveal the properties of endogenous neural stem cell proliferation in the adult mammalian forebrain. Development 1998; 125:2251–61.
20. Mirzadeh Z, Merkle FT, Soriano-Navarro M, et al. Neural stem cells confer unique pinwheel architecture to the ventricular surface in neurogenic regions of the adult brain. Cell Stem Cell 2008;3:265–78.
21. Tramontin AD, Garcia-Verdugo JM, Lim DA, et al. Postnatal development of radial glia and the ventricular zone (vz): A continuum of the neural stem cell compartment. Cereb Cortex 2003;13:580–7.
22. Alvarez-Buylla A, Garcia-Verdugo JM, Tramontin AD. A unified hypothesis on the lineage of neural stem cells. Nat Rev Neurosci 2001;2:287–93.
23. Lledo PM, Alonso M, Grubb MS. Adult neurogenesis and functional plasticity in neuronal circuits. Nat Rev Neurosci 2006;7: 179–93.
24. Sanai N, Tramontin AD, Quinones-Hinojosa A, et al. Unique astrocyte ribbon in adult human brain contains neural stem cells but lacks chain migration. Nature 2004;427:740–4.
25. Zhang RL, Zhang ZG, Zhang L, et al. Proliferation and differentiation of progenitor cells in the cortex and the subventricular zone in the adult rat after focal cerebral ischemia. Neuroscience 2001;105:33–41.
26. Jin K, Minami M, Lan JQ, et al. Neurogenesis in dentate subgranular zone and rostral subventricular zone after focal cerebral ischemia in the rat. Proc Natl Acad Sci U S A 2001;98:4710–15.
27. Parent JM, Vexler ZS, Gong C, et al. Rat forebrain neurogenesis and striatal neuron replacement after focal stroke. Ann Neurol 2002;52:802–13.
28. Iwai M, Sato K, Kamada H, et al. Temporal profile of stem cell division, migration, and differentiation from subventricular zone to olfactory bulb after transient forebrain ischemia in gerbils. J Cereb Blood Flow Metab 2003;23:331–41.
29. Ohab JJ, Fleming S, Blesch A, et al. A neurovascular niche for neurogenesis after stroke. J Neurosci 2006;26:13007–16.
30. Yamashita T, Ninomiya M, Hernandez Acosta P, et al. Subventricular zone-derived neuroblasts migrate and differentiate into mature neurons in the post-stroke adult striatum. J Neurosci 2006;26:6627–36.
31. Jin K, Wang X, Xie L, et al. Evidence for stroke-induced neurogenesis in the human brain. Proc Natl Acad Sci U S A 2006; 103:13198–202.
32. Macas J, Nern C, Plate KH, et al. Increased generation of neuronal progenitors after ischemic injury in the aged adult human forebrain. J Neurosci 2006;26:13114–19.
33. Minger SL, Ekonomou A, Carta EM, et al. Endogenous neurogenesis in the human brain following cerebral infarction. Regen Med 2007;2:69–74.
34. Curtis MA, Kam M, Faull RL. Neurogenesis in humans. Eur J Neurosci 2011;33:1170–4.
35. Marti-Fabregas J, Romaguera-Ros M, Gomez-Pinedo U, et al. Proliferation in the human ipsilateral subventricular zone after ischemic stroke. Neurology 2010;74:357–65.
36. Huttner HB, Bergmann O, Salehpour M, et al. The age and genomic integrity of neurons after cortical stroke in humans. Nat Neurosci 2014;17:801–3.
37. Zhang RL, Zhang ZG, Lu M, et al. Reduction of the cell cycle length by decreasing g(1) phase and cell cycle reentry expand neuronal progenitor cells in the subventricular zone of adult rat after stroke. J Cereb Blood Flow Metab 2006;26:857–63.
38. Zhang RL, Zhang ZG, Roberts C, et al. Lengthening the g(1) phase of neural progenitor cells is concurrent with an increase of symmetric neuron generating division after stroke. J Cereb Blood Flow Metab 2008;28:602–11.
39. Caviness VS Jr, Goto T, Tarui T, et al. Cell output, cell cycle duration and neuronal specification: A model of integrated mechanisms of the neocortical proliferative process. Cereb Cortex 2003;13:592–8.
40. Schultze B, Korr H. Cell kinetic studies of different cell types in the developing and adult brain of the rat and the mouse: A review. Cell Tissue Kinet 1981;14:309–25.
41. Zhang RL, Zhang ZG, Roberts C, et al. Lengthening the g(1) phase of neural progenitor cells is concurrent with an increase of symmetric neuron generating division after stroke. J Cereb Blood Flow Metab 2008;28:602–11.
42. Doetsch F, Garcia-Verdugo JM, Alvarez-Buylla A. Cellular composition and three-dimensional organization of the subventricular germinal zone in the adult mammalian brain. J Neurosci 1997;17:5046–61.
43. Gurok U, Steinhoff C, Lipkowitz B, et al. Gene expression changes in the course of neural progenitor cell differentiation. J Neurosci 2004;24:5982–6002.
44. Liu XS, Zhang ZG, Zhang RL, et al. Stroke induces gene profile changes associated with neurogenesis and angiogenesis in adult subventricular zone progenitor cells. J Cereb Blood Flow Metab 2007;27:564–74.
45. Lim DA, Suarez-Farinas M, Naef F, et al. In vivo transcriptional profile analysis reveals RNA splicing and chromatin remodeling as prominent processes for adult neurogenesis. Mol Cell Neurosci 2006;31:131–48.
46. Salim K, Guest PC, Skynner HA, et al. Identification of proteomic changes during differentiation of adult mouse subventricular zone progenitor cells. Stem Cells Dev 2007;16:143–65.
47. Maiorano D, Van Assendelft GB, Kearsey SE. Fission yeast cdc21, a member of the mcm protein family, is required for onset of s phase and is located in the nucleus throughout the cell cycle. EMBO J 1996;15:861–72.
48. Doetsch F, Verdugo JM, Caille I, et al. Lack of the cell-cycle inhibitor p27kip1 results in selective increase of transit-amplifying cells for adult neurogenesis. J Neurosci 2002;22: 2255–64.
49. Zhang R, Zhang Z, Tsang W, et al. Down-regulation of p27kip1 increases proliferation of progenitor cells in adult rats. Neuroreport 2004;15:1797–800.
50. Liu XS, Chopp M, Zhang RL, et al. Microrna profiling in subventricular zone after stroke: Mir-124a regulates proliferation of neural progenitor cells through notch signaling pathway. PLoS ONE 2011;6:e23461.
51. Liu XS, Chopp M, Wang XL, et al. MicroRNA-17/92 cluster mediates the proliferation and survival of neural progenitor cells after stroke. J Biol Chem 2013.
52. Xiao C, Srinivasan L, Calado DP, et al. Lymphoproliferative disease and autoimmunity in mice with increased miR-17-92 expression in lymphocytes. Nat Immunol 2008;9:405–14.

53. Gregorian C, Nakashima J, Le Belle J, et al. PTEN deletion in adult neural stem/progenitor cells enhances constitutive neurogenesis. J Neurosci 2009;29:1874–86.
54. Zheng H, Ying H, Yan H, et al. P53 and PTEN control neural and glioma stem/progenitor cell renewal and differentiation. Nature 2008;455:1129–33.
55. Bian S, Hong J, Li Q, et al. Microrna cluster miR-17-92 regulates neural stem cell expansion and transition to intermediate progenitors in the developing mouse neocortex. Cell Rep. 2013; 3:1398–406.
56. Nowakowski TJ, Fotaki V, Pollock A, et al. MicroRNA-92b regulates the development of intermediate cortical progenitors in embryonic mouse brain. Proc Nat Acad Sci U S A 2013;110: 7056–61.
57. de Pontual L, Yao E, Callier P, et al. Germline deletion of the mir-17 approximately 92 cluster causes skeletal and growth defects in humans. Nat Genet 2011;43:1026–30.
58. Sims JR, Lee SW, Topalkara K, et al. Sonic hedgehog regulates ischemia/hypoxia-induced neural progenitor proliferation. Stroke 2009;40:3618–26.
59. Northcott PA, Fernandez LA, Hagan JP, et al. The miR-17/92 polycistron is up-regulated in sonic hedgehog-driven medulloblastomas and induced by N-myc in sonic hedgehog-treated cerebellar neural precursors. Cancer Res 2009;69:3249–55.
60. Lim LP, Lau NC, Garrett-Engele P, et al. Microarray analysis shows that some microRNAs downregulate large numbers of target mRNAs. Nature 2005;433:769–73.
61. Cheng LC, Pastrana E, Tavazoie M, et al. MiR-124 regulates adult neurogenesis in the subventricular zone stem cell niche. Nat Neurosci 2009;12:399–408.
62. Jones PMG, Healy L, Brown J, et al. Stromal expression of jagged 1 promotes colony formation by fetal hematopoietic progenitor cells. Blood 1998;92:1505–11.
63. Gaiano NFG. The role of notch in promoting glial and neural stem cell fates. Annu Rev Neurosci 2002;25:471–90.
64. Wang LCM, Zhang RL, Zhang L, et al. The notch pathway mediates expansion of a progenitor pool and neuronal differentiation in adult neural progenitor cells after stroke. Neuroscience 2009;158:1356–63.
65. Zhao C, Sun G, Li S, et al. A feedback regulatory loop involving microRNA-9 and nuclear receptor tlx in neural stem cell fate determination. Nat Struct Mol Biol 2009;16:365–71.
66. Cai WY, Wei TZ, Luo QC, et al. Wnt-β-catenin pathway represses let-7 microRNAs expression via transactivation of Lin28 to augment breast cancer stem cell expansion. J Cell Sci 2013;126 (Pt 13):2877–89.
67. Dews M, Fox JL, Hultine S, et al. The myc-miR-17~92 axis blunts tgfβ signaling and production of multiple tgfβ-dependent antiangiogenic factors. Cancer Res 2010;70:8233–46.
68. Lim DA, Tramontin AD, Trevejo JM, et al. Noggin antagonizes BMP signaling to create a niche for adult neurogenesis. Neuron 2000;28:713–26.
69. Lie DC, Colamarino SA, Song HJ, et al. Wnt signalling regulates adult hippocampal neurogenesis. Nature 2005;437:1370–5.
70. Liu XS, Zhang ZG, Zhang RL, et al. Comparison of in vivo and in vitro gene expression profiles in subventricular zone neural progenitor cells from the adult mouse after middle cerebral artery occlusion. Neuroscience 2007;146:1053–61.
71. Morris DC, Zhang ZG, Wang Y, et al. Wnt expression in the adult rat subventricular zone after stroke. Neurosci Lett 2007;418: 170–4.
72. Zhang Z, Jiang Q, Jiang F, et al. In vivo magnetic resonance imaging tracks adult neural progenitor cell targeting of brain tumor. Neuroimage 2004;23:281–7.
73. Tran PB, Ren D, Veldhouse TJ, et al. Chemokine receptors are expressed widely by embryonic and adult neural progenitor cells. J Neurosci Res 2004;76:20–34.
74. Robin AM, Zhang ZG, Wang L, et al. Stromal cell-derived factor 1alpha mediates neural progenitor cell motility after focal cerebral ischemia. J Cereb Blood Flow Metab 2006;26: 125–34.
75. Imitola J, Raddassi K, Park KI, et al. Directed migration of neural stem cells to sites of cns injury by the stromal cell-derived factor 1alpha/CXC chemokine receptor 4 pathway. Proc Natl Acad Sci U S A 2004;101:18117–22.
76. Zhang RL, Zhang ZG, Chopp M. Ischemic stroke and neurogenesis in the subventricular zone. Neuropharmacology 2008;55: 345–52.
77. Thored P, Wood J, Arvidsson A, et al. Long-term neuroblast migration along blood vessels in an area with transient angiogenesis and increased vascularization after stroke. Stroke 2007; 38:3032–9.
78. Hou SW, Wang YQ, Xu M, et al. Functional integration of newly generated neurons into striatum after cerebral ischemia in the adult rat brain. Stroke 2008;39:2837–44.
79. Wang X, Mao X, Xie L, et al. Conditional depletion of neurogenesis inhibits long-term recovery after experimental stroke in mice. PLoS ONE 2012;7:e38932.
80. Franklin RJ. Why does remyelination fail in multiple sclerosis? Nat Rev Neurosci 2002;3:705–14.
81. Menn B, Garcia-Verdugo JM, Yaschine C, et al. Origin of oligodendrocytes in the subventricular zone of the adult brain. J Neurosci 2006;26:7907–18.
82. McTigue DM, Tripathi RB. The life, death, and replacement of oligodendrocytes in the adult cns. J Neurochem 2008;107:1–19.
83. Hughes EG, Kang SH, Fukaya M, et al. Oligodendrocyte progenitors balance growth with self-repulsion to achieve homeostasis in the adult brain. Nat Neurosci 2013;16:668–76.
84. Fancy SP, Chan JR, Baranzini SE, et al. Myelin regeneration: A recapitulation of development? Annu Rev Neurosci 2011;34: 21–43.
85. Dewar D, Underhill SM, Goldberg MP. Oligodendrocytes and ischemic brain injury. J Cereb Blood Flow Metab 2003;23: 263–74.
86. Lee Y, Morrison BM, Li Y, et al. Oligodendroglia metabolically support axons and contribute to neurodegeneration. Nature 2012;487:443–8.
87. Flygt J, Djupsjo A, Lenne F, et al. Myelin loss and oligodendrocyte pathology in white matter tracts following traumatic brain injury in the rat. Eur J Neurosci 2013;38:2153–65.
88. Rafalski VA, Ho PP, Brett JO, et al. Expansion of oligodendrocyte progenitor cells following sirt1 inactivation in the adult brain. Nat Cell Biol 2013;15:614–24.
89. Zhang RL, Chopp M, Roberts C, et al. Ascl1 lineage cells contribute to ischemia-induced neurogenesis and oligodendrogenesis. J Cereb Blood Flow Metab 2011;31:614–25.
90. Zhang RL, Chopp M, Roberts C, et al. Sildenafil enhances neurogenesis and oligodendrogenesis in ischemic brain of middle-aged mouse. PLoS ONE 2012;7:e48141.
91. Li L, Harms KM, Ventura PB, et al. Focal cerebral ischemia induces a multilineage cytogenic response from adult subventricular zone that is predominantly gliogenic. Glia 2010;58: 1610–19.
92. Zhang L, Chopp M, Zhang RL, et al. Erythropoietin amplifies stroke-induced oligodendrogenesis in the rat. PLoS ONE 2010; 5:e11016.
93. Zhao X, He X, Han X, et al. Microrna-mediated control of oligodendrocyte differentiation. Neuron 2010;65:612–26.
94. Dugas JC, Cuellar TL, Scholze A, et al. DICER1 and miR-219 are required for normal oligodendrocyte differentiation and myelination. Neuron 2010;65:597–611.
95. Budde H, Schmitt S, Fitzner D, et al. Control of oligodendroglial cell number by the miR-17-92 cluster. Development 2010;137: 2127–32.
96. de Faria O Jr, Cui QL, Bin JM, et al. Regulation of miRNA 219 and miRNA clusters 338 and 17-92 in oligodendrocytes. Front Genet 2012;3:46.
97. Buller B, Chopp M, Ueno Y, et al. Regulation of serum response factor by miRNA-200 and miRNA-9 modulates oligodendrocyte progenitor cell differentiation. Glia 2012.
98. Risau W. Development and differentiation of endothelium. Kidney Int Suppl 1998;67:S3–6.
99. Carmeliet P. VEGF gene therapy: Stimulating angiogenesis or angioma-genesis? [in process citation]. Nat Med 2000;6:1102–3.
100. Shen Q, Wang Y, Kokovay E, et al. Adult svz stem cells lie in a vascular niche: A quantitative analysis of niche cell-cell interactions. Cell Stem Cell 2008;3:289–300.
101. Tavazoie M, Van der Veken L, Silva-Vargas V, et al. A specialized vascular niche for adult neural stem cells. Cell Stem Cell 2008; 3:279–88.

102. Robertson PL, Du Bois M, Bowman PD, et al. Angiogenesis in developing rat brain: An in vivo and in vitro study. Brain Res 1985;355:219–23.
103. Zhang ZG, Zhang L, Jiang Q, et al. VEGF enhances angiogenesis and promotes blood–brain barrier leakage in the ischemic brain. J Clin Invest 2000;106:829–38.
104. Krupinski J, Kaluza J, Kumar P, et al. Role of angiogenesis in patients with cerebral ischemic stroke. Stroke 1994;25: 1794–8.
105. Garcia J, Cox J, Hudgins W. Ultrastructure of the microvasculature in experimental cerebral infarction. Acta Neuropathol 1971;18:273–85.
106. Zhang ZG, Zhang L, Tsang W, et al. Correlation of VEGF and angiopoietin expression with disruption of blood–brain barrier and angiogenesis after focal cerebral ischemia. J Cereb Blood Flow Metab 2002;22:379–92.
107. Li L, Jiang Q, Zhang L, et al. Ischemic cerebral tissue response to subventricular zone cell transplantation measured by iterative self-organizing data analysis technique algorithm. J Cereb Blood Flow Metab 2006;26:1366–77.
108. Jiang Q, Zhang ZG, Ding GL, et al. Investigation of neural progenitor cell induced angiogenesis after embolic stroke in rat using MRI. Neuroimage 2005;28:698–707.
109. Lin TN, Wang CK, Cheung WM, et al. Induction of angiopoietin and tie receptor mrna expression after cerebral ischemia-reperfusion. J Cereb Blood Flow Metab 2000;20:387–95.
110. Teng H, Chopp M, Liu X, et al. Stroke alters miRNA expression profiles in cerebral endothelial cells. Neuroscience 2012 2012; Poster: 58.06/K3.
111. Yin KJ, Olsen K, Hamblin M, et al. Vascular endothelial cell-specific microrna-15a inhibits angiogenesis in hindlimb ischemia. J Biol Chem 2012;287:27055–64.
112. Louissaint A Jr, Rao S, Leventhal C, et al. Coordinated interaction of neurogenesis and angiogenesis in the adult songbird brain. Neuron 2002;34:945–60.
113. Shen Q, Goderie SK, Jin L, et al. Endothelial cells stimulate self-renewal and expand neurogenesis of neural stem cells. Science 2004;304:1338–40.
114. Pereira AC, Huddleston DE, Brickman AM, et al. An in vivo correlate of exercise-induced neurogenesis in the adult dentate gyrus. Proc Natl Acad Sci U S A 2007;104:5638–43.
115. Lee SR, Kim HY, Rogowska J, et al. Involvement of matrix metalloproteinase in neuroblast cell migration from the subventricular zone after stroke. J Neurosci 2006;26:3491–5.
116. Robin A, Zhang Z, Wang L, et al. Stromal-derived factor 1a mediates neural progenitor cell motility after focal cerebral ischemia. Stroke 2004;35:272.
117. Teng H, Zhang ZG, Wang L, et al. Coupling of angiogenesis and neurogenesis in cultured endothelial cells and neural progenitor cells after stroke. J Cereb Blood Flow Metab 2008; 28:764–71.
118. Chopp M, Li Y. Treatment of neural injury with marrow stromal cells. Lancet Neurol 2002;1:92–100.
119. Chopp M, Li Y, Zhang J. Plasticity and remodeling of brain. J Neurol Sci 2008;265:97–101.
120. Cramer SC, Riley JD. Neuroplasticity and brain repair after stroke. Curr Opin Neurol 2008;21:76–82.
121. Parr AM, Tator CH, Keating A. Bone marrow-derived mesenchymal stromal cells for the repair of central nervous system injury. Bone Marrow Transplant 2007;40:609–19.
122. Chen J, Li Y, Wang L, et al. Therapeutic benefit of intravenous administration of bone marrow stromal cells after cerebral ischemia in rats. Stroke 2001;32:1005–11.
123. Zacharek A, Chen J, Cui X, et al. Angiopoietin1/TIE2 and VEGF/FLK1 induced by msc treatment amplifies angiogenesis and vascular stabilization after stroke. J Cereb Blood Flow Metab 2007;27:1684–91.
124. Chaudhary LR, Hruska KA. The cell survival signal AKT is differentially activated by PDGF-BB, EGF, and FGF-2 in osteoblastic cells. J Cell Biochem 2001;81:304–11.
125. Alessi DR, Andjelkovic M, Caudwell B, et al. Mechanism of activation of protein kinase B by insulin and IGF-1. EMBO J 1996; 15:6541–51.
126. Zhang R, Wang Y, Zhang L, et al. Sildenafil (viagra) induces neurogenesis and promotes functional recovery after stroke in rats. Stroke 2002;33:2675–80.
127. Zhang R, Zhang L, Zhang Z, et al. A nitric oxide donor induces neurogenesis and reduces functional deficits after stroke in rats. Ann Neurol 2001;50:602–11.
128. Chen J, Zhang ZG, Li Y, et al. Statins induce angiogenesis, neurogenesis, and synaptogenesis after stroke. Ann Neurol 2003; 53:743–51.
129. Wang L, Zhang Z, Wang Y, et al. Treatment of stroke with erythropoietin enhances neurogenesis and angiogenesis and improves neurological function in rats. Stroke 2004;35:1732–7.
130. Hossmann KA, Buschmann IR. Granulocyte-macrophage colony-stimulating factor as an arteriogenic factor in the treatment of ischaemic stroke. Expert Opin Biol Ther 2005;5: 1547–56.
131. Zhang L, Zhang Z, Zhang RL, et al. Tadalafil, a long-acting type 5 phosphodiesterase isoenzyme inhibitor, improves neurological functional recovery in a rat model of embolic stroke. Brain Res 2006;1118:192–98.
132. Chen J, Cui X, Zacharek A, et al. Niaspan increases angiogenesis and improves functional recovery after stroke. Ann Neurol 2007;62:49–58.
133. Nakano M, Satoh K, Fukumoto Y, et al. Important role of erythropoietin receptor to promote VEGF expression and angiogenesis in peripheral ischemia in mice. Circ Res 2007;100:662–9.
134. Tsai PT, Ohab JJ, Kertesz N, et al. A critical role of erythropoietin receptor in neurogenesis and post-stroke recovery. J Neurosci 2006;26:1269–74.
135. Chen ZY, Asavaritikrai P, Prchal JT, et al. Endogenous erythropoietin signaling is required for normal neural progenitor cell proliferation. J Biol Chem 2007;282:25875–83.
136. Iwai M, Cao G, Yin W, et al. Erythropoietin promotes neuronal replacement through revascularization and neurogenesis after neonatal hypoxia/ischemia in rats. Stroke 2007;38:2795–803.
137. Li Y, Lu Z, Keogh CL, et al. Erythropoietin-induced neurovascular protection, angiogenesis, and cerebral blood flow restoration after focal ischemia in mice. J Cereb Blood Flow Metab 2007; 27:1043–54.
138. Wang L, Zhang ZG, Zhang RL, et al. Matrix metalloproteinase 2 (MMP2) and MMP9 secreted by erythropoietin-activated endothelial cells promote neural progenitor cell migration. J Neurosci 2006;26:5996–6003.
139. Turchinovich A, Samatov TR, Tonevitsky AG, et al. Circulating miRNAs: Cell-cell communication function? Front Genet 2013; 4:119.
140. Hergenreider E, Heydt S, Treguer K, et al. Atheroprotective communication between endothelial cells and smooth muscle cells through mirnas. Nat Cell Biol 2012;14:249–56.
141. Shifrin DA Jr, Demory Beckler M, Coffey RJ, et al. Extracellular vesicles: Communication, coercion, and conditioning. Mol Biol Cell 2013;24:1253–9.
142. Li Y, Chen J, Zhang CL, et al. Gliosis and brain remodeling after treatment of stroke in rats with marrow stromal cells. Glia 2005;49:407–17.
143. Shen LH, Li Y, Chen J, et al. Intracarotid transplantation of bone marrow stromal cells increases axon-myelin remodeling after stroke. Neuroscience 2006;137:393–9.
144. Jiang Q, Zhang ZG, Ding GL, et al. MRI detects white matter reorganization after neural progenitor cell treatment of stroke. Neuroimage 2006;32:1080–9.
145. Ding G, Jiang Q, Li L, et al. Magnetic resonance imaging investigation of axonal remodeling and angiogenesis after embolic stroke in sildenafil-treated rats. J Cereb Blood Flow Metab 2008;28:1440–8.
146. Morris DC, Chopp M, Zhang L, et al. Thymosin beta4 improves functional neurological outcome in a rat model of embolic stroke. Neuroscience 2010;169:674–82.
147. Nedergaard M, Ransom B, Goldman SA. New roles for astrocytes: redefining the functional architecture of the brain. Trends Neurosci 2003;26:523–30.
148. Pekny M, Nilsson M. Astrocyte activation and reactive gliosis. Glia 2005;50:427–34.
149. Yiu G, He Z. Glial inhibition of cns axon regeneration. Nat Rev Neurosci 2006;7:617–27.
150. Shen LH, Li Y, Gao Q, et al. Down-regulation of neurocan expression in reactive astrocytes promotes axonal regeneration and facilitates the neurorestorative effects of bone marrow stromal cells in the ischemic rat brain. Glia 2008;56(16):1747-54.

12 Genetics and Vascular Biology of Angiogenesis and Vascular Malformations

Helen Kim, Ludmila Pawlikowska, Hua Su, William L. Young

KEY POINTS

- Cerebrovascular malformations are resource-intensive to manage, associated with serious neurologic morbidity, and poorly understood with respect to mechanisms and risk factors. Although rare, they are a major cause of intracranial hemorrhage in young adults and children.
- Most cases of brain arteriovenous malformations (AVMs) are sporadic but they can occur in Mendelian diseases, notably hereditary hemorrhagic telangiectasia (HHT), caused by autosomal dominant mutations in TGF-β signaling pathway genes.
- Animal models for brain AVM have been established through combining conditional deletion of HHT genes with angiogenic stimulation. Current models mimic aspects of the human disease and display arteriovenous shunting, a hallmark feature of AVMs.
- Cerebral cavernous malformations (CCM) are low-flow, angiographically occult lesions that can cause intracranial hemorrhage, seizures, neurological deficits, and death. CCM has sporadic and familial forms; familial CCM often displays multiple lesions, shows autosomal dominant inheritance, and is caused by loss-of-function mutations in three genes: *KRIT1*, *MGC4067*, and *PDCD10*.
- Somatic mutations occur in several cerebrovascular malformations, including CCM, vascular malformation-capillary malformation (VM-CM) and Sturge–Weber syndrome (SWS).
- Dural arteriovenous fistulae (DAVF) are acquired lesions, resulting from trauma and/or venous thrombosis, and characterized by venous hypertension.
- Different cerebrovascular malformations share commonalities in signaling pathways affecting angiogenesis, vascular remodeling, inflammation, and response to injury.

This chapter focuses on the vascular biology and genetics of brain arteriovenous malformations (AVMs) and cerebral cavernous malformations (CCMs); other cerebrovascular malformations are also discussed briefly. Despite their relative rarity, these malformations pose common challenges: they are resource-intensive to manage effectively, have high probability of serious neurological morbidity, and the biological mechanisms underlying them are poorly understood.

Each disease is characterized by distinct vascular malformations and a unique spectrum of clinical and phenotypic outcomes, for which biological risk factors are either poorly understood or completely unknown. The identification of these risk factors would improve patient surveillance and management. Since there are no specific medical therapies for these diseases, better understanding of the molecular etiology and pathophysiology holds promise for design of pharmacological treatments. Appropriate treatment (efficacy) trials will require risk stratification for selection and surrogate outcomes for trial development. Therefore, better biomarkers are needed, especially for assessing risk of hemorrhage.

BRAIN ARTERIOVENOUS MALFORMATIONS

Brain AVMs represent a rare but important source of neurological morbidity in young adults.[1] The population prevalence is 10–18 per 100,000 adults,[2,3] with a new detection rate of ~1.3 per 100,000 person-years.[4,5] The basic morphology is a vascular mass called the nidus, a complex tangle of abnormal, dilated channels, not clearly artery or vein, with intervening gliosis, that directly shunts blood from the arterial to venous circulations without a true capillary bed, typically with high flow.

Seizures, mass effect, and headache are causes of associated morbidity, but prevention of new or recurrent intracranial hemorrhage (ICH) is the primary rationale to treat AVMs, usually with some combination of surgical resection, embolization and stereotactic radiotherapy. The risk of spontaneous ICH has been estimated at 2–4% per year.[6] Other than nonspecific control of symptoms, e.g., headache and seizures, primary medical therapy is lacking.

Etiology and Pathogenesis

The genesis of AVMs has been enigmatic. There are no known environmental or epidemiological risk factors for AVM susceptibility, with the possible exception of essential hypertension.[7] Although AVMs have been detected in utero,[8] considering the high utilization of prenatal ultrasound, there is remarkably little evidence for the common belief that AVMs are congenital lesions arising during embryonic development (vein of Galen lesions are an interesting counterexample but probably represent a different disease process), and the etiological mechanism is likely more complex. In fact, the mean age at presentation (detection) is around 40 years of age, with a normal distribution. Epidemiological evidence suggests that the hemorrhagic behavior of most AVMs undergoes some fundamental change during childhood. Data from a large cohort of 1581 sporadic AVM cases suggest an increase in ICH rates around 10 years of age,[9] perhaps in response to changing hormonal levels. Others have noted higher ICH rates in women of childbearing age who harbor an AVM.[10]

There are multiple reports of AVMs that grow or regress and of local AVM regrowth after treatment, almost exclusively during childhood.[11] AVMs occasionally arise de novo after a normal angiogram and regrow after resection, either de novo, from a retained fragment,[12–14] or from a lesion treated with radiotherapy.[14,15] Although such events are relatively rare in clinical practice (1% to 5%; higher for radiotherapy), they support the hypothesis of active vascular changes in the lesion.[16] Perhaps these observations of regrowth or de novo appearance are extreme cases of a continuum of behaviors of actively, albeit slowly, growing lesions. Consistent with this hypothesis, endothelial proliferation in surgically resected AVM tissue was seven-fold higher than in control tissue (structurally normal temporal lobe).[16] The scarce data available on longitudinal assessment of AVM growth after detection suggest that approximately 50% of cases display interval growth.[16] Although the relationship of such growth with clinical risk profile (e.g., hemorrhagic risk) remains unknown, one plausible target for therapy might be to slow lesion growth over time. Factors that initiate AVM formation remain obscure. As discussed below, an underlying genetic predisposition may play a role, but some kind of inciting event(s) also appears necessary.

Mechanistic Hypotheses in Arteriovenous Malformation Pathobiology

Available evidence is more consistent with an active angiogenic and inflammatory lesion rather than with a static congenital anomaly. A prominent feature of the AVM phenotype is the relative overexpression of vascular endothelial growth factor (VEGF), at both the messenger RNA (mRNA) and protein levels.[17] Animal models suggest that VEGF may contribute to the hemorrhagic tendency.[18] Other upstream factors that may contribute to AVM formation include homeobox (HOX) transcription factors, such as excess expression of pro-angiogenic HOXD3, or deficient expression of anti-angiogenic HOXA5.[19,20] The vascular phenotype of AVM tissue may be explained, in part, by an inadequate recruitment of peri-endothelial support structures, which is mediated by angiopoietins and TIE-2 signaling. For example, angiopoietin-2 (ANG-2), which allows loosening of cell-to-cell contacts, is overexpressed in the perivascular region of AVMs.[21]

A key downstream consequence of VEGF and ANG-2 signaling, contributing to angiogenesis, is matrix metalloproteinase (MMP) expression. MMP-9 expression, in particular, is an order of magnitude higher in AVM than in control tissue,[22,23] and levels of naturally occurring MMP inhibitors, such as tissue inhibitor of metalloproteinases (TIMP)-1 and TIMP-3, are also increased. Additional inflammatory markers that are overexpressed include myeloperoxidase (MPO) and interleukin 6 (IL-6), which are highly correlated with MMP-9.[23,24] MMP-9 expression is correlated with the lipocalin-MMP-9 complex, which suggests neutrophils as a major source. In a subset of unruptured, non-embolized AVMs, neutrophils (MPO), macrophages/microglia (CD68) were prominent in the vascular wall and intervening stroma of AVM tissue, whereas T and B lymphocytes were present but rare.[25] Elevated immunoglobulin levels have also been reported in AVM tissue.[26]

Endothelial progenitor cells (EPCs) may incorporate into the AVM vessel wall, mediating pathologic angiogenesis and vascular remodeling.[27] EPCs, identified as CD133 and KDR double stained-positive cells, are increased in brain and spinal cord AVM nidus compared to epilepsy and basilar artery control tissue.[27] Increased expression of SDF-1 in AVM vessel wall could be responsible for the EPC homing.[27] In addition to EPCs, other bone-marrow (BM)-derived cells have also been implicated in AVM pathogenesis, such as CD68+ macrophages.[27] BM-derived monocytes/macrophages may provide critical repair functions in response to injury[28–30] and/or provide guidance involving Notch signaling during angiogenesis.[31,32]

Genetic Considerations Relevant to Arteriovenous Malformations

The majority of brain AVMs are sporadic; however, some evidence supports a familial component to the AVM phenotype, and that genetic variation is relevant to the disease course. Approximately 5% of AVMs occur in the context of rare inherited vascular disorders. A schematic of potentially relevant pathways[33–37] suggested by these Mendelian forms of the disease, human tissue investigations, and animal models is shown in Figure 12-1.

Mendelian Disease

AVMs in various organs, including the brain, are highly prevalent in patients with hereditary hemorrhagic telangiectasia (HHT, OMIM#187300), an autosomal dominant disorder of mucocutaneous fragility. The two main subtypes of HHT (HHT1 and 2) are caused by loss-of-function mutations in two genes[38] originally implicated in transforming growth factor-beta (TGF-β) signaling pathways (Fig. 12-1). The first is endoglin (*ENG*), which encodes an accessory protein of TGF-β receptor complexes. The second is activin-like kinase 1 (*ALK-1* or *ACVRL1*), which encodes a transmembrane kinase also thought to participate in TGF-β signaling. There are hundreds of reported mutations in the *ALK-1* and *ENG* genes;[39] the functional effect appears to be effective haploinsufficiency.

The signaling pathways for ALK-1 and ENG are complex and interrelated, and the relative importance and cellular

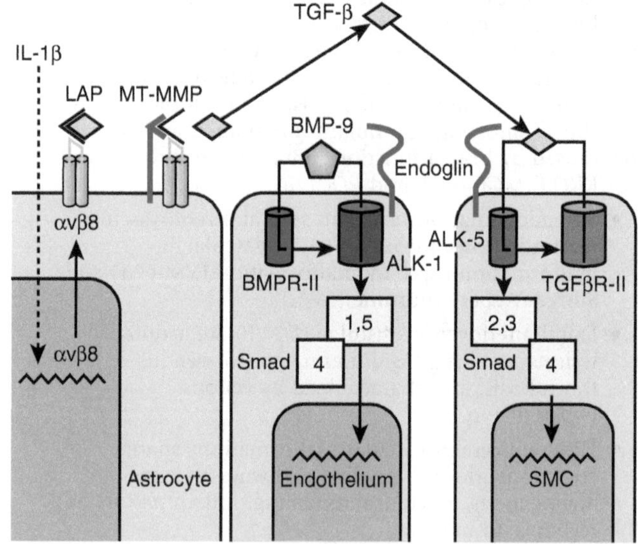

Figure 12-1. Transforming growth factor (TGF)-β superfamily signaling pathways relevant to arteriovenous malformation (AVM). Integrin αvβ8 is critical for liberation of TGF-β from latency-associated peptide (LAP); the β8-encoding gene, *ITGB8* has an interleukin (IL)-1β responsive element in its promoter in both humans and mice. TGF-β signaling involves both ALK-1 and ALK-5 receptors. ALK-5 receptors are expressed primarily on vascular smooth muscle cells, whereas ALK-1 is expressed in endothelial cells. BMP-9 may be an additional physiologic ligand for ALK-1 signaling. These signaling pathways have considerable cross-talk, the nature of which remains controversial. The ALK-1 signal is involved with endothelial cell migration and proliferation. Endoglin is an accessory receptor that can modulate both ALK-5 and ALK-1 signaling; ALK-1 and ALK-5 signal via distinct SMAD subtypes, all of which require the common co-SMAD, SMAD4, for translocation to the nucleus to effect downstream gene expression.

specificity are controversial.[34] ENG interacts with TGFBR2 (the type II TGF-β receptor) as well as with type I TGF-β receptors, ALK-1 and ALK-5,[40] and can bind ligands besides TGF-β, including activins and bone morphogenetic protein (BMP) family members.[41,42]

BMP-9 may be the physiologically relevant *endothelial* signaling ligand for ALK-1; ENG can potentiate the signal, which suggests a key interaction for HHT pathogenesis.[41,43,44] Mice lacking *Alk-1* (*Acvrl1*) form systemic arteriovenous fistulas (AVFs) from fusion of major arteries and veins in early vascular development.[45] Endothelial cell-specific ablation of *Alk-1* causes vascular malformations during development, whereas mice harboring an EC-specific knockout of *Alk-5* or *Tgfbr2* do not show any perturbation in vascular morphogenesis.[46]

A third gene implicated in AVM pathogenesis is *SMAD4*, encoding a downstream participant in TGF-β and BMP signaling. *SMAD4* is mutated in a combined syndrome of juvenile polyposis and HHT.[47] Two additional independent loci, termed HHT3 and HHT4, have been reported,[48,49] but the underlying genes have yet to be identified. More recently, mutations in *BMP9* have been reported to cause a vascular-anomaly syndrome with phenotypic overlap with HHT.[50]

Since defects in *ENG* or *ALK-1* signaling cause AVMs in HHT, by inference, this common pathway may also contribute to sporadic brain AVM development. A potential *mechanism* for the role of this pathway in AVM pathogenesis would include the requirement of ALK-1 for normal EC maturation.[51,52] Disruption of this signaling pathway would impair EC maturation, leading to inappropriate EC migration and proliferation. This is consistent with the view that aberrant EC migration and proliferation are an early stage in the development of an AVM. However, another view is that TGF-β/ALK-1 induces and TGF-β/ALK-5 inhibits cell migration and proliferation.[53] More work is needed with in vivo model systems to settle these apparent contradictions.

ENG and ALK-1 levels are reduced in HHT1 and HHT2 ECs.[54] Both ALK-1 and ENG are expressed predominantly in ECs,[55-57] but ENG is also expressed in other cell types, notably in monocytes.[58] Monocytic ENG appears to be critical for vascular repair in other organs, for example, the heart.[28] ENG expression appears grossly normal in both sporadic and HHT brain AVMs.[59] In one small series, ALK-1 expression was decreased in sporadic AVM.[60] The expression and functionality of these proteins in normal postnatal brain and in sporadic AVMs needs more elucidation.[33,34,46,61,62]

ENG and ALK1 may contribute to disease via mechanisms other than canonical TGF-β signaling in endothelium, smooth muscle or in BM-derived cells. ENG and ALK1 signaling may modulate endothelial nitric oxide synthase (eNOS) activation, thereby influencing local regulation of vascular tone and integrity.[63,64] Studies in $Eng^{+/-}$ mice suggest that impaired arterial myogenic responses and Eng-deficient ECs produce less nitric oxide (NO) and generate more eNOS-derived superoxide (O_2^-).[65] Treatment with an O_2^- scavenger reversed the vasomotor abnormalities in $Eng^{+/-}$ arteries, suggesting that uncoupled eNOS activity and the resulting impaired myogenic response represent early events in HHT1 pathogenesis related to oxidative stress. A loss of local microvascular flow regulation alone may lead to the development of arteriovenous shunts, as predicted by computational modeling studies.[66] There are conflicting data regarding the nature of the vasomotor response,[67] but this hemodynamic mechanism has been demonstrated in the pulmonary circulation.[68]

Soluble ENG (sENG; cleaved extracellular domain of ENG) is involved in preeclampsia pathogenesis[69] and might play roles in AVM development.[70] sENG is elevated in human AVM tissue, and sENG overexpression in the presence of VEGF stimulation induced vascular dysplasia in mice.[70] These findings suggest that increased sENG might compete with membrane-bound ENG for ligand binding, thus decreasing downstream signaling. It is not clear how sENG is formed. The soluble form of a related type III TGF-β receptor, betaglycan, appears to be shed by a process mediated by MMP-1.[71] Expression of several different MMPs is increased in AVM nidal tissue.[23,24,72] Thus, an MMP-mediated proteolytic mechanism may contribute to the formation of sENG.[69] AVMs seem to be characterized by a proinflammatory state.[23,24,73-75] Interestingly, TNF-α can induce release of sENG from normal placental villous explants.[76]

As a class, HHT AVMs have distinguishing morphologic characteristics such as smaller size, higher incidence of single hole fistulas, and higher incidence of cortical location. However, HHT and sporadic AVMs are generally similar and cannot be distinguished individually by their angioarchitecture.[77,78] Brain AVM multiplicity is highly predictive of HHT diagnosis, and rarely seen in sporadic disease.[79] HHT brain AVMs are also more frequently diagnosed before rupture, but this probably reflects more aggressive screening in HHT patients rather than any underlying biological difference.

Brain AVMs are approximately ten times more common in patients with HHT1/*ENG* mutations (≈20%) than those with HHT2/*ALK-1* mutations (≈2%).[80-82] Compared with the prevalence of sporadic lesions in the normal population, *ENG* or *ALK-1* mutation confers approximately a 1,000- and 100-fold increased risk, respectively, of developing a brain AVM. The greatly elevated risk of brain AVM in HHT suggests that germline *sequence variants* of these and other genes in shared pathways may likewise pose a significant risk for *sporadic* brain AVM development.

Because the population prevalence of HHT is roughly 1/10,000, and approximately 10% of all HHT cases harbor brain AVMs,[80] the population prevalence of HHT-AVMs should be approximately 1/100,000. Given the total AVM population prevalence of 10 to 18 per 100,000 adults,[2,3] the fraction of HHT-AVMs in large referral series might be expected to range from 5% to 10%. However, HHT accounts for less than 1% of the University of California San Francisco[6] and Columbia[83] AVM databases (unpublished data). These epidemiologic inconsistencies suggest systematic underestimation of undiagnosed HHT in the large sporadic AVM referral cohorts.

Familial Aggregation

Although rare, familial cases of brain AVM outside the context of HHT have been reported.[84-86] One literature review identified 53 non-HHT patients in 25 families with AVMs, mostly of first-degree relationships (79%).[85] While no clear pattern of inheritance emerged, the clinical characteristics did not differ significantly between familial and sporadic AVM except for a younger age at diagnosis, consistent with a genetic influence. Two small linkage studies in Japanese families with at least two affected relatives with non-HHT brain AVM have suggested an autosomal dominant mode of inheritance.[84,86] Linkage analysis revealed seven candidate regions, with the highest evidence on 6q25 (LOD = 1.88; $P = 0.002$),[84] but failed to identify the causative gene. These linkage regions did not overlap those found in the second study.[86]

Population-based estimates of recurrence risk for AVM are missing, but extrapolation from the above study[84] suggests a significant genetic component, with an estimated sibling recurrence risk of 16%.[87] Assuming a population prevalence of AVM of 18/100,000,[2] a sibling recurrence risk even as low as 0.05% would yield a relative risk to siblings of 2.78,[87] similar to that observed for ischemic stroke (2.0–5.0).[88]

Overall, there is modest evidence supporting familial aggregation for the AVM phenotype, although definitive proof is lacking. An increased relative risk to siblings would suggest a significant genetic influence, although this could also be the result of random chance, shared environmental factors and/or shared genetic factors. The challenge is identifying enough non-HHT families with imaging-confirmed AVM cases to perform classic familial aggregation and genetic studies.

GENETIC STUDIES OF NON-FAMILIAL ARTERIOVENOUS MALFORMATION

Candidate Gene Studies

Regardless of whether true familial non-HHT AVM cases exist, it is possible to evaluate whether genetic variants in candidate genes or genome-wide are *associated* with disease or disease progression. An important consideration in study design is the way one construes the nature of an "inherited disease".

The mechanism of AVM initiation is as yet unknown. However, even if it involves a structural aberration or mechanical insult - per se not a heritable trait - the subsequent growth and behavior of the lesion may still be influenced by genetic variation. For example, multiple genetic loci influence VEGF-induced angiogenesis.[89,90] Modifiers of TGF-β knockout phenotypes have been identified in mice, which may harbor genetic variation influencing HHT disease severity.[91] Genetic influences on AVM pathobiology may then be evaluated in a case-control study design (comparing affected patients to normal control subjects) or in cohort designs (cross-sectional or longitudinal), so that genetic influences on clinical course, such as propensity to rupture, can be investigated.

Candidate genes evaluated in brain AVM phenotypes include: (1) genes mutated in Mendelian cerebrovascular disorders (e.g., *ALK1* and *ENG* in HHT); (2) genes in pathways altered in AVM lesional tissue (e.g., inflammatory or angiogenic genes); (3) genes associated with relevant phenotypes in animal or in vitro models; and (4) genes which generally predispose to ICH, such as apolipoprotein E (*APOE*).[92,93] In all of these cases, common genetic polymorphisms may subtly alter protein function or expression, resulting in phenotypes relevant to AVM.

For example, a common intronic variant of *ALK-1*, IVS3-35A>G, is associated with AVM in US Caucasians.[94] This association was replicated in Germans,[95,96] but not in Dutch,[97] suggesting some population differences. The functionality of this variant is unknown but it could affect mRNA splicing or affect a regulatory element. Thus, common variation in a gene that, when mutated, causes HHT may also contribute to the sporadic AVM phenotype.

A candidate protein suggested by animal models is the astrocytic integrin αvβ8, an upstream regulator of TGF-β signaling. Integrin β8 abrogation in mice results in vascular instability and ICH.[98] Common genetic variants in *ITGB8* (encoding integrin β8) were associated with AVM susceptibility and correlated with decreased αvβ8 expression in resected AVM tissue.[99] Another candidate protein from animal models is G protein-coupled receptor 124 (*GPR124*), an orphan receptor that is highly expressed in CNS endothelium and mediates angiogenesis.[100] Common variants in *GPR124* were associated with AVM susceptibility, but no differences in GPR124 expression between AVM cases and controls were found.[101]

Polymorphisms in several inflammatory cytokine or receptor genes have also been associated with AVM susceptibility, including interleukin (*IL*)*-6* (-174 G>C) in US Hispanics,[102] *IL-1β* (-31 T>C and -511 C>T) in US Caucasians,[75] *IL-1α* (-889 C>T) in Italians,[103] and *IL-17A* (-875A>G) in Chinese.[104] Polymorphisms in *MMP3* (-707A>G),[105] and *TGRBR2*, a cytokine receptor (-875A>G),[104] have been reported to be associated with AVM susceptibility in Chinese populations, while polymorphisms in angiogenesis-related genes, *ANGPTL4* and *VEGFA*, have been associated with AVM susceptibility in US Caucasians and Chinese, respectively;[106,107] the latter is also associated with risk of ICH.[108] These studies illustrate the difficulty in conducting genetic association studies in populations of different race/ethnicity.[109]

Genetic influences on clinical course of AVM rupture resulting in intracranial hemorrhage have been reported in three settings: presentation with ICH,[73,110] new ICH after diagnosis,[74,75,111] and ICH after treatment.[112] The GG genotype of the *IL-6* -174G>C promoter polymorphism was associated with clinical presentation of ICH,[73] and with the highest IL-6 mRNA and protein levels in AVM tissue.[24] Polymorphisms in *EPHB4*, encoding a tyrosine kinase receptor involved in embryogenic arterial–venous determination, were also associated with increased risk of ICH presentation.[110]

Both *TNF-α* -238G>A[74] and *APOE* ε2[111] were independently associated with new hemorrhage in the natural history course of AVMs.[74] In addition, *APOE* ε2 and *TNF-α* -238 A alleles appear to confer greater risk for post-radiosurgical and post-surgical hemorrhage.[112] Finally, the *IL-1β* promoter variants associated with AVM susceptibility also appear to be associated with increased risk of new ICH after diagnosis.[75]

The majority of these genetic association results await replication in independent AVM cohorts. Because AVMs are rare, this requires international collaboration to accrue sufficiently large sample sizes for replication. There is indirect evidence of a genetic influence in that race/ethnic background appears to influence the risk of spontaneous ICH during the natural history course.[6] Further study is needed in this area as these associations could be explained by socio-economic and environmental factors, or a complex combination of these influences with genetics.

Beyond Candidate Gene Studies

A drawback of candidate gene studies is that, although they are hypothesis-driven, they represent, at best, an educated guess as to which genes are involved. An alternative is to conduct a genome-wide association study, which may also be designed as a case-control or a cohort study (GWAS). This hypothesis-free approach relies on scanning all common variation in the genome, utilizing microarrays that feature millions of variants selected based on human variation data from the International HapMap project (www.hapmap.org)[113] and the 1000 Genomes Project (www.1000genomes.org).[114] An advantage is that this approach can uncover completely novel biological mechanisms. A disadvantage is that a large sample size (preferably in the 1000s) and replication in two or more independent cohorts is needed to validate significant findings.[115] Furthermore, GWAS address the "common-disease, common-variant" hypothesis and cannot uncover rare variants associated with the disease (exome or whole-genome sequencing is needed to evaluate rare variants). Nonetheless, the first such studies are underway for sporadic AVMs.[116] A whole-genome scan did not identify common copy number variants associated with sporadic brain AVM.[117]

An Alternative Genetic Mechanism for Sporadic Arteriovenous Malformations

An alternative hypothesis for sporadic AVM pathogenesis posits that the relevant genes/pathways are disrupted by *somatic* rather than *germline* mutations, which are not inherited, but arise de novo in development in a subset of the cells in each affected individual. This genetic mechanism would parallel that found for venous malformations, where germline *TIE-2* mutations are found in autosomal dominant families with venous malformations,[118,119] but somatic mutations are found in *tissue* isolated from sporadic venous malformations,[120,121] and, as recently described, in Sturge–Weber syndrome, caused by somatic gain of function mutations in *GNAQ*.[122] The same pattern has also been demonstrated in CCM.[123] The somatic mutation mechanism might also explain the rarity of non-HHT families with AVMs. The occasional but rare familial occurrence of the usually sporadic AVM is similar to that found with other vascular traits such as Klippel–Trenaunay syndrome. This pattern has been termed *paradominant inheritance* and invokes both germline and somatic mutation for its underlying mechanism.[124,125] In the paradominant model, individuals heterozygous for a germline mutation are phenotypically normal, but germline homozygotes die during early embryogenesis. Thus the mutation rarely manifests as familial inheritance of a trait but instead is "silently" transmitted through generations. The trait becomes expressed when a second, somatic mutation occurs in the same gene, giving rise to a mutant cell population lacking a normal copy of the gene. This clone of mutant cells can now seed the development of the vascular anomaly. This intriguing hypothesis has yet to be explored for sporadic AVMs, and requires resequencing of DNA from AVM lesional tissue.

Insights from Experimental Arteriovenous Malformation Models

Animal model systems for AVM are needed to test mechanistic hypotheses and develop novel therapies. Early "AVM" models were largely based on extradural AVFs and used for study of hemodynamic changes, the development of platforms for technology,[126–144] investigating the pathophysiology of postoperative complications,[145] or to develop embolic or radiotherapeutic methods.[146] However, in these models a *parenchymal* nidus is not formed, and nidus growth and hemorrhage that mimic the human disease do not occur.

Manipulation of specific genes in mice has resulted in antenatal or perinatal ICH and, in some cases, vascular structures reminiscent of AVMs. Some of the mutated proteins may be related to AVM biology, e.g., integrin αvβ8, which is involved in modulating proteolytic cleavage of latency-associated peptide (LAP) from the TGF-β protein precursor to produce the mature TGF-β molecule.[98,99] Knockout of integrin αvβ8 (*Itgb8*) plus focal VEGF stimulation induced capillary dysplasia in the brain.[99] Endothelial expression of constitutively active Notch-4 elicited AVMs in mice.[147,148] In addition, homozygous knockout of matrix Gla protein (*Mgp*) also resulted in AVMs in the brain and multiple organs.[149]

Notch signaling is important for the determination of arterial and venous fate, a process dependent on local levels of VEGF.[150] Further, Notch influences endothelial tip and stalk phenotypes during angiogenesis.[151] Proteins involved in Notch signaling, including the receptor, its ligands, and downstream signals, are expressed in brain AVM tissue.[152,153] Overexpressing the tetracycline-controlled (tet-off) intracellular domain of Notch-4 (int3) in early post-natal mice induced a phenotype mimicking aspects of human AVMs.[148] Upon retreatment with doxycycline to stop int3 expression, the lesions regressed.[148,154] Although tetracyclines inhibit pathological angiogenesis and vascular remodeling,[18,155,156] the Notch pathway merits further exploration[157] because Notch activation is a fundamental part of the normal response to injury, which has also been shown in ischemia-induced neurogenesis.[158]

An important conceptual advance in modeling brain AVM has been to posit that HHT pathways can shed light on sporadic AVM pathogenesis, given the similarities in AVM phenotype.[38] Inactivating a single allele of *Eng* or *Alk1* reproduces aspects of the human disease in mouse models,[159,160] but spontaneous vascular lesions in the brain are rare and subtle, mostly in aged mice.[159,161] More pronounced cerebral microvascular dysplasia can be induced using VEGF stimulation in $Eng^{+/-}$ or $Alk1^{+/-}$ mice,[162–164] and enhanced by increasing tissue perfusion rates.[163] However, the dysmorphic vessels developed in $Eng^{+/-}$ or $Alk1^{+/-}$ mice are at the capillary level, and arteriovenous shunting is not detected.

Interestingly, the capillary level of cerebrovascular dysplasia seen in VEGF-stimulated $Eng^{+/-}$ mice is also seen in the brain of wild-type (WT) mice transplanted with $Eng^{+/-}$ BM following VEGF stimulation. In addition, the dysplasia in $Eng^{+/-}$ mice was partially rescued by transplantation of WT BM cells.[165] These findings suggest that Eng haploinsufficiency in BM-derived cells is sufficient to cause cerebrovascular dysplasia in the adult mouse after angiogenic stimulation.

Loss of both alleles of *Eng* or *Alk1* in mice is embryonic lethal.[45,166] Conditional deletion of *Alk1* from *Alk1* expressing cells resulted in arteriovenous fistulas in neonatal brain.[167] Brain and spinal cord AVMs also developed in mice with *SM22α*-Cre-mediated *Alk1* deletion during embryonic development,[168] most of which died shortly after birth.

The first adult-onset brain AVM model was developed using a combination of focal *Alk1* deletion mediated by adenoviral vectors expressing Cre-recombinase and VEGF stimulation.[169] This model mimics many aspects of human brain AVM lesions, such as arteriovenous shunting, microhemorrhage and macrophage infiltration (Fig. 12-2).[169–171] However, adenovirus-related inflammation complicates mechanistic analysis in this model.

Using Cre transgenic mouse lines, two more adult-onset and one developmental-onset brain AVM mouse model have been developed recently. Fully developed brain AVMs were detected in adult $Eng^{2f/2f}$;R26CreER mice 8 weeks after induction of global *Eng* gene deletion and brain angiogenesis[172] and $Alk1^{2f/2f}$;*Pdgfb*-iCre mice 4 weeks after induction of brain angiogenesis and 2 weeks after endothelial *Alk1* deletion.[173] Brain AVMs develop rapidly in $Alk1^{2f/2f}$;*Pdgfb*-iCre mice but the mice die within 10 to 14 days after tamoxifen-induced *Alk1* deletion. Brain AVM in $Eng^{2f/2f}$;R26CreER mice develop more slowly, and the mice survive more than 8 weeks after *Eng* deletion. Thus, this model is better suited for testing new therapies.

The developmental-onset brain AVM model was developed using the *SM22α*-Cre transgenic line to delete *Eng* during embryonic development.[172] Unlike conventional $Eng^{-/-}$ mice, which are embryonic lethal,[174–176] $Eng^{2f/2f}$;*SM22α*-Cre mice are born alive and develop various degrees of AVMs in the central nervous system (CNS) with more than 95% penetrance at 5 weeks of age.[172] They show important clinical aspects of the human lesion, including arteriovenous shunting and spontaneous hemorrhages. Further, AVM phenotypes were similar to those previously observed in $Alk1^{2f/2f}$;*SM22α*-Cre mice,[168] but with less lethality. Since brain AVMs develop spontaneously in this model without local manipulation, the lesion progression more closely mimics human disease, rendering this a better model for mechanistic studies and new drug testing.

Interestingly, homozygous knockout of matrix Gla protein (MGP), a BMP inhibitor, causes induction of Notch ligands, dysregulation of endothelial differentiation, and the development of brain AVMs in $Mgp^{-/-}$ mice.[149] Increased BMP activity in $Mgp^{-/-}$ endothelial cells induces expression of Alk1 in cerebrovascular endothelium, enhancing expression of Notch ligands, Jagged 1 and 2. As a consequence, Notch activity is increased, and expression of Ephrin B2 and Ephrin receptor B4 is altered.[149] These data suggest that changes in BMP (Alk1 activity) signaling alter Notch activity and lead to brain AVMs (see Fig. 12-4A).

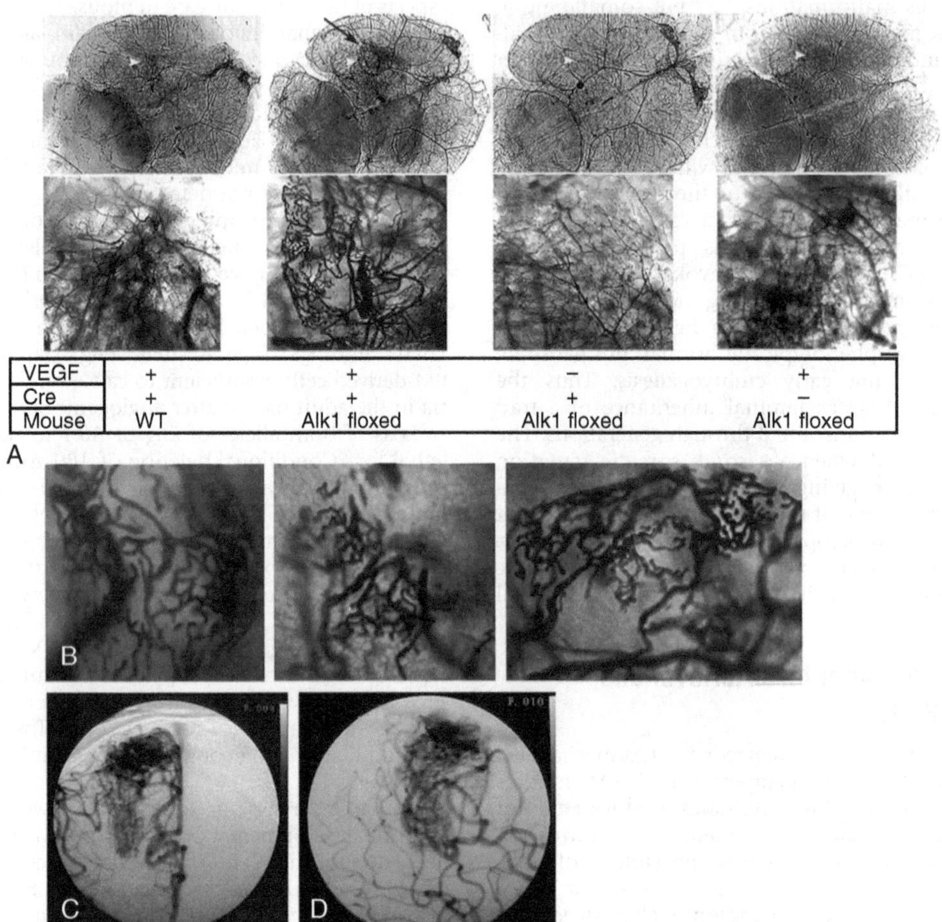

Figure 12-2. Vessel casting showing that VEGF stimulation induced distinct cerebrovascular abnormalities at the Alk1-deleted region that mimic many aspects of human brain arteriovenous malformation (AVM). A, Large tangled vessels resembling a brain AVM were detected at the injection site of Ad-Cre and AAV-VEGF in the brain of Alk1-floxed mice (black arrow). Alk1 deletion (Ad-Cre injection) without VEGF had no effect on the cerebrovascular structure. Overexpression of VEGF in the brain without ALK1 deletion (WT mice or Alk1 mice injected with control adenoviral vector) induced normal angiogenesis. The bottom images show the enlarged angiogenic foci of the images on top. Scale bar = 100 μm. Injection sites are indicated by white arrowheads. B, Abnormal vasculature from three different Alk1-floxed mice injected with Ad-Cre and AAV-VEGF. Scale bar = 100 μm. C and D, Right internal carotid artery anterior-posterior (C) and lateral (D) projections of an angiogram from an 18-year-old male who underwent microsurgical brain AVM resection. The brain AVM, supplied by the middle and anterior cerebral arteries, has a diffuse angioarchitecture, similar to the phenotype in the mouse model. *(Reprinted with permission from Walker EJ, Su H, Shen F, et al. Arteriovenous malformation in the adult mouse brain resembling the human disease.* Ann Neurol *69: 954–962, 2011.)*

Evidence obtained from modeling HHT brain AVM suggests that AVM initiation and progression require interplay between several factors, including (1) homozygous loss-of-function of causative genes in somatic endothelial cells, (2) angiogenic stimulation (response-to-injury), (3) participation of BM-derived cells, (4) alteration of monocyte/macrophage function, and (5) hemodynamic changes (Fig. 12-3).

First, genetic background may be important. It is reasonable to assume that (a) polymorphic variation in *ALK1* or *ENG*, or (b) an upstream or downstream component of the TGF-β/BMP9 signaling pathway, is affected. This is speculative, but rests on the high degree of similarity between HHT AVMs and sporadic AVMs. Second, an angiogenic phenotype seems likely. Clinically, environmental stimuli can result in an angiogenic response and fistula formation, i.e., trauma causing direct and indirect DAVF.[177-179] Venous hypertension (VH) can induce DAVF in rats,[132,135] and the fistulous material is angiogenic.[132] Resected human AVM specimens also induce angiogenesis in corneal transplant experiments.[180] This response almost certainly involves VEGF, which is expressed in human samples,[181] and in rat and mouse brain in the VH model.[182,183] Third, high flow rates and VH are present in human AVM nidal vessels.[184] Box 12-1 describes the components of an ideal AVM model.

Summary and Synthesis of Arteriovenous Malformation Etiology and Pathogenesis

A prevailing hypothesis is that AVM pathophysiology is governed by chronic hemodynamic derangements resulting from a congenital lesion. Recent findings suggest a set of alternative hypotheses where angiogenic and inflammatory pathways synergize with underlying structural defects or hemodynamic injury to produce the clinical phenotype, perhaps in conjunction with genetic or environmental influences (Fig. 12-4). Elucidating these mechanisms offers promise for developing innovative treatments and better risk stratification, and may provide insights into mechanisms of vascular biology.

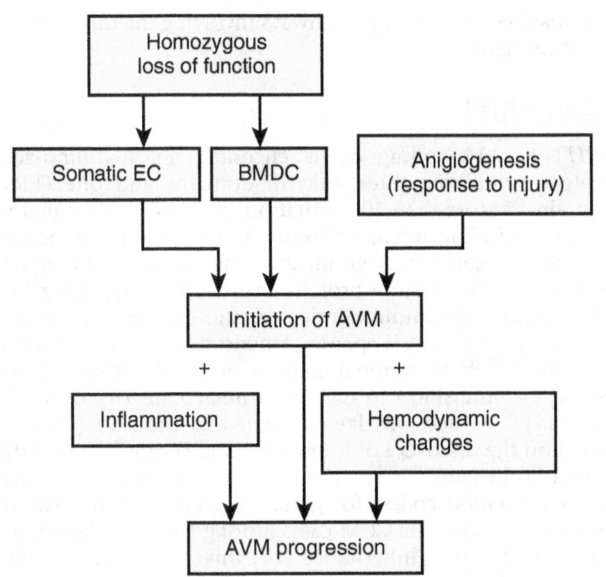

Figure 12-3. Novel theories of arteriovenous malformation (AVM) initiation and progression. EC: endothelial cell; BMDC: bone-marrow-derived cells.

BOX 12-1 Proposed Components of an Ideal Experimental AVM Model

ANATOMIC

Nidus of abnormal vessels of varying sizes
Both microcirculatory and macrocirculatory levels

PHYSIOLOGIC

Arteriovenous shunting
Hemodynamically significant (i.e., sufficient to decrease feeding artery or increase draining venous pressures)

BIOLOGICAL

Alterations in angiogenic and inflammatory protein expression
Involvement of, or intersection with, known genetic pathways

CLINICAL

Relative quiescence
Spontaneous hemorrhaging into the parenchyma or cerebrospinal fluid spaces

AVM, Arteriovenous malformation.

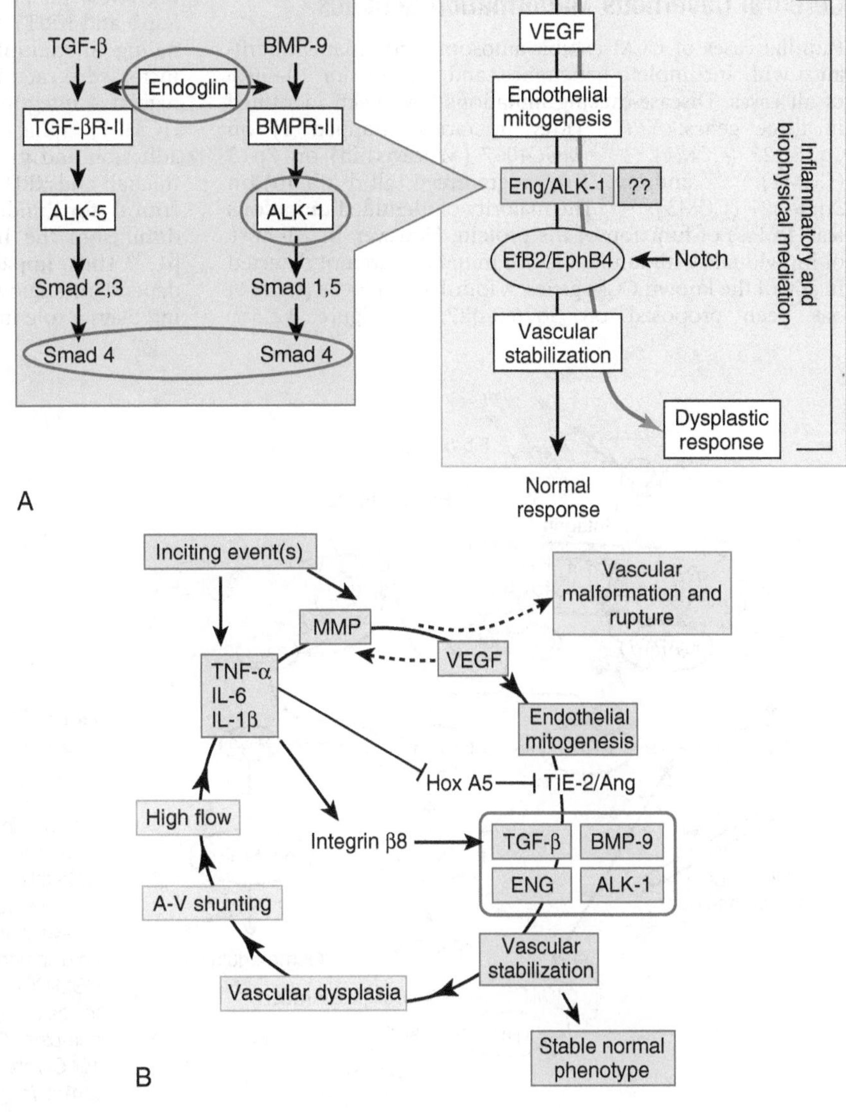

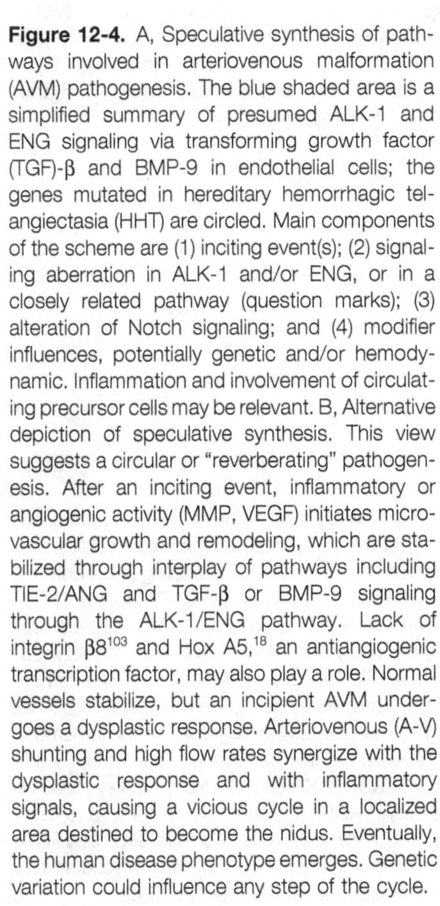

Figure 12-4. A, Speculative synthesis of pathways involved in arteriovenous malformation (AVM) pathogenesis. The blue shaded area is a simplified summary of presumed ALK-1 and ENG signaling via transforming growth factor (TGF)-β and BMP-9 in endothelial cells; the genes mutated in hereditary hemorrhagic telangiectasia (HHT) are circled. Main components of the scheme are (1) inciting event(s); (2) signaling aberration in ALK-1 and/or ENG, or in a closely related pathway (question marks); (3) alteration of Notch signaling; and (4) modifier influences, potentially genetic and/or hemodynamic. Inflammation and involvement of circulating precursor cells may be relevant. B, Alternative depiction of speculative synthesis. This view suggests a circular or "reverberating" pathogenesis. After an inciting event, inflammatory or angiogenic activity (MMP, VEGF) initiates microvascular growth and remodeling, which are stabilized through interplay of pathways including TIE-2/ANG and TGF-β or BMP-9 signaling through the ALK-1/ENG pathway. Lack of integrin β8[103] and Hox A5,[18] an antiangiogenic transcription factor, may also play a role. Normal vessels stabilize, but an incipient AVM undergoes a dysplastic response. Arteriovenous (A-V) shunting and high flow rates synergize with the dysplastic response and with inflammatory signals, causing a vicious cycle in a localized area destined to become the nidus. Eventually, the human disease phenotype emerges. Genetic variation could influence any step of the cycle.

CEREBRAL CAVERNOUS MALFORMATIONS

Overview

Cerebral cavernous malformations (CCMs) or cavernous angiomas (OMIM #116860) are vascular malformations that occur in the CNS, most often in the brain. In contrast to brain AVMs, CCMs are leaky, low-flow lesions that are angiographically occult. CCMs are clusters of enlarged capillary caverns lined with a single layer of endothelium without normal intervening brain parenchyma. Ultrastructural studies reveal abnormal or absent blood–brain barrier components, poorly formed tight junctions with gaps between EC, lack of astrocytic foot processes and few pericytes.[185]

The population prevalence of CCMs is estimated to be 0.1–0.5% based on MRI and autopsy studies;[186,187] CCMs represent 5–15% of all cerebral vascular malformations. CCMs can occur in a sporadic or familial form; familial cases often present with multiple lesions that grow in number and size over time, reflecting the dynamic nature of these lesions.[188–192] The most common clinical sequelae include seizures (40–70%) and ICH (32–59%), resulting in acute or permanent focal neurological deficits and even death.[190,193] Primary medical therapy for CCM is lacking, despite knowing the disease-causing genes and the signaling pathways involved.

Cerebral Cavernous Malformation Genetics

Familial cases of CCM exhibit autosomal dominant inheritance with incomplete penetrance, and account for 10–50% of all cases. Disease-causing mutations have been identified in three genes: *KRIT1* (Krev interaction trapped 1) on 7q21-q22 (CCM1),[194–199] *MGC4067* (Malcavernin) on 7p13 (CCM2),[200–202] and *PDCD10* (programmed cell death 10) on 3q26-q27 (CCM3).[200,203] The majority of identified mutations lead to loss-of-function of the protein. However, in 20–40% of individuals with familial CCM, mutations are not detected in any of the known CCM genes. A fourth CCM locus (CCM4) has been proposed on 3q26.3-q27.2.[204] Figure 12-5[205] summarizes the signaling pathways involving the three known CCM proteins.

CCM1/KRIT1

KRIT1 has 16 coding exons encoding a 736-amino-acid protein containing three ankyrin domains and one FERM domain.[206] More than 100 mutations have been identified in *KRIT1*, including micro-deletions, nonsense and frameshift mutations located throughout the gene. Most of these mutations lead to premature protein termination, suggesting loss of function. A common founder mutation has been identified in familial CCM1 Hispanic American cases of Mexican descent.[198,207,208] Mutational analysis originally identified this as a C-to-T transition in exon 6 at nucleotide 742 of *KRIT1* (Q248X),[207] which was later assigned to exon 10 (Q455X) based on the discovery of four additional coding exons at the 5′ end of the gene.[206,209,210] The mutation substitutes a premature termination codon for glutamine. Virtually all cases of familial and sporadic CCM cases among Hispanic Americans are due to the inheritance of this common founder mutation.[198,207]

KRIT1 was originally identified through a yeast two-hybrid screen as a novel binding partner of the Ras-family guanasine triphosphate (GTP)ase Rap1A,[211,212] and is a Rap1 binding protein regulating endothelial junction integrity by suppressing stress fibers and stabilizing cell–cell junctions.[213] Both Rap1 and KRIT1 act as inhibitors of canonical β-catenin signaling in multiple cell lineages, and loss of KRIT1 causes increased β-catenin signaling in mice.[214] Additionally, KRIT1 regulates integrin cytoplasmic domain-associated protein-1 (ICAP-1) alpha binding to integrin β1, which regulates cell adhesion and migration.[215,216] Both the integrin β1 cytoplasmic tail and KRIT1 N-terminus contain NPXY motifs that are critical for binding ICAP-1α.[215] Overexpression of KRIT1 diminishes the interaction between ICAP-1α and integrin β1.[216] Thus, impaired KRIT1 may interfere with integrin β1-dependent angiogenesis, which suggests that integrin signaling plays a role in CCM pathogenesis.

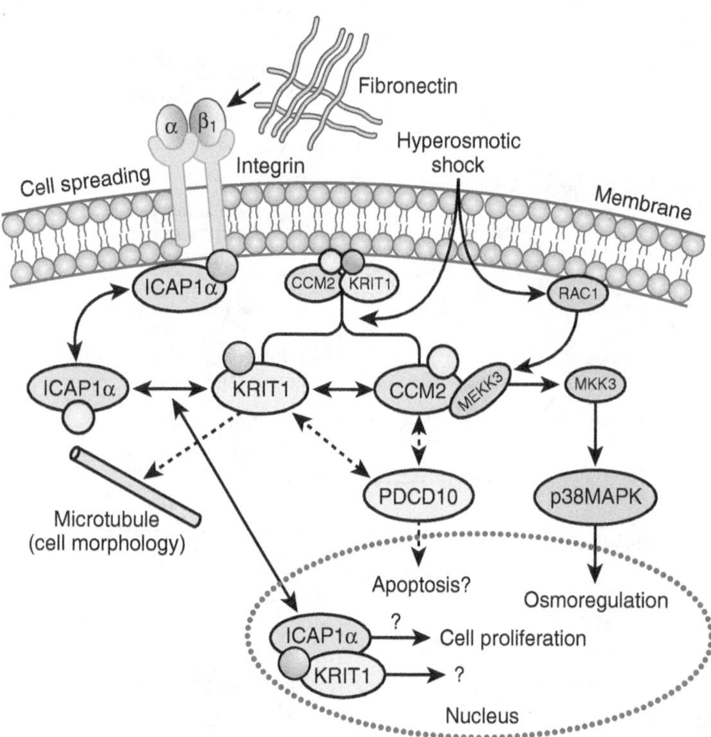

Figure 12-5. Schematic presentation of molecular pathways involving the cerebral cavernous malformation (CCM) proteins. • NPxY motif; ○ phosphotyrosine binding (PTB) domain; dashed lines, hypothetical interactions. ICAP1α interacts with the β1 integrin cytoplasmic domain and controls cell spreading/cell proliferation on fibronectin. KRIT1 could modulate this pathway. KRIT1/CCM2/ICAP1α can form a ternary complex. ICAP1α and KRIT1 can go to the nucleus. It is not known if they go separately or together. A hyperosmotic environment stimulates in mammalian cells the Rac1–OSM(CCM2)–MEKK3–MKK3–p38MAPK pathway leading to osmoregulation. KRIT1/CCM2/MEKK3 form a ternary complex. *(Reprinted with permission from Revencu N, Vikkula M. Cerebral cavernous malformation: new molecular and clinical insights.* J Med Genet *43:716–721, 2006.)*

KRIT1 mRNA and protein have been detected in astrocytes, neurons, and epithelial cells in adults, and in vascular ECs during early angiogenesis.[217–219] Mouse *Krit1*$^{-/-}$ knockouts die at mid-gestation due to abnormal vascular development associated with downregulation of arterial markers, such as *Efnb2*, *Dll4*, and *Notch4*.[220] In humans, NOTCH4 expression in arterioles associated with CCM is significantly reduced.[196,207] These results suggest that the basic defect in CCM1 involves abnormal arterial–venous specification, which, intriguingly, may also play a role in AVM pathogenesis as discussed above.[148]

CCM2/MGC4607

The *MGC4607* gene has ten exons encoding the malcavernin protein, named for cavernous malformations, and mutations in this gene cause CCM2.[201,202] Mutations identified to date include nonsense, missense, frameshift, and splicing mutations, and larger segmental deletions.

Ccm2 is expressed in the vasculature and is necessary for proper vacuolization leading to formation of endothelial tubes.[220,221] Kleaveland et al.[222] studied the interaction of Ccm2 with heart of glass (HEG1) receptor in zebrafish and found preserved EC vacuolization and lumenization but defects in endothelial cell–cell interaction. In mice and zebrafish, *Ccm2*$^{-/-}$ knockouts die early in embryonic development due to vascular defects.[223,224] Tissue-specific mutants show that selective deletion of *Ccm2* in the endothelium is sufficient to reproduce the vascular defects and timing in embryonic death seen in germline mutants, whereas mice lacking *Ccm2* in neural or smooth muscle cells develop normally.[225] Loss of Ccm2 results in activation of RhoA GTPase via loss of a CCM2–Smurf1 interaction, which localizes Smurf1 for RhoA degradation.[226] CCM2 also appears to mediate cell death signaling by tyrosine kinase (Trk) A receptor in neural cells (e.g., medulloblastoma or neuroblastoma).[227]

Malcavernin contains a phosphotyrosine binding domain (PTB), which interacts with KRIT1 to modulate the subcellular localization of KRIT1.[228] When overexpressed, malcavernin can sequester KRIT1 within the cytoplasm and form a molecular complex with MEKK3, a kinase involved in the activation of the p38 alpha pathway, and act as a scaffolding protein.[228] Mice deficient in Mekk3 or p38 Map kinase have significant defects in placental angiogenesis and blood vessel development, especially in the head region.[229,230] An in-frame deletion in *CCM2*, which leads to deletion of 58 amino acids encoded by exon 2, is critical for KRIT1 binding and for KRIT1–PDCD10 (CCM3) interaction.[231]

CCM3/PDCD10

PDCD10 has seven coding exons and three 5′ noncoding exons.[203] CCM3 mutations identified to date include nonsense and splice-site mutations, as well as larger macrodeletions including deletion of the entire gene.[203] The protein PDCD10 (Programmed Cell Death 10) has no known conserved functional domains or motifs. It was originally identified as a transcript showing increased expression in a myeloid cell line undergoing apoptosis[232] and, more recently, was shown to be both necessary and sufficient to induce apoptosis when overexpressed in cell culture.[233]

PDCD10 mRNA is highly expressed in cerebral arterial, but not venous, endothelium during both embryonic and postnatal brain development, as well as in neuronal cell layers.[234,235] Voss et al.[236] demonstrated that PDCD10 coprecipitated and colocalized with CCM2. They hypothesized that PDCD10 is part of the CCM1/CCM2 protein complex through its interaction with CCM2, and therefore may participate in CCM1-dependent modulation of integrin β1 signaling.[236] An in-frame deletion in *CCM2* was found to inhibit formation of a CCM1/CCM2/CCM3 complex.[231]

Cerebral Cavernous Malformation Pathogenesis

Several groups have hypothesized that the underlying pathogenesis of CCM might be due to somatic mutations in known CCM genes,[123,237,238] de novo germline mutations,[239] haploinsufficiency,[240,241] or paradominant inheritance as seen in other vascular malformations.[205] Evidence of Knudson's two-hit hypothesis has been demonstrated in both human CCM lesions[123,237,238] and murine models.[225,242,243] In the two-hit model, vascular cells with two mutations (either germline or somatic) would result in complete loss of functional protein; clonal expansion of the mutant cells would then seed formation of the CCM lesion. Both *Ccm1*$^{+/-}$ and *Ccm2*$^{+/-}$ heterozygous mice are viable and phenotypically normal.[223,242] However, *Ccm1*$^{+/-}$ or *Ccm2*$^{+/-}$ mice crossed with homozygous knockouts of the tumor suppressor gene *Trp53* or mismatch repair gene *Msh2* develop lesions resembling human CCM lesions with high penetrance.[242–244] *Trp53*$^{-/-}$ mice are highly susceptible to spontaneous mutations, suggesting that a second genetic hit is involved in CCM pathogenesis. In humans, biallelic germline and somatic mutations have been identified in lesions from all three forms of inherited CCMs,[123,237] with corresponding absence of CCM proteins in vascular EC lining the cavernous lesions.[245] The observation that de novo lesion formation can occur after radiation therapy also lends indirect support to the two-hit hypothesis.[246–248]

Abnormal inflammatory or immune response has been hypothesized to play a role in CCM pathogenesis and progression.[26,249] Microarray analysis of CCM lesions revealed upregulation of ten immunoglobulin (Ig) genes compared with AVM tissue and normal superficial temporal arteries.[250] B cells were detected in CCM lesions, as was an oligoclonal pattern of IgG that was not observed in AVM or control brain specimens.[249] Familial occurrence and more aggressive clinical behavior of cavernous angiomas were associated with higher expression of Ki-67, bcl-2, and TGF-β.[192] The perilesional brain parenchyma showed significantly higher expression of TGF-β, PDGF, and tenascin, a glycoprotein of the extracellular matrix that is absent in the normal brain, in more aggressive cavernomas with larger size (>2 cm), mass effect, documented growth, or significant extralesional symptomatic hemorrhage. Further, increased VEGF expression was reported in a case of multiple cavernomas with a progressive course.[251] In addition to providing clues to CCM pathogenesis, these proteins may also serve as biomarkers for disease severity.

Mutations in all three CCM genes give rise to phenotypically similar lesions, indicating that the three proteins work in the same pathway. Indeed, biochemical studies have revealed that the three proteins can physically form a ternary complex[252] but can also have independent functions. The CCM proteins do not have defined catalytic activity, and instead are thought to help scaffolding of protein complexes to regulate the cytoskeleton, including EC adherens junctions and vascular permeability. Loss of CCM1, CCM2 or CCM3 in ECs leads to RhoA activation and signaling through Rho kinase (ROCK), resulting in increased actin stress fibers, impaired cell–cell interactions and increased vascular permeability.[225,253,254] All of these functions were restored with treatment with either a RhoA inhibitor (statins or fasudil)[225,253,255] or RNAi knockdown.[254] CCM1 was also found to strongly induce DLL4-NOTCH signaling, and blocking NOTCH activity using the antiangiogenic drug Sorafenib, a multiple kinase inhibitor that targets VEGF receptors and the Raf/ERK pathway, rescued the abnormal vasculature in vitro and in vivo.[256] Although recent animal data show promising benefits of drug therapy, clinical trials testing efficacy in humans are still lacking.

Genotype–Phenotype Correlation

With the identification of the gene mutations underlying CCM1, CCM2, and CCM3, genotype–phenotype correlations between the three forms are emerging.[257] CCM1 mutation carriers appear to have a milder hemorrhage phenotype but may present with more seizures[258] and extraneurologic manifestations, such as cutaneous vascular malformations.[259,260] In a consecutive series of 417 patients with familial CCM, 9% displayed the cutaneous vascular malformation phenotype, including hyperkeratotic cutaneous capillary–venous malformations (CCM1), capillary malformations (CCM1), and venous malformations (both CCM1 and CCM3).[259] CCM3 patients may have a more aggressive clinical course with an earlier age of onset of symptoms and greater risk of ICH.[190] Retinal vascular malformations have been observed in all three familial forms with an estimated prevalence of 5%.[261] However, large prospective studies with better characterization and follow-up are needed to confirm these phenotypic differences. Towards this end, a cohort study of familial CCM1 patients, all with the same founder common Hispanic mutation (Q455X),[198,207] has been established as part of the NINDS Brain Vascular Malformation Consortium,[262,263] and should yield insight into modifiers of CCM disease severity and progression.

Summary of Cerebral Cavernous Malformation Biology and Pathogenesis

There has been remarkable progress in elucidating the molecular genetics and biology of CCM pathogenesis over the past decade. Now that the genes and proteins have been identified, the specific mechanisms of how these proteins interact and function to cause CCM are under intense investigation. Recent data from CCM animal models show promising benefits of drugs that target RhoA (statins and fasudil)[225,253,255] or Notch signaling (Sorafenib)[256] in ameliorating the abnormal vasculature, although clinical trials testing efficacy of these drugs in humans are lacking. Better clinical characterization of CCM patients is needed to obtain more accurate estimates of genotype–phenotype correlations, clinical penetrance, frequency and severity of symptoms, progression, and response to treatments. Longitudinal studies are needed to improve understanding of the progression of the disease in both sporadic and familial cases. Undoubtedly, additional modifier genes and other factors will emerge as important predictors explaining the variable expressivity of the disease, and may shed light on the progression of related vascular malformations that involve common downstream signaling pathways.

OTHER VASCULAR MALFORMATIONS

There exist several other types of vascular malformations affecting blood and lymphatic vessels including the brain vasculature. For some of these rare anomalies, a genetic cause has been identified offering biological insights of general relevance to vascular malformations, particularly where different malformations share similar signaling pathways or biological mechanisms, such as somatic mutations, which appear to be a contributing mechanism in several vascular disorders.

Patients with **capillary malformation-arteriovenous malformation (CM-AVM) syndrome**, an autosomal dominant disorder, have cutaneous capillary malformations (also known as *port-wine stain*) and AVFs or AVMs in organs including the brain (e.g., intracranial AVMs and carotid AVFs). CM-AVM is caused by heterozygous inactivating mutations in *RASA1* (encoding p120-RasGTPase-activating protein, p120RasGAP),[264] which can be inherited or arise de novo.[265] A recent comprehensive study found 58 distinct *RASA1* mutations in 68 CM–AVM patients but none in patients with other vascular malformation phenotypes,[266] suggesting that *RASA1* mutations are specific to the CM-AVM phenotype. p120RasGAP is a negative inhibitor of the Ras/MAPkinase signaling pathway in ECs, which mediates signaling from growth factor receptors and affects EC motility and apoptosis. *Rasa1*$^{-/-}$ mice die in embryo with defective angiogenesis and increased apoptosis, but heterozygotes are phenotypically normal.[267] Phenotypic variation and reduced penetrance of familial *RASA1* mutations suggest that a second hit, possibly a somatic mutation, may be required.[265] One instance of somatic loss of the wildtype allele (via a large deletion) in a lesion from a patient with a germline *RASA1* mutation has been reported.[266]

Venous anomalies are slow-flow lesions subclassified as **venous malformations (VMs), including cutaneomucosal VM (VMCMs) and glomuvenous malformations (GVMs)**. VMCMs show autosomal dominant inheritance and are caused by mutations in the gene encoding an EC-specific receptor tyrosine kinase, TIE2 (TEK).[118,119,268] TIE2 binds angiopoietins and signals via the PI3-kinase pathway and AKT to inhibit apoptosis, and via the MAP-kinase pathways to mediate EC proliferation. TIE2-mutant ECs are deficient in the production of PDGFB, apparently due to chronic, ligand-independent activation of AKT.[269] Somatic second-hit mutations have been identified in VMCM lesional tissue,[120,121] and in at least 50% of the more common, sporadic VM, with the same mutation appearing at multiple distant lesions in the same patient, suggesting a common developmental origin.[121] When overexpressed in vitro, all VM-causative mutations result in ligand-independent receptor hyperphosphorylation, but R849W, the most common VM-CM germline mutation, has a far weaker effect than the recurrent somatic mutation, L914F.[269]

Dural arteriovenous fistulas (DAVF) are rare neurovascular malformations comprising one or more arteriovenous shunts located in the dura mater.[270] DAVFs make up approximately one-tenth of intracranial vascular malformations. Like AVMs, DAVFs involve active shunting of blood from the arterial to venous circulations, but one principal difference is that DAVFs are typically supplied by extracranial arteries. DAVFs are associated with a high risk of ICH, primarily related to a change in hemodynamics when venous drainage is shifted from extracranial to intracranial routes. VH is a hallmark of the disease process,[270] and DAVFs can be induced in rodents by inducing VH.[131,132]

Another difference from AVMs is that DAVFs are thought to be acquired lesions, resulting from known or unrecognized trauma, and their pathophysiology may involve venous thrombosis.[177,271] Given this hypothesis, genetic variation contributing to susceptibility to thrombosis has been evaluated for association with DAVFs.[272–275] In several small case series, thrombophilic mutations, such as the factor V Leiden mutation and the prothrombin G20210A, were associated with DAVF.[272] However, overall these associations were not consistent between studies, and require replication in larger cohorts. Finally, the same *ALK-1* (IVS3-35A>G) polymorphism associated with brain AVMs[94] was also present at a higher frequency in DAVF cases compared with healthy controls.[95] Unlike for AVMs, this association has not yet been independently replicated for DAVFs, but suggests commonalities in AVM and DAVF etiology, especially given the presence of arteriovenous shunting in both malformations.

Sturge–Weber syndrome (SWS) is a sporadic congenital disorder characterized by a cutaneous port-wine stain in the distribution of the ophthalmic branch of the trigeminal nerve, abnormal venous vessels, glaucoma, seizures, stroke, and intellectual disability.[276] Vascular malformations in SWS consist of enlarged, tortuous leptomeningeal vessels and dilated deep venous vessels, resulting in impaired venous drainage and reduced arterial perfusion. Recently, somatic heterozygous activating mutations in *GNAQ* have been identified in SWS. *GNAQ* encodes Gαq, a G-protein alpha subunit that mediates signaling to downstream effectors. Interestingly, the same mutation, R183Q, was found in 88% of SWS patients and 92% of non-syndromic port-wine-stain samples tested;[122] the developmental timing of the somatic mutation likely determines whether SWS (early) or only the port-wine stain (late) develops. R183Q mutants demonstrated moderate constitutive hyper-phosphorylation of ERK and a trend toward increased phosphorylation of JNK. Gαq is associated with receptors including endothelin, angiotensin, and serotonin that can impact vascular development, remodeling, and function. Since many drugs target G-protein-coupled receptor signaling, the discovery of *GNAQ* mutations in SWS suggests immediate avenues for therapy development.

Summary of Other Vascular Malformations

Different cerebrovascular malformations have varying etiology but share commonalities in signaling pathways affecting angiogenesis, vascular remodeling, inflammation and response to injury. DAVF differ from other cerebrovascular malformations in that they are acquired lesions, resulting from known or cryptic trauma and/or venous thrombosis, and are characterized by VH. Somatic mutations have been identified in several cerebrovascular malformations, including CCM, VM-CM, SWS, and possibly in CM-AVM; whether this is a biological mechanism in AVMs remains to be determined.

Acknowledgments

This chapter is dedicated in memory of our collaborator and mentor, Dr. William L. Young, for his seminal contributions to brain AVM research. The authors gratefully acknowledge members of the UCSF Brain AVM Study Project <http://avm.ucsf.edu> and the Brain Vascular Malformation Consortium; NIH grant support (R01NS034949, R01NS027713, P01NS044155, U54NS065705); and Voltaire Gungab for assistance with manuscript preparation.

The complete reference list can be found on the companion Expert Consult website at www.expertconsult.inkling.com.

KEY REFERENCES

1. Arteriovenous Malformation Study Group. Arteriovenous malformations of the brain in adults. N Engl J Med 1999;340:1812–18.
2. Al-Shahi R, Fang JS, Lewis SC, et al. Prevalence of adults with brain arteriovenous malformations: a community based study in Scotland using capture-recapture analysis. J Neurol Neurosurg Psychiatry 2002;73:547–51.
3. Berman MF, Sciacca RR, Pile-Spellman J, et al. The epidemiology of brain arteriovenous malformations. Neurosurgery 2000;47:389–96.
6. Kim H, Sidney S, McCulloch CE, et al. Racial/ethnic differences in longitudinal risk of intracranial hemorrhage in brain arteriovenous malformation patients. Stroke 2007;38:2430–7.
9. Kim H, McCulloch CE, Johnston SC, et al. Comparison of 2 approaches for determining the natural history risk of brain arteriovenous malformation rupture. Am J Epidemiol 2010;171:1317–22.
14. Klimo P Jr, Rao G, Brockmeyer D. Pediatric arteriovenous malformations: a 15-year experience with an emphasis on residual and recurrent lesions. Childs Nerv Syst 2007;23:31–7.
15. Lindqvist M, Karlsson B, Guo WY, et al. Angiographic long-term follow-up data for arteriovenous malformations previously proven to be obliterated after gamma knife radiosurgery. Neurosurgery 2000;46:803–8.
17. Hashimoto T, Lawton MT, Wen G, et al. Gene microarray analysis of human brain arteriovenous malformations. Neurosurgery 2004;54:410–23.
22. Hashimoto T, Wen G, Lawton MT, et al. Abnormal expression of matrix metalloproteinases and tissue inhibitors of metalloproteinases in brain arteriovenous malformations. Stroke 2003;34:925–31.
25. Chen Y, Zhu W, Bollen AW, et al. Evidence of inflammatory cell involvement in brain arteriovenous malformations. Neurosurgery 2008;62:1340–9.
26. Shenkar R, Shi C, Check IJ, et al. Concepts and hypotheses: inflammatory hypothesis in the pathogenesis of cerebral cavernous malformations. Neurosurgery 2007;61:693–702.
27. Gao P, Chen Y, Lawton MT, et al. Evidence of endothelial progenitor cells in the human brain and spinal cord arteriovenous malformations. Neurosurgery 2010;67:1029–35.
28. van Laake LW, van den Driesche S, Post S, et al. Endoglin has a crucial role in blood cell-mediated vascular repair. Circulation 2006;114:2288–97.
29. Li Y, Hiroi Y, Ngoy S, et al. Notch1 in bone marrow-derived cells mediates cardiac repair after myocardial infarction. Circulation 2011;123:866–76.
30. Post S, Smits AM, van den Broek AJ, et al. Impaired recruitment of HHT-1 mononuclear cells to the ischaemic heart is due to an altered CXCR4/CD26 balance. Cardiovasc Res 2010;85:494–502.
33. ten Dijke P, Arthur HM. Extracellular control of TGFbeta signalling in vascular development and disease. Nat Rev Mol Cell Biol 2007;8:857–69.
34. ten Dijke P, Goumans MJ, Pardali E. Endoglin in angiogenesis and vascular diseases. Angiogenesis 2008;11:79–89.
38. Marchuk DA, Srinivasan S, Squire TL, et al. Vascular morphogenesis: tales of two syndromes. Hum Mol Genet 2003;12:R97–112.
39. Abdalla SA, Letarte M. Hereditary haemorrhagic telangiectasia: current views on genetics and mechanisms of disease. J Med Genet 2006;43:97–110.
40. Lux A, Attisano L, Marchuk DA. Assignment of transforming growth factor beta1 and beta3 and a third new ligand to the type I receptor ALK-1. J Biol Chem 1999;274:9984–92.
41. Scharpfenecker M, van Dinther M, Liu Z, et al. BMP-9 signals via ALK1 and inhibits bFGF-induced endothelial cell proliferation and VEGF-stimulated angiogenesis. J Cell Sci 2007;120:964–72.
42. Barbara NP, Wrana JL, Letarte M. Endoglin is an accessory protein that interacts with the signaling receptor complex of multiple members of the transforming growth factor-beta superfamily. J Biol Chem 1999;274:584–94.
43. David L, Mallet C, Mazerbourg S, et al. Identification of BMP9 and BMP10 as functional activators of the orphan activin receptor-like kinase 1 (ALK1) in endothelial cells. Blood 2007;109:1953–61.
45. Urness LD, Sorensen LK, Li DY. Arteriovenous malformations in mice lacking activin receptor-like kinase-1. Nat Genet 2000;26:328–31.
46. Park SO, Lee YJ, Seki T, et al. ALK5- and TGFBR2-independent role of ALK1 in the pathogenesis of hereditary hemorrhagic telangiectasia type 2 (HHT2). Blood 2008;111:633–42.
47. Gallione CJ, Richards JA, Letteboer TG, et al. SMAD4 Mutations found in unselected HHT patients. J Med Genet 2006;43:793–7.
50. Wooderchak-Donahue WL, McDonald J, O'Fallon B, et al. BMP9 mutations cause a vascular-anomaly syndrome with phenotypic overlap with hereditary hemorrhagic telangiectasia. Am J Hum Genet 2013;93:530–7.
52. David L, Mallet C, Vailhe B, et al. Activin receptor-like kinase 1 inhibits human microvascular endothelial cell migration: potential roles for JNK and ERK. J Cell Physiol 2007;213:484–9.
53. Goumans MJ, Valdimarsdottir G, Itoh S, et al. Balancing the activation state of the endothelium via two distinct TGF-beta type I receptors. EMBO J 2002;21:1743–53.
55. Seki T, Yun J, Oh SP. Arterial endothelium-specific activin receptor-like kinase 1 expression suggests its role in arterialization and vascular remodeling. Circ Res 2003;93:682–9.

56. Jonker L, Arthur HM. Endoglin expression in early development is associated with vasculogenesis and angiogenesis. Mech Dev 2002;110:193–6.
59. Matsubara S, Bourdeau A, terBrugge KG, et al. Analysis of endoglin expression in normal brain tissue and in cerebral arteriovenous malformations. Stroke 2000;31:2653–60.
63. Toporsian M, Gros R, Kabir MG, et al. A role for endoglin in coupling eNOS activity and regulating vascular tone revealed in hereditary hemorrhagic telangiectasia. Circ Res 2005;96: 684–92.
64. Jerkic M, Kabir MG, Davies A, et al. Pulmonary hypertension in adult Alk1 heterozygous mice due to oxidative stress. Cardiovasc Res 2011;92:375–84.
67. Jerkic M, Rivas-Elena JV, Prieto M, et al. Endoglin regulates nitric oxide-dependent vasodilatation. FASEB J 2004;18:609–11.
70. Chen Y, Hao Q, Kim H, et al. Soluble endoglin modulates aberrant cerebral vascular remodeling. Ann Neurol 2009;66:19–27.
73. Pawlikowska L, Tran MN, Achrol AS, et al. Polymorphisms in genes involved in inflammatory and angiogenic pathways and the risk of hemorrhagic presentation of brain arteriovenous malformations. Stroke 2004;35:2294–300.
74. Achrol AS, Pawlikowska L, McCulloch CE, et al. Tumor necrosis factor-alpha-238G>A promoter polymorphism is associated with increased risk of new hemorrhage in the natural course of patients with brain arteriovenous malformations. Stroke 2006;37:231–4.
75. Kim H, Hysi PG, Pawlikowska L, et al. Common variants in interleukin-1-beta gene are associated with intracranial hemorrhage and susceptibility to brain arteriovenous malformation. Cerebrovasc Dis 2009;27:176–82.
77. Matsubara S, Mandzia JL, ter Brugge K, et al. Angiographic and clinical characteristics of patients with cerebral arteriovenous malformations associated with hereditary hemorrhagic telangiectasia. AJNR Am J Neuroradiol 2000;21:1016–20.
78. Maher CO, Piepgras DG, Brown RD Jr, et al. Cerebrovascular manifestations in 321 cases of hereditary hemorrhagic telangiectasia. Stroke 2001;32:877–82.
80. Letteboer TG, Mager JJ, Snijder RJ, et al. Genotype-phenotype relationship in hereditary haemorrhagic telangiectasia. J Med Genet 2006;43:371–7.
81. Bayrak-Toydemir P, McDonald J, Markewitz B, et al. Genotype-phenotype correlation in hereditary hemorrhagic telangiectasia: mutations and manifestations. Am J Med Genet A 2006;140: 463–70.
83. Mast H, Young WL, Koennecke HC, et al. Risk of spontaneous haemorrhage after diagnosis of cerebral arteriovenous malformation. Lancet 1997;350:1065–8.
85. van Beijnum J, van der Worp HB, Schippers HM, et al. Familial occurrence of brain arteriovenous malformations: a systematic review. J Neurol Neurosurg Psychiatry 2007;78:1213–17.
87. Kim H, Marchuk DA, Pawlikowska L, et al. Genetic considerations relevant to intracranial hemorrhage and brain arteriovenous malformations. Acta Neurochir Suppl 2008;105:199–206.
94. Pawlikowska L, Tran MN, Achrol AS, et al. Polymorphisms in transforming growth factor-B-related genes ALK1 and ENG are associated with sporadic brain arteriovenous malformations. Stroke 2005;36:2278–80.
95. Simon M, Franke D, Ludwig M, et al. Association of a polymorphism of the ACVRL1 gene with sporadic arteriovenous malformations of the central nervous system. J Neurosurg 2006;104: 945–9.
97. Boshuisen K, Brundel M, de Kovel CG, et al. Polymorphisms in ACVRL1 and endoglin genes are not associated with sporadic and HHT-related brain AVMs in Dutch patients. Transl Stroke Res 2013;4:375–8.
98. Cambier S, Gline S, Mu D, et al. Integrin alpha(v)beta8-mediated activation of transforming growth factor-beta by perivascular astrocytes: an angiogenic control switch. Am J Pathol 2005;166: 1883–94.
99. Su H, Kim H, Pawlikowska L, et al. Reduced expression of integrin alphavbeta8 is associated with brain arteriovenous malformation pathogenesis. Am J Pathol 2010;176:1018–27.
100. Kuhnert F, Mancuso MR, Shamloo A, et al. Essential regulation of CNS angiogenesis by the orphan G protein-coupled receptor GPR124. Science 2010;330:985–9.
101. Weinsheimer S, Brettman AD, Pawlikowska L, et al. G protein-coupled receptor 124 *(GPR124)* gene polymorphisms and risk of brain arteriovenous malformation. Transl Stroke Res 2012;3: 418–27.
102. Kim H, Hysi PG, Pawlikowska L, et al. Population stratification in a case-control study of brain arteriovenous malformation in Latinos. Neuroepidemiology 2008;31:224–8.
103. Fontanella M, Rubino E, Crobeddu E, et al. Brain arteriovenous malformations are associated with interleukin-1 cluster gene polymorphisms. Neurosurgery 2012;70:12–17.
104. Jiang N, Li X, Qi T, et al. Susceptible gene single nucleotide polymorphism and hemorrhage risk in patients with brain arteriovenous malformation. J Clin Neurosci 2011;18:1279–81.
105. Zhao Y, Li P, Fan W, et al. The rs522616 polymorphism in the matrix metalloproteinase-3 (MMP-3) gene is associated with sporadic brain arteriovenous malformation in a Chinese population. J Clin Neurosci 2010;17:1568–72.
106. Mikhak B, Weinsheimer S, Pawlikowska L, et al. Angiopoietin-like 4 (ANGPTL4) gene polymorphisms and risk of brain arteriovenous malformations. Cerebrovasc Dis 2011;31:338–45.
107. Chen H, Gu Y, Wu W, et al. Polymorphisms of the vascular endothelial growth factor A gene and susceptibility to sporadic brain arteriovenous malformation in a Chinese population. J Clin Neurosci 2011;18:549–53.
108. Gong ZP, Qiao ND, Gu YX, et al. Polymorphisms of VEGFA gene and susceptibility to hemorrhage risk of brain arteriovenous malformations in a Chinese population. Acta Pharmacol Sin 2011;32:1071–7.
109. Sturiale CL, Puca A, Sebastiani P, et al. Single nucleotide polymorphisms associated with sporadic brain arteriovenous malformations: where do we stand? Brain 2013;136:665–81.
111. Pawlikowska L, Poon KY, Achrol AS, et al. Apoliprotein E epsilon2 is associated with new hemorrhage risk in brain arteriovenous malformation. Neurosurgery 2006;58:838–43, discussion 838–43.
112. Achrol AS, Kim H, Pawlikowska L, et al. Association of tumor necrosis factor-alpha-238G>A and Apolipoprotein E2 polymorphisms with intracranial hemorrhage after brain arteriovenous malformation treatment. Neurosurgery 2007;61: 731–9.
118. Vikkula M, Boon LM, Carraway KL 3rd, et al. Vascular dysmorphogenesis caused by an activating mutation in the receptor tyrosine kinase TIE2. Cell 1996;87:1181–90.
120. Brouillard P, Vikkula M. Genetic causes of vascular malformations. Hum Mol Genet 2007;16(Spec2):R140–9.
121. Limaye N, Wouters V, Uebelhoer M, et al. Somatic mutations in angiopoietin receptor gene TEK cause solitary and multiple sporadic venous malformations. Nat Genet 2009;41:118–24.
122. Shirley MD, Tang H, Gallione CJ, et al. Sturge-Weber syndrome and port-wine stains caused by somatic mutation in GNAQ. N Engl J Med 2013;368:1971–9.
123. Akers AL, Johnson E, Steinberg GK, et al. Biallelic somatic and germline mutations in cerebral cavernous malformations (CCM): evidence for a two-hit mechanism of CCM pathogenesis. Hum Mol Genet 2009;18:919–30.
125. Happle R. Klippel-Trenaunay syndrome: is it a paradominant trait? Br J Dermatol 1993;128:465–6.
147. Carlson TR, Yan Y, Wu X, et al. Endothelial expression of constitutively active Notch4 elicits reversible arteriovenous malformations in adult mice. Proc Natl Acad Sci U S A 2005;102: 9884–9.
148. Murphy PA, Lam MT, Wu X, et al. Endothelial Notch4 signaling induces hallmarks of brain arteriovenous malformations in mice. Proc Natl Acad Sci U S A 2008;105:10901–6.
149. Yao Y, Yao J, Radparvar M, et al. Reducing Jagged 1 and 2 levels prevents cerebral arteriovenous malformations in matrix Gla protein deficiency. Proc Natl Acad Sci U S A 2013;110: 19071–6.
150. Zhang G, Zhou J, Fan Q, et al. Arterial-venous endothelial cell fate is related to vascular endothelial growth factor and Notch status during human bone mesenchymal stem cell differentiation. FEBS Lett 2008;582:2957–64.
151. Benedito R, Roca C, Sorensen I, et al. The notch ligands Dll4 and Jagged1 have opposing effects on angiogenesis. Cell 2009;137: 1124–35.

152. ZhuGe Q, Zhong M, Zheng W, et al. Notch1 signaling is activated in brain arteriovenous malformation in humans. Brain 2009;132:3231–41.
153. Murphy PA, Lu G, Shiah S, et al. Endothelial Notch signaling is upregulated in human brain arteriovenous malformations and a mouse model of the disease. Lab Invest 2009;89:971–82.
154. Murphy PA, Kim TN, Lu G, et al. Notch4 normalization reduced blood vessel size in arteriovenous malformations. Sci Transl Med 2012;4:117ra118.
159. Srinivasan S, Hanes MA, Dickens T, et al. A mouse model for hereditary hemorrhagic telangiectasia (HHT) type 2. Hum Mol Genet 2003;12:473–82.
162. Xu B, Wu YQ, Huey M, et al. Vascular endothelial growth factor induces abnormal microvasculature in the endoglin heterozygous mouse brain. J Cereb Blood Flow Metab 2004;24: 237–44.
163. Hao Q, Su H, Marchuk DA, et al. Increased tissue perfusion promotes capillary dysplasia in the ALK1-deficient mouse brain following VEGF stimulation. Am J Physiol Heart Circ Physiol 2008;295:H2250–6.
167. Park SO, Wankhede M, Lee YJ, et al. Real-time imaging of de novo arteriovenous malformation in a mouse model of hereditary hemorrhagic telangiectasia. J Clin Invest 2009;119: 3487–96.
168. Milton I, Ouyang D, Allen CJ, et al. Age-dependent lethality in novel transgenic mouse models of central nervous system arteriovenous malformations. Stroke 2012;43:1432–5.
169. Walker EJ, Su H, Shen F, et al. Arteriovenous malformation in the adult mouse brain resembling the human disease. Ann Neurol 2011;69:954–62.
170. Guo Y, Saunders T, Su H, et al. Silent intralesional microhemorrhage as a risk factor for brain arteriovenous malformation rupture. Stroke 2012;43:1240–6.
171. Chen W, Guo Y, Walker EJ, et al. Reduced mural cell coverage and impaired vessel integrity after angiogenic stimulation in the *Alk1*-deficient brain. Arterioscler Thromb Vasc Biol 2013;33: 305–10.
174. Bourdeau A, Dumont DJ, Letarte M. A murine model of hereditary hemorrhagic telangiectasia. J Clin Invest 1999;104: 1343–51.
175. Li DY, Sorensen LK, Brooke BS, et al. Defective angiogenesis in mice lacking endoglin. Science 1999;284:1534–7.
177. Chaudhary MY, Sachdev VP, Cho SH, et al. Dural arteriovenous malformation of the major venous sinuses: an acquired lesion. AJNR Am J Neuroradiol 1982;3:13–19.
180. Konya D, Yildirim O, Kurtkaya O, et al. Testing the angiogenic potential of cerebrovascular malformations by use of a rat cornea model: usefulness and novel assessment of changes over time. Neurosurgery 2005;56:1339–45.
185. Clatterbuck RE, Eberhart CG, Crain BJ, et al. Ultrastructural and immunocytochemical evidence that an incompetent blood-brain barrier is related to the pathophysiology of cavernous malformations. J Neurol Neurosurg Psychiatry 2001;71:188–92.
187. Rigamonti D, Hadley MN, Drayer BP, et al. Cerebral cavernous malformations. Incidence and familial occurrence. N Engl J Med 1988;319:343–7.
190. Denier C, Labauge P, Bergametti F, et al. Genotype-phenotype correlations in cerebral cavernous malformations patients. Ann Neurol 2006;60:550–6.
192. Maiuri F, Cappabianca P, Gangemi M, et al. Clinical progression and familial occurrence of cerebral cavernous angiomas: the role of angiogenic and growth factors. Neurosurg Focus 2006;21:e3.
193. Denier C, Labauge P, Brunereau L, et al. Clinical features of cerebral cavernous malformations patients with KRIT1 mutations. Ann Neurol 2004;55:213–20.
194. Dubovsky J, Zabramski JM, Kurth J, et al. A gene responsible for cavernous malformations of the brain maps to chromosome 7q. Hum Mol Genet 1995;4:453–8.
195. Gunel M, Awad IA, Anson J, et al. Mapping a gene causing cerebral cavernous malformation to 7q11.2-q21. Proc Natl Acad Sci U S A 1995;92:6620–4.
196. Marchuk DA, Gallione CJ, Morrison LA, et al. A locus for cerebral cavernous malformations maps to chromosome 7q in two families. Genomics 1995;28:311–14.
197. Johnson EW, Iyer LM, Rich SS, et al. Refined localization of the cerebral cavernous malformation gene (CCM1) to a 4-cM interval of chromosome 7q contained in a well-defined YAC contig. Genome Res 1995;5:368–80.
198. Gunel M, Awad IA, Finberg K, et al. A founder mutation as a cause of cerebral cavernous malformation in Hispanic Americans. N Engl J Med 1996;334:946–51.
201. Liquori CL, Berg MJ, Siegel AM, et al. Mutations in a gene encoding a novel protein containing a phosphotyrosine-binding domain cause type 2 cerebral cavernous malformations. Am J Hum Genet 2003;73:1459–64.
202. Denier C, Goutagny S, Labauge P, et al. Mutations within the MGC4607 gene cause cerebral cavernous malformations. Am J Hum Genet 2004;74:326–37.
203. Bergametti F, Denier C, Labauge P, et al. Mutations within the programmed cell death 10 gene cause cerebral cavernous malformations. Am J Hum Genet 2005;76:42–51.
204. Liquori CL, Berg MJ, Squitieri F, et al. Low frequency of PDCD10 mutations in a panel of CCM3 probands: potential for a fourth CCM locus. Hum Mutat 2006;27:118.
205. Revencu N, Vikkula M. Cerebral cavernous malformation: new molecular and clinical insights. J Med Genet 2006;43: 716–21.
207. Sahoo T, Johnson EW, Thomas JW, et al. Mutations in the gene encoding KRIT1, a Krev-1/rap1a binding protein, cause cerebral cavernous malformations (CCM1). Hum Mol Genet 1999;8: 2325–33.
213. Glading A, Han J, Stockton RA, et al. KRIT-1/CCM1 is a Rap1 effector that regulates endothelial cell cell junctions. J Cell Biol 2007;179:247–54.
215. Zhang J, Clatterbuck RE, Rigamonti D, et al. Interaction between KRIT1 and ICAP1alpha infers perturbation of integrin beta1-mediated angiogenesis in the pathogenesis of cerebral cavernous malformation. Hum Mol Genet 2001;10:2953–60.
216. Zawistowski JS, Serebriiskii IG, Lee MF, et al. KRIT1 association with the integrin-binding protein ICAP-1: a new direction in the elucidation of cerebral cavernous malformations (CCM1) pathogenesis. Hum Mol Genet 2002;11:389–96.
217. Denier C, Gasc JM, Chapon F, et al. Krit1/cerebral cavernous malformation 1 mRNA is preferentially expressed in neurons and epithelial cells in embryo and adult. Mech Dev 2002;117: 363–7.
220. Whitehead KJ, Plummer NW, Adams JA, et al. Ccm1 is required for arterial morphogenesis: implications for the etiology of human cavernous malformations. Development 2004;131: 1437–48.
221. Boulday G, Blecon A, Petit N, et al. Tissue-specific conditional CCM2 knockout mice establish the essential role of endothelial CCM2 in angiogenesis: implications for human cerebral cavernous malformations. Dis Model Mech 2009;2:168–77.
225. Whitehead KJ, Chan AC, Navankasattusas S, et al. The cerebral cavernous malformation signaling pathway promotes vascular integrity via Rho GTPases. Nat Med 2009;15:177–84.
226. Crose LE, Hilder TL, Sciaky N, et al. Cerebral cavernous malformation 2 protein promotes smad ubiquitin regulatory factor 1-mediated RhoA degradation in endothelial cells. J Biol Chem 2009;284:13301–5.
228. Zawistowski JS, Stalheim L, Uhlik MT, et al. CCM1 and CCM2 protein interactions in cell signaling: implications for cerebral cavernous malformations pathogenesis. Hum Mol Genet 2005; 14:2521–31.
234. Petit N, Blecon A, Denier C, et al. Patterns of expression of the three cerebral cavernous malformation (CCM) genes during embryonic and postnatal brain development. Gene Expr Patterns 2006;6:495–503.
236. Voss K, Stahl S, Schleider E, et al. CCM3 interacts with CCM2 indicating common pathogenesis for cerebral cavernous malformations. Neurogenetics 2007;8:249–56.
237. Gault J, Shenkar R, Recksiek P, et al. Biallelic somatic and germ line CCM1 truncating mutations in a cerebral cavernous malformation lesion. Stroke 2005;36:872–4.
242. Plummer NW, Gallione CJ, Srinivasan S, et al. Loss of p53 sensitizes mice with a mutation in Ccm1 (KRIT1) to development of cerebral vascular malformations. Am J Pathol 2004;165: 1509–18.

243. McDonald DA, Shenkar R, Shi C, et al. A novel mouse model of cerebral cavernous malformations based on the two-hit mutation hypothesis recapitulates the human disease. Hum Mol Genet 2011;20:211–22.
245. Pagenstecher A, Stahl S, Sure U, et al. A two-hit mechanism causes cerebral cavernous malformations: complete inactivation of CCM1, CCM2 or CCM3 in affected endothelial cells. Hum Mol Genet 2009;18:911–18.
246. Detwiler PW, Porter RW, Zabramski JM, et al. Radiation-induced cavernous malformation. J Neurosurg 1998;89:167–9.
249. Shi C, Shenkar R, Batjer HH, et al. Oligoclonal immune response in cerebral cavernous malformations. Laboratory investigation. J Neurosurg 2007;107:1023–6.
250. Shenkar R, Elliott JP, Diener K, et al. Differential gene expression in human cerebrovascular malformations. Neurosurgery 2003; 52:465–78.
251. Jung KH, Chu K, Jeong SW, et al. Cerebral cavernous malformations with dynamic and progressive course: correlation study with vascular endothelial growth factor. Arch Neurol 2003;60: 1613–18.
252. Hilder TL, Malone MH, Bencharit S, et al. Proteomic identification of the cerebral cavernous malformation signaling complex. J Proteome Res 2007;6:4343–55.
253. Stockton RA, Shenkar R, Awad IA, et al. Cerebral cavernous malformations proteins inhibit Rho kinase to stabilize vascular integrity. J Exp Med 2010;207:881–96.
254. Borikova AL, Dibble CF, Sciaky N, et al. Rho kinase inhibition rescues the endothelial cell cerebral cavernous malformation phenotype. J Biol Chem 2010;285:11760–4.
255. McDonald DA, Shi C, Shenkar R, et al. Fasudil decreases lesion burden in a murine model of cerebral cavernous malformation disease. Stroke 2012;43:571–4.
256. Wustehube J, Bartol A, Liebler SS, et al. Cerebral cavernous malformation protein CCM1 inhibits sprouting angiogenesis by activating DELTA-NOTCH signaling. Proc Natl Acad Sci U S A 2010;107:12640–5.
258. Gault J, Sain S, Hu LJ, et al. Spectrum of genotype and clinical manifestations in cerebral cavernous malformations. Neurosurgery 2006;59:1278–84.
264. Eerola I, Boon LM, Mulliken JB, et al. Capillary malformation-arteriovenous malformation, a new clinical and genetic disorder caused by RASA1 mutations. Am J Hum Genet 2003;73: 1240–9.
265. Revencu N, Boon LM, Mulliken JB, et al. Parkes Weber syndrome, vein of Galen aneurysmal malformation, and other fast-flow vascular anomalies are caused by RASA1 mutations. Hum Mutat 2008;29:959–65.
268. Wouters V, Limaye N, Uebelhoer M, et al. Hereditary cutaneomucosal venous malformations are caused by TIE2 mutations with widely variable hyper-phosphorylating effects. Eur J Hum Genet 2010;18:414–20.
269. Uebelhoer M, Natynki M, Kangas J, et al. Venous malformation-causative TIE2 mutations mediate an AKT-dependent decrease in PDGFB. Hum Mol Genet 2013;22:3438–48.
270. Singh V, Smith WS, Lawton MT, et al. Risk factors for hemorrhagic presentation in patients with dural arteriovenous fistulae. Neurosurgery 2008;62:628–35.
272. van Dijk JM, TerBrugge KG, Van der Meer FJ, et al. Thrombophilic factors and the formation of dural arteriovenous fistulas. J Neurosurg 2007;107:56–9.
276. Thomas-Sohl KA, Vaslow DF, Maria BL. Sturge-Weber syndrome: a review. Pediatr Neurol 2004;30:303–10.

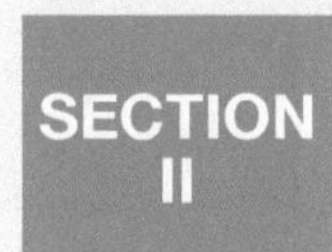

Epidemiology and Risk Factors

Ralph L. Sacco

Stroke continues to have a profound impact across the globe that is expanding given the aging of our population. Despite the concerning statistics, there are ample opportunities to intervene and prevent a stroke. Stroke and other vascular disorders have taken a centerstage in the increased efforts from the United Nations and the World Health Organization to reduce the burden of non-communicable diseases by 2025. The global focus on reducing these risks calls for an expanded understanding of the epidemiology, risk factors, determinants and outcomes of stroke and other vascular conditions that threaten brain health. In this sixth edition, the epidemiology and prevention section has been extensively updated and revised. New data from the Global Burden of Disease provide an extensive overview in the new chapter on the Global Burden of Stroke (Chapter 13) including temporal trends since 1990 and geographic variation in incidence, mortality, prevalence and disability. Stroke continues to affect certain population groups more than others and the new chapter on Stroke Disparities (Chapter 14) highlights important differences by race, ethnicity, geography, urban vs rural communities, and socioeconomic status. An overview of risk factors and determinants of incident and recurrent stroke is provided in the extensively updated chapters on Modifiable Risk Factors and Determinants of Stroke (Chapter 15) and Prognosis After Stroke (Chapter 16). The latter chapter also includes discussion of other outcomes including mortality, disability, quality of life, and depression. Another important outcome for stroke survivors and of growing concern for our aging population is cognitive impairment and dementia. The most recent definitions, criteria, imaging characteristics, and role of vascular risk factors are reviewed in the updated chapter on Vascular Dementia and Cognitive Impairment (Chapter 17). Our expanding knowledge of genetic determinants is discussed in the revised chapter on Genetic Basis of Stroke Occurrence, Prevention and Outcome (Chapter 18). We end the section with an updated review of the evidence on primary prevention in Preventing a First Stroke (Chapter 19) including the latest evidence-based recommendations on lifestyle modifications, blood pressure control, lipid lowering, oral anticoagulants for atrial fibrillation, and use of aspirin.

13 Global Burden of Stroke

Valery L. Feigin, Rita V. Krishnamurthi

KEY POINTS

- The GBD 2010 study shows that while mortality rates and mortality to incidence ratios for stroke have decreased, the global burden of stroke in terms of absolute numbers of incident strokes, survivors, stroke-related deaths and DALYs lost are high and have increased over the last two decades.
- While there has been a decline in stroke incidence, mortality, mortality to incidence ratios and DALYs in high-income countries, both the incidence and prevalence of stroke have increased in low- and middle-income countries in the past two decades. Low- and middle-income countries have had a lower rate of reduction in mortality rates and DALYs compared to high-income countries. Consequently, the burden of stroke is significantly higher in low- and middle-income countries than in high-income countries.
- While ischemic strokes comprise the highest number of strokes, most of the global burden of stroke measured in proportionate mortality and by DALYs is due to hemorrhagic stroke. The incidence of hemorrhagic stroke increased significantly worldwide over the last two decades by 18.5%, while there was no significant change in the incidence of ischemic stroke. Low- and middle-income countries endure 80% of deaths due to hemorrhagic stroke.
- The burden of stroke in people younger than 75 years has increased over the last two decades. Most of the ischemic stroke burden is in low- and middle-income countries, and both incident and fatal hemorrhagic and ischemic strokes occur at a younger age in these regions.
- Worldwide, there has been a startling 25% increase in the incidence of stroke among adults aged 20 to 64 years over the last 20 years. This study showed, for the first time, that more than 83,000 children and youths aged 20 years and younger are affected by stroke in the world annually. Children and youths (aged <20 years) and young and middle-aged adults (20–64 years) constitute a startling 0.5% and 31% of all people with incident stroke, respectively.
- Strategies to reduce burden at both population and individual levels to improve stroke awareness, implement targeted prevention strategies focussed on risk factors (such as high blood pressure, high cholesterol, smoking and unhealthy lifestyles) are essential to abate the currently alarming projections of stroke burden particularly in low- and middle-income countries and in younger people.

INTRODUCTION

Stroke is the second leading cause of death worldwide[1,2] and was responsible for 5.7 million deaths in 2005. Stroke is preventable to a large extent as many of the risk factors for stroke are modifiable. Modifiable risk factors for stroke include high blood pressure, smoking, obesity, lack of physical activity and unhealthy diets.[3] The largest proportion of the burden of stroke has previously been reported to be in low-income countries[2,4] and the majority of stroke-related deaths occurred in low- and middle-income countries.[1]

The Global Burden of Diseases, Injuries and Risk Factors Study (GBD 2010) is the most recent systematic analysis and update of global data on the comparative magnitude of health loss due to disease, risk factors and injuries from 1990 to 2010 by age, sex and geographical region.[5] Epidemiological data from the past two decades from 21 world regions were analyzed by the GBD 2010 investigators to provide the most recent and comprehensive estimates of the global burden of 291 diseases and injuries, including stroke. Statistical methods were developed to address incomplete epidemiologic data, particularly from low- and middle-income countries.[6] Stroke has a major health, economic and societal burden, particularly in the developing world, however it is highly preventable. Therefore, there is potential to dramatically reduce the impact of stroke by several means, including with adequate control of known risk factors. It is imperative to have a clear understanding of the global demographic pattern, distribution and temporal trends of the burden of stroke to best inform health policies to reduce its burden.

The latest estimates from the GBD 2010 studies reveal a shift in overall global disease burden from communicable, maternal, neonatal and nutritional causes towards non-communicable diseases.[7] This shift is likely to be a result of the world's population increasing in number and in age, reductions in deaths from communicable diseases, and decreasing death rates by age, sex, and cause of death in the past two decades.[7] Ischemic heart disease and stroke collectively resulted in 12.9 million (or one in four) deaths in 2010, compared with one in five deaths in 1990.[7] Previous estimates by the World Health Organization (WHO) showed that ischemic heart disease and stroke combined were the leading causes of adult mortality in 2004.[8] The latest GBD estimates show that stroke remained ranked the second most common cause of death after ischemic heart disease (Table 13-1).[7] While stroke has remained the second leading cause of death since 1990, the number of deaths from stroke has increased by 26%, from 4.7 million deaths in 1990 to 5.9 million deaths in 2010. This chapter provides an overview of the GBD 2010 stroke studies, with a brief description of the GBD methods and the most recent analysis of the global burden of stroke.

TABLE 13-1 Global Death Ranks for Top 10 Causes in 2010 and Percentage Change from 1990 and 2010

Disorder	Mean Rank (95% UI)	% Change (95% UI)
1. Ischemic heart disease	1.0 (1 to 1)	35 (29 to 39)
2. Stroke	2.0 (2 to 2)	25 (14 to 32)
3. Chronic obstructive pulmonary disease	3.4 (3 to 4)	−7 (−12 to 0)
4. Lower respiratory infections	3.6 (3 to 4)	−18 (−24 to −11)
5. Lung cancer	5.8 (5 to 10)	48 (24 to 61)
6. HIV/AIDS	6.4 (5 to 8)	396 (323 to 465)
7. Diarrhea	6.7 (5 to 9)	−42 (−49 to −35)
8. Road injury	8.4 (5 to 11)	47 (18 to 86)
9. Diabetes	9.0 (7 to 11)	93 (68 to 102)
10. Tuberculosis	10.1 (8 to 13)	−18 (−35 to −3)

(Partially reproduced from GBD Lancet, Lozano R, Naghavi M, Foreman K, et al. Global and regional mortality from 235 causes of death for 20 age groups in 1990 and 2000: a systematic analysis for the Global Burden of Disease Study 2010. Lancet *380:2133, Figure 4, 2012.)*

GLOBAL BURDEN OF DISEASE METHODS

GBD 2010 reported estimates for stroke incidence, mortality, mortality-incidence ratio, and DALYs lost for total stroke, and by ischemic and hemorrhagic stroke subtypes.[9,10] Multiple databases including Medline, EMBASE, LILACS, Scopus, PubMed and Science Direct, Global Health Database, WHO library and WHO regional databases, were searched to identify relevant studies published between 1990 and 2010. The Global Burden of Disease 2010 Study analytical tool (DisMod-MR) was used to calculate region-specific (including 95% confidence intervals [CI]) of IS incidence, mortality, mortality to incidence ratio (MIR) and disability-adjusted life years (DALYs) lost per 100,000 people by age groups (<75 years; ≥75 years; total) and country income level (HIC and LMIC) for 1990, 2005 and 2010.[11] Age-standardized incidence and mortality rates per 100,000 person-years and DALYs estimates per 100,000 people were computed using the direct method of standardization with the WHO standard population as a reference population. The studies included for data extraction and analysis were those that met the following criteria: studies that used the WHO definition of stroke,[12] reported methods for ascertaining stroke cases, distinguished between first-ever stroke and recurrent stroke (only incident strokes were included in these analyses), reported an age-specific epidemiologic parameter of interest and the population denominator (i.e., stroke incidence and/or prevalence in 5- or 10-year age bands) with sufficient detail to enable an estimate of age-adjusted parameters were included in the analysis. Incidence studies from HIC required complete stroke case ascertainment while less rigorous stroke case ascertainment was allowed for studies from LMIC in which no other relevant data were otherwise available. To estimate the mortality rate, the GBD mortality database and an ensemble cause of death modelling approach were used.[5,9,13]

Stroke burden in terms of DALYs for GBD 1990 was described in the World Development Report 1993,[14] as a means of estimating the years of healthy life lost due to poor health or disability. DALYs are used as a measure of population health, and are the sum of years of life lost due to death (YLL) and years lived with disability (YLD).[6] The detailed methodology for calculating DALYs in the GBD 2010 Project has been described elsewhere.[6] YLL is the product of the number of deaths at each age by a standard life expectancy at that age. YLD is the prevalence the disease multiplied by the disability weight for that disease. The disability weight is calculated in the basis of the level of health loss for the disease and reflects the severity of the disease on a scale from 0 (perfect health) to 1 (equivalent to death). Each DALY is a year of healthy life lost due to disease, impairment or death.

Overall Stroke Estimates

In 2010 there are 16.9 million cases of incident stroke worldwide, with 69% of these in low- and middle-income countries. Low- and middle-income countries had the greatest proportion of deaths with 71% of the 5.9 million stroke deaths. Country-specific variation in stroke incidence was noted in 2010 (Table 13-2), ranging from 60 cases in Kuwait to 504 cases per 100,000 person-years in Lithuania; mortality ranged from 27 cases in France to 264 cases per 100,000 person-years in Afghanistan; prevalence raged from 88 in Burundi to 1187 per 100,000 person-years in Canada; DALYs lost ranged from 398 in Australia to 5227 per 100,000 person-years in Afghanistan; mortality to incidence ratios ranged from 0.11 in Iran to 1.35 in Afghanistan. In terms of age at stroke, 50% of strokes in high-income countries and 32% of strokes in low- and middle-income countries were in people aged 75 years or older (Table 13-2). In high-income countries, 73% of stroke deaths occurred in people aged 75 year or older, while in low- to middle-income countries this proportion was lower, at 47%. Age standardized mortality was 33% higher in low- and middle-income countries than in high-income countries in people over 75 years, and 212% higher in people 75 years and younger. Mortality-to-incidence ratio was used as an ecological proxy estimation of stroke case fatality, calculated as the ratio of the number of deaths to the number of new cases of stroke within a specified period of time. The mortality to incidence ratio was 0.35 globally, and 0.32 and 0.36 in low- and middle-income and high-income countries, respectively.

Ischemic Stroke

In 2010 there were 11.6 million incident cases of ischemic stroke worldwide, and similar to total strokes, the majority (63%) occurred in low- and middle-income countries. There were 2.8 million ischemic stroke deaths and 57% of these were in low- to middle-income countries. Ischemic stroke resulted in a loss of 39.4 million DALYS with 64% of these in low- and middle-income countries. The age-standardized incidence of ischemic stroke per 100,000 person years ranged from 51.88 in Qatar to 433.97 in Lithuania (Table 13-3). Qatar also had the lowest age standardized mortality rate per 100,000 person years at 9.17, while Russia had the highest at 137.70. DALYs lost due to ischemic stroke ranged from 163.89 in Israel to 2032.11 in Afghanistan.

Hemorrhagic Stroke

There were 5.3 million cases of hemorrhagic stroke in 2010 and an even higher proportion (80%) of these, compared to ischemic stroke, occurred in low- and middle-income countries. There were over 3.0 million deaths (84% in low- and middle-income countries), and 62.8 million DALYs lost (86% in low- and middle-income countries) (Table 13-3). Age-adjusted incidence per 100,000 person years of hemorrhagic stroke was lowest in Qatar (14.55) and highest in China (159.81). The age-standardized mortality rate per 100,000 person years was lowest in the USA at 9.64, and highest in Mongolia at 210.56. DALYs lost due to hemorrhagic stroke ranged from 178.20 in Switzerland to 4118.9 in Mongolia.

Trends in Stroke Burden from 1990 to 2010

Globally, in the past two decades, there was an increase in the absolute numbers of people with incident stroke (68%); stroke survivors (84%); stroke-related deaths (26%); and DALYs lost (12%). Changes in stroke burden between 1990 and 2010 took differing directions by income level, with an increasing gap in the proportion of absolute numbers of incidence and prevalent strokes in the past two decades between low- and middle-income countries and high-income countries (Figs 13-1 and 13-2). In high-income countries, age-standardized rates of stroke decreased in the people 75 and older by 16% compared to a 9% decrease in those younger than 75 years. In contrast, there was an increase (non-significant) in age-standardized incidence and prevalence in both younger and older age groups in low- and middle-income countries. Age-standardized mortality rates in high-income countries decreased at similar rates (36–39%) in both younger and older age groups, whereas there was a greater reduction in DALYs lost in the older age group (63%), compared to people younger than 75 years (36%). High-income countries saw the greatest reduction in mortality-to-incidence ratios in people younger than 75 years (32% decrease) compared to people 75 years and older (21% decrease). In low-income countries there was a greater reduction in DALYs lost in people younger than 75 years (24% decrease) compared to the older age group (23% decrease). Similarly, in low- and middle-income countries, mortality-to-incidence ratio was also significantly reduced (32%) in people younger than 75 years (32%), and by 16% in the older age group.

The incidence of hemorrhagic stroke increased significantly worldwide over the last two decades by 18.5%, while there was no significant change in the incidence of ischemic stroke. There was a significant reduction (14.6%) globally in the incidence of hemorrhagic stroke in the older age group. However, in low- and middle-income countries, there was a significant increase (22%, 95%CI 5–30) in the incidence of hemorrhagic stroke, with a 19% (95%CI 5–30) increase in those younger than 75 years. In particular, in people aged 20–64 years, the incidence of both ischemic and hemorrhagic stroke in low- and middle-income countries increased significantly (12.6% and 33.8%, respectively).

Worldwide, a significant increase was seen in the mean age of incident, prevalent and fatal strokes. However, the mean age of incident and prevalent strokes was higher by at least 5 years in high-income countries than in low- and middle-income countries. The mean age of people for incident ischemic stroke in 2010 was 76.2 (0.13) years in high-income countries compared to 70.8 (0.12) years in low- and middle-income countries, and for hemorrhagic stroke the mean age in high-income countries was 69.1 (0.15) years compared to 63.8 (0.13) in low- and middle-income countries (Table 13-4). In 2010, the mean age at fatal stroke was also higher by 8 years in high-income countries than in low- and middle-income countries (higher by 6 years for hemorrhagic stroke and 5.6 years for ischemic stroke).

Geographical Variation

Significant geographical variations in stroke burden were noted (Fig. 13-3). In 2010 stroke incidence and DALYs lost were highest in Eastern Europe, east Asia and northern and sub-Saharan Africa, and lowest in Andean Latin America and Australasia. The incidence of ischemic stroke was also highest in Eastern Europe (particularly Russia at 23–416/100,000), as well as central and east Asia, North Africa, and the Middle East. The highest incidences of hemorrhagic stroke in 2010 were in central and east Asia (101–158/100,000) and east and southern sub-Saharan Africa (73–101/100,000) and the lowest rates were in high-income North America, central and Andean Latin America, western Europe, and Australasia (25–40/100,000).

In the past two decades, the greatest increases in stroke incidence were seen in sub-Saharan Africa, the Middle East, southeast Asia, central and Latin America, and south and east Asia, while stroke incidence decreased in high-income Asia Pacific countries. The greatest increases in ischemic stroke incidence were seen in Eastern Europe, central and east Asia, north and sub-Saharan Africa, and the Middle East. However, there were also significant reductions in ischemic stroke incidence in these regions (South Korea 44%, Chile 41%). The greatest increases in hemorrhagic stroke were seen in eastern and central Europe, north and sub-Saharan Africa and the Middle East, whereas significant reductions were noted in North America, western Europe, and tropical and southern Latin America.

Changes in DALYs lost per 100,000 people over the past two decades varied significantly between GBD regions, ranging from −50.4 to −0.74 (percent change) (Fig. 13-4). Interestingly, marked reductions in DALYs lost were in west and central sub-Saharan Africa, Eastern Europe, and Asia. Mortality-to-incidence ratios decreased in all GBD regions, but remained unchanged in Eastern Europe, south Asia and high-income Asia Pacific. Mortality-to-incidence ratios for ischemic stroke were lowest in high-income North America and east Asia (0.17–0.19), and for hemorrhagic stroke in high-income North America. Europe and the Caribbean had the highest mortality-to-incidence ratios for ischemic stroke (0.34–0.38) while Oceania had the highest for hemorrhagic stroke (0.94–1.27).

GLOBAL BURDEN OF STROKE COMMENTARY

The GBD 2010 study provides a detailed analysis of the global burden of stroke overall and by its pathological subtypes, in terms of incidence, prevalence, mortality and DALYs lost, across GDB regions and all countries in 1990, 2005, and 2010 and in all age groups. The studies add new insights to previous GBD studies with the aim of providing estimates of changes in stroke burden over the past two decades, by high-income and low- and middle-income countries, and for the first time by ischemic and hemorrhagic stroke subtypes. By current GBD estimates, ischemic heart disease and stroke remain the two most common causes of death worldwide.[7] Ischemic heart disease contributed to 13.3% of deaths followed closely by stroke, which resulted in 11% of deaths and 4% of DALYs lost worldwide in 2010.[7] Stroke deaths were spread roughly equally between ischemic and hemorrhagic strokes. Stroke and ischemic heart disease combined killed an estimated 12.9 million people in 2010. The proportion of deaths due to stroke and ischemic heart disease has risen from one-fifth of the world population in 1990 to one-quarter of the world population in 2010.

Globally, the absolute number of strokes and stroke survivors has increased in the past two decades, with the greatest increase in absolute numbers of incident strokes almost doubling in low- and middle-income countries. This increase could be attributed to the increase in the world population, in particular in the developing world, along with increasing life expectancies. According to the World Health Organization projections, stroke mortality is projected to rise faster in low- and middle-income countries.[1] The current studies showed that 53% of deaths occurred in the younger age group in low- and middle-income countries compared to 27% in high-income countries. Large geographic variations in the incidence of stroke are likely to be due to differences in the prevalence

TABLE 13-2 Absolute Number of Incident and Prevalent Strokes DALYs Lost and Mortality to Incidence Ratio (MIR) (Point Estimates and Corresponding 95% CIs) by Country in 1990 and 2010.

Ischemic Stroke

	1990					*2005*	
Country	***Prevalence***	***Incidence***	***MIR***	***Deaths***	***DALYs***	***Prevalence***	***Incidence***
Afghanistan	7,175 (4,148–11,325)	5,105 (3,268–7,354)	0.88 (0.49–1.54)	4,364 (3,144–6,587)	111,154 (78,389–164,790)	14,267 (8,082–22,988)	12,147 (7,938–17,422)
Albania	6,316 (3,707–10,333)	4,397 (2,884–6,325)	0.12 (0.08–0.18)	515 (466–551)	9,084 (8,221–9,812)	8,374 (4,917–13,149)	6,407 (4,250–9,207)
Algeria	22,963 (13,910–34,518)	13,308 (8,763–19,466)	0.58 (0.37–0.85)	7,485 (6,591–8,456)	134,658 (118,836–152,445)	40,522 (25,115–62,478)	23,673 (15,846–34,066)
Andorra	343 (212–516)	116 (77–169)	0.39 (0.24–0.58)	43 (34–52)	529 (431–617)	624 (388–976)	160 (105–227)
Angola	6,538 (3,902–10,529)	4,637 (3,070–6,534)	0.38 (0.23–0.64)	1,731 (1,291–2,426)	38,801 (28,600–53,893)	10,435 (6,231–16,077)	8,115 (5,316–11,733)
Antigua and Barbuda	147 (88–228)	66 (44–97)	0.25 (0.16–0.38)	16 (13–18)	276 (214–303)	298 (175–447)	98 (65–139)
Argentina	72,296 (68,201–76,544)	49,327 (31,644–73,053)	0.39 (0.24–0.60)	18,544 (14,170–19,975)	256,561 (201,877–273,649)	108,245 (101,603–115,248)	49,729 (32,308–72,056)
Armenia	8,956 (5,425–14,260)	5,478 (3,590–7,912)	0.23 (0.15–0.34)	1,216 (1,060–1,380)	18,511 (16,163–20,663)	11,650 (6,775–18,588)	8,235 (5,463–12,067)
Australia	75,794 (45,400–118,606)	21,784 (17,770–26,431)	0.43 (0.34–0.54)	9,277 (8,405–10,281)	98,977 (90,362–108,103)	121,588 (74,040–187,625)	26,067 (21,484–31,428)
Austria	45,288 (27,016–71,680)	17,892 (12,418–26,306)	0.45 (0.29–0.64)	7,763 (6,545–8,410)	80,989 (67,462–87,773)	68,814 (42,233–107,265)	17,132 (11,422–24,911)
Azerbaijan	13,140 (7,824–20,403)	8,368 (5,450–12,090)	0.21 (0.14–0.32)	1,713 (1,500–1,916)	31,668 (27,584–35,239)	20,087 (11,685–32,336)	14,211 (9,248–20,638)
Bahrain	554 (327–881)	85 (60–116)	0.64 (0.44–0.89)	53 (48–59)	1,135 (1,021–1,264)	1,169 (663–1,961)	160 (111–222)
Bangladesh	161,801 (96,377–258,964)	47,052 (30,773–66,710)	0.29 (0.17–0.47)	13,079 (9,963–17,594)	219,876 (170,773–293,831)	293,329 (172,530–476,212)	78,843 (50,894–116,363)
Barbados	985 (597–1,556)	542 (415–693)	0.30 (0.22–0.39)	160 (131–174)	1,954 (1,639–2,119)	1,566 (922–2,408)	647 (500–827)
Belarus	58,605 (34,863–90,570)	51,344 (42,561–61,193)	0.27 (0.22–0.34)	13,886 (11,947–15,150)	189,627 (163,635–204,416)	65,697 (39,721–102,614)	65,896 (54,467–78,752)
Belgium	64,027 (38,473–101,694)	23,101 (15,346–32,937)	0.49 (0.32–0.69)	10,823 (9,562–11,736)	115,081 (103,465–125,030)	92,130 (54,589–146,280)	22,443 (14,865–31,810)
Belize	341 (211–537)	133 (87–193)	0.31 (0.20–0.45)	39 (34–43)	579 (495–633)	617 (372–980)	192 (126–281)
Benin	2,604 (1,617–4,166)	2,533 (1,673–3,735)	0.33 (0.21–0.51)	814 (659–1,015)	16,433 (12,927–20,579)	3,916 (2,412–6,133)	4,104 (2,729–5,986)
Bhutan	919 (547–1,465)	240 (157–353)	0.22 (0.13–0.38)	52 (38–76)	1,021 (763–1,446)	1,359 (839–2,159)	395 (263–577)
Bolivia	5,157 (4,731–5,615)	2,799 (1,849–4,117)	0.42 (0.26–0.64)	1,132 (942–1,433)	22,881 (19,289–27,828)	7,865 (7,153–8,658)	4,098 (2,722–5,801)
Bosnia and Herzegovina	8,641 (5,222–13,747)	7,378 (4,941–10,835)	0.46 (0.30–0.66)	3,295 (3,037–3,492)	45,835 (42,052–48,682)	13,627 (8,233–21,693)	11,638 (7,830–17,201)
Botswana	1,015 (607–1,610)	687 (453–1,015)	0.27 (0.16–0.42)	181 (140–245)	3,302 (2,589–4,250)	1,616 (975–2,537)	1,350 (901–1,936)
Brazil	261,836 (163,633–405,461)	159,916 (123,886–204,565)	0.30 (0.23–0.39)	47,161 (42,132–49,950)	784,295 (707,847–829,197)	473,488 (287,235–726,055)	260,137 (192,745–337,035)

MIR	Deaths	DALYs	2010 Prevalence	Incidence	MIR	Deaths	DALYs
0.81 (0.47–1.29)	9,570 (7,094–14,685)	238,794 (170,781–352,521)	16,484 (9,406–26,449)	14,191 (9,527–20,277)	0.75 (0.44–1.23)	10,300 (7,962–14,683)	247,834 (187,725–346,249)
0.12 (0.08–0.18)	742 (640–806)	12,099 (10,323–13,214)	9,492 (5,661–15,123)	7,429 (4,960–10,679)	0.12 (0.08–0.18)	880 (693–1,009)	13,363 (10,769–15,224)
0.40 (0.27–0.59)	9,240 (8,221–10,210)	152,343 (135,593–168,347)	47,622 (30,107–74,617)	28,224 (18,714–40,953)	0.38 (0.25–0.56)	10,190 (9,065–11,256)	162,343 (144,995–176,806)
0.35 (0.23–0.54)	55 (43–67)	672 (555–811)	744 (449–1,145)	195 (130–281)	0.33 (0.20–0.51)	63 (49–79)	763 (612–928)
0.30 (0.18–0.49)	2,379 (1,751–3,207)	49,529 (36,332–64,759)	12,197 (7,450–19,143)	10,103 (6,545–14,872)	0.29 (0.17–0.47)	2,806 (2,021–3,842)	56,873 (41,174–74,552)
0.14 (0.09–0.22)	14 (12–18)	234 (205–297)	347 (208–550)	117 (79–173)	0.14 (0.09–0.21)	16 (13–21)	266 (229–344)
0.32 (0.20–0.52)	15,530 (13,417–23,523)	190,799 (169,891–271,125)	120,690 (113,311–128,124)	54,441 (36,031–78,699)	0.31 (0.19–0.51)	16,285 (13,587–24,831)	192,030 (167,832–273,593)
0.22 (0.14–0.33)	1,754 (1,472–1,972)	25,038 (21,095–27,930)	13,571 (8,231–21,657)	9,136 (6,064–13,147)	0.23 (0.14–0.34)	1,992 (1,600–2,303)	26,379 (21,296–30,104)
0.37 (0.29–0.47)	9,513 (8,446–11,319)	90,741 (81,002–104,617)	142,717 (84,450–221,907)	30,212 (24,781–36,614)	0.35 (0.27–0.44)	10,420 (8,731–12,671)	95,844 (82,266–113,125)
0.28 (0.17–0.43)	4,554 (3,954–6,518)	47,659 (40,658–63,357)	78,956 (48,716–119,590)	18,824 (12,827–27,677)	0.24 (0.15–0.38)	4,293 (3,556–6,657)	45,351 (38,032–63,208)
0.18 (0.12–0.28)	2,503 (2,126–2,768)	43,739 (37,320–48,041)	25,124 (15,060–38,832)	16,978 (10,978–24,877)	0.19 (0.12–0.29)	3,096 (2,395–3,527)	50,061 (39,133–56,386)
0.35 (0.24–0.48)	54 (47–59)	1,145 (995–1,281)	2,465 (1,329–4,035)	267 (182–364)	0.25 (0.17–0.36)	64 (56–71)	1,542 (1,307–1,779)
0.24 (0.14–0.38)	17,930 (12,717–24,753)	277,030 (205,961–370,787)	331,572 (199,099–528,163)	96,442 (61,708–139,555)	0.22 (0.13–0.37)	20,610 (14,153–29,074)	315,066 (234,823–438,736)
0.18 (0.13–0.29)	114 (95–182)	1,367 (1,167–2,040)	1,779 (1,035–2,781)	678 (527–878)	0.17 (0.12–0.28)	115 (93–184)	1,382 (1,147–2,056)
0.26 (0.20–0.32)	17,115 (13,396–18,578)	250,226 (202,420–271,669)	73,461 (43,923–119,183)	69,010 (57,590–83,117)	0.25 (0.17–0.30)	16,916 (12,269–19,034)	233,724 (174,994–260,070)
0.34 (0.21–0.55)	7,303 (6,278–10,437)	77,911 (67,085–102,525)	99,300 (59,190–155,143)	25,080 (16,768–36,635)	0.33 (0.20–0.50)	7,856 (6,622–10,133)	80,667 (69,650–101,594)
0.25 (0.16–0.37)	46 (42–52)	674 (612–761)	766 (470–1,197)	229 (155–324)	0.24 (0.17–0.35)	54 (48–63)	781 (700–891)
0.28 (0.17–0.42)	1,107 (862–1,387)	21,499 (16,525–26,452)	4,370 (2,607–6,986)	4,890 (3,229–7,100)	0.28 (0.17–0.42)	1,330 (1,028–1,640)	25,684 (19,811–30,988)
0.25 (0.14–0.40)	94 (68–133)	1,573 (1,184–2,190)	1,617 (945–2,623)	506 (338–724)	0.23 (0.13–0.37)	112 (81–156)	1,792 (1,337–2,462)
0.34 (0.23–0.54)	1,349 (1,107–1,854)	25,758 (21,756–31,873)	9,183 (8,309–10,100)	4,936 (3,140–7,308)	0.32 (0.20–0.49)	1,495 (1,245–2,077)	27,408 (23,477–34,054)
0.40 (0.26–0.58)	4,509 (3,741–5,129)	58,811 (48,367–67,103)	15,013 (8,639–24,173)	13,429 (8,798–19,686)	0.40 (0.25–0.59)	5,125 (4,147–5,936)	61,960 (50,144–71,882)
0.17 (0.10–0.27)	222 (147–289)	4,992 (3,594–6,198)	1,786 (1,119–2,796)	1,662 (1,088–2,422)	0.15 (0.08–0.25)	244 (149–322)	4,677 (3,166–5,872)
0.25 (0.18–0.33)	63,077 (58,610–75,024)	908,891 (852,606–1,060,891)	547,579 (326,396–856,688)	312,793 (237,502–403,776)	0.24 (0.17–0.32)	73,363 (66,926–86,298)	1,005,728 (930,464–1,168,006)

Continued

TABLE 13-2 Absolute Number of Incident and Prevalent Strokes DALYs Lost and Mortality to Incidence Ratio (MIR) (Point Estimates and Corresponding 95% CIs) by Country in 1990 and 2010.—cont'd

Ischemic Stroke

	1990					*2005*	
Country	***Prevalence***	***Incidence***	***MIR***	***Deaths***	***DALYs***	***Prevalence***	***Incidence***
Brunei	448 (272–704)	177 (117–256)	0.27 (0.15–0.42)	47 (30–56)	674 (474–791)	806 (493–1,277)	217 (144–323)
Bulgaria	28,502 (17,208–44,867)	31,499 (20,501–46,608)	0.55 (0.35–0.82)	16,581 (15,283–17,417)	217,788 (199,430–228,422)	32,279 (19,690–50,798)	33,659 (22,525–48,599)
Burkina Faso	5,733 (3,576–8,961)	3,628 (2,454–5,246)	0.18 (0.11–0.30)	644 (453–956)	15,440 (10,859–21,881)	6,115 (3,628–9,615)	5,668 (3,754–8,518)
Burundi	1,524 (902–2,414)	2,873 (1,917–4,279)	0.56 (0.26–1.06)	1,556 (805–2,629)	28,114 (14,527–49,034)	2,100 (1,238–3,295)	3,939 (2,622–5,702)
Cambodia	14,230 (8,292–22,621)	4,721 (3,113–6,985)	0.30 (0.18–0.50)	1,384 (1,081–1,886)	29,225 (23,005–39,553)	22,999 (13,742–35,866)	8,765 (5,878–12,875)
Cameroon	6,895 (4,240–10,856)	6,943 (4,329–10,096)	0.33 (0.21–0.52)	2,234 (1,868–2,738)	44,701 (37,142–55,042)	9,924 (5,961–15,350)	10,872 (7,217–15,657)
Canada	218,585 (132,423–335,129)	48,533 (31,489–70,899)	0.28 (0.18–0.42)	13,214 (11,931–14,759)	152,080 (136,290–172,880)	438,402 (269,153–706,065)	59,626 (40,527–86,488)
Cape Verde	208 (124–333)	261 (170–385)	0.49 (0.31–0.73)	123 (103–144)	1,999 (1,688–2,285)	309 (186–508)	416 (271–606)
Central African Republic	2,000 (1,223–3,249)	2,054 (1,311–2,981)	0.43 (0.26–0.70)	859 (624–1,188)	17,131 (12,283–22,881)	2,824 (1,740–4,394)	3,155 (2,011–4,688)
Chad	3,486 (2,139–5,556)	3,251 (2,123–4,777)	0.29 (0.17–0.46)	904 (707–1,199)	19,600 (15,364–26,132)	4,920 (2,840–7,860)	5,153 (3,312–7,587)
Chile	23,338 (14,365–35,568)	10,951 (8,384–14,012)	0.47 (0.35–0.62)	5,114 (4,432–5,557)	66,032 (57,073–70,470)	43,547 (26,016–66,535)	13,005 (9,894–16,933)
China	3,154,166 (1,897,932–4,941,783)	1,859,603 (1,399,273–2,421,600)	0.23 (0.15–0.36)	426,378 (304,427–639,742)	6,252,048 (4,408,024–9,652,909)	4,661,215 (2,666,891–7,330,800)	2,864,989 (2,137,087–3,740,780)
Colombia	40,680 (24,660–63,496)	17,160 (11,281–24,736)	0.38 (0.26–0.56)	6,250 (5,653–6,793)	96,288 (89,456–104,232)	69,163 (41,498–111,267)	27,462 (18,220–39,335)
Comoros	120 (72–184)	221 (149–319)	0.54 (0.33–0.81)	115 (90–141)	2,111 (1,643–2,598)	195 (120–311)	333 (223–482)
Congo	1,581 (928–2,535)	1,541 (1,017–2,189)	0.49 (0.31–0.75)	720 (576–891)	12,932 (10,507–15,554)	2,437 (1,477–3,885)	2,609 (1,748–3,779)
Costa Rica	5,331 (3,044–8,503)	1,794 (1,202–2,623)	0.19 (0.12–0.28)	332 (287–358)	5,119 (4,405–5,680)	9,719 (6,012–15,253)	3,089 (2,063–4,455)
Côte d'Ivoire	6,022 (3,595–9,613)	5,839 (3,845–8,497)	0.33 (0.22–0.51)	1,896 (1,644–2,234)	42,228 (36,478–49,165)	9,294 (5,509–14,672)	11,710 (7,796–17,534)
Croatia	15,468 (8,899–24,440)	13,876 (8,946–20,094)	0.41 (0.27–0.61)	5,460 (5,103–5,854)	70,124 (65,937–74,914)	22,295 (13,427–34,694)	17,259 (11,351–24,999)
Cuba	40,938 (36,790–45,129)	16,420 (11,059–23,811)	0.38 (0.25–0.54)	5,949 (5,247–6,515)	76,684 (68,443–81,554)	57,679 (52,652–63,328)	21,206 (13,675–30,803)
Cyprus	2,997 (1,816–4,682)	1,045 (690–1,499)	0.33 (0.21–0.50)	334 (272–391)	4,303 (3,627–4,906)	4,241 (2,548–6,601)	1,138 (749–1,703)
Czech Republic	35,333 (21,177–54,803)	35,852 (24,281–52,452)	0.58 (0.38–0.83)	20,139 (18,721–21,619)	246,472 (228,598–264,559)	51,186 (30,623–80,735)	38,015 (25,146–55,650)
Democratic Republic of the Congo	23,381 (13,697–35,806)	17,144 (11,360–24,967)	0.34 (0.21–0.53)	5,604 (4,566–7,626)	116,573 (94,460–157,295)	33,562 (19,942–54,906)	30,251 (19,641–44,945)
Denmark	35,442 (20,811–55,463)	14,653 (12,719–16,806)	0.26 (0.22–0.31)	3,801 (3,402–4,170)	43,175 (39,023–47,667)	38,624 (24,343–59,574)	12,707 (10,885–14,489)
Djibouti	169 (101–266)	241 (157–346)	0.39 (0.22–0.62)	90 (64–121)	1,830 (1,306–2,493)	301 (189–476)	452 (304–651)

			2010				
MIR	***Deaths***	***DALYs***	***Prevalence***	***Incidence***	***MIR***	***Deaths***	***DALYs***
0.26 (0.15–0.39)	54 (38–64)	771 (592–898)	1,058 (633–1,699)	276 (180–401)	0.25 (0.15–0.38)	67 (47–81)	942 (732–1,120)
0.54 (0.36–0.76)	17,442 (16,078–18,564)	218,984 (200,781–231,365)	33,377 (19,990–51,901)	35,568 (23,785–51,230)	0.55 (0.36–0.80)	18,942 (16,180–20,373)	223,658 (191,054–238,915)
0.23 (0.13–0.35)	1,240 (878–1,587)	27,098 (18,576–34,004)	6,178 (3,724–9,720)	7,174 (4,690–10,412)	0.27 (0.16–0.43)	1,902 (1,327–2,387)	39,841 (26,793–49,346)
0.44 (0.21–0.86)	1,645 (953–2,951)	29,899 (17,609–56,631)	2,413 (1,421–3,811)	4,878 (3,249–7,081)	0.42 (0.21–0.83)	1,951 (1,183–3,431)	35,649 (21,606–63,661)
0.31 (0.19–0.47)	2,616 (2,125–3,327)	51,977 (42,891–65,084)	27,381 (16,691–43,114)	11,233 (7,351–16,507)	0.28 (0.17–0.44)	3,045 (2,473–3,866)	59,753 (49,958–73,838)
0.26 (0.17–0.40)	2,775 (2,255–3,405)	53,508 (44,193–63,898)	10,566 (6,394–16,611)	12,905 (8,632–18,570)	0.26 (0.16–0.39)	3,266 (2,702–3,929)	62,020 (51,975–72,655)
0.24 (0.15–0.36)	13,709 (12,039–16,339)	170,868 (143,772–211,228)	519,746 (314,400–805,325)	67,280 (43,584–95,776)	0.23 (0.15–0.34)	14,925 (12,562–17,935)	185,245 (149,784–230,407)
0.38 (0.24–0.61)	153 (121–190)	2,251 (1,807–2,780)	375 (227–590)	502 (335–749)	0.38 (0.22–0.59)	183 (140–235)	2,544 (1,958–3,234)
0.34 (0.19–0.56)	1,025 (737–1,455)	18,711 (13,296–25,865)	2,998 (1,811–4,715)	3,666 (2,400–5,299)	0.34 (0.20–0.57)	1,211 (849–1,752)	21,563 (14,994–30,376)
0.25 (0.15–0.40)	1,262 (868–1,651)	26,860 (18,183–34,673)	5,364 (3,226–8,598)	6,010 (3,910–8,723)	0.25 (0.15–0.39)	1,434 (1,065–1,834)	30,408 (22,291–38,930)
0.38 (0.28–0.54)	4,839 (4,322–6,215)	56,810 (51,662–69,788)	54,829 (33,338–85,756)	15,321 (11,999–19,873)	0.34 (0.25–0.46)	5,092 (4,453–6,220)	60,474 (53,883–71,238)
0.20 (0.13–0.30)	567,582 (430,386–778,014)	8,013,519 (5,943,830–11,513,630)	5,401,942 (3,369,728–8,272,431)	3,307,909 (2,452,040–4,279,414)	0.19 (0.13–0.28)	609,570 (478,282–808,427)	8,383,821 (6,523,032–11,529,388)
0.31 (0.20–0.46)	8,193 (7,491–9,903)	111,671 (103,422–132,537)	84,925 (51,112–129,399)	33,409 (22,365–48,626)	0.29 (0.19–0.43)	9,446 (8,319–11,461)	125,058 (112,631–147,953)
0.40 (0.25–0.61)	128 (104–156)	2,254 (1,824–2,771)	213 (128–340)	408 (266–595)	0.38 (0.24–0.59)	149 (119–184)	2,665 (2,114–3,262)
0.38 (0.23–0.55)	950 (771–1,160)	16,920 (13,941–20,239)	2,633 (1,579–4,007)	3,182 (2,099–4,686)	0.37 (0.23–0.55)	1,121 (918–1,365)	19,855 (16,252–23,777)
0.15 (0.10–0.22)	434 (394–537)	6,159 (5,424–7,656)	12,450 (7,480–19,591)	3,712 (2,510–5,438)	0.14 (0.09–0.21)	490 (435–603)	6,920 (5,970–8,380)
0.31 (0.19–0.47)	3,461 (2,944–4,350)	72,592 (62,601–87,448)	10,048 (5,991–15,939)	14,094 (9,113–20,525)	0.32 (0.20–0.49)	4,336 (3,633–5,496)	85,971 (73,084–104,381)
0.34 (0.22–0.51)	5,699 (5,253–6,225)	67,994 (63,331–73,981)	25,356 (15,193–39,679)	19,246 (12,534–28,072)	0.32 (0.21–0.47)	5,930 (5,383–6,571)	67,075 (61,516–72,658)
0.38 (0.25–0.57)	7,715 (6,917–8,794)	87,996 (80,979–97,896)	68,604 (62,280–75,204)	24,336 (16,013–34,902)	0.35 (0.23–0.52)	8,250 (7,272–9,398)	92,844 (83,767–103,098)
0.29 (0.18–0.43)	311 (277–357)	4,084 (3,651–4,610)	4,593 (2,818–6,924)	1,190 (800–1,690)	0.25 (0.16–0.38)	287 (249–339)	3,813 (3,340–4,400)
0.43 (0.28–0.63)	15,603 (14,488–17,088)	174,519 (163,711–191,672)	60,587 (35,588–96,433)	42,841 (28,892–61,941)	0.35 (0.23–0.51)	14,474 (13,174–16,933)	157,334 (145,005–183,115)
0.29 (0.18–0.50)	8,539 (6,684–12,599)	170,572 (132,733–248,390)	37,429 (22,564–59,109)	37,433 (23,897–56,341)	0.30 (0.17–0.51)	10,691 (8,313–15,278)	214,220 (165,513–305,689)
0.26 (0.22–0.32)	3,348 (2,926–3,798)	35,622 (31,347–40,180)	42,106 (25,400–65,244)	13,697 (11,817–15,868)	0.24 (0.19–0.29)	3,221 (2,764–3,725)	34,058 (29,871–38,532)
0.30 (0.18–0.50)	133 (91–185)	2,490 (1,731–3,443)	363 (209–563)	571 (379–828)	0.28 (0.16–0.47)	154 (109–219)	2,843 (2,047–3,915)

Continued

TABLE 13-2 Absolute Number of Incident and Prevalent Strokes DALYs Lost and Mortality to Incidence Ratio (MIR) (Point Estimates and Corresponding 95% CIs) by Country in 1990 and 2010.—cont'd

Ischemic Stroke

	1990					*2005*	
Country	*Prevalence*	*Incidence*	*MIR*	*Deaths*	*DALYs*	*Prevalence*	*Incidence*
Dominica	191 (114–313)	73 (49–106)	0.28 (0.18–0.42)	20 (17–22)	307 (265–338)	274 (168–419)	86 (57–126)
Dominican Republic	13,062 (7,822–20,296)	5,185 (3,407–7,408)	0.25 (0.17–0.38)	1,262 (1,191–1,455)	24,148 (22,698–27,204)	24,378 (14,824–37,570)	9,556 (6,387–13,819)
Ecuador	11,010 (6,556–17,485)	4,720 (3,040–6,760)	0.21 (0.14–0.31)	934 (873–1,027)	19,245 (17,895–21,001)	19,608 (12,401–31,129)	7,629 (5,104–10,845)
Egypt	51,188 (47,339–55,845)	31,829 (21,309–45,294)	0.48 (0.32–0.73)	14,866 (13,638–18,354)	326,668 (299,175–411,039)	84,469 (77,777–91,756)	59,091 (39,604–85,479)
El Salvador	7,319 (4,361–11,728)	2,996 (2,008–4,304)	0.31 (0.17–0.47)	910 (575–1,026)	14,109 (8,965–15,914)	12,858 (7,783–20,674)	4,495 (3,113–6,494)
Equatorial Guinea	268 (160–428)	272 (180–398)	0.44 (0.26–0.77)	115 (85–174)	2,135 (1,583–3,208)	491 (293–775)	407 (270–601)
Eritrea	892 (533–1,426)	1,474 (989–2,106)	0.45 (0.25–0.75)	636 (428–861)	11,795 (8,172–16,018)	1,212 (709–1,850)	2,053 (1,325–3,010)
Estonia	8,824 (5,245–14,113)	10,277 (8,666–12,090)	0.29 (0.24–0.35)	2,968 (2,678–3,156)	38,996 (34,489–41,359)	12,454 (7,100–19,897)	12,303 (10,444–14,315)
Ethiopia	17,226 (15,865–18,665)	22,531 (14,757–32,423)	0.29 (0.17–0.47)	6,327 (4,556–8,854)	127,545 (92,666–176,307)	28,845 (26,689–31,185)	39,855 (26,311–59,055)
Federated States of Micronesia	86 (50–140)	68 (45–100)	0.52 (0.32–0.82)	34 (26–46)	737 (569–954)	109 (65–180)	77 (52–114)
Fiji	528 (295–854)	493 (321–736)	0.76 (0.36–1.21)	359 (182–431)	7,420 (3,475–9,005)	962 (546–1,517)	650 (427–960)
Finland	27,403 (16,653–43,411)	17,319 (15,067–20,073)	0.26 (0.21–0.30)	4,396 (3,796–4,796)	52,406 (46,017–56,464)	41,520 (25,374–63,595)	18,170 (15,767–21,003)
France	409,413 (250,284–615,601)	104,129 (87,481–121,230)	0.29 (0.24–0.36)	30,215 (26,072–33,292)	340,260 (302,497–380,731)	598,658 (363,757–942,833)	106,770 (90,277–126,830)
Gabon	849 (519–1,315)	824 (540–1,224)	0.44 (0.26–0.70)	350 (250–442)	5,815 (4,272–7,182)	1,202 (723–1,860)	1,227 (821–1,777)
Georgia	15,309 (9,153–23,875)	8,706 (6,489–11,251)	0.26 (0.17–0.35)	2,201 (1,665–2,505)	41,633 (31,757–47,445)	17,485 (10,540–27,077)	9,837 (7,343–12,842)
Germany	485,510 (453,867–519,099)	260,016 (223,138–301,668)	0.33 (0.25–0.39)	84,256 (67,589–91,362)	896,652 (750,259–957,077)	719,213 (669,767–770,470)	257,209 (220,748–301,930)
Ghana	8,223 (5,058–12,863)	7,273 (4,925–10,526)	0.35 (0.22–0.51)	2,484 (2,096–3,022)	50,710 (43,321–61,433)	11,041 (6,572–16,903)	14,058 (9,285–20,248)
Greece	48,540 (29,442–74,173)	19,811 (16,194–23,965)	0.58 (0.47–0.72)	11,456 (10,318–12,293)	121,654 (109,952–130,314)	62,855 (35,474–98,139)	22,096 (17,883–26,781)
Grenada	222 (138–340)	122 (79–181)	0.51 (0.32–0.77)	60 (48–66)	903 (709–985)	282 (168–445)	131 (87–190)
Guatemala	11,177 (6,614–17,365)	3,670 (2,387–5,476)	0.26 (0.16–0.39)	906 (827–1,153)	15,649 (14,242–19,505)	17,115 (10,165–26,937)	6,161 (4,022–8,791)
Guinea	3,064 (1,849–4,909)	3,017 (1,947–4,417)	0.33 (0.20–0.51)	967 (785–1,245)	21,835 (17,680–27,708)	4,747 (2,777–7,308)	5,299 (3,603–7,475)
Guinea-Bissau	559 (327–861)	572 (374–806)	0.35 (0.21–0.54)	194 (149–259)	4,319 (3,320–5,682)	686 (418–1,092)	832 (545–1,206)
Guyana	978 (582–1,535)	659 (437–931)	0.68 (0.46–0.99)	433 (370–462)	7,166 (6,079–7,624)	1,011 (596–1,580)	551 (366–786)
Haiti	7,561 (4,507–11,763)	4,797 (3,068–6,853)	0.65 (0.43–0.98)	2,992 (2,699–3,359)	59,554 (53,560–67,333)	11,532 (6,706–18,032)	6,417 (4,198–9,295)
Honduras	4,061 (2,392–6,558)	2,023 (1,333–2,935)	0.44 (0.29–0.65)	859 (737–933)	15,096 (12,828–16,282)	6,551 (3,967–10,371)	3,656 (2,444–5,301)

			2010				
MIR	***Deaths***	***DALYs***	***Prevalence***	***Incidence***	***MIR***	***Deaths***	***DALYs***
0.20 (0.13–0.30)	17 (15–19)	262 (236–298)	311 (188–492)	95 (61–137)	0.21 (0.14–0.32)	19 (17–22)	297 (263–335)
0.31 (0.19–0.46)	2,887 (2,201–3,144)	42,547 (33,445–46,191)	28,489 (17,025–46,464)	11,638 (8,055–15,996)	0.31 (0.20–0.45)	3,512 (2,633–3,886)	48,542 (38,534–53,405)
0.19 (0.13–0.27)	1,393 (1,226–1,501)	25,417 (22,048–27,605)	23,650 (14,474–36,757)	9,323 (6,159–13,798)	0.17 (0.11–0.25)	1,527 (1,356–1,669)	26,598 (23,614–29,191)
0.41 (0.27–0.60)	23,380 (19,794–24,728)	469,980 (392,457–496,898)	100,388 (92,327–108,864)	71,791 (48,083–104,420)	0.37 (0.24–0.54)	25,632 (22,018–27,363)	509,806 (433,652–544,852)
0.15 (0.09–0.24)	629 (543–955)	8,722 (7,476–12,341)	14,548 (8,734–23,777)	5,030 (3,280–7,346)	0.15 (0.09–0.24)	707 (599–1,039)	9,308 (7,926–12,850)
0.28 (0.15–0.45)	110 (74–157)	2,109 (1,443–2,866)	584 (344–918)	490 (328–718)	0.23 (0.11–0.40)	112 (59–167)	2,206 (1,252–3,150)
0.34 (0.21–0.54)	677 (522–893)	12,398 (9,612–16,234)	1,395 (842–2,151)	2,605 (1,678–3,730)	0.33 (0.20–0.52)	832 (652–1,090)	15,170 (11,978–19,813)
0.19 (0.16–0.23)	2,303 (2,153–2,561)	29,544 (27,665–32,910)	15,702 (9,183–25,859)	13,056 (11,008–15,190)	0.15 (0.12–0.20)	1,944 (1,723–2,480)	23,754 (21,200–29,107)
0.25 (0.15–0.37)	9,461 (7,299–12,321)	173,423 (135,411–229,598)	33,248 (30,811–36,085)	49,766 (33,157–72,931)	0.24 (0.15–0.37)	11,336 (8,991–14,631)	203,297 (161,851–262,290)
0.59 (0.35–0.92)	43 (32–58)	877 (650–1,137)	117 (67–191)	78 (51–113)	0.57 (0.33–0.95)	42 (31–57)	866 (632–1,159)
0.41 (0.26–0.63)	256 (227–318)	5,028 (4,500–5,965)	1,236 (727–1,988)	765 (497–1,130)	0.27 (0.16–0.52)	199 (161–354)	3,909 (3,241–6,565)
0.19 (0.16–0.24)	3,508 (3,146–4,164)	39,723 (35,697–46,169)	48,735 (30,308–76,159)	20,664 (17,830–23,774)	0.17 (0.14–0.21)	3,496 (3,078–4,210)	38,556 (34,343–45,324)
0.22 (0.18–0.30)	23,305 (20,653–30,736)	281,606 (239,476–348,933)	666,449 (396,940–1,048,330)	118,768 (99,321–140,730)	0.21 (0.16–0.27)	24,197 (20,787–30,793)	289,630 (244,310–359,259)
0.35 (0.21–0.54)	413 (294–520)	6,558 (4,879–7,996)	1,328 (813–2,072)	1,420 (927–2,041)	0.33 (0.21–0.51)	453 (325–566)	7,195 (5,393–8,806)
0.17 (0.12–0.22)	1,620 (1,485–1,779)	30,419 (27,511–33,243)	18,237 (10,965–28,659)	10,603 (7,901–13,998)	0.18 (0.13–0.24)	1,859 (1,608–2,028)	33,260 (29,025–36,270)
0.21 (0.17–0.25)	53,881 (49,209–61,134)	596,356 (545,343–646,632)	833,919 (772,954–899,201)	285,482 (242,243–333,496)	0.18 (0.15–0.23)	51,861 (46,614–60,020)	582,993 (538,128–644,823)
0.35 (0.23–0.54)	4,813 (4,180–5,713)	91,699 (80,279–105,286)	12,660 (7,632–19,473)	17,460 (11,590–25,474)	0.34 (0.22–0.51)	5,771 (4,962–6,766)	104,559 (91,783–119,452)
0.60 (0.48–0.76)	13,223 (12,193–14,691)	123,884 (115,195–137,331)	75,215 (42,778–120,497)	24,775 (20,321–30,186)	0.53 (0.42–0.66)	12,935 (11,631–15,313)	120,153 (109,165–141,263)
0.44 (0.29–0.66)	56 (50–65)	723 (659–850)	310 (188–483)	134 (91–191)	0.41 (0.26–0.60)	53 (46–66)	677 (603–834)
0.22 (0.14–0.33)	1,293 (1,145–1,446)	23,219 (19,984–25,221)	21,203 (12,451–33,616)	7,397 (4,995–10,878)	0.21 (0.14–0.31)	1,496 (1,338–1,720)	25,488 (22,558–28,294)
0.28 (0.17–0.42)	1,438 (1,159–1,847)	28,320 (23,229–35,182)	4,919 (3,031–7,754)	6,218 (4,094–9,072)	0.29 (0.18–0.45)	1,743 (1,402–2,254)	33,634 (27,433–41,414)
0.31 (0.18–0.49)	250 (193–343)	5,193 (4,055–6,943)	737 (437–1,142)	967 (638–1,383)	0.31 (0.18–0.49)	289 (225–398)	5,883 (4,670–7,920)
0.50 (0.33–0.73)	263 (243–309)	4,370 (4,011–5,360)	1,187 (734–1,896)	625 (414–899)	0.50 (0.32–0.73)	302 (268–362)	5,239 (4,609–6,570)
0.58 (0.38–0.86)	3,590 (3,264–3,995)	69,203 (62,988–76,469)	12,919 (7,827–20,373)	7,400 (4,785–11,066)	0.56 (0.36–0.83)	3,959 (3,541–4,522)	75,152 (66,970–85,652)
0.46 (0.30–0.67)	1,622 (1,365–1,879)	23,975 (20,450–27,152)	7,900 (4,715–13,076)	4,410 (2,958–6,347)	0.45 (0.29–0.68)	1,924 (1,576–2,270)	26,832 (22,444–31,478)

Continued

TABLE 13-2 Absolute Number of Incident and Prevalent Strokes DALYs Lost and Mortality to Incidence Ratio (MIR) (Point Estimates and Corresponding 95% CIs) by Country in 1990 and 2010.—cont'd

Ischemic Stroke

	1990					*2005*	
Country	***Prevalence***	***Incidence***	***MIR***	***Deaths***	***DALYs***	***Prevalence***	***Incidence***
Hungary	37,886 (22,348–58,065)	48,168 (39,808–57,546)	0.39 (0.31–0.47)	18,589 (16,772–19,655)	257,293 (228,181–271,118)	50,628 (30,516–79,312)	51,552 (43,024–60,927)
Iceland	1,375 (809–2,160)	432 (289–637)	0.26 (0.17–0.38)	107 (94–118)	1,265 (1,114–1,409)	2,146 (1,286–3,246)	456 (303–670)
India	1,166,573 (1,086,503–1,257,921)	540,113 (418,415–698,078)	0.26 (0.17–0.37)	136,610 (107,467–180,395)	2,535,000 (1,984,086–3,367,419)	1,830,341 (1,708,938–1,963,471)	886,911 (672,285–1,139,687)
Indonesia	325,649 (195,719–497,515)	115,952 (75,738–173,482)	0.50 (0.31–0.72)	55,285 (48,963–63,887)	970,615 (865,297–1,114,108)	451,268 (270,311–685,176)	205,565 (133,644–296,408)
Iran	56,071 (33,602–87,279)	116,527 (93,647–144,701)	0.09 (0.07–0.11)	10,608 (8,992–12,369)	246,975 (210,119–285,654)	117,486 (71,739–187,528)	246,679 (194,132–306,363)
Iraq	16,185 (9,813–24,994)	9,529 (6,398–13,864)	0.56 (0.36–0.81)	5,145 (4,353–5,806)	95,849 (80,967–108,923)	26,547 (15,751–42,243)	16,174 (10,702–22,782)
Ireland	17,248 (10,504–26,654)	6,196 (4,190–9,088)	0.37 (0.25–0.55)	2,234 (1,963–2,425)	25,224 (22,431–27,563)	25,361 (14,862–39,902)	6,090 (4,091–8,785)
Israel	21,510 (13,208–32,932)	6,819 (4,559–9,854)	0.16 (0.10–0.23)	1,043 (916–1,120)	15,283 (13,485–17,186)	40,285 (24,462–62,203)	8,722 (5,947–12,560)
Italy	345,766 (321,812–371,893)	91,355 (79,863–103,484)	0.73 (0.61–0.85)	66,452 (58,353–71,291)	693,889 (613,719–736,947)	525,365 (488,663–564,582)	98,866 (85,539–112,874)
Jamaica	5,810 (3,391–9,171)	2,832 (1,851–4,138)	0.53 (0.35–0.78)	1,448 (1,338–1,555)	21,723 (20,182–23,388)	8,585 (5,055–13,415)	3,380 (2,219–4,890)
Japan	801,869 (488,070–1,247,573)	316,473 (248,508–393,441)	0.26 (0.20–0.33)	80,283 (72,311–87,192)	957,225 (870,748–1,041,957)	1,529,148 (921,459–2,395,320)	393,478 (306,971–491,107)
Jordan	3,084 (1,873–4,865)	1,845 (1,218–2,695)	0.83 (0.54–1.21)	1,480 (1,314–1,666)	22,260 (20,140–25,040)	6,069 (3,475–9,578)	3,263 (2,192–4,783)
Kazakhstan	31,083 (18,572–48,742)	25,393 (16,732–37,948)	0.44 (0.28–0.66)	10,676 (9,895–11,811)	160,398 (150,539–176,830)	29,829 (17,871–47,603)	29,975 (19,398–43,717)
Kenya	8,143 (4,880–12,647)	10,461 (6,868–15,316)	0.32 (0.20–0.49)	3,206 (2,511–4,101)	53,008 (42,629–67,716)	14,740 (8,744–23,579)	17,008 (11,430–25,207)
Kiribati	51 (31–81)	38 (24–58)	0.64 (0.39–0.99)	23 (21–26)	623 (550–717)	69 (39–114)	46 (30–70)
Kuwait	2,403 (1,393–3,777)	222 (159–309)	0.91 (0.63–1.26)	198 (183–228)	4,679 (4,312–5,149)	3,803 (2,214–6,090)	457 (324–642)
Kyrgyzstan	6,715 (4,013–11,086)	5,897 (3,738–8,774)	0.62 (0.39–0.95)	3,485 (3,127–3,757)	51,459 (45,983–55,642)	7,552 (4,534–11,643)	7,363 (4,819–10,524)
Laos	7,237 (4,203–11,568)	2,633 (1,726–3,840)	0.34 (0.20–0.55)	855 (640–1,180)	17,272 (13,114–23,437)	9,952 (6,081–15,637)	4,241 (2,804–6,129)
Latvia	14,107 (8,339–21,898)	13,529 (9,044–19,705)	0.48 (0.32–0.70)	6,282 (5,909–6,652)	77,420 (73,048–81,709)	16,599 (9,779–26,277)	16,047 (10,372–23,193)
Lebanon	4,943 (2,814–7,909)	2,184 (1,502–3,154)	0.40 (0.26–0.58)	854 (729–1,008)	15,682 (13,174–18,226)	10,819 (6,007–17,965)	4,350 (2,917–6,357)
Lesotho	1,367 (820–2,077)	1,262 (829–1,814)	0.37 (0.24–0.58)	454 (369–595)	8,066 (6,596–10,429)	1,573 (903–2,457)	1,708 (1,135–2,463)
Liberia	1,043 (650–1,583)	916 (592–1,352)	0.26 (0.17–0.40)	243 (209–292)	6,156 (5,091–7,764)	1,514 (893–2,383)	1,548 (1,018–2,289)
Libya	3,749 (2,318–5,911)	912 (700–1,190)	0.88 (0.64–1.19)	803 (684–936)	18,562 (15,527–22,061)	7,381 (4,506–11,607)	1,961 (1,488–2,499)
Lithuania	25,074 (14,837–40,397)	19,981 (16,994–23,564)	0.21 (0.17–0.26)	4,208 (3,878–4,818)	55,073 (51,025–60,434)	29,469 (16,622–47,812)	25,680 (21,789–30,214)

			2010				
MIR	***Deaths***	***DALYs***	***Prevalence***	***Incidence***	***MIR***	***Deaths***	***DALYs***
0.29 (0.24–0.36)	14,672 (13,663–16,869)	189,064 (177,673–219,749)	56,942 (33,252–89,722)	54,800 (45,392–66,053)	0.25 (0.20–0.31)	13,490 (12,202–16,615)	165,829 (152,149–204,174)
0.21 (0.14–0.31)	94 (83–106)	1,116 (977–1,296)	2,530 (1,567–3,999)	522 (347–758)	0.20 (0.13–0.29)	98 (85–113)	1,169 (992–1,417)
0.27 (0.19–0.37)	234,363 (192,295–294,938)	3,994,367 (3,319,420–5,057,241)	2,141,072 (1,994,672–2,288,890)	1,097,876 (833,539–1,420,983)	0.24 (0.17–0.34)	263,604 (216,490–335,179)	4,301,051 (3,595,262–5,493,442)
0.51 (0.32–0.76)	99,711 (88,840–111,929)	1,687,047 (1,510,024–1,884,000)	524,970 (314,556–812,576)	245,360 (162,760–353,669)	0.48 (0.32–0.72)	114,184 (100,345–128,874)	1,889,364 (1,687,647–2,134,839)
0.07 (0.06–0.09)	17,830 (15,229–20,394)	290,058 (252,879–323,634)	137,942 (83,810–216,909)	288,458 (229,883–354,134)	0.07 (0.05–0.09)	19,870 (16,765–23,464)	304,573 (261,739–351,749)
0.49 (0.33–0.73)	7,709 (6,829–8,612)	131,744 (117,395–145,800)	28,901 (17,495–44,781)	17,680 (11,662–26,189)	0.45 (0.29–0.66)	7,687 (6,729–8,630)	139,363 (122,003–156,033)
0.28 (0.18–0.41)	1,619 (1,458–2,055)	17,536 (15,482–21,444)	28,202 (17,599–43,365)	6,693 (4,324–9,695)	0.25 (0.16–0.38)	1,587 (1,398–1,997)	16,910 (14,818–20,798)
0.12 (0.08–0.18)	1,041 (933–1,369)	15,710 (13,219–19,736)	47,778 (28,280–76,106)	9,749 (6,585–13,784)	0.11 (0.07–0.17)	1,060 (932–1,303)	16,234 (13,160–20,452)
0.58 (0.49–0.73)	57,498 (51,725–69,346)	523,605 (478,679–638,073)	591,593 (549,952–637,697)	110,797 (96,771–126,677)	0.55 (0.44–0.72)	60,523 (52,249–77,623)	539,236 (482,558–672,536)
0.42 (0.28–0.62)	1,377 (1,219–1,539)	19,300 (17,470–21,441)	9,065 (5,528–13,957)	3,741 (2,492–5,538)	0.44 (0.27–0.65)	1,571 (1,330–1,835)	21,656 (18,721–25,198)
0.26 (0.20–0.37)	101,801 (91,350–135,594)	1,081,206 (950,805–1,351,470)	1,821,535 (1,086,279–2,953,788)	457,623 (364,294–560,624)	0.26 (0.19–0.36)	115,652 (98,769–162,729)	1,171,966 (999,597–1,516,680)
0.47 (0.31–0.68)	1,480 (1,328–1,602)	23,621 (21,312–25,426)	7,500 (4,481–11,454)	4,057 (2,693–6,000)	0.42 (0.27–0.62)	1,634 (1,447–1,800)	26,025 (23,330–28,564)
0.47 (0.30–0.70)	13,626 (11,787–14,701)	220,036 (186,109–237,739)	34,780 (20,577–55,738)	30,971 (20,349–44,653)	0.40 (0.26–0.58)	11,841 (9,919–13,296)	190,384 (156,433–216,214)
0.23 (0.14–0.36)	3,758 (2,978–4,771)	62,893 (50,657–79,168)	16,206 (10,012–24,477)	20,679 (14,033–29,826)	0.23 (0.14–0.34)	4,522 (3,593–5,751)	74,089 (59,800–94,128)
0.76 (0.47–1.15)	34 (28–39)	915 (732–1,084)	83 (50–134)	52 (33–79)	0.69 (0.41–1.07)	34 (28–42)	924 (732–1,132)
0.74 (0.48–1.05)	329 (252–360)	6,921 (5,379–7,608)	3,912 (2,289–6,311)	525 (363–734)	0.86 (0.52–1.28)	437 (308–492)	8,549 (6,100–9,590)
0.53 (0.35–0.78)	3,747 (3,432–4,056)	60,915 (55,768–65,977)	8,329 (4,986–13,046)	7,338 (4,857–10,347)	0.47 (0.31–0.70)	3,350 (3,061–3,746)	54,103 (49,613–59,991)
0.33 (0.20–0.51)	1,354 (1,059–1,769)	25,416 (19,920–32,623)	11,389 (6,890–17,942)	5,040 (3,363–7,292)	0.31 (0.19–0.47)	1,491 (1,167–1,877)	27,472 (21,476–34,336)
0.41 (0.27–0.61)	6,264 (5,709–6,587)	78,555 (70,829–82,499)	20,273 (11,712–31,779)	16,812 (11,198–24,593)	0.33 (0.21–0.47)	5,287 (4,889–5,734)	62,824 (58,035–67,613)
0.24 (0.15–0.36)	999 (793–1,177)	17,434 (14,351–20,268)	12,065 (6,831–19,634)	4,977 (3,313–7,077)	0.22 (0.14–0.33)	1,058 (821–1,276)	17,874 (14,370–21,134)
0.40 (0.24–0.63)	650 (498–883)	12,020 (9,396–15,677)	1,467 (859–2,311)	1,855 (1,209–2,652)	0.38 (0.24–0.60)	677 (516–885)	11,512 (8,808–14,887)
0.23 (0.15–0.37)	352 (293–490)	7,533 (6,342–9,963)	1,810 (1,134–2,836)	2,099 (1,388–3,092)	0.24 (0.15–0.38)	491 (410–674)	10,186 (8,623–13,327)
0.76 (0.55–1.04)	1,463 (1,215–1,732)	27,216 (22,906–31,844)	8,842 (5,257–13,660)	2,471 (1,867–3,204)	0.74 (0.51–1.05)	1,796 (1,394–2,269)	31,865 (25,411–40,002)
0.20 (0.16–0.24)	5,126 (4,345–5,495)	66,533 (58,161–71,545)	34,529 (20,978–57,793)	27,484 (23,370–32,140)	0.17 (0.13–0.21)	4,747 (3,766–5,233)	59,011 (48,290–64,670)

Continued

TABLE 13-2 Absolute Number of Incident and Prevalent Strokes DALYs Lost and Mortality to Incidence Ratio (MIR) (Point Estimates and Corresponding 95% CIs) by Country in 1990 and 2010.—cont'd

Ischemic Stroke

	1990					2005	
Country	***Prevalence***	***Incidence***	***MIR***	***Deaths***	***DALYs***	***Prevalence***	***Incidence***
Luxembourg	1,957 (1,175–3,156)	767 (505–1,129)	0.32 (0.20–0.49)	238 (185–259)	2,893 (2,269–3,183)	3,021 (1,825–4,706)	782 (502–1,137)
Macedonia	3,748 (2,259–5,970)	3,895 (2,617–5,548)	0.60 (0.40–0.87)	2,244 (2,096–2,422)	29,848 (28,073–32,028)	5,270 (3,093–8,579)	5,632 (3,796–8,266)
Madagascar	3,021 (1,874–4,925)	6,443 (4,131–9,247)	0.65 (0.41–1.01)	4,039 (3,393–4,790)	73,810 (60,904–88,500)	4,898 (2,842–7,891)	10,736 (7,066–15,838)
Malawi	2,466 (1,504–3,793)	4,341 (2,885–6,205)	0.49 (0.28–0.77)	2,066 (1,419–2,733)	41,855 (28,657–55,538)	3,671 (2,188–5,984)	7,350 (4,860–10,515)
Malaysia	39,438 (36,153–42,851)	12,125 (7,951–17,416)	0.27 (0.18–0.41)	3,172 (2,857–3,564)	59,298 (54,041–66,182)	73,597 (64,989–83,346)	22,642 (15,066–32,961)
Maldives	493 (294–780)	117 (73–179)	0.33 (0.20–0.59)	38 (31–57)	912 (750–1,267)	1,061 (621–1,719)	239 (151–357)
Mali	4,094 (2,459–6,401)	4,075 (2,688–6,011)	0.33 (0.20–0.52)	1,305 (1,055–1,764)	29,429 (23,557–39,194)	5,098 (3,110–8,046)	5,533 (3,681–8,132)
Malta	1,648 (995–2,553)	559 (367–800)	0.33 (0.22–0.48)	176 (159–190)	2,352 (2,127–2,553)	2,517 (1,549–3,941)	677 (461–990)
Marshall Islands	39 (23–63)	24 (15–35)	0.45 (0.28–0.71)	11 (9–13)	263 (190–333)	50 (30–78)	30 (19–44)
Mauritania	911 (546–1,466)	853 (572–1,246)	0.30 (0.19–0.47)	252 (200–325)	5,695 (4,472–7,341)	1,445 (867–2,302)	1,493 (982–2,194)
Mauritius	2,200 (1,334–3,363)	892 (589–1,289)	0.56 (0.38–0.83)	482 (442–515)	8,263 (7,465–8,808)	4,442 (2,756–7,004)	1,640 (1,064–2,412)
Mexico	128,733 (76,265–202,909)	43,084 (28,132–64,064)	0.30 (0.19–0.46)	12,495 (11,259–13,722)	180,806 (165,869–197,906)	214,091 (129,324–323,216)	73,072 (50,264–106,135)
Moldova	18,255 (10,954–29,991)	14,426 (9,812–20,703)	0.29 (0.19–0.43)	4,088 (3,581–4,333)	60,955 (54,379–64,746)	21,207 (12,241–33,023)	18,083 (12,150–26,136)
Mongolia	2,754 (1,662–4,310)	2,266 (1,512–3,375)	0.06 (0.03–0.12)	127 (98–259)	3,461 (2,635–6,915)	2,858 (1,745–4,531)	2,751 (1,804–3,944)
Montenegro	1,690 (994–2,702)	1,361 (929–1,941)	0.13 (0.08–0.21)	169 (139–239)	2,551 (2,183–3,467)	2,136 (1,262–3,498)	1,787 (1,156–2,656)
Morocco	27,548 (16,206–43,476)	13,951 (9,222–20,694)	0.54 (0.34–0.81)	7,288 (6,438–8,425)	135,884 (119,443–161,485)	47,178 (28,373–74,282)	24,474 (15,584–34,863)
Mozambique	6,087 (3,604–9,862)	6,598 (4,277–9,618)	0.28 (0.17–0.45)	1,750 (1,305–2,423)	32,354 (23,778–44,674)	9,922 (5,947–15,649)	10,831 (7,060–15,820)
Myanmar	73,020 (44,345–117,640)	28,152 (18,578–40,937)	0.43 (0.25–0.73)	11,753 (8,491–17,119)	211,119 (151,701–307,128)	100,064 (61,206–156,686)	42,390 (26,984–62,640)
Namibia	993 (613–1,579)	922 (612–1,354)	0.39 (0.24–0.58)	344 (284–410)	6,320 (5,238–7,433)	1,473 (917–2,305)	1,497 (966–2,200)
Nepal	29,233 (17,499–47,250)	8,225 (5,254–11,951)	0.25 (0.14–0.40)	1,934 (1,385–2,735)	37,244 (27,133–52,656)	45,946 (27,538–73,194)	13,749 (8,864–19,807)
Netherlands	91,555 (55,847–142,365)	24,385 (19,946–29,865)	0.28 (0.22–0.36)	6,827 (6,063–7,470)	82,824 (75,296–92,742)	124,784 (76,017–198,059)	24,308 (19,495–29,709)
New Zealand	13,657 (12,900–14,478)	4,519 (3,676–5,512)	0.36 (0.28–0.46)	1,623 (1,489–1,816)	18,250 (17,002–19,837)	20,396 (19,169–21,587)	5,084 (4,159–6,238)
Nicaragua	3,548 (2,160–5,516)	1,595 (1,060–2,288)	0.45 (0.28–0.65)	686 (514–747)	11,302 (8,602–12,289)	5,847 (3,491–9,085)	2,741 (1,844–4,023)
Niger	3,258 (1,965–5,209)	2,726 (1,819–3,955)	0.29 (0.18–0.46)	795 (604–1,009)	22,853 (16,821–29,479)	5,792 (3,477–9,084)	5,483 (3,621–7,866)
Nigeria	53,936 (50,744–57,437)	49,410 (33,728–71,954)	0.28 (0.18–0.41)	13,379 (11,372–16,199)	297,509 (248,236–352,505)	83,200 (77,593–89,231)	79,836 (54,061–115,545)

			2010				
MIR	**Deaths**	**DALYs**	**Prevalence**	**Incidence**	**MIR**	**Deaths**	**DALYs**
0.17 (0.11–0.28)	130 (114–183)	1,658 (1,416–2,137)	3,703 (2,200–5,891)	886 (593–1,276)	0.16 (0.10–0.25)	135 (113–188)	1,723 (1,439–2,258)
0.58 (0.37–0.83)	3,131 (2,824–3,348)	40,403 (36,843–43,020)	5,916 (3,403–9,492)	6,282 (4,250–9,250)	0.56 (0.36–0.80)	3,363 (2,983–3,655)	41,506 (37,165–44,721)
0.55 (0.34–0.83)	5,682 (4,585–6,945)	101,018 (80,601–124,026)	5,701 (3,274–8,973)	13,401 (8,942–19,936)	0.53 (0.32–0.83)	6,847 (5,311–8,435)	119,346 (92,258–148,975)
0.49 (0.27–0.80)	3,431 (2,368–4,578)	65,202 (44,924–87,313)	4,041 (2,444–6,457)	8,986 (5,898–13,061)	0.44 (0.25–0.69)	3,797 (2,619–5,017)	69,482 (47,887–93,446)
0.20 (0.13–0.28)	4,254 (3,930–4,678)	81,753 (76,129–89,035)	91,156 (79,444–102,964)	28,608 (18,408–40,801)	0.19 (0.12–0.28)	5,081 (4,541–5,617)	97,725 (88,632–106,607)
0.19 (0.11–0.30)	44 (33–50)	833 (658–954)	1,277 (730–2,066)	299 (193–437)	0.19 (0.11–0.30)	55 (40–64)	1,011 (769–1,190)
0.29 (0.17–0.44)	1,530 (1,240–1,961)	34,124 (27,978–43,802)	5,611 (3,331–8,519)	6,496 (4,217–9,225)	0.27 (0.17–0.42)	1,700 (1,392–2,152)	38,128 (31,240–48,044)
0.31 (0.20–0.45)	204 (179–225)	2,459 (2,205–2,728)	2,900 (1,758–4,449)	781 (502–1,165)	0.29 (0.18–0.43)	214 (185–240)	2,494 (2,232–2,814)
0.53 (0.32–0.82)	15 (12–18)	375 (282–473)	62 (37–99)	35 (23–49)	0.46 (0.30–0.69)	16 (13–20)	391 (296–494)
0.25 (0.15–0.39)	357 (281–458)	7,812 (6,052–9,852)	1,615 (991–2,589)	1,823 (1,205–2,595)	0.24 (0.15–0.38)	425 (330–534)	9,210 (7,192–11,376)
0.38 (0.24–0.56)	593 (547–674)	8,287 (7,716–9,522)	5,563 (3,388–8,902)	1,963 (1,289–2,869)	0.30 (0.19–0.49)	571 (500–779)	7,619 (6,681–10,302)
0.24 (0.16–0.33)	16,630 (15,005–18,783)	232,251 (211,769–258,605)	252,666 (151,987–406,438)	88,775 (58,270–129,193)	0.24 (0.15–0.35)	20,117 (17,930–22,528)	283,453 (253,893–314,321)
0.26 (0.17–0.37)	4,474 (4,126–4,803)	68,197 (62,031–72,891)	22,678 (13,698–35,644)	18,446 (12,125–26,740)	0.24 (0.16–0.36)	4,291 (3,819–4,584)	64,499 (56,382–68,736)
0.07 (0.04–0.15)	182 (134–380)	5,094 (3,717–10,066)	3,508 (2,159–5,516)	3,188 (2,069–4,679)	0.06 (0.03–0.14)	195 (140–386)	5,403 (3,920–10,393)
0.18 (0.11–0.27)	301 (269–343)	4,251 (3,843–4,719)	2,497 (1,518–3,866)	1,945 (1,321–2,836)	0.17 (0.11–0.24)	314 (270–358)	4,418 (3,813–4,906)
0.40 (0.26–0.61)	9,430 (8,430–10,825)	161,592 (145,205–186,108)	55,235 (34,584–82,697)	29,080 (18,917–41,115)	0.38 (0.25–0.57)	10,657 (9,353–12,060)	176,134 (158,388–197,750)
0.28 (0.17–0.44)	2,887 (2,195–3,700)	52,450 (39,050–67,557)	11,066 (6,668–17,263)	13,311 (8,737–19,874)	0.28 (0.16–0.44)	3,571 (2,613–4,482)	63,363 (46,145–79,903)
0.41 (0.24–0.68)	16,594 (12,572–23,302)	284,844 (218,385–400,564)	112,173 (69,462–178,513)	49,209 (32,656–74,377)	0.38 (0.22–0.62)	17,983 (13,641–24,319)	308,777 (235,918–423,790)
0.41 (0.25–0.62)	581 (467–681)	10,764 (8,806–12,410)	1,611 (990–2,554)	1,816 (1,217–2,619)	0.34 (0.21–0.50)	588 (474–696)	10,408 (8,367–12,160)
0.27 (0.16–0.42)	3,519 (2,637–4,753)	61,972 (47,184–84,010)	52,339 (30,750–81,222)	17,266 (11,587–25,837)	0.25 (0.14–0.41)	4,155 (3,106–5,598)	71,010 (53,700–95,033)
0.25 (0.19–0.31)	5,901 (5,298–6,790)	75,071 (65,996–86,815)	143,299 (86,835–219,550)	27,292 (22,090–32,864)	0.21 (0.16–0.28)	5,655 (4,965–6,734)	72,108 (62,643–84,885)
0.32 (0.25–0.40)	1,612 (1,375–1,802)	16,200 (14,500–17,769)	24,470 (23,080–25,926)	5,881 (4,843–7,082)	0.28 (0.22–0.36)	1,637 (1,363–1,878)	16,441 (14,631–18,134)
0.34 (0.22–0.52)	906 (824–1,123)	12,554 (11,512–15,500)	7,018 (4,223–10,655)	3,395 (2,237–4,845)	0.34 (0.22–0.52)	1,109 (973–1,365)	14,345 (12,847–17,713)
0.23 (0.13–0.37)	1,208 (823–1,692)	29,799 (20,244–40,610)	6,360 (3,909–9,691)	6,833 (4,366–9,922)	0.23 (0.13–0.40)	1,558 (966–2,234)	37,638 (23,049–53,754)
0.21 (0.13–0.33)	16,559 (12,882–20,951)	336,926 (267,476–410,377)	91,600 (85,028–98,447)	95,529 (63,844–142,764)	0.21 (0.13–0.32)	19,698 (14,842–24,661)	392,333 (298,726–480,364)

Continued

TABLE 13-2 Absolute Number of Incident and Prevalent Strokes DALYs Lost and Mortality to Incidence Ratio (MIR) (Point Estimates and Corresponding 95% CIs) by Country in 1990 and 2010.—cont'd

Ischemic Stroke

	1990					*2005*	
Country	***Prevalence***	***Incidence***	***MIR***	***Deaths***	***DALYs***	***Prevalence***	***Incidence***
North Korea	51,733 (30,946–81,379)	19,392 (12,394–28,604)	0.24 (0.14–0.39)	4,369 (3,412–6,490)	81,306 (62,539–121,628)	84,997 (52,769–134,773)	38,284 (24,022–54,716)
Norway	29,201 (17,143–45,947)	11,005 (9,337–13,088)	0.27 (0.22–0.32)	2,943 (2,596–3,203)	33,137 (29,874–36,089)	37,278 (22,017–58,121)	9,881 (8,288–11,813)
Oman	1,533 (920–2,437)	681 (449–998)	0.52 (0.33–0.78)	353 (315–404)	7,697 (6,334–9,473)	3,024 (1,777–4,915)	1,245 (838–1,806)
Pakistan	178,569 (159,717–199,961)	55,807 (36,453–80,197)	0.31 (0.19–0.49)	16,393 (12,869–21,734)	282,181 (221,678–369,368)	243,114 (224,148–261,289)	93,422 (62,793–137,461)
Palestine	1,052 (631–1,716)	1,228 (959–1,571)	0.22 (0.16–0.34)	282 (240–396)	7,384 (6,023–9,439)	2,211 (1,334–3,459)	2,646 (2,052–3,261)
Panama	3,138 (1,870–5,143)	1,452 (941–2,132)	0.47 (0.30–0.70)	655 (582–711)	8,880 (7,765–9,517)	6,567 (4,024–10,296)	2,222 (1,435–3,240)
Papua New Guinea	5,622 (3,428–8,872)	1,872 (1,193–2,716)	0.17 (0.08–0.47)	303 (165–811)	8,787 (5,006–22,353)	8,676 (5,301–13,698)	2,703 (1,828–3,836)
Paraguay	6,703 (3,950–10,530)	3,194 (2,139–4,551)	0.33 (0.22–0.48)	1,019 (854–1,094)	16,071 (13,582–17,178)	10,187 (5,998–16,004)	5,134 (3,337–7,296)
Peru	24,198 (14,212–38,107)	9,832 (6,226–14,795)	0.42 (0.26–0.65)	3,970 (2,960–4,317)	66,587 (54,108–71,329)	40,748 (24,849–65,546)	15,378 (10,181–22,363)
Philippines	130,406 (77,706–206,935)	33,677 (21,790–49,040)	0.24 (0.15–0.35)	7,644 (6,795–8,246)	153,932 (139,990–168,142)	167,137 (99,086–260,217)	59,701 (39,328–86,339)
Poland	106,717 (63,776–165,019)	87,654 (72,499–104,584)	0.44 (0.35–0.53)	37,813 (34,304–39,826)	509,733 (457,476–536,749)	165,733 (96,967–268,154)	103,386 (85,318–123,896)
Portugal	36,896 (21,771–58,995)	22,747 (18,870–27,577)	0.77 (0.61–0.94)	17,376 (14,739–18,315)	189,595 (162,295–199,400)	62,971 (38,751–96,766)	23,927 (19,631–28,801)
Qatar	608 (330–1,038)	55 (39–75)	0.55 (0.26–0.81)	30 (15–37)	797 (441–993)	1,928 (1,006–3,408)	133 (93–185)
Romania	65,641 (39,099–108,178)	65,100 (43,267–94,358)	0.53 (0.35–0.77)	33,379 (30,477–35,086)	443,446 (406,470–465,634)	77,375 (45,125–123,273)	78,421 (53,902–115,080)
Russia	642,488 (387,614–1,038,613)	620,053 (529,487–723,055)	0.48 (0.38–0.57)	293,175 (247,399–317,539)	3,902,778 (3,245,332–4,243,775)	742,905 (430,934–1,171,628)	811,019 (697,729–934,819)
Rwanda	1,635 (943–2,559)	2,846 (1,878–4,145)	0.54 (0.33–0.88)	1,492 (1,089–1,909)	30,160 (22,233–39,111)	3,063 (1,833–4,737)	4,415 (2,897–6,423)
Saint Lucia	315 (193–483)	164 (109–236)	0.47 (0.31–0.68)	74 (64–80)	1,073 (929–1,147)	466 (285–720)	198 (128–279)
Saint Vincent and the Grenadines	225 (135–345)	111 (75–166)	0.41 (0.26–0.59)	44 (38–48)	627 (551–678)	330 (203–514)	129 (87–185)
Samoa	170 (101–268)	117 (77–172)	0.46 (0.28–0.69)	51 (41–62)	1,099 (849–1,351)	280 (164–451)	132 (86–186)
São Tomé and Príncipe	69 (42–109)	77 (49–114)	0.43 (0.27–0.65)	32 (28–37)	580 (513–661)	85 (51–133)	104 (68–151)
Saudi Arabia	14,805 (8,744–24,992)	4,412 (3,085–6,253)	0.83 (0.55–1.20)	3,568 (2,888–4,199)	58,521 (46,222–67,746)	27,609 (15,829–46,081)	8,900 (6,057–12,574)
Senegal	3,907 (2,348–6,067)	2,815 (1,898–4,186)	0.21 (0.13–0.32)	582 (471–722)	15,310 (12,312–18,859)	6,270 (3,740–9,628)	4,654 (3,123–6,742)
Serbia	27,756 (16,506–42,336)	25,892 (21,075–31,217)	0.53 (0.42–0.65)	13,555 (11,890–15,014)	187,003 (163,775–205,772)	36,714 (21,411–57,327)	36,487 (30,045–43,183)

			2010				
MIR	**Deaths**	**DALYs**	**Prevalence**	**Incidence**	**MIR**	**Deaths**	**DALYs**
0.25 (0.15–0.44)	9,326 (6,885–15,828)	150,514 (109,601–257,046)	91,642 (53,841–143,105)	44,052 (29,053–64,329)	0.26 (0.15–0.47)	11,049 (8,003–18,466)	170,366 (122,744–280,279)
0.22 (0.18–0.28)	2,187 (1,981–2,589)	23,502 (20,932–27,088)	40,054 (24,518–61,010)	10,483 (8,666–12,550)	0.21 (0.17–0.27)	2,164 (1,899–2,662)	22,780 (19,844–26,941)
0.33 (0.22–0.49)	401 (351–443)	7,603 (6,448–8,453)	2,570 (1,510–3,915)	1,495 (999–2,105)	0.28 (0.18–0.41)	404 (352–451)	7,012 (5,876–7,847)
0.33 (0.19–0.51)	29,527 (23,257–39,008)	479,505 (388,533–625,233)	273,906 (254,932–294,104)	114,089 (75,999–165,401)	0.29 (0.18–0.46)	31,786 (25,037–42,613)	514,264 (416,343–686,572)
0.21 (0.16–0.27)	554 (500–603)	12,384 (10,280–14,231)	2,615 (1,528–4,185)	3,371 (2,634–4,255)	0.24 (0.17–0.31)	798 (616–882)	16,417 (12,144–18,594)
0.35 (0.22–0.53)	744 (674–855)	9,389 (8,612–10,833)	6,961 (4,306–10,678)	2,771 (1,852–4,012)	0.36 (0.24–0.54)	966 (854–1,124)	12,244 (11,037–14,041)
0.19 (0.08–0.54)	489 (250–1,326)	13,846 (7,493–34,623)	10,158 (5,972–15,705)	3,271 (2,216–4,845)	0.18 (0.08–0.49)	571 (282–1,492)	16,103 (8,645–39,584)
0.31 (0.20–0.47)	1,549 (1,405–1,921)	22,434 (20,628–27,470)	11,666 (7,288–17,862)	6,235 (4,142–9,106)	0.32 (0.21–0.48)	1,918 (1,705–2,347)	27,224 (24,520–33,127)
0.26 (0.16–0.43)	3,897 (3,411–5,779)	61,220 (55,583–77,403)	48,233 (29,544–76,809)	18,267 (12,237–26,120)	0.25 (0.16–0.40)	4,461 (3,852–6,198)	66,905 (60,147–82,331)
0.27 (0.17–0.40)	15,658 (13,336–16,857)	312,922 (262,331–337,786)	190,678 (116,818–308,650)	73,236 (45,993–109,368)	0.27 (0.16–0.42)	18,689 (14,672–20,581)	373,866 (286,593–412,351)
0.35 (0.28–0.43)	35,744 (31,624–38,431)	449,027 (401,412–479,665)	188,509 (115,480–303,473)	115,771 (95,608–139,539)	0.34 (0.27–0.41)	38,437 (32,865–42,462)	457,740 (395,315–494,563)
0.48 (0.36–0.70)	11,326 (9,660–16,726)	112,035 (96,900–162,549)	69,145 (40,732–111,351)	26,503 (22,050–31,602)	0.46 (0.34–0.69)	11,995 (10,003–18,085)	114,495 (97,504–166,041)
0.14 (0.09–0.20)	18 (16–22)	660 (532–842)	3,998 (2,106–7,066)	242 (166–338)	0.11 (0.07–0.16)	26 (22–30)	1,135 (871–1,535)
0.53 (0.35–0.75)	40,016 (36,174–42,102)	512,190 (456,228–535,909)	84,205 (50,342–132,773)	83,276 (56,110–121,031)	0.50 (0.33–0.73)	40,343 (36,624–43,149)	489,334 (439,370–518,356)
0.47 (0.36–0.56)	375,356 (299,190–407,213)	5,192,635 (4,159,122–5,687,144)	894,544 (564,601–1,421,727)	847,367 (722,742–983,066)	0.40 (0.31–0.48)	339,779 (268,785–372,407)	4,373,350 (3,463,052–4,829,418)
0.34 (0.20–0.54)	1,438 (1,043–1,884)	26,595 (19,893–34,941)	3,428 (2,051–5,448)	5,620 (3,689–8,344)	0.34 (0.19–0.53)	1,816 (1,301–2,361)	32,405 (23,762–42,753)
0.43 (0.28–0.64)	81 (72–101)	889 (811–1,053)	518 (317–798)	211 (141–304)	0.42 (0.27–0.63)	85 (73–109)	915 (811–1,106)
0.30 (0.20–0.45)	37 (34–45)	525 (479–614)	344 (205–536)	135 (90–197)	0.28 (0.18–0.41)	36 (32–42)	509 (461–577)
0.36 (0.22–0.55)	45 (34–57)	859 (664–1,087)	331 (200–528)	144 (97–207)	0.31 (0.19–0.48)	42 (31–56)	773 (591–988)
0.35 (0.21–0.55)	35 (28–42)	601 (483–711)	88 (52–140)	111 (74–161)	0.35 (0.21–0.52)	37 (27–45)	620 (456–750)
0.53 (0.35–0.77)	4,594 (3,717–5,186)	77,945 (62,293–87,698)	36,397 (21,452–58,079)	10,426 (7,187–14,201)	0.54 (0.35–0.77)	5,447 (4,349–6,181)	87,891 (69,114–98,552)
0.14 (0.09–0.22)	650 (523–803)	15,672 (12,917–18,819)	6,509 (3,766–10,450)	5,372 (3,624–7,921)	0.15 (0.09–0.23)	771 (627–939)	18,525 (15,206–22,037)
0.57 (0.47–0.70)	20,680 (19,119–21,913)	263,642 (244,908–279,161)	42,059 (24,964–66,005)	38,872 (31,840–46,565)	0.50 (0.40–0.62)	19,327 (17,442–20,713)	229,296 (207,166–244,080)

Continued

TABLE 13-2 Absolute Number of Incident and Prevalent Strokes DALYs Lost and Mortality to Incidence Ratio (MIR) (Point Estimates and Corresponding 95% CIs) by Country in 1990 and 2010.—cont'd

Ischemic Stroke

	1990					2005	
Country	**Prevalence**	**Incidence**	**MIR**	**Deaths**	**DALYs**	**Prevalence**	**Incidence**
Seychelles	104 (63–165)	36 (23–51)	0.36 (0.23–0.54)	12 (10–14)	289 (224–333)	140 (83–221)	49 (32–72)
Sierra Leone	1,864 (1,104–2,993)	1,818 (1,159–2,687)	0.34 (0.22–0.53)	613 (518–742)	16,204 (13,557–19,755)	2,063 (1,241–3,203)	2,081 (1,338–3,051)
Singapore	8,535 (7,917–9,165)	3,188 (2,126–4,596)	0.21 (0.14–0.30)	640 (571–688)	11,478 (10,287–12,221)	17,716 (16,603–18,855)	4,108 (2,750–6,012)
Slovakia	17,433 (10,373–27,752)	14,693 (9,662–21,521)	0.42 (0.27–0.61)	5,913 (5,477–6,523)	79,448 (74,424–89,426)	23,749 (14,144–38,287)	16,441 (11,099–23,142)
Slovenia	7,337 (4,466–11,854)	6,035 (4,070–8,683)	0.50 (0.33–0.72)	2,895 (2,497–3,078)	35,864 (30,519–38,048)	12,952 (7,511–20,737)	7,391 (4,909–10,683)
Solomon Islands	237 (133–397)	186 (122–280)	0.55 (0.32–0.94)	99 (78–138)	2,249 (1,771–2,939)	355 (209–581)	257 (170–380)
Somalia	1,981 (1,190–3,160)	3,253 (2,164–4,757)	0.44 (0.24–0.74)	1,378 (922–2,019)	26,304 (17,852–39,465)	2,718 (1,626–4,277)	4,283 (2,820–6,293)
South Africa	27,342 (25,685–29,135)	24,202 (15,607–35,880)	0.34 (0.21–0.51)	7,854 (6,415–8,655)	146,679 (119,157–161,363)	41,376 (39,080–43,632)	41,352 (27,898–62,431)
South Korea	75,085 (44,653–120,007)	45,512 (30,419–66,096)	0.73 (0.48–1.07)	31,991 (26,840–33,719)	481,170 (410,922–505,567)	203,400 (123,144–319,965)	59,783 (39,754–87,340)
Spain	200,632 (186,462–215,561)	80,351 (52,823–114,566)	0.52 (0.34–0.77)	39,862 (32,745–42,993)	413,088 (354,648–438,931)	330,056 (305,713–354,100)	90,787 (57,641–132,916)
Sri Lanka	66,942 (39,908–104,659)	16,955 (11,053–25,091)	0.24 (0.15–0.36)	3,841 (3,371–4,142)	68,788 (60,799–74,914)	94,549 (55,692–148,316)	28,339 (18,875–40,749)
Sudan	10,431 (6,185–16,173)	13,375 (8,839–19,294)	0.32 (0.19–0.49)	4,081 (2,972–5,443)	72,863 (53,773–97,109)	20,102 (12,037–31,121)	22,400 (14,570–33,153)
Suriname	745 (440–1,175)	360 (242–526)	0.42 (0.27–0.60)	144 (133–164)	2,207 (2,050–2,522)	1,123 (695–1,806)	504 (332–729)
Swaziland	576 (358–917)	450 (297–663)	0.34 (0.22–0.51)	147 (125–178)	2,842 (2,434–3,398)	663 (385–1,053)	726 (470–1,065)
Sweden	70,195 (42,471–110,384)	27,663 (23,776–31,697)	0.30 (0.25–0.36)	8,294 (7,525–9,322)	88,498 (80,633–98,961)	81,765 (49,352–125,991)	25,339 (21,990–28,951)
Switzerland	48,373 (29,451–76,190)	15,305 (10,087–21,942)	0.35 (0.22–0.52)	5,099 (4,318–5,753)	53,571 (46,173–59,962)	71,093 (43,619–112,580)	15,451 (10,404–22,418)
Syria	11,168 (6,813–17,764)	6,080 (4,075–8,857)	0.30 (0.19–0.46)	1,764 (1,520–2,326)	35,876 (31,310–45,912)	20,797 (12,312–31,336)	11,441 (7,465–16,673)
Taiwan	66,882 (60,848–73,608)	25,756 (16,687–37,443)	0.23 (0.15–0.35)	5,756 (4,827–6,802)	90,318 (77,422–106,622)	140,957 (121,094–162,514)	46,117 (30,091–68,790)
Tajikistan	7,243 (4,180–11,832)	5,453 (3,572–8,135)	0.34 (0.22–0.51)	1,783 (1,566–2,005)	27,180 (24,000–30,245)	7,455 (4,465–11,922)	6,497 (4,272–9,360)
Tanzania	10,508 (9,382–11,738)	13,212 (10,019–17,497)	0.19 (0.13–0.28)	2,523 (2,024–3,265)	45,742 (36,678–59,578)	18,838 (16,811–21,138)	23,457 (17,909–30,479)
Thailand	196,998 (169,959–227,915)	45,757 (30,094–66,142)	0.09 (0.05–0.14)	3,801 (3,386–5,427)	91,968 (82,424–116,459)	341,118 (289,269–400,091)	93,407 (61,614–137,313)
The Bahamas	493 (304–752)	196 (133–285)	0.32 (0.21–0.46)	60 (51–66)	999 (833–1,088)	1,444 (814–2,348)	308 (202–457)
The Gambia	366 (220–582)	367 (237–531)	0.39 (0.22–0.62)	138 (100–183)	3,406 (2,396–4,531)	582 (359–914)	634 (412–933)

MIR	Deaths	DALYs	2010 Prevalence	Incidence	MIR	Deaths	DALYs
0.28 (0.16–0.42)	13 (9–15)	293 (209–346)	147 (88–235)	56 (36–81)	0.26 (0.15–0.40)	14 (10–17)	316 (222–378)
0.27 (0.16–0.43)	552 (425–703)	14,470 (11,025–18,048)	2,169 (1,279–3,478)	2,442 (1,591–3,627)	0.28 (0.16–0.43)	661 (501–841)	17,131 (12,856–21,376)
0.17 (0.11–0.25)	665 (590–736)	11,910 (11,015–12,983)	18,710 (17,700–19,673)	4,590 (3,095–6,650)	0.18 (0.12–0.26)	785 (662–933)	13,109 (11,621–14,991)
0.35 (0.23–0.50)	5,549 (5,059–6,034)	72,912 (66,355–78,324)	26,059 (15,664–40,324)	18,087 (12,083–26,602)	0.32 (0.21–0.47)	5,615 (5,002–6,144)	70,982 (62,636–76,493)
0.28 (0.18–0.41)	1,987 (1,832–2,339)	22,940 (21,157–27,188)	15,479 (9,134–24,401)	8,452 (5,577–12,083)	0.26 (0.18–0.39)	2,145 (1,939–2,427)	23,440 (21,473–26,467)
0.64 (0.39–1.02)	158 (128–216)	3,696 (3,013–4,661)	426 (251–708)	305 (193–446)	0.61 (0.37–0.99)	179 (145–240)	4,160 (3,347–5,214)
0.33 (0.19–0.55)	1,357 (965–1,905)	25,030 (17,987–36,454)	2,924 (1,761–4,662)	5,005 (3,376–7,186)	0.33 (0.19–0.54)	1,594 (1,121–2,281)	29,494 (20,543–43,044)
0.24 (0.15–0.34)	9,336 (8,455–10,820)	178,296 (164,114–211,324)	49,222 (46,195–52,252)	49,133 (32,414–71,730)	0.21 (0.13–0.32)	9,968 (8,601–11,640)	181,489 (161,620–214,655)
0.49 (0.32–0.75)	28,226 (25,667–36,216)	369,857 (339,085–461,177)	266,372 (158,771–407,827)	77,019 (49,965–111,609)	0.44 (0.28–0.68)	32,720 (28,548–44,547)	400,917 (356,266–525,361)
0.36 (0.23–0.59)	31,376 (27,230–44,917)	306,484 (273,421–416,354)	378,353 (351,022–407,918)	102,064 (68,344–144,786)	0.32 (0.20–0.51)	31,566 (26,480–47,045)	301,103 (263,517–418,358)
0.23 (0.15–0.35)	6,386 (5,298–7,463)	93,588 (78,732–108,137)	109,531 (66,315–172,308)	35,167 (22,311–51,257)	0.22 (0.13–0.33)	7,264 (5,764–8,554)	106,254 (86,380–124,801)
0.19 (0.11–0.31)	4,117 (3,019–5,510)	70,452 (52,453–93,547)	24,185 (14,361–37,060)	27,918 (18,717–41,029)	0.18 (0.10–0.27)	4,709 (3,465–6,344)	79,899 (59,452–107,510)
0.41 (0.26–0.60)	197 (156–215)	2,932 (2,333–3,185)	1,469 (906–2,322)	563 (377–810)	0.41 (0.26–0.60)	221 (170–247)	3,231 (2,537–3,597)
0.40 (0.25–0.61)	280 (230–330)	5,770 (4,829–6,669)	724 (436–1,159)	852 (561–1,259)	0.36 (0.22–0.53)	291 (241–344)	5,562 (4,671–6,474)
0.29 (0.24–0.35)	7,415 (6,571–8,350)	71,151 (63,523–80,541)	89,746 (54,418–143,080)	26,736 (23,413–30,624)	0.26 (0.22–0.32)	6,978 (6,077–8,087)	65,550 (57,809–76,044)
0.26 (0.17–0.39)	3,884 (3,345–4,694)	39,801 (34,199–47,337)	77,910 (45,933–122,967)	17,416 (11,705–25,083)	0.25 (0.16–0.37)	4,128 (3,464–4,999)	41,012 (34,655–49,021)
0.24 (0.15–0.38)	2,595 (2,179–3,397)	50,161 (42,639–65,181)	28,638 (17,364–44,969)	14,223 (9,352–20,714)	0.19 (0.12–0.30)	2,641 (2,205–3,494)	50,836 (43,158–66,809)
0.18 (0.11–0.26)	7,781 (6,563–9,164)	109,711 (97,273–123,492)	166,852 (143,815–192,436)	54,557 (35,608–79,942)	0.17 (0.11–0.26)	8,946 (7,330–10,625)	117,910 (103,355–132,036)
0.31 (0.20–0.47)	1,937 (1,676–2,169)	30,493 (26,689–34,000)	8,543 (5,148–13,242)	7,147 (4,529–10,402)	0.32 (0.20–0.49)	2,211 (1,850–2,538)	34,142 (29,210–38,619)
0.15 (0.11–0.21)	3,465 (2,874–4,394)	60,825 (50,795–76,964)	21,728 (19,249–24,362)	29,219 (22,227–37,800)	0.15 (0.10–0.21)	4,259 (3,421–5,393)	72,653 (59,009–91,693)
0.17 (0.08–0.25)	14,989 (8,655–17,189)	250,968 (162,721–280,359)	414,568 (351,060–491,437)	114,248 (72,996–165,145)	0.15 (0.08–0.24)	16,826 (9,915–19,583)	280,393 (191,206–315,876)
0.11 (0.07–0.16)	32 (27–37)	651 (550–797)	2,029 (1,136–3,375)	369 (246–527)	0.13 (0.08–0.21)	47 (38–58)	892 (744–1,097)
0.30 (0.18–0.47)	185 (139–240)	4,237 (3,104–5,415)	659 (404–1,051)	735 (485–1,069)	0.28 (0.15–0.44)	197 (144–253)	4,472 (3,205–5,651)

Continued

TABLE 13-2 Absolute Number of Incident and Prevalent Strokes DALYs Lost and Mortality to Incidence Ratio (MIR) (Point Estimates and Corresponding 95% CIs) by Country in 1990 and 2010.—cont'd

Ischemic Stroke

	1990					2005	
Country	**Prevalence**	**Incidence**	**MIR**	**Deaths**	**DALYs**	**Prevalence**	**Incidence**
Timor-Leste	1,089 (632–1,757)	293 (197–431)	0.25 (0.15–0.37)	71 (60–89)	1,738 (1,443–2,175)	1,645 (996–2,508)	549 (360–811)
Togo	1,757 (1,068–2,718)	1,808 (1,164–2,669)	0.36 (0.23–0.55)	623 (536–755)	12,861 (10,884–15,218)	2,764 (1,670–4,402)	3,144 (2,112–4,511)
Tonga	142 (85–221)	81 (54–119)	0.28 (0.18–0.44)	22 (18–27)	404 (341–477)	209 (126–326)	91 (59–135)
Trinidad and Tobago	2,481 (1,481–3,871)	1,205 (800–1,732)	0.41 (0.27–0.58)	470 (421–504)	7,467 (6,788–7,952)	4,011 (2,408–6,528)	1,485 (1,003–2,129)
Tunisia	10,223 (9,349–11,232)	5,420 (3,561–7,882)	0.43 (0.27–0.65)	2,280 (1,908–2,949)	44,058 (37,328–54,533)	18,518 (16,945–20,214)	10,544 (7,023–15,503)
Turkey	51,299 (32,323–77,868)	33,132 (21,437–48,253)	0.70 (0.45–1.03)	22,948 (20,031–26,047)	565,795 (480,551–651,841)	101,220 (60,670–157,024)	61,784 (40,631–89,279)
Turkmenistan	4,983 (2,989–8,046)	3,739 (2,468–5,367)	0.20 (0.12–0.32)	705 (588–939)	12,743 (10,821–17,303)	7,133 (4,289–11,209)	5,839 (3,970–8,281)
Uganda	6,263 (3,788–9,605)	7,784 (5,160–11,561)	0.34 (0.19–0.57)	2,532 (1,766–3,641)	47,689 (34,206–67,834)	9,236 (5,729–14,407)	12,985 (8,771–18,964)
Ukraine	283,975 (170,504–459,658)	375,387 (304,817–456,499)	0.28 (0.21–0.35)	102,846 (84,462–111,004)	1,348,855 (1,122,653–1,454,822)	335,320 (201,201–533,702)	446,114 (361,478–533,928)
United Arab Emirates	1,469 (797–2,450)	472 (311–693)	0.45 (0.28–0.71)	207 (170–240)	4,674 (3,490–5,639)	4,199 (2,392–7,008)	1,178 (735–1,799)
United Kingdom	377,495 (222,977–589,519)	115,470 (99,198–131,856)	0.50 (0.41–0.59)	57,183 (49,675–62,615)	602,507 (535,528–652,870)	477,105 (283,514–750,219)	104,468 (90,156–119,844)
United States	1,998,734 (1,878,241–2,126,999)	635,584 (496,882–794,447)	0.21 (0.16–0.27)	131,636 (118,711–147,064)	1,525,418 (1,415,367–1,680,948)	3,420,696 (3,301,067–3,540,781)	686,405 (546,497–864,089)
Uruguay	8,840 (5,386–13,981)	6,060 (3,954–8,690)	0.42 (0.28–0.61)	2,423 (2,227–2,701)	27,359 (25,532–30,154)	10,403 (6,238–16,983)	5,592 (3,589–8,200)
Uzbekistan	29,220 (17,809–46,618)	23,003 (15,056–33,257)	0.45 (0.29–0.66)	9,928 (8,904–11,133)	166,018 (149,546–182,866)	37,386 (22,772–58,517)	33,559 (22,225–49,207)
Vanuatu	136 (82–226)	110 (73–167)	0.58 (0.32–0.94)	61 (44–89)	1,296 (910–1,817)	172 (99–281)	132 (85–196)
Venezuela	22,098 (12,820–34,865)	9,016 (5,871–12,714)	0.33 (0.22–0.49)	2,877 (2,623–3,109)	49,703 (44,790–53,153)	41,654 (25,146–65,306)	16,702 (10,774–24,638)
Vietnam	129,288 (118,285–139,548)	46,713 (30,089–69,761)	0.10 (0.06–0.18)	4,449 (3,444–7,701)	96,175 (79,677–140,079)	196,148 (181,997–213,100)	76,960 (51,050–111,684)
Yemen	6,371 (3,842–10,125)	4,144 (2,790–6,119)	0.50 (0.30–0.82)	2,136 (1,575–3,057)	62,924 (43,869–90,542)	14,021 (8,523–21,499)	9,473 (6,320–14,022)
Zambia	2,546 (1,519–4,005)	3,796 (2,498–5,597)	0.41 (0.25–0.65)	1,507 (1,151–2,025)	26,654 (20,496–34,488)	3,576 (2,158–5,542)	6,363 (4,042–9,133)
Zimbabwe	9,428 (5,767–15,359)	5,753 (4,354–7,381)	0.24 (0.17–0.33)	1,359 (1,150–1,633)	24,052 (20,746–28,439)	10,391 (6,322–15,966)	9,073 (6,885–11,650)

Hemorrhagic Stroke

	1990					2005	
Country	**Prevalence**	**Incidence**	**MIR**	**Deaths**	**DALYs**	**Prevalence**	**Incidence**
Afghanistan	2,016 (1,152–3,185)	1,659 (1,032–2,476)	4.13 (2.07–7.15)	6,808 (3,760–10,675)	226,015 (119,685–359,390)	4,543 (2,564–7,391)	4,825 (3,082–7,400)
Albania	2,125 (1,254–3,508)	1,965 (1,258–2,901)	1.34 (0.85–1.99)	2,518 (2,354–2,852)	44,204 (40,977–49,445)	2,314 (1,368–3,622)	2,362 (1,509–3,503)

			2010				
MIR	**Deaths**	**DALYs**	**Prevalence**	**Incidence**	**MIR**	**Deaths**	**DALYs**
0.23 (0.14–0.35)	123 (103–153)	2,719 (2,284–3,297)	1,829 (1,099–2,842)	674 (440–977)	0.23 (0.14–0.35)	150 (126–186)	3,143 (2,649–3,831)
0.29 (0.18–0.44)	873 (735–1,109)	16,843 (14,176–20,443)	3,089 (1,871–4,773)	3,871 (2,529–5,651)	0.28 (0.17–0.43)	1,048 (877–1,313)	19,803 (16,535–24,077)
0.27 (0.17–0.43)	24 (19–30)	405 (330–479)	232 (139–363)	95 (60–140)	0.25 (0.15–0.41)	23 (17–29)	373 (302–448)
0.37 (0.25–0.55)	533 (490–632)	7,850 (7,260–9,240)	4,800 (2,853–7,659)	1,689 (1,124–2,450)	0.35 (0.22–0.51)	565 (501–654)	8,369 (7,489–9,593)
0.34 (0.21–0.51)	3,457 (2,891–4,461)	56,721 (48,333–70,089)	21,601 (19,588–23,558)	12,035 (8,033–17,968)	0.33 (0.20–0.51)	3,763 (3,102–4,794)	59,295 (49,995–72,592)
0.41 (0.26–0.59)	24,405 (21,591–27,443)	500,921 (428,197–566,570)	122,549 (75,511–195,953)	75,116 (49,652–108,728)	0.37 (0.24–0.54)	27,220 (23,588–31,191)	513,074 (437,888–603,371)
0.17 (0.11–0.27)	971 (816–1,296)	17,356 (14,893–23,467)	8,535 (5,153–13,330)	6,455 (4,241–9,537)	0.16 (0.10–0.25)	1,021 (846–1,336)	18,005 (15,160–23,670)
0.31 (0.18–0.49)	3,919 (2,774–5,311)	69,573 (50,444–93,839)	10,499 (6,360–16,711)	16,151 (10,699–23,397)	0.30 (0.17–0.48)	4,706 (3,223–6,346)	81,625 (57,306–109,083)
0.23 (0.18–0.29)	100,560 (86,500–109,784)	1,401,447 (1,214,543–1,527,250)	416,935 (247,901–663,911)	453,096 (368,222–553,580)	0.20 (0.16–0.25)	91,349 (76,006–102,070)	1,193,097 (997,898–1,319,896)
0.24 (0.14–0.39)	272 (204–330)	6,904 (4,753–8,808)	7,718 (4,447–12,948)	1,960 (1,204–3,129)	0.19 (0.10–0.30)	347 (239–433)	10,469 (6,694–13,540)
0.43 (0.36–0.52)	44,676 (40,039–50,841)	429,181 (387,856–488,727)	529,467 (316,612–833,362)	111,524 (96,216–128,839)	0.37 (0.30–0.46)	41,086 (35,601–48,291)	392,037 (346,388–457,352)
0.19 (0.14–0.24)	125,969 (112,278–152,947)	1,559,624 (1,425,267–1,750,410)	3,895,049 (3,762,823–4,032,319)	754,658 (593,952–934,666)	0.17 (0.13–0.22)	125,461 (108,957–150,304)	1,569,719 (1,428,604–1,756,141)
0.52 (0.33–0.79)	2,766 (2,471–3,228)	28,222 (25,801–31,166)	11,222 (6,628–17,662)	5,938 (3,886–8,731)	0.49 (0.31–0.75)	2,819 (2,421–3,313)	27,708 (24,739–31,030)
0.42 (0.26–0.62)	13,554 (11,348–14,724)	219,986 (190,523–235,552)	44,027 (26,386–69,237)	37,783 (24,987–55,410)	0.41 (0.26–0.61)	14,734 (11,780–16,832)	239,221 (191,444–269,056)
0.70 (0.40–1.17)	88 (62–126)	1,946 (1,365–2,784)	205 (117–337)	154 (105–227)	0.65 (0.38–1.07)	96 (68–139)	2,153 (1,491–3,022)
0.25 (0.16–0.37)	3,942 (3,645–4,495)	59,977 (56,166–68,181)	51,435 (30,583–81,646)	20,718 (13,753–30,708)	0.25 (0.16–0.37)	4,947 (4,469–5,577)	73,707 (67,739–82,573)
0.09 (0.05–0.16)	6,385 (5,089–10,255)	125,334 (108,556–171,226)	236,765 (219,166–254,654)	93,510 (61,276–135,784)	0.08 (0.05–0.13)	6,830 (5,491–10,632)	136,299 (119,491–178,314)
0.38 (0.23–0.60)	3,574 (2,825–4,787)	84,585 (66,434–109,487)	15,707 (9,557–24,793)	11,365 (7,711–16,215)	0.37 (0.23–0.57)	4,116 (3,300–5,631)	95,734 (76,353–124,905)
0.41 (0.25–0.65)	2,498 (1,910–3,288)	43,325 (33,329–56,457)	3,878 (2,269–6,280)	7,584 (4,936–10,916)	0.39 (0.24–0.64)	2,861 (2,165–3,756)	48,523 (37,543–62,381)
0.30 (0.20–0.44)	2,703 (2,048–3,604)	51,410 (40,429–65,114)	9,041 (5,505–14,196)	10,213 (7,860–12,905)	0.31 (0.21–0.47)	3,116 (2,305–4,393)	52,144 (39,334–71,521)

			2010				
MIR	**Deaths**	**DALYs**	**Prevalence**	**Incidence**	**MIR**	**Deaths**	**DALYs**
3.29 (1.64–5.94)	15,626 (8,417–24,028)	491,957 (249,627–773,109)	5,359 (3,069–8,668)	5,561 (3,582–8,548)	2.93 (1.48–4.98)	15,910 (9,308–23,393)	483,308 (272,348–732,139)
1.79 (1.11–2.69)	4,044 (3,544–4,335)	61,650 (54,287–65,991)	2,530 (1,516–4,005)	2,717 (1,681–4,092)	1.68 (1.04–2.62)	4,328 (3,721–4,885)	62,992 (54,380–70,980)

Continued

TABLE 13-2 Absolute Number of Incident and Prevalent Strokes DALYs Lost and Mortality to Incidence Ratio (MIR) (Point Estimates and Corresponding 95% CIs) by Country in 1990 and 2010.—cont'd

Hemorrhagic Stroke

	1990					*2005*	
Country	***Prevalence***	***Incidence***	***MIR***	***Deaths***	***DALYs***	***Prevalence***	***Incidence***
Algeria	5,581 (3,353–8,408)	4,309 (2,709–6,492)	1.94 (1.21–2.97)	8,137 (6,948–9,224)	212,231 (174,427–253,441)	11,456 (7,034–17,710)	9,346 (5,990–13,635)
Andorra	84 (52–127)	35 (23–52)	0.65 (0.39–1.04)	22 (18–27)	335 (279–405)	162 (101–253)	50 (33–75)
Angola	1,788 (1,071–2,897)	2,192 (1,415–3,306)	1.35 (0.75–2.43)	2,952 (2,003–4,356)	97,454 (63,054–150,007)	4,157 (2,480–6,461)	4,249 (2,778–6,256)
Antigua and Barbuda	37 (22–57)	33 (21–48)	1.33 (0.77–2.08)	42 (31–48)	781 (571–902)	80 (47–120)	46 (29–67)
Argentina	28,032 (26,648–29,326)	22,121 (14,275–34,431)	0.62 (0.38–0.94)	13,188 (11,071–14,317)	340,490 (281,854–368,141)	43,547 (41,341–45,920)	22,397 (14,337–32,654)
Armenia	3,236 (1,970–5,159)	3,078 (1,983–4,556)	0.59 (0.38–0.90)	1,742 (1,538–1,934)	32,458 (28,947–35,917)	3,790 (2,260–6,039)	4,338 (2,819–6,515)
Australia	19,346 (11,546–30,289)	6,540 (5,096–8,180)	0.61 (0.46–0.79)	3,905 (3,578–4,451)	73,470 (67,265–83,648)	31,407 (19,037–48,545)	7,589 (6,023–9,509)
Austria	11,097 (6,685–17,443)	5,192 (3,386–7,791)	0.90 (0.56–1.33)	4,476 (3,905–4,870)	68,231 (59,276–73,854)	18,044 (10,987–27,708)	5,193 (3,332–7,838)
Azerbaijan	5,189 (3,128–8,098)	4,950 (3,211–7,194)	0.71 (0.45–1.07)	3,373 (2,955–3,801)	75,150 (65,834–85,277)	7,766 (4,521–12,506)	8,325 (5,019–12,522)
Bahrain	174 (102–285)	25 (17–36)	2.96 (1.96–4.36)	72 (62–82)	2,005 (1,688–2,313)	400 (222–695)	63 (43–90)
Bangladesh	34,560 (20,813–55,481)	30,435 (19,918–45,013)	0.63 (0.36–1.02)	18,569 (11,675–23,724)	417,547 (268,540–533,603)	89,785 (53,190–145,526)	41,722 (25,914–64,581)
Barbados	213 (129–335)	210 (152–283)	0.80 (0.56–1.09)	164 (136–181)	2,504 (2,063–2,760)	384 (226–593)	278 (209–370)
Belarus	10,386 (6,271–15,785)	6,431 (4,886–8,406)	0.79 (0.59–1.05)	5,004 (4,530–5,814)	114,961 (103,786–126,866)	12,002 (7,187–18,771)	9,411 (7,140–12,220)
Belgium	15,770 (9,433–25,128)	6,466 (4,124–9,495)	0.44 (0.28–0.66)	2,721 (2,440–2,990)	54,935 (48,762–60,201)	23,827 (14,183–37,882)	6,827 (4,363–10,127)
Belize	92 (57–142)	54 (34–81)	0.89 (0.55–1.37)	47 (39–52)	1,057 (851–1,193)	186 (112–296)	83 (53–123)
Benin	655 (410–1,022)	1,421 (936–2,088)	0.91 (0.57–1.35)	1,373 (1,075–1,723)	46,881 (33,376–65,908)	1,369 (855–2,167)	2,429 (1,613–3,560)
Bhutan	201 (120–322)	133 (85–201)	0.66 (0.35–1.12)	85 (55–123)	2,305 (1,473–3,395)	417 (257–656)	190 (121–279)
Bolivia	1,261 (1,167–1,365)	1,539 (1,020–2,294)	1.42 (0.88–2.13)	2,152 (1,786–2,601)	62,157 (49,835–75,247)	2,694 (2,458–2,943)	2,018 (1,309–2,956)
Bosnia and Herzegovina	2,917 (1,773–4,646)	2,945 (1,922–4,536)	1.14 (0.72–1.67)	3,217 (2,875–3,487)	62,570 (55,777–68,254)	3,456 (2,078–5,485)	3,652 (2,366–5,395)
Botswana	409 (244–645)	374 (248–566)	0.74 (0.42–1.19)	264 (202–349)	6,793 (5,194–9,083)	734 (445–1,157)	830 (527–1,219)
Brazil	77,741 (48,329–120,209)	68,737 (51,480–91,706)	0.79 (0.56–1.04)	53,279 (46,248–57,430)	1,405,382 (1,210,701–1,516,668)	147,689 (89,309–227,487)	98,496 (72,076–130,492)
Brunei	280 (173–442)	82 (53–119)	0.65 (0.38–1.06)	51 (40–70)	1,291 (1,027–1,700)	483 (296–764)	105 (66–161)
Bulgaria	7,404 (4,462–11,846)	9,883 (6,246–15,151)	1.23 (0.76–1.84)	11,612 (10,251–12,515)	220,140 (193,242–235,861)	7,301 (4,440–11,483)	8,715 (5,466–12,931)
Burkina Faso	1,595 (994–2,447)	2,330 (1,564–3,393)	0.56 (0.32–0.90)	1,323 (964–1,930)	44,074 (30,228–65,588)	2,405 (1,435–3,789)	3,821 (2,518–5,764)

			2010				
MIR	***Deaths***	***DALYs***	***Prevalence***	***Incidence***	***MIR***	***Deaths***	***DALYs***
1.06 (0.66–1.60)	9,567 (8,056–10,713)	219,945 (183,160–248,755)	13,593 (8,544–21,828)	11,189 (6,993–16,615)	0.94 (0.58–1.44)	10,047 (8,468–11,230)	220,513 (184,757–246,371)
0.62 (0.38–0.95)	30 (24–36)	427 (356–501)	188 (113–288)	59 (37–87)	0.60 (0.36–0.94)	34 (27–42)	468 (382–573)
0.87 (0.50–1.40)	3,674 (2,511–5,046)	113,195 (78,242–159,407)	5,427 (3,302–8,394)	5,172 (3,199–7,641)	0.78 (0.46–1.26)	3,979 (2,927–5,269)	119,785 (87,274–160,890)
0.80 (0.48–1.38)	35 (28–48)	593 (488–809)	94 (57–148)	54 (35–83)	0.76 (0.43–1.26)	39 (30–57)	641 (507–917)
0.57 (0.36–0.87)	12,217 (11,060–14,455)	269,031 (243,646–327,589)	47,703 (45,230–50,210)	23,918 (15,172–35,244)	0.52 (0.33–0.81)	11,974 (10,486–14,701)	258,933 (226,145–329,878)
0.54 (0.33–0.81)	2,217 (1,925–2,524)	37,727 (32,728–42,733)	4,345 (2,656–6,963)	4,694 (3,019–6,911)	0.51 (0.32–0.78)	2,299 (1,916–2,709)	36,642 (30,552–43,008)
0.46 (0.36–0.59)	3,469 (2,994–3,872)	56,103 (49,511–62,314)	35,608 (21,202–56,035)	8,564 (6,684–10,806)	0.44 (0.33–0.58)	3,706 (3,015–4,386)	56,586 (48,898–63,314)
0.64 (0.39–0.97)	3,159 (2,778–3,829)	44,052 (39,055–53,461)	20,182 (12,395–30,133)	5,704 (3,734–8,654)	0.57 (0.34–0.84)	3,085 (2,593–3,813)	40,995 (35,274–50,977)
0.59 (0.36–0.94)	4,692 (3,761–5,271)	95,182 (76,951–105,998)	9,623 (5,770–14,820)	10,000 (6,338–15,149)	0.55 (0.33–0.85)	5,241 (4,047–6,112)	100,331 (79,526–116,229)
1.12 (0.73–1.62)	68 (60–77)	1,724 (1,506–1,935)	911 (481–1,523)	115 (76–166)	0.77 (0.50–1.16)	85 (73–96)	2,291 (1,936–2,578)
0.52 (0.26–0.90)	20,772 (13,008–29,543)	436,746 (279,189–623,988)	107,093 (64,850–170,754)	49,348 (30,452–73,264)	0.50 (0.27–0.89)	23,548 (14,864–33,748)	490,786 (310,847–703,340)
0.51 (0.35–0.76)	138 (113–189)	1,988 (1,675–2,597)	455 (266–714)	299 (220–391)	0.46 (0.31–0.69)	135 (106–190)	1,944 (1,596–2,545)
0.62 (0.46–0.81)	5,701 (5,151–6,450)	134,930 (119,395–149,045)	13,508 (8,141–21,347)	9,749 (7,474–12,473)	0.51 (0.38–0.66)	4,860 (4,320–5,602)	112,593 (99,159–125,571)
0.42 (0.25–0.65)	2,719 (2,024–3,181)	46,398 (37,822–51,917)	25,044 (15,003–38,702)	7,422 (4,872–11,210)	0.38 (0.22–0.61)	2,722 (1,902–3,425)	44,694 (35,587–51,463)
0.70 (0.44–1.06)	56 (49–63)	1,089 (969–1,260)	240 (146–377)	101 (66–150)	0.64 (0.40–0.93)	62 (54–72)	1,193 (1,061–1,399)
0.69 (0.42–1.06)	1,699 (1,350–2,141)	50,474 (37,492–66,342)	1,709 (1,010–2,794)	2,935 (1,902–4,267)	0.68 (0.42–1.06)	1,995 (1,603–2,480)	57,480 (44,196–74,888)
0.63 (0.36–1.05)	116 (83–169)	2,689 (1,892–3,961)	523 (307–854)	236 (149–345)	0.56 (0.32–0.92)	128 (92–183)	2,839 (1,992–4,132)
1.15 (0.74–1.76)	2,265 (1,879–2,832)	60,068 (49,336–73,333)	3,182 (2,894–3,493)	2,380 (1,492–3,648)	1.05 (0.62–1.62)	2,411 (1,987–3,172)	61,083 (49,296–76,601)
1.02 (0.63–1.54)	3,550 (2,884–4,247)	59,904 (47,863–70,618)	3,636 (2,086–5,804)	4,011 (2,581–5,901)	0.95 (0.58–1.47)	3,648 (2,950–4,494)	57,270 (45,196–69,750)
0.50 (0.30–0.81)	400 (296–570)	13,599 (10,262–19,238)	842 (522–1,314)	1,003 (643–1,460)	0.35 (0.20–0.59)	339 (232–496)	9,608 (6,951–13,900)
0.64 (0.46–0.87)	61,491 (55,932–70,478)	1,376,605 (1,271,044–1,603,858)	164,338 (97,428–253,411)	115,995 (85,474–155,314)	0.60 (0.43–0.80)	67,711 (61,359–77,487)	1,440,939 (1,314,664–1,673,676)
0.63 (0.37–1.00)	63 (51–82)	1,580 (1,299–2,013)	601 (361–965)	129 (80–197)	0.63 (0.36–1.00)	77 (61–100)	1,863 (1,499–2,383)
1.18 (0.73–1.89)	9,786 (8,649–12,249)	176,862 (157,667–217,882)	7,357 (4,370–11,421)	9,056 (5,714–12,905)	1.00 (0.61–1.61)	8,666 (7,215–11,370)	151,252 (128,501–196,982)
0.59 (0.36–0.91)	2,253 (1,732–2,890)	67,635 (50,248–89,393)	2,687 (1,633–4,237)	4,737 (3,057–7,029)	0.68 (0.42–1.05)	3,205 (2,480–4,143)	90,862 (68,308–120,433)

Continued

TABLE 13-2 Absolute Number of Incident and Prevalent Strokes DALYs Lost and Mortality to Incidence Ratio (MIR) (Point Estimates and Corresponding 95% CIs) by Country in 1990 and 2010.—cont'd

Hemorrhagic Stroke

	1990					*2005*	
Country	***Prevalence***	***Incidence***	***MIR***	***Deaths***	***DALYs***	***Prevalence***	***Incidence***
Burundi	342 (204–539)	1,456 (917–2,205)	2.02 (0.79–4.19)	2,854 (1,205–5,785)	75,302 (31,796–151,144)	701 (416–1,095)	2,705 (1,739–4,104)
Cambodia	3,960 (2,344–6,235)	2,713 (1,739–4,021)	1.48 (0.80–2.48)	3,934 (2,499–5,100)	111,440 (69,632–147,934)	9,200 (5,517–14,381)	5,789 (3,873–8,312)
Cameroon	1,727 (1,070–2,748)	3,787 (2,343–5,713)	0.90 (0.55–1.48)	3,517 (2,889–4,242)	112,012 (86,875–148,134)	3,349 (2,015–5,267)	6,163 (4,079–9,022)
Canada	51,865 (31,470–78,238)	12,034 (7,646–18,026)	0.37 (0.24–0.57)	4,278 (3,926–5,020)	95,144 (87,124–108,484)	107,311 (65,923–173,982)	15,006 (9,552–22,712)
Cape Verde	45 (27–71)	137 (88–203)	1.10 (0.67–1.70)	151 (126–184)	3,815 (2,904–4,806)	87 (53–140)	225 (146–336)
Central African Republic	479 (295–793)	863 (540–1,286)	1.66 (0.88–2.84)	1,397 (806–1,955)	41,608 (22,993–59,715)	983 (611–1,533)	1,479 (953–2,244)
Chad	886 (536–1,405)	1,886 (1,217–2,784)	0.85 (0.50–1.39)	1,672 (1,215–2,225)	56,076 (36,901–82,054)	1,724 (1,011–2,677)	3,141 (2,082–4,758)
Chile	10,124 (6,151–15,371)	5,940 (4,322–7,757)	0.75 (0.55–1.01)	4,357 (3,890–4,923)	91,680 (81,711–103,379)	18,888 (11,333–29,040)	7,652 (5,700–9,923)
China	929,124 (565,509–1,459,082)	1,041,778 (757,267–1,358,798)	0.90 (0.59–1.28)	914,249 (657,865–1,146,360)	18,624,716 (13,636,267–23,424,530)	1,550,525 (887,300–2,428,055)	1,992,340 (1,465,120–2,630,652)
Colombia	11,939 (7,218–18,534)	7,480 (4,870–11,358)	0.94 (0.59–1.40)	6,782 (6,141–7,560)	185,441 (166,812–206,857)	22,865 (13,654–36,994)	11,457 (7,392–17,461)
Comoros	27 (16–42)	114 (72–172)	1.80 (1.01–3.09)	200 (137–283)	5,294 (3,591–7,665)	67 (41–106)	235 (154–341)
Congo	386 (226–631)	648 (410–951)	1.51 (0.90–2.39)	948 (765–1,176)	25,119 (19,939–31,008)	878 (531–1,411)	1,222 (785–1,857)
Costa Rica	1,469 (843–2,331)	770 (495–1,144)	0.85 (0.52–1.30)	628 (522–692)	10,793 (9,012–11,684)	3,051 (1,894–4,789)	1,289 (844–1,919)
Côte d'Ivoire	1,672 (994–2,673)	3,569 (2,309–5,261)	0.95 (0.59–1.44)	3,560 (2,984–4,309)	125,290 (100,321–163,380)	3,159 (1,870–4,997)	7,085 (4,541–10,656)
Croatia	4,275 (2,475–6,772)	4,439 (2,833–6,659)	0.97 (0.61–1.44)	4,102 (3,718–4,609)	80,028 (72,115–90,308)	5,132 (3,125–8,016)	4,593 (2,904–6,769)
Cuba	9,421 (8,536–10,326)	5,120 (3,346–7,590)	0.48 (0.30–0.70)	2,339 (2,132–2,634)	64,936 (57,588–71,203)	14,487 (13,279–15,810)	7,330 (4,682–10,943)
Cyprus	797 (483–1,241)	352 (228–528)	0.86 (0.52–1.32)	296 (250–349)	5,192 (4,226–6,077)	1,211 (727–1,887)	390 (256–610)
Czech Republic	9,198 (5,508–14,274)	9,350 (6,112–13,978)	0.71 (0.45–1.06)	6,351 (5,280–6,934)	117,953 (96,385–129,062)	12,257 (7,457–19,266)	8,730 (5,458–13,730)
Democratic Republic of the Congo	6,263 (3,630–9,680)	8,326 (5,431–12,318)	1.25 (0.69–1.99)	10,411 (6,664–14,380)	330,744 (208,602–480,712)	13,079 (7,715–21,263)	16,608 (10,533–24,172)
Denmark	8,529 (5,018–13,248)	4,167 (3,294–5,141)	0.75 (0.58–0.96)	3,086 (2,721–3,531)	45,795 (41,430–51,775)	10,278 (6,487–15,882)	4,288 (3,408–5,253)
Djibouti	41 (25–65)	128 (81–191)	1.23 (0.68–2.03)	156 (110–223)	4,551 (3,201–6,582)	102 (64–161)	307 (204–447)
Dominica	48 (29–78)	33 (21–50)	0.88 (0.53–1.32)	28 (24–30)	500 (430–551)	74 (45–113)	41 (26–61)
Dominican Republic	3,786 (2,271–5,874)	2,419 (1,591–3,579)	1.03 (0.66–1.52)	2,412 (2,064–2,610)	55,688 (47,034–60,284)	6,819 (4,112–10,421)	4,026 (2,538–6,048)
Ecuador	2,566 (1,528–4,067)	2,536 (1,607–3,803)	1.14 (0.70–1.76)	2,784 (2,292–3,021)	62,149 (52,668–66,900)	6,238 (3,912–9,993)	3,510 (2,291–5,134)
Egypt	12,363 (11,424–13,436)	10,067 (6,655–15,087)	2.34 (1.35–3.78)	23,193 (18,855–32,332)	682,661 (505,159–1,033,373)	22,851 (21,015–24,665)	21,299 (13,863–31,684)

			2010				
MIR	**Deaths**	**DALYs**	**Prevalence**	**Incidence**	**MIR**	**Deaths**	**DALYs**
1.16 (0.46–2.75)	3,005 (1,413–6,380)	79,352 (36,515–176,816)	922 (543–1,450)	3,372 (2,229–5,018)	1.05 (0.44–2.11)	3,433 (1,683–6,860)	89,736 (43,365–183,709)
1.05 (0.62–1.62)	5,896 (4,303–7,331)	157,521 (115,025–198,702)	11,195 (6,814–17,433)	7,287 (4,723–10,648)	0.93 (0.52–1.48)	6,477 (4,985–8,007)	168,200 (131,023–208,494)
0.68 (0.43–1.02)	4,251 (3,484–5,137)	125,368 (99,264–157,706)	4,007 (2,418–6,370)	7,326 (4,874–10,959)	0.66 (0.41–1.01)	4,826 (3,939–6,034)	138,463 (110,895–173,315)
0.29 (0.18–0.44)	4,160 (3,512–4,666)	85,757 (74,035–97,034)	124,478 (75,369–193,678)	16,251 (10,260–24,615)	0.27 (0.16–0.42)	4,219 (3,442–4,902)	85,955 (73,218–99,060)
0.76 (0.47–1.21)	166 (135–215)	3,622 (2,821–4,580)	117 (72–184)	270 (177–405)	0.70 (0.41–1.08)	182 (147–243)	3,783 (2,995–4,805)
1.02 (0.47–1.77)	1,458 (803–2,193)	38,838 (20,882–58,526)	1,182 (714–1,845)	1,694 (1,103–2,487)	1.00 (0.49–1.71)	1,646 (907–2,485)	42,425 (22,837–65,234)
0.67 (0.38–1.08)	2,133 (1,457–2,902)	67,468 (43,011–97,370)	2,129 (1,280–3,439)	3,694 (2,397–5,426)	0.62 (0.36–0.97)	2,344 (1,674–3,143)	73,462 (49,427–103,231)
0.60 (0.44–0.80)	4,464 (3,960–5,172)	82,309 (73,402–95,515)	22,911 (13,836–35,787)	8,886 (6,680–11,646)	0.51 (0.37–0.69)	4,425 (3,837–5,243)	82,575 (71,844–96,891)
0.58 (0.40–0.81)	1,129,556 (891,918–1,347,241)	22,613,380 (18,122,641–26,505,967)	1,804,877 (1,116,209–2,796,425)	2,304,755 (1,700,626–3,050,617)	0.50 (0.33–0.68)	1,117,166 (887,089–1,359,056)	21,755,073 (17,436,164–25,934,576)
0.68 (0.43–1.02)	7,474 (6,850–8,716)	171,214 (157,234–202,443)	27,677 (16,692–41,764)	13,645 (8,814–20,072)	0.63 (0.40–0.95)	8,268 (7,432–9,786)	181,147 (163,002–216,210)
0.93 (0.53–1.58)	212 (147–322)	5,340 (3,700–8,308)	81 (49–127)	291 (184–437)	0.89 (0.50–1.57)	249 (171–385)	6,330 (4,364–10,101)
1.06 (0.63–1.58)	1,264 (1,023–1,516)	33,829 (26,737–41,222)	1,066 (639–1,635)	1,483 (986–2,205)	1.04 (0.61–1.61)	1,493 (1,197–1,843)	39,901 (31,294–50,219)
0.64 (0.41–0.95)	785 (700–965)	12,318 (11,176–14,600)	3,874 (2,335–6,080)	1,528 (1,007–2,293)	0.60 (0.37–0.91)	874 (763–1,091)	13,204 (11,863–15,715)
0.84 (0.50–1.31)	5,918 (4,650–7,596)	181,021 (138,512–227,290)	3,700 (2,191–5,851)	8,228 (5,295–12,359)	0.85 (0.51–1.37)	6,883 (5,291–9,060)	196,180 (146,534–250,753)
0.83 (0.53–1.27)	3,614 (3,218–4,046)	60,865 (54,611–68,437)	5,618 (3,383–8,786)	4,970 (3,148–7,525)	0.71 (0.45–1.09)	3,381 (2,953–3,805)	53,759 (47,890–61,071)
0.44 (0.27–0.67)	3,092 (2,661–3,364)	68,215 (61,200–77,895)	17,302 (15,763–18,953)	8,343 (5,167–12,476)	0.39 (0.25–0.62)	3,116 (2,666–3,464)	66,631 (59,239–77,555)
0.72 (0.43–1.05)	268 (232–302)	4,205 (3,672–4,663)	1,307 (805–1,962)	402 (257–582)	0.64 (0.41–0.99)	248 (215–286)	3,795 (3,316–4,330)
0.46 (0.27–0.70)	3,792 (3,451–4,476)	66,409 (60,431–79,329)	13,984 (8,146–22,101)	9,643 (6,167–14,429)	0.39 (0.25–0.62)	3,613 (3,160–4,316)	60,445 (53,206–73,311)
1.00 (0.52–1.63)	16,294 (9,556–22,788)	485,354 (276,489–702,019)	16,422 (9,916–25,772)	20,061 (12,702–30,237)	1.01 (0.52–1.68)	19,837 (11,595–28,700)	596,859 (343,700–892,683)
0.63 (0.48–0.80)	2,654 (2,280–3,021)	35,758 (30,765–39,598)	11,084 (6,735–17,111)	4,600 (3,651–5,704)	0.56 (0.42–0.73)	2,542 (2,126–2,977)	33,569 (28,623–37,740)
0.73 (0.40–1.24)	215 (141–316)	5,549 (3,687–7,910)	134 (77–210)	375 (248–551)	0.66 (0.37–1.12)	239 (160–345)	6,023 (4,027–8,511)
0.63 (0.40–0.94)	25 (22–28)	425 (374–471)	84 (51–134)	46 (29–68)	0.61 (0.38–0.94)	27 (23–31)	455 (388–510)
0.88 (0.55–1.36)	3,398 (3,065–3,834)	60,611 (54,316–68,243)	8,019 (4,819–13,049)	4,787 (3,178–6,928)	0.90 (0.56–1.33)	4,121 (3,620–4,593)	69,927 (61,930–79,676)
0.89 (0.57–1.34)	2,990 (2,714–3,634)	61,719 (56,323–70,927)	7,564 (4,596–11,789)	4,356 (2,781–6,412)	0.82 (0.52–1.21)	3,423 (3,062–4,005)	65,982 (58,988–74,420)
1.73 (1.08–2.61)	36,065 (29,542–39,423)	990,157 (767,654–1,123,166)	27,163 (25,076–29,525)	25,348 (16,554–37,954)	1.69 (1.02–2.58)	41,626 (33,666–46,488)	1,169,103 (871,382–1,374,828)

Continued

TABLE 13-2 Absolute Number of Incident and Prevalent Strokes DALYs Lost and Mortality to Incidence Ratio (MIR) (Point Estimates and Corresponding 95% CIs) by Country in 1990 and 2010.—cont'd

Hemorrhagic Stroke

	1990					*2005*	
Country	***Prevalence***	***Incidence***	***MIR***	***Deaths***	***DALYs***	***Prevalence***	***Incidence***
El Salvador	1,973 (1,181–3,123)	1,335 (862–1,903)	1.01 (0.61–1.53)	1,370 (981–1,579)	35,076 (23,583–42,389)	3,743 (2,286–6,077)	1,645 (1,082–2,458)
Equatorial Guinea	68 (39–108)	115 (74–172)	1.58 (0.84–2.94)	177 (111–283)	4,873 (2,969–7,921)	181 (109–289)	198 (131–295)
Eritrea	203 (121–322)	758 (495–1,138)	1.66 (0.91–2.79)	1,218 (712–1,664)	32,553 (18,609–44,807)	443 (263–674)	1,401 (917–2,072)
Estonia	1,505 (901–2,365)	1,139 (897–1,445)	0.62 (0.46–0.80)	695 (578–778)	14,909 (12,754–16,546)	2,052 (1,206–3,270)	1,564 (1,230–1,999)
Ethiopia	3,902 (3,595–4,237)	12,578 (7,908–18,905)	1.08 (0.60–1.85)	13,117 (8,225–17,734)	358,300 (220,680–483,440)	9,286 (8,575–10,022)	28,093 (18,412–41,756)
Federated States of Micronesia	20 (11–32)	24 (15–37)	1.60 (0.85–2.80)	37 (26–54)	908 (626–1,389)	26 (16–43)	25 (16–40)
Fiji	132 (73–217)	166 (102–254)	2.32 (1.13–4.13)	371 (224–496)	10,440 (5,981–14,759)	248 (141–393)	194 (118–302)
Finland	7,104 (4,331–11,172)	5,600 (4,499–6,757)	0.35 (0.27–0.44)	1,925 (1,697–2,110)	37,664 (33,250–41,372)	11,120 (6,851–16,961)	6,041 (4,917–7,366)
France	99,096 (60,457–147,665)	33,705 (26,136–42,460)	0.81 (0.61–1.04)	26,933 (23,509–30,042)	382,901 (339,018–425,579)	152,825 (92,116–240,201)	35,893 (27,825–45,489)
Gabon	182 (112–279)	316 (202–488)	1.19 (0.67–2.05)	367 (262–547)	9,166 (6,451–13,427)	400 (243–613)	533 (338–800)
Georgia	4,841 (2,928–7,594)	7,283 (5,365–9,608)	1.21 (0.87–1.63)	8,649 (7,840–9,976)	146,804 (132,023–168,374)	5,458 (3,288–8,406)	8,302 (6,106–10,878)
Germany	120,358 (112,994–128,316)	74,174 (60,065–89,320)	0.40 (0.32–0.51)	29,558 (26,361–32,951)	494,086 (423,961–531,820)	187,826 (176,266–200,465)	80,217 (64,685–99,580)
Ghana	2,219 (1,355–3,466)	4,279 (2,835–6,476)	0.96 (0.59–1.43)	4,242 (3,395–5,104)	134,772 (100,797–179,503)	3,774 (2,241–5,779)	8,319 (5,406–12,314)
Greece	12,273 (7,441–18,653)	6,618 (5,070–8,481)	1.68 (1.28–2.18)	10,925 (9,820–11,929)	141,872 (126,456–155,184)	16,508 (9,330–25,782)	7,331 (5,640–9,314)
Grenada	51 (32–78)	51 (33–78)	1.27 (0.78–1.93)	64 (49–72)	1,341 (1,004–1,550)	72 (43–112)	55 (35–83)
Guatemala	3,325 (1,978–5,124)	1,806 (1,199–2,702)	0.70 (0.41–1.10)	1,223 (1,061–1,671)	33,052 (28,356–45,746)	5,549 (3,319–8,643)	2,763 (1,863–4,110)
Guinea	805 (479–1,305)	1,775 (1,130–2,604)	1.00 (0.60–1.54)	1,908 (1,411–2,357)	69,193 (45,548–95,355)	1,622 (940–2,542)	3,167 (2,133–4,593)
Guinea-Bissau	142 (82–217)	331 (210–486)	1.00 (0.56–1.67)	350 (232–488)	12,237 (7,226–18,039)	237 (143–375)	504 (334–729)
Guyana	257 (153–404)	303 (192–443)	2.11 (1.35–3.24)	611 (509–664)	13,449 (10,939–14,736)	324 (191–507)	270 (175–400)
Haiti	2,204 (1,319–3,446)	2,898 (1,885–4,291)	2.21 (1.38–3.30)	6,245 (5,504–7,780)	158,529 (137,492–197,578)	3,645 (2,138–5,714)	4,174 (2,752–6,047)
Honduras	1,231 (728–1,994)	944 (603–1,383)	1.16 (0.74–1.75)	1,332 (1,143–1,512)	52,601 (42,900–64,577)	2,153 (1,307–3,378)	1,535 (1,005–2,287)
Hungary	9,718 (5,707–14,737)	13,454 (10,246–17,461)	0.64 (0.48–0.84)	8,491 (7,519–9,265)	159,031 (139,321–174,804)	11,644 (7,056–18,265)	11,751 (9,021–15,136)
Iceland	358 (211–562)	123 (79–187)	0.76 (0.46–1.12)	89 (77–100)	1,179 (1,027–1,306)	592 (354–896)	144 (91–220)

MIR	Deaths	DALYs	2010 Prevalence	Incidence	MIR	Deaths	DALYs
0.75 (0.47–1.16)	1,197 (1,046–1,584)	21,674 (19,264–28,062)	4,177 (2,517–6,759)	1,802 (1,117–2,698)	0.73 (0.45–1.20)	1,253 (1,068–1,651)	21,344 (18,728–27,583)
0.69 (0.40–1.12)	138 (101–199)	4,309 (3,050–6,302)	247 (146–387)	247 (162–367)	0.56 (0.30–0.98)	139 (88–215)	4,435 (2,838–7,064)
0.83 (0.47–1.33)	1,118 (779–1,430)	28,766 (20,146–37,327)	567 (338–869)	1,763 (1,133–2,567)	0.80 (0.47–1.27)	1,359 (952–1,781)	34,958 (24,391–46,667)
0.31 (0.23–0.41)	473 (432–552)	10,106 (9,168–11,779)	2,525 (1,482–4,171)	1,603 (1,229–2,014)	0.24 (0.18–0.33)	375 (332–468)	7,473 (6,639–9,005)
0.62 (0.34–0.98)	16,620 (11,139–21,520)	406,356 (274,930–529,424)	11,742 (10,840–12,743)	33,812 (22,468–50,182)	0.57 (0.34–0.90)	18,548 (12,476–24,348)	445,283 (303,921–583,753)
1.85 (0.99–3.21)	44 (31–64)	1,025 (704–1,522)	29 (17–47)	26 (16–39)	1.76 (0.94–3.20)	44 (30–63)	1,012 (674–1,545)
2.08 (1.22–3.28)	383 (346–445)	9,731 (8,697–11,275)	312 (186–503)	214 (130–322)	1.80 (1.02–3.13)	366 (290–487)	8,839 (6,965–11,716)
0.24 (0.19–0.31)	1,455 (1,311–1,685)	26,661 (24,071–31,041)	12,581 (7,784–19;551)	6,808 (5,554–8,460)	0.21 (0.17–0.27)	1,445 (1,266–1,651)	24,767 (22,182–28,212)
0.61 (0.46–0.85)	21,728 (18,712–27,718)	282,453 (250,880–344,983)	165,402 (99,208–260,550)	39,606 (31,217–48,875)	0.57 (0.42–0.78)	22,466 (18,770–28,562)	279,219 (244,399–337,026)
0.84 (0.48–1.40)	433 (324–578)	10,593 (7,804–14,213)	506 (312–792)	620 (393–911)	0.80 (0.48–1.28)	477 (367–625)	11,495 (8,806–15,157)
1.00 (0.74–1.35)	8,153 (7,247–8,812)	132,085 (116,632–143,266)	5,574 (3,390–8,670)	8,885 (6,604–11,660)	1.07 (0.78–1.44)	9,321 (7,797–10,167)	143,762 (118,753–157,200)
0.32 (0.23–0.41)	25,425 (19,675–28,791)	361,129 (288,796–399,054)	210,905 (195,321–226,455)	86,338 (69,991–104,819)	0.29 (0.21–0.37)	24,430 (18,763–28,128)	338,919 (271,243–375,988)
0.91 (0.57–1.38)	7,468 (6,101–8,736)	207,314 (167,266–246,088)	4,721 (2,890–7,307)	10,245 (6,518–14,822)	0.83 (0.51–1.29)	8,307 (6,610–9,976)	216,266 (171,659–261,203)
1.73 (1.30–2.27)	12,464 (10,968–13,958)	137,700 (121,686–154,353)	18,987 (10,867–30,330)	7,810 (5,991–9,733)	1.57 (1.19–2.14)	12,103 (10,543–14,386)	130,958 (117,117–151,266)
0.98 (0.62–1.51)	52 (46–63)	946 (844–1,150)	83 (51–129)	57 (37–84)	0.91 (0.57–1.38)	49 (42–62)	892 (781–1,127)
0.65 (0.41–0.97)	1,769 (1,400–1,977)	48,706 (35,727–55,948)	6,805 (4,023–10,861)	3,178 (2,081–4,690)	0.61 (0.38–0.92)	1,886 (1,606–2,145)	47,738 (39,550–53,954)
0.73 (0.45–1.12)	2,348 (1,794–2,887)	70,424 (49,448–91,729)	1,882 (1,147–2,990)	3,669 (2,368–5,455)	0.75 (0.46–1.16)	2,748 (2,114–3,347)	80,050 (57,741–104,785)
0.85 (0.48–1.41)	434 (307–646)	13,475 (8,695–19,546)	285 (167–445)	585 (377–838)	0.82 (0.48–1.41)	485 (346–709)	14,532 (9,767–20,857)
1.49 (0.95–2.29)	385 (346–474)	8,354 (7,292–10,701)	387 (239–621)	313 (196–463)	1.49 (0.91–2.42)	444 (381–567)	10,009 (8,382–13,173)
1.89 (1.21–2.81)	7,618 (6,214–8,452)	175,960 (145,077–195,895)	4,172 (2,525–6,578)	4,683 (3,040–6,925)	1.82 (1.11–2.72)	8,175 (6,677–9,225)	187,333 (153,847–212,720)
1.18 (0.75–1.77)	1,854 (1,564–2,169)	50,375 (41,470–62,075)	2,592 (1,552–4,259)	1,817 (1,197–2,626)	1.09 (0.69–1.62)	2,009 (1,693–2,328)	50,215 (41,620–61,564)
0.52 (0.38–0.71)	5,954 (5,322–7,458)	103,663 (93,524–128,958)	12,731 (7,484–20,350)	12,217 (9,304–15,749)	0.46 (0.33–0.64)	5,531 (4,747–7,003)	90,579 (79,954–115,194)
0.56 (0.33–0.85)	77 (65–88)	902 (780–1,006)	692 (428–1,092)	163 (101–248)	0.49 (0.30–0.76)	76 (64–90)	864 (759–980)

Continued

TABLE 13-2 Absolute Number of Incident and Prevalent Strokes DALYs Lost and Mortality to Incidence Ratio (MIR) (Point Estimates and Corresponding 95% CIs) by Country in 1990 and 2010.—cont'd

Hemorrhagic Stroke

	1990					*2005*	
Country	***Prevalence***	***Incidence***	***MIR***	***Deaths***	***DALYs***	***Prevalence***	***Incidence***
India	252,761 (236,816–270,620)	246,089 (180,752–326,132)	0.88 (0.58–1.27)	214,573 (161,185–271,086)	5,542,294 (4,184,895–7,022,119)	562,446 (527,449–602,764)	394,495 (286,108–517,980)
Indonesia	84,706 (50,711–130,160)	83,082 (53,624–126,191)	1.30 (0.81–1.95)	105,593 (90,695–124,226)	2,552,518 (2,142,988–3,082,318)	166,737 (100,076–258,297)	167,321 (109,386–247,480)
Iran	13,640 (8,154–21,344)	23,285 (17,073–30,399)	0.51 (0.35–0.73)	12,516 (10,252–15,574)	406,190 (323,880–514,414)	31,609 (19,335–50,382)	54,550 (40,363–71,378)
Iraq	3,761 (2,271–5,811)	2,607 (1,723–3,932)	1.85 (1.16–2.83)	5,027 (4,244–6,063)	141,798 (110,296–191,748)	7,402 (4,440–11,736)	5,406 (3,522–7,876)
Ireland	4,451 (2,754–6,929)	1,720 (1,088–2,573)	0.72 (0.45–1.09)	1,185 (1,060–1,353)	21,440 (19,215–24,384)	7,239 (4,221–11,313)	1,854 (1,178–2,723)
Israel	5,637 (3,471–8,640)	2,154 (1,370–3,184)	1.09 (0.69–1.63)	2,249 (1,944–2,476)	31,788 (27,913–34,747)	11,331 (6,926–17,552)	3,137 (2,060–4,639)
Italy	86,040 (80,369–92,233)	27,100 (22,812–31,844)	0.71 (0.59–0.86)	19,216 (17,423–21,677)	372,483 (334,003–414,470)	132,528 (123,964–142,121)	30,010 (25,184–35,428)
Jamaica	1,313 (777–2,068)	1,287 (820–1,946)	1.16 (0.73–1.78)	1,446 (1,313–1,612)	22,989 (20,956–25,430)	2,200 (1,301–3,446)	1,660 (1,086–2,452)
Japan	328,203 (200,396–507,084)	146,689 (112,553–189,850)	0.34 (0.25–0.45)	49,202 (44,871–56,536)	971,098 (888,060–1,108,996)	531,532 (323,352–825,746)	163,723 (122,716–211,693)
Jordan	719 (432–1,136)	465 (293–702)	1.65 (1.01–2.59)	741 (641–887)	16,955 (14,303–20,766)	1,772 (1,023–2,828)	1,043 (648–1,543)
Kazakhstan	11,144 (6,674–17,505)	15,098 (9,526–23,086)	0.82 (0.51–1.27)	11,762 (10,787–13,217)	231,999 (214,070–266,322)	11,084 (6,626–17,531)	16,711 (10,440–25,238)
Kenya	1,832 (1,099–2,838)	5,240 (3,416–7,725)	0.96 (0.56–1.57)	4,964 (3,473–6,832)	125,370 (85,981–180,558)	4,996 (2,948–7,942)	11,303 (7,461–16,761)
Kiribati	13 (8–21)	15 (9–24)	1.76 (1.01–2.76)	25 (22–30)	735 (625–871)	19 (11–30)	18 (12–29)
Kuwait	748 (433–1,178)	70 (46–99)	1.84 (1.21–2.71)	125 (107–140)	4,165 (3,595–4,723)	1,261 (737–2,036)	146 (94–217)
Kyrgyzstan	2,439 (1,455–3,965)	3,417 (2,130–5,077)	0.70 (0.43–1.07)	2,263 (2,045–2,599)	51,779 (47,232–59,545)	2,933 (1,756–4,541)	4,202 (2,677–6,277)
Laos	1,842 (1,067–2,928)	1,422 (906–2,121)	1.48 (0.77–2.47)	2,048 (1,277–2,878)	55,892 (33,765–79,808)	3,754 (2,299–5,943)	2,657 (1,742–3,852)
Latvia	2,382 (1,401–3,669)	1,643 (1,038–2,423)	0.89 (0.57–1.34)	1,395 (1,213–1,586)	28,529 (24,968–32,113)	2,751 (1,654–4,287)	2,243 (1,420–3,421)
Lebanon	1,076 (608–1,729)	509 (328–757)	1.59 (0.95–2.55)	791 (625–1,067)	20,496 (15,958–26,491)	2,689 (1,485–4,466)	1,192 (744–1,793)
Lesotho	470 (281–712)	677 (439–991)	1.11 (0.67–1.74)	722 (516–905)	17,006 (12,120–21,550)	646 (371–1,021)	1,036 (673–1,570)
Liberia	293 (183–451)	569 (367–867)	0.75 (0.46–1.17)	512 (409–646)	21,971 (15,297–32,195)	566 (331–905)	1,012 (656–1,508)
Libya	1,023 (625–1,623)	270 (194–370)	3.07 (2.03–4.69)	839 (673–1,205)	26,846 (20,546–37,968)	2,168 (1,318–3,443)	672 (488–910)
Lithuania	4,399 (2,602–7,110)	2,176 (1,683–2,779)	0.48 (0.35–0.64)	1,022 (892–1,165)	24,440 (21,362–27,953)	5,071 (2,852–8,199)	3,303 (2,553–4,169)
Luxembourg	507 (302–813)	286 (182–428)	1.40 (0.87–2.13)	382 (320–418)	4,997 (4,289–5,432)	832 (501–1,292)	299 (190–440)
Macedonia	1,163 (702–1,835)	1,531 (994–2,253)	1.34 (0.85–2.02)	1,954 (1,777–2,256)	35,062 (32,014–40,089)	1,386 (813–2,264)	1,920 (1,229–2,912)

			2010				
MIR	***Deaths***	***DALYs***	***Prevalence***	***Incidence***	***MIR***	***Deaths***	***DALYs***
0.84 (0.57–1.20)	324,310 (252,298–395,627)	7,683,201 (6,003,673–9,421,174)	684,407 (641,132–729,882)	472,153 (347,435–620,247)	0.74 (0.50–1.02)	342,284 (266,289–425,103)	7,782,365 (5,950,621–9,669,798)
1.07 (0.67–1.58)	172,250 (153,401–196,896)	3,936,253 (3,501,960–4,486,303)	197,243 (118,769–304,266)	195,052 (129,103–287,425)	1.02 (0.64–1.50)	191,509 (170,123–218,785)	4,271,284 (3,782,542–4,915,153)
0.30 (0.21–0.42)	15,987 (13,227–19,656)	321,829 (274,022–384,243)	37,770 (22,703–59,008)	63,321 (46,726–83,300)	0.27 (0.19–0.39)	17,003 (14,035–21,631)	325,297 (272,606–402,332)
1.36 (0.88–2.07)	7,447 (6,418–8,665)	185,268 (151,492–235,911)	8,586 (5,153–13,404)	6,113 (3,997–9,094)	1.24 (0.76–1.89)	7,712 (6,445–9,023)	203,295 (163,631–262,997)
0.50 (0.32–0.76)	892 (784–1,014)	15,329 (13,493–17,625)	8,009 (4,996–12,331)	2,058 (1,299–3,119)	0.47 (0.29–0.71)	913 (763–1,042)	15,096 (13,059–16,905)
0.77 (0.48–1.15)	2,317 (2,038–2,927)	29,143 (26,103–35,896)	13,325 (7,847–21,251)	3,458 (2,225–5,190)	0.66 (0.40–1.03)	2,187 (1,852–2,791)	26,547 (23,202–33,046)
0.60 (0.47–0.74)	17,816 (14,767–19,859)	272,494 (241,448–300,956)	144,424 (134,700–154,946)	32,776 (27,408–39,096)	0.57 (0.43–0.73)	18,536 (14,309–21,710)	267,792 (229,595–293,697)
0.80 (0.50–1.17)	1,276 (1,102–1,485)	19,026 (16,846–21,430)	2,400 (1,458–3,675)	1,832 (1,154–2,751)	0.81 (0.50–1.27)	1,428 (1,191–1,707)	20,860 (17,746–24,561)
0.37 (0.27–0.49)	58,699 (52,698–69,295)	964,412 (885,311–1,107,753)	583,004 (349,586–947,004)	179,795 (138,928–229,761)	0.37 (0.28–0.48)	64,737 (56,599–75,954)	955,449 (861,714–1,094,493)
0.71 (0.45–1.11)	705 (640–796)	15,690 (14,244–17,850)	2,173 (1,302–3,310)	1,270 (794–1,945)	0.64 (0.39–1.01)	772 (680–874)	16,772 (14,742–19,092)
0.91 (0.55–1.39)	14,490 (12,789–15,883)	314,009 (272,259–342,369)	13,214 (7,830–21,294)	17,713 (11,474–26,231)	0.72 (0.46–1.10)	12,262 (10,269–14,122)	261,444 (218,766–296,845)
0.51 (0.28–0.83)	5,598 (3,810–7,876)	143,859 (96,844–211,505)	6,126 (3,812–9,307)	13,690 (8,903–20,376)	0.47 (0.26–0.79)	6,296 (4,371–8,979)	153,861 (103,444–227,900)
2.05 (1.19–3.22)	36 (28–45)	1,023 (769–1,271)	22 (13–36)	21 (13–31)	1.88 (1.09–2.99)	37 (29–48)	1,038 (765–1,349)
1.07 (0.66–1.61)	150 (124–166)	4,817 (3,706–5,591)	1,336 (771–2,143)	165 (104–241)	1.14 (0.71–1.79)	180 (144–204)	5,620 (4,228–6,705)
0.72 (0.46–1.07)	2,905 (2,600–3,204)	73,525 (65,437–81,442)	3,382 (2,043–5,278)	4,253 (2,793–6,275)	0.67 (0.43–0.98)	2,722 (2,368–3,000)	69,713 (60,242–77,346)
1.06 (0.58–1.72)	2,729 (1,826–3,846)	69,847 (45,642–97,886)	4,500 (2,699–7,096)	3,162 (2,066–4,594)	0.93 (0.54–1.48)	2,853 (2,015–3,866)	71,456 (48,516–96,560)
0.52 (0.32–0.79)	1,111 (1,027–1,270)	22,974 (21,127–26,158)	3,311 (1,953–5,139)	2,240 (1,430–3,373)	0.38 (0.23–0.58)	818 (734–1,000)	16,028 (14,531–19,192)
0.76 (0.42–1.24)	871 (608–1,160)	19,461 (13,670–25,302)	3,038 (1,708–4,953)	1,347 (875–2,019)	0.69 (0.38–1.13)	887 (608–1,201)	19,038 (13,117–25,223)
1.08 (0.64–1.71)	1,077 (769–1,397)	30,575 (21,987–40,942)	647 (383–1,025)	1,130 (744–1,650)	0.90 (0.54–1.44)	983 (713–1,316)	24,827 (18,106–34,136)
0.63 (0.38–1.00)	655 (483–841)	20,995 (14,543–28,563)	746 (460–1,189)	1,356 (868–2,027)	0.63 (0.36–1.03)	877 (638–1,137)	27,173 (19,103–37,187)
2.06 (1.41–3.01)	1,361 (1,158–1,748)	33,359 (28,398–40,774)	2,562 (1,542–3,957)	832 (590–1,118)	1.95 (1.33–2.86)	1,594 (1,350–2,111)	37,257 (31,308–46,783)
0.29 (0.22–0.38)	957 (866–1,065)	22,426 (20,058–24,902)	5,797 (3,591–9,470)	3,461 (2,617–4,429)	0.23 (0.17–0.31)	787 (687–880)	17,755 (15,546–19,631)
1.01 (0.63–1.56)	288 (255–352)	3,586 (3,242–4,212)	1,000 (590–1,580)	332 (212–487)	0.89 (0.55–1.34)	283 (244–352)	3,344 (2,975–3,937)
1.42 (0.90–2.14)	2,595 (2,216–2,828)	43,945 (37,213–47,554)	1,515 (867–2,460)	2,100 (1,357–3,234)	1.31 (0.80–1.96)	2,614 (2,196–2,931)	42,200 (35,628–46,786)

Continued

TABLE 13-2 Absolute Number of Incident and Prevalent Strokes DALYs Lost and Mortality to Incidence Ratio (MIR) (Point Estimates and Corresponding 95% CIs) by Country in 1990 and 2010.—cont'd

Hemorrhagic Stroke

	1990					*2005*	
Country	***Prevalence***	***Incidence***	***MIR***	***Deaths***	***DALYs***	***Prevalence***	***Incidence***
Madagascar	657 (407–1,066)	3,234 (2,049–4,721)	2.14 (1.32–3.27)	6,696 (5,560–7,754)	182,600 (150,655–213,962)	1,566 (914–2,508)	6,918 (4,434–9,908)
Malawi	586 (354–900)	2,261 (1,477–3,305)	1.83 (0.90–3.04)	4,108 (2,476–5,499)	124,334 (72,416–174,589)	1,176 (699–1,905)	4,713 (3,116–6,988)
Malaysia	10,388 (9,559–11,222)	6,111 (3,856–9,023)	1.04 (0.64–1.59)	6,089 (5,271–6,842)	145,078 (123,115–163,202)	28,240 (24,949–32,106)	13,210 (8,230–19,138)
Maldives	132 (79–208)	69 (43–105)	0.46 (0.21–0.87)	37 (22–58)	1,387 (795–2,328)	390 (229–627)	137 (88–207)
Mali	1,096 (662–1,729)	2,427 (1,544–3,641)	1.09 (0.61–1.76)	2,747 (1,767–3,505)	92,676 (54,456–124,004)	1,985 (1,195–3,126)	3,538 (2,315–5,228)
Malta	464 (280–713)	173 (110–257)	0.73 (0.45–1.12)	121 (91–139)	1,972 (1,518–2,224)	727 (446–1,140)	213 (137–323)
Marshall Islands	10 (6–16)	9 (5–13)	1.35 (0.73–2.25)	11 (9–16)	324 (246–461)	13 (8–21)	10 (6–16)
Mauritania	260 (159–418)	525 (347–783)	0.94 (0.56–1.43)	494 (355–601)	15,808 (10,619–19,987)	552 (331–865)	964 (615–1,415)
Mauritius	557 (339–858)	418 (269–626)	1.38 (0.85–2.08)	548 (486–612)	12,818 (11,345–14,340)	1,518 (942–2,398)	854 (543–1,304)
Mexico	36,534 (21,590–57,560)	18,842 (12,014–28,076)	0.60 (0.38–0.92)	11,089 (9,996–12,707)	292,793 (263,454–339,196)	67,414 (40,688–101,394)	29,504 (19,600–44,262)
Moldova	3,656 (2,190–5,996)	2,143 (1,345–3,244)	1.33 (0.82–2.02)	2,710 (2,428–3,122)	62,890 (56,077–72,995)	4,278 (2,507–6,805)	3,132 (2,051–4,688)
Mongolia	1,041 (633–1,636)	1,614 (1,045–2,383)	1.45 (0.92–2.19)	2,293 (2,028–2,509)	50,822 (43,976–56,578)	1,237 (755–1,967)	2,031 (1,332–3,014)
Montenegro	493 (290–801)	552 (350–806)	1.52 (0.95–2.36)	804 (666–943)	13,405 (10,734–16,105)	537 (316–864)	635 (399–954)
Morocco	6,589 (3,914–10,430)	4,583 (2,912–6,967)	1.64 (0.98–2.55)	7,557 (6,260–9,135)	239,596 (176,773–318,349)	12,682 (7,503–20,027)	9,569 (5,964–14,093)
Mozambique	1,294 (769–2,084)	3,751 (2,390–5,629)	0.76 (0.42–1.19)	2,796 (1,894–3,777)	69,788 (45,650–96,412)	3,151 (1,889–4,997)	7,745 (4,907–11,599)
Myanmar	18,042 (10,981–28,359)	18,983 (12,427–27,704)	1.50 (0.70–2.50)	27,329 (13,943–39,716)	610,444 (307,098–908,114)	36,547 (22,555–57,060)	32,957 (20,485–49,477)
Namibia	368 (227–588)	484 (309–719)	1.14 (0.69–1.80)	527 (429–637)	13,176 (10,556–16,407)	659 (409–1,030)	917 (584–1,346)
Nepal	6,494 (3,906–10,471)	4,700 (3,017–6,952)	0.77 (0.43–1.24)	3,541 (2,335–4,716)	93,544 (60,940–127,036)	14,559 (8,718–23,369)	7,411 (4,588–11,154)
Netherlands	23,556 (14,420–36,716)	7,499 (5,821–9,654)	1.02 (0.76–1.32)	7,554 (6,665–8,503)	105,758 (94,620–118,521)	34,166 (20,860–54,378)	8,469 (6,533–10,670)
New Zealand	3,437 (3,257–3,614)	1,352 (1,069–1,736)	0.93 (0.71–1.19)	1,236 (1,123–1,392)	20,596 (18,558–22,854)	5,370 (5,085–5,644)	1,488 (1,167–1,858)
Nicaragua	1,091 (662–1,693)	816 (517–1,185)	1.01 (0.63–1.53)	793 (656–862)	19,305 (15,482–21,246)	1,944 (1,168–3,017)	1,205 (792–1,782)
Niger	979 (594–1,573)	1,818 (1,178–2,663)	1.03 (0.62–1.65)	2,040 (1,503–2,699)	88,633 (58,887–131,145)	2,225 (1,330–3,463)	3,826 (2,441–5,614)
Nigeria	14,212 (13,305–15,256)	29,133 (18,741–42,599)	0.74 (0.47–1.13)	23,042 (18,778–27,984)	827,394 (613,552–1,119,499)	28,762 (26,691–31,003)	48,461 (31,450–72,467)
North Korea	17,594 (10,526–27,409)	10,950 (6,853–16,344)	1.18 (0.65–1.90)	12,305 (8,538–16,139)	304,917 (211,930–400,190)	28,015 (17,559–44,150)	26,669 (16,732–40,256)

			2010				
MIR	Deaths	DALYs	Prevalence	Incidence	MIR	Deaths	DALYs
1.31 (0.79–2.07)	8,772 (6,593–10,940)	231,333 (172,132–293,722)	2,019 (1,147–3,135)	8,463 (5,487–12,584)	1.24 (0.74–1.95)	10,041 (7,360–12,824)	260,599 (190,620–336,867)
1.28 (0.63–2.03)	5,844 (3,438–8,015)	161,067 (94,471–225,933)	1,430 (864–2,278)	5,544 (3,682–8,234)	1.08 (0.56–1.84)	5,819 (3,463–7,976)	151,502 (88,383–216,252)
0.60 (0.38–0.93)	7,560 (6,757–8,566)	168,224 (151,014–191,790)	35,408 (31,205–39,991)	16,173 (10,183–23,841)	0.57 (0.36–0.88)	8,828 (7,795–9,902)	194,036 (171,370–218,902)
0.21 (0.12–0.34)	29 (22–35)	686 (538–821)	479 (275–775)	171 (106–256)	0.23 (0.11–0.40)	38 (25–51)	827 (561–1,082)
0.83 (0.48–1.30)	3,054 (2,176–3,893)	104,920 (67,517–143,659)	2,486 (1,464–3,780)	4,182 (2,686–6,000)	0.77 (0.47–1.20)	3,368 (2,428–4,206)	115,346 (75,842–157,035)
0.62 (0.38–0.91)	126 (103–142)	1,807 (1,545–2,014)	816 (496–1,245)	244 (157–368)	0.56 (0.34–0.87)	131 (106–150)	1,781 (1,503–2,010)
1.69 (0.96–2.78)	17 (12–22)	472 (365–631)	17 (10–27)	12 (7–18)	1.51 (0.86–2.51)	17 (13–23)	489 (372–661)
0.69 (0.42–1.07)	657 (529–802)	20,041 (15,381–24,581)	687 (420–1,100)	1,199 (772–1,761)	0.65 (0.41–1.00)	771 (641–942)	22,926 (18,447–28,078)
0.71 (0.43–1.09)	578 (513–680)	12,009 (10,699–14,129)	1,944 (1,169–3,065)	1,020 (653–1,527)	0.58 (0.36–0.90)	567 (488–756)	11,462 (9,903–15,372)
0.50 (0.32–0.75)	14,357 (12,410–15,915)	318,738 (276,229–352,944)	78,158 (47,042–125,703)	34,870 (22,535–52,072)	0.52 (0.33–0.78)	17,526 (14,555–19,395)	386,996 (328,061–430,008)
1.01 (0.63–1.52)	3,032 (2,702–3,369)	67,746 (60,210–75,884)	4,562 (2,748–6,976)	3,238 (2,052–4,764)	0.81 (0.51–1.24)	2,485 (2,274–2,864)	55,505 (50,683–64,207)
1.56 (0.99–2.35)	3,046 (2,607–3,353)	70,003 (59,353–77,528)	1,525 (939–2,416)	2,391 (1,497–3,620)	1.41 (0.88–2.16)	3,222 (2,720–3,592)	73,117 (61,335–81,560)
1.68 (1.04–2.57)	1,017 (885–1,149)	14,716 (12,892–16,342)	612 (373–947)	672 (414–996)	1.40 (0.88–2.18)	900 (796–1,056)	12,893 (11,595–14,921)
0.92 (0.57–1.46)	8,582 (7,577–10,204)	224,466 (190,144–266,249)	14,824 (9,185–22,176)	11,272 (7,004–16,835)	0.84 (0.52–1.33)	9,233 (8,110–10,922)	232,675 (193,981–277,306)
0.55 (0.32–0.89)	4,144 (3,079–5,412)	102,242 (75,182–135,697)	3,836 (2,290–5,954)	9,195 (5,960–13,661)	0.54 (0.31–0.86)	4,792 (3,596–6,286)	115,241 (85,382–152,941)
1.07 (0.50–1.95)	33,655 (18,201–49,875)	742,831 (393,884–1,130,223)	42,605 (26,268–68,115)	37,946 (24,114–58,490)	0.96 (0.46–1.64)	34,900 (19,766–50,769)	774,106 (421,939–1,152,560)
0.99 (0.60–1.55)	864 (710–1,028)	23,017 (19,019–27,697)	756 (467–1,183)	1,114 (731–1,650)	0.75 (0.47–1.15)	798 (650–949)	19,480 (15,880–23,275)
0.79 (0.44–1.32)	5,611 (3,850–7,396)	136,513 (92,966–181,341)	17,339 (10,209–26,795)	9,101 (5,886–13,797)	0.73 (0.42–1.17)	6,348 (4,382–8,511)	149,854 (101,946–201,092)
0.81 (0.60–1.05)	6,724 (5,795–7,809)	88,428 (77,615–99,118)	38,259 (23,101–58,535)	9,443 (7,371–12,051)	0.68 (0.50–0.92)	6,347 (5,507–7,510)	80,118 (72,041–92,064)
0.74 (0.56–0.96)	1,086 (906–1,212)	15,599 (13,427–17,052)	6,240 (5,929–6,569)	1,696 (1,323–2,176)	0.63 (0.46–0.83)	1,049 (851–1,227)	14,606 (12,324–16,295)
0.97 (0.62–1.43)	1,121 (1,006–1,289)	22,621 (20,556–26,379)	2,299 (1,379–3,518)	1,447 (931–2,198)	0.92 (0.58–1.39)	1,276 (1,126–1,483)	24,458 (21,937–28,679)
0.65 (0.38–1.07)	2,548 (1,872–3,414)	90,359 (61,043–127,812)	2,693 (1,650–4,113)	4,719 (3,002–6,925)	0.65 (0.37–1.10)	3,132 (2,202–4,451)	107,556 (70,902–153,612)
0.49 (0.29–0.76)	24,103 (19,322–30,392)	746,620 (567,621–976,195)	35,019 (32,480–37,641)	56,510 (37,726–83,571)	0.46 (0.28–0.72)	26,633 (21,064–34,175)	813,769 (601,900–1,107,500)
0.92 (0.52–1.51)	23,412 (15,965–31,266)	507,735 (347,028–668,423)	28,958 (17,071–45,359)	30,021 (19,482–43,785)	0.90 (0.51–1.45)	25,855 (17,461–34,473)	540,096 (362,718–712,940)

Continued

TABLE 13-2 Absolute Number of Incident and Prevalent Strokes DALYs Lost and Mortality to Incidence Ratio (MIR) (Point Estimates and Corresponding 95% CIs) by Country in 1990 and 2010.—cont'd

Hemorrhagic Stroke

	1990					*2005*	
Country	*Prevalence*	*Incidence*	*MIR*	*Deaths*	*DALYs*	*Prevalence*	*Incidence*
Norway	6,874 (4,028–10,809)	3,153 (2,487–3,917)	0.97 (0.74–1.26)	3,027 (2,625–3,358)	39,004 (34,329–43,070)	9,577 (5,657–15,016)	3,095 (2,464–3,871)
Oman	430 (256–693)	220 (142–330)	1.68 (0.94–2.97)	385 (303–568)	12,692 (9,320–19,409)	960 (563–1,619)	478 (301–707)
Pakistan	36,720 (33,029–40,686)	27,554 (17,908–40,602)	0.89 (0.52–1.39)	24,105 (17,190–30,037)	625,853 (427,983–808,104)	73,414 (68,271–78,566)	44,662 (29,283–66,699)
Palestine	299 (176–490)	525 (382–689)	1.76 (1.21–2.45)	942 (719–1,109)	23,633 (17,299–30,822)	682 (410–1,094)	1,315 (999–1,721)
Panama	873 (522–1,418)	658 (425–945)	0.98 (0.64–1.49)	618 (529–684)	12,542 (10,480–13,803)	2,072 (1,267–3,239)	1,047 (665–1,575)
Papua New Guinea	1,451 (883–2,310)	689 (429–1,027)	1.01 (0.32–2.69)	677 (279–1,608)	22,055 (8,438–53,636)	2,361 (1,438–3,720)	953 (597–1,419)
Paraguay	1,989 (1,168–3,144)	1,542 (1,014–2,287)	0.96 (0.62–1.42)	1,416 (1,227–1,528)	29,962 (26,084–32,330)	3,295 (1,956–5,142)	2,258 (1,421–3,271)
Peru	5,825 (3,467–9,198)	4,811 (3,067–7,131)	0.66 (0.42–1.01)	3,234 (2,794–3,574)	105,988 (91,914–116,949)	13,299 (8,126–21,241)	6,615 (4,245–9,906)
Philippines	34,915 (20,788–54,276)	17,524 (11,059–26,410)	0.91 (0.58–1.40)	15,430 (13,621–16,748)	459,409 (406,304–496,655)	66,135 (39,713–102,730)	36,611 (24,195–54,561)
Poland	29,605 (18,003–45,519)	30,287 (23,321–38,637)	1.66 (1.23–2.14)	49,396 (40,206–53,824)	742,491 (624,204–798,282)	40,837 (24,134–65,606)	29,585 (22,896–37,587)
Portugal	9,383 (5,478–15,062)	9,382 (7,320–11,843)	1.22 (0.92–1.60)	11,310 (9,337–12,305)	180,578 (150,640–194,382)	16,639 (10,201–25,622)	9,612 (7,387–12,270)
Qatar	215 (115–367)	21 (14–29)	2.37 (1.38–3.60)	48 (33–61)	1,619 (1,100–2,152)	733 (376–1,310)	55 (35–82)
Romania	18,177 (10,948–29,769)	21,784 (13,874–33,080)	1.17 (0.73–1.75)	24,281 (22,015–26,662)	458,871 (413,753–499,562)	18,547 (10,875–29,781)	22,064 (14,180–33,068)
Russia	118,329 (71,275–187,482)	78,646 (61,941–98,722)	1.16 (0.87–1.54)	89,843 (77,999–112,019)	1,920,833 (1,684,970–2,254,982)	141,980 (83,301–224,078)	119,911 (95,344–148,170)
Rwanda	398 (228–629)	1,556 (1,006–2,336)	1.91 (0.98–3.46)	2,896 (1,788–4,416)	84,520 (52,748–133,752)	1,054 (628–1,632)	3,084 (1,987–4,687)
Saint Lucia	73 (45–113)	73 (47–108)	1.27 (0.81–1.90)	89 (75–97)	1,696 (1,407–1,846)	122 (75–190)	92 (58–136)
Saint Vincent and the Grenadines	54 (32–84)	48 (31–73)	1.28 (0.79–1.92)	59 (48–65)	1,040 (856–1,146)	89 (55–139)	57 (36–83)
Samoa	39 (23–62)	44 (28–66)	1.43 (0.75–2.84)	60 (41–107)	1,463 (985–2,659)	66 (39–105)	47 (29–72)
São Tomé and Príncipe	16 (10–25)	43 (27–64)	1.01 (0.63–1.56)	45 (39–53)	1,458 (1,147–1,935)	27 (16–42)	60 (39–90)
Saudi Arabia	4,128 (2,407–6,939)	1,312 (864–1,902)	2.35 (1.47–3.60)	2,995 (2,519–3,553)	66,022 (54,819–81,888)	8,664 (4,898–14,447)	3,329 (2,200–4,734)
Senegal	1,111 (664–1,731)	1,830 (1,189–2,747)	0.66 (0.36–1.03)	1,219 (818–1,538)	43,533 (26,645–58,263)	2,404 (1,431–3,716)	3,118 (2,030–4,542)
Serbia	8,001 (4,747–12,306)	8,507 (6,682–10,857)	0.62 (0.46–0.82)	5,218 (4,422–6,134)	118,243 (99,913–139,810)	8,697 (5,149–13,414)	9,607 (7,444–12,378)
Seychelles	28 (17–44)	20 (13–29)	1.28 (0.82–1.96)	24 (21–29)	623 (534–741)	55 (33–87)	28 (18–42)
Sierra Leone	531 (316–848)	1,191 (775–1,761)	1.04 (0.63–1.59)	1,332 (1,077–1,640)	51,762 (38,505–69,432)	849 (509–1,324)	1,564 (1,039–2,305)

			2010				
MIR	***Deaths***	***DALYs***	***Prevalence***	***Incidence***	***MIR***	***Deaths***	***DALYs***
0.71 (0.54–0.95)	2,176 (1,923–2,619)	24,706 (22,299–28,926)	10,351 (6,306–15,865)	3,341 (2,646–4,126)	0.64 (0.48–0.85)	2,106 (1,780–2,603)	23,187 (20,667–27,259)
0.87 (0.53–1.40)	398 (336–529)	9,784 (8,163–12,539)	874 (508–1,383)	554 (358–834)	0.71 (0.43–1.13)	379 (317–500)	8,730 (7,217–11,070)
0.94 (0.56–1.45)	40,753 (31,210–50,740)	999,584 (745,493–1,261,981)	88,166 (82,623–94,369)	53,814 (34,792–79,721)	0.82 (0.50–1.26)	42,965 (32,992–53,999)	1,048,965 (783,882–1,335,269)
0.98 (0.68–1.31)	1,288 (1,055–1,426)	29,228 (23,481–34,199)	813 (479–1,326)	1,638 (1,229–2,142)	0.91 (0.65–1.22)	1,474 (1,200–1,627)	32,150 (25,789–36,743)
0.71 (0.43–1.07)	711 (624–802)	12,700 (11,203–14,479)	2,165 (1,336–3,302)	1,251 (788–1,845)	0.77 (0.49–1.18)	924 (798–1,092)	16,635 (14,557–20,124)
1.11 (0.33–2.98)	1,018 (387–2,564)	32,846 (11,916–84,158)	2,761 (1,629–4,252)	1,141 (719–1,727)	1.06 (0.31–2.85)	1,172 (444–2,833)	37,458 (13,509–93,173)
1.01 (0.65–1.57)	2,180 (1,980–2,614)	44,859 (40,564–52,888)	3,685 (2,320–5,583)	2,658 (1,685–3,907)	1.00 (0.63–1.51)	2,545 (2,250–3,018)	51,305 (44,960–60,338)
0.58 (0.36–0.89)	3,700 (3,178–4,117)	95,306 (76,892–106,575)	15,732 (9,739–25,023)	7,776 (4,991–11,584)	0.55 (0.34–0.83)	4,089 (3,357–4,688)	96,780 (75,800–111,626)
0.78 (0.50–1.16)	27,578 (23,750–30,351)	755,372 (647,900–831,338)	77,643 (47,548–126,185)	44,031 (28,059–65,766)	0.74 (0.46–1.13)	31,217 (25,720–34,481)	844,681 (690,138–942,650)
1.05 (0.76–1.56)	30,690 (26,128–42,334)	476,748 (424,093–612,134)	44,759 (27,062–71,716)	31,964 (24,324–40,717)	0.94 (0.63–1.53)	29,610 (23,555–44,937)	436,902 (373,013–594,766)
0.83 (0.56–1.29)	7,863 (6,340–11,054)	112,130 (93,381–150,730)	17,747 (10,480–28,562)	10,559 (8,129–13,316)	0.76 (0.53–1.14)	7,927 (6,340–10,837)	105,953 (87,443–139,737)
0.78 (0.49–1.19)	41 (36–51)	1,321 (1,133–1,615)	1,740 (904–3,153)	110 (73–163)	0.58 (0.35–0.87)	61 (49–71)	2,179 (1,690–2,613)
1.21 (0.75–1.88)	25,521 (23,704–29,183)	444,878 (413,327–506,909)	19,643 (11,722–31,053)	22,965 (15,194–33,894)	1.10 (0.70–1.66)	24,139 (21,867–27,949)	396,165 (361,450–462,620)
0.99 (0.77–1.31)	117,729 (103,657–141,334)	2,659,972 (2,363,651–3,038,866)	171,485 (107,781–263,304)	124,014 (98,442–155,249)	0.74 (0.55–0.98)	90,913 (78,034–114,574)	1,960,861 (1,698,099–2,310,172)
0.78 (0.42–1.30)	2,311 (1,541–3,418)	60,550 (39,660–91,760)	1,301 (781–2,092)	3,806 (2,520–5,538)	0.73 (0.40–1.22)	2,690 (1,823–4,009)	68,112 (44,966–102,984)
0.79 (0.50–1.20)	70 (62–82)	1,153 (1,040–1,375)	145 (88–222)	103 (66–155)	0.78 (0.47–1.22)	77 (66–95)	1,231 (1,074–1,592)
0.91 (0.58–1.38)	49 (44–60)	844 (754–1,001)	99 (59–153)	60 (39–89)	0.80 (0.51–1.21)	46 (41–56)	794 (702–955)
1.09 (0.58–1.98)	49 (34–82)	1,068 (744–1,800)	77 (47–121)	52 (32–78)	0.93 (0.47–1.81)	46 (30–77)	945 (636–1,622)
0.73 (0.45–1.09)	45 (37–54)	1,272 (1,016–1,601)	32 (19–51)	66 (43–95)	0.67 (0.41–1.02)	44 (36–55)	1,224 (963–1,514)
1.32 (0.83–1.97)	4,221 (3,527–4,775)	92,842 (77,076–104,743)	11,620 (6,858–18,697)	3,994 (2,680–5,772)	1.25 (0.79–1.81)	4,804 (3,976–5,458)	103,411 (85,575–118,076)
0.38 (0.21–0.60)	1,182 (764–1,574)	39,441 (23,680–52,245)	2,831 (1,643–4,573)	3,582 (2,342–5,487)	0.39 (0.21–0.63)	1,384 (908–1,820)	45,329 (27,699–59,270)
0.66 (0.49–0.87)	6,198 (5,669–6,893)	119,924 (109,843–134,191)	9,749 (5,851–15,136)	9,893 (7,536–12,765)	0.51 (0.38–0.67)	4,968 (4,502–5,775)	91,883 (83,439–108,834)
0.76 (0.47–1.18)	21 (18–25)	505 (439–593)	60 (36–96)	31 (21–47)	0.72 (0.44–1.10)	22 (18–26)	530 (455–627)
0.75 (0.45–1.15)	1,190 (936–1,536)	41,580 (31,472–56,098)	1,000 (587–1,593)	1,835 (1,175–2,749)	0.75 (0.44–1.15)	1,368 (1,070–1,755)	46,301 (35,650–59,877)

Continued

TABLE 13-2 Absolute Number of Incident and Prevalent Strokes DALYs Lost and Mortality to Incidence Ratio (MIR) (Point Estimates and Corresponding 95% CIs) by Country in 1990 and 2010.—cont'd

Hemorrhagic Stroke

	1990					*2005*	
Country	***Prevalence***	***Incidence***	***MIR***	***Deaths***	***DALYs***	***Prevalence***	***Incidence***
Singapore	4,527 (4,235–4,844)	1,288 (808–1,876)	0.68 (0.43–1.05)	836 (733–909)	18,910 (16,409–20,461)	8,829 (8,339–9,352)	1,669 (1,055–2,475)
Slovakia	4,818 (2,875–7,647)	3,665 (2,297–5,512)	0.66 (0.40–1.00)	2,299 (1,912–2,581)	47,473 (39,584–53,287)	6,058 (3,635–9,655)	3,443 (2,220–5,210)
Slovenia	2,031 (1,236–3,245)	1,589 (1,039–2,393)	0.33 (0.20–0.49)	499 (453–592)	12,519 (11,353–14,501)	3,055 (1,785–4,966)	1,774 (1,115–2,694)
Solomon Islands	57 (32–96)	70 (43–110)	1.90 (0.96–3.69)	126 (86–207)	3,214 (2,123–5,503)	93 (55–152)	94 (59–151)
Somalia	452 (270–729)	1,700 (1,092–2,565)	1.51 (0.74–2.64)	2,499 (1,494–3,894)	67,985 (40,490–107,022)	918 (549–1,463)	3,026 (1,980–4,527)
South Africa	10,601 (9,915–11,308)	12,041 (7,748–18,163)	1.08 (0.62–1.65)	12,453 (9,241–14,196)	325,705 (233,661–378,398)	18,357 (17,271–19,456)	25,061 (16,621–38,279)
South Korea	41,316 (24,816–65,609)	23,753 (15,012–34,950)	1.03 (0.65–1.56)	23,489 (19,672–25,188)	582,158 (484,610–626,104)	93,556 (56,815–147,227)	30,132 (18,802–45,111)
Spain	50,533 (47,222–54,066)	25,637 (16,671–37,189)	0.45 (0.30–0.68)	11,207 (10,180–12,889)	230,646 (205,879–260,156)	85,351 (79,559–91,026)	29,461 (18,612–45,010)
Sri Lanka	15,303 (9,089–23,454)	7,304 (4,420–11,017)	0.66 (0.41–1.06)	4,634 (4,076–5,178)	118,845 (103,677–131,691)	30,794 (18,161–48,004)	13,691 (8,713–20,734)
Sudan	2,341 (1,394–3,638)	6,754 (4,439–9,867)	0.99 (0.57–1.62)	6,573 (4,518–8,693)	169,730 (110,710–233,587)	6,407 (3,843–9,706)	14,610 (9,285–21,504)
Suriname	207 (124–325)	160 (102–237)	1.18 (0.74–1.81)	181 (165–210)	3,778 (3,458–4,328)	329 (202–532)	269 (174–392)
Swaziland	222 (139–354)	240 (154–364)	0.99 (0.59–1.54)	228 (178–278)	5,966 (4,625–7,325)	299 (173–474)	434 (285–652)
Sweden	16,132 (9,730–25,464)	6,986 (5,531–8,623)	0.49 (0.38–0.62)	3,357 (3,055–3,900)	52,866 (48,251–61,159)	20,385 (12,218–31,190)	6,985 (5,549–8,722)
Switzerland	11,859 (7,222–18,658)	4,473 (2,839–6,617)	0.62 (0.38–0.95)	2,651 (2,256–3,102)	37,967 (33,151–43,059)	18,576 (11,366–29,435)	4,572 (2,941–6,913)
Syria	2,699 (1,627–4,290)	1,591 (1,037–2,387)	3.02 (1.84–4.81)	4,701 (4,023–5,839)	136,096 (114,355–167,607)	5,802 (3,388–8,752)	3,792 (2,363–5,653)
Taiwan	20,055 (18,334–21,879)	11,955 (7,589–18,052)	0.80 (0.48–1.24)	9,096 (7,730–11,077)	203,945 (174,113–245,755)	42,421 (36,641–48,722)	26,595 (16,977–39,783)
Tajikistan	2,756 (1,614–4,459)	3,299 (2,085–4,863)	0.87 (0.54–1.34)	2,748 (2,259–3,052)	53,220 (44,688–58,395)	3,091 (1,847–4,914)	4,050 (2,686–5,930)
Tanzania	2,412 (2,156–2,699)	6,805 (4,993–9,106)	0.59 (0.38–0.86)	4,027 (2,905–5,165)	101,648 (72,317–134,076)	6,110 (5,429–6,875)	15,108 (11,254–20,130)
Thailand	48,038 (41,814–55,005)	22,683 (14,351–33,652)	0.84 (0.53–1.30)	18,246 (16,540–21,002)	444,447 (391,473–504,797)	110,195 (93,785–129,495)	57,618 (36,979–87,321)
The Bahamas	145 (89–220)	91 (59–135)	0.89 (0.57–1.31)	78 (69–87)	1,803 (1,560–1,993)	432 (243–703)	151 (97–226)
The Gambia	111 (67–179)	231 (147–343)	1.13 (0.57–1.92)	272 (173–388)	10,065 (5,851–14,958)	232 (142–367)	423 (273–623)
Timor-Leste	353 (204–571)	180 (115–269)	1.10 (0.66–1.72)	198 (155–251)	6,531 (5,117–8,566)	678 (405–1,038)	366 (234–537)
Togo	463 (279–712)	1,047 (654–1,555)	1.01 (0.63–1.58)	1,087 (912–1,293)	35,354 (27,485–45,558)	962 (583–1,535)	1,894 (1,261–2,870)

			2010				
MIR	***Deaths***	***DALYs***	***Prevalence***	***Incidence***	***MIR***	***Deaths***	***DALYs***
0.48 (0.30–0.75)	772 (690–893)	16,489 (14,931–19,173)	8,953 (8,526–9,353)	1,799 (1,107–2,687)	0.47 (0.29–0.74)	809 (701–930)	16,562 (14,526–18,889)
0.48 (0.30–0.74)	1,583 (1,451–1,845)	31,524 (28,854–36,938)	6,517 (3,932–10,150)	3,796 (2,350–5,665)	0.42 (0.26–0.63)	1,501 (1,350–1,732)	29,875 (26,517–34,203)
0.26 (0.15–0.41)	442 (346–493)	9,181 (7,631–10,070)	3,486 (2,067–5,592)	1,970 (1,244–3,032)	0.22 (0.13–0.35)	417 (306–483)	7,944 (6,470–8,831)
2.33 (1.23–4.45)	210 (147–360)	5,523 (3,748–9,830)	112 (66–186)	111 (70–169)	2.29 (1.14–4.65)	243 (166–442)	6,331 (4,231–11,869)
0.80 (0.42–1.37)	2,348 (1,373–3,569)	60,053 (35,546–92,496)	1,091 (651–1,744)	3,473 (2,366–5,221)	0.80 (0.42–1.40)	2,713 (1,574–4,092)	69,640 (40,305–107,310)
0.63 (0.39–0.95)	15,150 (13,504–19,224)	420,264 (369,516–565,979)	22,464 (21,174–23,871)	29,502 (19,082–43,599)	0.51 (0.32–0.78)	14,435 (12,444–18,567)	371,200 (317,890–499,846)
0.57 (0.35–0.91)	16,487 (14,685–20,692)	327,918 (294,933–405,264)	113,391 (67,661–174,215)	36,049 (22,752–53,014)	0.51 (0.32–0.80)	17,508 (14,889–22,207)	320,439 (279,197–406,054)
0.40 (0.25–0.63)	11,329 (9,674–12,579)	186,121 (165,231–207,833)	95,004 (88,724–101,864)	32,426 (21,252–47,896)	0.37 (0.22–0.56)	11,374 (8,897–13,451)	174,180 (150,233–193,600)
0.44 (0.27–0.67)	5,772 (4,881–6,776)	111,678 (95,085–128,744)	35,975 (21,746–55,633)	16,319 (10,054–24,725)	0.41 (0.25–0.64)	6,335 (5,201–7,515)	121,967 (101,178–143,221)
0.41 (0.24–0.67)	5,800 (4,327–7,504)	136,337 (99,164–179,522)	8,450 (5,037–13,062)	17,942 (11,778–26,838)	0.36 (0.21–0.57)	6,301 (4,827–8,171)	144,947 (109,967–189,286)
0.90 (0.52–1.40)	232 (163–265)	4,579 (3,252–5,242)	436 (269–686)	298 (200–444)	0.88 (0.51–1.32)	250 (178–293)	4,817 (3,467–5,598)
1.10 (0.65–1.68)	460 (365–549)	14,012 (11,040–17,097)	345 (207–546)	510 (329–759)	0.86 (0.51–1.32)	418 (331–497)	11,319 (8,989–13,634)
0.40 (0.30–0.50)	2,729 (2,396–3,076)	38,724 (34,080–43,123)	22,258 (13,418–35,167)	7,407 (5,877–9,079)	0.36 (0.28–0.46)	2,620 (2,265–2,987)	35,677 (31,532–40,292)
0.49 (0.29–0.75)	2,133 (1,775–2,544)	26,695 (22,965–31,192)	19,885 (11,767–31,334)	5,148 (3,330–7,698)	0.46 (0.28–0.71)	2,249 (1,852–2,726)	26,556 (22,347–31,041)
1.78 (1.08–2.88)	6,464 (5,164–8,014)	172,042 (139,238–208,797)	7,993 (4,853–12,690)	4,616 (2,960–6,837)	1.45 (0.85–2.28)	6,412 (4,934–8,173)	160,896 (124,879–202,308)
0.38 (0.24–0.58)	9,742 (8,530–11,192)	194,429 (169,080–221,444)	49,751 (42,966–57,067)	31,461 (19,550–47,027)	0.34 (0.21–0.52)	10,119 (8,750–11,686)	188,503 (162,715–215,548)
0.77 (0.46–1.16)	2,982 (2,335–3,361)	59,086 (47,136–66,647)	3,595 (2,164–5,674)	4,464 (2,823–6,718)	0.76 (0.46–1.19)	3,255 (2,468–3,757)	64,443 (49,435–75,421)
0.33 (0.21–0.47)	4,944 (3,572–6,445)	122,423 (87,369–164,279)	7,689 (6,750–8,656)	18,143 (13,687–24,202)	0.31 (0.21–0.45)	5,606 (4,096–7,470)	134,532 (96,855–181,745)
0.55 (0.34–0.82)	30,228 (25,163–33,923)	559,446 (463,558–618,369)	135,232 (114,313–161,110)	67,205 (42,255–102,211)	0.49 (0.30–0.75)	31,704 (26,733–36,778)	578,239 (476,660–653,008)
0.30 (0.18–0.47)	43 (37–50)	1,002 (885–1,164)	610 (343–998)	183 (118–273)	0.34 (0.21–0.51)	60 (49–72)	1,252 (1,062–1,489)
0.75 (0.40–1.27)	323 (206–454)	10,586 (6,279–15,143)	296 (182–471)	497 (323–751)	0.68 (0.35–1.11)	336 (219–460)	10,721 (6,607–14,730)
0.80 (0.49–1.28)	290 (238–369)	8,460 (6,878–10,744)	759 (455–1,171)	437 (282–648)	0.78 (0.47–1.18)	334 (275–424)	9,244 (7,472–11,763)
0.74 (0.45–1.14)	1,401 (1,140–1,720)	40,660 (31,835–50,815)	1,193 (725–1,857)	2,321 (1,500–3,422)	0.71 (0.45–1.11)	1,629 (1,317–2,037)	45,664 (35,608–57,344)

Continued

TABLE 13-2 Absolute Number of Incident and Prevalent Strokes DALYs Lost and Mortality to Incidence Ratio (MIR) (Point Estimates and Corresponding 95% CIs) by Country in 1990 and 2010.—cont'd

Hemorrhagic Stroke

	1990					*2005*	
Country	***Prevalence***	***Incidence***	***MIR***	***Deaths***	***DALYs***	***Prevalence***	***Incidence***
Tonga	31 (19–49)	24 (15–37)	0.91 (0.52–1.53)	21 (16–28)	421 (321–580)	46 (28–71)	25 (16–38)
Trinidad and Tobago	654 (392–1,017)	488 (313–711)	1.16 (0.74–1.74)	543 (474–590)	11,858 (10,294–12,915)	1,179 (708–1,907)	638 (402–933)
Tunisia	2,317 (2,122–2,534)	1,497 (961–2,275)	1.61 (0.89–2.61)	2,362 (1,733–3,206)	61,544 (43,474–81,954)	4,626 (4,249–5,042)	3,428 (2,189–5,224)
Turkey	12,379 (7,821–18,740)	10,088 (6,319–15,135)	2.74 (1.67–4.28)	27,833 (23,534–33,695)	958,025 (803,832–1,160,248)	26,930 (16,177–41,615)	21,522 (13,850–32,022)
Turkmenistan	1,967 (1,181–3,178)	2,194 (1,401–3,210)	1.06 (0.69–1.59)	2,260 (1,999–2,421)	53,652 (47,810–57,511)	2,951 (1,753–4,687)	3,379 (2,259–4,800)
Uganda	1,440 (869–2,201)	4,096 (2,623–6,132)	1.01 (0.48–1.78)	4,040 (2,285–5,981)	115,698 (65,710–174,014)	3,088 (1,920–4,846)	8,481 (5,451–12,520)
Ukraine	47,832 (28,900–77,865)	47,219 (35,197–61,595)	0.67 (0.50–0.89)	31,050 (28,165–35,893)	657,323 (595,450–733,798)	58,094 (34,611–89,992)	61,085 (46,370–79,514)
United Arab Emirates	539 (285–920)	175 (111–266)	1.33 (0.75–2.36)	224 (166–329)	7,320 (5,213–10,516)	1,863 (1,030–3,180)	568 (344–896)
United Kingdom	90,691 (53,840–140,256)	31,854 (26,074–38,874)	0.82 (0.65–1.02)	25,791 (23,318–28,778)	441,688 (399,515–491,907)	123,601 (73,069–193,910)	32,008 (26,540–39,133)
United States	447,917 (426,459–468,717)	149,313 (111,200–194,585)	0.31 (0.23–0.44)	46,138 (42,526–53,798)	1,045,410 (963,164–1,205,617)	832,652 (805,982–859,246)	171,722 (125,233–222,541)
Uruguay	3,176 (1,947–5,020)	2,710 (1,746–4,039)	0.77 (0.48–1.15)	1,992 (1,803–2,199)	40,430 (36,439–44,574)	3,865 (2,337–6,271)	2,633 (1,639–3,980)
Uzbekistan	11,084 (6,779–17,982)	12,158 (7,807–18,422)	0.70 (0.43–1.07)	8,076 (7,295–9,366)	173,718 (158,240–200,090)	15,138 (9,259–23,933)	17,873 (11,365–26,749)
Vanuatu	31 (19–51)	38 (25–60)	1.79 (0.92–3.12)	66 (46–99)	1,564 (1,056–2,521)	44 (25–71)	46 (28–69)
Venezuela	6,831 (3,991–10,766)	4,227 (2,719–6,074)	1.01 (0.65–1.52)	4,117 (3,608–4,523)	100,795 (87,377–110,047)	13,900 (8,395–21,813)	7,255 (4,591–11,257)
Vietnam	29,628 (27,280–32,044)	39,387 (25,481–58,443)	1.63 (0.98–2.52)	61,639 (46,786–70,258)	1,068,520 (789,785–1,238,382)	65,910 (61,356–71,291)	72,360 (48,625–104,530)
Yemen	1,764 (1,049–2,811)	1,309 (836–1,945)	2.38 (1.29–4.17)	3,422 (2,128–5,119)	143,936 (80,338–235,433)	4,253 (2,559–6,494)	3,593 (2,289–5,503)
Zambia	578 (344–893)	1,897 (1,203–2,875)	1.17 (0.69–1.88)	2,143 (1,556–2,735)	52,386 (37,745–67,893)	1,152 (687–1,813)	3,957 (2,565–5,867)
Zimbabwe	3,552 (2,148–5,808)	2,895 (2,102–3,792)	0.65 (0.46–0.91)	1,857 (1,563–2,234)	47,008 (39,606–57,764)	4,418 (2,706–6,801)	5,254 (3,943–6,931)

(From Feigin VL, Forouzanfar MH, Krishnamurthi R, et al. Global and regional burden of stroke in 1990–2010: incidence, mortality, prevalence, and disability-adjusted life-years lost. Lancet *382:Appendix, 2013.)*

			2010				
MIR	**Deaths**	**DALYs**	**Prevalence**	**Incidence**	**MIR**	**Deaths**	**DALYs**
0.87 (0.51–1.39)	21 (16–28)	390 (300–526)	51 (31–81)	26 (16–40)	0.80 (0.46–1.35)	20 (15–26)	355 (273–480)
0.91 (0.57–1.39)	555 (497–690)	11,068 (9,858–13,780)	1,435 (854–2,292)	734 (468–1,114)	0.82 (0.49–1.27)	573 (493–728)	11,362 (9,803–14,324)
0.98 (0.55–1.60)	3,199 (2,394–4,333)	65,178 (50,228–85,154)	5,460 (4,967–5,935)	3,862 (2,490–5,774)	0.90 (0.51–1.41)	3,327 (2,484–4,557)	65,040 (48,357–86,462)
1.24 (0.77–1.88)	26,197 (22,714–30,582)	731,341 (621,917–843,148)	32,362 (19,618–51,009)	25,552 (16,490–37,938)	1.10 (0.69–1.67)	27,589 (23,240–32,532)	715,112 (576,284–861,022)
0.93 (0.61–1.35)	3,011 (2,558–3,383)	69,748 (59,265–79,126)	3,594 (2,197–5,645)	3,802 (2,452–5,696)	0.84 (0.52–1.28)	3,042 (2,541–3,504)	69,858 (57,297–81,264)
0.61 (0.31–1.06)	5,054 (3,141–7,313)	131,165 (79,921–192,526)	3,926 (2,394–6,219)	10,306 (6,758–15,165)	0.56 (0.30–0.98)	5,649 (3,540–8,222)	142,056 (87,654–209,576)
0.53 (0.38–0.71)	31,594 (27,832–36,468)	697,055 (612,184–773,249)	72,060 (43,424–113,062)	60,926 (46,957–79,183)	0.41 (0.30–0.56)	24,705 (21,876–29,489)	516,501 (452,747–583,890)
0.60 (0.33–0.98)	324 (231–434)	10,827 (7,465–14,394)	3,624 (2,059–6,201)	1,032 (614–1,659)	0.48 (0.24–0.83)	469 (315–643)	17,111 (11,080–23,573)
0.62 (0.48–0.76)	19,654 (17,009–21,727)	301,205 (269,873–333,517)	135,404 (80,597–212,656)	34,176 (27,848–41,409)	0.55 (0.41–0.70)	18,603 (15,265–21,099)	272,521 (235,767–302,855)
0.29 (0.21–0.40)	48,394 (40,248–53,622)	1,045,515 (907,484–1,125,701)	941,780 (912,907–972,331)	188,036 (141,325–244,538)	0.25 (0.18–0.35)	46,858 (38,149–53,921)	1,004,258 (863,525–1,105,152)
0.73 (0.45–1.10)	1,822 (1,637–2,079)	33,589 (30,562–37,527)	4,098 (2,444–6,474)	2,725 (1,726–4,063)	0.66 (0.42–1.02)	1,719 (1,512–1,995)	30,912 (27,520–35,226)
0.62 (0.39–0.93)	10,576 (9,532–12,147)	219,929 (199,605–255,674)	18,069 (11,030–28,535)	20,442 (13,212–30,502)	0.58 (0.36–0.88)	11,353 (9,880–13,316)	238,179 (206,415–282,216)
2.21 (1.17–4.00)	97 (68–145)	2,447 (1,682–3,711)	53 (30–86)	54 (34–80)	2.05 (1.12–3.60)	106 (72–163)	2,679 (1,790–4,191)
0.77 (0.47–1.17)	5,296 (4,833–6,188)	115,861 (105,828–135,669)	16,765 (10,082–26,542)	8,619 (5,482–12,634)	0.77 (0.49–1.17)	6,330 (5,601–7,331)	134,275 (120,336–157,004)
1.13 (0.71–1.72)	78,336 (62,552–88,533)	1,219,395 (977,815–1,377,210)	82,809 (77,240–88,600)	84,962 (55,989–125,566)	0.99 (0.61–1.50)	80,833 (63,144–92,823)	1,251,752 (980,527–1,441,487)
1.37 (0.73–2.27)	4,975 (3,383–7,055)	158,579 (103,772–224,731)	4,937 (2,977–7,869)	4,314 (2,823–6,334)	1.32 (0.75–2.22)	5,701 (3,983–8,093)	176,748 (118,733–242,990)
0.88 (0.54–1.49)	3,364 (2,465–4,426)	79,382 (57,700–106,470)	1,378 (814–2,203)	4,589 (2,915–6,640)	0.79 (0.48–1.25)	3,497 (2,634–4,589)	79,977 (58,240–107,653)
0.80 (0.52–1.15)	4,116 (3,207–5,383)	122,890 (92,703–166,010)	3,974 (2,407–6,224)	5,798 (4,321–7,490)	0.73 (0.48–1.10)	4,169 (3,105–5,666)	102,485 (75,896–143,363)

TABLE 13-3 Age-Adjusted Annual Incidence and Mortality Rates (per 100,000 Person-years) Mortality to Incidence Ratio (MIR), and DALYs Lost for Ischemic Stroke and Hemorrhagic Stroke by Age Group in High-income, Middle-income and Low-income Countries and Gobally in 1990, 2005 and 2010

A. High-Income Countries

Age Group	Stroke Type		n	1990	n	2005	n	2010	P-value*
< 75 years	Ischemic	Incidence	1,640,887	110.80 (103.05; 118.54)	1,877,763	103.54 (97.10; 110.43)	1,956,205	100.47 (94.03; 107.16)	0.021
		MI Ratio		0.170 (0.145; 0.186)		0.154 (0.135; 0.169)		0.123 (0.108; 0.136)	< 0.001
		DALYs	6,635,623	451.36 (398.29; 474.50)	7,027,492	390.35 (346.79; 415.22)	6,020,126	310.82 (277.23; 332.68)	< 0.001
		Mortality	278,139	18.57 (16.07; 19.49)	289,631	15.43 (13.56; 16.38)	241,213	11.86 (10.47; 12.69)	< 0.001
	Hemorrhagic	Incidence	585,733	41.92 (38.89; 45.15)	651,199	38.83 (36.17; 41.79)	686,298	38.46 (35.68; 41.16)	0.038
		MI Ratio		0.508 (0.448; 0.565)		0.418 (0.371; 0.475)		0.332 (0.297; 0.384)	< 0.001
		DALYs	8,140,895	597.70 (536.34; 647.23)	7,497,665	459.56 (416.22; 505.24)	6,260,192	361.62 (326.30; 400.26)	< 0.001
		Mortality	297,404	20.95 (18.82; 22.83)	272,071	15.74 (14.28; 17.51)	227,485	12.29 (11.12; 13.74)	< 0.001
≥ 75 years	Ischemic	Incidence	1,751,254	2824.36 (2627.56; 3018.41)	2,031,829	2365.13 (2201.91; 2540.09)	2,297,052	2344.00 (2197.01; 2503.82)	< 0.001
		MI Ratio		0.537 (0.475; 0.584)		0.466 (0.428; 0.513)		0.422 (0.388; 0.466)	0.003
		DALYs	8,279,171	13354.53 (11987.70; 13857.29)	8,273,750	9660.42 (9191.97; 10223.96)	8,231,616	8434.88 (8041.62; 9048.47)	< 0.001
		Mortality	939,894	1511.37 (1353.61; 1565.14)	946,346	1082.75 (1031.81; 1161.73)	968,866	950.10 (905.53; 1030.62)	< 0.001
	Hemorrhagic	Incidence	258,372	417.51 (385.93; 450.79)	323,137	378.54 (349.89; 409.60)	364,687	380.14 (351.37; 409.58)	0.035
		MI Ratio		0.979 (0.882; 1.118)		0.820 (0.731; 0.954)		0.748 (0.664; 0.870)	< 0.001
		DALYs	2,359,112	3817.36 (3571.28; 4300.03)	2,342,929	2776.87 (2589.80; 3203.22)	2,309,063	2457.70 (2273.57; 2848.71)	< 0.001
		Mortality	252,454	407.10 (380.48; 462.06)	264,630	306.54 (285.54; 353.63)	272,324	275.06 (253.75; 320.33)	< 0.001
All ages	Ischemic	Incidence	3,392,142	193.02 (179.74; 205.88)	3,909,592	172.07 (161.23; 183.52)	4,253,257	168.45 (158.25; 179.52)	0.001
		MI Ratio		0.359 (0.316; 0.390)		0.316 (0.290; 0.343)		0.285 (0.263; 0.311)	< 0.001
		DALYs	14,914,794	842.32 (749.15; 875.30)	15,301,242	671.23 (618.65; 703.07)	14,251,741	556.98 (517.25; 588.11)	< 0.001
		Mortality	1,218,033	63.80 (56.45; 66.00)	1,235,978	47.77 (45.04; 50.41)	1,210,080	40.29 (38.23; 43.12)	< 0.001
	Hemorrhagic	Incidence	844,105	53.30 (49.44; 57.25)	974,336	49.12 (45.75; 52.84)	1,050,985	48.81 (45.44; 52.13)	0.032
		MI Ratio		0.652 (0.589; 0.729)		0.551 (0.492; 0.628)		0.476 (0.430; 0.546)	< 0.001
		DALYs	10,500,007	695.26 (629.69; 753.52)	9,840,594	529.78 (484.51; 582.25)	8,569,255	425.13 (385.67; 470.63)	< 0.001
		Mortality	549,858	32.65 (29.95; 35.68)	536,700	24.55 (22.67; 27.37)	499,809	20.25 (18.57; 22.91)	< 0.001

B. Low- to middle-income countries

Age Group	Stroke Type		n	1990	n	2005	n	2010	P-value*
< 75 years	Ischemic	Incidence	2,534,461	101.88 (89.20; 116.42)	3,890,497	104.98 (91.69; 120.90)	4,504,283	106.90 (93.62; 121.41)	0.318
		MI Ratio		0.177 (0.136; 0.243)		0.151 (0.121; 0.200)		0.136 (0.113; 0.176)	0.012

TABLE 13-3 Age-Adjusted Annual Incidence and Mortality Rates (per 100,000 Person-years) Mortality to Incidence Ratio (MIR), and DALYs Lost for Ischemic Stroke and Hemorrhagic Stroke by Age Group in High-income, Middle-income and Low-income Countries and Gobally in 1990, 2005 and 2010—cont'd

			B. Low- to middle-income countries						
Age Group	**Stroke Type**		***n***	***1990***	***n***	***2005***	***n***	***2010***	***P-value****
		DALYs	11,706,328	447.28 (367.62; 592.76)	15,093,667	397.26 (339.90; 509.02)	15,793,980	365.84 (324.72; 455.09)	< 0.001
		Mortality	448,265	18.08 (14.57; 24.39)	588,411	16.03 (13.47; 20.86)	612,409	14.71 (12.90; 18.75)	< 0.001
	Hemorrhagic	Incidence	1,592,786	61.64 (52.84; 71.54)	2,868,589	74.96 (64.23; 87.41)	3,322,839	75.68 (64.93; 88.74)	0.036
		MI Ratio		0.794 (0.612; 0.996)		0.551 (0.436; 0.673)		0.477 (0.373; 0.585)	< 0.001
		DALYs	37,509,020	1344.42 (1087.44; 1625.81)	45,236,696	1128.10 (956.71; 1309.70)	45,219,252	991.40 (839.24; 1153.66)	< 0.001
		Mortality	1,277,628	49.36 (39.54; 59.56)	1,584,138	41.59 (35.30; 48.41)	1,587,392	36.53 (31.01; 42.71)	< 0.001
≥ 75 years	Ischemic	Incidence	1,312,155	2367.54 (2026.74; 2735.51)	2,297,208	2537.52 (2202.95; 2941.36)	2,811,999	2575.40 (2240.67; 2950.24)	0.222
		MI Ratio		0.440 (0.355; 0.562)		0.384 (0.312; 0.480)		0.362 (0.298; 0.443)	0.046
		DALYs	5,507,099	9938.45 (8486.20; 12399.96)	8,176,998	9013.12 (7860.57; 10865.64)	9,343,686	8553.44 (7572.78; 10099.22)	0.001
		Mortality	574,779	1075.73 (915.74; 1336.49)	877,484	997.48 (870.23; 1204.49)	1,012,930	949.88 (838.56; 1128.36)	0.01
	Hemorrhagic	Incidence	403,286	713.83 (603.31; 847.38)	793,903	861.85 (735.11; 1020.98)	951,173	859.36 (729.17; 1012.58)	0.065
		MI Ratio		1.479 (1.090; 1.900)		1.094 (0.855; 1.356)		1.008 (0.784; 1.250)	0.002
		DALYs	5,873,138	10249.10 (7846.57; 12615.18)	8,302,502	8907.91 (7406.47; 10533.99)	9,054,390	8113.74 (6818.88; 9519.69)	0.002
		Mortality	591,886	1072.90 (819.30; 1329.49)	862,258	955.71 (789.22; 1138.04)	951,562	874.84 (736.84; 1026.62)	0.007
All ages	Ischemic	Incidence	3,846,616	170.53 (148.24; 195.28)	6,187,705	178.68 (156.28; 205.59)	7,316,281	181.70 (159.10; 206.78)	0.267
		MI Ratio		0.266 (0.213; 0.354)		0.238 (0.193; 0.303)		0.223 (0.186; 0.276)	0.051
		DALYs	17,213,426	734.86 (619.49; 948.36)	23,270,664	658.32 (571.81; 818.09)	25,137,666	613.93 (550.41; 748.03)	< 0.001
		Mortality	1,023,044	50.13 (42.02; 64.07)	1,465,895	45.77 (39.69; 56.27)	1,625,339	43.05 (38.25; 51.96)	< 0.001
	Hemorrhagic	Incidence	1,996,072	81.40 (69.54; 94.31)	3,662,492	98.80 (84.77; 115.66)	4,274,013	99.43 (85.37; 116.28)	0.040
		MI Ratio		0.932 (0.708; 1.177)		0.668 (0.534; 0.822)		0.595 (0.470; 0.729)	< 0.001
		DALYs	43,382,156	1614.23 (1292.98; 1946.36)	53,539,196	1363.83 (1154.83; 1580.73)	54,273,644	1207.21 (1024.82; 1408.04)	< 0.001
		Mortality	1,869,514	80.37 (63.72; 96.98)	2,446,397	69.29 (58.11; 81.26)	2,538,954	61.93 (52.53; 72.34)	< 0.001

			C. Globally						
Age Group	**Stroke Type**		***n***	***1990***	***n***	***2005***	***n***	***2010***	***P-value****
< 75 years	Ischemic	Incidence	4,175,349	105.14 (96.45; 114.89)	5,768,261	104.31 (94.65; 115.27)	6,460,488	104.68 (95.39; 114.91)	0.458
		MI Ratio		0.174 (0.149; 0.214)		0.152 (0.131; 0.184)		0.132 (0.116; 0.159)	< 0.001
		DALYs	18,341,950	453.01 (405.80; 539.58)	22,121,160	397.59 (361.73; 472.70)	21,814,106	350.60 (325.69; 415.40)	< 0.001

Continued

TABLE 13-3 Age-Adjusted Annual Incidence and Mortality Rates (per 100,000 Person-years) Mortality to Incidence Ratio (MIR), and DALYs Lost for Ischemic Stroke and Hemorrhagic Stroke by Age Group in High-income, Middle-income and Low-income Countries and Gobally in 1990, 2005 and 2010—cont'd

			C. Globally						
Age Group	**Stroke Type**		***n***	***1990***	***n***	***2005***	***n***	***2010***	***P-value****
		Mortality	726,404	18.34 (16.28; 21.99)	878,042	15.88 (14.36; 18.97)	853,622	13.83 (12.76; 16.64)	< 0.001
	Hemorrhagic	Incidence	2,178,519	54.07 (48.56; 60.22)	3,519,788	63.15 (55.91; 72.17)	4,009,137	64.07 (56.46; 73.33)	0.028
		MI Ratio		0.716 (0.586; 0.855)		0.525 (0.431; 0.626)		0.451 (0.366; 0.539)	< 0.001
		DALYs	45,649,912	1090.95 (916.03; 1280.24)	52,734,360	928.57 (807.58; 1061.56)	51,479,444	812.85 (701.43; 935.75)	< 0.001
		Mortality	1,575,032	39.04 (32.84; 45.93)	1,856,209	33.27 (28.92; 38.18)	1,814,877	29.07 (25.16; 33.70)	< 0.001
≥ 75 years	Ischemic	Incidence	3,063,410	2614.89 (2426.49; 2809.55)	4,329,037	2452.72 (2245.04; 2674.44)	5,109,051	2472.93 (2279.15; 2687.39)	0.176
		MI Ratio		0.495 (0.450; 0.547)		0.422 (0.379; 0.483)		0.389 (0.348; 0.450)	< 0.001
		DALYs	13,786,270	11766.13 (11034.98; 12688.85)	16,450,747	9314.39 (8699.15; 10498.56)	17,575,302	8509.08 (7979.52; 9562.85)	< 0.001
		Mortality	1,514,673	1313.55 (1225.05; 1407.29)	1,823,831	1040.14 (972.42; 1184.36)	1,981,797	952.73 (893.26; 1082.61)	< 0.001
	Hemorrhagic	Incidence	661,658	558.61 (503.36; 624.07)	1,117,040	630.25 (558.49; 712.17)	1,315,860	640.06 (569.10; 724.72)	0.046
		MI Ratio		1.280 (1.041; 1.542)		1.012 (0.841; 1.208)		0.934 (0.767; 1.107)	0.001
		DALYs	8,232,250	6899.22 (5819.05; 8101.89)	10,645,431	5985.97 (5185.38; 6900.83)	11,363,453	5544.55 (4848.87; 6377.47)	< 0.001
		Mortality	844,340	719.66 (605.91; 844.83)	1,126,888	638.52 (554.36; 736.04)	1,223,886	592.56 (517.87; 681.36)	< 0.001
All ages	Ischemic	Incidence	7,238,758	181.19 (167.30; 196.23)	10,097,297	175.46 (160.08; 192.26)	11,569,538	176.44 (161.46; 192.21)	0.324
		MI Ratio		0.310 (0.278; 0.352)		0.268 (0.237; 0.310)		0.245 (0.219; 0.285)	< 0.001
		DALYs	32,128,220	795.80 (733.54; 906.40)	38,571,908	667.77 (617.11; 774.20)	39,389,408	597.80 (559.75; 691.68)	< 0.001
		Mortality	2,241,077	57.59 (53.69; 63.97)	2,701,873	46.92 (43.58; 53.67)	2,835,419	42.27 (39.60; 48.71)	< 0.001
	Hemorrhagic	Incidence	2,840,177	69.36 (62.46; 77.18)	4,636,828	80.33 (71.40; 91.69)	5,324,997	81.52 (72.27; 92.82)	0.033
		MI Ratio		0.847 (0.692; 1.009)		0.643 (0.536; 0.766)		0.571 (0.471; 0.676)	< 0.001
		DALYs	53,882,164	1266.94 (1068.41; 1484.26)	63,379,792	1081.81 (935.41; 1234.23)	62,842,896	956.22 (827.57; 1104.44)	< 0.001
		Mortality	2,419,372	59.66 (50.61; 69.71)	2,983,097	51.61 (44.68; 59.07)	3,038,763	46.14 (40.13; 53.15)	< 0.001

*P-value considers the trend in rates between the 1990 and 2010 time points only.

(From Krishnamurthi RV, Feigin VL, Forouzanfar MH, et al. Global and regional burden of first-ever ischaemic and haemorrhagic stroke during 1990–2010: findings from the Global Burden of Disease Study 2010. The Lancet Global Health Vol 1, Issue 5, November 2013, Pages e259–e281.)

and significance of stroke risk factors,[3,15,16] as well as in the accessibility to adequate healthcare and management of risk factors.[17] Lower stroke mortality and DALYs lost in high-income countries are likely associated with higher stroke prevalence, and lower mortality-to-incidence ratios. This result is somewhat expected given high-income countries are more likely to have improved levels of acute stroke treatment, stroke-risk management and prevention.[18–21] However, the reduction in mortality rates in low- and middle-income countries was somewhat unexpected, but could be partially explained by the heterogeneity of the low- and middle-income regions in terms of improvements in stroke-risk management and healthcare.

The differential impact of stroke subtypes was seen in this study with the overall burden in terms of proportionate mortality and DALYs of hemorrhagic stroke being higher than that

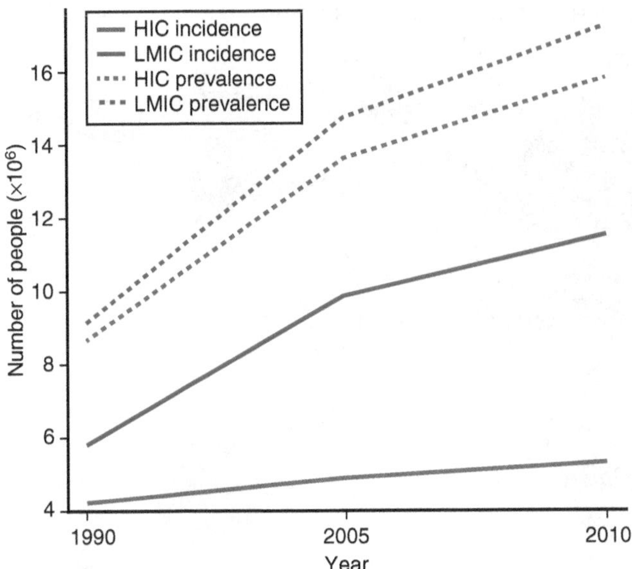

Figure 13-1. The gap in the absolute numbers of incident strokes and prevalence between HIC and LMIC increased on the last 2 decades, with a sharp increase in the absolute number of incident strokes in LMIC by 2010.

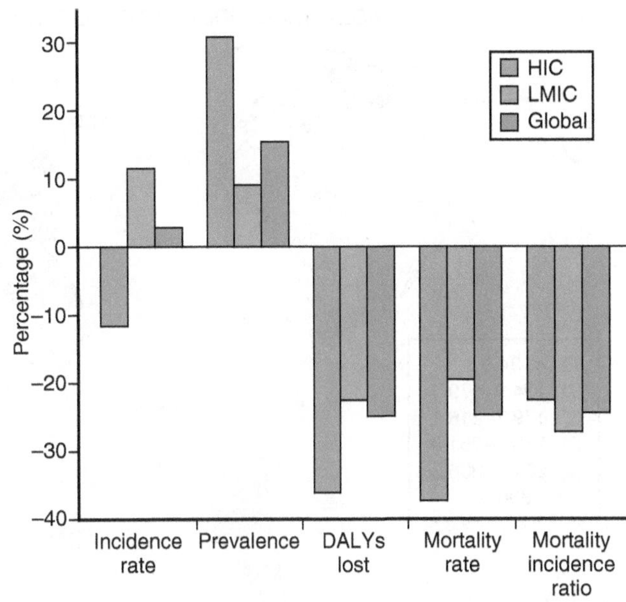

Figure 13-2. There was a significant decline in stroke incidence rates in HIC and non-significant increases in LMIC and globally, while prevalence of stroke increased across the globe. DALYs lost and mortality and MIR rates were reduced significantly in HIC LMIC and globally.

TABLE 13-4 Mean Age of Stroke by Stroke Type and Country Income Level in 1990, 2005 and 2010

	HIC				LMIC				Globally			
Mean age	*1990*	*2005*	*2010*	*P-value*	*1990*	*2005*	*2010*	*P-value*	*1990*	*2005*	*2010*	*P-value*
ISCHEMIC												
Incidence	75.4 (0.13)	75.9 (0.13)	76.2 (0.13)	<0.0001	69.6 (0.12)	70.6 (0.11)	70.8 (0.12)	<0.0001	72.9 (0.11)	73.0 (0.10)	73.1 (0.10)	<0.0079
Mortality	80.7 (0.12)	81.3 (0.22)	82.7 (0.21)	<0.0001	75.1 (0.32)	76.4 (0.27)	77.1 (0.26)	<0.0001	78.1 (0.27)	78.6 (0.20)	79.4 (0.19)	<0.0001
HEMORRHAGIC												
Incidence	67.6 (0.13)	68.7 (0.14)	69.1 (0.15)	<0.0001	62.8 (0.15)	63.7 (0.13)	63.8 (0.13)	<0.0001	64.7 (0.11)	65.0 (0.10)	65.1 (0.11)	<0.0001
Mortality	71.6 (0.29)	73.0 (0.30)	74.8 (0.32)	<0.0001	66.8 +/− 0.29	68.2 (0.28)	68.9 (0.31)	<0.0001	68.0 (0.23)	69.1 (0.25)	69.9 (0.30)	<0.0001

(From Krishnamurthi RV, Feigin VL, Forouzanfar MH, et al. Global and regional burden of first-ever ischaemic and haemorrhagic stroke during 1990–2010: findings from the Global Burden of Disease Study 2010. The Lancet Global Health Volume 1, Issue 5, November 2013, Pages e259–e281.)

of ischemic stroke, although the absolute number of ischemic strokes was twice that of hemorrhagic strokes. Low- and middle-income countries were disproportionately affected by hemorrhagic stroke burden. In high-income countries, overall incidence, mortality, DALYs, and mortality-to-incidence ratios for both ischemic and hemorrhagic strokes declined, whereas in low- and middle-income countries, the incidence of hemorrhagic stroke increased significantly, especially in the younger age groups.

There has been an increase in the mean age at stroke worldwide, however, there is now a substantial proportion of stroke in people under 65 years. Of concern is the finding that there has been a significant increase in the incidence of both ischemic and hemorrhagic stroke in the 20–64-year age group. Thus, these studies show for the first time a shift in the overall burden of stroke towards younger age groups, particularly in low- and middle-income countries. About half of all hemorrhagic strokes occur in people younger than 65 years, and over 80% of these are in low- and middle-income countries. These trends have been previously reported in other studies.[22,23] There has been an epidemic rise in diabetes[24,25] as well as other cardiovascular risk factors in young adults,[26,27] including excessive alcohol use in some regions such as Russia.[28] Over half of deaths in Russian men can be attributed to cardiovascular disease, with hypertension, hypercholesterolemia, tobacco use, inadequate diet, obesity, insufficient physical activity and alcohol being among the prevalent risk factors for death.[29] The high stroke burden in China, particularly of hemorrhagic stroke, might be attributable to the high prevalence of high blood pressure and smoking in this population.[30] Vascular causes are among the main contributors of death in India, with smoking as a major risk factor contributing to these deaths.[31]

Disparities in stroke burden were seen by GBD regions and income level. These disparities may be attributable to better health services and strategies for stroke prevention and

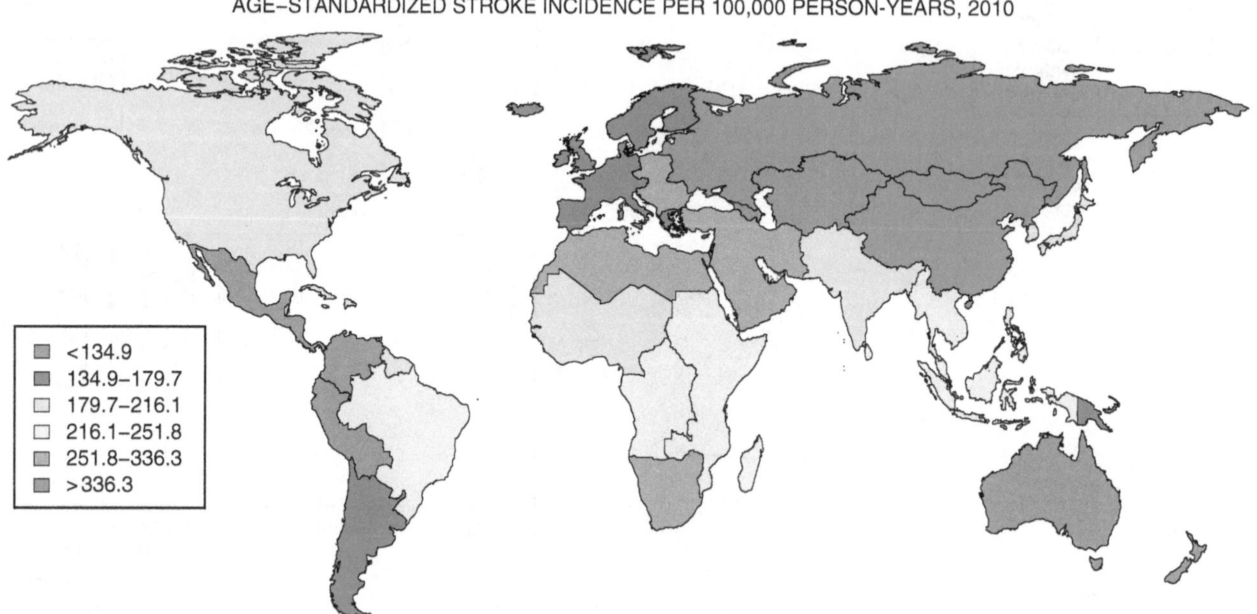

Figure 13-3. Significant geographical variations were seen in stroke burden by GBD region. Stroke incidence increased in sub-Saharan Africa (central, east, southern, and west), the Middle East, southeast Asia, central and Latin America, and south and east Asia, but decreased in high-income Asia Pacific.

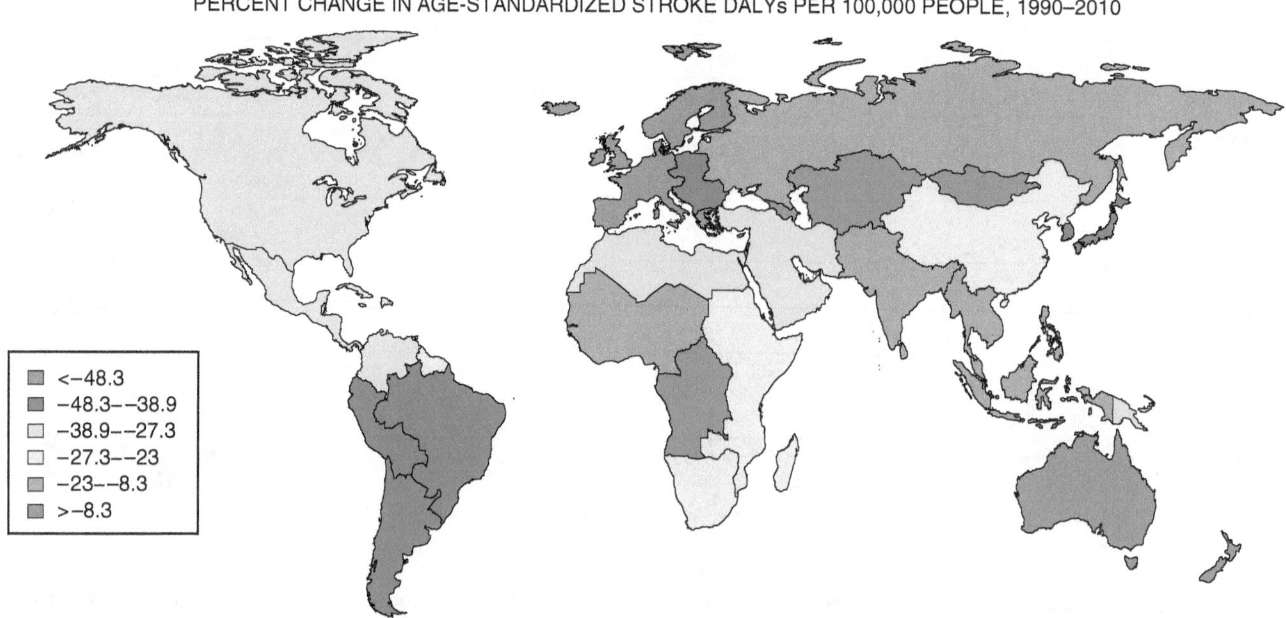

Figure 13-4. Percent change in DALYs lost per 100 000 people in GBD regions varied from –50·4% to –0·74%. The most marked reductions in DALYs lost were in west and central sub-Saharan Africa; eastern Europe; and central, south, and southeast Asia.

management in high-income countries, leading to lower levels of incidence, mortality, mortality-to-incidence ratios, and DALYs lost. In contrast, the increasing burden of stroke in economically underdeveloped regions could be attributed to lack of primary care treatment to screen patients for stroke risk and inadequate preventative measures to alleviate risk factors such as hypertension.[32] Encouragingly a trend towards a decrease in mortality rates, DALYs, and mortality-to-incidence ratios for both ischemic and hemorrhagic stroke was seen in low- and middle-income countries. This may reflect improvements in diagnosis, and more targeted healthcare in some developing regions, given the heterogeneity of socioeconomic development within regions of low- and middle-income countries.

The 2010 GBD study suggests that if current trends continue, by 2030 there will be an estimated 12 million stroke deaths, 70 million stroke survivors, and more than 200 million DALYs lost globally. Regional disparities by income level are likely to increase, due to the continuing shift from communicable diseases to non-communicable diseases in low- and middle-income countries.[13] Disparities in stroke burden are likely to be further exacerbated by lower access to medical management of risk factors and a lesser degree of emphasis on stroke prevention by governments in developing countries, whereas many high-income countries have implemented improved prevention strategies and more targeted and specialized healthcare for chronic conditions like stroke.[33] The alarming increase in stroke burden in younger age groups is likely to continue unless urgent preventative measures are undertaken, both at individual and governmental/organizational levels.

Strategies to reduce stroke burden should include at governmental levels population-based initiatives to improve stroke awareness, reduced salt content of manufactured products, and improve access to blood-pressure-lowering medications.[34,35] Education campaigns to reduce alcohol and tobacco use, increase physical activity and consumption of fruits and vegetables could also enhance the impact of prevention strategies.

The 2010 GBD study attempted to include data from as many low- and middle-income countries as possible. However, good-quality data, particularly from low-income countries, are scarce. These regions may also have had limitations in accurate diagnoses of stroke subtypes due to unavailability of brain imaging. There is also evidence of poor adherence to standardized methodology in stroke surveillance studies in low- and middle-income countries, where the incorporation of standardized procedures would enhance generalizability and improve the accuracy of stroke burden estimates.[36] Heterogeneity is likely to exist across large regions such as central Asia and sub-Saharan Africa, with some regions having the potential to conduct high-quality epidemiological studies in future. The establishment of sustainable systems to obtain stroke data shared by other non-communicable diseases, with a wide application of feasible and practical techniques is recommended in a systematic review, and may be adapted by low-income countries.[33] Hence, despite the inevitable limitations of a study such as the GBD 2010, the findings provide a valuable resource for the global perspective on stroke and by stroke subtype and can be used as a reliable reference for future stroke prevention strategies worldwide.

REFERENCES

1. Strong K, Mathers C, Bonita R. Preventing stroke: saving lives around the world. Lancet Neurol 2007;6:182–7.
2. Johnston SC, Mendis S, Mathers CD. Global variation in stroke burden and mortality: estimates from monitoring, surveillance, and modelling. Lancet Neurol [Research Support, Non-U.S. Gov't] 2009;8:345–54.
3. O'Donnell MJ, Xavier D, Liu L, et al. Risk factors for ischaemic and intracerebral haemorrhagic stroke in 22 countries (the INTERSTROKE study): a case-control study. Lancet 2010;376:112–23.
4. Feigin VL, Lawes CM, Bennett DA, et al. Worldwide stroke incidence and early case fatality reported in 56 population-based studies: a systematic review. Lancet Neurol 2009;8(4):355–69.
5. Murray CJL, Ezzati M, Flaxman AD, et al. GBD 2010: design, definitions, and metrics. Lancet 2012;380:2063–6.
6. Murray CJL, Vos T, Lozano R, et al. Disability-adjusted life years (DALYs) for 291 diseases and injuries in 21 regions, 1990–2010: a systematic analysis for the Global Burden of Disease Study 2010. Lancet 2012;380:2197–223.
7. Lozano R, Naghavi M, Foreman K, et al. Global and regional mortality from 235 causes of death for 20 age groups in 1990 and 2010: a systematic analysis for the Global Burden of Disease Study 2010. Lancet 2012;380:2095–128.
8. World Health Organization. The Global Burden of Disease: 2004 update. Geneva: WHO; 2004.
9. Feigin VL, Forouzanfar MH, Krishnamurthi R, et al. Global and regional burden of stroke in 1990-2010: incidence, mortality, prevalence, and disability-adjusted life-years lost. Lancet 382: 1–12, 2013.
10. Krishnamurthi RV, Feigin VL, Forouzanfar MH, et al. Global and regional burden of first-ever ischaemic and haemorrhagic stroke during 1990–2010: findings from the Global Burden of Disease Study 2010. Lancet 2013; Published Online <http://dx.doi.org/10.1016/S2214-109X(13)70089-5>.
11. Bennett DA, Anderson LM, Nair N, et al. Methodology of the global and regional burden of stroke study. Neuroepidemiol 2012;38(1):30–40.
12. Aho K, Harmsen P, Hatano S, et al. Cerebrovascular disease in the community: results of a WHO collaborative study. Bull World Health Organ 1980;58(1):113–30.
13. Wang H, Dwyer-Lindgren L, Lofgren KT, et al. Age-specific and sex-specific mortality in 187 countries, 1970-2010: a systematic analysis for the Global Burden of Disease Study 2010. Lancet 2012;380(9859):2071–94.
14. World Bank. World Health Development Report. Washington: 1993.
15. Lim SS, Vos T, Flaxman AD, et al. A comparative risk assessment of burden of disease and injury attributable to 67 risk factors and risk factor clusters in 21 regions, 1990–2010: a systematic analysis for the Global Burden of Disease Study 2010. Lancet 2012; 380(9859):2224–60.
16. Putaala JMDP, Yesilot NMD, Waje-Andreassen UMDP, et al. Demographic and geographic vascular risk factor differences in European young adults with ischemic stroke: The 15 Cities Young Stroke Study. Stroke 2012;43(10):2624–30.
17. WHO. Prevention of cardiovascular disease: Pocket guidelines for assessment and management of cardiovascular risk. World Health Organization; [updated 2007]; Available from:: <http://www.who.int/cardiovascular_diseases/resources/publications/en/index.html>.
18. Vaartjes IP, O'Flaherty MPMD, Capewell SPMD, et al. Remarkable decline in ischemic stroke mortality is not matched by changes in incidence. Stroke 2013;44(3):591–7.
19. Gillum RFMD, Kwagyan JP, Obisesan TOMD. Ethnic and geographic variation in stroke mortality trends. Stroke 2011; 42(11):3294–6.
20. Kunst AEP, Amiri MP, Janssen FP. The decline in stroke mortality: exploration of future trends in 7 western European countries. Stroke 2011;42(8):2126–30.
21. Redon J, Olsen MH, Cooper RS, et al. Stroke mortality and trends from 1990 to 2006 in 39 countries from Europe and Central Asia: implications for control of high blood pressure. Eur Heart J 2011;32(11):1424–31.
22. Kissela BM, Khoury JC, Alwell K, et al. Age at stroke: temporal trends in stroke incidence in a large, biracial population. Neurology 2012;79(17):1781–7.
23. Medin J, Nordlund A, Ekberg K. Increasing stroke incidence in Sweden between 1989 and 2000 among persons aged 30 to 65 years: evidence from the Swedish Hospital Discharge Register. Stroke 2004;35(5):1047–51.
24. Danaei G, Finucane M, Lin J, et al. National, regional, and global trends in systolic blood pressure since 1980: systematic analysis of health examination surveys and epidemiological studies with 786 country-years and 5.4 million participants. Lancet 2011;377: 568–77.
25. Norrving BMDPF, Kissela BMD. The global burden of stroke and need for a continuum of care. Neurology 2013;80(3 Suppl. 2):S5–12.
26. de los Rios FMD, Kleindorfer DOMD, Khoury JP, et al. Trends in substance abuse preceding stroke among young adults: a population-based study. Stroke 2012;43(12):3179–83.
27. Wolff V, Lauer V, Rouyer O, et al. Cannabis use, ischemic stroke, and multifocal intracranial vasoconstriction: A prospective study in 48 consecutive young patients. Stroke 2011;42(6): 1778–80.
28. Zaridze D, Brennan P, Boreham J, et al. Alcohol and cause-specific mortality in Russia: a retrospective case-control study of 48,557 adult deaths. Lancet [Research Support, Non-U.S. Gov't] 2009; 373(9682):2201–14.
29. Leon DA, Saburova L, Tomkins S, et al. lcohol consumption and public health in Russia. Lancet [Comment Letter] 2007; 370(9587):561.
30. Hu SS, Kong LZ, Gao RL, et al. Outline of the report on cardiovascular disease in China, 2010. Biomed Enviro Sci 2012;25(3): 251–6.
31. Jha P, Jacob B, Gajalakshmi V, et al. A nationally representative case-control study of smoking and death in India. New Eng J Med

[Research Support, N.I.H., Extramural Research Support, Non-U.S. Gov't] 2008;358(11):1137–47.
32. Norrving B, Kissela B. The global burden of stroke and need for a continuum of care. Neurology [Review] 2013;80(3 Suppl. 2):S5–12.
33. Yusuf S, Reddy S, Stephanie O, et al. Global Burden of Cardiovascular Diseases Part I: General Considerations, the Epidemiologic Transisiton, Risk Factors, and the Impact of Urbanization. Circulation 2001;104:2746–2753.
34. Gaziano TA, Galea G, Reddy KS. Scaling up interventions for chronic disease prevention: the evidence. Lancet [Review] 2007;370(9603):1939–46.
35. Mattei J, Malik V, Wedick NM, et al. A symposium and workshop report from the Global Nutrition and Epidemiologic Transition Initiative: nutrition transition and the global burden of type 2 diabetes. Br J Nutr [Congresses Research Support, Non-U.S. Gov't] 2012;108(7):1325–35.
36. Sajjad A, Chowdhury R, Felix JF, et al. A systematic evaluation of stroke surveillance studies in low- and middle-income countries. Neurology 2013;80(7):677–84.

14 Stroke Disparities

George Howard, Virginia J. Howard

KEY POINTS

- Despite dramatic temporal declines in stroke mortality for all race/ethnic groups, the black–white disparity in stroke has been persistent (or even perhaps growing).
- While the black–white disparity averages 40% across the age spectrum, this pooling across ages obscures a much larger (200% to 300%) excess mortality for blacks aged 45 to 65.
- Approximately one-half of the excess mortality in blacks appears to be attributable to "traditional" stroke risk factors and differences in socio-economic status, with a potentially differential and larger impact of hypertension also contributing to the disparity.
- Disparities in the Hispanic population are more complex, with lower stroke mortality in Hispanics than whites, but with evidence from two independent studies showing substantially higher incidence in Hispanics than whites.
- Despite a requirement for the National Institutes of Health to investigate urban–rural disparities in disease, there are strikingly few data describing this disparity for stroke. However, there appears to be approximately a 20% higher stroke mortality in rural than urban regions.
- The "stroke belt" region of higher stroke mortality in the southeastern US has existed for over a half-century, and persists with a stroke mortality as great as 300% higher in some regions.
- There is strong evidence that lower socio-economic status is associated with both higher incidence of stroke and poorer outcomes following stroke.

INTRODUCTION

While stroke has recently declined from the third to the fourth leading cause of death in the US,[1] the public health burden of the disease remains staggering, accounting for nearly 2 million years of life lost in 2010 (actually increasing from the 4th largest contributor to the 3rd largest contributor of years of life lost between 1990 and 2010)[2] and the lifetime cost of stroke is approximately $140,000 (in 1999 dollars).[3] Unfortunately, the burden of stroke does not fall equally across the population.[1] By law, the National Institutes of Health is required by the *Minority Health and Health Disparities and Education Act* (2000) to assess the impact and contributors to disparities in: (1) minority health and related activities, (2) rural health and related activities, and (3) other activities related to the socioeconomically disadvantaged in the urban setting.[4] All domains with substantial stroke disparities will be discussed in this chapter. In addition to the impact of geography by urban–rural exposures, we will also discuss the impact of regional differences in stroke risk in the US.

RACIAL AND ETHNIC DISPARITIES IN STROKE

One of the first descriptions of the racial disparity in stroke mortality was a 1970 publication providing nonwhite-to-white stroke mortality ratios, where the nonwhite-to-white mortality ratio between 1949 and 1950 was estimated to be 1.63 for men and 1.92 for women.[5] Using age-specific stroke mortality rates for 2010 available from the Centers for Disease Control and Prevention (CDC) WONDER,[6] and calculating age-adjusted rates standardized to the population distribution in 1950, the comparable nonwhite-to-white stroke mortality ratios for the year 2010 for ages 45+ are 1.96 for men and 2.04 for women. Hence, there has been no apparent decline in the overall (nonwhite-to-white) disparity in stroke mortality in over one half century.

In the more recent period from 1999 to 2010, the stroke mortality rates by specific race-ethnicity strata can also be described using data from the CDC WONDER system (Fig. 14-1). Here stroke mortality (ICD 10: I60–I69) is shown for non-Hispanic whites, blacks and Asians and for Hispanics of all races. Despite a dramatic 32% to 38% decline in stroke mortality across the race-ethnic strata (left panel), stroke mortality ratios contrasting each minority group with whites has remained relatively stable (right panel). There is some suggestion that the black-to-white stroke mortality ratio was increasing between 1999 and 2008 but decreasing after that. There is also a suggestion that the lower mortality for Hispanics relative to whites has been decreasing over time.

However, the black-to-white disparity in stroke mortality is disproportionately distributed across age groups, with a relative risk three times greater in blacks than whites for ages 45 to 54, but then a decreasing disparity with increasing age to the point of no increased risk for blacks relative to whites above the age of 85 years (Fig. 14-2). Other than for Native Americans aged 45 to 54, there were no other substantial racial/ethnic disparities in stroke mortality.

While the racial/ethnic differences in stroke mortality data are remarkably persistent, there are two possible concerns with these data. First, the numerator data of deaths from stroke and other diseases is from the vital statistics systems (information usually collected by physicians and funeral directors) while the denominator data on population is based on self-reported race/ethnicity from the Census, and it is possible that these two sources report race/ethnicity differently. The report by Arias and colleagues concluded this is of minimal concern for whites and blacks, only modest concern for Hispanic and Asian/Pacific-Islander populations, but may be substantial for Native American populations.[7] There could also be errors introduced by misclassification of causes of death; however, in a national cohort study, death certificates were found to have a sensitivity of 82% and a specificity of 96% relative to physician-adjudicated stroke events.[8] Hence, misclassification could be playing a potentially different role across the palette of diseases, particularly for the Native American population.

For blacks, the higher stroke mortality may be a result of either a higher incidence of stroke in blacks than whites, or a

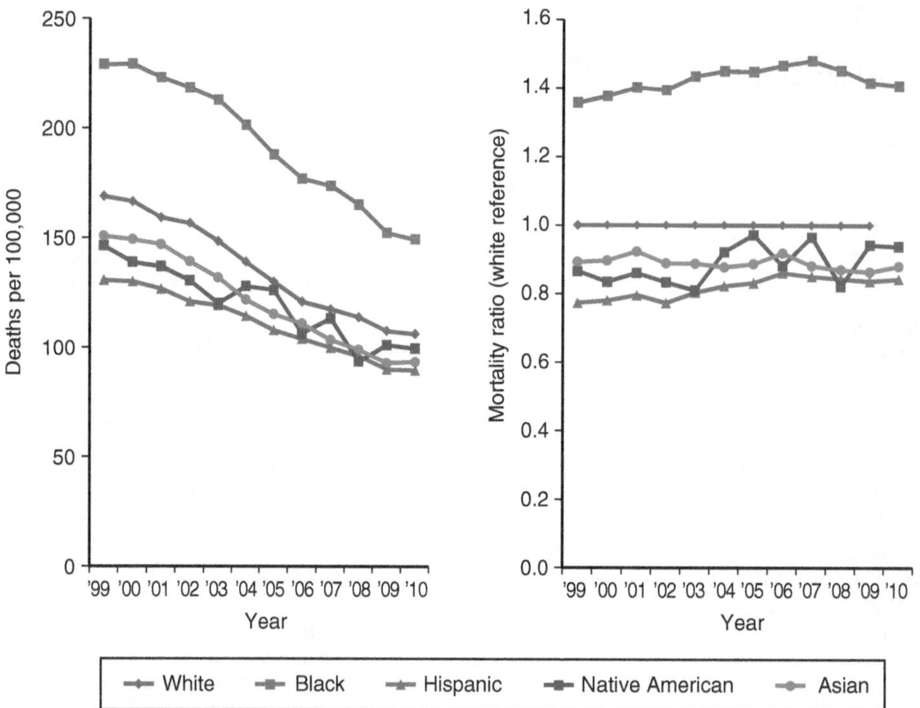

Figure 14-1 Race/ethnic differences in deaths from cerebrovascular disease (ICD 10: I60–I69) for US residents aged 45 and above for years 1999 through 2010. Left, shows the age-adjusted (year 2000 standard) death rate per 100,000 for mutually exclusive race/ethnic strata: non-Hispanic whites (White), non-Hispanic blacks (Black), Hispanic (all races), non-Hispanic Native American/Alaska Natives (Native American), and non-Hispanic Asians (Asian). Right, shows the cerebrovascular disease mortality ratio for minority groups relative to non-Hispanic whites.

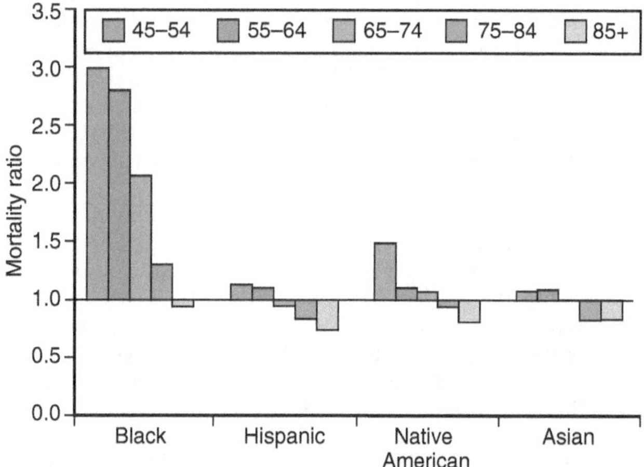

Figure 14-2 Mortality ratios for black, Hispanic, Native American and Asian populations by age strata (relative to white) for the year 2010.

higher case fatality among blacks suffering stroke than whites suffering stroke. There is strong evidence of a higher incidence of stroke in the black population than the white population, with both the Northern Manhattan Study (NOMAS)[9] and the Greater Cincinnati/Northern Kentucky Stroke Study (GCNKSS)[10] showing black-to-white incidence ratios of 2.0 and greater. In addition, the REasons for Geographic And Racial Differences in Stroke (REGARDS) study has shown a pattern of black-to-white incidence ratios strikingly similar to the black-to-white mortality ratios, with risk of incident stroke three times greater in blacks than whites for ages 45 to 54 and virtually no difference in stroke risk for those aged 85 years and over.[11,12] The Atherosclerosis Risk in Communities (ARIC) study showed a black-to-white incidence ratio of 2.77 (95%CI 1.37–5.62) for those aged 45–54 at baseline, and 2.23 (95%CI 1.66–3.00) for those aged 55–65 at baseline. In contrast, there is little evidence of a higher case fatality among blacks than whites. For example, the GCNKSS showed very similar 30-day, 90-day, and 1-year mortality following stroke for blacks and whites,[10] and this similarity has been remarkably consistent over time.[13] In general, studies have shown blacks to have lower or similar in-hospital mortality than whites.[14–18] In addition, data from the National Hospital Discharge Study has generally shown lower in-hospital mortality for blacks than whites after stroke,[14] while ARIC showed non-significantly higher stroke case-fatality in blacks compare to whites.[15] As such, it seems likely that the black-to-white disparity in stroke is largely attributable to a racial difference in stroke incidence.

Reflecting the temporal changes in mortality, the GCNKSS has also reported temporal decreases in stroke incidence rates, significant for whites, but non-significant for blacks.[19] While strokes among those aged 20 to 44 represent a relatively small portion of the total, there appears to be a disturbing increase in stroke incidence only in this age strata from 12/100,000 (95%CI 9–15) in 1993/1994 to 26/100,000 (95%CI 20–31) in whites (P = 0.02), and from 46/100,000 (95%CI 31–62) in 1993/1994 to 58/100,000 (95%CI 40–75) in blacks (P >0.05).[20]

Black–white differences in risk factors could be contributing to the racial disparity in stroke incidence through several pathways:

1. The possibility that a higher prevalence of major stroke risk factors could be contributing to a difference in stroke risk was first assessed using National Health and Nutrition Examination Survey (NHANES) data, showing that approximately one-third of the racial differences in risk for cerebral infarction could be attributed to racial differences in risk factor prevalence.[21] ARIC also showed that adjustment

for hypertension and diabetes attenuated the black-to-white stroke incidence ratio 60% from 2.41 (95%CI 1.85–3.15) to 1.57 (95%CI 1.18–2.09), and further adjustment for educational status attenuated the disparity an additional 13% to 1.38 (95%CI 1.01–1.89).[15] More recently, REGARDS showed that adjustment for the Framingham stroke risk factors[22] and socioeconomic status (SES) (as indexed by income and education) was associated with approximately a 50% mediation of the increased risk of stroke; for example, at age 45, the black-to-white increased risk of nearly threefold (HR = 2.90; 95%CI 1.72–4.89) was decreased to twofold the risk (HR = 2.01; 95%CI 1.1 –3.47).[12] In all of these analyses, however, the risk of stroke remained significantly elevated even after adjustment for differences in major stroke risk factors.

2. Both NHANES[23] and REGARDS[24] have documented that while blacks with hypertension are significantly more likely to know of their condition, and blacks who are aware of their hypertension are significantly more likely to be treated for it, blacks who are treated for hypertension are significantly less likely to have their blood pressure treated to guidelines. For example in REGARDS, after adjustment for SES and other risk factors, the odds of adequate control was 35% less in blacks than whites (OR = 0.65; 95%CI 0.57–0.72).[24]
3. Contributions of other or "novel" risk factors that are both more prevalent in the black population and strongly associated with stroke risk may be substantial contributors to disparities in stroke incidence. For example, blacks are at a disadvantage for many measures of SES, and lower SES has been shown to be strongly associated with stroke risk (and more weakly associated with case-fatality).[25–28] Much work remains to be done to investigate to what extent SES (and psychosocial factors such as stress, discrimination, etc.) attenuates the racial disparity in stroke, and whether it has a direct effect or whether its impact is through increasing the prevalence of traditional risk factors such as hypertension and diabetes. There could also be novel physiological risk factors, such as C-reactive protein (CRP) that have higher average levels in the black than the white population,[29] and have shown to be related to stroke risk;[30] however, much work also remains to assess whether such novel risk factors would attenuate the black-to-white disparities in stroke.
4. It is also possible that risk factors could be contributing to the disparities in stroke incidence through a mechanism where the impact of the same level of risk factors could have a larger impact in the black population than the white population. For example, REGARDS data have shown that a 10 mmHg difference in systolic blood pressure (SBP) is associated with an 8% (HR = 1.08; 95%CI 1.00–1.16) increased stroke risk in the white participants; however, a similar 10 mmHg difference in SBP in the black cohort was associated with a three-times larger, 24% increase in risk (HR = 1.24; 95%CI 1.14–1.35); this suggests that blacks are more susceptible to the failure to control elevated SBP.[31]

Disparities for the Hispanic population are more complex, as the mortality data described above show that in 1999, Hispanics were at approximately 30% lower risk of death from stroke than whites, an advantage that declined to approximately 15% lower risk by 2010 (see Fig. 14-1). This is in contrast to the Brain Attack Surveillance in Corpus Christi (BASIC) study showing that for ages 45–59 the risk of incident stroke was 1.94 (95%CI 1.67–2.25) times higher in the Hispanic population than the white, for ages 60–74, 1.50 (95%CI 1.35–1.67) times higher, and no difference in incident stroke risk for ages 75 and above (RR = 1.00; 95%CI 0.90–1.11).[32] NOMAS showed higher risk in Hispanics than whites for incident intracranial atherosclerotic strokes (RR = 5.00; 95%CI 1.69–14.76), extracranial atherosclerotic strokes (RR = 1.71; 95%CI 0.80–3.63), lacunar strokes (RR = 2.32; 1.48–3.63), cardioembolic strokes (RR = 1.42; 95%CI 0.97–2.09), cryptogenic stroke (RR = 1.44; 95%CI 1.09–1.92), and other strokes (RR = 2.27; 95%CI 0.42–51.91).[33]

The lower mortality but higher incidence in Hispanics could be a product of several factors. First, as described above, there could be misreporting of race/ethnicity in the vital statistics and census. However, it is also possible that there is confounding of ethnicity and geography. Alternatively, there is also the possibility that Hispanic–white *ethnic* differences in stroke mortality are also confounded with Hispanic–white *geographic* differences in stroke mortality. Specifically, New York County (largely Manhattan, the location of the NOMAS Study) was in the 9th percentile of counties reporting Hispanic stroke mortality but the 0th percentile of counties reporting white stroke mortality.[34] Likewise, Nueces County, Texas (the location of the BASIC Study) is in the 88th percentile of counties reporting Hispanic stroke mortality but the 53rd percentile of counties reporting white stroke morality.[34] Hence, another possible explanation of the paradox of high stroke incidence but low stroke mortality for Hispanics is that the NOMAS study is being conducted in a county with low Hispanic stroke mortality but strikingly lower white stroke mortality, while the BASIC study is being conducted in a county with high Hispanic stroke mortality but average white stroke mortality. With this uncertainty regarding the existence and magnitude of disparities in the Hispanic populations coupled with the remarkable growth in the Hispanic population in the US, it is critical to continue the efforts of studies such as BASIC and NOMAS and expand both surveillance and longitudinal efforts to understand Hispanic–white differences.

Similar to Hispanics, national mortality data suggest stroke mortality is lower for Native Americans than for whites; however, as noted the classification of race in these data is particularly problematic for Native Americans.[7] The relatively low reported stroke mortality for Native Americans stands in very stark contrast to reported stroke incidence from the Strong Heart Study, which estimated a stroke incidence rate of 384/100,000 for Native Americans at younger ages (45–54 years).[35] As the investigators report, this rate was 6.1-times higher than the rate for whites reported by the Rochester Epidemiological Program between 1985 to 1989, 2.8-times higher than whites in the GCNKSS in 1993, and 1.2 times higher than blacks in the GCNKSS. At older ages (55–64 and 65–74), Native Americans also had higher stroke incidence compared to whites and blacks in these studies, although the differences were much more modest. The interpretation of these observations is complex, since in addition to the racial differences in populations there is also the possibility that differences in incidence rates could be attributed to: (1) differences in study methods between the various sources, (2) confounding with geographic disparities in stroke, and (3) temporal changes in stroke risk. Regardless, this remarkable disparity in stroke risk (particularly at young ages) in Native Americans clearly warrants further study.

GEOGRAPHIC DISPARITIES IN STROKE

Urban-to-Rural Disparities in Stroke

Despite the call for NIH to investigate urban–rural disparities, there appears to be remarkably little in the literature describing potential disparities in this domain. While there is some literature regarding the care of stroke patients in urban vs. rural areas, including the availability of resources (such as

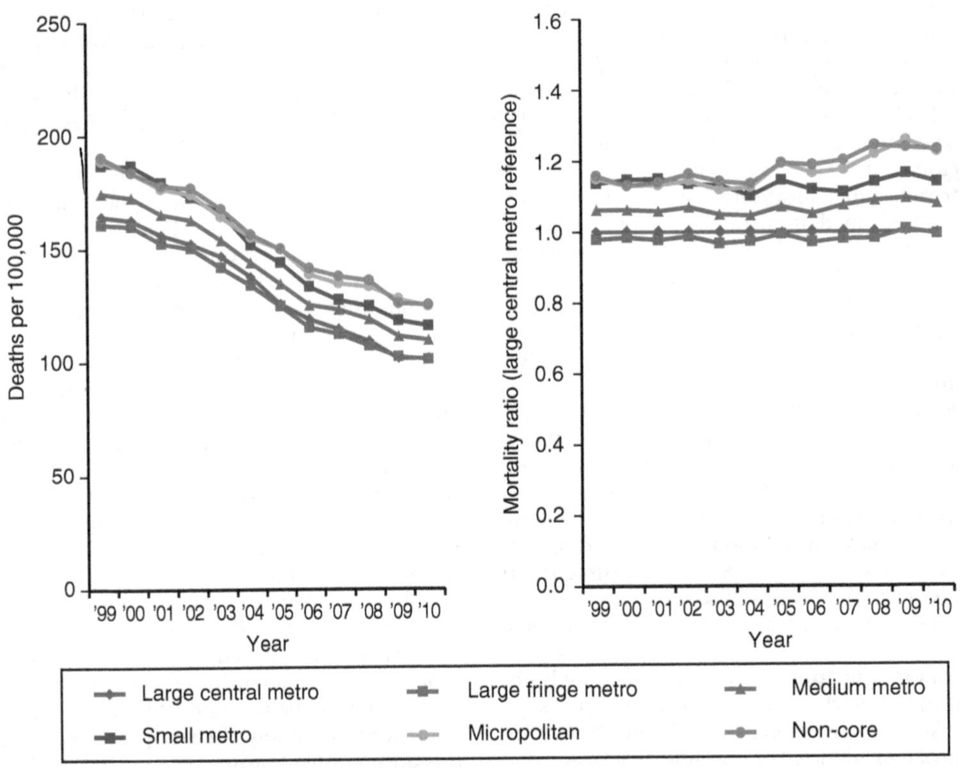

Figure 14-3 Urban–rural differences in deaths from cerebrovascular disease (ICD 10: I60–I69) for US non-Hispanic white residents aged 45 and above for the years 1999 to 2010. Left, shows the age-adjusted (year 2000 standard) death rate per 100,000 by the NCHS Urban-Rural Classification Scheme for counties classified as large central metro (most urban), large fringe metro, medium metro, small metro, micropolitan, or non-core (most rural). Right, shows the cerebrovascular disease mortality ratio for urban–rural groups relative to large central metro.

stroke centers),[36] there are no publications describing the impact of urban-to-rural residence on stroke incidence, and only a single publication documenting a 1.45-times higher prevalence of stroke in rural compared to urban areas.[37] Differences in a report described the rural-to-urban mortality ratio, reporting a mortality 1.37 times higher for states outside the stroke belt (no national data provided).[38]

Data were compiled to describe the urban–rural differences in stroke mortality, using CDC WONDER and the National Center for Health Statistics Urban-Rural Classification Scheme, a 6-point scale from the most urban *Large Central Metro* to the most rural *Non-Core*.[6] Estimates of urban–rural differences in stroke mortality for the non-Hispanic white population over age 45 are shown in Figure 14-3 (population restricted to avoid confounding with race). There is little difference in stroke mortality for the two most urban classifications (*Large Central Metro* and *Large Fringe Metro*), and there was higher stroke mortality in more rural areas with a trend for disparities to increase in the more recent years where data are available (2008–2010). Specifically, stroke mortality was approximately 6% higher in the *Medium Metro* regions, increasing to 8% higher in recent years (relative to *Large Central Metro*). The three more rural classifications (*Small Metro, Micropolitan*, and *Non-Core*) were approximately 15% higher than the *Large Central Metro*; however, in recent years the *Micropolitan* and *Non-Core* regions increased to a disparity of approximately 24% (while the *Small Metro* region remained relatively stable at a 15% disparity). While there is evidence of an increased mortality for the more rural areas, it is not clear whether the higher mortality in rural areas is a product of higher incidence (perhaps related to healthier habits in urban areas) or higher case fatality (perhaps related to better treatment of stroke and stroke centers in urban areas).

Regional Differences in Stroke

As noted in the previous chapter, the international differences in stroke mortality are striking, with approximately 300-times differences in crude death rates from stroke of 325/100,000 in women in the Russian Federation and 271/100,000 in men in Kazakhstan, compared to 1/100,000 in men and women in Papua New Guinea (Fig. 14-4).[39] While differences in reporting systems suggest that differences should be interpreted with caution, comparable age-adjusted incidence rates are available for 48 countries, with at most modest agreement between mortality (Fig. 14-4) and incidence (Fig. 14-5), underscoring the need for additional efforts to gather both more data and to standardize collection approaches.

There are also remarkable within-country disparities in stroke mortality, for example with a well-documented increased risk of stroke mortality in the more-rural regions referred to as the "stroke belt" in the Southeastern US, an area of higher stroke mortality that has been documented to have existed since at least the 1940s (Fig. 14-6).[40] There are not uniform definitions of the stroke belt region; however, most investigators include the states of North Carolina, South Carolina, Georgia, Tennessee, Alabama, Mississippi, Arkansas and Louisiana.[41–45] The increased risk in this region is surprisingly larger for the black population than the white;[46] and because the black population is over-represented in this region (these states include 13% of the US population but 25% of the US black population) confounding of geographic and racial effects may be contributing to the higher risk of stroke in blacks discussed in the previous section.[46, 47] The higher stroke mortality in the region has been remarkably persistent, with the most recent 12 years showing a 25% to 28% higher death rate from stroke in these states (Fig. 14-7).

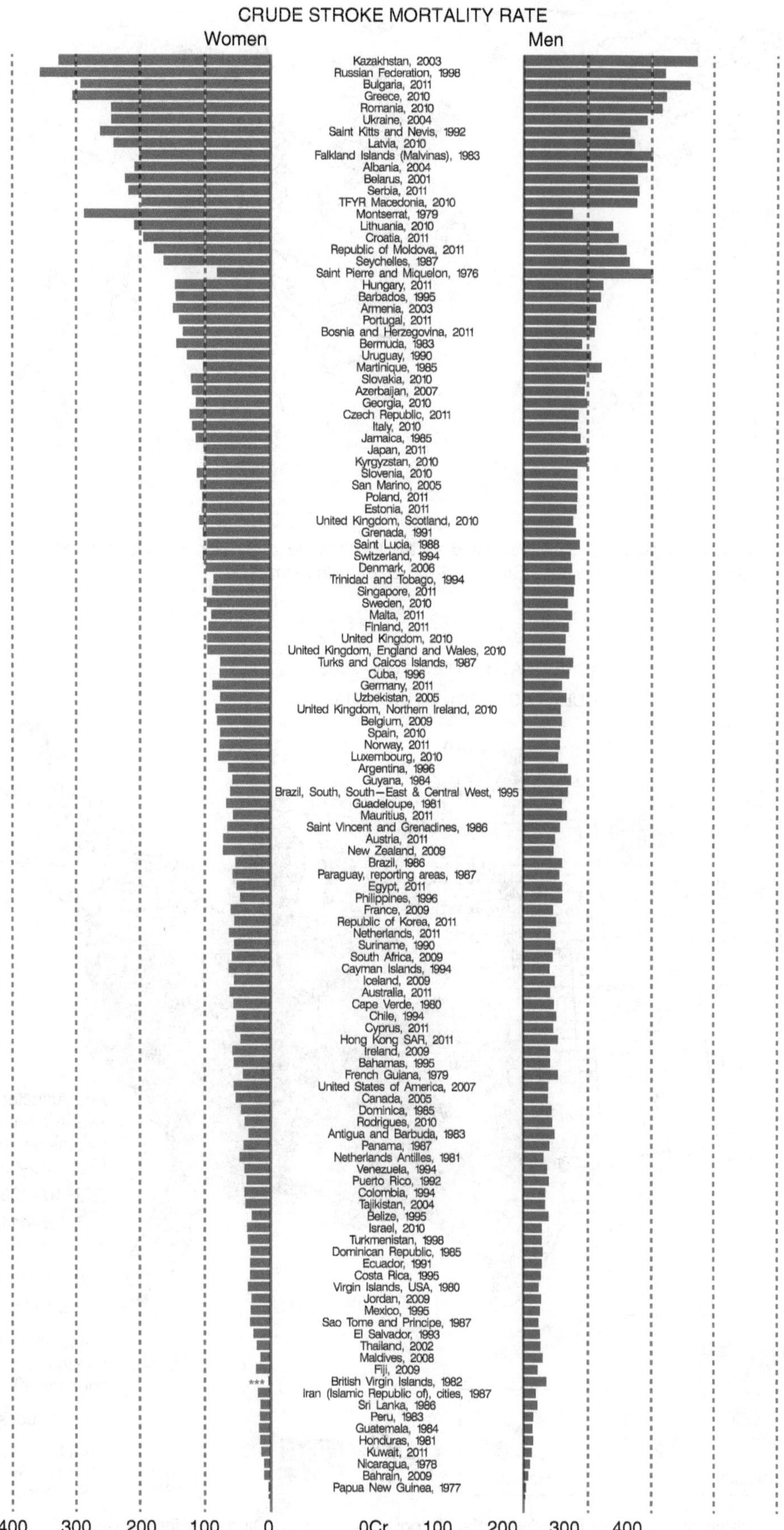

Figure 14-4 Crude mortality from stroke according to the proportion of the population aged at least 65 years and the year. These are for all countries that have reported mortality to the World Health Organization, and are for the most recent country year reported for each individual country. *(From Thrift AG, Cadilhac DA, Thayabaranathan T, et al. Global stroke statistics.* Int J Stroke *9:6–18, 2014, with permission.)*

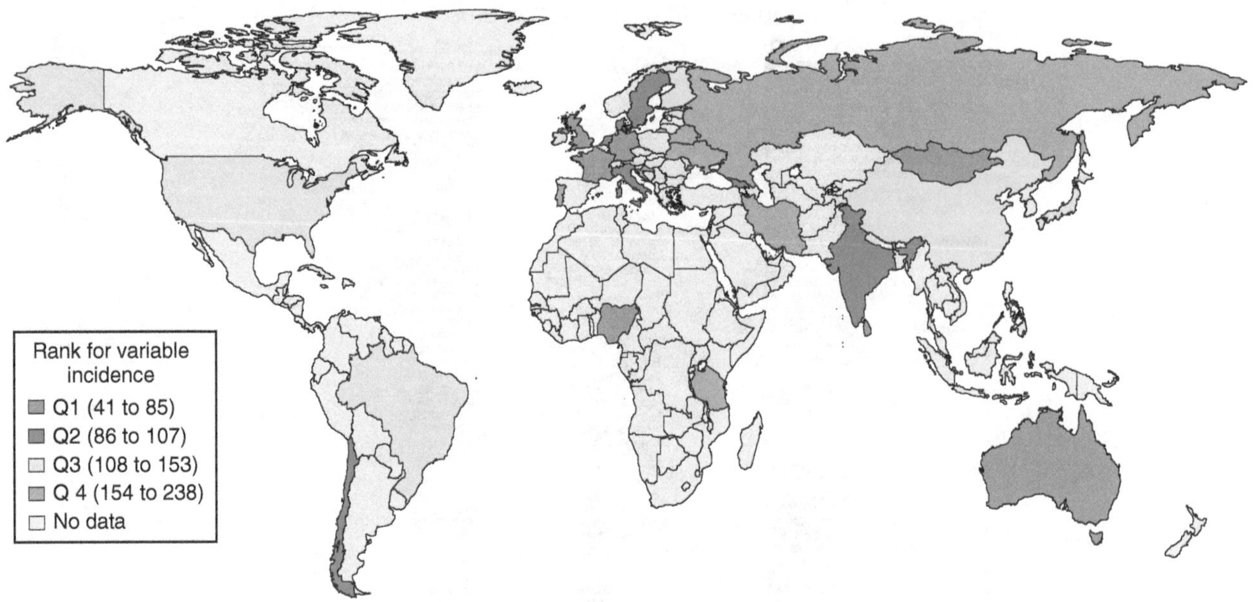

Figure 14-5 Heat map showing incidence of stroke adjusted to the WHO world population by quartiles. *(From Thrift AG, Cadilhac DA, Thayabaranathan T, et al. Global stroke statistics.* Int J Stroke *9:6–18, 2014, with permission.)*

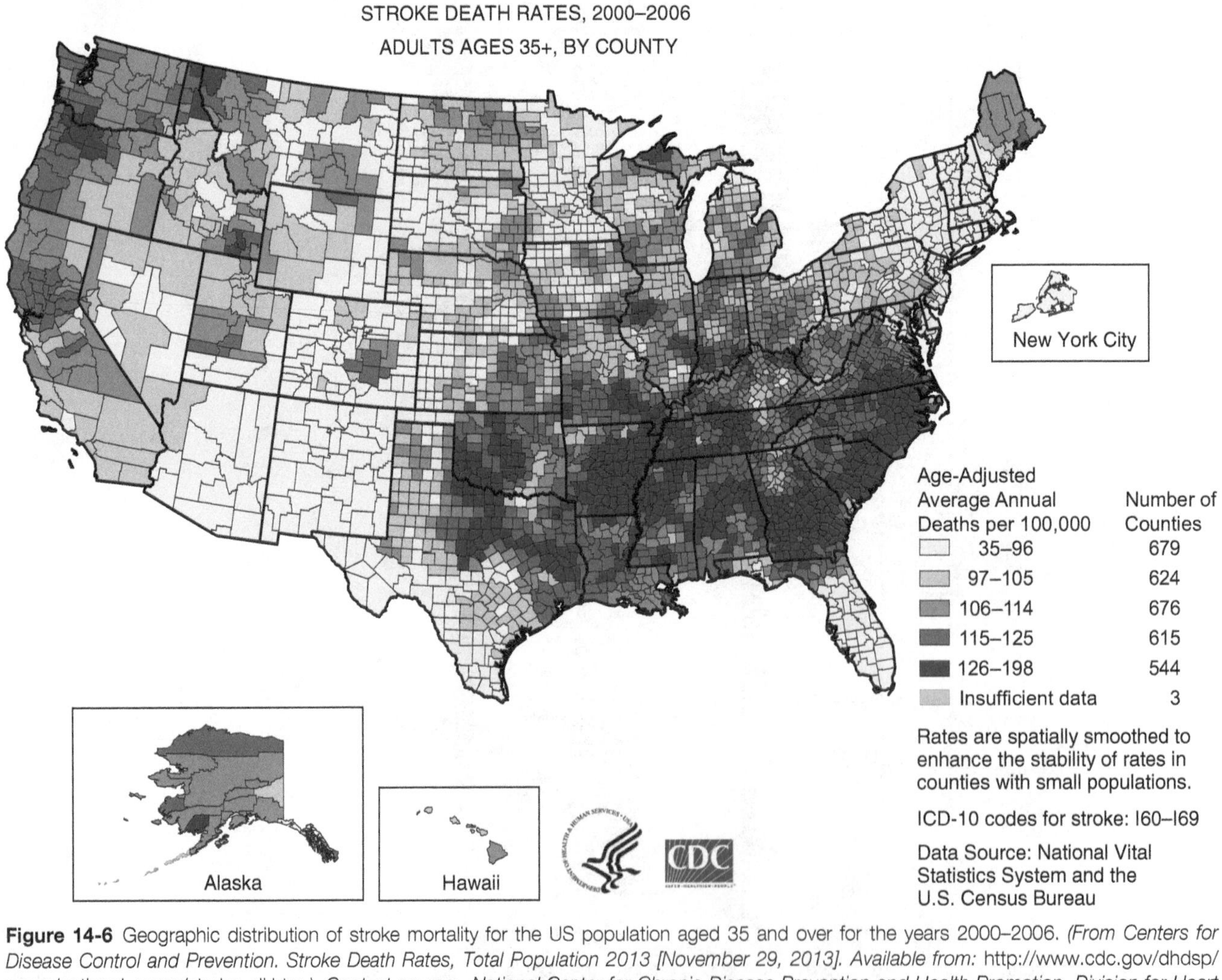

STROKE DEATH RATES, 2000–2006
ADULTS AGES 35+, BY COUNTY

New York City

Age-Adjusted Average Annual Deaths per 100,000 | Number of Counties

Age-Adjusted Average Annual Deaths per 100,000	Number of Counties
35–96	679
97–105	624
106–114	676
115–125	615
126–198	544
Insufficient data	3

Rates are spatially smoothed to enhance the stability of rates in counties with small populations.

ICD-10 codes for stroke: I60–I69

Data Source: National Vital Statistics System and the U.S. Census Bureau

Alaska

Hawaii

CDC

Figure 14-6 Geographic distribution of stroke mortality for the US population aged 35 and over for the years 2000–2006. *(From Centers for Disease Control and Prevention. Stroke Death Rates, Total Population 2013 [November 29, 2013]. Available from:* http://www.cdc.gov/dhdsp/maps/national_maps/stroke_all.htm.*). Content source: National Center for Chronic Disease Prevention and Health Promotion, Division for Heart Disease and Stroke Prevention.*

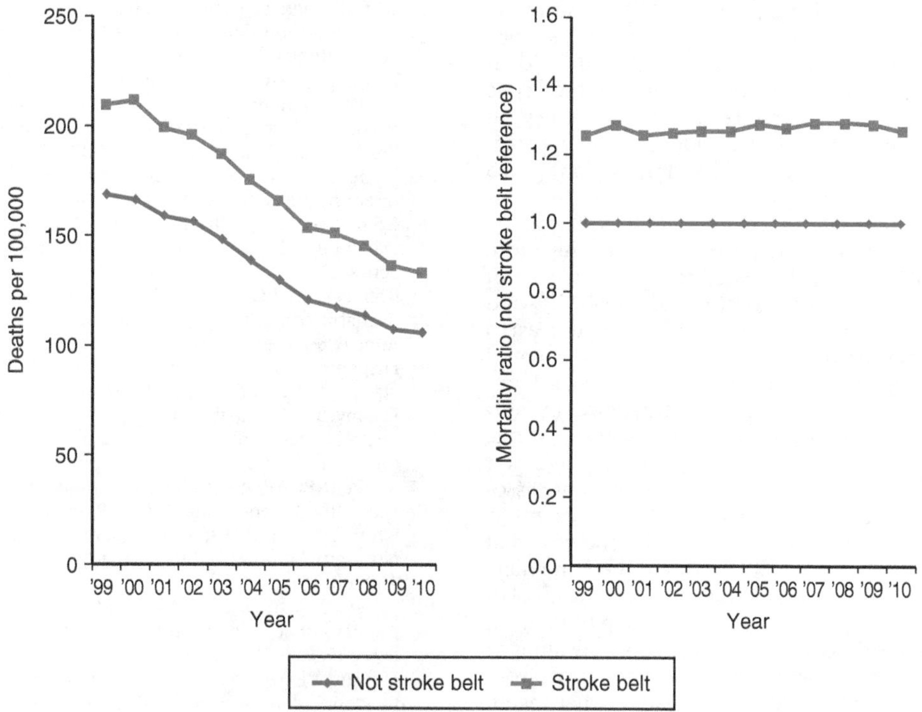

Figure 14-7 Stroke belt versus non-stroke belt differences in deaths from cerebrovascular disease (ICD 10: I60–I69) for non-Hispanic white US residents aged 45 and above, years 1999 through 2010. Left, shows the age-adjusted (year 2000 standard) death rate per 100,000 by the REGARDS defined stroke belt (states of North Carolina, South Carolina, Georgia, Tennessee, Alabama, Mississippi, Arkansas and Louisiana) and non-stroke belt regions (all states not included in the stroke belt). Right, shows the cerebrovascular disease mortality ratio for the stroke belt relative to the non-stroke belt.

While the stroke belt is most frequently described at the state level, there is considerable geographic heterogeneity both within the stroke belt (that includes relatively low-risk regions such as the Atlanta region and the mountain region of North Carolina) and outside of the stroke belt (that includes high-risk regions such as the Portland, Oregon area). Within the stroke belt a region of even higher stroke mortality along the coastal plain of North Carolina, South Carolina and Georgia, referred to as the "buckle of the stroke belt,"[48] has as much as a 300% higher stroke mortality than the lowest-risk regions in the non-belt (New York City, Miami, etc.).[49] Recently, a spatial analysis of the change over the decade between 1995–1996 and 2005–2006 in hospitalization of Medicare beneficiaries for stroke diagnoses showed while the stroke belt is persistent, there may be shifts where regions have newly joined the group with the highest admission rates (more in east-central Texas, South Central Georgia, central South Carolina, and western Pennsylvania), while other regions no longer are part of the group with the highest admission rates (central Tennessee and southeastern Georgia).[50]

The REGARDS study has a co-primary focus on advancing the understanding of the causes of the stroke belt. Initial examination of regional differences (i.e., stroke belt versus non-stroke belt) in incidence was non-significant;[11] however, additional analyses on the county level suggest that much of the geographic disparity in stroke mortality is attributable to geographic disparities in stroke incidence rather than stroke case-fatality.[51] In addition, a more rapid decline in cognitive function in the region may suggest a deficit of cerebrovascular health.[52] There has been an acknowledged need for a better understanding of the causes of the stroke belt,[44,53] with a higher prevalence of hypertension in the region being the most commonly hypothesized contributor.[42,54] More recent reports from REGARDS confirmed the geographic disparity in hypertension, but also established a higher prevalence of diabetes as an additional contributor to the increased stroke risk in the stroke belt; however, the geographic differences in the traditional risk factors were not sufficient to account for the geographic differences in projected risk of incident stroke.[55] Efforts in the REGARDS are currently investigating potential contributors to the geographic disparities in stroke risk including geographic differences in: (1) the prevalence of non-traditional risk factors, (2) the control of risk factors, (3) the role of nontraditional or novel risk factors, and (4) the susceptibility to risk factors.

In conclusion, the literature on urban-to-rural differences in stroke risk is quite scant but hopefully the recent mandate to investigate this potential difference will result in more reports. More progress is underway to understand the contributors to the stroke belt region of the US.

SOCIOECONOMIC STATUS AND STROKE

As early as 1992, documentation of higher stroke mortality in less affluent counties of the US was emerging; a finding that also showed a larger impact of lower SES on stroke mortality among blacks than whites, potentially contributing to the black-to-white disparities described above.[56] The literature documenting an association between SES and stroke has continued to steadily grow, and has been well-summarized in two recent review articles.[25,26]

Many of the reports in the US assessing the relationship of SES with stroke incidence have used neighborhood[57–59] rather than individual[15,60,61] measures of SES; the findings, generally in younger adults (<65 years), are that lower levels of SES were associated with approximately a doubling of risk for incident stroke. In addition, as many as seven international reports have reported similar magnitude of association (using either neighborhood or individual measures of SES) in Australia, France, Italy, United Kingdom, and Sweden.[26] Interestingly, efforts to examine the association between SES and incident stroke in older individuals have shown either a protective effect[60] or no association.[61] Despite this inconsistency in older ages, there appears to be strong evidence of an approximate doubling of incident stroke risk among lower SES populations.

The mechanism through which lower SES is associated with higher incident stroke risk requires further investigation. However, as low SES is strongly related to the prevalence of hypertension,[62] blood pressure control,[63] diabetes,[64,65] and cigarette smoking,[66] it seems highly likely that at least a portion of the harmful effect of low SES on stroke risk could be through a pathway of traditional risk factors.

Unlike racial disparities in stroke where differences in mortality appear to be associated with higher incidence of stroke rather than higher case fatality following stroke, there is a strong literature showing SES disparities in mortality are associated with poorer outcomes following stroke. For example, data from the Cardiovascular Health Study showed that despite relatively small mortality differences in the immediate post-stroke period, there was a 77% higher risk of death (HR = 1.77; 95%CI 1.17–2.68) following stroke among those from disadvantaged neighborhoods compared to more advantaged neighborhoods.[67] Very similar findings were reported from population-based registries in Ontario (Canada), where again the immediate post-stroke mortality was similar across neighborhoods, but there was an 18% (HR = 1.18; 95%CI 1.03–1.29) higher risk of death over 1 year post-stroke in the low versus high-income neighborhood regions.[68] Likewise, data from state-level discharge databases report that the odds of in-hospital mortality of those from poorer neighborhoods were 8% higher than those from more wealthy neighborhoods (OR = 1.08; 95%CI 1.02–1.15).[18] Additional research is also needed to better defined the mechanism for poorer outcomes after stroke, although it has been noted that the severity of stroke is greater in persons from poorer neighborhoods, perhaps because of lower medication compliance, less access to care, or as a proxy measure for undiagnosed diseases.[69]

In summary, while it appears clear that lower SES is associated with both higher risk of stroke incidence and poorer outcomes after stroke, much additional work is needed (particularly in the US) to focus on the impact of individual (rather than neighborhood) measures of SES and to further the understanding of the mechanisms where low SES is associated with higher incidence and mortality.

CONCLUSIONS

Despite remarkable temporal declines in stroke mortality that have been recognized as one of the great public health achievements of recent times,[70,71] there are large, persistent and costly disparities in stroke that must be addressed. While the racial disparities in mortality appear to be closely associated with racial disparities in incidence, the relative contribution of incidence versus case fatality to the geographic (both urban–rural and regional) and SES disparities remains unclear. Hence, we agree with current efforts of the National Institute for Neurological Disorders and Stroke that *"Identifying and implementing effective solutions to combat disparities in stroke will require sustained and concerted efforts from the research community."*[72]

REFERENCES

1. Go AS, Mozaffarian D, Roger VL, et al. Heart disease and stroke statistics – 2013 update: a report from the American Heart Association. Circulation 2013;127:e6–245.
2. U. S. Burden of Disease Collaborators. The state of US health, 1990–2010: burden of diseases, injuries, and risk factors. JAMA 2013;310:591–608.
3. Taylor TN, Davis PH, Torner JC, et al. Lifetime cost of stroke in the United States. Stroke 1996;27:1459–66.
4. S. 1880 – 106th Congress: Minority Health and Health Disparities Research and Education Act of 2000, 106–525 (2000).
5. Wylie CM. Death statistics for cerebrovascular disease: a review of recent findings. Stroke 1970;1:184–93.
6. Compressed Mortality File 1999–2009. CDC WONDER Online Database, compiled from Compressed Mortality File 1999–2009 Series 20 No. 2O, 2012: Centers for Disease Control and Prevention, National Center for Health Statistics; [November 20, 2013]. Available from: http://wonder.cdc.gov/.
7. Arias E, Schauman WS, Eschbach K, et al. The validity of race and Hispanic origin reporting on death certificates in the United States. Vital Health Stat 2008;148:1–23.
8. Halanych JH, Shuaib F, Parmar G, et al. Agreement on cause of death between proxies, death certificates, and clinician adjudicators in the Reasons for Geographic and Racial Differences in Stroke (REGARDS) study. Am J Epidemiol 2011;173:1319–26.
9. Sacco RL, Boden-Albala B, Gan R, et al. Stroke incidence among white, black, and Hispanic residents of an urban community: the Northern Manhattan Stroke Study. Am J Epidemiol 1998;147: 259–68.
10. Kissela B, Schneider A, Kleindorfer D, et al. Stroke in a biracial population: the excess burden of stroke among blacks. Stroke 2004;35:426–31.
11. Howard VJ, Kleindorfer DO, Judd SE, et al. Disparities in stroke incidence contributing to disparities in stroke mortality. Ann Neurol 2011;69(4):619–27. [Epub 2011/03/19. eng]; PubMed PMID: 21416498.
12. Howard G, Cushman M, Kissela BM, et al. Traditional risk factors as the underlying cause of racial disparities in stroke: lessons from the half-full (empty?) glass. Stroke 2011;42(12):3369–75. [Epub 2011/10/01. eng]; PubMed PMID: 21960581. Pubmed Central PMCID: 3226886.
13. Kleindorfer D, Broderick J, Khoury J, et al. The unchanging incidence and case-fatality of stroke in the 1990s: a population-based study. Stroke 2006;37(10):2473–8. PubMed PMID: 16946146.
14. Kennedy BS, Kasl SV, Brass LM, et al. Trends in hospitalized stroke for blacks and whites in the United States, 1980–1999. Neuroepidemiology 2002;21(3):131–41. PubMed PMID: 12006776.
15. Rosamond WD, Folsom AR, Chambless LE, et al. Stroke incidence and survival among middle-aged adults: 9-year follow-up of the Atherosclerosis Risk in Communities (ARIC) cohort. Stroke 1999;30(4):736–43. [Epub 1999/04/03. eng]; PubMed PMID: 10187871.
16. Qian F, Fonarow GC, Smith EE, et al. Racial and ethnic differences in outcomes in older patients with acute ischemic stroke. Circ Cardiovasc Qual Outcomes 2013;6(3):284–92. PubMed PMID: 23680966.
17. Xian Y, Holloway RG, Noyes K, et al. Racial differences in mortality among patients with acute ischemic stroke: an observational study. Ann Int Med 2011;154:152–9.
18. Hanchate AD, Schwamm LH, Huang W, et al. Comparison of ischemic stroke outcomes and patient and hospital characteristics by race/ethnicity and socioeconomic status. Stroke 2013; 44(2):469–76. PubMed PMID: 23306327. Pubmed Central PMCID: 3595403.
19. Kleindorfer DO, Khoury J, Moomaw CJ, et al. Stroke incidence is decreasing in whites but not in blacks: a population-based estimate of temporal trends in stroke incidence from the Greater Cincinnati/Northern Kentucky Stroke Study. Stroke 2010; 41(7):1326–31. [Epub 2010/05/22. eng]; PubMed PMID: 20489177. Pubmed Central PMCID: 2904073.
20. Kissela BM, Khoury JC, Alwell K, et al. Age at stroke: temporal trends in stroke incidence in a large, biracial population. Neurology 2012;79(17):1781–7. PubMed PMID: 23054237. Pubmed Central PMCID: 3475622.
21. Giles WH, Kittner SJ, Hebel JR, et al. Determinants of black-white differences in the risk of cerebral infarction. The National Health and Nutrition Examination Survey Epidemiologic Follow-up Study. Arch Int Med 1995;155(12):1319–24. [Epub 1995/06/26. eng]; PubMed PMID: 7778964.

22. Wolf PA, D'Agostino RB, Belanger AJ, et al. Probability of stroke: a risk profile from the Framingham Study. Stroke 1991;22(3):312–18. [Epub 1991/03/01. eng]; PubMed PMID: 2003301.
23. Hertz RP, Unger AN, Cornell JA, et al. Racial disparities in hypertension prevalence, awareness, and management. Arch Int Med 2005;165(18):2098–104. [Epub 2005/10/12. eng]; PubMed PMID: 16216999.
24. Howard G, Prineas R, Moy C, et al. Racial and geographic differences in awareness, treatment, and control of hypertension: the REasons for Geographic And Racial Differences in Stroke study. Stroke 2006;37(5):1171–8. [Epub 2006/03/25. eng]; PubMed PMID: 16556884.
25. Cox AM, McKevitt C, Rudd AG, et al. Socioeconomic status and stroke. Lancet Neurol 2006;5(2):181–8. PubMed PMID: 16426994.
26. Addo J, Ayerbe L, Mohan KM, et al. Socioeconomic status and stroke: an updated review. Stroke 2012;43(4):1186–91. PubMed PMID: 22363052.
27. Liu L, Xue F, Ma J, et al. Social position and chronic conditions across the life span and risk of stroke: a life course epidemiological analysis of 22 847 American adults in ages over 50. Int J Stroke 2013;8(Suppl. 100):50–5. PubMed PMID: 23231424. Pubmed Central PMCID: 3610802.
28. Hippisley-Cox J, Coupland C, Brindle P. Derivation and validation of QStroke score for predicting risk of ischaemic stroke in primary care and comparison with other risk scores: a prospective open cohort study. BMJ 2013;346:f2573. PubMed PMID: 23641033. Pubmed Central PMCID: 3641809.
29. Khera A, McGuire DK, Murphy SA, et al. Race and gender differences in C-reactive protein levels. J Am Coll Cardiol 2005; 46(3):464–9. PubMed PMID: 16053959.
30. Cao JJ, Thach C, Manolio TA, et al. C-reactive protein, carotid intima-media thickness, and incidence of ischemic stroke in the elderly: the Cardiovascular Health Study. Circulation 2003; 108(2):166–70. PubMed PMID: 12821545.
31. Howard G, Lackland DT, Kleindorfer DO, et al. Racial differences in the impact of elevated systolic blood pressure on stroke risk. JAMA 2013;173(1):46–51. PubMed PMID: 23229778. Pubmed Central PMCID: 3759226.
32. Morgenstern LB, Smith MA, Sanchez BN, et al. Persistent Ischemic stroke disparities despite declining incidence in mexican americans. Ann Neurol 2013;[Epub 2013, July 10]; PubMed PMID: 23868398.
33. White H, Boden-Albala B, Wang C, et al. Ischemic stroke subtype incidence among whites, blacks, and Hispanics: the Northern Manhattan Study. Circulation 2005;111(10):1327–31. PubMed PMID: 15769776.
34. Howard G. Ancel Keys Lecture: Adventures (and misadventures) in understanding (and reducing) disparities in stroke mortality. Stroke 2013;44(11):3254–9. PubMed PMID: 24029634.
35. Zhang Y, Galloway JM, Welty TK, et al. Incidence and risk factors for stroke in American Indians: the Strong Heart Study. Circulation 2008;118(15):1577–84. [Epub 2008/09/24. eng]; PubMed PMID: 18809797. Pubmed Central PMCID: 2754380.
36. Joubert J, Prentice LF, Moulin T, et al. Stroke in rural areas and small communities. Stroke 2008;39(6):1920–8. [Epub 2008/04/19. eng]; PubMed PMID: 18420955.
37. Adams PF, Hendershot GE, Marano MA, et al. Current estimates from the National Health Interview Survey, 1996. Vital Health Stat 10 1999;(200):1–203. [Epub 2005/03/24. eng]; PubMed PMID: 15782448.
38. Sergeev AV. Racial and rural-urban disparities in stroke mortality outside the Stroke Belt. Ethn Dis 2011;21(3):307–13. [Epub 2011/09/29. eng]; PubMed PMID: 21942163.
39. Thrift AG, Cadilhac DA, Thayabaranathan T, et al. Global stroke statistics. Int J Stroke 2014;9(1):6–18. PubMed PMID: 24350870.
40. Borhani NO. Changes and Geographic Distribution of Mortality from Cerebrovascular Disease. Am J Pub Health Nations Health 1965;55:673–81. [Epub 1965/05/01. eng]; PubMed PMID: 14287837. Pubmed Central PMCID: 1256296.
41. Centers for Disease C, Prevention. Regional and racial differences in prevalence of stroke–23 states and District of Columbia, 2003. MMWR Morb Mortal Wkly Rep 2005;54(19):481–4. [Epub 2005/05/20. eng]; PubMed PMID: 15902070.
42. Hall WD, Ferrario CM, Moore MA, et al. Hypertension-related morbidity and mortality in the southeastern United States. Am J Med Sci 1997;313(4):195–209. [Epub 1997/04/01. eng]; PubMed PMID: 9099149.
43. Lanska DJ. Geographic distribution of stroke mortality in the United States: 1939–1941 to 1979–1981. Neurology 1993;43(9): 1839–51. [Epub 1993/09/01. eng]; PubMed PMID: 8414045.
44. Perry HM, Roccella EJ. Conference report on stroke mortality in the southeastern United States. Hypertension 1998;31(6):1206–15. [Epub 1998/06/11. eng]; PubMed PMID: 9622131.
45. Howard G, Evans GW, Pearce K, et al. Is the stroke belt disappearing? An analysis of racial, temporal, and age effects. Stroke 1995;26(7):1153–8. [Epub 1995/07/01. eng]; PubMed PMID: 7604406.
46. Howard G, Labarthe DR, Hu J, et al. Regional differences in African Americans' high risk for stroke: the remarkable burden of stroke for Southern African Americans. Ann Epidemiol 2007;17(9):689–96. [Epub 2007/08/28. eng]; PubMed PMID: 17719482. Pubmed Central PMCID: 1995237.
47. Yang D, Howard G, Coffey CS, et al. The confounding of race and geography: how much of the excess stroke mortality among African Americans is explained by geography? Neuroepidemiology 2004;23(3):118–22. [Epub 2004/04/16. eng]; PubMed PMID: 15084780.
48. Howard G, Anderson R, Johnson NJ, et al. Evaluation of social status as a contributing factor to the stroke belt region of the United States. Stroke 1997;28(5):936–40. PubMed PMID: 9158628.
49. Casper MLBE, Williams GI Jr, Halverson JA, et al. Atlas of Stroke Mortality: Racial, Ethnic, and Geographic Disparities in the United States. Atlanta, GA: Department of Health and Human Services, Centers for Disease Control and Prevention; 2003.
50. Schieb LJ, Mobley LR, George M, et al. Tracking stroke hospitalization clusters over time and associations with county-level socioeconomic and healthcare characteristics. Stroke 2013;44(1): 146–52. PubMed PMID: 23192758.
51. Labarthe DR, Howard G, Peace F, et al. Incidence and Case Fatality at the County Level as Contributors to Geographic Disparities in Stroke Mortality: The REasons for Geographic And Racial Differences in Stroke (REGARDS) Study. International Stroke Conference [Internet]. ATMP44. Available from: http://stroke.ahajournals.org/gca?allch=&submit=Go&gca=strokeaha%3B44%2F2_MeetingAbstracts%2FATMP44.
52. Wadley VG, Unverzagt FW, McGuire LC, et al. Incident cognitive impairment is elevated in the stroke belt: the REGARDS study. Ann Neurol 2011;70(2):229–36. [Epub 2011/05/28. eng]; PubMed PMID: 21618586. Pubmed Central PMCID: 3152671.
53. Howard G. Why do we have a stroke belt in the southeastern United States? A review of unlikely and uninvestigated potential causes. Am J Med Sci 1999;317(3):160–7. [Epub 1999/04/01. eng]; PubMed PMID: 10100689.
54. Obisesan TO, Vargas CM, Gillum RF. Geographic variation in stroke risk in the United States. Region, urbanization, and hypertension in the Third National Health and Nutrition Examination Survey. Stroke 2000;31(1):19–25. [Epub 2000/01/08. eng]; PubMed PMID: 10625710.
55. Cushman M, Cantrell RA, McClure LA, et al. Estimated 10-year stroke risk by region and race in the United States: geographic and racial differences in stroke risk. Ann Neurol 2008;64(5):507–13. [Epub 2008/12/11. eng]; PubMed PMID: 19067365. Pubmed Central PMCID: 2802965.
56. Modan B, Wagener DK. Some epidemiological aspects of stroke: mortality/morbidity trends, age, sex, race, socioeconomic status. Stroke 1992;23(9):1230–6. PubMed PMID: 1519276.
57. Kleindorfer DO, Lindsell C, Broderick J, et al. Impact of socioeconomic status on stroke incidence: a population-based study. Ann Neurol 2006;60(4):480–4. PubMed PMID: 17068796.
58. Lisabeth LD, Diez Roux AV, Escobar JD, et al. Neighborhood environment and risk of ischemic stroke: the brain attack surveillance in Corpus Christi (BASIC) Project. Am J Epidemiol 2007;165(3): 279–87. PubMed PMID: 17077168.
59. Brown AF, Liang LJ, Vassar SD, et al. Neighborhood disadvantage and ischemic stroke: the Cardiovascular Health Study (CHS). Stroke 2011;42(12):3363–8. PubMed PMID: 21940966. Pubmed Central PMCID: 3781011.

60. Avendano M, Kawachi I, Van Lenthe F, et al. Socioeconomic status and stroke incidence in the US elderly: the role of risk factors in the EPESE study. Stroke 2006;37(6):1368–73. PubMed PMID: 16690902.
61. Avendano M, Glymour MM. Stroke disparities in older Americans: is wealth a more powerful indicator of risk than income and education? Stroke 2008;39(5):1533–40. PubMed PMID: 18436891. Pubmed Central PMCID: 3079499.
62. Grotto I, Huerta M, Sharabi Y. Hypertension and socioeconomic status. Curr Opin Cardiol 2008;23(4):335–9. PubMed PMID: 18520717.
63. Minor D, Wofford M, Wyatt SB. Does socioeconomic status affect blood pressure goal achievement? Curr Hyper Rep 2008;10(5):390–7. PubMed PMID: 18775118.
64. Agardh E, Allebeck P, Hallqvist J, et al. Type 2 diabetes incidence and socio-economic position: a systematic review and meta-analysis. Int J Epidemiol 2011;40(3):804–18. PubMed PMID: 21335614.
65. Espelt A, Arriola L, Borrell C, et al. Socioeconomic position and type 2 diabetes mellitus in Europe 1999–2009: a panorama of inequalities. Curr Diabetes Rev 2011;7(3):148–58. PubMed PMID: 21418003.
66. Freedman KS, Nelson NM, Feldman LL. Smoking initiation among young adults in the United States and Canada, 1998–2010: a systematic review. Prev Chron Dis 2012;9:E05. PubMed PMID: 22172172. Pubmed Central PMCID: 3277388.
67. Brown AF, Liang LJ, Vassar SD, et al. Neighborhood socioeconomic disadvantage and mortality after stroke. Neurology 2013;80(6):520–7. PubMed PMID: 23284071. Pubmed Central PMCID: 3589286.
68. Kapral MK, Fang J, Chan C, et al. Neighborhood income and stroke care and outcomes. Neurology 2012;79(12):1200–7. PubMed PMID: 22895592. Pubmed Central PMCID: 3440450.
69. Kleindorfer D, Lindsell C, Alwell KA, et al. Patients living in impoverished areas have more severe ischemic strokes. Stroke 2012;43(8):2055–9. PubMed PMID: 22773557. Pubmed Central PMCID: 3432858.
70. Centers for Disease C, Prevention. Ten great public health achievements–United States, 1900–1999. MMWR 1999;48(12): 241–3. [Epub 1999/04/29. eng]; PubMed PMID: 10220250.
71. Centers for Disease C, Prevention. Ten great public health achievements–United States, 2001–2010. MMWR 2011;60(19): 619–23. PubMed PMID: 21597455.
72. Pahigiannis K, Waddy SP, Koroshetz W. Toward solutions for minimizing disparities in stroke: National Institute of Neurological Disorders and Stroke update. Stroke 2013;44(10):e129–30. PubMed PMID: 24021681.

15 Modifiable Risk Factors and Determinants of Stroke

Sudha Seshadri, Philip A. Wolf

KEY POINTS

- This chapter briefly summarizes key evidence gathered over the past 50 years on the determinants of stroke, focusing on risk factors that are relatively common and modifiable, hence important for prevention of stroke.
- Data from large, prospective epidemiological cohort studies are summarized here, whereas clinical trial data are described in Chapter 19.
- Carotid bruits increase risk of stroke two- to threefold, but likely as markers of systemic atherosclerotic burden rather than local stenosis.
- Major risk factors for stroke include elevated blood pressure, diabetes, smoking, prior cardiovascular events or current cardiovascular diseases (coronary heart disease, heart failure, atrial fibrillation, peripheral vascular disease), obesity, low HDL cholesterol, low levels of physical activity, a positive family history of stroke before age 65, and several circulating biomarkers such as homocysteine levels and indices of inflammation.
- The metabolic syndrome, use of oral contraceptives and estrogen replacement after menopause, migraine, heavy alcohol use, obstructive sleep apnea syndrome, stress are other less firmly established stroke risk factors also discussed.
- Risk factors tend to cluster and need to be considered together in estimating stroke risk in individuals; the Framingham Stroke Risk Profile and other clinical risk predictors permit this to be done during an office visit.

Epidemiology is "the study of the distribution and determinants of disease frequency" in human populations. Population research for stroke is concerned with learning in what particulars those who go on to have a stroke differ from those who stay free of the condition over long periods of follow-up. It is concerned with assessment of risk and seeking predisposing risk factors. Consideration of the burden and distribution of stroke by geographic region, race-ethnicity, age, and gender has been dealt with in Chapters 13 and 14. We focus on the determinants of stroke: risk factors and predisposing conditions, including measures for stroke prevention. Although several medical and surgical therapies to reduce the damage from impending or recent-onset stroke have been shown to be effective in selected patients and deserve continued research and attention in practice, it seems likely that *prevention* will continue to be the most effective strategy for reducing the health and economic consequences of cerebrovascular disease. Prevention is facilitated by an understanding of predisposing host and environmental factors, particularly modifiable environmental factors. The relative impact of each of these factors has become clearer, chiefly through prospective epidemiologic investigation. Controlled clinical trials have demonstrated the effectiveness of some risk factor modifications in stroke prevention – addressed in Chapter 19. In this chapter, data obtained from a number of prospective observational studies of populations will be presented. In particular, assessment of risk factors measured systematically and prospectively in a variety of populations, before the appearance of disease, provides the least distorted picture of the influence of these host and environmental factors on stroke incidence.

MAGNITUDE OF THE PROBLEM

Stroke is the most common life-threatening neurologic disease and fourth leading cause of death in the US. Among the elderly, the segment of the population in whom stroke occurs most frequently, it is a major cause of disability requiring long-term institutionalization.

MORTALITY

Stroke accounted for about one of every 19 deaths in the US in 2010. About half of these deaths occurred out of hospital. The 2010 overall death rate per 100,000 for stroke was 39.1. Mortality rates per 100,000 were higher in black men and women (67.1) than in whites. Because women live longer than men, more women than men die of stroke each year. Women accounted for approximately 60% of US stroke deaths in 2010.[1]

Stroke case fatality rates are high: 8–12% of ischemic strokes and 37–38% of hemorrhagic strokes result in death within 30 days. From 2000 to 2010, the annual stroke death rate decreased 35.8%; however, because of the aging population, the actual number of stroke deaths declined only 22.8%.[1,2]

COST

The estimated direct and indirect cost of stroke for 2010 was $36.5 billion. The mean lifetime cost of ischemic stroke in the US is estimated at $140,048 in 1999 dollars. This includes inpatient care, rehabilitation, and follow-up care necessary for lasting deficits. Inpatient hospital costs for an acute stroke account for 70% of first-year post-stroke costs. Age, sex, and insurance status are unassociated with stroke cost. Severe strokes (National Institutes of Health Stroke Scale score, > 20) cost twice as much as mild strokes, despite similar diagnostic testing. Comorbidities such as ischemic heart disease and atrial fibrillation (AF) predict higher costs.[1]

INCIDENCE OF STROKE

The incidence of stroke should be ascertained by systematic evaluation of a population determined to be free of the disease at outset. Ideally, the population under study should be representative of a general population.

The incidence of stroke was ascertained from prospective study over 55 years of follow-up of 5184 men and women, ages 30–62, who were free of stroke at entry to the Framingham Study in 1950. The population has been examined every 2 years, and follow-up has been satisfactory in that approximately 85% of subjects have participated in each examination. After 55 years of follow-up in the Framingham Study, there were 893 cases of initial completed strokes and 152 instances of isolated transient ischemic attacks (TIA). The average annual incidence of stroke events increased with age and approximately doubled in successive decades. Overall, the annual age-adjusted (ages 35–94 years) total initial completed stroke event rates were 5.89/1000 in men and 4.91/1000 in women; a 20% excess was seen in men (Table 15-1). The annual age-adjusted (ages 35–94 years) incidence of isolated TIA also increased with age and was 1.2/1000 in men and 0.7/1000 in women. Perspective concerning incidence of symptomatic coronary heart disease (CHD) and stroke may be gained by a comparison of analogous manifestations, myocardial infarction (MI) (n = 1206), and ischemic stroke with no clear cardiac source for emboli, termed atherothrombotic brain infarction (ABI) (n = 536) (Fig. 15-1). When these two major manifestations of atherosclerotic disease are compared for men, the age-adjusted average annual incidence rate of MI was

TABLE 15-1 Annual Incidence of Atherothrombotic Brain Infarction (ABI) and Completed Strokes in Men and Women Aged 35 to 94 Years

	Men		Women		Men/Women Combined	
Age	*n*	*Rate/1000*	*n*	*Rate/1000*	*n*	*Rate/1000*
ABI						
35–44	1	0.12	1	0.1	2	0.11
45–54	15	0.97	13	0.67	28	0.81
55–64	37	1.94	35	1.4	72	1.64
65–74	80	5.14	68	3	148	3.87
75–84	79	9.06	119	7.52	198	8.07
85–94	16	8.64	72	13.79	88	12.44
Total	228	*3.60	308	*2.90	536	3.21
COMPLETED STROKE						
35–44	3	0.37	3	0.3	6	0.33
45–54	25	1.61	20	1.04	45	1.29
55–64	60	3.15	60	2.41	120	2.73
65–74	127	8.16	115	5.08	242	6.33
75–84	126	14.45	203	12.83	329	13.41
85–94	30	16.21	121	23.18	151	21.35
Total	371	*5.89	522	*4.91	893	5.35

*Age-adjusted.
Data from the Framingham Heart Study: 55-year follow-up.

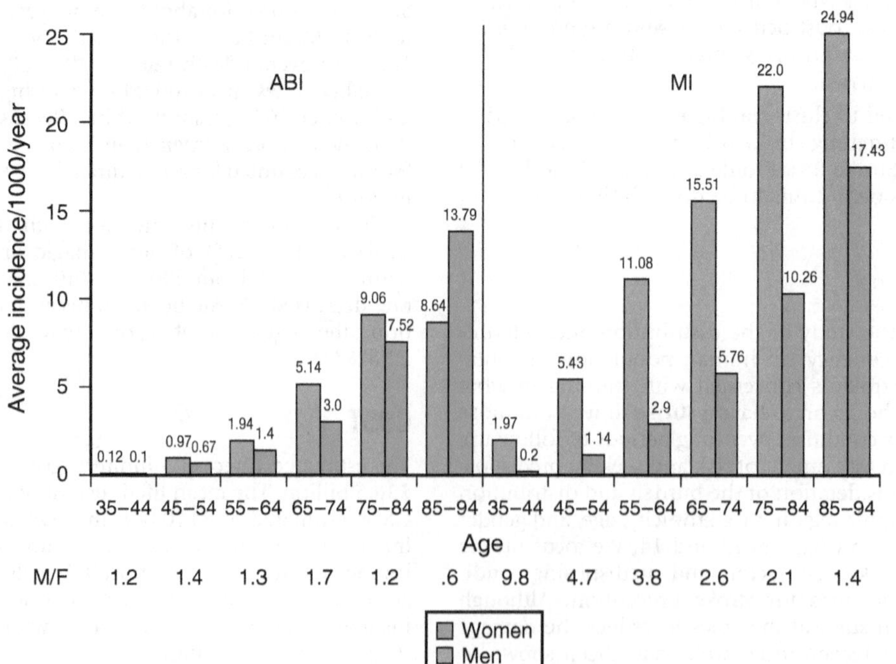

Figure 15-1. Incidence of atherothrombotic brain infarction (ABI) and myocardial infarction (MI); 50-year follow-up for the Framingham Heart Study. *(Data from the Framingham Heart Study.)*

4.1 times that of ABI; for women MI incidence was 1.6 times that of ABI. When the relative incidences are compared between the two genders, MI developed 2.6 times more often in men than in women, whereas ABI was approximately 1.24 times more frequent in men. In both sexes, rates doubled with each advancing decade. The 20-year lag in incidence of MI in women compared to men was not seen for ABI as age-specific rates were similar for both men and women.

FREQUENCY OF STROKE BY TYPE

The in-hospital assessment of stroke at Framingham by a study neurologist has helped document the stroke and determine stroke subtype as well as differentiate stroke from other neurologic diseases. Diagnosis of lacunar infarction was based on clinical and brain CT and MRI scan findings, whereas criteria for embolic infarction required a definite cardiac source for embolism. Distinction of cerebral infarction resulting from extracranial versus intracranial arterial disease was made on clinical grounds relying on non-invasive carotid studies and magnetic resonance angiography. Contrast angiography was requested only infrequently by the study subjects' personal physicians, chiefly in cases of extracranial carotid stenosis before endarterectomy or with subarachnoid hemorrhage (SAH). The occurrence of TIA was obtained by systematic routine questioning on each biennial examination since 1971 and by scrutiny of physician records and hospital notes. This surveillance for TIA has been comprehensive and systematic. In addition to the 15.1% of ABIs preceded by TIA, there were 148 persons whose initial cerebrovascular symptoms fulfilled criteria for TIA but who did not sustain a subsequent stroke. These isolated TIAs accounted for 14.8% of total cerebrovascular events in men and 12.7% of events in women.

The relative frequency of completed stroke by type was nearly identical in men and women (Table 15-2). ABI, which included infarction secondary to large vessel atherothrombosis, lacunar infarction, and infarct of undetermined cause, occurred most frequently: 61.5% in men and 60.0% in women. Intracranial hemorrhage accounted for 14.0% of completed strokes in men and 13.4% in women. Although a greater number of intracerebral hemorrhage (IH) and SAH occurred in women than in men, age-adjusted annual incidence rates of IH were higher in men than in women (0.52 vs 0.38 per 1000); rates of SAH were not appreciably different at 0.29 per 1000 in men and 0.28 in women. The relative frequency of IH and SAH varies according to the age of the population studied: SAH predominates below age 65 and is roughly equivalent at ages 65–74 years. At ages 75–84 years IH predominates: the incidence is 1.26 per 1000 annually compared with 0.29 per 1000 for SAH.

Covert (Silent) Stroke

It is now recognized that silent ischemic vascular insufficiency and infarction is a common occurrence in the peripheral and cerebral arterial vascular territories as well as in the heart. It is common to find CT scan or MRI evidence of a prior stroke without a history of such an event. In 1989, the Framingham Study reported the first population-based CT confirmation of the high prevalence (10–11%) of silent cerebral infarction that was later reported in the Stroke Data Bank investigation of hospitalized stroke patients from the National Institutes of Neurological and Communicative Disorders and Stroke.[3,4] MRI-defined infarcts were also similarly found to be associated with prevalent strokes in the population-based case-control Cardiovascular Health Study (CHS)[5] and in subsequent population-based data from the Framingham Heart Study,[6] the Northern Manhattan Study (NOMAS),[7] and the Rotterdam Study[8] among others; the MRI prevalence varied in the range of 10–20%, depending largely on the mean age of the study sample, the prevalence increasing with increasing age. The likely reason for their being unrecognized is their small size and location in brain areas likely to evoke minimal symptoms. They have been found in apparently healthy persons with hypertension, diabetes, elevated levels of plasma homocysteine and in patients with manifest atherosclerotic vascular disease.[6,9,10] Though the manifestations of these covert infarcts are clinically inapparent they are clearly not silent in that they are harbingers of future clinically manifest strokes and dementia and are associated with reduced executive function and depressed mood.[11,12] The risk of stroke is higher in Hispanic and Black communities than in Whites (Fig. 15-2). The impact of race and ethnicity on stroke risk are described in Chapters 13 and 14.

Recurrent Stroke

Recurrent stroke is common and likely to increase in frequency in the population as life expectancy increases and the stroke case fatality rates decline. The immediate period after a stroke is critical for recurrence. About one-third of recurrent strokes within 2 years recorded by the Stroke Data Bank occurred within the first month.[13] The reported long-term cumulative recurrence rate for stroke was 14.1% in the Stroke Data Bank, which is close to the 25% recurrence rate over 5 years reported in the Northern Manhattan Stroke Study.[14,15] Observed mortality from stroke recurrence exceeds that for an initial stroke. Compared with data on risk factors for an initial stroke, information on risk factors for recurrent ischemic stroke is limited, and the reported rates of stroke recurrence vary because of methodologic differences in analysis or differences in age, gender, or coexistent morbidities among the cohorts studied.

Many of the same risk factors that predispose to initial strokes increase risk of recurrences. Known modifiable stroke risk factors include hypertension, smoking, obesity, heavy alcohol consumption, impaired glucose tolerance, and physical inactivity.[16] Prognosis after stroke is addressed more completely in Chapter 16.

People who have just had their first ischemic stroke often have elevated inflammatory biomarkers in their blood that

TABLE 15-2 Frequency of Completed Stroke by Type in Men and Women Aged 35 to 94 Years

	Men		Women		Total	
Completed Stroke	*n*	%	*n*	%	*n*	%
Atherothrombotic brain infarction	228	61.5	308	59	536	60
Cerebral embolus	87	23.5	137	26.2	224	25.1
Subarachnoid hemorrhage	20	5.4	28	5.4	48	5.4
Intracerebral hemorrhage	32	8.6	42	8	74	8.3
Other	4	1.1	7	1.3	11	1.2
Total	371	100	522	100	893	100

Data from the Framingham Heart Study: 55-year follow-up.

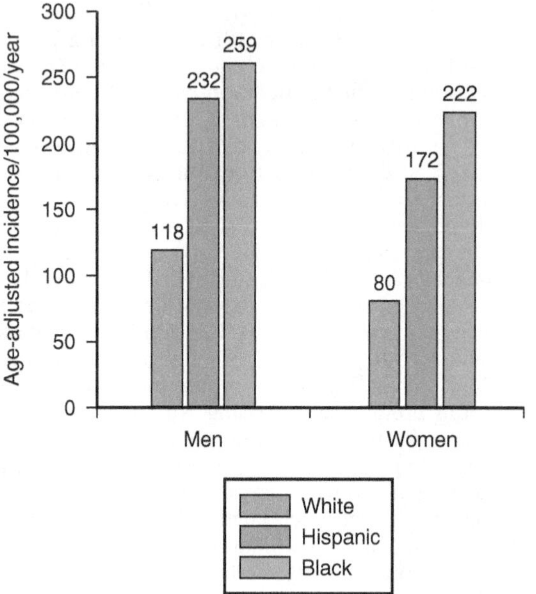

Figure 15-2. Stroke incidence according to race or ethnicity in the Northern Manhattan Stroke Study (NOMASS). *(From Sacco RL, Boden-Albala B, Gan R, et al: Stroke incidence among whites, blacks and Hispanics from the same community of Northern Manhattan.* Am J Epidemiol *147:260, 1998.)*

TABLE 15-3 Multivariable Risk Estimation of Stroke in Atrial Fibrillation: Framingham Study Cohorts – Predicted 5-Year Risk of Stroke

	Points*	Total Points	5-Year Risk (%)
Age (years)		*0–1*	*5*
50–59	0	2–3	6
60–62	1	4	7
63–66	2	5	8
67–71	3	6–7	9
72–74	4	8	11
75–77	5	9	12
78–81	6	10	13
82–85	7	11	14
86–90	8	12	16
91–93	9	13	18
>93	10	14	19
Diabetes		*15*	*21*
No	0	16	24
Yes	5	17	26
Prior stroke or TIA		*18*	*28*
No	0	19	31
Yes	6	20	34
Systolic BP (mm Hg)		*21*	*37*
<120	0	22	41
120–139	1	23	44
140–159	2	24	48
160–179	3	25	51
>179	4	26	55
Sex		*27*	*59*
Male	0	28	63
Female	6	29	67
		30	71
		31	75

*Add points to determine the 5-year risk of stroke as indicated in the total point score.

indicate an increased risk of dying or their likelihood of having another stroke.[17] The occurrence of an ischemic stroke usually signifies diffuse vascular atherosclerosis. Atherothrombotic brain infarctions are associated with about a twofold excess risk of cardiac failure and coronary disease, presumably on the basis of diffuse atherosclerosis. Cardiac failure occurs in about 15% of stroke patients over a period of 10 years, at virtually identical rates in men and women (Table 15-3). Coronary events can be expected in 44% of men and in 25% of women because of shared predisposing hypertension and diabetes. Various cardiac conditions increase the risk of developing a stroke.

Epidemiologic data indicate that development of a clinical atherosclerotic event in one arterial vascular territory is usually a hallmark of diffuse atherosclerosis and a heightened risk of clinical atherosclerotic events in other areas. The presence of cardiovascular risk factors common to all of the atherosclerotic cardiovascular disease outcomes suggests a universal pathogenesis promoting atherosclerosis in all vascular territories; however, some non-trivial differences exist. Although a better understanding of the reason for these differences is needed, it seems clear that measures taken against risk factors to prevent one atherosclerotic disease should carry a substantial bonus in also preventing atherosclerotic events in other vascular territories. Each of the standard risk factors has been shown to independently contribute to the occurrence of stroke and other atherosclerotic vascular disease, but the risk each imposes varies widely depending on the associated burden of other risk factors. This necessitates global risk evaluation with the use of multivariable risk formulations.

It is also important to recognize that the ultimate morbidity and mortality associated with a stroke are strongly affected by other cardiovascular events likely to make their appearance. For example, the risk of mortality is increased in persons with a stroke, but this mortality risk occurs not only from the stroke but also from cardiac failure and coronary disease. For example, not only do carotid bruits predict strokes, they also presage coronary disease, heart failure, and peripheral artery disease.

Vascular Bruits

Vascular bruits often signify the presence of diffuse as well as local vascular disease.[18] Because the femoral and carotid arteries are readily accessible for non-invasive assessment of the presence of obstructed blood flow, there is merit in detecting presymptomatic peripheral and cerebral arterial disease at a time when preventive measures can be effectively implemented to protect against occlusive clinical manifestations of atherogenesis in the brain. Although it is not surprising that femoral bruits are associated with a 20–30% prevalence of intermittent claudication, it is noteworthy that they are also associated with a significantly increased prevalence of atherothrombotic disease in other vascular territories.

Carotid bruits are indicators of vascular disease in the cerebral circulation and, as expected, are associated with a two- to threefold increase in the risk of stroke. However, they are also associated with a two- to threefold increase in the risk of developing peripheral artery disease (see Table 15-2). Detection of a carotid bruit is the most common finding leading to the diagnosis of asymptomatic carotid artery stenosis. A TIA is the most common expression of symptomatic carotid stenosis. Population-based data indicate that carotid bruits are present in 4–5% of persons older than 45 years and that its prevalence increases with age from 1% to 3% for those 45–54 years of age to 6–8% for persons older than 75 years.[18]

The Framingham Study population data indicate that it is associated with a stroke rate twice that expected for age and sex. However, more often than not, the brain infarction occurred in a vascular territory different from that of the carotid bruit, and lacunar infarction was the mechanism of stroke in nearly half the cases. Carotid bruit is clearly an indicator of increased risk of having a stroke, but largely as a consequence of systemic vascular disease and not necessarily as a direct effect of the local stenosis.[18]

RISK FACTORS FOR STROKE

It has been shown that risk factors differ between hemorrhagic and ischemic stroke and that the relative impact of risk factors operative in all ischemic stroke subtypes varies among its subtypes.[19] Identification of risk factors for stroke, awareness of the relative importance of each, and awareness of their interaction should facilitate stroke prevention. Because the pathogenetic process underlying the various stroke types differs, it is reasonable to expect that risk factors for infarction differ from risk factors for hemorrhage. Furthermore, precursors of intraparenchymatous bleeding are likely to differ from those for SAH. Risk factors for stroke from atherosclerosis of the carotid and vertebral arteries may well differ in their impact when compared with risk factors for stroke resulting from lacunar infarction. Precursors of embolic stroke are also likely to be different. Nevertheless, certain predisposing factors, particularly elevated blood pressure, are common to most stroke types.

Atherogenic Host Factors

The importance of the major atherogenic risk factors was assessed utilizing data from Framingham and other prospective epidemiologic studies. These risk factors include elevated blood pressure, blood lipid levels, diabetes, fibrinogen and other clotting factors, obesity, cardiac diseases (i.e., CHD, congestive heart failure [CHF], AF, left ventricular hypertrophy, and echocardiographic abnormalities), race, family history, and several circulating biomarkers, such as homocysteine levels and indices of inflammation.

Hypertension

Hypertension is the principal risk factor for ischemic stroke as well as for IH. Hypertension also predisposes to cardiac stroke precursors (notably MI and AF) that promote cerebral embolism. Elevated blood pressure also operates to increase the risk of SAH from aneurysm. Thus hypertension has the unique role of being a main risk factor for most types of stroke.

Hypertension and the Risk of Stroke. About 77% of people who have a first stroke, about 69% who have a first heart attack, and about 74% who have heart failure, have blood pressures higher than 140/90 mm Hg (National Heart, Lung and Blood Institute unpublished estimates from ARIC, CHS, and FHS). People with systolic blood pressures of 160 mm Hg or higher and/or diastolic blood pressures of 95 mm Hg or higher have a relative risk (RR) of stroke about four times greater than for those with normal blood pressures.[20,21] Hypertension is a powerful contributor to ABI in both sexes at all ages, including in persons 75–84 years of age.[22] It has been found to make a powerful and significant independent contribution to the incidence of ABI even after age and other pertinent risk factors had been taken into account (Fig. 15-3).[21,23] There is little support for the widely held belief of a stronger relation of hypertension to hemorrhagic than ischemic stroke.

Although hypertension increases the incidence of stroke and ABI, the level of risk is clearly related to the *height* of the blood pressure throughout its range. When the Framingham

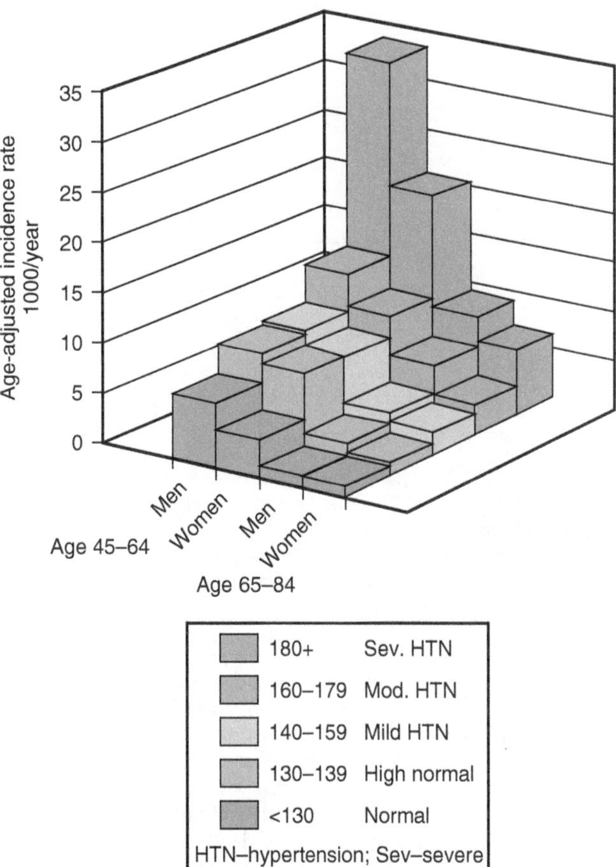

Figure 15-3. Incidence of stroke and systolic blood pressure level according to Joint National Committee VI categories; 50-year follow-up for the Framingham Study. *(From Wolf PA: Cerebrovascular risk. In Izzo JL, Black HR, editors:* Hypertension primer, the essentials of high blood pressure, *ed 3, Philadelphia, 2003, Lippincott Williams & Wilkins, pp 239–242.)*

cohort subjects are classified by the Joint National Committee seven systolic blood pressure categories, it is clear that the incidence of stroke increases with increasing blood pressure levels (see Fig. 15-3). However, more initial stroke events – hemorrhage as well as infarction – occurred in persons with Stage I (mild) hypertension (systolic blood pressure, 140 to 159 mm Hg) than in any other group (see Fig. 15-3). In fact, approximately half of the initial stroke events in Framingham occurred in subjects with pressures in the prehypertension/high normal (systolic pressure, 130–139 mm Hg) or in the mild hypertension categories (Fig. 15-4). On the basis of a combined analysis of nine major prospective (observational) studies of 420,000 individuals, a graded relationship between diastolic pressure and stroke and CHD incidence was apparent.[24]

Traditionally, greater importance has been ascribed to the diastolic than the systolic pressure level, although evidence for the ascendancy of diastolic blood pressure over systolic is lacking. The opposite is probably true. With advancing age, systolic blood pressure continues to rise into the 8th decade, whereas diastolic pressures decline after reaching a plateau in the early 50s. Systolic blood pressure level is clearly directly related to risk of stroke, particularly after age 65 years.[25]

Isolated Systolic Hypertension. In the elderly, isolated systolic hypertension (≥160/<90 mm Hg) becomes highly prevalent, affecting approximately 25% of persons older than 80 years. In Framingham, older subjects (65–84 years of age)

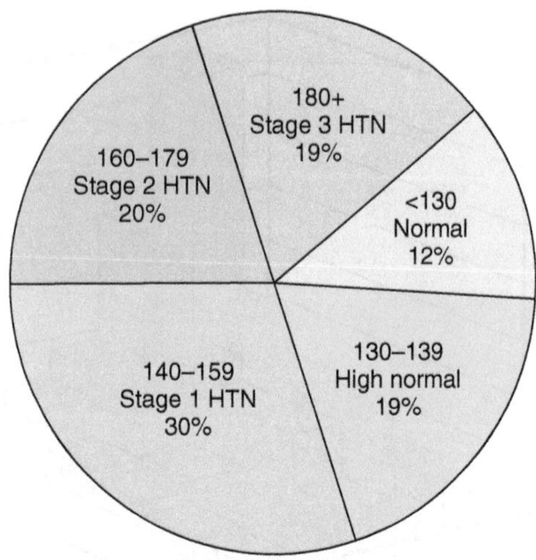

Figure 15-4. Percent of stroke by systolic blood pressure in subjects 45 to 64 years of age, the Framingham Study. *(From Wolf PA: Cerebrovascular risk. In Izzo JL, Black HR, editors:* Hypertension primer, the essentials of high blood pressure, *ed 3, Philadelphia, 2003, Lippincott Williams & Wilkins, pp 239–242.)*

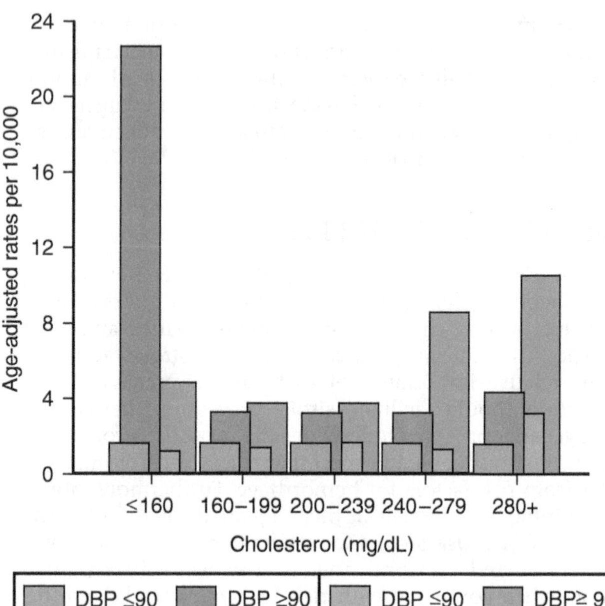

Figure 15-5. Ischemic stroke and intracerebral hemorrhage death rates in men with normal and elevated diastolic blood pressure (DBP) according to screening serum cholesterol level. *(From Wolf PA, Cobb JL, D'Agostino RB: Epidemiology of stroke. In Barnett HJM, Mohr JP, Stein BM, Yatsu FM, editors:* Stroke: Pathophysiology, diagnosis, and management, *ed 2, New York, 1992, Churchill Livingstone, p 16.)*

with isolated systolic hypertension had a high risk of stroke; the risk was doubled for men and increased by 1.5-fold for women. Antihypertensive therapy in the very elderly (i.e., persons 80 years or older) was beneficial: a 30% reduction in fatal and non-fatal strokes was seen after 2 years. This was associated with a 21% reduction in the rate of death from any cause, a 23% reduction in the rate of death from cardiovascular causes, and a 64% reduction in the rate of heart failure. Further, significantly fewer serious adverse events were reported in the active treatment group.[26]

Long-term Blood Pressure and Risk of Stroke. Blood pressure stroke risk predictions are generally based on the measurement of current blood pressure. Clearly, the duration of the blood pressure elevation, as well as its height and other host factors, contributes to its cardiovascular risk. When 50 years of blood pressure data from the Framingham Study are used, it is evident that elevated midlife blood pressure during the prior 10 years increases the RR of stroke by 1.7-fold per standard deviation increment in women and by 1.9-fold per standard deviation increment in men at age 60 years.[27] Similar increases in RR by elevated antecedent pressures were also seen at age 70. These data confirm clinical experience as well as prior prospective epidemiologic data that, at any level of pressure, persons with evidence of prior elevated blood pressure such as left ventricular hypertrophy by electrocardiography or increased left ventricular mass (LVM) on echocardiography are at increased risk of stroke.[28]

Blood Lipids

With increasing levels of total serum cholesterol, there is a steady increase in incidence of CHD in both sexes that declines with advancing age, but persists after accounting for other risk factors. However, for stroke generally and for non-embolic ischemic stroke in particular, there is no clear or consistent relationship of their incidence to antecedent blood lipid levels. A recent report from the ARIC study found only weak and inconsistent associations between ischemic stroke and each of five lipid factors in the 305 subjects who had ischemic stroke after 10 years of prospective investigation.[29] The authors noted that the lack of relationship of these lipid factors to ischemic stroke is at odds with their well-known association with CHD.[29] Furthermore, in a meta-analysis of 45 prospective epidemiologic studies comprising 450,000 subjects among whom 13,000 strokes occurred, no significant association between total serum cholesterol level and total stroke incidence was seen.[30] Possible exceptions were the Honolulu Heart Study of Hawaiian men of Japanese ancestry and the Multiple Risk Factor Intervention Trial (MRFIT) screenees.[31] In Honolulu, the level of total cholesterol measured years before was directly related to the incidence of thromboembolism.[32] In MRFIT, the incidence of ischemic stroke, diagnosed on death certificates, was greater in those with the highest levels of serum total cholesterol obtained 6 years before (Fig. 15-5).

Although the impact of blood lipids on ischemic atherothrombotic stroke differs from their relationship to coronary artery atherosclerosis, serum total cholesterol and low-density lipoprotein (LDL) cholesterol levels have been directly related to the extent of extracranial carotid artery atherosclerosis; high-density lipoprotein (HDL) cholesterol levels exert a protective effect. These relationships also apply to extracranial carotid artery wall thickness.[33-35] In a recent analysis of 6276 stroke-free FHS participants in whom we related serum total cholesterol, HDL, LDL and triglyceride levels to the 10-year risk of incident ischemic stroke (302 events over an average follow-up of 9 years), a low HDL (≤40) was associated with a 60% higher risk of ischemic stroke even after adjustment for other stroke risk factors, no associations were noted with total cholesterol or LDL levels. Triglyceride levels were associated with stroke risk in analyses adjusted only for age and sex, but not after additional adjustment for other stroke risk factors, such as diabetes, hypertension and prevalent cardiovascular disease. Despite the lack of association between LDL levels and stroke risk, the use of statins has been shown to reduce stroke risk (discussed in more detail in Chapter 19). It remains unclear as to what extent the beneficial effect of statins is mediated through lowering LDL, as statins can also act via other pathways, for example by reducing inflammation and C-reactive protein levels.

Low total serum cholesterol levels have been found to be related to an increased incidence of IH.[36] This was first noted after World War II among rural Japanese who had very low serum cholesterol levels by Western standards (i.e., <160 mg/dL).[37] As nutrition improved, intake of animal fat increased, and sodium chloride intake fell, an increase in total serum cholesterol levels was seen in this population.[37] In both sexes aged 40–49, the total serum cholesterol levels rose from 155 mg/dL in 1963–1966, to 175 mg/dL in 1972–1975, and to 181 mg/dL in 1980–1983. Total serum protein levels and relative weight also rose significantly during these 20 years, whereas systolic and diastolic blood pressures declined. Accompanying these major changes in risk factor levels were similar substantial declines in the incidence of IH, which fell 65% in men ($P < 0.05$) and 94% in women ($P < 0.001$) between 1964–1968 and 1979–1983.[37] An etiologic link has been suggested by the recent confirmation of this relationship in other Asian populations, as well as in white men in the US. In the 350,977 men aged 35–57 years who were screened for entry into the MRFIT, there were 83 deaths from IH and 55 deaths from SAH after 6 years of follow-up.[31] Compared with the lowest serum cholesterol category (<160 mg/dL), the risk-factor-adjusted RR of intracranial hemorrhage at all higher levels of serum cholesterol was approximately 0.32. Death rates per 10,000 were 23.07 in the lowest serum cholesterol category (<160 mg/dL) and ranged from 3.09 to 4.83 in the four higher categories.[31] The mechanism by which a very low serum cholesterol level accompanied by elevated diastolic blood pressure promotes IH has been suggested to be an alteration in the cell membranes that weakens the endothelium of intracerebral arteries. However, despite early concerns, significant increases in IH rates have not been noted in the many trials using statins to reduce total and LDL cholesterol levels.

Diabetes

Diabetic patients are known to have an increased susceptibility to coronary, femoral, and cerebral artery atherosclerosis. Up to 80% of type 2 diabetic patients will have macrovascular disease or die of it. Hypertension is common in diabetic patients, affecting approximately 60%. Surveys of stroke patients and prospective investigations have confirmed the increased risk of stroke in diabetic patients. The Honolulu Heart Program found that increasing degrees of glucose intolerance conferred an increasing risk of thromboembolic stroke that was independent of other risk factors, but found no relationship to hemorrhagic stroke (Fig. 15-6).[38,39] Evaluation of the impact of diabetes on stroke in a population-based cohort in Rancho Bernardo disclosed an RR of stroke that was 1.8 in men and 2.2 in women, even after adjustment for the effect of other pertinent risk factors.[39]

In the Framingham Study, peripheral artery disease with intermittent claudication occurs more than four times as often in diabetic patients; the coronary and cerebral arteries are also affected, but to a lesser extent.[40] For ABI, the impact of indicators of diabetes (i.e., physician-diagnosed diabetes, glycosuria, or a blood sugar level more than 150 mg/100 mL) was significant as an independent contributor to incidence only in older women. However, later follow-up indicated that both men and women with glucose intolerance at all ages have approximately double the risk of ABI of those without diabetes.[41]

Because it has been shown that persons on their way to developing diabetes are at twofold increased risk compared with persons without diabetes, interest is now focusing on the prediabetic insulin-resistant state. The Framingham Study found that the metabolic syndrome, an indicator of insulin resistance, carries a substantial risk of stroke.[41] Stroke risk was examined in men and women in relation to the metabolic syndrome alone, diabetes alone, and the presence of both. Over 14 years of follow-up, 75 men and 55 women had a first stroke; all but four events were ischemic. The RR of stroke in persons with both diabetes and metabolic syndrome (RR, 3.28; confidence interval [CI], 1.82–5.92) was higher than that for either condition alone (metabolic syndrome alone: RR, 2.10; CI, 1.37–3.22; diabetes alone: RR, 2.47; CI, 1.31–4.65). The population-attributable risk, because of its greater prevalence, was greater for metabolic syndrome alone than for diabetes alone (19% vs 7%), particularly in women (27% vs 5%). Thus, the metabolic syndrome is more prevalent than diabetes and a significant independent risk factor for stroke in people without diabetes. Prevention and control of the metabolic syndrome and its components, particularly the frequently associated hypertension, are likely to reduce stroke incidence (Fig. 15-7).

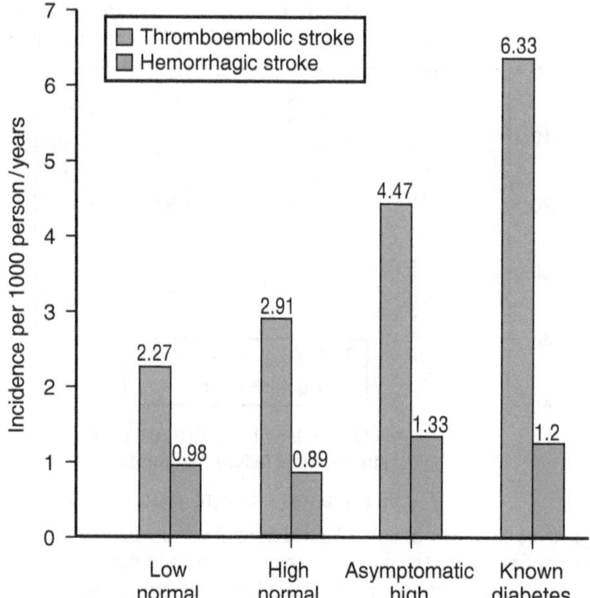

Figure 15-6. Incidence of stroke and glucose intolerance. Honolulu Heart Study; 22-year follow-up. *(From Burchfiel CM, Curb JD, Rodriguez BL, et al: Glucose intolerance and 22-year stroke incidence. The Honolulu Heart Program.* Stroke *25:951–957, 1994.)*

Obesity and Obstructive Sleep Apnea Syndrome

Obese persons have higher levels of blood pressure, blood glucose, and atherogenic serum lipids; on that account alone, they would be expected to have an increased risk of stroke. Obesity (relative weight ≥ 30% above the median) was a significant independent contributor to ABI incidence in younger men and older women in the Framingham original cohort. However, in all age groups and in both sexes, obesity exerts an adverse influence on health status that is probably mediated through elevated blood pressure, impaired glucose tolerance, insulin resistance, and other mechanisms. However, in the Honolulu Heart Study, obesity was a risk factor for stroke that was independent of associated hypertension, glucose intolerance, and other covariates. In the Nurses' Health Study, the incidence of stroke increased directly with body mass index in women aged 30–55 years after adjustment for other risk factors, but no such relationship was seen in men aged 40–75 years, comprising the Health Professionals Follow-up Study. Abdominal or central obesity seems more closely related to adverse cardiovascular outcomes including stroke

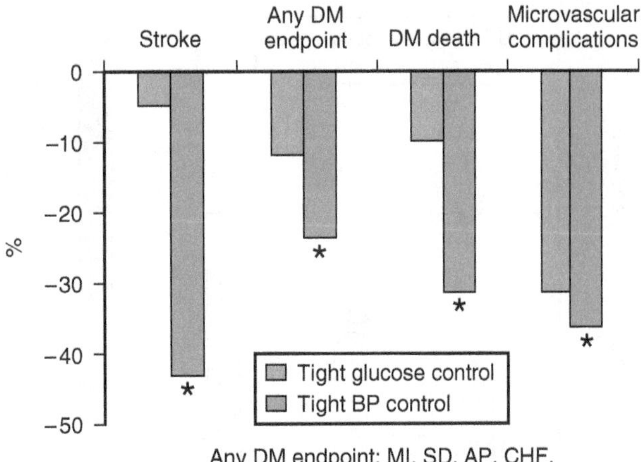

Figure 15-7. Effect of tight glucose control versus tight blood pressure control on cardiovascular disease outcomes in diabetic patients (United Kingdom Prospective Diabetes Study). *(From United Kingdom Prospective Diabetes Study Group: Tight blood pressure control and risk of macrovascular and microvascular complication in type 2 diabetes: UKPDS 38.* BMJ *317:703–713, 1998; and United Kingdom Prospective Diabetes Study Group: Efficacy of atenolol and captopril in reducing risk of macrovascular and microvascular complication in type 2 diabetes: UKPDS 39.* BMJ *317:713–720, 1998.)*

than overall elevated body mass index. In the NOMAS Study persons with a WHR equal to or greater than the median had an overall OR of 3.0 (95%CI, 2.1–4.2) for ischemic stroke even after adjustment for other risk factors and BMI, this was true in both sexes and all ethnic groups studied.[42] In 28,643 male health professionals, the RR of stroke was significantly greater (RR, 2.33; 95%CI, 1.25–4.37) in those men with a waist-to-hip ratio in the uppermost quintile. Obesity as reflected in the body mass index was less strongly related than waist circumference was to stroke incidence, likely as a result of its closer relationship to insulin resistance.[43]

Obstructive sleep apnea syndrome, frequently seen in obese patients, although it can occur in non-obese persons, has been independently associated with a doubling of stroke risk even after adjustment for age, sex, race, smoking status, alcohol-consumption status, body-mass index, and the presence or absence of diabetes mellitus, hyperlipidemia, atrial fibrillation, and hypertension (hazard ratio for association with a composite end-point of stroke or death:1.97; 95%CI, 1.12–3.48).[44]

Family History of Stroke

A family history of stroke is an important marker of increased stroke risk. Maternal history of death from stroke was significantly related to stroke incidence in a cohort of Swedish men born in 1913.[45] Maternal history of fatal stroke was independently related to stroke incidence in offspring, even after other significant risk factors such as hypertension, abdominal pattern of obesity, and fibrinogen level were taken into account.

In a study of familial predisposition to stroke in Framingham, there was no relationship between a *history* of stroke *death* in parents and documented stroke in subjects. However, definite non-fatal and fatal strokes in these cohort parents as determined by examination and systematic case review over decades were related to the observed *occurrence* of stroke in their children (members of the Framingham Offspring Study cohort). In these analyses, both maternal and paternal strokes by age 65 years were associated with approximately a threefold increased risk of stroke by age 65 years in their children, even after other risk factors were taken into account.[46]

These relationships were true for maternal and paternal strokes, total strokes, and ischemic stroke subtypes. This heritability strongly suggests a genetic propensity to stroke in addition to or in combination with environmental factors (see Chapter 18; Genetic basis of stroke occurrence, prevention and outcome).

Fibrinogen, Clotting Factors, and Inflammation

An elevated fibrinogen level has been implicated in atherogenesis and in arterial thrombus formation. A number of epidemiologic studies have found a significant independent increase in cardiovascular disease incidence, including stroke, in relation to fibrinogen level. In a prospective study of 54-year-old Swedish men, fibrinogen level in combination with elevated systolic blood pressure was found to be a potent risk factor for stroke.[47] Level of fibrinogen, measured on the tenth biennial examination in Framingham, was also significantly related to incidence of cardiovascular disease, including stroke.[48] In a large individual participant meta-analysis of 154,211 participants in 31 prospective studies, moderately strong associations and a continuous log-linear association were found between usual plasma fibrinogen level and the risks of stroke, as well as other CVD in a wide range of circumstances in healthy middle-aged adults.[49]

However, fibrinogen is associated with many other risk factors for stroke including age, hypertension, hematocrit level, obesity, and diabetes.[50] Fibrinogen is also an acute-phase reactant to inflammation, so it seems likely that the atherogenic and procoagulant effects of inflammation reflected by elevated fibrinogen levels are responsible for its association with cardiovascular disease incidence, including stroke. In the Framingham original cohort, CRP level was found to be an independent risk marker for stroke and TIA incidence over 14 years of follow-up. For men, those with CRP levels in the upper quartile had double the risk of stroke and TIA of men in the bottom quartile; for women, risk in the CRP upper quartile was increased nearly threefold after other pertinent risk factors were taken into account.[51] CRP was also a potent independent risk marker for cardiovascular disease in the Women's Health Study and was noted to be a stronger predictor than the LDL cholesterol level, making an independent contribution to cardiovascular disease risk prediction beyond that provided by the Framingham risk score.[52] Infections, especially periodontal, have been associated with an increased risk of stroke, perhaps by promoting systemic inflammation.[53]

Blood Homocysteine Levels

In a number of cross-sectional studies and case-control studies and in a meta-analysis, elevated levels of plasma homocysteine (tHcy) were found to be associated with a higher incidence of CHD (OR, 1.6 per 5 μmol/L tHcy) and an increased incidence of stroke (OR, 1.5 per 5 μmol/L tHcy).[54] Level of tHcy is also directly related to many of the major components of the cardiovascular risk profile: male sex, increasing age, cigarette smoking, increased blood pressure, elevated blood cholesterol level, and lack of exercise.[55] However, even after adjustment for these factors, the risk of stroke was independently related to non-fasting tHcy level in the original Framingham cohort after 9.9 years of follow-up: the RR of 1.82 (CI, 1.14–2.91) was seen in quartile 4 compared with quartile 1, and a significant linear trend was seen across the quartiles ($P < 0.001$).[56] A nested case-control study within the British Regional Heart Study cohort found a powerful and independent relationship

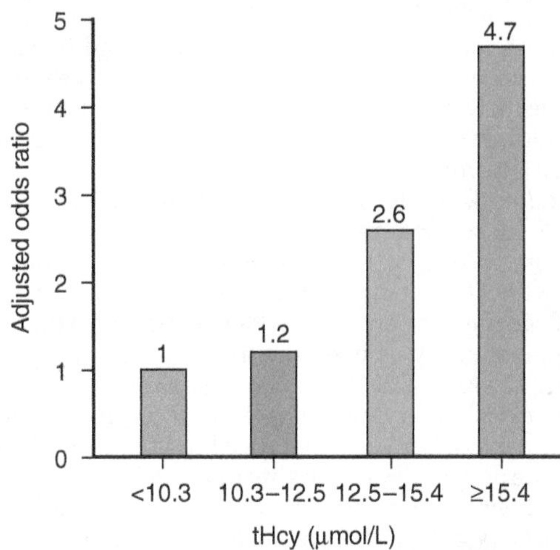

Figure 15-8. Homocysteine level and stroke risk in men; a case-control study. *(From Wolf PA: Epidemiology and risk factor management. In Welch M, Caplan LR, Reis DJ, et al, editors:* Primer on cerebrovascular disease, *San Diego, 1997, Academic Press, pp. 751–757.)*

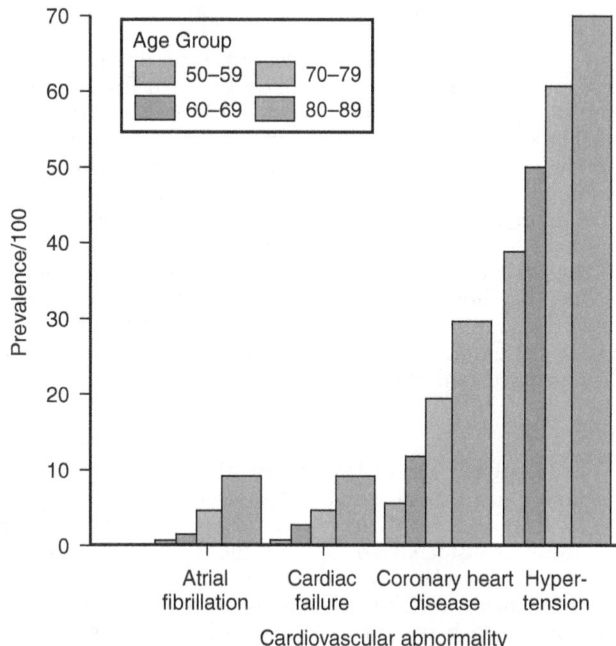

Figure 15-9. Prevalence of cardiovascular abnormality with increasing age, men and women combined; 34-year follow-up. *(Data from the Framingham Heart Study.)*

between non-fasting tHcy level and stroke incidence. There was a graded increase in risk with increasing quartile levels of tHcy (Fig. 15-8) from an OR of 1.2 (<10.3 μmol/L) to 4.7 (≈15.4 μmol/L) in successive quartiles of tHcy ($P = 0.03$ for trend). Risk in the uppermost quartile was 4.7-fold greater than in the lowest quartile. This graded response with no threshold occurred after adjustment for serum creatinine level (associated with increased tHcy levels), age, social class, blood pressure, and other pertinent risk factors.[57]

However, in some other large population studies (i.e., the ARIC study, Physicians Health Study, the Finnish Study, and MRFIT) no statistically significant relationship was found.[58] The ARIC study noted a strong independent relationship between fasting plasma tHcy concentrations and carotid artery intimal-medial wall thickening.[59] Increased levels of fasting plasma tHcy were also related to ultrasound-assessed extracranial common carotid artery stenosis of more than 25% in the Framingham cohort.[60] Plasma tHcy levels are inversely related to levels of dietary and plasma folic acid and vitamins B_{12} and B_6, which indicates a remedy for elevated tHcy levels.[61] The *fasting* tHcy level may miss persons with impaired tHcy metabolism because, in response to a methionine challenge, approximately 40% of persons with elevated tHcy levels, who are thought to be at increased cardiovascular risk, have normal fasting levels. Furthermore, tHcy level is like other physiologic measures such as blood pressure or serum cholesterol level in that it is a graded and continuous risk variable without a clear threshold effect. Nevertheless, a number of large-scale clinical trials in stroke survivors have not demonstrated a beneficial effect of folate (with B_6 and B_{12}) supplementation on risk of stroke recurrence.[62] Supplementation did reduce the level of tHcy in the serum, but did not result in lower rates of stroke or cardiovascular disease. Possible explanations for this puzzling finding include current universal supplementation of grains and cereals with folate in several countries and a relationship to level of vitamin B_{12}, among others.[63]

Heart Disease and Impaired Cardiac Function

Cardiac diseases and impaired cardiac function predispose to stroke. Although hypertension is the preeminent risk factor for strokes of all types, at each blood pressure level, persons with impaired cardiac function have a significantly increased stroke risk.[64] The prevalence of these cardiac contributors to stroke increases with age (Fig. 15-9). After 36 years of follow-up, the prevalence of cardiovascular disease among stroke cases in the Framingham Study was found to be high: 80.8% had hypertension; 32.7% had prior CHD; 14.5% had prior heart failure; 14.5% had AF; and only 13.6% had none of these. Cardiac disease is an important precursor of stroke and is also dealt with in detail in several other chapters.

Coronary Heart Disease

In Framingham, CHD was ascertained prospectively on biennial examination as well as by monitoring of hospitalizations. It predisposes to stroke as a source for embolism from the heart; by virtue of shared risk factors; as an untoward effect of medical and surgical treatments for coronary atherosclerotic disease; and, less commonly, as a consequence of pump failure. In the 2-week period after an acute MI, stroke occurs at an estimated rate of 0.7–4.7%.[65] As expected, older age and ventricular dysfunction (decreased ejection fraction) after MI increase stroke risk. Treatment with aspirin and, particularly, with warfarin anticoagulation decreased the incidence of stroke in a large group of MI survivors, which is consistent with an embolic mechanism.[65] Stroke occurs most frequently after *anterior* wall MI (2–6% of cases). The mechanism is cerebral embolism principally from a left ventricular mural thrombus, which is demonstrable on echocardiographic studies in 40% of cases. Inferior wall MI is an infrequent basis for mural thrombus or stroke. Often, however, the mechanism of stroke in persons with CHD is less apparent. Persons with uncomplicated angina pectoris, non-Q-wave infarction, and clinically silent MI also have an increased incidence of ischemic stroke. Data from Framingham suggest that silent or unrecognized MI survivors had a 10-year incidence of stroke of 17.8% in men and 17.3% in women, which is an incidence not that much less than the 19.5% in men and 29.3% in women seen after recognized MI.

Peripheral Artery Disease

The presence of peripheral artery disease often denotes widespread atherosclerotic vascular disease. In the Framingham study, 20% of persons 75 years or older had a low ankle brachial index (<0.9) denoting compromised peripheral arterial circulation. Among these, only 18% reported symptoms of intermittent claudication. In persons with a low ankle brachial index, cardiovascular disease was present in 50%, among whom 15% had experienced a stroke.

The prevalence of stroke and CHD increases continuously as the ankle brachial index decreases (see Fig. 15-1). A low ankle brachial index was shown to be associated with a 2.2-fold increase in risk of a stroke or TIA, even after adjustment for associated cardiovascular risk factors.[66]

Atrial Fibrillation

It has long been acknowledged that AF in association with rheumatic heart disease and mitral stenosis predisposes to stroke. Chronic AF without valvular heart disease, which was previously considered to be innocuous, has since been shown to be associated with approximately a fivefold increase in stroke incidence. This is ominous because AF is also the most prevalent persistent cardiac arrhythmia in the elderly. In the FHS, AF incidence has more than doubled in successive decades of follow-up. The incidence rises sharply with age from 0.2 per 1000 for ages 30–39 to 39.0 per 1000 for ages 80–89 years. AF is particularly important in the elderly because the proportion of total strokes associated with this arrhythmia increases steeply with age, reaching 36.2% for ages 80–89 years.[67, 68] Although the prevalence of other cardiac contributors to stroke also increases with age, the increased incidence of stroke in persons with AF is more likely to be a consequence of the AF and not the associated CHD or CHF. This becomes apparent when age trends in AF-associated risk of stroke are examined (Fig. 15-10). Whereas risk of stroke attributable to AF increases with age, risk of stroke attributable to cardiac failure, CHD, and hypertension decline with age.[67] Notably, in the oldest age group, 80–89 years, the percent of stroke attributable to AF was 23.5%, which approaches that of hypertension (33.4%), a far more prevalent disorder.

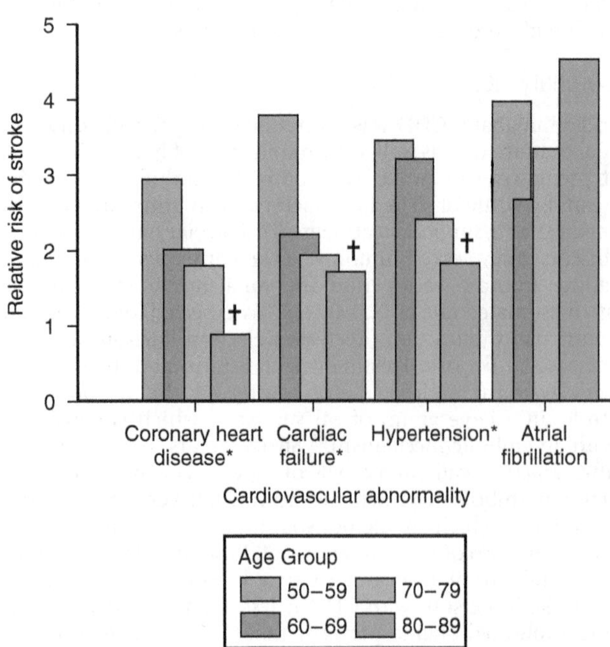

Figure 15-10. Estimated relative risk of stroke with advancing age according to the presence of coronary heart disease, cardiac failure, hypertension, and atrial fibrillation; 34-year follow-up. *Data from the Framingham Heart Study. *Significant inverse trend for age (P < 0.05); †no significant excess of strokes.*

A landmark study of untreated AF in 1983 by Sage et al. provided insight on the gravity of the condition. AF was present in 24.6% of patients with ischemic stroke. These strokes with AF were more often seen in women, persons 80 years of age or older, and more often associated with coronary or peripheral artery disease. Recurrent strokes were frequent, occurring at a rate of 20% per year regardless of age, sex, previous MI, or whether the AF is chronic or intermittent. AF strokes are major strokes that have a high (32.5%) 30-day case fatality rate and a 1-year mortality rate of 49.5%. They are also associated with a higher stroke recurrence rate within the first year (6.6% vs 4.4%). They tend to be severe or moderately severe strokes.[69,70]

Much of the morbidity associated with AF is attributable to the fivefold increased risk of stroke that it imposes. However, the risk is variable, which has stimulated numerous investigations designed to define clinical criteria useful for classifying AF persons at high or low risk of stroke or excess mortality and five risk factors were initially shown to increase AF stroke risk: increasing age, female sex, diabetes, hypertension, or a history of prior stroke or TIA.[71] The CHADS2 score, widely used as a simple clinical tool for predicting risk of stroke in persons with AF, assigns 1 point each for presence of congestive heart failure, hypertension (JNC-7 Stage I or II), age above 75 years and 2 points if the person has previously experienced a stroke or TIA. The 10-year risk of stroke in a person with AF ranges from 1.9% in persons with none of these risk factors to 18.2% in a person with all risk factors.[72] Such risk stratification is important for prognostication and the selection of candidates for anticoagulant therapy. (See Chapters 19 and 62 for more on this.)

Cardiac Failure

AF and CHF frequently occur together, but there has been limited information regarding their temporal relations and the combined influence of these conditions on mortality. The Framingham Study investigators studied participants with new-onset AF or CHF using multivariable Cox proportional hazards models with time-dependent variables to evaluate whether mortality after AF or CHF was affected by the occurrence and timing of the other condition. HRs were adjusted for time period and cardiovascular risk factors. During the study period, 1470 participants developed AF, CHF, or both. Among 382 individuals with both conditions, 38% had AF first, 41% had CHF first, and 21% had both diagnosed on the same day. The incidence of CHF among AF subjects was 33 per 1000 person-years, and the incidence of AF among CHF subjects was 54 per 1000 person-years. In AF subjects, the subsequent development of CHF was associated with increased mortality (men: HR, 2.7; 95%CI, 1.9–3.7; women: HR, 3.1; 95%CI, 2.2–4.2). Similarly, in CHF subjects, later development of AF was associated with increased mortality (men: HR, 1.6; 95%CI, 1.2–2.1; women: HR, 2.7; 95%CI, 2.0–3.6). Preexisting CHF adversely affected survival in individuals with AF, but preexisting AF was not associated with adverse chance of survival in those with CHF. Individuals with either AF or CHF who subsequently develop the other condition have a poor prognosis. Additional studies addressing the pathogenesis, prevention, and optimal management of the joint occurrence of AF and CHF appear warranted.[73]

Left Ventricular Hypertrophy

Left ventricular hypertrophy by electrocardiography increases in prevalence with age and blood pressure and the risk of ABI increases more than fourfold in men and sixfold in women with this electrocardiographic abnormality. The increased risk conferred persists even after the influence of age and other atherogenic precursors, including systolic blood pressure, are taken into account. The more sensitive and precise measure of cardiac hypertrophy, LVM, on echocardiography is also directly related to the incidence of stroke.[28] The estimated HR for stroke and TIA, when the uppermost quartile of LVM-to-height ratio is compared with the lowest, is 2.72 after adjustment for age, gender, and cardiovascular risk factors. There is a graded response with an HR of 1.45 for each quartile increment of LVM-to-height ratio. Clearly, echocardiography gives prognostic information beyond that provided by traditional risk factors.

Other Host Factors

Migraine

From clinical observations, case reports, and clinical series the notion evolved that migraine predisposes to stroke, particularly ischemic stroke. Complicated migraine with aura and migraine with neurologic concomitants seem to be the types most likely to be followed by stroke. Examples of the association between migraine and stroke occur in certain uncommon syndromes and instances. In cerebral autosomal dominant arteriopathy with subcortical infarcts and leukoencephalopathy (CADASIL), migraine headache is associated with white matter disease, dementia, and subcortical strokes.[74] Another migraine syndrome is seen in the antiphospholipid antibody syndrome. Atypical migraine syndromes such as hemiplegic migraine are also associated with stroke but are quite rare.

The relationship of stroke to the common migraine syndromes encompassing migraine with aura and migraine without aura has been investigated in two large case-control studies, the Italian National Research Council Study Group on Stroke in the Young and a substudy of the World Health Organization Collaborative Study of Cardiovascular Disease and Steroid Hormone Contraception.[93] Migraine as a predisposing factor for stroke was also investigated in the Physicians Health Study. Migraine was associated with an increased risk of ischemic stroke in these aforementioned studies, and RRs or ORs ranged from 2.0 to 3.8.[92] The studies that distinguished between migraine with or without aura usually detected a higher risk for migraine with aura. Concomitant presence of smoking and oral contraceptive use seem to increase the relative risk of stroke among women with migraine. The contribution of migraine to stroke risk decreases with increasing age. The mechanism of increased stroke risk in migraine sufferers in unclear and theories include the impact of a spreading electric depression that decreases local blood flow and an underlying patent foramen ovale (discussed in Chapter 43) that increases the risk of *both* migraine and stroke.

Environmental Factors

Cigarette Smoking

Cigarette smoking, a powerful risk factor for MI and sudden death, has been clearly linked to brain infarction, as well as to IH and SAH in both men and women.[75-77]

In the late 1970s, several studies of oral contraceptives (OCs) and stroke in young women identified cigarette smoking as an important risk factor. Surprisingly, the association between cigarette smoking, oral contraceptives, and stroke was primarily related to SAH. In the Royal College of General Practitioners Study of oral contraceptive use, the increased risk of SAH occurred principally in women older than 35 years, who were current or former OC users, and who smoked cigarettes.[78] In the Nurses' Health Study, a cohort of nearly 120,000 women, who were followed up prospectively for 8 years for the development of stroke, there was an increased risk of SAH as well as thrombotic stroke in cigarette smokers. The RR of SAH in smokers compared to non-smokers showed a dose–response relationship from fourfold in light smokers to 9.8-fold in smokers of 25 or more cigarettes daily. Of note, in each smoking category the RR of SAH, regardless of whether other associated risk factors were taken into account, was twice as great as for thromboembolic stroke (Table 15-4).

The association between cigarette smoking and SAH from aneurysm was also found in men (as well as women) in Framingham[79] and in New Zealand[80] in case-control analyses. In a case-control study of 114 patients with SAH in a defined region in Finland, cigarette smoking was significantly more prevalent in SAH patients than in control subjects matched for age, sex, and domicile.[81] The RR of SAH in smokers, as compared with non-smokers, was 2.7 in men and 3.0 in women. The authors suggested that smoking promoted a temporary

TABLE 15-4 Age-adjusted Relative Risks of Stroke (Fatal And Nonfatal Combined), by Daily Number of Cigarettes Consumed Among Current Smokers

Event	Never Smoked	Former Smoker	Current Smoker	No. of Cigarettes Smoked per Day among Current Smokers			
				1–14	*15–24*	*25–34*	*35 or More*
Total stroke	1.00	1.35 (0.98–1.85)	2.73 (2.18–3.41)	2.02 (1.29–3.14)	3.34 (2.38–4.70)	3.08 (1.94–4.87)	4.48 (2.78–7.23)
Subarachnoid hemorrhage	1.00	2.26 (1.16–4.42)	4.85 (2.90–8.11)	4.28 (1.88–9.77)	4.02 (1.90–8.54)	7.95 (3.50–18.07)	10.22 (4.03–25.94)
Ischemic stroke	1.00	1.27 (0.85–1.89)	2.53 (1.91–3.35)	1.83 (1.04–3.23)	3.57 (2.36–5.42)	2.73 (1.49–5.03)	3.97 (2.09–7.53)
Cerebral hemorrhage	1.00	1.24 (0.64–2.42)	1.24 (0.64–2.42)	1.68 (0.34–5.28)	2.53 (0.71–6.05)	1.41 (0.39–5.05)	

Numbers in parentheses are 95% confidence intervals.
Relative risk: Adjusted for age in 5-year intervals, follow-up period (1976–1978, 1978–1980, 1980–1982, 1982–1984, 1984–1986, or 1986–1988), history of hypertension, diabetes, high cholesterol levels, body mass index, past use of oral contraceptives, postmenopausal estrogen therapy, and age at starting smoking.
Adapted with permission from Kawachi I, Colditz GA, Stampfer MJ: Smoking cessation and decreased risk of stroke in women. JAMA *269:233, 1993, Table 1.*

increase in blood pressure, which, acting in concert with the "metastatic emphysema effect," was responsible for SAH from cerebral aneurysm. No more reasonable hypothesis has been promulgated to explain this powerful relationship.

The evidence that cigarette smoking increases the risk of thrombotic stroke and SAH is generally accepted, but the relationship of cigarette smoking to IH is less well-established. Data from the Honolulu Heart Program firmly link cigarette smoking in Hawaiian men of Japanese ancestry to stroke both "thromboembolic and hemorrhagic."[77] Risk of "hemorrhagic" stroke was significantly greater (RR, 2.5) in cigarette smokers than in nonsmokers, and this excess risk persisted at an RR of 2.8, even after adjustment for the other associated risk factors of age, diastolic blood pressure, serum cholesterol level, alcohol consumption, hematocrit, and body mass index.

A meta-analysis of 32 separate studies, including those already cited, indicates that cigarette smoking *is* a significant independent contributor to stroke incidence in both sexes at all ages and is associated with about a 50% increased risk overall when compared with the risk seen for non-smokers.[82] The risk of stroke generally, and of ABI specifically, rises as the number of cigarettes smoked per day increases, in both men and women.

Based on data from Framingham and the Nurses' Health Studies discussed earlier, it is clear that stroke risk in cigarette smokers is reduced by about 60% by stopping. This reduction in risk occurs in a remarkably short time and is similar to the reduction in CHD risk, which decreases by approximately 50% within 1 year of smoking cessation and reaches the level of those who never smoked within 5 years. In men and women in the Framingham Study, risk of stroke in former cigarette smokers did not differ from that of persons who never smoked by the end of 5 years. There was no interaction with age, which suggests that cigarette smoking exerted a precipitating effect on stroke regardless of age or duration of smoking. Similar findings from the Nurses' Health Study show a sizable reduction of risk within 2 years (a reduction to an RR of 0.4) by which the risk in former smokers approximated the risk in women who had never smoked (Fig. 15-11). Because smoking confers an increase in stroke risk of 40% in men and 60% in women after all other pertinent risk factors have been taken into account, smoking cessation deserves a high priority as it may be expected to significantly reduce the risk of stroke.

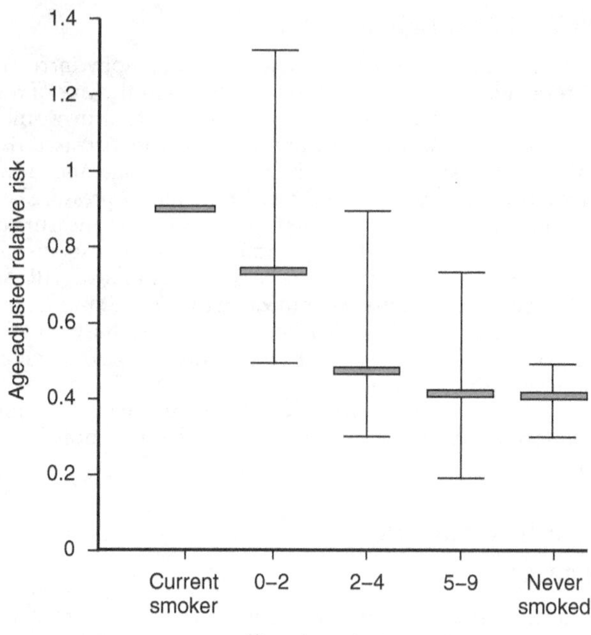

Figure 15-11. Smoking cessation and risk of stroke in women. *(From Kawachi I, Colditz GA, Stampfer MJ, et al: Smoking cessation and decreased risk of stroke in women. JAMA 269:232–236, 1993.)*

Oral Contraceptives

In the 1970s, risk of stroke was found to be increased fivefold in women using OCs. This increased risk was most marked in women older than 35 years and was seen predominantly in those with other cardiovascular risk factors, particularly hypertension and cigarette smoking.[83] The increased RR of stroke was seen in OC users and former users, and the risk was concentrated in cigarette smokers older than 35 years. However, the mechanism of stroke in OC users is unclear. Their cerebral infarctions are more likely to be due to thrombotic disease than to severity of atherosclerosis; it is known that clotting is enhanced by the OC-induced increased platelet aggregability and by its alteration of clotting factors to favor thrombogenesis. In young women with unexplained ischemic stroke, use of OCs is sometimes presumed to be the cause of the infarct; however, the stroke was attributed to OC use in no more than 10% of a series of carefully studied patients and such a diagnosis should only be arrived at after exclusion of other possible causes.[84]

There was no increase in stroke or other cardiovascular disease among former users of OCs in the Nurses' Health Study.[85] An international study of ischemic stroke and OC use assessed risk of stroke among women in Europe and in less developed countries.[86] Risk of stroke was increased for all OC users (OR, 2.99; 95%CI, 1.65–5.40) but was lowest in younger non-smokers without elevated blood pressure. Women with hypertension had an OR of 10.7 (95%CI, 2.04–56.6). In Europe, with current use of low-dose OCs (<50 μg estrogen), the OR was 1.53 (95%CI 0.71–3.31).[86] In the US, a population-based case-control study from California Kaiser Permanente Medical Care Program was conducted of OC use in women with stroke in which the OC preparations contained the current low dose of estrogen.[87] Comparing current to former and never-users of OCs, the OR for ischemic stroke was 1.18 (95%CI, 0.54–2.59) after adjustment for other risk factors for stroke.[87] Thus, the risk of ischemic stroke is quite low in women of childbearing age and is definitely not increased in non-smokers without hypertension.

A meta-analysis that included 16 studies published from 1960 to 1999 addressed the relationship of OC use with stroke. The overall RR of ischemic stroke across all preparations and study designs was 2.75 (95%CI, 2.24–3.38). The RR in population-based studies of low-dose estrogen preparations in which adjustment was made for both smoking and hypertension was 1.93 (95%CI, 1.35–2.74). If these latter results are true, then low-dose oral contraceptive pills might lead to one stroke for every 24,000 women users, or 425 ischemic strokes in the US each year. These results must be interpreted with caution because other studies did not find the same association between stroke and low-dose estradiol contraceptives.

With regard to SAH, of particular interest is the interaction between the older preparations of OCs (containing high doses of estrogens), cigarette smoking, and SAH. Prospective observation of more than 40,000 women, half of whom were taking OCs, showed an increased risk of fatal SAH (not cerebral infarction) in women taking OCs. The risk was increased fourfold in cigarette smokers older than 35 years, and most cases were confined to this group.[88]

The OR for hemorrhagic stroke in OC users in the California Kaiser Permanente Program study was not significantly increased.[87] There was a positive (non-significant) interaction for hemorrhage in current users who smoked (OR, 3.64;

95%CI, 0.95–13.87). In the World Health Organization collaborative study, risk of hemorrhagic stroke was not increased in younger women and was only slightly increased in older women.[89] The bulk of these hemorrhages were subarachnoid (200 of 248 in Europe), and the risk was significantly increased in women older than 35 years. The OR for hemorrhage among current OC users older than 35 years who were current cigarette smokers was 3.91 (95%CI, 1.54–9.89).

Hormone Replacement Therapy

Observational studies had largely either shown no influence of hormone replacement therapy (HRT) on stroke[90] or a weak protective effect with the notable exception of data from FHS, which showed a doubling of stroke risk among persons on HRT.[91] However, the Women's Health Initiative randomized controlled trial, the largest trial to date that examined the issue of HRT and cardiovascular disease in 16,608 subjects randomly assigned to conjugated estrogens plus progesterone or placebo, was stopped after 5.2 years because of a global statistic that indicated that the risks of treatment exceeded the benefit. Women taking HRT had an increased risk of stroke with an RR of 1.41 (CI, 1.07–1.85).[92] Pending further evidence to the contrary, HRT increases stroke and other negative outcomes and cannot be recommended as a measure to prevent cardiovascular disease.

Alcohol Consumption

As in MI, the impact of alcohol consumption on stroke risk is related to the amount of alcohol consumed. Heavy alcohol use, either habitual daily heavy alcohol consumption or binge drinking, seems to be related to higher rates of cardiovascular disease. Light or moderate alcohol consumption, on the other hand, is inversely related to the incidence of CHD.[93] Light and moderate alcohol use tend to raise the HDL cholesterol level, whereas high levels of alcohol intake are linked to hypertension and hypertriglyceridemia and may, in this way, predispose to fatal and nonfatal CHD, which is a high-risk condition for stroke.

The relationship of alcohol consumption to stroke occurrence per se is less clear.[94] Available evidence suggests that there is a U-shaped relationship between level of alcohol consumption and ischemic stroke risk. Minimal consumption or total abstinence and heavy alcohol consumption seem to increase ischemic stroke risk, whereas moderate alcohol use is associated with the lowest risk. Risk of stroke due to hemorrhage, however, increases linearly with the amount of alcohol consumed.[95]

In the Honolulu Heart Study of men of Japanese ancestry, there was a powerful dose–response relationship between alcohol consumption and incidence of IH and SAH. Increases in alcohol consumption were related to increasing levels of blood pressure, cigarette smoking, and to lower serum cholesterol levels, all of which are risk factors for IH. However, even after these factors were taken into account, alcohol consumption was independently related to the incidence of intracranial hemorrhage, both subarachnoid and intracerebral. The age-adjusted RR of IH for light drinkers (1 to 14 oz per month) as compared with non-drinkers was 2.1; for moderate drinkers (15 to 39 oz per month), 2.4; and for heavy drinkers (40+ oz per month), 4.0. After adjustment was made for the other associated risk factors, IH was 2.0, 2.0, and 2.4 times as frequent, respectively, in these alcohol consumption categories.[95] Data from the FHS also suggest an increased incidence of brain infarction and stroke with increased levels of alcohol use, but only in men.[94] There are a number of mechanisms by which heavy alcohol consumption may predispose to stroke and moderate alcohol consumption may protect from stroke.[96] Cigarette smoking is more frequent in heavy drinkers and contributes to the hemoconcentration accompanying heavy alcohol consumption, which increases hematocrit and viscosity. In addition, rebound thrombocytosis during abstinence has been observed. Cardiac rhythm disturbances, particularly AF, occur with alcohol intoxication, producing what has been termed *holiday heart*.[97] Acute alcohol intoxication has been invoked as a precipitating factor for thrombotic stroke and SAH in young people.[98] Others have found a relationship to acute intoxication, but a case-control study failed to find an effect that was independent of other risk factors, particularly cigarette smoking.[99]

Physical Activity

Vigorous exercise may exert a beneficial influence on risk factors for atherosclerotic disease by reducing elevated blood pressure, inducing weight loss, slowing the heart rate, raising HDL and lowering LDL cholesterol levels, improving glucose tolerance, and promoting a lifestyle conducive to favorably changing detrimental health habits, such as cigarette smoking. However, physical activity has also been found to be directly associated with reduced stroke incidence.[100,101] In the Framingham Study, physical activity in subjects with a mean age of 65 years was associated with a reduced stroke incidence.[101] In men, the RR was 0.41 ($P = 0.0007$) after the effects of potential confounders were taken into account, including systolic blood pressure, serum cholesterol level, glucose intolerance, vital capacity, obesity, left ventricular hypertrophy on electrocardiogram, AF, valvular heart disease, CHF, CHD, and occupation. However, there was no evidence of a protective effect of physical activity on the risk of stroke in women. As in CHD, moderate physical activity conferred no less benefit than heavy activity levels. In other studies, a beneficial effect of exercise has also been found in women.[100]

A graded response to exercise was found in male British civil servants: the greatest benefit in reduced stroke incidence was derived from the most intense level of exercise, and an intermediate protective effect was derived from medium levels.[102] In the Honolulu Heart Study of Japanese men, higher levels of physical activity, after adjustment for other risk factors, was associated with lower rates of both ischemic and hemorrhagic stroke.[103] Data from the National Health and Nutrition Examination Survey 1 (NHANES 1) epidemiologic follow-up study disclosed a consistent association of low levels of physical activity and an increased risk of stroke in women as well as in men and in both black people and white people.[104] In a meta-analysis of 31 studies, moderately intense physical activity lowered the risk of stroke when compared with inactivity (RR = 0.64; 95%CI, 0.48–0.87 for occupational activity and RR = 0.85; 95%CI, 0.78–0.93 for leisure time activity).[105] Moderate levels of activity tended to provide an intermediate level of protection.

Physical activity exerts a beneficial influence on standard risk factors for atherosclerotic disease by decreasing platelet aggregability, increasing insulin sensitivity, which improves glucose tolerance and HDL levels, and promoting a lifestyle conducive to a healthier diet and stopping cigarette smoking. Increased physical activity has now been convincingly associated with a reduced incidence of stroke. Moderate levels of recreational and non-recreational physical activity provide substantial benefits and may be recommended as a sensible lifestyle modification for reduction of the risk of cardiovascular disease, including stroke.

Diet

Consumption of grains, fruits, vegetables, and fish has been associated with a reduced incidence of stroke in a number of studies. In the Nurses' Health Study of more than 75,000 women, the RR of ischemic stroke in the uppermost quintile of grain consumption was 0.69 relative to the lowest quintile, after adjustment for other stroke risk factors.[106] In an analysis combining the Nurses' Health Study and the Health Professionals Follow-up Study, fruit and vegetable consumption was also associated with a decreased risk of stroke (RR, 0.69; 95%CI, 0.52–0.92).[107]

Nurses in the Nurses' Health Study who consumed five or more servings of fish per week had an adjusted RR for stroke of 0.38 compared with women consuming less than 1 serving per month, which suggests a protective effect of omega-3 fatty acids.[108] Consumption of fish, once a week or more frequently, was associated with an approximate 50% reduced stroke incidence in women and in black men. Stroke incidence was reduced by a non-statistically significant 15% in white men who consumed fish compared with those who never ate fish.[109] (See Chapters 17 and 19.) Vitamin C or E levels have been related to stroke incidence, but the findings have been inconsistent. Based on 20 years of follow-up in the Shibata study, a prospective cohort of 880 men and 1241 women, the RR of stroke adjusted for all other risk factors was 0.71 in the subjects with the highest vitamin C levels relative to those with the lowest levels. However, the Health Professionals Follow-up Study also examined this issue based on food frequency questionnaires administered to 43,738 men, aged 40–75 years. After 8 years of follow-up there were no significant relationships between consumption of vitamins C and E and the risk of stroke.[110]

Other putative stroke risk factors that have been explored include anger and psychological stress as well as job stress (highly demanding jobs where events were not under the person's control)[111] that have in a few studies been related to a higher risk of incident stroke.

Identification of High-risk Candidates for Stroke Prevention (see Chapter 19, "Primary Prevention of Stroke"). Multivariable analysis, initially employed to gain insight into the underlying atherogenic process, also generated a set of independent risk factors useful for crafting multivariable risk equations to predict cardiovascular disease events. For use as a multivariable risk tool, it is compelled by the availability of reliable non-invasive tests for candidate risk factors, cost, and whether the risk factors used can be safely modified with expectation of benefit. This methodology implicitly recognizes that no known risk factor either inevitably leads to development of disease or confers immunity. The risk factors chosen for prediction depend on the purpose for assigning risk and the costs entailed. Framingham Study CHD and stroke multivariable risk profiles have been tested in a variety of population samples and found to be reasonably accurate, except in those areas where the cardiovascular disease rates are very low.

However, even in these areas, high-risk persons can be distinguished from those at low risk, and if the intercept is adjusted (re-calibrated), the true absolute risk can be estimated. The Framingham Study has crafted multivariable risk profiles for risk assessment of candidates for cardiovascular disease in general and stroke in particular.[112] These facilitate estimation of the conditional probability of these initial events with the use of ordinary office procedures. Epidemiologic investigation has long contended that atherosclerotic cardiovascular disease is of multifactorial etiology. Risk factors are related to cardiovascular disease occurrence in a continuous graded fashion, extending down into the perceived normal range, without indication of a critical value where normal leaves off. At any level of each risk factor, cardiovascular disease risk varies widely in accordance with the burden of accompanying risk factors. National guidelines are now linking treatment goals to global CHD risk. It has long been recognized that for any risk factor, predisposition to cardiovascular disease is markedly influenced by the associated burden of other risk factors.

Cardiovascular disease risk factors seldom occur in isolation because they are metabolically linked, tending to cluster. It is postulated that an insulin resistance syndrome is the metabolic basis for other atherogenic risk factors clustering with each of the major risk factors. When confronted with a patient with any particular cardiovascular disease risk factor, it is essential to test for the others that are likely to coexist with it. Such coexistence can be expected over 80% of the time. Now that guidelines for dyslipidemia, hypertension, and diabetes recommend treating modest abnormality, candidates for treatment are best targeted by global risk assessment so that the number needed to treat to prevent one event is minimized.

To help identify persons at increased risk of stroke, a risk profile was developed, utilizing 36 years of follow-up data from Framingham, which allows physicians to determine a patient's conditional probability of having a stroke.[112] This can be done based only on information collected from a medical history and physical examination, plus an electrocardiogram. With the use of a risk factor scoring table that is sex-specific, the probability of a stroke occurring is determined, depending on the patient's age, systolic blood pressure, antihypertensive therapy use, and presence of diabetes, cigarette smoking, history of cardiovascular disease (CHD or CHF), and electrocardiographic abnormalities (left ventricular hypertrophy or AF). Stroke risk depending on the level of the aforementioned risk factors is distributed over a wide range and permits the physician to readily compare a particular patient's probability of stroke to that of an average person of the same age and sex. Similar stroke risk assessment tools have been developed by other investigators, but the FHS risk predictor has been most widely used.

This assessment of global stroke risk will help the physician to identify which patients with prehypertension warrant pharmacologic treatment by virtue of an increased probability of stroke attributable to the presence of several other risk factor abnormalities that often accompany elevated blood pressure (Fig. 15-12). With the use of stroke risk profiles of a man age 70 years with either a systolic blood pressure level of 120 mm Hg or 180 mm Hg, it can be seen that the probability of a stroke in 10 years ranges from less than half the average

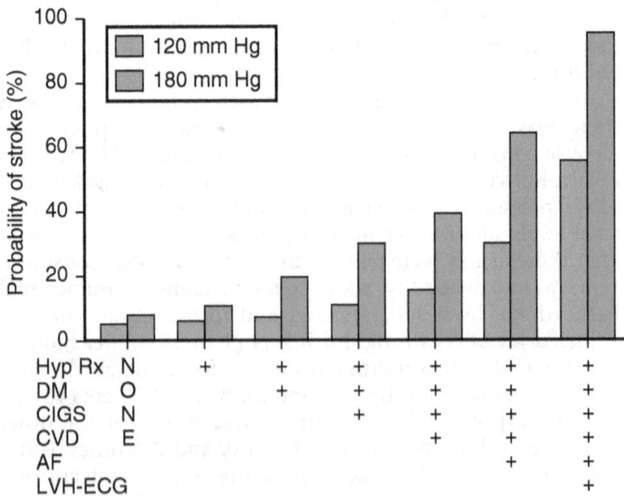

Figure 15-12. Probability of stroke in 10 years at two systolic blood pressure levels. Impact of other risk factors – 70-year-old man. *(From Wolf PA, D'Agostino RB, Belanger AJ, et al: Probability of stroke: A risk profile from the Framingham Study.* Stroke *22:312–318, 1991.)*

level to nearly 100% depending on the associated risk factor burden. In the presence of multiple risk factor abnormalities, the probability of a stroke may actually be higher in the presence of a normal systolic blood pressure of 120 mm Hg than in a man with a pressure of 180 mm Hg who is free of diabetes and cardiovascular disease and who is a non-smoker. The use of this risk profile thus provides a quantitative assessment of the level of risk and is particularly helpful in the presence of multiple borderline risk factor abnormalities. The graphic and percentage display provides the patient and his physician with a concrete estimate that the probability of stroke is below, at, or several-fold above average. It also can provide an illustration for patients of how treating certain of their risk factors that have been demonstrated to reduce stroke risk may be expected to result in a quantified decrease in stroke probability. Patients can be shown that reduction of their systolic blood pressure from 180 mm Hg to below 140 mm Hg by treatment, along with cessation of cigarette smoking and taking of warfarin anticoagulation if they have AF, may reduce their substantially elevated risk to nearly normal.[112]

The stroke profile may be used to select persons with prehypertension who warrant antihypertensive drug treatment. For example, by restricting drug treatment to persons with a borderline systolic blood pressure level (130–140 mm Hg) who have two or more other risk factor abnormalities (not including age and male sex), it is possible to identify a group consisting of 22% of the men and 14% of women at high risk.[112]

Clearly, there are other settings not considered here when a patient can be identified to be at substantially increased risk of stroke: recent TIA, particularly in the presence of internal carotid artery stenosis greater than 70%; recent-onset AF; recent MI; during and immediately after cardiac surgery and cerebral angiography; and other situations dealt with elsewhere in this book (see Chapters 22, 74 and Section IV).

Acknowledgments

Supported in part by grants 2R01 NS17950 (National Institute of Neurological Disorders and Stroke, National Heart, Lung, and Blood Institute) and Contract N01-HC-25195 (National Heart, Lung, and Blood Institute).

REFERENCES

1. Go AS, Mozaffarian D, Roger VL, et al. Heart disease and stroke statistics–2014 update: a report from the American Heart Association. Circulation 2014;129:e28–292.
2. Rosamond WD, Folsom AR, Chambless LE, et al. Stroke incidence and survival among middle-aged adults: 9-year follow-up of the Atherosclerosis Risk in Communities (ARIC) cohort. Stroke 1999;30:736–43.
3. Kase CS, Wolf PA, Chodosh EH, et al. Prevalence of silent stroke in patients presenting with initial stroke: the Framingham Study. Stroke 1989;20:850–2.
4. Chodosh EH, Foulkes MA, Kase CS, et al. Silent stroke in the NINCDS Stroke Data Bank. Neurology 1988;38:1674–9.
5. Manolio TA, Kronmal RA, Burke GL, et al. Magnetic resonance abnormalities and cardiovascular disease in older adults. The Cardiovascular Health Study. Stroke 1994;25:318–27.
6. Das RR, Seshadri S, Beiser AS, et al. Prevalence and correlates of silent cerebral infarcts in the Framingham offspring study. Stroke 2008;39:2929–35.
7. Prabhakaran S, Wright CB, Yoshita M, et al. Prevalence and determinants of subclinical brain infarction: the Northern Manhattan Study. Neurology 2008;70:425–30.
8. Vermeer SE, Koudstaal PJ, Oudkerk M, et al. Prevalence and risk factors of silent brain infarcts in the population-based Rotterdam Scan Study. Stroke 2002;33:21–5.
9. Giele JL, Witkamp TD, Mali WP, et al. Silent brain infarcts in patients with manifest vascular disease. Stroke 2004;35:742–6.
10. Vermeer SE, Den Heijer T, Koudstaal PJ, et al. Incidence and risk factors of silent brain infarcts in the population-based Rotterdam Scan Study. Stroke 2003;34:392–6.
11. Vermeer SE, Prins ND, den Heijer T, et al. Silent brain infarcts and the risk of dementia and cognitive decline. New Engl J Med 2003;348:1215–22.
12. Debette S, Beiser A, DeCarli C, et al. Association of MRI markers of vascular brain injury with incident stroke, mild cognitive impairment, dementia, and mortality: the Framingham Offspring Study. Stroke 2010;41:600–6.
13. Sacco RL, Foulkes MA, Mohr JP, et al. Determinants of early recurrence of cerebral infarction. The Stroke Data Bank. Stroke 1989;20:983–9.
14. Sacco RL, Wolf PA, Kannel WB, et al. Survival and recurrence following stroke. The Framingham study. Stroke 1982;13:290–5.
15. Sacco RL, Shi T, Zamanillo MC, et al. Predictors of mortality and recurrence after hospitalized cerebral infarction in an urban community: the Northern Manhattan Stroke Study. Neurology 1994;44:626–34.
16. Romano JG, Sacco RL. Progress in secondary stroke prevention. Ann Neurol 2008;63:418–27.
17. Elkind MS, Tai W, Coates K, et al. High-sensitivity C-reactive protein, lipoprotein-associated phospholipase A2, and outcome after ischemic stroke. Arch Intern Med 2006;166:2073–80.
18. Wolf PA, Kannel WB, Sorlie P, et al. Asymptomatic carotid bruit and risk of stroke. The Framingham study. JAMA 1981;245:1442–5.
19. Petty GW, Brown RD Jr, Whisnant JP, et al. Ischemic stroke subtypes: a population-based study of incidence and risk factors. Stroke 1999;30:2513–16.
20. MacMahon S, Rodgers A. Blood pressure, antihypertensive treatment and stroke risk. J Hypertens Suppl 1994;12:S5–14.
21. Kannel WB, Wolf PA, McGee DL, et al. Systolic blood pressure, arterial rigidity, and risk of stroke. The Framingham study. JAMA 1981;245:1225–9.
22. Kannel WB, Wolf PA, Verter J, et al. Epidemiologic assessment of the role of blood pressure in stroke. The Framingham study. JAMA 1970;214:301–10.
23. The sixth report of the Joint National Committee on prevention, detection, evaluation, and treatment of high blood pressure. Arch Intern Med 1997;157:2413–46.
24. Collins R, Peto R, MacMahon S, et al. Blood pressure, stroke, and coronary heart disease. Part 2, Short-term reductions in blood pressure: overview of randomised drug trials in their epidemiological context. Lancet 1990;335:827–38.
25. Kannel WB, Wolf PA, Verter J, et al. Epidemiologic assessment of the role of blood pressure in stroke: the Framingham Study. 1970. JAMA 1996;276:1269–78.
26. Beckett NS, Peters R, Fletcher AE, et al. Treatment of hypertension in patients 80 years of age or older. New Engl J Med 2008;358:1887–98.
27. Seshadri S, Wolf PA, Beiser A, et al. Elevated midlife blood pressure increases stroke risk in elderly persons: the Framingham Study. Arch Intern Med 2001;161:2343–50.
28. Bikkina M, Levy D, Evans JC, et al. Left ventricular mass and risk of stroke in an elderly cohort. The Framingham Heart Study. JAMA 1994;272:33–6.
29. Shahar E, Chambless LE, Rosamond WD, et al. Plasma lipid profile and incident ischemic stroke: the Atherosclerosis Risk in Communities (ARIC) study. Stroke 2003;34:623–31.
30. Cholesterol, diastolic blood pressure, and stroke: 13,000 strokes in 450,000 people in 45 prospective cohorts. Prospective studies collaboration. Lancet 1995;346:1647–53.
31. Iso H, Jacobs DR Jr, Wentworth D, et al. Serum cholesterol levels and six-year mortality from stroke in 350,977 men screened for the multiple risk factor intervention trial. New Engl J Med 1989;320:904–10.
32. Benfante R, Yano K, Hwang LJ, et al. Elevated serum cholesterol is a risk factor for both coronary heart disease and thromboembolic stroke in Hawaiian Japanese men. Implications of shared risk. Stroke 1994;25:814–20.
33. Wilson PW, Hoeg JM, D'Agostino RB, et al. Cumulative effects of high cholesterol levels, high blood pressure, and cigarette smoking on carotid stenosis. New Engl J Med 1997;337:516–22.

34. Fine-Edelstein JS, Wolf PA, O'Leary DH, et al. Precursors of extracranial carotid atherosclerosis in the Framingham Study. Neurology 1994;44:1046–50.
35. O'Leary DH, Anderson KM, Wolf PA, et al. Cholesterol and carotid atherosclerosis in older persons: the Framingham Study. Ann Epidemiol 1992;2:147–53.
36. Yano K, Reed DM, MacLean CJ. Serum cholesterol and hemorrhagic stroke in the Honolulu Heart Program. Stroke 1989;20: 1460–5.
37. Shimamoto T, Komachi Y, Inada H, et al. Trends for coronary heart disease and stroke and their risk factors in Japan. Circulation 1989;79:503–15.
38. Burchfiel CM, Curb JD, Rodriguez BL, et al. Glucose intolerance and 22-year stroke incidence. The Honolulu Heart Program. Stroke 1994;25:951–7.
39. Barrett-Connor E, Khaw KT. Diabetes mellitus: an independent risk factor for stroke? Am J Epidemiol 1988;128:116–23.
40. Kannel WB, McGee DL. Diabetes and cardiovascular disease. The Framingham study. JAMA 1979;241:2035–8.
41. Najarian RM, Sullivan LM, Kannel WB, et al. Metabolic syndrome compared with type 2 diabetes mellitus as a risk factor for stroke: the Framingham Offspring Study. Arch Intern Med 2006;166:106–11.
42. Suk SH, Sacco RL, Boden-Albala B, et al. Abdominal obesity and risk of ischemic stroke: the Northern Manhattan Stroke Study. Stroke 2003;34:1586–92.
43. Walker SP, Rimm EB, Ascherio A, et al. Body size and fat distribution as predictors of stroke among US men. Am J Epidemiol 1996;144:1143–50.
44. Yaggi HK, Concato J, Kernan WN, et al. Obstructive sleep apnea as a risk factor for stroke and death. New Engl J Med 2005; 353:2034–41.
45. Welin L, Svardsudd K, Wilhelmsen L, et al. Analysis of risk factors for stroke in a cohort of men born in 1913. New Engl J Med 1987;317:521–6.
46. Seshadri S, Beiser A, Pikula A, et al. Parental occurrence of stroke and risk of stroke in their children: the Framingham study. Circulation 2010;121:1304–12.
47. Wilhelmsen L, Svardsudd K, Korsan-Bengtsen K, et al. Fibrinogen as a risk factor for stroke and myocardial infarction. New Engl J Med 1984;311:501–5.
48. Kannel WB, Wolf PA, Castelli WP, et al. Fibrinogen and risk of cardiovascular disease. The Framingham Study. JAMA 1987;258: 1183–6.
49. Fibrinogen Studies C, Danesh J, Lewington S, et al. Plasma fibrinogen level and the risk of major cardiovascular diseases and nonvascular mortality: an individual participant meta-analysis. JAMA 2005;294:1799–809.
50. Kannel WB, D'Agostino RB, Belanger AJ. Fibrinogen, cigarette smoking, and risk of cardiovascular disease: insights from the Framingham Study. Am Heart J 1987;113:1006–10.
51. Rost NS, Wolf PA, Kase CS, et al. Plasma concentration of C-reactive protein and risk of ischemic stroke and transient ischemic attack: the Framingham study. Stroke 2001;32:2575–9.
52. Ridker PM, Rifai N, Rose L, et al. Comparison of C-reactive protein and low-density lipoprotein cholesterol levels in the prediction of first cardiovascular events. New Engl J Med 2002; 347:1557–65.
53. Wu T, Trevisan M, Genco RJ, et al. Periodontal disease and risk of cerebrovascular disease: the first national health and nutrition examination survey and its follow-up study. Arch Intern Med 2000;160:2749–55.
54. Boushey CJ, Beresford SA, Omenn GS, et al. A quantitative assessment of plasma homocysteine as a risk factor for vascular disease. Probable benefits of increasing folic acid intakes. JAMA 1995;274:1049–57.
55. Nygard O, Vollset SE, Refsum H, et al. Total plasma homocysteine and cardiovascular risk profile. The Hordaland Homocysteine Study. JAMA 1995;274:1526–33.
56. Bostom AG, Rosenberg IH, Silbershatz H, et al. Nonfasting plasma total homocysteine levels and stroke incidence in elderly persons: the Framingham Study. Ann Intern Med 1999;131:352–5.
57. Perry IJ, Refsum H, Morris RW, et al. Prospective study of serum total homocysteine concentration and risk of stroke in middle-aged British men. Lancet 1995;346:1395–8.
58. Verhoef P, Hennekens CH, Malinow MR, et al. A prospective study of plasma homocyst(e)ine and risk of ischemic stroke. Stroke 1994;25:1924–30.
59. Malinow MR, Nieto FJ, Szklo M, et al. Carotid artery intimal-medial wall thickening and plasma homocyst(e)ine in asymptomatic adults. The Atherosclerosis Risk in Communities Study. Circulation 1993;87:1107–13.
60. Selhub J, Jacques PF, Bostom AG, et al. Association between plasma homocysteine concentrations and extracranial carotid-artery stenosis. New Engl J Med 1995;332:286–91.
61. Selhub J, Jacques PF, Wilson PW, et al. Vitamin status and intake as primary determinants of homocysteinemia in an elderly population. JAMA 1993;270:2693–8.
62. Toole JF, Malinow MR, Chambless LE, et al. Lowering homocysteine in patients with ischemic stroke to prevent recurrent stroke, myocardial infarction, and death: the Vitamin Intervention for Stroke Prevention (VISP) randomized controlled trial. JAMA 2004;291:565–75.
63. Spence JD, Bang H, Chambless LE, et al. Vitamin Intervention For Stroke Prevention trial: an efficacy analysis. Stroke 2005;36: 2404–9.
64. Wolf PA, Kannel WB, McNamara PM, et al. The role of impaired cardiac function in atherothrombotic brain infarction: the Framingham study. Am J Public Health 1973;63:52–8.
65. Loh E, Sutton MS, Wun CC, et al. Ventricular dysfunction and the risk of stroke after myocardial infarction. New Engl J Med 1997;336:251–7.
66. Murabito JM, Evans JC, Larson MG, et al. The ankle-brachial index in the elderly and risk of stroke, coronary disease, and death: the Framingham Study. Arch Intern Med 2003;163: 1939–42.
67. Wolf PA, Abbott RD, Kannel WB. Atrial fibrillation as an independent risk factor for stroke: the Framingham Study. Stroke 1991;22:983–8.
68. Wolf PA, Abbott RD, Kannel WB. Atrial fibrillation: a major contributor to stroke in the elderly. The Framingham Study. Arch Intern Med 1987;147:1561–4.
69. Marini C, De Santis F, Sacco S, et al. Contribution of atrial fibrillation to incidence and outcome of ischemic stroke: results from a population-based study. Stroke 2005;36:1115–19.
70. Sage JI, Van Uitert RL. Risk of recurrent stroke in patients with atrial fibrillation and non-valvular heart disease. Stroke 1983;14: 537–40.
71. Wang TJ, Massaro JM, Levy D, et al. A risk score for predicting stroke or death in individuals with new-onset atrial fibrillation in the community: the Framingham Heart Study. JAMA 2003;290: 1049–56.
72. Rietbrock S, Heeley E, Plumb J, et al. Chronic atrial fibrillation: Incidence, prevalence, and prediction of stroke using the Congestive heart failure, Hypertension, Age >75, Diabetes mellitus, and prior Stroke or transient ischemic attack (CHADS2) risk stratification scheme. Am Heart J 2008;156:57–64.
73. Wang TJ, Larson MG, Levy D, et al. Temporal relations of atrial fibrillation and congestive heart failure and their joint influence on mortality: the Framingham Heart Study. Circulation 2003;107: 2920–5.
74. Chabriat H, Vahedi K, Iba-Zizen MT, et al. Clinical spectrum of CADASIL: a study of 7 families. Cerebral autosomal dominant arteriopathy with subcortical infarcts and leukoencephalopathy. Lancet 1995;346:934–9.
75. Wolf PA, D'Agostino RB, Kannel WB, et al. Cigarette smoking as a risk factor for stroke. The Framingham Study. JAMA 1988; 259:1025–9.
76. Colditz GA, Bonita R, Stampfer MJ, et al. Cigarette smoking and risk of stroke in middle-aged women. New Engl J Med 1988; 318:937–41.
77. Abbott RD, Yin Y, Reed DM, et al. Risk of stroke in male cigarette smokers. New Engl J Med 1986;315:717–20.
78. Hannaford PC, Croft PR, Kay CR. Oral contraception and stroke. Evidence from the Royal College of General Practitioners' Oral Contraception Study. Stroke 1994;25:935–42.
79. Sacco RL, Wolf PA, Bharucha NE, et al. Subarachnoid and intracerebral hemorrhage: natural history, prognosis, and precursive factors in the Framingham Study. Neurology 1984;34: 847–54.

80. Bonita R. Cigarette smoking, hypertension and the risk of subarachnoid hemorrhage: a population-based case-control study. Stroke 1986;17:831–5.
81. Fogelholm R, Murros K. Cigarette smoking and subarachnoid haemorrhage: a population-based case-control study. J Neurol Neurosurg Psychiatry 1987;50:78–80.
82. Shinton R, Beevers G. Meta-analysis of relation between cigarette smoking and stroke. BMJ 1989;298:789–94.
83. Stadel BV. Oral contraceptives and cardiovascular disease (second of two parts). New Engl J Med 1981;305:672–7.
84. Adams HP Jr, Butler MJ, Biller J, et al. Nonhemorrhagic cerebral infarction in young adults. Arch Neurol 1986;43:793–6.
85. Stampfer MJ, Willett WC, Colditz GA, et al. A prospective study of past use of oral contraceptive agents and risk of cardiovascular diseases. New Engl J Med 1988;319:1313–17.
86. Ischaemic stroke and combined oral contraceptives: results of an international, multicentre, case-control study. WHO Collaborative Study of Cardiovascular Disease and Steroid Hormone Contraception. Lancet 1996;348:498–505.
87. Petitti DB, Sidney S, Bernstein A, et al. Stroke in users of low-dose oral contraceptives. New Engl J Med 1996;335:8–15.
88. Further analyses of mortality in oral contraceptive users. Royal College of General Practitioners' Oral Contraception Study. Lancet 1981;1:541–6.
89. Haemorrhagic stroke, overall stroke risk, and combined oral contraceptives: results of an international, multicentre, case-control study. WHO Collaborative Study of Cardiovascular Disease and Steroid Hormone Contraception. Lancet 1996;348: 505–10.
90. Grodstein F, Stampfer MJ, Manson JE, et al. Postmenopausal estrogen and progestin use and the risk of cardiovascular disease. New Engl J Med 1996;335:453–61.
91. Wilson PW, Garrison RJ, Castelli WP. Postmenopausal estrogen use, cigarette smoking, and cardiovascular morbidity in women over 50. The Framingham Study. New Engl J Med 1985;313: 1038–43.
92. Rossouw JE, Anderson GL, Prentice RL, et al. Risks and benefits of estrogen plus progestin in healthy postmenopausal women: principal results From the Women's Health Initiative randomized controlled trial. JAMA 2002;288:321–33.
93. Stampfer MJ, Colditz GA, Willett WC, et al. A prospective study of moderate alcohol consumption and the risk of coronary disease and stroke in women. New Engl J Med 1988;319: 267–73.
94. Djousse L, Ellison RC, Beiser A, et al. Alcohol consumption and risk of ischemic stroke: The Framingham Study. Stroke 2002;33: 907–12.
95. Donahue RP, Abbott RD, Reed DM, et al. Alcohol and hemorrhagic stroke. The Honolulu Heart Program. JAMA 1986;255: 2311–14.
96. Camargo CA Jr. Moderate alcohol consumption and stroke. The epidemiologic evidence. Stroke 1989;20:1611–26.
97. Ettinger PO, Wu CF, De La Cruz C Jr, et al. Arrhythmias and the "Holiday Heart": alcohol-associated cardiac rhythm disorders. Am Heart J 1978;95:555–62.
98. Taylor JR, Combs-Orme T. Alcohol and strokes in young adults. Am J Psychiatry 1985;142:116–18.
99. Gorelick PB. The status of alcohol as a risk factor for stroke. Stroke 1989;20:1607–10.
100. Hu FB, Stampfer MJ, Colditz GA, et al. Physical activity and risk of stroke in women. JAMA 2000;283:2961–7.
101. Kiely DK, Wolf PA, Cupples LA, et al. Physical activity and stroke risk: the Framingham Study. Am J Epidemiol 1994;140: 608–20.
102. Wannamethee G, Shaper AG. Physical activity and stroke in British middle aged men. BMJ 1992;304:597–601.
103. Abbott RD, Rodriguez BL, Burchfiel CM, et al. Physical activity in older middle-aged men and reduced risk of stroke: the Honolulu Heart Program. Am J Epidemiol 1994;139:881–93.
104. Gillum RF, Mussolino ME, Ingram DD. Physical activity and stroke incidence in women and men. The NHANES I Epidemiologic Follow-up Study. Am J Epidemiol 1996;143:860–9.
105. Wendel-Vos GC, Schuit AJ, Feskens EJ, et al. Physical activity and stroke. A meta-analysis of observational data. Int J Epidemiol 2004;33:787–98.
106. Liu S, Manson JE, Stampfer MJ, et al. Whole grain consumption and risk of ischemic stroke in women: A prospective study. JAMA 2000;284:1534–40.
107. Joshipura KJ, Ascherio A, Manson JE, et al. Fruit and vegetable intake in relation to risk of ischemic stroke. JAMA 1999;282: 1233–9.
108. Iso H, Rexrode KM, Stampfer MJ, et al. Intake of fish and omega-3 fatty acids and risk of stroke in women. JAMA 2001;285: 304–12.
109. Gillum RF. Fish consumption and stroke incidence. Stroke 1996;27:1254.
110. Ascherio A, Rimm EB, Hernan MA, et al. Relation of consumption of vitamin E, vitamin C, and carotenoids to risk for stroke among men in the United States. Ann Intern Med 1999;130: 963–70.
111. Tsutsumi A, Kayaba K, Kario K, et al. Prospective study on occupational stress and risk of stroke. Arch Intern Med 2009;169: 56–61.
112. Wolf PA, D'Agostino RB, Belanger AJ, et al. Probability of stroke: a risk profile from the Framingham Study. Stroke 1991;22: 312–18.

16 Prognosis after Stroke

Tatjana Rundek, Ralph L. Sacco

KEY POINTS

- Stroke is the second most common cause of death in the world and a leading cause of long-term disability.
- In the US, stroke has declined from the third leading cause of death to the fourth leading cause of death. Despite this encouraging trend, there is a substantial ongoing race/ethnic and geographical disparity in stroke mortality.
- Strokes recur in 6–20% of patients, most commonly within the first year; after a transient ischemic attack (TIA) or minor stroke, most recurrences will occur within the first 90 days.
- Our ability to identify patients at high risk is poor and most recurrent strokes cannot be explained by traditional risk factors. However, the stroke prediction scales that combine neuroimaging with stroke severity and other clinical information hold promise of being reliable tools in predicting outcomes after stroke and are therefore useful in clinical practice.
- Stroke patients are faced with other risks, like cardiac events, disability and handicap, poor quality of life, depression, cognitive decline, and dementia.
- With the population aging, the need for timely and effective secondary prevention strategies is more pressing than ever.

INTRODUCTION

Stroke continues to be a common and debilitating disease with a great impact on the public health as the second most common cause of death in the world[1–3] and a leading cause of long-term disability.[2–5] In the US, stroke has declined from the third leading cause of death to the fourth leading cause of death.[3,6] In December of 2014, Centers for Disease Control and Prevention announced that stroke fell to the fifth cause of death in the US in 2013 (http://www.cdc.gov/nchs/data/databriefs/db178.htm). Despite this encouraging trend, there is substantial ongoing sex and race/ethnic disparities in stroke mortality.[3,4,7–9] Although interventions to reduce racial disparities in stroke risk factors hold promise to reduce these disparities in stroke mortality,[10–16] there are considerable geographic disparities in stroke mortality.[17–18]

In the US each year, about 800,000 people experience new or recurrent strokes.[4] About 610,000 of these are first strokes and 185,000 are recurrent strokes. Despite the expanding knowledge about novel strategies of stroke prevention, including the results from recent randomized clinical trials for secondary stroke prevention, e.g., novel oral anticoagulants for the risk reduction of initial and recurrent stroke,[10–16,20] the real challenge still remains to successfully implement evidence-based practices in secondary stroke prevention programs worldwide.

Overall, the global burden of stroke is likely to be substantially underestimated given the consequences of stroke that substantially affect well-being.[21] Overt and occult cerebrovascular disease contributes to depression, vascular dementia and Alzheimer's disease, and it is also a less recognized factor in gait disorders and oropharyngeal dysphagia, particularly in elderly, all of which can lead to poor quality of life (QOL). Inclusion of these outcomes in stroke preventive strategies and their implementation is urgently needed. How societies adapt to this anticipated burden of stroke and its consequences is vitally important.

The importance of recurrent stroke, functional disability, QOL, depression, and dementia after stroke will increase as more patients experience and survive a first stroke. Success of the secondary stroke prevention programs relies on understanding the outcomes of stroke, factors associated with increased risks for these outcomes, implementation of evidence-based preventive interventions and strategies, and a comprehensive public health approach.

The majority of strokes are cerebral infarcts. This chapter focuses on the prognosis after ischemic stroke and reviews evidence on ischemic stroke mortality, recurrence, functional disability, QOL, and depression after stroke. Cognitive impairment and dementia after stroke are discussed in Chapter 17.

MORTALITY AFTER ISCHEMIC STROKE

There has been a decline in stroke mortality over the past few decades. In the US, stroke has declined from the third to the fourth leading cause of death in recent years.[3] This major improvement has resulted from better risk-factor control, reduced stroke incidence and lower fatality rates. The hypertension control efforts seem to have had the most substantial effect on the decline in stroke mortality. In addition, control of diabetes, dyslipidemia, and smoking cessation also have contributed to the decline in stroke mortality.[22,23]

Stroke is the fourth leading cause of death, behind heart disease, cancer and chronic lower respiratory disease (CLRD) according to the latest published American Heart Association (AHA) statistics.[4] In 2010, the age-adjusted death rate for stroke as an underlying cause of death was 39.1 per 100,000.[24] From 2000 to 2010, the annual stroke death rate decreased 35.8% and the actual number of stroke deaths declined 22.8% according to the AHA analysis. Stroke death rates declined more in people aged 45 to 64 years (−51.7%) than in those ≥65 years of age (−48.3%) or those aged 18 to 44 years (−37.8%).[4]

Although stroke mortality also has decreased worldwide in the past two decades, stroke is still the second leading cause of death worldwide.[2] It is estimated that stroke caused 5.7 million deaths in 2005 and the number of global deaths is projected to rise to 6.5 million in 2015 and 7.8 million in 2030.[25]

Although rates of stroke mortality and morbidity differ greatly between countries, the overall burden of stroke is greater in low-income areas, where the stroke incidence and case fatality are rising.[26] The recent stroke mortality data available for over 50 countries have shown a significant country-specific disparity in crude stroke mortality, with greater mortality in Kazakhstan than any of the other countries reporting mortality data to WHO.[27] The Russian Federation, Bulgaria, Greece, and Romania also have reported very high stroke mortality while countries with lower mortality rates include Papua New Guinea, Bahrain, and Kuwait.

The absolute numbers of people with a new stroke, stroke survivors, related deaths, and the global burden of stroke are great and increasing. Despite overall declining stroke mortality, aging of the populations worldwide, improved prevention and stroke care will cause the prevalence of stroke to increase. The age, sex, race/ethnic, country-specific, regional and hospital-specific stroke disparities present major global challenges to reduce disparities in stroke mortality.

Early Mortality after Ischemic Stroke

The greatest risk of mortality for patients with cerebral infarction occurs in the first 30 days, and 1 month case-fatality for ischemic stroke in different country ranges from 8% to 23%.[3,4,26] In the Framingham Study the 30-day ischemic stroke case-fatality rate was 15%. It was similar in men and women and increased directly with age.[28] During this early period, death was more likely caused by the stroke itself or cardiopulmonary complications.[29] In the Atherosclerosis Risk in Communities (ARIC) study, 8% to 12% of ischemic strokes resulted in death within 30 days among persons 45 to 64 years of age.[30] In a study of persons older than 65 years recruited from a random sample of Health Care Financing Administration Medicare Part B eligibility lists in four U.S. communities, the 1-month ischemic stroke case-fatality rate was 8.1%.[31] In Rochester, Minnesota, the risk of death after first cerebral infarction was 7% at 7 days and 14% at 30 days.[26] In the Northern Manhattan Stroke Study (NOMASS), the 30-day mortality decreased from 7.7% in the 1980s (1983 to 1988) to 5.0% in the 1990s (1990 to 1997).[32] The 30-day cumulative mortality risk of 5% in NOMAS was lower than reported in other cohorts, likely due to exclusion of prior strokes, a higher proportion of lacunar infarcts, and less severe strokes at onset[33] (Table 16-1).

In the US, stroke hospitalization rates increased 18.6% between 1988 and 1997, and the increase was largely in elderly patients 65 years or older.[34] A decline, however, in the in-hospital case-fatality rate from stroke during the same time period was observed. The decline in the case-fatality rate suggested that there have been general improvements in the management of patients with acute stroke, decreases in the severity of strokes, or detection of milder cases of stroke secondary to greater use of neuroimaging technology. A decline in case-fatality rates was also observed in other countries.[2,35–37] "Jubilation" over the decline in stroke case-fatality rates should be tempered by the recognition that part of the decline may have been due to the shorter lengths of stay resulting in more out-of-hospital deaths.[34] In addition, new disparities in stroke mortality rates have emerged. Higher rates of in-hospital mortality were described for patients with acute strokes who arrived on weekends compared with regular workdays. In the Get With The Guidelines (GWTG) stroke program, which included data from 187,669 acute ischemic stroke admissions from 857 hospitals, the in-hospital case fatality rate was 6% for off-hour presentation compared with 5% for on-hour presentation.[38] Although this absolute effect was small, it was significantly associated with an increased risk of dying in-hospital, and it represents a potential target for quality improvement efforts. In the recent GWTG analysis among 502,036 ischemic stroke admissions from 1,256 hospitals from 2003 to 2009, the substantial temporal improvements in stroke mortality have been reported.[39] However, age-related treatment gap was observed. Older stroke patients had almost 30% greater in-hospital mortality for each 10-year age increase.

TABLE 16-1 Stroke Mortality and Recurrence Rates

	Stroke Mortality	Stroke Mortality in NOMASS	Stroke Recurrence	Stroke Recurrence in NOMASS
30-day	3–20%	5%	1–6%	2%
1-year	20–35%	16%	5–25%	8%
5-year	38–75%	41%	15–40%	16%

NOMASS, Northern Manhattan Stroke Study.

The decline in stroke mortality resulted from reduced incidence of stroke and lower case-fatality rates. These significant improvements in stroke outcomes are concurrent with improved risk factor control. The decline in stroke mortality can be attributed to a combination of improved and evidence-based stroke management and interventions, and implementation of these programs to the populations. The potential effects of implementations of stroke systems of care and telemedicine also may contribute to decline in stroke mortality, but they have not been in place long enough to be reliably evaluated for their effects on stroke mortality or other post-stroke outcomes.[3,40]

Causes of Early Death after Ischemic Stroke

The immediate cause of death in more than 60% of stroke cases was related to the stroke itself.[3,4,41–44] Death within 30 days after a first stroke due to incident stroke was found in 91% of patients in the Oxfordshire Community Stroke Project and in 85% of patients in the Perth Community Stroke Study.[45,46] After 30 days post stroke, cardiovascular pathology and conditions resulting from stroke were the causes of death in up to 80% of the patients, which is substantially greater than in the age- and gender-matched general population.[44] In the German Stroke Registry of 13,440 ischemic stroke patients from 104 academic centers, in-hospital mortality was 5%, and increased intracranial pressure had the highest attributable risk, accounting for 94% of deaths among these patients.[47] In the entire stroke population, pneumonia had the highest attributable risk of death, accounting for about one-third of all deaths.[48] Pneumonia has been associated with a threefold increased risk of in-hospital death in a study including 14,293 patients hospitalized for acute stroke[49] and with a fourfold increased early stroke mortality in a recent systematic review and meta-analysis of 87 studies involving 137,817 patients.[50] More than half of all in-hospital deaths were attributable to either serious medical or neurologic complications. Impaired consciousness on admission, posterior circulation infarcts, and transtentorial herniation are the most important neurologic causes of death during the first week after stroke onset. Thereafter, cardiac causes, pulmonary embolism, sepsis, and other medical complications account for the majority of deaths within the first month after stroke onset.[48] Excess mortality related to cardiovascular disease has also been described among young adults. Among the 30-day survivors from the Helsinki Young Stroke Registry of 711 patients, the cause of death was stroke in 21%, cardioaortic and other vascular causes in 36%, malignancies in 12%, and infections in 9%.[51] In NOMASS, the proportion of 30-day deaths after a first ischemic stroke was 75%.[43] Incident (53%) or recurrent (4%) stroke caused early deaths in 57% of patients. Cardiac causes of early death may be higher among blacks than among other races/ethnicities.[52–54] Excess early mortality related to cardiovascular disease has also been described among young black people and Caribbean-Hispanics.[3,35] In the International

Stroke Trial among 18,451 stroke patients, death within 14 days was more frequent in patients with AF (17% versus 8%) and more often attributed to neurological deterioration from the initial stroke (10% versus 4%).[55] Similarly in VISTA-Acute, an academic database containing standardized data for 28,131 stroke patients from 30 randomized-controlled acute stroke trials and one stroke registry,[56] AF was associated with over 40% increased risk of early mortality (OR 1.44, 95%CI 1.14–1.81) after adjusting for all baseline imbalances. In the GWTG program among 274,988 ischemic stroke patients enrolled between 2001 and 2007, characteristics associated with early in-hospital mortality included the NIHSS score, age, arrival mode (e.g., via ambulance versus other mode), history of atrial fibrillation, previous stroke, previous myocardial infarction, carotid stenosis, diabetes mellitus, peripheral vascular disease, hypertension, history of dyslipidemia, current smoking, and weekend or night admission.[57]

Late Mortality after Ischemic Stroke

Longitudinal studies among patients with ischemic stroke have demonstrated that the risk of death at 5 years ranged from 40% to 60%, including early fatalities.[35,41,58] The average annual mortality rate in 30-day stroke survivors ranges from 8% to 9%, and the risk of death is two to three times higher than that of the age- and sex-matched general population.[35,43,44] In the National Survey of Stroke, only 53% of stroke patients who survived the initial 6 months lived for 5 years.[59] The 5-year survival rate was 75% in those younger than 65 and fell to 23% in those 85 or older. In the Oxfordshire Community Stroke Project, the stroke mortality rate was 10% at 30 days, 23% at 1 year, and 51% at 5 years.[45] In Rochester, Minnesota, the risk of death after first cerebral infarction was 27% at 1 year and 53% at 5 years.[32] In the Monitoring Trends and Determinants in Cardiovascular Disease (MONICA) Project, the estimated cumulative risks of death were 41% at 1 year after stroke and 60% at 5 years.[60] In NOMASS the life table cumulative risk of ischemic stroke mortality was 5% at 30 days, 16% at 1 year, and 41% at 5 years after stroke (Table 16-1).[43] In the Framingham Study, 5-year mortality rates after atherothrombotic brain infarction were 44% for men and 36% for women and were similar to the standard population.[28] In the same cohort, however, stroke survivors for 20 years or more had a greater mortality rate than age- and sex-matched control subjects.[61] Among young adults, the overall cumulative mortality risks are low (i.e., 1% to 4.0% at 1 month, 3% to 6% at 1 year, and 10% to 12% at 5 years). However, those older than 45 years of age have lower probabilities of survival.

Despite the encouraging decline in stroke risk, there is evidence of a recent increase in mean blood pressure in young people in the US and UK, prompting concern that favorable trends in stroke risk may not be maintained.[62,63] Recent data from the Framingham Study suggest that the lifetime risk of stroke is very high.[64] The same has been observed in other Western countries; therefore monitoring cardiovascular risk factors in communities is of utmost importance for public health.

Causes of Late Death after Ischemic Stroke

Population-based epidemiological studies found that early mortality is more commonly related to the index or recurrent stroke, whereas later mortality is generally related to cardiovascular causes.[3,42,65]

In NOMASS patients with first ischemic stroke, 14% of long-term deaths were related to either incident or recurrent stroke.[43] Leukocyte counts at the time of incident ischemic stroke predicted outcomes including 5-year death after ischemic stroke in NOMAS,[66] indicating that underlying inflammation and acute infectious complications at time of index stroke could account for increased long-term stroke mortality. Recurrent stroke and a coronary event are also important causes of stroke mortality. The risk of a recurrent stroke is highest in the first month (4%) and the first year (12%) after a stroke, likely reflecting the presence of unstable and active atherosclerotic plaque.[67] After the first year, the risk of a recurrent cerebrovascular event falls to about 5% per year, similar to the risk of a coronary event. During years 1–5 after an ischemic stroke, cardiovascular disease increasingly becomes the major cause of death, reflecting the generalized nature of atherosclerosis. The most robust predictor of death within 1–5 years after stroke is increased age and heart failure. Additional baseline predictors of longer-term mortality include a history of previous ischemic stroke, peripheral arterial disease, and heart disease (myocardial infarction, heart failure, AF).

Predictors of Death after Ischemic Stroke

For early and late mortality, predictors of death after ischemic stroke may differ (Table 16-2). Most of them, however, affect both early and late mortality, and a clear distinction cannot be made. Early recognition of predictors of death after stroke

TABLE 16-2 Definite and Potential Predictors of Death and Poor Outcome after Ischemic Stroke

	Definite Predictors	Potential Predictors
Demographics	Age	Sex Race/ethnicity Socioeconomic status Region, country
Clinical parameters	Initial severity of stroke (NIHSS) Decreased consciousness Infarct size Large hemispheric or basilar syndrome Ischemic stroke subtype Fever Hypertension Atrial fibrillation Diabetes Congestive heart failure	Other cardiac disease Previous stroke Prestroke disability Prestroke depression Prestroke dementia Obstructive sleep apnea
Lifestyle parameters	Smoking Alcohol Obesity/diet	
Biochemical biomarkers	Hyperglycemia C-reactive protein	Cholesterol Erythrocyte sedimentation rate Fibrinogen White blood cell count Uric acid/creatinine Microalbuminuria/ albumin–globulin ratio LpPLA2 Homocysteine
Neuroimaging markers		White matter disease Silent brain infarcts Microbleeds
Systems of health care		Access to care Emergency response Telemedicine

LpPLA2, Lipoprotein-associated phospholipase A2.

onset is of special importance when relevant clinical variables are accounted for within the first 72 hours after a stroke. Although the prediction of stroke outcome could probably be improved by including variables that are assessed later, the practical value would be limited, as the prediction cannot be given as early. In addition, a development of early prediction models taking into account only variables that are evaluated within the first 6 hours after onset would be important for acute stroke interventional clinical trials. Stroke-related deaths continue to be a problem during the years after ischemic stroke, especially in patients who are functionally dependent at 6 months after onset.[68] Stroke risk factors and their control have a greater impact on long-term stroke outcome. Therefore, better short-term stroke treatments and interventions to reduce dependency and adequate secondary stroke prevention remain to be high priority in reducing stroke mortality and stroke burden.[22]

Age, Sex, and Race-Ethnicity

Non-modifiable factors such as age, sex, and race/ethnicity are important determinants of stroke outcomes. Age is an independent prognostic factor of both early and late stroke mortality.[69–75]Age has a significant role in the cause of death after a recurrent stroke, with a greater proportionate mortality attributable to recurrent stroke rather than cardiac causes of death. This may be enhanced by the greater mean age at stroke onset; that is, older people are more likely to die as a result of the event than younger people.[76] In the GWTG program, older stroke patients were more likely to die in hospital (adjusted OR 1.27; 95%CI 1.25–1.29) for each 10-year age increase.[77] Elderly patients have a higher risk of subsequent in-hospital complications after stroke and therefore lower chances of recovery from stroke.

More women than men die of stroke each year because of the larger number of elderly women. Women accounted for almost 60% of US stroke deaths in 2010.[24] There was a greater decline in stroke death rates in men than in women in the US, with the decrease in a male-to-female age-adjusted ratio from 1.11 to 1.05.[4] In men, stroke age-adjusted death rates fell by 28%, and stroke dropped from the third to the fifth leading cause of death after ischemic heart disease, lung cancer, accidents, and CLRD (Chronic Lower Respiratory Disease). Among women, although stroke age-adjusted death rates declined by 24%, stroke remained the second leading cause of death.[78] The age-standardized case-fatality rates are also greater for women than for men.[24] In the Framingham Study, 30-day case fatality declined significantly in men but not women.[79] Higher case fatality in women was reported in the International Stroke Trial,[80] which randomly assigned 8,003 women and 9,367 men to aspirin or heparin, or both; 14-day case fatality in women was 11.0% compared with 8.7% in men, and 6-month case fatality was 24.5% in women and 19.3% in men. However, after adjustment for age, stroke severity, AF, and blood pressure this difference disappeared, suggesting that baseline differences in age, stroke characteristics, and risk factors may account for much of the observed sex differences in case fatality. In the Danish MONICA study, women had a higher risk of death than men for up to 1 year after stroke, even after adjustment for age.[69] In contrast, in the Framingham Study, women had a better survival rate than men after stroke.[62] This sex-specific difference in stroke survival is age-dependent. Below the age of 45 years, stroke mortality for women and men is similar, but women aged 45–74 years have about 20–35% lower risk of stroke mortality than do men. This benefit for women declines in older age groups, such that women aged 85 years and older have 12–14% higher mortality than men.[81] Few studies have reported poorer stroke outcomes in women and suggested that women arrived later to the emergency departments than men, were less likely to receive thrombolytic therapy, lipid and other diagnostic testing and interventions, and were more likely to have more severe strokes at onset, and urinary tract infections.[80–83] In the GWTG program among 383,318 acute ischemic stroke patients from 1,139 US hospitals, women consistently received less care and had higher crude in-hospital mortality compared to men (6.0% versus 5.2%).[84] The greater burden of stroke deaths in women is predicted to be even higher in the future. Further studies are needed to specifically explore reasons for sex-specific differences in stroke mortality and plan effective interventions to reduce these sex-specific stroke mortality disparities.

Differences in stroke mortality rates between various race/ethnic groups have been reported.[85,85] Despite a decline in age-adjusted stroke death rates, stroke remained the second leading cause of death in blacks.[87] Among whites, however, the 26% decline in stroke age-adjusted death rates resulted in stroke moving from the second to the fourth leading cause of death after ischemic heart disease, lung cancer, and chronic lower respiratory disease (CLRD). In the GWTG program among 397,257 patients admitted with ischemic stroke to 1,181 hospitals from 2003 to 2008, black patients had greater in-hospital stroke mortality relative to white patients and received fewer evidence-based care processes than white or Hispanic patients.[88] Hispanic patients received similar care to their white counterparts and had similar in-hospital mortality. In the Cardiovascular Health Study (CHS) cohort of patients 65 years of age or older, black people had a greater risk of death after ischemic stroke than other groups.[89] In a cohort of veterans with stroke living in the southeastern United States, non-Hispanic black people had significantly higher mortality rates than did non-Hispanic white people 38 months after stroke.[90] In NOMASS, 5-year cumulative life table mortality estimates after stroke differed only slightly among the three race/ethnic groups.[43] Despite similar overall stroke mortality rates between race/ethnic groups in NOMASS, a higher incident stroke-related early mortality among Caribbean Hispanics was observed. In the REasons for Geographic And Racial Differences in Stroke (REGARDS) national cohort study among 27,744 patients enrolled between 2003 and 2007, national patterns of black–white and regional disparities in stroke incidence were similar to those for stroke mortality.[91] In the GWTG data linked with Medicare claims data set among 200,900 stroke patients, black and Hispanic patients had higher long-term mortality than white and Asian patients even after adjustment for stroke severity, other prognostic variables, and hospital characteristics.[92]

Disparities in the incidence of stroke risk factors (e.g., AF, diabetes mellitus, and hypertension) and socioeconomic status between black, Hispanic, and white patients may, in part, explain the disproportionate mortality rates among Hispanic, black, and white patients after stroke.[93] However, the majority of the excess burden of stroke mortality is borne by relatively young black people and by black people living in the southeastern US.[91,94,95]

While overall stroke mortality rates have been rapidly declining for both black people and white people, the magnitude of the relative increased risk of dying from a stroke among black people, as compared with white people, has remained largely unchanged. As such, coordinated efforts to reduce ethnic disparities in stroke mortality are still needed. Further studies are needed to determine how much of the race/ethnic disparities in stroke mortality may be explained by differences in stroke risk factors and ischemic stroke subtype as well as in differences in socioeconomic status, access to healthcare and deficiencies in the systems of healthcare.

Initial Stroke Severity

The initial severity of a stroke measured by the National Institutes of Health Stroke Scale (NIHSS),[70,96] remains one of the major predictors of mortality and poor outcomes after stroke.[70,96-99] In the TOAST trial, one additional point on the baseline NIHSS decreased the likelihood of survival and excellent outcomes at 7 days by 24% and at 3 months by 17%.[70] An NIHSS score of 16 or greater predicted a high probability of death or severe disability, whereas a score of 6 or less predicted a good recovery. In the GWTG program among 274,988 ischemic stroke patients between 2001 and 2007, the NIHSS score was the strongest predictor of in-hospital mortality and provided substantial incremental information on a patient's short-term mortality risk.[100] The NIHSS score is an important predictor for other stroke outcomes besides mortality such as recurrent stroke, complications after tPA, and functional outcome. The NIHSS score and age in various prediction schemes, are the two most potent predictors of stroke outcomes.[101] Markers of initial stroke severity such as depressed consciousness, infarct size, the severity of the neurologic deficit, the type of admitting syndrome and seizures have been reported as clinical predictors of early outcome after stroke.[102-106] Of the 1,754 prospectively collected records of patients with acute ischemic stroke in the German Stroke Database, orientation, limb paresis, trunk ataxia, and dysphagia were independent predictors of early death after stroke.[98]

The type of initial stroke syndrome has been found to be another important clinical determinant of mortality.[67] In NOMASS, patients seen with a major hemispheric or basilar syndrome had the worst early mortality rates, patients with minor hemispheric syndromes had an associated intermediate survival rate, and those with a lacunar syndrome had the best prognosis, as also reported previously. In the Oxfordshire cohort, patients with total anterior cerebral infarcts had the worst survival rate.[107] Mortality after posterior cerebral infarct seems to be low, but long-term behavioral and cognitive deficits are likely underestimated. In analyses from seven clinical trials of patients with a large representation of posterior strokes, stroke mortality ranged from 2% to 5%.[108] Amnesia and cortical blindness are the predictors of poor outcome after stroke in posterior infarcts.[109]

Fever/Pyrexia

Pyrexia after stroke onset is associated with a marked increase in morbidity and mortality. Admission body temperature is considered to be a major determinant of short-term as well as long-term mortality after stroke.[110-112] During the first days after acute stroke, a fever or subfebrile temperature elevation develops in one-fifth to almost one-half of patients.[113-114] Subfebrile temperatures (37.5 °C to 39 °C) and fever (>39 °C) after a stroke are associated with relatively large infarct volumes, high case-fatality rates, and poor functional outcomes, even after adjustment for initial stroke severity.[113-118] Hyperthermia within the first 12 or 24 hours after stroke onset may be more predictive of outcome than delayed fever.[117] The significant stroke prognostic influence of initial body temperature was confirmed by a meta-analysis of nine studies with 3,790 patients.[119] A fever of more than 38°C within 3 days after stroke was among the most important predictors of mortality or functional dependence after stroke.[113-120] In the recent pooled analyses covering 14,431 patients with stroke and other brain injuries, fever was consistently associated with worse outcomes across multiple outcome measures.[121]

In the Copenhagen Stroke Study, the mortality rate at 60 months after stroke was greater for patients with hyperthermia on admission (73% versus 59%).[112] A 1 °C increase of admission body temperature independently predicted a 30% relative increase (95%CI 4–57) in long-term mortality risk. An association between admission body temperature and stroke mortality was noted independent of stroke severity. Mortality 1 year after stroke for patients with admission hyperthermia was over threefold greater than for normothermic patients (RR 3.4, 95%CI 1.6–7.3).[110]

In patients with acute ischemic stroke, a pharmacologic reduction of body temperature or body cooling procedures may reduce mortality and improve functional outcome.[122-125] Promising therapeutic strategies include treatment of fever aiming to sustain normothermia and induced hypothermia, targeting core body temperatures below 36.5 °C.[126] Although supported by preclinical evidence, currently therapeutic hypothermia for acute stroke remains under study. In the Intravascular Cooling in the Treatment of Stroke (ICTuS) trial, awake acute stroke patients were successfully cooled using an endovascular cooling catheter and a novel anti-shivering regimen,[127] and further ICTuS phase II/III safety clinical study is underway.[128]

Ischemic Stroke Subtypes and Stroke Mortality

Ischemic stroke subtype is an important determinant of mortality in many prospective community stroke studies and clinical trials, including cohorts from Rochester, Minnesota, the NINDS Stroke Data Bank, Perth, Australia, Erlangen Stroke Project, German Stroke Registry, NOMASS, Oxfordshire Community Stroke Project, TOAST; CHS, ARIC, the Greater Cincinnati/Northern Kentucky Stroke Study and many other cohorts. The chance of survival was significantly better for patients with lacunar infarcts compared with non-lacunar infarcts.[67,129,130] In the northern Manhattan cohort, presentation with a lacunar syndrome was associated with a significantly better 5-year survival rate. Recent data on long-term outcomes in patients with lacunar stroke have shown that, for the first few years after lacunar infarct, the risk of death was similar or slightly increased to that of the general population.[131] However, a clear excess of death was observed later, indicating that the long-term prognosis in lacunar infarction appears less favorable than previously reported.[132] The trends towards an increased incidence of lacunar strokes have also been reported.[133] Recently, in a Beijing population in China, lacunar stroke was a common ischemic stroke subtype (about 40%), but with 1-year survival rates similar to non-lacunar stroke.[134] Therefore, lacunar infarcts show a paradoxical clinical course with a low early mortality but with an increased risk of death, stroke recurrence and dementia in the mid- and long term. Asymptomatic progression of small-vessel disease is a typical feature of the lacunar infarcts, and for this reason lacunar infarction should be regarded as a potentially severe condition that requires adequate and rigorous management.[135]

Ischemic stroke subtype according to the TOAST criteria[70] was a significant predictor of stroke survival after adjustment for age and sex.[136] The highest mortality rate was reported for cardioembolic and large atherothrombotic strokes, and the lowest was for lacunar strokes. In the Rochester Epidemiology Project,[137] the case-fatality rates for cardioembolic stroke at 1 month (30.3%), 1 year (53%), and 2 years (61.4%) were higher than reported in other cohorts, which was most likely due to the older patients in the cohort (mean age for cardioembolic stroke, 80 years). In CHS, the most lethal ischemic stroke subtype was also cardioembolic.[89] Patients with cardioembolic stroke were nearly four times more likely to be dead 30 days after the stroke than patients with stroke due to large-vessel atherosclerosis with stenosis and 2.5 times more likely to be dead 5 years later. Recently in ARIC, after adjustment for age, sex, and race, mortality was higher for cardioembolic stroke (HR 1.3; 95%CI 1.0–1.6) compared to other stroke subtypes.[138] Cardioembolic strokes present with greater stroke severity than other subtypes and with more vascular comorbidities that are likely the major factors responsible for the worse outcome of patients with cardioembolic stroke.[139]

In the New England Medical Center Posterior Circulation Registry, a low mortality rate at 30 days after stroke onset (3.6%) was observed among patients with vertebrobasilar occlusive strokes.[140] A poor outcome was associated with basilar artery involvement, embolic stroke mechanism, and multiple posterior circulation intracranial territory involvement. Increased mortality and poor functional outcome are significantly more frequent in the patients with intracranial large atherosclerotic stroke that in patients with extracranial large vessel disease, with vascular risk factors, particularly dyslipidemia, to be among the most important predictors of poor outcomes.[141] Interventions to improve outcome of patients with intracranial atherosclerotic strokes beyond medical treatment have recently failed to show benefit (i.e., SAMMPRIS) due to excessively high rate of death.[142] Carotid endarterectomy has significantly reduced poor outcome for patients with stroke due to extracranial disease, although the best intervention modality including best medical treatment is currently under investigations.[143]

Blood Pressure, Atrial Fibrillation, and Heart Failure

Elevated blood pressure was identified as being responsible for the largest number of stroke deaths.[3,144,145,146] The INTERSTROKE study reported that the contribution of various risk factors to the burden of stroke worldwide was 34.6% for hypertension.[147] The relationship between blood pressure and risk of stroke and stroke mortality has been consistently demonstrated over time and independent of other risk factors. The linear relationship holds true for all demographics, indicating that the higher the blood pressure, the greater the risk of stroke mortality.[3] Clinical trials have demonstrated that blood pressure reduction with the use of diuretics and/or angiotensin-converting enzyme inhibitors reduces stroke mortality and recurrence.[11,148–150]

Three-quarters of patients with acute ischemic stroke have elevated blood pressure at presentation.[151] Blood pressure declines spontaneously over the first week after stroke onset and returns to prestroke levels in two-thirds of patients. Most studies have found that high blood pressure, whether measured as casual or 24-hour ambulatory readings, in the acute phase of stroke is associated with a poor outcome,[152] and may promote early recurrence, hemorrhagic transformation, or cerebral edema.[153] Also, a U-shaped relation between the level of acute elevation in blood pressure and outcome has been introduced defining a middle area with better prognosis than patients with high as well as low blood pressure.[154] In the International Stroke Trial of 17,398 stroke patients, both high and low blood pressure were independent prognostic factors for 6-month poor outcome after stroke.[144] Early death increased by 3.8% for every 10 mm Hg above 150 mm Hg and by 17.9% for every 10 mm Hg below 150 mm Hg. In the Multicenter rt-PA Stroke Survey of 1,205 patients treated in routine clinical practice with intravenous rt-PA within 3 hours of stroke symptom onset, elevated pretreatment mean blood pressure was a main attribute associated with increased case-fatality and intracranial hemorrhage rates.[155] Admission blood pressure is also associated with long-term outcome after stroke. Low- or high-admission blood pressure indicates cardiac comorbidity or preexisting hypertension, where close monitoring and further examinations are requested to reduce mortality and prevent poorer outcome after stroke.[156]

Blood pressure management in acute ischemic stroke, however, remains problematic, with questions such as when to initiate antihypertensive agents, to what level of blood pressure reduction, and which class of agents should be used.[157] Ongoing clinical trials such as ENCHANTED, ATACH II, and ENOS are expected to provide evidence for blood pressure treatment in acute stroke, modify current guidelines for acute stroke, and potentially improve stroke clinical outcomes.[158]

Cardiac disease was a prominent predictor of survival after strokes in multiple studies. Heart failure is the most robust predictor of death within 1 to 5 years after stroke, secondary only to increasing age.[67,159–161] Patients with dilated cardiomyopathy have a high incidence of left ventricular thrombus formation and are at increased risk of embolic complications.[162] In the Framingham Study, heart failure was ranked second in cardiogenic stroke risk, with a two- to threefold relative risk.[163,164] Congestive heart failure is associated with high rates of mortality: a 15-year mortality rate is estimated at 39% for women and 72% for men.[165] In the Finland study, the presence of congestive heart failure doubled the age- and sex-adjusted risk of death from all causes, and quadrupled the risk of death from stroke and cardiovascular diseases during 4-year follow-up.[166] In the northern Manhattan cohort, congestive heart failure was an independent predictor of 5-year death among 30-day survivors. In Rochester, Minnesota, independent risk factors for death after first cerebral infarction were congestive heart failure, persistent AF, and ischemic heart disease.[32] In the Perth Community Stroke Study, predictors of death within 1 year included cardiac failure and AF.[41] In a 14-year follow-up study from Sweden, heart failure and history of diabetes were predictors of long-term mortality.[159] Stroke survivors with cardiac disease had a poorer 1-year survival rate in the Community Hospital-based Stroke Programs[9] and a decreased 10-year survival in Framingham.[164]

AF is the most prevalent chronic cardiac arrhythmia in the elderly and has a well-documented impact on the prognosis of first-ever stroke.[3,4,161] In the Framingham cohort, 30-day mortality and stroke severity in the AF subjects was 25% versus 14% in non-AF subjects.[167] The other studies reported 30-day mortality of 23% to 35% in AF subjects versus 7% to 14% in non-AF subjects.[161–166] The difference in mortality between AF and non-AF subjects was more evident in the extreme elderly. Half of the strokes in AF subjects 75 years of age or older were either severe or fatal because of the contribution of AF to death. Since 1989, numerous trials have shown a benefit of warfarin treatment over antiplatelet therapy among patients with AF.[168] The evidence is very strong that anticoagulation with warfarin for patients with AF reduces fatal and nonfatal stroke by ≈50%. There is a reduction in case-fatality rates in patients on warfarin compared to without.[169] New oral anticoagulants in treatment of AF have emerged as convenient agents with important advantages over warfarin in improving clinical outcomes including lower mortality and are now generally used as first-line treatment for stroke prevention in AF.[170] It will be important for post-marketing surveillance to monitor their use and clinical outcomes because available data suggest that they will have an even stronger effect than warfarin on reducing stroke mortality in AF.[22]

Hyperglycemia and Diabetes

Diabetes is common among patients with stroke and is associated with a poorer outcome. Post-stroke hyperglycemia is also recognized in up to half of the patients, and is independently associated with increased mortality and poorer functional outcomes in patients both with and without diabetes.[171–178] Hyperglycemia during acute ischemic stroke may augment brain injury, predispose to intracerebral hemorrhage, or both.[177] Alternatively, the effect of hyperglycemia may be confounded by the acute stress reaction secondary to an infarct. In the NINDS rt-PA Stroke Trial, higher admission glucose levels were associated with significantly lower odds for desirable clinical outcomes regardless of rt-PA treatment.[177] In northern Manhattan, admission glucose >140 mg/dl was associated with an increased mortality, independent of the size or severity of the ischemic stroke.[179] Diabetes mellitus was found to be a prognostic variable for death in several studies.[97-99] This could be due to greater preexisting comorbidity of diabetic patients as well as to greater neuronal damage of ischemic tissue in hyperglycemia. In the prospective observational study of 4,585 patients with type 2 diabetes in England, Scotland, and Northern Ireland, each 1% reduction in the mean HbA1c level was associated with reductions in risk of 21% for deaths related to diabetes, 14% for myocardial infarction (MI), and 37% for microvascular complications including stroke.[178] Early mortality after stroke in patients with type 2 diabetes was 28%. Recently, in a European Union Concerted Action involving seven countries and 4537 patients hospitalized for a first-time stroke (21% with diabetes), the case-fatality rates were not higher in the diabetic group in comparison with the non-diabetic group at 3 months after stroke onset.[180] A recent meta-analysis of five diabetes interventional trials has showed that tight glucose control provides benefit for reducing MI, but no consistent effect was found for stroke.[181] There was a suggestion that stroke mortality may be increased with tight glucose control, driven primarily by the Action to Control Cardiovascular Risk in Diabetes (ACCORD) trial results,[182] which, however, were primarily explained by insufficient blood pressure control in this trial.

Whether intensive glucose control (typically defined as a glucose goal ≤150 mg/dL) during the acute stroke hospitalization reduces stroke mortality and improves outcomes is an active area of investigation. The Stroke Hyperglycemia Insulin Network Effort (SHINE) trial, a large ongoing phase III clinical trial is aimed to determine the safety and efficacy of standard vs. intensive glucose control with insulin in hyperglycemic acute ischemic stroke patients.[183] At this time, there is insufficient evidence to know if reducing hyperglycemia is beneficial for reducing stroke mortality and the optimal management of hyperglycemia associated with acute stroke is unknown.[184]

Inflammatory Markers and Other Biochemical Blood Parameters

Inflammatory biomarkers, such as C-reactive protein (CRP) and lipoprotein-associated phospholipase A2 (Lp-PLA2), predict not only development of atherothrombotic events but also long-term mortality after acute ischemic stroke.[185-196] Elevated admission CRP levels within 12 to 72 hours of stroke were associated with an increased risk of death.[186,188,189] Individuals with increased CRP levels may have a twofold increased risk of death compared with those with low CRP levels after stroke.[189] In a recent study systematic review of five studies which met all inclusion criteria, CRP measured within 24 hours of symptom onset has been associated with unfavorable long-term mortality and functional outcome.[191] The relationship between CRP and post-stroke mortality may in part reflect inflammation-induced endothelial cell dysfunction and platelet activation. Also, levels of CRP increase with stroke severity and may be associated with mortality to a greater degree than recurrence, whereas Lp-PLA2 may be a stronger predictor of recurrent stroke risk.[197,198] Lp-PLA2 is a leukocyte-derived enzyme involved in the metabolism of low-density lipoprotein cholesterol to pro-inflammatory mediators and was shown to predict incident stroke[194] and recurrent stroke.[195] in addition, changes in immune and stress markers, for example a reduction in HLA-DR expression on monocytes or an increase in serum catecholamine levels, occur very early after stroke onset, and may explain the high susceptibility of stroke patients to infections and infectious complications resulting in increased mortality after stroke. Several soluble biomarkers have been identified as potential predictors of outcome and mortality after stroke including the stress marker copeptin and midregional pro-atrial natriuretic peptide.[199] The utility of these and other potential biomarkers (e.g., IL-6, fibrinogen, erythrocyte sedimentation rate, and leukocyte count)[185,187,200-204] and their ability to improve clinical decision-making in stroke patients require further studies.

Uric acid and other parameters of chronic kidney disease have been associated with poor long-term survival rates after stroke. There is a well-recognized link between serum urate levels and increased cardiovascular risk. The serum urate level was associated with a threefold increase in relative risk of cardiac death within 5 years after stroke.[205] Serum urate measured within the first 24 hours after hospital admission for acute stroke was an independent marker of poor outcome in a large study from Scotland.[206] In a systematic review and meta-analysis of 16 studies including 238,449 patients, hyperuricemia was associated with a significantly higher risk of stroke mortality (RR 1.26, 95%CI 1.12–1.39) independent of age, sex, hypertension, diabetes mellitus, and cholesterol.[207] Although the role of urate in stroke pathophysiology remains uncertain, intervention to lower urate levels may be worth considering.[208,209] Other measures of renal dysfunction, even to a subtle degree, have also been noted to be a prognostic indicator of overall mortality rates in many patient groups.[210-212] In a Scottish, 7-year follow-up study of 2,042 stroke patients, reduced admission creatinine clearance, raised serum creatinine and urea concentrations, and raised ratios of urea to creatinine were significant predictors of increased mortality.[210] In the recent analysis from the Get With The Guidelines-Stroke (GWTG-Stroke) program among 679,827 patients hospitalized with ischemic stroke from 1,564 US centers between 2009 and 2012, chronic kidney disease defined by glomerular filtration rate was associated with greater in-hospital mortality (adjusted OR 1.44, 95%CI 1.40–1.47), which progressively rose with more severe renal dysfunction.[213]

Soluble biomarkers may have a potential role in risk stratification, but their clinical utility and the clinical relevance of reducing their levels in reducing the risk of stroke outcomes require further investigation.

RECURRENCE AFTER ISCHEMIC STROKE

Recurrent stroke is a major cause of morbidity and mortality among stroke survivors. With aging of populations, improved survival rates after first ischemic stroke, and advances in rehabilitation and evidence-based secondary prevention strategies, stroke recurrence may account for a greater share of the future annual cost of stroke-related health care.[19] Recurrent stroke will continue to be the major threat to stroke survivors and their caregivers.

Recurrent strokes represent 23% of the 800,000 strokes that occur each year in the US.[4] Recurrent strokes are associated with higher mortality rates, greater levels of disability, and increased costs compared with first stroke events. Recurrent stroke rates within the first year have been shown to range from 4% to 15%.[3,4,179,214-220] In large prospective, community-based studies, the risk of recurrent stroke varies from 1% to 4% in the first 30 days, 6% to 13% in the first year, and 5% to 8% per year for the next 2 to 5 years, which a cumulative risk of recurrent stroke within 5 years of 19% to 42%.[4,215-217] Lower recurrent stroke rates have been observed among selected groups of patients in large clinical trials such as TOAST, International Stroke Trial (IST), WARSS, PRoFESS, SAMPRISS, and SPS3[13,101,103,142,218–220] and also in prospective community studies.[28,32,77,98,221–228] The reasons for the differences in recurrence rates between various studies may reflect the study design (hospital-based versus community), sociodemographics of the study populations, definitions of recurrent stroke, and the use of acute treatments/interventions and preventive medications. The 30-day case-fatality rate is almost double for a recurrent stroke compared with the index stroke.[67]

In Rochester, Minnesota, the risk of recurrent stroke after first cerebral infarction was 2% at 7 days, 4% at 30 days, 12% at 1 year, and 29% at 5 years.[28,221] In the Stroke Data Bank, 3.3% of the hospitalized cohort had a stroke recurrence within 30 days, and this accounted for 30% of the recurrent strokes in 2 years of follow-up.[224] In Framingham, cumulative recurrence rates at 5 years after an infarction were 42% for men and 24% for women.[28] Rates were lower in Rochester, Minnesota: 19.3% at 5 years and 28.8% at 10 years.[221] In the Perth Community Stroke Study of 343 patients with first-ever stroke, approximately one in six survivors (15%) of a first-ever stroke experienced a recurrent stroke over 5 years, of which 25% were fatal within 28 days.[228] The cumulative risks of first recurrent stroke were 23% at 5 years and 43% at 10 years.[224] In the northern Manhattan cohort of 992 patients with first-ever ischemic stroke, the cumulative life table estimated risks of recurrent stroke were 2.0% at 30 days, 8% at 1 year, and 16% at 5 years (Table 16-1).[223] At 30 days, the risk of recurrent stroke was approximately 2.5 times the risk of MI or fatal cardiac events, although this ratio fell to about twice the risk of MI or fatal cardiac event by 5 years.[229] Thus, risk of recurrent stroke predominated even at 5 years among stroke survivors. In the REGARDS cohort with 5 years of follow-up, participants with self-reported stroke symptoms, TIA, distant stroke, or recent stroke all had increased risk of future stroke compared with those with no symptoms.[230] After risk-factor adjustment, there was a monotonically increasing risk of subsequent stroke across this symptomatic spectrum.

Decline of Recurrent Stroke Rates

Recurrent stroke rates have been decreasing over time. In the control arms of randomized, controlled trials of secondary stroke prevention interventions, rates of recurrent stroke declined for an almost 50% in the 1990s and 2000s compared with the 1960s.[231] In a systematic review of 13 studies from hospital- or community-based stroke registries, there was a temporal reduction in 5-year risk of stroke recurrence from 32% to 16%, but with substantial differences across studies in terms of case mix and definition of stroke recurrence.[232] Clinical trials have demonstrated the benefit of secondary stroke prevention therapies including antihypertensive therapy, statins, and aspirin.[233–237] Further improvements in secondary prevention could reduce recurrent vascular events in stroke patients by as much as 80% if multiple approaches (e.g., dietary modification, exercise, aspirin, statin, and antihypertensives) in secondary prevention are combined.[238,239] Recent clinical trial evidence from Stenting Versus Aggressive Medical Therapy for Intracranial Arterial Stenosis (SAMMPRIS)[219] indicated a reduction of secondary stroke risk with aggressive medical management in patients with intracranial atherosclerotic stenosis. Results from the Secondary Prevention of Small Subcortical Strokes (SPS3) study showed a declining risk of recurrence of small-vessel disease compared with expected rates estimated from natural history studies [220] and findings from the prospective Oxford Vascular Study demonstrated declining risk of stroke caused by carotid stenosis.[240]

Predictors of Recurrence after Ischemic Stroke

Factors that have been associated with an increased risk of recurrent stroke in community-based and hospital-based series include: increasing age;[29,33,97,241,246,247] male sex;[242,243] female sex;[244] clinical stroke syndrome;[245] history of transient cerebral ischemic attack;[67,248,249] hypertension;[67,97,144,145,248,250–253] initial elevated blood pressure;[140,154,247,248] low blood pressure;[144,145,252] cigarette smoking;[245] alcohol abuse and diabetes mellitus;[173,174–178,225,247,248] elevated blood glucose levels;[171,172,177] history of coronary heart disease;[67,244,248] AF;[161,167,168–170,183,250,254] and other cardiac diseases such as valvular heart disease, congestive heart failure, patent foramen ovale (PFO), and aortic arch atheroma,[164–166,168,255–262] abnormal initial brain CT/CTA and MRI (DWI),[263,264] cerebral white matter disease,[265] cerebral microbleeds,[266] dementia after stroke,[97,267,268] and depression.[269] In addition, as with first strokes, the risk of recurrent stroke is affected by differences in geography, race/ethnicity, socioeconomic status, and type of care or systems of care.[3,270]

Recurrent stroke rates differ between individual subtypes of ischemic stroke.[136–139,159,271–278] In a recent study from Scandinavia of 600 stroke patients followed up for 2 years, recurrent stroke occurred in 19.2% of patients with index stroke caused by large-artery disease, 4.9% with small-vessel disease, 8.2% with cardioembolic cause, 5.6% with cryptogenic cause, and 12.8% of other and undetermined cause combined.[277] In the Rochester study, ischemic stroke due to atherosclerosis with stenosis was associated with fewer recurrent strokes than cardioembolic stroke,[32] whereas in NOMASS the late recurrence risk did not significantly differ between the large atherosclerotic and non-large atherosclerotic stroke subtype (Table 16-3).[223,224] In ARIC, lacunar infarcts had somewhat higher recurrence compared with thrombotic infarcts (HR 1.3; 95%CI 0.9–1.9), but lower all-cause readmission (HR, 0.8; 95%CI 0.7–1.0). Readmission was 40% higher for cardioembolic stroke relative to thrombotic stroke (HR, 1.4; 95%CI 1.1–1.7).[132] In addition, cryptogenic stroke as a common stroke subtype, is likely caused by thromboembolism from undetermined sources (cardiac or vascular) and therefore is a relevant clinical entity with potentially a high risk of recurrence. Randomized clinical trials testing direct-acting oral anticoagulants for secondary prevention of embolic strokes of undetermined source (ESUS), such as RE-SPECT ESUS, are currently underway.

Predictors of Early Stroke Recurrence

Predictors of recurrent stroke may be time-specific and therefore may differ between early and late recurrence. Early after stroke, recurrent stroke tends to predominate, whereas at later points cardiac events begin to increase in relative importance and are the major cause of mortality.[3,4,42] Ischemic stroke subtype was shown to be a predictor of early stroke recurrence. Higher early recurrence rates for ischemic stroke due to large-vessel atherosclerosis have been consistently reported.[96,136–141,223,224,279,280]

TABLE 16-3 Recurrence Risk by Ischemic Stroke Subtype in the Northern Manhattan Stroke Study

Stroke Subtype	30-Day	1-Year	5-Year
All stroke	2%	8%	16%
Extracranial atherosclerotic	9%	11%	23%
Intracranial atherosclerotic	8%	12%	16%
Cardioembolic	4%	7%	21%
Lacunar	1.4%	10%	14%
Cryptogenic	0.4%	6%	15%

In NOMASS, a high 30-day recurrence risk for stroke due to large artery atherosclerotic disease was also found (Table 16-3). Estimated rates of recurrent stroke were greater for extracranial atherosclerotic infarcts (9%) and intracranial atherosclerotic infarcts (8%) than for cardioembolic (4%), lacunar (1.4%), and cryptogenic infarcts (0.4%). Patients with large atherosclerotic infarcts were seven times more likely to have recurrence 30 days after the index stroke than those with other ischemic stroke subtypes.

Clinical trials have also provided indirect evidence that rates of recurrent stroke are higher among patients with carotid or intracranial atherosclerosis as a cause of the stroke, as compared with other mechanisms of stroke.[219,273,274,281] Although treatment effects likely will change these recurrent stroke rates, there are subgroups of patients who remain at high risk of recurrence with these subtypes despite aggressive medical or interventional therapy.[282] Stroke due to large-artery stenotic disease may be prone to procedure-related cerebral ischemia, which may in part account for the higher risk of early recurrent stroke in this stroke subtype.[219]

Early stroke recurrence in cardioembolic stroke appears to be low.[224] The frequent use of anticoagulants may prevent early cardioembolic events and, therefore, reduce the risk of early recurrence. However, patients with cardioembolic stroke who were unwilling or unable to take oral anticoagulants had the greatest risk of stroke recurrence, as recently reported by the Prevention Regimen for Effectively Avoiding Second Strokes (PRoFESS) trial.[283]

Infarct subtype is usually not yet determined on admission; rather it depends on the diagnostic in-patient evaluation. In formulating predictors of early recurrence the best method would be to rely on factors that can be classified readily on first encounter with the patient through the clinical history, examination, and initial neuroimaging and laboratory testing. In NOMASS, the most significant predictors associated with early stroke recurrence besides ischemic stroke subtype, were AF (RR, 4.0; 95%CI 1.1–14.6), alcohol consumption (2–4 drinks per day versus none; RR, 6.8; 95%CI 1.2–39.9), and hypercholesterolemia (RR, 0.15; 95%CI 0.1–0.7).[223] Other studies have also identified AF and the presence of a potential cardioembolic source as predictors of early recurrent stroke[255–257,284] as well as alcohol abuse, hypertension, valvular heart disease, nausea and vomiting, and previous cerebral infarction to be most prominent factor associated with an increased risk of early recurrent stroke.[284] In the IST, data from 17,398 patients with acute stroke and high or low systolic blood pressure were associated with increased stroke recurrence within 14 days after stroke onset.[144] The rate of recurrent ischemic stroke within 14 days increased by 4.2% for every 10-mm Hg increase in systolic blood pressure, and this association was present in both fatal and non-fatal recurrence. Also, relatively low blood pressure (systolic blood pressure, <120 mm Hg), although an uncommon clinical finding (5% of patients) was also associated with poor outcome. Both relationships appeared to be independent of age, stroke severity, level of consciousness, and AF. This may provide an explanation for a worsening of outcome after the use of calcium channel blockers in some of the acute ischemic stroke studies, most likely due to a reduction in cerebral perfusion,[285–287] which was not observed in clinical trials of ACE-Is and ARBs in ischemic stroke.[288] In addition, an increased risk of early, 30-day risk of recurrent events occurs following discontinuation of antiplatelet agents.[289]

Predictors of Late Stroke Recurrence

Some non-modifiable and modifiable predictors of late recurrence after ischemic stroke have been identified. Among non-modifiable predictors, age was the most important predictor of survival after stroke, but has not consistently been found to be a determinant of recurrence. The lack of a significant association between age and stroke recurrence has been observed in several studies.[32,225,228] Although some reported greater stroke recurrence rates for men than women,[283,290] there are important gaps in our understanding of sex differences in recurrent stroke events and other outcomes after stroke.[82,291] Fewer studies have evaluated stroke recurrence in different race/ethnic groups. Stroke recurrence was slightly more frequent among black people and Hispanics in northern Manhattan, but these differences failed to reach statistical significance.[42]

Modifiable predictors of late recurrence after ischemic stroke have not been uniformly established. Even the effect of *hypertension* has been a matter of continuous debate.[292,293] The relationship between hypertension and recurrent stroke has been less well studied, but is presumed to be similar to that of index stroke.[22] Some have found no effect of hypertension, while others have suggested that hypertension increased recurrence after stroke.[285–287,292,294–297] This failure to identify hypertension as a predictor of recurrence may reflect the phenomenon that the high risk among patients who already have the disease overwhelms any effect of a specific risk factor. Alternatively, it could serve as an indication that the thresholds for defining these risk factors dichotomously need to be adjusted for the population of patients who have already experienced stroke. In a sense, for a patient who has had a stroke, even a "normal" blood pressure may be too high.[287] Also, as hypertension is very prevalent among stroke patients, the degree of blood pressure control may be more important. High baseline, maximum, mean level, and variability of systolic blood pressure profiles were each inversely associated with favorable outcomes.[292] In PROGRESS, a randomized controlled trial among individuals with previous stroke or transient ischemic attack (TIA), a blood-pressure-lowering regimen with perindopril and indapamide reduced the risk of recurrent stroke by more than one-quarter.[11] Over 4 years, annual stroke recurrence was reduced from 3.8% to 2.7%. Importantly, stroke risk was also reduced among those patients classified as non-hypertensive. This is consistent with a meta-analysis of antihypertensive medication intervention trials in which blood-pressure-lowering drug interventions reduced the risk of stroke recurrence.[297,298] However, limited data specifically address the optimal BP targets for secondary stroke prevention. Evidence from recent randomized clinical trial and observational studies among high-risk patients with DM, CAD and recent ischemic stroke indicates that there is no benefit in achieving an aggressive blood pressure lowering (SBP of <120 mmHg) or that there may even be harm associated with treating SBP levels <120 mmHg.[299–302]

Lowering blood pressure after stroke remains a challenge, even in the context of clinical trials as recently shown in the Secondary Prevention of Small Subcortical Strokes (SPS3) trial.[303] SPS3 randomly assigned 3,020 patients with lacunar stroke to two blood pressure targets (SBP <150 versus <130 mm Hg) and reported greater primary outcome of recurrent stroke in patients assigned to the higher-target group (2.8% per year) versus those assigned to the lower-target group (2.3% per year; HR, 0.81; 95%CI 0.64–1.03). The AHA currently recommends starting therapy at a SBP ≥140 mm Hg or DBP ≥90 mm Hg for all adults with a history of stroke or TIA.[304] The treatment of BP in stroke patients remains challenging as evident by some discrepancies between recent reports on BP treatment between the new Joint National Committee 8 (JNC-8) blood pressure guidelines and recommendations by other professional organizations.[22,293]

Epidemiological data show only a modest link between high *serum LDL-C* and greater risk of stroke.[22] However, data from the Stroke Prevention by Aggressive Reduction in Cholesterol Levels (SPARCL) clinical trial and meta-analysis have shown that statins, which markedly reduce LDL-C levels, have proved efficacious in reducing recurrent stroke risk without any significant risk of ICH.[13,305] In addition, the achievement of nominal targets or a specific degree of LDL-C lowering may be beneficial and some ongoing stroke clinical trials will address these targets on recurrent events among patients with recent ischemic stroke.[306] The new ACC/AHA Guideline on the Treatment of Blood Cholesterol to Reduce Atherosclerotic Cardiovascular Risk in Adults released in 2013 moved away from reliance on cholesterol measurement to select individuals for therapy and guide drug dosage.[307] Instead, the ACC/AHA guidelines identify "statin benefit groups" for drug treatment to reduce risk for atherosclerotic CVD (ASCVD) including "Individuals with 1) clinical ASCVD, 2) primary elevations of LDL-C ≥190 mg/dL, 3) diabetes aged 40 to 75 years with LDL-C 70 to 189 mg/dL and without clinical ASCVD, or 4) without clinical ASCVD or diabetes and LDL-C 70 to 189 mg/dL and estimated 10-year ASCVD risk ≥7.5%." These guidelines include people with ischemic stroke or TIA presumed to be of atherosclerotic origin. However, the significant impact of index stroke on future events regardless of ischemic stroke etiology has led for the call to include ischemic stroke other than of large atherosclerotic origin to be included in cardiac risk assessment models.[308]

Cardiac disease has also been found to be a determinant of recurrence after ischemic stroke.[22,309] In Rochester, cardiac valvular disease and congestive heart failure were independent predictors of recurrent stroke.[32] In the Lehigh Valley, the odds ratio associated with stroke recurrence was approximately 8.0 for either MI or other coronary disease.[310] *Atrial fibrillation (AF)* continues to be a leading cause of cerebrovascular morbidity and mortality resulting from cardioembolic stroke. In FHS, only 10% of patients had AF without 2-year recurrence.[167] Compared with individuals without 2-year AF recurrences, the 10-year prognosis was worse for individuals with either sustained or recurrent AF.[311] In the Oxfordshire Community Stroke Project, AF was not associated with a recurrent stroke within the first 30 days and there was only a mild increase in the average annual risk of recurrent stroke from 8.2% with normal sinus rhythm to 11% with AF.[215] Thrombosis risk can be quantified using the CHADS2 or recently quantified CHA2DS2-VASc scores.[312,313] For CHADS2, patients with AF are classified according to awarded points for congestive heart failure (1 point), hypertension (1 point), age ≥75 years (1 point), DM (1 point), and prior stroke or TIA (2 points). The risk of stroke increases according to point score: 1.9% per year (0 points), 2.8% per year (1 point), 4.0% per year (2 points), 5.9% per year (3 points), 8.5% per year (4 points), 12.5% per year (5 points), and 18.2% (6 points). The CHA2DS2-VASc adds to stroke risk by reliably identifying patients at very low risk. Additional points are assigned for an additional age category of 65 to 74 years (1 point), female sex (1 point), and vascular disease other than cerebrovascular disease (1 point). Two points are awarded for age ≥75 years. The risk of stroke increases according to point score: 0.5% per year (0 points), 1.5% per year (1 point), 2.5% per year (2 points), 5% per year (3 points), 6% per year (4 points), and 7% per year (5–6 points). Both CHADS2 and CHA2DS2-VASc may underestimate stroke risk for patients with a recent TIA or ischemic stroke who have no other risk factors. Their risk for stroke may be closer to 7% to 10% per year.[314] Thus, treatment of AF among patients with prior ischemic stroke is a major focus in secondary stroke prevention programs. Fortunately, a large body of clinical trial research has demonstrated that anticoagulation therapy is very effective in prevention of first and recurrent stroke among patients with AF. Also, new direct oral anticoagulants, such as the direct factor Xa inhibitors rivaroxaban, apixaban, edoxaban, and the thrombin inhibitor dabigatran have been recently developed and overcome the limitations of the conventional anticoagulant drugs and showed a significant reduction of stroke risk.[315]

Diabetes has been found to be a determinant of stroke recurrence.[67] The data supporting diabetes as a risk factor for recurrent stroke, however, are sparse. In the Rochester study, age and diabetes mellitus were the only significant independent predictors of recurrent stroke.[32] In the Oxfordshire Stroke Project, diabetes was independently associated with stroke recurrence, and it was estimated that 9% of the recurrent strokes were attributable to diabetes.[215] In the Stroke Data Bank for 2-year stroke recurrence, patients at the lowest risk had no history of diabetes.[224] In a substudy of the Cardiovascular Health Study that enrolled patients with a first ischemic stroke, DM was associated with a 60% increased risk for recurrence.[316] In the recent reports from the population-based Monitoring Trends and Determinants of Cardiovascular Disease (MONICA) stroke incidence registry of 6,700 stroke survivors in Northern Sweden enrolled between 1995 and 2008, 14% patients had a recurrent stroke after 5 years of follow-up and beside age, diabetes was the most significant predictor of stroke recurrence (RR 1.34, 95%CI 1.15–1.57).[317] Because hyperglycemia at stroke onset is more common among diabetic patients and has been found to predict stroke recurrence, some of the effect of hyperglycemia may be dependent on the presence of diagnosed or undiagnosed diabetes.

No major trials for secondary prevention of stroke have specifically examined interventions for diabetes.[22] Among patients with a history of stroke who entered the Prospective Pioglitazone Clinical Trial in Macrovascular Events (PROactive) with a history of stroke, pioglitazone therapy was associated with a 47% RR reduction in recurrent stroke (HR, 0.53; 95%CI 0.34–0.85).[318] Currently the potential effectiveness of pioglitazone for secondary stroke prevention is being examined in the NINDS Insulin Resistance Intervention After Stroke (IRIS) trial.[319] Further clarification is needed to determine how much control of diabetes after stroke is associated with a reduction in stroke recurrence.

There is a paucity of data on the effect of *smoking and alcohol* on stroke recurrence; particularly because these risk factors were not well established during the design of earlier stroke epidemiologic studies. Whether smoking is a risk factor for recurrent stroke is still contradictory.[22,320] In the Cardiovascular Health Study (CHS), however, smoking was associated with a substantially increased risk for stroke recurrence in the elderly (HR, 2.06; 95%CI 1.39–3.56).[316] Cohort studies have suggested that cessation of smoking after MI is associated with a significant decrease in mortality.[321] Knowledge regarding modification of smoking habits after stroke is, nevertheless, scant.[322] No clinical trials have examined the effectiveness of smoking cessation for secondary prevention of stroke or TIA but given the overwhelming evidence on the harm of smoking and the result of observational studies on the benefits of cessation,[321–323] such trials are not likely to be conducted. Smoking cessation is the recommended strategy for secondary stroke prevention.[22]

Stroke recurrence was significantly increased among those with heavy alcohol use.[324–329] In the northern Manhattan cohort nearly half of those with a history of heavy alcohol use had a recurrent stroke within 5 years compared with 22% with no history of heavy alcohol use.[179] The effect of alcohol was observed in smokers, non-smokers, black people, and Hispanics, but not among white people. Ethanol could theoretically increase recurrent stroke risk through numerous mechanisms that include hypertension, hypercoagulable states, cardiac arrhythmias, cardiomyopathy, diabetes, and cerebral blood flow reduction.[329-331] Ethanol consumption rarely has been identified as a predictor of outcome after stroke except for aneurysmal subarachnoid hemorrhage.[325,329] In general, light-to-moderate alcohol consumption has been associated with a reduced risk of first-ever stroke and recurrent cardiovascular events.[22,332] There appears to be a J-shaped association between alcohol intake and risk of ischemic stroke, with a protective effect seen in light-to-moderate drinkers (up to ≈1 drink/d for women and up to ≈2 drinks/d for men) but elevated stroke risk with heavier alcohol use.

Because both alcohol and cigarette smoking are modifiable behaviors, it is important to determine their impact on stroke recurrence. In urban populations these behaviors may be more prevalent and may demand greater attention in stroke recurrence prevention programs.

Some other predictors of recurrent stroke have been suggested, including *rheumatic mitral valve disease*[259] *aortic atheromas,*[255,261,333,334] *PFO,*[257,258,260,335,336] and *cardiomyopathy,*[337] but inconsistently and they require further investigations.[22] Recurrent embolism occurs in 30% to 65% of patients with rheumatic mitral valve disease who have a history of a previous embolic event.[259] Between 60% and 65% of these recurrences develop within the first year, and most develop within 6 months. Mitral valvuloplasty does not seem to eliminate this risk; therefore these patients require long-term anticoagulation. In the French Study of Aortic Plaques in Stroke,[333] atherosclerotic plaques of 4-mm thick or more in the aortic arch were significant predictors of recurrent brain infarction and other vascular events. This association between aortic plaque and recurrent events has also been replicated in ethnically diverse populations of northern Manhattan.[261] In a large cohort of 360 stroke patients enrolled in the PFO in Cryptogenic Stroke Study (PICSS)[335] with a prevalence of PFO of 33.8%, there was no significant difference in the rate of recurrent stroke or death over 2 years between those with PFO (14.8%) of any size and those without PFO (15.4%). A recent meta-analysis of observational PFO studies reported an annual recurrent stroke rate of 2.53 events (95%CI 1.91–3.35) per 100 person-years among patients receiving medical therapy,[338] which was similar to the rate of outcomes in people aged <60 years. In recently completed clinical trials of PFO closure compared with medical therapy (e.g., CLOSURE, RESPECT, PC Trial), the rate of recurrent ischemic stroke among medically treated participants has ranged from 0.6% to 1.5% per year.[339,340,341] None of these PFO closure trials demonstrated a statistically significant finding for their primary end point in an intention-to-treat analysis. Predictors of high risk for recurrence among patients with PFO and cryptogenic stroke are uncertain and methods to develop a database to support modeling of PFO-attributable recurrence risk are currently underway as a part of the Risk of paradoxical Embolism (RoPE) Study.[342]

The evidence for the relationship between stroke recurrence and *inflammatory and hemostatic markers* has been accumulating.[22,343-351] Possible biochemical and clinical predictors of recurrent stroke include levels of CRP, Lp-PLA2, cholesterol, fibrinogen, hematocrit, protein C, lupus anticoagulant, anticardiolipin antibodies, and homocysteine and white blood cell count, the albumin–globulin ratio, free protein S deficiency, and obesity. Although some markers had some predictive ability, none of them demonstrated an added predictive power to a validated clinical model. The clinical usefulness of blood biomarkers for predicting prognosis in the setting of ischemic stroke secondary prevention has yet to be established.

STROKE OUTCOME PREDICTION MODELS

The discrepancies in identifying predictors of stroke outcome including mortality and recurrence have been observed across studies. They may result from the age and stroke subtype composition of the cohorts, the definition of the predictors used in the study, the duration of follow-up, the timing of the outcome of interest, and the relative contribution of other predictors. The great variability of outcome seen in stroke patients has led to an interest in identifying predictors of outcome with the use of prediction models. The combination of clinical and imaging variables as predictors of stroke outcome in a multivariable risk adjustment model may be a powerful approach. Clinical prediction models or scores combine multiple risk factors to estimate the absolute risk of a future clinical event. No estimate is perfect, but a model that predicted the risk of recurrent stroke just as well as, or better than, an experienced clinician might improve clinical practice.[352] Some prediction models are used widely in clinical practice to quantify risk of future vascular events such as the Framingham and CHADS scores.[312,313] None of the prediction models for recurrent events after stroke however, is in widespread use, either because their statistical performance is too poor or because the models are too hard to use. Age and the severity of the presenting clinical deficit are consistently found to be predictive of stroke outcome. Recently SPAN-100, the Stroke Prognostication using Age and NIH Stroke Scale (SPAN) index by combining age in years plus NIH Stroke Scale (NIHSS) ≥100, was proposed.[353]

Several stroke mortality prediction models have been reported. In a model of 1-year survival after ischemic stroke from the Perth Community Stroke Study, coma, urinary incontinence, cardiac failure, severe paresis, and AF were the most important predictors.[65] The sensitivity, specificity, and negative predictive value for predicting death were 90%, 83%, and 95%, respectively. In the northern Manhattan cohort, independent determinants of 5-year mortality among 30-day survivors were age, major hemispheric or basilar syndrome, congestive heart failure, and admission glucose level. In the Helsinki Young Stroke Registry of young adult patients of ages 15 to 49 years, increasing age, malignancy, heart failure, heavy drinking, infection, type 1 diabetes, and large artery atherosclerosis independently predicted 5-year mortality.[51] In the Randomized Trial of Tirilazad Mesylate in Acute Stroke (RANTTAS), the baseline NIHSS score, small-vessel infarct, history of previous stroke, history of diabetes, history of pre-stroke disability, and infarct volume at 7 to 10 days were significant predictors of survival and excellent outcome as determined by the NIHSS score of 1 at 3 months.[354] For very poor outcomes, including death, only infarct volume was a significant predictor of an NIHSS score of 20 or death at 3 months. Other studies have used brain imaging variables for predicting stroke outcomes. The Alberta Stroke Program Early CT score (ASPECTS) has been developed to predict stroke outcome using early ischemic changes on CT.[355] In addition, MR diffusion-weighted imaging (DWI), that identifies lesion volume in the acute setting may improve the ability to quickly predict stroke outcomes.[356-358] Recently, interest has focused on combining clinical and neuroimaging data to develop multivariable risk adjustment models of stroke outcome. Such models may provide greater discriminatory power to predict clinical outcomes than clinical or neuroimaging information alone. DWI is able to demonstrate areas of cerebral infarction within hours of symptom onset, and several studies of early DWI have found a strong association with stroke outcomes.[359-361] These studies have shown that combining quantitative MRI with the NIHSS score and other clinical information predicts good and poor

TABLE 16-4 The Barthel Index Activities of Daily Living

Domain Assessed	Score 0	5	10	15
Feeding	Unable	Requires assistance	Independent	
Bathing	Dependent	Independent		
Grooming	Needs help	Independent		
Dressing	Dependent	Needs some help	Independent	
Bowels	Incontinent	Occasional accident	Continent	
Bladder	Incontinent or catheterized	Occasional accident	Continent	
Toilet use	Dependent	Needs some help	Independent	
Transfers (bed to chair and back)	Unable	Major help	Minor help	Independent
Mobility (on level surface)	Immobile	Wheelchair independent >50 yards	Walks with help of one	Independent
Stairs	Unable	Needs help	Independent	

outcomes after acute stroke with high probability and is superior to the NIHSS score alone.

Stroke Prognostic Risk Scores

Risk stratification as a tool to determine optimal secondary prevention after a stroke requires consideration of levels of overall absolute vascular risk in patients with stroke rather than the risk of recurrent stroke alone. Those who experience a first ischemic stroke have a high relative risk as well as an absolute risk of a subsequent cardiovascular event. The subsequent event is more likely to be a stroke than an MI, but other manifestations of vascular disease, including MI and vascular death, are common potential outcomes. The risk of cardiovascular outcomes after TIA, even in the first 90 days, is as high as 25% and is not limited to stroke.[362] Predictive scores are important tools for stratifying patients based on the risk of future vascular events and for selecting potential prevention therapy. Several scores have been suggested for risk stratification in secondary stroke prevention including *Stroke Prognostic Instrument (SPI) II*,[363] and *Essen Stroke Risk Score* (ESRS), derived from cerebrovascular patients in the Clopidogrel versus Aspirin in Patients at Risk of Ischemic Events (CAPRIE) trial,[364] the Recurrence Risk Estimator at 90 days (RRE-90)[365] and the Life Long After Cerebral ischemia (LiLAC).[366] The ESRS and the SPI-II have four predictors in common (age, history of TIA or stroke, diabetes and blood pressure). ESRS was validated with the use of the data set of the ESPS-2 and in a large cohort of 15,605 outpatients with previous TIA or stroke from the REduction of Atherothrombosis for Continued Health (REACH) Registry.[367] In NOMASS, a weighted scoring system was developed using seven significant predictors of 5-year recurrent stroke (i.e., age, NIHSS, AF, peripheral artery disease, heavy alcohol use, physical inactivity, and high-density lipoprotein cholesterol level <40). In a recent systematic review and evaluation of recurrent stroke and MI prediction scales, four clinical prediction models were externally evaluated including the ESRS, the SPI-II, the RRE-90 and LiLAC.[368] The discriminative performances of all four models were similar to one another, but only modest at best, with the Area under the Receiver Operating Characteristic Curve values ranging from 0.60 to 0.72. Their performance was, therefore, modest and similar to experienced clinicians.

Some of the prediction scores include readily available patient demographic and clinical data and are, therefore, easy to calculate, and may be applicable to a broad population of stroke patients, and can aid in prediction of recurrent stroke and other vascular outcomes for direction of treatment strategies. However, a number of methodological decisions made in a various model development may lead to clinical prediction models that make less accurate predictions. An agreed set of guidelines and reporting in development of prognostic score models currently does not exist but would be helpful for future investigations as such studies are frequent and very likely may influence clinical practice.

TABLE 16-5 The Modified Rankin Scale (mRS)

Grade	Symptoms
Grade 0	No symptoms at all
Grade 1	No significant disability despite symptoms; able to carry out all usual duties and activities
Grade 2	Slight disability; unable to carry out all previous activities, but able to look after own affairs without assistance
Grade 3	Moderate disability; requiring some help, but able to walk without assistance
Grade 4	Moderately severe disability; unable to walk without assistance, unable to attend to needs without assistance
Grade 5	Severe disability; bedridden, incontinent, and requiring constant nursing care and attention
Grade 6	Dead

Note: The grade of mRS 6 was added for clinical trial purposes and was not part of the original scale.

FUNCTIONAL DISABILITY AND HANDICAP AFTER STROKE

Functional disability, the lack of ability to perform an activity or task in the range considered normal for an individual, is an important outcome after a non-fatal stroke. Reliable and valid scales have been developed to determine activities of daily living and other indices for measuring functional dependence. Two of the most used are the Barthel Activities of Daily Living (ADL) or the Barthel Index (BI)[369,370] and the modified Rankin Scale (mRS).[371] These instruments are simple, reliable, and reasonably sensitive for assessing disability (Tables 16-4 and 16-5). The approximate proportion of stroke survivors that is independent at 6 months ranges from 40% to 65%, depending on the characteristics of the study population. A high ADL score at hospital discharge is a good predictor of a favorable functional prognosis.[372] Day 5 seems to be the earliest time for making an optimal prediction of final outcome of activities of daily living using the BI.[373] Therefore, the BI should be measured at the end of the first week in hospital-based stroke units for early rehabilitation management.

Functional activity measured by ADL score has been often used as a primary outcome in randomized stroke clinical trials, showing functional independence 30–70% with the use of the ADL score (ADL of 95 to 100) and 20–50% with the use of the Rankin score (0 or 1) at 3 months after an acute onset of ischemic stroke, depending on the patient selection criteria for enrollment in these trials.[373–375]

Once the patient has survived the immediate stroke, the potential for recovery and the likelihood of long-term survival free of dependence on others are the concerns for stroke patients, their families, and healthcare professionals. This information should be based on predictive models derived from data sets that include complete follow-up of cases of first-ever stroke from large, community-based cohorts with the standard diagnostic criteria and clinical assessments of disease severity, comorbidities, and sociodemographic factors and standardized measures of functional outcome. There are several studies of long-term functional outcome after stroke, but only a few reliable estimates of the long-term functional outcome after first-ever ischemic stroke are available.[376–387] In a recent reliability study and systematic review of the literature, and despite the lack of uniformity of long-term outcome results among studies, the overall evidence supporting the use of the Barthel Index and modified Rankin Scale as prognostic tools is quite strong.[388]

One of the largest functional outcome studies was the Auckland Stroke Study, in which information on disability and health-related QOL (HRQOL) was available on nearly all of the 639 6-year survivors (36%) of the original cohort of 1761 patients registered in 1991 to 1992.[389] In this study, 42% of patients were dependent in at least one aspect of ADLs 6 years after stroke. In the Perth Community Stroke Study among 30-day survivors of initial stroke, one-third remained disabled, and one in seven were in permanent institutional care.[378] The major predictors of poor long-term outcome were a low level of activity before the stroke, subsequent recurrent stroke, older age, baseline disability defined by the Barthel Index score, and severe stroke at onset. In NOMASS among 359 stroke survivors, 35% were independent, 37% were moderately dependent, and 28% were dependent on the ADL scale at 7 to 10 days and 55% at 6 months after first ischemic stroke. In the multivariate model, only ADLs assessed at 7 to 10 days were predictive of 6-month functional independence, which indicates that long-term functional independence was strongly influenced by early functional recovery after stroke.

Handicap is the disadvantage for an individual resulting from an impairment or disability that limits or prevents the fulfillment of a role (depending on age, sex, and social and cultural factors) that is normal for that individual.[377,384] Although post-stroke disability has been the subject of much discussion in the literature, handicap has received little attention. Handicap is an important target of rehabilitation. Some domains of handicap are potentially modifiable, but knowledge of which aspects of handicap are most affected in stroke survivors is limited. In the Melbourne Stroke Study, stroke survivors were found to be handicapped over a wide range of domains.[390] Most disadvantages occurred in the domains of physical independence and occupation. Handicap increased with the severity of disability. Patients with total anterior circulation infarcts were the most disabled and handicapped 3 and 12 months after stroke.[388] Using the modified Rankin Scale, the Oxfordshire Community Stroke Project and the Perth Community Stroke Study found that patients with total anterior circulatory infarcts had a low likelihood of living independently 12 months after stroke.[379,380] Patients with lacunar infarcts were least disabled. Similarly, in the Rochester Epidemiology Project, patients with lacunar infarcts had the best functional outcomes: more than 80% had minimal or no functional impairment 1 year after stroke.[381] Patients with cardioembolic stroke had poorer pre-stroke functional status, more severe neurologic deficits at the time of stroke, and poorer functional outcomes compared with patients with other subtypes.

Some limitations of the ADL and Rankin scales need to be noted. One of them is the "ceiling effect" of the ADL scales. Patients who are functionally independent on the ADL scales (with the highest score) may continue to improve after stroke, and this improvement cannot be detected with the current ADL scales. The modified Rankin Scale, although easy to use and widely adopted as a measure of handicap in stroke clinical trials, is a fairly non-specific instrument that measures a mix of impairment, disability, and handicap when natural history data and the effects of interventions on outcomes are assessed.[376,377] Furthermore, summary scores based on aggregated data may hide wide intra-individual variations. Some patients make a rapid, early recovery; others have a more prolonged recovery. Continuing improvement may also be minimized by the effects of aging and the development of other disabilities that may or may not be stroke-related. Several new approaches to analysis of stroke outcome scales have recently been adopted, including the global statistic, responder analysis, and shift analysis.[383–387] Each of these approaches offers distinctive benefits and drawbacks. The choice of primary endpoint and analytical technique should be tailored to the study population, expected treatment response, and study purpose. Shift analysis, also known as analysis of distributions or rank analysis, generally provides the most comprehensive index of a treatment's clinical impact and has been a preferable choice of stroke outcome analysis in recent clinical trials.[385]

Numerous scales have been developed to assess specific domains of ADL, including the Motor Assessment Scale, the Fugl-Meyer Assessment, the Sodring Motor Evaluation for Stroke Patients, the Stroke Rehabilitation Assessment of Movement, the Motricity Index, and the Rivermead Motor Assessment.[386] They have been shown to be useful both in clinical practice and in terms of research. The most suitable scales in the clinical field seem to be the short versions of the Fugl-Meyer Assessment and the Stroke Rehabilitation Assessment of Movement.[387] A real consensus about the measurement of gross motor function in patients with stroke is not available in the recent literature.

Stroke disability outcome scales rate patients across multiple ranks; for example, the modified Rankin Scale divides global disability into seven strata, and the Barthel Index rates functional ADLs among 20 levels; stroke-related QOL scales have, however, finer gradations that substantially reduce ceiling and floor effects. The prognostic value of these scales and impaired cognition remains unclear, including the prognostic value of specific factors in the domains of emotional and communicative functioning that are rarely assessed.[388]

At the present time, the NIHSS, mRS, and BI are routine stroke scales because they have been routinely used for more than two decades and are well validated, and the results of most stroke clinical trials are driven using these scales presenting the basis for stroke management guidelines. A reliable prognosis soon after a stroke is highly relevant to patients who ultimately have a poor outcome, because it enables early planning of care tailored to their needs. Future research should focus on the selection of optimal screening instruments in multiple domains of functioning, including the timing of assessment and developing prediction tools stratified by more homogeneous, clinically distinguished stroke subtypes.

QUALITY OF LIFE AFTER STROKE

QOL is another important outcome after stroke. Recreational and social activities are reduced for most stroke survivors after they return home, regardless of whether they have made a complete functional recovery. There is no single accepted definition of HRQOL. It is assumed to be a broad, multidimensional construct that assesses some measurement of physical status, mental and psychological status, social activity status, and functional status. A substantial proportion of stroke survivors have very poor HRQOL.[389–394] In the community-based North East Melbourne Stroke Incidence Study (NEMESIS), 8% of patients had HRQOL assessed as equivalent to, or worse than, death and almost 25% had an overall poor outcome 2 years after stroke.[390]

Numerous instruments have been developed and applied to the evaluation of prognosis after stroke including the Stroke Impact Scale (SIS), Sickness Impact Profile, the Social Functioning subscale of the Short Form-36 (SF-36), the Nottingham Profile, EuroQol, and the Quality of Well Being (QWB).[391–396] All scales provide multidimensional assessment, but vary in the number and combination of dimensions. All include assessment of physical functioning and most incorporate concepts, such as psychological well-being, social well-being, and role activities. The assessment of outcomes including QOL in individuals after stroke is important for both clinical practice and research, yet there is no consensus on the best measures of stroke outcome in either clinical practice or research. Existing measures have not been sensitive to change in patients with mild strokes.[397] There are very few studies that have quantitated the impact of stroke on QOL. However, no stroke-specific outcome measure has been developed that assesses other dimensions of HRQOL (e.g., emotion, communication, memory and thinking, and social role function).

The SIS has been developed as a stroke-specific outcome measure, especially for mild-to-moderate strokes.[396] It was developed from the perspective input of both the patient and caregiver, and it incorporates contemporary standards of instrument development. This stroke-specific outcome measure seems to be comprehensive, reliable, valid, and sensitive to change. However, more studies are required to evaluate the SIS in larger and more heterogeneous populations and to evaluate the feasibility and validity of proxy responses for the most severely impaired patients.

In the northern Manhattan population-based case-control study of 207 patients older than 39 years with first cerebral infarction, the QWB scale was used to assess QOL after stroke. In the comparison with the pre-stroke QWB score, the 6-month QWB score decreased by 27%.[398] Even among those patients who were functionally independent at 6 months (the BI ≥ 70), there was still a 12% decrease in QWB. In the recent analysis from NOMAS using the Spitzer QOL index (QLI, a 10-point scale),[399] QOL declined annually up to 5 years after stroke (annual change −0.10, 95%CI −0.17 to −0.04) among survivors free of stroke recurrence or MI and independently of other risk factors or functional independence (BI of 95–100). QLI declined more among Medicaid patients and was associated with age, mood, stroke severity, urinary incontinence, functional status, cognition, and stroke laterality.

The SF-36 is the most widely used generic instrument for measuring QOL, although it is not specific to stroke patients.[400] The instrument is translated into numerous languages, and the validity of the eight subscales is confirmed in general populations and in a wide variety of patient groups in more than 2000 articles. In view of the current evidence that the subscales of the SF-36 are psychometrically sound for measuring QOL in a range of patient populations. Although the SF-36 may be a useful measure of QOL in stroke,[400,401] it has been validated for stroke patients in one study[402] and marked floor and ceiling effects limit its utility.[403]

EuroQol has been validated in stroke populations.[404] However, only a fraction of stroke survivors (61% in one study) could complete the scale without external assistance. Also, the stroke-specific QOL scale was developed based on interviews with stroke survivors.[405] It was validated in stroke populations with established values for "minimal detectable change" and "clinically important difference". [406] Its modification for patients with post-stroke aphasia is also described.[407]

Stroke-specific QOL scores and patient impairments predict patient-reported overall HRQOL after stroke.[408] Disease-specific HRQOL measures are more sensitive to meaningful changes in post-stroke HRQOL and may thus aid in identifying specific aspects of poststroke function that clinicians and "stroke trialists" can target to improve patients' HRQOL after stroke. In a recent review of the HRQOL scales, one generic (Sickness Impact Profile) and two stroke-specific scales (SIS and Stroke-Specific Quality of Life Scale) seemed most comprehensive.[388] Whether any of these assessments are sufficient to describe HRQOL after stroke is still unclear.

Several limitations of the QOL scales need to be emphasized. Most existing stroke QOL outcome measures suffer from floor and/or ceiling effects, and the summary scores may inadequately reflect the patient's physical and mental health. When traditional multi-item instruments such as the SF-36 are used, summated scores are dependent on the number of various items included in the different instruments; therefore, it is impossible to compare scores obtained on different instruments.[409] Furthermore, the clinical interpretation of summated scores is not straightforward. For example, the clinical meaning of a mean score of 47.6 on SF-36 in a stroke patient would be unclear for most neurologists. This problem is amplified by the ordinal nature of summated scores; that is, a given difference in scores at one point on the scale does not necessarily represent the same amount of functional change at another point on the scale. Following growing dissatisfaction with the classic scales, the alternative Item Response Theory (IRT) method has been introduced.[397,410] This statistical paradigm uses a logistic regression analysis to model the responses of the patients to the individual items. Therefore, the items can be placed on the same hierarchical continuous scale, which helps assessment and interpretation of the scales. Despite recent interest in IRT in clinical outcome measurement, these methods need to be developed in stroke research as a useful supplement to the traditional QOL approach. Debate continues as to the relative merits of various statistical techniques, including dichotomization and use of the complete range of a scale.[401,403,406]

No single outcome measure can describe or predict all dimensions of recovery and disability after stroke, and each scale has a potential role in patient care and outcome research. Composite measures and multiple scales may be useful in determining the multiple dimensions of outcomes after stroke (Fig. 16-1). In addition, ongoing attempts are being made to incorporate patients' perspectives to these scales, as these ultimately are critical measures of either a high QOL or failure.

Health-related quality of life assessments and interventions will become increasingly important for improving longer-term survival and functional outcomes following stroke. Evaluations of health-related QOL in stroke survivors can provide a rich description of the multifaceted effects of a stroke, providing insights above those recorded with traditional impairment and activity measures. Measuring health-related QOL in stroke, however, presents particular challenges and more research is needed in this area.

DEPRESSION AFTER STROKE

Major depression is a common occurrence after stroke.[411–414] Pooled estimates from a meta-analysis suggest an incidence of post-stroke depression of 33%.[413] This rate is relatively constant across the short and long term after stroke. The incidence, however, appears to vary widely across individual studies, ranging from 9% to 34% in the initial 3 to 6 months following stroke and 30% to 50% within the first year.[414] The studies that have compared the post-stroke incidence of depression with appropriately matched community control

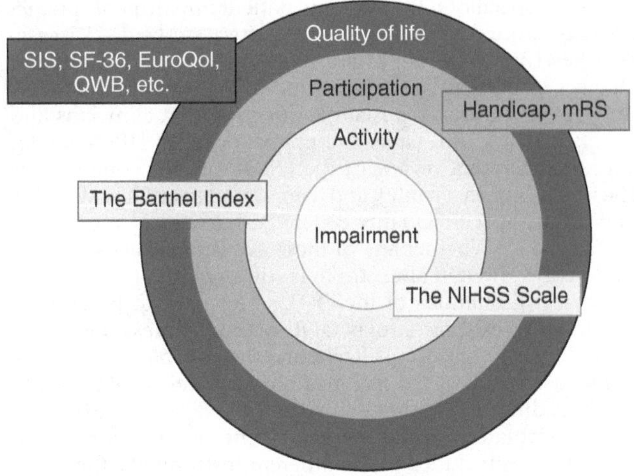

Figure 16-1 Multiple assessments of functional outcomes and quality of life after stroke.
SIS, Stroke Impact Scale; SF, Short Form; Qol, Quality of life; QWB; Quality of Well Being; mRS; modified Rankin Scale; NIHSS, National Institute of Health Stroke Scale

subjects have found that the risk of depression is at least doubled after stroke compared with what would be expected in the general population.[415,416] In addition to the emotional well-being of the stroke survivor, the recognition and treatment of depression is important because depression is associated with disability, cognitive impairment, suicide, and mortality.[417–419] Depression has been associated with excess stroke long-term disability,[415–420] poor rehabilitation outcomes[413,414,421] morbidity and mortality,[418–420] and suicidal thoughts and plans.[419–423] In the vast majority of patients the detection of depression during standard stroke care is still overlooked by treating physicians.[416]

If standard diagnostic criteria (either the *Diagnostic and Statistical Manual of Mental Disorders* [DSM] or Research Diagnostic Criteria) are used to establish the presence of a major depressive episode, depression occurs, at least temporarily, in up to 30% to 40% of stroke survivors.[414] Although, the term *post-stroke depression* has already been established in the literature, standardized criteria for this diagnosis do not exist. In most cases the DSM-IV or International Classification of Diseases system is applied. Other investigators used various psychiatric rating scales. In addition to diagnosis based on psychiatric interview and the DSM criteria, a variety of self-rating mood scales (e.g., Beck Depression Inventory [BDI])[424] and interviewer-administered scales (e.g., Hamilton Rating Scale for Depression [HRSD])[425] are used. These measures are not specifically designed for patients with stroke, who typically have a variety of physical and cognitive impairments that may introduce difficulties in the use of these instruments. The BDI and the HRSD in patients with stroke have been acceptable screening instruments in the assessment of post-stroke depression, but their specificity seems to be too low to provide a basis for diagnosis of depression.[426] Some scales have been developed and validated specifically for stroke patients. For example, the Post-stroke Depression Prediction Scale is a clinical prediction model for the early identification of stroke patients at increased risk for post-stroke depression.[427] The model included a medical history of depression or other psychiatric disorders, hypertension, angina pectoris, and the Barthel Index item dressing. The model had acceptable discrimination, based on an area under the receiver operating characteristic curve of 0.78 (0.72–0.85), and calibration (*P* value of the U-statistic, 0.96). Transforming the model to an easy-to-use risk-assessment table, the lowest-risk category (sum score, <−10) showed a 2% risk of depression, which increased to 82% in the highest category (sum score, >21). This clinical prediction model may help in the estimation of the degree of the depression risk for an individual patient within the first week after stroke.

It is generally acknowledged that there is a high prevalence of depression after stroke. The occurrence of depression after stroke is, however, underdiagnosed and often left untreated. In addition, little is known about the course of major depression after a stroke. Prevalence clearly varies over time; depression has an apparent peak 3 to 6 months after a stroke and a subsequent decline in prevalence at 1 year to about 50% of initial rates.[428]

Treatment or prevention of depression after stroke is greatly dependent on understanding the pathophysiologic mechanism linking stroke and depression. Even though the DSM-IV classification implies that strokes "cause" depression through a direct biological mechanism, the nature of the mechanism linking stroke and depression remains debated in the literature.[429] Some propose a primary biological mechanism according to which ischemic insults directly affect neural circuits involved in mood regulation, while others propose a psychosocial mechanism according to which the social and psychological stressors associated with a stroke are considered the primary cause of depression.[430]

Stroke survivors in active rehabilitation programs have been shown to have lower rates of depression.[431] It has also been reported that depressed stroke survivors with cognitive impairment had greater chronicity of depression than depressed stroke survivors without significant cognitive impairment.[432] Furthermore, left anterior ischemic lesions were associated with cognitive impairment in stroke survivors with major depression. This finding indicates that ischemic lesions in the area of the striatofrontal circuit identified on brain imaging are associated with increased cognitive impairment and chronicity of depression.[429]

As association between white matter hyperintensities on T2-weighted MRI with both depression and executive dysfunction has been reported.[433] The broader concept of vascular depression is hypothesized to result from disruption of prefrontal systems and lesions causing damage to the striatopallidothalamo-cortical pathways.[434] Emerging evidence has shown that vascular risk factors and vascular brain lesions impact the long-term course of depression, particularly among elderly patients.[435] Post-stroke depression occurs in stroke affecting not only medium or large vessels, but also to small vessel ischemic changes.[436] In essence, it seems that the vascular depression hypothesis includes the combined effects of small lesions located predominantly in brain white matter and due to small vessel ischemia and the effect of lesions that disrupt connectivity between gray matter assemblies that mediate mood.[437] This suggests that vascular dementia and vascular depression are related, as both entities can be seen in patients with extensive white matter disease and, therefore, vascular depression and vascular dementia may not be easily teased apart.[438]

Depression after stroke is a common occurrence associated with excess disability, cognitive impairment, and mortality. Post-stroke depression does not appear to be the result of "pure" biological versus psychological causes; instead it seems to be multifactorial in origin and consistent with the biopsychosocial model of mental illness.[439] The relative effects of disability and reduced neurotransmitter system activity on post-stroke depression remain uncertain. Similarly, although the role of antidepressants post-stroke has been demonstrated,[440] a better understanding of the pathomechanism, incidence, prevalence, and factors associated with depression after stroke is needed. The available data make a strong case for the prophylactic use and effectiveness of antidepressants post stroke, but precise timing of therapy, preferred agents, and optimal dosages remain to be determined.

The complete reference list can be found on the companion Expert Consult website at www.expertconsult.inkling.com.

KEY REFERENCES

1. Murray CJL, Lopez AD. Global mortality, disability and the contribution of risk factors: Global Burden of Disease Study. Lancet 1997;349:1436–42.
2. Feigin VL, Forouzanfar MH, Krishnamurthi R, et al. Global and regional burden of stroke during 1990–2010: findings from the Global Burden of Disease Study 2010. Lancet 2014;383: 245–55.
3. Lackland DT, Roccella EJ, Deutsch AF, et al. Factors influencing the decline in stroke mortality: a statement from the American Heart Association/American Stroke Association. Stroke 2014;45: 315–53.
4. Go AS, Mozaffarian D, Roger VL, et al. Executive summary: heart disease and stroke statistics – 2014 update: a report from the American Heart Association. Circulation 2014;129:399–410.
16. Romano JG, Sacco RL. Progress in secondary stroke prevention. Ann Neurol 2008;63(4):418–27.
19. Ovbiagele B, Goldstein LB, Higashida RT, Howard VJ, et al. Forecasting the future of stroke in the United States: a policy statement from the American Heart Association and American Stroke Association. Stroke 2013;44(8):2361–75.
22. Kernan WN, Ovbiagele B, Black HR, Bravata DM, et al. Guidelines for the prevention of stroke in patients with stroke and transient ischemic attack: a guideline for healthcare professionals from the American Heart Association/American Stroke Association. Stroke 2014;45(7):2160–236.
23. Centers for Disease Control and Prevention. Prevalence of stroke: United States, 2006–2010. MMWR Morb Mortal Wkly Rep 2012;61(20):379–82.
26. Thrift AG, Cadilhac DA, Thayabaranathan T, et al. Global stroke statistics. Int J Stroke 2014;9(1):6–18.
27. Feigin VL, Lawes CM, Bennett DA, et al. Worldwide stroke incidence and early case fatality reported in 56 population-based studies: a systematic review. Lancet Neurol 2009;8(4): 355–69.
28. Sacco RL, Wolf PA, Kannel WB, et al. Survival and recurrence following stroke. The Framingham study. Stroke 1982;13(3): 290–5.
30. Rosamond WD, Folsom AR, Chambless LE. Stroke incidence and survival among middle-aged adults: 9-year follow-up of the Atherosclerotic Risk in Communities (ARIC) cohort. Stroke 1999;30(4):736–43.
32. Petty GW, Brown RD Jr, Whisnant JP, et al. Survival and recurrence after first cerebral infarction: a population-based study in Rochester, Minnesota, 1975 through 1989. Neurology 1998; 50(1):208–16.
33. Sacco RL, Shi T, Zamanillo MC, et al. Predictors of mortality and recurrence after hospitalized cerebral infarction in an urban community: the Northern Manhattan Stroke Study. Neurology 1994;44(4):626–34.
40. Lahr MM, Luijckx GJ, Vroomen PC, et al. The chain of care enabling tPA treatment in acute ischemic stroke: a comprehensive review of organisational models. J Neurol 2013;260(4):960–8.
41. Hankey GJ, Jamrozik K, Broadhurst RJ, et al. Five-year survival after first-ever stroke and related prognostic factors in the Perth Community Stroke Study. Stroke 2000;31(9):2080–6.
42. Dhamoon MS, Sciacca RR, Rundek T, et al. Recurrent stroke and cardiac risks after first ischemic stroke: the Northern Manhattan Study. Neurology 2006;66(5):641–6.
43. Hartmann A, Rundek T, Mast H, et al. Mortality and causes of death after first-ischemic stroke: the Northern Manhattan Stroke Study. Neurology 2001;57(11):2000–5.
45. Dennis MS, Burn JP, Sandercock PA, et al. Long-term survival after first-ever stroke: the Oxfordshire Community Stroke Project. Stroke 1993;24(6):796–800.
46. Ward G, Jamrozik K, Stewart-Wynne E. Incidence and outcome of cerebrovascular disease in Perth, Western Australia. Stroke 1988;19(12):1501–6.
47. Heuschmann PU, Kolominsky-Rabas PL, Misselwitz B, et al. German Stroke Registers Study Group. Predictors of in-hospital mortality and attributable risks of death after ischemic stroke: the German Stroke Registers Study Group. Arch Intern Med 2004;164(16):1761–8.
51. Putaala J, Curtze S, Hiltunen S, et al. Causes of death and predictors of 5-year mortality in young adults after first-ever ischemic stroke: the Helsinki Young Stroke Registry. Stroke 2009; 40(8):2698–703.
57. Smith EE, Shobha N, Dai D, et al. Risk score for in-hospital ischemic stroke mortality derived and validated within the Get With the Guidelines-Stroke Program. J Am Heart Assoc 2013; 2(1):e005207.
60. Bronnum-Hansen H, Davidsen M, Thorvaldsen P. Danish MONICA Study Group. Long-term survival and causes of death after stroke. Stroke 2001;32(9):2131–6.
61. Gresham GE, Kelly-Hayes M, Wolf PA, et al. Survival and functional status 20 or more years after first stroke: the Framingham Study. Stroke 1998;29(4):793–7.
64. Seshadri S, Beiser A, Kelly-Hayes M, et al. The lifetime risk of stroke: estimates from the Framingham Study. Stroke 2006;37(2): 345–50.
65. Hankey GJ, Jamrozik K, Broadhurst RJ, et al. Five-year survival after first-ever stroke and related prognostic factors in the Perth Community Stroke Study. Stroke 2000;31(9):2080–6.
67. Hankey GJ. Long-term outcome after ischaemic stroke/ transient ischaemic attack. Cerebrovasc Dis 2003;16(Suppl. 1): 14–19.
68. Slot KB, Berge E, Sandercock P, et al. Causes of death by level of dependency at 6 months after ischemic stroke in 3 large cohorts. Stroke 2009;40(5):1585–9.
69. WHO MONICA Project (prepared by Thorvaldsen P, Asplund K, Kuulasmaa K, Rajakangas AM, Schroll M). Stroke incidence, case fatality, and mortality in the WHO MONICA Project: World Health Organization monitoring trends and determinants in cardiovascular disease. Stroke 1995;26(3):361–7.
70. Adams HP Jr, Davis PH, Leira EC, et al. Baseline NIH Stroke Scale score strongly predicts outcome after stroke: A report of the Trial of Org 10172 in Acute Stroke Treatment (TOAST). Neurology 1999;53(1):126–31.
71. Dhamoon MS, Tai W, Boden-Albala B, et al. Risk of myocardial infarction or vascular death after first ischemic stroke: the Northern Manhattan Study. Stroke 2007;38(6):1752–8.
74. Johnston KC, Connors AF, Wagner DP, et al. A predictive risk model for outcomes of ischemic stroke. Stroke 2000;31(2): 448–55.
77. Fonarow GC, Reeves MJ, Zhao X, Olson DM, et al. Age-related differences in characteristics, performance measures, treatment trends, and outcomes in patients with ischemic stroke. Circulation 2010;121(7):879–91.
79. Carandang R, Seshadri S, Beiser A, et al. Trends in incidence, lifetime risk, severity, and 30-day mortality of stroke over the past 50 years. JAMA 2006;296(24):2939–46.
81. Niewada M, Kobayashi A, Sandercock PA, et al. Influence of gender on baseline features and clinical outcomes among 17,370 patients with confirmed ischaemic stroke in the international stroke trial. Neuroepidemiology 2005;24(3):123–8.
85. Howard VJ, Kleindorfer DO, Judd SE, et al. Disparities in stroke incidence contributing to disparities in stroke mortality. Ann Neurol 2011;69(4):619–27.
89. Longstreth WT Jr, Bernick C, Fitzpatrick A, et al. Frequency and predictors of stroke death in 5,888 participants in the Cardiovascular Health Study. Neurology 2001;56(3):368–75.
94. Howard G, Howard VJ. REasons for Geographic And Racial Differences in Stroke (REGARDS) Investigators. Ethnic disparities in stroke: the scope of the problem. Ethn Dis 2001;11(4): 761–8.
97. Moroney JT, Bagiella E, Paik MC, et al. Risk factors for early recurrence after ischemic stroke: the role of stroke syndrome and subtype. Stroke 1998;29(10):2118–24.
98. Weimar C, König IR, Kraywinkel K, et al. German Stroke Study Collaboration, Age and National Institutes of Health Stroke Scale Score within 6 hours after onset are accurate predictors of outcome after cerebral ischemia: development and external validation of prognostic models. Stroke 2004;35(1):158–62.

101. Saposnik G, Guzik AK, Reeves M, et al. Stroke Prognostication using Age and NIH Stroke Scale: SPAN-100. Neurology 2013; 80(1):21–8.
112. Kammersgaard LP, Jorgensen HS, Rungby JA, et al. Admission body temperature predicts long-term mortality after acute stroke: the Copenhagen Stroke Study. Stroke 2002;33(7):1759–62.
121. Greer DM, Funk SE, Reaven NL, et al. Impact of fever on outcome in patients with stroke and neurologic injury: a comprehensive meta-analysis. Stroke 2008;39(11):3029–35.
128. Lyden PD, Hemmen TM, Grotta J, et al. Endovascular therapeutic hypothermia for acute ischemic stroke: ICTuS 2/3 protocol. Int J Stroke. 2014;9(1):117–25.
129. Sacco SE, Whisnant JP, Broderick JP, et al. Epidemiological characteristics of lacunar infarcts in a population. Stroke 1991;22(10):1236–41.
130. Schneider AT, Kissela B, Woo D, et al. Ischemic stroke subtypes: a population-based study of incidence rates among blacks and whites. Stroke 2004;35(7):1552–6.
132. Jones SB, Sen S, Lakshminarayan K, et al. Poststroke outcomes vary by pathogenic stroke subtype in the Atherosclerosis Risk in Communities Study. Stroke 2013;44(8):2307–10.
133. Bejot Y, Catteau A, Caillier M, et al. Trends in incidence, risk factors, and survival in symptomatic lacunar stroke in Dijon, France, from 1989 to 2006: a population-based study. Stroke 2008;39(7):1945–51.
136. Kolominsky-Rabas PL, Weber M, Gefeller O, et al. Epidemiology of ischemic stroke subtypes according to TOAST criteria. Incidence, recurrence, and long-term survival in ischemic stroke subtypes: a population-based study. Stroke 2001;32(12):2735–40.
137. Petty GW, Brown RD Jr, Whisnant JP, et al. Ischemic stroke subtypes: a population-based study of functional outcome, survival, and recurrence. Stroke 2000;31(5):1062–8.
138. Jones SB, Sen S, Lakshminarayan K, et al. Poststroke outcomes vary by pathogenic stroke subtype in the Atherosclerosis Risk in Communities Study. Stroke 2013;44(8):2307–10.
141. Lei C, Wu B, Liu M, et al. Risk factors and clinical outcomes associated with intracranial and extracranial atherosclerotic stenosis acute ischemic stroke. J Stroke Cerebrovasc Dis 2014;23(5): 1112–17.
144. Leonardi-Bee J, Bath PM, Phillips SJ, et al. Blood pressure and clinical outcomes in the International Stroke Trial. Stroke 2002;33(5):1315–20.
147. O'Donnell MJ, Xavier D, Liu L, et al. Risk factors for ischaemic and intracerebral haemorrhagic stroke in 22 countries (the INTERSTROKE study): a case-control study. Lancet 2010; 376(9735):112–23.
158. Alqadri SL, Sreenivasan V, Qureshi AI. Acute hypertensive response management in patients with acute stroke. Curr Cardiol Rep 2013;15(12):426.
161. Henriksson KM, Farahmand B, Johansson S, et al. Survival after stroke-The impact of CHADS(2) score and atrial fibrillation. Int J Cardiol 2010;141(1):18–23.
162. Gottdiener JS, Gay JA, VanVoorhees L, et al. Frequency and embolic potential of left ventricular thrombus in dilated cardiomyopathy: assessment by 2-dimensional echocardiography. Am J Cardiol 1983;52(10):1281–5.
164. Kannel WB, Wolf PA, Verter J. Manifestations of coronary disease predisposing to stroke. The Framingham Study. JAMA 1983; 250(21):2942–6.
167. Lin HJ, Wolf PA, Kelly-Hayes M, et al. Stroke severity in atrial fibrillation. The Framingham Study. Stroke 1996;27(10): 1760–4.
170. Granger CB, Armaganijan LV. Newer oral anticoagulants should be used as first-line agents to prevent thromboembolism in patients with atrial fibrillation and risk factors for stroke or thromboembolism. Circulation 2012;125(1):159–64.
171. Candelise L, Landi G, Orazio EN, et al. Prognostic significance of hyperglycemia in acute stroke. Arch Neurol 1985;42(7): 661–3.
179. Sacco RL, Shi T, Zamanillo MC, et al. Predictors of mortality and recurrence after hospitalized cerebral infarction in an urban community: the Northern Manhattan Stroke Study. Neurology 1994;44(4):626–34.
181. Ray KK, Seshasai SR, Wijesuriya S, et al. Effect of intensive control of glucose on cardiovascular outcomes and death in patients with diabetes mellitus: a meta-analysis of randomised controlled trials. Lancet 2009;373(9677):1765–72.
183. Bruno A, Durkalski VL, Hall CE, Juneja R, et al. The Stroke Hyperglycemia Insulin Network Effort (SHINE) trial protocol: a randomized, blinded, efficacy trial of standard vs. intensive hyperglycemia management in acute stroke. Int J Stroke. 2014;9(2):246–51.
196. Packard CJ, O'Reilly DS, Caslake MJ, et al. Lipoprotein-associated phospholipase A2 as an independent predictor of coronary heart disease. West of Scotland Coronary Prevention Study Group. N Engl J Med 2000;343(16):1148–55.
199. Katan M, Elkind MS. Inflammatory and neuroendocrine biomarkers of prognosis after ischemic stroke. Expert Rev Neurother 2011;11(2):225–39.
207. Kim SY, Guevara JP, Kim KM, et al. Hyperuricemia and risk of stroke: a systematic review and meta-analysis. Arthritis Rheum 2009;61(7):885–92.
213. Ovbiagele B, Schwamm LH, Smith EE, et al. Patterns of care quality and prognosis among hospitalized ischemic stroke patients with chronic kidney disease. J Am Heart Assoc 2014;3(3):e000905.
215. Burn J, Dennis M, Bamford J, et al. Long-term risk of recurrent stroke after a first-ever stroke. The Oxfordshire Community Stroke Project. Stroke 1994;25(2):333–7.
216. Hankey GJ, Jamrozik K, Broadhurst RJ, et al. Long-term risk of first recurrent stroke in the Perth Community Stroke Study. Stroke 1998;29(12):2491–500.
217. Matsumoto N, Whisnant JP, Kurland LT, et al. Natural history of stroke in Rochester, Minnesota, 1955 through 1969: an extension of a previous study, 1945 through 1954. Stroke 1973; 4(1):20–9.
222. Moroney JT, Bagiella E, Paik MC, et al. Risk factors for early recurrence after ischemic stroke: the role of stroke syndrome and subtype. Stroke 1998;29(10):2118–24.
224. Sacco RL, Foulkes MA, Mohr JP, et al. Determinants of early recurrence of cerebral infarction. The Stroke Data Bank. Stroke 1989;20(8):983–9.
226. Hardie K, Hankey GJ, Jamrozik K, et al. Ten-year risk of first recurrent stroke and disability after first-ever stroke in the Perth Community Stroke Study. Stroke 2004;35(3):731–5.
227. Peltonen M, Stegmayr B, Asplund K. Time trends in long-term survival after stroke: the Northern Sweden Multinational Monitoring of Trends and Determinants in Cardiovascular Disease (MONICA) study, 1985–1994. Stroke 1998;29(7): 1358–65.
229. Dhamoon MS, Sciacca RR, Rundek T, et al. Recurrent stroke and cardiac risks after first ischemic stroke: the Northern Manhattan Study. Neurology 2006;66(5):641–6.
230. Judd SE, Kleindorfer DO, McClure LA, et al. Self-report of stroke, transient ischemic attack, or stroke symptoms and risk of future stroke in the REasons for Geographic And Racial Differences in Stroke (REGARDS) study. Stroke 2013;44(1):55–60.
231. Hong KS, Yegiaian S, Lee M, et al. Declining stroke and vascular event recurrence rates in secondary prevention trials over the past 50 years and consequences for current trial design. Circulation 2011;123(19):2111–19.
244. Jorgensen HS, Nakayama H, Reith J, et al. Stroke recurrence: predictors, severity, and prognosis. The Copenhagen Stroke Study. Neurology 1997;48(4):891–5.
250. Rundek T, Chen X, Steiner MM. Predictors of 1-year stroke recurrence: the Northern Manhattan Stroke Study. Cerebrovasc Dis 1997;(Suppl. 7):1–88.
252. Alter M, Sobel E, McCoy RL, et al. Stroke in the Lehigh Valley: risk factors for recurrent stroke. Neurology 1987;37(3):503–7.
255. Amarenco P, Cohen A, Tzourio C, et al. Atherosclerotic disease of the aortic arch and the risk of ischemic stroke. N Engl J Med 1994;331(22):1474–9.
257. Di Tullio M, Sacco RL, Gopal A, et al. Patent foramen ovale as a risk factor for cryptogenic stroke. Ann Intern Med 1992;117(6): 461–5.
262. Dhamoon MS, Sciacca RR, Rundek T, et al. Recurrent stroke and cardiac risks after first ischemic stroke: the Northern Manhattan Study. Neurology 2006;66(5):641–6.
263. Coutts SB, Modi J, Patel SK, et al. CT/CT angiography and MRI findings predict recurrent stroke after transient ischemic attack

and minor stroke: results of the prospective CATCH study. Stroke 2012;43(4):1013–17.

265. Melkas S, Sibolt G, Oksala NK, et al. Extensive white matter changes predict stroke recurrence up to 5 years after a first-ever ischemic stroke. Cerebrovasc Dis 2012;34(3):191–8.

266. Thijs V, Lemmens R, Schoofs C, et al. Microbleeds and the risk of recurrent stroke. Stroke 2010;41(9):2005–9.

270. Allen NB, Holford TR, Bracken MB, et al. Geographic variation in one-year recurrent ischemic stroke rates for elderly Medicare beneficiaries in the USA. Neuroepidemiology 2010;34(2):123–9.

272. Paci M, Nannetti L, D'Ippolito P, et al. Outcomes from ischemic stroke subtypes classified by the Oxfordshire Community Stroke Project: a systematic review. Eur J Phys Rehabil Med 2011;47(1): 19–23.

275. Grau AJ, Weimar C, Buggle F, et al. Risk factors, outcome, and treatment in subtypes of ischemic stroke: the German stroke data bank. Stroke 2001;32(11):2559–66.

278. Hart RG, Diener HC, Coutts SB, Easton JD, et al. Embolic strokes of undetermined source: the case for a new clinical construct. Lancet Neurol 2014;13(4):429–38.

284. Arboix A, Alió J. Cardioembolic stroke: clinical features, specific cardiac disorders and prognosis. Curr Cardiol Rev 2010;6(3): 150–61.

289. Weimar C, Cotton D, Sha N, et al. Discontinuation of antiplatelet study medication and risk of recurrent stroke and cardiovascular events: results from the PRoFESS study. Cerebrovasc Dis 2013;35(6):538–43.

290. Elkind MS. Outcomes after stroke: risk of recurrent ischemic stroke and other events. Am J Med 2009;122(4 Suppl. 2):S7–13.

291. Bushnell C, McCullough LD, Awad IA, et al. Guidelines for the prevention of stroke in women: a statement for healthcare professionals from the American Heart Association/American Stroke Association. Stroke 2014;45(5):1545–88.

292. Yong M, Kaste M. Association of characteristics of blood pressure profiles and stroke outcomes in the ECASS-II trial. Stroke 2008;39(2):366–72.

293. James PA, Oparil S, Carter BL, et al. 2014 Evidence-based guideline for the management of high blood pressure in adults: report from the panel members appointed to the Eighth Joint National Committee (JNC 8). JAMA 2014;311(5):507–20.

295. Voko Z, Bots ML, Hofman A, et al. J-shaped relation between blood pressure and stroke in treated hypertensives. Hypertension 1999;34(6):1181–5.

298. Liu L, Wang Z, Gong L, et al. Blood pressure reduction for the secondary prevention of stroke: a Chinese trial and a systematic review of the literature. Hypertens Res 2009;32(11):1032–40.

301. Ovbiagele B, Diener HC, Yusuf S, Martin RH, et al. Level of systolic blood pressure within the normal range and risk of recurrent stroke. JAMA 2011;306(19):2137–44.

304. Go AS, Bauman M, King SM, et al. An effective approach to high blood pressure control: a science advisory from the American Heart Association, the American College of Cardiology, and the Centers for Disease Control and Prevention. Hypertension 2014;63(4):878–85.

308. Dhamoon MS, Elkind MS. Inclusion of stroke as an outcome and risk equivalent in risk scores for primary and secondary prevention of vascular disease. Circulation 2010;121(18):2071–8.

313. Lip GY, Nieuwlatt R, Pisters R, et al. Refining clinical risk stratification for predicting stroke and thromboembolism in atrial fibrillation using a novel risk factor-based approach: the euro heart survey on atrial fibrillation. Chest 2010;137(2):263–72.

315. Mani H, Lindhoff-Last E. New oral anticoagulants in patients with nonvalvular atrial fibrillation: a review of pharmacokinetics, safety, efficacy, quality of life, and cost effectiveness. Drug Des Devel Ther 2014;8:789–98.

317. Pennlert J, Eriksson M, Carlberg B, et al. Long-Term Risk and Predictors of Recurrent Stroke Beyond the Acute Phase. Stroke 2014;45(6):1839–41.

320. Bak S, Sindrup SH, Alslev T, et al. Cessation of smoking after first-ever stroke: a follow-up study. Stroke 2002;33(9):2263–9.

327. Sacco RL. Alcohol and stroke risk: an elusive dose-response relationship. Ann Neurol 2007;62(6):551–2.

328. O'Keefe JH, Bhatti SK, Bajwa A, et al. Alcohol and cardiovascular health: the dose makes the poison … or the remedy. Mayo Clin Proc 2014;89(3):382–93.

333. Atherosclerotic disease of the aortic arch as a risk factor for recurrent ischemic stroke. The French Study of Aortic Plaques in Stroke Group. N Engl J Med 1996;334(19):1216–21.

334. Di Tullio MR, Russo C, Jin Z, et al. Aortic arch plaques and risk of recurrent stroke and death. Circulation 2009; 119(17):2376–82.

339. Furlan AJ, Reisman M, Massaro J, et al. Closure or medical therapy for cryptogenic stroke with patent foramen ovale. N Engl J Med 2012;366(11):991–9.

342. Thaler DE, Di Angelantonio E, Di Tullio MR, et al. The risk of paradoxical embolism (RoPE) study: initial description of the completed database. Int J Stroke. 2013;8(8):612–19.

343. Di Napoli M, Papa F, Villa Pini Stroke Data Bank Investigators. Inflammation, hemostatic markers, and antithrombotic agents in relation to long-term risk of new cardiovascular events in first-ever ischemic stroke patients. Stroke 2002;33(7):1763–71.

346. Hankey GJ, Eikelboom JW. Homocysteine levels in patients with stroke: clinical relevance and therapeutic implications. CNS Drugs 2001;15(6):437–43.

351. Katan M, Elkind MS. Inflammatory and neuroendocrine biomarkers of prognosis after ischemic stroke. Expert Rev Neurother 2011;11(2):225–39.

353. Saposnik G, Guzik AK, Reeves M, et al. Stroke Prognostication using Age and NIH Stroke Scale: SPAN-100. Neurology 2013;80(1):21–8.

354. A randomized trial of tirilazad mesylate in patients with acute stroke (RANTTAS). The RANTTAS Investigators. Stroke 1996; 27(9):1453–8.

355. Pexman JH, Barber PA, Hill MD, et al. Use of the Alberta Stroke Program Early CT Score (ASPECTS) for assessing CT scans in patients with acute stroke. AJNR Am J Neuroradiol 2001;22(8): 1534–42.

358. Hand PJ, Wardlaw JM, Rivers CS, et al. MR diffusion-weighted imaging and outcome prediction after ischemic stroke. Neurology 2006;66(8):1159–63.

359. Johnston KC, Wagner DP, Wang XQ, Newman GC, et al. Validation of an acute ischemic stroke model: does diffusion-weighted imaging lesion volume offer a clinically significant improvement in prediction of outcome? Stroke 2007;38(6):1820–5.

362. Johnston SC, Gress DR, Browner WS, et al. Short-term prognosis after emergency department diagnosis of TIA. JAMA 2000; 284(22):2901–6.

363. Kernan WN, Viscoli CM, Brass LM, et al. The stroke prognosis instrument II (SPI-II): A clinical prediction instrument for patients with transient ischemia and nondisabling ischemic stroke. Stroke 2000;31(2):456–62.

365. Ay H, Gungor L, Arsava EM, et al. A score to predict early risk of recurrence after ischemic stroke. Neurology 2010;74(2):128–35.

367. Weimar C, Diener HC, Alberts MJ, Steg PG, et al. The Essen stroke risk score predicts recurrent cardiovascular events: a validation within the REduction of Atherothrombosis for Continued Health (REACH) registry. Stroke 2009;40(2):350–4.

368. Thompson DD, Murray GD, Dennis M, et al. Formal and informal prediction of recurrent stroke and myocardial infarction after stroke: a systematic review and evaluation of clinical prediction models in a new cohort. BMC Med 2014;12:58.

369. Wade DT, Collin C. The Barthel ADL Index: a standard measure of physical disability? Int Disabil Stud 1988;10(2):64–7.

371. Rankin J. Cerebral vascular accidents in patients over the age of 60. II. Prognosis. Scott Med J 1957;2(5):200–15.

372. Granger CV, Hamilton BB, Gresham GE, et al. The stroke rehabilitation outcome study: Part II. Relative merits of the total Barthel index score and a four-item subscore in predicting patient outcomes. Arch Phys Med Rehabil 1989;70(2):100–3.

374. Sacco RL, DeRosa JT, Haley EC Jr, et al. Glycine Antagonist in Neuroprotection Americas Investigators. Glycine antagonist in neuroprotection for patients with acute stroke: GAIN Americas: a randomized controlled trial. JAMA 2001;285(13):1719–28.

379. Hankey GJ, Jamrozik K, Broadhurst RJ, et al. Long-term disability after first-ever stroke and related prognostic factors in the Perth Community Stroke Study, 1989–1990. Stroke 2002;33(4): 1034–40.

380. Dennis MS, Burn JP, Sandercock PA, et al. Long-term survival after first-ever stroke: the Oxfordshire Community Stroke Project. Stroke 1993;24(6):796–800.

381. Dombovy ML, Basford JR, Whisnant JP, et al. Disability and use of rehabilitation services following stroke in Rochester, Minnesota, 1975–1979. Stroke 1987;18(5):830–6.
385. Saver JL. Novel end point analytic techniques and interpreting shifts across the entire range of outcome scales in acute stroke trials. Stroke 2007;38(11):3055–62.
388. van Almenkerk S, Smalbrugge M, Depla MF, et al. What predicts a poor outcome in older stroke survivors? A systematic review of the literature. Disabil Rehabil 2013;35(21):1774–82.
390. Sturm JW, Donnan GA, Dewey HM, et al. Quality of life after stroke: the North East Melbourne Stroke Incidence Study (NEMESIS). Stroke 2004;35(10):2340–5.
396. Duncan PW, Wallace D, Lai SM, et al. The stroke impact scale version 2.0. Evaluation of reliability, validity, and sensitivity to change. Stroke 1999;30(10):2131–40.
398. Sacco RL, Boden-Albala B, Kargman DE, et al. Quality of life after ischemic stroke: the Northern Manhattan Stroke Study. Ann Neurol 1995;38:322.
399. Dhamoon MS, Moon YP, Paik MC, et al. Quality of life declines after first ischemic stroke. The Northern Manhattan Study. Neurology 2010;75(4):328–34.
400. de Haan RJ. Measuring quality of life after stroke using the SF-36. Stroke 2002;33(5):1176–7.
406. Lin KC, Fu T, Wu CY, et al. Assessing the stroke-specific quality of life for outcome measurement in stroke rehabilitation: minimal detectable change and clinically important difference. Health Qual Life Outcomes 2011;9:5.
410. Saver JL, Gornbein J. Treatment effects for which shift or binary analyses are advantageous in acute stroke trials. Neurology 2009;72(15):1310–15.
413. Hackett ML, Yapa C, Parag V, et al. Frequency of depression after stroke: a systematic review of observational studies. Stroke 2005;36(6):1330–40.
420. Willey JZ, Disla N, Moon YP, et al. Early depressed mood after stroke predicts long-term disability: the Northern Manhattan Stroke Study (NOMASS). Stroke 2010;41(9):1896–900.
424. Beck AT, Ward CH, Mendelson M, et al. An inventory for measuring depression. Arch Gen Psychiatry 1961;4:561–71.
425. Hamilton M. A rating scale for depression. J Neurol Neurosurg Psychiatry 1960;23:56–62.
427. de Man-van Ginkel JM1, Hafsteinsdóttir TB, Lindeman E, et al. In-hospital risk prediction for post-stroke depression: development and validation of the Post-stroke Depression Prediction Scale. Stroke 2013;44(9):2441–5.
434. Alexopoulos GS, Meyers BS, Young RC, et al. Clinically defined vascular depression. Am J Psychiatry 1997;154(4):562–5.
436. Debette S, Beiser A, DeCarli C, et al. Association of MRI markers of vascular brain injury with incident stroke, mild cognitive impairment, dementia, and mortality. The Framingham Offspring Study. Stroke 2010;41(4):600–6.
438. Firbank MJ, Teodorczuk A, van der Flier WM, Gouw AA, et al. Relationship between progression of brain white matter changes and late-life depression:3-year results from the LADIS study. Br J Psychiatry 2012;201(1):40–5.
439. Flaster M, Sharma A, Rao M. Poststroke depression: a review emphasizing the role of prophylactic treatment and synergy with treatment for motor recovery. Top Stroke Rehabil 2013;20(2): 139–50.

17 Vascular Dementia and Cognitive Impairment

Sudha Seshadri, Alexis Economos, Clinton Wright

KEY POINTS

- Vascular dementia (VaD), as conventionally defined, is one of the most frequent forms of dementia. Further, when vascular contributions to other types of dementias are included, it is arguably the most common form of dementia.
- Criteria for the diagnosis of VaD have evolved to include a broader phenotype and memory impairment is not required for a diagnosis of vascular dementia.
- Vascular mild cognitive impairment (VaMCI) is a more recently recognized entity that includes mild cognitive deficits, which do not significantly impact function and hence cannot be categorized as dementia, and where the etiology is thought to be predominantly vascular rather than neurodegenerative.
- Newer, more sensitive imaging techniques, including high (3 and 7T) Tesla MRI, diffusion tensor imaging and susceptibility sequences, have increased the prevalence and range of subtle cerebrovascular damage that can be detected in persons with suspected VaMCI and VaD.
- A number of potentially modifiable risk factors for VaD have been identified and addressing these may help prevent the onset of clinical symptoms or slow the pace of decline in persons with VaMCI and VaD.

Current projections suggest that the US will have 72 million people older than 65 years of age by 2030, a greater than ten-fold increase in a century.[1] In this older population, having one or more vascular risk factors is the norm rather than the exception. Thus, in the community-based Framingham Heart Study (FHS) sample, the lifetime risk for development of hypertension is more than 90%.[2] Not surprisingly, the burden of age-related neurologic illness has increased in parallel with lengthening life expectancy. A 2006 analysis of data from the FHS sample predicted that one in three people currently aged 65 and free of stroke and dementia would experience one or both of these conditions during their lifetimes.[3] It is generally acknowledged that exposure to vascular risk factors adversely affects cognitive function, although there is uncertainty about the extent and the mechanisms. Observational studies show that vascular risk factors measured in midlife, but not those measured only in late life, predict later cognitive impairment and dementia.[4] The Cardiovascular Health Study identifies rates for Alzheimer disease and VaD to be 19.2 and 14.6 per 1000 person-years.[5] However, the concept of what constitutes "vascular dementia" remains in evolution.[6] There has been growing emphasis on identifying persons with early cognitive impairment due to vascular pathology, because these individuals are at maximal risk for development of vascular dementia (VaD) and might benefit the most from preventive measures.

HISTORICAL EVOLUTION OF THE CONCEPT OF VASCULAR DEMENTIA

The evolution of the concept of vascular dementia (VaD) has been elegantly summarized by Roman.[7] At the start of the 7th century, Saint Isadore, the Archbishop of Seville, used the term dementia (from the Latin root "demens," meaning out of one's mind) to describe a slowly progressive dullness or dotage. In 1672, Thomas Willis described the fairly sudden development of "dullness of mind and forgetfulness" accompanying a "half palsie" (hemiplegia) in his book *De Anima Brutorum*. Alzheimer's disease (AD) was described in 1904 but was considered a rare presenile form of dementia. In his 1910 *Lehrbuch der Psychiatrie*, Kraeplin, who has been called the Linnaeus of psychiatry, separated a presenile form of dementia from senile dementias and concluded that most senile dementia was arteriosclerotic insanity, which later became attributed to "progressive hardening of the arteries leading to slow ischemic neuronal loss." This remained a widely accepted viewpoint until 1970, when Blessed and Tomlinson established through careful autopsy studies that the pathology underlying most cases of dementia was, in fact, the plaques and tangles associated with Alzheimer's disease.[8] The definition of vascular dementia (VaD) became restricted to "multi-infarct" dementia; it was argued that vascular pathology resulted in dementia largely through the occurrence of multiple small or large cerebral infarcts.[9] In the next 20 years careful clinical studies did establish that single infarcts could result in dementia if they were strategically located, and CT scans showed that among persons with a similar number and location of strokes, concomitant cortical atrophy increased the risk of symptomatic dementia.[10] With the emergence of brain MRI, covert brain infarcts (CBIs) and white matter hyperintensities (WMHs) were found to be widespread and to be associated with an increased risk of cognitive impairment. With novel MRI imaging sequences and high- and ultra-high-strength MRI scans, the presence of cerebral microbleed, as well as subtle changes in white matter integrity and presence of microscopic infarcts can also be detected.[11,12] In recent decades the concept of mild cognitive impairment (MCI) as a prodromal stage of Alzheimer's disease (AD) has emerged, and, in parallel, a broader concept of vascular cognitive impairment (VCI) has solidified that includes all states of cognitive impairment associated with cerebrovascular disease (CVD), including VaD, AD with cerebrovascular disorder and mild cognitive impairment secondary to vascular pathology (VaMCI), which was previously also called VCI with no dementia (VCIND).[6,8,13–15]

DIAGNOSTIC CRITERIA FOR VASCULAR DEMENTIA

Since the 1970s, several sets of diagnostic criteria have been formulated in attempts to standardize the definition of VaD. Such criteria are essential for use as diagnostic tools in clinical practice, to compare prevalence and incidence in different population samples, to uncover risk factors, and to recruit homogeneous cohorts for drug trials. These criteria range from the entirely clinical Hachinski Ischemic Score (HIS) to the strict National Institute for Neurological Diseases and Stroke–Association Internationale pour la Recherche et l'Enseignement en Neurosciences (NINDS-AIREN) criteria,[16] formulated largely for use in research settings. They include the recent, inclusive, American Heart Association and American Stroke Association (AHA-ASA) vascular cognitive impairment criteria from 2011, the more epidemiologically applicable *Diagnostic and Statistical Manual* (DSM-III, IIIR, IV) criteria, the International Classification of Disease 10th revision (ICD-10) criteria, and the California Alzheimer's Disease Diagnostic and Treatment Centers (ADDTC) criteria.[17-19] In 2014, a further refinement of diagnostic criteria for vascular cognitive disorders were proposed by the International Society for Vascular Behavioral and Cognitive Disorders (VASCOG); the bewildering plurality of diagnostic criteria do, however, share a few core characteristics.[20]

The Hachinski Ischemic Score does not classify dementia, but seeks to predict the dominant underlying pathology. It is based entirely on the history of vascular risk factors and on the clinical signs; in an abbreviated version, a score of 7 or more out of a possible 12 points is considered diagnostic of VaD, whereas a score less than 4 is thought to exclude VaD. The NINDS-AIREN and ADDTC criteria additionally consider CT or MRI data. Each broadly requires clinical and/or imaging documentation of strokes or vascular brain injury (such as extensive WMH), a temporal profile linking the vascular damage and the dementia (for example, abrupt onset or onset within 3 months after stroke, a stuttering or stepwise progression) and focal neurologic signs if thought to be of vascular etiology, and assigns a degree of certainty to the diagnosis: "probable" or "possible." When each of the different criteria are applied to a single sample, a varying, only partially overlapping set of subjects are categorized as having VaD.[21] When pathology is used as a "gold standard," the sensitivities of the different clinical criteria have been noted to vary from 0.2 to 0.7 (possible VaD as defined by the ADDTC being the most sensitive criterion) and the specificities from 0.78 to 0.93 (probable VaD by the NINDS-AIREN criteria being the most specific). Thus, most of these criteria emphasize specificity over sensitivity; less than 50% of all persons with moderately severe vascular pathology at autopsy are diagnosed during life as having VaD.[22]

The criteria proposed in the AHA-ASA 2011 statement suggested that the term vascular cognitive impairment (VCI) be used for all cognitive disorders associated with any evidence of cerebrovascular disease and cerebrovascular brain dysfunction or injury, regardless of co-existing pathologies. Several of the criteria for VaD, including the AHA-ASA criteria, emphasize that a memory deficit is not required to diagnose VaD, only the presence of a cognitive deficit in one or more domains. Mild cognitive impairment of vascular origin (VaMCI) was also addressed, stipulating a decline in cognitive function in at least one cognitive domain, with normal or minimally affected activities of daily living. Like MCI, VaMCI includes four subtypes: amnestic, amnestic plus other domains, non-amnestic single domain and non-amnestic multiple domain. The term "unstable vascular MCI" was also introduced in this statement to describe patients who shift from an impaired to an unimpaired cognitive state. One limitation of these criteria is the lack of established sensitivity and specificity. The 2014 VASCOG criteria identify a continuum of vascular cognitive disorders, categorized into mild vascular cognitive disorder and major vascular cognitive disorder, following the DSM-V lead of renaming MCI and dementia as "minor" and "major" neurocognitive disorders, and detail neuroimaging, clinical, and/or pathologic criteria that may be considered supportive of these diagnoses. The various criteria for VaD have been summarized and compared in prior publications.[19,23] Table 17-1 compares the VASCOG, AHA-ASA and NINDS-AIREN VaD criteria. There is as yet no consensus on the best set of criteria to describe VaD.

COGNITIVE IMPAIRMENT AND DEMENTIA FOLLOWING STROKE

The risk of new-onset dementia in patients who have had stroke is approximately twice the risk in age- and sex-matched controls and averages about 10% after the first stroke,[24,25] depending on the location, volume of damaged brain tissue, clinical severity, and presence of early post-stroke complications (seizure, delirium, hypoxia, hypotension) as well as on pre-stroke cognitive status and concomitant imaging abnormalities such as covert or subclinical infarcts (CBI), cerebral microbleeds (CMB), WMH, and medial temporal lobe atrophy.[9,26-29] A 2009 review identified older age, less education, pre-stroke cognitive impairment, diabetes, and atrial fibrillation as factors that increased the risk, but the single strongest predictor of cognitive decline after an initial stroke was the occurrence of a second stroke.[26] In persons with recurrent stroke, the risk of dementia rose to approximately 30%, regardless of the number and severity of vascular risk factors. Whereas the occurrence of VaD in persons who have suffered large infarcts makes intuitive sense, VaD may also follow small infarcts. Among 1,636 participants with lacunar strokes in the Small Subcortical Strokes (SPS3) Trial, 47% were classified as having VaMCI with a diverse mix of subtypes: roughly one-third amnestic, one-third amnestic multidomain and one-third non-amnestic. The most frequently noted deficits were in the domains of episodic memory, language and executive function (verbal fluency) and motor speed and dexterity.[30] The Determinants of Dementia After Stroke (DEDEMAS) Study, an international multicenter observational prospective study aimed at identifying and characterizing the determinants of cognitive impairment after stroke, has been ongoing since 2013.[31]

Expanded Concept of Vascular Cognitive Impairment

The concept of VCI outlined in 2006 by the NINDS in collaboration with the Canadian Stroke Network (CSN), in a statement advising harmonization standards for data collection, and further elaborated upon in the 2011 AHA-ASA VCI statement, is broad.[32] It includes, but is not restricted to, dementia following stroke. The term "vascular cognitive impairment" may be used to describe any syndrome of cognitive and behavioral impairment that is thought to be due to vascular factors affecting the brain. Thus, it could range from the subtle cognitive deficits seen in persons with diabetes when compared with their non-diabetic peers, through the multifocal cognitive deficits that may accompany the presence of multiple brain infarcts or hemorrhages to clinical VaD. The last requires the presence of cognitive or behavioral problems severe enough to affect social or occupational functioning (i.e., amounting to "dementia"), the documentation of disease affecting the blood vessels or blood flow to part or all of the brain, and clinical or radiologic evidence of structural damage to the brain due to these vascular factors per the NINDS-CSN collaboration.[32] There have also been efforts to define diagnostic clinical criteria for subcortical VaD syndromes, conditions that have been described as Binswanger's syndrome: extensive WMHs and cognitive slowing in the absence of clinical strokes or CT/MRI

TABLE 17-1 Vascular Dementia Criteria – A Comparative Table*

Criterion	VASCOG (2014)[1]	AHA-ASA (2011)[2]	NINDS-AIREN (1993)[3]
Diagnosis of dementia	Decline in ≥1 cognitive domain that interferes with independence	≥2 cognitive domains that affect daily living[a]	Impairment of memory and decline in ≥2 cognitive domains that interfere with daily living[a]
Cognitive domains assessed	Attention and processing speed; frontal-executive function; learning and memory; language; visuoconstructional-perceptual; praxis-gnosis-body schema; social cognition	Executive/attention; memory; language: visuospatial functions	Orientation, attention, language, visuospatial functions, executive functions, motor control, praxis
Memory deficit required	No	No	Yes
Diagnostic categories	Major vascular cognitive disorder or VaD	Probable, possible VaD	Definite (histopathologically verified), probable, possible VaD
Temporal relationship between vascular event and cognitive deficits	Yes, OR frontal-executive, processing and attention decline WITH (1) early gait disturbance, (2) early urinary frequency, (3) personality/mood changes	Yes (probable); No (possible)	Yes (probable); No (possible)
Radiologic evidence of vascular disease	Yes	Yes (probable); No (possible)	Yes (probable); No (possible)
Co-existent neuro-degenerative diseases allowed	No	No (probable); Yes (possible)	No
Exclusions	Alternative neurologic diagnosis; other medical disorders	Delirium; active drug/alcohol abuse[b]	Disturbance of consciousness, delirium; psychosis, severe aphasia, major sensorimotor impairment

[1]VASCOG, International Society for Vascular Cognitive Disorders.
[2]AHA-ASA, American Heart Association/American Stroke Association Statement.
[3]NINDS-AIREN, National Institute of Neurological Disorders and Stroke and Association Internationale pour la Recherché et l'Enseignement en Neurosciences.
[a]Must be independent of motor/sensory sequelae of the vascular event.
[b]Must be free of any substance >3 months.
*Used with permission.

infarcts and hemorrhages.[33,34] The criteria proposed in the 5th edition of the *Diagnostic and Statistical Manual* (DSM5) replace the potentially stigmatizing term "dementia" with "major neurocognitive disorder," and the prodromal stage of MCI or VaMCI is called "minor neurocognitive disorder." The 2011 AHA/ASA scientific statement on vascular contributions to cognitive impairment and dementia defines VCI as "a syndrome with evidence of clinical stroke or subclinical vascular brain injury and cognitive impairment affecting at least one cognitive domain". The entire spectrum of cognitive disorders is included, with all forms of cerebral vascular brain injury, ranging from mild cognitive impairment to dementia. Importantly, memory impairment is not a requirement for diagnosis because unlike Alzheimer disease, which in most cases begins in the mesial temporal lobe structures and affects hippocampal – and thus memory – function, vascular damage is topographically heterogeneous and can involve deficits isolated to other domains.[35] The writing group emphasized the need for continued development and refinement of cognitive batteries for VCI, in addition to identification of biomarkers and pathological-radiological correlation.

OVERLAP OF VASCULAR AND NEURODEGENERATIVE PATHOLOGIES

The various criteria for VaD and AD define "probable AD" and "probable VaD," but do not address the large number of persons with mixed AD and VaD.[36–38] The current consensus among clinicians and epidemiologists is to independently decide on the presence or absence of clinically probable AD and VaD without requiring that the presence of one condition excludes the other diagnosis. There are two issues at play here. First, while a clinical diagnosis of AD is accurate roughly 90% of the time in autopsy studies,[39,40] clinicians are more likely to miss a diagnosis of a mixed dementia.[41–44] Second, a clinician's estimate of vascular pathology is only as good as the imaging modality (e.g., MRI) used for the assessment. Higher field strength MRI scanners at 7T are beginning to show microinfarcts that might not have been seen on older machines with less powerful magnetic fields. The degree to which microinfarctions may play a role in VCI and VaD is an active area of research.[45–47] AD and VCI may share pathogenic mechanisms, as evidenced by animal work[48,49] and the vascular risk factors associated with dementia are further discussed later in this chapter.

EPIDEMIOLOGY

When a similar set of criteria are used, the age-adjusted prevalence of VCI may be lower in low-to-middle-income countries that are early in the process of demographic transition.[50] However, it is these countries that may see the fastest *increase* in the prevalence of VCI. The incidence of VaD in the US among persons older than 65 years has been estimated at 14.6 per 1000 person-years.[51] The proportion of all cases of dementia that is vascular appears to vary by age, ethnicity, geography, and definition used.[52] Mixed AD and VaD may be the most common explanation for cognitive impairment in the elderly.[53] The ideal way to define the complete spectrum of cerebrovascular disease appears to be to prospectively follow epidemiologic cohorts exposed to vascular risk factors to define the full range of structural and cognitive changes associated with these

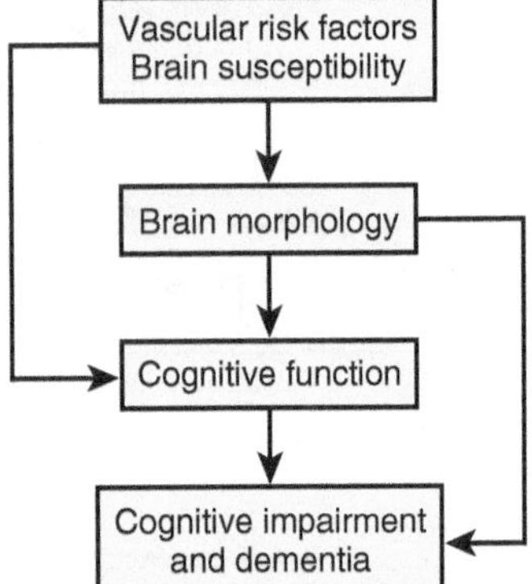

Figure 17-1. How to develop diagnostic and prognostic criteria and define the complete clinical spectrum.

vascular risk factors and also to determine which of these intermediate phenotypes results in clinical disease (Fig. 17-1). This approach is feasible because a number of studies of cardiovascular disease have incorporated brain imaging and cognitive testing in the past two decades,[54–59] and a few have additionally initiated brain banks to permit clinical-imaging–pathologic correlations.[60]

CLINICAL DIAGNOSIS

The VCI syndrome is best diagnosed and characterized by identifying the presence and quantifying the extent of (1) the cognitive deficits (and presence or absence of VaD and VaMCI) by clinical and formal neuropsychological testing *and* (2) the vascular brain injury through neuroimaging supplemented by cerebral and systemic vascular imaging as indicated. The term "VCI" can be used for cognitive disorders associated with varying forms of vascular brain injury: atherothrombotic, cardioembolic, hemorrhagic, and rare genetic vascular disorders. The role of other vascular pathologies, including white matter lesions and microbleeds, in VCI is unclear.[61] Recent research points to an association between asymptomatic carotid artery stenosis, defined as stenosis without a recognized neurologic deficit, and cognitive dysfunction primarily within the domains of processing speed and learning/memory. Further studies are needed to confirm this association and potential mechanisms.[61,62,63]

The clinical neurologic profile of VaD can be extremely varied depending on the underlying pathology, patient age and education, and presence or absence of concomitant AD pathology. However, patients with VaD are typically younger and more likely to be male. Some clinical symptoms and signs that are more frequently seen in persons with VaD than in persons with typical AD are a pattern of multifocal rather than global deficits, presence of focal neurologic signs (including gait abnormalities), an early and disproportionately severe involvement of executive dysfunction (unlike the early verbal memory loss in AD), and relatively preserved recognition (improved performance when categorical or phonemic clues are offered) in comparison with spontaneous recall.[64] Depression and emotional lability are also more frequently seen. The frequently considered differential diagnoses for VaD include AD, frontotemporal dementia, normal-pressure hydrocephalus, dementia with Lewy bodies, and dementia associated with cerebral infections such as HIV. The finding of cerebral vascular brain injury on CT or MRI can help establish a clinical diagnosis of VaD.

Vascular Mild Cognitive Impairment

Community-based data have shown that even before the occurrence of an initial stroke, persons who subsequently experience a stroke do worse on global tests of cognition such as the mini-mental state examination (MMSE) than do age- and sex-matched controls.[65] This feature may represent a subtle effect of cumulated exposure to vascular risk factors over the preceding years; indeed, a pattern of VCI can be defined that is associated with covert or subclinical brain injury and that doubles the risk of subsequent stroke.[66,67] Conversely, in a community-based series of subjects with MCI, a significant proportion has relative preservation of memory function and disproportionate involvement of attention, processing speed, and executive function domains. They are more likely to have vascular risk factors, imaging evidence of covert vascular brain injury, and a higher risk for subsequent stroke than persons with the predominantly amnestic MCI that seems to precede clinical AD; hence, these subjects were frequently considered to have VaMCI. However, the situation is likely more complex with MCI due to both neurodegenerative and vascular etiologies having multiple presentations. Thus all MCI may be categorized along multiple axes as single or multiple domain, predominantly amnestic or non-amnestic, and pathologically as likely vascular or neurodegenerative.[68–71] On follow-up, any sample of persons with VaMCI includes persons who revert to normal and are deemed to have "unstable MCI" (either they recover from the effects of a vascular insult such as a stroke or their clinical picture was due to a reversible cause such as depression), others who go on to demonstrate VaD, and yet others who have typical AD.[72,73] The MCI and subtype definitions are applied both in research studies and as a useful interim category for classifying patients in clinical practice.

NEUROPSYCHOLOGICAL ASSESSMENTS OF VASCULAR COGNITIVE IMPAIRMENT

The neuropsychological assessment of patients with suspected VCI requires a comprehensive cognitive battery, which should include tests sensitive to executive function abnormalities, a salient feature of the condition.[74] Thus, the Montreal Cognitive Assessment (MOCA) has been recommended in place of the MMSE, also called the Folstein test,[75] because the former is more sensitive for the detection of executive function abnormalities. The 2006 NINDS-CSN VCI harmonization guidelines described several neuropsychological test protocols of varying length (30 minutes and 60 minutes), each of which covers the domains of frontal executive function (animal naming and phonemic fluency, digit-symbol substitution +/– trail-making test), visual perception and organization (a figure-copying task such as using the Rey-Osterreith figure), a verbal learning and memory task (such as the Hopkins verbal learning test), a lexical retrieval task (such as the Boston naming test), and a questionnaire-based screen for neuropsychiatric and depressive symptoms (using the neuropsychiatric inventory [NPI] and the Center for Epidemiological Studies–Depression [CES-D] Scale). They also suggest the MOCA as a 5-minute battery for use in patients with suspected VCI.[32] Detailed discussion of these protocols is beyond the scope of this chapter, but the tests listed have been well standardized and are referenced in the NINDS-CSN guidelines. Other batteries that cover these domains have been used in existing

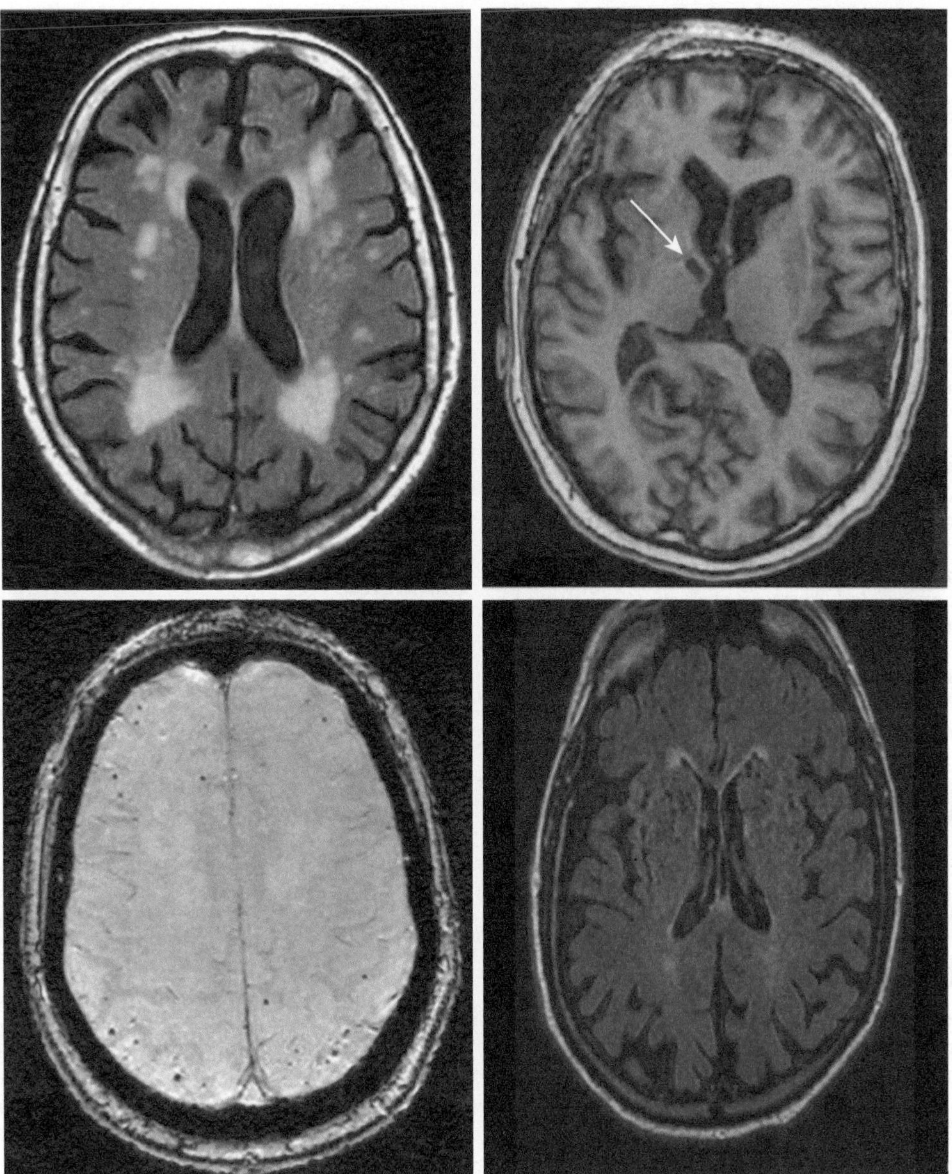

Figure 17-2. Brain MRI images showing typical examples of findings in persons with vascular cognitive impairment; clockwise from top left: white matter hyper intensities, lacunar infarct, cerebral microbleeds and enlarged perivascular (Virchow-Robin) spaces.

epidemiologic studies and in clinics.[54,56] The MOCA and trail-making test are also part of a cognitive test panel recommended by a National Human Genetics Research Institute (NHGRI) panel convened to suggest tests for use by phenotypic non-experts conducting genome-wide association studies (www.phenxtoolkit.org). The major limitation of neuropsychological testing geared toward identifying executive function abnormalities, such as the MOCA, is that deficits in executive function are not specific to cerebrovascular disease.[76] In a study of Framingham Heart Study subjects comparing new cognitive deficits that appeared in persons after stroke with cognitive deficits appearing over time in persons without stroke, persons with stroke had poorer cognitive function in multiple domains including immediate recall of verbal and visual memories, verbal learning and language as well as the more traditionally expected domains of executive function and visuospatial and motor skills.[77] The frequent co-existence of VaD and AD also makes reliance upon neuropsychological testing for diagnostic clarification difficult.

IMAGING CORRELATES OF VASCULAR COGNITIVE IMPAIRMENT (Fig. 17-2)

VCI may also be defined as a constellation of cognitive and functional impairments associated with the structural cerebrovascular brain injury (CVBI) noted on imaging (in vivo) or at autopsy. CVBI on imaging includes clinically symptomatic *large and small artery infarcts and hemorrhages*. However, clinically asymptomatic (covert) brain infarction is even more common, and the full spectrum of CVBI also includes *WMHs and total and regional brain atrophy*.[56,78,79,80] The relationship between CVBI on brain imaging and cognitive impairment is not simple or linear and remains inadequately understood. Partly, the prevalence and extent of CVBI detected vary with the imaging protocol used. Thus, subtle white matter injury in normal-appearing white matter can only be detected by diffusion tensor imaging (DTI) and some forms of cerebrovascular brain injury, such as microinfarcts, are not detectable by conventional 1.5 or 3T MRI imaging, although they can be detected by ultra-high-resolution 7T brain MRI imaging.[81,82] Furthermore, many changes that could be attributed to ischemia (such as generalized and lobar atrophy, hippocampal sclerosis, and, to a lesser extent, WMHs) have also been associated with AD and other neurodegenerative pathologies. Finally, in most elderly persons both vascular and non-vascular pathologies coexist, making it difficult to attribute the cognitive impairment or dementia detected to a specific etiology. Quantifying the extent of AD pathology through in vivo using newer amyloid imaging techniques with PET using the 11C-labeled Pittsburgh compound B (PiB) and other 18F containing amyloid labeling compounds are steps in that direction. Though rare, pure subcortical VaD has been identified using 11C-Pittsburgh compound B to rule out amyloid pathology.[83] Studies combining these modalities (volumetric MRI and amyloid PET) are underway in clinical and epidemiologic settings.[84]

Because of these caveats, neuroimaging is currently used to describe the vasculature and CVBI rather than to diagnose VCI or VaD. The NINDS-CSC VCI harmonization guidelines suggest that in a research setting, a minimal imaging dataset should include an MRI (≥1 T) with 3D T1-weighted, T2-weighted, fluid-attenuated inversion recovery (FLAIR), and gradient echo (GRE) sequences. Diffusion-weighted images (for acute stroke), diffusion tensor imaging (DTI) for assessing the state of the white matter tracts (abnormal DTI [lower fractional anisotropy] in normal-appearing white matter has been associated with poorer executive function and with vascular risk factors),[85] PET for β-amyloid, and non-invasive assessment of the cerebral vasculature (carotid ultrasound and/or MR angiogram) are encouraged. The minimum set of measurements recommended comprise: number, size and location of infarcts, and hemorrhages, extent on a quantitative or validated semiqualitative scale of WMH volume,[55,86,87] and measures of total brain (or ventricular) and hippocampal volumes.

Prevalence of Cerebrovascular Brain Injury

Covert or incidentally detected infarcts (CBIs) are five times as common as symptomatic infarcts. Estimates of the prevalence of MRI brain infarction (CBI) in community-based samples have varied between 5.8% and 17.7%, depending on age, ethnicity, presence of comorbidities, and imaging techniques.[88] On average, CBI is present in approximately 10–20% of individuals in middle or late life. Most have a single lesion, and the infarcts are most often located in the basal ganglia (52%), followed in frequency by other subcortical (35%) and cortical areas (11%).[95] Risk factors for CBI are generally the same as those for clinical stroke.[88,89] WMHs are present to some degree in most individuals older than 30 years[7] and increase in volume with increasing age and with exposure to vascular risk factors.[55,86,87,90] Age-specific definitions of extensive WMHs can be created and can be useful for defining persons at higher than average risk of VCI.[91] Cerebral microbleeds are also common with increasing age, and their prevalence rises with greater sensitivity of the imaging technique used.[92–95]

Association of Cerebrovascular Brain Injury with Cognitive Changes

The presence of CBI at baseline more than doubled the risk of dementia (and tripled the risk of stroke) at about 4 years of follow-up of Rotterdam study participants, even after adjustment of data for extent of WMHs and degree of atrophy.[11] Similar results were noted on follow-up of the younger FHS Offspring Study sample.[96] There are convincing data from population-based samples that a higher WMH volume is associated with poorer cognitive function in cross-sectional studies, and an enlargement of WMH on serial MRI is an even better predictor of cognitive decline than a single estimate of WMH.[91,97–99] The location of the WMH may also be important. A review found that periventricular locations are more frequently associated with decreased cognitive function, particularly in the domains of executive function and processing speed, compared with subcortical lesions.[100] Periventricular WMH have been found to be associated with an increased risk of dementia as well.[101] Interestingly, however, a study from the Washington Heights Inwood Columbia Aging Project found that parietal WMH were a stronger predictor of AD than hippocampal volume.[102] This supports the idea that WMH are heterogeneous in etiology and that some may be due to neurodegenerative changes rather than small-vessel damage. In addition to CBI and WMH, measures of cerebral gray matter and hippocampal volume have both been associated with decline in memory even among individuals clinically diagnosed with probable VaD according to NINDS-AIREN criteria.[103]

Summary

The clinical presentation and course of CVBI are highly variable, with the classic phenotype of stepwise decline seen in association with stroke being a relatively uncommon presentation for VCI. Structural MRI provides a fairly sensitive and specific marker for CVBI, but the relationship between CVBI and cognitive impairment is confounded by the frequent presence of AD changes of the brain. It is recommended that a careful record of the following aspects be made at baseline and at each follow-up imaging assessment: (1) description of the severity and type of extracranial and intracranial vessel disease; (2) definition of the volume and location of infarcts or hemorrhages (total volumes >100 mL, bilateral lesions, and lesions involving the thalamus, caudate, and basal forebrain being considered more likely to explain VCI and VaD), (3) the volume and location of white matter disease, and (4) the volume of total supratentorial brain parenchyma and of hippocampal lobes. In clinical situations, the same measures should be recorded qualitatively at baseline imaging, but the indications for follow-up imaging are unclear; such imaging might be indicated if sudden deterioration raises the possibility of an acute infarct or hemorrhage. How to integrate CVBI on brain MRI with PET and MRI measures of blood flow and amyloid burden remains under study.[32]

NEUROPATHOLOGIC ASPECTS

Defining the range and severity of pathologies underlying VCI has remained difficult. Infarcts and hemorrhages, the most obvious signs of vascular brain injury, can vary in size, location, and number (the number of infarcts, especially small infarcts, detected can vary depending on how carefully the brain is examined) and are prevalent among cognitively normal, community-dwelling persons. Such lesions may or may not have been accompanied by clinical symptoms or signs of a stroke, although covert and overt lesions may be equally significant in causing VCI. Further, there is associated AD pathology in a significant percentage of brains examined.[104–110]

Conceptually, it is generally acknowledged that the pathologic substrate of VCI and VaD likely includes focal infarction in key areas (both cortical and deep nuclear areas critical to aspects of cognition, and disrupting key association pathways in the white matter), high total volume of tissue damaged (again typically thought to be larger than 100 mL), and extent of demyelination and gliosis. However, defining a typical pattern of lesions or pathologic criteria for VaD that include a minimum amount of damage necessary for the diagnosis and/or a maximum amount sufficient to cause VCI has proved difficult because the pathologic substrate of VCI is highly heterogeneous.[32,111]

The most important cerebrovascular pathology that contributes to cognitive impairment is cerebral infarct.[112] Cerebral infarcts are discrete regions of tissue loss observed by the naked eye (macroscopic) or under the microscope (microscopic). Perimortem infarcts are of uncertain clinical significance, but chronic macroscopic infarcts occur in about one-third to one-half of older persons. Including other measures of vascular brain pathology, such as microscopic infarcts, small vessel disease, and white matter changes, increases the frequency of cerebrovascular disease in older persons to more than 75%.[53,109]

In clinical-pathologic studies, larger volumes[54,65] and higher numbers of macroscopic infarcts[13,16,54,68,69] are associated with an increased likelihood of dementia. However, determining a volume or number of CBIs *necessary* for a clinical diagnosis of VCI or dementia is difficult; and unlike AD and other neurodegenerative diseases, there are no currently accepted neuropathologic criteria to confirm a clinical diagnosis of VCI. Indeed, although Tomlinson et al.[8] described 100 mL of tissue loss as sufficient to cause VaD, persons with much lower volumes of infarcted tissue can have VaD. Infarcts, even small and single lesions, in certain locations, such as the thalamus, angular gyrus, and basal ganglia, are more likely to result in cognitive impairment. However, not all infarcts in these regions cause dementia, and small infarcts in other cortical and subcortical regions have also been associated with clinical dementia. Finally, multiple *microscopic* infarcts have been associated with an increased risk of dementia, even after the volume of macroscopic infarcts is accounted for.[106] This could be secondary to a cumulative large volume of tissue (neuronal and axonal pathway) damage from microscopic infarcts. However, it could just be a marker of other forms of vascular brain injury such as diffuse hypoxia or disruption in the blood–brain barrier. Other factors governing whether infarcts are related to impairment may include variation in cognitive reserve[113] and coexisting pathologies (see later).

Infarcts frequently coexist with AD pathology in the brains of older persons, and vascular disease may increase the risk of clinical dementia in two ways: (1) through an additive or synergistic effect of two pathologies on the clinical picture and (2) through a potentiation of the AD pathologic process. Snowdon et al.[114] showed that after adjustment of data for age and extent of AD pathology, persons with subcortical infarcts and, to a lesser extent, persons with large cortical infarcts were several-fold more likely to have clinical symptoms and signs of dementia than persons without concomitant vascular pathology. Further, in mouse models of AD, concomitant ischemia induced presenilin 1 (*ps1*) gene expression and levels of amyloid precursor protein.[115]

Other Vascular Pathologies

Other vascular pathologies commonly seen in the elderly include white matter degeneration, cerebral microbleeds, lipohyalinosis, atherosclerosis, and CAA, but there are few data on how to incorporate these additional pathologies into pathologic diagnostic criteria for VCI and VaD. Pathologic assessment in persons with suspected VCI/VaD is most useful in detecting and quantifying microscopic infarcts and in characterizing the extent and severity of neurodegenerative pathologies (AD and Lewy-body pathology, traumatic encephalopathy, argyrophilic grain disease, hippocampal sclerosis) that may be contributing to the cognitive status that was observed antemortem. These microinfarcts and neurodegenerative changes are not easy to detect antemortem. Prospective quantitative clinical–pathologic–neuroimaging studies are ongoing that should help clarify the complex interactions between vascular and AD pathologies in the evolution of VCI, VaD, and clinical AD.

PREVENTION OF VASCULAR COGNITIVE IMPAIRMENT

Association of Vascular Risk Factors with Vascular Cognitive Impairment and Vascular Dementia

Vascular risk factors and biomarkers that increase the risk of stroke would also be expected to increase the risk of VCI and VaD.[116] There are, however, several difficulties with interpreting data relating vascular risk factors with the risk of VCI and VaD. Cross-sectional studies cannot determine whether the observed association preceded or followed the onset of cognitive impairment. Further, epidemiologic studies cannot prove causality.

Genetic Factors

The apolipoprotein E ε4 (APOE-ε4) allele has been associated with an increased risk of all-cause dementia and VaD in some, but not all, studies. There are several other candidate genes, such as *MTHFR* and *VLDLR*, and recent genome-wide association studies have identified a locus on Chromosome X (near the androgen receptor gene) that was associated with VaD.[117] Specific genes have been identified through genome-wide association studies as being related to the risk of overt and covert brain infarcts and WMH,[118–120] but the role of these genes in determining the risk of VCI and VaD has not yet been studied.[121,122]

Modifiable Risk Factors

Those for VCI and VaD are listed in Box 17-1. These are based on findings from observational studies and, so far, clinical trials have not shown that modifying these reliably reduces the risk of VCI and VaD.

Lifestyle Factors

The following demographic and lifestyle factors affect the risk of VCI:

Lower **education** has been associated with an increased risk for VaD. However, cognitive test performance is generally better in persons with greater education. The concept of cognitive reserve (CR) in VCI is largely unstudied. One recent two-center study analyzed a cohort of CADASIL as a model of "pure" VCI and found that education had an independent impact in mild-to-moderate vascular pathology, whereas there was no influence of education on cognition in patients with

BOX 17-1 Modifiable Risk Factors for Vascular Cognitive Impairment and Vascular Dementia

Hypertension	Low education level
Insulin resistance	Diet
Diabetes mellitus	Sedentary lifestyle
Hyperlipidemia	Low vitamin D level
The metabolic syndrome	High homocysteine level
Alcohol intake	Systemic inflammatory markers
Smoking	

severe pathology.[123] Also, poor educational status may reflect lower socioeconomic status that is additionally associated with a less healthy lifestyle.

Several **dietary** factors have been associated with a lower risk of dementia in general, although few studies have specifically addressed the risk of VaD. These studies are difficult to perform because diet assessments are subject to recall bias and because dietary patterns rather than intake of individual items may be important.

Antioxidants (including vitamins E, C, and beta carotene, fruits, and vegetables) have been associated with a lower risk of cognitive impairment in some studies, but an interventional study showed no benefit.[124–126] A recent review of 14 studies evaluating the relationship between nutrition and VaD concluded that the best evidence of protective effect exists for oral micronutrient supplementation, however more research is needed.[127]

Intake of **n-3 polyunsaturated fatty acids (PUFAs)** found in fish oils and weekly intake of **fish** have been associated with better cognitive function and a lower risk of cognitive decline and dementia in most, but not all studies.[128,129] This is also true of circulating and red blood cell membrane levels of PUFAs.[130,131] PUFAs may be beneficial through their antioxidant and anti-inflammatory properties, but their levels as components of membrane phospholipids could also directly impact neuronal function. A 2012 Cochrane review found that there was no cognitive benefit in patients over the age of 60.[132] Though early randomized trials of fish oil did not show a benefit, larger trials are ongoing.[133]

Vitamin D deficiency is an emerging factor in increasing the risk of cardiovascular disease and stroke. Several studies have described an association of lower circulating vitamin D levels with poorer cognitive function, but there have been no randomized trials assessing the effect of vitamin D supplementation on cognitive decline.[134–137]

Homocysteine elevation is a risk factor for vascular damage.[138] Cross-sectional and longitudinal studies consistently show that rising levels of plasma total homocysteine (tHcy) are associated with poorer performance in global as well as multiple cognitive domains.[139–145] Elevated plasma tHcy values have also been associated with MRI evidence of CVBI and smaller brain volumes, suggesting that some of this cognitive decline is mediated through vascular pathways.[146–148] Folic acid and vitamins B_{12} and B_6 are key components of the pathways leading to the production and metabolism of homocysteine. Results of clinical trials on the impact of vitamin B supplementation on the risk of cognitive decline have been largely disappointing; a large meta-analysis of data from all these trials is ongoing.[149]

Physical activity may be beneficial in preventing strokes and maintaining cognitive function. Long-term regular physical activity has been consistently associated with higher levels of cognitive function and a lower risk of VCI and VaD.[150–153] There are few data on the type and frequency of physical activity required, although the American Heart Association recommends 30 minutes of moderate-intensity aerobic exercise at least five times a week and moderate to high muscle strength training two times a week. These benefits might accrue through improvements in vascular risk factor profiles (improved blood pressure [BP], weight, and insulin sensitivity), decreased inflammation, and increased levels of neurotrophic factors such as brain-derived neurotrophic factor (BDNF).[154,155] Several clinical trials of exercise intervention on cognitive function (as a primary or secondary outcome) are ongoing (http://www.clinicaltrials.gov).[152,156,157]

Although heavy drinking has been associated with smaller brain volumes and an increased risk of cognitive decline, moderate **alcohol intake** might be beneficial, perhaps because of an effect of resveratrol.[158–162] A few studies, however, did find that even moderate alcohol intake was associated with smaller brain volumes,[163,164] suggesting that the association needs to be explored in further detail; there may be subgroups (either genetic or based on gender or patterns of alcohol use) that are likely to benefit from mild-to-moderate alcohol intake, whereas others might be at risk of cognitive decline in relation to the same exposures.

Obesity, particularly midlife obesity, has been associated with an increased risk of dementia and separately with an increased risk of stroke.[165–168] Hence it is likely to also be associated with an increased risk of VCI. The association is stronger for central obesity (as assessed by the waist circumference, waist-to-hip ratio, or sagittal abdominal diameter) than for overall body mass index.[169] In the Framingham Offspring Study, waist-to-hip ratio was inversely associated with cognitive function as measured 12 years later; a synergistic interaction with hypertension was noted.[170] Abdominal CT scans showed an association of visceral, but not subcutaneous, fat with total brain volume assessed on MRI.[171] In the Health, Aging and Body Composition study, CT measures of total body fat were associated with global cognitive decline.[172] These associations persisted after adjustment of data for concomitant levels of BP but could be mediated by inflammation, insulin resistance, or lower physical activity or through the action of adipokines such as leptin and adiponectin.[173]

Smoking increases the risk of stroke[116] and atrial fibrillation, accelerates systemic atherosclerosis, and increases systemic inflammation and hence would be expected to raise the risk of VCI. However, nicotine is an agonist at acetylcholine receptors in the hippocampus and hence could also be expected to improve cognition. Although initial case-control studies suggested a possible beneficial effect of smoking on the risk of dementia, this suggestion was likely a bias related to survival.[174] Several prospective studies have shown a higher risk for cognitive decline and VaD in smokers than in nonsmokers.[175–177] Second-hand smoke may also be associated with cognitive decline.[178]

High **blood pressure** (BP), especially levels of systolic, mean, or pulse pressure, has long been recognized as a major modifier of stroke risk.[117] Midlife hypertension ranks as an important modifiable risk factor for late-life cognitive decline and VaD, an association that seems fairly consistent in a majority of observational studies, including cohort studies with follow-up spanning several decades.[179–186] Results of studies on BP measured in late life in relation to dementia are less consistent, most studies finding no association with hypertension or even a higher risk associated with lower systolic BPs.[187–189] This may be due to a parallel decrease in weight and BP in the decade preceding the onset of dementia and the impact of coexisting morbidities such as stroke and cardiovascular disease.

Of the **observational studies** on antihypertensive drugs and the risk of dementia, several longitudinal studies have assessed the impact of antihypertensive drug use on the risk of dementia and observed some benefit.[190] A longer duration of treatment and lower age at onset of treatment were associated with a stronger protective effect. Most studies suggest that it is the BP lowering rather than a particular class of drugs that is helpful. However, two population-based observational studies suggested that diuretics were more helpful than other antihypertensive drugs.[191,192] In a U.S. Veterans Affairs database study, men taking angiotensin receptor blockers (ARBs) were found to have a lower risk of dementia than those treated with lisinopril, an angiotensin-converting enzyme (ACE) inhibitor, and with other cardiovascular drugs.[193] These findings could represent bias by indication.

To date, nine large randomized **clinical trials** of antihypertensive medication have also assessed cognitive function; of these, only one suggested a tenuous benefit of treatment. The "negative" studies include: (1) the Systolic Hypertension in the Elderly Program (SHEP), which compared treatment with a diuretic and/or β-blocker to treatment with placebo;[194,195] (2) the Study on Cognition and Prognosis in the Elderly (SCOPE), which compared a combination of an angiotensin receptor blocker and a diuretic with usual treatment;[196] (3) the Perindopril Protection Against Recurrent Stroke Study (PROGRESS) trial, wherein patients with a prior stroke or transient ischemic attack (TIA) were randomly assigned to receive either an ACE inhibitor with a diuretic or a placebo (there was a benefit for the combined endpoint of stroke and dementia);[197] (4) the Hypertension in the Very Elderly–Cognitive Assessment (HYVET-COG) study, in which hypertensive persons older than 80 years were treated with slow-release indapamide and either perindopril or placebo;[198] (5) the Action in Diabetes and Vascular Disease: Preterax and Diamicron-MR Controlled Evaluation (ADVANCE) in which blood pressure lowering with perindopril/indapamide combination and a secondary outcome of dementia was examined;[199] (6) the Prevention Regimen for Effectively Avoiding Second Strokes trial (PRoFESS) wherein persons with recent ischemic stroke were treated with telmisartan;[200] (7) the Telmisartan Randomized Assessment Study in ACE Intolerant Subjects with Cardiovascular Disease (TRANSCEND) in which ramipril, telmisartan or a combination thereof was examined,[201] and (8) the Memory in Diabetes (MIND) substudy of the Action to Control Cardiovascular Risk in Diabetes (ACCORD) trial, which looked at intensive blood pressure control (systolic blood pressure <120 mmHg) among diabetics.[202] The only study that did suggest a benefit of BP lowering on dementia risk was the Systolic Hypertension in Europe (Syst-Eur) trial comparing nitrendipine treatment with placebo.[203] Other studies are ongoing. There is incontrovertible evidence that lowering BP prevents stroke and that initial and subsequent strokes increase the risk of VaD, whereas there is no compelling evidence that lowering BP increases the risk of dementia; hence antihypertensive treatment does appear to be indicated in persons with cognitive impairment if financial and logistic considerations permit its safe administration.

Hyperglycemia, insulin resistance, metabolic syndrome, and diabetes: Insulin resistance and hyperglycemia can lead to vascular and neuronal damage by promoting atherosclerosis and stroke, by directly promoting AD pathology, oxidative stress, and inflammation, and through other mechanisms. It may also, through an additive or synergistic effect with AD-related cognitive decline or through an ascertainment bias consequent to more frequent medical care, lead to earlier diagnosis. Diabetes itself and its component states of chronic hyperglycemia, insulin resistance, hyperinsulinemia, and the metabolic syndrome have each been associated with poorer cognitive function,[56,204–208] with cognitive decline in a pattern consistent with VCI,[206, 209–212] as well as with VaD in numerous studies.[213–219] This effect is accentuated by increased systemic inflammation.[220] Patients with a longer duration of diabetes were at highest risk of cognitive decline.

Careful control of hyperglycemia might reduce vascular damage but has not been shown to reduce the risk of stroke, cognitive decline, or VCI or VaD. Moreover there is a suggestion that repeated episodes of hypoglycemia may also cause persistent cognitive impairment, hence the need for caution when attempting aggressive glycemic control.[221] The results of the Action To Control Cardiovascular Risk in Diabetes–Memory in Diabetes (ACCORD-MIND) trial did not show any beneficial effect of tight diabetic control on cognitive function.[222] In the Action in Diabetes and Vascular Disease: Preterax and Diamicron Modified Release Controlled Evaluation (ADVANCE) trial, cognitive function status did not alter the benefit of controlling hypertension in reducing stroke and mortality risk.[223] Overall, the most beneficial intervention to reduce the risk of initial or continuing cognitive decline in persons with type 2 diabetes mellitus may remain the effective control of concomitant vascular risk factors such as hypertension, hypercholesterolemia, and smoking.

Lipids: In several large cohort studies and in the Kaiser Permanente database, midlife measures of total cholesterol predicted later cognitive impairment.[167,224–226] However, late-life or lifetime cumulated measures of serum cholesterol have not been consistently associated with an increased risk of clinical dementia in older cohorts.[227]

Treatment with *statins* has been associated with a lower risk of stroke and, in observational studies, with a lower risk of VCI and of dementia including VaD.[228,229] The Pravastatin in Older Persons at risk for cardiovascular disease (PROSPER) trial found no difference in cognitive decline between the placebo and treatment arms.[230] A recent Cochrane Database Systematic Review concluded that statins have no benefit on a primary outcome of cognitive decline.[231]

Inflammation and markers of endothelial function: Inflammation is a key process linking several cardiovascular risk factors to vascular and neuronal damage. It has been associated with an increased risk of stroke, smaller brain volumes, and an increased risk of dementia.[232,233] Plasma levels and peripheral blood monocyte production of inflammatory proteins, especially interleukin-6 (IL-6), α_1-antichymotrypsin, and C-reactive protein (CRP), were found to be increased prior to the onset of VaD in several studies,[234] and in the Conselice Study of Brain Aging, the combination of high CRP and high IL-6 was associated with a nearly threefold increase in the risk of VaD.[235–244] Plasma levels of asymmetric dimethyl arginine (ADMA), a modulator of endothelial function, have been associated with CBI on MRI and an increased risk of stroke and VCI.[245]

Please see Box 17-1 for a succinct list of modifiable risk factors for VCI and VaD.

Association of Vascular Disease Severity Measures with Vascular Cognitive Impairment

A number of imaging markers indicating the severity of systemic or cerebral *atherosclerosis* (such as coronary calcium, tonometric measures of aortic wall stiffness, carotid stenosis), of systemic *arteriosclerosis* (such as carotid intima-medial thickness [IMT]), and of cumulated exposure to higher BP or other vascular risk factors (such as echocardiographic left ventricular mass) have been associated with poorer cognitive function and a higher risk of VCI and VaD.

The relationship between carotid IMT and cognitive function has been analyzed cross-sectionally and longitudinally in a few studies.[246–249] Overall a significant inverse relationship was observed in each of these studies between carotid IMT and cognitive function – the greater the wall thickness, the poorer the cognitive performance. This relationship was significant after data were controlled for age, education, and, in some studies, concomitant levels of cardiovascular risk factors. It is not clear whether this association is mediated by a parallel impact of vascular risk factors on both the carotid wall and on the brain or it is a direct result of changes in the cerebral circulation secondary to changes in the carotid artery.

Aortic stiffness is best assessed by measuring the carotid-femoral pulse wave velocity (CFPWV) and more crudely by assessing pulse pressure (systolic BP – diastolic BP) or mean arterial pressure. An inverse association between CFPWV and cognitive function has been reported both cross-sectionally (for example, in the Maine-Syracuse study)[250] and longitudinally[251,252] and persists after adjustment of data for age and BP.[249,253] CFPWV has also been associated with WMH volume and smaller brain volumes.[254,255] Echocardiographic left ventricular mass, remodeling, and hypertrophy have been associated with a higher frequency and severity of subclinical brain injury and poorer cognition as well as an increased risk of dementia.[256,257]

Retinal vessels, assessed at fundoscopy or by scanning laser flowmetry, reflect cerebral arterioles, and narrowing of these vessels has been associated with increased arterial stiffness, cerebral small-vessel disease, stroke, and poorer cognitive function.[190,192]

Association of Common Clinical Disease States with Vascular Cognitive Impairment

Coronary Artery Disease

In the Cardiovascular Health Study (CHS)[258] and the Age, Gene/Environment Susceptibility Reykjavik Study,[259] CT coronary artery calcium (CAC), a measure of coronary atherosclerosis severity, was associated with a higher risk of cognitive impairment. There was a simultaneous increased risk of WMHs and CBIs in persons with higher CAC scores, and after adjustment of data for these lesions, cerebral microbleeds and brain volumes attenuated the observed association between CAC and cognition, implicating various vascular mechanisms. Coronary artery disease has also been identified as an independent risk factor for VaD.[260] Coronary artery bypass grafting (CABG) has been associated with poorer initial cognitive function and identified as a marker of late-life dementia risk. However, at 1-, 3-, and 6-year follow-up, the cognitive decline in these patients was no different from that observed in controls with an equivalent burden of CAD who opted for medical treatment or for percutaneous intervention.[261–263]

Chronic Kidney Disease

Severe chronic renal insufficiency has been associated with metabolic (uremic) and hypertensive encephalopathy, accelerated atherosclerosis, hyperhomocysteinemia, and an increased risk of stroke.[264] Data from the Heart Estrogen/Progestin Replacement Study (HERS), the Health Aging and Body Composition (Health ABC) Study, the Third National Health and Nutrition Examination Survey (NHANES III), the Reasons for Geographic and Racial Differences in Stroke (REGARDS) study, and the Maine-Syracuse study suggest that among all persons with severe and moderate CKD (estimated glomerular filtration rate [eGFR] less than 30 and less than 60 mL/min/1.73m^2, respectively) there is a graded continuous increase in the prevalence of cognitive impairment affecting the cognitive domains of attention and learning, memory, orientation, and visuospatial organization.[265–269] The Northern Manhattan Study (NOMAS) extended this observation to persons with mild renal dysfunction (eGFR higher than 60 but lower than 90 mL/min/1.73m^2) using a global measure of cognition, the modified Telephone Interview for Cognitive Status (TICS-m).[270] The Dijon 3C study, however, found no increased risk of cognitive decline or dementia with baseline low eGFR level, though faster decline of eGFR over the first 4-year period was associated with global cognitive decline and dementia with a vascular component.[271] The role of CKD in modifying the risk for clinical dementia is less certain; in the CHS, moderate CKD was related to risk of incident VaD but not to the risk of incident AD.[272] In a recent Japanese cohort study examining incident dementia, moderate-to-severe CKD was associated with VaD, and even mild CKD was associated with AD.[273]

Atrial Fibrillation

Atrial fibrillation, if not treated with adequate anticoagulation, is a strong risk factor for stroke.[116] In several large community-based samples and in a large prospectively studied registry of all persons undergoing cardiac catheterization within a geographic area, atrial fibrillation was found to be an independent risk factor for poorer cognitive performance and risk of VaD,[274–277] even after adjustment of data for associated cardiovascular risk factors and for interim clinical stroke. The mechanism may be through the independent association of atrial fibrillation with subclinical vascular brain injury (WMH and CBI) or hippocampal atrophy.[278,279] However, a few studies did not observe an association of atrial fibrillation with dementia.[280,281] Some of these differences could be related to age (effect being less consistent in older persons), sex (stronger effects were observed in men), and the prevalence and effectiveness of anticoagulation therapy.

Peripheral Arterial Disease

In the Honolulu–Asia Aging Study (HAAS) and the CHS, a low ankle-brachial index, a measure of peripheral arterial disease, was associated with an increased risk of VaD.[282,283]

Heart Failure and Cardiac Output

In case series, persons with clinical heart failure show deficits in attention and executive function and this appears to be an independent correlate of the severity of functional disability in these patients.[284–286] In persons with bradycardia, pacing has been shown to improve cognition in parallel with the observed improvement in cardiac output. In the Framingham Offspring Study it was shown that subclinical variation in cardiac output, insufficient to cause clinical heart failure, is also associated with a lower MRI brain volume and with lower cognitive function.[287] It is possible that this finding represents an early change and that on follow-up, subjects with a lower cardiac output will be at greater risk for clinical dementia, but this issue remains uncertain.

Depression

Depression has been associated with an increased risk of incident stroke and dementia, even after accounting for concomitant levels of vascular risk factors.[288–291] A recent meta-analysis examining 23 community cohort studies concluded that late-life depression does increase the risk of vascular dementia.[292] In addition, depression can impact cognitive performance. The effects may be mediated by poor effort, by residual effects of vascular risk factors, by lifestyle changes associated with depression such as decreased social networking and physical and cognitive activity, by changes in levels of neurotrophic factors, or through other mechanisms.

Thrombosis and Antiplatelets

Fibrinogen and D-dimer levels have been associated with an increased risk of stroke and VaD. Aspirin reduces stroke risk, and some observational studies have suggested an additional beneficial effect of a daily aspirin on cognition. In the Aspirin or Asymptomatic Atherosclerosis (AAA) trial, 3350 participants aged 50–75 years were randomly assigned to receive 100 mg of enteric-coated aspirin or placebo; over a 5-year follow-up, no difference in cognitive abilities was noted between the aspirin and the placebo arms.[293] In the Prevention Regimen for Effectively Avoiding Second Strokes (PRoFESS) trial, more than 20,000 patients with ischemic stroke were randomly assigned in a two-by-two factorial design to receive either 25 mg aspirin and 200 mg extended-release dipyridamole twice a day or 75 mg clopidogrel once a day, and either 80 mg telmisartan or placebo once per day, to assess effectiveness in preventing a second stroke. Cognitive decline was assessed as a secondary endpoint. After a median follow-up of 2.4 years, no difference was observed between the two antiplatelet regimens as to change in MMSE scores.[294]

TREATMENT OF PERSONS WITH CLINICAL VASCULAR DEMENTIA

Management of vascular risks and symptomatic pharmacotherapy targeting VaD has been the primary approach to treat patients with VaD.[295] Standardized screening and monitoring to document baseline status, disease trajectory, and treatment response are essential. This should be supplemented with a detailed medical history and assessment of social and daily functioning, and as appropriate with additional blood tests and vascular and brain imaging. Also, factors that exacerbate clinical disease manifestations (e.g., sleep disorders, pain, stress) should be addressed. Cognitive and behavioral interventions for the patient, social support, respite care, and caregiver support are as important for VaD as they are for AD, because these measures are critical to ensure optimal quality of life for patients and caregivers.

CONTROL OF VASCULAR RISK FACTORS

Currently, in the absence of definitive data or guidelines, clinicians should ideally use screening tools to detect cognitive impairment in persons with higher levels of vascular risk factors and in those who have had one or more strokes. The vascular risks should be treated according to nationally accepted guidelines for prevention of stroke and cardiac events.[296] There is some evidence that calcium channel blockers which cross the blood–brain barrier, for example nimodipine, may provide modest benefit in slowing cognitive decline in addition to their role in reducing blood pressure, although a study dedicated to this subject failed to reach its primary endpoint.[297] In individual patients, distinguishing the relative contributions of vascular and AD pathology to the observed cognitive deficits is difficult. It is advisable to accurately assess and record baseline cognitive function across multiple domains, detect and address all vascular risk factors, and monitor rate of decline, again in a global as well as domain-specific manner. Prevention of additional strokes is the most effective intervention to reduce risk and rate of cognitive decline.

PHARMACOLOGIC TREATMENT OF COGNITIVE IMPAIRMENT

There is pathologic and clinical evidence of cholinergic compromise in VCI as there is in AD, and double-blind, placebo-controlled, randomized clinical trials have tested the efficacy of cholinesterase inhibitors in improving cognitive, global, and daily functioning in patients with VaD, including the subgroup with VCI due to CADASIL.[298,299] Overall, the studies showed some benefit, particularly in tests of executive function, but a later meta-analysis concluded that the results were insufficient to recommend the routine use of these drugs in VCI.[300] Vascular dementia has not been approved by the U.S. Food and Drug Administration (FDA) as an indication for the use of these drugs. The presence of concomitant VaD need not, however, exclude a patient with AD from receiving a trial of these medications, unless there is a cardiac contraindication to their use, such as bradycardia or hypotension.

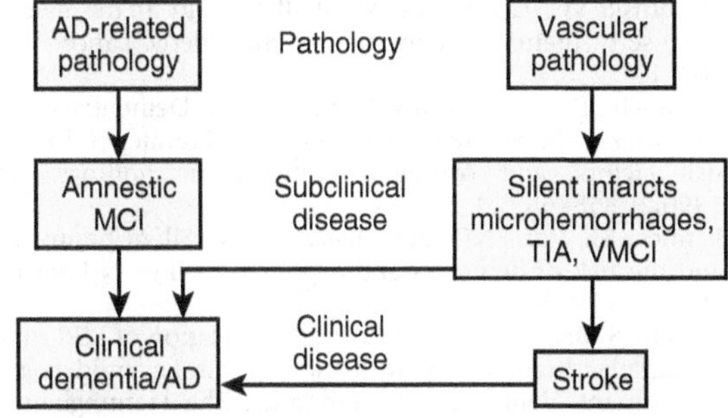

Figure 17-3. Markers of vascular brain injury related to vascular cognitive impairment.

Similarly studies of memantine, an *N*-methyl-D-aspartate (NMDA) antagonist, showed minimal cognitive improvement in a few domains insufficient to effect any functional benefit. Trials of other putative disease-modifying agents, such as gingko, piracetam, and huperzine A, have shown no benefit. Symptomatic treatment of apathy with selective serotonergic agents is based on anecdotal reports but has not been validated by clinical trials. Assessment and management of behavioral problems in patients are similar to those described for patients with AD.[300]

SUMMARY

Vascular risk factors contribute to the cognitive impairment and dementia that are common among older adults. A broad concept of VCI is currently used to describe the whole range of cognitive impairment that may be associated with various forms of CVBI, ranging from clinical VaD to mild cognitive difficulties that are evident only on cognitive testing, to VaMCI. Determining the contribution of vascular disease to an observed syndrome of cognitive impairment or dementia can be difficult and is greatly facilitated by sensitive neuroimaging studies such as MRI, which can show WMH and CBI. The neuropathology of cognitive impairment in later life is often a mixture of AD and vascular pathology, which may overlap and synergize to heighten risk of cognitive impairment (Fig. 17-3). Risk markers for VCI are largely the same as traditional risk factors for stroke. These risks include, but are not limited to, atrial fibrillation, hypertension, and diabetes. Currently, no specific treatments for VCI have been approved by the FDA. Neurobehavioral and psychiatric symptoms that may be common are treated by the usual drugs and supportive strategies. Finally, standard stroke preventive measures are recommended for most patients with VCI. There is a need for further prospective studies integrating genetic, risk factor, quantitative clinical, and neuroimaging and pathologic data to improve our understanding of the clinical syndromes of VCI and VaD.

The complete reference list can be found on the companion Expert Consult website at www.expertconsult.inkling.com.

KEY REFERENCES

4. Whitmer RA, Sidney S, Selby J, et al. Midlife cardiovascular risk factors and risk of dementia in late life. Neurology 2005;64:277–81.
5. Kuller LH, Ives DG, Lopez OL, et al. Incidence and prevalence of dementia in the Cardiovascular Health Study. J Am Geriatr Soc 2004;52:195–204.
6. Gorelick PB. AHA/ASA Scientific Statement Vascular Contributions to Cognitive Impairment and Dementia. Stroke 2011;42:2672–713.

9. Hachinski VC, Lassen NA, Marshall J. Multi-infarct dementia. A cause of mental deterioration in the elderly. Lancet 1974;2: 207–10.
10. Tatemichi TK, Foulkes MA, Mohr JP, et al. Dementia in stroke survivors in the Stroke Data Bank cohort. Prevalence, incidence, risk factors, and computed tomographic findings. Stroke 1990;21:858–66.
11. Vermeer SE, Prins ND, den Heijer T, et al. Silent brain infarcts and the risk of dementia and cognitive decline. N Engl J Med 2003;348:1215–22.
12. Debette S, Beiser A, Decarli C, et al. Association of MRI markers of vascular brain injury with incident stroke, mild cognitive impairment, dementia, and mortality: The Framingham Offspring Study Stroke. Stroke 2010;41:600–6.
13. Petersen RC, Smith GE, Waring SC, et al. Mild cognitive impairment: Clinical characterization and outcome. Arch Neurol 1999; 56:303–8.
14. Farooq MU, Gorelick PB. Vascular cognitive impairment. Curr Atheroscler Rep 2013;15:330.
15. Pendlebury ST, Rothwell PM. Prevalence, incidence, and factors associated with pre-stroke and post-stroke dementia: a systematic review and meta-analysis. Lancet Neurol 2009;8:1006–18.
16. Roman GC, Tatemichi TK, Erkinjuntti T, et al. Vascular dementia: diagnostic criteria for research studies. Report of the NINDS-AIREN International Workshop. Neurology 1993;43:250–60.
17. Chui HC, Victoroff JI, Margolin D. Criteria for the diagnosis of ischemic vascular dementia proposed by the State of California Alzheimer's Disease Diagnostic and Treatment Centers. Neurology 1992;42:473–80.
18. Wetterling T, Kanitz RD, Borgis KJ. The ICD-10 criteria for vascular dementia. Dementia 1994;5:185–8.
19. American Psychiatric Association. Diagnostic and statistical manual of mental disorders (DSM-IV). Washington, DC: American Psychiatric Association; 1994.
20. Sachdev P, Kalaria R, O'Brien J, et al. Diagnostic criteria for vascular cognitive disorder: a VASCOG statement. Alzheimer Dis Assoc Disord 2014;28(3):206–18.
21. Pohjasvaara T, Mantyla R, Ylikoski R. Comparison of different clinical criteria (DSM-III, ADDTC, ICD-10, NINDS-AIREN, DSM-IV) for the diagnosis of vascular dementia. National Institute of Neurological Disorders and Stroke-Association Internationale pour la Recherche et l'Enseignement en Neurosciences. Stroke 2000;31:2952–7.
22. Gold G, Bouras C, Canuto A, et al. Clinicopathological validation study of four sets of clinical criteria for vascular dementia. Am J Psychiatry 2002;159:82–7.
23. Erkinjuntti T. Vascular dementia: Challenge of clinical diagnosis. Int Psychogeriatr 1997;9(Suppl. 1):51–8.
24. Ivan CS, Seshadri S, Beiser A, et al. Dementia after stroke: The Framingham Study. Stroke 2004;35:1264–8.
25. Kokmen E, Whisnant JP, O'Fallon WM. Dementia after ischemic stroke: A population-based study in Rochester, Minnesota (1960–1984). Neurology 1996;46:154–9.
26. Henon H, Pasquier F, Durieu I. Medial temporal lobe atrophy in stroke patients: Relation to pre-existing dementia. J Neurol Neurosurg Psychiatry 1998;65:641–7.
27. Henon H, Durieu I, Guerouaou D. Poststroke dementia: Incidence and relationship to prestroke cognitive decline. Neurology 2001;57:1216–22.
29. Tatemichi TK, Desmond DW, Mayeux R, et al. Dementia after stroke: Baseline frequency, risks, and clinical features in a hospitalized cohort. Neurology 1992;42:1185–93.
30. Jacoba C, Pearce LA, Costello R, et al. Cognitive impairment in lacunar strokes: The SPS3 Trial. Ann Neurol 2012;72:351–62.
31. Wollenweber FA. The determinants of dementia after stroke study: protocol and pilot data. Int J Stroke 2014;9(3):387–92.
32. Hachinski V, Iadecola C, Petersen RC, et al. National Institute of Neurological Disorders and Stroke-Canadian Stroke Network vascular cognitive impairment harmonization standards. Stroke 2006;37:2220–41.
33. Roman GC. Senile dementia of the Binswanger type. A vascular form of dementia in the elderly. JAMA 1987;258:1782–8.
34. Mathers SE, Chambers BR, Merory JR, et al. Subcortical arteriosclerotic encephalopathy: Binswanger's disease. Clin Exp Neurol 1987;23:67–70.
35. Human BT, Van Hoesen GW, Damasio AR. Memory-related neural systems in Alzheimer's disease: an anatomic study. Neurology 1990;40:1721–30.
36. Chui HC, Victoroff JI, Margolin D. Criteria for the diagnosis of ischemic vascular dementia proposed by the State of California Alzheimer's Disease Diagnostic and Treatment Centers. Neurology 1992;42:473–80.
38. Roman GC, Tatemichi TK, Erkinjuntti T, et al. Vascular dementia: diagnostic criteria for research studies. Report of the NINDS-AIREN International Workshop. Neurology 1993;43:250–60.
39. Kazee AM, Eskin TA, Lapham LW, et al. Clinicopathologic correlates in Alzheimer disease: assessment of clinical and pathologic diagnostic criteria. Alzheimer Dis Assoc Disord 1993;3(3): 152–64.
40. Dubois B, Feldman HH, Jacoba C, et al. Research criteria for the diagnosis of Alzheimer's disease: revising the NINCDS-ADRDA criteria. Lancet Neurol 2007;6(8):734–46.
41. Zekry D, Duyckaerts C, Belmin J, et al. Alzheimer's disease and brain infarcts in the elderly: agreement with neuropathology. J Neurol 2002;249:1529–34.
42. Moroney JT, Bagiella E, Desmond DW, et al. Meta-analysis of the Hachinski Ischemic Score in pathologically verified dementias. Neurology 1997;49(4):1095–105.
43. White L, Small BJ, Petrovitch H, et al. Recent clinical-pathologic research on the causes of dementia in late life: update from the Honolulu-Asia Aging Study. J Geriatr Psychiatry Neurol 2005; 18(4):224–7.
45. Arvanitakis Z, Leurgans SE, Barnes LL, et al. Microinfarct pathology, dementia, and cognitive systems. Stroke 2011;42: 722–7.
46. Brayne C, Richardson K, Matthews FE, et al. Neuropathological correlates of dementia in over-80-year-old brain donors from the population-based Cambridge city over-75s cohort (CC75C) study. J Alzheimers Dis 2009;18:645–58.
47. Smith EE, Schneider JA, Wardlaw JM, et al. Cerebral microinfarcts: the invisible lesions. Lancet Neurol 2012;11(3):272–82.
48. Iadecola C. The pathobiology of vascular dementia. Neuron 2013;80(4):844–66.
49. Iadecola C, Gorelick PB. Converging pathogenic mechanisms in vascular and neurodegenerative dementia. Stroke 2003;34: 335–7.
51. Fitzpatrick AL, Kuller LH, Ives DG, et al. Incidence and prevalence of dementia in the Cardiovascular Health Study. J Am Geriatr Soc 2004;52:195–204.
53. Schneider JA, Aggarwal NT, Barnes L, et al. The neuropathology of older persons with and without dementia from community versus clinic cohorts. J Alzheimers Dis 2009;18:691–701.
54. Au R, Seshadri S, Wolf PA, et al. New norms for a new generation: cognitive performance in the Framingham Offspring cohort. Exp Aging Res 2004;30:333–58.
55. Decarli C, Massaro J, Harvey D, et al. Measures of brain morphology and infarction in the Framingham Heart Study: Establishing what is normal. Neurobiol Aging 2005;2:491–510.
56. Seshadri S, Wolf PA, Beiser A, et al. Stroke risk profile, brain volume, and cognitive function: The Framingham Offspring Study. Neurology 2004;63:1591–9.
58. Harris TB, Launer LJ, Eiriksdottir G, et al. Age, Gene/Environment Susceptibility-Reykjavik Study: Multidisciplinary applied phenomics. Am J Epidemiol 2007;165:1076–87.
59. Hofman A, Breteler MM, van Duijn CM, et al. The Rotterdam Study: Objectives and design update. Eur J Epidemiol 2007;22: 819–29.
60. White L, Petrovitch H, Hardman J, et al. Cerebrovascular pathology and dementia in autopsied Honolulu-Asia Aging Study participants. Ann N Y Acad Sci 2002;977:9–23.
61. Lorius N, Locascio JJ, REntz DM, et al. Vascular disease and risk factors are associated with cognitive decline in the Alzheimer disease spectrum. Alzheimer Dis Assoc Disord 2014;[epub ahead of date].
62. Dux MC, Kowalewski G, Zhao L, et al. Asymptomatic carotid stenosis is associated with cognitive dysfunction. AAN 66th Annual Meeting Abstract, April 2014.
64. Lopez OL, Kuller LH, Becker JT, et al. Classification of vascular dementia in the Cardiovascular Health Study Cognition Study. Neurology 2005;64:1539–47.

65. Kase CS, Wolf PA, Kelly-Hayes M. Intellectual decline after stroke: The Framingham Study. Stroke 1998;29:805–12.
69. Petersen RC, Stevens JC, Ganguli M. Practice parameter: early detection of dementia: Mild cognitive impairment (an evidence-based review). Report of the Quality Standards Subcommittee of the American Academy of Neurology. Neurology 2001;56: 1133–42.
70. Winblad B, Palmer K, Kivipelto M, et al. Mild cognitive impairment—beyond controversies, towards a consensus: Report of the International Working Group on Mild Cognitive Impairment. J Intern Med 2004;256:240–6.
73. Maioli F, Coveri M, Pagni P, et al. Conversion of mild cognitive impairment to dementia in elderly subjects: A preliminary study in a memory and cognitive disorder unit. Arch Gerontol Geriatr 2007;44(Suppl. 1):233–41.
74. O'Brien JT, Erkinjuntti T, Reisberg B, et al. Vascular cognitive impairment. Lancet Neurol 2003;2:89–98.
76. Reed BR, Mungas DM, Kramer JH, et al. Profiles of neuropsychological impairment in autopsy-defined Alzheimer's disease and cerebrovascular disease. Brain 2007;130:731–9.
80. Massaro JM, D'Agostino RB Sr, Sullivan LM, et al. Managing and analysing data from a large-scale study on Framingham Offspring relating brain structure to cognitive function. Stat Med 2004;23:351–67.
81. Maillard P, Seshadri S, Beiser A, et al. Effects of systolic blood pressure on white-matter integrity in young adults in the Framingham Heart Study: a cross-sectional study. Lancet Neurol 2012;11:1039–47.
83. Lee JH, Kim SH, Kim GH, et al. Identification of pure subcortical vascular dementia using 11C-Pittsburgh compound B. Neurology 2011;77:18–25.
85. Vernooij MW, Ikram MA, Vrooman HA, et al. White matter microstructural integrity and cognitive function in a general elderly population. Arch Gen Psychiatry 2009;66:545–53.
86. Manolio TA, Kronmal RA, Burke GL, et al. Magnetic resonance abnormalities and cardiovascular disease in older adults. The Cardiovascular Health Study. Stroke 1994;25:318–27.
87. Scheltens P, Erkinjuntti T, Leys D, et al. White matter changes on CT and MRI: an overview of visual rating scales. European Task Force on Age-Related White Matter Changes. Eur Neurol 1998; 39:80–9.
91. Au R, Massaro JM, Wolf PA, et al. Association of white matter hyperintensity volume with decreased cognitive functioning: The Framingham Heart Study. Arch Neurol 2006;63: 246–50.
96. Debette S, Beiser A, Decarli C, et al. Association of MRI markers of vascular brain injury with incident stroke, mild cognitive impairment, dementia, and mortality. The Framingham Offspring Study. Stroke 2010;41:600–6.
98. Mosley TH Jr, Knopman DS, Catellier DJ, et al. Cerebral MRI findings and cognitive functioning: The Atherosclerosis Risk in Communities study. Neurology 2005;64:2056–62.
99. Prins ND, van Dijk EJ, den Heijer T, et al. Cerebral small-vessel disease and decline in information processing speed, executive function and memory. Brain 2005;128:2034–41.
102. Brickman AM, Provenzano FA, Muraskin J, et al. Regional white matter hyperintensity volume, not hippocampal atrophy, predicts incident Alzheimer disease in the community. Arch Neurol 2012;69(12):1621–7.
104. Kalaria RN, Kenny RA, Ballard CG. Towards defining the neuropathological substrates of vascular dementia. J Neurol Sci 2004;226:75–80.
105. Esiri MM, Wilcock GK, Morris JH. Neuropathological assessment of the lesions of significance in vascular dementia. J Neurol Neurosurg Psychiatry 1997;63:749–53.
108. Savva GM, Wharton SB, Ince PG. Age, neuropathology, and dementia. N Engl J Med 2009;360:2302–9.
109. Schneider JA, Arvanitakis Z, Bang W, et al. Mixed brain pathologies account for most dementia cases in community-dwelling older persons. Neurology 2007;69:2197–204.
110. Schneider JA, Aggarwal NT, Barnes L. The neuropathology of older persons with and without dementia from community versus clinic cohorts. J Alzheimers Dis 2009;18:691–701.
113. Greenberg SM. Cerebral amyloid angiopathy: Prospects for clinical diagnosis and treatment. Neurology 1998;51:690–4.
115. Sadowski M, Pankiewicz J, Scholtzova H, et al. Links between the pathology of Alzheimer's disease and vascular dementia. Neurochem Res 2004;29:1257–66.
117. Schrijvers EM, Schurmann B, Koudstaal PJ, et al. Genome-wide association study of vascular dementia. Stroke 2012;43: 315–19.
118. Schmidt H, Zeginigg M, Wiltgen M, et al. Genetic variants of the NOTCH3 gene in the elderly and magnetic resonance imaging correlates of age-related cerebral small vessel disease. Brain 2011;134:3384–97.
119. Fornage M, Debette S, Bis JC, et al. Genome-wide association studies of cerebral white matter lesion burden: the CHARGE consortium. Ann Neurol 2011;69:928–39.
120. Debette S, Bis JC, Fornage M, et al. Genome-wide association studies of MRI-defined brain infarcts: meta-analysis from the CHARGE Consortium. Stroke 2010;41:210–17.
121. Ikram MA, Seshadri S, Bis JC, et al. Genome wide association studies of stroke. N Engl J Med 2009;360:1718–28.
124. Morris MC, Evans DA, Tangney CC. Associations of vegetable and fruit consumption with age-related cognitive change. Neurology 2006;67:1370–6.
127. Perez L, Heim L, Sherzai A, et al. Nutrition and vascular dementia. J Nutr Health Aging 2012;16:319–24.
131. Schaefer EJ, Bongard V, Beiser AS, et al. Plasma phosphatidylcholine docosahexaenoic acid content and risk of dementia and Alzheimer disease: The Framingham Heart Study. Arch Neurol 2006;63:1545–50.
132. Sydenham E, Dangour AD, Lim WS. Omega 3 fatty acid for the prevention of cognitive decline and dementia. Cochrane Database Syst Rev Published June 2012.
133. van de Rest O, Geleijnse JM, Kok FJ, et al. Effect of fish oil on cognitive performance in older subjects: A randomized, controlled trial. Neurology 2008;71:430–8.
135. Llewellyn DJ, Langa KM, Lang IA. Serum 25-hydroxyvitamin D concentration and cognitive impairment. J Geriatr Psychiatry Neurol 2009;22:188–95.
137. Annweiler C, Schott AM, Allali G, et al. Association of vitamin D deficiency with cognitive impairment in older women: Cross-sectional study. Neurology 2010;74:27–32.
139. Wright CB, Lee HS, Paik MC. Total homocysteine and cognition in a tri-ethnic cohort: The Northern Manhattan Study. Neurology 2004;63:254–60.
140. Miller JW, Green R, Ramos MI, et al. Homocysteine and cognitive function in the Sacramento Area Latino Study on Aging. Am J Clin Nutr 2003;78:441–7.
141. Elias MF, Sullivan LM, D'Agostino RB, et al. Homocysteine and cognitive performance in the Framingham offspring study: Age is important. Am J Epidemiol 2005;162:644–53.
142. Prins ND, den Heijer T, Hofman A, et al. Homocysteine and cognitive function in the elderly—The Rotterdam Scan Study. Neurology 2002;59:1375–80.
145. Seshadri S, Beiser A, Selhub J, et al. Plasma homocysteine as a risk factor for dementia and Alzheimer's disease. N Engl J Med 2002;346:476–83.
149. Hankey GJ, Ford AH, Yi Q, et al. Effect of B vitamins and lowering homocysteine on cognitive impairment in patients with previous stroke or transient ischemic attack: a prespecified secondary analysis of a randomized, placebo-controlled trial and meta-analysis. Stroke 2013;44(8):2232–9.
150. Larson EB, Wang L, Bowen JD, et al. Exercise is associated with reduced risk for incident dementia among persons 65 years of age and older. Ann Intern Med 2006;144:73–81.
151. Scarmeas N, Luchsinger JA, Schupf N, et al. Physical activity, diet, and risk of Alzheimer disease. JAMA 2009;302:627–37.
153. Verghese J, Lipton RB, Katz MJ, et al. Leisure activities and the risk of dementia in the elderly. N Engl J Med 2003;348: 2508–16.
156. Etgen T, Sander D, Huntgeburth U. Physical activity and incident cognitive impairment in elderly persons: The INVADE study. Arch Intern Med 2010;170:186–93.
157. Liu-Ambrose T, Eng JJ, Boyd LA, et al. Promotion of the mind through exercise (PROMoTE): A proof-of-concept randomized controlled trial of aerobic exercise training in older adults with vascular cognitive impairment. BMC Neurol 2010; 10:14.

159. Ganguli M, Vander BJ, Saxton JA. Alcohol consumption and cognitive function in late life: A longitudinal community study. Neurology 2005;65:1210–17.
160. Elias PK, Elias MF, D'Agostino RB. Alcohol consumption and cognitive performance in the Framingham Heart Study. Am J Epidemiol 1999;150:580–9.
162. Takahashi PY, Caldwell CR, Targonski PV. Effect of alcohol and tobacco use on vascular dementia: a matched case control study. Vasc Health Risk Manag 2011;7:685–91.
167. Kivipelto M, Ngandu T, Fratiglioni L, et al. Obesity and vascular risk factors at midlife and the risk of dementia and Alzheimer disease. Arch Neurol 2005;62:1556–60.
168. Whitmer RA, Gunderson EP, Quesenberry CP Jr. Body mass index in midlife and risk of Alzheimer disease and vascular dementia. Curr Alzheimer Res 2007;4:103–9.
169. Whitmer RA, Gustafson DR, Barrett-Connor E. Central obesity and increased risk of dementia more than three decades later. Neurology 2008;71:1057–64.
172. Kanaya AM, Lindquist K, Harris TB, et al. Total and regional adiposity and cognitive change in older adults: The Health, Aging and Body Composition (ABC) study. Arch Neurol 2009;66: 329–35.
173. Lieb W, Beiser AS, Vasan RS, et al. Association of plasma leptin levels with incident Alzheimer disease and MRI measures of brain aging. JAMA 2009;302:2565–72.
176. Ott A, Slooter AJ, Hofman A, et al. Smoking and risk of dementia and Alzheimer's disease in a population-based cohort study: The Rotterdam Study. Lancet 1998;351(9119):1840–3.
179. Elias MF, Wolf PA, D'Agostino RB. Untreated blood pressure level is inversely related to cognitive functioning: The Framingham Study. Am J Epidemiol 1993;138:353–64.
180. Kivipelto M, Helkala EL, Hanninen T, et al. Midlife vascular risk factors and late-life mild cognitive impairment: A population-based study. Neurology 2001;56:1683–9.
181. Launer LJ, Masaki K, Petrovitch H. The association between midlife blood pressure levels and late-life cognitive function. The Honolulu-Asia Aging Study. JAMA 1995;274:1846–51.
182. Petrovitch H, White LR, Izmirilian G, et al. Midlife blood pressure and neuritic plaques, neurofibrillary tangles, and brain weight at death: The HAAS. Honolulu-Asia Aging Study. Neurobiol Aging 2000;2:57–62.
185. Launer LJ, Hughes T, Yu B, et al. Lowering midlife levels of systolic blood pressure as a public health strategy to reduce late-life dementia: Perspective from the Honolulu Heart Program/ Honolulu Asia Aging Study. Hypertension 2010;55:1352–9.
186. Muller M, Sigurdsson S, Kjartansson O, et al. Joint effect of mid- and late-life blood pressure on the brain: The AGES-Reykjavik Study. Neurology 2014;82(24):2187–95.
187. Skoog I, Lernfelt B, Landahl S, et al. 15-year longitudinal study of blood pressure and dementia. Lancet 1996;347(9009): 1141–5.
190. in't Veld BA, Ruitenberg A, Hofman A. Antihypertensive drugs and incidence of dementia: The Rotterdam Study. Neurobiol Aging 2001;22:407–12.
194. Di Bari BM, Pahor M, Franse LV, et al. Dementia and disability outcomes in large hypertension trials: Lessons learned from the Systolic Hypertension in the Elderly Program (SHEP) trial. Am J Epidemiol 2001;153:72–8.
195. Prevention of stroke by antihypertensive drug treatment in older persons with isolated systolic hypertension: Final results of the Systolic Hypertension in the Elderly Program (SHEP). SHEP Cooperative Research Group. JAMA 1991;265:3255–64.
196. Lithell H, Hansson L, Skoog I, et al. The Study on Cognition and Prognosis in the Elderly (SCOPE): principal results of a randomized double-blind intervention trial. J Hypertens 2003;21: 875–86.
197. Tzourio C, Anderson C. Blood pressure reduction and risk of dementia in patients with stroke: rationale of the dementia assessment in PROGRESS (Perindopril Protection Against Recurrent Stroke Study). PROGRESS Management Committee. J Hypertens Suppl 2000;18:S21–4.
198. Peters R, Beckett N, Forette F, et al. Incident dementia and blood pressure lowering in the Hypertension in the Very Elderly Trial Cognitive Function Assessment (HYVET-COG): A double-blind, placebo controlled trial. Lancet Neurol 2008;7:683–9.
199. ADVANCE Collaborative Group. Effects of a fixed combination of perindopril and indapamide on macrovascular and microvascular outcomes in patients with type 2 diabetes mellitus (the ADVANCE trial): a randomised controlled trial. Lancet 2007;370: 829–40.
200. Yusuf S, Diener HC, Sacco RL, PRoFESS Study Group, et al. Telmisartan to prevent recurrent stroke and cardiovascular events. N Engl J Med 2008;359:1225–37.
201. Anderson C, Teo K, Gao P, for the ONTARGET and TRANCEND Investigators, et al. Renin-angiotensin system blockade and cognitive function in patients at high risk of cardiovascular disease: analysis of data from the ONTARGET and TRANSCEND studies. Lancet Neurol 2010.
202. Williamson JD, Launer LJ, Bryan RN, et al. Cognitive function and brain structure in persons with type 2 diabetes mellitus after intensive lowering of blood pressure and lipid levels – a randomized control trial. JAMA Intern Med 2014; 174(3):324–33.
203. Forette F, Seux ML, Staessen JA, et al. Prevention of dementia in randomised double-blind placebo-controlled Systolic Hypertension in Europe (Syst-Eur) trial. Lancet 1998;352(9137): 1347–51.
213. Hebert R, Lindsay J, Verreault R. Vascular dementia: Incidence and risk factors in the Canadian study of health and aging. Stroke 2000;31:1487–93.
214. Ott A, Stolk RP, Hofman A. Association of diabetes mellitus and dementia: The Rotterdam Study. Diabetologia 1996;39: 1392–7.
217. Hassing LB, Johansson B, Nilsson SE, et al. Diabetes mellitus is a risk factor for vascular dementia, but not for Alzheimer's disease: A population-based study of the oldest old. Int Psychogeriatr 2002;14:239–48.
218. MacKnight C, Rockwood K, Awalt E, et al. Diabetes mellitus and the risk of dementia, Alzheimer's disease and vascular cognitive impairment in the Canadian Study of Health and Aging. Dement Geriatr Cogn Disord 2002;14:77–83.
220. Solfrizzi V, Scafato E, Capurso C, et al. Metabolic syndrome and the risk of vascular dementia: the Italian longitudinal study on ageing. J Neurol Neurosurg Psychiatry 2010;81:433–40.
221. Whitmer RA, Karter AJ, Yaffe K. Hypoglycemic episodes and risk of dementia in older patients with type 2 diabetes mellitus. JAMA 2009;301:1565–72.
222. Cukierman-Yaffe T, Gerstein HC, Williamson JD, et al. Relationship between baseline glycemic control and cognitive function in individuals with type 2 diabetes and other cardiovascular risk factors: The Action to Control Cardiovascular Risk in Diabetes-Memory in Diabetes (ACCORD-MIND) trial. Diabetes Care 2009;32(2):221–6.
223. de Galan BE, Zoungas S, Chalmers J, et al. Cognitive function and risks of cardiovascular disease and hypoglycaemia in patients with type 2 diabetes: The Action in Diabetes and Vascular Disease: Preterax and Diamicron Modified Release Controlled Evaluation (ADVANCE) trial. Diabetologia 2009;52:2328–36.
224. Solomon A, Kivipelto M, Wolozin B. Midlife serum cholesterol and increased risk of Alzheimer's and vascular dementia three decades later. Dement Geriatr Cogn Disord 2009;28:75–80.
228. Jick H, Zornberg GL, Jick SS. Statins and the risk of dementia. Lancet 2000;356(9242):1627–31.
230. Trompet S, van VP, de Craen AJ, et al. Pravastatin and cognitive function in the elderly. Results of the PROSPER study. J Neurol 2010;257:85–90.
231. McGuiness B, Craig D, Bullock R, et al. Statins for the treatment of dementia. Cochrane Database Syst Rev 2014;(7):CD007514.
239. Ravaglia G, Forti P, Maioli F, et al. Blood inflammatory markers and risk of dementia: The Conselice Study of Brain Aging. Neurobiol Aging 2007;28:1810–20.
241. van Dijk EJ, Prins ND, Vermeer SE, et al. C-reactive protein and cerebral small-vessel disease: The Rotterdam Scan Study. Circulation 2005;112:900–5.
251. Scuteri A, Tesauro M, Appolloni S, et al. Arterial stiffness as an independent predictor of longitudinal changes in cognitive function in the older individual. J Hypertens 2007;25:1035–40.
260. Kuller LH, Lopez OL, Jagust WJ, et al. Determinants of vascular dementia in the Cardiovascular Health Cognition Study. Neurology 2005;64:1548–52.

281. Miyasaka Y, Barnes ME, Petersen RC, et al. Risk of dementia in stroke-free patients diagnosed with atrial fibrillation: Data from a community-based cohort. Eur Heart J 2007;28:1962–7.
282. Laurin D, Masaki KH, White LR, et al. Ankle-to-brachial index and dementia: The Honolulu-Asia Aging Study. Circulation 2007;116:2269–74.
283. Newman AB, Fitzpatrick AL, Lopez O, et al. Dementia and Alzheimer's disease incidence in relationship to cardiovascular disease in the Cardiovascular Health Study cohort. J Am Geriatr Soc 2005;53:1101–7.
294. Diener HC, Sacco RL, Yusuf S, et al. Effects of aspirin plus extended-release dipyridamole versus clopidogrel and telmisartan on disability and cognitive function after recurrent stroke in patients with ischaemic stroke in the Prevention Regimen for Effectively Avoiding Second Strokes (PRoFESS) trial: a double-blind, active and placebo-controlled study. Lancet Neurol 2008; 7:875–84.
298. Dichgans M, Markus HS, Salloway S, et al. Donepezil in patients with subcortical vascular cognitive impairment: a randomised double-blind trial in CADASIL. Lancet Neurol 2008;7:310–18.
299. Burns A, O'Brien J, Auriacombe S, et al. Clinical practice with anti-dementia drugs: a consensus statement from British Association for Psychopharmacology. J Psychopharmacol 2006;20: 732–55.
300. Kavirajan H, Schneider LS. Efficacy and adverse effects of cholinesterase inhibitors and memantine in vascular dementia: a meta-analysis of randomised controlled trials. Lancet Neurol 2007;6:782–92.

18 Genetic Basis of Stroke Occurrence, Prevention and Outcome

James F. Meschia, Daniel Woo, David Werring

KEY POINTS

- Fabry disease is an X-linked recessive disorder caused by reduced alpha-galactosidase activity for which enzyme replacement therapy is available.
- CADASIL is a small-vessel stroke disorder caused by mutations in the *NOTCH3* gene.
- CARASIL is a stroke disorder caused by mutations in the *HTRA1* gene.
- Homocysteinemia, commonly due to cystathionine-beta-synthase deficiency, can be treated with restriction in dietary methionine and vitamin B6 supplementation.
- Mitochondrial mutations can lead to a syndrome of encephalopathy, lactic acidosis, and stroke-like episodes known as MELAS.
- In children with sickle cell disease, transcranial Doppler ultrasound can define populations at high risk of stroke and transfusion therapy can dramatically reduce the risk of stroke.
- Mutations in *COL4A1* can cause small-vessel stroke, cerebral hemorrhage, and the HANAC syndrome.
- Several single-gene disorders cause cerebral amyloid angiopathy.
- Several single-gene disorders cause cerebral cavernous malformations.
- Genome-wide association studies have identified risk loci for large-vessel and cardioembolic stroke.

INTRODUCTION

The basic terms and concepts of modern genetic epidemiology, reviewed in this introductory section, provide a framework for the chapter. One of the most important accomplishments of the late 20th century was completion of the Human Genome Project. With the identification of millions of genetic variations comes the possibility of identifying genetic risk associations for numerous complex traits.

A simple trait refers to a disease (or phenotype) that has a Mendelian (i.e., autosomal recessive, autosomal dominant, X-linked recessive, or X-linked dominant) or mitochondrial pattern of inheritance. Typically, a mutation in a single gene is both necessary and sufficient for a Mendelian disorder like Huntington disease to occur. A complex trait, however, refers to a disease (or phenotype) that does not follow a simple pattern of inheritance and is the result of multiple factors, including genes. Stroke, cancer, and many other common diseases are highly complex, with multiple interacting genetic and environmental risk factors. Other features of complex traits include genetic heterogeneity in which different genes lead to the same disease and phenotypic variation in which the same disease gene causes different phenotypes.

The central dogma of genetics is that DNA is transcribed into RNA, which is then translated into proteins. The genome refers to all the genetic information of an organism stored in DNA. Analogously, the transcriptome refers to all the messenger RNA transcribed from DNA; the proteome, to all the expressed proteins. Autosomes (non-sex chromosomes) are characterized by size, from largest (chromosome 1) to smallest (chromosome 22).

At any given location (locus) in the genome, a genotype may refer to the sequences on the paternal and maternal chromosomes. A polymorphism indicates a genetic variation, and the different variations are called alleles. Numerous types of polymorphisms occur, including single base pair changes called single nucleotide polymorphisms (SNPs) as well as insertions, deletions, or translocations of a single base pair or sections of DNA. Other types of polymorphisms include variable numbers of tandem repeats (VNTRs), which refer to consecutive repeats of the same nucleotide sequence. Examples of VNTR polymorphisms are trinucleotide repeats such as those seen in Huntington disease. These are also called *microsatellites.* Although most microsatellites are non-pathogenic, they occur frequently and have multiple alleles. Thus, microsatellites are useful both for forensic identification of individuals and as markers for linkage analysis.

Copy number variations refer to sections of DNA that are copied onto the same section for variable numbers of times. A classic example in neurology occurs at the peripheral myelin protein 22 (*PMP22*) gene, in which the loss of one copy of the gene leads to hereditary neuropathy with liability to pressure palsies; the gain of one copy, Charcot-Marie-Tooth disease. Several hundred thousand copy number variations have been identified in the genome, although their use as markers for disease has not yet been established.

Two classic methods of identifying risk genes are association studies and linkage studies. Association refers to a polymorphism and a particular phenotype occurring together more often than expected by chance alone. Association is not synonymous with causation, however, and a genetic marker may be associated with a disease due to chance, confounding, or linkage, with a causal variant. The major advantages of association studies are the ability to identify risks of small effect, and the ease of collecting cases relative to collecting families.

The other major method for identifying risk genes is through linkage analysis (Fig. 18-1). Mendel's law of independent assortment states that the inheritance pattern of one trait is independent of the inheritance of another. This is true for traits that are on different chromosomes or appreciably separated in physical space on the same chromosome. However, loci that are physically close to one another on the same chromosome will not segregate independently and will instead be inherited together more often than expected by chance.

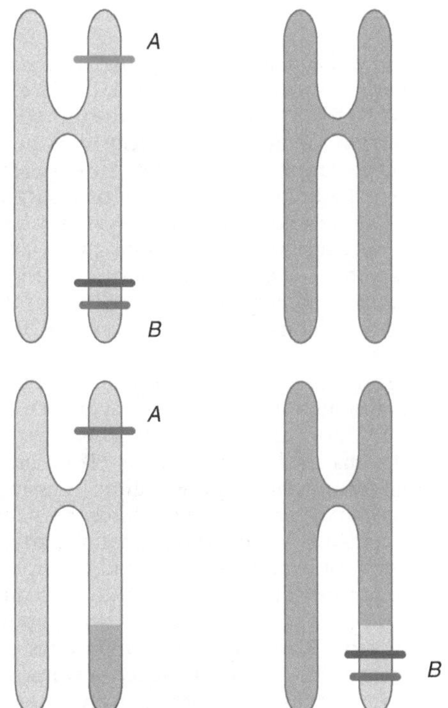

Figure 18-1. Parental chromosomes are shown above, and chromosomes after recombination are shown below. The assumption in this figure is that a stroke mutation occurs on the purple band, but it has not yet been identified. The locations of markers *A* and *B* are known. Because *B* is so much closer to the disease-causing locus than *A*, it will be inherited along with the trait of stroke more often than *A* will. Only a recombination event between *B* and the stroke mutation will lead to the marker not being linked with stroke. A classic example of linkage of traits is hemophilia and color blindness. Neither trait causes the other to occur, but they occur in the same individual more often than expected by chance because the genes responsible for each trait are physically adjacent to one another on the same chromosome. Using this basic phenomenon, one can examine a series of markers across the genome. Even if the marker itself does not lead to disease, if it is close enough to the actual disease-causing gene, it will be inherited more often than expected by chance alone.

EVIDENCE FOR HERITABILITY FOR STROKE AND ITS SUBTYPES

Many lines of evidence support a familial component to stroke risk. A meta-analysis of 53 independent studies found that monozygotic twins were 65% more likely to be concordant for stroke (i.e., both twins having stroke) than dizygotic twins.[1] However, the confidence intervals were broad, and twin studies often failed to differentiate ischemic from hemorrhagic stroke. Case–control studies showed that a positive family history of stroke increased the risk of stroke by 76%. One limitation of case–control studies is that patients with severe strokes may not have survived long enough to be included in the study (survivor bias). Furthermore, patients might have had recall bias in which experiencing a stroke might trigger memories about family members who had a similar affliction (information bias). Finally, there may have been a tendency not to publish negative results (publication bias). Cohort studies have the advantage of not having the same risk of survivor or information biases as case-control studies. It is thus reassuring that cohort studies show that family history of stroke increases the risk of stroke by about 30%.

TABLE 18-1 Physical Examination Findings that are Clues to Inherited Disorders Associated with Cerebrovascular Diseases

System	Disease	Findings
Ophthalmologic findings	MELAS	Bilateral cataracts
	Fabry disease	Whorl-like corneal dystrophy
	RVCL	Retinal vascular malformations
	Homocystinuria	Ectopia lentis, glaucoma
	Moyamoya disease	Morning glory optic disc
Dermatologic	Fabry disease	Angiokeratoma ("swim trunk" distribution)
	Vascular Ehlers–Danlos	Thin translucent skin and excessive bruising
Otologic	MELAS	Progressive bilateral sensorineural hearing loss

RVCL, retinal vasculopathy with cerebral leukodystrophy; MELAS, mitochondrial encephalopathy, lactic acidosis, and stroke-like episodes.

Probands have a nearly linear increased risk of having a sibling history of stroke with age of the proband at the time of stroke from 55 to 80 years.[2] However, family history of stroke seems to be a greater risk factor for stroke in individuals younger than 70 years of age.[1] A positive maternal history of stroke increases the risk in women by nearly 50% relative to a positive paternal history.[3] Whether these observations are attributable to genetic, epigenetic, or non-genetic factors is uncertain.

Inherited risk may differ depending on the type of ischemic stroke. A review of two population-based studies from Oxfordshire and three hospital-based studies found that family history of stroke was least frequent in patients with cardioembolic stroke compared with patients with large- or small-vessel stroke or stroke of unknown etiology.[4] Heritability seemed comparable among non-cardioembolic etiologies of ischemic stroke. Notably, however, comparable rates of family history of conditions like large-vessel stroke and small-vessel stroke give insight into the magnitude of the heritable component to stroke risk, but these rates do not address whether genetic factors for the various types of ischemic stroke might differ qualitatively; that is, different genetic variants might predispose to different types of ischemic stroke.

DISORDERS ASSOCIATED WITH ISCHEMIC OR HEMORRHAGIC STROKE

Several disorders have cerebrovascular disease as a prominent feature. Stroke is common and typically not associated with an obvious genetic disorder. This, combined with the fact that genetic disorders are so diverse, makes the task of precise diagnosis seem daunting. Targeted gene testing should be done after considering the constellation of physical findings (Table 18-1) and considering patterns of inheritance consistent with the findings of a detailed family history (Table 18-2).

Fabry Disease

Fabry disease (Anderson-Fabry disease or angiokeratoma corporis diffusum) is an X-linked recessive disorder caused by reduced activity of the enzyme α-galactosidase. This enzyme is essential to the biodegradation of lipids, and its decreased activity leads to accumulation of lipids in lysosomes in endothelial and vascular smooth muscle cells, where cellular damage may lead to stroke.

TABLE 18-2 Patterns of Inheritance for Diseases or Conditions Associated with Cerebrovascular Diseases

Patterns of Inheritance	Disease/Condition
Autosomal dominant	CADASIL
	RVCL
	Vascular Ehlers–Danlos syndrome
	Cerebral cavernous malformations
	CCM1
	CCM2
	CCM3
	Cerebral amyloid angiopathy
	HCHWA-Dutch type
	HCHWA-Icelandic type
	FAP
	Polycystic kidney disease
	ADPKD 1
	ADPKD 2
Autosomal recessive	Sickle cell disease
	CARASIL
	Homocystinuria
X-linked recessive	Fabry disease
Mitochondrial	MELAS

ADPKD, Autosomal dominant polycystic kidney disease; CADASIL, cerebral autosomal dominant arteriopathy with subcortical infarcts and leukoencephalopathy; CARASIL, cerebral autosomal recessive arteriopathy with subcortical infarcts and leukoencephalopathy; CCM, cerebral cavernous malformation; FAP, familial amyloid polyneuropathy; HCHWA, hereditary cerebral hemorrhage with amyloidosis; MELAS, mitochondrial encephalopathy, lactic acidosis, and stroke-like episodes; RVCL, retinal vasculopathy with cerebral leukodystrophy.

Early in life, patients with Fabry disease may present with burning pain or acroparesthesia due to small-fiber sensory neuropathy, corneal clouding (cornea verticillata), or angiokeratomas. Because peripheral neuropathy typically involves only small fibers, it may be missed on nerve conduction studies and electromyography. Later in life, the major sequelae of Fabry disease are symptoms of stroke, heart disease, and kidney disease from blood vessel ectasia. Grewal[5] reported a stroke prevalence of 24% in patients with cerebrovascular complications, and six of eight patients had strokes occur before 40 years of age.

Although Fabry disease has traditionally been classified as an X-linked recessive disorder in which males showed complete penetrance and women were carriers, the epidemiology of the disease may be more complex than originally thought. Among 721 German adults aged 18 to 55 years with cryptogenic stroke, 4.9% of male patients and, surprisingly, 2.4% of female patients had a biologically significant mutation of the α-galactosidase (*GLA*) gene.[6] Among the male patients with stroke, 38.1% demonstrated the typical dolichoectatic vertebrobasilar vessels. Fewer than half the patients had angiokeratomas, acroparesthesia, or cornea verticillata, which suggests wide phenotypic variation. In a study of 103 young patients with cryptogenic stroke in a Belgian population, only three patients had low α-galactosidase activity, and none was found to have a mutation of the α-galactosidase gene.[7]

Diagnosis of Fabry disease can be made by different methods but is done most commonly by measurement of α-galactosidase activity. In some patients, the α-galactosidase level may be normal, and identification of abnormally low activity of the enzyme is essential to the diagnosis. Two recombinant enzyme preparations have been approved for treatment of Fabry disease: agalsidase alpha and agalsidase beta. Although some benefits accrue from treatment, trials have yet to show that enzyme replacement reduces the risk of stroke.

CADASIL

Cerebral autosomal dominant arteriopathy with subcortical infarcts and leukoencephalopathy (CADASIL) is caused by mutations of the *NOTCH3* receptor gene on chromosome 19. *NOTCH3* expression occurs almost exclusively in smooth muscle cells, and mutations of the receptor lead to accumulation of the protein. Pathologically, granular osmiophilic material accumulates in the smooth muscle of vessels, which leads to smooth muscle degeneration and, ultimately, subcortical leukoencephalopathy. Magnetic resonance imaging (MRI), positron emission tomography, and transcranial Doppler (TCD) studies have demonstrated reduced cerebral blood flow in the white matter.[8–11]

The mean age of onset of symptoms is in the later part of the 4th decade, although the condition may be detectable by MRI years earlier.[12] More than 85% of patients have migraine headaches, and transient ischemic attacks (TIAs) and mood disorders are also common at presentation. Classic lacunar stroke syndromes may occur in two-thirds of patients. A patient with progressive leukoencephalopathy, particularly a young patient without hypertension, should prompt a search for CADASIL. In northeast England, CADASIL has a minimum prevalence of 1 to 25 in 50,000 in the general population.[13] Brain MRI scans show T2-weighted hyperintensities occurring symmetrically in the white matter and deep gray nuclei. Small lacunar lesions immediately subcortical in the anterior temporal lobes (O'Sullivan sign) have been reported to be 100% specific and 59% sensitive for CADASIL.[14]

Genetic testing is available but may require extensive sequencing of the large *NOTCH3* gene, which contains 33 exons. Identification of granular osmiophilic material in vascular tissue from biopsy specimens from skin, muscle, or peripheral nerves in the appropriate clinical setting of premature white matter ischemic strokes, dementia, and migraine may be sufficient for diagnosis.

Donepezil at a daily dose of 10 mg causes significant improvements in Trail-Making Tests, parts A and B, and on the Executive Interview 25 (EXIT25), but the clinical significance of the modest improvements is limited.[15] Anecdotally, acetazolamide at doses of 125 to 500 mg may help prevent migraines.[16]

CARASIL

Cerebral autosomal recessive arteriopathy with subcortical infarcts and leukoencephalopathy (CARASIL), also called Maeda syndrome, is a distinct clinical entity that predominantly affects individuals of Japanese ancestry; although, Chinese and Caucasian pedigrees have been reported.[17] CARASIL is caused by mutations in the *HTRA1* gene encoding HtrA serine peptidase/protease 1.[18] Subcortical encephalopathy leads to psychomotor deterioration when patients are in their 20s and 30s. Migraine is not a feature. Distinctive extracerebral manifestations of the disease that often predate the neurologic presentation include premature alopecia and bouts of lumbago with herniation of vertebral disks and spondylosis deformans. T2-weighted MRI shows extensive areas of hyperintensity in the hemispheric white matter and less dramatic changes in the thalami and pons.[19] The white matter changes occur without significant hypertension. Pathologically, there is severe widespread loss of arterial medial smooth muscle cells. Sclerotic changes are infrequent compared with CADASIL.[20] Also, unlike CADASIL, abnormal vessels are not periodic acid-Schiff-stain positive.[19]

Homocystinuria

The most common inherited form of elevated homocystine is attributable to cystathionine β-synthase deficiency and is referred to as homocystinuria. The trait is inherited in an autosomal recessive pattern; thus, both parents are typically asymptomatic carriers. It was first described in 1962 when elevated homocystine levels were identified in the serum and urine of mentally retarded patients; the enzymatic defect was reported several years later.[21–23]

Patients with homocystinuria are typically divided between those who respond to vitamin B_6 (pyridoxine) supplementation and those who do not. In 1985, Mudd et al.[24] reported on 629 patients with homocystinuria; by the age of 10 years, 55% of vitamin-B_6-responsive patients and 82% of vitamin-B_6-unresponsive patients had dislocated lenses. Along with Marfan syndrome, syphilis, and trauma, homocystinuria is one of the major diagnostic considerations in a patient with dislocation of the lens of the eye.[24] Also similar to patients with Marfan syndrome, those with homocystinuria may develop skeletal abnormalities such as long limbs, tall height, pectus excavatum (caved chest) or pectus carinatum (pigeon chest), and arachnodactyly. Classically, homocystinuria patients have the dermatologic features of thin blonde hair, a malar flush, and livedo reticularis. Affected young adults with stroke may lack the classic phenotype.[25] Without treatment, mental retardation may occur in two-thirds of patients.[24] Elevated homocystine levels are associated with both thrombotic and embolic strokes, which occur by the age of 15 years in 12% of vitamin-B_6-responsive patients and in 27% of vitamin-B_6-unresponsive patients.[24] Stroke occurs in more than 60% of patients with homocystinuria by the age of 40 years.[24]

Homocystinuria is screened for by measuring plasma homocysteinemia and confirmed by gene testing. Routine testing at birth can identify patients at an early age. Restriction of dietary methionine and supplementation of vitamin B_6 are recommended.

MELAS

The syndrome of mitochondrial encephalopathy, lactic acidosis, and stroke-like episodes (MELAS) is caused by mutations in mitochondrial DNA. As with other mitochondrial disorders, it is inherited in a maternal pattern. Clinical criteria for making the diagnosis include stroke before the age of 40 years, encephalopathy characterized by seizures or dementia, and blood lactic acidosis or ragged red fibers on skeletal muscle pathologic examination.[26] Brain MRI typically shows lesions involving the occipital lobes. The lesions often do not respect the boundaries of named vascular territories. MELAS mutations cause impairment in respiratory chain enzymes, particularly complex I. Eighty percent of cases are caused by a substitution mutation (A3243G) in the gene encoding for transfer RNA $(tRNA)^{Leu(UUR)}$. Other substitution mutations and deletions have also been described.[27,28]

There is no proven treatment for MELAS. However, seizures should not be treated with valproic acid because patients can have a paradoxical reaction.[29]

Sickle Cell Anemia

Sickle cell anemia is vital to recognize because there are clearly efficacious therapies. It is an autosomal recessive disorder, whereby valine is substituted for glutamic acid at position 6 of the β-polypeptide chain of hemoglobin.

The mutation causes polymerization or aggregation of abnormal hemoglobin within red blood cells, inducing the sickling change in the shape of the red cells. Patients typically have compensated hemolytic anemia, mild jaundice, and vaso-occlusive crises that cause excruciating pain in the back, chest, and extremities. Stroke is also a major complication of sickle cell disease.

The condition is most prevalent among patients of African origin. In untreated populations, sickle cell disease can cause stroke, typically in elementary-school-aged patients. In the Cooperative Study of Sickle Cell Disease (CSSCD), a multicenter study of approximately 4000 patients followed from the late 1970s to the late 1980s, the first incidence peak for stroke was between the ages of 2 and 5 years.[30] The cumulative risks of the first stroke were 11% by the age of 20 years and 24% by the age of 45 years. In patients younger than 20 years, most strokes are ischemic; after the age of 20 years, most are hemorrhagic.

Sickle cell disease is associated with Moyamoya syndrome. The vasculopathy of Moyamoya, causing proximal intracranial arterial stenosis, shows elevated blood flow velocities on transcranial Doppler (TCD). The CSSCD identified dactylitis, severe anemia, and leukocytosis in very young children as risk factors for adverse outcomes, including stroke, death, and pain crises. However, these risk factors, when tested in a more current series of newborns and young children in the Dallas Newborn Cohort (DNC), were found to have poor clinical utility.[31] All children in the DNC received prophylactic penicillin, which may account for the different findings. Stroke remained the most frequent adverse event documented in both the DNC and the CSSCD. Neither cohort reflects the effects of TCD screening on natural history.

The Stroke Prevention in Sickle Cell Disease trial, known as the STOP trial, definitively established that transfusion therapy dramatically reduces the risk of recurrent stroke in high-risk patients, where "high risk" was defined predominately by values on TCD studies.[32] In STOP, approximately 2000 children between the ages of 2 and 6 years old underwent TCD screening to detect blood flow velocities consistent with intracranial stenosis. Approximately 9% of those screened had time-averaged mean blood flow velocities in excess of 200 cm/s in either the middle cerebral artery or the internal carotid artery on either the right or the left side. Patients were randomly assigned to episodic blood transfusion according to standard practice or to long-term transfusion therapy, intended to reduce hemoglobin S levels to a target of less than 30% of total hemoglobin. The aggressive transfusion protocol was so overwhelmingly efficacious that the study was stopped early.

In the follow-up, STOP2, patients whose TCD blood-flow velocities normalized after a 30-month transfusion program had a high rate of stroke and reversion to abnormal velocities with discontinuation of transfusion. Despite clear stroke prevention benefits, long-term aggressive transfusion therapy is not easily tolerated. Children must receive transfusions approximately once monthly to achieve the target hemoglobin S level consistent with STOP (<30% of total hemoglobin). Long-term transfusion therapy puts patients at risk of iron overload. Because of the complexities of transfusion therapy, a pediatric neurologist and a pediatric hematologist with experience in treating patients with sickle cell disease typically monitor patients. The efficacy of long-term transfusion therapy for preventing recurrent stroke has been less well studied than primary prevention. However, in defense of transfusion therapy as a means of secondary prevention, the STOP trial showed that transfusion therapy lowered the risk of new silent infarction or stroke in the 37% of patients who had clinically silent cerebral infarctions on baseline brain MRI.[33]

Therapies other than transfusion have been tested with variable success. Myeloablative stem-cell transplantation is an appealing alternative therapy.[34] In a series of 87 patients treated with allogeneic hematopoietic stem-cell transplant, no individual who had successful engraftment developed stroke or silent ischemic lesions. Of further encouragement, arterial velocities were significantly reduced 1 year after transplantation. It should be noted, however, that patients who undergo such transplants are at risk of seizures and posterior reversible leukoencephalopathy due to the adverse effects of cyclosporine and corticosteroid therapy, and female children are at risk of ovarian failure.

Hydroxyurea has also been tested. Long-term observational follow-up in the multicenter study of hydroxyurea in sickle cell anemia showed that the risk of stroke was not substantially altered by treatment of hydroxyurea in adults with sickle cell anemia.[35] In contrast, hydroxyurea has been shown to reduce TCD velocities in children with sickle cell anemia.[36]

Fibromuscular Dysplasia

Fibromuscular dysplasia (FMD) is usually regarded as sporadic and often subclinical. Cerebral angiography often shows the so-called stack-of-coins or string-of-beads appearance of the cervical and petrous segments of the carotid artery. Among children with stroke and FMD, focal stenosis is far more common than string-of-beads or angiography.[37] FMD can lead to carotid dissection and stroke along with renovascular hypertension. In the US Registry for Fibromuscular Dysplasia, hypertension, headache, and pulsatile tinnitus were the most common presenting symptoms among the first 447 patients enrolled.[38] Segregation analysis of pedigrees with renovascular FMD using echotracking of the carotid arteries found evidence supporting autosomal inheritance.[39] In one pediatric stroke series, FMD was associated with 7% of stroke cases. FMD may be a risk factor for both carotid dissection and its recurrence.[40] Stenting can be performed with minimal risk, but the long-term benefits of such a procedure remain to be established.[41]

FMD is also part of Grange syndrome. In the originally described pedigree with Grange syndrome, patients had stenosis or occlusion of renal, abdominal, and cerebral arteries, congenital cardiac defects, brachydactyly (particularly of the second and fifth digits), syndactyly, bone fragility, and learning disabilities.[42]

Vascular Ehlers–Danlos Syndrome

Vascular Ehlers–Danlos syndrome (EDS), also known as Type IV EDS, is an autosomal dominant disorder caused by mutations in the collagen III, alpha-1 polypeptide gene (*COL3A1*). Individuals can develop cervical and intracranial arterial dissections and aneurysms and carotid-cavernous sinus fistula, although thoracic and abdominal vessels are more commonly affected.[43] EDS is associated with <2% of cervical arterial dissections.[44] Phenotypic clues to the condition include thin lips, lobeless ears, fragile skin, so-called cigarette paper scars, and easy bruisability. In addition to neurologic complications, life-threatening complications include bowel rupture and uterine rupture in pregnancy. Patients have high complication rates with surgery and with endovascular treatments, which should, therefore, only be used in case of life-threatening emergencies.[45]

Collagen Type IV Alpha 1 Mutations

Mutations in the collagen type IV alpha 1 (*COL4A1*) gene can cause an autosomal dominant stroke syndrome causing small-vessel disease and cerebral hemorrhage.[46] The mutations appear to exert an effect through haploinsufficiency.[47] In addition to the stroke syndrome, mutations are associated with infantile spasms and porencephaly. As in patients with CADASIL, brain MRI findings include leukoaraiosis, microbleeds on gradient imaging, and lacunes. Dilated perivascular spaces can also be prominent in *COL4A1* disorders. Recurrent intracranial hemorrhages have been observed.[48] Additional features include retinal arteriolar tortuosities and retinal hemorrhages. *COL4A1* mutations can also cause the HANAC syndrome (hereditary angiopathy, nephropathy, aneurysms and cramps).[49] Early diagnosis may be clinically advantageous because patients can be advised to avoid behaviors that would put them at risk of cerebral hemorrhage. Putative risk factors for hemorrhage include parturition, sports-related head trauma, and anticoagulation therapy.

Hypercoagulable Disorders

Well-recognized thrombophilias, including deficiencies of protein C, protein S, and antithrombin III; the factor V Leiden point mutation; and the prothrombin G20210A point mutation have been studied in relation to stroke. Primary protein C, protein S, and antithrombin III deficiencies are challenging to diagnose in patients immediately after stroke. Measurements in the acute stroke setting can be misleading. Warfarin and vitamin K deficiency lower protein C and protein S blood levels. Heparin lowers antithrombin III levels. Levels that are found to be low initially in the early post-stroke period should be verified as persistently low >1 month after the stroke and in the absence of an active infection. Primary protein C, protein S, and antithrombin III deficiencies are uncommon and have only a tenuous association with adult ischemic stroke. Factor V Leiden (the most common cause of activated protein C deficiency) and prothrombin G20210A, determined by gene tests, can be measured with equal validity in the acute or chronic phases of stroke. A meta-analysis of candidate gene association studies shows that these genes likely impart a modest increased risk of ischemic stroke.[50]

No clear guidelines describe the most appropriate time to perform these tests when a patient with stroke is evaluated. It is likely that the tests are overused. The tests have the highest yields in cases of pediatric stroke and cerebral venous thrombosis.[51]

Moyamoya Disease

Moyamoya disease, also known as spontaneous occlusion of the circle of Willis, is characterized by stenosis or occlusion of the terminal portions in the internal carotid artery bilaterally in the presence of an abnormal vascular network near the arterial occlusion. The disease is most prevalent in Japan. An epidemiologic study of Moyamoya disease in Washington state and California found an overall incidence of 0.086 per 100,000 individuals.[52] Although this incidence was lower than the 0.35 per 100,000 rate found in the National Japanese Survey,[53] the incidence was comparable for Asian Americans in California and native Japanese. At least five chromosomal regions have been linked to Moyamoya disease in Japanese populations: 3p24.2-p26, 6q25, 8q23, 12p12, and 17q25.[54] The *RNF213* gene is responsible for the 17q25 locus. A founder mutation p.R4859K dramatically increases the risk of Moyamoya disease (OR 190.8).[55]

Moyamoya disease is diagnosed on the basis of conventional angiographic findings. Other radiologic studies are helpful in delineating the extent of neovascularization and pathophysiologic disturbances in blood flow. High-field imaging such as 3.0-T time-of-flight magnetic resonance angiography (MRA) appears more sensitive in the detection of Moyamoya vessels than 1.5-T imaging.[56] Steno-occlusive arteries show proliferation of smooth muscle cells and permanently tortuous, often-duplicated internal elastic lamina.[57]

MRI techniques can detect asymptomatic microbleeding in >40% of individuals with Moyamoya disease.[58] Surgical pathology specimens of microbleeding indicate a correspondence to arteries and some arterioles with disrupted internal elastic lamina surrounding a small hemorrhage.[59] Computed tomographic angiography (CTA) can reveal a false "spot sign" in patients with Moyamoya disease.[60]

Clinically, Moyamoya causes infarcts, hemorrhages, and headaches. Severe headache is a prominent symptom in younger patients.[61] The number of microbleeds detected on 3-T MRI successfully predicts the likelihood of subsequent intracranial hemorrhaging.[62]

Surgical management consists of two different approaches: direct and indirect revascularization. Direct techniques include superficial temporal artery-to-middle cerebral artery bypass. Indirect techniques include pial synangiosis. Pial synangiosis generally carries a favorable prognosis in patients with recurrent stroke and in pediatric patients with transient ischemic attack.[63]

No randomized trial of surgical intervention has been reported. In a consecutive series that involved 450 revascularization procedures performed at Stanford University Medical Center, surgical morbidity was 3.5%, and mortality was 0.7% per treated hemisphere.[64]

In addition to Moyamoya disease, there is Moyamoya syndrome that occurs secondary to a systemic condition. Conditions associated with Moyamoya vascular abnormalities include neurofibromatosis, tuberous sclerosis, and sickle cell anemia. In addition to these single-gene disorders, children with exposure to external-beam radiotherapy are at risk of developing Moyamoya syndrome.[65]

Moyamoya syndrome roughly doubles the risk of cerebrovascular events in sickle-cell disease.[66] Consensus does not exist regarding the screening of first-degree relatives of patients with Moyamoya disease. A small study in Japan argued in favor of MRA screening of asymptomatic relatives of patients with Moyamoya disease.[67] A multicenter Japanese study has shown that asymptomatic Moyamoya disease is not benign; the study showed an annual stroke risk of 3.2%.[68]

Asymptomatic patients may be seen with so-called morning glory disc anomaly, which is characterized by spoke-like vessels radiating outward from the edge of an anomalous optic disc. Typically, morning glory disc is seen unilaterally and is twice as common in females as it is in males. It has been argued that MRA or CTA should be performed in any patient with this ophthalmologic finding, typically a child between the ages of 2 and 12 years, to detect vascular or structural brain abnormalities, including Moyamoya disease.[69]

Mendelian Cerebral Amyloid Angiopathys

Cerebral amyloid angiopathy (CAA) is the chief manifestation of some rare single-gene disorders. Hereditary cerebral hemorrhaging with amyloidosis of the Dutch type (HCHWA-D) is an autosomal dominant condition caused by a mutation in the amyloid precursor protein *(APP)* gene. A glutamine (Q) is substituted for glutamic acid (E) at position 22 of *APP*, which is the result of a point mutation at base position number 693. About two-thirds of HCHWA-D patients are seen with intracerebral hemorrhage, and the remainder is seen with vascular dementia. Four Italian families have been described with HCHWA due to a mutation in the same APP codon 693, but that causes an (E) to lysine (K) substitution.[70] Patients present with recurrent headaches and multiple strokes leading to cognitive decline and epilepsy.

A mutation substituting glutamine for leucine at position 68 (C68Q) in the cystatin C (*CST3*) gene causes hereditary cerebral hemorrhage with amyloidosis of the Icelandic type (HCHWA-I).[71] This amino acid substitution destabilizes α-helical structures, exposing tryptophan residue to a more polar environment. This mutant protein with a more open structure is more prone to form insoluble β-pleated sheets.[72] About 17% of patients in Iceland who have stroke before the age of 35 years have stroke due to HCHWA-I.[73] Most HCHWA-I patients experience their first stroke before the age of 30 years and die before the age of 50 years.

Mutations in the transthyretin (*TTR*) gene usually manifest as small fiber sensory and autonomic familial polyneuropathy. In rare instances, point mutations can result in cerebral hemorrhage. Mutation Phe64Ser causes oculoleptomeningeal amyloidosis and cerebral hemorrhage.[74,75] Mutation Val30Met has caused intracerebral hemorrhage in one autopsy-confirmed case.[76] Gly53glu caused recurrent subarachnoid hemorrhage in siblings of one family.[77]

Mendelian Cerebral Cavernous Malformation Syndromes

Cerebral cavernous malformations (CCMs) can be sporadic or dominantly inherited. They have a prevalence of 0.1% to 0.5% in the general population. These lesions are often detected incidentally on MRI studies. They can act as an ictal focus or a nidus for cerebral hemorrhage. Three familial CCM syndromes have been defined molecularly.

CCM1 is caused by various mutations in the *KRIT1* gene, which encodes for the Krev interaction trapped 1 protein. *KRIT1* mutations include frame shift, nonsense, missense, and splice-junction mutations. Frame shifts account for half the observed mutations. *KRIT1* is thought to be a tumor suppressor gene. The *KRIT1* mutations have high rates of incomplete clinical and radiographic penetrance. In a study of 33 *KRIT1* mutation carriers from several families, 57.6% had no symptoms.[78] Of symptom-free carriers, 82.3% had CCM lesions detected on MRI.

CCM2 is caused by mutations in the *CCM2* gene, which encodes for malcavernin, a phosphotyrosine binding protein. There is an intriguing potential pathophysiologic link between CCM1 and CCM2. Malcavernin binds to two NPXY motifs in the KRIT1 protein. NPXY stands for an amino acid motif of asparagine, proline, an undetermined/variable amino acid, and tyrosine.

CCM3 is caused by mutations in the programmed cell death 10 (*PDCD10*) gene.[79] A case of CCM3 with cerebral and multiple spinal cavernous malformations has been described.[80]

Autosomal Dominant Polycystic Kidney Disease

Patients with autosomal dominant polycystic kidney disease (ADPKD) are at substantially increased risk of intracranial aneurysms relative to the general population. The prevalence of intracranial aneurysms in patients with ADPKD is 4% to 12%. Furthermore, segregation analysis suggests that ADPKD is a risk factor for aneurysmal subarachnoid hemorrhage.[81] A consensus does not exist on the optimal imaging protocol for aneurysm screening. A study of Japanese patients with ADPKD found that serial MRA studies detected new intracranial aneurysms in two of 15 patients over the course of 18 to 72 months of follow-up.[82]

Hereditary Hemorrhagic Telangiectasia

The clinical triad of epistaxis, telangiectasia, and a positive family history characterizes hereditary hemorrhagic telangiectasia (HHT), also known as Osler-Weber-Rendu syndrome. HHT is inherited as an autosomal dominant condition. HHT causes vascular malformations of the lung, liver, brain, and gastrointestinal tract. Two types of HHT have been defined. HHT1 is caused by mutations in the endoglin (*ENG*) gene. HHT2 is caused by mutations in the activin-A-receptor-type-II-like 1 (*ACVRL1*) gene. Endoglin and *ACVRL1* are cell surface receptors involved in the transforming growth factor-β

pathway. Both types of HHT appear to be the result of haploinsufficiency. Mutations in the genes lead to a reduction in the number of wild-type receptors on vascular endothelial cells.

Interestingly, although HHT causes vascular malformations, ischemic cerebrovascular disease is more common than hemorrhage. In a series of more than 300 patients, just over 2% were seen with intracranial hemorrhages.[83] In contrast, nearly 30% had experienced either cerebral infarction or TIA. Acute ischemic cerebrovascular disease in this setting is often attributed to paradoxic embolism of thrombi or septic emboli by way of pulmonary arteriovenous malformations. Patients with infarction or TIA should be screened for pulmonary arteriovenous malformations, and if detected, ablation should be considered for these lesions.

Retinal Vasculopathy with Cerebral Leukodystrophy

Patients with retinal vasculopathy with cerebral leukodystrophy (RVCL) usually present with visual impairment and renal dysfunction.[84] Findings on ophthalmologic examination include macular edema with capillary dropout and perifoveal microangiopathic telangectasias. Urinalysis may detect hematuria and proteinuria. Neurologically, patients can experience migraine headaches, strokes, and psychiatric symptoms. Contrast-enhancing subcortical lesions can be seen on brain imaging. Inheritance is autosomal dominant. The disease is caused by mutations in the 3′-5′ DNA endonuclease *TREX1*.[85] Sometimes patients present with evolving tumor-like lesions.[86]

NON-MENDELIAN RISK FACTORS

Genome-wide association studies (GWASs) use markers along the entire genome to identify risk genes and are known as hypothesis-free approaches. SNPs make up about 90% of all human genetic variation and occur frequently throughout the genome (1 in every 200 to 300 bases). SNPs on the same chromosome in physical proximity are more likely to be inherited together than SNPs that are farther apart. Linkage disequilibrium is a measure of this non-random association between markers. Thus, if a disease-predisposing polymorphism is close to a SNP used as a marker, then the marker is associated with the disease proportional to the degree of linkage disequilibrium between them. With current technology, more than 90% of the genome among people of European and African origin is within a reasonable degree of linkage disequilibrium to available markers on standard genotyping sets.

GWASs aim to identify regions of interest throughout the genome that may harbor disease-predisposing polymorphisms, by comparing genotypes of case patients and control subjects at specific marker SNPs distributed across the genome. GWASs are based on two assumptions: (1) a patient with disease will carry a disease-predisposing polymorphism more commonly than will a control individual; and (2) specific alleles at nearby marker SNPs, inherited in conjunction with this disease-predisposing polymorphism, will also be more common in case patients than in control subjects.

Ischemic Stroke

Genome-wide association studies have made inroads in understanding the genetic underpinnings of ischemic stroke risk. A recurring finding is that genetic risk factors tend to associate with ischemic stroke subtypes. In a multistage study supported by the Wellcome Trust, a genome-wide association study was performed with 3548 cases of ischemic stroke and 5972 controls.[87] Stage 2 consisted of replication of top associations in 5859 cases and 6281 controls. SNPs near *PITX2* and *ZFHX3* genes were associated with cardioembolic stroke. A9p21 locus and *HDAC9* on chromosome 7p21.1 were associated with large-vessel stroke. Subsequently, a meta-analysis of 12,389 individuals with ischemic stroke and 62,004 controls of European ancestry showed that *PITX2* and *ZFHX3* are associated with cardioembolism via their association with atrial fibrillation.[88] A locus on chromosome 9p21 and *HDAC9* is associated with large-vessel stroke. A three-stage study of end-stage coagulation and the structure and function of fibrinogen was done to assess associations with ischemic stroke and its subtypes, and a SNP in the *ABO* gene (rs505922) was associated with large-vessel and cardioembolic stroke, but not small-vessel stroke.[89] A genome-wide association study of 1162 cases of ischemic stroke and 1244 population controls from an Australian population found a locus at chromosome 6p21.1 to be associated with large-vessel stroke.[90] The association replicated when tested in an independent population of 1715 cases and 52,695 population controls.

Association studies have been done to gain better insight into the relationship of a gene with intermediate phenotypes that may be along the causal pathway to subtypes of ischemic stroke. For example, the lead SNPs in the *HDAC9* gene associated with large-vessel stroke were found to associate with common carotid intima-media thickness (tested in 31,210 individuals) and with the presence of asymptomatic carotid plaque (tested in 25,179 individuals).[91] These findings support the theory that the *HDAC9* association with large-vessel stroke is related to atherosclerosis. A genome-wide association study of leukoaraiosis assessed by MRI of the stroke-free hemisphere of 2588 patients with ischemic stroke found an association between hyperintensity volume and a locus on chromosome 17q25.[92] Perhaps surprisingly, this locus was not found to associate with small-vessel stroke. The lack of co-association may point to diverging mechanisms behind leukoaraiosis and small-vessel stroke.

Studies have attempted to assess the degree of overlap of the genetic risk factors of stroke with various clinical conditions. For example, a study was done to understand the commonalities and differences between coronary artery disease and ischemic stroke. A study of 42 genome-wide significant SNPs associated with coronary artery disease found that three were associated with ischemic stroke and five were associated with large-vessel stroke.[93] Fifteen loci reached genome-wide significance for ischemic stroke or coronary artery disease and 17 loci reached genome-wide significance for large-vessel stroke or coronary artery disease.

Genetic association studies have also generated insights into trials of stroke prevention. For example, a meta-analysis of the *MTHFR* C677T mutation and ischemic stroke showed greater association in regions with low dietary folate than in regions with high dietary folate.[94] The authors hypothesize that the negative trials of folate supplementation may have been negative because they were generally conducted in regions with high dietary folate. Another meta-analysis of the same mutation and randomized trials of folate supplementation suggested that the randomized trials may have been negative because they were performed in populations where co-treatment with daily aspirin is routine.[95]

Intracerebral Hemorrhage

Once considered a rare cause of lobar hemorrhaging, CAA is now recognized as an important cause of lobar hemorrhage in the elderly.[96–98] Its principal pathologic feature is the deposition of amyloid protein in the media and adventitia of leptomeningeal arteries, arterioles, capillaries, and, less often, veins.[99,100] CAA occurs in 50% to 79% of patients with AD.[101,102] A number of studies have associated apolipoprotein (Apo)E2, ApoE4, or both with CAA or lobar intracerebral hemorrhage. McCarron and Nicoll[103] reported that the risk of ApoE2 with CAA occurred among subjects with and without AD, while the association of ApoE4 with CAA correlated with concomitant AD. This finding suggested that ApoE2 is a specific risk factor for CAA-related hemorrhage, while ApoE4 is related to CAA in general.

When APP is cleaved by α-secretase, a transmembrane portion of the protein is left, ranging in length from 37 to 42 amino acids. Researchers have found that the β-amyloid 42 level is significantly elevated in AD patients and their first-degree relatives.[104] McCarron et al.[105] reported that patients with CAA-related hemorrhage were more reactive to β-amyloid 42. Rosand et al.[106] reported an association of ApoE2 among 41 patients with warfarin-related intracerebral hemorrhage compared with 66 control subjects in which seven of 11 subjects had pathologic evidence of CAA. In animal models, knock-in mice with human ApoE4 developed amyloid plaques as well as CAA, whereas ApoE3 knock-in mice developed almost no CAA or parenchymal plaques.[107]

Initial reports suggested that as many as 60% of lobar hemorrhage cases may have evidence of petechial hemorrhage on gradient-echo MRI.[108] In addition, the technique detects new hemorrhages in 47% of cases of probable CAA.[109] Roob et al.[110] found petechial hemorrhages in 6.4% of otherwise healthy elderly individuals, suggesting a means of early detection of CAA. In a study of 1062 people from Rotterdam, the overall prevalence of microbleeds ranged from 17.8% among those aged 60 to 69 years to 38.3% for those older than 80 years, and ApoE4 carriers had more strictly lobar microbleeds than non-carriers.[111]

A meta-analysis found that ApoE alleles reached genome-wide levels of significance in their relationship to lobar ICH, and it is suggested that ApoE4 may be associated with deep ICH.[112] In addition, ApoE2 has been associated with a larger volume of hemorrhage and higher mortality (no association was identified for ApoE4).[113]

Changes in management based on the results of genetic testing are not currently recommended, although some studies suggest that an increased risk of intracerebral hemorrhage with anticoagulant treatment may occur.[106]

INTRACRANIAL ANEURYSMS

Intracranial aneurysms (IA) are found in about 2% to 5% of the healthy general population, depending on the method used to detect them.[114] In about 25% of cases there are multiple aneurysms.[115] The mean age of detection of unruptured IA is about 50 years. Although the vast majority of IA remains asymptomatic, annually, about 1% to 2% of cases rupture,[114] causing subarachnoid hemorrhage. Subarachnoid hemorrhage accounts for about 5% of all strokes, but because it affects people at a younger age than other stroke types and has very high morbidity and mortality, it has a socio-economic effect similar to that of ischemic stroke. Over 80% of IAs are in the anterior circulation, mostly on the circle of Willis. The commonest sites are the anterior communicating artery, posterior communicating artery, and the middle cerebral artery. In the posterior circulation, aneurysms affect the top of the basilar artery; and superior, anterior inferior, or posterior inferior cerebellar arteries. Aneurysms more commonly affect females, especially in those over 50 years of age, when they may outnumber males by up to 2:1.

Evidence for a Genetic Component in Intracranial Aneurysms. For such a common and devastating disease, the cause of IA and subarachnoid hemorrhage remains enigmatic. Although modifiable risk factors are known to contribute to IA, particularly smoking, hypertension, and alcohol intake,[116,117] a genetic component to IA has long been recognized. Initial evidence came from reports of clustering within families, and the well-described occurrence of IA in known genetic diseases (including Ehlers–Danlos syndrome and pseudoxanthoma elasticum, autosomal dominant adult polycystic kidney disease, and Moyamoya disease). First-degree relatives of patients with IA have an about fourfold higher risk of harboring an IA than the general population, even without evidence of any known hereditary syndrome.[118] For example, in European studies (Finland and the Netherlands), the prevalence of IAs in first-degree relatives was 4% to 9%.[119,120] In familial IA, the modes of inheritance are mixed, suggesting heterogeneous genetic factors. Familial aneurysms tend to rupture earlier in life and at smaller sizes than sporadic aneurysms,[119,121] and IA in siblings may rupture in the same decade of life. Aneurysms tend to occur at similar locations within families, suggesting that a specific anatomical vulnerability may be inherited.[122] However, only about between 5% and 20% of all IA is familial, and families with more than two affected individuals are rare. There has thus been great interest in studying the role of genetics in sporadic IA.

A recent systematic review and meta-analysis confirmed a substantial genetic contribution to the occurrence of sporadic IA, implicating multiple pathophysiologic pathways relating to vascular endothelial maintenance, extracellular matrix integrity and inflammation.[123] The identified studies included 60 candidate gene association studies (CGAS) and six genome-wide association studies (GWAS). Selected loci showing robust associations in at least two studies are shown in Table 18-3.

Candidate Gene Association Studies. Candidate gene association studies (CGAS) of sporadic IA have tested associations

TABLE 18-3 Selected Genetic Variants Associated with Intracranial Aneurysms

Gene or Locus	SNP	Cases/Controls	Odds Ratio (95%CI; FE)	Potential Biological Mechanism
CDKN2B (9p21.3)	rs1333040	11949/29014	1.24 (1.20–1.29)	Vascular endothelium
ANRIL (9p2121.3)	rs10757278	3394/17075	1.29 (1.21–1.38)	Vascular endothelium
SOX17 (8q11)	rs9298506	9246/26331	1.21 (1.15–1.27)	Vascular endothelium
	rs10958409	9873/27029	1.20 (1.15–1.26)	
EDNRA (4p31.23)	rs6841581	4370/14181	1.22 (1.14–1.31)	Vascular endothelium
BOLL (2q33)	rs1429412	2675/7632	1.20 (1.12–1.30)	? Endothelial development
	rs700651	4283/13236	1.11 (1.03–1.19)	
SERPINA3	rs4934	892/1029	2.22 (1.68–2.94)	Extracellular matrix
COL1A2	rs42524	812/806	1.77 (1.14–2.75)	Extracellular matrix
COL3A1	rs1800255	546/2235	1.55 (1.21–2.00)	Extracellular matrix
HSPG2	rs3767137	1316/1742	1.22 (1.08–1.39)	Extracellular matrix
Versican	rs251124	1316/1742	1.22 (1.08–1.39)	Extracellular matrix

of variants in genes plausibly linked to aneurysm development or rupture. CGAS have identified numerous potential risk loci, but these studies have been limited by small sample sizes and lack of replication. Nevertheless, a recent systematic review found that eight SNPs from CGAS were significantly associated with IAs in at least two studies. These SNPs relate to genes with potential relevance to IA biology, including those important for extracellular matrix integrity, vascular endothelium maintenance, and inflammatory mediators. *SERPINA3* (rs4934), which codes for a plasma protease inhibitor, and two variants relating to collagen genes (*COL1A2* [rs42524 G.C] and *COL3A1* [rs1800255 G.A]) showed the most robust associations with IA. The remaining significantly associated CGAS SNPs included heparan sulfate proteoglycan 2 (rs3767137), versican (rs251124 and rs173686), and interleukin 6 (IL6) G572C.[123] Extracellular matrix gene variants may predispose to IA development by weakening arterial walls. For example, the *COL1A2* rs42524 SNP is located on chromosome 7q22.1 close to the elastin gene, a key protein component of arterial walls. Another potential mechanism of aneurysm development or rupture is through the effect of circulating inflammatory mediators on vascular remodeling, which may have a genetic component; this mechanism is of particular interest due to the potential for therapeutic blockade if specific targets could be identified. However, currently available data are inconclusive: although the pro-inflammatory cytokine IL6 G572C SNP had an overall protective association with IAs in a recessive model, there was significant statistical heterogeneity, and sensitivity analysis revealed no association once one Chinese study in only unruptured aneurysms was excluded.[124] IL-6 may injure vessel walls by inhibiting collagen synthesis, thus increasing wall fragility and increasing the risk of aneurysmal dilatation and has been shown to influence prognosis for abdominal aneurysms,[125] but further studies of genes relevant to inflammation in larger populations of unruptured and ruptured IA are required.

Genome-Wide Association Studies. The first GWAS in IA was published in 2008, and included a European (Finnish and Dutch) population for discovery, followed by Japanese replication cohorts (a total of 2196 cases; 8085 controls).[126] The loci associated with IA were 2q33.1, 8q11.23, and 9p21.3. A subsequent replication study in 5891 cases and 14,181 controls confirmed the association of IAs with the loci on chromosomes 8 and 9.[127] In the recent meta-analysis, the most robust association was confirmed for the 9p21.3 locus, with a total of 11,949 cases and 29,014 controls showing an odds ratio of 1.24 (1.20–1.29).[123] The SNP rs1333040, located on chromosome 9p21.3, is in the cyclin-dependent kinase inhibitor 2B antisense gene (*CDKN2B*), which plays a role in cell cycle signaling. Intriguingly, this locus is associated with a wide spectrum of arterial disorders, including coronary artery disease and abdominal aortic aneurysms,[128] raising the possibility of an as yet unidentified common pathogenic arterial process. The association of IA with this locus is independent of smoking and hypertension,[129] and showed preferential association with posterior communicating artery aneurysms, providing preliminary evidence that IA site could be related to genetic factors.

Another SNP close by on chromosome 9p21.3 (rs10757278), in a non-coding RNA region called *ANRIL* (antisense noncoding RNA in the INK4 locus) showed robust association with IAs; its function remains unclear, but it may also influence the regulation of cell-cycle genes.[130] In the most recent GWAS in a Caucasian population of familial and sporadic IA[131], six SNPs, also in the 9p21.3 region, were associated with IA; one of these (rs6475606) achieved GWAS-level statistical significance for association with sporadic and familial IAs.

Two SNPs on chromosome 8q (rs10958409 and rs9298506), surrounding the *SOX17* gene – critical to the maintenance of stem cells of endothelial and hematopoietic lineages and the formation and maintenance of vascular endothelium – were studied in European and Japanese populations; rs10958409 was associated in both populations, but the rs9298506 SNP was associated with IA only in the European population. The heterogeneity observed emphasizes the potentially different genetic effects across populations. Further support implicating chromosome 8 *SOX17* loci was shown by identification of a new locus in a recent GWAS in a Caucasian cohort[131] (rs1072737: OR 1.22; 95%CI 1.07–1.39), independent of, but interacting with, smoking.

Another new potential IA mechanism is suggested by another recent GWAS,[132] which discovered a locus (rs6841581) coding for the endothelin receptor type A (*EDNRA*) gene, to be significantly associated with IA (OR 1.22; 95%CI 1.14–1.31; $p = 2.2 \times 10^{-8}$). Another GWAS[133] also found a locus near the *EDNRA* gene (rs6842241) to be significantly associated with IA. *EDNRA* is a G-protein-coupled receptor for endothelins, which modulate vasoconstriction and vasodilatation after hemodynamic insult, pathways which are activated at the site of vascular injury.

Gene Expression Studies. Gene expression studies using microarrays have investigated the transcription profiles of sporadic IAs and found abnormal transcription of proteins related to arterial wall integrity or remodeling including collagens, matrix metalloproteinases, and cell adhesion molecules.[134–137] Genes related to inflammatory signaling have also been implicated in other studies.[138] However, challenges remain in designing and interpreting studies of gene expression in IA due to the difficulty of obtaining the appropriate healthy control tissue, and the difficulty of attributing causality direction (i.e., whether gene expression alterations are causative or reactive).

Summary and Future Directions. IA genetic studies have generated many new exciting risk loci in a short space of time. These have clear potential to illuminate disease mechanisms for IA, and as further information is available, the most robust associations will emerge. The available studies still do not explain the majority of genetic risk, and many loci remain un-replicated, or have conflicting data. There is also evidence of heterogeneity of risk across populations,[123] emphasizing the need for studies in large cohorts of patients of different ancestries. Full incorporation of known strong environmental risk factors, as well as aneurysm phenotype (location, size, multiplicity) is needed to better understand the complexity of genetic risk on different groups. Studies of genetic associations with outcome after SAH (e.g. vasospasm and physical recovery) are also needed. Perhaps the most exciting potential for genetics in IA is in predicting rupture risk, which will require comparison of genetic variants in ruptured vs unruptured aneurysms, but may open up future possibilities for understanding and ultimately preventing IA rupture by not only endovascular or surgical but also rational biological therapies.

REFERENCES

1. Flossmann E, Schulz UG, Rothwell PM. Systematic review of methods and results of studies of the genetic epidemiology of ischemic stroke. Stroke 2004;35:212–27.
2. Meschia JF, Atkinson EJ, O'Brien PC, et al. Familial clustering of stroke according to proband age at onset of presenting ischemic stroke. Stroke 2003;34:e89–91.
3. Touze E, Rothwell PM. Sex differences in heritability of ischemic stroke: a systematic review and meta-analysis. Stroke 2008; 39:16–23.

4. Schulz UG, Flossmann E, Rothwell PM. Heritability of ischemic stroke in relation to age, vascular risk factors, and subtypes of incident stroke in population-based studies. Stroke 2004;35:819–24.
5. Grewal RP. Stroke in Fabry's disease. J Neurol 1994;241:153–6.
6. Rolfs A, Bottcher T, Zschiesche M, et al. Prevalence of Fabry disease in patients with cryptogenic stroke: a prospective study. Lancet 2005;366:1794–6.
7. Brouns R, Sheorajpanday R, Braxel E, et al. Middelheim Fabry Study (MiFaS): a retrospective Belgian study on the prevalence of Fabry disease in young patients with cryptogenic stroke. Clin Neurol Neurosurg 2007;109:479–84.
8. Chabriat H, Pappata S, Ostergaard L, et al. Cerebral hemodynamics in CADASIL before and after acetazolamide challenge assessed with MRI bolus tracking. Stroke 2000;31:1904–12.
9. Tuominen S, Miao Q, Kurki T, et al. Positron emission tomography examination of cerebral blood flow and glucose metabolism in young CADASIL patients. Stroke 2004;35:1063–7.
10. van den Boom R, Lesnik Oberstein SA, Ferrari MD, et al. Cerebral autosomal dominant arteriopathy with subcortical infarcts and leukoencephalopathy: MR imaging findings at different ages - 3rd–6th decades. Radiology 2003;229:683–90.
11. Liebetrau M, Herzog J, Kloss CU, et al. Prolonged cerebral transit time in CADASIL: a transcranial ultrasound study. Stroke 2002;33(2):509–12.
12. Dichgans M, Mayer M, Uttner I, et al. The phenotypic spectrum of CADASIL: clinical findings in 102 cases. Ann Neurol 1998;44(5):731–9.
13. Narayan SK, Gorman G, Kalaria RN, et al. The minimum prevalence of CADASIL in northeast England. Neurology 2012; 78(13):1025–7.
14. van Den Boom R, Lesnik Oberstein SA, van Duinen SG, et al. Subcortical lacunar lesions: an MR imaging finding in patients with cerebral autosomal dominant arteriopathy with subcortical infarcts and leukoencephalopathy. Radiology 2002;224(3): 791–6.
15. Dichgans M, Markus HS, Salloway S, et al. Donepezil in patients with subcortical vascular cognitive impairment: a randomised double-blind trial in CADASIL. Lancet Neurol 2008;7(4): 310–18.
16. Donnini I, Nannucci S, Valenti R, et al. Acetazolamide for the prophylaxis of migraine in CADASIL: a preliminary experience. J Headache Pain 2012;13(4):299–302.
17. Mendioroz M, Fernandez-Cadenas I, Del Rio-Espinola A, et al. A missense HTRA1 mutation expands CARASIL syndrome to the Caucasian population. Neurology 2010;75(22):2033–5.
18. Fukutake T. Cerebral autosomal recessive arteriopathy with subcortical infarcts and leukoencephalopathy (CARASIL): from discovery to gene identification. J Stroke Cerebrovasc Dis 2011;20(2): 85–93.
19. Yanagawa S, Ito N, Arima K, et al. Cerebral autosomal recessive arteriopathy with subcortical infarcts and leukoencephalopathy. Neurology 2002;58(5):817–20.
20. Oide T, Nakayama H, Yanagawa S, et al. Extensive loss of arterial medial smooth muscle cells and mural extracellular matrix in cerebral autosomal recessive arteriopathy with subcortical infarcts and leukoencephalopathy (CARASIL). Neuropathology 2008;28(2):132–42.
21. Carson NA, Neill DW. Metabolic abnormalities detected in a survey of mentally backward individuals in Northern Ireland. Arch Dis Child 1962;37:505–13.
22. Gerritsen T, Vaughn JG, Waisman HA. The identification of homocystine in the urine. Biochem Biophys Res Commun 1962;9:493–6.
23. Mudd SH, Finkelstein JD, Irreverre F, et al. Homocystinuria: An enzymatic defect. Science 1964;143(3613):1443–5.
24. Mudd SH, Skovby F, Levy HL, et al. The natural history of homocystinuria due to cystathionine beta-synthase deficiency. Am J Hum Genet 1985;37(1):1–31.
25. Kelly PJ, Furie KL, Kistler JP, et al. Stroke in young patients with hyperhomocysteinemia due to cystathionine beta-synthase deficiency. Neurology 2003;60(2):275–9.
26. Hirano M, Pavlakis SG. Mitochondrial myopathy, encephalopathy, lactic acidosis, and strokelike episodes (MELAS): current concepts. J Child Neurol 1994;9(1):4–13.
27. Goto Y, Nonaka I, Horai S. A new mtDNA mutation associated with mitochondrial myopathy, encephalopathy, lactic acidosis and stroke-like episodes (MELAS). Biochim Biophys Acta 1991;1097(3):238–40.
28. Ciafaloni E, Ricci E, Shanske S, et al. MELAS: clinical features, biochemistry, and molecular genetics. Ann Neurol 1992;31(4): 391–8.
29. Lam CW, Lau CH, Williams JC, et al. Mitochondrial myopathy, encephalopathy, lactic acidosis and stroke-like episodes (MELAS) triggered by valproate therapy. Eur J Pediatr 1997;156(7): 562–4.
30. Ohene-Frempong K, Weiner SJ, Sleeper LA, et al. Cerebrovascular accidents in sickle cell disease: rates and risk factors. Blood 1998;91(1):288–94.
31. Quinn CT, Lee NJ, Shull EP, et al. Prediction of adverse outcomes in children with sickle cell anemia: a study of the Dallas Newborn Cohort. Blood 2008;111(2):544–8.
32. Adams RJ, McKie VC, Hsu L, et al. Prevention of a first stroke by transfusions in children with sickle cell anemia and abnormal results on transcranial Doppler ultrasonography. N Engl J Med 1998;339(1):5–11.
33. Pegelow CH, Wang W, Granger S, et al. Silent infarcts in children with sickle cell anemia and abnormal cerebral artery velocity. Arch Neurol 2001;58(12):2017–21.
34. Bernaudin F, Socie G, Kuentz M, et al. Long-term results of related myeloablative stem-cell transplantation to cure sickle cell disease. Blood 2007;110(7):2749–56.
35. Steinberg MH, Barton F, Castro O, et al. Effect of hydroxyurea on mortality and morbidity in adult sickle cell anemia: risks and benefits up to 9 years of treatment. JAMA 2003;289(13): 1645–51.
36. Zimmerman SA, Schultz WH, Burgett S, et al. Hydroxyurea therapy lowers transcranial Doppler flow velocities in children with sickle cell anemia. Blood 2007;110(3):1043–7.
37. Kirton A, Crone M, Benseler S, et al. Fibromuscular dysplasia and childhood stroke. Brain 2013;136(Pt 6):1846–56.
38. Olin JW, Froehlich J, Gu X, et al. The United States Registry for Fibromuscular Dysplasia: results in the first 447 patients. Circulation 2012;125(25):3182–90.
39. Perdu J, Boutouyrie P, Bourgain C, et al. Inheritance of arterial lesions in renal fibromuscular dysplasia. J Hum Hypertens 2007;21(5):393–400.
40. de Bray JM, Marc G, Pautot V, et al. Fibromuscular dysplasia may herald symptomatic recurrence of cervical artery dissection. Cerebrovasc Dis 2007;23(5–6):448–52.
41. Assadian A, Senekowitsch C, Assadian O, et al. Combined open and endovascular stent grafting of internal carotid artery fibromuscular dysplasia: long term results. Eur J Vasc Endovasc Surg 2005;29(4):345–9.
42. Grange DK, Balfour IC, Chen SC, et al. Familial syndrome of progressive arterial occlusive disease consistent with fibromuscular dysplasia, hypertension, congenital cardiac defects, bone fragility, brachysyndactyly, and learning disabilities. Am J Med Genet 1998;75(5):469–80.
43. Pepin MG, Schwarze U, Rice KM, et al. Survival is affected by mutation type and molecular mechanism in vascular Ehlers-Danlos syndrome (EDS type IV). Genet Med 2014;doi:10.1038/gim.2014.72; [Epub ahead of print].
44. Debette S, Leys D. Cervical-artery dissections: predisposing factors, diagnosis, and outcome. Lancet Neurol 2009;8(7): 668–78.
45. Bergqvist D, Bjorck M, Wanhainen A. Treatment of vascular Ehlers-Danlos syndrome: a systematic review. Ann Surg 2013; 258(2):257–61.
46. Gould DB, Phalan FC, van Mil SE, et al. Role of COL4A1 in small-vessel disease and hemorrhagic stroke. N Engl J Med 2006;354(14):1489–96.
47. Lemmens R, Maugeri A, Niessen HW, et al. Novel COL4A1 mutations cause cerebral small vessel disease by haploinsufficiency. Hum Mol Genet 2013;22(2):391–7.
48. Vahedi K, Alamowitch S. Clinical spectrum of type IV collagen (COL4A1) mutations: a novel genetic multisystem disease. Curr Opin Neurol 2011;24(1):63–8.
49. Plaisier E, Chen Z, Gekeler F, et al. Novel COL4A1 mutations associated with HANAC syndrome: a role for the triple

helical CB3[IV] domain. Am J Med Genet A 2010;152A(10): 2550–5.

50. Casas JP, Hingorani AD, Bautista LE, et al. Meta-analysis of genetic studies in ischemic stroke: thirty-two genes involving approximately 18,000 cases and 58,000 controls. Arch Neurol 2004;61(11):1652–61.
51. Rahemtullah A, Van Cott EM. Hypercoagulation testing in ischemic stroke. Arch Pathol Lab Med 2007;131(6):890–901.
52. Uchino K, Johnston SC, Becker KJ, et al. Moyamoya disease in Washington State and California. Neurology 2005;65(6): 956–8.
53. Fukui M. Current state of study on moyamoya disease in Japan. Surg Neurol 1997;47(2):138–43.
54. Meschia JF, Ross OA. Heterogeneity of Moyamoya disease: after a decade of linkage, is there new hope for a gene? Neurology 2008;70(24 Pt 2):2353–4.
55. Kamada F, Aoki Y, Narisawa A, et al. A genome-wide association study identifies RNF213 as the first Moyamoya disease gene. J Hum Genet 2011;56(1):34–40.
56. Fushimi Y, Miki Y, Kikuta K, et al. Comparison of 3.0- and 1.5-T three-dimensional time-of-flight MR angiography in moyamoya disease: preliminary experience. Radiology 2006;239(1):232–7.
57. Fukui M, Kono S, Sueishi K, et al. Moyamoya disease. Neuropathology 2000;20(Suppl.):S61–4.
58. Fukui M. Guidelines for the diagnosis and treatment of spontaneous occlusion of the circle of Willis ('moyamoya' disease). Research Committee on Spontaneous Occlusion of the Circle of Willis (Moyamoya Disease) of the Ministry of Health and Welfare, Japan. Clin Neurol Neurosurg 1997;99(Suppl. 2): S238–40.
59. Kikuta K, Takagi Y, Nozaki K, et al. Histological analysis of microbleed after surgical resection in a patient with moyamoya disease. Neurol Med Chir (Tokyo) 2007;47(12):564–7.
60. Gazzola S, Aviv RI, Gladstone DJ, et al. Vascular and nonvascular mimics of the CT angiography "spot sign" in patients with secondary intracerebral hemorrhage. Stroke 2008;39(4):1177–83.
61. Okada Y, Kawamata T, Kawashima A, et al. The efficacy of superficial temporal artery-middle cerebral artery anastomosis in patients with moyamoya disease complaining of severe headache. J Neurosurg 2012;116(3):672–9.
62. Kikuta K, Takagi Y, Nozaki K, et al. The presence of multiple microbleeds as a predictor of subsequent cerebral hemorrhage in patients with moyamoya disease. Neurosurgery 2008;62(1): 104–11, discussion 11–2.
63. Scott RM, Smith JL, Robertson RL, et al. Long-term outcome in children with moyamoya syndrome after cranial revascularization by pial synangiosis. J Neurosurg 2004;100(2 Suppl. Pediatrics):142–9.
64. Guzman R, Lee M, Achrol A, et al. Clinical outcome after 450 revascularization procedures for moyamoya disease. Clinical article. J Neurosurg 2009;111(5):927–35.
65. Ullrich NJ, Robertson R, Kinnamon DD, et al. Moyamoya following cranial irradiation for primary brain tumors in children. Neurology 2007;68(12):932–8.
66. Dobson SR, Holden KR, Nietert PJ, et al. Moyamoya syndrome in childhood sickle cell disease: a predictive factor for recurrent cerebrovascular events. Blood 2002;99(9):3144–50.
67. Houkin K, Tanaka N, Takahashi A, et al. Familial occurrence of moyamoya disease. Magnetic resonance angiography as a screening test for high-risk subjects. Childs Nerv Syst 1994;10(7): 421–5.
68. Kuroda S, Hashimoto N, Yoshimoto T, et al. Radiological findings, clinical course, and outcome in asymptomatic moyamoya disease: results of multicenter survey in Japan. Stroke 2007; 38(5):1430–5.
69. Lenhart PD, Lambert SR, Newman NJ, et al. Intracranial vascular anomalies in patients with morning glory disk anomaly. Am J Ophthalmol 2006;142(4):644–50.
70. Bugiani O, Giaccone G, Rossi G, et al. Hereditary cerebral hemorrhage with amyloidosis associated with the E693K mutation of APP. Arch Neurol 2010;67(8):987–95.
71. Revesz T, Holton JL, Lashley T, et al. Sporadic and familial cerebral amyloid angiopathies. Brain Pathol 2002;12(3):343–57.
72. Calero M, Pawlik M, Soto C, et al. Distinct properties of wild-type and the amyloidogenic human cystatin C variant of hereditary cerebral hemorrhage with amyloidosis, Icelandic type. J Neurochem 2001;77(2):628–37.
73. Olafsson I, Grubb A. Hereditary cystatin C amyloid angiopathy. Amyloid 2000;7(1):70–9.
74. Uitti RJ, Donat JR, Rozdilsky B, et al. Familial oculoleptomeningeal amyloidosis. Report of a new family with unusual features. Arch Neurol 1988;45(10):1118–22.
75. Uemichi T, Uitti RJ, Koeppen AH, et al. Oculoleptomeningeal amyloidosis associated with a new transthyretin variant Ser64. Arch Neurol 1999;56(9):1152–5.
76. Sakashita N, Ando Y, Jinnouchi K, et al. Familial amyloidotic polyneuropathy (ATTR Val30Met) with widespread cerebral amyloid angiopathy and lethal cerebral hemorrhage. Pathol Int 2001;51(6):476–80.
77. Ellie E, Camou F, Vital A, et al. Recurrent subarachnoid hemorrhage associated with a new transthyretin variant (Gly53Glu). Neurology 2001;57(1):135–7.
78. Battistini S, Rocchi R, Cerase A, et al. Clinical, magnetic resonance imaging, and genetic study of 5 Italian families with cerebral cavernous malformation. Arch Neurol 2007;64(6):843–8.
79. Guclu B, Ozturk AK, Pricola KL, et al. Mutations in apoptosis-related gene, PDCD10, cause cerebral cavernous malformation 3. Neurosurgery 2005;57(5):1008–13.
80. Lee ST, Choi KW, Yeo HT, et al. Identification of an Arg35X mutation in the PDCD10 gene in a patient with cerebral and multiple spinal cavernous malformations. J Neurol Sci 2008; 267(1–2):177–81.
81. Belz MM, Hughes RL, Kaehny WD, et al. Familial clustering of ruptured intracranial aneurysms in autosomal dominant polycystic kidney disease. Am J Kidney Dis 2001;38(4):770–6.
82. Nakajima F, Shibahara N, Arai M, et al. Intracranial aneurysms and autosomal dominant polycystic kidney disease: followup study by magnetic resonance angiography. J Urol 2000;164(2): 311–13.
83. Maher CO, Piepgras DG, Brown RD Jr, et al. Cerebrovascular manifestations in 321 cases of hereditary hemorrhagic telangiectasia. Stroke 2001;32(4):877–82.
84. Jen J, Cohen AH, Yue Q, et al. Hereditary endotheliopathy with retinopathy, nephropathy, and stroke (HERNS). Neurology 1997;49(5):1322–30.
85. Richards A, van den Maagdenberg AM, Jen JC, et al. C-terminal truncations in human 3′-5′ DNA exonuclease TREX1 cause autosomal dominant retinal vasculopathy with cerebral leukodystrophy. Nat Genet 2007;39(9):1068–70.
86. Mateen FJ, Krecke K, Younge BR, et al. Evolution of a tumor-like lesion in cerebroretinal vasculopathy and TREX1 mutation. Neurology 2010;75(13):1211–13.
87. International Stroke Genetics C, Wellcome Trust Case Control C, Bellenguez C, et al. Genome-wide association study identifies a variant in HDAC9 associated with large vessel ischemic stroke. Nat Genet 2012;44(3):328–33.
88. Traylor M, Farrall M, Holliday EG, et al. Genetic risk factors for ischaemic stroke and its subtypes (the METASTROKE Collaboration): a meta-analysis of genome-wide association studies. Lancet Neurol 2012;11(11):951–62.
89. Williams FM, Carter AM, Hysi PG, et al. Ischemic stroke is associated with the ABO locus: the EuroCLOT study. Ann Neurol 2013;73(1):16–31.
90. Holliday EG, Maguire JM, Evans TJ, et al. Common variants at 6p21.1 are associated with large artery atherosclerotic stroke. Nat Genet 2012;44(10):1147–51.
91. Markus HS, Makela KM, Bevan S, et al. Evidence HDAC9 genetic variant associated with ischemic stroke increases risk via promoting carotid atherosclerosis. Stroke 2013;44(5):1220–5.
92. Adib-Samii P, Rost N, Traylor M, et al. 17q25 Locus is associated with white matter hyperintensity volume in ischemic stroke, but not with lacunar stroke status. Stroke 2013;44(6):1609–15.
93. Dichgans M, Malik R, Konig IR, et al. Shared genetic susceptibility to ischemic stroke and coronary artery disease: a genome-wide analysis of common variants. Stroke 2014;45(1):24–36.
94. Holmes MV, Newcombe P, Hubacek JA, et al. Effect modification by population dietary folate on the association between MTHFR genotype, homocysteine, and stroke risk: a meta-analysis of genetic studies and randomised trials. Lancet 2011;378(9791): 584–94.

95. Wald DS, Morris JK, Wald NJ. Reconciling the evidence on serum homocysteine and ischaemic heart disease: a meta-analysis. PLoS ONE 2011;6(2):e16473.
96. Okazahi H, Whisnant JP. Clinical pathology of hypertensive intracerebral hemorrhage. In: Mizukami M, Kogure K, Kanaya H, et al., editors. Hypertensive Intracerebral Hemorrhage. New York: Raven Press; 1983. p. 177–80.
97. Vinters HV. Cerebral amyloid angiopathy. A critical review. Stroke 1987;18(2):311–24.
98. Vonsattel JP, Myers RH, Hedley-Whyte ET, et al. Cerebral amyloid angiopathy without and with cerebral hemorrhages: a comparative histological study. Ann Neurol 1991;30(5):637–49.
99. Mandybur TI, Bates SR. Fatal massive intracerebral hemorrhage complicating cerebral amyloid angiopathy. Arch Neurol 1978;35(4):246–8.
100. Maruyama K, Ikeda S, Ishihara T, et al. Immunohistochemical characterization of cerebrovascular amyloid in 46 autopsied cases using antibodies to beta protein and cystatin C. Stroke 1990;21(3):397–403.
101. Olichney JM, Hansen LA, Galasko D, et al. The apolipoprotein E epsilon 4 allele is associated with increased neuritic plaques and cerebral amyloid angiopathy in Alzheimer's disease and Lewy body variant. Neurology 1996;47(1):190–6.
102. Glenner GG, Henry JH, Fujihara S. Congophilic angiopathy in the pathogenesis of Alzheimer's degeneration. Ann Pathol 1981;1(2):120–9.
103. McCarron MO, Nicoll JA. High frequency of apolipoprotein E epsilon 2 allele is specific for patients with cerebral amyloid angiopathy-related haemorrhage. Neurosci Lett 1998;247(1): 45–8.
104. Jensen M, Schroder J, Blomberg M, et al. Cerebrospinal fluid A beta42 is increased early in sporadic Alzheimer's disease and declines with disease progression. Ann Neurol 1999;45(4): 504–11.
105. McCarron MO, Nicoll JA, Stewart J, et al. Amyloid beta-protein length and cerebral amyloid angiopathy-related haemorrhage. Neuroreport 2000;11(5):937–40.
106. Rosand J, Hylek EM, O'Donnell HC, et al. Warfarin-associated hemorrhage and cerebral amyloid angiopathy: a genetic and pathologic study. Neurology 2000;55(7):947–51.
107. Fryer JD, Simmons K, Parsadanian M, et al. Human apolipoprotein E4 alters the amyloid-beta 40:42 ratio and promotes the formation of cerebral amyloid angiopathy in an amyloid precursor protein transgenic model. J Neurosci 2005;25(11):2803–10.
108. Greenberg SM, Finklestein SP, Schaefer PW. Petechial hemorrhages accompanying lobar hemorrhage: detection by gradient-echo MRI. Neurology 1996;46(6):1751–4.
109. Greenberg SM, O'Donnell HC, Schaefer PW, et al. MRI detection of new hemorrhages: potential marker of progression in cerebral amyloid angiopathy. Neurology 1999;53(5):1135–8.
110. Roob G, Schmidt R, Kapeller P, et al. MRI evidence of past cerebral microbleeds in a healthy elderly population. Neurology 1999;52(5):991–4.
111. Vernooij MW, van der Lugt A, Ikram MA, et al. Prevalence and risk factors of cerebral microbleeds: the Rotterdam Scan Study. Neurology 2008;70(14):1208–14.
112. Biffi A, Sonni A, Anderson CD, et al. Variants at APOE influence risk of deep and lobar intracerebral hemorrhage. Ann Neurol 2010;68(6):934–43.
113. Biffi A, Anderson CD, Jagiella JM, et al. APOE genotype and extent of bleeding and outcome in lobar intracerebral haemorrhage: a genetic association study. Lancet Neurol 2011;10(8): 702–9.
114. Rinkel GJ, Djibuti M, Algra A, et al. Prevalence and risk of rupture of intracranial aneurysms: a systematic review. Stroke 1998;29(1):251–6.
115. Stehbens WE. Aneurysms and Anatomical Variation of Cerebral Arteries. Arch Pathol 1963;75:45–64.
116. Feigin VL, Rinkel GJ, Lawes CM, et al. Risk factors for subarachnoid hemorrhage: an updated systematic review of epidemiological studies. Stroke 2005;36(12):2773–80.
117. Clarke M. Systematic review of reviews of risk factors for intracranial aneurysms. Neuroradiology 2008;50(8):653–64.
118. Vlak MH, Algra A, Brandenburg R, et al. Prevalence of unruptured intracranial aneurysms, with emphasis on sex, age, comorbidity, country, and time period: a systematic review and meta-analysis. Lancet Neurol 2011;10(7):626–36.
119. Ronkainen A, Hernesniemi J, Puranen M, et al. Familial intracranial aneurysms. Lancet 1997;349(9049):380–4.
120. Raaymakers TW. Aneurysms in relatives of patients with subarachnoid hemorrhage: frequency and risk factors. MARS Study Group. Magnetic Resonance Angiography in Relatives of patients with Subarachnoid hemorrhage. Neurology 1999;53(5):982–8.
121. Broderick JP, Brown RD Jr, Sauerbeck L, et al. Greater rupture risk for familial as compared to sporadic unruptured intracranial aneurysms. Stroke 2009;40(6):1952–7.
122. Mackey J, Brown RD Jr, Moomaw CJ, et al. Familial intracranial aneurysms: is anatomic vulnerability heritable? Stroke 2013; 44(1):38–42.
123. Alg VS, Sofat R, Houlden H, et al. Genetic risk factors for intracranial aneurysms: a meta-analysis in more than 116,000 individuals. Neurology 2013;80(23):2154–65.
124. Sun H, Zhang D, Zhao J. The interleukin-6 gene -572G>C promoter polymorphism is related to intracranial aneurysms in Chinese Han nationality. Neurosci Lett 2008;440(1):1–3.
125. Jones KG, Brull DJ, Brown LC, et al. Interleukin-6 (IL-6) and the prognosis of abdominal aortic aneurysms. Circulation 2001; 103(18):2260–5.
126. Bilguvar K, Yasuno K, Niemela M, et al. Susceptibility loci for intracranial aneurysm in European and Japanese populations. Nat Genet 2008;40(12):1472–7.
127. Yasuno K, Bilguvar K, Bijlenga P, et al. Genome-wide association study of intracranial aneurysm identifies three new risk loci. Nat Genet 2010;42(5):420–5.
128. Helgadottir A, Thorleifsson G, Magnusson KP, et al. The same sequence variant on 9p21 associates with myocardial infarction, abdominal aortic aneurysm and intracranial aneurysm. Nat Genet 2008;40(2):217–24.
129. Nakaoka H, Takahashi T, Akiyama K, et al. Differential effects of chromosome 9p21 variation on subphenotypes of intracranial aneurysm: site distribution. Stroke 2010;41(8):1593–8.
130. Olsson S, Csajbok LZ, Jood K, et al. Association between genetic variation on chromosome 9p21 and aneurysmal subarachnoid haemorrhage. J Neurol Neurosurg Psychiatry 2011; 82(4):384–8.
131. Foroud T, Koller DL, Lai D, et al. Genome-wide association study of intracranial aneurysms confirms role of Anril and SOX17 in disease risk. Stroke 2012;43(11):2846–52.
132. Yasuno K, Bakircioglu M, Low SK, et al. Common variant near the endothelin receptor type A (EDNRA) gene is associated with intracranial aneurysm risk. Proc Natl Acad Sci U S A 2011;108(49): 19707–12.
133. Low SK, Takahashi A, Cha PC, et al. Genome-wide association study for intracranial aneurysm in the Japanese population identifies three candidate susceptible loci and a functional genetic variant at EDNRA. Hum Mol Genet 2012;21(9):2102–10.
134. Peters DG, Kassam AB, Feingold E, et al. Molecular anatomy of an intracranial aneurysm: coordinated expression of genes involved in wound healing and tissue remodeling. Stroke 2001;32(4):1036–42.
135. Li L, Yang X, Jiang F, et al. Transcriptome-wide characterization of gene expression associated with unruptured intracranial aneurysms. Eur Neurol 2009;62(6):330–7.
136. Shi C, Awad IA, Jafari N, et al. Genomics of human intracranial aneurysm wall. Stroke 2009;40(4):1252–61.
137. Pera J, Korostynski M, Krzyszkowski T, et al. Gene expression profiles in human ruptured and unruptured intracranial aneurysms: what is the role of inflammation? Stroke 2010;41(2): 224–31.
138. Roder C, Kasuya H, Harati A, et al. Meta-analysis of microarray gene expression studies on intracranial aneurysms. Neuroscience 2012;201:105–13.

19 Preventing a First Stroke

Larry B. Goldstein, Ralph L. Sacco

KEY POINTS

- Poor dietary habits (high salt, low fruits and vegetables), smoking, and physical inactivity are among the leading modifiable behaviors accounting for the rising global burden of deaths and disability from cardiovascular diseases and stroke, and other non-communicable diseases.
- Smoking cessation is associated with a reduction in the risk of stroke within 2 to 5 years to a level that approaches the risk of those who never smoked.
- Physical inactivity is a well-established and modifiable risk factor for stroke. The protective effects of physical activity are present across different age groups, for men and women, and among different race-ethnic groups.
- Hypertension is one of the most important modifiable risk factors for prevention of a first stroke.
- Careful treatment of hypertension and treatment with an HMG-CoA reductase inhibitor (statin) reduces the risk of a first stroke in persons with diabetes.
- Warfarin, dabigatran, apixaban, and rivaroxaban are all indicated for the prevention of a first and recurrent stroke in patients with non-valvular atrial fibrillation, depending on specific patient characteristics.
- Aspirin is indicated for cardiovascular (including, but not specific to, stroke) prophylaxis for persons who have a 10-year risk of cardiovascular events of 6% to 10% or greater.

Primordial and primary prevention remain the most effective means for reducing stroke's public health burden. Primordial prevention is a population-based approach that aims to reduce the likelihood of the development of disease risk factors, usually through environmental changes. Primary prevention can also include community or individual interventions aimed at reducing the probability of a stroke event. The identification of the high-risk, stroke-prone individual helps select persons for general and specific risk factor modification interventions. Numerous randomized clinical trials have been conducted that inform comprehensive, evidence-based guidelines for the management of risk factors to prevent a first stroke.[1]

This chapter provides an overview of primordial and primary prevention of stroke. Approaches to improve the identification of the stroke-prone individual are reviewed including the use of stroke-risk prediction models. The major focus is given to discussion of the management of modifiable stroke risk factors including lifestyle behaviors such as smoking, alcohol use, physical inactivity, diet, and obesity, and the management of hypertension, diabetes, dyslipidemia, atrial fibrillation, sleep-disordered breathing and the use of platelet antiaggregants in primary stroke prevention. Carotid artery stenosis is addressed in Chapter 74 and sickle cell disease in Chapters 26, 42, and 56. The discussion of less well-documented risk factors such as inflammation, infection, migraine, patent foramen ovale, and hypercoagulable disorders are not discussed here.

PRIMORDIAL PREVENTION

Although stroke has a variety of etiologies, atherosclerosis is one of the major causes of stroke. Autopsies conducted in children and young adults who died of unrelated causes find pathologic evidence of atherosclerosis in the form of intimal lesions in the aorta of all 15–19-year-olds and in the coronary arteries of more than half.[2] Among 12–19-year-olds in the US, 14% have prehypertension or hypertension, 22% have borderline or high low-density lipoprotein cholesterol levels, and 15% have pre-diabetes or diabetes, all risk factors for stroke.[3] The evidence of disease and risk factors in the young supports the need for population-based approaches to reduce the development of risk factors beginning at the earliest ages. Population-based approaches contributed significantly to the dramatic reduction in cardiovascular mortality in both the US and in other industrialized nations over the last decade.[4] Environmental approaches to risk reduction are not only cost-effective, but may, at least in some cases, be cost-savings.[5]

Virtually no American adults and a very low proportion of children have ideal cardiovascular health.[6] Poor dietary habits (high salt, low fruits and vegetables), smoking, and physical inactivity are among the leading modifiable behaviors accounting for the rising global burden of deaths and disability from cardiovascular diseases and stroke and other non-communicable diseases.[7] Population-based approaches are a main component of policies targeting the American Heart Association's 2020 goal of improving cardiovascular health of all Americans by 20%.[8] Environmental strategies include reducing tobacco use and exposure to environmental tobacco smoke, consuming a diet low in sodium, low in sugar, and rich in grains, fruits and vegetables, and encouraging physical activity.[8] These goals can be addressed through a variety of public policy interventions. Examples include support of tobacco control legislation, clean indoor air regulations, providing nutrition information in restaurants, encouraging programs to bring fruits and vegetables to inner cities and to provide healthy food options in schools, mandating physical education in schools, and devoting public land to parks and other recreational centers to promote physical activity.

ASSESSING THE RISK FOR A FIRST STROKE

Although primordial prevention aims to lower risk on a population basis, primary prevention strategies target individuals at increased stroke risk owing to their personal behaviors and characteristics. Approaches to predict an individual's stroke risk can aid healthcare professionals in identifying the stroke-prone individual and help motivate patient lifestyle modification and compliance with medical interventions. Many factors can contribute to stroke risk, and most individuals have more

TABLE 19-1 Modified Framingham Stroke Risk Profile[16]

Risk Factor Points	0	1	2	3	4	5	6	7	8	9	10
Age (years)	54–56	57–59	60–62	63–65	66–68	69–71	72–74	75–77	78–80	81–83	84–86
SBP (mmHg)	95–105	106–116	117–126	127–137	138–148	149–159	160–170	171–181	182–191	192–202	203–213
SBP Rx	No		Yes								
DM	No		Yes								
CS	No			Yes							
CHD	No			Yes							
AF	No				Yes						
LVH	No						Yes				

SBP, systolic blood pressure; SBP Rx, treated systolic blood pressure; DM, diabetes mellitus; CS, cigarette smoking; CHD, coronary heart disease; AF, atrial fibrillation; LVH, left ventricular hypertrophy on EKG.

than one such factor. A variety of specific stroke risk assessment tools are available to use for primary stroke prevention screening programs.[9] It should be recognized, however, that risk assessment for primary stroke prevention should not be conducted in isolation and needs to be considered in the context of global vascular risk that includes the risks of myocardial infarction and vascular death.[10,11] For example, although controversial because of possible overestimation of risk, a prediction tool has been developed to inform guideline-based statin therapy for prevention of a first atherosclerotic vascular event, including stroke.[12,13]

Stroke-specific risk estimation tools are generally focused on combining several major vascular risk factors to compute a predicted risk probability. The Framingham Stroke Profile (FSP) is among the most widely utilized for predicting the risk of a first stroke.[14,15] It includes age, systolic blood pressure, hypertension, diabetes mellitus, current smoking, established cardiovascular disease (any one of myocardial infarction [MI], angina or coronary insufficiency, congestive heart failure, or intermittent claudication), atrial fibrillation, and left ventricular hypertrophy on electrocardiogram. The FSP provides sex-specific 1-, 5-, or 10-year cumulative stroke risks and was updated to include the use of antihypertensive therapy and the risk of stroke or death among individuals with AF (Table 19-1).[16] Despite its widespread use, the validity of the FSP among individuals of different age ranges and race/ethnic groups has not been fully studied. Although alternative risk prediction models have been developed in other cohorts, their validity has not been well tested.[10,17,18]

American Heart Association (AHA) Guidelines for the Primary Prevention of Stroke indicate that the use of a risk assessment tool such as the AHA/ACC CV Risk Calculator (http://my.americanheart.org/cvriskcalculator) is reasonable because they can help identify individuals who could benefit from therapeutic interventions, but might not be treated on the basis of any one risk factor.[1] Despite the existence of risk tools, none have been widely used in clinical settings. Validation of stroke risk assessment tools is needed in different age, gender, and race/ethnic groups. Emerging risk factors also may need to be considered. There is a need for simple risk scores that can be easily integrated in primary care settings and within electronic health records to help healthcare providers predict risk and monitor the effects of changing risk behaviors. The ultimate public health benefit, however, will depend on not only identification of specific stroke risk, but on the assessment and reduction of global vascular risk.[10]

LIFESTYLE MODIFICATION

Modification of a variety of lifestyle factors can lower the risk of stroke (Table 19-2). Persons who follow these five lifestyle factors have an 80% lower risk of a first stroke compared to persons who don't with a dose effect for the number followed.[19] The benefits are similar for men and women. Moreover, similar dose-dependent lowering risks of global cardiovascular events have been observed across white, black and Hispanic/Latino race/ethnic groups with increasing numbers of ideal cardiovascular health factors.[20]

Cigarette Smoking

Cigarette smoking is a well-recognized, modifiable risk factor for ischemic and hemorrhagic stroke.[21–24] The risk of ischemic stroke has been estimated to be twofold higher for smokers vs. nonsmokers and threefold higher for subarachnoid hemorrhage.[25] The risk of stroke is reduced among those who quit.[22] Smoking cessation is associated with a reduction in the risk of stroke within 2 to 5 years to a level that approaches the risk of those who never smoked.[26,27] Exposure to environmental tobacco smoke carries a risk similar to that of smokers.[1]

Effective smoking cessation programs often require a combination of social support, behavioral treatments such as hypnosis, and pharmacotherapies including nicotine replacement (Table 19-2).[28] Three major pharmacotherapies that have demonstrated efficacy, especially when combined with behavioral support, are nicotine replacement therapy (NRT), bupropion, and varenicline.[29] Multiple commercially available forms of NRT (gum, transdermal patch, nasal spray, inhaler, and sublingual tablets/lozenges) are helpful in smoking cessation, increasing quitting rates by 50–70%.[30] Bupropion improves smoking cessation rates relative to placebo for both confirmed 7-day point-prevalence abstinence and self-reported prolonged abstinence.[31] Varenicline is a novel smoking-cessation agent that acts as a partial nicotinic receptor agonist, and is superior to the current standard patch in achieving abstinence and in reducing withdrawal phenomena such as urges to smoke and withdrawal symptoms.[32,33] Further studies of varenicline are needed to evaluate long-term efficacy of smoking cessation, and the use of the drug can be associated with a variety of side effects, including depression and suicidal ideation. The Centers for Disease Control and Prevention (CDC) has online support tools to help persons quit (http://betobaccofree.hhs.gov/quit-now/index.html). The most effective preventive measure is to never smoke, as well as to minimize exposure to environmental tobacco smoke.

Physical Activity

Physical inactivity is a well-established and modifiable risk factor for stroke.[34–36] The protective effects of physical activity are present across different age groups, for men and women, and among different race/ethnic groups.[37,38] In the Northern Manhattan Stroke Study, a protective effect was noted with

TABLE 19-2 AHA Management Recommendations for Lifestyle Risk Factors[1]

Factor	Goal	Recommendation
Cigarette smoking	Cessation	Abstention from cigarette smoking and (for current smokers) smoking cessation are recommended (*Class I; Level of Evidence B*). Counseling in combination with drug therapy using nicotine replacement, bupropion, or varenicline is recommended for active smokers to assist in quitting smoking (*Class I; Level of Evidence A*)
Physical activity	≥ 40 min a day 3 to 4 d/wk	Healthy adults should perform at least moderate- to vigorous-intensity aerobic physical activity at least 40 min a day 3 to 4 d/wk
Obesity	BMI < 25 kg/m^2	Among overweight (body mass index = 25 to 29 kg/m^2) and obese (body mass index >30 kg/m^2) individuals, weight reduction is recommended for reducing the risk of stroke (*Class I; Level of Evidence B*)
Diet/nutrition	Well-balanced diet	A Mediterranean diet supplemented with nuts may be considered in lowering the risk of stroke (*Class IIb; Level of Evidence B*)
Alcohol	Moderation	For those who consume alcohol, a recommendation of ≤2 drinks per day for men and ≤1 drink per day for non-pregnant women best reflects the state of the science for alcohol and stroke risk (*Class IIb; Level of Evidence B*)
Drug abuse	Cessation	Referral to an appropriate therapeutic program is reasonable for patients who abuse drugs that have been associated with stroke, including cocaine, khat, and amphetamines (*Class IIa; Level of Evidence C*)

Please refer to page xvii in the front matter for explanations of the levels and classes of evidence.

a dose–response relationship showing more intensive physical activity had additional benefits compared to light-to-moderate physical activity.[38,39] In women, however, even a program of walking is associated with lower risks of both ischemic and hemorrhagic stroke.[40] The protective effect is likely partially mediated through the control of other vascular risk factors including blood pressure, body weight, lipids, and diabetes.[41]

Although no clinical trials have specifically addressed the effects of physical activity for stroke prevention, the evidence from epidemiologic studies and from a few clinical trials in other chronic diseases is very supportive of a beneficial effect. Clinical trials show that exercise reduced the risk of falls resulting in injury among the elderly, as well as reduced systolic blood pressure, diastolic blood pressure, and had beneficial effects on blood lipids without any reported harm.[42] The benefits of physical activity have been highlighted in CDC, National Institutes of Health, and American Heart Association guidelines that recommend moderate exercise for at least 30 minutes per day (Table 19-2).[43–45] Despite these recommendations, over 45% of adults in the US engage in no regular moderate or vigorous physical activity.[6] Increasing physical activity could yield major public health gains in the prevention of cardiovascular disease and stroke.

Weight Management and Diet

Obesity is a risk factor for both stroke and cardiovascular disease and is associated with multiple other stroke risk factors including hypertension, dyslipidemia, hyperinsulinemia, and glucose intolerance. Greater weight during young adulthood and weight gain thereafter are associated with an increased stroke risk.[46] Measures of abdominal obesity, such as waist-to-hip ratio or waist circumference, are also stroke risk factors.[47] Increased waist circumference is a component of the metabolic syndrome.[48] In 2010, it was estimated that 32% of children in the US were overweight (body mass index, BMI 25–30 kg/m^2) and 154.7 million adults were obese (BMI ≥ 30 kg/m^2).[6] What makes obesity of even greater public health concern is its alarming increase in prevalence. By 2030, it is estimated that 51% of the population will be obese and 11% will have severe obesity.[6]

Losing weight is associated with a reduction of other vascular risk factors, possibly leading to a reduction in stroke risk. Although specific clinical trials evaluating the effects of weight reduction on stroke risk are lacking, the beneficial effects of weight reduction on blood pressure are well-documented. In a meta-analysis of 25 clinical trials, blood pressure was reduced by 3.6–4.4 mmHg with an average weight loss of 5.1 kg.[49] Weight reduction is a key component of the lifestyle measures recommended by JNC 7 and American College of Cardiology/American Heart Association guidelines for control of high blood pressure and dyslipidemia, respectively.[50,51]

Multiple dietary components are associated with the risk of stroke. Diets with increased fruit and vegetable content are associated with a dose-related reduction in the risk of stroke.[52] The risk of stroke was reduced by 6% in the Nurses' Health Study and the Health Professionals' Follow-Up Study for each 1-serving/day increment in fruit and vegetable intake.[53] A Mediterranean dietary pattern, which incorporates the consumption of fruits and vegetables, whole grains, folate, and fatty fish, as well as legumes and olive oil, may also prevent stroke.[54,55] Multiple prospective studies have demonstrated lower cardiovascular and stroke risks among those who follow Mediterranean-pattern diets.[56,57] Dietary consumption of excess salt is associated with hypertension and increased rates of cardiovascular disease and stroke.[58,59]

Randomized trials have assessed the effects of diets rich in fruits and vegetables on lowering blood pressure, but have not had sufficient follow-up to evaluate clinical events. The Dietary Approaches to Stop Hypertension (DASH) diet, which includes high consumption of fruits, vegetables, low-fat dairy products, and reduced intake of total and saturated fat reduces blood pressure.[60,61] Among high-cardiovascular-risk Spanish subjects, groups randomized to a Mediterranean-style diet enriched with nuts or extra-virgin olive oil had significantly lower risks of cardiovascular events, especially stroke, compared to control diets.[62] The American Heart Association recommends that an ideal cardiovascular diet includes 4 to 5 of the following components: (1) fruits and vegetables: ≥4.5 cups per day; (2) fish (preferably oily): ≥2 × 3.5-oz servings per week; (3) fiber-rich whole grains (1.1 g fiber per 10 g carbohydrate): ≥3 × 1-oz-equivalent servings per day; (4) sodium: <1500 mg per day; and (5) sugar-sweetened beverages: ≤450 kcal (36 oz) /week.[63]

Alcohol and Drug Abuse

Epidemiological evidence associating alcohol consumption and stroke risk has suggested a J-shaped relationship.[64] For ischemic stroke, as compared to non-drinkers, moderate drinkers (one to two drinks a day) have between a 0.3 and 0.5 stroke risk, whereas persons consuming three or more drinks per day have a greater risk.[65] Among Chinese, protective effects from moderate alcohol consumption have been less apparent for ischemic stroke and excessive alcohol use is deleterious for hemorrhagic stroke. In a meta-analysis of 35 observational studies, consumption of less than one drink per day (one drink defined as 12 g of alcohol), but not abstention, was associated with a 20% reduced risk of stroke. Consumption of one to two drinks per day was associated with a 28% risk reduction.[66] As compared with non-drinkers, those who drank more than five drinks per day had a 69% increased stroke risk. No protective relationship has been found for hemorrhagic stroke with a relative increased risk varying from two to four.[67] The deleterious consequences of heavy alcohol consumption include hypertension, hypercoagulability, reduced cerebral blood flow, and a greater likelihood of atrial fibrillation and other arrythmias.[68]

Despite the potential benefit of moderate alcohol consumption, there are other adverse health consequences related to excess alcohol use. Alcoholism remains a major public health problem in the US. Given the health risks associated with excessive alcohol use, it is not prudent to recommend alcohol consumption for stroke prevention among those who do not drink. For those who drink alcohol, suggested consumption is no more than two drinks per day for men and no more than one drink per day for non-pregnant women (Class IIb, Level of Evidence B; Table 19-2).

Drug abuse including heroin, cocaine, and amphetamines is associated with an increased risk of ischemic and hemorrhagic stroke.[69–71] These drugs can cause hematologic and metabolic derangements including increased platelet aggregation, fluctuations in blood pressure, vasculopathy, and cause cerebral embolization from secondary cardiac conditions or endocarditis.[72] Identification and management of drug abuse can be very challenging. When a patient is identified as having a drug-addiction problem, referral for appropriate counseling is recommended.[73] Various strategies are needed and often require a long-term commitment, medication and psychological counseling. Community outreach programs are needed to prevent drug abuse and reduce the prevalence of drug dependency.

MANAGEMENT OF MODIFIABLE RISK FACTORS TO PREVENT FIRST STROKE

Detailed, evidence-based guidelines are available for the management of several modifiable risk factors for a first stroke.[1] Selected risk factors are discussed below. AHA guideline recommendations are given in Tables 19-3 and 19-4.

Hypertension

Hypertension is one of the most important modifiable risk factors for prevention of a first stroke.[1] The most comprehensive review of evidence-based treatment of hypertension is

TABLE 19-3 AHA Recommendations for Management of Selected Risk Factors for Preventing a First Stroke[1,125]

Factor	Recommendation
Hypertension	Regular BP screening and appropriate treatment of patients with hypertension, including lifestyle modification and pharmacological therapy, are recommended (*Class I; Level of Evidence A*)
Diabetes	Control of BP to a target of <140/90 mm Hg is recommended in patients with type 1 or type 2 diabetes mellitus (*Class I; Level of Evidence A*). Treatment of adults with diabetes mellitus with a statin, especially those with additional risk factors, is recommended to lower the risk of first stroke (*Class I; Level of Evidence A*)
Non-valvular atrial fibrillation (anticoagulation candidates)	For patients with nonvalvular atrial fibrillation, a CHA2DS2-VASc score of ≥2, and acceptably low risk for hemorrhagic complications, oral anticoagulants are recommended (*Class I*). Options include warfarin (INR, 2.0 to 3.0) (*Level of Evidence A*), dabigatran (*Level of Evidence B*), apixaban (*Level of Evidence B*), and rivaroxaban (*Level of Evidence B*)
Non-valvular atrial fibrillation (not anticoagulation candidates)	Closure of the left atrial appendage may be considered for high-risk patients with atrial fibrillation who are deemed unsuitable for anticoagulation if performed at a center with low rates of periprocedural complications and the patient can tolerate the risk of at least 45 d of postprocedural anticoagulation (*Class IIb; Level of Evidence B*)
Sleep disordered breathing	Treatment of sleep apnea to reduce stroke risk might be reasonable, although its effectiveness is unknown (*Class IIb; Level of Evidence C*)

Please refer to page xvii in the front matter for explanations of the levels and classes of evidence.

TABLE 19-4 AHA Recommendations for the Use of Selected Treatments/Assessments for Preventing a First Stroke[1]

Treatment/Assessment	Recommendation
Risk Assessment	The use of a risk assessment tool such as the AHA/ACC CV Risk Calculator (http://my.americanheart. org/cvriskcalculator) is reasonable because they can help identify individuals who could benefit from therapeutic interventions, but might not be treated on the basis of any one risk factor
Aspirin	The use of aspirin for cardiovascular (including but not specific to stroke) prophylaxis is reasonable for people whose risk is sufficiently high (10-y risk >10%) for the benefits to outweigh the risks associated with treatment. A cardiovascular risk calculator to assist in estimating 10-y risk can be found online at http://my.americanheart. org/cvriskcalculator (*Class IIa; Level of Evidence A*). Aspirin is not indicated for preventing a first stroke in persons with diabetes or diabetes plus asymptomatic peripheral artery disease in the absence of other established cardiovascular disease (*Class III; Level of Evidence B*)
Statins	In addition to therapeutic lifestyle changes, treatment with an HMG coenzyme-A reductase inhibitor (statin) medication is recommended for primary prevention of ischemic stroke in patients estimated to have a high 10-y risk for cardiovascular events (*Class I; Level of Evidence A*)

Please refer to page xvii in the front matter for explanations of the levels and classes of evidence.

TABLE 19-5 Classification and Treatment of Blood Pressure Based on JNC 7[50]

Classification	Blood Pressure mm Hg	No Convincing Anti-hypertensive Indication*	With Convincing Anti-hypertensive Indication*
Normal	<120/80	No drug	No drug
Pre-hypertension	<139/90	No drug	Drugs for the compelling indication
Stage 1 hypertension	<159/99	Thiazide-type diuretics. May consider ACEIs, ARBs, β-blockers, calcium channel blockers, or combination	Drugs for the compelling indication. Other drugs (diuretics, ACEIs, ARBs, β-blockers, calcium channel blockers) as needed
Stage 2 hypertension	≥160/100	Two-drug combination for most (usually thiazide-type diuretic and ACEI or ARB or β-blocker or calcium channel blocker)	Drugs for the compelling indication and other drugs as needed

*Lifestyle modifications are encouraged for all and include (1) weight reduction if overweight, (2) limitation of ethyl alcohol intake, (3) increased aerobic physical activity (30–45 minutes daily), (4) reduction of sodium intake (<2.34 g), (5) maintenance of adequate dietary potassium (>120 mmol/d), (6) smoking cessation, and (7) DASH diet (rich in fruit, vegetables, and low-fat dairy products and reduced in saturated and total fat). Compelling indications include (1) congestive heart failure, (2) MI, (3) diabetes, (4) chronic renal failure, and (5) prior stroke

Initial combined therapy should be used cautiously in those at risk for orthostatic hypotension.

ACEI, Angiotensin converting enzyme inhibitor;ARB, Angiotensin receptor blocker.

provided in the Seventh Report of the Joint National Committee on Prevention, Detection, Evaluation, and Treatment of High Blood Pressure (JNC 7).[74] The classification and treatment scheme for elevated blood pressure is outlined in Table 19-5.

The risk of stroke associated with increasing blood pressure is continuous;[75] even prehypertension increases the risk of incident stroke.[76] JNC 7 guidelines recommend lowering blood pressure to <140/90 mm Hg (or <130/80 mm Hg in individuals with diabetes). JNC 8 guidelines have been more controversial and recommended 140/90 mm Hg as the target BP for individuals <60 and diabetics, and a different target of 150/90 mm Hg for persons 60 years and older.[77] In failing to recommend a level of SBP of 140 for persons over age 60, the JNC 8 panel relied on evidence from two lower-quality trials that setting a goal SBP of lower than 140 mm Hg in this age group demonstrated no added benefit compared with a higher goal SBP of 140 to 160 mm Hg or 140 to 149 mm Hg.[78,79] Prospective epidemiological data and most randomized trials, however, have shown linear relationships between SBP and stroke risk without substantial interactions by age.

Meta-analysis shows a 35–44% reduction in the incidence of stroke across various antihypertensive regimens.[80] There are several classes of antihypertensive medications that have been evaluated for reducing stroke, including thiazide diuretics, angiotensin-converting enzyme inhibitors (ACEIs), angiotensin receptor blockers (ARBs), β-adrenergic receptor blockers, and calcium channel blockers. In JNC-7 thiazide-type diuretics are often recommended as the preferred initial drugs for treatment of hypertension in most patients.[81] Differential efficacy of some of these classes of antihypertensive agents has been suggested by individual trials, as well as meta-analyses.[80] Recent data suggest that, in addition to absolute blood pressures, increasing blood pressure variability may increase stroke risk.[82] The effects of anti-hypertensives on stroke risk may in part depend on their effects on blood pressure variability.[83] In this regard, β-adrenergic receptor blockers are associated with greater blood pressure variability and a higher risk of stroke compared to other anti-hypertensives. Selection of a specific anti-hypertensive regimen also needs to be based on other comorbidities. For example, the use of an ACEI or an ARB is associated with greater survival in patients with chronic kidney disease who are not dialysis-dependent.[84]

Some individual trials provide evidence on the efficacy of anti-hypertensives for stroke prevention in specific patient subgroups. For patients with isolated systolic hypertension over age of 60 years, the Systolic Hypertension in the Elderly Program (SHEP) found a 36% reduction in the incidence of stroke with treatment with a thiazide diuretic with or without a β-blocker.[85] ALLHAT (The Antihypertensive and Lipid-Lowering Treatment to Prevent Heart Attack Trial) demonstrated the superiority of diuretic-based over a-blocker-based antihypertensive treatment for the prevention of stroke and cardiovascular events in a randomized, double-blind, active, controlled clinical trial including 24,316 participants.[86]

There is conflicting evidence regarding the efficacy of calcium channel blockers for stroke prevention. In the Systolic Hypertension in Europe (Syst-Eur) Trial, a 42% stroke risk reduction was found among patients with isolated systolic hypertension treated with a calcium channel blocker (nitrendipine) compared to placebo.[87] Data from the CONVINCE (Controlled ONset Verapamil INvestigation of Cardiovascular Endpoints) trial, however, did not find benefit for cardiovascular risk reduction for another calcium channel blocker (verapamil) compared with a diuretic or beta-blocker treatment.[88] In the ASCOT-BPLA trial, a combination of atenolol (β-blocker) with a thiazide prevented more major cardiovascular events and was associated with less diabetes than amlodipine (a calcium channel blocker) with perindopril (an ACEI).[89]

Some of the most convincing evidence regarding the benefits of ACE-I comes from the Heart Outcomes Prevention Evaluation (HOPE) study that demonstrated that ramipril (an ACEI) reduced the risk of cardiovascular events by approximately 20% compared with placebo in patients at risk for cardiovascular events without heart failure.[90] A substudy, the Study to Evaluate Carotid Ultrasound Changes in Patients Treated with Ramipril and Vitamin E (SECURE), also found that ramipril reduced carotid atherosclerosis.[91] Other ACEIs have not fared as well. Among 10,985 patients in the Captopril Prevention Project (CAPPP), no difference in efficacy was found between an ACE-inhibitor-based therapeutic regimen (captopril) compared to conventional anti-hypertensive therapy (diuretics, β-blockers) in preventing cardiovascular morbidity and mortality.[92]

Angiotensin II type 1 receptor antagonists (ARBs) have been proposed as being better tolerated than ACEIs. The LIFE (Losartan Intervention for Endpoint Reduction in Hypertension) study found a substantial reduction in stroke risk among 9,193 participants aged 55–80 years with essential hypertension treated with an ARB compared to conventional therapy with atenolol (β-blocker) for a similar reduction in blood pressure.[93]

The hypothesis that combined treatment with both an ACEI and ARB may be beneficial was assessed in the Ongoing Telmisartan Alone and in Combination with Ramipril Global

Endpoint Trial (ONTARGET).[94] This large trial compared the benefits of ACE inhibitor treatment, ARB treatment, and treatment with an ACE inhibitor and ARB together. In the parallel study, TRANSEND (Telmisartan Randomized Assessment Study in ACEI Intolerant Patients with Cardiovascular Disease), patients unable to tolerate an ACE inhibitor were randomized to receive an ARB (telmisartan) or placebo. The results of these landmark trials show that telmisartan, a second-generation ARB, was as effective as the current standard, ramipril (ACEI), in reducing the risk of stroke, myocardial infarction, cardiovascular death, and hospitalization for congestive heart failure in a broad spectrum of high-risk cardiovascular patients. The combination of an ACEI (ramipril) and an ARB (telmisartan), however, did not show any advantages compared to single blockade.

Combinations of an ACEI and calcium channel blocker have also been assessed. In the Avoiding Cardiovascular events through Combination therapy in Patients Living with Systolic Hypertension (ACCOMPLISH) trial, the effects of two forms of antihypertensive combination therapy (benazepril plus hydrochlorothiazide and amlodipine plus benazepril) were compared for the reduction of major fatal and non-fatal cardiovascular events in 11,454 hypertensive patients at high cardiovascular risk.[95] The study was terminated early because combination ACEI plus the calcium channel blocker was more effective than combination treatment with ACEI plus the diuretic.

Treatment of hypertension is beneficial for younger, as well as older, patients. In the Hypertension in the Very Elderly Trial (HYVET), among 3,845 individuals 80 years of age or older with a sustained systolic blood pressure of 160 mmHg or more, a 30% reduction in the rate of fatal or non-fatal stroke and a 39% reduction in the rate of death from stroke was achieved on active treatment (the diuretic indapamide with addition of ACEI perindopril if needed to achieve the target blood pressure of 150/80 mmHg) in comparison to placebo.[96] In another meta-analysis of 31 trials, among 190,606 participants, the benefits of blood pressure reduction were found in younger (<65 years) and older (≥65 years) adults with no strong evidence that protection against stroke and other vascular events varies substantially with age.[97]

It is well established that blood pressure lowering is effective for the primary prevention of stroke and other cardiovascular disorders. Although pharmacotherapies have helped achieve blood pressure control in most patients, the majority require combination therapy, often with more than two antihypertensive medications.[98] Despite the evidence from clinical trials, blood pressure levels are adequately controlled in less than 25% of the hypertensive population worldwide.[99] Many more strokes could be prevented with more effective treatment of hypertension. Lack of diagnosis and inadequate treatment are of particular importance among minority populations and in the elderly.[81,100]

Current AHA guidelines for primary stroke prevention call for regular screening for hypertension and appropriate management (*Class I; Level of Evidence A*), including dietary changes, lifestyle modification, and pharmacological therapy.[1]

Diabetes

Diabetes increases the risk of stroke nearly threefold and disproportionately affects the elderly and minority populations.[101] Moreover, the duration of diabetes increases the risk of ischemic stroke risk 3% each year, and triples with those who have had diabetes for 10 years or more.[102] Although generally considered a disease having pathophysiological effects related to impaired blood glucose control, there remains no evidence that tight control of blood glucose levels reduces the risk of stroke or cardiovascular events in diabetic patients. The hypothesis was directly tested in several clinical trials.

The Action to Control Cardiovascular Risk in Type 2 Diabetes (ACCORD) study randomized 10,251 patients with a median glycated hemoglobin of 8.1% to intensive blood glucose control (target glycated hemoglobin less than 6%) or standard control (glycated hemoglobin 7.0 to 7.9%).[103] The study was stopped because of higher mortality rates in the intensive control group (hazard ratio = 1.22, 95%CI 1.01–1.46, $P = 0.04$). There was no difference in the risk of non-fatal stroke (hazard ratio = 1.06, 95%CI 0.75–1.50, $P = 0.74$). The Action in Diabetes and Vascular Disease: Preterax and Diamicron Modified Release Controlled Evaluation (ADVANCE) trial randomized 11,140 patients with diabetes to intensive blood glucose control (target glycated hemoglobin less than 6.5%) or standard therapy.[104] Although there was a treatment-related reduction in nephropathy, there was no reduction in macrovascular events (hazard ratio = 0.94, 95%CI 0.84–1.06, $P = 0.32$) including no reduction in non-fatal stroke (relative risk reduction −2%, 95%CI −24–15%). The United Kingdom Prospective Diabetes Study (UKPDS) had also found that newly diagnosed patients with type 2 diabetes had a lower risk of microvascular complications with intensive therapy.[105] Post-trial 10-year follow-up found that, although the initial difference in glycated hemoglobin was not evident after the first year, reduction in microvascular complications persisted and reductions in the rate of myocardial infarction and death emerged over time.[106] There was, however, not a significant reduction in stroke (risk ratio 0.80, 95%CI 0.50–1.27, $P = 0.35$). The Veterans Affairs Diabetes Trial (VADT) randomized 1,791 veterans who had diabetes for a mean of 11.5 years, but who had a suboptimal response to treatment (40% had a cardiovascular event) to intensive blood glucose control or standard therapy.[107] There was no effect of intensive control (mean glycated hemoglobin 6.9% vs. 8.4%) on the occurrence of major cardiovascular events (hazard ratio = 0.88, 95%CI 0.74–1.05, $P = 0.14$), again including no impact on stroke (hazard ratio = 0.78, 95%CI 0.48–1.28, $P = 0.32$). Therefore, evidence that intensive blood glucose control decreases the risk of stroke, or other cardiovascular events, in persons with diabetes is lacking.

Despite these disappointing results, treatments other than intensive blood glucose control have been associated with reductions in the risk of stroke in patients with diabetes. The UKPDS compared the effects of tight blood pressure control (target <150/85 mm Hg, mean achieved 144/82mm Hg) with less tight control (mean 154/87 mm Hg) in 1148 hypertensive patients with type 2 diabetes finding that tight control led to a 44% reduction (relative risk = 0.56, 95%CI 0.35–0.89, $P = 0.01$) in the risk of stroke over a median of 8.4 years.[108] The between-group difference in blood pressures became insignificant after the trial was completed with benefits decreasing over time; by 10 years the reduction in stroke was reduced by half and no longer significant (relative risk = 23%, $P = 0.12$), suggesting that tight blood pressure control needs to be sustained.[109] The Systolic Hypertension in the Elderly Program (SHEP) found that anti-hypertensive treatment of elderly diabetic patients led to a 34% (relative risk = 0.66, 95%CI 0.46–0.94) reduction in major cardiovascular events that included a 22% (relative risk = 0.78, 95%CI 0.45–1.034) reduction in stroke.[110] A substudy of 3,577 diabetic patients with a previous cardiovascular event or an additional cardiovascular risk factor enrolled in the Heart Outcomes Prevention Evaluation (HOPE) trial (of a total population of 9,541 participants in the HOPE study) found the addition of an ACEI to other antihypertensive drugs reduced a combined outcome of MI, stroke and cardiovascular death by 25% (95%CI 12–36, $P = 0.0004$) and stroke by 33% (95%CI 10–50; $P = 0.0074$).[90] A prespecified subanalysis of the Losartan Intervention for Endpoint (LIFE) reduction in hypertension study compared the effects of an angiotensin II type-1 receptor blocker with β-adrenergic receptor blocker in diabetic patients with essential hypertension (160–200/95–115 mmHg) and electrocardiographically determined left ventricular hypertrophy.[111] There was a 24% (relative risk = 0.76, 95%CI 0.58–0.98) reduction in major vascular events and a non-significant 21% (relative risk = 0.79, 95%CI 0.55–1.14) reduction in stroke among those treated with the angiotensin receptor blocker. The available data suggest careful treatment of hypertension in people with diabetes can reduce the risk of a first stroke. Control of blood pressures in patients with either type 1 or type 2 diabetes is recommended (*Class I; Level of Evidence A*).[1]

Persons with diabetes may also benefit from treatment with an HMG-CoA reductase inhibitor (statin). The MRC/BHF Heart Protection Study (HPS) found the addition of a statin to existing treatments resulted in a 22% (95%CI 13–30%) reduction in major vascular events (regardless of cholesterol levels) and a 24% (95%CI 6–39%, $P = 0.01$) reduction in strokes among 5,963 patients with diabetes.[112] Consistent with these results, the Collaborative Atorvastatin Diabetes Study (CARDS) found that treatment with a statin in subjects with type 2 diabetes, an LDL-C less than 160 mg/dL and at least one additional risk factor (retinopathy, albuminuria, current smoking, or hypertension) led to a 48% (95%CI 11–69%) reduction in the risk of a first stroke.[113] Treatment of adults with diabetes with a statin is recommended to lower risk of a first stroke (*Class I; Level of Evidence A*).[1]

Atrial Fibrillation

Non-valvular atrial fibrillation is an important, treatable risk factor for stroke. Depending on patient age, the population-attributable risk varies from 1.5% to 23.5% with relative risks varying from approximately 2.5 to 4.5.[1] A systematic literature review identified 29 randomized trials including over 28,000 subjects evaluating the impact of antithrombotic therapy in patients with atrial fibrillation.[114] Treatment with antiplatelet drugs reduced the risk of stroke by 22% (95%CI 6–35%) whereas dose-adjusted warfarin reduced risk by 64% (95%CI 49–74%) with warfarin more efficacious than antiplatelet therapy (relative risk reduction 39%, 95%CI 22–52%). These reductions included the risk of antithrombotic-related intracranial hemorrhage.

The risk of stroke, and therefore the benefits vs risks of antithrombotic therapy, is not uniform for all patients with non-valvular atrial fibrillation. As noted above, the population-attributable and relative risks of atrial fibrillation-related stroke increases with advancing age. A systematic review assessed the impact of a series of potential factors on the risk of stroke in patients with atrial fibrillation based on studies using multivariable regression analyses.[115] Increasing age (relative risk = 1.5 per decade, 95%CI 1.3–1.7; absolute rate 1.5–3% per year for age over 75), a history of hypertension (relative risk = 2.0, 95%CI 1.6–2.5; absolute rate 1.5 to 3% per year), and diabetes mellitus (relative risk = 1.7, 95%CI 1.4–2.0; absolute rate 2.0 to 3.5% per year) were the strongest, most consistent independent risk factors.

There have been more than 12 schemes developed and published that stratify the stroke risk of patients with atrial fibrillation.[18] The rates of stroke predicted by these various schemes vary widely. This systematic review found that observed rates for those categorized as low risk ranged from 0% to 2.3% per year with rates for those categorized as being at high risk ranging from 2.5% to 7.9% annually.[18] When these schemes were applied to the same cohorts, the proportions of patients categorized as low risk varied from 9% to 49% and those categorized as high risk varied from 11% to 77%.[18] Although the $CHADS_2$ (congestive heart failure, hypertension, age >75 years, diabetes, 1 point each; stroke or TIA, 2 points) score is commonly used and predicts stroke risk (score = 0–1, low risk, stroke rate ~ 1% per year; score = 2, moderate risk, 2.5% per year; score ≥3, high risk, >5% per year), it includes a history of prior stroke or TIA.[116] In the absence of specific contraindications, the benefits of warfarin generally outweigh the risks when the predicted annual stroke rate is more than 4%.[1] The systematic review, however, concluded that, "additional research to identify an optimum scheme for primary prevention."[18]

In addition to the limitations of the $CHADS_2$ score discussed above, approximately 60% receive a score = 1, corresponding to a 2.8% annual stroke risk, a rate for which the risks and benefits of anticoagulation are balanced leading to uncertainty regarding treatment. The CHA_2DS_2VASc includes additional risk prediction variables (congestive heart failure/left ventricular dysfunction, hypertension, diabetes, prior stroke or TIA, other vascular disease, and sex) and when applied to the same cohort, identifies fewer patients as having intermediate level risk.[117] The calibrations of the two scores, however, are similar ($CHADS_2$, c = 0.59, 95%CI 0.48–0.70 vs CHA_2DS_2VASc, c = 0.61, 95%CI 0.51–0.70).[117]

There is commonly concern among physicians about the risks of warfarin among the elderly. Advancing age, however, is associated with increasing risk of atrial-fibrillation-related stroke. A small, open label, safety study in patients with atrial fibrillation age 80 to 89 years found dose-adjusted warfarin was better tolerated than 300 mg of aspirin daily.[118] The Birmingham Atrial Fibrillation Treatment of the Aged (BAFTA) study was an open label, randomized comparison of dose-adjusted warfarin vs 75 mg of aspirin daily in patients with atrial fibrillation over 75 year of age.[119] Based on a treatment-masked assessment of outcomes, the risk of stroke was reduced by nearly half with warfarin (annual risk 1.8% vs 3.8%; relative risk = 0.48, 95%CI 0.28–0.80, $P = 0.003$). The annual risks of extracranial hemorrhage were 1.4% for warfarin compared to 1.6% for aspirin. These results suggest that concern about the risk of warfarin-associated hemorrhage in the elderly may be overestimated with the benefits outweighing the risks in the absence of specific contraindications.

Because of concerns about drug interactions, food interactions, the need for monitoring and the risk of bleeding complications, there was a clear clinical need for anticoagulant alternatives to warfarin. Several novel oral anticoagulants have now been evaluated in randomized trials in comparison to warfarin. In comparison to warfarin, dabigatran, a direct thrombin inhibitor was studied in the Randomized Evaluation of Long-Term Anticoagulation Therapy (RE-LY) trial.[120] There have also been trials of three factor Xa inhibitors. Rivaroxaban was evaluated in the ROCKET AF trial,[121] apixaban in the ARISTOTLE trial,[122] and edoxaban in the ENGAGE AF trial.[123] A detailed discussion of each of these alternatives to warfarin for patients with atrial fibrillation is beyond the scope of this chapter. Each is not inferior to warfarin for the prevention of stroke/systemic embolization and associated with a lower risk of intracranial hemorrhage. Direct comparative studies among the novel oral anticoagulants have not been conducted. There are presently no clinically proven reversal agents to be used in the setting of bleeding complications, although dialysis or the administration of activated prothrombin-concentrate may be useful for patients receiving dabigatran and 4-factor prothrombin-concentrate (factors II, VII, IX, X) may be helpful for those receiving rivaroxaban, apixaban, and presumably edoxaban.[124] Each may or may not prolong the prothrombin or activated thromboplastin times. At present, there are no available assays to determine the level of anticoagulation with these agents for use in emergency situations, such as determining suitability for treatment with intravenous r-tPA in the setting of acute ischemic stroke. There can be clinically important interactions with p-glycoprotein inhibitors such as verapamil, quinidine and amiodarone, and with CYP3A4 inhibitors and inducers.[125] Doses need to be adjusted in patients with moderate renal impairment, and depending on the agent, certain other conditions; in addition these drugs are contraindicated in patients with severe renal impairment.[125] They are contraindicated in patients with mechanical heart valves. Warfarin *(Class I; Level of Evidence A)*, dabigatran *(Class I; Level of Evidence B)*, apixaban *(Class I; Level of Evidence B)*, and rivaroxaban *(Class IIa; Level of Evidence B)* are all indicated for the prevention of a first and recurrent stroke in patients with non-valvular atrial fibrillation, depending on specific patient characteristics.[125] Data on edoxaban were not available at the time of the most recent guideline review and has not yet been FDA approved.

Aspirin is commonly used for stroke prevention in patients with atrial fibrillation who are thought unsuitable or who are unable to take warfarin. Aspirin alone is indicated for patients unable to take oral anticoagulants *(Class I; Level of Evidence A)*.[125] The ACTIVE trial compared aspirin versus aspirin plus clopidogrel in this population.[126] The combination is associated with a reduction in the risk of stroke, systemic embolization or vascular death (relative risk = 0.89, 95%CI 0.81–0.98), but an increase in major bleeding (relative risk = 1.57, 95%CI 1.29–1.92) with no overall benefit (relative risk = 0.97, 95%CI 0.89–1.06). Dual antiplatelet therapy with aspirin and clopidogrel might be reasonable as it offers more stroke protection than aspirin, but with an increased risk of major bleeding *(Class IIb; Level of Evidence B)*.[125]

Apixaban versus aspirin for patients with atrial fibrillation who were unsuitable or refused warfarin was evaluated in the AVERROES trial.[127] The trial was terminated early for efficacy. Apixaban was associated with similar rates of bleeding complications, but lower rates of stroke or systemic embolization (hazard ratio = 0.45, 95%CI 0.32–0.62) compared to aspirin. Apixaban is useful as an alternative to aspirin in selected patients with non-valvular atrial fibrillation who are unsuitable for warfarin *(Class I; Level of Evidence B)*.[125]

Sleep-Disordered Breathing

Sleep apnea is associated with an increased risk of cardiovascular disease and stroke. For example, a longitudinal prospective study found that sleep apnea more than doubled the risk of developing a first stroke (hazard ratio = 2.52, 95%CI 1.04–6.01).[128] Another found that severe sleep apnea was associated with a three- to fourfold increase in stroke risk in patients with established coronary heart disease (hazard ratio = 3.56, 95 CI 1.56–8.16).[129] There are, however, no prospective trials showing that treatment of sleep apnea reduces stroke risk. AHA Primary Stroke Prevention Guidelines indicate that treatment of sleep apnea to reduce stroke risk might be reasonable, although its effectiveness is unknown *(Class IIb; Level of Evidence C)*.[1]

OTHER PREVENTIVE THERAPIES

Aspirin

The use of aspirin in the setting of non-valvular atrial fibrillation was reviewed in the previous section. There is no evidence that platelet anti-aggregants reduce the risk of stroke in persons without atrial fibrillation at otherwise low stroke risk. [130–132] Because the risk of coronary heart disease generally outweighs the risk of stroke, coronary heart risk generally drives recommendations for the use of aspirin. The U.S. Preventive Services Task Force recommends 75 mg of aspirin per day for cardiac prophylaxis for persons whose 5-year coronary heart disease risk is ≥3%.[130] American Heart Association Guidelines for the primary prevention of cardiovascular disease and stroke recommends aspirin if the patient has ≥10% risk per 10 years, rather than >3% risk over 5 years.[133] This excludes patients with atrial fibrillation (discussed above) and patients who have had a carotid endarterectomy.[134]

The majority of patients included in the aspirin prevention studies were men. The Women's Health Study (WHS) randomized 39,876 initially asymptomatic women 45 years of age or older to receive 100 mg of aspirin on alternate days or placebo (combined primary endpoint was non-fatal MI, non-fatal stroke or cardiovascular death).[135] There was a non-significant reduction in the primary endpoint with aspirin (relative risk = 0.91, 95%CI 0.80–1.03, *P* = 0.13), but a significant reduction in the risk of stroke (relative risk = 0.83, 95%CI 0.69–0.99, *P* = 0.04; 0.11% per year in aspirin-treated patients and 0.13% per year in placebo-treated patients, absolute risk reduction = 0.02% per year, Number Needed to Treat = 5,000). Gastrointestinal hemorrhage requiring transfusion was more frequent in the aspirin group (relative risk = 1.40, 95%CI 1.07–1.83, *P* = 0.02). Subgroup analyses showed the most consistent benefit with treatment in women having a 10-year cardiovascular risk ≥10% (relative risk = 0.54; 95%CI 0.30–0.98; *P* = 0.04). Similar to the previous recommendations, the 2007 Update of the AHA Evidence-Based Guidelines for Cardiovascular Disease Prevention in Women recommended that women be considered for aspirin therapy for primary stroke prevention depending on the balance of risks and benefits.[136]

Although diabetes is a coronary heart disease equivalent, there is a paucity of data supporting the use of aspirin in patients with diabetes and no other symptomatic vascular disease. Meta-analysis of trials of aspirin for cardiovascular prevention found no definite benefit of aspirin among those with diabetes, but the possibility of benefit could not be excluded (rate ratio = 0.88, 95%CI 0.67–1.15).[137] The POPADAD trial found no benefit of aspirin in patients with diabetes and asymptomatic peripheral vascular disease (combined risk of death from coronary heart disease or stroke, non-fatal MI or stroke, or amputation for critical limb ischemia, hazard ratio = 0.98, 95%CI 0.76–1.26), including no reduction in fatal (hazard ratio = 0.89, 95%CI 0.34–2.30) or non-fatal (hazard ratio = 0.71, 95%CI 0.44–1.14) stroke.[138]

AHA Primary Stroke Prevention Guidelines recommend the use of aspirin for cardiovascular (including but not specific to stroke) prophylaxis for persons whose risk is sufficiently high for the benefits to outweigh the risks associated with treatment (i.e., a 10-year risk of cardiovascular events of at least 10%) *(Class IIa; Level of Evidence A)*.[1] Aspirin is not indicated for preventing a first stroke in persons with diabetes or diabetes plus asymptomatic peripheral artery disease in the absence of other established cardiovascular disease *(Class III; Level of Evidence B)*.[1]

Lipid-Lowering Therapy

Unlike coronary heart disease, there is only a weak relationship between lipid levels and stroke risk,[139] however, lipids may have a more specific relationship with carotid atherosclerosis and atherosclerotic stroke subtypes.[140,141] Meta-analysis finds no significant reduction in stroke risk with a variety of lipid-lowering therapies including diet (ten trials, risk ratio, relative risk = 0.99, 95%CI 0.85–1.15), fibrates (11 trials, relative risk = 1.04, 95%CI 0.92–1.19), resins (four trials, relative risk = 1.03, 95%CI 0.54–2.00), or omega-3 fatty acids (eight trials, relative risk = 0.91, 95%CI 0.56–1.48).[142] In contrast, meta-analysis shows that treatment of patients with a history of coronary heart disease or other high-risk conditions with statins reduces the risk of a first non-fatal or fatal stroke by 19% (relative risk = 0·81, 95%CI 0·75–0·87) with a trend for a similar reduction in hemorrhagic stroke (relative risk = 0·81, 95%CI 0·60–1·08).[143] Statin treatment is recommended for primary prevention of ischemic stroke in patients with coronary heart disease or other high-risk conditions such as diabetes (*Class I; Level of Evidence A*).[1]

The Justification for the use of Statins in Primary Prevention: an Interventional Trial Evaluating Rosuvastatin (JUPITER) trial randomized 17,802 cardiovascular disease-free men over age 55 and women over age 65 with an LDL-C less than 130 mg/dL, but evidence of systemic inflammation based on an elevated high-sensitivity C reactive protein more than 2 mg/L to statin therapy or placebo.[144] Treatment resulted in a 44% (hazard ratio = 0.56, 95%CI 0.46–0.69, $P < 0.00001$) reduction in the time to a combined cardiovascular endpoint that included a 48% (hazard ratio = 0.52, 95%CI 0.34–0.79, $P = 0.002$) reduction in the risk of stroke. Further work will need to be done to determine the usefulness of widescale population screening to identify patients who might benefit from statin treatment.[145]

REFERENCES

1. Meschia JF, Bushnell C, Boden-Albala B, et al. Guidelines for the primary prevention of stroke. Stroke 2014;45:3754–832.
2. Strong JP, Malcom GT, McMahan C, et al. Prevalence and extent of atherosclerosis in adolescents and young adults: Implications for prevention from the pathobiological determinants of atherosclerosis in youth study. JAMA 1999;281:727–35.
3. May AL, Kuklina EV, Yoon PW. Prevalence of cardiovascular disease risk factors among US adolescents, 1999-2008. Pediatrics 2012;129:1035–41.
4. Ford ES, Capewell S. Proportion of the decline in cardiovascular mortality disease due to prevention versus treatment: public health versus clinical care. Annu Rev Public Health 2011;32: 5–22.
5. Chokshi DA, Farley TA. The cost-effectiveness of environmental approaches to disease prevention. N Engl J Med 2012;367: 295–7.
6. Go AS, Mozaffarian D, Roger VL, et al. Heart Disease and Stroke Statistics—2013 Update A Report From the American Heart Association. Circulation 2012;127:e6–245.
7. Ezzati M, Riboli E. Behavioral and dietary risk factors for noncommunicable diseases. N Engl J Med 2013;369:954–64.
8. Pearson TA, Palaniappan LP, Artinian NT, et al. American Heart Association Guide for Improving Cardiovascular Health at the Community Level, 2013 update: a scientific statement for public health practitioners, healthcare providers, and health policy makers. Circulation 2013;127:1730–53.
9. Grundy SM, Pasternak R, Greenland P, et al. Assessment of cardiovascular risk by use of multiple-risk-factor assessment equations: A statement for healthcare professionals from the American Heart Association and the American College of Cardiology. J Am Coll Cardiol 1999;34:1348–59.
10. Sacco RL. The 2006 William Feinberg Lecture: shifting the paradigm from stroke to global vascular risk estimation. Stroke 2007;38:1980–7.
11. Sacco RL, Khatri M, Rundek T, et al. Improving global vascular risk prediction with behavioral and anthropometric factors. The multiethnic NOMAS (Northern Manhattan Cohort Study). J Am Coll Cardiol 2009;54:2303–11.
12. Goff DC Jr, Lloyd-Jones DM, Bennett G, et al. 2013 ACC/AHA Guideline on the Assessment of Cardiovascular Risk: A Report of the American College of Cardiology/American Heart Association Task Force on Practice Guidelines. J Am Coll Cardiol 2013.
13. Ridker PM, Cook NR. Statins: new American guidelines for prevention of cardiovascular disease. Lancet 2013.
14. Wolf PA, D'Agostino RB, Belanger AJ, et al. Probability of stroke: a risk profile from the Framingham Study. Stroke 1991;22: 312–18.
15. D'Agostino RB, Wolf PA, Belanger AJ, et al. Stroke risk profile: adjustment for antihypertensive medication. The Framingham Study. Stroke 1994;25:40–3.
16. Wang TJ, Massaro JM, Levy D, et al. A risk score for predicting stroke or death in individuals with new-onset atrial fibrillation in the community: The Framingham Heart Study. JAMA 2003; 290:1049–56.
17. Lumley T, Kronmal RA, Cushman M, et al. A stroke prediction score in the elderly: validation and web-based application. J Clin Epidemiol 2002;55:129–36.
18. Hart RG, Pearce LA, Halperin JL, et al. Comparison of 12 risk stratification schemes to predict stroke in patients with nonvalvular atrial fibrillation. Stroke 2008;39:1901–10.
19. Chiuve SE, Rexrode KM, Spiegelman D, et al. Primary prevention of stroke by healthy lifestyle. Circulation 2008;118:947–54.
20. Dong C, Rundek T, Wright CB, et al. Ideal cardiovascular health predicts lower risks of myocardial infarction, stroke, and vascular death across whites, blacks, and hispanics: the northern Manhattan study. Circulation 2012;125:2975–84.
21. Wolf PA, D'Agostino RB, Kannel WB, et al. Cigarette smoking as a risk factor for stroke. The Framingham Study. JAMA 1988; 259:1025–9.
22. Manolio TA, Kronmal RA, Burke GL, et al. Short-term predictors of incident stroke in older adults: The Cardiovascular Health Study. Stroke 1996;27:1479–86.
23. Broderick JP, Viscoli CM, Brott T, et al. Major risk factors for aneurysmal subarachnoid hemorrhage in the young are modifiable. Stroke 2003;34:1375–81.
24. Surgeon General of the United States. The Centers for Disease Control. The Surgeon General's 1989 Report on Reducing the Health Consequences of Smoking: 25 Years of Progress. MMWR Morb Mortal Wkly Rep 1989;38:(Suppl. 2): 1-32.
25. Shinton R, Beevers G. Meta-analysis of relation between cigarette smoking and stroke. BMJ 1989;298:789–94.
26. Fagerstrom K. The epidemiology of smoking: health consequences and benefits of cessation. Drugs 2002;62(Suppl. 2): 1–9.
27. Kawachi I, Colditz GA, Stampfer MJ, et al. Smoking cessation and decreased risk of stroke in women. JAMA 1993;269: 232–6.
28. Fiore MC. U.S. Public Health Service Clinical Practice Guideline: treating tobacco use and dependence. Respir Care 2000;45: 1200–62.
29. Galanti LM. Tobacco smoking cessation management: integrating varenicline in current practice. Vasc Health Risk Manag 2008;4:837–45.
30. Stead LF, Perera R, Bullen C, et al. Nicotine replacement therapy for smoking cessation. Cochrane Database Syst Rev 2008; (23):CD000146.
31. McCarthy DE, Piasecki TM, Lawrence DL, et al. A randomized controlled clinical trial of bupropion SR and individual smoking cessation counseling. Nicotine Tob Res 2008;10:717–29.
32. Aubin H-J, Bobak A, Britton JR, et al. Varenicline versus transdermal nicotine patch for smoking cessation: results from a randomised open-label trial. Thorax 2008;63:717–24.
33. Cahill K, Stead LF, Lancaster T. Nicotine receptor partial agonists for smoking cessation. Cochrane Database Syst Rev 2008; (16):CD006103.
34. Fletcher GF. Exercise in the prevention of stroke. Health Rep 1994;6:106–10.
35. Wendel-Vos GCW, Schuit AJ, Feskens EJM, et al. Physical activity and stroke. A meta-analysis of observational data. Intern J Epidemiol 2004;33:787–98.
36. Lee CD, Folsom AR, Blair SN. Physical activity and stroke risk: a meta-analysis. Stroke 2003;34:2475–81.
37. Gillum RF, Mussolino ME, Ingram DD. Physical activity and stroke incidence in women and men: The NHANES I Epidemiologic Follow-up Study. Am J Epidemiol 1996;143: 860–9.
38. Sacco RL, Gan R, Boden-Albala B, et al. Leisure-time physical activity and ischemic stroke risk: The Northern Manhattan Stroke Study. Stroke 1998;29:380–7.
39. Willey JZ, Moon YP, Paik MC, et al. Physical activity and risk of ischemic stroke in the Northern Manhattan Study. Neurology 2009;73:1774–9.

40. Sattelmair JR, Kurth T, Buring JE, et al. Physical activity and risk of stroke in women. Stroke 2010;41:1243–50.
41. Shinton R, Sagar G. Lifelong exercise and stroke. Br Med J 1993;307:231–4.
42. Karmisholt K, Gyntelberg F, Gøtzche PC. Physical activity for primary prevention of disease. Systematic reviews of randomised clinical trials. Dan Med Bull 2005;52:86–9.
43. NIH develops consensus statement on the role of physical activity for cardiovascular health. Am Fam Physician 1996;54: 763–7.
44. Pate RR, Pratt M, Blair SN, et al. Physical activity and public health: a recommendation from the Centers for Disease Control and Prevention and the American College of Sports Medicine. JAMA 1995;273:402–7.
45. Eyre H, Kahn R, Robertson RM, et al. Preventing cancer, cardiovascular disease, and diabetes: a common agenda for the American Cancer Society, the American Diabetes Association, and the American Heart Association. Circulation 2004;109: 3244–55.
46. Heyden S, Hames CG, Bartel A, et al. Weight and weight history in relation to cerebrovascular and ischemic heart disease. Arch Intern Med 1971;128:956–60.
47. Suk S-H, Sacco RL, Boden-Albala B, et al. Abdominal obesity and risk of ischemic stroke: The Northern Manhattan Stroke Study. Stroke 2003;34:1586–92.
48. Boden-Albala B, Sacco RL, Lee H-S, et al. Metabolic syndrome and ischemic stroke risk: Northern Manhattan Study. Stroke 2008;39:30–5.
49. Neter JE, Stam BE, Kok FJ, et al. Influence of weight reduction on blood pressure: a meta-analysis of randomized controlled trials. Hypertension 2003;42:878–84.
50. Chobanian AV, Bakris GL, Black HR, et al. The Seventh Report of the Joint National Committee on Prevention, Detection, Evaluation, and Treatment of High Blood Pressure: The JNC 7 Report. JAMA 2003;289:2560–71.
51. Stone NJ, Robinson J, Lichtenstein AH, et al. 2013 ACC/AHA Guideline on the Treatment of Blood Cholesterol to Reduce Atherosclerotic Cardiovascular Risk in Adults: A Report of the American College of Cardiology/American Heart Association Task Force on Practice Guidelines. Circulation 2013.
52. Steffen LM, Jacobs DR, Stevens J, et al. Associations of whole-grain, refined-grain, and fruit and vegetable consumption with risks of all-cause mortality and incident coronary artery disease and ischemic stroke: the Atherosclerosis Risk in Communities (ARIC) Study. Am J Clin Nutr 2003;78:383–90.
53. Joshipura KJ, Ascherio A, Manson JE, et al. Fruit and vegetable intake in relation to risk of ischemic stroke. JAMA 1999; 282:1233–9.
54. Ding EL, Mozaffarian D. Optimal dietary habits for the prevention of stroke. Semin Neurol 2006;26:11–23.
55. Serra-Majem L, Roman B, Estruch R. Scientific evidence of interventions using the Mediterranean Diet: a systematic review. Nutr Rev 2006;64:S27–47.
56. Gardener H, Wright CB, Gu Y, et al. Mediterranean-style diet and risk of ischemic stroke, myocardial infarction, and vascular death: the Northern Manhattan Study. Am J Clin Nutr 2011;94: 1458–64.
57. Misirli G, Benetou V, Lagiou P, et al. Relation of the traditional Mediterranean diet to cerebrovascular disease in a Mediterranean population. Am J Epidemiol 2012;176:1185–92.
58. Gardener H, Rundek T, Wright CB, et al. Dietary sodium and risk of stroke in the Northern Manhattan study. Stroke 2012; 43:1200–5.
59. Kotchen TA, Cowley AW Jr, Frohlich ED. Salt in health and disease – a delicate balance. N Engl J Med 2013;368:1229–37.
60. Appel LJ, Moore TJ, Obarzanek E, et al. A clinical trial of the effects of dietary patterns on blood pressure. N Engl J Med 1997;336:1117–24.
61. John JH, Ziebland S, Yudkin P, et al. Effects of fruit and vegetable consumption on plasma antioxidant concentrations and blood pressure: a randomised controlled trial. Lancet 2002;359: 1969–74.
62. Estruch R, Ros E, Salas-Salvado J, et al. Primary prevention of cardiovascular disease with a Mediterranean diet. N Engl J Med 2013;368:1279–90.
63. Whelton PK, Appel LJ, Sacco RL, et al. Sodium, blood pressure, and cardiovascular disease: further evidence supporting the American Heart Association sodium reduction recommendations. Circulation 2012;126:2880–9.
64. Elkind MS, Sciacca R, Boden-Albala B, et al. Moderate alcohol consumption reduces risk of ischemic stroke: The Northern Manhattan Study. Stroke 2006;37:13–19.
65. Bazzano LA, Gu D, Reynolds K, et al. Alcohol consumption and risk for stroke among Chinese men. Ann Neurol 2007;62: 569–78.
66. Reynolds K, Lewis LB, Nolen JDL, et al. Alcohol consumption and risk of sroke: a meta-analysis. JAMA 2003;289:579–88.
67. Berger K, Ajani UA, Kase CS, et al. Light-to-moderate alcohol consumption and the risk of stroke among U.S. male physicians. N Engl J Med 1999;341:1557–64.
68. Djoussé L, Levy D, Benjamin EJ, et al. Long-term alcohol consumption and the risk of atrial fibrillation in the Framingham Study. Am J Cardiol 2004;93:710–13.
69. Brust JCM. Neurological Aspects of Substance Abuse. Philadelphia: Butterworth-Heinemann; 2004.
70. Levine SR, Brust JC, Futrell N, et al. Cerebrovascular complications of the use of the "crack" form of alkaloidal cocaine. N Engl J Med 1990;323:699–704.
71. Sloan MA, Marc F. Illicit drug use/abuse and stroke. Handbook of Clinical Neurology. Elsevier; 2008. p. 823–40.
72. Neiman J, Haapaniemi HM, Hillbom M. Neurological complications of drug abuse: pathophysiological mechanisms. Eur J Neurol 2000;7:595–606.
73. Cami J, Farre M. Drug addiction. N Engl J Med 2003;349: 975–86.
74. Chobanian AV, Bakris GL, Black HR, et al. The Seventh Report of the Joint National Committee on Prevention, Detection, Evaluation, and Treatment of High Blood Pressure: The JNC 7 Report. JAMA 2003;289:2560–71.
75. Prospective Studies Collaboration. Blood cholesterol and vascular mortality by age, sex, and blood pressure: a meta-analysis of individual data from 61 prospective studies with 55,000 vascular deaths. Lancet 2007;370:1829–39.
76. Lee M, Saver JL, Chang B, et al. Presence of baseline prehypertension and risk of incident stroke. Neurology 2011;77:1330–7.
77. James PA, Oparil S, Carter BL, et al. 2014 evidence-based guideline for the management of high blood pressure in adults: report from the panel members appointed to the eighth Joint National Committee (JNC 8). JAMA 2013.
78. JATOS Study Group. Principal results of the Japanese trial to assess optimal systolic blood pressure in elderly hypertensive patients (JATOS). Hypertens Res 2008;31:2115–27.
79. Ogihara T, Saruta T, Rakugi H, et al. Target blood pressure for treatment of isolated systolic hypertension in the elderly: valsartan in elderly isolated systolic hypertension study. Hypertension 2010;56:196–202.
80. Law MR, Morris JK, Wald NJ. Use of blood pressure lowering drugs in the prevention of cardiovascular disease: meta-analysis of 147 randomised trials in the context of expectations from prospective epidemiological studies. BMJ 2009;338:b1665.
81. Expert Panel on Detection E, Treatment of high blood cholesterol in adults. Executive summary of the Third Report of the National Cholesterol Education Program (NCEP) Expert Panel on Detection, Evaluation, and Treatment of High Blood Cholesterol in Adults (Adult Treatment Panel III). JAMA 2001;285: 2486–97.
82. Rothwell PM. Limitations of the usual blood-pressure hypothesis and importance of variability, instability, and episodic hypertension. Lancet 2010;375:938–48.
83. Webb AJS, Fischer U, Mehta Z, et al. Effects of antihypertensive-drug class on interindividual variation in blood pressure and risk of stroke: a systematic review and meta-analysis. Lancet 2010; 375:906–15.
84. Molnar MZ, Kalantar-Zadeh K, Lott EH, et al. ACE inhibitor and angiotensin receptor blocker use and mortality in patients with chronic kidney disease. J Am Coll Cardiol 2013.
85. SHEP Cooperative Research Group. Prevention of stroke by antihypertensive drug treatment in older persons with isolated systolic hypertension. Final results of the Systolic Hypertension in the Elderly Program (SHEP). JAMA 1991;265:3255–64.

86. ALLHAT Collaborative Research Group. Major outcomes in high-risk hypertensive patients randomized to angiotensin-converting enzyme inhibitor or calcium channel blocker vs diuretic: The Antihypertensive and Lipid-Lowering Treatment to Prevent Heart Attack Trial (ALLHAT). JAMA 2002;288: 2981–97.
87. Staessen JA, Fagard R, Thijs L, et al. Randomised double-blind comparison of placebo and active treatment for older patients with isolated systolic hypertension. Lancet 1997;350: 757–64.
88. Black HR, Elliott WJ, Grandits G, et al. Principal results of the Controlled Onset Verapamil Investigation of Cardiovascular End Points (CONVINCE) Trial. JAMA 2003;289:2073–82.
89. Dahlöf B, Sever PS, Poulter NR, et al. Prevention of cardiovascular events with an antihypertensive regimen of amlodipine adding perindopril as required versus atenolol adding bendroflumethiazide as required, in the Anglo-Scandinavian Cardiac Outcomes Trial-Blood Pressure Lowering Arm (ASCOT-BPLA): a multicentre randomised controlled trial. Lancet 2005;366: 895–906.
90. Heart Outcomes Prevention Evaluation Study Investigators. Effects of ramipril on cardiovascular and microvascular outcomes in people with diabetes mellitus: results of the HOPE study and MICRO-HOPE substudy. Lancet 2000;355: 253–9.
91. Lonn EM, Yusuf S, Dzavik V, et al. Effects of ramipril and vitamin E on atherosclerosis: The Study to Evaluate Carotid Ultrasound Changes in Patients Treated With Ramipril and Vitamin E (SECURE). Circulation 2001;103:919–25.
92. Hansson L, Lindholm LH, Niskanen L, et al. Effect of angiotensin-converting-enzyme inhibition compared with conventional therapy on cardiovascular morbidity and mortality in hypertension: the Captopril Prevention Project (CAPPP) randomised trial. Lancet 1999;353:611–16.
93. Dahlöf B, Devereux RB, Kjeldsen SE, et al. Cardiovascular morbidity and mortality in the Losartan Intervention For Endpoint reduction in hypertension study (LIFE): a randomised trial against atenolol. Lancet 2002;359:995–1003.
94. The ONTARGET Investigators. Telmisartan, ramipril, or both in patients at high risk for vascular events. N Engl J Med 2008; 358:1547–59.
95. Weber MA, Bakris GL, Dahlöf B, et al. Baseline characteristics in the Avoiding Cardiovascular events through Combination therapy in Patients Living with Systolic Hypertension (ACCOMPLISH) trial: a hypertensive population at high cardiovascular risk. Blood Press 2007;16:13–19.
96. Beckett NS, Peters R, Fletcher AE, et al. Treatment of hypertension in patients 80 years of age or older. N Engl J Med 2008; 358:1887–98.
97. Blood Pressure Lowering Treatment Trialists' Collaboration. Effects of different regimens to lower blood pressure on major cardiovascular events in older and younger adults: meta-analysis of randomised trials. Br Med J 2008;336:1121–3.
98. Cushman WC, Ford CE, Cutler JA, et al. Success and predictors of blood pressure control in diverse North American settings: the antihypertensive and lipid-lowering treatment to prevent heart attack trial (ALLHAT). J Clin Hypertens (Greenwich) 2002;4: 393–404.
99. Cutler DM, Long G, Berndt ER, et al. The value of antihypertensive drugs: a perspective on medical innovation. Health Aff 2007;26:97–110.
100. Douglas JG, Bakris GL, Epstein M, et al. Management of high blood pressure in African Americans: consensus statement of the Hypertension in African Americans Working Group of the International Society on Hypertension in Blacks. Arch Intern Med 2003;163:525–41.
101. Air EL, Kissela BM. Diabetes, the metabolic syndrome, and ischemic stroke: epidemiology and possible mechanisms. Diabetes Care 2007;30:3131–40.
102. Banerjee C, Moon YP, Paik MC, et al. Duration of diabetes and risk of ischemic stroke: the Northern Manhattan Study. Stroke 2012;43:1212–17.
103. Action to Control Cardiovascular Risk in Diabetes Study Group. Effects of intensive glucose lowering in type 2 diabetes. N Engl J Med 2008;358:2545–59.
104. Advance Collaborative Group. Intensive blood glucose control and vascular outcomes in patients with type 2 diabetes. N Engl J Med 2008;358:2560–72.
105. UK Prospective Diabetes Study Group. Intensive blood-glucose control with sulphonylureas or insulin compared with conventional treatment and risk of complications in patients with type 2 diabetes (UKPDS 33). Lancet 1998;352:837–53.
106. Holman RR, Paul SK, Bethel MA, et al. 10-year follow-up of intensive glucose control in type 2 diabetes. N Engl J Med 2008;359:1577–89.
107. Duckworth W, Abraira C, Moritz T, et al. Glucose control and vascular complications in veterans with type 2 diabetes. N Engl J Med 2009;360:129–39.
108. UK Prospective Diabetes Study Group. Tight blood pressure control and risk of macrovascular and microvascular complications in type 2 diabetes: UKPDS 38. BMJ 1998;317:703–13.
109. Holman RR, Paul SK, Bethel MA, et al. Long-term follow-up after tight control of blood pressure in type 2 diabetes. N Engl J Med 2008;359:1565–76.
110. Curb JD, Pressel SL, Cutler JA, et al. Effect of diuretic-based antihypertensive treatment on cardiovascular disease risk in older diabetic patients with isolated systolic hypertension. Systolic Hypertension in the Elderly Program Cooperative Research Group. JAMA 1996;276:1886–92.
111. Lindholm LH, Ibsen H, Dahlof B, et al. Cardiovascular morbidity and mortality in patients with diabetes in the Losartan Intervention For Endpoint reduction in hypertension study (LIFE): a randomised trial against atenolol. Lancet 2002;359: 1004–10.
112. Heart Protection Study Collaborative Group. MRC/BHF Heart Protection Study of cholesterol-lowering with simvastatin in 5963 people with diabetes: a randomized placebo-controlled trial. Lancet 2003;361:2005–16.
113. Colhoun HM, Betteridge DJ, Durrington PN, et al. Primary prevention of cardiovascular disease with atorvastatin in type 2 diabetes in the Collaborative Atorvastatin Diabetes Study (CARDS): multicentre randomised placebo-controlled trial. Lancet 2004;364:685–96.
114. Hart RG, Pearce LA, Aguilar MI. Meta-analysis: antithrombotic therapy to prevent stroke in patients who have nonvalvular atrial fibrillation. Ann Intern Med 2007;146:857–67.
115. Hart RG, Pearce LA, Albers GW, et al. Independent predictors of stroke in patients with atrial fibrillation: a systematic review. Neurology 2007;69:546–54.
116. Gage BF, Waterman AD, Shannon W, et al. Validation of clinical classification schemes for predicting stroke: results from the National Registry of Atrial Fibrillation. JAMA 2001;285: 2864–70.
117. Lip GY, Nieuwlaat R, Pisters R, et al. Refining clinical risk stratification for predicting stroke and thromboembolism in atrial fibrillation using a novel risk factor-based approach: the Euro Heart Survey on Atrial Fibrillation. Chest 2010;137: 263–72.
118. Rash A, Downes T, Portner R, et al. A randomised controlled trial of warfarin versus aspirin for stroke prevention in octogenarians with atrial fibrillation (WASPO). Age Ageing 2007;36:151–6.
119. Mant J, Hobbs FD, Fletcher K, et al. Warfarin versus aspirin for stroke prevention in an elderly community population with atrial fibrillation (the Birmingham Atrial Fibrillation Treatment of the Aged Study, BAFTA): a randomised controlled trial. Lancet 2007;370:493–503.
120. Connolly SJ, Ezekowitz MD, Yusuf S, et al. Dabigatran versus warfarin in patients with atrial fibrillation. N Engl J Med 2009; 361:1139–51.
121. Patel MR, Mahaffey KW, Garg J, et al. Rivaroxaban versus warfarin in nonvalvular atrial fibrillation. N Engl J Med 2011; 365:883–91.
122. Granger CB, Alexander JH, McMurray JJV, et al. Apixaban versus warfarin in patients with atrial fibrillation. N Engl J Med 2011;365:981–92.
123. Giugliano RP, Ruff CT, Braunwald E, et al. Edoxaban versus warfarin in patients with atrial fibrillation. N Engl J Med 2013.
124. Siegal DM, Cuker A. Reversal of novel oral anticoagulants in patients with major bleeding. J Thromb Thrombolysis 2013; 35:391–8.

125. Furie KL, Goldstein LB, Albers GW, et al. Oral antithrombotic agents for the prevention of stroke in nonvalvular atrial fibrillation. Stroke 2012;43:3442–53.
126. The ACTIVE Investigators. Effect of clopidogrel added to aspirin in patients with atrial fibrillation. N Engl J Med 2009;360: 2066–78.
127. Connolly SJ, Eikelboom J, Joyner C, et al. Apixaban in patients with atrial fibrillation. N Engl J Med 2011;364:806–17.
128. Munoz R, Duran-Cantolla J, Martinez-Vila E, et al. Severe sleep apnea and risk of ischemic stroke in the elderly. Stroke 2006;37:2317–21.
129. Valham F, Mooe T, Rabben T, et al. Increased risk of stroke in patients with coronary artery disease and sleep apnea: a 10-year follow-up. Circulation 2008;118:955–60.
130. Hayden M, Pigone M, Phillips C, et al. Aspirin for the primary prevention of cardiovascular events: a summary of the evidence for the US Preventive Services Task Force. Ann Intern Med 2002;136:161–72.
131. Antiplatelet Trialists' Collaboration. Collaborative overview of randomised trials of antiplatelet therapy – I: Prevention of death, myocardial infarction, and stroke by prolonged antiplatelet therapy in various categories of patients. BMJ 1994;308: 81–106.
132. Hart RG, Halperin JL, McBride R, et al. Aspirin for the primary prevention of stroke and other major vascular events: meta-analysis and hypotheses. Arch Neurol 2000;57:326–32.
133. Pearson TA, Blair SN, Daniels SR, et al. AHA guidelines for primary prevention of cardiovascular disease and stroke: 2002 update. Circulation 2002;106:388–91.
134. Taylor DW, Barnett HJM, Haynes RB, et al. Low-dose and high-dose acetylsalicylic acid for patients undergoing carotid endarterectomy: a randomised controlled trial. Lancet 1999;353: 2179–84.
135. Ridker PM, Cook NR, Lee I-M, et al. A randomized trial of low-dose aspirin in the primary prevention of cardiovascular disease in women. N Engl J Med 2005;352:1293–304.
136. Mosca L, Benjamin EJ, Berra K, et al. Effectiveness-based guidelines for the prevention of cardiovascular disease in women–2011 update: a guideline from the american heart association. Circulation 2011;123:1243–62.
137. Antithrombotic Trialists' Collaboration. Aspirin in the primary and secondary prevention of vascuar disease: collaborative meta-analysis of individual participant data from randomized trials. Lancet 2009;373:1849–60.
138. Belch J, MacCuish A, Campbell I, et al. The prevention of progression of arterial disease and diabetes (POPADAD) trial: factorial randomised placebo controlled trial of aspirin and antioxidants in patients with diabetes and asymptomatic peripheral arterial disease. Br Med J 2008;337:a1840.
139. Willey JZ, Xu Q, Boden-Albala B, et al. Lipid profile components and risk of ischemic stroke: the Northern Manhattan Study (NOMAS). Arch Neurol 2009;66:1400–6.
140. Sacco RL, Benson RT, Kargman DE, et al. High-density lipoprotein cholesterol and ischemic stroke in the elderly – The Northern Manhattan Stroke Study. JAMA 2001;285: 2729–35.
141. Gardener H, Della Morte D, Elkind MS, et al. Lipids and carotid plaque in the Northern Manhattan Study (NOMAS). BMC Cardiovasc Disord 2009;9:55.
142. Briel M, Studer M, Glass TR, et al. Effects of statins on stroke prevention in patients with and without coronary heart disease: a meta-analysis of randomized controlled trials. Am J Med 2004;117:596–606.
143. Amarenco P, Labreuche J. Lipid management in the prevention of stroke: review and updated meta-analysis of statins for stroke prevention. Lancet Neurol 2009;8:453–63.
144. Ridker PM, Danielson E, Fonseca FAH, et al. Rosuvastatin to prevent vascular events in men and women with elevated C-reactive protein. N Engl J Med 2008;359:2195–207.
145. Goldstein LB. JUPITER and the world of stroke medicine. Lancet Neurol 2009;8:130–1.

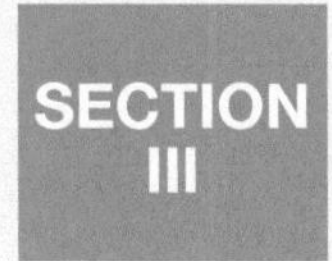

Clinical Manifestations

Lawrence K.S. Wong

This section continues the attempt to cover the major syndromes of stroke, and, where possible, to point to issues of pathophysiology that bear on the diagnosis of stroke subtype, both ischemic and hemorrhagic.

Evolving imaging information is offering insight into the pathophysiology of different stroke subtypes. There have been advances in the classification of stroke and transient ischemic attack based on imaging criteria. Stroke scales are important in assessing stroke severity and stratifying patients for different treatments, especially for acute stroke. More advanced cardiac monitoring, high-resolution MRI and wall imaging provide a clearer description of the pathophysiology of strokes related to large-artery occlusive disease such as carotid stenosis, anterior cerebral, middle cerebral, posterior cerebral and vertebrobasilar arteries. The clinical manifestations and treatments might be different with different stroke etiology.

The classification of small-artery disease has been clarified with detailed imaging as well as many prospective studies. Clinical lacunar syndromes may be caused by other mechanisms than small-artery disease in one-third or more of all cases. More importantly, lacunar infarcts are part of the spectrum of cerebral small-vessel disease that manifested as silent cerebral infarcts, white matter lesions, and cerebral microbleeds. Cerebral small-vessel disease has an important role in cerebrovascular disease and is a leading cause of cognitive decline and functional loss in the elderly. Clinicians are fascinated by the various syndromes of the clinical signs and symptoms of stroke in the posterior circulation. The topographic pattern of a lesion provides insight into the underlying etiology.

In the past decade, we have come to understand more about the evolution and progression of the intracerebral hemorrhage. Intracerebral hemorrhage associated with the use of thrombolysis, anticoagulation and antiplatelet treatment is commonly encountered in clinical practice. New findings of the importance of hematoma expansion and the presence of "spot sign" on enable clinicians to plan treatment. Subarachnoid hemorrhage commonly presents as severe and sudden headache. Clinicians should look out for neurological complications such as hydrocephalus, delayed cerebral ischemia, rebleeding, seizures, and hyponatremia. Spontaneous bleeding from arteriovenous malformation is less common than other causes of hemorrhagic stroke. The risk factors of bleeding from an arteriovenous malformation include history of prior hemorrhage and morphological characteristics such as deep location and the pattern of venous drainage.

20 Classification of Ischemic Stroke

Hakan Ay

KEY POINTS

- Extensive etiologic heterogeneity in ischemic stroke necessitates categorizing patients into homogeneous classes with discrete phenotypic, pathophysiologic, therapeutic, and prognostic features.
- Phenotypic classification provides a summary of abnormal test findings organized in major etiologic categories without weighting toward the most likely cause in the presence of multiple etiologies. Its advantage is that it retains as much patient information as possible. Its shortcoming is that it assigns strokes to a vast number of categories.
- Causative classification identifies the most likely cause of stroke through a decision-making process that requires integration of clinical, laboratory and imaging information. Its advantage is that it assigns stroke etiologies into a small number of mutually exclusive categories. Its shortcoming is that collapsing individual etiologies into categories may result in loss of information on an individual basis.
- Identification of an abnormality in stroke work-up does not necessarily mean that it is the cause. Newer probabilistic classification systems take into account the relative strength of causal connections and determine the most likely causative etiology in the presence of multiple competing etiologies.
- An etiology that has potential to cause another stroke in the short term is called an unstable etiology. Infarct characteristics on brain imaging, such as size, age, location, and pattern of infarcts can help identify an unstable etiology.

More than 100 pathological conditions can play a role in etiopathogenesis of ischemic stroke.[1,2] Etiologic heterogeneity of this magnitude requires an effective way of sorting patients into classes. The main goal of etiologic classification is to generate homogeneous subtypes with discrete phenotypic, pathophysiologic, therapeutic, and prognostic features. The challenge is attaining consistent subtype assignments among different raters. Consistency ensures unity among physicians and comparability among studies. Reliable etiologic subtype information can be used to select patients in clinical trials, determine the phenotype genetic and epidemiological studies, assess treatment response, code for administrative purposes, and predict prognosis. Additionally, stroke subtypes are predictors of the future risk of recurrent stroke.[3–6] Hence, in-depth evaluation to identify the etiologic mechanism of stroke is imperative for effective secondary prevention.

HISTORY

Infarct subtype used to be determined chiefly on clinical grounds, relying heavily on the clinical syndrome, neurologic findings, and coexisting risk factors. For patients who died, autopsy confirmation was often the basis of the classification. With the widespread application of brain imaging, extracranial and intracranial vascular imaging, cardiac ultrasonography, long-term cardiac monitoring, and other diagnostic studies, clinical impressions have been refined and supported by laboratory confirmation of the stroke subtype.

The origin of major traditional subtypes such as large artery atherosclerosis, cardiac embolism, or cryptogenic stroke is a report from an expert committee appointed by the National Institute for Neurological Disorders and Blindness (NINDB) in 1958.[7] The goal of the NINDB project was "to place in classified form all of the known types of cerebrovascular diseases, and to give meaning to such classification by defining all terms so clearly that they can be employed interchangeably by all investigators in various parts of the country", highlighting one of the most important and challenging aspects of etiologic classification: reliability.

The NINDB classification had four major etiologic categories: "thrombosis with atherosclerosis," "cerebral embolism," "other causes", and "cerebral infarction of undetermined origin." The category of cerebral embolism included a subcategory, "cerebral emboli of undetermined origin," referring to cases where diagnosis of cerebral embolism was made at autopsy without evidence of a clear source for embolism. Stroke subtypes in the NINDB classification were determined on clinical grounds. Stroke that began during sleep or within 1 hour of awakening suggested thrombosis with atherosclerosis, whilst a rapid onset of symptoms and a lack of warning symptoms indicated embolism from a cardiac source. For example, hemorrhagic infarction within the territory of middle cerebral artery (MCA) in the absence of bruit in the ipsilateral carotid artery suggested cardiac embolism.

Heavy reliance on the clinical syndrome began to diminish in the 1960s and early 1970s due to the increased use of computerized brain tomography and catheter angiography. In addition, description of clinic-anatomic correlates of deep and brainstem-penetrating artery infarcts allowed for diagnosis of lacunar infarcts.[8–11] The Harvard Cooperative Stroke Registry classification devised in 1978 incorporated these advances, sorting stroke etiology into the categories of "large artery thrombosis," "lacunar infarcts," and "embolism."[12] Concurrent use of brain and vascular imaging led to more frequent detection of embolic events characterized by an imaging-confirmed infarction in the absence of occlusion in the clinically relevant artery than previously published rates based on clinical criteria and autopsy (31% vs 3–15%).[13,14] It is now well-known that embolism is indeed a very common mechanism accounting for approximately two-thirds of strokes.[15,16]

In the 1980s and 1990s, brain imaging, echocardiography, and Doppler ultrasonography for extracranial vessel imaging were more readily available for clinical use. These tools led to frequent detection of lacunar infarcts, extracranial large artery atherosclerosis, and cardiac emboli sources. Stroke Data Bank classification[17] in 1986 and TOAST[18] classification in 1993 further revised subtype definitions by incorporating findings from diagnostic technologies of the time. Stroke Data Bank classification separated ischemic strokes into "large artery thrombosis," "infarct with tandem arterial pathology or arterial embolism," "embolism attributed to cardiac or transcardiac source," "lacunar infarction," "infarct of undetermined cause," and "infarct with normal angiogram." The last category was similar to "cerebral embolism of undetermined origin" in the original NINDB classification and designated cases without an obvious stroke etiology in which there was no occlusion in angiogram. The Causative Classification of Stroke System (CCS) devised in 2007 carried on this subtype in the form of "cryptogenic embolism," which denoted angiographic evidence of abrupt cut-off in an otherwise normal looking artery, or subsequent complete recanalization of a previously occluded artery.[1,19]

TOAST stratified ischemic strokes into "large artery atherosclerosis," "cardiac embolism," "small artery occlusion," "stroke of other determined etiology," and "stroke of undetermined etiology."[18] This system categorized every stroke patient into one of the five subtypes. It was different from prior systems where etiologic categories did not necessarily accommodate every stroke patient (subtypes added up to 100% in TOAST but not in others). This feature provided utility to TOAST in clinical trials and epidemiological studies.

CHALLENGES IN THE DIAGNOSIS OF ETIOLOGIC SUBTYPES

Even when strenuous efforts are made to establish the exact mechanism of infarction, current diagnostic technologies are far from precise. Available vascular imaging technologies cannot always differentiate whether a given arterial stenosis or occlusion is due to atherosclerosis. In addition, when a significant carotid stenosis is found, judging whether the clinical syndrome arises from an embolic or hemodynamic mechanism is often difficult. Vascular imaging during the acute stage might suggest an abrupt occlusion of an intracranial large artery, but the presence of abrupt occlusion does not always settle the problem of the underlying source of embolus. The sensitivity of available vascular imaging technologies is not sufficient to visualize the pathology in deep, cortical, and brainstem penetrating arteries that leads to small artery occlusion. Identifying early signs of parenchymal damage and brain edema, proven to be useful as a prognostic index is not as helpful in differentiating etiologic mechanisms.[20-24]

Causation is difficult to infer in the absence of a gold-standard test to demonstrate the true cause of stroke. Earlier systems heavily relied on clinical criteria, but clinical grounds alone – age, risk factors, and so forth – are not sufficient to classify patients by different mechanism of cerebral infarction. Common risk factors such as hypertension and diabetes mellitus lack specificity for stroke subtypes and are not distinctive enough to infer the cause.[1] Likewise, the presenting clinical syndrome has little value to suggest a stroke subtype. This is even more apparent in the acute setting, where the common cognitive impairment, agitation, and poor cooperation of patients can hinder a thorough assessment of neurologic functions. Relying on clinical criteria alone becomes even more problematic when risk factors or clinical syndromes are consistent with more than one etiologic subtype. Sorting such complex cases into one etiologic category based on clinical criteria alone injects uncertainty and introduces disagreement into stroke classification.

The use of CT, MRI, non-invasive vascular imaging, echocardiography, and long-term cardiac monitoring has greatly improved our ability to diagnose the etiologic subtype but has still left large issues unresolved. Reliance on only abnormal test results to determine causative etiology is problematic because identification of an abnormality does not necessarily mean that it is the cause. In the National Institute of Neurological Disorders and Stroke – Stroke Genetics Network Study (NINDS – SiGN),[25] which included approximately 17,000 patients with ischemic stroke, the cause of stroke could be attributed to large artery atherosclerosis with a high level of confidence in 54% of patients who had an atherosclerotic lesion causing ≥50% stenosis in the cerebral circulation. Likewise, only 45% of those with a major cardiac source of embolism, and 40% of those with a typical lacunar infarct on brain imaging, could be classified into the same causative category with high confidence.

ALGORITHMIC APPROACH TO STROKE

Confidence in attributing an etiology to the cause of stroke is determined by coexisting clinical and radiographic stroke features and the extent to which diagnostic investigations are completed. For instance, the causal mechanism can be attributed to atrial fibrillation with a high level of confidence only when diagnostic investigations for alternative etiologies are done and fail to reveal any source. Atrial fibrillation, on the other hand, is assigned as the cause of stroke with low probability when alternative etiologies coexist or tests for alternative etiologies are not obtained. In a complex patient with atrial fibrillation and stroke features that strongly suggest an underlying vascular pathology such as recurrent unilateral transient retinal or hemispheric ischemic symptoms, or unilateral internal borderzone infarcts on MRI, an ipsilateral vascular lesion needs to be ruled out before attributing atrial fibrillation to the cause of stroke with high confidence. The probabilistic approach does not require a minimum level of investigations for etiologic subtyping. Determining causal connections with high probability, however, requires a thorough diagnostic evaluation. In clinical settings where diagnostic investigations are stopped when a positive finding is obtained, the quality of etiologic subtype information is expected to be low.

Current diagnostic technologies allow for frequent identification of multiple abnormalities. At least one cardiac source of embolism can be detected in about 50–70% of patients with stroke by echocardiography.[25-27] Likewise, about one-quarter of patients with a lacunar infarction harbor ipsilateral large artery atherosclerosis causing stenosis ≥50%.[25,28] Overall, approximately one-half of patients with stroke exhibit one or more etiology, and around 20% of those harbor multiple major etiologies, such as intra-cardiac thrombus and acute arterial dissection.[25] Non-probabilistic classification systems lack the objective criteria to identify the most likely cause in the presence of multiple competing etiologies. Cases with multiple etiologies are grouped into the heterogeneous category of "undetermined etiology" along with cryptogenic strokes and strokes with unknown etiology due to incomplete evaluation. This practice inflates the size of the undetermined category. If such cases with competing etiologies are assigned into a known subtype based on best clinical guess, instead of being classified in the undetermined category, then the size of the undetermined category becomes smaller, but at the expense of losing inter-rater reliability because personal opinion varies from one rater to another. Reports from independent investigators consistently demonstrate no better than moderate reliability, with agreement rates that hover around 50% for conventional etiologic classification sytems.[29–33]

Newer probabilistic classification systems use several criteria to determine the most likely etiology in the presence of multiple competing etiologies.[1,19] These criteria include: (1) consideration of relative potential of each etiology to cause a stroke, (2) the use of clinical and imaging stroke features that support one mechanism over others, and (3) consideration of the relationship between the etiology and the brain infarct in time and space.

Relative potential to cause stroke is based on risk estimates for first-ever stroke associated with each etiology in the absence of effective treatment. This criterion has proven useful to stratify cardiac sources of embolism. Abnormalities such as left ventricular hypertrophy and mitral annulus calcification convey low or uncertain risk of stroke and are, therefore, considered a minor etiology. On the other hand, abnormalities such as atrial fibrillation pose a substantial risk and are considered major. Box 20-1 lists minor and major cardiac sources using a 2% annual or one-time primary stroke risk as cut-off.[1] Atherosclerotic stenosis in the cerebral arteries causing ≥50% stenosis is also considered a major etiology. A cardiac source cannot compete with ≥50% atherosclerotic stenosis as another stroke mechanism unless the annual or one-time primary stroke risk associated with its presence exceeds 2%. According to this criterion, the etiologic subtype is classified as large artery atherosclerosis when ≥50% atherosclerotic stenosis coexists with a minor cardiac source, and undetermined when it coexists with a major cardiac source.

Assigning stroke patients with more than one major etiology to known subtypes (instead of undetermined category) depends on capability to establish the strength of causal connections. Certain clinical and imaging stroke features might support one mechanism over others. A recent examination of previously published features associated with etiologic subtypes revealed eight that exhibited discriminative value:[1]

- Three features for large artery atherosclerosis, including prior history of one or more transient monocular blindness, TIA, or stroke in the territory of index atherosclerotic artery within the last month; ipsilateral and unilateral internal watershed infarction; and multiple, temporally separate infarcts exclusively within the territory of the stenotic artery.
- Two features for cardiac embolism, including evidence of concurrent systemic embolism; and multiple acute and subacute ischemic lesions in right and left anterior or anterior and posterior circulations, or both, in the absence of non-embolic occlusion or near occlusive stenosis of all relevant vessels.
- Three features for small artery occlusion, including stereotypic lacunar transient ischemic attacks that started within the week preceding the index stroke; presentation with a lacunar syndrome; and single acute infarct within the territory of penetrating arteries in the brainstem, deep gray matter, or internal capsule that is ≤20 mm in the largest diameter.

In the presence of more than one major etiology, the causative subtype can be inferred with a moderate level of confidence based on presence or absence of supportive stroke features. For instance, the presence of unilateral internal watershed infarcts makes an ipsilateral atherosclerotic stenosis in the internal carotid artery a more likely cause of stroke than atrial fibrillation when they both coexist.

BOX 20-1 Cardiac and Aortic Sources of Cerebral Embolism

SOURCES WITH HIGH PRIMARY RISK OF ISCHEMIC STROKE

Left atrial thrombus
Left ventricular thrombus
Atrial fibrillation
Paroxysmal atrial fibrillation
Sick sinus syndrome
Sustained atrial flutter
Recent myocardial infarction (within 1 month)
Mitral stenosis or rheumatic valve disease
Bioprosthetic and mechanical heart valves
Chronic myocardial infarction together with low ejection fraction <28%
Dilated cardiomyopathy
Non-bacterial thrombotic endocarditis
Infective endocarditis
Papillary fibroelastoma
Left atrial myxoma
Patent foramen ovale and concurrent systemic embolism

SOURCES WITH LOW OR UNCERTAIN PRIMARY RISK OF ISCHEMIC STROKE

Mitral annular calcification
Patent foramen ovale
Atrial septal aneurysm
Left ventricular aneurysm without thrombus
Isolated left atrial smoke (no mitral stenosis or atrial fibrillation)
Complex atheroma in the ascending aorta or proximal arch
Symptomatic congestive heart failure with ejection fraction <30%
Wall motion abnormalities (hypokinesia, akinesia, dyskinesia)
Hypertrophic cardiomyopathy
Left ventricular hypertrophy
Left ventricular hypertrabeculation/non-compaction
Other rare sources (atrial or ventricular septal defect, preexcitation syndromes, left atrial dilation)

To identify the causative subtype, clinicians frequently consider the relationship between the etiology and the brain infarct in time and space. Temporal relationship implies stroke following an antecedent and clearly discernible event that is closely related in time to the index stroke. Examples include stroke following acute arterial dissection, acute myocardial infarction, or a vascular or cardiac procedure. Spatial relationship refers to the ability to align an etiology to the territory where the infarct has occurred. Spatial relationship is generally harder to establish than temporal relationship because it requires identification of the clinically relevant artery; a challenging process with complex occlusion patterns. For instance, an internal carotid artery stenosis might be judged to be responsible for acute ischemic lesions within both the middle and the posterior cerebral artery territories if the ipsilateral posterior cerebral artery has fetal origin. Likewise, internal carotid artery stenosis might be responsible for bilateral anterior circulation infarcts when the contralateral internal carotid artery is occluded or when there is an azygous A2 segment or aplasia of the contralateral A1 segment. In the presence of multiple competing etiologies, the mechanism that bears temporal or spatial relationship is considered more likely to be the cause of stroke.

CCS is an example for a probabilistic algorithm. It establishes causal associations by incorporating clinical, laboratory, imaging, and other stroke work-up information on a case-by-case basis (available at https://ccs.mgh.harvard.edu).[1,19,26] CCS

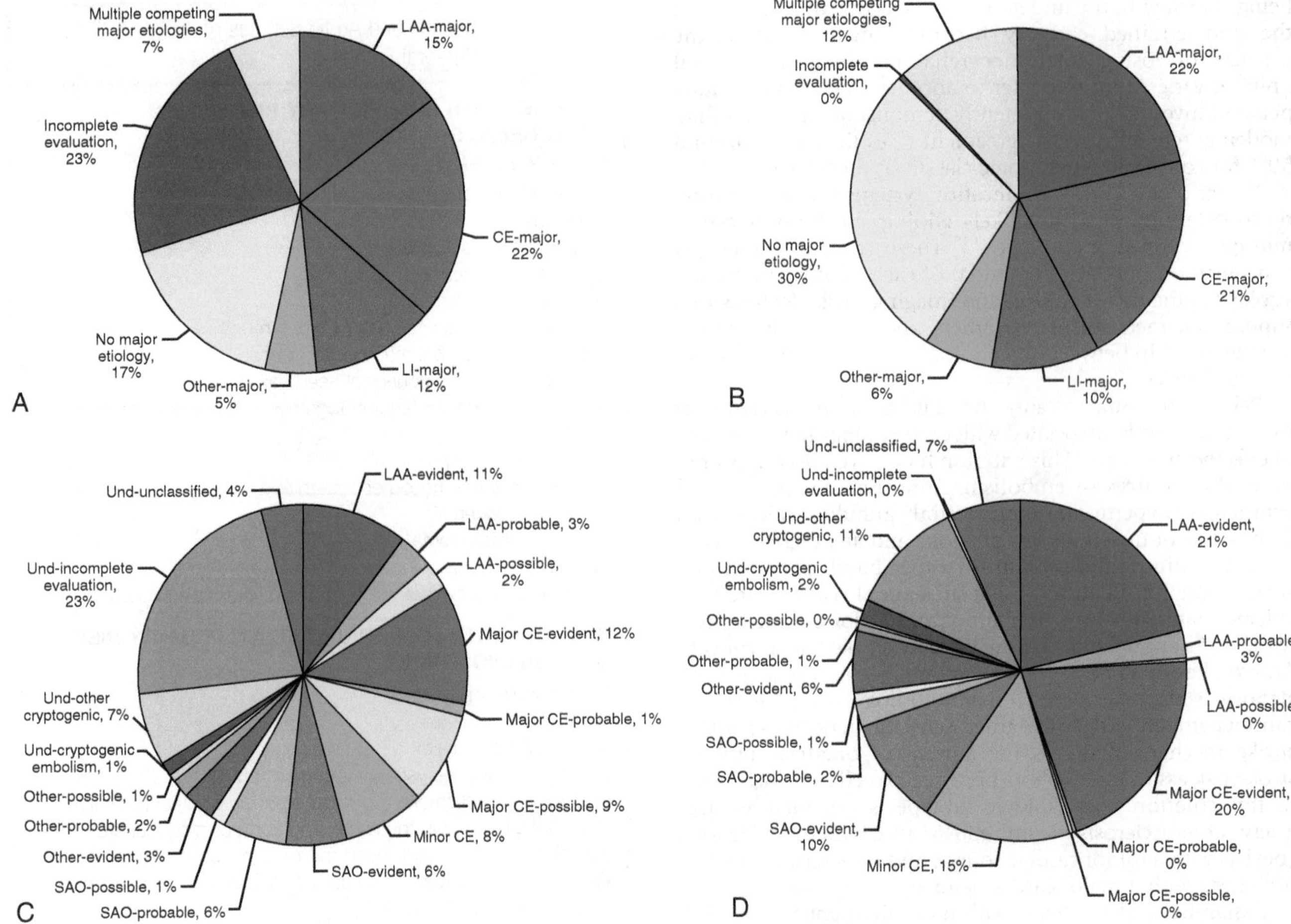

Figure 20-1. Distribution of phenotypic and causative stroke subtypes in the NINDS Stroke Genetics Network. A, Phenotypic subtypes in the entire population (n = 16954); B, phenotypic subtypes in the subset with complete vascular and cardiac investigation (n = 7748); C, causative subtypes in the entire population; and D, causative subtypes in the subset with complete vascular and cardiac investigation. Please note that the category of incomplete evaluation in A and C designates an etiologic subgroup that is considered when diagnostic investigations are not performed in the absence of an identified etiology. According to this definition, a case with atrial fibrillation in history is not classified as incomplete evaluation when vascular and cardiac investigations are not done. The term complete investigation in the title of B and D, however, is solely based on availability of diagnostic tests indicating that brain imaging, vascular imaging, and cardiac evaluation are available. Evident denotes a sole and important mechanism of stroke; probable, the most likely mechanism of stroke when there are more than one evident mechanism; and possible, an evident mechanism with missing tests for alternative etiologies or an etiology that is diagnosed solely based on the clinical syndrome (19). Major CE indicates cardiac sources with high risk of stroke and minor CE, cardiac sources with low or uncertain risk of stroke (Box 20-1). CE, cardiac embolism; LAA, large artery atherosclerosis; LI, lacunar infarction; SAO, small artery occlusion. *(With permission from Ay H, Arsava EM, Andsberg G, et al. Pathogenic ischemic stroke phenotypes in the National Institute of Neurological Disorders and Stroke – Stroke Genetics Network. Stroke 2014: Nov 6.pii: STROKEAHA.114.007362.)*

categorizes ischemic strokes into the same major etiologic groups as TOAST (Fig. 20-1). Definitions for subtypes are, however, different between TOAST and CCS. The latter incorporates newer diagnostic technologies such as non-invasive intracranial angiography, diffusion- and perfusion-weighted imaging, and cardiac imaging into subtype definitions. A study that included 13,596 patients with ischemic stroke participating in the NINDS-SiGN Study demonstrated moderate agreement (kappa = 0.59) between TOAST and CCS.[34] Agreement was highest for large-artery atherosclerosis (kappa = 0.71) and lowest for small-artery occlusion (kappa = 0.56). Several studies have assessed the reliability of CCS revealing agreement rates ranging from 80% to 95%.[1,19,25,26] Those studies have also shown, however, that even with an automated evidence- and rule-based algorithm, disagreements can occur in etiologic classification due to lack of data, ambiguities in the source data such as medical record notes, raters who overlook important etiologic data, and differences in interpreting test results, such as distinguishing atherosclerosis from other causes of vascular stenosis or whether a given infarct described in a radiology report is lacunar.

CAUSATIVE VERSUS PHENOTYPIC CLASSIFICATION

There are two forms of etiologic classification in stroke: phenotypic and causative. *Phenotypic* classification documents abnormal test findings without weighting toward the most likely cause in the presence of multiple etiologies. There are no trade-offs among different etiologies. Abnormal test findings are mapped onto one or more of the four following major etiologic categories: large-artery atherosclerosis, cardiac embolism, lacunar infarction, and other uncommon causes. Thus, a patient can be placed into more than one etiologic category. For instance, a patient with a typical lacunar infarction, ≥50% atherosclerotic stenosis, and dilated cardiomyopathy is classified as "lacunar infarction plus large-artery atherosclerosis plus cardiac embolism." Baltimore-Washington Classification,[35] CCS,[1,19] and the Atherothrombosis - Small vessel disease - Cardiac causes - Other uncommon causes (ASCO)[36] system are phenotypic classification systems. Phenotypic classification might be useful for selecting patients in large-scale epidemiologic and genetic studies and coding for administrative purposes. Its main advantage is that it retains as much patient information as possible. Its shortcoming is that is assigns strokes into a vast number of categories. For example, a three-category phenotypic system where each category is defined in four possible states (such as major, minor, absent, and unknown) could result in 81 possible subtypes (4th power of 3). There are 257 subtypes in Baltimore-Washington Classification, 96 in the phenotypic version of CCS, and 625 in ASCO. The number of etiologic categories inversely correlates with statistical power in research studies dealing with etiologic subtypes.

It is imperative, therefore, to reduce the number of subtypes, which can be done with *causative* classification. Unlike phenotypic classification, where etiologies can be mapped on more than one etiologic category, causative classification assigns etiologies into mutually exclusive categories. As outlined in the prior section, designation of the causative subtype is a decision-making process that requires integration of multiple aspects of ischemic stroke evaluation including clinical and imaging stroke characteristics. TOAST and CCS are causative systems. Causative classification's ability to unambiguously assign the cause of stroke is limited, however, because of the lack of a gold standard. Collapsing individual etiologies into categories results in loss of information on an individual basis, but, as previously mentioned, this loss is compensated by the gain in statistical power in research studies.

IDENTIFICATION OF UNSTABLE CAUSATIVE ETIOLOGY

The primary goal of identifying the underlying causative mechanism is to institute the most effective treatment for secondary prevention. Nevertheless, the majority of patients with a major causative mechanism do not develop a subsequent stroke in the short term even without treatment. It is important to differentiate the causative etiology that has potential to cause another stroke (unstable etiology) from the etiology that does not (stable etiology). The concept of unstable etiology is important because it urges the identification of high-risk patients who benefit from timely institution of preventive treatments, such as carotid endarterectomy or acute anticoagulation, in specialized stroke centers that have the infrastructure for prompt evaluation. Predictive models developed to quantify stroke risk associated with individual etiologies, such as a CHA2DS2-VASc[37] score for atrial fibrillation, can be used for this purpose. Although none of the individual etiology-based prognostic algorithms has been validated for predicting stroke risk during the critical 90-day period, they could still provide a useful estimate. The challenge is that acquiring predictor variables requires additional investigation, time, resources, and sometimes prolonged hospitalization.

Stroke etiologies appear to leave different footprints in the brain depending on their potential to cause another stroke in the short term.[3] Infarct characteristics on brain imaging that correlate with increased risk for recurrent stroke include the presence of simultaneous acute infarcts in both hemispheres or in both anterior and posterior circulations, multiple acute or subacute infarcts, and isolated cortical location.[38–40] An instrument that incorporated these imaging data generated 90-day stroke risk estimates ranging from 1% to 40%, depending on the number of predictors.[3]

SUBTYPES OF ISCHEMIC STROKE

Large-Artery Atherosclerosis

Many of the descriptions leading to the definition of large-artery atherosclerosis stem from pathologic studies of the past.[13] Atherosclerotic lesions were found at bifurcations and curves of the larger vessels; the more proximal the location in the vascular tree, the more severe the atherosclerotic lesions.[41,42] Primary occlusion of the arteries distally located over the cerebral surface was less frequent.[43,44] Atherosclerotic plaque usually led to progressive stenosis, and the final large-artery occlusion was due to thrombosis of the narrowed lumen. The occurrence of intraplaque hemorrhage sometimes led to accelerated occlusion,[45] although the frequency of this condition is more often a matter of speculation rather than confirmed in pathologic specimens.[46,47]

Infarct Mechanism

Perfusion Failure. Stroke in the patient with large-artery atherosclerosis can be caused by perfusion failure distal to the site of severe stenosis or occlusion of the major vessel.[44,48] In some instances, the major vessel occlusion is rather proximal in the arterial tree, and some degree of collateral flow is interposed between the occlusion and the cerebral territory at risk of infarction.[49] Some cases with interposed collateral are spared infarction of any kind, whereas in others the infarct is located mainly along the most distal brain regions originally supplied by the occluded vessel.[44,50–53] In the carotid territory, these regions are the supra-Sylvian frontal, central, and parietal portions of the hemisphere, and in the vertebrobasilar territory, they are the bilateral occipital poles. Internal borderzone regions have also been demonstrated in the white matter of the corona radiata supplied by both superficial MCA pial penetrators and lenticulostriate arteries.

The usually accepted mechanism of perfusion failure is more readily recognized in occlusive disease, but becomes more difficult to define when the extracranial vessel is patent but highly stenotic. Positron-emission-tomography-based studies demonstrate that selective hemodynamic impairment does not always develop among patients with transient ischemic attacks (TIAs) and severe carotid stenosis.[54,55] The development of borderzone ischemia probably depends on multiple factors, not just on the severity of stenosis.[53,56,57]

Artery-to-Artery Embolism. Infarcts can be produced by emboli arising from atheromatous lesions situated proximally to otherwise healthy branches located more distal in the arterial tree.[58] Embolic fragments may arise from extracranial arteries affected by stenosis or ulcer,[50,59–66] from the stump of the occluded internal carotid artery (ICA),[67] and even from the intracranial tail of the anterograde thrombus atop an occluded carotid.[68,69] Nowadays embolism from a carotid source has become recognized as another, perhaps more common, cause of stroke in a setting of arterial stenosis and even occlusion.[70–72] In later stroke series, borderzone infarcts appear to be less common than previously thought, which has led to the presumption that embolism was the actual mechanism even in the presence of tight stenoses or occlusions. To add to the difficulty in distinguishing between these two mechanisms of infarction, cases of perfusion failure due to embolism have been demonstrated. Internal borderzone infarcts have been reported after embolic occlusion of MCA pial branches.[73] This finding may be an example of an embolic stroke with a possible local hemodynamic effect as the final mechanism of the infarct.

Distinguishing between the infarct mechanisms (hemodynamic versus embolism) in patients with large-artery disease can be quite difficult. The sudden mode of onset may suggest, but does not confirm, a diagnosis of embolism.[74] Other clinical features may not enable such a distinction. Moreover, it is even more difficult to discriminate between emboli from a cardiac source and those from an arterial source. One study reported that isolated superficial infarcts were more common in artery-to-artery embolism whereas decreased consciousness at stroke onset was associated with cardiac embolism.[21] Clinical features are in general not reliable enough to lead to a definite diagnosis without confirmatory laboratory data. CT and MRI are of help in supporting a diagnosis of arterial embolism when (1) a large territorial infarct is detected,[75] (2) a hyperdense spot along the course of the MCA is seen on non-contrast CT,[51] (3) a scattered infarct pattern is seen on diffusion-weighted MRI[76,77] (4) no obvious cardioembolic source is present and the extent of stenosis is less than 80% (which would not explain the stroke on the grounds of hemodynamic insufficiency), or (5) there is an ulcerative or thrombotic plaque regardless of the degree of stenosis. The more widespread use of perfusion imaging techniques such as SPECT,[78] xenon-enhanced CT,[79] regional cerebral blood flow measurements,[80] MRI,[81–83] and positron emission tomography[54,84,85] in patients with atherosclerotic stenosis or occlusive disease should allow for more accurate distinction between embolism and perfusion failure in the clinical setting.

Clinical Features

Discriminating among etiologic subtypes on clinical grounds alone is difficult. Fractional arm weakness (shoulder different from the hand), hypertension, diabetes, and male gender can occur more frequently with atherosclerotic than with cardioembolic infarcts, but their discriminative value is limited.[1] Prior history of one or more ischemic events (transient monocular blindness, TIA, or stroke) in the territory of index atherosclerotic artery within the month preceding the stroke strongly suggests a diagnosis of large-artery atherosclerosis.[86–88] Limb-shaking TIAs, characterized by involuntary, unilateral, trembling, shaking, twisting, or jerking movements of limbs lasting for a few minutes, can be a manifestation of contralateral carotid occlusive disease.[89,90] Differentiating these spells from focal seizures is of practical importance. Limb-shaking spells are not associated with epileptiform activity in the interictal electroencephalography, lack response to antiepileptic medications, and can sometimes be precipitated by maneuvers that lead to carotid compression.

Results of Diagnostic Tests

Brain Imaging. Abnormalities on MRI or CT that are attributable to cerebral infarction from carotid artery atherosclerosis are those that can be interpreted to reflect the distal field effect along the external and internal borderzones. External borderzone infarcts due to atherosclerotic stenosis occur between middle and anterior cerebral territories, especially on the middle cerebral side.[44,48,50,91] This topographic pattern involves the supra-Sylvian frontal and central regions, shading toward normal in the parietooccipital region, sparing the region of the Sylvian fissure (operculum, insula) and the penetrating territories of the lenticulostriates. The centripetal spreading in more severe cases may involve so much of the hemisphere that a differentiation from embolism to the MCA stem is impossible. Internal watershed infarcts occur between superficial and deep penetrating arteries located in the centrum semiovale or corona radiata and are characterized by rosary-like pattern of infarcts (often three or more, each ≥3 mm in diameter) that are arranged in a linear fashion parallel to the lateral ventricle.[92,93] Both external and internal watershed infarcts can occur as a result of micro-embolism from a proximal (cardiac, aortic, or venous) source.[94–97] Bilateral borderzone infarcts may suggest a proximal source. In contrast, unilateral borderzone infarcts, in particular, unilateral internal borderzone infarcts, indicate an ipsilateral carotid artery disease.[92,93] A combination of acute, subacute, and chronic infarcts exclusively located in one hemisphere also suggests an underlying carotid artery disease.[92,98] Likewise, multiple temporally separate infarcts confined to a single arterial territory indicate repetitive ischemic injury most likely from an ipsilateral arterial source.

Vascular Imaging. In the clinical setting, angiography, magnetic resonance angiography (MRA), computed tomographic angiography (CTA), and Doppler ultrasonography remain the most important laboratory tests for a diagnosis of large-artery atherosclerotic occlusive disease. On a conventional cerebral angiogram, the occlusion of the internal carotid artery at its origin or in the siphon has the appearance of a pencil point, blunt end, smooth end, or shoulder, and the intracranial portion of the internal carotid or major cerebral artery stems and branches are open.[99] Spiral occlusions of the extracranial portion of the internal carotid beyond 2 cm of its origin (a finding consistent with dissection)[100] indicate that the carotid lesion may be the source of the stroke but not by means of atherosclerosis. Because of the risks of cerebral angiography,[101–103] there has been increased reliance on extracranial duplex Doppler and transcranial Doppler ultrasonography techniques to show no or highly resistant flow in the extracranial carotid with dampened pulsatility in the ipsilateral MCA.[104–109] MRA and CTA have become reliable diagnostic tools for the detection of extracranial and intracranial large-artery stenosis,[110,111] which has led to less reliance on conventional angiography.[60]

Intracranial stenoses or occlusions may be due to arteriosclerosis, but are often difficult to distinguish from emboli of any extracerebral source.[112–114] If one or more appropriate TIAs occurred within the past 30 days, the diagnosis of large-artery atherosclerosis may be correct, but the matter can be settled only if a widely patent lumen is subsequently found by serial vascular imaging.[115] The latter is diagnostic of embolism, whereas persistence of the occlusion leaves the mechanism unsettled.

Basilar occlusion on angiography is usually considered the mechanism for brainstem stroke even though, in many such cases, the clinical syndrome fits the criteria for lacune resulting from occlusion of a penetrating artery by the major basilar atheroma.[116–119] As for the carotid artery, the finding of stenosis of the basilar artery prevents a definite diagnosis regarding the mechanism of infarction because infarcts more distal in the vertebrobasilar territory might well be the result of distal embolization.[112,120] Atheromatous disease of the basilar artery often affects the vessel at sites where local branches directly supply brain tissue.[119,121] When the clinical syndrome of basilar stroke can be localized to the point of the stenosis, infarction may be caused by mural atheroma that only slightly stenoses the basilar artery, but totally occludes a small penetrator departing from the basilar artery at that location.

Embolism Attributed to Cardiac Sources

Embolism from any source probably accounts for up to 70% of all cases of ischemic stroke,[70,122–125] many of which occur from embolism into the territory of the MCA. Although the subject of embolism seems clear enough, in that a particle is swept through the bloodstream until it jams in an artery too small to allow it to pass, the many complexities of the embolic process make it anything but easy to account for on a case-by-case basis.

The biggest clinical problem in arriving at a diagnosis of embolism is identifying the source. Embolism was diagnosed in earlier studies mainly when a cardiac source was obvious.[51] The results of later studies have shown that emboli, diagnosed angiographically from isolated branch occlusions, may occur despite all efforts to identify the source. Given the many possibilities and given the traditional use of the term embolism to refer to a cardiac source, the following discussion is limited to that subject.

Properties of Emboli

The instability of the embolic material is a point of prime importance in clinical and angiographic analysis of cases of embolism. Mural thrombi and platelet aggregates are the materials most commonly embolized to the brain. These materials are remarkably evanescent, as has been repeatedly inferred from findings on angiography. Embolic fragments are found in more than 75% of cases studied by angiography within 8 hours of the onset of the stroke,[70,126,127] whereas embolic occlusion is demonstrated in 40% of clinically identical cases in which angiography is delayed for up to 72 hours after the clinical onset of the stroke[128] and in only 15% of cases studied more than 72 hours after the onset. These decreasing proportions imply that embolic occlusions are liable to spontaneously recanalize in a sizable number of cases. Serial studies with transcranial Doppler ultrasonography demonstrated a recanalization of MCA mainstem or branch occlusions in up to 52% of cases within the first 48 hours of stroke.[129–133] Second angiographic evaluations, performed in subsets of patients in whom arterial occlusion was demonstrated by an earlier angiogram, showed recanalization in 30–60% of cases.[17,115] During recanalization, a column of blood develops between the embolus and the arterial wall, enlarges, and erodes the embolus until the lumen is finally cleared. The exact sequence of events is not fully understood in human material, but cases documented at different stages during the process make it clear that recanalization is accomplished within periods as short as hours to days.[134–136] The angiographic appearance of the gradually eroding embolus is indistinguishable from that of atherosclerotic stenosis. During this process, the lumen may appear stenotic.[137–139]

No reliable means have been developed thus far to identify which embolic occlusions will persist and which will disappear, although it is inferred that the more friable materials will disperse more rapidly. In one of the TCD ultrasonography studies mentioned, patients with an arterial source of emboli experienced recanalization of the vessel less frequently than those with a cardiac source, which suggests a different composition or size of emboli.[130] Thrombi have a complex architecture that is composed of fibrin, erythrocytes, leukocytes, and platelets. In one study, histopathologic examination of cardiac thrombus obtained during valve replacement surgery or embolectomy from 22 patients with atrial fibrillation showed platelets and fibrin.[140] Embolized thrombi exhibited twice as much platelet content as compared to in situ cardiac thrombi suggesting that the platelet component increased propensity for embolization. The size of the emboli is also probably responsible, at least in part, for high frequency of both spontaneous[130,131,133] and pharmacologic[141–143] recanalization in cases of distal MCA occlusion.

The distribution of embolic material within a vascular tree depends on angulation of bifurcations, direction of gravity, relative flow within each vascular branch, and physical properties of the embolic material.[144,145] Small embolic particles (<250 microns in diameter) are distributed to branch arteries according to volumetric flow distribution. Larger embolic particles tend to favor wider-diameter branches at bifurcations beyond the distribution of volumetric flow.[146–148] The size of the embolic material determines the site at which it initially comes to rest in the circulation, but does not determine its final point of arrest. Embolic material stops where the lumen diameter is too small to permit it to pass. Bifurcations or foci of atheroma at curves in the artery are the two sites where emboli arrest. Fibrin–platelet complexes and those also laden with bacteria vary considerably in size; some are so huge that they have obstructed the stem of the MCA,[149] and others have been so small they have lodged asymptomatically in a sensitive region such as the rolandic branch of the MCA. Calcific plaques have only rarely been described as producing large embolic strokes.[61,62,150] For non-compressible objects such as shotgun pellets, the site of embolus can easily be predicted from its size.[129] For the more common fibrin–platelet complexes, however, other factors are involved, especially the poorly understood compressibility of the mass and the time required to transit a certain point of narrowing in the arterial tree. The few cases that document the passage of fibrin–platelet emboli through the arterial tree[135] show considerable alteration in the length and width of the material at different points, which indicates that it possesses a remarkable elasticity and friability. What is sufficient lumen reduction to arrest the material may not be enough to keep it from changing shape or fragmenting within minutes to hours, leaving the site of the original embolic occlusion widely patent.

Clinical Features

It was once thought that the sudden onset of a clinical deficit was typical of embolism and that a non-sudden onset would be more typical of thrombosis. Numerous case examples have now amply demonstrated that onset may be sudden in either condition. Non-sudden or fluctuating onset occurs in 5–6% of documented embolic strokes; the syndrome often requires about 36 hours to evolve.[44,151] Occasionally, a clinical diagnosis of multiple, sometimes stereotypic, TIAs, is entertained. The re-establishment of flow, presumed further migration of embolic material, and subsequent repetition of these events are thought to be the mechanisms involved. Embolic material has even been documented to go to the same site on repeated occasions,[152] which is the opposite of traditional predictions.

One syndrome seems to have held its own as a sign of embolism, although it is met only rarely. A spectacular shrinking deficit can occur when the embolus is introduced into the ICA, causing a profound full hemispheral syndrome, after which it passes up the artery to its final resting place in, for example, the angular branch of the MCA, leaving only a mild aphasia after a few days or a week.[153] Especially characteristic of the MCA migratory embolism is the syndrome of fading hemiparesis with Wernicke's aphasia: the embolus lodges initially at the stem of the MCA, occluding the penetrating lenticulostriate branches long enough to produce scattered foci of infarction through the basal ganglia and internal capsule, of which the involvement of the latter produce the hemiparesis. Distal migration of the embolus then occurs, finally occluding the lower division of the MCA at the superior temporal plane and beyond. This infarct yields Wernicke's aphasia.

Two separate foci of infarction occur, but they result from the same embolic event.

The cardiac history of the patient often provides important clues about a potential embolic source. Besides a greater frequency of cardiac disease, patients with cardioembolic infarction more often present with reduced consciousness, non-fractional arm weakness, a history of systemic embolism, and an abrupt onset.[21,88,154] These clinical features with the exception of concurrent systemic embolism have limited ability to distinguish the cardioembolic group from other subtypes alone.[1,155] Systemic embolism occurring immediately before or soon after an ischemic stroke strongly suggests the presence of a cardiac, aortic, or paradoxical source of embolism.[156] A careful evaluation for the signs and symptoms of embolism to the limbs, lungs, spleen, kidneys, and gastrointestinal system may help infer cardiac embolism as the likely mechanism of stroke.

Results of Diagnostic Tests

Simultaneous infarcts involving branches of different divisions of major cerebral arteries, particularly distributed across both hemispheres or both anterior and posterior circulations, strongly suggest that cardiac embolism is the cause of at least some of the clinical strokes that have occurred.[157,158] A diagnosis of embolism is suggested by a large zone of low density that encompasses the entire territory of a major cerebral artery or its main divisions. Only when the infarction is confined to the cerebral surface territory of a single branch can embolism be inferred from a scan or image. Embolism is also the leading diagnosis when hemorrhagic infarction is seen on brain imaging.[159,160] This assumption is plausible in the presence of a more or less extended hematoma, but it may not be true for other cases displaying petechial, scattered high density along the margins or in the infarct zone.[161] In some 30–50% of cases, the CT scan (or MRI) may show the occlusion itself, as the presence of the hyperdense vessel sign. Finally, as mentioned previously, a scattered infarct pattern on diffusion-weighted MRI may suggest embolism.[76,77,162] Angiography was once considered sufficient to diagnose embolism if the angiogram showed branch occlusion in the absence of other occlusive disease elsewhere.[163-165] This rule still holds for practical purposes, but isolated branch occlusions may also occur in arteritis.

The cardiac diagnostic evaluation starts with careful review of cardiac history and electrocardiography for identifying atrial fibrillation, acute myocardial infarction, or other arrhythmias. Holter monitoring for 24 hours is sometimes necessary to detect paroxysmal atrial fibrillation. Identification of the cardiac source depends most on transthoracic and transesophageal echocardiography. Cardiac investigation is considered to be incomplete when clinical history, physical examination, and electrocardiography do not reveal a cardiac pathology and further cardiac evaluation by echocardiography is not performed. Occasionally, embolic material large enough to produce a focal stroke can be so small that it may escape detection by echocardiography and all too often eludes all efforts at diagnosis.

Small-Artery Occlusion

This category denotes single infarcts within the territory of penetrating arteries in the paramedian regions of the brainstem, deep gray matter, or internal capsule that are ≤20 mm in their greatest diameter on acutely obtained imaging and there is no known pathology such as embolus, focal protruding atheroma, parent vessel dissection, or vasospasm in the parent artery at the site of the origin of the penetrating artery.[1,19] The infarct must be exclusively limited to the territory of deep or brainstem penetrating arteries and should not be accompanied by additional acute infarcts or perfusion defects in other territories or a visible non-chronic arterial cut-off on angiogram. The term "small-artery occlusion" is limited to infarcts within the territory of deep and brainstem penetrators. Anteromedial, anterolateral, and posteromedial thalamic infarcts deserve special consideration as some reports suggest that arteries supplying these regions are more amenable to occlusion via embolism as compared to other deep penetrators.[166–168] Occasionally, in patients with a typical lacunar infarct, careful examination of DWI may reveal additional hyperintense small lesions consistent with infarctions. These subsidiary lesions often lay within the pial artery territories and are frequently associated with an identifiable cause of stroke, suggesting an embolic etiology.[169]

The exact vascular pathology causing lacunar infarction is not known. Lacunar infarcts often occur as a common set of clinical syndromes, angiographic findings are usually normal, and the zone of ischemia is confined to the territory of a single vessel, usually quite small. Only a handful have been studied by autopsy, and an even smaller number have been subjected to serial section.[170] The most common lesion is a tiny focus of microatheroma or lipohyalinosis stenosing one of the deep penetrating arteries. Less frequent causes are parent artery disease or thrombotic occlusion,[171,172] increased vascular permeability leading to leaks of blood and fluid into the perivascular space,[173] and, as mentioned before, microembolization to penetrating arterial territories.[9,169]

Clinical Features

The diagnosis of lacunar infarcts has long been based on clinical characteristics alone. The term *lacunar syndrome* refers to the constellation of clinical features that may indicate, although not invariably, a lacune. The characteristic features of all these syndromes are their relative purity and their failure to involve higher cerebral functions such as language, praxis, behavior controlled by the non-dominant hemisphere, memory, and vision.[174] The classic lacunar syndromes include pure motor, pure sensory, and sensorimotor syndromes; ataxic hemiparesis; and clumsy hand dysarthria. However, other combinations of findings may be attributed to small, deep infarcts due to a lacunar mechanism. Efforts to expand the diagnosis into new formulas that account for the presence of cognitive changes have shaken the earlier purity and confounded the appealing simplicity of the initial syndromes,[175] leading some to question the separate nosologic identity of lacunar infarcts.[176,177] Some skeptics have suggested the abolition of terms like *lacunar syndrome, lacune,* and *lacunar infarction* because of confusion. However, most of the investigations that have included analyses of clinical syndromes, results of diagnostic imaging, etiopathophysiologic correlations, and treatment implications justify the continued use of the term *lacunar infarct.* Lacunar infarcts were slow to gain clinical acceptance, but they are now considered to account for between 10% and 20% of all cases of stroke (see Fig. 20-1).[25,52,122,124,178]

Investigators have used the term *lacunar hypothesis* to refer to the clinicopathophysiologic correlation of the condition. The hypothesis consists of two parts: (1) symptomatic lacunes are usually present with a small number of distinct lacunar syndromes and (2) lacunes are caused by a characteristic disease of the penetrating artery.[179] After satisfying both parts of the hypothesis, the stroke can be classified as a lacunar infarction. The correspondence between lacunar syndrome and lacunar infarction depends on the timing of presentation and examination. The concordance is greatest among patients examined up to 96 hours after stroke onset[179,180] and is much less when patients are tested in the first few hours of stroke onset.[71,123,181]

One study concluded that lacunar syndromes, especially pure sensory syndrome and ataxic hemiparesis, were highly predictive of small deep infarcts;[182] however, about one in four patients seen with lacunar syndromes may ultimately be proved to have a non-lacunar infarct mechanism. A complete diagnostic evaluation of large vessels and potential cardiogenic sources of embolism is warranted in these patients.

Stuttering lacunar syndrome or capsular warning syndrome strongly suggests an underlying small-artery occlusion. This syndrome is characterized by a cluster of repetitive, stereotypic, and typically short-lasting events.[13,183,184] Between attacks, patients may be completely normal (lacunar TIA) or may return to near normal with a mild residual deficit. In almost half of the patients with repetitive lacunar spells, the cluster period ends with a persistent deficit, usually hemiparesis.[184] MRI typically shows a lacunar infarct in deep or brainstem locations when persistent deficit develops.

Results of Diagnostic Tests

Because the vascular lesion lies in vessels that are only 200 to 400 µm in diameter, it is no surprise that conventional cerebral angiographic and MRA findings are normal. Incidental parent artery disease may be found in approximately 20% of cases,[25] but whether it is causally related to the site of infarction is often unclear. An angiogram with normal findings could also be expected if microembolism was the cause of the deep infarction. CT is positive only for roughly half of cases of even the most common form of lacunar infarct: pure motor stroke.[64] MRI is clearly superior to CT in evaluating lesions, especially in the posterior fossa.[185] Nevertheless, even a diffusion-weighted MRI may sometimes miss a definite lesion in patients presenting with a lacunar syndrome.[186–188] This might be especially evident in the brainstem location. A repeat MRI 1 or 2 days later often demonstrates the lacunar infarct.

Large deep infarcts, some of which have been called *super lacunes* or *giant lacunes,* may be seen on CT or MRI as a focal deep infarct without involvement of the cerebral surface.[189] A problem arises in the interpretation of these deep lesions because an embolus may initially be arrested in the stem of the MCA, causing a large swath of infarction scattered through the lenticulostriate territories. When accompanied by a separate cerebral surface low-density area, such large deep infarcts are easily reclassified as examples of embolism, nonthrombotic infarction, or infarction of other cause. Therefore, most of these large, deep infarcts are really not lacunes.

BOX 20-2 Uncommon Causes of Stroke

- Acute arterial dissection
- Cerebral vascular abnormalities (chronic dissection, dolichoectasia, post-radiation arteriopathy, arteriovenous malformation)
- Cerebral vasculitis
- Cerebral venous thrombosis
- Acute disseminated intravascular coagulation
- Drug-induced stroke
- Fibromuscular dysplasia
- Heparin-induced thrombocytopenia type II
- Cerebral autosomal dominant arteriopathy with subcortical infarcts and leukoencephalopathy
- Hyperviscosity syndromes (multiple myeloma and other monoclonal gammapathies, polycytemia, leukemia, essential thrombocytosis, myelodysplastic disorders)
- Hypoperfusion syndromes (sepsis, severe hypotension, cardiogenic shock)
- Iatrogenic causes
- Partially thrombosed cerebral aneurysm
- Mitochondrial and metabolic causes of stroke
- Meningitis
- Migraine-induced stroke
- Moyamoya disease
- Primary antiphospholipid antibody syndrome
- Primary infection of the arterial wall
- Sickle cell disease
- Sneddon's syndrome
- Thrombotic thrombocytopenic purpura – hemolytic uremic syndrome
- Segmental vasoconstriction or vasospasm (subarachnoid hemorrhage, reversible cerebral vasoconstriction syndromes, benign angiopathy of the central nervous system, drugs)
- Abnormalities of thrombosis and hemostasis
- Other causes (neurosarcoidosis, Fabry disease, stroke secondary to compression by intracranial mass lesion, cancer-related stroke)

Uncommon Causes of Stroke

This category consists of a cluster of miscellaneous disorders that are difficult to further categorize into more homogeneous groups (Box 20-2). Collectively, uncommon causes account for about 3–7% of ischemic strokes.[25] A more detailed description for each disorder in this category is provided in relevant sections of this book.

Stroke of Undetermined Etiology

Despite efforts to arrive at a diagnosis, the cause of the infarction may remain undetermined. A number of explanations can be offered. The first of the three major reasons for the failure is easily understood: no appropriate laboratory studies are performed. Advanced age, limited resources, coexisting severe disease with a poor prognosis, and patients' or physicians' unwillingness are only a few of the many reasons for deferring an evaluation. Brain imaging, imaging of the extra- and intra-cranial circulation, cardiac evaluation, and specific blood and CSF tests based on the level of suspicion of a particular cause are warranted in every stroke patient. Failure to perform etiologic investigations in the absence of a positive test result is considered "incomplete evaluation". Failure to investigate for an etiology in the presence of clinical or imaging stroke features suggestive of that etiology is also incomplete evaluation. For instance, diagnostic evaluation is incomplete in a patient with atrial fibrillation who has temporally separate infarcts exclusively in one hemisphere (a suggestive feature for large-artery atherosclerosis), but no angiographic evaluation.

A second common reason for failure to classify stroke etiology into a determined subtype is due to multiple competing etiologies. Assigning patients with more than one etiology into a distinct undetermined category enhances the homogeneity of other determined etiologic categories. However, as previously mentioned, without a rule-based approach, frequent detection of multiple competing etiologies with present-day stroke work-up results in categorization of approximately one-half of stroke patients into the undetermined category.[25,27,28]

The third category includes normal or inconclusive findings that are reached despite appropriate laboratory studies performed at the appropriate time. In the SiGN study, a rigorous diagnostic scheme (brain imaging, imaging of the extra- and intra-cranial circulation, and cardiac evaluation with echocardiography when necessary) resulted in classifying 13% of the study population as having infarcts of unknown or cryptogenic cause (Fig. 20-1).[25] An additional 15% had a minor or uncertain-risk cardiac source. Inadequate sensitivity and improper timing of diagnostic tests are partially responsible for inability to identify the cause of stroke. The latter is particularly important because stroke etiologies are dynamic abnormalities that can transform or disappear in time. A flap or double lumen associated with acute arterial dissection may disappear on repeat angiography, a critical stenosis may regress as a result of dissolution of the overlying thrombus, an intracardiac thrombus may vanish within hours to days after stroke, or an underlying hematologic or immunologic abnormality may not be detected when the disease is in remission. Angiography for embolism performed more than 48 hours after the ictus has a yield as low as 15% for evidence of the responsible occlusion.[126] Brain scans performed once only within a few hours of the onset of an ischemic stroke have a similarly low yield. In summary, performing diagnostic studies too early or too late may increase false-negative diagnoses. Optimal timing of evaluation for each etiology is unknown. In general, the probability of finding an abnormality increases as the time from stroke onset to diagnostic evaluation decreases.

Angiography may be normal or may show a distal branch occlusion or occlusion of a major cerebral artery stem in cryptogenic strokes. Because arterial occlusions can have thrombotic or embolic causes, their demonstration does not settle the mechanism in all cases, particularly among black, Asian, and Hispanic patients, in whom intracranial atheroma has been more frequently detected.[178] In white patients, on the other hand, pathologic examination of occlusions has rarely demonstrated an organized thrombus,[190] so the angiographic identification of an intracranial occlusion can usually be considered typical for embolism provided that there is no other explanation for arterial occlusion, such as hypercoagulability disorders, or inflammatory, infectious, or other disorders of the vessel wall. As previously mentioned, this mechanism of stroke is called cryptogenic embolism and implies catheter-, CT-, or MR-angiographic evidence of abrupt vessel cut-off in an otherwise normal-appearing artery.[1] Complete recanalization of a prior occlusion by angiographic methods or ultrasound further supports an embolic etiology. A less stringent definition for cryptogenic embolism that does not require angiographic evidence of abrupt cut-off and recanalization has been proposed.[191] According to this definition, embolic stroke of undetermined source or ESUS is diagnosed when there is a non-lacunar brain infarct without proximal arterial stenosis or cardioembolic or other uncommon sources.[191] Cryptogenic embolism or ESUS as a distinct category can be expected to allow studying new emboli sources in a more refined way.

Efforts should be made in each case to establish the existence of uncommon causes of stroke. Emerging technologies have led to the suggestions that some of the cases of cryptogenic infarct may still be explained by cardiac embolism and large-artery atherosclerosis. Long-term (30 days to 6 months) non-invasive ECG monitoring leads to detection of atrial fibrillation in approximately 10% of patients who have had cryptogenic strokes within the previous 6 months.[192,193] Symptomatic atherosclerotic lesions causing less than 50% stenosis are typically classified in the cryptogenic category unless they are associated with apparent superimposed thrombus or ulceration. Recent studies with MR plaque imaging show that a great deal of such lesions exhibit complicated plaque characteristics, such as ruptured fibrous cap and intraplaque hemorrhage, suggesting that plaques causing mild stenosis may not be incidental.[194,195]

The complete reference list can be found on the companion Expert Consult website at www.expertconsult.inkling.com.

KEY REFERENCES

1. Ay H, Furie KL, Singhal A, et al. An evidence-based causative classification system for acute ischemic stroke. Ann Neurol 2005;58:688–97.
2. Amarenco P, Bogousslavsky J, Caplan LR, et al. Classification of stroke subtypes. Cerebrovasc Dis 2009;27:493–501.
3. Ay H, Gungor L, Arsava EM, et al. A score to predict early risk of recurrence after ischemic stroke. Neurology 2010;74:128–35.
4. Sacco RL, Foulkes MA, Mohr JP, et al. Determinants of early recurrence of cerebral infarction. The Stroke Data Bank. Stroke 1989;20:983–9.
5. Moroney JT, Bagiella E, Paik MC, et al. Risk factors for early recurrence after ischemic stroke: the role of stroke syndrome and subtype. Stroke 1998;29:2118–24.
6. Petty GW, Brown RD Jr, Whisnant JP, et al. Ischemic stroke subtypes: a population-based study of functional outcome, survival, and recurrence. Stroke 2000;31:1062–8.
7. Ad hoc Committee by the Advisory Council for the National Institute of Neurological Diseases and Blindness. A classification and outline of cerebrovascular diseases. Neurology 1958;8:395–4343.
8. Fisher CM. Capsular infarcts. The underlying vascular lesions. Arch Neurol 1979;36:65–73.
9. Fisher CM. The arterial lesions underlying lacunes. Acta Neuropathol (Berl) 1969;12:1–15.
10. Fisher CM. Lacunes: Small, deep cerebral infarcts. Neurology 1965;15:774–84.
11. Fisher CM, Caplan LR. Basilar artery branch occlusion: a cause of pontine infarction. Neurology 1971;21:900–5.
12. Mohr JP, Caplan LR, Melski JW, et al. The harvard cooperative stroke registry: A prospective registry. Neurology 1978;28:754–62.
13. Aring CD, Meritt HH. Differential diagnosis between cerebral hemorrhage and cerebral thrombosis. Arch Intern Med 1935;56:435–56.
14. Kannel WB, Dawber TR, Cohen MS, et al. Vascular disease of the brain – epidemiologic aspects: The Framingham study. Am J Public Health 1965;55:1355–66.
15. Williams GR, Jang JG, Matchar DB, et al. Incidence and occurrance of total (first-ever and recurrent) stroke. Stroke 1999;30:2523–8.
16. Kolominsky-Rabas PL, Weber M, Gefeller O, et al. Epidemiology of ischemic stroke subtypes according to TOAST criteria: Incidence, recurrence, and long-term survival in ischemic stroke subtypes: A population-based study. Stroke 2001;32:2735–40.
17. Mohr JP, Barnett HJM. Classification of Ischemic Strokes. In: Stroke: Pathophysiology, diagnosis, and management. 1986. p. 281–91.
18. Adams HP Jr, Bendixen BH, Kappelle LJ, et al. Classification of subtype of acute ischemic stroke. Definitions for use in a multicenter clinical trial. Toast. Trial of org 10172 in acute stroke treatment. Stroke 1993;24:35–41.
19. Ay H, Benner T, Arsava EM, et al. A computerized algorithm for etiologic classification of ischemic stroke: the Causative Classification of Stroke System. Stroke 2007;38:2979–84.
20. Hacke W, Kaste M, Fieschi C, et al. Safety and efficacy of intravenous thrombolysis with a recombinant tissue plasminogen activator in the treatment of acute hemispheric stroke. JAMA 1995;27:1017–25.
21. Timsit S, Sacco RL, Mohr JP, et al. Brain infarction severity differs according to cardiac or arterial embolic source: The NINDS Stroke Data Bank. Neurology 1993;43:728–33.
22. Toni D, Fiorelli M, Gentile M, et al. Progressing neurological deficit secondary to acute ischemic stroke: Study on predictability, pathogenesis and prognosis. Arch Neurol 1995;52:670–5.
23. von Kummer R, Meyding-Lamadi U, Forsting M, et al. Sensitivity and prognostic value of early CT in occlusion of the middle cerebral artery trunk. AJNR Am J Neuroradiol 1994;15:9–15.

24. Pexman JH, Barber PA, Hill MD, et al. Use of the Alberta Stroke Program Early CT Score (ASPECTS) for assessing CT scans in patients with acute stroke. AJNR Am J Neuroradiol 2001;22: 1534–42.
25. Ay H, Arsava EM, Andsberg G, et al. Pathogenic ischemic stroke phenotypes in the National Institute of Neurological Disorders and Stroke – Stroke Genetics Network. Stroke 2014;45:3589–96.
26. Arsava EM, Ballabio E, Benner T, et al. The Causative Classification of Stroke system: an international reliability and optimization study. Neurology 2010;75:1277–84.
27. Comess KA, DeRook FA, Beach KW, et al. Transesophageal echocardiography and carotid ultrasound in patients with cerebral ischemia: prevalence of findings and recurrent stroke risk. J Am Coll Cardiol 1994;23:1598–603.
28. Tejada J, Diez-Tejedor E, Hernandez-Echebarria L, et al. Does a relationship exist between carotid stenosis and lacunar infarction? Stroke 2003;34:1404–11.
29. Goldstein LB, Jones MR, Matchar DB, et al. Improving the reliability of stroke subgroup classification using the Trial of ORG 10172 in Acute Stroke Treatment (TOAST) criteria. Stroke 2001;32:1091–8.
30. Gordon DL, Bendixen BH, Adams HP Jr, et al. Interphysician agreement in the diagnosis of subtypes of acute ischemic stroke: implications for clinical trials. The TOAST Investigators. Neurology 1993;43:1021–7.
31. Atiya M, Kurth T, Berger K, et al. Women's Health Study. Interobserver agreement in the classification of stroke in the Women's Health Study. Stroke 2003;34:565–7.
32. Meschia JF, Barrett KM, Chukwudelunzu F, et al. Siblings with Ischemic Stroke Study (SWISS) Investigators. Interobserver agreement in the trial of org 10172 in acute stroke treatment classification of stroke based on retrospective medical record review. J Stroke Cerebrovasc Dis 2006;15:266–72.
33. Selvarajah JR, Glaves M, Wainwright J, et al. Classification of minor stroke: intra- and inter-observer reliability. Cerebrovasc Dis 2009;27:209–14.
34. McArdle PF, Kittner SJ, Ay H, et al. Agreement between TOAST and CCS ischemic stroke classification: The NINDS SiGN Study. Neurology 2014;83:1653–60.
35. Johnson CJ, Kittner SJ, McCarter RJ, et al. Interrater reliability of an etiologic classification of ischemic stroke. Stroke 1995;26: 46–51.
36. Amarenco P, Bogousslavsky J, Caplan LR, et al. New approach to stroke subtyping: the A-S-C-O (phenotypic) classification of stroke. Cerebrovasc Dis 2009;27:502–8.
37. Lip GY, Nieuwlaat R, Pisters R, et al. Refining clinical risk stratification for predicting stroke and thromboembolism in atrial fibrillation using a novel risk factor-based approach: the euro heart survey on atrial fibrillation. Chest 2010;137(2):263–72.
38. Sylaja PN, Coutts SB, Subramaniam S, et al. VISION Study Group. Acute ischemic lesions of varying ages predict risk of ischemic events in stroke/TIA patients. Neurology 2007;68:415–19.
39. Wen HM, Lam WW, Rainer T, et al. Multiple acute cerebral infarcts on diffusion-weighted imaging and risk of recurrent stroke. Neurology 2004;63:1317–19.
40. Bang OY, Lee PH, Heo KG, et al. Specific DWI lesion patterns predict prognosis after acute ischaemic stroke within the MCA territory. J Neurol Neurosurg Psychiatry 2005;76:1222–8.
41. Fisher CM, Gore I, Okabe N, et al. Atherosclerosis of the carotid and vertebral arteries: Extracranial and intracranial. J Neuropathol Exp Neurol 1965;24:455.
43. Fisher CM. Cerebral thromboangiitis obliterans. Medicine (Baltimore) 1957;36:169.
45. Ogata J, Masuda J, Yutani C, et al. Rupture of atheromatous plaque as a cause of thrombotic occlusion of stenotic internal carotid artery. Stroke 1990;21:1740–5.
46. Lennihan L, Kupsky WJ, Mohr JP, et al. Lack of association between carotid plaque hematoma and ipsilateral cerebral symptoms. Stroke 1987;18:879–81.
47. Ballotta E, Da Giau G, Renon L. Carotid plaque gross morphology and clinical presentation: A prospective study of 457 carotid artery specimens. J Surg Res 2000;89:78–84.
48. Bogousslavsky J, Regli F. Borderzone infarctions distal to internal carotid artery occlusion: Prognostic implications. Ann Neurol 1986;20:346–50.
49. Pessin MS, Hinton RC, Davis KR, et al. Mechanisms of acute carotid stroke: A clinicoangiographic study. Ann Neurol 1979;6: 245.
50. Tsiskaridze A, Devuyst G, de Freitas GR, et al. Stroke with internal carotid artery stenosis. Arch Neurol 2001;58:605–9.
51. Ring BA. Diagnosis of embolic occlusions of smaller branches of the intracerebral arteries. Am J Roentgenol Radium Ther Nucl Med 1966;97:575.
53. Torvick A. The pathogenesis of watershed infarcts in the brain. Stroke 1984;15:221–3.
54. Powers WJ. Cerebral hemodynamics in ischemic cerebrovascular disease. Ann Neurol 1991;29:231–40.
55. Carpenter DA, Grubb RL Jr, Powers WJ. Borderzone hemodynamics in cerebrovascular disease. Neurology 1990;40: 1587–92.
57. Powers WJ, Tempel LW, Grubb RL Jr. Influence of cerebral hemodynamics on stroke risk: One year follow up of 30 medically treated patients. Ann Neurol 1989;25:325–30.
58. Fisher CM, Karnes WE. Local embolism. J Neuropathol Exp Neurol 1965;24:174.
60. Masuda J, Ogata J, Yutani C, et al. Artery to artery embolism from a thrombus formed in stenotic middle cerebral artery: Report of an autopsy case. Stroke 1987;18:680–4.
61. Beal MF, Williams RS, Richardson EP, et al. Cholesterol embolism as a cause of transient ischemic attacks and cerebral infarction. Neurology 1981;31:860.
62. David NJ, Gordon KK, Friedberg SJ, et al. Fatal atheromatous cerebral embolism associated with bright plaques in the retinal arterioles. Neurology 1963;13:708.
67. Barnett HJM, Peerless SJ, Kaufmann JCE. "Stump" of internal carotid artery – a source for further cerebral embolic ischemia. Stroke 1978;9:448.
68. El-Mitwalli A, Saad M, Christou I, et al. Clinical and sonographic patterns of tandem internal carotid artery/middle cerebral artery occlusion in tissue plasminogen activator-treated patients. Stroke 2002;33:99–102.
72. Imparato AM, Riles TS, Gorstein F. The carotid bifurcation plaque: Pathologic findings associated with cerebral ischemia. Stroke 1979;10:238.
73. Angeloni U, Bozzao L, Fantozzi L, et al. Internal border zone infarction following acute middle cerebral artery occlusion. Neurology 1990;40:1196–8.
74. Fieschi C, Sette G, Fiorelli M, et al. Clinical presentation and frequency of potential sources of embolism in acute ischemic stroke patients: The experience of the Rome Acute Stroke Registry. Cerebrovasc Dis 1995;5:75–8.
75. Ringelstein EB, Koschorke S, Holling A, et al. Computed tomographic patterns of proven embolic brain infarctions. Ann Neurol 1989;26:759–65.
76. Ay H, Oliveira-Filho J, Buonanno FS, et al. Diffusion-weighted imaging identifies a subset of lacunar infarction associated with embolic source. Stroke 1999;30:2644–50.
77. Koennecke HC, Bernarding J, Braun J, et al. Scattered brain infarct pattern on diffusion-weighted magnetic resonance imaging in patients with acute ischemic stroke. Cerebrovasc Dis 2001;11:157–63.
78. Heiss WD, Herholz K, Podreka I, et al. Comparison of 99mTc HMPAO SPECT with 18F fluoromethane PET in cerebrovascular disease. J Cereb Blood Flow Metab 1990;10:687–97.
79. Johnson DW, Stringer WA, Marks MP, et al. Stable xenon CT cerebral blood flow imaging: Rationale for and role in clinical decision making. AJNR Am J Neuroradiol 1991;12: 201–13.
83. Nasel C, Azizi A, Wilfort A, et al. Measurement of time-to-peak parameter by use of a new standardization method in patients with stenotic or occlusive disease of the carotid artery. AJNR Am J Neuroradiol 2001;22:1056–61.
84. Baron JC, Frackowiak RS, Herholz K, et al. Use of PET methods for measurement of cerebral energy metabolism and hemodynamics in cerebrovascular disease. J Cereb Blood Flow Metab 1989;9:723–42.
86. Donders RC, Dutch TMB Study Group. Clinical features of transient monocular blindness and the likelihood of atherosclerotic lesions of the internal carotid artery. J Neurol Neurosurg Psychiatry 2001;71:247–9.

88. Timsit SG, Sacco RL, Mohr JP, et al. Early clinical differentiation of cerebral infarction from severe atherosclerotic stenosis and cardioembolism. Stroke 1992;23:486–91.
89. Fisher CM. Occlusion of the internal carotid artery. AMA Arch Neurol Psychiatry 1951;69:346–77.
90. Yanagihara T, Klass DW. Rhythmic involuntary movement as a manifestation of transient ischemic attacks. Trans Am Neurol Assoc 1981;106:46–8.
91. Ringelstein EB, Zeumer H, Angelou D. The pathogenesis of strokes from internal carotid artery occlusion: Diagnostic and therapeutic implications. Stroke 1983;14:867.
92. Hennerici M, Daffertshofer M, Jakobs L. Failure to identify cerebral infarct mechanisms from topography of vascular territory lesions. AJNR Am J Neuroradiol 1998;19:1067–74.
93. Chaves CJ, Silver B, Schlaug G, et al. Diffusion- and perfusion-weighted MRI patterns in borderzone infarcts. Stroke 2000;31: 1090–6.
94. Torvik A, Skullerud K. Watershed infarcts in the brain caused by microemboli. Clin Neuropathol 1982;1:99–105.
95. Pollanen MS, Deck JH. Directed embolization is an alternate cause of cerebral watershed infarction. Arch Pathol Lab Med 1989;113:1139–41.
98. Bogousslavsky J. Double infarction in one cerebral hemisphere. Ann Neurol 1991;30:12–18.
99. Pessin MS, Duncan GW, Davis KR, et al. Angiographic appearance of carotid occlusion in acute stroke. Stroke 1980; 11:485.
100. Quisling RG, Friedman WA, Rhoton AL. High cervical dissection: Spontaneous resolution. AJNR Am J Neuroradiol 1980;1:463.
103. Leow K, Murie JA. Cerebral angiography for cerebrovascular disease: The risks. Br J Surg 1988;75:428–30.
106. Grolimund P, Seiler RW, Aaslid R, et al. Evaluation of cerebrovascular disease by combined extracranial and transcranial Doppler sonography: Experience in 1,039 patients. Stroke 1987;18:1018–24.
110. Hirai T, Korogi Y, Ono K, et al. Prospective evaluation of suspected stenoocclusive disease of the intracranial artery: Combined MR angiography and CT angiography compared with digital subtraction angiography. AJNR Am J Neuroradiol 2002; 23:93–101.
111. Romero JM, Ackerman RH, Dault NA, et al. Noninvasive evaluation of carotid artery stenosis: Indications, strategies, and accuracy. Neuroimaging Clin N Am 2005;15:351–65.
113. Castaigne P, Lhermitte F, Gautier J-C, et al. Internal carotid artery occlusion: A study of 61 instances in 50 patients with postmortem data. Brain 1970;93:231.
115. Dalal PM, Shah PM, Aiyar RR. Arteriographic study of cerebral embolism. Lancet 1965;2:358.
117. Caplan LR. "Top of the basilar" syndrome. Neurology 1980; 30:72.
118. Castaigne P, Lhermitte F, Buge A, et al. Paramedian thalamic and midbrain infarcts: Clinical and neuropathological study. Ann Neurol 1981;10:127.
119. Fisher CM. Bilateral occlusion of basilar artery branches. J Neurol Neurosurg Psychiatry 1977;40:1182.
120. Voetsch B, DeWitt LD, Pessin MS, et al. Basilar artery occlusive disease in the New England Medical Center Posterior Circulation Registry. Arch Neurol 2004;61:496–504.
121. Caplan LR. Intracranial branch atheromatous disease: A neglected, understudied, and underused concept. Neurology 1989;39:1246–50.
122. Foulkes MA, Wolf PA, Price TR, et al. The Stroke Data Bank: Design, methods, and baseline characteristics. Stroke 1988;19: 547–54.
123. Droste DW, Dittrich R, Kemeny V, et al. Prevalence and frequency of microembolic signals in 105 patients with extracranial carotid artery occlusive disease. J Neurol Neurosurg Psychiatry 1999;67:525–8.
125. Babikian VL, Caplan LR. Brain embolism is a dynamic process with variable characteristics. Neurology 2000;54:797–801.
126. Bozzao L, Fantozzi LM, Bastianello S, et al. Ischaemic supratentorial stroke: Angiographic findings in patients examined in the very early phase. J Neurol 1989;236:340–2.
127. del Zoppo GJ, Higashida RT, Furlan AJ, et al. PROACT: A phase II randomized trial of recombinant pro-urokinase by direct arterial delivery in acute middle cerebral artery stroke. Stroke 1998;29:4–11.
128. Fieschi C, Bozzao L. Transient embolic occlusion of the middle cerebral and internal carotid arteries in cerebral apoplexy. J Neurol Neurosurg Psychiatry 1969;32:236–40.
129. Kase CS, White L, Vinson L, et al. Shotgun pellet embolus to the middle cerebral artery. Neurology 1981;31:458.
130. Zanette EM, Roberti C, Mancini G, et al. Spontaneous middle cerebral artery reperfusion in ischemic stroke: A follow-up study with transcranial Doppler. Stroke 1995;26:430–3.
133. Molina CA, Montaner J, Abilleira S, et al. Timing of spontaneous recanalization and risk of hemorrhagic transformation in acute cardioembolic stroke. Stroke 2001;32:1079–84.
134. Ringelstein EB, Biniek R, Weiller C, et al. Type and extent of hemispheric brain infarctions and clinical outcome in early and delayed middle cerebral artery recanalization. Neurology 1992;42:289–98.
135. Liebeskind A, Chinichian A, Schechter MM. The moving embolus seen during serial cerebral angiography. Stroke 1971;2:440.
137. Irino T, Tandea M, Minami T. Angiographic manifestations in postrecanalized cerebral infarction. Neurology 1977;27:471.
138. Little JR, Shawhan B, Weinstein M. Pseudo-tandem stenosis of the internal carotid artery. Neurosurgery 1980;7:574.
140. Wysokinski WE, Owen WG, Fass DN, et al. Atrial fibrillation and thrombosis: immunohistochemical differences between in situ and embolized thrombi. J Thromb Haemost 2004;2:1637–44.
143. del Zoppo GJ, Poeck K, Pessin MS, et al. Recombinant tissue plasminogen activator in acute thrombotic and embolic stroke. Ann Neurol 1992;32:78–86.
144. Bushi D, Grad Y, Einav S, et al. Hemodynamic evaluation of embolic trajectory in an arterial bifurcation: An in-vitro experimental model. Stroke 2005;36:2696–700.
145. Liebeskind D, Babikian V, Llanes J, et al. CT angiography reveals anatomic features that account for the distribution of emboli in the anterior cerebral circulation. Stroke 2001;32:335.
147. Pollanen MS. Behaviour of suspended particles at bifurcations: implications for embolism. Phys Med Biol 1991;36:397–401.
148. Carr IA, Nemoto N, Schwartz RS, et al. Size-dependent predilections of cardiogenic embolic transport. Am J Physiol Heart Circ Physiol 2013;305:H732–9.
149. Friedlich AL, Castleman B, Mohr JP. Case records of the Massachusetts General Hospital. N Engl J Med 1968;278:1109.
151. Fisher CM, Pearlman A. The non-sudden onset of cerebral embolism. Neurology (Minneap) 1967;17:1025.
152. Whisnant JP. Multiple particles injected may all go to the same cerebral artery branch. Stroke 1982;13:720.
153. Minematsu K, Yamaguchi T, Omae T. Spectacular shrinking deficit: Rapid recovery from a full hemispheral syndrome by migration of an embolus. Neurology 1991;41(Suppl.):329.
154. Kittner SJ, Sharkness CM, Price TR, et al. Infarcts with a cardiac source of embolism in the NINDS Stroke Data Bank: Historical features. Neurology 1990;40:281–4.
156. Clergeau MR, Hamon M, Morello R, et al. Silent cerebral infarcts in patients with pulmonary embolism and a patent foramen ovale: a prospective diffusion-weighted MRI study. Stroke 2009; 40(12):3758–62.
157. Kang DW, Chalela JA, Ezzeddine MA, et al. Association of ischemic lesion patterns on early diffusion-weighted imaging with TOAST stroke subtypes. Arch Neurol 2003;60:1730–4.
158. Roh JK, Kang DW, Lee SH, et al. Significance of acute multiple brain infarction on DWI. Stroke 2000;31:688–94.
159. Beghi E, Bogliun G, Cavaletti G, et al. Hemorrhagic infarction: Risk factors, clinical and tomographic features, and outcome: A case-control study. Acta Neurol Scand 1989;80:226–31.
161. Hornig CR, Dorndorf W, Agnoli AL. Hemorrhagic cerebral infarction – a prospective study. Stroke 1986;17:179–85.
163. Bladin PF. A radiologic and pathologic study of embolism of the internal carotid-middle cerebral arterial axis. Radiology 1964;82:614.
165. David DO, Rumbaugh CL, Gilson JM. Angiographic diagnosis of small-vessel cerebral emboli. Acta Radiol Diagn (Stockh) 1969; 9:264.
166. Bogousslavsky J, Regli F, Uske A. Thalamic infarcts: clinical syndromes, etiology, and prognosis. Neurology 1988;38: 837–48.

167. Kim J, Choi HY, Nam HS, et al. Mechanism of tuberothalamic infarction. Eur J Neurol 2008;15(10):1118–23.
168. Perren F, Clarke S, Bogousslavsky J. The syndrome of combined polar and paramedian thalamic infarction. Arch Neurol 2005;62: 1212–16.
169. Ay H, Oliveira-Filho J, Buonanno FS, et al. Diffusion-Weighted Imaging Identifies a Subset of Lacunar Infarction Associated with Embolic Source. Stroke 1999;30:2644–50.
170. Tohgi H, Kawashima M, Tamura K, et al. Coagulation fibrinolysis abnormalities in acute and chronic phases of cerebral thrombosis and embolism. Stroke 1990;21:1663–7.
171. Hinton RC, Mohr JP, Ackerman RA, et al. Symptomatic middle cerebral artery stem stenosis. Ann Neurol 1979;5:152.
172. Nishida N, Ogata J, Yutani C, et al. Cerebral artery thrombosis as a cause of striatocapsular infarction: A histopathological case study. Cerebrovasc Dis 2000;10:151–4.
173. Wardlaw JM, Dennis MS, Warlow CP, et al. Imaging appearance of the symptomatic perforating artery in patients with lacunar infarction: Occlusion or other vascular pathology? Ann Neurol 2001;50:208–15.
174. Nelson RF, Pullicino P, Kendall BE, et al. Computed tomography on patients presenting with lacunar syndromes. Stroke 1980; 11:256.
175. Fisher CM. Lacunar strokes and infarcts: A review. Neurology 1982;32:871.
176. Landau WM. Clinical neuromythology VI. Au clair de lacune: Holy wholly, holey logic. Neurology 1989;39:725–30.
177. Millikan C, Futrell N. The fallacy of the lacunar hypothesis. Stroke 1990;21:1251–7.
179. Bamford JM, Warlow CP. Evolution and testing of the lacunar hypothesis. Stroke 1988;19:1074–82.
180. Bamford J, Sandercock P, Dennis M, et al. Classification and natural history of clinically identifiable subtypes of cerebral infarction. Lancet 1991;337:1521–6.
181. Chimowitz MI, Furlan AJ, Sila CA, et al. Etiology of motor or sensory stroke: A prospective study of the predictive value of clinical and radiological features. Ann Neurol 1991;30:519–25.
182. Gan R, Sacco RL, Kargman DE, et al. Testing the validity of the lacunar hypothesis: The Northern Manhattan Stroke Study experience. Neurology 1997;48:1204–11.
184. Donnan GA, O'Malley HM, Quang L, et al. The capsular warning syndrome: pathogenesis and clinical features. Neurology 1993;43:957–62.
185. Hommel M, Besson G, Le Bas JF, et al. Prospective study of lacunar infarction using magnetic resonance imaging. Stroke 1990;21:546–54.
187. Singer MB, Chong J, Lu D, et al. Diffusion-weighted MRI in acute subcortical infarction. Stroke 1998;29:133–6.
188. Ay H, Koroshetz WJ, Buonanno FS, et al. Negative diffusion-weighted MR imaging with stroke-like focal deficits. Neurology 1999;51:1369–76.
189. Rascol A, Clanet M, Manelfe C. Pure motor hemiplegia: CT study of 30 cases. Stroke 1982;13:11.
190. Jorgensen L, Torvik A. Ischaemic cerebrovascular diseases in an autopsy series. Part I: Prevalence, location and predisposing factors in verified thromboembolic occlusions, and their significance in the pathogenesis of cerebral infarction. J Neurol Sci 1966;3:490–5.
191. Hart RG, Diener HC, Coutts SB. Embolic strokes of undetermined source: the case for a new clinical construct. Lancet Neurol 2014;13:429–38.
192. Gladstone DJ, Spring M, Dorian P, et al. Atrial fibrillation in patients with cryptogenic stroke. N Engl J Med 2014;370: 2467–77.
193. Sanna T, Diener HC, Passman RS, et al. Cryptogenic stroke and underlying atrial fibrillation. N Engl J Med 2014;370:2478–86.
194. Kwee RM, van Oostenbrugge RJ, Prins MH, et al. Symptomatic patients with mild and moderate carotid stenosis: plaque features at MRI and association with cardiovascular risk factors and statin use. Stroke 2010;41:1389–93.
195. Esposito L, Saam T, Heider P, et al. MRI plaque imaging reveals high-risk carotid plaques especially in diabetic patients irrespective of the degree of stenosis. BMC Med Imaging 2010;10:27.

21 Clinical Scales to Assess Patients with Stroke

Harold P. Adams, Jr.

KEY POINTS

- Several scales are used to assess patients with ischemic or hemorrhagic stroke.
- These scales ease communication among healthcare professionals, facilitate stroke care, and are crucial for stroke research.
- The scales are used in a variety of settings and include systems to screen for the presence of a stroke in an emergency setting, to describe the severity of neurological impairments, to differentiate hemorrhagic and ischemic stroke, to determine the most likely subtype of ischemic stroke, to monitor neurological improvement or worsening, to assess responses to therapy, and to describe outcomes including disability, handicap, and quality of life.
- Both clinicians and investigators should become familiar and use those scales that have the best face validity.
- The most widely used scales are the Glasgow Coma Scale, National Institutes of Health Stroke Scale, modified Rankin Scale, and the Barthel Index.

Several clinical stroke scales are used to expedite clinical research, management of patients, and communication among healthcare providers. Some scales are widely accepted and are now used extensively. As a result, it is important for physicians to have a working knowledge of the most commonly used rating instruments. Physicians also should be aware of the limitations of each of the scales; they cannot describe all the variations and nuances of the broad spectrum of the clinical manifestations of stroke. All the stroke rating instruments involve some element of combining patients with some differences in findings into groups. Thus, any stroke scale should be considered as an adjunct to a carefully performed history and neurological examination. The scales discussed in this chapter are based primarily on clinical findings and those instruments that are scored on the findings of brain imaging or other diagnostic tests are not discussed.

Some clinical rating instruments aid emergency medical services (EMS) personnel and emergency medicine physicians in their diagnosis of stroke (Box 21-1). Additional scales are used to distinguish hemorrhagic from ischemic stroke or to define the subtype of ischemic stroke; differentiation may be made by vascular territory, size of the stroke, location of the brain injury, or by the presumed etiology. Clinical scales are used to rate the types and severity of neurological impairments, which, in turn reflect the extent of the brain injury. These scales also are used to monitor neurological worsening or improvement and they provide prognostic information. Some modality-specific scales, which are most commonly used by rehabilitation personnel, rate very specific functions and responses to local interventions. Other scales are used to assess a patient's status after stroke including disability, handicap, global outcome, and quality of life. Many scales are complementary and patients may be assessed at different points of their illness by the use of several rating instruments. The most frequently used stroke scales are those that rate impairments, disability, and global outcomes or handicap. Physicians, other healthcare providers, and the public have a reasonable understanding of the meanings of these terms, which are used in this chapter. However, the World Health Organization has developed different terms (body dimension, activities dimension, and participation dimension) that generally correspond to the terms of impairment, disability, and handicap.

DESIRED QUALITIES OF STROKE SCALES

Most of the currently used scales were developed to describe subjects enrolled in clinical trials, but their use has been expanded to a spectrum of clinical settings. The result or score of a stroke scale should be clinically relevant and should be obvious to the healthcare providers that will use the scale (face validity.)[1–4] The aim of the scale should be clear. For a stroke scale to be useful, it should be able to provide a numerical score of some other categorization that is clinically relevant. The results should provide a clear impression that provides a mental image of the patient's status to a clinician. The derived information may affect decisions in diagnosis, treatment, or counseling. The purpose of the scale and the proper time for its use should be obvious. For example, using an outcome scale such as the modified Rankin Scale (mRS) at the time of admission for treatment of a stroke is not appropriate because the scale emphasizes functional outcomes that cannot be accurately assessed in the setting of an acute stroke.[5,6] Some scales provide quantitative items that may be calculated with scores of individual items added to form a total scale; the National Institutes of Health Stroke Scale (NIHSS) is a widely used example.[7] Some scores involve the addition of points to achieve a total score. In other instances, the score entails subtraction from an initial baseline score; in such a case a low score reflects a serious brain injury. In either instance, the total score of a numerical system is important because it usually provides information about prognosis, which, in turn, may affect decisions about treatment.[8] Thus, the clinician needs to understand the scoring system that is used for each individual rating instrument.

Scales should be examined in a manner that is similar to that used to validate a diagnostic test because, in fact, a stroke scale is an ancillary instrument even if it is based on clinical findings. The scale should be sensitive; it should be able to detect those findings that are of most interest. The scale should be specific; it should permit recognition and scoring of only those abnormalities that are important. As much as possible,

BOX 21-1 Types and Goals of Stroke Scales

Emergency recognition of stroke
  Emergency medical services personnel
  Emergency medicine physicians
Differentiation of hemorrhagic from ischemic stroke
Differentiation of ischemic stroke syndromes
Determination of the most likely etiology of ischemic stroke
Quantify the types and severity of neurological impairments (stroke) to provide prognostic information and guide treatment decisions
  Ischemic stroke
  Hemorrhagic stroke
Monitor for neurological improvement or worsening
Measure modality-specific responses to specific rehabilitation therapies
Rate outcomes after stroke
  Disability
  Handicap
  Quality of life

the scale should not have high rates of false-positive or false-negative results that would affect patient care. In summary, if possible, both the positive and negative predictive values of the scale should be determined with comparisons to a standard. These features are especially important for those clinical scales that are used to differentiate stroke from other acute neurological illnesses, hemorrhagic from ischemic stroke, or the subtype of ischemic stroke. The standards to which these diagnoses are compared include subsequent clinical diagnoses, outcomes and the results of diagnostic studies such as brain imaging. In summary, a scale must be accurate. Unfortunately, some scales, such as those differentiating hemorrhagic from ischemic stroke, have not met these criteria.

There is no single scale that provides information about the gamut of the clinical aspects of stroke. In most circumstances, patients are assessed by combinations of rating instruments that are performed at different times. All the scales have individual strengths and weaknesses. For example, the widely used NIHSS has a bias towards higher scores being calculated with strokes affecting the left hemisphere.[9] Practitioners need to know the limitations and idiosyncrasies of each scale.

A clinically used scale should be easy to perform and germane to the clinical situation. In addition, scales that are used in an emergency situation should be able to be performed rapidly. Some rating instruments use components based on history obtained from the patient or observers; information may reflect performance, demographic findings (i.e., age), or the presence of risk factors for stroke or accelerated atherosclerosis. Other scales are based solely on findings detected by direct physical examination and place an emphasis on the neurological assessment. Many scales, especially those used to rate the severity of neurological impairments, include gradations in scoring; for example, different scores for the severity of motor signs or levels of consciousness. Other scales use a numeric system of rating but these numbers are not based on computation of points from items contained within the scale. For example, the Hunt-Hess Scale for subarachnoid hemorrhage has five defined grades that do not include scoring of components to reach that grade.[10]

Weighting of different items is included in some scales. For example, in the Canadian Stroke (Neurological) Scale (CNS) the item scoring consciousness is given more points than individual items rating language or arm motor function.[11,12] An even more elaborate system (the Japan Stroke Scale) was developed by Gotoh et al.;[13] they selected ten variables ranging from consciousness to pupillary changes. The weighted factors ranged from consciousness (49.8%) to plantar reflex (2.2%) to sensory impairment (2.1%). The utility of this very complex approach that results in a wide range of scores is not established. Regardless of the rating instrument, the bottom line for the success of the scale is its credibility. Healthcare providers need to recognize the utility of the scale in their assessment and care of patients with stroke. A few scales that have been used for several years have considerable cachet. For example, the Glasgow Coma Scale (GCS), which was originally developed to define the severity of brain injury among patients with craniocerebral trauma, has become a worldwide standard for assessing a wide variety of critically ill patients with impairments of consciousness including those with stroke.[8]

A valid scale must have attributes of strong inter-rater agreement and intra-rater reproducibility in scoring. These features are especially important for scales that describe subtypes of stroke, that measure the severity of neurological impairments, or that rate outcomes. The goal is to achieve an accurate measure of the patient's condition. A lack of agreement in diagnoses or assessments of the clinical findings is a potential disaster for multicenter clinical trials and also weakens the applicability of the data obtained from these trials. For example, during the development of the Trial of Org 10172 in Acute Stroke Treatment (TOAST) classification, the researchers found that physicians often disagreed about the subtype of ischemic stroke despite being presented by the same information.[14] Agreement was very high when assessing a straightforward case, but was disappointingly low for those cases that had multiple potential explanations or when important supporting data were missing. Thus, the researchers found that the kappa statistic (the degree of improvement about chance) was reasonably good for some subtypes of stroke but less acceptable for others. Measures to improve the agreement of the scales can be undertaken but both researchers and clinicians should recognize that no scale will ever achieve unanimity or perfection when a complex, multifactorial disease such as stroke is being evaluated.

To improve agreement and reproducibility, developers of scales use arbitrary rules to define the various grades of scored items. For instruments that are based on historical information, specific questions to ask and specific answers that are sought are explained. For those scales based primarily on findings on an examination, the steps in the performance of the assessment and the methods to rate the findings are described. Some scales include scoring responses for contingencies such as an absent limb or the presence of a severe comorbid disease. The scales that perform the best included detailed definitions for all the potential scores for items that are being assessed. Still, even these definitions are open to interpretation by the rater and they may not address the wide range of potential scenarios that may be found in a large group of patients with stroke. As an additional step to improve validity, researchers and other groups created programs to train clinicians on the use of several scales. The programs usually are supplemented by a certification process that tests the clinician's ability to accurately use the rating instrument. Because the mRS and the NIHSS are the most widely used rating instruments in clinical trials, they have the most extensive educational and certification programs, which have become a critical quality component of clinical trials.[15-17]

Because of marked differences between measurements of scales and among investigators in multicenter studies, some trials used central adjudication or scoring as an additional quality control measure.[18] This approach is most commonly used to assess outcome data. The relevant information is sent to an individual or panel that reviews a videotape of the patient's performance. This tactic improves consistency of scoring in the trial and may be accompanied by a reduction in the size of the trial that usually would be needed to compensate for differences in scoring among raters.

SCALES USED BY EMERGENCY MEDICAL SERVICES

The GCS was developed to quantify the severity of neurological impairments with head injuries[8] (Table 21-1). Potential scores range from 3 to 15 points and are based on the patient's best verbal response, best motor response, and eye movement. For example, a patient with hemiparetic but volitional movement on the left and flexor posturing on the right would be rated as having 5 or 6 points on the motor item. In general, patients with scores less than 8 have a very serious brain injury and a poor prognosis. Although the GCS has not been tested for inter-rater agreement and intra-rater reproducibility, it has strong predictive power. It is used widely by EMS personnel, physicians, and other healthcare providers. The rating system is most useful in assessment of patients with alterations in consciousness. Thus, its value generally is greater among persons with hemorrhagic stroke than among those with cerebral infarction.[19] Although the GCS usually is not helpful in evaluation of cases of suspected ischemic stroke because consciousness usually is not disturbed, it may be a strong predictor of outcomes among patients with severe strokes affecting the brainstem.[20] A pared down ("slim") version of the GCS has been developed to expedite its use by non-physicians; unfortunately, it has not been found to be useful.[21] The World Federation of Neurological Surgeons (WFNS) Scale for measuring the severity of subarachnoid hemorrhage is a derivative of the GCS.[22,23] The GCS score also is included in scales to rate the severity of intracerebral hemorrhage.[24] Overall, the GCS continues to be an important component of assessment of patients in multiple care settings. The Japan Coma Scale also may be used to assess patients with impaired consciousness due to a variety of neurological illnesses including subarachnoid hemorrhage.[25]

Rating systems are used by EMS personnel to determine if it is likely that a patient has had a stroke.[26-30] A variation of the Cincinnati Pre-Hospital Stroke Scale (CPHSS) called the FAST (Face, Arm, and Speech Test) scale is used in the UK.[31] Another derivative of the CPHSS is the Medic prehospital Assessment for Code Stroke; it contains all the components of the CPHSS but adds assessments of gaze and leg function. Besides screening the patient at the scene, these scales are used to transmit information to a hospital emergency department. The Miami Emergency Neurologic Deficit (MEND) scale has two versions; one involves a brief examination that is performed on the scene and the second includes a more extensive examination that is done in the ambulance as the patient is being transported to the hospital.[29] The scales include a limited number of findings obtained by history or examination. The MEND scale includes information about severe headache or a stiff neck, information that points towards an intracranial hemorrhage.[29] The MEND scale also includes questions that are directly related to possible exclusions for treatment with recombinant tissue plasminogen activator (rtPA) including the use of medications such as warfarin.[29] Screening for marked disturbances in blood glucose levels (hyperglycemia or hypoglycemia) is used to detect these possible causes of acute neurological signs that could mimic a stroke.[26] The most commonly assessed features of the emergency scales are language, facial weakness, and arm weakness; which is based on the assumption that unilateral weakness or speech/language trouble points to a stroke (Tables 21-2, 21-3, Box 21-2). These scales can be rated quickly with a reasonable degree of accuracy. Kothari et al.[28] compared the scores obtained by paramedics using the CPHSS with those obtained by physicians using the NIHSS. They found that an abnormality in any of the three scale items was associated with 66%

TABLE 21-1 Glasgow Coma Scale#

Best Response – Eye Opening	(Range of Scores 1–4 Points)
Eyes open spontaneously, not necessarily aware of environment	4 points
Eyes open to speech, not necessarily in response to command	3 points
Eyes open in response to painful stimuli	2 points
No eye opening in response to painful stimuli	1 point
Best Response – Motor	**(Range of Scores 1–6 Points)**
Follows simple commands, may have paresis or hemiplegia	6 points
Responds to painful stimuli by attempting to remove source of pain	5 points
Withdraws to painful stimuli	4 points
Flexor (decorticate) posturing in response to painful stimuli	3 points
Extensor (decerebrate) posturing in response to painful stimuli	2 points
No motor response to painful stimuli	1 point
Best Response – Verbal	**(Range of Scores 1–5 Points)**
Oriented to time, place, and person	5 points
Responds to conversation but is confused	4 points
Intelligible speech but no sustained sentences	3 points
Incomprehensible sounds, moans, groans, but no words	2 points
No verbal response	1 point

Cannot be scored if a patient is intubated

Adapted from Jennett B, Teasdale G, Braakman R, et al. Prognosis of patients with severe head injury. Neurosurgery, *1979; 4: 283–289*

TABLE 21-2 Los Angeles Prehospital Stroke Scale

General Screening			
Age > 45 years	Yes__	No__	Unsure__
No history of seizures	Yes__	No__	Unsure__
Symptoms < 24 hours	Yes__	No__	Unsure__
Not in wheelchair/ bedridden	Yes__	No__	Unsure__
Blood glucose > 60 mg/Dl and < 400 mg/Dl	Yes__	No__	Unsure__
Neurological Examination			
Facial smile	Normal__	Right droop__	Left droop__
Grip	Normal__	Right weak__	Left weak__
		Right absent__	Left absent__
Arm strength	Normal__	Right drift__	Right falls__
		Left drift__	Left falls__
Has only unilateral weakness	Yes__	No__	

Adapted from Kidwell CS, Starkman S, Eckstein M, et al. Identifying stroke in the field: Prospective validation of the Los Angeles Prehospital Stroke Screen (LAPSS) Stroke, *2000; 31: 71–76*

TABLE 21-3 Miami Emergency Neurologic Deficit (MEND) Prehospital Check List

HISTORY			
BASIC DEMOGRAPHIC INFORMATION:			
name, age, sex			
WITNESS INFORMATION (CONTACT TELEPHONE NUMBERS)			
DATE AND TIME OF ONSET OF STROKE (last normal)			
EXCLUSIONS FOR TREATMENT WITH rtPA:			
head injury, use of warfarin, past history of bleeding, brain hemorrhage			
EXAMINATION			
Blood pressure, heart rate, heart rhythm	Normal__	Abnormal__	
Mental Status			
Level of consciousness	Normal__	Abnormal__	
Speech (slurred or wrong words)	Normal__	Abnormal__	
Questions (age and month)	Normal__	Abnormal__	
Commands (close and open eyes)	Normal__	Abnormal__	
Cranial Nerves			
Facial droop (show teeth or smile)	Normal__	Abnormal right__	Abnormal left __
Visual Fields (Four Quadrants)	Normal	Abnormal right__	Abnormal left__
Limbs			
Arm drift (hold out both arms)	Normal__	Abnormal right__	Abnormal left__
Left drift (lift each leg)	Normal__	Abnormal right__	Abnormal left __
Sensory (Feels Touch or Pinch)	Normal__	Abnormal right__	Abnormal left__
Coordination (Touch Finger to Nose)	Normal__	Abnormal right__	Abnormal left__

Adapted from Gordon DL, Issenberg SB, Gordon MS, et al. Stroke training of prehospital providers. An example of simulation-enhanced blended learning and evaluation. Med Teach, *2005; 2&: 114–121*

BOX 21-2 Cincinnati Prehospital Scale

FACIAL WEAKNESS (patient is asked to smile or show teeth)
- Normal – both sides of the face move equally
- Abnormal – one side of the face does not move as well as the other

ARM DRIFT (patient extends both arms straight out for 10 seconds, eyes closed)
- Normal – both arms do the same or do not move at all
- Abnormal – one arm either does not move or drifts downward compared with the other

SPEECH (patient is asked to repeat a sentence of at least seven words)
- Normal – says correct words without slurring
- Abnormal – slurs words, says wrong words, or does not speak

Adapted from Kothari RU, Pancioli A, Liu T, et al. Cincinnati Prehospital Stroke Scale: Reproducibility and validity. Ann Emerg Med, *1999; 33: 373–378*

sensitivity and 87% specificity for identifying a stroke; the sensitivity was much higher for vascular events in the anterior circulation than for strokes in the posterior circulation. The diagnoses of paramedics using the FAST scale were compared with diagnoses by vascular neurologists; agreement was best for detection of arm weakness but acceptable levels of concurrence were noted for both facial weakness and speech disturbance.[32] These scales have been validated by in-field tests and educational programs are available to train EMS personnel. In another study, Studnek et al.[33] compared the CPHSS with the Medica Prehospital for Code Stroke system; they compared assessments by EMS personnel with hospital discharge diagnoses of stroke. While the CPHSS was the more sensitive instrument, they concluded that the specificity was marginal. The CPHSS probably is the most widely used scale in the US. Its advantages are its ease of use and limited information that is required. The MEND scale does require a reasonably high level of sophistication, which may limit its use to only highly trained paramedics and emergency medical services specialists. This scale may not be as applicable for use by volunteer community services that often exist in smaller communities or rural areas. Much of the information in MEND is similar to that collected as part of the assessment for the NIHSS and an alternative to MEND is to train EMS in the use of the NIHSS itself; for example, a potential scenario would be its use during air evacuation.

The Recognition of Stroke in the Emergency Room (ROSIER) Scale was developed to assist emergency medicine physicians in their rapid diagnosis of stroke.[34] The goal is to differentiate stroke from stroke mimics including seizures, syncope, or other acute neurological illnesses and to facilitate the selection of patients who may be treated with emergency therapies such as intravenous rtPA. The scale includes seven items with a total score ranging from −2 to +5 (Table 21-4). In general, a stroke is unlikely if the total score is less than 0; scores of 4 or 5 are strongly correlated with the diagnosis of stroke. The ROSIER scale was tested in a prospective study and showed a sensitivity of 93% (95% confidence interval [CI], 89–97%), specificity of 83% (95%CI, 77–89%), positive predictive value of 90% (95%CI, 85–95%), and negative predictive value of 88% (95%CI, 83–93%.) Information about the utility and implementation of the ROSIER Scale is not available. Whiteley et al.[35] compared the ROSIER scale with the FAST scale and found that the sensitivity and specificity of the two scales were similar. They concluded that the FAST system, which is quicker and easier to perform, probably is sufficient for screening in an emergency department. In another study that tested the utility of the FAST and ROSIER systems for diagnosis in stroke in children, the investigators concluded that these scales had reasonable sensitivity in pediatric patients.[36] Singer et al.[37] developed a simple system involving measurement of consciousness, gaze, and motor function. Each of the items is scored from 0 (normal) to 2 (severe). They found that scoring would predict an occlusion of the proximal middle cerebral artery with reasonable accuracy and that the tool could be used for triage of patients with suspected stroke.

TABLE 21-4 Recognition of Stroke in the Emergency Room (ROSIER) Scale

General Information		
Time of onset of symptoms	Date___	Time ___
Time of examination	Date___	Time ___
Glasgow Coma Scale Score		
Eye movement ___	Motor response___	Verbal response
Blood Pressure		___/___
Blood Glucose Level		___
Correct glucose urgently if level is < 3.5 mmol/L, then reassess		
Scale		
Loss of consciousness/ syncope	Yes: minus 1	No: zero
Presence of seizure activity	Yes: minus 1	No: zero
New onset impairments (including upon awakening)		
Asymmetrical facial weakness	Yes: plus 1	No: zero
Asymmetrical arm weakness	Yes: plus 1	No: zero
Asymmetrical leg weakness	Yes: plus 1	No: zero
Speech disturbance	Yes: plus 1	No: zero
Visual field defect	Yes: plus 1	No: zero

Adapted from Nor AM, Davis J, Sen B, et al. The Recognition of Stroke In the Emergency Room (ROSIER) scale. Development and validation of a stroke recognition instrument. Lancet Neurol, *2005; 4: 727–734*

SCALES TO DIFFERENTIATE HEMORRHAGIC STROKE FROM ISCHEMIC STROKE

Clinical rating instruments to distinguish hemorrhagic from ischemic stroke have been constructed to provide a diagnosis that would obviate the need for brain imaging before treatment, in particular emergency administration of intravenous rtPA. These scales usually include historical information, blood pressure measurements, and findings on the neurological examination. These instruments have not reached adequate levels of either sensitivity or specificity for use in either clinical trials or patient care.[38–40] As a result, the use of these scales should not be considered as a substitute for modern brain imaging, particularly if decisions about emergency treatment of stroke, such as the administration of intravenous rtPA are under consideration.

DIFFERENTIATION OF ISCHEMIC STROKE SYNDROMES

In ischemic stroke, the findings on neurological examination generally reflect the location and size of the brain injury. Still, the clinical manifestations of stroke are diverse and often idiosyncratic to individual patients. Each patient has her or his own individual pattern of impairments. Still, there are features that are common to all and that may be aggregated and correlated with specific patterns or stroke syndromes. These general features may be classified into groupings that could be useful in addressing questions about prognosis, etiology of stroke, acute treatment, and long-term management. For example, most isolated infarctions affecting the cerebral cortex are secondary to branch occlusions from emboli that arise either in the heart or from proximal segments of major extracranial or intracranial arteries. Generally, patients with cortical infarctions have a good prognosis for survival. Those patients with small deep infarctions (lacunes) restricted to deep hemispheric structures (basal ganglia, thalamus, or internal capsule) usually have diseases of small penetrating arteries and their acute prognosis for survival also is good. On the other hand, those patients with major hemispheric infarctions with involvement of both cortical and deep structures often have occlusions of major intracranial or extracranial arteries, in particular the middle cerebral artery or internal carotid artery. These patients are at greatest risk for malignant brain edema and death. The clinical features of ischemic strokes affecting the brainstem and cerebellum may differ from those seen with events affecting the cerebral hemispheres. The prognosis of patients with cerebellar and/or brainstem lesions generally reflects the extent of the ischemic lesion, which in turn is manifested by the pattern of neurological impairments.

The Oxford Community Stroke Project (OCSP) Classification is the most widely used system to categorize patterns of ischemic strokes based on the types of neurological impairments found on examination.[41] It divides events into four groups: (1) total anterior circulation infarction (TACI) – a large cerebral infarction that usually is the result of an occlusion of a major intracranial or extracranial artery, (2) partial anterior circulation infarction (PACI) – smaller cerebral infarction that affects primarily the cortex and/or adjacent (lobar) white matter and that is usually due to embolic occlusion of a pial or cortical branch artery, (3) lacunar infarction (LACI) – a small infarction restricted to the structures deep in the cerebral hemisphere and secondary to occlusion of a small penetrating artery, and (4) posterior circulation infarction (POCI) – an infarction involving primarily the brainstem and/or cerebellum (Box 21-3). There is some uncertainty about some of the definitions for the categories. For example, an isolated homonymous hemianopia, presumably due to embolic occlusion of the calcarine or posterior cerebral artery, is categorized as POCI because these arteries are usually derived from the basilar artery. It also could be considered to be a PACI event because it is restricted to the cerebral cortex and patients with this infarction are more likely to behave similarly to patients with anterior circulation events than those patients with brainstem strokes. The definition of pure motor hemiparesis for the LACI category does not include dysarthria while many patients with these strokes do have mild-to-moderate impairments in circulation. Although the OCSP was developed for differentiating patterns of cerebral infarction, Barber et al.[42] used the system to define patterns of clinical findings among patients with intracerebral hemorrhage. This approach has not been implemented widely.

Lindley et al.[43] tested the inter-rater agreement of the OCSP and found it was moderate-to-good (kappa: 0.54; 95%CI, 0.39–0.68). Another group that tested the OCSP classification among nurses and physicians found only moderate agreement (95%CI, kappa: 0.31–0.45). Because the features of the classification are straightforward and the number of categories is limited, the relatively low rate is surprising. Pittock et al.[44] found that the primary utility of the OCSP was to differentiate the patients with TACI from the other three groups because those with TACI had poor outcomes. This finding is not unexpected given the extensive nature of the brain injury that occurs in this group of patients. The pattern diagnosis achieved by the OCSP was compared to the results of brain imaging in another study; the classification predicted the site of stroke in 80 of 91 patients (88%; 95%CI, 77–92%).[45] The system was most successful for cases of large hemispheric infarctions and did least well among small subcortical lesions. In a study using magnetic resonance imaging (MRI), Mead et al.[46] found that the OCSP classification successfully predicted the site of the lesion. In another study that focused on classification when done in an emergency setting, Smith et al.[47] found that the subtype diagnosis was correct in approximately 65% of cases.

BOX 21-3 Oxford Community Stroke Project Classification of Ischemic Stroke Syndromes

TOTAL ANTERIOR CIRCULATION INFARCTION (TACI)

Presence of the following:

Contralateral weakness of face, arm, and leg
Contralateral homonymous hemianopia
Behavioral or cognitive impairments (aphasia, neglect, etc.)

PARTIAL ANTERIOR CIRCULATION INFARCTION (PACI)

Presence of two of the following:

Contralateral restricted weakness or sensory loss (face, arm, or leg)
Contralateral homonymous hemianopia
Behavioral or cognitive impairments (aphasia, neglect, etc.)

LACUNAR INFARCTION (LACI)

Presence of one of the following:

Pure motor stroke
- Contralateral weakness of the face, arm, and leg
- No other impairments

Pure sensory stroke
- Contralateral sensory loss of the face, arm, and leg
- No other impairments

Ataxic hemiparesis
- Coexistent cerebellar and motor signs
- May have dysarthria
- No visual or cognitive impairments

Sensorimotor stroke
- Contralateral sensory loss and motor signs of face, arm, and leg
- No visual or cognitive impairments

POSTERIOR CIRCULATION INFARCTION (POCI)

Presence of one or more of the following:

Bilateral weakness or sensory loss
Crossed (ipsilateral face and contralateral body) weakness or sensory loss
Ipsilateral incoordination (cerebellar sign) not explained by weakness
Diplopia with or without extraocular palsy
Isolated homonymous hemianopia

Adapted from Bamford J, Sandercock P, Dennis M, et al Classification and natural history of clinically identifiable subtypes of cerebral infarction. Lancet, *1991; 337: 1521–1526*

The sensitivity and specificity were highest for the POCI category (1.00 and 0.97, respectively) and lowest for the LACI category (0.33 and 0.88, respectively). While the early use of vascular and brain imaging may improve the accuracy of the classification system, it seems that the reliance on MRI or other imaging to make the OCSP subtype diagnosis partially defeats the original intent of the scale that was based solely on clinical findings. Although Zhang et al.[48] found that narrowing of the extracranial segment of the internal carotid artery was correlated with the TACI category, a finding that is not surprising, the OCSP classification categories may not be associated with either the site or presence of a demonstrated occlusion of an intracranial artery.

Despite some limitations, the OCSP is widely used in both clinical trials and epidemiological studies. It also is an excellent way to teach the basic principles of neurological localization in stroke to medical students and other trainees. The OCSP system has advantages. It mimics the process that physicians use when they are assessing their patients. It is relatively simple and it gives general information about localizing the stroke. The TACI category forecasts a poor prognosis. When compared to scales that quantify the severity of neurological impairments following stroke, the OCSP classification is not as robust in forecasting outcomes. The OCSP does not predict the location of arterial pathology with sufficiently high frequency to be useful. It does not distinguish the etiology of stroke; for example, patients with the PACI pattern may have an embolus arising from either the heart or an extracranial artery and subsequent management of these underlying causes differs considerably.

TABLE 21-5 Intracerebral Hemorrhage Score

GLASGOW COMA SCALE SCORE	
3–4 points	2 points
5–12 points	1 point
13–15 points	0 points
AGE	
80 years or older	1 point
Younger than 80	0 points
INFRATENTORIAL LOCATION OF HEMATOMA	
Yes	1 point
No	0 points
VOLUME OF HEMORRHAGE	
30 cm^3 or greater	1 point
Smaller than 30 cm^3	0 points
INTRAVENTRICULAR HEMORRHAGE	
Yes	1 point
No	0 points

Adapted from Hemphill, JC, Bonovich DC, Besmertis L, et al. The ICH score. A simple, reliable grading scale for intracerebral hemorrhage. Stroke, *2001; 32: 891–897*

SCALES TO QUANTIFY THE SEVERITY OF INTRACEREBRAL HEMORRHAGE

Scales to quantify the severity of intracerebral hemorrhage differ from most systems that rate the severity of subarachnoid hemorrhage or ischemic stroke, in that they include both clinical information and the results of ancillary studies, usually brain imaging. Several scales are available and all have limitations.[49] The Unified Neurological Stroke Scale was developed to be used in patients with either hemorrhagic or ischemic stroke; it incorporates components from the Scandinavian Stroke Scale (SSS) and the Middle Cerebral Artery Neurological Scale.[50] It includes assessments of consciousness, language, eye movements, tone, and power of the face, arm, hand, leg, and foot. The Intracerebral Hemorrhage (ICH) Scale is the most widely implemented instrument; it contains the following features: GCS score, age, infratentorial location of the hematoma, volume of the hemorrhage, and the presence of intraventricular bleeding[24,51] (Table 21-5). The range of scores is 0–6. In one study, all patients with a score of 5 or 6 died and the mortality was 0 among those with a score of 0.[52] This observation was confirmed in a study by Appelboom et al.[53] who reported that the ICH score was strongly correlated with findings using the standard measures of stroke outcomes including the mRS. A variation of the ICH score involves the substitution of the GCS with the NIHSS score; in a comparison study, the modified scale was equal to the traditional ICH score in predicting mortality and was slightly better in forecasting favorable outcomes.[54] Another variation of the instrument, called the ICH-GS, includes an expanded range of

TABLE 21-6 Essen Intracerebral Hemorrhage Scale

AGE	
< 60 years	0 points
60–69 years	1 point
70–79 years	2 points
80 years or older	3 points
TOTAL NIHSS SCORE	
0–5 points	0 points
6–10 points	1 point
11–15 points	2 points
16–20 points	3 points
Greater than 20 or coma	4 points
NIHSS LEVEL OF CONSCIOUSNESS	
Alert	0 points
Drowsy	1 point
Stupor	2 points
Coma	3 points

NIHSS, National Institutes of Health Stroke Scale

Adapted from Weimar C, Beneman J, Diener H-C, et al. Development and validation of the Essen Intracerebral Hemorrhage Score. J Neurol, Neurosurg, Psychiatry, *2005; 77: 601–605*

TABLE 21-7 World Federation of Neurological Surgeons Subarachnoid Hemorrhage Scale

GRADE I	
Glasgow Coma Scale score	15
Focal signs	Absent
GRADE II	
Glasgow Coma Scale score	13–14
Focal signs	Absent
GRADE III	
Glasgow Coma Scale score	13–14
Focal signs	Present
GRADE IV	
Glasgow Coma Scale score	7–12
Focal signs	Present or absent
GRADE V	
Glasgow Coma Scale score	3–6
Focal signs	Present or absent

Adapted from Ogungbo B: The World Federation of Neurological Surgeons Scale for subarachnoid hemorrhage. Surg Neurol, *2003; 25: 236–238*

points and results in an improved ability to predict both mortality and functional outcomes.[55] The severity of neurological impairments after intracerebral hemorrhage also has been examined through the use of the CNS, SSS, or the NIHSS.[42,54,56] Smith et al.[57] concluded that the NIHSS could be used effectively to predict in-hospital mortality among patients with intracerebral hemorrhage. Weimar et al.[58] developed the Essen ICH score based on the patient's age, the score on the consciousness item of the NIHSS and an aggregate score based on the range of total NIHSS scores (Table 21-6). The scores range from 0 to 10 with favorable outcomes predicted among patients with scores less than 3 and mortality being high among those with more than 7 points. In one study that compared the prognostic utility of the several scales, the Essen ICH score was the best to discriminate for different outcome measures.[59] An advantage of the Essen ICH scale is that it is based solely on clinical variables and the score may be calculated without the results of brain imaging studies being available.

SCALES TO QUANTIFY THE SEVERITY OF SUBARACHNOID HEMORRHAGE

Scales are used to rate the severity of aneurysmal subarachnoid hemorrhage (SAH). The Hunt and Hess scale consists of five grades ranging from minimally symptomatic to coma[10] (Box 21-4). It is most useful in forecasting outcomes among patients with severe neurological impairments or coma.[60] Although this scale is used widely by both clinicians and researchers, the interobserver agreement is relatively low and it is poorer than for the WFNS Scale.[61] There also are concerns about the ability of the milder scores to forecast outcomes.

Because of the perceived limitations of the Hunt-Hess Scale, the WFNS Scale was created. Scoring is largely based on the severity of neurological impairments as rated by the GCS[22,23,62,63] (Table 21-7). The scale has five grades that range from normal consciousness to major impairments and coma. It has a strong predictive value and it has largely replaced the Hunt-Hess Scale for evaluation of patients in clinical trials.[63] Some investigators have used only the scoring of the GCS in the prediction of outcomes after SAH and found that the scores were superior to either the WFNS scale or the Hunt-Hess Scale.[64] On the other hand, Lagares et al.[65] concluded that scales that include factors besides level of consciousness had the best predictive function.

BOX 21-4 Hunt-Hess Classification of Aneurysmal Subarachnoid Hemorrhage

Grade 1

Asymptomatic, mild headache, or possibly nuchal rigidity

GRADE 2

Moderate-to-severe headache, nuchal rigidity, oculomotor nerve palsy but normal consciousness

GRADE 3

Drowsy or confused, mild focal neurological signs

GRADE 4

Stupor, moderate-to-severe motor signs

GRADE 5

Coma, moribund, and extensor posturing

Adapted from Hunt WE, Hess RM Surgical risk as related to time of intervention in repair of intracranial aneurysms. J Neurosurg, *1968; 28: 14–20*

Smith et al.[57] found that the total score on the NIHSS also was a robust predictor of in-hospital mortality among patients with aneurysmal subarachnoid hemorrhage. The NIHSS is also useful in providing supplemental information among patients with milder SAH.[66] Recently, Naval et al.[67] reported on the utility of a scale that combined GCS scores, age of the person and the presence of medical comorbidities.

Scales that are based on imaging findings are also used to help forecast the development of complications of subarachnoid hemorrhage, such as vasospasm and ischemic stroke, or to predict clinical outcomes. Another system is based on the patient's age, the Hunt-Hess grade, the imaging findings on CT that predict vasospasm, and the size of the aneurysm to forecast outcomes.[68] Starke et al.[69] proposed adding the Hunt-Hess scale and the score on the GCS for further defining the severity of SAH among critically ill patients; they found that the combination was helpful in predicting outcomes. These additions add complexity of the assessment and the modifications have not yet been widely accepted.

SCALES TO QUANTIFY THE SEVERITY OF ISCHEMIC STROKE

Several scales are available for assessing the severity of neurological impairments among patients with ischemic stroke. These scales generally are similar because they are based on findings detected on the neurological examination and they have gradations of scoring of the items to reflect the severity of the neurological impairments. A few scales have been tested for validity, inter-rater agreement, and intra-rater reproducibility. The most important scales, which are the focus of this section, are the CNS, SSS, and NIHSS. However, some of the other scales that have been used to assess the severity of ischemic strokes are mentioned. The Mathew Scale includes most of the components of the other scales, but it also has items such as scoring of muscle stretch reflexes that appears to have limited prognostic information.[70] It also has a global rating item that is not clearly described and that appears to have limited usefulness in an acute setting. The Mathew Scale has not undergone the testing of other rating instruments. The Orgogozo Scale corresponds to other stroke scales but it has not undergone the testing of the other rating instruments.[71,72] While it does evaluate level of consciousness, language, proximal and distal motor strength and motor tone, it does not test vision or articulation. The Japanese Stroke Scale also is not used widely.[13] The European Stroke Scale is a multi-item clinical rating instrument that includes assessment of gait, which is a component of the neurological examination that usually cannot be performed in the acute care situation and as a result it is also not widely used.[73] While the Orpington Prognostic Scale is used to predict outcomes after rehabilitation, it also has been used in the first week after stroke.[74] The usefulness of this scale in the evaluation of acutely ill patients within the first hours after stroke is not known.

The CNS has two variations that are scored based on the patient's ability to understand commands[11,12] (Table 21-8). It meets the criteria of validity, reliability, and reproducibility and as a result, it has been used in several clinical trials.[12,75–77] It includes assessments of consciousness, language, and motor function. An advantage is that it tests proximal and distal strength in one version. On the other hand, vision, articulation, sensation, and right hemisphere cognitive impairments such as neglect are not tested. The scores of the individual items are added with a high score generally predicting a favorable outcome. A total score less than 6.5 points strongly predicts mortality at both 1 month and 1 year.[72,76] It also underestimates some functional impairments in persons that survive stroke.[72] The conversion of the scores on the CNS to other rating scales is uncertain, particularly among patients with severe stroke or aphasia. Still, Nilanont et al.[78] concluded that the score on the CNS may be converted to a NIHSS score by use of the following formula NIHSS score = 23 − 2 × CNS score. Although it is not used as extensively as the SSS or the NIHSS, the CNS remains an option for both clinicians and researchers.

TABLE 21-8 Canadian Neurological (Stroke) Scale

Level of Consiousness	
Alert	3 points
Drowsy	1.5 points
Oriented	1 point
Disoriented/not applicable	0 points
Language	
Normal	1 point
Expressive deficit	0.5 point
Receptive deficit	0 points
Motor Function (Scoring if Normal Comprehension)	
Face	
No facial weakness	0.5 point
Facial weakness present	0 points
Proximal Arm	
No weakness	1.5 points
Mild weakness	1 point
Significant weakness	0.5 point
Paralysis	0 points
Distal Arm	
No weakness	1.5 points
Mild weakness	1 point
Significant weakness	0.5 point
Paralysis	0 points
Proximal Leg	
No weakness	1.5 points
Mild weakness	1 point
Significant weakness	0.5 point
Paralysis	0 points
Distal Leg	
No weakness	1.5 points
Mild weakness	1 point
Significant weakness	0.5 point
Paralysis	0 points
Motor Function (Scoring if Impaired Comprehension)	
Face	
Symmetrical	0.5 point
Asymmetrical	0 points
Arms	
Equal	1.5 points
Unequal	0 points
Legs	
Equal	1.5 points
Unequal	0 points

Adapted from Cote R, Hachinski VC, Shurvell BL, et al. The Canadian Neurological Scale. A preliminary study in acute stroke. Stroke, *1986; 17: 731–737*

The SSS has two different versions, an acute prognostic scale that has a range of 0–22 points and a convalescent scale that has a range of 0–48 points.[79] The two versions are used to examine patients at different time points in the course of stroke (Table 21-9). The acute prognosis version of the SSS has reasonable validity and reliability. It has been adapted for multiple languages and cultures and as a result the SSS has been used in both clinical trials and epidemiological studies.[80–82] A low score on the prognostic version of the SSS predicts neurological worsening, poor outcomes, and a high mortality within 30 days of stroke.[83,84] The SSS score also has been combined with other factors to predict mortality at 1 year. The score on the SSS also correlates strongly with the diagnosis of a lacunar infarction.[85] The SSS has been used to describe neurological findings in studies testing the utility of early brain imaging in the evaluation of patients with suspected stroke.[86] The convalescent SSS has not been tested extensively. The aphasia component of the SSS was tested by Davalos et al.; they found the item had reasonable sensitivity and specificity but that the positive predictive value was low. This observation was confirmed in another study.[87] Low scores on the SSS (poor prognosis) can be compared with high scores on the NIHSS. Ali et al.[88] created an equation for conversion of the two scales; the SSS score = 50 − 2 times the NIHSS score. Another conversion system was developed by Gray et al.

The NIHSS was developed to rate the severity of several individual components as found by the neurological examination.[7,89] Originally, the scale was not designed to calculate a total score but initial testing found a strong correlation between the size of the ischemic lesion on brain imaging and the total score.[89] Subsequently, the NIHSS has become the most widely used instrument for rating the severity of stroke,

TABLE 21-9 Scandinavian Stroke Scales

ACUTE PROGNOSIS SCALE	SCORES RANGE 0–22 POINTS
Consciousness	
Fully conscious	6 points
Somnolent but can be awakened	4 points
Reacts to verbal command	2 points
Eye Movements	
No gaze palsy	4 points
Gaze palsy present	2 points
Conjugate eye deviation	0 points
Affected Arm Power	
Raises arm with normal strength	6 points
Raises arm but reduced strength	5 points
Raises arm with elbow flexion	4 points
Can move arm but not against gravity	2 points
Paralysis of the arm	0 points
Affected Leg Power	
Raises leg with normal strength	6 points
Raises leg but reduced strength	5 points
Raises leg with knee flexion	4 points
Can move leg but not against gravity	2 points
Paralysis of the leg	0 points
LONG-TERM CONVALESCENCE SCALE	**SCORES RANGE 0–48 POINTS**
Orientation	
Correct for time, place and person	6 points
2 of the above correct	4 points
1 of the above correct	2 points
Completely disoriented	0 points
Language	
No aphasia	10 points
Limited vocabulary	6 points
Say more than yes/no but no sentences	3 points
Can say only yes/no	0 points
Affected Arm Power	
Raises arm with normal strength	6 points
Raises arm but reduced strength	5 points
Raises arm with elbow flexion	4 points
Can move but not against gravity	2 points
Paralysis	0 points
Affected Hand Power	
Normal hand strength	6 points
Reduced strength in full range	4 points
Some finger movement	2 points
Paralysis	0 points
Affected Leg Power	
Raises leg with normal strength	6 points
Raises leg but reduced strength	5 points
Raises leg with knee flexion	4 points
Can move but not against gravity	2 points
Paralysis	0 points
Facial Palsy	
None or uncertain	2 points
Facial palsy present	0 points
Gait	
Walks 5 meters without aids	12 points
Walks with aids	9 points
Walks with person helping	6 points
Sits without support	3 points
Wheelchair or bedridden	0 points

Adapted from Scandinavian Stroke Study Group. Multicenter trial of hemodilution in ischemic stroke. Background and study protocol. Stroke, *1985; 16: 885–889.*

for monitoring for neurological improvement or worsening, for forecasting outcomes, and for rating outcomes after stroke. While the potential range of scores is from 0 (best possible) to 42 points; the latter score cannot be achieved because some items are not assessed in severely affected patients. The worst possible score is 38. The NIHSS may be done in a few minutes, which is a major advantage.[7,90] The instrument includes 15 independently scored items[7] (Table 21-10). The scale includes items to test function of both the right (non-dominant) and left (dominant) hemispheres, the brain stem, and cerebellum. It has excellent inter-rater agreement and intra-rater reproducibility, particularly if the user has been trained in the use of the instrument; it can be used by a broad spectrum of health-care professionals. The scale may be calculated through assessment of patients using telemedicine or modern communication technology.[91] A score also may be estimated based on the review of medical record; which is a particular attribute for epidemiological research. The NIHSS is accompanied by a detailed description of scoring and includes definitions for each of the assessed items. It has been translated into a number of languages and cultures. In order to improve compliance with the administration of the scale, instruction and certification programs have been developed.[92,93] These programs are widely available on the internet.[15]

The NIHSS may function differently with strokes in the right hemisphere than with lesions in the left hemisphere.[9,94–96] In general, scores are higher with vascular events in the left hemisphere and comparable scores are associated with larger lesions in the right hemisphere; this discrepancy may affect the impact of the scoring on prognosis and decisions about acute management. In addition, the NIHSS appears to be weighted more towards hemispheric infarctions than with strokes affecting the brain stem and cerebellum. The pattern of the changes on the NIHSS also can be used to predict the subtype of ischemic stroke; in particular the presence of neglect, visual field defects, language impairments, or prominent arm weakness point against the diagnosis of a lacunar infarction.[97] Some components of the scale do not perform as well as others. For example, rating of the severity of limb ataxia, articulation, and facial weakness is difficult; inter-rater agreement may be poor.[98] In an attempt to increase inter-rater agreement, elimination of these items has been proposed.[96] However, these modifications have not been widely implemented and may affect the robust prognostic features of the NIHSS. An abbreviated version of the NIHSS, which could be used by non-physician providers, is not useful.[21]

The total score on the NIHSS, when it is calculated within the first hours after stroke, is strongly predictive of the location of an arterial occlusion among patients with events in the carotid circulation; in general, the baseline scores are greater than 8.[99] The total score on the NIHSS also is a robust predictor of outcomes after stroke.[4,94,100] It predicts both acute and longer-term outcomes and forecasts the likelihood of major complications such as malignant brain edema and increased intracranial pressure. In general, a patient with a score less than 5 has a high likelihood of a favorable outcome, whereas a score greater than 20 is associated with a high probability of either death or very severe disability. Patients with multilobar infarctions generally have a score greater than 15. Between the range of 5 and 15 points, the probability of a favorable outcome declines approximately 5% per point.

A discrepancy between a high NIHSS score that usually is associated with a large infarction and the finding of a small lesion on CT or MRI (clinical-imaging mismatch) may influence decisions about emergency treatment because it may predict those patients that may have growth in the size of the infarction and/or neurological worsening.[101] The utility of this potential relationship is not established and it may not predict

TABLE 21-10 National Institutes of Health Stroke Scale

Level of Consciousness	
Alert	0 points
Drowsy	1 point
Stupor	2 points
Coma	3 points
Orientation (Responses to Two Questions)	
Knows age and current month	0 points
Answers one question correctly	1 point
Cannot answer either question correctly	2 points
Commands (Responses to Two Commands)	
Follows two commands correctly	0 points
Follows one command	1 point
Cannot follow either command	2 points
Best Gaze (Movement of Eyes to Left and Right)	
Normal full range of eye movements	0 points
Partial gaze paresis to one side	1 point
Forced gaze (deviation) to one side	2 points
Visual Fields	
No visual field loss	0 points
Partial homonymous hemianopia	1 point
Complete homonymous hemianopia	2 points
Bilateral visual loss	3 points
Facial Motor Function	
No facial muscle weakness	0 points
Minor unilateral facial weakness	1 point
Partial unilateral facial weakness	2 points
Complete paralysis of one or both sides	3 points
Upper Extremity Motor Function (Arm Extension)	
Right and Left Upper Extremities Scored Independently (Range of 0–8 Points)	
Normal movement	0 points
Drift of arm with extension	1 point
Some effort against gravity	2 points
No effort against gravity but moves limb	3 points
No movement of the arm	4 points
Lower Extremity Motor Function (Leg Extension)	
Right and Left Lower Extremities Scored Independently (Range of 0–8 Points)	
Normal movement	0 points
Drift of leg with extension	1 point
Some effort against gravity	2 points
No effort against gravity but moves limb	3 points
No movement of the leg	4 points
Limb Ataxia (Cannot Be Tested in the Presence of Motor Weakness)	
No limb ataxia	0 points
Ataxia present in one limb	1 point
Ataxia present in two limbs	2 points
Sensory Function	
No sensory loss	0 points
Mild-to-moderate sensory loss	1 point
Severe-to-total sensory loss	2 points
Language	
Normal language	0 points
Mild-to-moderate aphasia	1 point
Severe aphasia	2 points
Mute	3 points
Articulation	
Normal articulation	0 points
Mild-to-moderate dysarthria	1 point
Severe dysarthria	2 points
Extinction or Inattention (Neglect)	
No neglect or extinction	0 points
Visual or sensory inattention or extinction	1 point
Profound visual and sensory inattention	2 points

Adapted from Brott T, Adams HP Jr, Olinger CP et al. Measurements of acute cerebral infarction. A clinical examination scale. Stroke, *1989; 20: 864–870*

responses to early reperfusion therapy. On the other hand, the baseline NIHSS score does predict responses to acute treatment including intravenous thrombolysis or endovascular interventions.[102,103] While the NIHSS score is inversely associated with the likelihood of a favorable outcome, no individual item or combination of items is predictive of outcomes; as a result, the types of neurological impairments, as detected by the NIHSS, should not be used as a criterion for withholding emergency reperfusion therapy.[102] The baseline score on the NIHSS also forecasts the likelihood of hemorrhagic complications following administration of intravenous thrombolysis or other agents that affect coagulation.[104,105] The severity of stroke as measured by the NIHSS score also helps to predict responses to treatment with thrombolytic therapy.

In an attempt to improve the predictive power of the NIHSS, several investigators combined the results with other forecasters of outcome including the patient's age and the interval from onset of stroke.[106,107] The most common is the iScore that combines the score on either the NIHSS or CNS; the patient's age and sex; the stroke subtype; the presence of the risk factors of atrial fibrillation, congestive heart failure, previous myocardial infarction, and current smoking; the presence of comorbid diseases including cancer or renal failure; the pre-stroke disability, and the blood glucose on admission. This combination score was useful in predicting outcomes after stroke and responses to thrombolysis.[108,109] In some instances, the NIHSS score was combined with imaging and epidemiological variables.[110,111]

Changes in the NIHSS score upon sequential examinations are used to monitor for alterations of patients' neurological status.[112] Early improvement in the score is predictive of a higher likelihood of a favorable outcome while worsening is associated with increased risk of mortality or poor outcomes. Generally, a change of 2–4 points is used as a marker of important neurological change.[113] One trial used either a deterioration of 4 or more points on the total score or a decline of 1 or more points on the consciousness item as the clinical criterion for diagnosing symptomatic hemorrhagic transformation after reperfusion therapy.[114] The score on the NIHSS also is used as a long-term outcome measure of impairment in clinical trials.[112] There are some limitations to this strategy because, generally, patients who die are given the maximum score of 42 points and this tactic may skew the data. In addition, regardless of treatment, many patients have some improvement in their NIHSS scores in the weeks following stroke.

The total NIHSS score is employed as a criterion for enrollment in clinical trials.[103,114–122] Enrollment of patients with milder strokes (generally at total score < 5) is restricted because of a generally favorable prognosis and demonstration of a benefit from treatment may be difficult, while patients with very high scores (usually a total score > 20) also are not entered because of a very poor prognosis and a limited likelihood of success with treatment.[121,123] Unfortunately, it is not clear that this strategy is necessary and it is possible that clinical trials may be excluding patients who might respond to treatment. Another tactic involves the use of the baseline NIHSS score as a stratification variable in treatment assignments. Responses to treatment are judged as per the baseline score.[114,124–127] A favorable outcome for a patient with a low score might be complete recovery, whereas a favorable response for a patient with a severe stroke may be avoidance of severe disability.[126,127] The NIHSS is utilized in epidemiological and population studies. Use of the scale also is recommended in guidelines for treatment of stroke; in particular it is used for the selection of patients who should be treated with thrombolytic therapy.[128]

Although the NIHSS does have limitations, it is a robust clinical rating instrument that is used effectively to assess a broad range of neurological impairments among patients with stroke. The validity of the scale is established and inter-rater agreement and intra-rater reproducibility are quite high. Given the diversity of clinical findings with stroke, the ability to score a variety of components of the neurological examination with the NIHSS is an attribute. The scale only includes items that are based on the findings on examination. With training, it can be performed with a reasonable degree of accuracy in a community setting by a broad spectrum of healthcare professionals. Educational programs are available for instruction and certification in the scale. With multiple uses, practitioners can do the assessment quickly. The rules for its use are straightforward and it has been adapted to multiple languages and cultures. The NIHSS now is the standard way to quantify the severity of stroke in research and clinical settings. Its value is recognized by governmental and regulatory bodies.

Because of the perceived limitations of the previously described scales for evaluating patients with strokes affecting the brainstem and cerebellum, Israeli investigators developed a scale specific for testing impairments in this situation.[129] This scale has been subjected to limited testing but it appears to correlate well with scores of the mRS and NIHSS.

SYSTEMS TO FORECAST THE RISK OF STROKE AMONG PATIENTS WITH TRANSIENT ISCHEMIC ATTACK

Transient ischemic attacks (TIA) are considered as an important risk factor for ischemic stroke. Rather than being a true risk factor, a TIA is indeed an ischemic stroke that is clear, spontaneous and complete. The difference between a TIA and a minor stroke is really minimal and the modern definition of TIA has been modified from a primarily time-associated phenomenon that uses the presence of an ischemic lesion detected by imaging, with a TIA being diagnosed if no relevant ischemic lesion is seen.[130] Research has focused on those factors associated with the diagnosis of TIA that are correlated with an especially high risk of stroke and scales to identify the highest-risk patients.[131] The most commonly used instrument is the ABCD score that is based on the patient's age, blood pressure level at the time of presentation, clinical features of the TIA, and the duration of symptoms. Some variations have included the addition of the presence of diabetes and imaging findings. These scales are being used in clinical research and they are being implemented in clinical practice.

SCALES USED TO ASSESS PATIENTS WITH ATRIAL FIBRILLATION

While not truly scales used to assess patients' neurological impairments, disability, outcomes, or quality of life, a number of rating scales are being used to assess the risk of ischemic stroke, systemic embolization or hemorrhagic complications among patients with atrial fibrillation. Because atrial fibrillation has emerged as a leading cause of ischemic stroke, especially among older women, the scores obtained on these scales are of clinical relevance for neurologists and other physicians who assess patients with ischemic cerebrovascular disease. The results do influence decisions about the selection of treatments to prevent stroke, in particular the use of traditional oral anticoagulants or the newer oral antithrombotic agents.

The CHADS2 scale is the most commonly used rating instrument to predict the risk of thromboembolic events. The maximum score is 6, with a score of 2 or greater being associated with sufficiently high risk of thromboembolism to justify the use of oral anticoagulants.[132] Patients receive one point each for the presence of C (congestive heart failure), H (hypertension), A (age > 75), and D (diabetes). The presence of stroke (S) is calculated as 2 points (S2), thus all patients with ischemic neurological symptoms have reached the threshold for anticoagulation. The risk of thromboembolism in 1 year is 1.7% among those patients with a score of 0 and 22.4% among those persons who have a score of 6 or greater.[133] A modification of the CHADS 2 scale is the CHA2DS2-VASc Score that divides some of the previous categories and includes additional variables to calculate a score that can reach 9.[134] The scoring for congestive heart failure/left ventricular dysfunction, diabetes mellitus, hypertension, and previous thromboembolism is unchanged. The scoring for age is divided into 1 point for age 65–74 and 2 points for age 75 and above. A point also is added for being a woman. The changes reflect the higher risk of thromboembolism among older women. Either of these scales is acceptable for use in patient care.

A number of scales to forecast bleeding complications also have been created. The most commonly used is the HAS-BLED scale. It uses nine variables in calculating the risk of bleeding, with a rapid escalation of risk with higher scores. Points (1 each) are given for an elevated systolic blood pressure, abnormal renal function, abnormal hepatic function, age greater than 64, history of stroke in the past, history of bleeding in the past, the use of other medications, alcohol use, and the presence of a labile INR.[135]

SYSTEMS TO DIFFERENTIATE THE CAUSE OF ISCHEMIC STROKE (STROKE SUBTYPE)

Ischemic stroke is secondary to a broad variety of diseases. Arterial diseases include large-artery atherosclerosis, diseases of small penetrating arteries or arterioles, and non-atherosclerotic vasculopathies. The latter may be infectious, inflammatory but not infectious, or non-inflammatory. Several cardiac diseases predispose to embolism to the brain and a variety of inherited or acquired pro-thrombotic disorders may also lead to stroke. In some cases, no specific underlying cause for stroke may be identified (cryptogenic stroke). The cause of the stroke is important clinically. It affects both acute and long-term prognosis and, in particular, influences decisions about measures to prevent recurrent stroke.

Several factors affect the diagnosis of the subtype of ischemic stroke. The presence of multiple risk factors for accelerated atherosclerosis may be obtained from the patient's past medical history and supports the diagnosis of large-artery atherosclerosis. A history of heart disease, such as atrial fibrillation, often buttresses the diagnosis of cardioembolic stroke. A family or personal history of recurrent thromboembolic events, including venous thrombosis, may provide evidence that a hypercoagulable disorder is present. The general medical and neurological examinations provide clues to the cause. For example, the presence of an ipsilateral carotid bruit supports large-artery atherosclerosis, while evidence of embolization to multiple organs provides information buttressing the diagnosis of a cardiac etiology. The neurological manifestations of the stroke (OCSP scale) may not be specific for the etiology. For example, the findings of branch cortical infarction (PACI) may be found with an embolic event of either arterial or cardiac origin. The location and size of the ischemic brain injury as detected by imaging provide clues about the likely etiology. A small, deep lesion in the hemisphere or brainstem suggests small-vessel disease. A multilobar infarction portends occlusion of a major artery, which often is affected by atherosclerosis. Multiple infarctions affecting different vascular territories point to cardioembolic events. Branch cortical infarctions restricted to the cerebral cortex are often attributed to emboli that arise in the heart or from a proximal extracranial or intracranial artery. In most cases, the accurate diagnosis of the subtype of ischemic stroke requires the performance of ancillary studies including electrocardiography, cardiac imaging, vascular imaging, coagulation tests, and assessment of metabolic risk factors or immunologic tests.

Investigators in the TOAST study developed a classification system to facilitate the diagnosis of subtypes of ischemic stroke; it is based on the clinical findings, the results of brain imaging, and the findings on ancillary diagnostic studies[136] (Box 21-5). The categories are: (1) large-artery atherosclerosis, (2) cardiac embolism, (3) small-artery occlusion, (4) other cause (most commonly non-atherosclerotic vasculopathy or a hypercoagulable disorder), or (5) stroke undetermined cause. The latter category is used if the patient did not have ancillary diagnostic studies done, if the evaluation did not demonstrate a likely cause, or if the assessment found two or more potential etiologies that were equally likely to have caused the stroke. The diagnosis of the subtype is influenced by the perceived risk from the identified potential cause. For example, atrial fibrillation complicated with myocardial infarction is considered as a "high-risk" source for emboli whereas a patent foramen ovale is considered as a lower-risk lesion. Some of the definitions are arbitrary; for example, the diagnosis of large-artery atherosclerosis requires imaging demonstration of an occlusion or stenosis of the relevant artery. Thus, a fracture atherosclerotic plaque that does not lead to a narrowing greater than 50% of the lumen is not considered as providing sufficient evidence for the diagnosis of stroke secondary to large-artery atherosclerosis. Because of the relatively rigid requirements for diagnosis, especially for the diagnosis of stroke secondary to large-artery atherosclerosis, the proportion of stroke with undetermined etiology is relatively large in both clinical trials and epidemiological studies. While the original definitions in the TOAST classification were developed prior to the development of several modern imaging studies, the results of transcranial Doppler ultrasonography, computed tomographic angiography, MRA, and modern MRI sequences can be incorporated easily into the system.

This classification system is implemented extensively in both epidemiological and clinical studies of stroke performed around the world.[137] The system is also used to help researchers to examine special populations, such as young adults with stroke, study the impact of common risk factors for stroke, evaluate genetic markers for stroke, validate brain imaging studies, forecast long-term prognosis, and affect decisions for treatment.[138,139]

The validity, inter-rater agreement, and intra-rater reproducibility of the TOAST classification have been tested.[14,138,140] The use of DWI and MRA improves the likelihood of agreement in the TOAST subtype classification.[141] Inter-rater agreements are highest for the subtypes of large-artery atherosclerosis and cardioembolism. Fure et al.[142] found that the classification was particularly helpful in differentiating stroke with small-vessel disease from stroke with other causes when it was applied in an emergency setting; they found the sensitivity of the diagnosis of 0.93 and the specificity to be 0.83. On the other hand, the TOAST classification is not easily used in the first hours after stroke when the results of ancillary diagnostic studies may not be available.[143] As a result, clinical trials testing interventions for acute stroke treatment should not use either the TOAST or another subtype classification to restrict enrollment of stroke subtypes. Some patients, who are truly eligible, will be excluded. Other ineligible patients will be enrolled. Fortunately, advances in brain and vascular imaging, in particular CTA and MRA may have eased some of these problems.

Ay et al.[144,145] developed a classification system that is a direct derivative of the TOAST system (SSS-TOAST). They made adjustments including a description called evidence that is based largely on the strength of current natural history data that shows the annual risk of stroke. The revised classification also places aortic causes of embolism, including complex atherosclerotic plaques in the category of cardioembolism because the clinical findings overlap with those emboli arising in the heart. The SSS-TOAST also includes cryptogenic embolism in the category of stroke of undetermined etiology. This classification has been converted to a computer-based

BOX 21-5 Trial of ORG 10172 in Acute Stroke Treatment (TOAST) Classification of Subtypes of Ischemic Stroke[#]

LARGE-ARTERY ATHEROSCLEROSIS

Clinical evidence of cerebral cortical or cerebellar infarction
Cerebral cortical, cerebellar, brain stem, or subcortical infarction on CT or MRI
- Infarction is >1.5–2 cm in size

Stenosis or occlusion of major intracranial or extracranial artery relevant to the stroke
- Stenosis is >50%
- Stenosis ≤50% if ulceration or thrombus is present at site
- Occlusion

No high-risk cardiac lesion found (for evident or probable diagnosis)

SMALL-ARTERY OCCLUSION

Clinical evidence of one of the traditional lacunar syndromes
Subcortical or brain stem infarction on CT or MRI
- Infarction is < 1.5–2.0 cm in size

No ipsilateral large-artery atherosclerotic lesion found (for evident or probable diagnosis)
No high-risk cardiac lesion is found (for evident or probable diagnosis)

CARDIOEMBOLISM

Clinical evidence of cerebral cortical or cerebellar infarction
Cerebral cortical, cerebellar, or brain stem infarction on CT or MRI
- Infarction is > 1.5–2.0 cm in size

Cardiac source for embolism is found (high versus medium risk)
No ipsilateral large-artery atherosclerotic lesion found (for evident or probable diagnosis)

OTHER DEMONSTRATED CAUSE

Evaluation demonstrates another cause for stroke
Presence of a specific vascular disease in appropriate cerebral artery
Presence of a specific hypercoagulable disorder
Other causes of stroke have been excluded (for evident or probable diagnosis)

UNDETERMINED CAUSE (CRYPTOGENIC STROKE)

Two or more causes identified and most likely cause is not obvious
No abnormality is found on evaluation
- Includes cases of presumed cryptogenic embolism

Evaluation incomplete

[#]Includes modifications from Ay et al.
Adapted from Adams HP Jr, Bendixen BH, Kappelle LJ et al. Classification of subtype of acute ischemic stroke. Definitions for use in a multicenter clinical trial. TOAST. Trial of Org 10172 in Acute Stroke Treatment. Stroke, *1993; 24: 35–41 and Ay H, Furie KL, Singhal A, et al. An evidence-base causative classification system for acute ischemic stroke.* Ann Neurol, *2005; 58: 688–697*

algorithm titled the Causative Classification of Stroke (CCS).[146] One of the major advantages of this system is its availability on the internet so that physicians and investigators can enter data into a form that automatically leads to the classification of stroke subtype. When compared to the TOAST system, the CCS appears to reduce the number of cases of stroke that are classified as undetermined etiology and increases the number of cases in the other categories.[147] Overall, the two systems give similar data.

The TOAST and CCS systems have been criticized, in particular, for the relatively high percentage of strokes classified as being of undetermined etiology.[148] The combination of non-atherosclerotic vasculopathies and pro-thrombotic disorders, both of which are relatively uncommon causes of stroke, into one category is also disconcerting. Suggestions have been made to discard these classifications.[149] Still, critics have not developed a superior alternative. Han et al.[150] developed a classification system that has not been used extensively. Hoffmann et al.[148] expanded the classification into a large number of categories including (1) large-vessel cerebrovascular disease (presumably due to atherosclerosis), (2) small-vessel cerebrovascular disease, (3) cardiogenic, (4) dissection, (5) hypercoagulable disorders, (6) migraine-induced, (7) cerebral venous sinus thrombosis, (8) vasculitis, (9) other vasculopathy, (10) miscellaneous, and (11) unknown. This classification includes several categories and, as a result, it will be likely associated with a decline in inter-rater agreement and intra-rater reproducibility. Besides having a different clinical profile than acute ischemic stroke secondary to arterial occlusive disease, cerebral venous sinus thrombosis is also the result of several etiologies, including hypercoagulable disorders. This new system needs considerable testing but it is unlikely that it will be superior to the TOAST or CCS systems. The Chinese Ischemic Stroke Subclassification is another program for distinguishing subtypes of stroke.

Because of the perceived limitations of TOAST and CCS systems and in order not to neglect any information when diagnoses were made, investigators created another classification scheme titled ASCO (atherosclerosis, small-vessel disease, cardiac source, and other cause). One of the goals was to reduce the number of strokes that were classified as undetermined etiology. This phenotype-based classification employs the same criteria as the TOAST program. The assumption is that treatment may be adapted to the observed phenotype and most likely etiology. In the system, the rater classifies the likelihood of a causative relationship as (1) definitely a potential cause for stroke, (2) causality is uncertain, (3) unlikely a direct cause of stroke but disease may be present, (4) disease completely absent, and (5) grading not possible due to insufficient evaluation. More recently, the classification system was revised to ASCOD with the category of stroke due to arterial dissections being made a distinct category.[151] All five categories are scored independently, which results in more than 3000 possible combinations. One study that evaluated ASCO ratings at two different epochs found that the data changed in approximately 65% of cases.[152] The inter-rater reliability of the ASCO system appears to be moderate.[153] The relative utility of the TOAST and ASCO classifications has been tested.[154,155] The spectrum of subtype diagnoses is similar using the classifications but with a reduction in the number of stroke of undetermined etiology in ASCO. In general, the cases that are assigned a specific subtype by TOAST and rated as having a category 1 for a specific group in ASCO are comparable.[147,156] Because it is a phenotype-based system, its future role may be primarily in epidemiological and genetic research studies.

The TOAST classification has gained international acceptance. The CCS system contains some modifications in the definitions included in TOAST that have strengthened the scale. The availability of computer algorithms when using the CCS is an advantage. Nam et al.[157] developed a handheld computerized system that allows for accurate subtype determination on the basis of answers of six questions. This system could greatly expedite the use of the TOAST classification. Until another clinical rating instrument is developed that is superior to TOAST/CCS, these scales will continue to be used in a wide range of stroke-related research projects.

The applicability of the TOAST/CCS classifications to stroke in children appears limited. As a result, Wraige et al [158] proposed modifications for a subtype classification system for the causes of stroke in childhood. These changes reflect the differences in diseases that lead to brain ischemia in children versus those that are found in adults. The proposed categories for pediatric ischemic stroke are: (1) sickle cell disease, (2) cardioembolism, (3) moyamoya, (4) cervical arterial dissection, (5) steno-occlusive cerebral arteriopathy, (6) other determined cause, (7) multiple possible causes, and (8) undetermined cause. While this system has great potential, it has not been tested extensively. This system may be useful for categorizing subtypes in both epidemiological studies and clinical trials of ischemic stroke in children.

SCALES AND MEASURES TO ASSESS RESPONSES TO REHABILITATION INTERVENTIONS

Rehabilitation specialists employ a wide range of rating instruments to assess the severity of neurological impairments or disabilities and to rate responses to modality-specific interventions.[159] An in-depth assessment of these scales is beyond the scope of this chapter. Some scales use assistive devices or computer technology to rate responses.[160,161] In other circumstances, combinations of rating instruments are used.[162] These measures are instruments to rate the severity of fatigue or apathy after stroke.[163,164]

The Fugl-Myer scale is used primarily by physical therapists and physiatrists to assess primarily motor recovery after stroke.[165] This scale has been used to monitor responses among patients receiving medications to augment recovery after stroke.[166] Still, most non-rehabilitation physicians do not use these scales nor are they familiar with the nuances of the results of these instruments. The development of measures and scales to assess specific patterns of recovery after stroke remains a very vibrant area for research.

The most commonly used scales to assess cognitive impairments after stroke are the Mini-Mental State Examination (MMSE) and the Montreal Cognitive Assessment.[167-169] The Montreal scale may be performed via the telephone as well as by direct contact. These scales are used during the period of recovery and rehabilitation after stroke; they are also performed to assess for the presence of vascular dementia in stroke survivors. The Montreal battery appears to perform better than the MMSE among persons with stroke.[170] While these scales have not been used regularly in a patient-care setting, their implementation in clinical trials in stroke, especially those for stroke recovery, is increasing.

Depression is a common complication of stroke; it has a major impact on outcomes. Because of its effects on recovery after stroke, scales to assess the severity of depression are being developed to help expedite both patient care and research. While the most commonly used scale is the Hamilton Rating Scale for Depression,[171-173] other options include the Beck Depression Inventory and the Patient Health Questionnaire-2 and -9.[174] All the scales appear to function in similar ways. Because of its limited number of items and its availability, the

Patient Health Questionnaire-2 may be the most useful screening tool in stroke.[175]

SCALES TO RATE OUTCOMES (DISABILITY) AFTER STROKE

Disability following stroke is evaluated by a variety of rating tools. The purposes are to monitor responses to rehabilitation and other interventions, to provide prognostic information and to judge outcomes of early and subsequent therapies. Some outcome scales include assessments of the patient's ability to perform the activities of daily living (ADLs.) Some scales are based on historical information shared by the patient, family, or other observers. The instruments usually have a series of relatively straightforward questions that can be asked during a telephone conversation or in-person interview. Patients' self-reporting of perceived impairments appears to be valid.[176] Scales also involve direct observation of the patient's performance; in some instances, the scale includes evaluations of complex tasks or activities. Some scales emphasize physical independence and are weighted towards motor activities; others include observations of cognition and other brain function. In general, the scales appear to have similar clinometric behavior.[177] The most commonly used scales are the BI, the Functional Independence Measure (FIM) and the Frenchay Activities Index.[4,178–182]

The BI may evaluate disability and performance of ADLs in a broad spectrum of patients with acute or chronic diseases[4,178] (Table 21-11). Presently, it is the most widely used clinical rating instrument to assess stroke-related disability.[115,183–186] The BI has been translated and adapted for use in multiple languages and countries. The patient or caregiver is asked a series of questions about ten different aspects of the ADLs. Priority is given to mobility and continence.[187] Potential responses are independent, partially independent, or dependent. Definitions for each score are straightforward. The BI is easy to administer and scores are easy to calculate. The range is 0–100 points. Generally, a score of 60 or greater is associated with functional independence; although it is possible that a patient with a score of 100 may not be completely independent.[185,186,188,189] Higher scores associated with shorter courses of acute hospitalization and less need for intensive rehabilitation after stroke. The score on the BI also predicts long-term outcomes including mortality. A variation of the BI called the Extended BI has been used to examine patients with recent stroke.[190]

A minimally important difference in scores on the BI appears to be approximately 10 points. Dichotomous or trichotomous divisions in scoring, most commonly at 0–55, 60–90 and 95–100, have been used to define poor, good and excellent outcomes.[115,183] Song et al.[191] recommended that mean values of the BI be included along with the distribution of outcome scores so that results of multiple trials can be combined in meta-analyses of the future. Another group proposed that the psychometric properties of the BI could be improved by focusing on the motor components of the scale.[192] The BI does have limitations. Because of its emphasis on motor recovery, patients with aphasia or neglect may achieve relatively good scores and still not be independent. It does have floor and ceiling effects.[193] These limitations mean that the BI may not be the primary best outcome measure to assess responses in clinical trials. Martinsson and Eksborg[194] recommended that additional measures of ADLs be added to refine outcomes.

TABLE 21-11 Barthel Index

Component	Independent	Partially Independent	Dependent
Walking	15 points	5 or 10 points	0 points
Climbing stairs	10 points	5 points	0 points
Chair/bed transfers	15 points	5 or 10 points	0 points
Toilet transfers	10 points	5 points	0 points
Grooming	5 points	0 points	0 points
Dressing	10 points	5 points	0 points
Bathing	5 points	0 points	0 points
Eating	10 points	5 points	0 points
Bowel control	10 points	5 points	0 points
Bladder control	10 points	5 points	0 points

Adapted from Mahoney FI, Barthel DW. Functional evaluation. The Barthel Index. Med State Med J, *1965; 14: 61–65*

Despite its limitations, the BI has high levels of agreement for the entire scale and its constituents.[195] It has high inter-rater agreement, internal consistency and validity.[186,196] It has good agreement with other measures of disability.[193] A BI score of 95 generally correlates with a mRS score of 1, a BI score of 90 is comparable to a mRS score of 2 and a BI score of 75 is approximately the same as a mRS score of 3.[197] Because of its simplicity and utility of the score on the BI, it is widely recognized by physicians treating patients with stroke. At present, the BI is the most important and commonly used measure to assess disability among patients enrolled in clinical trials testing therapies for acute stroke.

The 17-item FIM tests a broad range of cognitive and motor functions; it is used extensively in rehabilitation research and clinical care. Each item is scored from 1 to 4 (total 17–68 points).[198–200] The results of the FIM, which is often measured sequentially during rehabilitation, are correlated with quality-of-life outcomes.[200] A FIM score less than 40 predicts a low likelihood of independence. The FIM has demonstrated validity, reliability, and strong psychometric measures.[201] Overall, the FIM functions similarly to the BI and it appears to have little advantage over the BI. The FIM has not been used in acute stroke trials.

SCALES TO RATE OUTCOMES (GLOBAL OR HANDICAP) AFTER STROKE

Several scales to rate global (handicap) outcomes after stroke are available. These scales are relatively brief and include a few well-defined clinical grades. The most frequently used scales are the mRS and the Glasgow Outcome Scale (GOS).[5,6,202] They are efficient and effective ways to assess outcomes in clinical trials and epidemiological studies.[183,203] The scales have shown a high degree of validity and intra-rater reproducibility is strong.[204]

The mRS is judged as the best currently available scale to assess outcomes after stroke.[17] It should not be considered a pure handicap scale, but rather a global outcome measure. It does have limitations. Definitions are somewhat arbitrary. The score of 0 on the mRS may be difficult to achieve because a patient must not have any residual symptoms related to stroke (Table 21-12). This strict definition is problematic because a patient may have made an excellent recovery but if minimal problems persist, a score of 1 must be rated. As a result, the score of 1 covers a broad spectrum of patients. Generally, clinical trials have used a dichotomous or trichotomous division of scores with scores of 0–1 being considered as very favorable outcomes, 2–3 as favorable, and 4–6 as unfavorable. In some cases a score of 2 is considered a positive response and in others, it may be rated as unfavorable. Inter-rater agreement in differentiating adjacent scores, particularly among mildly affected patients, may be difficult.[205] The mRS has shown moderate inter-rater reliability that improves with structured

TABLE 21-12 Modified Rankin Scale

Score	Definition
0	No symptoms present at all
1	No disability despite some symptoms
2	Slight disability but does not require assistance
3	Moderate disability but can walk
4	Moderately severe disability
5	Severe disability, usually bedridden
6	Dead

Adapted from van Swieten JC, Koudstaal PJ, Visser MC et al. Interobserver agreement for the assessment of handicap in stroke patients. Stroke, *1988; 19: 604–607*

Table 21-13 Glasgow Outcome Scale

GRADE 5	**GOOD RECOVERY**
A	Full recovery, without symptoms or signs
B	Capable of resuming normal activities but has minor complaints
GRADE 4	**MODERATE DISABILITY**
	Independent but Disabled
A	Signs present but can resume most former activities
B	Independent in activities of daily living but cannot resume previous activities
GRADE 3	**SEVERE DISABILITY**
	Conscious but Dependent
A	Partial independence in activities of daily living but cannot return to previous activities
B	Total or almost total dependency for activities of daily living
GRADE 2	**VEGETATIVE STATE**
GRADE 1	**DEATH**

Adapted from Jennett B, Bond M. Assessment of outcome after severe brain damage. A practical scale, Lancet, *1975; 305: 480–484*

interviews.[204] Training in the use of the scales that lead to certification also improves their reliability.[206] The use of central adjudication of outcomes through the transmission of videotapes is another strategy that increases the robustness of the scales.[16,207,208] The construct validity of the mRS is demonstrated by its strong relationship with other indicators of stroke severity including NIHSS scores and brain imaging.[204] Adams et al.[126] proposed adjusting the definitions of favorable outcomes on the mRS by the baseline severity of neurological impairments rated on the NIHSS. Saver[209] advocated that a change in the distribution of scores on the mRS be used as a way to judge success of a treatment. This latter approach has been criticized.[210] Mandava et al.[211] found that the use of dichotomizations of endpoints were more reliable than the use of the distribution strategy.

The GOS was designed to rate outcomes among patients with head injuries but now, it is used to rate outcomes among patients with stroke, in particular hemorrhages.[202,212,213] It consists of five grades with subdivisions within the three highest categories (Table 21-13). Separating the scores of 2 (moderate disability) and 3 (severe disability) may be difficult. Still, the GOS has good inter-rater agreement and intra-rater reproducibility. The utility of the GOS seems to be best suited for patients with subarachnoid hemorrhage because of the link of the GCS with the WFNS scale. The spectrum of grades on the GOS may reflect serious diffuse or multi-focal brain injury, which may occur with subarachnoid hemorrhage. The GOS includes the grade of a permanent vegetative state that does not occur very often among survivors of ischemic stroke. In addition, the GOS does not differentiate between some of the more mildly affected patients. Thus, the use of the GOS has declined in ischemic stroke trials as the mRS has become more wildly used.

All global outcome measures involve some lumping of groups of patients with a wide spectrum of neurological sequelae; they may not adequately define many of the subtle or diverse but important neurological sequelae of stroke. However, the scales are relatively simple to use, educational and certification programs are available to improve their validity and reliability, and they have been used successfully in numerous clinical trials. The scales are used by clinicians and increasingly by groups that certify or monitor the quality of care at medical centers. Physicians dealing with stroke patients are familiar with these instruments and they are used commonly. Other outcome scales have been proposed but they are not used extensively.[214] Pediatric stroke outcome scales also have been evaluated.[215] Until better rating instruments become available, the mRS or the GOS should continue to be used.[17]

SCALES TO ASSESS THE QUALITY OF LIFE AFTER STROKE

Because of the many long-term sequelae, stroke produces many problems that are seen among persons with other chronic conditions. Outcomes affect not only the patient but also families and society at large, thus, determination of the quality of life is important. Although the term quality of life is difficult to define, McKevitt et al.[216] concluded that the term might be translated to happiness and contentment. However, the term probably covers more than emotional responses and includes many other areas of functioning that are intact. Because stroke is a life-changing disease, most patients do not consider themselves as being better off after having had a stroke.[217] In addition, a stroke affects relationships among family members and may affect the family's fiscal status. Many stroke survivors complain of a lack of meaningful activity, severe depression, or a sense that their health is poor.[218] Reductions in quality of life may be expected among stroke survivors of all age groups. The cause of stroke does not seem to have a major impact but the severity of the neurological impairments is a major predictor of an unsatisfactory quality of life.[219] Not surprisingly, those patients with severe impairments that require assistive devices or the help of family members or friends rate their quality of life as poor.[220] Quality of life measures also are lower among women than among men, which may reflect older age and the higher likelihood of a woman living alone.[220] Other predictors of quality of life include overall functional status, the presence of residual upper extremity dysfunction, and educational level. After a severe stroke, many survivors need the assistance of family members or caregivers, which also affects their lives.[221,222]

Several scales to differentiate health-related quality of life (HRQL) are used to complement assessments of handicap and disability.[217,221,223,224] The scales are designed to address symptoms, conditions, and social roles that are important for patients with stroke and that could be affected either positively or negatively by an intervention or the disease.[223] Components include ratings of physical, social, psychological, and overall health as affected by the individual person's beliefs, perceptions, experiences, and expectations. This is a difficult task because there probably is no scale that is able to define all these components but scales that assess most of these issues are designated as having good coverage. Most of the currently available HRQL scales have not been evaluated extensively for sensitivity, specificity, reliability, reproducibility, or validity in patients with stroke.

21

TABLE 21-14 Stroke Specific Quality Of Life Scale

Tested items	Number of questions
Energy	4
Family role	8
Language	7
Mobility	12
Mood	8
Personality	4
Self-care	8
Social roles	7
Thinking	4
Upper extremity function	9
Vision	4
Work and productivity	3

Adapted from Williams LS, Weinberger M, Harris LE, et al. Measuring quality of life in a way that is meaningful to stroke patients. Neurology, *1999; 53: 1839–1843*

Some stroke-specific HRQL scales have been created.[203,219,225-230] Other scales have been adapted from instruments used to rate outcomes of patients with other chronic diseases, including the Nottingham Health Profile, the Medical Outcomes Short Form - 36 (SF-36,) the Sickness Impact Profile (SIP), and the World Health Organization Quality of Life measure.[72,214,231-235] Hobart et al.[234] found that five of the eight sections of the SIP had limited validity in evaluating the quality of life among survivors of stroke. Conversely, another study noted that the SIP30 had satisfactory performance for evaluation of physical and psychosocial dimensions.[236] The SIP30 has been modified to form the Stroke-Adapted Sickness Impact Profiles (SA-SIP).[50] Among patients with mild strokes, the emotional well-being and activity participation components of the SA-SIP effectively detect the most obvious quality-of-life problems.[237]

The Stroke Specific Quality of Life (SS-QOL) scale is available in American and European versions.[238] It measures a wide range of sequelae from stroke including language and behavior problems (Table 21-14). It has been validated and is shown to have a good association with scores on the NIHSS and the BI, and with the severity of depression. It has been used successfully to assess outcomes among patients with aneurysmal subarachnoid hemorrhage.[239] An abbreviated version of the SSQOL that consists of 12 items also has been developed.[240] It is a reliable instrument for measuring self-reported HRQL outcomes among persons with mild-to-moderate stroke. The SS-QOL is becoming one of the more widely used tools for rating quality of life among persons who have had a stroke.[217]

The EuroQOL scale is used widely to rate the quality of life in patients with a wide variety of diseases, including stroke.[241-243] The scale consists of two components. Patients are asked about mobility, self-care, usual activities, pain or discomfort, or symptoms of anxiety or depression. For each category, patients are given a choice of three responses: no problem, moderate problem, or severe problem. In addition, the patient is asked to rate the state of his/her health on a range from 0 (worst) to 100 (best.) Dorman et al.[240,242] found that the EuroQOL has an acceptable validity for measurement of HRQL among patients with stroke and that it functioned similarly to the SF-36. Because many patients with stroke might not be able to give information directly, Dorman et al. evaluated the utility of proxy assessments. While the patients actually scored their quality of life better than did the proxies, the tactic of using proxy report was considered acceptable. Because it contains a limited survey of questions and because it can be performed by either patients or proxies, the EuroQOL is increasingly used for the assessment of HRQL among survivors of stroke.

The Stroke Impact Scale (SIS) is another valid assessment tool to rate the quality of life after stroke.[217,244,245] It tests a range of 16 items including activities of daily living, instrumental activities of daily living, mobility, strength, physical parameters, and participation.[246] It can be administered to the patient or be answered by a proxy.[247] It functions similarly to the SF-36.[248] Another recently developed scale is the Neuro-QOL, which has been developed to test the HRQL outcomes in children and adults with a variety of neurological disorders including stroke.[249] The purpose is to examine the well-being of patients with a wide variety of diseases through the use of 13 measures of physical, mental, and social health. The future role of the NeuroQOL is unclear.

The complete reference list can be found on the companion Expert Consult website at www.expertconsult.inkling.com. 

KEY REFERENCES

1. Lyden PD, Lau GT. A critical appraisal of stroke evaluation and rating scales. Stroke 1991;22:1345–52.
2. Boysen G. Stroke scores and scales. Cerebrovasc Dis 1992;2: 239–47.
3. Harrison JK, McArthur KS, Quinn TJ. Assessment scales in stroke: Clinimetric and clinical considerations. Clin Interv Aging 2013;8: 201–11.
4. Kasner SE. Clinical interpretation and use of stroke scales. Lancet Neurol 2006;5:603–12.
5. Rankin J. Cerebral vascular accidents in patients over the age of 60. Scott Med J 1957;2:200–15.
6. van Swieten JC, Koudstaal PJ, Visser MC, et al. Interobserver agreement for the assessment of handicap in stroke patients. Stroke 1988;19:604–7.
7. Brott T, Adams HP Jr, Olinger CP, et al. Measurements of acute cerebral infarction: A clinical examination scale. Stroke 1989;20: 864–70.
8. Jennett B, Teasdale G, Braakman R, et al. Prognosis of patients with severe head injury. Neurosurgery 1979;4:283–9.
10. Hunt WE, Hess RM. Surgical risk as related to time of intervention in the repair of intracranial aneurysms. J Neurosurg 1968;28: 14–20.
11. Cote R, Hachinski VC, Shurvell BL, et al. The Canadian Neurological Scale: A preliminary study in acute stroke. Stroke 1986; 17:731–7.
12. Cote R, Battista RN, Wolfson SK, et al. The Canadian Neurological Scale: Validation and reliability assessment. Neurology 1989;39:638–43.
14. Gordon DL, Bendixen BH, Adams HP Jr, et al. Interphysician agreement in the diagnosis of subtypes of acute ischemic stroke: Implications for clinical trials. The TOAST investigators. Neurology 1993;43:1021–7.
15. Lyden P, Raman R, Liu L, et al. NIHSS training and certification using a new digital video disk is reliable. Stroke 2005;36: 2446–9.
17. Lees KR, Bath PM, Schellinger PD, et al; European Stroke Organization Outcomes Working G. Contemporary outcome measures in acute stroke research: Choice of primary outcome measure. Stroke 2012;43:1163–70.
18. Quinn TJ, Dawson J, Walters MR, et al. Variability in modified Rankin scoring across a large cohort of international observers. Stroke 2008;39:2975–9.
22. Oshiro EM, Walter KA, Piantadosi S, et al. A new subarachnoid hemorrhage grading system based on the Glasgow Coma Scale: A comparison with the Hunt and Hess and World Federation of Neurological Surgeons scales in a clinical series. Neurosurgery 1997;41:140–7.
23. Ogungbo B. The World Federation of neurological surgeons scale for subarachnoid hemorrhage. Surg Neurol 2003;25: 236–8.
24. Hemphill JC, Bonovich DC, Besmertis L, et al. A simple, reliable grading scale for intracerebral hemorrhage. Stroke 2001;32: 891–7.

26. Kidwell CS, Saver JL, Schubert GB, et al. Design and retrospective analysis of the Los Angeles Prehospital Stroke Screen (LAPSS). Prehosp Emerg Care 1998;2:267–73.
27. Kidwell CS, Starkman S, Eckstein M, et al. Identifying stroke in the field. Prospective validation of the Los Angeles Prehospital Stroke Screen (LAPSS). Stroke 2000;31:71–6.
28. Kothari RU, Pancioli A, Liu T, et al. Cincinnati Prehospital Stroke Scale: Reproducibility and validity. Ann Emerg Med 1999;33: 373–8.
29. Gordon DL, Issenberg SB, Gordon MS, et al. Stroke training of prehospital providers: An example of simulation-enhanced blended learning and evaluation. Med Teach 2005;27:114–21.
30. Bray JE, Coughlan K, Barger B, et al. Paramedic diagnosis of stroke: Examining long-term use of the Melbourne Ambulance Stroke Screen (MASS) in the field. Stroke 2010;41: 1363–6.
31. Harbison J, Hossain O, Jenkinson D, et al. Diagnostic accuracy of stroke referrals from primary care, emergency room physicians, and ambulance staff using the Face Arm Speech Test. Stroke 2003;34:71–6.
32. Nor AM, McAllister C, Louw SJ, et al. Agreement between ambulance paramedic- and physician-recorded neurological signs with Face Arm Speech Test (FAST) in acute stroke patients. Stroke 2004;35:1355–9.
34. Nor AM, Davis J, Sen B, et al. The Recognition of Stroke in the Emergency Room (ROSIER) Scale: Development and validation of a stroke recognition instrument. Lancet Neurol 2005;4: 727–34.
35. Whiteley WN, Wardlaw JM, Dennis MS, et al. Clinical scores for the identification of stroke and transient ischaemic attack in the emergency department: A cross-sectional study. J Neurol Neurosurg Psychiatry 2011;82:1006–10.
39. Badam P, Paik M, Solao V, et al. Poor accuracy of the Siriraj and Guy's Hospital Stroke Scores in distinguishing haemorrhagic from ischaemic stroke in a rural, tertiary care hospital. Natl Med J India 2003;16:8–12.
41. Bamford J, Sandercock P, Dennis M, et al. Classification and natural history of clinically identifiable subtypes of cerebral infarction. Lancet 1991;337:1521–6.
45. Wardlaw JM, Dennis MS, Lindley RI, et al. The validity of a simple clinical classification of acute ischaemic stroke. J Neurol 1996;243:274–9.
46. Mead GE, Lewis SC, Wardlaw JM, et al. How well does the Oxfordshire Community Stroke Project Classification predict the site and size of the infarct on brain imaging? J Neurol Neurosurg Psychiatry 2000;68:558–62.
50. Edwards DF, Chen Y-W, Diringer MN. Unified Neurological Stroke Scale is valid is ischemic and hemorrhagic stroke. Stroke 1995;26:1852–8.
51. Hemphill JC, Bonovich DC, Besmertis L, et al. The ICH score: A simple, reliable grading scale for intracerebral hemorrhage. Stroke 2001;32:891–7.
55. Ruiz-Sandoval JL, Chiquete E, Romero-Vargas S, et al. Grading scale for prediction of outcome in primary intracerebral hemorrhages. Stroke 2007;38:1641–4.
58. Weimar C, Benemann J, Diener HC. Development and validation of the Essen Intracerebral Hemorrhage Score. J Neurol Neurosurg Psychiatry 2006;77:601–5.
64. St Julien J, Bandeen-Roche K, Tamargo RJ. Validation of an aneurysmal subarachnoid hemorrhage grading scale in 1532 consecutive patients. Neurosurgery 2008;63:204–10.
66. Leira EC, Davis PH, Martin CO, et al. Improving prediction of outcome in "good grade" subarachnoid hemorrhage. Neurosurgery 2007;61:470–4.
67. Naval NS, Kowalski RG, Chang TR, et al. The SAH score: A comprehensive communication tool. J Stroke Cerebrovasc Dis 2014; 23:902–9.
68. Ogilvy CS, Cheung AC, Mitha AP, et al. Outcomes for surgical and endovascular management of intracranial aneurysms using a comprehensive grading system. Neurosurgery 2006;59: 1036–42.
69. Starke RM, Komotar RJ, Kim GH, et al. Evaluation of a revised Glasgow Coma Score scale in predicting long-term outcome of poor grade aneurysmal subarachnoid hemorrhage patients. J Clin Neurosci 2009;16:894–9.
72. De Haan R, Horn J, Limburg M, et al. A comparison of five stroke scales with measures of disability, handicap, and quality of life. Stroke 1993;24:1178–81.
73. Hantson L, De Keyser J. Neurological scales in the assessment of cerebral infarction. Cerebrovasc Dis 1994;4(Suppl. 2):7–14.
74. Wright CJ, Swinton LC, Green TL, et al. Predicting final disposition after stroke using the Orpington Prognostic Score. Can J Neurol Sci 2004;31:494–8.
76. Stavem K, Lossius M, Ronning OM. Reliability and validity of the Canadian Neurological Scale in retrospective assessment of initial stroke severity. Cerebrovasc Dis 2003;16:286–91.
78. Nilanont Y, Komoltri C, Saposnik G, et al. The Canadian Neurological Scale and the NIHSS: Development and validation of a simple conversion model. Cerebrovasc Dis 2010;30: 120–6.
80. Barber M, Fail M, Shields M, et al. Validity and reliability of estimating the Scandinavian Stroke Scale score from medical records. Cerebrovasc Dis 2004;17:224–7.
84. Davalos A, Toni D, Iweins F, et al. Neurological deterioration in acute ischemic stroke: Potential predictors and associated factors in the European Cooperative Acute Stroke Study (ECASS). Stroke 1999;30:2631–6.
85. Sprigg N, Gray LJ, Bath PM, et al. Stroke severity, early recovery and outcome are each related with clinical classification of stroke: Data from the 'Tinzaparin in Acute Ischaemic Stroke Trial' (TAIST). J Neurol Sci 2007;254:54–9.
88. Ali K, Cheek E, Sills S, et al. Development of a conversion factor to facilitate comparison of National Institute of Health Stroke Scale scores with Scandanavian Stroke Scale scores. Cerebrovasc Dis 2007;24:509–15.
89. Brott T, Marler JR, Olinger CP, et al. Measurements of acute cerebral infarction: Lesion size by computed tomography. Stroke 1989;20:871–5.
92. Albanese MA, Clarke WR, Adams HP Jr, et al. Ensuring reliability of outcome measures in multicenter clinical trials of treatments for acute ischemic stroke. The program developed for the Trial of Org 10172 in Acute Stroke Treatment (TOAST). Stroke 1994;25:1746–51.
93. Lyden P, Brott T, Tilley B, et al. Improved reliability of the NIH Stroke Scale using video training. NINDS TPA Stroke Study Group. Stroke 1994;25:2220–6.
97. Leira EC, Adams HP Jr, Rosenthal GE, et al. Stroke Scale responses estimate the probability of each particular stroke subtype. Cerebrovasc Dis 2008;26:573–7.
99. Heldner MR, Zubler C, Mattle HP, et al. National Institutes of Health Stroke Scale score and vessel occlusion in 2152 patients with acute ischemic stroke. Stroke 2013;44:1153–7.
100. Adams HP Jr, Davis PH, Leira EC, et al. Score strongly predicts outcome after stroke. Neurology 1999;53:126–31.
105. Derex L, Hermier M, Adeleine P, et al. Clinical and imaging predictors of intracerebral haemorrhage in stroke patients treated with intravenous tissue plasminogen activator. J Neurol Neurosurg Psychiatry 2005;76:70–5.
106. Saposnik G, Guzik AK, Reeves M, et al. Stroke Prognostication using Age and NIH Stroke Scale: SPAN-100. Neurology 2013;80: 21–8.
109. Park TH, Saposnik G, Bae HJ, et al. The I-score predicts functional outcome in Korean patients with ischemic stroke. Stroke 2013;44:1440–2.
122. Weimar C, Ho TW, Katsarava Z, et al. German Stroke Study C. Improving patient selection for clinical actue stroke trials. Cerebrovasc Dis 2006;21:386–92.
124. DeGraba TJ, Hallenbeck JM, Pettigrew KD, et al. Progression in acute stroke: Value of the initial NIH Stroke Scale score on patient stratification in future trials. Stroke 1999;30: 1208–12.
125. Savitz SI, Lew R, Bluhmki E, et al. Shift analysis versus dichotomization of the modified Rankin Scale outcome scores in the NINDS and ECASS-II trials. Stroke 2007;38:3205–12.
126. Adams HP Jr, Leclerc JR, Bluhmki E, et al. Measuring outcomes as a function of baseline severity of ischemic stroke. Cerebrovasc Dis 2004;18:124–9.
128. Jauch EC, Saver JL, Adams HP, et al. Guidelines for the early management of patients with acute ischemic stroke: A guideline for healthcare professionals from the American

Heart Association/American Stroke Association. Stroke 2013;44: 870–947.

131. Johnston SC, Rothwell PM, Nguyen-Huynh MN, et al. Validation and refinement of scores to predict very early stroke risk after transient ischaemic attack. Lancet 2007;369:283–92.
132. Gage BF, Waterman AD, Shannon W, et al. Validation of clinical classification schemes for predicting stroke. Results of the National Registry of Atrial Fibrillation. JAMA 2001;385: 2864–70.
133. Olesen JB, Lip GY, Hansen ML, et al. Validation of risk stratification schemes for predicting stroke and thromboembolism in patients with atrial fibrillation. Nationwide cohort study. BMJ 2011;342:d124.
134. Lip GY, Nieuwlaat R, Pisters R, et al. Refining clinical risk stratification for predicting stroke and thromboembolism in atrial fibrillation using a novel risk factor-based approach. The Euro Heart Survey on Atrial Fibrillation. Chest 2010;137:263–72.
135. Pisters R, Lane DA, Nieuwlaat R, et al. A novel user-friendly score (HAS-BLED) to assess 1-year risk of major bleeding in patients with atrial fibrillation. The Euro Heart Survey. Chest 2010;138: 1093–100.
136. Adams HP Jr, Bendixen BH, Kappelle LJ, et al. Classification of subtype of acute ischemic stroke. Definitions for use in a multicenter clinical trial. TOAST. Trial of Org 10172 in Acute Stroke Treatment. Stroke 1993;24:35–41.
138. Meschia JF, Barrett KM, Chukweudelunzu F, et al. Interobserver agreement in the Trial of Org 10172 in Acute Stroke Treatment classification of stroke based on retrospective medical record review. J Stroke Cerebrovasc Dis 2006;15:266–72.
144. Ay H, Furie KL, Singhal A, et al. An evidence-based causative classification system for acute ischemic stroke. Ann Neurol 2005;58:688–97.
145. Ay H, Benner T, Arsava EM, et al. A computerized algorithm for etiologic classification of ischemic stroke: The Causative Classification of Stroke system. Stroke 2007;38:2979–84.
147. Marnane M, Duggan CA, Sheehan OC, et al. Stroke subtype classification to mechanism-specific and undetermined categories by TOAST, A-S-C-O, and Causative Classification System: Direct comparison in the North Dublin Population Stroke Study. Stroke 2010;41:1579–86.
151. Amarenco P, Bogousslavsky J, Caplan LR, et al. The ASCOD phenotyping of ischemic stroke (updated asco phenotyping). Cerebrovasc Dis 2013;36:1–5.
155. Amort M, Fluri F, Weisskopf F, et al. Etiological classifications of transient ischemic attacks: Subtype classification by TOAST, CCS, and ASCO–a pilot study. Cerebrovasc Dis 2012;33:508–16.
156. Cotter PE, Belham M, Martin PJ. Towards understanding the cause of stroke in young adults utilising a new stroke classification system (A-S-C-O). Cerebrovasc Dis 2012;33:123–7.
158. Wraige E, Pohl KR, Ganesan V. A proposed classification for subtypes of arterial ischaemic stroke in children. Dev Med Child Neurol 2005;47:252–6.
162. Baker K, Cano SJ, Playford ED. Outcome measurement in stroke: A scale selection strategy. Stroke 2011;42:1787–94.
164. Mayo NE, Fellows LK, Scott SC, et al. A longitudinal view of apathy and its impact after stroke. Stroke 2009;40:3299–307.
165. Hsieh YW, Hsueh IP, Chou YT, et al. Development and validation of a short form of the Fugl-Meyer Motor Scale in patients with stroke. Stroke 2007;38:3052–4.
167. Toglia J, Fitzgerald KA, O'Dell MW, et al. The Mini-Mental State Examination and Montreal Cognitive Assessment in persons with mild subacute stroke: Relationship to functional outcome. Arch Phys Med Rehabil 2011;92:792–8.
170. Pendlebury ST, Cuthbertson FC, Welch SJV, et al. Underestimation of cognitive impairment by Mini-Mental State Examination versus the Montreal Cognitive Assessment in patients with transient ischemic attack and stroke: A population-based study. Stroke 2010;41:1290–3.
171. Hamilton MA. A rating scale for depression. J Neurol Neurosurg Psychiatry 1960;23:56–62.
174. Williams RT, Heinemann AW, Bode RK, et al. Improving measurement properties of the Patient Health Questionnaire-9 point rating scale analysis. Rehabil Psychol 2009;54:198–203.
175. Turner A, Hambridge J, White J, et al. Depression screening in stroke: A comparison of alternative measures with the structured diagnostic interview for the Diagnostic and Statistical Manual of Mental Disorders, Fourth Edition (major depressive episode) as criterion standard. Stroke 2012;43:1000–5.
178. Mahoney FI, Barthel DW. Functional evaluation: The Barthel Index. Md State Med J 1965;14:61–5.
179. Katz S, Ford AB, Moskowitz RW, et al. The index of ADL: A atandardized measure of biological and psychosocial function. JAMA 1963;185:914–19.
180. Granger CV, Hamilton BB, Linacre JM, et al. Performance profiles of the Functional Independence Measure. Am J Phys Med Rehabil 1993;72:84–9.
181. Sulter G, Steen C, De Keyser J. Use of the Barthel Index and Modified Rankin Scale in acute stroke trials. Stroke 1999;30: 1538–41.
182. Appelros P. Characteristics of the Frenchay Activities Index one year after a stroke: A population-based study. Disabil Rehabil 2007;29:785–90.
194. Martinsson L, Eksborg S. Activity index-a complementary adl scale to the Barthel Index in the acute stage in patients with severe stroke. Cerebrovasc Dis 2006;22:231–9.
195. de Caneda MA, Fernandes JG, de Almeida AG, et al. Reliability of neurological assessment scales in patients with stroke. Arq Neuropsiquiatr 2006;64:690–7.
208. Quinn TJ, Dawson J, Walters MR, et al. Reliability of the modified Rankin Scale: A systematic review. Stroke 2009;40:3393–5.
213. Wahlgren NG, Romi F, Wahlgren J. Glasgow Outcome Scale and Global Improvement Scale were at least as sensitive as the Orgogozo, Mathew and Barthel scales in the Intravenous Nimodipine West Stroke Trial (INWEST). Cerebrovasc Dis 1995; 5:235.
214. Essink-Bot M, Krabbe P, Bonsel B, et al. An empirical comparison of four generic health status measures. The Nottingham Health Profile, the Medical Outcomes Study 36-item Short-Form health survey, the COOP/WONCA charts, and the EURO/QOLl intstrument. Med Care 1997;35:522–37.
242. Dorman PJ, Waddell F, Slattery J, et al. Is the EUORQOL a valid measure of health-related quality of life after stroke? Stroke 1997;28:1876–82.
243. King JT Jr, Tsevat J, Roberts MS. Measuring preference-based quality of life using the EUROQOL EQ-5D n patients with cerebral aneurysms. Neurosurgery 2009;65:565–72.
245. Duncan PW, Lai SM, Bode RK, et al. Stroke Impact Scale-16: A brief assessment of physical function. Neurology 2003;60: 291–6.
248. Lai SM, Perera S, Duncan PW, et al. Physical and social functioning after stroke: Comparison of the Stroke Impact Scale and Short Form-36. Stroke 2003;34:488–93.
249. Gershon RC, Lai JS, Bode R, et al. Neuro-QOL: Quality of life item banks for adults with neurological disorders: Item development and calibrations based upon clinical and general population testing. Qual Life Res 2012;21:475–86.

22 Carotid Artery Disease

Leo H. Bonati, Martin M. Brown

KEY POINTS

- Carotid disease is a common manifestation of focal atherosclerosis most often located at the origin of the internal carotid artery, and accounts for 10–20% of ischemic strokes.
- Intracranial carotid disease is more common than extracranial disease in Asian, black and Hispanic populations.
- The most common mechanism of stroke involves rupture of the atherosclerotic plaque with subsequent embolism to the brain hemisphere or eye.
- Carotid stenosis can reliably be detected by non-invasive imaging, including CT and MR angiography as well as ultrasound. MRI and ultrasound are increasingly used to measure the composition of the atherosclerotic plaque which, together with clinical risk factors, may give clues to the risk of stroke and the necessity of invasive revascularizations.
- Stroke risk in patients with carotid disease has been lowered with better medication, notably with widespread use of statins.

EPIDEMIOLOGY

The most common disease of the carotid artery is atherosclerosis occurring at the carotid artery bifurcation, typically involving the distal common carotid and the proximal internal carotid artery, and to a lesser extent the proximal external carotid artery. Carotid artery disease accounts for between 10% and 20% of ischemic stroke, depending on the method of classification.[1] The carotid arteries provide about 80% of the blood supply to the brain and thus the majority of emboli from the heart and the proximal aorta also pass through the carotid circulation, which makes it difficult to distinguish between carotid disease and these other sources as the cause for carotid territory stroke. Thus a carotid source for stroke or TIA tends to be inferred from the imaging finding of disease of the carotid artery in association with ipsilateral carotid territory symptoms in the absence of any other obvious cause. Most studies have required the finding of at least 50% stenosis of the carotid artery as indicating significant carotid disease, partly because detection of lesser degrees of stenosis was unreliable on Doppler ultrasound, and partly because mild disease of the carotid artery is very common. However, this does not mean that lesser degrees of disease will not necessarily cause stroke. Modern methods of carotid plaque imaging described below may alter this situation in the future.

Atherosclerotic carotid disease is more common in men than in women and its prevalence increases with age; ultrasound screening studies in Central and Northern European and North American populations have shown a prevalence of, at least a moderate degree of asymptomatic carotid stenosis narrowing the lumen by 50% or more of 2.3% in 60–69-year-old men, 6% in 70–79-year-old men, and up to 7.5% in ≥80-year-old men; in women the prevalence rates were 2%, 3.6%, and 5%, in the same age groups, respectively.[2] Severe carotid stenosis measuring 70% or more was present in 0.8%, 2.1%, and 3.1% in the same age groups in men, and in 0.2%, 1.0%, and 0.9% in women. Despite the high prevalence of carotid disease in the community, only a small proportion of these patients will develop TIA and stroke. Symptomatic carotid stenosis is less common in women, presumably reflecting the difference in prevalence in the community, and is more common in white Caucasian races than in black, Asian, or other races.[3] Among white Caucasians, there appears to be considerable heritability of carotid plaque characteristics and individual gene variants promoting carotid atherosclerosis in stroke patients have been identified.[4,5]

Risk factors for carotid atherosclerosis are similar to atherosclerosis at other sites and include raised cholesterol, systolic hypertension, and smoking, as well as increasing age. However, after adjustment for other risk factors, it appears that diabetes is not a strong risk factor.[6] Among stroke survivors, smoking appears to be more strongly associated with the presence of carotid stenosis than other risk factors for atherosclerosis such as hypertension, diabetes mellitus, and hypercholesterolemia.[7]

CAROTID ANATOMY AND LESION DEVELOPMENT

Lesion Location

The anatomy of the cerebral artery tree is presented in Figure 22-1. The bifurcation lies at the level of C3–4 in 55% of cases; the locations of the remainder are scattered from as high as C2–3 to as low as C5–6. In 85% the bifurcations are located at the same height on both sides.[8] On average, women have smaller carotid arteries with a diameter of the internal carotid artery of 4.7 mm, compared with 5.1 mm in men.[9]

Atherosclerotic deposits are usually greatest in the distal common carotid artery, the bifurcation and the first few centimeters of the internal carotid artery, leaving the proximal common carotid artery and distal extracranial segment of the internal carotid artery relatively unaffected.[10] In contrast, spontaneous or traumatic dissection typically occurs more distally along the course of the internal carotid artery close to the basis of the skull, where the artery is more vulnerable to traction during neck movement.[11] Dissection is discussed in detail in Chapter 35. Atherosclerosis is also seen at the origin of the common carotid artery and in the intracranial carotid syphon and cavernous portions of the internal carotid artery (Fig. 22-2). The predilection for areas of flow disturbance supports the concept that wall shear stress plays an important role in the pathogenesis of atherosclerosis.[12] Only about 30% of patients with stenosis of one carotid artery will have significant stenosis of the other carotid artery. When asymmetry of

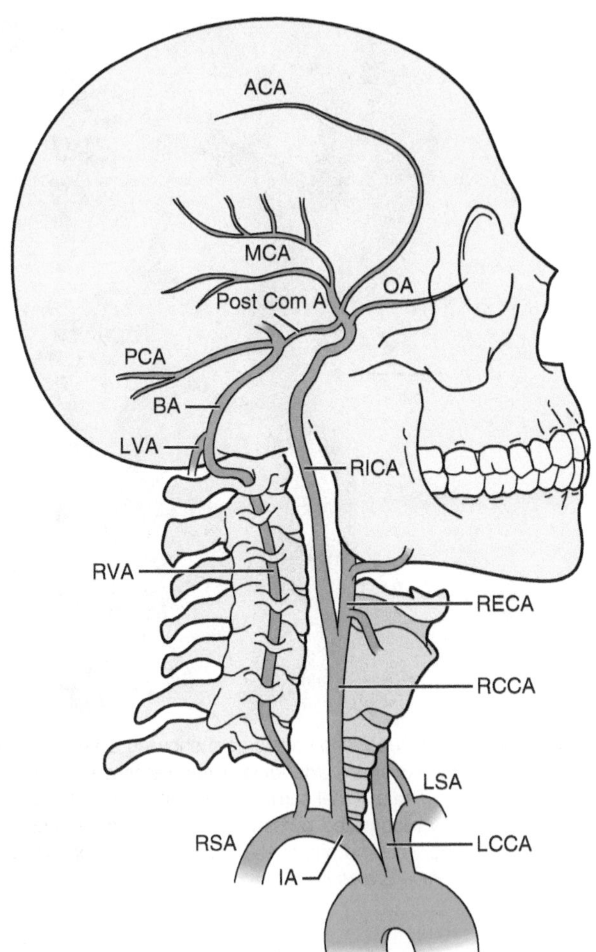

Figure 22-1. Anatomy of the extracranial cerebral-bound arteries and their main intracranial supplies, lateral view from the right. ACA, anterior cerebral artery; BA, basilar artery; IA, innominate artery; LCCA, left common carotid artery; LSA, left subclavian artery; LVA, left vertebral artery; MCA, middle cerebral artery; OA, ophthalmic artery; PCA, posterior cerebral artery; Post Com A, posterior communicating artery; RCCA, right common carotid artery; RECA; right external carotid artery; RICA, right internal carotid artery; RSA, right subclavian artery; RVA, right vertebral artery. The anterior choroidal artery is not depicted. *(From Gautier JC, Mohr JP: Ischemic stroke. In Mohr JP, Gautier JC, editors:* Guide to clinical neurology, *New York, 1995, Churchill Livingstone, p 543.)*

atheroma severity is found, the atheroma is more common in the smaller carotid,[13] the one more angulated,[14] and the one in which flow separation is more easily demonstrated.[15-18]

Tempo of Development of Carotid Stenosis

Atherosclerotic stenosis may on occasions be shown to develop swiftly over a few months by digital subtraction angiography,[19] conventional angiography,[20] or non-invasive techniques.

Sudden stenosis can also develop very rapidly as a result of hemorrhage into the plaque. An apparent sudden progression of stenosis or the development of occlusion is, however, more commonly caused by thrombosis on the ruptured plaque surface. In general, the development of carotid stenosis from atherosclerosis is a very slow process, stretching over 50 to 60 years or more, starting with fatty streaks early in adolescent or adult life and progressing to atheroma formation, and finally atherosclerosis and stenosis in middle or old age. Significant

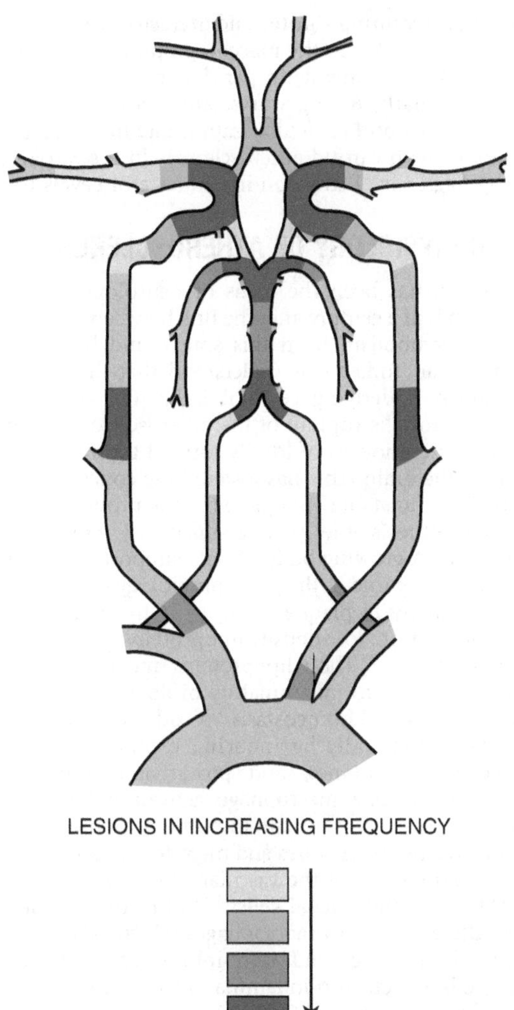

Figure 22-2. Distribution of atherosclerotic lesions in the carotid and vertebrobasilar territories.

stenosis from atherosclerosis is rare under the age of 40, but earlier atheroma might still have a role to play in some younger cases of stroke. In many cases, atherosclerotic stenosis may even remain static, especially if the lesion is heavily calcified despite being hemodynamically significant.[21]

In the Asymptomatic Carotid Stenosis and risk of Stroke (ACSRS) Study involving 1121 patients with asymptomatic carotid disease who were followed with 6-monthly duplex ultrasound examination for a mean duration of 4 years, the degree of stenosis remained unchanged in 76% of patients, stenosis progressed in 20% of patients, and regression of stenosis was observed in only 4% of patients.[22] Male sex, diabetes mellitus, and active smoking were among the clinical predictors of progression identified in prospective ultrasound studies.[22,23]

Statins reduce the progression of early-stage carotid atherosclerosis measured by intima-media-thickness on ultrasound.[24] Small case-control and prospective cohort studies with ultrasound and magnetic resonance imaging (MRI) showed that statins reduce the lipid content, but not the total volume of developed plaques.[25-27] However, patients not receiving lipid-lowering therapy in the ACSRS study were at increased risk of stenosis progression.[22] Further, indirect evidence that intensive statin therapy slows plaque progression stems from randomized placebo-controlled secondary prevention trials: among patients with a history of cerebrovascular disease, the proportion requiring carotid endarterectomy or stenting was reduced from 2.3% in the placebo group to 1% in the group receiving 40 mg simvastatin per day in the Heart Protection Study.[28] Similarly, 80 mg atorvastatin per day versus placebo reduced the carotid revascularization rate from 7.2% to 3.2% in patients with carotid atherosclerosis in the Stroke Prevention by Aggressive Reduction in Cholesterol Levels trial.[29]

PATHOPHYSIOLOGY OF ATHEROSCLEROSIS

The carotid has been the focus of neurologic attention for more than half a century after the link between stenosis, occlusion, and embolism from this source and brain infarction became clear. Today, it is understood that the predominant mechanism underlying cerebral ischaemia associated with carotid stenosis is rupture of the atherosclerotic plaque with subsequent embolism of locally formed thrombus or plaque debris to the brain. This has fostered the concept of the "vulnerable" or "unstable" plaque which is prone to rupture, as opposed to the "stable" plaque which may remain inert over many years. A growing body of data supports that inflammation plays a key role in the pathophysiology of atherosclerosis and particularly in plaque rupture.[30-32] In the early phase of plaque formation, low-density lipoproteins (LDL) accumulate in the vessel wall.[33] These lipoproteins undergo oxidation and thereby acquire pro-inflammatory biological functions unrelated to cholesterol homeostasis.[34] Oxidized lipoproteins activate endothelial cells by inducing expression of adhesion molecules, chemokines, and pro-inflammatory cytokines. They also facilitate macrophage activation by triggering a variety of receptors of innate immune responses. Monocytes are attracted by chemokines and migrate into the plaque facilitated by expression of the vascular cell adhesion molecule-1 (VCAM-1) on endothelial cells.[35] Within the plaque, monocytes differentiate into macrophages which take up oxidized lipoprotein particles and turn into so-called foam cells.[36] Foam cells secrete pro-inflammatory cytokines and a large array of proteases, including matrix metalloproteases (MMPs), serine proteases, elastases, and cysteine proteases, that contribute to degradation of elastin and collagen in advanced lesions leading to destabilization of the plaque, thinning of its fibrous cap, and – ultimately – plaque rupture.[37,38] If the plaque surface ruptures, platelets are exposed to sub-endothelial collagen, von Willebrand factor (vWF), and local agonists such as adenosine diphosphate (ADP). Activated platelets bind to fibrinogen and secrete various pro-coagulatory and pro-inflammatory factors, which mediate the binding of leukocytes and enhance fibrin formation. A local thrombus may form on the plaque surface, leading to embolization and occlusion of arteries in the eye or the brain manifesting as amaurosis fugax, transient ischemic attack (TIA), or stroke.

EVALUATION OF EXTRACRANIAL CAROTID STENOSIS

Auscultation

A bruit in the neck is commonly encountered in routine clinical examination, found in as many as 4–5% of the population aged 45–80 years.[39,40] A local cervical bruit can be detected in approximately 70–89% of patients with an internal carotid stenosis of greater than or equal to 75% stenosis or less than or equal to 2 mm residual lumen.[41,42] In a population-based study of a stroke-free cohort of 686 subjects with a mean age of 68.2 years, the prevalence of carotid stenosis ≥60% detected by ultrasound was 2.2%; bruits had a prevalence of 4.1%. Bruit detection by auscultation had a sensitivity of 56%, a specificity of 98%, a positive predictive value of 25%, and a negative predictive value of 99%; the overall accuracy was 97.5%.[43] Similar values demonstrating high specificity but low sensitivity were reported in a more recent meta-anlysis of 26 studies.[44] Modern practice, therefore, dictates immediate imaging of the carotid as well as the brain in any patient with symptoms suggestive of ocular or cerebral ischemia, regardless of whether or not a carotid bruit is present.

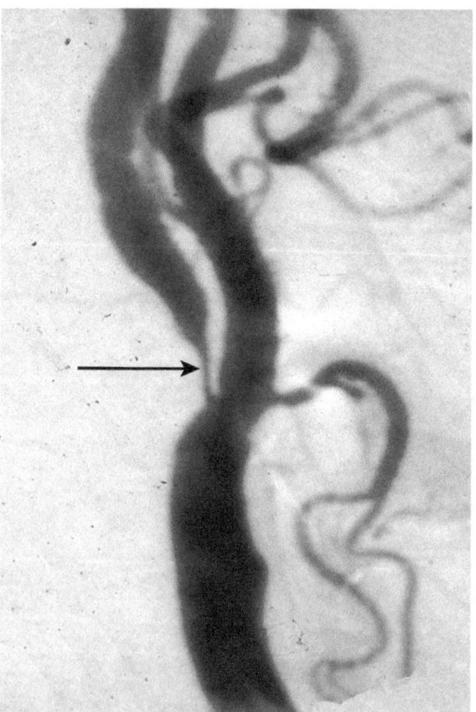

Figure 22-3. Digital subtraction angiogram showing severe stenosis of the internal carotid artery extending a few centimeters from the carotid bifurcation. The external carotid artery arising from the carotid bifurcation is easily recognized by its multiple branches. In contrast, internal carotid artery has no branches in the neck. *(Reproduced with permission from M.M. Brown.)*

Degree of stenosis

The degree of luminal narrowing has traditionally been the most common parameter used to grade the severity of carotid disease. The standard method to determine degree of stenosis before the widespread availability of modern non-invasive techniques was the radiographic measurement of the diameter reduction of the carotid artery lumen on photographic film obtained after intra-arterial injection of contrast (catheter-based angiography). After the introduction of computerized imaging, the native radiographic X-ray image was subtracted from the contrast-enhanced view (digital subtraction angiography, DSA). An example of a very severe carotid stenosis shown by DSA is shown in Figure 22-3. Importantly, the two clinical trials that were pivotal in demonstrating efficacy of endarterectomy to prevent stroke in symptomatic carotid stenosis, the European Carotid Surgery Trial (ECST) and the North American Carotid Endarterectomy Trial (NASCET), used catheter-based angiography and DSA to measure stenosis severity. As atherosclerotic narrowing does not typically develop in a concentric way around the lumen, at least two perpendicular views, and often a third, oblique projection, were used in the trials as well as in clinical practice to show the maximum degree of narrowing. NASCET and ECST initially used different sites to measure the normal reference

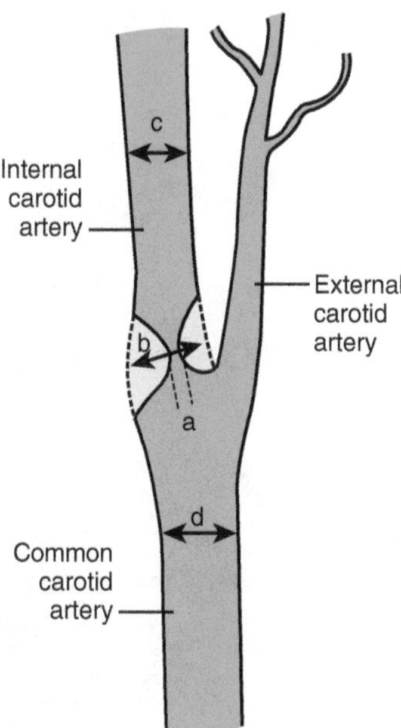

Figure 22-4. Position of measurements for stenosis. a, Site of maximum stenosis (regardless of whether in the carotid bulb); b, original internal carotid lumen; c, internal carotid distal to the stenosis; d, common carotid lumen. *(From Young GR, Humphrey PR, Nixon TE, et al: Variability in measurement of extracranial internal carotid artery stenosis as displayed by both digital subtraction and magnetic resonance angiography: An assessment of three caliper techniques and visual impression of stenosis.* Stroke *1996;27:467, with permission.)*

diameter of the artery against which the diameter of the lumen at the site of maximum stenosis was compared: NASCET defined the diameter of the non-diseased ICA distal to the stenosis at a point where the artery became uniform in diameter as the reference,[45] whereas ECST estimated the normal vessel diameter at the site of the stenosis by visual estimation of the likely normal diameter of the carotid bulb.[46] The degree of stenosis was expressed as percentage in diameter reduction by the formula ([1 – minimum residual lumen/normal ICA diameter] × 100). A third trial, the Carotid And Vertebral Artery Transluminal Angioplasty Study (CAVATAS) compared the diameter at the site of the stenosis to the diameter of the common carotid artery. The different reference sites to measure the normal carotid diameter are shown in Figure 22-4. A lesion occurring in a typical location in the carotid bulb will result in a higher degree of stenosis using the ECST method than using the NASCET method, as the reference diameter of the normal artery is wider at the bulb than more distally along its cervical course. On average, 50% and 70% stenosis measured by the NASCET method are equivalent to 65% and 82% stenosis, respectively, measured by the ECST method.[47] This methodological difference partly explained the seemingly different long-term results of the two trials reported in 1998, with NASCET showing benefit of carotid endarterectomy for patients with 50% stenosis or greater,[48] and ECST for patients with 80% stenosis or greater.[46] However, re-assessment of angiograms in ECST by the method used in the NASCET trial demonstrated that, in fact, the results of the two trials were broadly similar, the pooled analysis showing 4.6% absolute reduction in 5-year ipsilateral stroke-risk patients with symptomatic, moderate carotid stenosis (50–69% NASCET narrowing), and 15.3% risk reduction in patients with symptomatic, severe stenosis (70–99% NASCET narrowing, excluding patients with near-occlusion defined by collapsed lumen distal to the stenosis).[47] Subsequently, the NASCET method

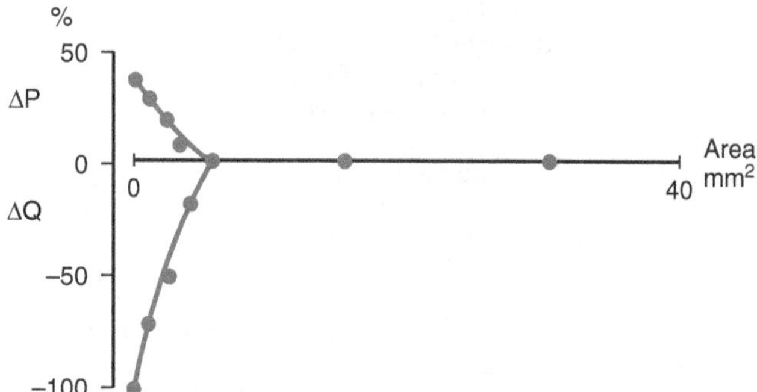

Figure 22-5. Effect of progressive in-vivo reduction in cross-sectional area (horizontal axis) in a carotid artery on mean pressure gradient (ΔP) and flow (ΔQ) across the applied constriction. *(From Brice JG, Dowsett DJ, Lowe RD. Haemodynamic Effects of Carotid Artery Stenosis. BMJ 1964;2:1363-1366, with permission.)*

has become widely accepted as the standard method to measure stenosis severity throughout the cerebral circulation, using any technique of direct visualization of the vessel lumen.

Since the time these trials were done, non-invasive imaging methods have largely superseded DSA in measuring degree of carotid stenosis. Using Doppler ultrasound and duplex sonography, the degree of stenosis is determined by a set of flow velocity criteria, most importantly the peak systolic and end-diastolic velocity in the ICA.[49] Contrast-enhanced (CE) magnetic resonance or computer tomography angiography (MRA and CTA) after injections of intravenous contrast provide an anatomical image of the artery, albeit at lower resolution than DSA. It is standard practice to report the degree of stenosis measured by these non-invasive tests using measures regarded as giving results equivalent to the NASCET method used for DSA. Ultrasound laboratories use standard criteria that were originally calibrated against catheter-based angiographic measurements using the NASCET method. However, it should be borne in mind that few laboratories regularly audit the accuracy of their stenosis measurements given the risks of catheter-based angiography and there is a tendency for radiologists to believe they can simply "eyeball" a stenosis and report its severity, which can lead to errors in interpretation.

In a systematic review published in 2006, ultrasound, CTA, and MRA all had high sensitivity and specificity for diagnosing severe, 70–99% carotid stenosis, with CEMRA appearing superior to ultrasound, CTA, and non-contrast MRA.[50] In the interval since this report, the introduction of superior multislice CT machines has improved the resolution of cross-sectional CTA to the extent that, unless there is heavy calcification of the carotid plaque, the resolution of the lumen now exceeds that of standard CEMRA. None of the non-invasive techniques is entirely reliable and all suffer from technical limitations. Therefore, we recommend confirming the degree of stenosis by consistent findings from two different non-invasive tests in patients being considered for carotid revascularization, DSA being reserved for patients in whom the non-invasive tests disagree or do not differentiate between total occlusion, near-occlusion, or high-grade stenosis.

The fact that the focus of carotid imaging has been limited to measuring the degree of stenosis for a long time is partly explained by the historical concept of flow impairment as the main mechanism of cerebral ischemia. Reduced cross-sectional area is the main factor in causing hemodynamic impairment.[51-53] Other factors include the length of the stenosis,[51] blood flow velocity,[54] and blood viscosity.[55] Limitation of intracranial flow requires a cross-sectional area of 4 mm^2 to 5 mm^2 along a length of 3 mm (Fig. 22-5); this area corresponds to less than

2 mm in the smallest 2D profile seen on an angiogram[52] and occurs when 84% diameter stenosis and 96% area stenosis are achieved.[56] Until these severities of stenosis are reached, any reduction in diameter is compensated for by an increase in blood flow velocity across the stenosis, which is the basis of using Doppler ultrasound to determine stenosis severity. It is important to note that flow in the carotid artery is predominantly the result of a bolus of a column of blood ejected from the heart and is influenced by the distensibility of the arterial wall, thus it is not laminar and does not obey Poiseuille's law defining the relationship between flow velocity and radius. Only a small minority, even among symptomatic patients with carotid disease, has such severely narrowed arteries that significant impairment of cerebral blood flow can be inferred, suggesting that other mechanisms may play a part in the strong association between stenosis severity and risk of recurrent stroke in medical-treated patients.

Another piece of evidence arguing against impairment of blood flow being the main mechanism of stroke associated with carotid stenosis is that in ECST and NASCET, patients with near-occlusion or collapse of the carotid artery beyond the stenosis (generally patients with at least 95% stenosis), had a lower rate of stroke on medical therapy than patients with lesser degrees of stenosis and did not benefit from endarterectomy.[47] This might in part reflect selection of patients in the trial who had sufficient intracranial collateral supply to the ipsilateral carotid territory to protect them against major stroke: major stroke was an exclusion criteria for the trials. An alternative explanation for these somewhat contradictory findings is that rather than directly affecting blood flow to the brain, increasing stenosis is associated with increasing turbulence beyond the stenosis, hence activating platelets and contributing to thrombus formation in symptomatic patients.[57] In near-occlusion, flow velocity in the carotid artery is very low and hence might not activate platelets in the same way.

Despite the observation that the degree of stenosis was an important predictor of stroke risk under medical therapy and, hence, benefit from carotid endarterectomy in patients with recently symptomatic stenosis,[47] the same relationship could not be demonstrated in trials of carotid endarterectomy for patients with asymptomatic disease.[58,59] Some authors explained this by the fact that mostly ultrasound instead of DSA was used for inclusion of patients in these trials, which is less accurate in determining the degree of stenosis.[60] Certainly in a large community study of the prevalence of carotid stenosis there was a strong association between the severity of carotid stenosis measured on ultrasound and a history of previous stroke or TIA.[6]

Plaque Surface Irregularity and Ulceration

Given our current understanding that arterio-arterial embolism is the most important mechanism causing stroke in patients with extracranial carotid stenosis, it is counterintuitive that luminal narrowing should be the only or, in fact, the most important determinant of stroke risk. Indeed, early studies already seemed to suggest that TIAs could be attributable to any degree of stenosis by means of microembolization.[61–64] Evidence in support of this view arose from individual case reports, to which whole series of cases were later added.[61,65–70] In more recent research, carotid imaging has, therefore, focussed on the morphology of the lesion and the composition of the atherosclerotic plaque. Already at the time of NASCET and ECST, irregular or ulcerated plaque surface was identified as an important predictor of stroke risk under medical therapy.[71] Fig. 22-6 shows a large ulcer within a carotid plaque shown using the early catheter-based angiography technique common at that time. Ulcers are often found in surgical specimens.[66–68,72]

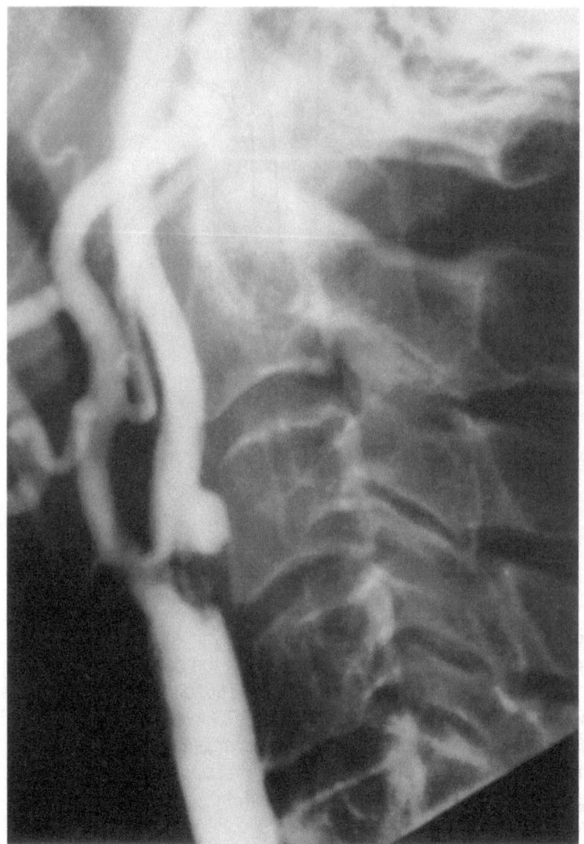

Figure 22-6. Internal carotid artery with combined stenosis and large ulceration shown using the early technique of catheter-based angiography without digital subtraction of the structures seen on a non-contrast X-ray.

Small ulcers are difficult to demonstrate angiographically, and considerable interobserver variation exists in the diagnosis of ulceration.[73] As many as 40% of small ulcers may be missed on routine angiograms,[67] but whether these are clinically relevant is uncertain.

After the introduction of ultrasound and non-invasive angiography as the methods of imaging carotid atherosclerosis, the importance of ulceration was neglected and often not reported routinely, probably because earlier techniques had a low resolution and, therefore, were not very sensitive to ulceration. However, modern ultrasonography using B-mode imaging may be as sensitive as conventional angiography to the presence of plaque irregularity and ulceration[74] (Fig. 22-7). The use of a bolus of micro-bubble contrast during the examination increases the sensitivity of ultrasound to ulceration, while the yield of modern CTA is better than either conventional angiography or ultrasound because of the ability to view the entire circumference and length of the plaque.[75] However, CEMRA remains poorly sensitive to ulceration compared to the other techniques.

Plaque Composition and Inflammation

One advantage of the non-invasive diagnostic modalities in contrast to DSA is their ability to image the arterial wall and composition of the atherosclerotic plaque itself. On B-mode ultrasound of carotid bifurcation plaques, parts appearing dark (echolucent) correspond to necrotic areas with increased lipid content and plaque hemorrhage in histological examination.[76,77] Interrater reliability on qualitative interpretation of

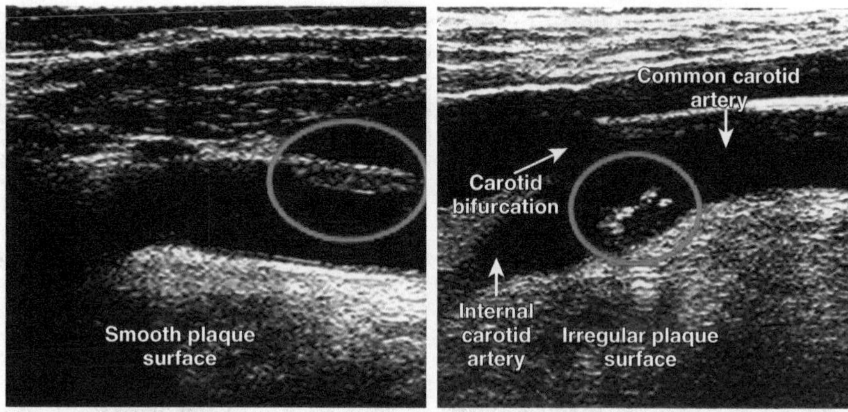

Figure 22-7. Left panel, Regular carotid plaque surface. Right panel, Irregular carotid plaque surface. *(Reproduced with permission from Prabhakaran S, Rundek T, Ramas R, et al: Carotid plaque surface irregularity predicts ischemic stroke: The Northern Manhattan Stroke Study.* Stroke *2006;37:2696-2701.)*

carotid plaque morphology has in the past been poor.[78] More recently, computerized analysis of B-mode ultrasound images has allowed for normalization against reference tissues and, therefore, a quantitative and objective assessment of plaque echolucency. The most common quantitative measure of plaque morphology on ultrasound is the so-called grayscale median (GSM), i.e., the median grayscale value in the plaque.[79–81] Several prospective studies have demonstrated that patients with echolucent plaques[82,83] and low GSM[84,85] are at increased risk of stroke, independently from degree of stenosis. More recently, an Echographic Risk Index based on a combination of degree of stenosis and proportion of echolucent area near the plaque surface, has been demonstrated to be superior to degree of stenosis and GSM alone in predicting cerebrovascular ischemic events and brain infarction on MRI.[86] Echolucent plaque area at the surface also independently predicted stroke in the ACSRS study.[87]

MRI is able to visualize key structural correlates of carotid bifurcation plaque instability, including lipid-rich necrotic core, intra-plaque hemorrhage (IPH), and disruption of the luminal surface (Fig. 22-8).[88,89] These findings are more common in patients with symptomatic than with asymptomatic stenosis.[90] The presence of these features fundamentally alters the biology and natural history of carotid atherosclerosis:[91] plaques with MRI evidence of IPH may exhibit rapid progression despite statin therapy,[92–94] and are associated with a six- to tenfold increase in risk of ipsilateral cerebrovascular events compared to plaques without IPH.[95,96] In one of these studies, IPH was a better predictor of recurrent events in recently symptomatic patients than stenosis severity.[95] Plaques with a disrupted luminal surface (DLS) were found to have a 17-fold higher risk for cerebrovascular events.[97]

Positron emission tomography (PET) studies have shown that radiolabeled 18F-fluorodeoxyglucose (FDG) accumulates in carotid plaques, particularly at sites with high inflammatory activity.[98–100] In a recent prospective cohort study of 60 patients with symptomatic carotid stenosis higher plaque FDG uptake at baseline was associated with increased risk of recurrent stroke, independently from degree of stenosis.[101]

Cerebrovascular Reserve

On a physiological level, hemodynamic impairment resulting from carotid stenosis may best be understood as a reduced capacity of the cerebral vasculature to increase flow when required, rather than as a reduction in blood flow per se. This autoregulatory capacity can be assessed as the so-called cerebrovascular reserve, i.e., the increase in blood flow to stimuli such as carbon dioxide (CO_2). This has been most often assessed by measuring blood flow in the middle cerebral artery by transcranial Doppler (TCD) or single photon emission CT (SPECT), before and after induction of hypercapnia by breath-holding, inhalation of hyperbaric CO_2, or administration of acetazolamide. PET can also be used to directly identify patients with exhausted cerebrovascular reserve by demonstrating increased oxygen extraction in areas of impaired blood flow. Prospective cohort studies demonstrated that reduced cerebrovascular reserve measured by TCD was associated with an increased risk of recurrent stroke or TIA independently from degree of stenosis, both among patients with symptomatic and asymptomatic carotid stenosis.[102,103] A meta-analysis of 13 prospective studies found that reduced cerebrovascular reserve was associated with an almost four-fold increase in stroke risk (odds ratio [OR], 3.9; 95% confidence interval [CI], 2.0–7.5), without material differences in the strength of this association between patients with symptomatic and asymptomatic carotid stenosis.[104] However, it has not been shown that measuring cerebrovascular reserve consistently identifies patients who will benefit from revascularization. In the most recent trial of extracranial–intracranial bypass surgery, patients with symptomatic carotid occlusion and exhausted cerebral reserve identified by PET scanning had no improvement in cognitive function after bypass surgery and had a significantly higher rate of stroke than those treated with medical therapy alone.[105,106]

Microembolization

TCD is able to detect emboli passing along the insonated portion of the middle cerebral artery as short, high-intensity signals (HITS) which are characterized by a chirping sound.[107,108] The presence of these so-called microembolic signals during a 1-hour TCD recording at baseline predicted the risk of stroke, and stroke and TIA combined, in a cohort of 200 patients with symptomatic carotid stenosis.[109] The association with cerebrovascular events was independent from other risk factors including degree of stenosis. A systematic literature review and meta-analysis published in 2009 found that the presence of HITS increased the risk of stroke in patients with symptomatic carotid stenosis by an odds ratio of 9.6 (95%CI, 1.5–59.4) and in patients with asymptomatic carotid stenosis by an odds ratio of 7.5 (2.2–24.9).[110] This finding was later confirmed in a large prospective cohort of patients with asymptomatic carotid stenosis (Asymptomatic Carotid Emboli Study, ACES).[111]

Thus, qualitative, quantitative and functional imaging of the carotid plaque and assessment of microembolization hold

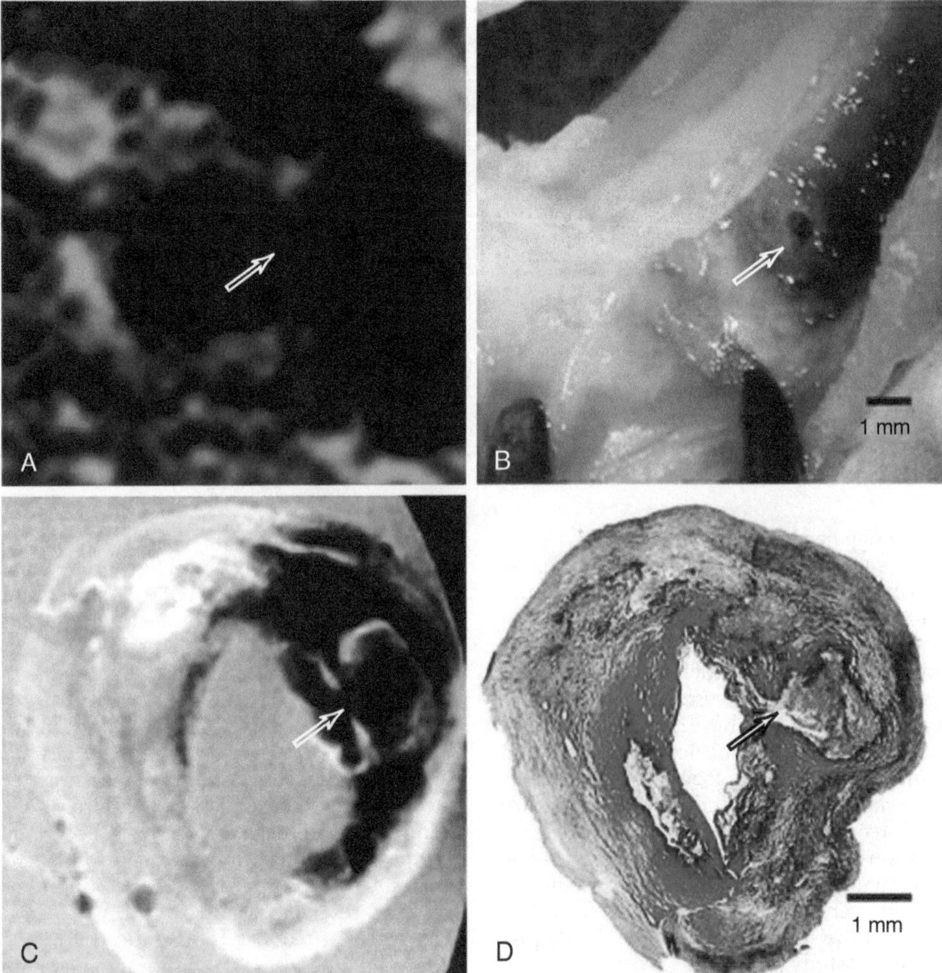

Figure 22-8. Rupture of an ulcerated left internal carotid artery atherosclerotic stenosis. A, In vivo T1-weighted MRI at 3T showing the area of maximal luminal reduction communicating with an ulcer crater (arrow). The widening of the more normal lumen is seen at the top of the image. B, Gross inspection of the carotid endarterectomy specimen. C, Ex vivo T1-weighted MRI at 11.7 T of the specimen showing rupture of the thinned fibrous cap (arrow), the slit-like lumen of the artery (crossed by the arrowhead), and areas of hemorrhage and lipid-rich core within the plaque (dark areas of low signal). D, Trichrome-stained specimen showing matched histology.

promise of identifying patients with carotid disease at risk for stroke. This evidence is further discussed in the section "Stroke risk in patients with carotid artery disease" below. Whether these tests add to clinical decision making in improving the selection of patients who benefit from carotid revascularization, remains to be proven in randomized controlled trials.

INTRACRANIAL CAROTID ARTERY DISEASE

In ethnically mixed populations, relevant stenosis of large intracranial arteries (including the intracranial internal carotid, middle cerebral and vertebrobasilar arteries) has been identified as the cause of acute ischemic stroke in as many as 8% of patients.[112] The intracranial ICA, especially the cavernous part, is the second site of predilection of carotid atherosclerosis, but in Western populations, the extent and severity of the lesions are far behind those of the extracranial bifurcation. In contrast, symptomatic intracranial atherosclerosis is generally reported as being much more common among Asians, Hispanics, and blacks than among white Caucasian patients, and its incidence exceeds that of symptomatic extracranial atherosclerosis in those populations.[112-115] Although recognized as an important cause of stroke in white Caucasians in post-mortem studies performed early in the 20th century, intracranial atherosclerosis, therefore, came to be considered a rare cause of stroke in white Caucasian races compared to carotid stenosis. However, recent post-mortem studies and community imaging studies have once again drawn attention to the frequent finding of intracranial carotid atherosclerosis in white Caucasian patients with stroke, suggesting that it may be a more common cause of stroke than currently recognized.[116,117] Metabolic syndrome and diabetes mellitus as risk factors are more strongly associated with intracranial disease than with extracranial disease.[114,115]

There is no clear evidence to indicate that a siphon stenosis (tandem stenosis) increases the risk of occlusive thrombosis of a stenosis at the ICA origin or vice versa,[118-120] nor do tandem stenoses appear to raise the risk involved in carotid endarterectomy,[121] although one has to acknowledge that most trials of carotid revascularization excluded patients with significant tandem lesions.

Anterograde and retrograde secondary thromboses of the intracranial ICA are subjects for which only scanty literature exists. In general, occlusive thrombus arising on atheromatous plaque at the carotid bifurcation extends rapidly from the origin of the internal carotid artery at least to the origin of the ophthalmic artery, the first branch beyond the bifurcation. The distal intracranial internal carotid may then remain patent

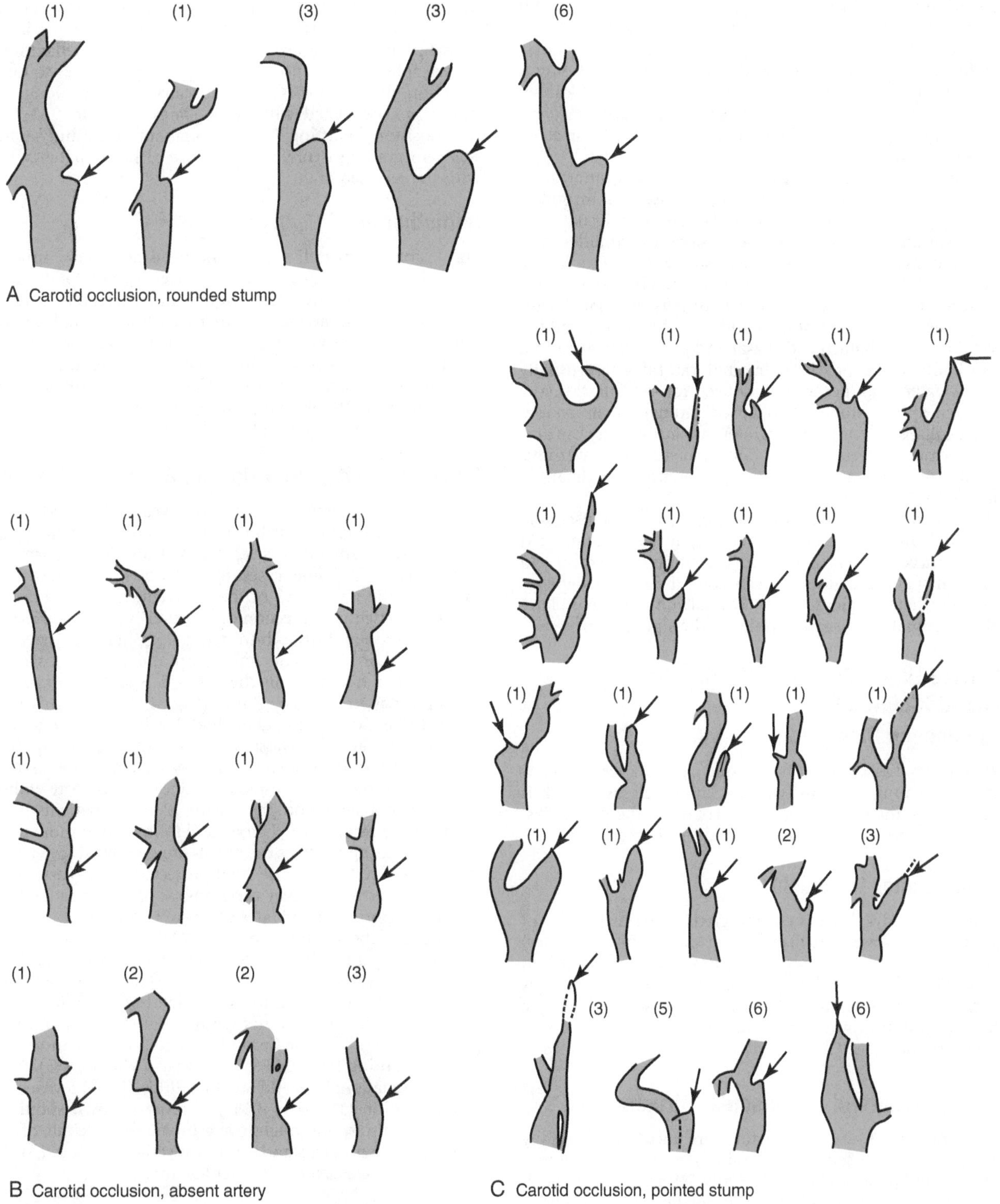

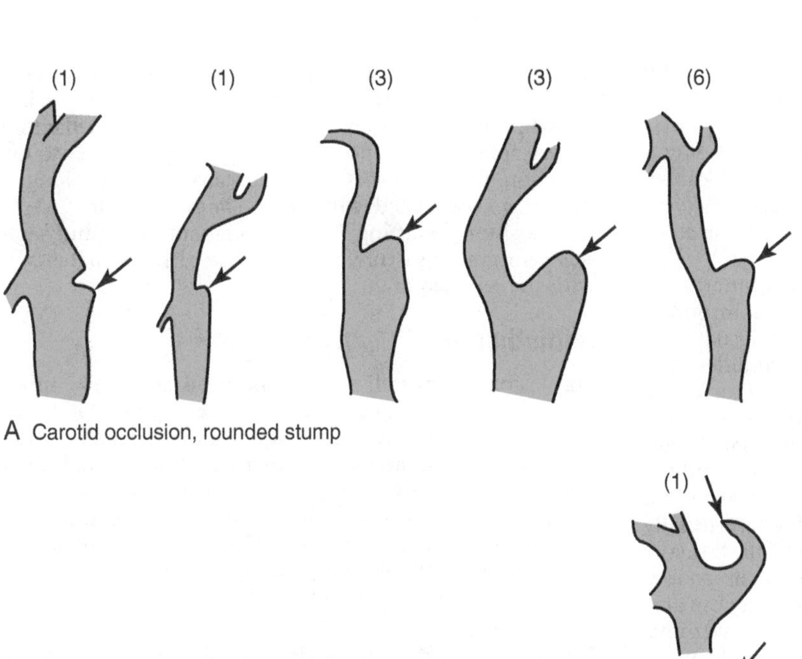

A Carotid occlusion, rounded stump

(1) (1) (1) (1)
(1) (1) (1) (1)
(1) (2) (2) (3)

B Carotid occlusion, absent artery

(1) (1) (1) (1) (1)
(1) (1) (1) (1) (1)
(1) (1) (1) (1) (1)
(1) (1) (1) (2) (3)
(3) (5) (6) (6)

C Carotid occlusion, pointed stump

Figure 22-9. Angiographic appearance of different types of internal carotid artery occlusion. Numbers in parentheses indicate days between stroke onset and angiography.

either as a result of reversed flow in the ophthalmic artery maintained by external carotid artery collaterals or reversed flow down the distal internal carotid artery to the ophthalmic artery. However, in many cases, angiography will show an occlusion extending all the way from the bifurcation to the tip of the intracranial carotid artery and even beyond into the middle cerebral artery. It is then difficult in such a case to know whether the thrombosis started at the bifurcation and extended intracranially or vice versa. Pathologically well-studied instances of intracranial ICA thrombotic occlusion are rare, and the role of anterograde or retrograde extension of an associated thrombus is unclear.[118,122–124] Retrograde thrombi developing down to the ICA origin are probably not rare, and the angiographic appearance of the proximal end of carotid occlusion does not predict the age of the occlusion, at least within the first 6 days after stroke onset (Fig. 22-9).[125]

Discontinuous occlusions (i.e., the presence of a patent segment of the ICA between the extracranial occluded ICA and the intracranial ICA) have been reported at autopsy, and it may be difficult or impossible to decide whether the distal plug is the result of local thrombosis or embolic, the lack of knowledge of which poses some difficulties for surgeons or interventionalists attempting removal of what is inferred to be an acute occlusion at the origin or the siphon of the ICA.[118,123,124,126]

Progressive occlusion of the siphon and distal intracranial ICA has been reported in a setting of essential thrombocythemia[127] and in mucormycosis, and encasement by nasopalatine carcinoma (carcinoma of the fossa of Rosenmüller) and inflammatory pseudotumors[128] is also well-known. Progressive occlusion of the distal intracranial ICA, often bilateral, is also a feature of moyamoya disease, where it is associated with contiguous involvement of the middle cerebral artery and the development of characteristic basal and pial collateralization. In such cases, the proximal internal carotid artery usually remains patent, but because of reduced run-off intracranially will often appear small or collapsed throughout its course. Similar collapse of the proximal internal carotid artery can also occur in cases of severe atheromatous stenosis of the cavernous carotid artery. Moyamoya disease is described in detail in Chapter 40.

Described in more detail in Chapters 46–48, transcranial ultrasound and non-invasive angiography (MRA and CTA) have advanced enough to allow investigation of the orbit and siphon in many individuals, decreasing the former dependency on catheter angiography.[129] The calcium score correlates with atheromatous disease severity in the siphon.[117,130]

CAROTID DISEASE OTHER THAN ATHEROSCLEROSIS

Spontaneous Dissection

Spontaneous dissection of the internal carotid artery typically occurs in young patients without atherosclerosis, and is located along the distal extracranial course of the vessel. Dissections of cervical arteries are covered in Chapter 35.

Fibromuscular Dysplasia

Fibromuscular dysplasia is encountered in less than 0.6% of cases of ICA disease.[131] It may explain some kinks (see later) and is associated with separate intracranial aneurysm in almost 25% of cases of fibromuscular dysplasia (see later). Its clinical importance is unclear, but the disease has been the subject of publication often enough that it is discussed in a separate chapter (see Chapter 35).

Primary Tumors of the Vascular Structures

Primary tumors of vascular structures are uncommon, usually arising from mesoblastic and neural elements such as chemodectomas and paragangliomas.[132] Only 5% are bilateral. Such masses grow slowly, manifesting as dysphagia and hoarseness, although dyspnea, Horner's syndrome, and facial pain may also occur.[133] The lesions produce metastases in only about 2% of cases. Local recurrence is uncommon and is usually delayed for many years. They are not usually associated with stroke, except as a result of surgery to remove the tumor.

Complications of Head and Neck Cancer

Involvement of the extracranial carotid artery by direct extension of a local tumor is distinctly uncommon.[134] However, this complication occurs often enough in hospitals with a large oncology caseload to warrant consideration here. Direct tumor invasion of the arterial wall from an extracranial site is well known,[135] but only rarely has involvement of parasellar tumors in the siphon been reported.[136] Surgical approaches to tumor resection that involve taking the carotid artery along with tumor are associated with stroke rates of up to 25%.[137,138] Interpositional grafting[139] is the usual approach, but saphenous vein grafting is preferred because of better patency than with the reversed graft.[140]

Radiotherapy

The lesions from radiation to the head and neck, although typically delayed in onset, affect a longer segment of the artery than that affected by conventional atherosclerosis.[141] Radiation can induce or accelerate atherosclerosis, generally after an interval of several years,[135,142] and in some cases delays have been as long as 25 years.[143] Recurrence after stenting is higher in radiation-related stenoses.[144] Carotid rupture is a serious late complication of nasopharyngeal cancer and radiation treatment; management options are limited.[145]

Restenosis after Prior Carotid Revascularization

Restenosis occurring up to about 2 years after endarterectomy is commonly attributed to neointimal hyperplasia, whereas recurrent atherosclerosis is thought to cause later restenosis.[146–148] Some cases of restenosis characteristically located at the upper end of the endarterectomy field are the result of inadequate resection of an extensive plaque. Neointimal formation and smooth-muscle cell proliferation have also been found in a patient with symptomatic restenosis after endovascular treatment in the Carotid And Vertebral Artery Transluminal Angioplasty Study (CAVATAS).[149] In this randomized trial, 30.7% of patients had developed severe residual or recurrent carotid stenosis on ultrasound follow-up (here commonly termed restenosis) following endovascular treatment, which mostly consisted of balloon angioplasty without insertion of a stent, compared with 10.5% of patients in the endarterectomy group.[150] Ultrasound follow-up in more recent trials comparing primary carotid stenting showed lower long-term rates of restenosis. The Stent-protected Angioplasty versus Carotid Endarterectomy in symptomatic patients trial (SPACE) trial also reported higher rates of severe restenosis 2 years after treatment in the stenting group (10.7%) than in the endarterectomy group (4.6%).[151] In contrast, there was no significant difference in severe restenosis between stenting and endarterectomy in the Endarterectomy vs Stenting in Patients with Symptomatic Severe Carotid Stenosis trial (EVA-3S) at 3 years (3.3% vs 2.8%),[152] in the Carotid Revascularization Endarterectomy vs Stenting Trial (CREST) at 2 years (6% vs 6.3%),[153] nor in the International Carotid Stenting Study (ICSS) 5 years after randomization (11.8% vs 8.6%),[154] respectively. It should be noted that ultrasound might overestimate the true rate of restenosis after stenting if standard velocity criteria are used, owing to changes in elasticity of the stented artery.[155]

PATHOPHYSIOLOGY OF CAROTID ARTERY ISCHEMIA

The clinical syndromes of TIA and stroke that occur from disease involving the carotid artery itself result from three basic mechanisms: (1) embolism of thrombosis formed on a proximal lesion in the carotid artery, usually atheromatous, to a distal intracranial artery receiving blood from the ICA; (2) propagation of thrombus from an occluded ICA into its intracranial branches; and (3) hemodynamic ischemia, i.e., a reduction in perfusion pressure below the threshold for ischemia due to inadequate collateral pathways distal to a hemodynamically significant stenosis or occlusion of the ICA. A combination of mechanisms may be operative in the same patient.[156,157]

Collateral Pathways

When the ICA is unable to supply its usual intracranial territory via its direct anterograde route, six major potential sources of collateral flow may develop, individually or in combination (Fig. 22-10).[158–160] The extent of such collateral pathways mirrors the severity of the carotid stenosis for which they are intended to compensate, at least in patients who have presented with only TIA or minor stroke.[161]

Extracranial Pathways

Internal Carotid–Ophthalmic. The most readily recognized *extracranial* source is an anastomosis *via the external carotid artery (ECA) through the orbit.* Anterograde blood flow up the ECA via its facial branches to the orbit provides a ready link through the floor and roof of the orbit to the ophthalmic branch of the intracranial ICA. When blood flow is available in sufficient force, the direction of the ophthalmic artery flow can reverse, which provides a path to the siphon and thence, now anterograde, to the ipsilateral circle of Willis. These specific paths of anastomoses occur mainly between the maxillary branch of the ECA and the ophthalmic artery in the floor of the orbit. Smaller anastomoses occur over the roof of the orbit between the facial and frontal branches of the ECA and the supratrochlear and supraorbital branches of the ophthalmic artery. Collateral flow to the ophthalmic artery may come from meningeal branches of the ECA; rarely, the ophthalmic artery is not a branch of the ICA, and instead receives its entire flow from the meningeal artery, which is a linkage that offers little intracranial supply to the circle of Willis.

Intracranial Pathways

The most important source of collateral circulation for a hemisphere comes from the *contralateral ICA via the circle of Willis.* In this case, blood flows anterograde up the opposite ICA and then across the circle of Willis via the anterior communicating artery, from which it has several potential paths to the affected hemisphere. The most useful is straight across the affected side of the circle directly into the middle cerebral artery (MCA). In addition, or, barring the patency of the path to the MCA, collateral flow may ascend along the cortical branches of the anterior cerebral artery (ACA), lacking direct supply from its own ICA, and then over the hemisphere and through the pial collaterals linking the ACA to the MCA in the cortical borderzone between their territories, filling these MCA branches retrogradely.

In like fashion, collateral supply around the circle can also come from the vertebrobasilar circulation via either or both posterior cerebral arteries. This source can be sufficient to supply both carotid territories in patients with severe bilateral carotid disease.

The circle of Willis, an arterial polygon, has many minor variations in its degree of completeness; in the most severe cases it has no links to the threatened ICA territory via either the contralateral ACA or ipsilateral PCA. In such instances the territory of the affected ICA can be isolated; this is especially so if its ipsilateral ACA is not linked to the opposite side via the circle of Willis and its ipsilateral PCA is also supplied by the ICA (so-called fetal PCA, representing persistence of the early embryologic links between these two vessels). In extreme cases, the ACA of the affected territory may have an azygous

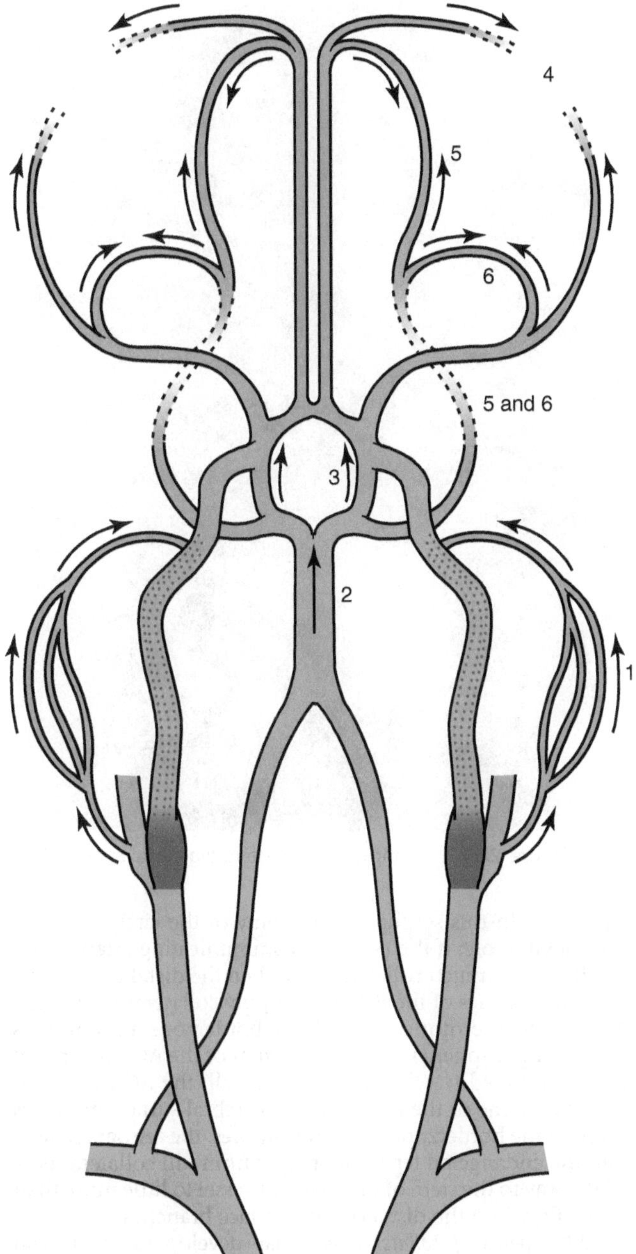

Figure 22-10. Sources of collateral flow for occlusion of the internal carotid territory (purple, site of occlusion; stippled, distal flow failure) showing external carotid collateral to the ophthalmic (1) and intracranial collaterals via the basilar (2) through the posterior communicating arteries (3), the borderzone vessels linking the distal branches of the anterior-middle cerebral arteries (4) and posterior cerebral to anterior (5) and middle cerebral arteries (6). *(From Gautier JC, Mohr JP: Ischemic stroke. In Mohr JP, Gautier JC, editors:* Guide to clinical neurology, *New York, 1995, Churchill Livingstone, p 543.)*

supply to both ACA territories, adding a portion of the fourth contralateral ACA territory to the areas at risk.

Rarely, the flow into the ICA territory from the basilar artery is by way of a persisting trigeminal artery, which usually reaches the ICA near the base of the skull (Fig. 22-11).

Borderzone Collaterals. Flow retrograde from cerebral arteries *through the borderzones over the brain surface* may spare some or all of the cortical surface branches of the endangered arterial

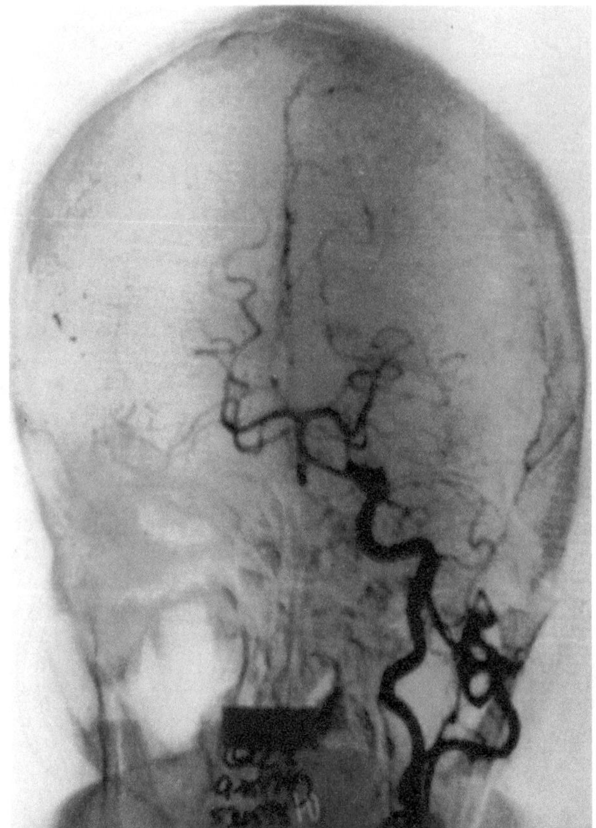

Figure 22-11. Example of a persistent trigeminal artery.

territories. In this setting, the anatomy of the circle of Willis plays a vital role: if the posterior communicating artery is too small to carry much collateral flow, then the distal ends of the cortical branches of the PCA may supply collateral flow to the ACA or MCA territories through the borderzone anastomoses over the hemisphere surface. If the stem of the ACA ipsilateral to the occluded ICA is likewise too small, the ACA may collateralize some or the entire middle cerebral surface branches through the borderzone. In such instances, the retrograde flow into the endangered territories ranges from full collateral flow all the way to the stem of the recipient vessel to little more than feeble flow into the distal cortical surface branches.

Other paths of collateral flow may develop under special circumstances, usually in patients with childhood occlusive arteriopathy, such as moyamoya disease. It would be exceptional to see these rarer routes after the onset of carotid disease in adult life. Thus, cerebral surface vessels may anastomose with an extracranial arterial source via meningeal arteries penetrating the dura or via a craniotomy site and extremely rare instances have been described in which the deep penetrating arteries (the lenticulostriate arteries) have linked through the deep white-matter borderzones to the cerebral convexity resulting in reversed flow in the cortical penetrating vessels.

It has long been obvious that the mere angiographic demonstration of collateral flow bears little relationship to its physiologic effect. Using PET measurements (CBF, blood volume, and oxygen extraction fraction) Powers et al.[162] found that neither the percent stenosis nor the residual lumen diameter of the extracranial ICA was a reliable predictor of the hemodynamic state of the cerebral circulation in patients. Hemodynamic insufficiency of the hemisphere correlated best with angiographic patterns of meningeal and ophthalmic arterial collateral paths. Similarly, transcranial Doppler (TCD) ultrasonography has shown that ophthalmic collateral flow is an insufficient source of supply to the brain and that its presence indicates that the more common sources of collateral flow are unavailable or incompetent. Prominent ophthalmic collateral flow is usually a poor prognostic sign, not a favorable one.[163,164]

Mechanisms of Ischemic Stroke and Transient Ischemic Attack

The challenges in the diagnosis and management of carotid artery disease lie mainly in (1) identifying the mechanism of symptoms at work in a given case, (2) confirming the nature and severity of associated carotid disease, (3) predicting the likely rate of future events, and (4) deciding whether the patient would benefit from revascularization. The key to answering these questions, as in most medical conditions, is a careful history of the symptoms, focusing on the precipitants and timing of the events, combined with appropriate investigations. It is important to recognize that, although a CT scan may identify larger cerebral infarcts and duplex ultrasound detect significant carotid stenosis, a proper understanding of the consequences of the carotid stenosis and likely mechanisms of symptoms, requires brain MRI and detailed vascular imaging of both the extracranial cervical vessels and the intracranial circulation with MRA or CTA and sometimes catheter angiography. Determining the nature of the stenosis may require cross-sectional imaging of the vessel lumen and wall, e.g., to identify atheromatous plaque or a mural hematoma or free intimal flap in carotid dissection.

Previous editions of this chapter to which the interested reader is referred, provide an interesting perspective on the history of the early controversies surrounding the mechanisms by which disease of the carotid artery might be associated with clinical manifestations of transient symptoms and stroke. In the first half of the last century, TIAs and even stroke were often attributed to spasm, although there were sporadic reports of carotid occlusion and thrombosis associated with stroke. C. Miller Fisher is credited with drawing attention to the association between carotid disease and TIAs, including transient monocular blindness, as well as stroke, during the 1950s.[165] However, at the time much of the thinking about carotid disease concentrated on carotid occlusion and a presumed hemodynamic origin for symptoms or the continued assumption that occlusion in some way precipitated intracranial spasm. Embolism was thought to be only an occasional cause of stroke, and was thought unlikely to explain TIAs. Nowadays, it is generally accepted that embolism is the major cause of both TIA and stroke in patients with *carotid stenosis*. Much of the evidence indicating the importance of plaque rupture, local thrombosis, and embolism as the main mechanism of stroke in association with carotid stenosis is reviewed above, and includes the direct visualization of embolization in association with recent stroke and TIAs using TCD. Direct visualization of distal artery occlusion at the time of carotid artery stenting associated with typical symptoms of stroke or TIA provided additional "proof of concept" concerning the mechanism of embolization from plaque rupture. In the current age of mechanical thrombectomy as a treatment for acute stroke, the re-emergence of catheter-based angiography in the first few hours after onset of stroke (which was often avoided for fear of making the patient worse until intra-arterial treatments for stroke became practical) frequently demonstrates a combination of carotid stenosis or acute occlusion and more distal arterial occlusion consistent with embolism as the main mechanism of stroke.[166,167] However, there still remains a proportion of cases where a hemodynamic origin of symptoms is likely and many more where it is likely that hemodynamic impairment of flow contributes to infarction.

Although most cases of carotid territory ischemia are broadly attributed to embolism from atherosclerosis, a variety of embolic material from the atheromatous plaque may be responsible. Histology of emboli extracted from an intracranial artery during mechanical thrombectomy for acute stroke has shown varying proportions of platelets and fibrin strands with intervening masses of erythrocytes.[168] Emboli arising from atherosclerosis appear less likely to have clots incorporating a large number of white cells than cardiogenic sources.[169] Cholesterol crystals or other components of the atheromatous plaque appear to be rare components of emboli causing stroke, although during carotid stenting the embolic material caught by distal protection filters during stent deployment includes cholesterol clefts and foam cells, as well as thrombi.[170] Rarely, we have seen cases of symptomatic carotid stenosis in which an acutely occluded segment of an intracranial artery has such high attenuation on CT that calcific material must be responsible. It is less easy to demonstrate that emboli are responsible for TIAs, although the fact that many TIAs are associated with small cortical lesions on diffusion-weighted MRI that are not located in the borderzones lends support to this likely mechanism. Acute infarction on diffusion-weighted MRI (DWI) is more likely to be seen in patients with TIA and minor stroke whose carotid plaque shows one or more features of unstable plaque, including intraplaque hemorrhage, surface rupture, and luminal thrombosis.[171] It is probable that TIAs from carotid disease result in most cases from small thrombo-emboli that lyse rapidly because of their small size or composition.

Fisher[172] and, independently, Ross Russell[173] observed material passing through the retinal circulation during attacks of transient monocular blindness, documenting that migrating particles could be associated with transient symptoms, but the nature of the material was uncertain. Certainly, the size of embolic material sufficient to cause retinal ischemia (0 to 100 microns) is likely to be much smaller than those causing hemisphere symptoms since, such a size of embolus would be too small to affect or block any but the tiny pial surface branches in the hemisphere. Either this very small size or perhaps the different composition of emboli causing transient monocular blindness (TMB) might account for the fact that TMB is much less likely to be followed by stroke than hemisphere TIA.[71] The observation of refractile material in the walls of retinal arteries (Hollenhorst plaques[174]) has been attributed to cholesterol emboli lodging in the walls of arteries, although histological proof of the association with emboli is scanty and many cases do not have a history of associated TMB or retinal infarction.[175,176]

The spectrum of the clinical effects of *carotid artery occlusion* is wide, ranging from no symptoms to disastrous outcomes.[177] Only about one in ten patients with documented carotid artery occlusion have associated clinical symptoms, demonstrating the adequacy of collateral supply in the majority of individuals. The features compatible with a *hemodynamic* origin for symptoms in carotid occlusion are discussed below. Other mechanisms include *anterograde propagation of carotid thrombosis,* which is the easiest of the effects of carotid artery occlusion to understand, although it is quite uncommon. Extension distally from the siphon to and beyond the circle of Willis involving the stems of the ACA and MCA usually creates devastating cerebral infarction (see below).[157,178] Carotid occlusion could also lead to *embolization,* via ECA collaterals, arising from the *stump of the ICA* that remains emanating from the bifurcation of the CCA at the bottom end of the thrombus.

Hemodynamic ischemia or *perfusion failure with distal insufficiency* as it was referred to in previous editions is a major mechanism that may account for or contribute to symptoms in patients with severe carotid stenosis or occlusion. Although characteristic precipitants and features of transient ischemic attacks may suggest a hemodynamic mechanism, as described in the next section, the distribution of acute infarction on brain imaging provides the strongest evidence for a hemodynamic mechanism of underlying symptoms associated with carotid insufficiency. Characteristically, infarction associated with hemodynamic mechanisms is located in the borderzones of the arterial territory of the middle cerebral artery, the main destination for blood flowing up the carotid artery.[179] This distribution reflects decreased vascular perfusion in those areas of the brain parenchyma located at the greatest distance from the site of severe stenosis or occlusion. In addition to impaired perfusion from low arterial pressure, stagnation thrombus has been observed in vessels at these distant sites,[180] and infarction follows. For the carotid system, if one assumes that collateral flow is available from the posterior cerebral for the lateral occipital and superior parietal areas, the borderzone regions at risk include the most distal segments of the cortical branches of the ACA and MCA, in particular the superior frontal and paracentral lobules (the superficial anterior borderzone).[181] The posterior superficial borderzone between the cortical branches of the MCA and the PCA are also at risk in some patients. However, it is difficult to be certain that a superficial infarct in the borderzone has not been caused by embolism to an MCA branch, especially given the variability in anatomical and angiographic studies of the portion of the hemisphere supplied by the MCA. However, infarction in the deep borderzone located in the centrum semiovale between the territories supplied by the arterioles penetrating through the cortex to the underlying white matter from the MCA and the ACA or PCA is much more specific for hemodynamic distal field ischemia. This may be associated with contiguous superficial borderzone infarcts, but may also occur as an isolated finding on imaging. In the latter case the infarction is often distributed in a linear fashion along the deep borderzone like a string of beads or rosary. This finding, when unilateral is virtually diagnostic of severe ipsilateral carotid stenosis or occlusion to the extent that in the odd strictly unilateral case when the carotid is found only to have mild or moderate plaque, it is tempting to speculate that the carotid was temporarily occluded by thrombus that has lysed spontaneously. Typical examples of superficial and deep borderzone infarction are shown in Fig. 22-12.

Perfusion imaging studies, ranging from CT[182,183] – including xenon CT – to positron emission tomography (PET) and MRI (Fig. 22-12C), have confirmed the correlation of a distal field borderzone topography with high-grade carotid stenosis or occlusion.[179,184–192] Quantitative TCD ultrasonography has also been used to assess perfusion failure in carotid occlusive disease. Low reactivity of middle cerebral blood vessels in a setting of hypercapnia, a sign of fully dilated collateral vessels, has been documented by a number of groups to have a significant relationship ($P = 0.04$) to high-grade carotid stenosis[193–195] and is also associated with an increased risk of future TIA or stroke.[196]

Although hemodynamic ischemia and embolism have been considered completely separate mechanisms, it has been suggested that both mechanisms operate to produce infarction, particularly in the deep borderzones, in patients with severe carotid disease, and that impaired perfusion leads to less washout of small emboli from the borderzones.[197]

CLINICAL SYNDROMES

Ischemic Stroke from Carotid Artery Disease

Ocular Infarction

In natural history studies of transient monocular blindness (TMB, also known as amaurosis fugax),[198] retinal infarction

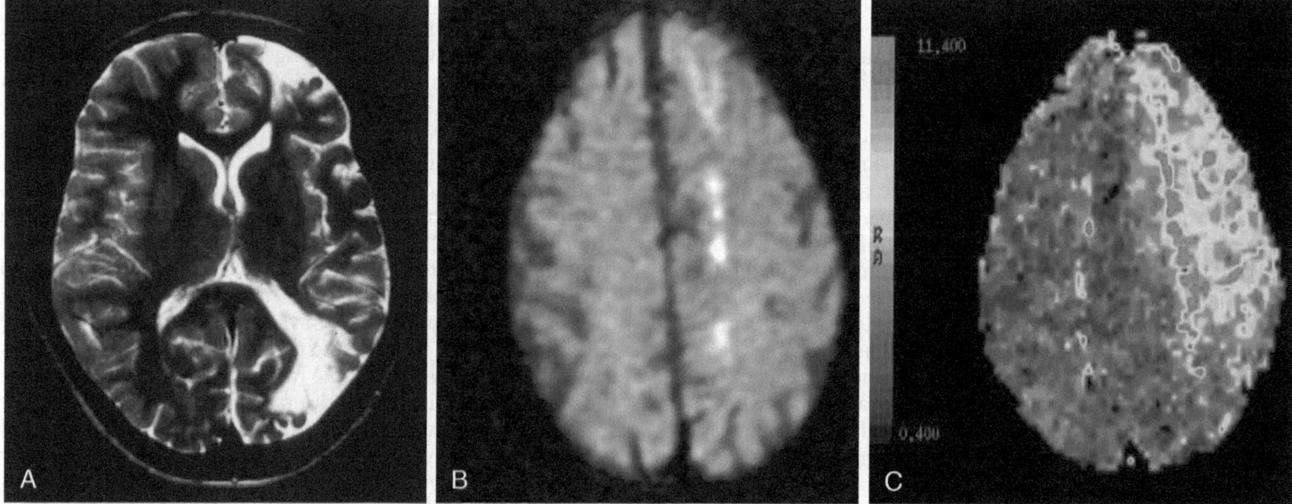

Figure 22-12. MR imaging showing (A) anterior and posterior superficial borderzone infarction in the left hemisphere shown on a T2 sequence, (B) deep borderzone infarction in the left hemisphere of a different patient shown as bright signal on diffusion-weighted imaging in a linear string-of-beads (rosary) pattern, and (C) perfusion MRI time to peak images showing impaired perfusion throughout most of the left middle cerebral artery territory (yellow and red colors) in a patient with severe ipsilateral carotid stenosis. The maximum impairment of flow is within the deep borderzone (red color). This image is from the same patient and at the same level as shown in (B) and demonstrates the concordance between hemodynamic impairment and borderzone infarction. *(Reproduced with permission from M.M. Brown.)*

occurs in only a small percentage of patients monitored over the long term. The presumed mechanism is embolic occlusion of either a retinal branch or the central retinal artery. Several large series of patients with central retinal artery occlusion who underwent cerebral angiography have documented ipsilateral carotid artery disease (i.e., ulcerative non-stenotic, stenotic without ulceration or irregularity, or occlusive) consistent with an embolic source in 50–70% of cases.[199,200] Carotid territory TIAs, including TMB, had occurred in many patients before central retinal artery occlusion.

Ischemic Optic Neuropathy and Ischemic Retinopathy

This disorder is widely acknowledged to be related to ischemia at the optic nerve head[201] and has a wide range of causes, including giant-cell arteritis, carotid dissection, Takayasu's disease, and carotid cavernous fistula, and many sources of embolism. The characteristic ocular abnormalities are severely reduced visual acuity with reduced pupillary reaction to light and papilloedema on fundoscopy. Significant visual loss sometimes ending in blindness with optic atrophy makes this a serious condition. Ischemic optic neuropathy needs to be distinguished from an ischemic retinopathy in which there is pupillary dilatation with light reaction: (1) neovascularization of the iris (rubeosis iridis), (2) elevated intraocular pressure with secondary glaucoma, and (3) proliferative retinopathy (Fig. 22-13) with microaneurysms, scattered flame-shaped hemorrhages, and prominent venous stasis, often secondary to diabetes or venous occlusion.[202-206] Carotid stenosis is not a common cause of these ophthalmological syndromes, affecting only 5% of cases in one early series[202] and 1.6% in a more recent series.[207] In these minority of cases severe carotid stenosis and occlusion cause a low-flow ischemic retinopathy with similar (but unilateral) fundal features to other causes of ischemic retinopathy.

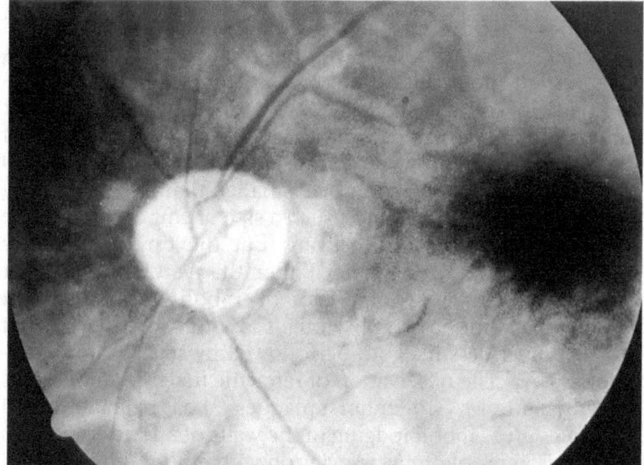

Figure 22-13. Chronic ischemic retinopathy with attenuated retinal vessels and a pale disc.

The Anterior Choroidal Artery

The anterior choroidal artery (AChA) is a branch of the intracranial internal carotid, arising distal to the ophthalmic artery but below the circle of Willis. Its size compares with that of cerebral surface artery branches, but its location makes it an uncommon site of occlusion that causes stroke. The AChA supplies the posterior two-thirds of the posterior limb of the internal capsule, the retrolenticular fibers posterior to the internal capsule, the medial aspect of the pallidum, the uncus, the posterior portion of the optic tract, the tail of the caudate nucleus, the lateral choroid plexus, the posterior and superficial areas of the thalamus, the anterior portion of the cerebral peduncle, and the lateral geniculate body.[208-214] AChA infarction may arise from embolism, or local microatheroma.

There is increasing awareness of the variety of syndromes from infarction in the AChA vascular territory, although for decades it was rarely considered among carotid artery syndromes.

Helgason et al. postulated a hemihypesthetic–ataxic syndrome,[215,216] drawing on the CT maps created by Damasio,[217] which prompted challenges from other authors. Based on these considerations, some reports argued such infarcts should be considered as the small, deep types labeled as *lacunes.*[218]

Ambiguities in the location of the regions of supply prompted challenges from others concerned that infarcts long inferred to affect the lateral lenticulostriates – MCA origin – might be commingled with and considered due to occlusion of the AChA.[219] MRI of the infarct unambiguously, angiographically documented that AChA infarction affects the uncus, amygdaloid nucleus, genu and posterior limb of the internal capsule, globus pallidus, lateral geniculate body, and tail of the caudate nucleus.[220,221] Others consider that they have demonstrated the AChA as a cause of infarction affecting the posterior leg of the internal capsule and extending upward into the paraventricular corona.[222] The matter continues to attract interest and was discussed in detail as separate chapters in prior editions of this book.[223,224] Considering the spectrum of sites affected by the AChA, it is perhaps no surprise that a wide range of syndromes have been attributed to occlusion along its course. These include pure motor stroke,[215] pure sensory stroke, sensorimotor stroke,[225] pseudobulbar state,[226] mutism,[227] possibly a form of neglect,[228] and remarkable visual field disturbances including homonymous hemianopia,[229] homonymous scotoma,[230] and quadrantic defects and sectoranopia.[231]

Cerebral Infarction

On clinical grounds of severity and topography of cerebral infarction, there appears to be no essential difference between the type and severity of the embolic syndromes associated with carotid and cardiac sources.[157,182] The clinical details of these stroke syndromes are discussed in the chapters on ACA and MCA disease (see Chapter 23 and 24). Carotid disease is also a rare cause of posterior cerebral artery occlusion in the small percentage of individuals in whom the posterior cerebral artery is supplied only by a dominant posterior communicating branch of the ipsilateral internal carotid artery.

In some patients, the timing of the onset of symptoms may point to ICA thrombus propagation rather than cardiac embolism as a likely mechanism, for example if there is gradual progression of ischemic hemispheric symptoms over more than a few hours. However, such a symptom course can also arise from hemodynamic failure of collaterals associated with more distal MCA occlusion or the development of malignant MCA edema.

The clinical syndromes from cerebral infarction from hemodynamic ischemia with distal field insufficiency are characterized by a prominent visual field defect, aphasia, or hemi-inattention features (from dominant or non-dominant hemisphere involvement, respectively), and variable degrees of contralateral sensorimotor deficit. Based on now somewhat outmoded classic clinicopathologic correlations of the homunculus,[232] the latter should affect the proximal more than the distal segments of the upper limb, reflecting the location of the infarct along the upper portions of the frontal–parietal convexity borderzone.[233] Although the preceding constellation of symptoms is commonly found (bilaterally) in cases of cardiac arrest and hypotension with resulting bilateral distal field infarction, its unilateral occurrence from ICA atherothrombosis was not documented by CT scanning until the mid-1980s.[181] Of diagnostic importance is that these hemodynamic syndromes are generally *less severe* than those attributed to embolism on account of their location in the borderzones and feature a higher frequency of premonitory TIAs.[157]

Dementia and Cognitive Impairment

It is generally accepted that dementia risk is increased in patients with arteriosclerosis in general[234] and, in a setting of stroke from occult repeated emboli,[235] showing high convexity, "distal field" infarction with high-grade carotid stenosis[236–238] or extracranial carotid disease and MRI evidence of brain infarction (this last from the Framingham Study).[239] However, a recent epidemiological study in Japan has suggested that while carotid stenosis was associated with an increased incidence of subsequent dementia, the association disappeared after correction for age and sex.[240] Whether there is a nonspecific effect of reduction in cerebral perfusion pressure in the absence of infarction causing cognitive impairment is open to doubt. Individual case reports of patients recovering cognitive function after revascularization continue to appear, but overall the conclusion from a review of 32 studies reporting tests of cognitive function before and after carotid revascularization is that it has no significant overall early benefit to cognitive function.[241] Any late benefit in preventing dementia, which is yet to be shown, can be expected to result only from the prevention of infarction.

TRANSIENT ISCHEMIC ATTACKS

TIAs are defined as a focal, ischemic neurologic deficit of brief duration. For carotid territory TIAs in a setting of high-grade stenosis, their duration is typically 5–15 minutes.[242,243] There is ample evidence to support TIA as a strong marker of stroke risk, mechanism, and source, namely – albeit not exclusively – embolism from the carotid arteries. For carotid stroke, the prognostic significance of TIA indicating stroke risk is clearly evident from the carotid surgery trials showing an almost tenfold higher risk of stroke in patients presenting with TIA and carotid stenosis as compared with cases with asymptomatic arterial narrowing.[47,59] Further, recurrent TIAs with similar or identical clinical presentation clearly hint of an arterial obstruction, most frequently of the carotids. Most TIAs caused by carotid artery obstruction arise from embolism; however, hemodynamic failure presenting as brief spells of focal neurologic symptoms are well-known, and TIAs are not exclusively related to the carotid arteries. Cardiac embolism as well as lacunar syndromes may also present as abrupt-onset focal cerebral deficits lasting less than 24 hours. Last, but not least, other disease entities may present as brief spells of circumscribed cerebral dysfunction, the most frequent of which are migrainous aura and partial seizure.

The typical carotid territory TIAs are brief, typically lasting only some 7–10 minutes, as stated by patients in retrospective interviews. In early reports, the prognosis for subsequent stroke appeared to be the same regardless of whether the spell is brief or long,[244,245] but more recent studies suggested that spells longer than 60 minutes in duration have a higher risk of subsequent stroke without taking into account the presence of carotid disease.[246] Nevertheless, among all causes of TIA, the presence of carotid stenosis is associated with a significant increase in early risk of recurrence, especially in the first 48 hours.[247] More important, evidence has been demonstrated in the literature of brain infarction on DWI in patients whose syndromes lasted longer than an hour,[248] as well as disturbed MR spectroscopy findings in the ipsilateral hemisphere,[249] giving rise to calls for a new definition of TIA. A committee of the American Heart Association and other organizations concluded that a proposed 1-hour definition for TIA was not helpful because this did not clearly demarcate events with and without tissue infarction.[250] Instead, the following revised definition of TIA was endorsed: "a transient episode of neurological dysfunction caused by focal brain, spinal cord, or retinal ischemia, without acute infarction." A subsequent very large study of nearly 2,000 patients has confirmed that, although about 11% of all TIAs were associated with cerebral infarction on MRI, the presence of infarction did not correlate with duration of symptoms of 1 hour or longer.[251] Although the finding of infarction on MRI in a patient with TIA is indicative of an increased risk of early stroke recurrence, the finding of carotid stenosis (or an intracranial occlusion) on CTA in an acute stroke is equally predictive of increased early risk.[252]

The importance of carotid TIAs is highlighted when they are viewed from the perspective of carotid stroke. Patients who have a carotid stroke from extracranial carotid artery occlusive disease have a known prior TIA incidence of 50–75%.[253-256] This situation contrasts sharply with the low incidence of TIAs (approximately 10%) associated with all types of stroke considered as a group and reinforces the strong relationship between these transient events and underlying atherothrombotic occlusive disease. The available data, both prospective and retrospective, indicate that TIAs may be impressive warnings of stroke in some patients, and their recognition provides the opportunity for therapeutic intervention.

The old argument that the outlook for TIA cases was too benign for endarterectomy to influence outcome favorably[21,257-259] was settled by the dramatic results of the studies for symptomatic patients: both the NASCET and ECST, which both showed a clear advantage of surgery over medical (aspirin) therapy in patients with TIA, especially hemisphere TIA. The most striking of the positive findings were in those patients whose stenosis exceeded 70%. Over a period of 18 months in NASCET, of patients who were symptomatic with TIAs and who were found to have stenosis of 70–90%, 7% of the 300 who underwent surgery had a stroke or died, mostly in the peri-operative period, whereas 24% of the 295 undergoing aspirin therapy had a stroke or died. This difference favoring surgery was highly significant ($P < 0.001$).[260] The risk of stroke was higher in patients with brain imaging showing "leukoaraiosis" than in those without such findings.[256] The outcomes and best management plans for those whose stenosis was in the 30–70% range were less striking in both trials: only modest benefit was seen with moderate stenosis (50–69%) with surgery, minimal benefits were seen with mild stenosis (30–49%), while harm accrued from surgery in patients with less than 30% stenosis.[47] More recent large cohort studies of management for TIA in a setting of intervention-eligible carotid stenosis support the long-standing bias toward intervention to avoid infarction.[261]

Transient Monocular Blindness

TMB, also known as amaurosis fugax, has been recognized as an important manifestation of carotid artery disease since early reports.[262] TMB may be considered a brief monocular visual obscuration described by patients as a fog, blur, cloud, mist, and so forth. A shade or curtain effect occurs in only a minority of cases, approximately 15–20%, and is no more predictive of carotid artery disease than other variations of monocular visual loss.[263] The duration of visual impairment is brief, usually less than 15 minutes and rarely exceeding 30 minutes, and most patients are affected for only 1–5 minutes.[173,264-267]

The symptom of hemodynamic TMB secondary to low retinal perfusion is characteristically described by the patient as a "white out" or as a checkerboard distortion of vision like looking through frosted glass, in contrast to embolic TMB where the visual loss is described as blackness or darkness. The symptoms may be precipitated by going from a dark room into bright sunlight or even by looking at a bright light inside.[268,269] In such cases, bright light has been shown to precipitate impairment of visual-evoked responses.[270] The mechanism is thought to involve failure of the ischemic retina to regenerate rhodopsin at the usual rate. In such cases, fundal examination may show poor perfusion pressure in the

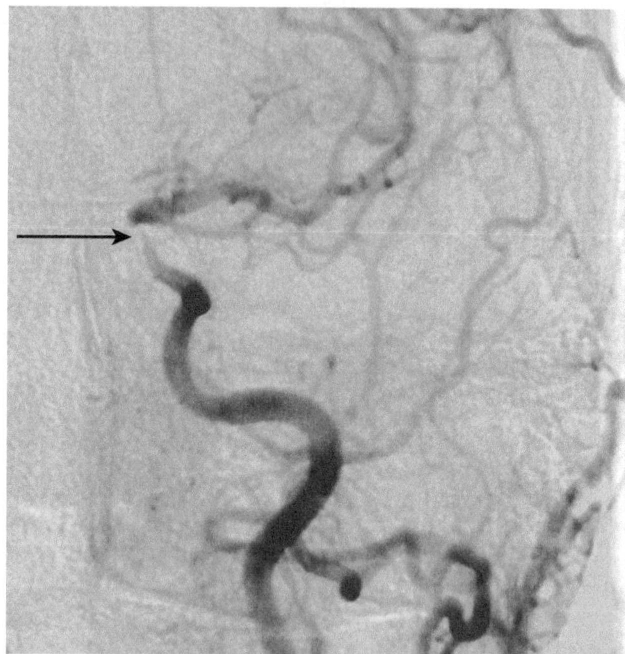

Figure 22-14. Digital subtraction angiogram showing severe distal internal carotid artery stenosis (arrow). This patient also had a moderate stenosis at the carotid bifurcation and presented with a low-pressure ischemic retinopathy. The carotid artery subsequently occluded and the patient became blind in that eye. *(Reproduced with permission from M.M. Brown.)*

retinal arterioles, which can be seen to pulsate and collapse in diastole in response to a slight pressure on the eyeball. In severe cases, fundoscopy may also show the features of a low-pressure ischemic retinopathy, with dilated veins, peripheral microaneurysms, and blot hemorrhages.[271] This is usually associated with very severe stenoses of the carotid bifurcation and/or distal internal carotid artery (Fig. 22-14).

Flashing lights, scintillations, colors, and fortification spectra rarely occur as TIA manifestations and usually signify a migrainous event.[267] However, the presence of visual phenomena during TMB in patients with greater than 75% stenosis has been recorded by Goodwin et al.,[272] which makes differentiation from retinal migraine difficult on clinical grounds alone in some cases.

Compared with hemisphere TIAs (see below), TMB secondary to carotid stenosis has a less malevolent prognosis for stroke; for the 198 cases of TMB in the non-surgical treatment arm of the NASCET, the 3-year ipsilateral stroke rate was half that for the 417 medically treated cases of hemisphere TIA (adjusted hazard ratio, 0.53; 95% CI, 0.30 to 0.94).[273] Similar findings were reported in ECST.[274]

Hemisphere Transient Ischemic Attacks

The symptoms reported for TIAs involving the carotid territory within the ipsilateral hemisphere generally match those found in stroke involving these territories, except for their briefer duration. The commonest symptoms are weakness or numbness (or both) of part or all of the side of the body contralateral to the affected hemisphere, with the presence or absence of a speech disturbance, depending on whether the dominant hemisphere is affected.[275-278]

The most common constellation of symptoms involves motor and sensory dysfunction of the contralateral limbs, followed by pure motor dysfunction, pure sensory dysfunction, and lastly, isolated dysphasia.[253] The contralateral distal arm and hand are the body parts that most consistently suffer in the attack, and their symptoms may be the only manifestation. The deficit presumably reflects ischemia to a portion of the motor cortex in the distal field of the carotid circulation.

Like the occurrences of TMB, hemisphere TIAs are typically brief in duration (<15 minutes, with most lasting for 1 to 10 minutes). In one study, patients with hemisphere TIAs lasting for 1 hour or more tended to have wide-open carotid arteries with evidence of intracranial branch occlusion, which suggests that the hemisphere TIAs reflected a short-lived cerebral embolus.[253] Patients may have one or many hemisphere TIAs before coming to medical attention; a few have 20 or more.[253] Most patients have hemisphere TIAs over several weeks to a few months, but some may have a history spanning months to a year or, rarely, longer.

It may be difficult to distinguish the symptoms of *hemodynamic hemisphere TIA* from embolic TIA in the absence of imaging showing infarction in a borderzone territory or measurements of cerebrovascular reactivity. However, an association with very severe internal carotid artery stenosis (>95%) or occlusion should lead to consideration of hemodynamic mechanisms, while symptoms precipitated by documented hypotension or precipitants likely to cause peripheral or core vasodilatation, e.g., orthostasis, a hot bath, or a large meal are likely to be hemodynamic in origin. One distinctive if uncommon form of hemodynamic hemisphere TIA involves *limb shaking*.[276,279-284] Typically associated with severe carotid stenosis or occlusion, the attacks feature recurrent, involuntary, irregular, wavering movements of the contralateral arm or leg. Rarely, in cases of severe bilateral carotid disease, the shaking occurs on both sides of the body simultaneously. The movements are described as shaking, trembling, twitching, flapping, or wavering. Limb shaking may be the presenting symptom of a hemisphere TIA, making the distinction from focal epilepsy an important differential point. The demonstration of severe carotid stenosis or occlusion associated with ipsilateral impairment of cerebral blood flow or reactivity is important in confirming the diagnosis. Furthermore, hemodynamic TIAs do not respond to anticonvulsants. The symptoms are abolished by endarterectomy.

STROKE RISK IN PATIENTS WITH CAROTID DISEASE

Symptomatic Carotid Stenosis

The bulk of evidence to estimate stroke risk under conservative management (medical therapy) of symptomatic carotid stenosis stems from the medical arms of randomized controlled trials evaluating the benefit of endarterectomy more than two decades ago. In a pooled analysis of ECST,[46] NASCET[48] and a third, smaller trial (the Veterans Affairs trial, VA309[285]) including 6092 patients and 35000 patient-years of follow-up, the cumulative risk of ipsilateral stroke in patients with recently symptomatic severe carotid stenosis (70–99% narrowing according to the NASCET method of measuring stenosis, excluding near-occlusion) randomized to continue on medical therapy alone, was approximately 26% at 5 years after randomization.[47] This risk was reduced by an absolute difference of 16% among patients randomised to undergo endarterectomy. In patients with moderate, 50–69% stenosis the 5-year risk of ipsilateral stroke was about 18% and reduced by only 4.6%.[48] Importantly, 55% of patients in the NASCET trial were randomized more than 30 days after the qualifying event (TIA or minor stroke), and in ECST this proportion was 65%. These data, therefore, do not allow estimating stroke risk in the first days after initial symptoms. In large prospective registries of patients presenting with TIA, up to 20% of those with large-artery atherosclerosis as the underlying cause had a stroke within 90 days of the TIA, the bulk of events occurring in the first 7–14 days.[286,287]

ECST recruited patients between 1981 and 1994, and NASCET between 1988 and 1996. Medical therapy in these trials mainly consisted of taking aspirin. In the NASCET trial, only 14% of patients were under lipid-lowering therapy at the time of randomization. It is reasonable to assume that with more widespread use of statins and more aggressive antiplatelet regimens, the risk of early recurrent stroke in symptomatic carotid stenosis is lower today than reported in these earlier trials and TIA cohorts. Indeed, data from a recent large TIA cohort presented at the 2014 European Stroke Conference showed 90-day stroke risk after TIA caused by larger-artery atherosclerosis to be as low as 6%.

Clinical risk modelling and imaging allow further differentiation of stroke risk in patients with symptomatic carotid stenosis. A score was developed based on variables associated with risk of ipsilateral stroke in patients with symptomatic carotid stenosis randomized to medical therapy in ECST, which included age, sex, degree of stenosis, type (retinal ischemia, transient ischemic attack, or stroke) and time since presenting event, as well as presence of irregular or ulcerated plaque surface.[274] This score accurately predicted the risk of ipsilateral stroke in an independent group of patients with symptomatic carotid stenosis who were included in the medical group of the NASCET trial, while having no effect on the risk on peri-procedural stroke in patients treated with endarterectomy[288] (Fig. 22-15).

In a systematic review and meta-analysis, the presence of microembolic signals detected during TCD monitoring increased the risk of stroke by an odds ratio of 9.6 (95%CI, 1.50–59.4) in patients with symptomatic carotid stenosis.[110]

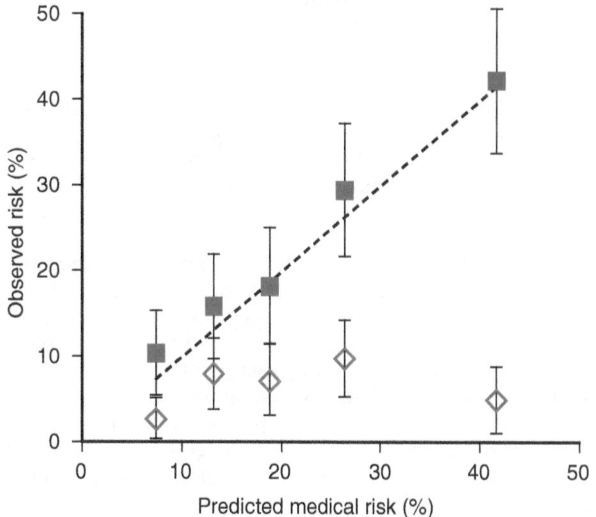

Figure 22-15. Graph showing the reliability of the model derived from the European Carotid Surgery Trial predicting the 5-year risk of ipsilateral stroke in patients with 50–99% carotid stenosis treated with medical therapy alone. The filled squares show the 5-year risk of stroke observed in the North American Symptomatic Carotid Endarterectomy Trial (NASCET) plotted against the predicted risk. The open diamonds plot the risk of stroke or death within 30 days of carotid endarterectomy observed in NASCET showing that patients with a high predicted risk of stroke when treated with medical therapy alone did not have an increased risk from surgery. *(Reprinted from Rothwell PM, Mehta Z, Howard SC, et al. Treating individuals 3: from subgroups to individuals: general principles and the example of carotid endarterectomy. Lancet 2005;365(9455):256–65, with permission from Elsevier.)*

Several studies have also reported on an increased risk of cerebrovascular events associated with intra-plaque hemorrhage visible on MRI; a meta-analysis pooling data from studies on symptomatic carotid stenosis reported the risk of the combined endpoint of TIA and stroke to be elevated by an odds ratio of 11.7 (5.2–26.5) among patients with intra-plaque hemorrhage.[96] Unfortunately, most included studies combined recurrent stroke or TIA for reasons of increasing statistical power; therefore, no reliable estimates of increase in stroke risk based on the presence of IPH can be made at present.

Asymptomatic Carotid Stenosis

Two large randomized trials, the Asymptomatic Carotid Atherosclerosis Study (ACAS), which recruited 1662 patients between 1987 and 1993, and the Asymptomatic Carotid Surgery Trial (ACST), which recruited 3120 patients between 1993 and 2003, consistently demonstrated an 11% 5-year risk of ipsilateral stroke in patients with asymptomatic carotid stenosis of 60% or higher who were assigned to initial medical management.[58,289] This risk was reduced by 6% in ACAS and 4% in ACST in patients assigned to immediate endarterectomy. Of note, fewer than 10% of patients in ACST were on lipid-lowering therapy at the beginning of recruitment in 1993, and this proportion steadily increased to more than 80% at termination of follow-up in 2008.

In the ACSRS study, which included 1121 patients with asymptomatic carotid stenosis who were studied at baseline using ultrasound imaging of plaque echolucency between 1998 and 2002, the risk of ipsilateral stroke after a mean duration of 4 years' follow-up was 4.1% among patients with <70% carotid stenosis equivalent to the NASCET method and 6.3% among those with ≥70% stenosis.[85] Twenty-five percent of patients were on lipid-lowering therapy at baseline at the beginning of the study, and this proportion increased to 85% at the end. The 22% of patients with ≥8 mm echolucent plaque area near the lumen at baseline had 3.2–5% annual ipsilateral stroke rates, while the remainder only faced 0.4–1.4% annual risk.[87] In a separate analysis of this cohort, progression of stenosis observed in 6-monthly duplex ultrasound examinations was an independent predictor of ipsilateral stroke.[22] However, only 7% of patients with ≥70% stenosis at baseline and further progression of stenosis during follow-up had 2.6% annual ipsilateral stroke risk; in the remainder, stroke risk was lower.

ACES included 482 patients with at least 70% asymptomatic carotid stenosis between 1999 and 2007. In 77 of 467 patients with evaluable TCD recordings, microembolic signals were detected in the ipsilateral middle cerebral artery at baseline during two 1-hour recording sessions. These patients had an increased risk of ipsilateral stroke at a hazard ratio of 5.6 (95%CI, 1.6–19.3) compared with patients who did not have microembolic signals.[111] Two-year ipsilateral stroke risk was 3.6% in patients with microembolic signals and 0.7% in those without.

Data from prospective cohorts of asymptomatic patients investigated with plaque MRI show an increased risk of ipsilateral stroke or TIA by presence of intra-plaque hemorrhage at a hazard ratio of 3.5 (2.6–4.7), but as in symptomatic patients, no pooled data on stroke risk alone are available.

A meta-regression analysis of data from medical arms of randomized trials and prospective cohorts suggested that the risk of ipsilateral stroke associated with asymptomatic carotid stenosis has declined over the past 20 years and may now be only 1% or lower,[290] most likely attributable to advances in medical therapy. Indeed, under modern medical management of atherosclerosis, only a minority of patients with asymptomatic carotid disease may currently benefit from invasive revascularization. The existing literature suggests that this minority may be identified by detection of microemboli on TCD and echolucent area at the plaque surface on ultrasound. However, it is uncertain if these investigations are still capable of identifying patients at high risk of stroke under current management of atherosclerosis. Plaque imaging with MRI detects strong structural correlates of clinically manifest embolic events, but larger prospective cohort studies and pooling of individual patient data from these studies are necessary to produce reliable estimates of stroke risk and investigate if MRI adds to existing clinical risk models in predicting stroke. However, screening of the population with MRI is unlikely to be cost-effective, given the low rate of stroke associated with asymptomatic stenosis and the large number of patients that would need to be screened to detect patients at higher risk.

The changes in stroke risk in patients with symptomatic and asymptomatic carotid stenosis stress the need to reassess the benefit of endarterectomy (or stenting) in the context of modern medical therapy. Several trials addressing this issue are currently ongoing.

Carotid Artery Occlusion

The documentation of asymptomatic carotid artery occlusion by a non-invasive study or angiography is fairly common, and the literature dates back several decades.[291] A series of studies attempted to use the case-control method to estimate stroke risk, the first and still the dominant of which was that conducted by Furlan and Whisnant,[292] in which the annual rate of 2% was derived from six cases among 138 that were evaluated angiographically and studied retrospectively. Similar event rates have been reported in other series from angiography.[156,293] The cohort studies reported by Sacquegna et al.[294] consisted of a consecutive series of 100 patients with angiographically proven ICA occlusion, 68 of whom were monitored from 17 to 69 months; seven of the patients had new strokes, only three of which were in the territory of the occluded carotid artery, and four had TIAs during follow-up. The observed stroke rate was 4.7% at 1 year, 12.2% at 3 years, and 17.1% at 5 years.

Non-invasive Doppler ultrasonography provided the database for other studies. The early study by Bernstein and Norris[295] documented an annual stroke rate of 3.8%. A higher rate was reported in the original EC-IC bypass study, where the annual stroke rate was 13% per patient-year, perhaps indicating referral bias.[296] A more recent series followed 117 patients with symptomatic carotid artery occlusion initially presenting with TIA, retinal ischemia, or stroke for a median of 10 years and reported an annual ischemic stroke risk of 2.4%.[297]

Intracranial Stenosis

Evidence on stroke risk in symptomatic intracranial atherosclerosis can be gathered from medical treatment arms of randomized controlled trials. In the Warfarin–Aspirin Symptomatic Intracranial Disease trial (WASID), 569 patients with symptomatic intracranial stenosis were randomly assigned to high-dose aspirin (1300 mg daily) or treatment with warfarin to a target international normalized ratio of 2.0–3.0 between 1999 and 2003. About 60% of patients were on statin therapy at the time of randomization. The cumulative incidence of recurrent stroke was about 20% after 2 years, and did not differ significantly between treatment groups. The trial was stopped because patients in the warfarin group had a significant excess of major bleeding events, most of which occurred extracranially.[298] The Stenting and Aggressive Medical Management for

Preventing Recurrent Stroke in Intracranial Stenosis trial (SAMMPRIS), therefore, investigated whether treatment of intracranial stenosis with stents lowers the risk of recurrent stroke compared with aggressive medical therapy.[299] Four hundred and fifty-one patients with 70–99% symptomatic intracranial stenosis were enrolled between 2008 and 2011. However, this trial was also stopped early because patients treated with stents had more strokes than those receiving medication alone. This unfavorable outcome was in part attributable to a higher than expected procedural stroke risk associated with intracranial stenting (15% within 30 days of procedure), and in part to a lower than expected recurrent stroke risk in the medical therapy group (14% risk of stroke in the territory of the stenotic artery at 2 years). Medical therapy in this trial consisted of dual antiplatelet therapy with clopidogrel and aspirin for the first 3 months, rosuvastatin titrated to achieve LDL-C levels <70 mg/dl (1.81 mmol/L) and lowering of blood pressure to normal levels. In both the WASID and the SAMMPRIS trials, the intracranial section of the internal carotid artery was the index vessel in just over 20% of patients, the remainder of patients having stenoses in other intracranial arteries. The SAMMPRIS trial reported outcomes by type of affected artery; cumulative 2-year stroke rates were highest in patients with intracranial carotid disease (23% in the medical group and 29% in the stenting group). The comparison of recurrent stroke rates between the WASID study population and the medical therapy arm of SAMMPRIS thus yields further evidence that aggressive medical therapy lowers stroke risk in patients with symptomatic large-artery atherosclerosis.[300]

The complete reference list can be found on the companion Expert Consult website at www.expertconsult.inkling.com.

KEY REFERENCES

1. Flaherty ML, Kissela B, Khoury JC, et al. Carotid artery stenosis as a cause of stroke. Neuroepidemiology 2013;40:36–41.
2. de Weerd M, Greving JP, Hedblad B, et al. Prevalence of asymptomatic carotid artery stenosis in the general population: an individual participant data meta-analysis. Stroke 2010;41(6): 1294–7.
5. Markus HS, Mäkelä K-M, Bevan S, et al. Evidence HDAC9 genetic variant associated with ischemic stroke increases risk via promoting carotid atherosclerosis. Stroke 2013;44:1220–5.
6. Mathiesen EB, Joakimsen O, Bønaa KH. Prevalence of and risk factors associated with carotid artery stenosis: the Tromsø Study. Cerebrovasc Dis 2001;12:44–51.
9. Krejza J, Arkuszewski M, Kasner SE, et al. Carotid artery diameter in men and women and the relation to body and neck size. Stroke 2006;37:1103–5.
12. Dhawan SS, Avati Nanjundappa RP, Branch JR, et al. Shear stress and plaque development. Expert Rev Cardiovasc Ther 2010;8(4): 545–56.
18. Zarins CK, Giddens DP, Balasubramanian K, et al. Carotid plaques localized in regions of low flow velocity and shear stress. Circulation 1981;64:44.
19. Schneidau A, Harrison MJ, Hurst C, et al. Arterial disease risk factors and angiographic evidence of atheroma of the carotid artery. Stroke 1989;20:1466–71.
20. Javid H, Ostermiller WE Jr, Hengesh JW, et al. Natural history of carotid bifurcation atheroma. Surgery 1970;67:80–6.
22. Kakkos SK, Nicolaides AN, Charalambous I, et al. Predictors and clinical significance of progression or regression of asymptomatic carotid stenosis. J Vasc Surg 2014;59(4):956–67.
23. Jahromi AS, Clase CM, Maggisano R, et al. Progression of internal carotid artery stenosis in patients with peripheral arterial occlusive disease. J Vasc Surg 2009;50(2):292–8.
24. C Bedi US, Singh M, Singh PP, et al. Effects of statins on progression of carotid atherosclerosis as measured by carotid intimal–medial thickness: a meta-analysis of randomized controlled trials. J Cardiovasc Pharmacol Ther 2010;15:268–73.
25. Zhao XQ, Yuan C, Hatsukami TS, et al. Effects of prolonged intensive lipid-lowering therapy on the characteristics of carotid atherosclerotic plaques in vivo by MRI: a case-control study. Arterioscler Thromb Vasc Biol 2001;21(10):1623–9.
26. Yamada K, Yoshimura S, Kawasaki M, et al. Effects of atorvastatin on carotid atherosclerotic plaques: a randomized trial for quantitative tissue characterization of carotid atherosclerotic plaques with integrated backscatter ultrasound. Cerebrovasc Dis 2009;28(4):417–24.
27. Underhill HR, Yuan C, Zhao XQ, et al. Effect of rosuvastatin therapy on carotid plaque morphology and composition in moderately hypercholesterolemic patients: a high-resolution magnetic resonance imaging trial. Am Heart J 2008;155(3): 584–8.
28. Collins R, Armitage J, Parish S, et al. Effects of cholesterol-lowering with simvastatin on stroke and other major vascular events in 20536 people with cerebrovascular disease or other high-risk conditions. Lancet 2004;363(9411):757–67.
29. Sillesen H, Amarenco P, Hennerici MG, et al. Atorvastatin reduces the risk of cardiovascular events in patients with carotid atherosclerosis: a secondary analysis of the Stroke Prevention by Aggressive Reduction in Cholesterol Levels (SPARCL) trial. Stroke 2008;39(12):3297–302.
30. Ross R. Atherosclerosis–an inflammatory disease. N Engl J Med 1999;340(2):115–26.
31. Glass CK, Witztum JL. Atherosclerosis. the road ahead. Cell 2001;104(4):503–16.
32. Libby P, Ridker PM, Maseri A. Inflammation and atherosclerosis. Circulation 2002;105(9):1135–43.
43. Ratchford EV, Jin Z, Di Tullio MR, et al. Carotid bruit for detection of hemodynamically significant carotid stenosis: The Northern Manhattan Study. Neurol Res 2009;31:748–52.
44. McColgan P, Bentley P, McCarron M, et al. Evaluation of the clinical utility of a carotid bruit. QJM 2012;105:1171–7.
45. North American Symptomatic Carotid Endarterectomy Trial. Methods, patient characteristics, and progress. Stroke 1991;22(6): 711–20.
46. Randomised trial of endarterectomy for recently symptomatic carotid stenosis: final results of the MRC European Carotid Surgery Trial (ECST). Lancet 1998;351(9113):1379–87.
47. Rothwell PM, Eliasziw M, Gutnikov SA, et al. Analysis of pooled data from the randomised controlled trials of endarterectomy for symptomatic carotid stenosis. Lancet 2003;361(9352): 107–16.
48. Barnett HJ, Taylor DW, Eliasziw M, et al. Benefit of carotid endarterectomy in patients with symptomatic moderate or severe stenosis. North American Symptomatic Carotid Endarterectomy Trial Collaborators. N Engl J Med 1998;339(20): 1415–25.
49. von Reutern GM, Goertler MW, Bornstein NM, et al. Grading carotid stenosis using ultrasonic methods. Stroke 2012;43(3): 916–21.
50. Wardlaw JM, Chappell FM, Best JJ, et al. Non-invasive imaging compared with intra-arterial angiography in the diagnosis of symptomatic carotid stenosis: a meta-analysis. Lancet 2006; 367(9521):1503–12.
53. Shipley RE, Gregg DE. The effect of external constriction of a blood vessel on blood flow. Am J Physiol 1944;141:389–92.
56. Archie JP, Feldtman RW. Critical stenosis of the internal carotid artery. Surgery 1981;89:67–72.
57. Kinsella J, Tobin WO, Tierney S, et al. Increased platelet activation in early symptomatic vs. asymptomatic carotid stenosis and relationship with microembolic status: results from the Platelets and Carotid Stenosis Study. J Thromb Haemost 2013; 11:1407–16.
58. Endarterectomy for asymptomatic carotid artery stenosis. Executive Committee for the Asymptomatic Carotid Atherosclerosis Study. JAMA 1995;273(18):1421–8.
59. Halliday A, Harrison M, Hayter E, et al. 10-year stroke prevention after successful carotid endarterectomy for asymptomatic stenosis (ACST-1): a multicentre randomised trial. Lancet 2010;376(9746):1074–84.
61. Moore WS, Hall AD. Ulcerated atheroma of the carotid artery: A major cause of transient cerebral ischemia. Am J Surg 1968; 116:237–41.

64. Toole JF, Janeway R, Choi K, et al. Transient ischemic attacks due to atherosclerosis: A prospective study of 160 patients. Arch Neurol 1975;32:5–12.
71. Rothwell PM, Eliasziw M, Gutnikov SA, et al. Endarterectomy for symptomatic carotid stenosis in relation to clinical subgroups and timing of surgery. Lancet 2004;363(9413):915–24.
72. Imparato AM, Riles TS, Gorstein F. The carotid bifurcation plaque: Pathologic findings associated with cerebral ischemia. Stroke 1979;10:238–45.
74. Comerota AJ, Katz ML, White JV, et al. The preoperative diagnosis of the ulcerated carotid atheroma. J Vasc Surg 1990;11: 505–10.
75. ten Kate GL, van Dijk AC, van den Oord SCH, et al. Usefulness of contrast-enhanced ultrasound for detection of carotid plaque ulceration in patients with symptomatic carotid atherosclerosis. Am J Cardiol 2013;112:292–8.
77. Carotid artery plaque composition–relationship to clinical presentation and ultrasound B-mode imaging. European Carotid Plaque Study Group. Eur J Vasc Endovasc Surg 1995;10(1): 23–30.
79. Biasi GM, Sampaolo A, Mingazzini P, et al. Computer analysis of ultrasonic plaque echolucency in identifying high risk carotid bifurcation lesions. Eur J Vasc Endovasc Surg 1999;17(6): 476–9.
82. Polak JF, Shemanski L, O'Leary DH, et al. Hypoechoic plaque at US of the carotid artery: an independent risk factor for incident stroke in adults aged 65 years or older. Cardiovascular Health Study. Radiology 1998;208(3):649–54.
83. Mathiesen EB, Bonaa KH, Joakimsen O. Echolucent plaques are associated with high risk of ischemic cerebrovascular events in carotid stenosis: the tromso study. Circulation 2001;103(17): 2171–5.
84. Gronholdt ML, Nordestgaard BG, Schroeder TV, et al. Ultrasonic echolucent carotid plaques predict future strokes. Circulation 2001;104(1):68–73.
85. Nicolaides AN, Kakkos SK, Kyriacou E, et al. Asymptomatic internal carotid artery stenosis and cerebrovascular risk stratification. J Vasc Surg 2010;52(6):1486–96.
86. Momjian-Mayor I, Kuzmanovic I, Momjian S, et al. Accuracy of a novel risk index combining degree of stenosis of the carotid artery and plaque surface echogenicity. Stroke 2012;43(5): 1260–5.
87. Kakkos SK, Griffin MB, Nicolaides AN, et al. The size of juxtaluminal hypoechoic area in ultrasound images of asymptomatic carotid plaques predicts the occurrence of stroke. J Vasc Surg 2013;57(3):609–18.
88. Yuan C, Kerwin WS, Ferguson MS, et al. Contrast-enhanced high resolution MRI for atherosclerotic carotid artery tissue characterization. J Magn Reson Imaging 2002;15(1):62–7.
90. King-Im JM, Tang TY, Patterson A, et al. Characterisation of carotid atheroma in symptomatic and asymptomatic patients using high resolution MRI. J Neurol Neurosurg Psychiatry 2008;79(8):905–12.
91. Saam T, Hatsukami TS, Takaya N, et al. The vulnerable, or high-risk, atherosclerotic plaque: noninvasive MR imaging for characterization and assessment. Radiology 2007;244(1):64–77.
94. Sun J, Underhill HR, Hippe DS, et al. Sustained acceleration in carotid atherosclerotic plaque progression with intraplaque hemorrhage: a long-term time course study. JACC Cardiovasc Imaging 2012;5(8):798–804.
95. Hosseini AA, Kandiyil N, Macsweeney ST, et al. Carotid plaque hemorrhage on magnetic resonance imaging strongly predicts recurrent ischemia and stroke. Ann Neurol 2013;73(6):774–84.
96. Saam T, Hetterich H, Hoffmann V, et al. Meta-analysis and systematic review of the predictive value of carotid plaque hemorrhage on cerebrovascular events by magnetic resonance imaging. J Am Coll Cardiol 2013;62(12):1081–91.
97. Takaya N, Yuan C, Chu B, et al. Association between carotid plaque characteristics and subsequent ischemic cerebrovascular events: a prospective assessment with MRI–initial results. Stroke 2006;37(3):818–23.
99. Rudd JH, Narula J, Strauss HW, et al. Imaging atherosclerotic plaque inflammation by fluorodeoxyglucose with positron emission tomography: ready for prime time? J Am Coll Cardiol 2010;55(23):2527–35.
101. Marnane M, Merwick A, Sheehan OC, et al. Carotid plaque inflammation on 18F-fluorodeoxyglucose positron emission tomography predicts early stroke recurrence. Ann Neurol 2012; 71(5):709–18.
104. Gupta A, Chazen JL, Hartman M, et al. Cerebrovascular reserve and stroke risk in patients with carotid stenosis or occlusion: a systematic review and meta-analysis. Stroke 2012;43(11): 2884–91.
105. Marshall RS, Festa JR, Cheung Y-K, et al. Randomized evaluation of carotid occlusion and neurocognition (RECON) trial. Neurology 2014;82:744–51.
106. Powers WJ, Clarke WR, Grubb RL, et al. Extracranial-Intracranial bypass surgery for stroke prevention in hemodynamic cerebral ischemia: the Carotid Occlusion Surgery Study: a randomized trial. JAMA 2011;306:1983–92.
109. Markus HS, MacKinnon A. Asymptomatic embolization detected by Doppler ultrasound predicts stroke risk in symptomatic carotid artery stenosis. Stroke 2005;36(5):971–5.
110. King A, Markus HS. Doppler embolic signals in cerebrovascular disease and prediction of stroke risk: a systematic review and meta-analysis. Stroke 2009;40(12):3711–17.
111. Markus HS, King A, Shipley M, et al. Asymptomatic embolisation for prediction of stroke in the Asymptomatic Carotid Emboli Study (ACES): a prospective observational study. Lancet Neurol 2010;9(7):663–71.
115. Rincon F, Sacco RL, Kranwinkel G, et al. Incidence and risk factors of intracranial atherosclerotic stroke: the Northern Manhattan Stroke Study. Cerebrovasc Dis 2009;28(1):65–71.
117. Bos D, Portegies MLP, van der Lugt A, et al. Intracranial carotid artery atherosclerosis and the risk of stroke in whites: the Rotterdam Study. JAMA Neurol 2014;71:405–11.
121. Schuler JJ, Falnigan DP, Lim LT, et al. The effect of carotid siphon stenosis on stroke rate, death, and relief of symptoms following elective carotid endarterectomy. Surgery 1982;92:1058–67.
125. Pessin MS, Duncan GW, Davis KR, et al. Angiographic appearance of carotid occlusion in acute stroke. Stroke 1982;11: 485–90.
126. Baud JM, De Bray JM, Delanoy P, et al. Reproductibilité ultrasonore dans la caractérisation des plaques carotidiennes. J Echograph Med Ultrason 1996;17:377.
127. Mosso M, Georgiadis D, Baumgartner RW. Progressive occlusive disease of large cerebral arteries and ischemic events in a patient with essential thrombocythemia. Neurol Res 2004;26:702–3.
128. Lu CH, Yang CY, Wang CP, et al. Imaging of nasopharyngeal inflammatory pseudotumours: Differential from nasopharyngeal carcinoma. Br J Radiol 2010;83:8–16.
130. Taoka T, Iwasaki S, Nakagawa H, et al. Evaluation of arteriosclerotic changes in the intracranial carotid artery using the calcium score obtained on plain cranial computed tomography scan: Correlation with angiographic changes and clinical outcome. J Comput Assist Tomogr 2006;30:624–8.
131. Croft RJ, Ellam LD, Harrison MJG. Accuracy of carotid angiography in the assessment of atheroma of the internal carotid artery. Lancet 1980;315:997–1003.
136. Spallone A. Occlusion of the internal carotid artery by intracranial tumors. Surg Neurol 1981;15:51–7.
138. Snyderman CH, D'Amico F. Outcome of carotid artery resection for neoplastic disease: A meta-analysis. Am J Otolaryngol 1992;13:373–80.
141. Shichita T, Ogata T, Yasaka M, et al. Angiographic characteristics of radiation-induced carotid arterial stenosis. Angiology 2009;60: 276–82.
143. Levinson SA, Close MB, Ehrenfeld WK, et al. Carotid artery occlusive disease following external cervical irradiation. Arch Surg 1973;107:395–7.
144. Shin SH, Stout CL, Richardson AI, et al. Carotid angioplasty and stenting in anatomically high-risk patients: Safe and durable except for radiation-induced stenosis. J Vasc Surg 2009;50: 762–7.
149. Crawley F, Clifton A, Taylor RS, et al. Symptomatic restenosis after carotid percutaneous transluminal angioplasty. Lancet 1998;352(9129):708–9.
150. Bonati LH, Ederle J, McCabe DJ, et al. Long-term risk of carotid restenosis in patients randomly assigned to endovascular treatment or endarterectomy in the Carotid and Vertebral Artery

Transluminal Angioplasty Study (CAVATAS): long-term follow-up of a randomised trial. Lancet Neurol 2009;8(10):908–17.
151. Eckstein HH, Ringleb P, Allenberg JR, et al. Results of the Stent-Protected Angioplasty versus Carotid Endarterectomy (SPACE) study to treat symptomatic stenoses at 2 years: a multinational, prospective, randomised trial. Lancet Neurol 2008;7(10): 893–902.
152. Arquizan C, Trinquart L, Touboul PJ, et al. Restenosis is more frequent after carotid stenting than after endarterectomy: the EVA-3S study. Stroke 2011;42(4):1015–20.
153. Lal BK, Beach KW, Roubin GS, et al. Restenosis after carotid artery stenting and endarterectomy: a secondary analysis of CREST, a randomised controlled trial. Lancet Neurol 2012;11(9): 755–63.
154. Bonati LH, Dobson J, Featherstone RL, et al. Long-term outcome after stenting versus endarterectomy for treatment of symptomatic carotid stenosis in the International Carotid Stenting Study (ICSS): primary analysis of a randomised trial. Lancet 2015;385:529–38.
155. Nederkoorn PJ, Brown MM. Optimal cut-off criteria for duplex ultrasound for the diagnosis of restenosis in stented carotid arteries: review and protocol for a diagnostic study. BMC Neurol 2009;9:36.
162. Powers WJ, Press GA, Grubb RL, et al. The effect of hemodynamically significant carotid artery disease on the hemodynamic status of the cerebral circulation. Ann Intern Med 1987; 106:27–35.
165. Estol CJ. Dr C. Miller Fisher and the history of carotid artery disease. Stroke 1996;27:559–66.
168. Marder VJ, Chute DJ, Starkman S, et al. Analysis of thrombi retrieved from cerebral arteries of patients with acute ischemic stroke. Stroke 2006;37:2086–93.
169. Boeckh-Behrens T, Schubert M, Förschler A, et al. The Impact of Histological Clot Composition in Embolic Stroke. Clin Neuroradiol Sep 27, 2014;doi:10.1007/s00062-014-0347-x; [Epub ahead of print].
170. Angelini A, Reimers B, Della Barbera M, et al. Cerebral protection during carotid artery stenting: collection and histopathologic analysis of embolized debris. Stroke 2002;33:456–61.
171. Lindsay AC, Biasiolli L, Lee JM, et al. Plaque features associated with increased cerebral infarction after minor stroke and TIA: a prospective, case-control, 3-T carotid artery MR imaging study. JACC Cardiovasc Imaging 2012;5:388–96.
173. Russell RW. Observations on the retinal blood vessels in monocular blindness. Lancet 1961;278:1422–8.
177. Macchi C, Molino LR, Miniati B, et al. Collateral circulation in internal carotid artery occlusion: A study by duplex scan and magnetic resonance angiography. Minerva Cardioangiol 2002; 50(695):695–700.
179. Kumral E, Bayülkem G, Sağcan A. Mechanisms of single and multiple borderzone infarct: transcranial Doppler ultrasound/ magnetic resonance imaging correlates. Cerebrovasc Dis 2004; 17:287–95.
180. Fisher CM. Cerebral thromboangiitis obliterans. Medicine (Baltimore) 1957;36:169–209.
182. Ringelstein EB, Zeumer H, Angelou D. The pathogenesis of strokes from internal carotid artery occlusion. Stroke 1983;14: 867–75.
184. Carpenter DA, Grubb RL Jr, Powers WJ. Borderzone hemodynamics in cerebrovascular disease. Neurology 1990;40:587–92.
185. Leblanc R, Yamamoto YL, Tyler JL, et al. Borderzone ischemia. Ann Neurol 1987;22:707–13.
189. Yamauchi H, Fukuyama H, Kimura J, et al. Hemodynamics in internal carotid artery occlusion examined by positron emission tomography. Stroke 1990;21:1400–6.
190. Del Sette M, Eliasziw M, Streifler JY, et al. Internal borderzone infarction: a marker for severe stenosis in patients with symptomatic internal carotid artery disease. For the North American Symptomatic Carotid Endarterectomy (NASCET) Group. Stroke 2000;31:631–6.
191. Chaves CJ, Silver B, Schlaug G, et al. Diffusion- and perfusion-weighted MRI patterns in borderzone infarcts. Stroke 2000;31: 1090–6.
192. Lin W, Celik A, Derdeyn C, et al. Quantitative measurements of cerebral blood flow in patients with unilateral carotid artery occlusion: A PET and MR study. J Magn Reson Imaging 2001; 14:659–67.
195. Markus H, Cullinane M. Severely impaired cerebrovascular reactivity predicts stroke and TIA risk in patients with carotid artery stenosis and occlusion. Brain 2001;124:457–67.
196. Gupta A, Chazen JL, Hartman M, et al. Cerebrovascular reserve and stroke risk in patients with carotid stenosis or occlusion: a systematic review and meta-analysis. Stroke 2012;43:2884–91.
197. Caplan LR, Wong KS, Gao S, et al. Is hypoperfusion an important cause of strokes? If so, how? Cerebrovasc Dis 2006;21: 145–53.
198. Marshall J, Meadows S. The natural history of amaurosis fugax. Brain 1968;91:419–34.
202. Kearns TP, Hollenhorst RW. Venous-stasis retinopathy of occlusive disease of the carotid artery. Proc Staff Meet Mayo Clin 1963;38:304–12.
207. McCullough HK, Reinert CG, Hynan LS, et al. Ocular findings as predictors of carotid artery occlusive disease: Is carotid imaging justified? J Vasc Surg 2004;40:279–86.
215. Helgason C, Capalan LR, Goodwin J, et al. Anterior choroidal artery-territory infarction. Arch Neurol 1986;43:681–6.
216. Helgason C, Wilbur AC. Capsular hypesthetic ataxic hemiparesis. Stroke 1990;21:24–33.
222. Hupperts RMM, Lodder J, Heuts-van Raak EPM, et al. Infarcts in the anterior choroidal artery territory. Anatomical distribution, clinical syndromes, presumed pathogenesis and early outcome. Brain 1994;117:825–34.
232. Mohr JP, Foulkes MA, Polis AB, et al. Infarct topography and hemiparesis profiles with cerebral convexity infarction: The Stroke Data Bank. J Neurol Neurosurg Psychiatry 1993;56:344–51.
238. Hashiguchi S, Mine H, Ide M, et al. Watershed infarction associated with dementia and cerebral atrophy. Psychiatry Clin Neurosci 2000;54:163–8.
239. Romero JR, Beiser A, Seshadri S, et al. Carotid artery atherosclerosis, MRI indices of brain ischemia, aging, and cognitive impairment: The Framingham study. Stroke 2009;40:1590–6.
240. Kitagawaa K, Miwab K, Yagitab Y, et al. Association between carotid stenosis or lacunar infarction and incident dementia in patients with vascular risk factors. Eur J Neurol 2015;22(1): 187–92.
241. De Rango P, Caso V, Leys D, et al. The role of carotid artery stenting and carotid endarterectomy in cognitive performance: a systematic review. Stroke 2008;39:3116–27.
246. Johnston SC, Rothwell PM, Nguyen-Huynh MN, et al. Validation and refinement of scores to predict very early stroke risk after transient ischaemic attack. Lancet 2007;369:283–92.
247. Ois A, Cuadrado-Godia E, Rodríguez-Campello A, et al. High risk of early neurological recurrence in symptomatic carotid stenosis. Stroke 2009;40:2727–31.
248. Kidwell CS, Alger JR, Di Salle F, et al. Diffusion MRI in patients with transient ischemic attacks. Stroke 1999;30:1174–80.
249. Bisschops RH, Kappelle LJ, Mali WP, et al. Hemodynamic and metabolic changes in transient ischemic attack patients: A magnetic resonance angiography and (1)H-magnetic resonance spectroscopy study performed within 3 days of onset of a transient ischemic attack. Stroke 2002;33:110–15.
250. Easton JD, Saver JL, Albers GW, et al. Definition and Evaluation of Transient Ischemic Attack. Stroke 2009;40:2276–93.
251. Al-Khaled M, Matthis C, Münte TF, et al. The incidence and clinical predictors of acute infarction in patients with transient ischemic attack using MRI including DWI. Neuroradiology 2013;55:157–63.
252. Coutts SB, Modi J, Patel SK, et al. CT/CT angiography and MRI findings predict recurrent stroke after transient ischemic attack and minor stroke: results of the prospective CATCH study. Stroke 2012;43:1013–17.
253. Pessin MS, Duncan GW, Mohr JP, et al. Clinical and angiographic features of carotid transient ischemic attacks. N Engl J Med 1977;296:358–62.
256. Streifler JY, Eliasziw M, Benavente OR, et al. Prognostic importance of leukoaraiosis in patients with symptomatic internal carotid artery stenosis. Stroke 2002;33:1651–5.
260. Haynes RB, Taylor DW, Sackett DL, et al. Prevention of functional impairment by endarterectomy for symptomatic

high-grade carotid stenosis: North American Symptomatic Carotid Endarterectomy Trial Collaborators. JAMA 1994;271: 1256–9.
268. Furlan AJ, Whisnant JP, Kearns TP. Unilateral visual loss in bright light: An unusual symptom of carotid artery occlusive disease. Arch Neurol 1979;36:675–6.
269. Wiebers DO, Swanson JW, Cascino TL, et al. Bilateral loss of vision in bright light. Stroke 1989;20:554–8.
270. Donnan GA, Sharbrough FW, Whisnant JP. Carotid occlusive disease: Effect of bright light on visual evoked responses. Arch Neurol 1982;39:687–9.
271. Russell RW. Page NGR: Critical perfusion of brain and retina. Brain 1983;106:419–34.
272. Goodwin JA, Gorelick PB, Helgason CM. Symptoms of amaurosis fugax in atherosclerotic carotid artery disease. Neurology 1987;37:829–32.
273. Benavente O, Eliasziw M, Streifler JY, et al. Prognosis after transient monocular blindness associated with carotid-artery stenosis. N Engl J Med 2001;345:1084–90.
274. Rothwell PM, Warlow CP. Prediction of benefit from carotid endarterectomy in individual patients: a risk-modelling study. European Carotid Surgery Trialists' Collaborative Group. Lancet 1999;353(9170):2105–10.
279. Baquis GD, Pessin MS, Scott RM. Limb shaking—a carotid TIA. Stroke 1985;16:444–8.
281. Tatemichi TK, Young WL, Prohovnik I, et al. Perfusion insufficiency in limb shaking transient ischemic attacks. Stroke 1990; 21:341–7.
283. Klempen NL, Janardhan V, Schwartz RB, et al. Shaking limb transient ischemic attacks: Unusual presentation of carotid artery occlusive disease: Report of two cases. Neurosurgery 2002; 51:483–7.
285. Mayberg MR, Wilson SE, Yatsu F, et al. Carotid endarterectomy and prevention of cerebral ischemia in symptomatic carotid stenosis. Veterans Affairs Cooperative Studies Program 309 Trialist Group. JAMA 1991;266(23):3289–94.
286. Lovett JK, Coull AJ, Rothwell PM. Early risk of recurrence by subtype of ischemic stroke in population-based incidence studies. Neurology 2004;62(4):569–73.
287. Purroy F, Montaner J, Molina CA, et al. Patterns and predictors of early risk of recurrence after transient ischemic attack with respect to etiologic subtypes. Stroke 2007;38(12):3225–9.
288. Rothwell PM, Mehta Z, Howard SC, et al. Treating individuals 3: from subgroups to individuals: general principles and the example of carotid endarterectomy. Lancet 2005;365(9455): 256–65.
289. Halliday A, Mansfield A, Marro J, et al. Prevention of disabling and fatal strokes by successful carotid endarterectomy in patients without recent neurological symptoms: randomised controlled trial. Lancet 2004;363(9420):1491–502.
290. Abbott AL. Medical (nonsurgical) intervention alone is now best for prevention of stroke associated with asymptomatic severe carotid stenosis: results of a systematic review and analysis. Stroke 2009;40(10):e573–83.
292. Furlan AJ, Whisnant JP. Long-term prognosis after carotid artery occlusion. Neurology 1980;30:986–8.
294. Sacquegna T, DeCarolis P, Pazzaglia P, et al. The clinical course and prognosis of carotid artery occlusion. J Neurol Neurosurg Psychiatry 1982;45:1037–9.
295. Bernstein NM, Norris JW. Benign outcome of carotid occlusion. Neurology 1989;39:6–8.
296. Wade JPH, Wong W, Barnett HJM, et al. Bilateral occlusion of the internal carotid arteries: Presenting symptoms in 74 patients and a prospective study of 34 medically treated patients. Brain 1987;110:667–82.
297. Persoon S, Luitse MJ, de Borst GJ, et al. Symptomatic internal carotid artery occlusion: a long-term follow-up study. J Neurol Neurosurg Psychiatry 2011;82(5):521–6.
298. Chimowitz MI, Lynn MJ, Howlett-Smith H, et al. Comparison of warfarin and aspirin for symptomatic intracranial arterial stenosis. N Engl J Med 2005;352(13):1305–16.
299. Derdeyn CP, Chimowitz MI, Lynn MJ, et al. Aggressive medical treatment with or without stenting in high-risk patients with intracranial artery stenosis (SAMMPRIS): the final results of a randomised trial. Lancet 2014;383(9914):333–41.
300. Chimowitz MI. The Feinberg Award Lecture 2013 Treatment of Intracranial Atherosclerosis: Learning From the Past and Planning for the Future. Stroke 2013;44:2664–9.

23 Anterior Cerebral Artery Disease

John C.M. Brust, Angel Chamorro

KEY POINTS

- Anterior cerebral artery (ACA) territory infarction can be the result of carotid artery atherosclerosis and embolism, cardioembolism, local ACA atherosclerosis, or ACA dissection.
- Considerable variation describes the anatomy of the ACA and the brain regions it supplies.
- Neurological impairments following ACA territory infarction include weakness, sensory loss, apraxia and callosal disconnection signs, akinetic mutism and motor neglect, language disturbance, and urinary incontinence.

Infarction in the territory of one or both anterior cerebral arteries (ACAs) can follow vasospasm after rupture of saccular aneurysms of the ACA or the anterior communicating artery (ACoA). When such cases are excluded, ACA infarcts represent 0.6% to 3% of acute ischemic strokes.[1-5] In most reports, ACA territory infarction is more often associated with internal carotid artery (ICA) atherosclerosis than with primary stenosis or thrombosis of the ACA itself.[6] In a series of 100 consecutive Korean patients with ACA infarction, however, 68 had local atherosclerosis of the vessel.[7] In a series of 51 Spanish patients with ACA territory infarction, 45% were cardioembolic, 29% were atherothrombotic, 12% were lacunar, and 12% were of unknown cause.[8] In a series of 27 Swiss patients, 17 (63%) had probable emboli from the ICA or the heart; other causes were isolated proximal ACA occlusion, paraneoplastic disseminated intravascular coagulation, ICA dissection with embolic occlusion of the opposite ACA, acute ethanol intoxication, and hypertensive occlusion of a small penetrating branch of the ACA. Six patients with no obvious cause were older than 50 years, five of whom had risk factors for atherosclerotic stroke.[2] In an autopsy series of 55 patients with ACA infarcts, ten had probable cardiac emboli and only five had atherosclerosis primarily involving the ACA itself.[9] ACA territory infarction has resulted from vessel compression during transfalcial herniation.[10,11]

Dissecting aneurysms of the ACA affect either proximal or distal segments, produce both infarction and subarachnoid hemorrhage, and occur either spontaneously or after head trauma.[12-20] In two reports from Japan, ACA dissection accounted for 43% and 64% of infarcts in isolated ACA territory.[21,22] Case reports suggest embolic occlusion from small aneurysms of the distal ICA.[23]

A patient with transient ischemic attacks had fibromuscular dysplasia of both pericallosal arteries.[24] In another report, bilateral ACA infarction occurred in a patient with sickle cell trait during acute ethanol intoxication and withdrawal.[25] ACA infarction has also resulted from intracranial extension of Wegener's granulomatosis,[26] arteritis secondary to subarachnoid neurocysticercosis,[27,28] tuberculous meningitis,[28,29] and radiation vasculitis 19 years after cranial irradiation for acute lymphoblastic leukemia.[30] ACA territory infarction is also described in association with moyamoya disease,[31-33] migraine,[34] Takayasu disease,[35] and Susac's syndrome[36] and as a complication of intraarterial recombinant tissue plasminogen activator.[37]

Symptoms and signs, including weakness, sensory loss, and behavioral disturbance, vary widely among patients with ACA infarcts. To understand this variety, one must be familiar with the relevant anatomy.

ANATOMY

The ACA can be divided into a proximal or A1 segment, from its origin as the medial component of the internal carotid bifurcation to its junction with the ACoA, and a distal or postcommunicating artery segment (Fig. 23-1).[38-40] The distal segment has been variably subdivided by different authorities;[39,41-50] for example, into an A2 segment beginning at the ACoA and passing in front of the lamina terminalis as far as the junction of the rostrum and genu of the corpus callosum, an A3 segment passing around the genu of the corpus callosum, an A4 segment from above the corpus callosum to just beyond the coronal suture, and an A5 segment extending to the artery's termination.[44] The A2 and A3 segments have together been referred to as the *ascending segment*, and the A4 and A5 segments have been referred to as the *horizontal segment.*[40]

The A1 segment passes over the optic chiasm (in 70% of cases) or optic nerve (30%), varying in length from 7.2 to 18 mm (average, 12.7 mm).[39] Its diameter ranges from 0.9 to 4.0 mm (average, 2.6 mm) and is greater than 1.5 mm in 90% of brains. In 74% of brains, both A1 segments are larger than the ACoA, the diameter of which ranges from 0.2 to 3.4 mm (average, 1.5 mm).[39]

The ACAs pass over the corpus callosum side by side in only a minority of cases, so the ACoA is most often directed obliquely or even anteroposteriorly; thus, it is often best seen with angiography on oblique projections.[39]

The recurrent artery of Heubner[51] arises either at the level of the ACoA or just proximal or distal to it; in different series, it was described as arising most often from the A1 segment,[52] from the A2 segment,[39] or at the level of the ACoA.[53-66] Usually the largest branch of the A1 or proximal A2 segment, Heubner's artery doubles back on the ACA for a variable distance and then, either as a single trunk or with as many as 12 branches, penetrates the anterior perforated substance above the ICA bifurcation or lateral to it in the sylvian fissure; some branches enter the olfactory sulcus, the gyrus rectus, or more lateral inferior frontal areas.[39,57] Of obvious importance to the neurosurgeon[58-60] is the fact that Heubner's artery most consistently supplies the head of the caudate, the anterior inferior part of the internal capsule's anterior limb, the anterior globus pallidus, and parts of the uncinate fasciculus, olfactory regions, and anterior putamen and hypothalamus.[39,43,52,54,57,61-63]

In addition to Heubner's artery, the A1 and A2 segments give off smaller basal perforating branches, up to 15 from each A1 segment[39,64,54] and up to ten from each A2 segment.[39,40,58] One of these, called the short central artery, is considered more

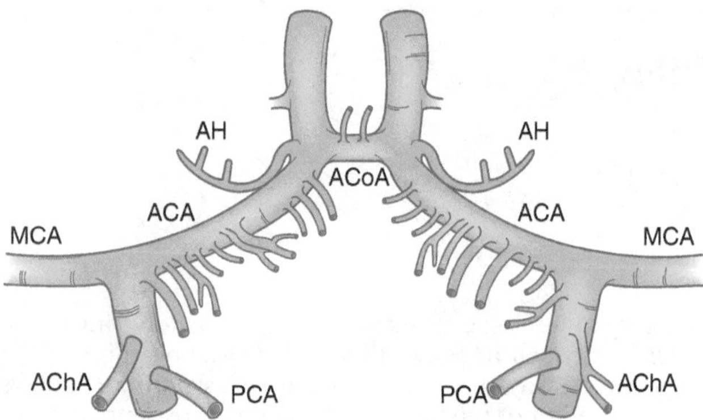

Figure 23-1. Diagram of the dorsal surface of the anterior circle of Willis, showing branches from the A1 segment of the anterior cerebral artery and from the anterior communicating artery. ACA, Anterior cerebral artery; AChA, anterior choroidal artery; ACoA, anterior communicating artery; AH, Heubner's artery; MCA, middle cerebral artery; PCA, posterior communicating artery. *(From Dunker RO, Harris AB. Surgical anatomy of the proximal anterior cerebral artery.* J Neurosurg *44:359, 1976.)*

consistent than others, in some people supplying part of the caudate nucleus and anterior limb of the internal capsule.[65,66] Other proximal branches penetrate the anterior perforated substance and the optic tract and supply, variably, parolfactory structures, the medial anterior commissure, globus pallidus, caudate and putamen, and the anterior limb of the internal capsule; these vessels also commonly supply the genu and contiguous posterior limb of the internal capsule, part of the anterior nucleus of the thalamus, and most of the anterior hypothalamus.[54] More distal A1 penetrating branches are smaller and supply the optic nerve, chiasm, and tract;[54,67] gyrus rectus and inferior frontal lobe; anterior perforated substance; and suprachiasmatic area.[39] Additional supply to the anterior inferior striatum and anterior hypothalamus comes from A2 segment branches, which can arise either separately or from a larger common trunk (the precallosal artery).[40] Similar penetrating branches from the ACoA, 13 or fewer in number,[54,68] supply the suprachiasmatic and parolfactory areas, dorsal optic chiasm, anterior perforated substance, inferior frontal lobe, septum pellucidum, columns of the fornix, corpus callosum, septal region, and anterior hypothalamus and cingulum.[38,39,67,68]

Vascular anastomoses are less functional in the diencephalon and basal ganglia than elsewhere in the cerebral hemispheres, and the territories supplied by these ACA penetrating end-zone arteries are no exception. Capillary anastomoses, which are difficult to demonstrate by standard perfusion techniques, exceed arterial anastomoses.[42,69–73]

The distal ACAs, deep in the interhemispheric fissure, are the only example of major cerebral arteries running side by side, although, as noted, one (usually the left) is often posterior to the other, and because of crossover of branches to the other hemisphere, occlusion of either artery can cause contralateral or bilateral infarction.[40] Beyond the lamina terminalis, the main trunk of the ACA – the pericallosal artery – runs above the corpus callosum in the pericallosal cistern (or, less often, over the cingulate gyrus or in the cingulate sulcus[41]), passes around the splenium of the corpus callosum, and terminates in the choroid plexus of the third ventricle; its posterior extent depends on the anterior extent of the posterior cerebral artery (PCA).[40,74] Except most posteriorly, the pericallosal artery lies below the free edge of the falx cerebri and can, therefore, shift across the midline.

The pericallosal artery has been variably defined as beginning at the ACoA[50] or at the point where the ACA gives off the callosomarginal artery; however, the callosomarginal artery is absent in 18% to 60% of brains.[40,49] The callosomarginal artery has been defined as that branch of the ACA traveling in or near the cingulate sulcus and giving off at least two major cortical branches. It originates from just beyond the ACoA to the genu of the corpus callosum, most often from the A3 segment,[40] and can be of the same diameter, larger, or smaller than the pericallosal artery.[40] Any or all of the callosomarginal artery's usual branches can arise from the pericallosal artery;[40] these branches supply the inferior frontal lobe (including the gyrus rectus, the orbital part of the superior frontal gyrus, the medial part of the orbital gyri, and the olfactory bulb and tract), the medial surface of the hemisphere (including the cingulate gyrus, the superior frontal gyrus, the paracentral lobule, and the precuneus), and the superior 2 cm of the lateral convexity (including the superior frontal, precentral, central, and postcentral gyri), anastomosing there with branches of the middle cerebral artery (MCA).[41] (These border zones of shared arterial territory are of clinical importance: In a radionuclide study of 365 consecutive patients with stroke, infarction occurred in the "watershed" between the ACA and the MCA in 5% of patients compared with the MCA territory in 28% and the ACA territory in 1%.)[75–77] The band of lateral convexity supplied by the ACA is wider anteriorly than posteriorly and may extend into the middle frontal gyrus.

Although variable in number and in whether they arise directly from the pericallosal artery or from its callosomarginal branch, eight major cortical branches of the distal ACA can usually be defined.[40] The orbitofrontal artery arises from the A2 segment except, infrequently, when it shares a common trunk with the frontopolar artery or arises just proximal to the ACoA.[39] Running forward in the floor of the anterior fossa as far as the planum sphenoidale, the orbitofrontal artery supplies the gyrus rectus, olfactory bulb and tract, and orbital surface of the frontal lobe. The frontopolar artery arises from the A2 segment (or, uncommonly, from the callosomarginal artery), passes to the frontal pole along the medial hemispheric surface, and supplies parts of the medial and lateral surfaces of the frontal pole.

The anterior, middle, and posterior frontal arteries arise separately from the A2, A3, and A4 segments of the pericallosal artery or from the callosomarginal artery; infrequently they arise from a common stem.[40,49] They supply the anterior, middle, and posterior parts of the superior frontal gyrus and the cingulate gyrus. The paracentral artery, arising from A4 or the callosomarginal artery, supplies premotor areas and the paracentral lobule.

The superior parietal artery, arising anterior to the splenium of the corpus callosum from A4, A5, or the callosomarginal artery, passes through the marginal limb of the cingulate sulcus and supplies the superior part of the precuneus. The inferior parietal artery, subdivided by some authorities into the precuneal and parietooccipital arteries,[41,43] is the most commonly absent cortical branch of the ACA (36% of brains in one series[40]); it arises from the A5 segment (or rarely from the callosomarginal artery) just above the splenium of the corpus callosum and supplies the posterior inferior part of the precuneus and portions of the cuneus.

The rostrum, genu, body, and splenium of the corpus callosum are supplied by short callosal arteries, pericallosal artery branches that pass through the callosum to supply, additionally, the septum pellucidum, anterior pillars of the fornix, and anterior commissure.[40,41] Posteriorly, the pericallosal artery extends around the splenium of the corpus callosum (the posterior pericallosal artery) and then passes forward, ending

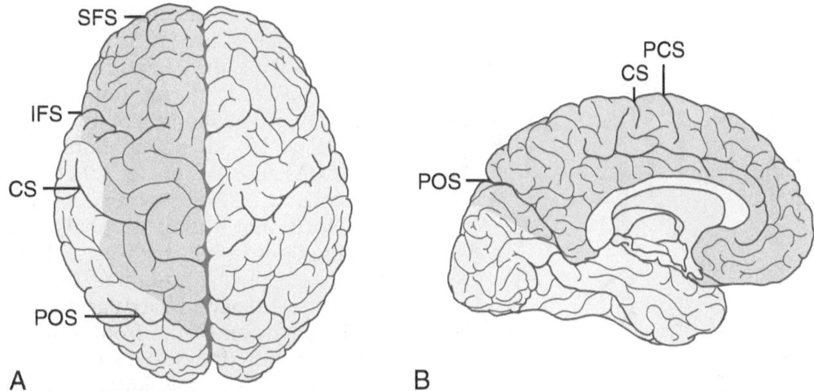

Figure 23-2. Cortical distribution of the anterior cerebral artery. A, Area of variation on the cerebral convexity. B, Area of variation on the cerebral medial surface. Combined pink and gray areas represent a composite of maximal extent. Gray areas represent a composite of minimal extent. CS, Central sulcus; IFS, inferior frontal sulcus; PCS, precentral sulcus; POS, parietooccipital sulcus; SFS, superior frontal sulcus. *(From Van der Zwan A, Hillen B, Tulleken CAF, et al. Variability of the territories of the major cerebral arteries.* J Neurosurg *77:927, 1992.)*

on the inferior surface of the splenium or extending all the way to the foramen of Monro.[78]

Of obvious importance in interpreting symptoms and signs is the normal variability of the boundaries (or border zones) between the anterior, middle, and posterior cerebral arteries. Figure 23-2, which is based on postmortem injection studies of 25 healthy brains, illustrates the range of cortical distribution of the ACA.[79] In those with the most extensive ACA distribution, the primary motor and sensory cortices were supplied by the ACA, not only medially but also over the convexity as far as the inferior frontal sulcus. In those with the least extensive ACA distribution, the ACA supplied little or none of the primary motor cortex, even medially.

Anomalies and Species Differences

The anatomy of the anterior circle of Willis is so varied among otherwise healthy people that whether a variation should be called an anomaly is sometimes difficult to define. Especially common are hypoplastic A1 segments, from mildly narrow to non-functionally threadlike, with both distal ACAs filling from the larger A1 segment.[58,80-85] In one study, 7% of brains had a stringlike A1 segment, and 6% had a hypoplastic ACoA.[86] In another study, 22% of brains had A1 segment hypoplasia, which was severe in 8% of cases and was associated with additional anomalies of the ACA or the posterior cerebral, posterior communicating, or basilar arteries in 82%.[87] Such anomalies are associated with a greater frequency of saccular aneurysms, and ACA occlusion secondary to cardiac embolism is often accompanied by proximal hypoplasia of the contralateral ACA.[83,88-90]

A smaller ACA often occurs on the same side as a smaller ICA,[91] and a hypoplastic A1 segment tends to be associated with an ACoA of larger diameter than usual.[39,92] Small A1 segments are several times more common among patients with symptomatic cerebrovascular disease than in the general population.[63] Cerebral angiography in one young man with episodic vertigo, loss of consciousness, and left leg weakness showed absence of the ACAs; the MCAs and one intracavernous carotid artery provided collateral vessels to the patient's medial cerebral hemispheres.[93]

In 50 adult autopsy specimens, 60% had one ACoA, 30% two, and 10% three;[39] other investigators have also found doubling and tripling of this vessel, and some have found absence of the ACoA.[43,94,95] A1 segment duplication also occurs,[39] as well as a third or median ACA arising from the ACoA (arteria termatica), which is sometimes as large as the two other ACAs and may be the major supplier to the posterior medial hemispheres.[43,54,96]

The recurrent artery of Heubner rarely arises from the ICA at its bifurcation, from the MCA, from the ACoA, or from the orbitofrontal or frontopolar branches of the ACA.[39,97-99] Such anomalies increase the risk of infarction in the territory of the recurrent artery of Heubner during surgical treatment of aneurysms arising from the anterior circle of Willis.[100] Absence or doubling of Heubner's artery occurs.[57,101] Embryologically, this artery is a remnant of the primitive olfactory artery; thus a patient with a persistent primitive olfactory artery has no Heubner's artery.[102]

Another well-recognized anomaly is a supernumerary vessel arising from the ICA at the level of the ophthalmic artery, coursing below the optic nerve, ascending in front of the optic chiasm, and terminating on the ipsilateral ACA near the ACoA. The A1 segment may be normal, hypoplastic, or absent;[103-107] in one instance both ACAs were absent.[108] Such an anomaly, which may be bilateral,[109] is commonly associated with ACA saccular aneurysm[104,106,108,110] and with other anomalies, such as duplication of the MCA,[111] median corpus callosum artery, distal moyamoya, aortic coarctation,[112] facial congenital defects, cerebral lipoma,[52] and absence of the ICA (in which the remaining carotid artery gives off a branch that passes beneath the optic nerve and divides into two ACAs while the other MCA arises from the PCA).[113] The anomalous vessel itself can cause visual symptoms from compression of the optic nerve or chiasm.[114]

The infraoptic ACA has been considered a remnant of the embryonic primitive maxillary artery, present in 3- to 4-mm embryos as an ICA branch and normally becoming a cavernous carotid branch, the inferior hypophyseal artery.[103,104,114-116] (The ACA normally arises from the primitive olfactory artery, eventually becoming the dominant vessel.)

Other anomalies, reported in an autopsied infant, include unilateral absence of the proximal MCA, ACA, and anterior choroidal artery, with much of the ipsilateral inferior frontal lobe supplied by branches from the opposite ACA, and secondary porencephaly of the orbital frontal lobe.[117] Autopsy of a neurologically healthy man showed a plexiform anterior communicating system connected to the left ICA by an anomalous vessel arising from the ICA near the ophthalmic artery, a single distal ACA, marked right A1 segment hypoplasia, and right plexiform vessels in the area of Heubner's artery, along with other anomalies of the posterior circulation.[118] Such

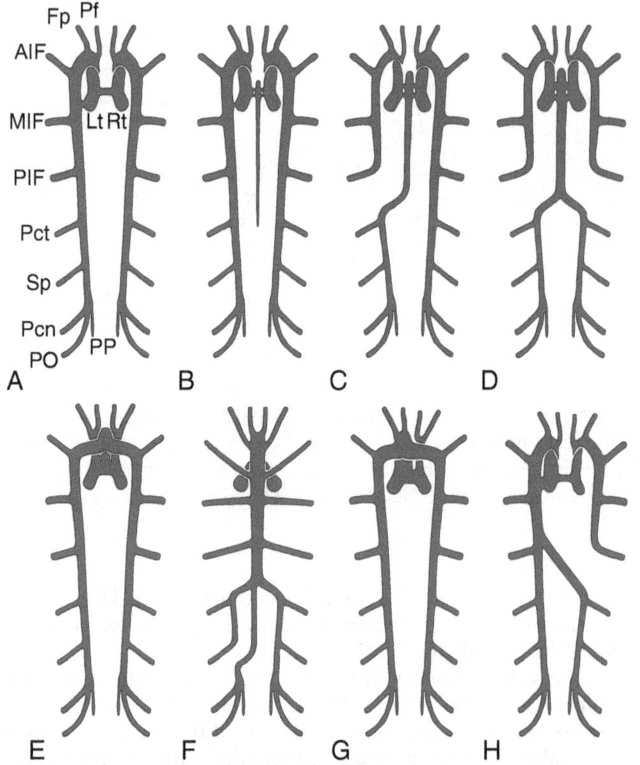

Figure 23-3. Variations in the distal anterior cerebral artery including patterns without (A) and with (B) a medial artery of the corpus callosum and variously developed accessory (C to E), unpaired (F), and bihemispheric lateral arteries (G and H). AIF, Anterior internal frontal; Fp, frontopolar; MIF, middle internal frontal; Pcn, precuneal; Pct, paracentral; Pf, prefrontal (orbitofrontal); PIF, posterior internal frontal; PO, parietooccipital; PP, posterior pericallosal; Sp, superior parietal. *(From Baptista AG. Studies on the arteries of the brain. II: The anterior cerebral artery: Some anatomic features and their clinical implications.* Neurology *13:825, 1963.)*

anomalies, rare in combination, are not unusual individually. For example, in a series of 1250 consecutive autopsies, a plexiform anterior communicating system was found in 15% of subjects, hypoplastic ACAs were found in 4%, and fused distal ACAs were found in 4%; a plexiform Heubner artery was much less common.[118] An ophthalmic artery arising from the ACA has also been reported,[78,119–121] as has an accessory MCA arising from the A2 segment of the ACA.[122]

In a study of 381 brains, distal ACA anomalies were found in 25%.[41] Such anomalies include pericallosal artery triplication, absence of ACA pairing, branches from one ACA to the other hemisphere, and bihemispheric branches (Fig. 23-3).[40,43,80,94,96,123,124] Triplicate ACAs with a variably developed midline accessory artery arising from the ACoA and supplying little, much, or most of either or both hemispheres have been observed in up to 22% of autopsy specimens.[41,66,94,125–129] Also, a long callosal artery (medial artery of the corpus callosum, anterior MCA) can arise from the pericallosal artery and pass parallel to it, giving off callosal perforating branches.[40,41] At angiography these anomalies, like a hypoplastic A1 segment, produce apparent bilateral ACA filling after unilateral injection of a carotid artery.[42,48,130–132] Bihemispheric ACAs, with either ACA taking over the supply of part or all of the other hemisphere, have been reported in up to 64% of brains.[40,42,129] (The highest value comes from a study in which any contralateral supply, however small, was included; brains in which most of both hemispheres are supplied by one of two ACAs are less common.[40])

In the fetus, there is gradual embryonic transition from one to two ACAs.[125,133] An unpaired or azygous ACA, arising through proximal union of the ACAs without an ACoA, occurs in 5% or less of adult brains.[41,94,95,125–128,134,135] Sometimes, the ACAs fuse for up to 3.9 cm, and an ACoA is absent.[93] Azygous ACAs are associated with a variety of other anomalies, including hydranencephaly, septum pellucidum defects, meningomyelocele, hydroencephalodysplasia, and vascular malformations,[136] and, like other ACA anomalies, with a higher frequency of saccular aneurysm.[137,138] In holoprosencephaly (fusion of the frontal neocortex and absence of the interhemispheric fissure), an azygous ACA courses just beneath the inner table of the skull.[112]

As noted, ACA anomalies are associated with an increased frequency of saccular aneurysms, especially at the ACoA, but also on distal or anomalous branches.[57,102,139–155] The embryonic prominence of the interhemispheric arterial plexus that develops into the ACoA is the most common site for the development of intracranial aneurysms.[156] Of 206 patients with ACoA aneurysms in one study, 44 (21.4%) had ACA anomalies, especially a median artery of the corpus callosum and duplication of the ACoA.[144] Ruptured fusiform aneurysm of the A1 segment of the ACA has been reported.[157] Giant aneurysms have been found on azygous ACAs.[158,159] After subarachnoid hemorrhage, a congenitally narrow A1 segment may be mistaken for vasospasm. Furthermore, proximal ACA ligation in patients with surgically unclippable ACoA aneurysms is not a valid option if one A1 segment fills both distal ACAs or if, in the absence of cross-compression, the aneurysms fill well from either side.[81,160–163]

Dolichoectasia – pathological elongation, tortuosity, and dilatation of an artery – most often affects the vertebrobasilar system and rarely the ACA.[164] The cause can be either acquired (e.g., trauma or atherosclerosis) or congenital. Headache, seizure, visual field defects, dementia with hydrocephalus, subarachnoid hemorrhage, and mania are described in patients with dolichoectatic ACAs.

A common anomaly, ACA fenestration has no clinical significance except when it is mistaken for an aneurysm on angiography.[165] Vestibulocochlear symptoms developed in a 22-year-old patient with fenestration and ectasia of the left ACA and persistence of the right trigeminal artery.[166]

Species differences in the anatomy of the ACA (and other cerebral vessels) must be kept in mind when one is interpreting animal studies of cerebral ischemia and stroke. For example, birds, amphibians, and anteaters have paired arteries without an ACoA or other left-to-right anastomoses.[43] In most mammals, the two ACAs join to form a single pericallosal (azygous) artery, which may or may not bifurcate distally, and there is no ACoA.[43] In subhuman primates, several recurrent medial striate arteries (the equivalent of Heubner's artery in humans) supplying the anterior caudate, putamen, and globus pallidus have rich preparenchymal anastomoses with lateral lenticulostriate arteries from the MCA; the orbitofrontal artery, supplying most of the orbital surface of the frontal lobe, arises from the MCA and anastomoses with branches of the ACA, and extensive anastomoses exist between the ACA and the proximal MCA in the sylvian fissure.[62,167–170] In cats, the presence of an ACoA has been both claimed[171,172] and denied.[173] The feline ACA supplies the medial hemispheric cortex containing hindlimb motor representation, but cerebral arterial occlusion tends to cause smaller and deeper infarcts than in higher primates.[174] In rats the rostral caudatoputamen is supplied by penetrating ACA branches and a vessel running alongside the lateral olfactory tract, and this area accounts for 25% of strokes in stroke-prone, spontaneously hypertensive rats.[175,176]

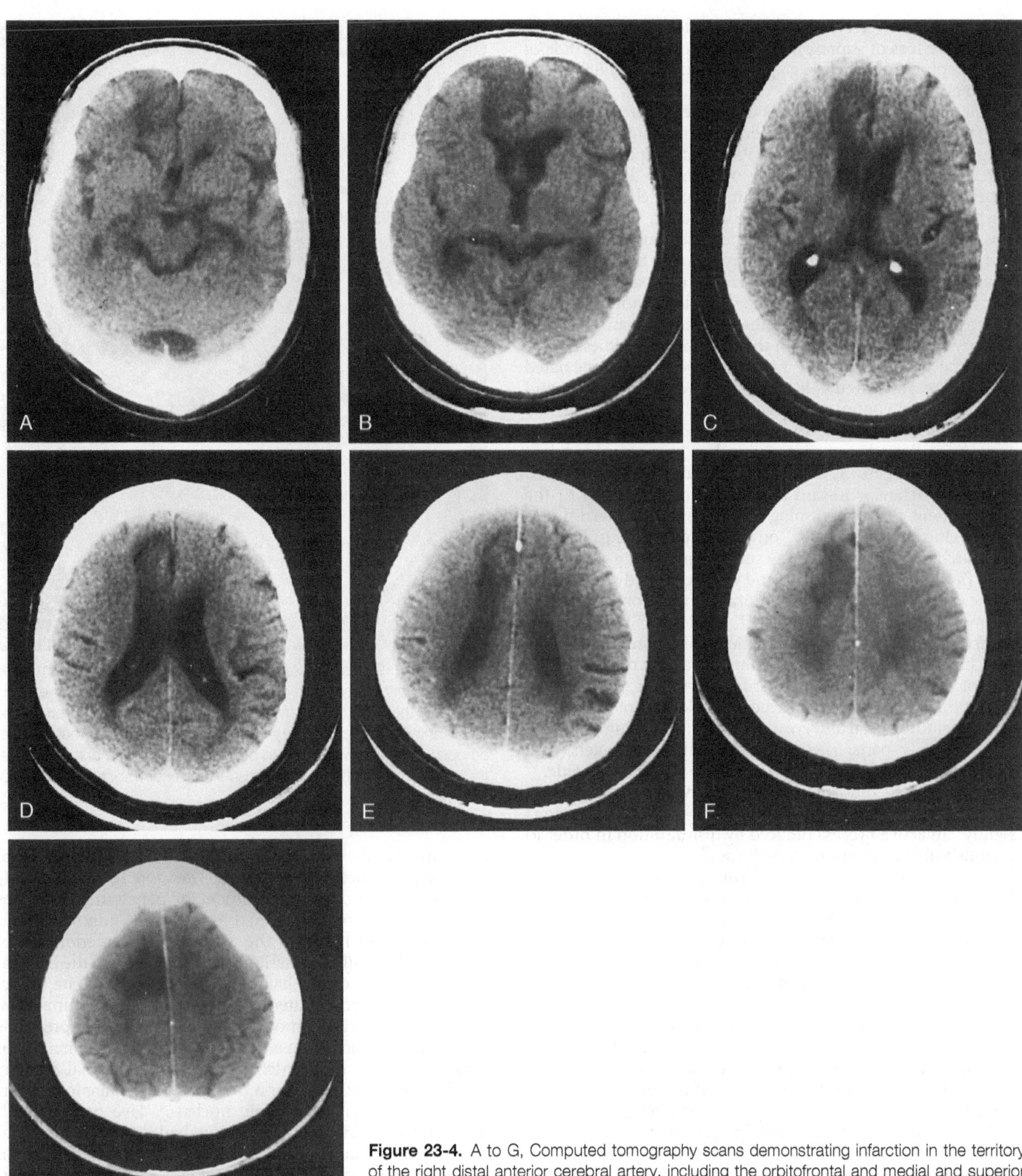

Figure 23-4. A to G, Computed tomography scans demonstrating infarction in the territory of the right distal anterior cerebral artery, including the orbitofrontal and medial and superior frontoparietal lobes. Diencephalic structures supplied by proximal anterior cerebral artery penetrating branches are not involved.

SYMPTOMS AND SIGNS

Weakness and Sensory Loss

ACA occlusion causes infarction of the paracentral lobule and, as a result, weakness and sensory loss in the contralateral leg (Fig. 23-4).[177-182] The deficit is usually greatest distally for the following two reasons: (1) the proximal leg is represented on the primary sensorimotor cortex either superiorly on the medial hemisphere or on the high convexity with, therefore, richer collateral vessels from the MCA and (2) proximal muscles have substantial representation in the ipsilateral hemisphere.[183] If infarction extends to the upper convexity, there may be proximal arm weakness or, as is usual with cortical lesions, clumsiness or slowness out of proportion to the actual loss of strength.

Paretic muscles are initially most often flaccid, becoming spastic over days or weeks; at the outset, tendon reflexes may be decreased, normal, or increased. (This common early dissociation between tone and tendon reflexes has been attributed to the loss of supraspinal influence on different kinds of muscle spindle afferents [e.g., phasic versus tonic].) Babinski's sign may be present.

The sensory modalities most often affected are discriminative (two-point discrimination, localization, stereognosis) and proprioceptive (position sense). Pain and temperature sensation and gross touch are usually only mildly decreased; the patient can tell sharp from dull, but the pinprick does not feel as sharp or as "normal" as on the unaffected side. Vibratory loss is variable. Depending on the posterior extent of the ACA and collaterals from the PCA, sensory loss may be mild or even absent in the presence of marked crural hemiparesis.[43] Sensation may be similarly spared when occlusion is not of the ACA or the pericallosal artery but of the paracentral branch.[43,184–187] Sensory loss can also occur in the absence of weakness.[188,189]

In the acute phase, the head and eyes may be deviated toward the side of the lesion.[43,190,191] Forced grasping and groping of the contralateral hand, regardless of whether it is weak, follows damage to the posterior superior frontal gyrus.[43,192–194] Such forced grasping has been considered "a type of limb-kinetic apraxia" and "only one aspect of a total change in behavior toward a compulsive exploration of the environment";[195] foot grasping[196] can cause the lower limb to seem "glued to the floor"[195] on attempted walking. Patients with such findings also display sucking and biting,[188] "ansaugen" (a movement of the lips and tongue toward stimulation of the skin near the lower lip),[193] bradykinesia (or an "absence of movement intention"),[43,197,198] catalepsy,[199] and "tonic innervation" ("amorphous movements of a pseudospontaneous character")[43] on attempted voluntary action of the affected arm or leg.[196–198] During the first few days after ACA territory infarction, two patients displayed "hyperkinetic motor behaviors" (including head and eye movements, grimacing, chewing, rubbing body parts, rhythmically moving the fingers, and flexing and extending the thigh) on the non-paralyzed side.[200] It was suggested that such movements (which also occurred contralateral to hemiplegia after MCA territory infarction) signify "an active process induced by disinhibition in order to establish new compensatory pathways."

The "pusher syndrome", a disturbed control of upright body posture in which the patient suffers from a severe misperception of his body's orientation in the coronal plane, was described in a patient with a right ACA infarction, severe left hemiparesis, spatial neglect, visual and auditory extinction, and forced contraversive pushing away from the non-paralyzed side.[201,202]

Pronounced weakness of the arm and face in the presence of ACA occlusions has been attributed to involvement of Heubner's artery and its supply to the anterior limb and genu of the internal capsule (Fig. 23-5).[43,203] If the circle of Willis is complete, such proximal thrombosis must extend as far as the ACoA to produce complete hemiplegia, or the contralateral ACA takes over the supply of both medial hemispheres and weakness is limited to the face and arm. Paralysis of the right arm, paresis of the right face, and only slight weakness of the right leg occurred in a man who at autopsy was found to have infarction of the left putamen, caudate, and anterior limb of the internal capsule, plus a "shrunken and occluded artery of Heubner."[43] (The leg weakness was attributed to additional softening in the territories of the ACA's middle and posterior internal frontal branches.) "Capsular warning syndrome", with recurrent attacks of left face, arm, and leg weakness followed by fixed hemiplegia, was attributed to atherosclerotic stenosis of Heubner's artery, verified angiographically.[204]

Later anatomic studies have shown, however, that Heubner's artery supplies only the most anterior striatum and anterior limb of the internal capsule and is, therefore, probably uncommonly the responsible vessel when brachial or facial palsy accompanies ACA occlusion. The more likely possibility in such a situation is involvement of penetrating branches arising from the most proximal ACA and the internal carotid bifurcation, which supply the genu and the anterior part of the internal capsule's posterior limb in addition to the hypothalamus and the rostral thalamus.[54] Moreover, caudate infarction can cause contralateral limb bradykinesia, clumsiness, and loss of associated movements mistakenly interpreted as weakness.[65] Dysarthria has followed unilateral infarction of either the left or right anterior limb of the internal capsule, and in one report, dysarthria occurred after infarction apparently confined to the caudate nucleus.[65] Five patients with unilateral capsular genu infarction had contralateral facial and lingual weakness with dysarthria, three had unilateral mastication-palatal-pharyngeal weakness, and one had unilateral vocal cord paresis; the only limb involvement was mild hand weakness in three patients.[205]

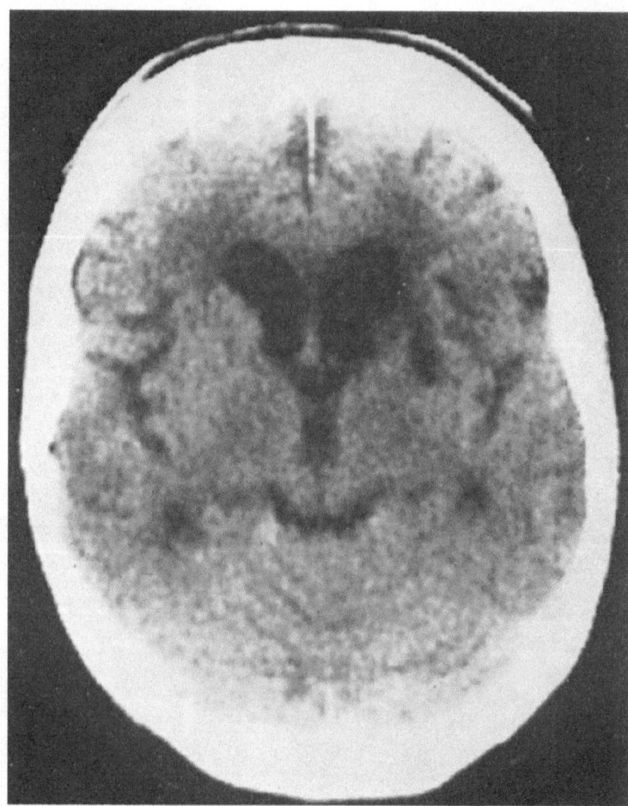

Figure 23-5. Computed tomography scan showing infarction in the territory of either the left artery of Heubner or another penetrating branch of the proximal anterior cerebral artery. Brain supplied by the distal anterior cerebral artery was radiographically normal, and at autopsy, infarction was found to be limited to the head of the caudate, the anterior part of the internal capsule's anterior limb, and the anterior putamen.

As previously noted, the ACA territory in some individuals encompasses a considerable portion of the upper cerebral convexity; in such a situation, infarction would include arm and hand representations on the primary motor (and sensory) cortex.[79,206] Conversely, in subjects with a smaller than usual ACA territory, leg weakness can be a consequence of MCA or PCA territory infarction. Of 63 patients in one series with acute stroke and "leg-predominant weakness," infarction occurred in 12 in the ACA territory, in nine in the MCA territory, in two in both territories (not "watershed"), in 18 in the internal capsule, in ten in the brainstem, and in two in the thalamus.[207] Leg weakness was more lasting when infarction involved the motor cortex than when it involved the premotor cortex or supplementary area and spared the motor cortex.

Of 36 consecutive patients with isolated pericallosal artery territory infarction, 29 had hemiparesis with leg predominance, yet only five had abnormal motor-evoked potential recordings, indicating preserved corticospinal tracts. The weakness was attributed to supplementary motor area (SMA) damage.[208]

Of 100 patients with "ataxic hemiparesis" after a first stroke, four had infarction of the contralateral ACA territory.[209] Pyramidal weakness was greatest in the leg, and ataxia of the cerebellar type was seen in the ipsilateral arm. Such ataxia has been attributed to involvement of frontopontocerebellar projections and also, on the basis of single-photon emission computed tomography (SPECT) studies, to transsynaptic dysfunction of the contralateral cerebellum (diaschisis).[210,211] A problem with the ataxic hemiparesis syndrome - regardless of the lesion's location - is that upper motor neuron lesions, as a rule, produce clumsiness out of proportion to weakness; determining whether the "ataxia" is qualitatively or quantitatively sufficient to label it "cerebellar" can be difficult.

The transient ischemic attack syndrome of limb shaking of the leg was described in a woman with an acute infarction on the right corpus callosum and cingulate gyrus secondary to focal stenosis of the right ACA. She had episodic shaking movements of the left leg one to 15 times per day, preceded by a brief sensation of weakness and elicited only when she arose from a sitting position.[212]

Infarction in the territories of both ACAs causes paraparesis, with or without sensory loss.[213] Paraparesis occurs most often as a consequence of bilateral ACA vasospasm after rupture of an ACA or ACoA aneurysm.[214,215] In thrombotic or embolic infarction, paraparesis is especially likely when there is a vascular anomaly, such as a hypoplastic A1 segment or an azygous distal ACA.[39,133,183,216-222] Particularly when symptoms are stutteringly progressive, spinal cord disease may be erroneously suspected.[40,41,223,224] Even if weakness is mild or absent, there may be severe gait disturbance, with inability to initiate the first step with either foot, to lift either foot off the ground, or to turn to either side ("slipping clutch syndrome").[225-227] Grasp reflexes of the feet (or hands) are not present in all affected patients, and although some can move their legs freely in the air (e.g., bicycling motions),[227] others cannot.[225] When severe, such medial prefrontal damage can produce a pronounced immobility of all four limbs, from bradykinesia to catatonic (perseverative) posturing with gegenhalten, sucking, and biting.[227] In one such report the patient had unexplained vertical gaze palsy (upward and downward), suggesting midbrain localization.[228]

The gait disability bears an obvious resemblance to that found with hydrocephalus and with the paraplegia in flexion of degenerative disease that mainly affects the frontal lobes;[229] in these conditions, the pathophysiology is not understood, and the possible roles of descending frontal and prefrontal fibers[230,231] or the globus pallidus[232] are uncertain. Pulsatile flow in the ACAs is decreased in infantile hydrocephalus,[233] and some researchers have suggested that secondary ACA ischemia may be the cause of lower-extremity spasticity in hydrocephalic infants and may contribute to the gait disturbance seen in adult normal-pressure hydrocephalus.[234]

A man whose anomalous ACAs resulted in bilateral infarction restricted to the supplementary motor areas had what was considered gait apraxia; he had difficulty standing from a chair on command, rolling over in bed, starting or stopping walking, and maintaining stance. There were no elementary motor abnormalities, and the authors considered his disorder a "loss of monitoring of the automatic implementation of gait mechanisms."[235] Drop attacks and right-sided limb-shaking TIAs occurred in a man with left ICA stenosis and a left A1 segment of the ACA supplying both medial frontal lobes; symptoms resolved after endarterectomy.[236]

Callosal Disconnection Signs

In addition to either right or left leg weakness, ACA occlusion can cause left-sided apraxia, agraphia, and tactile anomia.[46,80,193,197,237-240] Early cases, however, are difficult to interpret.[241,242] For example, the patient reported by Liepmann and Maas[46] had right hemiplegia, including his arm, so it is uncertain whether the agraphia and apraxia were truly unilateral. The patient described by Goldstein[197] had left-sided weakness, greatest in the leg, with a pronounced left hand grasp reflex, which was itself another possible reason for left-sided motor difficulty.[227,243] Agraphia, apraxia, and tactile anomia have occurred, however, in otherwise normal left limbs of patients with ACA occlusion, right leg weakness, and normal right arms.[238,239,244,245]

After surgical occlusion of the left ACA, a patient described by Geschwind and Kaplan[241] had right hemiparesis that was worse in the leg, a marked grasp reflex in the right hand, and mild right proprioceptive loss. He also had left-handed agraphia, writing incorrectly and paragraphically both spontaneously and to dictation, and he could not perform written calculations with his left hand. He could not name objects, letters, or numbers placed in his left hand out of his sight, but he could identify them afterward with his left hand by pointing to them or demonstrating their use. Using either hand, he could not correctly select from a group of objects placed out of sight in the other hand. Finally, he had difficulty performing verbal commands with his left hand (e.g., draw a square, point to the examiner, show how to brush teeth). Despite the grasp reflex, his right hand could write normally, and his left hand could slavishly copy writing. Either hand could imitate the examiner's movements or manipulate objects. Following the lead of earlier investigators,[46] Geschwind and Kaplan[241] attributed their findings to anterior callosal destruction, with disconnection of the right hemisphere from the left hemisphere or, more specifically, of the right sensorimotor cortex from the left language areas. (Earlier writers who claimed that callosal lesions could cause left astereognosis[197,246] were undoubtedly observing tactile anomia rather than true agnosia, although the ability of a patient to identify objects but not letters placed in the left hand is less easily explained.[247]) Preservation of the posterior corpus callosum was manifested by the ability of Geschwind and Kaplan's[241] patient to read words presented to either visual field. Retained ability to perform tasks requiring both hands, such as threading a needle, suggested that the two hemispheres could cooperate like two individuals on such visually guided activities.

A left-handed patient had a stroke with weakness of the right leg but not the right arm, plus loss of ability to write with the right but not the left hand; if he is presumed to have had right cerebral language dominance, callosal disconnection might explain the agraphic right hand.[248] Another patient, considered to have pure agraphia, may represent a similar example of ACA occlusion.[249]

Some patients with presumed ACA occlusion and anterior callosal damage have had difficulty not only in performing verbal commands with the left hand but also in imitating the examiner and using actual objects.[192,199,246,250] Inaccessibility of verbal information to the right sensorimotor cortex would not explain this type of apraxia. Some investigators have suggested that, in right-handed people, engrams for skilled movements (space–time or visuokinesthetic engrams)[251] reside in the left hemisphere and that callosal apraxia with impaired imitation and object use is the result of disconnection between these motor engrams and the right hemisphere.[251,252] In support of such a view is the observation, in a left-handed person, that dominance for language and dominance for skilled motor acts appeared to be in different hemispheres.[242] That some patients with ACA occlusion have impaired imitation and object use and some do not has been explained by the hypothesis that verbal motor programs may be transmitted to the right hemisphere across the genu of the corpus callosum, whereas visuokinesthetic engrams may be transmitted across the body.[251]

The alien hand syndrome consists of apparently purposeful movements of an upper extremity that a patient cannot control.[252–257] Different forms are described. A review of published cases concluded that damage to the medial prefrontal cortex of the dominant hemisphere and the anterior corpus callosum resulted in intermanual conflict and inability to perform bimanual tasks.[253] In another report, interfering movements of the alien hand were triggered by movements of the other hand and often had a mischievous quality. For example, a patient was about to hit a nail on a block with a hammer when his left hand pushed the block away, causing the hammer to miss the target. In that report patients with chronic symptoms had lesions of both the anterior corpus callosum and the contralateral medial frontal cortical and subcortical regions.[258] Patients express astonishment and frustration when conflict occurs, and they adopt avoidance behavior such as sitting on the alien hand. Involuntary masturbation by the alien hand has followed both unilateral and bilateral ACA territory infarction.[259,260]

The alien hand phenomenon is possibly related to other bizarre signs associated with callosal and/or medial frontal damage, including diagonistic apraxia (as one hand attempts to perform a voluntary action, the other performs the opposite; e.g., the patient puts on his glasses with his right hand, but his left hand then takes them off)[261] and utilization behavior (the patient cannot refrain from picking up and using an object, such as a toothbrush, placed in front of him).[262–264] A patient developed severe utilization behavior after bilateral infarcts that damaged both supplementary motor areas but spared the rest of the premotor cortices, the cingulate gyri, and the corpus callosum. The authors speculated that utilization behavior, reflecting disinhibition of responses to environmental stimuli, might be viewed as a bilateral alien hand syndrome.[265]

A woman with left ACA territory infarction had difficulty naming her left fingers and moving her named left fingers; she also had difficulty pointing to her own body parts with her left hand.[266] It was suggested that the patient's "body schema" was organized principally in her left cerebral hemisphere and was, therefore, as a consequence of callosal infarction, disconnected from her right hemisphere.

Occlusion of an ACA that extends around the splenium of the corpus callosum can produce pure alexia in the left visual field or other visual anomic or agnostic problems.[40,251]

A problem in evaluating these patients is the extent to which they differ from those who have undergone surgical callosectomy. Left-sided apraxia to verbal commands occurs immediately after complete section of the corpus callosum and anterior commissure, usually with preserved ability to carry out the act in imitation of the examiner.[267,268] Right-sided movements, when governed by the right hemisphere (e.g., drawing an object seen only in the left visual field), are also impaired.[269] Such deficits tend to improve over days, however,[268] unless severe extracallosal brain damage is present.[267] A lasting deficit after callosal and commissural section is most likely to affect homolateral control of fingers (e.g., moving the left fingers to identify areas corresponding to regions stimulated on the right fingers or mimicking with the left hand postures shown pictorially to the right visual field). When left hemispheric damage occurs early in life, the minor hemisphere can comprehend spoken or written names of familiar objects[270–273] but, except in the setting of prolonged stimulus exposure[274] or in rare instances of unusual plasticity in speech organization,[275,276] usually cannot comprehend verbs or action nouns.[271,277,278] Such lack of comprehension accounts for the inability of a patient who has callosectomy to follow verbal commands with either hand when the information is given to the minor hemisphere. Recovery of all but the most distal and subtle apraxia when commands are given to the language hemisphere is explained by each hemisphere's control over homolateral as well as contralateral limbs.

A patient with anterior callosal hemorrhage and bilateral ACA vasospasm had alexia in the left hemifield, anomia for objects held in the left hand, and left-handed agraphia and apraxia (including imitation and object use).[279] She also had bilateral pseudoneglect: visual or tactile line bisection produced left hemineglect with the right hand in the left hemispace and right hemineglect with the left hand in the right hemispace. A proposed explanation was disconnection of "the hemisphere important for directing attention–intention into the contralateral hemispace" from "the hemisphere important for controlling sensory motor processing of the limb."[279] By contrast, left hemispatial neglect "confined to right-hand and verbal responses" occurred in a patient with infarction of the posterior genu and whole trunk of the corpus callosum plus the left medial frontal and temporooccipital lobes.[280] These findings were consistent with the hypothesis that "the left hemisphere is only concerned with attending to the contralateral hemispace," whereas "the right hemisphere is specialized for attending to both sides of space." Also consistent with previous reports, hemineglect does not seem to occur with lesions restricted to the corpus callosum but requires additional destruction (e.g., medial frontal lobe) that blocks transmission through extracallosal commissures.[254,281]

In a right-handed patient who had undergone callosectomy but displayed unusually rich right hemispheric verbal comprehension, there was no left-sided apraxia to verbal information presented to the right hemisphere.[278] This finding argues against the notion that motor engrams reside solely in one hemisphere, language-dominant or not.[246,282–287] In other patients undergoing callosectomy, visual nonverbal stimulation has also produced normally coordinated contralateral motor acts.[288]

Consistent with the view that extracallosal damage is probably crucial to the appearance of anterior callosal disconnection syndrome after ACA occlusion is the finding that left tactile anomia, apraxia for verbal commands, and agraphia did not occur in two patients who underwent sectioning of the anterior commissure and only the anterior two-thirds of the corpus callosum.[268] These patients, moreover, performed a variety of non-verbal cross-integration tasks, matching visual or tactile stimuli directed separately to each hemisphere.[289] Conversely, selective sectioning of the splenium, sparing the genu and body, does produce verbal deficits for left visual field and tactile stimuli[247,290] as well as for tactile-motor tasks requiring interhemispheric integration.[287,288] It appears that "the anterior commissure and the rostral callosum do not transfer either lateralized visual images that elicit motor activity or the specific motor program needed to carry out the appropriate movement."[288] An isolated 3-cm midcallosal section impairs interhemispheric transfer of tactile data but not of information obtained visually.[291] Section of the most posterior 1.5 cm of the callosum disrupts naming of visual stimuli in the left visual field,[290,292–294] and an additional 1.5-cm section further impairs sensorimotor integration and tactile naming.[288,295] What information is transferred across the rostral callosum (the part most often damaged after ACA occlusion) is unclear; it has been suggested that the anterior callosum transfers information after processing it into higher order abstraction.[288,296] Tomaiuolo et al.[297] performed simple reaction times for interhemispheric transfer tasks in a patient with callosal lesions sparing the splenium and rostrum. They measured unimanual responses to simple lateralized visual displays presented tachistoscopically. The impaired responses, when compared with those of a patient with complete callosal section, led to the conclusion that "specific callosal channels mediate the basic visuomotor interhemispheric transfer times (ITTs), and these do not include the rostrum and/or the splenium of the corpus callosum." (After posterior callosal section, interhemispheric transfer of sensory information from the right hemisphere is lost, but transfer of semantic information is still possible; after complete section, neither sensory nor semantic information can be transferred.)[296]

Akinetic Mutism (Abulia)

Akinetic mutism is "a state of limited responsiveness to the environment in the absence of gross alteration of sensorimotor mechanisms operating at a more peripheral level."[298] Neither paralysis nor coma accounts for the symptoms. Patients may open their eyes and seem alert, and brief movement, speech, or even agitation may follow powerful stimuli; however, patients are otherwise "indifferent, detached, frozen, and apathetic."[298] The term *akinetic mutism* was used by Cairns et al.[299] to describe such a state in association with a tumor of the third ventricle. Patients with such lesions often have ophthalmoparesis and fluctuating or continuous somnolence.[300,301]

Akinetic mutism also occurs with lesions of the anteromedial frontal lobes, including infarction.[296,302–308] Ophthalmoparesis (except for early gaze preference) is then not present, and the patient, whose open eyes may follow objects, is more obviously alert than the patient with mesencephalic or thalamic lesions; the patient may make brief, monosyllabic, but appropriate responses to questions. Striking dissociation occurs between spontaneous verbal communication, which is often totally absent, and solicited communication, which is often retained although restricted.[302] *Abulia* refers to a continuum of such abnormalities, from mild to severe, having in common decreased spontaneous movement and speech, latency in responding to verbal and other stimuli, and impersistence in responses and tasks.[112,306] Although verbal responses are "late, terse, incomplete, and emotionally flat," the patient who is sufficiently prodded sometimes reveals a cognitive capacity much more normal than expected.[65] When the patient is literally akinetic and mute, however, the condition must be differentiated from true stupor or coma, a locked-in state, extrapyramidal akinesia, catatonia, hysteria, and a persistent vegetative state. The two structures most often implicated in the production of abulia are the cingulate gyrus and the supplementary motor area (SMA).

Abulia has occurred after bilateral cingulate gyrus lesions. A woman had a sudden headache and then "lay staring at the ceiling, not asking for water or food, and never speaking spontaneously."[309] She was incontinent of urine, ate and drank when food or water was brought, comprehended spoken speech, answered questions monosyllabically, and did not display any emotional reaction. Right-sided hyperreflexia and bilateral Babinski's signs were present. At autopsy, embolic hemorrhagic infarction of the cingulate gyri bilaterally and of the corpus callosum was seen. A clinically and pathologically similar patient showed Babinski's signs but no hypertonus, and there were "no visible reactions to pain."[310] Inability to walk despite normal strength has been specifically mentioned in other reports.[311] In another report, however, unilateral cingulate infarction in two patients was followed by seizures in one and personality change in another, with no reduction in motor activity.[311] Akinetic mutism occurred in one patient with presumed unilateral cingulate (and pontine) damage, but autopsy findings were incomplete.[312] A patient with hemorrhage into the right medial frontal lobe had marked bradykinesia of the left limbs that improved when the limbs were placed in his right hemispace.[313] This disturbance was considered motor neglect ("a failure of the intentional systems that lead to preparation and activation of movement"), possibly secondary to SMA damage.[313] It is not unusual for patients with unilateral ACA territory infarction (or medial frontal lobe surgical ablation) to have several days of abulia followed by return of verbal and ipsilateral motor responses, persistence of weakness in the contralateral leg, and a disinclination to move the contralateral arm. Motor neglect thus might be viewed as unilateral abulia.[43,196,314–317]

Chamorro et al.[182] demonstrated that motor neglect explains some of the apparent hemiparesis affecting the face, arm, and leg in infarction in the ACA territory, as revealed by computed tomography (CT) or magnetic resonance imaging (MRI) and, in one case, by autopsy correlation (Fig. 23-6). Before the report of these cases, the usual explanation for such face–arm–leg hemiparesis had been involvement of the primary motor cortex or the deeper pathways, neither of which was involved in this series of eight patients. Instead, defective supramotor planning, unilateral hypokinesia, and motor neglect were due to damage of medial premotor areas. Five of the patients had a total lack of voluntary movement in the contralateral limbs that prevented adequate testing of motor praxis and performance of bimanual tasks. Movement could not be elicited by the examiner despite strong verbal and gestural commands. Pain reaction was also defective or absent in the limbs contralateral to the lesion. Transcranial motor stimulation demonstrated absence of responses to cortical stimulation in the lower limbs of the affected side, interpreted as a sign of functional interruption of the corticospinal tract. In the upper limbs, the response to transcranial motor stimulation was normal; this finding indicated that the impaired voluntary function reflected impairment of circuits involved in motor planning or in the initiation of motor action.

With further improvement, signs can become increasingly subtle (e.g., difficulty with sequential movements involving different joints or coordinating the movements of both arms).[317,318] In one report there was inability to reproduce rhythms from memory,[319] and in another, in patients with bilateral SMA lesions, there was inability to perceive as separate two successive tactile stimuli applied to the body.[320] Observations such as these have led to the hypotheses that the SMA (and perhaps other premotor structures) is responsible for generating "sequences from memory that fit into a precise timing plan."[319]

Patients with abulia or motor neglect often display relative preservation of reflexic (externally stimulated) movements, in contrast to anticipated or willed movements. (A comparable dissociation is seen in parkinsonism.) Disinhibition of unanticipated complex motor movements as a result of SMA damage has been invoked to explain such phenomena as alien hand syndrome, diagonistic apraxia, and utilization behavior.[321]

A man with akinetic mutism after bilateral ACA territory infarction had bilateral independent periodic lateralized epileptiform discharges (BIPLEDs) frontally on electroencephalography (EEG).[322] A woman with akinetic mutism after bilateral infarcts that included the cingulate gyri and orbitofrontal structures had reduced striatal dopamine uptake that returned to normal as her symptoms resolved.[323] Anecdotal

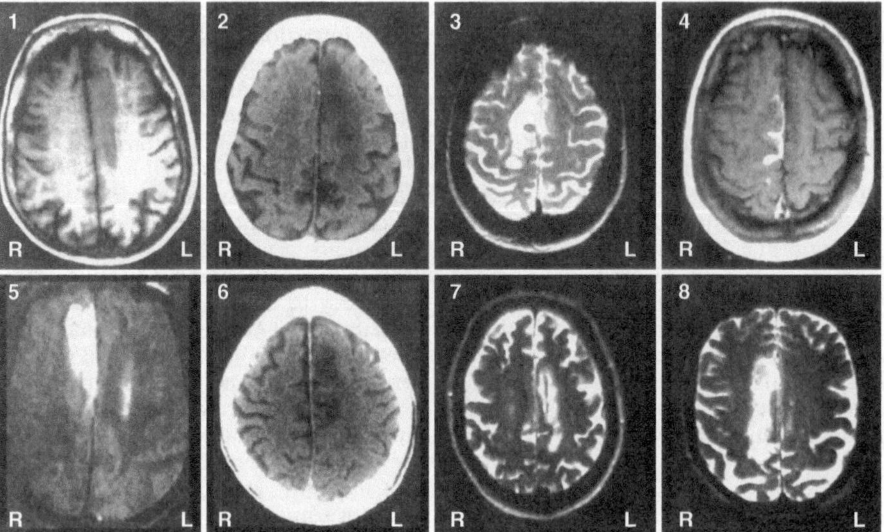

Figure 23-6. Representative axial magnetic resonance (MR) images and computed tomography (CT) scans of the brains of eight patients with anterior cerebral artery (ACA) infarctions. 1, T1-weighted axial MR image; 2, CT scan; 3, T2-weighted MR image; 4, T1-weighted MR image; 5, proton-density MR image; 6, CT scan; 7, T2-weighted MR image; 8, T2-weighted MR image. *(From Chamorro A, Marshall RS, Valls-Sole J, et al. Motor behavior in stroke patients with isolated medial frontal ischemic infarction.* Stroke *28:1755, 1997.)*

reports describe improvement in akinetic mutism from frontal lobe damage after treatment with levodopa.[324]

Cingulectomy in monkeys caused reduction of motor activity and "loss of social conscience"; the animals treated their fellows as inanimate objects not to be feared.[170] Monkeys in which the medial temporal lobes were removed and with Klüver–Bucy syndrome (quietness, no fear, and increased curiosity with compulsive nosing and smelling of all objects) showed gradual clearing of symptoms, which returned after bilateral cingulectomy.[325] In cingulectomized cats, motor signs suggested catatonia.[325] The consequences of surgical cingulate ablation for psychiatric disturbance in humans are difficult to interpret because the amount of cingulate removed is usually small.[326]

The full syndrome of akinetic mutism or abulia has thus not been produced in animals by experimental cingulectomy or in humans by surgical cingulectomy, and even bilateral ACA ligation in humans has on occasion failed to cause the syndrome.[303] In an autopsy report of eight patients with akinetic mutism and bilateral cingulate destruction, no difference was seen in the clinical picture regardless of whether additional lesions existed in the medial orbital cortex or septal region.[311] Most reports, however, have emphasized additional lesions or diffuse compressive cerebral injury,[302,303] and electroencephalograms usually show bilateral cerebral slowing.[303] An angiographic study of patients with subarachnoid hemorrhage showed correlation of unilateral or bilateral ACA vasospasm with akinetic mutism, but it was unclear whether brain damage was limited to one hemisphere in the patients with unilateral vasospasm.[327]

Abulia has also followed unilateral or bilateral caudate infarction (most likely from occlusion of the recurrent artery of Heubner). In one series of unilateral caudate infarction in 17 patients, abulia was the most prominent feature in ten patients (six left, four right).[65] In four patients, CT showed the lesions to be restricted to the caudate; in others, the anterior limb of the internal capsule was involved. Three abulic patients had alternating restlessness and hyperactivity, and in four others, hyperactivity was present without abulia. In another report it was proposed that abulia resulted from damage to the dorsolateral caudate (which connects to the dorsolateral frontal lobe) and disinhibition from damage to the ventromedial caudate (which connects to orbitofrontal areas).[328]

After surgical partial section of the anterior corpus callosum, acute akinetic mutism is often seen, but patients tend to recover over days.[329,330] Positron emission tomography studies in baboons showed that the procedure causes transient depression of cortical metabolism in widespread areas of both frontal lobes (diaschisis).[331]

Language Disturbance

Unilateral ACA occlusion can produce language disturbance, but whether the disturbance is aphasic is uncertain.[332–334] Details are often lacking in case reports. In some patients, "reduction of spontaneous verbal expression"[314] or muteness, often in association with more global psychomotor bradykinesia,[314,335] seems to be a manifestation of abulia; in such patients' comprehension of spoken speech may be untestable.[336] Some investigators describe true impairment of speech comprehension,[337] word-finding difficulty, alexia,[46] and phonemic or verbal paraphasias on spontaneous speech, reading aloud, or writing.[337,338] Others, however, emphasize the absence of paraphasias[335,339,340] or consider the difficulty "partly defects of an aphasic order and partly those of a dysarthria."[43] A number of reports describe impairment of spontaneous speech with normal repetition and sometimes echolalia (transcortical aphasia),[336,339,341–344] and in one instance, echolalia and palilalia occurred without other evidence of aphasia.[190] A man with transcortical motor aphasia, although lacking echolalia and echopraxia, could not refrain from completing the sentences of others.[345] Some patients have had transcortical aphasia, with relative preservation of speech repetition and a strikingly greater impairment of list naming than of naming to confrontation,[339] or particularly impaired speech initiative, as in attempts to narrate stories or describe complex pictures.[345]

A patient with transcortical mixed aphasia had infarction of both the medial frontal and the medial parietal lobes, whereas two other patients with transcortical motor aphasia had infarction of only the medial frontal lobe.[344] After a large left ACA infarction, a patient had transcortical motor aphasia and mirror writing.[334] Another, who was right-handed, had left-handed mirror writing after infarction of the right medial frontal cortex sparing the corpus callosum, leading to the conjecture that the SMA is "responsible for nonmirror transformation of motor programs originating in the left hemisphere before execution by the primary motor area in the right hemisphere."[346] A woman with aphasia that included impairment of comprehension, repetition, reading, and writing had medial frontal infarction plus an old infarct over the rolandic convexity.[347]

In some patients, speech disturbance was transient, whereas paucity of other movements, including writing, persisted.[337] *Strategic infarct dementia* is a term also used to describe the paucity of speech and motor behavior, accompanied by long delays in response and poor scores on tests involving narrative and naming response. Deep infarcts in the anterior limb of the internal capsule or anterior thalamus are associated with this syndrome.[348,349]

Nearly all reports of severe language impairment after pathologically documented ACA occlusion have involved left-sided lesions[334] with one exception:[350] a right-handed woman with left hemiparesis, diffuse bradykinesia, speech limited to short replies to questions, and a tendency to echolalia; naming and comprehension of spoken or written language seemed impaired in this patient but were difficult to test. At autopsy, infarction was found in the territory of the right ACA, including the head of the caudate, the anterior limb of the internal capsule, the anterior putamen, the anterior cingulate and superior frontal gyri, and the entire SMA (Fig. 23-7). Several reports describe language disturbance after bilateral ACA occlusion,[336,351,352] including stuttering;[353] in one report with neither postmortem examination nor disclosure of the patient's handedness, the patient had occlusion of the right ACA.[354] Another report described two right-handed women with transient verbal output loss, normal writing and ability to comprehend spoken language, and infarction of the right

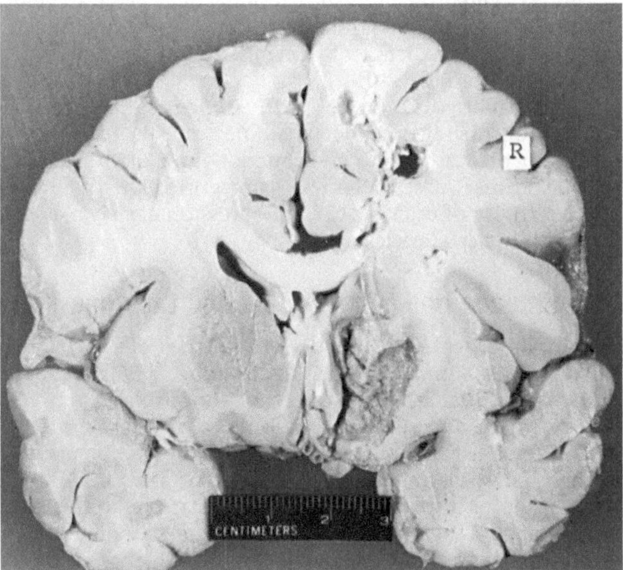

Figure 23-7. Autopsy specimen showing a coronal section of the anterior frontal and temporal lobes. There is infarction in the territories of both the proximal and distal portions of the right anterior cerebral artery. Affected areas include the caudate, putamen, internal capsule's anterior limb, cingulate gyrus, and supplementary motor area. *(From Brust JCM, Plank C, Burke A, et al. Language disorder in a right-hander after occlusion of the right anterior cerebral artery.* Neurology *32:492, 1982.)*

anterior cingulate cortex. In these cases, impaired speech initiation was attributed to disruption of a signal transmission through the right anterior corpus callosum to the left language network.[354] A man with right SMA infarction had "aphemia": impaired articulation with normal repetition, auditory comprehension, reading, and writing. The author proposed that both SMAs participate in the initiation of articulatory movements, but only the left SMA affects linguistic aspects of speech.[355]

Most investigators, regardless of whether they consider these abnormalities to be truly aphasic, attribute them to damage to the SMA on the medial surface of the frontal lobe, anterior to the paracentral lobule, and between the cingulate and superior frontal gyri (i.e., the medial hemispheric part of Brodmann's area 6).[332,356–358] Of ten right-handed patients with left ACA territory infarcts described in one report, four had transcortical motor aphasia, and in each, the SMA was involved. Three other patients with sparing of the SMA but involvement of the cingulate had only "alterations of verbal memory."[359] In monkeys, stimulation of this area causes arm and leg movements and head turning, and there seems to be rostral–caudal forelimb–hindlimb somatotopy.[360–366] Unilateral ablation of the SMA in monkeys produces a deficit in tasks of bimanual coordination.[367] In humans, SMA stimulation induces bodily postures (e.g., turning of the head and eyes toward a contralaterally uplifted arm) or repetitive movements (e.g., stepping or hand-waving).[358] Such responses are often bilateral and can occur after ablation of area 4 (the primary motor cortex). SMA stimulation can also cause speech and movement arrest or vocalization.[368]

Although stimulation of the face region of area 4 causes vocalization of continuous vowel sounds,[368] SMA stimulation on either hemisphere[183] produces intermittently repeated words, syllables, or meaningless combinations of syllables (saccadic vocalization).[368] The repeated word might be a palilalia of what was being said at the onset of stimulation. Rhythmic mouth and jaw movements sometimes accompany the vocalization. Speech arrest, hesitation, or slowing also occurs, sometimes with mouth movements suggesting attempted speech or with arrest of other voluntary movement. Speech comprehension is usually preserved, but anomia and paraphasias have occurred.[183]

Such symptoms, with or without other motor, sensory, or autonomic phenomena, may be the manifestation of seizures caused by structural lesions affecting the SMA, especially meningiomas.[348,351,369–373] Although experimental stimulation of either the right or left SMA can cause speech arrest or repetition, seizures causing altered speech have only rarely occurred in right-handed persons with lesions of the right SMA.[374] Both stimulation and seizure phenomena raise the question of whether true aphasia is occurring and which brain structures are, in fact, responsible.

Destructive lesions, including infarction, are similarly problematic. Medial hemispheric structural lesions such as neoplasm, vascular malformation, subdural empyema, surgical ablation, and trauma not only can directly affect more regions than the SMA, but also produce distant effects from edema or brain distortion. SMA excision for the treatment of epilepsy has led to language disturbance, but interpretation of such cases has varied. One group found that excision of the language hemisphere's SMA back to area 4 caused muteness, whereas excision of the language hemisphere's anterior SMA or the non-language hemisphere's entire SMA produced "no specific deficit."[375] Others found, after excision of either SMA, more lasting speech disturbances, although they seemed nonaphasic and secondary to bradykinesia.[376] Bilateral ideomotor apraxia without aphasia affected two patients with ACA infarction involving both the left SMA and the corpus callosum.[377]

The SMA receives afferents from the ipsilateral primary and secondary somatosensory cortex and has reciprocal connections to ipsilateral area 4, posterior parietal cortex, upper convexity premotor cortex (area 6), several thalamic nuclei, and, across the corpus callosum, the contralateral SMA and convexity area 6.[378–380] It has been suggested, therefore, that the SMA is "an area of sensory convergence."[360] Efferents project bilaterally to the cingulate gyrus and striatum;[291,335,381,382] ipsilaterally to the red nucleus, pontine nuclei, and dorsal column nuclei;[349] and contralaterally to area 4 and the midconvexity premotor region (area 8).[335] There are also SMA neurons that project to the spinal cord.[361,383,384] Regional cerebral blood flow (rCBF) increases in the SMA during automatic speech and during repetitive finger movement but not during isometric hand muscle contraction.[385–387] Cerebral blood flow also increases in the SMA during planning of sequential movements.[388–390] (By contrast, the cerebral blood flow of area 4 increases only during execution of such movements.[389]) In monkeys, medullary pyramidal section did not affect movements produced by SMA stimulation,[391] increased discharge of SMA neurons preceded stereotyped learned motor tasks of either the ipsilateral or contralateral extremities, and SMA neurons fired in response to sensory signals "only when the signal called for a motor response."[365] Neurons in the SMA are, however, less responsive to peripheral stimuli than those in area 4,[360,365] which suggests that part of the SMA's function may be "to 'gate' or suppress the afferent influences on area 4"[187] (perhaps accounting for the transient contralateral grasp reflex commonly seen after SMA ablation).[183,339,358,366,392] Such suppression would convert area 4's activity from a closed loop to an open loop mode,[365,393] consistent with the further notion that the SMA develops "a preparatory state" for impending movement[364,394] or that it elaborates "programs for motor subroutines necessary in skilled voluntary motion,"[395] including, with its "sequences of fast isolated muscular contraction", human speech.[389]

The often-cited case described by Bonhoeffer[199] in 1914 may represent ACA occlusion causing language disturbance by a different mechanism. The patient experienced right hemiplegia, with the leg weaker than the arm, plus reduction of speech to one or two words, relatively preserved comprehension of spoken speech, alexia, agraphia, and apraxia (difficulty following commands, imitating, and handling objects) that was greater on the left than the right. Abnormalities at autopsy included infarction of the posterior left middle and superior frontal gyri, the anterior four-fifths of the corpus callosum, the anterior limb of the left internal capsule, and a small part of the left posterior inferior parietal lobule. Bonhoeffer[199] (and Geschwind,[246] reviewing the case 50 years later) explained the left apraxia as that resulting from the callosal lesion and the aphasia from the combined callosal and capsular lesions, which in effect isolated Broca's area; the posterior parietal lesion probably contributed to the alexia, agraphia, and right apraxia. Neither writer discussed the possible contribution of SMA destruction to the language disturbance, which theoretically could have occurred without it.

Other Mental Abnormalities

Besides abulia, apraxia, and language impairment, patients with ACA occlusion can have a variety of other emotional or intellectual disturbances, usually attributed to involvement of structures supplied by branches of the proximal ACA (A1 segment or ACoA).[60,370,396] Anxiety, fear, insomnia, talkativeness, or agitation have occurred with or without weakness, bradykinesia, or grasp and suck reflexes.[43,190,311,370] A young woman, awakening from a coma after ACoA aneurysm rupture, had severe withdrawal with unprovoked agitation and screaming; autopsy demonstrated bilateral infarction of the orbital gyri, gyri recti, septal nuclei, cingulate gyri, hippocampal formations, and right amygdala.[397] Damage to hypothalamic or other limbic structures has also been considered responsible for these symptoms,[54] which, when they predominate, can suggest nonstructural neurotic or psychotic illness.[41] In any event, the notion that apathy and poor motivation predictably follow dorsolateral frontal lesions and that orbitofrontal damage causes disinhibited behavior appears to be an oversimplification.[313,398]

Confusion, disorientation, and memory loss, sometimes severe, also occur.[40,82,351,399–402] Retrograde and anterograde amnesia after ACoA aneurysm rupture may be subtle or severe,[403–406] with variable denial or confabulation.[195,407–409] In one report, a patient with bilateral infarction of both medial frontal lobes as well as the right inferior temporal lobe and pole had severely impaired recognition of previously presented words or pictures yet could spontaneously recall them.[410] In another report, five patients with lesions restricted to basal forebrain structures (sparing the hippocampus and temporal lobes) were able to recall particular stimuli (e.g., someone's name or face) but could not bring such differently learned components together as an integrated memory.[411] Structures that have been implicated in these amnestic syndromes include the hypothalamus, medial forebrain bundle, septum, nucleus basalis of Meynert, nucleus accumbens, and fornix, with possible secondary dysfunction of medial temporal regions.[412–414] Bilateral infarction of the caudate nucleus and fornix resulted in impaired verbal working memory and "delayed recall."[415] Left caudate infarction in five patients resulted in impairment of both declarative memory and motor procedural memory.[416]

Functional neuroimaging studies implicate medial frontal structures in the ability of humans to attribute mental states to others ("mentalizing," "Theory of Mind").[417] Such a role was questioned in a study of a woman with bilateral ACA territory infarction who had impairments in planning and memory but who performed normally on Theory of Mind tasks.[418]

Of 251 patients examined 3 months after acute ischemic stroke, 66 had dementia. Infarction in the territory of the left ACA was more predictive of dementia than infarction in the MCA or PCA territory.[419]

Visuospatial disturbance with difficulty in dressing, drawing, or copying or with left hemineglect has occurred after infarction of the caudate and anterior limb of the internal capsule. Primary dyscalculia was also reported after infarction in the territory of the left ACA.[420] Depression has been associated with left caudate lesions.[421]

Incontinence and Other Autonomic Changes

Urinary (and, less often, fecal) incontinence can occur with either unilateral or bilateral ACA occlusion.[41,43,63] Involvement of the paracentral lobule (presuming homuncular representation of motor and sensory components of micturition) has been offered as an explanation,[40,109] even though paracentral stimulation was found to produce only contralateral sensation without motor response in the penis.[422] Damage to the superior medial frontal lobe, especially the midportion of the superior frontal gyrus, the cingulate, and the white matter in between, is a more likely cause, because such damage (e.g., from frontal leukotomy) causes transient or permanent disturbance of urination and defecation, including urgency and incontinence.[229,423–425]

Cardiorespiratory alterations are common after stroke, regardless of whether limbic structures are specifically damaged.[426,427] Such changes seen after ACA occlusion are therefore open to interpretation, but it is not unreasonable to incriminate damage to the hypothalamus, cingulate gyrus, or other limbic areas. Fever not always related to infection, tachycardia, and unexpected death have followed cingulate infarction in humans.[310,311] Human and animal cingulate stimulation can produce altered respiration, bradycardia, temporary respiratory or cardiac arrest, hypertension or hypotension, pupillary dilatation, and piloerection.[310,428,429] Diabetes insipidus, perhaps from anterior hypothalamic infarction, has occurred after surgical occlusion of a proximal ACA for ACoA aneurysm.[43,60] Gastrointestinal bleeding after ACoA aneurysm rupture has also been blamed on hypothalamic damage.[430]

Miscellaneous Symptoms

Visual loss has followed compression of the optic nerve or chiasm by an ACA aneurysm or dolichoectasia.[431,432] Bitemporal hemianopia occurred from compression of the optic chiasm by an elongated right ACA.[433]

Inability to close the left eye on verbal command with otherwise preserved movement of left facial muscles followed right ACA territory infarction. The authors suspected an apraxia of eye closure from damage to the anterior corpus callosum.[434]

Generalized tonic-clonic seizures during menses arose from a region of the left frontal lobe supplied by an aberrant contralateral orbitofrontal artery. The authors speculated that increased progesterone levels during the luteal phase lowered blood pCO_2, leading to ischemia in the tenuously supplied region.[435]

Periventricular Leukomalacia of Infancy

Brains of infants dying within hours or months of birth may have necrotic foci along the lateral ventricles, considered by some investigators to be infarcts at border zones between the territories of the ACA, MCA, and PCA.[436] Others have stressed that the periventricular areas are more properly called end zones and are not in anastomotic areas but rather within a few millimeters of the ventricular wall "between the terminal distributions of ventriculopetal and ventriculofugal branches of small arteries that penetrate deeply into the brain,"[37] including those from the ACA passing through the cingulate gyrus.[438] Such lesions usually spare the cerebral cortex because the fetus has rich meningeal anastomoses between pial vessels and because the white matter in newborns has a relatively higher metabolic rate.[437] Hypotensive newborn dogs develop decreased white matter blood flow and lesions resembling those of periventricular leukomalacia.[439] Autopsy in infants with periventricular leukomalacia and no apparent perinatal asphyxia has shown poorly developed ventriculofugal branches.[438,440] Affected infants display lethargy, hypotonia, difficulty feeding, and seizures; survivors are usually intellectually disabled, with spastic quadriparesis.

Because cerebral autoregulation is impaired in neonates with asphyxia, periventricular hemorrhage in the newborn may be the result of capillary dilatation and rupture in these same deep end zones.[436]

The complete reference list can be found on the companion Expert Consult website at www.expertconsult.inkling.com.

KEY REFERENCES

1. Bogousslavsky J, Regli F. Anterior cerebral artery territory infarction in the Lausanne Stroke Registry: Clinical and etiological patterns. Arch Neurol 1990;47:144.
2. Moussouttas M, Boland T, Chung L, et al. Prevalence, timing, risk factors, and mechanisms of anterior cerebral artery infarctions following subarachnoid hemorrhage. J Neurol 2013; 260:21.
3. Gacs G, Fox AJ, Barnett HJM, et al. Occurrence and mechanism of occlusion of the anterior cerebral artery. Stroke 1983;14:952.
5. Hollander M, Bots ML, Del Sol AI, et al. Carotid plaques increase the risk of stroke and subtypes of cerebral infarction in asymptomatic elderly: The Rotterdam study. Circulation 2002; 105:2872.
6. Rodda RA. The arterial patterns associated with internal carotid disease and cerebral infarcts. Stroke 1986;17:69.
7. Kang SY, Sim JS. Anterior cerebral artery infarction. Stroke mechanism and clinical-imaging study in 100 patients. Neurology 2008;70:2386.
8. Arboix A, Garcia-Eroles L, Sellares N, et al. Infarction in the territory of the anterior cerebral artery: clinical study of 51 patients. BMC Neurol 2009;9:30.
9. Castaigne P, Lhermitte F, Escourelle R, et al. Étude anatomopathologique de 74 infarcts de l'artère cérébrale antérieure (55 observations). Rev Med Toulouse 1975;(Suppl.):339.
19. Kodera T, Hirose S, Takeuchi H, et al. Radiological findings for arterial dissection of the anterior cerebral artery. J Clin Neurosci 2007;14:77.
32. Lim SM, Chae EJ, Kim MY, et al. Steal phenomenon through the anterior communicating artery in Moyamoya disease. Eur Radiol 2007;17:61.
37. King S, Khatri P, Carrozella J, et al. Anterior cerebral artery emboli in combined intravenous and intra-arterial rtPA treatment of acute ischemic stroke in the IMS I and II trials. AJNR Am J Neuroradiol 2007;28:1890.
38. Czochra M, Kozniewska H, Muszynski A, et al. Surgical treatment of aneurysms of the anterior communicating artery using Yasargil's approach. Neurol Neurochir Pol 1979;13:71.
39. Perlmutter D, Rhoton AL. Microsurgical anatomy of the anterior cerebral-anterior communicating-recurrent artery complex. J Neurosurg 1976;45:259.
40. Perlmutter D, Rhoton AL. Microsurgical anatomy of the distal anterior cerebral artery. J Neurosurg 1978;49:204.
42. Beevor CE. The cerebral arterial supply. Brain 1907;30:403.
43. Critchley M. The anterior cerebral artery and its syndromes. Brain 1930;53:120.
45. Lazorthes G, Bastide G, Gomes FA. Les variations du trajet de la carotide interne d'après une étude artériographe. Arch Anat Pathol 1961;9:129.
47. Marino R. The anterior cerebral artery. I: Anatomico-radiological study of its cortical territories. Surg Neurol 1976;5:81.
51. Heubner O. Zur Topographie der Ernährungsgebiete der einzelnen Hirnarterien. Zentralbl Med Wissenschaften 1872;10: 817.
52. Ostrowski AZ, Webster JE, Gurdjian ES. The proximal anterior cerebral artery: An anatomic study. Arch Neurol 1960;3:661.
54. Dunker RO, Harris AB. Surgical anatomy of the proximal anterior cerebral artery. J Neurosurg 1976;44:359.
55. Gomes F, Dujouny M, Umansky F, et al. Microsurgical anatomy of the recurrent artery of Heubner. J Neurosurg 1984;60:130.
61. Alexander MP, Freedman M. Amnesia after anterior communicating artery aneurysm rupture. Neurology 1983;33(Suppl. 2): 104.
64. Ghika JA, Bogousslavsky J, Regli F. Deep perforators from the carotid system: Template of the vascular territories. Arch Neurol 1990;47:1097.
65. Caplan LR, Schmahmann JD, Kase CS, et al. Caudate infarcts. Arch Neurol 1990;47:133.
71. Cobb S. The cerebral circulation. 13: The question of "end-arteries" of the brain and the mechanism of infarction. Arch Neurol Psychiatry 1931;25:273.
72. Shellshear JC. The basal arteries of the forebrain and their functional significance. J Anat 1920;55:27.
73. Van den Bergh R, Vander Eecken H. Anatomy and embryology of cerebral circulation. Prog Brain Res 1968;30:1.
78. Lasjaunias P, Vignaud J, Clay C. Radioanatomie de la vascularisation artérielle de l'orbite, à l'éxception du tronc de l'artère ophtalmique. Ann Radiol 1975;18:181.
79. Van der Zwan A, Hillen B, Tulleken CAF, et al. Variability of the territories of the major cerebral arteries. J Neurosurg 1992; 77:927.

84. Uchino A, Nomiyama K, Takase Y, et al. Anterior cerebral artery variations detected by MR angiography. Neuroradiology 2006;46: 647.
88. Kirgis HD, Fisher WL, Llewellyn RC, et al. Aneurysms of the anterior communicating artery and gross anomalies of the circle of Willis. J Neurosurg 1966;25:73.
95. Kapoor K, Singh B, Dewan LI. Variations in the configuration of the circle of Willis. Anat Sci Int 2008;83:96.
97. Pearce JMS. Heubner's artery. Eur Neurol 2005;54:112.
111. Milenkovic Z. Anastomosis between internal carotid artery and anterior cerebral artery with other anomalies of the circle of Willis in a fetal brain. J Neurosurg 1981;55:701.
115. Padget DH. The development of the cranial arteries in the human embryo. Contrib Embryol 1948;32:205.
124. Kahilogullari G, Comert A, Arslan M, et al. Callosal branches of the anterior cerebral artery: An anatomical report. Clin Anat 2008;21:383.
126. Fawcett E, Blachford JV. The circle of Willis: An examination of 700 specimens. J Anat Physiol 1905/06;40:63a.
128. Lazorthes G, Gaubert J, Poulhes J. La distribution centrale et corticale de l'artère cérébrale antérieure: Étude anatomique et incidences neuro-chirurgicales. Neurochirurgie 1956;2: 237.
129. Van der Eecken H. Discussion of "collateral circulation of the brain". Neurology 1961;11:16.
131. Ruggiero G. Factors influencing the filling of the anterior cerebral artery in angiography. Acta Radiol 1952;37:87.
136. Niizuma H, Kwak R, Uchida K, et al. Aneurysms of the azygous anterior cerebral artery. Surg Neurol 1980;15:225.
144. Ogawa A, Suzuki M, Sakurai Y, et al. Vascular anomalies associated with aneurysms of the anterior communicating artery: Microsurgical observations. J Neurosurg 1990;72: 706.
146. Schick RM, Rumbaugh CL. Saccular aneurysm of the azygous anterior cerebral artery. AJNR Am J Neuroradiol 1989;10(Suppl.): S73.
152. Bikmaz K, Erdem E, Kright A. Arteriovenous fistula originating from proximal part of the anterior cerebral artery. Clin Neurol Neurosurg 2007;109:589.
153. Lehecka M, Lehto H, Niemela M, et al. Distal anterior cerebral artery aneurysms. Treatment and outcome analysis of 501 patients. Neurosurgery 2008;62:590.
158. Hashizume K, Nukui H, Horikoshi T, et al. Giant aneurysm of the azygous anterior cerebral artery associated with acute subdural hematoma: Case report. Neurol Med Chir (Tokyo) 1992; 32:693.
165. Ito J, Washiyama K, Kim CH, et al. Fenestration of the anterior cerebral artery. Neuroradiology 1981;21:277.
170. Ward AA. The anterior cingulate gyrus and personality. Res Publ Assoc Nerv Ment Dis 1948;27:438.
171. Hayakawa T, Waltz AG. Immediate effects of cerebral ischemia: Evolution and resolution of neurological deficits after experimental occlusion of one middle cerebral artery in conscious cats. Stroke 1975;6:321.
175. Rieke GK, Bowers DE, Penn P. Vascular supply pattern to rat caudatoputamen and globus pallidus: Scanning electron microscopic study of vascular endocasts of stroke-prone vessels. Stroke 1981;12:840.
179. Tichy F. The syndromes of the cerebral arteries. Arch Pathol 1949;48:475.
182. Chamorro A, Marshall RS, Valls-Sole J, et al. Motor behavior in stroke patients with isolated medial frontal ischemic infarction. Stroke 1997;28:1755.
183. Penfield W, Jasper H. Epilepsy and the functional anatomy of the human brain. Boston: Little, Brown; 1954.
186. Wilson G. Crural monoplegia. Arch Neurol Psychiatry 1923;10: 699.
191. Foix C, Hillemand P. Les syndromes de l'artère cérébrale antérieure. Encephale 1925;20:209.
192. Lhermitte J, Schiff P, Curtois A. Le phénomène de la préhension forcée, expression d'un ramollissement complet de la première convolution frontale. Rev Neurol 1907;15:1218.
201. Bonhoeffer K. Klischer U. anatomischer Befund zur Lehre von der Apraxie und der motorischen Sprachbahn. Monatsschr Psychiatr Neurol 1914;35:113.
202. Ghika J, Bogousslavsky J, van Melle G, et al. Hyperkinetic motor behaviors contralateral to hemiplegia in acute stroke. Eur Neurol 1995;35:27.
204. Karnath H-O, Suchan J, Johannsen L. Pusher syndrome after ACA territory infarction. Eur J Neurol 2008;15:e84.
205. Bogousslavsky J, Regli F. Capsular genu syndrome. Neurology 1990;40:1499.
213. Stuss DT, Benson DF. Neuropsychological studies of the frontal lobes. Psychol Bull 1984;95:3.
223. Marie P, Foix C. Paraplégie en flexion d'origine cérébrale par nécrose sous épendymaire progressive. Rev Neurol 1920;27:1.
225. Meyer JS, Barron DW. Apraxia of gait: A clinicophysiological study. Brain 1960;83:261.
226. Ueno E. Clinical and physiological study of apraxia of gait and frozen gait. Rinsho Shinkeigaku 1989;29:275.
241. Geschwind N, Kaplan E. A human cerebral disconnection syndrome: A preliminary report. Neurology 1962;12:675.
244. Geschwind N. The apraxias: Neural mechanisms of disorders of learned movement. Am Sci 1975;63:188.
246. Geschwind N. Disconnection syndromes in animals and man. Brain 1965;88:237.
250. Luria AR, Tsvetkova LS. Towards the mechanism of "dynamic aphasia". Acta Neurol Belg 1967;67:1045.
251. Watson RT, Heilman KM. Callosal apraxia. Brain 1983;106:391.
252. Goldberg G, Mayer NH, Toglia JU. Medial frontal cortex infarction and the alien hand sign. Arch Neurol 1981;38:683.
253. Feinberg TE, Schindler RJ, Flanagan NG, et al. Two alien hand syndromes. Neurology 1992;42:19.
254. Gasquoine PG. Alien hand sign. J Clin Exp Neuropsychol 1993; 15:653.
264. Lhermitte F, Pillon B, Serdaru M. Human anatomy and the frontal lobes. Part I: Imitation and utilization behavior: A neuropsychological study of 75 patients. Ann Neurol 1986;19:326.
267. Gazzaniga MS, Bogen JE, Sperry RW. Some functional effects of sectioning the cerebral commissures in man. Proc Natl Acad Sci U S A 1962;48:1765.
269. Bogen JE, Gazzaniga MS. Cerebral commissurotomy in man: Minor hemisphere dominance for certain visuo-spatial functions. J Neurosurg 1965;23:394.
271. Gazzaniga MS, Sperry RW. Language after section of the cerebral commissures. Brain 1967;90:131.
278. Gazzaniga MS, LeDoux JE, Wilson DH. Language, praxis, and the right hemisphere: Clues to some mechanisms of consciousness. Neurology 1977;27:1144.
282. Heilman KM, Coyle JM, Gonyea EF, et al. Apraxia and agraphia in a left-hander. Brain 1973;96:21.
284. Kimura D, Archibald Y. Motor functions of the left hemisphere. Brain 1974;97:337.
288. Volpe BT, Sidtis JJ, Holzman JD, et al. Cortical mechanisms involved in praxis: Observations following partial and complete section of the corpus callosum in man. Neurology 1982;32: 645.
298. Segarra JM. Cerebral vascular disease and behavior. I: The syndrome of the mesencephalic artery (basilar artery bifurcation). Arch Neurol 1970;22:408.
300. Castaigne P, Buge A, Cambier J, et al. Démence thalamique d'origine vasculaire par ramollissement bilateral, limité au territoire du pedicule retromammilaire. Rev Neurol 1966; 114:89.
309. Nielsen JM, Jacobs LL. Bilateral lesions of the anterior cingulate gyri. Bull Los Angeles Neurol Soc 1951;16:231.
313. Meador KJ, Watson RT, Bowers D, et al. Hypometria with hemispatial and limb motor neglect. Brain 1986;109:293.
319. Halsband U, Ito N, Tanji J, et al. The role of premotor cortex and the supplementary motor area in the temporal control of movement in man. Brain 1993;116:243.
326. Whitty CWM, Duffield JE, Tow PM, et al. Anterior cingulectomy in the treatment of mental disease. Lancet 1952;1:475.
328. Mendez MF, Adams NL, Lewandowski KS. Neurobehavioral changes associated with caudate lesions. Neurology 1989;39:349.
335. Damasio AR, Van Hoesen GW. Structure and function of the supplementary motor area. Neurology 1980;30:359.
337. Masdeu JC, Schoene WC, Funkenstein H. Aphasia following infarction of the left supplementary motor area: A clinical pathological study. Neurology 1978;28:1220.

342. Damasio AR, Kassel NF. Transcortical motor aphasia in relation to lesions of the supplementary motor area. Neurology 1978;28: 396.
350. Brust JCM, Plank C, Burke A, et al. Language disorder in a right-hander after occlusion of the right anterior cerebral artery. Neurology 1982;32:492.
358. Penfield W, Welch K. The supplementary motor area of the cerebral cortex: A clinical and experimental study. Arch Neurol Psychiatry 1951;66:289.
375. Penfield W, Rasmussen T. The Cerebral Cortex of Can: a Clinical Ctudy of Localization of Function. New York: Macmillan; 1950.
377. Watson RT, Fleet S, Gonzalez-Rothi L, et al. Apraxia and the supplementary motor area. Arch Neurol 1986;43:787.
385. Ingvar DH, Schwartz MS. Blood flow patterns induced in the dominant hemisphere by speech and reading. Brain 1974;97:273.
386. Larson B, Skinhoj E, Larsen NA. Variations in regional cortical blood flow in the right and left hemispheres during automatic speech. Brain 1978;101:193.
389. Roland PE, Larsen B, Lassen NA, et al. Supplementary motor areas in organization of voluntary movements in man. J Neurophysiol 1980;43:118.
397. Faris AA. Limbic system infarction. J Neuropathol Exp Neurol 1967;26:174.
398. Grafman J, Vance SC, Weingartner H, et al. The effects of lateralized frontal lesions on mood regulation. Brain 1986;109:1127.
399. Davison C, Goodhart SP, Needles W. Cerebral localization in cerebrovascular disease. Res Publ Assoc Res Nerv Ment Dis 1934;13:435.
404. Parkin AJ, Leng NRC, Stanhope N, et al. Memory impairment following ruptured aneurysm of the anterior communicating artery. Brain Cogn 1988;7:231.
411. Damasio AR, Graff-Radford NR, Eslinger PJ, et al. Amnesia following basal forebrain lesions. Arch Neurol 1985;42:263.
413. Wolfe N, Linn R, Babikian VL, et al. Frontal system impairment following multiple lacunar infarcts. Arch Neurol 1990;47:129.
414. Moudgil SS, Azzouz M, Al-Azzaz A, et al. Amnesia due to fornix infarction. Stroke 2000;31:1418.
416. Mizuta H, Motomura N. Mental dysfunction in caudate infarction caused by Heubner's recurring artery occlusion. Brain Cogn 2006;61:133.
419. Tatemichi TK, Desmond DW, Patik M, et al. Clinical determinants of dementia related to stroke. Ann Neurol 1993;33:568.
422. Penfield W, Boldrey E. Somatic motor and sensory representation in cerebral cortex of man as studied by electrical stimulation. Brain 1937;60:384.
423. Andrew J, Nathan PW. Lesions of the anterior frontal lobes and disturbances of micturition and defecation. Brain 1964;87:233.
429. Segundo JP, Naquet R, Buser P. Cortical stimulation in monkeys. J Neurophysiol 1955;18:236.
437. De Reuck J, Chatta AS, Richardson EP. Pathogenesis and evolution of periventricular leukomalacia in infancy. Arch Neurol 1972;27:229.
439. Young RSK, Hernandez MJ, Yagel SK. Selective reduction of blood flow to white matter during hypotension in newborn dogs: A possible mechanism of periventricular leukomalacia. Ann Neurol 1982;12:445.

24 Middle Cerebral Artery Disease

Vijay K. Sharma, Lawrence K.S. Wong

KEY POINTS

- The middle cerebral artery (MCA) is the largest cerebral artery and it is the most commonly affected intracranial vessel in cerebrovascular accident. It supplies most of the outer convex brain surface, nearly all the basal ganglia, and the anterior and posterior internal capsules.
- Infarcts that occur within the vast distribution of MCA territory lead to diverse neurologic sequelae. In general, the clinical features depend on the site of MCA occlusion. More distal blockages tend to produce milder deficits while the proximal occlusions result in widespread effects that could even be fatal.
- Contralateral hemiparesis and hemisensory loss of the face, upper and lower extremities is the most common presentation of MCA syndrome. Lower extremity function is more spared than that of the faciobrachial region.
- Aphasia is a common feature when the cortical areas of the dominant hemisphere are involved. In comparison, involvement of homologous regions in the nondominant hemisphere often results in impaired awareness of the deficit.
- Advances in modern parenchymal, vascular, molecular and functional imaging techniques have enhanced our understanding of the pathophysiology of various neurological deficits observed in MCA disease and carry potential to predict the extent of expected recovery as well as influence the results of various therapeutic strategies to improve outcome.

The middle cerebral artery (MCA), the largest of the branches of the internal carotid artery (ICA), is also the most commonly affected artery in stroke syndromes.[1–6] The MCA supplies most of the convex surface of the brain, leaving to other cerebral arteries the frontal pole and its immediately adjacent lateral gyro, the extremes of the high parietal and very posterolateral aspects of the occipital gyri, and occipital pole. In the brain parenchyma, its branches irrigate almost all of the basal ganglia and capsules (internal, external, and extreme capsule), claustrum, putamen, the upper parts of the globus pallidus, parts of the substantia innominata of Reichert, the posterior portion of the head and all of the body of the caudate nucleus, and all but the very lowest portions of the anterior and posterior limbs of the internal capsule. Supply to any portion of the thalamus has only rarely been demonstrated.[7]

The internal capsule, classically the MCA territory, has a complex arterial supply. Its anterior limb has some supply from a large branch of the anterior cerebral artery known as Heubner's artery, yet the MCA supplies the anterior limb in one third of cases. Most of the posterior limb of the internal capsule and corona radiata are fed by the deep, lenticulostriate branches of the MCA, whereas the lowest portion of the posterior limb is supplied by the anterior choroidal artery, which usually arises from the internal carotid artery just proximal to the circle of Willis.[8]

DESCRIPTIVE TERMS

The anatomy of the MCA tree has been described by named branching and by the relationship between the vessel and the anatomic landmarks of the cerebral surface.

Names of Stem, Divisions, and Branches

The traditional terminology analogizes the vessel as a tree with a trunk and branches (Fig. 24-1), a clinically useful descriptive method that we employ throughout this chapter. The MCA regularly begins as a single trunk or stem. Its length varies from 18 to 26 mm. The diameter at its origin is roughly 3 mm (range 2.5 mm to 4.9 mm).[9,10] The stem gives rise to most of the lenticulostriate branches, so named because they supply the lentiform nucleus (putamen and pallidum), body of the caudate nucleus, and the internal capsule.[9] The claustrum and external capsule are supplied by vessels from the surface, penetrating through the insula.[11] The lenticulostriate arteries are five to 17 branches, each of them end arteries that supply cones of varying size of adjacent tissue in their curvilinear (on coronal view) course to end in the corona radiata near the lateral ventricular wall. Some smaller lenticulostriate arteries may arise from the distal internal carotid artery.[10]

No clear correlations between the length of the MCA stem and the pattern or number of the lenticulostriate arteries has been shown, nor does the pattern on one side predict that on the other.[10] The lenticulostriate arteries arising more medially on the MCA stem are the smaller vessels (50 to 150 μm), whereas those arising more laterally are larger (some as large as 500 μm). Three patterns of origin of the lenticulostriate arteries from the MCA have been described.[10] In the most common variant (49%), one or more of the larger lenticulostriate branches arise just beyond the major bifurcation (in the territory of the upper division). The next most common permutation (39%) features all the larger lenticulostriate arteries arising from the stem just proximal to its bifurcation. In the least commonly encountered pattern, some of the larger penetrators arise from the medial portion of the stem. These variations may explain differing patterns of infarction from occlusion of the MCA stem alone or its main divisions. One important anatomic feature of these arteries is the lack of anastomoses among themselves.

The cerebral surface, centrum semiovale, claustrum, external capsule, hemispheral cortex, and white matter are supplied by those MCA branches that originate beyond the lenticulostriate arteries. These cortical surface branches usually number 12 to 15. They arise from the MCA stem in a variety of patterns, and by far the most common (78%) is

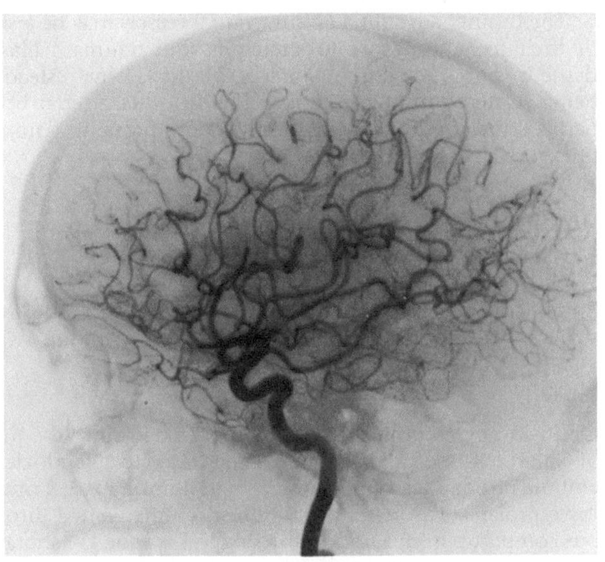

Figure 24-1. Lateral view of the middle cerebral artery anatomy.

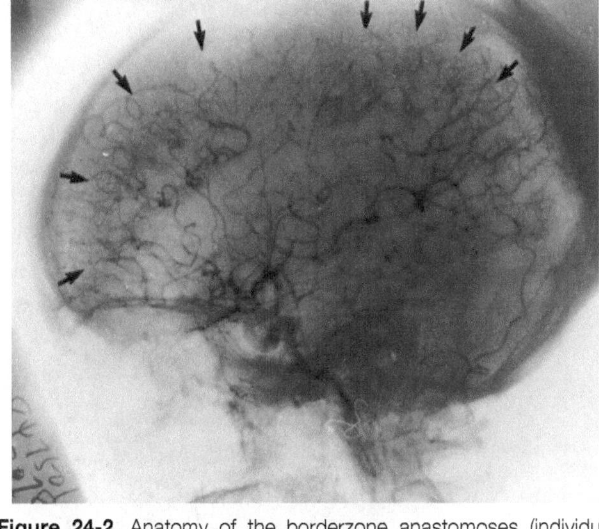

Figure 24-2. Anatomy of the borderzone anastomoses (individual anastomoses shown by *arrows*).

two large branches (bifurcation pattern).[9] Less often (12%) the 12 branches arise from three major trunks (trifurcation pattern). The least differentiated and least common (10% of cases) is the continuation of the stem with no major divisions, and each of the surface branches arises in turn from the common trunk until the primary vessel has given off 11 of the usual 12 branches, after which it terminates as the angular artery.[6]

In the bifurcation pattern, the two main branches are called the superior and inferior division. The superior division supplies insula, frontal lobe, and rolandic regions and always contains the orbitofrontal and prefrontal branches. The inferior division supplies the temporal polar, anterior temporal, and middle temporal branches. Although the central (rolandic) branch is almost always in the upper division, in a few cases it is included in the lower. Likewise, the posterior temporal branch is almost always in the lower division. The upper division is usually the source of the anterior parietal, posterior parietal and angular branches. No branch arising from the upper division irrigates brain regions that would be expected to be supplied from a branch of the lower division or vice versa.

In the trifurcation pattern, the orbitofrontal, prefrontal, and precentral branches supplying the frontal lobe are regularly represented in the upper division. The middle division is made up of the central (rolandic), the anterior parietal, and the angular branches. Less often, the precentral branch is a member of this trunk on the frontal side, and in a few other instances, the temporooccipital and superior temporal branches are added on the inferior side. The inferior division regularly contains the temporal polar, anterior, and middle temporal branches, to which the posterior temporal and temporooccipital branches are less often added.

Other Anatomic Features

Regardless of the brain regions supplied by each branch, remarkable variations have been found in the position over gyri and sulci of individual branches within their section of the convexity. Variation in length is orderly: the smallest and the shortest branches supply the frontal lobe; the longest, the high parietal and lateral occipital.[12] Only 27% of the orbital frontal branches are as large as 1 mm in diameter.[9] The largest artery is usually the artery of the central (rolandic) sulcus. The more posterior regions of the brain are supplied by fewer arteries, which are larger in diameter, give off fewer major branches, and have the longest course from the circle of Willis to their termination in a borderzone (Fig. 24-2). The temporooccipital artery is 1 mm in diameter in 90% of cases and more than 1.5 mm in up to 63% of cases. This large diameter and the ease with which it can be followed on the surface for long distances helps surgeons to use this branch for the extracranial–intracranial anastomosis operation. The three vessels with the longest course on the cortical surface are the angular, posterior parietal, and temporooccipital arteries. Intraluminal diameters greater than 1 mm have been encountered in up to 86% of angular arteries, in 68% of temporooccipital arteries, and in 52% of posterior parietal arteries but in only 14% of central sulcus arteries.[13]

Arterial Segments in Relation to Anatomic Landmarks

Another method of classifying the MCA branches is based on the relationship of the artery with the major landmarks on the brain, especially the Sylvian fissure, the operculum, and the convex surface. This scheme, which has found its greatest use in angiographic descriptions divides the MCA into four major segments (Fig. 24-3).[9,14] The first sphenoidal segment (M1) occupies the space from the origin of the MCA to the limen insulae. The second segment (M2) encompasses the branches of the upper and lower divisions that overlie the insula. The M3 segments are the continuation of these branches as they curve caudally along the undersurface of the operculum, most of which are upper division branches. The M4 segments describe those portions of the branches of the MCA over the convex surface of the brain.

The MCA branches that constitute the M3 or opercular segment follow the curve of the operculum back over the surface of the insula. Some of these branches reverse course over as much as 180°.[6] The branches passing over the parietal and temporal operculum make less striking reversals of direction, some turning only a few degrees before reaching the convex surface of the temporal and parietal regions. M4 branches of the MCA emerge from the Sylvian fissure beyond the operculum and course along the sulci and gyri of the cerebral convexity. Considerable variation is noted in their path. Upper division M4 branches typically follow a path mainly along the depths of a given sulcus and a few of them pass long

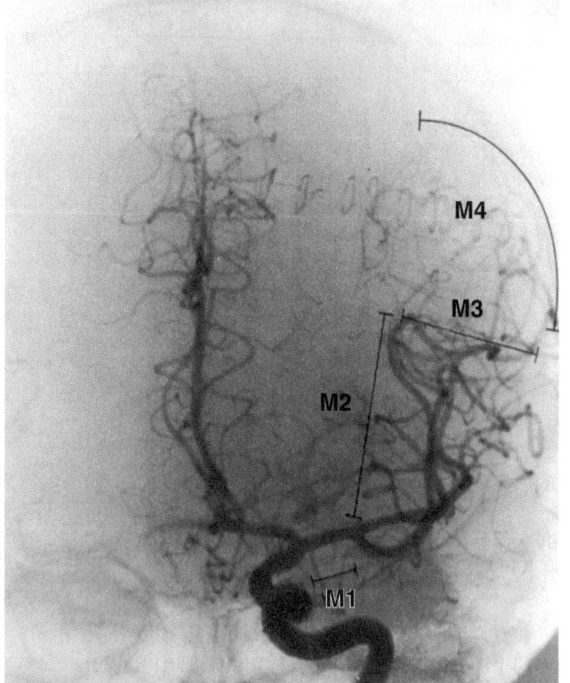

Figure 24-3. Classification of the middle cerebral artery by segments.

distances over the surface of a gyrus, making them also suitable for extracranial-intracranial bypass surgery.

Anomalies

Anomalies of the MCA occur in no more than 3% of cases.[9,15,16] Some writers even dispute their occurrence.[10] Duplication of the MCA is more common, usually arising from the internal carotid artery and supplying the same regions that would otherwise have been supplied by the original MCA. An accessory MCA has also been described,[17] arising from the anterior cerebral artery and runs through the Sylvian fissure along with the normal MCA, usually supplying frontal polar areas. It has been reported in 0.3–4.0% of the general population.[18,19] Previous reports mainly focused on the association of the accessory MCA with cerebral aneurysms and the role of the accessory MCA as a collateral blood supply in the event of MCA occlusion.[20-21] Rarely, an accessory MCA may develop atherosclerosis and present with ischemic symptoms.[22]

Borderzone Anastomoses

For each cerebral surface branch of the major cerebral arteries, the terminal twigs end in a narrow network of vessels that form the borderzone (see Fig. 24-2) between the major arterial territories.[23-25]

HISTOLOGY

The MCA contains the same intima, media, and adventitia as other arteries, but the relative thicknesses of these component parts differ from those in peripheral arteries of comparable size.[26] Compared with extracranial vessels of similar size, the MCA has a narrower adventitia with little elastic tissue and few perivascular supporting structures; the media is also thinner, with some 20 circular muscle layers.[27,28] The internal elastic lamina is thicker[29] and finely fenestrated. The intima, although somewhat thin, seems essentially the same as that of comparably sized vessels elsewhere.[28] No vasa vasorum has been demonstrated in MCA.[28-30]

The thinner adventitia of intracranial vessels may be a sign of their lower exposure to stretching and trauma.[31] Elastic tissue is concentrated in the internal elastic lamina instead of being scattered through the vessel as in other arterial beds, perhaps making intracranial arteries more prone to dampen pulse waves.[29]

PATHOLOGY

Embolism

Embolism exceeds atheroma and accounts for 15–30% of strokes,[32-34] most of which occur in the territory of the MCA.

Etiology

Occlusion by embolism has been appreciated since the time of Chiari.[35] These large ones have been traced to "paradoxical" embolus from a leg vein source,[36,37] atrial fibrillation,[38] mitral valve prolapse,[39,40] marantic embolus,[42-44] fragmented thrombus complexes from a nonobstructing ICA plaque,[42,44] shotgun pellet,[45] metal fragment from a penetrating neck wound,[46] traumatic dissection of the ICA,[47] ICA of various causes,[48] and automobile accident with angiographically normal ipsilateral ICA.[34,47] Recent striking images support aortic arch embolism, even in a setting of clinically important carotid stenosis.[49]

Embolism to one or more branches of the MCA may occur from almost any of the above as well as other less well documented sources.[50,51] Sources include calcific material from the ipsilateral ICA (although Chiari's famous case also had a patent cardiac foramen ovale),[35] spontaneous dissection of the ICA from fibromuscular hyperplasia,[52] traumatic ICA dissection,[53] mucin and emulsified fat from breast metastasis,[54] endocarditis due to candida,[55] mitral valve prolapse,[39] cardiac myxoma,[56] marantic embolus,[41] arterial wall fragments after resuscitation,[57] giant fusiform MCA aneurysm,[58] ICA occlusion from various causes, and various types of transcardiac emboli via a patent cardiac foramen ovale.

Particle Size and Composition

An embolus of merely a few millimeters may occlude the MCA stem. Some calcific plaques[59] may also embolize to the MCA but are too small to block the stem.[60] Carotid plaque rupture as a cause of major middle cerebral stem occlusion has been difficult to demonstrate.[61,62]

Accumulating evidence indicates that inflammation is of key importance in atherosclerotic plaque destabilization, thrombo-embolism and stroke. Inflammatory cells within plaque, particularly macrophages, are increasingly recognized as key mediators of lipid oxidation, plaque remodeling, and fibrous cap erosion and rupture, leading to acute thromboembolic events. Imaging with 18-fluorodeoxyglucose [18-FDG] positron-emission tomography (PET) has significant potential for non-invasive imaging of atherosclerotic inflammation, providing information about plaque biology associated with clinical events independently of the effect of the plaque on narrowing of the arterial lumen.[63] In a recent study, carotid plaque PET 18-FDG uptake predicted early recurrent stroke.[64] This study found that the predictive utility of 18-FDG plaque uptake was independent of age and degree of lumen stenosis (categorized as 50–69% and 70–99%, adjusted hazard ratio [HR], 6.1; confidence interval [CI], 1.3–28.8; $P = 0.02$).

Although, molecular imaging (FDG-PET) can help in imaging plaque inflammation, it is difficult to apply in intracranial stenosis due to high uptake of FDG by surrounding brain parenchyma. Recently sodium fluoride (18F-NaF) PET/CT imaging was applied in coronary artery diseases to facilitate understanding of plaque calcification. The same radiotracer might help to determine calcification in intracranial arterial stenosis. Furthermore, combining 18F-NaF with Gd-enhanced vessel wall imaging could further elucidate the link between local hemorrhage, microcalcification, progression to plaque rupture, and potential cerebrovascular event.[65]

Most of the embolic material is a small fragment of a vessel or cardiac wall thrombus or vegetation.[4] Being compressible,[66] such embolic fragments may alter their length and width as they pass through the arterial tree. Rarely, large-particle embolism may occur from fibrocartilaginous material.[67]

Distribution in the Middle Cerebral Artery Territory

Emboli follow preferential paths through the MCA system.[34,68] The lower division receives the larger share of the emboli. In the upper division, the serial arrangement of the major branches allows the entire division to be occluded by a large embolus blocking the first branch point. Small emboli often pass by the anterior branches to lodge in the more posterior branches. The sharply angulated orbitofrontal branch is rarely occluded.[34,68–70] The lower division remains a single vessel until it reaches the superior temporal plane, where it gives off its three main branches within the space of 1 cm or less. As a result, even small emboli may result in simultaneous occlusion of more than one or even all the branches.

Persistence of Material

Autopsies commonly show no occlusion, despite stem, division or branch occlusion typical of embolism. Many emboli must be poorly organized and may undergo spontaneous dissolution. For vessels with persisting occlusion, the functional prognosis for the infarct is worse.[48,71–73] By imaging alone, such persistent occlusions may have all the features of in situ thrombi.[74] Transcranial Doppler (TCD) studies are often useful in demonstrating rapid recanalization as well as persistent occlusion.[47,75]

Effects of Collateral Flow on Embolic Infarct Patterns

Unless adequate collateral flow is present, embolic occlusion of the MCA yields a gigantic infarct. On the contrary, in patients with good collateral flow, the brain parenchyma may be remarkably spared.[76]

Intracranial collateral pathways are important for the perfusion of brain regions affected by an intracranial occlusion.[77] These channels may be pre-existing or develop de novo. The collateral status correlates well with final infarct volume and functional outcome.[78] Collaterals can also predict the effectiveness of intravenous thrombolysis as well as various endovascular intervention.[79] Furthermore, good collaterals are believed to reduce hemorrhagic complications of various therapeutic strategies in acute ischemic stroke.[79]

Clinical Syndromes of Embolism

A variety of clinical profiles occur in embolism to MCA branches (Fig. 24-4). In some instances, the deficits are only transient, even with angiographic persisting occlusion, which raises the possibility that the nature of the embolic material may play a role in the severity of the infarct.[80,81] In the days of polymeric silicone (Silastic) pellet therapy for arteriovenous malformations (AVMs), aberrant embolism was a well-recognized risk,[82] usually occurring near the end of the embolization procedure.[82–83]

Emboli initially occluding the MCA stem and then migrating to the distal branches may lead to discontinuous multifocal infarction. The lack of collateral branches to the lenticulostriates makes these deep territories especially vulnerable to infarction. The initial major hemispheral clinical syndrome may ameliorate to that of deep infarction affecting the penetrating vessels of the MCA stem. This clinical picture, dubbed spectacular shrinking deficit (SSD),[76] appears to be the consequence of thrombolysis or distal migration of the fragmented clot and its residual particles. Such cases often leave two separate foci of infarction, assumed to be from the same embolic event[84] (Fig. 24-5). Syndromes of nonsudden

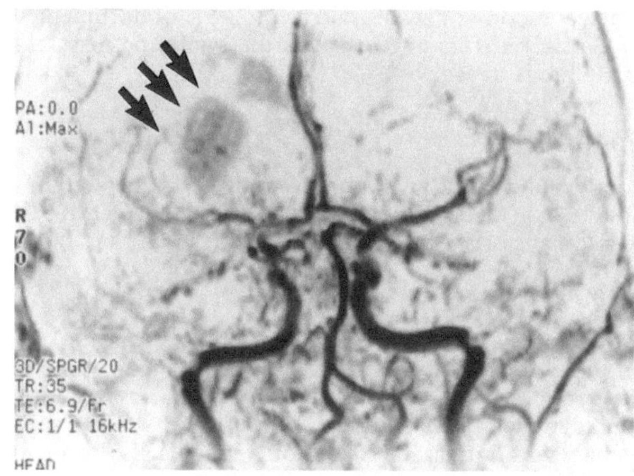

Figure 24-4 Hemorrhagic infarction *(arrows)* shown in the deep (lenticulostriate) territories of the middle cerebral artery on a coronal magnetic resonance image. *(From Gautier JC, Mohr JP: Ischemic stroke. In Mohr JP, Gautier JC, editors:* Guide to clinical neurology, *New York, 1995, Churchill Livingstone, p 543.)*

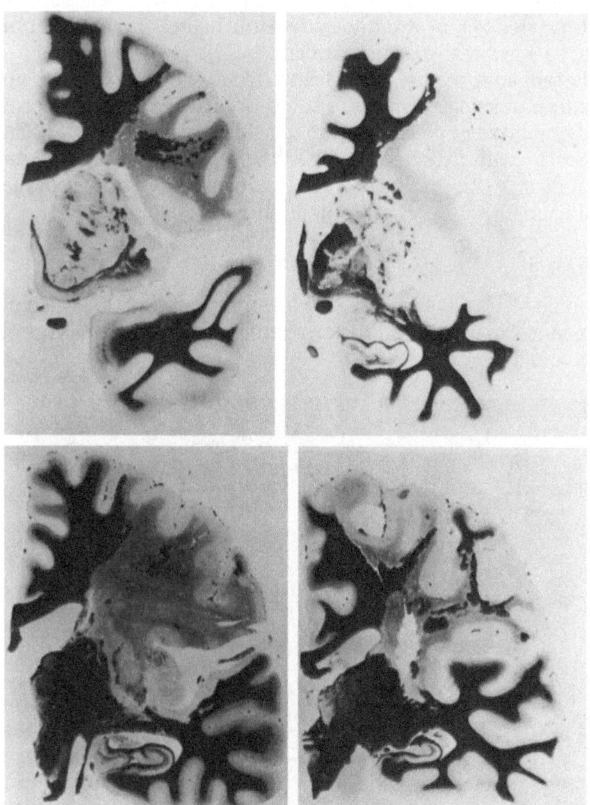

Figure 24-5 Deep and superficial infarction from the same embolic occlusion (myelin stain of celloidin section). *(From Friedlich AL, Castleman B, Mohr JP: Case records of the Massachusetts General Hospital.* N Engl J Med *278:1109, 1968.)*

or fluctuating onset may also occur in 5–6% of documented embolic strokes. In some instances the syndrome may take upto 36 hours to evolve.[34,85]

Thrombosis

Autopsy studies indicate that thrombotic occlusion accounts for only 2% of cases of ischemic events in the MCA territory.[34] Asymptomatic occlusion of the MCA stem is rare.[86,87]

Atherosclerosis

Primary arteriosclerotic occlusive thrombosis is an uncommon cause of symptomatic MCA disease.[34,88-91] However, it is more common in Asians, Hispanics and Africans. In acute ischemic stroke, angiographically demonstrated MCA stenosis found above a normal internal carotid artery is also compatible with recanalizing embolism.[73,92,93]

Although small, deep infarcts known as lacunes are usually explained by local microatheroma, some infarcts affecting the subinsula, external and extreme capsule, and upper corona radiata, which lie in the territory of several lateral lenticulostriates, create a curvilinear appearance on coronal imaging. They often spare the putamen, globus pallidus, capsule, and even the entry zone for the corona radiata (Fig. 24-6). Local atheromatous stenosis of the upper division is the usual cause but is not always easily demonstrated.[94]

Recent advancements in MRI technology enable direct visualization of vessel lumen and steno-occlusive plaque. A recent study reported good correlation of MRI measurements of MCA stenosis with digital subtraction angiography.[95] High-resolution MRI provides crucial information about plaque characteristics.[96-98] An example is shown in Figure 24-7.

Stenosis

Lunmen stenosis of the MCA is commonly found in the stem. In Asians, Hispanics and Africans, atherosclerosis is a common cause of MCA stenosis. However, other causes such as moyamoya disease, dissection, postradiation effects, metastatic tumors (including atrial myxoma), and infection may also cause stenotic lesions. The clinical syndromes range from minor pure motor stroke,[99,100] minor focal hemispheral syndrome, TIA;[87,92,99,101,102] to severe disability.[103,104]

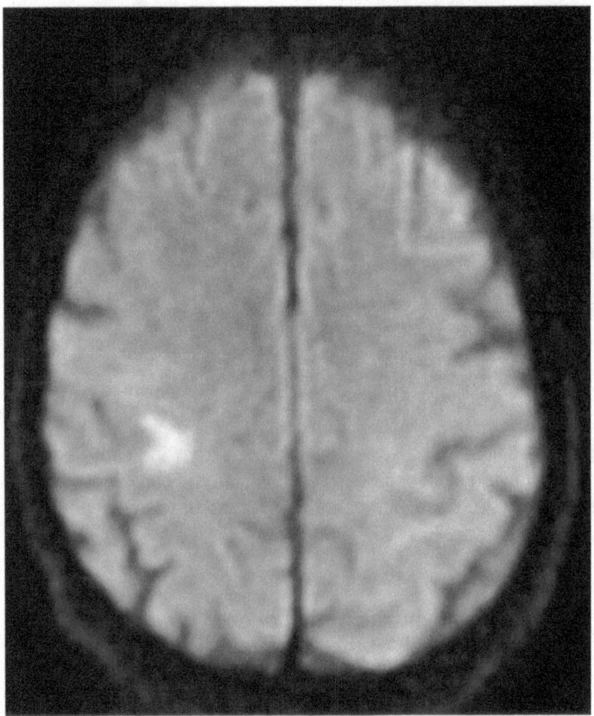

Figure 24-6 Brain imaging showing a high rolandic focal infarct in a patient with acute distal brachial plagia, normal after 1 month.

Dissection

Autopsy diagnosis of MCA dissection has been rare. A wide variety of conditions that may result in dissection include trauma,[105] strenuous physical exertion,[106] surgery,[107] fibromuscular hyperplasia,[108] atherosclerosis,[100] mucoid degeneration of the media,[105] moyamoya disease,[109] split or frayed internal elastic lamina,[110] congenital defect of the media,[111] syphilis,[112] and even migraine.[113] The disorder has been most often reported in younger patients. The usual site is a short section of the stem, although adjacent branches may also be affected.[114] In some, symptoms have been delayed for minutes,[114] hours,[111] or many days.[115]

Capsular Warning Syndrome

Capsular warning syndrome was first described in 1993 in patients who presented with stereotypic recurrent episodes of TIA.[116] This syndrome is associated with a high risk of developing a completed stroke.[117] Although, the exact pathogenesis of this syndrome remains debatable, small perforator artery disease is believed to be the most common mechanism. Recent developments in high-resolution MR imaging enable evaluation of arterial wall characteristics. Accordingly, recent studies suggest eccentric atherosclerosis of a non-stenosing segment of MCA as the underlying pathophysiology.[118]

Other Diseases

MCA may be affected by arteritis, fibromuscular hyperplasia, altered coagulation states, delayed effects of radiation, and other conditions.

An important condition that has been described recently is reversible cerebral vasoconstriction syndrome (RCVS). It is characterized by recurrent thunderclap headache, seizures, stroke, and non-aneurysmal subarachnoid hemorrhage. Reversibility of vasoconstriction within 3 months is the hallmark of RCVS. Common conditions associated with RCVS include post-partum state, use of vasoactive agents and immunosuppressive agents.[119-121] The clinicoradiological features are often dynamic in nature. Nimodipine, a calcium channel blocker, seems to reduce thunderclap headaches. However, it has no proven effect on hemorrhagic and ischemic complications. Corticosteroids are avoided since they may worsen the clinical course.[122]

CLINICAL SYNDROMES OF MIDDLE CEREBRAL ARTERY TERRITORY INFARCTION

The textbook accounts, briefly reviewed here, assume total infarction in the territory at risk. Uncollateralized occlusion of the main trunk of the MCA causes softening of the basal ganglia and internal capsule within the substance of the hemisphere as well as a large portion of the cerebral surface and subcortical white matter.[4,123-126] The large infarct produces contralateral hemiplegia, deviation of the head and eyes toward the side of the infarct, hemianesthesia, and hemianopia. Foix and Levy[4] detailed the clinical elements almost a century ago. Major disturbances also occur in behavior. Global aphasia occurs when the hemisphere dominant for speech and language is involved, whereas impaired awareness of the

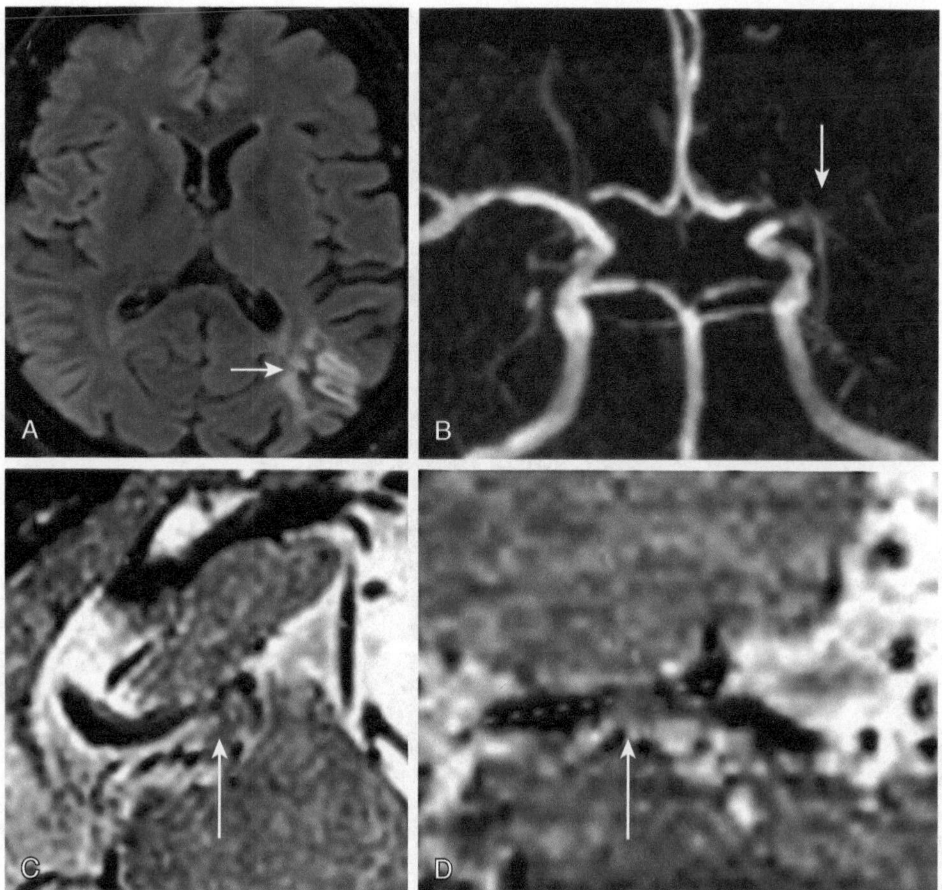

Figure 24-7 High-resolution MRI in a patient with left posterior watershed infarction (A) due to severe stenosis of the left middle cerebral artery (B). Although time-of-flight MR angiogram showed an occlusion of proximal left MCA, high-resolution MRI showed an atherosclerotic plaque and severe stenosis (C) that resulted in complete occlusion of the distal MCA (D).

stroke is expected when the nondominant hemisphere is affected. When the infarct is large, the hemianopia may be due to involvement of the visual radiations. More often, hemianopia is part of a syndrome of hemineglect for the opposite side of the space and is accompanied by failure to turn toward the side of the hemiplegia in response to sounds from that side.

A variant of the syndrome of MCA stem occlusion, colorfully named malignant infarction,[127] applies mainly to those experiencing subsequent herniation. The time to severe decline is brief (2–5 days). Advances in treatment have allowed survival for some; however, most of the syndrome elements persist (Fig. 24-8).[128] Results of a pooled analysis of the three European randomized controlled trials demonstrated better clinical outcome in patients that underwent decompressive surgery within 48 hours of stroke onset. Compared to the best medical therapy, more patients in the decompressive-surgery group achieved modified Rankin score (mRS) 0-3 (43% vs 21%) and mRS 0-4 (75% vs 24%).[129]

When the occlusion is restricted to the upper division, the sensorimotor syndrome mimics that from occlusion of the main trunk. Added to it is aphasia when the dominant hemisphere is involved or impaired awareness of the deficit when the other hemisphere is affected. However, the hemiparesis usually affects the face and arm more heavily than the leg. Because the occlusions usually affect the upper division, aphasia from dominant hemisphere infarction is usually of the motor (Broca's) type (Figs 24-9, 24-10), whereas the disturbance in behavior from nondominant hemisphere infarction may be mild.

In the lower division syndromes, infarction typically spares the rolandic region, hemiparesis is mild, head and eye deviations are rarely encountered, and even disorders of sensation are infrequent. When the infarct affects the dominant hemisphere, pure aphasia (Wernicke's type) is the rule, whereas in nondominant hemisphere infarction, the behavior disturbances may appear in relative isolation. Hemianopia may be a prominent sign.

When the involvement is limited to the territory of a small penetrating artery branch of the main stem, a small, deep infarct (lacune) occurs, affecting part or the entire internal capsule and producing a syndrome of pure hemiparesis unaccompanied by sensory, visual, language, or behavior disturbances.

CLINICAL SYNDROMES FROM INFARCTION OF EITHER HEMISPHERE

Loss of Consciousness

Transient loss of consciousness is rare in MCA territory infarction. It occurs at onset in only 8.4% of carotid ischemic strokes.[130] Delayed loss of consciousness is more common, often occurring 36 hours to 4 days after hemispherical infarcts ranging in size from the entire MCA territory to only the frontotemporal region.[131] The decline in consciousness is usually part of a larger clinical picture of impending cerebral herniation and seems not to be due to an injury to a specific brain region in the MCA territory controlling consciousness (see Fig. 24-11).

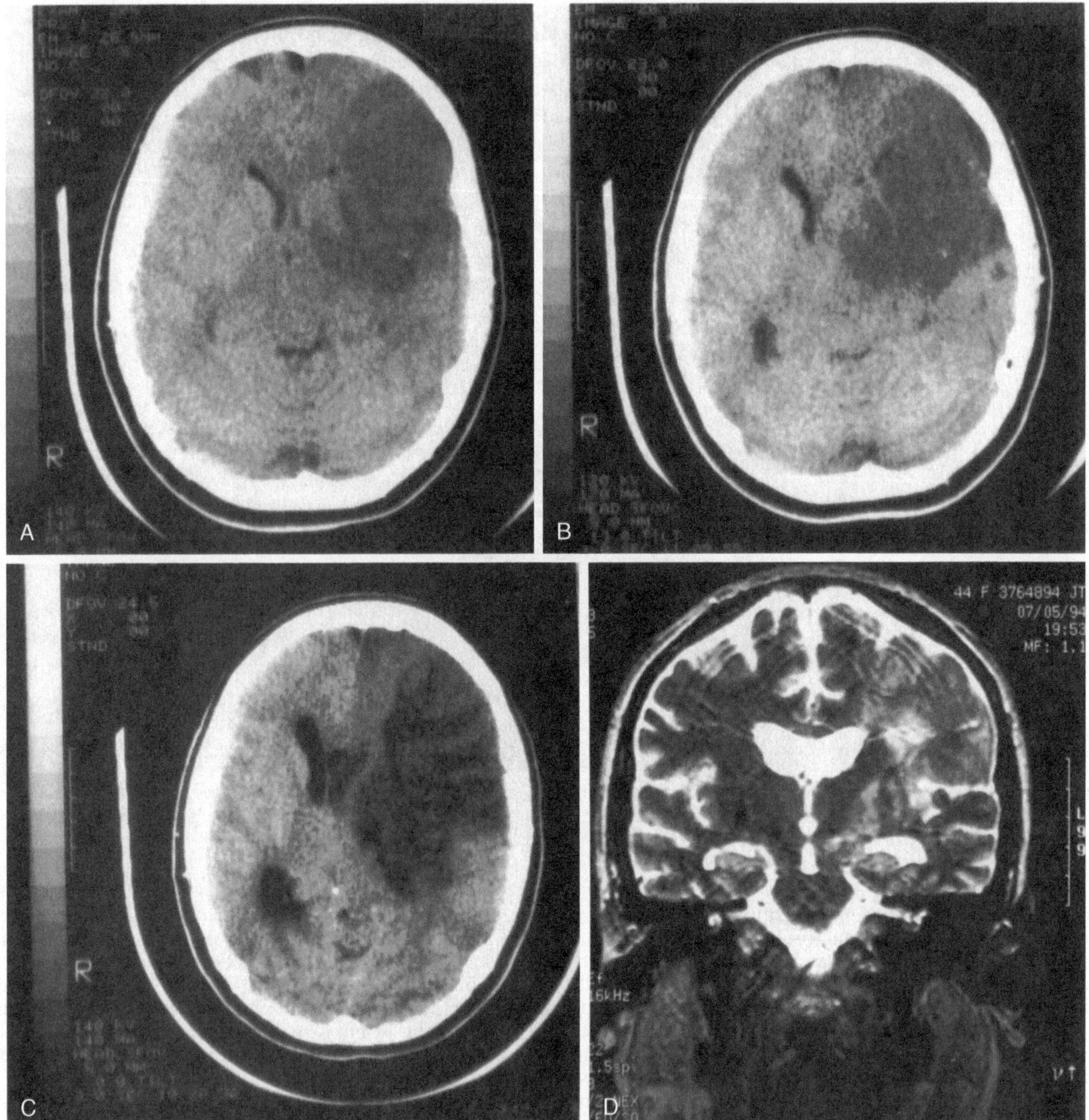

Figure 24-8 Four stages of midbrain compression. A, Viewed from an axial CT scan, the large middle cerebral artery (MCA) territory infarction has just begun to produce slight displacement a few hours after the acute stroke. B, By the second day, edema and "mass effect" have displaced the midbrain and thalamic structures slightly across the midline. C, By the fourth day, at the height of compression, the midline structures have been rotated and displaced considerably, during which time the patient appeared in a state of uncal herniation. D, A week later, a coronal T2-weighted MR image shows the midline structures back at their normal positions, and no lasting damage is evident from the displacement. *(From Gautier JC, Mohr JP: Ischemic stroke. In Mohr JP, Gautier JC, editors:* Guide to clinical neurology, *New York, 1995, Churchill Livingstone, p 543.)*

Hemiplegia and Hemiparesis

The terms hemiplegia and hemiparesis have been used rather loosely in the literature, which makes a clear correlation between the severity of weakness and a given site of infarction difficult. The number of cases that correlate the hemiparesis formula and imaging or autopsy findings remains disappointingly small, and some of them, despite an autopsy study, lack credibility.[132] Henschen's[133] massive review of the published autopsy literature on higher cerebral function before 1920 was typical of most writers. The literature remains frustrating because of many surprising instances in which the motor deficit showed considerable improvement. MCA stem occlusions affecting either side of the brain appear to produce the same basic motor deficit and can be described under the same heading. Such were the findings in the 488 cases of MCA territory infarction published in the pilot phase of the National Institute of Neurological and Communicative Disorders and Stroke (NINCDS) Stroke Data Bank project.[134]

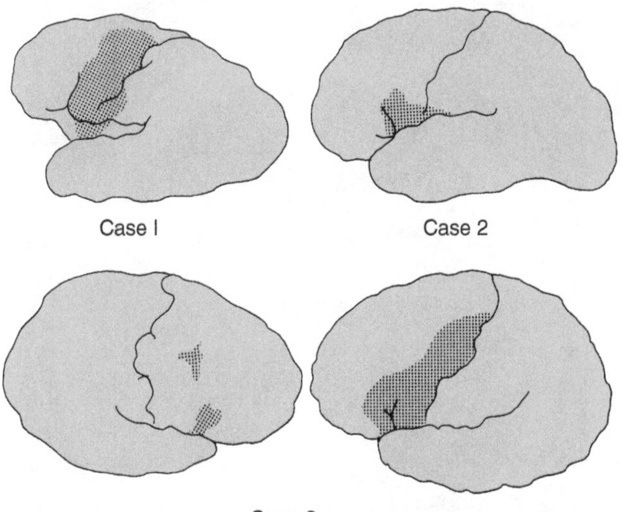

Figure 24-9 Three examples of embolic infarction of Broca's area and surrounding cerebrum. *(From Mohr JP. Broca's area and Broca's aphasia. In: Whitaker H, editor.* Studies in neurolinguistics. *New York, 1976, Academic Press, p 201.)*

Hemiplegia

The most reliable occurrence of hemiplegia follows complete occlusion of the MCA at its stem (Figs 24-10 and 24-11). The typical picture consists of dense contralateral hemiplegia, hemianesthesia, homonymous hemianopia, and conjugate gaze deviation to the contralateral side.[4] The syndrome is more severe when the stem is affected.[4,87,135,136] Among the patients who die within days, contralateral hemiplegia is usually accompanied by hemianesthesia and hemianopia.[137]

The syndrome among survivors without hemicraniectomy seems similar.[93] While some have had only mild facial paresis,[138] distal functions of the limbs are much impaired, and hand and finger movements and the foot are often paralyzed. In some patients, movement of the shoulder and elbow may allow the arm to lift, and movement of the hip and knee may suffice for walking.

Hemiplegia from deep infarction alone features several different syndromes. Foix and Levy[4] described two types. In the first, massive hemiplegia occurred, and the appearance was the same as that observed when the infarct involved both the superficial and deep territories. Initial hemiplegia gave way to marked contractures. No involuntary movements, choreoathetosis, parkinsonism or disturbances in balance were

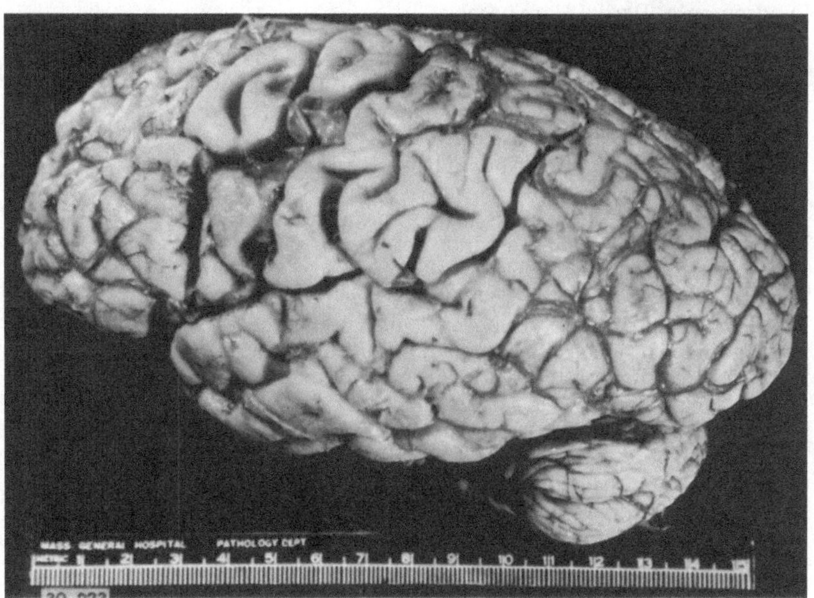

Figure 24-10 Small upper rolandic infarction. The pia-arachnoid has been stripped away to show the infarct. *(Courtesy of J.M.C. Pearce.)*

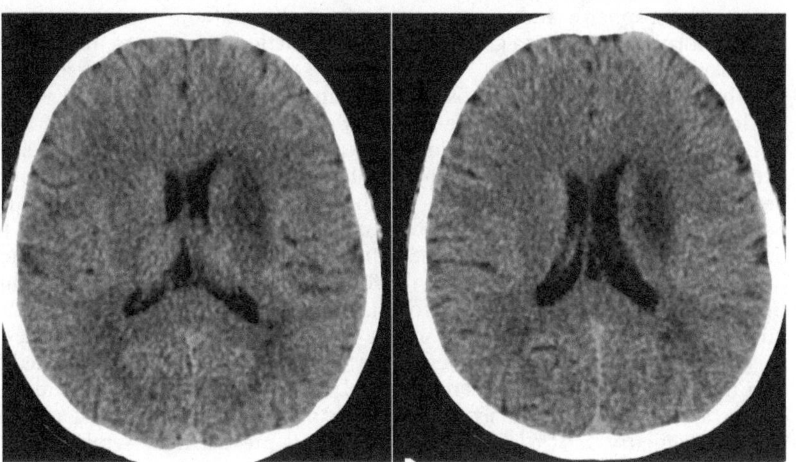

Figure 24-11 Large deep infarction of the middle cerebral artery lenticulostriate territories shown by CT scan.

described. The second type involved a more marked hemiplegia in the leg than in the arm, rendering the patient unable to walk. Contracture in this syndrome was more common in the leg and was often associated with a permanently flaccid hemiplegia. Later studies[139-141] and CT scans have reported a range of weakness, from profound hemiplegia to mild weakness, which underwent striking improvement despite persistence of the deep infarct.[142,143]

Hemiplegia from surface infarction is the third type. Infarction of the entire surface territory produces a syndrome essentially identical to a deep territory infarction. Surface infarcts confined to the cortical surface of insula and operculum cause hemiplegia with faciobrachial predominance that soon fades to a facial plegia with mild, predominantly distal paresis of the arm.[144]

Individual branch occlusions uncommonly produce hemiplegia.[4] In most cases, either hemiparesis occurs or the syndrome of paralysis is incomplete and confined to one or more body parts. The most reliable deficit is encountered among patients with occlusion of the ascending frontal branch.[55] Dramatic improvements within weeks are reported.[39] A large number of variables affect the outcome.[145] Efforts are under way to study a variety of treatment options, among them constraint therapy, transcranial magnetic stimulation[146] and transcranial direct current stimulation.[147]

Syndromes of Partial Hemiparesis

The most commonly encountered pattern of hemiparesis is weakness of the hand, shoulder, foot, and hip. This type was described in 71.2% of the 488 unilateral hemisphere strokes studied during the pilot phase of the NINCDS Stroke Data Bank project.[134] A few other types of hemiparesis are also well known. Among them are the classic syndromes of distal predominance of the hemiparesis (often attributed to Broadbent,[148] although we have found no source among his writings), a faciobrachial paresis, and monoplegia. The main phase of the NINCDS Stroke Data Bank study provided data for 183 of 1276 patients with convexity infarction in the MCA territory and is still the largest reported cohort. Infarct size did not differ according to side, but the location of the main site of the infarct did. On the left side, the infarct was centered in the inferior parietal region, but on the right, it was midfrontal. There was a good correlation between infarct size and extent of weakness as estimated by overall motor function. There was poor correlation for lesion location (lower third, middle third, or upper third on either side of the rolandic fissure) and any of the specific syndromes of focal weakness; no two cases shared the same lesion for the same syndrome, and several cases shared the same lesion with a different syndrome. The findings indicated a difference in weakness syndromes between the two hemispheres and great individual variation of the acute syndrome caused by a given site of focal infarction along the rolandic convexity.[134]

When hemiparesis features distal predominance, it affects the lower face, fingers, forearm, toes and lower leg, with relative sparing of the forehead, shoulder, upper arm, hip, thigh, neck, and trunk. This lower facial and distal predominance of hemiparesis is believed to represent the density of the homuncular representation over the hemispheral surface,[149,150] but occurred in only 23.5% of the 488 patients with unilateral weakness affecting the cerebrum in the Stroke Data Bank.[134] In addition, it occurred with approximately the same frequency regardless of whether the infarct was confined to a single lobe or was as large as several lobes and whether the area involved was frontal, parietal, temporal, or opercular.

The syndrome of faciobrachial paresis also has a widely varying frequency.[87,144,150-152] Obvious weakness is present in the jaw muscles. Movements of the tongue and oropharynx show impairment of swallowing and occasionally impairment of vocalization. These lower face and oral pharyngeal disturbances may persist long after forehead movement has been restored. The initial appearance is sometimes similar to Bell's palsy, but the upper deviation of the eyes characteristic of peripheral facial palsy (Bell's phenomenon) is typically not present, even in the earliest stages. The involvement of the upper extremity is usually more obvious in the form of impaired movement of the fingers and hand.

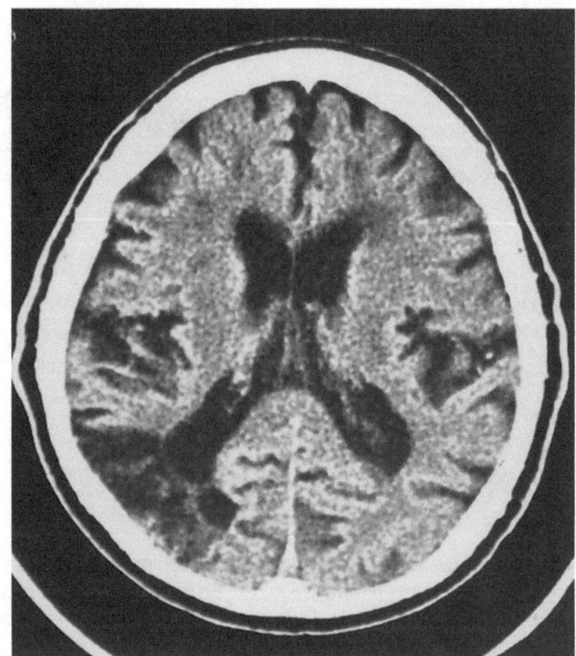

Figure 24-12 Axial CT scan showing a left parietal infarct in a patient with right inferior quadrantanopia.

Monoplegia

Although described in standard texts, detailed case reports of monoplegia are not easily found in the literature. von Monakow[153] made reference to the possibility of an isolated brachial plegia arising from a lesion confined to the middle of the second frontal gyrus, provided that the lesion is acute and does not extend too deeply into the white matter ("wenn sie akut einsetzt und nicht zu tief in das subcorticale Mark übergrieft"). Dejerine and Regnard[154] found a case with weakness limited to the muscles of the thenar, hypothenar and interosseous muscles; they did not mention confirmation of the presumed vascular nature of the lesion. Garcin[155] described a monoparesis with weakness predominating in the flexor movements, mimicking median nerve palsy; the locus of the lesion was inferred in the absence of autopsy data. The only case of focal upper rolandic infarction with autopsy documentation (Fig. 24-12) of an elderly woman, whose examination within hours of onset revealed normal power in the upper extremity. The only clinical signs were slight right facial weakness with initial mutism. She was monitored for months, during which time the initial deficit improved, but no disturbance of limb power occurred at any time. Among recent publications was a well-documented example of "hand knob" infarction.[156]

Isolated brachial monoplegia has often been described as a clinical sign in carotid territory TIAs. It has also been encountered as a transient syndrome in aberrant emboli during pellet embolization in the treatment of AVMs. These findings are of great interest but must be interpreted with caution because the setting (an angiogram suite with the patient under a drape) does not lend itself to detailed evaluation of the leg and axial structures during the frantic period when the physicians are striving to reverse the acute deficit. Schneider and Gautier,[157] in an extensive review of 1575 patients with acute stroke and predominance of leg weakness, found that only 63 had predominance of leg weakness. Although 41 patients had hemispheric convexity lesions, the MCA territory was affected in only one. The NINCDS Pilot Stroke Data Bank project contained a mere 31 cases of monoplegia involving the arm among the 488 patients with cerebral stroke,[134] yet even this small number showed a significant correlation with infarct of a single lobe rather than multiple lobes ($P < 0.002$).

Recovery from Hemiparesis

The means by which improvement occurs in hemiparesis remains unclear but is persistently described as recovery, a term suggesting a restoration of the original function. Such may not be the case, but the term is too well embedded in usage for us to constantly point out the ambiguities and force readers to face alternative terms throughout this chapter.

"Recovery" after stroke-induced hemiparesis is the rule rather than the exception. Clinical and imaging factors have been put forward to predict who is likely to recover and to what extent. The degree and nature of recovery depends critically on the outcome measure chosen. Several commonly cited observational studies have demonstrated, for example, that the initial severity of hemiparesis and lesion volume are reasonably good at predicting scores on disability scales at 3 or 6 months.[158–162] Neurologic impairment can dissociate from disability assessments, however, allowing a patient to be deemed recovered by a disability score while still harboring a substantial, unaddressed neurologic deficit.[163] Because the approach of most stroke rehabilitation programs is to teach compensation for deficits, such as the nonparetic hand accomplishing a motor task, rather than to reverse the neurologic impairment, recovery may be reported after a course of rehabilitation; however, at the level of impairment, recovery may not have occurred. Other studies have used impairment of motor function as the primary outcome measure and have shown varying correlations with their independent variables.[164–166] Duncan et al.[164] ran a widely cited study that serially evaluated the course of motor recovery among 104 hemiparetic stroke patients. Stratifying by severity of the motor impairment as measured by the standardized Fugl-Meyer (FM) stroke scale at day 1, the investigators followed the course of motor recovery at 5 days and at 1, 3, and 6 months. The investigators showed that the FM scores at day 1 accounted for only half of the variance in 6-month motor function ($r^2 = 0.53$, $P < 0.001$).[164]

Alternatively, if one defines recovery as the change in impairment score from the initial time point to 90 days later, prediction of recovery is more consistent. Newer evidence suggests that for patients who have mild-to-moderate deficits, there is a remarkably consistent course of recovery, and all patients achieve a specific proportion (approximately 70%) of the potential total remaining recovery.[167] For patients with severe deficits at onset, prediction of recovery is much more difficult. To distinguish those likely to recover from those who are not likely to recover, investigators recently showed that expression of a "recovery pattern" on functional magnetic resonance imaging (fMRI), obtained in the first few days after stroke, correlated well with the degree of subsequent recovery that then occurred.[168]

Functional imaging has also begun to reveal the dynamic process of brain reorganization after stroke. Neuronal activity in regions outside primary motor cortex after stroke-induced hemiparesis may appear both in the opposite hemisphere and in secondary motor areas in the ipsilesional hemisphere as early as 24 hours after stroke onset.[169,170] The appearance of this task-related activity suggests that alternative brain regions participate in the performance of motor function when a deficit is present, then revert to a more typical, contralateral pattern as recovery proceeds.[171–174] Physiologic measures of white matter tracts such as transcranial magnetic stimulation (TMS) also support the idea that a changing balance of cross-callosal inhibition between the two hemispheres plays a role in recovery. Loss of inhibition from the stroke hemisphere to the contralesional hemisphere may interfere with recovery of motor function through the increased inhibition back on the hemisphere with the stroke.[175] This competitive inhibition between hemispheres after stroke has led to the proposal of rehabilitation measures that restore physiologic balance between hemispheres through the use of TMS[146,176] and transcranial direct current stimulation (tDCS).[147,177]

Infarcts without Hemiparesis

Infarction confined to the lower division of the MCA is not expected to produce hemiparesis in any form because the site of the infarct lies so far posterior to the rolandic sulcus. This point also seems to apply to the postrolandic branches of the upper division. Occlusion of the ascending parietal branch is uncommonly reported, but the few cases documented have been remarkably free of focal motor deficit.[178] The pilot phase of the NINCDS Stroke Data Bank study[134] documented a handful of instances of hemiparesis after opercular infarction. Several notable cases exist with autopsy correlation in which weakness did not occur in the face or the limbs at any time during an acute infarction affecting the inferior frontal region's anterior operculum.[179] Reports of infarction confined to the orbital frontal branch of the upper division are exceedingly rare. In one case,[13] a man's only motor deficit consisted of the grasp reflex and contralateral extensive planar response. The case was studied by angiography only.

Movement Disorders

Temporary or permanent movement disorders, including hemichorea, athetosis and dystonia, are uncommon sequelae of MCA territory infarcts. Despite a large body of literature on the subject in children, few reports have appeared on adults.[180] Only one adult has been described with chorea.[181] Recently, hemichorea was reported to be the presenting feature of stroke in diabetic patients. The hypothesis was that the slow-flow hypoxic–ischemic insult due to severe ICA stenosis provided a fertile ground for neuronal damage secondary to hyperglycemia. Perhaps, the reduced 'wash-out' of hyperglycemic blood led to the accumulation of reactive oxygen species and other neurotoxic glycosylated end products of hyperglycemia, aggravating injury to the involved basal ganglia.[182]

Dystonia has also been the subject of some reports. The one adult described in the series reported by Demierre and Rondot[142] was a 17-year-old with left hemiplegia that improved slightly within 4 weeks, by which time signs of dystonia had appeared. A large hypodensity affecting the putamen, anterior capsule and caudate was seen on CT. Some similar cases have also been reported.[180]

Contraversive Eye and Head Deviation

Prevost[178] first described deviation of the head and eyes after a unilateral lesion in 1896. Ocular deviation is included as part of the National Institutes of Health Stroke Scale (NIHSS) but is rarely cited with clinical correlation of the infarct focus.[183–186] It has long been held that deviation of the eyes represents disruption of the frontal eye fields in and around area 8 alpha, located in the premotor region of the superior frontal lobe,[183,184,187–189] but few examples exist.[190,191] In most cases, deviation of the head or eyes has been associated with large lesions more centrally located in the deeper MCA territory near the operculum or insula.

Types of Head and Eye Deviation

De Renzi et al.[192] encountered three types of deviation in their 120 patients with ocular motility disorders. In the first group, the head and eyes were midline and moved spontaneously to either side in response to stimulus, but were less complete to the side of the space served by the damaged hemisphere. In the second group, the head and eyes were found completely to one side with absence of spontaneous movements to the contralateral side and only fleeting voluntary deviation of the eyes into the side of the space served by the damaged hemisphere. In the most severely affected group, the head, eyes, or both were completely deviated away from the side of the space served by the damaged hemisphere and failed to turn in response to verbal or sensory stimuli; no spontaneous or voluntary movements were observed to the midline or beyond. Hemi-inattention or neglect of the contralateral side of the space usually accompanied cases with head and eye deviation.

Eye Deviation and Infarct Topography

Eye deviation is the expected finding after massive infarction of the entire MCA territory.[87] For upper division syndromes encountered in studies of Broca's aphasia, ten autopsy cases from the Massachusetts General Hospital files[193] were described; all of the patients had experienced head and eye deviation to the site of the lesion that persisted for days and cleared within a week. Less frequent eye deviation has been found in opercular infarction. Ocular deviation with deep infarction has been reported in individual cases with autopsy correlation and has occurred from hemorrhage (thalamus, frontal, or frontotemporal location) and subdural hematoma.[131,186] From CT scan studies and in the NINCDS Stroke Data Bank study,[194] 86 cases (16%) of supratentorial-type conjugate ocular deviation occurred among the 531 cases of hemispheral stroke diagnosed according to clinical or radiologic criteria. The occurrence of ocular deviation was significantly correlated with larger infarcts, but among the infarcts confined to single lobes, those involving the right side were more commonly associated with ocular deviation.[192] A frontal predominance over parietal infarcts was not found, and a parietal location was not the explanation for the effect of the right-sided stroke. The prevalence of frontal or parietal lobe location did not differ significantly in single-lobe infarcts. Ocular deviation occurred from infarction as low on the surface as the operculum.

Duration of the Deviation and Severity of Infarct

In the NINCDS Stroke Data Bank, gaze deviation of less than 5 days' duration did not correlate with lesion side, size, site, cause or positive initial CT findings. However, the larger lesions predominated among the nine patients whose ocular deviation persisted beyond 20 days.

Some infarcts affecting the operculum and insula can cause pseudoophthalmoplegia for the first few days after the stroke.[144] Conjugate deviation of the head and eyes lasts for several days and then disappears. The lesion causing this condition is far away from area 8 and considered a reliable feature of infarcts of the insula and operculum.

Infarction with No Eye Movement Disturbances

De Renzi et al[192] reported one patient who was completely free of any gaze disturbance and who had a cortical–subcortical lesion (a frontal hematoma) on the left involving the areas of the rolandic fissure. The few cases with focal infarction confined to the superior frontal region, near area 8 alpha, have not confirmed the hypothesis that this region is vital for ocular motility.

Dizziness and Vertigo

Hemispheral infarcts have long been assumed to have a vertiginous component. A unique case reported by Brandt et al.[195] provides a contrasting view. The patient had "well-demarcated infarction" in the right posterior insular region and had rotational vertigo, among other signs, for almost a week.

Sensory Disturbances

Although sensory disturbances have been assumed to be part of the hemispheral infarct syndrome, few details have been published concerning the syndrome elements, their lesion correlation and duration. On the basis of the NINCDS Stroke Data Bank material, a disturbance in sensation carries an important indication of a large lesion when it accompanies hemiparesis; it is highly significant for infarcts greater than a single lobe in size ($P < 0.001$).[134]

Hemispherectomies and Sensory Disturbances

Late after surgery, a relative preservation of sensory function in the face seems common, whereas more blunted sensation to several modalities has been reported.[138] Complete astereognosia is common. Vibration and position sense are heavily affected, but not definite alteration of the body scheme. Recent reports focus on hemiplegia and hemianopia; mention of hemisensory changes is infrequent.[196] We await more detailed reports of the sensory disturbances in the massive "malignant" infarcts treated with hemicraniectomy.

Pure Sensory Deficits

Focal sensory deficits have been described in detail in only a handful of cases with autopsy correlation. One syndrome is a pseudoradicular pattern of sensory loss, with impairment of joint position sense, stereognosis, graphesthesia and two-point discrimination.[152] The hand is the most severely affected, but two cases have been described with both hand and foot disturbances. Hemianesthesia has also been described in a few other cases.[4,13,197] One recent case described contralateral loss of cold, pain and pinprick perception; other sensory modalities were reported as normal.[198]

Hemisensory Deficits and Lesion Topography

Foix et al.[199] are credited with describing an infarct affecting the anterior parietal region that produced a profound hemisensory loss (pseudothalamic syndrome) with little or no accompanying hemiparesis. Their patient had a large anterior parietal infarct that was so deep that it created almost a cleft in the hemisphere to the ventricular wall. Only a few subsequent reports have appeared[197,200,201] and are in general agreement with the original publication.

Correlation of Sensory Disturbances with Motor Deficits

The few cases reported suggest that, for the same size lesion, the sensory disturbance may affect a far more circumscribed area of the face, limbs, or trunk than that affected by the accompanying motor disturbance.[202]

Visual Field Disturbances

There is little doubt that hemianopia to confrontation clinical testing accompanies the huge infarcts.[4] Before modern imaging provided ample contradictory evidence, hemianopia was often ascribed to involvement of the visual radiation, through a mechanism of edema, even though the MCA supplies only the upper half of the radiation.[203] For less global infarcts, hemianopia has been described with infarcts involving the frontal region, and some have been as low as the Sylvian fissure.[150] However, hemianopia has been absent in some instances of focal infarction, even when impaired opticokinetic nystagmus (OKN) was found.

It is difficult to sustain the notion that edema involving the radiations explains hemianopia when the infarct is far away from these structures. It is likely that hemianopia may actually be a disturbance in hemispatial response that is part of a hemineglect syndrome.[204] In such cases, other faulty responses to spatial stimuli are noted, such as the patient with a left hemispheral infarction turning toward the left in response to a voice from the right and a patient showing failure to blink in response to threat stimuli from the right.

Quadrantanopia

Parietal infarction deep enough to affect the fibers of the upper half of the visual radiation is presumably responsible for the infrequently described inferior quadrantanopia of MCA territory infarction (Fig. 24-13).[205] Case reports with lower quadrantanopia have eluded our search to date. The syndrome should indicate a deep cleft of infarction reaching the visual radiation, but it remains unsettled whether it may occur in a more superficial infarct.

The inferior bundle of fibers in the optic radiation, commonly called Meyer's loop, courses in and around the ventricular system into the anterior pole of the temporal lobe to the cortical area below the calcarine fissure.[206] These fibers are nourished by the anterior choroidal artery and other MCA branches. Ischemia of this portion of the optic radiations may result in a homonymous, wedge-shaped, superior quadrant visual field defect commonly known as "pie-in-the-sky.[206,207]

Impairment of Opticokinetic Nystagmus

A test for OKN is assumed to detect disorders of the gaze mechanism mild enough that conjugate ocular gaze deviation is not present at rest. Considering the number of patients tested for OKN, it is remarkable that there is still considerable controversy over the usual locus of the lesion, the pathways injured, and even the nature of the disturbance. The early view was that OKN was a reflex activity of the cerebral cortex, that the slow component was initiated from the occipital region and the fast corrective phase from the frontal region, and that the OKN response was blunted by lesions at any point in the pathway.[208,209] However, the higher prevalence of abnormal OKN in parietal lesions has supported another view that the slow component from the occipital region passed directly to the brainstem through a pathway adjacent to the visual radiations organized in ipsilateral pathways.[210,211] Still another approach has argued that the pathway runs deep through the parietal region to the frontal lobe, crosses the posterior limb of the corpus callosum, and controls fast-phase components generated in the opposite frontal lobe.[208] Other arguments have been put forward for separate mechanisms controlling foveal and full-field pursuit.[212] These studies have shown the main disturbance to be in the slow component when targets were moved into the field of vision from the side of space served by the damaged hemisphere.

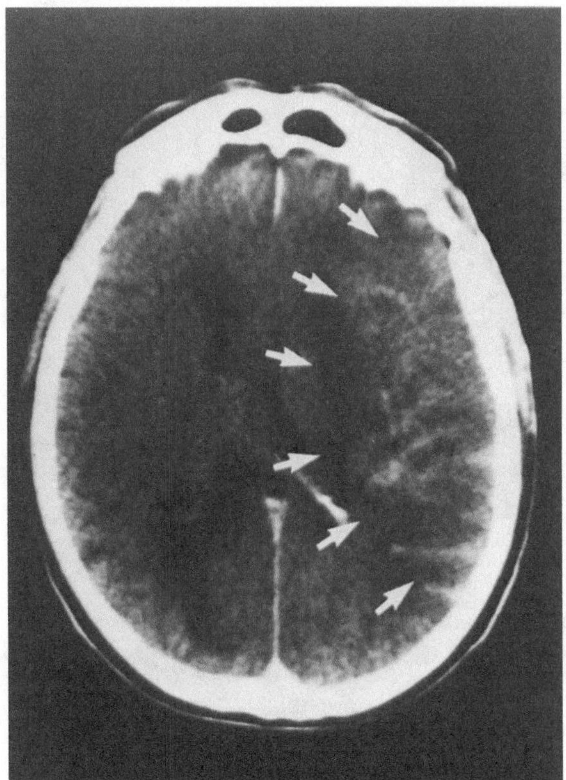

Figure 24-13 Coronal view of insular and upper opercular infarction from embolism to the upper division of the middle cerebral artery. (Myelin stain of celloidin section.)

The actual documented sites vary considerably (and are not all in the parietal lobe) and demonstrate that clinically evident hemianopia need not occur. Impairment of OKN has been encountered in at least one patient with a small, high rolandic infarct whose visual fields were intact (see Fig. 24-12).[150] Baloh et al.[212] also reported a patient with a large infarct apparently involving the posterior cerebral artery territory, accompanied by right hemianopia and alexia, but no language disturbance.

Autonomic Disturbances

Excessive sweating contralateral to an MCA territory infarction is rarely encountered. Case reports show that patients have major syndromes of hemiparesis, hemisensory problems, hemianopia, and altered behavior states, indicating a large lesion affecting both the superficial and deep territories of the MCA (Fig. 24-14).[213] Sweating in these few cases affected the face, neck, axilla and upper trunk contralateral to the infarct and faded to normal within days. Appenzeller[214] published an autopsy case for which the patient was described clinically as showing hyperhidrosis on the contralateral side of the body. The published photographs show a site of small hemorrhagic infarction in the upper bank of the insula and adjacent orbital surface of the operculum. An MRI series described

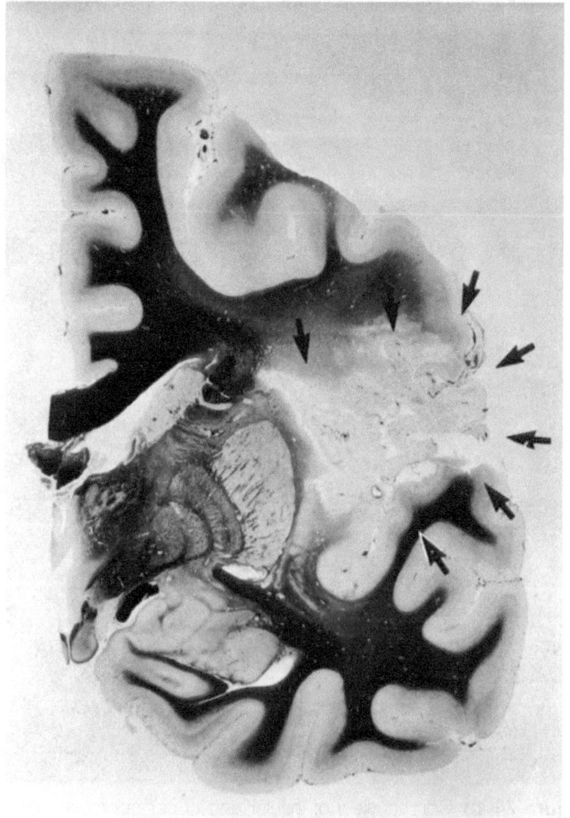

Figure 24-14 Non-contrast-enhanced CT scan showing hemorrhagic infarction of the entire middle cerebral artery territory *(arrows)*. Hemi-hyperhidrosis and distal arm edema were part of the clinical picture.

hypertensive episodes in patients with infarcts restricted to the right insular cortex.[215] Contralateral rubbery edema of the affected hands and feet may also occur from large MCA territory infarction (Fig. 24-15). The syndrome usually becomes evident within a few hours and persists for up to 2 weeks. The exact anatomic correlates are unknown.

SYNDROMES REFERABLE TO LANGUAGE-DOMINANT (USUALLY LEFT) HEMISPHERE INFARCTION

Aphasia

The cerebrum irrigated by the left MCA is of prime importance in language function. This function can be defined as a symbolic system in which the relations between meaningful elements (sounds, print, gestural signs) are purely arbitrary. Aphasia (or its more commonly less severe variant known as dysphasia) is thus regarded as a disorder caused by acquired brain injury that results in dysfunctional use of rule-governed, symbolic behavior.[216,217] The Sylvian fissure of the hemisphere dominant (for speech and language) is most likely to cause symptoms of dysphasia after a focal brain lesion. More than 95% of right-handed people and even most left-handed people have dominance for speech and language in the left hemisphere. Right hemisphere dominance for speech and language in a right-handed person is distinctly uncommon.

Many of the traditional clinicopathologic correlations of brain and language function have undergone revisions in the last few decades under the influence of modern imaging.[218,219] Among them has been that smaller focal brain lesions once thought to produce the major syndromes of aphasia are now known to cause less severe, minor, or even transient disturbances in production or comprehension of speech, sounds, and shapes. Much larger lesions are necessary to produce the lasting major disruptions in language function. Furthermore, it is apparent that deeper structures, especially the thalamus,

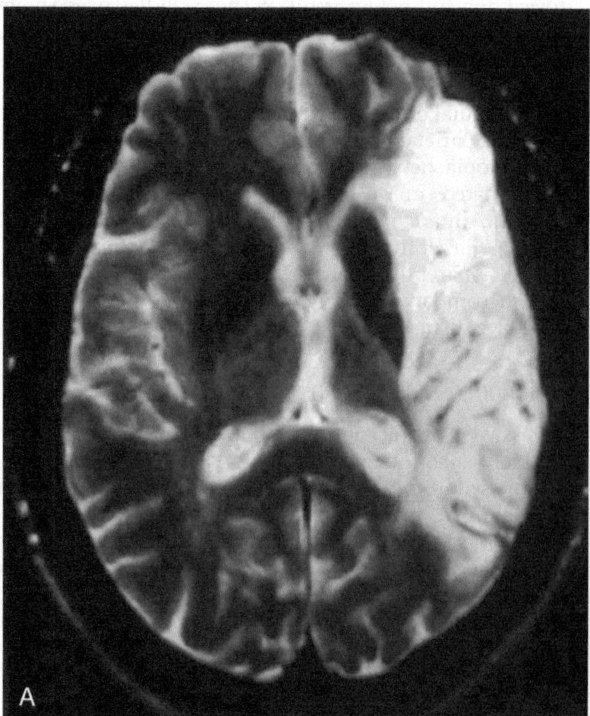

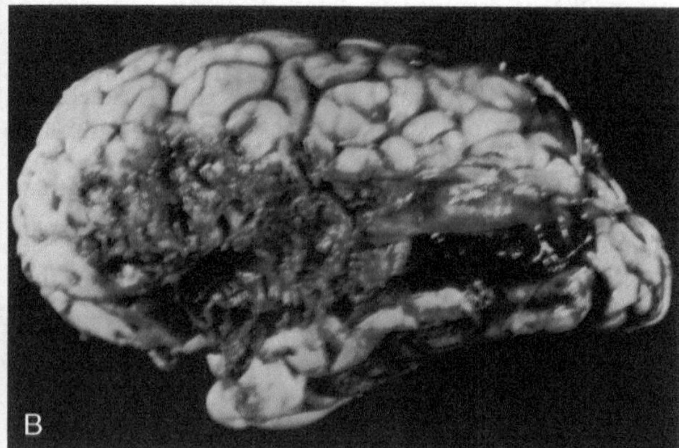

Figure 24-15 A, Complete infarction of the surface territory of the middle cerebral artery after occlusion of the middle cerebral artery. B, Appearance of another similar case at a later stage.

play vital roles in speech and language.[220] Most new studies show that lesion location is still the main determinant of the language syndrome. The contributions of new work have centered on insights achieved with functional imaging during the course of stroke recovery, and the pharmacologic challenge has been targeted toward restitution of function.

Global or Total Aphasia

Few studies have indicated the different types of aphasia expected in a setting of acute stroke. In a survey of 850 patients, Brust et al.[221] found that 177 (21%) had acute aphasia. Fifty-seven (32%) had "fluent" aphasia, and 120 (68%) had "nonfluent". Nonfluency was significantly correlated ($P < 0.01$) with a poor prognosis for mortality. Even highly significant mortality was found for patients with fluent and nonfluent aphasia who showed hemiparesis or a visual field disturbance. Similarly, Marquardson[222] reported 769 patients with acute stroke, 133 (33%) of whom showed aphasia in the acute state; hemiplegia was less likely to improve if accompanied by aphasia, and aphasia had a better outlook when unaccompanied by hemiplegia.

Clinical Features. Occlusion of the MCA trunk or its upper division produces a global disruption of language function. The initial disturbance can be profound (total aphasia). After the early period, clinicians and family sometimes observe some improvement in the patient's capacity to both understand context-related information (e.g., "Are you feeling better?") and participate in the give-and-take of simple communication. Within weeks or months, comprehension improves, especially for nongrammatical forms, and the patient shows more disturbances in speaking and writing than in listening and reading.[223] This kind of dysphasia is known as Broca's aphasia or major motor aphasia.

Lesion Size. With the advent of CT and MRI, a volumetric measure of the lesion permits estimation of the lesion size associated with the syndrome.[46,224] Naeser and Hayward[225] documented the lesion volume in patients with mixed aphasia and global aphasia. The site of the lesion in seven cases of mixed aphasia reflected a large infarct affecting the Sylvian region and beyond, but in a few instances, Broca's or Wernicke's areas proper were not mapped in the scanned lesion. The lesion size in these cases was approximately 3.9 × 3.9 cm, and such a lesion was usually seen on five CT slices. The lesion volume in five cases of global aphasia was considerably larger (5.8 × 5.8 cm). As with the mixed aphasia cases, the site of the minimal lesion lay in the Sylvian region and the major contribution to the larger volume was its centrifugal spreading into the adjacent frontal, parietal, and temporal regions (Fig. 24-16). With time, such lesions may evolve, leaving a major syndrome associated with considerable postinfarction atrophy.

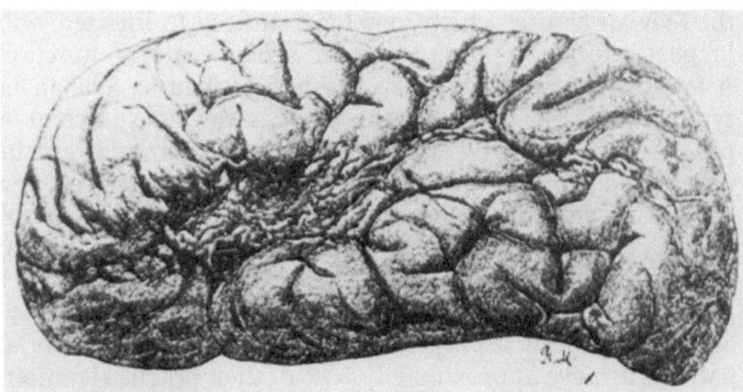

Figure 24-16 One of Broca's original cases.

Advances in MRI have shown that "lesion" size is actually the total region of hemodynamically compromised tissue, encompassing areas of infarction and nearby ischemic zones.[226,227] Asymmetries of Broca's area recording the left side have still not reliably been demonstrated.[228] Hillis et al. have shown that aphasia severity correlates more strongly with the volume of abnormality on perfusion-weighted imaging (PWI) than the volume of abnormality on diffusion-weighted imaging (DWI).[229] This group also demonstrated that the volume of left-sided subcortical infarcts can underrepresent the extent of cortical hypoperfusion. Of 37 patients in one study with strictly left-sided subcortical strokes on DWI, 25 had aphasia with cortical hypoperfusion in the distal left MCA territory demonstrated on PWI. Six of these patients with cortical hypoperfusion and subcortical infarction then underwent treatment to restore blood flow, which resulted in at least partial cortical reperfusion after repeated PWI. Repeated language testing showed improvement in all of the subjects who had cortical reperfusion.[230]

Motor Aphasia

For more than 100 years, a syndrome has been recognized in which the ability to communicate by speaking or writing seems far more impaired than the comprehension of words heard or seen.[70] Although Boulliaud[231] deserves credit for popularizing the notion that a lesion of both frontal lobes disrupts the power of spoken speech, the surgeon Paul Broca has received most of the credit for documenting that a left-sided Sylvian infarct more reliably causes the syndrome. Broca described two patients who appeared to have lost their memory of how to speak. Considerable controversy has persisted concerning whether this characterization is suitable for the findings and for the locus of the minimal lesion to precipitate the major syndrome and whether the effects are the same when the lesion is confined to the third frontal convolution, which Broca took to be the site causing the syndrome that bears his name. The actual lesion sizes were far larger, encompassing most of the Sylvian region and adjacent superior temporal lobe; lesions of this size nowadays would be expected to be associated with a syndrome of total aphasia (Fig. 24-17). Recent studies using MRI for Broca's two important cases confirm the large size of the lesions.[232] Efforts continue to explain the basis for the syndrome.[233]

Major Motor Aphasia. In its usual form, major motor aphasia appears to be an improvement of a syndrome of total

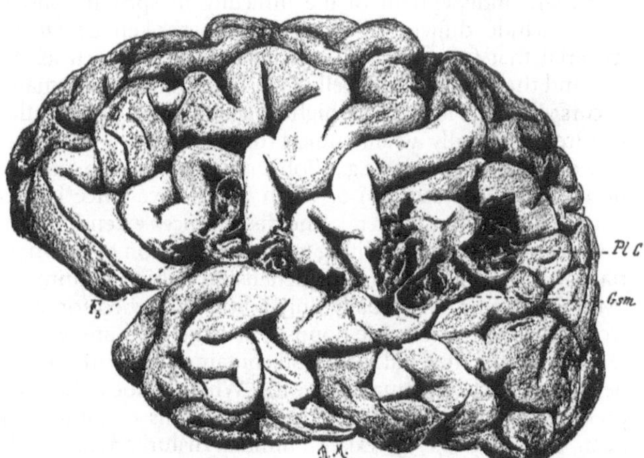

Figure 24-17 Lithograph of an example of infarction limited to the Sylvian lip. *(From Moutier F:* L'aphasie de Broca. *Paris, 1908, Thèse Médicine.)*

aphasia and is a late sign in the course of the major Sylvian cerebral infarct. In such patients, there is a sharp contrast between the hesitant, agrammatical speech and the relatively better comprehension evident in conversational tests as long as the examiner keeps the sentences and questions simple.

In the initial period after the acute infarction, the speech and language disturbances are too severe to allow a distinction between speech and language comprehension.[150,152,193,234–236] With the passage of a few months with some improvement, Broca's aphasia begins to appear.

Whether the motor aphasia that emerges is a disturbance confined to speaking and writing or contains a global disturbance in the brain's capacity to deal with grammatical functions has been argued for almost 150 years. Part of the argument stems from the terms used to substitute for Broca's aphasia: expressive dysphasia, efferent motor dysphasia,[237] motor dysphasia,[238] verbal dysphasia,[239] and, simply, nonfluency.[235] Despite the semantics, most investigators echo the impression of Liepmann[240] that symptoms of motor aphasia predominate and the limited capacity for spoken expression conceals the deeper language disturbances that persist but are less obvious.

The speech disturbance is evident to a similar degree whether the utterances are produced in spontaneous conversation or during efforts to repeat aloud or read aloud. The spoken responses are hesitant, demonstrating impairment of skilled interaction (dyspraxia) between the settings of the oropharynx and the respiratory elements that permit smooth vocalization.[241] In the production of individual words, the transitions from sound to sound are accomplished only with difficulty,[237] which is especially obvious with polysyllabic words. The disturbance disrupts the usual clustering of words to form phrases, interfering with the normal melodic intonation that serves to indicate differences among exclamations, questions, and declarative statements. There is a high correlation between the degree of buccolingual dyspraxia and the extent of speech loss in patients with Broca's aphasia.[242]

Apart from these signs of speech dyspraxia, the structure of the spoken phrases may show a simplification of grammar, in that the language content consists largely of single words that function as predicative elements (formerly known as telegraphic speech). These grossly condensed utterances have also been labeled agrammatism. In some cases, the utterances have been limited to a single word or phrase,[243] characterized as verbal stereotypes. The more limited the range of utterances, the more discouraging the prognosis for improvement.

Other disorders of language usage are part of the syndrome and seem independent of the difficulty in speaking aloud. They include difficulties responding to spoken or written material that features small grammatical words such as the, are, and then or involves spelling.[244] The poorest performance occurs when the meaning is highly dependent on grammatical features, especially when subject–object relations are based less on simple nouns (e.g., "John saw Jane") than on pronouns (e.g., "He saw it") or when the passive voice is used (e.g., "He was seen by her"). The disturbances extend beyond the acts of speaking or writing to comprehension of the material itself. Silent reading comprehension, which requires no overt vocalization, is usually only a little disturbed for single words that are pictureable nouns, but difficulties are encountered when the material to be read contains a particularly high density of such grammatical words. When it does, the comprehension may be strikingly abnormal. This condition has been termed deep dyslexia.[243] Similar disturbances can be documented in tests requiring the patient to point to visual displays containing single letters or grammatical words in response to hearing the names of the letters. Some have even shown faulty selection of a single letter among a visually presented display of letters when the test stimulus was a printed word whose pronounced sound (homophone) is identical to that of a given letter (i.e., "eye" to "I").[223]

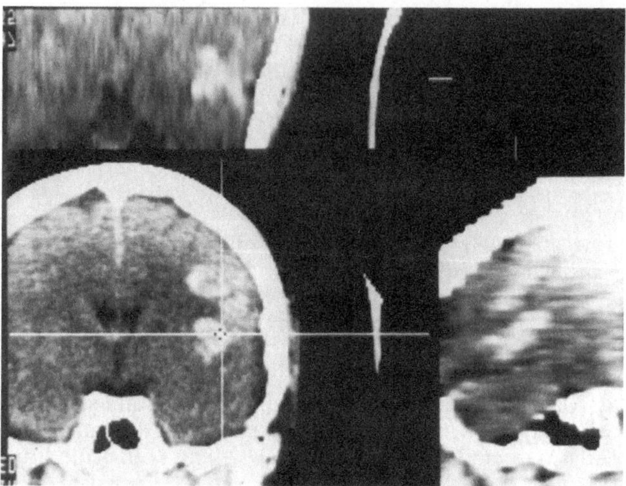

Figure 24-18 CT scan showing three views of an inferior frontal infarct, presenting as minor motor aphasia.

The clinicopathologic correlation for aphasia has evolved over the last century. Major motor or Broca's aphasia is not expected from infarction restricted to Broca's area. It usually reflects a major infarction involving most of the territory supplied by the upper division of left MCA (actually shown in Broca's original cases).[193] Accompanying disturbances in motor, sensory, and visual function usually makes the diagnosis easy. The usually large size of the Sylvian infarct sets the stage for contralateral hemiplegia.[245] At times, however, the main weight of the lesion may fall on the Sylvian region alone, which produces a surprisingly slight hemiparesis and profound language dysfunction (Fig. 24-18).[246] Ideomotor dyspraxia of the unaffected left upper extremity is the rule, as is bilateral buccofacial dyspraxia, which has been reported in 90% of patients.[242,247] Contralateral hemineglect to the right is the rule in the early stage.

Autopsy documentation of the Broca's aphasia comes largely from the older literature.[167] Living patients with the syndrome have been studied extensively by CT and MRI. [248–250] The imaged lesions in patients with persistent Broca's aphasia were largely opercular and insular[251] and fronto-Sylvian, sparing the temporal lobe. The larger Sylvian lesions were associated with persistent nonfluency.[237]

A few notable exceptions to the usual clinical picture accompanying Broca's aphasia may occur when the lesion is confined to the insula and adjacent operculum. Moutier's[252] patient had hemiplegia in the early period that improved to mild motor deficit at chronic stage. A remarkably circumscribed infarct was found along the lip of the upper bank of the Sylvian fissure, which may have sufficed to interfere with language function and not with sensory motor function. A few cases of this type have been described as Sylvian lip syndrome.[243] The issue of the smallest lesion sufficient to produce the persisting syndrome of Broca's aphasia remains unresolved. To date, no known case of an infarct confined to Broca's area alone has produced lasting, severe Broca's aphasia,[253] save for the tersely described case cited by Van Gehuchten.[254]

Like motor recovery, impairment reversal in aphasia appears to follow a proportional recovery pattern: nearly all patients achieve approximately 70% of their potential remaining recovery.[255] Work with metabolic imaging points to activation of tissue adjacent to the lesion site as instrumental in

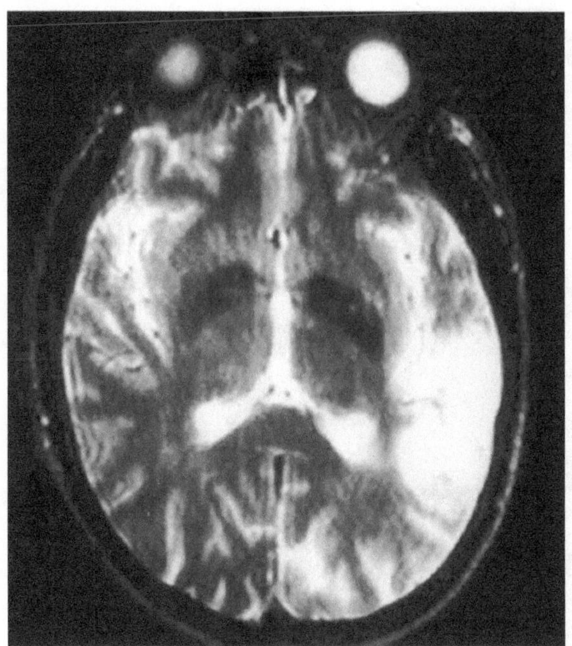

Figure 24-19 Large posterior hemispheral infarct with syndrome of major sensory (Wernicke's) aphasia.

recovery, whereas activation in the opposite hemisphere, while supportive in the first few weeks,[256] is associated with a worse outcome when the activity is persistent.

Minor Motor Aphasia. Focal infarcts affecting the operculum produce a rather circumscribed syndrome lacking the full elements of Broca's aphasia.[150,183,224,253,257] In the acute stages, complete mutism with ideomotor and buccofacial dyspraxia is commonly encountered. Auditory and visual comprehension for language is virtually intact, and some patients are capable of writing properly with the unaffected left hand. Improvement from the initial mutism begins within hours or, at the least, days and, rarely, weeks later.[250,258] Any language deficit evident in speaking and writing is extremely transitory and often disappears before it can be tested in full detail. In some cases, the dyspraxic disturbance in respiration interferes with the smooth flow of sounds and transition from syllable to syllable in running speech; this pattern has variously been called aphemia, oral–verbal apraxia, and apraxia of speech.[259]

The initial mutism is usually accompanied by contralateral hemiparesis. Head and eye deviation have also been documented.[150] A few cases of Broca's infarction have manifested with no hint of motor paresis.[179,260] In those reports using the term nonfluency,[235] a similarly transient disturbance has been seen in the smaller lesions found on CT (Fig. 24-19).

The clinicopathologic correlation has shown few exceptions to the rule that Broca's area infarction does not precipitate either the acute or the chronic forms of Broca's aphasia[261] and confirmed many times since.[193,250,262,263] Van Gehuchten[254] described a 60-year-old man with sudden total loss of speech accompanied by paresis of the right upper limb and a small amount of facial involvement. The paresis diminished progressively, but the speech disturbance persisted unchanged until the man's death 1 year later. Van Gehuchten described the clinical picture as "pure motor aphasia with agraphia with no word blindness or deafness."[254] The patient was incapable of speaking. He uttered only a few sounds and sometimes a word or two. However, he could express himself adequately by gestures and writing some letters or ordinary words in response to dictation but was unable to write spontaneously or from dictation under more demanding circumstances. Autopsy revealed an infarct affecting the inferior half of the middle frontal gyrus from the top to the bottom of what was described as Broca's area.

Kleist[264] believed that the rare instances of a persistent and severe deficit associated with Broca's area infarction could be explained by an extension of the infarct deep into the hemisphere, disrupting the white matter fibers that serve as projection and association pathways for Broca's area. Foix[265] made a similar inference earlier, referring to infarcts affecting the deeper branches of the MCA. Goldstein[238] also made similar suggestions but did not specify the vascular territory involved in these larger lesions.

Speech Disturbances with Lower Rolandic Infarction. Few cases of lower rolandic infarction have been reported since the days of Moutier,[252] whose studies suggested that infarcts in the region did not cause motor aphasia.[257,258] Levine and Sweet[266] cited a third case of rolandic infarction involving most of the precentral gyrus. The patient was only able to vocalize grunting or moaning sounds for the 10 days she was testable before her death. Autopsy disclosed a highly focal hemorrhage involving the midportion of the precentral gyrus that spared the frontal region in Broca's area.

The overlap of this syndrome with cases producing predominantly literal paraphasias has been described by Luria[237] as afferent motor aphasia, attributed to faulty sensory feedback from a postrolandic lesion, leading to inaccurate anatomic settings of the oropharynx, with resultant mispronunciations.

Speech Disturbances from Deep Infarcts. Infarcts affecting the motor outflow of both sides have produced mutism as part of a syndrome of paralysis of both sides of the face, oropharynx, and tongue. However, a more interesting syndrome occurs from a single deep infarct that can cause enough disturbance in speech and language. Bonhoeffer's[57] classic patient, unable to speak anything more than a few poorly formed vowels, had a large, deep infarct of the type described as a "giant lacune."[267] This prevented innervation of the bulbar apparatus from ipsilateral pathways as well as transcallosal projections. The basic pathophysiology is supported by a handful of other autopsy reports[264] or CT studies.[268,269] Altogether the studies suggest that the disorder may be explained by damage to thalamofrontal pathways, and the diminished verbal behavior forms part of the syndrome of abulia.[270,271]

Sensory Aphasia

The syndrome known as Wernicke's aphasia is most commonly explained by occlusion of the lower division of the MCA and its branches. Because the lower division gives off its branches over an extremely short distance just at or distal to the posterior end of the Sylvian fissure, the occlusion at or near the point of takeoff of these branches may give rise to several distinct variants. There is a rough correlation between the extent of the language deficit and its intensity as a function of the lesion size.

Major Sensory Aphasia. An occlusion that blocks the trunk or branches of the lower division of MCA causes a large infarct encompassing the whole posterior temporal, inferior parietal, and lateral temporooccipital regions (Fig. 24-20). Infarcts of such huge size generate a profound deficit in language function, classically known as Wernicke's aphasia but here described as major sensory aphasia.

In the early phase, in contrast to motor aphasia, patients with any degree of sensory aphasia show little or no disturbance in the ability to vocalize; they even make smooth transitions between syllables, assembling utterances in the form of

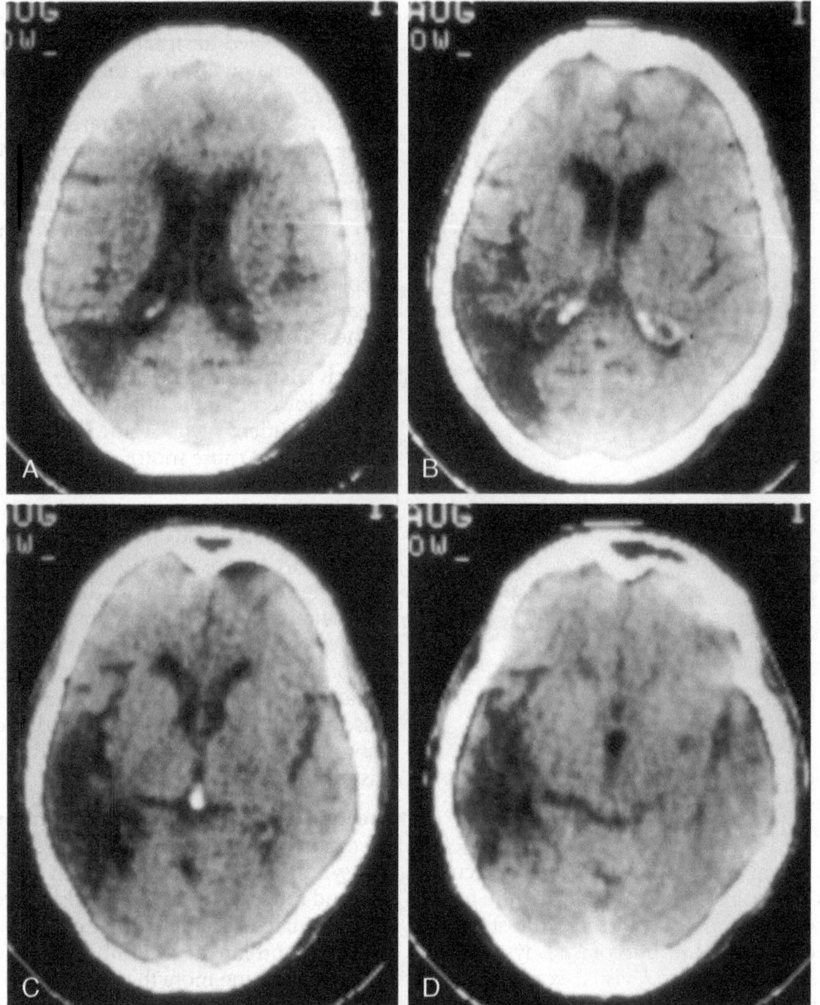

Figure 24-20 A–D, CT evidence of large infarct involving the lower division of the middle cerebral artery in a right-handed woman who had no aphasia.

phrases, and usually achieve intonations of utterances that sound like questions, replies, and declarative statements.[234]

The extent of the language disturbance may often require prolonged conversation to document the full range of errors. The casual or hurried examiner may find that the patient speaks easily, engages in simple conversational exchanges, and even appears to be making an effort at communication. At the extreme, the normal-appearing expressive tone during spontaneous discourse is such that if the patient were assumed to be speaking in an unfamiliar language, the listener might infer intact linguistic function. However, attempts to engage the patient in testing often fail to yield much evidence that the patient has understood the task and is attempting to respond. When the patient does not respond properly, the examiner is faced with the difficulty of deciding whether the fault lies in comprehension, in praxis, or in his/her own failure to make clear to the patient what is required.[272]

For the large infarcts, the disturbance in language content manifests as such gross disturbance in the content of spoken speech as to contain no understandable words, often occurring as isolated single or multiple syllables, a condition known as jargon paraphasia, word salad or gibberish. The specific words expected to be uttered – the target words – are often distorted (but recognizable) in their phonetic structure (literal paraphasia) both in vowels and consonants or comprise other words in the same class (verbal paraphasias). In addition, these errors are occasionally accompanied by unwanted suffixes (e.g., "cold-ing"; less often prefixes) and are often also contaminated by the recurrence (perseverations) of previously uttered words or word fragments. The speech that is understandable is filled with small grammatical words but is missing the key words (the predicative elements) that contain the essence of the message (e.g., "I...you well"; the expected "know" is absent from the sentence).

Writing is usually disturbed in content but not in form, much like spoken speech. The cursive script is usually legible, but the language content in the written letters and words has little communicative value. In some cases, writing and oral naming show striking differences in the severity of the language disorder, which some researchers have argued means that the two forms of expression are not under the same control.[273,274] The disturbance in comprehension of language for words heard or seen has long been assumed to be of the same type as that observed in spoken and written speech, claimed to be a sign of the essentially unitary nature of the disorder.[247] However, despite the assumption that the brain lesion on the superior temporal plane interferes with auditory comprehension, it has been difficult to demonstrate any such disturbance in phonemic processing.[258] Instead, the problem lies at the level of determining the linguistic significance of the adequately discriminated auditory stimuli.[275] It has likewise proved difficult to determine the extent to which disturbances in reading comprehension parallel those of auditory comprehension.[273]

The phenomenology of major sensory aphasia has always been of interest to students of language abnormality, but the severe comprehension deficits during the acute syndrome usually preclude study[276] and often represent the insensitivity of the observer's methods.[277]

The clinicopathologic correlation in Wernicke's aphasia, as in Broca's aphasia, has been with a rather large lesion.[225,278] Some correlation exists between lesion size and performance in special language studies comparing the spoken and written response to auditory and visual presentation of words, pictures, and sounds: patients with small lesions are no better at oral response to words, sounds, or pictures of the same items (i.e., the disturbance was just as severe for words heard as words seen or for sounds heard as pictures seen). Other patients with smaller lesions may show limited disturbance in either auditory or visual comprehension but not both to the same degree.[273] Patients with protracted and exaggerated spontaneous speaking (logorrhea) suffered from larger infarcts; those with smaller infarcts rarely show this sign.

Exceptions exist: some patients with a large lesion across the lower division may not show a full clinical picture of Wernicke's aphasia. In some, the syndrome has been conduction aphasia.[279,280] In these cases, comprehension is so satisfactory that the main finding is difficulty in repeating aloud. A few cases have been reported in which either no detectable initial deficit in language occurred or the deficit was at most only slight and transient,[281–283] even though the patient had an infarct affecting the posterior superior temporal region that was large enough to have been expected to produce Wernicke's aphasia. Dr. JP Mohr described a similar case of an elderly right-handed woman whose cerebral embolism occurred while she was walking in her garden in the company of her internist son. She was immediately tested: she could read aloud and write correctly and could repeat and converse normally, but she experienced signs of right hemianopia. Examination within days also failed to disclose language disturbance (Fig. 24-21). Such cases indicate the limitations of our understanding of language organization in the brain.

Minor Sensory Aphasia and Variants. Retrograde collateral flow established from the branches of the posterior cerebral artery may reduce the total infarct size; the ischemic zone may shrink in centripetal fashion toward the site of occlusion.

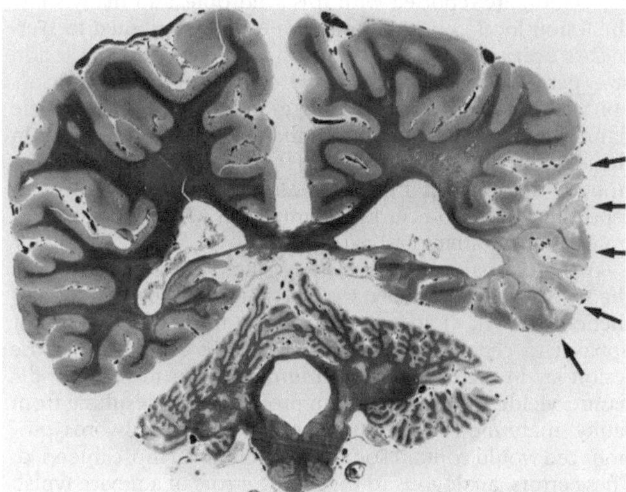

Figure 24-21 Coronal section from the posterior half of the brain in a patient with Wernicke's aphasia that evolved over years toward a syndrome of dyslexia with dysgraphia.

An associated issue is the precise location and size of Wernicke's area.[284,285] Lesion mapping by CT or MRI has led to a Venn diagram of overlaps,[286] but may be misleading because the site common to all cases is the posterior superior temporal plane, the usual site of the embolic vascular occlusion causing the syndrome. Cases of the fully developed, major Wernicke's aphasia with an isolated lesion of superior temporal plane appear to be remarkably rare.[133,237,251,265,287–289] The literature search shows that only three superior temporal plane lesions have been found with Wernicke's aphasia among 89 published cases with autopsy correlation. Two of the cases are subject to criticisms[109] and the third is described too briefly to permit much analysis.[264] Henschen,[133] in a review of the literature up to the mid-1920s, concluded that a superior temporal plane lesion does not cause the full picture of Wernicke's aphasia (both "pure word deafness" and "alexia"). He based this opinion on a review of 35 patients with temporal lobe lesions, 20 of whom had "pure word deafness." In none was alexia present. Earlier, Bastian[290] had found alexia and sensory (Wernicke's) aphasia in only five of 16 cases of temporal lobe lesions, and in most, the lesion was large. Studies based on imaging have added no qualitatively new cases.[224,269]

Pure Word Deafness. More than 40 cases with CT or autopsy correlation of pure word deafness have been reported. According to the classic formulations, the only deficit should be auditory; spontaneous speech should be normal, as should reading comprehension and writing.[291] Eight well-known cases exist in which a unilateral lesion is confined to the superior temporal plane in the dominant hemisphere. In seven of them, paraphasic speaking was prominent, which is a clinical picture not permitted in the formulation of pure word deafness, which, by definition, should be free of a disturbance in speaking. In many cases, the elements of paraphasic speech cleared later.[292,293]

Many of the patients with bilateral lesions also experienced paraphasic speaking with poor comprehension during the early phase of the stroke.[279,294] In the famous case reported by Pick,[295] bilateral lesions, including a large left temporal plane lesion, rendered the patient paraphasic for 4 years.[279]

There is not much evidence that unilateral infarcts of the left temporal lobe can create a state of impaired auditory discrimination.[234] The spontaneous speech contains many paraphasic errors, especially in the acute stages; the errors are frequent enough that the listener may make a preliminary diagnosis of Wernicke's aphasia. In addition, when tasked with reading aloud or comprehension tasks, patients with such lesions make enough errors that the notion of a pure disorder in auditory comprehension is not easily maintained.

Cortical Deafness. At least one case report exists of an autopsied patient who was well studied clinically and was found to have deafness from an infarct confined to Heschl's transverse gyrus.[296] Bilateral infarcts affecting the temporal plane are a well-recognized cause of deafness, even though only a few reports have appeared.[297,298]

Alexia with Agraphia. Alexia with agraphia as an isolated syndrome, with absent aphasic errors in speech or in auditory comprehension, is extremely rare. Henschen[133] found five "pure" cases among the more than 250 patients who had dyslexia and dysgraphia as part of larger clinical syndromes, noting that almost all patients suffering alexia with agraphia have some degree of aphasia which ranges from a minimal degree of word-finding difficulty. The disturbance in reading comprehension and in the morphology and language content of writing far exceeds. but does not occur in the absence of, a

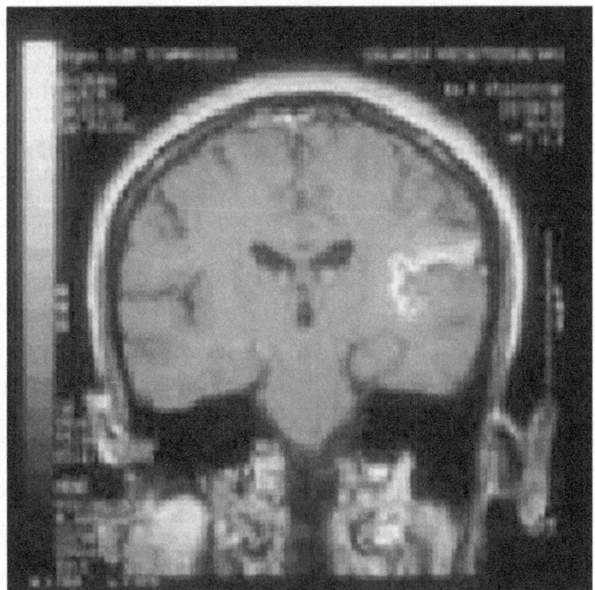

Figure 24-22 Coronal T1-weighted MR image with contrast enhancement showing a posterior insular cortex infarct in a patient with conduction aphasia featuring semantic errors.

disturbance in auditory comprehension or in spontaneous speech.[152,278,288,299,300] Sidman et al.[301,302] studied such a patient for many years; autopsy eventually showed a large lesion affecting much of the posterior left hemisphere (Fig. 24-22). His deficit began as sensory aphasia, affecting all forms of language and all conditions of testing. As time passed, the spoken response to auditory language stimuli improved, but the written response to any tests and the response to printed words remained impaired, which is a disturbance that could be classified grossly as dyslexia with dysgraphia.

The clinical problem is not whether dyslexia with dysgraphia exists, but whether it is only a transient, acute disorder or one that occurs mainly as a long-term condition of an initially more severe Wernicke's aphasia. For the syndrome to be dyslexia and dysgraphia, classic doctrine would require a circumscribed infarction beyond the superior temporal plane. Embolism is the only reliable source of such an infarct, apart from the focal form of vasculitis. In the unusual case in which the posterior cerebral artery takes its origin from the carotid artery, the main weight of the distal infarction could fall on the parietooccipital lobe, which happened in the case reported by Sidman et al.[302] The cases in the literature suggest that it is a late development from an earlier syndrome of more extensive deficits.

Conduction Aphasia

Conduction aphasia occupies a special position in aphasiology, mainly because of its theoretical prediction rather than its isolated occurrence as a clinical entity. It was described by Wernicke[303] as the interruption of fiber pathways connecting the sensory language zone of the posterior half of the brain with the motor language zone in the frontal lobe. For Goldstein,[238] the disorder also represented disruption of a brain region that mediated the interaction between the major sensory and motor centers. Neither theory accounts for the clinical features.[304] Modern efforts with tensor MR tractography have also not settled the issue,[305] and examples even exist with the syndrome and a left thalamic infarct by MRI.[306]

The term conduction aphasia is applied to patients with poor repetition, mostly of phonemic errors (substitutions of one sound for the target sound), especially for unfamiliar material, and far better auditory and visual comprehension of language than that evident in their spontaneous spoken and written efforts. That spontaneous speech is often contaminated by paraphasic utterances is not emphasized. Although auditory and visual language comprehension is relatively preserved, neither function is normal at any stage of the disorder.[269] The disturbance in repeating aloud, on which great stress has been laid,[244,307] is not so useful a distinguishing point in the early stage of the syndrome because it also occurs in Wernicke's aphasia. In assessing the deficits in conversation, Burns and Canter[308] found a higher incidence of unwanted phonemes and intrusion of semantically related words among those patients classified as having Wernicke's aphasia than among those with conduction aphasia. Patients with conduction aphasia are also said to have a greater tendency to attempt self-correction than those with Wernicke's aphasia.[288] For ordinary clinical purposes, the distinction between the error patterns in speaking in the two types is not an easy one, except that semantic word substitutions are rare in conduction aphasia.[309,310] The syndrome often proves surprisingly evanescent when seen in an acute setting. More often, the initial syndrome is Wernicke-type aphasia, evolving later into the picture of greater difficulty with pronunciation of words.[280]

Disturbances in eye movements and visual fields are minor or not present. Bucco-linguo-facial dyspraxia is a common accompaniment, as is bimanual ideomotor dyspraxia. The dyspraxia of the latter state is different in the two limbs: the disorder in the limb served by the infarcted hemisphere takes the form of a de-afferentation[200] and that in the other limb conforms more to the picture expected in ideomotor dyspraxia.

The clinicopathologic correlation is also at odds with the theory. The classic hypothesis envisioned interruption of the arcuate fasciculus as the mechanism for the errors.[244,307] The interruption presumably prevents adequate control by the auditory system over the speech apparatus. Because the lesion interrupts arcuate fasciculus, the findings expected on brain imaging or autopsy would be mainly subcortical. However, autopsy evidence in support of this hypothesis is surprisingly slight. The documented lesions have all been superficial infarcts whose penetration into the subcortical white matter has varied considerably.[243] In only a few has it been profound enough to produce a cleft deep enough to injure the arcuate fasciculus.[279] More than 20 cases with CT, MRI, or autopsy correlation are reported with this syndrome, and many show the lesion located in the same area usually attributed to Wernicke's aphasia. Naeser[251] found no difference in the lesion size per CT slice in cases with conduction or Wernicke's aphasia, but the mean percentage of left hemispheral tissue damage was larger in patients with Wernicke's aphasia than in those with conduction aphasia ($P < 0.01$). Electrical stimulation of the exposed brain has also shown disturbances in repeating aloud from surface stimulation of the superior temporal and supramarginal gyri.[311]

Another major hypothesis of the conduction aphasia theory considers the deficit to represent a disturbance in kinesthetic feedback. Luria[237] coined the term afferent motor aphasia to characterize this behavior. He assumed that the lesion lay in the Sylvian operculum posterior to the rolandic fissure, yielding a disturbance in pronunciation resulting from faulty anatomic oropharyngeal positioning. The words pronounced would contain sounds different from those intended. These errors, analogous to the typing errors of a novice typist, require considerable listener training for their detection, rather like the recognition of typing errors by those familiar with the typewriter keyboard. The novice listener may easily mistake them for language errors (paraphasias) and may assume that

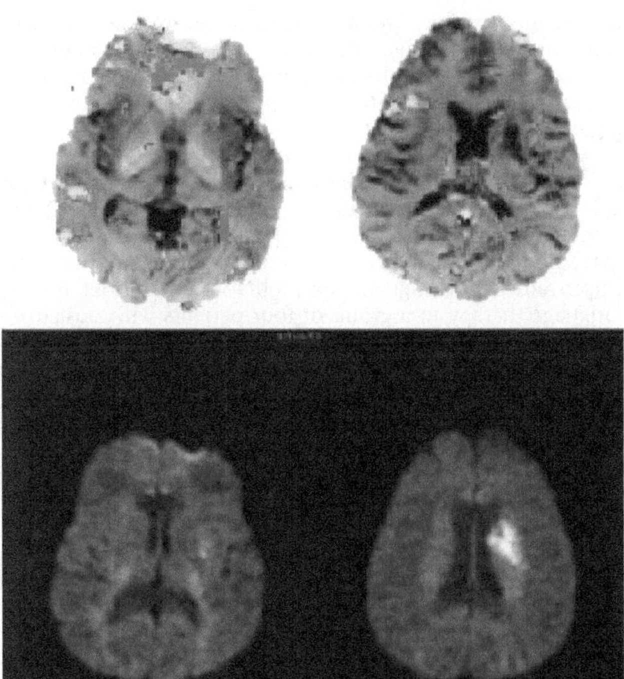

Figure 24-23 Aphasia recovery. Activation seen in the right frontal and temporal lobes in regions homologous to Broca's and Wernicke's areas. Infarct in left basal ganglia and periventricular white matter seen on diffusion-weighted MR image.

the speaker has a language disorder. Such an interpretation may be inaccurate, but it remains common medical practice to refer to errors of this type as "literal paraphasias." The major difficulty experienced by affected patients in repeating aloud can be considered to represent a disturbance in encoding accompanied by a disturbance in short-term memory.[312]

Whether the impairment in conduction aphasia represents mere phonologic mistargeting or is truly language-based is debatable. A patient experienced a syndrome of fluent conversational speech, normal auditory and reading comprehension. However, repetition was halting and effortful.[313] Nearly all the paraphasic errors (naming, repetition, reading aloud and writing) were semantic substitutions. For example, "The quarterback threw the football down the field on Saturday" became "The quarterback through the baseball into the field." High-resolution MRI identified an infarct restricted to the posterior left insular cortex and intra-Sylvian parietal operculum (Fig. 24-23). As a result of the more modern studies using brain imaging, it has been recognized that the syndrome may occur from infarction in the lower division of the MCA.[264] The disturbance is often considered merely a mild form of sensory aphasia.[314]

"Transcortical" Aphasia

The observation of an aphasic syndrome with relatively intact ability to repeat dictated material aloud is attributed to Wernicke,[303,315] but Goldstein[238,316] has been recognized for his attempt to establish a separate entity characterized by an "isolation of the speech area." The traditional inference has been that the Sylvian region is preserved, as demonstrated by intact repetition skills, and that the responsible lesion for the aphasic disorder is elsewhere. The exact anatomic basis is less well-established than the term transcortical suggests, but three syndrome subsets have been described–motor, sensory, and mixed.[317,318] Recent reports of such cases have shown some very large lesions.[319]

Transcortical motor aphasia (TCMA) resembles major motor aphasia (limited spontaneous speech and good comprehension) with relatively intact repetition.[304] The language of some patients matches the classic behavioral description, but lesions have been found in the white matter anterolateral to the left frontal horn. They demonstrate that the expected lesion location for TCMA produces varying degrees of impaired articulation, mild deficits in auditory comprehension, and stuttering. TCMA has also been described as a phase during the evolution of Broca's syndrome. It has also been observed that motor language syndromes with good repetition occur during the recovery process after infarction in the territory of the anterior cerebral artery, usually involving the supplementary motor area in the paramedian region of the frontal lobe.

Transcortical sensory aphasia (TCSA) resembles a major sensory syndrome consisting of fluent speech, impaired comprehension, alexia with agraphia, and paraphasic errors, but relatively preserved repetition ability.[320] Patients often display compulsive repetition (echolalia). The responsible lesion is usually large, occurring in the territory of the posterior cerebral artery and involving the temporoparietooccipital junction.[321] The broad range of cognitive deficits often seen in conjunction with TCSA, including amnestic and attention disturbances.[322]

Mixed transcortical aphasia is the entity to which Goldstein[316] made reference in 1917 as "isolation of the speech." These patients have a global aphasia, except for retention of good repetition and virtually no other capacity for receptive or expressive propositional language. This is a very unusual syndrome and only a small number of cases have been reported.[307] In the setting of acute stroke with no prior language disturbance, mixed transcortical aphasia has been said to occur from occlusion of the left internal carotid artery, resulting in simultaneous embolism in the anterior pial territory and perfusion failure in the terminal branches of MCA and PCA.[323]

Functional Imaging in Aphasia

Regional changes in cerebral blood flow and metabolism can be identified by single-photon emission CT (SPECT), PET, or ultrafast MRI. Hypoperfusion and hypometabolism may extend into the peri-infarct area or may be seen at a site distant from the lesion itself.[324]

Patients with moderate to severe aphasia often show regions of hypometabolism encompassing large frontoparietal or temporoparietal areas, even in the presence of modest cortical or subcortical structural lesions.[276,317,325,326] Larger metabolic defects in the early phase of hemispheral stroke that extend beyond the borders of infarction[327,328] correlate with a worse initial clinical state and appear to predict poorer recovery from aphasia.[329,330] Reversal of cortical hypometabolism may correlate with clinical improvement when lesions are deep,[279,331] although in some cases of subcortical stroke, cortical hypometabolism may persist for at least 3 months despite good clinical recovery.[332]

A PET study by Metter et al.[327] suggested that different aphasias may share common regions of hypometabolism regardless of lesion site. These researchers studied 44 aphasic patients with FDG-PET. Metabolic decreases were found in the left angular gyrus in 97% of patients, in the left supramarginal gyrus in 87%, and in the left posterior superior temporal gyrus in 85%. Taken all together, 100% of the patients had PET abnormalities in the left parietotemporal region. A greater degree of hypometabolism in the prefrontal region was the only imaging feature that distinguished patients with Broca's aphasia from those with Wernicke's aphasia. In functional imaging studies of normal control subjects performing language tasks, hyperperfusion or hypermetabolism has been demonstrated in certain brain regions. The superior temporal gyrus has been implicated both in the early acoustic processing of words and nonwords[333–335] and in the word-retrieval process required to generate verbs from noun stimuli.[336] The prefrontal region and supplementary motor area may also play a role in word selection and output.[335]

Cappa et al.[337] showed that, in two right-handed aphasic patients with right-sided lesions (periventricular corona radiata and lentiform nucleus), there was not only widespread hypometabolism in right cortical and subcortical structures, but also decreased metabolism in the left frontal and parietal cortex, suggesting that the left hemisphere played a role in the aphasia even though the structural lesion was restricted to the right. When structural damage has unexpectedly included the left peri-Sylvian region, SPECT and 133Xe regional cerebral blood flow studies have revealed extensive hypoperfusion throughout the left hemisphere but increased blood flow in the contralateral right temporal lobe.[317] Finally, in a patient with a conduction aphasia in which the paraphasic errors were nearly all semantic substitutions, MRI showed an infarct restricted to the posterior left insular cortex and intra-Sylvian parietal operculum, but SPECT revealed hypometabolism in the inferomedial and lateral left temporal lobe, suggesting a physiologic role for these regions in the syndrome.[338]

Various advanced imaging studies have begun to elucidate the functional reorganization that is associated with recovery of stroke-induced deficits. Although some investigators have reported that contrahemispheral mirror locations correlate with the recovery process in mildly affected aphasic patients, others claim that peri-infarct and other ipsilateral regions are crucial for recovery and that activation in the contralateral hemisphere may correlate with persistence of aphasia.[339] Most of the evidence suggests that the right hemisphere contributes to recovery from aphasia, particularly in the early phase and ultimate recovery depends on return of function in the left hemisphere.[256] In a PET study of 12 aphasic patients with strokes in the left MCA territory, Heiss et al.[340] observed unique activation during a word-repetition task 3–4 weeks after the patients had experienced stroke in the right supplementary motor area (SMA); this activation was not seen in ten roughly age-matched control subjects. In follow-up PET performed 18 months after the stroke, return of left superior temporal activity was shown to be associated with good performance on an auditory comprehension task, which suggests that it was the return of left hemisphere function over time that was important in good recovery. Additional evidence that right hemisphere involvement in language was only the second-best mediator of recovery was demonstrated by the findings that (1) persistence of the right SMA activity was inversely correlated with performance on the language comprehension task and (2) persistence of right temporal activation was inversely correlated with recovery of left temporal activity. In a follow-up study, the same investigators performed PET imaging at 1 week and 8 weeks after cortical or subcortical stroke in 23 aphasic patients. They observed unique activation in the right inferior frontal region at 1 week. Good recovery of language correlated with activity in the left superior temporal region at 1 week, 8 weeks, or both and also with a disappearance of the right hemisphere activation. Patients with stroke whose original infarcts destroyed the left superior temporal region were not able to incorporate Wernicke's area back into a language network, and this was the reason, the investigators argued, that these patients had a worse prognosis for language recovery.[340]

Timely recanalization in acute ischemic stroke often results in good clinical outcomes. However, sudden recanalization and increased blood flow into the ischemic brain tissue may be harmful in some patients. Impaired cerebral autoregulation during the first few days after acute stroke may occasionally result in "luxury perfusion", due to excessive vasodilatation of collaterals, with neurological worsening in some patients.[341] An example of this interesting phenomenon is shown in Figure 24-24.

Functional significance of brain reorganization after stroke can be understood better by imaging before and after a specific rehabilitative intervention. Only a few studies of this type have been done to date. The right superior temporal gyrus and left precuneus were reported to be associated with improvements in language comprehension after brief, intense language therapy in a group of four patients with poststroke Wernicke's aphasia.[342] Ipsihemispheral translocation of language function has also been demonstrated in patients with AVM in the posterior, dominant hemisphere,[343] but contralesional extension of function has been seen in right frontal AVM.[276]

Epidemiology and Natural History of Aphasia

According to NINCDS, there are more than 1 million aphasia survivors in the US.[344] Acquired disorders of language can arise from many causes, such as cerebrovascular disease, trauma, tumor, and most other causes of cerebral dysfunction,[343] but stroke represents by far the most frequent etiology of language-based disorders. Among those with acute stroke, 21–38% of patients are seen with aphasia,[345] and an ischemic event is the cause in about 80%.[346] As a group, 79% of patients with poststroke aphasia still have aphasic deficits at the end of 12 months. Engelter et al.[347] showed that there is increasing risk of developing poststroke aphasia with advancing age. In their population-based study of first-ever stroke patients, the risk of aphasia increased by 1–7% per each year of age. Whereas every seventh patient younger than 65 years had aphasia, subjects older than 85 years were three times more likely to develop aphasia. Depression is common after stroke,[348] but studies have confirmed that 30–40% of patients with left hemisphere stroke and a nonfluent aphasia experienced profound depressive symptoms.[349]

Most patients who have had a stroke improve in function at least to some degree.[350] Although most improvement is detected within the first 3 months after a stroke,[351,352] longer-term follow-up has shown that motor function improvement continues well beyond 6 months[353] and after 2 years for aphasia.[223,354] Pedersen et al.[346] showed that different initial syndromes appear to improve at different rates. In their series of 203 first-time stroke patients with aphasia, 32% had global aphasia and 25% had anomic aphasia. By the end of 1 year, nearly 40% of patients had anomic syndromes, and about one-fourth had Wernicke's and Broca's aphasias, respectively. In general, older patients were likely to be seen with focal aphasias, whereas younger patients were more likely to be seen with global syndromes that evolved to more focal features. The greatest degree of spontaneous improvement appears to occur within the first 3 months after a stroke.[355–358] Among the factors purported to determine language improvement after stroke, initial syndrome severity and lesion size have been reported to be important predictors.[359–363]

Many studies of the course of aphasia, however, did not collect baseline data until several weeks after admission, did not exclude patients with prior strokes, and reported data as mean values for patient groups based on initial aphasia diagnosis, which obscures potential variability across individual patients. The advantage of evaluating individual deficits rather than global characterizations (Wernicke's and Broca's aphasias) is that within each of these syndromes is a wide range of profiles and that disturbances can be highly idiosyncratic, especially when the lesions are smaller. Moreover, it has been

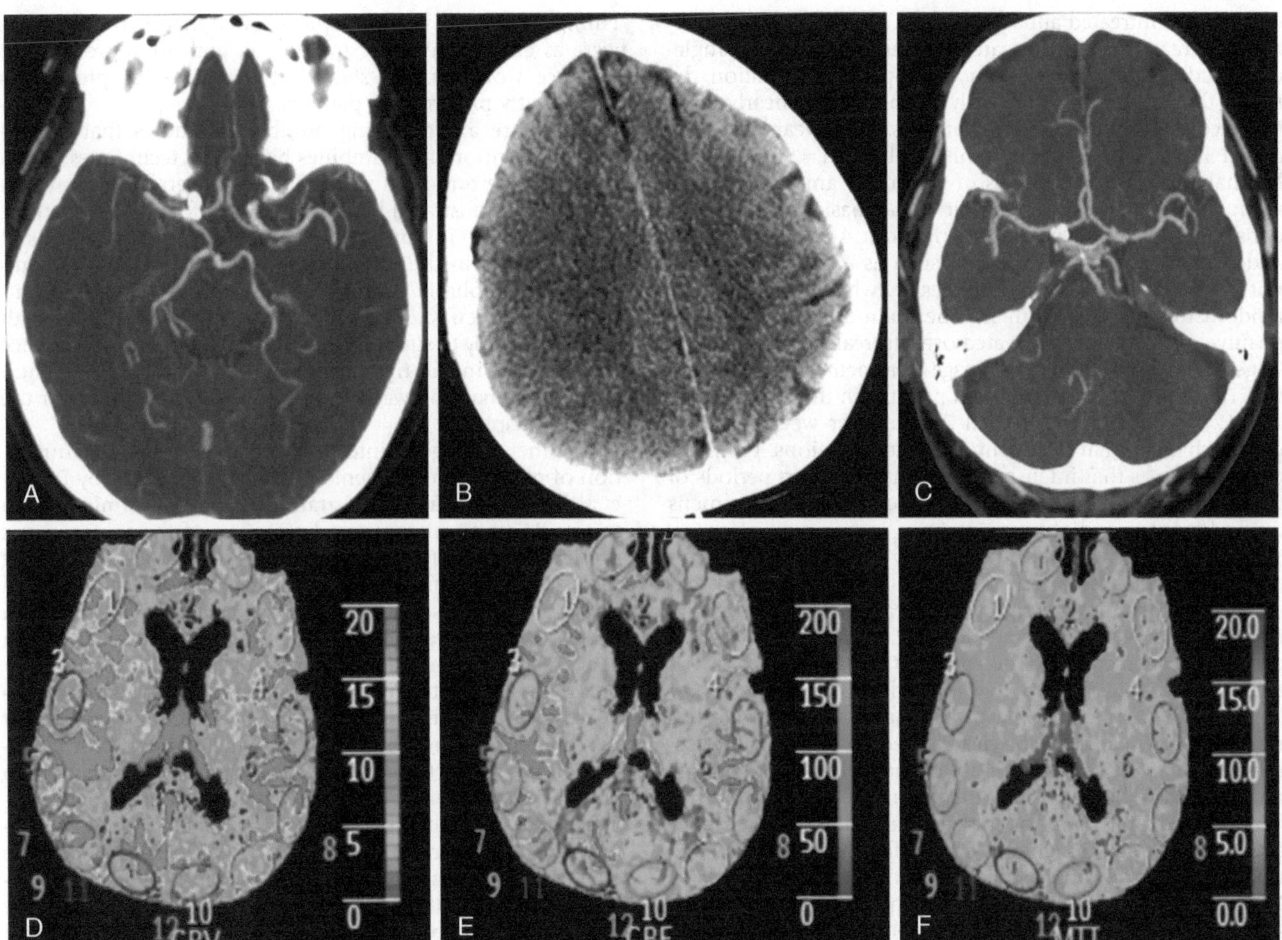

Figure 24-24 A, Pre-thrombolysis CT angiography shows an occlusion of right MCA. This patient achieved complete recovery within 25 minutes of initiating intravenous thrombolysis. However, she deteriorated rapidly about 2 hours later. Repeat CT of the brain did not show any intracranial hemorrhage. However, diffuse swelling of the right hemisphere was noted (B). CT angiogram showed complete recanalization of the right MCA (C). CT-perfusion revealed increased cerebral blood volume (D), cerebral blood flow (E) and normal mean transit time (F), suggestive of cerebral hyperperfusion syndrome.

shown in large studies of acute poststroke aphasia that only slightly more than half of patients have the classic syndrome of aphasiology.[363]

The evolution of language was followed up in the Columbia Performance and Recovery in Stroke (PARIS) study, a prospective database of first-ever stroke patients.[364] Comprehension, naming, and repetition were chosen because of their sensitivity to deficits that can arise from anterior or posterior lesions and because of their objectivity in measurement. The major aim of this study was to characterize the nature and extent of recovery of aphasic deficits from 24–72 hours after stroke-onset through a 90-day follow-up. Twenty-two of 91 patients had language disorders. Initial syndrome scores were positively correlated with 90-days scores ($r = 0.60$) and negatively correlated with the change in score from baseline to follow-up ($r = -0.66$). Lesion size, age or education did not show correlation with initial syndrome severity or performance at 90 days. A multiple regression model that combined lesion size, age and initial syndrome was significant ($P = 0.03$) but only explained 29% of the variance. Patients with severe deficits at baseline in individual language domains could improve close to normal, improve to a less severe deficit, or not improve at all. These data suggest that other factors have not yet been identified that account for functional stroke recovery.

Efficacy of Aphasia Therapy

It is widely agreed that in the clinical practice of speech-language pathology a comprehensive examination is appropriate.[358] Some of the commonly used aphasia batteries include the Boston Diagnostic Aphasia Examination[365] and the Western Aphasia Battery,[366] both of which assess functions such as spontaneous speech, comprehension, naming, reading, writing, and repetition. There are also more functionally based evaluation batteries, such as the Porch Index of Communicative Abilities[367] and the Communicative Abilities in Daily Living.[368]

An evaluation of aphasia therapy depends on the choice of outcome measurements and the language assessment methodology. Two considerations include whether there should be a single outcome measure of global function (the Aphasia Severity Score of the Western Aphasia Battery) or a focus on particular outcome skills (Visual Confrontation Naming on the Boston Diagnostic Aphasia Examination). Outcomes can also be based on a group-design format or the use of single subjects as their own controls. Regardless of the analytic approach, more than 600 articles have appeared in the literature examining treatment approaches.[369]

Among the first meta-analyses in the aphasia literature was Robey's inclusion of 21 studies that evaluated three classes of effect sizes: untreated aphasia recovery, treated aphasia recovery, and treated versus untreated recovery.[370] Excluding single-case studies and reports with incomplete information, he found that treatment in the early period yielded nearly twice the recovery of untreated individuals. Four years later, he added 34 additional studies to his database (n = 55) in which he analyzed four dimensions of treatment: amount of treatment, type of treatment, severity of aphasia, and type of aphasia.[356] To his inclusion criteria from 4 years earlier, he added quasiexperimental designs such as patients who were not randomly selected and studies in which there was no random treatment assignment. The main findings showed a positive outcome for (1) treated over untreated patients at all stages of recovery, with an average treatment effect size that was 1.83 times that for untreated patients in the early period, and (2) treatment longer than 2 hours per week inducing greater changes than treatment of shorter durations. The main conclusion was that intensive treatment over short periods of time provides better outcomes than less intensive regimens over a longer period of time.

Bhogal et al. evaluated the intensity of aphasia therapy in a meta-analytic evaluation of ten studies.[371] They found that studies demonstrating a significant treatment effect required 8.8 hours per week of therapy for 11.2 weeks. In a Cochrane review, Greener et al. examined 60 RCTs in which only 12 satisfied selection criteria.[372] It was concluded that "speech and language therapy for people with aphasia after a stroke has not been shown either to be clearly effective or clearly ineffective within an RCT. Decisions about management of patients must therefore be based on other forms of evidence." It has been argued that many of the studies included by Greener et al. were not well-designed to draw definite conclusions.[369,373] Using analysis for single-subject treatment effects, Moss and Nicholas[374] evaluated 23 studies that met criteria identifying subjects who received direct continuous therapy for spoken language deficits and whose changes in response to therapy were measurable. Thus treatment was capable of demonstrating benefit even years after stroke onset.

All language-based therapies, whether analyzed on an individual or group basis, occur in patients who have an admixture of factors that mediate the outcomes of intervention.[358] Factors such as nonlanguage cognitive status, affective status (depression), physical illness, concomitant medications, and support system have all been shown to affect long-term aphasia outcomes.

Innovative Aphasia Therapies

New therapies hold promise for increased benefits for patients with postinjury aphasia. Rather than being based on the traditional notion of compensating for deficits, more recent approaches have been based on principles of human learning and on theories of neural plasticity.

Based on the success of constraint-induced therapy for hemiparesis,[375] constraint-induced language therapy (CILT) involves the forced use of spoken communication with restraint of other modalities of communication, including gestures.[376,377] To determine whether there are corresponding neurophysiologic changes that would provide a mechanistic basis for improvement in behavioral function, Breier et al.[377] showed that five patients who responded well to CILT exhibited a greater degree of late magnetoencephalographic (MEG) activation in posterior language areas of the left hemisphere and homotopic areas of the right hemisphere before therapy than those who did not respond well. Analogously, probes with TMS have also demonstrated functional reorganization after therapy.[378] Errorless learning procedures, derived from principles of operant conditioning, have also been studied.[379] Fillingham et al.,[380] for example, showed that such techniques were as effective as more traditional, errorful approaches to enhance word-retrieval skills but that errorless procedures were greatly preferred by patients.

There are an increasing number of studies that suggest that intervention that combines behavioral techniques with a biological perturbation might improve overall outcomes, as was first demonstrated by Feeney et al. studying the effects of amphetamines in an animal model of motor deficits.[381] Some efficacy in the administration of amphetamines combined with aphasia remediation to improve language outcomes has been shown.[382] TMS has also been paired with aphasia therapy to suppress the presumed inhibitory influence of activation in the right hemisphere. Naeser et al.[383] found that picture naming was enhanced with stimulation over the right hemisphere.

Another biological intervention involves the administration of pharmacologic agents. Early animal studies by Feeney et al.[381] showed that administration of D-amphetamines given to rats 24 hours after surgical resection of the motor cortex produced acceleration of function. Later studies reproduced the facilitating effects in rats after experimenter-induced stroke.[384,385] After several pilot investigations in patients with poststroke weakness had positive results,[386,387] Walker-Batson et al.[382] showed, in a double-blind, placebo-controlled study of 21 patients with aphasia, that dextroamphetamine produced greater improvement in language scores at 1 week, but the differences were not significant when corrected for multiple comparisons. Unfortunately, a recent review of ten human poststroke studies involving 287 patients did not provide evidence that amphetamine treatment improved either neurologic function or activities of daily living.[388] Indeed, Gladstone et al. showed in a large double-blind study that amphetamines coupled with physical therapy given to patients in the early poststroke period provided no additional benefit in motor recovery compared with physiotherapy alone.[389] A concern regarding the use of amphetamines is their effect on blood pressure and heart rate during treatment compared with placebo.[390,391] Perhaps such safety issues contribute to the lack of a sustainable amphetamine effect, in addition to the reluctance to increase the dose higher than 10 mg in human treatment protocols.

Others have sought to administer pharmacologic agents that target specific transmitter systems. There is some evidence that cholinergic mechanisms may also be important in stroke and that such agents may work both as neuroprotectant and independent promoters of functional recovery.[392] While acetylcholine appears to induce plasticity as a facilitator of other mechanisms, such as N-methyl-D-aspartate-receptor-dependent long-term potentiation, it has also been shown to be an independent initiator of plasticity in rats.[393] There are reports suggestive of the restorative effects of cholinergic therapy for the treatment of poststroke aphasia.[394-396] A recent small clinical trial of 26 patients compared aphasia recovery for those taking donepezil versus placebo. At the end of the 12-week treatment period, those taking active drug had greater language recovery, which, unfortunately, was not sustained 1 month after drug cessation.[397]

The administration of dopaminergic agents has a role that combines controlling functions for both motor performance and cognition.[398] Studies in animals and humans reported that the dopamine agonist bromocriptine improves aphasia (left hemisphere function) and left hemineglect (right hemisphere function). With regard to restoration of language after stroke, bromocriptine has been extensively studied for treatment of motor (nonfluent) aphasias. Positive results in the initial study[399] were followed by negative findings in a second study,[124] although the patients in the latter study were described only as "brain-injured." Later work with a higher dose of bromocriptine in the first double-blind study involving stroke patients (more than 1 year before recruitment) showed statistically significant improvement in verbal latency, repetition, reading comprehension, dictation, and free speech.[400,401] Bragoni et al.[401] proposed that these findings result from dopamine's active role in neuronal projections from the midbrain to frontal brain regions, including SMAs and the cingulate gyrus.

Once a function has significantly improved after infarction, former stroke or TIA deficits can be transiently reinduced with a targeted sedating agent. The short-acting gamma-aminobutyric acid A (GABAA) agonist midazolam was administered to eight poststroke patients.[125] Those with left cerebral injury demonstrated reemergence of aphasia, right-sided weakness, or both but never left-sided weakness or left hemineglect. Conversely, patients who had had a right cerebral stroke demonstrated left-sided weakness, hemineglect, or both but no aphasia or right-sided paresis. Later, in a series of seven recovered aphasic patients, a double-blinded study showed that midazolam reinduced former aphasia deficits, whereas the sedative scopolamine had no impact on language function in the same group of patients.[402] Moreover, neither midazolam nor scopolamine had any statistical effect on the language behavior of age-matched, healthy control subjects. A recent double-blind, placebo-controlled trial showed that Fluoxetine (20 mg once a day), in patients recruited within 5–10 days after stroke-onset and Fugl-Meyer motor scale (FMMS) scores of 55 or less, resulted in better outcome as compared to placebo. In a study of 118 patients, FMMS improvement at day 90 was significantly greater in the fluoxetine group (adjusted mean 34.0 points [95%CI, 29.7–38.4]) than in the placebo group (24.3 points [19.9–28.7]; $P = 0.003$).[403]

The data seem to suggest that remediation for aphasia is most effective when outcomes are specific and intervention is tailored to the nature of the deficits. Therapy appears most effective when initiated earlier rather than later, but there is evidence to indicate that therapy may be useful even when initiated years after stroke.

Apraxias

Apraxias are acquired disorders of execution. They represent an inability to perform a previously learned, skilled act that is unexplained by weakness, visual loss, incoordination, dementia, sensory loss, or aphasia. Liepmann[404,405] described apraxia as the "incapacity for purposive movement despite retained mobility." Because these deficits in skilled movement are rarely complete, the term dyspraxia is often used. Apraxic deficits may affect movements of the body, face, or limbs. Liepmann proposed that the left hemisphere possesses the motor engrams necessary for skilled movements, just as it possesses the linguistic engrams necessary for speech. A left hemisphere dominance for skilled motor activity has been proposed,[406] in part based on the overwhelming proportion of left hemisphere lesions in right-handed patients with motor apraxia,[407] and the absence of motor apraxia in those with right retrorolandic lesions.[408]

Ideomotor Apraxia

The most common type of motor apraxia, ideomotor apraxia, was speculated by Liepmann[404,405] to be a dissociation between the brain areas that contain the "ideas" for movements and the "motor" areas responsible for execution. The examiner tests for the disturbance by asking patients to show how they would salute, wave goodbye, hammer a nail, saw wood, and perform various other actions; only crude left-sided movement is observed in the most severe cases. In milder cases, the actions are clumsy and lack precision. Performance may improve on imitation but typically is abnormal.[409] The best performance is elicited on actual use of the object.[247] Although aphasia commonly accompanies ideomotor apraxia, there is no close relationship between ideomotor apraxia and either the severity or the type of aphasia.[410–412] Heilman[413] suggested that the motor programs for skilled motor movements are stored in the left superior parietal lobe. Skilled motor activity would then depend on the transmission of these programs to the premotor area in the left frontal lobe. Ideomotor apraxia may then arise from either (1) direct destruction of motor programs in the left superior parietal lobe or (2) destruction of the pathways from the left superior parietal lobe to the premotor area of the left frontal lobe (i.e., disconnection).[414] Although ideomotor apraxia is more common with superficial than with deep lesions, large, deep lesions may produce ideomotor apraxia.[262] Ideomotor apraxia does not occur with smaller or deeper infarcts of the lacunar type. Little is known about the course of improvement, but it can be rapid in some cases.[247] Frontal lesions have a better prognosis than do posterior lesions.[410]

Ideational Apraxia

Ideational apraxia, a disorder of the sequencing and planning of complex motor acts,[415] bears an uncertain relation to ideomotor apraxia. The examiner can elicit it by asking the patient to demonstrate complex motor tasks, such as lighting a candle or mailing a letter. The literature is sparse in cases of stroke.[409] Sittig[416] believed that ideational apraxia is only a severe form of ideomotor apraxia, but others hold that they are distinct entities.[417,418] Ideational apraxia is generally observed after dominant hemisphere parietal lobe lesions. Bilateral parietal lesions are present in some cases,[408,419] but isolated right parietal lesions seem to produce ideational apraxia only in individuals with anomalous cerebral dominance.[420] Little is known about the improvement over time and whether there is "recovery" or simply a new strategy in responding.

Limb-Kinetic Apraxia

Limb-kinetic (also innervational or melokinetic) apraxia is manifested as a lack of rapidity, skill, and delicacy in the performance of learned motor movements.[407] Liepmann held that in limb-kinetic apraxia "the virtuosity which practice lends to movement is lost. Therefore the movements are...clumsy, without precision" (quoted by Kertesz[421]). The patient is clumsy in the execution of common motor acts, such as the manipulation of objects (eating with utensils, combing, brushing, using saws and hammers, and playing cards). Limb-kinetic apraxia is unilateral and affects the limb contralateral to the cerebral lesion. It may be difficult to distinguish between limb-kinetic apraxia and paresis in some cases. Commonly associated neurologic signs are ataxia, choreoathetosis, grasping, spasticity, weakness, and dystonic posturing. However, the clumsiness in using objects is out of proportion to these other deficits. Performance may improve slightly with the use of the object, but patients often act as if they were somewhat unfamiliar with its use.

Limb-kinetic apraxia may occur after injury to either the right or left premotor cortex or subjacent white matter.[287] Slight weakness is usually present, which suggests that injury to the pyramidal pathways is an essential feature of limb-kinetic apraxia. Patients with pure motor hemiplegia due to lacunar infarction in the internal capsule do not manifest limb-kinetic apraxia. Thus, the elicitation of this sign is a useful indicator that the surface cortex or subjacent white matter has been injured. The diagnosis of limb-kinetic apraxia is rarely made.

Callosal Apraxia

Callosal apraxia (sympathetic apraxia) represents a restricted form of ideomotor apraxia in which the apraxia is limited to the nondominant arm. Liepmann and Maas[314] first described a patient with right hemiplegia who was unable to perform skilled movements with his nonparetic left arm. Similar patients have been described.[422,423] Critical to the syndrome is disruption of the anterior portions of the corpus callosum. Infarction of the medial or anterior left frontal lobe with Broca's aphasia and right hemiplegia is often present, but these elements are not critical to the genesis of the apraxia.

The syndrome is unilateral and limited to the nondominant arm. The disturbance is similar to the bilateral apraxia that characterizes ideomotor apraxia: the movements are slow and lacking "lithness."[424] Two somewhat similar hypotheses have been offered to explain callosal apraxia; both cite a form of "disconnection": one from the dominant hemisphere's "speech area"[307,422] and the other[413] from the "motor engram centers" in the left hemisphere.

The lesion producing callosal apraxia is rare, given the low frequency of an isolated lesion of the corpus callosum. More commonly, the crossing callosal fibers are disrupted in the mesial left hemisphere by an infarction either in the left anterior cerebral artery territory or in the distribution of the anterior division of the left MCA. Injury to the corpus callosum rather than to the left supplementary motor cortex is critical to the syndrome.[425]

Oral-Bucco-Lingual Apraxia

Orofacial or oral-bucco-lingual apraxia is the inability to perform skilled movements with the oral and facial musculature on command.[245,415] Oral apraxia is unusual in cases of anomic or Wernicke's aphasia. Although oral apraxia is common in global aphasia, testing for oral apraxia may be difficult because of comprehension disturbances.[426] Oral-bucco-lingual apraxia generally results from an inferior frontal lesion in the premotor cortex adjacent to the face area on the motor strip. Most lesions are cortical and superficial,[427] but some have been from large, deep lesions.[7]

SYNDROMES OF INFARCTION IN THE HEMISPHERE NONDOMINANT FOR SPEECH AND LANGUAGE

A wide variety of behavioral abnormalities may follow stroke in the hemisphere nondominant for speech and language; this is the right hemisphere in most left-handed people. (For brevity of text, this hemisphere is referred to as the right in this chapter.)

The clinical syndromes observed are governed in general by several unifying observations. First, despite some rudimentary capacity to comprehend language, language plays no important role in the activities subserved by the right hemisphere. Second, the commitment of the cerebral cortex to a specific "higher cortical" function is less precise in the right hemisphere than in the left hemisphere. Higher cortical functions of the right hemisphere appear to be governed by far-flung "networks."

The right hemisphere is dominant for certain aspects of attention,[428] including directed attention, focused attention, and vigilance. This specialization for attention may be reflected in a variety of right hemisphere deficits, such as neglect, extinction, and impersistence. Many spatial and quasispatial operations are performed by the right hemisphere. This specialization for spatial operations may be reflected in such right hemisphere deficits as prosopagnosia,[429] topographic disorientation, constructional apraxia, and dressing apraxia. Confabulatory behaviors are more common after right than left hemisphere injury.[307] Both reduplicative paramnesia and anosognosia may be considered forms of confabulation that occur after right hemisphere stroke.

Patients lacking the syndromes from right hemispheral infarction fare better in rehabilitation than do patients with these deficits. Although some patients show a steady improvement (Fig. 24-25), others are left with persistent and disabling behavioral abnormalities, including constructional and dressing apraxias, left neglect, and motor impersistence. The size of the lesion, rather than its exact location, is a better predictor of behavioral deficits after right hemisphere damage (Fig. 24-26).

Neglect and Extinction

Extinction and neglect are two forms of impaired response to contralateral space, labeled hemi-inattention, and may occur after right hemisphere stroke. Extinction implies that a "stimulus is not perceived only when a second stimulus is presented simultaneously–usually but not necessarily on the opposite side of the body."[430] Unilateral spatial neglect (USN) is a restricted syndrome in which patients fail to copy one side (usually the left) of a figure, fail to read one side of words or sentences, and bisect lines far to the right of center.

The term neglect indicates disturbances shown by patients in their responses to stimuli from the right side of space, including impairment of OKN, turning to the left in response to auditory stimuli from the right, and faulty performance in reading aloud or naming objects in the right side of space.[431,432]

Neglect is often trimodal (auditory, visual, and tactile). In left-sided neglect, the patient may not explore the left side of space; the eyes and body may be turned tonically to the right.[210] Neglect is characterized by "a lack of responsivity to stimuli on one side of the body, in the absence of any sensory or motor deficit severe enough to account for the imperception,"[433] seen more often from right than left hemispheral lesions.[434–436] Marked neglect of the left side tends to occur in conjunction with other markers of severe right hemisphere damage, including anosognosia (implicit unawareness of illness and its clinical manifestations)[204] and motor impersistence. By contrast, USN may occur with smaller right hemisphere strokes, which usually have a good prognosis (Fig. 24-27). Failure to bisect a line using an opticokinetic tape appears to be a common finding in posterior hemispheral lesions.[437,438]

Neglect has been traditionally attributed to injury in the vicinity of the right parietal lobe. However, neglect may follow injury to the right frontal lobe,[439] right cingulum,[440] right lenticular nucleus, or right thalamus.[437,441] Mesulam has postulated a "network" model to account for the lesions of a variety of cortical and subcortical structures that produce left neglect,[442] consisting of a reticular element (providing arousal and vigilance), a parietal element (providing sensory and spatial mapping), a frontal element (providing the motor programs for exploration), and a limbic element.

Neglect from Frontal Lesion

It has long been appreciated that a parietal lesion (from infarct or hemorrhage or even other causes) may be associated with an impaired response to stimuli from the opposite side of space, whether from a visual, auditory, or even somatosensory

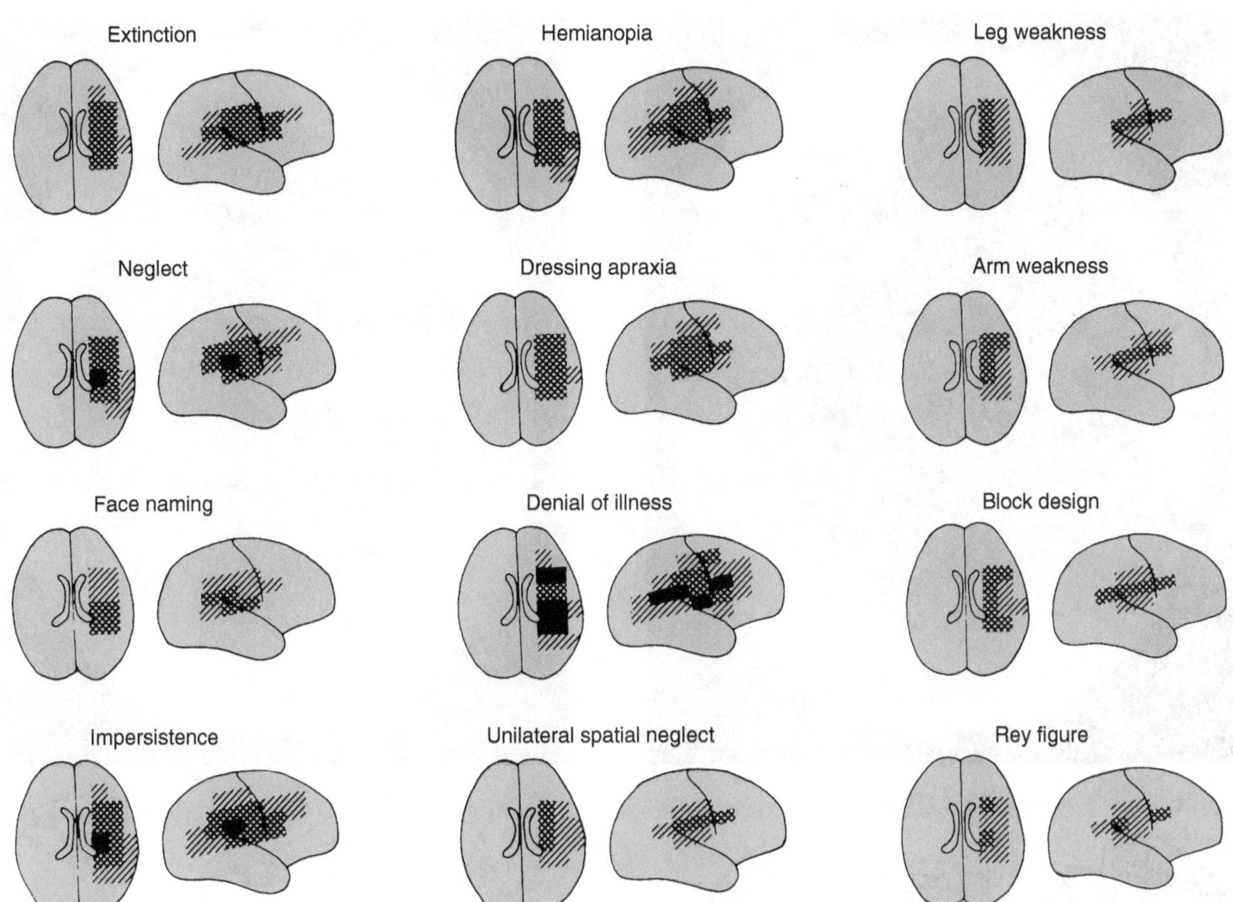

Figure 24-25 Topography of infarction as documented by CT scan for patients with nondominant hemisphere deficits. *(From Hier DB, Mondlock J, Caplan LR: Behavioral abnormalities after right hemisphere stroke.* Neurology [NY] *33:337, 1983.)*

source.[443,444] These deficits are thought to reflect impaired input from sensory to motor regions. However, a similar disturbance occurs from frontal lesions as well,[439,445] whether cortical or subcortical.[446] Using PET scanning, Deuel and Collins[447] found widespread metabolic suppression in the basal ganglia and thalamus after a unilateral frontal lesion, with little evidence of cortical hypometabolism. Their findings suggest that part of the syndrome might result from impaired activation of subcortical structures involved in planning motor movements. Corbetta et al., using fMRI, showed that the spatial attention deficits in neglect (rightward bias and reorienting) after right frontal damage correlated with abnormal activation of structurally intact dorsal and ventral parietal regions that mediate related attentional operations in the normal brain.[448] In the human, the signs of neglect from frontal lesions are remarkably transient, usually fading within a week in all patients except those with the largest infarcts.[449]

Motor Neglect

Motor neglect, said to be characterized by underutilization of one side without defects in strength reflex or sensibility, has been described by LaPlane and Degos.[450] It is characterized as underutilization of the opposite side of the body.[451] The patient with this syndrome appears to have a hemiparesis; with special efforts on examination, however, normal strength and dexterity can be demonstrated.

The usual features are: (1) a lack of spontaneous placing reaction, such as failure to place the hand in the lap or on the arm of a chair when sitting, letting it instead drag down beside the body; (2) delayed or insufficient assumption of correct postures, resulting in heavy falls to the affected side with no attempts to minimize the effect of the fall by reaching out or correcting the balance; (3) impairment of automatic withdrawal reaction to pain; and (4) lack of excursions of the limb necessary to achieve a movement such as touching the nose; for example, the patient instead leans the head forward to compensate for failure to bring the finger far enough up. This disturbance may occur in the absence of a sensory disturbance or demonstrable hemiparesis. Hartmann[452] described an autopsy case with similar disturbances secondary to an infarct affecting the second frontal gyrus of the right frontal lobe. Animal studies in the monkey have demonstrated a similar transitory disturbance observed high over the prefrontal region after selective research.[453]

Neglect for Verbal Material

Leicester et al.[454] described a form of visual neglect in which the occurrence and frequency of errors were determined by the verbal content of the test materials. When the patient was required to select from an array of choices displayed directly in front, errors were seen with those materials that the patient found the most difficult to name or write; in such instances, responses were made less frequently to choices on the right-hand side of the display. When the test materials were easily named, little or no evidence of neglect for the right side of space was noted.

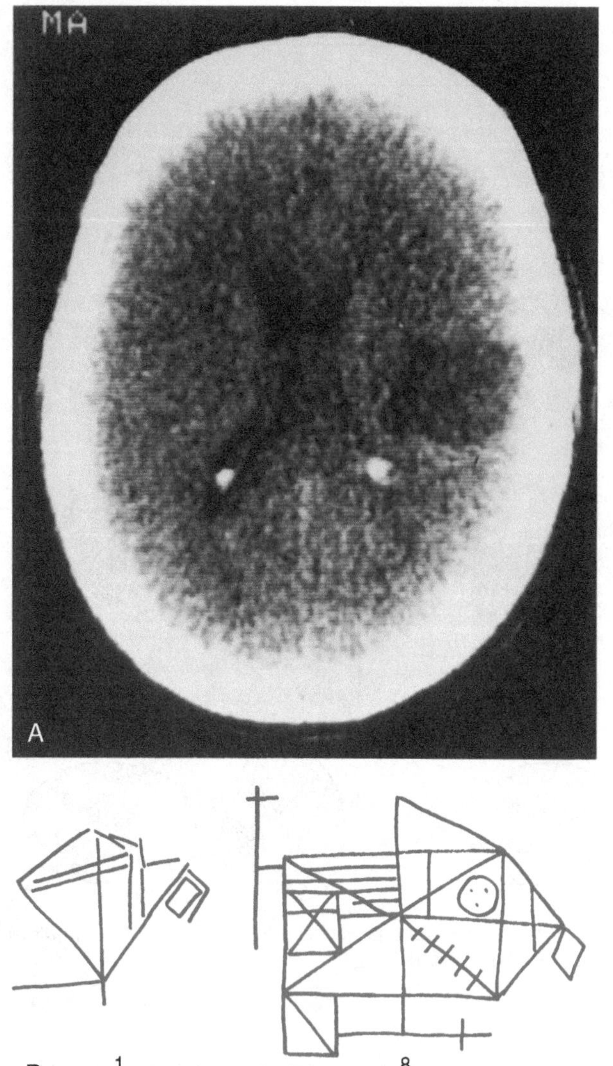

Figure 24-26 A, CT scan of small right middle cerebral artery territory infarct. B, Drawings made by the patient with the infarct shown in A at 1 and 8 weeks after stroke.

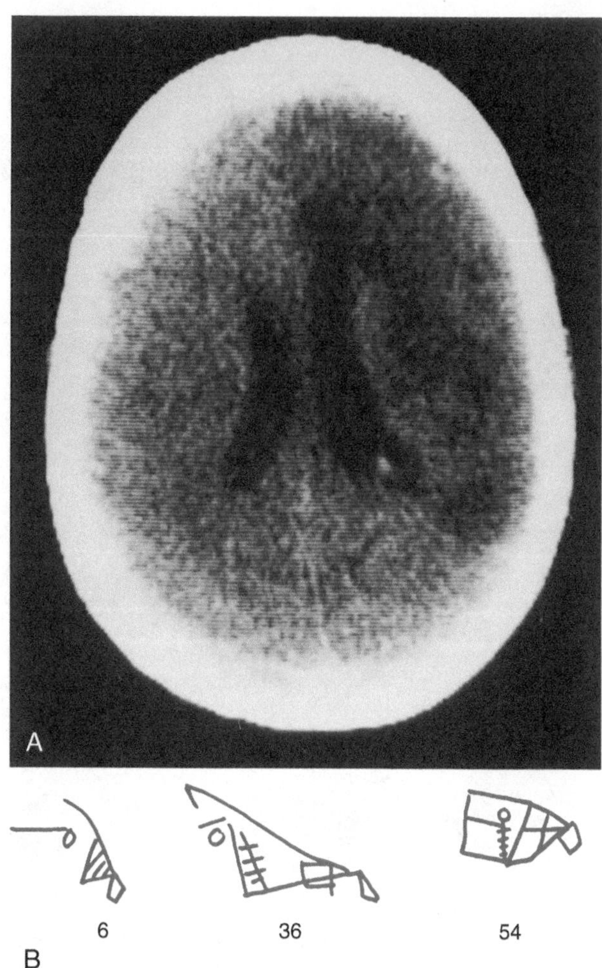

Figure 24-27 A, CT scan of large right middle cerebral artery territory infarct. B, Drawings done by the patient with the infarct shown in A at 6, 36, and 54 weeks after stroke.

Anosognosia

This syndrome (unawareness of illness or its clinical manifestations) is more likely to be associated with severe as opposed to mild hemiparesis.[455-457] Anosognosia for either hemianopia or hemiparesis can be dissociated from elementary[126] neurologic deficits or neglect. Nonpersistence of the syndrome was evidenced in studies showing improvement toward normal within 22 weeks.[455,458] The lesion producing anosognosia is usually large.[455] Involvement of the insula plays an important role.[459] Although a hemispheral site is classic, a pontine infarct has reportedly caused such disturbance.[460]

Gerstmann[461] has viewed anosognosia as a disorder of a hypothetical "body image." Although he believed that this body image is "mapped" into the left parietal lobe, input from the right parietal lobe is essential in updating the left parietal lobe as to the condition of the left side of the body. Injury to the right parietal lobe or to connecting pathways between the right and left parietal lobes could lead to anosognosia. It may be viewed as a variation of "neglect" or "inattention" in that the patient with anosognosia fails to "attend" to the hemiplegia.

Impersistence

In 1956, Fisher[462] introduced the term impersistence to characterize ten patients with left hemiplegia who were unable to persist at a variety of willed acts, including eye closure, breath-holding, conjugate gaze deviation, tongue protrusion, and hand gripping. He noted that "mental impairment of some degree was always present" and that impersistence was "encountered almost exclusively in association with left hemiplegia." Many of the patients had accompanying left neglect, constructional apraxia, and anosognosia. Subsequent studies have found impersistence with both left and right hemispheral lesions individually.[458,463-466]

Impersistence has been correlated with the severity of hemiparesis and with a poor prognosis for rehabilitation efforts, as well as with a variety of other deficits, including prosopagnosia, dressing apraxia, constructional apraxia, left neglect, and anosognosia.[455]

Dressing Apraxia

Brain[467] described "apraxia for dressing" in 1941. The syndrome appears with difficulty in the orientation of clothing during dressing.[468] There is a close association with constructional apraxia.[469] In a setting of stroke, the syndrome occurs almost exclusively with lesions of the right hemisphere.

Loss of Topographic Memory and Disorientation for Place

This disorder is shown by an inability of patients to find their way in familiar surroundings, to recognize familiar surroundings, and to learn new routes in unfamiliar surroundings. Loss of topographic memory is somewhat different from disorientation to place, which refers to confusion about current location.[470–471] In milder cases, patients recognize surroundings as familiar; in more severe cases, even very familiar surroundings may seem strange. Loss of topographic memory is uncommon.[472] Although this is often considered a parietal lobe syndrome, right medial temporoparietal lesions may be the most common and may be in the territory of the posterior cerebral artery.[473] It can occur with unilateral stroke in either hemisphere.[474] The mechanism underlying loss of topographic memory is uncertain.[475,476]

Disorders of Spatial Localization

The right hemisphere plays a special role in the spatial localization of both visual and auditory stimuli. The most severe syndromes occur after posterior right hemisphere damage.[477,478] Short-term spatial memory (a skill analogous to the auditory short-term memory task of digit span) is a dominant function of the posterior right hemisphere.[477] Auditory localization of sounds in space also depends on an intact posterior right hemisphere.[126]

Confusion and Delirium

Acute confusion and delirium are characterized by impaired orientation, diminished attention, and aberrant perception. Alertness is usually well-maintained, clarity and speed of thinking are diminished, and memories are poorly formed. Inattentiveness, poor concentration, and awareness of irrelevant stimuli are present. There is overlap between confusional and delirious states, and some investigators regard delirium as a subset of confusion.

Acute confusional states have been reported after right MCA infarctions[479–481] and may be accompanied by retropulsion, unsteady gait, incontinence, difficulty in using common objects, and lack of concern for the illness. The disorder has been found in conjunction with parietal as well as temporal lesions.[440] Hallucinations, delusions, and agitation have also been described.[430,482,483]

Caplan et al.[484] found that posterior right temporal lesions were more likely to produce acute confusion than posterior right parietal lesions. The propensity of temporal lesions to produce confusional states may be explained by the proximity of these lesions to the underlying limbic system. Recently, we described a case that showed an excellent recovery after intravenous thrombolysis for an acute right MCA stroke. A 73-year-old man presented left-sided weakness (NIHSS 19 points). CT angiography revealed right MCA occlusion. Continuous TCD monitoring revealed complete recanalization of right MCA at 14 minutes after treatment-onset. This was accompanied by rapid and persistent clinical recovery (NIHSS score 1-point at 1 hour). However, despite brilliant clinical recovery, he displayed severe suicidal ideations on day 3. He had never suffered from depression or psychiatric illness in the past. Brain MRI showed an acute lacunar infarction in the putamen. TCD and CT perfusion were suggestive of right MCA hyperperfusion. Interestingly, electroencephalography (EEG) showed considerable slowing over the right hemisphere, even in the absence of any parenchymal damage. Head-up position, fluid restriction and aggressive blood pressure control (120/80 mmHg) resulted in rapid improvement in psychiatric features during the next 2 days. CT perfusion, TCD and EEG abnormalities resolved completely within a few days. We hypothesize that neurovascular uncoupling due to acute stroke resulted in these transient findings.[485] Post-stroke depression has been described in patients with small subcortical infarcts, suggesting that cerebral blood perfusion may play an important role in the development of PSD.[486]

Confabulation and Reduplicative Paramnesia

Confabulation, the unintentional production of inappropriate and fabricated information, is often associated with a failure to inhibit incorrect responses, poor error awareness, and poor self-correction abilities. Although impairment of memory is often associated with confabulation, the two behaviors vary independently in severity.[487,488]

Reduplication is a special form of confabulation. It appears to reflect an attempt of brain-injured patients to fuse experiences from two disparate periods in their lives. In instances of reduplication for place, patients hold an inaccurate belief that two versions of a geographic location exist. Hospitalized patients may persist in believing that they are at home or at another hospital despite repeated attempts to orient them to current location.[489] Environmental reduplication occurs most commonly after right frontoparietal lobe injury. Reduplication of person, a restricted form of confabulation (a false belief that two versions of an individual exist) may also occur after right hemisphere injury.

Constructional Apraxia

In 1934, Kleist[264] defined constructional apraxia as "a disturbance which appears in formative activities (arranging, building, drawing) and in which a spatial part of the task is missed, although there is no apraxia of single movements." Clinically, the patients fail at tasks that require the manipulation of objects in space. A variety of tests have been utilized to identify constructional apraxia, including the copying of block designs, the copying of simple and complex figures, puzzle constructions, mental rotations, and 3D model building. Constructional apraxia is synonymous with apractognosia, constructional disability, and visual-spatial agnosia.

Constructional apraxia occurs after injury to either cerebral hemisphere.[490,491] Most lesions are parietal. The nature of constructional apraxia differs according to the hemisphere injured. Patients with left-sided lesions improve their drawings when aided by visual cues, whereas patients with right-sided lesions do not.[492] It is widely believed that the drawings of patients with left hemisphere damage are oversimplified and have reduced detail, whereas left unilateral neglect characterizes the drawings of patients with right hemisphere damage; however, Gainotti et al.[493,494] were not able to distinguish right-sided from left-sided constructional apraxia. Lazar et al.[495] reported a 66-year-old woman with infarction in the right caudate nucleus and putamen who was tested for perception, attention, and constructional apraxia, followed by the presentation of matching-to-sample procedures. She showed severe constructional apraxia without hemineglect; the matching procedures then provided demonstrable evidence that she could not copy Greek letter forms that she could otherwise match with perfect accuracy.

Allesthesia

Allesthesia (also "allochiria") is the referral of a sensory stimulus (visual, tactile, or auditory) from one side of the body to the other.[17,444] Right hemisphere involvement with left-sided neglect is usually present. When the left side is touched, the sensation may be reported by the patient as occurring on the right side.

Amusia

Amusia (loss of musical ability secondary to brain disease) has been an elusive deficit to study.[496–498] Brust[499] concluded that no simple relationship exists between the location of a lesion and the extent of musical disability. Case reports of expressive amusia after right hemisphere lesions are numerous. Affected patients are unable to sing or whistle, but their language function and melody recognition are preserved. Receptive amusia may also occur with right hemisphere lesions. The neural basis of music remains obscure. Amusia is often an isolated phenomenon. A remarkable case of a blind organist who had left hemispheral infarction with aphasia, but without amusia (some of his poststroke compositions were published) suggests that a clear separation between the two entities is possible.[500]

Aprosody and Affective Agnosia

Monrad-Krohn[501] defined prosody as the musical quality of speech produced by "variations in pitch, rhythm, and stress of pronunciation." Buck and Duffy[502] reported that after right hemisphere damage, some patients are unable to intone affect into their speech; this deficit is known as aprosody. On the basis of their work and that of Heilman et al.,[503] Ross and Mesulam[504] proposed that the right hemisphere was dominant for the modulation of affective language and that this modulation was organized in a fashion analogous to left hemisphere organization for propositional language. In a subsequent study, Ross[505] provided additional confirmatory evidence of the functional–anatomic organization of the affective components of language in the right hemisphere.

Ross[505] proposed the existence of motor, sensory, global, conduction, and transcortical aprosodias. In motor aprosody, the patient is unable to utilize prosody to inject affect into speech, nor is the patient able to repeat the affect-laden prosody of others. However, the patient can comprehend the affect conveyed by the prosody of other speakers. The patient with sensory aprosody shows poor comprehension of affective prosody and cannot repeat affective prosody; however, the patient has normal spontaneous affective prosody in speech. Global aprosody is reflected in the drawing errors of apraxias. Heilman and Van Den Abell,[506] noting that right temporoparietal lesions cause defects in the comprehension of affective speech, term this disorder affective agnosia. Tucker et al.[507] observed that right temporoparietal lesions caused deficits both in affective comprehension and in evoking emotional intonation in a speech repetition task.

Treatment of Hemineglect

Proposed approaches to treat hemineglect have largely failed to show positive results. For those whose neglect does not fade spontaneously, global inattention may impede necessary cooperation with treatment regimens. Most treatment trials have focused on altering the asymmetry of attention. One approach (called "top-down") uses external cues and guidance to engage the conscious and purposeful involvement of the patient. These treatments rely heavily on the participation of a therapist who provides continuous feedback, encouragement, and training. Treatments that follow such an approach include visual scanning training,[448,508,509] sustained attention training,[510,511] and mental imagery training.[512] Alternatively, "bottom-up" approaches attempt to alter the attentional system by manipulating endogenous components of the neural axis. This has been tried with prism glasses,[513] trunk rotation,[514,515] or by stimulation of the contralateral body with neck vibration,[516] limb movements,[517] or opticokinetic stimulation.[518,519] Combined top-down and bottom-up approaches include the moderately successful prism adaptation[520] method in which the patient wears prism glasses that shift the visual world further to the right (away from the neglected side). Training follows to move the attention leftward using a line bisection paradigm. Removal of the glasses may then produce a lasting shift of attention toward the neglected field.[521] A final approach has been to try to alter brain function directly, for example, with TMS to decrease overactive input from the contralateral parietal lobe.[522] Although this approach can result in an improved symmetry of attention at the time of the stimulus, the behavior reverts back to the hemiinattentive state once the stimulation stops.

The complete reference list can be found on the companion Expert Consult website at www.expertconsult.inkling.com.

KEY REFERENCES

15. Teal JS, Rumbaugh CL, Bergeron RT, et al. Anomalies of the middle cerebral artery: Accessory artery, duplication, and early bifurcation. Am J Roentgenol Radium Ther Nucl Med 1973; 118:567.
19. Reis CV, Zabramski JM, Safavi-Abbasi S, et al. The accessory middle cerebral artery: anatomic report. Neurosurgery 2008;63: 10–14.
30. Clower BR, Sullivan DM, Smith RR. Intracranial vessels lack vasa vasorum. J Neurosurg 1984;61:44.
34. Lhermitte F, Gautier JC, Derouesne C. Nature of occlusions of the middle cerebral artery. Neurology (Minneap) 1970;20:82.
48. Pessin MS, Duncan GW, Mohr JP, et al. Clinical and angiographic features of carotid transient ischemic attacks. N Engl J Med 1977;296:358.
63. Marnane M, Merwick A, Sheehan OC, et al. Carotid plaque inflammation on ^{18}FDG-PET predicts early stroke recurrence – the Dublin Carotid Atherosclerosis Stroke Study. Ann Neurol 2012;71:709–18.
77. Liebeskind DS. Stroke: the currency of collateral circulation in acute ischemic stroke. Nat Rev Neurol 2009;5:645–6.
80. Donnan GA, Bladin PF, Berkovic SF, et al. The stroke syndrome of striatocapsular infarction. Brain 1991;114:51.
81. Pessin MS, Hinton RC, Davis KR, et al. Mechanisms of acute carotid stroke. Ann Neurol 1979;6:245.
86. Fisher CM. Capsular infarcts. Arch Neurol 1979;36:65.
93. Irino T, Tandea M, Minami T. Angiographic manifestations in postrecanalized cerebral infarction. Neurology 1977;27:471.
94. Kumral E, Ozdemirkiran T, Alper Y. Strokes in the subinsular territory: clinical, topographical, and etiological patterns. Neurology 2004;63:2429–32.
95. Liu Q, Huang J, Degnan AJ, et al. Comparison of high-resolution MRI with CT angiography and digital subtraction angiography for the evaluation of middle cerebral artery atherosclerotic steno-occlusive disease. Int J Cardiovasc Imaging 2013;29:1491–8.
97. Xu WH, Li ML, Gao S, et al. In vivo high-resolution MR imaging of symptomatic and asymptomatic middle cerebral artery atherosclerotic stenosis. Atherosclerosis 2010;212:507–11.
98. Li ML, Xu WH, Song L, et al. Atherosclerosis of middle cerebral artery: evaluation with high-resolution MR imaging at 3T. Atherosclerosis 2009;204:447–52.
103. Corston RN, Kendall BE, Marshall J. Prognosis in middle cerebral artery stenosis. Stroke 1984;15:237.
116. Donan GA, O'Malley HMM, Quang L, et al. The capsular warning syndrome. Neurology 1993;43:957–62.
117. Paul NL, Simoni M, Chandratheva A, et al. Population-based study of capsular warning syndrome and prognosis after early recurrent TIA. Neurology 2012;79:1356–62.
118. Zhou L, Ni J, Xu W, et al. High-resolution MRI findings in patients with capsular warning syndrome. BMC Neurol 2014; 14:16.

119. Calabrese LH, Dodick DW, Schwedt TJ, et al. Narrative review: Reversible cerebral vasoconstriction syndromes. Ann Intern Med 2007;146:34–44.
120. Boughammoura A, Touze E, Oppenheim C, et al. Reversible angiopathy and encephalopathy after blood transfusion. J Neurol 2003;250:116–18.
121. Staykov D, Schwab S. Posterior reversible encephalopathy syndrome. J Intensive Care Med 2012;27:11–24.
122. Singhal AB, Hajj-Ali RA, Topcuoglu MA, et al. Reversible cerebral vasoconstriction syndromes: analysis of 139 cases. Arch Neurol 2011;68:1005–12.
127. Hacke W, Schwab S, Horn M, et al. 'Malignant' middle cerebral artery territory infarction: Clinical course and prognostic signs. Arch Neurol 1996;53:309.
128. Steiner T, Ringleb P, Hacke W. Treatment options for large hemispheric stroke. Neurology 2001;57(Suppl. 2):S61.
129. Vahedi K, Hofmeijer J, Juettler E, et al. DECIMAL, DESTINY and HAMLET investigators. Early decompressive surgery in malignant infarction of the middle cerebral artery: a pooled analysis of three randomised controlled trials. Lancet Neurol 2007;6: 215–22.
134. Mohr JP, Foulkes MA, Polis AT, et al. Infarct topography and hemiparesis profiles with cerebral convexity infarction: The Stroke Data Bank. J Neurol Neurosurg Psychiatry 1993;56: 344.
147. Marquez J, van Vliet P, McElduff P, et al. Transcranial direct current stimulation (tDCS): Does it have merit in stroke rehabilitation? A systematic review. Int J Stroke 2013;doi: 10.1111/ijs.12169; [Epub ahead of print]; PubMed PMID: 24148111.
161. Johnston KC, Barrett KM, Ding YH, et al. Clinical and imaging data at 5 days as a surrogate for 90-day outcome in ischemic stroke. Stroke 2009;40:1332–3.
168. Marshall RS, Zarahn E, Alon L, et al. Early imaging correlates of subsequent motor recovery after stroke. Ann Neurol 2009;65: 596–602.
170. Dijkhuizen RM, Singhal AB, Mandeville JB, et al. Correlation between brain reorganization, ischemic damage, and neurologic status after transient focal cerebral ischemia in rats: A functional magnetic resonance imaging study. J Neurosci 2003; 23:510–17.
173. Feydy A, Carlier R, Roby-Brami A, et al. Longitudinal study of motor recovery after stroke: recruitment and focusing of brain activation. Stroke 2002;33:1610–17.
176. Khedr EM, Ahmed MA, Fathy N, et al. Therapeutic trial of repetitive transcranial magnetic stimulation after acute ischemic stroke. Neurology 2005;65:466–8.
190. Bender MB. Brain control of conjugate horizontal and vertical eye movements: A survey of the structural and functional correlates. Brain 1980;103:23.
192. De Renzi E, Colombo A, Faglioni P, et al. Conjugate gaze paresis in stroke patients with unilateral damage. Arch Neurol 1982; 39:42.
224. Mazzocchi F, Vignolo LA. Localization of lesions in aphasia: Clinical-CT scan correlations in stroke patients. Cortex 1979; 15:627.
226. Quast MJ, Huang NC, Hillman GR, et al. The evolution of acute stroke recorded by multimodal magnetic resonance imaging. Magn Reson Imaging 1993;11(4):465–71.
227. Schlaug G, Benfield A, Baird AE, et al. The ischemic penumbra: operationally defined by diffusion and perfusion MRI. Neurology 1999;53(7):1528–37.
230. Lee A, Kannan V, Hillis AE. The contribution of neuroimaging to the study of language and aphasia. Neuropsychol Rev 2006;16(4):171–83.
255. Lazar RM, Minzer B, Antoniello D, et al. Improvement in aphasia scores after stroke is well predicted by initial severity. Stroke 2010;41:1485–8.
256. Saur D, Lange R, Baumgaertner A, et al. Dynamics of language reorganization after stroke. Brain 2006;129:1371–84.
258. Tonkonogy J, Goodglass H. Language function, foot of the third frontal gyrus, and rolandic operculum. Arch Neurol 1981;38:486.
262. Agostini E, Coletti A, Orlando G, et al. Apraxia in deep cerebral lesions. J Neurol Neurosurg Psychiatry 1983;46:804.
263. Levine DN, Mohr JP. Language after bilateral cerebral infarctions: Role of the minor hemisphere and speech. Neurology 1979;29: 927.
280. Rothi LJ, McFarling D, Heilman KM. Conduction aphasia, syntactic alexia, and the anatomy of syntactic comprehension. Arch Neurol 1982;39:272.
305. Yamada K, Nagakane Y, Mizumo T, et al. MR tractography depicting damage to the arcuate fasciculus in a patient with conduction aphasia. Neurology 2007;68:789. and Geldmacher DS, Quigg M, Elias WJ. MR tractography depicting damage to the arcuate fasciculus in a patient with conduction aphasia (letter). *Neurology* 2007;69:321–22.
318. Grossi D, Trohano L, Chiacchio L, et al. Mixed transcortical aphasia: Clinical features and neuroanatomical correlates: A possible role of the right hemisphere. Eur Neurol 1991;31: 204.
321. Kertesz A, Sheppard A, MacKenzie R. Localization in transcortical sensory aphasia. Arch Neurol 1982;39:475.
324. Rango R, Candelise L, Perani D, et al. Cortical pathophysiology and clinical neurologic abnormalities in acute cerebral ischemia. Arch Neurol 1989;46:1318.
329. Bushnell DL, Gupta S, Mlcoch AG, et al. Prediction of language and neurologic recovery after cerebral infarction with SPECT imaging using N-isopropyl-p-(I 123) iodoamphetamine. Arch Neurol 1989;46:665.
331. Vallar G, Perani D, Cappa SF, et al. Recovery from aphasia and neglect after subcortical stroke: Neuropsychological and cerebral perfusion study. J Neurol Neurosurg Psychiatry 1988;51: 1269.
332. Demeurisse G, Capon A, Verhas M, et al. Pathogenesis of aphasia in deep-seated lesions: Likely role of cortical diaschisis. Eur Neurol 1990;30:67.
344. NIDCDS. Aphasia 2007;<http://www.aphasia.org/>.
347. Engelter ST, Gostynski M, Papa S, et al. Epidemiology of aphasia attributable to first ischemic stroke: Incidence, severity, fluency, etiology, and thrombolysis. Stroke 2006;37(6): 1379–84.
350. Gresham GE, Phillips TF, Wolf PA, et al. Epidemiologic profile of long-term stroke disability: The Framingham Study. Arch Phys Med Rehabil 1979;60:487–91.
351. Kelly-Hayes M, Wolf PA, Kase C, et al. Time course of functional recovery after stroke. J Neurol Rehabil 1989;3:65–70.
352. Skilbeck CE, Wade DT, Hewer RL, et al. Recovery after stroke. J Neurol Neurosurg Psychiatry 1983;46(1):5–8.
353. Ferrucci L, Bandinelli S, Guralnik JM, et al. Recovery of functional status after stroke. A postrehabilitation follow-up study. Stroke 1993;24:200–5.
355. Demeurisse G, Demol O, Derouck M, et al. Quantitative study of the rate of recovery from aphasia due to ischemic stroke. Stroke 1980;11(5):455–8.
356. Robey RR. A meta-analysis of clinical outcomes in the treatment of aphasia. J Speech Lang Hear Res 1998;41(1):172–87.
357. Laska AC, Hellblom A, Murray V, et al. Aphasia in acute stroke and relation to outcome. J Intern Med 2001;249(5): 413–22.
358. Berthier ML. Poststroke aphasia: Epidemiology, pathophysiology and treatment. Drugs Aging 2005;22(2):163–82.
360. Mark VW, Thomas BE, Berndt RS. Factors associated with improvements in global aphasia. Aphasiology 1992;6: 121–34.
362. Mohr JP, Lazar RM, Marshall RS, et al. Middle cerebral artery disease. In: Mohr JP, Choi DW, Grotta JC, et al., editors. Stroke: Pathophysiology, diagnosis, and management. ed 4. Philadelphia: Churchill-Livingstone; 2004. p. 123–66.
365. Goodglass H, Kaplan E. Boston diagnostic aphasia examination. Philadelphia: Lea & Febiger; 1983.
366. Kertesz A. Western Aphasia Battery-Revised. San Antonio, Tex: Harcourt Assessment; 2006.
370. Robey RR. The efficacy of treatment for aphasic persons: A meta-analysis. Brain Lang 1994;47(4):582–608.
371. Bhogal SK, Teasell R, Speechley M. Intensity of aphasia therapy, impact on recovery. Stroke 2003;34(4):987–93.
372. Greener J, Enderby P, Whurr R. Speech and language therapy for aphasia following stroke. Cochrane Database Syst Rev 2000;(2):CD000425.

392. Fisher M, Finklestein S. Pharmacological approaches to stroke recovery. Cerebrovasc Dis 1999;9(Suppl. 5):29–32.
397. Berthier ML, Green C, Higueras C, et al. A randomized, placebo-controlled study of donepezil in poststroke aphasia. Neurology 2006;67(9):1687–9.
399. Albert ML, Bachman DL, Morgan A, et al. Pharmacotherapy for aphasia. Neurology 1988;38:877.
403. Chollet F, Tardy J, Albucher JF, et al. Fluoxetine for motor recovery after acute ischaemic stroke (FLAME): a randomized placebo-controlled trial. Lancet Neurol 2011;10:123–30.
430. Mori E, Yamadori A. Acute confusional state and acute agitated delirium: Occurrence after infarction in the middle cerebral artery territory. Arch Neurol 1987;4:1139.
470. Fisher CM. Topographic disorientation. Arch Neurol 1982;19:33.
490. Piercy M, Hecaen H, de Ajuriaguerra J. Constructional apraxia associated with unilateral cerebral lesions: Left and right cases compared. Brain 1960;83:225.
491. Arrigoni G, De Renzi E. Constructional apraxia and hemispheric locus of lesion. Cortex 1964;1:170.
509. Fanthome Y, Lincoln NB, Drummond A, et al. The treatment of visual neglect using feedback of eye movements: A pilot study. Disabil Rehabil 1995;17:413–17.
511. Wilson FC, Manly T, Coyle D, et al. The effect of contralesional limb activation training and sustained attention training for self-care programmes in unilateral spatial neglect. Restor Neurol Neurosci 2000;16:1–4.

25 Posterior Cerebral Artery Disease

Jong S. Kim

KEY POINTS

- Large-artery atherothrombosis, cardiac embolism and small-artery disease are important stroke mechanisms of posterior cerebral artery territory infarction.
- The clinical features of thalamic infarction vary according to vascular topography: the inferolateral, tuberothalamic, paramedian, and posterior choroidal arteries
- Inferolateral territory infarction is the most common type of thalamic infarction, and the main clinical features are hemisensory deficits.
- The main clinical features of tuberothalamic and paramedian territory infarctions are neuropsychiatric disturbances including somnolence, memory deficits, etc.
- The most important clinical feature of cortical posterior cerebral artery infarction is visual field defect, especially homonymous hemianopia.
- Memory deficits and various types of cognitive dysfunction associated with visual disturbances are encountered in patients with cortical PCA infarction.
- The prognosis of pure PCA territory infarction is relatively good, but sensory dysfunction and visual field defect may remain as troublesome sequelae.

ANATOMY

The posterior cerebral artery (PCA) originates at the terminal bifurcation of the basilar artery (BA). Both PCAs arise from the BA in 70% of cases, the PCA arises from the posterior communicating arteries in 20%, and the origin is mixed in 10%[1] (Figs 25-1 and 25-2).

In the proximal portion of the PCA, the penetrating branches arise and supply the deep structures such as the midbrain and thalamus. The initial portion of the PCA – the segment between the top of the BA and the origin of the posterior communicating artery – is referred to as the P1 segment. P2 refers to the segment after the communicating artery. In patients with fetal PCA, the P1 segment is hypoplastic or absent.

The main branches of the P1 segment include the paramedian arteries that supply the medial portion of the rostral midbrain (mesencephalic arteries) and the thalamic arteries (thalamic-subthalamic artery). The perforating arteries are 200 and 400 µm in diameter, respectively. The anterior and anterolateral portions of the thalamus are usually supplied by the tuberothalamic arteries (polar or premammillary), which generally arise from the posterior communicating arteries; however, in some patients, the tuberothalamic arteries are absent, and these areas are supplied by the paramedian arteries.[2]

In the segment distal to the posterior communicating artery (P2 portion), there arise peduncular perforating arteries that supply the lateral midbrain, and thalamogeniculate (inferolateral) arteries supplying the ventrolateral portion of the thalamus.[3] These arteries measure between 320 µm and 800 µm in diameter and contain between eight and ten branches. The thalamogeniculate, posterior thalamic, and pulvinarian branches curve upward into the posterior portions of the thalamus to supply the posterolateral nuclei and pulvinar. There are also several medial and lateral branches in the posterior choroidal artery. The choroidal arteries supply the choroid plexus of the lateral ventricle, pulvinar, the posterior part of dorsolateral nucleus, lateral geniculate body, hippocampus, and mesial temporal lobe.[4,5]

P3 and P4 segments refer to the distal, superficial segments of PCA with cortical branches. Distal to the peduncle, the PCA initially courses downward and backward in to the ambient cistern immediately below the tentorium cerebelli, just above and slightly lateral to the superior cerebellar artery, then curves upward and medially to the quadrigeminal cistern. After crossing above the medial edge of the tentorium, the PCA reaches the medial surface of the occipital lobe near the anterosuperior border of the lingual gyrus just below the splenium of the corpus callosum. As it reaches the surface, it divides into two major divisions: one angling sharply forward and the other continuing posteriorly to become the calcarine artery.

Anterior division gives rise to the two inferior temporal arteries: the anterior and posterior. These branches supply the ventral surface of the temporal and occipital lobes. They anastomose with the middle cerebral artery (MCA) via a borderzone network that runs roughly along the margin of the hemisphere, where the ventral surfaces become convex. The anterior, inferior, and posterior temporal arteries usually originate from a single trunk; less often, these and the occipitotemporal branch arise from a common trunk.

The posterior division yields three major branches in sequence: the occipitotemporal, calcarine, and occipitoparietal arteries. The occipitotemporal branch supplies the undersurface of the occipital lobe, including the posterior portion of the fusiform and lingual gyri.

The calcarine artery, which may be single or double, supplies the calcarine cortex and medial surface of the occipital lobe as far distal as the occipital pole,[6] anastomosing with terminal branches of the MCA. The branches of the occipitoparietal artery supply the splenium and portions of the precuneus and cuneus, and along a borderzone network, the terminal vessels anastomose with branches of the anterior cerebral artery (ACA).

PATHOLOGY AND STROKE MECHANISMS

PCA territory infarction is caused by large-artery disease, small-artery disease, cardiogenic embolism, and other uncommon etiologies (Table 25-1). The prevalence of stroke mechanism differs according to the characteristics of studies; some were based on autopsy findings[7] while others used imaging data.[8–16] Imaging quality (e.g., CT vs. MRI, sonography vs. angiogram) and the extent of vascular or cardiac work-up would affect the final results. In addition, inclusion criteria were often heterogeneous. Some defined PCA infarction only when the superficial PCA territory (i.e., the occipital area) was

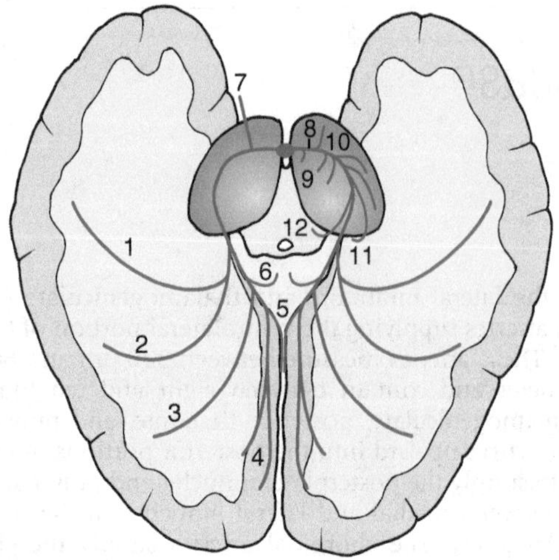

Figure 25-1. Schematic diagram of the posterior cerebral artery and its branches: 1, anterior inferior temporal artery; 2, posterior inferior temporal artery; 3, occipitotemporal artery; 4, calcarine arteries; 5, occipitoparietal artery; 6, splenial artery; 7, posterior communicating artery; 8, tuberothalamic arteries; 9, thalamoperforating arteries; 10, thalamogeniculate and posterior thalamic arteries; 11, posterolateral choroidal artery; 12, posteromedial choroidal artery.

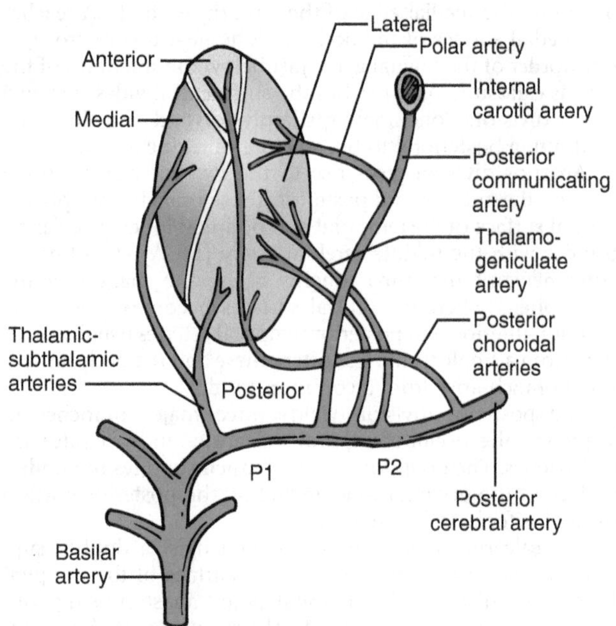

Figure 25-2. Schematic representation of the blood supply to the thalamus, including the polar artery, thalamosubthalamic arteries, thalamogeniculate artery and posterior choroidal arteries. *(From Carrera E, Caplan LR, Mechel P. Thalamic infarcts and hemorrhages. In Caplan LR, van Gijn eds, Stroke Syndromes. ed 3. pp. 387–396.)*

involved,[8,10,11,16] while others also considered infarcts restricted to deep structures.[14,15] Some papers even considered the patients with superficial PCA territory involvement only.[12] Moreover, some studies considered infarcts that occur only in the PCA territory[8,12,15] whereas others included infarcts that occur in extra-PCA territories.[11,14] Ethnicity may further complicate this issue because Asians develop intracranial atherosclerosis and small-artery disease more often, and cardiogenic embolism less often, than Caucasians.[17,18] These heterogenic aspects should be considered when evaluating the literature.

Large-artery Disease

The main pathology of large-artery disease consists of thromboses that are superimposed on atherosclerosis. In posterior circulation, atherosclerosis often occurs in the proximal vertebral artery (VA), distal intracranial VA, the lower-middle portion of the BA, and proximal PCA.[17,19] Detailed stroke mechanisms include artery-to-artery embolism, branch occlusion, in situ thrombotic occlusion, hemodynamic impairment, and their various combinations.

Artery-to-artery Embolism

Large-artery atherothrombosis is an important cause of PCA territory infarction. The main mechanism of infarction related to proximal (VA, BA, subclavian artery, and aorta) artery atherosclerosis is artery-to-artery embolism. Ulcerative plaques generate emboli that occlude the PCA and/or its branches (Fig. 25-3).[20,21] Artery-to-artery embolism accounts for 11–32% of PCA territory infarctions (see Table 25-1). VA disease (either extracranial or intracranial) is the most common source of embolism, followed by BA atherosclerosis.[11–13] It seems that posterior fossa hypoperfusion due to bilateral VA disease and contralateral VA hypoplasia predisposes the formation of emboli.[11,13] Although uncommon, internal carotid artery (ICA) disease can produce embolic PCA infarction in patients with fetal-type PCA.[11,12,22]

The role of intrinsic PCA atherosclerosis as a cause of PCA territory infarction remains uncertain, even though the proximal PCA is a predilection site of atherosclerosis.[17] Previous studies report a low (<10%) prevalence of intrinsic PCA disease in patients with PCA infarction.[8,10–12] (see Table 25-1). However, this may be due to insufficient vascular examination. Recent studies in Turkey[13] and Korea,[14] where MR angiogram (MRA) was performed on all the cases, identified PCA atherosclerosis as a cause of PCA territory infarction in 20–25% of cases. These results suggest that PCA atherosclerosis may be at least as important as proximal-artery diseases for the development of PCA territory infarction. Ethnic differences and the inclusion of isolated deep infarction may also explain the different prevalences of PCA disease among studies.

Whatever the prevalence, PCA atherosclerosis also results in artery-to-artery embolism; Doppler-monitoring[23] and diffusion-weighted MRI (DWI)[14] studies describe artery-to-artery embolism (from the proximal PCA to distal branches) as an important mechanism of occipital infarction in patients with PCA disease (Fig. 25-4C). As expected, unlike proximal-artery disease, embolic infarction that originates from PCA atherosclerosis is always confined to the PCA territory.[11]

Branch Occlusion

Atherosclerotic plaques in an intracranial artery can occlude the orifice of one or several perforators, causing infarction that is limited to the perforator territory (Fig. 25-4D).[24] This so-called "atheromatous branch occlusion"[25,26] seems to be a more important stroke mechanism in Asians, who demonstrate prevalent intracranial atherosclerosis.[17,27] Branch occlusion is more often observed in posterior than anterior circulation stroke, and is an important stroke mechanism of deep PCA territory (midbrain and thalamus) infarction associated with atherosclerosis in the P1 and P2 portions of the PCA.[17,28,29] A recent Korean study showed that branch occlusion was the most important stroke mechanism in patients with intrinsic PCA atherosclerosis and that the thalamus was the most commonly involved region.[14] Asian studies have reported that branch occlusion in association with PCA atherosclerosis accounts for 7–22% of lateral thalamic infarction.[29,30] Generally, arterial stenosis associated with branch

TABLE 25-1 Mechanism of Posterior Cerebral Artery Territory Infarction in Published Studies

Authors	Pessin et al.	Moriyasu et al.	Steinke et al.	Yamamoto et al.	Cals et al.	Kumral et al.	Lee et al.	Arboix et al.	Ntaios et al.
Published year	1987	1995	1997	1999	2002	2004	2009	2011	2011
Country	USA	Japan	Germany	USA	Switzerland	Turkey	Korea	Spain	Greece
Number of patients	35	85 (72*)	74	79	117	137	126	232	122
Diagnostic imaging	CT	CT/MRI	CT/MRI	CT/MRI	CT/MRI	CT/MRI	DWI	CT/MRI	CT/MRI
Vascular imaging									NM
MR angiography	None	None	31 (42%)	40 (51%)	15 (13%)	137 (100%)	126 (100%)	33%	
Conventional angiography	23 (66%)	72 (85%)	22 (30%)	28 (35%)	36 (31%)	NM	NM	10%	
Included topography	cortical, cortical + deep	NM	cortical, cortical + deep	cortical, cortical + deep	cortical only	cortical, cortical + deep	cortical, cortical + deep, deep	cortical, cortical + deep, deep	cortical, cortical + deep
Stroke mechanism									
Large artery disease	6 (17%)	11 (15%)	22 (31%)	32 (41%)	15 (13%)	69 (50%)	51 (41%)	68 (29%)	31 (25%)
PCA atherothrombosis	None	2 (3%)	6 (8%)	7 (9%)	2 (2%)	36 (26%)	38 (19%)	NM	15 (12%)
VA, BA atherothrombosis	6 (17%)	9 (11%)	16 (22%)	25 (32%)	13 (11%)	33 (24%)	10 (5%)	NM	16 (13%)
PCA+VB atherothrombosis	NM	NM	NM	NM	NM	NM	36 (18%)	NM	NM
Cardiac embolism	10 (29%)	12 (17%)	23 (31%)	32 (41%)	51 (44%)	29 (21%)	20 (16%)	50 (22%)	58 (48%)
Small artery disease	NM	NM	NM	NM	NM	NM	41 (33%)	80 (35%)	NM
Cause undetermined	11 (31%)	NM	18 (24%)	NM	38 (32%)	22 (16%)	14 (11%)	20 (9%)	25 (20%)
Uncommon causes	8 (22%)	5 (6%)	11 (15%)	7 (9%)	8 (7%)	16 (12%)	NM	14 (6%)	8 (7%)

PCA, posterior cerebral artery; VA, vertebral artery; BA, basilar artery; NM, not mentioned.
*Analysis of mechanism was performed only in 72 patients who underwent angiography.

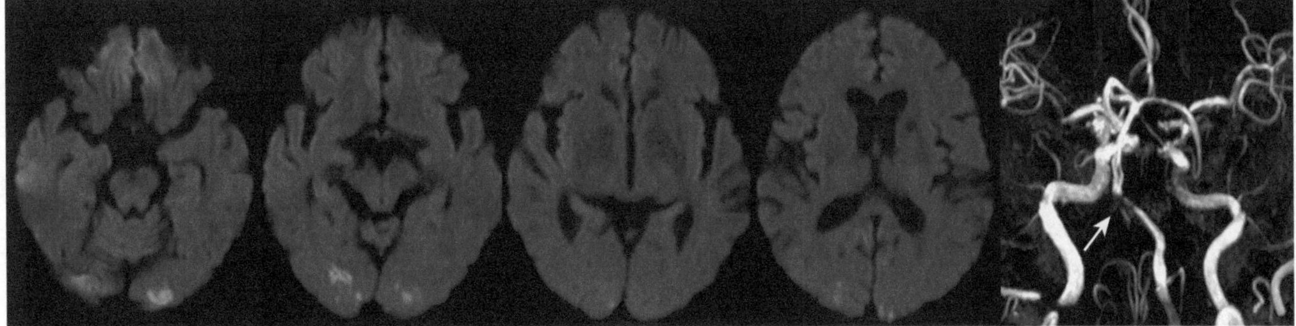

Figure 25-3. A 70-year-old woman who had hypertension and diabetes mellitus suddenly complained of dim vision. She also reported that there were several dark spots in the visual field. The symptoms disappeared in 3 days. Diffusion weighted MRI (first four images) show bilateral, scattered occipital infarcts. MR angiogram (right image) shows a severe, focal atherosclerotic stenosis in the left vertebro-basilar artery junction (arrow) that probably generates artery-to-artery embolism. There was a hypoplasia in the right vertebral artery.

occlusion is milder in degree than that causing artery-to-artery embolism or in situ thrombotic occlusion.[31] However, small thalamic infarcts may occur in patients with complete PCA occlusion who probably have well-developed collateral circulation (Fig. 25-5).

Lateral thalamic infarcts associated with PCA stenosis (branch occlusion) tend to enlarge over time, and are associated with complex symptoms (ataxia and/or hemiparesis in addition to sensory disturbances) and worse clinical outcomes than infarcts associated with small-artery disease (Fig. 25-6).[29] Branch occlusion may also play a role in the pathogenesis of thalamic infarction in other perforator territories (Figs 25-7 and 25-8), although this issue has not been sufficiently investigated. A DWI and MRA study reported that among 37 patients with pure midbrain infarction, branch occlusion in association with either BA or PCA atherosclerosis was the presumed stroke mechanism in 17 patients.[32]

In situ Thrombotic Occlusion

In patients with PCA atherosclerosis, thrombus formation in areas of plaque can result in total vascular occlusion, leading to infarction.[14,17] Occlusion of the proximal PCA may not produce significant infarction if the posterior communicating artery is well developed. On the other hand, P2 and P3 occlusions can produce relatively extensive infarction in the

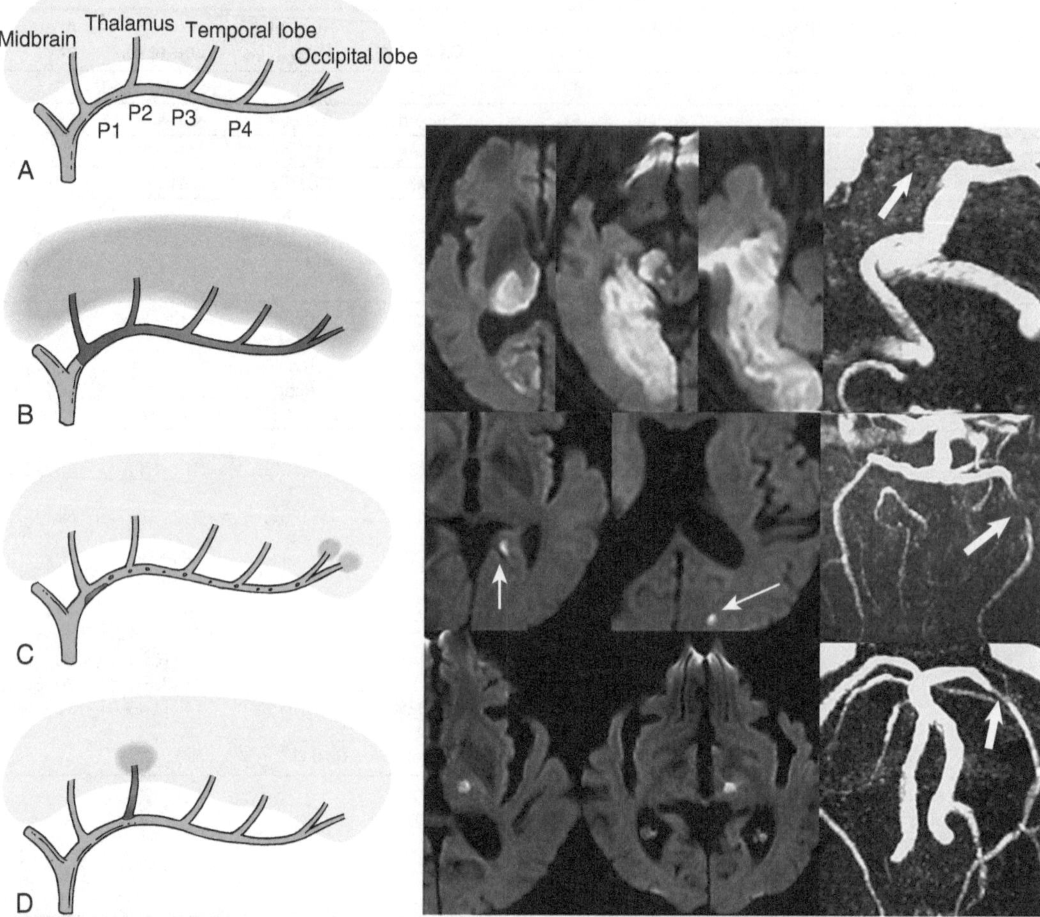

Figure 25-4. Schematic drawing and illustrative examples of the diverse patterns of posterior cerebral artery (PCA) territory infarction due to PCA atherothrombosis, as assessed by diffusion weighted MRI and MR angiography. The stenosis or occlusion of PCA shown in these patients was persistent on follow-up MR angiography. A, Schematic drawing illustrating PCA branches supplying midbrain, thalamus and temporo-occipital area. B, In situ thrombotic occlusion; whole right PCA territory infarction is produced by the right P1 occlusion (arrow). C, Artery to artery embolism; the severe atherosclerotic stenosis in the left P2 portion of the PCA P2 (thick arrow) presumably generates emboli that cause multiple small infarcts (thin arrows) scattered in the occipital lobe. D, Branch occlusion; mild atherosclerotic stenosis in the left P2 portion of the PCA (arrow) causes the left lateral thalamic infarction probably by occluding the orifice of the thalamogeniculate artery.

occipital lobe, medial temporal lobe, and thalamus. However, unlike cardiogenic embolism, in situ thrombotic occlusion less often produces sudden whole-territory infarction because of the relatively well-developed collateral circulation in the setting of the chronic atherosclerotic process.[33] The initial infarct frequently grows with persistent occlusion, leading to progressive neurological worsening (Figs 25-4B–25-9). Thus, the ultimate size of the infarct varies according to collateral circulation, the speed of arterial occlusion, and the hemodynamic stability of the patient.

Hemodynamic Disturbance

In patients with severe, bilateral VA, BA, or PCA steno-occlusive disease, hemodynamic mechanisms probably play a role in the development of ischemic lesions, especially when collateral circulation is insufficient (e.g., absent posterior communicating artery, inadequate compensation via leptomeningeal anastomoses form MCA or ACA).[3] However, hemodynamic disturbance has not been discussed as a stroke mechanism in previous studies on PCA infarction.[8,12,14,15,34]

There are anecdotal reports that described hemodynamic failure as a stroke mechanism for bilateral infarcts that occurs in the borderzone area between the MCA and PCA territories, thereby resulting in Balint's syndrome (see the following section on Bilateral infarction and associated syndromes).[35,36] However, embolism in the borderzone area cannot be ruled out, and PCA infarction solely due to hemodynamic failure seems to be rare. More often, hypoperfusion plays an additive role together with other major stroke mechanisms that may eventually determine the extent of infarction. Hemodynamic insufficiency may be a mechanism of transient ischemic attack (TIA) that occurs in the PCA territory (see the following section on Transient ischemic attack).

Small (penetrating)-artery Disease

Penetrating arteries in association with small subcortical or brainstem infarction demonstrate disorganized vessel walls, fibrinoid material deposition, and hemorrhagic extravasation through the arterial walls: this combination of findings was first called "segmental arterial disorganization" and then

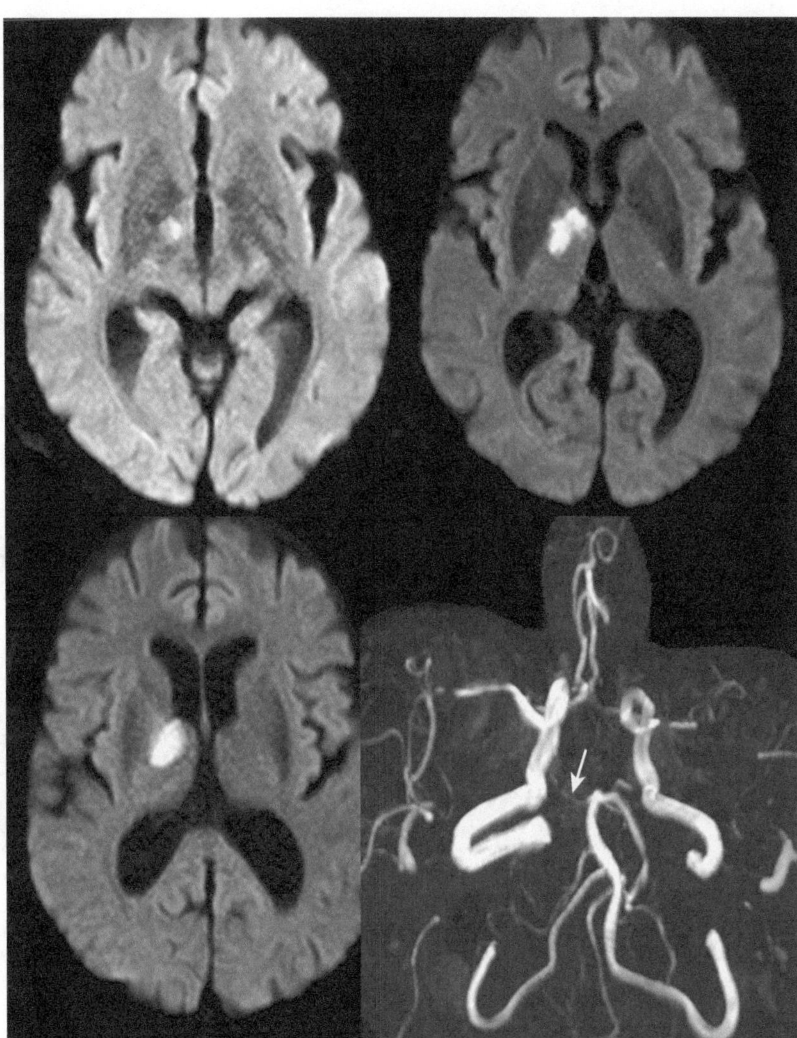

Figure 25-5. A 76-year-old woman developed confusion and memory loss. Diffusion weighted MRI showed an infarct in the anterior part of the right thalamus. MR angiogram showed complete occlusion of the P1 portion of the posterior cerebral artery (arrow). There was bilateral MCA atherosclerotic stenosis. Follow-up MR angiogram, performed 4 days later showed identical findings (not shown).

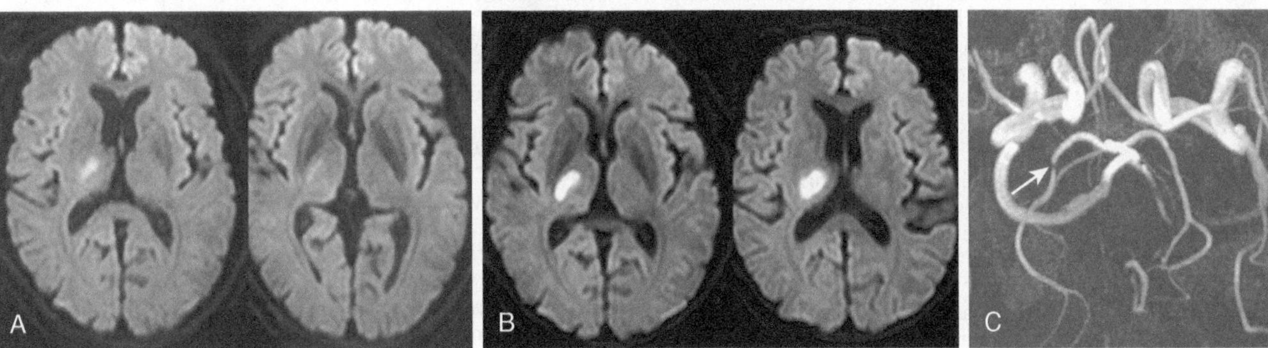

Figure 25-6. A 66-year-old hypertensive man developed tingling sensation in the left cheek and fingers. Examination showed slightly decreased perception of pain and touch in those areas, but without motor function abnormality. Diffusion weighted MRI showed a small lateral thalamic infarction (A). After admission the neurologic deficits progressively worsened, and 4 days later he had severe sensory deficits of all sensory modalities in the left face and limbs. There developed mild left hemiparesis and ataxia. Follow-up MRI showed enlargement of the lesion (B). MR angiogram showed a focal atherosclerotic stenosis in the right P2 portion of the posterior cerebral artery (arrow) (C) that resulted in branch occlusion.

"lipohyalinosis" by Fisher.[26,37–43] These vascular changes develop in arteries or arterioles that are 40–400 µm in diameter and frequently affect the perforating arteries from the PCA that supply the thalamus and midbrain (Fig 25-10).

Although small-artery disease has been neglected as a potential cause of PCA territory infarction (see Table 25-1), recent series that included infarcts limited to the deep territory found that small-artery disease is the most or the second-most important cause of PCA territory infarction.[14,15]

Cardiac Embolism

Cardiac embolism accounts for 18–41% of PCA territory infarction.[8–11,13,14] Atrial fibrillation is the most important

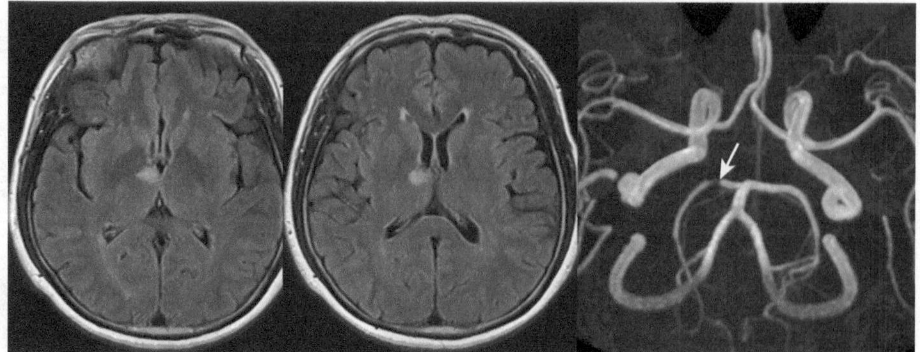

Figure 25-7. A 56-year-old hypertensive woman suddenly had memory loss. Examination showed severe anterograde amnesia. Flair MRI showed right anterior thalamic infarct (first two images). MR angiogram showed focal stenosis in the P1 portion of the right posterior cerebral artery (arrow) that probably produced branch occlusion (occlusion of the paramedian artery). The posterior communicating artery was not visible.

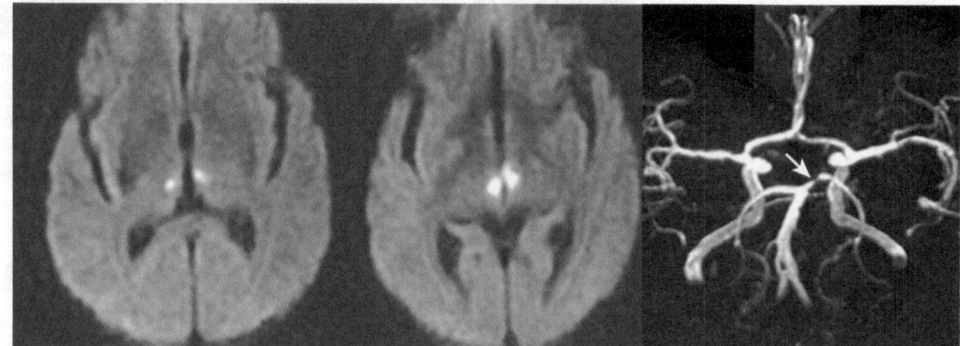

Figure 25-8. A 64-year-old hypertensive woman became stuporous. Examination showed severe vertical gaze limitation and confused mentality. Diffusion weighted MRI showed bilateral paramedian midbrain and thalamic infarcts. MR angiogram showed focal atherothrombotic stenosis in the P1 portion of the left posterior cerebral artery (arrow). The focal thrombus at this portion probably occluded the pedicle of a paramedian artery (branch occlusion) that branches off to supply both parts of the paramedian midbrain and thalamus. There was a fenestration of the lower basilar artery.

etiology. The occluded artery is usually spontaneously recanalized, and the angiographic findings are often normal if angiography is not performed early. The hemorrhagic transformation of an infarct often occurs in association with recanalization and worsens patients' headaches and other neurologic symptoms (Fig. 25-11). In one series, hemorrhagic infarction occurred in 44% of patients with PCA infarction due to cardioembolic stroke.[10]

Patent foramen ovale (PFO) with a large amount of right-to-left shunting may be an etiology of embolic infarction (e.g., paradoxical embolism), especially in young patients without an evident cause of stroke.[44,45] As discussed in Chapter 26, posterior circulation seems to be a predilection site for embolism in patients with PFO,[46,47] and PFO probably is an important cause of stroke in the previously described "cryptogenic embolism" group of patients.[8,11,12] It seems that PFO should be suspected and investigated in young patients with PCA territory infarction due to unclear etiology.[10,12]

Uncommon Causes

Dissection

In posterior circulation, dissection most commonly develops in the VA, either extracranially[48,49] or intracranially.[50] Headache and neck pain may be the only complaints. Ischemic symptoms and signs may develop concomitantly or after a delay of hours or days. The lateral medulla and cerebellum are the most susceptible to ischemia due to VA dissection.[48,49] Although uncommon, VA dissection can be a possible donor site for distal embolism that leads to PCA infarction.[11,13] Dissection in the PCA is rare. In a review of 40 patients with PCA dissection, 15 had ischemia, 15 had subarachnoid hemorrhage, and six had aneurysmal mass effects (Fig. 25-12).[51]

Migraine

Migraine is considered closely related to posterior circulation ischemia,[52–56] and previous studies described migraine as a cause of PCA infarction in 3–14% of patients.[8,12,13] However, there are controversies over whether migraine is the real cause of PCA infarction in these patients. Angiograms of patients with migrainous stroke occasionally show thrombotic arterial occlusion, and extensive investigations often reveal hidden embolic sources such as PFO with a large amount of shunting.[8,10,53,57] As discussed above, posterior circulation is a predilection site of embolism in patients with PFO. Therefore, the diagnosis of migraine stroke should be made very cautiously, and thorough etiological examination should be performed even when PCA infarction develops in patients with migraine.

Moyamoya Disease

Moyamoya disease is characterized by the progressive occlusion of the distal ICA or proximal MCA and the development of fine meshworks of basal collateral vessels. Cerebral hypoperfusion is the predominant stroke mechanism in these patients, and repeated TIAs are observed when patients are dehydrated or hyperventilating. Less often, cerebral infarction due to embolism or thrombotic occlusion is encountered.[58]

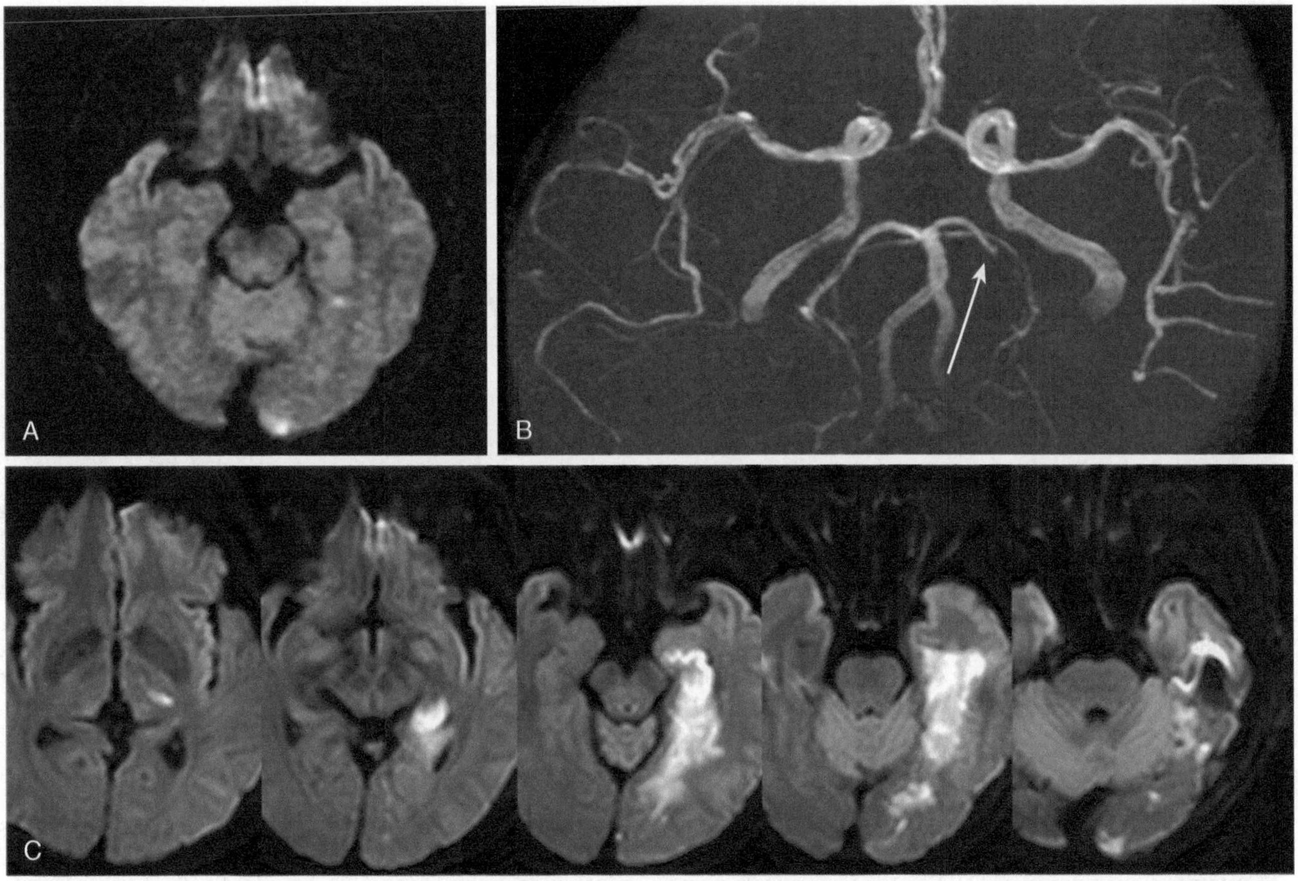

Figure 25-9. A 60-year-old man with a history of hypertension, diabetes and coronary heart disease had sudden blurred vision which was followed by clumsiness of the left hand. On examination, he showed right homonymous hemianopia, and slight weakness and moderately decreased sensation in the left arm and leg. Initial diffusion weighted MRI showed a few scattered, tiny infarcts in the left medial temporal and occipital area (A). Initial MR angiogram showed occlusion of the P2 portion of the left posterior cerebral artery (B). Diffusion MRI taken 1 day later showed expansion of the lesion to the left lateral thalamus, medial temporal area and occipital area (C). A mild stenosis was also observed in the right middle cerebral artery. A follow-up MR angiogram 6 days later showed persistent occlusion of the left posterior cerebral artery. This patient showed normal vertebral artery and normal echocardiographic findings and thus was considered to have infarction due to intrinsic posterior cerebral artery atherosclerotic occlusion. *(From Caplan LR, Amarenco P. Kim JS. Posterior circulation disorders. In, Kim JS, Caplan LR, Wong KSL ed. Intracranial Atherosclerosis, pp 83–99, with permission.)*

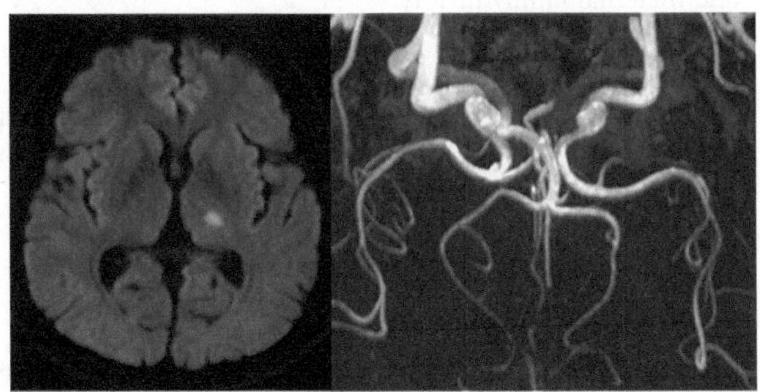

Figure 25-10. A 55-year-old hypertensive man suddenly felt a tingling sensation in the left face and distal limbs. Pinprick and touch sensation were mildly decreased in these areas. Diffusion weighted MRI showed a small, left lateral thalamic infarction. MR angiogram findings were normal.

Posterior circulation stroke has been considered uncommon and appears in the late stage of moyamoya disease associated with widespread vascular involvement including PCA.[59] However, a recent study reported that PCA involvement is present in 29% of patients, with 17% demonstrating PCA territory infarction.[60] There were no differences in the prevalence of PCA involvement and PCA territory infarction between pediatric and adult patients. These results suggest that PCA infarction may be more common in moyamoya disease than previously recognized, especially in young patients. Occipital infarction in moyamoya patients often includes a part of the posterior MCA territory, probably because vascular collaterals from the PCA supply a part of the MCA territory in these patients (Fig. 25-13).

Fibromuscular Dysplasia

Fibromuscular dysplasia (FMD) is a vasculopathy of unknown cause that is characterized by hyperplasia of the intima and media of the arteries, adventitial sclerosis, and breakdown of the normal elastic tissue without inflammation. Thickened septa and ridges protrude into the lumen. The most common angiographic finding is the "string of beads" appearance: segments of constriction alternate with normal or dilated segments. The ICA is most often affected in patients with cervicocranial artery involvement (95%), and extracranial VA involvement has been reported in 12–43% of affected patients. VA FMD may cause infarction via artery-to-artery embolism, hemodynamic insufficiency, or the combination of the two.[61]

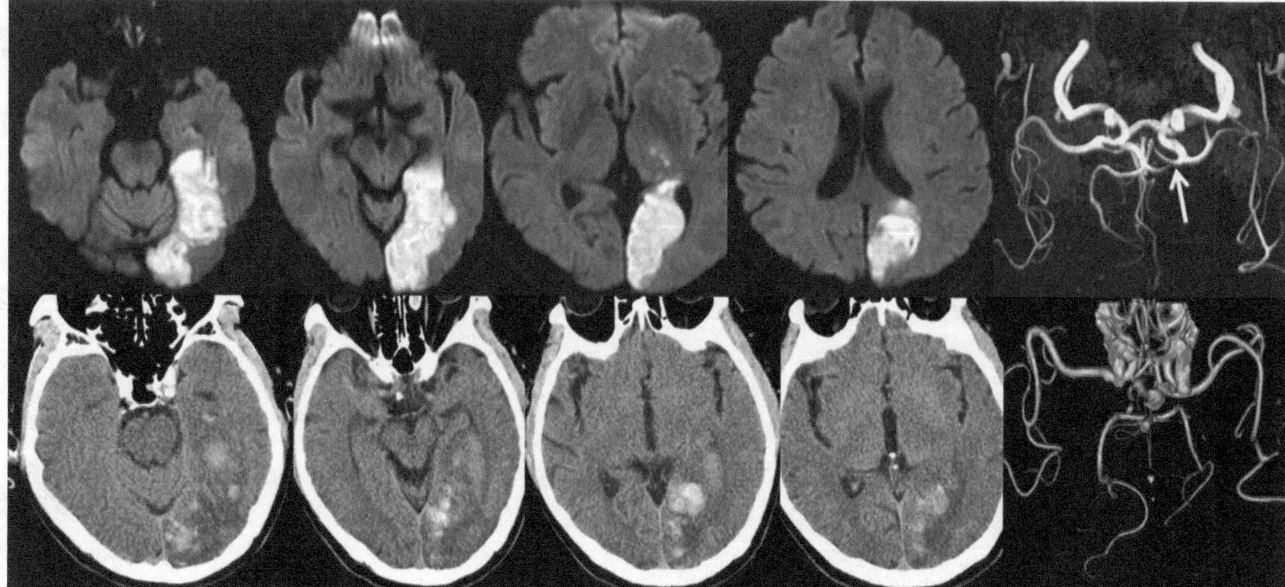

Figure 25-11. A 75-year-old man with atrial fibrillation suddenly developed occipital headache followed by visual field defect and tingling sensation in the right limbs. Examination showed mild sensory deficits in the right face and limbs, dense right homonymous hemianopia. He was able to write but could not read what he wrote (alexia without agraphia). Diffusion weighted MRI showed acute infarcts in the left occipital lobe and the lateral thalamus (upper row). MR angiogram showed occlusion of the left posterior cerebral artery (arrow) (last image in the upper row). During admission, the patient complained of progressively worsening occipital headache. CT performed 7 days later showed hemorrhagic transformation (lower row). CT angiogram revealed recanalized posterior cerebral artery (last image in the lower row).

Although rare, FMD may occur in the intracranial arteries such as BA[62–64] or PCA[65] resulting in posterior circulation TIA,[63] and PCA territory infarctions[62,65] FMD in association with dissection in the ICA may produce PCA infarction in patients with persistent fetal-type circulation.[66]

Reversible Cerebral Vasoconstriction Syndrome

Reversible cerebral vasoconstriction syndrome is characterized by severe headache with or without additional neurological symptoms and the "string and beads" appearance in cerebral arteries; cerebral vasoconstriction generally resolves in 1–3 months.[67] Cerebral infarction occurs in 4–31% of patients, usually after hemorrhagic events (during the second week).[67] Occipital infarction resulting in visual field defects is common in patients who develop stroke.[67] Previously described conditions, such as postpartum cerebral angiopathy and migraine stroke with vasospasm, are now considered parts of reversible cerebral vasoconstriction syndrome.[68]

Arterial Compression

Arterial compression (or secondary thrombus formation) may produce PCA territory infarction. The most commonly observed example is PCA infarction that develops at the time of transtentorial brain herniation. The PCA is usually compressed in its course around the midbrain, medial to the herniated temporal lobe and lateral to the tentorium.[69,70] Compression may also occur contralateral to the herniation because of the lateral displacement of the brainstem against the contralateral tentorium. Surgery or endovascular intervention on the posterior communicating artery or BA aneurysm may result in the occlusion of the PCA or perforating arteries.[71]

Mitochondrial Disease

Mitochondrial encephalomyopathy, lactic acidosis, and stroke-like episodes (MELAS) present with infarction-like lesions, most frequently in the occipital area.[72,73] In a study on 38 young patients (≤45 years old) who presented with occipital infarction, four patients (10%) received a clinical or molecular diagnosis of mitochondrial disorder: two patients had A3243G mitochondrial DNA mutation.[74] Therefore, MELAS should be considered an etiology of young-age occipital infarction. The pathogenesis of stroke-like lesions seems to be associated with endothelial damage in the small arteries associated with mitochondrial dysfunction[75] and metabolic derangement[76] rather than large-artery occlusion. Therefore, stroke-like lesions often do not exactly conform to the usual PCA territory (Fig. 25-14).[77,78] Patients generally present with other features of MELAS, such as short stature, hearing impairments, seizures, and maternal family history.

Other Miscellaneous Causes

Hypercoagulopathy, central nervous system infection, and immunologic vasculitis may result in PCA infarction, and usually involve other vascular territories as well.

PREVALENCE AND FREQUENCY OF INVOLVED STRUCTURES

According to registry studies, pure PCA territory infarction accounts for about 5–10% of cerebral infarctions.[15,79] Patients with PCA infarction have concomitant infarcts in other vascular territories in 34–39% of cases (PCA plus).[11,14,16] According to a study that investigated 205 patients using DWI, 79 patients had infarcts in other vascular territories, including the posterior (n = 39), anterior (n = 29), or both territories (n = 11).[14] The cerebellum is the most common site of extra-PCA territory infarction[11,14] followed by the MCA territory.[14] Superior cerebellar artery and posterior inferior cerebellar artery infarction present at equal frequencies among cerebellar infarcts, while anterior inferior cerebellar artery infarction is uncommon.[14] Pontine and medullary infarcts are also encountered.

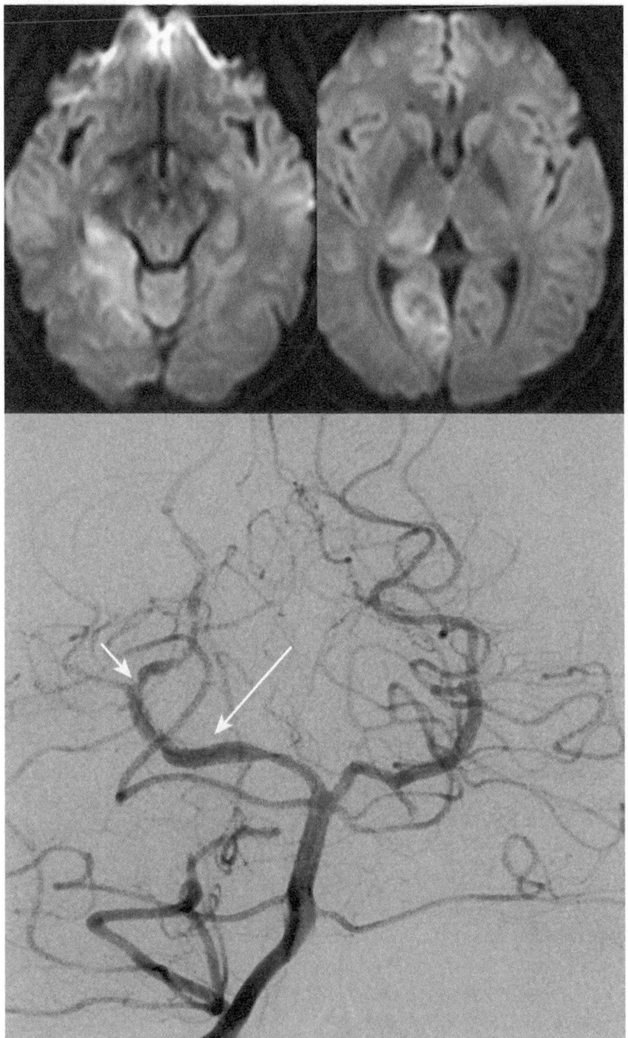

Figure 25-12. A 32-year-old woman suddenly developed tingling sensation in the left limbs and visual field defect. Examination showed impaired sensory perception in the left face and limbs, mild ataxia and dense left homonymous hemianopia. Diffusion weighted MRI showed acute infarcts in the right lateral thalamus and occipital lobe (upper row). Conventional angiogram showed diffuse, fusiform dilatation (long arrow) and stenosis (short arrow) of the posterior cerebral artery (lower row). The angiographic findings were unchanged after 3 months. Vasculitis work ups were all negative, and the most likely diagnosis was dissection.

Among patients with pure PCA territory infarction, the proportion of infarcts located in deep structures only ranges between 34% and 64%,[13-15,34] and the proportion of cortical infarcts varies between 14% and 51%.[14,15,34] Asians appear to develop deep infarction more often than Caucasians.[13,14] In addition, the use of advanced brain imaging such as DWI may increase the detection of small, deep infarcts.[14] In deep structures, the thalamus is involved approximately six times as often as the midbrain.[14] The most frequently involved deep structure is the ventrolateral thalamus.[14,34]

Among patients with only cortical PCA territory infarction, the frequency of involvement is 60% occipital, 20% occipito-temporal, 7% occipito-parietal, 4% occipito-temporal-parietal, 2% temporal, and 7% bilateral.[12] The relatively uncommon involvement of the temporal lobe may be due to the acute angle of the anterior temporal division from the PCA stem that prevents emboli from occluding this branch.

CLINICAL–TOPOGRAPHICAL CORRELATION

Midbrain Infarction

Occlusion of the mesencephalic branches from the P1 segment of the PCA results in paramedian rostral midbrain infarction, while occlusion of the peduncular perforating arteries from the P2 portion results in anterolateral midbrain infarction. Paramedian infarction frequently results in oculomotor and pupillary disturbances, while anterolateral midbrain infarction results in hemiparesis or ataxic hemiparesis due to the involvement of the descending motor tracts in the crus cerebri. Involvement of the midbrain is one of the causes of hemiparesis in patients with PCA territory infarction.[80,81] The clinical features and the role of PCA disease in the pathogenesis of midbrain infarction are described in Chapter 26.

Thalamic Infarction

The arteries that supply the thalamus branch from the P1 and P2 portions of the PCA and the posterior communication artery. Thalamic infarction generally follows the topography according to four major thalamic vascular territories: the inferolateral, tuberothalamic, paramedian, and posterior choroidal arteries[2,82] (see Fig. 25-2).

Inferolateral (Thalamogeniculate) Artery Territory Infarction

The inferolateral (thalamogeniculate) arteries are composed of 5–10 arteries that arise from the P2 portion of the PCA.[83] These arteries mainly supply the ventrolateral thalamus, which includes the ventrolateral (VL) and ventroposterior (VP) nuclear groups. Inferolateral artery territory infarction is the most common type of thalamic infarction (see Figs 25-6, 25-10).

The clinical features of inferolateral artery infarction were described as "thalamic syndrome" by Dejerine and Roussy.[84] The most frequent and important symptom/sign is hemisensory disturbance.[82,85] Small lateral thalamic stroke that selectively involves the VP nucleus is the most common etiology of pure sensory stroke.[86-88] Although both spinothalamic and lemniscal sensation are usually simultaneously impaired, small lesions may produce only paresthesias or selective impairment of lemniscal or spinothalamic sensation.

The sensory topography includes half of the face, arms, trunk, and legs in > 50% of patients.[89] Occasionally, sensory symptoms are restricted to the acral body parts from onset: the most frequent form is cheiro-oral syndrome.[87,90] More commonly, initial hemisensory disturbance is gradually restricted to the most vulnerable areas, usually the distal part of the limbs. Cheiro-oral-pedal and cheiro-pedal syndrome are also observed, though much less frequently. Occasionally, the thumb and index finger are preferentially or selectively involved.[90,91] Restricted acral sensory syndrome is explained by (1) the anatomical proximity of the sensory fibers to the acral body parts (in primates, the representative areas of the thumb and index finger are located in the most medial portion of the VP lateral, adjacent to the lip area of the VP medial),[92] (2) the increased vulnerability of the acral body parts in association with disproportionately large representative areas in the human sensory system, and (3) the lack of interhemispheric connections.[93]

In patients with hemisensory deficits, intraoral regions are occasionally involved (e.g., the gums, hard palate, tongue).

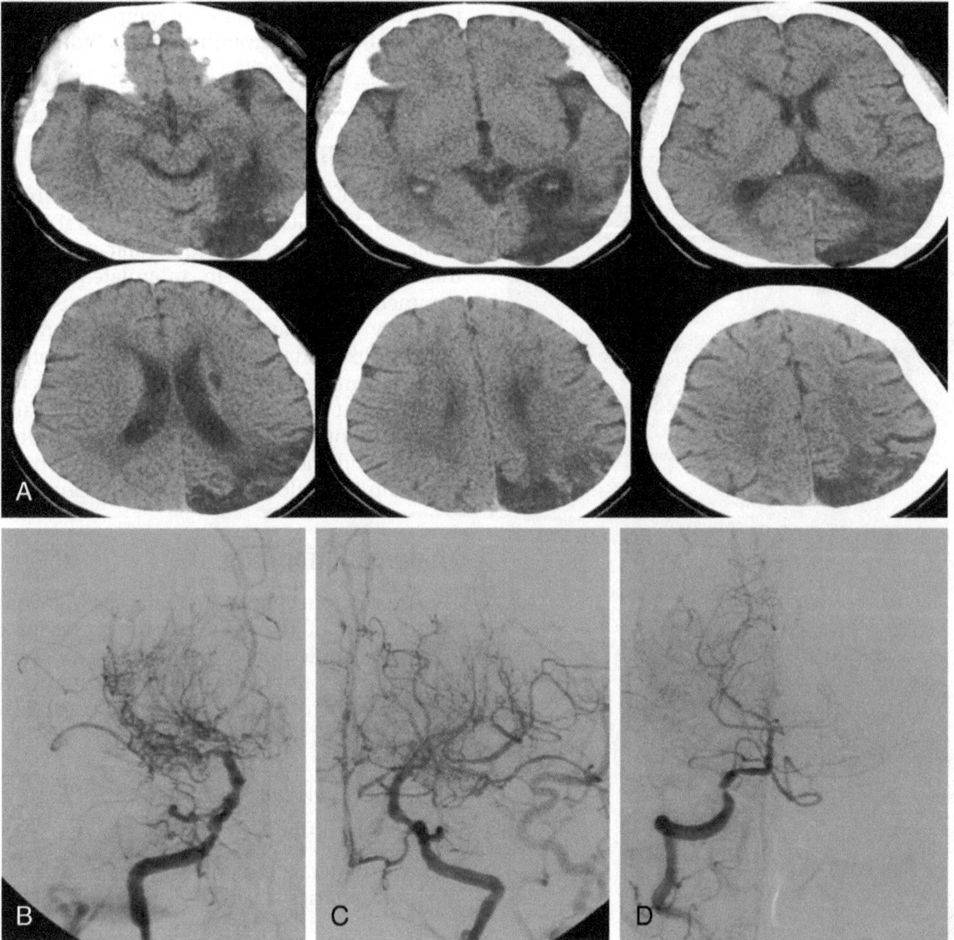

Figure 25-13. A 64-year-old woman developed a visual field defect on the right side. CT shows an infarct in the left occipital area that extends to the borderzone area between the posterior cerebral artery and middle cerebral artery. Asymptomatic subcortical infarcts are also shown on the left side (A). Angiogram showed bilateral occlusion of distal internal carotid arteries and numerous basal moyamoya vessels. Posterior circulation was also involved and left posterior cerebral artery was occluded (B–D). *(From Miyamoto S, Takahashi JC, Kim JS, Moyamoya disease. In, Kim JS, Caplan LR, Wong KSL ed. Intracranial Atherosclerosis, pp 246–258, with permission.)*

The loss of taste sensation may also occur. Rarely, sensory symptoms restricted to the proximal limbs and trunk that spare the face and distal limbs are observed.[94] Isolated trigeminal sensory loss is reportedly due to tiny lesions that presumably involve the most medial parts of the VP nucleus.[95] Thalamic pure sensory syndrome is a lacunar syndrome that is primarily caused by the lipohyalinotic penetrating artery disease (see Fig. 25-10).[87,88] However, other etiologies, such as atherosclerosis of the PCA, cardiogenic embolism, and hypertensive hemorrhage, may also produce pure sensory syndromes.[89,90]

A relatively large lesion that concomitantly involves the adjacent internal capsule can result in sensorimotor stroke, and additional involvement of the cerebellothalamic fibers at the VL nucleus may result in "hypesthetic ataxic hemiparesis" syndrome. Although uncommon, a small infarction limited to the VL nucleus may produce hemiataxia and dysarthria without sensory loss. Neuropsychological and cognitive deficits are generally absent.

Tuberothalamic (Polar) Artery Territory Infarction

The tuberothalamic artery originates from the middle-third of the posterior communicating artery. In approximately one-third of the normal population, this territory is supplied by the paramedian artery that arises from the P1 portion of the PCA (see Fig. 25-7).[96] The tuberothalamic arteries mainly supply the ventral anterior nucleus (VA), rostral part of the VL, and the ventral pole of the medial dorsal nucleus (MD). It seems that the anterior nuclear group is supplied by both the tuberothalamic and choroidal arteries.

The main clinical syndromes that result from tuberothalamic infarction include neuropsychological deficits. In the early stages of infarction, patients exhibit fluctuating levels of consciousness and appear withdrawn. Patients show impaired recent memory formation, which is more prominent when left-sided lesions are present. Visual memory impairments more often develop with right-sided lesions.[96,97] Amnestic syndrome seems to be caused by the disconnection of memory circuitry (e.g., between the VA and the hippocampal formation or amygdala).[98,99]

Language disturbances also occur in patients with left-side infarction. This is characterized by anomia with decreased verbal output and impaired fluency, impaired comprehension, and paraphasic speech. Reading and repetition are relatively preserved. Left thalamic lesions are also associated with acalculia. Constructional, buccofacial, and limb apraxia may present (more often with left-sided lesions), whereas hemineglect may present in patients with right-side infarction. Patients may develop persistent personality changes, including

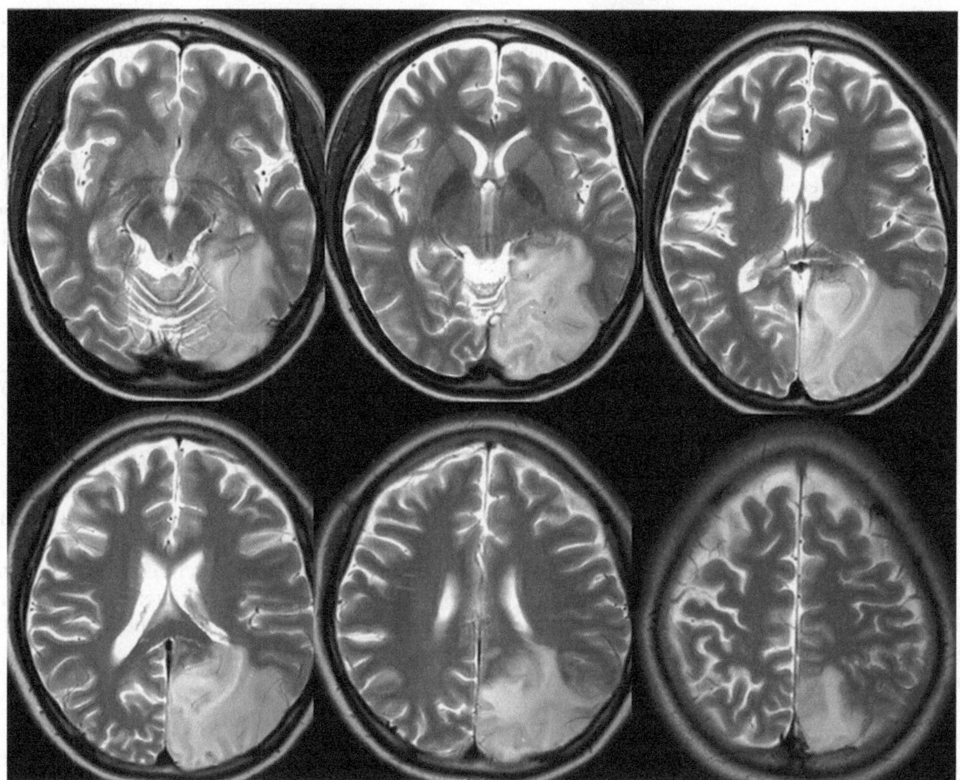

Figure 25-14. A 17-year-old girl felt that she could not clearly see objects on the right side 2 months before admission. She had had hearing difficulty and recurrent episodes of generalized seizures. Examination showed dense right homonymous hemianopia. There was serum lactic acidosis, and genetic studies revealed mitochondrial gene (3243A>G) mutation. She was diagnosed as having MELAS (mitochondrial encephalomyopathy, lactic acidosis, and stroke-like episodes). T2 weighted MRI showed a large left occipital infarction that extended beyond the usual posterior cerebral artery territory.

euphoria, lack of insight, apathy, and lack of spontaneity.[97,100,101] Hypometabolism in the posterior cingulate cortex of these patients, as assessed by positron-emission tomography, suggests that these behavioral changes may be related to thalamocortical disconnection.[101]

Paramedian (Thalamic-subthalamic) Artery Territory Infarction

The paramedian arteries supply the paramedian parts of the upper midbrain and thalamus, including the intralaminar nuclear group and most of the dorsomedial nucleus. Involvement of the paramedian territory is very common in patients with occlusion of the top of the basilar artery (top of the basilar artery syndrome; see Chapter 26). Other commonly involved structures include the occipital lobe, cerebellum, and brainstem. Infarction limited to the paramedian territory is uncommon in this condition.

The most characteristic clinical feature of paramedian territory infarction is prominent neuropsychological disturbance, particularly disturbances that affect arousal and memory (without or with minimal sensorimotor dysfunction). The significant somnolence and fluctuating levels of consciousness are a conspicuous feature during the early stages, and can last for hours or days. This is probably related to involvement of the rostral portion of the brainstem reticular activating system. Confusion, agitation, aggression, and apathy may be present.[82,102,103] In patients with left-sided lesions, speech and language impairment often present, which are characterized by hypophonia, reduced verbal fluency, perseveration, and occasionally paraphasic errors, but preserved repetition.[104] Apraxia may also be observed.[105]

Another characteristic of paramedian artery territory infarction is the common occurrence of bilateral infarction.[82] This is because a single pedicle arising from the P1 portion of the PCA on one side may branch off and supply the paramedian territory on both sides (see Fig. 25-8).[83] Generally, bilateral infarction results in more severe clinical symptoms: patients demonstrate stupor, disorientation, and dementia. Patients are unresponsive, unable to speak, and apathetic. Severe memory impairment and confabulation are also observed.[102,103,106] Even after the acute stage, patients may show long-lasting neuropsychologic problems such as inappropriate social behaviors, impulsiveness, aggressive outbursts, and emotional blunting.

The pathogenic mechanism of memory loss and other behavioral syndromes in thalamic infarction remains unclear, but disconnection syndrome has been suggested. Two neuronal networks relevant to learning and memory include: (1) the mammillothalamic tract, which connects the anterior thalamic nucleus with the hippocampus via the fornix (lesions in these systems may result in memory-encoding deficits that are similar to the effects of hippocampal lesions), and (2) the ventral amygdalofugal pathway, which links the amygdala to the medial dorsal nucleus of the thalamus and prefrontal cortex. Medial thalamic lesions may interrupt this pathway.[98] Recent blood flow studies using SPECT illustrate that decreased blood flow in the frontal lobe or limbic cortex is correlated with the degree of memory and cognitive dysfunction in patients with left thalamic infarction, which explains both memory disturbance and behavioral dysfunction.[107]

Ocular motor disturbances are commonly accompanied by neuropsychiatric symptoms, that include vertical gaze palsy (upgaze, downgaze or both), convergence failure, pseudo-sixth-nerve palsy, pupillary changes, internuclear ophthalmoplegia, and ocular tilt reaction.[82,102,103,106] These abnormalities are due to the concomitant involvement of the rostral midbrain structures involved in ocular motor control, and result in symptoms such as diplopia, dizziness, and gait difficulty. This issue will be further discussed in Chapter 26. Other clinical features include sensorimotor symptoms, which are uncommon and usually transient. Asterixis may develop in the acute phase of infarction.[82,108]

Posterior Choroidal Artery Territory Infarction

The posterior choroidal arteries arise from the P2 segment of the PCA distal to the origin of the posterior communicating artery. The posterior choroidal arteries are divided into two groups: 1–2 medial branches and 1–10 lateral branches (Fig. 25-15). These arteries supply the lateral geniculate body (LGB), the inferolateral region of the pulvinar, the lateral dorsal nucleus, and the lateral posterior nucleus. The LGB may also receive blood supply from the anterior choroidal artery.

Infarction limited to the posterior choroidal artery territory area is uncommon and accounts for 9.5% of thalamic infarcts.[109] The two most prominent clinical manifestations are visual field defects and hemisensory deficits. Visual field defects include homonymous hemianopia (either congruent or incongruent), quadrantanopia, and sectoranopia.[110] It has been shown that the lower retinal quadrant is represented in the anterolateral part of the LGB, the upper quadrant occupies the anteromedial part, and the macula is represented by the posterior pole of the LGB.[111,112] Horizontal sectoranopia usually indicates the involvement of the central part of the LGB. The fact that the anterior choroidal artery supplies a part of the LGB may explain the diverse pattern of visual field defects in patients with posterior choroidal artery infarction.[109] Spontaneous nystagmus or impaired fast-phase optokinetic response to the opposite side of the lesion has also been observed, which could be attributed to the involvement of the smooth pursuit pathways in the LGB.[113]

Hemisensory dysfunction is another common clinical manifestation. Involvement of the VP nucleus, which is often supplied by the lateral posterior choroidal artery at least its caudal section, explains this feature. The sensory manifestations are essentially the same as those observed in patients with inferolateral territory infarction. Concomitant mild motor dysfunction may be present due to the involvement of the adjacent internal capsule.

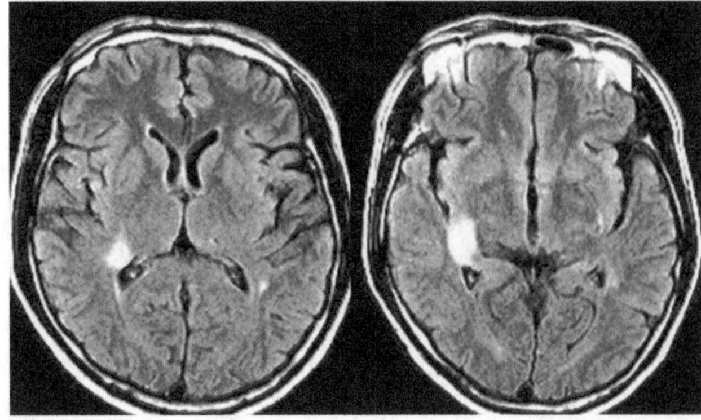

Figure 25-15. A 55-year-old man with diabetes suddenly developed a visual field defect on his left side. On examination, there was a dense left homonymous hemianopia. Diffusion weighted MRI showed an infarct in the posterior choroidal artery territory that probably involved the lateral geniculate body.

Neuropsychiatric symptoms may also present, although not as prominently as paramedian or tuberothalamic infarction. Left-sided lesions may produce aphasia, paraphasia, and word-finding difficulty, usually with normal repetition and comprehension due to the involvement of the pulvinar.[114,115] Spatial neglect is associated with right pulvinar lesions.[116] Visual and verbal memory disturbances and temporal disorientation are rare and may be related to the involvement of the hippocampus, parahippocampal gyrus, or pulvinar.[109,117]

Combined Polar and Paramedian Territory Infarction

Because of the variability in the vascular supply to the thalami, some infarcts do not exactly correlate with the alleged topography. Most notably, because the territory of the polar thalamic artery is often taken over (either unilaterally or bilaterally) by the paramedian thalamic artery, combination polar and paramedian artery infarction is not uncommon. The clinical picture of these patients includes (1) amnesia, which is often severe and presents in combination with various neuropsychological deficits, (2) altered consciousness and frontal lobe dysfunction, and (3) eye movement disturbances (most frequently vertical gaze palsy).[118]

Cortical (Superficial) Infarction

Hemispheric infarction due to PCA occlusion involves the occipital, posterior temporal, and parietal lobes, and clinical manifestations vary according to the location and extent of infarction. The most frequent clinical finding is visual field defects, which occur in > 90% of patients with cortical PCA infarction.[8,12,13] Various types of cognitive abnormalities have been described. According to a study on patients with only cortical PCA infarction, memory impairment and aphasia affect 18% and 15% of patients, respectively.[12] Although the cognitive deficits associated with visual function have been intensively studied in order to understand the human nature of cognitive visual function, they are actually uncommon in clinical practice. In the cited study, the following frequencies were reported: visual hallucination (10%), visual neglect (9%), visual agnosia (8.5%), prosopagnosia (5.5%), color dysnomia (5%), palinopsia (3%), and color agnosia (3%).

Visual Field Defects

The lower portion of visual radiation belongs to the PCA territory through the entire course while most of the upper portion, which runs through the upper wall of the ventricle, receives some supply from the branches of the MCA (especially the angular and posterior temporal branches). Visual field defects occur in >90% of patients with infarcts involving the cortical PCA territory.[12,13] The most common type of visual field disturbance is homonymous hemianopia, which occurs in approximately three-quarters of patients.[13] Homonymous hemianopia is usually congruent, but may spare or selectively involve the ipsilateral temporal crescent of vision depending on the location of the lesion.[119,120]

Previous studies have shown that neurons subserving central visual field occupy a larger portion of the striate cortex than those responsible for the peripheral visual field. The area representing the central field corresponds to the posterior half of the medial striate including occipital pole whereas the peripheral visual field corresponds to the anterior half.[121–125] The visual field defect tends to be more complete in occipital pole lesions, suggesting the higher concentration of fibers in this region.[125] The pattern and severity of visual field defect may vary according to the lesion location and extension, which is in part related to the status of collateral flows (e.g., flows from the MCA);[126] patients may have macula sparing[127] or isolated central hemianopia (infarction is confined to the occipital pole).[125,128]

Field defects may be limited to quadrantanopia. Superior quadrantanopia is caused by lesions that involve the lower bank of the striate cortex or inferior optic radiation in the temporal lobe, and inferior quadrantanopia is due to infarction in the upper calcarine bank or involvement of the upper optic radiation in the inferior parietal lobe. Superior quadrantanopia occurs more than three times as often as inferior quadrantanopia in patients with PCA infarction.[12] Hemianopia may evolve into quadrantanopia during the recovery phase.

About half of patients are unaware of their unilateral visual problems. Patients may report their problems as grayness, spots, voids and focusing difficulties.[52] They may bump into things and may hit their head (superior quadrantanopia) or leg (inferior quadrantanopia) on objects. Old patients may complain of dizziness in association with the deprivation of visual sensory inputs.

Cognitive Disturbances Related to Visual Function

Visual Hallucination

In patients with PCA infarction, visual hallucination is uncommon and tends to occur in the recovery phase than the acute stage. Symptoms may develop on either side after infarction.[12] Hallucinations are either elementary (e.g., simple streaks, patterns, or blurs of color)[129] or complex (e.g., detailed images of animals or people).[130] Pathogenesis is considered a release phenomenon in the presence of impaired visual function. Most patients are aware that the hallucinations are not real and do not feel that they are threatening. These hallucinations differ from peduncular hallucination, which develops following midbrain-thalamic lesions and is vivid, occasionally perceived as real, and not accompanied by visual field defects (see Chapter 26).

Palinopsia

Palinopsia is the visual perseveration of images over time, i.e., a recent image either persists after the object leaves the visual field or recurs after minutes, hours, or even days.[131,132] In the latter case, the palinoptic images may be incorporated into the visual stimuli in the present environment, such as a cigar or beard appearing on the faces of all persons at a party. Palinopsia usually occurs in patients with impaired vision who are not entirely blind.[133] Hallucinations and the illusion of visual movement are common.[134]

One autopsied patient with palinopsia had a subcortical infarct that undermined the right lingual and fusiform gyri.[132] It seems that both left- and right-sided lesions may produce palinopsia.[135] Palinopsia is a reported cause of brain tumors, arteriovenous malformation, inflammation, and the use of anticonvulsants.[136] In patients with stroke, palinopsia tends to occur transiently during the progression or resolution of visual field defect,[133] although symptoms may persist for years.[137]

Other Visual Perception Disorders

Other visual perception disorders caused by occipital infarction include cerebral polyopia (multiple images),[138,139] micropsia (objects appear smaller than they are),[140] and macropsia (objects appear larger than they are).[141] Metamorphopsia is another unusual condition: objects, faces, and, rarely, other visual stimuli appear distorted in size[142] or even look like monsters.[143] The specific locations of the lesions and pathogeneses of these visual perception disorders remain obscure. Most patients have visual field defects.

Visual Agnosia

Visual agnosia is the inability to recognize visually presented objects despite the preservation of elementary sensory functions. Visual agnosia is diagnosed by assessing the patient's ability to name, describe uses for, and pantomime the use of visually presented objects. Extensive occipital damage due to anoxic insult or severe infarction is the usual cause of this rare syndrome.[144–146]

Theoretically, there are two forms of visual agnosia: the "apperceptive" form that is caused by impaired visual processing that results in the poor perception of the object, and the "associative" form that is caused by disorders that affect the associative cortex and results in the correctly formed visual percepts being poorly matched with previously processed sensory data and recognition.[147,148] Most patients with visual agnosia present with both aspects, although one type may predominate.

There appear to be multiple pathophysiological mechanisms that result in apperceptive visual agnosia. These may be related to the misperception of shapes due to defects in representing the elementary properties of curvature, surface and volume[149] or failure to integrate multiple elements into a perceptual whole.[150] Patients with severe apperceptive agnosia usually have extensive and diffuse occipital lesions and tend to have residual field defects.[151]

Closely related to the associative form of visual agnosia is optic aphasia, in which patients are unable to name visually presented objects but otherwise show relatively intact knowledge about objects and are, thereby, able to categorize and demonstrate their use through pantomime.[152,153] Visual agnosia and optic aphasia may simply represent a continuum with varying deficits in knowledge retrieval.[154,155] Patients typically present with large left PCA territory infarction with right homonymous hemianopia.[152–154,156,157] It has been suggested that there is a functional disconnection between visual perception and language systems.

Prosopagnosia

Prosopagnosia is the inability to recognize previously familiar faces.[158] The deficit is mostly restricted to the identification of faces, but some patients have difficulty recognizing other objects such as animals, cars, buildings, food, or clothing.[159–163] Many patients can perceive gender, age, and recognize facial expressions.[164,165] Some patients are unable to process the general features of objects, such as curved surfaces and spatial configurations, which is particularly important when discriminating faces.[166–168] When object agnosia is also present, the stimulus classes that are mostly affected include perceptually similar members, such as cars, flowers, and buildings.[160,169,170] Poor discrimination between similar members in the same category, whether at a perceptual or semantic level, may be the crucial deficit of prosopagnosia.[160,168]

Prosopagnosia is usually caused by lesions that damage the ventrotemporal or temporooccipital areas that involve the lingual and fusiform gyri.[160,171,172] This localization is consistent with functional imaging studies that show that the right posterior fusiform gyrus, superior temporal sulcus, and temporal pole are involved in facial recognition.[173–175] Although earlier studies report that bilateral lesions are required to produce prosopagnosia, recent studies using MRI show that unilateral right PCA territory infarction may suffice.[160,171,176–179] It was previously hypothesized that right occipitotemporal lobe lesions may damage the structures needed to perceive faces and thereby cause apperceptive prosopagnosia, whereas bilateral anterior temporal lesions may impair facial memory and thereby cause associative prosopagnosia: patients can perceive the face but cannot remember who the face belongs to.[180]

Prosopagnosia is often accompanied by visual field defects (bilateral upper quadrantanopia in bilateral infarction and left hemi- or quadrantanopia in unilateral infarction), and other visual symptoms such as achromatopsia or topographical disorientation.[160,176,178]

Topographagnosia (Topographical Disorientation)

Patients with topographical disorientation are unable to find their way around their surroundings.[181] This syndrome consists of several heterogeneous conditions. First, patients may have difficulty identifying familiar environmental landmarks such as buildings and street corners (topographical or landmark agnosia).[182–184] This deficit is associated with the right posterior parahippocampal gyrus and the anterior part of the lingual and fusiform gyri, which are critical for acquiring information and identifying buildings and landscapes.[183] Second, landmarks are "recognized" but do not evoke a sense of direction (i.e., directional or heading disorientation). The patient fails to utilize previously learned routes when traveling from one landmark to another. This may be caused by posterior cingulate lesions.[185] Third, patients have cognitive deficits that limit the development of a mental map of their environment. The lesions typically involve the hippocampus and retrosplenial cortex.[186]

Alexia

Reading difficulties (alexia or dyslexia) occur to varying degrees in the majority of patients with dominant (mostly left-sided)-hemisphere PCA infarction (see Fig. 25-11).[187] Writing, speaking, and other language functions are typically spared.[188] The spectrum ranges from global alexia, in which patients cannot read single letters or numbers, to spelling dyslexia or letter-by-letter reading, a less severe deficit.[188,189] In the latter case, the patient needs to depend on the sequential identification of letters, and the time needed to read a word increases with word length.[189–193]

The prevailing theory that explains alexia asserts that in patients with left PCA infarction, visual information can be only received by the right visual cortex. If there is concomitant damage to the splenium or callosal fibers, visual information cannot be conveyed to the language-processing area, notably the left angular gyrus, and patients cannot read what they see. Because the language-processing area itself is spared, language functions unrelated to visual information are spared.[187,194,195] In patients with extensive infarction that damages the left angular gyrus, alexia with agraphia will develop but oral language functions are still preserved.[194]

Although the majority of patients with alexia present with right homonymous hemianopia, alexia may not be associated with visual field defects if the lesions selectively disconnect the fibers in the white matter that underlie the angular gyrus.[196–199] In this case, patients usually have mild deficits, such as slowed or hesitant reading that rapidly improves.

It should be noted that reading difficulties may also occur with conditions other than pure alexia. Patients with macular hemianopia may have reading difficulties because they have trouble locating the beginning of the next line (hemianopic dyslexia) that lies in their blind visual field.[200] Patients with biparietal lesions may have reading difficulties due to impaired fixation or saccades (see below, Balint's syndrome).[201] Hemineglect may also result in reading errors on the neglected (left) side (neglect dyslexia).[202]

Achromatopsia

Achromatopsia is the inability to perceive color following brain injury.[203] The total absence of color perception is uncommon.[204] Objects look gray, pale, or are tinged.[205–207] Patients with less severe symptoms have difficulty distinguishing color hues and/or intensity and demonstrate impaired performance on color-discrimination tests (e.g., Ishihara color plates, Farnsworth-Munsell 100-hue test). Infarctions associated with achromatopsia are usually located inferior to the calcarine cortex and involve the fusiform or lingual gyri. The lesion may be bilateral or unilateral on either side.[205,208] Impairment may occur in the unilateral (hemidyschromatopsia) or quadrantic field.[206] Prosopagnosia and topographagnosia are often accompanied, particularly in patients with bilateral lesions.[205,206,209–211]

Cognitive Disorders not Primarily Associated with Visual Function

Aphasia

Aphasia is uncommon in patients with PCA infarction. However, patients with an infarct that involves the left temporal or parietal lobe may develop anomic or transcortical sensory aphasia.[212,213]

Anomic (amnestic) aphasia is characterized by word-finding and naming difficulties, but these patients retain normal repetition and comprehension abilities. Commonly, patients pause and hesitate as if the name is about to be produced momentarily ("tip of the tongue" phenomenon). Instead of the correct name, attributes of the item are often described, indicating the patient's familiarity with the item in question. The independence of the deficit from the modality of the sensory inputs distinguishes anomic aphasia from optic aphasia, in which anomia occurs only when the object is visually presented. Anomic aphasia is often non-specifically observed during the recovery phase of more severe forms of aphasia (e.g., global or sensory). However, prominent or isolated anomia during the acute stage of stroke is usually observed in patients with infarction in the left posterior inferior/middle temporal lobe.[214,215]

Transcortical sensory aphasia is an uncommon form of aphasia. It is similar to Wernicke's sensory aphasia, but repetition is spared. Echolalia is occasionally accompanied. Infarctions are usually present in the posterior parieto-occipital region of the PCA territory or MCA-PCA borderzone area, thereby sparing Wernicke's area.[212,213] Hemianopia and visual object agnosia are often concomitant.[212,216] However, this aphasic syndrome does not have a localizing value because it is also observed in patients with infarction in the thalamus[114] or the frontal lobe of the MCA territory.[217–220] Wherever the location of lesion, the outcomes of transcortical sensory aphasia are usually good.[212]

Memory Impairment

Bilateral or unilateral left PCA infarction produces significant memory impairment by damaging the hippocampus, parahippocampus, and connecting fibers.[52,117,221,222] Patients demonstrate the impaired acquisition of new memories (anterograde amnesia) with relatively little effect on the retrieval of memories that were encoded prior to onset of the infarction (retrograde amnesia).

Memory impairment is reportedly present in 11–55% of patients with PCA infarction.[8,10,34,223] In a recent DWI study, the hippocampus was involved in about one-fifth of PCA territory infarctions.[79] All of these patients had concomitant infarcts in other PCA territory. Although clinically evident memory deficits were present in only 19% of patients, neuropsychological examination showed deficits in verbal episodic memory and nonverbal episodic memory due to left- and right-sided infarcts, respectively. These results suggest that mild amnestic dysfunction that is not detected on routine examination may actually be more common than realized.

As previously discussed, thalamic infarction in the territory of the tuberothalamic or paramedian arteries also results in memory impairment. Although uncommon, patients with infarction involving the posteromedial thalamus or temporal lobe may show amnesia, but only for visually presented materials (visual amnesia).[224]

Emotional and Behavioral Disturbances

Patients with bilateral (or less often unilateral) PCA infarction occasionally show restless, hyperactive behaviors. Patients become easily agitated and aggressive, especially when stimulated. They respond to solicitations by relatives and medical personnel by shouting obscenities, hitting, and biting. This agitated delirium occurs in about 7% of patients with superficial PCA infarction,[12] and seems to be attributed to the limbic system involvement in patients with bilateral or, less often, unilateral inferior temporal lobe infarction.[52,225,226] Hemianopia commonly accompanies the neurological symptoms and signs.

Conversely, some patients may present with visual hypoemotionality, which refers to reduced affective response to visual stimuli.[227,228] People, landscapes, and erotic pictures do not elicit the expected response, whereas non-visual stimuli such as words, music, and touch do. This is attributed to visual-limbic disconnection secondary to bilateral or right temporo-occipital lesions.

Bilateral Infarction and Associated Syndromes

Bilateral PCA infarction occurs in 6–13% of patients.[10,12,13,34] Bilateral infarction can occur simultaneously, but more often, infarction on one side precedes the other. The hallmark clinical feature is cortical blindness.[229] On examination, there is the absence of blinking in response to visual threats and optokinetic reflex. Pupillary reflexes and fundus examination are normal. Although uncommon, patients may not recognize their deficits and do not admit that they cannot see (visual anosognosia or Anton's syndrome).[13] It has been hypothesized that the visual association area in the parietal lobe is concomitantly affected in these patients, which causes the lack of awareness of deficits.[230] Patients may demonstrate confabulation or increased verbosity, possibly to compensate for the lack of visual input.[231]

In patients who are not completely blind, the degree of visual disturbance varies according to infarction severity, which is in part related to the size of the occluded arteries and the variability in compensatory blood supply (e.g., from posterior temporal, parieto-occipital branches, and MCA).[6] In these patients, visual field defects may develop in various patterns, including bilateral (yet incomplete) homonymous hemianopia or bilateral altitudinal hemianopia, both of which result in various difficulties in daily life activities.[229,232,233] In some, the visual disturbances are mild and transient (Fig. 25-3). Conversely, extensive bilateral PCA infarction may result in severe edema or herniation that may lead to death.[234]

As previously discussed, bilateral PCA infarction tends to produce severe amnesia and a variety of other cognitive dysfunctions. It has been reported that structures located below the calcarine fissure contain a specialized neural network that can identify the nature, shape, and morphology of objects – the so-called ventral "what" pathway – whereas structures in the superior bank belong to the dorsal "where" pathway and assess the direction and spatial relationship of visually perceived objects.[235] Infarction in the ventral pathway often involves the temporal lobe and produces symptoms such as achromatopsia, apperceptive visual agnosia, prosopagnosia and agitated delirium.

Infarcts that primarily involve the dorsal pathway produce a variety of syndromes. Simultanagnosia is the inability to form a panoramic view, although patients can perceive individual items in the scene.[236] Patients see objects piecemeal and have to use head and eye movements to perceive and understand the whole picture. Tests are required to show that this difficulty is not caused by hemineglect or visual field defects. Optic ataxia is the inability to direct hand movements under visual guidance – i.e., the lack of coordination between visual input and hand motions. Typically, patients have difficulty touching a visually presented target (either stationary or moving) using their hands, but show relatively good accuracy when touching their own body or pointing to auditory targets.[237] Intention tremors and dysdiadochokinesia are absent.

Gaze apraxia (psychic paralysis of gaze) is the inability to directly focus on a specific object. Patients have difficulty initiating saccades to visual targets on command, although they can make spontaneous scanning saccades. Even when they make saccades, accuracy is frequently impaired.[238,239] Because of the scanning failure patients have reading difficulties that should be differentiated from alexia. Gaze problems are often associated with simultanagnosia.[240] The triad of simultanagnosia, optic ataxia and apraxia of gaze is referred to as "Balint's syndrome",[241,242] although there have been arguments on the independency of the three components.[243,244] Balint's syndrome is most often caused by bilateral lesions that involve the inferior parietal lobe and lateral occipital cortex.[35,36] Because this area corresponds to the PCA–MCA borderzone, hemodynamic disturbance has been suggested as a pathogenic mechanism.

Transient Ischemic Attack

PCA infarction is preceded by TIA in 13–24% of patients (usually by 1 day to several months).[11–13,15] Frequency does not differ between patients with superficial infarction and patients with both superficial and deep infarction.[13] Patients with TIA appear to present with large-artery disease more often than those without.[11,13] The manifestations of TIA associated with PCA atherosclerosis are mainly visual or sensory symptoms, although TIAs associated with proximal artery disease (VA or BA) may include other symptoms such as vertigo, dizziness, dysarthria, diplopia, and the loss of consciousness. Sensory and visual TIAs are described here because these are relatively specific to PCA territory ischemia.

Sensory Transient Ischemic Attack

In 1982, Fisher described 42 patients with pure sensory TIA, in whom the face, arms, and legs were involved in 33 patients (79%), the face and arms in three patients (7%), the arms and legs in four patients (9%), and only the face in two patients (5%).[245] The pathological findings in one patient indicated lateral thalamic infarction. More recently, Kim described patients with repeated, pure or predominantly sensory TIAs with or without PCA stenosis.[246] The presumed mechanism was repeated hemodynamic compromise of the thalamogeniculate artery associated with thrombus within the perforating artery or at the stenotic portion of the PCA (Fig. 25-16). These patients may or may not eventually develop lateral thalamic infarction. In addition, the author observed patients who developed occipital infarction following sensory TIAs in association with PCA stenosis, which suggests subsequent development of artery-to-artery emboli that arise from atherosclerotic PCA diseases.

Of note is that somatosensory TIAs are not necessarily caused by posterior circulation diseases. Recurrent sensory TIAs are occasionally observed in patients with middle cerebral artery atherosclerosis, which may even herald a large middle cerebral artery territory infarction.[247]

Visual Transient Ishemic Attack

Visual TIA is not uncommon. According to a recent TIA registry study that examined 2398 patients, 826 patients (34.5%) had transient visual symptoms, including 422 patients (17.6%) with isolated transient visual symptoms.[248] Transient monocular blindness was the most frequent symptom (36.3%), followed by diplopia (13.4%), homonymous hemianopia (12.3%), bilateral positive visual phenomena (10.8%), and bilateral blindness (4.5%). The latter three symptoms seem to be associated with PCA territory TIA (Fig. 25-17). However, transient visual field defects may go unnoticed by patients, and the prevalence of visual field defects may be underestimated in TIA patients. According to a study wherein all TIA patients were examined using perimetry, asymptomatic visual field defects (more often upper than lower field defects) were found in as many as 29% of patients.[249] These results suggest that hemivisual field defects are actually more common in TIA patients than previously realized.

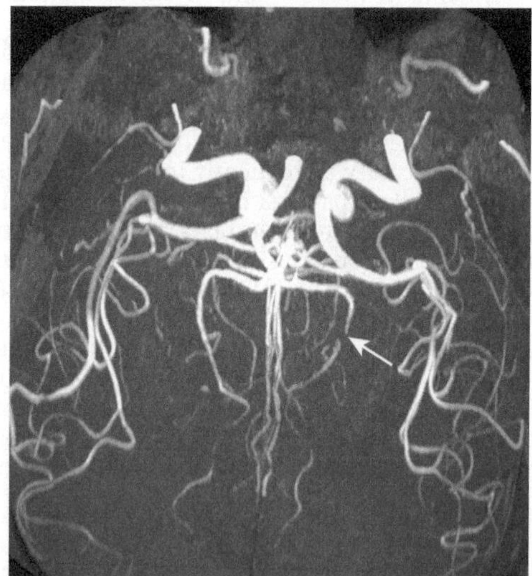

Figure 25-16. A 72-year-old hypertensive woman developed recurrent episodes of tingling sensation in the right face and arm, when she had clumsiness in using the arm. The episodes occurred once in a few days and lasted for a few minutes. MRI showed no abnormality. MR angiogram showed a focal stenosis of P2 portion of the posterior cerebral artery (arrow).

Transient bilateral blindness may be caused by the sudden decrease in the perfusion of both occipital areas (either due to hypoperfusion or embolism), and is usually associated with severe vertebrobasilar occlusive disease or heart disease. Because the embolic source is more likely to be the arteries that are proximal to the PCA, the visual symptoms are often associated with the symptoms such as vertigo, ataxia, diplopia, and motor dysfunction. The presentation of bilateral visual field defects as the only symptom of TIA is rare, and other etiologies such as migraine or syncope should also be considered. In one study, six patients presented with transient, isolated bilateral blindness.[250] All patients had vascular risk factors, and two subsequently developed TIAs. Therefore, the symptoms were considered a TIA that affected the bilateral occipital areas probably related to embolic events. However, only one patient had severe BA stenosis and one patient had atrial fibrillation.

PROGNOSIS

General Prognosis

Unlike MCA territory infarction, unilateral occipital infarction alone seldom results in massive edema or herniation. Extensive bilateral PCA infarction may produce fatal herniation, but this is uncommon.[234] Therefore, the prognosis of PCA territory infarction is favorable. In-hospital mortality was 3.9% according to the Barcelona registry, which was lower than MCA (17.3%) and ACA infarction (7.8%). Herniation, sudden unexplained death, or pneumonia were the causes of death.[15]

It seems that patients with infarction limited to the superficial territory do better than those with extensive involvement in deep structures. In one study, six of 82 patients (7%) died during the initial hospitalization, all of whom demonstrated deep structure involvement.[34] Concomitant involvement of the extra-PCA territory (PCA plus), especially the brainstem,

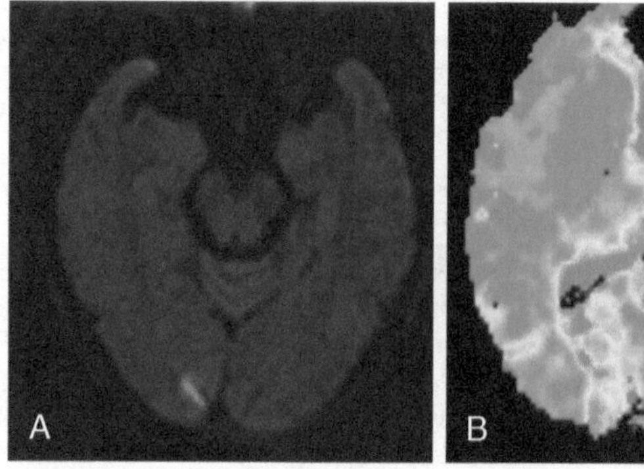

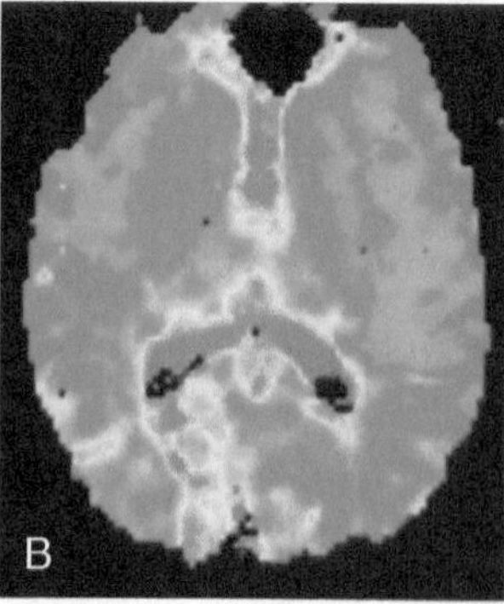

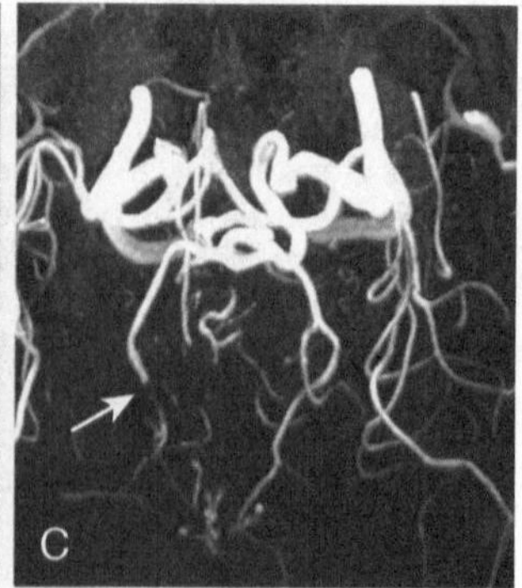

Figure 25-17. A 78-year-old hypertensive woman suddenly could not clearly see television and people around her. She reported that there was general dimness in her vision, although she could recognize people and color. However, she did not attempt to cover one eye during the episodes. The episodes lasted usually for a few minutes, and recurred several times a day. Two days later, when she visited our clinic, neurologic examination revealed left homonymous hemianopia. Diffusion and perfusion weighted MRIs showed a small infarct (A) and decreased perfusion (B) in the right occipital area. MR angiogram showed a focal severe stenosis in the right posterior cerebral artery (arrow) (C). *(From Kim JS, Symptoms of Transient Ischemic Attack. In Uchiyama S, Amarenco P, Minematsu K, Wong KSL. (eds) TIA as Acutee Cerebrovascular Syndrome. Front Neurol Neurosci. Basel, Karger 2014; vol 33, pp 82–102.)*

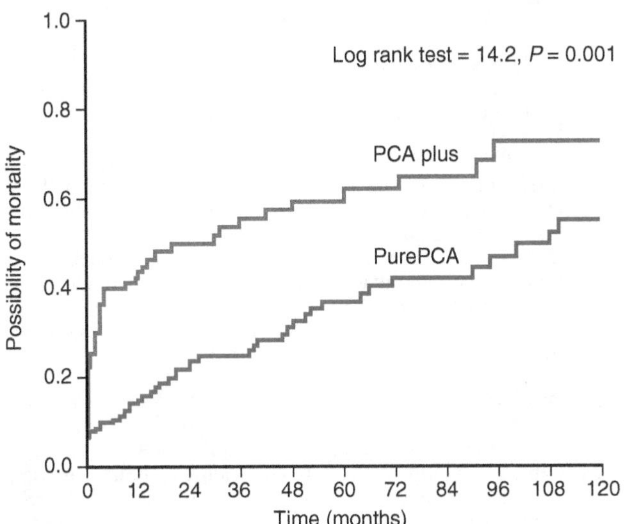

Number at risk

Pure PCA	122	97	80	66	50	42	31	28	21	19	14
PCA plus	63	35	28	25	21	15	13	12	7	5	4

Figure 25-18. Kaplan–Meier estimates of 10-year mortality in patients with pure posterior cerebral artery (PCA) (blue line) and PCA-plus (red line) stroke. *(From Ntaiosa G, et al. Long-term outcome in posterior cerebral artery stroke.* Eur J Neurol *2011, 18: 1074–1080.)*

also results in a worse prognosis. Ntaios et al. studied the clinical outcomes of 185 patients with PCA infarction for a mean follow-up period of 50 months.[16] In-hospital neurological complications, such as brain edema and infection, were significantly more common in PCA-plus patients than in patients with pure PCA infarction. Mortality was also significantly higher in PCA-plus patients at 1 month, 6 months, and 10 years (Fig. 25-18).

Recurrent stroke and cardiac disease are important causes of morbidity and mortality.[8,13] It seems that the presence of extensive atherothrombosis predicts the high risk of recurrence.[8] Patients with proximal large-artery disease (e.g., BA disease) demonstrate a higher risk of stroke recurrence and worse clinical outcomes than patients with intrinsic PCA atherosclerosis.[13]

Sequelae

Remaining deficits include residual motor dysfunction, ataxia, and ocular motor dysfunction. Cognitive dysfunction may persist in patients with initially severe symptoms. Here, sequelae related to sensory and visual field defects are described, because they are common and relatively specific for PCA territory infarction.

Sequelae Related to Sensory Dysfunction

Sensory Deficit-related Functional Disability. Lateral thalamic infarction is relatively common, and sensory symptoms and deficits are the most prominent manifestations. Therefore, the sequelae related to sensory dysfunction are relatively common. Clinical and evoked potential studies report that post-stroke sensory dysfunction can improve to a certain degree, usually within 3 months after onset.[52] However, patients with dense sensory abnormalities may develop residual sensory perception disorder, which leads to a variety of problems including frequent falls, hand swelling, shoulder subluxation, burns, and other injuries.[53] In addition, patients who lose proprioceptive function often have considerable difficulty executing manual tasks, especially those that require complex movement coordination between several joints (pseudoparesis); this is most likely due to the loss of sensory feedback in the sensory–motor circuitry.[8] Patients may also present with motor incoordination (sensory ataxia) or dystonic/athetoid postures.[73]

Central Post-stroke Pain One of the most troublesome post-stroke sensory sequelae is the development of uncomfortable, distressful, and sometimes painful paresthesias.[54] Once considered a typical sequela of thalamic strokes (thalamic syndrome of Dejerine and Roussy),[84] it is now recognized that strokes occurring anywhere in the sensory tracts can produce similar symptoms.[7,55,56] Lateral thalamic infarction and hemorrhage are the most common causes of central post-stroke pain (CPSP);[251,252] 25% of patients reportedly developed CPSP if the VP nucleus was involved.[82]

Symptoms are variably described as burning, aching, squeezing, pricking, cold, lacerating, etc., and are frequently aggravated by cold temperatures, psychological stress, heat, and fatigue.[55,56] Dysesthesia and allodynia are common.[55] Symptoms usually develop weeks or months after the onset of stroke. They usually develop in the areas where the sensory deficits are the most severe; accordingly, the areas of CPSP are often restricted to certain body parts such as the distal limbs.[56] The pathogenesis of CPSP probably involves the hyperexcitation of damaged sensory pathways, damage to the central inhibitory pathways, or the combination of the two. The detailed mechanisms, however, remain unclear.[253,254]

Involuntary Movements. Some patients with thalamic stroke demonstrate involuntary movements, such as asterixis, dystonia, chorea/athetosis, tremors, and myoclonus.[84,108,255–260] Except for asterixis, these movement disorders develop months (or even years) after onset and tend to occur in combination. Patients often show complex hyperkinetic movements, including ataxia, tremors, dystonia, chorea, and myoclonus.[261–263] These complex movements are sometimes referred to as "jerky dystonic unsteady hand"[264] or "delayed onset mixed involuntary movements".[263]

These involuntary movements are usually associated with posterior-lateral thalamic infarction in the thalamogeniculate or posterior choroidal artery territories.[264] Sensory deficits are commonly accompanied. There have been efforts to correlate each movement disorder with specific thalamic nuclei (e.g., dystonia and athetoid movements to the ventral intermediate [Vim] and ventral caudal nuclei).[262] However, the symptoms are usually mixed, and the clinical features tend to evolve over time. Moreover, the lesions are often large and destructive (i.e., hemorrhage more often than infarction) lesions causing severe neurologic symptoms, including hemiparesis, hemiataxia, and dense sensory deficits.[263]

Dystonia and choreoathetosis seem to be related to severe positional sensory deficits, while tremor/myoclonus is related to severe cerebellar ataxia probably associated with the cerebello-rubro-thalamic tract involvement. Mixed movement disorders tend to start with the successful recovery of paralyzed limbs, but with persistently impaired proprioceptive sensory and cerebellar functions. Thus, these mixed movement disorders may, at least in part, be related to abnormally organized motor circuitry due to unbalanced recovery in the motor, cerebellar, and sensory systems.[263] Although rare, delayed-onset palatal myoclonus may occur after unilateral thalamic infarction.[265]

Visual Field Defect. Visual field defect is one of the most important and disabling sequelae of PCA infarction. The impact of visual field defects on daily activities is significant, contributing to poor mobility, collisions, and impaired reading and driving. During the acute stage of stroke, patients may develop rapid improvement (e.g., from hemianopia to quadrantopia) or the complete resolution of visual field defects if the infarction is not large (see Fig. 25-3). Improvement is still possible even in patients with a sizable lesion, most likely due to the resolution of cerebral edema, restitution of perfusion in the penumbral tissue surrounding the infracted area, resolution of diaschisis, and the recovery of neurotransmission.[266]

Generally, 27–38% of patients demonstrate visual field improvements.[267,268] The probability of improvement seems to be related to the time that has elapsed since brain injury. In one study, there was a reported 50–60% chance of improvement in patients who were tested within 1 month after brain injury, but this decreased to approximately 20% among patients who were tested at 6 months after injury.[268] The initial severity of symptoms is another factor that influences recovery; in one study improvement in visual field defects was observed in 17% of patients who had complete hemianopia, while 72% of patients improved who initially presented with partial hemianopia.[267] In addition, lesion extension, collateral circulation, and the early recanalization of the occluded PCA seem to be related to the outcome of visual function. In most cases, improvement occurs within the first 3 months. Spontaneous improvement after 6 months is rare, although patients may demonstrate improvement in functional ability despite persistent defects.

The complete reference list can be found on the companion Expert Consult website at www.expertconsult.inkling.com.

KEY REFERENCES

1. Cereda C, Carrera E. Posterior cerebral artery territory infarctions. Front Neurol Neurosci 2012;30:128–31.
2. Schmahmann JD. Vascular syndromes of the thalamus. Stroke 2003;34:2264–78.
3. Brandt T, Steinke W, Thie A, et al. Posterior cerebral artery territory infarcts: clinical features, infarct topography, causes and outcome. Multicenter results and a review of the literature. Cerebrovasc Dis 2000;10:170–82.
4. Takahashi S, Goto K, Fukasawa H, et al. Computed tomography of cerebral infarction along the distribution of the basal perforating arteries. Part II: Thalamic arterial group. Radiology 1985;155:119–30.
6. Smith CG, Richardson WF. The course and distribution of the arteries supplying the visual (striate) cortex. Am J Ophthalmol 1966;61:1391–6.
7. Castaigne P, Lhermitte F, Gautier JC, et al. Arterial occlusions in the vertebro-basilar system. A study of 44 patients with postmortem data. Brain 1973;96:133–54.
8. Pessin MS, Lathi ES, Cohen MB, et al. Clinical features and mechanism of occipital infarction. Ann Neurol 1987;21:290–9.
9. Moriyasu H, Yasaka M, Minematsu K, et al. The pathogenesis of brain infarction in the posterior cerebral artery territory. Rinsho Shinkeigaku 1995;35:344–51.
10. Steinke W, Mangold J, Schwartz A, et al. Mechanisms of infarction in the superficial posterior cerebral artery territory. J Neurol 1997;244:571–8.
11. Yamamoto Y, Georgiadis AL, Chang HM, et al. Posterior cerebral artery territory infarcts in the New England Medical Center Posterior Circulation Registry. Arch Neurol 1999;56(7):824–32.
12. Cals N, Devuyst G, Afsar N, et al. Pure superficial posterior cerebral artery territory infarction in The Lausanne Stroke Registry. J Neurol 2002;249(7):855–61.
13. Kumral E, Bayulkem G, Atac C, et al. Spectrum of superficial posterior cerebral artery territory infarcts. Eur J Neurol 2004; 11(4):237–46.
14. Lee E, Kang DW, Kwon SU, et al. Posterior cerebral artery infarction: diffusion-weighted MRI analysis of 205 patients. Cerebrovasc Dis 2009;28(3):298–305.
15. Arboix A, Arbe G, Garcia-Eroles L, et al. Infarctions in the vascular territory of the posterior cerebral artery: clinical features in 232 patients. BMC Res Notes 2011;4:329.
16. Ntaios G, Spengos K, Vemmou AM, et al. Long-term outcome in posterior cerebral artery stroke. Eur J Neurol 2011;18(8): 1074–80.
17. Kim JS, Nah HW, Park SM, et al. Risk factors and stroke mechanisms in atherosclerotic stroke: intracranial compared with extracranial and anterior compared with posterior circulation disease. Stroke 2012;43(12):3313–18.
19. Ueda K, Toole JF, McHenry LC Jr. Carotid and vertebrobasilar transient ischemic attacks: clinical and angiographic correlation. Neurology 1979;29(8):1094–101.
22. Pessin MS, Kwan ES, Scott RM, et al. Occipital infarction with hemianopsia from carotid occlusive disease. Stroke 1989; 20(3):409–11.
23. Diehl RR, Sliwka U, Rautenberg W, et al. Evidence for embolization from a posterior cerebral artery thrombus by transcranial Doppler monitoring. Stroke 1993;24(4):606–8.
24. Caplan LR. Intracranial branch atheromatous disease: a neglected, understudied, and underused concept. Neurology 1989;39(9):1246–50.
27. Kim JS, Yoon Y. Single subcortical infarction associated with parental arterial disease: important yet neglected sub-type of atherothrombotic stroke. Int J Stroke 2013;8(3):197–203.
29. Kwon JY, Kwon SU, Kang DW, et al. Isolated lateral thalamic infarction: the role of posterior cerebral artery disease. Eur J Neurol 2012;19(2):265–70.
30. Wang X, Fan YH, Lam WW, et al. Clinical features, topographic patterns on DWI and etiology of thalamic infarcts. J Neurol Sci 2008;267(1–2):147–53.
32. Kim JS, Kim J. Pure midbrain infarction: clinical, radiologic, and pathophysiologic findings. Neurology 2005;64(7):1227–32.
33. Wong KSCL, Kim JS. Stroke mechanisms. In: Kim JS, Caplan LR, Wong KS, editors. Intracranial Atherosclerosis. 2008. p. 57–68.
34. Milandre L, Brosset C, Botti G, et al. A study of 82 cerebral infarctions in the area of posterior cerebral arteries. Rev Neurol (Paris) 1994;150(2):133–41.
35. Montero J, Pena J, Genis D, et al. Balint's syndrome. Report of four cases with watershed parieto-occipital lesions from vertebrobasilar ischemia or systemic hypotension. Acta Neurol Belg 1982;82(5):270–80.
42. Fisher CM. Pure Sensory Stroke Involving Face, Arm, and Leg. Neurology 1965;15:76–80.
45. Lamy C, Giannesini C, Zuber M, et al. Clinical and imaging findings in cryptogenic stroke patients with and without patent foramen ovale: the PFO-ASA Study. Atrial Septal Aneurysm. Stroke 2002;33(3):706–11.
47. Kim BJ, Sohn H, Sun BJ, et al. Imaging Characteristics of Ischemic Strokes Related to Patent Foramen Ovale. Stroke 2013;44(12): 3350–56.
48. Chiras J, Marciano S, Vega Molina J, et al. Spontaneous dissecting aneurysm of the extracranial vertebral artery (20 cases). Neuroradiology 1985;27(4):327–33.
49. Mokri B, Houser OW, Sandok BA, et al. Spontaneous dissections of the vertebral arteries. Neurology 1988;38(6):880–5.
50. Huang YC, Chen YF, Wang YH, et al. Cervicocranial arterial dissection: experience of 73 patients in a single center. Surg Neurol 2009;72(Suppl. 2):S20–7, discussion S7.
51. Caplan LR, Estol CJ, Massaro AR. Dissection of the posterior cerebral arteries. Arch Neurol 2005;62(7):1138–43.
52. Fisher CM. The posterior cerebral artery syndrome. Can J Neurol Sci 1986;13(3):232–9.
53. Broderick JP, Swanson JW. Migraine-related strokes. Clinical profile and prognosis in 20 patients. Arch Neurol 1987; 44(8):868–71.
56. Caplan LR. Migraine and vertebrobasilar ischemia. Neurology 1991;41(1):55–61.
59. Kim JM, Lee SH, Roh JK. Changing ischaemic lesion patterns in adult moyamoya disease. J Neurol Neurosurg Psychiatry 2009;80(1):36–40.
60. Hishikawa T, Tokunaga K, Sugiu K, et al. Assessment of the difference in posterior circulation involvement between pediatric

and adult patients with moyamoya disease. J Neurosurg 2013; 119(4):961–5.

65. Frens DB, Petajan JH, Anderson R, et al. Fibromuscular dysplasia of the posterior cerebral artery: report of a case and review of the literature. Stroke 1974;5(2):161–6.
67. Ducros A, Boukobza M, Porcher R, et al. The clinical and radiological spectrum of reversible cerebral vasoconstriction syndrome. A prospective series of 67 patients. Brain 2007;130 (Pt 12):3091–101.
68. Calabrese LH, Dodick DW, Schwedt TJ, et al. Narrative review: reversible cerebral vasoconstriction syndromes. Ann Intern Med 2007;146(1):34–44.
69. Sato M, Tanaka S, Kohama A, et al. Occipital lobe infarction caused by tentorial herniation. Neurosurgery 1986;18(3): 300–5.
73. Goto Y, Horai S, Matsuoka T, et al. Mitochondrial myopathy, encephalopathy, lactic acidosis, and stroke-like episodes (MELAS): a correlative study of the clinical features and mitochondrial DNA mutation. Neurology 1992;42(3 Pt 1):545–50.
74. Majamaa K, Turkka J, Karppa M, et al. The common MELAS mutation A3243G in mitochondrial DNA among young patients with an occipital brain infarct. Neurology 1997;49(5):1331–4.
75. Sakuta R, Nonaka I. Vascular involvement in mitochondrial myopathy. Ann Neurol 1989;25(6):594–601.
79. Szabo K, Forster A, Jager T, et al. Hippocampal lesion patterns in acute posterior cerebral artery stroke: clinical and MRI findings. Stroke 2009;40(6):2042–5.
80. Hommel M, Besson G, Pollak P, et al. Hemiplegia in posterior cerebral artery occlusion. Neurology 1990;40(10):1496–9.
82. Bogousslavsky J, Regli F, Uske A. Thalamic infarcts: clinical syndromes, etiology, and prognosis. Neurology 1988;38(6): 837–48.
83. Percheron G. The anatomy of the arterial supply of the human thalamus and its use for the interpretation of the thalamic vascular pathology. Z Neurol 1973;205(1):1–13.
84. Déjerine JRG. La syndrome thalamique. Rev Neurol (Paris) 1906;14:521.
85. Caplan LR, DeWitt LD, Pessin MS, et al. Lateral thalamic infarcts. Arch Neurol 1988;45(9):959–64.
86. Kim JS. Pure sensory stroke. Clinical-radiological correlates of 21 cases. Stroke 1992;23(7):983–7.
87. Arboix A, Garcia-Plata C, Garcia-Eroles L, et al. Clinical study of 99 patients with pure sensory stroke. J Neurol 2005; 252(2):156–62.
88. Fisher CM. Thalamic pure sensory stroke: a pathologic study. Neurology 1978;28(11):1141–4.
89. Paciaroni M, Bogousslavsky J. Pure sensory syndromes in thalamic stroke. Eur Neurol 1998;39(4):211–17.
90. Kim JS. Restricted acral sensory syndrome following minor stroke. Further observation with special reference to differential severity of symptoms among individual digits. Stroke 1994; 25(12):2497–502.
96. Bogousslavsky J, Regli F, Assal G. The syndrome of unilateral tuberothalamic artery territory infarction. Stroke 1986; 17(3):434–41.
97. Ghika-Schmid F, Bogousslavsky J. The acute behavioral syndrome of anterior thalamic infarction: a prospective study of 12 cases. Ann Neurol 2000;48(2):220–7.
98. von Cramon DY, Hebel N, Schuri U. A contribution to the anatomical basis of thalamic amnesia. Brain 1985;108(Pt 4): 993–1008.
99. Graff-Radford NR, Tranel D, Van Hoesen GW, et al. Diencephalic amnesia. Brain 1990;113(Pt 1):1–25.
101. Clarke S, Assal G, Bogousslavsky J, et al. Pure amnesia after unilateral left polar thalamic infarct: topographic and sequential neuropsychological and metabolic (PET) correlations. J Neurol Neurosurg Psychiatry 1994;57(1):27–34.
102. Castaigne P, Lhermitte F, Buge A, et al. Paramedian thalamic and midbrain infarct: clinical and neuropathological study. Ann Neurol 1981;10(2):127–48.
103. Graff-Radford NR, Eslinger PJ, Damasio AR, et al. Nonhemorrhagic infarction of the thalamus: behavioral, anatomic, and physiologic correlates. Neurology 1984;34(1):14–23.
104. Guberman A, Stuss D. The syndrome of bilateral paramedian thalamic infarction. Neurology 1983;33(5):540–6.
105. Warren JD, Thompson PD. Diencephalic amnesia and apraxia after left thalamic infarction. J Neurol Neurosurg Psychiatry 2000;68(2):248.
107. Meguro K, Akanuma K, Ouchi Y, et al. Vascular dementia with left thalamic infarction: neuropsychological and behavioral implications suggested by involvement of the thalamic nucleus and the remote effect on cerebral cortex. The Osaki-Tajiri project. Psychiatry Res 2013;213(1):56–62.
108. Kim JS. Asterixis after unilateral stroke: lesion location of 30 patients. Neurology 2001;56(4):533–6.
109. Neau JP, Bogousslavsky J. The syndrome of posterior choroidal artery territory infarction. Ann Neurol 1996;39(6):779–88.
111. Frisen L, Holmegaard L, Rosencrantz M. Sectorial optic atrophy and homonymous, horizontal sectoranopia: a lateral choroidal artery syndrome? J Neurol Neurosurg Psychiatry 1978; 41(4):374–80.
112. Luco C, Hoppe A, Schweitzer M, et al. Visual field defects in vascular lesions of the lateral geniculate body. J Neurol Neurosurg Psychiatry 1992;55(1):12–15.
115. Bruyn RP. Thalamic aphasia. A conceptional critique. J Neurol 1989;236(1):21–5.
116. Karnath HO, Himmelbach M, Rorden C. The subcortical anatomy of human spatial neglect: putamen, caudate nucleus and pulvinar. Brain 2002;125(Pt 2):350–60.
117. Mohr JP, Leicester J, Stoddard LT, et al. Right hemianopia with memory and color deficits in circumscribed left posterior cerebral artery territory infarction. Neurology 1971;21(11):1104–13.
119. Benton S, Levy I, Swash M. Vision in the temporal crescent in occipital infarction. Brain 1980;103(1):83–97.
120. Lepore FE. The preserved temporal crescent: the clinical implications of an "endangered" finding. Neurology 2001;57(10):1918–21.
121. McFadzean R, Brosnahan D, Hadley D, et al. Representation of the visual field in the occipital striate cortex. Br J Ophthalmol 1994;78(3):185–90.
122. Horton JC, Hoyt WF. The representation of the visual field in human striate cortex. A revision of the classic Holmes map. Arch Ophthalmol 1991;109(6):816–24.
124. Wong AM, Sharpe JA. Representation of the visual field in the human occipital cortex: a magnetic resonance imaging and perimetric correlation. Arch Ophthalmol 1999;117(2):208–17.
125. Ogawa K, Ishikawa H, Suzuki Y, et al. Clinical study of the visual field defects caused by occipital lobe lesions. Cerebrovasc Dis 2014;37(2):102–8.
126. Lister WT, Holmes G. Disturbances of vision from cerebral lesions, with special reference to the cortical representation of the macula. Proc R Soc Med 1916;9(Sect Ophthalmol):57–96.
129. Kolmel HW. Coloured patterns in hemianopic fields. Brain 1984;107(Pt 1):155–67.
130. Lance JW. Simple formed hallucinations confined to the area of a specific visual field defect. Brain 1976;99(4):719–34.
133. Bender MB, Feldman M, Sobin AJ. Palinopsia. Brain 1968; 91(2):321–38.
134. Critchley M. Types of visual perseveration: "Palinopsia" and "illusory visual spread". Brain 1951;74:267.
135. Michel EM, Troost BT. Palinopsia: cerebral localization with computed tomography. Neurology 1980;30(8):887–9.
137. Cummings JL, Syndulko K, Goldberg Z, et al. Palinopsia reconsidered. Neurology 1982;32(4):444–7.
144. Benson DF, Greenberg JP. Visual form agnosia. A specific defect in visual discrimination. Arch Neurol 1969;20(1):82–9.
147. Rubens AB, Benson DF. Associative visual agnosia. Arch Neurol 1971;24(4):305–16.
151. Sparr SA, Jay M, Drislane FW, et al. A historic case of visual agnosia revisited after 40 years. Brain 1991;114(Pt 2):789–800.
152. Coslett HB, Saffran EM. Preserved object recognition and reading comprehension in optic aphasia. Brain 1989;112(Pt 4):1091–110.
153. Lhermitte F, Beauvois MF. A visual-speech disconnexion syndrome. Report of a case with optic aphasia, agnosic alexia and colour agnosia. Brain 1973;96(4):695–714.
154. Schnider A, Benson DF, Scharre DW. Visual agnosia and optic aphasia: are they anatomically distinct? Cortex 1994;30(3): 445–57.
156. Carlesimo GA, Casadio P, Sabbadini M, et al. Associative visual agnosia resulting from a disconnection between intact visual memory and semantic systems. Cortex 1998;34(4):563–76.

160. Damasio AR, Damasio H, Van Hoesen GW. Prosopagnosia: anatomic basis and behavioral mechanisms. Neurology 1982;32(4):331–41.
161. Farah MJ, Levinson KL, Klein KL. Face perception and within-category discrimination in prosopagnosia. Neuropsychologia 1995;33(6):661–74.
162. Barton JJ, Hanif H, Ashraf S. Relating visual to verbal semantic knowledge: the evaluation of object recognition in prosopagnosia. Brain 2009;132(Pt 12):3456–66.
164. Tranel D, Damasio AR, Damasio H. Intact recognition of facial expression, gender, and age in patients with impaired recognition of face identity. Neurology 1988;38(5):690–6.
165. Sergent J, Poncet M. From covert to overt recognition of faces in a prosopagnosic patient. Brain 1990;113(Pt 4):989–1004.
170. De Haan EH, Young AW, Newcombe F. Covert and overt recognition in prosopagnosia. Brain 1991;114(Pt 6):2575–91.
171. Meadows JC. The anatomical basis of prosopagnosia. J Neurol Neurosurg Psychiatry 1974;37(5):489–501.
173. Nakamura K, Kawashima R, Sato N, et al. Functional delineation of the human occipito-temporal areas related to face and scene processing. A PET study. Brain 2000;123(Pt 9):1903–12.
174. Leveroni CL, Seidenberg M, Mayer AR, et al. Neural systems underlying the recognition of familiar and newly learned faces. J Neurosci 2000;20(2):878–86.
175. Kanwisher N, McDermott J, Chun MM. The fusiform face area: a module in human extrastriate cortex specialized for face perception. J Neurosci 1997;17(11):4302–11.
177. De Renzi E, Perani D, Carlesimo GA, et al. Prosopagnosia can be associated with damage confined to the right hemisphere – an MRI and PET study and a review of the literature. Neuropsychologia 1994;32(8):893–902.
180. Damasio AR, Tranel D, Damasio H. Face agnosia and the neural substrates of memory. Annu Rev Neurosci 1990;13:89–109.
181. Aguirre GK, D'Esposito M. Topographical disorientation: a synthesis and taxonomy. Brain 1999;122(Pt 9):1613–28.
183. Takahashi N, Kawamura M. Pure topographical disorientation – the anatomical basis of landmark agnosia. Cortex 2002;38(5):717–25.
185. Takahashi N, Kawamura M, Shiota J, et al. Pure topographic disorientation due to right retrosplenial lesion. Neurology 1997;49(2):464–9.
188. Binder JR, Mohr JP. The topography of callosal reading pathways. A case-control analysis. Brain 1992;115(Pt 6):1807–26.
190. Warrington EK, Shallice T. Word-form dyslexia. Brain 1980;103(1):99–112.
192. Coslett HB, Saffran EM, Greenbaum S, et al. Reading in pure alexia. The effect of strategy. Brain 1993;116(Pt 1):21–37.
193. Leff AP, Spitsyna G, Plant GT, et al. Structural anatomy of pure and hemianopic alexia. J Neurol Neurosurg Psychiatry 2006;77(9):1004–7.
194. Geschwind N. Disconnexion syndromes in animals and man. I. Brain 1965;88(2):237–94.
195. Damasio AR, Damasio H. The anatomic basis of pure alexia. Neurology 1983;33(12):1573–83.
196. Vincent FM, Sadowsky CH, Saunders RL, et al. Alexia without agraphia, hemianopia, or color-naming defect: a disconnection syndrome. Neurology 1977;27(7):689–91.
199. Leff AP, Crewes H, Plant GT, et al. The functional anatomy of single-word reading in patients with hemianopic and pure alexia. Brain 2001;124(Pt 3):510–21.
201. Pierrot-Deseilligny C, Gray F, Brunet P. Infarcts of both inferior parietal lobules with impairment of visually guided eye movements, peripheral visual inattention and optic ataxia. Brain 1986;109(Pt 1):81–97.
202. Behrmann M, Moscovitch M, Black SE, et al. Perceptual and conceptual mechanisms in neglect dyslexia. Two contrasting case studies. Brain 1990;113(Pt 4):1163–83.
203. Zeki S. A century of cerebral achromatopsia. Brain 1990;113(Pt 6):1721–77.
205. Damasio A, Yamada T, Damasio H, et al. Central achromatopsia: behavioral, anatomic, and physiologic aspects. Neurology 1980;30(10):1064–71.
206. Meadows JC. Disturbed perception of colours associated with localized cerebral lesions. Brain 1974;97(4):615–32.
207. Rizzo M, Smith V, Pokorny J, et al. Color perception profiles in central achromatopsia. Neurology 1993;43(5):995–1001.
212. Kertesz A, Sheppard A, MacKenzie R. Localization in transcortical sensory aphasia. Arch Neurol 1982;39(8):475–8.
213. Servan J, Verstichel P, Catala M, et al. Aphasia and infarction of the posterior cerebral artery territory. J Neurol 1995;242(2):87–92.
215. DeLeon J, Gottesman RF, Kleinman JT, et al. Neural regions essential for distinct cognitive processes underlying picture naming. Brain 2007;130(Pt 5):1408–22.
221. De Renzi E, Zambolin A, Crisi G. The pattern of neuropsychological impairment associated with left posterior cerebral artery infarcts. Brain 1987;110(Pt 5):1099–116.
222. Benson DF, Marsden CD, Meadows JC. The amnesic syndrome of posterior cerebral artery occlusion. Acta Neurol Scand 1974;50(2):133–45.
223. Brandt T, Thie A, Caplan LR, et al. Infarcts in the brain areas supplied by the posterior cerebral artery. Clinical aspects, pathogenesis and prognosis. Nervenarzt 1995;66(4):267–74.
225. Botez SA, Carrera E, Maeder P, et al. Aggressive behavior and posterior cerebral artery stroke. Arch Neurol 2007;64(7):1029–33.
229. Symonds C, Mackenzie I. Bilateral loss of vision from cerebral infarction. Brain 1957;80(4):415–55.
235. Levine DN, Warach J, Farah M. Two visual systems in mental imagery: dissociation of "what" and "where" in imagery disorders due to bilateral posterior cerebral lesions. Neurology 1985;35(7):1010–18.
236. Luria AR. Disorders of "simultaneous perception" in a case of bilateral occipito-parietal brain injury. Brain 1959;82:437–49.
237. Holmes G. Disturbances of visual orientation. Br J Ophthalmol 1918;2(10):506–16.
238. Cogan DG. Ophthalmic manifestations of bilateral non-occipital cerebral lesions. Br J Ophthalmol 1965;49:281–97.
241. Hecaen H, De Ajuriaguerra J. Balint's syndrome (psychic paralysis of visual fixation) and its minor forms. Brain 1954;77(3):373–400.
245. Fisher CM. Pure sensory stroke and allied conditions. Stroke 1982;13(4):434–47.
246. Kim JS. Pure or predominantly sensory transient ischemic attacks associated with posterior cerebral artery stenosis. Cerebrovasc Dis 2002;14(2):136–8.
248. Lavallee PC, Cabrejo L, Labreuche J, et al. Spectrum of transient visual symptoms in a transient ischemic attack cohort. Stroke 2013;44(12):3312–17.
249. Falke P, Abela BM Jr, Krakau CE, et al. High frequency of asymptomatic visual field defects in subjects with transient ischaemic attacks or minor strokes. J Intern Med 1991;229(6):521–5.
250. Krasnianski M, Bau V, Neudecker S, et al. Isolated bilateral blindness as the sole manifestation of transient ischaemic attacks. Acta Ophthalmol Scand 2006;84(3):415–18.
251. Bowsher D, Leijon G, Thuomas KA. Central poststroke pain: correlation of MRI with clinical pain characteristics and sensory abnormalities. Neurology 1998;51(5):1352–8.
254. Kim JS. Post-stroke pain. Expert Rev Neurother 2009;9(5):711–21.
256. Lee MS, Marsden CD. Movement disorders following lesions of the thalamus or subthalamic region. Mov Disord 1994;9(5):493–507.
258. Bastian AJ, Thach WT. Cerebellar outflow lesions: a comparison of movement deficits resulting from lesions at the levels of the cerebellum and thalamus. Ann Neurol 1995;38(6):881–92.
262. Lehericy S, Grand S, Pollak P, et al. Clinical characteristics and topography of lesions in movement disorders due to thalamic lesions. Neurology 2001;57(6):1055–66.
263. Kim JS. Delayed onset mixed involuntary movements after thalamic stroke: clinical, radiological and pathophysiological findings. Brain 2001;124(Pt 2):299–309.
264. Ghika J, Bogousslavsky J, Henderson J, et al. The "jerky dystonic unsteady hand": a delayed motor syndrome in posterior thalamic infarctions. J Neurol 1994;241(9):537–42.
266. Romano JG. Progress in rehabilitation of hemianopic visual field defects. Cerebrovasc Dis 2009;27(Suppl. 1):187–90.
268. Zhang X, Kedar S, Lynn MJ, et al. Natural history of homonymous hemianopia. Neurology 2006;66(6):901–5.

26 Vertebrobasilar Disease

Jong S. Kim, Louis R. Caplan

KEY POINTS

- Large-artery atherothrombosis, cardiac embolism and small-artery disease are the important mechanisms of infarction in vertebrobasilar artery territory.
- In lateral medullary infarction, clinical manifestations vary according to rostro-caudal and ventro-dorsal topography. Rostral-ventral infarcts are associated with severe dysphagia, dysarthria and contralateral trigeminal sensory involvement whereas caudal-lateral lesions are characterized by severe gait ataxia, absent dysphagia and sensory symptoms worse in the lower extremities.
- Medial medullary infarction occurs mostly in the rostral medulla, and presents with unilateral motor, sensory and ocular motor disturbances depending on ventro-dorsal topographic involvement.
- Branch occlusion associated with intracranial vertebral artery disease is the most important cause of medullary infarction.
- Unilateral paramedian infarction is the most common pattern of pontine infarction. Basal involvement is associated with motor syndromes such as pure motor stroke, ataxic hemiparesis, dysarthria clumsy hand, while tegmental lesions produce sensory symptoms and/or ocular motor disturbances, notably internuclear ophthalmoplegia.
- Bilateral pontine infarcts result in quadriparesis, horizontal gaze palsy and locked in syndrome, and are usually associated with significant basilar artery thrombotic occlusion.
- The most common topographic pattern of midbrain infarction is anteromedial followed by anterolateral; the former is characterized by ocular motor dysfunction (the 3rd nerve palsy or internuclear ophthalmoplegia), whereas the latter lesions produce various motor syndromes.
- Cerebellar infarcts generally follow the topography of three major arteries: posterior inferior cerebellar artery, superior cerebellar artery and anterior inferior cerebellar artery.
- Basilar top occlusion is mostly embolic and results in peculiar syndromes associated with paramedian midbrain, and diencephalic infarctions, with occasional involvement of the occipital and cerebellar regions

ANATOMY

Vertebral Artery

The two vertebral arteries (VAs), which often differ in size, are traditionally divided into four segments (Fig. 26-1). In the first segment, the artery courses directly cephalad from its origin as the first branch of the subclavian artery, riding anterior to the transverse foramen until it enters the costotransverse foramen usually at C6 or C5. The second segment runs entirely within the transverse foramina from C5–6 to C2. The third segment emerges from the transverse foramen of C2 and has a complex course posteriorly and laterally toward the costotransverse foramen of the atlas. There it circles the posterior arch of C1 and passes between the atlas and occiput within the suboccipital triangle. During its course, the third segment of the VA is covered by muscles and nerves and is pressed against bone while being covered by the atlanto-occipital membrane. Its intracranial portion constitutes the fourth segment of the VA. It pierces the dura mater to enter the foramen magnum, where its adventitial and medial coats become less thick, and there is a gross reduction in elastic lamina.[1]

At the level of the pontomedullary junction, the two VAs merge to form the basilar artery (BA), but the exact site varies; the site is sometimes high enough on the brainstem for the VA to supply the middle and lower pons. The BA becomes somewhat smaller as it travels distally, frequently curving slightly away from the larger VA. It divides near the pontomesencephalic junction to form the two posterior cerebral arteries (PCAs).

Variations are relatively common. In approximately 8% of humans, the left VA originates directly from the aortic arch and not from the subclavian artery. Rarely, the right VA arises as a separate branch from the innominate artery and not from the subclavian artery. The VAs are commonly asymmetrical. Depending on the criteria, the prevalence of a hypoplastic VA ranges from 1.9% to 7.8%.[2-4] In 45% of people the left VA is larger, in 21% the right VA is larger, and in 24% the arteries are of equal size.

Cerebellar Arteries

The cerebellum is mainly supplied by the three long, circumferential arteries (Figs 26-2, 26-3).

Posterior Inferior Cerebellar Artery

The posterior inferior cerebellar artery (PICA), usually the largest branch of the VA, arises from its intradural segment approximately 10–20 mm from the origin of the BA. This site is an average of 8.6 mm above the foramen magnum, but variations occur: it may originate from the VA as low as 24 mm below the foramen magnum.[5] Sometimes, the PICA arises extracranially and courses cephalad within the spinal canal.[6]

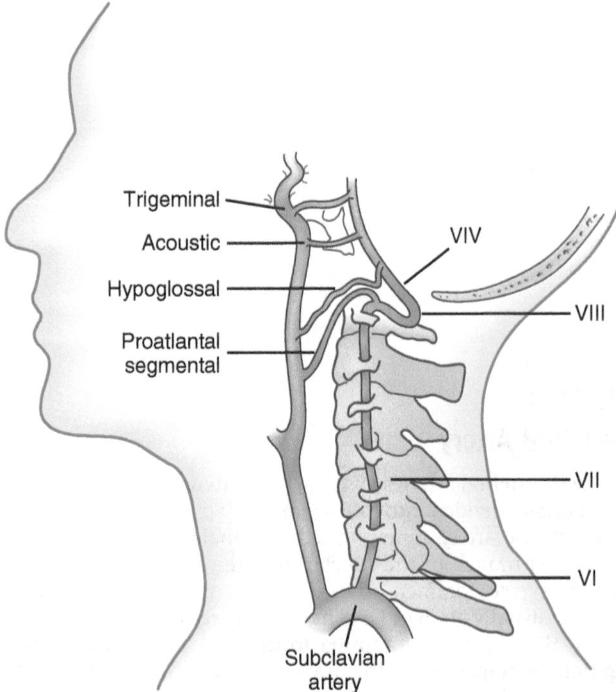

Figure 26-1. Vertebral artery segments and persisting primitive anastomotic connections within the carotid arterial tree (VI to VIV denote vertebral artery segments 1 to 4).

In some subjects, PICAs are a branch of the ascending pharyngeal artery.[7]

Although a branch of the VA, the PICA may be its termination, in which case the VA segment distally is a hypoplastic link to the BA or even non-existent. When the VA ends in the PICA, it is smaller than the contralateral VA. The PICA has a medial branch, which also arises directly from the VA. Its lateral branch may be from the BA or, more commonly, from the anterior inferior cerebellar artery (AICA).

In 10–20% of individuals, PICA is hypoplastic or absent, typically accompanied by a prominent ipsilateral AICA. The PICA and AICA are often reciprocally related in size; a large PICA may supply most of the inferior surface of the cerebellum, and the AICA on the same side is quite small with little cerebellar supply. When the AICA on one side is large, the ipsilateral PICA is frequently small. Duplication of the PICA and double origin with distal arterial convergence of the PICA may occur.[8] Other variations included posterior spinal arteries taking their origin from the PICA instead of the VA.[9] The lateral medulla is primarily supplied by direct lateral medullary branches of the VA rather than PICA.[10] The only part of the medulla which is constantly supplied by the medial PICA branches, together with the posterior spinal arteries, is the dorsal tegmental area.[10]

The PICA course encircles the medulla and supplies the suboccipital surface in the caudal part of the cerebellum. The PICA has a sinuous course with several loops (see Fig. 26-3). It travels dorsally, lateral to the medulla, below the roots of the ninth and tenth cranial nerves. From there, it courses inferiorly, makes the first (caudal) loop at a variable level, and goes up onto the posterior surface of the medulla in the sulcus, separating the medulla and the tonsil. At the top of the tonsil, the PICA makes a second (cranial) loop around the tonsil and then goes downward to the inferior part of the vermis. Sometimes the second loop occurs at the midpoint of the tonsil. Thus, the PICA has lateral medullary, dorsal medullary (ventral tonsillar), superior tonsillar, and dorsal tonsillar segments.

The PICA divides into two main branches, the medial and the lateral PICA. The medial PICA climbs along the inferior and dorsal surface of the vermis and the internal part of the hemispheres, making a third loop. The lateral PICA most often arises from the upper part of the dorsal medullary segment of the parent trunk, between the first and second loops, and then gives rise to several terminal branches to the caudal hemisphere. Sometimes it arises from the first loop. The caudal loop is usually found at the level of the foramen magnum. It can be found below this level, but rami from the lateral PICA that supply the tonsil are always above the foramen magnum. Rami from the cranial loop supply the choroid plexus of the fourth ventricle.

Two main areas of supply can be distinguished within the PICA territory. The dorsomedial area is supplied by the medial PICA, whose territory includes the dorsolateral portion of the medulla. The anterolateral area is supplied by the lateral PICA, which does not supply the medulla (see Fig. 26-2).

Anterior Inferior Cerebellar Artery

The AICA arises from the caudal third of the BA in 74% of people,[11] sometimes from the middle third and occasionally from its inferior limit. The AICA is absent in 4% of individuals, and can arise from the VA or the BA by a common trunk together with the PICA. Rarely, several small vessels arising directly from the BA or from the internal auditory artery may replace the AICA. The AICA winds around the lower pons and supplies the middle cerebellar peduncle, flocculus, and a small portion of the anterior inferior cerebellum.[12] Proximal branches of the AICA usually supply the lateral portion of the pons, including the facial, trigeminal, vestibular and cochlear nuclei, the root of the seventh and eighth cranial nerves, and the spinothalamic tract (Fig. 26-2).[13]

Superior Cerebellar Artery

The superior cerebellar artery (SCA) takes its origin from the rostral BA just before its bifurcation into the PCAs. In some individuals there are two parallel SCAs rather than a single artery.

Each SCA has a short trunk that divides into two main branches, a medial branch and a lateral branch. They follow the pontomesencephalic sulcus and pass around the superior cerebellar peduncle to ramify onto the rostral cerebellum (Fig. 26-3). The SCA courses along the anterosuperior margin of the cerebellum. The medial SCA starts with a course parallel to that of the lateral SCA but turns medially to reach the lateral surface of the mesencephalon and the inferior colliculus; from there, the medial SCA makes a rostral loop along the superior margin of the colliculus and then courses over the superior vermis (see Fig. 26-3). The SCA supplies the rostral half of the cerebellar hemispheres as well as the dentate nucleus.[14] Along the course of the SCA, branches supply the laterotegmental portion of the rostral pons (see Fig. 26-2).

These three major arteries (the PICA, AICA, and SCA) and their branches are connected by numerous anastomoses, which limit infarct size in patients who have VA or BA occlusions. Drawings of the territory of each cerebellar artery and their branches conform to the computed tomographic (CT) and magnetic resonance imaging (MRI) horizontal axial sections (Fig. 26-4).

Basilar Artery and its Main Branches

The BA extends from the unification of the two VAs at the pontomedullary junction to the terminal bifurcation of the PCAs at the rostral midbrain. The length of BA is approximately 25–35 mm, and the diameter is about 2.7–4.3 mm at

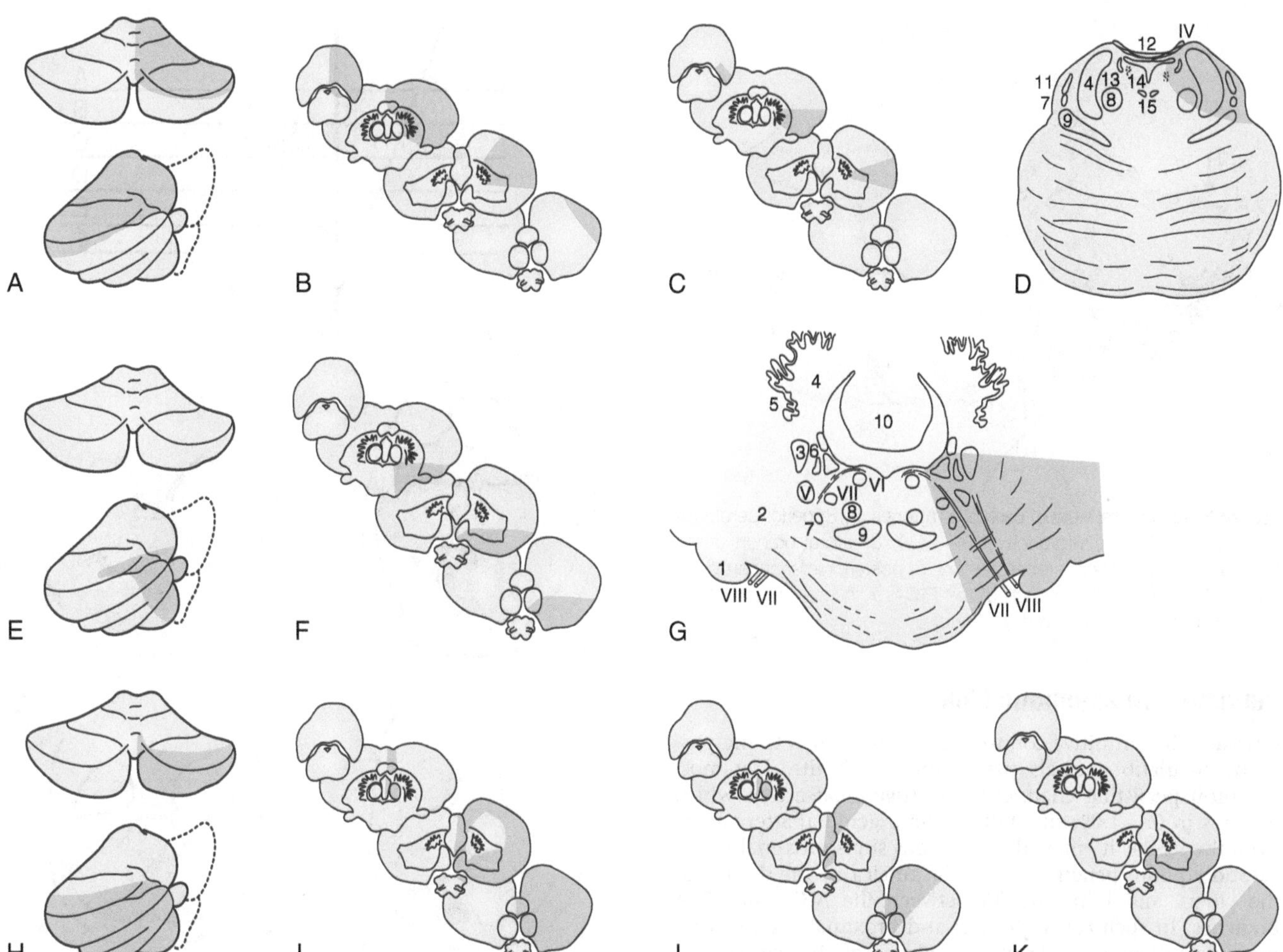

Figure 26-2. Anatomic drawings of the territory of cerebellar arteries and their branches at autopsy. A, Superior cerebellar artery (SCA) territory (superior, dorsal view; inferior, lateral view). B, SCA territory (sections from the rostral to the caudal cerebellum). C, Lateral SCA territory. D, Brainstem territory of SCA. E, Anterior inferior cerebellar artery (AICA) territory (dorsal and lateral views). F, AICA territory. G, Brainstem territory of AICA. H, Posterior inferior cerebellar artery territory (PICA) (dorsal and lateral views). I, PICA territory. J, Medial PICA territory. K, Lateral PICA territory. 1, Flocculus; 2, middle cerebellar peduncle; 3, inferior cerebellar peduncle; 4, superior cerebellar peduncle; 5, dentate nucleus; 6, vestibular nuclei; 7, spinothalamic tract; 8, central tegmental tract; 9, medial lemniscus; 10, nodulus; 11, lateral lemniscus; 12, decussation of trochlear nerve; 13, mesencephalic trigeminal tract; 14, locus ceruleus; 15, medial longitudinal fasciculus. *(Data from Amarenco P, Hauw J-J: Cerebellar infarction in the territory of the anterior and inferior cerebellar artery: A clinicopathological study of 20 cases.* Brain *113:139, 1990; Amarenco P, Hauw J-J: Anatomie des artères cérébelleuses.* Rev Neurol *145:267, 1989; and Amarenco P, Roullet E, Goujon C, et al: Infarction in the anterior rostral cerebellum (the territory of the lateral branch of the superior cerebellar artery).* Neurology *41:253, 1991.)*

the proximal portion.[15] The luminal diameter tends to taper towards the distal end. The largest branches of the BA are SCA and AICA. In addition, there are numerous smaller perforating arteries.

The three groups of arterial penetrators (Fig. 26-5) are (1) median arteries, which usually take a slightly caudal course and then penetrate the brainstem and supply the paramedian basal and tegmental regions, (2) short lateral circumferential arteries, which give rise to branches that penetrate the brainstem and supply the intermediate tegmental and basal regions, and (3) long lateral circumferential arteries, which course around the brainstem and supply the lateral basal and tegmental regions. There are also posterior branches, which arise from the long lateral circumferential cerebellar vessels (the SCA, PICA, and AICA), course in a horizontal and dorsoventral direction, and supply the lateral tegmentum (see Fig. 26-5). Penetrating vessels are usually less than 100 μm in diameter, and their size is roughly proportional to their length. The medial penetrating vessels arise from the VA, BA as well as from the AICA and PCA; lateral penetrators frequently enter the brainstem along the laterally emerging nerve roots and arise from the VA, PICA, AICA, BA, SCA, and posterior choroidal arteries.

The distal basilar segments are also the source of occasional variations. During early fetal life, the internal carotid artery (ICA) supplies the posterior hemispheres and brainstem via posterior communicating arteries. In one-third of humans, this primitive vascular pattern persists, and the connecting segment from the BA to the PCA remains vestigial.[16] In these patients, the PCA may fill from carotid injection and not after VA opacification. In 2% of humans, this primitive circulatory pattern is bilateral; the BA may be hypoplastic in its distal segment and end in the SCAs.[16] Penetrating branches from the posterior communicating artery, SCA, and proximal PCA supply the paramedian midbrain and thalamus; details are described in Chapter 25.

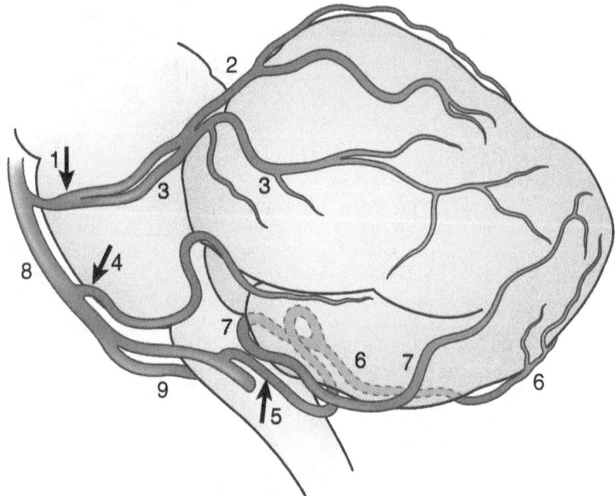

Figure 26-3. Lateral view of cerebellar arteries. 1, Superior cerebellar artery (SCA); 2, medial branch of the SCA; 3, lateral branch of the SCA; 4, anterior inferior cerebellar artery; 5, posterior inferior cerebellar artery (PICA); 6, medial branch of the PICA; 7, lateral branch of the PICA; 8, basilar artery; 9, vertebral artery.

Persistent Anastomotic Links

Occasionally, primitive connections from the ICA to the posterior circulation vessels persist into adult life. The most common persisting channel is the trigeminal artery, which remains in 0.1–1.0% of adults.[17] The trigeminal artery arises from the ICA as it enters the cavernous sinus proximal to the carotid siphon, penetrates the sella turcica or the dura near the clivus, and joins the BA between the AICA and SCA branches. In such cases, the VAs and proximal BA are commonly small or hypoplastic. Persistence of the hypoglossal artery is the next most common variant.[18] This vessel originates from the ICA in the neck, usually between C1 and C3, and courses posteriorly to enter the hypoglossal canal, from which it joins the BA.[19]

A persistent otic artery is a rarer anomaly; this vessel leaves the ICA within the petrous bone and enters the posterior fossa with the seventh and eighth cranial nerves at the internal acoustic meatus, later to join the mid-BA. The rarest fetal communicating channels are persistent proatlantal intersegmental arteries, which originate from the nuchal internal or external carotid artery at C2 and C3 and join the horizontal (third) segment of the VA suboccipitally.[20] Isolated reports describe communications between the common or proximal ICA and the lower VAs.[21]

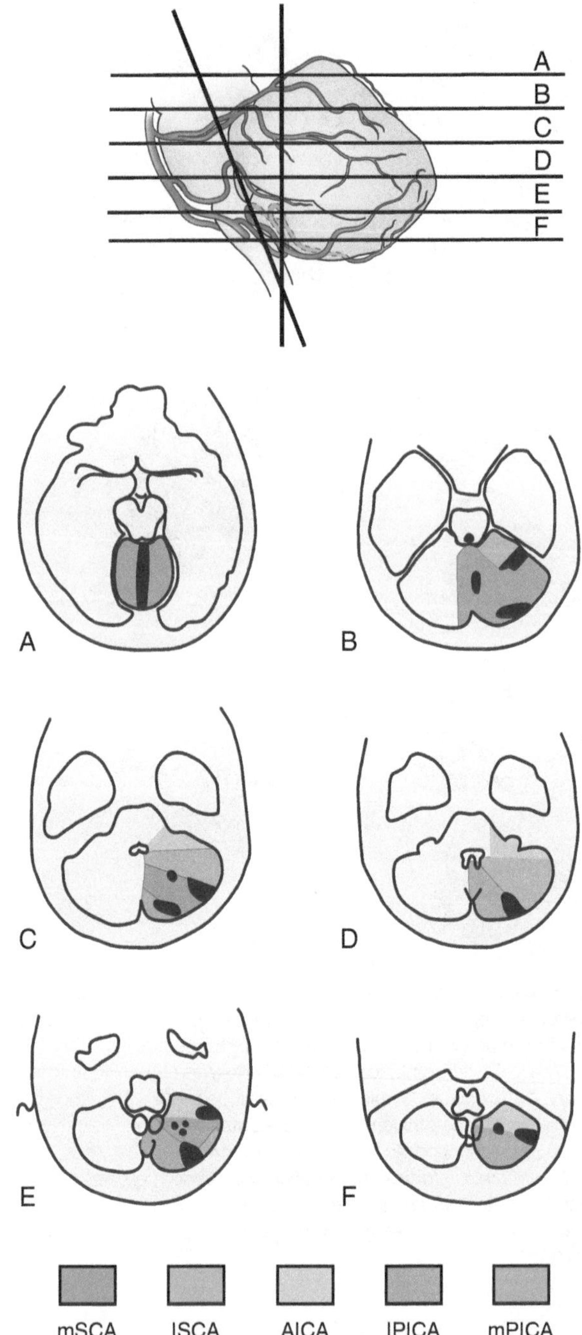

Figure 26-4. Anatomic drawings (A to F) of the territory of branches of the cerebellar arteries as they appear on computed tomography and magnetic resonance imaging. AICA, Anterior inferior cerebellar artery; lPICA, lateral branch of the posterior inferior cerebellar artery; lSCA, lateral branch of the SCA; mPICA, medial branch of the PICA; mSCA, medial branch of the superior cerebellar artery. *(Data from Amarenco P, Kase CS, Rosengart A, et al: Very small [border zone] cerebellar infarcts: Distribution, mechanisms, causes and clinical features.* Brain *116:161, 1993.)*

PATHOLOGY AND STROKE MECHANISMS

Vertebro-basilar artery territory ischemia is caused by large-artery disease, small-artery disease, cardiogenic embolism, and other uncommon diseases.

Large-Artery Disease

The main pathology of large-artery disease consists of thrombosis superimposed on atherosclerosis. In the posterior circulation, atherosclerosis is prone to occur in the proximal extracranial VA (ECVA), distal intracranial VA (ICVA), lower-middle portion of the BA, and proximal PCA[22,23]. The histologic features of posterior circulation atherosclerosis do not differ qualitatively from atherosclerosis elsewhere.[24,25]

Thrombosis occurring within the ECVA seldom forms a long anterograde or retrograde extension, which differs from thrombus in the ICA. Extensive collateral channels in the VA system may explain the difference. Thrombus formed within the ICVA, however, frequently extends into the proximal BA.[26] Within the BA, atherosclerotic stenosis is common in the proximal 2 cm, more often seen on the ventral than on the dorsal side.[24,26] Thrombi within the BA tend to have

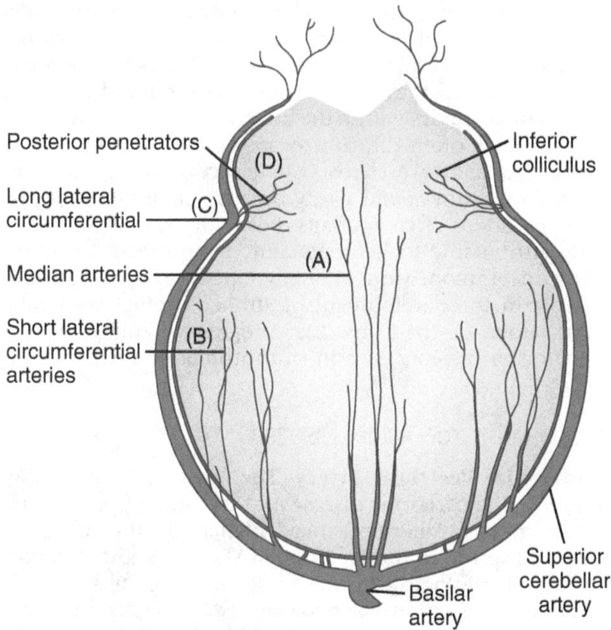

Figure 26-5. Rostral pons with the usual arterial distribution. A, Median penetrating arteries. B, Short lateral circumferential arteries. C, Long lateral circumferential artery. D, Posterior penetrating arteries.

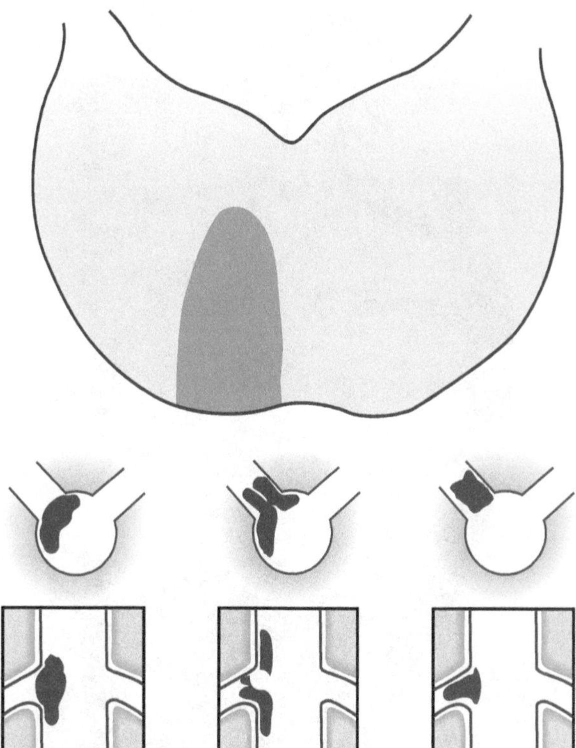

Figure 26-6. Diagrammatic representation of types of branch occlusion. *Left to right,* Luminal plaque blocking the orifice of a branch, junctional plaque spreading into a branch, and a clot in the proximal part of a branch.

limited propagation,[27] occasionally extending only to the orifice of the next long circumferential cerebellar artery (the AICA or SCA).

Mechanisms of Stroke in Large-Artery Disease

Detailed stroke mechanisms of large-artery disease include artery-to-artery embolism, in situ thrombotic occlusion, branch occlusion, hypoperfusion and their combinations.

Artery-to-Artery Embolism. Atherosclerotic plaques with erosion and ulceration often generate embolism.[28,29] Emboli arising from the ECVA occlude distal arteries such as the PCA, SCA, PICA and distal BA.[30] Stenoses in the ICVA or BA also produce embolism, although they more often cause infarction by way of branch occlusion.[31,32] Embolism seems to occur more frequently in the setting of posterior fossa hypoperfusion associated with significant bilateral VA occlusive disease, due in part to ineffective washout of emboli in hypoperfused areas.[33] Embolisms may develop from more proximal arteries, such as the subclavian artery, the ascending aorta and aortic arch.[34]

In situ Thrombotic Occlusion. In patients with intracranial artery atherosclerosis, thrombus formation in areas of plaque can result in total arterial occlusion, leading to infarction. In the posterior circulation, in situ thrombotic occlusion is often observed in the territories of PCA, and BA branches such as AICA or PICA.[22,35] In situ thrombotic occlusion produces relatively large territorial infarction. However, unlike cardiogenic embolism, it less often produces "malignant" infarction because of relatively well-developed collateral circulation in the setting of the chronic atherosclerotic process.[36] With persistent occlusion, the initial infarct frequently grows, leading to progressive neurological worsening. Thus, the ultimate size of the infarct varies according to the status of the collateral circulation, the speed of arterial occlusion, and hemodynamic stability in these patients.

Branch Occlusion. Atherosclerotic plaques in an intracranial artery can occlude the orifice of one or several perforators, causing infarcts limited to the perforator territory[37] (Figs 26-6, 26-7A). Pathological features of this "atheromatous branch occlusion" were described.[38,39] Branch occlusions are more often observed in posterior than in anterior circulation stroke and are the major mechanism of thalamic, pontine and medullary infarctions.[31,32,40–42]

Brainstem infarcts associated with branch occlusion tend to extend to the basal surface (Fig. 26-7A,B), whereas those caused by small-artery lipohyalinotic disease (see below) produce a small island of infarction within the parenchyma (Fig. 26-7C). The former is more often associated with atherosclerotic characteristics,[43] larger lesion volume, and an unstable and unfavorable clinical course than the latter.[32,44,45] Compared with arterial lesions producing embolism, branch occlusion is related to less severe degrees of stenosis.[46] Now, high-resolution vessel wall MRI (HR–MRI) can identify the small plaque that occludes the perforator, even in patients with normal MRA findings.[47,48]

Hypoperfusion. In patients with severe vascular stenosis/occlusion and insufficient collaterals, hemodynamic TIAs can occur. Typically, symptoms such as dizziness, diplopia, and visual disturbances occur briefly and stereotypically in patients who are dehydrated or fatigued or at the time they suddenly stand up. When stroke develops, the symptoms may fluctuate widely according to the degree of hydration, blood pressure and the position of the patient's head. Revascularization therapies, such as angioplasty/stenting may rapidly relieve these symptoms (Fig. 26-8).

Unlike anterior circulation diseases, MRI lesion patterns of hemodynamic infarction are not clearly established in the posterior circulation, due in part to considerable normal variations and collateral patterns that influence perfusion. Small

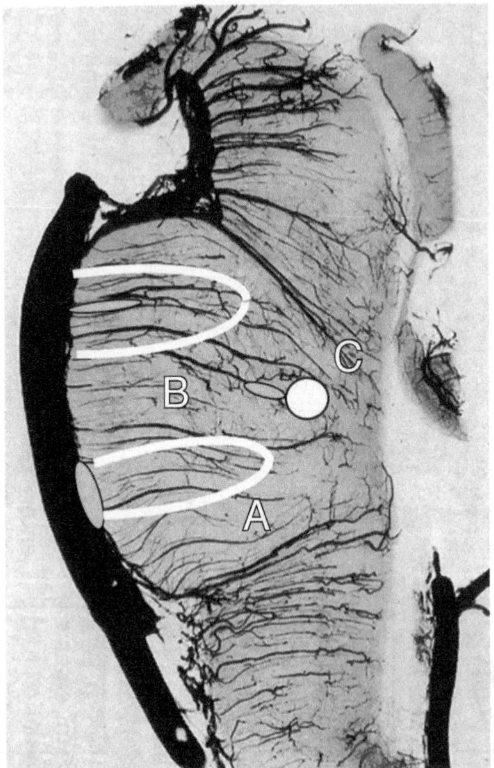

Figure 26-7. Schematic drawing of the mechanism of brainstem infarction. A, Atherothrombosis occurring in the basilar artery obliterates the orifice of the perforator. B, Atherosclerotic occlusion of the proximal portion of the perforator. C, Lipohyalinotic distal small-artery occlusion. A and B are referred to as "branch atheromatous disease". They produce infarcts abutting on the basal surface whereas C (lipohyalinotic disease) produces an island-like deep infarction.

infarcts occurring in the cerebellar borderzone (areas bordering PICA, AICA and SCA) may be attributed to hypoperfusion associated with cardiac arrest or severe VA or BA occlusive disease. However, these infarcts are also produced by embolism to small arteries within the borderzone areas.[49] The stroke mechanism is often difficult to assess partly because severe vertebrobasilar atherosclerosis can induce both hemodynamic and embolic strokes and partly because the territory of each cerebellar artery often overlaps. Posterior circulation infarcts solely attributable to hemodynamic failure seem to be distinctly uncommon. More often, hypoperfusion plays an additive role in the development of stroke, together with other major stroke mechanisms, e.g., progressive enlargement of infarction in patients with in situ thrombotic occlusion (see above).

Location of Large-Artery Disease

Extracranial Vertebral Artery. The most frequent location for ECVA atherosclerotic disease is at the origin from the subclavian arteries. Atheromas may originate in the subclavian artery and spread to the proximal ECVA. ECVA atherosclerosis shares epidemiologic features with its close cousin, atherosclerosis of the ICA origin; the two sites are frequently affected in the same individuals. Despite the high incidence of ECVA atherosclerosis, serious posterior circulation strokes are relatively uncommon in this condition.[50] When stroke does develop, it is almost always related to embolism from thrombi formed in the proximal ECVA.[9,30,52–54] Compared to unilateral VA lesions, bilateral lesions (contralateral occlusion or hypoplasia) seem to generate embolism more often, probably related to hypoperfusion in the posterior fossa, that may promote thrombus generation, and inefficient washout of emboli. Hypoperfusion in turn is related to the effective development of collateral circulation, especially when the VA occlusion occurs gradually. Important sources of collaterals include occipital branches of the external carotid artery, the ascending cervical and transverse cervical branches of the thyrocervical trunk, and retrograde flow from the contralateral VA or from the posterior communicating system.

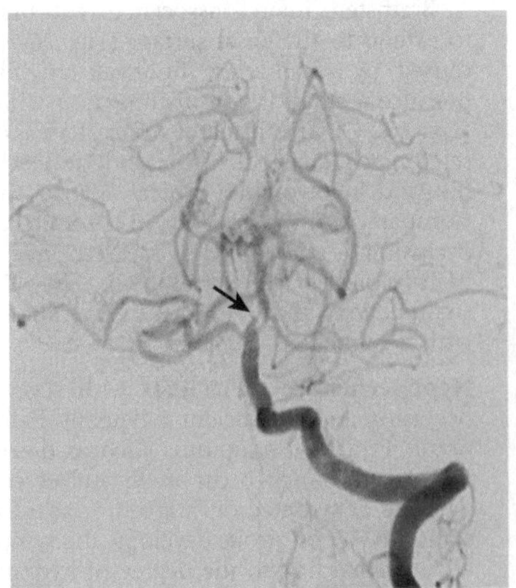

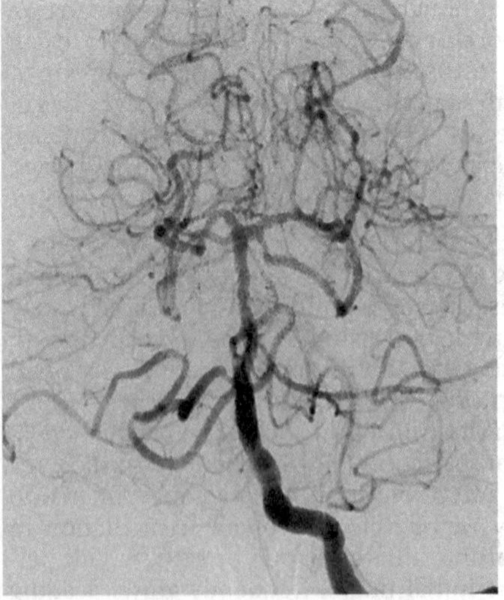

Figure 26-8. An example of recurrent vertebrobasilar artery territory transient ischemic attacks attributed to hypoperfusion. Left image: A 68-year-old woman with hypertension, diabetes and a history of coronary heart disease developed recurrent, brief attacks of dizziness, diplopia, dysarthria and gait instability that lasted for seconds or a few minutes. The episodes more often occur when patients are working and exhausted. MRI showed no abnormal findings. Angiogram showed severe stenosis of the basilar artery just above the right anterior inferior cerebellar artery and below the left anterior cerebellar artery (arrow). Right image: Angioplasty and stenting were performed and the stenosis was improved. The patient no longer developed such symptoms during 6 months of follow-up.

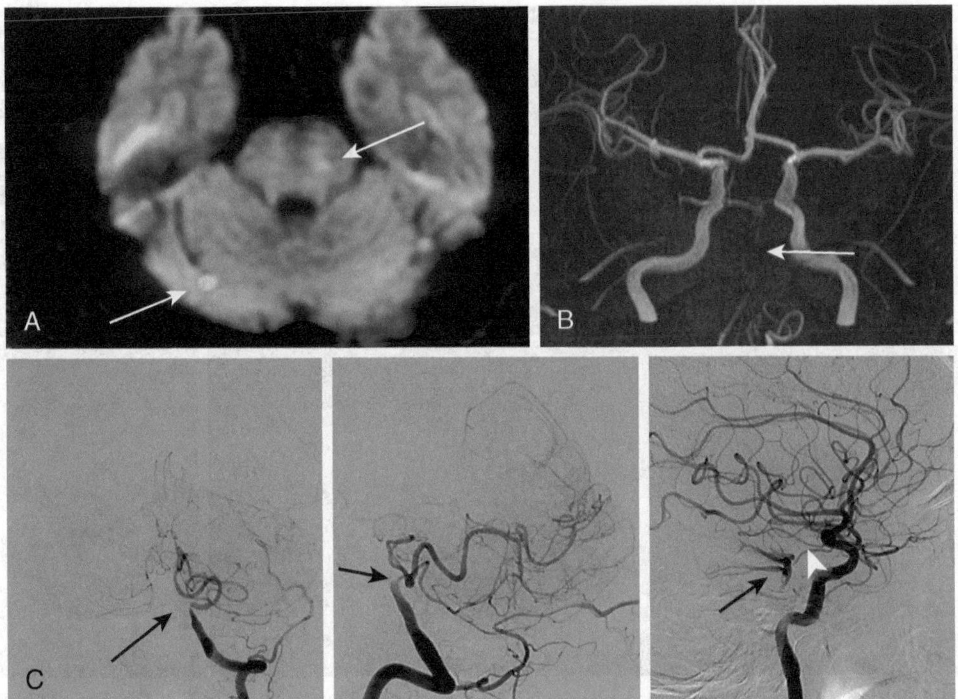

Figure 26-9. An example of a patient with basilar artery occlusion with benign outcome. A 66-year-old man with hypertension and diabetes mellitus developed sudden dizziness and dysarthria that lasted for 10 minutes. Neurologic examination showed no abnormal signs. Diffusion-weighted MRI shows two small recent infarcts in the left pons and right cerebellum (A, arrows). MR angiogram shows non-visualization of the basilar artery due to thrombotic occlusion (B, arrow). Conventional angiogram 4 days later shows occlusion of the vertebrobasilar junction on both sides. AP view (C) and lateral view (D) show occlusion of the distal left vertebral artery (arrows). The left posterior inferior cerebellar artery is well developed to supply much of the left cerebellum. Right cerebellum is also supplied by vermian branches from left posterior inferior cerebellar artery. Lateral view of the carotid system shows that an upper portion of the posterior circulation system (posterior cerebral artery, superior cerebellar artery and upper portion of the basilar artery) (E, arrow) is supplied by posterior communicating artery (arrowhead). *(From Caplan LR, Amarenco P, Kim JS. Posterior circulation disorders. In, Kim JS, Caplan LR, Wong KSL ed.* Intracranial Atherosclerosis, *pp 83–99, with permission.)*

Intracranial Vertebral Artery. Generally, ICVA occlusive disease is a more serious condition than ECVA disease. Unilateral ICVA disease may produce medullary infarction or PICA cerebellar infarction through branch occlusion, i.e., occlusion of the medullary perforators and the ostium of the PICA, respectively. Thrombi within the stenosed ICVA may also generate emboli that occlude distal vessels (artery-to-artery embolism). Bilateral ICVA occlusion is less well tolerated and often leads to TIAs or cerebellar and brainstem infarction,[51–53] although some patients who have adequate collateral circulation may survive without major infarction.[53]

Basilar Artery. Pathologically[54] and angiographically[55] documented BA occlusion often leads to catastrophic bilateral pontine infarction, but some patients have only limited or transient deficits.[56–59] The variable outcome depends on extensiveness of the thrombus and the status of collateral circulation (e.g., backward flow from the well-developed posterior communicating artery) (Fig. 26-9). The collateral status may in turn be influenced by the extent of the thrombotic occlusion. For example, collateral circulation through the PICA would be poor when the ICVA is also obstructed. When thrombus propagates to the distal BA, collateral circulation from the SCAs and the posterior communicating arteries becomes limited. The speed of BA occlusion also matters; BA embolism and dissection result in sudden coma and quadriparesis, while progression of brainstem ischemia related to atherothrombosis is slow, progressive and earns time for collateral development. Early plaques associated with mild stenosis generally produce unilateral pontine infarcts through the mechanism of branch occlusion.

Small-Artery (Penetrating Artery) Disease

A single subcortical or brainstem infarct usually results from disease of penetrating arteries[60] (Fig. 26-7C). Its pathological hallmarks include irregular cavities, less than 15–20 mm in size, located in subcortical, brainstem, and cerebellar areas. Penetrating arteries associated with these lesions have disorganized vessel walls, fibrinoid material deposition and hemorrhagic extravasation through arterial walls, first called "segmental arterial disorganization" and then lipohyalinosis by Fisher.[39,60–66] These vascular changes develop in arteries or arterioles 40–400 μm in diameter, and frequently affect the perforating arteries from the PCA or BA. Penetrating artery disease is the main mechanism of brainstem infarction, although brainstem infarctions may also be caused by atheromatous branch occlusion[37] as discussed before (Fig. 26-7A,B).

Cardiac Embolism

A thrombus arising in the heart more often travels to the anterior circulation than to the posterior circulation system. Nevertheless, previous studies showed that about one-fifth of posterior circulation infarcts result from cardiogenic embolism.[67] These emboli commonly occlude the PCA, rostral BA, SCA, PICA and the ICVA. Infarcts are typically larger than those associated with large-artery atherosclerotic

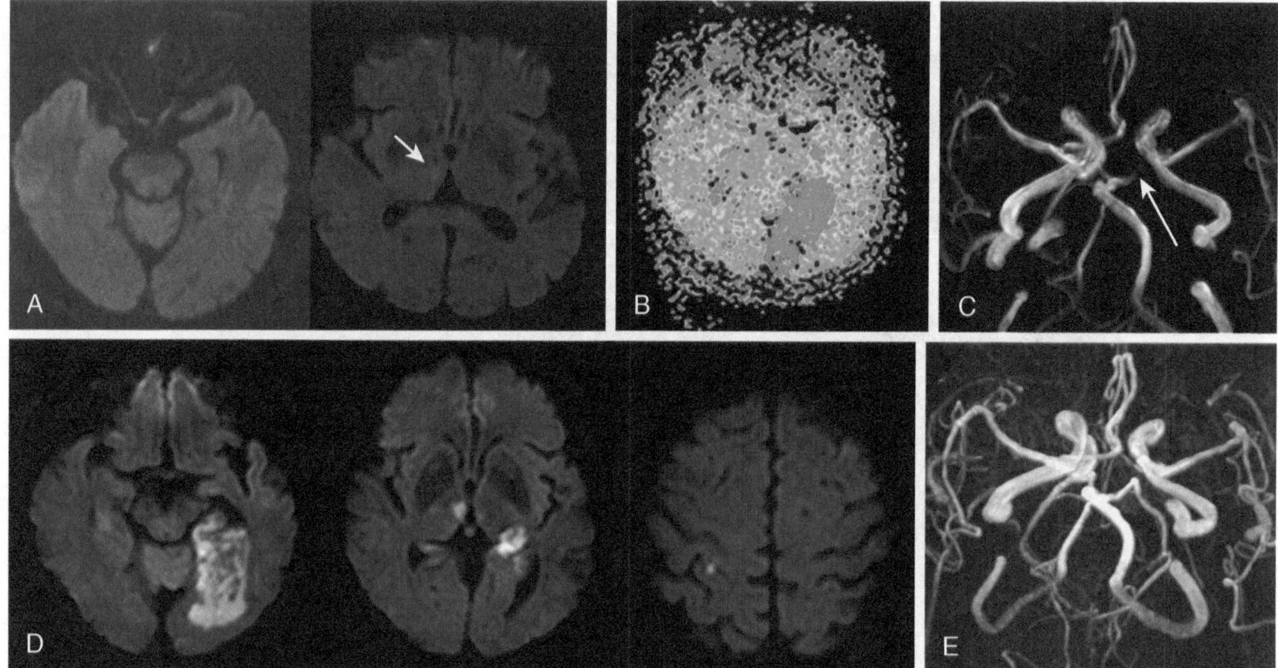

Figure 26-10. A 71-year-old woman with atrial fibrillation suddenly developed confusion. A, Initial diffusion-weighted MRI (DWI) showed right medial thalamic infarction (short arrow) without definite lesion on the occipital area. B, Perfusion-weighted MRI (MTT map) showed decreased perfusion in the left occipital area. C, MR angiography showed occlusion of the left posterior cerebral artery (long arrow). D, Follow-up DWI 4 days later showed hemorrhagic infarction in the left occipital area, and an infarct in the right thalamus. A small infarct is also shown in the right cortical area of middle cerebral artery territory. E, MR angiography showed complete recanalization of the posterior cerebral artery.

disease, partly because the clots are larger and partly because of the insufficiently developed collateral circulation.[68] The onset is usually abrupt. Additional infarcts may be seen in the anterior circulation as well. The occluded artery is often spontaneously recanalized, and hemorrhagic transformation of an infarct is common, which may cause worsening headache or neurological deterioration (Fig 26-10). Atrial fibrillation is the most common cause of embolic infarction, and among stroke patients with atrial fibrillation, slightly less than one-quarter develop infarction in the vertebrobasilar territory.[69]

Although there still are debates,[70] patent foramen ovale (PFO) with a large amount of shunt may be an etiology of embolic infarcts (paradoxical embolism).[71,72] The posterior circulation seems to be a predilection site for embolism in patients with PFOs.[69,73] A recent study showed that embolic infarctions associated with PFO more often occurred in the vertebrobasilar artery territory than those associated with atrial fibrillation (44.4% vs 22.9%).[69] Relatively poor adrenergic innervation in the vertebrobasilar circulation, and inefficient response to sympathetic stimuli at the time of Valsalva maneuvers may explain the increased chance of blood clot traveling to the vertebrobasilar system. Embolic infarction associated with cardiac catheterization also occurs preferentially in the posterior circulation.[74,75]

Less Common Causes

Dissection

Cervicocranial artery dissections occur in 1–2% of patients with ischemic strokes, but are one of the major causes (10–25%) of stroke in young patients.[76] In the posterior circulation, dissection most commonly develops in the VA. Although ECVA dissection has been traditionally emphasized,[77,78] recent reports from Asia suggest that ICVA dissection may be equally prevalent.[79]

Dissection of the ECVA is often associated with trauma associated with rotating neck motion such as chiropractic procedures or other neck manipulations.[80] Some arise from very minor trauma such as riding on a rollercoaster, coughing, falling on the back and turning the head to back a car.[80–84] VA dissections are associated with conditions such as Marfan's syndrome, Ehlers-Danlos syndrome, pseudoxanthoma elasticum, systemic lupus erythematosus, fibromuscular dysplasia, and congenital bicuspid aortic valves.[85–89] Patients with a family history of dissection have a higher risk of recurrent dissection.[89,90]

The most common symptom of ECVA dissection is pain in the posterior head or neck. Ischemic symptoms and signs may develop at the same time or after a delay of hours to a few days. The lateral medulla and cerebellum are the regions most susceptible to ischemia from ECVA dissection[77,78] (Fig. 26-11). ICVA dissections present either as ischemia, subarachnoid hemorrhage (SAH) or headache and most often occur near the origin of the PICA. The dissection often extends into the BA. Less commonly, a dissecting aneurysm forms and acts as a mass lesion compressing the brainstem, cranial nerves or other vessels.[91] In one study, among 31 patients with ICVA dissections, 55% had headache, 48% had brainstem or cerebellar infarction, and 10% presented with SAH.[92]

BA dissections are very uncommon and carry a graver prognosis than VA dissections. They often produce extensive, bilateral pontine infarction presenting with altered consciousness and quadriparesis.[93] In a review of 38 patients with BA dissections, 27 had brainstem infarctions, five had SAH, and six patients had both. Thirty patients (79%) died.[94] However, a more recent study emphasized that unilateral pontine infarctions with a relatively favorable outcome are relatively common.[95] Dissections occurring in the PCA are uncommon, and present with PCA territory infarction, SAH and mass

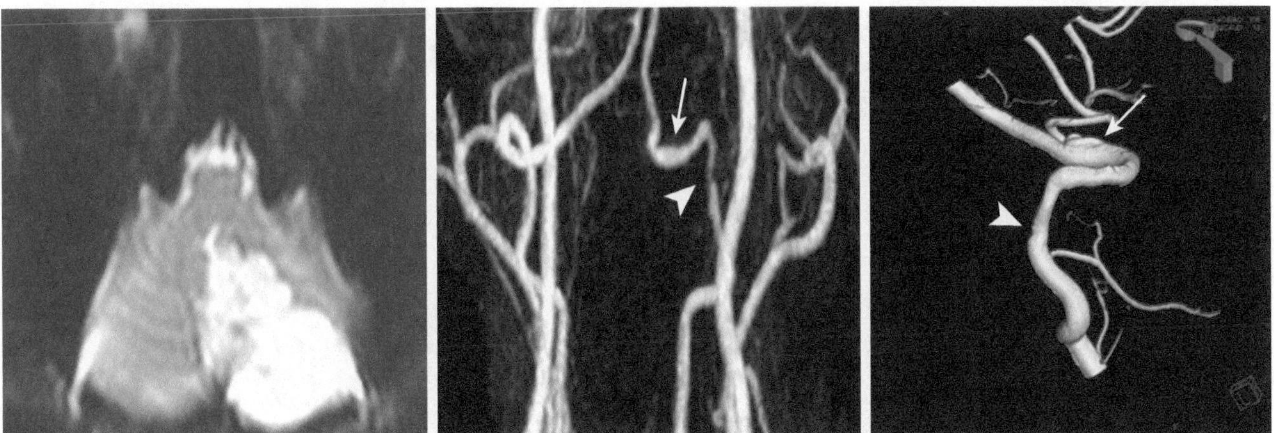

Figure 26-11. A 33-year-old man without vascular risk factors suddenly developed right nuchal and occipital pain, which was followed by severe dizziness and vertigo. Diffusion-weighted MRI showed an infarct in the left medial posterior inferior cerebellar artery territory (left image). MR angiogram showed stenosed distal vertebral artery (arrowhead) and aneurysmal dilatation (arrow), consistent with arterial dissection (middle image). 3D reconstruction angiogram showed the vascular lesions more clearly (right image).

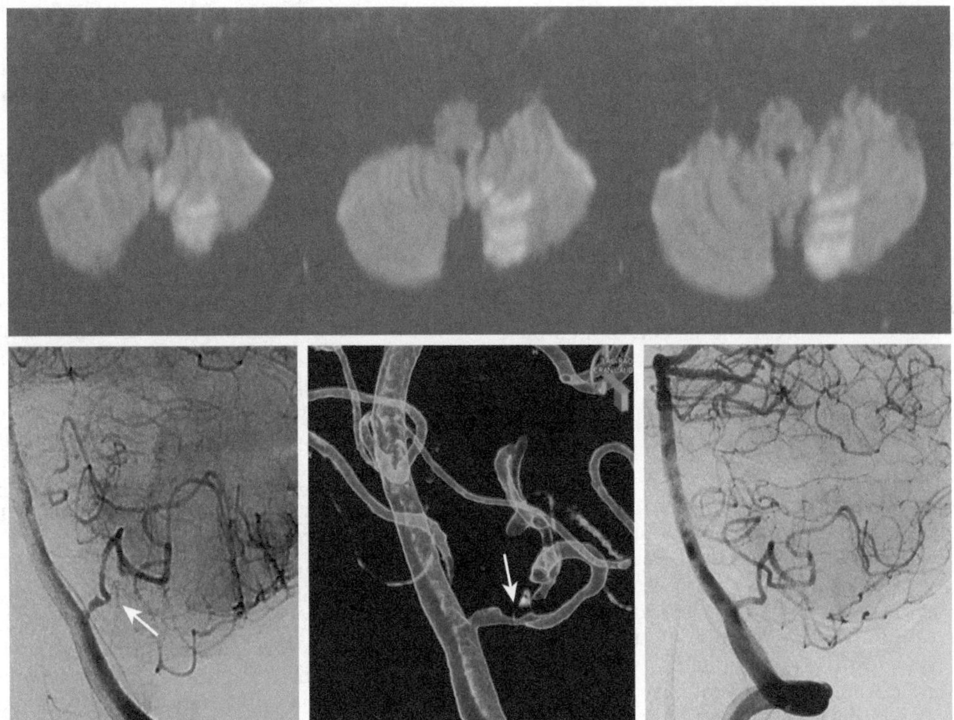

Figure 26-12. A 53-year-old woman suddenly developed vertigo and gait instability. Neurological examination showed gait ataxia, left trigeminal sensory deficit and left Horner sign. Diffusion-weighted MRI showed left medial posterior inferior cerebellar artery (PICA) territory infarction involving the cerebellum and dorsal lateral medulla (upper images). Angiogram showed dilatation and focal stenosis (arrow) in the proximal part of the PICA consistent with dissection (lower, left and middle images). Repeat angiogram 1 month later showed that the vascular abnormality improved (lower right image).

effect.[96] Isolated dissections of the PICA are rare and present with either SAH or infarctions[97,98] (Fig. 26-12). Dissections occurring in the proximal PICA appear to produce ischemic symptoms, while those in the distal portion tend to cause SAH.[99] Dissection occurring in the SCA is also very rare, and seems to produce SAH more often than infarction.[100]

Fusiform (Dolichoectatic) Dilatation

With the advent of imaging techniques, fusiform, tortuous, elongated, ectatic arteries (dolichoectasia) are increasingly recognized. They are found in the distal ICA and MCA, but are most often observed in the BA.[101] The ICVA may also be affected.

The etiologies of fusiform arterial dilatation remain unclear, but may involve degenerative processes under genetic influences that lead to structural arterial defects characterized by fibrous dysplasia, internal elastic lamina degeneration, and fibrous and collagen replacement of the media.[102] In adults, atherosclerotic changes in the vessels may interact with congenital structural defects to augment fusiform dilatation. A genetic deficiency in α-glucosidase was found in patients with fusiform BA aneurysms.[103] In some, the arterial

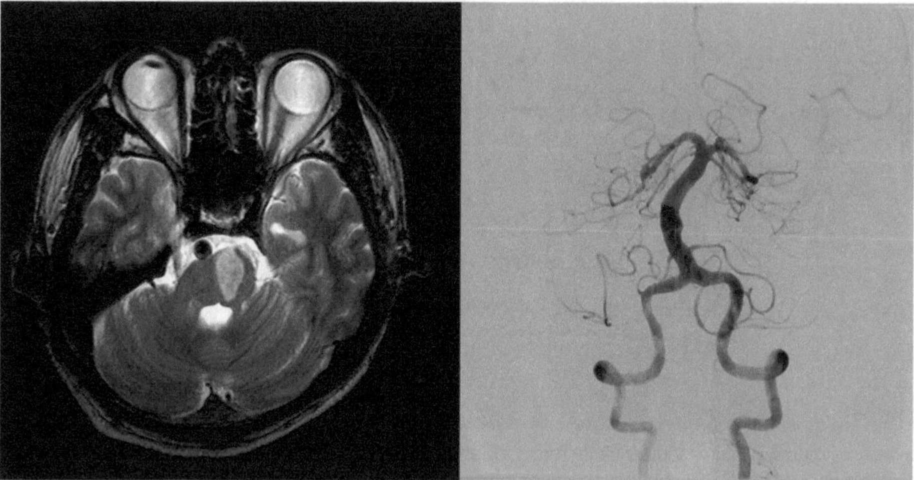

Figure 26-13. A 37-year-old hypertensive man suddenly developed right hemiparesis and dysarthria. MRI showed a left pontine base infarction. MR angiogram showed dolichoectatic basilar artery.

abnormalities are widespread, and affect other vessels such as the abdominal aorta.[101,104]

In the dilated vessel, blood flow is slowed, which predisposes to thrombus formation. Artery-to-artery embolism or branch occlusion may lead to infarction[105–107] (Fig. 26-13). One recent study reported that vertebrobasilar dolichoectasia was present in 6.4% of patients with cerebral infarction.[108] Symptoms may occur due to compression and traction on posterior fossa structures.[106,109] Occipital–nuchal pain is common, and cranial nerve damage may result in seventh and eighth cranial nerve palsies, hemifacial spasms, tinnitus, deafness, vertigo, trigeminal pain, and hypoglossal paralysis.[104,110,111] Large BA aneurysms can compress the cerebellar peduncle leading to hydrocephalus,[112] or may manifest as cerebellopontine angle masses.[113] ICVA aneurysms may compress the medulla resulting in hemiparesis and other deficits.[114]

Arterial Compression

Spondylitic osteophytes that project from the vertebral joints adjacent to the transverse foramina can compress the VA, usually at C1,2 level on neck rotation, and lead to recurrent TIAs or even strokes. In many cases, the contralateral VA is hypoplastic, ends at PICA or is previously occluded, rendering the compressed VA the major supply to the posterior circulation.[115–120] Symptoms are precipitated by turning or rotation of the neck, during which the VA may become temporarily occluded. According to the recent series of 21 patients with this "rotational VA occlusion" syndrome, all patients developed vertigo accompanied by tinnitus (38%), fainting (24%), or blurred vision (19%).[121] The induced nystagmus was mostly downbeat with horizontal and torsional components beating toward the compressed vertebral artery side. Artery-to-artery embolism arising from stenosed VA was proposed,[120] but more recent studies suggest that symptoms are attributed to asymmetrical excitation of the bilateral labyrinth induced by transient ischemia or by disinhibition from inferior cerebellar hypoperfusion.[121,122] The prognosis is benign, contrary to what was previously thought, and conservative treatment is usually sufficient.

Posterior fossa ischemic strokes may occur during or after surgical or interventional procedures, such as aneurysm clipping, stenting or surgical removal of tumor. In patients with aneurysms, blockage of the orifice of tributary vessels due to embolization from a clot within the aneurysm[123] may be responsible for ischemic stroke. Other mechanisms include: (1) forceful retraction of the artery or interventional procedure may induce dissection or intimal tear, (2) sudden decompression of the artery by tumor removal, which had been encased and compressed for a long time, may result in turbulent blood flow and subsequent thrombus formation,[124] (3) vasospasm due to localized SAH secondary to vessel injury.

Fibromuscular Dysplasia

Fibromuscular dysplasia (FMD) is a vasculopathy of unknown cause characterized by hyperplasia of the intima and media of arteries, adventitial sclerosis, breakdown of normal elastic tissue, without inflammation. Thickened septa and ridges protrude into the lumen. The most common angiogram findings are a "string of beads" appearance: segments of constriction alternating with normal or dilated segments. Renal arteries and cervicocranial arteries are the two sites most commonly involved. In patients with cervicocranial artery involvement, lesions are present in the ICA in 95% and are bilateral in 60–85% of cases. ECVA involvement has been reported in 12–43% of affected patients.

FMD affecting the ECVA may cause TIA or stroke via artery-to-artery embolism, hemodynamic insufficiency or their combination.[125] Although rare, FMD may occur in the intracranial arteries such as BA[126–128] or PCA[129] resulting in posterior circulation TIA[127] and infarctions.[126,129] Intracranial FMDs are often associated with dissection[130] or pseudoaneurysm formation[129,131] and carry a relatively poor prognosis. Hypertension secondary to the renal involvement also contributes to the development of stroke in patients with FMD.

Moyamoya Disease

Moyamoya disease is characterized by progressive occlusion of the distal ICA or proximal MCA, with the development of fine meshworks of basal collateral vessels.[132] Posterior circulation stroke is rarely a presenting manifestation of moyamoya disease, except for PCA infarction in patients with PCA involvement[133] (for details, see Chapter 25).

Giant Cell (Temporal) Arteritis

Giant cell arteritis is a systemic vasculitis characterized by subacute granulomatous inflammation of the aorta and its major branches (large and medium-sized vessels) with particular tropism for the extracranial carotid artery branches. Headache and visual loss, the most common clinical manifestations, are caused by involvement of the superficial temporal arteries and ophthalmic branches/central retinal arteries, respectively. Stroke is a rare complication of giant cell arteritis, occurring in about 3% of patients.[134,135] Giant cell arteritis may involve ECVA usually in its V3 portion, and produce TIAs or brainstem/cerebellar infarctions.[136–138] Occasionally, the subclavian arteries become occluded. Because this condition is treatable, and the prognosis is poor if untreated, this possibility should be suspected in elderly patients with extensive ECVA steno-occlusive disease when they have prolonged unexplained fever, headache, malaise, anemia and ESR, and/or CRP elevation.

Infectious or Immunologic Vasculitis

Vasculitis may be caused by infectious (e.g., bacterial, tuberculous, spirochetal, fungal, viral) and immunologic (e.g., lupus, polyarteritis nodosa) disorders. Vasculitis more often involves the anterior circulation, but involvement of the posterior circulation is not an exception.[49] Takayasu's disease primarily involves the aorta and its branches, and involvement of the subclavian artery and ECVA may produce subclavian steal syndrome or vertebrobasilar ischemia.[139,140]

Persistent Anastomotic Links

A persistent trigeminal artery (PTA) is the most common embryonic carotid-basilar anastomosis, occurring in 0.1–1.0% of general population. It usually forms a connection between the cavernous part of the ICA and the upper third of the BA.[17] A high incidence (85%) of VA hypoplasia or atresia is associated. The severe VA hypoplasia may lead to vertebrobasilar ischemic symptoms when collaterals are insufficient. In addition, brainstem TIA or infarction may occur due to emboli that originate from an ICA plaque[141] or diseased heart[142] and traverse through the PTA.

VASCULAR TOPOGRAPHIC SYNDROMES

Medullary Infarction

The medulla is mainly supplied by a number of penetrating arteries arising from the ICVAs. The dorsal tegmental area is also supplied by branches arising from the medial PICA and posterior spinal artery. The most rostral part may be supplied by branches from the BA or AICA. The caudal part of the anterior medulla is supplied by penetrating arteries arising from the anterior spinal artery (ASA).

Lateral Medullary Infarction

Since the first description of Wallenberg's syndrome more than 100 years ago,[143] clinical[144–147] and pathological[10] findings of lateral medullary infarction (LMI) have been reported. However, pre-mortem lesion identification became possible only after MRI was introduced.[148] Recent studies using MRI[31,149–152] have rapidly expanded our understanding of LMI syndromes. One study reported that LMI represents 1.9% of all admitted acute stroke.[144]

Clinical Manifestations

The onset may be sudden, but in more than half of the patients, symptoms/signs develop progressively or stutteringly; the first symptoms/signs are usually headache, vertigo, nausea/vomiting or gait instability whereas hiccup tends to occur later.[31] Occasionally, some of these symptoms/signs develop days or even weeks after the onset. The progressive onset is probably related to enlargement of ischemic area associated with progressive thrombosis. Symptoms/signs of LMI are summarized in Table 26-1.

TABLE 26-1 Neurologic Symptoms and Signs Published in the Largest Series

Items	N = 130
Sensory symptoms/signs	125 (96)
Ipsilateral trigeminal	34 (26)
Contralateral trigeminal	32 (25)
Bilateral trigeminal	18 (14)
Isolated limb/body	27 (21)
Isolated trigeminal	13 (10)
Gait ataxia	120 (92)
Severe gait ataxia*	79 (61)
Dizziness	119 (92)
Horner sign	114 (88)
Hoarseness	82 (63)
Dysphagia	84 (65)
Severe dysphagia**	52 (40)
Dysarthria	28 (22)
Vertigo	74 (57)
Nystagmus	73 (56)
Limb ataxia	72 (55)
Nausea/vomiting	67 (52)
Headache	67 (52)
Neck pain	9 (7)
Skew deviation of eyes	53 (41)
Diplopia	41 (32)
Hiccup	33 (25)
Facial palsy	27 (21)
Forced gaze deviation	8 (6)

Data are expressed as number (%).
*Unable to stand or walk alone.
**Requires naso-gastric feed for feeding.
From Kim JS. Pure lateral medullary infarction: clinical-radiological correlation of 130 acute, consecutive patients. Brain *2003;126:1864–1872.*

Dizziness, Vertigo and Ataxia. A dizzy sensation and gait instability are the most common symptoms occurring in more than 90% of patients. Whirling vertigo, a symptom attributed to involvement of vestibular nuclei and their connections, occurs in approximately 60%.[31] Vertigo is an early sign that usually improves within days or weeks, even if dizziness and gait instability persist. Vertigo is usually accompanied by nystagmus and vomiting.

Gait instability and dizziness can be attributed either to dysfunctional vestibular or cerebellar system. In the acute stage, approximately 60% of patients are unable to stand or walk. Gait ataxia is usually more common and severe than limb incoordination.[31,153] Lateropulsion (forced to sway when patients stand or sit) seems to be attributed to lesions affecting the vestibular nuclei and vestibulospinal projections,[154] while limb and gait ataxia are related to damage to the inferior cerebellar peduncle, spinocerebellar fibers or the cerebellum itself.[153,155] Occasionally, patients fall to any direction, which may be related to involvement of the ventral spinocerebellar tract, which conveys proprioceptive information from both sides.[155] Limb ataxia is usually milder than that shown in SCA territory cerebellar infarction, and may be described as "weakness" or "clumsiness" by the patient.

Nystagmus and Ocular Motor Abnormality. Involvement of the vestibular nuclei and their connections lead to nystagmus. The nystagmus is mostly horizontal or horizontal-rotational to the side opposite to the lesions.[10,147] It improves over time but rarely can be permanent. Although forced conjugate eyeball deviation to the lesion side (ocular lateropulsion)[156] is uncommon, a milder degree of eyeball deviation is frequently observed when patients are ordered to close and then open the eyes, when correctional eyeball movements occur. Skew deviation, with the ipsilateral eye going down, is also frequent, and ocular torsion is often accompanied by head tilt (ocular tilt reaction).[154] Most often, lateral gaze is characterized by hypermetric saccades to the side of the lesion and hypometric saccades to the opposite side.[157] These ocular manifestations are caused by dysfunctional vestibulo-ocular reflex pathways and can present clinically as blurred vision, diplopia, oscillopsia (a sense of moving objects) or tilting of visual images.[147,154]

Nausea/Vomiting. Nausea/vomiting is usually an initial and transient symptom closely associated with vertigo, nystagmus and gait instability,[31] and is probably caused by involvement of vestibular nuclei and their connections. It may also be caused by involvement of a putative vomiting center near the nucleus ambiguus or the tractus solitaries.[147,153]

Horner Syndrome. Elements of Horner syndrome are frequent, occurring in about 90% of patients. This is caused by involvement of the descending sympathetic fibers in the lateral reticular substance. A constricted pupil with ipsilateral palpebral fissure narrowing is more frequently observed than facial anhidrosis.

Dysphagia, Dysarthria, Hoarseness. Involvement of the nucleus ambiguus results in paralysis of the ipsilateral palate, pharynx and larynx producing dysphagia, dysarthria and hoarseness. Dysarthria may also be attributed to the concomitant involvement of the cerebellum. Dysphagia is present in approximately two-thirds of LMI patients, among whom about 60% require a nasogastric tube for feeding.[31,153] Swallowing difficulty usually improves within days or months, but rare patients require persistent assistance in feeding. Dysphagia in LMI is more often associated with problems in the range of, than timing of, hyolaryngeal excursion.[158] During eating, foods are often stuck in the piriform recess of the pharynx, and patients attempt to extricate the material by a crowing-like cough. Hoarseness is equally common, while dysarthria is less common, occurring in about one-quarter of patients with pure LMI patients.[31] Some patients may show paralysis of the ipsilateral vocal cord.

Hiccup. Approximately one-quarter of patients develop hiccup,[31,153] often days after stroke onset. Hiccup usually goes away within a few days, but can persist for weeks or even months when it becomes a quite annoying symptom. Involvement of the dorsal motor nucleus of the vagus, solitary tract, and neurons related to expiration and inspiration in the reticular formation near the nucleus ambiguous may be responsible for hiccup.[31,147]

Sensory Symptoms/Signs

Sensory symptoms/signs are one of the most common manifestations of LMI. In the largest series, sensory function was intact in only 4% of patients.[31] Sensory symptoms/signs occur more frequently in the contralateral body/limbs (in approximately 85%) than in the face (58–68%),[149,151] and the sensory defect in the face usually clears more quickly than that on the body/limbs. Although a selective loss of spinothalamic sensation is a rule, vibration sensation is occasionally involved as well in the hypalgic body/limbs,[151] due probably to the fact that some of vibratory sensations are carried through the lateral column.[159]

Crossed (ipsilateral trigeminal-contralateral limb/body) sensory changes have been considered a typical sensory pattern in LMI. However, recent studies have identified that sensory findings are much more diverse in the acute stage.[151] In the largest series,[31] the patterns included ipsilateral trigeminal-contralateral limb/body in 26%, contralateral trigeminal-contralateral limb/body in 25%, bilateral trigeminal-contralateral limb/body in 14%, limb/body involvement without trigeminal involvement in 21% and trigeminal involvement without limb/body involvement in 10%. Although the arm and leg are usually equally involved, in approximately 30% of the patients, there is a discrepancy; some have more severe sensory deficits in the arm while others have more severe deficits in the leg.[151] The latter occasion is more common, and some may have a sensory level on the trunk mimicking a spinal cord syndrome.[160]

These diverse sensory manifestations are related to the varied patterns of involvement of the spinothalamic tract, descending trigeminal tract and ascending secondary trigeminal fibers (Fig. 26-14). In addition, approximately 7% of LMI patients have additional ipsilateral tingling sensation often associated with lemniscal sensory deficits, more marked in the arm than in the leg. Due to the leminscal sensory impairment, these patients often have a feeling of "clumsiness" or "weakness" in the ipsilateral extremities. This sensory pattern is related to involvement of the lower-most medulla, and explained by partial involvement of lemniscal sensory fibers at the upper-most part of the fasciculus cuneatus or crossing fibers to the medial lemniscus.[161]

In the descending trigeminal tract, the V3-representing area is located most dorsally and V1 most anteriorly, but in the ascending secondary trigeminal tracts, V3 is located most medially and V1 most laterally. Therefore, trigeminal sensory involvement is often inhomogeneous, more so on the contralateral side than ipsilateral side. On both sides, the inhomogeneity is either divisional or segmental (onion-skin) pattern.[146,147,151] Bilateral perioral paresthesia, often observed in patients with large infarcts extending medially,[151] may be caused by the simultaneous involvement of the descending and ascending V3 pathways near its decussation.[162,163] The perioral or V3 area is usually spared or less markedly involved

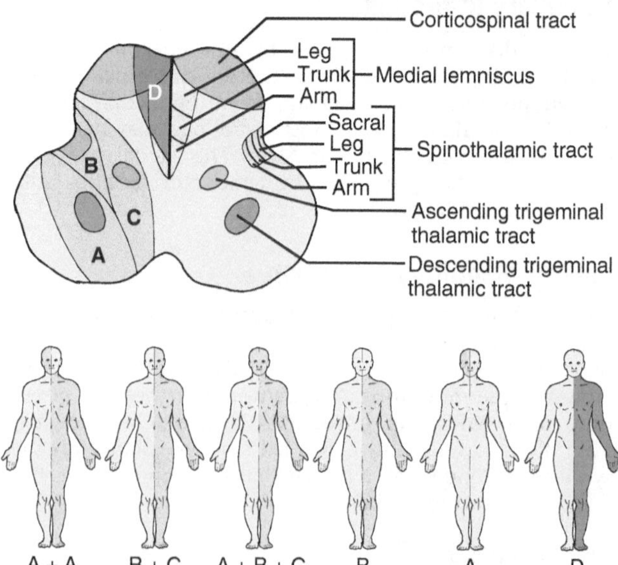

Figure 26-14. Anatomic structures of the medulla and various patterns of sensory dysfunction caused by medullary infarction. Yellow areas represent patterns of lateral medullary infarcts and red area represents the pattern of medial medullary infarction (see text for details). *(From Kim JS, Sensory abnormalities, In Caplan LR, van Gijn J, eds,* Stroke Syndrome *3rd ed, Cambridge University Press, 2012, pp. 11–20)*

on the side contralateral to the lesion, probably because the V3 area is located most medially in the secondary ascending trigeminal tract, and so less often affected by the lesion primarily involving the lateral part of the medulla.[151]

Finally, patients occasionally complain of facial pain. The pain usually appears at onset and heralds other symptoms and signs.[147] It is described as sharp, stinging, stabbing, or burning, tingling, and uncomfortably numb. The eyeball and surrounding area is the most commonly affected, but the entire face including the lips and inside the mouth may be involved. The reason for the occurrence of spontaneous pain, almost exclusively in the face, remains uncertain. Perhaps, involvement of the sensory nucleus of the descending tract of the 5th cranial nerve may explain the facial pain.

Headache. Headache occurs in about half of the patients.[31,153] It usually begins at onset or a few days before other symptoms/signs and subsides within several days. It most often occurs in the ipsilateral occipital or upper nuchal area followed by the frontal region, and is usually described as dull, aching or throbbing. Considering that headache occurs before other symptoms, and is not related to any symptoms/signs of LMI,[31] headache seems to be caused by an ICVA pathology, possibly related to dilatation of VA or collateral vessels after VA stenosis/occlusion,[153] rather than the medullary lesion itself. Involvement of the descending spinal tract of the fifth cranial nerve and its nucleus may also be responsible for frontal headache. Prominent and persistent nuchal pain may be a manifestation of VA dissection.

Facial Palsy. Facial palsy, usually mild and upper neuron type, is present in one-fifth to one-quarter of patients.[31] It is presumably caused by involvement of aberrant corticobulbar fibers that loop caudally before travelling rostrally toward the facial nucleus.[164] In patients with an upper-most medullary (or pontomedullary junction) lesion, there occurs relatively severe peripheral-type facial palsy due to direct involvement of facial nerve fascicles.[165]

Respiratory Difficulty and Other Autonomic Signs

The medullary reticular formation contains neurons related to the control of respiration, and patients may show respiratory arrest or decreased respiratory drive especially during sleep (Ondine's curse).[166] Severe respiratory abnormalities calling for medical attention are uncommon unless patients have bilateral or extensive lesions.[153] In pure LMI, aspiration pneumonia associated with dysphagia is the most common reason for respiratory care, in which case it is usually unclear how much respiratory control abnormality contributes to the patient's condition. Other autonomic disturbances such as tachycardia, bradycardia, sweating, orthostatic hypotension, gastric motility dysfunction, urinary retention are sporadically observed.

Ipsilateral Hemiparesis. Ipsilateral hemiparesis may be associated with other typical symptoms of LMI.[167]

The pathogenic mechanism of this so-called Opalski syndrome remains debatable. Recent imaging techniques such as diffusion-weighted MRI (DWI) and diffusion tensor imaging (DTI) showed that infarcts occurring at the lower-most medullary area or the medulla–spinal cord junction involve the ipsilateral corticospinal tract after the pyramidal decussation.[168,169] This observation corroborates with Opalski's original patients who showed hyperreflexia and Babinski signs. Concomitant infarcts in the spinal cord[170] may also produce Opalski syndrome.

In addition, patients with ipsilateral ataxia or lemniscal sensory dysfunction (see above) may complain of "clumsiness" or "weakness" in their limbs.[161] In view of transient motor deficits and absent reflex abnormalities in these patients, Kim suggested that most of the patients with ipsilateral "weakness" may be a pseudoparesis unrelated to pyramidal damage.[161] It seems that ipsilateral weakness in LMI patients may have diverse causes, and the term Opalski syndrome should be cautiously used.[168]

Clinical-topographical Correlation

The symptoms/signs of LMI are diverse and differ according to the topography of lesions. Currier et al.[147] was the first to divide the lesion topography into ventral, superficial, and dorsal, suggesting that clinical features vary according to the pattern. More recently, Kim et al.[31,152] analyzed the MRI-identified lesions in a 3D manner and made a clinical-topographical correlation.

Generally, rostral lesions tend to involve ventral, deep areas while caudal lesions involve lateral-superficial region[31,152] (Figs 26-15–26-18). This is probably related to the anatomical course of the ICVA; the ICVAs are located adjacent to the lateral surface at a caudal medulla level (Fig. 26-16), which ascend ventrorostrally (Fig. 26-18) to fuse into the BA at the pontomedullary junction. The rostral-ventral lesions tend to produce ipsilateral trigeminal sensory symptoms, whereas caudal-lateral superficial lesions tend to produce sensory levels with a gradient worse in the leg. A large, wide lesion is associated with a bilateral trigeminal sensory pattern[31] (Fig. 26-19), which is quite uncommon in patients with caudal lesions.

The more important rostrocaudal difference is dysphagia, which is distinctly more prevalent and severe in patients with rostral than in caudal lesions[31,152] (Figs 26-16, 26-18) This may be explained by: (1) caudal medullary lesions are usually thin (Fig. 26-16) and do not extend deeply as to involve the nucleus ambiguus, and (2) the lower part of the nucleus ambiguus is not directly related to pharyngeal muscle motility.[171] Facial palsy is also more common in rostral lesions.[31] In patients with most rostral lesions, often at the pontomedullary junction, dysphagia is slight or absent because the nucleus ambiguus is spared at this level.[172]

The caudal lesions are closely associated with severe lateropulsion and gait ataxia probably due to frequent involvement of the latero-dorsally located spinocerebellar tract and vestibular nuclei (Fig. 26-16). Dissection and headache are also more common in this group.

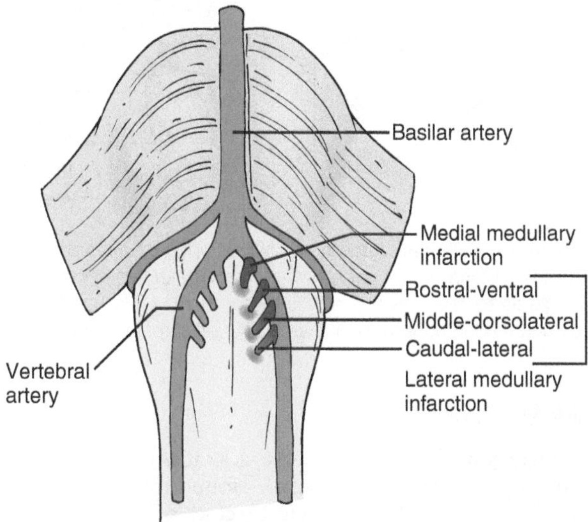

Figure 26-15. Schematic drawing indicating pathogenesis of various patterns of lateral medullary infarction and medial medullary infarction due to intracranial vertebral artery disease.

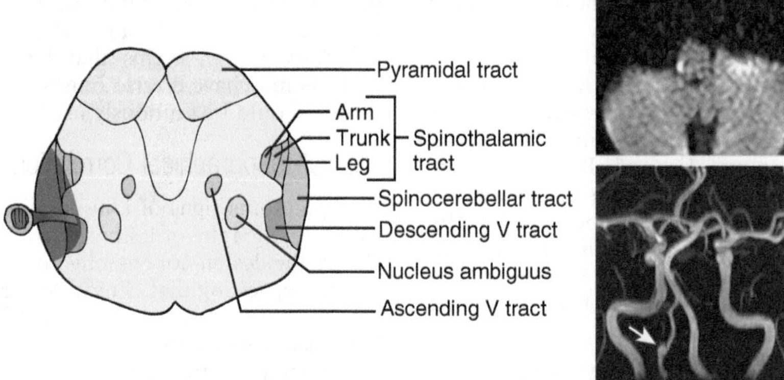

Figure 26-16. Schematic drawing showing important structures in the lower medulla and explaining caudal-lateral type of lateral medullary infarction (left image). Diffusion-weighted MRI shows a right caudal-lateral-type lateral medullary infarction (right upper image). This 46-year-old man had vertigo, headache, severe gait instability, Horner sign and right periorbital pain. Sensory deficits were detected below T4 level on the left side. He did not have dysphagia or dysarthria. The infarct was caused by right distal vertebral artery dissection (arrow, right lower image).

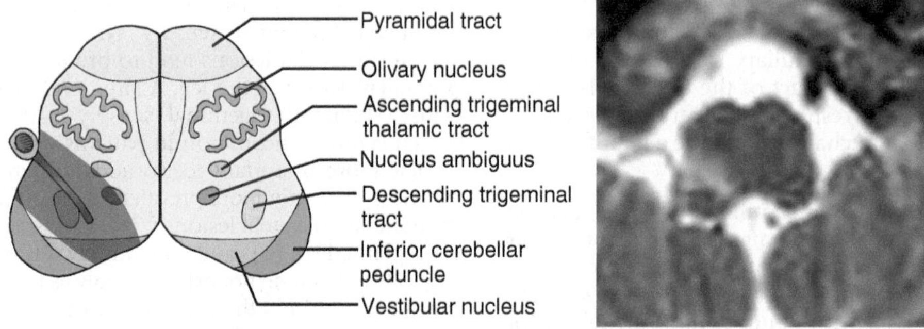

Figure 26-17. Schematic drawing showing important structures in the medulla and explaining middle-dorsolateral type of lateral medullary infarction (left image). MRI shows a right middle-dorsolateral type of lateral medullary infarction (right image). The patient had vertigo, gait ataxia, Horner sign and moderate degree of dysphagia, dysarthria and hoarseness. Sensory deficits were found in the right trigeminal area and left limbs and trunk.

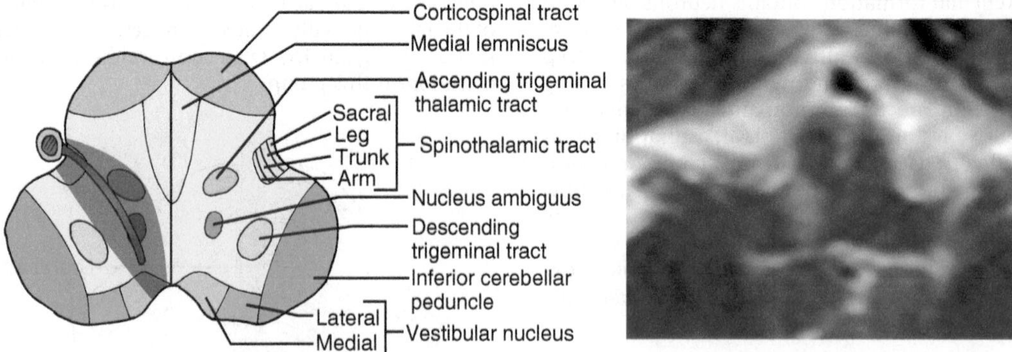

Figure 26-18. Schematic drawing showing important structures in the medulla and explaining rostral-ventral type of lateral medullary infarction (left image). MRI shows a right rostral-ventral type of lateral medullary infarction (right image). The patient had severe dysarthria, hoarseness and dysphagia as to need naso-gastric tube for feeding. He had mild dizziness, transient gait ataxia, and partial Horner sign. Sensory deficit was detected in the left right trigeminal area and left limbs and trunk.

Stroke Mechanisms

Wallenberg considered PICA disease as a cause of LMI.[143] More than half a century later, Fisher et al.[10] found sole involvement of the PICA in only two of their 17 cases of LMI. Fourteen patients showed ICVA steno-occlusion. Although the medial PICA gives rise to branches supplying the dorsal medulla, PICA disease producing pure LMI is uncommon. The most common cause of LMI is occlusion of penetrating branches associated with intracranial ICVA steno-occlusive disease.[10] In a large series that investigated 123 LMI patients,[31] ipsilateral ICVA steno-occlusive disease was present in 83 (67%) (33 distal ICVA disease, 34 whole ICVA disease and five proximal ICVA disease) and PICA disease in 12 (10%) patients. Atherothrombosis is a dominant pathology, while dissection of the ICVA or PICA is the cause of steno-occlusive lesions in

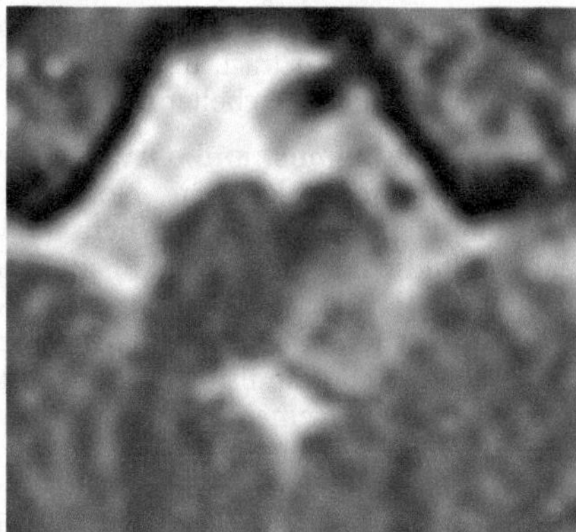

Figure 26-19. An example of large infarction encompassing both the dorsal and ventral parts of the lateral medulla that produces sensory disturbances in bilateral trigeminal areas and left limbs and trunk.

approximately 14–33% of cases.[31,149,150] In patients with normal angiographic findings, perforating artery disease seems to be the mechanism of infarction. Patients with large-artery disease either due to atherothrombosis or dissection more often show perfusion abnormalities than those with perorating artery disease.[173] Embolic occlusion of the PICA or distal ICVA from diseased heart or proximal artery atherosclerosis may also produce LMI,[26,59] but concomitant brainstem or cerebellar infarcts are usually present in these patients.

Prognosis

In patients with concomitant infarcts in other areas, the prognosis strongly depends on the location and extent of the extramedullary lesions. In patients with large PICA territory cerebellar infarction, massive edema and consequent herniation may yield a poor prognosis (see PICA infarction).

The prognosis of pure LMI is benign mainly due to the absence of significant motor dysfunction. The hospital mortality ranges from 0.8% to 11.6%.[31,144–146] Patients with large, rostral lesions tend to have severe dysphagia, aspiration pneumonia, requiring ICU care. Sudden respiratory (Ondine's curse) or other autonomic failure may produce respiratory-cardiac arrest, and physicians may have to keep this possibility in mind. Nevertheless, recent studies have shown very low hospital mortality, which is probably related to improved care for respiration, infection and dysphagia.[31]

Despite the benign overall outcome, the majority of survivors have at least one remaining sequelae. The most important one is sensory symptoms/signs followed by dizziness and dysphagia.[174] Usually, the most persistent and disturbing sequela correlates with the most severe initial symptom. Patients with rostral lesions tend to have dysphagia as a main sequela whereas those with caudal lesions tend to have long-standing dizziness. Approximately one-quarter of the patients develop uncomfortable painful paresthesia (central post-stroke pain, CPSP),[175] that is described as numb, burning or cold.[174] The symptoms usually occur in the body parts where the initial sensory perception deficit was most severe.

Patients with severe and extensive VA diseases more often develop recurrent cerebral infarction or coronary disease than those without.[144] The presence of posterior fossa hypoperfusion may also predict poor prognosis.[176]

Medial Medullary Infarction

Medial medullary infarction (MMI) was initially described by Spiller in 1908.[177] Dejerine later proposed a triad of symptoms: contralateral hemiplegia sparing the face, contralateral loss of deep sensation, and ipsilateral hypoglossal paralysis.[178] Pathological findings were first reported by Davison in 1937, who described thrombotic occlusion of the anterior spinal artery (ASA) and the adjacent ICVA.[179]

TABLE 26-2 Neurologic Symptoms and Signs Published in the Largest Series

Symptoms and Signs (n = 86)	
Motor dysfunction	78 (91)
	hemiparesis 68, quadriparesis 8, monoparesis 2
Facial paresis	21 (24)
Sensory dysfunction	59 (73)
	paresthesia 55
	impairment of objective sensory perception
	vibration 48
	position 41
	touch 32
	pinprick 17
	cold 22
Limb ataxia	36 (42)
Dysarthria	54 (63)
Dysphagia	25 (29)
Ipsilateral hypoglossal palsy	3 (3)
Contralateral tongue deviation	9 (10)
Vertigo/dizziness	51 (59)
Nausea/vomiting	14 (16)
Nystagmus	38 (44)
Diplopia	7 (8)
Headache	9 (10)

Number in parenthesis indicates percentage.
From Kim JS, Han Y, Medial medullary infarction: clinical, imaging, and outcome study in 86 consecutive patients. Stroke. *2009;40: 3221–3225*

With the advent of MRI, the pre-mortem diagnosis of MMI can easily be made, and understanding of the MMI syndrome has dramatically improved. Kim et al.[180] compared their own series of 17 patients diagnosed by MRI, with 26 previously reported patients (22 of them diagnosed by autopsy). They found that in the former group, bilateral lesions (1/17 vs 13/26), quadriparesis (none vs 11/26), lingual paresis (2/17 vs 12/26), and respiratory difficulty (none vs 7/26) were much rarer, and the prognosis was much better (all vs 6/26 survived). MMI is an example of concepts rapidly changing after the advent of modern brain imaging. Recent studies using MRI showed that bilateral lesions occur only in 0–18% of patients,[41,180–183] and that patients usually present with relatively benign, unilateral sensori-motor stroke.[180]

Clinical Manifestations

Symptoms and signs of MMI are summarized in Table 26-2.

Limb Weakness. Contralateral hemiparesis sparing the face is the most characteristic sign of MMI.[184] Quadriparesis occurs in less than 10% of patients.[31,41] When the weakness is severe, muscle tone may be initially flaccid, which becomes spastic overtime. Although rare, hemiparesis may occur on the ipsilateral side due to the lower-most lesion involving the crossed pyramidal tract.[180] The degree of motor dysfunction is variable; in one study,[41] it was severe (Medical Research Council scale ≤3) in 37%, two-thirds of whom had gradual progression of weakness during several days after onset.

Facial Palsy. Facial paresis is usually mild and transient; it occurs in one-quarter to one-half,[41,153] probably related to involvement of yet-uncrossed corticobulbar fibers directed to the contralateral cranial nuclei at the level of the upper medulla.[164]

Dysarthria, Dysphagia. In patients with quadriparesis, dysarthria and dysphagia are severe, whereas a nasogastric tube is required in less than 10% of those with unilateral lesions. However, a study using video fluoroscopic swallowing tests showed that dysphagia in MMI is not less frequent than LMI and is associated with delayed timing rather than reduced range of hyolaryngeal excursion.[158] Dysphagia in MMI may be attributed to damage to the corticobulbar tract or adjacent pattern generator regulating the nucleus ambiguus rather than direct involvement of this structure.

Ipsilateral Hypoglossal Nerve Palsy. Ipsilateral hypoglossal nerve palsy was one of the Dejerine symptom triad, and has been considered an important localizing sign. [178] Its prevalence is reported extremely variably, from 3% to 82%.[41,152,180–183] Recent MRI-based studies found a lower prevalence of ipsilateral hypoglossal palsy than earlier studies; a large series showed that definite ipsilateral hypoglossal paresis occurred in only 3% of patients while clumsy tongue movements with occasional contralateral tongue deviation were more common.[41] MRI-based studies emphasized that MMI lesions most often involve the rostral medulla, and the hypoglossal nerve nucleus and fasciculus, located in the lower medulla, are frequently spared.

Sensory Dysfunction. Sensory dysfunction is the second most important symptom/sign of MMI. Unlike LMI patients, MMI patients typically complain of tingling sensation from the onset. The involved area is usually hemibody/limbs below the ear or neck. However, sensory symptoms may extend to the face, probably due to additional involvement of the ascending trigeminal sensory tract. The facial sensory symptoms are usually mild, incomplete and transient. Occasionally, the sensory abnormality is restricted to a certain body part such as the lower leg.[185] Dermatomal distribution sensory abnormalities are also reported.[186] Although lemniscal sensory deficits are characteristic, mild and transient impairment of pain/temperature perception is occasionally present due possibly to involvement of the spinoreticulothalamic system that regulates the spinothalamic sensory system.[41,181,182]

Ataxia. Limb incoordination is occasionally noted[42,186] and is usually attributed to involvement of pontocerebellar fibers and/or associated proprioceptive sensory dysfunction. Gait instability or body lateropulsion may be related to involvement of the vestibulocerebellar tract, inferior olivary nucleus or more laterally located spinocerebellar tract.[182]

Vertigo/Dizziness, Nystagmus and Ocular Motor Disturbances. These symptoms/signs are closely related to involvement of the dorsal medulla,[41,187] where the vestibular nuclei, medial longitudinal fasciculus (MLF), and the nucleus prepositus hypoglossi (NPH) are located. In contrast to LMI, nystagmus is mostly ipsilesional, and ocular lateropulsion is to the contralateral side (contrapulsion).[188] Ocular lateropulsion may be related to involvement of neural pathways connecting the inferior olivary nucleus, cerebellar Purkinje cells, fastigial nucleus, and paramedian pontine reticular formation. Damage to the climbing fibers before (MMI) or after (LMI) decussation explains the opposite direction of ocular pulsion.[187,188] Upbeat nystagmus is observed in one-tenth to one-fifth of patients,[41,187] which may be explained by involvement of the VOR pathways from both anterior semicircular canals.[189] Unilateral lesions may also produce upbeat nystagmus[41] by damaging the decussating fibers from both anterior semicircular canals to ocular motor nuclei at the MLF in the rostral medulla.[189]

Emotional Disturbances. Previous reports have described patients presenting with pathological crying and laughing, depression and psychotic behaviors.[190,191] A recent study showed that emotional incontinence in MMI patients is as common as in those with pontine base infarction.[192]

Clinical-topographical Correlation

The majority of MMI lesions involve the rostral part of the medulla, and lesions limited to the caudal medulla are rare.[41] Ventro-dorsally, ventral lesions are closely related to motor dysfunction, middle lesions to sensory symptoms, and dorsal lesions are associated with vertigo, ataxia and ocular motor dysfunction (Fig. 26-20). The symptom correlation according to ventro-dorsal distribution is similar to that of pontine base infarction. Unlike pontine infarction, the face is mostly spared because the lesions are below the level of the facial nerve nucleus/fascicles. Sensory abnormalities are mostly lemniscal because lemniscal and spinothalamic tracts are separated in the medulla. In a large series, the lesion patterns included ventral in 20%, ventral+middle in 33% and ventral+middle+dorsal in 41%.[41]

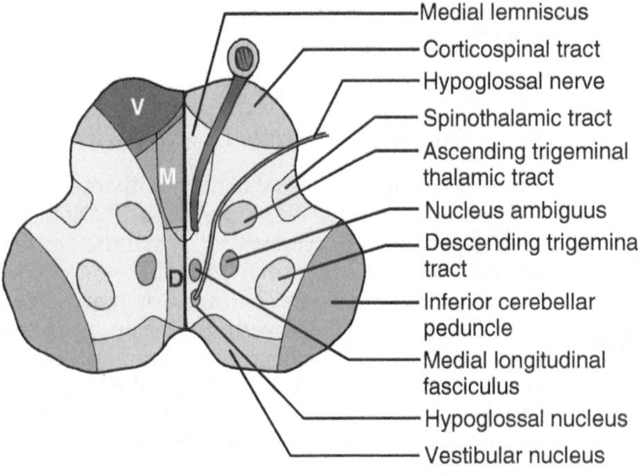

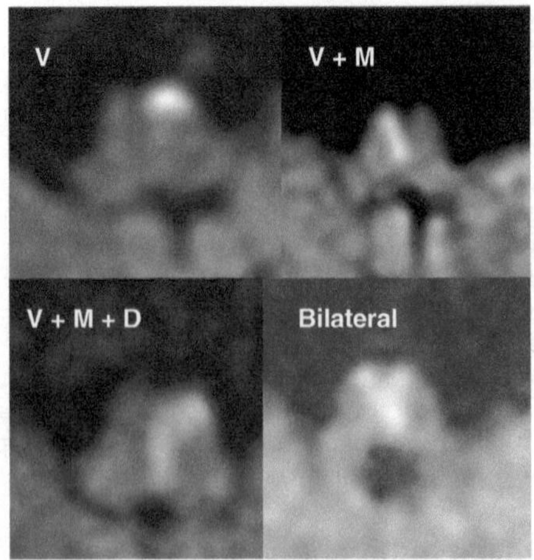

Figure 26-20. Left image: Schematic diagram showing structures in the rostral medulla, and the topographic patterns of medial medullary infarction, the ventral (V), middle (M), and dorsal (D) portions. Right image: MRI findings of representative patients (see text for details). *(Modified from Kim JS, Han YS. Medial Medullary Infarction: Clinical, Imaging, and Outcome Study in 86 consecutive patients.* Stroke *2009;40:3211–3225)*

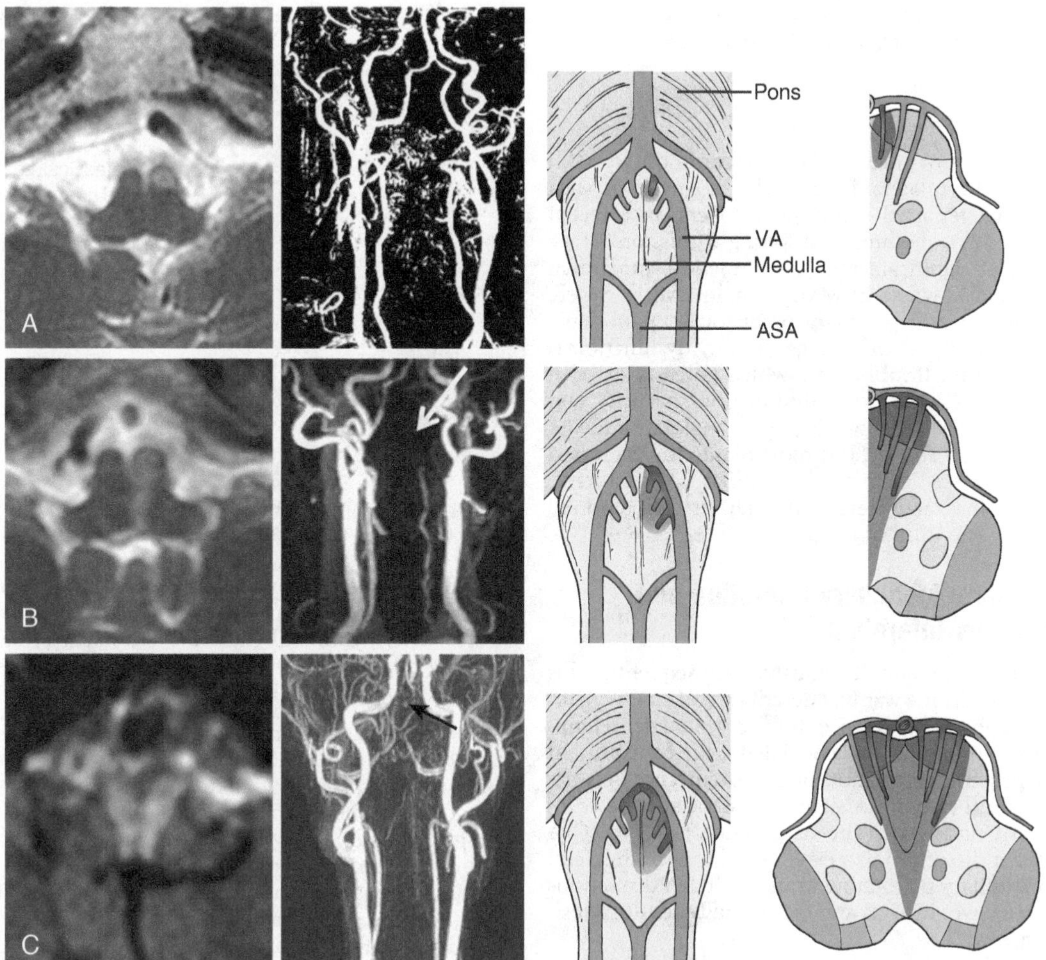

Figure 26-21. Illustrative patients and schematic drawings illustrating pathogenic mechanism of medial medullary infarction. Diagrams on the right show presumed stroke mechanism of small-vessel disease (upper) and branch occlusion resulting in unilateral (middle) and bilateral (low) infarcts. A, Small-artery disease. T2-weighted MRI (left image) shows an infarct involving the "V" portion only (V type), which produced pure motor stroke. MR angiogram (MRA) of the patient shows normal vertebral arteries (right image). B, Branch occlusion associated with vertebral artery disease causing unilateral infarction. T2-weighted MRI shows an infarct involving the V, M, and D (VMD type), which produced hemisensori-motor dysfunction, dizziness, and horizontal nystagmus (left image). MRA shows distal vertebral artery atherothrombotic occlusion (arrow) (right image). C, Branch occlusion associated with vertebro-basilar junction atherosclerosis causing bilateral infarction. Diffusion-weighted MRI shows bilateral infarcts, producing severe dysarthria, quadriparesis, and upbeat nystagmus (left image). MRA shows severe stenosis in the vertebrobasilar artery junction (arrow) (right image). VA, vertebral artery; ASA, anterior spinal artery. *(Modified from Kim JS, Han YS. Medial medullary infarction: clinical, imaging, and outcome study in 86 consecutive patients. Stroke 2009;40:3211–3225)*

Bilateral Medial Medullary Infarction

Bilateral MMI is uncommon. In one study, bilateral lesions occurred in 14%. Because the lesion on the one side is occasionally small and asymptomatic, quadriparesis was observed in 9%.[41] In patients with quadriparesis, MRI lesions are usually symmetrical and heart-shaped (Figs 26-20, 26-21). Patients have severe bulbar palsy and sensory symptoms, mimicking pontine locked in syndrome (see below, pontine infarction). Unless the dorsal pons is concomitantly involved, gaze is generally preserved. Nystagmus is common and patients usually suffer from prolonged dizziness.

Stroke Mechanism

Although ASA occlusion has traditionally been emphasized,[177–179] recent studies showed that MMI is more often caused by ICVA or ICVA-BA junction atherothrombotic diseases that obliterate perforating branches[193] (Figs 26-15, 26-21). In one series, relevant ICVA atherosclerotic disease was present in 62% of patients while perforator occlusion without ICVA disease (small artery disease) occurred in 28% of patients.[41] VA dissection may cause MMI, but is less common than in LMI. Infarcts associated with distal ICVA atherothrombotic disease tend to extend deeper and wider (occasionally resulting in bilateral lesions) than those of single perforator disease (Fig. 26-21), perhaps associated with either multiple perforator occlusion or more extensive hypoperfusion in the medulla.

ASA occlusion, although uncommon, may produce caudal MMI infarction. Rarely, embolic occlusion of ASA branches by talc[194] or fibrocartilaginous material,[195] or syphilitic arteritis[196,197] can cause MMI. Embolism from the diseased heart or proximal ECVA or ICVA disease is an uncommon cause of pure MMI.

Bilateral MMI may be caused by occlusion of one ASA supplying both parts of the medulla. However, a recent study[41] showed that bilateral MMIs are generally located rostrally in the territory of the distal ICVA or proximal BA. It seems that bilateral MMIs are usually caused by ICVA-BA atherothrombotic disease that obliterates multiple perforators bilaterally (Fig. 26-21).

Prognosis

Unlike LMI, aspiration pneumonia is uncommon in MMI except for those with bilateral lesions. The prognosis of MMI is better than that reported in the pre-MRI era; in a recent series of 86 patients, only three died during admission.[41] Due to the presence of significant motor dysfunction, functional outcome is generally worse in MMI than in LMI.[174] Severe initial motor dysfunction is a main predictor for poor functional outcome.[41] In the chronic stage, sensory dysfunction is equally prevalent and troublesome, which consists of both joint pain associated with motor dysfunction/spasticity and CPSP. In one study, CPSP defined by visual analogue scale ≥4 was present in 36%.[41] The CPSP is most frequently expressed as numb followed by aching, and unlike LMI patients, "burning" sensation is rarely described.[174] Dizziness is reported in approximately one-third of the patients.[41]

Combined Lateral Medullary Infarction and Medial Medullary Infarction

LMI and MMI may occur simultaneously or consequently. This hemimedullary syndrome was first described in 1894 by Reinhold[198] and by Babinski and Nageotte[199] 8 years later. Hemimedullary infarction is usually associated with concomitant infarcts in the posterior circulation, and its occurrence in isolation is rare. Clinical symptoms/signs are essentially the combination of LMI and MMI. The usual etiologies are ICVA atherosclerosis or dissection that extends to block both lateral and medial medullary perforating branches. ICVA dissections tend to produce lower infarcts and occasionally result in ipsilateral hemiparesis.[200]

Pontine Infarcts

Pontine infarction may occur in isolation or in association with other posterior circulation infarction. Hospital registry studies showed that patients with isolated pontine infarcts account for 2.6–3% of ischemic stroke and 12–15% of patients with posterior circulation infarcts.[201–203] One study from Asia showed a higher prevalence; 7.6% of cerebral infarcts and 28% of vertebrobasilar artery territory infarcts.[204]

Clinical Features

Motor Dysfunction (including Dysarthria and Ataxia). The pontine base contains fibers regulating motor function including descending corticospinal, corticopontocerebellar, and corticobulbar tracts (Fig. 26-22). Accordingly, pontine base infarction easily produces motor system dysfunction. Although limb weakness is the most common symptom, the clinical features depend upon the degree of involvement of each fiber tract. Fisher and his colleagues described pure motor stroke,[193] ataxic-hemiparesis,[63] dysarthria clumsy hand syndromes[61] as "lacunar" syndromes. However, other combinations are observed such as dysarthria-hemiataxia or dysarthria-facial paresis.[205] The categorization is not strict as patients with ataxic hemiparesis may evolve into pure motor stroke as the limb weakness progresses over time, or vice versa. Although uncommon, patients with ataxic hemiparesis may have additional ataxia on the side ipsilateral to the lesion;[205–207] this is attributable to involvement of the crossing corticopontocerebellar tracts.[207] Patients having bilateral ataxia frequently feel a sense of heaviness or weakness on both sides and have marked gait difficulty.[205]

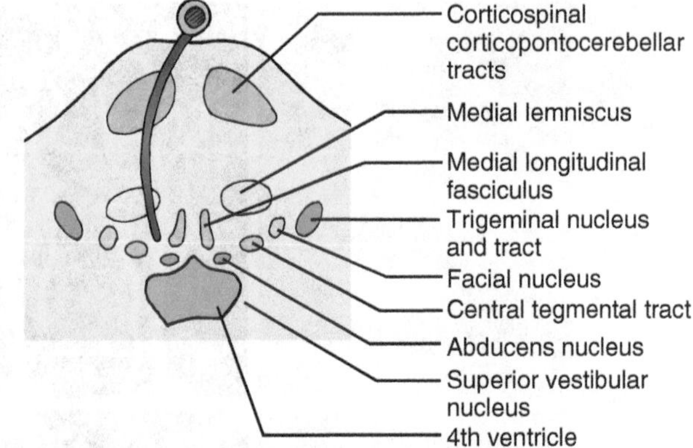

Figure 26-22. Schematic drawing showing structures in the pons and paramedian branch occlusion leading to pontine infarction.

Severe hemiparesis is usually associated with large lesions affecting the ventral surface of the caudal or middle pons, whereas similar-sized lesions tend to produce milder limb weakness but relatively prominent dysarthria (producing dysarthria clumsy hand) when they are located in the rostral pons; here, pyramidal tract fibers are sparsely arranged and located relatively laterally, and are, therefore, not extensively damaged by paramedian lesions.[205]

Sensory Dysfunction. Small tegmental pontine infarcts or hemorrhages that selectively involve sensory tracts (medial lemniscus and spinothalamic tract) produce a pure or predominant hemisensory deficit without other neurological dysfunctions[208,209] (Fig. 26-22). Although both the spinothalamic and lemniscal sensations are simultaneously involved, lemniscal sensations are usually more severely affected, probably because small infarcts tend to occur in the paramedian area where the medial lemniscus is located. Occasionally, patients have hemi-paresthesias without objectively detectable sensory deficits.

In the pontine medial lemniscal tract, the sensory projections from the arm, trunk and leg are arranged from a medial to lateral direction. Therefore, a medially located lesion preferentially affects the face and arm, causing a cheiro-oral syndrome whereas laterally located lesions produce leg-dominant sensory symptoms.[208] The most medially located lesions sometimes produce bilateral facial or perioral sensory symptoms due to involvement of trigemino-thalamic fibers bilaterally.[208] Occasionally, patients complain of bilateral "salt and pepper"-like sensations on the face,[162] which may herald significant neurological symptoms due to progressive BA occlusion. Cheiro-oral-pedal,[210] and oro-crural[211] sensory distribution patterns are also reported. Although these sensory manifestations are similar to those associated with lateral thalamic lesions, patients with a pontine pure sensory stroke more often have dizziness/gait ataxia, predominant lemniscal sensory involvement, and bilateral perioral involvement.[208]

Trigeminal sensory deficits are often noticed in patients with infarcts affecting the lateral pons usually accompanied by other symptoms of AICA territory infarction. Isolated trigeminal sensory symptoms without other neurological deficits may occur in patients with small strokes affecting the trigeminal fascicles or nucleus in the lateral pons.[212] Trigeminal sensory symptoms may be restricted to the intraoral area. This may be explained by an alleged functional anatomy that the most rostral part of the trigeminal tract/nucleus represents sensory fibers from the intraoral area.[213] Isolated involvement of taste sensation[214] or facial pains indistinguishable from idiopathic trigeminal neuralgia[215] have been reported in patients with small pontine infarction.

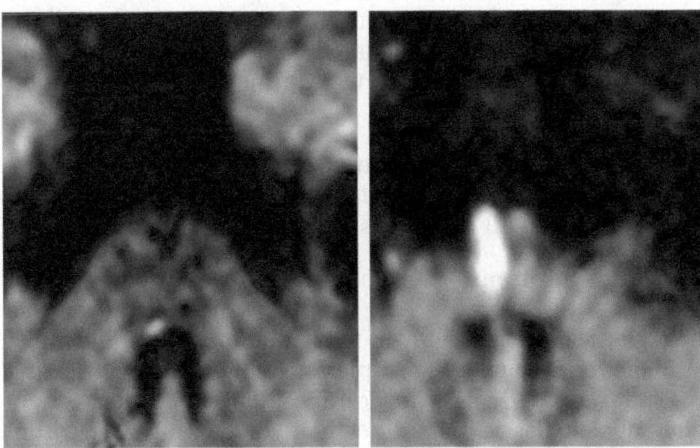

Figure 26-23. Diffusion-weighted MRI shows an infarct in the right lower pons (or pontomedullary junction). The patient showed right 6th and 7th nerve palsy and left hemiparesis (Millard-Gubler syndrome).

Ocular Motor Dysfunction. Structures related to ocular motor function such as abducens nucleus and fascicles, paramedian pontine reticular formation (PPRF) and medial longitudinal fasciculus (MLF) are located in the paramedian, dorsal pontine tegmentum (Fig. 26-22). Infarcts affecting this region cause various ocular motor dysfunctions.

6th Nerve Palsy. The abducens nucleus is located in the paramedian, dorsal, lower pons. Although rare, isolated 6th nerve palsy can result from a small pontine infarct that damages the abducens fascicles.[216–218] Because the abducens nucleus is surrounded by facial nerve fascicles, dorsal lesions involving the lower pons often produce both 6th and 7th nerve palsies, occasionally associated with contralateral hemiparesis (Millard-Gubler syndrome) (Fig. 26-23).

Internuclear Ophthalmoplegia. Internuclear ophthalamoplegia (INO) due to involvement of the MLF is much more common in patients with pontine infarction than 6th nerve palsy, probably because the MLF is a vertically long structure located in the paramedian area (Fig. 26-22), easily involved by deep, paramedian pontine infarcts. In the largest series that included 30 patients with INO with minimal neurologic deficits, authors found that they account for 0.47% of all ischemic stroke patients.[219] If the adjacent medial lemniscus or pontocerebellar fibers are involved, sensory symptoms, ataxia, and dysarthria are added. The lesions that extend laterally produce additional facial paresis.

The symptoms of INO are characterized by: (1) paralysis of adduction (or slowed adductive saccade when symptoms are mild) of the ipsilateral eye for all conjugate eye movements, (2) nystagmus in the contralateral eye when this eye is in abduction. Convergence is more often preserved than impaired. In pontine infarction, INO is usually unilateral whereas bilateral INO is more often caused by demyelinating diseases.[220] Although early authors attempted to separate posterior INO (normal convergence) from anterior INO (impaired convergence),[220] the difference in localization has not been proved. Some argue that the presence or absence of convergence may simply reflect the extent of the infarct.

The nystagmus appears to reflect an adaptive mechanism involving quick phases.[221] Occasionally, the contralateral eye is exotropic on neutral gaze, which is called "paralytic pontine exotropia". The exotropic gaze deviation is attributed to the unopposed tonic activity of the spared PPRF on the side opposite to a unilateral lesion. Although less common, some patients with bilateral INO show bilateral exotropia, a phenomenon referred to as "wall-eyed bilateral internuclear ophthalmoplegia (WEBINO)".[222] The mechanism of WEBINO is uncertain since bilaterally involved PPRF (no excessive activity of PPRF) cannot theoretically produce bilateral pontine esotropia. WEBINO may be caused by a lesion in the midbrain involving the medial rectus subnuclei,[223] as well as the MLF bilaterally.

The INO is frequently associated with contraversive ocular tilt reaction (OTR) (subjective visual vertical, ocular torsion or skew deviation), probably because graviceptive pathways join the MLF after crossing between the vestibular and abducens nuclei.[224] OTR improves faster than INO, suggesting that vestibular tone imbalance is more easily compensated by central vestibular adaptation mechanisms.

Conjugate Horizontal Gaze Palsy. Fibers from the frontal eye fields affecting conjugate lateral gaze cross at or near the level of the abducens nucleus in the pons and end in the reticular gray region called PPRF adjacent to the contralateral abducens nucleus.[225] Involvement of the PPRF leads to the absence of voluntary lateral gaze to the side of the lesion, including the quick phase of nystagmus. Patients' eyes remain at the midline in attempted ipsilateral saccade, or when they begin in a position contralateral to the lesion, return to the midline slowly.[226] The vestibular ocular reflex and ipsilateral smooth pursuit usually remain intact because relevant pathways do not pass through the PPRF. Bilateral lesions involving the abducens nucleus and PPRF produce paralysis of all horizontal eye movements. Although vertical gaze is mediated at a more rostral level, patients with bilateral horizontal gaze palsies may show slow vertical gaze saccades or limitation of upgaze. This is probably related to the fact that the omnipause neurons that modulate saccadic triggering are also involved in vertical saccades via sending signals to the rostral interstitial MLF (riMLF).[227] Vertical gaze palsy improves faster than horizontal palsy.[228]

One-and-a-Half Syndrome. Fisher[229] introduced the term one-and-a-half syndrome to refer to "a paralysis of eye movements in which one eye lies centrally and fails completely to move horizontally while the other eye lies in an abducted position and cannot be adducted past the midline." A unilateral pontine lesion involving the PPRF produces an ipsilateral conjugate gaze palsy and also affects the MLF on the same side, which leads to paralysis of adduction of the ipsilateral eye on conjugate gaze to the opposite side.[230] Lesions that produce one-and-a-half syndrome are usually larger than those producing INO, and are more often accompanied by other neurological deficits. Patients who initially present with one-and-a-half syndrome occasionally evolve into INO over time as the symptoms improve.

Ocular Bobbing and Other Related Signs. Fisher[231] introduced the term ocular bobbing: "The eyeballs intermittently dip briskly downward through an arc of a few millimeters and then return to the primary position in a kind of bobbing action." Ocular bobbing is an ominous sign, usually associated with extensive, bilateral pontine infarcts or hemorrhages.[231,232] Quadriparesis and decreased consciousness are usually present. Bobbing is usually bilateral and symmetric, but can be predominantly unilateral or asymmetric.[229,233] Asymmetric bobbing is common in patients in whom there is an asymmetric paralysis of either conjugate gaze or ocular abduction. When bobbing is asymmetric, usually the eye ipsilateral to the side of limited gaze bobs when gaze is directed to that side.[229,231] In patients with extensive pontine lesions, horizontal gaze is lost, but vertical gaze is preserved; the vertical vector of gaze may be accentuated so that the eyes "bob" down.[232,234] A unilateral bob when the affected eye is pointed toward the direction of paralytic lateral gaze, further supports this hypothesis.

In patients with bilateral pontine infarcts, ptosis of the upper eyelids is also frequent,[234] usually attributed to involvement of descending sympathetic fibers in the lateral pontine tegmentum. The pupils become small (pinpoint pupil),[229] but pupillary response to light is usually preserved if examined by magnifying glass.

Involuntary Movements.

Palatal Myoclonus. Palatal myoclonus is a rhythmic involuntary jerking movement of the soft palate and pharyngopalatine arch, often involving the diaphragm and laryngeal muscles.[235]

Palatal myoclonus does not appear in the acute stage of stroke, but develops several months later. Occasionally, rhythmic, jerky movements are also observed in the face, eyeballs, tongue, jaw, vocal cord or extremities (mostly hands); they may not be synchronous with palatal movements. The movements of the palate vary in rate between 40 and 200 beats per minute. The movements may involve the Eustachian tube and make a click that the patient can hear.

The posited anatomical lesion involves the "Guillain-Mollaret triangle" which includes the dentate nucleus of the cerebellum, the red nucleus in the midbrain, and the inferior olivary nucleus in the medulla and their interconnections.[236] The pathologic lesion most often seen in these patients is hypertrophic degeneration of the inferior olive. Enlarged neurons and diffuse gliosis are observed. In patients with pontine strokes, damage on the central tegmental tract, and consequent hypertrophic degeneration of the inferior olive is considered to be a mechanism related to palatal myoclonus (Fig. 26-24).

Periodic Limb Movements and Restless Legs. Periodic limb movements or restless legs are involuntary movements associated with sleep disturbances. Periodic limb movements[237] and restless-leg-like symptoms[238] may occur after unilateral pontine base infarction. The presumed mechanisms are disinhibited propriospinal/segmental spinal reflexes or dopaminergic fibers involvement due to pontine reticular formation lesions.[237,239]

Other Cranial Nerve Dysfunction. 5th, 7th, and 8th nerve nerves or fascicles are involved when lesions are laterally situated. This issue will be discussed in the AICA syndrome.

Auditory Symptoms. After entering into the cochlear nucleus some auditory fibers ascend directly while others traverse through the trapezoid body to the contralateral lateral lemniscus. Due to the bilateral, complex auditory pathways, hearing loss is rare in patients with pontine infarction unless the 8th nerve nucleus/fascicles are directly involved in AICA territory infarction.

However, extensive and destructive lesions involving the tegmental area may produce auditory symptoms. Bilateral total deafness was reported in a patient with extensive tegmental hemorrhage.[240] More often, tinnitus and auditory hallucination, usually associated with a certain degree of hearing impairment, are found in patients with pontine strokes.[241–243] The auditory hallucinations are considered a central "release phenomenon" in the setting of peripheral input deficiency. The hallucination often disappears as the hearing loss improves.[243] For unclear reasons, hallucinations are mostly musical, i.e., songs, drum sound, etc. Contralateral hyperacousis has also been observed in a patient with unilateral pontine tegmental stroke,[244] possibly attributed to hypersensitization phenomenon similar to CPSP after damage on the sensory tract.

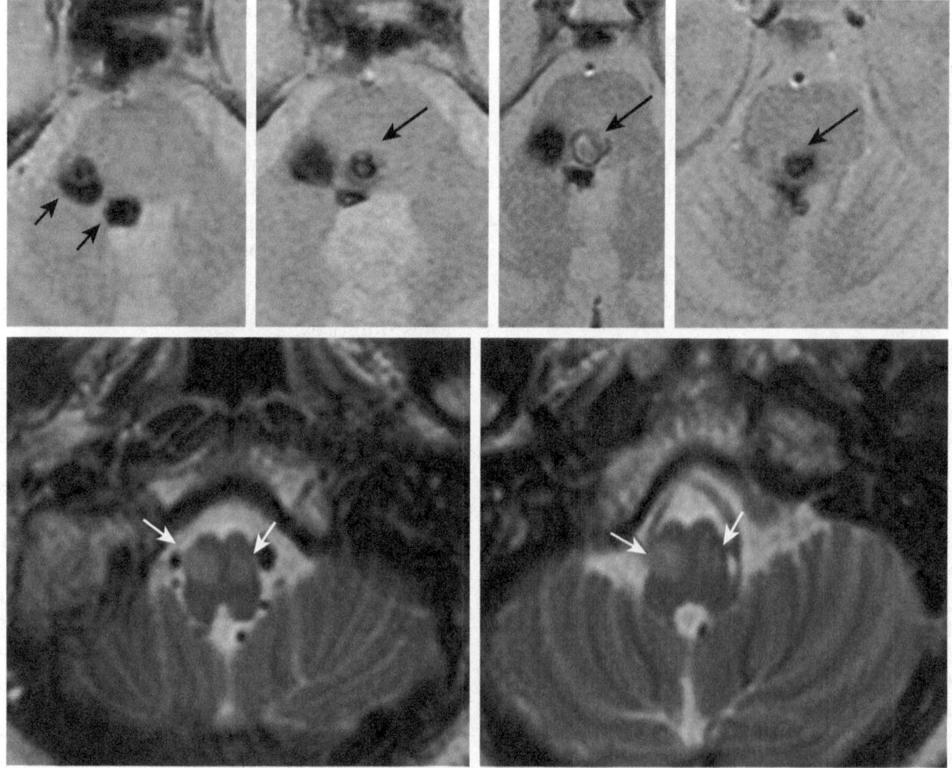

Figure 26-24. A 56-year-old woman developed right facial numbness. Three months later she developed tingling sensation on the left limbs. Neurological examination showed sensory deficits on the left face and limbs. MRI showed two previous, old hemorrhages on the right middle cerebellar peduncle (short, black arrows) and a recent hemorrhage (long, black arrows) on the right pontine tegmentum. They were considered to be due to multiple carvernous malformation. Four months later she started to experience dizziness and a regular clicking sound in the ear. Neurological examination showed newly developed right beating, horizontal and rotational nystagmus and palatal myoclonus. MRI showed bilateral olivary nuclei hypertrophy in the medulla (white arrows).

Consciousness Disturbances or Coma. Patients with bilateral, extensive pontine infarcts caused by sudden BA occlusion often present with decreased consciousness or even coma, probably related to involvement of brainstem reticular activating structures responsible for the regulation of alertness.

Abnormalities of Respiration. Abnormalities of respiration are also common, but their mechanism is difficult to determine because of the extensiveness of the infarction and the presence of general medical factors (e.g., aspiration, fever, and hypoventilation). Apneustic breathing with a hang-up of the inspiratory phase and grossly irregular breathing (ataxic respirations) occasionally occur terminally in patients with BA occlusion and indicate an ominous prognosis.[245]

Emotional Disturbances. Pathological laughing or crying occasionally occur in patients with pontine infarction.[204–206,246] Patients with bilateral pontine lesions have more frequent and severe symptoms. Recent studies[192,247] focusing on poststroke emotional symptoms showed that excessive or inappropriate laughing/crying is fairly common, occurring in 33–50% of the patients with unilateral pontine base infarction. Depression was less common, occurring in 16%.[192] Patients with tegmental lesions rarely showed emotional disturbances.

The relatively frequent emotional disturbances in pontine base infarction may be attributed to involvement of profuse serotonergic fibers from the brainstem raphe nuclei projecting to the basal ganglia or the cerebellum.[192,248,249] Another closely related emotional symptom, anger proneness (excessive or inappropriate anger) is equally common in patients with pontine base infarction.[247] Mania[250] and psychotic behaviors[251,252] are also observed, but are distinctly uncommon.

Clinical-topographical Correlation

Old reports extensively described bilateral pontine infarcts; however, in the era of MRI, unilateral pontine infarct is much more common, occupying approximately 90% of isolated pontine infarction.[201,202]

Unilateral Infarcts

In one study examining 49 patients with unilateral paramedian infarcts, 27 patients had basal infarcts, 15 basal-tegmental infarcts and seven had infarcts limited to the tegmental area.[204]

Unilateral Paramedian Basal Infarcts

Paramedian infarction involving mainly the pontine base is the most common pattern occurring in 54–58% of isolated pontine infarctions.[201,203,204] Motor dysfunction is the main symptom (Fig. 26-25A). Lesions extending dorsally to involve the tegmentum produce sensory symptoms as well (Fig. 26-25B). According to a study that evaluated 37 patients with acute, unilateral infarcts that mainly involved the pontine base,[205] the clinical presentations included pure motor hemiparesis in 17, sensorimotor stroke in three, ataxic hemiparesis in four, and dysarthria-clumsy hand syndrome in six patients. One patient had dysarthria-hemiataxia, two had quadrataxic-hemiparesis, and four had dysarthria-facial paresis.

Acute or subacute neurologic progression occurs in upto one-quarter of patients with pontine base infarction, along with subacute lesion volume increase.[32] It seems that infarcts in the lower pons are more often associated with progressive

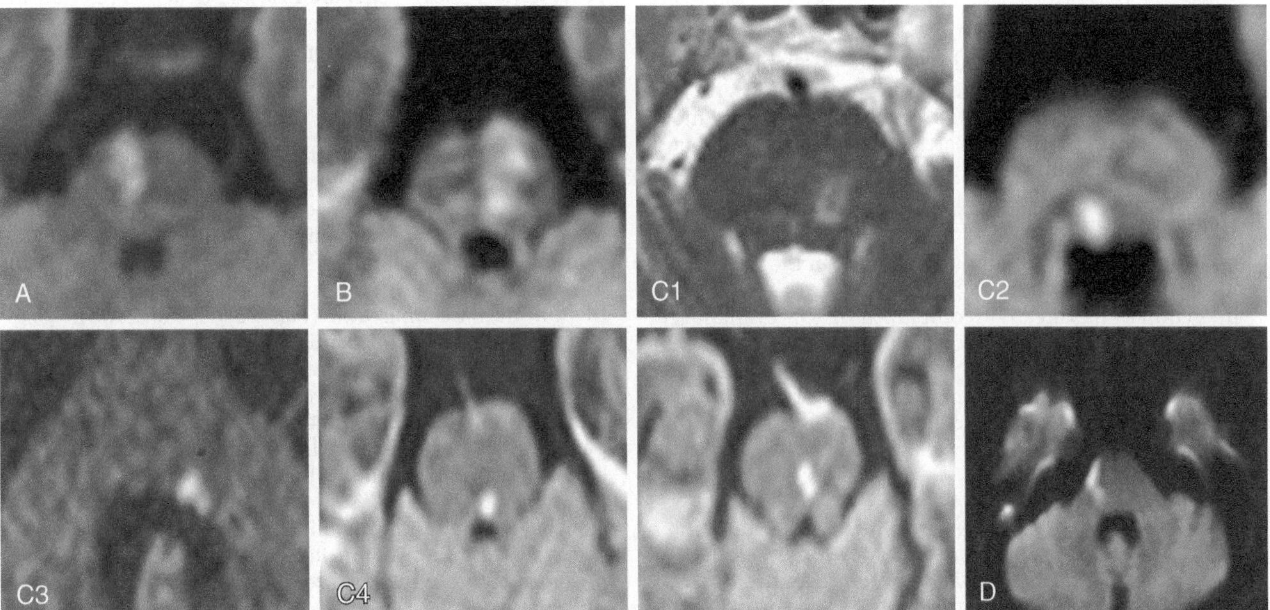

Figure 26-25. Patterns of unilateral pontine infarction. A, Paramedian basal infarction. The patient had pure motor stroke (left hemiparesis, facial palsy and dysarthria) due to involvement of the corticospinal and corticobulbar tracts. B, Combined basal-tegmental infarction. The patient had sensorimotor stroke (right hemiparesis, facial palsy and sensory deficit) due to involvement of both the descending corticospinal tract and ascending medial lemniscus. C, Paramedian tegmental infarction. C1, The infarct restricted to the pontine tegmentum produced right hemisensory deficit (pure sensory stroke), probably due to selective involvement of the medial lemnscus. C2, The infarct involving the most dorsal part of the tegmentum produced isolated internuclear ophthalmoplegia due to selective involvement of the medial longitudinal fasciculus. C3, Dorsally located and slightly laterally extended infarct produced left internuclear ophthalmoplegia and peripheral-type facial palsy, due probably to involvement of the medial longitudinal fasciculus and the genu portion of the facial nerve fascicle. C4, A dorsal tegmental infarct (left image) slightly extending ventrally (right image) produced internuclear ophthalmoplegia and right hemisensory disturbances, due to involvement of both the medial longitudinal fasciculus and the medial lemniscus. D, Circumferential artery territory (ventroloateral) infarcts. The patient had left hemisensory disturbances associated with mild and transient left hemiparesis.

worsening and poorer functional outcome than upper pontine lesions.[204]

Unilateral Paramedian Tegmental Infarction

Unilateral tegmental infarction is the second most common pattern of pure pontine infarction, occurring in 12–31% of patients.[201,202,204] Unilateral tegmental infarcts frequently produce hemisensory syndromes[208] (Fig. 26-25, C1), while more dorsally located lesions produce ocular motor dysfunction. The most common ocular motor dysfunction is an INO[219] (Fig. 26-25, C2), but one-and-a-half syndrome and horizontal gaze palsy also occur.[204] Involvement of adjacent structures such as facial nerve/fascicules may produce INO plus peripheral-type facial palsy (Fig. 26-25, C3). Relatively large lesions result in both hemisensory syndromes and ocular motor dysfunction (Fig. 26-25, C4).

Combined Basal–tegmental Infarction

Paramedian pontine base infarction may extend dorsally to involve the tegmental portion (Fig. 26-25, B). The clinical features are essentially a combination of basal and tegmental syndromes.

Unilateral Circumferential Artery Territory (Ventrolateral) Infarcts

Ventrolateral territory infarcts were reported to occur in 17–25% of patients with isolated pontine infarction.[201,202] However, it is often difficult to clearly differentiate the ventrolateral from the ventromedial group, and some studies did not separate them.[203,204] Follow-up DWI examinations often show that small, laterally placed infarcts evolve into larger ones involving the ventromedial area as well. Therefore, infarcts strictly limited to the ventrolateral area may be less common. Clinical features are similar to those of paramedian infarcts. However, hemiparesis is relatively mild, probably because pyramidal motor fibers located in the paramedian area are generally spared (Fig. 26-25, D). Accordingly patients more often present with ataxic hemiparesis, dysarthria clumsy hand syndrome, or predominant hemisensory symptoms.

Unilateral Dorso-lateral Infarcts

The dorsolateral areas are supplied by AICA in the lower pons and SCA in the upper pons.

Infarction of this area is accompanied by concomitant cerebellar infarcts and rarely involved in isolation. Trigeminal sensori-motor dysfunction, 6th nerve palsy, 7th nerve palsy, auditory disturbances and contralateral sensory dysfunction are usually observed. Contralateral hemiparesis is rare or mild when present.

Bilateral Infarcts

Bilateral infarcts are usually associated with BA occlusion and result in grave neurological symptoms. As the bilateral lesions almost always involve the ventral part, involving the corticospinal tracts, quadriparesis is usual.[54,251,253] The quadriparesis may start from the beginning; more often, the initial motor dysfunction is lateralized to one side and then progresses.[254] Hemiparetic patients with BA occlusion often show some motor or reflex abnormalities on the non-paretic side such as clumsiness, ataxia, hyperreflexia and extensor plantar reflex. Occasionally, there are abnormal movements such as shivering, twitching, shaking or jerking of the relatively spared side which may be precipitated by painful stimuli.[255] Unless successful therapy (e.g., recanalization) is quickly performed, asymmetrical motor disturbances often progress to severe quadriplegia. The progression usually occurs within 24 hours,[256] but may be delayed up to several days (Fig. 26-26).

Ataxia or incoordination is another common finding, observed in the limbs that are not severely paretic. The ataxia is invariably bilateral but is frequently asymmetric. Dysarthria and dysphagia due to bilateral bulbar muscle paresis are also common, associated with bilateral facial weakness, tongue weakness and limited jaw movements. Some patients become totally unable to speak, open their mouth, or protrude their tongue. The jaw, face, and pharyngeal reflexes may be hyperactive and even clonic. Secretions pool in the pharynx and are an important cause of aspiration pneumonia. Somatosensory abnormalities should also be common, but they are usually overshadowed by motor dysfunction and cannot be precisely assessed in patients with a severe condition. Occasionally, patients complain of uncomfortable paresthesias or CPSP.

Because large bilateral pontine infarcts frequently involve the dorsal tegmental area, ocular motor dysfunction is also common, including INO, horizontal gaze palsy, one-and-a-half syndrome, and sixth nerve palsies. Ocular bobbing, ptosis and pinpoint pupils strongly suggest extensive, bilateral tegmental lesions (see above). Symptoms such as tinnitus, hearing loss and auditory hallucination are related to involvement of the central auditory tracts or the 8th nerves/fascicles. Some may develop delayed-onset palatal myoclonus.

Altered consciousness is an important sign in patients with sudden BA occlusion and is related to bilateral medial tegmental pontine ischemia. Usually, the level of consciousness improves over time even if other neurological deficits persist. Patients may show pathological crying and laughing spells that are triggered by minimal social-emotional stimuli. When all voluntary movements are lost, the deficit is referred to as the "locked-in" syndrome. Vertical eye movements are usually spared, and are used for simple communication.

Stroke Mechanisms

Unilateral infarcts involving the ventral pons are caused either by large-artery disease or penetrating artery disease. Studies primarily using MRA revealed BA atherosclerotic stenosis was associated with 23% of pontine infarction,[201] and 39–50% of pontine base infarction.[32,202,204] Therefore, branch occlusion associated with BA stenosis is an important stroke mechanism of pontine base infarction (Figs 26-7A, 26-25A,B). Even in patients without MRA-identified BA stenosis, small plaques that obstruct the orifice of perforating branches are occasionally seen if high-resolution vessel wall MRI is used.[47] Pontine infarcts limited to the tegmental area are mostly caused by penetrating artery disease (lipohyalinosis) (Figs 26-7C, 26-25C) unassociated with BA disease.[201,204,208] Although uncommon, however, the most dorsally located infarcts may be associated with significant, bilateral ICVA or BA steno-occlusive disease. Restoration of BA flow through collaterals (e.g., the posterior communicating artery) explains the sparing of most of the pons.[219]

In patients with bilateral pontine infarction, significant BA steno-occlusive disease is usually present.[251] Bilateral ICVA occlusion is often accompanied (Fig. 26-26). Pathologically, the vast majority is atherothrombosis, and dissection is uncommon as compared to medullary infarction. Occasional patients with bilateral pontine infarcts have sequential infarcts caused by occlusion of BA branches on both sides. In these patients, a hemiparesis is followed days, weeks, or months later by another event that leads to paresis on the other side of the body. Embolism is a less common cause of isolated pontine infarction.

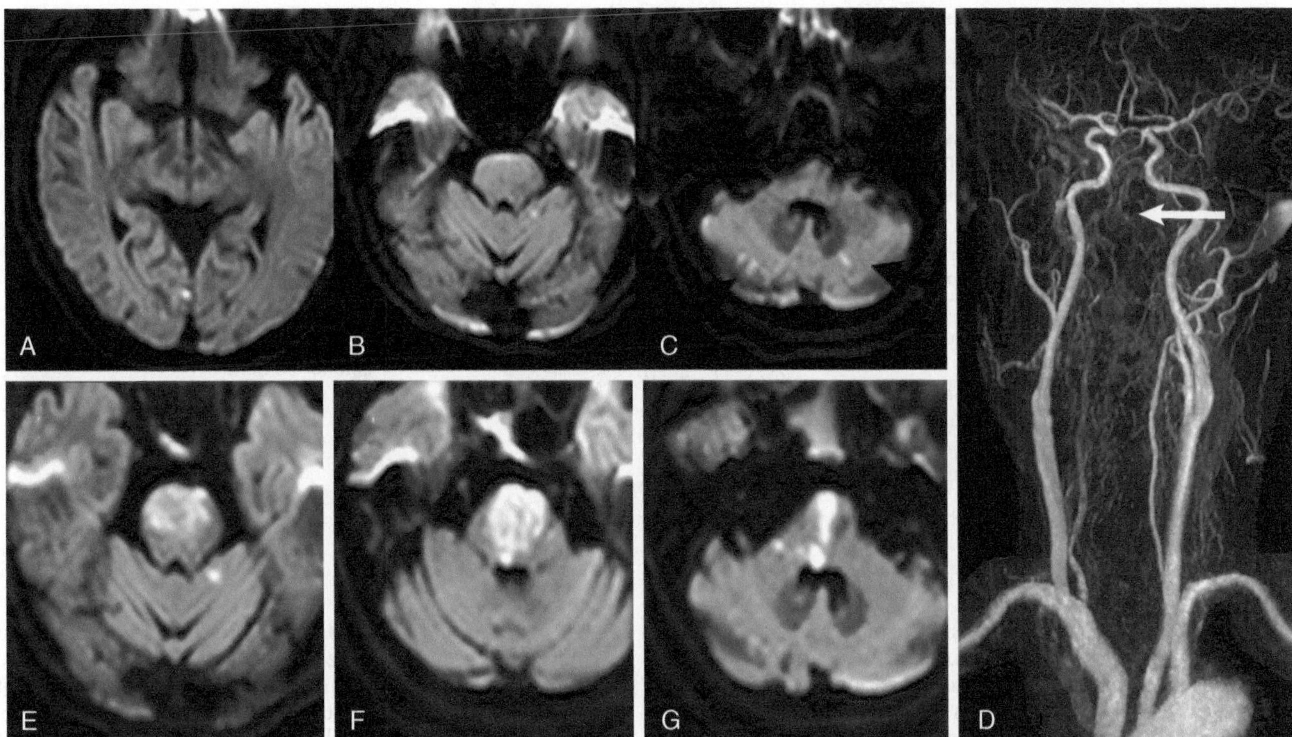

Figure 26-26. A 73-year-old man with hypertension and a history of cigarette smoking developed recurrent episodes of dizziness followed by left hemiparesis that progressed to quadriparesis 10 days later. Initial diffusion-weighted MRI showed tiny, scattered infarcts involving the right occipital area and the cerebellum (A, B, and C). No definite lesions were identified in the pons. MR angiogram showed thrombotic occlusion of both distal vertebral arteries and basilar artery (D, arrow). Intra-arterial thrombolysis was attempted, but failed to recanalize the vessel (not shown). Follow-up diffusion-weighted MRI showed bilateral pontine infarction (E, F, and G). MR angiogram showed persistent occlusion of the basilar artery (not shown). The patient remained in a locked-in state. *(From Caplan LR, Amarenco P, Kim JS. Posterior circulation disorders. In, Kim JS, Caplan LR, Wong KSL ed.* Intracranial Atherosclerosis, *pp 83–99, with permission.)*

Prognosis

Unless accompanied by infarcts in other areas, the prognosis of unilateral pontine infarction is relatively favorable. Most patients survive the acute stage. Their functional deficits depend upon residual neurologic severity. Patients with initially severe hemiparesis, progressive worsening, bilateral ataxia, and with lower pontine lesion have relatively unfavorable functional outcomes.[201,204,205] The prognosis of patients with tegmental lesions is even better. However, patients with severe sensory deficits may have difficulty in performing fine movements due to sensory deficits. More problematic is the development of CPSP, which usually remains persistent once it develops. When patients have INO as an isolated symptom, INO mostly improves.[219] However, in patients with more extensive ocular dysfunction associated with other major neurologic sequelae, residual ocular motor dysfunction frequently remains, and patients suffer from diplopia and dizziness. The prognosis of bilateral pontine infarcts presenting with quadriparesis is ominous. Most patients die or remain bed-ridden. Some have persistent diplopia, dizziness or palatal myoclonus.

Midbrain Infarction

The midbrain is mainly supplied by branches arising from the PCA, upper BA, SCA, and the anterior choroidal artery (Fig. 26-27). It is often affected in patients with embolic stroke occurring in the posterior circulation usually with the concomitant involvement of other structures such as the pons, thalamus and cerebellum.[257] According to New England Medical Center Registry, midbrain infarction is tenfold more likely to be accompanied by ischemia of neighboring structures than it is to occur in isolation.[258] Isolated midbrain infarcts account for 0.2–2.3% of admitted ischemic strokes.[40,259,260] While one study showed that pure midbrain infarct occupied only 0.7% of posterior circulation ischemic stroke,[258] another reported that it represented 8% of posterior circulation infarcts.[259]

Clinical Features

The 3rd nerve palsy has been considered the most important clinical feature indicating midbrain stroke. However, with the advent of MRI, it has been recognized that non-localizing "lacunar" syndromes are actually quite common. In the largest series assessed by MRI,[40] clinical manifestations included gait ataxia (68%), dysarthria (55%), limb ataxia (50%), sensory symptoms (43%), third nerve palsy (35%), limb weakness (≤ IV/V) (23%), and INO (13%).

Ocular Motor Dysfunction. Ocular motor dysfunction in patients with midbrain infarcts includes 3rd nerve palsy, INO, vertical gaze disturbances, skew deviation, and rarely, 4th nerve palsy. As the 3rd nerve nuclei, fascicles and the MLF are all located in the paramedian area, paramedian lesions tend to produce ocular motor disturbances. The lesions often involve adjacent pyramidal or cerebellar tracts resulting in additional contralateral hemiparesis (Weber syndrome) or hemiataxia (Claude syndrome). Small infarcts may produce isolated ocular motor dysfunction.[218]

Third Nerve Palsy. Although 3rd nerve palsy has been considered a clinical hallmark of midbrain infarction, it occurs in

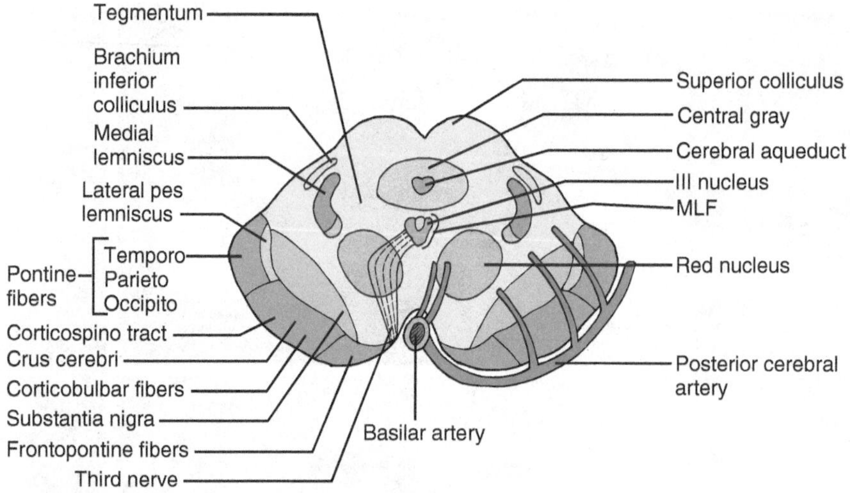

Figure 26-27. Schematic drawing showing important structures in the midbrain and main vascular supply.

only 33–50%[40,259,261] of patients with pure midbrain infarction. Third nerve palsy can be caused by involvement of either the 3rd nerve fascicles or the nucleus. Lesions that affect the 3rd nerve nucleus often cause bilateral ptosis and upgaze deficits; this is attributed to involvement of the caudal subnucleus supplying both levator palpebrae, and the crossing fibers from the contralateral subnucleus of the superior rectus, repectively, within the 3rd nucleus complex.[262]

The 3rd nerve palsy is frequently incomplete, and certain ocular muscles may be selectively involved. For example, divisional oculomotor paresis was reported to be caused by midbrain lesions involving the fascicle suggesting the functional separation of superior (subserving levator palpebrae, superior rectus) and inferior (subserving inferior and medical rectus and inferior oblique) divisions within the brainstem in the fascicular portion of the nerve.[263] Patients with a tiny lesion within the 3rd nucleus may even produce weakness of a single extraocular muscle such as the inferior rectus[218]) or medial rectus.[264] A very small infarct was reported to produce isolated inferior rectus palsy due to selective involvement of the relevant fascicle.[265]

Internuclear Ophthalmoplegia. The lesions producing an INO are located in the paramedian, dorsal lower midbrain, involving the MLF. A detailed description of INO was included with the topic of pontine infarction. Some patients have abnormal control of head and eye posture in the roll plane (OTR).[266]

Vertical Gaze Disturbances. Involvement of the most rostral part of the midbrain produces vertical gaze paresis (see below, top of the Basilar artery syndrome).

Fourth Nerve Palsy. The trochlear nucleus lies in the lower midbrain caudal to the oculomotor nuclear complex. Unlike 3rd nerve fascicles that travel in the paramedian area, the 4th nerve fascicles run dorsally around the aqueduct to decussate in the anterior medullary velum just caudal to the inferior colliculus. Because this dorsolateral part of the lower midbrain is mainly supplied by the SCA, 4th nerve palsy is almost always accompanied by concomitant SCA infarction (see below, SCA infarction); 4th nerve palsy is extremely uncommon in pure midbrain stroke.[218,267] Because the lesions mostly damage the trochlear nucleus or the fascicle before decussation, superior oblique palsy usually develops in the eye contralateral to the midbrain stroke. The etiology is more often vascular malformation than ischemic stroke.

Hemiparesis and Other Motor Dysfunction. Although limb weakness is found in more than half of patients, a severe hemiparesis is present in only approximately one-quarter of patients when the pyramidal tract at the crus cerebri was heavily and densely involved.[40] The uncommon occurrence of severe hemiparesis may at least in part be due to sparsely arranged pyramidal fibers in the crus cerebri as compared to the lower brainstem.[205] Dysarthria is invariably present, and hemiataxia is usually obvious in patients without severe hemiparesis.

Sensory Symptoms/Signs

Unlike the pons, where the sensory tracts are located in the paramedian area, the sensory tracts are located at the dorsolateral portion of the midbrain, in which the medial lemniscal fibers are situated medio-ventrally, and the spinothalamic tracts, dorso-laterally within the so-called sensory lemniscus (Fig. 26-27). In one study, sensory disturbances were observed in 43% of pure midbrain infarction.[40] However, because infarcts preferentially involve the paramedian area, sensory tracts are more often spared or partially involved; symptoms are usually minor and often restricted to certain body parts. Cheiro-oral distribution is relatively common,[40] probably because face and finger representation areas are located medially in the sensory tract, being vulnerable to paramedian infarction. Mesencephalic pure hemisensory syndrome is rare, and is caused by small infarcts or hemorrhages affecting the dorso-lateral area.[40,208] Sensory symptoms may be limited to trigeminal areas, which usually are accompanied by a 3rd or 4th nerve palsy.[268]

Ataxia. Ataxia is one of the most frequently observed symptoms/signs in midbrain infarction,[40] probably related to the presence of abundant neuronal fibers connecting with the cerebellum in the midbrain: the descending cortico-ponto-cerebellar fibers at the crus cerebri and ascending cerebello-rubro-thalamic tracts in the paramedian area (see Fig. 26-29).

In the cerebral peduncle, descending cerebellar fibers are rarely involved in isolation, and concomitant involvement of the pyramidal tracts or corticobulbar tracts lead to syndromes such as ataxic hemiparesis or dysarthria with ataxia. Paramedian lesions affecting ascending cerebello-rubro-thalamic tracts at or near the red nucleus may produce ataxia without significant other motor dysfunction. Because paramedian lesions usually also involve the oculomotor nucleus or fasci-

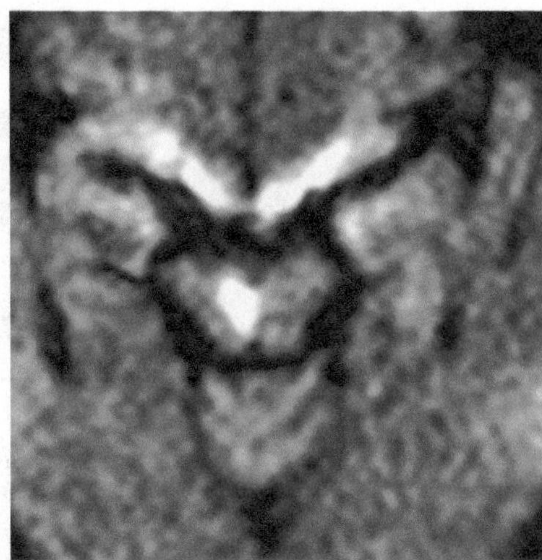

Figure 26-28. An 80-year-old hypertensive woman suddenly developed dysarthria and gait difficulty. Neurological examination showed severe, cerebellar-type dysarthria and bilateral limb and gait ataxia worse on the left side. Diffusion-weighted MRI showed a paramedian infarct in the right lower midbrain that probably involved ascending cerebello-rubro-thalamic tracts bilaterally.

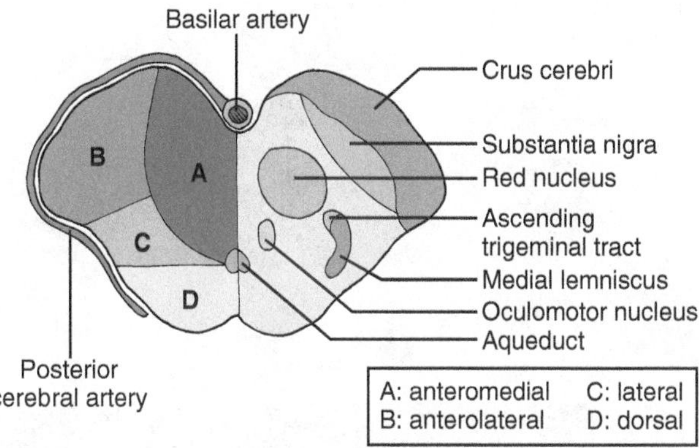

Figure 26-29. Schematic drawing of midbrain indicating important structures, supplying vessels and four topographic subgroups. A, Anteromedial; B, anterolateral; C, lateral; D, posterior. *(Modified from Kim JS, Kim J. Pure midbrain infarction: Clinical, radiologic, and pathophysiologic findings.* Neurology *2005;64;1227–1232).*

cles, ipsilateral 3rd nerve palsy is often combined with contralateral ataxia (Claude syndrome).

Patients with a unilateral lower midbrain lesion may have bilateral ataxia usually worse on the contralateral side.[40,259] This is attributed to bilateral involvement of crossing efferent dentato-rubral fibers at the lower midbrain level (Fig. 26-28) by lesions located in the paramedian area. Bilateral ataxia caused by a single lesion is a localizing sign for paramedian lower midbrain infarction. The outcome of such patients is unfavorable; they have marked dysarthria and long-lasting gait instability.

Involuntary Movements

Holmes Tremor. Patients with midbrain strokes occasionally develop tremor, referred to as "rubral tremor" or "Holmes' tremor". The characteristics of the tremor are as follows:[269]

1. Intention and resting tremor, but some may show postural tremor as well.

The tremor may not be as regular as other tremors, and occasionally shows jerky components.

2. Tremor is of low frequency, mostly below 4.5 Hz.
3. There is a variable delay (mostly 2 weeks to 2 years) between the onset of the lesion and the appearance of tremor. There may be a gradual increase in amplitude after the development.

The tremor is predominantly unilateral, and mainly affects the hands and the proximal arm.

The responsible lesions are usually situated at the superior and external part of the red nucleus affecting the rubrothalamic pathways. Lesions affecting the thalamus, the central tegmental tract in the pons or deep nuclei of the cerebellum or their outflow tracts may cause similar movement disorders.

Recent dopaminergic PET imaging studies showed striatal dopaminergic dysfunction in these patients, probably due to the involvement of the nigrostriatal system.[270,271] Holmes tremor was reported to develop after the onset of Parkinson disease in a patient with a previous cerebellar lesion[272] and in a patient with a previous Parkinson disease after the onset of cerebellar infarction.[273] These pieces of evidence suggest that combined damage of the cerebellothalamic and nigrostriatal system may be required to generate Holmes tremor.

Third nerve palsy accompanied by contralateral ataxia and tremor is referred to as Benedict syndrome.

Parkinsonism. Midbrain strokes may produce hemiparkinsonism due to involvement of the substantia nigra.[274–276] The prevalence is very low, probably because parkinsonian symptoms are masked by other major deficits such as hemiparesis or ataxia. However, if carefully tested, subtle symptoms such as micrographia[277] or hypokinetic dysarthria and palilalia[278] are observed. Dopaminergic system dysfunction is documented by PET imaging in these patients.

Dystonia. Unilateral dystonia may be observed in patients with extensive ponto-mesencephalic tegmental lesions,[279] usually associated with sensori-motor dysfunction and other involuntary movements such as rubral tremor or excessive twitching.

Asterixis. Paramedian midbrain infarcts may produce asterixis in the contralateral limbs,[280] probably related to the involvement of the rubrospinal or cerebellar-rubral tracts that are involved in the regulation of postural/tonic control of extremities.

Neuropsychiatric and Emotional Disturbances

Symptoms such as emotional incontinence,[192] agitation, and impulsive behavior[281] have been reported in patients with midbrain infarction. These features may be related to serotonergic or limbic dopaminergic system involvement.

Clinical-topographic Correlation

According to MRI findings, the lesions are categorized as the following groups (Fig. 26-29).

Anteromedial (or Paramedian) Lesion. This is the most common pattern; approximately 50–60% of pure midbrain infarction belong to this group[40,261] (Figs 26-29A, 26-30A1, A2). The lesions usually involve the 3rd nerve fascicles or nucleus (at the upper midbrain), the MLF (at the lower midbrain), the red nucleus and the medial part of the cerebral peduncle. The clinical features are characterized by ocular motor disturbances (3rd nerve palsy or INO), contralateral mild hemiparesis and ataxia. Ataxia may be bilateral when the paramedian lesion is located in the lower midbrain (Fig. 26-28). Sensory deficits, when present, are usually mild and often present in restricted body parts such as the perioral or perioral-hand areas.

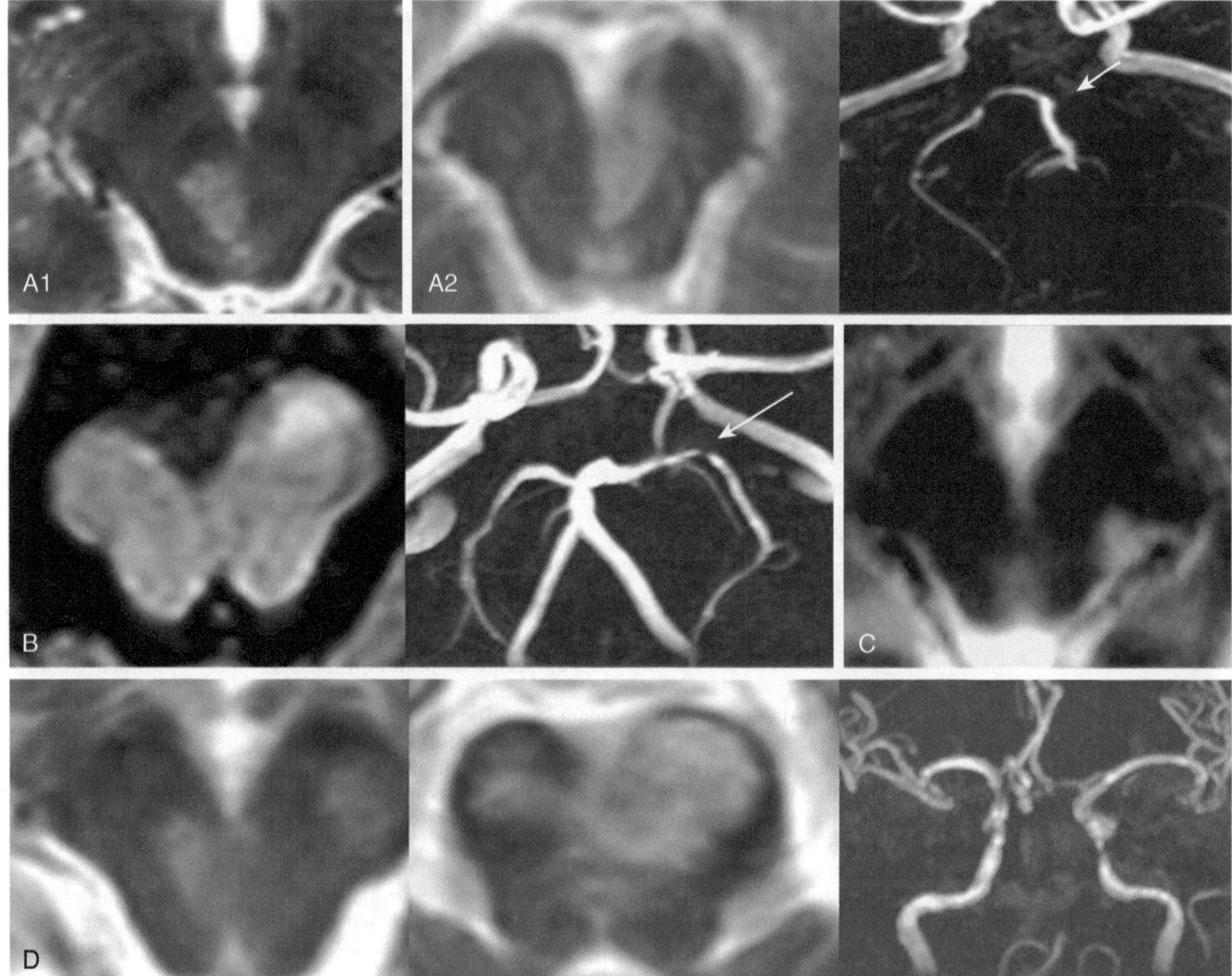

Figure 26-30. Patients A (A1 and A2) represent the anteromedial group. Both had oculomotor disturbances and mild contralateral ataxia. Patient A1 had a small deep infarct. The lesion of patient A2 was similar, but extended to the medial surface. MR angiography (MRA) findings of A1 patient were normal (not shown), but those of A2 showed occlusion of the left posterior cerebral artery (arrow). Patient B represents the anterolateral group. The patient had dysarthria clumsy hand syndrome. He did not have oculomotor disturbances. MRA showed stenosis in the P2 portion of the left posterior cerebral artery (arrow). Patient C represents the lateral group. The patient presented with pure sensory stroke. Patient D represents the bilateral group. The patients had quadriparesis and bilateral oculomotor paresis. MRA showed occlusion of the basilar artery. *(Modified from Kim JS, Kim J. Pure midbrain infarction: Clinical, radiologic, and pathophysiologic findings.* Neurology *2005;64;1227–1232)*

Anterolateral Lesion. Approximately one-quarter of patients belong to this group[40,261] (Figs 26-29B, 26-30B). Because the crus cerebri is primarily involved, the patients' main symptom is hemiparesis. Although severe motor dysfunction in uncommon (see above), some patients may have progressively worsening hemiparesis. In patients who do not have severe hemiparesis, ataxic hemiparesis, dysarthria-clumsy hand syndrome, pure dysarthria, dysarthria-ataxia may develop. If adjacent sensory tracts are involved, sensory deficits may be added. Ocular motor disturbances are not present.

Combined Lesions. Some patients have lesions in both anteromedial and anterolateral areas. Clinical features are the combination of the two; ocular motor disturbances, ataxia and various motor syndromes.

Lateral Lesion. Although quite uncommon, lesions may be confined to the lateral part of the midbrain (Figs 26-29C, 26-30C). The clinical features are characterized by hemisensory deficits caused by involvement of the laterally located sensory lemniscus. The clinical features are not distinguishable from thalamic pure sensory stroke (see Chapter 25).

Dorsolateral Lesion. This area is supplied by the SCA (Fig. 26-29D) and infarcts occurring in this area are almost always accompanied by concomitant involvement of the cerebellum. Fourth nerve palsy, INO, ataxia and partial sensory disturbances may be present (see below, SCA infarction syndrome).

Bilateral Lesions. Bilateral midbrain infarctions are almost always accompanied by extensive infarcts in the other parts of the posterior circulation. Pure bilateral midbrain infarctions are very rare[40,261] (Fig. 26-30D). Patients develop altered consciousness, quadriparesis, severe dysarthria, dysphagia and ultimately, a locked-in state. Patients may have bilateral oculomotor palsy,[261] but ocular movements may remain intact if dorsal areas are spared.[282,283]

Stroke Mechanism

Approximately two-thirds of pure midbrain infarction is caused by large-artery atherosclerotic disease. Anteromedial, anterolateral and combined-type lesions are usually caused by branch occlusion associated with PCA or rostral BA atherothrombosis[40] (Fig. 26-30A2,B,D). Small penetrating artery disease explains stroke in approximately one-quarter of the patients who have deep-seated lesions (Fig. 26-30A1). Cardiac embolism is rare in patients with isolated midbrain infarction.[40,261] The stroke mechanism of the lateral group is uncertain, but artery-to-artery embolization from tightly stenosed BA was reported.[40] Dorsolateral infarcts are almost always caused by SCA occlusion.

Prognosis

In patients with pure midbrain infarction, the lesions are mostly unilateral and prognosis is relatively good. Initial severe motor dysfunction may predict worse prognosis. However, 36 out of 40 patients were functionally independent after 2 years of follow-up in one study.[40] The functional outcome of patients with bilateral ataxia (Fig. 26-28) is unfavorable because they usually have persistent gait difficulty and dysarthria. As in patients with medullary or pontine infarction, underlying vascular diseases (BA or PCA) probably affect the future outcome of these patients. Patients with bilateral infarction have a grave prognosis; they often die due to aspiration pneumonia and frequently remain locked-in.

Cerebellar Infarcts

Cerebellar infarction accounts for 1–4% of brain infarctions.[284–288] However, because small infarcts may produce symptoms mimicking vestibulopathy, the prevalence is likely to be underestimated. Cerebellar infarction usually follows the vascular topography, i.e., SCA, PICA and AICA territories, or their combination. In studies using CT or MRI,[284,285,289] PICA territory infarction is slightly more common than SCA infarction. AICA territory infarction is distinctly uncommon.

Clinical Manifestations

The clinical manifestations depend on the location and the extent of the lesion (Table 26-3).

Patients with lesions in other parts of the brain such as the brainstem will have additional symptoms/signs, such as limb weakness, sensory deficits and cranial nerve palsies in addition to classic cerebellar syndromes.

Classic Cerebellar Syndromes. In patients who had infarcts solely or predominantly in the cerebellum, the most common symptoms are dizziness. Vertigo is less common.[285,290] Because dizziness and vertigo may occur in other common diseases such as vestibulopathy, differential diagnosis is important. Nausea/vomiting is usually accompanied by dizziness/vertigo and occurs in more than half of the patients.[285] Nystagmus is present in about half of the patients, usually horizontal, and occasionally vertical.

Headache occurs in the ipsilateral nuchal-occipital area in 30–50% of cases,[284,285,290] presumably related to acute distention or stretch on the intracranial pain-sensitive structures including cerebral vessels. Increasing severity of headache is a sign suggesting expanding edema or hemorrhagic transformation. Severe headache occurring in the nuchal area may indicate VA dissection. Limb incoordination is an important sign, occurring in 60–70% of patients.[284,285,290] Patients may describe incoordination as limb weakness or clumsiness, and appropriate examination is necessary to define the nature of the problem. Dysarthria is common and mainly due to involvement of the superior paravermal region.

TABLE 26-3 Clinical Manifestations of Pontine Infarction by Study

	Macdonell et al.	Kase et al.	Tohgi et al.
Country	Australia	USA	Japan
Published year	1987	1993	1993
Diagnosis	CT based	CT/MRI based	CT/MRI based
Number of patients	30	66	293
Symptoms			
Dizziness/vertigo	80	50 (vertigo)	70
Nausea/vomiting	63	52	56
Gait difficulty (or truncal ataxia)	77	71	40
Headache	40	53	32
Dysarthria	60		20
Signs			
Limb ataxia	70	61	59
Truncal ataxia	67	62	45
Nystagmus	53	64	38
Decreased consciousness	36		34
Ocular movement disorder	27		
Hemi(mono)paresis	7		20
Facial palsy	13		8

One of the most serious concerns in cerebellar infarction is progressive edema and enlargement of the lesion, and subsequent herniation (pseudotumoral presentation). After the first day or so, patients develop increasingly severe headache, vomiting, and decreased consciousness; they become drowsy and then stuporous. Bilateral Babinski signs and brainstem ocular motor abnormalities develop, such as conjugate gaze paresis or bilateral 6th nerve palsy. Development of ocular bobbing is a sign suggestive of significant brainstem dysfunction. Coma, respiratory and cardiac arrest will follow if patients are not adequately treated. Surgical decompression, if done early enough, frequently improves the condition (Fig. 26-31).

Cognitive Dysfunction. The cerebellum contributes to the regulation of cognitive function. Certain parts of the cerebellum are anatomically linked with the cerebral cortex concerning cognitive function such as prefrontal cortex, posterior parietal cortex, superior temporal cortex, cingulate gyrus and posterior paprahippocampal area.[291] Functional MRI studies also show that performance of cognitive tasks activates certain parts of the cerebellar posterior lobe.[292]

Cerebellar infarction may produce various cognitive-emotional dysfunctions, the so-called "cerebellar cognitive affective syndrome."[293] Findings include: impairment of executive function (planning, set-shifting, abstract reasoning, verbal fluency, working memory) often with perseveration, distractibility, or inattention; visuospatial disorganization, and impaired visuospatial memory; personality change with blunting of affect or disinhibited and inappropriate behavior; and difficulties with language production including dysprosodia, agrammatism and mild anomia. These symptoms are more pronounced in patients with bilateral, large infarcts. Posterior (as opposed to anterior) lobe lesions appear to be more important in the generation of these symptoms.

Emotional Disturbances. In humans, cerebellar areas around the vermis appear to be involved in the formation of fear memory traces.[294] One of the authors (JSK) observed patients who showed phobic attacks after cerebellar infarction. In clinical practice, however, emotional incontinence (excessive or inappropriate laughing/crying) is much more frequently observed. The cerebellum has a role in adjusting the

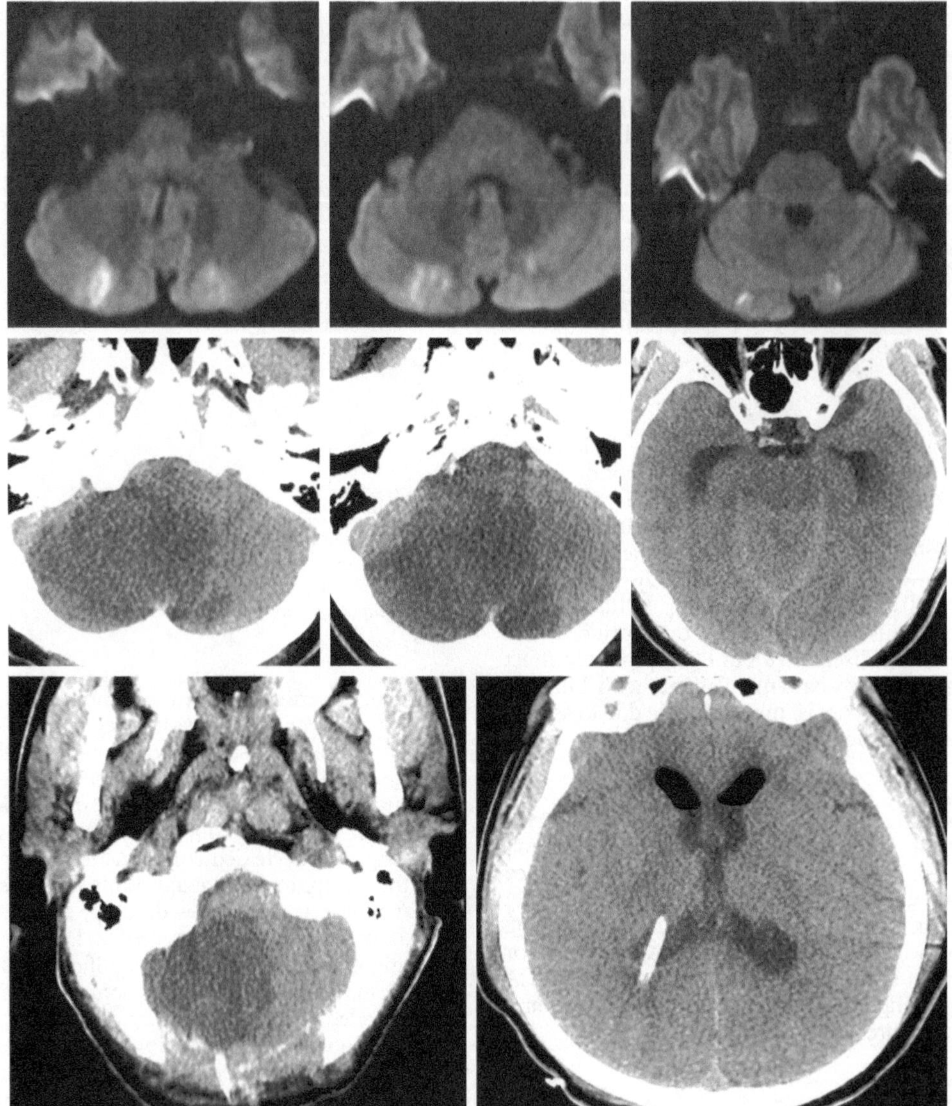

Figure 26-31. A 51-year-old hypertensive man sudden developed vertigo and gait ataxia. On admission, diffusion-weighted MRI showed small infarcts in both posterior inferior cerebellar artery (PICA) territories (upper row). The next day, he complained of severe generalized headache and dysarthria which was followed by stuporous mentality. CT showed a large PICA infarction in the right side. Left medial PCA territory was also involved. There was effacement of perimesencephalic space, and hydrocephalus due to aqueduct compression (middle row). Decompressive craniectomy and ventriculotomy were performed (lower row). The patient became alert and survived, although he had persistent gait and limb ataxia.

execution of laughter and crying to the cognitive or emotional context of a stimulus.[295] A study reported that approximately one-fifth of patients with cerebellar infarction showed emotional incontinence.[192] Depression was uncommon, suggesting that the cerebellum plays a role mainly on the expression side of human emotional behaviors.

Clinical-topographic Correlation

Posterior Inferior Cerebellar Artery Infarction. PICA territory infarction is more frequent than SCA territory infarction.[284,285,289] According to Kumral et al.[296] PICA infarction accounts for 2% of all ischemic strokes. However, PICA infarctions are probably underdiagnosed because they occasionally present with isolated vertigo mimicking peripheral vestibulopathy.[297]

The symptoms of LMI concomitantly occur in approximately 10%[296] to 33%[284] of the patients with PICA infarction. The syndromes can be either complete or partial. In these patients, MRI usually shows concomitant involvement of the medulla (Fig. 26-12). However, medullary lesions may not be seen or detected only after repeated MRI scans. In patients with partial LMI syndromes, ipsilateral trigeminal sensory loss is more common than other components or may be an early sign heralding more extensive LMI symptoms, probably because the descending trigeminal tracts are located in the dorsal medullary area primarily supplied by the PICA (Fig. 26-14). The co-occurrence of the LMI is usually due to involvement of medullary perforators in the presence of proximal PICA occlusion. However, it is also possible that ICVA atherothrombosis simultaneously occludes both the PICA and medullary perforators. Although much less common, MMI may occur together with PICA cerebellar infarction,[296] supporting the latter argument.

Manifestations of PICA territory infarction include vertigo, headache, gait ataxia, limb ataxia, and nystagmus.[284] Headache is usually unilateral, occurring in cervical, occipital, or both regions. In the series of Kase et al. [284] nystagmus was common (75%) and was either horizontal (ipsilateral in 47% of patients, contralateral in 5%, bilateral in 11%) or vertical (11% of patients). Another striking finding in PICA territory infarction is axial lateropulsion, a phenomenon suggestive of a lateral displacement in the representation of the center of gravity.[287] A patient's attempts to stand or walk are usually associated with falling to one or either side.

PICA territory infarction can affect the full territory, but partial (medial or lateral) territory involvement is more common, occurring in two-thirds[298] to three-quarters[284] of PICA cerebellar infarctions. In one series,[296] medial PICA infarctions (n = 23) outnumbered lateral PICA (n = 9) or whole PICA (n = 9) infarctions. Medial PICA infarctions (Figs 26-11, 26-12) present with isolated vertigo, with or without axial lateropulsion and dysmetria. LMI symptoms may be combined. [289,299] The isolated acute vertigo from PICA territory infarction mimicks labyrinthitis;[300–302] the vertigo may be aggravated (or relieved) on certain head positions and patients may describe recurrent vertigo symptoms. These patients usually have medial and caudal cerebellar infarction involving the uvulonodular complex of the vermis. This area corresponds to the vestibular portion of the cerebellum and is exclusively supplied by medial PICA. In a series describing small infracts limited to the nodule,[303] all patients presented with isolated vertigo, unilateral ipsilesional nystagmus and falling to the opposite direction. However, head impulse and bithermal caloric tests were normal, which may distinguish this condition from peripheral vestibulopathy.

In patients with lateral PICA territory cerebellar infarction, the most common symptom at onset is acute unsteadiness, gait ataxia, and unilateral limb ataxia (Fig. 26-32). Compared with medial PICA infarction, lateral PICA territory infarctions rarely produce acute rotatory vertigo and lateropulsion,[304] and are less often associated with LMI. Unlike SCA territory infarcts, dysarthria is absent or mild in these patients. The clinical manifestation of whole PICA territory infarction is the combination of medial and lateral PICA infarction. While infarcts limited to a branch territory almost never become edematous, progressive herniation occasionally occurs in patients with whole PICA territory infarction (Fig. 26-31).

Occasionally, PICA territory cerebellar infarctions occur bilaterally (Fig. 26-31). Several hypotheses have been put forth to explain the pathogenesis:[305–307] (1) unilateral supply to both medial PICA territories, (2) both PICAs arising from an occluded BA, (3) pressure effect is caused by a large PICA infarct, (4) hemodynamic mechanism with hypoperfusion in the most peripheral branches, and (5) double, simultaneous embolic strokes. Among them, the first one seems to be the most frequent mechanism.[308] The contralateral PICA infarct is usually small and limited within the medial PICA territory (Fig. 26-31). The clinical manifestations, vertigo and gait imbalance, are similar to those shown in patients with unilateral PICA infarction. The prognosis is not worse than unilateral PICA infarction.

Stroke Mechanisms

Occlusion of the ICVA or PICA itself can produce PICA territory infarction. The etiology of occlusion is either cardiogenic embolism or atherosclerotic disease. According to previous studies, while SCA occlusions are most commonly cardioembolic, PICA occlusions are equally divided between in situ atherothrombosis and cardioembolism.[309,310] Other less common causes include dissection (either VA or PICA itself) (Figs 26-11, 26-12) thromboembolism from the PFO or the aortic arch.

Prognosis

Clinical series have shown that PICA territory infarctions have a relatively benign outcome. Kase et al.[284] found signs of brainstem compression in one-quarter of their 36 patients (all of whom had full PICA territory infarctions) and acute hydrocephalus in seven patients; only four patients died from cerebellar swelling. Patients with large infarction may have long-standing dizziness or gait instability. Partial PICA territory infarctions almost always show a benign course;[284,298,299,304] vertigo or dizziness often go away within several days or weeks. PICA territory infarctions accompanied by AICA or SCA infarctions are more severe in clinical presentation,[287] and more often manifest as a pseudotumoral pattern. In patients with PICA territory infarction associated with brainstem infarction, the prognosis mostly depends upon the extent of brainstem infarction.

Superior Cerebellar Artery Territory Infarction

Since early in the 20th century, a constellation of syndromes was reported to be caused by SCA territory infarction, that includes ipsilateral limb ataxia, ipsilateral Horner's syndrome, contralateral loss of pain and temperature sensation of the face, arm, leg, and trunk, paralysis of emotional expression of in the face, unilateral or bilateral hearing loss and contralateral fourth nerve palsy.[311] The symptoms other than ipsilateral ataxia are caused by involvement of the lateral tegmental area of the upper pons or lower midbrain; involved structures include: ascending spinothalamic/medical lemniscus for contralateral sensory deficits; lateral lemniscus for unilateral or bilateral hearing difficulty; sympathetic fibers for Horner sign, and 4th nerve nucleus or fascicles before decussation for

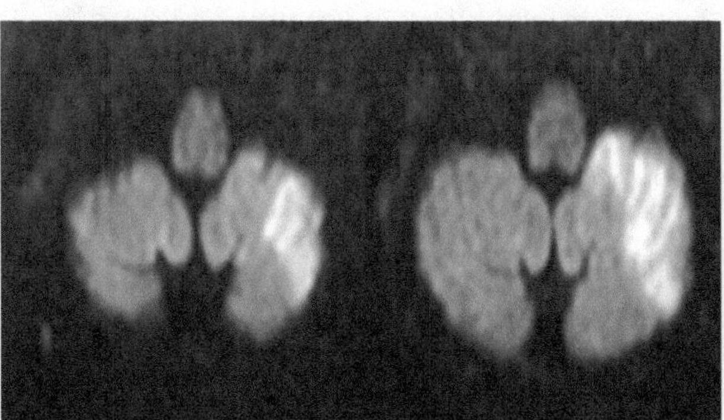

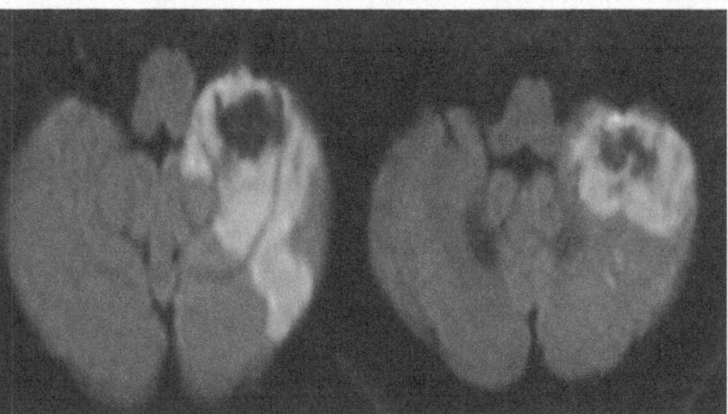

Figure 26-32. A 70-year-old woman with atrial fibrillation suddenly developed dizziness, gait instability, and headache. Neurologic examination showed ataxia and disadokinesia in the left limb. Diffusion-weighted MRI showed an infarct with hemorrhagic transformation (dark signals inside the infarct) in the left lateral posterior cerebellar artery territory.

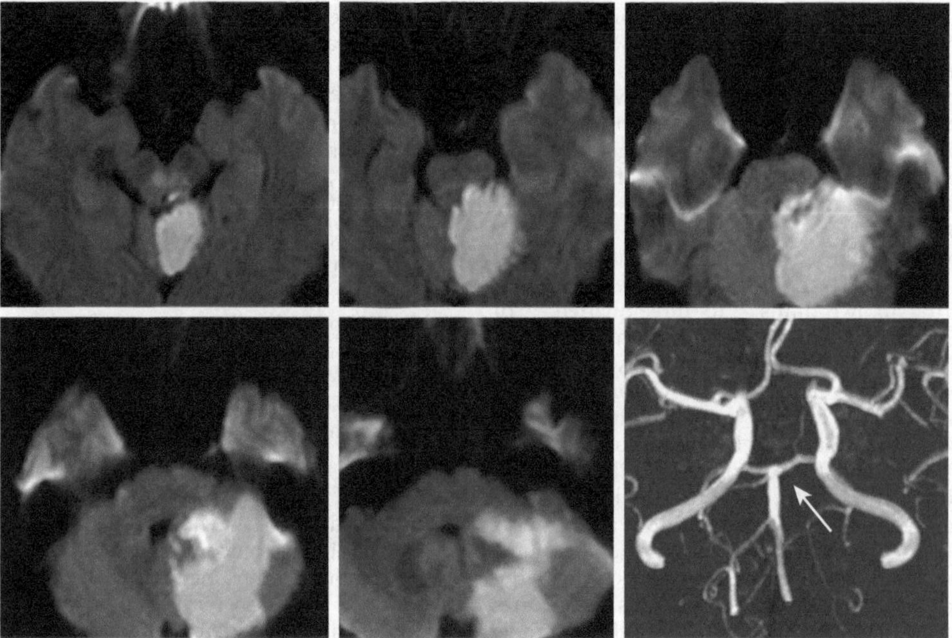

Figure 26-33. A 53-year-old man developed dizziness, diplopia, right tinnitus, and hearing difficulty. There were left Horner sign, right hearing loss, decreased pain and temperature sensory perception in right face and limbs, limb ataxia on the left, and right superior oblique palsy. Diffusion-weighted MRI showed an infarct in the left superior cerebellar artery territory. MR angiography showed non-visualization of the left superior cerebellar artery (arrow).

contralateral 4th nerve palsy (see above, Midbrain infarction) (Fig. 26-33). However, this so-called "classic" SCA syndrome is actually very rare in either autopsy[310] or imaging-based studies.[284] Most patients show symptoms and signs of cerebellar dysfunction only, i.e., gait imbalance, ipsilateral limb ataxia and cerebellar-type dysarthria.

Kase et al.[284] compared symptoms between PICA and SCA territory infarcts and found that vertigo (78% vs 37%), vomiting (61% vs 40%), nystagmus (75% vs 50%) and headache (64% vs 40%) were more common in the former. This difference is probably related to the fact that the flocculonodular lobe that has rich vestibular connections is mainly supplied by PICA. However, according to a recent study that used video-oculography,[312] approximately half of the patients with SCA territory infarction had true vertigo early in the course. Limb ataxia and dysarthria are distinctly more common and prominent in SCA than in PICA territory infarction.[284,289] Dysarthria in SCA territory infarction is characterized by irregularly distributed articulatory deficits, monotonous and scanning speech, and is localized to the paravermal segments of the rostral cerebellar hemisphere,[313] an area supplied by the medial branch of SCA. Tiny lesions occurring in this area may produce cerebellar dysarthria as a sole manifestation of cerebellar infarction.[314]

Although uncommon, patients may show ipsilateral involuntary movements including tremor, choreiform or athetoid movements.[284,310] They appear while patients move or use the limbs and are aggravated with emotional upset. These movement disorders may be attributed to involvement of the cerebellar outflow tract: dentate nucleus or the superior cerebellar peduncle (see above, Midbrain infarction). Damage to the dentate nucleus may lead to delayed-onset palatal myoclonus associated with contralateral hypertrophy of the inferior olivary nucleus.[315]

SCA territory cerebellar infarctions more often occur in limited (medial or lateral) SCA territories than in full territory.[284,289,316] Infarction limited to the medial SCA branch territory occurs in four of 33 patients in autopsy series[310] and 14 of 47 (30%) patients in a recent MRI-based series.[317] The main clinical symptoms are ataxia and dysarthria in both medial and lateral SCA territory infarctions, but patients with medial SCA infarcts have more prominent truncal ataxia or lateropulsion and less severe limb incoordination because the rostral vermis is specialized for gait and postural control while the lateral part is related to limb coordination. Isolated lateropulsion as a sole clinical manifestation was reported in patients with infarction selectively involving the central portion of the rostral vermis.[318] While the prognosis is good for patients with both medial[317] and lateral[319] SCA territory infarctions, pseudotumoral presentation resulting in herniation or hydrocephalus is occasionally seen in whole SCA territory infarction.

Unlike PICA infarcts, bilateral SCA infarcts are uncommon. Only one of 15 patients in one series[316] and five of 23 patients in another[310] had bilateral SCA territory infarcts.

Stroke Mechanism

Most SCA territory infarctions are caused by embolism from heart disease such as atrial fibrillation or PFO, and less commonly from proximal large-artery atherosclerosis.[284,310,316] Arterial occlusions are occasionally observed in the distal tip of the BA, the ICVA, and, less frequently, the SCA itself. Spontaneous recanalization is common in patients with cardiac embolism. Less common causes include atherothrombosis in the rostral BA or the proximal SCA. Uncommon etiologies include dissection, fibromuscular dysplasia, and migraine.[125,320,321]

Prognosis

SCA territory infarctions have a pseudotumoral presentation in 21% of autopsy cases.[310] However, the outcome was much better in studies using CT and MRI.[284,285,289] According to Kase et al.[284] 7% of patients had a pseudotumoral presentation leading to coma and, occasionally, death. In most patients, the lesions involve partial SCA territory, and the prognosis is benign in both medial SCA and lateral SCA infarctions, although patients often have residual limb incoordination and dysarthria.

Anterior Inferior Cerebellar Artery Infarction

The AICA syndrome is strikingly different from SCA and PICA territory infarctions in that brainstem symptoms/signs are prominent. Autopsy reports[13] and imaging studies[322] indicate that most AICA infarctions involve the lateral region of the caudal pons, middle cerebellar peduncle (100% of cases) and flocculus (69% of cases). Infarctions often affect other cerebellar lobules (75% of cases), but usually remain limited in size. The infarction sometimes extends up to the middle third of the lateral pons and down to the superior part of the lateral medulla. When the AICA is large (usually associated with hypoplastic PICA), AICA occlusion may produce infarction encompassing the whole anterior inferior cerebellum.

AICA territory infarctions are accompanied by PICA and SCA territory infarcts in 35% of autopsy cases, when tonsillar herniation may occur.[13] Among 23 patients with AICA territory infarction identified by MRI, six had isolated lesions in the AICA territory, six had additional PICA territory infarcts and 11 had multiple infarcts in the posterior circulation.[12]

The classic syndrome of the AICA territory infarction, first described by Adams,[323] includes vertigo, vomiting, tinnitus, dysarthria, ipsilateral facial palsy, hearing loss, trigeminal sensory loss, Horner's syndrome, appendicular dysmetria, and contralateral temperature and pain sensory loss over the limbs and trunk (Fig. 26-34). The AICA syndrome may also include ipsilateral conjugate gaze palsy due to involvement of the flocculus, dysphagia due to extension of the infarction to the upper lateral medulla, and limb weakness due to involvement of the corticospinal tract in the pons or midbrain.[13] Although some signs are similar to those observed in LMI, the presence of severe facial palsy, deafness, tinnitus, and multimodal sensory impairment over the face, allow accurate diagnosis.

The internal auditory artery is most often a branch of AICA. Symptoms of inner ear ischemia such as tinnitus, hearing loss and vertigo may occur in isolation in AICA infarction.[301] In some patients, especially diabetics, ischemia of the inner ear structures supplied by the internal auditory artery heralds a full AICA territory infarction.[324]

Stroke Mechanism

AICA territory infarction is often associated with lower BA (or, ICVA + BA) atherosclerotic disease.[13,309] Significant ICVA or BA occlusive disease is usually associated with infarcts in other posterior circulation territories. When the infarcts are limited completely to AICA-supplied territory, patients are often diabetic and AICA itself is the likely site of occlusion. Embolism is distinctly uncommon in patients with isolated AICA territory infarction. According to Kumral et al.,[12] large-artery disease was the cause of stroke in 52%, cardiac embolism in 4%, while 17% had both etiologies.

Prognosis

In one autopsy series,[13] coma with tetraplegia occurred in 20% of patients with AICA territory infarction, due to massive ventromedial involvement of the basis pontis. However, CT- or MRI-based studies showed that AICA territory infarction does not produce massive edema, and patients generally show a benign outcome, unless other territories are concomitantly involved.[12,322] However, it should be kept in mind that because AICA territory infarction is often associated with significant lower BA atherosclerosis, AICA syndrome may herald massive BA thrombotic infarction.[322] The surviving patients usually have residual deficits such as peripheral facial palsy, trigeminal sensory symptoms or hearing loss.

Top of the Basilar Artery Syndrome

Infarction of rostral brainstem and cerebral hemispheral regions fed by the distal BA causes a clinically recognizable syndrome characterized by visual, ocular motor, and behavioral abnormalities, often without significant motor dysfunction. Caplan[257] described this as "top of the basilar artery syndrome". Typically, there are bilateral, multiple infarcts in the paramedian midbrain, medial thalamus, medial temporal areas and occipital lobes (Fig. 26-35). The clinical features vary greatly and depend on the topography of damaged brain. Below are the symptoms most commonly encountered. In rare occasions, bilateral SCA infarctions are the only manifestation of basilar tip occlusion when bilateral fetal-type PCAs are present without anastomosis between the anterior and posterior circulations.[325]

Clinical Features

Ocular Motor Dysfunction

Vertical Gaze Palsy. Vertical voluntary eye movements are generated by bilaterally simultaneous activation of the frontal and parietal occipital conjugate gaze centers. Vertical gaze pathways then converge on the periaqueductal region beneath the collicular plate, near the interstitial nucleus of Cajal and the

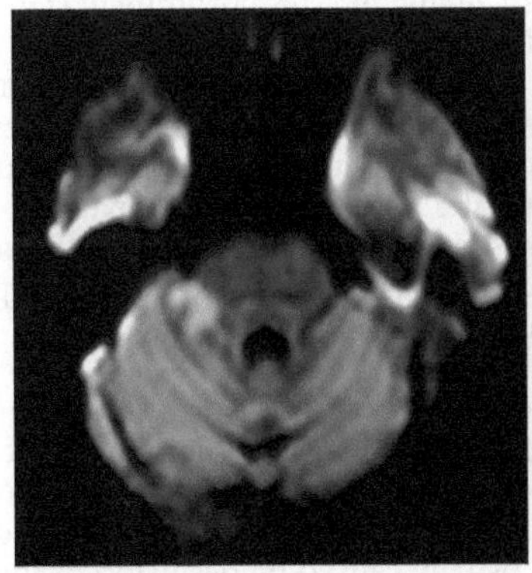
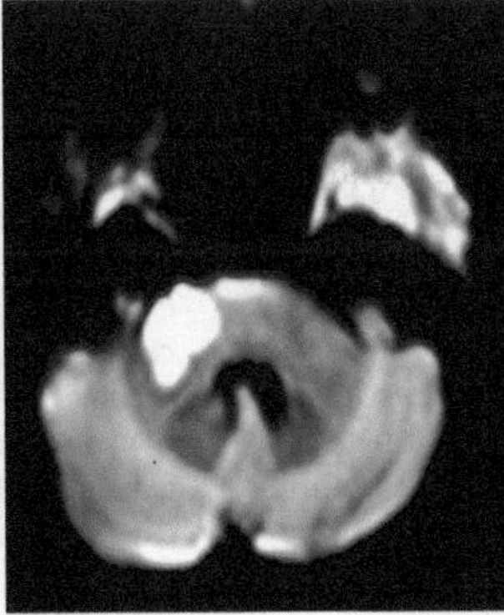
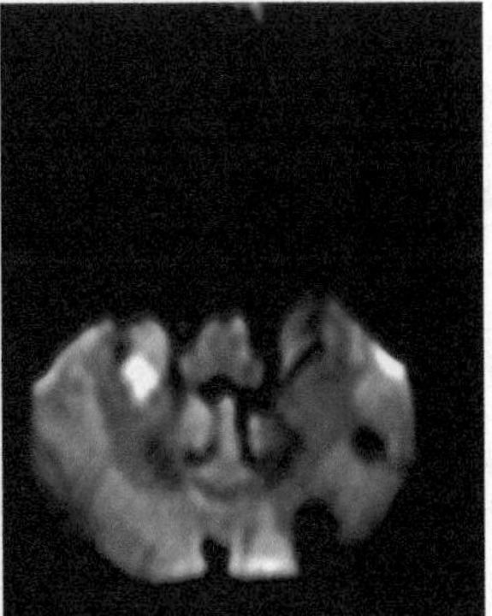

Figure 26-34. A 72-year-old hypertensive and diabetic man suddenly developed dizziness, right tinnitus, hearing impairment and gait difficulty. Neurologic examination showed sensory perception impairment in the right face, right facial palsy, right hearing loss, dysarthria, right limb ataxia and gait ataxia. Diffusion-weighted MRI showed infarcts in the right anterior inferior cerebellar artery territory.

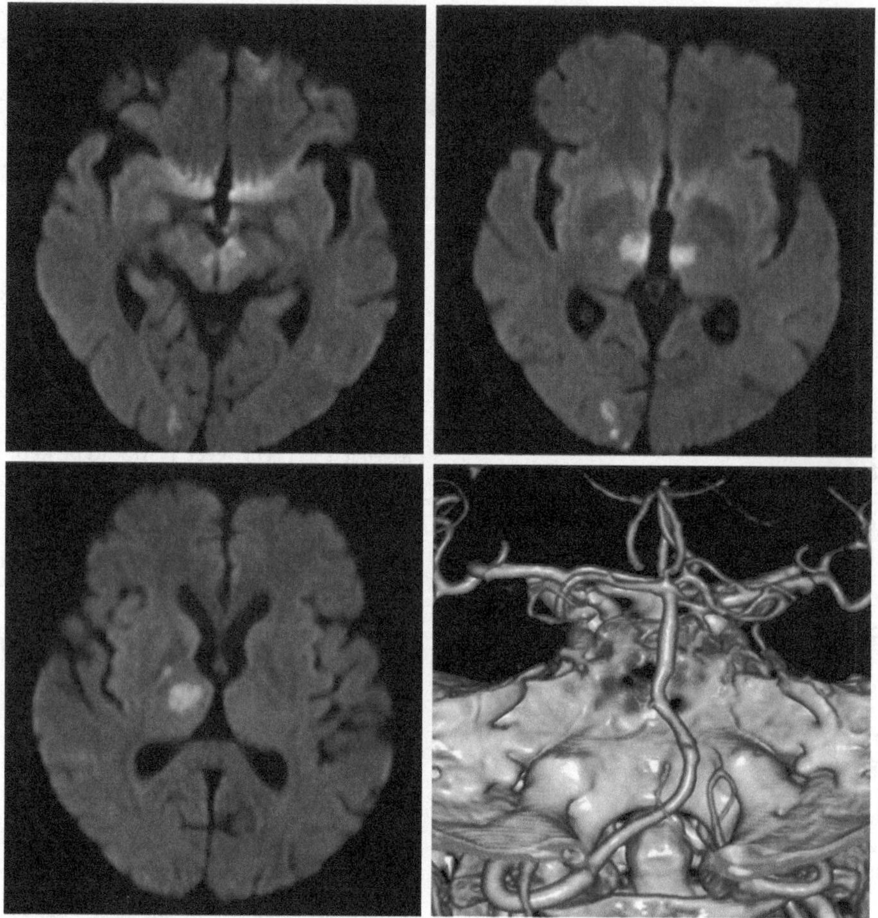

Figure 26-35. A 72-year-old woman with atrial fibrillation became drowsy and confused. Examination showed confused mentality, anterograde memory impairment and vertical gaze failure. Diffusion-weighed MRI showed multiple infarcts in the bilateral paramedian midbrain and thalalmus, and right occipital area. CT angiogram performed 2 days later showed normal basilar and posterior cerebral arteries suggesting spontaneous recanalization of occluded basilar tip.

posterior commissure. In this region, there is a cluster of neurons important in vertical gaze, referred to as rostral interstitial MLF (riMLF).[326,327]

The riMLF, interstitial nucleus of Cajal and posterior commissures are closely integrated structures related to vertical gaze. Extensive lesions occurring in the rostral midbrain result in both upgaze and downgaze failure. Vertical VOR is usually preserved. A unilateral lesion affecting the posterior commissure can cause upward saccadic failure due probably to the fact that fibers involved in upward saccades decussate through the posterior commissure which connects the riMLF on both sides.[328,329] Bilateral damage to the riMLF is required to produce downgaze paresis, probably because the riMLF involved in downward saccades includes both a direct projection onto the ipsilateral oculomotor and trochlear nuclei and an indirect projection onto the contralateral nuclei. Therefore, isolated upgaze palsy is much more commonly observed than isolated downgaze paresis.[330,331]

If the connections from the riMLF to the 3rd nuclei are selectively damaged just above the nucleus on one side, monocular upgaze palsy may occur.[332–334] A vertical one-and-half syndrome (upward gaze paresis with monocular downward gaze paresis or downward gaze paresis with monocular upward gaze paresis) is also observed.[335,336]

Convergence, Eyelid and Pupillary Abnormalities. Ocular convergence is probably controlled in the medial midbrain tegmentum, although there is debate as to whether the nucleus of Perlia specifically subserves this function. Convergence vectors are frequently evident on attempted upward gaze. Rhythmic convergence nystagmus may be elicited if patients are told to follow a downgoing opticokinetic target with their eyes. Convergence vectors may modify lateral gaze, and patients may have limiting abduction and present with pseudo-sixth nerve palsy.[257] Lid abnormalities are also a sign of rostral brainstem infarction. Unilateral infarction of the 3rd cranial nerve nucleus can lead to complete bilateral ptosis.[234] Retraction of the upper lid, giving the eye a prominent stare (Collier's sign), is observed in patients with tectal lesions.[337] When ischemia affects the medial midbrain tegmentum or diencephalon, pupillary reactivity is often abnormal. If the lesion affects only the Edinger-Westphal nucleus, the pupils are usually fixed and dilated, but if the lesion involves sympathetic fibers, the pupil size becomes smaller.[338] Midbrain pupils are occasionally eccentric (corectopia iridis) and may shift position from a central to an eccentric one intermittently.[339]

Somnolence and Loss of Attention. The medial mesencephalon and diencephalon contain the most rostral portions of the reticular activating system. Infarcts in these regions frequently produce excessive sleep, and lack of attention. Infarcts are usually caused by occlusion of the mesencephalic artery (from the proximal PCA) and its perforating branches[27,340] (see Chapter 25, Thalamic infarction). Because the reticular gray matter is adjacent to the third nerve nuclei, riMLF and

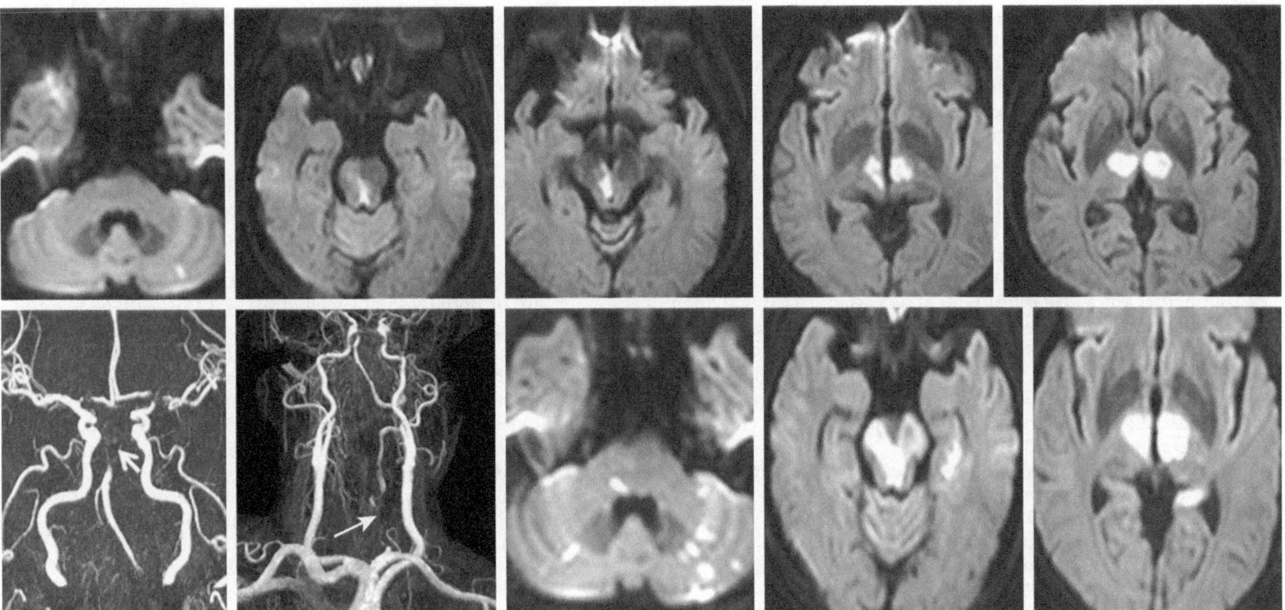

Figure 26-36. A 66-year-old woman suddenly became drowsy and confused. Examination showed drowsy mentality, dysarthria, bilateral ptosis and vertical gaze limitation. Diffusion-weighted MRI (DWI) showed bilateral paramedian midbrain and thalamic infarcts. A small infarct in the left cerebellum was also seen (upper row). MR angiography showed occlusion of the distal basilar artery (arrow, first image of lower row) that probably was caused by artery-to-artery embolism arising from the left extracranial vertebral artery atherothrombosis (arrow, second image of the lower row), that could not be recanalized by interventional therapy (not shown). The next day, she became stuporous and quadriplegic. Follow-up DWI showed newly developed cerebellar infarcts and bilateral ponto-midbrain infarction and enlarged previous paramedian thalamic lesions (last three images, lower row).

the posterior commissure, somnolence is frequently associated with relevant ocular motor disturbances.

Hallucinations. Patients with rostral brainstem infarction often have hallucination (peduncular hallucinosis).[341] The hallucinations tend to occur at twilight or during the night, and such patients usually have sleep disorders (nocturnal insomnia or daytime hypersomnolence).[257] Symptoms such as oculomotor disturbances, dysarthria and ataxia are frequently associated. The hallucinations are usually vivid, mostly visual, and contain multiple colors, objects, and scenes. Occasionally, auditory or tactile hallucinations are associated.

The structure responsible for hallucinations may be located near the substantia nigra. Bilateral infarcts confined to the medial substantia nigra pars reticulata are reported to cause peduncular hallucinosis.[342] However, similar hallucinations are observed in patients with infarcts that involve the pons or the posterior thalamus.[343] Neuropsychological testing in patients with hallucination shows impairments of episodic memory, confabulation, attention deficits, confusion, delusion, and misidentification for persons and places. It seems that brainstem hallucinosis may be related with dysfunctional ascending reticular system and thalamocortical circuits.[344]

Confabulations. Confabulations are often reported in patients with rostral brainstem infarcts.[257] The features are similar to what were described as Wernicke-Korsakoff psychosis.

Hemiballism and Abnormal Movements. Hemichorea or hemiballism may occur from infarcts affecting the subthalamic nucleus (corpus Luysii).[345] Other movement disorders related to midbrain involvement are described above (see Midbrain infarction).

Other Symptoms and Signs

Occipital and thalamic infarcts are common and relevant symptoms and signs are described in Chapter 25. Embolism may produce infarcts in the pons, cerebellum, and rarely medulla. The relevant symptoms and signs are described in the early part of this chapter.

Stroke Mechanisms and Prognosis

Occlusions of the BA tip are generally embolic,[257] more often from the heart than proximal artery atherothrombosis. Although uncommon, atherothrombosis occurring in the distal BA can also result in this syndrome.[346] In patients with embolic occlusion, the emboli may also occlude other vessels such as the PICA, SCA or pontine branches before they abut on the top of BA. PCA territory infarcts are also commonly found. In patients with cardiac embolism, embolus is frequently evanescent, and at the time of angiographic study, it is already gone (Fig. 26-35). In this case, the patient's prognosis is generally fair, although they may have residual deficits depending on already-damaged structures. Although uncommon, the occlusion persists and may lead to downward extension of thrombi to result in catastrophic bilateral midbrain or pontine infarction (Fig. 26-36). The recent advent of interventional treatment is occasionally of great help in preventing this event by early and successful recanalization of the occluded BA.

The complete reference list can be found on the companion Expert Consult website at www.expertconsult.inkling.com. 

KEY REFERENCES

1. Wilkinson IM. The vertebral artery. Extracranial and intracranial structure. Arch Neurol 1972;27:392–6.
5. Lister JR, Rhoton AL Jr, Matsushima T, et al. Microsurgical anatomy of the posterior inferior cerebellar artery. Neurosurgery 1982;10:170–99.
10. Fisher CM, Karnes WE, Kubik CS. Lateral medullary infarction-the pattern of vascular occlusion. J Neuropathol Exp Neurol 1961;20:323–79.
11. Rhoton AL Jr. The cerebellar arteries. Neurosurgery 2000; 47(3 Suppl.):S29–68.

12. Kumral E, Kisabay A, Atac C. Lesion patterns and etiology of ischemia in the anterior inferior cerebellar artery territory involvement: a clinical – diffusion weighted – MRI study. Eur J Neurol 2006;13(4):395–401.
13. Amarenco P, Hauw JJ. Cerebellar infarction in the territory of the anterior and inferior cerebellar artery. A clinicopathological study of 20 cases. Brain 1990;113(Pt 1):139–55.
14. Hardy DG, Peace DA, Rhoton AL Jr. Microsurgical anatomy of the superior cerebellar artery. Neurosurgery 1980;6(1):10–28.
15. Brassier G, Morandi X, Riffaud L, et al. Basilar artery anatomy. J Neurosurg 2000;93(2):368–9.
17. Suttner N, Mura J, Tedeschi H, et al. Persistent trigeminal artery: a unique anatomic specimen–analysis and therapeutic implications. Neurosurgery 2000;47(2):428–33, discussion 433–4.
22. Kim JS, Nah HW, Park SM, et al. Risk factors and stroke mechanisms in atherosclerotic stroke: intracranial compared with extracranial and anterior compared with posterior circulation disease. Stroke 2012;43(12):3313–18.
26. Castaigne P, Lhermitte F, Gautier JC, et al. Arterial occlusions in the vertebro-basilar system. A study of 44 patients with post-mortem data. Brain 1973;96(1):133–54.
27. Castaigne P, Lhermitte F, Buge A, et al. Paramedian thalamic and midbrain infarct: clinical and neuropathological study. Ann Neurol 1981;10(2):127–48.
30. Caplan LR, Amarenco P, Rosengart A, et al. Embolism from vertebral artery origin occlusive disease. Neurology 1992;42(8):1505–12.
31. Kim JS. Pure lateral medullary infarction: clinical-radiological correlation of 130 acute, consecutive patients. Brain 2003;126(Pt 8):1864–72.
33. Caplan LR, Hennerici M. Impaired clearance of emboli (washout) is an important link between hypoperfusion, embolism, and ischemic stroke. Arch Neurol 1998;55(11):1475–82.
34. Amarenco P, Cohen A, Tzourio C, et al. Atherosclerotic disease of the aortic arch and the risk of ischemic stroke. N Engl J Med 1994;331(22):1474–9.
35. Lee E, Kang DW, Kwon SU, et al. Posterior cerebral artery infarction: diffusion-weighted MRI analysis of 205 patients. Cerebrovasc Dis 2009;28(3):298–305.
36. Wong KS, Caplan LR, Kim JS. Stroke mechanisms. In: Kim JS, Caplan LR, Wong KS, editors. Intracranial Atherosclerosis. 2008. p. 57–68.
37. Caplan LR. Intracranial branch atheromatous disease: a neglected, understudied, and underused concept. Neurology 1989;39(9):1246–50.
39. Fisher CM, Caplan LR. Basilar artery branch occlusion: a cause of pontine infarction. Neurology 1971;21(9):900–5.
40. Kim JS, Kim J. Pure midbrain infarction: clinical, radiologic, and pathophysiologic findings. Neurology 2005;64(7):1227–32.
41. Kim JS, Han YS. Medial medullary infarction: clinical, imaging, and outcome study in 86 consecutive patients. Stroke 2009;40(10):3221–5.
42. Kim JS, Yoon Y. Single subcortical infarction associated with parental arterial disease: important yet neglected subtype of atherothrombotic stroke. Int J Stroke. 2013;8(3):197–203.
44. Bang OY, Joo SY, Lee PH, et al. The course of patients with lacunar infarcts and a parent arterial lesion: similarities to large artery vs small artery disease. Arch Neurol 2004;61(4):514–19.
45. Kwon JY, Kwon SU, Kang DW, et al. Isolated lateral thalamic infarction: the role of posterior cerebral artery disease. Eur J Neurol 2012;19(2):265–70.
47. Klein IF, Lavallee PC, Schouman-Claeys E, et al. High-resolution MRI identifies basilar artery plaques in paramedian pontine infarct. Neurology 2005;64(3):551–2.
49. Amarenco P, Kase CS, Rosengart A, et al. Very small (border zone) cerebellar infarcts. Distribution, causes, mechanisms and clinical features. Brain 1993;116(Pt 1):161–86.
51. Caplan LR. Bilateral distal vertebral artery occlusion. Neurology 1983;33(5):552–8.
52. Shin HK, Yoo KM, Chang HM, et al. Bilateral intracranial vertebral artery disease in the New England Medical Center, Posterior Circulation Registry. Arch Neurol 1999;56(11):1353–8.
53. Bogousslavsky J, Gates PC, Fox AJ, et al. Bilateral occlusion of vertebral artery: clinical patterns and long-term prognosis. Neurology 1986;36(10):1309–15.
54. Kubik CS, Adams RD. Occlusion of the basilar artery; a clinical and pathological study. Brain 1946;69(2):73–121.
62. Fisher CM. Lacunar strokes and infarcts: a review. Neurology 1982;32(8):871–6.
69. Kim BJ, Sohn H, Sun BJ, et al. Imaging characteristics of ischemic strokes related to patent foramen ovale. Stroke 2013;44:3350–6.
71. Mas JL, Arquizan C, Lamy C, et al. Recurrent cerebrovascular events associated with patent foramen ovale, atrial septal aneurysm, or both. N Engl J Med 2001;345(24):1740–6.
76. Schievink WI. Spontaneous dissection of the carotid and vertebral arteries. N Engl J Med 2001;344(12):898–906.
78. Mokri B, Houser OW, Sandok BA, et al. Spontaneous dissections of the vertebral arteries. Neurology 1988;38(6):880–5.
88. Rubinstein SM, Peerdeman SM, van Tulder MW, et al. A systematic review of the risk factors for cervical artery dissection. Stroke 2005;36(7):1575–80.
90. Schievink WI, Mokri B, O'Fallon WM. Recurrent spontaneous cervical-artery dissection. N Engl J Med 1994;330(6):393–7.
91. Caplan LR, Baquis GD, Pessin MS, et al. Dissection of the intracranial vertebral artery. Neurology 1988;38(6):868–77.
92. Hosoya T, Adachi M, Yamaguchi K, et al. Clinical and neuroradiological features of intracranial vertebrobasilar artery dissection. Stroke 1999;30(5):1083–90.
95. Ruecker M, Furtner M, Knoflach M, et al. Basilar artery dissection: series of 12 consecutive cases and review of the literature. Cerebrovasc Dis 2010;30(3):267–76.
104. Nishizaki T, Tamaki N, Takeda N, et al. Dolichoectatic basilar artery: a review of 23 cases. Stroke 1986;17(6):1277–81.
105. Kwon HM, Kim JH, Lim JS, et al. Basilar artery dolichoectasia is associated with paramedian pontine infarction. Cerebrovasc Dis 2009;27(2):114–18.
107. Passero S, Filosomi G. Posterior circulation infarcts in patients with vertebrobasilar dolichoectasia. Stroke 1998;29(3):653–9.
116. Rosengart A, Hedges TR 3rd, Teal PA, et al. Intermittent downbeat nystagmus due to vertebral artery compression. Neurology 1993;43(1):216–18.
120. Kuether TA, Nesbit GM, Clark WM, et al. Rotational vertebral artery occlusion: a mechanism of vertebrobasilar insufficiency. Neurosurgery 1997;41(2):427–32, discussion 432–3.
121. Choi KD, Choi JH, Kim JS, et al. Rotational vertebral artery occlusion: mechanisms and long-term outcome. Stroke 2013;44(7):1817–24.
122. Strupp M, Planck JH, Arbusow V, et al. Rotational vertebral artery occlusion syndrome with vertigo due to "labyrinthine excitation". Neurology 2000;54(6):1376–9.
129. Frens DB, Petajan JH, Anderson R, et al. Fibromuscular dysplasia of the posterior cerebral artery: report of a case and review of the literature. Stroke 1974;5(2):161–6.
133. Hishikawa T, Tokunaga K, Sugiu K, et al. Assessment of the difference in posterior circulation involvement between pediatric and adult patients with moyamoya disease. J Neurosurg 2013;119(4):961–5.
135. Gonzalez-Gay MA, Vazquez-Rodriguez TR, Gomez-Acebo I, et al. Strokes at time of disease diagnosis in a series of 287 patients with biopsy-proven giant cell arteritis. Medicine (Baltimore) 2009;88(4):227–35.
136. Ruegg S, Engelter S, Jeanneret C, et al. Bilateral vertebral artery occlusion resulting from giant cell arteritis: report of 3 cases and review of the literature. Medicine (Baltimore) 2003;82(1):1–12.
144. Norrving B, Cronqvist S. Lateral medullary infarction: prognosis in an unselected series. Neurology 1991;41(2 Pt 1):244–8.
145. Lewis GLN, Littman A, Foley EF. The syndrome of thrombosis of the posterior inferior cerebellar artery: a report of 28 cases. Ann Intern Med 1952;36(2:2):592–602.
146. Peterman AF, Sieker TR. The lateral medullary (Wallenberg) syndrome: clinical features and prognosis. Med Clin North Am 1960;44:887–96.
147. Currier RD, Giles CL, DeJong RN. Some comments on Wallenberg's lateral medullary syndrome. Neurology 1961;1:778–92.

149. Sacco RL, Freddo L, Bello JA, et al. Wallenberg's lateral medullary syndrome. Clinical-magnetic resonance imaging correlations. Arch Neurol 1993;50(6):609–14.
150. Vuilleumier P, Bogousslavsky J, Regli F. Infarction of the lower brainstem. Clinical, aetiological and MRI-topographical correlations. Brain 1995;118(Pt 4):1013–25.
151. Kim JS, Lee JH, Lee MC. Patterns of sensory dysfunction in lateral medullary infarction. Clinical-MRI correlation. Neurology 1997; 49(6):1557–63.
152. Kim JS, Lee JH, Suh DC, et al. Spectrum of lateral medullary syndrome. Correlation between clinical findings and magnetic resonance imaging in 33 subjects. Stroke 1994;25(7):1405–10.
154. Dieterich M, Brandt T. Wallenberg's syndrome: lateropulsion, cyclorotation, and subjective visual vertical in thirty-six patients. Ann Neurol 1992;31(4):399–408.
158. Kwon M, Lee JH, Kim JS. Dysphagia in unilateral medullary infarction: lateral vs medial lesions. Neurology 2005;65(5): 714–18.
160. Matsumoto S, Okuda B, Imai T, et al. A sensory level on the trunk in lower lateral brainstem lesions. Neurology 1988;38(10): 1515–19.
161. Kim JS. Sensory symptoms in ipsilateral limbs/body due to lateral medullary infarction. Neurology 2001;57(7):1230–4.
162. Caplan L, Gorelick P. "Salt and pepper on the face" pain in acute brainstem ischemia. Ann Neurol 1983;13(3):344–5.
165. Fisher CM, Tapia J. Lateral medullary infarction extending to the lower pons. J Neurol Neurosurg Psychiatry 1987;50(5):620–4.
166. Bogousslavsky J, Khurana R, Deruaz JP, et al. Respiratory failure and unilateral caudal brainstem infarction. Ann Neurol 1990;28(5):668–73.
168. Hermann DM, Jung HH, Bassetti CL. Lateral medullary infarct with alternating and dissociated sensorimotor deficits: Opalski's syndrome revisited. Eur J Neurol 2009;16(4):e72–4.
169. Nakamura S, Kitami M, Furukawa Y. Opalski syndrome: ipsilateral hemiplegia due to a lateral-medullary infarction. Neurology 2010;75(18):1658.
174. Kim JS, Choi-Kwon S. Sensory sequelae of medullary infarction: differences between lateral and medial medullary syndrome. Stroke 1999;30(12):2697–703.
175. MacGowan DJ, Janal MN, Clark WC, et al. Central poststroke pain and Wallenberg's lateral medullary infarction: frequency, character, and determinants in 63 patients. Neurology 1997; 49(1):120–5.
178. Dejerin J. Semiologie des affections du système nerveux. Paris, France: Masson; 1914. p. 226–30.
179. Davison C. Syndrome of the anterior spinal artery of the medulla oblongata. Arch Neurol Psychiatry 1937;37:91–107.
180. Kim JS, Kim HG, Chung CS. Medial medullary syndrome. Report of 18 new patients and a review of the literature. Stroke 1995;26(9):1548–52.
181. Toyoda K, Imamura T, Saku Y, et al. Medial medullary infarction: analyses of eleven patients. Neurology 1996;47(5):1141–7.
182. Bassetti C, Bogousslavsky J, Mattle H, et al. Medial medullary stroke: report of seven patients and review of the literature. Neurology 1997;48(4):882–90.
183. Kumral E, Afsar N, Kirbas D, et al. Spectrum of medial medullary infarction: clinical and magnetic resonance imaging findings. J Neurol 2002;249(1):85–93.
187. Kim JS, Choi KD, Oh SY, et al. Medial medullary infarction: abnormal ocular motor findings. Neurology 2005;65(8): 1294–8.
188. Kim JS, Moon SY, Kim KY, et al. Ocular contrapulsion in rostral medial medullary infarction. Neurology 2004;63(7): 1325–7.
192. Kim JS, Choi-Kwon S. Poststroke depression and emotional incontinence: correlation with lesion location. Neurology 2000; 54(9):1805–10.
193. Fisher CM, Curry HB. Pure Motor Hemiplegia of Vascular Origin. Arch Neurol 1965;13:30–44. Dtsch Zeit Nervenheilk. 1894;5: 351–74.
199. Babinski J, Nageotte J. Hdmiasynergie, lateropulsion et myosis bulbaires avec hemianesthesie et hemiplegie croisees. Rev Neurol (Paris) 1902;10:358–65.
201. Bassetti C, Bogousslavsky J, Barth A, et al. Isolated infarcts of the pons. Neurology 1996;46(1):165–75.
202. Kumral E, Bayulkem G, Evyapan D. Clinical spectrum of pontine infarction. Clinical-MRI correlations. J Neurol 2002;249(12): 1659–70.
203. Erro ME, Gallego J, Herrera M, et al. Isolated pontine infarcts: etiopathogenic mechanisms. Eur J Neurol 2005;12(12): 984–8.
204. Kataoka S, Hori A, Shirakawa T, et al. Paramedian pontine infarction. Neurological/topographical correlation. Stroke 1997;28(4): 809–15.
205. Kim JS, Lee JH, Im JH, et al. Syndromes of pontine base infarction. A clinical-radiological correlation study. Stroke 1995;26(6): 950–5.
208. Kim JS, Bae YH. Pure or predominant sensory stroke due to brain stem lesion. Stroke 1997;28(9):1761–4.
210. Kim JS. Restricted acral sensory syndrome following minor stroke. Further observation with special reference to differential severity of symptoms among individual digits. Stroke 1994; 25(12):2497–502.
213. Graham SH, Sharp FR, Dillon W. Intraoral sensation in patients with brainstem lesions: role of the rostral spinal trigeminal nuclei in pons. Neurology 1988;38(10):1529–33.
218. Kim JS, Kang JK, Lee SA, et al. Isolated or predominant ocular motor nerve palsy as a manifestation of brain stem stroke. Stroke 1993;24(4):581–6.
219. Kim JS. Internuclear ophthalmoplegia as an isolated or predominant symptom of brainstem infarction. Neurology 2004;62(9): 1491–6.
220. Smith JW, Cogan DG. Internuclear ophthalmoplegia; a review of fifty-eight cases. AMA Arch Ophthalmol 1959;61(5): 687–94.
221. Zee DS, Hain TC, Carl JR. Abduction nystagmus in internuclear ophthalmoplegia. Ann Neurol 1987;21(4):383–8.
224. Zwergal A, Cnyrim C, Arbusow V, et al. Unilateral INO is associated with ocular tilt reaction in pontomesencephalic lesions: INO plus. Neurology 2008;71(8):590–3.
229. Fisher CM. Some neuro-ophthalmological observations. J Neurol Neurosurg Psychiatry 1967;30(5):383–92.
230. Pierrot-Deseilligny C, Chain F, Serdaru M, et al. The 'one-and-a-half' syndrome. Electro-oculographic analyses of five cases with deductions about the Physiological mechanisms of lateral gaze. Brain 1981;104(Pt 4):665–99.
231. Fisher CM. Ocular Bobbing. Arch Neurol 1964;11:543–6.
233. Newman N, Gay AJ, Heilbrun MP. Disjugate ocular bobbing: its relation to midbrain, pontine, and medullary function in a surviving patient. Neurology 1971;21(6):633–7.
235. Tahmoush AJ, Brooks JE, Keltner JL. Palatal myoclonus associated with abnormal ocular and extremity movements. A polygraphic study. Arch Neurol 1972;27(5):431–40.
239. Lee SJ, Kim JS, Song IU, et al. Poststroke restless legs syndrome and lesion location: anatomical considerations. Mov Disord 2009;24(1):77–84.
241. Cascino GD, Adams RD. Brainstem auditory hallucinosis. Neurology 1986;36(8):1042–7.
245. Fisher CM. The neurological examination of the comatose patient. Acta Neurol Scand 1969;45(Suppl. 36):1–56.
247. Kim JS, Choi S, Kwon SU, et al. Inability to control anger or aggression after stroke. Neurology 2002;58(7):1106–8.
249. Choi-Kwon S, Han SW, Kwon SU, et al. Fluoxetine treatment in poststroke depression, emotional incontinence, and anger proneness: a double-blind, placebo-controlled study. Stroke 2006;37(1):156–61.
251. Ferbert A, Bruckmann H, Drummen R. Clinical features of proven basilar artery occlusion. Stroke 1990;21(8):1135–42.
253. Voetsch B, DeWitt LD, Pessin MS, et al. Basilar artery occlusive disease in the New England Medical Center Posterior Circulation Registry. Arch Neurol 2004;61(4):496–504.
257. Caplan LR. "Top of the basilar" syndrome. Neurology 1980;30(1): 72–9.
258. Martin PJ, Chang HM, Wityk R, et al. Midbrain infarction: associations and aetiologies in the New England Medical Center Posterior Circulation Registry. J Neurol Neurosurg Psychiatry 1998;64(3):392–5.
259. Bogousslavsky J, Maeder P, Regli F, et al. Pure midbrain infarction: clinical syndromes, MRI, and etiologic patterns. Neurology 1994;44(11):2032–40.

260. Kumral E, Bayulkem G, Akyol A, et al. Mesencephalic and associated posterior circulation infarcts. Stroke 2002;33(9):2224–31.
261. Ogawa K, Suzuki Y, Oishi M, et al. Clinical study of twenty-one patients with pure midbrain infarction. Eur Neurol 2012;67(2): 81–9.
263. Ksiazek SM, Repka MX, Maguire A, et al. Divisional oculomotor nerve paresis caused by intrinsic brainstem disease. Ann Neurol 1989;26(6):714–18.
266. Halmagyi GM, Brandt T, Dieterich M, et al. Tonic contraversive ocular tilt reaction due to unilateral meso-diencephalic lesion. Neurology 1990;40(10):1503–9.
270. Remy P, de Recondo A, Defer G, et al. Peduncular 'rubral' tremor and dopaminergic denervation: a PET study. Neurology 1995; 45(3 Pt 1):472–7.
274. Morgan JC, Sethi KD. Midbrain infarct with parkinsonism. Neurology 2003;60(12):E10.
280. Kim JS. Asterixis after unilateral stroke: lesion location of 30 patients. Neurology 2001;56(4):533–6.
282. Zakaria T, Flaherty ML. Locked-in syndrome resulting from bilateral cerebral peduncle infarctions. Neurology 2006;67(10):1889.
284. Kase CS, Norrving B, Levine SR, et al. Cerebellar infarction. Clinical and anatomic observations in 66 cases. Stroke 1993; 24(1):76–83.
285. Tohgi H, Takahashi S, Chiba K, et al. Cerebellar infarction. Clinical and neuroimaging analysis in 293 patients. The Tohoku Cerebellar Infarction Study Group. Stroke 1993;24(11):1697–701.
287. Amarenco P. The spectrum of cerebellar infarctions. Neurology 1991;41(7):973–9.
289. Barth A, Bogousslavsky J, Regli F. The clinical and topographic spectrum of cerebellar infarcts: a clinical-magnetic resonance imaging correlation study. Ann Neurol 1993;33(5):451–6.
290. Macdonell RA, Kalnins RM, Donnan GA. Cerebellar infarction: natural history, prognosis, and pathology. Stroke 1987;18(5): 849–55.
293. Schmahmann JD, Sherman JC. The cerebellar cognitive affective syndrome. Brain 1998;121(Pt 4):561–79.
295. Parvizi J, Anderson SW, Martin CO, et al. Pathological laughter and crying: a link to the cerebellum. Brain 2001;124(Pt 9): 1708–19.
296. Kumral E, Kisabay A, Atac C, et al. Spectrum of the posterior inferior cerebellar artery territory infarcts. Clinical-diffusion-weighted imaging correlates. Cerebrovasc Dis 2005;20(5): 370–80.
298. Amarenco P, Levy C, Cohen A, et al. Causes and mechanisms of territorial and nonterritorial cerebellar infarcts in 115 consecutive patients. Stroke 1994;25(1):105–12.
299. Amarenco P, Roullet E, Hommel M, et al. Infarction in the territory of the medial branch of the posterior inferior cerebellar artery. J Neurol Neurosurg Psychiatry 1990;53(9):731–5.
300. Duncan GW, Parker SW, Fisher CM. Acute cerebellar infarction in the PICA territory. Arch Neurol 1975;32(6):364–8.
303. Moon IS, Kim JS, Choi KD, et al. Isolated nodular infarction. Stroke 2009;40(2):487–91.
304. Barth A, Bogousslavsky J, Regli F. Infarcts in the territory of the lateral branch of the posterior inferior cerebellar artery. J Neurol Neurosurg Psychiatry 1994;57(9):1073–6.
308. Kang DW, Lee SH, Bae HJ, et al. Acute bilateral cerebellar infarcts in the territory of posterior inferior cerebellar artery. Neurology 2000;55(4):582–4.
309. Amarenco P, Hauw JJ, Gautier JC. Arterial pathology in cerebellar infarction. Stroke 1990;21(9):1299–305.
310. Amarenco P, Hauw JJ. Cerebellar infarction in the territory of the superior cerebellar artery: a clinicopathologic study of 33 cases. Neurology 1990;40(9):1383–90.
311. Mills CK. Preliminary note on a new symptom complex due to lesion of the cerebellum and crebello-rubro-thalamic system, the main symptoms being ataxia of the upper and lower extremities of one side, and the other side deafness, paralysis of emotional expression in the face, and loss of the senses of pain, heat, and cold over the entire half of the body. J Nerv Ment Dis 1912;39: 73–6.
312. Lee H, Kim HA. Nystagmus in SCA territory cerebellar infarction: pattern and a possible mechanism. J Neurol Neurosurg Psychiatry 2013;84(4):446–51.
316. Chaves CJ, Caplan LR, Chung CS, et al. Cerebellar infarcts in the New England Medical Center Posterior Circulation Stroke Registry. Neurology 1994;44(8):1385–90.
317. Sohn SI, Lee H, Lee SR, et al. Cerebellar infarction in the territory of the medial branch of the superior cerebellar artery. Neurology 2006;66(1):115–17.
319. Amarenco P, Roullet E, Goujon C, et al. Infarction in the anterior rostral cerebellum (the territory of the lateral branch of the superior cerebellar artery). Neurology 1991;41(2 Pt 1):253–8.
322. Amarenco P, Rosengart A, DeWitt LD, et al. Anterior inferior cerebellar artery territory infarcts. Mechanisms and clinical features. Arch Neurol 1993;50(2):154–61.
327. Buttner-Ennever JA, Buttner U, Cohen B, et al. Vertical glaze paralysis and the rostral interstitial nucleus of the medial longitudinal fasciculus. Brain 1982;105(Pt 1):125–49.
329. Bhidayasiri R, Plant GT, Leigh RJ. A hypothetical scheme for the brainstem control of vertical gaze. Neurology 2000;54(10): 1985–93.
334. Thomke F, Hopf HC. Acquired monocular elevation paresis. An asymmetric upgaze palsy. Brain 1992;115(Pt 6):1901–10.
335. Bogousslavsky J, Regli F. Upgaze palsy and monocular paresis of downward gaze from ipsilateral thalamo-mesencephalic infarction: a vertical "one-and-a-half" syndrome. J Neurol 1984;231(1): 43–5.
337. Collier J. Nuclear ophthalmoplegia with special reference to retraction of the lids and ptosis and to lesions of the posterior commissure. Brain 1927;50:488.
339. Selhorst JB, Hoyt WF, Feinsod M, et al. Midbrain corectopia. Arch Neurol 1976;33(3):193–5.
340. Segarra JM. Cerebral vascular disease and behavior. I. The syndrome of the mesencephalic artery (basilar artery bifurcation). Arch Neurol 1970;22(5):408–18.
344. Benke T. Peduncular hallucinosis: a syndrome of impaired reality monitoring. J Neurol 2006;253(12):1561–71.
345. Martin JP. Hemichorea resulting from a local lesion of the brain (the syndrome of the body of Luys). Brain 1927;50:637–42.
346. Mehler MF. The rostral basilar artery syndrome: diagnosis, etiology, prognosis. Neurology 1989;39(1):9–16.

27 Lacunar Syndromes, Lacunar Infarcts, and Cerebral Small-vessel Disease

Bo Norrving

KEY POINTS

- Lacunar infarcts are small (<15 mm diameter) subcortical infarcts that result from occlusion of a single penetrating artery.
- Lacunar infarcts account for about one-quarter of all ischemic strokes.
- Lacunar infarcts are associated with clinical lacunar syndromes, but the specificity of the syndromes is only moderate: lacunar syndromes may be caused by other mechanisms than small-artery disease in one-third or more of all cases.
- Lacunar infarcts presenting with stroke or transient symptoms are part of the spectrum of cerebral small-vessel disease that also include silent cerebral infarcts, white matter lesions, and cerebral microbleeds.
- Whereas the short-term prognosis after lacunar infarcts is benign, the long-term prognosis is serious with a high risk of cumulative vascular events, cognitive decline, and increased risk of death.
- Cerebral small-vessel disease has an important role in cerebrovascular disease and is a leading cause of cognitive decline and functional loss in the elderly.
- Thrombolytic therapy with tPA is of similar benefit and carries similar risks in patients with acute lacunar infarct as in patients with other mechanisms of acute ischemic stroke.
- Most aspects of secondary prevention after acute lacunar ischemic stroke are similar to principles that apply to ischemic stroke in general.

The term cerebral small-vessel disease refers to a group of pathological processes with various etiologies that affect the small arteries, arterioles, venules, and capillaries of the brain.[1] Age-related and hypertension-related small-vessel diseases and cerebral amyloid angiopathy are the most common forms. The small blood vessels are found in the surface of the brain or in the inner or deep cerebral tissue. These are the small cortical arteries and arterioles and the penetrating arteries, including superficial or medullary and deep penetrating arteries. Deep penetrating arteries include lenticulostriate, thalamoperforating, and brainstem paramedian branches.

Brain areas mainly supplied by microcirculation are cortical and subcortical areas; distal zones of frontier territories; centrum semiovale; central and deep encephalic areas, such as the caudate nucleus, internal capsule, globus pallidus, putamen, and the middle line of the brainstem; and the cerebellum.

Of all small-vessel diseases resulting from angiopathies that affect microcirculation, the most widely recognized clinical entity is lacunar infarct, traditionally defined as an ischemic stroke caused by occlusion of a single penetrating artery.[2] Lacunar infarcts account for up to about one-quarter of all ischemic strokes, constitute one of the classical stroke subtypes, and are included as a separate entity in all major stroke classification algorithms, like the Oxfordshire Stroke Classification,[3] the TOAST classification,[4] and its later derivatives,[5,6] and the ASCO classification.[7]

In the majority of cases, small-vessel disease is due to arteriolosclerosis related to vascular risk factors (see below). However, several other disease processes may also affect the cerebral small vessels.[1] These include sporadic and hereditary cerebral amyloid angiopathy, inherited or genetic small-vessel diseases distinct from cerebral amyloid angiopathy (such as CADASIL, CARASIL, hereditary multi-infarct dementia of the Swedish type, MELAS, Fabry's disease, hereditary cerebroretinal vasculopathy, hereditary endotheriopathy with retinopathy, nephropathy and stroke, small-vessel diseases caused by COL4A1 mutations). Small-vessel disease may also be caused by inflammatory and immunological mechanisms (e.g., Wegener's granulomatosis, Churg-Strauss syndrome, microscopic polyangitis, Henoch-Schönlein purpura, cryoglobulinemic vasculitis, cutaneous leucocytoclastic angiitis, primary angiitis of the brain, Sneddon's syndrome, nervous system vasculitis secondary to infections, nervous system vasculitis associated with connective tissue disorders such as systemic lupus erythematosus, Sjögren's syndrome, rheumatoid vasculitis, scleroderma, and dermatomyositis). Other examples of causes of cerebral small-artery disease are post-radiation angiopathy and non-amyloid microvessel degeneration in Alzheimer's disease.[1]

These more rare causes of cerebral small-vessel disease are further detailed in other chapters of this book. The focus of the present chapter is a delineation of cerebral vessel disease as it presents with acute ischemic stroke, lacunar infarcts in the context of the spectrum of cerebral small-vessel disease, risk factors, imaging features, and prognosis.

HISTORICAL ASPECTS

In 1838, Dechambre[8] used the term *lacune* for the first time with pathologic criteria. The entity was confused with other cavity lesions in the brain such as état criblé (small bilateral, multiple lesions in the white matter described by Durand-Fardel[9] in 1842; Fig. 27-1), residual necrotic tissue of small infarcts or hemorrhages, enlarged perivascular spaces (Fig. 27-2), and porosis due to postmortem bacterial autolysis.

In 1901, Pierre Marie[10] used *lacune* as his descriptive term for 50 cases of capsular infarction and clearly established the concept and classification of different small cavities in the brain, writing:

> *One could therefore picture the anatomo-pathological process of formation of lacunes in the following manner: the influence of the general causes of atherosclerosis, the vessels which irrigate the brain change, the nutrition of the brain*

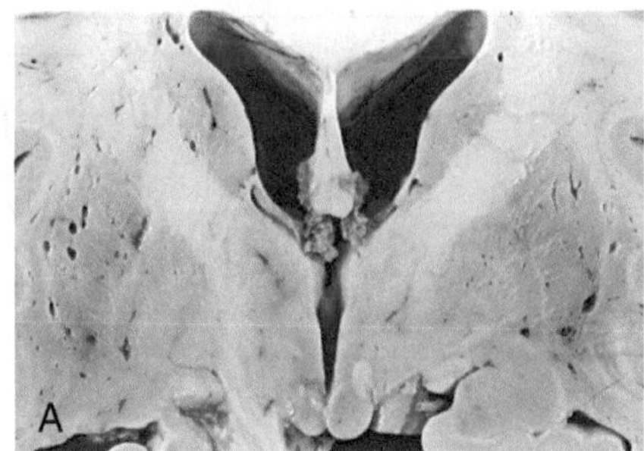

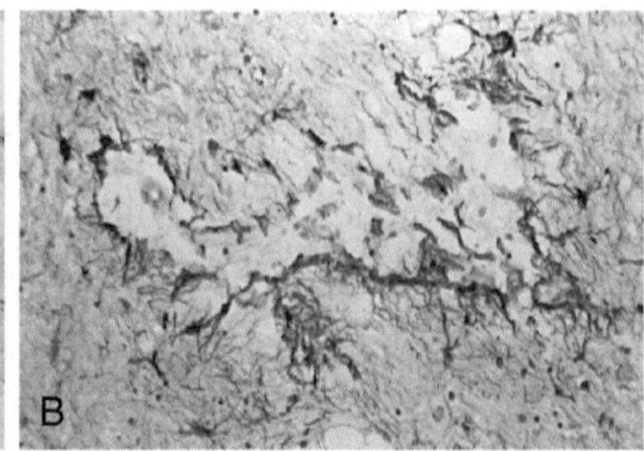

Figure 27-1. État criblé. A, Macroscopic coronal section. B, Microscopic pathologic specimen. (Glial fibrillary acidic protein [GFAP] stain.)

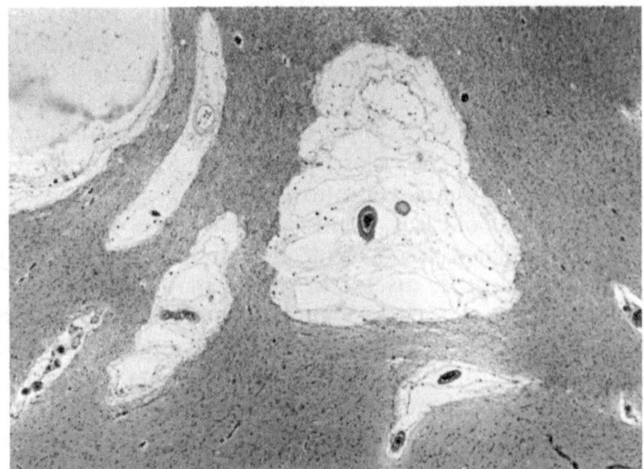

Figure 27-2. Multiple enlarged perivascular spaces in the putamen of a patient with marked small blood vessel disease. (Hematoxylin and eosin, ×40.) *(From Garcia JH, Ho KL: Pathology of hypertensive arteriopathy.* Neurosurg Clin N Am *3:487, 1992.)*

diminishes, its parts become atrophied, which contributes to the dilatation of the ventricles of the perivascular spaces. As the vascular lesions progress, one or more small vessels break or are obliterated, hence the production of one or more lacunes. In effect, it is known that in the central areas of the brain the blood vessels are terminal, that is, there are no astomoses, so that the whole territory is irrigated by the blood vessel which is obliterated is inevitably infarcted.

Marie emphasized a capsular and lenticular location for the syndrome.

Ferrand[11] claimed the next year that the same syndrome occurred whether the lesion was capsular or pontine in location. During the first quarter of the 20th century, the German pathologists Cecil and Oscar Vogt[12] firmly established the ischemic etiology.

Lacunes began their modern comeback almost entirely through the efforts of C. Miller Fisher. Fisher described pure motor hemiplegia,[13] pure sensory stroke,[14] homolateral ataxia and crural paresis (known mainly thereafter as ataxic hemiparesis),[15] dysarthria-clumsy hand syndrome,[16] sensorimotor stroke,[17] basilar branch syndromes,[18] and the vascular pathology underlying lacunes.[19] The position was so thoroughly developed that it triggered companion studies, of which many corroborated[17,20] and others enlarged on the clinical entities, vascular pathology, and clinicoradiological correlations.[21–23] Other researchers attacked the basic principles:[24–26] some argued for other causes including embolism[27] and others recommended that the concepts be abandoned altogether.[28] Numerous studies have claimed that the syndromes may have causes other than hypertensive arteriopathy.[15,29–32]

Studies on lacunar infarcts causing acute stroke and TIA changed direction dramatically with the advent of modern imaging techniques. Problems with low resolution and low detection rates of lacunar infarcts with CT were largely resolved by MRI techniques, in particular diffusion-weighted MRI which permits identification of acute ischemic lesions in the vast majority of patients. Through DW-MRI, much more precise clinic-imaging correlative studies became possible, changing the perspective of the precision of diagnosing lacunar stroke from clinical and CT features alone. A further dramatic change in our concepts of cerebral small-vessel disease was the recognition that the majority of parenchymal manifestations of cerebral small-vessel disease (such as silent cerebral infarcts, microbleeds, white matter abnormalities) did not present with acute stroke, but has been found to have other important consequences of brain function (cf. below).

LACUNAR INFARCTS IN THE SPECTRUM OF CEREBRAL SMALL-VESSEL DISEASE

For a long time it was commonly thought that most arterial occlusions in the brain presented clinically with acute neurological dysfunction and that the majority could be clinically diagnosed. Lacunar infarcts cause clinical symptoms when they affect the long motor and sensory tracts in the subcortical areas, linked to their clinical presentation. However, MRI studies of the general population, the reporting of which began in the 1990s, have shown that most lacunar infarcts do not produce acute stroke symptoms but are clinically unrecognized or "silent".[33–40] Silent cerebral infarcts (95% of which are "lacunar") are at least five times as common as symptomatic ones. Silent infarcts are not innocent; they have been shown to increase the risk of vascular events (including stroke), cognitive decline and dementia. They are "silent" only in the aspect that they have not caused acute cerebral dysfunction. Silent cerebral infarcts have the same pathological appearance as lacunar infarcts that cause acute stroke symptoms.[41]

Diagnosing a visualized infarct as "silent" is challenging, and several potential sources of error should be recognized. A previous clinical symptom, and even hospital admissions resulting in a diagnosis of TIA or stroke, may not be adequately recalled in a patient's self-report. Careful questioning may reveal that symptoms possibly related to the location of a SCI were actually present but ignored due to a lack of awareness of stroke symptoms in the elderly and in the families.[42] Furthermore, clinical symptoms may fail to be recognized as TIA or stroke even when brought to medical attention. There is a long list of "stroke chamelions", i.e., uncommon presentations of stroke that may be missed.[43]

Silent cerebral infarcts are closely linked to ischemic white matter lesions (WMLs). WMLs are even more prevalent in the elderly population than SCIs and the two conditions share most risk factors and show a high degree of covariance. The distinction between the two conditions may be less clear than previously thought.

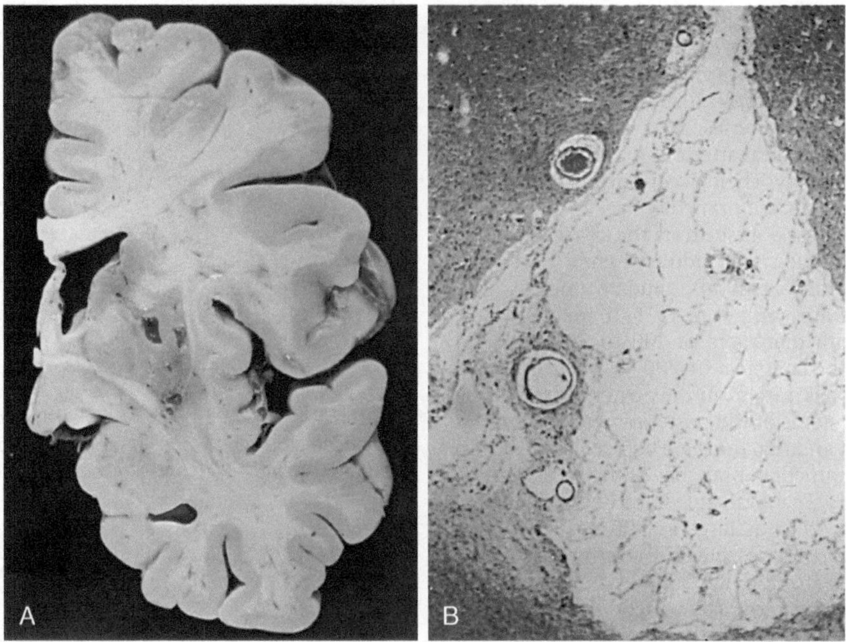

Figure 27-3. Lacunes in the basal ganglia. A, Macroscopic coronal section. B, Microscopic pathologic specimen. (Hematoxylin and eosin stain.)

A recent addition to the spectrum of silent brain infarcts is the cerebral microinfarct, very small (<1 mm) often a cortical infarct, that is not detected on conventional structural MRI.[44] Cerebral microinfarcts may be up to 15 times more frequent than "conventional" SCIs. Their role in contributing to clinical features and prognosis is currently unclear and merits further study.

Another component of the spectrum of cerebral small-vessel disease is the cerebral microbleed (CMB). CMBs are small (2 to 5 mm) hypointense lesions on paramagnetic sensitive MR sequences such as T2*-weighted gradient-echo (GRE) or susceptibility-weighted sequences. They are most often located in the cortico-subcortical junction, deep gray or white matter in the cerebral hemispheres, brainstem, and cerebellum. The common occurrence of CMB has only been recognized since the mid-1990s,[45,46] as CMBs are generally not visualized on CT or FLAIR, T1- or T2-weighted MR sequences. There has been substantial progress made in the understanding of CMBs during recent years (recently summarized in a comprehensive monograph),[47] but there are several areas in need of further study. CMBs localized to the deep hemispheric regions, brain stem and cerebellum have been closely linked to traditional vascular risk factors similar to lacunar infarcts, whereas multiple, strictly lobar CMBs, have been shown to be highly specific for severe cerebral amyloid angiopathy, and are prerequisites in establishing a diagnosis of cerebral amyloid angiopathy.[46,47]

DEFINITIONS

Precise definitions of several terms related to cerebral small-vessel disease have been lacking. A large number of terms have been used which has created confusion, in particular for the use of "lacune". In a paper late in his career, C. Miller Fisher wrote: "Historically, the original small vessel disease feature was the lacune (hole), which derived from French for a small fluid-filled cavity that was thought to mark the healed stage of a small deep brain infarct. The term was adopted into English. By a process of medico-linguistic evolution, the precavitary phase became the lacunar infarct, the associated clinical entity became the lacunar stroke and the neurological features became the lacunar syndrome".[48] Thus, the term lacune is a neuropathological term that refers to a finding of a cavitation (Fig. 27-3). Lacunar infarct refers to an infarct that is presumably related to a single penetrating artery occlusion. When causing acute stroke symptoms, a lacunar infarct most commonly presents clinically as a lacunar syndrome (see below). Lacunar syndromes can more rarely (in about 5% of cases) be caused by a small hemorrhage.

PATHOANATOMY

Most pathological studies on lacunar infarcts were performed before or in the early CT era, whereas later reports are scarce. The paucity of autopsy reports overall in lacunar infarcts is, however, not surprising: the early mortality rates after lacunar infarcts are very low, and if an autopsy examination is carried out it is usually performed months or years after a stroke event, making inference of etiology very difficult. The pathological reports on lacunes should be read with these limitations in mind.

Most autopsy-documented lacunar infarcts are small, ranging from 0.2 to 15 mm^3 in size.[49] They vary according to the territory supplied by the occluded vessel feeding the infarct. In general, vessels are 100 to 400 μm[10] in size and serve territories varying from little more than a cylinder the size of the vessel itself to wedges as large as 15 mm on a side. Deep infarcts of larger size than 15 mm at autopsy were in some early reports labeled as "super lacunes" and found to be associated with occlusion (usually embolic) of the middle cerebral artery affecting multiple lenticulostriate branches; they are today classified as striatocapsular infarcts and constitute a distinct stroke entity separate from lacunar infarct.[50] However, it should be noted that partial striatocapsular infarcts occur, and that they can shrink with time to less than 15 mm in diameter.

Lacunes predominate in the basal ganglia, especially the putamen, the thalamus, and the white matter of the internal capsule and pons; they also occur occasionally in the white matter of the cerebral gyri. They are rare in the gray matter of the cerebral surface, as well as in the corpus callosum, visual radiations, centrum semiovale of the cerebral hemispheres, medulla, cerebellum, and spinal cord.[51] Most lacunes occur in the territories of the lenticulostriate branches of the anterior and middle cerebral arteries, the thalamoperforating branches of the posterior cerebral arteries, and the paramedian branches of the basilar artery. Their occurrence is rare in the territories of the cerebral surface branches.

The lenticulostriate vessels arise from the circle of Willis and the stems of the anterior and middle cerebral arteries to supply the putamen, globus pallidus, caudate nucleus, and internal capsule. They are composed of two main groups: those more medial, with diameters of 100 to 200 μm, and those more lateral, with diameters of 200 to 400 μm.[49] The thalamoperforating vessels arise from the posterior half of the circle of Willis and the stems of the posterior cerebral arteries to supply the midbrain and thalamus.[52] Their size varies from 100 to 400 μm. The paramedian branches of the basilar artery mainly supply the pons. Few branches have been measured, but sizes ranging from 40 to as large as 500 μm have been observed.[19,53] What these arteries have in common is a tendency to arise directly from much larger arteries and an unbranching end-artery anatomy. The penetrators are all less than 500 μm in size and arise directly from the larger, 6- to 8-mm, internal carotid or basilar artery. Their small size and their points of origin rather proximal in the arterial network are thought to expose these vessels to forces that scarcely reach other arteries of similar size in the cerebral cortex.[54] These latter arteries are apparently protected by a gradual step-down in size from the 8-mm internal carotid, to the 3- to 4-mm middle cerebral, to the 1- to 2-mm surface branches, from which the intracortical vessels whose diameters are less than 500 μm arise. Perhaps this difference explains the low frequency of lacunes in the cerebral surface vessels.[55,56]

The lack of collateral circulation for the penetrators results in an infarct that spreads distally from the point of occlusion through the entire territory of the vessel affected. The exact volume of tissue supplied by each penetrating artery varies enormously.[19] Some arteries supply little more than a territory of the same diameter as the vessels,[49] whereas others arborize widely and leave an infarct shaped like a wedge or cone.[19] Most capsular infarcts arise from arteries 200–400 μm in size and produce infarcts of about 2–3 mm^3. These small infarcts are found regularly only on MRI with 1.5-Tesla strength, are commonly missed on CT scanning, and are easily overlooked at autopsy.[22] The arterial occlusion usually occurs in the first half of the course of the penetrating vessel, which ensures that most such occlusions are quite small.

Several distinct but related arteriopathies cause lacunes. Microatheroma is believed to be the most common mechanism of arterial stenosis underlying symptomatic lacunes (Fig. 27-4).[19,49,57] The artery is usually involved in the first half of its course. Microatheroma stenosing or occluding a penetrating artery was found in six of 11 capsular infarcts in the only published pathologic study on the cause of capsular infarcts,[49] and it was the cause of the only published case of a thalamic lacune.[14] The histologic characteristics of the microatheroma are identical to those affecting the larger arteries.

These tiny foci of atheromatous deposits are commonly encountered in chronic hypertension. In the usual nonhypertensive case, atheroma appears mostly in the extracranial internal carotid and basilar arteries but only rarely in the stems of the major cerebral arteries.[58,59] In hypertension, however, the lesions not only are more advanced for the patient's age, but also are spread more distally in the arterial system, at times involving even some of the cerebral surface arteries. In patients with advanced hypertension, miniature foci of typical atherosclerotic plaques are found even in arteries as small as

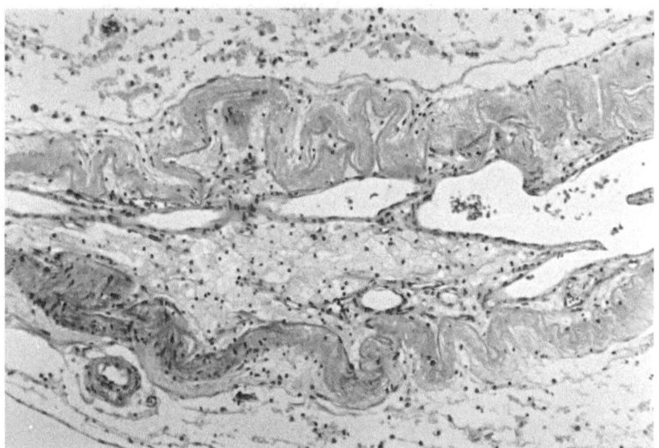

Figure 27-4. Intimal deposit of lipid-laden macrophages in a penetrating intracerebral artery that shows partial occlusion of the lumen. (Hematoxylin and eosin, ×100.) *(Courtesy of J.H. Garcia, MD.)*

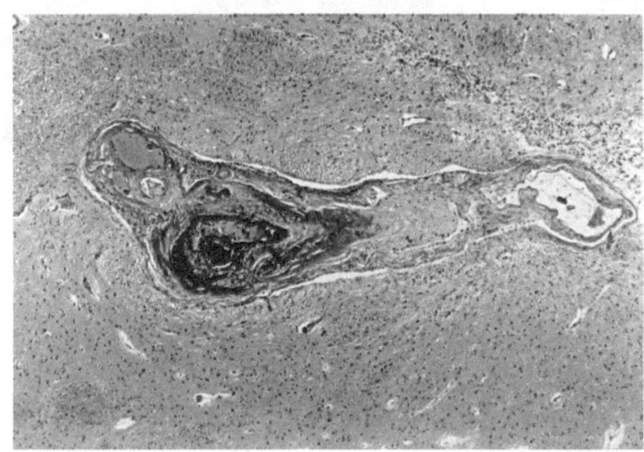

Figure 27-5. Terminal segment of a lenticulostriate artery showing marked mural changes (hyalinization and fibrinoid change) as well as occlusion of the lumen. (Hematoxylin and eosin, ×60.) *(From Garcia JH, Ho KL: Pathology of hypertensive arteriopathy.* Neurosurg Clin N Am *3:487, 1992.)*

100–400 μm in diameter, resulting in a stenosis or occlusion that sets the stage for a lacune. In a retrospective autopsy study of 70 brains with microscopic evidence of small-vessel disease, the morphology of the vessel disease, the arteriolosclerosis, was similar in normotensive and hypertensive subjects. Lacunes were as prevalent in normotensive subjects (36%) as in hypertensive patients (40%), which would suggest that the control of hypertension has modified the pathology of small-vessel disease.[60]

Other arterial disorders seem less common. Lipohyalinosis, formerly considered the most frequent cause of lacunes, affects penetrating arteries in a segmental fashion in chronic hypertension.[54] It was the cause attributed to 40 of 50 lacunes studied in serial section by Fisher[19] in four cases of stroke. It seems to occur most often in the smaller penetrating arteries, that is, in those less than 200 μm in diameter, and accounts for many of the smaller lacunes, especially those that are clinically asymptomatic. Lipohyalinosis has been thought to be an intermediate stage between the fibrinoid necrosis of severe hypertension and the microatheroma associated with more long-standing hypertension.[19,53,56]

Fibrinoid necrosis is a related condition found in arterioles and capillaries of the brain (Fig. 27-5), retina, and kidneys in a setting of extremely high blood pressure.[61] It appears histopathologically as a brightly eosinophilic, finely granular, or homogeneous deposit involving the connective tissue of blood vessels.[62] The mechanism is believed to involve disordered cerebrovascular autoregulation[63,64] and has a necrotizing consequence.[55] Fibrinoid necrosis shares some of the histochemical, electron microscopic,[30,65] and immunofluorescent[66] characteristics of lipohyalinosis,[67] another cause of lacunes.

Microembolism has been inferred in a few serially sectioned lacunes shown to have normal arteries leading to the infarct.[49] However, such cases have been examined with autopsy years after the stroke, which makes inference on mechanisms of injury in the acute phase spurious.

RISK FACTORS

Lacunar infarctions share many risk factors with other types of ischemic stroke, of which the most common are hypertension and diabetes mellitus. These two risk factors for lacunar disease have been present with comparable frequencies in larger clinical series of lacunar infarcts: 75% and 29%, respectively, of lacunar cases diagnosed in the Harvard Cooperative Stroke Registry;[68] and 72% and 28%, respectively, of the Barcelona series reported by Arboix et al.[69] There has been considerable debate in the past about whether these two risk factors are more prevalent, and characteristic, for lacunar infarcts compared to other subtypes. A problem with the TOAST classification,[4] used in many of the risk factor studies, is that hypertension and diabetes have been included in the definition of the small-vessel disease (lacunar) subtype, creating a potential bias for risk factor analyses. In a systematic review of studies Jackson and Sudlow found only a marginal excess of hypertension in lacunar versus non-lacunar infarcts.[70] In a later study[71] pooling individual data on 2875 patients with first-ever ischemic stroke from five collaborating prospective stroke registers that used similar, unbiased methods to define risk factors and classify stroke subtypes, a lower prevalence of cardioembolic source (adjusted odds ratio, 0.33; 95% confidence interval [CI], 0.24–0.46), ipsilateral carotid stenosis (odds ratio [OR], 0.21; 95%CI, 0.14–0.30), and ischemic heart disease (OR, 0.75; 95%CI, 0.58–0.97) were noticed in lacunar compared with non-lacunar patients, but no differences for hypertension, diabetes, or any other risk factors were searched for. Results were robust to sensitivity analyses and largely confirmed in our meta-analysis. Thus, hypertension and diabetes appear equally common in lacunar and non-lacunar ischemic stroke, but lacunar stroke is less likely to be caused by embolism from the heart or proximal arteries, and the lower prevalence of ischemic heart disease in lacunar stroke provides additional support for a non-atherosclerotic arteriopathy causing many lacunar ischemic strokes.

Atrial fibrillation, one of the hallmarks of embolism, has a low frequency of small, deep infarcts (5%),[72] similar to the frequency in the general population older than 60 years. In very elderly patients (older than 85 years), there is a high frequency of atrial fibrillation (28%) as a consequence of age. Several other risk factors for vascular disease, such as smoking, obesity, low physical activity, are also frequently present in patients with lacunar infarcts, but appears as a general risk factor for stroke rather than being specific for lacunar infarction.

More advanced genetic studies on specific stroke subtypes have been reported only recently. A genetic risk of stroke may be mediated through already-known risk factors, such as cholesterol and blood pressure levels.[73] In earlier study on specific SNPs the angiotensin-converting enzyme gene and the angiotensinogen gene were found to be associated with the presence of neurologic manifestations in lacunar infarctions.[74] Homozygosity for the G allele of the Glu298Asp polymorphism in the endothelial constitutive nitric oxide synthetase gene was associated with brain infarction and, especially, with lacunar stroke.[75] The TPA-7351C/T polymorphism appeared as an independent risk factor for lacunar stroke.[76] AGT gene M235T polymorphism may represent a risk factor for lacunar infarction.[77] An association between lacunar infarction and the genotype of the interleukin-6 polymorphism was also reported.[78]

However, it is notable that in GWAS studies on ischemic stroke[79] no specific variants have been found in patients of white ethnic origin with small-vessel ischemic stroke, possibly because of the high heterogeneity in phenotype ascertainment (i.e., many definitions of small-vessel ischemic stroke can be used) and the fairly small sample sizes. Research is ongoing to improve phenotyping in these cases. With new classification schemes, the aim is to standardize nomenclature used in small-vessel stroke and related imaging findings and to reduce the number of diseases that mimic small-vessel disease and lead to misclassification.

IMAGING STUDIES

Computed Tomography

Technical limitations of even the most modern CT scanners prevent the resolution of most lacunes smaller than 2 mm in the internal capsule and almost all of those in the thalamus and brainstem[26,80] because of an obscuring artifact. For the lacunar syndromes documented in the NINCDS Stroke Data Bank, a lesion was found in 35% of cases on the first CT scan; most lesions were located in the posterior limb of the internal capsule and corona radiate.[81] Repeated CT scans increased the yield to 39%. Brainstem lesions were not often visualized. The mean infarct volume in this cohort was greater in pure motor and sensorimotor stroke syndromes than in ataxic hemiparesis, dysarthria-clumsy hand, and pure sensory stroke syndromes. In those patients with pure motor stroke and posterior capsule infarction, there was a correlation between lesion size and severity of hemiparesis, except for the small number of patients whose infarcts involved the lowest portion of the capsule, supplied by the anterior choroidal artery, where severe deficits occurred without regard for lesion size.

Magnetic Resonance Imaging

MRI has greatly changed the frequency with which small infarcts are demonstrated.[82] Although CT is still used in clinical practice as the first (and often only) imaging technique, MRI has now surpassed it in sensitivity for the detection of lacunes.[83,84] In their study of 227 patients with lacunar infarcts, Arboix et al.[69] found that CT findings were positive in 100 patients (44%), whereas MRI findings were positive in 35 of 45 (78%). MRI was significantly better ($P < 0.001$) than CT for imaging lacunes, especially those located in either the pons ($P < 0.005$) or the internal capsule ($P < 0.001$). Motor stroke, pure or sensorimotor, has the highest positive rate on MRI, and pure sensory stroke has the lowest. This finding corresponds to the main volumes of the classic lacunar syndromes on MRI: sensorimotor, 1.7 mL; pure motor, 1.2 mL; ataxic hemiparesis, 0.6 mL; and pure sensory, 0.2 mL. Hommel et al.[84] used MRI for 100 patients hospitalized with lacunar infarct syndrome and also found it more sensitive. MRI detected at least one lacune appropriate to the symptoms in 89 patients in whom 135 lacunes were found on imaging. MRI was more effective when it was performed a few days after the stroke. However, it should be recognized that MR-negative cases exist: in one study up to 30% of patients with symptomatic lacunar stroke syndromes no infarct was in the subcortex or elsewhere in the brain.[85]

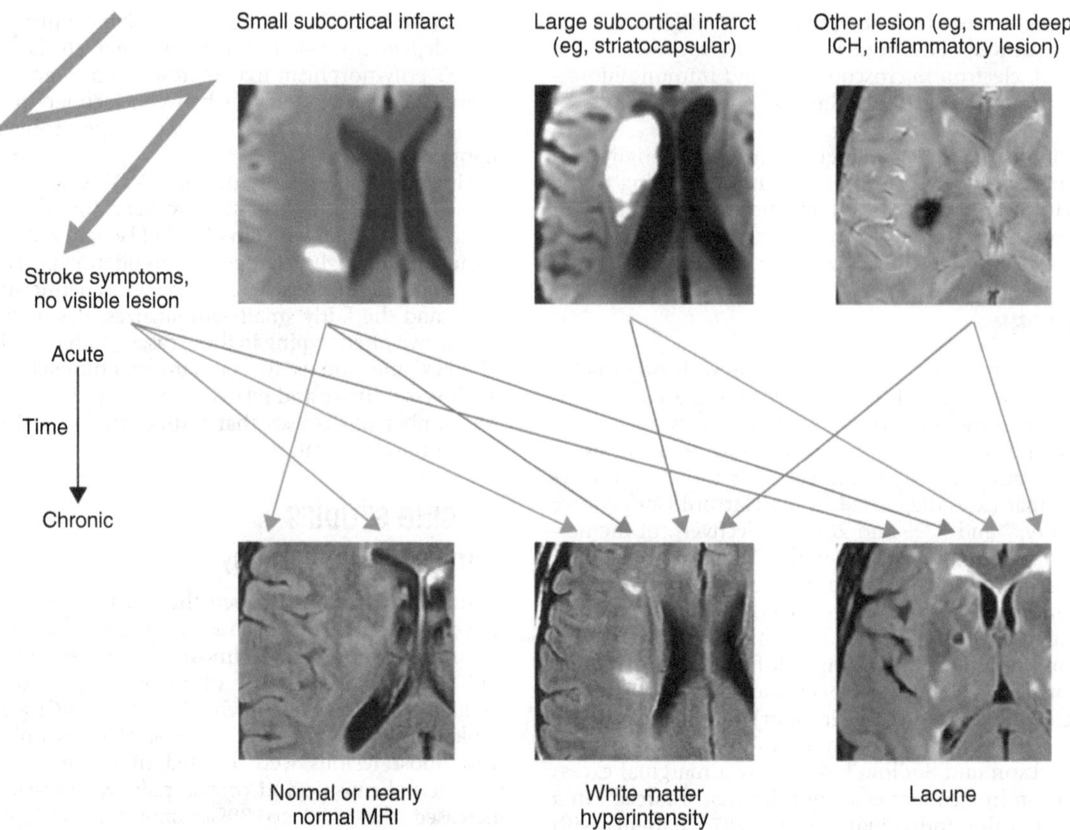

Figure 27-6. Variable fates of lesions related to small-vessel disease and the convergence of acute lesions with different causes but similar late appearances on MRI. *(From Wardlaw JM, Smith EE, Biessels GJ, et al. Neuroimaging standards for research into small vessel disease and its contribution to ageing and neurodegeneration.* Lancet Neurology *2013;12:822–38).*

Diffusion-weighted (DW) MRI is the most sensitive and specific imaging method for detection of acute subcortical ischemic lesions and can differentiate acute from non-acute lesions. Acute lacunar infarcts appear on DW-MRI as a bright area of decreased apparent diffusion coefficient (ADC); a subacute lacunar infarct is seen as an area of decreased or normal ADC, and a chronic infarct is seen as with a normal or increased ADC.[86] In several reports, all or almost all patients with clinical acute subcortical infarction had focal areas of high intensity appeared on DW MRI that correlated with all or part of the patient's clinical syndromes.[87,88]

MRI criteria for cerebral small-vessel disease infarcts have been imprecise. Recently, a report on neuroimaging standards for research into small-vessel disease and its contribution to aging and neurodegeneration was published.[89] Studies have shown that not all (symptomatic) acute small deep infarcts cavitate with time and appear as "lacunes": some appear as white matter hyperintensities, whereas some are not visualized at all with time. As a consequence, the distinction between previous symptomatic cerebral infarcts, silent brain infarcts and white matter hyperintensities of presumed vascular origin is less sharp than previously recognized, or reported in scientific studies, as interpreted from late neuroimaging findings alone. Estimates of the proportion of acute small deep infarcts that cavitate are variable and range from 28% to 94%.[90,91] Cavitation may be related to time and size of the lesion, but also to neuroimaging methods such as MRI sequences.[92] It should be recognized that a very small proportion of cavitated lesions appearing as a silent cerebral infarct may have been caused by a previous small bleed. The variable fates of small-vessel disease-related lesions and convergence of etiologically different lesions to result in similar late appearances on MRI are illustrated in Figure 27-6.

Presumed silent cerebral infarcts need to be carefully separated from prominent perivascular spaces (Virchow-Robin spaces), a distinction which may have been overseen in early reports. Perivascular spaces are fluid-filled spaces that follow a typical course of a vessel penetrating/transversing the brain through gray or white matter.[89] They will appear linear when imaged parallel to the course of the vessel, and round or ovoid (with a diameter less than 2 mm) when imaged perpendicular to the course of the vessel.

Magnetic resonance angiography (MRA) can detect intracranial large-artery diseases, stenoses, or occlusions in 21% of patients meeting clinical and radiologic criteria for lacunar infarcts, but only in 10% is the artery disease related to the affected penetrating vessel.[93] In one study MRA disclosed a basilar artery stenosis in four of 11 patients with paramedian pontine infarction of lacunar type and a clinical lacunar syndrome (ten with pure motor hemiparesis and one with ataxic hemiparesis).[94] Microvasculature of the brain as lenticulostriate arteries can be observed by 7.0-Tesla MRA.[95]

CLINICAL SYNDROMES

When symptomatic, lacunar infarcts are associated with clinical "lacunar" syndromes, five of which are well recognized: pure motor hemiparesis, pure sensory stroke, sensorimotor stroke, dysarthria-clumsy hand syndrome, and ataxic hemiparesis. Face, arm, and leg involvement are characteristic of the first three syndromes. The most important clinical feature for lacunar syndromes is the absence of cognitive symptoms or signs and visual field defects.

Pure Motor Stroke

Pure motor stroke is undoubtedly the most common of any lacunar form, accounting for between one-half and two-thirds of cases, depending on the series.[69,96–98] It was the first lacunar syndrome recognized clinically,[10,13] and its features have been the most thoroughly explored. Fisher and Curry defined the syndrome in their original report:[13] "… a paralysis complete or incomplete of the face, arm and leg on one side not accompanied by sensory signs, visual field defect, dysphasia, or apractognosia. In the case of brainstem symptoms the hemiplegia will be free of vertigo, deafness, tinnitus, diplopia, cerebellar ataxia, and gross nystagmus. … This definition applies to the acute phase of the vascular insult and does not include less recent strokes in which other signs were present at the beginning, but faded with the passage of time …"

Clinicoanatomic Correlations

Pure motor stroke, also known as pure motor hemiparesis, has been reported from autopsied cases with focal infarction involving the corona radiate,[99] internal capsule,[13,92] pons,[18] and medullary pyramid.[13,24,100] The most common correlations have been with capsular locations. Of the two ends of the capsule, the greater number of lacunes has been reported in the posterior limb (Fig. 27-7).

Posterior limb capsular lacunes usually involve the globus pallidus and posterior limb of the capsule,[101] which are supplied by the lenticulostriate branches of the middle cerebral artery. The vessels occluded vary in size from small, medially placed penetrators to the larger lateral lenticulostriate vessels. The infarcts range in location from the genu to the back of the posterior limb. It is in this group that most of the data referable to the classic views of a homunculus in the internal capsule are to be found. Lesions in this region, especially those affecting the corona radiata, have also produced the syndrome of ataxic hemiparesis.

Anterior limb capsular lacunes constitute a smaller number of cases and are smaller infarcts that may affect the caudate in addition to the anterior limb of the capsule.[22] Some of them are in the territory of supply of the anterior cerebral artery, including the largest of the penetrating vessels, the recurrent artery of Heubner. Syndromes of hemiparesis constitute only one of the many permutations of anterior capsular infarcts,[101,102] which also include ataxic hemiparesis.[103]

Other Causes of Pure Motor Syndromes

Not all pure motor syndromes are due to a lacunar infarct. Non-lacunar locations are found in a proportion of patients (as discussed below) indicating a mechanism different from small-vessel occlusion. Also, a small proportion (5%) of patients with pure motor stroke have an intracerebral hemorrhage as the cause. Pure motor stroke has also, in rare cases, been reported in patients with non-vascular lesions such as brain tumor or abscess.

Clinical Features

Pure motor stroke is most easily diagnosed when the stroke affects the face, arm, and leg equally on the same side, sparing sensation, vision, language, and behavior.[13] The complete syndrome, however, is somewhat uncommon. As a clinical rule, as long as the syndrome is purely motor, the diagnosis applies when the affected side involves one part more than the other. Some cases have been described in which the face is essentially spared; the best known is from pyramidal infarction.[104] In a series of 22 patients with a brachiofacial pure motor stroke, four had a cortical infarct in the superficial middle cerebral artery.[105] Pure motor monoparesis is almost never due to a lacunar infarct.[106] The term *pure motor stroke* was initially used to draw attention to the lack of expected accompanying sensory, visual, or behavior disturbances, especially considering the severity of the weakness. In this sense only is it "pure".

Pure motor stroke has been described in both capsular and pontine locations, producing a clinical picture essentially identical to that first suggested by Ferrand.[11] Despite earlier opinions expressed by Ferrand[11] and by Foix and Levy,[107] it has become clear that pure motor stroke may be associated with considerable variations among the syndromes involving the face, arm, and leg. Fisher and Curry[13] found the arm severely affected in all 50 of their cases of pure motor stroke, but the lower the lesion occurred in the neuraxis, the less the face was involved.

Most of the initial imaging studies were based on CT scans. Donnan et al.[21] found hemiplegia involving the face, arm, and

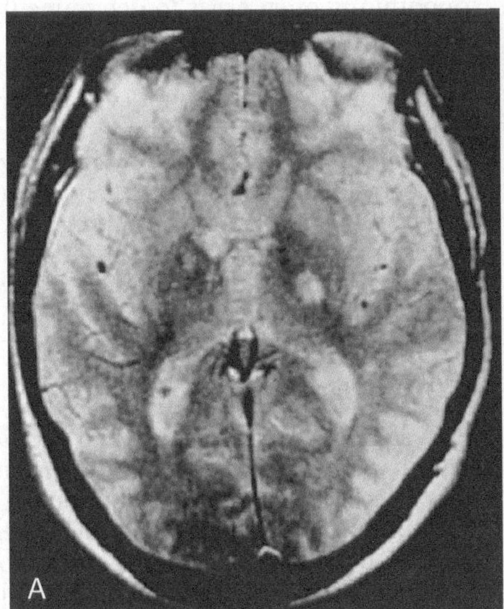

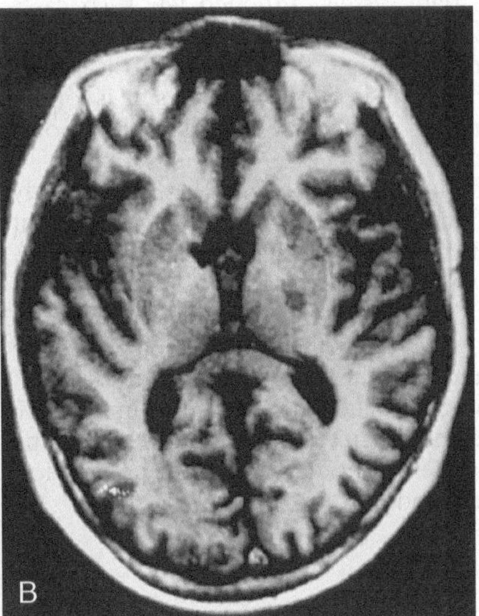

Figure 27-7. Axial (A) T2-weighted and (B) T1-weighted magnetic resonance images showing a lacunar infarct in the posterior limb of the internal capsule.

leg in equivalent fashion in all 36 patients with infarction involving the capsule, but 22 other patients in the same series had incomplete syndromes, the most common of which was paresis of the arm and leg that spared the face. The inferred lacunar infarct in these latter cases occurred more often in the fibers of the corona radiata or at the extreme ends of the capsule. One lacunar infarct with pure facial weakness was located at the genu, whereas another associated with pure leg weakness lay at the extreme posterior end of the capsule. Rascol et al.[101] also found a spectrum of syndromes of hemiparesis that varied at one end from equal involvement of the face, arm, and leg to partial syndromes of faciobrachial weakness, and a few cases were purely crural; similar incomplete formulas of hemiparesis occurred in the smaller capsule-pallidal cases and also in the anterior capsulocaudate infarct cases. In both the NINCDS Pilot Stroke Data Bank project[98] and the population-based study of stroke conducted in southern Alabama,[108] lacunes located more posteriorly in the capsule produced a deficit greater in the leg than in the arm, but several varieties were encountered, including some in which the arm was worse than the leg. Lesions affecting the anterior limb and genu have also been a source of syndromes of partial hemiparesis, and a few cases have featured greater weakness of the face than of the leg.[21] In cases studied in the Stroke Data Bank, lesions seen in the corona radiata were associated with hemiparesis that took highly variable forms, whereas those located lower in the capsule produced a wide variety of syndromes (Fig. 27-8).[81] Taken together, the CT scan correlations with the syndromes of hemiparesis showed only slight support for the classic view of a homunculus in the internal capsule with the face, arm, and leg displayed in an anteroposterior distribution.

Although the main elements of the pure motor stroke syndromes are motor, other complaints are not rare, especially sensory disturbances, which occur initially in as many as 42% of cases.[21] These complaints usually are seen as numbness, heaviness, and loss of feeling. Only scant abnormalities are found on clinical examination. Given their vague character, they are all too easily brushed aside or ignored. However, complaints of undue coldness, at times confined to the distal arm, are less easily ignored, and, in a few cases personally observed by the author, they have lasted for years.[68] The anatomic disorder of these complaints has not been resolved. These sensory complaints are thought to reflect slight involvement of the projections to the sensory cortex from occlusion of the larger lateral striate vessels, although few such cases have actually been documented by autopsy. When the perception threshold for temperature and thermal pain is measured, a significant thermal hypesthesia on the affected side is found. This semiologic finding has also been reported in pure motor and sensorimotor stroke.[109]

Preceding TIAs occur in about 25% of all cases, usually only shortly before the infarct occurs. Sometimes patients present with a burst of dramatic TIAs with dense hemiparesis for 5–15 minutes alternating with normal function - the "capsular warning syndrome". About half of these patients go on to develop a lacunar infarct within the first 1–2 days, despite routine antiplatelet and even heparin therapies. Initial progression of the neurological deficit is observed in up to 40% of all cases, making lacunar infarct the most common subtype of progressive stroke. The exact mechanisms of the progression are still not well understood.[110]

Clinical Course

Compared with the sudden onset more typical of infarction in other territories, a leisurely mode of onset has occurred in many lacunar strokes, delayed over enough time that an opportunity often exists to determine the effects of intervention. In contrast to major atheromatous or embolic stroke, in which a gradual onset is encountered in less than 5% of cases, as many as 30% of lacunes develop over a period of up to 36 hours.[14,49,111,112] During this time, a mild weakness may evolve into total paralysis, usually by intensifying the initial deficit but occasionally by spreading into limbs not affected initially.[14] At clinical onset, the progression of the neurologic deficit is frequent, and lacunar infarct is the major cause of progressive motor dysfunction.[113] This smooth onset occurs with equal frequency in all types of lacunar syndromes.

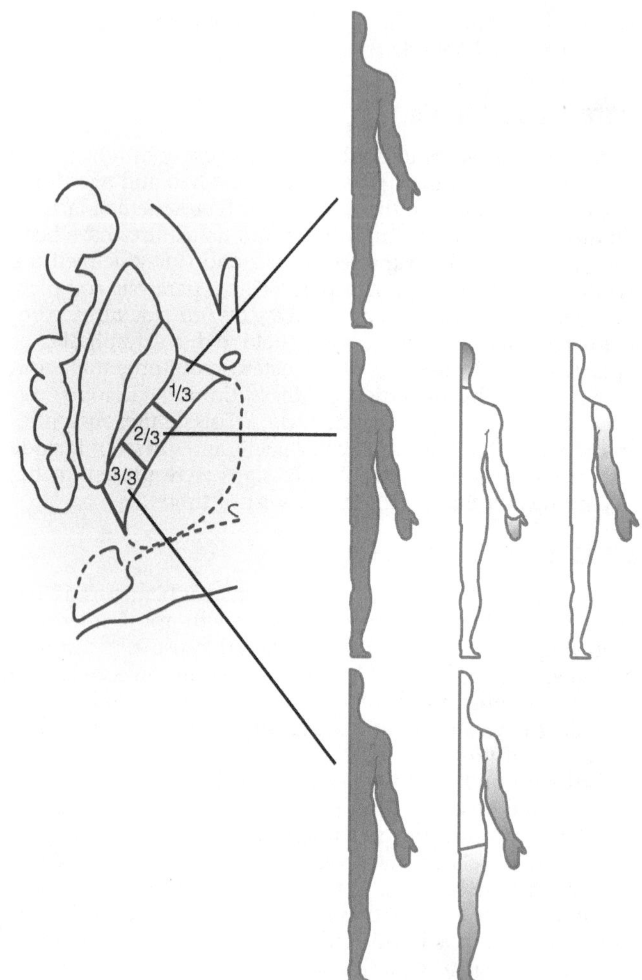

Figure 27-8. Hemiparesis formulas for capsular lesions of the anterior, middle, and posterior thirds of the posterior limb of the internal capsule. *(From Chamorro AM, Saco RL, Mohr JP, et al: Lacunar infarction: Clinical–CT correlations in the Stroke Data Bank.* Stroke *22:175, 1991.)*

Pure Sensory Stroke

Pure sensory stroke is assumed to be due to infarction of the sensory pathway of the brainstem, thalamus, or thalamocortical projections. The thalamus is supplied by very small arteries susceptible to the effects of chronic hypertension.[52] In the few autopsy-documented cases, the most common location was the thalamus,[14,17,114] mostly in the ventral posterior tier nuclei, which is the main sensory relay nuclei to the cerebrum.[114] The only autopsied case with pure sensory stroke from a lesion outside the thalamus[115] consisted of a small hemorrhage that involved the corona radiata of the posterior limb of the internal capsule.

CT has been the basis of identification of the other sites associated with pure sensory stroke (Fig. 27-9). One case, inferred to be due to a lacune because of the small size of the lesion, affected the centrum semiovale, presumably with involvement of the thalamocortical projection area.[116] Caution is necessary in this interpretation because lacunes in the centrum semiovale are distinctly uncommon in series based on autopsy data.[29,99] Involvement of subthalamic brainstem pathways has not yet been reported to be associated with pure sensory stroke. Pure sensory stroke due to a pontine tegmentum lesion can cause ipsilateral impairment of the smooth pursuit eye movements, which can be differentiated to thalamic topography.[117]

Observations of the underlying arterial pathology are confined to two cases. In one, a microatheroma was found narrowing the lumen of a small artery to the posterior thalamus,[19] which led to a lacunar infarct. The report did not mention whether the lacune was symptomatic. In the other case, a pure sensory syndrome was described clinically.[14] The 54-year-old patient was recovering from a right-sided pure motor hemiplegia when a feeling of pins and needles developed in the left lower lip, the left side of the mouth, and the fingers of the left hand; the sole of the left foot tingled and felt numb, dull, and swollen many hours later. No sensory deficit was evident on examination. Unpleasant paresthesias affected the left side of the face and the left foot. The CT scan findings were normal on the fourth day. At autopsy 6 months later, a lacune measuring 2 × 2 × 3.7 mm was found in the right ventral posterior nucleus, fed by four tiny arteries that arose from a single artery destroyed by lipohyalinosis.

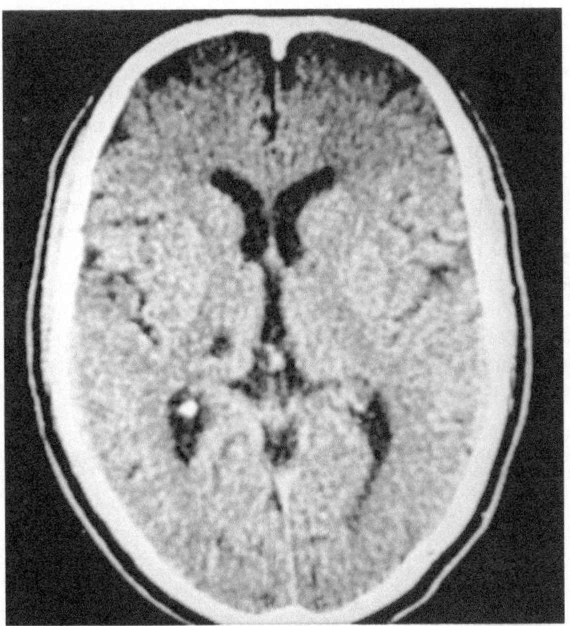

Figure 27-9. CT scan showing thalamic lacunar infarct.

The lacunes in both of the reported autopsied cases were quite small. If they are typical, it is easy to understand why many thalamic lacunes have thus far escaped detection by CT and require the higher-grade image provided by MRI. Larger lesions may be seen with both techniques (Fig. 27-10). In a clinical series of 99 patients with pure sensory stroke that accounted for 17.4% of lacunar syndromes, a lacunar infarct on CT or MRI studies was observed in 84% of cases.[118]

Typically, the disturbance in sensation extends over the entire side of the body, involving the face, proximal as well as distal limbs, and axial structures including the scalp, neck, trunk, and genitalia right to the midline, even splitting the two sides of the nose, tongue, penis, and anus.[68,114] This remarkable midline split, especially when the trunk or abdomen is involved, may be unique to thalamic or thalamocortical pathway lesions. This type of hemisensory syndrome affected one patient with a thalamic infarction measuring 4 × 4 × 2 mm.

Variants in the topography of pure sensory stroke have been reported that involve less than the entire side of the body. One patient, reported with autopsy correlation (case 9 in Fisher's original collection of pure sensory stroke),[114] suffered only TIAs affecting at one time the right fingers and at another time the right upper and lower lips, right side of the tongue, and the two medial toes of the right foot. At autopsy, a lacune 7 mm in diameter was found in the left ventral posterior nucleus. The complaints in other cases without autopsy documentation have involved the face, arm, and leg; head, cheek, lips, and hand; unilateral intraoral and perioral sites and fingers, the so-called cheiro-oral syndrome; face, fingers, and foot; shoulder tip and lower jaw; distal forearm alone; fingers alone; and leg alone.[51,114] How many permutations exist is a subject of some interest because establishing them might serve

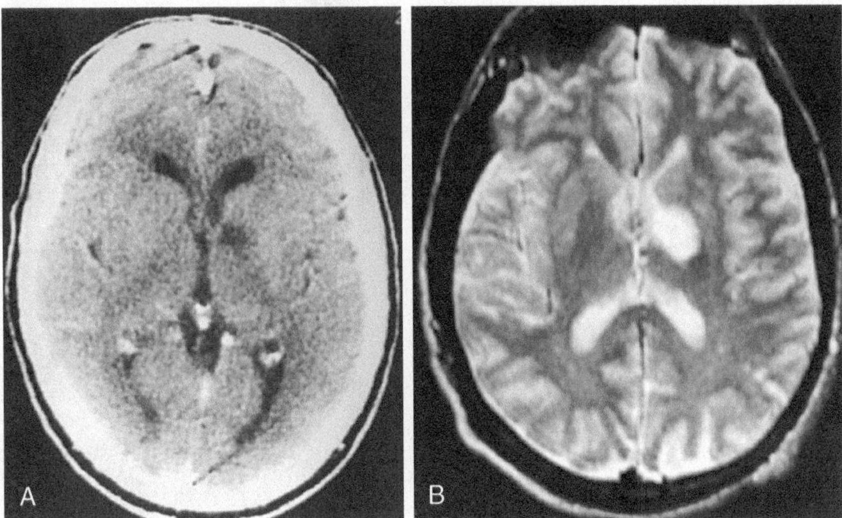

Figure 27-10. Anterior thalamic infarct seen on (A) CT scan and (B) MRI of the same patient.

to determine the organization of a sensory homunculus in the ventral tier nuclei.

Lapresle and Haguenau[119] found partial sensory syndromes involving the face, the arms, the leg, the oral cavity, the peribuccal area and forearm, and the peribuccal area and radial edge of the forearm, of which all were from focal thalamic softening of lacunar size. As already mentioned, the patient in Fisher's case 9 suffered only TIAs affecting the right fingers at one time, and the right upper and lower lips, the right side of the tongue, and the two medial toes of the right foot at another time.[14] A lacune 7 mm in diameter affecting the left ventral posterior nucleus was found at autopsy. In another autopsied case also previously described, a 54-year-old patient recovering from a right pure motor hemiplegia experienced a feeling of pins and needles in the left lower lip, the left side of the mouth, and the fingers of the left hand; the sole of the left foot tingled and felt numb, dull, and became swollen many hours later. No sensory deficit was evident on examination. Unpleasant paresthesias affected the left side of the face and the left foot. CT scan results were normal on the fourth day. At autopsy 6 months later, a 2 × 2 × 3-mm lacune was found in the right ventral posterior thalamus.[14] The complaints in other cases without autopsy documentation have involved the face, arm, and leg; head, cheek, lips, and hand; face, fingers, and foot; shoulder tip and lower jaw; distal forearm alone; fingers alone; and leg alone. The full array of permutations has been subject to considerable study.[120] Incomplete hemisensory syndrome was present in 19 of 99 patients with pure sensory stroke (cheiro-oral in 12, cheiro-oral-pedal in six, and isolated oral in one).[118]

Nature of the Sensory Complaints

The patients complain of striking alterations in spontaneous sensations.[114,121] The parts feel stretched, hot, and sunburned, as if being stuck by pins, larger, smaller, or heavier. Contacts with the skin from eyeglasses, bedclothes, rings, watches, and sheets feel heavier on the affected side and may transiently aggravate the sensory disturbance. The stimulus seems to persist for a few seconds after its removal. In the patients with severe disturbances, the occurrence of a stimulus is better reported than its exact location. In a series of 21 cases, impairment of all sensory types (touch, pinprick, vibration, and position sense) was usually associated with large lacunes in the lateral thalamus; restricted sensory complaints suggest small lacunes at any level of the sensory pathway.[122]

Central post-stroke pain (sometimes called the Dejerine-Roussy syndrome)[123] is an uncommon accompaniment of lacunar infarction of the thalamus, although dysesthetic accompaniments are common in pure sensory stroke, as described previously. The full syndrome was originally described as the effect of occlusion of the thalamogeniculate branch of the posterior cerebral artery, with infarction of the ventral posterolateral and ventral posteromedial nuclei, largely sparing the remaining nuclei of the thalamus. Cases documented only by CT have shown a lesion small enough to qualify for a clinical diagnosis of lacunar infarction.[124] The initial deficit usually consists of hemiparesis and a hemisensory syndrome. The pain, which is an inconstant feature in cases with such infarcts, may begin at the onset of the syndrome or appear only later; delays of up to several months are common. The pains are intermittent or constant, appear spontaneously, or at other times are provoked by contact with the affected parts. The severity may range from mild to severe; it is a common misperception that all central post stroke pain is of high intensity.[125] They are usually accompanied by many other disturbances in sensation, including tingling, feelings of excessive weight, and feelings of cold, although a few cases exist in which the sensory function is normal on clinical testing. The special disturbance known as hyperpathia is particularly characteristic, but not common: after a sensory stimulus, a disagreeable response occurs that is usually delayed in onset, may spread over a large area, persists after removal of the stimulus, and may even increase in intensity over several seconds. The syndrome may outlast other features of the original stroke syndrome and may even become permanent.

Clinical Course

Improvement, often to normal within weeks, appears to be the rule.[120] The topography of the shrinking deficit may be rather unusual. Improvement in the trunk with persistence of deficit in the distal extremities, a pattern common in hemispheral disease, is only occasionally encountered. In one case, the deficit shrank to a vertical band from the axilla down the lateral trunk to the thigh.[111]

Sensorimotor Stroke

Three autopsied cases of sensorimotor stroke have been reported,[17,126,127] but only one of which was published with "sensorimotor stroke" in the title.[17] Such cases, although rare, are important because they attest to the occurrence of a combined motor and sensory deficit from a small, deep infarct. Their vascular anatomy also helps clarify the vascular supply to the thalamus and adjacent internal capsule (Fig. 27-11). The rarity of these cases should obviate any casual assumption that small, deep infarcts cause most cases of sensorimotor stroke.

Initially it was thought that sensorimotor stroke could not be caused by a lacunar infarct, because the vascular supply to the internal capsule was believed to be wholly separate from that to the thalamus. The lenticulostriate branches of the middle cerebral artery presumably supplied the capsule, and the thalamus was the artery presumed to receive its supply from the perforating branches of the posterior cerebral

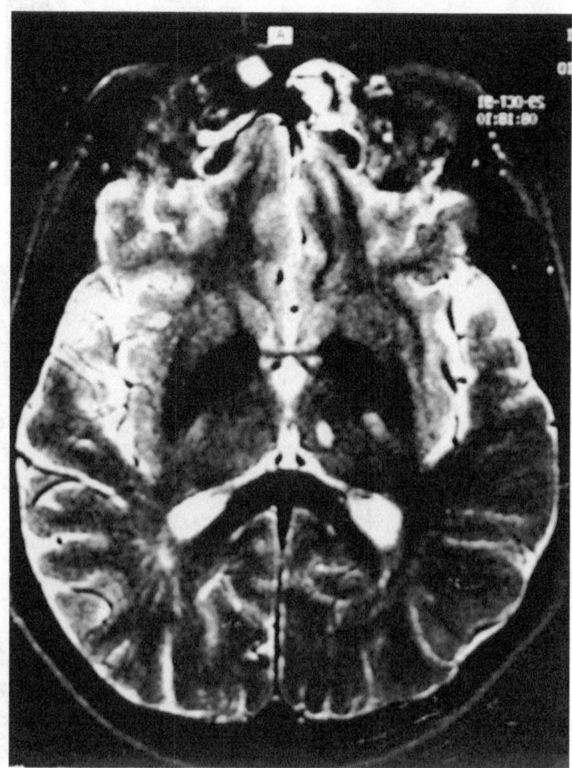

Figure 27-11. MRI showing a small thalamic lacune.

artery.[128] The extreme posterior nuclei of the thalamus received a few branches from the choroidal arteries.[52] However, cases now exist showing that a single infarct may involve both the thalamus and the adjacent internal capsule. These cases suffice to overturn earlier claims and to reopen the issues of the boundary line between the middle and posterior cerebral artery territories.

Several clinical examples of sensorimotor stroke have been documented by CT.[21,98,23,129] In these cases, the lesions were fairly large within the spectrum for lacunar infarcts. Donnan et al.[21] described one extending from the left putamen to the corona radiata, not obviously involving the thalamus. This pattern was the reverse of the author's autopsy-documented case of sensorimotor stroke.

The proportion of sensorimotor stroke among all cases with lacunar infarct is variable across cohorts reported, ranging from 13% in one cohort[81] to 40% of all patients with lacunar syndromes in the Oxfordshire Community Stroke Project.[130] The varying proportions may relate to the well-known problems with the sensory examination, which is one of the least reliable items in the neurological examination.

Ataxic Hemiparesis

The syndrome of ataxic hemiparesis has both cerebellar and pyramidal elements.[58] It was initially described as homolateral ataxia with crural paresis, which is its most familiar form.[15,131] The investigators of the original report speculated that the lesion might lie either in the anterior limb of the internal capsule or in the adjacent corona radiata. However, the first autopsied cases showed a pontine lesion of the small size typical of lacunar infarction.[58]

Since these early observations, numerous case reports have shown a low-density CT lesion lying in the corona radiate[132] or the posterior limb of the internal capsule, thalamus, lentiform nucleus, cerebellum, and frontal cortex.[58,112,99,23,133,134] These lesions have not been in the same site in each case and have been encountered as far forward as the head of the caudate and as far posterior as the posterior limb of the internal capsule.[99] Because the lesions in all these cases have been documented by CT scan alone, their exact correlation with the syndrome has been called into question by an illustrative case reported by Kistler et al.[135] The CT scan showed a corona radiata lesion; a MR scan revealed a recent pontine lesion that better explained the deficit. The pontine lesion was not seen on CT scanning because of the difficulty in averaging the bone densities adjacent to the brainstem. Because this effect prevents all but the largest pontine infarcts from being seen on CT scans, other cases may also have had a similar second lesion. In the series reported by Gorman et al.,[136] 3% of patients with stroke fulfilled criteria for a diagnosis of ataxic hemiparesis. In another series, ataxic hemiparesis accounted for 4.1% of all lacunar infarcts, and the internal capsule was the most frequent lesional topography, followed by pons (13%) and corona radiata (9%).[137] In a series of 29 patients, diffusion-weighted MRI carried out within the first 4 days of stroke onset identified infarcts in 97% of patients; pontine lesions were the main topography followed by the internal capsula and corona radiate.[138]

The clinical features have been rather similar from case to case. The usual form manifests as a mild-to-moderate weakness of the leg, especially the ankle, with little or no weakness of the upper limb and face, accompanied by an ataxia of the arm and leg on the same side. In a few cases, a mild and transient hemisensory deficit may initially accompany the motor findings.[132,139,140] In one series of 100 patients with ataxic hemiparesis, sensory disturbances were frequently associated with the capsular location.[133] The syndrome commonly develops only gradually, requiring from hours to a day or more to reach its peak.[132] There are a few instances of a chronic state, but some degree of improvement within days or months is usual. In some cases, the syndrome changes: the hemiparesis clears but the ataxia remains.[132]

Efforts to separate a hemispheral location from a brainstem location have met with only limited success.[15,132] In most instances, no distinctive features separate the cases of capsular or radiation origin from those involving the pons. The extent of weakness accompanying the ataxia is no guide to the location. In both the capsular and pontine cases, weakness may involve more structures than the leg, at times affecting the face and arm to almost the same extent. In all cases, the severity of ataxia is more striking than the weakness and exceeds that attributable to weakness alone.

Dysarthria-Clumsy Hand Syndrome

In patients seen with the syndrome, the dysarthria and the ataxia of the upper limb appear to be the prominent components of the clinical deficit, but they do not occur in isolation. The syndrome usually also includes facial weakness, which at times may be profound; dysphagia; and some weakness of the hand and even of the leg. The reflexes on the affected side are usually exaggerated, and the plantar response is extensor. The clinical picture usually develops suddenly. The cases with autopsy correlation have shown no sensory deficit. In one case, the facial weakness was accompanied by impaired strength in opening the jaw.[149]

Some researchers have equated the dysarthria-clumsy hand syndrome with ataxic hemiparesis,[141] whereas Fisher,[139] the originator, has come to the view that it is a variant. The best-recognized association has been with lacunes of the anterior limb of the internal capsule.[29] Other sites have been reported less often: Spertell and Ransom[142] described a case with a low-density lesion near the genu, and two of Fisher's patients with anterior capsular infarcts had combinations of mild ataxia and dysarthria. In a few other cases, the lesion has been in the basis pontis or corona radiate.[143,144] The syndrome has also been reported from hemorrhage of the pons.[145] The outlook for functional recovery is good. Of 2500 acute stroke patients included in a hospital-based prospective stroke registry, 35 were identified as having dysarthria-clumsy hand syndrome, which accounted for 1.6% of all acute stroke, 1.9% of acute ischemic stroke, and 6.1% of lacunar syndromes.[144]

Other Stroke Syndromes Associated with Lacunar Infarcts

Apart from the five classical lacunar syndromes outlined above, several other more rare clinical syndromes may also be caused by occlusion of single penetrating arteries, but the clinicopathological evidence for this is more limited. Descriptions include movement disorders such as chorea, dystonia, hemibalismus and asterixis. Brainstem syndromes (such as internuclear ophthalmoplegia, horizontal gaze palsy, Bendikt's syndrome, Claude's syndrome, pure motor hemiplegia plus sixth nerve palsies) and isolated cranial nerve palsies (most often third nerve palsies) may be caused by a micro-infarct in the brainstem (visualized only by MRI), presumably most often due to occlusion of a small penetrating artery, though the mechanism is likely to vary. The old doctrine that isolated vascular cranial nerve syndromes were usually caused by affection of vasa vasorum to the peripheral nerve outside the brainstem is probably incorrect.[146]

Several types of movement disorders have been described with small, deep infarcts. Although the exact vascular occlusion has not been demonstrated in many of these cases, the small size of the infarct and its occurrence in territories supplied by small penetrating arteries suggest that the majority is caused by penetrating small-artery disease. The movement disorder may appear as the only sign of the infarct or may develop later, after an initial syndrome, different in character, has resolved.

Hemichorea–hemiballismus is the most commonly documented form of movement disorder, accounting for 68% in a series of 22 patients with movement disorders of vascular origin; lacunar infarct was proposed as the most frequent cause.[147] The infarcts found in different parts of the striatum have been of lacunar size,[148,149] including those in the head of the caudate nucleus and adjacent corona radiate,[150] the subthalamic nucleus,[138,21,151] and the thalamus.[111,149,152] The onset is typically abrupt and is usually unaccompanied by other complaints. The chorea usually involves the forearm, hand, and fingers. In one case, it was accompanied by hemiparesis that faded within 3 months even though the chorea persisted unchanged.[150] In some cases, chorea has been delayed by some weeks or months after the initial occurrence of hemiparesis. One patient whose putaminal lesion was documented only by CT scan,[153] suffered choreic movements of the distal parts of the arm and leg that interfered with normal activity and prevented easy walking for more than 4 weeks. In this case, the chorea improved, only to relapse a few weeks later. Rare ballistic movements were superimposed. The examination revealed normal strength, sensation, and reflexes.

Two types of dystonia have been described in cases of lacunes; action-induced and focal dystonia. Action-induced rhythmic dystonia has been documented by an autopsy study. In the case reported, the syndrome began as a sensorimotor stroke.[154] Both of the deficits improved within a month. By 3 months, the movement disorder began in the left leg, which had been the most severely affected part in the initial stroke. The disorder spread to involve the patient's entire left side. The fingers of the affected hand became flexed into the palm, leaving only the thumb free. When the patient was examined 4 years later, the hand was unchanged, but strength was otherwise normal. Voluntary movements of any parts of the body, including even eye closure, precipitated rhythmic dystonic extension and rotation of the left arm and leg (sparing the trunk) that subsided a few seconds after the voluntary movements ceased. Clonazepam and 5-hydroxytryptophan were successful in suppressing the involuntary movement disorder. At autopsy, an infarct 5 × 1 × 2 mm was found straddling the ventral posterolateral nucleus and the adjacent posterior limb of the internal capsule. Focal dystonia occurred in one patient whose CT scan showed a low density in the right lenticular nucleus.[155] As with the cases of hemichorea and hemiballismus, the deficit appeared abruptly, unaccompanied by weakness or sensory disturbances. Only the distal end of the upper extremity was affected. Although it was described as dystonic, the disorder featured changing postures: "The movements were slow and caused the patient's fingers to assume unusual positions. Activity exacerbated the movements ... the left hand and forearm showed involuntary movements that produced an unusual posture, with hyperpronation and flexion at the wrist, extension of the fingers, and opposition of the thumb."

Speech and Language Disorders, and Other Disorders of Higher Cerebral Function

Bilateral capsular lacunar infarctions have been a cause of mutism in the absence of any disturbance in language or praxis. One patient reported by Fisher,[49] in whom infarction was documented by microscopic vascular pathology, had no difficulty with speech after his first infarct but became mute with the second infarct, which involved the left internal capsule. The left capsular lacune was 4 × 4 × 5 mm and lay at the genu. More recently, several cases with mutism, anarthria, or severe dysphonia have been described in association with a new lacunar infarct occurring in a patient with a previous lacunar infarct contralaterally and with residual symptoms.[98,97,156,157]

The earlier literature up to the MR era includes debates as to if small deep infarcts may cause language dysfunction. A few such case reports claim such an association, but it should be recognized that CT has a limited precision to visualize the full extent of an ischemic lesion or identify multiple lesions (see below). Similarly, there has been debate as to if lacunar infarcts may cause disorders of higher cortical dysfunction. It has been reported that symptomatic supratentorial lacunar infarction, even single, could cause neuropsychological impairment, decreased performance for mental capacities, and, more often than in control subjects, emotional disturbances.[158] A prospective series of 40 lacunar stroke patients studied within 1 month after stroke onset found mild neuropsychological disturbances in 57% of the patients.[159] It is presently uncertain whether such neuropsychological findings are related to the recent stroke, to preexisting mild cognitive dysfunction, silent cerebral infarcts and white matter lesions – or combinations thereof. Cognitive effects of stroke are described in another chapter in this textbook.

Specificity of the Clinical Lacunar Syndromes for Small-Vessel Disease. Several early studies tested the diagnostic validity of subtyping ischemic stroke into the lacunar infarct subtype based on correlation between clinical features (lacunar syndromes) and findings on CT scan (for which patients with a visualized small deep infarct usually were lumped together with patients with no imaging abnormality). Some studies included presence of extracranial large-artery disease and cardiac findings. In general the findings supported the "lacunar hypothesis", i.e., that the clinical lacunar syndromes were quite highly suggestive of a small-vessel disease as the likely underlying cause. A possible exception was demonstrated in patients with sensorimotor stroke in which one-third were reported to have findings indicating a non-lacunar pathogenesis.[160]

The research field entered a new era with the advent of MRI, and in particular DW-MRI, which highly reliably can identify acute ischemic abnormalities and separate acute from old lesions. In two smaller studies, DW-MRI visualized multiple regions of ischemia not compatible with lacunar infarcts in 16%[161] and 29%.[162] Another study[163] reported the finding of a single subcortical ischemic area in only 59% of patients, whereas 22% had large or scattered lesions in one territory and 19% had multiple lesions in multiple territories. Potter et al.[164] studied associations of clinical stroke misclassifications ("clinical-imaging dissociation") in 137 patients with an acute ischemic stroke presenting with a mild cortical or lacunar syndrome; 21/93 (23%) patients with a cortical syndrome had an acute lacunar infarct, whereas 7/44 (16%) patients with a lacunar syndrome had an acute cortical infarct. Another study[165] compared the lacunar syndrome subtype of the Oxfordshire Community Stroke Project classification with DW-MRI findings, and reported a positive predictive value for the LACI subtype of only 40–60%.

Conversely, the imaging finding of a subcortical or brainstem small ischemic abnormality does not always present as a lacunar syndrome. In one study,[166] only 44% of such patients examined with DW-MRI within 7 days from the onset of stroke symptoms presented clinically with a lacunar syndrome according to the OSCP criteria.

These findings indicate the uncertainty that surrounds conclusions on stroke pathophysiology based on clinical findings for the lacunar infarct subtype. MRI (including DW-MRI) is clearly the preferred imaging modality in investigations for cerebral small-vessel disease – as well as for TIA or stroke in general.

PROGNOSIS

In general, the patient with a lacunar infarction has a good early prognosis, which is a finding that Pierre Marie and Miller Fisher noted as one of the characteristics of lacunes. In comparison with other vascular processes (ischemic or hemorrhagic, hemispheric or in the brainstem), lacunes have the best early prognosis (not always, however, as good as we expect). The prognosis of lacunes is influenced by several factors. The presence of TIAs before the infarct indicates a poor prognosis, more recurrence, and coronary artery disease in the clinical evolution. Generally, when the motor or sensory deficit is complete (affecting the face, arm, and leg), the prognosis is worse than with an incomplete deficit. The size of the lacunar infarction on CT or MRI is usually correlated with prognosis and is better for smaller lesions. Hyperglycemia, which is associated with a poor outcome in acute ischemic strokes because of large-vessel atherothrombotic or cardioembolic disease, does not affect the prognosis in acute lacunar cerebral infarction.[167,168]

The prognosis in such vascular processes as lacunes implies four aspects: survival, recovery of deficits, general or neurologic complications in the acute phase, and recurrence. Survival is the rule during the acute phase. The possibility of death in this phase is related to other complications rather than the lacunar infarct itself. The risk of death after the acute phase is no different from that in the general population within the first few years after a lacunar infarct. However, during longer follow-up periods (5 years or more) a clear excess of deaths is seen also in a cohort with lacunar infarcts.[169]

Early neurologic deterioration in lacunar infarction, as well as a poor outcome, has been associated with a high blood concentration of inflammatory markers such as interleukin-6, tumor necrosis factor-α, and intercellular adhesion molecule-1.[170] Recovery of deficits is generally good in the first few weeks after onset. Related functional outcomes of 94% of patients at 6 months[171] are independent. Complications in the acute phase occur in 18% of patients, and urinary infections are the most common.[171] The prognosis for recurrence of stroke in lacunar infarcts at 1 year in hospital studies or community series is about 10%. The rate of recurrence in following years is similar;[172] the rate is 23.5%, however, with a follow-up of 10 years, as shown in one series of pure motor stroke from presumed lacunar infarction.[169] A comparison of recurrence rates after lacunar infarcts compared to non-lacunar infarcts showed similar rates of recurrent stroke in the two groups; hence lacunar infarcts are not more benign in this respect.[173]

Hypertension, diabetes mellitus, leukoaraiosis, and high hematocrit levels are the main risk factors associated with recurrence and multiple lacunar infarcts.[174,175] Recurrent strokes were more likely to be lacunar if the first event was lacunar.[173]

An important concern long term after lacunar infarcts is the development of mild cognitive impairment and dementia. Symptomatic lacunar infarcts, silent lacunar brain infarcts and white matter disease have synergistic effects on cognitive dysfunction after stroke. The risks of dementia after stroke, and the role of small-vessel disease are covered by Chapter 17.

In summary, lacunar infarcts have been considered to be the most benign stroke subtype, but recent studies have modified this view. It still holds true that the prognosis is more favorable in terms of survival and disability than other subtypes during the first years, which is probably explained simply by the small lesion size. For the first 5 years the average annual recurrence rate is about 5%, and may decrease somewhat after that. Among recurrent strokes, new lacunar infarcts are most common but the pattern is heterogeneous and almost half are due to other mechanisms. This is not surprising because the major risk factors that predispose to vascular occlusions in small brain arteries also promote atherosclerosis in the coronary arteries, aorta, and cervico-cranial arteries. At 10 years after onset one-third or less of the patients are alive and free of recurrent stroke, and a large proportion of survivors are disabled, have cognitive impairment, or are demented. Thus, there is little support that lacunar infarcts should carry a more benign prognosis than other ischemic stroke subtypes.

There is a growing body of evidence that vascular risk factor and extent of asymptomatic small-vessel disease (silent infarcts and white matter ischemic abnormalities) at the time of the index stroke have significant prognostic implications for almost all outcomes.[176] Patients with both multiple risk factors and advanced cerebral small-vessel disease already at the time of the first stroke appear to have a several-fold higher risk of a disabling outcome and death. A lacunar infarct may also act synergistically with silent small-vessel disease and incipient Alzheimer changes in promoting dementia. Silent cerebral infarcts, as well as microbleeds, are more prevalent at stroke onset in patients with lacunar infarction than in those with atherothrombotic or cardioembolic infarcts, and appear to negatively influence recovery of function, probably by limiting the possibilities of plastic brain rescue mechanisms. Furthermore, in the long term, asymptomatic progression of cerebral small-vessel disease is several-fold more common than new strokes, and is likely to be detrimental to brain function with time.[177,178]

Aspects on Therapy in Lacunar Infarcts

There is a separate extensive section in the present textbook on acute therapy and secondary prevention of stroke. However, there have been controversies as to whether therapies used in ischemic stroke in general apply equally for lacunar infarcts, as the pathophysiology of small-vessel disease is different than large-artery atherosclerosis or cardiac embolism to the brain. Most trials on acute therapies and secondary prevention in TIA and ischemic stroke have been performed in patients with heterogeneous stroke mechanisms and not specifically in patients with well-proven smal-vessel disease. At present there is only one trial (SPS3)[179] that specifically has included a cohort of recent lacunar infarcts assessed for secondary prevention, but several other trials (acute as well as secondary preventive) have reported subgroup analyses on lacunar infarcts. Some aspects on therapeutic issues in lacunar infarcts are, therefore, included in this chapter.

Thrombolysis in Acute Ischemic Stroke

Thrombolytic therapy is the firmly established standard for acute ischemic stroke. The pivotal NINDS study[180] showed that intravenous tPA was effective for all subtypes including small-vessel disease; a favorable outcome was observed for 63% in the tPA group versus 40% in the placebo group. However, the assignment of stroke subtype in the NINDS study was largely based on initial clinical features and CT scan findings, an uncertain diagnostic principle for lacunar stroke as discussed earlier in this chapter. However, several later studies using more refined diagnostic criteria have demonstrated similar effectiveness and risks of tPA in patients with acute lacunar infarcts.[181–183] There is likely a component of thrombosis in intrinsic disease of small penetrating cerebral arteries when occlusion occurs and presents with acute stroke symptoms, and the small amount of total thrombus mass may actually make acute lacunar stroke especially suitable for intravenous tPA.

There is a concern that the presence of white matter hyperintensities, silent cerebral infarcts, and microhemorrhages (all of which are more common in the lacunar infarct subgroup than in other ischemic stroke subtypes) may imply a greater risk for hemorrhagic cerebral complications in lacunar stroke. However, there is at present no such evidence from clinical trials, and current guidelines recommends not to exclude patients with acute lacunar stroke from thrombolytic therapy.

The Capsular Warning Syndrome Dilemma

Worsening in acute lacunar stroke is common (see above), and a fluctuating course with initial TIAs followed by a fixed deficit (the capsular warning syndrome) is regularly seen in clinical practice. The mechanism of fluctuations and progressive symptoms in acute lacunar stroke is not well established but may include progressive branch occlusion, altered hemodynamics, peri-infarct edema, excitotoxicity, or inflammation.[184] At present, no therapy has been firmly shown to affect fluctuations or progression in acute lacunar stroke (not in ischemic stroke in general). Limited experience from intravenous tPA in patients with the capsular warning syndrome suggests that thrombolytic therapy may be of benefit and safe,[185] but further studies are much needed.

Secondary Prevention of Lacunar Infarcts

Antiplatelet Therapy. Almost all studies on antiplatelet therapy have been performed on mixed populations of patients with TIA and ischemic stroke not limited to any specific subtype. Lacunar stroke patients have even been overrepresented in most secondary prevention trials as such patients may be easier to recruit as they do not present with aphasia and reduced levels of consciousness that may limit the ability to give consent. From 1983 to 2012, 11 stroke secondary prevention trials have reported results by index event mechanism.[186] Overall results show that antiplatelet therapy is superior to placebo in preventing recurrent stroke in lacunar patients, and that the response is similar to the overall results in the studies. However, it should be recognized that the diagnostic precision of lacunar stroke in these studies is limited as it is usually based on clinical features and CT scan findings. The group labeled lacunar stroke may be contaminated by other pathophysiologies than small-vessel disease in up to half of the patients.

The Small Subcortical Stroke (SPS3) Study is the only randomized trial that has included well-defined patients with imaging-supported symptomatic lacunar infarcts.[179] In a factorial design patients were randomized to two interventions: (a) antiplatelet therapy with aspirin 325 mg vs aspirin 325 mg + clopidogrel 75 mg, and (b) two target levels of blood pressure control "higher" 130–149 mmHg vs "lower" <130 mmHg. The antiplatelet part of the study was stopped early due to lack of benefit and excess of mortality for those assigned to combination therapy.[187] Major hemorrhage rates were doubled in the combination group. Hence, dual antiplatelet therapy with aspirin and clopidogrel should not be used for long-term secondary prevention in patients with acute lacunar stroke. Recommended options are aspirin in doses between 75 and 325 mg per day, aspirin 25 mg plus extended-release dipyridamole 200 mg twice daily, or clopidogrel 75 mg daily.

Statin Therapy. Current guidelines recommend statin therapy in patients with ischemic stroke with few exclusion criteria (see section on statin therapy in this book). In the only study that has reported specifically on a lacunar stroke subgroup (the SPARCLE trial), no difference in benefit or risk of intracerebral hemorrhage was reported for this subgroup.[188,189]

Blood Pressure Lowering. Two target levels of blood pressure were tested in the SPS3 trial: "higher" 130–149 mmHg versus "lower" <130 mmHg.[179] After a mean follow-up of 3.7 years, a 19% non-significant reduction in all recurrent stroke was seen in those assigned to the lower group (HR 0.81; 95%CI, 0.64–1.03).[190] However, ICH was reduced significantly by 63% (HR 0.37; 95%CI 0.15–0.95; $P < 0.03$). Blood pressure lowering to both target levels was well tolerated, and serious side effects were uncommon (3%) and did not differ between groups. The demonstration of a significant benefit for reduction of hemorrhagic stroke and a trend towards reduction of all recurrent stroke supports the targeting of blood pressure reduction to a systolic pressure of 130 mmHg in patients with lacunar stroke. In SPS3 there was not a preferential use of one particular antihypertensive agent or combination of agents.

Concurrent Potential Causes of Ischemic Stroke

Concurrent potential mechanisms of ischemic stroke, such as cardioembolic sources (in particular atrial fibrillation) and ipilateral carotid stenosis, are not rare in patients with acute lacunar stroke, by any definition, and may appear also even in those in whom neuroimaging has confirmed the symptomatic ischemic lesion to be confined to the territory of a single penetrating arteriole. In individual patients it may be difficult or even impossible to firmly determine one of several potential concurrent mechanisms as the causative one.

For patients with atrial fibrillation and a previous ischemic stroke, current treatment algorithms stratify such patients as having an indication for anticoagulant therapy (see therapy section in this textbook). The risk stratification schemes do not specify further details on likely subtype of the ischemic stroke nor verification of the ischemic lesion by neuroimaging. Hence, patients with a lacunar stoke and concurrent atrial fibrillation should normally be treated with anticoagulants unless there is a contraindication. Studies on the potentially increased risk of intracerebral haemorrhage in patients with microbleeds treated with anticoagulants are currently ongoing.

Similarly, the co-existence of an ipsilateral carotid stenosis in patients with acute lacunar stroke may occur, and it may be impossible to determine if the carotid stenosis is symptomatic or not. However, the North American Symptomatic Carotid Endarterectomy Trial (NASCET) showed that carotid endarterectomy still reduced stroke occurrence in patients who appeared to have a lacunar infarct, although the benefit was less than in patients with non-lacunar events.[191]

The complete reference list can be found on the companion Expert Consult website at www.expertconsult.inkling.com.

KEY REFERENCES

1. Pantoni L. Cerebral small vessel disease: from pathogenesis and clinical characteristics to therapeutic challenges. Lancet Neurol 2010;9:689–701.
2. Donnan GA, Norrving B, Bamford J, et al. Subcortical infarction: classification and terminology. Cerebrovasc Dis 1993;3:248–51.
3. Bamford J, Sandercock P, Dennis M, et al. Classification and natural history of clinically identifiable subtypes of cerebral infarction. Lancet 1991;337:1521–6.
4. Adams HP, Bendixen BH, Kappelle LJ, et al. Classification of subtype of acute ischemic stroke. Definitions for use in a multicenter clinical trial. Stroke 1993;24:35–41.

5. Ay H, Benner T, Arsava EM, et al. A computerized algorithm for etiologic classification of ischemic stroke: the Causative Classification of Stroke System. Stroke 2007;38:2979–84.
7. Amarenco P, Bogousslavsky J, Caplan LR, et al. New approach to stroke subtyping: The a-s-c-o (phenotypic) classification of stroke. Cerebrovasc Dis 2009;27:502–8.
8. Dechambre A. Mémoire sur la curabilité du ramollissement cérébral. Gaz Med (Paris) 1838;6:305.
9. Durand-Fardel M. Mémoire sur une alteration particulière de la substance cérébrale. Gaz Med (Paris) 1842;10:23.
10. Marie P. Des foyers lacunaire de désintegration et de différents autres états cavitaires du cerveau. Rev Med 1901;21:281.
11. Ferrand J. Essai sur l'hémiplegie des vieillards, les lacunes de désintegrations cérébrale, [thesis]. Paris: Rousset; 1902.
12. Vogt C, Vogt O. Zur Lehre der Erkrankungen des striaren Systems. J Psychol Neurol 1920;25:627.
13. Fisher CM, Curry HB. Pure motor hemiplegia of vascular origin. Arch Neurol (Chic) 1965;13:30.
14. Fisher CM. Thalamic pure sensory stroke: A pathologic study. Neurology 1978;28:1141.
15. Fisher CM, Cole M. Homolateral ataxia and crural paresis: A vascular syndrome. J Neurol Neurosurg Psychiatry 1965;28:48.
16. Fisher CM. A lacunar stroke: The dysarthria-clumsy hand syndrome. Neurology (Minneap) 1967;17:614.
17. Mohr JP, Kase CS, Meckler RJ, et al. Sensorimotor stroke. Arch Neurol 1977;34:739.
18. Fisher CM, Caplan LR. Basilar artery branch occlusion: A cause of pontine infarction. Neurology (Minneap) 1971;21:900.
19. Fisher CM. The arterial lesions underlying lacunes. Acta Neuropathol 1969;12:1.
21. Donnan GA, Tress BM, Bladin PF. A prospective study of lacunar infarction using computerized tomography. Neurology 1982;32:49.
22. Pullicino P, Nelson RF, Kendall BE, et al. Small deep infarcts diagnosed on computed tomography. Neurology 1980;30:1090.
23. Weisberg LA. Computed tomography and pure motor hemiparesis. Neurology 1979;29:490.
24. Chokroverty S, Rubino FA, Haller C. Pure motor hemiplegia due to pyramidal infarction. Arch Neurol 1975;2:647.
27. Michel D, Laurent B, Foyatier N, et al. Infarctus thalamique paramedian gauche. Rev Neurol (Paris) 1982;138:6.
29. Fisher CM. Lacunes: Small deep cerebral infarcts. Neurology (Minneap) 1965;15:774.
31. Nelson RF, Pullicino P, Kendall BE, et al. Computed tomography on patients presenting with lacunar syndromes. Stroke 1980; 11:256.
33. Vermeer S, Longstreth WT Jr, Koudstaal PJ. Silent brain infarcts: a systematic review. Lancet Neurol 2007;6:611–19.
34. Bryan RN, Wells SW, Miller TJ, et al. Infarctlike lesions in the brain: prevalence and anatomic characteristics at MR imaging of the elderly – data from The Cardiovascular Health Study. Radiology 1997;202:47–54.
35. Price TR, Manolio TA, Kronmal RA, et al. Silent brain infarction on magnetic resonance imaging and neurological abnormalities in community-dwelling older adults. The Cardiovascular Health Study CHS Collaborative Research Group. Stroke 1997;28: 1158–64.
36. Howard G, Wagenknecht LE, Cai J, et al. Cigarette smoking and other risk factors for silent cerebral infarction in the general population. Stroke 1998;29:913–17.
37. Bryan RN, Caj J, Burke G, et al. Prevalence and anatomic characteristics of infarct-like lesions on MR images of middle-aged adults: the atherosclerosis risk in communities study. AJNR 1999;20:1273–80.
38. Vermeer SE, Koudstaal PJ, Oudkerk M, et al. Prevalence and risk-factors of silent brain infarcts in the population-based Rotterdam Scan Study. Stroke 2002;33:21–5.
39. DeCarli C, Massaro J, Harvey D, et al. Measures of brain morphology and infarction in the Framingham Heart Study: establishing what is normal. Neurobiol Aging 2005;26:491–510.
40. Das RR, Seshadri S, Beiser AS, et al. Prevalence and correlates of silent cerebral infarcts in the Framingham offspring study. Stroke 2008;39:2929–35.
41. Bailey EL, Smith C, Sudlow CLM, et al. Pathology of lacunar ischemic stroke in humans: a systematic review. Brain Pathol 2012;22:583–91.
42. Saini M, Ikram K, Hilal S, et al. Silent stroke: not listened to rather than silent. Stroke 2012;11:3102–4.
43. Edlow JA, Selim MH. Atypical presentations of acute cerebrovascular syndromes. Lancet Neurol 2011;10:550–60.
44. Smith EE, Schneider JA, Wardlaw JM, et al. Cerebral microinfarcts: the invisible lesions. Lancet Neurol 2012;11:272–82.
45. Offerbacher H, Fazekas F, Schmidt R, et al. MR of cerebral abnormalities concomitant with primary intracerebral hematomas. AJNR 1996;17:573–8.
46. Greenberg SM, Vernooij MW, Cordonnier C, et al., for the Microbleed Study Group. Cerebral microbleeds: a guide to detection and interpretation. Lancet Neurol 2009;8:165–74.
47. Werring DJ, editor. Cerebral Microbleeds. Pathophysiology to Clinical Practice. Cambridge: Cambridge University Press; 2011.
48. Fisher CM. Lacunar infarcts – a review. Cerebrovasc Dis 1991; 1:311–20.
49. Fisher CM. Capsular infarcts. Arch Neurol 1979;36:65.
50. Donnan GA, Bladin PF, Berkovic SF, et al. The stroke syndrome of striatocapsular infarction. Brain 1991;114:51–70.
52. Percheron SMJ. Les artères du thalamus humain. Rev Neurol 1976;132:297.
56. Chester EM, Agamanolis DP, Banker Q, et al. Hypertensive encephalopathy: A clinicopathologic study of 20 cases. Neurology 1978;28:928.
57. Fisher CM. Bilateral occlusion of basilar artery branches. J Neurol Neurosurg Psychiatry 1977;40:1182.
58. Fisher CM. Ataxic hemiparesis. Arch Neurol 1978;35:126.
59. Fisher CM, Gore I, Okabe N, et al. Atherosclerosis of the carotid and vertebral arteries: Extracranial and intracranial. J Neuropathol Exp Neurol 1965;24:455.
60. Lammie GA, Brannan F, Slattery J, et al. Nonhypertensive cerebral small-vessel disease: An autopsy study. Stroke 1997;28: 2222.
68. Mohr JP, Caplan LR, Melski JW, et al. The Harvard Cooperative Stroke Registry. Neurology 1978;28:754.
69. Arboix A, Marti-Vilalta JL, Garcia JH. Clinical study of 227 patients with lacunar infarcts. Stroke 1990;21:842.
70. Jackson C, Sudlow C. Are lacunar strokes really different? A systematic review of differences in risk factor profiles between lacunar and nonlacunar infarcts. Stroke 2005;36:891–901.
71. Jackson CA, Hutchison A, Dennis MS, et al. Differing risk factor profiles of ischemic stroke subtypes: evidence for a distinct lacunar arteriopathy? Stroke 2010;41:624–9.
72. Arboix A, Garcia-Eroles L, Massons J, et al. Lacunar infarcts in patients aged 85 years and older. Acta Neurol Scand 2000; 101:25.
73. Matarin M, Brown WM, Scholtz S, et al. A genome-wide genotyping study in patients with ischaemic stroke: Initial analysis and data release. Lancet Neurol 2007;6:414–20.
74. Zhang J, Kohara K, Yamamoto Y, et al. Genetic predisposition to neurological symptoms in lacunar infarction. Cerebrovasc Dis 2004;17:273–9.
75. Elbaz A, Poirier O, Moulin T, et al. Association between the Glu298Asp polymorphism in the endothelial constitutive nitric oxide synthase gene and brain infarction. The GENIC investigators. Stroke 2000;31:1634–9.
76. Jannes J, Hamilton-Bruce MA, Pilotto L, et al. Tissue plasminogen activator -7351C/T enhancer polymorphism is a risk factor for lacunar stroke. Stroke 2004;35:1090–4.
77. Nakase T, Mizuno T, Harada S, et al. Angiotensinogen gene polymorphism as a risk factor for ischemic stroke. J Clin Neurosci 2007;14:943–7.
78. Chamorro A, Revilla M, Obach V, et al. The -174G/C polymorphism of the interleukin 6 gene is a hallmark of lacunar stroke and not other ischemic stroke phenotypes. Cerebrovasc Dis 2005;19:91–5.
79. Falcone GJ, Malik R, Dichgans M, et al. Current concepts and clinical applications of stroke genetics. Lancet Neurol 2014;13: 405–18.
81. Chamorro AM, Sacco RL, Mohr JP, et al. Lacunar infarction: Clinical–computed tomographic correlations in the Stroke Data Bank. Stroke 1991;22:175.
82. Arboix A, Marti-Vilalta JL, Pujol J, et al. Lacunar infarct and nuclear magnetic resonance: A review of sixty cases. Eur Neurol 1990;30:47.

83. Barinagarrementeria F, Del Brutto OH. Lacunar syndrome due to neurocysticercosis. Arch Neurol 1989;46:415.
84. Hommel M, Besson G, Le Bas JF, et al. Prospective study of lacunar infarction using magnetic resonance imaging. Stroke 1990;21:546.
85. Hommel M, Besson G, Le Bas JF, et al. Prospective study of lacunar infarction using magnetic resonance imaging. Stroke 1990;21:546.
86. Noguchi K, Nagayoshi T, Watanabe N, et al. Diffusion-weighted echo-planar MRI of lacunar infarcts. Neuroradiology 1998;40: 448.
87. Schonewille WJ, Tuhrim S, Singer MB, et al. Diffusion-weighted MRI in acute lacunar syndromes: A clinical-radiological correlation study. Stroke 1999;30:2066.
88. Singer MB, Chong J, Dongfeng L, et al. Diffusion-weighted MRI in acute subcortical infarction. Stroke 1998;29:133.
89. Wardlaw JM, Smith EE, Biessels GJ, et al. Neuroimaging standards for research into small vessel disease and its contribution to ageing and neurodegeneration. Lancet Neurol 2013;12:822–38.
90. Potter G, Doubal FN, Jackson CA, et al. Counting cavitating lacunes underestimates the burden of lacunar infarction. Stroke 2010;41:267–72.
91. Moreau F, Patel S, Lauzon ML, et al. Cavitation after acute symptomatic lacunar stroke depends on time, location, and MRI sequence. Stroke 2012;43:1837–42.
92. Bokura H, Kobayashi S, Yamaguchi S. Distinguishing silent lacunar infarction from enlarged Virshow-Robin spaces: a magnetic resonance imaging and pathological study. J Neurol 1998; 245:116–22.
95. Cho Z-H, Kang CK, Han J-Y, et al. Observation of the lenticulostriate arteries in the human brain in vivo using 7.0T MR angiography. Stroke 2008;39:1604–6.
96. Reimers J, de Wytt C, Seneviratne B. Lacunar infarction: A 12 month study. Clin Exp Neurol 1987;24:28.
97. Tuszynski MH, Petito CK, Levy DE. Risk factors and clinical manifestations of pathologically verified lacunar infarctions. Stroke 1989;20:990.
98. Mohr JP, Kase CS, Wolf PA, et al. Lacunes in the NINCDS Pilot Stroke Data Bank [abstract]. Ann Neurol 1982;12:84.
99. De Reuck J, van der Eecken H. The topography of infarcts in the lacunar state. In: Meyer JS, Lechner H, Reivich M, editors. Cerebral Vascular Disease: 7th International Conference. Salzburg. New York: Thieme Edition/Publishing Sciences Group; 1976. p. 162.
101. Rascol A, Clanet M, Manelfe C, et al. Pure motor hemiplegia: CT study of 30 cases. Stroke 1982;13:11.
102. Weisberg LA. Lacunar infarcts. Arch Neurol 1982;39:37.
103. Iragui VJ, McCutchen CB. Capsular ataxic hemiparesis. Arch Neurol 1982;39:528.
104. Robinson RK, Richey ET, Kase CS, et al. Somatosensory evoked potentials in pure sensory stroke and allied conditions [abstract]. Neurology 1984;34:231.
105. Fraix V, Besson G, Hommel M, et al. Brachiofacial pure motor stroke. Cerebrovasc Dis 2001;12:34.
106. Melo TP, Bogousslavsky J, Van Melle G, et al. Pure motor stroke: A reappraisal. Neurology 1992;42:789.
108. Gross CR, Kase CS, Mohr JP, et al. Stroke in south Alabama: Incidence and diagnostic features. Stroke 1984;15:249.
109. Samuelsson M, Samuelsson L, Lindell D. Sensory symptoms and signs and results of quantitative sensory thermal testing in patients with lacunar infarct syndromes. Stroke 1994;25:2165.
110. Staaf G, Geijer B, Lindgren A, et al. Diffusion-weighted MRI findings in patients with capsular warning syndrome. Cerebrovasc Dis 2004;17:1–8.
111. Hyland HH, Forman DM. Prognosis in hemiballismus. Neurology (Minneap) 1957;7:381.
112. Ichikawa K, Tsutsumishita A, Fujioka A. Capsular ataxic hemiparesis: A case report. Arch Neurol 1982;39:585.
113. Steinke W, Ley SC. Lacunar stroke is the major cause of progressive motor deficit. Stroke 2002;33:1510–16.
114. Fisher CM. Pure sensory stroke involving face, arm and leg. Neurology (Minneap) 1965;15:76.
115. Groothius DR, Duncan GW, Fisher CM. The human thalamocortical sensory path in the internal capsule: Evidence from a capsular hemorrhage causing a pure sensory stroke. Ann Neurol 1977;2:328.
116. Rosenberg NL, Koller R. Computerized tomography and pure sensory stroke. Neurology 1981;31:217.
117. Jokura K, Matsumoto S, Komiyama A, et al. Unilateral saccadic pursuit in patients with sensory stroke: Sign of pontine tegmentum lesion. Stroke 1998;29:2377.
118. Arboix A, García C, Massons J, et al. Clinical study of 99 patients with pure sensory stroke. J Neurol 2005;252:156–62.
120. Fisher CM. Pure sensory stroke and allied conditions. Stroke 1982;13:434.
121. Mohr JP. Lacunes. Neurol Clin 1983;1:201.
122. Kim JS. Pure sensory stroke: Clinical-radiological correlates of 21 cases. Stroke 1992;23:983.
123. Dejerine J, Roussy G. La syndrome thalamique. Rev Neurol (Paris) 1906;14:521.
124. Manfredi M, Cruccu G. Thalamic pain revisited. In: Loeb C, editor. Studies in Cerebrovascular Disease. Milano: Masson Italiano; 1981. p. 73.
125. Klit H, Finnerup NB, Jensen TS. Central post-stroke pain: clinical characteristics, pathophysiology, and management. Lancet Neurol 2009;8:857–68.
126. Misra UK, Kalita J. Putaminal haemorrhage leading to pure motor hemiplegia. Acta Neurol Scand 1995;91:283.
128. Plets C, De Reuck J, Vander Eecken H, et al. The vascularization of the human thalamus. Acta Neurol Belg 1970;70:685.
129. Gursahani RD, Khadilkar SV, Surya N, et al. Capsular involvement and sensorimotor stroke with posterior cerebral artery territory infarction. J Assoc Physicians India 1990;38:939.
130. Bamford J, Sandercock P, Jones L, et al. The natural history of lacunar infarction: The Oxfordshire community stroke project. Stroke 1987;18:545–51.
132. Huang CY, Lui FS. Ataxic hemiparesis: Localization and clinical features. Stroke 1984;15:363.
133. Moulin T, Bogousslavsky J, Chopard JL, et al. Vascular ataxic hemiparesis: A re-evaluation. J Neurol Neurosurg Psychiatry 1995;58:422.
134. Sage JI. Ataxic hemiparesis from lesions of the corona radiata. Arch Neurol 1983;40:449.
135. Kistler JP, Buonanno FS, DeWitt LD, et al. Vertebral basilar posterior cerebral territory stroke delineation by proton nuclear magnetic resonance imaging. Stroke 1984;15:417.
136. Gorman MJ, Dafer R, Levine SR. Ataxic hemiparesis: Critical appraisal of a lacunar syndrome. Stroke 1998;29:2549.
137. Arboix A. Clinical study of 23 patients with ataxic hemiparesis. Med Clin (Barc) 2004;122:342–4.
138. Hiraga A, Uzawa A, Kamitsukasa I. Diffusion weighted imaging in ataxic hemiparesis. J Neurol Neurosurg Psychiatry 2007;78: 1260–2.
139. Fisher CM. Lacunar strokes and infarcts: A review. Neurology 1982;32:871.
140. Sakai T, Murakami S, Ito K. Ataxic hemiparesis with trigeminal weakness. Neurology 1981;31:635.
141. Tuhrim S, Yang WC, Rubinowitz H, et al. Primary pontine hemorrhage and the dysarthria-clumsy hand syndrome. Neurology 1982;31:635.
142. Spertell RB, Ransom BR. Dysarthria-clumsy hand syndrome produced by capsular infarct. Ann Neurol 1979;6:268.
143. Glass JD, Levey AI, Rothstein JD. The dysarthria-clumsy hand syndrome: A distinct clinical entity related to pontine infarction. Ann Neurol 1990;27:487.
144. Arboix A, Bell Y, García-Eroles L, et al. Clinical study of 35 patients with dysarthria-clumsy hand syndrome. J Neurol Neurosurg Psychiatry 2004;75:231–4.
145. Tjeerdsma HC, Rinkel GJE, van Gijn J. Ataxic hemiparesis from a primary intracerebral haematoma in the precentral area. Cerebrovasc Dis 1996;6:45.
146. Thömke F, Gutmann L, Stoeter P, et al. Cerebrovascular brainstem diseases with isolated cranial nerve palsies. Cerebrovasc Dis 2002;13:147–55.
147. D'Olhaberriague L, Arboix A, Marti-Vilalta JL, et al. Movement disorders in ischemic stroke: Clinical study of 22 patients. Eur J Neurol 1995;2:553.
148. Goldblatt D, Markesbery W, Reeves AG. Recurrent hemichorea following striatal lesions. Arch Neurol 1974;31:51.
149. Martin JP. Hemichorea (hemiballismus) without lesions in the corpus Luysii. Brain 1957;80:1.

150. Saris S. Chorea caused by caudate infarction. Arch Neurol 1983; 40:590.
151. Meyers R. Ballismus. In: Vinken PJ, Bruyn GW, editors. Handbook of Clinical Neurology, vol. 6. Amsterdam: North Holland; 1968. p. 476.
152. Antin SP, Prockop LD, Cohen SM. Transient hemiballismus. Neurology (Minneap) 1967;17:1068.
153. Kase CS, Maulsby GO, de Juan E, et al. Hemichorea hemiballism and lacunar infarction in the basal ganglia. Neurology 1981; 31:454.
155. Russo LS. Focal dystonia and lacunar infarction of the basal ganglia. Neurology 1983;40:61.
156. Croisile B, Henry E, Trillet M, et al. Loss of motivation for speaking with bilateral lacunes in the anterior limb of the internal capsule. Clin Neurol Neurosurg 1989;91:325.
158. Van Zandvoort MJE, Kappelle LJ, Algra A, et al. Decreased capacity for mental effort after single supratentorial lacunar infarct may affect performance in everyday life. J Neurol Neurosurg Psychiatry 1998;56:697.
159. Grau-Olivares M, Arboix A, Bartrés-Faz D, et al. Neuropsychological abnormalities associated with lacunar infarction. J Neurol Sci 2007;257:160–5.
160. Arboix A, Oliveres M, García-Eroles L, et al. Risk factors and clinical features of sensorimotor stroke. Cerebrovasc Dis 2003;16: 448–51.
161. Ay H, Oliveira-Filho J, Buonanno FS, et al. Diffusion-weighted imaging identifies a subset of lacunar infarction associated with embolic stroke. Stroke 1999;30:2644.
162. Caso V, Budak K, Georgiadis D, et al. Clinical significance of detection of multiple acute brain infarcts on diffusion weighted magnetic resonance imaging. J Neurol Neurosurg Psychiatry 2005;76:514–18.
163. Wessels T, Röttger C, Jauss M, et al. Identification of embolic stroke patterns by diffusion-weighted MRI in clinically defined lacunar stroke syndromes. Stroke 2005;36:757–61.
164. Potter G, Doubal F, Jackson C, et al. Associations of clinical stroke misclassification ("clinical-imaging dissociation") in acute ischemic stroke. Cerebrovasc Dis 2010;29:395–402.
165. Asdaghi N, Jeerakathil T, Hameed B, et al. Oxfordshire community stroke project classification poorly differentiates small cortical and subcortical infarcts. Stroke 2011;42:2143–8.
166. Seifert T, Enzinger C, Storch MK, et al. Acute small subcortical infarctions on diffusion weighted MRI: clinical presentation and aetiology. J Neurol Neurosurg Psychiatry 2005;76:1520–4.
167. Bruno A, Biller J, Adams HP Jr, et al. Acute blood glucose level and outcome from ischemic stroke. Neurology 1999;52: 280.
168. Chan RKT, Chong PN. Hyperglycemia is not associated with adverse outcome in patients with lacunar infarcts. Neurology 1999;52(Suppl. 2):301.
169. Staaf G, Lindgren A, Norrving B. Pure motor stroke from presumed lacunar infarct: Long-term prognosis for survival and risk of recurrent stroke. Stroke 2001;32:2592.
170. Castellanos M, Castillo J, García MM, et al. Inflammation-mediated damage in progressing lacunar infarctions. A potential therapeutic target. Stroke 2002;33:982–7.
171. Boiten J. Lacunar stroke: A prospective clinical and radiological study, [thesis]. Maastricht: 1991.
172. Hier DB, Foulkes MA, Swiontoniowski M, et al. Stroke recurrence within 2 years after ischaemic infarction. Stroke 1991; 22:155.
173. Jackson C, Sudlow C. Comparing risks of death and recurrent vascular events between lacunar and non-lacunar infarction. Brain 2005;128:2507–17.
174. Arauz A, Murillo L, Cantú C, et al. Prospective study of single and multiple lacunar infarcts using magnetic resonance imaging. Risk factors, recurrence, and outcome in 175 consecutive cases. Stroke 2003;34:2453–8.
175. Arboix A, Font A, Garro C, et al. Recurrent lacunar infarction following a previous lacunar stroke: A clinical study of 122 patients. J Neurol Neurosurg Psychiatry 2007;78:1392–4.
176. Samuelsson M, Söderfelt B, Olsson GB. Functional outcome in patients with lacunar infarction. Stroke 1996;27:842–6.
177. Norrving B. Long-term prognosis after lacunar infarction. Lancet Neurol 2003;2:238–45.
178. Norrving B. No black holes in the brain are benign. Pract Neurol 2008;8:222–8.
179. Benavente OR, White CL, Pearce L, et al. The Secondary Prevention of Small Subcortical Stroke (SPS3) study. Int J Stroke 2011;6:164–75.
180. National Institute of Neurological Disorders and Stroke rt-PA Stroke Study Group. Tissue plasminogen activator for acute ischemic stroke. New Engl J Med 1995;333:1581–7.
181. Hsia AW, Sachdev HS, Tomlinson J, et al. Efficacy of IV tissue plasminogen activator in acute stroke: does stroke subtype really matter? Neurology 2003;61:71–5.
182. Cocho D, Belvis R, Marti-Fabregas J, et al. Does thrombolysis benefit patients with lacunar syndrome? Eur Neurol 2006;55: 70–3.
183. Fluri F, Hatz F, Rutgers MP, et al. Intravenous thrombolysis in patients with stroke attributable to small artery occlusion. Eur J Neurol 2010;17:1054–60.
184. Del Bene A, Palumbo V, Lamassa M, et al. Progressive lacunar stroke: review of mechanisms, prognostic features, and putative treatments. Int J Stroke 2012;7:321–9.
185. Vivanco-Hidalgo RM, Rodriguez-Campello A, Ois A, et al. Thrombolysis in capsular warning syndrome. Cerebrovasc Dis 2008;25:508–10.
186. Nakajima M, Field T, Benavente O. Treatment approaches for lacunar strokes. In: Pantoni L, Gorelick P, editors. Cerebral Small Vessel Disease. Cambridge: Cambridge University Press; 2014. p. 323–35.

28 Intracerebral Hemorrhage

Carlos S. Kase, Ashkan Shoamanesh, Steven M. Greenberg, Louis R. Caplan

KEY POINTS

- Intracerebral hemorrhage (ICH) accounts for 10–35% of stroke cases depending on the population studied.
- Its incidence has remained stable over the past three decades despite improvements in primary prevention measures, such as blood pressure management.
- ICH can result from a number of mechanisms, the predominant one being hypertension, while others include vascular malformations, brain tumors, sympathomimetic drugs, anticoagulant and fibrinolytic agents, cerebral amyloid angiopathy, vasculitis, and hemorrhagic transformation of ischemic infarction.
- Hemorrhagic transformation of ischemic infarction occurs spontaneously as part of the natural history of cerebral embolism, but its presence and severity can be enhanced by agents that alter blood coagulation, especially therapeutic thrombolysis.
- The acute phase of ICH is characterized by a high frequency of hematoma expansion in the early hours after onset, and this phenomenon is highly associated with neurological deterioration. The imaging counterpart of this phenomenon is the "spot sign" detected in computerized tomography angiography, a finding that results from ongoing blood extravasation at the site of the hematoma.
- The clinical aspects of ICH in the various brain locations often include the combination of features of increased intracranial pressure (headache, vomiting, depressed level of consciousness), along with the neurological deficits that result from the specific site of the hematoma in the brain.
- Novel neuroimaging markers such as cerebral microbleeds, superficial siderosis and remote small diffusion-weighted imaging hyperintense lesions are encountered frequently in individuals with ICH. However, many unanswered questions remain pertaining to their clinical significance and ability to guide individual patient care.
- The management of ICH requires monitoring and treatment in an ICU setting, and treatment decisions regarding conservative versus surgical treatment are highly individualized and depend on the size and location of the hematoma, presence of associated hydrocephalus, intraventricular hemorrhage, and increased intracranial pressure.

Intracerebral hemorrhage (ICH) occurs as a result of bleeding from an arterial source directly into the brain substance. Although its relative frequency in patients with stroke is subject to geographic and racial variations, values between 5% and 10% are most commonly quoted in Western populations.[1-3] In a consecutive series of 938 patients with stroke entered into the National Institute of Neurological and Communicative Disorders and Stroke (NINCDS) Data Bank, primary ICH accounted for 10.7% of the cases.[4] Similar figures were obtained in population or community studies from Denmark (10.4%),[5] Holland (9%),[6] Oxfordshire, England (10%),[7] southern Alabama (8%),[8] Italy (13.5%),[9] France (11%),[10] and Iran (12.7%).[11] However, within the INTERSTROKE study, which recruited 3000 participants from 22 countries, ICH accounted for 22% of the cases. This higher proportion was largely driven by ICH in African, South American and South East Asian populations where ICH accounted for 22–34% of cases (n = 2578) in comparison to 9% in designated 'high-income' countries (n = 422).[12]

The incidence rates are relatively constant in predominantly white populations: rates range between 7 and 11 cases per 100,000 (Table 28-1).[13-17] The figures were higher in a U.S. population (southern Alabama) with a mixture of white and black people because the former had an incidence rate of 12 per 100,000; in black people, the rate was 32 per 100,000.[8] Similar comparisons between white and black people in Cincinnati, Ohio, yielded an overall age- and sex-adjusted incidence of ICH that was 1.4-fold higher in black people.[13] The difference in ICH incidence was even higher (2.3-fold) for black persons who were younger than 75 years. In addition, a Hispanic population in New Mexico had a high incidence of ICH (34.9), whereas non-Hispanic Whites from the same population had an incidence rate (16.6) comparable to that of Whites in other geographic locations.[18] Some series from Asian countries, such as that from Shibata, Japan,[19] report severalfold higher incidence rates of ICH (61). A recent systematic review suggests that these racial differences may in part be attributed to regional environmental factors.[20] In reviewing incidence rates among 36 studies encompassing roughly 9 million people from 21 countries, van Asch et al. observed an overall ICH incidence of 24.6/100,000, and within pooled analyses, global incidence rates (per 100, 000) were comparable between white persons (24.2), black persons (22.9), Hispanics (19.6), Indian people (21.4) and Maoris (22.2), but increased twofold in East and South East Asian people (51.8). When examining regional differences however, they observed that incidence of ICH was higher in black persons in Northern Manhattan (49.5), in comparison to those in Martinique (23.1), south London (14.9), and Barbados (17.6). The same was true when comparing Hispanic people in Manhattan (24.0) to those in Chile and Brazil (14.5), whereas the incidence of ICH among white people in Manhattan (22.6) was comparable to that of white people in other populations. Similarly, in Auckland they observed that the incidence rate of ICH in East and South East Asian

TABLE 28-1 Incidence of Intracerebral Hemorrhage in Studies from Various Geographic Locations

Location	Chapter Reference	No. of Cases	Rate*
Rochester, Minnesota	13	81	7
Framingham, Massachusetts	3	58	10
Southern Alabama	8	13	12
Cincinnati, Ohio	14	154	11
Giessen, Germany	15	100	11
Shibata, Japan	17	97	61
L'Aquila, Italy	10	588	16
Bernalillo Co., New Mexico	16		
Non-Hispanic Whites		47	17
Hispanics		39	35

*Per 100,000 population.

immigrants (20.7) was similar to that of white (18.6) and Maori people (22.2) in the same region, but lower than values reported in Asian people living in China and Japan (57.6).[20] Regional differences in incidence rates were confirmed by the European Registers of Stroke which found ICH incidence rates ranging from 7.3–25.2/100,000 when comparing population-based stroke registers in six European countries.[21]

Prior reports had noted a general trend toward declining rates of ICH, starting in the 1960s with the initial observation in Göteborg, Sweden[22] and subsequently confirmed in the US in a population from Rochester, Minnesota.[14,23] From analysis of data encompassing a 32-year period (1945 to 1976), Furlan et al.[14] showed a significant decrease in incidence between the first and second parts of this period: 13.3 per 100,000 for 1945 to 1960 and 6.7 per 100,000 for 1961 to 1976. These figures correlated with a similar decline in the frequency and severity of hypertension in the population studied. A similarly declining trend in the incidence of ICH had been reported from Hisayama, Japan,[24] where it was also related to a decrease in the frequency of hypertension. However, figures from Gothenburg, Sweden, documented no changes in ICH incidence in men and women when comparing years 1987 to 1989, 1990 to 1994, and 1995 to 1999, and van Asch et al. did not detect a significant decrease in incidence of ICH between 1980 and 2008 in their comprehensive systematic review.[20]

The incidence of ICH increases with advancing age,[3,13,20,25] which is a feature that applies to all types of stroke, both ischemic and hemorrhagic. A publication from the Dijon Stroke Registry (Dijon, France) found that, although incidence of ICH appeared stable between 1985 and 2008, the incidence had decreased 50% in individuals below 60. Conversely, it had increased roughly 80% in people aged ≥ 75 years. This increased incidence was driven largely by lobar ICH and coincided with an increase in use of antithrombotic therapy. These results suggest that the beneficial effects of primary prevention measures over previous decades, such as blood pressure control, might be offset by antithrombotic-induced ICH in older individuals who are more vulnerable to bleeding-prone vasculopathies such as cerebral amyloid angiopathy (CAA).[10] This potential association is supported by a hospital-based study that documented a fivefold increase in the incidence of anticoagulant-associated ICH in greater Cincinatti/Northern Kentucky from 1988 to 1999. The incidence among persons age ≥ 80 increased 18-fold during this time.[26] However, data from a similar time period (1993–2008) from Northern Ostrobothnia, Finland, showed a decrease in anticoagulant-associated ICH despite a 3.6-fold increase in warfarin use. This paradox was attributed to a high initial rate of ICH at the beginning of the study period and subsequent decline with improved patient selection for warfarin therapy and INR monitoring.[27] There also appears to be an 'age-by-race interaction', whereby white persons are particularly more prone to increasing ICH incidence with increasing age in comparison to black persons. The REasons for Geographic and Racial Differences in Stroke (REGARDS) study reported that ICH risk in Blacks is roughly 5.4-fold greater than Whites at age 45, but only one-third that of Whites at age 85. Whites were found to have an adjusted ICH hazard ratio of 2.03 for each subsequent decade of life, whereas rates did not differ significantly with age in Blacks.[28] The underlying contributors to the observed 'age-by-race interaction' remain unclear. In assessing demographic trends in our aging population, Stein and colleagues project that by the year 2050, the proportion of all patients with ICH ≥ 80 years will be 2.5-fold higher than in 2009, with substantial increases in ICH cases (35.2% increase), severe disability (36.8%), and in-hospital mortality (60.2%).[29]

The role of hypertension as a leading risk factor is well-established, and its frequency has been estimated to be between 72%[2,14,30] and 81%.[2,14,30] The causative role of hypertension is supported by the high frequency of left ventricular hypertrophy in autopsy cases of ICH[31–33] and the significantly higher admission blood pressure readings in patients with ICH than in those with other forms of stroke.[34] The autopsy study by McCormick and Rosenfield[35] challenged the view that hypertension represents the main causative factor in ICH. Their series included a large number of cases of ICH due to blood dyscrasias, vascular malformations, and tumors, and hypertension was regarded as the sole basis for the bleeding in only 25% of the total. This difference from most reported series of ICH may reflect a referral pattern bias in this series as well as more stringent criteria for establishing a causal relationship between hypertension and ICH. However, clinical series have also questioned the validity of the concept of ICH as a condition most commonly related to hypertension. Brott et al.[16] found a history of hypertension in only 45% of 154 patients, which is a figure that rose to only 56% when electrocardiographic or chest radiographic evidence of cardiomegaly was added to criteria for the diagnosis of hypertension. Similarly, Schütz et al.[17] labeled only 59% of their cases of ICH as due to hypertension. Certain subgroups of hypertensive patients, however, appear to be at particularly high risk of ICH. They include subjects who are 55 years or younger, smokers, and those who have stopped taking their antihypertensive medications.[36] In the INTERSTROKE study, hypertension (self-reported history or mean blood pressure >160/90) was the strongest risk factor for ICH, accounting for 73.6% of the population-attributable risk.[12]

A number of other risk factors in addition to advancing age, hypertension, and race have been evaluated, including cigarette smoking, alcohol consumption, and serum cholesterol levels. Abbott et al.[37] showed a higher risk of intracranial hemorrhage (both ICH and subarachnoid hemorrhage [SAH]) in cigarette-smoking Hawaiian men of Japanese ancestry. The risk of "hemorrhagic stroke" was 2.5 times higher in smokers, which was an effect that was independent of other risk factors. However, the diagnosis of ICH was often made on clinical grounds, without verification by imaging or autopsy findings. In a study based on computed tomography (CT) diagnosis of ICH in Finland, Juvela et al.[38] found that smoking was not an independent risk factor for ICH. However, recent data from the Physicians' Health Study and the Women's Health Study[39] documented a significant association between cigarette smoking and both SAH and ICH risk in men and women.[39,40] After controlling for a number of vascular risk factors, investigators found that smoking 20 or more cigarettes per day was an independent risk factor for SAH (relative risk [RR] = 3.22; 95% confidence interval [CI], 1.26–8.18) and ICH (RR = 2.06; 95%CI, 1.08–3.96) in a cohort of predominantly white male physicians.[40] Corresponding figures for women who smoked 15 or more cigarettes per day were RR of 4.02 (95%CI, 1.63–9.89) for SAH and 2.67 (95%CI, 1.04–6.90) for ICH in the Women's Health Study.[39]

The series reported by Donahue et al.[41] and Juvela et al.[38] also documented an increased risk of ICH in relation to alcohol ingestion, which was an effect that operated independently of other risk factors. Both studies showed a strong dose–response relationship between alcohol use and ICH. Juvela et al.[38] documented a similar effect for alcohol ingestion within 24 hours and within 1 week before onset of ICH. Moreover, there are data that suggest that ICH occurs at a younger age in heavy alcohol users.[42] Low serum cholesterol level, defined as serum cholesterol less than 160 mg/dL, has been shown to be associated with a higher risk of ICH in Japanese men[19] as well as in Hawaiian men of Japanese origin.[43] Similar results were documented in a population-based study in Rotterdam, Netherlands.[44] Increased risk of ICH in relation to excessive smoking (>20 cigarettes per day), alcohol intake, and low cholesterol levels (particularly non-HDL cholesterol) were confirmed in the INTERSTROKE study.[12] Increased ICH risk was also observed with increased waist-to-hip ratio, psychosocial stress, unhealthy diet (red meat, organ meat, egg, salty or fried food consumption and cooking with lard), whereas increased physical activity, and consumption of fruit and fish were protective. These modifiable risk factors combined with hypertension, smoking status and alcohol intake accounted for 90.8% of the population-attributable ICH risk.[12] The risk of ICH attributable to statin therapy is controversial. In the Stroke Prevention by Aggressive Reduction in Cholesterol Levels (SPARCL) study,[45] the overall benefit of active treatment with atorvastatin in secondary stroke prevention included an approximate 70% increase in risk of ICH.[46] Initially, pooled analysis from a systematic review encompassing 8832 participants from four studies confirmed an approximate 70% increase in risk of ICH among statin users with prior cerebrovascular disease.[47] However, a subsequent larger meta-analyses encompassing > 90,000 participants did not show a significant association between statin therapy and increased rates of ICH.[48,49] The discrepancy likely reflects the populations being studied, with the more recent negative analyses being largely comprised of data from primary prevention studies or populations without known cerebrovascular disease. The suggested increased rate of ICH in persons with prior cerebrovascular disease seems to be independent of the cholesterol-lowering effects of statin therapy, and has been postulated to result from possible antifibrinolytic and/or antiplatelet properties of statins.[46,47]

Additional risk factors have been suggested in some studies. Cirrhosis was highly represented (15.5%) in the autopsy series of Boudouresques et al.,[50] but its significance could not be assessed because comparison with a control autopsy series of the general population was not available. The occasional association of ICH with cirrhosis has been linked to thrombocytopenia and other abnormalities in coagulation.[51] Interestingly, in a nationwide multicenter case-control study, the risk of ICH increased by 30% per each number of childbirths, an association that persisted following adjustment for multiple covariates. The biological mechanism of this observation is uncertain but may be due to hormonal influences, physical and environmental factors during pregnancy, such as the increased risk of pregnancy-induced hypertension with increasing parity, and psychosocial stress and adverse lifestyle factors attributed to the rearing of multiple children.[52]

The role of aspirin use in the risk of ICH is controversial. The Physicians' Health Study, which evaluated the effect of low-dose aspirin (325 mg every other day) in comparison with placebo in the primary prevention of coronary events, documented a borderline-significant increase in the relative risk of hemorrhagic stroke (ICH and SAH) in the aspirin group.[53] Similarly, the Swedish Aspirin Low-Dose Trial (SALT), a secondary stroke prevention trial, documented a significantly higher frequency of hemorrhagic stroke in the group assigned to aspirin (75 mg/day) than in the group given placebo.[54] These data contrast with those from other secondary stroke prevention trials, in which various doses of aspirin did not lead to a higher risk of ICH.[55–60]

CAA is a diagnosis being recognized with increasing frequency. The difficulty of diagnosing CAA in living subjects makes precise figures on disease incidence or prevalence hard to ascertain. CAA *without* ICH is clearly a common phenomenon in the elderly brain. A review of published autopsy series suggests a prevalence for CAA of approximately 10% to 30% among unselected brains and 80% to 100% among brains with accompanying Alzheimer's disease (AD).[61] When these figures are compared with the annual rate for *all* types of ICH, approximately 0.1% among North American and European elderly,[14,17,18] it is clear that only a minority of pathologically advanced CAA results in hemorrhagic stroke.

Despite the low frequency of hemorrhage, those produced by CAA account for a substantial proportion of all spontaneous ICHs in elderly patients. Estimated rates of 11% to 15% emerged from autopsies of elderly patients with ICH (age ≥ 60 years) at the Japanese Yokufukai Geriatric Hospital between 1979 and 1990[62] and the Hawaiian Kuakini Hospital between 1965 and 1976.[63] Analysis of consecutively encountered clinical patients at the Massachusetts General Hospital (MGH) between 1994 and 2001 suggests an even greater proportion of hemorrhages, approximately 34%, attributable to CAA (Table 28-2). The apparently higher frequency of CAA in the MGH cohort might reflect either a lower incidence of hypertensive ICH in this Western population or secular improvements in blood pressure control as well as the methodologic differences between autopsy-based and clinic-based studies.

Examination of the clinical characteristics that predispose to CAA-related ICH (Box 28-1) suggests that its incidence is likely to rise with the aging of the population and is unlikely to be reduced through control of modifiable risk factors. *Advancing age* is the strongest clinical risk factor for CAA-related ICH, as predicted by the age dependence of the underlying disease.[61,64–66] There is no marked predilection for *gender* in either clinical (54% men, 46% women)[2] or pathologic (49% men, 51% women)[67] series.

Dementia has generally been considered a major risk factor for CAA-related ICH because of the close molecular relationship between CAA and AD. A pathologic study of 117 consecutive brains with AD demonstrated advanced CAA to be common; moderate-to-severe CAA was found in 25.6% of specimens and CAA-related hemorrhages were found in 5.1%.[68] Despite the frequent overlap of AD with CAA, approximately 60% to 80% of patients given diagnoses of CAA-related

TABLE 28-2 Estimated Prevalence of CAA-Related ICH in a Clinical Series of Elderly Patients

ICH Location (n = 355)	Percentage of Total*
Lobar	45.9 × 74%† = 34% of all primary ICHs in elderly due to CAA
Deep hemispheric	41.1
Brainstem	3.7
Cerebellum	8.5
Intraventricular	0.9

CAA, Cerebral amyloid angiopathy; ICH, intracerebral hemorrhage.
*Data from 355 consecutive patients age ≥55 presenting to Massachusetts General Hospital with spontaneous ICH.
†The estimated proportion of primary lobar ICH in the elderly caused by CAA, based on detection of advanced CAA in 29 of 39 consecutive pathology specimens of lobar ICH.

BOX 28-1 Risk Factors for CAA-Related ICH

RISK FACTORS FOR CAA

Advanced age
ApoE ε2 or ε4
Alzheimer's disease

RISK FACTORS FOR LOBAR ICH (NOT SPECIFICALLY LINKED TO CAA)

Family history of ICH
Frequent use of alcohol
Previous ischemic stroke
Low serum cholesterol

CAA, Cerebral amyloid angiopathy; ICH, intracerebral hemorrhage; ApoE, apolipoprotein E.

ICH do *not* show clinical symptoms of dementia before their initial hemorrhagic stroke.[67,69,70] It is thus unclear from a clinical standpoint whether the presence or absence of dementia is useful in making the diagnosis of CAA. The association of CAA and AD appears to be due in part to the shared genetic risk factor apolipoprotein E (ApoE) ε4, although there are substantial differences between the roles of ApoE in the two disorders.

Despite the clear importance of *hypertension* in promoting necrosis and rupture of the deep penetrating vessels,[71] there is little evidence for a similar role in CAA-related ICH. The estimated prevalence of hypertension in CAA is in the range of 32% (determined from pathologic cases[67]) to 49% (measured in clinical subjects[2]), which are figures not much greater than the expected rate of hypertension for the general elderly population. Hypertension is significantly less common in lobar ICH than in ICH of the deep hemispheres, cerebellum, or pons in most[17,70,72,73] though not all[36,74] studies of the elderly. Among other vascular factors, neither *diabetes mellitus* nor *coronary atherosclerosis* has demonstrated an elevated frequency in CAA.

Other clinical risk factors have been suggested for lobar ICH without specific evidence linking them to CAA. Midpoint analysis of the population-based Greater Cincinnati/Northern Kentucky study identified *family history of ICH, previous ischemic stroke*, and *frequent alcohol use* in addition to ApoE genotype as predictors of lobar ICH in a multivariable model.[75] *Low serum cholesterol* has been found to be associated with ICH in several other population-based studies.[76-78] The few studies that have analyzed ICH according to location or presumed etiology have not indicated a specific relationship of cholesterol to CAA-related hemorrhages.[79]

CAA can also present clinically with non-hemorrhagic features. These include the following:

1. There are accumulating data to suggest that advanced CAA may sufficiently affect blood flow (possibly by the effects on vascular reactivity)[80] to cause *ischemic brain injury* as well as ICH. Various types of ischemic lesions are reported in association with CAA, including punctate areas of gliosis in the cerebral cortex[81] and regions of myelin loss and focal gliosis in the white matter, termed microinfarcts.[82] Although microinfarcts are conventionally reported on pathology, asymptomatic small diffusion-weighted imaging hyperintense lesions are being increasingly recognized on MRIs of persons with CAA, and may be a radiographic marker for the formation of these lesions.[83,84] A histopathologic study of 73 postmortem brains found a correlation between white matter lesions and the proportion of amyloid-positive vessels but not with age or severity of Alzheimer pathology.[76] Similarly, magnetic resonance imaging (MRI) analysis of subjects with probable CAA demonstrated significantly greater volume of white matter T2-hyperintensity (median normalized volume, 19.8 cm^3) than similar-aged subjects with AD (11.1 cm^3) or mild cognitive impairment (10.0 cm^3).[77] Furthermore, it has been shown that Pittsburgh compound B (PiB) - a ligand that labels both vascular and parenchymal amyloid - retention on positron emission tomography (PET) is strongly correlated with degree of white matter T2-hyperintensity in individuals with CAA.[85,86] Radiographic markers of white matter lesions in CAA appear to correlate with cognitive impairment,[78] which suggests that ischemic brain injury may be an important contributor to neurologic disability in these patients.
2. A subset of patients with CAA is seen with clinical and radiographic features related to *vascular inflammation*. Although some increase in inflammatory cells may be a common feature of advanced CAA,[69,87] a minority of patients demonstrate more robust reactions ranging from perivascular giant cells to frank vasculitis.[79,87,88] These patients are more likely to be seen with subacute cognitive decline or seizures than with symptomatic ICH. MRI often shows T2-hyperintensity that is asymmetrical, extends to subcortical white matter and the overlying cortex, and improves dramatically with courses of immunosuppressive agents such as high-dose corticosteroids or cyclophosphamide.[89] The clinical and radiographic response of many subjects to treatment suggests that CAA-related inflammation may be an important subtype to diagnose during life.
3. CAA can also manifest as *transient neurologic symptoms*,[90-92] another syndrome for which diagnosis during life is of particular practical importance. A multicenter retrospective cohort study observed transient neurological symptoms to be a common occurrence in CAA (14.5% of 172 cases).[93] The neurologic symptoms can include focal weakness, numbness, paresthesias, or language abnormalities, often occurring in a recurrent and stereotyped pattern. Spells typically last for minutes and may spread smoothly from one contiguous body part to another during a single spell. Transient neurologic symptoms in CAA appear to be related to the hemorrhagic rather than the ischemic component of the disease because gradient-echo MRI commonly demonstrates otherwise asymptomatic hemorrhage in the cortical region corresponding to the spell.[90] Superficial siderosis and cerebral microbleeds have also been visualized at neuroanatomical sites that correspond with the presenting symptoms.[93,94] Spells often cease with anticonvulsant treatment. The major practical issue is to differentiate these episodes by clinical or radiographic means from true transient ischemic attacks because administering anticoagulant

agents in this setting may severely increase the risk of major ICH. A systematic review has shown the future risk of ICH at 2 months following an episode of transient neurological symptoms to be approximately 17%.[93]

GENETICS

The study of the genetics of cerebrovascular disease has focused mainly on ischemic stroke, but some researchers have also addressed ICH.[95] Alberts et al.[96] addressed the issue of familial aggregation of cases of ICH. Their prospective study in North Carolina found that 10% of probands had a history of ICH. No significant clinical or demographic differences separated those with and without family history of ICH. Data reported by Woo et al.[75] indicated that the presence of a first-degree relative is a risk for ICH of the lobar variety. These investigators also documented that the occurrence of lobar ICH is associated with the ε2 and ε4 alleles of the ApoE gene. These alleles, particularly ε4, have been identified as factors related to an increased risk of lobar ICH, presumably owing to the presence of CAA.[70] In addition, the presence of the ε4 allele was found to determine an earlier age of onset of ICH in its carriers compared with the age of presentation of CAA-related ICH in those without the allele.[70]

A potential association between a point mutation in codon 34 of exon 2 for factor XIII Val34Leu and ICH was suggested by Catto et al.[97] The suggested association was based on the known protective effect of this mutation for myocardial infarction (MI), as a result of its interfering with the formation of cross-linked fibrin. This last feature suggested the hypothesis that the mutation may result in an increased risk of ICH via the formation of weak fibrin structures. The study, which involved a large cohort of patients with stroke of both ischemic and hemorrhagic varieties, suggested that the mutation was significantly more common in subjects with ICH than in controls and in those with cerebral infarction.[97] However, a similar study from Korea did not show an association between factor XIII Val34Leu polymorphism and ICH.[98] These inconsistent observations may simply reflect the differences in the cohorts studied, and further data from other population samples will be required before a definitive statement can be made about the potential role of this mutation in the risk of ICH. A study in Chinese people of Han ancestry suggested an association between the 1425G/A single nucleotide polymorphism in the *PRKCH* gene in chromosome 14q22-q23 and increased incidence of ICH.[99] Growing literature also suggests that angiotensin-converting enzyme (ACE) gene polymorphism, resulting in hypertension and possible vessel wall remodeling by way of higher ACE levels and activity, increases ICH risk.[100] Similarly, genetic risk scores devised to assess burden of risk alleles related to hypertension, suggest that larger burdens of risk alleles for hypertension are associated with risk of ICH, particularly in deep regions, larger hematoma volume and worse outcome.[101,102]

Dominant mutations in the gene encoding type IV collagen α1 (COL4A1), a basement membrane protein, confer a highly penetrant genetic predisposition to familial cerebral small-vessel disease, characterized by retinal vascular tortuosity, T2-white matter hyperintensities, cerebral microbleed formation and predominantly deep ICH.[103,104] Recently, novel COL4A1 mutations have also been identified in cases of sporadic (non-familial) ICH.[105]

Familial Cerebral Amyloid Angiopathy

Several familial forms of CAA have been identified in which a protein entirely unrelated to amyloid beta (Aβ) accumulates in vessels, assumes amyloid conformation, and promotes vascular dysfunction. The clinical presentation of these familial CAAs differs from mutation to mutation, suggesting that each protein deposit provokes its own specific reaction. Substitution of glutamine for leucine at position 68 in the protease inhibitor cystatin C results in Icelandic CAA, which is characterized by very early deposition of a mutant protein fragment in vessel walls and symptomatic ICH by the third or fourth decades.[106] ICH is much less prominent in familial British dementia, a disorder caused by mutation in the *BRI* gene.[107] A single nucleotide substitution in the BRI stop codon causes cerebrovascular deposition of an abnormal carboxyl-terminus peptide fragment and a clinical syndrome of dementia and ataxia.[108] A third clinical presentation is associated with mutations in the transthyretin gene. When these mutations affect the central nervous system, they favor leptomeningeal and subependymal deposition, causing varying combinations of SAH, seizures, hydrocephalus, cognitive changes, ataxia, and hearing loss.[109]

The other major forms of familial CAA are caused by mutations or duplications of the *APP* gene. Interestingly, the APP mutations associated with CAA cluster within the Aβ-coding region of *APP* (Fig. 28-1) rather than flanking the Aβ-coding segment like the AD-associated mutations.[110] The Dutch-type hereditary CAA caused by substitution of glutamate to glutamine at Aβ position 22[111,112] manifests as recurrent lobar ICH in the fifth or sixth decades and progresses to an early mortality.[113] A similar clinical picture is produced by the Italian substitution of lysine at this position.[114,115] Dementia and AD-like neuritic pathology are more prominent features of duplication of the APP locus[116] and of two other CAA-associated APP mutations, the Flemish substitution of glycine at Aβ position 21[117] and the Iowa asparagine for aspartate substitution at residue 23.[118] Although differences have emerged among the various mutations in their effects on APP

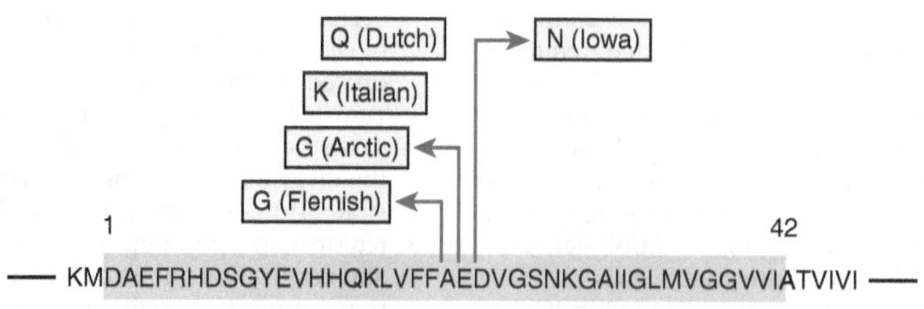

Figure 28-1. Mutations of the APP (β-amyloid precursor protein) gene associated with familial cerebral amyloid angiopathy (CAA). The boxed segment of APP contains the region representing Aβ42 as well as the amino acid substitutions at positions 21 to 23 associated with familial CAA (see text for references). Asterisks indicate the positions of some of the mutations linked with early-onset Alzheimer's disease.

processing and Aβ bioactivity,[119,120] the precise mechanisms by which they predispose toward specific combinations of CAA and AD pathology remain unclear.

Sporadic Cerebral Amyloid Angiopathy

The genes associated with familial CAA do not appear to play major roles as risk factors for sporadic CAA. Among 55 patients with sporadic CAA-related ICH examined for the cystatin C Icelandic mutation,[121,122] only one positive finding has been reported. Similar searches for APP mutations at Aβ position 22 or 23 have yielded no instances in 111 reported patients with sporadic CAA.[118,121] ApoE has emerged as the strongest predictor of risk for sporadic CAA-related ICH. The ApoE ε2 and ε4 alleles appear to promote CAA-related ICH at two distinct steps in the disease's pathogenesis, as previously described.[123-125] Each of these alleles was over-represented more than twofold among 182 reviewed pathologic cases of CAA-related ICH.[126] The general importance of ApoE to lobar ICH was further supported by the midpoint analysis of the Greater Cincinnati/Northern Kentucky cohort, in which the presence of ApoE ε2 or ε4 was associated with an adjusted odds ratio for lobar ICH of 2.3.[75] The ApoE alleles had an attributable risk for lobar ICH of 29% in this study, which is the largest proportion for any risk factor examined. ApoE ε2 and ε4 appear to associate with not only greater risk of ICH occurrence,[123] but also a younger age at first hemorrhage[125] and a shorter time until ICH recurrence (see later).[127] The ApoE ε2 allele in particular has also been associated with intrahematomal contrast extravasation during CT angiography (CTA), termed 'spot sign', in lobar and CAA-related ICH, hematoma expansion, larger hematoma volumes, as well as poor functional outcomes and mortality at 90 days.[128,129] ApoE polymorphism may also influence the risk of lobar ICH attributable to treatment for the secondary prevention of ischemic stroke, such as statin therapy, by way of a 'gene-by-drug effect'.[130]

PATHOLOGIC FEATURES AND PATHOGENESIS

Spontaneous ICH occurs predominantly in the deep portions of the cerebral hemispheres. Its most common location is the putamen; this site accounts for 35% to 50% of the cases.[2,4,14,131-133] The second site of preference varies in different series; in most, it is the subcortical white matter,[2,14,32,132] and the frequency is 30%. The thalamus follows, with a uniform frequency of 10% to 15%.[2,4,14,132-136] Pontine hemorrhage accounts for 5% to 12% of cases of ICH.[2,4,14,132,134] The distribution figures in a series of 100 unselected cases of ICH are shown in Table 28-3.

The hemorrhages of putaminal, thalamic, and pontine location occur in the vascular distribution of small, perforating intracerebral arteries: the lenticulostriate, thalamoperforating, and basilar paramedian groups, respectively. Cerebellar hemorrhage occurs in the area of the dentate nucleus,[137,138] which is supplied by small branches of both the superior and the posterior-inferior cerebellar arteries.[137] Thus, most ICHs originate from the rupture of small, deep arteries[71] with diameters between 50 and 200 μm. The same arteries are recognized to be those occluded in cases of lacunar infarcts,[139] a form of stroke correlated primarily with chronic hypertension and diabetes.[140,141] Thus, it is apparent that these various groups of small arteries, located in well-defined anatomic areas, become the targets of chronic hypertension, and the result can be either occlusion or rupture, leading to lacunar infarcts or ICH, respectively.

TABLE 28-3 Distribution by Site of 100 Cases of ICH at the University of South Alabama Medical Center

Type	No. of Cases
Putaminal	34
Lobar	24
Thalamic	20
Cerebellar	7
Pontine	6
Miscellaneous	
Caudate	5
Putaminothalamic	4

ICH, Intracerebral hemorrhage.

Vascular Rupture

The actual mechanism of vascular rupture leading to ICH has been the subject of considerable interest, and several detailed pathologic studies[142-144] have addressed this point. Because hypertension is one of its main causative factors,[145] arterial changes associated with it have been commonly implicated in its pathogenesis. Since Charcot and Bouchard[146] described "miliary aneurysms" in brain specimens from patients with hypertensive ICH in 1868, these lesions have been the subject of extensive interest. Initially, they were thought to represent true dilatations of the arterial wall, and their preferential location deep in the hemispheres lent support to their pathogenic role. In the early twentieth century, however, with the use of a more precise histologic technique, Ellis[147] was able to show that miliary aneurysms represent "false aneurysms" and are actually made of blood collected outside the vessel wall, as "masses of blood" surrounded by either "remains of the vessel wall" or fibrin. His view of the pathogenesis of ICH implied a primary intimal lesion, with or without secondary involvement of the media and adventitia, and the former often led to passage of blood into the vessel wall and formation of a dissecting aneurysm. Either form of vascular abnormality (dissecting aneurysm or simple "weakening" of the vessel wall by extension of the primary intimal lesion into the media and adventitia) would then be responsible for rupture and hemorrhage.

Over the following years, miliary aneurysms in the brains of hypertensive patients were shown through the use of thick frozen sections[148] and x-ray imaging of brain specimens injected with radiopaque media.[149] Green[148] demonstrated three such lesions, two of which were associated with a fresh hemorrhage in the pons and frontal lobe. His view was that these lesions were mainly related to atherosclerosis and that they "may be responsible for some cases of cerebral hemorrhage." However, the definitive work that established the relationship between hypertension and miliary aneurysms was performed by Ross Russell,[149] who combined postmortem angiography with routine histologic study of brain specimens. He found miliary aneurysms in 15 of 16 brains of hypertensive patients and in ten of 38 normotensive patients. The aneurysms were found mostly in the basal ganglia, internal capsule, and thalamus and less commonly in the centrum semiovale and cortical gray matter. Ross Russell[149] regarded these lesions as most likely acquired, strongly related to hypertension, and possibly causally related to ICH. He rejected the notion that aneurysms may be consequences rather than causes of ICH, as they were present in brains of hypertensive patients without ICH.

This study was followed by a series of observations reported by Cole and Yates[142,143,150] in a systematic analysis of 100 brains from hypertensive patients and an equal number of brains from normotensive persons. Miliary aneurysms were found in 46% of hypertensive brains but only in 7% of normotensive brains; furthermore, they occurred in 85% of the hypertensive patients with massive ICH and in all of those with small "slit" hemorrhages, which suggested that small hemorrhages probably result from microaneurysmal "leaks."[142] These researchers did not, however, establish a relationship between microaneurysms and bleeding sites, thereby failing to prove that these leaks had a causal role in ICH.

In 1971, Fisher[71] reported the study of two brains containing three ICHs, one pontine and two putaminal, by serial sections of blocks of tissue containing the hemorrhage. In both putaminal hemorrhages, the primary arterial bleeding sites were identified along with multiple sites of secondary bleeding. The latter was thought to result from mechanical disruption and tearing of smaller vessels at the periphery of the enlarging hematoma. In the pontine ICH, only the secondary bleeding sites were recognized. No instances of microaneurysm formation were found in immediate relationship to the hematomas, whereas "lipohyalinosis" was a common abnormality of the walls of small arteries harboring the bleeding sites. Miliary aneurysms were identified in both hemorrhages, although not in relation to the bleeding points. Fisher[71] thought the aneurysms were unlikely to be sources of major hemorrhage and more probably the end result of old small sites of arterial rupture ("the end stage of a limited extravasation"). A year later, Fisher[151] reported a detail of the types of microaneurysms found in brains of hypertensive patients. He described "saccular," "lipohyalinotic," and "fusiform" varieties of microaneurysms and suggested that the lipohyalinotic form may be the process underlying ICH (as well as lacunar infarcts). He regarded the saccular and fusiform varieties as less likely to be important factors in the pathogenesis of ICH. On the basis of these two studies, Fisher[71,151] concluded that hypertensive ICH most likely results from rupture of one or two lipohyalinotic arteries, followed by secondary arterial ruptures at the periphery of the enlarging hematoma in a cascade or avalanche fashion.

Active Bleeding

Early studies conducted before the wide availability of CT scanning suggested that the period of active bleeding in ICH is rather brief (<1 hour),[152] and the observation of clinical deterioration after admission was frequently attributed to the effects of brain edema,[2,152] although instances of continuous bleeding were occasionally reported.[153] A number of subsequent CT studies of the early phases of ICH have helped to clarify these concepts.

Broderick et al.[154] evaluated eight patients with ICH by CT within 2.5 hours of onset and again several hours later (within 12 hours of onset in seven patients), documenting a substantial increase in hematoma size (mean percentage increase, 107%) (Fig. 28-2). This increase in the volume of the hemorrhage was accompanied by clinical deterioration in six of the eight patients, all of whom had a 40% increase in hematoma volume. In five patients, the clinical deterioration occurred with blood pressure measurements of 195 mm Hg or higher. These investigators suggested that a prolongation of active bleeding for several hours (up to 5 or 6 hours) after onset may not be uncommon as a mechanism of early clinical deterioration in ICH. Similarly, Fehr and Anderson[155] reviewed 56 cases of hypertensive ICH in the basal ganglia and thalamus and documented enlargement of the hematoma with CT in four (7%); in two of the four, the increase in hematoma size was documented within 24 hours from onset, and in the other two, it was documented on days 5 and 6. Three of the patients had neurologic deterioration. In two who experienced deterioration within 24 hours, it occurred in the setting of poorly controlled hypertension, whereas the others had adequate blood pressure control. One of two patients with adequate blood pressure control was a chronic alcoholic, leading the investigators to suggest that alcoholism may be a risk factor for delayed progression of ICH.

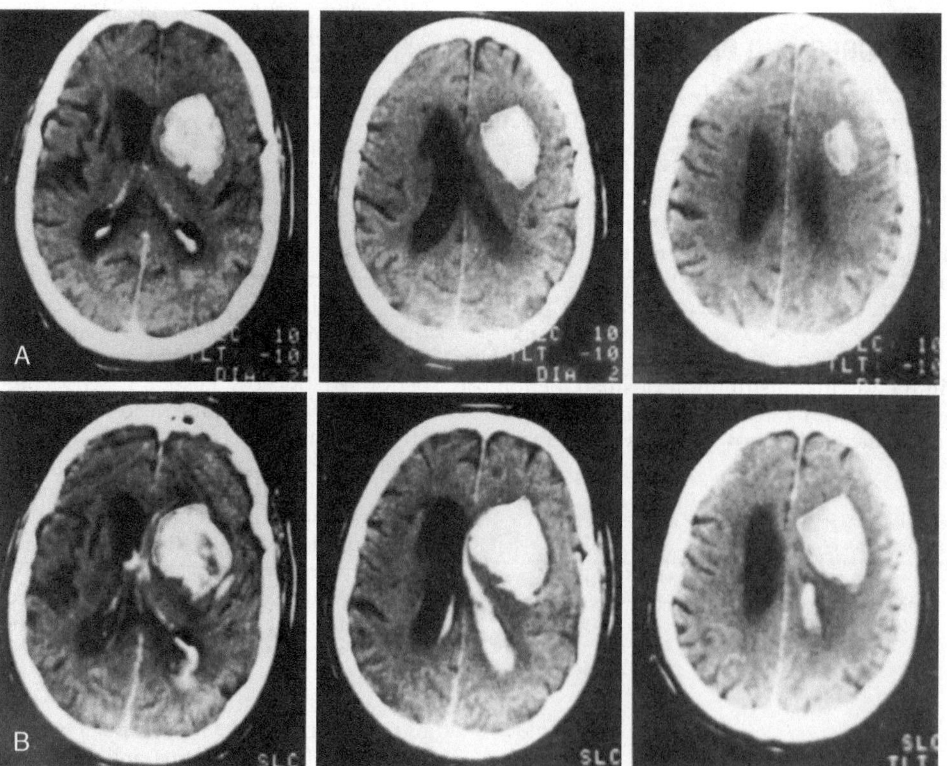

Figure 28-2. Enlargement of left putaminal hemorrhage (A) from 25 mL on CT scan performed 35 minutes after onset, to (B) 44 mL on scan obtained 70 minutes later (105 minutes after onset). *(Reprinted with permission from Broderick JP, et al. Ultra early evaluation of intracerebral hemorrhage,* J Neurosurg, *72, 2, February, p 195–9, 1990.)*

Three subsequent studies further clarified the patterns of early enlargement of ICH. Fujii et al.[156] studied 419 patients with ICH, in whom they performed the first CT within 24 hours of onset and the follow-up CT within 24 hours of admission, which showed hematoma enlargement in 60 patients (14.3%). Kazui et al.[157] conducted sequential CT evaluations in 204 patients with acute ICH, documenting enlargement of at least 12.5 cm^3, or by 40% of the original volume, in 20% of the cases. The highest frequency of detection of hematoma enlargement was seen in patients in whom the initial CT scan was performed within 3 hours of stroke onset (36%); the detection of enlargement declined progressively as the time from ICH onset to first CT increased, and there was no documentation of enlargement in those first scanned more than 24 hours after onset. These observations suggest that the period of hematoma enlargement can extend for a number of hours from onset as a result of active bleeding, which is a phenomenon that is frequently, but not always, associated with clinical deterioration. The study reported by Brott et al.[158] involved 103 patients in whom first CT scans were obtained within 3 hours of ICH onset and follow-up CT scans were obtained 1 hour and 20 hours after the initial scans. ICH enlargement (>33% volume increase) was detected in 26% of patients at the 1-hour follow-up scan, and an additional 12% showed enlargement between the 1-hour and 20-hour CT scans. The change in hematoma volume was often associated with clinical deterioration, but there were exceptions. These researchers found no predictors of ICH enlargement, evaluating age, hemorrhage location, severity of initial clinical deficit, systolic and diastolic blood pressure at onset or history of hypertension, use of antiplatelet drugs, platelet counts, prothrombin time, and partial thromboplastin time.

Recent data suggest that the presence of small foci of contrast extravasation (the "spot sign"[159]) during CTA in patients with acute ICH may predict subsequent hematoma enlargement.[159,160] The documentation of active bleeding by this technique (Fig. 28-3), especially when CTA is performed within the first few hours from symptom onset, has been correlated with a high frequency of hematoma enlargement (in up to 77% of patients with the spot sign) in comparison with patients without the sign (with only 4% showing hematoma expansion).[159] In the PREDICT (predicting haematoma growth and outcome in intracerebral haemorrhage using contrast bolus CT) study, a multicenter prospective observational cohort study, 30% of 268 ICH cases presenting within 6 hours of symptom onset were spot sign positive. Presence of spot sign within this cohort had a positive predictive value of 61% and negative predictive value of 78% for hematoma expansion (sensitivity 51%, specificity 85%).[161] Similar figures have also been reported in ICH cases where the spot sign was visualized greater than 6 hours from symptom onset.[162] Spot sign independently predicts 3-month disability (defined by the modified Rankin scale) and mortality.[161,163] The following criteria for the definition of the spot sign have been outlined:[164] a spot-like or serpiginous focus of enhancement located within a parenchymal hematoma without connection to vessels outside the ICH, with a diameter greater than 1.5 mm, and with Hounsfield units (HU) at least double that of the background hematoma density. Further evidence for the value of the spot sign for predicting hematoma expansion includes its correlation with features such as number of spot signs (≥ 3), maximal diameter (≥ 5 mm), and maximal attenuation (HU ≥ 180), all of which were found to be independent predictors of hematoma expansion.[165] Of these, the number of spot signs has been suggested as most predictive of hematoma expansion.[166]

Further studies are needed to identify potential risk factors of early ICH enlargement so that attempts can be made to prevent its associated neurologic morbidity and mortality. Promising additional markers for early ICH enlargement currently under investigation include spot sign visualized on CT perfusion source images,[167] visualization of a striate artery feeding the point of CTA contrast extravasation (termed 'spot and tail' sign),[168] postcontrast CT extravasation,[169] irregular hematoma shape and heterogeneous density on non-contrast CT,[170,171] as well as the presenting average hematoma growth rate, estimated as the baseline ICH volume divided by the time from symptom onset to baseline neuroimaging.[172] These studies should be facilitated with the use of techniques of hematoma volume measurement that are easy to apply.[173-175] The "abc method"[174] uses the formula $(a \times b \times c)/2$, in which *a* is the largest diameter of the hematoma in the CT slice with

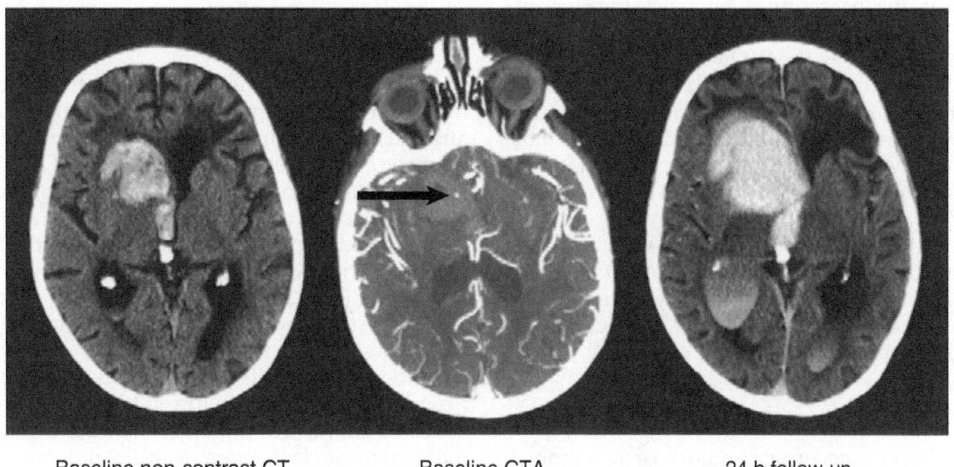

Baseline non-contrast CT (total hematoma volume 19.6 mL) | Baseline CTA (single spot-sign positive) | 24 h follow-up non-contrast CT (total hematoma volume 110.8 mL)

Figure 28-3. Computed tomographic angiogram (CTA) scan demonstrating intrahematomal contrast extravasation – "spot sign" – corresponding to ongoing bleeding at that site, and subsequent hematoma expansion on 24 hours follow-up CT scan. *(Reprinted with permission from Demchuk AM et al. Prediction of haematoma growth and outcome in patients with intracerebral haemorrhage using the CT-angiography spot sign (PREDICT): a prospective observational study,* Lancet Neurology, *11, 4, April, pp. 307–14, 2012.)*

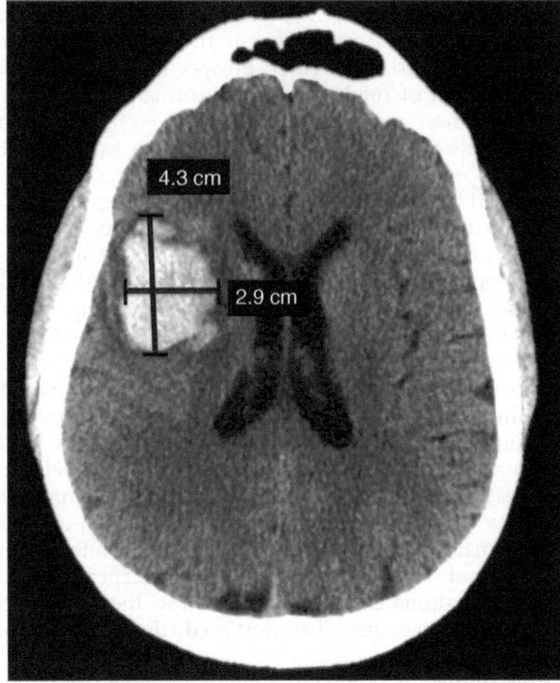

Figure 28-4. Method of calculating hematoma volume on CT, in which *a* is the largest diameter, *b* is the largest diameter perpendicular to *a*, and *c* is the number of slices with hematoma times the slice thickness in centimeters. The formula [(a × b × c)/2] gives the hematoma volume in cubic centimeters.

the largest area of ICH; *b* is the largest diameter of the hemorrhage perpendicular to line *a*; and *c* is the number of slices with hematoma times the slice thickness; this formula yields hematoma volume in cubic centimeters (Fig. 28-4). The use of these volumetric measurements of ICH should improve our understanding of the clinical consequences of early changes in hematoma size and their risk factors so that we may better define clinical and CT patterns of ICH evolution. The use of volumetric measurements of ICH in the early phase, along with neuroimaging techniques used to predict ongoing bleeding, should serve as the background for new strategies of management of ICH and their eventual testing in randomized clinical trials; one such trial is the STOP-IT trial, which will evaluate hematoma growth in patients with ICH and a CTA-detected spot sign at baseline, with randomized treatment allocation to activated factor VII or placebo. It is expected that the study of patients with ICH at high risk of hematoma expansion will help identify treatments with potential for arresting this process.

Lastly, whether MRI markers of cerebral small-vessel disease, such as cerebral microbleeds or white matter hyperintensities (indicating possible underlying vascular fragility vulnerable to Fisher's aforementioned 'avalanche theory'), are helpful in predicting hematoma growth remains to be confirmed.[176–178]

Secondary Brain Injury

In contrast to the immediate primary injury of hematoma formation, which ensues from mechanical damage to surrounding brain tissue during expansion, secondary injury of ICH is believed to result from the potentiation of various parallel cascades (namely inflammation, coagulation, and red cell lysis) resulting in cerebral edema and neuronal death.[179]

Extravasated blood exposes perihematomal brain tissue to blood components including red blood cells, leukocytes, and plasma proteins, which in turn activate surrounding microglia and astrocytes.[180] Activated microglia/macrophages serve a major protective role in clearing the hematoma and tissue debris. However, experimental models suggest that they also increase blood–brain barrier permeability and promote surrounding brain tissue damage by releasing inflammatory cytokines, reactive oxygen species, and proteases, which contribute to ICH-induced secondary brain injury.[180] Astrocytes play both a neuroprotective role, by promoting neurotrophic factors and cascade modulation, and a neurotoxic one, through the secretion of inflammatory cytokines and metalloproteinases in concert with migroglia, and by promoting reactive gliosis. Attempts at minimizing ICH-induced neurotoxicity through the use of anti-microglial therapies, such as minocycline,[181,182] have proven to reduce ICH-induced edema and neuronal injury in murine models. However, the apparent combined neurotoxic and neuroprotective actions of microglia/macrophages and astrocytes in response to ICH require further characterization in order to better identify therapeutic targets within their cascades that minimize neurotoxicity while preserving neuroprotective actions.

Red blood cell lysis occurs within 3 days of ICH, causing the release of hemoglobin and heme, which are then phagocytized and degraded by microglia/macrophages by way of heme-oxygenases.[179] Heme degradation products – carbon monoxide, biliverdin, and iron – are believed to contribute to oxidative stress, edema formation, and neuronal death. The role of iron in ICH-induced secondary injury is supported by the neuroprotective role of the iron-chelator deferoxamine in experimental ICH models.[183] These observations have led to ongoing clinical trials aimed at reducing post-ICH iron-mediated toxicity.[184]

Thrombin formation, resulting from activation of the coagulation cascade in order to limit hematoma expansion, can also initiate several deleterious pathways at high concentrations that promote cerebral edema formation, and both neuronal and astrocytic death, serving as another potential therapeutic target.[185,186]

Gross Pathologic Anatomy

The gross pathologic anatomy of ICH includes a number of features peculiar to the various locations of the hematomas.

Putaminal Hemorrhage

The common *putaminal* variety originates at the posterior angle of this nucleus and spreads in a concentric fashion but generally extends more in the anteroposterior than the transverse diameter.[134] The result is an ovoid mass of maximal anteroposterior diameter collected in the putamen and the structures located laterally to it, the external capsule and claustrum. The insular cortex is pushed laterally, whereas the internal capsule is either displaced medially or involved directly by the hematoma (Fig. 28-5). The origin of this form of ICH in the lateral–posterior aspect of the putamen is bleeding from a lateral branch of the striate arteries.[134] The lumens of these laterally placed middle cerebral artery perforating branches are between 200 μm and 400 μm wide at their entry to the brain,[149] and they supply the putamen, internal capsule, and head of the caudate nucleus. From its initial putaminal–claustral location, a sufficiently large hematoma may extend to other structures in the vicinity: medially into the internal capsule and lateral ventricle, superiorly into the corona radiata, and inferolaterally into the white matter of the temporal lobe (Fig. 28-6).

These variations in the pattern of extension result in clinical variants of putaminal hemorrhage. The extension of the hemorrhage from its site of origin can follow several patterns, of

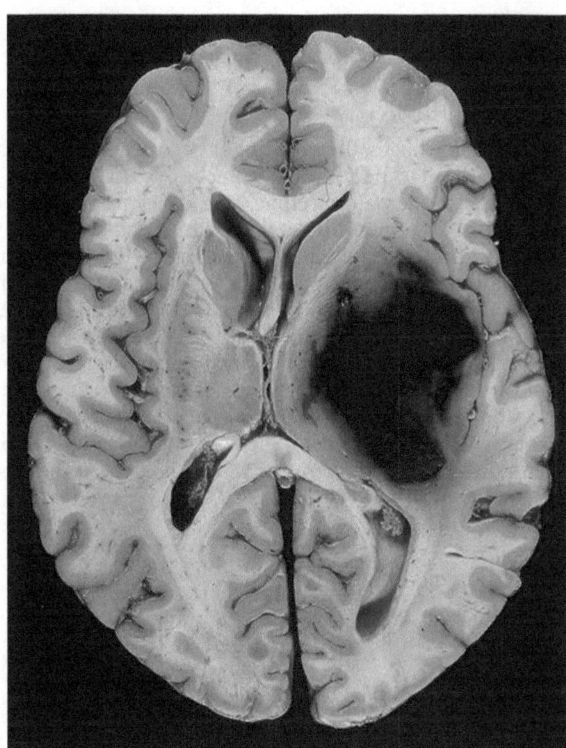

Figure 28-5. Massive left putaminal hemorrhage involving the posterior half of the putamen, globus pallidus, posterior limb of the internal capsule, and claustral area. Effacement of the ipsilateral lateral ventricle and midline shift is present.

which the most common is dissection along the course of adjacent white matter fibers. The common medial extension of the hematoma leads to communication with the lateral ventricle, through a process of slow leakage of blood rather than as direct communication between active bleeding site and ventricular system.[134] Direct communication of the hematoma with the ventricular system, at times with associated hydrocephalus, is more likely to result from bleeding at sites adjacent to the ventricular space, such as the thalamus[128] and the head of the caudate nucleus.[187] A putaminal hematoma that extends directly into the ventricle is usually large and thus is associated with high mortality.[188]

Caudate Hemorrhage

A variant of striatal hematomas is that occurring in the head of the *caudate* nucleus. Although the bleeding source is thought to be the same as in putaminal hemorrhage (the lateral group of striate arteries), this form of ICH is less common.[187] The recognized low frequency of this type of striatal hemorrhage in hypertensive patients leads the clinician to search for a different underlying cause, such as an arteriovenous malformation (AVM) or aneurysm. This variation in the frequency of two types of striatal bleeding (putaminal and caudate) from the same arterial source is unexplained and may reflect a higher rate of arterial rupture at the more proximal segments of these arteries. This higher rate, in turn, may correlate with a higher frequency of "lipohyalinosis" or "microatheroma" at the more proximal segments of these vessels, as shown by Fisher[189] in serial studies of the underlying vascular lesions in cases of capsular infarcts. Fisher implied that the same basic vascular abnormality (lipohyalinosis or microatheroma) may be the basis for both lacunar infarcts and ICH in hypertensive patients.[134] The predominantly proximal location of these

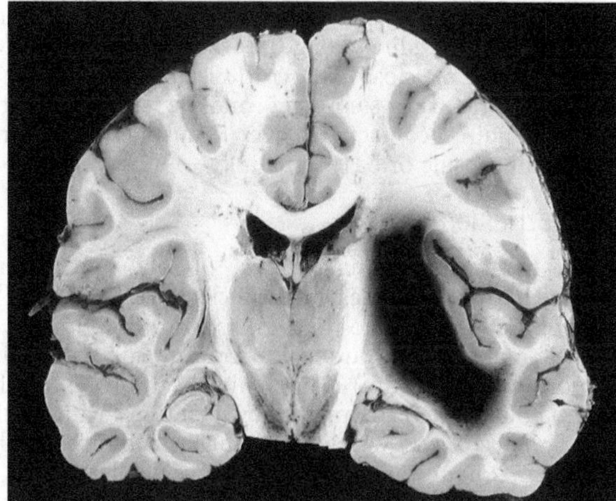

Figure 28-6. Large left putaminal–capsular hemorrhage, with tracking into the white matter of the temporal lobe.

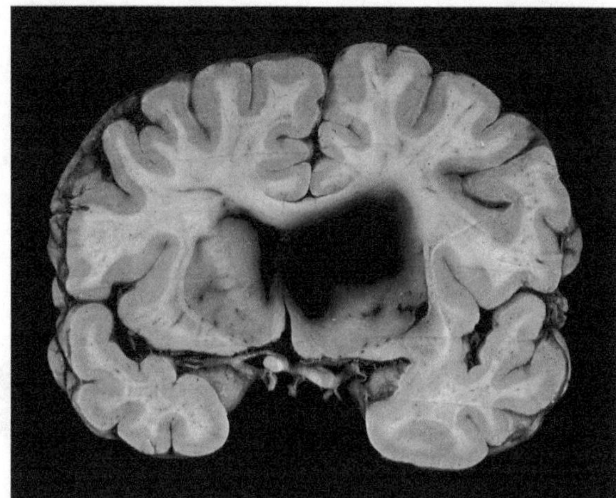

Figure 28-7. Hemorrhage originating from the head of the left caudate nucleus, with involvement of the anterior limb of the internal capsule and direct ventricular extension with formation of a ventricular cast.

lesions could therefore explain the low frequency of caudate hemorrhage because it originates from the distal ends of these lateral striate branches. Caudate hemorrhage occurs most commonly in the head of this nucleus (Fig. 28-7), and ventricular entry is an early event; this component is sometimes many times larger than the parenchymal hematoma.[188] Involvement of the anterior limb of the internal capsule is the rule.

Thalamic Hemorrhage

Thalamic hemorrhages can involve most or the entire nucleus, and their extension is mostly in the transverse direction, into the third ventricle medially and the posterior limb of the internal capsule laterally (Fig. 28-8). Because the hemorrhage commonly extends transversely, it produces a pressure effect or extends directly inferiorly into the tectum and tegmentum of the midbrain. Moderate-sized and large thalamic hematomas often extend superiorly into the corona radiata and parietal white matter, following the orientation of their fibers.

Lobar (White Matter) Hematoma

White matter (*lobar*) hematomas collect along the fiber bundles of the cerebral lobes, most commonly at the parietal and occipital levels (Fig. 28-9).[132,190] Blood usually collects between the cortex and underlying white matter, separating them and often extending along the white matter pathways. These hematomas are close to the cortical surface, at a distance from the ventricular system and midline structures, and usually not in direct contact with deep hemispheric structures (e.g., internal capsule or basal ganglia).

Cerebellar Hemorrhage

Cerebellar hemorrhages usually occur on one hemisphere, originating in the area of the dentate nucleus (Fig. 28-10).[137,138] From here they extend into the hemispheric white matter as well as the cavity of the fourth ventricle. The adjacent brainstem (pontine tegmentum) is rarely involved directly by the hematoma but is often compressed by it, at times with resultant pontine necrosis. A variant of cerebellar hemorrhage, the midline hematoma originating from the cerebellar vermis is virtually always in direct communication with the fourth ventricle through its roof and frequently extends into the pontine tegmentum bilaterally. The bleeding artery in this variety usually corresponds to distal branches of the superior cerebellar artery. These two forms of cerebellar hemorrhage have distinct clinical and prognostic features.

Pontine Hemorrhage

In *pontine* hemorrhages, the bleeding sites correspond to small paramedian basilar perforating branches.[71] The result is a medially placed hematoma that extends symmetrically to involve the basis pontis bilaterally, with variable degrees of tegmental extension (Fig. 28-11). Tracking of the hematoma into the middle cerebellar peduncle is rarely seen. A partial unilateral variety of pontine hematoma, predominantly tegmental in location, is recognized clinically and documented by CT scans.[191,192] These hypertensive hemorrhages result from rupture of distal tegmental segments of long circumferential branches of the basilar artery.[192] The hematomas usually communicate with the fourth ventricle, and they extend laterally and ventrally into the tegmentum and upper part of the basis pontis on one side.

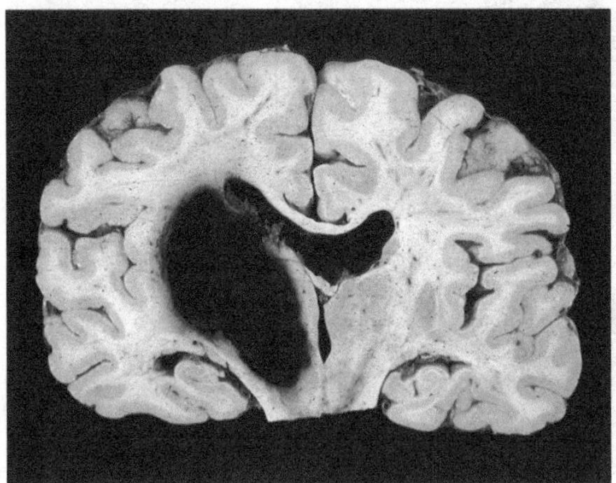

Figure 28-8. Right thalamic hemorrhage, involving most of this nucleus, with extension into the corona radiata as well as inferiorly into the subthalamic area, with compression of the dorsal midbrain.

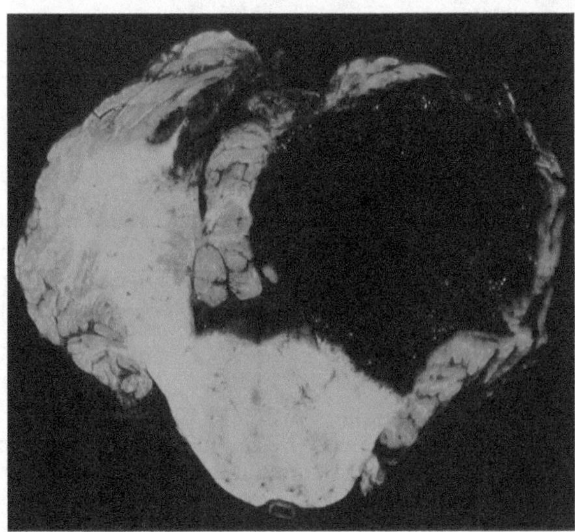

Figure 28-10. Left cerebellar hemorrhage with mass effect on the pontine tegmentum. *(Reprinted with permission from Kase CS: Cerebellar hemorrhage, Kase CS, Caplan LR, editors:* Intracerebral hemorrhage, *Boston, 1994, Butterworth-Heinemann, p 425.)*

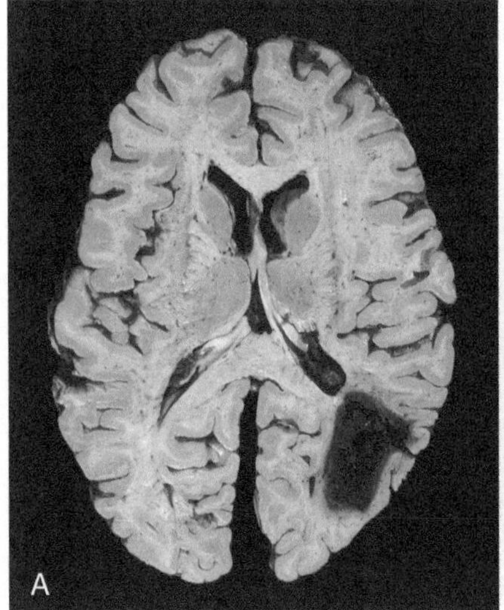

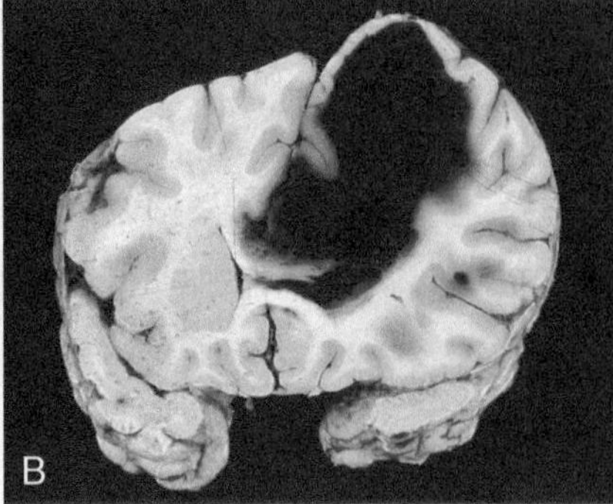

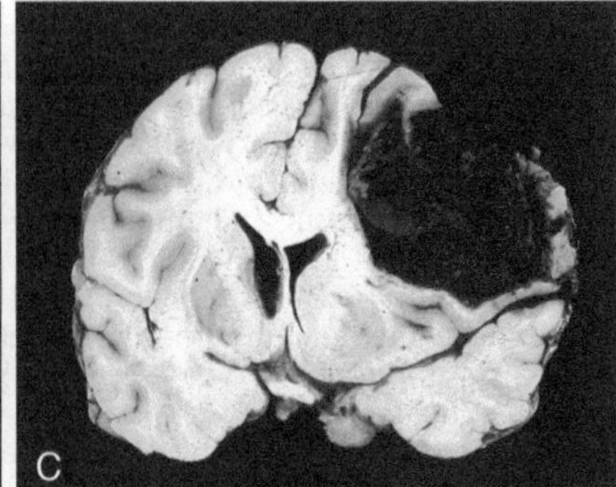

Figure 28-9. A, Left subcortical (white matter) occipital lobe hemorrhage, without extension into the ventricular system or midline shift. B, Large left frontal subcortical hemorrhage, with extension into the lateral ventricle and marked midline shift. C, Large left frontoparietal lobar hemorrhage, with cortical involvement and communication with the subarachnoid space; marked mass effect and midline shift.

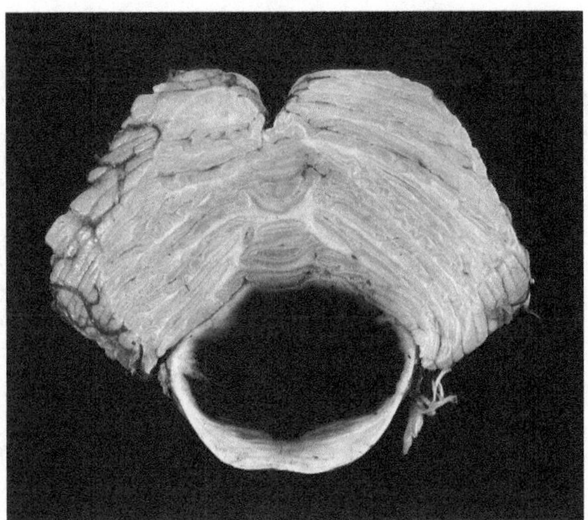

Figure 28-11. Massive midline basal pontine hemorrhage, with bilateral destruction of basis and tegmentum.

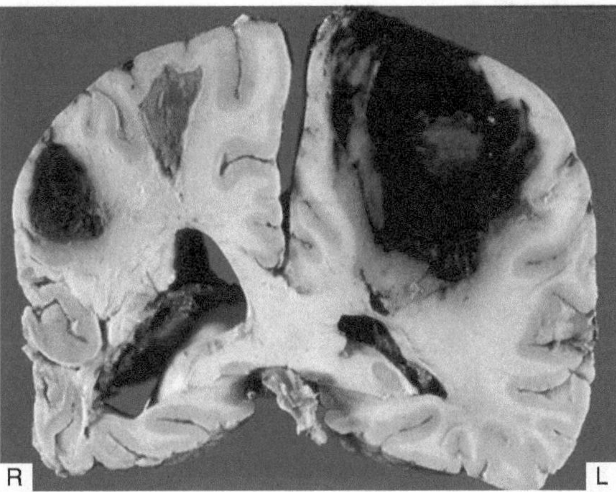

Figure 28-12. Multiple intracerebral hemorrhages of different ages in a patient with autopsy-documented cerebral amyloid angiopathy: acute fatal left lobar, subacute right lateral parietal, and chronic (with ocher discoloration) right upper parietal locations.

Recurrence of Intracerebral Hemorrhage

The ICH of hypertensive patients is often a one-time event: in a group of 101 patients with ICH entered into the NINCDS Stroke Data Bank,[4] history of a prior hemorrhage was documented in only one instance. Long-term follow-up studies in patients with ICH have found a low frequency of recurrent bleeding,[193] which clearly differentiates ICH from aneurysms and AVMs, in which rebleeding is a prominent feature. In a study reported by Gonzalez-Duarte et al.,[194] however, data showed ICH recurrence in approximately 6% of an unselected series of patients with ICH. Among hypertensive patients, the pattern of recurrence was that of repeated episodes of basal ganglionic ICH, whereas recurrence of lobar ICH was observed more often in non-hypertensive subjects, in whom the predominant putative mechanism of ICH was CAA. A similar rate of recurrence (5.4%) was documented by Bae et al.[195] within a median interval of about 2 years from the first episode of ICH. The risk of ICH recurrence was significantly increased by poor hypertension control, which stresses the value of hypertension treatment in the prevention of ICH.

Occasionally, multiple simultaneous ICHs can occur.[196,197] In a series of 600 consecutive cases of ICH diagnosed by CT scan, Weisberg[189] found 12 patients (2%) with multiple hematomas. These double lesions were probably simultaneous (because of equal CT attenuation values) in 11 instances, and they occurred in the same intracranial compartment (supratentorial or infratentorial) in all patients but one, in whom thalamic and cerebellar hematomas coexisted. The incidence of hypertension was unusually low (two of 12 patients) in this series, which suggests that cases of multiple spontaneous ICHs may frequently have other causative factors.

Cerebral Amyloid Angiopathy

Among the survivors of CAA-related ICH, the major neurologic risk is hemorrhage recurrence. A pooled analysis of patients monitored after lobar ICH reported a recurrence rate of 4.4% per year.[198] The value for cumulative ICH recurrence rate among the consecutive patients followed up at MGH was approximately 10% per year,[127] perhaps reflecting a higher prevalence of CAA among the patients with lobar ICH in this population. Recurrent hemorrhages, like the initial hemorrhages, are typically lobar, although generally at a site distinct from that of the initial ICH (Fig. 28-12).

The strongest risk factors for CAA-related ICH recurrence are a history of previous recurrences, ApoE genotype, antithrombotic exposure, posterior predominant white matter changes and number of hemorrhages (microbleeding plus macrobleeding) detected by gradient-echo MRI.[126,127,199] The prognosis for good functional outcome after a second CAA-related ICH appears to be relatively poor.[127] These observations highlight secondary hemorrhage prevention as an important treatment goal in CAA.

Histopathologic Studies

The studies on the histopathology of ICH have been mostly concerned with pathogenic issues. However, the main features of the microscopic anatomy of ICH and its changes with time are well-documented. The initial arterial rupture leads to local accumulation of blood, which in part destroys the parenchyma locally, displaces nervous structures in the vicinity, and dissects at some distance from the initial focus. The bleeding sites are at times difficult to locate, and serial sections are needed to show them.[55] The bleeding sites appear as round collections of platelets admixed with and surrounded by concentric lamellae of fibrin, so-called bleeding globes or fibrin globes.[71] These fibrin or bleeding globes at the primary and secondary sites are histologically identical, except that the fibrin globes are larger. The bulk of the hematoma is formed by a compact mass of red blood cells, and the bleeding sites are characteristically found at its periphery.

García et al.[200] have described in detail the sequential histologic changes that take place in the hematoma. After hours or days, extracellular edema develops at the periphery of the hematoma, resulting in pallor and vacuolation of myelin sheaths. After 4 to 10 days, the red blood cells begin to lyse, eventually turning into an amorphous mass of methemoglobin. Cellular infiltration by polymorphonuclear leukocytes appears at the periphery of the hematoma as early as 2 days after onset, and the number of leukocytes peaks at 4 days.[201] This event is followed by the arrival of microglial cells, which become foamy macrophages after the ingestion of cellular debris, including products of disintegration of myelin as well as blood-derived pigments, especially hemosiderin. The final stages of this process consist of the proliferation of astrocytes at the periphery of the hematoma, where these cells become enlarged and display prominent eosinophilic cytoplasm (gemistocytes), which at times contains hemosiderin granules.

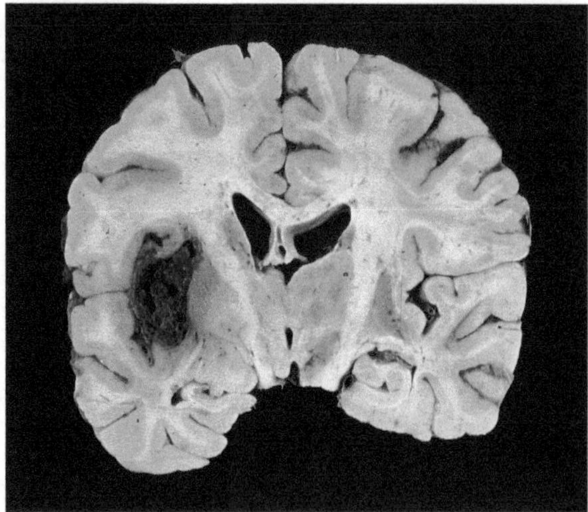

Figure 28-13. A 2-month-old right putaminal–insular hemorrhage, with partial cavitation, good demarcation from the adjacent parenchyma, and lack of signs of mass effect.

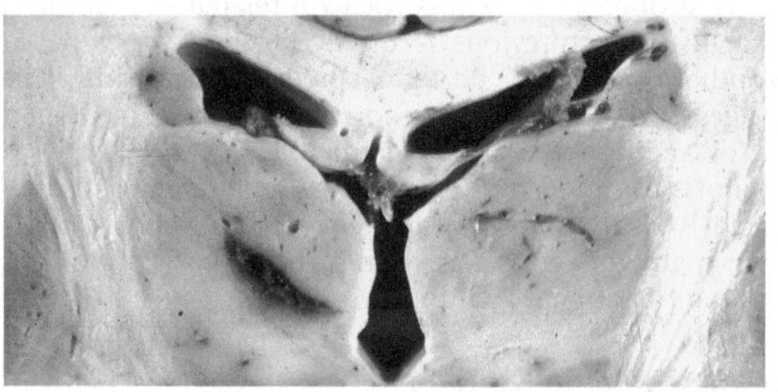

Figure 28-14. Old right thalamic hemorrhage reduced to a slit with hemosiderin-stained edges.

Once the late stage of hematoma reabsorption and repair has been reached, the astrocytes are replaced by abundant glial fibrils.

This histologic process is correlated with macroscopic changes in the hematoma, which initially becomes a soft, spongy mass of brick-red, altered blood (Fig. 28-13). After many months of slowly progressing phagocytosis, the residua of the hematoma is confined to a flat, collapsed cavity lined by reddish orange discoloration resulting from the accumulation of hemosiderin-laden macrophages (Fig. 28-14).[33]

Cerebral Amyloid Angiopathy

CAA appears on pathologic analysis as a variable combination of vascular amyloid deposition and vessel wall breakdown (Fig. 28-15). Affected vessels are the capillaries, arterioles, and small- and medium-sized arteries primarily of the cerebral cortex, overlying leptomeninges, and cerebellum; the white matter and deep gray structures are largely spared. The distribution of CAA is typically patchy and segmental, such that heavily involved vessel segments may alternate with essentially amyloid-free regions (see Fig. 28-15C).[88] In its mildest detectable form, congophilic material accumulates at the border of the vessel's media and adventitia (see Fig. 28-15A). Amyloid-lined vacuoles often seen at this stage[88] may represent former sites of vascular smooth muscle cells that have died in apparent response to the surrounding amyloid. In moderately severe segments of CAA, vascular amyloid extends throughout the media to replace essentially the entire smooth muscle cell layer (see Fig. 28-15B).

The most advanced extent of CAA is marked by not only severe amyloid deposition but also pathologic changes in the amyloid-laden vessel wall. These vasculopathic changes can include microaneurysms, concentric splitting of the vessel wall (see Fig. 28-15D), chronic perivascular or transmural inflammation, fibrinoid necrosis (see Fig. 28-15E), and even perivascular giant-cell reaction (Fig. 28-15F).[69,87–89] CAA-related vasculopathic changes are often associated with paravascular red cells or hemosiderin deposits, which suggests ongoing leakage of blood. It is this combination of extensive amyloid deposition and breakdown of the amyloid-laden vessel walls that appears to act as the substrate for symptomatic hemorrhagic strokes.[69,88,116,123]

The principal constituent of both vascular amyloid in CAA and plaque amyloid is the β-amyloid peptide (Aβ). The Aβ peptides are 39- to 43-amino-acid proteolytic fragments of the 695- to 770-residue β-amyloid precursor protein (APP). The subset of Aβ peptides with carboxyl termini extending to positions 42 or 43 (denoted Aβ42) appears to be an important trigger to amyloid aggregation in both vessels and plaques.[202] In support of Aβ42 deposition as an early step in initiation of CAA is the observation that mildly affected vessels can stain positive for Aβ42 but stain negative for the more common Aβ fragments terminating at positions 39 or 40 (Aβ40).[203] It is Aβ40, however, that appears to be the predominant species in more heavily involved vessel segments.[204–206] Quantitative analysis of brains with mild and severe CAA suggests a progressive addition of Aβ40 to previously seeded vessel segments.[206] A variety of other proteins or protein fragments can also be detected as components of vascular amyloid, although the pathogenic role in the breakdown of the vessel wall is not known. These CAA-associated proteins include apoE, cystatin C, α-synuclein, heparan sulfate proteoglycan, amyloid P component, and several complement proteins.[207,208]

The relationship of the pathology of CAA and ApoE genotype provides an interesting insight into the importance of both Aβ deposition and vessel breakdown to the pathogenesis of CAA-related ICH. The ApoE ε2 and ε4 alleles, each a suggested risk factor for CAA-related ICH, appear to act at these two distinct stages of CAA to promote hemorrhage. ApoE ε4 associates in a dose-dependent manner with increased deposition of Aβ in vessels as it does in plaques;[124] ApoE ε2 appears instead to promote the CAA-related vasculopathic changes such as concentric vessel splitting and fibrinoid necrosis.[123,125] The mechanism for this unexpected effect of ApoE ε2 on vascular breakdown is unknown. The domain of the ApoE protein containing the ε2 determinant is present in both vessel and plaque amyloid deposits[208] but has not been linked to any specific pathogenic function.

One experimental approach to clarifying pathogenic mechanisms for CAA has been to study the effects of Aβ on vessel components in vitro. Aβ exerts toxic effects on a variety of vascular cells in culture, including cerebrovascular smooth muscle cells, endothelial cells, and pericytes.[119,209] Cell death is enhanced when the Aβ peptide used is either wild-type Aβ42 or mutant Aβ40 containing one of the amino acid substitutions associated with hereditary CAA,[114,120,210] which suggests that particular chemical properties of Aβ can specifically promote toxicity. Death of the cultured cerebrovascular smooth muscle cells appears to require a series of events on the cell surface, including assembly of Aβ into amyloid fibrils (Fig. 28-16) and accumulation of the secreted amino-terminal portion of APP.[211] Another in vitro property of Aβ is to stimulate tissue-type plasminogen activator (t-PA),[212] which raises the intriguing possibility that CAA might promote ICH through direct effects on the coagulation–thrombolysis cascade as well as on the integrity of the vessel wall.

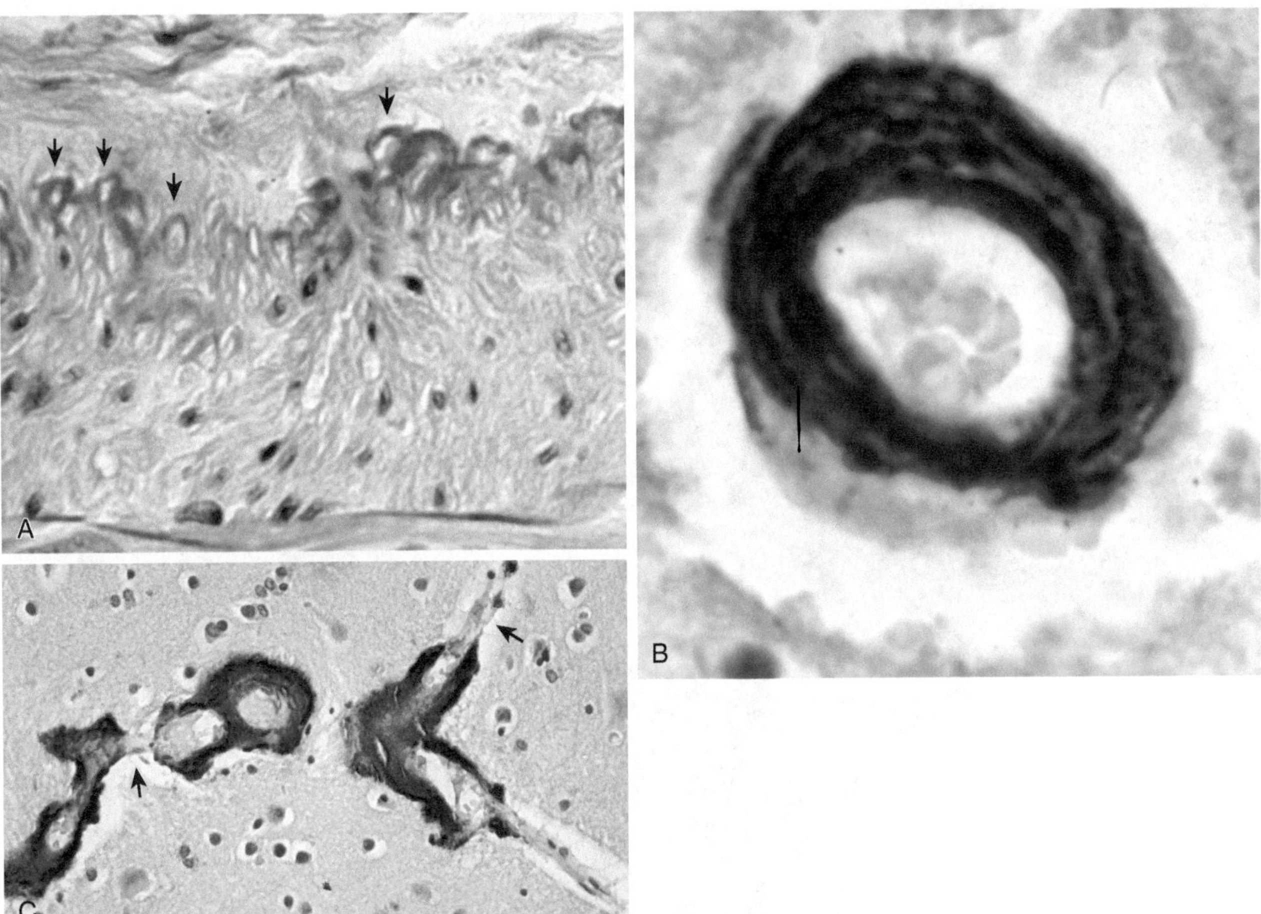

Figure 28-15. Pathologic appearances of cerebral amyloid angiopathy (CAA). A, Vessel in longitudinal section. In mild stages of disease, amyloid appears at the outer edge of the vessel media, creating vesicle-like structures *(arrows)* at sites believed to be previously occupied by smooth muscle cells. B, Further amyloid deposition replaces the media and all smooth muscle cells. C, Specimen taken from a brain with the Iowa APP mutation. Amyloid deposits can cause marked thickening of vessel wall segments that alternate with skipped areas of normal caliber *(arrows)*. Further vasculopathic changes in amyloid-laden vessels include concentric splitting of the vessel wall, creating a vessel-in-vessel appearance.

The pathogenesis of CAA has also been studied in transgenic mouse models (Fig. 28-17). Substantial CAA develops at advanced ages in lines of mice expressing high levels of mutant APP.[205,206] Affected vessels in these animals can demonstrate several pathologic features reminiscent of human CAA, including disruption or loss of the vascular smooth muscle, microaneurysms, and perivascular cerebral hemorrhages.[213-215] Because the expression of human APP in these animals is virtually all neuronal, the occurrence of CAA demonstrates that Aβ produced by neurons is capable of reaching vascular sites of deposition, possibly via the interstitial fluid drainage pathway.[216] Once produced, Aβ may be cleared by proteolytic enzymes such as neprilysin[17,62] or insulin-degrading enzyme[63] or may exit the brain by receptor-mediated efflux across the blood–brain barrier.[64]

A further insight to come from these transgenic studies is the possibility that Aβ may have specific effects on vessel physiology. Investigations in mouse models of CAA using a variety of techniques to measure blood flow have indicated blunted vasodilatory response to pharmacologic or functional stimulation.[65-67] These hints of altered vascular physiology, raised as well by earlier studies of isolated vessel segments exposed to Aβ, have found important parallels in studies of vascular reactivity to visual stimulation in humans with CAA.[68]

Other Causes of Non-traumatic Intracerebral Hemorrhage

There are a number of instances in which ICH occurs. These mechanisms of ICH are (1) vascular malformations and angiopathies such as Moyamoya disease (discussed elsewhere), (2) sympathomimetic drugs, (3) brain tumors, (4) hemorrhagic diathesis (discussed elsewhere), (5) anticoagulants, (6) fibrinolytic agents, (7) vasculitides (discussed elsewhere), and (8) hemorrhagic infarction. In a consecutive series of 378 surgical samples from patients with non-traumatic ICH, the majority of which were supratentorial and superficial, vascular pathologies (33.5%) prevailed in cases where a putative origin of ICH was determined, with arteriolosclerosis (15.6%) and CAA (10.1%) being the most frequent. Vascular malformations were encountered in 7.1%, hemorrhagic infarction in 1.6%, and brain tumor in 2.4%. These figures differed widely from preoperative assumptions where brain tumors, vascular malformations, and hemorrhagic infarctions were overestimated, while arteriolosclerosis and CAA were underestimated.[217]

Sympathomimetic Drugs

ICH related to the use of *amphetamines* has been documented in several publications.[218-221] The preparation most commonly

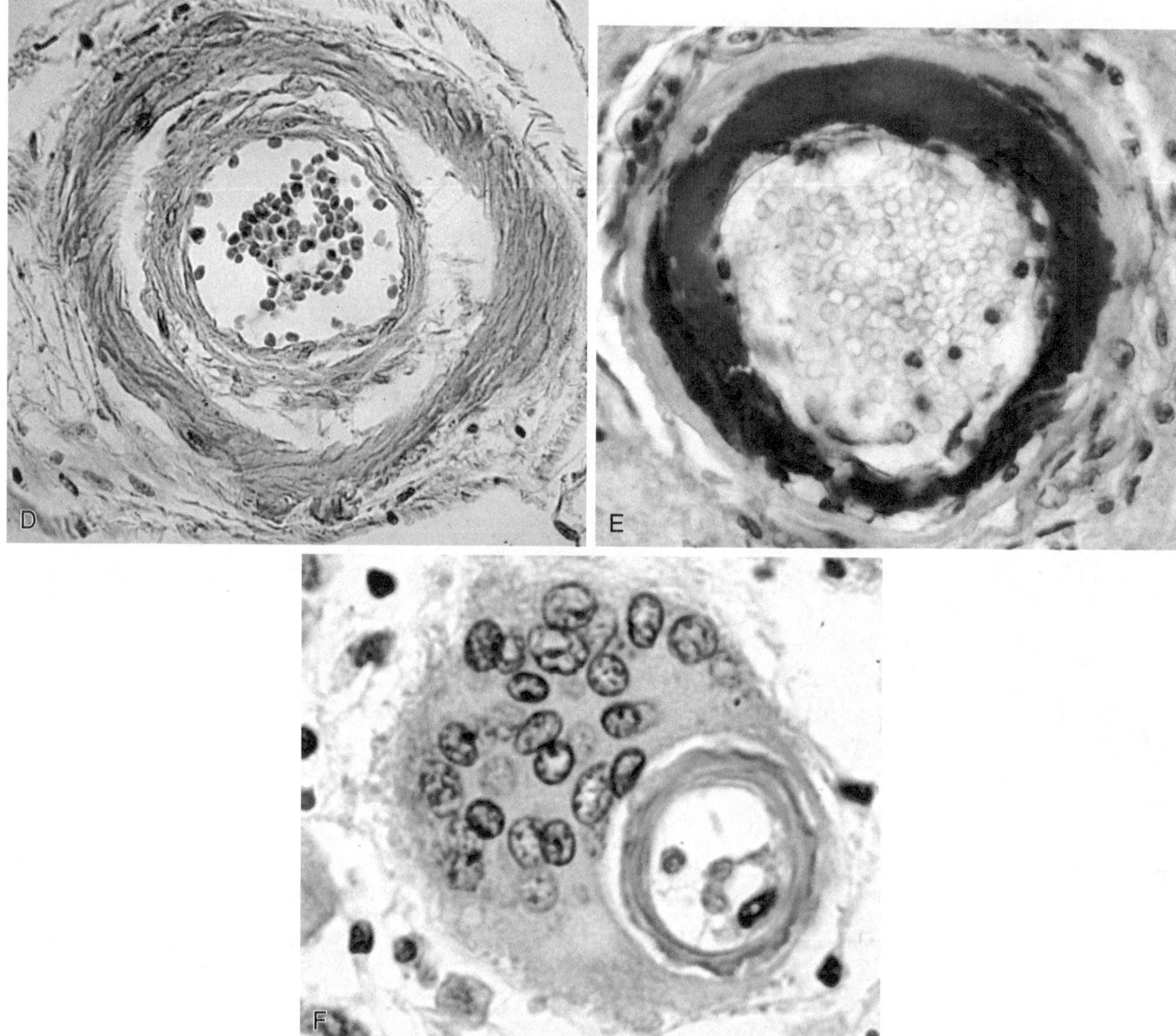

Figure 28-15, cont'd (D) and fibrinoid necrosis (E), signifying entry of plasma components into the wall. F, Some instances of advanced CAA are accompanied by visible inflammatory changes such as perivascular giant cell reaction. (A, D, and F stained by Luxol fast blue–hematoxylin-eosin; B and C by anti-β-amyloid immunostain with hematoxylin counterstain; and E with phosphotungstic acid–hematoxylin.)

implicated has been intravenous methamphetamine,[210] but cases related to intranasal[220] or oral[219] use of this drug and amphetamine have also been reported. Another sympathomimetic drug, *pseudoephedrine*, has been associated with one reported instance of ICH.[221] In these cases, ICHs have developed usually within minutes (20 to 40) to a few hours (4 to 6) after the use of the drug; frequently, the ICH represents an established pattern of drug abuse for months beforehand, but at times it has followed a first-time use.[219] An association with transiently elevated blood pressure has been noticed in about 50% of cases, and most of the hematomas have been of lobar location.[220,221] Their pathogenesis has been related to either transient drug-induced elevation in blood pressure[219] or an arteritis-like vascular change histologically similar to periarteritis nodosa.[222] The latter is considered either a direct "toxic" effect of the drug on cerebral blood vessels or a hypersensitivity reaction to the drug or its vehicle.

The cerebral "arteritis" related to use of these drugs is characterized angiographically by beading (multiple areas of focal arterial stenosis or constriction) of medium-sized and large intracranial arteries,[220,221,223-225] which is an effect that has been shown to be reversible after use of steroids and discontinuation of drug abuse.[225] However, it is likely that these reversible vascular changes correspond not to a true vasculitis but rather to a nonspecific phenomenon of multifocal spasm related to the effects of the sympathomimetic drug on the vessel wall. In isolated instances, intravenous use of methamphetamine precipitated an ICH from a Sylvian-region AVM,[226] and oral use of dextroamphetamine was associated with SAH in the presence of a small middle cerebral artery aneurysm.[227] Most other reports of amphetamine-related ICH and SAH have not documented preexisting vascular malformations or mycotic aneurysms.

Other sympathomimetic agents have been related to episodes of ICH. *Phenylpropanolamine* (PPA) has been associated with instances of ICH and SAH. Most affected patients have been young (median age in the third decade), have been women more often than men, and generally have lacked other

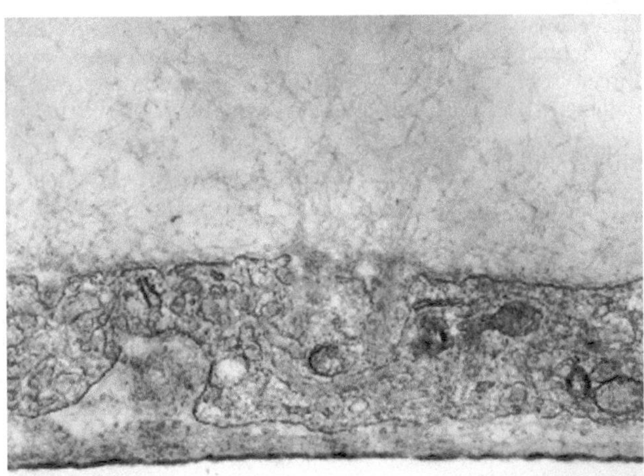

Figure 28-16. Deposition of β-amyloid (Aβ) on cerebrovascular smooth muscle cell. This transmission electron micrograph shows a cultured human cerebrovascular smooth muscle cell treated with Dutch-type mutant Aβ40 for 6 days. Under these conditions, Aβ assembles into amyloid fibrils on the cell surface (seen at top). *(Courtesy of William E. Van Nostrand.)*

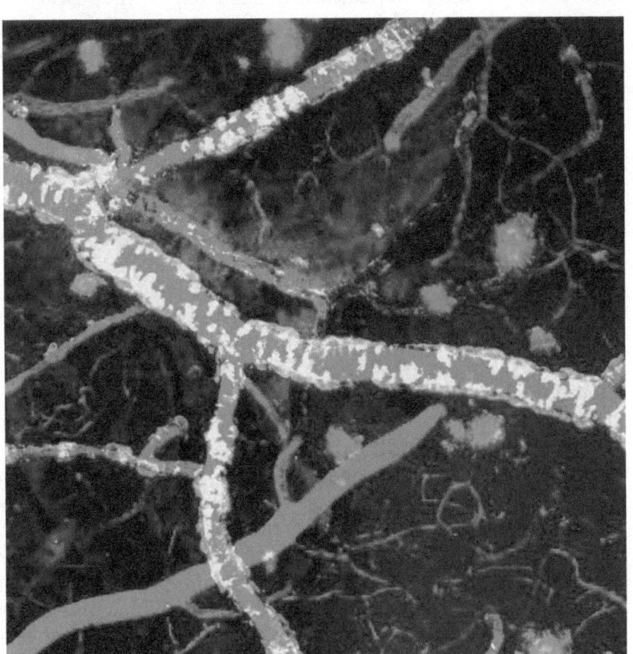

Figure 28-17. Cerebral amyloid angiopathy in a transgenic mouse (Tg2576). Vascular and parenchymal amyloid deposits are identified by systemic administration of methoxy-XO4 (blue) and vessel lumens with intravenous Texas red-labeled dextran (red). In vivo imaging is performed by multiphoton fluorescent microscopy. *(Courtesy of Michal Arbel-Ornath and Brian Bacskai.)*

risk factors for ICH.[228] Results of a case-control study reported by Kernan et al.[221] have suggested the potential association between PPA and ICH. These investigators found that women who used appetite suppressants containing PPA had a significantly higher risk of intracranial hemorrhage (odds ratio [OR], 16.58; 95%CI, 1.51–182.21; *P* = 0.02). The hemorrhages occur shortly after PPA ingestion (most between 1 and 8 hours).[228–234] The ICHs are most commonly of lobar location, and about two-thirds of the patients that have undergone angiography have shown widespread beading of intracranial arteries (Fig. 28-18), without documentation of other vascular lesions responsible for bleeding, such as AVM and aneurysm. Histologic examination of blood vessels from biopsy material has been nondiagnostic, except for one instance in which changes consistent with vasculitis were found.[235]

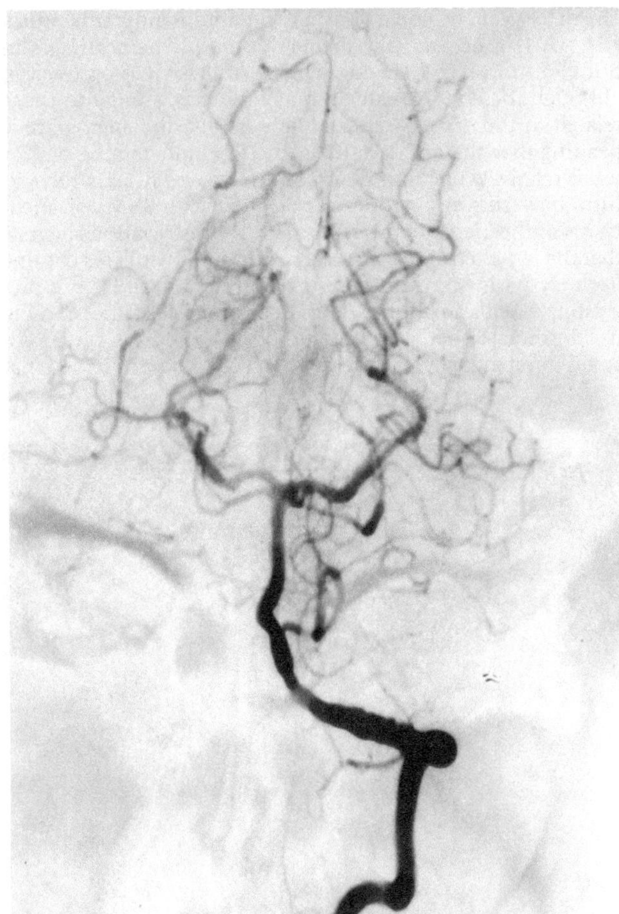

Figure 28-18. Multifocal areas of arterial constriction and dilatation ("beading") in the vertebrobasilar system after an episode of severe headache and transient hypertension (200/110 mm Hg), shortly after the ingestion of a phenylpropanolamine-containing nasal decongestant. *(Reprinted with permission from Kase CS, et al. Intracerebral hemorrhage and phenylpropanolamine use,* Neurology, *37, 3, March, pp. 399–404, 1987.)*

The pathogenesis of these PPA-related hemorrhages is obscure. Although rare patients have been previously hypertensive, transient hypertension was noted at presentation in about 50% of the reported cases.[228] This finding suggests that a possible mechanism of vascular rupture is drug-induced transient hypertension associated with multifocal arterial changes due to vasospasm or, less commonly, vasculitis. However, transient hypertension alone is an unlikely explanation for these hemorrhages because the hypertension has generally been modest, even in comparison with blood pressure rises documented under physiologic conditions.[236] These observations suggest that mechanisms other than transient hypertension must be present in order for intracranial hemorrhage to occur under these circumstances.

Cocaine is being increasingly reported as a cause of cerebral hemorrhage in young individuals, especially in its precipitate form, known as "crack." Instances of ICH and SAH have occurred within minutes to 1 hour from use of crack cocaine.[237]

The ICHs can be lobar, but are predominantly subcortical (Fig. 28-19); occasionally there are multiple hemorrhages in both locations.[238,239] The mechanism of these ICHs is unclear, although these lesions are, in many respects, similar to those related to the use of amphetamine or PPA; the angiographic beading that characterizes ICHs due to amphetamine or PPA use is relatively uncommon in cocaine-related ICHs, which, in turn, have shown a stronger association with AVMs or aneurysms as the bleeding mechanism.[237] This association suggests that the hypertensive response that commonly follows cocaine use may act in some instances as a precipitant of ICH in preexisting vascular malformations. In one case, ICH after cocaine use was related to pathologically documented vasculitis of a small intraparenchymal artery.[240] A recent report observed that patients with cocaine-associated ICH had higher rates of intraventricular hemorrhage, worse functional outcome, and a threefold increase in in-hospital mortality in comparison with patients with ICH unrelated to cocaine use.[239]

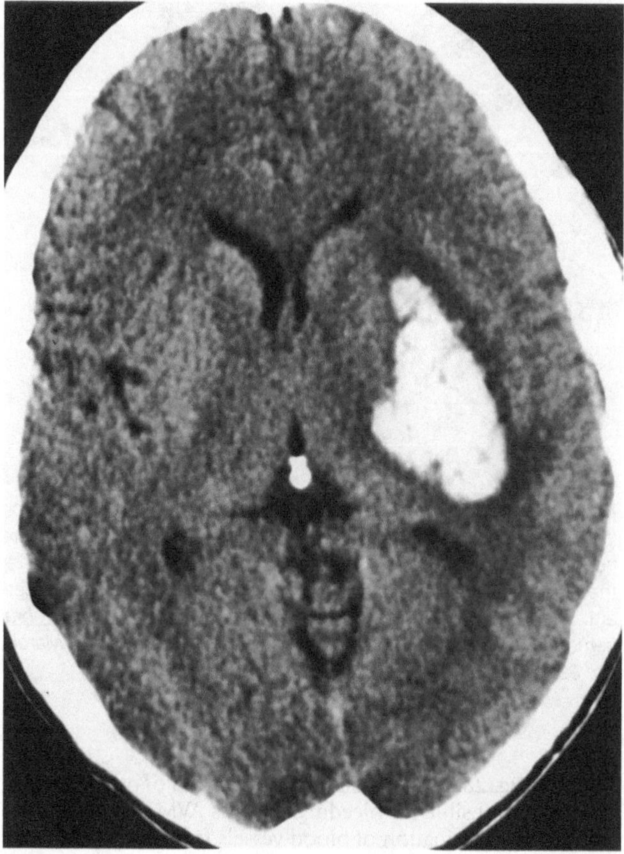

Figure 28-19. Left putaminal hemorrhage secondary to use of crack cocaine.

Intracranial Tumors

Intracranial tumors are a well-recognized but uncommon cause of ICH. Underlying tumors have accounted for 1% to 2% of cases of ICH in autopsy series,[32] whereas rates of 6% to 10% have been found in clinical-radiologic series.[241,242] The great majority of the underlying neoplasms have been malignant, either primary or metastatic, but rarely, meningiomas[243] or oligodendrogliomas[241] have manifested as ICH. An example of a generally benign tumor with relatively high tendency to bleed is pituitary adenoma, which was associated with bleeding in 15% of the cases in one large series of brain tumors.[244] Among the primary malignant brain tumors causing ICH, glioblastoma multiforme predominates;[241] the metastatic tumors have been melanoma, choriocarcinoma, renal cell, and bronchogenic carcinoma.[242,245–248] The frequency of hemorrhagic metastases was estimated at 60% for germ cell tumors, 40% for melanoma, and 9% for bronchogenic carcinoma.[249]

The bleeding tendency in neoplasms is thought to be directly related to the richness of their vascular components and their pathologic, neoplastic character.[250] In the case of metastatic choriocarcinoma, these features are enhanced by the normal biological tendency of trophoblastic tissue to invade the walls of blood vessels.[246,251] The location of the hemorrhage relates to some extent to the type of neoplasm involved: hemorrhages occurring in glioblastoma multiforme are frequently deep into the hemispheres, basal ganglia, or corpus callosum.[241] Hemorrhages due to metastatic tumors occur more often in the subcortical white matter (Fig. 28-20)[245] because metastatic nodules commonly deposit at the gray–white matter junction.

In approximately half of the reported instances of ICH within an intracerebral tumor, the hemorrhage was the first clinical manifestation of the neoplasm. The radiologic diagnosis by CT can be established easily in instances of multiple metastatic lesions,[245] but cases of ICH into a single tumor can be more difficult to diagnose. Such a diagnosis should be suspected with the finding of large areas of low-density edema surrounding the hematoma (Fig. 28-21) of an area of contrast enhancement at the periphery of the hematoma, frequently forming a ring pattern on initial presentation with ICH.[241,245] Because ring enhancement is not expected on presentation of spontaneous, hypertensive ICH,[251–254] its presence should strongly suggest the possibility of an underlying, previously asymptomatic primary or metastatic brain tumor. Other features suggesting ICH into a brain tumor are: (1) finding of

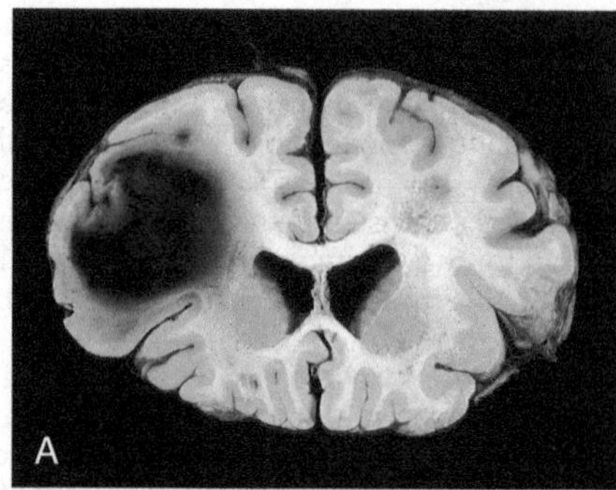

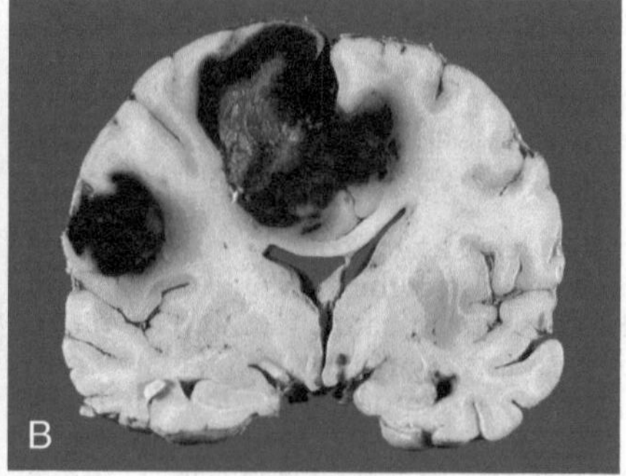

Figure 28-20. A, Large hemorrhage into a metastatic lesion (from bronchogenic carcinoma) in the right frontal subcortical white matter. A second, nonhemorrhagic metastasis is present in the white matter of the left frontal lobe. B, Hemorrhagic metastases from melanoma, with visible necrotic tumor at the center of the larger hemorrhage, extending into both medial parietal lobes.

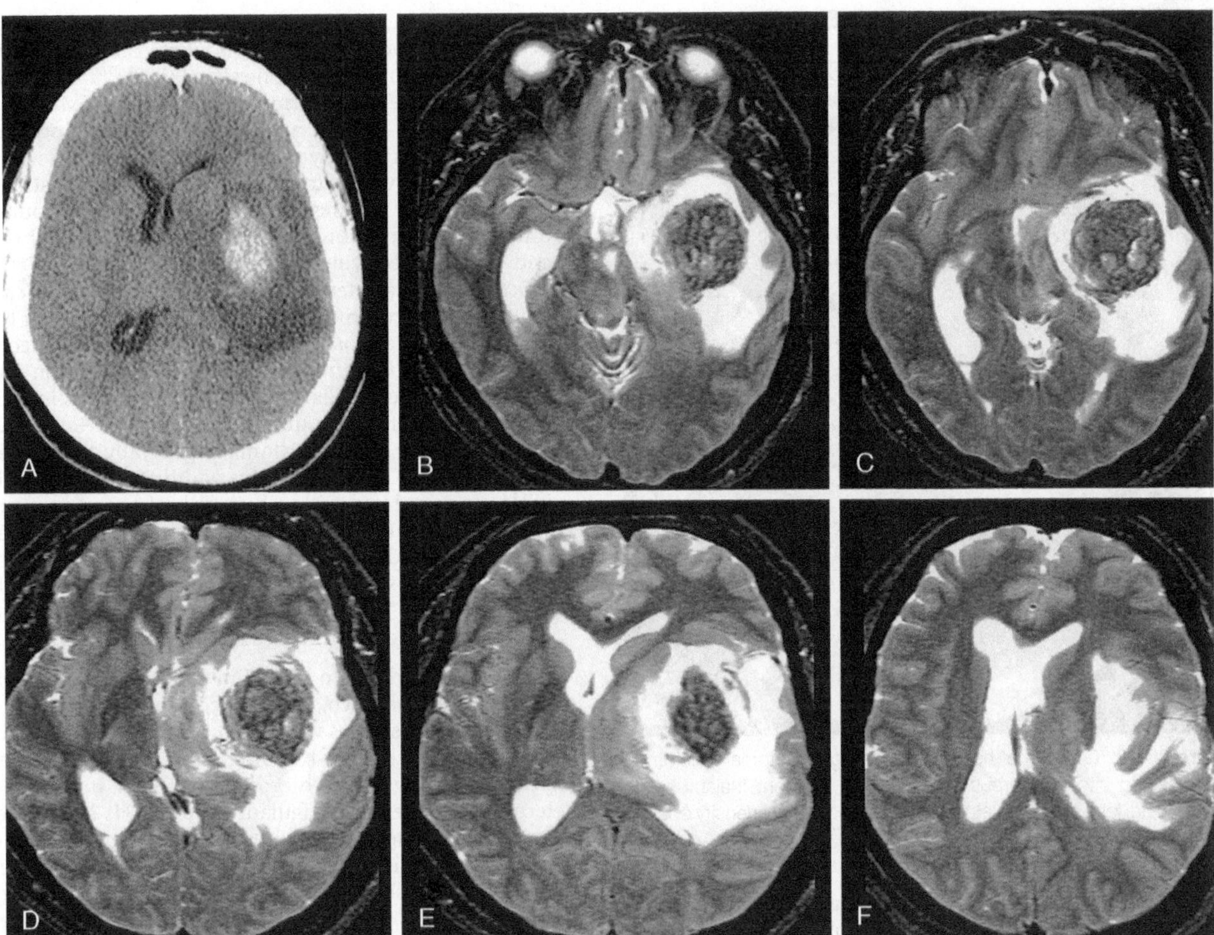

Figure 28-21. CT scan (A) and T2-weighted MR images (B to F) of acute hemorrhage into glioblastoma multiforme, showing the acute hematoma with marked edema extending well beyond the immediate vicinity of the acute hemorrhage.

papilledema at presentation with acute ICH; (2) atypical location of the ICH, in areas such as the corpus callosum, which is rarely the site of "spontaneous" ICH and is commonly involved by malignant gliomas (Fig. 28-22); and (3) a ringlike high-density area corresponding to blood around a low-density center, resulting from bleeding by tumor vessels at the junction of tumor and adjacent brain parenchyma.[255] In addition, Iwama et al.[256] have suggested that a low-density indentation of the periphery of an ICH on CT should raise the suspicion of an underlying tumor nodule. These clinical and radiologic features should prompt a search for a primary or metastatic brain tumor with MRI and cerebral angiography. If the results of these studies are inconclusive, biopsy of the hematoma cavity should be considered to establish the diagnosis of an underlying brain tumor because the therapeutic options and prognosis are radically different from those for spontaneous or hypertensive ICH.

Anticoagulant and Thrombolytic Therapy

Warfarin. Long-term oral anticoagulation with warfarin is often listed among the causes of ICH. In a consecutive series of 100 cases of ICH that Kase et al.[257] observed over a 3-year period, warfarin anticoagulation was a factor in 9% of the cases. Boudouresques et al.[50] reported that in their autopsy series of 500 cases of ICH, anticoagulation was implicated in 11%. After excluding cases due to trauma, ruptured aneurysm, or concomitant brain tumor, Rådberg et al.[258] documented an anticoagulant-related mechanism in 14% of 200 consecutive patients with ICH. Furthermore, anticoagulation is second only to hypertension as a causative factor in series of cerebellar[259] and lobar[190] locations. The risk of ICH in patients undergoing long-term oral anticoagulation has been shown to be eight to 11 times that in patients of similar age who are not receiving anticoagulants.[260–263]

The incidence of ICH in patients receiving warfarin after MI is approximately 1% per year.[253] A number of factors are known to contribute to a higher risk of ICH in these patients, including advanced age (>70 years),[264,265] hypertension,[257,263,264,266–268] and concomitant use of aspirin, which has been estimated to double the rate of ICH in comparison with individuals taking oral anticoagulants alone.[261,269]

Other features related to ICH in patients receiving anticoagulants are as follows:

Duration of anticoagulation therapy before onset of ICH. In two series, most ICHs (70%,[257] 54%[258]) occurred during the first year after the start of treatment. In another report, only one third of ICHs occurred after that period of time;[260] the other two-thirds appeared between 2 and 18 years after the start of treatment.

Relationship between intensity of anticoagulant effect and risk of ICH. Excessive anticoagulant effect is now well-established as a powerful risk factor for ICH.[247,263–266,268,270] Hylek and Singer,[264] reporting data from an anticoagulant therapy unit, showed that the risk of ICH doubled with each 0.5-point increase in the prothrombin time ratio above the recommended limit of 2.0. Data from the Stroke Prevention in

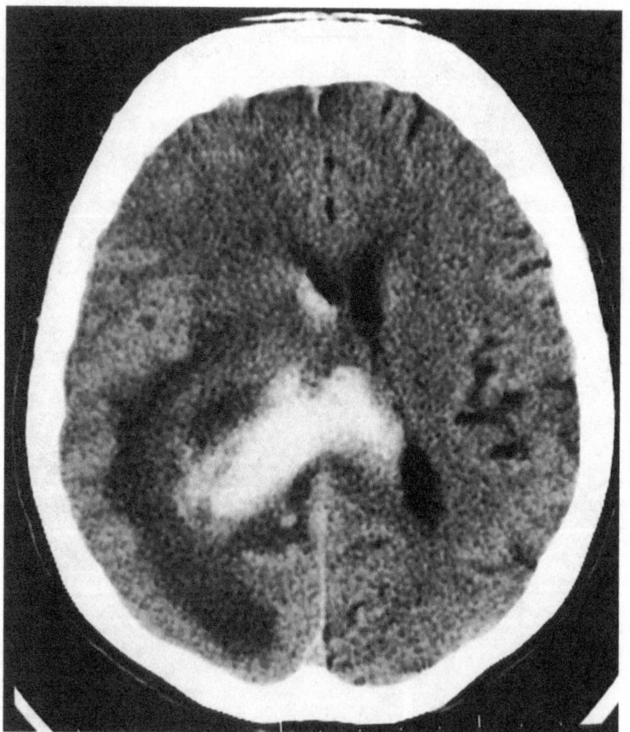

Figure 28-22. CT scan of hemorrhage into glioblastoma multiforme, with bleeding into the corpus callosum and adjacent thalamus and deep parietal lobe as well as extensive surrounding low-density edema.

Reversible Ischemia Trial,[271] a secondary stroke prevention trial in which patients with transient ischemic attack or minor ischemic stroke were randomly assigned to receive either aspirin (30 mg/day) or warfarin (to achieve an international normalized ratio [INR] of 3.0 to 4.5), add further evidence of the effect of excessive anticoagulation and frequency of ICH: the trial was stopped early, after the occurrence of 24 ICHs (14 fatal) in the warfarin group in comparison with only three ICHs (one fatal) in the aspirin group; there was a strong relationship between bleeding complications and rise in INR values. A relationship between increasing INR values and large ICH volume has also been reported.[272,273]

Presence of leukoaraiosis. Severe and confluent areas of leukoaraiosis were associated with a higher risk of ICH in warfarin-anticoagulated subjects in the Stroke Prevention in Reversible Ischemia Trial.[271] Similarly, data reported by Smith et al.[268] documented CT-detected leukoaraiosis as an independent risk factor (OR, 12.9; 95%CI, 28–59.8) for ICH in subjects receiving anticoagulation therapy with warfarin after an episode of ischemic stroke.

Presence of cerebral microbleeds. Cerebral microbleeds (CMBs), represent remnants of previous blood degradation in the form of hemosiderin-laden macrophages,[274] and are believed to result from underlying bleeding-prone microangiopathy. The largest study to date investigating the association of CMBs and antithrombotic-related ICH (antiplatelet or warfarin), prospectively followed 908 stroke patients presenting to a regional stroke center in Hong Kong for an average period of 2.2 years, and noted a dose-dependent independent relationship between the number of CMBs on baseline MRI and subsequent ICH while on antithrombotic therapy, reaching a hazard ratio of 9.81 (95%CI, 2.76–34.83) in individuals with five or more CMBs.[275] Although the majority of antithrombotic use was in the form of antiplatelet therapy in this study, its findings were subsequently supported by two additional cohorts where CMBs strongly correlated with anticoagulation-related ICH.[276,277] Additional data are required to determine the utility of CMBs on MRI within the risk–benefit analysis of implementing chronic anticoagulation therapy at an individual patient level.

Location of ICH. A high frequency of cerebellar location was found in some studies,[257,258,278] whereas others found no differences in location of ICH between patients who were and were not receiving anticoagulation therapy.[260,261,263]

Characteristics. Characteristics of these hemorrhages include a tendency to occur in the absence of signs of systemic bleeding, lack of relationship between the ICH and preceding cerebral infarction, frequent leisurely progression of the focal neurologic deficits (at times over periods as long as 48 to 72 hours), and high mortality (46% to 68%) related to hematoma size (the hematoma is generally larger than in hypertensive ICH).[258,260,261] In addition, warfarin-related ICHs are associated with a high risk of hematoma expansion,[279] which in turn correlates with clinical deterioration (Fig. 28-23) and increased mortality. On CT scan, the hemorrhages often show blood-fluid levels, which result from "sedimentation" of red blood cells in a hematoma that does not clot because of the anticoagulation effect (Fig. 28-24).

The actual mechanism of ICH in patients undergoing anticoagulation is unknown, in part because of the lack of adequate pathologic studies with serial histologic sections aimed at identifying the type of bleeding vessel and the histopathologic abnormality at the bleeding site. Such studies should determine whether anticoagulant-related ICHs have different microscopic pathologic features from that of spontaneous ICH, in terms of the type of affected vessel as well as the eventual presence of local vascular disease (i.e., microaneurysm, fibrinoid necrosis, lipohyalinosis, or CAA) at the rupture site as a possible substrate for this complication of warfarin anticoagulation. Hart et al.[261] have hypothesized that ICH in patients undergoing anticoagulation could result from enlargement of small, spontaneous hemorrhages that would otherwise occur without clinical consequence in individuals with normal coagulation function. The contributing role of local vascular disease, such as CAA, is favored by observation of a high frequency of this angiopathy in individuals with warfarin-related ICH. Rosand et al.[280] documented CAA in brain tissue samples from seven of 11 patients with warfarin-related ICH. In addition, these investigators found an over-representation of the ApoE ε2 allele, a marker of CAA, in patients with warfarin-related ICH in comparison with a control group.

Heparin. The occurrence of ICH during intravenous heparin anticoagulation represents a different situation because this complication generally occurs in the setting of preceding acute cerebral infarction (because ICH is extremely uncommon in patients receiving intravenous heparin for noncerebrovascular indications, such as deep vein thrombosis and MI[281,282]). Thus, a recent cerebral infarction with local ischemic blood vessels is a likely site for the occurrence of secondary ICH, especially in embolic infarcts, which tend to become hemorrhagic as part of their natural history.[283] ICH in this setting occurs within 24 to 48 hours of the start of heparin treatment,[284] and excessive prolongation of the activated partial thromboplastin time (aPTT) is common.[285,286] Other risk factors for ICH in the setting of intravenous heparin therapy for acute cerebral infarction are infarcts of large size and uncontrolled hypertension (blood pressure exceeding 180 mm Hg systolic/100 mm Hg diastolic).[287]

These findings have led to recommendations that the immediate use of intravenous heparin anticoagulation in acute nonseptic cerebral infarction be limited to those patients

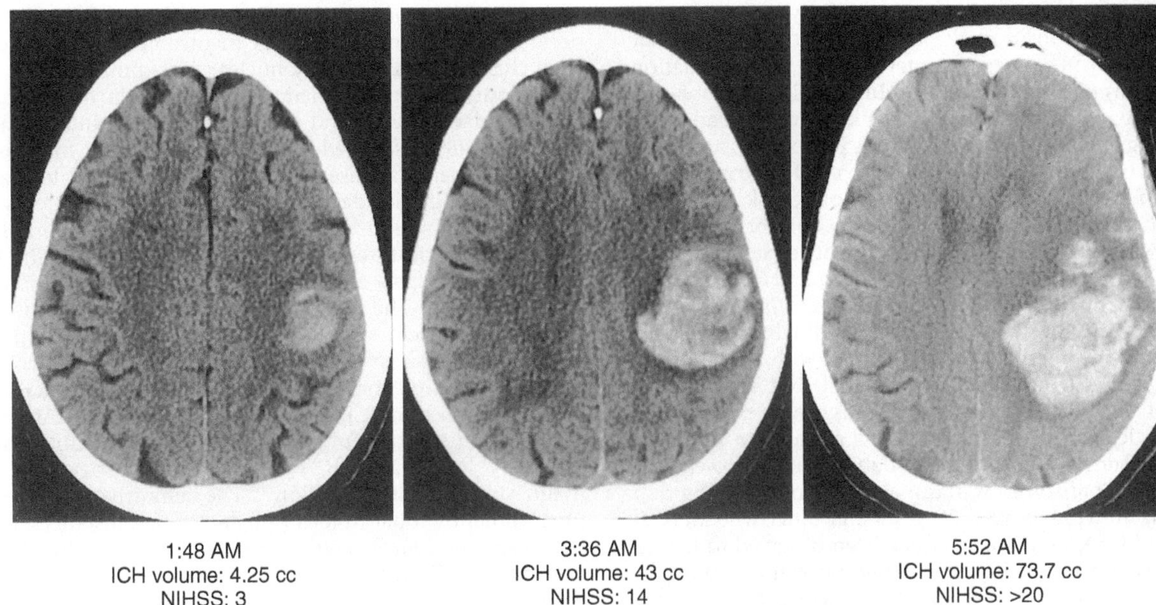

Figure 28-23. Gradual enlargement of hematoma in patient receiving anticoagulation with warfarin, showing progression over time of the volume of the hematoma and the corresponding neurologic deterioration, as measured by the National Institutes of Health Stroke Scale (NIHSS) score.

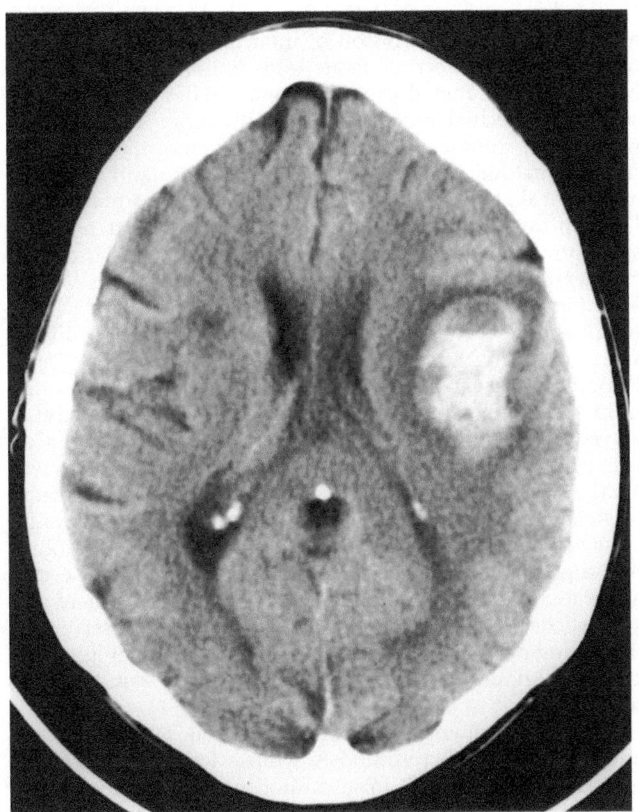

Figure 28-24. CT of acute intracerebral hemorrhage in left frontal white matter, with blood-fluid level.

with subtotal infarcts in a given vascular territory but without uncontrolled hypertension (i.e., blood pressure <180/100 mm Hg) and that it be accompanied by close adherence to a prolongation of the aPTT value within the recommended therapeutic range (1.5 times the control value).[286] However, the immediate use of intravenous heparin after cerebral infarction has been questioned in view of the lack of data supporting the value of any parenteral antithrombotic agents in this setting.[288] Because intravenous heparin has not been properly tested in patients with acute ischemic stroke of nonlacunar type, a prospective, randomized clinical trial, the Rapid Anticoagulation Prevents Ischemic Damage (RAPID) trial,[289] was performed in Europe. The design involved the comparison between aspirin and unfractionated heparin (administered within 12 hours of stroke symptom onset) given for 1 week, with regard to the primary endpoint of rate of favorable outcome, measured as a modified Rankin Scale (mRS) score of 2 or less at 90 days. Although the sample size for the study was 592 patients, the trial was stopped early because of low recruitment (only 67 patients had been recruited after 30 months from study onset). An analysis of the small sample of 67 patients showed no significant differences between the groups in terms of mRS, National Institutes of Health Stroke Scale (NIHSS) score < 1, mortality, ischemic stroke worsening, or stroke worsening related to hemorrhage, whereas a trend ($P = 0.09$) in favor of unfractionated heparin was detected for the secondary endpoint of ischemic stroke recurrence.[290] Based on these limited data, the authors planned to conduct a larger multicenter trial to test the hypothesis that early administration of unfractionated intravenous heparin may have a neuroprotective effect in patients with acute ischemic stroke.

Anticoagulation and cerebral amyloid angiopathy. Iatrogenic ICH occurring during anticoagulation or thrombolysis is an especially important manifestation of CAA. Anticoagulation is hypothesized to promote ICH by allowing small leakages of blood to expand into large symptomatic hemorrhages and might thus be particularly risky in the setting of advanced CAA. This possibility is supported by demonstration of advanced CAA in individuals who have ICH after thrombolysis or during warfarin therapy. CAA may also have a role in ICH occurring with antiplatelet treatment.[75,199] These observations raise the important possibility that an individual's risk for CAA could ultimately be incorporated into the decision whether to treat with thrombolytic or anticoagulant therapy.

Novel oral anticoagulants. In recent years a number of randomized controlled trials have compared novel oral anticoagulants to warfarin therapy for the prevention of stroke and systemic embolism in the management of nonvalvular atrial fibrillation. These agents interfere with the coagulation cascade by way of either direct thrombin (dabigatran) or factor Xa (apixaban, edoxaban, rivaroxaban) inhibition. In addition to providing at least non-inferior stroke prevention, an attractive benefit of these agents is lower rates of ICH in comparison to warfarin therapy, with significant absolute risk reductions (ARR) in hemorrhagic stroke of 0.23% for apixaban,[291] 0.31% and 0.21% for the 30 mg and 60 mg dose of edoxaban, respectively,[292] 0.26% and 0.28% for the 110 mg and 150 mg dose of dabigatran, respectively,[293] and an ARR in intracranial hemorrhage of 0.20% for rivaroxaban.[294] Accordingly, these agents offer a promising alternative to individuals with atrial fibrillation who are also at higher risk of ICH, but whether the benefits of these novel oral anticoagulants can be extrapolated to this particular subgroup of patients remains to be determined. Reassuringly, in the case of dabigatran the lower rates of ICH in comparison to warfarin also occurred in subgroup analysis of individuals aged 75 years and older who were at high risk of CAA, and apixaban has been observed to have a similar ICH rate as aspirin, while being superior to aspirin for stroke prevention.[295,296] The specific targeting of the novel agents of a single factor within the coagulation cascade (factor Xa or IIa [thrombin]), rather than the inhibition of four vitamin-K-dependent factors (II, VII, IX and X) by warfarin, has been speculated to account for these differences.[297]

Fibrinolytic agents. Fibrinolytic agents, especially t-PA, are used in the treatment of coronary, arterial, and venous thromboses in the limbs and pulmonary circulation. The ability of these agents to produce clot lysis and a relatively low level of systemic hypofibrinogenemia makes them ideal choices for the treatment of acute thrombosis. However, their most feared complication is ICH, which has been reported in 0.4% to 1.3% of patients with acute MI treated with the single-chain t-PA alteplase.[298] The clinical and CT features of ICHs related to coronary thrombolysis with t-PA have been extensively reviewed.[299-303] The hemorrhages tend to occur early after the start of t-PA treatment: in one study, 40% of the hemorrhages started during the infusion, and another 25% occurred within 24 hours of the onset of treatment.[299] In 70% to 90% of cases, the hemorrhages are lobar, in about 30% of cases are multiple,[300] the latter being associated with a mortality of 44% to 66%.[299-302]

The mechanism of bleeding in this setting is unknown. On occasions, patients have had excessively prolonged aPTT values at the time of onset of intracranial hemorrhage as a result of the use of intravenous heparin (aimed at preventing reocclusion of reperfused coronary arteries).[300-302] Other factors suggested as significant in raising the risk of ICH after the use of t-PA in acute MI are advanced age (>65 years), history of hypertension, and the use of aspirin before t-PA therapy;[302] in one study, however, none of these factors was found to be significantly different in patients with or without ICH.[301] A possible role for local cerebral vascular disease has been considered because examples of pretreatment head trauma[301] and concomitant CAA[303-305] have been documented in association with ICH after the use of t-PA. Other coagulation defects related to this treatment, such as hypofibrinogenemia and thrombocytopenia, have not been found to correlate with this complication.

Vasculitis

The cerebral vasculitides generally result in arterial occlusion and cerebral infarction and are only rarely responsible for ICH. Most of these unusual examples of ICH secondary to cerebral arteritis have been secondary to *granulomatous angiitis of the nervous system* (GANS).[306] This primary cerebral vasculitis occurs in the absence of systemic involvement. Histologically, it is characterized by mononuclear inflammatory exudates with giant cells in the media and adventitia of small and medium-sized arteries and veins. This vascular inflammation is occasionally associated with the formation of microaneurysms. The cerebral disease evolves with chronic headache, progressive cognitive decline, seizures, and recurrent episodes of cerebral infarction.[291] Because of its primary cerebral location, systemic features such as malaise, fever, weight loss, arthralgias, myalgias, anemia, and elevated sedimentation rate are absent.[307,308] The diagnosis is favored by the finding of lymphocytic cerebrospinal fluid (CSF) pleocytosis with elevated protein levels, and angiography may show a beading pattern in multiple medium-sized and small intracranial arteries. The instances of ICH reported in patients with GANS have occurred in the setting of progressive encephalopathy or myelopathy,[309,310] although ICH has occasionally been the first manifestation of the condition.[311] The hemorrhages have been predominantly lobar in location, and in rare instances, histologic examination of cerebral vessels has shown the association of GANS with CAA,[312,313] which suggests that either vascular lesion could have been responsible for the episode of ICH.

HEMORRHAGIC INFARCTION

Hemorrhagic infarction (HI) differs pathologically from ICH as it results from reperfusion of infarcted tissue. Restoration of blood flow to necrotic tissue leads to the extravasation of blood through altered capillaries and arterioles resulting in scattered petechial blood-staining, with more advanced HI resulting in confluent petechial areas of hemorrhage or even frank hematoma. This process occurs predominantly in deep and cortical gray matter, owing to the higher density of capillaries in these regions in comparison to white matter.[314] The spectrum of HI severity has been categorized by the European Cooperative Acute Stroke Study (ECASS) investigators[315] into HI-1 (small petechiae along the margins of the infarct), HI-2 (confluent petechiae within the infarcted area but without space-occupying effect), parenchymal hematoma 1 (PH)-1 (blood clot not exceeding 30% of the infarcted area with some mild space-occupying effect) and PH-2 (dense blood clot[s] exceeding 30% of the infarct volume with significant space-occupying effect or hematoma remote from the infarcted area). As the bleeding predominantly occurs in areas of already infarcted tissue, most cases of HI are asymptomatic, with only a subset being accompanied by neurological deterioration. Although the occurrence of PH-2 is often a symptomatic event associated with acute neurological deterioration,[316] there are suggestions that worse 90-day outcomes can be observed in the setting of HI-2 and PH-1,[317] leading to questioning of the often-held notion of clinical irrelevance of these less dramatic forms of HI.[318]

The most frequent causes of HI are embolic ischemic stroke and cerebral venous thrombosis, while a less common cause is global hypoperfusion from cardiogenic shock followed by reinstitution of cerebral perfusion resulting in hemorrhagic transformation of borderzone infarcts (Fig. 28-25). In the case of embolic stroke, reperfusion is believed to result from fragmentation and distal migration of arterial emboli or by way of leptomeningeal collateral blood flow, the former tending to cause HI at the initial site of occlusion and the latter in a purely distal gyral pattern.[283,319,320] HI is part of the natural history of ischemic stroke, and occurs in approximately 40% of cases,[321,322] however HI rates in the literature have ranged widely from 5% to 50% when examining all ischemic strokes irrespective of particular subtype.[323] The majority of cases of

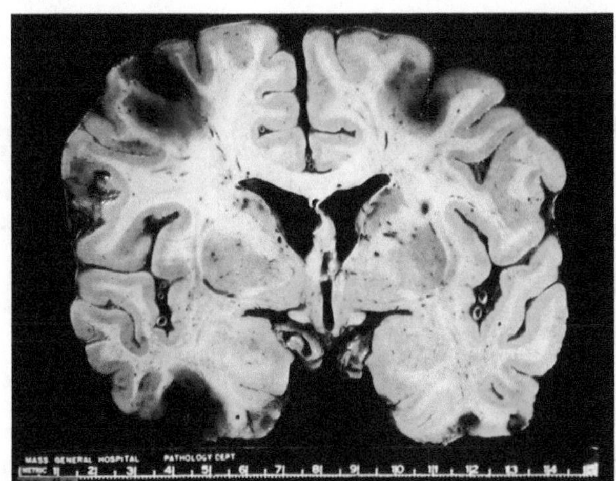

Figure 28-25. Gross pathology demonstrating bilateral cortical borderzone hemorrhagic infarctions following cardiac arrest. *(Image courtesy of Dr. Robert H. Ackerman, Massachusetts General Hospital, Boston, MA.)*

HI occur within 3–14 days of symptom onset.[322,324] In the absence of thrombolytic therapy, the strongest predictors of hemorrhagic transformation of an ischemic infarct have been large infarct volume, detection of focal hypodensity on early CT (<5 hours), worse neurological status on admission, cardioembolic or cryptogenic stroke subtype, hyperthermia, hyperglycemia, hypertension, albuminuria, as well as high baseline matrix metalloproteinase-9 (MMP-9) and cellular fibronectin levels.[323,325]

In addition to their role in the treatment of acute MI, intravenous thrombolytic agents (t-PA) are the only approved therapy for patients with acute ischemic stroke. HI is a common phenomenon that follows thrombolysis of patients with acute ischemic stroke. T-PA is believed to increase the rates of HI by way of increased recanalization rates, fibrinolysis, and possibly indirect upregulation of MMP-9.[326] Initial pilot studies with the use of intra-arterial agents, mainly urokinase and t-PA, yielded encouraging rates of reperfusion, in the order of 55% of patients treated, and hemorrhagic complications (i.e., HI and ICH) and neurologic deterioration occurred in about 11% of patients.[327] The initial experience with intravenous thrombolytics administered within 8 hours of stroke onset, reported by del Zoppo et al.,[328] yielded angiographically documented rates of reperfusion at a disappointingly low level, in the range of 26% to 38%. Despite this low level of recanalization, hemorrhagic changes with neurologic deterioration occurred in 9% of patients. In addition, the study showed that the rate of hemorrhagic complications was significantly higher in patients in whom t-PA was administered more than 6 hours after stroke onset, in comparison with patients treated within 6 hours.[329]

Nonangiographic studies of intravenous t-PA in acute stroke, the ECASS[315] and the National Institute of Neurological Diseases and Stroke (NINDS) rt-PA Stroke Study,[330] used entry windows (time after onset during which patients could be entered into the study) of 6 hours and 3 hours, respectively, and doses of alteplase of 1.1 mg/kg (to a maximum of 100 mg) and 0.9 mg/kg (to a maximum of 90 mg), respectively. Results of both studies were positive, especially those of the NINDS study, which showed an improved functional outcome at 3 months in the group treated with t-PA without a higher mortality due to hemorrhagic complications. Despite a tenfold increase in symptomatic ICH during the first 36 hours in patients treated with t-PA (6.4% versus 0.6% for the placebo group), a net benefit accrued for the t-PA-treated group as measured by three functional scales 3 months after treatment. The intracranial hemorrhages in the t-PA group occurred in both the lobar white matter and the deep gray nuclei (Fig. 28-26), and they carried a high mortality (45%).[331] The risk factors for intracranial hemorrhage after thrombolysis with intravenous t-PA within 3 hours of acute ischemic stroke onset include the severity of the neurologic deficit (as measured by the NIHSS score), the presence of edema and mass effect in the baseline CT scan, degree of early ischemic changes on CT as measured by the ASPECTS (Alberta Stroke Program Early CT Score) score, and antiplatelet use (particularly dual therapy with aspirin and clopidogrel).[331-333] When intravenous t-PA was given between 3 and 6 hours from stroke onset, the baseline DWI lesion volume, history of atrial fibrillation, 24-hour weighted average systolic blood pressure, and evidence of early post-t-PA reperfusion were independent predictors of the risk of HI.[334,335] Higher risk has also been reported in individuals with infective endocarditis,[336] severe renal impairment (glomerular filtration rate < 30 mL/min),[337] severity of leukoaraiosis,[338] degree of hypoperfusion and very low regional cerebral blood volume on perfusion imaging,[339,340] and fluid-attenuated inversion recovery hyperintensity within the acute ischemic territory on MRI.[341] Other potential factors associated with increased risk of postintravenous t-PA bleeding include hyperglycemia at baseline[342] and elevated serum levels of biomarkers indicative of vascular fragility or abnormal permeability of the blood–brain barrier such as MMP-9,[343,344] cellular fibronectin,[345] endogenous activated protein C,[346] vascular adhesion protein-1/semicarbazide-sensitive amine oxidase activity,[347] and markers of endogenous fibrinolysis.[348]

The Safe Implementation of Treatment in Stroke-Monitoring Study (SITS-MOST)[349] identified nine independent risk factors for symptomatic ICH (defined as PH-2 accompanied by ≥4-point worsening on the NIHSS score or death) among 31,267 ischemic stroke patients treated with IV alteplase: baseline NIHSS score, serum glucose, systolic blood pressure, history of hypertension, age, body weight, stroke onset to treatment time, aspirin monotherapy, and dual antiplatelet therapy with aspirin and clopidogrel. From these data, they devised a 12-point score (SITS SICH risk score) with good discriminatory ability in the identification of stroke patients at high risk of symptomatic ICH following IV alteplase.[350]

Three clinical trials of intravenous streptokinase in acute ischemic stroke found an alarmingly high rate of ICH and mortality.[351-353] The use of 1.5 million IU of streptokinase within 4[351] or 6[352,353] hours from stroke onset resulted in rates of symptomatic ICH between 6%[283] and 21.2%,[351] with mortality rates of 19%[352] and 34%[353] at 10 days and 43.4%[351] at 90 days, resulting in the termination of the trials. It is possible that the higher rates of ICH after streptokinase therapy than after t-PA therapy in acute ischemic stroke patients may reflect a dose of streptokinase that is too high for this indication (as opposed to its safer profile in the treatment of patients with acute MI[354]). Additional possible reasons for such observations include a more pronounced and longer-lasting systemic fibrinolytic effect with streptokinase than with t-PA.[355]

The use of intra-arterial recombinant prourokinase (proUK) was tested in the PROlyse in Acute Cerebral Thromboembolism (PROACT) I[356] and II trials.[357] When given directly into a middle cerebral artery clot, proUK was associated with a recanalization rate of 66% (compared with 18% for the control group) in the PROACT II study.[357] This rate correlated with a significantly better functional outcome at 3 months for the treated group, without differences in mortality, even though the rate of symptomatic ICH was 10% in treated patients and only 2% in the control subjects. Virtually all proUK-related

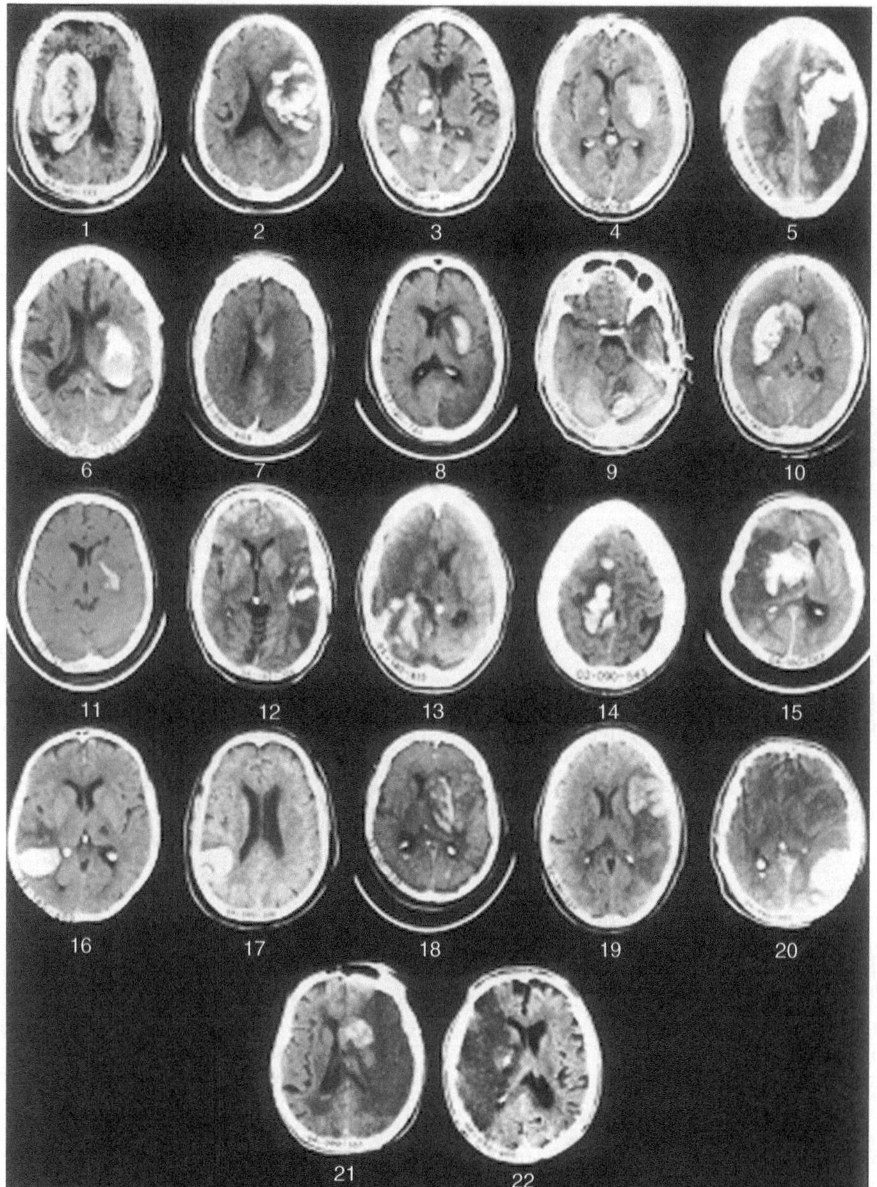

Figure 28-26. CT scans of hemorrhages from the National Institutes of Neurological Diseases and Stroke (NINDS) trial of tissue-type plasminogen activator (t-PA). Cases 3 through 22 are from the t-PA-treated group; cases 1 and 2 are from the control group. *Reprinted with permission from The NINDS t-PA Stroke Study Group, Intracerebral hemorrhage after intravenous t-PA therapy for ischemic stroke, Stroke, 28, 11, November, pp. 2109–18, 1997.)*

ICHs were massive (Fig. 28-27), and all occurred in the area of the qualifying acute infarct in the middle cerebral artery distribution.[358] Among a number of possible risk factors for post-proUK symptomatic ICH, only hyperglycemia at baseline was identified as being potentially associated with a higher risk.[358]

Concerns regarding whether individuals with CMBs are at higher risk of ICH following thrombolysis have been raised, particularly following reports of post-thrombolysis ICH occurring at sites of previous CMBs remote from areas of acute infarction.[359] Although a number of nonrandomized observational studies have yet to produce a significant association between CMBs and post-thrombolysis ICH, they were all limited by small sample size, and pooled data from two recent systematic reviews suggest possibly higher rates of post-thrombolysis ICH in individuals with CMBs,[360,361] and particularly in those with high CMB burden.[360] The pooled data were, however, largely unadjusted, stressing the need for larger well-designed trials. Additionally, whether CMBs in purely lobar regions, suggestive of CAA, confer additional risk for post-thrombolysis ICH remains to be determined.

BRAIN IMAGING

The imaging aspects of ICH are discussed in Chapters 45, 46, and 47. This section only briefly highlights developments in this area.

The view that CT is superior to MRI for the diagnosis of acute ICH has been challenged by new observations. With the use of susceptibility-weighted (also known as gradient-echo) MRI sequences, Linfante et al.[362] were able to document acute ICHs within periods as short as 30 minutes after symptom onset. Their observations, along with those of others,[363,364] suggest that in the early phase of ICH, MRI protocols that

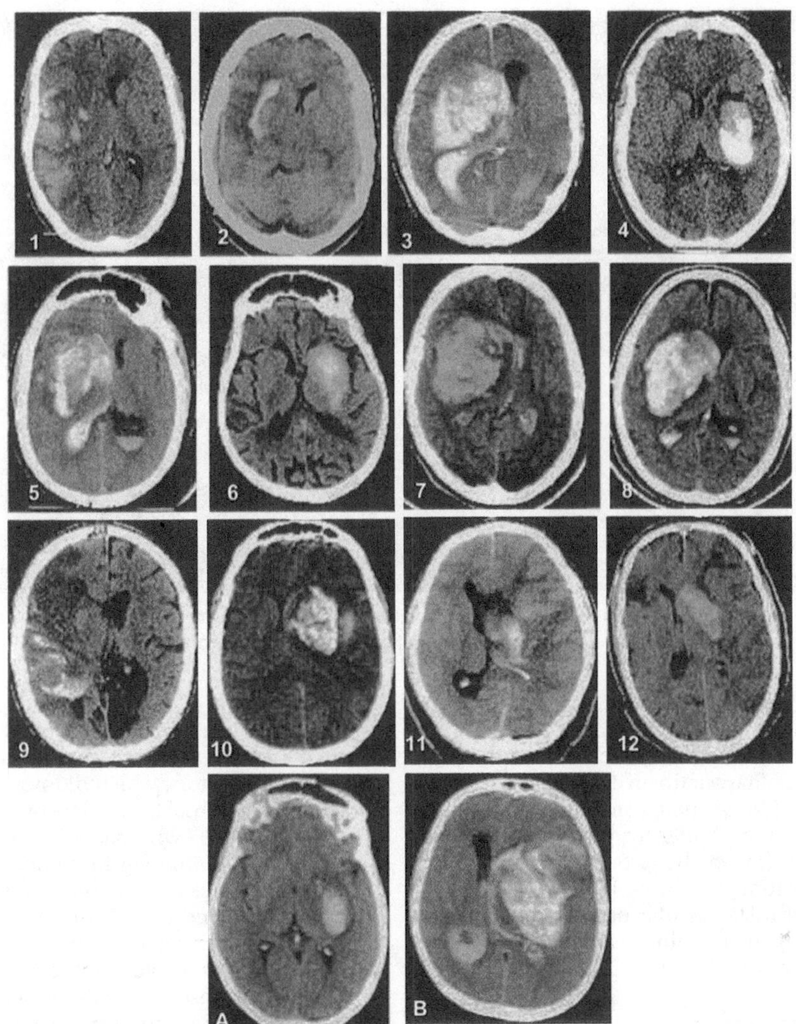

Figure 28-27. CT scans of hemorrhages from the PROlyse in Acute Cerebral Thromboembolism (PROACT) II trial. Cases 1 through 12 are from the recombinant pro-urokinase (r-proUK) group, and cases A and B are from the control group. *(Reprinted with permission from Kase CS, et al. Symptomatic intracerebral hemorrhage after intra-arterial thrombolysis with prourokinase in acute ischemic stroke: The PROACT II trial,* Neurology, *57, 9, November, p 1603–10, 2001.)*

include susceptibility-weighted sequences are as reliable as CT for diagnosis.

Cerebral Microbleeds

An additional value of these MRI sequences is their ability to document areas of CMBs, detected as areas of low signal of up to 10 mm in diameter (Fig. 28-28), that correspond to deposits of hemosiderin as a sequelae from past episodes of minor bleeding.[274,365–369] CMBs are visualized on MRI in 5% of neurologically healthy individuals, and their prevalence increases with age and history of cerebrovascular disease, reaching 60% in individuals with ICH.[370] Their presence is considered to reflect an underlying bleeding-prone microangiopathy, most commonly in the form of hypertensive vasculopathy or CAA, with CMBs located in the deep gray/white matter and brainstem favoring hypertension as their mechanism while those located in superficial lobar regions favor CAA.[371–374] The importance of these lesions stems from their potential role in instances of major hemorrhage in subjects receiving anticoagulants or after treatment with thrombolysis. The potential association between CMBs and ICH after use of anticoagulants or thrombolytics, as outlined above, is still controversial. Although the known correlation between CMBs, especially those located in lobar regions, and subsequently increased risk of spontaneous ICH[375–377] raises a potential concern about the use of oral anticoagulants in patients with a heavy burden of CMBs, the currently available data suggest that a balance between this risk, on the one hand, and the expected benefits in the prevention of ischemic stroke, on the other, should drive this clinical decision in individual patients.[378] The data on antiplatelet agents use derived from a population-based study in Rotterdam, The Netherlands, indicate that CMBs may be more prevalent in subjects receiving aspirin and clopidogrel monotherapy than in those not receiving these agents.[379,380] Data from observational studies[199,381,382] further suggest a relationship between antiplatelet treatment, CMBs, and risk of ICH, but additional prospectively collected data are required before these observations can be applied to clinical decisions in individual patients.

Moreover, although once assumed to be asymptomatic, several case reports have suggested that strategically placed CMBs may result in focal neurological deficits in themselves,[94,383,384] and there is a growing evidence implying that their overall burden may contribute to vascular cognitive impairment,[385–390] as well as gait,[391,392] and mood

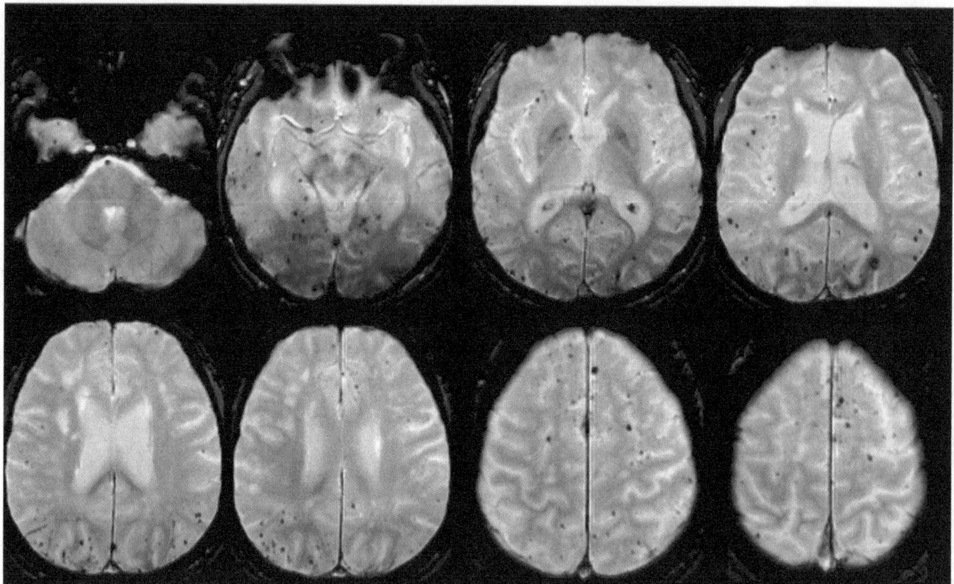

Figure 28-28. MRI, gradient-echo sequence, showing multiple microbleeds as small black round foci corresponding to hemosiderin deposits. The microbleeds predominate in the cortical and subcortical areas in this patient suggestive of underlying cerebral amyloid angiopathy.

disturbances.[393,394] CMBs were also found to be predictive of overall, cardiovascular-related, and stroke-related mortality in the PROspective Study of Pravastatin in the Elderly at Risk (PROSPER) study.[395] In view of their consistent association with vascular risk factors, in particular hypertension,[396] future studies aimed at reducing the evolving burden of CMBs by way of risk factor modification may prove beneficial in reducing the overall burden of microvascular neuronal injury and functional deficit in individuals with cerebral small-vessel disease, in addition to the risk of future ICH.

DIFFUSION-WEIGHTED IMAGING HYPERINTENSITIES

Recently, with the increasing use of MRI in the assessment of ICH, diffusion-weighted imaging hyperintense lesions (DWIHL) have been recognized to occur concurrently with acute ICH at remote sites in 15% to 41% of individuals.[83,397–403] In the absence of direct radiographic-pathologic concordance studies, these lesions are presumed to be ischemic in nature. DWIHLs are typically small (< 15 mm) and occur either ipsilateral or contralateral to the presenting ICH in cortical-subcortical and deep regions. They have been observed to occur more frequently in individuals with higher CMB burden,[83,398,399,402] white matter changes,[398,399] larger hematoma volumes,[402] intraventricular extension of hematoma,[402] prior history of stroke,[397,402] rapid therapeutic reductions in mean arterial pressure,[397,401,402] and in individuals who had undergone surgical evacuation of ICH.[397]

DWIHLs are likely an inherent manifestation of the underlying cerebral small-vessel disease as they have been observed to continue to occur at a lower rate outside of the acute post-ICH period.[400,402] In view of their association with degree of blood pressure lowering, the triggering event for the higher rates observed in the acute post-ICH period has been hypothesized to be related to hypoperfusion from aggressive blood pressure management that is aggravated by impaired cerebral autoregulation.[402] However, this association may be attributed to residual confounding from increased admission blood pressures observed within these individuals - possibly as a manifestation of the degree of underlying hypertensive vasculopathy in a proportion of cases - rather than a treatment effect.[403] In line with this view are results reported by the ICH ADAPT investigators, which did not show a clinically relevant reduction in cerebral blood flow or blood volume in individuals with acute ICH who had rapid reduction of systolic blood pressure to <150 mmHg in comparison to <180 mm Hg.[404] An alternate plausible explanation is that the rapid release of cytokines resulting from acute ICH create a prothrombotic/inflammatory central nervous system milieu that promotes microthrombosis in vulnerable cerebral vessels afflicted by small-vessel disease. Associations between DWIHLs and larger hematoma volume, intraventricular extension, and surgical evacuation, all of which could exacerbate the inflammatory response, support this notion. Indeed, serum C-reactive protein has been reported to markedly increase over the first 48–72 hours following ICH and is proportional to ICH volume.[405] Moreover, although DWIHLs are largely considered to be ischemic, a recent report suggests that at least subsets of these lesions in the acute post-ICH period are acute/subacute CMBs captured in evolution.[406] If confirmed in large prospective studies, the concurrent development of both small ischemic and hemorrhagic lesions at sites distant from the primary ICH would favor inflammatory cascades inciting both microthrombosis and increased vascular permeability at sites of diseased small vessels over hemodynamic fluctuations as the causative trigger.

HYPERACUTE INJURY MARKER (HARM)

Further evidence of global alterations in blood–brain barrier permeability following ICH comes from the novel observation from one retrospective cohort analysis of 46 cases of ICH who had undergone post-gadolinium MRI within 5 days of symptom onset. It was noted that in 85% of cases, some degree of sulcal enhancement was present on post-gadolinium FLAIR sequences at sites that were noncontiguous with the hematoma, a finding termed Hyperacute Injury Marker (HARM).[407] Although confirmation of these findings and further research into the clinical relevance of HARM following ICH is required in additional cohorts, HARM may ultimately prove useful in participant selection for targeted therapeutic trials aimed at reducing the secondary injury of ICH.[179]

PERIHEMATOMAL EDEMA

Perihematomal edema can be visualized on both CT and MRI. It is believed to occur initially from clot-retraction followed by neurotoxicity and blood–brain barrier dysfunction, predominantly as a result of cascades triggered by erythrocyte degradation products. Recent longitudinal studies have shown that, although maximal within the first 48 hours, perihematomal edema formation continues until approximately 1–2 weeks post-ICH.[408–410] The perihematomal region is characterized on MRI by delayed perfusion and increased diffusivity (vasogenic edema), with admixed areas of reduced diffusion suggestive of cytotoxic edema.[411] However, artifacts from magnetization gradients induced by the paramagnetic properties of erythrocyte degradation products need to be considered when interpreting MRI signal characteristics in the perihematomal border, and conclusions regarding the underlying physiologies at play must be derived cautiously. If the reduced diffusion is indeed representative of cytotoxic edema, however, data suggest that the mechanism may be inflammatory/mechanical cellular injury rather than ischemia.[404]

The most consistent predictor of larger absolute perihematoma edema volume is larger hematoma volume.[409,410] A predictor of late perihematomal edema growth is high admission serum hematocrit, implying that a higher dose of erythrocytes and their ensuing degradation products may have a role in prolonging edema formation.[410] Erythrocyte heme iron content is believed to play a key role in triggering cellular cascades that promote such edema formation, and serves as one of many targets in current trials aimed at minimizing the secondary injury that ensues from ICH.[179]

GENERAL CLINICAL AND LABORATORY FEATURES

The different forms of ICH share a number of clinical features that result from the progressive accumulation of a mass of blood in the parenchyma. These features include mode of onset as well as clinical manifestations reflecting increased intracranial pressure. ICH occurs characteristically during activity,[71,138] and its onset during sleep is extremely rare.[412] It occurred in only one instance in the series reported by Fisher,[412] and in only 3% of ICH cases included in the NINDS Data Bank.[4] The type of onset, studied in 70 cases of ICH prospectively included in the Harvard Cooperative Stroke Registry, was found to be one of gradual and smooth progression in two-thirds of the cases; the deficit was maximal at onset in the remainder.[2] No cases showed a regressive course in the early phase, which supports the clinical dictum that a definite improvement in the early hours of a stroke syndrome rules out ICH.[413] Along with a gradual onset over periods of 5 to 30 minutes, patients with ICH frequently show some decrease in alertness at the time of admission. The frequency and severity of this sign vary to some extent according to the location of the hemorrhage, but when all forms are considered, a decrease in alertness is present in at least 60% of cases;[2,188] in two-thirds of them, the decrease is to a level of coma.[2,101] Coma has been correlated with ventricular extension of the hemorrhage,[133,365] large hematoma,[135] and poor vital prognosis.[133,188,414,415]

The clinical features of ICH associated with increased intracranial pressure are headache and vomiting. Although these features also vary widely in frequency with the location of hemorrhage, their overall diagnostic value at the onset of ICH is limited.[2] Of 54 patients alert enough to report the symptom, only 36% reported headache in the study by Mohr et al.[2]; in Aring's[416] series, the frequency of headache was 23%. The reporting of vomiting at onset follows similar frequencies: 44%[2] and 22%[416] in two series. These findings stress the important clinical point that absence of a headache or vomiting does not rule out ICH. On the other hand, when present, these signs suggest ICH (or SAH) as the most likely diagnosis because they are present in less than 10% of ischemic strokes.[2]

Seizures at the onset of ICH are uncommon. They have been reported at rates as low as 7%,[2] 11%,[14] and 14%[416,417] when all forms of ICH are considered together. In some groups, such as in patients with lobar hemorrhages, seizures have been reported with a frequency as high as 32%.[132] Previous ICH, cortical involvement, younger age and worse neurological deficit are factors that have been reported as independent predictors of seizures at onset.[417]

In the general physical examination, a common abnormality is hypertension, found in as many as 91% of the cases in some series.[2] The high frequency of elevated blood pressure on admission in all forms of ICH correlates with other physical signs indicative of hypertension, such as left ventricular hypertrophy[418] and hypertensive retinopathy.[412] The examination of the ocular fundi in a case of suspected ICH serves the dual purpose of detecting signs of hypertensive retinopathy and allowing careful search for subhyaloid hemorrhages. The latter represent blood collections in the preretinal space, and their presence is virtually diagnostic of SAH[406] because they rarely occur in primary ICH.[190,259,413] Although an occasional case of massive primary ICH does show this sign,[419] its presence has a high correlation with ruptured aneurysm as the cause of the intracranial hemorrhage. The neurologic findings permit the differentiation of the different topographic varieties of ICH (see later).

Communication of the hematoma with the ventricular space accounts for the presence of bloody or xanthochromic CSF in 70% to 90% of cases.[2,14,133,259,412,416,420] A somewhat lower frequency of bloody CSF (63%) has been reported in hematomas of lobar location,[190] probably reflecting the less frequent communication with the ventricular system[132] due to the subcortical location of the hematoma. The small percentages of cases with clear CSF in all series of ICH reflect hematomas of small size that do not reach the ventricular system even though located close to it. Furthermore, on account of the small size of such hematomas, the clinical presentation may not clearly indicate ICH; signs of increased intracranial pressure may be lacking in such cases, so differentiating them from ischemic strokes is difficult. It is in this particular group of strokes that CT scan has had its most dramatic impact.

In addition to simple inspection of the CSF for bloody or xanthochromic aspect, spectrophotometric CSF analysis can disclose blood products in virtually 100% of cases.[421] However, this technique is not routinely used because the two widely available anatomic means of diagnosis (CT and MRI) have made CSF examination unnecessary in establishing the presence of an ICH. Moreover, the uncommon but well-recognized precipitation of uncal or tonsillar herniation by lumbar puncture in supratentorial ICH[134,413,422] has contributed to the abandonment of this test for the diagnosis of ICH.

The use of angiography in the evaluation of cases of ICH has similarly declined since the introduction of CT and MRI. Angiography most commonly shows the nonspecific signs of mass effect at the site of the hematoma[423] and occasionally has detected extravasation of contrast medium.[424,425] The study by Mizukami et al.[426] correlated the angiographic pattern of displacement of the lenticulostriate arteries with functional prognosis in putaminal hemorrhage. Because of the obvious advantages of CT and MRI in disclosing most of the anatomic features of ICH, angiography is now used only in selected instances. Its main role at present is in the evaluation of nonhypertensive forms of ICH, multiple ICHs, and ICHs located in atypical sites, to look for AVM, aneurysm, or tumor as the possible cause of the hemorrhage. Even this role for angiography is steadily diminishing with improvements in noninvasive brain imaging.

SUPRATENTORIAL INTRACEREBRAL HEMORRHAGE

Most cases of ICH occur in the supratentorial compartment, usually involving the deep structures of the cerebral hemispheres, the basal ganglia, and the thalamus.[2,14,34,128,132,133] In addition, a substantial number of hemispheral ICHs occur in the subcortical white matter of the cerebral lobes, the so-called lobar hemorrhages.[132,190] These various forms of ICH have distinctive features in terms of clinical presentation, CT aspects, course, and therapy.

Putaminal Hemorrhage

The several clinical subtypes of putaminal hemorrhage, which is the most common form of ICH, are determined by the size and pattern of extension of the hematoma. Each of these variables in turn determines the prognosis. Overall, a mortality of 37% is expected,[188] which is a value that is far lower than those quoted in the pre-CT literature,[427] which did not include the undiagnosed smaller cases.

The classic presentation of massive putaminal hemorrhage (Fig. 28-29) is with rapidly evolving unilateral weakness accompanied by sensory, visual, and behavioral abnormalities. Headache is common, as is vomiting, within a few hours of onset.[2] Although the onset is abrupt, there is often a gradual worsening of both the focal deficit and the level of consciousness in the following minutes or hours.[412,413] A "maximal from the onset" deficit is uncommon. Whether with sudden or gradual onset, medium-sized or large hematomas are invariably accompanied by a decreased level of alertness correlated with hematoma size. Once the syndrome is well developed, neurologic examination shows a dense flaccid hemiplegia with a hemisensory syndrome and homonymous hemianopia, with global aphasia if the hematoma is in the dominant hemisphere and hemi-inattention if it is in the nondominant hemisphere.[412,413] A horizontal gaze palsy, with the eyes conjugately deviated toward the side of the lesion, is usually found, which can be reversed momentarily by doll's head maneuver or ice-water caloric testing.[415] The pupillary size and reactivity are normal unless uncal herniation has occurred; if it has, signs of an ipsilateral third cranial nerve palsy are present.[412] These abnormalities in oculomotor function have a poor prognosis.[188] Total unilateral motor deficit, coma, and clinical progression after admission all correlate with large hematoma size and poor functional and vital prognosis, as does ventricular extension of the hematoma by CT scan.[188]

The presence of two hypertensive putaminal hemorrhages, one recent and one old, has been described in pathologic material.[32,51,71,135] The occurrence of simultaneous fresh bilateral putaminal hemorrhages (Fig. 28-30), although occasionally reported,[428] is distinctly uncommon: it was observed in only two of 86 cases in Fisher's series[128] and in none of 42 hypertensive ICH cases from the series reported by McCormick

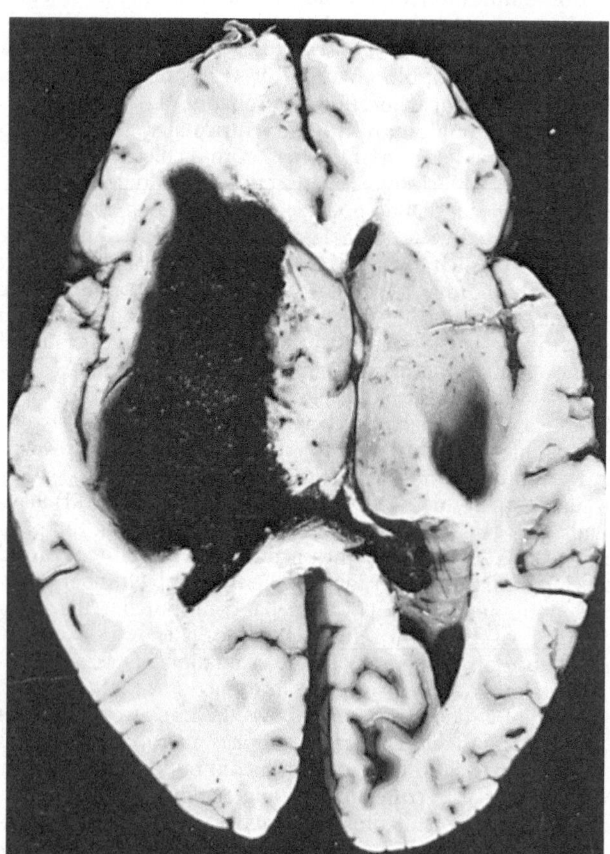

Figure 28-29. Massive right putaminal hemorrhage with ventricular extension. Incidental finding of a small hemorrhage on the posterior corner of the contralateral (left) putamen.

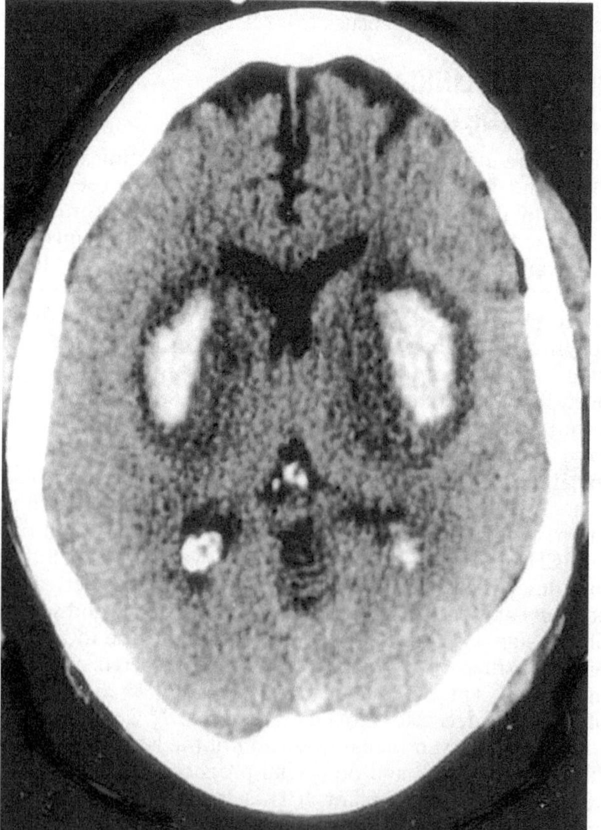

Figure 28-30. CT scan of bilateral, symmetric putaminal hemorrhages in a hypertensive subject. *(Reprinted with permission from Silliman S, et al. Simultaneous bilateral hypertensive putaminal hemorrhages,* J Stroke Cerebrovasc Dis, *12, 1, January, p 44–6, 2003.)*

and Schochet.[51] Multiple ICHs are rare unless due to bleeding diathesis associated with thrombocytopenia,[128,429] metastatic tumor,[245] or CAA.[430]

Syndromes Due to Small Hemorrhages

The availability of CT and MRI allows the diagnosis of a number of variations in the presentation of small putaminal ICHs, which in the pre-CT era would have been clinically diagnosed as small infarcts. They are as follows:

Pure motor stroke. Instances of pure motor stroke due to small putaminal–capsular hemorrhages have been rarely documented.[431,432] The clinical presentation in such cases has consisted of a mild and transient pure motor syndrome affecting the face and limbs, and the small hematomas originated from the posterior angle of the putamen, with impingement of the posterior limb of the internal capsule. At times, a small capsular hemorrhage has manifested as pure motor stroke and dysarthria,[433] although the clinical syndrome has been more properly that of a "pure sensory-motor" stroke, related to a component of lateral thalamic compression accompanying the capsular lesion.

Pure sensory stroke. The syndrome of pure sensory stroke, related to thalamic lacunar infarction, has rarely been due to a small putaminal ICH. Three such cases were reported among a group of 152 patients with putaminal ICH.[434] All three patients had posteriorly located putaminal hemorrhages that were adjacent to the posterior limb of the internal capsule and the adjacent thalamus. The clinical syndrome was a contralateral hemisensory syndrome involving both superficial and deep sensory modalities, with more severe involvement of the leg than the arm and face. The imaging studies demonstrated involvement of the dorsolateral thalamus or the ascending thalamocortical projections located in the posterior ("retrolenticular") portion of the posterior limb of the internal capsule.

Hemichorea–hemiballism. A unilateral dyskinetic syndrome, hemichorea–hemiballism is most commonly due to lacunar infarction in the basal ganglia, thalamus, or subthalamic nucleus but can rarely result from a small putaminal hemorrhage.[435,436] In both series reporting such cases, a right, laterally placed putaminal hemorrhage manifested as contralateral chorea and ballism in the absence of hemiparesis, hemisensory loss, gaze paresis, and hemineglect. The prognosis was excellent in both cases.

Clinical Syndromes in Relationship to the Location of Putaminal Hemorrhage

In a study of 100 patients with putaminal hemorrhage, Weisberg et al.[437] established the following clinicoanatomic correlations:

1. *Medial hemorrhages* extended medially from the putamen and involved the genu and posterior limb of the internal capsule. This finding correlated with a contralateral hemisensory syndrome, but there were no abnormalities of ocular motility, visual fields, or level of consciousness. Affected patients generally had full clinical recovery.
2. *Lateral hemorrhages* originated from the lateral putamen and extended anteriorly along the external capsule. They produced a contralateral hemiplegia and sensory deficits. More than half the patients showed delayed neurologic deterioration, and persistent deficits were more common than full recovery.
3. *Putaminal hemorrhages with extension to the internal capsule and subcortical white matter* extended medially through the internal capsule and superiorly into the corona radiata, causing a more severe syndrome of hemiplegia and hemianesthesia, often but not always with homonymous hemianopia and conjugate ocular deviation. Most patients were left with persistent neurologic sequelae.
4. *Putaminal hemorrhages with subcortical and hemispheric extension* were large hematomas that extended into the white matter of adjacent cerebral lobes, causing mass effect on the lateral ventricle and frequently extending into the ventricular system. They were clinically similar to those of the preceding group, except for having more prominent aphasia or parietal lobe findings and causing impaired consciousness. The mortality rate in this group was 16%, and the majority of the survivors had deficits that interfered with independent living.
5. *Putaminal–thalamic hematomas,* the largest group, extended from the putamen into the thalamus (through the internal capsule) and into the subcortical white matter. They all were accompanied by intraventricular hemorrhage. The clinical picture included impaired consciousness in all patients, frequently associated with hemiplegia, abnormalities of horizontal more than vertical gaze, and homonymous hemianopia. The mortality rate in this group was 79%.

These clinical–CT correlations allowed Weisberg et al.[437] to characterize a number of clinically useful patterns as follows: (1) intraventricular hemorrhage was seen with large hematomas, and both features were associated with high mortality rates; (2) all patients had combined motor and sensory deficits; (3) the best functional outcome was seen in patients with medial or lateral putaminal hematomas that did not involve the internal capsule or the corona radiata; and (4) delayed neurologic deterioration occurred only in patients with hematomas that extended into the cerebral hemisphere or the thalamus.

Chung et al.[433] analyzed the clinicoanatomic correlations in 192 patients with putaminal hemorrhage. They divided their cases into five anatomic types - middle, posteromedial, posterolateral, lateral, and massive - and related the outcomes to the presumed ruptured arterial branches leading to hematoma formation. The *middle* type (Fig. 28-31) was caused by rupture of medial lenticulostriate arteries, with bleeding into the medial putamen and globus pallidus; the result was a benign syndrome of mild contralateral hemiparesis and hemisensory loss, with a low frequency of impairment of consciousness and with transient conjugate ocular deviation toward the side of the hematoma. Intraventricular extension of the hemorrhage did not occur, and all patients survived. This group of lesions was equivalent to the medial putaminal hemorrhages described by Weisberg et al.[437]

The *posteromedial* type (Fig. 28-32) corresponded to small hematomas confined to the posterior limb of the internal capsule ("capsular" hemorrhages) and were associated with contralateral hemiparesis, hemisensory loss, and dysarthria. The small hematomas, which did not reach the ventricular system, were associated with excellent functional outcome and no mortality. The bleeding vessel in this type of hemorrhage is a branch of the anterior choroidal artery, which supplies a portion of the posterior limb of the internal capsule.[438]

The *posterolateral* type (Fig. 28-33) was a putaminocapsular hemorrhage caused by rupture of posterior branches of the lateral lenticulostriate arteries. These larger hematomas occasionally ruptured into the lateral ventricle and produced a more severe syndrome consisting of impaired consciousness, frequent conjugate ocular deviation toward the affected hemisphere, and constant and generally severe contralateral hemiparesis and hemisensory loss, along with aphasia or hemineglect, depending on hematoma location in the dominant or nondominant hemisphere, respectively.

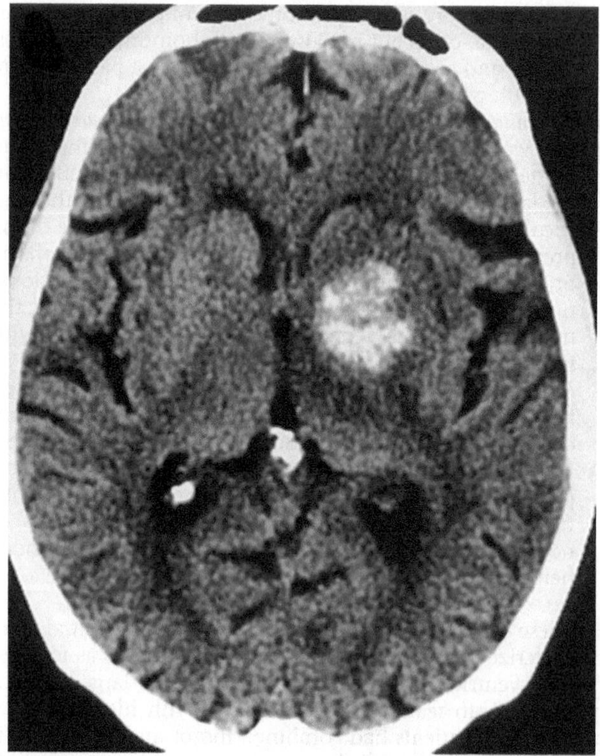

Figure 28-31. CT scan of the medial variety of striatocapsular (putaminal) hemorrhage with minimal mass effect on the frontal horn of the lateral ventricle. *(Reprinted with permission from Chung C, et al, Striatocapsular haemorrhage.* Brain, *123, Pt 9, p 1850–62, 2000.)*

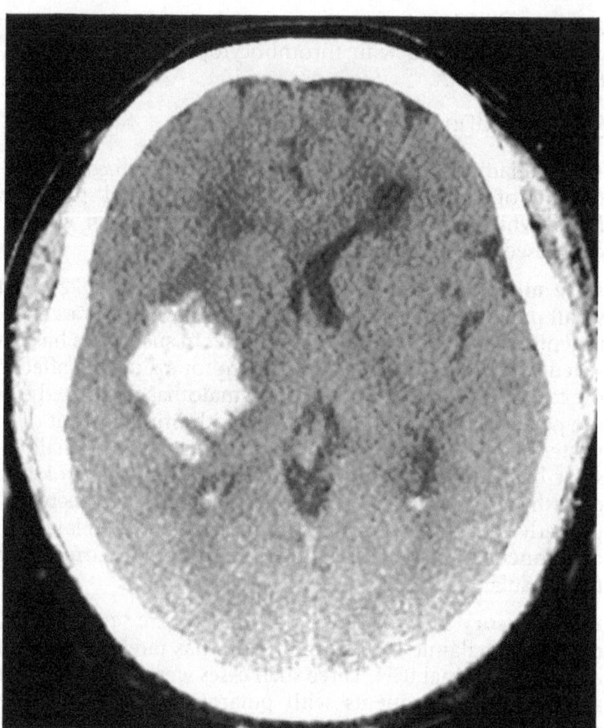

Figure 28-33. CT scan of posterolateral putaminal hemorrhage. Moderate-sized hematoma originating in the posterior putamen, with compression and medial displacement of the posterior limb of the internal capsule but without ventricular extension.

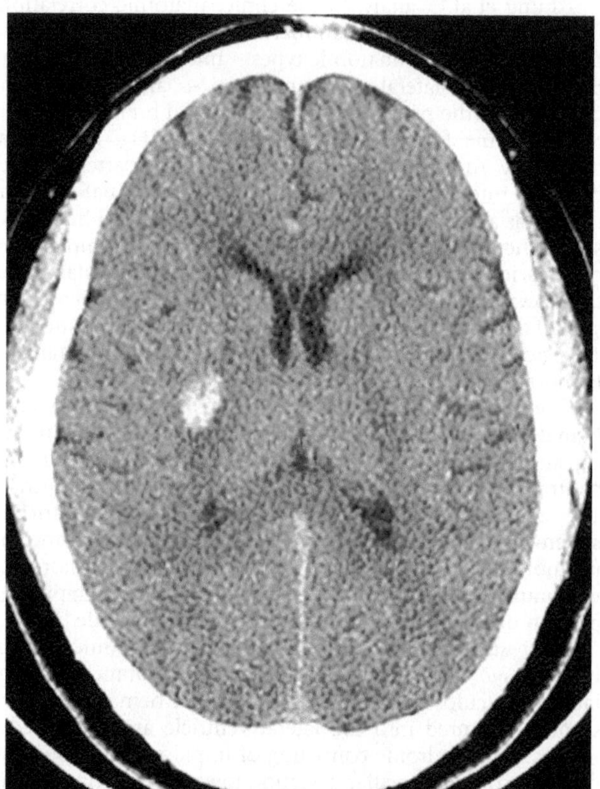

Figure 28-32. CT scan of posteromedial ("capsular") form of putaminal hemorrhage. This small hemorrhage is limited to the posterior limb of the internal capsule.

The *lateral* type of hematoma (Fig. 28-34) originated from rupture of the most lateral branches of the lenticulostriate arteries. It remained confined to an elliptical hematoma collected between the putamen and the insular cortex, producing contralateral hemiparesis, often without an associated hemisensory loss but frequently with either aphasia or hemineglect, depending on the side of the brain involved. The outcome was generally excellent, except in cases of large hematomas, which frequently ruptured into the ventricular system and often required surgical treatment, which in turn was generally associated with a good outcome. This lateral type of putaminal ICH in the dominant hemisphere is occasionally the cause of the syndrome of conduction aphasia.[439]

The *massive* type (Fig. 28-35) involved the entire striatocapsular area and probably resulted from rupture of the same branches (posteromedial branches of the lateral lenticulostriate arteries) that cause the posterolateral type of putaminal ICH. Affected patients had a depressed level of consciousness and hemiparesis, frequently associated with ipsilateral conjugate eye deviation, and often progressed to coma with brainstem involvement and death despite treatment with surgical drainage of the hematoma. This group corresponds to the "putaminal–thalamic" group described by Weisberg et al.[437]

In a separate study, Weisberg et al.[440] analyzed 14 cases of massive putaminal–thalamic hemorrhage. All of their patients were young black people with hypertension who were seen with headache several hours before the onset of the focal deficit, and all became hemiplegic and comatose over periods of 4 to 12 hours. The hematomas were large, with marked mass effect and intraventricular extension. All patients died within 72 hours of onset of symptoms despite treatment of hypertension and increased intracranial pressure.

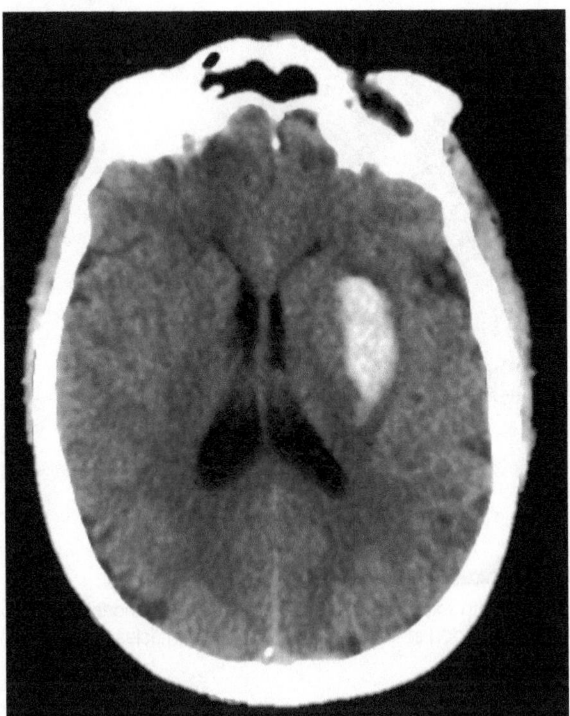

Figure 28-34. CT scan of lateral variety of putaminal hemorrhage. The lens-shaped hematoma has collected between the insula and the putamen without ventricular extension.

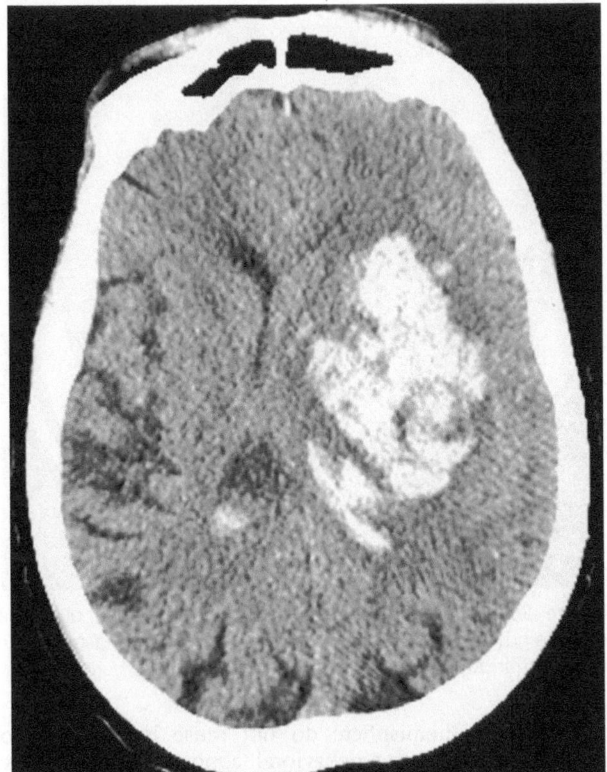

Figure 28-35. CT scan of massive type of putaminal hemorrhage, showing marked mass effect with midline shift and effacement of the lateral ventricle as well as intraventricular extension.

Caudate Hemorrhage

Caudate hemorrhage represents approximately 5% to 7% of cases of ICH (see Table 28-3).[134] Most of the published series on caudate ICH have identified hypertension as the leading cause.[187,441,442] However, other causes not generally associated with deep spontaneous ICH are frequently identified, including cerebral aneurysms,[443] arteriovenous malformations,[444,445] and the basal vascular abnormalities associated with moyamoya disease.[441,446] The last mechanism is thought to lead to ICH through rupture of the anastomotic channels that develop in the area of the basal ganglia, including the head of the caudate, as a result of the progressive occlusion of trunks of the circle of Willis.[447]

The bleeding vessels correspond to deep penetrating branches of the anterior and middle cerebral arteries, which are vessels similar in diameter to those that supply the putamen and thalamus.[448] Because of its paraventricular location, the caudate also receives blood supply from ependymal arteries that flow outward from the ventricular surface into the parenchyma. These arteries originate beneath the ependymal surface as terminal branches of the anterior choroidal artery, posterior choroidal artery, and striatal rami of the middle cerebral artery.[449]

A number of reported cases of spontaneous hemorrhage in the caudate nucleus have delineated a relatively consistent clinical picture.[187,441–443,450,451] The onset has generally been abrupt, with headache and vomiting commonly followed by variably decreased level of consciousness, resembling the onset of SAH from aneurysmal rupture. Seizures at onset have been reported rarely[444] and were not encountered in the series of 12 patients reported by Stein et al.[187] Consistent physical findings have included neck stiffness and various types of behavioral abnormalities, of which the latter are most commonly abulia, impairment of memory (both short-term and long-term), and abnormalities of speech, especially verbal fluency.[187,441] These deficits are thought to occur as a result of interruption of cortical–subcortical tracts between the caudate nucleus and the frontal cortex.[441]

The neuropsychological abnormalities of caudate hemorrhage have been described in detail by Fuh and Wang[441] and by Kumral et al.[442] A common pattern is that of presentation with abulia, confusion, and disorientation at onset, followed by the development of a prominent amnestic syndrome, at times accompanied by language disturbances. The latter have most often included a nonfluent aphasia,[442] and occasional examples of transcortical motor aphasia have also been recorded.[438] Hematomas in the nondominant hemisphere generally do not produce unilateral disturbances of attention,[187,438] although one patient reported by Kumral et al.[442] developed visuospatial neglect.

In approximately 50% of cases, the common clinical features are accompanied by others, which most often take the form of transient gaze paresis and contralateral hemiparesis and, rarely, features of an ipsilateral Horner's syndrome.[187] The abnormalities described in gaze mechanisms have most often been horizontal gaze palsies with conjugate deviation or preference toward the side of the hemorrhage, with full correction by oculocephalic maneuvers. Less commonly, vertical gaze palsy has been described, either combined with a horizontal gaze palsy or, more commonly, as an isolated phenomenon. Occasionally, the motor deficit is accompanied by a transient hemisensory syndrome. In those cases in which hemiparesis is a feature, the weakness tends to be slight (never to the point of hemiplegia) and transient, resolving within days of the onset.[187,450] The generally small size and the localized character of caudate hemorrhage are the reasons why focal neurologic deficits such as transient hemiparesis are relatively uncommon

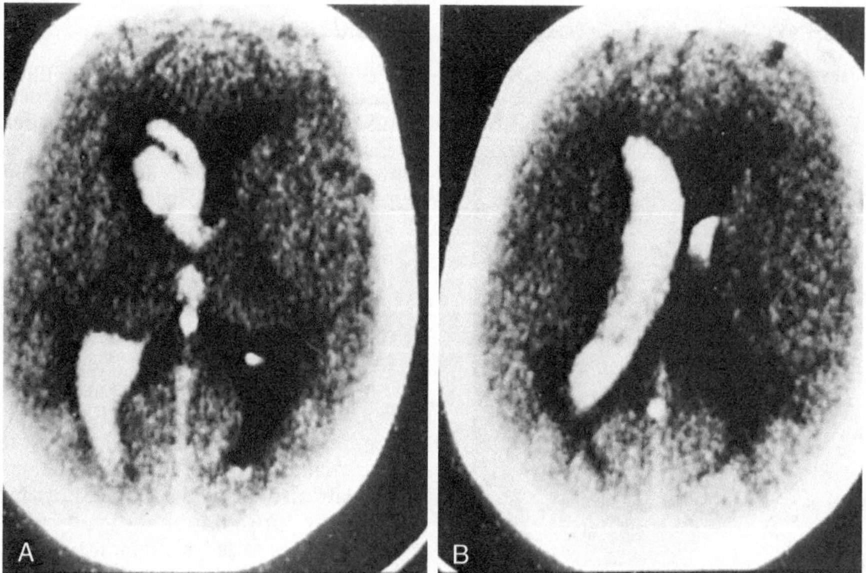

Figure 28-36. A, Hemorrhage originating in the head of the right caudate nucleus with extension into the anterior limb of the internal capsule and into the lateral ventricle and third ventricle. B, Extensive amount of intraventricular blood in the body of the lateral ventricles, primarily on the right side, associated with moderate hydrocephalus.

(in 30% of the 23 cases studied by Chung et al.[433]). The virtually consistent extension into the ventricular system accounts for the high frequency of headache and meningeal signs, which resemble those seen in SAH. Rare instances of bilateral caudate ICH[452] or hemorrhage associated with intraventricular extension with acute hydrocephalus[187] can have a more dramatic presentation, with coma and ophthalmoplegia; the latter is presumably due to oculomotor nuclei involvement as a result of aqueductal dilatation.[453]

In typical cases, a CT scan shows a hematoma located in the area of the head of the caudate nucleus (Fig. 28-36). Ventricular extension into the frontal horn of the ipsilateral ventricle is an invariable feature.[187] In approximately 75% of cases, mild-to-moderate hydrocephalus of the body and temporal horns of the lateral ventricles has been present.

Hemorrhages that are medium-sized or large are frequently accompanied by transient gaze palsies and hemiparesis, and those accompanied by an ipsilateral Horner's syndrome extend more inferiorly and laterally. Occasionally, the hematomas extend from the region of the head of the caudate nucleus into the anterior portions of the thalamus (Fig. 28-37). In those instances, the clinical syndrome has featured a prominent but transient short-term memory defect.[134] Before the introduction of CT, these cases of caudate ICH with consistent extension into the ventricular system may have been diagnosed as "subarachnoid hemorrhage with negative arteriography" or even as "primary intraventricular hemorrhage."[449] The latter is probably a rare condition,[34] in most instances reflecting a lack of documentation of the parenchymal or meningeal (in cases of ruptured aneurysm) site of origin of the hemorrhage rather than a hemorrhage truly confined to the ventricular space.

Caudate hemorrhage can be separated from putaminal and thalamic hemorrhage clinically and radiographically. Headache, nausea, vomiting, and stiff neck regularly accompany caudate hemorrhage,[187] but are less common manifestations in putaminal hemorrhage.[188] Disorders of language are regular features of putaminal and thalamic hemorrhage in the dominant hemisphere,[136,188,454] whereas hemorrhages that remain confined to the caudate nucleus are only rarely associated with aphasia.[442] Furthermore, caudate hemorrhages in the

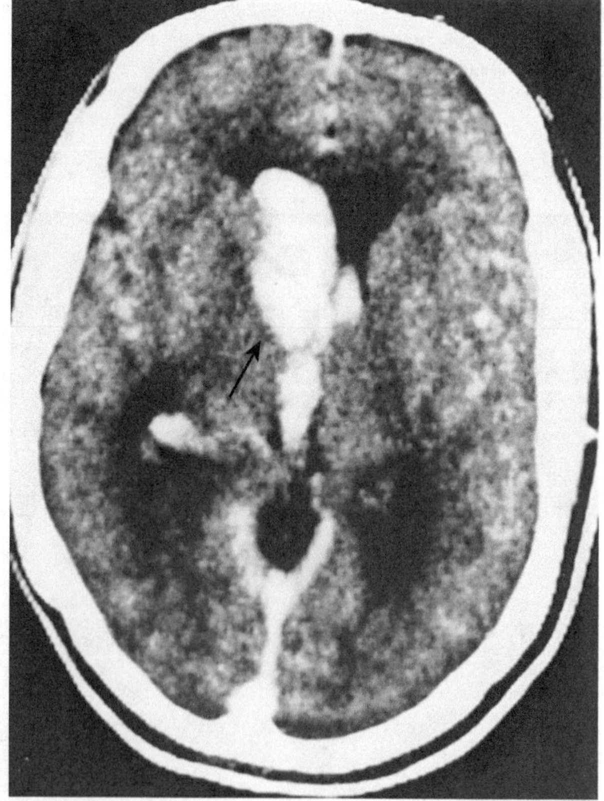

Figure 28-37. Hemorrhage originating from the head of the left caudate nucleus with extension into the anterior-dorsal aspect of the thalamus *(arrow)*, lateral ventricle, and third ventricle.

nondominant hemisphere do not cause hemi-inattention and anosognosia, the behavioral abnormalities associated with thalamic[455–457] and putaminal[188] hemorrhages in that hemisphere.

Caudate hemorrhage must be distinguished from anterior communicating artery aneurysms that bleed into the brain parenchyma. In primary caudate hemorrhage, there is no accumulation of blood in the interhemispheric fissure, and most of the blood is located in the lateral ventricle adjacent to the involved caudate nucleus. In addition, extension of the hemorrhage into the basal frontal region, a feature invariably seen when hemorrhage into the parenchyma results from ruptured anterior communicating aneurysm, is rarely present in caudate ICH.[187]

The outcome in caudate hemorrhage is usually benign, and most patients recover fully, without permanent neurologic deficits.[187] The accompanying hydrocephalus characteristically tends to disappear as the hemorrhage resolves, and ventriculoperitoneal shunting for persistent hydrocephalus is rarely required.[187] This generally benign outcome in caudate ICH occurs despite the virtually consistent ventricular extension of the hemorrhage.

Thalamic Hemorrhage

The thalamic form of ICH accounts for 10% to 15% of parenchymatous hemorrhages.[2,4,128,132,133,135,136] Its clinical and pathologic characteristics are well-recognized, and the spectrum of clinical variations reflects the size and pattern of extension of the hematoma. The mass originates in the thalamus and, if it enlarges, extends laterally (into the internal capsule), medially (into the third ventricle), inferiorly (into the subthalamus and dorsal midbrain), upward, and into the parietal white matter.[413,456,458]

The main cause of thalamic hemorrhage is hypertension, which accounts for 74% to 83% of cases.[458–460] Other reported mechanisms are the use of anticoagulant and thrombolytic agents,[461] use of cocaine,[458] rupture of posterior cerebral artery aneurysm,[462] and cavernous malformations.[463] The hemorrhages due to these mechanisms are not clinically different from those caused by hypertension, except for (1) the tendency toward recurrent bleeding in those due to cavernous angioma[463] and (2) the potential for multiple ICHs after use of cocaine[238] and after thrombolysis.[461]

The clinical picture has several distinctive features. They are listed in Table 28-4 which summarizes data from a total of 41 patients in two series.[136,464] A typical mode of presentation features a rapid onset of unilateral sensorimotor deficit, frequent occurrence of vomiting (about half the cases) but a low frequency of headache (less than one third of cases). In some, the onset was signaled by coma.[136] A slowly progressive initial course with headache preceding the focal deficits is distinctly uncommon,[413] and only four of 13 patients in the series reported by Walshe et al.[136] experienced symptoms for 1 to 2 hours before hemiparesis occurred. In a few cases, unilateral sensory symptoms (numbness) precede the onset of hemiparesis and stupor.[136,465]

The physical findings include hemiparesis or hemiplegia in 95% of cases,[136,454,455,464] virtually all of which have an associated severe hemisensory syndrome (see Table 28-4). This syndrome usually appears as a decrease or loss of all sensory modalities over the contralateral limbs, face, and trunk.[460] The severity and distribution of the motor and sensory symptoms are similar to those of putaminal hemorrhage and therefore are not useful differentiating points. Homonymous hemianopia is an uncommon finding and tends to be transient,[134,412] probably reflecting the location of the lateral geniculate body below and lateral to the hematoma. This sign would be expected in large hemorrhages with extrathalamic extension, but these lesions also affect consciousness severely, generally precluding detection of the visual field defect.

The clinical presentation of thalamic hemorrhage has distinctive oculomotor findings. The most characteristic combination is one of upward gaze palsy with miotic, unreactive pupils[134,136,412,465] and elements of Parinaud's syndrome caused when the enlarging mass presses on the upper midbrain. The upward gaze palsy determines the ocular position at rest of conjugate downward deviation, sometimes associated with convergence, as if the eyes were peering at the tip of the nose.[134] In addition, nystagmus retractorius on attempted upward gaze and skew deviation are commonly present.[134,412] Other, less common oculomotor abnormalities reported in thalamic hemorrhage are downward gaze palsy;[134,412] anisocoria with ipsilateral miosis, sometimes associated with palpebral ptosis;[412] transient opsoclonus;[466] and ipsilateral[136,464] or contralateral[464,467] horizontal ocular deviation.

TABLE 28-4 Clinical Features of Thalamic Hemorrhage

	Walshe et al.[136] (n = 18)	Barraquer-Bordas et al.[464] (n = 23)
History		
Age (years) (mean)	64	68
Headache	22%	30%
Vomiting	77%	48%
Physical Findings		
Level of consciousness		
Alert	6%	21%
Drowsy	33%	40%
Stuporous	33%	18%
Comatose	28%	21%
Hemiplegia-hemiparesis	100%	100%
Hemisensory deficit	100%	100%
Homonymous hemianopia	–	18%
Aphasia	4/7*	4
Mutism	1	1
Anosognosia	2/3*	2
Upward gaze palsy	94%	35%
Horizontal ocular deviation		
Toward side of lesion	6	3
Opposite side of lesion	3	6
Pupillary abnormalities		
Miosis	100%	70%
Absence of light reflex	62%	13%
Mortality	50%	39%

*Number of patients with deficit/number of patients tested.

The classic combination of upward gaze palsy with miotic unreactive pupils has high diagnostic value, and it is due to compressive or destructive effects of the thalamic hematoma on the underlying midbrain tectum.[134,412,419,464] The precise anatomic structures involved in these oculomotor abnormalities have been delineated by experimental studies in monkeys[468,469] and a number of observations in humans.[470,471] The experimental observations of Pasik et al.[469] established that involvement of the posterior commissure and the "nucleus interstitialis of the posterior commissure" were consistently associated with upward gaze palsy. Areas that were not essential for the development of the gaze palsy included the superior colliculi, the nucleus of Darkschewitsch and the interstitial nucleus of Cajal, and the medial thalamus. Christoff et al.,[470,472] from their observations in human clinicopathologic material, concluded that most lesions producing upward gaze palsy required bilateral or midline involvement of the midbrain tectum, particularly when loss of pupillary light reflex was also present.[470] Denny-Brown and Fischer,[468] however, performed unilateral midbrain tegmental lesions in monkeys, which resulted in upward gaze palsy, skew deviation (with the ipsilateral eye in a higher position than the contralateral eye), and head tilt. In addition, after performing unilateral stereotactic lesions of the dorsolateral midbrain tegmentum in humans for the treatment of pain syndromes, Nashold and Seaber[471] recorded symmetrical upward gaze palsy in 13 of 16 subjects. In ten subjects, downward gaze was also impaired but never without upward gaze palsy. Of their 16 patients, 15 had miotic nonreactive pupils, 11 had convergence paralysis, and ten showed skew deviation; the ipsilateral eye was in a lower position in two-thirds.

In summary, virtually all the oculomotor findings observed in thalamic hemorrhage have been described after unilateral tegmental midbrain lesions in humans. This fact supports the view that the oculomotor findings in this condition are due to compression or extension of the hemorrhage into the midbrain tegmentum. However, other observations suggest that CSF hypertension and hydrocephalus associated with the hemorrhage may play an additional role in the production of the oculomotor findings because ventricular shunting has been shown to reverse these manifestations.[465,473,474] In conclusion, a compressive effect on the tegmental–tectal portion of the midbrain, either directly from unilateral compression by the hematoma or indirectly through hydrocephalus, results in the classic oculomotor and pupillary abnormalities of thalamic hemorrhage.

Contralateral Conjugate Eye Deviation

Some patients with thalamic hemorrhage may show horizontal eye deviation, with or without the characteristic downward deviation at rest. This horizontal eye deviation is more commonly ipsilateral (toward the side of the lesion),[136] as is routinely observed in putaminal hemorrhage, but a contralateral conjugate deviation (toward the side of the hemiplegia) is occasionally observed.[136,464] This eye deviation occurs in the direction opposite that is expected in a supratentorial lesion and is thus labeled the "wrong-way eye deviation."[475] Although this peculiar sign has been recorded in instances of unilateral subarachnoid–Sylvian hemorrhage with frontal and insular extension[476] and in frontoparietal subcortical hematoma,[477] most reported cases have occurred in association with thalamic hemorrhage. The mechanism of the sign is obscure. Postdecussation involvement of horizontal oculomotor pathways by compression by the hematoma at the midbrain level has been suggested, and support exists from autopsy data.[477]

Aphasia in Dominant Hemisphere Thalamic Hemorrhage

Occasionally, left thalamic hemorrhages have been associated with a peculiar form of language disturbance.[136,412,464] The relatively low frequency reported for this disturbance is probably because its detection is restricted to cases of small dominant hemisphere hemorrhages, as large ones are likely to be accompanied by stupor or coma.[474] A detailed analysis of three cases by Mohr et al.[454] stressed the main feature of this syndrome: fluctuating performance in language function from almost normal to a profusely paraphasic, fluent speech akin to a delirium. The almost "uncontrollable" character of the paraphasias, in conjunction with intact repetition, led these investigators to postulate the removal by the thalamic lesion of a controlling influence of that structure over the intact cerebral surface speech areas. Similar clinical observations were reported by Reynolds et al.,[474] who commented on the frequency of aphasic abnormalities after left stereotactic thalamotomy and suggested that language disorders occurring after acute thalamic lesions may, to some extent, be mediated by disturbances in attention and recent memory.

A study by Alexander and LoVerme[478] involved nine cases of aphasia in left thalamic hematomas, in which the speech profile was a fluent, relatively well-articulated speech with poor naming, relatively good repetition, and prominent paraphasias. These researchers commented on the lack of distinctive features in aphasias from putaminal and thalamic hemorrhages. They also suggested a prominent role for memory and attention deficits in the production of the language disturbances.

Neglect in Thalamic Hemorrhage of the Nondominant Lobe

Syndromes of hemineglect are classically associated with lesions of the nondominant parietal lobe. Other areas, such as the frontal lobe, can rarely give rise to a similar set of symptoms.[479] Among ICHs, those in the putamen can be associated with this syndrome.[188] The occurrence of the syndrome in thalamic hemorrhage is rare. Reports by Walshe et al.[136] and Barraquer-Bordas et al.[464] each described two patients with anosognosia from right thalamic hemorrhages. Watson and Heilman[455] reported hemineglect in three patients with right thalamic hemorrhages. These patients exhibited prominent anosognosia and hemispatial agnosia, and two of them (cases 1 and 2) showed limb akinesia, manifested as lack of spontaneous movements of the left limbs despite only mild weakness. The patients in this study, particularly the two with limb akinesia, had relatively small thalamic hemorrhages that disrupted sensation only partially in case 1 and affected motor function partially, to a level of weakness only, in cases 1 and 2. In the third patient, a larger hemorrhage was associated with arm paralysis, marked leg weakness, absence of sensation, bilateral Babinski signs, and drowsiness, whereas patients 1 and 2 were alert and cooperative. These three cases illustrated a neglect syndrome similar to that observed in nondominant cortical surface disease, from documented medium-sized and small right thalamic hematomas.

Clinical Syndromes Related to the Topography of Thalamic Hemorrhage

Both Kumral et al.[459] and Chung et al.[458] delineated the clinical syndromes related to specific areas of involvement of the thalamus by hemorrhage. These two groups divided the thalamic hematomas into anterior, posteromedial, posterolateral, dorsal, and global, and related each location to the presumed arterial rupture within the thalamus.[458] The clinical features of hemorrhages in these various locations were as follows:

Anterior. Hematomas located in the most anterior portion of the thalamus, in the territory of the polar or tuberothalamic artery (Fig. 28-38), are often associated with ventricular extension and are clinically characterized by memory impairment and apathy, preservation of alertness, rare and transient sensory motor deficits, and absence of ophthalmologic findings.

Posteromedial. Posteromedial hemorrhages occur from rupture of thalamoperforating arteries. Hematomas are located in the medial aspect of the thalamus, with frequent rupture into the third ventricle and hydrocephalus, along with extension into the midbrain (Fig. 28-39). Small, localized hematomas result in memory disturbances and behavioral abnormalities, whereas larger lesions with downward extension into the midbrain are associated with early stupor or coma along with severe motor deficits and oculomotor disturbances.

Posterolateral. Posterolateral hemorrhages are due to rupture of thalamogeniculate arteries (Fig. 28-40). They are generally large and commonly extend into the internal capsule and ventricular space. Clinical features are severe sensory motor deficits as well as aphasia or hemineglect. Large hematomas also cause ipsilateral Horner's syndrome, a depressed level of consciousness, and ophthalmologic abnormalities.[459] Approximately one-third of patients with posterolateral

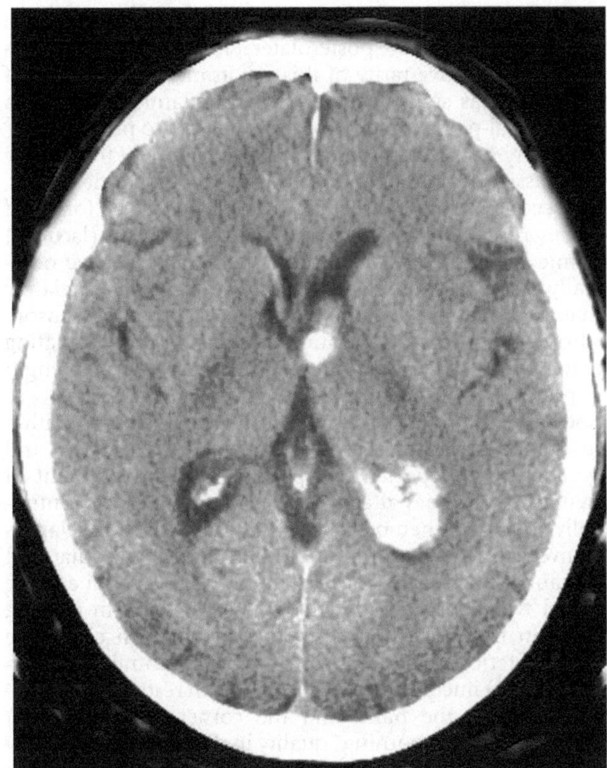

Figure 28-38. CT scan of anterior type of thalamic hemorrhage. Small hematoma confined to the most anterior aspect of the thalamus, with ventricular extension (blood in the atrium of the ipsilateral lateral ventricle).

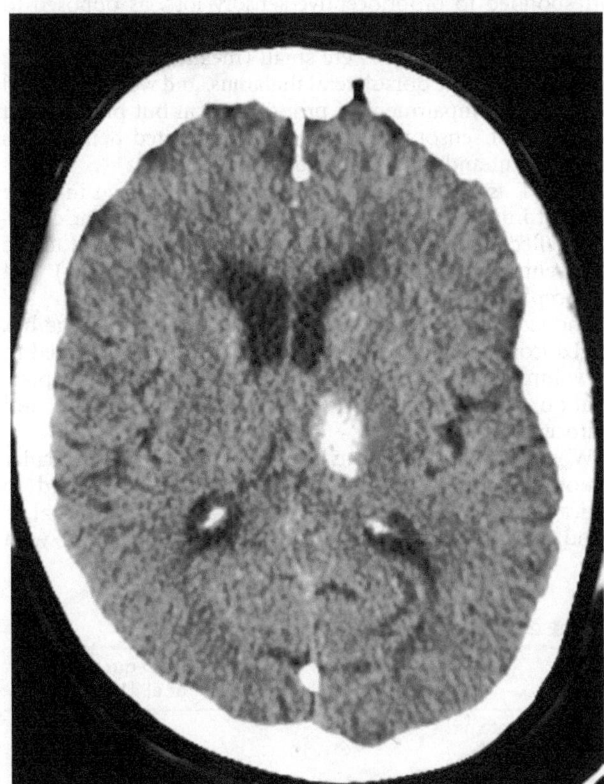

Figure 28-39. CT scan of posteromedial type of thalamic hemorrhage, with small hematoma along the medial aspect of the thalamus that does not extend into the third ventricle.

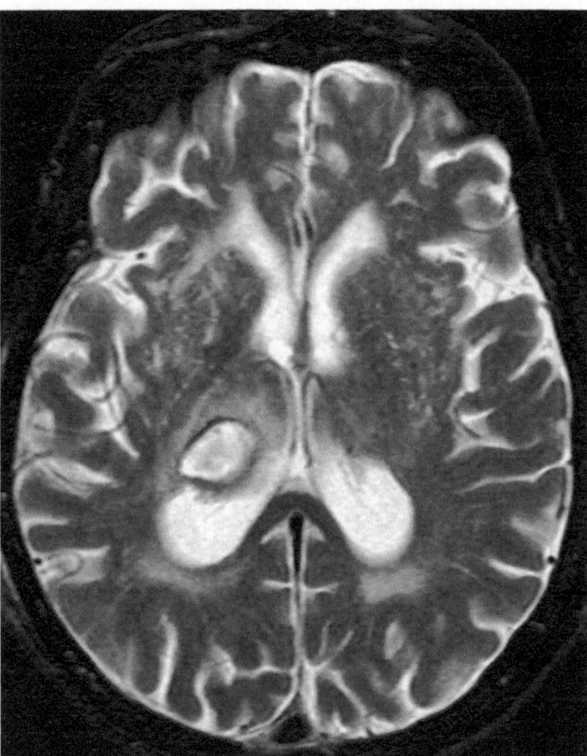

Figure 28-40. T2-weighted MR image of posterolateral form of thalamic hemorrhage, in which hematoma abuts the atrium of the lateral ventricle without ventricular extension.

thalamic hemorrhage reported by Chung et al.[458] showed delayed onset of a "thalamic pain syndrome." The aphasia of dominant posterolateral thalamic hematomas has been most often described as "transcortical motor" type,[459,480] although in hematomas of the pulvinar nucleus, the aphasia can be so markedly paraphasic that it becomes jargon.[454] The syndromes of hemi-inattention in nondominant thalamic hemorrhage have included marked anosognosia,[480] in one instance with prominent associated mania,[481] and examples of motor neglect or "inertia" manifested as lack of use of limbs with normal strength.[482]

Dorsal. Rupture of branches of the posterior choroidal artery causes hematomas located high in the thalamus, with frequent extension into the parietal white matter and the ventricular space (Fig. 28-41). They are characterized clinically by mild and transient sensory motor deficits, generally without oculomotor disturbances, with rare confusion and memory abnormalities in hemorrhages located most posteriorly (in the area of the pulvinar nucleus).

Global. The global type corresponds to involvement of the whole thalamus by a large hematoma that commonly enters the ventricular system (with associated hydrocephalus) and extends into the suprathalamic hemispheric white matter (Fig. 28-42). The clinical features are stupor or coma, severe sensory motor deficits, and paralysis of upward more than downward gaze, skew deviation, and small and unreactive pupils.

Unusual Sensory Syndromes

Unusual sensory syndromes are infrequently encountered in thalamic hemorrhage. The best recognized is the *thalamic pain syndrome* described by Dejerine and Roussy,[483] which is usually regarded as a feature of thalamic infarction in the distribution of the perforating branches of the posterior cerebral artery.[484,485] The profoundly distressing dysesthesias and spontaneous pain characteristically arise days to weeks after onset. The occurrence of this syndrome after thalamic hemorrhage is variable: Alexander and LoVerme[478] commented on the presence of a central pain syndrome in six of their nine patients with thalamic hemorrhages; Chung et al.[458] reported it in one-third of their patients with the posterolateral form of thalamic hemorrhage. The relative rarity of this syndrome in the setting of hemorrhage has suggested that partial thalamic lesions of a precise lateral-posterior location are necessary to produce it.[485] This sensory syndrome is an uncommon feature of the usually more massive thalamic destruction due to hematoma.

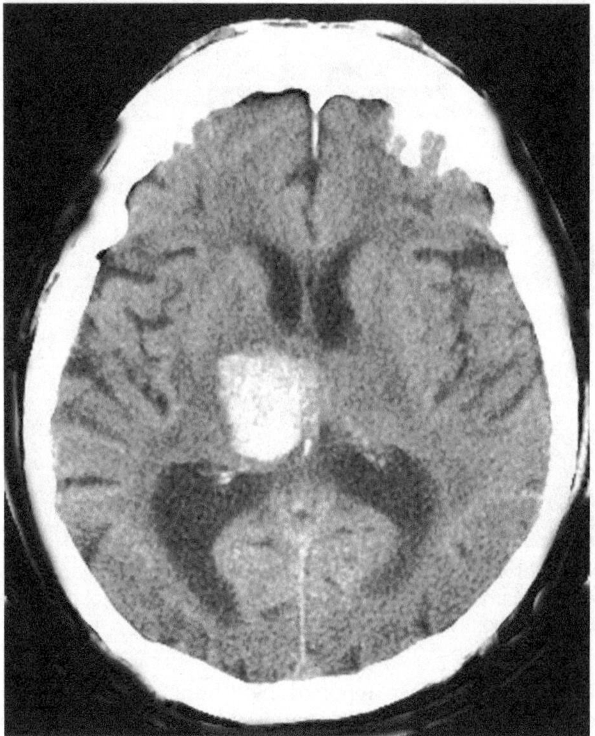

Figure 28-41. CT scan of dorsal thalamic hemorrhage, located in the medial portion of the upper thalamus, without ventricular extension.

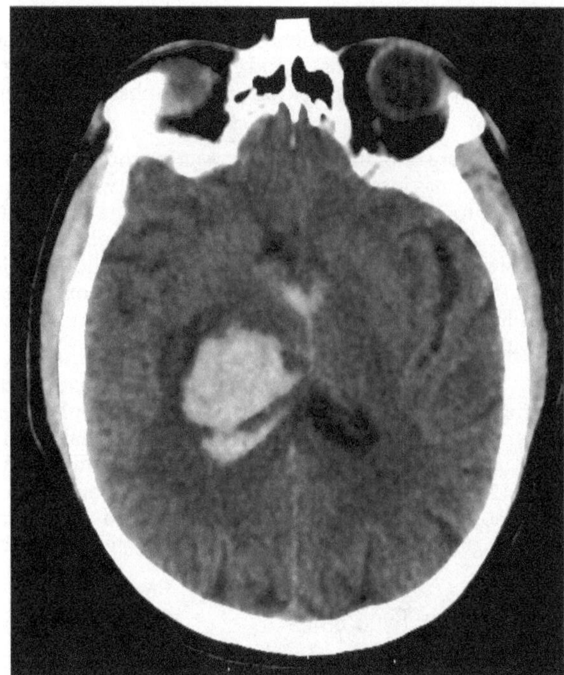

Figure 28-42. CT scan of large, global type of thalamic hemorrhage, with mass effect on the third ventricle and extension into the third and lateral ventricles.

A second unusual sensory syndrome is a form of *pure sensory stroke,* classically associated with small (lacunar) thalamic infarcts.[486] Small thalamic hemorrhages have occasionally presented as pure sensory stroke.[487–489] Thalamic hematomas of dorsal location have caused a pure hemisensory syndrome, with loss of sensation to pinprick predominating over that of vibration and joint position sense; motor strength was preserved, but coordination in the affected arm was abnormal with the eyes closed, reflecting the "sensory" rather than cerebellar character of the ataxia.[487] Paciaroni and Bogousslavsky[488] reported two patients with involvement of all sensory modalities affecting the face, arm, and leg contralaterally to a small hemorrhage in the center of the thalamus that involved all the ventral nuclei and the parvocellular and dorsocaudal nuclei but sparing the pulvinar. Shintani et al.[489] reported two patients with sensory loss in the arm and leg more than the face, with contralateral lesions in either the ventral-posterior-lateral (VPL) nucleus or the ventral-posterior-medial (VPM) nucleus; another patient with restricted "cheiro-oral" (affecting the hand and the corner of the mouth) dysesthesias with a "burning" quality in the absence of sensory loss to superficial or deep modalities had a small hematoma in the border between the VPL and VPM.

The syndrome of sensory ataxic hemiparesis has also been reported in the setting of small thalamic hemorrhages.[490] The clinical presentation differed from that of lacunar ataxic hemiparesis,[491] in that the ataxia of the patients with hemorrhages corresponded to proprioceptive sensory loss, as opposed to the cerebellar character of the ataxia in lacunar ataxic hemiparesis. The hematomas were small (mean volume, 7.2 mL), were located in the dorsolateral thalamus, and were associated with marked impairment of proprioception but preservation of superficial sensory modalities; the associated hemiparesis was transient and predominated in the leg.

The *CT aspects of thalamic hemorrhage* are shown in Table 28-5. Of interest are the high frequency of ventricular extension (reflecting the location of the hematoma adjacent to the third ventricle) and the resulting high rate (about 25%)[363] of hydrocephalus.

The *mortality rate* reported after thalamic hemorrhage has ranged from 25% to 52%,[458–460] and it is closely correlated to the volume of the hematoma, level of consciousness at presentation, and presence of intraventricular hemorrhage and hydrocephalus.[459,460,492]

When comparing patients with or without intraventricular hemorrhage who were otherwise comparable in regard to clinical features with prognostic significance, Steinke et al.[460] found a significantly higher mortality rate for those with

TABLE 28-5 CT Aspects of Thalamic Hemorrhage

	Walshe et al.[136] (n = 18)	Barraquer-Bordas et al.[484] (n = 23)
Side of hematoma		
Right/left	8/10	17/6
Size of hematoma		
<3.3 cm	11	–
>3.3 cm	7	–
Ventricular extension	66%	50%
Hydrocephalus	27%	21%

intraventricular extension. The finding suggests that this factor is an independent predictor of mortality. In addition, the different locations of hemorrhage within the thalamus have been associated with outcome: anterior and dorsal hematomas had a benign course, whereas posterolateral, posteromedial, and global hemorrhages were associated with higher mortality rates and higher levels of disability.[458] The functional motor outcome in survivors after thalamic hemorrhage is compromised by extension of the hematoma into the internal capsule, midbrain, or putamen. Cognitive impairment as a sequela correlates with initial disturbance of consciousness and ventricular extension of the hematoma.[492] Performance in activities of daily living is influenced by advanced age and hematoma size[492] as well as by the presence of unilateral spatial neglect, aphasia, and severity of paresis of the lower limb.[493]

White Matter (Lobar) Hemorrhage

The main clinical features of lobar hemorrhage were delineated in the early 1980s,[132,190] and still there are no reliable criteria for a choice of therapy.[175,494]

Anatomy

Lobar hemorrhages occur in the subcortical white matter of the cerebral lobes, usually extending longitudinally in a plane parallel to the overlying cortex. As they become larger, their shape changes into the more common oval or round one. They occur in all cerebral lobes but have a predilection for the parietal, temporal, and occipital lobes (Table 28-6).[132,190] This predilection for the posterior half of the brain in lobar ICH is unexplained and is probably not a reflection of differences in relative lobe size because the ratio of 3 : 1 between parietotemporooccipital and frontal hematomas[132] is larger than the anatomic volumetric ratio between these two areas, which is 2 : 1 or 3 : 2. A possible explanation for this finding is the predilection of intracerebral microaneurysms for the parietooccipital area found by Cole and Yates.[150] These investigators found that the junction of cortical gray matter and white matter contained about 30% of the microaneurysms, and the diagrams included in their article show a higher concentration of these lesions on the parietooccipital areas and proportionately smaller numbers of them in the frontal and temporal poles. Although the causal relationship between microaneurysms and ICH has not been established, these anatomic correlations in lobar ICH lend some support to it. Alternatively this posterior predominance can be attributed to underlying CAA as, for yet to be determined reasons, there also exists a posterior predilection for pathological and neuroimaging changes related to this microangiopathy.[495]

TABLE 28-6 Location of Lobar ICH

Location	No.	
Frontal	4	
Parietal	3	18 (82%)
Temporoparietal	8	
Parietooccipital	2	
Parietotemporooccipital	1	
Parietofrontal	2	
Occipital	2	
Total	**22**	

From Kase CS, Williams JP, Wyatt DA, et al: Lobar intracerebral hematoma: Clinical and CT analysis of 22 cases. Neurology *32:1146, 1982.*
ICH, Intracerebral hemorrhage.

Etiology

The etiologic factors in lobar ICH may be somewhat different from those in other forms of ICH, particularly with regard to a less significant role of hypertension.[32,35,132,190,252] Ropper and Davis[190] reported chronic hypertension in only 31% of their cases of lobar ICH, and in the series reported by Kase et al.,[132] only 50% of the patients had elevated blood pressure on admission; in half of this group high blood pressure had been documented before the hemorrhage. In Weisberg's[252] study, only 33% of the patients with lobar ICH had hypertension compared with 81% of the patients with deep (ganglionic–thalamic) ICHs. However, data reported by Broderick et al.[74] suggest that hypertension contributes to lobar hemorrhage as much as it does to deep hemispheric, cerebellar, or pontine hemorrhages. These authors found hypertension to be the likely explanation of ICH in 67% of their patients with lobar ICHs and in 73% with deep hemispheric, 73% with cerebellar, and 78% with pontine hemorrhages. This predominance of the hypertensive mechanism in lobar ICH remained unchanged with advancing age, which argues against the notion that nonhypertensive mechanisms such as CAA may be the predominant cause of lobar ICH in elderly patients.

Etiologic factors other than hypertension that are relevant in lobar ICH include (1) AVMs, which occur at rates between 7% and 14%, (2) tumors, which occur in 7% to 9%, and (3) blood dyscrasias or anticoagulation, in 5% to 20% of the hemorrhages.[313] There is a large group of patients (22% in one series[132]) in whom the mechanism for ICH remains unknown. This fact raises the possibility that some etiologic factors may exist for white matter (lobar) ICH that are more common than in other forms of ICH. One such factor is CAA, which is being increasingly recognized as the substrate of recurrent, sometimes multiple ICHs in elderly nonhypertensive patients. In this CAA-related category of lobar hemorrhage, O'Donnell et al.[127] found that the presence of ε2 or ε4 alleles of the ApoE gene was associated with a high risk of recurrent ICH (28% at 2 years compared with 10% in patients with lobar ICH who did not have the ε2/ε4 alleles). An additional factor that is highly correlated with the risk of lobar ICH recurrence is the presence and number of microhemorrhages detected at the time of presentation with the initial lobar ICH.[375]

Clinical Features

The clinical manifestations of lobar ICH have been extensively analyzed, and a number of differences from other types of ICH have been noted.[73,132,190,496] The circumstances at onset are listed in Table 28-7, which compares series of lobar ICH with those including all forms of ICH.[2,73,132,190,496–498] The distinguishing features of lobar ICH are lower frequency of hypertension and coma on admission and higher frequency of headache and seizures. The higher frequency of headache at onset may reflect the larger number of patients with lobar ICH who are awake and can give a history. Ropper and Davis[190] described the headaches as located in and around the ipsilateral eye in occipital hematomas, around the ear in temporal hemorrhages, anteriorly in frontal hemorrhage, and anterior temporal (temple) in parietal lobe hematomas. The low incidence of coma on admission in lobar ICH is probably related to the peripheral location of the hematoma, at a distance from midline structures.[190]

Seizure as a common event at the onset of lobar ICH has been well-documented.[73,132,496,499–503] The mechanism of seizures in lobar hematomas may reflect the location of the hemorrhage in the gray matter–white matter interface, which creates a situation similar to the surgical isolation of cortex by

TABLE 28-7 Comparison of Clinical Features of Lobar ICH with all Forms of ICH

	*All Forms of ICH (%)**			*Lobar ICH (%)**		
Feature	*HCSR*[2]	*Lausanne*[3]	*Kase et al*[132]	*Ropper and Davis*[190]	*Weisberg*[496]	*SDB*[73]
Hypertension						
History	72		22	31	30	55
On admission	91	55†	66	46	56	?
Headache	33	40	61	46	72	60
Vomiting	51	?	33	61	32	29
Seizures	6	7	33	0	28	16
Coma	24	22	18	0.4	?	19

From Kase CS: Lobar hemorrhage. In Kase CS, Caplan LR, editors: Intracerebral hemorrhage. *Boston, 1994, Butterworth-Heinemann, p 363.*
*Percentages rounded to the closest whole number (decimals from the original omitted).
†Not specified whether hypertension was diagnosed by history or at entry examination. HCSR, Harvard Cooperative Stroke Registry; ICH, intracerebral hemorrhage; SDB, Stroke Data Bank; ?, information not provided.

subcortical injury that results in sustained paroxysmal activity from the isolated cortex.[504]

The neurologic deficits seen with lobar ICH depend on the location and size of the hematoma.[190] They include (1) sudden hemiparesis, worse in the arm, with retained ability to walk, in frontal hematoma, (2) combined sensory and motor deficits, the former predominating, and visual field defects in parietal hemorrhage, (3) fluent paraphasic speech with poor comprehension and relative sparing of repetition in left temporal lobe hematomas, and (4) homonymous hemianopia, occasionally accompanied by mild sensory changes (extinction to double simultaneous stimulation), in occipital lobe hemorrhages. In the group of 24 patients described by Kase et al.,[132] hemiparesis and visual field defects were the most common abnormality, found in 60% and 30% of patients who were not comatose on admission, respectively. Those patients in whom the two signs coexisted had larger and more anteriorly placed hematomas, whereas those with hemianopia and no hemiparesis had posterior hemorrhages. From these data, the clinical presentation in a lobar parietooccipital hematoma emerges as sudden onset of headache, sometimes associated with vomiting, not uncommonly associated with seizure activity, with state of consciousness in the alert or obtunded level, associated with mild contralateral hemiparesis and visual field defect. Specific deficits in speech or spatial function are seen when the hematomas are of dominant frontotemporal or nondominant parietal location, respectively, mimicking the deficits seen with infarction.[505,506]

Cerebral Amyloid Angiopathy and Lobar Hemorrhage

The best recognized clinical manifestation of CAA is spontaneous ICH. The hemorrhages largely follow the distribution of the vascular amyloid, appearing with highest frequency in the corticosubcortical or lobar regions and less commonly in cerebellum, generally sparing the brainstem and deep hemispheric structures.[62,67] Lobar ICH in CAA is more likely to dissect into the subarachnoid space than into the lateral ventricles.[62,507,508] Despite extensive involvement of the leptomeningeal vessels, symptomatic subarachnoid hemorrhage due to CAA is rare.[507,509] Conversely, MRI studies have shown a high prevalence of hemosiderin staining within the sulci of individuals with CAA ranging from 40% to 60%, suggestive of previous small occult subarachnoid hemorrhage.[510,511] Subdural hematomas (SDH) have been recently reported to occur in 20% of primary lobar ICH and be predictive of mortality. The vast majority of SDHs are contiguous with the underlying presenting ICH. Accordingly, this occurrence has been hypothesized to result from rupture of an amyloid-laden leptomeningeal artery adjacent to the dura with bleeding into both the underlying parenchyma and overlying subdural space.[512]

CAA-related lobar ICH presents much like other types of lobar ICH,[498] with early onset of neurologic symptoms and a variable combination of headache, seizures, and decreased consciousness according to hemorrhage size and location. Hemorrhagic lesions in CAA can also be small and clinically silent.[81] These small corticosubcortical "microbleeds" are well-visualized by gradient-echo or T2*-weighted MRI techniques, which enhance the signal dropout associated with deposited hemosiderin.[513] By detecting even old hemorrhagic lesions, gradient-echo MRI provides a clinical method for demonstrating an individual's lifetime history of hemorrhage and thus for identifying the pattern of multiple lobar lesions characteristic of CAA (Fig. 28-43). CAA-related microbleeds, like symptomatic "macrobleeds," occur typically in corticosubcortical locations[54] or at the superficial cortical surface.[71]

The Boston criteria for CAA codify the typical features of CAA-related ICH into the diagnostic categories "definite," "probable," and "possible" disease, as listed in Table 28-8.[70,514] Although diagnosis of definite CAA requires demonstration of advanced disease through postmortem examination, a clinical diagnosis of probable CAA can be reached during life through radiographic demonstration of at least two strictly lobar or corticosubcortical hemorrhagic lesions (either large symptomatic macrobleeds or smaller microbleeds) without other definite hemorrhagic process. In a small clinical-pathologic validation study, 13 of 13 subjects given a clinical diagnosis of probable CAA also had pathologic evidence of CAA,[514] which suggests that the criteria may be sufficiently specific to be useful in practice. In the same study, gradient-echo MRI detected the diagnostic pattern in eight of 11 patients (73%) with pathologically documented CAA, providing an estimate for the sensitivity of the diagnosis. The Boston criteria propose a separate category of *probable CAA with supporting pathology* for patients with lobar ICH and an antemortem brain sample containing evidence of CAA (see Table 28-8). A validation study for this diagnosis suggested that CAA of at least moderate severity in a random tissue sample was a reasonably specific marker for severe CAA in the brain as a whole.[61]

For reasons that are poorly understood, CAA pathology[72,73] and CAA-related hemorrhagic lesions localize preferentially to posterior (parietooccipital or temporooccipital) cortical brain regions. In a study of 321 macrobleeds and microbleeds detected by gradient-echo MRI among 59 subjects with probable CAA, 26.5% of the lesions were in occipital cortex and 30.5% were in temporal cortex, which was significantly greater than the proportions (18.3% and 22.3%, respectively)

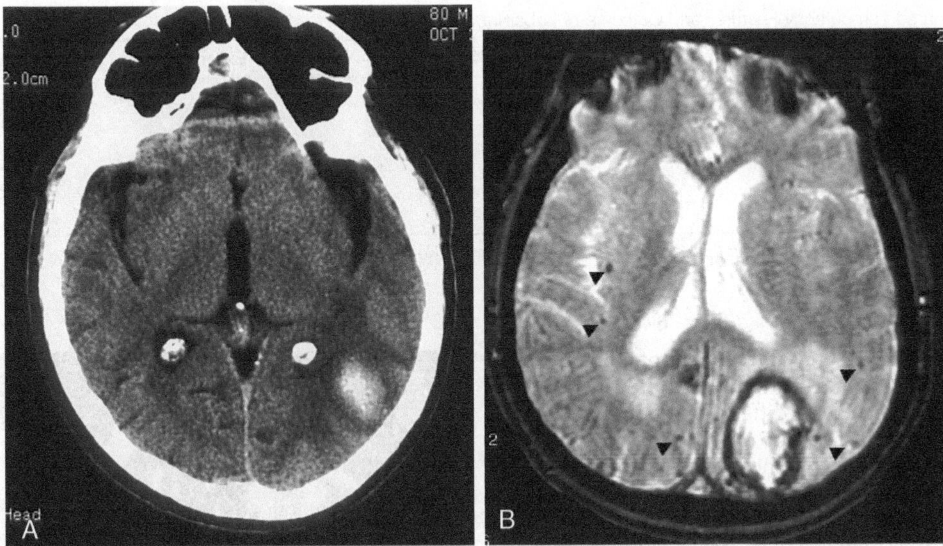

Figure 28-43. Recurrent intracerebral hemorrhage (ICH). A, The CT scan shows a left temporal ICH in an 80-year-old man with a history of previous cognitive decline. B, A gradient-echo MRI sequence obtained 2 years later demonstrates recurrent ICH in the left parietal lobe as well as multiple punctate hypointense lesions *(arrowheads)* consistent with chronic asymptomatic hemorrhages. The presence of two or more strictly lobar hemorrhagic lesions is consistent with a diagnosis of probable cerebral amyloid angiopathy (see Table 28-8).

TABLE 28-8 Boston Criteria for Diagnosis of CAA–Related ICH

Definite CAA	Full postmortem examination of brain shows lobar ICH, severe CAA (Vonsattel et al.),[88] and no other diagnostic lesion
Probable CAA with supporting pathology	Clinical data and pathologic tissue (evacuated hematoma or cortical biopsy specimen) showing some lobar CAA in pathologic specimen, and no other diagnostic lesion
Probable CAA	Clinical data and MRI or CT demonstration of two or more hemorrhagic lesions restricted to lobar regions (cerebellar hemorrhage allowed), patient age ≥55 years, and no other cause of hemorrhage*
Possible CAA	Clinical data and MRI or CT demonstration of single lobar ICH, patient age ≥55 years, and no other cause of hemorrhage*

CAA, Cerebral amyloid angiopathy; CNS, central nervous system; CT, computed tomography; ICH, intracerebral hemorrhage; INR, international normalized ratio; MRI, magnetic resonance imaging.
*Other causes of ICH defined as excessive anticoagulation (INR > 3.0), antecedent head trauma or ischemic stroke, CNS tumor, vascular malformation or vasculitis, blood dyscrasia or coagulopathy. INR > 3.0 or other nonspecific laboratory abnormalities permitted for diagnosis of *possible* CAA.

predicted by the volumes of these cortical regions.[54] The posterior predilection of CAA has been further corroborated by the distribution of the amyloid-ligand Pittsburgh Compound B detected by positron emission tomographic imaging in subjects with probable CAA but without dementia.[36,74]

Prognosis for Lobar Hemorrhage

The prognosis in lobar hematomas is usually less grave than in other forms of ICH. The mortality rates reported have been between 11.5% and 29%,[132,190,253,515] all of which are lower than the rates for the other varieties of ICH. A low frequency (6%) has been reported in an autopsy series,[135] whereas in clinical series, the frequency is between 10% and 32%.[132,190,253] In addition, the functional outcome for survivors is generally better than in those with deep hemispheric ICHs; a good outcome was reported in 57% to 85% of patients.[515–517]

Computed Tomography Aspects

After the early phase of the ICH, lobar hematomas can adopt a number of residual patterns, as analyzed by Sung and Chu.[518] Frequently (27% of the time), the ICH leaves no CT-demonstrated residual, although a slit and a round cavity (34%) are the most common CT sequelae; rarely (3%), only calcification at the ICH site remains.

Ropper and Davis[190] provided two-dimensional measurements of 26 hematomas and commented on the tendency of these lesions to enlarge mostly in the transverse and anteroposterior planes of the CT section. In Weisberg's[252] series of 45 patients with lobar ICH, ten were found to have intraventricular extension, a factor that did not affect the mortality rates in this group.

The CT features of the 22 cases reported by Kase et al.[132] are shown in Table 28-9. The hematomas could be divided by volume into three main groups, which in turn correlated with the presence and severity of mass effect. Ventricular extension was a factor that correlated with location (proximity to ventricular system) rather than size of the hematoma. The outcome was in part a function of hematoma size; no patient with a hematoma larger than 60 mL survived, whereas all those with small hematomas (<20 mL) did. In the group with moderate-sized hematomas, 75% survived, and the functional level was, in general, poorer than in the group with small hematomas. In a subsequent analysis of Mayo Clinic data, Flemming et al.[519] reported observations on 81 patients with lobar ICH. Volume larger than 40 mL on CT was associated with poor outcome; in patients with hemorrhage smaller than 40 mL, interval from symptom onset to hospital presentation of less than 17 hours and a Glasgow Coma Scale (GCS) score of 13 or less were predictive of a poor outcome. These data stress the importance of hematoma enlargement as a factor in the deterioration of patients who are seen early after the onset of lobar ICH.

These figures, in addition, give some indication of the possible role of surgical drainage as a therapeutic option in lobar ICH. The Surgical Trial in Intracerebral Hemorrhage (STICH)

TABLE 28-9 Computed Tomography Features and Outcome of Lobar Intracerebral Hematomas

Hematoma Size	No. of Cases	Midline Shift	Ventricular Extension	Outcome/Operated
Small (<20 mL)	5	1	0	5 improved/0
Moderate (20–40 mL)	7	6	1	6 improved/3 1 died/0
Massive (>40 mL)	10	10	7	4 improved/2 6 died/1
Total	22	17	8	

From Kase CS, Williams JP, Wyatt DA, et al: Lobar intracerebral hematomas: Clinical and CT analysis of 22 cases. Neurology *32:1146, 1982.*

compared surgical and nonsurgical treatment of patients with both deep and lobar ICH in a randomized multicenter international study and detected no difference among groups.[520] However, in a prespecified subgroup analysis a favorable trend towards surgical management was noted in cases of lobar ICH located at 1 cm or less from the cortical surface. Based on this observation, the subsequent STICH II trial examined the benefit of conservative management versus surgical therapy within 48 hours of ictus in patients with lobar ICH located at 1 cm or less from the cortical surface with a volume of between 10 mL and 100 mL, and without intraventricular extension.[521] Again, there were no significant differences found between early surgical and initial conservative medical management. However, 21% of participants randomly assigned to the conservative management group underwent surgery following randomization according to the clinical judgment of treating physicians. Despite this methodological limitation, post hoc analyses observed that patients deemed to have baseline characteristics that put them in a poor prognostic category (calculated by an algorithm derived from patient age, Glasgow Coma Scale, and ICH volume at randomization) were more likely to have favorable outcome with early surgery (OR, 0.49, 95%CI, 0.26 to 0.92; $P = 0.02$), implying a target population that may possibly benefit from early surgical treatment. Moreover, almost all patients in STICH II underwent conventional craniotomy, and currently on-going trials are assessing the benefit of promising minimally invasive procedures for hematoma evacuation in patients with ICH[522] which, if successful, may provide additional reasons for considering special subsets of patients with ICH for early evacuation of the hematoma.

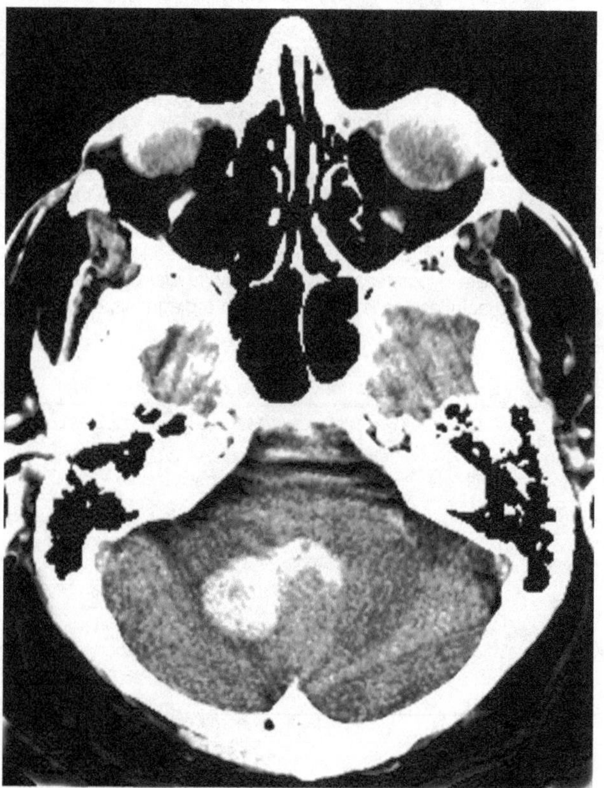

Figure 28-44. CT scan of right cerebellar hemorrhage originating in the area of the dentate nucleus, with extension into the adjacent fourth ventricle.

HEMORRHAGE AFFECTING THE BRAINSTEM AND CEREBELLUM

Cerebellar Hemorrhage

In a landmark article in 1959, Fisher et al.[138] described the main clinical features of cerebellar hemorrhage. Especially important diagnostic features were the inability to walk, gaze palsy without hemiplegia, and the absence of unilateral limb paresis. These investigators found that surgical decompression could be lifesaving, occasionally even in patients in deep coma before surgery. More important, patients who had been treated surgically were often able to return to active lives without the overwhelming disability often retained by survivors of basal ganglionic hemorrhages. Although these diagnostic formulations were initially subject to dispute, CT scanning and MRI have made the detection of smaller cerebellar hematomas possible,[523,524] essentially confirming the initial observations of Fisher et al.[138]

Cerebellar hemorrhage appears at a rate variously quoted as between 5% and 15%.[128,137,525-528] The average rate is about 10%, which is also approximately the percentage of brain weight accounted for by the cerebellum. Although 10% is a relatively low frequency, the importance of establishing the diagnosis resides in the good prognosis after prompt surgical treatment.[128,259,529] Cerebellar hemorrhage usually occurs in one of the hemispheres, generally originating in the region of the dentate nucleus, from distal branches of the superior cerebellar artery[138] or occasionally the posterior–inferior cerebellar artery.[226] In the study by Fisher et al.,[138] the left hemisphere was affected twice as often as the right. McKissock et al.[530] also commented on a left hemisphere preponderance in cerebellar hemorrhage. Most other series do not report hemorrhage laterality.

The hematoma collects around the dentate and spreads into the hemispheral white matter, commonly extending into the cavity of the fourth ventricle as well (Fig. 28-44). The adjacent brainstem (pontine tegmentum) is rarely involved directly by the hematoma but is often compressed by it, which, at times, leads to pontine necrosis. The midline variant of cerebellar hemorrhage originates from the vermis and represents only about 5% of the cases.[138] It virtually always communicates directly with the fourth ventricle through its roof and frequently extends into the pontine tegmentum bilaterally (Fig. 28-45). The bleeding vessel in this variety corresponds to

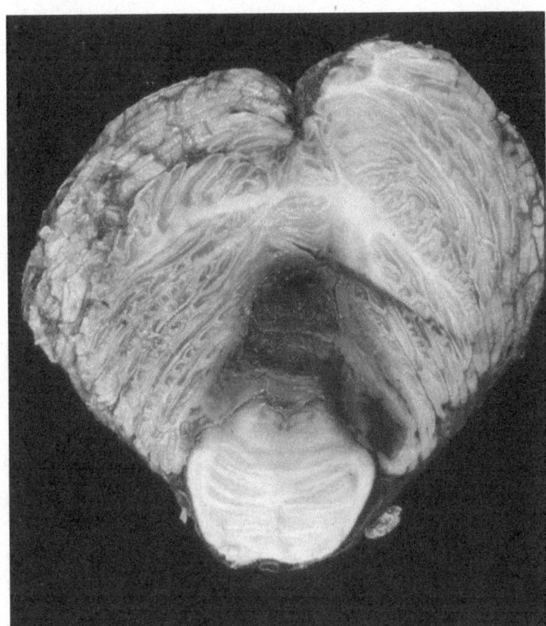

Figure 28-45. Vermian cerebellar hemorrhage with pressure on the pontine tegmentum.

TABLE 28-10 Neurologic Findings in Cerebellar Hemorrhage for Noncomatose Patients

Neurologic Finding	No.	%
Appendicular ataxia	17/26	65
Truncal ataxia	11/17	65
Gait ataxia	11/14	78
Dysarthria	20/32	62
Gaze palsy	20/37	54
Cranial nerve findings		
Peripheral facial palsy	22/36	61
Nystagmus	18/35	51
Miosis	11/37	30
Decreased corneal reflex	10/33	30
Abducens palsy	10/36	28
Loss of gag reflex	6/30	20
Skew deviation	4/33	12
Trochlear palsy	0/36	–
Hemiparesis	4/35	11
Extensor plantar response	23/36	64
Respiratory irregularity	6/28	21
Nuchal rigidity	14/35	40
Subhyaloid hemorrhage	0/34	–

From Ott KH, Kase CS, Ojemann RJ, et al: Cerebellar hemorrhage: Diagnosis and treatment. Arch Neurol *31:160, 1974.*

distal branches of the superior or the posterior–inferior cerebellar artery. These two forms of cerebellar hemorrhage have distinctive clinical and prognostic features.

Distribution of etiologic factors in cerebellar hemorrhage is similar to that in other forms of ICH, and hypertension is the leading cause.[138,259] AVMs are said to be common in the cerebellum:[527,430] they accounted for five out of 15 cerebellar hematomas in the autopsy series reported by McCormick and Rosenfield;[35] in other series,[259] lower rates of AVMs (4%), similar to those for ICH at other sites, have been reported.[190] Anticoagulation is an important etiologic factor in cerebellar hemorrhage and was the second most common cause reported by Ott et al.[259] Among 24 ICHs in patients undergoing oral anticoagulation therapy,[257] nine occurred in the cerebellum. Three of these were of the less common vermian or midline variety. Fisher et al.[138] commented on a relative female preponderance in their series (13 : 8); in other series, the female-to-male ratio was reported as 26 : 30,[530] 6 : 6,[137] 5 : 14,[531] and 17 : 17.[530]

Symptoms usually develop while the patient is active. Occasionally a single prodromal episode of dizziness or facial numbness may precede the hemorrhage. The most common symptom is *an inability to stand or walk,* which in many patients has been dramatic in onset. One man leaned against a fence while painting and could not right himself; another bumped downstairs on his bottom to call for help. Crawling or propelling oneself prone on the floor to get to the bathroom to vomit has been mentioned. Rare patients maintain their ability to walk a few steps, but scarcely any patient with a sizable hemorrhage (>2 cm) walks into the emergency room or physician's office.

Vomiting is also very common, being present in 42 of 44 patients,[259] 12 of 12 patients,[529] and 14 of 18 patients[138] in various series. Vomiting usually occurs soon after the onset in cerebellar and subarachnoid hemorrhage but often develops later, after other symptoms, in putaminal hemorrhage. *Dizziness* is also common, occurring in 24 of 44 patients,[259] eight of 21 patients,[138] and four of 12 patients[529] in various series. More often the feeling is one of insecurity, a "drunken feeling," or wavering rather than true rotational vertigo.

Headache is also very common, occurring in 32 of 44 patients,[259] ten of 21 patients,[138] and 12 of 12 patients[137] in various series. Most often the pain is occipital, but occasionally it can occur on the side of the head or frontally. At times the headache is abrupt and excruciating, closely mimicking SAH. In other patients the pain is located primarily in the neck or shoulder. Dysarthria, tinnitus, and hiccups occur but are less common. Loss of consciousness at onset is unusual,[259,532] and only one-third of patients are obtunded by the time they reach the hospital.[259] Most patients show gradual worsening over 1 to 3 hours, as in other forms of ICH.[2]

The classic physical findings are a combination of a unilateral cerebellar deficit with variable signs of ipsilateral tegmental pontine involvement. These are detailed in Table 28-10, from an analysis of 38 noncomatose patients in the series reported by Ott et al.[259] Appendicular and gait ataxia occurred in 65% and 78%, respectively, of patients who were alert enough to cooperate for cerebellar function testing. Other patients lean to the side when placed upright. On the side of the hemorrhage, there usually is overshoot or inability to brake the limb quickly; this sign is more common than finger-to-nose or finger-to-object ataxia. Signs of involvement of the ipsilateral pontine tegmentum include peripheral facial palsy, ipsilateral horizontal gaze palsy, sixth cranial nerve palsy, depressed corneal reflex, and miosis. In some patients the hemorrhage presses laterally in the area of the cerebellopontine angle, producing peripheral facial palsy, deafness, and diminished corneal response.

From analysis of the relative frequency of signs in noncomatose patients reported by Ott et al.,[259] a characteristic triad consisting of appendicular ataxia, ipsilateral gaze palsy, and peripheral facial palsy was suggested; at least two of the three signs were present in 73% of the patients tested for all three. Ocular skew deviation is also common.[525] Additional findings useful in differential diagnosis are hemiplegia and subhyaloid hemorrhages, both of which are uncommon enough in cerebellar hemorrhage that their presence essentially rules out the diagnosis.[259] The frequency of unilateral limb weakness in cerebellar hemorrhage has been a matter of controversy. In the study by Fisher et al.,[138] hemiplegia was observed only in the setting of a prior stroke, and similar findings were recorded by Ott et al.[259] In two autopsy series, however, hemiplegia was reported in 50% and 20% of the cases,[527,529] and Richardson[528] noted contralateral hemiplegia in more than 50% of cases in his clinical series. Although in some instances reports of ipsilateral hemiplegia may have corresponded to decreased mobility of grossly ataxic limbs or decreased spontaneous movement, a contralateral hemiplegia cannot be explained on those bases, so one must assume involvement of the corticospinal tract in the ipsilateral basis pontis.

Other neurologic findings add little specific diagnostic data: the pupils are commonly small and reactive to light, dysarthria is present in two-thirds of cases, and the respiratory rhythm is usually unaffected.[259] Unilateral involuntary eye closure has been occasionally observed,[475,533] the involved eye usually being contralateral to the hematoma. This sign has been interpreted as eye closure for avoidance of diplopia, but this interpretation is probably not always correct because the sign occurs in the absence of diplopia, in both infratentorial and supratentorial strokes.[475] Other less common oculomotor abnormalities, such as ocular bobbing, have occasionally been reported in cerebellar hemorrhage[259,534,535] but with a lower frequency than in pontine hemorrhage and infarction. Some patients have a head tilt. Neck stiffness and unwillingness to move the head or neck either actively or passively probably signify increased pressure in the posterior fossa.

Along with these focal neurologic manifestations, patients with cerebellar hemorrhage may be seen with variable levels of decreased alertness. Of the 56 cases reported by Ott et al.,[259] 14 (25%) were alert, 22 (40%) were drowsy, five (9%) were stuporous, and 15 (26%) were comatose. That two-thirds of the patients are responsive (alert or drowsy) on admission justifies the intensive efforts to diagnose this condition early because the surgical prognosis largely depends on the preoperative level of consciousness.

The clinical course in cerebellar hemorrhage is notoriously unpredictable: some patients who are alert or drowsy on admission can deteriorate suddenly to coma and death without warning,[138,259,536] whereas others with similar clinical status have an uneventful course with complete recovery of function. Of those patients who were not comatose on admission, only 20% had a smooth, uneventful recovery in the series reported by Ott et al.;[259] 80% deteriorated to coma, and in one-fourth of these patients, this occurred within 3 hours of onset (Fig. 28-46). A similar frequency was observed in the study by Fisher et al.,[138] in which only two of 18 patients had a benign course; the other 16 deteriorated to coma at variable intervals, mostly within a few hours after onset. Most patients deteriorate early in the course, but occasional patients have shown fatal decompensation at a later stage, even a month later, after being stable in the interim.[537]

Because prediction of the clinical course cannot be made on the basis of clinical variables on admission, Ott et al.[259] recommended that surgical evacuation of the hematoma should be undertaken whenever the diagnosis is made within 48 hours of onset.[259] They justified the need for prompt diagnosis and emergency surgery by pointing to poor surgical outcome with worsening preoperative mental status: the surgical mortality was 17% for responsive and 75% for unresponsive patients.[259] These figures have proved generally accurate, despite occasional reports of good surgical results in comatose patients.[538]

The use of CT and MRI in cerebellar hemorrhage has permitted the recognition of many different aspects of these lesions, some of which are useful early predictors of clinical course.[523,524,539] Little et al.[523] reported two groups of patients with cerebellar hemorrhage: one group had abrupt onset, a more severely depressed level of consciousness, and a tendency toward progressive deterioration, and the other had a more benign, stable course. The first group required surgical treatment, whereas the second group did well with a medical program. CT scans of the first group showed hematomas 3 cm or more in diameter, obstructive hydrocephalus, and ventricular extension of the hemorrhage; in the second group of patients, all of whom had hematomas less than 3 cm in diameter, the other two features were absent. These observations, along with those of others,[540] have identified a group of cerebellar hemorrhages with a benign course. It may be possible to make accurate predictions from the combined analysis of clinical and CT data at the time of onset. Especially important is careful monitoring of the status of the patient. The development of obtundation and extensor plantar responses is ominous and is virtually always followed by a fatal outcome unless surgery is performed.

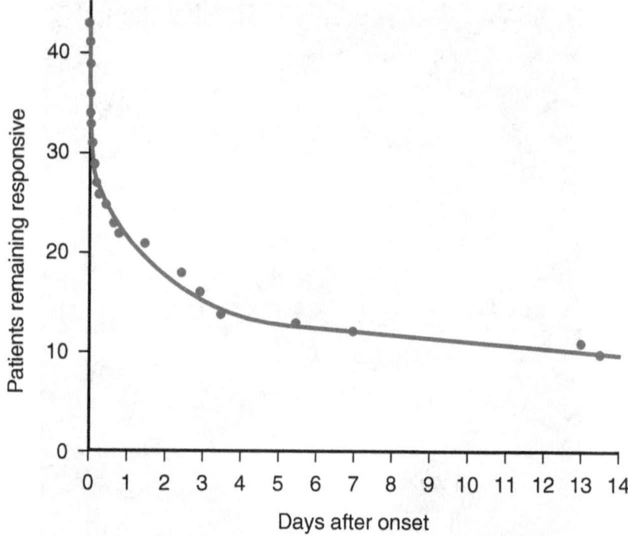

Figure 28-46. Coma in patients with cerebellar hemorrhage as a function of time after onset. *(Reprinted with permission from Ott KH, et al., Cerebellar hemorrhage: Diagnosis and treatment,* Arch Neurol, *31, 3, September, pp. 160–7, 1974.)*

In an attempt to identify predictors of neurologic deterioration, St. Louis et al.[536] analyzed a series of 72 patients with cerebellar hemorrhage. For the 33 patients (46%) with deterioration, independent predictors of such a course were a vermian location of the hemorrhage and hydrocephalus. On the basis of these data, St. Louis et al.[536] suggested that patients with these features are likely to require neurosurgical treatment. The same group analyzed clinical factors predictive of poor outcome in a group of 94 patients. Poor outcome was predicted by admission systolic blood pressure higher than 200 mm Hg, hematoma diameter more than 3 cm, brainstem distortion, and acute hydrocephalus, and death was predicted by abnormal brainstem reflexes (corneal and oculocephalic), GCS score less than 8, acute hydrocephalus, and intraventricular hemorrhage.[541]

Kirollos et al.[542] have made further refinements in the approach to the treatment of cerebellar hemorrhage. They evaluated 50 consecutive patients and used the level of mass effect in the fourth ventricle (graded as absent, compression, or complete obliteration), size of hematoma, GCS score, and hydrocephalus as the variables correlated with type of management and outcome. Their findings indicated that patients with an obliterated fourth ventricle, even if conscious on admission, had a high rate of subsequent neurologic deterioration (43%) and that surgical treatment with posterior fossa craniectomy for clot evacuation was recommended before

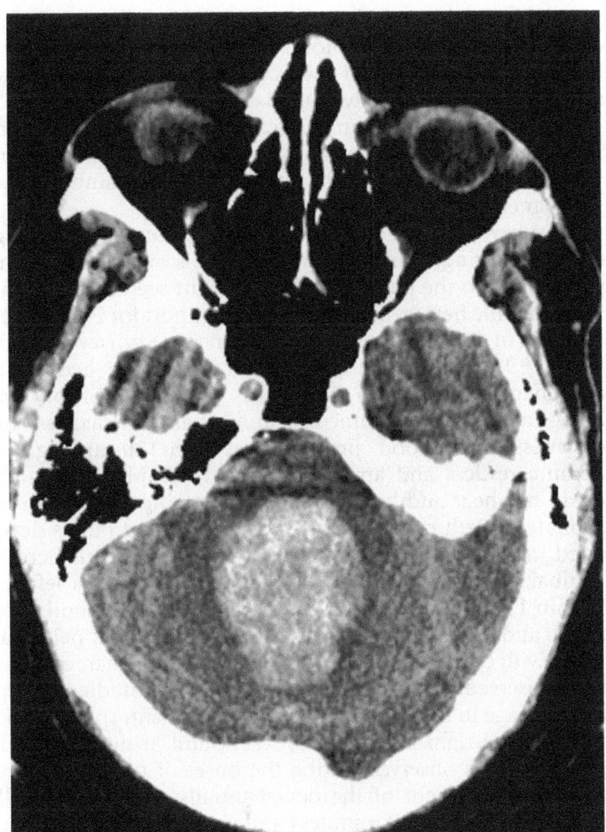

Figure 28-47. CT scan of large midline (vermian) cerebellar hemorrhage with extension into the fourth ventricle and compression of the tegmentum of the pons.

these patients experienced neurologic deterioration. Of interest, 60% of subjects in whom hematoma diameter was more than 3 cm but who had only moderate compression or normal size of the fourth ventricle did not require surgery for clot evacuation.

The uncommon midline (vermian) cerebellar hematoma still represents a serious diagnostic challenge, and its outcome is generally poor. Its frequency in autopsy series has been 6% of all cerebellar hemorrhages.[137] Our experience has documented syndromes featuring relatively early onset of coma, ophthalmoplegia, and respiratory abnormalities, and the severity of bilateral limb weakness has been variable. Early extension of the vermian hematoma into the midline pontine tegmentum is probably responsible for the abrupt onset of coma and bilateral oculomotor signs (Fig. 28-47). This variant of cerebellar hematoma carries a poor prognosis, similar to that of primary pontine hemorrhage. At times, a relatively small hematoma in this location results in fatal brainstem compression.

Midbrain Hemorrhage

Spontaneous, nontraumatic mesencephalic hemorrhage is rare. In most instances, the hemorrhage has dissected down from the thalamus or putamen, is part of a lesion originating in the cerebellum or pons, or arises from blood dyscrasias or AVMs.

Mesencephalic AVMs generally produce a stepwise progressive deterioration. Ataxia and ophthalmoplegia (especially third cranial nerve palsy and paralysis of upward gaze) are common. Aqueductal or third ventricular blockage or

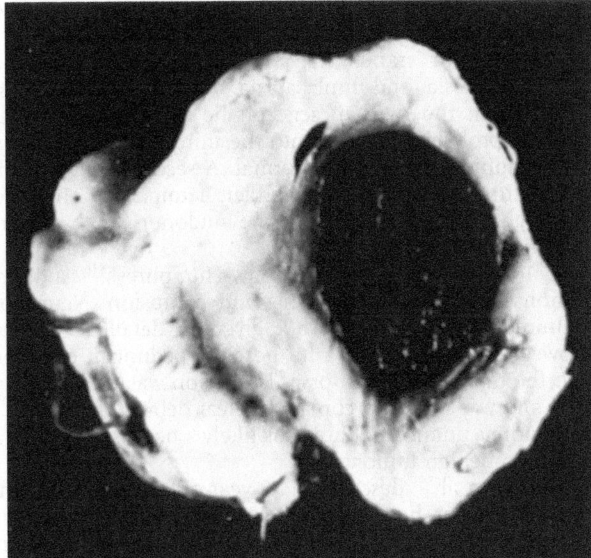

Figure 28-48. Midbrain hemorrhage in a patient with bleeding diathesis.

distension often leads to hydrocephalus. Bleeding diathesis can lead to isolated midbrain hemorrhage, as shown in Figure 28-48, a brain tissue specimen from an elderly woman with leukemia in whom a third cranial nerve palsy and contralateral intention tremor developed shortly before death. Hypertensive primary mesencephalic hemorrhage is very rare but does occur. One might predict that the hemorrhage would be in the tegmentum in the territory supplied by branches of the superior cerebellar arteries, as in the hypertensive patients reported by several groups.[543–545] The details of these cases follow.

Durward et al.[544] described two patients with mesencephalic hematomas. Their first patient was a 71-year-old hypertensive man (blood pressure 230/130 mm Hg) who suddenly could not stand or open his eyes. Signs included bilateral third cranial nerve paralysis, bulbar weakness, and extensor plantar responses. CT scan revealed a 1-cm hematoma in the ventral tegmentum of the midbrain with rupture into the third ventricle. He experienced obstructive hydrocephalus, which was treated with a ventriculoperitoneal shunt, and survived with bilateral third cranial nerve palsies and poor balance with a tendency to fall backward. Arteriographic findings were normal. Although there was no pathologic confirmation, this case may represent a primary hypertensive mesencephalic tegmental hematoma. The second patient was a normotensive young man who experienced Weber's syndrome (crossed third cranial nerve palsy and hemiparesis) after a week of prodromal headache. The CT scan showed a right midbrain hematoma. After further deterioration, the hematoma was surgically decompressed, and microscopic examination of the wall of the hematoma revealed an AVM. The patient survived but was grossly ataxic.

A 71-year-old patient reported by Morel-Maroger et al.[545] had midbrain hemorrhage due to hypertension. After being treated for hypertension for 5 years, he suddenly lost consciousness and awakened confused and dizzy. He had a diffuse headache and vomited. Clinical findings included a right third cranial nerve palsy, left hemiparesis, and a cerebellar-type ataxia of the right limbs. Blood pressure was 290/110 mm Hg. CT scan documented a 12 × 16-mm hematoma in the right superior cerebellar peduncle. The patient recovered after antihypertensive therapy without surgical intervention.

Roig et al.[543] described two patients with hypertensive mesencephalic hematomas detected on CT. One patient had an ipsilateral third cranial nerve paralysis with contralateral hemihypesthesia and limb ataxia. The hyperdense lesion was high in the right mesencephalic tegmentum near the midline, probably draining into the third ventricle. Vertebral angiographic findings were normal. A second patient had a right third cranial nerve palsy and left hemiparesis. The lesion was high in the right side of the midbrain. Both patients survived.

A 10-year-old boy reported by Humphreys[546] suddenly demonstrated right hemiparesis and confusion. Neuroophthalmologic findings were not given in detail. A CT scan showed a large hematoma in the basis pedunculi extending into the interpeduncular fossa. The lesion was drained surgically and was found to contain nuclear debris. The nature of the lesion is unknown, but it was likely a hemorrhage into an AVM or a benign tumor.

LaTorre et al.[547] described a 38-year-old woman who, after complaining of headache and intermittent diplopia for 2 years, vomited and demonstrated bilateral sixth cranial nerve palsies and paralysis of upward gaze. CSF was found to contain blood, and ventriculography visualized a beaded aqueduct and hydrocephalus. Surgical exploration of the midbrain discovered an AVM of the quadrigeminal plate with a blood clot embedded in the aqueduct.

A single patient was reported by Scoville and Poppen.[548] The 44-year-old woman experienced an ataxic right hemiparesis in stepwise fashion over 1.5 years. Vomiting, bilateral third cranial nerve paralysis, stupor, and pinpoint pupils suddenly supervened. After a blood clot was drained from her left cerebral peduncle, the patient awakened. Normal blood pressure and coagulation values and the gradual onset favored an AVM in this patient.

A number of further observations have stressed the presentation of small midbrain hemorrhages with features of isolated forms of ophthalmoplegia.[549–551] These have included isolated fourth[549] and third[550,551] nerve palsies as well as various combinations of a dorsal midbrain syndrome.[552,553] Most of these cases were remarkable for the absence or paucity of signs of long-tract involvement, stressing the fact that small midbrain ICHs can present with isolated ophthalmoplegia.

Pontine Hemorrhage

The early clinicopathologic observations in pontine hemorrhage correspond to those made by Fang and Foley[554] and later by Dinsdale,[137] who reviewed the necropsies at Boston City Hospital and found 511 ICHs among 19,093 autopsies, of which 30 were pontine (6%). Two-thirds of the patients in this autopsy series had been comatose when first seen, 13% vomited, and 78% were dead within 48 hours. One patient who survived for 23 days had a small hemorrhage in the right pontine tegmentum. All of the remainder had massive hemorrhages, usually in the midpons at the junction of the basis pontis and tegmentum that frequently spread rostrally into the midbrain; the hemorrhages almost never spread caudally to the medulla but frequently ruptured into the fourth ventricle.

In 1971 Fisher,[71] using serial sections from a patient with a massive fatal pontine hemorrhage, identified numerous small vessels with "fibrin globes," which he thought were related to the vascular rupture causing the hemorrhage. "From the gaping end of each of these torn vessels there protruded a large mass of platelets partially encircled by thin concentric layers of fibrin." He suggested that the primary hemorrhage led to pressure on surrounding vessels, which subsequently ruptured, causing a cascade or avalanche effect and producing gradual enlargement of the hematoma. Ross Russell[149] had demonstrated large asymptomatic fusiform enlargements on the penetrating vessels of the pons in patients with "atherosclerosis" and hypertensive vascular disease. Cole and Yates,[142] Rosenblum,[144] Fisher,[71] and Caplan[555] all explained bleeding in hypertensive patients as leakage from tiny penetrating vessels damaged by lipohyalinosis and containing small microaneurysms.

Kornyey[556] reported a patient whose pontine hemorrhage occurred during clinical observation; the slow march of signs was similar to the pattern of development seen in ganglionic and thalamic hemorrhages, providing support for Fisher's postulation of the slowly evolving avalanche. Kornyey's patient was a 39-year-old man referred for admission because of malignant hypertension. While his admission history was being taken, he complained of numb hands, weakness, and dizziness. His blood pressure was 245/170 mm Hg. He became restless and apprehensive and complained that he could not hear and had difficulty swallowing and breathing. A bilateral sixth cranial nerve palsy and dilated pupils developed, and his corneal reflexes disappeared. Speech became "bulbar," he was deaf, and he could not move his left leg. Within 15 minutes, the patient was comatose; the pupils were small, and the eyes were converged. Bilateral bulbar palsy, stiff limbs with exaggerated reflexes, and extensor plantar responses were observed. Two hours after onset, the patient died. A large hemorrhage in the tegmentum of the pons, with some spreading into the right basis pontis, was found at necropsy.[556] In other patients observed during the onset of pontine hemorrhage, development of the deficit usually evolved gradually over minutes (1 to 30 minutes) and was not as instantaneous as aneurysmal SAH.

In the pons, the largest penetrating arteries enter medially, arise perpendicular to the basilar artery, and course from the base to the tegmentum. Other small penetrating arteries originate from the short and long circumferential vessels and enter more laterally, also coursing from base to tegmentum. Some arteries enter the tegmentum laterally and course horizontally across it.[192] Because vessels in all of these sites are potentially susceptible to hypertensive damage and lipohyalinosis, they could theoretically also be sites for pontine bleeding. Silverstein[557,558] reviewed the pathologic material from Philadelphia General Hospital and confirmed that these sites (Fig. 28-49) were the usual regions of pontine hemorrhage. Of 50 cases, 28 were massive central hemorrhages presumably arising from large paramedian penetrators; 11 were more lateralized,

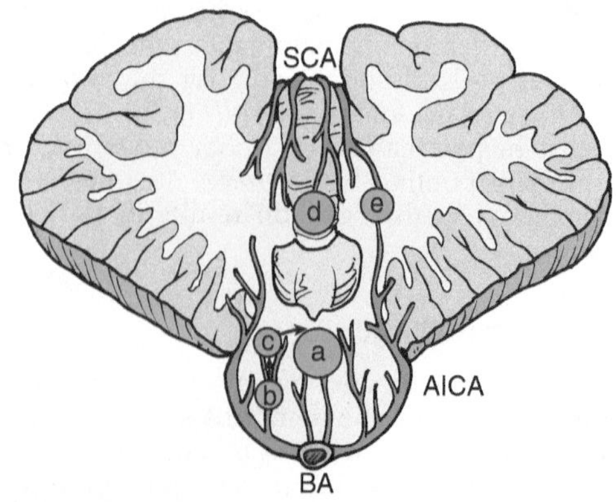

Figure 28-49. Schematic representation of common sites of hypertensive pontine and cerebellar hemorrhages: *a*, massive, paramedian pontine; *b*, basal pontine; *c*, lateral tegmental pontine; *d*, cerebellar vermian; *e*, cerebellar hemispheral. AICA, anterior–inferior cerebellar artery; BA, basilar artery; SCA, superior cerebellar artery.

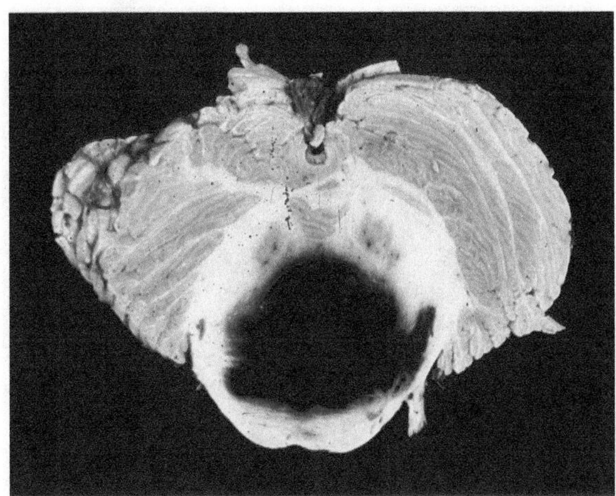

Figure 28-50. Massive pontine hemorrhage with dissection into brachium pontis and fourth ventricle.

usually spreading from base to tegmentum; and 11 had a tegmental location, of which four remained unilateral and seven involved the tegmentum bilaterally.

Not until the mid-1970s, when CT became available, was it possible to diagnose smaller nonfatal pontine hemorrhages accurately and to separate them positively from pontine infarction during life. MRI data, acquired through the use of gradient-echo sequences, indicate that pontine microhemorrhages tend to adopt a distribution similar to that of the large, symptomatic hemorrhages,[559] favoring the dorsal aspect of the basis pontis.

Large Paramedian Pontine Hemorrhage

Massive pontine hemorrhage results from rupture of parenchymal midpontine branches originating from the basilar artery. The bleeding vessel is thought to be a paramedian perforator in its distal portion,[137] causing initial hematoma formation at the junction of tegmentum and basis pontis,[137,558] from which the mass grows into its final round or oval shape and replaces most of both subdivisions of the pons (Fig. 28-50). The lesion usually begins in the middle of the pons and extends along the longitudinal axis of the brainstem into the lower midbrain. The hematoma may track into the middle cerebellar peduncles but usually does not extend caudally beyond the pontomedullary junction.[137] In the process of rapid hematoma expansion, destruction of tegmental and ventral pontine structures results, with the classic combination of signs caused by involvement of cranial nerve nuclei, long tracts, autonomic centers, and structures responsible for maintenance of consciousness. Large pontine hematomas also regularly rupture into the fourth ventricle.[137,557,558]

The classic form of pontine hemorrhage, bilateral and massive, is almost exclusively of hypertensive origin. Other etiologies, such as cryptic vascular malformation, account for 10% or less of the cases in most series.[137,558] Russell[560] regarded pontine hemorrhage as a form of ICH most likely to occur in patients with so-called malignant hypertension or hypertension associated with chronic nephropathy. Clinical presentation is characteristically one of rapid development of coma (80% of cases) without warning signs. Dana[561] recognized that some patients were conscious when first examined; in three different series, four of 19 patients (22%),[554] ten of 30 patients (33.3%),[137] and five of 50 patients (10%)[557,558] were alert when initially seen. By 48 hours, approximately 80% were dead.[137,554] In some patients (30%), a complaint of severe occipital headache preceded by minutes the catastrophic onset of coma.[557,562] Vomiting was noted in four of 30 (13%)[137] and four of 19 (22%)[554] patients in two series, occasionally being a prominent early symptom.

The frequency of seizures at onset, estimated to be as high as 22%,[557] probably represents a combination of true convulsive phenomena in rare instances, along with episodes of spasmodic decerebrate posturing and even the sometimes violent shivering associated with autonomic dysfunction and rapidly evolving hyperthermia. Some patients are seen before the development of coma with focal pontine signs, such as facial or limb numbness, deafness, diplopia, bilateral leg weakness, or progressive hemiparesis. Physical examination often reveals an abnormal respiratory rhythm or apnea.[137,558,563] Steegmann[563] analyzed these respiratory abnormalities in detail and reported a variety of abnormal respiratory patterns, including "inspiratory gasps of apneustic respiration," Cheyne-Stokes rhythm, slow and labored respirations, "gasping" respiration, and apnea. Two-thirds of his 17 patients exhibited either apnea or severely abnormal patterns of hypoventilation. Hyperthermia frequently coexisted, with temperatures above 39 °C in more than 80% of the patients,[562] in one-fourth of whom it reached levels of 42 °C to 43 °C,[557] usually in the preterminal stages. Neurologic findings characteristically result from involvement of cranial nerve nuclei and long tracts; they include quadriplegia with decerebrate posturing, bilateral Babinski signs, absence of corneal reflexes, pinpoint miotic pupils, and various forms of ophthalmoplegia.[184,562,563]

The oculomotor findings include miotic pinpoint pupils, absence of horizontal eye movements, and ocular bobbing. *Miotic pinpoint pupils* are usually about 1 mm in diameter. They react to light if a strong light source is used, and a tiny constriction can be detected with a magnifying lens.[475,532] Pontine hemorrhage can be confused with opiate poisoning.[563] The pupillary abnormality probably results from bilateral interruption of descending sympathetic pupillodilator fibers.[475,532] Because pupillary dilatation preceded miosis in Kornyey's[556] patient, it is possible that early stimulation of these fibers could lead to transient pupillary dilatation.

Absence of horizontal eye movements, detected with reflex testing with the doll's head maneuver or ice-water caloric stimulation, reflects bilateral injury of the paramedian pontine reticular formation. This sign occurs in partial forms or variants such as the *one-and-a-half syndrome*,[475] also referred to as *paralytic pontine exotropia*,[564] which represents a combination of unilateral horizontal gaze palsy plus ipsilateral internuclear ophthalmoplegia, resulting in one immobile eye and abduction preserved only in the contralateral one. It is more commonly seen in the smaller unilateral lesions from infarcts,[475,564] partial hematomas,[191,565,566] AVMs,[564] or tumors,[564] which result in unilateral involvement of the paramedian pontine reticular formation and the dorsally located ipsilateral medial longitudinal fasciculus. In one of our patients with a hematoma limited to the basis pontis, there was no voluntary horizontal gaze, but reflex movements were preserved. This situation, which has been described by Halsey et al.,[567] reflects damage to supranuclear fibers traveling with corticobulbar fibers in the pontine basis before they reach the tegmental paramedian pontine reticular formation.

Described by Fisher,[535] *ocular bobbing* denotes brisk movements of conjugate ocular depression, followed within seconds by a slower return to midposition. It occurs most commonly from a pontine lesion, either hemorrhage or infarction, although it has also been described in cerebellar hemorrhage.[259,535,568] Typically, it affects both eyes simultaneously and is accompanied by bilateral paralysis of horizontal gaze.[535] Atypical varieties include unilateral or markedly asymmetrical forms and those occurring when horizontal eye movements are still present.[535,568] The latter form is less strictly localizing to pontine disease, as it can be seen in cerebellar hemorrhage, SAH, and even coma of nonvascular mechanism.[535]

Weakness of pontine and bulbar musculature is invariable in the larger median hemorrhages but is difficult to assess because patients with bilateral tegmental damage are always comatose. Puffing of the cheeks with expiration, diminished eyelid tone, and pooling of secretions in the oropharynx are commonly observed. Deafness, dysarthria, dizziness, and facial numbness occasionally precede the development of coma. Facial weakness is often asymmetrical and may be associated with a crossed hemiplegia at the time the patient is first seen.[569]

Limb motor abnormalities are also always present in large tegmental–basal hemorrhages; usually it is quadriplegia with stiffness of all limbs. Hemiplegia was noted in four of 15 tegmental–basal hemorrhages by Goto et al.,[569] but was present in only three of 28 cases of bilateral hemorrhages reviewed by Silverstein.[557,558] The motor abnormality is usually bilateral with minor asymmetries. Asymmetries in decerebrate posturing, reflexes, or clonus are commonly detected. Tremor, shivering, restless limb movements, and dystonic postures have been common in our experience; patients may suddenly stiffen, giving the false impression of convulsive phenomena. Shivering occurs as the patient's condition worsens and can indicate failing motor function. Decerebrate posturing was noted in 12 of 15 patients reported by Goto et al.[569] Surprisingly, only two of the 28 patients in Silverstein's[557,558] series of large bilateral pontine hematomas were reported to have decerebrate rigidity, but 13 had flaccid quadriplegia, and ten had "generalized flaccidity."

Massive pontine hemorrhages are always fatal, although death does not come instantaneously. Steegmann[556] noted no deaths among 17 patients in less than 2 hours. Death usually occurs between 24 and 48 hours.[137,554,558,563] Survival for 2 to 10 days is not unusual and depends on the vigor of nursing and supportive care and the presence of complicating respiratory or urinary sepsis. Factors found to be early predictors of mortality include hyperthermia (temperature > 39 °C), tachycardia (heart rate > 110 beats/min), CT evidence of extension into midbrain and thalamus, and acute hydrocephalus.[570] Some patients with medium-sized hemorrhages survive.[570,571] On rare occasions, a patient has survived the surgical removal of a pontine and fourth ventricular clot,[565,572] which usually has been due to bleeding from a pontine AVM. Because the development of such lesions is so rapid, it is unlikely that surgical treatment could be provided early enough in the larger hemorrhages to be helpful. No other medical or surgical therapy seems likely to help these grave lesions.

Unilateral Basal or Basotegmental Hemorrhages

Unilateral basal or basotegmental hemorrhages are less common than the large paramedian lesions already discussed. In his autopsy-based series, Silverstein[558] described 11 such lesions (22%); three were limited to the base, and eight were basotegmental. The larger lesions ruptured into the fourth ventricle. Reports based on CT scans have shown more restricted syndromes,[524,573] increasing the range of causes of a pure motor syndrome. Gobernado et al.[574] described a hypertensive woman with the gradual development over 3 days of a pure motor hemiplegia affecting the right arm and leg, sparing the face. A CT scan defined a small hematoma limited to the base of the left pons. Another patient with a small hematoma confined to the right basis pontis had an "ataxic hemiparesis" of the left limbs.[575] Small unilateral hematomas limited to the base manifest as syndromes indistinguishable from lacunar infarction in the same region (Fig. 28-51). Tuhrim et al.[576] reported a patient with dysarthria, limb ataxia, and extensor plantar response due to a small basal pontine hematoma; although they labeled this case dysarthria–clumsy hand syndrome, it more closely resembles ataxic hemiparesis.[141]

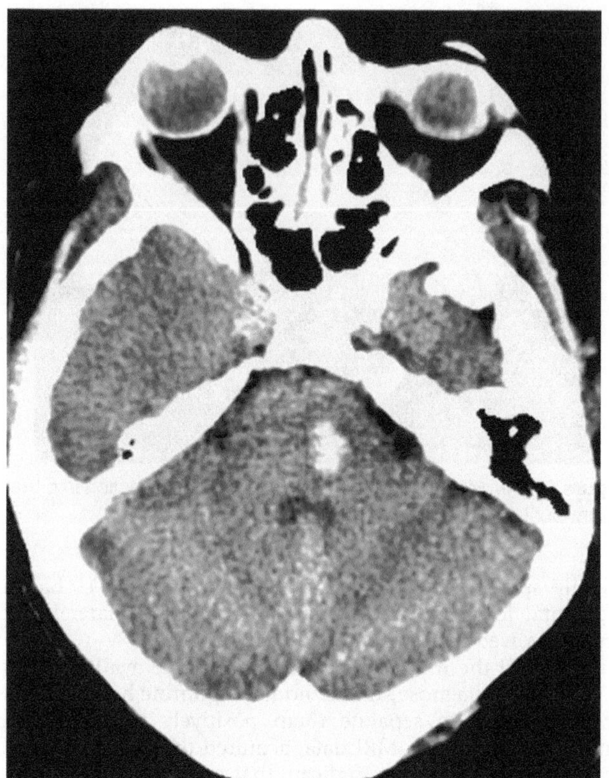

Figure 28-51. CT scan of a small left basal paramedian pontine hemorrhage.

Bleeding originating from a pontine penetrating artery may start in the basis pontis but also frequently dissects dorsally into the tegmentum. When the lesion spreads to the tegmentum, an ipsilateral facial palsy and conjugate gaze or sixth cranial nerve palsy often accompanies the contralateral hemiplegia.[577] Larger unilateral lesions may rupture into the fourth ventricle after spreading within the tegmentum (Fig. 28-52). In Silverstein's series,[558] these larger unilateral basotegmental lesions usually lead to hemiplegia, coma, and death.

Lateral Tegmental Brainstem Hematomas

Lateral tegmental brainstem hematomas usually originate from vessels penetrating into the brainstem from long circumferential branches. They enter the tegmentum laterally and course medially. Small hematomas remain confined to the lateral tegmentum, and larger lesions spread across to the opposite side and can destroy the entire tegmentum. Neurologic examination reveals a predominantly unilateral tegmental lesion with variable degrees of basilar involvement.[191,192] Oculomotor abnormalities, especially the "one-and-a-half syndrome," horizontal gaze palsy, internuclear ophthalmoplegia, partial involvement of vertical eye movements, and ocular bobbing, have been described.[191,192,571,577–579] The tegmental location of the spinothalamic tract makes sensory symptoms common. Ataxia, either unilateral or bilateral, may also accompany the oculomotor signs.[191,192] Action tremor has developed as the transient hemiparesis improves; this observation can be possibly explained by involvement of the red nucleus or its connections.[192] Facial numbness, ipsilateral miosis, and hemiparesis have also been noted.[191,192] Two

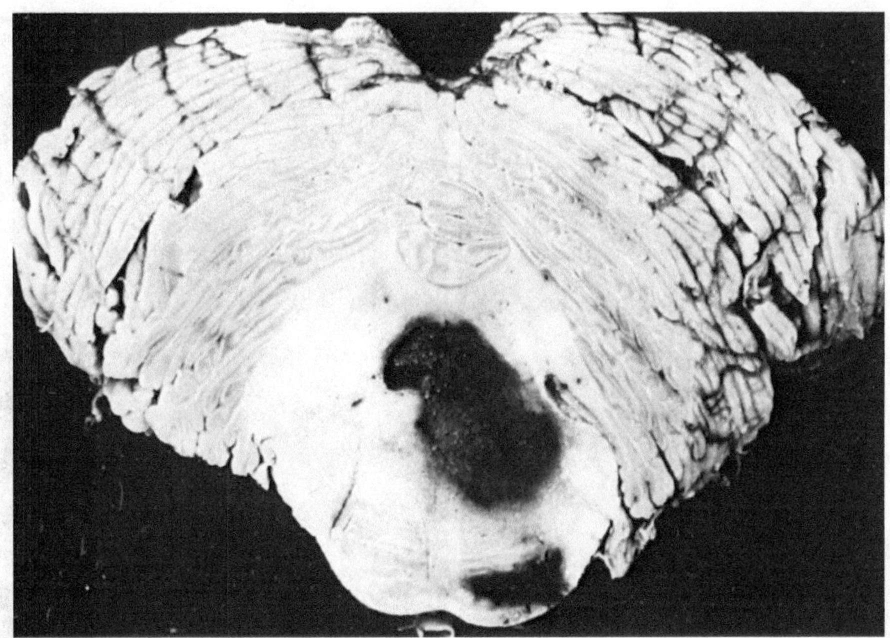

Figure 28-52. Unilateral basotegmental pontine hemorrhage with rupture into the fourth ventricle.

TABLE 28-11 Tegmental Pontine Hemorrhages

Study	Extraocular Movements	Motor	Sensory	Other Cranial Nerves	Cerebellar
		Computed Tomography Diagnosis			
Caplan and Goodwin[192]	No vertical, R gaze, R 6th, bilat. INO	L ↑ toe	L ↓ pin	R 7th, dysarthria, ptosis	Ataxia R > L
Caplan and Goodwin[192]	"1½," vertical nystagmus	L hemip, ↑ ↑ toes	L ↓ pin	R 7th, 8th, ptosis, dysarthria	Ataxia L > R
Müller et al.[524]	R INO	L hemip, ↑ ↑ toes	L ↓ pin	R 5th, 7th	–
Kase et al.[191]	"1½," No ↑ gaze	R hemip	R ↓ pin and joint position sense	Dysarthria, L 7th	Ataxia L
Kase et al.[191]	L INO and 6th, R 4th, bobbing	R hemip	R ↓ pin	Dysphagia, L 7th	Ataxia R & L
		Autopsy Cases			
Caplan and Goodwin[192]	"1½," bobbing, OD ↓ & inward	L hemip, Babinski	L ↓ pin	Dysarthria	Ataxia R>L
Tyler and Johnson[578]	No horizontal or ↑ gaze, bobbing, skew	L hemip, ↑ ↑ toes	L ↓ pin	R 5th, 7th, dysarthria, dysphagia, ptosis	R tremor
Dinsdale[137]	R gaze palsy	L hemip	L ↓ pin	R 7th, 8th	–
Silverstein[558]	R gaze palsy	L hemip, ↑ ↑ toes	L ↓ pin	R 7th, ptosis, dysphagia	–
Pierrott-Deseilligny et al.[566]	"1½"	L hemip, ↑ ↑ toes	L hemis	R 5th, 7th, 8th	Ataxia R arm

Hemip, hemiparesis; hemis, hemisensory syndrome; INO, internuclear ophthalmoplegia; OD, right eye; "1½" the "one-and-one-half" syndrome; R, right; L, left.

patients[191] developed Cheyne-Stokes respirations, one of the short-cycle type,[415,532] the other of the classic variety. Table 28-11 reviews some reported examples of tegmental pontine hematomas.[137,191,192,534,558,566,578]

We examined two patients with tegmental pontine hemorrhage, and Lawrence and Lightfoote[580] studied a patient with a pontine AVM; all three patients showed vertical pendular ocular oscillations with dizziness and vertical oscillopsia weeks after the hemorrhage. Delayed pain in the contralateral limbs, as in the thalamic pain syndrome, began during recovery from a unilateral tegmental hemorrhage in another patient. We have also observed "palatal myoclonus" as a sequela of lateral tegmental hematomas.

Medullary Hemorrhage

Hemorrhage into the medulla oblongata (Fig. 28-53) is even less frequent than hemorrhage into the midbrain.

Arseni and Stanciu[581] described a 40-year-old woman with dizziness, vomiting, and headache with diplopia and right limb paresthesias. She suddenly became somnolent and ataxic, with a stiff neck, left hemiparesis, diminished pain and temperature sensation on the left side of the face, left limb ataxia, nystagmus, dysphonia, and dysphagia. Surgical exploration found a hematoma on the floor of the fourth ventricle laterally. After drainage of the clot, the patient was said to do well.

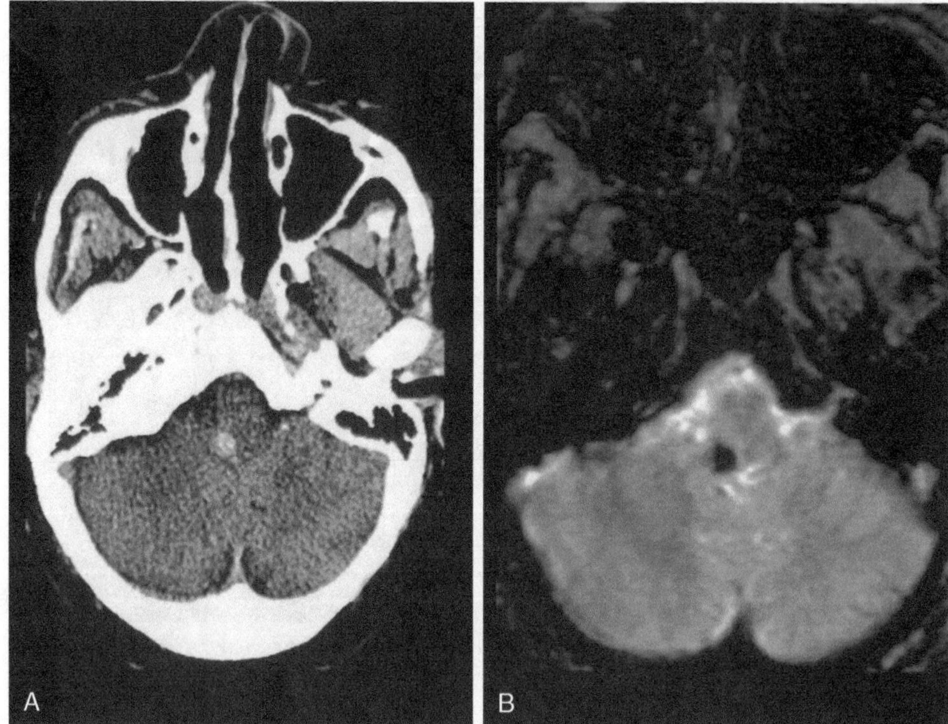

Figure 28-53. Right dorsolateral medullary hemorrhage on CT scan (A) and gradient-echo MR image (B).

Kempe[582] reported on a similar patient who had a lateral medullary hematoma. The 25-year-old woman noted diminished hearing on the left and then suddenly became ill with headache, vomiting, vertigo, and hiccups. She was ataxic and fell to the left. Findings included left nystagmus, diminished pain and temperature sensation on the left side of the face, and left facial weakness; the left ear was deaf and unreactive to caloric stimuli. Pneumoencephalography documented a defect in the rhomboid fossa of the fourth ventricle, which at surgical exploration was found to be a clot bulging through the floor of the fourth ventricle medial to the restiform body. Both this patient and the one described by Arseni and Stanciu[581] had findings similar to those in patients with lateral medullary infarcts, and each had a stepwise course. Arteriography was not performed, and CT and MRI were not available. We suspect that the underlying process in both patients was a cavernous angioma.

In another patient,[415] the explanation was an AVM. At age 37, the woman experienced weakness and decreased position sense in her left arm and leg. Right vocal cord and hypoglossal paralysis developed at age 60, and 2 years later, she became gradually and then abruptly worse and was hypertensive. Necropsy revealed a hemorrhage in the medial medullary tegmentum with spreading into the dorsal medulla and right lateral medulla.

Mastaglia et al.[583] reported two cases of medullary hemorrhage with quite different clinical features. In one case, an 87-year-old hypertensive woman was found unconscious with a right gaze palsy, right facial weakness, and left hemiplegia. The hemorrhage was largest in the lateral pons and descended into the medullary pyramid. The cause seems to have been a pontine basal–tegmental hemorrhage with unusual caudal dissection, but its clinical picture did not differ from that already described in unilateral pontine hemorrhage. The other patient was hypertensive and had been undergoing anticoagulation with warfarin. She demonstrated an unusual clinical picture consisting of markedly decreased postural sensation and incoordination of her left arm and leg, diminished left arm reflexes, numbness over the right eye, and subjective numbness of the right limbs. Autopsy showed a hemorrhage into the rostral spinal cord with dissection into the left medullary pyramid. The most likely etiologic factor in this patient was anticoagulation, perhaps compounded by hypertension.

There is one well-documented case of medullary hemorrhage due to hypertension, but whether the hemorrhage arose in the medulla or arose in the caudal pontine tegmentum and dissected into the medulla is not certain.[540] The patient, a 56-year-old, previously hypertensive man, experienced difficulty swallowing, and examination found paralysis of the left side of the face, soft palate, vocal cord, and tongue. A left Horner's syndrome, deafness in the left ear, and paresthesias of the right limbs were also found. CT scan showed a left medullary tegmental hematoma, but the signs of deafness and facial palsy might indicate some pontine involvement.

Barinagarrementeria and Cantú[584] described four cases of their own and reviewed 12 others from the literature. The characteristic profile was one of sudden onset of headache, vertigo, dysphagia, dysphonia or dysarthria, and limb incoordination. Common findings on examination were palatal weakness (88%); nystagmus, cerebellar ataxia, or both (75%); limb weakness (68%); and hypoglossal nerve palsy (56%). Less common signs were facial palsy and Horner's syndrome. The mechanism of the medullary hemorrhage could be determined in only seven of the 16 patients, corresponding to ruptured vascular malformation (three), hypertension (three), and anticoagulation treatment (one). The mortality rate for the group was 19% (three of 16), and in most of the survivors, residual neurologic deficits were either mild (56%) or absent (19%).

Unusual presentations of medullary hemorrhage have included a patient with isolated hiccups from a small dorsal ICH,[585] and a second patient with dorsolateral hemorrhage into an area of infarction[586] who was seen initially with features of Wallenberg's syndrome.

The complete reference list can be found on the companion Expert Consult website at www.expertconsult.inkling.com.

KEY REFERENCES

2. Mohr JP, Caplan LR, Melski JW, et al. The Harvard Cooperative Stroke Registry: A prospective registry. Neurology 1978;28:754.
7. Bamford J, Sandercock P, Dennis M, et al. A prospective study of acute cerebrovascular disease in the community: The Oxfordshire Community Stroke Project, 1981–86. 2: Incidence, case fatality rates and overall outcome at one year of cerebral infarction, primary intracerebral and subarachnoid haemorrhage. J Neurol Neurosurg Psychiatry 1990;53:16.
12. O'Donnell MJ, Xavier D, Liu L, et al. Risk factors for ischaemic and intracerebral haemorrhagic stroke in 22 countries (the INTERSTROKE study): a case-control study. Lancet 2010;376:112.
13. Broderick J, Brott T, Tomsick T, et al. The risk of subarachnoid and intracerebral hemorrhages in blacks as compared with whites. N Engl J Med 1992;326:733.
16. Brott T, Thalinger K, Hertzberg V. Hypertension as a risk factor for spontaneous intracerebral hemorrhage. Stroke 1986;17:1078.
20. van Asch CJ, Luitse MJ, Rinkel GJ, et al. Incidence, case fatality, and functional outcome of intracerebral haemorrhage over time, according to age, sex, and ethnic origin: a systematic review and meta-analysis. Lancet Neurol 2010;9:167.
30. Qureshi AI, Suri MAK, Safdar K, et al. Intracerebral hemorrhage in blacks: Risk factors, subtypes, and outcomes. Stroke 1997;28:961.
38. Juvela S, Hillbom M, Palomaki H. Risk factors for spontaneous intracerebral hemorrhage. Stroke 1995;26:1558.
39. Kurth T, Kase CS, Berger K, et al. Smoking and risk of hemorrhagic stroke in women. Stroke 2003;34:2792.
40. Kurth T, Kase CS, Berger K, et al. Smoking and the risk of hemorrhagic stroke in men. Stroke 2003;34:1151.
45. Amarenco P, Bogousslavsky J, Callahan A 3rd, et al. High-dose atorvastatin after stroke or transient ischemic attack. N Engl J Med 2006;355:549.
61. Greenberg SM, Vonsattel J-PG. Diagnosis of cerebral amyloid angiopathy: Sensitivity and specificity of cortical biopsy. Stroke 1997;28:1418.
65. Vinters HV, Gilbert JJ. Cerebral amyloid angiopathy: Incidence and complications in the aging brain. II: The distribution of amyloid vascular changes. Stroke 1983;14:924.
67. Vinters HV. Cerebral amyloid angiopathy: A critical review. Stroke 1987;18:311.
70. Greenberg SM, Briggs ME, Hyman BT, et al. Apolipoprotein E ε4 is associated with the presence and earlier onset of hemorrhage in cerebral amyloid angiopathy. Stroke 1996;27:1333.
71. Fisher CM. Pathological observations in hypertensive cerebral hemorrhage. J Neuropathol Exp Neurol 1971;30:536.
73. Massaro AR, Sacco RL, Mohr JP, et al. Clinical discriminators of lobar and deep hemorrhages: The Stroke Data Bank. Neurology 1991;41:1881.
74. Broderick J, Brott T, Tomsick T, et al. Lobar hemorrhage in the elderly: The undiminishing importance of hypertension. Stroke 1993;24:49.
75. Woo D, Sauerbeck LR, Kissela BM, et al. Genetic and environmental risk factors for intracerebral hemorrhage: Preliminary results of a population-based study. Stroke 2002;33:1190.
83. Kimberly WT, Gilson A, Rost NS, et al. Silent ischemic infarcts are associated with hemorrhage burden in cerebral amyloid angiopathy. Neurology 2009;72:1230.
84. Smith EE, Schneider JA, Wardlaw JM, et al. Cerebral microinfarcts: the invisible lesions. Lancet Neurol 2012;11:272.
85. Greenberg SM, Grabowski T, Gurol ME, et al. Detection of isolated cerebrovascular beta-amyloid with Pittsburgh compound B. Ann Neurol 2008;64:587.
88. Vonsattel JP, Myers RH, Hedley-Whyte ET, et al. Cerebral amyloid angiopathy without and with cerebral hemorrhages: A comparative histological study. Ann Neurol 1991;30:637.
90. Greenberg SM, Vonsattel JP, Stakes JW, et al. The clinical spectrum of cerebral amyloid angiopathy: Presentations without lobar hemorrhage. Neurology 1993;43:2073.
91. Smith DB, Hitchcock M, Philpott PJ. Cerebral amyloid angiopathy presenting as transient ischemic attacks: Case report. J Neurosurg 1985;63:963.
93. Charidimou A, Peeters A, Fox Z, et al. Spectrum of transient focal neurological episodes in cerebral amyloid angiopathy: multicentre magnetic resonance imaging cohort study and meta-analysis. Stroke 2012;43:2324.
95. Alberts MJ. Stroke genetics update. Stroke 2003;34:342.
103. Gould DB, Phalan FC, van Mil SE, et al. Role of COL4A1 in small-vessel disease and hemorrhagic stroke. N Engl J Med 2006;354:1489.
116. Natte R, Vinters HV, Maat-Schieman ML, et al. Microvasculopathy is associated with the number of cerebrovascular lesions in hereditary cerebral hemorrhage with amyloidosis, Dutch type. Stroke 1998;29:1588.
118. Grabowski TJ, Cho HS, Vonsattel JPG, et al. Novel amyloid precursor protein mutation in an Iowa family with dementia and severe cerebral amyloid angiopathy. Ann Neurol 2001;49:697.
122. McCarron MO, Nicoll JA, Stewart J, et al. Absence of cystatin C mutation in sporadic cerebral amyloid angiopathy-related hemorrhage. Neurology 2000;54:242.
124. Olichney JM, Hansen LA, Galasko D, et al. The apolipoprotein E epsilon 4 allele is associated with increased neuritic plaques and cerebral amyloid angiopathy in Alzheimer's disease and Lewy body variant. Neurology 1996;47:190.
125. Greenberg SM, Vonsattel JP, Segal AZ, et al. Association of apolipoprotein E epsilon2 and vasculopathy in cerebral amyloid angiopathy. Neurology 1998;50:961.
127. O'Donnell HC, Rosand J, Knudsen KA, et al. Apolipoprotein E genotype and the risk of recurrent lobar intracerebral hemorrhage. N Engl J Med 2000;342:240.
128. Fisher CM. The pathology and pathogenesis of intracerebral hemorrhage. In: Fields WS, editor. Pathogenesis and Treatment of Cerebrovascular Disease. Springfield, IL: Charles C Thomas; 1961. p. 295.
130. Biffi A, Anderson CD, Jagiella JM, et al. APOE genotype and extent of bleeding and outcome in lobar intracerebral haemorrhage: a genetic association study. Lancet Neurol 2011;10:702.
132. Kase CS, Williams JP, Wyatt DA, et al. Lobar intracerebral hematomas: Clinical and CT analysis of 22 cases. Neurology 1982;32:1146.
136. Walshe TM, Davis KR, Fisher CM. Thalamic hemorrhage: A computed tomographic-clinical correlation. Neurology 1977;27:217.
138. Fisher CM, Picard EH, Polak A, et al. Acute hypertensive cerebellar hemorrhage: Diagnosis and surgical treatment. J Nerv Ment Dis 1965;140:38.
142. Cole FM, Yates PO. Intracranial microaneurysms and small cerebrovascular lesions. Brain 1967;90:759.
146. Charcot JM, Bouchard C. Nouvelles recherches sur la pathogénie de l'hémorragie cérébrale. Arch Physiol Norm Pathol 1868;1:110.
149. Ross Russell RW. Observations on intracerebral aneurysms. Brain 1963;86:425.
153. Kelley RE, Berger JR, Scheinberg P, et al. Active bleeding in hypertensive intracerebral hemorrhage: Computed tomography. Neurology 1982;32:852.
154. Broderick JP, Brott TG, Tomsick T, et al. Ultra-early evaluation of intracerebral hemorrhage. J Neurosurg 1990;72:195.
156. Fujii Y, Tanaka R, Takeuchi S, et al. Hematoma enlargement in spontaneous intracerebral hemorrhage. J Neurosurg 1994;80:51.
158. Brott T, Broderick J, Kothari R, et al. Early hemorrhage growth in patients with intracerebral hemorrhage. Stroke 1997;28:1.
159. Wada R, Aviv RI, Fox AJ, et al. CT angiography "spot sign" predicts hematoma expansion in acute intracerebral hemorrhage. Stroke 2007;38:1257.
160. Goldstein JN, Fazen LE, Snider R, et al. Contrast extravasation on CT angiography predicts hematoma expansion in intracerebral hemorrhage. Neurology 2007;68:889.
161. Demchuk AM, Dowlatshahi D, Rodriguez-Luna D, et al. Prediction of haematoma growth and outcome in patients with intracerebral haemorrhage using the CT-angiography spot sign (PREDICT): a prospective observational study. Lancet Neurol 2012;11:307.
163. Romero JM, Brouwers HB, Lu J, et al. Prospective validation of the computed tomographic angiography spot sign score for intracerebral hemorrhage. Stroke 2013;44:3097.
164. Thompson AL, Kosior JC, Gladstone DJ, et al. Defining the CT angiography "spot sign" in primary intracereberal hemorrhage. Can J Neurol Sci 2009;36:456.
165. Delgado Almandoz JE, Yoo AJ, Stone MJ, et al. Systematic characterization of the computed tomography angiography spot sign

in primary intracerebral hemorrhage identifies patients at highest risk for hematoma expansion: the spot sign score. Stroke 2009;40:2994.
173. Broderick J, Brott TG, Duldner JE, et al. Volume of intracerebral hemorrhage: A powerful and easy-to-use predictor of 30-day mortality. Stroke 1993;24:987.
174. Kothari RU, Brott T, Broderick JP, et al. The ABCs of measuring intracerebral hemorrhage volumes. Stroke 1996;27:1304.
179. Ziai WC. Hematology and inflammatory signaling of intracerebral hemorrhage. Stroke 2013;44:S74.
187. Stein RW, Kase CS, Hier DB, et al. Caudate hemorrhage. Neurology 1984;34:1549.
190. Ropper AH, Davis KR. Lobar cerebral hemorrhages: Acute clinical syndromes in 26 cases. Ann Neurol 1980;8:141.
191. Kase CS, Maulsby GO, Mohr JP. Partial pontine hematomas. Neurology 1980;30:652.
192. Caplan LR, Goodwin JA. Lateral tegmental brainstem hemorrhages. Neurology 1982;32:252.
194. González-Duarte A, Cantú C, Ruiz-Sandoval JL, et al. Recurrent primary cerebral hemorrhage: Frequency, mechanisms, and prognosis. Stroke 1802;29:1998.
197. Weisberg L. Multiple spontaneous intracerebral hematomas: Clinical and computed tomographic correlations. Neurology 1981;31:897.
198. Bailey RD, Hart RG, Benavente O, et al. Recurrent brain hemorrhage is more frequent than ischemic stroke after intracranial hemorrhage. Neurology 2001;56:773.
199. Biffi A, Halpin A, Towfighi A, et al. Aspirin and recurrent intracerebral hemorrhage in cerebral amyloid angiopathy. Neurology 2010;75:693.
200. García JH, Ho KL, Caccamo DV. Intracerebral hemorrhage: Pathology of selected topics. In: Kase CS, Caplan LR, editors. Intracerebral Hemorrhage. Boston: Butterworth-Heinemann; 1994. p. 45.
205. Mann DM, Iwatsubo T, Ihara Y, et al. Predominant deposition of amyloid-beta 42(43) in plaques in cases of Alzheimer's disease and hereditary cerebral hemorrhage associated with mutations in the amyloid precursor protein gene. Am J Pathol 1996;148:1257.
206. Alonzo NC, Hyman BT, Rebeck GW, et al. Progression of cerebral amyloid angiopathy: Accumulation of amyloid-β40 in already affected vessels. J Neuropathol Exp Neurol 1998;57:353.
208. Cho HS, Hyman BT, Greenberg SM, et al. Quantitation of apoE domains in Alzheimer disease brain suggests a role for apoE in Abeta aggregation. J Neuropathol Exp Neurol 2001;60:342.
216. Weller RO, Massey A, Newman TA, et al. Cerebral amyloid angiopathy: Amyloid beta accumulates in putative interstitial fluid drainage pathways in Alzheimer's disease. Am J Pathol 1998;153: 725.
218. Delaney P, Estes M. Intracranial hemorrhage with amphetamine abuse. Neurology 1980;30:1125.
228. Kase CS, Foster TE, Reed JE, et al. Intracerebral hemorrhage and phenylpropanolamine use. Neurology 1987;37:399.
229. Kernan WN, Viscoli CM, Brass LM, et al. Phenylpropanolamine and the risk of hemorrhagic stroke. N Engl J Med 1826;343: 2000.
237. Levine SR, Brust JCM, Futrell N, et al. Cerebrovascular complications of the use of the "crack" form of alkaloid cocaine. N Engl J Med 1990;323:699.
241. Little JR, Dial B, Bellanger G, et al. Brain hemorrhage from intracranial tumor. Stroke 1979;10:283.
242. Scott M. Spontaneous intracerebral hematoma caused by cerebral neoplasms: Report of eight verified cases. J Neurosurg 1975; 42:338.
257. Kase CS, Robinson RK, Stein RW, et al. Anticoagulant-related intracerebral hemorrhage. Neurology 1985;35:943.
258. Rådberg JA, Olsson JE, Rådberg CT. Prognostic parameters in spontaneous intracranial hematomas with special reference to anticoagulant treatment. Stroke 1991;22:571.
259. Ott KH, Kase CS, Ojemann RG, et al. Cerebellar hemorrhage: Diagnosis and treatment. Arch Neurol 1974;31:160.
260. Franke CL, deJonge J, van Swieten JC, et al. Intracerebral hematomas during anticoagulant treatment. Stroke 1990;21:726.
261. Hart RG, Boop BS, Anderson DC. Oral anticoagulants and intracranial hemorrhage. Stroke 1995;26:1471.
264. Hylek EM, Singer DE. Risk factors for intracranial hemorrhage in outpatients taking warfarin. Ann Intern Med 1994;120:897.
268. Smith EE, Rosand J, Knudsen KA, et al. Leukoaraiosis is associated with warfarin-related hemorrhage following ischemic stroke. Neurology 2002;59:193.
271. The Stroke Prevention In Reversible Ischemia Trial (SPIRIT) Study Group. A randomized trial of anticoagulants versus aspirin after cerebral ischemia of presumed arterial origin. Ann Neurol 1997;42:857.
274. Shoamanesh A, Kwok CS, Benavente O. Cerebral microbleeds: histopathological correlation of neuroimaging. Cerebrovasc Dis 2011;32:528.
275. Soo YO, Yang SR, Lam WW, et al. Risk vs benefit of antithrombotic therapy in ischaemic stroke patients with cerebral microbleeds. J Neurol 2008;255:1679.
279. Filibotte JJ, Hagan N, O'Donnell J, et al. Warfarin, hematoma expansion, and outcome of intracerebral hemorrhage. Neurology 2004;63:1059.
280. Rosand J, Hylek EM, O'Donnell HC, et al. Warfarin-associated hemorrhage and cerebral amyloid angiopathy: A genetic and pathologic study. Neurology 2000;55:947.
283. Fisher CM, Adams RD. Observations on brain embolism with special reference to the mechanism of hemorrhagic infarction. J Neuropathol Exp Neurol 1951;10:92.
286. Chamorro A, Villa N, Saiz A, et al. Early anticoagulation after large cerebral embolic infarction: A safety study. Neurology 1995;45:861.
290. Chamorro A, Busse O, Obach V, et al. The Rapid Anticoagulation Prevents Ischemic Damage study in acute stroke: Final results from the Writing Committee. Cerebrovasc Dis 2005;19:402.
297. Lauer A, Pfeilschifter W, Schaffer CB, et al. Intracerebral haemorrhage associated with antithrombotic treatment: translational insights from experimental studies. Lancet Neurol 2013;12:394.
299. Gore JM, Sloan M, Price TR, et al. Intracerebral hemorrhage, cerebral infarction, and subdural hematoma after acute myocardial infarction and thrombolytic therapy in the Thrombolysis in Myocardial Infarction Study: Thrombolysis in myocardial infarction, phase II, pilot and clinical data. Circulation 1991;83:448.
301. Kase CS, Pessin MS, Zivin JA, et al. Intracranial hemorrhage following coronary thrombolysis with tissue plasminogen activator. Am J Med 1992;92:384.
303. Sloan MA, Price TR, Petito CK, et al. Clinical features and pathogenesis of intracerebral hemorrhage after rt-PA and heparin therapy for acute myocardial infarction: The Thrombolysis in Myocardial Infarction (TIMI) II pilot and randomized clinical trial combined experience. Neurology 1995;45:649.
314. Alvarez-Sabin J, Maisterra O, Santamarina E, et al. Factors influencing haemorrhagic transformation in ischaemic stroke. Lancet Neurol 2013;12:689.
315. Hacke W, Kaste M, Fieschi C, et al. Intravenous thrombolysis with recombinant tissue plasminogen activator for acute hemispheric stroke: The European Cooperative Acute Stroke Study (ECASS). JAMA 1995;274:1017.
319. Ogata J, Yutani C, Imakita M, et al. Hemorrhagic infarct of the brain without a reopening of the occluded arteries in cardioembolic stroke. Stroke 1989;20:876.
326. Wang X, Tsuji K, Lee SR, et al. Mechanisms of hemorrhagic transformation after tissue plasminogen activator reperfusion therapy for ischemic stroke. Stroke 2004;35:2726.
327. Pessin MS, del Zoppo GJ, Estol CJ. Thrombolytic agents in the treatment of stroke. Clin Neuropharmacol 1990;13:271.
328. del Zoppo GJ, Poeck K, Pessin MS, et al. Recombinant tissue plasminogen activator in acute thrombotic and embolic stroke. Ann Neurol 1992;32:78.
330. The National Institute of Neurological Disorders and Stroke rt-PA Stroke Study Group. Tissue plasminogen activator for acute ischemic stroke. N Engl J Med 1995;333:1581.
331. The NINDS: t-PA Stroke Study Group. Intracerebral hemorrhage after intravenous t-PA therapy for ischemic stroke. Stroke 1997; 28:2109.
342. Bruno A, Levine SR, Frankel MR, et al. Admission glucose level and clinical outcomes in the NINDS rt-PA stroke trial. Neurology 2002;59:669.
343. Montaner J, Molina CA, Monasterio J, et al. Matrix metalloproteinase-9 pretreatment level predicts intracranial

hemorrhagic complications after thrombolysis in human stroke. Circulation 2003;107:598.
345. Castellanos M, Leira R, Serena J, et al. Plasma cellular-fibronectin concentration predicts hemorrhagic transformation after thrombolytic therapy in acute ischemic stroke. Stroke 2004;35:1671.
346. Mendioroz M, Fernández-Cadenas I, Alvarez-Sabín J, et al. Endogenous activated protein C predicts hemorrhagic transformation and mortality after tissue plasminogen activator treatment in stroke patients. Cerebrovasc Dis 2009;28:143.
348. Ribo M, Montaner J, Molina CA, et al. Admission fibrinolytic profile is associated with symptomatic hemorrhagic transformation in stroke patients treated with tissue plasminogen activator. Stroke 2004;35:2123.
356. Del Zoppo GJ, Higashida RT, Furlan AJ, et al. PROACT: A phase II randomized trial of recombinant pro-urokinase by direct arterial delivery in acute middle cerebral artery stroke. Stroke 1998; 29:4.
357. Furlan A, Higashida R, Wechsler L, et al. Intra-arterial prourokinase for acute ischemic stroke: The PROACT II Study: A randomized controlled trial. JAMA 2003;282:1999.
358. Kase CS, Furlan AJ, Wechsler LR, et al. Symptomatic intracerebral hemorrhage after intra-arterial thrombolysis with prourokinase in acute ischemic stroke: The PROACT II trial. Neurology 2001; 57:1603.
359. Kidwell CS, Saver JL, Villablanca JP, et al. Magnetic resonance imaging detection of microbleeds before thrombolysis: an emerging application. Stroke 2002;33:95.
360. Shoamanesh A, Kwok CS, Lim PA, et al. Postthrombolysis intracranial hemorrhage risk of cerebral microbleeds in acute stroke patients: a systematic review and meta-analysis. Int J Stroke 2013;8:348.
362. Linfante I, Llinas RH, Caplan LR, et al. MRI features of intracerebral hemorrhage within two hours from symptom onset. Stroke 1999;30:2263.
368. Fazekas F, Kleinert R, Roob G, et al. Histopathologic analysis of foci of signal loss on gradient-echo T2*-weighted MR images in patients with spontaneous intracerebral hemorrhage: evidence of microangiopathy-related microbleeds. AJNR Am J Neuroradiol 1999;20:637.
370. Cordonnier C, Al-Shahi Salman R, Wardlaw J. Spontaneous brain microbleeds: systematic review, subgroup analyses and standards for study design and reporting. Brain 2007;130:1988.
371. Greenberg SM, Finklestein SP, Schaefer PW. Petechial hemorrhages accompanying lobar hemorrhage: Detection by gradient-echo MRI. Neurology 1996;46:1751.
375. Greenberg SM, Eng JA, Ning MM, et al. Hemorrhage burden predicts recurrent intracerebral hemorrhage after lobar hemorrhage. Stroke 2004;35:1415.
378. Koenneke H-C. Cerebral microbleeds on MRI: Prevalence, associations, and potential clinical implications. Neurology 2006;66: 165.
379. Vernooij MW, Haag MDM, van der Lugt A, et al. Use of antithrombotic drugs and the presence of cerebral microbleeds: The Rotterdam Scan Study. Arch Neurol 2009;66:714.
404. Butcher KS, Jeerakathil T, Hill M, et al. The Intracerebral Hemorrhage Acutely Decreasing Arterial Pressure Trial. Stroke 2013;44: 620.
408. Gebel JM Jr, Jauch EC, Brott TG, et al. Natural history of perihematomal edema in patients with hyperacute spontaneous intracerebral hemorrhage. Stroke 2002;33:2631.
409. Staykov D, Wagner I, Volbers B, et al. Natural course of perihemorrhagic edema after intracerebral hemorrhage. Stroke 2011;42: 2625.
410. Venkatasubramanian C, Mlynash M, Finley-Caulfield A, et al. Natural history of perihematomal edema after intracerebral hemorrhage measured by serial magnetic resonance imaging. Stroke 2011;42:73.
415. Tuhrim S, Dambrosia JM, Price TR, et al. Prediction of intracerebral hemorrhage survival. Ann Neurol 1988;24:258.
433. Chung C, Caplan LR, Yamamoto Y, et al. Striatocapsular haemorrhage. Brain 2000;123:1850.
437. Weisberg LA, Stazio A, Elliott D, et al. Putaminal hemorrhage: Clinical-computed tomographic correlations. Neuroradiology 1990;32:200.
442. Kumral E, Evyapan D, Balkir K. Acute caudate vascular lesions. Stroke 1999;30:100.
443. Weisberg LA. Caudate hemorrhage. Arch Neurol 1984;41:971.
458. Chung CS, Caplan LR, Han W, et al. Thalamic haemorrhage. Brain 1973;119:1996.
459. Kumral E, Kocaer T, Ertubey NO, et al. Thalamic hemorrhage: A prospective study of 100 patients. Stroke 1995;26:964.
460. Steinke W, Sacco R, Mohr JP, et al. Thalamic stroke: Presentation and prognosis of infarcts and hemorrhages. Arch Neurol 1992;49:703.
467. Keane JR. Contralateral gaze deviation with supratentorial hemorrhage: Three pathologically verified cases. Arch Neurol 1975;32:119.
475. Fisher CM. Some neuro-ophthalmological observations. J Neurol Neurosurg Psychiatry 1967;30:383.
476. Pessin MS, Adelman LS, Prager RJ, et al. "Wrong-way eyes" in supratentorial hemorrhage. Ann Neurol 1981;9:79.
480. Karussis D, Leker RR, Abramsky O. Cognitive dysfunction following thalamic stroke: A study of 16 cases and review of the literature. J Neurol Sci 2000;172:25.
483. Dejerine J, Roussy G. Le syndrome thalamique. Rev Neurol 1906;12:521.
484. Percheron SMJ. Les artères du thalamus humain. Rev Neurol 1976;132:297.
497. Bogousslavsky J, Van Melle G, Regli F. The Lausanne Stroke Registry: Analysis of 1,000 consecutive patients with first stroke. Stroke 1988;19:1083.
501. Sung C-Y, Chu N-S. Epileptic seizures in intracerebral hemorrhage. J Neurol Neurosurg Psychiatry 1989;52:1273.
514. Knudsen KA, Rosand J, Karluk D, et al. Clinical diagnosis of cerebral amyloid angiopathy: Validation of the Boston criteria. Neurology 2001;56:537.
519. Flemming KD, Wijdicks EF, Li H. Can we predict poor outcome at presentation in patients with lobar hemorrhage. Cerebrovasc Dis 2001;11:183.
520. Mendelow AD, Gregson BA, Fernandes HM, et al. Early surgery versus initial conservative treatment in patients with spontaneous supratentorial intracerebral haematomas in the International Surgical Trial in INtracerebral Haemorrhage (STICH): A randomized trial. Lancet 2005;365:387.
521. Mendelow AD, Gregson BA, Rowan EN, et al. Early surgery versus initial conservative treatment in patients with spontaneous supratentorial lobar intracerebral haematomas (STICH II): a randomised trial. Lancet 2013;382:397.
532. Fisher CM. The neurological examination of the comatose patient. Acta Neurol Scand Suppl 1969;45:44.
535. Fisher CM. Ocular bobbing. Arch Neurol 1964;11:543.
536. St. Louis EK, Wijdicks EF, Li H. Predicting neurologic deterioration in patients with cerebellar hematomas. Neurology 1998;51: 1364.
541. St. Louis EK, Wijdicks EF, Li H, et al. Predictors of poor outcome in patients with a spontaneous cerebellar hematoma. Can J Neurol Sci 2000;27:32.
542. Kirollos RW, Tyagi AK, Ross SA, et al. Management of spontaneous cerebellar hematomas: A prospective treatment protocol. Neurosurgery 2001;49:1378.
566. Pierrott-Deseilligny C, Chain F, Serdaru M, et al. The "one-and-a-half" syndrome: Electro-oculographic analysis of five cases with deductions about the physiological mechanisms of lateral gaze. Brain 1981;104:665.
570. Wijdicks EF, St. Louis E. Clinical profiles predictive of outcome in pontine hemorrhage. Neurology 1997;49:1342.
584. Barinagarrementeria F, Cantú C. Primary medullary hemorrhage: Report of four cases and review of the literature. Stroke 1994; 25:1684.
586. Jung HH, Baumgartner RW, Hess K. Symptomatic secondary hemorrhagic transformation of ischemic Wallenberg's syndrome. J Neurol 2000;247:463.

29 Aneurysmal Subarachnoid Hemorrhage

José I. Suarez, Eric M. Bershad

KEY POINTS

- Subarachnoid hemorrhage (SAH) is a neurological emergency. Severe and sudden headache is the most common presentation but patients can experience loss of consciousness or seizures at onset.
- Most patients with non-traumatic SAH will harbor a ruptured cerebral aneurysm.
- Patients with SAH need to be evaluated immediately and admitted to an intensive care unit environment.
- The most frequent and dreaded neurological complications associated with SAH include hydrocephalus, delayed cerebral ischemia, rebleeding, seizures, and hyponatremia. Practitioners must be aware and monitor and treat patients for these complications.
- SAH outcome is still dismal with a 50% mortality rate and dependency in one third of survivors.

A woman, of forty years of age, and much given to drinking, was seiz'd with an apoplexy. From this she became paralytic in both sides, and was brought into the hospital at Padua, and there she soon died.... The vessels of the pia mater were so distended with blood that the larger ones were almost black; and the smallest made a very beautiful appearance, as if injected with red wax.... [T]he trunk of that artery into which the vertebrals are conjoin'd, exhibited a small white elliptical spot.... I found it was not of that kind, which is generally us'd to be the beginning of an ossification, as I had thought; but somewhat soft in the parietes of the artery itself, and rather in the interior coat.

G. Morgagni, De Sedibus et Causis Morborum (1761)[1]

Subarachnoid hemorrhage (SAH) refers to the extravasation of blood into the spaces filled with cerebrospinal fluid (CSF). In the absence of trauma, aneurysmal rupture is the most common cause of SAH. Often aneurysms remain silent until the cataclysmic rupture. Our understanding of the machinations underlying this condition has evolved; however, many issues remain unresolved. Despite advances in diagnosis and management, the mortality rate for SAH remains unacceptably high. The future holds promise, but there are obstacles to overcome.

HISTORICAL ASPECTS

Our concept of aneurysms began in ancient times. The Egyptian Papyrus of Ebers (c.1550 BC) contains an early description of an arterial aneurysm;[2] however, the first definite report of an intracranial aneurysm came later. Our modern understanding that the anatomic framework gives rise to intracranial aneurysms began in 1664 when Sir Christopher Wren, under the direction of Thomas Willis, illustrated the collateral arterial circulation at the base of the brain (circle of Willis).[3-4] In 1761, Morgagni[1] published *De sedibus et causis morborum* (*The Seats and Causes of Diseases*), a collection of detailed clinicopathologic observations that may have included the earliest pathologically confirmed case of aneurysmal SAH. About 50 years later, in 1812, Cheyne[5] published *Cases of Apoplexy and Lethargy...*, which included an illustration of SAH presumably due to a ruptured aneurysm at the intracranial carotid artery bifurcation. In 1859, William Gull[6] detailed a series of 62 cases of intracranial aneurysms that included thorough clinicopathologic descriptions. He astutely suggested that the presence of an acute severe headache should raise the suspicion of SAH. The promulgation of lumbar puncture by Quincke[7] in 1891 paved the way for the routine premortem diagnosis of SAH. A major breakthrough came in 1927, when Moniz[8] first applied cerebral angiography to a living person to diagnose tumor; in 1933 he reported the successful visualization of an intracranial internal carotid aneurysm.[9] The successful clipping of an intracranial aneurysm by Dandy[10] in 1937 marked the beginning of an era in which active intervention for SAH superseded the nihilistic approach. The history of SAH continues with the advent of sophisticated neuroimaging techniques, multimodality brain monitoring, and endovascular therapy.

EPIDEMIOLOGY

Aneurysmal SAHs cause 2% to 7% of all strokes[11,12] but disproportionately account for 27% of stroke-related years of life lost before age 65. The incidence of SAH varies substantially by region, ranging from 2 per 100,000 population per year in Beijing, China, up to 27 per 100,000 population per year in Japan.[13-14] Finland has a relatively high incidence of SAH, 22 per 100,000 population per year.[13] The worldwide aggregate incidence of SAH is 10.5 per 100,000 per year, which is about the same as the incidence in North America (United States and Canada), and has remained stable over approximately 40 years.[15,16] There is ethnic variability in the incidence of SAH, with a higher age-adjusted incidence among Mexican-Americans than in non-Hispanic Whites.[12] The incidence of SAH increases with age. The mean age at presentation is 49 to 55 years.[11,13] There is a relative risk of SAH of 1.6 : 1 for women in comparison with men.[17] In North America, the relative risk of SAH is 2.1 : 1 for black in comparison with white persons.[18]

The prevalence of intracranial aneurysms in the general population is between 1% and 6% on the basis of autopsy studies, and 0.5% to 1% on the basis of angiographic data.[19] Of these, about 20% to 50% rupture during the person's lifetime. About 12% to 45% of patients with aneurysmal SAH have multiple aneurysms.[11,16] The risk for development of a new (de novo) aneurysm after diagnosis of SAH may be about 2% per year, according to results of a study using serial angiographic screenings.[20]

The case fatality rate for SAH has been gradually decreasing, by about 0.5% per year.[21] Between 1945 and 1974 in Rochester, Minnesota, the case fatality rate was 57%; it declined to 42% between 1974 and 1984.[22] A recent analysis of the Nationwide Inpatient Sample showed that between 2004 to 2008, the case fatality rate decreased to 20%, compared to 30% in the years from 1979 to 1983.[23] Overall, approximately 10% to 20% of patients with SAH die before reaching the hospital, and about 25% die within 24 hours of the ictus.[11,16]

There are diurnal and seasonal variations in the occurrence of SAH.[14,24] In two Japanese studies, peaks of SAH occurred from 7 to 10 am and from 5 to 8 pm, an effect attributed to circadian changes in blood pressure (BP).[14] The nadir diurnal occurrence was between 10 pm and 6 am.[24] A seasonal variation in the incidence of SAH is not consistent in all studies.[14,24] Other factors that may influence SAH occurrence include changes in the ambient temperature, barometric pressure, and humidity.[25]

Risk Factors

Many potential risk factors for SAH have been studied, but only a few have been convincingly identified.[11,16,26–38] Risk factors are categorized as modifiable or non-modifiable. The most important modifiable risk factors are cigarette smoking and hypertension; other modifiable risk factors for SAH include heavy alcohol use, cocaine abuse, caffeine and nicotine intake in pharmaceutical products, and use of nonsteroidal anti-inflammatory drugs, but these are less well established. Contrary to traditional beliefs, oral contraceptive use, hypercholesterolemia, and exercise are probably not associated with an increased risk of SAH.[27,28]

Cigarette smoking is a robust modifiable risk factor for aneurysmal SAH. In 1996, Teunissen and colleagues systematically reviewed studies evaluating risk factors for aneurysmal SAH.[28] Among two longitudinal and seven case-control studies that evaluated smoking as a possible risk factor, the aggregate relative risk (RR) and odds ratio (OR) for SAH were 1.9 and 3.5, respectively, with smoking. At least five subsequent retrospective studies found that active cigarette smoking was an independent risk factor for SAH.

Hypertension is another robust modifiable risk factor for SAH. In the review by Teunissen and colleagues[28] of seven case-control studies and three longitudinal studies, hypertension had an aggregate OR of 2.9 and an RR of 2.8.

Heavy alcohol use is an inconsistently reported risk factor for SAH.[28–31,36,37] In the pooled analysis of SAH risk factors by Teunissen and colleagues,[28] which included two longitudinal series and three case-control series, heavy alcohol use (>150 g/day) was a statistically significant risk factor, with an RR of 4.7 and an OR of 1.5. In contrast, several other studies found that heavy alcohol use was not an independent predictor for SAH.[28,29] Non-modifiable risk factors for SAH include a family history of SAH in a first-degree relative, female sex, low educational achievement, low body mass index, and undetermined genetic factors.[11,16,27,38] Some known inherited conditions associated with SAH and/or intracranial aneurysms include adult dominant polycystic kidney disease (ADPKD), Ehlers–Danlos disease (type IV), alpha$_1$-antitrypsin deficiency, sickle cell disease, pseudoxanthoma elasticum, hereditary hemorrhagic telangiectasia, neurofibromatosis type I, tuberous sclerosis, fibromuscular dysplasia, and coarctation of the aorta.[11,16,39–41]

A family history of SAH in a close relative is an important non-modifiable risk factor.[11,16,27,38] People with a first-degree relative with SAH have a relative risk of 3 to 7 for SAH in comparison with the general population; however, having a second-degree relative with SAH does not significantly increase the risk over that of the general population. Regarding the increased risk of SAH in patients with a family history of SAH, the clinical implications for screening are controversial. For example, a prospective observational study found that routine screening for aneurysms in first-degree relatives of patients with SAH did not translate into a hypothetical clinical benefit, owing to the anticipated postoperative disability that was expected to outweigh the reduction in mortality from the repair of asymptomatic aneurysms at low risk for rupture.[42]

Female gender is another important non-modifiable risk factor for SAH. Women have 1.6 times the risk for SAH that men have, and the higher risk in women may increase further with advancing age.[43] The reasons for gender-related differences in SAH may be related to menstrual and hormonal influences.[44]

Adult dominant polycystic kidney disease is a known risk factor for SAH.[11,16,45] Intracranial aneurysms are present in 5% to 40% of patients. Patients with the disease who also have SAH tend to be younger, male, and have a higher proportion of middle cerebral artery aneurysms than the general population of patients with SAH.[46]

Causes of Subarachnoid Hemorrhage

Excluding trauma, rupture of a saccular (berry) aneurysm is the most common cause (85%) of SAH. Perimesencephalic hemorrhage (10%) is the next most common cause, followed by myriad uncommon etiologies including arteriovenous malformations (AVMs), intracranial arterial dissections, and others (5%) (Table 29-1).[16]

Perimesencephalic non-aneurysmal subarachnoid hemorrhage (PNSH) is a distinct form of non-aneurysmal SAH. The pathophysiology is not well known but may be associated with venous anomalies.[47] Clinically, patients present similarly to those with aneurysmal SAH; however, patients with PNSH are generally alert, without loss of consciousness at onset, and have no risk factors for aneurysms (i.e., hypertension and smoking). The standard CT definition of PNSH dictates that the blood is located mainly anterior to midbrain, in the interpeduncular cistern, or anterior to the pons, in the prepontine cistern, but may extend to the anterior ambient cistern, quadrigeminal cistern, or basal Sylvian fissure. Also, there should be no involvement of the anterior hemispheric fissure, lateral Sylvian fissure, or intraventricular hemorrhage (IVH). By definition, angiography reveals no aneurysm. Angiographic vasospasm is not uncommon; however, delayed cerebral ischemia (DCI) is rare. Some patients may experience hydrocephalus and may rarely require a permanent shunt.[48] The

TABLE 29-1 Less Common Causes of Spontaneous SAH

Category	Cause
Inflammatory	Vasculitis
Vascular	Perimesencephalic hemorrhage, cerebral arteriovenous malformation (AVM), intracranial arterial dissection, carotid-cavernous fistula, cerebral sinus venous thrombosis, eclampsia, spinal AVM, spinal artery aneurysms, moyamoya disease*
Infectious	Mycotic aneurysms, gnathostomiasis (parasitic), Lyme vasculitis
Neoplastic	Pituitary apoplexy (adenoma), carcinomatous meningitis
Hematologic	Coagulopathy, thrombocytopenia, sickle cell disease
Drugs	Cocaine, amphetamines
Other	Eclampsia

*Mechanism thought to be rupture of transdural anastomotic vessels.

prognosis is usually excellent, and the risk of rebleeding is extremely low.

PATHOPHYSIOLOGY

The processes preceding catastrophic aneurysm rupture occur on a continuum that involves aneurysm formation, growth, and ultimate rupture. The dynamic interactions among inflammatory, hemodynamic, hormonal, and genetic contributors that drive this insidious process are gradually being elucidated.

Distribution and Types of Aneurysms

The saccular (berry) aneurysm is responsible for 85% of cases of aneurysmal SAH.[16] Less commonly, aneurysms may be fusiform or mycotic. Fusiform aneurysms are dilatations of the entire arterial circumference, usually related to atherosclerosis. Mycotic (infectious) aneurysms are rare, may be saccular or fusiform, are usually associated with bacteremia, are typically seen in distal branches of the anterior circulation, and are found in the systemic arterial circulation.

Intracranial aneurysms are usually solitary (70% to 75%) but may be multiple in some patients (25% to 50%).[11,16] The majority of saccular aneurysms arise from the circle of Willis and occur in the anterior circulation. The most common distribution for intracranial aneurysms includes the following arteries: anterior communicating (30%), posterior communicating (25%), middle cerebral (20%), internal carotid bifurcation (7.5%), and top of the basilar artery (7%).[49]

Aneurysm Development

The origin of intracranial aneurysms stems from insidious and dynamic processes that slowly erode the structure of arterial wall. Traditionally, it was believed that congenital defects in the tunica media at arterial bifurcations gave rise to intracranial aneurysms; however, this hypothesis has been largely refuted.[50] First, because aneurysms form during life, it is likely that acquired factors rather than congenital abnormalities are implicated in the pathogenesis.[51] Next, the distribution of saccular aneurysms, predominantly in the anterior circulation, does not correlate well with the distribution of tunica media defects in the posterior circulation. Also, tunica media defects may be present without evidence of aneurysms.[52] Additionally, pathologic specimens of aneurysms show a distinct pattern of sclerosis, ischemia, and degenerative changes, which suggests that atherosclerotic processes are involved. Finally, the site of rupture of aneurysms on pathologic studies occurs distal to the supposed defects.

During cerebral aneurysm pathogenesis, the arterial wall undergoes characteristic changes. Early on, hemodynamic factors such as hypertension result in endothelial cell injury as well as associated histopathologic findings of balloon-like protrusions and crater-like concavities, cytoplasmic swelling, and subendothelial fibrin and cellular infiltration.[51,52] Other changes include degeneration of the arterial basement membrane and internal elastic lamina. Eventually, degeneration of the muscular tunica media occurs, possibly mediated by an apoptotic mechanism.[53] Hemodynamic stressors may occlude the vasa vasorum, resulting in smooth muscle ischemia. Alternatively, impaired diffusion of nutrients across a damaged internal elastic lamina and basement membrane may result in tunica media degeneration.

In addition to hemodynamic factors, defects in arterial connective tissue structure (i.e., elastin and collagen) via either inherited or acquired conditions may predispose one to aneurysm development. Some evidence supporting this is the known association between certain diseases that affect connective tissue and aneurysms (i.e., collagen type III deficiency, alpha$_1$-antitrypsin).[54] Furthermore, inflammatory processes may also contribute to aneurysm development; however, it is unclear whether the inflammation is a primary cause of, or a compensatory response to, arterial wall stress.[55] Moreover, cigarette smoking may induce a proteolytic state by increasing the ratio of plasma and arterial wall elastase levels to alpha$_1$-antitrypsin activity.[51] Finally, hormonal factors such as estrogen are implicated in aneurysm development and SAH. Estrogen may exert beneficial effects on the cerebral blood vessels through mechanisms such as increased endothelial nitric oxide, mitochondrial production, and collagen strengthening.[43,56] Therefore, the decrease in estrogen levels in postmenopausal women may have an adverse effect on the vasculature and possibly increase the risk for SAH; however, this issue requires further study.

Aneurysm Rupture

The pathophysiology associated with aneurysm rupture is still being elucidated. Some clinical factors that may be useful to determine the risk of rupture of an unruptured aneurysm are the size and location of the aneurysm and a previous history of SAH (Table 29-2).[57]

Several investigators have evaluated the histology of saccular aneurysms to identify features that may be associated with rupture. The most important factors are decellularization, apoptosis, matrix degeneration, loss of endothelialization, thrombus formation, and inflammatory infiltration.[58] In addition, some anatomic features of the aneurysm may increase the risk of rupture; they include a smaller neck-to-body ratio and smaller caliber of associated draining arteries.

There may be specific genetic factors predisposing an aneurysm to rupture. In one study, a specific polymorphism in the endothelial nitric oxide synthase gene was found significantly more often in patients with aneurysmal SAH than in community controls and patients with unruptured aneurysms.[59]

CLINICAL PRESENTATION

Signs and Symptoms

The classic presentation of SAH is an acute and severe headache, often described as the "worst ever." The time to peak

TABLE 29-2 Cumulative (5-Year) Risk of Rupture for Unruptured Saccular Aneurysms

Size of Aneurysm (mm)	No History of SAH and Anterior Circulation Aneurysm	No History of SAH and Posterior Circulation or PCOM Aneurysm	History of SAH and Incidental Aneurysm
<7	0	2.5	1.5 anterior circulation; 3.5 posterior circulation (including PCOM)
7–12	2.6	14.5	n/a
13–24	14.5	18.4	n/a
>25	40	50	n/a

Data derived from Wiebers DO, Whisnant JP, Huston J III, et al: Unruptured intracranial aneurysms: Natural history, clinical outcome, and risks of surgical and endovascular treatment. Lancet *362:103–110, 2003.*

n/a, not available; PCOM, posterior communicating artery; SAH, subarachnoid hemorrhage.

headache intensity is usually seconds.[11,16] However, occasionally the headache may be mild and may respond to over-the-counter analgesics. Only a minority of patients have a warning "sentinel" headache days to weeks before an aneurysmal SAH, which probably represents a small aneurysmal leak.

Syncope occurs in 50% of patients, a phenomenon that may be due to an abrupt rise in intracranial pressure (ICP), which exceeds the mean arterial pressure (MAP), thus resulting in a critically low cerebral perfusion pressure (CPP) and global cerebral ischemia. Seizures occur acutely in 6% to 16% of patients.[16]

Other common manifestations are nausea, vomiting, neck stiffness, photophobia, and phonophobia. Retinal or preretinal hemorrhages (Terson's syndrome) are seen on funduscopy in about 17% of patients, in relation to an acute rise in ICP and are associated with poor outcome.[11] Occasionally, meningeal signs are present owing to the chemical meningitis associated with SAH. A depressed level of consciousness (LOC) is very common and ranges from mild drowsiness to coma.

Focal neurologic deficits related to aneurysm rupture may include intracerebral hemorrhage (ICH), aneurysmal mass effect, and postictal paralysis after complex partial seizures. Classically, one may observe a third nerve palsy with pupillary dilation, which is related to extrinsic compression of the oculomotor nerve by a posterior communicating (PCOM) artery aneurysm. This syndrome may also be seen with posterior cerebral artery and superior cerebellar artery aneurysms. The finding of sixth nerve palsy may be a "false localizing sign," representing elevated ICP. Additionally, one may observe impaired upgaze, which is seen in association with hydrocephalus and is related to pressure on the dorsal midbrain vertical gaze centers. Other focal neurologic deficits may be related to anterior communicating (ACOM) artery or middle cerebral artery (MCA) aneurysms.

Misdiagnosis of Subarachnoid Hemorrhage

The clinical presentation of aneurysmal SAH is usually straightforward; however, in the community, initial misdiagnosis occurs in 23% to 51% of patients.[60] Occasionally, patients present with seizure, acute confusional state, subdural hematoma, or head trauma, making the underlying diagnosis of aneurysmal SAH more elusive. A delayed diagnosis often has a disastrous outcome.[60,61] The most common misdiagnoses are migraine headache and headache of unknown cause; other misdiagnoses include meningitis, influenza, hypertensive crisis, myocardial infarction, arthritis, and psychiatric disease. In addition, the most frequent reasons for misdiagnoses of SAH are failure to obtain appropriate imaging study and misinterpretation of, or failure to perform, a lumbar puncture.

RADIOGRAPHIC AND DIAGNOSTIC TESTING

The most appropriate initial diagnostic test for SAH is a non-contrast-enhanced head CT scan. The sensitivity of CT for acute SAH is very high initially but diminishes with increasing delay between the onset of symptoms and imaging. Newer CT scanners (third-generation or later) are reported to be 98% to 100% sensitive for detecting subarachnoid blood within 12 hours of onset of symptoms when compared with the "gold standard," lumbar puncture.[62,63] However, the sensitivity of CT drops to 93% at 24 hours and 50% at 7 days. The accuracy of CT for SAH also depends on expert interpretation from a radiologist, because a preliminary reading by a non-expert interpreter may be inaccurate. Classically, the head CT reveals hyperintense signal in the basal subarachnoid cisterns. Other locations include the Sylvian fissures, interhemispheric fissure, interpeduncular fossa, and suprasellar, ambient, and quadrigeminal cisterns. There may also be associated intracerebral hemorrhage, intraventricular hemorrhage, subdural hematoma, cerebral edema, and hydrocephalus (Fig. 29-1A). The pattern of blood seen on head CT scans may suggest a certain location of the underlying aneurysm; however, the accuracy of this approach is poor and thus has little diagnostic value.

Lumbar puncture (LP) is considered the gold standard for detection of SAH. In patients with suspected SAH in whom head CT scan results are non-definitive, it is absolutely essential to obtain an LP.[11] LP may be contraindicated in patients suspected to have focal mass lesions, elevated ICP, and herniation. The presence of xanthochromia in the CSF strongly suggests SAH. Several hours after SAH, the lysing of red blood cells releases oxyhemoglobin, with subsequent formation of bilirubin, which has a yellowish appearance. This process may take up to 12 hours, so results of an LP performed too early after SAH may be falsely negative. One should evaluate CSF for xanthochromia with spectrophotometry rather than visual examination, which is not as sensitive. Most institutions rely on visual inspection of CSF. It may be difficult to differentiate a "traumatic tap" from SAH. The finding of a serially decreasing red blood cell count from the first to the last CSF tube may suggest a traumatic tap, but because this decrement may also be seen with aneurysmal SAH, it is not definitive. In contrast, xanthochromia is usually absent with a traumatic tap if the CSF is promptly analyzed.

MRI is not indicated as an initial diagnostic test for SAH; however, it may be useful if the head CT findings are negative, but results of the LP are abnormal. Mitchell and coworkers[64] found that gradient-echo T2-weighted MRI was 94% and 100% sensitive for detecting subarachnoid blood in the acute and subacute phases, respectively. Additionally, the fluid-attenuated inversion recovery (FLAIR) MRI sequence may detect SAH as well as non-contrast-enhanced head CT in the acute setting and better in the subacute to chronic phase.

The combination of normal CT and LP findings safely rules out SAH and thus should obviate cerebral angiography. In a prospective cohort study of patients with suspected SAH in whom CT and LP findings were negative, no SAH was observed in any patient during a 3-year follow-up.[65] Consequently, angiography is not routinely indicated in these patients, because the possibility of SAH is remote. Furthermore, the finding of a small incidental intracranial aneurysm does not imply that it has ruptured and may lead to unnecessary surgical or endovascular interventions that may result in perioperative morbidity and mortality. Applying clinical rules may supplement the imaging in patients suspected of SAH. Accordingly, Perry et al.[66] reported clinical decision-making rules developed in a large Canadian cohort study that had 100% sensitivity to detect SAH, which includes any of the following: age >40, neck pain or stiffness, witnessed loss of consciousness, or onset during exertion PLUS thunderclap headache (instant headache) and pain on neck flexion.

SEARCHING FOR THE ANEURYSM

After diagnosis of SAH, the next step is to promptly identify an aneurysm. Current practice dictates the early treatment of ruptured intracranial aneurysms. Delayed treatment of aneurysms increases the risk of rebleeding and may prohibit aggressive hemodynamic management of DCI.

Cerebral (Catheter) Angiography

Cerebral angiography has remained the gold standard for diagnosis of intracranial aneurysms.[11,16,67] Advances in this technique have improved the diagnostic accuracy and

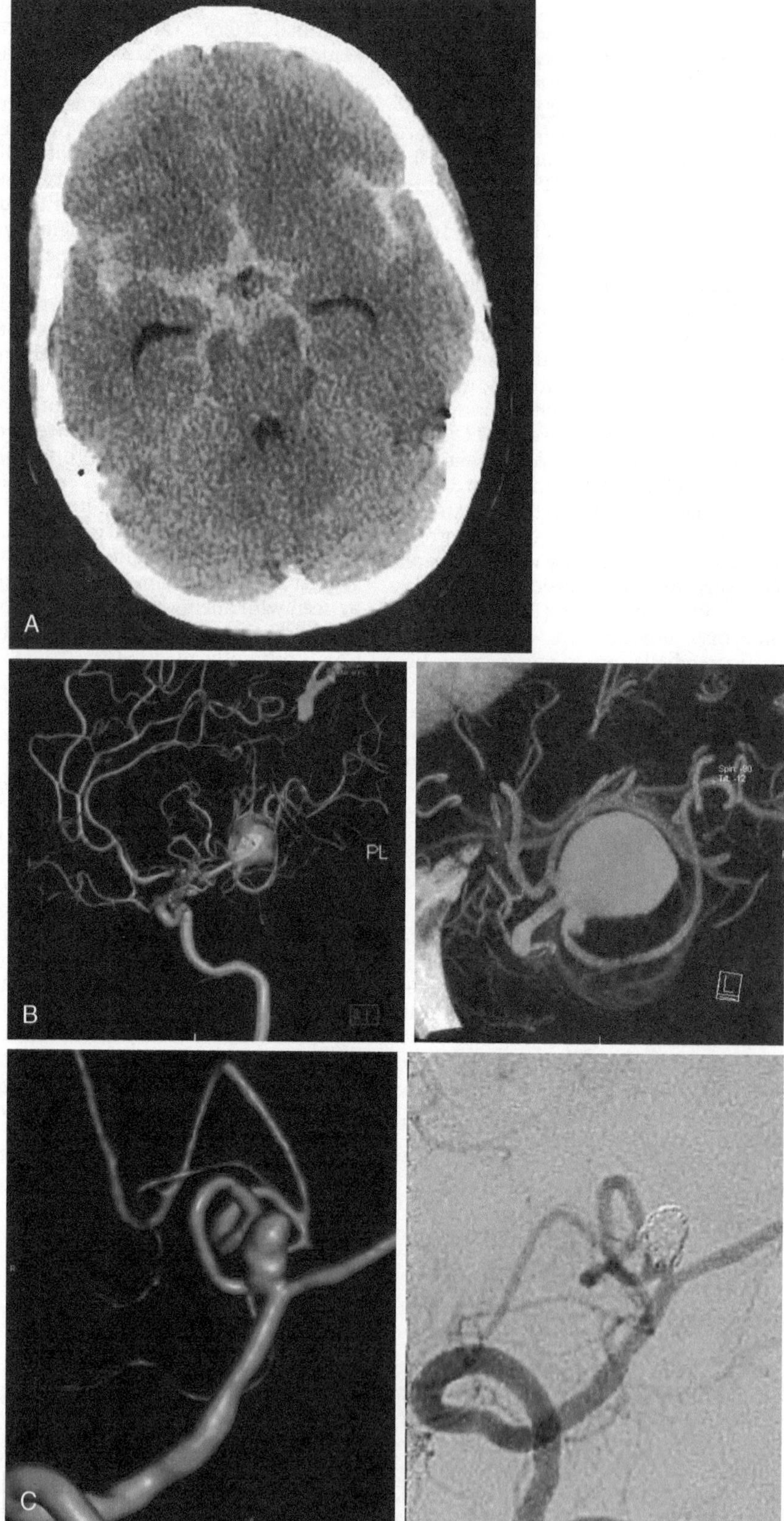

Figure 29-1. Neuroimaging evaluation of patients with subarachnoid hemorrhage (SAH). A. A non-contrast-enhanced head CT scan reveals extensive SAH in the basal cisterns, Sylvian fissures, and anterior interhemispheric fissure in a patient with a ruptured left posterior communicating artery aneurysm. There is also prominence of the temporal horns of the lateral ventricles, suggesting hydrocephalus **B.** *Left,* Three-dimensional reconstruction angiogram (oblique anterolateral view) showing giant left middle cerebral artery bifurcation aneurysm, with several branches arising from the aneurysm body. *Right,* CT angiogram of the same aneurysm (left lateral view). **C.** *Left,* Three-dimensional reconstruction angiogram showing a multilobed right posterior inferior cerebellar artery aneurysm. *Right,* Angiogram (AP right vertebral injection) showing coil occlusion of a posterior inferior cerebellar artery aneurysm.

decreased procedural morbidity. A "four-vessel" evaluation of the bilateral internal carotid arteries and vertebral arteries is necessary. The standard, digital subtraction angiography (DSA), may be supplemented by 3D rotational angiography (3DRA) (Figs 29-1B and 29-1C).

Catheter angiography carries significant risks. Neurologic complications may include arterial dissection or rupture, ischemic stroke, and seizures. Non-neurologic complications include groin or retroperitoneal hematoma, contrast agent nephropathy, allergic reaction to contrast agent, and femoral artery dissection. With an experienced operator, there is about a 1.0% to 2.5% risk of neurologic complications, and 0.1% to 0.5% risk of permanent neurologic injury. However, these complication rates apply to patients with various neurologic indications; patients who specifically have an angiogram for SAH may have different rates of complications.

CT Angiography

CT angiography (CTA) is emerging as an alternative diagnostic test for SAH; however, the diagnostic accuracy may be less than that of standard angiography.[68] The accuracy of CTA for detecting aneurysms varies widely in different studies. The sensitivity and specificity of CTA in comparison with those for DSA range from 77% to 100%, and 87% to 100%, respectively (see Fig. 29-1B).[69]

Advantages of CTA include a quick procedural time, excellent anatomic rendering, and a low risk of complications. CTA reconstructed in 3D provides anatomically accurate relationships between the vascular structures and bone, which may be useful for surgical planning. CTA poses less risk for iatrogenic complications than DSA because contrast agent is given intravenously for CTA. Some important limitations of CTA include a lower sensitivity for smaller aneurysms (<4 mm) and posterior circulation distribution aneurysms in comparison with DSA. Furthermore, the large bolus of contrast agent needed for CTA may increase the risk of contrast-induced nephropathy, especially if performed in conjunction with DSA.

Magnetic Resonance Angiography

Magnetic resonance angiography (MRA) is not appropriate to diagnose aneurysms in patients with suspected aneurysmal SAH. The sensitivity and specificity value for MRA for aneurysms in comparison with that for DSA ranges from 69% to 99%;[67] however, these studies were performed mostly in patients with unruptured aneurysms. The sensitivity for detecting small (<4 mm) aneurysms is poor. Some other limitations of MRA are the prolonged time required for scanning, susceptibility to motion artifact, and inability to be performed in patients who carry metallic objects such as pacemakers.

Angiographically "Negative" Subarachnoid Hemorrhage

In about 15% of patients with spontaneous SAH, results of the initial angiogram are negative; however, a second angiogram may reveal abnormalities in 2% to 24% of patients.[70] Thus, it is usual practice to obtain a second angiogram during initial hospitalization to exclude aneurysm and other vascular sources of SAH. The chance of finding an aneurysm is higher in patients in whom the initial CT scan showed a typical pattern for aneurysmal SAH than in patients in whom CT findings were negative but LP results positive. Rarely, angiographically "negative" SAH may be due to spinal artery aneurysms or arteriovenous malformations; thus, MRI of the spinal cord should be considered.[11,16]

Grading Scales for Subarachnoid Hemorrhage

Numerous clinical and radiologic scales have been used to predict outcome after SAH.[71–73] Some of the clinical scales are Hunt and Hess, Glasgow Coma Scale (GCS), World Federation of Neurological Surgeons (WFNS) scale, and Prognosis on Admission of Aneurysmal Subarachnoid Hemorrhage (PAASH) scale (Table 29-3). Radiologic grading scales include the Fisher scale, modified Fisher scale, and head CT grading scale (Table 29-3).

The Hunt and Hess scale is the most widely used clinical scale, but its validity and reliability are suboptimal. The reason is the difficulty in grading subjective clinical symptoms and signs such as headache and level of consciousness. Some newer scales (WFNS and PAASH) are more objective because they are largely based on the Glasgow Coma Scale (GCS), which is known to have good validity and reliability. Radiologic scales have attempted to relate the amount of initial hemorrhage to the risk of DCI. In 1980, Fisher and coworkers[73] reported a scale that related the amount of SAH on initial head CT to subsequent risk of symptomatic vasospasm. The presence of thick SAH and vertical layering of blood in cisterns predicts the highest risk for development of symptomatic vasospasm; however, the Fisher scale has several limitations. First, the measurements used to determine blood thickness are based on printed CT images but have no relationship to true measurements. Second, an ascending grade does not correlate well with an increased risk of symptomatic vasospasm, because grade III rather than grade IV carries the highest risk. Third, ventricular blood is disregarded on the scale. Finally, the scale predicts DCI rather than long-term outcomes. A modified Fisher scale has been proposed that better accounts for ventricular blood and contains a more linear association between ascending grade and DCI.[72]

MANAGEMENT

Initial management of the patient with SAH begins with the stabilization of the airway, breathing, and circulation. Then attention turns to the institution of general supportive and neuroprotective measures, in anticipation of the known complications of SAH. Concurrently, one should make expeditious plans to secure the aneurysm.

Several new and revised guidelines have become available over the last several years regarding aneurysmal SAH issued by both the Neurocritical Care Society (NCS) 2011 and the American Heart Association (AHA) 2012 update.[74,75] A summary of these can be reviewed in Table 29-4. For the AHA update, only class I recommendations are listed. For the NCS guidelines, only the strong recommendations are listed. The guidelines from each society have some overlap, and mostly agree with each other. The NCS guidelines take a more pragmatic approach with regards to the acute management, and use a different grading methodology, based on the GRADE system, which allowed for strong recommendations to be made with less evidence, compared to the AHA guidelines.

General Measures

Given the high likelihood of acute deterioration, one should manage patients with SAH in the intensive care unit (ICU). Admission to a specific neurologic ICU is preferable, because there is evidence that care of critically ill neurologic patients by a neurointensive care team may enhance outcomes.[76,77]

Blood Pressure Management

The optimal BP target for patients with SAH is unknown and may vary among individuals or at different points during the

TABLE 29-3 Clinical and Radiological Grading Scales for SAH

	Clinical Scales*		
Grade	**Hunt and Hess Scale**¥	**World Federation of Neurological Surgeons Scale**	**Prognosis on Admission of Aneurysmal Subarachnoid Hemorrhage Scale**
1	Asymptomatic, mild headache, slight neck rigidity	GCS score 15	GCS score 15
2	Moderate-to-severe headache, neck rigidity, cranial nerve palsy	GCS score 13 or 14, without focal deficit	GCS score 11 to 14
3	Drowsiness, confusion, mild focal deficit	GCS score 13 or 14, with focal deficit	GCS score 8 to10
4	Stupor, moderate to severe hemiparesis	GCS score 7 to12	GCS score 4 to 7
5	Coma, decerebrate posturing	GCS score 3 to 6	GCS score 3

	Radiological Scalesᵠ	
Grade	**Fisher Scale**	**Modified Fisher Scale**
1	No visualization of blood	Diffuse thin SAH with no IVH
2	Diffuse thin layer <1 mm thick in vertical layers	Any IVH with thin or no visualized SAH
3	Localized clots and/or vertical layers <1 mm thick	Diffuse or localized thick SAH without IVH
4	Diffuse blood, but intraventricular or intracerebral clots	Diffuse or localized thick SAH with IVH

*Data from Hunt WE, Hess RM: Surgical risk as related to time of intervention in the repair of intracranial aneurysms. *J Neurosurg* 28:14–20, 1968; Report of World Federation of Neurological Surgeons Committee on a Universal Subarachnoid Hemorrhage Grading Scale. *J Neurosurg* 68:985–986, 1988; and Takagi K, Tamura A, Nakagomi T, et al: How should a subarachnoid hemorrhage grading scale be determined? A combinatorial approach based solely on the Glasgow Coma Scale. *J Neurosurg* 90: 680–687, 1999.
GCS, Glasgow Coma Scale.
¥Severe systemic conditions, including hypertension, diabetes mellitus, chronic obstructive pulmonary disease, coronary artery disease, and angiographically detected vasospasm, require advancing classification by one grade.
ᵠData from Fisher CM, Kistler JP, Davis JM: Relation of cerebral vasospasm to subarachnoid hemorrhage visualized by computerized tomographic scanning. *Neurosurgery* 6:1–9, 1980; and Frontera JA, Claassen J, Schmidt JM, et al: Prediction of symptomatic vasospasm after subarachnoid hemorrhage: The modified Fisher scale. *Neurosurgery* 59: 21–27; discussion 21–27, 2006.
IVH, intraventricular hemorrhage; SAH, subarachnoid hemorrhage.

disease course. Some of the factors that may influence BP management include the aneurysm status (secured or unsecured), presence of elevated ICP, integrity of the autoregulatory mechanism of cerebral vessels, and presence of vasospasm, DCI, or end-organ dysfunction.[74,75,78]

Cerebral autoregulation refers to the process of maintaining a constant cerebral blood flow (CBF) despite large fluctuations in CPP. Normally, CBF remains stable, with CPP values ranging from 50 to 150 mm Hg.[78] The CPP is the difference between the MAP and the ICP. The autoregulatory mechanism may be impaired after SAH. Thus, it is prudent to maintain CPP within a narrow range. Although not routinely used, several methods are available to check the integrity of the autoregulatory response. One can assess the mean CBF velocity change induced by changes in the MAP using transcranial Doppler (TCD) monitoring.[79] Another method is to evaluate changes in brain tissue oxygen pressure in response to changes in the CPP in patients with SAH. Those who had impaired autoregulation, defined as a significant change in brain tissue oxygenation for a given change in CPP, had a significantly higher incidence of DCI.

Unsecured aneurysms are at risk for rebleeding; however, the literature has not conclusively identified hypertension as an independent predictor.[80] Nevertheless, the general consensus is that extreme elevations of BP should be reduced to below systolic BP of 160 mm Hg or mean BP < 110 mmHg in patients with unsecured aneurysms.[74,75] Care should be taken in the process, because excessive lowering may increase the risk of DCI in the setting of elevated ICP, vasospasm, or impaired cerebral autoregulation. Furthermore, intraoperatively induced hypotension is not advocated because of the possibility of harm from cerebral ischemia in patients who may have impaired cerebral autoregulation.

The presence of symptomatic vasospasm and DCI usually indicates a need to increase the BP to above the point at which symptoms resolve. Induced hypertension may require vasopressors to elevate the MAP above a certain threshold to improve the symptoms. The maximum BP target that is safe has not been well established, but generally the limit is a systolic BP of 200 to 220 mm Hg.[78]

The presence of end-organ dysfunction, such as hypertensive encephalopathy, aortic dissection, myocardial ischemia, pulmonary edema, or acute renal failure, may necessitate lowering the BP; however, there are no specific guidelines regarding this issue in patients with SAH. In patients with ischemic stroke, the usual goal is to reduce the BP by no more than 15% to avoid worsening ischemia.

In the case of symptomatic vasospasm and DCI, it may be necessary to induce hypertension. However, important systemic complications associated with induced hypertension include acute heart failure, myocardial ischemia, cardiac arrhythmias, and acute respiratory distress syndrome (ARDS). Some preferred choices for antihypertensive therapy are intravenous (IV) labetalol, esmolol, and nicardipine drip. Nitroprusside should be avoided because it can increase ICP.

Fluid Management

The fluid management strategy in SAH depends on myriad factors, including the status of the aneurysm (secured or unsecured), and presence of vasospasm, DCI, cerebral edema, cerebral salt wasting, syndrome of inappropriate antidiuretic hormone (secretion) (SIADH), and diabetes insipidus. However, it is generally agreed that hypovolemia should be avoided, and that euvolemia is achieved by keeping the central venous pressure (CVP) between 5 and 8 mm Hg with crystalloids or colloids. In general, hypotonic fluids such as 0.45% saline, 5% dextrose in water (D_5W), and lactated Ringer's injection should be avoided because they may worsen cerebral edema.

Text continued on p. 527

TABLE 29-4 Neurocritical Care Society and American Heart Association Guidelines on the Diagnosis and Treatment of Aneurysmal SAH[74,75]

	Neurocritical Care Society Guidelines 2011[74]	American Heart Association Guidelines 2012[75]
Diagnosis of Aneurysmal SAH		**aSAH is a medical emergency that is frequently misdiagnosed. A high level of suspicion for aSAH should exist in patients with acute onset of severe headache** *(Class I; Level of Evidence B)* **Acute diagnostic workup should include non-contrast head CT, which, if non-diagnostic, should be followed by lumbar puncture** *(Class I;Level Evidence B)* Digital subtraction angiography with 3D rotational angiography is indicated for aneurysm treatment planning *(Class I, Level Evidence B)* **The initial clinical severity of aSAH should be determined rapidly by use of simple validated scales (e.g., Hunt and Hess, World Federation of Neurological Surgeons), because it is the most useful indicator of outcome after aSAH** *(Class I; Level of Evidence B)*
Securing Ruptured Aneurysm	Early aneurysm repair should be undertaken, when possible and reasonable, to prevent rebleeding (High-Quality Evidence; Strong Recommendation)	**The risk of early aneurysm rebleeding is high, and rebleeding is associated with very poor outcomes. Therefore, urgent evaluation and treatment of patients with suspected aSAH is recommended** *(Class I; Level of Evidence B)* **After any aneurysm repair, immediate cerebrovascular imaging is generally recommended to identify remnants or recurrence of the aneurysm that may require treatment** *(Class I; Level of Evidence B)*. **Surgical clipping or endovascular coiling of the ruptured aneurysm should be performed as early as feasible in the majority of patients to reduce the rate of rebleeding after aSAH** *(Class I; Level of Evidence B)* **Complete obliteration of the aneurysm is recommended whenever possible** *(Class I; Level of Evidence B)* **Determination of aneurysm treatment, as judged by both experienced cerebrovascular surgeons and endovascular specialists, should be a multidisciplinary decision based on characteristics of the patient and the aneurysm** *(Class I; Level of Evidence C)* **For patients with ruptured aneurysms judged to be technically amenable to both endovascular coiling and neurosurgical clipping, endovascular coiling should be considered** *(Class I; Level of Evidence B)* **In the absence of a compelling contraindication, patients who undergo coiling or clipping of a ruptured aneurysm should have delayed follow-up vascular imaging (timing and modality to be individualized), and strong consideration should be given to retreatment, either by repeat coiling or microsurgical clipping, if there is a clinically significant (e.g., growing) remnant** *(Class I; Level of Evidence B)*
Blood Pressure Goals (Unsecured Aneurysm)	Treat extreme hypertension in patients with an unsecured, recently ruptured aneurysm. Modest elevations in blood pressure (mean blood pressure <110 mmHg) do not require therapy. Pre-morbid baseline blood pressures should be used to refine targets; hypotension should be avoided (Low-Quality Evidence; Strong Recommendation)	**Between the time of aSAH symptom onset and aneurysm obliteration, blood pressure should be controlled with a titratable agent to balance the risk of stroke, hypertension-related rebleeding, and maintenance of cerebral perfusion pressure** *(Class I; Level of Evidence B)*
Antifibrinolytic Agents	Delayed (>48 hour after the ictus) or prolonged (>3 days) antifibrinolytic therapy exposes patients to side effects of therapy when the risk of rebleeding is sharply reduced and should be avoided (High-Quality Evidence; Strong Recommendation) Antifibrinolytic therapy is relatively contraindicated in patients with risk factors for thromboembolic complications (Moderate-Quality Evidence; Strong Recommendation) Patients treated with antifibrinolytic therapy should have close screening for deep venous thrombosis (Moderate-Quality Evidence; Strong Recommendation)	

Continued

TABLE 29-4 Neurocritical Care Society and American Heart Association Guidelines on the Diagnosis and Treatment of Aneurysmal SAH[74,75]—cont'd

	Neurocritical Care Society Guidelines 2011[74]	American Heart Association Guidelines 2012[75]
Hospital/System Characteristics	Patients with SAH should be treated at high-volume centers (Moderate-Quality Evidence; Strong Recommendation) High-volume centers should have appropriate specialty neurointensive care units, neurointensivists, vascular neurosurgeons and interventional neuroradiologists to provide the essential elements of care (Moderate-Quality Evidence; Strong Recommendation) Monitoring for neurological deterioration, and specifically DCI, should take place in an environment with substantial multidisciplinary expertise in the management of SAH (Moderate-Quality Evidence; Strong Recommendation) SAH clinical trials should use only radiographic evidence of cerebral infarction and functional outcome as the primary outcome measures (Moderate-Quality Evidence; Strong Recommendation)	Low-volume hospitals (e.g., ten aSAH cases per year) should consider early transfer of patients with aSAH to high-volume centers (e.g., >35 aSAH cases per year) with experienced cerebrovascular surgeons, endovascular specialists, and multidisciplinary neurointensive care services *(Class I; Level of Evidence B)*
Fluid Management	Intravascular volume management should target euvolemia and avoid prophylactic hypervolemic therapy. In contrast, there is evidence for harm from aggressive administration of fluid aimed at achieving hypervolemia (High-Quality Evidence; Strong Recommendation) The goal should be maintaining euvolemia, rather than attempting to induce hypervolemia (Moderate-Quality Evidence; Strong Recommendation)	**Maintenance of euvolemia and normal circulating blood volume is recommended to prevent DCI** *(Class I; Level of Evidence B).* (Revised recommendation from previous guidelines)
Nimodipine	Oral nimodipine (60 mg every 4 h) should be administered after SAH for a period of 21 days (High-Quality Evidence; Strong Recommendation)	**Oral nimodipine should be administered to all patients with aSAH** *(Class I; Level of Evidence A).* (It should be noted that this agent has been shown to improve neurological outcomes but not cerebral vasospasm. The value of other calcium antagonists, whether administered orally or intravenously, remains uncertain)
Magnesium	Inducing hypermagnesemia is NOT recommended pending the conclusion of current randomized trials (Moderate-Quality Evidence; Strong Recommendation) Hypomagnesemia should be avoided (Moderate-Quality Evidence; Strong Recommendation)	
Imaging Studies and Monitoring of Vasospasm and DCI	Imaging of vascular anatomy and/or perfusion can be used to confirm a diagnosis of DCI in monitored good-grade patients who show a change in neurologic exam. A strategy for detection and confirmation of DCI should be employed. This should first and foremost involve frequent repeat neurological assessment by qualified providers. Intermittent screening or more continuous monitoring methods may additionally be used • TCD may be used for monitoring and detection of large-artery vasospasm with variable sensitivity. Thresholds of mean blood flow velocities <120 cm/second for absence and >200 cm/second and/or MCA/ICA ratio >6 for presence are reasonable (Moderate-Quality Evidence; Strong Recommendation) DSA is the gold standard for detection of large-artery vasospasm (High-Quality Evidence; Strong Recommendation) In high-risk patients who have a clinical picture strongly suggestive of DCI, and in whom elective screening CTA/CTP or DSA has already demonstrated vasospasm/DCI, it is reasonable to initiate medical therapy without further investigations (Moderate-Quality Evidence; Strong Recommendation) In patients where there is clinical uncertainty regarding the cause of neurological deterioration, DSA is indicated if an endovascular intervention is planned (Moderate-Quality Evidence; Strong Recommendation)	

TABLE 29-4 Neurocritical Care Society and American Heart Association Guidelines on the Diagnosis and Treatment of Aneurysmal SAH[74,75]—cont'd

	Neurocritical Care Society Guidelines 2011[74]	American Heart Association Guidelines 2012[75]
INDUCED HYPERTENSION	Patients clinically suspected of DCI should undergo a trial of induced hypertension (Moderate-Quality Evidence; Strong Recommendation) The choice of vasopressor should be based on the other pharmacologic properties of the agents (e.g., inotropy, tachycardia) (Moderate-Quality Evidence; Strong Recommendation) Blood pressure augmentation should progress in a stepwise fashion with assessment of neurologic function at each MAP level to determine if a higher blood pressure target is appropriate (Poor-Quality Evidence; Strong Recommendation) If nimodipine administration results in hypotension, then dosing intervals should be changed to more frequent lower doses. If hypotension continues to occur, then nimodipine may be discontinued (Low-Quality; Strong Recommendation) If patients with DCI do not improve with blood pressure augmentation, a trial of inotropic therapy may be considered (Low-Quality Evidence, Strong Recommendation) Inotropes with prominent b-2 agonist properties (e.g., dobutamine) may lower MAP and require increases in vasopressor dosage (High-Quality Evidence; Strong Recommendation) Hemodilution in an attempt to improve rheology should not be undertaken except in cases of erythrocythemia (Moderate-Quality Evidence; Strong Recommendation)	**Induction of hypertension is recommended for patients with DCI unless blood pressure is elevated at baseline or cardiac status precludes it** *(Class I; Level of Evidence B)*
ENDOVASCULAR THERAPY AND VASOSPASM	Endovascular treatment using intra-arterial vasodilators and/or angioplasty may be considered for vasospasm-related DCI (Moderate-Quality Evidence; Strong Recommendation) The timing and triggers of endovascular treatment of vasospasm remain unclear, but generally rescue therapy for ischemic symptoms that remain refractory to medical treatment should be considered. The exact timing is a complex decision which should consider the aggressiveness of the hemodynamic intervention, the patient's ability to tolerate it, prior evidence of large-artery narrowing, and the availability of and the willingness to perform angioplasty or infusion of intra-arterial agents (Moderate-Quality Evidence; Strong Recommendation) The use of routine prophylactic cerebral angioplasty is not recommended (High-Quality Evidence; Strong Recommendation) Mechanical augmentation of cardiac output and arterial blood flow (e.g., intra-aortic balloon counter-pulsation) may be useful (Low-Quality Evidence; Weak Recommendation)	Cerebral angioplasty and/or selective intra-arterial vasodilator therapy is reasonable in patients with symptomatic cerebral vasospasm, particularly those who are not rapidly responding to hypertensive therapy. *(Class IIa; Level of Evidence B)*
PATIENTS WITH DCI WHO HAVE UNSECURED ANEURYSMS	If the aneurysm thought to have ruptured is unsecured when a patient develops DCI, cautious blood pressure elevation to improve perfusion might be attempted, weighing potential risks and benefits (Low-Quality Evidence; Strong Recommendation) Unsecured aneurysms which are not thought to be responsible for the acute SAH should not influence hemodynamic management (Moderate-Quality Evidence; Strong Recommendation)	
HYDROCEPHALUS		aSAH-associated acute symptomatic hydrocephalus should be managed by cerebrospinal fluid diversion (external ventricular drainage or lumbar drainage, depending on the clinical scenario) *(Class I; Level of Evidence B)* aSAH-associated chronic symptomatic hydrocephalus should be treated with permanent cerebrospinal fluid diversion *(Class I; Level of Evidence C)*

Continued

TABLE 29-4 Neurocritical Care Society and American Heart Association Guidelines on the Diagnosis and Treatment of Aneurysmal SAH[74,75]—cont'd

	Neurocritical Care Society Guidelines 2011[74]	American Heart Association Guidelines 2012[75]
Seizure Prophylaxis and Monitoring	Routine use of anticonvulsant prophylaxis with phenytoin is not recommended after SAH (Low-Quality Evidence; Strong Recommendation) Continuous EEG monitoring should be considered in patients with poor-grade SAH who fail to improve or who have neurological deterioration of undetermined etiology (Low-Quality Evidence; Strong Recommendation)	
	Medical Complications	
Cardiac	Baseline cardiac assessment with serial enzymes, electrocardiography, and echocardiography is recommended, especially in patients with evidence of myocardial dysfunction (Low-Quality Evidence; Strong Recommendation) Monitoring of cardiac output may be useful in patients with evidence of hemodynamic instability or myocardial dysfunction (Low–Quality Evidence; Strong Recommendation) Patients on statins prior to presentation with aneurysmal SAH should have their medication continued in the acute phase (Low-Quality Evidence; Strong Recommendation)	
Fever	Temperature should be monitored frequently; infectious causes of fever should always be sought and treated (High-Quality Evidence; Strong Recommendation) During the period of risk for DCI control of fever is desirable; intensity should reflect the individual patient's relative risk of ischemia (Low-Quality Evidence; Strong Recommendation) While the efficacy of most antipyretic agents (acetaminophen, ibuprofen) is low, they should be used as the first line of therapy (Moderate-Quality Evidence; Strong Recommendation) Surface cooling or intravascular devices are more effective and should be employed when antipyretics fail in cases where fever control is highly desirable (High-Quality Evidence; Strong Recommendation) Use of these devices should be accompanied by monitoring for skin injury and venous thrombosis (Low-Quality Evidence; Strong Recommendation) Patients should be monitored and treated for shivering (High-Quality Evidence; Strong Recommendation)	
Anemia	Measures should be taken to minimize blood loss from blood drawing (Low-Quality Evidence; Strong Recommendation) Transfusion criteria for general medical patients should not be applied to decisions in SAH patients Patients should receive packed RBC transfusions to maintain hemoglobin concentration above 8–10 g/dl (Moderate-Quality Evidence; Strong Recommendation) Higher hemoglobin concentrations may be appropriate for patients at risk for DCI, but whether transfusion is useful cannot be determined from the available data (No Evidence; Strong Recommendation)	The use of packed red blood cell transfusion to treat anemia might be reasonable in patients with aSAH who are at risk of cerebral ischemia. The optimal hemoglobin goal is still to be determined *(Class IIb; Level of Evidence B)*. (New recommendation)
Serum Sodium and Fluids	Fluid restriction should not be used to treat hyponatremia (Low-Quality Evidence; Strong Recommendation) Mild hypertonic saline solutions can be used to correct hyponatremia (Very Low-Quality Evidence; Strong Recommendation) Extreme caution to avoid hypovolemia is needed if vasopressin-receptor antagonists are used for treatment of hyponatremia (Low-Quality Evidence; Strong Recommendation) Free water intake via intravenous and enteral routes should be limited (Very Low-Quality Evidence; Strong Recommendation)	

TABLE 29-4 Neurocritical Care Society and American Heart Association Guidelines on the Diagnosis and Treatment of Aneurysmal SAH[74,75]—cont'd

	Neurocritical Care Society Guidelines 2011[74]	American Heart Association Guidelines 2012[75]
Endocrine	Hypoglycemia (serum glucose <80 mg/dl) should be avoided (High-Quality Evidence; Strong Recommendation) Serum glucose should be maintained below 200 mg/dl (Moderate-Quality Evidence; Strong Recommendation)	
DVT Prophylaxis	Measures to prevent deep venous thrombosis should be employed in all SAH patients (High-Quality Evidence; Strong Recommendation) Sequential compression devices, should be routinely used in all patients (High-Quality Evidence; Strong Recommendation) The use of low-molecular-weight heparin or unfractionated heparin for prophylaxis should be withheld in patients with unprotected aneurysms and expected to undergo surgery (Low-Quality Evidence; Strong Recommendation) The use of unfractionated heparin for prophylaxis could be started 24 h after undergoing surgery (Moderate-Quality Evidence; Strong Recommendation) Unfractionated heparin and low-molecular-weight heparin should be withheld 24 h before and after intracranial procedures (Moderate-Quality Evidence; Strong Recommendation)	Heparin-induced thrombocytopenia and deep venous thrombosis are relatively frequent complications after aSAH. Early identification and targeted treatment are recommended, but further research is needed to identify the ideal screening paradigms *(Class I; Level of Evidence B)*
Risk Factors for Recurrent SAH and Aneurysm		In addition to the size and location of the aneurysm and the patient's age and health status, it might be reasonable to consider morphological and hemodynamic characteristics of the aneurysm when discussing the risk of aneurysm rupture *(Class IIb; Level of Evidence B)* Consumption of a diet rich in vegetables may lower the risk of aSAH *(Class IIb; Level of Evidence B)*

For more details refer to the 'AHA Evidence box index' in the FM

SAH, subarachnoid hemorrhage; aSAH, aneurysmal subarachnoid hemorrhage; CT, computed tomography; DCI, delayed cerebral ischemia; TCD, transcranial Doppler; MCA, middle cerebral artery; ICA, internal carotid artery; DSA, digital subtraction angiography; CTA, CT angiography; CTP, CT perfusion; MAP, mean arterial pressure; EEG, electroencephalogram; RBC, red blood cellSAH, subarachnoid hemorrhage; aSAH, aneurysmal subarachnoid hemorrhage; CT, computed tomography; DCI, delayed cerebral ischemia; TCD, transcranial Doppler; MCA, middle cerebral artery; ICA, internal carotid artery; DSA, digital subtraction angiography; CTA, CT angiography; CTP, CT perfusion; MAP, mean arterial pressure; EEG, electroencephalogram; RBC, red blood cell.

Temperature Control

Fever is common in patients with SAH and is associated with a poor outcome.[81,82] Fever is associated with exacerbation of cerebral edema, elevated ICP, and vasospasm. Infection is the most common reason for fever in patients with SAH; however, noninfectious etiologies, including venous thromboembolism, intraventricular hemorrhage, drug effect, and central fever, should be considered if results of the diagnostic work-up are unrevealing. Some predictors of fever in patients with SAH include intraventricular hemorrhage and poor Hunt and Hess grade.[82]

Maintenance of normothermia can be achieved by antipyretic administration (i.e., acetaminophen), ice packs, water-circulating cooling blankets, adhesive surface cooling, or endovascular heat exchange catheters. The optimal method is unknown. Furthermore, despite retrospective data showing a strong association between fever and poor outcome, there are no prospective data to support routine prophylaxis to maintain normothermia in patients with SAH.

Avoiding Hyperglycemia

Hyperglycemia is associated with poor outcome in aneurysmal patients with SAH.[83,84] In a retrospective study of 352 patients with SAH, Badjatia and colleagues[83] found that higher mean inpatient serum glucose levels were significantly associated with a longer ICU stay, symptomatic vasospasm, and poor neurologic outcome at hospital discharge. Additionally, Lanzino and associates[84] found that elevated admission and inpatient serum glucose values independently predicted increased mortality and worse neurologic outcome as measured on the Glasgow Outcome Scale (GOS). In two large randomized controlled trials by Van den Berghe and coworkers,[85,86] intensive insulin therapy in critically ill patients to maintain blood glucose between 80 and 110 mg/dL reduced duration of both ICU and hospital stays, chance of renal failure, and duration of mechanical ventilation. In the first of the two studies, which enrolled patients in surgical ICUs, strict glucose control also reduced mortality;[86] however, this finding was not seen in the subsequent study of patients in medical ICUs.[85] A post hoc analysis of patients with acute brain injury who were enrolled in the first of these two randomized trials found that intensive insulin therapy was associated with fewer seizures, lower ICP, and better neurologic outcomes.[87] Currently, there are no large randomized trials specifically evaluating patients with SAH.

In the absence of good-quality prospective data, the optimal target for blood glucose in SAH is uncertain. A reasonable goal is to keep blood glucose less than 200 mg/dL.[74,75] Intravenous infusion of insulin may be necessary. One should be cautious to avoid hypoglycemia, which could potentially worsen outcome. Therefore, a well-designed insulin protocol with defined treatment for hypoglycemia may be helpful.

Nutrition

Acute brain injury induces a hypercatabolic state. Early institution of nutrition is associated with enhanced outcomes in patients with traumatic brain injury;[88,89] however, there are currently no specific data evaluating early nutrition for patients with SAH. The enteral route is generally preferred.

Neuroprotective Agents

Myriad agents have been tested for neuroprotection in patients with aneurysmal SAH. Some of the agents tested include calcium antagonists (i.e., nimodipine, nicardipine, AT877), aminosteroids (i.e., tirilazad), antioxidants (i.e., nicaraven and ebselen), and antiplatelet agents (i.e., aspirin, dipyridamole, nizofenone, ozagrel sodium, and OKY-46).[16] The only agent that has definitely improved outcome in randomized controlled trials is nimodipine.

Nimodipine and Other Calcium Antagonists. A 2007 *Cochrane Database Systematic Review* evaluated 16 randomized trials of calcium antagonists in SAH involving 3361 patients.[90] The investigators found that oral nimodipine was associated with a significantly reduced relative risk (RR) of poor outcome (0.67; 95% confidence interval [CI], 0.55–0.81) in comparison with controls. This beneficial effect was not seen for intravenous nimodipine or other calcium antagonists. The beneficial results were strongly influenced by the largest of the trials (n = 544), which randomly assigned patients to oral nimodipine 60 mg every 4 hours for 21 days or placebo. Although generally safe, nimodipine has the potential to produce hypotension.

Steroids. There is no evidence to support the routine use of steroids in patients with aneurysmal SAH. A 2005 *Cochrane Database Systematic Review* evaluated three randomized trials with 256 patients with aneurysmal SAH; however, because of the small number of patients, there was insufficient evidence to suggest either a beneficial or a harmful effect of steroids.[91]

Magnesium. Traditionally, IV magnesium was thought to have favorable effects on the arterial vasculature, vasospasm, and that it may be neuroprotective for SAH. However, a large meta-analysis, and randomized phase III clinical trial of magnesium in SAH patients (IMASH) were recently reported, and unfortunately did not show any benefit of IV magnesium for up to 10–14 days in SAH patients compared to placebo.[92,93]

Statins. There has been interest in statins as possible neuroprotective agents in SAH. The physiologic rationale for using statins in SAH includes enhancement of nitric oxide production and reduction of free radical formation, which may attenuate vasospasm.[94,95] However, there is currently a paucity of evidence from randomized controlled trials to support the routine use of statins in patients with SAH.

Antiplatelets. DCI with subsequent infarction after aneurysmal SAH is a major source of long-term disability. Although the mechanism of infarction may be related to symptomatic vasospasm, thromboembolism may also be involved.[96] A 2007 *Cochrane Database Systematic Review* evaluated seven randomized trials involving 1385 patients with SAH. There was a trend toward better outcomes with antiplatelet drugs but a higher rate of intracranial hemorrhages; neither of these differences attained statistical significance.[97] Therefore, there is currently no solid evidence to support the routine use of antiplatelet drugs after aneurysmal SAH.

Venous Thromboembolism Prophylaxis

Patients with SAH are at high risk for venous thromboembolism (VTE), either deep vein thrombosis (DVT) or pulmonary embolism. The safety of anticoagulant use for prophylaxis of venous thromboembolism in patients with SAH is not firmly established. There is some indirect evidence from randomized trials that low-molecular-weight heparin may be relatively safe after the aneurysm has been secured. Siironen and coworkers[98] evaluated the efficacy of enoxaparin on mortality and neurologic outcome in patients with aneurysmal SAH. Although they were not specifically looking at VTE in this trial, the researchers found that enoxaparin, 40 mg SC daily for 10 days, did not significantly increase bleeding complications or affect neurologic outcomes. In patients who have contraindications to anticoagulant prophylaxis, mechanical prophylaxis with sequential pneumatic compression devices and thigh-high elastic compression hose is advocated.

Stress Ulcer Prophylaxis

Gastric stress ulcers are common in critically ill patients and are associated with worse outcome.[99] Important risk factors for stress ulcers include acute brain injury, mechanical ventilation, and coagulopathy. Measures that may help reduce the risk of ulcers include early feeding and administration of H_2 receptor antagonists (e.g., ranitidine, famotidine), proton pump inhibitors (PPIs) (e.g., pantoprazole, omeprazole), or sucralfate. Unfortunately, there are no randomized data to guide the optimal regimen in patients with SAH.

Ventilator Management

Many patients with aneurysmal SAH require mechanical ventilation, and improper ventilator management increases patient mortality.[100] Some indications for mechanical ventilation in patients with SAH are respiratory failure due to impaired oxygenation or inadequate ventilation, elevated ICP, need for surgery, and inadequate airway protection.

The mode of ventilation is probably not important so long as the patient maintains good oxygenation and ventilation and does not receive excessive tidal volumes. The plateau pressure, as determined by a short end-inspiratory hold, should be less than 30 cm H_2O to help minimize the risk of ventilator-induced alveolar injury. The patient should be made comfortable with ample sedation and analgesia.

One should closely monitor carbon dioxide (PCO_2) levels in ventilated patients with SAH to avoid hypercarbia and excessive hypocarbia. The CBF increases linearly in response to changes in the PCO_2 level; an increase in PCO_2 can significantly increase the CBF and cerebral blood volume and lead to exacerbation of the ICP. In contrast, hyperventilation may do harm by reducing CBF and thus lowering the threshold for cerebral ischemia.

A critical concept in ventilator management is that patients should receive lower tidal volumes than traditionally used. There are compelling data from two randomized controlled trials demonstrating that traditional (high) tidal volumes (12 mL/kg) increase mortality over that seen with lower tidal volumes (6 mL/kg). Although these studies were not specifically conducted in neurologic patients, it would be prudent to err on the side of lower tidal volumes, so long as the PCO_2 can be controlled. If the ICP is an issue, the respiratory rate can be set to a higher level to facilitate PCO_2 clearance.

The application of positive end-expiratory pressure (PEEP) may reduce ventilator-induced lung injury by preventing alveolar derecruitment at end-expiration. Although there is a theoretical concern that positive end-expiratory pressure may increase the ICP by impairing venous return or lowering cardiac output, the data do not necessarily support this possibility.[101]

Sedation and Analgesia

One should adequately control agitation and pain in the patient with SAH, because they may exacerbate hypertension and ICP and potentially increase the risk of aneurysmal rebleeding. However, one should start with low doses and carefully titrate upward to avoid oversedation, which will obscure neurologic findings.

The optimal agents are short-acting and free of significant hemodynamic effects. For sedation, some reasonable choices include intermittent doses of lorazepam or midazolam, either orally or intravenously. In patients undergoing mechanical ventilation who require sedation, propofol or midazolam intravenous infusion is appropriate; both are easily titratable, although midazolam may require longer clearance time with prolonged use. Propofol characteristically lowers the BP, so supportive vasopressors may be needed.

Some initial analgesic choices include acetaminophen and codeine; however, these are usually inadequate.[102] Opiates such as morphine and fentanyl are usually needed but may lower the BP or contribute to delirium. Meperidine and tramadol are best avoided because they can trigger seizures. Diclofenac has antiplatelet effects and should be avoided. Continuous infusion of fentanyl is convenient for intubated patients; patient-controlled analgesia may be appropriate for awake and alert patients.

Nausea and vomiting may be problematic and can be controlled with ondansetron, which has minimal sedating effects. Alternatively, one can use metoclopramide, keeping in mind the potential for dystonic reactions.

Securing the Aneurysm: Surgical versus Endovascular Treatment

Early treatment of the aneurysm has largely replaced the traditional "wait and see" approach. The potential benefits of securing the aneurysm early include reducing the risk of rebleeding and allowing aggressive hemodynamic management.[103] Endovascular therapy has now become the preferred treatment modality for the majority of aneurysms over surgical clipping. There has been debate regarding the best modality to repair a given aneurysm. Some of the factors that are important to consider in choosing the best approach are aneurysm anatomy, patient characteristics, and institutional expertise. For example, surgical clipping is preferred in patients with wide-neck aneurysms, giant aneurysms, and aneurysms located in the middle cerebral artery. The International Subarachnoid Hemorrhage Aneurysm Treatment Trial (ISAT) attempted to determine the optimal aneurysm therapy.[104,105] This was a European multicenter, randomized controlled trial of 2143 patients with aneurysmal SAH. The patients were randomly assigned to surgical clipping (n = 1070) or endovascular therapy (EVT) with coiling (n = 1073). The primary outcome was death or dependency at 1 year, as measured by the modified Rankin scale. EVT yielded a significantly lower rate of death or dependency than did surgical clipping (23.7% vs. 30.6%, respectively; $P = 0.0019$). The risk of early rebleeding was modestly higher in the EVT group.

There are some criticisms of the International Subarachnoid Hemorrhage Aneurysm Treatment Trial. First, prior to enrollment, there had to be agreement between the neurosurgeon and interventionalist that either treatment modality was acceptable for the given aneurysm. Consequently, a large number of patients were excluded from enrollment owing to the perception that one modality was superior. Second, the risk of early rebleeding (within 30 days) was found to be higher with EVT. In fact, a long-term follow-up study of patients enrolled in the trial revealed that retreatment of aneurysms after EVT was necessary in 17.4% of patients, compared with 3.8% in the surgically treated patients. The EVT retreatment occurred throughout the follow-up period and was more likely to be used in patients who were younger, had incomplete aneurysm occlusion, or had a wide aneurysm lumen. However, the long-term risk of rebleeding was rare and not significantly higher in the EVT group than in the surgically treated patients. Even though a higher proportion of patients required retreatment after EVT, the benefit in outcome was maintained in comparison with that in surgically treated patients in long-term follow-up.

Neurologic Complications

One must remain vigilant to anticipate the myriad conditions that can lead to neurologic deterioration after SAH. A systematic approach can be helpful (Fig. 29-2). Some neurologic complications are aneurysmal rebleeding, hydrocephalus, seizures, vasospasm and DCI, and cerebral infarction. Systemic complications may also contribute to apparent neurologic deterioration and are discussed later in the chapter.

Aneurysmal Rebleeding

One of the most devastating early complications after SAH is aneurysmal rebleeding, which increases mortality up to 80%.[106] The risk of rebleeding peaks at 4% on the first day and is 1.5% per day for the next 2 weeks. One study cites a risk of rebleeding of up to 17% on the first day after the ictus. The cumulative risk of rebleeding is about 15% to 20% in the first 2 weeks and about 50% by 6 months. Some patients may have rebleeding before seeking medical attention, so the true rate is unknown. Some known predictors of rebleeding are a history of sentinel headache, female gender, larger aneurysm size, higher Hunt and Hess clinical grade on admission, and time to surgery. Some authorities speculate that placement of an external ventricular drain or lumbar puncture may increase the risk of rebleeding, but the literature does not support this proposition.

Clinically, rebleeding may manifest as an acute or worsening headache, decrease in the level of consciousness, loss of brainstem reflexes, posturing, respiratory arrest, or seizures. Other manifestations include BP changes and elevated ICP. Rebleeding may manifest visually as an acute increase in external ventricular drainage or a change in the color of CSF from clear to red. One can confirm the diagnosis of rebleeding by urgent non-contrast-enhanced head CT. Definitive treatment of the aneurysm with EVT or surgical clipping markedly reduces the risk of rebleeding.

Before definitive treatment of the aneurysm, medical measures may help attenuate the risk of rebleeding. General measures, which are based mainly on common sense, include bed rest, maintaining a quiet and peaceful environment, treating pain, avoiding constipation, and controlling hypertension.[107] Antifibrinolytic therapy with tranexamic acid or ε-aminocaproic acid (Amicar) reduces the risk of rebleeding but carries significant risks.[108] These agents inhibit plasminogen activation, which helps protect fibrin clots from degradation. There is some evidence from randomized trials that short-term use of these agents (less than 72 hours) before definitive aneurysm treatment significantly reduces the risk of rebleeding without increasing the risk of ischemia; however, it is uncertain whether long-term outcome is improved. A 2003 *Cochrane Database Systematic Review*, which included 1399 patients from nine trials, concluded that antifibrinolytic agents reduced the risk of rebleeding (odds ratio [OR], 0.55; 95%CI, 0.42–0.71) but increased the risk of thromboembolism (OR, 1.39; 95%CI, 1.07–1.82) and did not improve neurologic outcome or mortality.[108] However, on the basis of current recommendations, a short course of antifibrinolytics before securing the aneurysm, or in patients deemed to be at low risk for vasospasm or in whom surgical delay is beneficial, is considered reasonable.[74,75] The usual

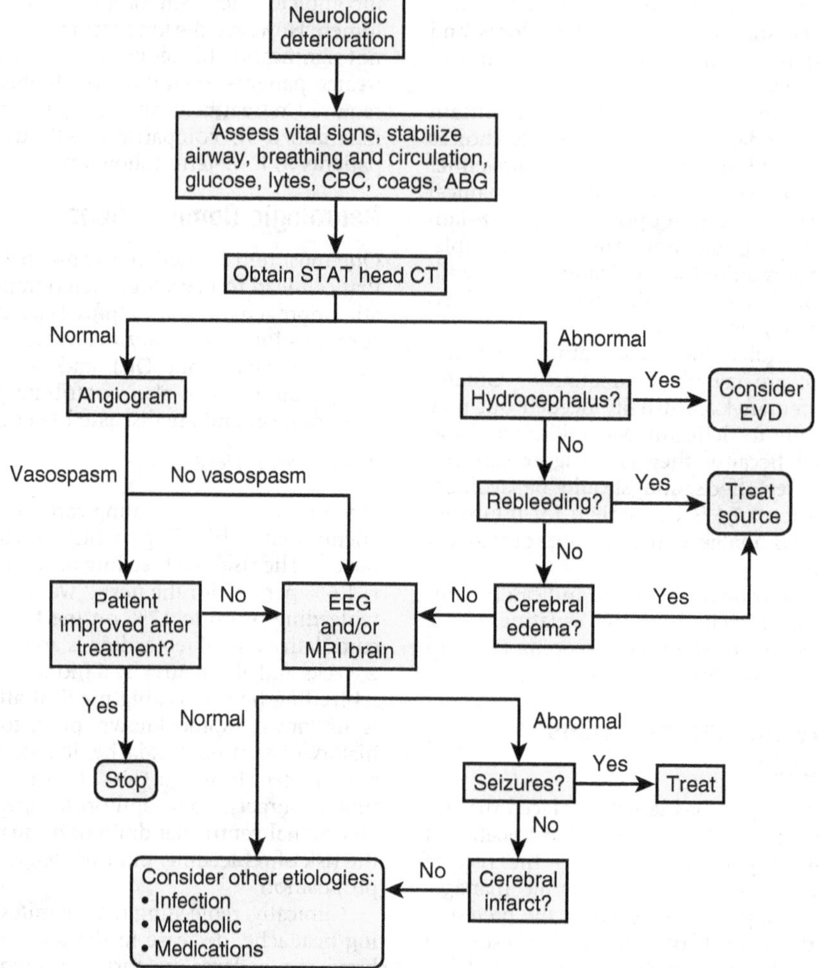

Figure 29-2. An approach to neurologic deterioration after subarachnoid hemorrhage. ABG, arterial blood gas analysis; CBC, complete blood count; coags, coagulation studies; EEG, electroencephalography; EVD, external ventricular drain; lytes, electrolytes.

dose of aminocaproic acid is a 5-g IV bolus, followed by an infusion of 1.5 g/hour for 24 to 48 hours. A regimen for tranexamic acid is 1 g every 4 hours, with no bolus. In addition to increasing the risk of ischemic stroke, other complications of antifibrinolytic therapy include venous thromboembolism, rhabdomyolysis, and acute renal failure.

Hydrocephalus

Acute hydrocephalus occurs in about 20% of patients within 72 hours and is predicted by the demonstration of intraventricular blood rather than cisternal blood on head CT.[109] Acute hydrocephalus after SAH is associated with significantly increased mortality and neurologic impairment.

The usual clinical findings in hydrocephalus include a progressively worsening level of consciousness and small, poorly reactive pupils in comatose patients. Impaired upgaze due to dysfunction of the dorsal midbrain vertical gaze centers may be evident. Diagnosis is made from non-contrast-enhanced head CT showing increased ventricular size. Urgent external ventricular drainage may be life-saving. A clinically dramatic response is often witnessed in comatose patients with SAH, who become alert and responsive shortly after placement of the external ventricular drain.

About 20% of patients with aneurysmal SAH require permanent shunting for chronic hydrocephalus. The mechanism is not well determined but may be related to impairment of CSF absorption due to fibrosis of arachnoid villi in response to blood breakdown products and CSF inflammation. Some retrospective data suggest that neurosurgical fenestration of the lamina terminalis to facilitate CSF drainage significantly reduces the occurrence of shunt dependence,[110] but a randomized controlled trial is needed to confirm the benefits of this approach.

Seizures

The incidence of seizures after aneurysmal SAH is 21% to 26%;[111] furthermore, the presence of seizures at the onset of SAH is an independent risk factor for poor outcome. Risk factors for seizures after SAH include poor-grade WFNS scale score on admission, thick cisternal blood clots, and aneurysmal rebleeding. The efficacy of anticonvulsant prophylaxis of seizures after SAH is an area of controversy. Traditionally, patients with SAH were started on anticonvulsants upon hospital admission and remained on the regimen for months to years. Later evidence suggests that long-term (>1 week) anticonvulsant prophylaxis may not be necessary and may even be harmful. Anticonvulsant use is independently associated with worse outcome and may increase in-hospital complications.[112] Additionally, there is evidence that most seizures after SAH occur at the ictus rather than during hospitalization, the long-term risk of epilepsy is relatively low in survivors, and early prophylaxis does not prevent the long-term risk of epilepsy. If anticonvulsant prophylaxis is used, there seems to be no benefit for an extended regimen. Chumnanvej and associates[113] retrospectively compared two different anticonvulsant regimens using phenytoin, evaluating seizure incidence and adverse effects. The traditional regimen consisted of phenytoin prophylaxis until hospital discharge, whereas the short regimen involved only 3 days of prophylaxis. The seizure incidences for the traditional and short prophylaxis regimens were not statistically different, 1.3% and 1.9%, respectively; however, the risk of hypersensitivity reaction was significantly higher in the traditional group (8.8% and 0.5%, respectively).

Vasospasm, Delayed Cerebral Ischemia, and Infarction

One of the most feared complications after SAH is DCI and subsequent infarction, which is a source of major long-term disability. Although DCI is an anticipated complication, our treatment arsenal remains limited. One should understand an important distinction among radiologic vasospasm, symptomatic (clinical) vasospasm, and DCI. Radiologic evidence of vasospasm on angiography is found in about 66% of patients, whereas DCI occurs in about 32% to 46% of patients.[114,115] Symptomatic vasospasm is the most common cause of DCI; however, it has become clear that not all DCI is caused by vasospasm.

The pathophysiology of DCI after SAH requires further elucidation. The instigating factor is thought to be related to extravasation of arterial blood, because the amount of subarachnoid blood in the basal subarachnoid cisterns correlates with the risk of DCI.[116-119] Second, the source of bleeding (i.e., arterial or venous) may be important. For example, it is known that the risk of vasospasm is exceedingly low after perimesencephalic hemorrhage, which may have a venous origin. Oxyhemoglobin is implicated as the main trigger for vasospasm; however, this issue needs further confirmation. Some of the subsequent mediators may be excess intracellular calcium, free radical production, neurogenic vascular dysfunction, inflammatory infiltration of blood vessels, and imbalances in vasoconstrictor and vasodilatory substances.

DCI is usually related to vasospasm; however, attention has now turned to other etiologies, such as microthrombosis due to activation of the coagulation cascade and prolonged cortical spreading depression.[119] Stein and colleagues,[96] autopsying patients with SAH who died with or without DCI, found that patients with DCI had a much higher microclot burden, suggesting that thromboembolism played an important role in development of DCI in these patients. Interestingly, it was reported that patients with SAH who were undergoing aspirin therapy before aneurysmal rupture had a significantly lower risk of cerebral infarction.[120] Another interesting observation is that nimodipine, which improves outcome after SAH without affecting vasospasm, exerts fibrinolytic activity through a decrease in plasminogen-activator inhibitor-1 (PAI-1) levels.[121] Another potential cause for DCI that has gained attention is recurrent prolonged cortical spreading depression.[122] Dreier and associates[122] recorded spreading depolarization with electrocorticography in 18 patients with SAH who underwent surgical repair of an aneurysm. Recurrent spreading depolarizations were observed in 72% (n = 13) of cases and were closely correlated with subsequent DCI, with positive and negative predictive values of 86% and 100%, respectively.

The time course of vasospasm is usually predictable, with an onset beginning after 72 hours, a peak between days 6 to 8, and gradual resolution in 2 to 4 weeks.[1] It is unusual for vasospasm to begin within 72 hours after initial SAH. Evidence of vasospasm may be observed on TCD ultrasonography up to 4 weeks after the ictus.

Clinically, DCI may manifest subtly as worsening headache, confusion, decreasing level of consciousness, and eventual progression to a focal neurologic deficit.

The diagnosis of DCI is confirmed by urgently ruling out other causes of acute neurologic deterioration and demonstrating narrowing of the cerebral blood vessels on angiography (see Fig. 29-1). TCD monitoring is a useful noninvasive, bedside screening test for vasospasm. There is a good correlation between TCD evidence and angiographic demonstration of vasospasm. Vora and coworkers[123] demonstrated that mean CBF velocities less than 120 cm/second and greater than or equal to 200 cm/second had negative and positive predictive values of 94% and 87%, respectively, for demonstration of moderate to severe vasospasm on angiography; however, in most (57%) patients, CBF velocities were in the indeterminate range (120 to 199 cm/second).[123] Other TCD measures that suggest vasospasm include an increase in flow velocity greater than 50 cm/second in 24 hours and an elevated "Lindegaard" ratio. The Lindegaard ratio, which helps differentiate global hyperemia from vasospasm, is calculated as the ratio of the flow velocities in the middle cerebral artery and the ipsilateral *extracranial* internal carotid artery.[124] Ratios greater than 3 and greater than 6 are consistent with mild and severe vasospasm, respectively, whereas a ratio less than 3 in the setting of elevated blood flow velocities is consistent with global hyperemia, because the extracranial internal carotid artery does not have vasospasm but will increase with systemic hemodynamic factors. Although TCD evidence of vasospasm correlates well with angiographic demonstration of vasospasm, the sensitivity of TCD for DCI is less robust. Suarez and associates[124] found that the sensitivity of TCD evidence of vasospasm for detection of DCI was 73% for the anterior circulation; interestingly, angiography was only 80% sensitive. This finding is consistent with the notion that there are other causes for DCI than strictly angiographic narrowing of the blood vessels. TCD has several limitations, including dependence on operator technique, patient-specific anatomic factors (i.e., abnormal bone window anatomy), and inability for insonation of distal arterial branches. Additionally, TCD blood flow velocities may be influenced by factors other than vasospasm, including BP, ICP, PCO_2, hematocrit, and patient age. Furthermore, TCD is more accurate in the anterior circulation than in the posterior circulation. Perfusion CT of the head with or without CTA has shown promise for assessing the presence of symptomatic vasospasm.[125] Findings on perfusion CT that are consistent with DCI due to vasospasm include increases in cerebral blood volume, mean transit time, and time to peak and decreased CBF.

Treatment of symptomatic vasospasm consists of medical and endovascular therapy. Trasitionally, the cornerstone of medical management is triple-H therapy.[126] The hypertensive component of this therapy often requires a vasopressor such as phenylephrine, norepinephrine, or dopamine. Hypervolemia and hemodilution are achieved with aggressive crystalloid and colloid administration aimed at lowering hematocrit to about 30% to decrease blood viscosity. Endpoints of hypervolemia include targeting the central venous pressure to 8 to 12 mm Hg or pulmonary capillary wedge pressure to 14 to 18 mm Hg. Despite the widespread use of triple-H therapy, there are few prospective data supporting its efficacy. Potential complications of the approach include pulmonary edema, myocardial infarction, arrhythmias, acute respiratory distress syndrome, dilutional hyponatremia, and exacerbation of cerebral edema.[127] Additionally, there may be significant complications associated with the hemodynamic monitoring devices, either Swan-Ganz or central venous catheters, used to guide triple-H therapy. Current recommendations are to institute normovolemia along with induced hypertension.[74,75] Patients with DCI that is refractory to induced hypertension may benefit from augmentation of cardiac output. However, a recent prospective trial comparing prophylactic intra-aortic balloon pump to standard hypervolemic therapy, did not show any benefit with regards to improving cerebral blood flow, or clinical outcomes.[128]

There had previously been interest in an endothelin receptor antagonist to prevent vasospasm, reduce the risk of DCI, and improve outcomes.[129,130] As such, prospective randomized trials, CONSCIOUS-2 and CONSCIOUS-3, were conducted comparing clazosentan versus placebo in SAH patients. The CONSCIOUS-2 study investigators reported that, although clazosentan 15 mg per hour significantly reduced post-SAH vasospasm-related morbidity and all-cause mortality, none of the doses improved outcome on the extended Glasgow Outcome Scale. As a result, the CONSCIOUS-3 trial was terminated.

EVT for DCI is evolving, but large randomized trials of its use are lacking. EVT can be used alternatively or in conjunction with induced hypertension. The two main approaches for EVT are intra-arterial injection of vasodilators and/or transluminal balloon angioplasty.

Some IA vasodilators that have been used are papaverine, verapamil, nimodipine, and nicardipine. Advantages of intra-arterial vasodilators include immediate action and ability to alleviate distal arterial vasospasm; however, the effects of these agents are transient, and a second intervention may be necessary. Papaverine use has diminished owing to the observation that it may be neurotoxic.[131] Furthermore, intra-arterial nicardipine may be longer-acting than papaverine. Although intra-arterial vasodilators are generally safe, some possible complications of their use are hypotension, bradycardia, and elevation of ICP.

Balloon angioplasty has also been used to treat vasospasm. A pooled analysis of balloon angioplasty for DCI showed about a 60% response overall.[132] Clinical response is associated with increased CBF and decreased TCD-detected flow velocities. Typically, balloon angioplasty involves gentle inflation of the balloon to successively larger volumes. A limitation of angioplasty is that the relatively large balloon size precludes dilation of smaller distal arteries. Possible complications of balloon angioplasty include those associated with angiography, such as arterial dissection, stroke, contrast allergy, and renal nephropathy, as well as catastrophic arterial rupture. After EVT, one can monitor blood flow velocities with TCD ultrasonography. A subsequent increase in TCD-detected flow velocities toward the level that previously produced symptoms can be used as a trigger for repeating EVT.

Cerebral Edema

The formation of cerebral edema after SAH occurs in 8% to 20% of patients and independently predicts poor outcome.[133,134] Cerebral edema may be present on admission or may develop subacutely. Predictors of acute cerebral edema include loss of consciousness at ictus and poor-grade Hunt and Hess scale value; late predictors include vasopressor use, large aneurysm size (>10 mm), and loss of consciousness at ictus. Cerebral edema after SAH can be cytotoxic, vasogenic, hydrocephalic, or osmotic in origin. Cytotoxic edema may occur early, as a result of transient global cerebral ischemia due to the abrupt rise in ICP after aneurysmal rupture, or late, because of DCI. Hydrocephalic edema arises from impairment of CSF drainage and involves transependymal CSF flow. Vasogenic edema may occur from impairment of cerebral autoregulation, resulting in increased CBF and cerebral blood volume. Finally, osmotic edema may result from hyponatremia.

Cerebral edema is reliably diagnosed from the presence of severe effacement of hemispheric sulci and basal cisterns, and blurring or finger-like extension of the gray–white matter junction at the level of the centrum semiovale.

Medical Complications of Subarachnoid Hemorrhage

Multiorgan systemic disturbances are frequent after SAH and may be life-threatening. Some of the medical complications are those seen in any critically ill patient receiving intensive care, and others are more specific to patients with SAH. Cardiac complications include neurogenic stunned myocardium, heart failure, myocardial infarction, and arrhythmias. Pulmonary complications include pneumonia, acute lung injury (ALI), ARDS, and pulmonary embolism. Endocrinologic disturbances include disorders of the hypothalamic–pituitary axis, cerebral salt wasting, and adrenal insufficiency. Infectious complications other than pneumonia include urinary tract infections, sepsis, and ventriculitis. Other medical complications are acute renal failure, electrolyte disturbances, DVT, gastrointestinal bleeding, and pressure ulcers.

Cardiac Complications

Cardiac dysfunction following SAH is common, occurring in 50% to 100% of patients, and includes arrhythmias, electrocardiographic abnormalities, neurogenic stunned myocardium, troponin elevation, heart failure, and myocardial infarction.[135,136] There may be genetic polymorphisms that predispose to development of cardiac dysfunction after SAH.[137]

Cardiac arrhythmias are frequent and range in severity from benign to life-threatening. Presence of serious arrhythmias occurs in about 4% of patients with SAH and independently predicts increased ICU length of stay, death, and poor neurologic outcome.[135] However, the cause of death in these patients is not usually related to the arrhythmia.[138]

Neurogenic stunned myocardium refers to acutely decreased left ventricular function that occurs shortly after aneurysmal rupture. On echocardiography, one observes a pattern of global or regional ventricular wall hypokinesis that is not usually referable to a distinct vascular territory.[139,140] Cardiac catheterization usually reveals normal-appearing coronary arteries.[140] Pathologic studies show a characteristic "contraction band necrosis."[141] The pathophysiology is thought to be related to sudden catecholamine surge. Ventricular function usually improves to normal spontaneously within a few weeks.

Troponin elevation after SAH is also frequent. Multiple studies report that an elevated troponin-I value on admission is common after SAH and that it predicts cardiac dysfunction and poor outcome.[142] There is some evidence that β-blockade may have a beneficial effect on outcome in SAH; however, this possibility requires confirmation.[143]

Pulmonary edema is reported in about 29% of patients and may be related to both systolic and diastolic dysfunction after SAH. The finding of elevated brain natriuretic peptide (BNP) after SAH may correlate with ventricular dysfunction and myocardial necrosis.[144]

Pulmonary Complications

Disturbances in pulmonary function may occur in SAH because of pulmonary edema, pneumonia, pulmonary embolism, and ALI or ARDS. Abnormalities in oxygen exchange have been seen in 80% of patients with SAH and are associated with poor outcome. In addition, pulmonary dysfunction has been associated with increased risk of DCI, thought to be due to the preclusion of aggressive hemodynamic therapy by tenuous lung function.[145]

Infection

Nosocomial infections are common after SAH. In a series of 573 consecutive patients with SAH, the following infections were identified: pneumonia (20%), urinary tract infection (13%), bloodstream infection (8%), and meningitis or ventriculitis (5%).[146] In this study, pneumonia or bloodstream infection independently predicted death or severe disability at 3 months.

Endocrine Disturbances

One should consider disorders of the hypothalamic–pituitary axis after SAH, which are likely under-recognized.[147] The most common hormonal abnormalities are deficiencies in growth hormone and adrenocorticotropic hormone. Acutely, patients may also have abnormalities in thyroid hormones that are compatible with euthyroid sick syndrome. Deficiency in adrenocorticotropic hormone has direct clinical relevance because hypotension may increase the risk of DCI in the setting of vasospasm or elevated ICP. Similarly, central diabetes insipidus due to vasopressin deficiency has been described after clipping of anterior communicating artery aneurysms, which could lead to rapid intravascular volume depletion and hypotension. Chronic endocrine disturbances occur in up to 55% of patients with SAH. Patients with growth hormone deficiency after SAH may experience significant weight gain.

Electrolyte Abnormalities

Abnormalities in serum electrolyte values are common after SAH and may be associated with poor outcome.[148] Thus, careful attention to electrolyte replacement is essential. Some of these disturbances are hyponatremia or hypernatremia, hypomagnesemia, hypokalemia, hypocalcemia, and hypophosphatemia.

Hyponatremia should raise suspicion of cerebral salt-wasting syndrome (CSWS) or SIADH.[149] Hyponatremia may exacerbate cerebral edema and ICP. Hypernatremia may represent underlying central diabetes insipidus and is associated with a poor outcome. Hypomagnesemia is associated with increased DCI. Hypokalemia may contribute to life-threatening ventricular arrhythmias and prolongation of the QT interval.

CSWS following neurologic injury has gradually gained widespread acceptance.[149] Traditionally, hyponatremia after aneurysmal SAH was presumed to be due to SIADH; however, it has become clear that many cases of hyponatremia are due to renal sodium loss and have associated intravascular volume depletion. The differentiation of SIADH from CSWS is essential because the treatments vary markedly: SIADH requires fluid restriction, whereas CSWS requires aggressive volume replacement. Inappropriate fluid restriction in patients with CSWS may lead to dehydration and hypotension, which potentially increase the risk of DCI and cerebral infarction. The pathophysiology leading to CSWS is unclear but may be related to elevations of brain natriuretic peptide and depressed levels of aldosterone.

The diagnosis of CSWS requires a determination of volume depletion. Volume depletion may be difficult to determine, and one should not rely on a single measure. The most accurate methods use radionuclide scanning with albumin or chromium-labeled red blood cells but are expensive and not generally practical. Some bedside indicators of volume depletion may include a central venous pressure less than 5 mm Hg, negative fluid balances, increased urine output, decreasing body weight, and low skin turgor. Laboratory tests are not generally useful to differentiate SIADH from CSWS. Treatment of CSWS involves aggressive volume and sodium replacement. Recommended regimens include various combinations of normal saline or hypertonic saline (3%) infusion, oral sodium replacement, and exogenous mineralocorticoids such as hydrocortisone and fludrocortisone. Fludrocortisone is usually given at a dose of 0.1 mg daily up to 0.2 mg twice daily. Serious hypokalemia may result. Treatment is gradually tapered over several weeks.

OUTCOMES

Despite advances in diagnosis and management of SAH, the outcome for most patients with aneurysmal SAH remains suboptimal. The case mortality rate is 40% to 50%; 10% to 20% of patients survive with severe disability, and 40% with independent function.[11,12,16] Some independent predictors of mortality and long-term disability include worse neurologic grade on admission, age, increasing systolic BP, fever, rebleeding, DCI and cerebral infarction, large aneurysm size (>10 mm), and elevated SAH Physiologic Derangement score.[150] The SAH Physiologic Derangement score combines a number of physiologic parameters – the arterioalveolar gradient and serum bicarbonate, glucose, and mean arterial pressure values – to create a score ranging from 0 to 8; a rising score strongly predicts neurologic disability and death. Patients with a score of 8 have a mortality approaching 80%, compared with about 10% for a score of 0.

Long-term neurologic sequelae may be under-recognized. Hackett and coworkers,[151] interviewing 230 patients with SAH 1 year after onset, found that 46% reported impairment in cognitive function or mood. The most common areas of impairment were memory (50%), mood (39%), speech (14%), and self-care (10%). Thus, quality of life after SAH may be impaired. Furthermore, there is about a 7% risk of epilepsy, which is associated with severe disability and reduced quality of life.[11,16]

REFERENCES

1. Morgagni G. On the seats and causes of diseases investigated by anatomy. London; 1761.
2. Haas LF. Papyrus of Ebers and Smith. J Neurol Neurosurg Psychiatry 1999;67:578.
3. Willis T. Cerebri anatome: cui accessit nervorum descriptio et usus. London: J Flesher; 1664.
4. Flamm ES. History of diagnosis and treatment of aneurysmal subarachnoid hemorrhage. Neurosurg Clin N Am 2001;12:23–35, vii.
5. Cheyne J. Cases of apoplexy and lethargy: with observations upon the comatose diseases. London: Thomas Underwood; 1812.
6. Gull W. Cases of aneurism of the cerebral vessels. Guys Hospital Reports 1859;5:281–304.
7. Quincke H. Verhandlungen des Congresses für Innere Medizin, vol. 10. Wiesbaden: Zehnter Congress; 1891. p. 321–31.
8. Moniz E. L'encephalographie arterielle, son importance dans la localisation des tumerus cerebrales. Rev Neurol (Paris) 1927;2.
9. Moniz E. Cerebral angiography. Its application in clinical practice and physiology. Lancet 1933;225:1144–7.
10. Dandy W. Intracranial aneurysm of the internal carotid artery cured by operation. Ann Surg 1938;107:654–9.
11. Suarez JI, Tarr RW, Selman WR. Aneurysmal subarachnoid hemorrhage. N Engl J Med 2006;354:387–96.
12. Go AS, Mozaffarian D, Roger VLK, et al. Heart disease and stroke statistics – 2014 update: A report from the American Heart Association Statistics Committee and Stroke Statistics Subcommittee. Circulation 2014;129:e28–292.
13. Ingall T, Asplund K, Mahonen M, et al. A multinational comparison of subarachnoid hemorrhage epidemiology in the WHO MONICA stroke study. Stroke 2000;31:1054–61.
14. Kozak N, Hayashi M. Trends in the incidence of subarachnoid hemorrhage in Akita Prefecture, Japan. J Neurosurg 2007;106: 234–8.

15. King JT Jr. Epidemiology of aneurysmal subarachnoid hemorrhage. Neuroimaging Clin N Am 1997;7:659–68.
16. van Gijn J, Rinkel GJ. Subarachnoid haemorrhage: Diagnosis, causes and management. Brain 2001;124:249–78.
17. Anderson C, Anderson N, Bonita R, et al. Epidemiology of aneurysmal subarachnoid hemorrhage in Australia and New Zealand: incidence and case fatality from the Australasian Cooperative Research on Subarachnoid Hemorrhage Study (ACROSS). Stroke 2000;31:1843–50.
18. Broderick JP, Brott T, Tomsick T, et al. The risk of subarachnoid and intracerebral hemorrhages in blacks as compared with whites. N Engl J Med 1992;326:733–6.
19. Schievink WI. Intracranial aneurysms. N Engl J Med 1997;336: 28–40.
20. Juvela S, Porras M, Heiskanen O. Natural history of unruptured intracranial aneurysms: A long-term follow-up study. J Neurosurg 1993;79:174–82.
21. Hop JW, Rinkel GJ, Algra A, et al. Case-fatality rates and functional outcome after subarachnoid hemorrhage: A systematic review. Stroke 1997;28:660–4.
22. Ingall TJ, Whisnant JP, Wiebers DO, et al. Has there been a decline in subarachnoid hemorrhage mortality? Stroke 1989;20: 718–24.
23. Rincon F, Rossenwasser RH, Dumont A. The epidemiology of admissions of nontraumatic subarachnoid hemorrhage in the United States. Neurosurgery 2013;73:217–22, discussion 12–13.
24. Inagawa T, Takechi A, Yahara K, et al. Primary intracerebral and aneurysmal subarachnoid hemorrhage in Izumo City, Japan. Part I: Incidence and seasonal and diurnal variations. J Neurosurg 2000;93:958–66.
25. Jehle D, Moscati R, Frye J, et al. The incidence of spontaneous subarachnoid hemorrhage with change in barometric pressure. Am J Emerg Med 1994;12:90–1.
26. Qureshi AI, Suri MF, Yahia AM, et al. Risk factors for subarachnoid hemorrhage. Neurosurgery 2001;49:607–12, discussion 612–13.
27. Broderick JP, Viscoli CM, Brott T, et al. Major risk factors for aneurysmal subarachnoid hemorrhage in the young are modifiable. Stroke 2003;34:1375–81.
28. Teunissen LL, Rinkel GJ, Algra A, et al. Risk factors for subarachnoid hemorrhage: A systematic review. Stroke 1996;27: 544–9.
29. Fogelholm R, Murros K. Cigarette smoking and subarachnoid haemorrhage: A population-based case-control study. J Neurol Neurosurg Psychiatry 1987;50:78–80.
30. Juvela S, Hillbom M, Numminen H, et al. Cigarette smoking and alcohol consumption as risk factors for aneurysmal subarachnoid hemorrhage. Stroke 1993;24:639–46.
31. Longstreth WT Jr, Nelson LM, Koepsell TD, et al. Cigarette smoking, alcohol use, and subarachnoid hemorrhage. Stroke 1992;23:1242–9.
32. Kawachi I, Colditz GA, Stampfer MJ, et al. Smoking cessation and decreased risk of stroke in women. JAMA 1993;269: 232–6.
33. Okamoto K, Horisawa R, Ohno Y. The relationships of gender, cigarette smoking, and hypertension with the risk of aneurysmal subarachnoid hemorrhage: A case-control study in Nagoya, Japan. Ann Epidemiol 2005;15:744–8.
34. Jimenez-Yepes CM, Londono-Fernandez JL. Risk of aneurysmal subarachnoid hemorrhage: The role of confirmed hypertension. Stroke 2008;39:1344–6.
35. Iso H, Jacobs DR Jr, Wentworth D, et al. Serum cholesterol levels and six-year mortality from stroke in 350,977 men screened for the multiple risk factor intervention trial. N Engl J Med 1989; 320:904–10.
36. Stampfer MJ, Colditz GA, Willett WC, et al. A prospective study of moderate alcohol consumption and the risk of coronary disease and stroke in women. N Engl J Med 1988; 319:267–73.
37. Donahue RP, Abbott RD, Reed DM, et al. Alcohol and hemorrhagic stroke. The Honolulu Heart Program. JAMA 1986;255: 2311–14.
38. Okamoto K, Horisawa R, Kawamura T, et al. Family history and risk of subarachnoid hemorrhage: A case-control study in Nagoya, Japan. Stroke 2003;34:422–6.
39. Putman CM, Chaloupka JC, Fulbright RK, et al. Exceptional multiplicity of cerebral arteriovenous malformations associated with hereditary hemorrhagic telangiectasia (Osler-Weber-Rendu syndrome). AJNR Am J Neuroradiol 1996;17:1733–42.
40. Schievink WI, Riedinger M, Maya MM. Frequency of incidental intracranial aneurysms in neurofibromatosis type 1. Am J Med Genet 2005;134A:45–8.
41. Brill CB, Peyster RG, Hoover ED, et al. Giant intracranial aneurysm in a child with tuberous sclerosis: CT demonstration. J Comput Assist Tomogr 1985;9:377–80.
42. Magnetic Resonance Angiography in Relatives of Patients with Subarachnoid Hemorrhage Study Group. Risks and benefits of screening for intracranial aneurysms in first-degree relatives of patients with sporadic subarachnoid hemorrhage. N Engl J Med 1999;341:1344–50.
43. Kongable GL, Lanzino G, Germanson TP, et al. Gender-related differences in aneurysmal subarachnoid hemorrhage. J Neurosurg 1996;84:43–8.
44. Okamoto K, Horisawa R, Kawamura T, et al. Menstrual and reproductive factors for subarachnoid hemorrhage risk in women: A case-control study in Nagoya, Japan. Stroke 2001;32: 2841–4.
45. Oken BS. Intracranial aneurysms in polycystic kidney disease. N Engl J Med 1983;309:927–8.
46. Gieteling EW, Rinkel GJ. Characteristics of intracranial aneurysms and subarachnoid haemorrhage in patients with polycystic kidney disease. J Neurol 2003;250:418–23.
47. Yamakawa H, Ohe N, Yano H, et al. Venous drainage patterns in perimesencephalic nonaneurysmal subarachnoid hemorrhage. Clin Neurol Neurosurg 2008;110:587–91.
48. Rinkel GJ, Wijdicks EF, Vermeulen M, et al. The clinical course of perimesencephalic nonaneurysmal subarachnoid hemorrhage. Ann Neurol 1991;29:463–8.
49. Brisman JL, Song JK, Newell DW. Cerebral aneurysms. N Engl J Med 2006;355:928–39.
50. Stehbens WE. Heredity and the etiology of intracranial berry aneurysms. Stroke 1996;27:2338–40.
51. Juvela S, Poussa K, Porras M. Factors affecting formation and growth of intracranial aneurysms: A long-term follow-up study. Stroke 2001;32:485–91.
52. Krex D, Schackert HK, Schackert G. Genesis of cerebral aneurysms – an update. Acta Neurochir (Wien) 2001;143:429–48, discussion 448–9.
53. Kondo S, Hashimoto N, Kikuchi H, et al. Apoptosis of medial smooth muscle cells in the development of saccular cerebral aneurysms in rats. Stroke 1998;29:181–8, discussion 189.
54. Majamaa K, Myllyla VV. A disorder of collagen biosynthesis in patients with cerebral artery aneurysm. Biochim Biophys Acta 1993;1225:48–52.
55. Chyatte D, Bruno G, Desai S, et al. Inflammation and intracranial aneurysms. Neurosurgery 1999;45:1137–46, discussion 1146–7.
56. Stirone C, Duckles SP, Krause DN, et al. Estrogen increases mitochondrial efficiency and reduces oxidative stress in cerebral blood vessels. Mol Pharmacol 2005;68:959–65.
57. Wiebers DO, Whisnant JP, Huston J 3rd, et al. Unruptured intracranial aneurysms: Natural history, clinical outcome, and risks of surgical and endovascular treatment. Lancet 2003;362: 103–10.
58. Frösen J, Piippo A, Paetau A, et al. Remodeling of saccular cerebral artery aneurysm wall is associated with rupture: Histological analysis of 24 unruptured and 42 ruptured cases. Stroke 2004;35:2287–93.
59. Khurana VG, Meissner I, Meyer FB. Update on genetic evidence for rupture-prone compared with rupture-resistant intracranial saccular aneurysms. Neurosurg Focus 2004;17:E7.
60. Edlow JA, Caplan LR. Avoiding pitfalls in the diagnosis of subarachnoid hemorrhage. N Engl J Med 2000;342:29–36.
61. Mayer PL, Awad IA, Todor R, et al. Misdiagnosis of symptomatic cerebral aneurysm: Prevalence and correlation with outcome at four institutions. Stroke 1996;27:1558–63.
62. van der Wee N, Rinkel GJ, Hasan D, et al. Detection of subarachnoid haemorrhage on early CT: Is lumbar puncture still needed after a negative scan? J Neurol Neurosurg Psychiatry 1995;58: 357–9.

63. Sames TA, Storrow AB, Finkelstein JA, et al. Sensitivity of new-generation computed tomography in subarachnoid hemorrhage. Acad Emerg Med 1996;3:16–20.
64. Mitchell P, Wilkinson ID, Hoggard N, et al. Detection of subarachnoid haemorrhage with magnetic resonance imaging. J Neurol Neurosurg Psychiatry 2001;70:205–11.
65. Perry JJ, Spacek A, Forbes M, et al. Is the combination of negative computed tomography result and negative lumbar puncture result sufficient to rule out subarachnoid hemorrhage? Ann Emerg Med 2008;51:707–13.
66. Perry JJ, Stiell IG, Sivilotti ML, et al. Clinical decision rules to rule out subarachnoid hemorrhage for acute headache. JAMA 2013;310:1248–55.
67. Bederson JB, Awad IA, Wiebers DO, et al. Recommendations for the management of patients with unruptured intracranial aneurysms: A statement for healthcare professionals from the Stroke Council of the American Heart Association. Stroke 2000;31: 2742–50.
68. Anderson GB, Findlay JM, Steinke DE, et al. Experience with computed tomographic angiography for the detection of intracranial aneurysms in the setting of acute subarachnoid hemorrhage. Neurosurgery 1997;41:522–7, discussion 527–8.
69. Chappell ET, Moure FC, Good MC. Comparison of computed tomographic angiography with digital subtraction angiography in the diagnosis of cerebral aneurysms: A meta-analysis. Neurosurgery 2003;52:624–31, discussion 630–1.
70. Schwartz TH, Solomon RA. Perimesencephalic nonaneurysmal subarachnoid hemorrhage: Review of the literature. Neurosurgery 1996;39:433–40, discussion 440.
71. Rosen DS, Macdonald RL. Subarachnoid hemorrhage grading scales: A systematic review. Neurocrit Care 2005;2:110–18.
72. Frontera JA, Claassen J, Schmidt JM, et al. Prediction of symptomatic vasospasm after subarachnoid hemorrhage: The modified Fisher scale. Neurosurgery 2006;59:21–7, discussion 21–7.
73. Fisher CM, Kistler JP, Davis JM. Relation of cerebral vasospasm to subarachnoid hemorrhage visualized by computerized tomographic scanning. Neurosurgery 1980;6:1–9.
74. Diringer MN, Bleck TP, Claude Hemphill J 3rd, et al. Critical care management of patients following aneurysmal subarachnoid hemorrhage: recommendations from the Neurocritical Care Society's Multidisciplinary Consensus Conference. Neurocrit Care 2011;15:211–40.
75. Connolly ES Jr, Rabinstein AA, Carhuapoma JR, et al. Guidelines for the management of aneurysmal subarachnoid hemorrhage: a guideline for healthcare professionals from the American Heart Association/american Stroke Association. Stroke 2012;43:1711–37.
76. Bershad EM, Feen ES, Hernandez OH, et al. Impact of a specialized neurointensive care team on outcomes of critically ill acute ischemic stroke patients. Neurocrit Care 2008;9:287–92.
77. Suarez JI, Zaidat OO, Suri MF, et al. Length of stay and mortality in neurocritically ill patients: Impact of a specialized neurocritical care team. Crit Care Med 2004;32:2311–17.
78. Mocco J, Rose JC, Komotar RJ, et al. Blood pressure management in patients with intracerebral and subarachnoid hemorrhage. Neurosurg Clin N Am 2006;17(Suppl. 1):25–40.
79. Tseng MY, Czosnyka M, Richards H, et al. Effects of acute treatment with pravastatin on cerebral vasospasm, autoregulation, and delayed ischemic deficits after aneurysmal subarachnoid hemorrhage: A phase II randomized placebo-controlled trial. Stroke 2005;36:1627–32.
80. Naidech AM, Janjua N, Kreiter KT, et al. Predictors and impact of aneurysm rebleeding after subarachnoid hemorrhage. Arch Neurol 2005;62:410–16.
81. Oliveira-Filho J, Ezzeddine MA, Segal AZ, et al. Fever in subarachnoid hemorrhage: Relationship to vasospasm and outcome. Neurology 2001;56:1299–304.
82. Fernandez A, Schmidt JM, Claassen J, et al. Fever after subarachnoid hemorrhage: Risk factors and impact on outcome. Neurology 2007;68:1013–19.
83. Badjatia N, Topcuoglu MA, Buonanno FS, et al. Relationship between hyperglycemia and symptomatic vasospasm after subarachnoid hemorrhage. Crit Care Med 2005;33:1603–9, quiz 1623.
84. Lanzino G, Kassell NF, Germanson T, et al. Plasma glucose levels and outcome after aneurysmal subarachnoid hemorrhage. J Neurosurg 1993;79:885–91.
85. van den Berghe G, Wilmer A, Hermans G, et al. Intensive insulin therapy in the medical ICU. N Engl J Med 2006;354:449–61.
86. van den Berghe G, Wouters P, Weekers F, et al. Intensive insulin therapy in the critically ill patients. N Engl J Med 2001;345: 1359–67.
87. van den Berghe G, Schoonheydt K, Becx P, et al. Insulin therapy protects the central and peripheral nervous system of intensive care patients. Neurology 2005;64:1348–53.
88. Hartl R, Gerber LM, Ni Q, et al. Effect of early nutrition on deaths due to severe traumatic brain injury. J Neurosurg 2008; 109:50–6.
89. Taylor SJ, Fettes SB, Jewkes C, et al. Prospective, randomized, controlled trial to determine the effect of early enhanced enteral nutrition on clinical outcome in mechanically ventilated patients suffering head injury. Crit Care Med 1999;27:2525–31.
90. Dorhout Mees SM, Rinkel GJ, Feigin VL, et al. Calcium antagonists for aneurysmal subarachnoid haemorrhage. Cochrane Database Syst Rev 2007;(3):CD000277.
91. Feigin VL, Anderson N, Rinkel GJ, et al. Corticosteroids for aneurysmal subarachnoid haemorrhage and primary intracerebral haemorrhage. Cochrane Database Syst Rev 2005;(3):CD004583.
92. Suarez JI, Participants in the International Multidisciplinary Consensus Conference on the Critical Care Management of Subarachnoid H. Magnesium sulfate administration in subarachnoid hemorrhage. Neurocrit Care 2011;15:302–7.
93. Dorhout Mees SM, Algra A, Vandertop WP, et al. Magnesium for aneurysmal subarachnoid hemorrhage (MASH-2): a randomized placebo-controlled trial. Lancet 2012;380:44–9.
94. Trimble JL, Kockler DR. Statin treatment of cerebral vasospasm after aneurysmal subarachnoid hemorrhage. Ann Pharmacother 2007;41:2019–23.
95. Chou SH, Smith EE, Badjatia N, et al. A randomized, double-blind, placebo-controlled pilot study of simvastatin in aneurysmal subarachnoid hemorrhage. Stroke 2008;9:2891–3.
96. Stein SC, Browne KD, Chen XH, et al. Thromboembolism and delayed cerebral ischemia after subarachnoid hemorrhage: An autopsy study. Neurosurgery 2006;59:781–7, discussion 787–8.
97. Dorhout Mees SM, van den Bergh WM, Algra A, et al. Antiplatelet therapy for aneurysmal subarachnoid haemorrhage. Cochrane Database Syst Rev 2007;(4):CD006184.
98. Siironen J, Juvela S, Varis J, et al. No effect of enoxaparin on outcome of aneurysmal subarachnoid hemorrhage: A randomized, double-blind, placebo-controlled clinical trial. J Neurosurg 2003;99:953–9.
99. Stollman N, Metz DC. Pathophysiology and prophylaxis of stress ulcer in intensive care unit patients. J Crit Care 2005;20:35–45.
100. Ventilation with lower tidal volumes as compared with traditional tidal volumes for acute lung injury and the acute respiratory distress syndrome. The Acute Respiratory Distress Syndrome Network. N Engl J Med 2000;342:1301–8.
101. Apuzzo JL, Wiess MH, Petersons V, et al. Effect of positive end expiratory pressure ventilation on intracranial pressure in man. J Neurosurg 1977;46:227–32.
102. Roberts GC. Post-craniotomy analgesia: Current practices in British neurosurgical centres – a survey of post-craniotomy analgesic practices. Eur J Anaesthesiol 2005;22:328–32.
103. Whitfield PC, Kirkpatrick PJ. Timing of surgery for aneurysmal subarachnoid haemorrhage. Cochrane Database Syst Rev 2001; (2):CD001697.
104. Molyneux A, Kerr R, Stratton I, et al. International Subarachnoid Aneurysm Trial (ISAT) of neurosurgical clipping versus endovascular coiling in 2143 patients with ruptured intracranial aneurysms: a randomised trial. Lancet 2002;360:1267–74.
105. Molyneux AJ, Kerr RS, Yu LM, et al. International Subarachnoid Aneurysm Trial (ISAT) of neurosurgical clipping versus endovascular coiling in 2143 patients with ruptured intracranial aneurysms: A randomised comparison of effects on survival, dependency, seizures, rebleeding, subgroups, and aneurysm occlusion. Lancet 2005;366:809–17.
106. Rosenorn J, Eskesen V, Schmidt K, et al. The risk of rebleeding from ruptured intracranial aneurysms. J Neurosurg 1987;67: 329–32.
107. Lee K. Aneurysm precautions: A physiologic basis for minimizing rebleeding. Heart Lung 1980;9:336–43.

108. Roos YB, Rinkel GJ, Vermeulen M, et al. Antifibrinolytic therapy for aneurysmal subarachnoid haemorrhage. Cochrane Database Syst Rev 2003;(3):CD001245.
109. van Gijn J, Hijdra A, Wijdicks EF, et al. Acute hydrocephalus after aneurysmal subarachnoid hemorrhage. J Neurosurg 1985;63: 355–62.
110. Komotar RJ, Hahn DK, Kim GH, et al. The impact of microsurgical fenestration of the lamina terminalis on shunt-dependent hydrocephalus and vasospasm after aneurysmal subarachnoid hemorrhage. Neurosurgery 2008;62:123–32, discussion 132–4.
111. Lin CL, Dumont AS, Lieu AS, et al. Characterization of perioperative seizures and epilepsy following aneurysmal subarachnoid hemorrhage. J Neurosurg 2003;99:978–85.
112. Rosengart AJ, Huo JD, Tolentino J, et al. Outcome in patients with subarachnoid hemorrhage treated with antiepileptic drugs. J Neurosurg 2007;107:253–60.
113. Chumnanvej S, Dunn IF, Kim DH. Three-day phenytoin prophylaxis is adequate after subarachnoid hemorrhage. Neurosurgery 2007;60:99–102, discussion 102–3.
114. Hijdra A, van Gijn J, Nagelkerke NJ, et al. Prediction of delayed cerebral ischemia, rebleeding, and outcome after aneurysmal subarachnoid hemorrhage. Stroke 1988;19:1250–6.
115. Solenski NJ, Haley EC Jr, Kassell NF, et al. Medical complications of aneurysmal subarachnoid hemorrhage: A report of the multicenter, cooperative aneurysm study. Participants of the Multicenter Cooperative Aneurysm Study. Crit Care Med 1995;23: 1007–17.
116. Macdonald RL, Weir BK. A review of hemoglobin and the pathogenesis of cerebral vasospasm. Stroke 1991;22:971–82.
117. Weir B, Macdonald RL, Stoodley M. Etiology of cerebral vasospasm. Acta Neurochir Suppl 1999;72:27–46.
118. Kolias AG, Sen J, Belli A. Pathogenesis of cerebral vasospasm following aneurysmal subarachnoid hemorrhage: Putative mechanisms and novel approaches. J Neurosci Res 2008;87:1–11.
119. Vergouwen MD, Vermeulen M, Coert BA, et al. Microthrombosis after aneurysmal subarachnoid hemorrhage: An additional explanation for delayed cerebral ischemia. J Cereb Blood Flow Metab 2008;28:1761–70.
120. Juvela S. Aspirin and delayed cerebral ischemia after aneurysmal subarachnoid hemorrhage. J Neurosurg 1995;82:945–52.
121. Roos YB, Levi M, Carroll TA, et al. Nimodipine increases fibrinolytic activity in patients with aneurysmal subarachnoid hemorrhage. Stroke 2001;32:1860–2.
122. Dreier JP, Woitzik J, Fabricius M, et al. Delayed ischaemic neurological deficits after subarachnoid haemorrhage are associated with clusters of spreading depolarizations. Brain 2006;129: 3224–37.
123. Vora YY, Suarez-Almazor M, Steinke DE, et al. Role of transcranial Doppler monitoring in the diagnosis of cerebral vasospasm after subarachnoid hemorrhage. Neurosurgery 1999;44:1237–47, discussion 1247–8.
124. Suarez JI, Qureshi AI, Yahia AB, et al. Symptomatic vasospasm diagnosis after subarachnoid hemorrhage: Evaluation of transcranial Doppler ultrasound and cerebral angiography as related to compromised vascular distribution. Crit Care Med 2002;30: 1348–55.
125. van der Schaaf I, Wermer MJ, van der Graaf Y, et al. CT after subarachnoid hemorrhage: Relation of cerebral perfusion to delayed cerebral ischemia. Neurology 2006;66:1533–8.
126. Kassell NF, Peerless SJ, Durward QJ, et al. Treatment of ischemic deficits from vasospasm with intravascular volume expansion and induced arterial hypertension. Neurosurgery 1982;11:337–43.
127. Lee KH, Lukovits T, Friedman JA. Triple-H" therapy for cerebral vasospasm following subarachnoid hemorrhage. Neurocrit Care 2006;4:68–76.
128. Bulters DO, Birch AA, Hickey E, et al. A randomized controlled trial of prophylactic intra-aortic balloon counterpulsation in high-risk aneurysmal subarachnoid hemorrhage. Stroke 2013;44: 224–6.
129. Macdonald RL, Higashida RT, Keller E, et al. Randomized trial of clazosentan in patients with aneurysmal subarachnoid hemorrhage undergoing endovascular coiling. Stroke 2012;43: 1463–9.
130. Vajkoczy P, Meyer B, Weidauer S, et al. Clazosentan (AXV-034343), a selective endothelin A receptor antagonist, in the prevention of cerebral vasospasm following severe aneurysmal subarachnoid hemorrhage: results of a randomized, double-blind, placebo-controlled, multicenter phase IIa study. J Neurosurg 2005;103:9–17.
131. Smith WS, Dowd CF, Johnston SC, et al. Neurotoxicity of intra-arterial papaverine preserved with chlorobutanol used for the treatment of cerebral vasospasm after aneurysmal subarachnoid hemorrhage. Stroke 2004;35:2518–22.
132. Hoh BL, Ogilvy CS. Endovascular treatment of cerebral vasospasm: Transluminal balloon angioplasty, intra-arterial papaverine, and intra-arterial nicardipine. Neurosurg Clin North Am 2005;16:501–16, vi.
133. Mocco J, Prickett CS, Komotar RJ, et al. Potential mechanisms and clinical significance of global cerebral edema following aneurysmal subarachnoid hemorrhage. Neurosurg Focus 2007; 22:E7.
134. Claassen J, Carhuapoma JR, Kreiter KT, et al. Global cerebral edema after subarachnoid hemorrhage: Frequency, predictors, and impact on outcome. Stroke 2002;33:1225–32.
135. Frontera JA, Parra A, Shimbo D, et al. Cardiac arrhythmias after subarachnoid hemorrhage: Risk factors and impact on outcome. Cerebrovasc Dis 2008;26:71–8.
136. Andreoli A, di Pasquale G, Pinelli G, et al. Subarachnoid hemorrhage: Frequency and severity of cardiac arrhythmias. A survey of 70 cases studied in the acute phase. Stroke 1987;18:558–64.
137. Zaroff JG, Pawlikowska L, Miss JC, et al. Adrenoceptor polymorphisms and the risk of cardiac injury and dysfunction after subarachnoid hemorrhage. Stroke 2006;37:1680–5.
138. Zaroff JG, Rordorf GA, Newell JB, et al. Cardiac outcome in patients with subarachnoid hemorrhage and electrocardiographic abnormalities. Neurosurgery 1999;44:34–9, discussion 39–40.
139. Kono T, Morita H, Kuroiwa T, et al. Left ventricular wall motion abnormalities in patients with subarachnoid hemorrhage: neurogenic stunned myocardium. J Am Coll Cardiol 1994;24:636–40.
140. Mayer SA, Fink ME, Homma S, et al. Cardiac injury associated with neurogenic pulmonary edema following subarachnoid hemorrhage. Neurology 1994;44:815–20.
141. Wu DJ, Fujiwara H, Matsuda M, et al. Clinicopathological study of myocardial infarction with normal or nearly normal extracardiac coronary arteries: Quantitative analysis of contraction band necrosis, coagulation necrosis, hemorrhage, and infarct size. Heart Vessels 1990;6:55–62.
142. Naidech AM, Kreiter KT, Janjua N, et al. Cardiac troponin elevation, cardiovascular morbidity, and outcome after subarachnoid hemorrhage. Circulation 2005;112:2851–6.
143. Hamann G, Haass A, Schimrigk K. Beta-blockade in acute aneurysmal subarachnoid haemorrhage. Acta Neurochir (Wien) 1993;121:119–22.
144. Tung PP, Olmsted E, Kopelnik A, et al. Plasma B-type natriuretic peptide levels are associated with early cardiac dysfunction after subarachnoid hemorrhage. Stroke 2005;36:1567–9.
145. Vespa PM, Bleck TP. Neurogenic pulmonary edema and other mechanisms of impaired oxygenation after aneurysmal subarachnoid hemorrhage. Neurocrit Care 2004;1:157–70.
146. Frontera JA, Fernandez A, Schmidt JM, et al. Impact of nosocomial infectious complications after subarachnoid hemorrhage. Neurosurgery 2008;62:80–7, discussion 87.
147. Schneider HJ, Kreitschmann-Andermahr I, Ghigo E, et al. Hypothalamopituitary dysfunction following traumatic brain injury and aneurysmal subarachnoid hemorrhage: A systematic review. JAMA 2007;298:1429–38.
148. Qureshi AI, Suri MF, Sung GY, et al. Prognostic significance of hypernatremia and hyponatremia among patients with aneurysmal subarachnoid hemorrhage. Neurosurgery 2002;50:749–55, discussion 755–6.
149. Kurokawa Y, Uede T, Ishiguro M, et al. Pathogenesis of hyponatremia following subarachnoid hemorrhage due to ruptured cerebral aneurysm. Surg Neurol 1996;46:500–7, discussion 507–8.
150. Claassen J, Vu A, Kreiter KT, et al. Effect of acute physiologic derangements on outcome after subarachnoid hemorrhage. Crit Care Med 2004;32:832–8.
151. Hackett ML, Anderson CS. Health outcomes 1 year after subarachnoid hemorrhage: An international population-based study. The Australian Cooperative Research on Subarachnoid Hemorrhage Study Group. Neurology 2000;55:658–62.

30 Arteriovenous Malformations and Other Vascular Anomalies

Christian Stapf

KEY POINTS

- Intracerebral vascular malformations constitute an important cause of intracranial hemorrhage, especially in younger patients. The spectrum ranges from sporadic congenital lesions (such as brain AVMs) to genetically determined familial disorders that may progress over time.
- Arterial aneurysms, moyamoya disease, and arteriovenous dural fistulas are considered acquired lesions, and developmental venous anomalies represent a variant of physiological venous drainage.
- Among the "true" vascular malformations, only cerebral cavernous malformations and arteriovenous malformations are of clinical relevance, while capillary telangiectasias constitute asymptomatic, incidental imaging findings.
- Surgical treatment indications for cerebral cavernous malformations are controversial since longitudinal population-based data suggest that neurological long-term outcome may be better without intervention.
- Brain arteriovenous malformations are usually eradicated after hemorrhagic complications. Preventive eradication of unruptured lesions, however, appears scientifically unjustified as interventions are associated with a higher risk of stroke and neurological deficits during both, short-term and long-term follow-up.

INTRODUCTION

Intracerebral vascular malformations constitute an important cause of intracranial hemorrhage, especially in younger patients. However, this group of pathologies is quite heterogeneous and comprises a large spectrum ranging from sporadic congenital lesions (such as brain AVMs) to genetically determined familial disorders that may progress over time (e.g., hereditary hemorrhagic telangiectasia, familial cerebral cavernous malformations, etc.).

Currently, no defined strategies exist for the diagnostic workup after acute intracerebral hemorrhage (ICH), and no diagnostic criteria have so far been established or prospectively validated. Therefore, the timing and use of currently available diagnostic tools (such as angio-CT, MRI, MRA, MRV, and cerebral angiography) vary depending on individual attitudes, local routine, regional traditions, and national health care plans. Data from a recent prospective series suggested that cerebral angiography may have a low yield in identifying an underlying vascular malformation in ICH patients older than 45 years with a history of hypertension and presenting with a thalamic, putaminal, or posterior fossa bleed.[1] Current recommendations favor angiography for all cases without a clear cause of hemorrhage, particularly for young, normotensive patients.[2,3] Nonetheless, timing of cerebral angiography after acute ICH depends usually on the patient's clinical state and the neurosurgeon's judgment about the need for surgical intervention. Consequently, the underlying pathology may be missed in those who die or who have severe morbidity at initial presentation. In other cases, an underlying AVM or aneurysm may be compressed by mass effect of the initial hematoma and only be visible on follow-up angiography. Cavernous malformations presenting with hemorrhage beyond the limits of the actual malformations may only be identified on MRI after hematoma resorption, i.e., several months after the index bleed. The outdated concept of so-called "primary intracerebral hemorrhage" adds to the possibility that intracranial vascular malformations may still be under-diagnosed in ICH patients.[4] Whatever the actual cause of the hemorrhagic complication, patients hospitalized for hemorrhagic stroke have better functional outcomes if managed acutely in a stroke unit or ICU.[5] Therefore, admission to a dedicated treatment unit is now recommended.[6]

In principle, vascular malformations may arise from any segment of the different functional units of the brain vasculature, including arteries, arterioles, capillaries, venules, and veins. This may be due to either developmental derangement during the time of the vessel formation, or may occur later in time based on external risk factors and genetic predisposition (Fig. 30-1). Many of these anomalies are associated with an increased risk of hemorrhage, as structural changes of the vascular wall lead to often progressive hemodynamic changes and lower resistance to intraluminal volume and pressure. As a general rule, the average risk of spontaneous hemorrhage appears to be rather low if the vascular malformation is diagnosed unruptured. Most types have been associated with higher bleeding rates if hemorrhage occurred at initial presentation.

ANOMALIES OF THE ARTERIAL WALL

Aneurysms

Aneurysms do not constitute vascular malformations sensu stricto, but their formation represents the most frequently observed structural anomaly of intracranial arteries after endoluminal changes due to atherosclerosis. Aneurysm rupture constitutes the principal cause of non-traumatic subarachnoid hemorrhage (SAH) with an overall crude annual incidence between 10 and 15 in 100,000 in the Western world and up to 30 in 100,000 in high-risk populations such as Asia or Finland.[7] Both, aneurysm development and growth. Depend on familial predisposition and additional risk factors such as increasing age, female sex, smoking, and alcohol consumption. Looking at age alone, most prospective and retrospective studies have independently demonstrated an almost steady increase of annual incidence rates with age, with values ranging from below 5 per 100,000 for those younger than 35 years and rates between 30 and 40 per 100,000 for individuals aged 75 or older.[8,9] Morphological factors favoring hemorrhage from previously unruptured aneurysm include increasing aneurysm size and location in the posterior (i.e. vertebrobasilar) circulation.[10]

Recent US population estimates suggest an overall mortality rate of 2.77 per 100,000 person-years attributable to aneurysm rupture.[11] Most of the larger outcome studies indicate that roughly one-third of patients who suffer a first-ever SAH die in the acute state, another one-third will survive with a disabling deficit, and only one-third will not be disabled from the event. The probability of survival seems to be lower in women[11] and has been shown to depend on the degree of initial neurologic impairment,[12] commonly graded according to the Glasgow Coma Scale[13] or by the grading system as proposed by Hunt and Hess.[14]

In some instances, rupture of an intracranial aneurysm may lead to intraparenchymatous cerebral hemorrhage, particularly if located on MCA branches, or in distinct etiological subtypes, such as dissecting or mycotic aneurysms (Fig. 30-2). Therefore, whenever an intracerebral hematoma reaches down to the level of the carotid tip or circle of Willis arteries, or if ICH is associated with subarachnoid bleeding into the basal cisterns, an underlying aneurysm should be excluded by MRA, CTA or conventional angiography in the acute phase, as re-rupture rates seem to be similarly high as in cases with isolated SAH. Some arterial aneurysms develop in the context of an arteriovenous malformation and may add to the potential hazard of intracranial hemorrhage associated with such lesions (see below).

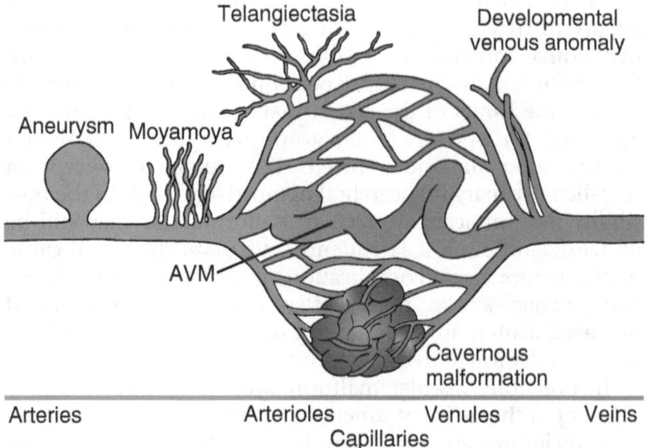

Figure 30-1. Synopsis of intracerebral vascular anomalies. Only arteriovenous malformations (AVMs), cavernous malformations and capillary telangiectasias are considered true malformations.

No systematic data exist on whether endovascular or surgical techniques are preferred after intracerebral (i.e., intraparenchymatous) aneurysm bleeding. Recent outcome data on aneurysm treatment after subarachnoid hemorrhage favor endovascular embolization.[15,16] Individual treatment decisions should be based on a multidisciplinary consideration of the patient's age and clinical condition, aneurysm anatomy, and the indication for additional hematoma evacuation or placement of a ventricular drain. More detailed data on aneurysm rupture and management are available in Chapters 29, 66, and 69.

Telangiectasias

At the level of the arterioles, telangiectasias may develop as clusters of pencil-like vessels located mainly in the brain stem or cerebellum. Even though considered true vascular malformations, they have long been considered curiosities for the pathologist and are of only minor clinical significance, as they may not be an actual source of symptomatic bleeding.[17] They may demonstrate small microhemorrhages on histologic examination, but the size of the hemorrhage does not appear to be massive enough to create a clinical syndrome. Nowadays, telangiectasias may be detected on MRI with and without contrast injection (Fig. 30-3).

So-called familial hemorrhagic telangiectasia or Weber-Osler-Rendu syndrome is an autosomal dominant disorder associated with multiple "telangiectasias" elsewhere in the body, which actually constitute tiny vascular nodules with

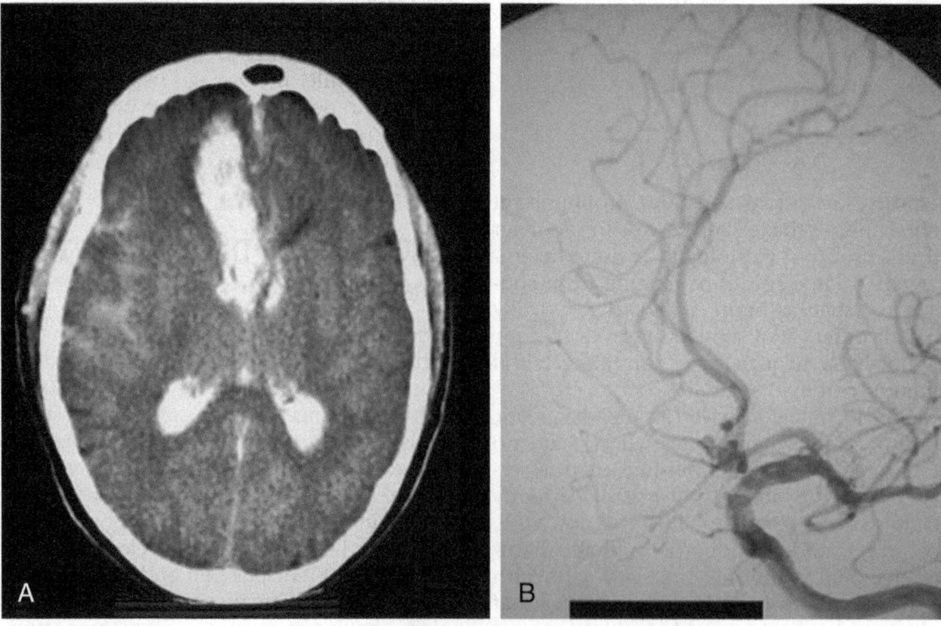

Figure 30-2. Right frontal hematoma with ventricular extension and subarachnoid hemorrhage (A, non-contrast CT scan) due to rupture of an aneurysm of the anterior communicating artery (B, diagnostic angiography with left carotid injection).

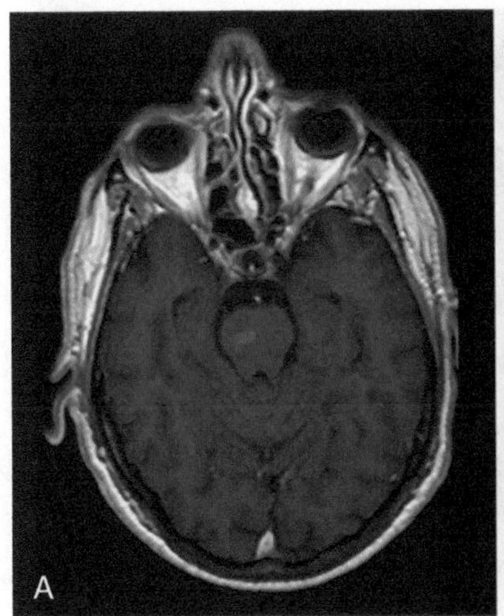

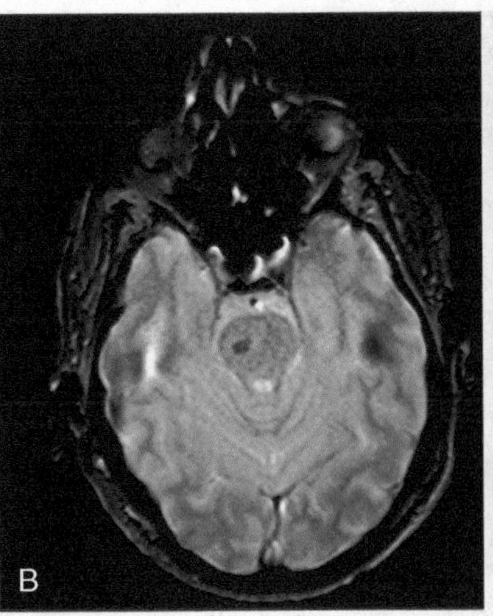

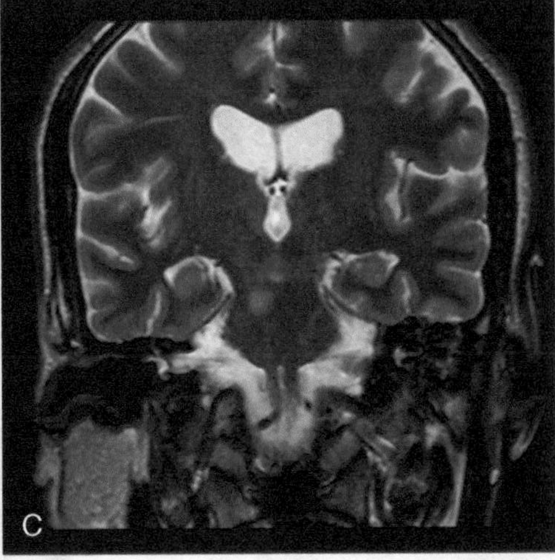

Figure 30-3. Asymptomatic pontine telangiectasia with hyperintense signal on T1-weighted images after contrast injection (A), hemosiderin staining on gradient echo (B), and a spontaneously hyperintense signal on standard T2 imaging (C).

arteriovenous shunting. Their number may increase during lifetime with the mostly affected organs being the mucosa, skin, and lungs. If located in the brain, these lesions may behave similar to sporadic arteriovenous malformations and may cause spontaneous rupture with intracranial hemorrhage (see below).[18]

Moyamoya

Moyamoya is a rare form of chronic cerebrovascular occlusive disease with angiographic findings of progressive stenosis or occlusion of the circle of Willis arteries together with a network of dilated perforating neo-vessels in the vicinity of the occlusion.[19] The initial description arose from the angiographic appearance of this pathological vascularization at the base of the brain: The tiny size and large number of vessels imaged made the combination look like a cloud or a puff of smoke instead of single arteries.[20] The numerous, dilated small neo-vessels have also been termed "rete mirabile".

In the vascular network of perforating arteries (the so-called moyamoya vessels), various histological changes can be observed: the distal portion of the carotid arteries as well as those constituting the circle of Willis often show fibrocellular intimal thickening, waving of the internal elastic lamina, and attenuation of the media. Dilated neo-vessels are found around the circle of Willis, and reticular conglomerates of small vessels may appear in the pia mater. With hemodynamic stress or aging, the dilated arteries with attenuated walls may predispose to the formation of microaneurysms, and their rupture is considered one of the mechanisms leading to parenchymatous hemorrhages in moyamoya patients.

Annual incidence estimates of symptomatic moyamoya range between 0.06 per 100,000 in Caucasians and 0.54 per 100,000 in Japan, but seem to be almost twice as high in women, and show two age distribution peaks around 10–20 and 40–50 years.[21–24] Clinically, ischemic and hemorrhagic symptoms are encountered. The ischemic type dominates in childhood, and clinically transient ischemic events occur more often than infarctions with persistent neurological deficits. Hemorrhagic complications are more frequent in adult patients. Bleeding occurs often in repetitive intervals, and massive bleeding, although infrequent, is the principal cause of death.

Hereditary factors and ethnic origins may play a role in the occurrence or susceptibility to idiopathic moyamoya disease, as suggested by the occasional familial occurrence (12% in Japanese cases).[24] A secondary moyamoya syndrome may be seen in association with other congenital diseases such as sickle cell anemia, von Recklinghausen disease (neurofibromatosis type 1), and Down syndrome (trisomy 21).[25] However, the clinical manifestation and disease progression are not congenital and may also be seen as a secondary complication of early-onset intracranial atherosclerosis, autoimmune disease, vasculitis, meningitis, post-radiation changes, cranial trauma, and brain neoplasm.[19,26]

Typical angiographic findings were considered indispensable for the diagnosis of moyamoya, but as the quality of MRI and MRA greatly improved, the diagnosis was also made if they clearly demonstrated all the findings indicative of moyamoya (Fig. 30-4).[19]

In advanced stages of moyamoya, some degree of early venous drainage may be seen on angiograms suggesting arteriovenous shunting at the level of the neo-vessel network. On the other hand, moyamoya-type vascular changes have been observed on high-flow feeding arteries in brain AVMs. Whether the two entities are linked biologically, or whether the moyamoya type vascular pathology observed in AVM patients merely results from hemodynamic changes associated with the AVM remains yet unclear.

More data on the management of moyamoya are available in Chapter 40.

ANOMALIES OF THE CAPILLARY JUNCTION

Brain Arteriovenous Malformations

Among vascular malformations causing intracranial hemorrhage, brain arteriovenous malformations (AVMs) are among the most frequently encountered. Brain AVMs commonly affect distal arterial branches and in roughly half of the cases, the malformation is found in the borderzone region shared by the distal anterior, middle, and/or posterior cerebral arteries.[15] Morphologically, they resemble tortuous agglomerations of abnormally dilated arteries with drainage into deep and/or superficial veins. In its core region or "nidus", the AVM lacks a capillary bed, thereby allowing high-flow arteriovenous shunting through one or more fistulae. The lack of capillary resistance turns an AVM into a high-flow and low-pressure lesion that may not directly depend on the systemic blood pressure (explaining why AVMs tend not to rupture in a context of physical exercise).

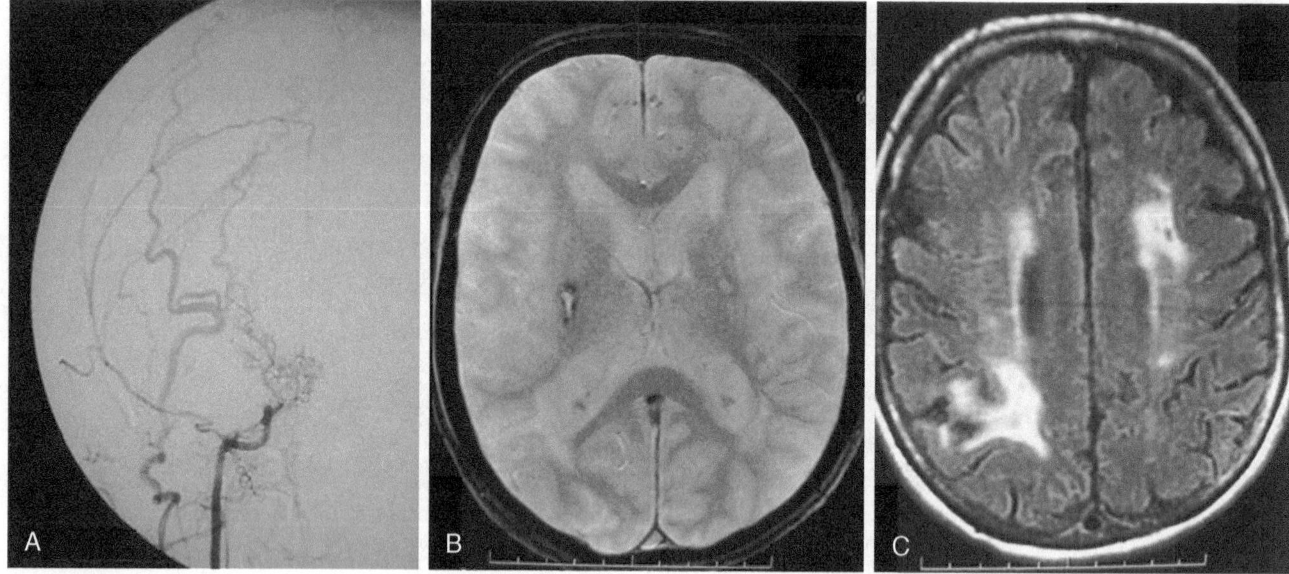

Figure 30-4. Moyamoya disease with typical angiographic and MR imaging features: After injection of the right common carotid artery (A) visualization of distal internal carotid artery occlusion with filling of dilated neo-vessels (moyamoya vessels). The gradient echo (T2*) MR shows subacute ICH at the level of the right lateral lenticulostriate arteries (B). Old ischemic lesions in the distal right MCA and deep left MCA territory can be seen on FLAIR (C).

History and Pathogenetic Concepts

The pathologic case material provides the earliest examples of what we call today a brain AVM. The 1846 publication by Viennese pathologist Rokitansky[27] may be the first to mention the existence of such lesions. He did not provide a detailed morphologic description of what he called "vascular brain tumors in pial tissue", but he was puzzled by the structural analogy between their "cavernous textures" and the "gaps, windows or canals in certain blastemas of the vascular system" that he had noted in embryonic tissue. This observation led him to the idea that a developmental derangement was the most likely underlying cause for this type of lesion. Half a century later Carl Emanuel, a pathologist working at Heidelberg University, published one of the first detailed histopathologic case studies.[28] He had already described "substantial enlargement of the microcirculatory pathways" reflecting the lack of a capillary bed in the angioma arteriale racemosum. Emanuel's report is noteworthy because he appears to be the first researcher considering three possible causes of such lesions: congenital, secondary development from an innate telangiectasia, or a sequel to trauma. His landmark proposal drafted the three major etiologic concepts – embryologic derangement, dynamic development, and vascular trauma – upon which most future theories were built and further elaborated.[29]

Thanks to now routinely applied fetal ultrasound screening, an increasing number of vein of Galen aneurysmal malformations has been detected during gestation, and a few patients have been studied by prenatal magnetic resonance imaging (MRI).[30,31] Information on comparable cases with an intrauterine diagnosis of a brain AVM, however, are lacking; none has yet been reported from studies on routine fetal ultrasound evaluations, which are commonly performed between the 20th and 22nd gestational weeks.[32,33] Probably the youngest individual so far reported may be a preterm neonate (born at 32 weeks' gestation) who died during the second postnatal day from acute hemorrhage of an infratentorial AVM that was fed by the superior cerebellar artery.[34] The lack of observed cases in which a brain AVM was detected at earlier fetal stages hence challenges the widespread assumption that these lesions also arise from an embryonic disturbance at the time of the vessel formation.[35]

The vascular topography in many AVMs also argues against a genuine embryonic disorder. Brain AVMs commonly affect distal arterial branches, and in roughly half the cases, the malformation is found in the borderzone region shared by the distal anterior, middle, and posterior cerebral arteries.[36] These "watershed areas" constitute anatomic remnants of the manifold artery-to-artery links that once covered the brain surface at its lissencephalic state. With the onset of cortical gyration (29th gestational week), the original arterial mesh regresses, giving rise eventually to the defined arterial territories of the leptomeningeal arteries. In the distal fields of these arterial territories, pial anastomoses between otherwise separated brain arteries persist, even though the number, size, and exact location of the leptomeningeal anastomoses show numerous inter-individual variations.[37,38] This possibility suggests that the initial lesion may actually arise with a timely link to the formation of the arterial borderzones, that is, at some point after the 29th gestational week.[39] In one case report in which the interplay between cortical gyration and borderzone formation was disturbed by a primary migration disorder such as schizencephaly, an AVM had developed at the site where the neural defect straddled the arterial borderzone territory.[40]

Epidemiology

Based on large-scale imaging data involving healthy volunteers, one brain AVM may be found in every 2,000 MRI scans, leading to an estimated prevalence of about 50 (95%CI, 10–100) cases per 100,000.[41] Improved access to diagnostic MR brain imaging may also explain the increasing detection rates of unruptured AVMs, while the incidence of AVM rupture appears remarkably stable across different population-based surveys (see Table 30-1). The annual incidence of AVM hemorrhage in the general population is 0.5 per 100,000, but with the increasing availability of MR brain imaging, even more unruptured AVMs are diagnosed every year in the Western world and typical symptoms include seizures or headaches.

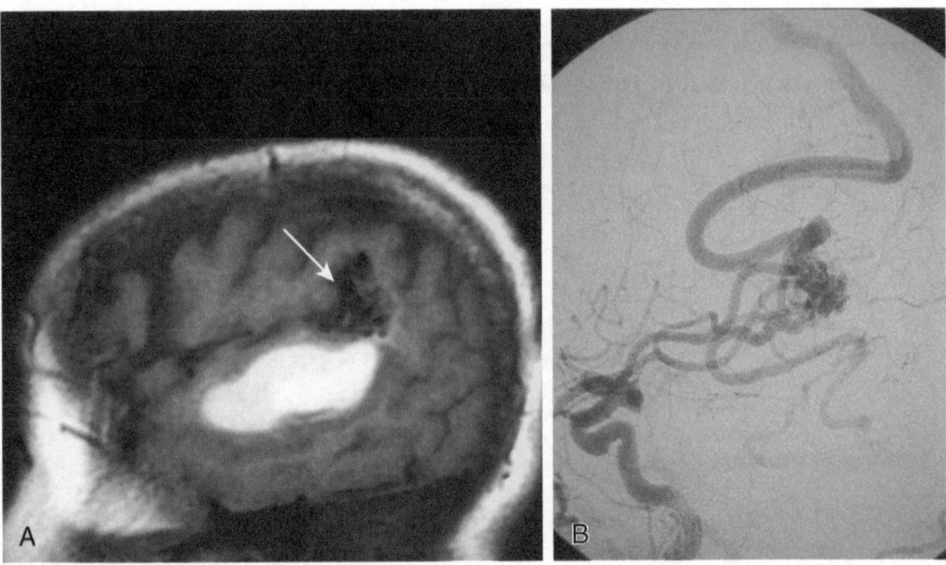

Figure 30-5. Intracerebral hemorrhage due to an arteriovenous malformation. T1-weighted MRI (A) showing a hyperintense left temporal hematoma with an AVM nidus (arrow) visualized in the vicinity of the hemorrhage. Carotid artery angiography confirms the presence of a brain AVM fed by cortical MCA branches and with superficial venous drainage (B).

Some present with progressive or fluctuating neurological deficits without signs of hemorrhage. An increasing number of patients are diagnosed with an incidental finding of an asymptomatic malformation. Overall, women and men are equally affected with a mean age at diagnosis around 40 years.[42] Women do not show higher rupture rates during pregnancy and the puerperium.[43] Familial AVMs are extremely rare and have been described in only 25 pedigrees world-wide.[44] Therefore, the low prevalence of familial brain AVMs does not justify systematic screening of first-degree family members.[45]

Overall, clinical deficits after AVM rupture may be more benign as compared to intracranial hemorrhage from other sources,[46] but population data also suggest that patients with prior AVM rupture show excess long-term mortality rates if left untreated.[47] Preventive interventions for unruptured AVMs, however, are associated with a higher risk of stroke and neurological deficits during both short-term (3 years)[48,49] and long-term (12-years) follow-up.[50] For patients with AVM-associated epilepsy, population-based data do not confirm a long-term benefit of AVM eradication on future seizure occurrence.[51]

Diagnosis and Risk Evaluation

Even though many AVMs can be detected on MR brain imaging, diagnostic four-vessel angiography remains the gold standard for the correct diagnosis on anatomic characterization of these malformations (see Fig. 30-5). Cerebral angiography may also help to differentiate brain AVMs from other types of intracranial anomalies with arteriovenous shunting (Table 30-2). In a standard description of a newly diagnosed brain AVM, important morphological baseline variables include the maximal AVM diameter, the topographic nidus location in the brain, the arterial supply (number and type of feeding artery), the presence of associated (i.e., feeding-artery or intranidal) aneurysms, arterial stenosis with or without moyamoya-type changes, deep and/or superficial venous drainage, as well as the presence of any venous outflow stenosis and/or ectasia.

Risk factors for spontaneous bleeding include mainly a history of prior hemorrhage, but also morphological characteristics such as deep AVM location and exclusive deep venous drainage (Table 30-1, Fig. 30-6).[52] Brain AVMs without these risk factors seem to carry a rather low hemorrhage risk (<1% per year). Additional risk factors favoring future rupture include increasing patient age, Hispanic ethnicity, exclusive deep venous drainage, deep AVM location, and neuroradiological evidence of old AVM hemorrhage, whereas the independent effects of the nidus size, infratentorial AVM location, associated unruptured aneurysms, and venous dilatations have as yet not been confirmed during prospective follow-up of untreated patients.[52–55] When acute rupture occurs, the clinical deficits tend to be less severe and the associated mortality to be far lower, as compared to ICH from other causes.[56]

Treatment Strategy

As a complex neurovascular disorder, brain AVMs are ideally managed by a multidisciplinary team of vascular neurologists, neuroradiologists, neurosurgeons, and radiotherapists. Seizures, headaches, and chronic disability require symptomatic treatment and follow-up by a neurologist, while people with AVMs that have bled need appropriate monitoring in a dedicated neuroscience or stroke unit.[57] Current interventional treatment options comprise any combination of endovascular embolization (interventional neuroradiology), microsurgical removal (neurosurgery), and/or stereotactic radiotherapy (radiosurgery).[58] Despite technical advances in these treatments during recent decades, none has been tested in a controlled study. A recent systematic meta-analysis of published (2000–2011) treatment data on 13,698 AVM patients (including 46,314 patient-years of follow-up) suggests interventional AVM therapy remains associated with considerable risks and incomplete efficacy (Table 30-3).[59] The best possible treatment strategy should be discussed in view of the topographical and morphological characteristics and possible risk factors for natural history and treatment risk. Intervention seems justified in many ruptured brain AVMs, mainly to prevent subsequent hemorrhage. No systematic data exist on the best timing for intervention (early versus late after AVM rupture), but recent series suggest the risk of re-rupture seems particularly high (18% within the first year after the initial hemorrhage).[60] Increasing AVM size has a negative effect on technical treatment success (eradication) and clinical outcome for any of the

TABLE 30-1 Epidemiology of Arteriovenous Malformations (literature data 2002–2014)

	Detection rates n/100,000 per year (95% CI)			Spontaneous rupture rates Observed crude annual rates (95% CI)		
	Ruptured *at diagnosis*	***Unruptured*** *at diagnosis*	*Total*	***Ruptured*** *at diagnosis*	***Unruptured*** *at diagnosis*	*Total*
Prospective Population-Based Data						
New York Islands AVM Study[a]	0.51 (0.41–0.61)	0.83 (0.77–0.88)	1.34 (1.18–1.49)	n.a.	n.a.	n.a.
SIVMS[b]	0.51 (0.37–0.69)	0.61 (0.52–0.68)	1.12 (0.90–1.37)	n.a.	n.a.	n.a.
NOMASS[c]	0.55 (0.11–1.61)	n.a.	n.a.	n.a.	n.a.	n.a.
Retrospective Population-Based Data						
California[d,e]	0.70 (0.60–0.80)	0.72 (0.63–0.83)	1.42 (1.29–1.57)	3.3% (2.9–3.6)	0.7% (0.4–1.0)	4.0% (3.8–4.2)
Finland[f]	n.a.	n.a.	n.a.	2.8 (2.4–3.2)	1.6 (1.1–2.0)	2.4 (1.9–2.8)
Patient Level Meta-Analysis, Randomized Trial Data						
MARS[g]	n.a.	n.a.	n.a.	4.8% (3.9–5.9)	1.3% (1.0–1.7)	2.3% (2.0–2.7)
ARUBA[h]	n.a.	n.a.	n.a.	n.a.	2.2% (0.9–4.5)	n.a.

[a]Stapf C, Mast H, Sciacca RR, Berenstein A, Nelson PK, Gobin YP, Pile-Spellman J, Mohr JP; New York Islands AVM Study Collaborators. The New York Islands AVM Study: design, study progress, and initial results. *Stroke* 2003;34:e29–33.
[b]Al-Shahi R, Bhattacharya JJ, Currie DG, Papanastassiou V, Ritchie V, Roberts RC, Sellar RJ, Warlow CP; Scottish Intracranial Vascular Malformation Study Collaborators. Prospective, population-based detection of intracranial vascular malformations in adults: the Scottish Intracranial Vascular Malformation Study (SIVMS). *Stroke* 2003;34:1163–1169.
[c]Stapf C, Labovitz DL, Sciacca RR, Mast H, Mohr JP, Sacco RL. Incidence of adult brain arteriovenous malformation hemorrhage in a prospective population-based stroke survey. *Cerebrovasc Dis* 2002;13:43–46.
[d]Gabriel RA, Kim H, Sidney S, McCulloch CE, Singh V, Johnston SC, Ko NU, Achrol AS, Zaroff JG, Young WL. Ten-year detection rate of brain arteriovenous malformations in a large, multiethnic, defined population. *Stroke* 2010;41:21–26.
[e]Halim AX, Johnston SC, Singh V, McCulloch CE, Bennett JP, Achrol AS, Sidney S, Young WL. Longitudinal risk of intracranial hemorrhage in patients with arteriovenous malformation of the brain within a defined population. *Stroke* 2004;35:1697–1702.
[f]Hernesniemi JA, Dashti R, Juvela S, Väärt K, Niemelä M, Laakso A. Natural history of brain arteriovenous malformations: a long-term follow-up study of risk of hemorrhage in 238 patients. *Neurosurgery* 2008;63:823–829
[g]Kim H, Al-Shahi Salman R, McCulloch CE, Stapf C, Young WL; MARS Coinvestigators. Untreated brain arteriovenous malformation: patient-level meta-analysis of hemorrhage predictors. *Neurology* 2014;83:590–597.
[h]Mohr JP, Parides MK, Stapf C, Moquete E, Moy CS, Overbey JR, Al-Shahi Salman R, Vicaut E, Young WL, Houdart E, Cordonnier C, Stefani MA, Hartmann A, von Kummer R, Biondi A, Berkefeld J, Klijn CJ, Harkness K, Libman R, Barreau X, Moskowitz AJ; international ARUBA investigators. Medical management with or without interventional therapy for unruptured brain arteriovenous malformations (ARUBA): a multicentre, non-blinded, randomised trial. *Lancet* 2014;383:614–621.

TABLE 30-2 Brain Arteriovenous Malformation Differential Diagnosis: Intracranial Arteriovenous Fistulae

Entity	Pathogenesis	Clinical characteristics
Vein of Galen aneurysmal malformation[a,b]	Persistent dilated embryonic vein of the prosencephalon, posterior choroidal artery affected	Congestive heart failure in neonates, intracranial hemorrhage in infants
Dural arteriovenous fistula[c]	Different types (traumatic, secondary to venous occlusion, etc.)	Arterial supply through meningeal arterial branches. High recurrence rate
Hereditary hemorrhagic telangiectasia (Rendu-Osler-Weber)	Capillary regression leads to multiple small AV-shunts in various tissues.	Vascular abnormalities in nose, skin, lung, brain, and gastro-intestinal tract
Encephalo-trigeminal syndrome (Sturge-Weber)[d]	Phakomatosis	Neurocutaneous syndrome affecting the meninges, not the brain
Cerebro-retinal angiomatosis (von Hippel-Lindau)[d]	Phakomatosis	Associated malignancy
Wyburn-Mason (or Bonnet-Dechaume-Blanc) syndrome[e,f]	Phakomatosis	Neurocutaneous syndrome with metameric brainstem AVM in newborns
Neovascular collaterals	Venous thrombosis or arterial occlusion may lead to focal angioneogenesis with early arteriovenous shunting	Postthrombotic syndrome, moyamoya syndrome, etc.

[a]Raybaud CA, Strother CM, Hald JK. Aneurysms of the vein of Galen: embryonic considerations and anatomical features relating to the pathogenesis of the malformation. *Neuroradiology* 1989;31:109–128.
[b]Lasjaunias P. *Vascular diseases in neonates, infants and children. Interventional neuroradiology management.* 1st edition. Berlin, Germany: Springer-Verlag; 1997.
[c]Cognard C, Gobin YP, Pierot L, Bailly AL, Houdart E, Casasco A, Chiras J, Merland JJ. Cerebral dural arteriovenous fistulas: clinical and angiographic correlation with a revised classification of venous drainage. *Radiology* 1995; 194: 671–680.
[d]Alberts MJ. Intracerebral hemorrhage and vascular malformations. In: Alberts MJ, ed. *Genetics of cerebrovascular disease.* Armonk, NY, USA: Futura Publishing Company. 1999:209–236.
[e]Patel U, Gupta SC. Wyburn-Mason syndrome. A case report and review of the literature. *Neuroradiology* 1990;31:544–546.
[f]Ponce FA, Han PP, Spetzler RF, Canady A, Feiz-Erfan I. Associated arteriovenous malformation of the orbit and brain: a case of Wyburn-Mason syndrome without retinal involvement. Case report. *J Neurosurg* 2001;95:346–349

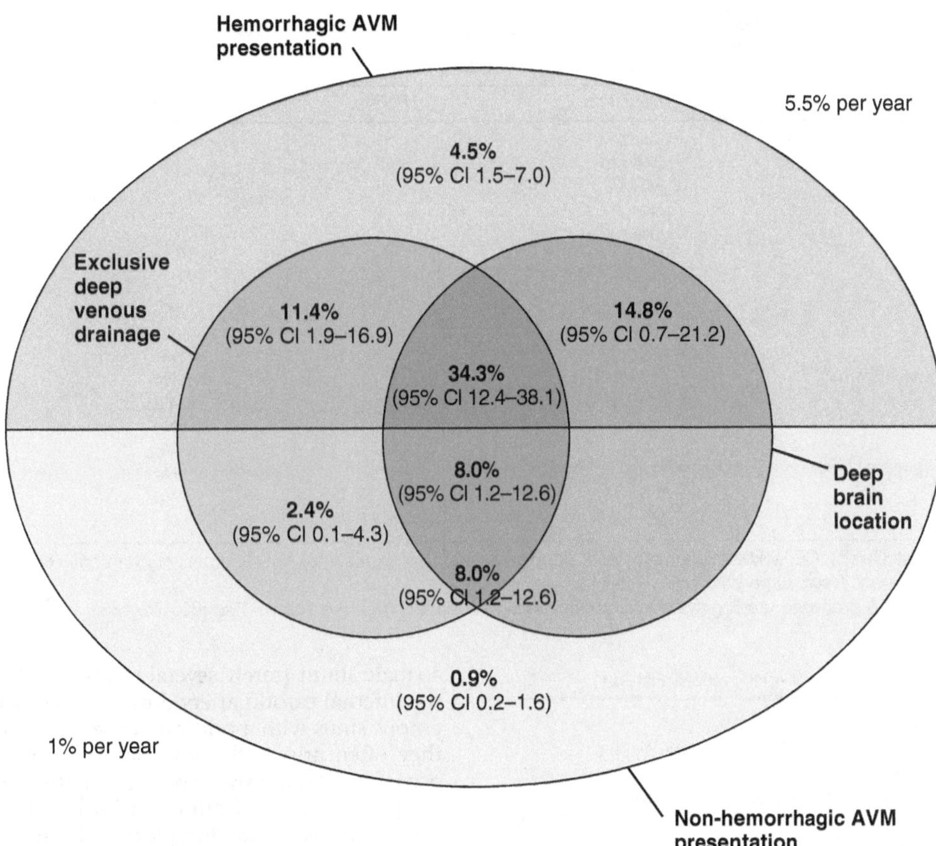

Figure 30-6. The Columbia AVM Hemorrhage Risk Model has been widely used: The plot summarizes observed crude annual hemorrhage rates in overlapping risk groups based on prospective observational data from n=622 untreated AVM patients. *(Modified after data from Zhu XL, Chan MS, Poon WS. Spontaneous intracranial hemorrhage: which patients need diagnostic cerebral angiography? A prospective study of 206 cases and a review of literature.* Stroke *28:1406–1409, 1997.)*

TABLE 30-3 Reported treatment complications and occlusion rates based on a systematic meta-analysis of the available literature (2000–2011)

Treatment Modality	Any Treatment Complication median (range)	Severe Treatment Complications median (range)	Complete Arteriovenous Malformation Occlusion median (range)
Endovascular therapy	25% (7.6–55%)	6.6% (0–28%)	13% (0–94%)
Neurosurgery	29% (1.5–54%)	7.4% (0–40%)	96% (0–100%)
Stereotactic radiotherapy	13% (0–63%)	5.1% (0–21%)	38% (0–75%)

three treatment modalities. There may also be a negative interaction between stereotactic radiotherapy and prior embolization.[61] The surgical risk may be higher in older patients, those showing a diffuse AVM nidus, and in unruptured AVMs; hence the proposal of Lawton's 5-point "supplementary scale" in addition to the established 5-point Spetzler/Martin grading system (Table 30-4), which increased significantly the accuracy of the surgical risk prediction.[62]

While there is usually an indication for complete lesion eradication after AVM rupture, preventive interventions for unruptured AVMs cannot be justified based on recent outcome data since interventions are associated with a higher risk of stroke and neurological deficits in population-based studies with both short-term (3 years)[48] and long-term (12-years) follow-up.[50] In addition, a randomized controlled trial (ARUBA) showed a more than fivefold increased risk of death and stroke for patients undergoing invasive therapy (hazard ratio, 5.26; 95%CI, 2.63–11.11), and a significantly increased risk of major neurological deficits (relative risk, 2.77; 95%CI, 1.20–6.25).[49]

For patients with AVM-associated epilepsy, population-based data do not confirm a long-term benefit of AVM eradication on future seizure occurrence,[51] neither do the secondary outcome data in the randomized ARUBA trial.[49] From a scientific standpoint, treatment indications remain mainly limited to secondary hemorrhage prevention in patients whose AVM has already bled.

More detailed descriptions of surgical and endovascular treatment options and techniques are available as part of Chapters 67 and 72.

Dural Arteriovenous Fistulae

Dural arteriovenous fistulae (DAVFs) constitute arteriovenous shunts at the level of the meninges that are usually supplied by branches of the external carotid and/or vertebral artery. They are generally considered acquired lesions due to trauma or venous occlusion and have an extracerebral location. Often they present with pulse-synchronic bruits, headaches, and signs of increased intracranial pressure, but they may also

TABLE 30-4 Risk Prediction Grading Scales for Surgical Arteriovenous Malformation Resection, After[ab]

	Spetzler/Martin Grading Scale		Lawton Supplementary Scale	
Variable	*Definition*	*Points*	*Definition*	*Points*
AVM size	<3 cm	1		
	3–6 cm	2		
	>6 cm	3		
Deep venous drainage (any)	No	0		
	Yes	1		
Eloquence	No	0		
	Yes	1		
Patient age			<20 years	1
			20–40 years	2
			>40 years	3
Unruptured AVM presentation			No	0
			Yes	1
Diffuse AVM nidus			No	0
			Yes	1
Perforating artery supply			No	0
			Yes	1
Total Grade		1–5		1–5

[a]Lawton MT, Kim H, McCulloch CE, Mikhak B, Young WL. A supplementary grading scale for selecting patients with brain arteriovenous malformations for surgery. *Neurosurgery* 2010;66:702–713.
[b]Spetzler RF, Martin NA. A proposed grading system for arteriovenous malformations. *J Neurosurg* 1986;65:476–483.

TABLE 30-5 Classification of Dural Arteriovenous Fistulae

BORDEN CLASSIFICATION	
1	Venous drainage directly into dural venous sinus or meningeal vein
2	Venous drainage into dural venous sinus with CVR
3	Venous drainage directly into subarachnoid veins (CVR only)
MERLAND-COGNARD CLASSIFICATION	
I	Venous drainage into dural venous sinus with antegrade flow
IIa	Venous drainage into dural venous sinus with retrograde flow
IIb	Venous drainage into dural venous sinus with antegrade flow and CVR
IIa&b	Venous drainage into dural venous sinus with retrograde flow and CVR
III	Venous drainage directly into subarachnoid veins (CVR only)
IV	Type III with venous ectasias of the draining subarachnoid veins
V	Venous drainage into medullary veins

CVR: Cerebral venous reflux.

cause progressive neurological deficits and intracranial bleeding, including ICH. Those with direct or retrograde venous outflow into cerebral veins have been associated with hemorrhagic presentation or progressive neurological symptoms at initial diagnosis, but no controlled longitudinal data exist on the actual longitudinal risk of these lesions. Nonetheless, the most widely used classification as proposed by Merland and Cognard is mainly based on the venous outflow pattern as these characteristics may also impact on the endovascular treatment approach: In type I fistulas, meningeal branches shunt directly into a dural sinus without retrograde venous filling. Type II lesions are similar to type I but show venous reflux from the dural sinus into subarachnoid veins. Type III fistulas connect directly to cortical veins. If the latter type shows venous ectasias, it is labeled type IV. The rare infratentorial type V lesions show retrograde venous drainage into the spinal venous system.[63] The Borden classification mainly stratifies DAVFs according to the presence of cerebral venous reflux, but does not include the Merland-Cognard DAVF type V (Table 30-5).

A common presentation of a dural arteriovenous shunt is the carotid-cavernous fistula. This subtype consists of mainly a single shunt (rarely several trans-dural feeders) which links the internal carotid artery during its passage through the cavernous sinus with a portion of the cavernous sinus. Although they often arise following trauma, they are also known to occur spontaneously, especially in the elderly. The classic symptom complex features an injected sclera of the affected eye, chemosis, ophthalmoplegia, a bruit, and, in severe cases, even loss of vision.[64]

Quite commonly, DAVFs are missed on standard CT, MRI, and MRA images, and their definite diagnosis is mainly based on diagnostic cerebral angiography after obligatory injection of the common carotid and vertebral arteries (Fig. 30-7).

Most often, DAVFs are treated using an endovascular approach, either via the feeding artery system, or via retrograde occlusion of the draining veins. Depending on the topographic location, direct embolization via transcranial puncture or neurosurgical occlusion of the venous draining system constitutes an alternative therapeutic strategy.

More details on endovascular and surgical techniques in the treatment of DAVFs are available as part of Chapters 68 and 72.

ANOMALIES OF CEREBRAL VEINS

Cavernous Malformations

Cerebral cavernous malformations (CCMs) or cavernomas constitute abnormally enlarged capillary cavities without intervening brain parenchyma. The lesions may occur anywhere including the cortical surface, white matter pathways, basal ganglia, or deep in the brain stem. They rarely occupy a clinically significant amount of space in the brain, but may be located in clinically important regions and are occasionally multiple. Their cavernous channels often show multiple areas of thrombosis and hemosiderin deposits as remnants of prior intra-cavernomatous (less often extra-cavernomatous) hemorrhage. Blood flow through these lesions is minimal, and, therefore, they are generally not seen on diagnostic angiograms.

They may be recognized as round, slightly hyperdense lesions on non-contrast head CT showing some ring enhancement after injection (Figs. 30-8A and B). In most cases, the diagnosis is easily established on brain MRI with a typical popcorn-shaped, mixed hyper- and hypointense appearance,

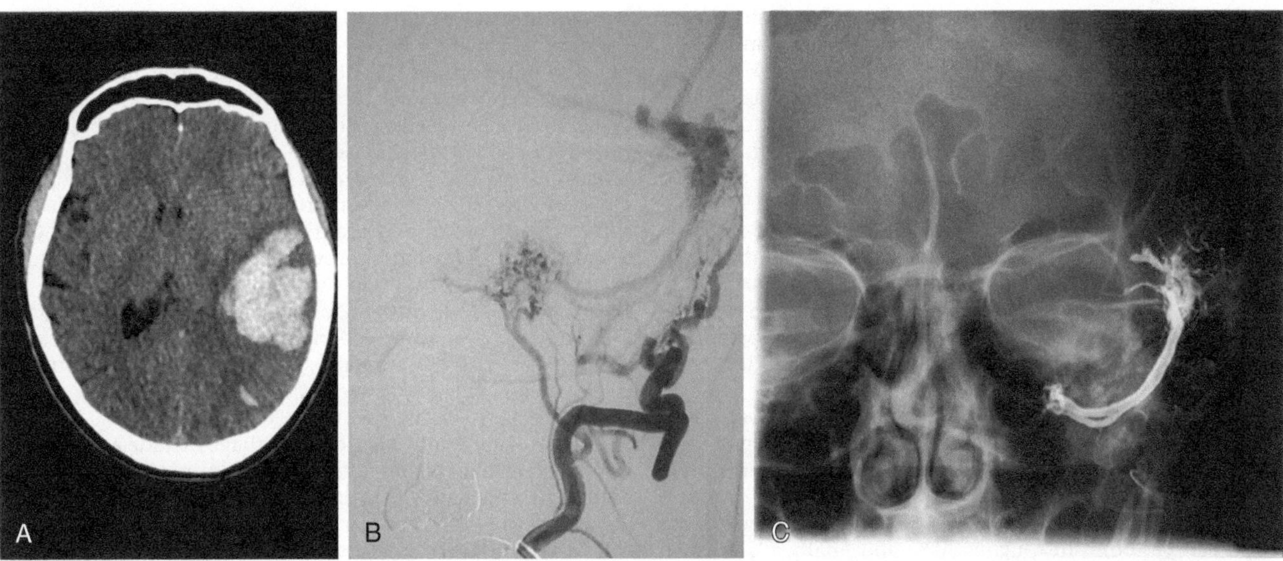

Figure 30-7. Dural arteriovenous fistula with initial hemorrhagic manifestation (A). Angiography after injection of the left external carotid artery showing arteriovenous shunting with retrograde venous outflow into the cerebral venous system (B). After successful embolization, the remaining cast permanently blocks arterial flow through the fistula (C).

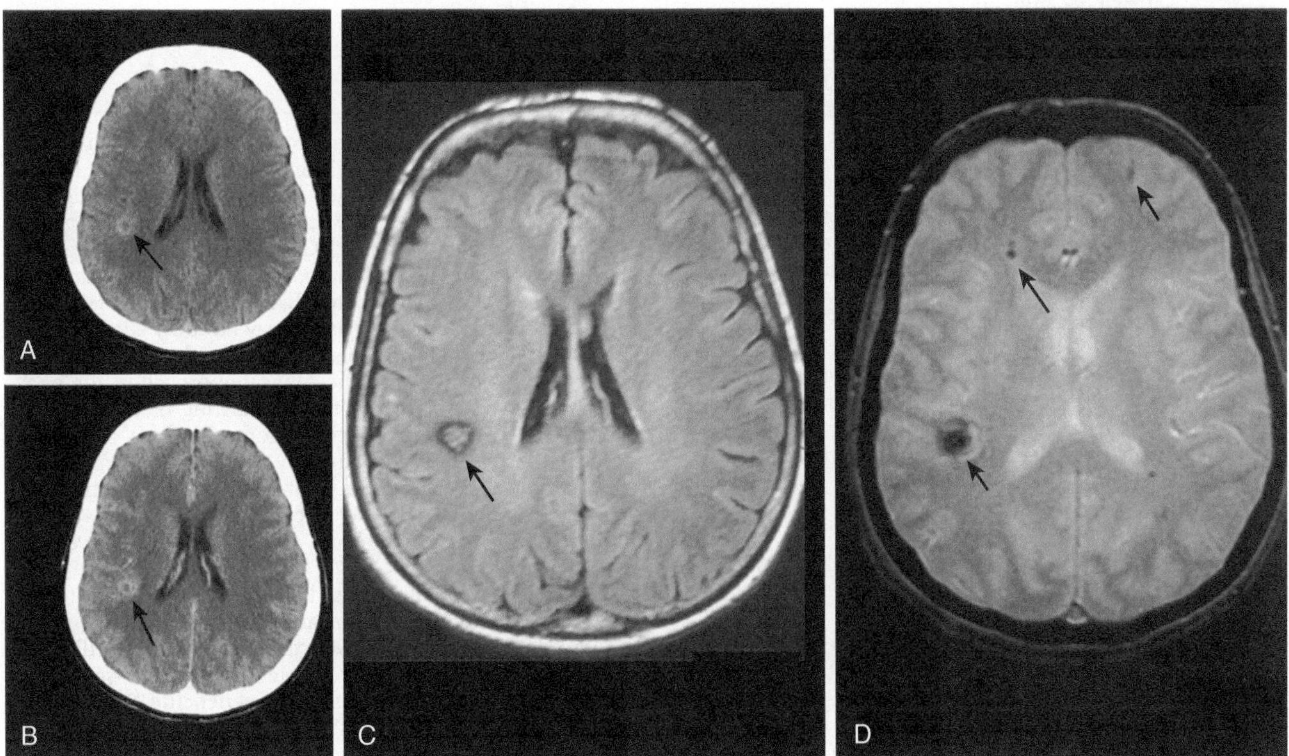

Figure 30-8. Multiple cerebral cavernomatosis in a patient with proven with CCM1/KRIT1 mutation. A subcortical right hemispheric CCM with hyperdense "ring" can be appreciated on non-contrast (A, arrow) and post-contrast (B, arrow) cranial CT. Brain MR imaging shows the same malformation with a mixed hyperintense/hypointense "popcorn" signal and a hypointense perilesional rim on FLAIR (C, arrow) and presence of multiple hypointense CCMs using the T2*-weighted (gradient echo) sequence (D, arrows).

and usually a hypointense perilesional signal on FLAIR and T2-weighted images (Fig. 30-8C). Gradient echo (T2*-weighted) imaging carries the highest sensitivity for the detection of CCM revealing intralesional paramagnetic hemosiderin deposits as hypointense signals (Fig. 30-8D). Extracerebral manifestations may affect cranial nerves (rare, but most commonly the trigeminal, optic or oculomotor nerves), the spinal cord, the retina (in up to 5% of familial CCM cases), and the skin (visible as isolated hyperkeratotic cutaneous capillary venous malformations, so far described in cases with familial CCMs only).

Based on autopsy data, prevalence estimates for CCMs in the general population range between 100 and 500 per 100,000; similar figures have been found in a meta-analysis of routine MR imaging in healthy individuals.[41] Women and men appear to be equally affected. The mean age at diagnosis spreads around age 30 in most recent series with an estimated annual detection rate of 0.56 per 100,000.[65] The proportion of familial cases ranges between 10% and 40% in most Western populations, but the highest frequency (50%) has been reported in Hispanic Americans, suggesting a genetic founder effect.[66] Patients harboring multiple CCMs have a high likelihood of carrying a genetic mutation, as do those with a positive familial history.

Clinically, it is often difficult to determine a one-to-one relationship between lesion and symptoms. At initial diagnosis, the latter include epileptic seizures in 45%, symptomatic hemorrhage in 40%, and headaches or other/unrelated symptoms leading to diagnostic imaging in 15%. Among patients with familial CCMs, 60% will become symptomatic. The proportion of symptomatic patients among sporadic cases remains as yet unknown. Three different gene loci have been defined so far, all leading to an autosomal dominant pattern of inheritance: CCM 1 or KRIT 1 is located on chromosome 7q and accounts for over 40% of familial cases (up to 70% in Hispanic Americans); CCM 2 or MGC4607 is on chromosome 7p and can be found in roughly 30%; and finally, CCM3 or PDCD10 has been mapped to chromosome 3q and is the underlying defect in 15%. Another 15% of familial cases show no mutation in the three loci, which is why at least one more gene defect can be suspected.[66]

Diagnosis and Risk Stratification

In routine clinical practice, the diagnosis of CCMs should be stratified by patient history (symptomatic versus asymptomatic, family history), MR imaging data (anatomic location, single versus multiple CCMs, hemorrhagic versus non-hemorrhagic, with or without associated developmental venous anomaly), and genetic test results (if performed). Ideally, the hemorrhage status is specified based on extra- versus intra-cavernomatous bleeding, and whether the MRI signal suggests acute blood or chronic hemosiderin deposits (Table 30-6, Fig. 30-8). In the early days of MR imaging in surgical CCM patients, an initial morphological classification has been proposed based on their appearance on T1- and T2-weighted sequences: Type 1 cavernomas are hyperintense lesions indicating recent hemorrhage. Type 2 malformations are those most often seen in daily practice; they harbor mixed hyper- and hypointense signals suggestive of mixed subacute and chronic hemorrhage signs or calcifications. Type 3 lesions are hypointense and mostly asymptomatic. Type 4 CCMs are also assumed to be asymptomatic and can be detected on gradient echo (T2*) imaging alone. The latter group, however, may be difficult to differentiate from other causes of cerebral microbleeds, such as amyloid angiopathy, arteriolosclerotic small-vessel disease, CADASIL, vasculitis, and others.[67] Therefore, the Angioma Alliance has defined reporting standards for CCM hemorrhage, allowing a consistent approach to clinical and brain imaging classification of CM hemorrhage in hopes to improve the external validity of future CM research.[68]

On longitudinal patient follow-up, the number of CCM may increase over time, especially in genetic CCM types. A given cavernoma may remain stable, increase in volume or even regress.[69] The crude average hemorrhage risk of a cavernoma seems to be as low as 0.6% per year (Table 30-7).[70] Factors favoring symptomatic hemorrhage include a history of prior cavernoma hemorrhage, strategic locations such as the brainstem and basal ganglia, and anticoagulation therapy.[71] Pregnancy as a risk factor for cavernoma hemorrhage remains controversial. There is, however, increasing evidence that neither antiplatelet therapy nor oral anticoagulation have a negative impact on the bleeding risk in CCM patients.[72,73] Overall, even in genetically determined cases, the long-term prognosis is favorable with 80% preserved long-term autonomy, with less favorable outcome seen in patients with brainstem CCM.[66]

TABLE 30-6 Neurological Classification of Cerebral Cavernous Malformation

	Parameter	
Clinical	Symptomatic • Seizures • Hemorrhage • Headache	Asymptomatic
Family history	Positive • Pedigree • Pattern of inheritance	Negative
Imaging	MRI (T1 +/− contrast, T2 or FLAIR, T2*)	
Number	Multiple • Anatomic location	Single • Anatomic location
Size	Maximum cavernoma diameter	
Hemorrhage	Acute bleeding Extra-cavernomatous	Chronic hemosiderin Intra-lesional
DVA	Present	Absent
Genetic testing	Positive • CCM 1 (KRIT 1) • CCM 2 (MGC4607) • CCM 3 (PDCD10)	Negative

Treatment Strategy

If indicated, neurosurgical excision is the treatment of choice as outcome after stereotactic radiotherapy appears to have less favorable results.[74,75] The decision for intervention is ideally based on a multidisciplinary discussion considering the overall profile of the patient (see Table 30-2). Surgery is generally limited to symptomatic CCMs associated with therapy-resistant epilepsy, progressive CCM enlargement, or after symptomatic CCM hemorrhage. If extra-lesional CCM bleeding has occurred, surgical excision may not only eliminate the risk of subsequent hemorrhage, but the risk of intervention itself may also be lower as the surgical approach in the post-acute phase is facilitated by the pre-existing bleeding cavity. Due to the progressive multiplication of lesions over time, surgical intervention is not generally recommended in patients with familial CCM. Resection of an associated developmental venous anomaly (see below) is contraindicated as its occlusion may lead to venous stasis, brain edema, and eventual hemorrhage.

In a recent population-based study of 134 CCM patients, the risk of persistent neurological deficits was twice as high in the group undergoing CCM excision (adjusted HR, 2.2; 95%CI, 1.1–4.2). Similarly, the patients who underwent CCM excision endured a higher risk of experiencing ICH or new focal neurological deficits following CCM excision (HR, 3.6; 95%CI, 1.3–10.0).[76] Contrary to prior conventional wisdom that selected symptomatic patients should undergo surgery, this study is one of the first to show worsened outcomes in those who do. Therefore, surgical cavernoma excision cannot be routinely recommended, especially not in asymptomatic patients, until a clinical trial provides more evidence in favor of surgical interventions.

More details on surgical treatment of CCMs are provided in Chapter 73.

Developmental Venous Anomaly

A developmental venous anomaly (DVA) is found in up to 30% of CCM patients.[77] In the pre-MRI era, so-called "venous

TABLE 30-7 Crude Annual Rates of Symptomatic Intracerebral Hemorrhage in Patients with Cerebral Cavernous Malformations

Initial Cerebral Cavernous Malformation Presentation	Mayo Clinic[a]	SIVMS[b]	*Lariboisière CCM Databank*[cd]
With symptomatic hemorrhage	6.2% per year	6% per year	***15.2%*** *per patient-year* ***9.2%*** *per lesion-year*
Without symptomatic hemorrhage	0.3–2.2% per year	0.5% per year	***1.5%*** *per person-year* ***0.2%*** *per lesion-year*

[a]Flemming KD, Link MJ, Christianson TJ, Brown RD Jr. Prospective haemorrhage risk of intracerebral cavernous malformations. *Neurology* 2012;78:632–636.
[b]Al-Shahi Salman R, Hall JM, Horne MA, Moultrie F, Josephson CB, Bhattacharya JJ, Counsell CE, Murray GD, Papanastassiou V, Ritchie V, Roberts RC, Sellar RJ, Warlow CP; Scottish Audit of Intracranial Vascular Malformations (SAIVMs) collaborators. Untreated clinical course of cerebral cavernous malformations: a prospective, population-based cohort study. *Lancet Neurol* 2012;11:217–224.
[c]Schneble HM, Soumare A, Hervé D, Bresson D, Guichard JP, Riant F, Tournier-Lasserve E, Tzourio C, Chabriat H, Stapf C. Antithrombotic therapy and bleeding risk in a prospective cohort study of patients with cerebral cavernous malformations. *Stroke* 2012;43:3196–3199.
[d]Flemming KD, Link MJ, Christianson TJ, et al. Use of antithrombotic agents in patients with intracerebral cavernous malformations. *J Neurosurg* 2013;118:43–46.
(Data From Three Independent Datasets)

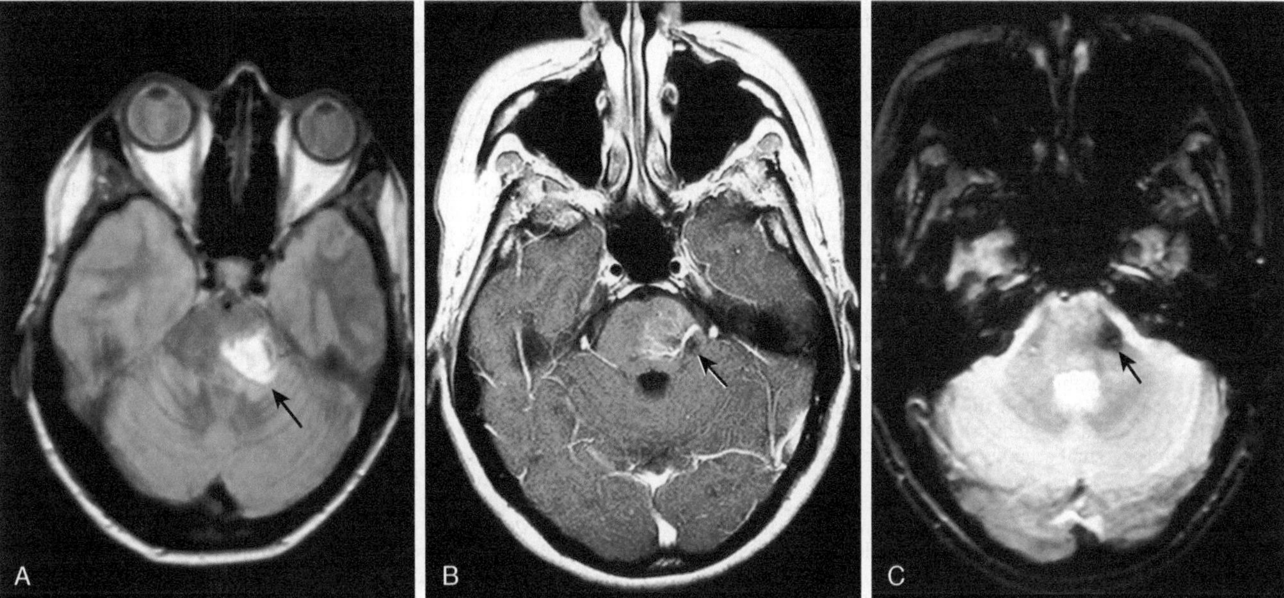

Figure 30-9. Subacute pontine hemorrhage on non-contrast T1-weighted MR imaging in a 32-year-old patient without significant prior medical history (A). Follow-up imaging after hematoma resorption reveals a developmental venous anomaly (B, T1 after gadolinium injection) with an associated cavernous malformation (C, hypointense on T2*-weighted image).

malformations" were considered a possible cause of ICH. The term is now obsolete, as DVAs constitute mainly asymptomatic variants of the physiological white matter or tectal venous drainage system. They constitute physiological drainage pathways of normal brain tissue. They are represented by a deep prominent vein that appears late on the venous phase of an arteriogram or in post-contrast MRI or CT, and are associated with a finger-like projection from the main vein, resembling a broom or caput medusae. Hemosiderin staining along the DVA wall may be seen on T2*- or SWI-weighted images, and the lack of an arterial component in DVAs distinguishes them from AVMs. Recent studies suggest altered hemodynamics as one possible link to cavernoma formation.[78] An associated cavernoma constitutes the actual bleeding source, if hemorrhage occurs in the vicinity of a DVA (Fig. 30-9).

Clinically, DVAs are usually asymptomatic, and only rarely may a cortical DVA lead to seizure activity.[79] Another, extremely rare complication is symptomatic thrombosis of the DVA, leading to focal edema and potential hemorrhagic transformation.[80] Their role in the physiological drainage of normal brain tissue usually precludes any surgical or endovascular intervention.

REFERENCES

1. Zhu XL, Chan MS, Poon WS. Spontaneous intracranial hemorrhage: which patients need diagnostic cerebral angiography? A prospective study of 206 cases and a review of literature. Stroke 1997;28:1406–9.
2. Broderick JP, Adams HP, Barsan W, et al. Guidelines for the management of spontaneous intracerebral hemorrhage. A statement for healthcare professionals from a special writing group of the Stroke Council, American Heart Association. Stroke 1999;30: 905–15.
3. The European Stroke Initiative (EUSI) Writing Committee Writing Committee for the EUSI Executive Committee: Recommendations for the diagnosis and management of intracranial haemorrhage. Cerebrovasc Dis 2006;22:294–316.
4. Stapf C, Van der Worp HB, Steiner T, et al. Stroke research priorities for the next decade – a supplement statement on intracranial haemorrhage. Cerebrovasc Dis 2007;23:318–19.
5. Langhorne P, Fearon P, Ronning OM, et al; Stroke Unit Trialists' Collaboration. Stroke unit care benefits patients with intracerebral hemorrhage: systematic review and meta-analysis. Stroke 2013;44:3044–9.
6. Steiner T, Al-Shahi Salman R, Beer R, et al. European Stroke Organisation (ESO) guidelines for the management of spontaneous intracerebral hemorrhage. Int J Stroke 2014;9:840–55.

7. Stapf C, Mohr JP. Aneurysms and subarachnoid hemorrhage – epidemiology. In: Le Roux PD, Winn RH, editors. Management of Cerebral Aneurysms. Philadelphia, USA: Saunders; 2004. p. 183–7.
8. Phillips LH, Whisnant JP, O'Fallon M, et al. The unchanging pattern of subarachnoid hemorrhage in a community. Neurology 1980;30:1034–40.
9. The ACROSS Group. Epidemiology of aneurysmal subarachnoid hemorrhage in Australia and New Zealand. Incidence and case fatality from the Australasian Cooperative Research on Subarachnoid Hemorrhage Study (ACROSS). Stroke 2000;31:1843–50.
10. International Study of Intracranial Aneurysms Investigators. Unruptured intracranial aneurysms: natural history, clinical outcome, and risks of surgical and endovascular treatment. Lancet 2003;362:103–10.
11. Johnston SC, Selvin S, Gress DR. The burden, trends, and demographics of mortality from subarachnoid hemorrhage. Neurology 1998;50:1413–18.
12. Longstrength WT Jr, Nelson LM, Koepsell TD, et al. Subarachnoid hemorrhage and hormonal factors in women: a population-based case-control study. Ann Int Med 1994;121:168–73.
13. Jennett B, Teasdale G. Management of head injuries. Philadelphia: FA Davis; 1981.
14. Hunt WE, Hess RM. Surgical risk as related to time of intervention in the repair of intracranial aneurysms. J Neurosurg 1968;28:14.
15. Johnston SC, Wilson CB, Halbach VV, et al. Endovascular and Surgical Treatment of Unruptured Cerebral Aneurysms: Comparison of Risks. Ann Neurol 2000;48:11–19.
16. International Subarachnoid Aneurysm Trial (ISAT) Collaborative Group. International Subarachnoid Aneurysm Trial (ISAT) of neurosurgical clipping versus endovascular coiling in 2143 patients with ruptured intracranial aneurysms: a randomised trial. Lancet 2002;360:1267–74.
17. Farrell DF, Forno LS. Symptomatic capillary telangiectasis of the brainstem without hemorrhage. Report of an unusual case. Neurology 1970;20(4):341–6.
18. Jessurun GA, Kamphuis DJ, van der Zande FH, et al. Cerebral arteriovenous malformations in The Netherlands Antilles. High prevalence of hereditary hemorrhagic telangiectasia-related single and multiple cerebral arteriovenous malformations. Clin Neurol Neurosurg 1993;95(3):193–8.
19. Fukui M. Members of the Research Committee on Spontaneous Occlusion of the Circle of Willis (Moyamoya Disease) of the Ministry of Health and Welfare, Japan. Guidelines for the diagnosis and treatment of spontaneous occlusion of the circe of Willis ('moyamoya' disease). Clin Neurol Neurosurg 1997;99(Suppl. 2):S238–40.
20. Suzuki J. Moyamoya disease. Berlin: Springer-Verlag; 1986.
21. Goto Y, Yonekawa Y. Worldwide distribution of moyamoya disease. Neurol Med Chir 1992;32:883–6.
22. Kuroda S, Ishikawa T, Houkin K, et al. Incidence and Clinical Features of Disease Progression in Adult Moyamoya Disease. Stroke 2005;36:2148–53.
23. Uchino K, Johnston CS, Becker KJ, et al. Moyamoya disease in Washington State and California. Neurology 2005;65:956–8.
24. Kuriyama S, Kusaka Y, Fujimura M, et al. Prevalence and clinicoepisemiological features of moyamoya disease in Japan. Findings from a nationwide epidemiological survey. Stroke 2008;39: 42–7.
25. Merkel KH, Ginsberg PL, Parker JC Jr, et al. Cerebrovascular disease in sickle cell anemia: a clinical, pathological and radiological correlation. Stroke 1978;9:45–52.
26. Ullrich NJ, Robertson R, Kinnamon DD, et al. Moyamoya following cranial irradiation for primary brain tumors in children. Neurology 2007;68:932–8.
27. Rokitansky C. Handbuch der allgemeinen pathologischen Anatomie. Wien, Austria: Braumüller & Seidel; 1846. p. 276–7.
28. Emmanuel C. Ein Fall von Angioma arteriale racemosum des Gehirns. Deutsche Zeitschr Nervenheilk 1899;14:288–318.
29. Stapf C, Mohr JP, Mast H. History of concepts on the etiology of brain arteriovenous malformations. Neurology 2002;58(Suppl. 3): A342.
30. Yuval Y, Lerner A, Lipitz S, et al. Prenatal diagnosis of vein of Galen aneurysmal malformation: Report of two cases with proposal for prognostic indices. Prenat Diagn 1997;17:972–7.
31. Campi A, Scotti G, Filippi M, et al. Antenatal diagnosis of vein of Galen aneurysmal malformation: MR study of fetal brain and postnatal follow-up. Neuroradiology 1996;38:87–90.
32. Pschyrembel W, Dudenhausen JW. Praktische Geburtshilfe mit geburtshilflichen Operationen. 17th ed. Berlin: Walter de Gruyter; 1991.
33. Weaver DD, Brandt IK. Catalog of Prenatally Diagnosed Conditions. 3rd ed. Baltimore: Johns Hopkins University Press; 1999.
34. Baird WF, Stitt DG. Arteriovenous aneurysm of the cerebellum in a premature infant. Pediatrics 1959;24:455–7.
35. Padget DH. The development of the cranial arteries in the human embryo. (Carnegie Inst Wash Pub. 575.) Contrib Embryol 1948; 32:205.
36. Stapf C, Mohr JP, Sciacca RR, et al. Incident hemorrhage risk of brain arteriovenous malformations located in the arterial borderzones. Stroke 2000;31:2365–8.
37. van den Bergh R, van der Eecken H. Anatomy and embryology of the cerebral circulation. Prog Brain Res 1968;30:1–25.
38. Van der Eecken HM, Fisher CM, Adams RD. The anatomy and functional significance of the meningeal arterial anastomoses of the human brain. J Neuropathol Exp Neurol 1953;12:132–57.
39. Nelson MD, Gonzalez-Gomez I, Gilles FH. The search for human telencephalic ventriculofugal arteries. AJNR Am J Neuroradiol 1991;12:215–22.
40. Hung PC, Wang HS, Yeh YS, et al. Coexistence of schizencephaly and intracranial arteriovenous malformation in an infant. AJNR Am J Neuroradiol 1996;17:1921–2.
41. Morris Z, Whiteley WN, Longstreth WT Jr, et al. Incidental findings on brain magnetic resonance imaging: systematic review and meta-analysis. BMJ 2009;339:b3016.
42. Stapf C, Mast H, Sciacca RR, et al. The New York Islands AVM Study: Design, study progress and initial results. Stroke 2003;34: E29–33.
43. van Beijnum J, van der Worp HB, Algra A, et al. Prevalence of brain arteriovenous malformations in first-degree relatives of patients with a brain arteriovenous malformation. Stroke 2014;45: 3231–5.
44. Van Beijnum J, van der Worp HB, Schippers HM, et al. Familial occurrence of brain arteriovenous malformations: a systematic review. J Neurol Neurosurg Psychiatry 2007;78:1213–17.
45. Liu XJ, Wang S, Zhao YL, et al. Risk of cerebral arteriovenous malformation rupture during pregnancy and puerperium. Neurology 2014;82:1798–803.
46. van Beijnum J, Lovelock CE, Cordonnier C, et al; SIVMS Steering Committee and the Oxford Vascular Study. Outcome after spontaneous and arteriovenous malformation-related intracerebral haemorrhage: population-based studies. Brain 2009;132: 537–43.
47. Laakso A, Dashti R, Seppänen J, et al. Long-term excess mortality in 623 patients with brain arteriovenous malformations. Neurosurgery 2008;63(2):244–53.
48. Wedderburn CJ, van Beijnum J, Bhattacharya JJ, et al, SIVMS Collaborators. Outcome after interventional or conservative management of unruptured brain arteriovenous malformations: a prospective, population-based cohort study. Lancet Neurol 2008;7:223–30.
49. Mohr JP, Parides MK, Stapf C, et al, international ARUBA investigators. Medical management with or without interventional therapy for unruptured brain arteriovenous malformations (ARUBA): a multicentre, non-blinded, randomised trial. Lancet 2014;383:614–21.
50. Al-Shahi Salman R, White PM, Counsell CE, et al, Scottish Audit of Intracranial Vascular Malformations Collaborators. Outcome after conservative management or intervention for unruptured brain arteriovenous malformations. JAMA 2014;311:1661–9.
51. Josephson CB, Bhattacharya JJ, Counsell CE, et al, Scottish Audit of Intracranial Vascular Malformations (SAIVMs) steering committee and collaborators. Seizure risk with AVM treatment or conservative management: prospective, population-based study. Neurology 2012;79:500–7.
52. Stapf C, Mast H, Sciacca RR, et al. Predictors of hemorrhage in patients with untreated brain arteriovenous malformation. Neurology 2006;66:1350–5.
53. Kim H, Al-Shahi Salman R, McCulloch CE, et al; MARS Coinvestigators. Untreated brain arteriovenous malformation:

patient-level meta-analysis of hemorrhage predictors. Neurology 2014;83:590–7.
54. Kim H, Sidney S, McCulloch CE, et al; UCSF BAVM Study Project. Racial/Ethnic differences in longitudinal risk of intracranial hemorrhage in brain arteriovenous malformation patients. Stroke 2007;38:2430–7.
55. Guo Y, Saunders T, Su H, et al, University of California, San Francisco Brain Arteriovenous Malformation (UCSF bAVM) Study Project. Silent intralesional microhemorrhage as a risk factor for brain arteriovenous malformation rupture. Stroke 2012;43: 1240–6.
56. Choi JH, Mast H, Sciacca RR, et al. Clinical outcome after first and recurrent hemorrhage in patients with untreated brain arteriovenous malformation. Stroke 2006;37:1243–7.
57. Al-Shahi R, Stapf C. The prognosis and treatment of arteriovenous malformations of the brain. Practical Neurology 2005;5: 194–205.
58. Ogilvy CS, Stieg PE, Awad I, et al. Recommendations for the management of intracranial arteriovenous malformations: a statement for healthcare professionals from a special writing group of the stroke council, american stroke association. Stroke 2001;32: 1458–71.
59. van Beijnum J, van der Worp HB, Buis DR, et al. Treatment of brain arteriovenous malformations: a systematic review and meta-analysis. JAMA 2011;306:2011–19.
60. Mast H, Young WL, Koennecke HC, et al. Risk of spontaneous hemorrhage after diagnosis of cerebral arteriovenous malformations. Lancet 1997;350:1065–8.
61. Andrade-Souza YM, Ramani M, Scora D, et al. Embolization before radiosurgery reduces the obliteration rate of arteriovenous malformations. Neurosurgery 2007;60:443–51.
62. Lawton MT, Kim H, McCulloch CE, et al. A supplementary grading scale for selecting patients with brain arteriovenous malformations for surgery. Neurosurgery 2010;66:702–13.
63. Cognard C, Gobin YP, Pierot L, et al. Cerebral dural arteriovenous fistulas: clinical and angiographic correlation with a revised classification of venous drainage. Radiology 1995;194:671–80.
64. Theaudin M, Saint-Maurice JP, Chapot R, et al. Diagnosis and treatment of dural carotid-cavernous fistulas: a consecutive series of 27 patients. J Neurol Neurosurg Psychiatry 2007;78:174–9.
65. Al-Shahi R, Bhattacharya JJ, Currie DG, et al; Scottish Intracranial Vascular Malformation Study Collaborators. Prospective, population-based detection of intracranial vascular malformations in adults: The Scottish Intracranial Vascular Malformation Study (SIVMS). Stroke 2003;34:1163–9.
66. Labauge P, Denier C, Bergametti F, et al. Genetics of Cavernous Angiomas. Lancet Neurol 2007;6:237–44.
67. Viswanathan A, Chabriat H. Cerebral microhemorrhage. Stroke 2006;37:550–5.
68. Al-Shahi Salman R, Berg MJ, Morrison L, et al; Angioma Alliance Scientific Advisory Board. Hemorrhage from cavernous malformations of the brain: definition and reporting standards. Angioma Alliance Scientific Advisory Board. Stroke 2008;39:3222–30.
69. Clatterbuck RE, Moriarity JL, Elmaci I, et al. Dynamic nature of cavernous malformations: a prospective magnetic resonance imaging study with volumetric analysis. J Neurosurgery 2000;93: 981–6.
70. Labauge P, Brunerau L, Laberge S, et al. Prospective follow-up of 33 asymptomatic patients with familial cerebral cavernous malformations. Neurology 2001;57:1825–8.
71. Lehnhardt FG, von Smekal U, Rückriem B, et al. Value of gradient-echo magnetic resonance imaging in the diagnosis of familial cerebral cavernous malformation. Arch Neurol 2005;62:653–8.
72. Schneble HM, Soumare A, Hervé D, et al. Antithrombotic therapy and bleeding risk in a prospective cohort study of patients with cerebral cavernous malformations. Stroke 2012;43:3196–9.
73. Flemming KD, Link MJ, Christianson TJ, et al. Use of antithrombotic agents in patients with intracerebral cavernous malformations. J Neurosurg 2013;118:43–6.
74. Mathiesen T, Edner G, Kihlström L. Deep and brainstem cavernomas: a consecutive 8-year series. J Neurosurgery 2003;99:31–7.
75. Pollock BE, Garces YI, Stafford SL, et al. Stereotactic radiosurgery for cavernous malformations. J Neurosurg 2000;93:987–91.
76. Moultrie F, Horne MA, Josephson CB, et al, Scottish Audit of Intracranial Vascular Malformations (SAIVMs) steering committee and collaborators. Outcome after surgical or conservative management of cerebral cavernous malformations. Neurology 2014;83:582–9.
77. Rabinov JD. Diagnostic imaging of angiographically occult vascular malformations. Neurosurg Clin N Am 1999;10:419–32.
78. Sharma A, Zipfel GJ, Hildebolt C, et al. Hemodynamic effects of developmental venous anomalies with and without cavernous malformations. AJNR Am J Neuroradiol 2013;34:1746–51.
79. Töpper R, Jürgens E, Reul J, et al. Clinical significance of intracranial developmental venous anomalies. J Neurol Neurosurg Psychiatry 1999;67:234–8.
80. Brasse G, Stammel O, Siemens P, et al. Thrombosis of developmental venous anomaly and consecutive venous infarction. Nervenarzt 2008;79:703–5.

31 Stroke and Other Vascular Syndromes of the Spinal Cord

Joshua Z. Willey

KEY POINTS

- Spinal cord stroke presents with painless paraparesis with urinary retention.
- The majority of spinal cord stroke can be attributed to diseases of the aorta.
- Spinal cord infarction occurs most frequently as a complication of aortic dissection and surgery for diseases in the aorta.
- Prevention of spinal cord infarction may occur with lumbar drainage at the time of aortic surgery.
- Immobility and urinary retention are the principal sources of morbidity after spinal cord infarction.

INTRODUCTION

Vascular syndromes of the spinal cord, including stroke and vascular malformations, are significantly less common than those occurring in the brain and retina. Because of the tight arrangement of the pathways in the cord, small infarcts are usually associated with more obvious symptoms and signs than similar lesions in the brain.[1] These diseases are rarely studied outside of the cardiovascular and neurological surgery literature, where significant attention has been given to causes and prevention strategies. In the neurology literature many of the discussions stem from small case series and case reports. The incidence of vascular syndromes in the spinal cord is unknown, and large epidemiologic stroke studies have generally not included spinal cord stroke. Advances in imaging techniques, including magnetic resonance imaging (MRI), have led to improved diagnosis of vascular syndromes in the spinal cord and updated recognition of the underlying causes. With improved diagnosis prevention and acute treatment strategies may eventually emerge. Until that time the cornerstone of management is prevention of the associated medical complications that arise from paraplegia and urinary bladder dysfunction.

HISTORICAL ASPECTS

The clinical syndrome of paraparesis with urinary retention due to disease in the aorta was known by the late nineteenth and early twentieth centuries, with the initial cases describing atherosclerotic and syphilitic diseases of the aorta as the predominant causes.[2,3] In the early twentieth century diseases of the spinal cord venous system were also first described, notably the syndrome of Foix-Alajouanine with progressive necrotizing myelopathy due to venous occlusion.[4] For much of the past century the literature on vascular diseases of the spinal cord was primarily in the form of case reports and short case series describing a wide range of presumed etiologies. In the last two to three decades substantial literature has emerged on spinal cord stroke, particularly in relation to surgery in diseases of the aorta, and on the diagnosis and management of vascular malformations.

ANATOMY: BLOOD SUPPLY TO THE SPINAL CORD

The pattern of arterial blood supply to the spinal cord consists of three families of arteries with a specific anatomic location: longitudinal vessels that extend in a cranial–caudal direction from the upper cervical cord to the conus medullaris, radicular tributary vessels feeding into longitudinal vessels across multiple spinal segments, and numerous feeder (intrinsic) arteries that enter the parenchyma[5–7] (Figs 31-1–31-3). Anastomoses between the longitudinal and radicular vessels lead to the formation of a rich vascular plexus from which medullary vessels penetrate both white and gray matter. These vessels are end arteries and do not anastomose further.

The venous supply to the spinal cord exhibits greater variability but can be subdivided into the extrinsic and intrinsic systems.[8]

Longitudinal Arteries

There are three longitudinal arteries, the anterior spinal artery and the two posterior spinal arteries. The single *anterior spinal artery* forms rostrally from the union of the two anterior spinal branches of each vertebral artery at the level of the foramen magnum. From here it descends up to the tip of the conus medullaris. The caliber of the artery is largest in the region of the lower thoracic and upper lumbar enlargement and smallest in the midthoracic region.[2] The anterior spinal artery is reinforced by successive feeder arterial branches, which enter the artery in a caudal direction and supply the spinal cord below the point of entry. At the conus medullaris and along the filum terminale, the anterior spinal artery communicates through anastomotic branches with the posterior spinal arteries.[2]

The two *posterior spinal arteries* originate directly from the vertebral arteries (see Figs 31-1–31-3). Each vessel descends on the posterior surface of the spinal cord along the posterolateral sulcus. Throughout its course, each posterior spinal artery gives off branches that penetrate the cord to supply the posterior columns, dorsal gray matter, and superficial dorsal aspect of the lateral columns.[2]

Radicular Tributary Arteries

Thirty-one pairs of radicular arteries penetrate the spinal canal through the intervertebral foramina. Usually the 62 radicular branches contribute to the vascularization of the spinal cord and define three major spinal arterial territories – cervicothoracic, midthoracic, and thoracolumbar.[9] These radicular tributaries may be further subdivided according to their origin. The

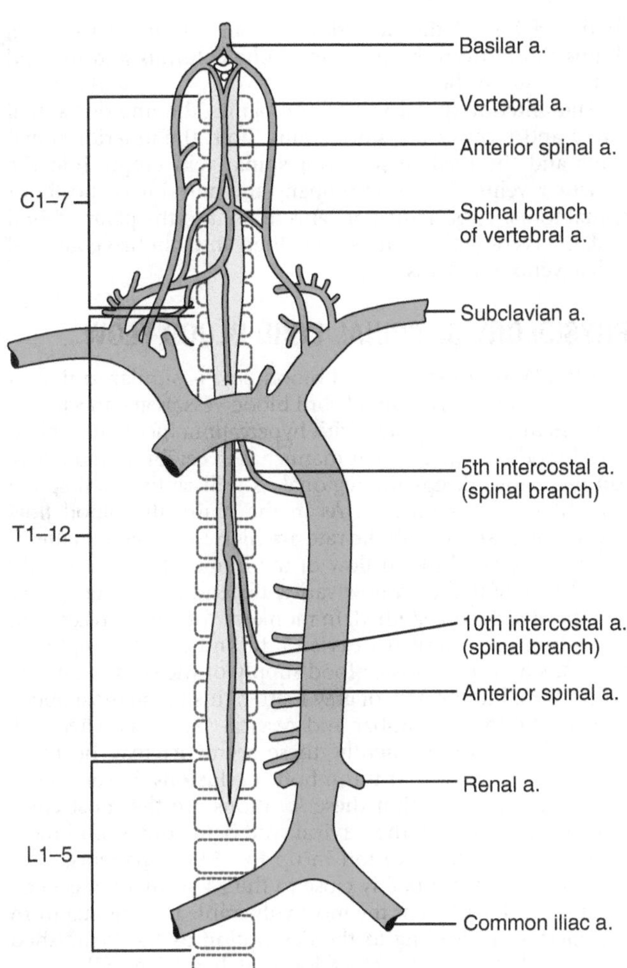

Figure 31-1. Extrinsic vascular supply of the spinal cord. Schematic representation of the anterior spinal artery. *(Adapted from Gray H: Development and gross anatomy of the human body. In Clemente CD, editor:* Anatomy of the human body, *ed 30 (American ed), Philadelphia, 1984, Lea & Febiger; and Benavente OR, Barnett HJM: Spinal cord infarction. In Carter LP, Spetzler RF, editors:* Neurovascular surgery, *New York, 1995, McGraw-Hill, p 1229.)*

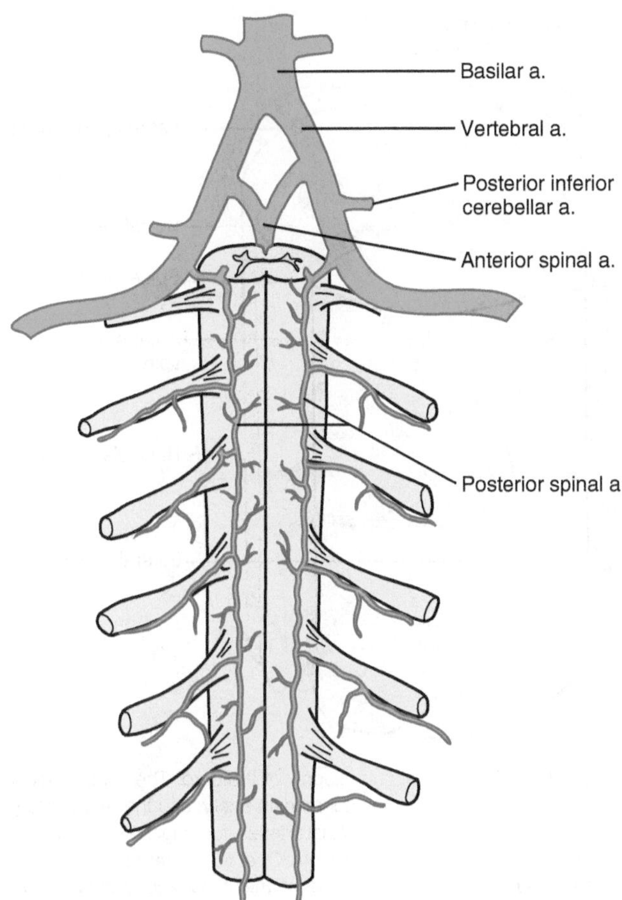

Figure 31-2. Extrinsic vascular supply of the spinal cord. Schematic representation of the posterior spinal arteries. *(Adapted from Gray H: Development and gross anatomy of the human body. In Clemente CD, editor:* Anatomy of the human body, *ed 30 (American ed), Philadelphia, 1984, Lea & Febiger; and Benavente OR, Barnett HJM: Spinal cord infarction. In Carter LP, Spetzler RF, editors:* Neurovascular surgery, *New York, 1995, McGraw-Hill, p 1229.)*

first group consists of those derived from the subclavian artery; the second group is supplied directly from the aorta. At the level of the second thoracic spinal cord segment the arterial supply changes from the subclavian artery to supply directly from the aorta.[10]

The *cervicothoracic* territory consists of the cervical spinal cord, its brachial plexus enlargement, and the first two or three thoracic segments. This territory is richly supplied by the anterior spinal artery arising from the intracranial vertebral arteries, the midcervical radicular branches of the vertebral artery, and the branches of the costocervical trunk. In the *midthoracic* territory, the radicular arteries supplying the middle and lower thoracic cord are less prominent.[5] This territory is usually supplied by a radicular branch arising at about the T7 level; it comprises the fourth to eighth segments of the thoracic cord.

The lower thoracic and upper lumbar segments, which contain the lumbar enlargement and lumbosacral plexus receives its blood supply from the artery of Adamkiewicz, which variably arises from T8 to T12 and exhibits notable differences in size between individuals.[6,9] The artery of Adamkiewicz may be fed by collateral segmental arteries in the setting of chronic occlusive disease, which may have implications for the development for spinal cord infarction in the setting or aortic surgery. These collaterals may be further visualized by magnetic resonance angiography.[10]

Intrinsic (Feeder) Arteries

When the radicular arteries reach the surface of the spinal cord, they form two distinct systems of intrinsic blood supply (see Fig. 31-3). The first is the posterolateral and peripheral plexus formed by the two posterior spinal arteries, which are interconnected by anastomotic channels. This plexus, a centripetal vascular territory, is formed by radial arteries directed inward as branches from the coronal arterial plexus surrounding the spinal cord. It supplies from one-third to one-half of the outer rim of the cord, including the lateral and ventral spinothalamic tracts. These radial arteries are longer in the posterior white columns than in the anterior and lateral columns. The second arterial system to the spinal cord is a centrifugal system formed by the sulcal arteries, which arise from the anterior spinal artery and pass backward in the anterior medial sulcus. These arteries enter the gray commissure and, turning left or right, supply the gray matter and adjacent white matter. The corticospinal tract is nourished by both arterial systems.[11]

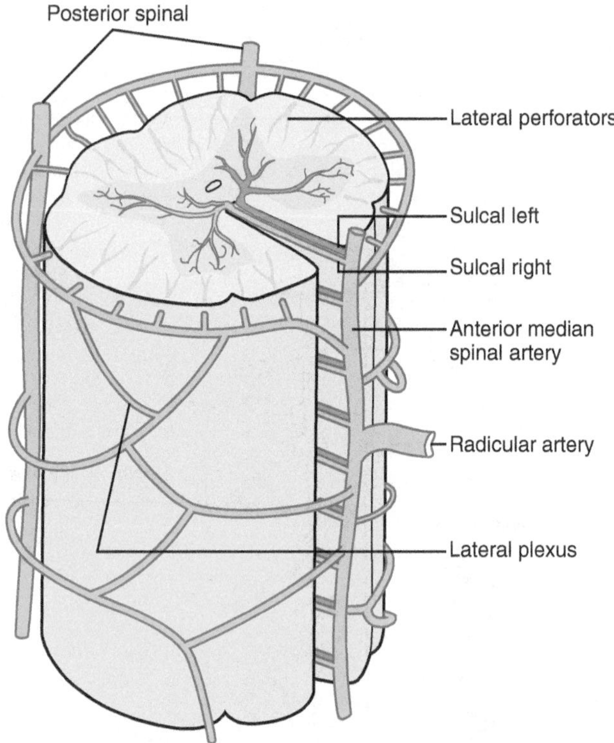

Figure 31-3. Intrinsic vascular supply of the cord. The central sulcal artery is supplied from the anterior median artery, and the lateral artery from the anterior and posterior spinal arteries, forming the vasa corona. *(From Lazorthes G, Gouaze A, Zadeh JO, et al. Arterial vascularization of the spinal cord: Recent studies of the anastomotic substitution pathways.* J Neurosurg *35(3):253–262, 1971.)*

Both arterial systems are interconnected by a capillary anastomosis in the spinal cord. The number of sulcal arteries supplying each segment of the spinal cord varies with the region of the cord. They are most numerous in the thoracolumbar segment and least numerous in the upper thoracic segment.[5]

Venous System

The intrinsic venous system can be classified into two groups based on the pattern of drainage in the anterior and posterior directions.[8] The anterior median group (central veins) collects blood from both halves of the medial aspects of the anterior horns, anterior gray commissure, and white matter of the anterior funiculus. The central veins also drain adjacent levels above and below through intersegmental anastomoses. They commonly anastomose with other veins within the fissure. Finally, the central veins empty into the anterior median spinal vein. The second group consists of radial veins that arise from capillaries near the periphery of the gray matter or from the white matter. They are radially oriented and directed outward toward the surface of the spinal cord, where they join the superficial plexus of veins surrounding the cord and form a venous vasa corona or corona plexus. These veins are more numerous in the white matter of the posterior and lateral funiculi, but they are also found in the anterior funiculus. The radial veins are more prominent at certain cervical and thoracic levels; they drain laterally from the gray matter of the lateral horns as well as posteriorly from the dorsal nucleus of Clark.

The extrinsic venous system is conspicuous on the posterior aspect of the spinal cord and is especially prominent in the lumbosacral region. There is a rich anastomosis between the large venous trunks. The median posterior spinal vein descends in the region of the posterior median septum. This vessel drains blood from the posterior white columns and the end of the posterior horns.

The anterior spinal vein accompanies the anterior spinal artery and receives the sulcal veins. Both the anterior spinal veins and the median posterior spinal vein empty into the radicular veins, which accompany the anterior or posterior spinal roots. These radicular veins drain into the paravertebral and intervertebral plexuses, and then into the azygous and pelvic venous systems.

PHYSIOLOGY OF SPINAL CORD BLOOD FLOW

The regulation of spinal cord blood flow is similar to that of brain blood flow. The spinal cord blood vessels are affected by changes in pO_2 and pCO_2, with hypercapnia increasing spinal cord blood flow in a similar manner as in cerebral blood flow. Autoregulation keeps the regional as well as the total spinal cord blood flow constant. As in the brain, the blood flow requirement and metabolic rate are high in the gray matter.[12] The total cerebral blood flow of the human brain is 50 mL/min/100 g. Spinal cord flow varies, depending on the species and the area of cord studied. In monkeys, total flow in cervical, upper trunk, and lumbar areas is 15, 10, and 20 mL/min/100 g, respectively. The intrinsic blood supply of the cord is directly proportional to the area of gray matter, this being most abundant in the thoracolumbar and cervical segments where the cord enlarges. Consequently, these segments may be more vulnerable to emboli or thrombotic occlusions; in case series of spinal cord infarction these locations are the most commonly involved, with the cervical cord being the second most commonly affected location in up to 25% of patients.[1] The mid-thoracic cord, notably close to the T4 segment, has been commonly described as the most vulnerable to ischemia from hypoperfusion, leading to the description as the "watershed territory",[11] though the exact location has been called into question by some radiological studies.[13,14]

Another important consideration is that the cord is contained within the spinal canal, which has fixed dimensions. Akin to the changes observed with elevated intracranial pressure, a rise in intraspinal canal pressure can cause a lowering of spinal cord blood flow and subsequent ischemia. The parallel of this process is the potential therapeutic benefit of lowering spinal pressure with cerebral spinal fluid drainage to prevent peri-operative spinal cord stroke in aortic surgery.[15]

The blood flow of the spinal cord has a different pattern in the anterior and posterior systems. Flow in the anterior spinal artery is mainly caudal and unidirectional. Infarcts are most likely to be located in the anterior spinal artery distribution.[16] Flow in the posterior spinal arteries is bidirectional, caudal in the cervical and thoracic regions, and rostral in the lumbosacral region.[17]

Pathology of Spinal Cord Infarction

Occlusion of any vessels supplying the spinal cord stemming from a wide range of etiologies may lead to infarction in the cord, while systemic or local hypoperfusion may lead to ischemia in the spinal cord "watershed" territory.[18] The final pathological processes appear to be similar regardless of the etiology (Fig. 31-4).

The cellular events in spinal cord infarction are similar to those seen in cerebral infarction. Depending on the intensity of tissue damage, the infarct can be complete or incomplete. In complete infarction, all cellular elements die rapidly. In incomplete infarction blood vessels and, to a lesser extent, astrocytes are unaffected, while neurons undergo delayed cell death that is likely mediated through apoptosis.[19] An initial

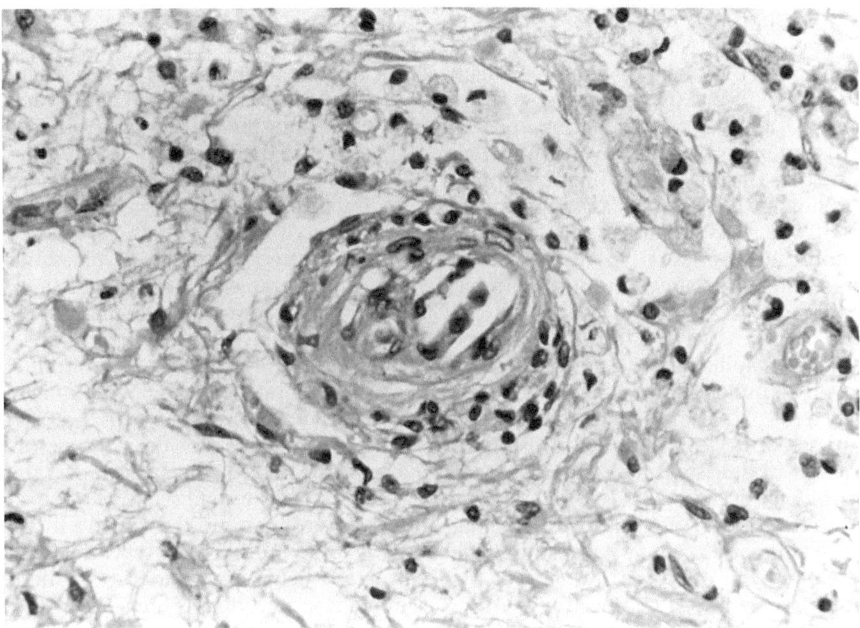

Figure 31-4. Obstruction of a small medullary artery within the spinal cord by atheromatous debris, including cholesterol clefts. The material came from a severely diseased thoracic aorta removed surgically after aneurysmal rupture. Many similar lesions, found at postmortem, caused this patient's total paraplegia at the T8 level.

ischemic and inflammatory cascade is triggered,[20] including n-methyl-D-aspartate-mediated excitotoxic neuronal injury.[21] Microglial cell activation through activation of toll-like receptor 4 mechanisms has been noted in animal models of spinal cord ischemia similar to cerebral ischemic injury models.[22] Subsequent cell death, delayed up to 2 days after the initial ischemic injury, occurs due to apoptic cell death via activation of caspases; this delay after the initial injury may in turn be mediated after the failure of initial endogeneous neuroprotective mechanisms.[23] Post-ischemia activation of inflammatory and apoptosis pathways may further worsen injury to the cord and could be an explanation of delayed-onset paraplegia that can be observed after surgery on the aorta.[19,24] The presence of heat-shock proteins, which can be observed in a range of ischemic injuries, has been noted in cerebro-spinal fluid samples of patients undergoing aortic surgery with subsequent spinal cord stroke.[25] The presence of edema association with spinal cord infarction is mediated in part by varying expression of aquaphorin-4.[26] The pathological changes observed at autopsy in the spinal cord mirror those seen with cerebral infarction.

BOX 31-1 Causes of Spinal Cord Ischemia

SPONTANEOUS ETIOLOGIES

Diseases of the Aorta

Dissection
Coarctation
Atherosclerosis
Thoraco-abdominal aortic aneurysm[100]

Vasculitis

Polyarteritis nodosa[101]
Behçet's[102]
Giant cell arteritis[103,104]

Embolic

Atrial fibrillation
Atrial myxoma[29]
Bacterial endocarditis
Fibrocartilaginous emboli[33]

Infection

Syphilis
Bacterial meningitis[105]
Mucormycosis[106]

Other

Cardiac arrest/systemic hypotension[14]
Cocaine[107,108]
Sickle cell disease[109]
Vertebral dissection[110]

IATROGENIC

Non-Aortic Surgery

Aortography[111]
Spinal anesthesia[47]
Retroperitoneal lymph node dissection[112]
Repair of spinal vascular malformation
Lumbar spine surgery[51]
Epidural steroid injection[50]
Tuberculous spondylodiscitis repair[113]

Aortic Surgery

Repair of aortic dissection
Abdominal aortic aneurysm repair
Repair of coarctation

ETIOLOGY

Infarction of the spinal cord involving the territory supplied by the anterior spinal artery may result from interruption of arterial flow in any vessel from the aorta to the intramedullary vasculature from either local occlusive disease or embolic phenomena; systemic hypoperfusion presents another possible etiology. Several conditions have been identified as leading to spinal cord infarction, with most descriptions originating from single case reports or small series (Box 31-1). In broad terms the etiology can be divided into spontaneous and iatrogenic.

Spontaneous Spinal Cord Ischemia

Syphilitic arteritis was one of the initially described causes of spinal cord infarction, though in contemporary series this is rarely described or seen. In recent series the most common etiologies are related to disease of the aorta, either from atherosclerotic disease, or complications arising from surgical repair in the aorta. In small case series, cardiothoracic surgery is the leading identified cause of spinal cord ischemia, though overall a definite cause is not identified in many cases.[13,16,27] Infarction of the spinal cord secondary to emboli has been described due to many of the same reasons as in cerebral infarction, including atypical etiologies such as bacterial endocarditis,[28] atrial myxoma,[29] and paradoxical embolism secondary to patent foramen ovale or pulmonary arteriovenous malformation.[30] Other rare presentations include upper cervical and brainstem infarction due to vertebral artery dissection with presumed occlusion of the anterior spinal artery,[31] and surfer's myelopathy.[32] Fibrocartilaginous emboli from herniated inter-vertebral discs are also a rare but well-recognized phenomenon causing spinal infarction.[33] The mechanisms of FCE are poorly understood. Proposed mechanisms for fibrocartilaginous emboli include that fragments from herniated nucleus pulposus may be forced in a retrograde manner into the anterior spinal artery segments, or into the venous plexus, though an underlying spinal vascular malformation may also play a role.[34,35] The patient usually experiences sudden onset of back or neck pain, which is followed by spinal cord dysfunction including paraparesis or quadriparesis with urinary emptying dysfunction. The diagnosis is suspected in patients with this clinical syndrome with imaging excluding diseases of the aorta and compressive lesions. The infarction is typically central, with major involvement of the anterior and lateral horns. The etiology had been previously made on post-mortem examination of the spinal cord showing embolic matter that appeared histologically similar to the fibrocartilaginous material in the nucleus pulposus.[36] In more recent case series the cause of spinal cord ischemia is presumed to be fibrocartilaginous emboli based on the lack of available evidence for other causes,[35,37] though evidence on MRI of cord edema with a collapsed intervertebral disc space at the appropriate level without compression of the cord is suggestive.

Primary thrombosis of the anterior spinal artery as a cause of spinal infarction has not been well documented and is considered rare.[38]

Diseases of the Aorta

Thoracic aortic aneurysm is a life-threatening disorder with a lifetime incidence of 10 per 100,000, with dissection and rupture incidence of 3.5 per 100,000 and in-hospital mortality close to 60% in medically managed patients, and 26% in those treated surgically.[39] Neurologic complications of aortic aneurysms occur at different levels of the nervous system in the setting of rupture, and are more likely to occur in the territory of the cerebral vasculature; spinal cord ischemic stroke is present in a small minority of patients before surgery.[40] There are wide reports of neurological symptoms present at the time of a type A aortic dissection (17–40%), though cerebral infarction (10%) seems to be more common than spinal cord infarction (1%).[40,41] Among patients with aortic aneurysms, those with thoracoabdominal dilatations tend to have a higher incidence of spinal cord infarction.[42]

Aortic dissection is characterized by hemorrhage into the tunica media of the aorta, which separates the aortic wall into two layers. The dissection may extend up or down along the media narrowing the lumen, and impairing blood flow. This condition is most commonly associated with arteriosclerosis, in which hypertension and aneurysmal dilatation of the aorta predispose to dissection.[43] Less often, dissecting aortic aneurysms occur in Marfan's syndrome and other collagen vascular disorders. Dissecting aortic aneurysms can produce spinal cord ischemia when an important intercostal or lumbar artery is sheared or occluded at its origin. The dissection may involve one or several of the intercostal and lumbar arteries. The severity of impairment of blood flow determines the extent of spinal infarction. The other factor of importance is whether a large or small tributary artery is affected. In general, the midthoracic to lower thoracic cord is the region most often damaged, because it is supplied by the intercostal arteries that are most frequently affected by aortic dissection.[16] If the artery of Adamkiewicz is involved, the area of maximal damage extends from the T10 to L1 levels. The midthoracic cord (T4 to T6) is also susceptible to injury as it lies in between the blood supply of the upper and lower parts of the cord, thereby representing a probable watershed territory.[11] The upper part of the cervical cord, which is supplied from branches of the vertebral arteries, is rarely involved in aortic dissection. Acute onset of paraplegia or paraparesis with a thoracic sensory level can be a dramatic presentation in dissection of the aorta. Dissection is usually heralded by the sudden onset of severe pain in the chest or back, or in both regions. However, a few cases of spinal cord infarction have been associated with painless dissecting aneurysms.[44] Coarctation of the aorta is a congenital stenosis of the isthmus of the aorta. Coarctation has been divided into two types, infantile and adult. In the infantile type, a small segment of narrowing can occur before, at, or (most commonly) beyond the origin of the left subclavian artery. In the adult type, there is a vast anastomotic circulation between the arteries of the upper trunk and limbs and those beyond the stenosis in the lower trunk and legs. Arteries from the spinal cord form an important part of this anastomosis. In most case series cerebrovascular complications are more common, and occur in those older than age 10.[45]

Systemic Hypoperfusion

A profound and sustained drop in perfusion pressure may lead to an ischemic myelopathy involving primarily the watershed area of the midthoracic cord, with predominant involvement in the gray matter. In an early case series of 14 patients with spinal infarction secondary to hypoperfusion, a sensory level was present in the thoracic region in 13/14. Spinal cord infarction occurred most often in the midthoracic region. In other case series, however, the spinal cord in the lumbosacral region was most commonly involved. All of the lesions in this series were symmetrical and limited to the gray matter.

Iatrogenic Ischemia of the Spinal Cord

In recent case series from the Mayo Clinic of 115 patients over 17 years, 45% of all spinal cord infarcts were perioperative, with close to 70% occurring with surgery on the aorta.[46] Spinal cord ischemia has been associated with a number of other surgical and diagnostic procedures, with a common thread of ligation of a segmental artery. Usual procedures associated with spinal cord infarction include repair of a variety of pathological processes in the aorta, as well as treatment of vascular malformations in the spinal cord. Other unusual iatrogenic causes have been described (see Box 31-1). Cardiac catheterization, aortography, vertebral angiography, and diagnostic spinal cord angiography have also been described.[47–50] Lumbar spine surgery with subsequent thoracic cord ischemia has also been described as a consequence of micro-embolization of disc material,[51] while one group described a case of conus medullaris infarction following lumbar discectomy from an occult dural arterio-venous fistula.[52] The treatment of spinal arterio-venous malformations and dural arterio-venous fistulas[53] has also been associated with spinal cord ischemia, though the actual risk of ischemic injury from the treatment is difficult to establish, as is whether the ischemia represents an arterial or venous thrombosis.

The replacement, by grafts, of segments of the thoracic or abdominal aorta and its transitory clamping are one of the principal and well-characterized causes of iatrogenic spinal cord ischemia. The anterior spinal artery syndrome, the most common neurologic complication after aortic surgery, was first reported in 1962,[54] and in early case series, paraplegia associated with unruptured aortic aneurysm repair was present in 5% of 101 patients who underwent surgery.[55]

Subsequent case series also noted rates of 6% of permanent paraparesis or paraplegia after surgery, though more recent estimates place the risk closer to 3%.[56] Risk factors for the development of ischemic myelopathy include extent of the aneurysm (higher incidence of paraplegia in large ruptured aneurysms with involvement of the entire descending aorta), the presence of previous dissection or prior surgery for an abdominal aortic aneurysm, prior cerebrovascular disease, and duration of clamping (which is longer in complicated operations).[56] In the various case series the mechanism of stroke is hypothesized to be ligation, resection, or embolization of the artery of Adamkiewicz or sustained hypotension during clamping with associated watershed involvement. Other mechanisms of action have been proposed, including increased intrathecal pressure and impairment of spinal blood perfusion during aortic cross-clamping, and obstruction of intraspinal arterioles from showers of atheromatous debris precipitated by the surgical handling of an ulcerated atherosclerotic plaque.

CLINICAL PRESENTATION OF SPINAL CORD INFARCTION

Spinal cord infarction has many similarities to cerebral infarction in that the presentation varies depending on the vascular territory, the size of the lesion, cause, and collateral circulation. If the neurologic manifestations are attributable to a specific spinal cord arterial territory, the diagnosis of a vascular myelopathy is most likely. Motor, sensory, and autonomic signs may be present in spinal cord infarction, but these findings are common to most causes of myelopathy. These findings may include paraparesis, tetraparesis, paraplegia, and loss of sphincter control depending on the level of vascular territory involved. Transient ischemic attacks (TIAs) can theoretically involve the spinal cord. These focal neurologic deficits, which were previously defined by duration of less than 24 hours, rarely precede spinal cord infarctions; it is unclear to what degree the new definition of TIA requiring no imaging evidence of acute infarction will affect the prevalence of TIA.[57] Spinal TIA was reported in one case report of a patient with an AVM, with the underlying mechanism as either steal phenomenon, in which blood is shunted through a low-pressure AVM, or compression of the cord by the vascular malformation;[58] other case reports have described associated polycythemia vera and other hypercoagulable states.[59]

The term *claudication of the cord* was introduced by Dejerine; it was thought to be a result of impaired blood flow.[60] The term refers to transitory symptoms in the legs that are associated with exercise and disappear with rest. Many of the early cases were attributed to syphilitic arteritis of the radicular arteries, though in older series atherosclerosis and pronounced lumbar spondylosis or thoracic disc protrusion were also described.[61]

The initial complaints in spinal claudication are consistent with exercise-induced myelopathy, with symptoms including heaviness in one or both legs, along with pain and occasional sphincter dysfunction which are relieved by rest. Intermittent symptoms have also been described in patients with lumbar spinal cord stenosis. The episodic neurologic dysfunction in lumbar stenosis with involvement in the cauda equina has been attributed to a vascular origin,[62] supported by the frequent association of peripheral arterial disease with lumbar spine disease.[63] A primary vascular etiology has been called into question in contemporary reviews.[64] The condition is more common in males, is characterized by pain, numbness, and paresthesias with exercise and relief with rest. Symptoms begin in the lower back and buttocks and spread down the legs. Neurologic findings in a patient at rest are generally normal, but after exercise, minor motor and sensory disturbances may be found. The syndrome has been associated with spinal stenosis and disc protrusion. Symptoms develop with actions or postures that involve extension of the lumbar spine, and relief occurs when the patient leans forward or sits.[65]

Anterior Spinal Artery Syndrome

The territory supplied by the anterior spinal artery is the most common location of ischemic lesions of the spinal cord. Occlusion of this artery results in infarction of the anterior two-thirds of the spinal cord. Involved structures are the anterior horns of the gray matter, the spinothalamic tracts, and the pyramidal tracts.[66] The clinical syndrome is further defined by the spinal level of where the infarction occurs.

In the cervical spine syndrome there is sudden onset of quadriparesis that may be associated with pain depending on the underlying etiology. Because of spinal shock, the paraplegia may remain flaccid for several days to weeks, with absence of reflexes. Disturbances in the control of bowel and bladder function are common. The sensory loss is marked and involves pain, temperature, and pinprick, below the segmental or dermatomal level of the lesion. Due to sparing of the posterior columns proprioception, light touch, and vibration senses are almost always spared, except in high cervical lesions where there may be involvement of medial lemniscus. This dissociation is more predictive of a vascular etiology of myelopathy, as opposed to compressive syndromes.[67] Motor neuron signs may develop in the upper extremities after the initial period of spinal shock: spasticity of the legs, hyper-reflexia and extensor plantar responses.[38]

Infarction of the spinal cord is most common at the thoracic and upper lumbar levels and manifests as paraparesis or paraplegia (with or without pain) with the arms spared, urinary and rectal incontinence or retention, and a sensory loss to pain and temperature at a specific spinal level. The initial spinal shock gives way to hypertonia, hyper-reflexia, and extensor plantar responses below the level of the lesion.

Occlusion of a central sulcal artery could produce small lesions in half the spinal cord leading to an incomplete Brown-Séquard syndrome. This is a rare phenomenon, attributed to embolic or thrombotic or iatrogenic occlusion of the perforating branches of sulcal arteries.[68,69]

Posterior Spinal Artery Syndrome

Posterior spinal artery infarctions are less common than anterior infarctions and have been noted in single case reports,[70] or as a complication of spine procedures.[71] The lesion mainly involves posterior columns and horns. This syndrome manifests as a suspended pattern of total anesthesia at the affected level. The tendon and cutaneous reflexes for that specific spinal segment are reduced, and vibration and position senses are impaired below the affected level out of proportion to other sensory alterations. Paralysis, if present, is minimal.

Venous Infarction

Venous infarction of the spinal cord is less common than arterial infarction, and most cases are diagnosed postmortem.[72] The most common causes of venous infarction in the spinal cord are vascular malformations of the spinal cord and acute compression by epidural processes such as hematomas and abscess. Venous infarctions can be classified as hemorrhagic or non-hemorrhagic. The hemorrhagic type has a sudden onset, with severe pain in the back and sometimes in the legs and abdomen. Lower-extremity weakness, producing a flaccid paraplegia or quadriplegia, follows. The paralysis may be progressive over hours or days. Sensation is impaired in the legs and may involve the trunk or upper limbs, depending on the extent of the lesion. Bowel and bladder dysfunction invariably occurs.

Venous infarcts tend to be more extensive in longitudinal and cross-sectional areas than anterior cord arterial infarctions. Hemorrhagic venous infarction has also been associated with sepsis and tuberculosis.[73] Non-hemorrhagic infarctions evolve slowly with leg paralysis, sphincter dysfunction, and sensory loss without back pain. Survival time is longer than in hemorrhagic infarction. These types of infarctions are commonly associated with underlying vascular malformations, but at least one report described a complication following sclerotherapy for esophageal varices.[74]

BOX 31-2 Differential Diagnosis of Myelopathy

COMPRESSIVE
- Degenerative spine disease
- Trauma
- Hemorrhage
- Abscess
- Metastases
- Meningioma

INFECTION
- HTLV-1
- HIV
- Varicella zoster
- PML

INFLAMMATORY
- Multiple sclerosis
- Transverse myelitis
- Neuromyelitis optica

NUTRITIONAL DEFICIENCIES
- Vitamin B12
- Copper

OTHER
- Adrenomyeloneuropathy
- Intramedullary spinal cord tumor

DIFFERENTIAL DIAGNOSIS

The differential diagnosis of spinal cord infarction is broad and includes all conditions that can manifest as an acute-incomplete myelopathy or as early Guillain-Barré syndrome. Box 31-2 lists common conditions associated with myelopathy.

DIAGNOSTIC TESTING

Sudden neurologic deficit of spinal cord origin requires immediate investigation. Initial investigations must be designed to rule out a compressive myelopathy due to the potential for therapeutic intervention. The most important diagnostic aid in assessing vascular disease of the cord, or any patient with myelopathy, is MRI (Fig. 31-5). CT scan may show spinal cord swelling or a compressive lesion, but because of its poor spatial discriminations, tends to have limited utility in ischemia; CT myelography may provide more subtle details on intramedullary space-occupying lesions. Hemorrhagic infarctions may be seen on CT.

On MRI, the infarcted cord can have an increased diameter. Infarcts can be first seen on diffusion-weighted imaging (DWI) with high sensitivity within 8 hours of cord infarction.[75–77] Within 1 week after infarction the DWI changes will normalize, while T2 hyperintensity will become more prominent.[75] Once the blood–cord barrier becomes affected, enhancement of the ischemic or infarcted tissue can be seen after administration of gadolinium. In the subacute phase, high-intensity lesions are seen on T2-weighted images. A highly suggestive pattern for ischemia rather than another etiology of T2 hyperintensity in the spinal cord is intervertebral disk and vertebral body infarction in the adjacent level,[78,79] and is particularly suggestive of aortic pathology.[80] Sometimes the infarcts can be better visualized on contrast-enhanced T1-weighted MR images. There are instances of combined cord and cerebellar infarction with bilateral vertebral artery occlusion.[81]

Although MRI is a highly sensitive tool for detecting infarction of the spinal cord, a definitive diagnosis is not always possible, because the presence of other conditions, such as transverse myelitis, intramedullary tumors, and multiple sclerosis, cannot be entirely excluded.

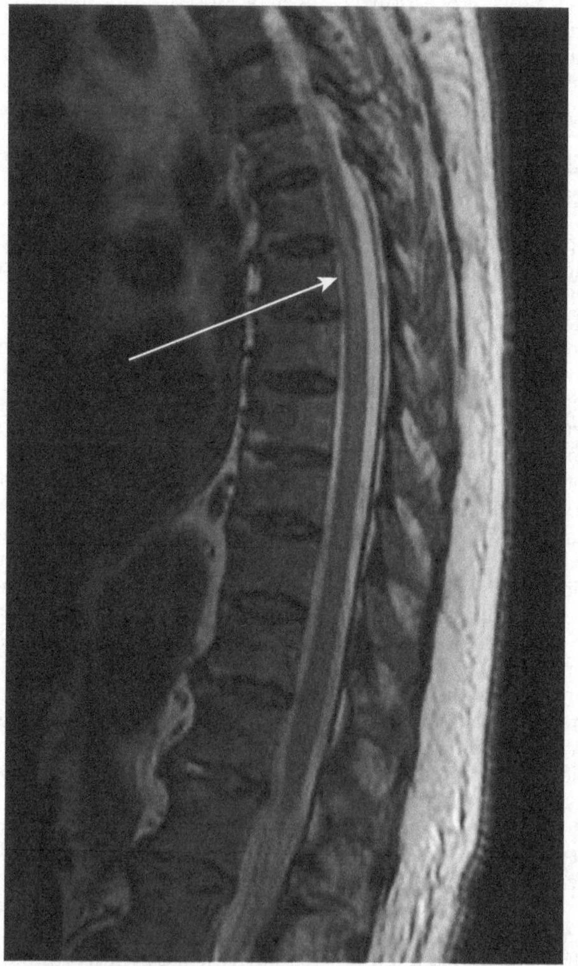

Figure 31-5. MRI of the thoracic spine representing (arrow) spinal cord infarction at the level of T6 after surgical repair of an acutely ruptured thoracic aortic aneurysm. *(From Benavente OR, Barnett HJM: Spinal cord infarction. In Carter LP, Spetzler RF, editors:* Neurovascular surgery, *New York, 1995, McGraw-Hill, p 1229.)*

TREATMENT

No data are available regarding specific therapeutic regimens in patients who have suffered spinal cord infarction. There have been few reported case series of systemic thrombolysis with spinal cord infarction, likely due to the rare nature of the condition and usually associated exclusion criteria (such as aortic dissection). Multiple pharmacological agents have been tested in animal models of spinal cord ischemia, including ketamine, carbamezepine, and inhibitors of the ischemic cascade – none have been tested prospectively yet in humans. One case report points to the successful use of hyperbaric oxygen,[82] but this therapy remains completely unproven to date and has not been successful in cerebral infarction or other spinal cord injury mechanisms.[83] Another case report documented treatment for an iatrogenic spinal cord infarct after coil embolization of the vertebral artery for a cervical spine osseous metastasis. The patient underwent a combination of intravenous and intra-arterial tissue plasminogen activator, hyperbaric oxygen, and hypothermia. The patient made significant clinical improvement after treatment with hyper-baric oxygen, though the proximal vertebral artery had already been recanalized with the thrombolytic agents, and it is difficult to establish which treatment modality helped.[84]

Prevention of spinal cord ischemia during surgical treatment of aortic dissections remains the most active area of research. The development of endovascular procedures for aortic dissection appears to carry a lower risk of spinal cord ischemia in traumatic aortic injury.[85] Preventing prolonged and profound hypotension during aortic surgery is essential for reducing the incidence of perioperative cord ischemia. The use of bypass with distal perfusion remains one of the better studied methods for preventing spinal cord ischemia, while the use of surgical techniques to re-attach ligated spinal arteries may not affect the risk of spinal cord ischemia. The most widely used and studied strategy for preventing post-operative spinal cord ischemia has been CSF shunting with the use of a lumbar drain under the premise that reducing CSF volume will improve spinal cord perfusion pressure. Case series from multiple sites have shown reduced rates of spinal ischemia after the introduction of placing a lumbar drain for CSF drainage in all patients compared to the historical experience before this protocol.[86] The combination of distal perfusion therapy and CSF drainage may be particularly effective in reducing the risk of spinal cord ischemia,[56] and has in some centers virtually eliminated spinal cord ischemia.[87] The mode of CSF drainage remains controversial as excess CSF drainage may be associated with the development of sub-dural hemotomas.[15,88] Lumbar CSF drainage may even be safe in patients receiving extra-corporeal membrane oxygen.[89] The use of spinal somatosensory-evoked potentials during surgery for a thoracoabdominal aneurysm has been shown to be a valuable guide in detecting whether or not the spinal cord is at risk and thereby allowing measures to be taken to prevent cord ischemia.[90] Motor-evoked potentials, with demonstration of the presence of the artery of Adamkiewicz, may also help guide surgical treatment to minimize spinal cord ischemia.[91] In experimental animal models, selective hypothermia has proved to be efficacious in reducing paraplegia after prolonged aortic clamping, and increasingly protocols using spinal fluid cooling after CSF diversion are being used which may be clinically effective.[92]

The combined use of elevating the mean arterial pressure, diverting CSF, and using hypothermia may account for much of the reduction in rates of spinal cord ischemia after surgical repairs.[93]

Correction of underlying pathogenic factors and modification of the usual risk remains important regardless of the underlying etiology. Treatment is supportive, and special attention must be given to bowel and bladder function as well as to skin integrity. Though methylprednisolone reduces the extent of disability after spinal cord trauma[94] and is commonly used with inflammatory conditions, its efficacy in cord ischemia has not been established. Clinicians often use steroids in the acute period if the MRI makes it difficult to distinguish vascular from inflammatory conditions. In selected cases when spinal cord ischemia occurs due to a vascular malformation, surgical options using a combined endovascular and open approach are an option.

PROGNOSIS

The prognosis of spinal cord infarction is variable and depends on the extent of parenchymal damage and the cause. Long-term outcome studies are few and restricted to small case series, though in the largest contemporary study of 115 patients, 42% required a wheelchair and 54% required bladder catherization over a mean follow-up of 3 years.[46] The presence of chronic pain is a common and disabling feature for these patients in the long term,[1] but the greatest morbidity stems from complications arising due to incontinence and immobility. Similar to other causes of myelopathy, preventive strategies are required to prevent urinary tract infections including measuring post-void residuals, implementing intermittent straight catherization protocols, and antibiotics as needed. These patients also require aggressive bowel care, careful monitoring and prevention of deep venous thrombosis, as well as therapy for the prevention of contractures. The most significant predictor of recovery appears to be the severity of the initial impairment, though the initial presence of bladder dysfunction is also important.[95-97] The degree of impairment after spinal cord trauma is defined by the American Spinal Injury Association scoring system, which, along with peripheral artery disease and age, correlates with prognosis in spinal cord stroke.[46] There has also been emerging literature on the long-term risk of other adverse health outcomes after spinal cord trauma, including diabetes and cerebral infarction,[98,99] and it is likely that this is also the case after spinal cord infarction. The underlying etiology of spinal cord infarction in itself is likely to influence the risk of future vascular events, emphasizing the need for surveillance and aggressive preventive interventions.

REFERENCES

1. Masson C, Pruvo JP, Meder JF, et al. Spinal cord infarction: clinical and magnetic resonance imaging findings and short term outcome. J Neurol Neurosurg Psychiatry 2004;75:1431–5.
2. Woollam HM, Millen JW, Blackwood W, et al. Discussion on vascular disease of the spinal cord. Proc R Soc Med 1958;51:540–50.
3. Hughes JT, Brownell B. Spinal cord ischemia due to arteriosclerosis. Arch Neurol 1966;15:189–202.
4. Ferrell AS, Tubbs RS, Acakpo-Satchivi L, et al. Legacy and current understanding of the often-misunderstood Foix-Alajouanine syndrome. Historical vignette. J Neurosurg 2009;111:902–6.
5. Gillilan LA. The arterial blood supply of the human spinal cord. J Comp Neurol 1958;110:75–103.
6. Brockstein B, Johns L, Gewertz BL. Blood supply to the spinal cord: anatomic and physiologic correlations. Ann Vasc Surg 1994;8:394–9.
7. Sliwa JA, Maclean IC. Ischemic myelopathy: a review of spinal vasculature and related clinical syndromes. Arch Phys Med Rehabil 1992;73:365–72.
8. Gillilan LA. Veins of the spinal cord. Anatomic details; suggested clinical applications. Neurology 1970;20:860–8.
9. Lazorthes G, Gouaze A, Zadeh JO, et al. Arterial vascularization of the spinal cord. Recent studies of the anastomotic substitution pathways. J Neurosurg 1971;35:253–62.
10. Backes WH, Nijenhuis RJ, Mess WH, et al. Magnetic resonance angiography of collateral blood supply to spinal cord in thoracic and thoracoabdominal aortic aneurysm patients. J Vasc Surg 2008;48:261–71.
11. Henson RA, Parsons M. Ischaemic lesions of the spinal cord: an illustrated review. Q J Med 1967;36:205–22.
12. Marcus ML, Heistad DD, Ehrhardt JC, et al. Regulation of total and regional spinal cord blood flow. Circ Res 1977;41:128–34.
13. Cheshire WP, Santos CC, Massey EW, et al. Spinal cord infarction: etiology and outcome. Neurology 1996;47:321–30.
14. Duggal N, Lach B. Selective vulnerability of the lumbosacral spinal cord after cardiac arrest and hypotension. Stroke 2002;33:116–21.

15. Estrera AL, Sheinbaum R, Miller CC, et al. Cerebrospinal fluid drainage during thoracic aortic repair: safety and current management. Ann Thorac Surg 2009;88:9–15.
16. Novy J, Carruzzo A, Maeder P, et al. Spinal cord ischemia: clinical and imaging patterns, pathogenesis, and outcomes in 27 patients. Arch Neurol 2006;63:1113–20.
17. Hughes JT. The Pathology of Vascular Disorders of the Spinal Cord. Paraplegia 1965;2:207–13.
18. Imaizumi H, Ujike Y, Asai Y, et al. Spinal cord ischemia after cardiac arrest. J Emerg Med 1994;12:789–93.
19. Kakinohana M, Kida K, Minamishima S, et al. Delayed paraplegia after spinal cord ischemic injury requires caspase-3 activation in mice. Stroke 2011;42:2302–7.
20. Akuzawa S, Kazui T, Shi E, et al. Interleukin-1 receptor antagonist attenuates the severity of spinal cord ischemic injury in rabbits. J Vasc Surg 2008;48:694–700.
21. Jellish WS, Zhang X, Langen KE, et al. Intrathecal magnesium sulfate administration at the time of experimental ischemia improves neurological functioning by reducing acute and delayed loss of motor neurons in the spinal cord. Anesthesiology 2008;108:78–86.
22. Bell MT, Puskas F, Agoston VA, et al. Toll-like receptor 4-dependent microglial activation mediates spinal cord ischemia-reperfusion injury. Circulation 2013;128:S152–6.
23. Sakurai M, Nagata T, Abe K, et al. Survival and death-promoting events after transient spinal cord ischemia in rabbits: induction of Akt and caspase3 in motor neurons. J Thorac Cardiovasc Surg 2003;125:370–7.
24. Smith PD, Puskas F, Meng X, et al. The evolution of chemokine release supports a bimodal mechanism of spinal cord ischemia and reperfusion injury. Circulation 2012;126:S110–17.
25. Hecker JG, Sundram H, Zou S, et al. Heat shock proteins HSP70 and HSP27 in the cerebral spinal fluid of patients undergoing thoracic aneurysm repair correlate with the probability of postoperative paralysis. Cell Stress Chaperones 2008;13:435–46.
26. Xu WB, Gu YT, Wang YF, et al. Bradykinin preconditioning modulates aquaporin-4 expression after spinal cord ischemic injury in rats. Brain Res 2008;1246:11–18.
27. Cheng MY, Lyu RK, Chang YJ, et al. Spinal cord infarction in Chinese patients. Clinical features, risk factors, imaging and prognosis. Cerebrovasc Dis 2008;26:502–8.
28. Greenlee JE, Mandell GL. Neurological manifestations of infective endocarditis: a review. Stroke 1973;4:958–63.
29. Hirose G, Kosoegawa H, Takado M, et al. Spinal cord ischemia and left atrial myxoma. Arch Neurol 1979;36:439.
30. Espinosa PS, Pettigrew LC, Berger JR. Hereditary hemorrhagic telangectasia and spinal cord infarct: case report with a review of the neurological complications of HHT. Clin Neurol Neurosurg 2008;110:484–91.
31. Machnowska M, Moien-Afshari F, Voll C, et al. Partial anterior cervical cord infarction following vertebral artery dissection. Can J Neurol Sci 2008;35:674–7.
32. Chang CW, Donovan DJ, Liem LK, et al. Surfers' myelopathy: a case series of 19 novice surfers with nontraumatic myelopathy. Neurology 2012;79:2171–6.
33. Roshal D, Gutierrez C, Brock D, et al. Pearls & Oy-sters: fibrocartilaginous embolism myelopathy. Neurology 2010;74: e21–3.
34. Srigley JR, Lambert CD, Bilbao JM, et al. Spinal cord infarction secondary to intervertebral disc embolism. Ann Neurol 1981;9: 296–301.
35. Raghavan A, Onikul E, Ryan MM, et al. Anterior spinal cord infarction owing to possible fibrocartilaginous embolism. Pediatr Radiol 2004;34:503–6.
36. Case records of the Massachusetts General Hospital. Weekly clinicopathological exercises. Case 5-1991. A 61-year-old woman with an abrupt onset of paralysis of the legs and impairment of the bladder and bowel function. N Engl J Med 1991;324: 322–32.
37. Han JJ, Massagli TL, Jaffe KM. Fibrocartilaginous embolism – an uncommon cause of spinal cord infarction: a case report and review of the literature. Arch Phys Med Rehabil 2004;85: 153–7.
38. Foo D, Rossier AB. Anterior spinal artery syndrome and its natural history. Paraplegia 1983;21:1–10.
39. Chau KH, Elefteriades JA. Natural history of thoracic aortic aneurysms: size matters, plus moving beyond size. Prog Cardiovasc Dis 2013;56:74–80.
40. Gaul C, Dietrich W, Erbguth FJ. Neurological symptoms in aortic dissection: a challenge for neurologists. Cerebrovasc Dis 2008;26: 1–8.
41. Gaul C, Dietrich W, Friedrich I, et al. Neurological symptoms in type A aortic dissections. Stroke 2007;38:292–7.
42. Lynch DR, Dawson TM, Raps EC, et al. Risk factors for the neurologic complications associated with aortic aneurysms. Arch Neurol 1992;49:284–8.
43. Braunstein H. Pathogenesis of dissecting aneurysm. Circulation 1963;28:1071–80.
44. Gerber O, Heyer EJ, Vieux U. Painless dissections of the aorta presenting as acute neurologic syndromes. Stroke 1986;17: 644–7.
45. Jenkins NP, Ward C. Coarctation of the aorta: natural history and outcome after surgical treatment. QJM 1999;92:365–71.
46. Robertson CE, Brown RD Jr, Wijdicks EF, et al. Recovery after spinal cord infarcts: long-term outcome in 115 patients. Neurology 2012;78:114–21.
47. LaFerlita BW. Postoperative paraplegia coincident with single shot spinal anaesthesia. Anaesth Intensive Care 2007;35: 605–7.
48. Lyders EM, Morris PP. A case of spinal cord infarction following lumbar transforaminal epidural steroid injection: MR imaging and angiographic findings. AJNR Am J Neuroradiol 2009.
49. Glaser SE, Falco F. Paraplegia following a thoracolumbar transforaminal epidural steroid injection. Pain Physician 2005;8: 309–14.
50. Muro K, O'Shaughnessy B, Ganju A. Infarction of the cervical spinal cord following multilevel transforaminal epidural steroid injection: case report and review of the literature. J Spinal Cord Med 2007;30:385–8.
51. Burbank SA, Vaccaro AR, Goins ML, et al. Thoracic paraparesis following an embolic vascular event during lumbar spinal surgery. J Spinal Disord Tech 2006;19:68–72.
52. Stevens EA, Powers AK, Morris PP, et al. Occult dural arteriovenous fistula causing rapidly progressive conus medullaris syndrome and paraplegia after lumbar microdiscectomy. Spine J 2009;9:e8–12.
53. Lee SH, Kim KT, Kim SM, et al. Extensive spinal cord infarction after surgical interruption of thoracolumbar dural arteriovenous fistula presenting with subarachnoid hemorrhage. J Korean Neurosurg Soc 2009;46:60–4.
54. Mehrez IO, Nabseth DC, Hogan EL, et al. Paraplegia following resection of abdominal aortic aneurysm. Ann Surg 1962;156: 890–8.
55. Hollier LH, Symmonds JB, Pairolero PC, et al. Thoracoabdominal aortic aneurysm repair. Analysis of postoperative morbidity. Arch Surg 1988;123:871–5.
56. Estrera AL, Miller CC 3rd, Chen EP, et al. Descending thoracic aortic aneurysm repair: 12-year experience using distal aortic perfusion and cerebrospinal fluid drainage. Ann Thorac Surg 2005;80:1290–6.
57. Easton JD, Saver JL, Albers GW, et al. Definition and evaluation of transient ischemic attack: a scientific statement for healthcare professionals from the American Heart Association/American Stroke Association Stroke Council; Council on Cardiovascular Surgery and Anesthesia; Council on Cardiovascular Radiology and Intervention; Council on Cardiovascular Nursing; and the Interdisciplinary Council on Peripheral Vascular Disease. The American Academy of Neurology affirms the value of this statement as an educational tool for neurologists. Stroke 2009;40: 2276–93.
58. Taylor JR, Van Allen MW. Vascular malformation of the cord with transient ischemic attacks. Case Report. J Neurosurg 1969;31: 576–8.
59. Costa S, Marques J, Barradas A, et al. Transient spinal cord ischemia as presenting manifestation of polycythemia vera. Case Rep Neurol 2011;3:284–8.
60. Zulch KJ, Kurth-Schumacher R. The pathogenesis of "intermittent spinovascular insufficiency" ("spinal claudication of Dejerine") and other vascular syndromes of the spinal cord. Vasc Surg 1970;4:116–36.

61. Bergmark G. Intermittent spinal claudication. Acta Med Scand Suppl 1950;246:30–6.
62. Brish A, Lerner MA, Braham J. Intermittent claudication from compression of cauda equina by a narrowed spinal canal. J Neurosurg 1964;21:207–11.
63. Ain DL, Slovut DP, Kamath R, et al. The association between peripheral artery and lumbar spine disease: a single-center study. Am J Med 2012;125:411–15.
64. Siebert E, Pruss H, Klingebiel R, et al. Lumbar spinal stenosis: syndrome, diagnostics and treatment. Nat Rev Neurol 2009;5: 392–403.
65. Suri P, Rainville J, Kalichman L, et al. Does this older adult with lower extremity pain have the clinical syndrome of lumbar spinal stenosis? JAMA 2010;304:2628–36.
66. Laguna J, Cravioto H. Spinal cord infarction secondary to occlusion of the anterior spinal artery. Arch Neurol 1973;28:134–6.
67. Sandson TA, Friedman JH. Spinal cord infarction. Report of 8 cases and review of the literature. Medicine (Baltimore) 1989;68: 282–92.
68. Fernandez-Torron R, Palma JA, Riverol M, et al. Brown-sequard syndrome after endovascular embolization of vertebral hemangioma. Spinal Cord 2012;50:636–7.
69. Kuga A, Mitani M, Funakawa I, et al. Posterior spinal cord infarction presenting Brown-Sequard syndrome. Rinsho Shinkeigaku 2005;45:730–4.
70. Petruzzellis M, Fraddosio A, Giorelli M, et al. Posterior spinal artery infarct due to patent foramen ovale: a case report. Spine (Phila Pa 1976) 2010;35:E155–8.
71. Hughes JT. Thrombosis of the posterior spinal arteries. A complication of an intrathecal injection of phenol. Neurology 1970; 20:659–64.
72. Hughes JT. Venous infarction of the spinal cord. Neurology 1971;21:794–800.
73. Kim RC, Smith HR, Henbest ML, et al. Nonhemorrhagic venous infarction of the spinal cord. Ann Neurol 1984;15:379–85.
74. Heller SL, Meyer JR, Russell EJ. Spinal cord venous infarction following endoscopic sclerotherapy for esophageal varices. Neurology 1996;47:1081–5.
75. Kuker W, Weller M, Klose U, et al. Diffusion-weighted MRI of spinal cord infarction – high resolution imaging and time course of diffusion abnormality. J Neurol 2004;251:818–24.
76. Loher TJ, Bassetti CL, Lovblad KO, et al. Diffusion-weighted MRI in acute spinal cord ischaemia. Neuroradiology 2003;45: 557–61.
77. Thurnher MM, Bammer R. Diffusion-weighted MR imaging (DWI) in spinal cord ischemia. Neuroradiology 2006;48:795–801.
78. Amoiridis G, Ameridou I, Mavridis M. Intervertebral disk and vertebral body infarction as a confirmatory sign of spinal cord ischemia. Neurology 2004;63:1755.
79. Bornke C, Schmid G, Szymanski S, et al. Vertebral body infarction indicating midthoracic spinal stroke. Spinal Cord 2002;40: 244–7.
80. Cheng MY, Lyu RK, Chang YJ, et al. Concomitant spinal cord and vertebral body infarction is highly associated with aortic pathology: a clinical and magnetic resonance imaging study. J Neurol 2009;256:1418–26.
81. Reich P, Muller-Schunk S, Liebetrau M, et al. Combined cerebellar and bilateral cervical posterior spinal artery stroke demonstrated on MRI. Cerebrovasc Dis 2003;15:143–7.
82. Tofuku K, Koga H, Yamamoto T, et al. Spinal cord infarction following endoscopic variceal ligation. Spinal Cord 2008;46: 241–2.
83. New P. Inappropriate suggestion of benefit from hyperbaric oxygen for spinal cord injury. Spinal Cord 2008;46:824.
84. Lee K, Strozyk D, Rahman C, et al. Acute spinal cord ischemia: treatment with intravenous and intra-arterial thrombolysis, hyperbaric oxygen and hypothermia. Cerebrovasc Dis 2009;29: 95–8.
85. Xenos ES, Abedi NN, Davenport DL, et al. Meta-analysis of endovascular vs open repair for traumatic descending thoracic aortic rupture. J Vasc Surg 2008;48:1343–51.
86. Cina CS, Abouzahr L, Arena GO, et al. Cerebrospinal fluid drainage to prevent paraplegia during thoracic and thoracoabdominal aortic aneurysm surgery: a systematic review and meta-analysis. J Vasc Surg 2004;40:36–44.
87. Hnath JC, Mehta M, Taggert JB, et al. Strategies to improve spinal cord ischemia in endovascular thoracic aortic repair: Outcomes of a prospective cerebrospinal fluid drainage protocol. J Vasc Surg 2008;48:836–40.
88. Wynn MM, Mell MW, Tefera G, et al. Complications of spinal fluid drainage in thoracoabdominal aortic aneurysm repair: a report of 486 patients treated from 1987 to 2008. J Vasc Surg 2009;49:29–34.
89. Cheung AT, Pochettino A, Guvakov DV, et al. Safety of lumbar drains in thoracic aortic operations performed with extracorporeal circulation. Ann Thorac Surg 2003;76:1190–6.
90. Shine TS, Harrison BA, De Ruyter ML, et al. Motor and somatosensory evoked potentials: their role in predicting spinal cord ischemia in patients undergoing thoracoabdominal aortic aneurysm repair with regional lumbar epidural cooling. Anesthesiology 2008;108:580–7.
91. Ogino H, Sasaki H, Minatoya K, et al. Combined use of adamkiewicz artery demonstration and motor-evoked potentials in descending and thoracoabdominal repair. Ann Thorac Surg 2006;82:592–6.
92. Tabayashi K, Motoyoshi N, Saiki Y, et al. Efficacy of perfusion cooling of the epidural space and cerebrospinal fluid drainage during repair of extent I and II thoracoabdominal aneurysm. J Cardiovasc Surg (Torino) 2008;49:749–55.
93. Acher CW, Wynn M. A modern theory of paraplegia in the treatment of aneurysms of the thoracoabdominal aorta: An analysis of technique specific observed/expected ratios for paralysis. J Vasc Surg 2009;49:1117–24.
94. Bracken MB, Shepard MJ, Holford TR, et al. Administration of methylprednisolone for 24 or 48 hours or tirilazad mesylate for 48 hours in the treatment of acute spinal cord injury. Results of the Third National Acute Spinal Cord Injury Randomized Controlled Trial. National Acute Spinal Cord Injury Study. JAMA 1997;277:1597–604.
95. de Seze M, de Seze M, Joseph PA, et al. Functional prognosis of paraplegia due to cord ischemia: a retrospective study of 23 patients. Rev Neurol (Paris) 2003;159:1038–45.
96. Nedeltchev K, Loher TJ, Stepper F, et al. Long-term outcome of acute spinal cord ischemia syndrome. Stroke 2004;35:560–5.
97. Salvador de la Barrera S, Barca-Buyo A, Montoto-Marques A, et al. Spinal cord infarction: prognosis and recovery in a series of 36 patients. Spinal Cord 2001;39:520–5.
98. Cragg JJ, Noonan VK, Krassioukov A, et al. Cardiovascular disease and spinal cord injury: results from a national population health survey. Neurology 2013;81:723–8.
99. Wu JC, Chen YC, Liu L, et al. Increased risk of stroke after spinal cord injury: a nationwide 4-year follow-up cohort study. Neurology 2012;78:1051–7.
100. Ki YJ, Jeon BH, Bang HJ. Spinal cord infarction caused by non-dissected and unruptured thoracoabdominal aortic aneurysm with intraluminal thrombus. Ann Rehabil Med 2012;36:297–302.
101. Ojeda VJ. Polyarteritis nodosa affecting the spinal cord arteries. Aust N Z J Med 1983;13:287–9.
102. Akman-Demir G, Serdaroglu P, Tasci B. Clinical patterns of neurological involvement in Behcet's disease: evaluation of 200 patients. The Neuro-Behcet Study Group. Brain 1999;122: 2171–82.
103. Fruchter O, Ben-Ami H, Schapira D, et al. Giant cell arteritis complicated by spinal cord infarction: a therapeutic dilemma. J Rheumatol 2002;29:1556–8.
104. Galetta SL, Balcer LJ, Lieberman AP, et al. Refractory giant cell arteritis with spinal cord infarction. Neurology 1997;49: 1720–3.
105. Haupt HM, Kurlinski JP, Barnett NK, et al. Infarction of the spinal cord as a complication of pneumococcal meningitis. Case report. J Neurosurg 1981;55:121–3.
106. Giuliani A, Mettimano M, Viviani D, et al. An uncommon case of systemic Mucormycosis associated with spinal cord infarction in a recently diagnosed diabetic. Int J Immunopathol Pharmacol 2010;23:355–8.
107. Di Lazzaro V, Restuccia D, Oliviero A, et al. Ischaemic myelopathy associated with cocaine: clinical, neurophysiological, and neuroradiological features. J Neurol Neurosurg Psychiatry 1997; 63:531–3.

108. Sawaya GR, Kaminski MJ. Spinal cord infarction after cocaine use. South Med J 1990;83:601–2.
109. Sarnaik SA, Lusher JM. Neurological complications of sickle cell anemia. Am J Pediatr Hematol Oncol 1982;4:386–94.
110. Stevinson C, Honan W, Cooke B, et al. Neurological complications of cervical spine manipulation. J R Soc Med 2001;94: 107–10.
111. Killen DA, Foster JH. Spinal cord injury as a complication of aortography. Ann Surg 1960;152:211–30.
112. Leibovitch I, Nash PA, Little JS Jr, et al. Spinal cord ischemia after post-chemotherapy retroperitoneal lymph node dissection for nonseminomatous germ cell cancer. J Urol 1996;155:947–51.
113. Weber P, Vogel T, Bitterling H, et al. Spinal cord infarction after operative stabilisation of the thoracic spine in a patient with tuberculous spondylodiscitis and sickle cell trait. Spine (Phila Pa 1976) 2009;34:E294–7.

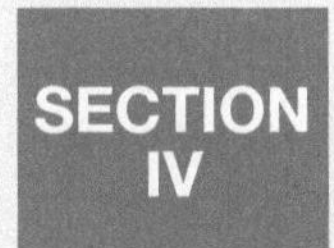

SECTION IV Specific Conditions and Stroke

Scott E. Kasner

For this edition of *Stroke: Pathophysiology, Diagnosis, and Management,* this section has been updated, augmented, and reorganized. The authors provide in-depth reviews of the most prevalent specific causes and conditions related to stroke, including diseases of the heart, arteries, and veins, as well as systemic disorders and exogenous factors. One notable addition is a detailed summary of infectious diseases and stroke. We have also launched two new chapters, one on stroke related to surgery and invasive procedures, and the other on the elusive but rapidly evolving topic of cryptogenic stroke.

There are seemingly innumerable factors that contribute to the pathophysiology of stroke. This section presents the most common and most studied. Ongoing research will inevitably yield new tools for the diagnosis and management of these other disorders, and therefore this section will continue to expand in future editions of this book.

32 Cardiac Diseases

David M. Greer, Shunichi Homma, Karen L. Furie

KEY POINTS

- Stroke due to cardiac embolism is commonly of sudden onset, and more prone to hemorrhagic transformation.
- The etiologic work up for stroke due to a cardiogenic source is crucial in determining appropriate secondary prevention.
- Anticoagulation is the mainstay of therapy for patients with cardioembolic stroke secondary to atrial fibrillation, absent any contraindications.
- Some cardioembolic sources, including infective endocarditis and some intracardiac tumors, present a contraindication to treatment with anticoagulation.

Embolism is the major mechanism of stroke in the United States, accounting for 60% of all ischemic strokes.[1] Up to 25% of these embolic strokes have a readily identifiable specific cardioembolic cause, atrial fibrillation (AF).[1] AF affects 9% of men aged 65 years and older.[2–4] In addition, approximately 25% to 30% of strokes in the young (younger than 45 years) can be attributed to cardiac embolism.[5,6] Table 32-1 estimates the prevalence of various cardiac conditions in embolic ischemia and infarction.[7] The economic toll of stroke in the United States amounts to $39 billion annually in both direct and indirect healthcare costs.[8,9,10]

In comparison with other subtypes of stroke, the prognosis after a cardioembolic stroke is poor.[11] There is up to a 6.5% risk of stroke recurrence within 7 days, and the in-hospital mortality rate is 27.3%.[11] The 5-year mortality rate for cardioembolic stroke has been reported as high as 80%.[11,12]

CLINICAL FEATURES OF CARDIOEMBOLIC TRANSIENT ISCHEMIC ATTACK OR STROKE

Cardioembolism as a cause of stroke can be inferred as the diagnosis and distinguished from other stroke subtypes on the basis of (1) *absence* of a large-artery stenosis or occlusion in the vessel supplying the involved vascular territory, (2) a clinical syndrome or radiographic appearance *inconsistent* with a small-vessel (lacunar) stroke, (3) *absence* of unusual precipitants of stroke (e.g. vasculitis), and (4) *absence* of an atheroma of the aortic arch larger than 4 mm.

Clinical features of cardioembolic stroke are summarized in Box 32-1. The onset of symptoms due to cardioembolism is often sudden, as observed in 25% to 82% of possible cardioembolic strokes, but the rapidity of onset has low specificity, inasmuch as the onset is sudden in 66% of strokes from other mechanisms.[13,14] Sudden onset and loss of consciousness are also insensitive for determining that symptoms are due to embolism.[11,13,15] In 1967, Fisher and Pearlman[16] described "non-sudden" cerebral embolism with stuttering progression, which they attributed to vacillating flow around an embolus lodged in the intracranial circulation. Seizures related to acute stroke are more common in patients with cardiac embolism.[17] There may be fluctuations in symptoms as the embolus lyses and fragments move downstream.[18] In addition, early clinical improvement or recovery may be due either to the recruitment of collateral sources of blood flow or to distal migration of the embolus.

Repetitive stereotyped transient ischemic attacks (TIAs) are unusual in embolic stroke. Less than one-third of patients experience transient ischemic symptoms before the stroke.[13,14,19,20]

The size of the emboli partially determines which vessels are affected. Small emboli can cause retinal ischemia.[21–25] In a balloon catheter model of embolism, the majority of emboli were found to occlude the middle cerebral artery or one of its branches; the next most commonly affected vessel was the basilar artery and its branches, and then the anterior cerebral artery.[26] The size and composition of the embolus vary according to the underlying cardiac disorder (Table 32-2). Valvular lesions may result in the embolization of calcified particles. Atrial myxomas can cause tumor emboli. In nonbacterial thrombotic endocarditis (NBTE), platelets are the main component of the embolic material, whereas emboli from left ventricular aneurysms contain mainly fibrinous material.[27]

Patients at high risk for cardioembolism are more likely to have large infarcts that involve both deep and superficial structures and are frequently visible on initial head CT (Fig. 32-1).[15,20,28,29] Strokes caused by cardioembolism from AF commonly lead to a significant neurologic disability.[30] A pattern of multiple infarctions involving multiple vascular territories is distinctive for cardioembolism.[20,30–32] Cerebral or cerebellar surface branch occlusion by an embolus may lead to focal infarctions causing specific syndromes of focal motor deficits, isolated aphasia, hemiataxia, or hemianopia.[20,33,34] Posterior cerebral artery territory infarcts, in particular, are commonly caused by cardiac embolism.[35,36] Embolic strokes are believed to be more prone to hemorrhagic conversion, a complication detected on follow-up CT in approximately 20% of cardioembolic strokes.[37] Hemorrhagic conversion occurs when there is spontaneous lysis of the thrombus with reperfusion into infarcted tissue.

Between 30% and 60% of patients with ischemic stroke have a possible source of cardiac embolism.[27,38] The detection of a potential cardiac source of embolism depends, to a large extent, on the thoroughness of the evaluation. For example, one study demonstrated that 15% of potential embolic sources were detected only after cardiac monitoring

TABLE 32-1 Cardiac Conditions Strongly Associated with Cerebral Emboli

Source	Percentage of All Cardiogenic Emboli
Non-valvular atrial fibrillation	45
Acute myocardial infarction	15
Ventricular aneurysm	10
Rheumatic heart disease	10
Prosthetic cardiac valve	10
Other	10

TABLE 32-2 Characteristics of Emboli by Source

Source	Type	Size
Atrial fibrillation	Fibrin	Large
Left ventricular thrombus	Fibrin	Large
Myxoma	Myxomatous	Small or large
Infective endocarditis	Septic debris	Small or large
Degenerative valvular disease	Calcium	Small

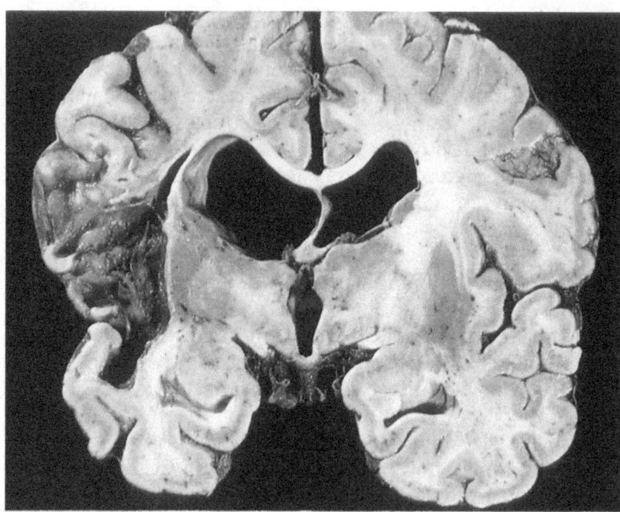

Figure 32-1. Middle cerebral artery (MCA) territory infarction. A complete MCA territory infarction due to stem occlusion is common in embolic stroke. *(From Rosenberg R, editor:* Atlas of clinical neurology, *Philadelphia, 1998, Current Medicine.)*

BOX 32-1 Clinical Characteristics of Cardioembolic Stroke

CLINICAL FEATURES

Neurologic history and findings
Sudden onset
Isolated focal deficit
Seizure at onset
Loss of consciousness at onset
Peak of deficit at onset
Involvement of more than one vascular territory
Evidence of systemic embolization

NEUROIMAGING FINDINGS

Multiple infarcts in more than one vascular territory
Deep and superficial infarctions
Hemorrhagic conversion
Absence of large-artery stenosis or occlusion in parent vessels
Rapid recanalization of intracranial vessels on transcranial Doppler ultrasonography

and 2D transthoracic echocardiography.[39] In addition, ascribing a stroke to a definite cardioembolic cause can be difficult because of a coexistent mechanism involving a potential noncardiac source of embolus (e.g., large-vessel atherosclerosis in approximately 30% of cases).[20,27,40–43]

DIAGNOSTIC STUDIES

A thorough cardiac assessment of patients with stroke is necessary for accurate diagnosis of the mechanism of cerebral ischemia and to help establish prognosis. A standard 12-lead electrocardiogram (ECG) can identify patients who are in sustained AF and can detect acute myocardial ischemia; however, a 24- to 48-hour cardiac monitor is essential to detect paroxysmal AF, and the result is not always positive despite numerous such studies in the same patient.[40] More extended cardiac monitoring may be more sensitive to the detection of AF, and in a patient in whom the index of suspicion is high, this testing should be considered.[44–47] A clinical history of angina pectoris or abnormal electrocardiography findings (e.g., anterior wall myocardial infarction [MI], left ventricular hypertrophy, or inverted T waves) has associated hazard ratios of 1.6 to 3.2 for nonfatal MI or cardiac death in patients with TIA or minor stroke.[48]

Transthoracic echocardiography (TTE) is an essential part of the embolic evaluation. M-mode and 2D echocardiography can define the cardiac chambers, valves, and left ventricular function. The use of agitated saline allows for detection of an intracardiac shunt, such as a patent foramen ovale (PFO). The proper detection of a shunt with this procedure requires an adequate Valsalva maneuver, with crossing of the bubbles from the right atrium to the left atrium seen upon release of the Valsalva maneuver after two to four cardiac cycles. The more delayed appearance of bubbles is suggestive of a pulmonary source of shunting, such as a pulmonary arteriovenous malformation (AVM). TTE may be insensitive for masses and thrombi in the left atrium and upon the mitral valve, requiring further studies.[49,50]

Transesophageal echocardiography (TEE) is more sensitive than TTE in detecting abnormalities in the left atrium and appendage, atrial septum, mitral valve, and aortic arch.[51–53] The cost-effectiveness of performing TEE in all patients with stroke remains controversial.[54,55] This evaluation is recommended for patients with a suspected embolic stroke in whom cardiac monitoring and TTE findings are unremarkable and in young patients without a clear other cause of stroke. It may be less sensitive for the detection of a PFO with agitated saline, as patients who are sedated for the procedure are less able to perform an adequate Valsalva maneuver.

Embolus detection by *transcranial Doppler* (TCD) ultrasonography can be used to identify microemboli due to a variety of potential cardiac sources (AF, infectious endocarditis, cardiomyopathy, aortic stenosis, mitral stenosis, and PFO).[56] The frequency of high-intensity transient signals (HITS) did not appear to vary according to echocardiographic diagnosis in one study, but another demonstrated a higher rate (33%) of microembolization in patients with high-risk sources of embolism (e.g., prosthetic valves) compared with patients with other, lower-risk cardiac conditions (e.g., AF [15%]).[56,57]

APPROACH TO MANAGEMENT

Box 32-2 summarizes potential cardiac conditions according to the strength of indication for anticoagulation for stroke prevention. Although the early period after stroke appears to be the highest risk period for recurrent embolization, it is also

BOX 32-2 Classification of Cardioembolic Cerebral Ischemic Events

DEFINITE CARDIOEMBOLISM

Antithrombotic therapy considered the standard of practice
- Left ventricular thrombus
- Left atrial thrombus
- Recent transmural anterior myocardial infarction
- Rheumatic valvular disease
- Mechanical prosthetic valve
- Atrial fibrillation

Antithrombotic therapy may be of value
- Nonbacterial thrombotic endocarditis

Antithrombotic therapy contraindicated
- Bacterial endocarditis
- Atrial myxoma

POSSIBLE CARDIOEMBOLISM

- Mitral annular calcification
- Mitral valve prolapse
- Cardiomyopathy
- Patent foramen ovale
- Atrial flutter
- Sick sinus syndrome
- Valve strands
- Left atrial spontaneous echo contrast seen on transesophageal echocardiogram

the period of greater risk of hemorrhagic conversion. One study examining the utility of immediate anticoagulation for a stroke due to any presumed mechanism but occurring in a patient with AF did not demonstrate a benefit of anticoagulation in the first 2 weeks.[58] However, in patients at higher risk for embolism, such as those with mechanical prosthetic valves or left ventricular thrombi, immediate anticoagulation should be considered.[59]

For long-term prevention of stroke, AF is the only condition for which anticoagulation has been conclusively shown to be superior to aspirin.[59] Still, anticoagulation is often used in situations with the potential for recurrent embolization. In the Warfarin Aspirin Recurrent Stroke Study (WARSS), warfarin was weakly (absolute risk reduction, 9%) superior to aspirin therapy in patients in whom an embolic stroke was suspected but there was no evidence of a definite cardiac source; this difference was not statistically significant, however.[60]

SPECIFIC CARDIAC CONDITIONS CAUSING CEREBRAL EMBOLISM

The numerous structural and functional cardiac conditions associated with transient cerebral symptoms and infarction are described here in greater detail (see Table 32-1). Although cardiac testing can reveal a potential source, the clinician must determine whether the symptoms, physical findings, and results of neuroimaging support the causal relationship.

Structural Cardiac Defects

Cardiomyopathy

In patients with cardiomyopathy, the reported annual stroke rates (1.3% to 3.5% per year) that were derived from cardiac trials likely underestimate the actual risk of stroke.[7,61-65] The risk of stroke is inversely related to the ejection fraction (EF), with as much as a 58% increase in thromboembolic events for every 10% decrease in EF, but not to the functional classification (New York Heart Association [NYHA] Functional Class).[64,66] There is a fourfold risk of stroke in patients who are 50 to 59 years old and have congestive heart failure.[4,67] The annual rate of stroke in patients with nonischemic dilated cardiomyopathy is approximately 1.5% to 3.5%.[62,68] In patients with cardiomyopathy, AF is often a complicating factor that further raises the risk of stroke. Other factors include decreased apical flow and a possible intracardiac hypercoagulable state. Patients with CHF have been found to have increased sympathetic activity, which may lead to increased platelet activation as well as increased levels of β-thyroid-binding globulin, D dimer, von Willebrand factor, fibrinopeptide A, thrombin-antithrombin complexes, β-thromboglobulin, and P-selectin; they also have impaired vascular endothelial function, which impairs the release of nitric oxide, further contributing to platelet adhesion. In the Survival and Ventricular Enlargement (SAVE) study, patients with EF values of 29% to 35% (mean 32%) had a stroke rate of 0.8% per year; the rate in patients with EF values of ≤28% (mean 23%) was 2.5% per year.[64] The Warfarin and Antiplatelet Therapy in Chronic Heart Failure (WATCH) trial was a prospective, three-arm randomized trial comparing warfarin (international normalized ration [INR] goal 2.0 to 3.0), aspirin (162 mg/day), and clopidogrel (75 mg/day) in patients with an EF ≤35% and NYHA class II to IV. The study was stopped early at 1587 patients after poor enrollment rates and without showing a significant difference between the treatment arms, although there was a suggestion of a benefit for warfarin in reducing nonfatal stroke compared to aspirin (0.7% vs. 2.1%; $P = 0.06$) as a secondary endpoint.[69] Compared with placebo, warfarin has been shown to significantly reduce the relative risk of stroke by 40% to 55% in patients with ischemic and non-ischemic cardiomyopathy.[70,71] However, the Sixty Plus Reinfarction Study failed to show a significant risk reduction in stroke using an INR value as high as 2.7 to 4.5.[72] In the Warfarin versus Aspirin in Reduced Cardiac Ejection Fraction (WARCEF) trial,[73] patients with a reduced left ventricular ejection fraction (≤35%) without atrial fibrillation were randomized to receive warfarin adjusted to an INR of 2.0–3.5 vs aspirin 325 mg daily. The composite outcome of ischemic stroke, intracerebral hemorrhage or death from any cause was not different between the groups. Ischemic strokes were significantly reduced with the use of warfarin (0.72 vs 1.36 events per 100 patient-years, warfarin compared to aspirin), but the rate of major hemorrhage was significantly increased with warfarin (1.78 vs 0.87 events per 100 patient-years). Interestingly, the rates of intracerebral and intracranial hemorrhage did not differ between the groups.

Acute Myocardial Infarction

Within 2 to 4 weeks of acute MI, 2.5% of patients suffer a stroke.[74,75] Stroke is more common with an anterior wall MI (4% to 12% of cases) than with an inferior wall MI (1%) and usually occurs within the first 2 weeks.[74,75] Left ventricular thrombi develop in up to 40% of patients with an anterior wall MI, usually in those first 2 weeks, and can be detected with TTE.[74-76] However, there have been reports of development of a left ventricular thrombus as a late complication of anterior wall MI, and patients with low EF due to MI have a cumulative stroke risk of 8.1% after 5 years.[64,77] Clinicians commonly choose to administer anticoagulation immediately and then maintain it for at least 3 to 6 months in patients in whom a left ventricular thrombus is detected. The thrombus may resolve with anticoagulant therapy or may persist for several months. Intravenous recombinant tissue plasminogen activator (t-PA) has been used safely in patients with acute ischemic stroke and left ventricular thrombus.[78] After MI, warfarin alone (INR 2.8–4.2) or warfarin (INR 2.0–3.0) in combination with

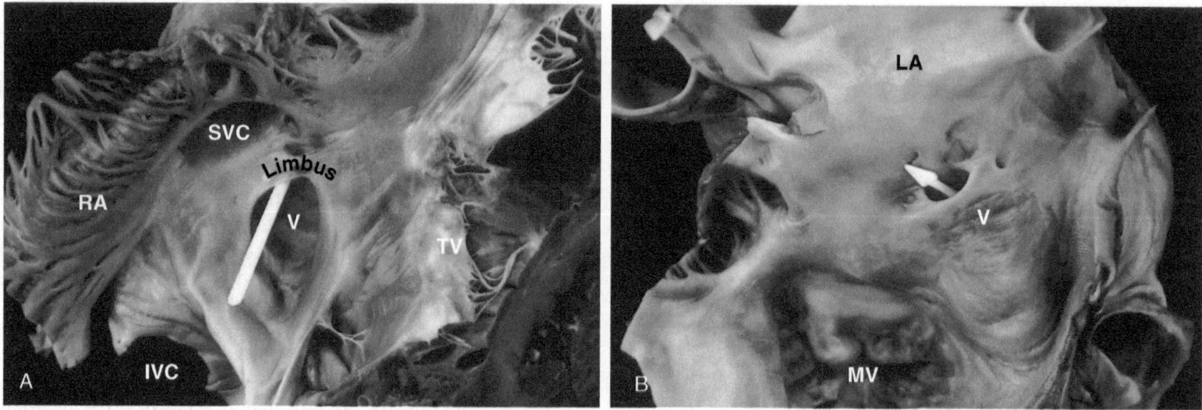

Figure 32-2. Patent foramen ovale, shown in autopsy specimen. A, Right atrial (RA) view shows a probe in the foramen ovale, between limbus and valve (V) of fossa ovalis. B, Left atrial (LA) view shows the probe exiting through the ostium secundum, the prominent fenestration in the valve. Normally, when left atrial pressure exceeds right atrial pressure, the valve of the fossa ovalis is impressed against the limbus and closes the foramen ovale. IVC, inferior vena cava; MV, mitral valve; SVC, superior vena cava; TV, tricuspid valve. *(From Hagen PT, Scholz DG, Edwards WD: Incidence and size of patent foramen ovale during the first 10 decades of life: An autopsy study of 965 normal hearts.* Mayo Clin Proc *59:17, 1984.)*

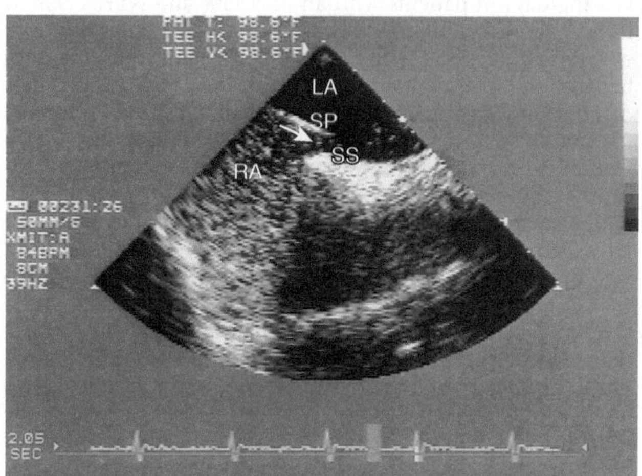

Figure 32-3. Vertical transesophageal echocardiographic view of fossa ovalis area demonstrating the passage of microbubbles through the patent foramen ovale (*arrow*) from right atrium (RA) into left atrium (LA). Separation of septum primum (SP) from septum secundum (SS) is clearly visualized. *(From Homma S, DiTullio MR, Sacco RL: Patent foramen ovale and ischemic stroke. In Barnett HJM, et al, editors:* Stroke: Pathophysiology, diagnosis, and management, *ed 3, New York, 1998, Churchill Livingstone.)*

aspirin at 75 mg daily resulted in fewer reinfarctions, thromboembolic events, and deaths compared with aspirin (162 mg day) alone. However, the warfarin-treated patients had a fourfold higher risk of major hemorrhage.[79]

Patent Foramen Ovale

Paradoxic embolism, or crossing of a venous thrombus into the arterial system, can occur in a patient with a PFO (Fig. 32-2).[80] The resultant right-to-left shunt may appear only in the setting of elevated right heart pressures, as occurs with a Valsalva maneuver or with pulmonary hypertension (Fig. 32-3). PFO is common in the general population (20% to 25%),[81] so care should be taken to establish a causal relationship of PFO with cerebral ischemic symptoms before PFO-specific treatment is initiated for secondary prevention of stroke.[80,82]

Thrombus is believed to emanate from either a leg or pelvic vein. The latter should not be overlooked in the search for venous thrombus in the patient with a PFO and cerebral ischemic symptoms.[83,84] In addition, there is conjecture that microthrombi can form within the PFO itself, particularly when there is a coexistent atrial septal aneurysm.[85]

In the French PFO Study,[86] the risk of recurrent stroke after 4 years of follow-up was 2.3% in patients with PFO alone (95%CI, 0.3%–4.3%), 15.2% among patients with both patent foramen ovale and atrial septal aneurysm (95%CI, 1.8%–28.6%), and 4.2% in patients with neither (95%CI, 1.8%–6.6%). These investigators found no recurrent strokes in patients with atrial septal aneurysms alone. The principal author continues to emphasize uncertainties in risk factors and management.[87] A later report described a high prevalence of PFO in older patients with cryptogenic stroke, but methodologic issues obscure the significance of the findings.[88]

Larger defects with a higher degree of shunting, as measured by the number of microbubbles crossing into the left atrium, have been associated with cryptogenic embolism.[89,90] Whether the mean diameter of a PFO affects the risk of embolism remains unsettled.[91,92,93] In the PFO in the Cryptogenic Stroke Study, there was no difference in rates of recurrent stroke or death between those with PFO (14.8%) and those without (15.4%) in the entire population or the subset with a cryptogenic mechanism (14.3% versus 12.7%). Neither PFO size nor the association of an atrial septal aneurysm increased the risk of stroke or death. These patients were randomized as part of the Warfarin Aspirin Recurrent Stroke Study (WARSS) to receive either aspirin (325 mg daily) or warfarin (INR 1.4 to 2.8) for 2 years. Treatment did not affect time to primary endpoints in patients with PFO.[94]

TEE with color Doppler may be more sensitive than TTE with use of a contrast agent in detecting a PFO.[95] However, TTE is risk-free, and positive findings may eliminate the need for additional invasive testing.[96] TEE measurement of PFO size may be more accurate than the traditionally used contrast agent technique.[97] Patients with cerebral ischemic symptoms and a PFO should undergo noninvasive studies of the legs to rule out deep vein thrombosis, and a pelvic vein MR venogram (MRV) or CT venogram (CTV) should be considered.[96]

Optimal treatment for stroke prevention in this context is unclear. Clinical trial data argue against anticoagulation but have not been definitive. Transcatheter closure of PFO is available and observational data have suggested a benefit but also raised concerns for safety,[98] including device-related thrombosis, delayed-onset atrial fibrillation,[99] and cardiac erosions.[100,101–105,106,107] Uncertainty about the need for closure led to a call for further clinical trials comparing best medical therapy with closure.[108] The PC Trial in 2013 randomized patients with cryptogenic embolic events and PFO to closure with the Amplatzer PFO Occluder device vs best medical therapy.[109] The mean duration of follow up was 4.1 years, and there was no statistical difference in the rates of recurrent embolic events or death. The RESPECT trial in 2013 randomized 980 patients with cryptogenic stroke and PFO to closure vs medical therapy (antiplatelet agents, 74.8%, or warfarin 25.2%).[110] The primary intention-to-treat analysis showed no statistical difference between the groups, but per-protocol and as-treated analyses suggested superiority of closure over medical therapy. The CLOSURE 1 Trial in 2012 randomized 909 patients in an open-label trial of closure vs. medical therapy for patients ages 18–60 with cryptogenic stroke or TIA with a PFO.[111] Again, patients did not have a statistical benefit of closure over medical therapy, and in patients who did have a recurrent neurological event, a cause other than paradoxical embolism was often found.

Intracardiac Tumors

An embolic event occurs in up to 3% to 50% of patients with atrial myxoma. Atrial myxoma is the most common primary cardiac tumor, but is found in only 75 out of 1 million autopsies.[112–114] Papillary fibroelastoma is another embologenic tumor that is less common. Multiple events have been reported, some separated in time by months to years. The friability of the tumor lends itself to embolism of tumor fragments and/or superimposed thrombus (Fig. 32-4).[115,116] Cardiac tumors can be detected on TTE or TEE. The treatment is surgical resection.

Spontaneous Echo Contrast

Spontaneous echo contrast (SEC), a marker of disordered flow and hemostatic activation in the left atrium, is often seen on TEE in patients with AF.[54,117,118] SEC is associated with a higher risk of thromboembolism in mitral valve disorders.[119,120] Numerous studies have established an association between SEC and intracardiac thrombus formation, but SEC has not been established as an independent risk factor for embolic stroke.[119–122]

Mitral Valve Strands

Lambl's excrescences, or mitral valve strands, are filamentous processes on the ventricular surface of the aortic valve or the atrial surface of the mitral valve; they are detectable on TEE. Histologically, the strands are composed of endothelialized connective tissue. One study found that mitral valve strands were more common in patients with a history of recent cerebral ischemic events (6.3%) than in control subjects who had neither (0.3%). In young patients in whom cardioembolic stroke was suspected, 16% were found to have mitral valve strands, often without another identifiable cardiac source.[123] Other retrospective studies have shown that mitral valve strands are found more commonly in younger patients and in patients with a recent embolic event (10.6% to 53%) than in patients referred because of findings on TEE performed for other reasons (2.3% to 15%).[124–126]

Dysrhythmias

Atrial Fibrillation

Thrombi in AF arise from the left atrium and atrial appendage. The combination of rheumatic heart disease (RHD) and AF carries a stroke risk 17 times that of normal controls (who have neither AF nor RHD).[3] Of all the mechanisms of cardioembolic stroke, AF has been the most extensively studied.[127–132] It is the most common cause of embolic stroke, accounting for 25% to 30% of all embolic strokes.[7] The incidence of AF-related stroke rises with age.[3,4] Younger patients with AF who are free of cardiac disease, diabetes, and hypertension have an extremely low rate of stroke (1.3% per 15 years).[127,133] Beginning at age 65 years, however, the annual risk of stroke is 3% to 5% per year; the risk increases to 10% per year or higher by age 80, with women predominating.[4] The age-related risk is independent of other major risk factors (diabetes, hypertension, previous stroke, and congestive heart failure).[127] Multiple grading schemes are available for quantifying the risk of stroke in patients with non-valvular atrial fibrillation. These consistently find a prior stroke or TIA to be the highest risk for another event, but otherwise may give variable rates of prediction based on other risk factors.[134]

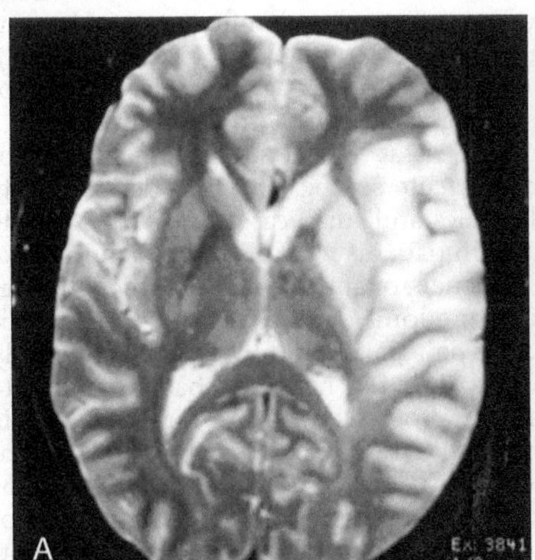

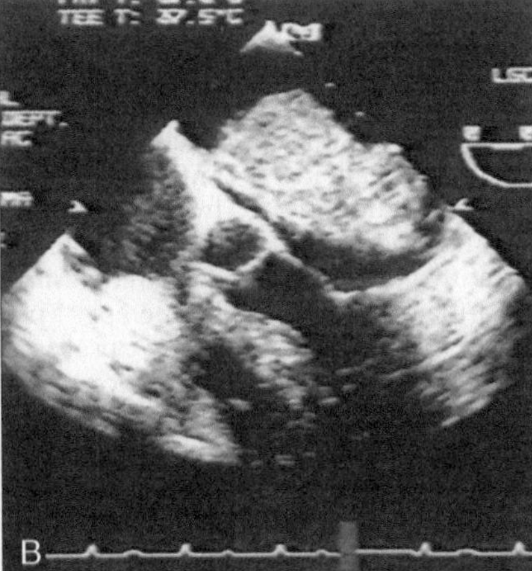

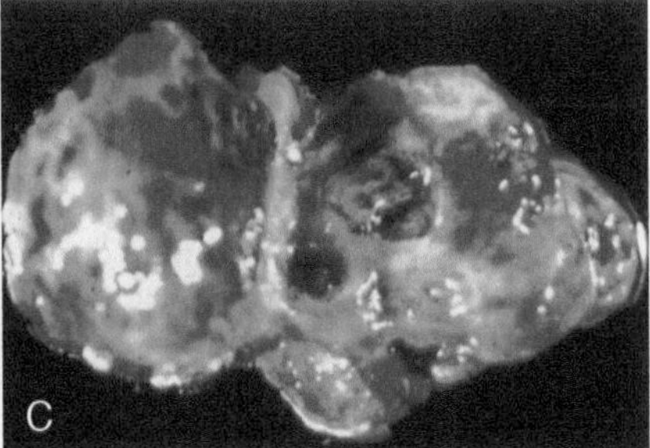

Figure 32-4. A, T2-weighted MR image of the brain in a patient with left middle cerebral artery territory infarction due to atrial myxoma embolization. B, Echocardiogram showing a large atrial myxoma above the mitral valve during systole. C, Pathologic specimen showing a gelatinous atrial myxoma with numerous cysts. *(From Rosenberg R, editor:* Atlas of clinical neurology, *Philadelphia, 1998, Current Medicine.)*

The aforementioned randomized primary and secondary prevention trials have demonstrated the efficacy and safety of warfarin in preventing AF-related stroke.[127–132,135] Pooled data from these trials demonstrated a 68% reduction in ischemic stroke (95%CI, 50%–79%) and an intracerebral hemorrhage rate of less than 1% per year. The data for aspirin suggest a much more modest effect. One European study randomly assigned patients with stroke or TIA with AF to aspirin (300 mg daily) vs placebo, and found a non-significant 16% relative risk reduction.[132] The Stroke Prevention in Atrial Fibrillation (SPAF) III study suggested that patients with low-risk AF (without prior stroke/TIA, hypertension, low EF, or advanced age and female sex) may be treated as safely with aspirin as with warfarin, the rates of thromboembolism being similar.[135]

Newer antithrombotic agents have been developed recently, and offer an alternative therapy to warfarin. The RE-LY study randomized 18,133 patients with AF and an additional risk factor for stroke to warfarin (goal INR 2.0–3.0, unblinded) vs the direct thrombin inhibitor, Dabigatran, at two separate blinded doses, 110 mg twice daily and 150 mg twice daily.[136] Both doses were found to be non-inferior to warfarin in preventing stroke or systemic embolism, and the 150 mg twice daily dose was superior to warfarin, without an increase in major bleeding. The ARISTOTLE study evaluated the direct factor Xa inhibitor, apixaban vs warfarin in 18,201 AF patients, and achieved both non-inferiority and superior for stroke or systemic embolism, with a reduction in intracerebral hemorrhage by 49%.[137] The ROCKET AF study evaluated 14,264 AF patients with the direct factor Xa inhibitor rivaroxaban vs warfarin, also achieving non-inferiority for stroke or systemic embolism, with lower rates of intracerebral hemorrhage and fatal bleeding.[138] The ENGAGE-AF study randomized 21,105 AF patients to high- or low- dose once-daily edoxaban, another factor Xa inhibitor, or warfarin, and showed edoxaban to be non-inferior in preventing stroke or systemic embolism, with lower risks of major bleeding.[139] The direct thrombin inhibitors and the Xa inhibitors are predominantly renally metabolized, and are not readily reversed in the setting of hemorrhagic events.

The combination of aspirin and clopidogrel has been evaluated in the atrial fibrillation population. The Atrial Fibrillation Clopidogrel Trial with Irbesartan for Prevention of Vascular Events (ACTIVE W) randomly divided patients with AF and at least one stroke risk factor to receive either warfarin or the combination of aspirin (75–100 mg daily) and clopidogrel (75 mg daily). The trial was terminated early because of a lack of comparative efficacy in preventing embolic events in the aspirin plus clopidogrel arm, even though the agents caused equivalent rates of hemorrhage (INR goal, 2–3).[140] Among patients with AF who cannot take warfarin, the combination of aspirin and clopidogrel was not found to be superior to aspirin alone.[141] The ACTIVE A study found, in patients with AF who could not take warfarin and who were randomly assigned to either the combination of aspirin and clopidogrel or aspirin alone, ischemic events were significantly prevented, but at a cost of relatively the same number of major hemorrhagic events.[142] In contrast, the factor Xa inhibitor apixaban was compared to aspirin in the AVERROES trial which enrolled 5600 patients with AF who were deemed unsuitable for warfarin or other vitamin K antagonist therapy. Apixaban was associated with a remarkable 54% relative risk reduction compared to aspirin, without excess bleeding.[143]

Oral anticoagulation for secondary stroke prevention in patients with AF is associated with a small but definite risk of hemorrhage, particularly intracerebral hemorrhage, which is more common in elderly patients (>75 years).[127] Despite the increased risk of intracerebral hemorrhage in patients aged older than 85, there continues to be a benefit of anticoagulation for AF, and care should be taken to ensure that these patients' INR values stay within the target range, as higher values significantly increase the risk.[144]

Independent risk factors associated with a higher risk of stroke include age older than 65, previous history of stroke or TIA, hypertension, and diabetes mellitus. Impaired left ventricular function was identified as an additional risk factor in the SPAF study population. In a pooled analysis of seven separate studies conducted by the SPAF study investigators, AF with a prior stroke or TIA carried the strongest risk for future stroke, an estimated rate of 6% to 9% per year.[145] Despite these findings, only 30% to 60% of patients with AF receive appropriate anticoagulation therapy.[146] Long-term oral anticoagulation is recommended for patients with AF and a recent stroke or TIA.[147]

An alternative approach in the future may include complete isolation of the left atrial appendage, perhaps obviating the need for anticoagulation. Because the vast majority (estimated at 90%) of thrombi in AF form in the left atrial appendage, mechanical isolation of this compartment is an attractive theoretical approach. The PROTECT AF (Watchman Left Atrial Appendage System for Embolic Protection in Patients with Atrial Fibrillation) Trial randomized 707 patients with nonvalvular AF to left atrial appendage closure vs warfarin, and found non-inferiority of the device implantation to warfarin.[148] In patients who are unable to be anticoagulated, this approach may be particularly attractive.

TTE findings can also be factored into risk stratification. Moderate-to-severe impairment of left ventricular function is associated with a 2.5-fold greater risk of stroke. A left atrial antero-posterior diameter greater than 2.5 cm/m^2 was also found to be a predictor of cerebral embolism. In the SPAF study, 26% of patients had no clinical risk factors and normal TTE findings. These patients had a low risk of stroke (<1% per year). Approximately one-third of patients considered at low risk according to clinical criteria are reclassified as having a high risk on the basis of echocardiographic findings.[149–152]

TEE has greater sensitivity for detecting abnormalities in the left atrium. SEC, reduced left atrial appendage emptying, and left atrial thrombi are markers of higher stroke risk. In addition, TEE is better able to visualize aortic plaque.[153,154] In patients with high-risk clinical factors, the presence of any left atrial abnormality or an aortic arch atheroma larger than 4 mm on TEE was found to raise the risk of stroke by as much as 20% per year.[155]

The use of anticoagulation for acute cardioembolic stroke due to AF is controversial. There is a significant risk of hemorrhagic conversion of the acute infarction (1.7% to 4.4%), particularly with larger strokes.[156–159] Conversely, the risk of recurrent embolism ranges from 0.1% to 1.3% in the first 2 weeks.[58,160,161] There are meager data supporting the use of anticoagulation in the acute setting, and they derive mostly from non-blinded studies and small case series.[162,163] A study of immediate therapy in patients with AF and ischemic stroke appeared to show no benefit of anticoagulation over antiplatelet therapy;[58] patients randomly assigned within 30 hours of stroke onset to receive dalteparin (100 IU/kg subcutaneously [SC] twice daily) or aspirin (160 mg daily) had a higher rate of stroke recurrence or progression, death, or symptomatic intracerebral hemorrhage (24.6% vs 16.9%; $P = 0.048$) and of extracerebral hemorrhages (5.8% vs 1.8%; $P = 0.028$). Major limitations of this study were that a significant proportion of the strokes in this study were characterized as lacunar, suggesting that the mechanism of stroke may not have been cardioembolic, and higher-risk patients may not have been enrolled in this trial, as it was left to the treating physicians' discretion.

Sick Sinus Syndrome

Sick sinus syndrome (SSS), also referred to as tachycardia-bradycardia syndrome, is more common in older patients and is often attributed to ischemia, degeneration, or neuromuscular disease. Patients may experience atrial flutter and AF as part of this syndrome.[164] SSS has been associated with a higher risk of stroke; systemic embolism occurs in 16% of patients with SSS, in comparison with only 1.9% of patients with complete heart block.[165,166] The treatment of choice is surgical insertion of an atrial on-demand pacemaker.[167] Antithrombotic therapy has not been directly compared with antiplatelet therapy in this population, although clearly, in patients with paroxysmal AF, warfarin is recommended. An atrial pacemaker, of course, does not prevent the occurrence of AF, and thus antithrombotic therapy is still warranted.

Atrial Flutter

Atrial flutter is an unstable rhythm that belies underlying atrial disease and commonly degenerates into AF. In a study examining a large Medicare database, the stroke risk in patients with atrial flutter (relative risk [RR], 1.41) was determined to be higher than in a control group but lower than in patients with AF (RR, 1.64). Patients with atrial flutter who subsequently experienced an episode of AF had a higher risk of stroke (RR, 1.56) than patients with atrial flutter who never had a subsequent episode of AF (RR, 1.11).[168] Left atrial appendage velocities are similar in patients with AF and patients with AF-flutter (an intermediate form with elements of both AF and atrial flutter); thus, the risk of left atrial thrombus formation should be comparable in the two conditions.[169]

Largely because of the risk of intermittent AF in patients with atrial flutter, it is appropriate to consider anticoagulation in patients who present with atrial flutter and coexistent cardiac disease that predisposes to left atrial thrombi.[160]

Valvular Disease

Mitral Annular Calcification

Mitral annular calcification (MAC) has been associated with a higher risk of ischemic stroke.[170–172] This disorder is associated with aging, ischemic heart disease, and cardiac arrhythmias. Because patients with MAC are also at risk of stroke by other mechanisms, it is unclear whether there is a causal relationship (i.e., that thrombus calcific debris embolizes from the degenerated valve) or merely whether mitral annulus calcification is a marker of systemic atherosclerosis and intrinsic cardiac dysfunction.

Prosthetic Valves

The rate of embolism in patients with mechanical prosthetic valves who are receiving anticoagulation approximates that of patients with bioprosthetic valves who are not, approximately 3% to 4% annually for mitral valves and 1.3% to 3.2% for aortic valves.[173–175] It is recommended that patients with bioprosthetic valves undergo anticoagulation either for the first 3 months or on a long-term basis if there is evidence of AF, a left atrial thrombus, or previous emboli.[176] Adding aspirin to warfarin therapy in patients with mechanical valves and high-risk bioprosthetic valves is superior to warfarin alone in reducing rates of vascular mortality and systemic embolism (1.9% per year versus 8.5% per year, respectively) without a significant increase in major bleeding complications.[177] Current data do not support the use of newer anticoagulants in patients with prosthetic valves.

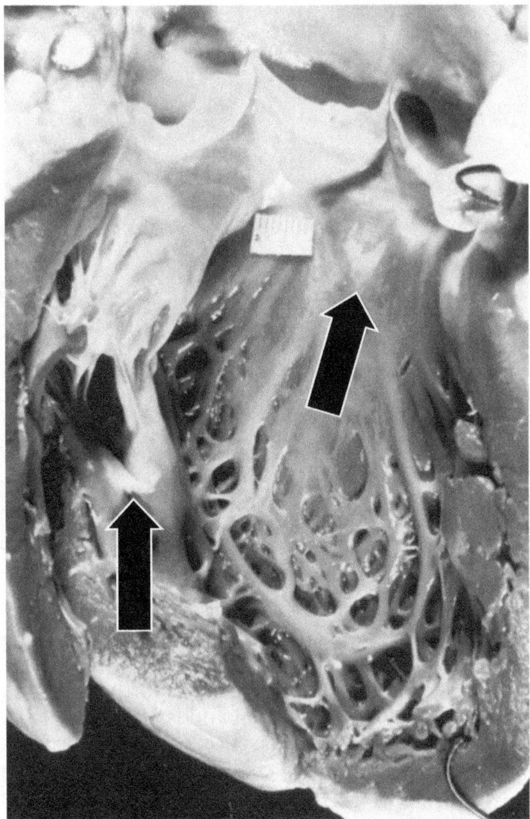

Figure 32-5. Pathologic specimen showing mitral stenosis resulting from rheumatic heart disease with "jet lesions" (*arrows*) on the wall of the left ventricle. *(From Hinchey JA, Furlan AJ, Barnett HJM: Cardiogenic brain embolism: Incidence, varieties, and treatment. In Barnett HJM, editors:* Stroke: Pathophysiology, diagnosis, and management, *ed 3, New York, Churchill Livingstone, 1998.)*

Mitral Stenosis

Mitral stenosis, often related to rheumatic heart disease, is associated with left atrial thrombi in 15% to 17% of cases in autopsy series, and 'jet' lesions may appear in the left ventricle (Fig. 32-5).[178,179] The annual rate of stroke is approximately 2% in patients with mitral stenosis, and recurrent embolism is common. Warfarin should be considered when there is a strong suspicion of coexistent AF.[180]

Infective Endocarditis

Stroke occurs in 15% to 20% of patients with infective endocarditis, usually within the first 48 hours (Fig. 32-6). Appropriate antibiotic therapy dramatically reduces the risk of stroke, and late embolism occurs in less than 5% of cases.[180,181] An elevated erythrocyte sedimentation rate in the setting of cerebral ischemic symptoms and fever or a new heart murmur should trigger a diagnostic evaluation, including serial blood cultures, a transthoracic echocardiogram, and, if a high level of suspicion remains, TEE. Neurologic complications of infective endocarditis, including ischemic and hemorrhagic infarctions, toxic encephalopathy, arteritis, meningitis, and subarachnoid hemorrhage, contribute to the high mortality rate (15% to 20%) associated with this condition despite antibiotic therapy.[182,183] Infective endocarditis can be complicated by mycotic aneurysms, which can rupture, causing subarachnoid hemorrhage. Mycotic aneurysms can be differentiated from berry aneurysms on the basis of their location in the distal cerebral vasculature (third or fourth branches from the

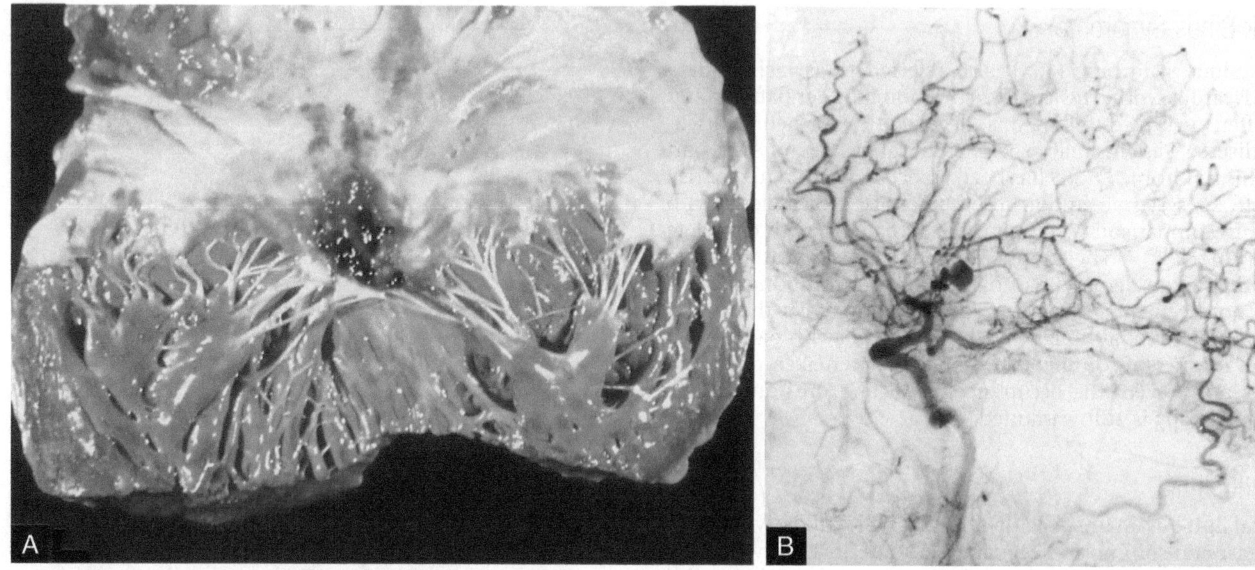

Figure 32-6. A, Pathologic specimen showing a large hemorrhagic vegetation. B, Left common carotid angiogram showing an aneurysm of a proximal branch of the left middle cerebral artery. *(From Rosenberg R, editor:* Atlas of clinical neurology, *Philadelphia, 1998, Current Medicine.)*

circle of Willis). When subarachnoid hemorrhage occurs in this setting, it is typically superficial and is not generally complicated by vasospasm. The presence of strokes or hemorrhages, even if small, poses a challenge in this population, because definitive therapy often requires surgical valve replacement. This procedure requires large doses of anticoagulation, so it should be delayed if possible in the acute setting to let the lesions heal. It is commonly recommended to wait a minimum of 2 weeks after an ischemic or hemorrhagic cerebral event and longer if possible (4 to 6 weeks), although no strong prospective studies have evaluated the most appropriate waiting periods.

The most common organisms causing native valve endocarditis are streptococci, staphylococci, and enterococci. More rarely, other species of bacteria, fungi, spirochetes, and rickettsiae can infect valves.[184] Echocardiography has not been shown to be useful in predicting risk of embolism, and early antibiotic therapy is still the mainstay of treatment.[182,185] The risk of subarachnoid hemorrhage is considered by many authorities to represent a contraindication to the use of anticoagulation in infectious endocarditis. Noninvasive MR angiography or CT angiography have largely replaced conventional angiography in screening for mycotic aneurysms.[186]

Nonbacterial Thrombotic Endocarditis

Also known as marantic endocarditis, NBTE is associated with malignancy, often in combination with Trousseau's syndrome (Fig. 32-7).[187] The clinical manifestation may be one of focal deficits referable to one or more vascular territories, or a nonfocal encephalopathy.[188] NBTE should be suspected in all cases of stroke in patients with an underlying malignancy, and is best diagnosed with echocardiography, either TEE or TTE.[187] Some clinicians recommend anticoagulation to prevent recurrent embolism, especially in a patient with a coexistent hypercoagulable state; however, the efficacy of anticoagulation in this setting has not been proven.

Libman-Sacks endocarditis represents an atypical form of NBTE associated with systemic lupus erythematosus.[189–191] It is often associated with an antiphospholipid antibody-mediated systemic hypercoagulable state. There are no proven treatment strategies for Libman-Sacks endocarditis and the antiphospholipid antibody syndrome.[190] Although anticoagulation is often used, particularly in patients with transient ischemic symptoms or stroke, the target INR range is debated.

Other Valvular Disorders

Mitral regurgitation is associated with a higher risk of stroke, largely because of coexistent AF in many cases.[192,193] *Aortic stenosis* can also cause stroke, mainly through embolization of calcific material.[194] One case-control study demonstrated that *mitral valve prolapse* is considerably less common among young patients with stroke or transient ischemic symptoms than previously reported.[195]

Cardiac Procedures

Coronary Artery Bypass Surgery-Related Embolism

Approximately 3% to 6% of patients undergoing coronary artery bypass grafting or valve replacement surgery experience a perioperative stroke.[196,197] The mechanism of stroke may be cardioembolism, low flow (distal field or watershed hypotensive ischemia), or artery-to-artery emboli from the aortic arch.[198] Most delayed strokes are due to postoperative AF, particularly in the setting of low EF.[196,199] Clinical factors such as age more than 75 years, recent MI or unstable angina, history of previous stroke, carotid artery disease, hypertension, diabetes, previous coronary artery surgery, postoperative AF, low EF, and history of pulmonary or renal insufficiency are associated with a higher risk of stroke.[196,200,201] Diffusion-weighted MRI is more sensitive than CT for visualizing these acute infarcts, which are often multiple and may manifest as encephalopathy.[202] There appears to be a posterior circulation predominance to the pattern of infarction after coronary artery bypass grafting.[203]

Cardiac Catheterization

Cardiac catheterization can result in ischemic stroke, usually embolic. The embolus may occur secondary to an artery-to-artery cause from the disruption of atherosclerotic plaque in the aorta or due to cardiac injury during the procedure. The risk of stroke has been found to be significantly associated with the severity of coronary artery disease (OR, 1.96) and the duration of fluoroscopy (OR, 1.65). Diffusion-weighted MRI

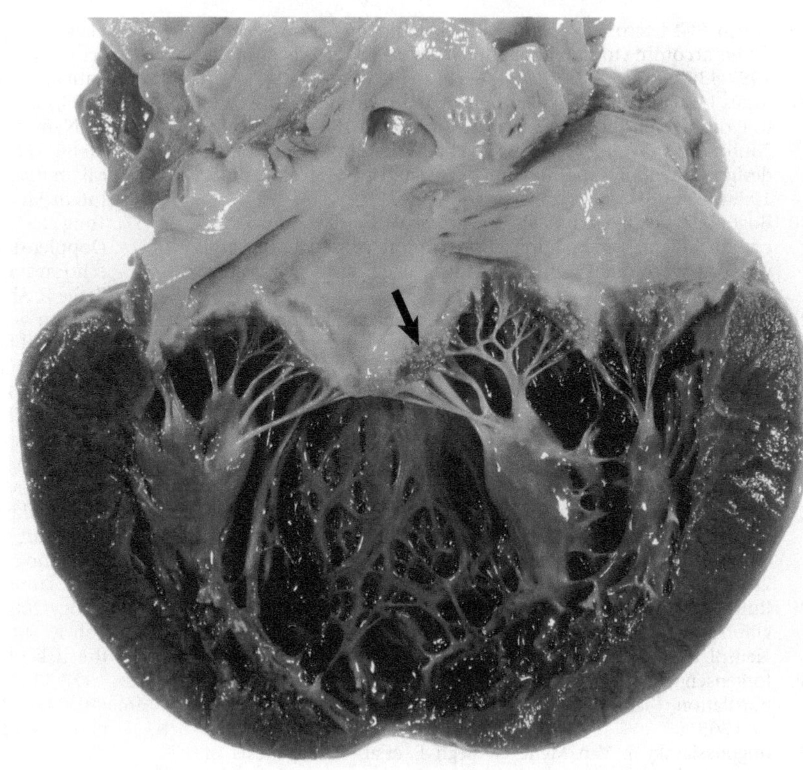

Figure 32-7. Mitral valve vegetations of nonbacterial thrombotic endocarditis (*arrow*). *(From Rogers LR, Cho ES, Kempin S, Posner JB: Cerebral infarction from nonbacterial thrombotic endocarditis: Clinical and pathological study including the effects of anticoagulation.* Am J Med *83:746, 1987.)*

was shown to be sensitive for detecting multiple silent infarcts and small-vessel infarcts.[204] Hypertension, age more than 60 years, peripheral vascular disease, emergency performance of the procedure and angioplasty raise the risk of catheterization-related thromboembolic complications.[205]

Cardiac Embolism and the Hemostatic System

Atrial fibrillation, a model for embolic stroke, has been linked to alterations in the hemostatic system.[206–210] Local hemostatic factors in the endocardium are likely responsible for the development of left atrial thrombi.[211] As in other vascular beds, the regulation of this signaling is under genetic control, although a variety of external stimuli modulate the expression. In patients with AF, the level of prothrombin fragment F1+2, a byproduct of the conversion of prothrombin to thrombin and thus a measure of thrombin generation, increases with age in parallel with the rate of stroke.[212] The overwhelming majority of patients experience a dramatic reduction in stroke risk with warfarin, which correlates well with a reduction in the level of activity of the hemostatic system. In addition, aspirin has little effect on F1+2, corresponding to its relative lack of efficacy in stroke prevention in patients with AF. Other studies have confirmed that levels of prothrombotic factors are increased in AF (factor VIII, fibrinogen, thrombin-antithrombin complex), as are levels of those involved in fibrinolysis (tissue plasminogen activator, D dimer).[206–210,213] Von Willebrand factor levels are a marker of endothelial damage associated with AF as well.[209,210] Platelet activation has been shown to play a role in AF. Elevations in platelet factor 4, β-thromboglobulin, and P-selectin have been demonstrated in patients with AF.[206,209] This increased hemostatic activity is not unique to AF and suggests a common mechanism of stroke among other cardiac conditions associated with risk of embolism – left ventricular aneurysm,[214] mitral stenosis,[215] and heart failure.[216]

Therefore, it appears that aberrant flow in the heart secondary to structural disease may result in endothelial disruption, triggering local thrombus formation. The stability of the thrombus is mediated by the integrity of fibrin cross-linking. The genetic control regulating the interaction between the endothelium and the coagulation system may, in part, explain why some high-risk patients remain free of embolic events. These genetic influences may also be at play in cases of high-risk patients who experience emboli while undergoing therapeutic anticoagulation. The interaction between the endocardial surface and the coagulation system requires additional study.

The complete reference list can be found on the companion Expert Consult website at www.expertconsult.inkling.com.

KEY REFERENCES

1. Sacco RL, Ellenberg JH, Mohr JP, et al. Infarcts of undetermined cause: the NINCDS Stroke Data Bank. Ann Neurol 1989; 25:382–90.
3. Wolf PA, Dawber TR, Thomas HE Jr, et al. Epidemiologic assessment of chronic atrial fibrillation and risk of stroke: the Framingham study. Neurology 1978;28:973–7.
4. Wolf PA, Abbott RD, Kannel WB. Atrial fibrillation: a major contributor to stroke in the elderly. The Framingham Study. Arch Intern Med 1987;147:1561–4.
5. Kittner SJ, Stern BJ, Wozniak M, et al. Cerebral infarction in young adults: the Baltimore-Washington Cooperative Young Stroke Study. Neurology 1998;50:890–4.
7. Cerebral Embolism Task Force. Cardiogenic brain embolism. Arch Neurol 1986;43:71–84.
9. Lloyd-Jones D, Adams RJ, Brown TM, et al. Heart disease and stroke statistics – 2009 update: a report from the American Heart Association Statistics Committee and Stroke Statistics Subcommittee. Circulation 2009;119:e21–181.
10. Go AS, Mozaffarian D, Roger VL, et al. Heart disease and stroke statistics – 2013 update: a report from the American Heart Association. Circulation 2013;127:e6–245.
12. Petty GW, Brown RD Jr, Whisnant JP, et al. Ischemic stroke subtypes : a population-based study of functional outcome, survival, and recurrence. Stroke 2000;31:1062–8.
14. Caplan LR, Hier DB, D'Cruz I. Cerebral embolism in the Michael Reese Stroke Registry. Stroke 1983;14:530–6.

15. Timsit SG, Sacco RL, Mohr JP, et al. Brain infarction severity differs according to cardiac or arterial embolic source. Neurology 1993;43:728–33.
17. Kraus JA, Berlit P. Cerebral embolism and epileptic seizures-the role of the embolic source. Acta Neurol Scand 1998;97:154–9.
19. Foulkes MA, Wolf PA, Price TR, et al. The Stroke Data Bank: design, methods, and baseline characteristics. Stroke 1988; 19:547–54.
20. Bogousslavsky J, Cachin C, Regli F, et al. Cardiac sources of embolism and cerebral infarction-clinical consequences and vascular concomitants: the Lausanne Stroke Registry. Neurology 1991;41:855–9.
23. Hankey GJ, Slattery JM, Warlow CP. Prognosis and prognostic factors of retinal infarction: a prospective cohort study. BMJ 1991;302:499–504.
25. Murkin JM. Etiology and incidence of brain dysfunction after cardiac surgery. J Cardiothorac Vasc Anesth 1999;13:12–17, discussion 36–7.
27. The second report of the Cerebral Embolism Task Force. Cardiogenic brain embolism. Arch Neurol 1989;46:727–43.
28. Kittner SJ, Sharkness CM, Sloan MA, et al. Features on initial computed tomography scan of infarcts with a cardiac source of embolism in the NINDS Stroke Data Bank. Stroke 1992; 23:1748–51.
29. Ringelstein EB, Koschorke S, Holling A, et al. Computed tomographic patterns of proven embolic brain infarctions. Ann Neurol 1989;26:759–65.
30. Jorgensen HS, Nakayama H, Reith J, et al. Acute stroke with atrial fibrillation. The Copenhagen Stroke Study. Stroke 1996; 27:1765–9.
32. Bogousslavsky J, Van Melle G, Regli F, et al. Pathogenesis of anterior circulation stroke in patients with nonvalvular atrial fibrillation: the Lausanne Stroke Registry. Neurology 1990; 40:1046–50.
33. Horowitz DR, Tuhrim S. Stroke mechanisms and clinical presentation in large subcortical infarctions. Neurology 1997;49: 1538–41.
34. Bogousslavsky J, Van Melle G, Regli F. Middle cerebral artery pial territory infarcts: a study of the Lausanne Stroke Registry. Ann Neurol 1989;25:555–60.
35. Yamamoto Y, Georgiadis AL, Chang HM, et al. Posterior cerebral artery territory infarcts in the New England Medical Center Posterior Circulation Registry. Arch Neurol 1999;56:824–32.
38. Mast H, Thompson JL, Voller H, et al. Cardiac sources of embolism in patients with pial artery infarcts and lacunar lesions. Stroke 1994;25:776–81.
39. Rem JA, Hachinski VC, Boughner DR, et al. Value of cardiac monitoring and echocardiography in TIA and stroke patients. Stroke 1985;16:950–6.
41. Tayal AH, Tian M, Kelly KM, et al. Atrial fibrillation detected by mobile cardiac outpatient telemetry in cryptogenic TIA or stroke. Neurology 2008;71:1696–701.
43. Moncayo J, Devuyst G, Van Melle G, et al. Coexisting causes of ischemic stroke. Arch Neurol 2000;57:1139–44.
45. Bogousslavsky J, Regli F, Maeder P, et al. The etiology of posterior circulation infarcts: a prospective study using magnetic resonance imaging and magnetic resonance angiography. Neurology 1993;43:1528–33.
46. Seet RC, Friedman PA, Rabinstein AA. Prolonged rhythm monitoring for the detection of occult paroxysmal atrial fibrillation in ischemic stroke of unknown cause. Circulation 2011;124: 477–86.
47. Higgins P, MacFarlane PW, Dawson J, et al. Noninvasive cardiac event monitoring to detect atrial fibrillation after ischemic stroke: a randomized, controlled trial. Stroke 2013;44: 2525–31.
48. Pop GA, Koudstaal PJ, Meeder HJ, et al. Predictive value of clinical history and electrocardiogram in patients with transient ischemic attack or minor ischemic stroke for subsequent cardiac and cerebral ischemic events. The Dutch TIA Trial Study Group. Arch Neurol 1994;51:333–41.
51. Pop G, Sutherland GR, Koudstaal PJ, et al. Transesophageal echocardiography in the detection of intracardiac embolic sources in patients with transient ischemic attacks. Stroke 1990;21:560–5.
52. Hata JS, Ayres RW, Biller J, et al. Impact of transesophageal echocardiography on the anticoagulation management of patients admitted with focal cerebral ischemia. Am J Cardiol 1993;72:707–10.
54. McNamara RL, Lima JA, Whelton PK, et al. Echocardiographic identification of cardiovascular sources of emboli to guide clinical management of stroke: a cost-effectiveness analysis. Ann Intern Med 1997;127:775–87.
57. Tong DC, Bolger A, Albers GW. Incidence of transcranial Doppler-detected cerebral microemboli in patients referred for echocardiography. Stroke 1994;25:2138–41.
58. Berge E, Abdelnoor M, Nakstad PH, et al. Low molecular-weight heparin versus aspirin in patients with acute ischaemic stroke and atrial fibrillation: a double-blind randomised study. HAEST Study Group. Heparin in Acute Embolic Stroke Trial. Lancet 2000;355:1205–10.
60. Mohr JP, Thompson JL, Lazar RM, et al. A comparison of warfarin and aspirin for the prevention of recurrent ischemic stroke. N Engl J Med 2001;345:1444–51.
61. Katz SD, Marantz PR, Biasucci L, et al. Low incidence of stroke in ambulatory patients with heart failure: a prospective study. Am Heart J 1993;126:141–6.
63. Pullicino PM, Halperin JL, Thompson JL. Stroke in patients with heart failure and reduced left ventricular ejection fraction. Neurology 2000;54:288–94.
64. Loh E, Sutton MS, Wun CC, et al. Ventricular dysfunction and the risk of stroke after myocardial infarction. N Engl J Med 1997;336:251–7.
66. Dries DL, Rosenberg YD, Waclawiw MA, et al. Ejection fraction and risk of thromboembolic events in patients with systolic dysfunction and sinus rhythm: evidence for gender differences in the studies of left ventricular dysfunction trials. J Am Coll Cardiol 1997;29:1074–80.
67. Kannel WB, Wolf PA, Verter J. Manifestations of coronary disease predisposing to stroke. The Framingham study. JAMA 1983; 250:2942–6.
69. Massie BM, Collins JF, Ammon SE, et al. Randomized trial of warfarin, aspirin, and clopidogrel in patients with chronic heart failure: the Warfarin and Antiplatelet Therapy in Chronic Heart Failure (WATCH). Trial Circulation 2009;119:1616–24.
70. Anticoagulants in the Secondary Prevention of Events in Coronary Thrombosis (ASPECT) Research Group. Effect of long-term oral anticoagulant treatment on mortality and cardiovascular morbidity after myocardial infarction. Lancet 1994; 343:499–503.
72. Sixty Plus Reinfarction Study Research Group. A double-blind trial to assess long-term oral anticoagulant therapy in elderly patients after myocardial infarction. Report of the Sixty Plus Reinfarction Study Research Group. Lancet 1980;2:989–94.
73. Homma S, Thompson JL, Pullicino PM, et al. Warfarin and aspirin in patients with heart failure and sinus rhythm. N Engl J Med 2012;366:1859–69.
76. Asinger RW, Mikell FL, Elsperger J, et al. Incidence of left-ventricular thrombosis after acute transmural myocardial infarction. Serial evaluation by two-dimensional echocardiography. N Engl J Med 1981;305:297–302.
77. Stratton JR, Resnick AD. Increased embolic risk in patients with left ventricular thrombi. Circulation 1987;75:1004–11.
78. Derex L, Nighoghossian N, Perinetti M, et al. Thrombolytic therapy in acute ischemic stroke patients with cardiac thrombus. Neurology 2001;57:2122–5.
79. Hurlen M, Abdelnoor M, Smith P, et al. Warfarin, aspirin, or both after myocardial infarction. N Engl J Med 2002; 347:969–74.
80. Sacco RL, Homma S, Di Tullio MR. Patent foramen ovale: a new risk factor for ischemic stroke. Heart Dis Stroke 1993; 2:235–41.
81. Lechat P, Mas JL, Lascault G, et al. Prevalence of patent foramen ovale in patients with stroke. N Engl J Med 1988;318: 1148–52.
82. Di Tullio M, Sacco RL, Gopal A, et al. Patent foramen ovale as a risk factor for cryptogenic stroke. Ann Intern Med 1992; 117:461–5.
83. Cramer SC, Rordorf G, Maki JH, et al. Increased pelvic vein thrombi in cryptogenic stroke: results of the Paradoxical Emboli

from Large Veins in Ischemic Stroke (PELVIS) study. Stroke 2004;35:46–50.
85. Hanna JP, Sun JP, Furlan AJ, et al. Patent foramen ovale and brain infarct. Echocardiographic predictors, recurrence, and prevention. Stroke 1994;25:782–6.
86. Mas JL, Arquizan C, Lamy C, et al. Recurrent cerebrovascular events associated with patent foramen ovale, atrial septal aneurysm, or both. N Engl J Med 2001;345:1740–6.
88. Handke M, Harloff A, Olschewski M, et al. Patent foramen ovale and cryptogenic stroke in older patients. N Engl J Med 2007;357:2262–8.
89. Steiner MM, Di Tullio MR, Rundek T, et al. Patent foramen ovale size and embolic brain imaging findings among patients with ischemic stroke. Stroke 1998;29:944–8.
90. Homma S, Di Tullio MR, Sacco RL, et al. Characteristics of patent foramen ovale associated with cryptogenic stroke. A biplane transesophageal echocardiographic study. Stroke 1994; 25:582–6.
92. Kutty S, Brown K, Qureshi AM, et al. Maximal potential patent foramen diameter does not correlate with the type or frequency of the neurologic event prior to closure. Cardiology 2009; 113:111–15.
93. Serena J, Marti-Fàbregas J, Santamarina E, et al. Recurrent stroke and massive right-to-left shunt: results from the prospective Spanish multicenter (CODICIA) study. Stroke 2008;39:3131–6.
94. Homma S, Sacco RL, Di Tullio MR, et al. Effect of medical treatment in stroke patients with patent foramen ovale: patent foramen ovale in Cryptogenic Stroke Study. Circulation 2002; 105:2625–31.
96. Lethen H, Flachskampf FA, Schneider R, et al. Frequency of deep vein thrombosis in patients with patent foramen ovale and ischemic stroke or transient ischemic attack. Am J Cardiol 1997;80:1066–9.
97. Schuchlenz HW, Weihs W, Beitzke A, et al. Transesophageal echocardiography for quantifying size of patent foramen ovale in patients with cryptogenic cerebrovascular events. Stroke 2002;33:293–6.
98. Mohr JP, Homma S. Patent cardiac foramen ovale: stroke risk and closure. Ann Intern Med 2003;139:787–8.
100. Hung J, Landzberg MJ, Jenkins KJ, et al. Closure of patent foramen ovale for paradoxical emboli: intermediate-term risk of recurrent neurological events following transcatheter device placement. J Am Coll Cardiol 2000;35:1311–16.
101. Buscheck F, Sievert H, Kleber F, et al. Patent foramen ovale using the Premere device: the results of the CLOSEUP trial. J Interv Cardiol 2006;19:328–33.
102. Mullen MJ, Hildick-Smith D, De Giovanni JV, et al. BioSTAR Evaluation STudy (BEST): a prospective, multicenter, phase I clinical trial to evaluate the feasibility, efficacy, and safety of the BioSTAR bioabsorbable septal repair implant for the closure of atrial-level shunts. Circulation 2006;114:1962–7.
103. Taaffe M, Fischer E, Baranowski A, et al. Comparison of three patent foramen ovale closure devices in a randomized trial (Amplatzer versus CardioSEAL-STARflex versus Helex occluder). Am J Cardiol 2008;101:1353–8.
106. Lakkireddy D, Rangisetty U, Prasad S, et al. Intracardiac echo-guided radiofrequency catheter ablation of atrial fibrillation in patients with atrial septal defect or patent foramen ovale repair: a feasibility, safety, and efficacy study. J Cardiovasc Electrophysiol 2008;19:1137–42.
108. O'Gara PT, Messe SR, Tuzcu EM, et al. Percutaneous device closure of patent foramen ovale for secondary stroke prevention: a call for completion of randomized clinical trials: a science advisory from the American Heart Association/American Stroke Association and the American College of Cardiology Foundation. Circulation 2009;119:2743–7.
109. Meier B, Kalesan B, Mattle HP, et al. Percutaneous closure of patent foramen ovale in cryptogenic embolism. N Engl J Med 2013;368:1083–91.
110. Carroll JD, Saver JL, Thaler DE, et al. Closure of patent foramen ovale versus medical therapy after cryptogenic stroke. N Engl J Med 2013;368:1092–100.
111. Furlan AJ, Reisman M, Massaro J, et al. Closure or medical therapy for cryptogenic stroke with patent foramen ovale. N Engl J Med 2012;366:991–9.
113. Muir KW, McNeish I, Grosset DG, et al. Visualization of cardiac emboli from mitral valve papillary fibroelastoma. Stroke 1996;27:1133–4.
115. Sandok BA, von Estorff I, Giuliani ER. CNS embolism due to atrial myxoma: clinical features and diagnosis. Arch Neurol 1980;37:485–8.
117. Zotz RJ, Muller M, Genth-Zotz S, et al. Spontaneous echo contrast caused by platelet and leukocyte aggregates? Stroke 2001;32:1127–33.
119. Castello R, Pearson AC, Labovitz AJ. Prevalence and clinical implications of atrial spontaneous contrast in patients undergoing transesophageal echocardiography. Am J Cardiol 1990; 65:1149–53.
120. Daniel WG, Nellessen U, Schröder E, et al. Left atrial spontaneous echo contrast in mitral valve disease: an indicator for an increased thromboembolic risk. J Am Coll Cardiol 1988; 11:1204–11.
121. Comess KA, DeRook FA, Beach KW, et al. Transesophageal echocardiography and carotid ultrasound in patients with cerebral ischemia: prevalence of findings and recurrent stroke risk. J Am Coll Cardiol 1994;23:1598–603.
123. Tice FD, Slivka AP, Walz ET, et al. Mitral valve strands in patients with focal cerebral ischemia. Stroke 1996;27:1183–6.
124. Freedberg RS, Goodkin GM, Perez JL, et al. Valve strands are strongly associated with systemic embolization: a transesophageal echocardiographic study. J Am Coll Cardiol 1995; 26:1709–12.
125. Orsinelli DA, Pearson AC. Detection of prosthetic valve strands by transesophageal echocardiography: clinical significance in patients with suspected cardiac source of embolism. J Am Coll Cardiol 1995;26:1713–18.
126. Roberts JK, Omarali I, Di Tullio MR, et al. Valvular strands and cerebral ischemia. Effect of demographics and strand characteristics. Stroke 1997;28:2185–8.
127. [No authors listed]. Risk factors for stroke and efficacy of antithrombotic therapy in atrial fibrillation. Analysis of pooled data from five randomized controlled trials. Arch Intern Med 1994;154:1449–57.
128. [No authors listed]. Warfarin versus aspirin for prevention of thromboembolism in atrial fibrillation: Stroke Prevention in Atrial Fibrillation II Study. Lancet 1994;343:687–91.
130. The Boston Area Anticoagulation Trial for Atrial Fibrillation Investigators. The effect of low-dose warfarin on the risk of stroke in patients with nonrheumatic atrial fibrillation. N Engl J Med 1990;323:1505–11.
131. [No authors listed]. Stroke Prevention in Atrial Fibrillation Study. Final results. Circulation 1991;84:527–39.
132. EAFT (European Atrial Fibrillation Trial) Study Group. Secondary prevention in non-rheumatic atrial fibrillation after transient ischaemic attack or minor stroke. Lancet 1993;342:1255–62.
133. Nabavi DG, Allroggen A, Reinecke H, et al. Absence of circulating microemboli in patients with lone atrial fibrillation. Neurol Res 1999;21:566–8.
134. Stroke Risk in Atrial Fibrillation Working Group. Comparison of 12 risk stratification schemes to predict stroke in patients with nonvalvular atrial fibrillation. Stroke 2008;39:1901–10.
135. The SPAF III Writing Committee for the Stroke Prevention in Atrial Fibrillation Investigators. Patients with nonvalvular atrial fibrillation at low risk of stroke during treatment with aspirin: Stroke Prevention in Atrial Fibrillation III Study. JAMA 1998; 279:1273–7.
136. Connolly SJ, Ezekowitz MD, Yusuf S, et al. Dabigatran versus warfarin in patients with atrial fibrillation. N Engl J Med 2009;361:1139–51.
137. Granger CB, Alexander JH, McMurray JJ, et al. Apixaban versus warfarin in patients with atrial fibrillation. N Engl J Med 2011;365:981–92.
138. Patel MR, Mahaffey KW, Garg J, et al. Rivaroxaban versus warfarin in nonvalvular atrial fibrillation. N Engl J Med 2011; 365:883–91.
140. ACTIVE Writing Group of the ACTIVE Investigators1, Connolly S, Pogue J, et al. Clopidogrel plus aspirin versus oral anticoagulation for atrial fibrillation in the Atrial fibrillation Clopidogrel Trial with Irbesartan for prevention of Vascular Events (ACTIVE W): a randomised controlled trial. Lancet 2006;367:1903–12.

141. Hart RG, Bhatt DL, Hacke W, et al. Clopidogrel and aspirin versus aspirin alone for the prevention of stroke in patients with a history of atrial fibrillation: subgroup analysis of the CHARISMA randomized trial. Cerebrovasc Dis 2008;25:344–7.
144. Fang MC, Chang Y, Hylek EM, et al. Advanced age, anticoagulation intensity, and risk for intracranial hemorrhage among patients taking warfarin for atrial fibrillation. Ann Intern Med 2004;141:745–52.
145. Stroke Risk in Atrial Fibrillation Working Group. Independent predictors of stroke in patients with atrial fibrillation: a systematic review. Neurology 2007;69:546–54.
146. Albers GW, Bittar N, Young L, et al. Clinical characteristics and management of acute stroke in patients with atrial fibrillation admitted to US university hospitals. Neurology 1997;48: 1598–604.
147. Albers GW, Amarenco P, Easton JD, et al. Antithrombotic and thrombolytic therapy for ischemic stroke: American College of Chest Physicians Evidence-Based Clinical Practice Guidelines. Chest 2008;133:630S–669S.
148. Reddy VY, Doshi SK, Sievert H, et al. Percutaneous left atrial appendage closure for stroke prophylaxis in patients with atrial fibrillation: 2.3-Year Follow-up of the PROTECT AF (Watchman Left Atrial Appendage System for Embolic Protection in Patients with Atrial Fibrillation). Trial Circulation 2013;127: 720–9.
151. The Stroke Prevention in Atrial Fibrillation Investigators. Predictors of thromboembolism in atrial fibrillation: II. Echocardiographic features of patients at risk. Ann Intern Med 1992; 116:6–12.
152. [Not author listed]. Echocardiographic predictors of stroke in patients with atrial fibrillation: a prospective study of 1066 patients from 3 clinical trials. Arch Intern Med 1998;158: 1316–20.
153. Abe Y, Asakura T, Gotou J, et al. Prediction of embolism in atrial fibrillation: classification of left atrial thrombi by transesophageal echocardiography. Jpn Circ J 2000;64:411–15.
154. Fagan SM, Chan KL. Transesophageal echocardiography risk factors for stroke in nonvalvular atrial fibrillation. Echocardiography 2000;17:365–72.
155. The Stroke Prevention in Atrial Fibrillation Investigators Committee on Echocardiography. Transesophageal echocardiographic correlates of thromboembolism in high-risk patients with nonvalvular atrial fibrillation. Ann Intern Med 1998; 128:639–47.
156. Babikian VL, Kase CS, Pessin MS, et al. Intracerebral hemorrhage in stroke patients anticoagulated with heparin. Stroke 1989;20:1500–3.
157. Rothrock JF, Dittrich HC, McAllen S, et al. Acute anticoagulation following cardioembolic stroke. Stroke 1989;20:730–4.
158. Bogousslavsky J, Regli F. Anticoagulant-induced intracerebral bleeding in brain ischemia. Evaluation in 200 patients with TIAs, emboli from the heart, and progressing stroke. Acta Neurol Scand 1985;71:464–71.
161. Sacco RL, Foulkes MA, Mohr JP, et al. Determinants of early recurrence of cerebral infarction. The Stroke Data Bank. Stroke 1989;20:983–9.
162. Cerebral Embolism Study Group. Immediate anticoagulation of embolic stroke: a randomized trial. Stroke 1983;14:668–76.
163. Chamorro A, Vila N, Ascaso C, et al. Heparin in acute stroke with atrial fibrillation: clinical relevance of very early treatment. Arch Neurol 1999;56:1098–102.
167. Santini M, Alexidou G, Ansalone G, et al. Relation of prognosis in sick sinus syndrome to age, conduction defects and modes of permanent cardiac pacing. Am J Cardiol 1990;65:729–35.
168. Biblo LA, Yuan Z, Quan KJ, et al. Risk of stroke in patients with atrial flutter. Am J Cardiol 2001;87:346–9, A9.
169. Santiago D, Warshofsky M, Li Mandri G, et al. Left atrial appendage function and thrombus formation in atrial fibrillation-flutter: a transesophageal echocardiographic study. J Am Coll Cardiol 1994;24:159–64.
172. de Bono DP, Warlow CP. Mitral-annulus calcification and cerebral or retinal ischaemia. Lancet 1979;2:383–5.
173. Chesebro JH, Adams PC, Fuster V. Antithrombotic therapy in patients with valvular heart disease and prosthetic heart valves. J Am Coll Cardiol 1986;8:41B–56B.
174. Kuntze CE, Ebels T, Eijgelaar A, et al. Rates of thromboembolism with three different mechanical heart valve prostheses: randomised study. Lancet 1989;1:514–17.
175. Kuntze CE, Blackstone EH, Ebels T. Thromboembolism and mechanical heart valves: a randomized study revisited. Ann Thorac Surg 1998;66:101–7.
177. Turpie AG, Gent M, Laupacis A, et al. A comparison of aspirin with placebo in patients treated with warfarin after heart-valve replacement. N Engl J Med 1993;329:524–9.
181. Salgado AV, Furlan AJ, Keys TF, et al. Neurologic complications of endocarditis: a 12-year experience. Neurology 1989;39: 173–8.
182. Hart RG, Foster JW, Luther MF, et al. Stroke in infective endocarditis. Stroke 1990;21:695–700.
183. Pruitt AA, Rubin RH, Karchmer AW, et al. Neurologic complications of bacterial endocarditis. Medicine (Baltimore) 1978; 57:329–43.
184. Karchmer A. Infective Endocarditis. In: Braunwald E, editor. Harrison's principles of internal medicine. New York: McGraw-Hill, Medical Publishing Division; 2001.
185. Buda AJ, Zotz RJ, LeMire MS, et al. Prognostic significance of vegetations detected by two-dimensional echocardiography in infective endocarditis. Am Heart J 1986;112:1291–6.
187. Lopez JA, Ross RS, Fishbein MC, et al. Nonbacterial thrombotic endocarditis: a review. Am Heart J 1987;113:773–84.
188. Rogers LR, Cho ES, Kempin S, et al. Cerebral infarction from non-bacterial thrombotic endocarditis. Clinical and pathological study including the effects of anticoagulation. Am J Med 1987;83:746–56.
190. Futrell N, Millikan C. Frequency, etiology, and prevention of stroke in patients with systemic lupus erythematosus. Stroke 1989;20:583–91.
191. Gorelick PB, Rusinowitz MS, Tiku M, et al. Embolic stroke complicating systemic lupus erythematosus. Arch Neurol 1985;42: 813–15.
194. Kapila A, Hart R. Calcific cerebral emboli and aortic stenosis: detection of computed tomography. Stroke 1986;17: 619–21.
195. Gilon D, Buonanno FS, Joffe MM, et al. Lack of evidence of an association between mitral-valve prolapse and stroke in young patients. N Engl J Med 1999;341:8–13.
196. Roach GW, Kanchuger M, Mangano CM, et al. Adverse cerebral outcomes after coronary bypass surgery. Multicenter Study of Perioperative Ischemia Research Group and the Ischemia Research and Education Foundation Investigators. N Engl J Med 1996;335:1857–63.
197. Barbut D, Caplan LR. Brain complications of cardiac surgery. Curr Probl Cardiol 1997;22:449–80.
198. Salazar JD, Wityk RJ, Grega MA, et al. Stroke after cardiac surgery: short- and long-term outcomes. Ann Thorac Surg 2001;72:1195–201, discussion 1201–2.
199. Hogue CW Jr, Murphy SF, Schechtman KB, et al. Risk factors for early or delayed stroke after cardiac surgery. Circulation 1999;100:642–7.
200. Newman MF, Wolman R, Kanchuger M, et al. Multicenter preoperative stroke risk index for patients undergoing coronary artery bypass graft surgery. Multicenter Study of Perioperative Ischemia (McSPI) Research Group. Circulation 1996;94:II74–80.
201. Stamou SC, Corso PJ. Coronary revascularization without cardiopulmonary bypass in high-risk patients: a route to the future. Ann Thorac Surg 2001;71:1056–61.
202. Wityk RJ, Goldsborough MA, Hillis A, et al. Diffusion- and perfusion-weighted brain magnetic resonance imaging in patients with neurologic complications after cardiac surgery. Arch Neurol 2001;58:571–6.
204. Segal AZ, Abernethy WB, Palacios IF, et al. Stroke as a complication of cardiac catheterization: risk factors and clinical features. Neurology 2001;56:975–7.
207. Lip GY, Lowe GD, Rumley A, et al. Fibrinogen and fibrin D-dimer levels in paroxysmal atrial fibrillation: evidence for intermediate elevated levels of intravascular thrombogenesis. Am Heart J 1996;131:724–30.
208. Lip GY, Lowe GD, Rumley A, et al. Increased markers of thrombogenesis in chronic atrial fibrillation: effects of warfarin treatment. Br Heart J 1995;73:527–33.

209. Gustafsson C, Blomback M, Britton M, et al. Coagulation factors and the increased risk of stroke in nonvalvular atrial fibrillation. Stroke 1990;21:47–51.
210. Mitusch R, Siemens HJ, Garbe M, et al. Detection of a hypercoagulable state in nonvalvular atrial fibrillation and the effect of anticoagulant therapy. Thromb Haemost 1996;75:219–23.
211. Rosenberg RD, Aird WC. Vascular-bed-specific hemostasis and hypercoagulable states. N Engl J Med 1999;340:1555–64.
212. Kistler JP, Singer DE, Millenson MM, et al. Effect of low-intensity warfarin anticoagulation on level of activity of the hemostatic system in patients with atrial fibrillation. BAATAF Investigators. Stroke 1993;24:1360–5.
213. Lip GY, Rumley A, Dunn FG, et al. Plasma fibrinogen and fibrin D-dimer in patients with atrial fibrillation: effects of cardioversion to sinus rhythm. Int J Cardiol 1995;51:245–51.
215. Yamamoto K, Ikeda U, Seino Y, et al. Coagulation activity is increased in the left atrium of patients with mitral stenosis. J Am Coll Cardiol 1995;25:107–12.
216. Jafri SM, Ozawa T, Mammen E, et al. Platelet function, thrombin and fibrinolytic activity in patients with heart failure. Eur Heart J 1993;14:205–12.

33 Atherosclerotic Disease of the Proximal Aorta

Marco R. Di Tullio, Shunichi Homma

KEY POINTS

- Large atherosclerotic plaques in the proximal segment of the aorta are a potential cause of ischemic stroke in individuals over age 60.
- The magnitude of the risk depends on the morphologic characteristics of the plaque (thickness, ulceration, presence of mobile components).
- Transesophageal echocardiography (TEE) is the most widely used and sensitive diagnostic technique; MRI, CT or PET/CT are also used.
- Unsuspected proximal aortic plaques increase the stroke risk during cardiac catheterization or cardiac surgery, requiring screening before the procedure and possibly alteration of the technique used to perform it.
- Hypercoagulability may increase the possibility of superimposed thrombus formation on a plaque and therefore the associated stroke risk.
- The best preventive treatment to decrease the risk of embolic events in patients with proximal aortic plaques is still controversial.
- The relative benefit of antiplatelet agents versus systemic anticoagulation requires further investigation; anticoagulation appears indicated in the case of documented mobile superimposed thrombus.
- Surgical aortic endarterectomy carries great risk of embolization and should be reserved to highly selected cases.

The presence of atherosclerotic plaques in the aorta is a risk factor for ischemic stroke. The proximal portion of the aorta, where the blood vessels that supply the brain originate, may become the source for cerebral embolism. The present chapter will review the principal studies on the association between aortic plaques and ischemic stroke, and the related diagnostic and therapeutic issues.

FREQUENCY OF AORTIC PLAQUES IN THE GENERAL POPULATION

Atherosclerosis in the aorta develops throughout life, becoming especially evident after the 4th decade of life; the prevalence and number of atherosclerotic lesions increases continuously thereafter. In the Stroke Prevention: Assessment of Risk in a Community (SPARC) study,[1] the prevalence of "simple" (less than 4 mm in thickness, without ulceration or mobile debris) or "complex" (≥4 mm thick, or with complex features) atherosclerotic lesions was evaluated by transesophageal echocardiography (TEE) in 588 volunteers over the age of 44 years. Aortic atherosclerosis of any degree and complex atherosclerosis in any aortic segment were present in 51.3% and 7.6% of subjects, respectively. Atherosclerosis of any degree was identified in the ascending aorta, aortic arch and descending aorta in 8.4%, 31.0%, and 44.9%, respectively. Corresponding figures for complex atherosclerosis were 0.2%, 2.2%, and 6.0%. Any atherosclerosis prevalence increased from approximately 17% in the 45–54 years subgroup to over 80% in subjects older than 75. Complex atherosclerosis was virtually absent in the younger subgroup, but present in over 20% of subjects after age 75. In a TEE study on healthy volunteers over the age of 59,[2] the prevalence of simple plaques in the aortic arch was 22%, that of complicated plaques (≥5 mm in thickness or with irregular, ulcerated surface) 4%. The prevalence of aortic atherosclerosis in the general population varies with the characteristics, and especially risk factors distribution, of the sample studied. In the tri-ethnic study group of the Aortic Plaque and Risk of Ischemic Stroke (APRIS) study, the prevalence of aortic arch atherosclerosis of any degree in 209 stroke-free volunteers over age 55 undergoing TEE was 62.2%, that of large (≥ 4 mm) arch plaques 23.9%.[3] These figures, considerably higher than those of the other studies, were associated with a greater burden of atherosclerotic risk factors. Compared with SPARC, the APRIS study group had higher frequencies of diabetes (23.0% vs 8.9%), hypertension (69.4% vs 55.2%), past and current smoking history (60.3% vs 39.0% and 16.1% vs 8.2%, respectively).

AORTIC PLAQUES AND ISCHEMIC STROKE: PATHOLOGY STUDIES

A strong association between aortic arch plaques and ischemic stroke was first reported by Amarenco and colleagues in an autopsy case-control study.[4] A much greater frequency of ulcerated aortic plaques was observed in elderly patients who had died from a stroke than in patients who had died from other neurological diseases (26% vs 5%; age-adjusted odds ratio [OR] 4.0; 95% confidence interval [CI], 2.1–7.8). Importantly, the highest frequency of ulcerated plaques was observed in patients with unexplained (cryptogenic) stroke (61% vs 28%, adjusted OR 5.7, 95%CI, 2.4–13.6), providing a potential mechanism for the stroke. The lack of association between ulcerated plaques and significant carotid artery stenosis or atrial fibrillation, important sources for brain embolism, suggested an independent role of aortic plaques on stroke risk. Among patients with ulcerated plaques, only 3% were younger than 60 years.

In another necropsy study on 120 unselected patients,[5] Khatibzadeh and colleagues found evidence of arterial embolization in 40 (33%). Complicated aortic arch plaques were significantly associated with arterial embolism (OR 5.8, 95%CI, 1.1–31.7), independent of and with similar strength as severe ipsilateral carotid artery disease and atrial fibrillation.

IN VIVO STUDIES: TRANSESOPHAGEAL ECHOCARDIOGRAPHY

TEE is the most sensitive and widely used technique for examining the proximal portion of the aorta, and allowed to study the association between aortic plaques and ischemic stroke in vivo. The proximity of the esophagus to the aorta and the absence of interposed structures allow the use of high-frequency ultrasound transducers, providing high-resolution images of the vessel. When searching for plaques possibly related to stroke, the portion of aorta proximal to the take-off of the left subclavian artery is the focus of the examination. The ascending aorta can be accurately visualized by TEE from the aortic valve level to the initial curvature of the arch (Fig. 33-1). The mid and distal portions of the aortic arch are also visualized in all patients (Fig. 33-2). A small portion of the vessel (proximal arch) may not be visualized due to the interposition of the trachea, and may be a "blind spot" of the examination, although modern multiplane transducers allow a more complete visualization of the vessel in most patients. By TEE, an accurate assessment is possible of the presence and thickness of plaques (Fig. 33-3), as well as the presence of ulcerations (Fig. 33-4) or superimposed thrombus (Figs 33-5–33-7). TEE has been shown to be highly sensitive and specific in the detection of aortic plaques.[6,7] Its diagnostic accuracy for the presence of thrombus is high (sensitivity 91%, specificity 90%).[7] However, the sensitivity of TEE for detecting small ulcerations of the plaque surface, which may carry additional risk for embolic events,[2,8,9] is less than optimal (approximately 75%). Reproducibility of TEE measurements of aortic plaque thickness is very good, with agreement of 84% to 88% for the diagnosis of large (≥4 mm) plaques.[10]

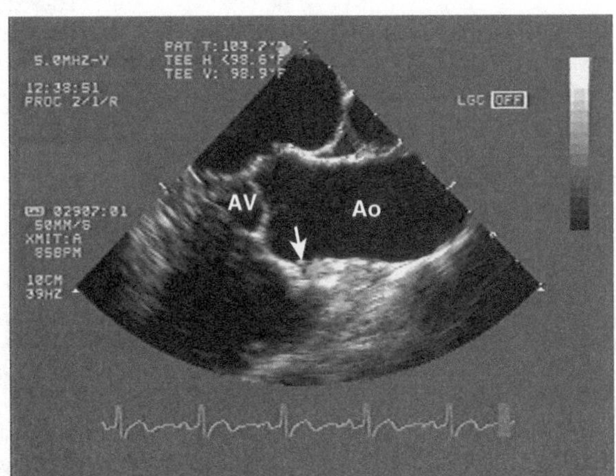

Figure 33-1. Longitudinal view of the ascending aorta (AO) by transesophageal echocardiography (TEE). The entire ascending aorta is visualized, from the aortic valve (AV) to the initial curvature of the aortic arch. The takeoff of the right coronary artery is visible (*arrow*).

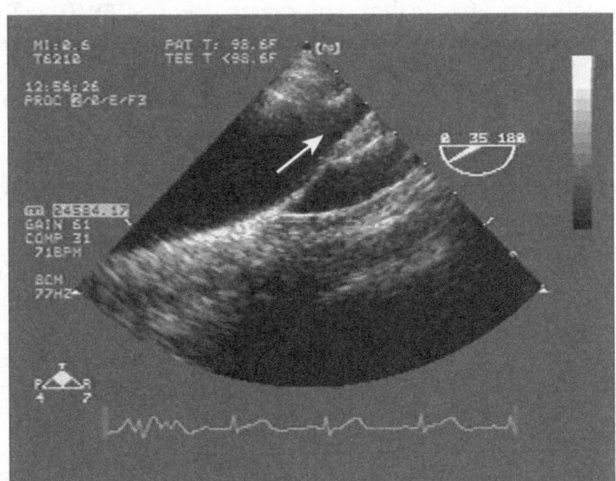

Figure 33-2. TEE visualization of the mid to distal portion of the aortic arch. The takeoff of the left subclavian artery is visible (*arrow*).

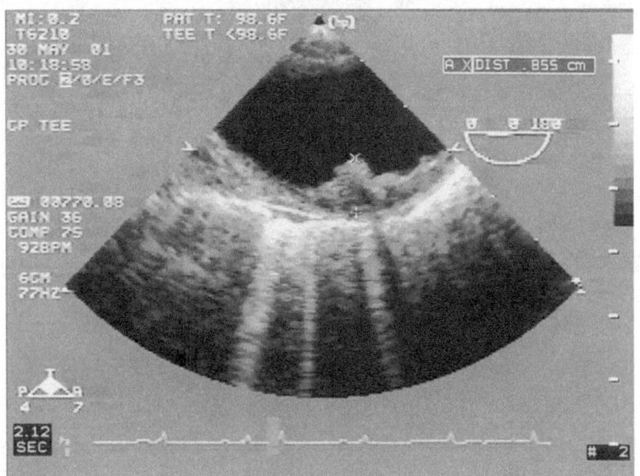

Figure 33-3. Protruding atherosclerotic plaque in the distal aortic arch. Measurement of plaque thickness, perpendicular to the major axis of the aortic lumen, is shown. Plaque thickness (0.855 cm) is displayed in the upper right corner.

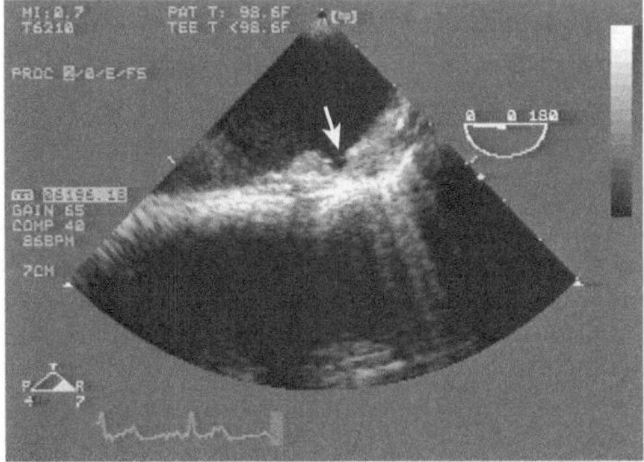

Figure 33-4. Complex plaque in the distal aortic arch. A large ulceration (*arrow*) is visible.

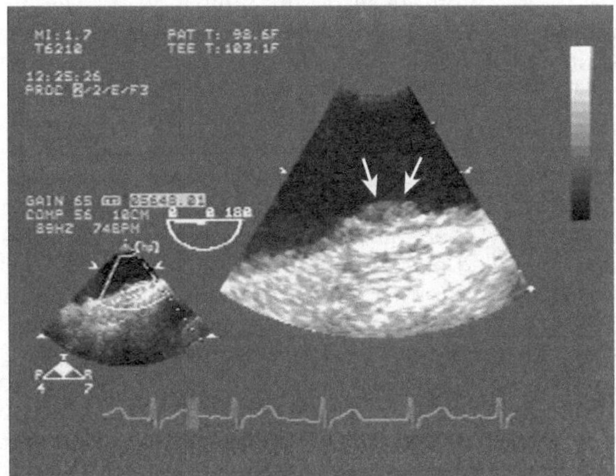

Figure 33-5. Enlarged view of a plaque in the mid portion of the aortic arch. Hypoechoic material suggestive of thrombus (*arrows*) appears superimposed to the brightly echogenic plaque.

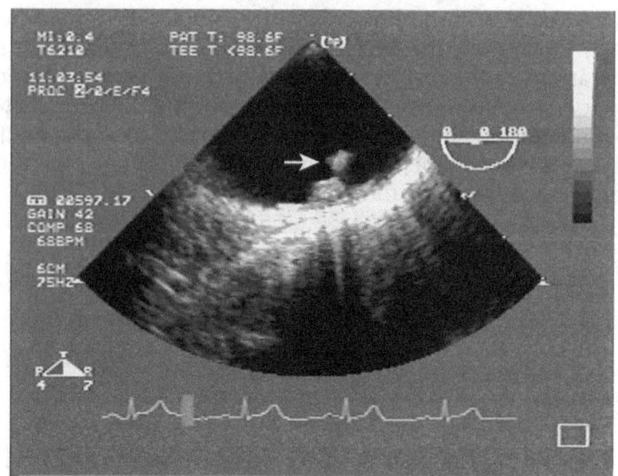

Figure 33-6. Complex plaque in the mid portion of the aortic arch. A large pedunculated portion is seen (*arrow*), which was highly mobile in real time imaging.

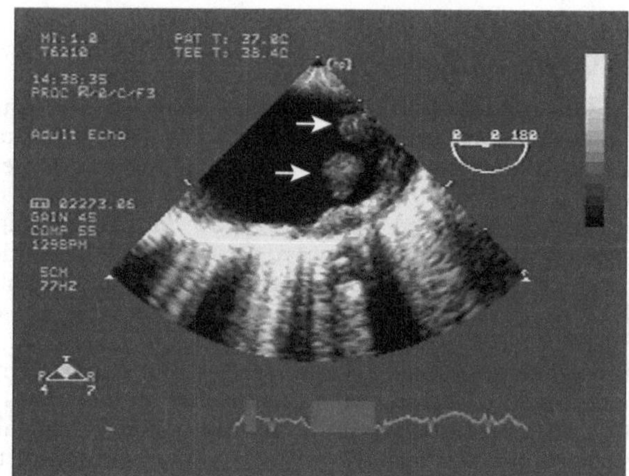

Figure 33-7. Complex atherosclerotic plaque of the distal aortic arch. Two large thrombi (*arrows*) are visible.

TABLE 33-1 Association between Proximal Aortic Plaques and Ischemic Stroke: Transesophageal Echocardiographic Case-Control Studies

Study (Reference No.)	Cases/ Controls (N)	Age (Years)	Type of Atheroma	Controls (%)	Patients with Stroke (%)	Adjusted Odds Ratio* (95% CI)
Amarenco et al.[17]	250/250	≥60	1–3.9 mm	22	46	4.4 (2.8–6.8)
			≥4 mm	2	14	9.1 (3.3–25.2)
Jones et al.[2]	215/202	≥60	<5 mm, smooth	22	33	2.3 (1.2–4.2)
			≥5 mm, complex	4	22	7.1 (2.7–18.4)
Di Tullio et al.[8]	106/114	≥40	≥5 mm	13	26	2.6 (1.1–5.9)
	30/36	<60		3	3	1.2 (0.7–20.2)
	76/78	≥60		18	36	2.4 (1.1–5.7)
Di Tullio et al.[20]	255/209	≥55	≥4 mm	24	49	2.4 (1.3–4.6)

CI, confidence interval.
*Adjusted for conventional stroke risk factors (also see text).

TEE is a safe, although semi-invasive, diagnostic test. Major complications are uncommon and mainly due to unsuspected pre-existing esophageal disease. In over 10,000 patients,[11] one death was observed. In an additional 2.7%, the test was not performed due to unsuccessful intubation (1.9%) or patient intolerance (0.8%). Similar results were obtained in 15,381 consecutive patients, with two deaths (0.01%) and an overall incidence of complications of 1.7%.[12] In 901 patients,[13] intubation was unsuccessful in 1.2% of cases, with no deaths and a low incidence (0.6%) of major complications. Our experience in stroke patients has shown no increased frequency of patient discomfort, unsuccessful intubation or significant complications.[14] Moreover, the test can be safely performed even in patients of very advanced age.[15]

Case-Control Studies

Using TEE, Tunick and colleagues[16] first reported on an increased frequency of aortic plaques ≥5 mm in 122 patients with a history of arterial embolism compared with 122 age- and sex-matched patients with other diagnoses (27% vs 9%, OR 3.2, 95%CI, 1.6–6.5). This retrospective study, not adjusted for other potential embolic sources, was followed by other case-control studies which are summarized in Table 33-1. Amarenco and colleagues studied 250 patients with acute ischemic stroke over the age of 60 and 250 controls.[17] Arch plaques between 1 mm and 3.9 mm in thickness were associated with stroke after adjustment for conventional stroke risk factors (adjusted OR 4.4), but a sharp increase in risk was present for plaques ≥4 mm (adjusted OR 9.1, 95%CI, 3.3–25.2). Also, the stroke risk associated with plaques ≥4 mm was independent of the presence of carotid stenosis and atrial fibrillation.[17] The authors speculated that the sharp increase in risk observed for larger plaques might depend on a more frequent presence of superimposed thrombus, which would be included in the measurement of plaque thickness, and to higher frequency of mobile components, a circumstance confirmed in other studies.[18] Plaques ≥4 mm were significantly more frequent in patients with cryptogenic stroke than in patients with stroke of determined origin (28.2% vs 8.1%; OR 4.7, 95%CI, 2.2–10.1).

Similar results, except for the association with cryptogenic stroke, were obtained by Jones et al.,[2] who studied 215 stroke patients and 202 healthy volunteers over age 59 (see Table 33-1). Plaques ≥5 mm or with ulcerated/mobile components were associated with much greater stroke risk (adjusted OR 7.1, 95%CI, 2.7–18.4) vs no plaque than smaller, smooth plaques (adjusted OR 2.3, 95%CI, 1.2–4.2). However, the frequency of large or complex plaques was similar in patients with cryptogenic stroke (20%) and patients with stroke of determined origin (23%).

We studied 106 stroke patients over the age of 40 and 114 age- and gender-matched controls,[8] detecting an increased risk of stroke associated with aortic plaques ≥5 mm (adjusted OR 2.6, 95%CI, 1.1–5.9). The risk was entirely due to the subgroup of patients over age 59, while the prevalence of large plaques was very low (3%) below that age in both stroke patients and controls (see Table 33-1).

Using epiaortic ultrasonography, Davila-Roman and colleagues studied the prevalence of aortic plaques in 1,200 subjects over the age of 49 years undergoing cardiac surgery, 158 of them with a previous embolic event.[19] They found plaques

≥3 mm in 26.6% of patients with a previous cerebrovascular event and in 18.1% of those without it. Aortic plaques, arterial hypertension, atrial fibrillation and carotid artery stenosis were independently associated with neurological events.

More recently, we reported similar results in 255 stroke patients and 209 age-, gender- and race/ethnicity-matched controls of APRIS. Large aortic arch plaques (≥4 mm) were again found to be associated with an increased stroke risk after adjustment for other stroke risk factors (adjusted OR 2.4, 95%CI, 1.3–4.6; see Table 33-1).[20] Complex plaque morphology and coexisting hypercoagulability increased the stroke risk, as will be discussed later.

Retrograde embolization to the brain from the proximal segment of the descending aorta has been known to occur,[21] although its actual involvement as a stroke mechanism is difficult to quantify. Retrograde flow from aortic segments containing large plaques was visualized by MRI in 28 of 94 stroke patients (29.8%), potentially affecting all brain territories.[22]

Prospective Studies

The role of aortic arch plaques as a risk factor for peripheral and cerebral embolization has also been confirmed prospectively (Table 33-2), following patients who had a first stroke or other embolic event, and comparing the embolic recurrence rate in patients with and without plaques. After a mean follow-up of 14 months, Tunick and colleagues noted a significantly greater incidence of cerebral or peripheral embolic events in 42 patients with protruding aortic atheromas compared with control subjects matched for age, gender, and hypertension (33% vs. 7%; relative risk [RR] 4.3, 95%CI, 1.2–15.0).[23] Similar results were reported by Mitusch and colleagues in 47 patients with large or mobile arch plaques and 136 patients with small or no plaque.[24] Recurrence rate of embolic events was 13.7%/year in the former group, 4.1%/year in the latter (RR 4.3, 95%CI, 1.5–12.0). In a French multicenter study on 331 stroke patients 60 years or older,[25] arch plaques ≥4 mm were associated with an almost fourfold increase in risk of recurrent stroke after adjusting for carotid stenosis, atrial fibrillation, peripheral artery disease, and conventional risk factors (see Table 33-2). The recurrence rate was highest in patients whose index stroke was cryptogenic (16.4 per 100 person-years). The incidence of vascular events was also significantly greater in patients with large plaques (RR 3.5; see Table 33-2). In 236 patients with ischemic stroke, Tanaka and colleagues observed an increased risk of recurrent stroke or myocardial infarction in patients with arch plaques ≥3.5 mm followed for 42 months (see Table 33-2).[26] Fujimoto and colleagues followed 283 patients with embolic stroke and no significant occlusive lesion in their cerebral arteries for a mean of 3.4 years.[27] Patients who experienced a recurrent stroke (32, or 11.3%) had significantly increased prevalence of arch plaques ≥4 mm (41% vs 22%) and of plaque extension to the cephalic branches (63% vs 39%), and the combination of these two features had the highest recurrence risk (see Table 33-2). We more recently reported on the incidence of recurrent stroke and death in 516 patients with acute ischemic stroke treated with aspirin or warfarin as part of the Patent Foramen Ovale in Cryptogenic Stroke Study (PICSS). Over a follow-up of 2 years, large plaques (≥4 mm) remained associated with an increased risk of events (adjusted HR 2.1, 95%CI, 1.04–4.3), especially those with complex morphology (HR 2.6, 95%CI, 1.1–5.8; see Table 33-2). The risk was highest among cryptogenic stroke patients, for both large plaques (HR 6.42, 95%CI, 1.62–25.46) and large-complex plaques (HR 9.50, 95%CI, 1.92–47.10)[28] Finally, large plaques were detected in 14% of patients with a history of transient ischemic attacks (TIA), and increased their risk of recurrent vascular events at 1 year (6.6%, vs 2.2% in patients without plaque; $P = 0.003$).[29]

In a report from the SPARC study,[1] the association between aortic atherosclerosis and cerebrovascular events was questioned. In 581 community-derived subjects undergoing TEE, large (≥4 mm), ulcerated or mobile plaques were associated with a history of coronary artery disease (OR 2.35, 95%CI, 1.1–5.0) but not ischemic stroke (OR 1.37, 95%CI, 0.44–4.3). The inclusion in that study of younger subjects (age cutoff 45 years) may have diluted the strength of the association between aortic plaques and stroke. Also, the prevalence of severe plaques in the proximal aorta was low (2.4%). However, we more recently reported similar findings from the follow-up of the APRIS control group (age over 54 years), in which large arch plaques were also not associated with stroke and vascular events (hazard ratio [HR] 1.05, 95%CI, 0.37–3.03).[3] These observations suggest that the risk of stroke from arch plaques incidentally detected in healthy subjects may be lower than that generally reported in the literature, which was obtained in subjects with previous stroke or peripheral embolic events, or referred for TEE because of other coexisting conditions.

PLAQUE MORPHOLOGY AND STROKE RISK

The role of aortic plaques as a risk factor for stroke has been mainly established measuring the thickness of the plaque, with

TABLE 33-2 Recurrence Rate of Embolic Events and Stroke in Patients with and Without Proximal Aortic Plaques: Transesophageal Echocardiographic Prospective Studies

Study (Reference No.)	Aortic Plaque Present/ Aortic Plaque Absent (N)	Follow-up (Months)	Type of Plaque	Aortic Plaque Absent (%)	Aortic Plaque Present (%)	Adjusted* Relative Risk (95% CI)
Tunick et al.[23]	42/42	14	≥4 mm	7	33	4.3 (1.2–15.0)
Mitusch et al.[24]	47/136	16	≥5 mm/mobile vs <5 mm	4.1/year	13.7/year	4.3 (1.5–12.0)
FAPS[25†]	45/286	24–48	≥4 mm vs <4 mm	3.2/year	11.9/year	3.8 (1.8–7.8)
				7.5/year	26.0/year	3.5 (2.1–5.9)
Tanaka et al.[26]	97/139	42	≥3.5 mm	not reported	not reported	2.1 (1.2–3.7)
Fujimoto et al.[27]	51/232	40	≥4 mm, extending to branches	2.9/person-year	9.8/person-year	2.4 (1.1–5.2)
Di Tullio et al.[28**]	101/415	24	≥4 mm	5.1/year	13.4/year	2.1 (1.04–4.3)
	44/415	24	≥4 mm, complex	5.1/year	13.7/year	2.6 (1.1–5.9)

*Adjusted for conventional stroke risk factors (also see text).
†Only study conducted on patients with ischemic stroke. Data in first row refer to recurrence rate of stroke; data in second row refer to recurrence rate of all embolic events.
**All patients treated with warfarin or aspirin.

TABLE 33-3 Effect of Aortic Plaque Morphology on the Risk of Ischemic Stroke

	Patients with Stroke (n = 152)		Control Subjects (n = 152)		Unadjusted Odds Ratio* (95% CI)	Adjusted Odds Ratio* (95% CI)
	n	%	*n*	%		
No plaque	28	18.4	55	36.2	–	–
Small plaque (<4 mm)†	56	36.8	68	44.7	1.6 (0.9–2.9)	1.9 (1.0–3.6)
Large plaque (≥4 mm)	68	44.8	29	19.1	4.6 (2.5–8.6)	4.3 (2.1–8.7)
Noncomplex plaque	34	22.4	25	16.5	2.7 (1.3–5.3)	2.4 (1.1–5.1)
Complex plaque	34	22.4	4	2.6	16.7 (5.4–51.8)	17.1 (5.1–57.3)
Ulcerated	24	15.8	3	2.0	15.7 (4.4–56.7)	15.8 (4.1–61.4)
Mobile	10	6.6	1	0.7	19.6 (2.4–161.3)	21.3 (2.4–193.2)

CI, confidence interval.
*Adjusted for age, gender, arterial hypertension, diabetes mellitus, and hypercholesterolemia.
†No complex forms were present among small plaques.

either 4 mm or 5 mm chosen as the threshold for increased risk. It is unclear, however, whether plaque thickness is directly related to the stroke mechanism, or is rather a marker of diffuse atherosclerosis, with the latter being in fact responsible for the increased risk. We demonstrated differences in plaque-related stroke risk between genders.[30] Aortic plaques ≥4 mm were significantly more frequent in men than in women (31.5% vs 20.3%; $P = 0.025$), and were associated with ischemic stroke in both men (adjusted OR 6.0, 95%CI, 2.1–16.8) and women (adjusted OR 3.2, 95%CI, 1.2–8.8) after adjusting for other stroke risk factors. Plaques 3 to 3.9 mm in thickness, however, were significantly associated with stroke in women (adjusted OR 4.8, 95%CI, 1.7–15.0), but not in men (adjusted OR 0.8, 95%CI, 0.2–3.0). This observation suggests that plaque thickness, rather than identifying the actual culprit lesion for the stroke, may be a marker of diffuse atherosclerosis, including intracranial atherosclerosis, or of other conditions that may differ between genders, and are possibly related to the stroke mechanism.[25] In any case, plaque progression, defined as increase in thickness over time, was found to be associated with increased incidence of vascular events. Among 117 patients with stroke or TIA, those who showed plaque progression over 1 year were significantly more likely to experience a vascular event (stroke, TIA, myocardial infarction or death) than those with no plaque progression over a median follow-up of 1.7 years (51% vs 11%; $P < 0.0001$).[31]

The complex morphology of a plaque may be more directly related to the stroke mechanism. As mentioned earlier, morphologic features of the plaque, such as ulceration or mobility, have been linked with an increased stroke risk,[1,5–9,18] especially for cryptogenic stroke. Stone and colleagues[9] initially showed significantly greater frequency of ulcerated plaques in 23 patients with cryptogenic stroke than in 26 patients with stroke of determined origin (39% versus 8%; $P < 0.001$). In our experience on 152 elderly stroke patients and 152 age-matched controls,[18] ulcerated or mobile plaques were found to be a much stronger risk factor for stroke than large but non-complex plaques (Table 33-3). The study confirmed that plaques ≥4 mm were indeed associated with increased stroke risk (adjusted OR 4.3, 95%CI, 2.1–8.7); however, when they were divided on the basis of the presence or absence of ulceration (a discrete indentation of at least 2 mm in width and depth) or mobile components, the stroke risk associated with those complex features was exceedingly high (adjusted OR 17.1), while large but non-complex plaques only carried a modest risk increase (adjusted OR 2.4; see Table 33-3). The same remained true even after excluding patients with other stroke sources such as atrial fibrillation, carotid stenosis ≥60%, or intracranial atherosclerosis. Cohen and colleagues studied the impact of plaque morphology (ulceration, hypoechoic

TABLE 33-4 Prevalence of Mobile Thrombi Superimposed on Proximal Aortic Plaques in Patients with Ischemic Stroke

Study	Patients (n)	Mobile Thrombi	
		n	%
Toyoda et al.[6]	62	3	4.8
Nihoyannopoulos et al.[35]	152	3	2.0
Jones et al.[2]	202	11	5.4
Amarenco et al.[17]			
Unselected	250	7	2.8
Cryptogenic	78	6	7.7
Stone et al.[9]			
Unselected	49	2	4.1
Cryptogenic	23	2	8.7
Di Tullio et al.[18]	152	10	6.6
Ueno et al.[36]	167	12	7.2
Di Tullio et al.[20]	255	4	1.6

components or calcification) on the risk of recurrent vascular events in a prospective study on 334 stroke patients over the age of 60 followed for 2 to 4 years.[32] In patients with plaques ≥4 mm, the presence of ulcerations or hypoechoic components did not increase the risk of vascular events. However, the absence of calcification was associated with the strongest increase in risk (adjusted RR 10.3, 95%CI, 4.2–25.2), while the presence of calcification decreased the risk (adjusted RR 1.2, 95%CI, 0.6–2.1), possibly signaling a more stable lesion. These observations suggest that, although plaque thickness represents the most readily available marker of embolic risk, the plaque's morphologic features strongly affect its embolic potential, possibly calling for different therapeutic approaches in individual patients. It should be remembered that, whenever TEE identifies a protruding, mobile component on a plaque, this represents thrombus superimposed to atherosclerotic material, and usually occurs on ulcerated plaques. This observation has been confirmed by several studies that correlated the TEE findings with the histopathologic examination of the aorta.[5,33,34] Mobile components superimposed to an aortic plaque are infrequently seen in elderly stroke patients, ranging from 1.6% to 8.7% in different studies[2,6,9,17,18,20,35,36] (Table 33-4). When present, however, they represent a very strong risk factor for brain embolization. In our study,[18] mobile components superimposed to a plaque were present in 6.6% of elderly stroke patients, and were associated with a more than 20-fold increase in the risk of stroke, after adjusting for other stroke risk factors (see Table 33-3). Occasionally, mobile thrombi without severe atherosclerosis can be seen in patients younger than 60 years who present with an embolic

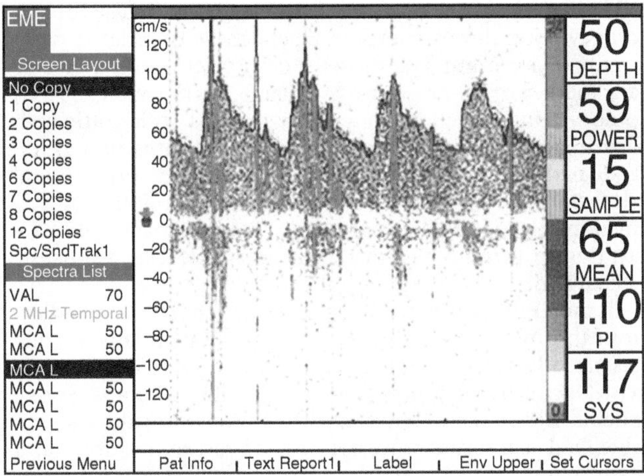

Figure 33-8. Transcranial Doppler examination of the middle cerebral artery. High-intensity transient signals (HITS) are visualized as vertical high-amplitude signals with narrow spectrum superimposed to the normal blood flow.

event (23 cases out of 27,855 TEE examinations in a multicenter cardiology study).[37] These thrombi usually have insertion on small atherosclerotic plaques, and appear to represent a rare variant of atherosclerotic disease in younger patients.[37]

The potential for brain embolism from large plaques, and even more from complex plaques, has been confirmed using transcranial Doppler monitoring. Continuous monitoring of the blood flow into the middle cerebral arteries is obtained, which can be performed simultaneously on both sides, and maintained for prolonged periods of time. The passage of small particles produces characteristic high-intensity transient signals, or HITS (Fig. 33-8), the identification of which can be enhanced through the application of appropriate filters. Using this technique for 30 minutes in 46 patients with acute ischemic stroke, Rundek and colleagues demonstrated the presence of HITS in a much larger proportion of stroke patients with plaques ≥4 mm than with small or no plaques, even in the absence of other TEE-detected possible embolic sources (70% vs 18%; $P = 0.007$).[38] Moreover, all patients with large and complex plaques were found to have HITS, compared with 39% of patients with large but non-complex plaques ($P = 0.005$). Similar results for plaques ≥4 mm and HITS were obtained in cryptogenic stroke patients in a study by Castellanos et al.,[39] in which data on plaque complexity were not reported.

In summary, aortic plaque thickness ≥4 mm has been shown to be associated with increased stroke risk and remains a useful tool for risk stratification, although part of the risk may come from superimposed thrombus included in the measurement. Plaque thickness is also a marker of diffuse atherosclerosis, which may also play an important role in the stroke mechanism. The presence of complex morphologic features of a plaque, and especially mobile components, appears more directly related to the stroke mechanism in individual patients. Overall, the incidence of recurrent embolic events in patients with large or mobile aortic plaques has been estimated at up to 14% per year, underscoring the need for effective secondary prevention strategies.[40]

NATURAL HISTORY OF AORTIC PLAQUES

The natural history of atherosclerotic plaques in the proximal aorta has not been extensively studied. However, it appears that plaque size and morphology are important in determining the evolution of a plaque over time. Montgomery and colleagues[41] followed 30 patients who had aortic atherosclerosis (12 with plaque <5 mm, eight with plaques ≥5 mm, and ten with mobile components) on an initial TEE, and a repeat TEE performed at 12 months. While subjects with smaller plaques showed no significant changes, four of eight patients with plaques ≥5 mm had developed a new mobile lesion. In patients who initially had a mobile lesion, such a lesion had resolved in 70% of cases, but a new mobile lesion was observed in another 70%. Overall, although 20 of 30 patients (67%) had no change in degree of atherosclerosis, substantial changes were observed in plaque morphology. In a study on 78 patients with stroke or TIA, plaque progression over 9 months was observed in 37% of cases, and was more frequent in the arch than in other aortic segments.[42] Using transthoracic echocardiographic imaging from a suprasternal window, Geraci and Weinberger[43] studied plaque progression in 89 patients followed for up to 18 months (mean 7.7). While only 23% of plaques <4 mm at baseline showed thickness changes, 52% of plaques ≥4 mm showed thickness changes, upward or downward. It therefore appears that large aortic plaques are extremely dynamic lesions, whose appearance may change considerably over a relatively short period of time.

AORTIC PLAQUES IN STROKE PATIENTS OF DIFFERENT RACE-ETHNICITY

Most studies on aortic atherosclerotic plaques and ischemic stroke were conducted in Caucasian populations. Some information, however, is available for Blacks and Hispanics that allows a comparison of plaque frequency, which is important in the light of the different prevalence of risk factors for atherosclerosis in different race/ethnic groups. In a retrospective study on 1,553 ischemic stroke patients (889 Whites, 664 Blacks), Gupta and colleagues[44] found a higher prevalence of aortic plaques in Whites than in Blacks in the ascending aorta (14.7% vs 11.1%; $P = 0.04$), aortic arch (67.7% vs 62.2%; $P = 0.03$) and descending aorta (58.4% vs 50.3%; $P = 0.002$). The plaque burden (sum of maximum plaque thickness at the three locations) was also significantly higher in Whites (4.97 mm vs 4.28 mm; $P = 0.007$), and so was, but only in the aortic arch, the prevalence of plaques ≥4 mm (25.9% vs 18.7%; $P < 0.001$) and of complex plaques, defined as protruding, ulcerated, mobile or calcified regardless of plaque thickness (26.3% vs 19.0%; $P < 0.001$). These findings were observed despite a higher prevalence of arterial hypertension and diabetes mellitus in the Black subgroup, and cannot therefore be explained by differences in conventional atherosclerotic risk factors. In our case-control study in ischemic stroke patients over age 59 from the tri-ethnic community of Northern Manhattan,[18] plaques ≥4 mm had similar frequency in Whites, Blacks, and Hispanics (24.1%, 20.0%, and 22.5%, respectively). However, complex plaques were twice as frequent in Whites (32.3%) as in Blacks (15.6%) and Hispanics (16.3%). Complex plaques were associated with a strong increase in stroke risk in all three race/ethnic subgroups. Similar to Gupta's study, the frequency of arterial hypertension and diabetes mellitus was significantly lower in Whites than in the other two race/ethnic subgroups, and that of hypercholesterolemia was significantly lower in Whites than in Blacks. The prevalence of plaques ≥4 mm in the overall study population (44.8%) was much higher than in a similar study from France (14.4%),[17] and also higher than the frequency of plaques ≥5 mm or complex in a similar study from Australia (22%).[2] Therefore, even though the stroke risk associated with large or complex plaques appeared similar across the studies, the attributable risk of stroke from proximal aortic plaques may be greater in the American population, underscoring the need for effective preventive measures and risk factors reduction.

FACTORS ASSOCIATED WITH AORTIC PLAQUES IN STROKE PATIENTS

Although traditional risk factors do not seem to explain the race/ethnic differences in the frequency of aortic plaques, some of these risk factors are indeed associated with plaque presence. Age is the strongest predictor of aortic atherosclerosis.[1,2,4,5,8,17–19,45,46] Cigarette smoking has consistently been shown to be associated with aortic atherosclerosis,[2,17,19,45,46] and appears as the most important modifiable risk factor. Arterial hypertension is also associated with proximal aortic atherosclerosis,[4,46] especially in the case of ulcerated lesions.[4] In the SPARC study, systolic and pulse pressure variables (office and ambulatory), but no diastolic variables were associated with any atherosclerosis and complex atherosclerosis in the aorta after adjusting for age and smoking history.[46] Using ambulatory blood pressure monitoring, we recently reported that systolic variables (24-hour, daytime and night-time blood pressure) were independently associated with arch atherosclerosis, and that night-time systolic blood pressure variability was independently associated with the presence of large plaques.[47] The association between diabetes mellitus and aortic atherosclerosis has been supported in some studies,[2] and negated in others,[45,46] at least after adjusting for other risk factors.[45] Hypercholesterolemia was associated with aortic atherosclerosis in some studies,[19,45,48] and treatment with 3-hydroxy-3-methylglutaryl coenzyme A (HMG-CoA) reductase inhibitors (statins) has been shown to induce regression of aortic atherosclerotic lesions in humans.[49–51]

Besides traditional risk factors, other variables have been identified as associated with aortic atherosclerosis, and possibly as cofactors in increasing the embolic risk of aortic plaques. As mentioned earlier, the plaque embolic potential is related at least in part to the presence of superimposed thrombus. It is therefore conceivable that the coexistence of a hypercoagulable state may increase the likelihood of thrombus formation, and enhance the plaque's embolic potential. Procoagulant properties have been demonstrated in atherosclerotic aortas; increased tissue factor expression and activity has been observed in the atherosclerotic intima that may lead to thrombus formation as the result of its exposure to the flowing blood.[52] Among coagulation factors, fibrinogen level has been shown to be a risk factor for cardiovascular disease and ischemic stroke,[53,54] and to be associated with degree of carotid stenosis,[55–57] abdominal aortic atheromas[55] and peripheral atherosclerotic disease.[58,59] Atherogenic effects of fibrinogen have been described, possibly as the result of its interactions with some lipoproteins. In fact, fibrinogen has been shown to modulate the atherogenic effects of lipoprotein (a),[60] and to increase the risk of severe carotid atherosclerosis and stroke in patients with low levels of HDL cholesterol.[61] The association between fibrinogen and carotid artery disease was particularly strong in the elderly.[62] Moreover, inter-racial differences have been reported in the levels of fibrinogen, with Blacks having higher levels than Whites[63] and both groups having higher levels than Asians.[64] Fibrinogen has also been shown to be independently associated with aortic atherosclerosis in a group of 148 patients undergoing TEE for valvular heart disease.[45] In that study, there was a relation between fibrinogen levels and severity of aortic atherosclerosis and of coronary artery disease.

Plasma homocysteine has been found to be independently associated with aortic atherosclerosis diagnosed by TEE. In a multivariate analysis in 82 cardiac patients, Tribouilloy and colleagues[65] found that age, male gender, LDL cholesterol and homocysteine levels were independently associated with severity of aortic atherosclerosis. Homocysteine may therefore be a marker of atherosclerosis in large arterial vessels. Also, homocysteine was independently associated with aortic arch atheroma progression over a period of 9 months in a group of 78 patients with stroke or TIA, whereas no conventional risk factor had similar independent effect.[42] Endothelial dysfunction causing plaque progression, or hypercoagulable state resulting in thrombus deposition was invoked as a possible mechanism.

In the APRIS study, prothrombin fragment F 1.2, an indicator of thrombin generation, was associated with large plaque presence in stroke patients ($P = 0.02$), but not in control subjects. Over a mean follow-up of 55.1 ± 37.2 months, stroke patients with large plaques and F1.2 levels over the median value had significantly higher risk of recurrent stroke and death than those with similar plaques but lower F 1.2 levels (230/1000 person-years versus 85/1000 person-years; $P = 0.05$).[20] This observation suggests that, in patients presenting with acute ischemic stroke, large aortic plaques are associated with blood hypercoagulability, suggesting a role for coagulation activation in the stroke mechanism.

The embolic potential of an aortic atheroma is also related to its lipid content. Cholesterol crystal emboli have been observed in peripheral arteries of patients with large atheromas seen on TEE.[66–68] However, total cholesterol, or even low-density lipoprotein (LDL) levels may not be the best predictors of arch atherosclerosis. In the APRIS study, low high-density lipoprotein (HDL) level and high apolipoprotein ratio Apo B/A1 ratio were better predictors of aortic atherosclerosis than LDL cholesterol, and HDL and Apo A1 levels were also inversely associated with plaque thickness ≥4 mm.[69] Lipoprotein (a) has been shown to be an independent marker of aortic atherosclerosis.[70] Lipoprotein (a) is a complex between LDL and apoprotein (a). In spite of the close structural resemblance between LDL and Lp (a), these particles have very different metabolic properties. Serum Lp (a) levels are under strong genetic influence and are mainly determined by the synthetic rate of apo (a), a protein with remarkable similarities to plasminogen, which has prompted the speculation that Lp (a) may be an important risk factor for both atherosclerosis and thrombosis. In addition, Lp (a) has been detected in atherosclerotic plaques, where it combines with fibrin and attenuates the clearance of this protein, promoting atherogenesis and vascular dysfunction.[71]

In addition to the control of traditional cardiovascular risk factors such as hypertension and dyslipidemia, other nonpharmacologic measures may be associated with lower aortic arch atherosclerotic burden. Light to moderate alcohol consumption was associated with decreased risk of any (adjusted OR 0.45, 95%CI, 0.29–0.68) or large (adjusted OR 0.51, 95%CI, 0.34–0.77) arch plaque in APRIS,[72] suggesting a possible mechanism for the decreased stroke risk associated with this level of alcohol consumption described in observational studies.[73]

PROXIMAL AORTIC PLAQUES AND CAROTID ARTERY DISEASE

The relation between proximal aortic plaques and carotid artery disease has been investigated in several studies. In Amarenco's autopsy study,[4] ulcerated aortic plaques were as frequent in patients with carotid stenosis ≥75% as in patients without it. In the same author's case-control TEE study,[17] no correlation was observed between aortic plaques ≥4 mm and carotid stenosis ≥70%. We observed that the frequency of carotid stenosis ≥60% increased with increasing aortic plaque thickness;[8] however, the positive predictive value of carotid stenosis ≥60% for arch plaque ≥5 mm was only 16%. Jones and colleagues[2] obtained similar results, reporting a positive predictive value of carotid disease for aortic plaque of 57%. In 62 cardiac patients, Kallikazaros and colleagues[74] reported that carotid plaque presence had good positive predictive value (83%) and acceptable sensitivity (75%) and specificity (74%) for aortic plaque presence, but lower negative predictive value (63%). In summary, a general correlation exists between carotid and aortic atherosclerosis, but one cannot be reliably predicted based on the presence of the other, with the possible exception of cardiac patients, in whom the relation appears to be tighter.[74]

PROXIMAL AORTIC PLAQUES AND CORONARY ARTERY DISEASE

The relation between aortic atherosclerosis and coronary artery disease has been extensively studied. In a TEE study on 61 patients who had undergone coronary angiography, Fazio and colleagues[75] found atherosclerotic plaques in the thoracic aorta in 37 of 41 patients (90%) with obstructive coronary disease (≥50% left main coronary artery stenosis or ≥70% stenosis in the left anterior descending, circumflex or right coronary arteries), but in only two of 20 patients (10%) with no or non-obstructive coronary disease. The presence of aortic plaque on TEE had 90% sensitivity and 90% specificity for obstructive coronary artery disease. In 153 consecutive patients, Khoury and colleagues[76] detected plaques in the aortas of 90 out of 97 patients (93%) with coronary stenosis ≥50% in ≥1 major branch versus 12 of 55 patients (22%) with normal coronaries. In the SPARC study,[1] aortic plaques were independently associated with history of myocardial infarction and coronary bypass surgery. In the population-based Rotterdam Coronary Calcification Study,[77] coronary calcification, assessed by electron beam computed tomography in 2,013 subjects, showed a graded association with aortic calcification, considered a marker of atherosclerosis. The association was stronger than that between coronary calcification and carotid disease.

The strength of the association between coronary disease and aortic atherosclerosis appears somewhat lower in elderly patients. In Khoury's study,[76] the specificity of aortic plaque presence for the diagnosis of coronary artery disease was decreased in patients over 63 years of age compared with younger patients (64% versus 90%). In another study on 84 cardiac patients,[78] the presence of aortic plaques failed to predict significant coronary artery disease in patients over 69 years of age, while it was a strong predictor in younger patients.

AORTIC PLAQUES AND ATHEROEMBOLISM

Besides being the site of origin of thromboembolism, the atherosclerotic aorta can also give origin to atheroembolic phenomena, in which cholesterol crystal emboli are sent to the arterial circulation. Atheroembolism is generally characterized by small embolic particles that lodge in arterioles (less than 200 μm in diameter),[79] and may occur spontaneously or following vascular surgery, arteriography or anticoagulation.[80,81] The clinical consequences of atheroembolism vary depending on the location of the target organ and the number and frequency of embolic episodes. Therefore, atheroembolism has a wide spectrum of clinical presentations, from clinically silent episodes only recognized during diagnostic procedures[82–84] to complex clinical pictures characterized by multiple organ involvement (brain, retina, kidneys, gastrointestinal tract, lower limbs).[85,86] The simultaneous or sequential involvement of different body segments may greatly facilitate a correct diagnosis in case of subtle or subacute clinical presentation.

Older age appears as the strongest risk factor for atheroembolism from an aortic source. All 16 cases of atheroembolism reported by Gore and Collins[85] were over age 60. In that study, 12 of 13 autopsied patients had evidence of embolism to multiple sites. Older age and aortic atherosclerosis have a major impact on the risk of atheroembolism following cardiac surgery, as will be discussed in the next section.

Proximal Aortic Plaques and Cardiac Surgery

Aortic atherosclerosis is widely recognized as a strong risk factor for atheroembolic events, and especially stroke, after cardiac surgery. As the population ages and indications for cardiac surgery expand, an ever-increasing number of elderly patients undergo open-heart surgery, raising the number of individuals at high risk for atheroembolic events. Blauth and colleagues[87] studied the autopsies of 221 subjects who had undergone cardiac surgery, and identified embolic disease in 69 (31%), atheroembolic in over two-thirds of cases. The brain was the most common target organ (16%), followed by spleen (11%), kidney (10%) and pancreas (7%). Atheroembolism was multiple in 63% of subjects, and was more common after coronary than after valvular procedures (26% versus 9%; P = 0.008). Atheroembolic events occurred in 37% of patients with severe ascending aortic atherosclerosis, but only in 2% of patients without significant aortic disease ($P < 0.0001$); 96% of patients who had evidence of atheroemboli had severe atherosclerosis of the ascending aorta. In that study, there was a strong relation between age, severe aortic atherosclerosis, and atheroembolism.

The consequences of atheroembolism during or after cardiac surgery may be devastating. In an autopsy study,[88] in six of 29 patients (21%) with evidence of atheroemboli, death was directly attributed to the embolic event (intraoperative cardiac failure due to coronary embolization in three, massive stroke in two, and extensive gastrointestinal embolization in one). Proximal aortic atherosclerosis is also associated with severe post-operative neurological complications. In a multicenter prospective study on 2,108 patients from 24 U.S. institutions,[89] the most severe cerebral complications (focal injury, or stupor or coma at discharge) after coronary bypass surgery were predicted by proximal aortic atherosclerosis, history of neurological disease and older age. In 921 consecutive patients undergoing cardiac surgery,[90] the incidence of post-operative stroke was 8.7% in patients with atherosclerotic disease of the ascending aorta and 1.8% in patients without it ($P < 0.0001$). Multivariate analysis indicated aortic atherosclerosis as the strongest predictor of perioperative stroke. Aortic atherosclerosis predicted both early (immediately after surgery) and delayed (after initial uneventful recovery) stroke after cardiac surgery in 2,972 patients.[91] In that study, 82% of early strokes and 71% of delayed strokes occurred in patients ≥65 years of age. In a recent study on 190 patients undergoing aortic arch surgery under deep hypothermic circulatory arrest and antegrade selective cerebral perfusion, a 7.0% incidence of intraoperative complications was observed (1.1% death, 5.9% stroke), and high-grade atheroma was the strongest predictor, especially for multiple-embolism stroke.[92]

The increased risk of stroke during coronary artery bypass has been linked to the cannulation of the aorta to establish extracorporeal circulation. Ura and colleagues[93] performed epiaortic echocardiography before cannulation and after decannulation in 472 patients undergoing cardiac surgery. A new lesion in the intima of the ascending aorta after decannulation was found in 16 patients (3.4%). In ten of the 16 (63%), the new lesions were severe, with mobile components

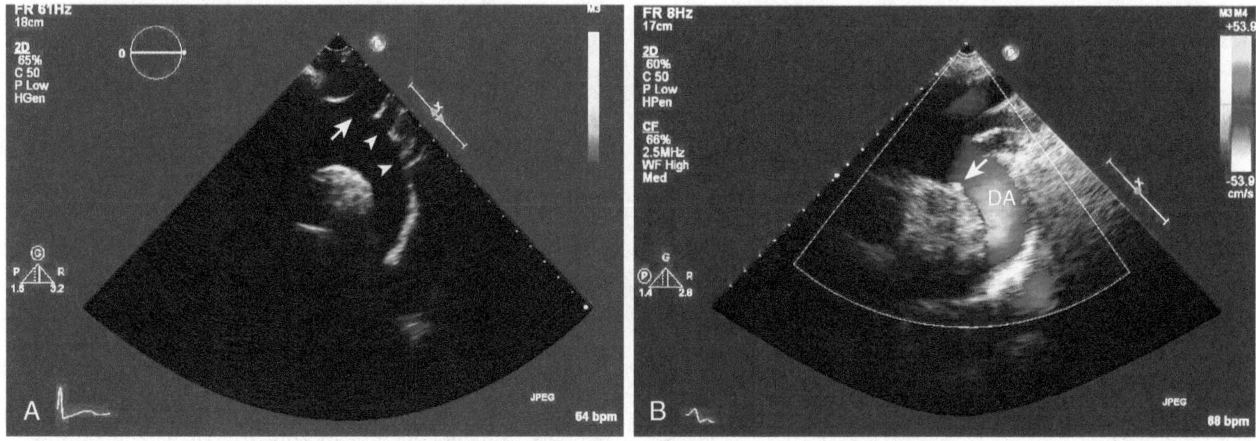

Figure 33-9. A, Imaging of the aortic arch by transthoracic echocardiography from a suprasternal window. The takeoff of the innominate artery (*large arrow*) and of the left carotid and left subclavian arteries (*small arrows*) is visualized. B, in the same view from a different patient, an atherosclerotic plaque (*arrow*) is visualized. Systolic flow into the innominate artery (red) and into the other branch vessels and the descending aorta (DA; blue) is seen by color flow Doppler.

or disruption of the intimal layer. Three patients in this group had a post-operative stroke. Thickness of the plaque near the site of aortic manipulation was associated with the development of a new lesion. The frequency of new lesion was 33.3% with plaque thickness ≥4 mm, 11.8% with thickness 3–4 mm, and only 0.8% with thickness <3 mm. It has been suggested that the incidence of peri-operative stroke and vascular events in patients with severe proximal aortic atherosclerosis can be reduced by modifications in surgical approach. Trehan and colleagues[94] performed TEE in 3,660 patients scheduled for coronary artery bypass surgery, and found proximal aortic atheromas with mobile components in 104 (2.84%). In those patients, they modified the surgical approach, the most frequent change being off-pump surgery (88 of 104 patients). The incidence of stroke and of vascular events at 1 week after surgery was 0.96% and 1.92%, respectively, and there were no embolic events in the 88 patients who had undergone off-pump surgery. Therefore, pre-operative TEE evaluation of the proximal aorta and modification of surgical techniques may decrease the incidence of stroke associated with cardiac surgery.

Proximal Aortic Plaques and Cardiac Catheterization

A high risk of embolism to the brain exists in subjects undergoing catheter-based diagnostic or therapeutic procedures involving the aortic arch who have severe atherosclerosis, often unbeknownst to the operator. This is especially important in elderly patients, and awareness of the presence of aortic plaques can be of great importance in reducing the risk of embolic sequelae. Karalis and colleagues[95] performed cardiac catheterization via the usual femoral approach in 59 patients with aortic atherosclerosis and in 71 control patients. The incidence of embolic events was 17% in the former group and 3% in the latter ($P = 0.01$). No embolic events occurred in 11 patients with aortic atherosclerosis in whom the femoral approach was replaced by a brachial approach. It is therefore evident that the identification of subjects at high risk of atheroembolism (elderly, with history of prior embolic events or evidence of atherosclerosis in other body segments, or with multiple risk factors for atherosclerosis) can be invaluable in selecting patients to refer for TEE before intra-aortic procedures, and could drastically reduce the incidence of embolic complications. Transthoracic echocardiography from a suprasternal window (Figs 33-9A, 33-9B) may often provide adequate visualization of the arch and therefore be used for screening purposes.

Obviously, the same considerations just discussed for diagnostic cardiac catheterization also apply to therapeutic procedures. Keeley and Grines[96] evaluated the frequency of aortic debris retrieved during placement of guiding catheters in 1,000 consecutive patients undergoing percutaneous revascularization procedures. In more than 50% of cases, guiding catheter placement was associated with scraping debris from the aorta. Allowing debris to exit the back of the catheter was essential to prevent the injection of atheromatous debris into the bloodstream. Karalis and colleagues[95] also compared the results of intra-aortic balloon pump placement in ten patients with aortic atherosclerosis and in 12 patients without it. An embolic event related to the procedure was observed in five patients (50%) in the former group, and in none in the latter ($P = 0.02$). Therefore, replacing femoral with brachial catheterization and avoiding placement of an intra-aortic balloon pump may reduce the risk of embolism.

Atherosclerosis of Aortic Arch Branch Vessels and Ischemic Stroke Risk

The innominate artery and left subclavian artery, which depart from the aortic arch, represent potential sites of origin of embolism to the brain. Frequently, aortic plaques may extend from the aorta into the proximal portion of these vessels. In a series of 283 patients with brain embolism, Fujimoto and colleagues found arch plaques ≥4 mm in 67 (25.3%); extension into the origin of the arch branches was observed in 51 of them (76.1%).[27] Over a mean follow-up of 3.4 years, 32 of 283 patients (11.3%) had recurrent cerebral ischemic events. Large plaques and extension to the branches were significantly more frequent in patients with recurrence (38% vs 16%; $P < 0.01$), and were associated with a 2.4-fold increase of recurrence after adjustment for age and hypertension (see Table 33-2).[27] In another study, out of 347 patients with recent ischemic stroke undergoing TEE (mean age 69 years), one-third had plaque visualized at the origin of the left subclavian artery. However, posterior circulation infarcts, which could be conceivably associated with embolism from the artery, were not more frequent in these patients.[97]

Subclavian steal syndrome is a condition in which the subclavian artery is stenosed or occluded, and blood flow in the ipsilateral vertebral artery is reversed, potentially leading to ischemia in the posterior brain circulation. The left subclavian artery, which is more often affected by atherosclerosis than its contralateral, is the most frequent location for the condition. Because subclavian steal is often asymptomatic, its prevalence in the general population is unknown. In a recent study on 7881 patients undergoing carotid duplex scan, blood pressure arm differential of >20 mmHg, a clue to possible subclavian stenosis, was observed in 514 (6.5%), affecting the left arm in over 80% of cases. Further diagnostic work-up revealed complete subclavian steal in 61%, partial steal in 23%.[98] Symptoms were present in 38 patients (7.4%), involving the posterior circulation in 32 of them, and were associated with higher blood pressure differential (>40–50 mmHg). In the end, only seven patients required intervention, either subclavian-carotid bypass or transluminal angioplasty with stenting.[98] Therefore, subclavian steal syndrome is a possible but probably rare cause of stroke in the posterior circulation, and clinically relevant ischemia tends to occur only when stenoses in the other cerebral arteries are also present.

TREATMENT OF PROXIMAL AORTIC PLAQUES

Although the role of proximal aortic plaques as a risk factor for cerebral and peripheral embolism has become increasingly evident, the best treatment options to reduce the risk of embolism are not yet clearly defined. Several preventive and therapeutic possibilities have been suggested, which will be reviewed in this section.

Systemic Anticoagulation

As most embolic events associated with large or complex proximal aortic plaques are thought to be thromboembolic, systemic anticoagulation has been suggested to reduce their incidence, especially in patients with superimposed thrombus. Dressler and colleagues[99] reported on the frequency of recurrent vascular events in 31 subjects presenting with a systemic embolic event and a mobile aortic plaque on TEE, according to the use of warfarin. Treatment was not randomized, and while 79% patients (11 of 14) with medium or large mobile components received warfarin, only 53% (nine of 17) of those with small mobile components (diameter ≤1 mm) did. Overall, 45% of patients not receiving warfarin had a vascular event over a mean follow-up of approximately 10 months, compared with 5% of those on warfarin. Corresponding figures for stroke were 27% and 0%, respectively. The authors concluded that warfarin was protective against recurrent embolic events in patients with mobile plaques, and that the dimension of the mobile component should not be used to assess the need for anticoagulation. Prospective results from the Stroke Prevention of Atrial Fibrillation (SPAF) study[100] showed a significant reduction of embolic events in patients with protruding atheromas treated with adjusted-dose warfarin (international normalized ratio, 2 to 3) compared with patients treated with low-intensity warfarin (international normalized ratio, 1.2 to 1.5) plus aspirin (325 mg/d). Overall, patients with complex aortic plaques had a fourfold increase in stroke incidence compared with patients without plaques, and adjusted-dose warfarin decreased the risk by 75% ($P = 0.005$). All patients had non-valvular atrial fibrillation, which precludes the direct extrapolation of the results to the general population.

While the use of oral anticoagulation in patients with mobile plaques appears logical, its use in patients with large but non-mobile lesions is more controversial. In 50 patients with atheromas ≥4 mm, but without mobile components followed for 22 ± 10 months, Ferrari et al.[101] found a substantial incidence of stroke in patients treated with aspirin or ticlopidine (5/23, or 21.7%), compared with no stroke in 27 patients on warfarin ($P = 0.01$). This study was small, however, and the treatment was not randomized. In the earlier-mentioned PICSS, medical treatment with warfarin or aspirin did not seem to affect the significance of the association between large arch plaques and recurrent events.[28] Although event rates tended to be lower in the warfarin than in the aspirin group (2-year event rate in patients with large plaques: 23.0% and 30.2%, respectively; $P = 0.21$), the difference was not statistically significant.[28] Further studies with larger patient populations are needed to evaluate the possibility of different efficacy between warfarin or newer anticoagulants and aspirin or other antiplatelet agents in specific patient subgroups, such as patients with cryptogenic stroke.

The safety of systemic anticoagulation in patients with aortic plaques has traditionally been questioned,[102] as anticoagulation might induce bleeding within the plaque, with consequent ulceration and risk of embolization. Moreover, anticoagulation might remove the thrombin coating from ulcerated atheromas and facilitate microembolization of cholesterol crystals.[103,104] Atheroembolism is a real clinical entity, and its sequelae[78-85] and association with anticoagulation[80,81] in patients with aortic atherosclerosis have been discussed earlier. However, its incidence after systemic anticoagulation appears to be rather low. In the SPAF study,[105] adjusted-dose treatment with warfarin (international normalized ratio, 2 to 3) was associated with an incidence of cholesterol embolization of 0.7% per year.

Antiplatelet Medications

As mentioned earlier, antiplatelet therapy with aspirin or ticlopidine has been reported to be less protective against recurrent embolic events than warfarin therapy in patients with large or complex plaques,[99,101,106] but generally in small studies without treatment randomization. The only data from a randomized study came from PICSS,[28] and were summarized earlier. The combination of aspirin and clopidogrel was tested against adjusted-dose warfarin in stroke patients with large (≥4mm) plaques enrolled in the Aortic arch Related Cerebral Hazard (ARCH) trial. Primary endpoint was a composite of recurrent stroke, myocardial infarction, peripheral embolism vascular death or intracerebral hemorrhage. Unfortunately, insufficient enrollment (349 patients enrolled of the anticipated 744) and lower than expected event rates during the follow-up resulted in the termination of the trial before adequate statistical power could be achieved. On the available data, over a median follow up of 3.4 years the primary endpoint occurred in 7.6 % of patients on combination therapy vs. 11.3% of those on warfarin therapy (log-rank, $P = 0.2$); adjusted HR was 0.76 (95% CI, 0.36 to 1.61, $P = 0.5$). Combination therapy was associated with a reduction in vascular deaths (0% vs. 3.4%; log-rank, $P = 0.013$), but this result was based on a very low number of events (0 and 6, respectively).[107] Therefore, additional data are needed to assess the role of antiplatelet agents in the prevention of aortic plaque-related embolic events, their relative efficacy in comparison with warfarin or newer anticoagulants, and the selection of patients suitable for either treatment.

Thrombolysis

Thrombolysis has been occasionally used to treat large mobile plaques with seemingly very high embolic potential.[108] A high risk of major hemorrhagic complications, especially in elderly patients, and the questionable advantages over anticoagulation make thrombolysis an unlikely therapeutic choice in patients with mobile plaques, and it should be reserved for selected cases. Like systemic anticoagulation, thrombolysis has also been associated with atheroembolic complications in patients with aortic atherosclerosis,[109] although the incidence of these complications is probably rather low.[110]

Statins

The use of statins to prevent embolic events in patients with large or complex aortic plaques has a powerful rationale, as statins may induce plaque stabilization through the reduction of the lipid content, with consequent reduced frequency of ulceration and superimposed thrombus formation. As mentioned earlier, statins have been shown to induce plaque regression in humans.[49–51] To date, no randomized trial has assessed the efficacy of statins for this indication. Nonrandomized data were reported by Tunick and colleagues,[111] who retrospectively identified 519 patients with severe thoracic aortic plaques and looked at the incidence of embolic events by treatment status (statins, warfarin, or antiplatelet medications). Patients taking each class of medication were matched with patients of similar age and embolic risk profile not taking that medication. Over an average follow-up of 34 ± 26 months, embolic events occurred in 111 patients (21%). In multivariate analysis, statin treatment was independently protective against recurring events (P = 0.0001). In the matched analysis, the relative risk reduction was 59%. No protective effect was found for warfarin or antiplatelet medication. Although with the limitations of the retrospective, non-randomized design, this study provided preliminary evidence on the efficacy of statins in preventing embolic events in patients with severe aortic plaques. Randomized controlled trials would be needed for confirmation, which are unlikely to be conducted since statins are now indicated after stroke, and a placebo-treated comparison group could be considered unethical.

Surgery

Aortic endarterectomy was proposed for patients with large mobile plaques in the proximal aorta at impending risk of embolism. However, this surgical procedure carries high risks, for the potential to dislodge parts of the plaque and precipitate an embolic event. Stern et al.[112] performed intraoperative TEE in 3,404 patients undergoing heart surgery, finding complex plaques (≥5 mm, or mobile) in 268 (8%). Arch endarterectomy was performed in 43 patients. The intra-operative stroke rate in the 268 patients was high (15.3%), as was mortality (14.9%). In multivariate analysis, age and arch endarterectomy were independently associated with intraoperative stroke (OR for arch endarterectomy: 3.6; P = 0.01). Therefore, the use of arch endarterectomy should be considered only in carefully selected cases.

Resection and graft replacement of a severely atherosclerotic segment of ascending aorta was performed by Rokkas and Kouchoukos in 81 patients (mean age 71) undergoing coronary bypass surgery.[113] The 30-day mortality was 8.6%. Perioperative strokes occurred in four patients (4.9%), and TIA in two (2.5%). During the follow-up, only one stroke occurred 4 months after the procedure. However, 3-year survival was only 40%, with mortality mainly secondary to complications from generalized atherosclerosis. In 17 patients undergoing graft replacement of severely atherosclerotic ascending aorta during coronary bypass grafting, King and colleagues[114] reported an in-hospital mortality of 23.5%, compared with only 2.3% in 89 patients undergoing replacement for ascending thoracic aortic aneurysm (P = 0.006). Cerebrovascular event rates were 17.6% and 3.4%, respectively (P = 0.05). Nonfatal post-operative complications were observed in 53% of the patients with atherosclerosis, compared with 20% of others (P = 0.01).

From the cumulative evidence presented, surgical procedures on a severe atherosclerotic proximal aorta are associated with substantial morbidity and mortality, and should be reserved for carefully selected cases.

PROXIMAL AORTIC PLAQUES AND ISCHEMIC STROKE: FUTURE DIRECTIONS

As the population ages, the proportion with atherosclerotic disease will increase, and identifying individuals at high risk of embolic events will become increasingly important for prevention. Better non-invasive ways to identify high-risk aortic plaques will be needed. More accurate assessment of plaque morphology and attempts to identify plaques more likely to rupture and give origin to embolic events (vulnerable plaques) will become important.

Plaque Morphology: Newer Imaging Modalities

The assessment of stroke risk in patients with proximal aortic plaques has been based on plaque thickness and morphology. Plaque thickness, although helpful for risk stratification, is a mono-dimensional measurement of a tri-dimensional lesion, and may, therefore, not convey the entire information on the plaque embolic potential. Also, plaque thickness and morphology are usually evaluated by TEE, a semi-invasive technique unsuitable for screening in asymptomatic individuals. Transthoracic echocardiography from a suprasternal or supraclavicular approach would be an easier and widely applicable technique, provided questions on its sensitivity in comparison with TEE can be addressed, especially for identification of complex plaque morphology. Real-time 3D echocardiography might prove useful in the non-invasive evaluation of the aortic arch. Figure 33-10 displays an example of an ulcerated plaque in the distal portion of the

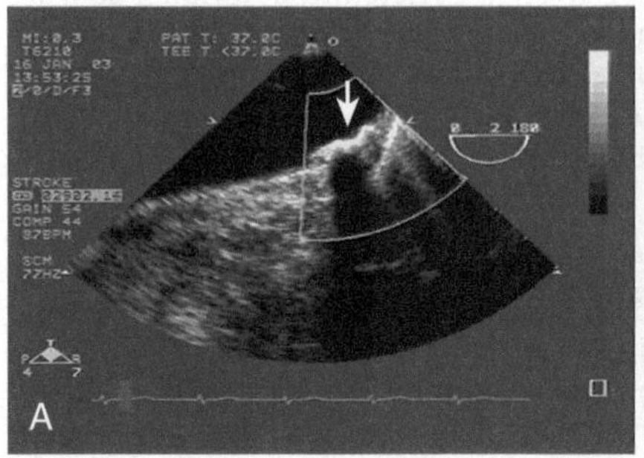

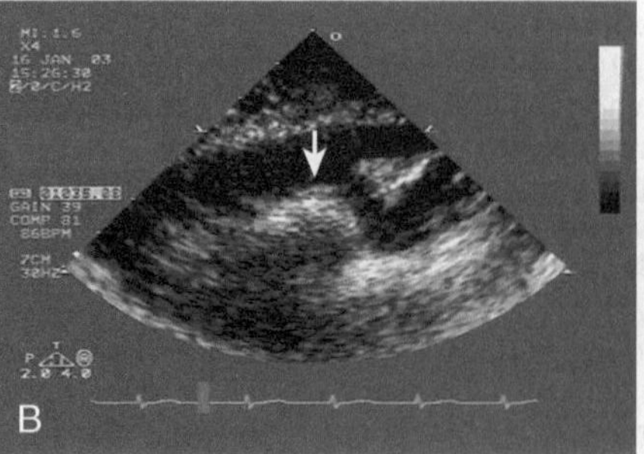

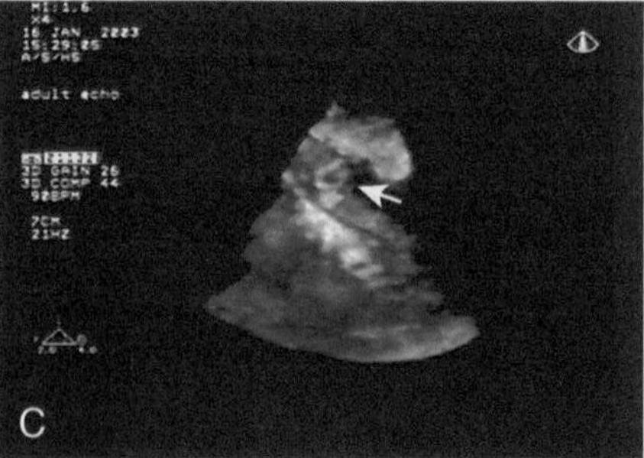

Figure 33-10. A, Transesophageal echocardiographic visualization of a calcified plaque in the distal aortic arch. A large ulceration (*arrow*) is seen. B, Same plaque as in A, visualized by suprasternal transthoracic approach. No definite ulceration is visible. C, Transthoracic 3D imaging of the same plaque. Rotation of transducer plane has allowed a better visualization of the plaque, and the entire area of ulceration (*arrow*) is now visible.

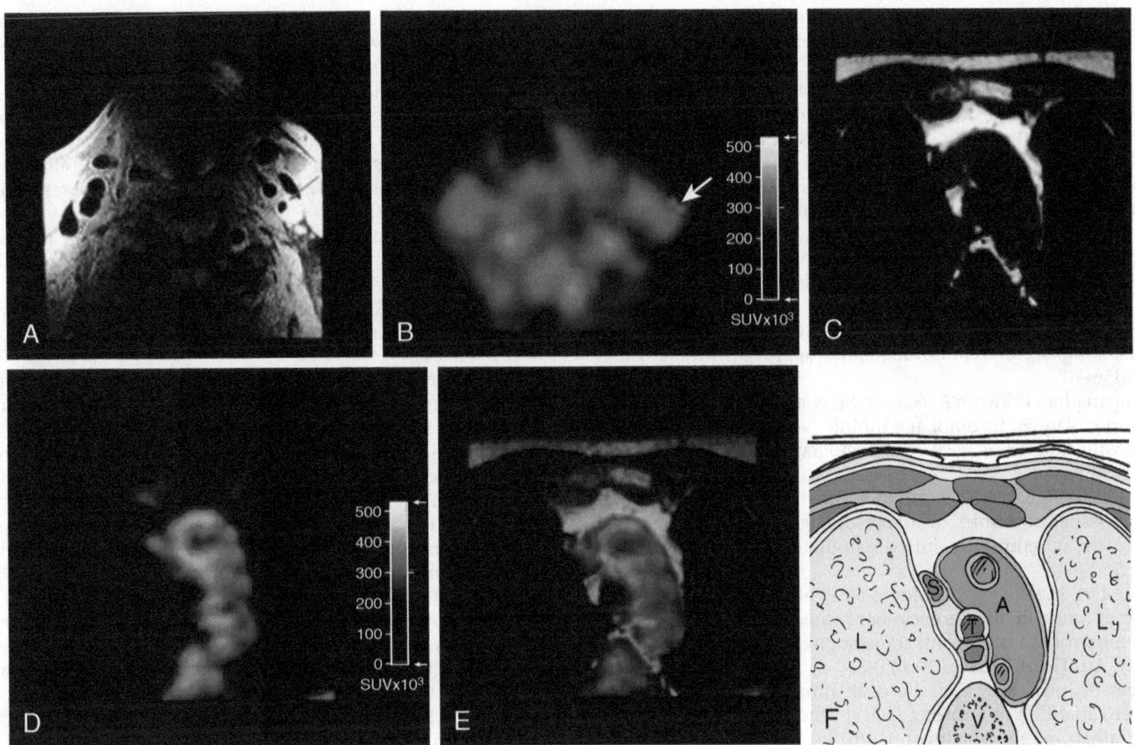

Figure 33-11. Co-registered axial fludeoxyglucose F 18 (FDG) positron emission tomography scan and MR image of the neck (*A* and *B*) and chest (*C* to *E*), showing minimal tracer uptake in the ipsilateral carotid artery (*arrow*) and high uptake into an eccentric plaque in the arch of the aorta. *F*, Schematic of chest MR images, showing the aortic arch (A) with plaque, lungs (L), superior vena cava (S), trachea (T), and vertebral body (V). *(Reprinted with permission from Moustafa RR, Azquierdo D, Weissberg PL, et al: Neurological picture: Identifying aortic plaque inflammation as a potential cause of stroke.* J Neurol Neurosurg Psychiatry *2008;79:236. ©BMJ Publishing Group Ltd.)*

aortic arch, visualized by TEE (A), traditional 2D transthoracic echocardiography (B), and 3D echocardiography (C). The advantages of 3D in displaying the extension of the plaque and its ulceration are apparent, with representation of plaque morphology that appears similar to that obtained by TEE. Further technical refinements, including transducers with smaller footprint to better fit into the suprasternal or supraclavicular notch, and assessment of diagnostic accuracy by comparison with TEE will be needed.

Besides echocardiography, other non-invasive techniques have been shown to have excellent accuracy for the detection of proximal aortic plaques. Magnetic resonance imaging (MRI) correlated well with TEE,[115] and accurately quantified the fibrotic and lipidic plaque components in animal models.[116] Compared with TEE, dual-helical computerized tomography (CT) showed sensitivity of 87%, specificity of 82% and overall accuracy of 84% for the detection of aortic plaques.[117] A combination of different techniques, such as positron emission tomography (PET) and MRI, has been successfully applied to the imaging of plaques in the aortic arch (Fig. 33-11).

Identification of the Vulnerable (High-Risk) Plaque

The non-invasive identification of the vulnerable plaque, or plaque that is at higher risk of rupture and consequent superimposed thrombus formation, would be of great importance to prevent embolic sequelae. MRI has shown potential for identifying components of a plaque;[116] newer contrast agents, such as those targeting iron-laden macrophages in the aortic subendothelium,[118] or activated matrix metalloproteinases (enzymes that have been implicated in the propensity of a plaque to rupture)[119] may enhance this capability. PET or PET/CT with18F-fluorodeoxyglucose is a promising tool to visualize inflammation in the plaque and statin-induced reduction in its degree.[120] Advantages of MRI over CT and PET/CT for vessel wall imaging include the absence of ionizing radiation and of need for exogenous contrast agents, as well as its being unaffected by severe calcification. However, MRI has lower spatial resolution and longer imaging time than CT, and lower sensitivity for depicting contrast agents than PET.[121] The further development of these techniques may improve their ability to identify those plaques that are more likely to become sources for cerebral embolization.

SUMMARY

Large and complex plaques in the proximal portion of the thoracic aorta are a risk factor for ischemic stroke, especially cryptogenic, and peripheral embolic events in patients over the age of 60 years. The frequency of embolic events, spontaneous or precipitated by diagnostic or therapeutic procedures on the aorta, has been defined. Data on treatments to decrease the embolic risk have been obtained, although further investigation remains to be done. Further advancement may come from improved imaging of high-risk plaques, and from the results of randomized treatment trials.

REFERENCES

1. Agmon Y, Khandheria BK, Meissner I, et al. Relation of coronary artery disease and cerebrovascular disease with atherosclerosis of the thoracic aorta in the general population. Am J Cardiol 2002;89:262–7.

2. Jones EF, Kalman JM, Calafiore P, et al. Proximal aortic atheroma. An independent risk factor for cerebral ischemia. Stroke 1995;26:218–24.
3. Russo C, Jin Z, Rundek T, et al. Atherosclerotic disease of the proximal aorta and the risk of vascular events in a population-based cohort: the Aortic Plaques and Risk of Ischemic Stroke (APRIS) study. Stroke 2009;40:2313–18.
4. Amarenco P, Duyckaerts C, Tzourio C, et al. The prevalence of ulcerated plaques in the aortic arch in patients with stroke. N Engl J Med 1992;326:221–5.
5. Khatibzadeh M, Mitusch R, Stierle U, et al. Aortic atherosclerotic plaques as a source of systemic embolism. J Am Coll Cardiol 1996;27:664–9.
6. Toyoda K, Yasaka M, Nagata S, et al. Aortogenic embolic stroke: a transesophageal echocardiographic approach. Stroke 1992; 23:1056–61.
7. Vaduganathan P, Ewton A, Nagueh SF, et al. Pathologic correlates of aortic plaques, thrombi and mobile "aortic debris" imaged in vivo with transesophageal echocardiography. J Am Coll Cardiol 1997;30:357–63.
8. Di Tullio MR, Sacco RL, Gersony D, et al. Aortic atheromas and acute ischemic stroke: a transesophageal echocardiographic study in an ethnically mixed population. Neurology 1996; 46:1560–6.
9. Stone DA, Hawke MW, LaMonte M, et al. Ulcerated atherosclerotic plaques in the thoracic aorta are associated with cryptogenic stroke: a multiplane transesophageal echocardiographic study. Am Heart J 1995;130:105–8.
10. Weber A, Jones EF, Zavala JA, et al. Intraobserver and interobserver variability of transesophageal echocardiography in aortic arch atheroma measurement. J Am Soc Echocardiogr 2008;21: 129–33.
11. Daniel WG, Erbel R, Kasper W, et al. Safety of transesophageal echocardiography. A multicenter survey of 10,419 examinations. Circulation 1991;83(3):817–21.
12. Oh JK, Seward JB, Tajik AJ. Transesophageal echocardiography. *The Echo Manual*. ed 2. Lippincott Williams & Wilkins; 1999. p. 23–36.
13. Chee TS, Quek SS, Ding ZP, et al. Clinical utility, safety, acceptability and complications of transoesophageal echocardiography (TEE) in 901 patients. Singapore Med J 1995;36(5):479–83.
14. Weslow RG, Di Tullio MR, Sacco RL. Safety and tolerability of transesophageal echocardiography in stroke patients. Cerebrovasc Dis 1995;5:243.
15. Zabalgoitia M, Gandhi DK, Evans J, et al. Transesophageal echocardiography in the awake elderly patient: its role in the clinical decision-making process. Am Heart J 1990;120(5): 1147–53.
16. Tunick PA, Perez JL, Kronzon I. Protruding atheromas in the thoracic aorta and systemic embolization. Ann Intern Med 1991;115(6):423–7.
17. Amarenco P, Cohen A, Tzourio C, et al. Atherosclerotic disease of the aortic arch and the risk of ischemic stroke. N Engl J Med 1994;331(22):1474–9.
18. Di Tullio MR, Sacco RL, Savoia MT, et al. Aortic atheroma morphology and the risk of ischemic stroke in a multiethnic population. Am Heart J 2000;139(2 Pt 1):329–36.
19. Davila-Roman VG, Barzilai B, Wareing TH, et al. Atherosclerosis of the ascending aorta. Prevalence and role as an independent predictor of cerebrovascular events in cardiac patients. Stroke 1994;25(10):2010–16.
20. Di Tullio MR, Homma S, Jin Z, et al. Aortic atherosclerosis, hypercoagulability and stroke: the Aortic Plaques and Risk of Ischemic Stroke (APRIS) Study. J Am Coll Cardiol 2008; 52(10):855–61.
21. Tenenbaum A, Motro M, Feinberg MS, et al. Retrograde flow in the thoracic aorta in patients with systemic emboli: a transesophageal echocardiographic evaluation of mobile plaque motion. Chest 2000;118(6):1703–8.
22. Harloff A, Nussbaumer A, Bauer S, et al. In vivo assessment of wall shear stress in the atherosclerotic aorta using flow-sensitive 4D MRI. Magn Reson Med 2010;63(6):1529–36.
23. Tunick PA, Rosenzweig BP, Katz ES, et al. High risk for vascular events in patients with protruding aortic atheromas: a prospective study. J Am Coll Cardiol 1994;23(5):1085–90.
24. Mitusch R, Doherty C, Wucherpfennig H, et al. Vascular events during follow-up in patients with aortic arch atherosclerosis. Stroke 1997;28(1):36–9.
25. Atherosclerotic disease of the aortic arch as a risk factor for recurrent ischemic stroke. The French Study of Aortic Plaques in Stroke Group. N Engl J Med 1996;334(19):1216–21.
26. Tanaka M, Yasaka M, Nagano K, et al. Moderate atheroma of the aortic arch and the risk of stroke. Cerebrovasc Dis 2006; 21(1–2):26–31.
27. Fujimoto S, Yasaka M, Otsubo R, et al. Aortic arch atherosclerotic lesions and the recurrence of ischemic stroke. Stroke 2004;35(6):1426–9.
28. Di Tullio MR, Russo C, Jin Z, et al. Aortic arch plaques and risk of recurrent stroke and death. Circulation 2009;119(17): 2376–82.
29. Guidoux C, Mazighi M, Lavallee P, et al. Aortic arch atheroma in transient ischemic attack patients. Atherosclerosis 2013; 231(1):124–8.
30. Di Tullio MR, Sacco RL, Savoia MT, et al. Gender differences in the risk of ischemic stroke associated with aortic atheromas. Stroke 2000;31(11):2623–7.
31. Sen S, Hinderliter A, Sen PK, et al. Aortic arch atheroma progression and recurrent vascular events in patients with stroke or transient ischemic attack. Circulation 2007;116(8): 928–35.
32. Cohen A, Tzourio C, Bertrand B, et al. Aortic plaque morphology and vascular events: a follow-up study in patients with ischemic stroke. FAPS Investigators. French Study of Aortic Plaques in Stroke. Circulation 1997;96(11):3838–41.
33. Tunick PA, Culliford AT, Lamparello PJ, et al. Atheromatosis of the aortic arch as an occult source of multiple systemic emboli. Ann Intern Med 1991;114(5):391–2.
34. Tunick PA, Lackner H, Katz ES, et al. Multiple emboli from a large aortic arch thrombus in a patient with thrombotic diathesis. Am Heart J 1992;124(1):239–41.
35. Nihoyannopoulos P, Joshi J, Athanasopoulos G, et al. Detection of atherosclerotic lesions in the aorta by transesophageal echocardiography. Am J Cardiol 1993;71(13):1208–12.
36. Ueno Y, Kimura K, Iguchi Y, et al. Mobile aortic plaques are a cause of multiple brain infarcts seen on diffusion-weighted imaging. Stroke 2007;38(9):2470–6.
37. Laperche T, Laurian C, Roudaut R, et al. Mobile thromboses of the aortic arch without aortic debris. A transesophageal echocardiographic finding associated with unexplained arterial embolism. The Filiale Echocardiographie de la Societe Francaise de Cardiologie. Circulation 1997;96(1):288–94.
38. Rundek T, Di Tullio MR, Sciacca RR, et al. Association between large aortic arch atheromas and high-intensity transient signals in elderly stroke patients. Stroke 1999;30(12):2683–6.
39. Castellanos M, Serena J, Segura T, et al. Atherosclerotic aortic arch plaques in cryptogenic stroke: a microembolic signal monitoring study. Eur Neurol 2001;45(3):145–50.
40. Zavala JA, Amarrenco P, Davis SM, et al. Aortic arch atheroma. Int J Stroke 2006;1(2):74–80.
41. Montgomery DH, Ververis JJ, McGorisk G, et al. Natural history of severe atheromatous disease of the thoracic aorta: a transesophageal echocardiographic study. J Am Coll Cardiol 1996; 27(1):95–101.
42. Sen S, Oppenheimer SM, Lima J, et al. Risk factors for progression of aortic atheroma in stroke and transient ischemic attack patients. Stroke 2002;33(4):930–5.
43. Geraci A, Weinberger J. Natural history of aortic arch atherosclerotic plaque. Neurology 2000;54(3):749–51.
44. Gupta V, Nanda NC, Yesilbursa D, et al. Racial differences in thoracic aorta atherosclerosis among ischemic stroke patients. Stroke 2003;34(2):408–12.
45. Tribouilloy C, Peltier M, Colas L, et al. Fibrinogen is an independent marker for thoracic aortic atherosclerosis. Am J Cardiol 1998;81(3):321–6.
46. Agmon Y, Khandheria BK, Meissner I, et al. Independent association of high blood pressure and aortic atherosclerosis: A population-based study. Circulation 2000;102(17):2087–93.
47. Iwata S, Jin Z, Schwartz JE, et al. Relationship between ambulatory blood pressure and aortic arch atherosclerosis. Atherosclerosis 2012;221(2):427–31.

48. Di Tullio MR, Savoia MT, Sacco RL. Aortic arch atheromas and ischemic stroke in patients of different race-ethnicity. Neurology 1996;46:A441.
49. Pitsavos CE, Aggeli KI, Barbetseas JD, et al. Effects of pravastatin on thoracic aortic atherosclerosis in patients with heterozygous familial hypercholesterolemia. Am J Cardiol 1998;82(12):1484–8.
50. Corti R, Fayad ZA, Fuster V, et al. Effects of lipid-lowering by simvastatin on human atherosclerotic lesions: a longitudinal study by high-resolution, noninvasive magnetic resonance imaging. Circulation 2001;104(3):249–52.
51. Corti R, Fuster V, Fayad ZA, et al. Lipid lowering by simvastatin induces regression of human atherosclerotic lesions: two years' follow-up by high-resolution noninvasive magnetic resonance imaging. Circulation 2002;106(23):2884–7.
52. Sueishi K, Ichikawa K, Nakagawa K, et al. Procoagulant properties of atherosclerotic aortas. Ann N Y Acad Sci 1995;748:185–92.
53. Qizilbash N. Fibrinogen and cerebrovascular disease. Eur Heart J 1995;16(Suppl. A):42–5.
54. Kannel WB, D'Agostino RB, Belanger AJ. Update on fibrinogen as a cardiovascular risk factor. Ann Epidemiol 1992;2(4):457–66.
55. Levenson J, Giral P, Razavian M, et al. Fibrinogen and silent atherosclerosis in subjects with cardiovascular risk factors. Arterioscler Thromb Vasc Biol 1995;15(9):1263–8.
56. Heinrich J, Schulte H, Schonfeld R, et al. Association of variables of coagulation, fibrinolysis and acute-phase with atherosclerosis in coronary and peripheral arteries and those arteries supplying the brain. Thromb Haemost 1995;73(3):374–9.
57. Agewall S, Wikstrand J, Suurkula M, et al. Carotid artery wall morphology, haemostatic factors and cardiovascular disease. An ultrasound study in men at high and low risk for atherosclerotic disease. Blood Coagul Fibrinolysis 1994;5(6):895–904.
58. Smith FB, Lowe GD, Fowkes FG, et al. Smoking, haemostatic factors and lipid peroxides in a population case control study of peripheral arterial disease. Atherosclerosis 1993;102(2):155–62.
59. Lassila R, Peltonen S, Lepantalo M, et al. Severity of peripheral atherosclerosis is associated with fibrinogen and degradation of cross-linked fibrin. Arterioscler Thromb 1993;13(12):1738–42.
60. Willeit J, Kiechl S, Santer P, et al. Lipoprotein(a) and asymptomatic carotid artery disease. Evidence of a prominent role in the evolution of advanced carotid plaques: the Bruneck Study. Stroke 1995;26(9):1582–7.
61. Szirmai IG, Kamondi A, Magyar H, et al. Relation of laboratory and clinical variables to the grade of carotid atherosclerosis. Stroke 1993;24(12):1811–16.
62. Willeit J, Kiechl S. Prevalence and risk factors of asymptomatic extracranial carotid artery atherosclerosis. A population-based study. Arterioscler Thromb 1993;13(5):661–8.
63. Folsom AR, Wu KK, Conlan MG, et al. Distributions of hemostatic variables in blacks and whites: population reference values from the Atherosclerosis Risk in Communities (ARIC) Study. Ethn Dis 1992;2(1):35–46.
64. Iso H, Folsom AR, Sato S, et al. Plasma fibrinogen and its correlates in Japanese and US population samples. Arterioscler Thromb 1993;13(6):783–90.
65. Tribouilloy CM, Peltier M, Iannetta Peltier MC, et al. Plasma homocysteine and severity of thoracic aortic atherosclerosis. Chest 2000;118(6):1685–9.
66. Katz ES, Tunick PA, Kronzon I. Observations of coronary flow augmentation and balloon function during intraaortic balloon counterpulsation using transesophageal echocardiography. Am J Cardiol 1992;69(19):1635–9.
67. Coy KM, Maurer G, Goodman D, et al. Transesophageal echocardiographic detection of aortic atheromatosis may provide clues to occult renal dysfunction in the elderly. Am Heart J 1992;123(6):1684–6.
68. Koppang JR, Nanda NC, Coghlan C, et al. Histologically Confirmed Cholesterol Atheroemboli with Identification of the Source by Transesophageal Echocardiography. Echocardiography 1992;9:379–83.
69. Kohsaka S, Jin Z, Rundek T, et al. Relationship between serum lipid values and atherosclerotic burden in the proximal thoracic aorta. Int J Stroke 2010;5(4):257–63.
70. Peltier M, Iannetta Peltier MC, Sarano ME, et al. Elevated serum lipoprotein(a) level is an independent marker of severity of thoracic aortic atherosclerosis. Chest 2002;121(5):1589–94.
71. Rabbani LE, Loscalzo J. Recent observations on the role of hemostatic determinants in the development of the atherothrombotic plaque. Atherosclerosis 1994;105(1):1–7.
72. Kohsaka S, Jin Z, Rundek T, et al. Alcohol consumption and atherosclerotic burden in the proximal thoracic aorta. Atherosclerosis 2011;219(2):794–8.
73. Thun MJ, Peto R, Lopez AD, et al. Alcohol consumption and mortality among middle-aged and elderly U.S. adults. N Engl J Med 1997;337(24):1705–14.
74. Kallikazaros IE, Tsioufis CP, Stefanadis CI, et al. Closed relation between carotid and ascending aortic atherosclerosis in cardiac patients. Circulation 2000;102(19 Suppl. 3):III263–8.
75. Fazio GP, Redberg RF, Winslow T, et al. Transesophageal echocardiographically detected atherosclerotic aortic plaque is a marker for coronary artery disease. J Am Coll Cardiol 1993;21(1):144–50.
76. Khoury Z, Gottlieb S, Stern S, et al. Frequency and distribution of atherosclerotic plaques in the thoracic aorta as determined by transesophageal echocardiography in patients with coronary artery disease. Am J Cardiol 1997;79(1):23–7.
77. Oei HH, Vliegenthart R, Hak AE, et al. The association between coronary calcification assessed by electron beam computed tomography and measures of extracoronary atherosclerosis: the Rotterdam Coronary Calcification Study. J Am Coll Cardiol 2002;39(11):1745–51.
78. Matsumura Y, Takata J, Yabe T, et al. Atherosclerotic aortic plaque detected by transesophageal echocardiography: its significance and limitation as a marker for coronary artery disease in the elderly. Chest 1997;112(1):81–6.
79. Soloway HB, Aronson SM. Atheromatous emboli to central nervous system. Report of 16 cases. Arch Neurol 1964;11:657–67.
80. Ben-Horin S, Bardan E, Barshack I, et al. Cholesterol crystal embolization to the digestive system: characterization of a common, yet overlooked presentation of atheroembolism. Am J Gastroenterol 2003;98(7):1471–9.
81. Theriault J, Agharazzi M, Dumont M, et al. Atheroembolic renal failure requiring dialysis: potential for renal recovery? A review of 43 cases. Nephron Clin Pract 2003;94(1):c11–18.
82. Bruno A, Russell PW, Jones WL, et al. Concomitants of asymptomatic retinal cholesterol emboli. Stroke 1992;23(6):900–2.
83. Bruno A, Jones WL, Austin JK, et al. Vascular outcome in men with asymptomatic retinal cholesterol emboli. A cohort study. Ann Intern Med 1995;122(4):249–53.
84. Mouradian M, Wijman CA, Tomasian D, et al. Echocardiographic findings of patients with retinal ischemia or embolism. J Neuroimaging 2002;12(3):219–23.
85. Gore I, Collins DP. Spontaneous atheromatous embolization. Review of the literature and a report of 16 additional cases. Am J Clin Pathol 1960;33:416–26.
86. Hauben M, Norwich J, Shapiro E, et al. Multiple cholesterol emboli syndrome – six cases identified through the spontaneous reporting system. Angiology 1995;46(9):779–84.
87. Blauth CI, Cosgrove DM, Webb BW, et al. Atheroembolism from the ascending aorta. An emerging problem in cardiac surgery. J Thorac Cardiovasc Surg 1992;103(6):1104–11.
88. Doty JR, Wilentz RE, Salazar JD, et al. Atheroembolism in cardiac surgery. Ann Thorac Surg 2003;75(4):1221–6.
89. Roach GW, Kanchuger M, Mangano CM, et al. Adverse cerebral outcomes after coronary bypass surgery. Multicenter Study of Perioperative Ischemia Research Group and the Ischemia Research and Education Foundation Investigators. N Engl J Med 1996;335(25):1857–63.
90. van der LJ, Hadjinikolaou L, Bergman P, et al. Postoperative stroke in cardiac surgery is related to the location and extent of atherosclerotic disease in the ascending aorta. J Am Coll Cardiol 2001;38(1):131–5.
91. Hogue CW Jr, Murphy SF, Schechtman KB, et al. Risk factors for early or delayed stroke after cardiac surgery. Circulation 1999;100(6):642–7.
92. Okada T, Shimamoto M, Yamazaki F, et al. Insights of stroke in aortic arch surgery: identification of significant risk factors and

surgical implication. Gen Thorac Cardiovasc Surg 2012;60(5): 268–74.
93. Ura M, Sakata R, Nakayama Y, et al. Ultrasonographic demonstration of manipulation-related aortic injuries after cardiac surgery. J Am Coll Cardiol 2000;35(5):1303–10.
94. Trehan N, Mishra M, Kasliwal RR, et al. Reduced neurological injury during CABG in patients with mobile aortic atheromas: a five-year follow-up study. Ann Thorac Surg 2000;70(5): 1558–64.
95. Karalis DG, Quinn V, Victor MF, et al. Risk of catheter-related emboli in patients with atherosclerotic debris in the thoracic aorta. Am Heart J 1996;131(6):1149–55.
96. Keeley EC, Grines CL. Scraping of aortic debris by coronary guiding catheters: a prospective evaluation of 1,000 cases. J Am Coll Cardiol 1998;32(7):1861–5.
97. Kuwashiro T, Toyoda K, Yoshimura S, et al. Atheromatous plaques at the origin of the left subclavian artery in patients with ischemic stroke. Cerebrovasc Dis 2010;29(3):290–6.
98. Labropoulos N, Nandivada P, Bekelis K. Prevalence and impact of the subclavian steal syndrome. Ann Surg 2010;252(1): 166–70.
99. Dressler FA, Craig WR, Castello R, et al. Mobile aortic atheroma and systemic emboli: efficacy of anticoagulation and influence of plaque morphology on recurrent stroke. J Am Coll Cardiol 1998;31(1):134–8.
100. Transesophageal echocardiographic correlates of thromboembolism in high-risk patients with nonvalvular atrial fibrillation. The Stroke Prevention in Atrial Fibrillation Investigators Committee on Echocardiography. Ann Intern Med 1998;128(8):639–47.
101. Ferrari E, Vidal R, Chevallier T, et al. Atherosclerosis of the thoracic aorta and aortic debris as a marker of poor prognosis: benefit of oral anticoagulants. J Am Coll Cardiol 1999;33(5): 1317–22.
102. Moldveen-Geronimus M, Merriam JC Jr. Cholesterol embolization. From pathological curiosity to clinical entity. Circulation 1967;35(5):946–53.
103. Hollier LH, Kazmier FJ, Ochsner J, et al. "Shaggy" aorta syndrome with atheromatous embolization to visceral vessels. Ann Vasc Surg 1991;5(5):439–44.
104. Hilton TC, Menke D, Blackshear JL. Variable effect of anticoagulation in the treatment of severe protruding atherosclerotic aortic debris. Am Heart J 1994;127(6):1645–7.
105. Blackshear JL, Zabalgoitia M, Pennock G, et al. Warfarin safety and efficacy in patients with thoracic aortic plaque and atrial fibrillation. SPAF TEE Investigators. Stroke Prevention and Atrial Fibrillation. Transesophageal echocardiography. Am J Cardiol 1999;83(3):453–5, A9.
106. Transesophageal echocardiographic correlates of thromboembolism in high-risk patients with nonvalvular atrial fibrillation. The Stroke Prevention in Atrial Fibrillation Investigators Committee on Echocardiography. Ann Intern Med 1998;128(8):639–47.
107. Amarenco P, Davis S, Jones EF, et al. Clopidogrel plus aspirin versus warfarin in patients with stroke and aortic arch plaques. Stroke 2014;45(5):1248–57.
108. Hausmann D, Gulba D, Bargheer K, et al. Successful thrombolysis of an aortic-arch thrombus in a patient after mesenteric embolism. N Engl J Med 1992;327(7):500–1.
109. Geraets DR, Hoehns JD, Burke TG, et al. Thrombolytic-associated cholesterol emboli syndrome: case report and literature review. Pharmacotherapy 1995;15(4):441–50.
110. Aggarwal K, Tjahja IE. Atheroembolic disease following administration of tissue plasminogen activator (TPA). Clin Cardiol 1996;19(11):906–8.
111. Tunick PA, Nayar AC, Goodkin GM, et al. Effect of treatment on the incidence of stroke and other emboli in 519 patients with severe thoracic aortic plaque. Am J Cardiol 2002;90(12): 1320–5.
112. Stern A, Tunick PA, Culliford AT, et al. Protruding aortic arch atheromas: risk of stroke during heart surgery with and without aortic arch endarterectomy. Am Heart J 1999;138(4 Pt 1): 746–52.
113. Rokkas CK, Kouchoukos NT. Surgical management of the severely atherosclerotic ascending aorta during cardiac operations. Semin Thorac Cardiovasc Surg 1998;10(4):240–6.
114. King RC, Kanithanon RC, Shockey KS, et al. Replacing the atherosclerotic ascending aorta is a high-risk procedure. Ann Thorac Surg 1998;66(2):396–401.
115. Fayad ZA, Nahar T, Fallon JT, et al. In vivo magnetic resonance evaluation of atherosclerotic plaques in the human thoracic aorta: a comparison with transesophageal echocardiography. Circulation 2000;101(21):2503–9.
116. Helft G, Worthley SG, Fuster V, et al. Atherosclerotic aortic component quantification by noninvasive magnetic resonance imaging: an in vivo study in rabbits. J Am Coll Cardiol 2001;37(4):1149–54.
117. Tenenbaum A, Garniek A, Shemesh J, et al. Dual-helical CT for detecting aortic atheromas as a source of stroke: comparison with transesophageal echocardiography. Radiology 1998; 208(1):153–8.
118. Litovsky S, Madjid M, Zarrabi A, et al. Superparamagnetic iron oxide-based method for quantifying recruitment of monocytes to mouse atherosclerotic lesions in vivo: enhancement by tissue necrosis factor-alpha, interleukin-1beta, and interferon-gamma. Circulation 2003;107(11):1545–9.
119. Lancelot E, Amirbekian V, Brigger I, et al. Evaluation of matrix metalloproteinases in atherosclerosis using a novel noninvasive imaging approach. Arterioscler Thromb Vasc Biol 2008;28(3): 425–32.
120. Tahara N, Kai H, Ishibashi M, et al. Simvastatin attenuates plaque inflammation: evaluation by fluorodeoxyglucose positron emission tomography. J Am Coll Cardiol 2006;48(9): 1825–31.
121. Makowski MR, Botnar RM. MR imaging of the arterial vessel wall: molecular imaging from bench to bedside. Radiology 2013;269(1):34–51.

34 Stroke Related to Surgery and Other Procedures

Steven R. Messé, Michael T. Mullen

KEY POINTS

- Periprocedural stroke accounts for at least 5% of the ~800,000 strokes that occur each year in the US.
- Stroke can occur after a wide range of surgeries, and when it occurs it is associated with substantial morbidity, mortality, and cost.
- Surgeries with high risk of periprocedural stroke include carotid revascularization, intracranial vascular procedures, cardiac valve surgery, thoracic aortic procedures, and coronary artery bypass grafting.
- Predictors of periprocedural stroke are similar to predictors of stroke in the general population and include advanced age, history of prior stroke, and/or history of other vascular disease.
- Carotid screening prior to high-risk surgeries, including coronary artery bypass grafting, should be limited to selected high-risk patients. The utility of pre-operative or simultaneous carotid revascularization is uncertain, but is not likely to be beneficial unless the patient is recently symptomatic or has severe bilateral asymptomatic disease.
- Stopping antithrombotic therapy in the periprocedural period may be associated with an increased risk of stroke. For dental and dermatologic procedures continuation of antithrombotic therapy, including aspirin and warfarin, is likely safe. Optimal management for more invasive procedures is less certain.
- Major surgery within 14 days is a contra-indication to intravenous rt-PA. Patients who have had minor procedures at a readily compressible site, such as percutaneous coronary intervention, may still be treated. Endovascular therapy should be considered after more invasive procedures.

INTRODUCTION

Many surgical and endovascular procedures place the central nervous system at direct risk of ischemic injury, and any procedure requiring anesthesia or with the possibility of significant blood loss has the potential to cause neurologic injury, particularly in high-risk patients. When they occur, periprocedural strokes are associated with a dramatic increase in morbidity, mortality, and healthcare costs. For example, stroke complicating cardiac surgery has been reported to double the duration and cost of hospitalization, increase the mortality rate 5–10-fold, and leave the majority of survivors with significant disability.[1-4]

The risk of periprocedural stroke depends in part on the particular intervention being performed. Stroke after general surgery and vascular surgery (excluding the carotid and thoracic aorta) is estimated to be less than 1%.[5-8] Stroke risk after cardiac catheterization is also low, with estimates ranging from 0.1 to 0.4%, although rates are likely higher after valvuloplasty and electrophysiologic ablation procedures.[9-22] The risk of stroke is significantly higher during cardiac surgery, carotid revascularization, cerebrovascular procedures, and thoracic or thoracoabdominal aortic repairs.[1,4,23-36] Among cardiac procedures, valve procedures are higher risk than coronary artery bypass graft (CABG) and multivalve or combined CABG plus valve replacement are highest of all.[37] In general, endovascular procedures in the heart or cervicocephalic vessels are higher risk for stroke than comparable open surgical procedures. Multiple randomized trials of carotid revascularization have demonstrated a higher risk of stroke but a lower risk of myocardial infarction with stenting than endarterectomy.[27,38-40] Compared to traditional surgical aortic valve replacement, randomized trials of transcutaneous aortic valve replacement (TAVR) have yielded mixed results, with one study finding similar risk of stroke and another suggesting that TAVR had double the risk of stroke.[41,42] A notable exception to the apparent increased risk of stroke in endovascular cardiac procedures, relative to open procedures, is percutaneous coronary intervention (PCI), which has a significantly lower risk of stroke than CABG. Although CABG patients are more likely to have multivessel coronary disease and diffuse atherosclerosis, observed differences are not explained solely by patient selection.[13] Table 34-1 presents a list of common cardiovascular and cerebrovascular procedures, a range of risks for neurologic ischemia quoted from the literature, and an estimated number of procedures performed annually in the US. Taken together, these estimates suggest that periprocedural stroke accounts for at least 5% of the ~800,000 strokes that occur each year in the US.

PERIOPERATIVE RISK ASSESSMENT

Numerous patient-level predictors of peri-operative stroke have been identified. Not surprisingly, risk factors for peri-operative stroke are similar to stroke risk factors in the general population including advanced age, history of prior stroke, diabetes, and a history of vascular disease. A multicenter prospective study of patients undergoing coronary artery bypass grafting surgery found that age, history of previous neurological disease, diabetes, history of vascular disease, previous coronary artery surgery, unstable angina, and history of pulmonary disease were independent predictors of neurologic complications.[43] Another study of 2,792 patients with a history of cerebrovascular disease or over age 65 undergoing CABG and/or cardiac valve surgery found that independent predictors of early stroke (upon awakening from anesthesia) included female sex, prior neurological event, aortic atherosclerosis, and duration of cardiopulmonary bypass.[44] Delayed stroke was independently associated with female sex, prior neurological event, diabetes, aortic atherosclerosis, and the combined end points of low cardiac output and atrial fibrillation. Another prospective study including over 16,000 patients undergoing a variety of cardiac surgeries identified the following risk factors: history of cerebrovascular disease, peripheral vascular disease, diabetes, hypertension, previous cardiac

TABLE 34-1 Common Procedures and the Reported Risk for Neurologic Ischemic Complications

Procedure	Ischemic Neurologic Complication Rate	Estimated Annual Number of Procedures in the US[99]
Cardiac catheterization[11,100]	Stroke in 0.2–0.5%	1,000,000
Coronary artery bypass grafting (CABG)[23,24]	Stroke in 1–4%	450,000
Asymptomatic carotid endarterectomy (CEA) or stenting[25–27]	Stroke in 1–3%	100,000
Symptomatic CEA or stenting[27–29,65]	Stroke in 4–10%	70,000
Cerebral aneurysm clipping or coiling[30]	Stroke in 6–10%	20,000
Intracranial stenting[31,32]	Stroke in 9–15%	500
Cardiac valve replacement[4,33,34]	Stroke in 2–17%	100,000
Descending thoracic aorta and thoracoabdominal aorta repair[1,4,35]	Stroke in 1.4–8.7% Spinal infarct in 3.8–23%	20,000

surgery, pre-operative infection, urgent operation, cardiopulmonary bypass time more than 2 hours, need for intra-operative hemofiltration, and high transfusion requirement.[37] Multiple risk prediction scores have been developed for the prediction of stroke after CABG.[43,45] The CHADS2 and CHADS2-VaSC scores, which were originally developed to predict the risk of stroke in patients with atrial fibrillation, also predict the risk of stroke after CABG.[46,47] Existing risk prediction models have moderate discriminatory ability. Unfortunately, most identified risk factors are not modifiable and there are no therapies proven to reduce the risk of stroke in high-risk individuals or procedures. For high-risk patients the relative risks/benefits of surgery should be carefully considered to determine whether the procedure is necessary, and the patient should be monitored closely for signs and symptoms of stroke in the perioperative period. Specific interventions for perioperative stroke are discussed below.

As noted, prior stroke is a strong predictor of peri-operative risk. Optimal timing of elective surgery in patients who have had a recent stroke is unknown. Cerebrovascular autoregulation is dysfunctional following stroke, and data suggest that cerebral autoregulation may remain impaired for up to 10 days after stroke.[48–50] During this period, peri-operative blood pressure changes have the potential to impact cerebral blood flow, placing the brain at risk for further ischemia if pressure drops and hemorrhage if pressure rises. Discontinuation of antithrombotic therapy in anticipation of surgery may also increase the risk of stroke.[51–54] In many cases, the risk of recurrent stroke is highest in the weeks and months immediately following a stroke, and discontinuation of antithrombotic therapy may be particularly risky during this period. For all of these reasons, elective surgery should be delayed, when possible, for at least 2–4 weeks and up to 90 days for truly elective procedures. The major exception to this rule is carotid revascularization after stroke from a symptomatic carotid stenosis. The benefit of carotid revascularization is maximized when performed within 2 weeks from symptom onset, and current guidelines from the American Heart Association support early revascularization in selected patients.[55,56]

Another potential exception is valve surgery following stroke due to endocarditis, although ideal timing is uncertain. A small randomized trial of 76 patients, 29% of whom had a cerebral embolism, found that in patients with vegetations >10 mm and severe valvular dysfunction, surgery within 48 hours reduced the rates of in-hospital death and embolic events within 6 weeks (3% vs 23%).[57] An observational study of 198 patients suggested that early surgery is safe in endocarditis patients with a recent ischemic stroke, although there may be significant selection bias in this non-randomized study.[58] For patients with small or clinically silent infarcts who otherwise require valve surgery it may be safe to proceed to early surgery. For patients with larger infarcts, those with mycotic aneurysms, and certainly for patients who present with an intracerebral hemorrhage, the risk of early surgery is likely higher and treatment decisions must be individualized. It is not known whether unruptured mycotic aneurysms should be secured prior to surgery or if antibiotic therapy alone is sufficient therapy.

Prior studies have identified certain intra-operative factors that may impact periprocedural stroke risk. Maintaining a higher intra-operative goal for mean arterial pressure (MAP) has been associated with fewer areas of diffusion restriction on MRI after carotid endarterectomy.[59] Similarly, a randomized trial of a high (80–100 mm Hg) versus low (50–60 mm Hg) MAP goal during CABG found that the higher MAP goal was associated with reduced cardiac and cerebrovascular complications.[60] A series of 98 patients with clinical stroke after cardiac surgery found that a drop in MAP of greater than 10 mm Hg from preoperative baseline to intra-operative MAP was associated with the development of bilateral watershed infarct, which was seen in almost half of the patients and was associated with poor short-term outcome.[61] Among patients undergoing procedures that require cardiopulmonary bypass, longer duration of time on bypass is associated with increased risk of stroke.[4,37,62,63] Finally, based on non-randomized studies of carotid endarterectomy, local anesthesia may have a reduced likelihood of stroke compared to general anesthesia.[64]

CAROTID ASSESSMENT PRIOR TO CARDIAC AND OTHER SURGERY

As noted in Chapter 74, there is robust evidence that carotid revascularization for symptomatic moderate-to-severe carotid stenosis is beneficial.[65] However, it remains controversial whether neurologically asymptomatic patients should be screened for extracranial carotid atherosclerosis prior to undergoing cardiovascular surgery or other interventions. Although a carotid bruit has been associated with an increased risk of post-surgical encephalopathy and stroke, the presence of a bruit is not strongly associated with carotid stenosis.[3,66] Among patients in the North American Symptomatic Carotid Endarterectomy Trial (NASCET), the presence of a carotid bruit had a sensitivity of 63% and a specificity of 61% for ipsilateral high-grade stenosis.[67] Carotid ultrasonography has a sensitivity and specificity of more than 90% for the detection of moderate to severe carotid stenosis.[68] However, most patients undergoing surgery will not have concomitant severe carotid atherosclerosis, so screening unselected patients is likely a poor use of healthcare resources. When severe carotid stenosis is identified, it is unclear whether or not to attempt revascularization, and if revascularization is considered, it is unclear by what means (stenting or open endarterectomy) and in what order it should occur (before, during, or after the cardiac procedure).

While the data are limited, there does not appear to be a strong association between peri-operative stroke and presence of an asymptomatic carotid stenosis. A retrospective cohort study of 4,335 patients who underwent CABG identified stroke in 1.8%, but the stroke was attributable to a significant carotid stenosis in only 5% of these events.[69] In contrast, patients who underwent combined carotid and cardiac operations had a greatly increased risk of post-operative stroke compared to patients with a similar degree of carotid stenosis who underwent cardiac surgery alone (15.1% vs 0%; $P = 0.004$). A 2011 meta-analysis demonstrated that the risk of peri-operative stroke after cardiac surgery was increased among those with ≥50% carotid stenosis.[70] Patients with prior stroke/TIA or complete occlusion of the carotid artery were at particularly high risk. Patients with carotid stenosis and no recent stroke/TIA were not at an increased risk of peri-operative stroke. Another retrospective study of carotid duplex ultrasound prior to CABG compared 117 patients with severe asymptomatic carotid stenosis (≥75%) to 761 patients without severe carotid stenosis and reported similar rates of in-hospital stroke (3.4 vs 3.6%) and mortality (3.4 vs 4.2%) in both groups.[71] Published guidelines from the American Heart Association and American College of Cardiology recommend limiting carotid screening prior to CABG to patients who are >65 years old, have left main coronary disease, peripheral vascular disease, history of tobacco use, history of prior stroke/TIA, or a carotid bruit.[72,73] In general, carotid revascularization should only be considered in patients with a recently symptomatic carotid stenosis >50%, bilateral asymptomatic carotid stenosis ≥70%, or unilateral asymptomatic carotid stenosis ≥70% with a contralateral carotid occlusion.[72,73] There is insufficient evidence to make firm recommendations about the timing of carotid revascularization and the relative merits of carotid artery stenting (CAS) versus carotid endarterectomy (CEA). Treatment decisions must be individualized, but given the greater risk of myocardial infarction after CEA and the high complication rate with combined CEA and CABG, CAS is an appealing alternative in patients who require carotid revascularization before CABG, if dual antiplatelet therapy is not contraindicated.

PERIPROCEDURAL ANTITHROMBOTIC MANAGEMENT IN PATIENTS WITH CEREBROVASCULAR DISEASE

Neurologists are frequently asked to provide guidance on the management of antithrombotic medication in patients with prior stroke who are planning interventional, surgical, or dental procedures. For most patients, the absolute risk of recurrent stroke in the setting of a brief suspension of antithrombotic medication for a procedure is not high. However, when peri-operative stroke occurs there may be devastating long-term consequences whereas most peri-procedural bleeding complications do not have persistent sequelae.

It is tempting to estimate the risk of a brief cessation of antithrombotic medication by prorating the estimated annual risk of an untreated stroke patient. However, this approach likely underestimates the actual risk as surgery is thought to contribute to a procoagulable milieu via inflammation, dehydration, and immobility, which may transiently increase the risk of myocardial infarction and/or stroke. Further, there may be a rebound effect in response to cessation of antithrombotic therapy, resulting in a disproportionately elevated short-term risk. In 2013 the American Academy of Neurology (AAN) performed a systematic review of the risks and benefits of stopping antithrombotic medication before invasive procedures.[34] Several informative studies were identified. A double-blind study randomized 109 patients to continue aspirin and 111 to discontinue aspirin prior to non-cardiac surgery.[74] Twelve patients (5.4%) had major adverse cardiac events (MACE), defined as acute myocardial infarction, cardiac arrest, cardiovascular death, or severe arrhythmia. Although the number of events was low, treatment with aspirin resulted in a 7.2% absolute risk reduction (95% confidence interval [CI], 1.3–13%) for post-operative MACE. No significant differences in bleeding complications were seen between the two groups. Another case control study compared 309 stroke patients who had been previously prescribed aspirin for secondary prevention and 309 matched controls without recent stroke.[53] Patients with recent stroke were significantly more likely to have recently discontinued aspirin, adjusted OR 3.4 (95%CI, 1.08–10.63; $P < 0.005$). A primary care database in the UK identified patients taking aspirin for secondary prevention and followed them for a mean of 3.4 years to assess predictors of stroke and TIA.[52] Cerebrovascular events were more common among those who discontinued aspirin 31–180 days before the index date (RR 1.40; 95%CI, 1.03–1.92). The risk was even greater among those who had discontinued use in the 2 weeks prior to the event (RR 1.97; 95%CI, 1.24-3.12). A prospective observational study described 1,293 episodes of patients who stopped taking Coumadin prior to a planned procedure; 80% of patients had warfarin therapy withheld for 5 days or fewer.[51] Peri-operative bridging heparin or low-molecular-weight heparin was used in 8.3% of cases overall. Peri-procedural thromboembolism occurred in 0.7% (95%CI, 0.3–1.4%), none of whom had received bridging therapy. Six patients (0.6%; 95%CI, 0.2–1.3%) experienced major bleeding, whereas an additional 17 patients (1.7%; 95%CI, 1.0–2.6%) experienced a clinically significant, non-major bleeding episode. Of the 23 patients who had bleeding episodes, 14 received peri-procedural heparin or low-molecular-weight heparin.

A large randomized trial comparing perioperative aspirin to placebo in 10,010 subjects undergoing in-hospital, non-cardiac surgery was published shortly after the AAN review.[75] In this study the risk of death or non-fatal myocardial infarction was similar in the aspirin and placebo groups (7.0% vs 7.1%, HR = 0.99, 95%CI, 0.86–1.15). Aspirin use was associated with a small absolute increase in the risk of major bleeding (4.6% vs 3.8%, HR = 1.23, 95%CI, 1.01–1.49). Stroke was rare, occurring in 0.3% of the aspirin group and 0.4% of the placebo group ($P = 0.62$). Most of the patients (78%) were undergoing major surgery, defined as intra-peritoneal, intrathoracic, retro-peritoneal, or major orthopedic surgery. A history of vascular disease was present in 33% of the subjects and only 5% had a prior history of stroke. Although these findings may not be generalizable to patients with a prior history of stroke or patients undergoing minor surgeries, these data suggest that it is likely appropriate to discontinue antiplatelet therapy before major non-cardiac open surgical procedures.

The comprehensive literature review performed by the AAN identified some less invasive procedures in which the risk of clinically significant bleeding with continued antithrombotic medication is very low.[34] In particular, there is strong evidence that aspirin has a very low risk of major bleeding complications during dental procedures and thus, it is reasonable to continue aspirin in the vast majority of patients.[34] There is moderate evidence supporting a very low risk for meaningful bleeding complications in patients who continue aspirin and undergo invasive ocular anesthesia, cataract surgery, dermatologic procedures, transrectal ultrasound-guided prostate biopsy, spinal/epidural procedures, and carpal tunnel surgery.[34] There is weak evidence that the risk of bleeding is low in patients taking aspirin prior to vitreoretinal surgery, EMG, transbronchial lung biopsy, colonoscopic polypectomy, upper endoscopy, and abdominal ultrasound-guided biopsies. It is unknown if the AAN recommendations can be extrapolated to other antiplatelet agents, such as clopidogrel or prasugrel. Dual antiplatelet therapy is likely to be higher risk.

Similar to aspirin, there is strong evidence that warfarin has a very low risk of major bleeding complications during dental procedures and it is likely reasonable to continue warfarin in most patients.[34] For warfarin, there is moderate evidence suggesting a very low risk for bleeding in patients who continue warfarin prior to a dermatologic procedure. Warfarin may increase the risk of bleeding after colonoscopic polypectomy and so it is likely reasonable to temporarily discontinue anticoagulation for this procedure.[34] There are, unfortunately, limited or no data assessing the risk of bleeding due to use of warfarin during other more invasive procedures. Although it may be safe to continue aspirin during a range of procedures, warfarin likely poses an unacceptably high risk of bleeding for most procedures. Similarly, the risk of periprocedural bleeding while on a novel oral anticoagulant, none of which are reversible at this time, is likely to be unacceptably high. Clinical judgment should be informed by the expected cerebrovascular risk for each individual patient and the bleeding risk associated with the planned procedure. General recommendations for peri-operative antithrombotic management are summarized in Table 34-2. There are little data that bridging therapy with heparin, low-molecular-weight heparin, or a novel oral anticoagulant reduces perioperative stroke; although, there is biologic plausibility. Some, but not all, studies have suggested an increased risk of bleeding with bridging therapy; although, the existing studies are likely biased and there is insufficient evidence to make a recommendation about the use of routine bridging therapy.[76–79]

Neurologists are often asked to provide neurologic "clearance" for patients prior to invasive procedures. Although there are existing guidelines for peri-operative cardiovascular clearance, no such guidelines exist for neurologic clearance.[80] Evaluations should account for the indications for surgery, the risk of the procedure, and individual patient risk factors. As detailed above, antithrombotic therapy can be continued for many minor procedures. For other procedures, the period of time off antithrombotic therapy should be minimized. Based on studies of intra-operative stroke risk factors noted above, neurologists should recommend that surgeons, interventionalists, and anesthesiologists be vigilant about blood pressure management and avoid hypotension when possible. In addition, patients should be carefully monitored in the peri-operative period for signs and symptoms of stroke.

ACUTE STROKE THERAPY

Acute stroke therapies, including intravenous (IV) recombinant tissue plasminogen activator (rt-PA), intra-arterial thrombolysis, and/or mechanical thrombectomy, have the potential to recanalize occluded arteries, restore blood flow to ischemic brain tissue, and reduce disability after stroke when they are delivered rapidly after symptom onset. Peri-operative stroke occurs intra-operatively in about 40–50% of cases and in the immediate post-operative period in many more.[81,82] Because post-operative strokes typically occur while patients are hospitalized, they present an opportunity for early identification and treatment within established windows.[83] Medical management of ischemic stroke, including thrombolytic therapy, antiplatelet therapy, and permissive hypertension, will be reviewed in other chapters. In peri-operative patients the risks and benefits of these therapies must be carefully considered, as there may be increased risk in this population. This is particularly true for thrombolytic therapy. Although thrombolytic therapy has the potential to reverse a serious

TABLE 34-2 Antiplatelet Management in the Perioperative Period

Antithrombotic Agent	Perioperative Management	Notes
Aspirin*	• Continue for low-risk procedures such as dental procedures, dermatologic procedures, prostate biopsy, EMG, anterior chamber ophthalmologic procedures, colonoscopy with polypectomy • Uncertain if continuation is necessary for more invasive surgeries. It is likely appropriate to stop aspirin before most major open surgical procedures, but decisions will need to be individualized • Discontinue for 7–10 days prior to intracranial, posterior chamber of the eye, intramedullary spine, and other procedures where a small amount of hemorrhage could be devastating	• Dual antiplatelet therapy likely carries a higher risk of hemorrhage than single antiplatelet therapy • Patients with recent coronary artery stent should delay discontinuation of antiplatelet therapy, if possible, according to guidelines by stent type
Warfarin	• Continue for dental procedures • May be able to continue for dermatologic procedures, EMG, prostate procedures • Discontinue for 5 days prior to more invasive procedures, including colonoscopy with polypectomy	• PT/INR to monitor drug activity
Dabigatran	<u>Manufacturer recommendations:</u> • 1–2 days if CrCl ≥ 50 mL/min* • 3–5 days if CrCl <50 mL/min* Consider longer time periods for major surgery, spinal puncture*	• Ecotrin clotting time monitors activity • A low normal aPTT may provide evidence for little or no anticoagulation effect[101]
Rivaroxaban	<u>Manufacturer recommendations:</u> • 24 hours prior	• Anticoagulant activity can be monitored with a factor Xa level[102]
Apixaban	<u>Manufacturer recommendations:</u> • 24 hours prior to low-risk procedures • 48 hours prior to moderate- to high-risk procedures	• Anticoagulant activity can be monitored with a factor Xa level[102]
Edoxaban	<u>Manufacturer recommendations:</u> • At least 24 hours prior to surgery	• Anticoagulant activity can be monitored with a factor Xa level

*It is unknown if these recommendations can be extrapolated to patients treated with other antiplatelet agents such as aspirin plus extended-release dipyridamole, clopidogrel, or prasugrel.

neurologic deficit, treatment decisions must also consider the risk of devastating bleeding at the operative site.

Intravenous rt-PA has been proven to reduce disability after stroke and guidelines support its use up to 4.5 hours after ischemic stroke.[84–89] Major surgery within 14 days is a strong relative contra-indication to IV rt-PA.[87] Fibrin at the surgical site could be disrupted by rt-PA, leading to clinically significant bleeding. The risks associated with rt-PA use after surgeries have not been well studied, and "major" surgery has not been defined in existing guidelines. It is likely that the risk of systemic bleeding varies considerably with the extent of the surgery and with the time from the procedure. Patients who have had minor procedures at readily compressible sites are not excluded from IV rt-PA. Examples of such procedures include cardiac catheterization or digit amputation. A small case series consisting of seven patients with stroke complicating cardiac catheterization who were safely treated with IV rt-PA reported no major systemic bleeding and no increase in minor puncture site bleeding.[90] More invasive procedures, in which surgical site bleeding is likely to be serious, should be excluded from IV rt-PA up to 14 days post-operatively. In some instances the risk of bleeding complications with IV rt-PA may extend beyond 14 days, as illustrated by a case of hemopericardium reported in a patient treated with IV rt-PA 16 days after coronary artery bypass surgery.[91] After particularly invasive surgeries, or surgeries in which a small amount of peri-operative bleeding could have catastrophic complications, such as cardiac surgery, neurosurgery, organ transplant, or laryngeal surgery, it may be prudent to avoid IV rt-PA beyond 14 days. Neurosurgical procedures are likely to be particularly high risk. Other forms of cerebral injury, such as prior stroke or severe head trauma, are strong contra-indications to IV rt-PA within 90 days and it may be reasonable to exclude neurosurgical patients for an equivalent length of time. For all cases of peri-operative stroke, clinical decision making should be individualized, and both the severity of the stroke and the potential for clinically significant bleeding at the operative site should be carefully considered.

For acute stroke patients who have had major surgery within 14 days, endovascular therapy with intra-arterial thrombolysis (IAT) and/or mechanical thrombectomy is the preferred therapeutic modality when available.[92–96] These therapies are generally used within 6–8 hours of symptom onset, although data suggest that they are most effective when reperfusion, not initiation of therapy, is achieved within 7 hours.[97] Although these targeted interventions should be associated with lower rates of systemic bleeding than IV rt-PA, there may still be risk. A retrospective case series of 36 patients who received IAT within 2 weeks of surgery reported surgical site bleeding in nine patients (25%).[98] This was minor in six patients and major in three. Major bleeding occurred in two of three neurosurgical patients (intracranial hemorrhage) and in one of 18 cardiac surgery patients (hemopericardium). Although the number of neurosurgical patients was small, the concerning rate of ICH suggests that neurosurgical patients should be considered particularly high risk. Mechanical thrombectomy without the use of thrombolytic drugs should theoretically have a lower risk of intracerebral hemorrhage and is the preferred therapeutic intervention in post-neurosurgical patients.

CONCLUSION

Stroke is a common and feared complication of a wide range of surgical and interventional procedures. It is particularly common after carotid revascularization, cardiothoracic, neurosurgical, and endovascular procedures. Overall, iatrogenic stroke comprises a small but meaningful portion of the total strokes that occur in the US each year. Unfortunately, most risk factors for perioperative stroke, such as age, prior stroke, diabetes, and history of vascular disease, are not modifiable, so decisions to pursue elective surgery must balance the risk of stroke against the need for surgery. There is not a clear link between asymptomatic carotid stenosis and peri-operative stroke risk, so screening carotid ultrasound is not recommended in unselected patients; however, there may be a role in selected patients preparing to undergo coronary artery bypass graft (CABG). Continued use of aspirin or warfarin before minor interventions such as dental and dermatologic procedures is likely safe and may be beneficial for high-risk patients. Finally, when a peri-operative stroke does occur aggressive interventions are available, which may be able to reverse acute neurologic deficits with an acceptable bleeding risk in appropriately selected patients.

REFERENCES

1. McKhann GM, Grega MA, Borowicz LM Jr, et al. Stroke and encephalopathy after cardiac surgery: An update. Stroke 2006;37: 562–71.
2. John R, Choudhri AF, Weinberg AD, et al. Multicenter review of preoperative risk factors for stroke after coronary artery bypass grafting. Ann Thorac Surg 2000;69:30–5, discussion 35–36.
3. Puskas JD, Winston AD, Wright CE, et al. Stroke after coronary artery operation: Incidence, correlates, outcome, and cost. Ann Thorac Surg 2000;69:1053–6.
4. Messe SR, Acker MA, Kasner SE, et al. Stroke after aortic valve surgery: Results from a prospective cohort. Circulation 2014;129: 2253–61.
5. Axelrod DA, Stanley JC, Upchurch GR Jr, et al. Risk for stroke after elective noncarotid vascular surgery. J Vasc Surg 2004;39: 67–72.
6. Bateman BT, Schumacher HC, Wang S, et al. Perioperative acute ischemic stroke in noncardiac and nonvascular surgery: Incidence, risk factors, and outcomes. Anesthesiology 2009;110: 231–8.
7. Kam PC, Calcroft RM. Peri-operative stroke in general surgical patients. Anaesthesia 1997;52:879–83.
8. Sharifpour M, Moore LE, Shanks AM, et al. Incidence, predictors, and outcomes of perioperative stroke in noncarotid major vascular surgery. Anesth Analg 2013;116:424–34.
9. Brown DL, Topol EJ. Stroke complicating percutaneous coronary revascularization. Am J Cardiol 1993;72:1207–9.
10. Dukkipati S, O'Neill WW, Harjai KJ, et al. Characteristics of cerebrovascular accidents after percutaneous coronary interventions. J Am Coll Cardiol 2004;43:1161–7.
11. Fuchs S, Stabile E, Kinnaird TD, et al. Stroke complicating percutaneous coronary interventions: Incidence, predictors, and prognostic implications. Circulation 2002;106:86–91.
12. Noto TJ Jr, Johnson LW, Krone R, et al. Cardiac catheterization 1990: A report of the registry of the society for cardiac angiography and interventions (sca&i). Cathet Cardiovasc Diagn 1991; 24:75–83.
13. Serruys PW, Morice MC, Kappetein AP, et al. Percutaneous coronary intervention versus coronary-artery bypass grafting for severe coronary artery disease. N Engl J Med 2009;360:961–72.
14. Wong SC, Minutello R, Hong MK. Neurological complications following percutaneous coronary interventions (a report from the 2000-2001 new york state angioplasty registry). Am J Cardiol 2005;96:1248–50.
15. McKay RG. The mansfield scientific aortic valvuloplasty registry: Overview of acute hemodynamic results and procedural complications. J Am Coll Cardiol 1991;17:485–91.
16. [No authors listed]. Percutaneous balloon aortic valvuloplasty. Acute and 30-day follow-up results in 674 patients from the nhlbi balloon valvuloplasty registry. Circulation 1991;84: 2383–97.
17. Bhargava M, Marrouche NF, Martin DO, et al. Impact of age on the outcome of pulmonary vein isolation for atrial fibrillation using circular mapping technique and cooled-tip ablation catheter. J Cardiovasc Electrophysiol 2004;15:8–13.

18. Chen SA, Chiang CE, Tai CT, et al. Complications of diagnostic electrophysiologic studies and radiofrequency catheter ablation in patients with tachyarrhythmias: An eight-year survey of 3,966 consecutive procedures in a tertiary referral center. Am J Cardiol 1996;77:41–6.
19. Hindricks G. The Multicentre European Radiofrequency Survey (MERFS): Complications of radiofrequency catheter ablation of arrhythmias. The Multicentre European Radiofrequency Survey (MERFS) Investigators of the Working Group on Arrhythmias of the European Society of Cardiology. Eur Heart J 1993;14: 1644–53.
20. Kay GN, Epstein AE, Dailey SM, et al. Role of radiofrequency ablation in the management of supraventricular arrhythmias: Experience in 760 consecutive patients. J Cardiovasc Electrophysiol 1993;4:371–89.
21. Scheinman MM, Huang S. The 1998 NASPE prospective catheter ablation registry. Pacing Clin Electrophysiol 2000;23:1020–8.
22. Zhou L, Keane D, Reed G, et al. Thromboembolic complications of cardiac radiofrequency catheter ablation: A review of the reported incidence, pathogenesis and current research directions. J Cardiovasc Electrophysiol 1999;10:611–20.
23. Likosky DS, Leavitt BJ, Marrin CAS, et al. Intra- and postoperative predictors of stroke after coronary artery bypass grafting. Ann Thorac Surg 2003;76:428–34.
24. Salazar JD, Wityk RJ, Grega MA, et al. Stroke after cardiac surgery: Short- and long-term outcomes. Ann Thorac Surg 2001;72: 1195–201.
25. Young B, Moore WS, Robertson JT, et al. An analysis of perioperative surgical mortality and morbidity in the asymptomatic carotid atherosclerosis study. Acas investigators. Asymptomatic carotid artheriosclerosis study. Stroke 1996;27:2216–24.
26. MRC Asymptomatic Carotid Surgery Trial (ACST) Collaborative Group. Prevention of disabling and fatal strokes by successful carotid endarterectomy in patients without recent neurological symptoms: Randomised controlled trial. Lancet 2004;363: 1491–502.
27. Brott TG, Hobson RW 2nd, Howard G, et al. Stenting versus endarterectomy for treatment of carotid-artery stenosis. N Engl J Med 2010;363:11–23.
28. Ferguson GG, Eliasziw M, Barr HW, et al. The north american symptomatic carotid endarterectomy trial: Surgical results in 1415 patients. Stroke 1999;30:1751–8.
29. Rothwell PM, Gutnikov SA, Warlow CP. Reanalysis of the final results of the european carotid surgery trial. Stroke 2003;34: 514–23.
30. Ross IB, Dhillon GS. Complications of endovascular treatment of cerebral aneurysms. Surg Neurol 2005;64:12–18.
31. Zaidat OO, Klucznik R, Alexander MJ, et al. The NIH registry on use of the wingspan stent for symptomatic 70-99% intracranial arterial stenosis. Neurology 2008;70:1518–24.
32. Chimowitz MI, Lynn MJ, Derdeyn CP, et al. Stenting versus aggressive medical therapy for intracranial arterial stenosis. N Engl J Med 2011;365:993–1003.
33. Vasques F, Messori A, Lucenteforte E, et al. Immediate and late outcome of patients aged 80 years and older undergoing isolated aortic valve replacement: A systematic review and meta-analysis of 48 studies. Am Heart J 2012;163:477–85.
34. Armstrong MJ, Gronseth G, Anderson DC, et al. Summary of evidence-based guideline: Periprocedural management of antithrombotic medications in patients with ischemic cerebrovascular disease: Report of the guideline development subcommittee of the american academy of neurology. Neurology 2013;80: 2065–9.
35. Coselli JS, Bozinovski J, LeMaire SA. Open surgical repair of 2286 thoracoabdominal aortic aneurysms. Ann Thorac Surg 2007;83:S862–4.
36. Messe SR, Bavaria JE, Mullen M, et al. Neurologic outcomes from high risk descending thoracic and thoracoabdominal aortic operations in the era of endovascular repair. Neurocrit Care 2008;9:344–51.
37. Bucerius J, Gummert JF, Borger MA, et al. Stroke after cardiac surgery: A risk factor analysis of 16,184 consecutive adult patients. Ann Thorac Surg 2003;75:472–8.
38. Ringleb PA, Allenberg J, Bruckmann H, et al. 30 day results from the space trial of stent-protected angioplasty versus carotid endarterectomy in symptomatic patients: A randomised non-inferiority trial. Lancet 2006;368:1239–47.
39. Mas JL, Chatellier G, Beyssen B, et al. Endarterectomy versus stenting in patients with symptomatic severe carotid stenosis. N Engl J Med 2006;355:1660–71.
40. Ederle J, Dobson J, Featherstone RL, et al. Carotid artery stenting compared with endarterectomy in patients with symptomatic carotid stenosis (international carotid stenting study): An interim analysis of a randomised controlled trial. Lancet 2010; 375:985–97.
41. Leon MB, Smith CR, Mack M, et al. Transcatheter aortic-valve implantation for aortic stenosis in patients who cannot undergo surgery. N Engl J Med 2010;363:1597–607.
42. Adams DH, Popma JJ, Reardon MJ, et al. Transcatheter aortic-valve replacement with a self-expanding prosthesis. N Engl J Med 2014.
43. Newman MF, Wolman R, Kanchuger M, et al. Multicenter preoperative stroke risk index for patients undergoing coronary artery bypass graft surgery. Multicenter study of perioperative ischemia (mcspi) research group. Circulation 1996;94:II74–80.
44. Hogue CW Jr, Murphy SF, Schechtman KB, et al. Risk factors for early or delayed stroke after cardiac surgery. Circulation 1999; 100:642–7.
45. Charlesworth DC, Likosky DS, Marrin CA, et al. Development and validation of a prediction model for strokes after coronary artery bypass grafting. Ann Thorac Surg 2003;76:436–43.
46. Hornero F, Martin E, Paredes F, et al. Stroke after coronary artery bypass grafting: Preoperative predictive accuracies of CHADS2 and CHA2DS2VASc stroke risk stratification schemes. J Thorac Cardiovasc Surg 2012;144:1428–35.
47. Hornero F, Martin E, Rodriguez R, et al. A multicentre spanish study for multivariate prediction of perioperative in-hospital cerebrovascular accident after coronary bypass surgery: The PACK2 score. Interact Cardiovasc Thorac Surg 2013;17:353–8, discussion 358.
48. Dawson SL, Panerai RB, Potter JF. Serial changes in static and dynamic cerebral autoregulation after acute ischaemic stroke. Cerebrovasc Dis 2003;16:69–75.
49. Olsen TS, Larsen B, Herning M, et al. Blood flow and vascular reactivity in collaterally perfused brain tissue. Evidence of an ischemic penumbra in patients with acute stroke. Stroke 1983; 14:332–41.
50. Hillis AE, Ulatowski JA, Barker PB, et al. A pilot randomized trial of induced blood pressure elevation: Effects on function and focal perfusion in acute and subacute stroke. Cerebrovasc Dis 2003;16:236–46.
51. Garcia DA, Regan S, Henault LE, et al. Risk of thromboembolism with short-term interruption of warfarin therapy. Arch Intern Med 2008;168:63–9.
52. Garcia Rodriguez LA, Cea Soriano L, Hill C, et al. Increased risk of stroke after discontinuation of acetylsalicylic acid: A uk primary care study. Neurology 2011;76:740–6.
53. Maulaz AB, Bezerra DC, Michel P, et al. Effect of discontinuing aspirin therapy on the risk of brain ischemic stroke. Arch Neurol 2005;62:1217–20.
54. Patel MR, Hellkamp AS, Lokhnygina Y, et al. Outcomes of discontinuing rivaroxaban compared with warfarin in patients with nonvalvular atrial fibrillation: Analysis from the ROCKET AF trial (rivaroxaban once-daily, oral, direct factor Xa inhibition compared with vitamin K antagonism for prevention of stroke and embolism trial in atrial fibrillation). J Am Coll Cardiol 2013;61:651–8.
55. Rothwell PM, Eliasziw M, Gutnikov SA, et al. Endarterectomy for symptomatic carotid stenosis in relation to clinical subgroups and timing of surgery. Lancet 2004;363:915–24.
56. Furie KL, Kasner SE, Adams RJ, et al. Guidelines for the prevention of stroke in patients with stroke or transient ischemic attack: A guideline for healthcare professionals from the american heart association/american stroke association. Stroke 2011;42: 227–76.
57. Kang DH, Kim YJ, Kim SH, et al. Early surgery versus conventional treatment for infective endocarditis. N Engl J Med 2012; 366:2466–73.
58. Barsic B, Dickerman S, Krajinovic V, et al. Influence of the timing of cardiac surgery on the outcome of patients with

infective endocarditis and stroke. Clin Infect Dis 2013;56: 209–17.
59. Kobayashi M, Ogasawara K, Yoshida K, et al. Intentional hypertension during dissection of carotid arteries in endarterectomy prevents postoperative development of new cerebral ischemic lesions caused by intraoperative microemboli. Neurosurgery 2011;69:301–7.
60. Gold JP, Charlson ME, Williams-Russo P, et al. Improvement of outcomes after coronary artery bypass. A randomized trial comparing intraoperative high versus low mean arterial pressure. J Thorac Cardiovasc Surg 1995;110:1302–11, discussion 1311–1304.
61. Gottesman RF, Sherman PM, Grega MA, et al. Watershed strokes after cardiac surgery: Diagnosis, etiology, and outcome. Stroke 2006;37:2306–11.
62. Brown WR, Moody DM, Challa VR, et al. Longer duration of cardiopulmonary bypass is associated with greater numbers of cerebral microemboli. Stroke 2000;31:707–13.
63. Filsoufi F, Rahmanian PB, Castillo JG, et al. Incidence, imaging analysis, and early and late outcomes of stroke after cardiac valve operation. Am J Cardiol 2008;101:1472–8.
64. Rerkasem K, Rothwell PM. Local versus general anaesthesia for carotid endarterectomy. Cochrane Database Syst Rev 2008; CD000126.
65. Rothwell PM, Eliasziw M, Gutnikov SA, et al. Analysis of pooled data from the randomised controlled trials of endarterectomy for symptomatic carotid stenosis. Lancet 2003;361:107–16.
66. McKhann GM, Grega MA, Borowicz LM Jr, et al. Encephalopathy and stroke after coronary artery bypass grafting: Incidence, consequences, and prediction. Arch Neurol 2002;59:1422–8.
67. Sauve JS, Thorpe KE, Sackett DL, et al. Can bruits distinguish high-grade from moderate symptomatic carotid stenosis? The north american symptomatic carotid endarterectomy trial. Ann Intern Med 1994;120:633–7.
68. Grant EG, Benson CB, Moneta GL, et al. Carotid artery stenosis: Grayscale and doppler ultrasound diagnosis – society of radiologists in ultrasound consensus conference. Ultrasound Q 2003;19: 190–8.
69. Li Y, Walicki D, Mathiesen C, et al. Strokes after cardiac surgery and relationship to carotid stenosis. Arch Neurol 2009;66:1091–6.
70. Naylor AR, Bown MJ. Stroke after cardiac surgery and its association with asymptomatic carotid disease: An updated systematic review and meta-analysis. Eur J Vasc Endovasc Surg 2011;41: 607–24.
71. Mahmoudi M, Hill PC, Xue Z, et al. Patients with severe asymptomatic carotid artery stenosis do not have a higher risk of stroke and mortality after coronary artery bypass surgery. Stroke 2011;42:2801–5.
72. Brott TG, Halperin JL, Abbara S, et al. 2011 ASA/ACCF/AHA/AANN/AANS/ACR/ASNR/CNS/SAIP/SCAI/SIR/SNIS/SVM/SVS guideline on the management of patients with extracranial carotid and vertebral artery disease: executive summary. A report of the American College of Cardiology Foundation/American Heart Association Task Force on Practice Guidelines, and the American Stroke Association, American Association of Neuroscience Nurses, American Association of Neurological Surgeons, American College of Radiology, American Society of Neuroradiology, Congress of Neurological Surgeons, Society of Atherosclerosis Imaging and Prevention, Society for Cardiovascular Angiography and Interventions, Society of Interventional Radiology, Society of NeuroInterventional Surgery, Society for Vascular Medicine, and Society for Vascular Surgery. Circulation 2011;124:489–532.
73. Hillis LD, Smith PK, Anderson JL, et al. 2011 ACCF/AHA guideline for coronary artery bypass graft surgery: A report of the American College of Cardiology Foundation/American Heart Association Task Force on Practice Guidelines. Circulation 2011; 124:e652–735.
74. Oscarsson A, Gupta A, Fredrikson M, et al. To continue or discontinue aspirin in the perioperative period: A randomized, controlled clinical trial. Br J Anaesth 2010;104:305–12.
75. Devereaux PJ, Mrkobrada M, Sessler DI, et al. Aspirin in patients undergoing noncardiac surgery. N Engl J Med 2014;370: 1494–503.
76. Gerson LB, Michaels L, Ullah N, et al. Adverse events associated with anticoagulation therapy in the periendoscopic period. Gastrointest Endosc 2010;71:1211–17, e1212.
77. Jaffer AK, Brotman DJ, Bash LD, et al. Variations in perioperative warfarin management: Outcomes and practice patterns at nine hospitals. Am J Med 2010;123:141–50.
78. Krane LS, Laungani R, Satyanarayana R, et al. Robotic-assisted radical prostatectomy in patients receiving chronic anticoagulation therapy: Role of perioperative bridging. Urology 2008;72: 1351–5.
79. McBane RD, Wysokinski WE, Daniels PR, et al. Periprocedural anticoagulation management of patients with venous thromboembolism. Arterioscler Thromb Vasc Biol 2010;30:442–8.
80. Fleisher LA, Beckman JA, Brown KA, et al. ACC/AHA 2007 guidelines on perioperative cardiovascular evaluation and care for noncardiac surgery: a report of the American College of Cardiology/American Heart Association Task Force on Practice Guidelines (Writing Committee to Revise the 2002 Guidelines on Perioperative Cardiovascular Evaluation for Noncardiac Surgery): developed in collaboration with the American Society of Echocardiography, American Society of Nuclear Cardiology, Heart Rhythm Society, Society of Cardiovascular Anesthesiologists, Society for Cardiovascular Angiography and Interventions, Society for Vascular Medicine and Biology, and Society for Vascular Surgery. Circulation 2007;116:e418–99.
81. Tarakji KG, Sabik JF 3rd, Bhudia SK, et al. Temporal onset, risk factors, and outcomes associated with stroke after coronary artery bypass grafting. JAMA 2011;305:381–90.
82. Likosky DS, Marrin CA, Caplan LR, et al. Determination of etiologic mechanisms of strokes secondary to coronary artery bypass graft surgery. Stroke 2003;34:2830–4.
83. Alberts MJ, Brass LM, Perry A, et al. Evaluation times for patients with in-hospital strokes. Stroke 1993;24:1817–22.
84. The National Institute of Neurological Disorders and Stroke RT-PA Stroke Study Group. Tissue plasminogen activator for acute ischemic stroke. N Engl J Med 1995;333: 1581–7.
85. Hacke W, Kaste M, Bluhmki E, et al. Thrombolysis with alteplase 3 to 4.5 hours after acute ischemic stroke. N Engl J Med 2008; 359:1317–29.
86. Lees KR, Bluhmki E, von Kummer R, et al. Time to treatment with intravenous alteplase and outcome in stroke: An updated pooled analysis of ecass, atlantis, ninds, and epithet trials. Lancet 2010;375:1695–703.
87. Jauch EC, Saver JL, Adams HP Jr, et al. Guidelines for the early management of patients with acute ischemic stroke: A guideline for healthcare professionals from the american heart association/american stroke association. Stroke 2013;44: 870–947.
88. Lansberg MG, O'Donnell MJ, Khatri P, et al. Antithrombotic and thrombolytic therapy for ischemic stroke: Antithrombotic therapy and prevention of thrombosis, 9th ed: American College of Chest Physicians evidence-based clinical practice guidelines. Chest 2012;141:e601S–636S.
89. American College of Emergency Physicians, American Academy of Neurology. Clinical policy: Use of intravenous tpa for the management of acute ischemic stroke in the emergency department. Ann Emerg Med 2013;61:225–43.
90. Khatri P, Taylor RA, Palumbo V, et al. The safety and efficacy of thrombolysis for strokes after cardiac catheterization. J Am Coll Cardiol 2008;51:906–11.
91. Kasner SE, Villar-Cordova CE, Tong D, et al. Hemopericardium and cardiac tamponade after thrombolysis for acute ischemic stroke. Neurology 1998;50:1857–9.
92. Penumbra Pivotal Stroke Trial Investigators. The penumbra pivotal stroke trial: Safety and effectiveness of a new generation of mechanical devices for clot removal in intracranial large vessel occlusive disease. Stroke 2009;40:2761–8.
93. Smith WS, Sung G, Saver J, et al. Mechanical thrombectomy for acute ischemic stroke: Final results of the multi merci trial. Stroke 2008;39:1205–12.
94. Smith WS, Sung G, Starkman S, et al. Safety and efficacy of mechanical embolectomy in acute ischemic stroke: Results of the merci trial. Stroke 2005;36:1432–8.
95. Furlan A, Higashida R, Wechsler L, et al. Intra-arterial prourokinase for acute ischemic stroke. The proact ii study: A randomized controlled trial. Prolyse in acute cerebral thromboembolism. JAMA 1999;282:2003–11.

96. Saver JL, Jahan R, Levy EI, et al. Solitaire flow restoration device versus the merci retriever in patients with acute ischaemic stroke (swift): A randomised, parallel-group, non-inferiority trial. Lancet 2012;380:1241–9.
97. Khatri P, Abruzzo T, Yeatts SD, et al. Good clinical outcome after ischemic stroke with successful revascularization is time-dependent. Neurology 2009;73:1066–72.
98. Chalela JA, Katzan I, Liebeskind DS, et al. Safety of intra-arterial thrombolysis in the postoperative period. Stroke 2001;32: 1365–9.
99. National hospital discharge survey, 2014: National Hospital Discharge Survey Data Highlights. Retrieved March 6th, 2014, from http://www.cdc.gov/nchs/nhds/nhds_tables.htm#detailed.
100. Aggarwal A, Dai D, Rumsfeld JS, et al. Incidence and predictors of stroke associated with percutaneous coronary intervention. Am J Cardiol 2009;104:349–53.
101. van Ryn J, Stangier J, Haertter S, et al. Dabigatran etexilate – a novel, reversible, oral direct thrombin inhibitor: Interpretation of coagulation assays and reversal of anticoagulant activity. Thromb Haemost 2010;103:1116–27.
102. Samama MM, Guinet C. Laboratory assessment of new anticoagulants. Clin Chem Lab Med 2011;49:761–72.

35 Arterial Dissections and Fibromuscular Dysplasia

Richard M. Zweifler, Gerald Silverboard

KEY POINTS

- Cervicocerebral arterial dissection constitutes 2% of strokes occurring most frequently in young and middle-aged populations.
- Medical interventions depending on the timing and severity of initial presentation and site of dissection may include thrombolytics, antiplatelet agents, or anticoagulation.
- Clinical prognosis of extracranial dissection is associated with excellent outcome in 70–85% of cases with mortality less than 5%.
- Fibromuscular dysplasia (FMD) is an uncommon non-atheromatous, non-inflammatory vasculopathy that may be associated with cervicocerebral dissection or ischemia.
- Most cases are asymptomatic although symptomatic FMD may be treated with antithrombotic therapy depending on the clinical presentation.

Cervicocerebral arterial dissection constitutes 2% of strokes, occurring most frequently in young and middle-aged populations. The site of cervicocerebral dissection dictates differences in clinical presentation, complications, and prognosis. Diagnostic modalities including MRI, MRA, and CTA are the most direct non-invasive modalities for confirmation. Medical interventions depending on the timing and severity of initial presentation and site of dissection may include thrombolytics, antiplatelet agents, or anticoagulation. Neuroendovascular interventional therapy has increasingly been utilized when conventional medical therapy fails or is contraindicated. Clinical prognosis of extracranial dissection is associated with excellent outcome in 70–85% of cases with mortality less than 5%. Fibromuscular dysplasia (FMD) is an uncommon non-atheromatous, non-inflammatory vasculopathy that may be associated with cervicocerebral dissection or ischemia. FMD most commonly affects extracranial vessels, especially carotids, but may also involve the intracranial carotids and vertebrobasilar vessels. Most cases are asymptomatic, although symptomatic FMD may be treated with antithrombotic therapy depending on the clinical presentation.

ARTERIAL DISSECTIONS

Epidemiology

Cervicocerebral arterial dissections account for approximately 2% of all ischemic strokes but they are among the more common causes of stroke in young and middle-aged patients.[1–6] Most patients with dissection are between 30 and 50 years of age, with a mean age of approximately 40 years.[3,4] In patients younger than 45 years, arterial dissection is the second leading cause of stroke, accounting for 10–25% of ischemic strokes.[6–9] Although older studies reveal no overall gender predilection in adults, a 2006 study of 696 patients with spontaneous cervicocerebral dissection found a preponderance in males.[10] Females with arterial dissection are approximately 5 years younger at the time of dissection.[3,10] Childhood arterial dissections are unique in that they occur more commonly in boys.[11,12]

Population-based studies have reported the incidence of dissection as ranging from 2.6 to 2.9 cases per 100,000 per year.[2,3] The true incidence of cervicocerebral arterial dissection is likely higher than these estimates, however, because asymptomatic patients and patients with pain but no neurologic symptoms are underdiagnosed.[13] The annual incidence of cervical internal carotid artery (ICA) dissection was 3.5 per 100,000 in those older than 20 years in a Mayo Clinic series.[3] Seventy percent of cervical internal carotid dissections occur in patients between 35 and 50 years of age, with a mean age at presentation of 44 years; there is no sex predilection.[14] Patients with intracranial carotid dissection tend to be younger than those with cervical dissections. In a review of 59 cases of intracranial carotid dissection, the mean age at onset was 30 years and there was a slight male predominance.[15] The annual incidence of spontaneous vertebral artery dissection is one third of ICA dissections,[5,16–18] with estimates of 1 to 1.5 per 100,000.[19] Extracranial vertebral artery dissection accounts for up to 15% of cervicocerebral dissections, whereas dissection of the intracranial vertebral artery accounts for only 5%.[20] The mean age at onset of intracranial vertebral dissection is the late 40s for isolated and the late 30s for dissection with extension to the basilar artery.[21–24] In contrast to extracranial dissections, intracranial vertebral artery dissections are more common in men than in women.[21,25]

Pathology

Arterial dissections usually arise from an intimal tear that allows the development of an intramural hematoma (false lumen) (Figs 35-1, 35-2). In some patients, no communication between the true and false lumens can be demonstrated, suggesting that some dissections are the result of a primary intramedial hematoma. Furthermore, intimal disruption could occur as a result of rupture of a primary intramural hematoma into the intima. Although it is likely that the former mechanism is more common, both could occur.

The intramural hematoma is located within the layers of the tunica media but may be eccentric towards the intima (subintimal dissection) or adventitia (subadventitial dissection). Subintimal dissections are more likely to cause luminal stenosis, whereas subadventitial dissections may cause arterial dilatation (aneurysm). These aneurysms are often referred to as "false aneurysms" or "pseudo-aneurysms" but they are true aneurysms because their walls contain blood vessel elements (i.e., media and adventitia);[19] they are better termed "dissecting" aneurysms.[26,27] The absence of an external elastic lamina and a thin adventitia makes intracranial arteries prone to subadventitial dissection and subsequent subarachnoid hemorrhage (SAH). SAH is reported in about one-fifth of intracranial ICA dissections and in more than one-half of intracranial vertebral artery dissections.[11,21,23,24, 28–32]

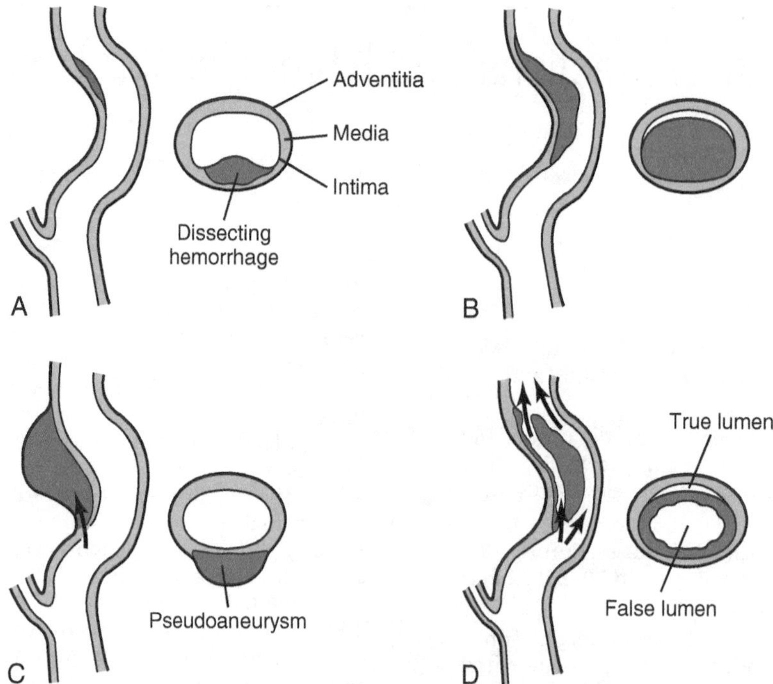

Figure 35-1. Anatomy of dissections. A, Lateral *(left)* and cross-sectional *(right)* schematic views of internal carotid artery demonstrate initial phase of intramedial and subintimal dissecting aneurysm; the three basic arterial layers (intima, media, and adventitia) are delineated. B, Comparable views of the progression of intramedial hemorrhage; the arterial lumen is reduced in size. C, Comparable views of an intramedial hemorrhage that dissects into the subadventitial rather than the subintimal plane, as in A and B; a large pseudoaneurysm results. D, Dissecting hemorrhage ruptures through the intima, establishing communication with the true lumen; recanalization may occur, enlarging the true or false lumen. *(From Friedman AH, Day AL, Quisling RGJ, et al: Cervical carotid dissecting aneurysms.* Neurosurgery *7:207, 1980.)*

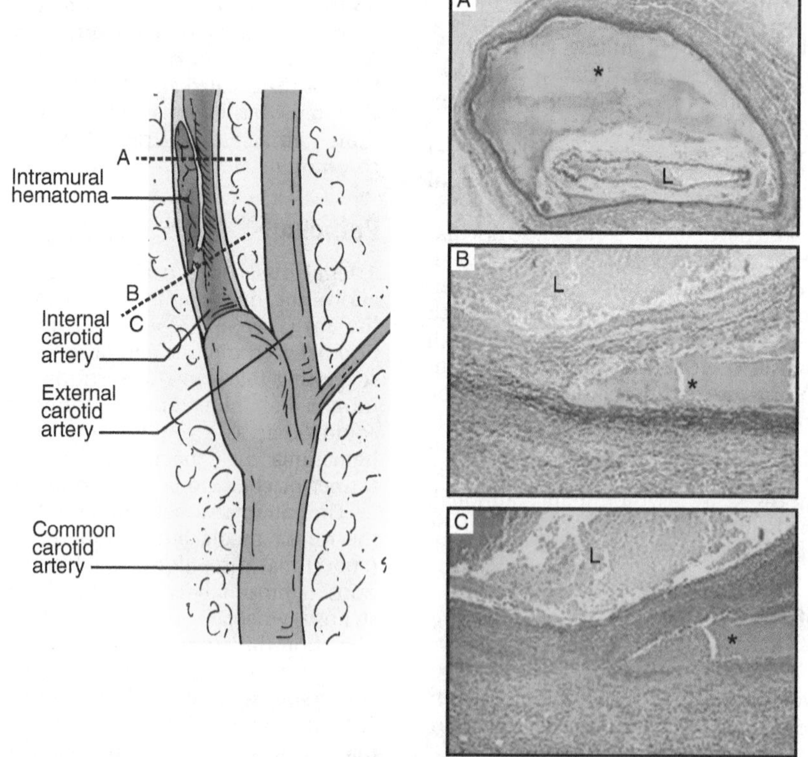

Figure 35-2. Pathologic findings in a 37-year-old woman with a dissection of the internal carotid artery. Photomicrographs of the right extracranial internal carotid artery (A through C) show a dissection within the outer layers of the tunica media, resulting in stenosis of the arterial lumen (L). The *dashed lines* on the left indicate the sites of the photomicrographs. A, The intramural hemorrhage (*) extends almost entirely around the artery (van Gieson stain, ×4). B and C, Higher-power views of the internal carotid artery at the point of dissection show fragmentation of elastic tissue (B; van Gieson stain, ×25), with the accumulation of pale ground-glass substance in the tunica media, indicated by the blue-staining mucopolysaccharides (C; Alcian blue, ×25). These changes are consistent with a diagnosis of cystic medial necrosis. *(From Schievink WI: Spontaneous dissection of the carotid and vertebral arteries.* N Engl J Med *344:898, 2001.)*

Pathogenesis

The pathogenesis of most spontaneous arterial dissections is unknown. Dissections can be iatrogenic or due to severe trauma, in which cases the causes are obvious, but most occur spontaneously or are associated with antecedent trivial trauma. Precipitating events reported to antedate dissection include sudden head movement, coughing, vomiting, sneezing, chiropractic manipulation, performing yoga, painting a ceiling, vigorous nose blowing, sexual activity, anesthesia administration, resuscitation, and many types of sports activity.[33-49] Such activities may cause arterial injury due to mechanical stretching. A prospective study found that 81% of dissections were associated with some form of sudden neck movement.[36] Estimates of dissection risk following chiropractic manipulation vary widely based on study methodology but range from 1 in 5.85 million manipulations[37] to as many as 1 in 20,000 manipulations.[50] One study found connective tissue disorders in one-fourth of patients with cervical artery dissection after chiropractic manipulation.[51]

An underlying arteriopathy has been postulated to lead to structural instability of the arterial wall. Fibromuscular dysplasia (FMD) is found in approximately 15–20% of all patients with cervicocephalic dissection and is seen in more than half of those with bilateral carotid involvement.[3,52-57] From 1% to 5% of patients have an identifiable heritable connective tissue disorder,[58] such as Ehlers–Danlos syndrome type IV,[59-61] Marfan's syndrome,[54,55,62,63] autosomal dominant polycystic kidney disease,[55] osteogenesis imperfecta type I,[55] pseudoxanthoma elasticum,[55,64] type I collagen point mutation,[65] or α_1-antitrypsin deficiency.[66] Dissection has also been associated with other arteriopathies such as cystic medial necrosis[3,67] and moyamoya disease.[68-70] The association with arterial redundancies (e.g., coils, kinks, and loops),[71,72] increased arterial distensibility,[73] widened aortic root,[74] and intracranial aneurysms[75,76] provide indirect evidence of an underlying arteriopathy.

Five percent of patients with spontaneous cervicocephalic dissection have at least one family member with a spontaneous dissection of the aorta or its main branches, including the vertebral and carotid arteries.[77] Atherosclerosis does not appear to be a risk factor.[27] Other reported risk factors for dissection include migraine,[78-81] recent infection,[82-84] pregnancy,[85,86] hyperhomocyst(e)inemia,[87,88] smoking,[27,89] hypertension,[27,90] and oral contraceptive use.[27] The possibility of an infectious etiology is supported by the reported seasonal variation of cervical artery dissection, with a 58% increase in frequency in the autumn.[56] Schievink and colleagues[91,92] have reported familial associations between dissection and multiple cutaneous lentigines and bicuspid aortic valves, suggesting an underlying neural crest defect.

Ultrastructural aberrations of dermal collagen fibrils and elastic fibers have been reported in 54–68% of patients with spontaneous cervical artery dissection in whom there is no clinical evidence of a known connective tissue disorder,[93-95] suggesting a molecular defect in the biosynthesis of the extracellular matrix.[96] Evidence of a generalized arteriopathy was reported[97] in an ultrastructural study of superficial temporal artery specimens in patients with spontaneous cervicocephalic dissection. A study of skin biopsies from healthy relatives of patients with dissection indicates a familial occurrence of connective tissue abnormalities.[98] No genetic mutation responsible for the majority of patients with cervical artery dissection has been identified.[94] Results of screening for mutations in the genes for type V procollagen (*COL5A1*),[99] type III collagen (*COL3A1*),[100,101] and tropoelastin (*ELN*)[102] have been negative.

Despite an association with many disorders (Box 35-1), the precise cause of cervicocephalic dissection remains unknown in most cases. The pathogenesis is likely multifactorial with mechanical factors and underlying arteriopathy, possibly genetic or infectious, playing roles.

BOX 35-1 Predisposing Factors for Cervicocephalic Dissection

- Trauma
  - Mild or trivial
  - Major
  - Iatrogenic
- Arteriopathies
  - Fibromuscular dysplasia
  - Cystic medial necrosis
  - Ehlers–Danlos syndrome type IV
  - Marfan's syndrome
  - Type I collagen point mutation
  - Alpha$_1$-antitrypsin deficiency
  - Osteogenesis imperfecta type I
  - Pseudoxanthoma elasticum
  - Autosomal-dominant polycystic kidney disease
  - Moyamoya disease
  - Redundancies (e.g., coils, kinks, and loops)
  - Intracranial aneurysms
- Migraine
- Family history
- Recent infection
- Hyperhomocyst(e)inemia
- Less well established
  - Hypertension
  - Pregnancy and post-partum (e.g., post-partum angiopathy)
  - Smoking
  - Oral contraceptives

Sites of Dissection

Dissection of the extracranial carotid and vertebral arteries accounts for approximately 80% to 90% of all cervicocephalic dissections.[103,104] This disparity may be explained by the greater mobility of the extracranial segments and the potential for injury by contact with bony structures such as the transverse processes of the upper cervical vertebrae or the styloid process, either normal or pathologically elongated (Eagle syndrome) (Fig. 35-3).[14,105] Extracranial ICA dissection typically occurs at least 2 cm distal to the bifurcation, near the C2–C3 vertebral level, and extends superiorly for a variable distance. It usually terminates before the artery enters the petrous bone, where mechanical support appears to limit further dissection in the majority of cases.[14] This location is distinct from that of atherosclerosis, which most commonly affects the ICA origin or the siphon. The vertebral artery is most mobile, and most susceptible to mechanical injury, at the C1–C2 level, as it leaves the transverse foramen of the axis and abruptly turns to enter the intracranial cavity (the V3 segment) (Fig. 35-4). The C1–C2 site is involved in one-half to two-thirds of all vertebral artery dissections and in 80–90% of rotation-related dissections.[17,106-109]

Intracranial arterial dissection is more common in children and adolescents than in adults, although intracranial dissection in children usually affects the anterior circulation, and intracranial posterior circulation dissection is more common in adults.[11] The most commonly involved intracranial sites are the supraclinoid segment of the ICA and the middle cerebral artery stem.[110,111] The most common site of intracranial vertebral artery dissection is the V4 segment at or near the origin

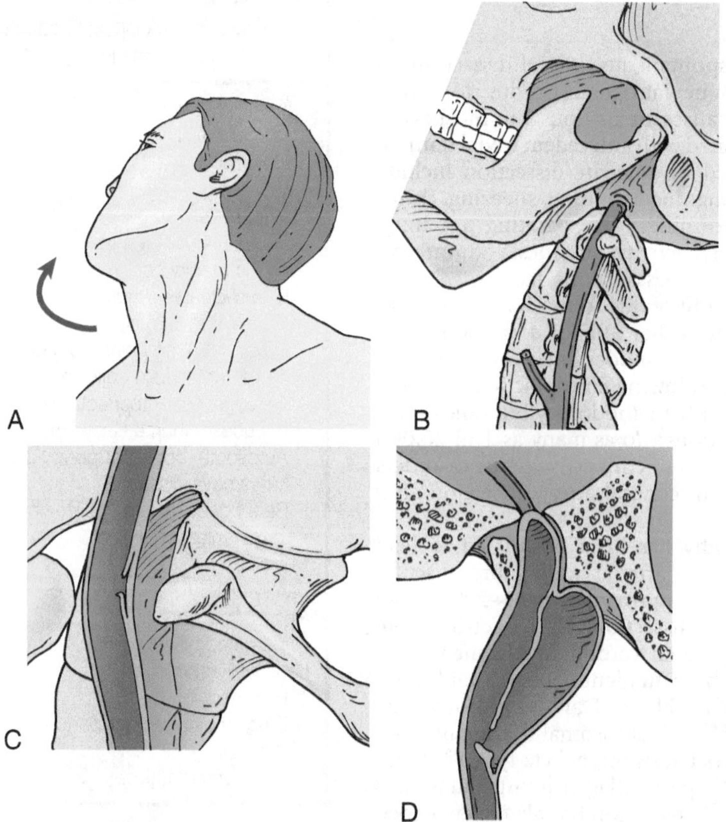

Figure 35-3. Presumed mechanism of carotid injury induced by neck rotation. A, Direction of hyperextension. B, Impingement of artery on the process of the vertebra. C, Intimal tear caused by impingement. D, Progression of intimal tear to dissection. *(From Stringer WL, Kelly DLJ: Traumatic dissection of the extracranial internal carotid artery.* Neurosurgery *6:123, 1980.)*

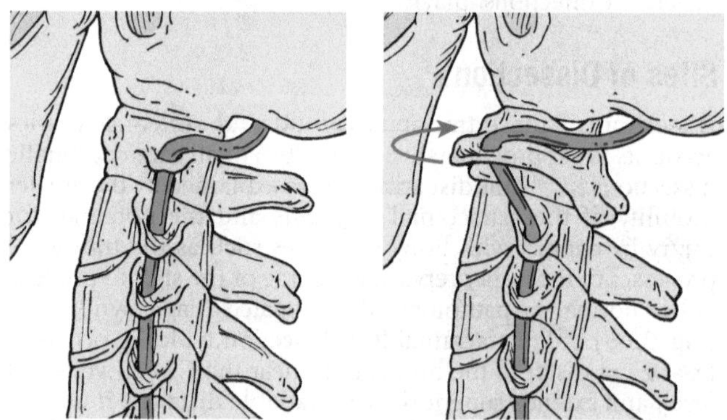

Figure 35-4. Vertebral artery injury with abrupt cervical rotation. The vertebral artery is subject to stretch and mechanical trauma between C1 and C2 when the neck is vigorously rotated and extended. *(From Barnett HJM: Progress towards stroke prevention.* Neurology [NY] *30:1212, 1980.)*

of the posterior inferior cerebellar artery. At this level the artery may be compressed during head maneuvers, the media and adventitia diminish in size and elastic components, and the external elastic lamina terminates. Approximately 20% of vertebral artery dissections involve both the extra- and intracranial segments.[112]

Mechanisms of Ischemia

Cervicocephalic dissection can cause ischemic symptoms due to hemodynamic compromise secondary to luminal narrowing or occlusion, thromboembolism, or both. Several reports investigating the pattern of infarction in patients with carotid dissection indicate that most strokes are the result of distal embolization.[113-117] A high incidence of middle cerebral artery microemboli correlating with stroke symptoms has been found in patients with carotid artery dissection, further supporting a thromboembolic mechanism.[118]

Clinical Manifestations

Extracranial Carotid Artery Dissection

Local Signs and Symptoms. The major presenting features of extracranial carotid dissection are pain in the ipsilateral head, face, or neck associated with focal ischemic symptoms (cerebral or retinal). In about one-third of cases, partial Horner's syndrome is present[20] (Table 35-1).

Pain (in head, face, or neck) is the most common overall symptom, present in more than 80% of symptomatic cases, and is the initial presenting symptom in one-half to two-thirds of patients.[11,20,52,115,117,119-127]

Headache, present in 60% to 75% of patients, may precede other signs or symptoms by hours or weeks.[113,117,120,123,126,128] The pain is typically ipsilateral over the anterior head but may be more diffuse or bilateral, even with unilateral dissection.[79,126,129] Onset of headache is usually gradual, although sudden "thunderclap" headache has been reported.[126,129] The headache is usually non-throbbing and severe, and ipsilateral scalp tenderness may occur.[79,126,129] Unilateral neck pain is present in 20–30% of patients and may involve the anterior neck with radiation toward the ear, scalp, jaw, face, or pharynx.[113,117,126] Facial or orbital pain has been reported in more than 50% of cases.[126]

TABLE 35-1 Clinical Features of Extracranial Carotid Dissection

No. of cases	635
Age	Mean 44.4 year Range 4–74 year
Sex	
Male	53%
Female	47%
Laterality	
Unilateral	86%
Left	60%
Right	40%
Bilateral	14%
Major presenting complaint*	
Cerebral infarction	46%
Transient ischemic attack	30%
Neck or head pain	21%
Pulsatile tinnitus only	2%
Asymptomatic bruit only	2%
Associated features at diagnosis	
Symptoms	
Neck pain	20%
Headache	64%
Neck or head pain	67%
Tinnitus or subjective bruit	3%
Signs	
Partial Horner's syndrome	32%
Cervical bruit	18%
Linguinal paresis	6%
Early outcome	
Angiographic	
Normal or mildly stenotic vessel on follow-up imaging	70%
Clinical	
Neurologically normal	50%
Mild deficits only	21%
Moderate to severe deficits	25%
Death	4%

Data from Schievink et al. 1994,[11] Saver et al. 1998,[20] Ast et al. 1993,[119] Cox et al. 1991,[121] Early et al. 1991,[122] Mulges et al. 1992,[124], Ramadan et al. 1991,[125], Sue et al 1992,[127] Hennerici 1989,[194]

*Major presenting complaint leading to evaluation, not necessarily the initial symptom.

Ipsilateral partial oculosympathetic paresis (Horner's syndrome), present in approximately one-third of patients, results from involvement of sympathetic fibers of the internal carotid plexus.[117,123,126] Ptosis and miosis are seen, but facial sweating remains intact (except for a focal area of the ipsilateral forehead) because the majority of sympathetic fibers supplying the face travel with the external carotid artery.[27]

Cranial nerve palsies have been reported in 12% of patients with spontaneous ICA dissection.[130] Lower cranial nerve palsies are most common and are found in approximately 5–10% of patients.[117,126,130] Figure 35-5 displays the anatomic relationship of the lower cranial nerves and the carotid artery. The most commonly affected cranial nerve is CN XII, followed in frequency by nerves IX, X, XI, and V.[126,130–136] Cranial nerves III, IV, VI, or VII may also be involved.[126,130,137] Dysguesia is reported in about 10%.[126] Pulsatile tinnitus or a subjective bruit is reported in up to one-fourth of patients, and an objective bruit may be heard in nearly one-fifth.[52,64,126,138]

Ischemic Signs and Symptoms. Ischemic manifestations have been reported in 50% to 95% of patients,[117,120,126] although the highest rates were reported in older studies. At the time of the earlier reports, the diagnosis of dissection was typically suspected only in the presence of ischemic signs, and non-invasive diagnostic techniques were not available.[120] Most ischemic symptoms occur within 1 week of the onset of pain;[120,126,128] one study reported a median delay in the appearance of other symptoms of 4 days.[126] A 1998 case report describes a disabling stroke occurring 5 months after traumatic ICA dissection, although the patient did suffer a silent stroke at the time of the dissection.[139] Most infarctions are territorial (as opposed to borderzone) supporting an emboligenic etiology.[113–117] Transient ischemic attacks (TIAs) are common, being reported in about 50% of patients, and they are recurrent in one-half of the cases.[120] Of patients with stroke, approximately 75% report at least one preceding TIA.[120] Transient monocular blindness occurs in one-fourth of cases.[126] Other ischemic ocular syndromes such as central retinal artery occlusion and anterior ischemic optic neuropathy are rare.[103,140,141]

Dissections causing ischemic events are more often associated with occlusions and stenosis greater than 80%, and dissections that do not cause ischemic events are more often associated with Horner's syndrome and lower cranial nerve palsies.[117]

Intracranial Carotid and Middle Cerebral Artery Dissection

Dissection of the intracranial ICA and its branches is almost universally associated with severe unilateral headache, and ischemic symptoms typically occur with a much shorter delay (within minutes or hours) compared with extracranial dissection. Seizures or syncope can be the presenting symptom, and half the patients have altered level of consciousness.[20] Three-quarters of cases involve the supraclinoid ICA or the middle cerebral artery stem; the anterior cerebral artery is infrequently involved.[11,142] Although reported, bilateral dissections occur less commonly in the intracranial circulation than in the extracranial circulation.[70,111,143,144] SAH, resulting from subadventitial hematoma rupture through the external vessel wall, occurs in approximately 20% of cases.[15,111,145]

Extracranial Vertebral Artery Dissection

The clinical features and course of 174 cases of extracranial vertebral dissection are summarized in Table 35-2.[20]

Local Signs and Symptoms. Headache occurs in one-half to two-thirds of patients with extracranial vertebral dissection and is typically ipsilateral and occipital.[20,108,112,126,146,147,148] The pain can be either throbbing or pressure-like.[126] Neck pain occurs in approximately half of patients and is typically gradual in onset.[20,108,112,126,146–149] The pain is usually unilateral, but is bilateral in one-third of cases.[126] Pulsatile tinnitus occurs less commonly with extracranial vertebral compared with extracranial ICA dissection.[112,138]

Ischemic Signs and Symptoms. The majority of patients with vertebral artery dissection have ischemic symptoms, although this may reflect an underdiagnosis of cases without ischemic manifestations. The median interval between onsets of neck pain and headache and the development of ischemic symptoms is 2 weeks and 15 hours, respectively.[126] TIA has been reported to precede stroke in 13% of cases.[109] Lateral medullary signs and symptoms may be seen in isolation or in combination with other brainstem, posterior cerebral artery distribution, or upper cervical spinal cord findings.[14,52,109,126,150–154] Cervical radiculopathy (most commonly at C5–C6) has been reported, although it is unclear if the etiology is ischemic or mechanical.[151,152]

Intracranial Vertebral and Basilar Artery Dissections

Intracranial vertebral artery dissection is distinguished clinically from extracranial dissection by the association with

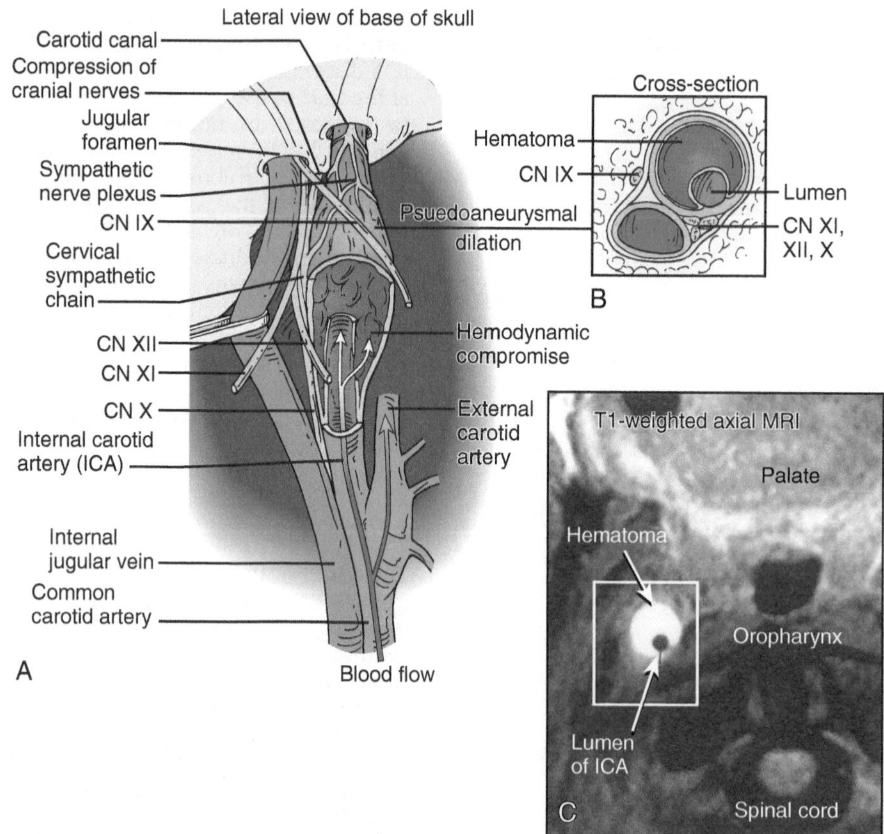

Figure 35-5. Anatomy of carotid artery dissection. A, Diagram demonstrating hematoma tracking into the vessel wall, resulting in a long segment of narrowing distal to the carotid artery bifurcation. B, Pseudoaneurysmal dilatation of the carotid artery at the base of the skull due to dissection may injure adjacent lower cranial nerves. C, T1-weighted axial magnetic resonance image of the upper neck. The hematoma in the wall of the internal carotid artery appears as a bright crescent around the residual vessel lumen (appearing as a dark flow void in the center of the vessel). CN, cranial nerve. *(From Wityk RJ: Stroke in a healthy 46-year-old man.* JAMA *285:2757, 2001.)*

subarachnoid hemorrhage. Coexistent subarachnoid hemorrhage has been reported to occur in as many as one-half to two-thirds of adult cases[21,23,24,28–32] but the association has not been reported in children.[11] Basilar artery dissections are rare. They may be isolated (primary) or associated with concomitant vertebral artery dissection. Clinical manifestations vary according to the extent of involvement. Primary basilar dissection typically manifests as rapidly progressive brainstem signs, although it can manifest as headache and more slowly developing focal signs or as a mass lesion due to intravascular hematoma.[25,29,111,112,145,155–180] Like other intracranial dissections, basilar dissections can manifest as subarachnoid hemorrhage and dissecting aneurysm if the dissection plane is subadventitial or transmural.[29,111,145,161,156,157,165,166,174]

Diagnosis

When clinical presentation suggests cerebrovascular arterial dissection, whether spontaneous or traumatic in occurrence, an aggressive diagnostic approach is immediately warranted. The combination of magnetic resonance imaging (MRI) and magnetic resonance angiography (MRA) or computerized tomography angiography (CTA) are the best non-invasive modalities for confirmation of arterial dissection.[19,181–188] When MRA or CTA are not possible, carotid ultrasonography (US), transcranial Doppler ultrasonography (TCD), or both, can provide direct or indirect evidence of dissection.[189–195] Conventional angiography is the definitive test for accurately defining the exact level and arterial territory of dissection and for imaging complications associated with dissection, such as pseudoaneurysm, double lumen, and presence of intraluminal or distal clot, but is seldom necessary for extracranial dissections.[9,31,104,185,196]

Ultrasonography

The combination of extracranial carotid B-mode imaging and carotid color-flow Doppler ultrasonography combined with TCD offers the most reliable systematic ultrasound investigation.[118,124,128,189–195,197] Extracranial vertebral artery dissection may also be diagnosed using a multimodal ultrasound approach.[197] Indirect rather than direct evidence of extracranial carotid artery dissection is often more prominent on ultrasound because extracranial carotid artery dissection typically occurs 2 cm or more distal to the carotid bulb and, therefore, above the typical field of insonation.[20,190] Decrease or absence of flow velocities in the affected vessel, retrograde flow in supraorbital vessels, or bidirectional ICA flow suggests more distal obstruction or stenosis resulting from dissection.[198] Direct ultrasound visualization of tapering of ICA lumen may be achieved, as well as presence of a true and false lumen with an intraluminal flap in 15% of cases (Figs 35-6, 35-7).[190,193]

Extracranial color-flow duplex ultrasonography has been effective in detecting abnormalities in extracranial vertebral artery dissection, similarly demonstrating indirect evidence of absence, reduction, or reversal of flow in the vertebral artery or, rarely, direct evidence of intimal hemorrhage.[191,192,197] The severity of stenosis and the presence of occlusion and site of dissection significantly affect the sensitivity and specificity of ultrasound in extracranial carotid and vertebral artery dissection.[190] Insonating the high cervical (retromandibular) region in extracranial carotid artery dissection and stepwise segmental insonation of the vertebral artery in extracranial vertebral artery dissection improve detection of suspected dissection.[20,190] TCD delineates flow abnormalities distal to vascular luminal narrowing or occlusion by dissection, including signs of carotid–carotid collateral cross-flow; artery-to-artery embolic middle cerebral artery stem occlusion is suggested when the middle cerebral artery signal is absent and the ipsilateral anterior cerebral and posterior cerebral artery velocities are increased.[20,195] Serial examinations of extracranial carotid and vertebral artery dissection for spontaneous or therapy-based recanalization with these US techniques allows outpatient monitoring and the use of clinical decision algorithms.[190–193,197,199]

TABLE 35-2 Clinical Features of Extracranial Vertebral Dissection

No. of cases	174
Age	Mean 38.9 year Range 3–67 year
Sex	
Male	43%
Female	57%
Laterality	
Unilateral	69%
Left	56%
Right	44%
Bilateral	31%
Clinical features at presentation*	
Cerebral infarction	75%
At onset	17%
Delayed	83%
Transient ischemic attack	25%
Neck pain	55%
Headache	53%
Head or neck pain	75%
Lateral medullary symptoms	33%
Associated conditions	
Hypertension	25%
Migraine	13%
Oral contraceptives (among women)	24%
Fibromuscular dysplasia	17%
Early outcome	
Angiographic	
Normal or mildly stenotic vessel on follow-up imaging	78%
Clinical	
Neurologically normal or mild deficits only	83%
Moderate to severe deficits	11%
Death	6%

Data from references Saver et al. 2001,[20] De Bray et al. 1977,[146] Provenzale et al. 1996,[147] Takis and Saver 1997.[148]

*Major presenting complaint leading to evaluation, not necessarily the initial symptom.

Magnetic Resonance Imaging

MRI coupled with MRA currently offers sophisticated noninvasive imaging of cerebrovascular arterial dissection. Simultaneous definition of the brain and the major cervical and intracranial arteries are achieved with conventional T1- and T2-weighted and fluid attenuation inversion recovery (FLAIR) axial MRI with 3Dl time-of-flight (TOF) MRA (Fig. 35-8). The typical abnormalities associated with dissection are most easily defined in extracranial carotid (Fig. 35-9) and vertebral artery dissection, whereas intracranial arterial dissection imaging often shows less specific abnormalities.[20] Characteristic imaging findings on MRI in extracranial carotid artery dissection include diminution or absence of signal flow void and a crescent sign, owing to narrowing of the vessel by intramural dissection of blood appearing in a semilunar fashion as a spiraling periarterial rim of intramural hematoma in cross-section on T1-weighted and fluid attenuation inversion recovery axial MR images (see Figs 35-5C, 35-8, 35-9).[19,20,181–188,200–203]

The intensity of the hematoma on T1- and T2-weighted images depends on the age of the dissection, because the hyperintense signal corresponds to intramural hematoma with methemoglobin signal intensity; in some dissections, all or part of the intramural hematoma appears hypointense on T2-weighted images as a result of acute clot deoxyhemoglobin or hemosiderin in the chronic type.[118] Subtle abnormalities also include (1) high signal intensity from the entire vessel, (2) significant compromise of the vessel lumen by adjoining tissue with abnormally increased signal, (3) enlargement of

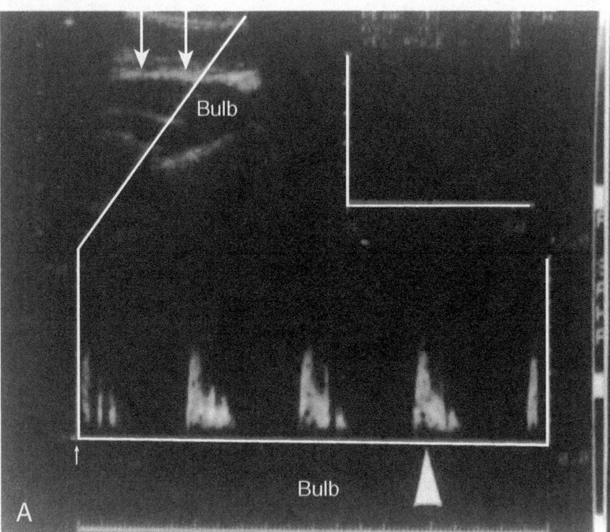

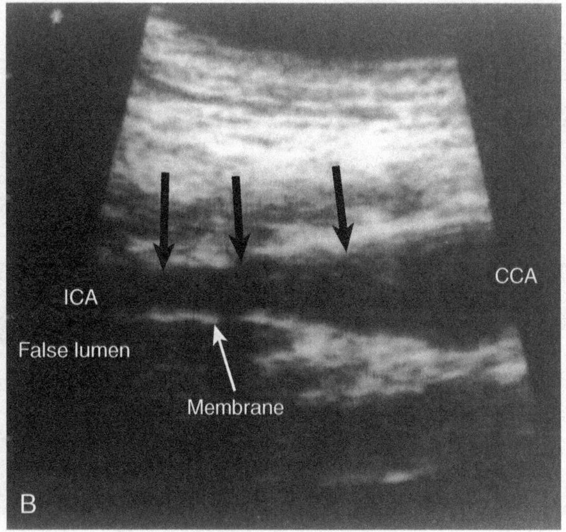

Figure 35-6. A, Duplex ultrasonogram demonstrates a patent bulb without atherosclerotic wall changes *(arrows)*. Doppler sample in the bulb demonstrates only short systolic flow signal without diastolic flow (stump flow) *(arrowhead)*. B, B-mode ultrasonogram of bulb and proximal internal carotid artery shows tapering luminal narrowing *(black arrows)* and a membrane *(white arrow)* separating true from false lumen. *(From Sturzenegger M: Spontaneous internal carotid artery dissection: Early diagnosis and management in 44 patients.* J Neurol *242:231, 1995.)*

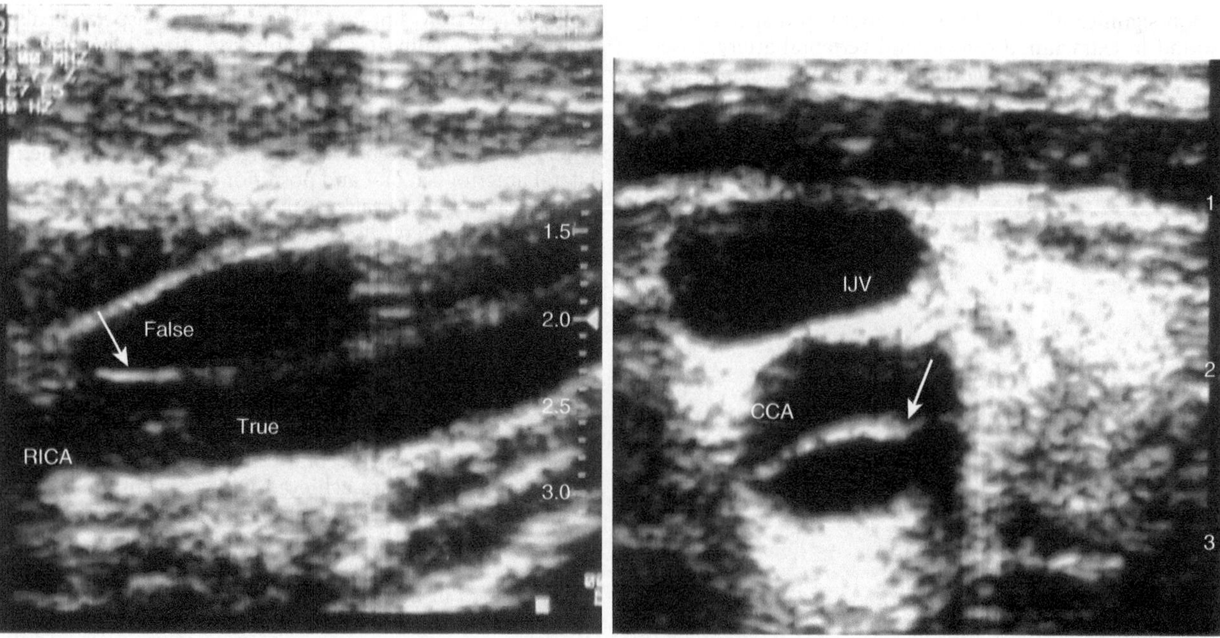

Figure 35-7. B-mode ultrasonography images of a carotid artery dissection demonstrating the true (True) and false (False) lumens separated by a membrane *(arrows)*. CCA, cervical carotid artery; IJV, internal jugular vein; RICA, right internal carotid artery. *(Courtesy of Christine Miles, RVT.)*

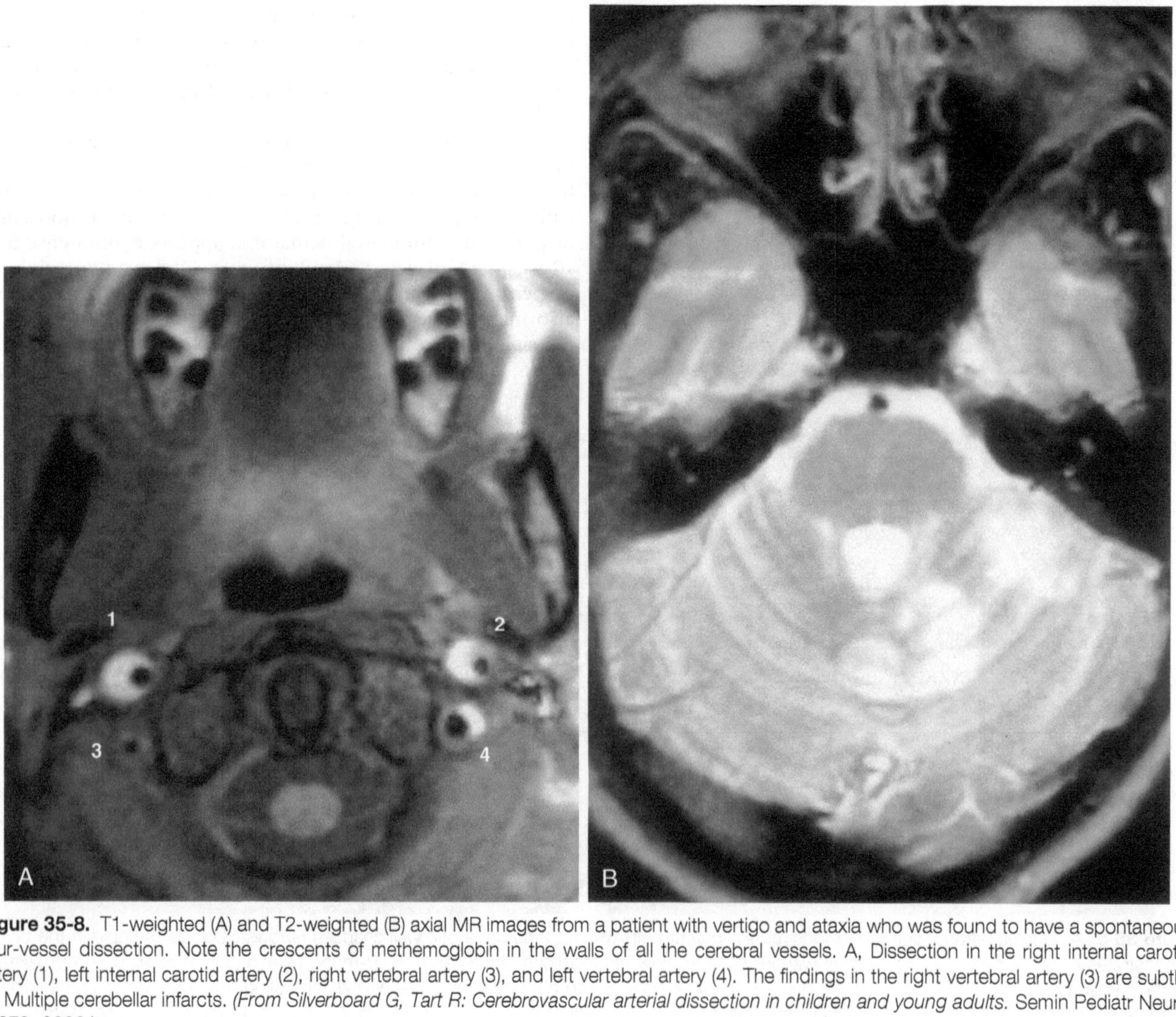

Figure 35-8. T1-weighted (A) and T2-weighted (B) axial MR images from a patient with vertigo and ataxia who was found to have a spontaneous four-vessel dissection. Note the crescents of methemoglobin in the walls of all the cerebral vessels. A, Dissection in the right internal carotid artery (1), left internal carotid artery (2), right vertebral artery (3), and left vertebral artery (4). The findings in the right vertebral artery (3) are subtle. B, Multiple cerebellar infarcts. *(From Silverboard G, Tart R: Cerebrovascular arterial dissection in children and young adults.* Semin Pediatr Neurol *7:278, 2000.)*

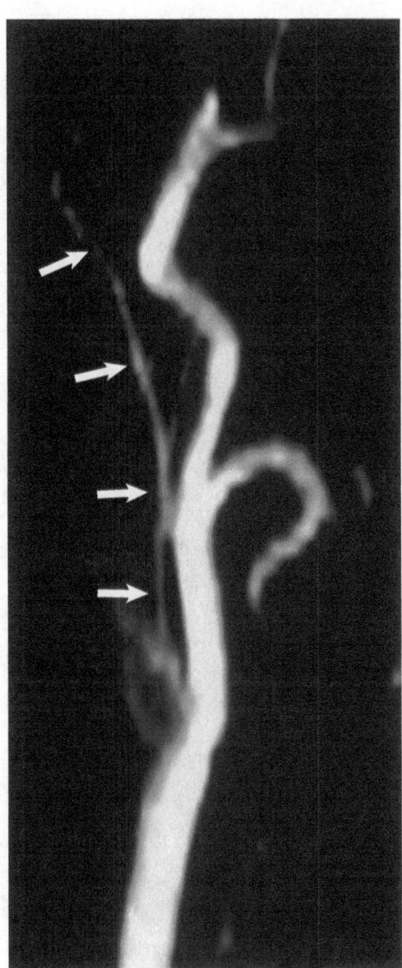

Figure 35-9. Lateral projection from an MR angiogram of a segmented cervical carotid artery, demonstrating complete occlusion of the high cervical portion of the internal carotid artery *(arrows)*. This spontaneous dissection manifested as a minor stroke. The patient made a near-complete recovery with anticoagulation therapy. *(From Silverboard G, Tart R: Cerebrovascular arterial dissection in children and young adults.* Semin Pediatr Neurol *7:278, 2000.)*

the vessel diameter, and (4) poor or no visualization of the vessel. Fat suppression techniques are important to differentiate small intramural hematomas from surrounding soft tissues.[19] In the absence of significant luminal stenosis or compromise, MRI may detect carotid dissection missed by conventional angiography; however, MRI may fail to demonstrate mural hematoma even though associated vessel wall thickening is present.

The pattern of stroke associated with extracranial carotid artery dissection is predominantly cortical (83%) and subcortical (60%) with the middle cerebral artery territory affected in 99%, anterior cerebral artery territory in 4%, and the posterior cerebral artery territory in 3%, with border zone infarcts in 5% of cases.[116,117] In extracranial carotid artery dissection, MRA in tandem with MRI provide sensitivity and specificity of 95% and 99%, respectively, for MRA and 84% and 99%, respectively, for MRI.[20,186] Dissecting aneurysms may be missed in the acute stage by 3D time-of-flight MRA if the hematoma is isointense.[185]

Intracranial carotid arterial dissection produces less specific abnormalities on non-invasive studies, although MRI may demonstrate intramural hematoma.[20,204,205] The presence of SAH, occurring in one-fifth of cases, is notable and may clinically suggest dissection; however, cerebral angiography rather than MRI–MRA is the standard for diagnosis of intracranial carotid artery dissection.[20,31,104,112]

The extracranial vertebral artery distribution is the second most common site of dissection, typically at the C1–C2 site. Although unilateral extracranial vertebral artery dissection may go unrecognized owing to collateral flow by the uninvolved vertebral artery, bilateral vertebral artery dissection is well recognized. It may be associated with cerebellar, brainstem, or hemispheric infarction which is demonstrated on routine MRI; concurrent carotid artery dissections may also occur.[20,112,206,207] The entire spectrum of MRI–MRA findings seen in extracranial carotid artery dissection may occur in extracranial vertebral artery dissection, although these two modalities are not as sensitive in extracranial vertebral artery dissection. One study reported sensitivity and specificity for MRI of 60% and 98% in extracranial carotid artery dissection and extracranial vertebral artery dissection respectively, for MRI and 20% and 100%, respectively, for MRA.[186] CTA or conventional angiography is warranted if MRI–MRA findings are non-diagnostic in spite of a high clinical index of suspicion for extracranial vertebral artery dissection.

Intracranial vertebral artery dissection occurs at or near the origin of the posterior inferior cerebellar artery. Although the presentation is similar to that of extracranial vertebral artery dissection, with brainstem, cerebellar or hemispheric infarction, intracranial vertebral artery dissection may be distinguished on the basis of its association with SAH.[20,21,23,24,28,29] MRI–MRA may demonstrate a crescent sign or suggestion of dissecting aneurysm.

Computed Tomography

CTA has gained acceptance as a diagnostic option and is particularly suited for investigation of dissection (Fig. 35-10).[208] CTA is rapid, allowing unstable patients to be imaged without compromising patient monitoring. CTA is an excellent diagnostic option as it compares favorably with other diagnostic modalities including catheter angiography.[208–212]

Angiography

Although the complementary use of MRI, MRA, CTA, and US is usually sufficient for the diagnosis of extracranial carotid artery dissection and some instances of extracranial vertebral artery dissection, angiography is the most definitive test for investigation of intracranial dissection as well as extracranial vertebral artery dissection. Angiography, although invasive, yields excellent delineation of abnormalities associated with dissection (Fig. 35-11), including intimal flaps, intraluminal clots, flame-shaped tapering occlusion, double lumen, vessel stenosis with string sign, and dissecting aneurysm formation. Double lumen and intimal flaps are the most specific angiographic findings in dissection. More often, angiographic features of intracranial dissection are not definitive but suggest dissection by demonstrating irregular or scalloped stenoses, a "string of beads," or complete vessel occlusion.[185] With intracranial dissection, angiography may delineate cerebral aneurysm from dissection causing SAH. The finding at angiography of aneurysmal formation at a non-bifurcation location suggests dissection. Irregular narrowing of the affected artery may give a wavy ribbon appearance. The presence of FMD (Fig. 35-12) in 15% of cases may be associated with multi-vessel dissections.[213–215] Atherosclerotic disease should be suspected in lesions seen proximal to and within 2 cm of the carotid bifurcation.

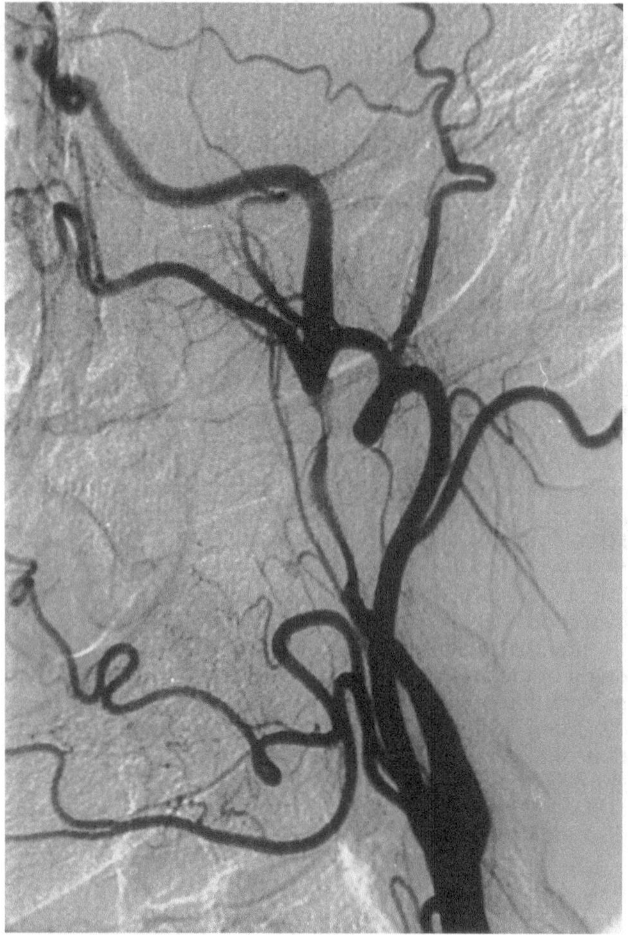

Figure 35-10. Digital subtraction angiogram (lateral view) showing irregular narrowing of the left internal carotid artery beginning approximately 3 cm distal to the bifurcation in a 38-year-old woman who presented with expressive aphasia and right hemiparesis. Note that the dissection terminates at the skull base, with a normal-appearing intracranial internal carotid artery.

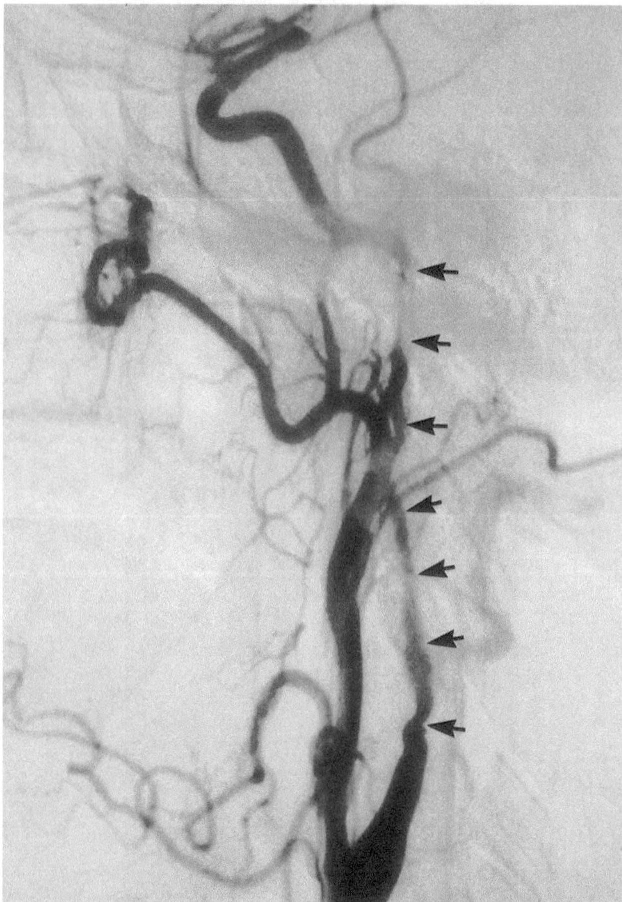

Figure 35-11. Lateral view from a digital subtraction angiogram showing the high cervical internal carotid artery. In this patient with fibromuscular dysplasia (more prominently seen on the opposite side; not shown), there is a long, irregular narrowing of the internal carotid artery. The dissection involves nearly the entire cervical portion of the internal carotid artery *(black arrows)*, starting just beyond the cervical bifurcation and ending in the petrous portion of the internal carotid artery with a normal carotid siphon. *(From Silverboard G, Tart R: Cerebrovascular arterial dissection in children and young adults.* Semin Pediatr Neurol *7:278, 2000.)*

Treatment

Medical Therapy

Acute thrombolysis with tissue plasminogen activator (tPA), given both intravenously and intra-arterially, has been administered safely after dissection-related stroke.[216-224] Increased intramural hemorrhage with exacerbation of dissection-related stenosis has not been observed. A meta-analysis of individual patient data of 180 patients with cervical dissection treated with intravenous tPA found no safety concerns.[225]

Although antithrombotic treatment of extracranial cerebrovascular dissection is controversial and large controlled clinical trials are lacking, treatment is based both on empiric and clinical observations that most cerebral injuries, at least acutely, result from secondary thrombotic events, particularly artery-to-artery embolism.[20] Whether anticoagulation is superior to antiplatelet therapy remains an open question. A 2011 *Cochrane Review* on the use of antithrombotic drugs for carotid artery dissection found no evidence that anticoagulants were better than aspirin for the treatment of extracranial carotid artery dissection[226] and a 2012 meta-analysis found no evidence of superiority of anticoagulants over antiplatelet agents.[227] The 2014 American Stroke Association (ASA) stroke prevention guidelines recommend that for patients with ischemic stroke or TIA and extracranial carotid or vertebral arterial dissection, antithrombotic treatment for at least 3 to 6 months is reasonable (Class IIa; Level B) and the relative efficacy of antiplatelet therapy compared with anticoagulation is unknown (Class IIb; Level B).[228] An international prospective, randomized controlled trial compared anticoagulation to antiplatelet therapy in patients with cervicocephalic dissection, The Cervical Artery Dissection in Stroke Study (CADISS), found no difference in the rate of ipsilateral stroke or death provided by antiplatelets and anticoagulants in patients with carotid or vertebral artery dissections.[229,299a]

Historically, anticoagulation has typically been avoided in the presence of intracranial dissection because of the perceived increased risk of SAH. A published series of 81 intracranial dissection patients suggests that anticoagulation may be safe in patients without associated aneurysm, however.[230] Other relative contraindications to anticoagulation are the presence of a large infarct with mass effect, hemorrhagic transformation of the infarcted arterial territory or presence of an intracranial aneurysm.[26]

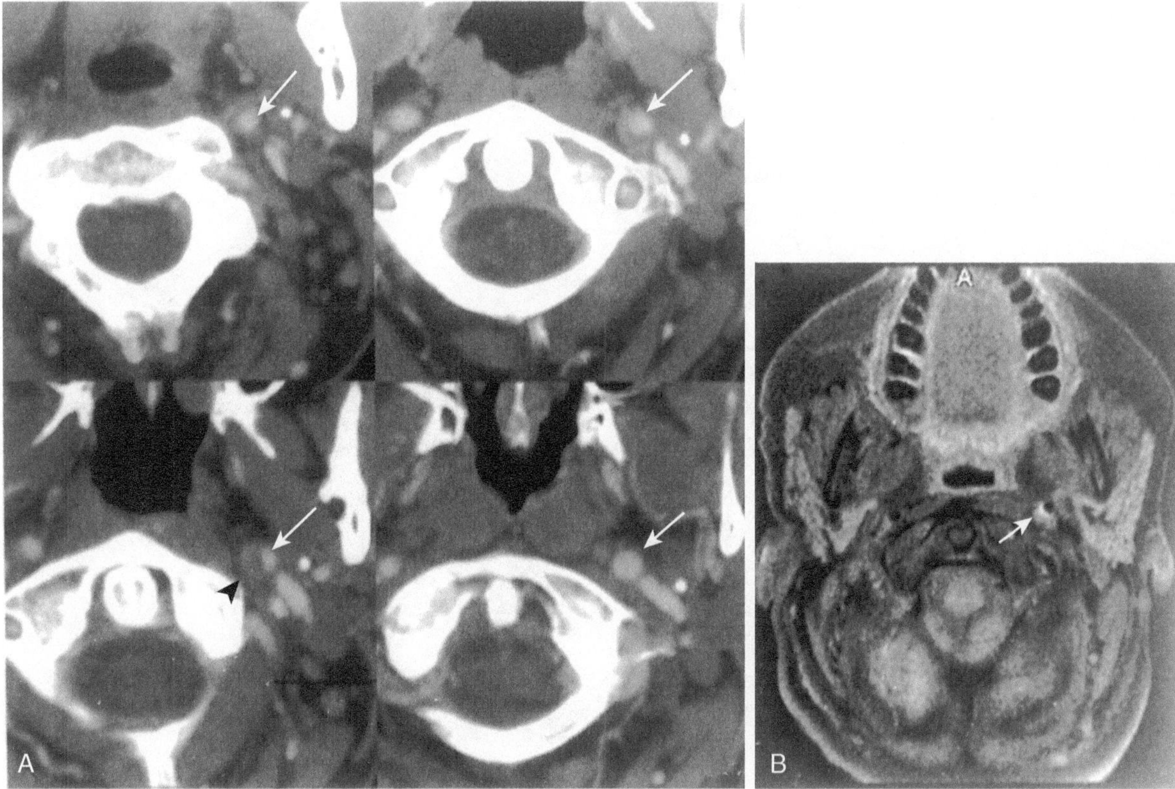

Figure 35-12. A, Axial multiplanar volume reconstruction CT angiograms obtained because of the possibility of acute carotid dissection shows that the caudal configuration of the internal carotid artery (ICA) is normal *(upper left, arrow)*. Moving rostrally in the neck *(upper right, lower left)*, the caliber of the ICA narrows *(arrows)*. A crescent-shaped intraluminal thrombus is visible *(lower left, arrowhead)*. Superior to the lesion *(lower right)*, the ICA is enlarged abnormally, suggesting a post-dissection pseudoaneurysm *(arrow)*. B, The next day, a fat-saturated, T1-weighted axial MR image through the lesion shows a crescent-shaped area of abnormally high signal intensity *(arrow)* consistent with intramural thrombus related to the acute dissection. *(From Fredenberg P, Forbes K, Toye L, et al: Assessment of cervical vascular injury with CT angiography.* BNI Q *17:44, 2001.)*

Neuroendovascular Interventional Therapy

Neurovascular intervention is increasingly being employed in patients for whom medical therapy has failed and who have (1) recurrent ischemic symptoms, (2) contraindications to anticoagulation, (3) surgically inaccessible lesions, (4) limited reserve due to involvement of other vessels, or (5) persistent or expanding dissecting aneurysm.[231] For both spontaneous and traumatic dissections, endovascular therapy in appropriate circumstances allows reestablishment of the true lumen, resulting in the obliteration of the false lumen and restoration of hemodynamic flow in the true lumen and thereby reducing the risk of artery-to-artery embolism (Fig. 35-13).[26,30,172,231–250] Through the use of a covered stent or coil embolization placed through the interstices of the stent where necessary, obliteration of dissecting aneurysms in both the extracranial carotid and vertebral arteries may be accomplished (see Fig. 35-15).[30,236,238,239,241,245,247,248,251] Endovascular therapy can re-establish hemodynamic flow in severely stenotic or totally occluded true lumens in select cases (Figs 35-14, 35-15); sequential reconstruction of the true lumen is accomplished by means of stents that provide gradual radial force, permitting apposition of the dissected segment to the vessel wall and thereby obliterating the false lumen and resolving the consequent loss of vascular continuity.[241,252] Extracranial and intracranial components of dissection can be addressed simultaneously if necessary.

When intracranial extension has occurred, endovascular techniques are also applicable and may be of particular benefit for balloon occlusion of intracranial dissection of the vertebral artery if temporary occlusion studies suggest adequate collateral blood flow. Long-term efficacy and endovascular therapy-related complications are still being assessed.[216,251,253–256] Complications of endovascular intervention include intracranial and retroperitoneal hemorrhage, vasospasm which may be treated with angioplasty during the endovascular procedure, and the possibility of recurrent stenosis and distal embolism if there is large thrombus burden.[252] Because the risk of recurrent embolization is low and dissecting aneurysms do not usually rupture, stenting as an initial therapy is not warranted and should be reserved for cases in which medical therapy has failed.[26,252,257] When stenting is performed, antiplatelet agents are administered for at least 4 weeks to prevent stent occlusion.[252] There is a lack of prospective, randomized data evaluating stenting for cervicocephalic dissection. Menon and colleagues[258] systematically reviewed the available literature prior to 2008 and reported a relatively low technical failure rate (5%) and a low perioperative complication rate (3.1%). A 2013 meta-analysis of non-randomized studies comparing endovascular and conservative treatment found a higher rate of good recovery with endovascular therapy in patients with ruptured dissection.[259]

Surgical Therapy

With the advent of endovascular techniques, the need for surgical intervention as the treatment for symptomatic dissecting aneurysm or post-dissection stenosis has significantly

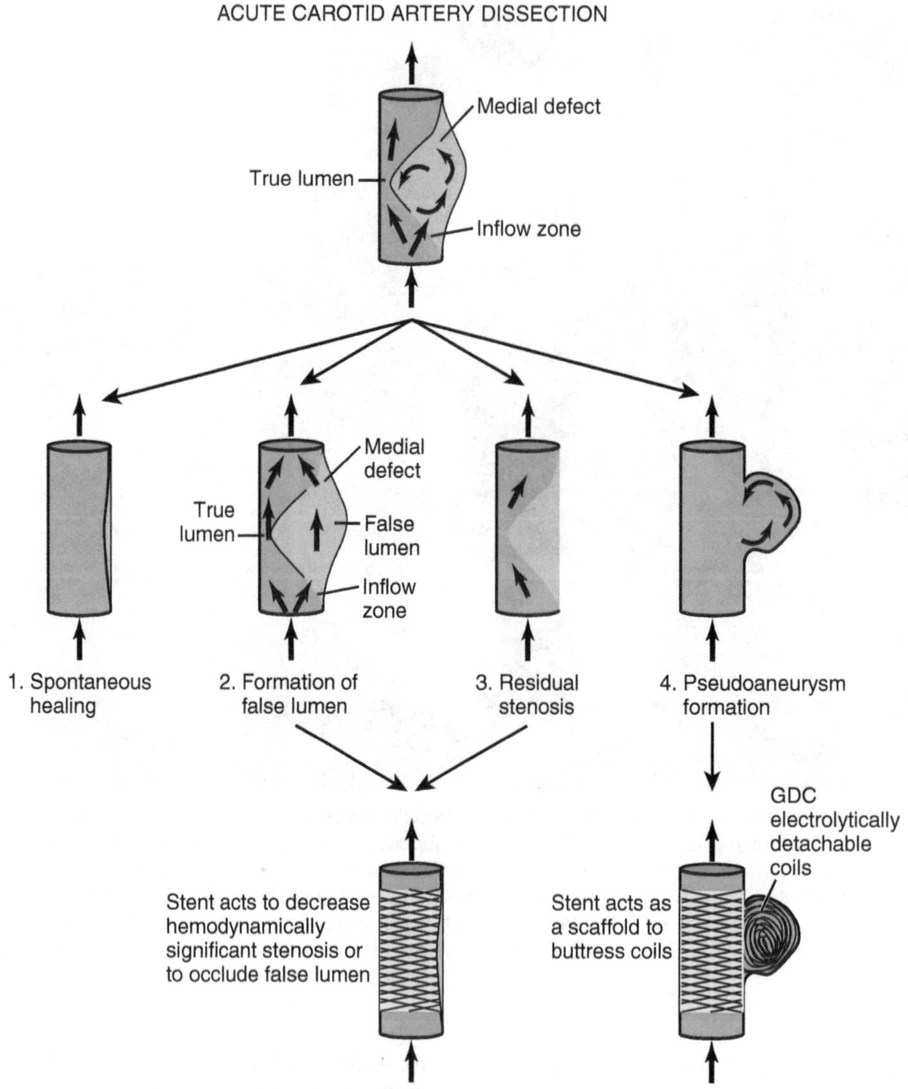

Figure 35-13. Simplified schematic illustration of the pathophysiologic process of carotid artery dissection proceeding from the acute stage to spontaneous healing (1), formation of false lumen (2), residual stenosis of varying degree or complete occlusion (3), or formation of a pseudoaneurysm (4). A stent is used in cases that have not responded to medical therapy, to relieve a hemodynamically significant stenosis, to occlude a false lumen, or to serve as a scaffold to enable coil embolization of a wide-necked pseudoaneurysm. GDC, Guglielmi detachable coil (Boston Scientific Corporation, Boston). *Arrows* indicate direction(s) of blood flow. *(From Malek AM, Higashida RT, Phatouros CC, et al: Endovascular management of extracranial carotid artery dissection achieved using stent angiography.* AJNR Am J Neuroradiol *21:1380, 2000.)*

decreased. Formerly, aneurysms accounted for 0.3% of extracranial ICA operations performed at the Cleveland Clinic[260] and 0.2% of those performed by the neurovascular surgical service at the Mayo Clinic.[252,261] Surgery is now reserved for patients who are symptomatic despite optimal medical therapy and who are not candidates for endovascular intervention.[26,252,262] Patients with impaired cerebral vasoreactivity who are at increased risk for stroke may benefit from surgical revascularization.[26,263]

Surgical treatment consists of carotid ligation, aneurysmal resection with carotid reconstruction, and cervical-to-intracranial ICA bypass (supraclinoid or petrous ICA). Aneurysmal clipping is usually not an option because of the fusiform configuration usually found at surgery. Extracranial dissecting aneurysms rarely necessitate surgery; they often resolve spontaneously, particularly those that are not traumatic in origin.[252,264] Surgical excision of the symptomatic dissecting aneurysm with reconstruction of the ICA to eliminate the aneurysm and maintain the artery's hemodynamic flow may be accomplished with interposition of a saphenous vein graft or primary reanastomosis (Fig. 35-16).[26] Because the majority of carotid dissecting aneurysms occur in the distal carotid artery near the skull base, surgery may cause pharyngeal and superior laryngeal branch injuries of the vagus nerve and resultant, although usually transient, dysphonia or dysphagia.

Carotid artery ligation, provided that adequate collateral flow is documented, has been performed. Complications include delayed ischemia due to embolization in the immediate post-operative period or long-term potential occurrence of cerebral ischemia or cerebral aneurysms.[26] Because of the risk of recurrent dissection in another vessel, preservation of vessel integrity is a practical and potentially critical consideration. Schievink[26] favors cervical-to-intracranial ICA bypass using a saphenous vein graft between the cervical carotid artery and the petrous or supraclinoid portion of the ICA or, less often, the proximal middle cerebral artery.

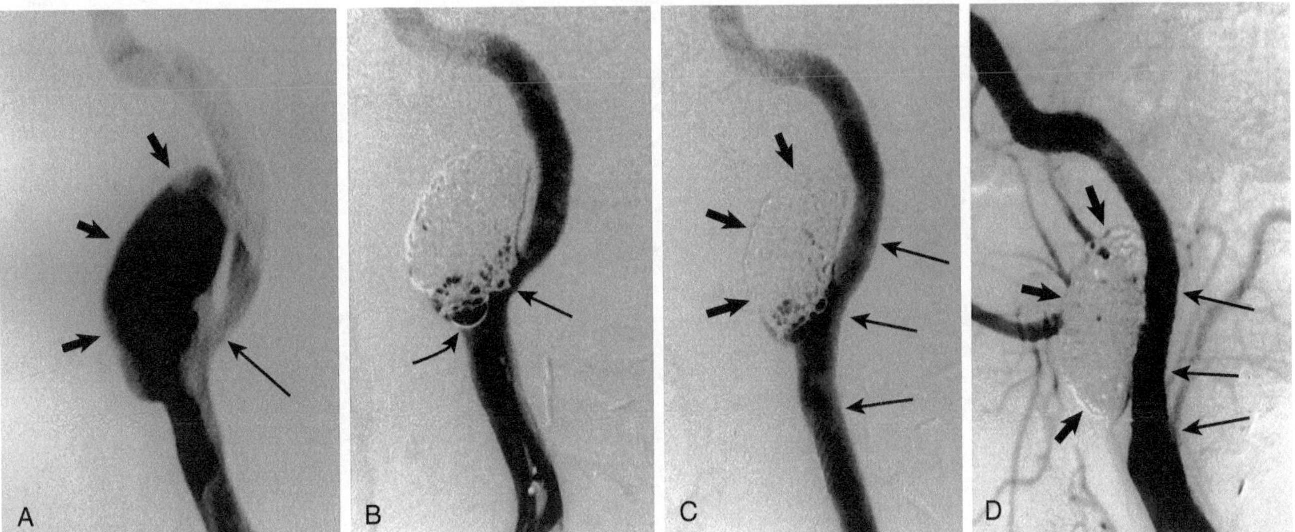

Figure 35-14. A 30-year-old woman with a left cervical internal carotid artery (ICA) pseudoaneurysm. A, Left internal carotid injection, lateral view, shows pseudoaneurysm *(short arrows)* and narrowed ICA *(long arrow)*. B, Left ICA angiogram after embolization with Guglielmi detachable coils shows the coils protruding into the parent artery *(arrows)*. C, Left ICA angiogram after embolization and stent placement shows the occluded pseudoaneurysm *(short arrows)* and the remodeled, stented carotid artery *(long arrows)*. D, At 6-month follow-up, a left common carotid angiogram shows total occlusion of the pseudoaneurysm *(short arrows)* and normal width and patency of the stented segment of the ICA *(long arrows)*. *(From Klein GE, Szolar DH, Raith J, et al: Post-traumatic extracranial aneurysm of the internal carotid artery: Combined endovascular treatment with coils and stents.* AJNR Am J Neuroradiol *18:1261, 1997.)*

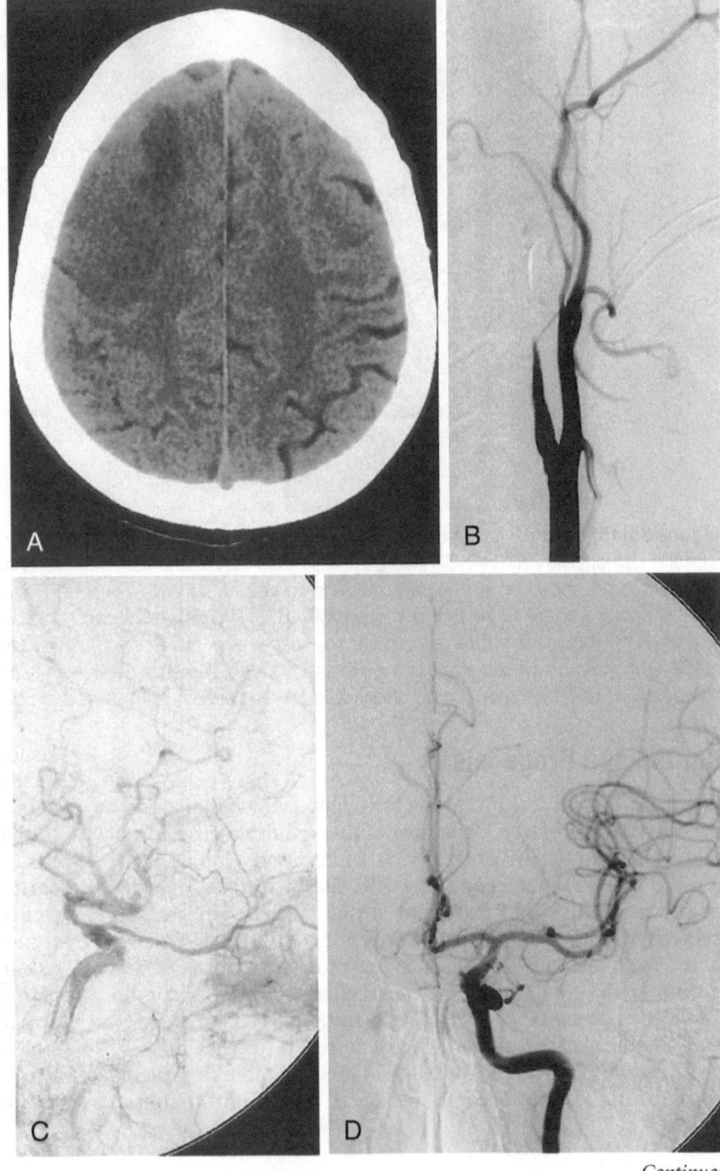

Figure 35-15. A 45-year-old woman noted to have left hemiparesis after diagnostic angiography. A, CT scan of the head shows evidence of a previous focal infarct as well as diffuse edema in the right posterior frontal lobe. B, Digital subtraction angiogram of the right common carotid artery reveals tapering of the right internal carotid artery (ICA) to a complete occlusion, with appearance consistent with dissection. C, Injection of the right external carotid artery shows retrograde collateral flow through the right ophthalmic artery, with filling of the cavernous segment of the right ICA. D, Injection of the left ICA shows no significant flow across the anterior communicating artery.

Continued

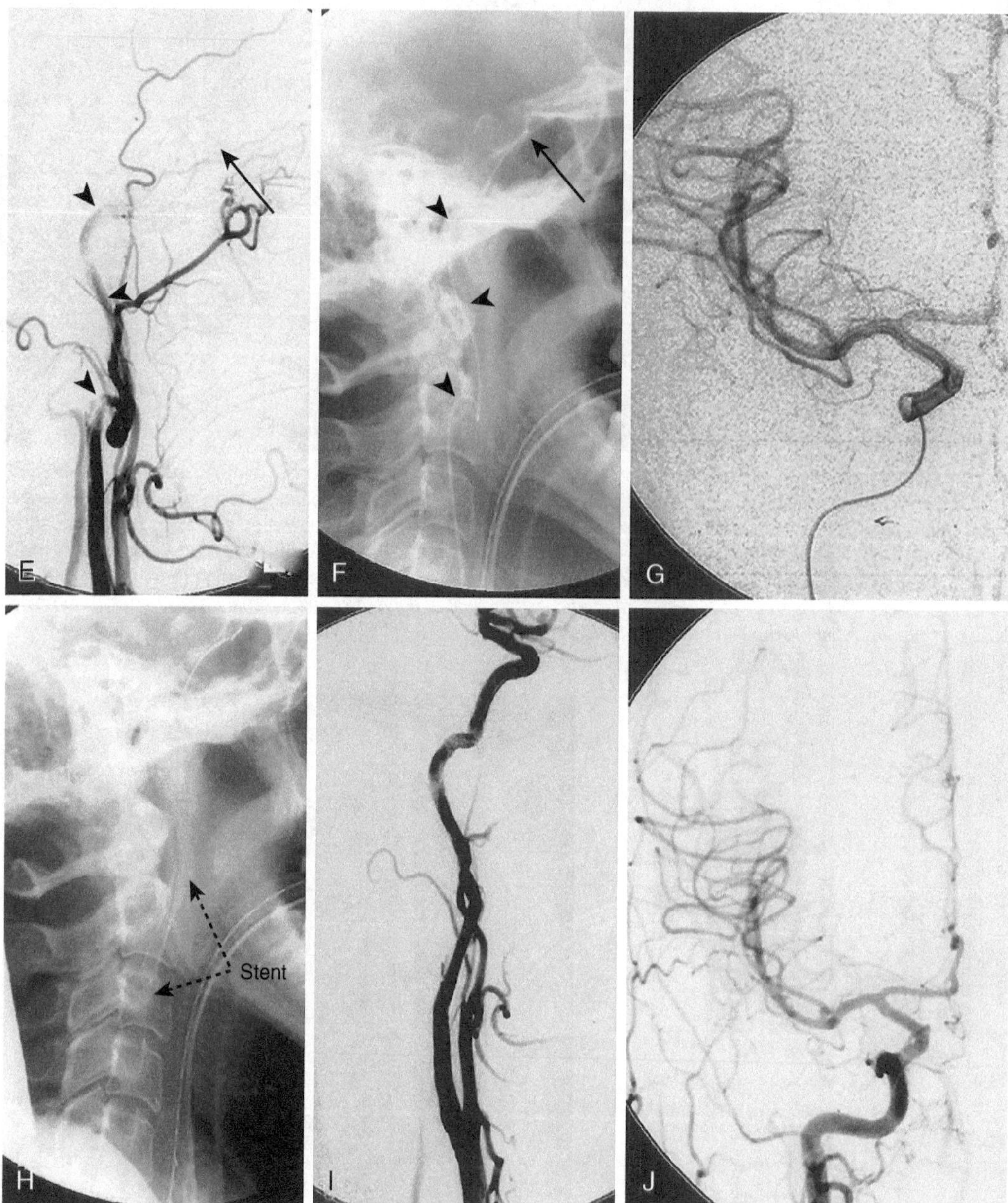

Figure 35-15, cont'd The treatment approach consisted of initial recanalization of the dissected right ICA, achieved by entering the true lumen with the use of a RAPIDTRANSIT Microcatheter (Codman & Shurtleff, Inc, Raynham, Mass) and Instinct-10 Microguidewire (E and F; *arrowheads*), which were advanced up to the cavernous portion of the right ICA (E and F; *arrow*). G, Superselective injection shows a patent right middle and anterior cerebral artery. H, An 8 mm × 2 cm WALLSTENT (Boston Scientific Corporation) was then deployed at the dissection site over a STABILIZER exchange Microguidewire (Cordis Corporation, Bridgewater, NJ) at the C2 level. The reconstitution of the lumen of the right ICA is shown by injection of the right common carotid artery (I), with resumption of intracranial perfusion (J). *(From Malek AM, Higashida RT, Phatouros CC, et al: Endovascular management of extracranial carotid artery dissection achieved using stent angiography.* AJNR Am J Neuroradiol *21:1380, 2000.)*

Course and Prognosis

Although the clinical prognosis following extracranial carotid or vertebral dissection depends on the severity of the initial neurologic injury, in general it is quite good (Tables 35-1, 35-2).[20] The CADISS reported a 2% rate of ipsilateral stroke or death.[229a] Risk of subsequent stroke is higher in patients presenting with ischemic symptoms (i.e., stroke or TIA) compared to those with only local symptoms (e.g., Horner's syndrome, pain, etc.). Complete or excellent recovery occurs in 70–85% of patients.[27,109,112,113,265,266] Mortality is less than 5%[123] and significant neurologic deficits persist in only 5–10% of patients.[27,112] Neurologic outcome is less favorable in patients with carotid as opposed to vertebral dissection,[266] arterial occlusion,[140,267–269] traumatic dissections,[265] or intracranial dissection;[15,270] especially when it is associated with subarachnoid hemorrhage.[29,150,230,271] For example, 50% of survivors of intracranial carotid artery dissection have major residual deficits.[12,15,270] The prognosis of basilar artery dissection is particularly poor, with mortality exceeding 60%.[272] The risk of recurrent stroke more than 2 weeks after the diagnosis of dissection is exceedingly low (0.4% per year) with the highest risk in the first year.[20] Persistent recurrent headaches or neck pain are not uncommon and tend to occur more commonly in patients with traumatic dissections.[27,265,273]

Recurrent dissection in a previously involved extracranial artery is rare,[3–5,140,274,275] whereas the risk of recurrence in a previously uninvolved artery is low but not insignificant.[276]

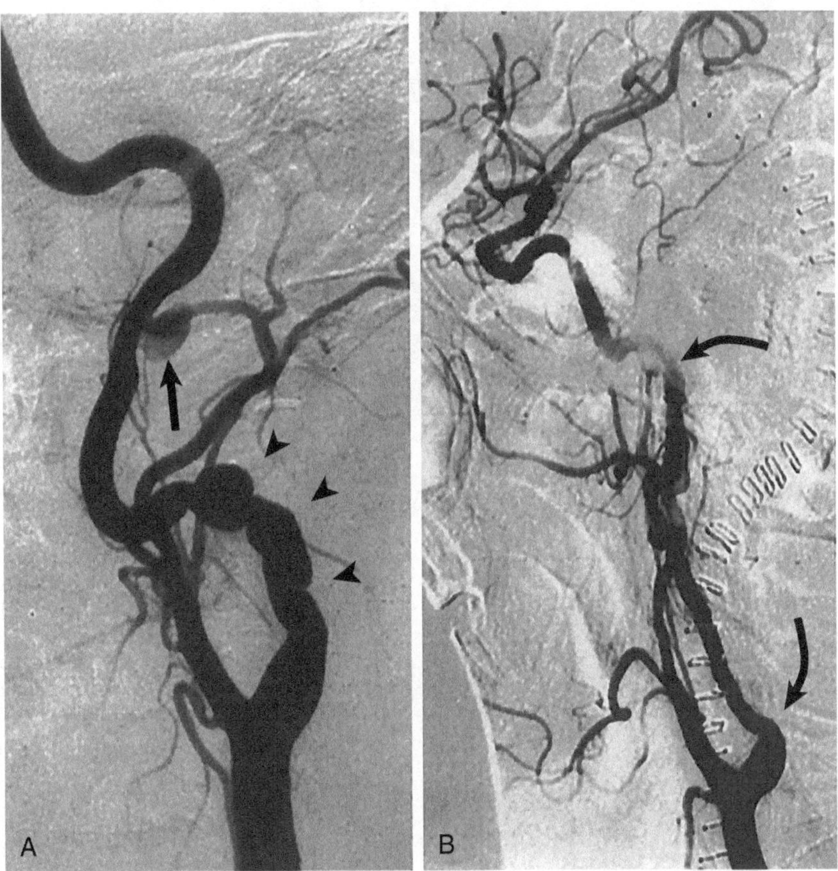

Figure 35-16. A, A lateral left common carotid angiogram reveals a spontaneous dissecting aneurysm (*arrow*) of the internal carotid artery and evidence of fibromuscular dysplasia (*arrowheads*). B, A lateral left common carotid angiogram obtained after resection of the abnormal segment of artery and reconstruction with an interposition saphenous vein graft; *arrows* indicate the location of the anastomoses. *(From Schievink WI: Spontaneous dissection of the carotid and vertebral arteries.* N Engl J Med *344:898, 2001.)*

Schievink and colleagues[3] reported a 2% recurrence risk in the first month with a 1% annual risk thereafter, and other series have reported similar figures, with equal rates for carotid and vertebral dissections.[4,5,20] A 24-center study of 459 patients by Touze and colleagues[275] reported a stroke recurrence rate of only 0.3% per year and a small study of 11 patients with triple or quadruple extracranial dissection reported no recurrence over 4 years.[277] In the Schievink series, risk declined with advancing age; the 10-year recurrence rate was 17% for patients younger than 45 years, and only 6% for patients older than 45 years (Fig. 35-17).[3] A family history of arterial dissection increased the risk of recurrence six times.[77] Presence of an underlying arteriopathy likewise increases the risk of recurrence.[4,5] Prognosis following intracranial dissection is more variable. After a mean follow-up of 46 months, Kim and colleagues reported no ruptures in a series of 191 patients.[278] All patients presenting with headache alone had good outcomes and 92 of 102 (90%) presenting with ischemic symptoms had good outcomes. Prognosis following ruptured intracranial dissection is not as benign. A Japanese series found 35 of 37 (95%) patients who presented with hemorrhage had hemorrhagic recurrence within 4.8 days.[279]

The angiographic prognosis of cervicocephalic dissection is favorable, although no correlation between angiographic and clinical prognosis has been found.[113,280] Angiographic stenoses improve or resolve in 80–90% of cases, with the rate of complete resolution averaging approximately 50–65% in published series.[27,112,113,182,184,196,265,280,281] Arterial occlusions recanalize in more than one-half of cases.[112,113,140,182,184,265] Complete resolution is seen in more than 20% of dissecting aneurysms,[112,181,184,196,265,282,283] and resolution or improvement in approximately 50%.[112,181,184,196,265,280,283] Angiographic improvement occurs within the first 2–3 months after the dissection and is rare after 6 months.[19,20,113,128,140,187,190,284] Rupture of extracranial dissecting aneurysms is not commonly described; rather, thromboembolism from dissecting aneurysms or expansion of the aneurysm compressing adjacent structures merits continued monitoring.[11,181,252,282,285]

FIBROMUSCULAR DYSPLASIA

Epidemiology

Fibromuscular dysplasia (FMD) is an uncommon non-atheromatous, non-inflammatory vasculopathy characterized by alternating fibrotic thickening and atrophy of the vessel wall. It affects women more commonly than men at a ratio of 2:1 and is more common in white persons.[286,287] Although commonly diagnosed in middle age (20–50 years), FMD can be found at any age. Population data regarding prevalence are lacking, although a single autopsy study reported histologically confirmed FMD of the internal carotid artery in 0.02% of 20,244 cases between 1968 and 1992.[286]

Pathology

FMD is classified based on the arterial layer that is primarily affected (intima, media, or adventitia). *Medial dysplasia* is the most common type of FMD and is further subdivided into three histologic types (medial fibroplasia, perimedial fibroplasia,

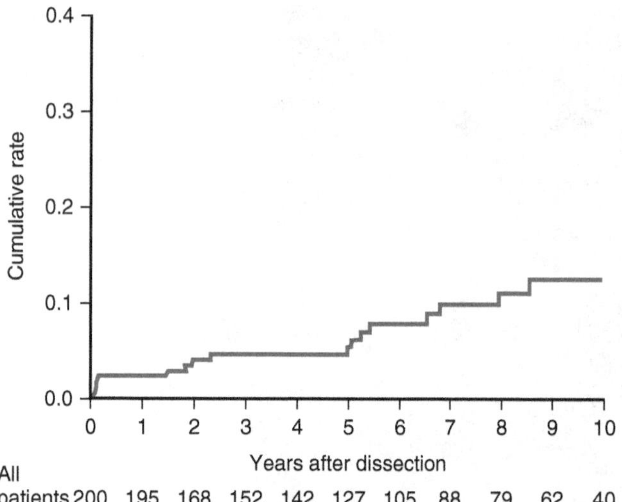

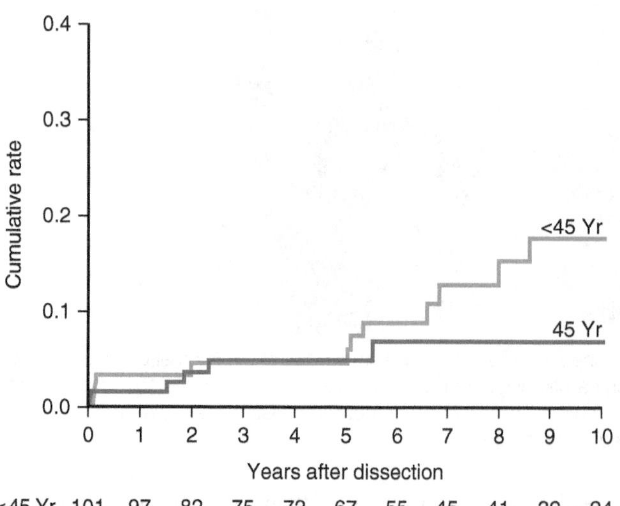

Figure 35-17. Cumulative rate of recurrent arterial dissection in all patients (*upper panel*) and according to age (*lower panel*). The numbers shown below each panel are the numbers of patients at risk for recurrent dissection at each point. *(From Schievink WI, Mokri B, O'Fallon M: Recurrent spontaneous cervical artery dissection.* N Engl J Med *330:393, 1994.)*

and medial hyperplasia). Medial fibroplasia is the most common form (75–80%) leading to the classic "string of beads" appearance, in which the beads are larger than the normal vessel diameter. Perimedial fibroplasia accounts for less than 10% of FMD cases and occurs most commonly in girls between 5 and 15 years old. Histologically, there is extensive collagen deposition in the outer half of the media. Medial hyperplasia is rare and is characterized by smooth muscle cell hyperplasia without fibrosis. *Intimal fibroplasia* affects fewer than 10% of patients with FMD and is characterized by focal concentric stenosis, long, smooth narrowing, or an arterial loop. The rarest form, *adventitial (periarterial) fibroplasia,* is characterized by sharply localized, tubular areas of stenosis. Histologically, dense collagen replaces the fibrous tissue of the adventitia.

Pathogenesis

Although several risk factors have been identified (e.g., tobacco use and hypertension[288]), the etiology of FMD remains unknown. As with dissection, genetic factors likely play a role because FMD is more common in first-degree relatives of patients with renal artery FMD[289] and individuals with the angiotensin converting enzyme allele ACE-I.[290] Other associated conditions include Ehlers–Danlos syndrome (type IV) and α_1-antitripsin deficiency.[56,291–293] Additional hypotheses regarding pathogenesis have been proposed, including ischemic, mechanical, toxic, hormonal, metabolic and immunological factors.[294–297] It remains most likely that the cause of FMD is multifactorial. Irrespective of the specific type and pathoetiology of FMD, the histopathologic changes are due to a fibroblast-like transformation of smooth muscle cells that allows them to produce extracellular matrix proteins, particularly collagen.[298]

Sites

FMD more commonly affects the extracranial vessels with a predilection for the carotid artery.[299] Carotid involvement is typically bilateral[57,299] and adjacent to the C1–C2 interspace.[287,300] Vertebral involvement occurs in roughly 10% of cervicocephalic cases,[287,300] is typically randomly distributed[299] and often coexists with carotid involvement.[300] Intracranial carotid or vertebral involvement occurs in up to 20% of cases and is typically limited to the intrapetrosal ICA or carotid siphon, although other vessels may be affected.[299,301,302]

Clinical Manifestations and Diagnosis

FMD is often asymptomatic but may present as nonspecific symptoms (e.g., Horner's syndrome) or cause a stroke syndrome via hemodynamic compromise,[303,304] secondary thromboembolism[299,305,306] or by direct complication (e.g., dissection,[3,53–55,269,307,308] aneurysm,[309] arteriovenous fistula[310,311]).

The diagnosis of cervicocephalic FMD may be made in asymptomatic patients undergoing evaluation of another disorder or in patients with ischemic and/or non-ischemic (e.g., bruit) symptoms. Imaging findings of cervicocephalic FMD typically fall into one of three categories. The most common is the typical string of beads pattern of alternating narrowing and dilation, most typically seen with the medial type (see Figs 35-16, 35-18). Unifocal or multifocal tubular narrowing is less common and not specific for any one histopathological subtype. Finally, imaging may reveal less common associated phenomena such as diverticula, aneurysms, and arterial webs.

There are no published studies comparing different imaging techniques in the diagnosis of cervicocephalic FMD. Digital subtraction angiography has been long considered the gold standard but non-invasive imaging techniques have been relied upon with increasing frequency. Duplex ultrasonography may reveal irregular patterns of stenosis suggestive of FMD,[312] but is a non-specific modality limited to evaluating the carotid bifurcation. MRA and CTA have become increasingly popular due to their non-invasive characteristics and abilities to image the complete cerebrovascular system. MRA artifact may mimic FMD;[313] when combined with MRI, MRA has the additional benefit of evaluation for associated ischemia.

Treatment

The prognosis of cervicocephalic FMD is typically fairly benign, and there are no prospective, randomized controlled trials to guide therapy. Studies of stroke rates in patients with cervicocephalic FMD suffer from poor design, but typically report low rates, even without therapy.[299,314–316] Corrin and associates,[315] for example, reported a recurrent stroke rate of 3.8% over 60 months. For this reason, treatment should

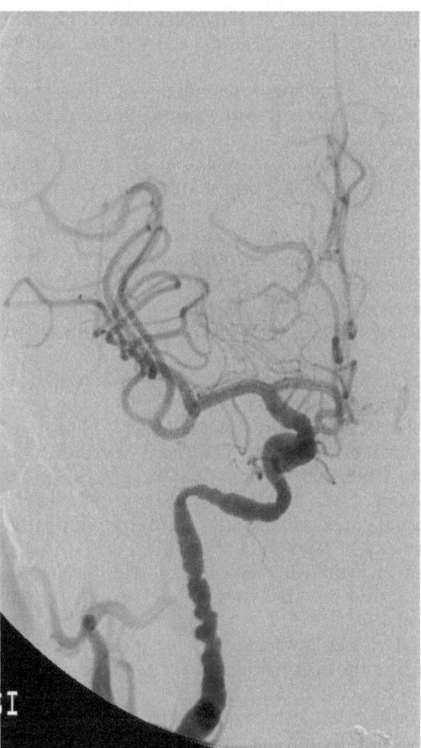

Figure 35-18. Digital subtraction angiogram of the carotid artery (lateral view) showing the typical string of beads pattern of alternating narrowing and dilation in fibromuscular dysplasia. *(Image courtesy of John Agola, MD.)*

generally be conservative in nature, especially in asymptomatic patients.

For the majority of symptomatic FMD cases, initial medical therapy, typically with antiplatelet agents, is recommended. In patients with cerebral aneurysms, antithrombotic therapy should be withheld until endovascular or surgical obliteration is achieved. For patients who fail to respond to antithrombotic therapy, consideration of percutaneous transluminal angioplasty with or without endovascular stenting may be appropriate, especially if there is hemodynamic compromise.[317,318] Surgical intervention is reserved for progressive clinical cases not amenable to endovascular therapy. Surgical procedures for FMD have included graduated internal dilatation, resection with end-to-side anastomosis or interposition graft and extracranial to intracranial (EC–IC) bypass in patients with hemodynamic compromise.[319–321]

The complete reference list can be found on the companion Expert Consult website at www.expertconsult.inkling.com.

KEY REFERENCES

1. Chan MT, Nadareishvili ZG, Norris JW. Diagnostic strategies in young patients with ischemic stroke in Canada. Can J Neurol Sci 2000;27:120.
3. Schievink WI, Mokri B, O'Fallon M. Recurrent spontaneous cervical artery dissection. New Engl J Med 1994;330:393.
4. Leys D, Moulin T, Stojkovic T, et al. Follow-up of patients with history of cervical artery dissection. Cerebrovasc Dis 1995; 4:43.
5. Bassetti C, Carruzzo A, Sturzenegger M, et al. Recurrence of cervical artery dissection: a prospective study of 81 patients. Stroke 1996;27:1804.
10. Arnold M, Kappeler L, Georgiadis D, et al. Gender differences in spontaneous cervical artery dissection. Neurology 2006;67: 1050–2.
11. Schievink WI, Mokri B, Jackers G. Spontaneous dissections of cervicocephalic arteries in childhood and adolescence. Neurology 1994;44:1607.
12. Fullerton HJ, Johnston SC, Smith WS. Arterial dissection and stroke in children. Neurology 2001;57:1155.
13. Leys D, Lucas C, Govert M, et al. Cervical artery dissections. Eur Neurol 1997;37:3.
15. Bassetti C, Bogousslavsky J, Eskenasy-Cottier AC, et al. Spontaneous intracranial dissection in the anterior circulation. Cerebrovasc Dis 1994;4:170.
16. Caplan LR, Zarins CK, Hemmat M. Spontaneous dissection of the extracranial vertebral arteries. Stroke 1996;16:1030.
19. Schievink WI. Spontaneous dissection of the carotid and vertebral arteries. New Engl J Med 2001;344:898.
21. Caplan LR, Baquis GD, Pessin MS, et al. Dissection of the intracranial vertebral artery. Neurology 1988;38:868.
22. Kawaguchi S, Sakaki T, Tsunoda S. Management of dissecting aneurysms of the posterior circulation. Acta Neurochir (Wien) 1994;131:26.
23. Kitanaka C, Sasaki T, Eguchi T, et al. Intracranial vertebral artery dissections: clinical, radiological features and surgical considerations. Neurosurgery 1994;34:620.
24. Sasaki O, Ogawa H, Koike T, et al. A clinicopathologic study of dissecting aneurysms of the intracranial vertebral artery. J Neurosurg 1991;75:874.
25. Bogousslavsky J. Dissections of the cerebral arteries clinical effects. Curr Opin Neurol Neurosurg 1988;1:63.
26. Schievink WI. The treatment of spontaneous carotid and vertebral artery dissections. Curr Opin Cardiol 2000;15:318–21.
27. Mokri B, Sundt TM, Houser OW, et al. Spontaneous dissection of the cervical internal carotid artery. Ann Neurol 1986;19:126.
28. Berger MS, Wilson CB. Intracranial dissecting aneurysms of the posterior circulation. Neurosurgery 1984;61:882.
34. Haldeman S, Kohlbeck F, McGregor M. Risk factors for vertebrobasilar artery dissection following cervical spine manipulation: a review of 60 cases. Neurology 1996;46:A440.
36. Norris JW, Beletsky V, Nadareishvili ZG, et al. Sudden neck movement and cervical artery dissection. CMAJ 2000;163:38.
41. Rothwell DM, Bondy SJ, Williams JI. Chiropractic manipulation and stroke: a population-based case-control study. Stroke 2001; 32:1054.
51. Schievink WI, Mokri B, Piepgras DG, et al. Cervical artery dissections associated with chiropractic manipulation of the neck; the importance of pre-existing arterial disease and injury. J Neurol 1996;243:S92.
52. Fisher CM, Ojemann RG, Robertson GH. Spontaneous dissection of cervicocerebral arteries. Can J Neurol Sci 1978;5:9–19.
54. Schievink WI, Bjornsson J, Piepgras DG. Coexistence of fibromuscular dysplasia and cystic medial necrosis in a patient with Marfan's syndrome and bilateral carotid artery dissections. Stroke 1994;25:2492–6.
55. Schievink WI, Michels VV, Piepgras DG. Neurovascular manifestations of heritable connective tissue disorders – a review. Stroke 1994;25:889.
56. Schievink WI, Mokri B, Piepgras DG. Fibromuscular dysplasia of the internal carotid artery associated with alpha-1-antitrypsin deficiency. Neurosurg 1998;43:229.
57. Stanley JC, Fry WJ, Seeger JF, et al. Extracranial internal carotid and vertebral artery fibrodysplasia. Arch Surg 1974;109:215–22.
58. Schievink WI, Wijdicks EFM, Michels VV, et al. Heritable connective tissue disorders in cervical artery dissections: a prospective study. Neurol 1998;50:1166.
59. North KN, Whiteman DAH, Pepin MG, et al. Cerebrovascular complications in Ehlers-Danlos syndrome type IV. Ann Neurol 1995;38:960.
60. Schievink WI, Limburg M, Dorthuys JE, et al. Cerebrovascular disease in Ehlers-Danlos syndrome type IV. Stroke 1990;21:626.
61. Ulbricht D, Diederich NJ, Hermanns-Le T, et al. Cervical artery dissection: An atypical presentation with Ehlers-Danlos-like collagen pathology? Neurology 2004;63:1708–10.
66. Schievink WI, Prakash UBS, Piepgras DG, et al. α-Antitrypsin deficiency in intracranial aneurysms and cervical artery dissection. Lancet 1994;343:452.
67. Brice JG, Crompton MR. Spontaneous dissecting aneurysms of the cervical internal carotid artery. BMJ 1964;2:790.

73. Guillon B, Tzourio C, Biousse V, et al. Arterial wall properties in carotid artery dissection: An ultrasound study. Neurology 2000; 55:663–6.
74. Tzourio C, Cohen A, Lamisse N, et al. Aortic root dilatation in patients with spontaneous cervical artery dissection. Circulation 1997;95:2351.
75. Schievink WI, Mokri B, Michels VV, et al. Familial association of intracranial aneurysms and cervical artery dissections. Stroke 1991;22:1426–30.
76. Schievink WI, Mokri B, Piepgras DG. Angiographic frequency of saccular intracranial aneurysms in patients with spontaneous cervical artery dissection. J Neurosurg 1992;76:62–6.
77. Schievink WI, Mokri B, Piepgras DG, et al. Recurrent spontaneous arterial dissections: risk in familial versus nonfamilial disease. Stroke 1996;27:622.
79. Fisher CM. The headache and pain of spontaneous carotid dissection. Headache 1982;22:60–5.
81. Rist PM, Diener HC, Kurth T, et al. Migraine, migraine aura, and cervical artery dissection: a systematic review and meta-analysis. Cephalalgia 2011;31:886–96.
85. Wiebers DO, Mokri B. Internal carotid artery dissection after childbirth. Stroke 1985;16:956.
91. Schievink WI, Michels VV, Piepgras DG, et al. A familial syndrome of arterial dissections with lentiginosis. New Engl J Med 1995;332:579.
93. Brandt T, Hausser I, Orberk E, et al. Ultrastructional connective tissue abnormalities in patients with spontaneous cervicocerebral artery dissections. Ann Neurol 1998;44:281.
94. Brandt T, Orberk E, Weber R, et al. Pathogenesis of cervical artery dissections: association with connective tissue abnormalities. Neurol 2001;57:24.
95. Dunac A, Blecic S, Jeangette S, et al. Stroke due to artery dissection: role of collagen disease. Cerebrovasc Dis 1998;8:18.
96. Brandt T, Grond-Ginsbach C. Spontaneous cervical artery dissection: from risk factors toward pathogenesis (editorial). Stroke 2002;33:657.
97. Volker W, Besselmann M, Dittrich R, et al. Generalized arteriopathy in patients with cervical artery dissection. Neurology 2005;64:1508–13.
98. Grond-Ginsbach C, Weber R, Hausser I, et al. Familial connective tissue alterations in patients with spontaneous cervical artery dissections. Cerebrovasc Dis 2000;10:37.
99. Grond-Ginsbach C, Weber R, Haas J, et al. Mutations in the COL5A1 coding sequence are not common in patients with cervical artery dissections. Stroke 1999;30:1887.
100. Kiuvaniemi H, Prockop DJ, Wu Y, et al. Exclusion of mutations in the gene for type III collagen (COL3A1) as a common cause of intracranial aneurysms or cervical artery dissections: results from sequence analysis of the coding sequences of type III collagen from 55 unrelated patients. Neurol 1993;43: 2652.
101. van den Berg JS, Limburg M, Kappelle LJ, et al. The role of type III collagen in spontaneous cervical arterial dissections. Ann Neurol 1998;43:494.
102. Grond-Ginsbach C, Thomas-Feles C, Weber R, et al. Mutations in the tropoelastine gene (ELN) were not found in patients with spontaneous cervical artery dissection. Stroke 2000;31: 1935.
105. Renard D, Azakri S, Arquizan C, et al. Styloid and hyoid bone proximity is a risk factor for cervical carotid artery dissection. Stroke 2013;44:2475–9.
106. Frisoni GB, Anzola GP. Vertebrobasilar ischemia after neck motion. Stroke 1991;22:1452.
107. Josien E. Extracranial vertebral artery dissection: nine cases. J Neurol 1992;239:327.
108. Bin Saeed A, Shuaib A, Al-Sulaiti G, et al. Vertebral artery dissection: warning symptoms, clinical features and prognosis in 26 patients. Can J Neurol Sci 2000;27:292.
109. Arnold M, Bousser MG, Fahrni G, et al. Vertebral Artery Dissection: Presenting Findings and Predictors of Outcome. Stroke 2006;37(10):2499–503.
113. Desfontaines P, Despland A. Dissection of the internal carotid artery: aetiology, symptomatology, clinical and neurosonological follow-up and treatment in 60 consecutive cases. Acta Neurol Psych Belg 1995;94:226.
114. Weiller C, Mullges W, Ringelstein EB, et al. Patterns of brain infarction in internal carotid artery dissections. Neurosurg Rev 1991;14:111.
115. Steinke W, Schwartz A, Hennerici M. Topography of cerebral infarction associated with carotid artery dissection. J Neurol 1996;243:323.
116. Lucas C, Moulin T, Deplanque D, et al. Stroke patterns of internal carotid artery dissection in 40 patients. Stroke 1998;29: 2646.
117. Baumgartner RW, Arnold M, Baumgartner I, et al. Carotid dissection with and without ischemic events: local symptoms and cerebral artery findings. Neurol 2001;57:827.
120. Biousse V, D'Anglejean-Chatillon J, Touboul P-J, et al. Time course of symptoms in extracranial carotid artery dissections. Stroke 1995;26:235.
123. Mokri B. Spontaneous dissections of internal carotid arteries. Neurologist 1997;3:104.
124. Mullges W, Ringelstein EB, Leibold M. Non-invasive diagnosis of internal carotid artery dissections. J Neurol Neurosurgery Psychiatry 1992;55:98.
125. Ramadan NM, Tietjen GE, Levine SR, et al. Scintillating scotomata associated with internal carotid artery dissection. Neurology 1991;41:1084.
126. Silbert PL, Mokri B, Schievink WI. Headache and neck pain in spontaneous internal carotid and vertebral artery dissections. Neurol 1995;45:1517.
127. Sue DE, Brant-Zawadzki MN, Chance J. Dissection of cranial arteries in the neck: correlation of MRI and arteoriography. Neuroradiology 1992;34:273.
128. Sturzenegger M. Spontaneous internal carotid artery dissection: early diagnosis and management in 44 patients. J Neurol 1995; 242:231.
129. Biousse V, D'Anglejean-Chatillon J, Touboul P-J, et al. Head pain in non-traumatic carotid artery dissections. Cephalgia 1994;14: 33.
130. Mokri B, Silbert PL, Shievink WI, et al. Cranial nerve palsy in spontaneous internal carotid and vertebral artery dissections. Neurol 1996;46:356.
131. Francis KR, Williams DP, Troost BT. Facial numbness and dysesthesia: new features of carotid artery dissection. Arch Neurol 1987;44:345.
132. Goodman JM, Zink WL, Cooper DF. Hemilingual paralysis caused by carotid artery dissection. Arch Neurol 1983;653.
133. Guidetti D, Pisanello A, Giovanardi F, et al. Spontaneous carotid dissection presenting lower cranial nerve palsies. J Neurol Sci 2001;184:203–7.
134. Panisset M, Eidelman BH. Multiple cranial neuropathy as a feature of internal carotid artery dissection. Stroke 1990;21:141.
135. Sturzenegger M, Huber P. Cranial nerve palsies in spontaneous carotid artery dissection. J Neurol Neurosurg Psychiatry 1993;56: 1191.
138. Pelkonen O, Tikkakoski T, Luotonen J, et al. Pulsatile tinnitus as a symptom of cervicocephalic arterial dissection. J Laryngol Otol 2004;118:193–8.
145. Adams HPJ, Aschenbrener CA, Kassell NF, et al. Intracranial hemorrhage produced by spontaneous dissecting intracranial aneurysm. Arch Neurol 1982;39:773.
152. Crum B, Mokri B, Fulgham J. Spinal manifestations of vertebral artery dissection. Neurology 2000;55:304.
153. Weidauer S, Claus D, Gartenschlager M. Spinal sulcal artery syndrome due to spontaneous bilateral vertebral artery dissection. J Neurol Neurosurg Psychiatry 1999;67:550.
154. Goldsmith P, Rowe D, Jager R, et al. Focal vertebral artery dissection causing Brown-Sequard's syndrome. J Neurol Neurosurg Psychiatry 1998;64:415.
161. Woimant F, Spelle L. Spontaneous basilar artery dissection: contribution of magnetic resonance imaging to diagnosis. J Neurol Neurosurg Psychiatry 1995;58:540.
166. Hosoda K, Fujita S, Kawaguchi T, et al. Spontaneous dissecting aneurysms of the basilar artery presenting with subarachnoid hemorrhage. J Neurosurg 1991;75:628.
171. Pasquier B, N'Golet A, Pasquier D, et al. Vertebro-basilar dissecting aneurysm. Sem Hop Paris 1979;55:487–8.
174. Pozzati E, Andreoli A, Padovani R, et al. Dissecting aneurysms of the basilar artery. Neurosurgery 1995;36:254.

181. Djouhri H, Guillon B, Brunereau L, et al. MR angiography for the long-term follow-up of dissecting aneurysms of the extracranial internal carotid artery. Am J Roentgenol 2000;174:1137.
188. Mascalchi M, Bianchi MC, Mangiafico S, et al. MRI and MRI angiography of vertebral artery dissection. Neuroradiol 1997;39: 329.
189. de Bray JM, Lhoste P, Dubas F, et al. Ultrasonic features of extracranial carotid dissections: 47 cases studied by angiography. J Ultrasound Med 1994;13:659.
190. Sturzenegger M, Mattle HP, Rivoir A, et al. Ultrasound findings in carotid artery dissection: analysis of 43 patients. Neurology 1995;45:691.
192. Sturzenegger M, Mattle HP, Rivoir A, et al. Ultrasound findings in spontaneious extracranial vertebral artery dissection. Stroke 1993;24:1910.
193. Steinke W, Rautenberg W, Schwartz A, et al. Noninvasive monitoring of internal carotid artery dissection. Stroke 1994;25:998.
195. Baumgartner RW, Baumgartner I, Mattle HP, et al. Transcranial color-coded duplex sonography in the evaluatin of collateral flow througt the circle of Willis. Am J Neuroradiol 1997;18:127.
197. Lu C-J, Sun Y, Jeng J-S, et al. Imaging in the diagnosis and follow-up evaluation of vertebral artery dissection. J Ultrasound Med 2000;19:263.
198. Alecu C, Fortrat JO, Ducrocq X, et al. Duplex scanning diagnosis of internal carotid artery dissections. A case control study. Cerebrovasc Dis 2007;23:441–7.
202. Stapf C, Elkind SV, Mohr JP. Carotid artery dissection. Annu Rev Med 2001;51:329.
203. Silverboard G, Tart R. Cerebrovascular arterial dissection in children and young adults. Sem Pediatr Neurol 2000;7:4, 278.
208. Fredenberg P, Forbes K, Toye L, et al. Assessment of cervical vascular injury with CT angiography. BNI Q 2001;17:44.
209. Elijovich L, Kazmi K, Gauvrit J, et al. The emerging role of multidetector row CT angiography in the diagnosis of cervical arterial dissection: preliminary study. Neuroradiology 2006;48: 606–12.
210. Chen CJ, Tseng YC, Lee TH, et al. Multisection CT Angiography Compared with Catheter Angiography in Diagnosing Vertebral Artery Dissection. AJNR Am J Neuroradiol 2004;25:769–74.
211. Vertinsky AT, Schwartz NE, Fischbein NJ, et al. Comparison of Multidetector CT Angiography and MR Imaging of Cervical Artery Dissection. AJNR Am J Neuroradiol 2008;29:1753–60.
212. Provenzale JM, Sarikaya B. Comparison of test performance characteristics of MRI, MR angiography, and CT angiography in the diagnosis of carotid and vertebral artery dissection: a review of the medical literature. AJR Am J Roentgenol 2009;193: 1167–74.
213. Osborn AG, Anderson RE. Angiographic spectrum of cervical and intracranial fibromuscular dysplasia. Stroke 1997;8:617.
217. Derex L, Nighoghossian N, Turjman F, et al. Intravenous tPA in acute ischemic stroke to internal carotid artery dissection. Neurology 2000;54:2159.
218. Arnold M, Nedeltchev K, Sturzzenegger M, et al. Thrombolysis in patients with acute stroke caused by cervical artery dissection: analysis of 9 patients and review of the literature. Arch Neurol 2002;59:549.
222. Georgiadis D, Lanczik O, Schwab S, et al. IV thrombolysis in patients with acute stroke due to spontaneous carotid dissection. Neurology 2005;64:1612–14.
223. Lavallee PC, Mazighi M, Saint-Maurice JP, et al. Stent-assisted endovascular thrombolysis versus intravenous thrombolysis in internal carotid artery dissection with tandem internal carotid and middle cerebral artery occlusion. Stroke 2007;38:2270–4.
224. Engelter ST, Rutgers MP, Hatz F, et al. Intravenous thrombolysis in stroke attributable to cervical artery dissection. Stroke 2009; 40(12):3772–6.
225. Zinkstok SM, Vergouwen MDI, Engelter ST, et al. Safety and Functional Outcome of Thrombolysis in Dissection-Related Ischemic Stroke: A Meta-Analysis of Individual Patient Data. Stroke 2011;42(9):2515–20.
226. Lyrer P, Engelter S. Antithrombotic drugs for carotid artery dissection. Cochrane Coll 4-13-2011.
227. Kennedy F, Lanfranconi S, Hicks C, et al. Antiplatelets vs anticoagulation for dissection: CADISS nonrandomized arm and meta-analysis. Neurology 2012;79:686–9.
228. Kurnan WN, Ovbiagele B, Black HR, et al. Guidelines for the prevention of stroke in patients with stroke and transient ischemic attack: a guideline for healthcare professionals from the American Heart Association/American Stroke Association. Stroke 2014;45:2160–236.
229. The CADISS Trial Investigators. Antiplatelet therapy vs. anticoagulation in cervical artery dissection: rationale and design of the Cervical Artery Dissection in Stroke Study (CADISS). Int J Stroke 2007;2(4):292–6.
229a. Markus HS. The Cervical Artery Dissection in Stroke Study (CADISS), International Stroke Conference, Nashville, 2015.
230. Metso TM, Metso AJ, Helenius J, et al. Prognosis and safety of anticoagulation in intracranial artery dissections in adults. Stroke 2007;38(6):1837–42.
234. Malek AM, Higashida RT, Phatouros CC, et al. Endovascular management of extracranial carotid artery dissection achieved using stent angioplasty. Am J Neuroradiology 2000;21:1380.
251. Scavee V, DeWispelaere JF, Mormont E, et al. Psuedoaneurysm of the internal carotid artery: Treatment with a covered stent. Cardiovasc Intervent Radiol 2001;24:283.
252. Schievink WI, Piepgras DG, McCaffrey TV, et al. Surgical treatment of extracranial internal carotid artery dissecting aneurysms. Neurosurgery 1994;35:809.
258. Menon R, Kerry S, Norris JW, et al. Treatment of cervical artery dissection: a systematic review and meta-analysis. J Neurol Neurosurg Psychiatry 2008;79:1122–7.
259. Chen Y, Guan J-J, Liu A-H, et al. Outcome of cervicocranial artery dissection with different treatments: a systematic review and meta-analysis. J Stroke Cerebrovasc Dis 2014;23:e177–86.
266. von Babo M, De Marchis GM, Sarikaya H, et al. Differences and similarities between spontaneous dissections of the internal carotid artery and the vertebral artery. Stroke 2013;44:1537–42.
268. Milhaud K, de Freitas GR, van Melle G, et al. Occlusion due to carotid artery dissection. Arch Neurol 2002;59:557.
269. Dziewas R, Konrad C, Drager B, et al. Cervical artery dissection – clinical features, risk factors, therapy and outcome in 126 patients. J Neurol 2003;250(10):1179–84.
270. de Bray JM, Pennison-Besnier I, Dubas F, et al. Extracranial and intracranial vertebrobasilar dissections: diagnosis and prognosis. J Neurol Neurosurgery Psychiatry 1997;63:46.
275. Touze E, Gauvrit JY, Moulin T, et al. Risk of stroke and recurrent dissection after a cervical artery dissection: A multicenter study. Neurology 2003;61:1347–51.
276. Dittrich R, Nassenstein I, Bachmann R, et al. Polyarterial clustered recurrence of cervical artery dissection seems to be the rule. Neurology 2007;69(2):180–6.
277. Arnold M, De Marchis GM, Stapf C, et al. Triple and quadruple spontaneous cervical artery dissection: presenting characteristics and long-term outcome. J Neurol Neurosurg Psychiatry 2009;80: 171–4.
278. Kim BM, Kim SH, Kim DJ, et al. Outcomes and prognostic factors of intracranial unruptured vertebrobasilar artery dissection. Neurology 2011;76:1735–41.
279. Ono H, Nakotomi H, Tsutsumi K, et al. Symptomatic recurrence of intracranial arterial dissections. Stroke 2013;44:126–31.
280. Engelter ST, Lyrer PA, Kirsch EC, et al. Long-term follow-up after extracranial internal carotid artery dissection. Eur Neurol 2000; 44:199.
281. Arauz A, Marquez JM, Artigas C, et al. Recanalization of vertebral artery dissection. Stroke 2010;41:717–21.
282. Guillon B, Brunereau L, Biousse V, et al. Long-term follow-up of aneurysms developed during extracranial internal carotid dissection. Neurol 1999;53:117.
283. Touze E, Randoux B, Meary E, et al. Aneurysmal forms of cervical artery dissection: associated factors and outcome. Stroke 2001;32: 418.
284. Treiman GS, Treima RL, Foran RF, et al. Spontaneous dissection of the internal carotid artery: a nineteen-year clinical experience. J Vasc Surg 1996;24:597.
285. Benninger DH, Gandjour J, Georgiadis D, et al. Benign long-term outcome of conservatively treated cervical aneurysms due to carotid dissection. Neurology 2007;69(5):486–7.
286. Schievink WI, Bjornsson J. Fibromuscular dysplasia of the internal carotid artery: A clinicopathological study. Clin Neuropathol 1996;15(1):2–6.

287. Mettinger KL. Fibromuscular dysplasia and the brain II: current concept of disease. Stroke 1982;13(1):53–8.
291. Solder B, Streif W, Ellemunter H, et al. Fibromuscular dysplasia of the internal carotid artery in a child with alpha-1-antitrypsin deficiency. Dev Med Child Neurol 1997;39(12):827–9.
292. Schievink WI, Bjornsson J, Parisi JE, et al. Arterial fibromuscular dysplasia associated with severe alpha 1-antitrypsin deficiency. Mayo Clin Proc 1994;69(11):1040–3.
299. So EL, Toole JF, Dalal P, et al. Cephalic fibromuscular dysplasia in 32 patients: clinical findings and radiologic features. Arch Neurol 1981;38(10):619–22.
300. Osborn AG, Anderson RE. Angiographic spectrum of cervical and intracranial fibromuscular dysplasia. Stroke 1977;8(5):617–26.
307. Grotta JC, Ward RE, Flynn TC, et al. Spontaneous internal carotid artery dissection associated with fibromuscular dysplasia. J Cardiovasc Surg 1982;23(6):512–14.
308. de Bray JM, Marc G, Pautot V, et al. Fibromuscular dysplasia may herald symptomatic recurrence of cervical artery dissection. Cerebrovasc Dis 2007;23(5–6):448–52.
309. Kimura H, Hosoda K, Hara Y, et al. A very unusual case of fibromuscular dysplasia with multiple aneurysms of the vertebral artery and posterior inferior cerebellar artery. J Neurosug 2008;109(6):1108–12.
312. Arning C, Grzyska U. Color doppler imaging of cervicocephalic fibromuscular dysplasia. Cardiovasc Ultrasound 2004;2:7.
313. Heiserman JE, Drayer BP, Fram EK, et al. MR angiography of cervical fibromuscular dysplasia. AJNR Am J Neuroradiol 1992;13(5):1454–7.
314. Sandok BA. Fibromuscular dysplasia of the internal carotid artery. Neurological Clinics. Philadelphia, PA: WB Saunders; 1983. p. 17–26.
315. Corrin LS, Sandok BA, Houser OW. Cerebral ischemic events in patients with carotid artery fibromuscular dysplasia. Arch Neurol 1981;38(10):616–18.
316. Wells RP, Smith RR. Fibromuscular dysplasia of the internal carotid artery: a long term follow-up. Neurosurgery 1982;10(1):39–43.
317. Wilms GE, Smits J, Baert AL, et al. Percutaneous transluminal angioplasty in fibromuscular dysplasia of the internal carotid artery: one year clinical and morphological follow-up. Cardiovasc Intervent Radiol 1985;8(1):20–3.
318. Curry TK, Messina LM. Fibromuscular dysplasia: when is intervention warranted? Semin Vasc Surg 2003;16(3):190–9.
320. Collins GJ Jr, Rich NM, Clagett GP, et al. Fibromuscular dysplasia of the internal carotid arteries. Clinical experience and follow-up. Ann Surg 1981;194(1):89–96.
321. Wesen CA, Elliott BM. Fibromuscular dysplasia of the carotid arteries. Am J Surg 1986;151(4):448–51.

36 Collagen Vascular and Infectious Diseases

Jose Gutierrez, Mira Katan, Mitchell S.V. Elkind

KEY POINTS

- Primary angiitis of the CNS (PACNS) is an inflammatory arterial disease restricted to the cerebral circulation that can afflict patients of any age, and often responds poorly to steroids alone.
- Patients with PACNS commonly present with a combination of headache, encephalopathy, seizure, and ischemic or hemorrhagic stroke.
- PACNS can be associated with lymphoma, AIDS, leukemia, sarcoidosis, varicella zoster virus infection, and cerebral amyloid angiopathy.
- The most consistent cerebrospinal fluid (CSF) abnormality in PACNS is an increase in protein, and many patients have a moderate lymphocytic pleocytosis.
- Neurological symptoms associated with giant cell arteritis (GCA) include the new onset of a persistent headache, jaw claudication, visual symptoms (such as diplopia, scotoma, amaurosis fugax, or blindness), and rarely stroke.
- Almost all patients with giant cell arteritis-associated strokes have a significant acute-phase response with elevated ESR and C-reactive protein.
- Visual loss is one of the most feared complications of giant cell arteritis, and anterior ischemic optic neuropathy is its most common cause.
- Once the diagnosis of GCA is suspected, the patient should be started on steroid therapy and biopsy performed as soon as possible.
- Although vasculitis is frequently mentioned as an important cause of stroke in patients with systemic lupus erythematosus, documented vasculitic changes on postmortem examination are actually quite rare.
- All patients with neurosyphilis should also be tested for HIV.
- The most common parasitic illnesses that cause stroke are Chagas disease and neurocysticercosis.
- *Aspergillus fumigatus* is a highly angiotrophic fungus that causes stroke in immunocompromised patients, but it can affect immunocompetent patients as well.
- Because not all patients with vasculitis due to varicella zoster virus report prior exposure to VZV infection or rash, VZV should be considered in cases of cryptogenic arteriopathy and stroke.

Stroke is a common complication of many inflammatory, collagen vascular, and infectious diseases. This chapter reviews the clinical findings, diagnosis, and treatment of stroke associated with some of the most common inflammatory and infectious diseases.

VASCULITIDES OF THE CENTRAL NERVOUS SYSTEM

Vasculitides comprise a heterogeneous group of diseases characterized by inflammation of the blood vessel wall.[1] The central nervous system (CNS) can be a target of both primary and secondary CNS vasculitis. Causes of secondary CNS vasculitis include systemic vasculitides, such as giant-cell arteritis and Takayasu arteritis, as well as several infectious agents (Box 36-1). Secondary causes of vasculitis need to be excluded before primary CNS vasculitis, also often called primary angiitis of the CNS, can be diagnosed.

Primary Vasculitis of the Central Nervous System

Primary angiitis of the CNS (PACNS) is an inflammatory arterial disease restricted to the cerebral circulation. PACNS afflicts patients of any age, preferentially involves smaller arteries and veins, and often responds poorly to steroids alone. The diagnosis is difficult, and because it has often been made without pathological confirmation, the true extent and characteristics of the disease are poorly understood.[2,3] The incidence of PACNS has been estimated to be 2.4 cases per 1,000,000 person-years.[4]

The pathologic process in PACNS is segmental, and a negative biopsy therefore does not exclude the diagnosis. Any of the vessels of the brain and spinal cord may be involved, but most report a predilection for the small leptomeningeal vessels. Precapillary arterioles are most often affected, but some have noted venular involvement.[5] Three main histopathological patterns are seen: granulomatous, lymphocytic, and necrotizing vasculitis.[6] The etiology of PACNS is unknown. Basic research suggests that memory T cells are associated with its pathogenesis, and that it can result from an antigen-specific immune response occurring in the wall of cerebral arteries.[7,8] Cases have been reported in association with Hodgkin lymphoma, acquired immunodeficiency syndrome (AIDS),[9] primary intracerebral lymphoma, leukemia, sarcoidosis, varicella zoster virus infection, and cerebral amyloid angiopathy (CAA).[10,11] In a subset of patients with amyloid-β (Aβ) deposition, vascular inflammation is present, with features of a true vasculitis, most frequently granulomatous (Aβ-related angiitis or ABRA).[12] It is likely that PACNS encompasses a spectrum of different diseases characterized by a vascular inflammatory reaction to antigens rather than a single nosologic entity.

The presentation of PACNS is heterogeneous. Patients range in age widely, from 3 to 96 years. The duration of illness is variable. Death may occur within days after presentation in some patients, whereas others have an indolent course lasting years.[13,14] The two most common clinical manifestations at presentation are headache and altered cognition.[4] Multifocal neurologic symptoms and signs may develop in a stepwise, progressive fashion. Seizures are common. Ischemic or hemorrhagic stroke may occur.[15–17] When rapidly progressive, PACNS may be fatal.[4] Some patients have spinal cord involvement (either alone or with brain involvement), including progressive or acute myelopathy.[18,19]

BOX 36-1 Etiologies for Secondary Central Nervous System Vasculitides

Large, medium, small and variable vessel vasculitides
- Giant cell arteritis
- Takayasu arteritis
- Polyarteritis nodosa
- Kawasaki disease
- Granulomatosis with polyangitis (formerly Wegener disease)
- Cryoglobulinemic vasculitis
- Behçet disease
- Eosinophilic granulomatosis with polyangiitis (formerly Churg–Strauss)

Vasculitides associated with systemic diseases/connective tissue diseases
- Systemic lupus erythematosus
- Rheumatoid arthritis
- Sjögren syndrome
- Scleroderma

Others
- Drug-induced (cocaine, amphetamine) antiphospolipid antibody syndrome
- Lymphoma
- Graft-versus-host disease
- Paraneoplastic
- Bacterial endocarditis

INFECTIOUS AGENTS

Viral
- HIV
- Varicella zoster virus
- Cytomegalovirus
- Parvovirus B19
- Others

Bacterial
- *Treponema pallidum*
- *Mycobacterium tuberculosis*
- *Borrelia burgdorferi*
- Others

Fungal
- *Cryptococcus*
- Aspergillosis
- Mucormycosis
- Coccidioidmycosis
- Candidiasis
- Others

Parasitic
- Chagas disease
- Cysticercosis
- Malaria
- Schistosomiasis
- Others

Systemic symptoms, such as fever and weight loss, are uncommon, distinguishing this entity from most systemic inflammatory diseases that cause stroke, such as giant cell arteritis (GCA) or systemic lupus erythematosus. The erythrocyte sedimentation rate (ESR) is usually not increased, and when abnormal, it is not as high as in GCA. Blood cell counts, electrolyte levels, and results of serologic tests for collagen vascular disease are usually normal. The most consistent cerebrospinal fluid (CSF) abnormality is an increase in protein (abnormal in 80–90% and frequently >100 mg/dL), although CSF may be normal. Many patients have a moderate lymphocytic pleocytosis (usually <150 cells/mL) and thus manifest as a chronic meningitis.[20]

Computed tomography (CT) and MRI findings are heterogeneous and non-specific, but PACNS is unlikely if MRI is normal (Figs 36-1A–C). Cerebral angiographic results are usually abnormal, with alternating segments of concentric arterial narrowing and dilatation. However, cerebral angiographic findings may be normal when smaller blood vessels are affected, and abnormal constrictions found in vessels may also be due to a host of other causes, making reliance on angiography alone for the diagnosis problematic. The sensitivity of angiography varies between 40% and 90%[4,25–27] and cerebral angiograms have specificity as low as 30%.[26] One increasingly recognized mimic of primary CNS vasculitis is the reversible cerebral vasoconstriction syndrome, which may also present with severe headache, subarachnoid hemorrhage, focal deficits and infarcts, and evidence of vasculopathy on angiography (see Chapter 37). It may be distinguished, however, by the normal CSF and benign clinical course.[21]

The most common pathologic finding in PACNS is multiple small foci of infarction, followed by multiple foci of hemorrhage ("brain purpura," "petechiae", Fig. 36-1D). Large infarcts and, less often, large confluent intraparenchymal hemorrhages may be present.[5,15–17] Occlusion of large or medium-sized vessels by thrombus is uncommon,[15,22] but vessel wall thickening and intramural inflammation of large arteries is quite specific.[23] Brain and leptomeningeal biopsy demonstrating angiitis remains the gold standard for the diagnosis of PACNS.[6,28–30] A biopsy, ideally taken from a region of brain enhancement on neuroimaging, is the best test for the diagnosis of PACNS[30,31] and is necessary to distinguish among tumor (especially lymphoma or intravascular malignant lymphomatosis), infection, and other mimics. However, biopsy results have been negative in several subsequently autopsy-proven cases, presumably due to the segmental nature of the disease.[32]

No controlled therapeutic trials for CNS angiitis have been performed, and there is no generally accepted standard treatment. Remissions have been reported with the use of prednisone, in some cases combined with cyclophosphamide.[28] Methotrexate has also been used as a steroid-sparing agent.[33] In a recent cohort of 101 patients, glucocorticoids alone or the combination with cyclophosphamide resulted in a favorable outcome in most, though 26% of patients had recurrences. Patients with relapsing disease needed therapy for longer than did those with non-relapsing disease, but otherwise had outcomes similar to those without relapses.[4]

Secondary Vasculitis of the Central Nervous System

Secondary causes of CNS vasculitis include systemic large-, medium-, and small-vessel vasculitides due to connective tissue diseases, drugs, neoplasms, and some infectious agents. In a recent national epidemiological study in Sweden, several immune-mediated diseases increased the risk of hospitalization for both ischemic and hemorrhagic stroke. The relative risk of ischemic and hemorrhagic stroke during the first year after hospitalization with systemic inflammatory diseases (including systemic vasculitides but also other diseases) was even higher than the risks associated with many traditional risk factors for ischemic and hemorrhagic stroke.[34] Identification of these secondary causes of CNS vasculitis is important, since they may be treated differently, including removal of the offending antigen, and antimicrobial therapy. Prognosis in these cases also depends on the underlying disease, and other causes, especially infectious causes, must be excluded before treating patients with immunosuppressants.

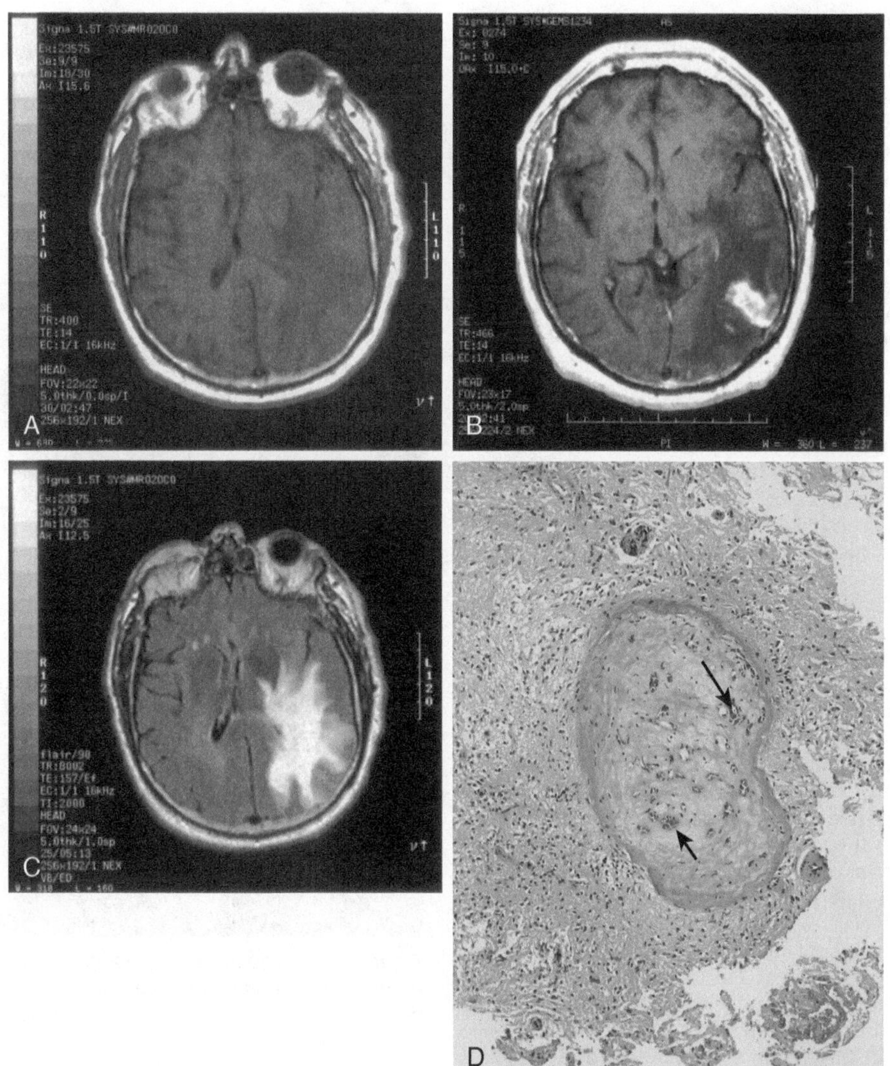

Figure 36-1. Cerebral vasculitis manifesting as a mass lesion. T1-weighted MR images before (A) and after (B) administration of contrast agent, showing the enhancement of a left temporoparietal mass lesion. C, T2-weighted MR image showing extensive edema around the lesion. D, Pathologic specimen from brain biopsy demonstrates an intraparenchymal blood vessel with chronic occlusive changes, mural fibrosis, and recanalization by small, thin-walled vessels (*arrows*). The gray matter surrounding the blood vessel shows extensive gliosis and loss of neurons. Leukocytes, primarily lymphocytes, infiltrate the arterial adventitia and, to a lesser extent, the media, findings consistent with a chronic vasculitic process.

Large-vessel Vasculitides

Giant Cell Arteritis. Giant cell arteriitis (GCA) is the most common of the vasculitic syndromes and, being a disease of the elderly, its incidence is increasing with the aging of the population.[35] GCA, also known as temporal arteritis, is an inflammatory disease affecting medium and large arteries throughout the body, including the aorta and most of its major branches.[36,37]

Current incidence rates vary between 1 and 30/100,000 people aged ≥50 years. The highest frequencies have been reported from Scandinavian countries and populations of predominantly Scandinavian descent; rates in southern Europe are intermediate, and they are still lower in people of African, Asian, and Hispanic descent. There is an almost threefold greater incidence in women than in men.[38] The incidence may be up to seven times higher among Whites than Blacks, possibly in relation to the lower frequency of HLA-DR4 (D-related human leukocyte antigen) among Blacks.[39,40]

Inflammation of the vessel wall is characterized by infiltration of T-cells and macrophages, the presence of giant cells, granulomatous lesions, intimal hyperplasia, and destruction of elastic fibers.[41] Circulating immune complexes[42] and immunoglobulins[43] in the sera of patients with biopsy-proven GCA have been demonstrated. The etiology is unknown. Geographical differences as well as occasional familial clustering suggest environmental, infectious, or genetic factors may play a role.[35]

Clinically, GCA may present with symptoms related to the involved cranial vessels, with the signs of a systemic illness (fever, malaise, and weight loss), or with polymyalgia rheumatica. Neurological symptoms include the new onset of a persistent headache, jaw claudication, visual symptoms such as diplopia, scotoma, amaurosis fugax, or blindness, or, rarely, stroke.[3] Almost all patients with GCA-associated strokes have a significant acute-phase response with elevated ESR and C-reactive protein (CRP). The most common presentation of GCA is headache.[44]

Visual loss is one of the most feared complications of GCA. Anterior ischemic optic neuropathy is the most common cause.[45] Posterior ischemic optic neuropathy and central retinal artery occlusion may cause visual loss. Less often, the visual loss takes the form of homonymous hemianopia, or even cortical blindness, as a result of posterior circulation infarction. Visual loss due to GCA rarely improves, despite treatment with corticosteroids.[45] Visual loss occurs in 40% to 50% of patients.[46] Before fixed visual deficits develop, 10% to 20% of patients experience transient loss of vision (transient monocular blindness).[46] Bilateral involvement occurs in 33% of patients. Afferent pupillary defects are common. Field defects are usually altitudinal and inferior.[45]

In a recent cohort study of 781 patients suffering from polymyalgia rheumatica (PMR), which is associated with GCA, 113 had a stroke within 3 years follow-up. The hazard ratio of stroke for patients with PMR was 2.09 times that of age- and sex-matched controls (95%CI, 1.63–2.66, $P < 0.001$), after adjusting for sociodemographic characteristics and comorbidities.[47] Mortality with GCA has been reported to be as high as 75%.[48]

Post-mortem examinations usually document involvement of the extradural segments of the vessels only,[49,50] although some have shown evidence of intradural involvement as well.[51-53] Thrombotic occlusion due to arteritis in internal carotid arteries has also been described, although GCA-associated stroke is more common in the vertebral artery territories.[54] Other patients have had artery-to-artery embolism with hemorrhagic infarction.[54]

When GCA is suspected, ESR and CRP should be obtained to confirm evidence of inflammation, but biopsy of an artery showing the typical histological features provides the definitive diagnosis. Because of its easy accessibility and frequent involvement, the temporal artery is usually chosen as the biopsy site.[38] The sensitivity and specificity of temporal artery biopsy have been reported to be approximately 75% and 90%, respectively.[55] Due to the possibility of skip-lesions, however, sensitivity depends on obtaining a sufficient length of the biopsy sample, and bilateral biopsies may be performed.[56] In one study, CRP levels >2.45 mg/dL and platelet counts >400,000 were the strongest laboratory predictors of a positive temporal artery biopsy, whereas ESR was not significant in models already including CRP and platelet count.[57]

Modern imaging including ultrasound, positron emission tomography, and MRI has begun to play a role as a broadly applicable and non-invasive tool to establish the diagnosis of GCA. Using color duplex ultrasonography, a typical dark halo has been reported around the lumen of the superficial temporal artery in 73% of patients, an abnormality that disappears with treatment.[58] The vertebral arteries may also show this abnormality (Figs 36-2A,B).[59] Assessing 18F-fluoro-2-deoxy-D-glucose (FDG) uptake by PET appears helpful to assess vasculitic involvement of intrathoracic vessels that cannot be readily visualized by duplex ultrasound, and in cases of non-specific signs and symptoms compatible with large-vessel vasculitis. Sensitivity and specificity of PET/CT to detect large-vessel vasculitis in untreated patients are about 85% and 95%, respectively.[60] Brain magnetic resonance imaging (MRI) may show multifocal dural enhancement and temporalis muscle enhancement.[61,62]

Once the diagnosis of GCA is suspected, the patient should be started on steroid therapy and biopsy performed as soon as possible. Initiating treatment prior to biopsy is unlikely to significantly influence results if the biopsy is not delayed beyond 1 week.[63] Symptoms usually respond promptly to steroids, although visual loss and stroke may occur after initiation of treatment. When ischemic complications – such as visual impairment or stroke – are present, 0.5–1 g of methylprednisolone can be administered intravenously for 3 days. Based on a metaanalysis of the published evidence, current EULAR (European League Against Rheumatism) guidelines suggest that the initially prescribed dose of prednisolone should be maintained for 4 weeks and tapered gradually thereafter. In the absence of evidence for relapsing disease, the dose should reach 10–15 mg/d by month 3, and 5 mg/d by month 6; this dose should be maintained for at least 12 month after diagnosis.[64]

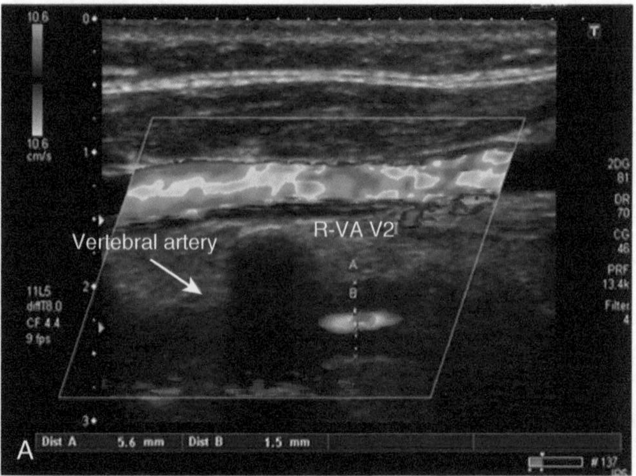

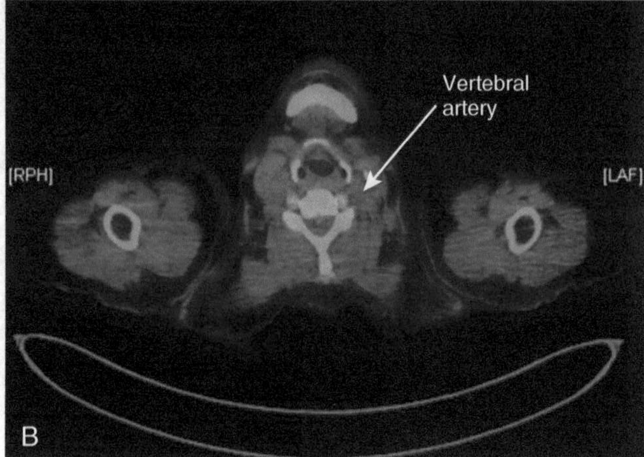

Figure 36-2. Vertebral artery involvement in giant cell arteritis (GCA). A 79-year-old patient presented with a transient ischemic attack with dysarthria and double vision. Her color duplex ultrasonography study showed a typical dark halo, which can be seen around the lumen of the vertebral artery (A). In the FDG-PET study, vasculitic involvement was seen in both vertebral arteries (B). The biopsy of the superficial temporal artery was suggestive for GCA and the patient had typical symptoms of polymyalgia rheumatica.

Because complications due to steroid therapy are very common, Steroid-sparing/Disease Modifying Anti-Rheumatic Drugs (DMARD) have been tested in various studies aiming to optimize outcome while reducing glucocorticoid toxicity. However, with the exception of methotrexate, no DMARD has been shown to be unequivocally effective in the treatment of GCA.[65,66-68]

Randomized controlled clinical trials are needed to clarify the usefulness of aspirin in primary prevention of GCA-associated vascular complications, but low-dose aspirin should be considered for all patients without contraindications.[64]

Takayasu Arteritis. Takayasu arteritis (pulseless disease, idiopathic aortitis) is a large-vessel arteritis that affects the aorta, its main branches, and, occasionally, the pulmonary artery. Although pathologic changes in the arteries are similar to those found in GCA, Takayasu arteritis (TA) affects younger people, particularly women. The disease is found worldwide.[69] As in GCA, constitutional symptoms and increased ESR are common in the acute phase. Symptoms such as arm claudication and syncope are common. Brachial pressures and pulses are frequently asymmetrical, and there may be differences between blood pressures in the arms and legs.

Cerebrovascular complications occur in patients with more advanced disease.[70] Cerebral infarction and retinal ischemia may occur subsequent to stenosis or occlusion of the extracranial carotid or vertebral arteries, but the intracranial arteries are rarely involved. Among a retrospective cohort of 190 TA patients, hemodynamic compromise due to large-artery stenosis and thromboembolic mechanisms were the most important causes of ischemic stroke associated with TA.[71]

Conventional angiography remains the most reliable investigation for the diagnosis of TA, but MRA, PET/CT, and high-resolution ultrasound are being used more frequently.[72] Gadolinium-enhanced MRI shows delayed hyperenhancement in the aortic wall in patients with TA, and this correlates with ESR and CRP.[73,74] FDG-PET can detect metabolic activity in vasculitis because of increased FDG uptake in inflammatory cells in the vessel wall, including larger vessels such as the aorta, its main branches, and the femoral and pulmonary arteries.[75]

Treatment consists of corticosteroids, cytotoxic agents (cyclophosphamide), anti-tumor necrosis factor (TNF) agents, surgery, or a combination of these modalities. Tocilizumab and rituximab have been shown to lead to reduced disease activity in small numbers of patients, including those refractory to anti-TNF treatment.[76] Fifty percent of patients respond to corticosteroids alone.[77] Antiplatelet agents are recommended in secondary prevention. A recent retrospective multicenter study found that in 79 consecutive patients with TA who underwent 166 vascular procedures, the overall 5-year arterial complication rate was 44% and biological inflammation at the time of revascularization increased by seven times the likelihood of complications.[78]

Medium- to Small-vessel Vasculitides

CNS involvement is infrequent (<15%) in small-to-medium-size vessel vasculitis, including polyarteritis nodosa, Kawasaki disease, antineutrophil cytoplasmic antibody (ANCA)-associated vasculitides, eosinophilic granulomatosis with polyangiitis (formerly Churg-Strauss syndrome), immune complex vasculitis (such as cryoglobulinemic vasculitis), and variable vessel vasculitis (such as Behçet disease).

Polyarteritis Nodosa. Polyarteritis nodosa (PAN) is a necrotizing angiitis of the medium to small muscular arteries throughout the body. The peripheral nervous system is more commonly involved than the CNS. In a series of 348 patients diagnosed with PAN over a 42-year period, only 4.6% presented with CNS-related abnormalities.[79] Three major clinical presentations related to CNS involvement have been described in earlier studies: (1) diffuse encephalopathy characterized by cognitive impairment, disorientation or psychosis; (2) seizures (focal or generalized); and (3) focal neurologic deficits including strokes.[80]

Ischemic or hemorrhagic strokes occurred as late CNS manifestations in 19% (22/114) of PAN patients in one series.[81] Lacunar infarcts were the most frequent (73%) stroke type, consistent with the medium-to-small-size vessel involvement, though this could also be due to the association of PAN with arterial hypertension.[82] Whether PAN-associated strokes are caused by atherosclerosis-like mechanisms or by segmental inflammation of the arterial wall remains unclear.

In PAN with negative hepatitis serology, induction treatment is started with prednisone and cyclophosphamide. In emergency situations plasmapheresis may be tried. In hepatitis-virus-associated PAN, prednisone is combined with virustatics like lamivudine (for hepatitis B) or interferon-alpha and ribavirin (for hepatitis C).[2]

Granulomatosis with Polyangiitis (Formerly Wegener Granulomatosis). Wegener granulomatosis is an ANCA-associated necrotizing granulomatous vasculitis involving the respiratory tract, kidney, and other organ systems. The prevalence of CNS manifestations ranges from 3% to 9% in large series of patients. Neurological involvement may occur through three major mechanisms: (1) vasculitis involving CNS vessels; (2) granulomatous lesions located in the brain, meninges, or cranial nerves; and (3) direct extension of destructive granulomatous tissue from nasal or paranasal structures.[83–85]

Granulomatosis with polyangiitis should be suspected when stroke patients have evidence of other manifestations of neurological inflammatory disease, such as meningeal disease, cranial neuropathies, and mononeuritis multiplex; concomitant constitutional symptoms, such as fever, malaise, weight loss, or migratory arthralgias; or involvement of the ear and nasal passages, pulmonary airways or parenchyma, or kidneys, especially glomerulonephritis. Diagnosis can be challenging, as the signs and symptoms are variable and may mimic infectious or malignant disease. Anti-neutrophil cytoplasmic antibodies should be tested, as approximately 90% of patients are ANCA-positive. Patients with proteinase 3 (PR3) ANCA may have a reduced vascular risk compared to myeloperoxidase ANCA or negative ANCA (about 10% of patients) status.[86] In addition, the diagnosis should be confirmed by biopsy of involved tissue, often lung or kidney. Chest CT and renal evaluation should be undertaken to assess for involvement of those organs.

Therapy for granulomatosis with polyangiitis includes initial immunosuppressive therapy followed by maintenance therapy. The mainstay of initial therapy is glucocorticoids and either cyclophosphamide or rituximab. Plasma exchange may be used in severe disease. Once remission has been achieved, maintenance therapy with less toxic immunosuppressive medications, such as azathioprine, mycophenolate mofetil, or methotrexate, may be used. Patients should also receive prophylaxis against opportunistic infections.

Eosinophilic Granulomatosis with Polyangiitis (Formerly Churg-Strauss Syndrome). Eosinophilic granulomatosis with polyangiitis is a rare systemic ANCA-associated vasculitis.[87] In a series of 14 patients, 12 had some type of neuropathy and only two patients had a stroke.[88] The central nervous system is involved in 8–14% of patients, and cerebral infarction is one of the most frequently reported manifestations.[89–91]

Cyclophosphamide and glucocorticoids are the main therapy for induction of remission in patients with generalized or severe ANCA-associated vasculitides. Dose reductions and avoidance of prolonged use of these agents have also been successfully implemented, although less-toxic regimens are still required. For patients without organ-threatening disease, methotrexate can be used. Rituximab is as effective as cyclophosphamide for remission induction.[92]

Cryoglobulinemia. Cryoglobulinemia may be associated with systemic vasculitis.[93] Cryoglobulinemic vasculitis (CV) is a small-vessel systemic vasculitis resulting from deposition of cryoglobulins in vessel walls, activating the complement cascade. CNS involvement, while uncommon, may include diffuse encephalopathic syndromes with focal signs, seizures, myelopathy, and, occasionally, ischemic stroke. In a retrospective series of 29 patients, CNS involvement occurred in three.[94] Clinical features of CNS involvement in cryoglobulinemia include encephalopathy, stroke, TIA, and hemorrhage. Most cases are associated with hepatitis C infection.[95,96] Hyperviscosity syndrome due to high cryoglobulin levels is another rare but life-threatening complication of CV and is seen mainly in patients with lymphoproliferative disorders, chiefly Waldenström macroglobulinemia.[97] Angiographic findings include narrowing of the major cerebral arteries with development of a moyamoya pattern of collateral vessels.[95] Favorable outcome has been reported after treatment with corticosteroids, cyclophosphamide, and, in some cases, interferon.[98]

Behçet Disease. Vasculitis occurring in patients with Behçet disease (BD) can affect arteries or veins. According to the Chapel Hill Consensus Claasification, BD belongs to the group of variable vessel vasculitides. BD is characterized by recurrent oral and/or genital aphthous ulcers accompanied by cutaneous, ocular, articular, gastrointestinal, and/or CNS inflammatory lesions. Small-vessel vasculitis, arteritis, arterial aneurysms, and venous and arterial thromboangiitis and thrombosis may occur.[1] CNS involvement is more common in young male patients. CNS complications usually occur in patients who have established cutaneous or ocular disease.[99] In less than 6% the first signs of BD are CNS symptoms.[100] CNS involvement occurs through two major mechanisms: (1) meningoencephalitis and (2) cerebrovascular disease. The most common manifestation of vascular neuro-Behçet is central venous thrombosis with signs and symptoms of intracranial hypertension, including papilledema. Intracranial aneurysms and ischemic stroke occur less frequently. Combined parenchymal and vascular involvement may be seen in 20% of patients.[100]

Patients with neuro-Behçet are treated with high-dose glucocorticoids and cyclophosphamide. Infliximab or etanercept may be useful in refractory patients.[100,101] For the treatment of sinus thrombosis, corticosteroids in combination with anticoagulation are recommended.[102]

Systemic Lupus Erythematosus. Reports on the neurologic manifestations of systemic lupus erythematosus (SLE) have long emphasized the relatively high frequency of CNS complications, including stroke. The American College of Rheumatology (ACR) established a case definition for 19 central and peripheral nervous system syndromes, including stroke, TIA, and cerebral venous thrombosis.[103] In a recent cohort study of SLE patients with no previous history of CNS involvement, the proportion of major CNS manifestations (including chorea, aseptic meningitis, psychosis, seizures, myelopathy, demyelinating syndrome, acute confusional state, and stroke) was 16/370 (4.3%) within 3 years (incidence 7.8/100 person years).[104] The proportion of patients with SLE in whom stroke develops is difficult to estimate. The frequency of stroke assessed in several studies varied from 2% to 19%. The large range reflects differences in study design and definition of stroke.[105–108]

Strokes usually occur within the first 5 years of the onset of SLE, generally in the setting of clinically and serologically active SLE.[109] About 6% of patients with SLE die of stroke.[110] In the Hopkins lupus cohort, the overall risk of cardiovascular events associated with SLE was 2.66 times higher than expected based on Framingham risk score.[111] Increased prevalence of premature atherosclerosis in patients with SLE has been well established by autopsy series, but a prospective study failed to show a strong association between SLE activity and duration with carotid plaque.[112]

Although vasculitis is frequently mentioned as an important cause of stroke in patients with SLE, documented vasculitic changes on postmortem examination are actually quite rare.[113,114] One study found that microembolic signals detected on transcranial Doppler ultrasonography testing, possibly indicating embolic material, were more common in patients with SLE who had neuropsychiatric symptoms than in those who had no CNS symptoms, raising the possibility that microemboli may play an even broader role in SLE than previously suspected.[115] Cardiac sources of emboli should be sought in patients with SLE and stroke. Thrombotic thrombocytopenic purpura (thrombocytopenia, microangiopathic hemolytic anemia, fever, renal failure, CNS signs) is another mechanism of stroke in the terminal stages of SLE, and was found in 14% of patients in one autopsy series.[113] Additional possible causes of infarction in patients with SLE are hypertension and hyperlipidemia, both of which are overrepresented among these patients.[116]

Antiphospholipid antibodies, including anticardiolipin antibodies (aCL) and the lupus anticoagulant, are associated with cerebrovascular disease, systemic thrombotic events, spontaneous abortion, and thrombocytopenia.[117–119] These phenomena may be associated with antiphospholipid antibodies either in the setting of SLE or as a "primary" antiphospholipid syndrome (APS). In one cohort of 132 patients with focal cerebral ischemia (112 ischemic stroke and 20 transient ischemic attack), those with positive immunoglobulin G (IgG) anticardiolipin antibody had a risk ratio for recurrent stroke of 1.98 (95% CI, 0.68–5.76).[120] In patients with documented SLE, an association of anti-phospholipid antibodies with both transient ischemic attack and stroke has also been found.[121]

In a cohort study of 1795 SLE patients, with a total of 193 thrombotic events over 10,508 person-years of follow up (rate 18.4/1000 person-years), hydroxychloroquine was protective against thrombosis in SLE patients.[122] A consensus panel has recommended the use of low-dose aspirin in SLE patients with antiphospholipid antibody for primary thrombosis prevention.[123]

Rheumatoid Arthritis. CNS manifestations of rheumatoid arthritis are rare and tend to occur in the setting of long-established disease, with either clinical signs (fever, weight loss, active arthritis) or laboratory evidence (increase in rheumatoid factor titer or ESR) of disease activity. Systemic inflammation and its interplay with traditional cardiovascular risk factors appear to have a major role, through direct and indirect effects on the vasculature.[124] Proinflammatory cytokines such as interleukin (IL)-1, IL-6, and TNF-α produced within locally affected joints in RA may promote both traditional (e.g., dyslipidemia, insulin resistance) and non-traditional (e.g., oxidative stress) systemic cardiovascular risk factors.[125] CNS vasculitis, either isolated or in association with systemic rheumatoid vasculitis,[126] has been documented on rare occasions. A feared neurologic complication of rheumatoid arthritis is compressive myelopathy secondary to C1–C2 vertebral subluxation, and a potential complication of C1–C2 subluxation is massive vertebrobasilar territory infarction due to vertebral artery thrombosis from pinching of the vertebral artery.[127] Formation of vertebral artery pseudoaneurysms has also been reported.[128]

INFECTIOUS DISEASES AND STROKE

Infections may cause stroke through several mechanisms, including contributions to atherosclerosis, platelet aggregability, and endothelial dysfunction (Box 36-2). Some mechanisms may involve direct infection of the arterial wall, leading to dysfunction, smooth-muscle-cell proliferation, or increased levels of cytokines.[129] Alternatively, infections may affect cells remote from the vascular wall, with indirect consequences to the artery from systemic inflammation.

Bacterial/Spirochetal Infections

Treponema pallidum

Neurosyphilis is a well-known consequence of *Treponema pallidum* infection, and syphilitic meningoencephalitis has long

BOX 36-2 Potential Mechanisms by which Infections may Contribute to Stroke Risk

- Direct infection of the arterial wall, leading to dysfunction, smooth muscle cell proliferation, or increase in levels of cytokines
- Induction of peripheral blood monocytes to produce pro-inflammatory cytokines (TNF-alpha, IL-1beta, IL-6, IFN-gamma)
- Induction of tissue factor production by monocytes
- Lipopolysaccharide induction of cytokines
- Facilitation of conversion of macrophages to foam cells
- Increasing macrophage oxidative metabolism of LDL
- Increase CRP
- Hypersensitivity reaction on re-exposure to organism
- Autoimmune mechanisms: molecular mimicry with heat shock proteins
- NF-kappaB activation
- Induction of plasminogen activator inhibitor (PAI-1) expression
- Platelet activation
- Platelet–leukocyte interactions
- Impair endothelium-dependent relaxation
- Association with socioeconomic status or other risk factors

been recognized as a cause of stroke.[130] The prevalence of seropositivity to *T. pallidum* using the fluorescent treponemal antibody absorbed (FTA-ABS) test in patients admitted with acute stroke was 38% 30 years ago, but dropped to 4% in the last decade.[131,132] Among those with neurosyphilis as determined by cerebrospinal fluid (CSF) evidence of *T. pallidum* infection, stroke occurs in 14–23%.[133,134] Although the incidence of neurosyphilis has decreased in the US and other developed countries, it remains important among immunocompromised patients and in developing countries where access to diagnostic testing and treatment may not be available.[132,133,135–137]

The mean age at time of stroke among patients with neurosyphilis is 53–72 years, the majority comprises men, and 71% have concomitant vascular risk factors.[131,133,137] There are no specific criteria to suggest syphilis in the general population admitted with stroke. Some authors advocate testing all patients with stroke for syphilis, with special emphasis on those who migrate from developing countries, have evidence of meningoencephalitis, or are immunosuppressed.[131,133,136] Imaging findings suggestive of neurosyphilis include arteriopathy (50% of cases when vascular imaging is obtained), nonspecific white matter lesions (20%), and cerebral gummas or meningeal enhancement (6%). One-third of all patients with neurosyphilis had normal neuroimaging.[132] The CDC Sexually Transmitted Disease Treatment Guidelines recommends that when syphilis is suspected, non-treponemal (Venereal Disease Research Laboratory [VDRL] and RPR) and treponemal tests (FTA-ABS and *T. pallidum* passive particle agglutination [TP-PA] assay) are performed to reduce the chances of false-negative results.[138] To diagnose neurosyphilis, both VDRL and FTA-ABS in CSF are recommended. The VDRL is highly specific but less sensitive while FTA-ABS is not very specific but highly sensitive.[138] In patients with suspected neurosyphilis and stroke, a negative CSF FTA-ABS effectively rules out the disease and a positive VDRL effectively confirms it. In patients with a positive CSF FTA-ABS and a negative VDRL, CSF protein and cell count and clinical judgment might be needed to decide on the treatment. The treatment of choice for neurosyphilis remains intravenous penicillin G 18–24 million units per day for 10–14 days.[138,139] All patients with neurosyphilis should also be tested for HIV.

Mycobacterium tuberculosis

Tuberculous meningitis can cause significant permanent disability and high mortality, despite prompt administration of therapy.[140] Seven percent of patients with tuberculosis develop tuberculous meningitis,[141] and among these, between 20% and 45% will have a stroke on admission or during follow-up.[140,142–144] Stroke tends to be more frequent in those with tuberculous meningitis at advanced stages of the disease, older individuals, and those with HIV.[141,143–145] Although stroke predominantly occurs among patients with tuberculous meningitis, evidence exists to support an increased risk of ischemic stroke and coronary events in individuals infected with TB without CNS involvement compared to the general population.[146]

Strokes can be either single or, more frequently, multiple.[147,148] They are often localized in the anterior thalamus and caudate nucleus, and appear as lacunar infarctions, but they can also present as large-artery infarction.[147–149] The most affected artery is the middle cerebral artery (MCA) and its penetrating branches followed by the posterior cerebral artery thalamoperforators.[144,147] Enhanced brain MRI or CT will be abnormal in 95% of patients with tuberculous meningitis and strokes. The most common abnormalities include hydrocephalus, parenchymal enhancement, and cisternal enhancement with exudates.[147,150] In 50% of cases MRA shows vessel abnormalities, and in those with abnormal MRA, 62% have a corresponding infarct either at baseline or during follow-up.[147] The treatment is mainly focused on the administration of antibiotics, and the length of therapy, based on expert opinion, should be between 9 and 12 months. The use of concomitant dexamethasone is strongly recommended.[151] Stroke portends a poor prognosis: mortality among those with tuberculous meningitis and stroke reaches 17% despite treatment compared to 5% among those with tuberculous meningitis without stroke.[24–25,143]

Parasitic Infections

Parasites can infect the central nervous system and on occasion, cause stroke. Many parasites can directly invade the brain parenchyma and cause inflammation and focal findings, without necessarily causing a vascular lesion. However, inflammation can spread to neighboring arteries or meninges and cause a stroke.[152–155] Parasites may also affect immunoregulation, contributing to vasculitis.[156,157]

The most common parasitic illnesses that cause stroke are Chagas disease and neurocysticercosis. However, strokes have been reported in malaria,[158–160] free-living amoebic meningoencephalitis,[152] neurotoxocariosis,[161] cardiac echinococcosis,[162,163] sparganosis (caused by *Spirometra mansoni*),[155,164,165] schistosomiasis,[166,167] and others.[168] In the modern era of globalization, physicians should be aware of these potential, though rare, causes of stroke, and consider them in the differential diagnosis in individuals from endemic areas in whom unexplained vasculitis, meningitis, or cerebritis is observed in association with stroke.

Chagas Disease

Chagas disease is widely spread in the Americas. It is the third most common parasitosis in the world, after malaria and schistosomiasis.[169] The disease is caused by *Trypanosoma cruzi*, a parasite that gets transmitted to humans by blood-sucking triatomine bugs. Other methods of spread include vertical transmission and transfusion.[170] The prevalence of seropositivity in endemic areas ranges from 0.1% to 30%.[171] The primary infection commences with fever, headache, and myalgias, but up to 40% of acutely infected individuals develop myocarditis.[172] The disease becomes chronic in about one-third of these individuals, who later in life develop chronic cardiac disease.[169]

Stroke is a common complication of chagasic cardiomyopathy. The impact of Chagas disease on public health is not only limited to endemic areas in Central and South America, but to developed countries with immigrants from these areas.[173] The seroprevalence of *T. cruzi* among patients with stroke in endemic areas is as high as 55%.[174,175] Some of the more common cardiac consequences in patients with Chagas disease and stroke include left ventricle apical aneurysm, left atrial dilatation, left ventricle hypokinesia and right bundle branch block.[176] In a prospective population-based study of individuals >60 years old, one-third were found to have evidence of *T. cruzi* infection. Among these patients, stroke-related mortality was significantly higher compared to those without infection (hazard ratio (HR) 2.35, 95% CI 1.25–4.44), even after controlling for demographics and vascular risk factors.[175] Cardioembolism is the most common mechanism of stroke attributable to Chagas disease, although the aging population with Chagas disease might have alternative mechanisms of stroke attributable to traditional vascular risk factors.[175,176] Further evidence of the cardiac role of stroke in Chagas patients comes from studies suggesting that in patients with atrial fibrillation and high brain natriuretic peptide (a marker of congestive heart failure), the stroke-related mortality is almost 12 times higher than in those without either of these.[175] Additionally, emboli detection protocols with TCD have demonstrated that microembolic signals are more frequent in patients with Chagas than in those without it.[177] The treatment is directed to the underlying cardiac disease and follows the guidelines for each specific condition. An ongoing trial is testing the hypothesis that treating the parasite even when the cardiomyopathy has already developed reduces the risk of stroke and cardiovascular events.[178]

Neurocysticercosis

The prevalence of stroke among individuals with neurocysticercosis (NCC) varies from 2% to 10%.[154,179-181] Few studies, however, have addressed systematically the confounding effects of vascular risk factors. In one of the largest studies, investigators from a tertiary care center analyzed whether the coexistence of NCC with other central nervous system (CNS) comorbidities, among them stroke, was incidental or causal. Brain MRIs that were performed in 10,350 subjects for any indication were retrospectively reviewed. The prevalence of NCC was 7%; only two of 515 cases with infarction had NCC while 701 of 8465 controls without infarction had NCC (0.4 vs 8.3%, unadjusted relative ratio (RR) 0.05, 95% CI, 0.01–0.19, $P =< 0.001$).[182] This study highlights the need for studies that systematically include controls without NCC in samples that represent the general population.

Ischemic stroke is more frequently reported than intracranial hemorrhage.[153,183] Because inflammation around the parasite as evidenced by contrast enhancement has been cited concomitantly with the presence of stroke, it is plausible to think that strokes can occur more in the colloidal and granulomatous stages when active inflammation occurs, rather than in stages with a viable or calcified cyst where inflammation is not as prominent.[184-187] Of note, in patients with multiple lesions (the most common presentation in Latin America), cysts at difference stages can coexist.[184] Enhancement of the brain arteries has been cited as arteritis related to NCC.[185] The vasculitis presumably occurs due to arachnoiditis, contiguous spreading of parenchymal inflammation, or direct contact of the cyst with the culprit artery.[188-190] NCC can affect large arteries in the form of occlusion or stenosis,[153,186,189,191] or more frequently it presents as a lacunar stroke affecting penetrating arteries.[154,192,193] Other presumed mechanisms of stroke include mechanical compression of large arteries in the basal cisterns or in the subarachnoid space.[191,194] The dramatic recovery of treated patients with presumed strokes due to NCC suggests that some of those patients might have had imaging and clinical changes associated with NCC rather than a true ischemic stroke.[153]

Fungal Infections

Fungal infections tend to occur in patients with immunosuppression.[195] Among the most common infections in this group that have been associated with strokes include cryptococcal meningitis, aspergillosis, and mucormycosis.

Cryptococcal Meningitis

Cerebrovascular events in the setting of cryptococcal meningitis have been described in individuals with HIV or other types of immunosuppression, although it can also occur in immunocompetent hosts.[196,197] In patients with HIV and stroke, 3–10% will have cryptococcal meningitis as the etiology of their stroke.[198,199] In those without HIV, approximately one-fifth of all patients with cryptococcal meningitis will develop a stroke.[200,201] Strokes are predominantly of lacunar type, and they can affect the anterior or posterior circulation.[201] The diagnosis usually requires evidence of cryptococcal antigen in the CSF. Stroke adds to the poor prognosis of these patients, underlying the importance of promptly considering *Cryptococcus* in the differential diagnosis of unexplained stroke in immunosuppressed patients, and particularly in those with meningitis.[201]

Aspergillosis

Aspergillus fumigatus is a highly angiotrophic fungus that frequently causes stroke. Individuals at risk of developing aspergillosis include those with transplants, patients on immunosuppressive drugs, or individuals with AIDS, diabetes, or blood malignancies, but it can occur in immunocompetent patients as well.[202-204] The majority of patients present with headache or symptoms related to sinusitis.[205,206] Strokes can occur in up to 65% of cases. Although the majority of patients have concurrent pulmonary infections, about 11% have isolated neuroaspergillosis.[204] Systemic aspergillosis can also cause stroke due to embolism from infected distant vessels.[207-209] Brain lesions tend to be multiple, and some present with ring enhancement.[210,211] About one-half of these lesions have a "target-like" appearance with central and peripheral hypodensities on DWI and corresponding hyperintensities in apparent diffusion coefficient (ADC) sequences.[211] Arteritis and aneurysmal dilatation of the affected arteries are also common findings.[205,212] Pathological studies demonstrated hemorrhagic infarction in the majority of patients with focal findings.[204] Clusters of *Aspergillus fumigatus* are found in atherosclerotic plaques of affected vessels accompanied by a heavy granulomatous reaction.[213] Among the most commonly used therapeutic agents are amphotericin, itraconazole and, more recently, voriconazole.[203,213,214] Early treatment appears the key to improve survival; however, initial responses to treatment can be followed by recurrence and death.[205,212,213] The localization of the fungus in dead tissue might decrease the efficacy of antifungals by impairing their penetration, so treating it early may decrease the rate of tissue damage and enhance the efficacy of therapy.[215] Prognosis is poor for those with advanced neuroaspergillosis, and it is worse among those with strokes.[203,214]

Mucormycosis

This life-threatening infection is caused by multiple fungi belonging to the order Mucorales, which includes the genera Rhizopus, Mucor, Rhizomucor, Absidia, Apophysomyces, Saksenaea, Cunninghamella, Cokeromyces, and Syncephalastrum.[216] Most affected patients with mucormycosis are diabetic or have blood malignancies.[217,218] Typically, patients with rhinocerebral mucormycosis complain of symptoms like headache and fever, although crusting of the nasal mucosa can be observed, which aids in the diagnosis.[219] Visual symptoms can include progressive or sudden blindness due to compression of the chiasm or embolism to ophthalmic arteries.[220,221] Ischemic or hemorrhagic strokes can occur in the brain or spine, usually associated with heavily damaged arteries, large-artery occlusion or artery-to-artery embolism.[222–224,225] Supportive MRI findings include arterial enhancement, aneurysmal arteriopathy, bone destruction, or central hypodensities in the paranasal sinuses.[225,226] On occasion, peripheral serpiginous and radial strand-like enhancement can be appreciated.[227] Pathological examination of affected tissue universally discloses vascular invasion by the fungus with extensive necrosis.[228,229] Treatment with antifungals is recommended early, but the outcome is frequently fatal.[217,230]

Viral Infections

HIV

Individuals with HIV are at a higher risk of cardiac and cerebrovascular disease compared to non-HIV populations, though modern antiretroviral (ARV) therapy may have changed this risk.[231–233] In individuals with HIV and persistent immunosuppression, opportunistic infections and neoplasms appear to be the most common causes of stroke.[200,236–238] The stroke in these situations is attributable to direct effects of the pathological agent.[238,239] Among the most common infectious causes of stroke in immunosuppressed individuals with HIV are varicella zoster virus (VZV), cryptococcal meningitis, tuberculosis, syphilis and toxoplasmosis.[199,238,240] Cardioembolism has also been reported in this population.[200,238] A more elusive-to-diagnose form of arteriopathy has been attributed to HIV infection. HIV vasculopathy presumably affects between 5% and 20% depending on the definition and evaluation for differential diagnosis.[200,237] It has been reported in children and adults.[241,242] This arteriopathy presents usually in immunosuppressed individuals as an aneurysmal dilatation of large arteries that leads to hemispheric, large infarcts more often than to small infarcts.[243–245] Multiple hypotheses have been invoked to explain the development of HIV vasculopathy, but small sample sizes of the reported studies hamper a firm conclusion. Some of these hypotheses include direct infection of the smooth muscle cells by HIV,[246] perhaps leading to a thinner media layer and subsequent dilatation of the arteries,[247,248] mineralization and fragmentation of the intima,[237] and increased elastolytic activity induced by matrix metalloproteinase overexpression.[249]

In the post ARV-era, most individuals in the developed world who are aware of their HIV infection are treated with ARV and now live longer.[235] In this population, cardiac and cerebrovascular disease is among the most common causes of death.[233,250–252] As individuals with HIV age, traditional vascular risk factors become more common. In fact, there is evidence suggesting that compared to their non-HIV peers and after adjusting for demographic and clinical confounders, individuals with HIV might have a higher-then-expected prevalence of vascular risk factors.[232,234,253,254] The single most important modifiable risk of increased vascular disease in the population with HIV is smoking.[233,255] Additionally, comorbidities such as co-infection with hepatitis C, cocaine or intravenous drug use, inadequate healthcare access, or lack of exercise may influence the increased vascular risk.[251,253,256–258] ARV related to myocardial infarction (MI) has been better studied than in stroke. The increased risk of MI, although partially mediated by cholesterol levels, persists after adjusting for dyslipidemia.[235,259–261] There are no data showing direct evidence of increased stroke risk with ARV, or in particular with protease inhibitors. On the contrary, stroke appears more common in those with detectable viral HIV levels and lower CD4 counts, presumably a consequence of not taking ARV.[231]

The discrepancy between cardiac and cerebrovascular outcomes suggests different factors influencing each disease and calls for studies dedicated to the mechanisms underlying the increased incidence of stroke in the population with HIV infection.

Herpesviruses

Herpesviruses induce atherosclerotic-like changes in animal models.[262] An avian herpesvirus, Marek's disease virus, causes atherosclerosis in normocholesterolemic chickens, while without this pathogen, even hypercholesterolemic chickens do not develop atherosclerosis.[263] Herpes simplex virus was also found in human early aortic atherosclerotic lesions.[264] There are less data to support a direct effect of herpes simplex virus in the development of stroke.

Cytomegalovirus

Cytomegalovirus (CMV) has been recognized as a contributor to vasculopathy after heart transplantation.[265] Recent data suggest that elevated titers against CMV are associated with early and late carotid atherosclerotic changes.[266] Prospective studies have shown that those in the upper quintile of CMV titers have twice the risk of developing cardiac disease as those in the lowest.[267] Restenosis after coronary angioplasty occurs more frequently in those positive for CMV.[268] CMV has also been detected by PCR in atherosclerotic plaques of those with coronary disease more frequently than in those without atherosclerosis.[269] Other prospective studies have not confirmed that elevated titers predict increased clinical events.[270]

Varicella Zoster Virus

Arterial infection by VZV is a well-known but underdiagnosed cause of arteriopathy and vascular events, including stroke (Fig. 36-3).[243,271–273] Although the prevalence of VZV-related cerebrovascular disease is not well known, in an institutional report of acute stroke cases, VZV arteriopathy was present in about 9% of non-atherosclerotic strokes.[274] Some populations, like diabetics and individuals infected with HIV, are particularly prone to develop VZV arteriopathy in the setting of immunosuppression.[243,275,276] In patients with diabetes, pathology studies have demonstrated intimal proliferation in large arteries suggesting a role of VZV infection in the development of stroke in this population.[277] The association of VZV with arterial stenosis affecting multiple segments of an artery is the underlying explanation to the typical "beading" pattern observed in angiographic studies of patients with VZV arteriopathy.[273,278] Small-artery stenosis has also been reported in pathology studies.[279] These stenoses might explain the relative tendency of VZV to present with small-artery occlusions more often than with pure large-artery disease.[243,271]

The diagnosis of VZV vasculitis is established by clinical suspicion, exclusion of known causes of stroke and evidence of intrathecal production of VZV antibodies or evidence

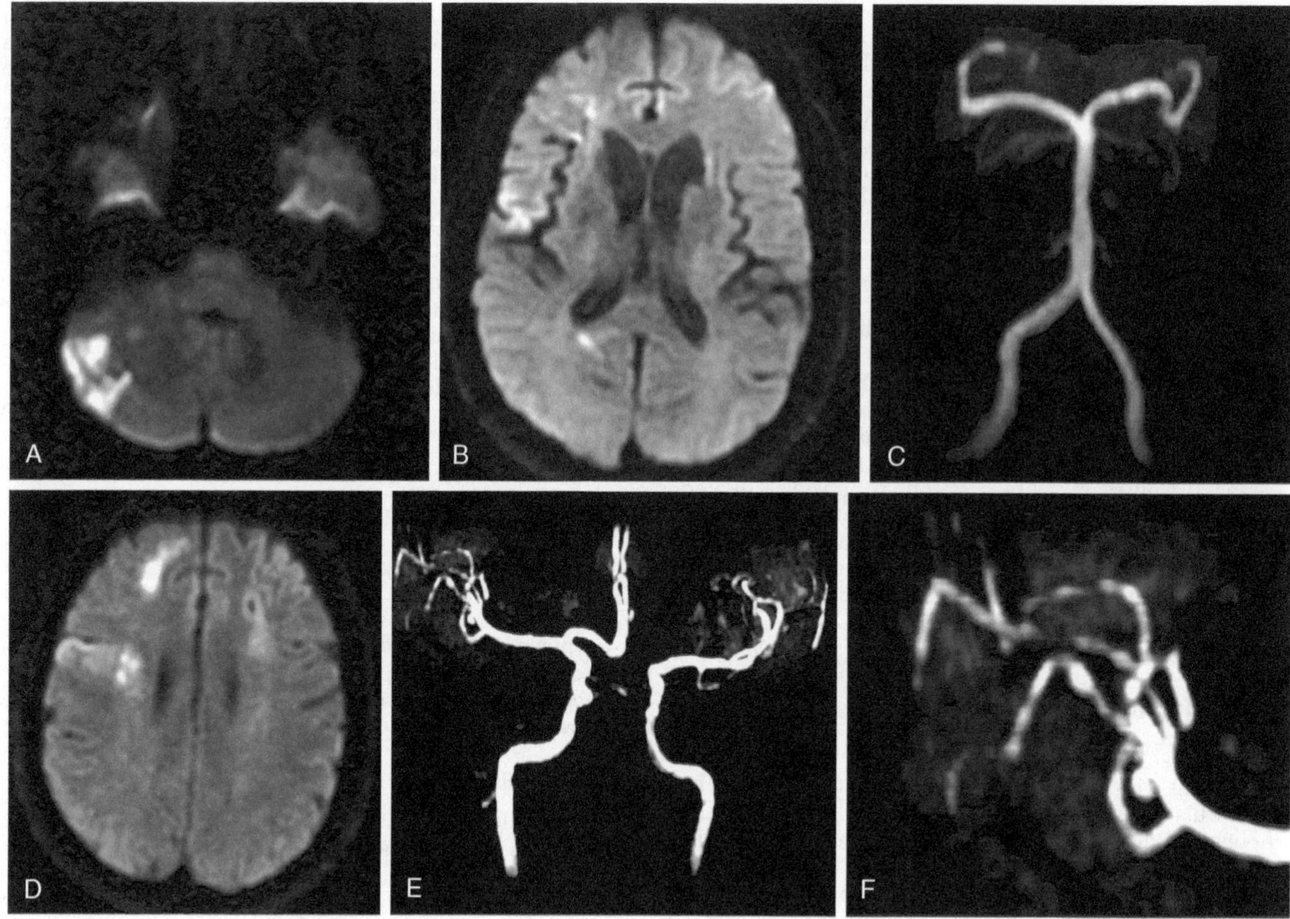

Figure 36-3. Varicella zoster virus reactivation in brain arteries as a cause of stroke. A 47-year-old man was admitted with left-sided weakness and headache. His brain MRI showed right cerebellar (A) and right pulvinar acute infarcts. The vertebrobasilar system arteries showed evidence of vasculopathy (C) (MRA). Additionally, bilateral acute infarcts were found in the frontal lobes (B, D) (MRI). The arteries of the anterior circulation showed beading throughout (E) (MRA), but it was more evident on the right compared to the left (F).

of VZV DNA by PCR.[271,280] Because not all patients with VZV-related vasculitis report prior exposure to VZV infection or rash, VZV should be considered in cases of cryptogenic arteriopathy and stroke.[281] Although there have been no randomized trials to test the most effective therapy for patients with VZV vasculitis, intravenous acyclovir is recommended by most investigators.[271,275,282,283] Observational data suggest that adding steroids to the acyclovir regimen might lead to a better outcome.[271] Stroke recurrence rates of up to 45% have been reported in children with treated VZV vasculitis.[284] The majority of adults with VZV vasculitis improve after administration of antivirals, but mortality in treated patients has been reported at 13% and up to 18% in those with HIV, underscoring the seriousness of this disease.[271,285]

Parvovirus B19

Single case reports of infection by parvovirus B19 and stroke have been published.[286,287] Retrospective review of cases with aplastic crisis in children with sickle cell anemia suggests that the risk of stroke is increased substantially in the 5 weeks following a B19-induced aplastic crisis.[288] Among published cases with parvovirus B19 infection and central nervous system complications, stroke is reported in 9%, the majority in children with sickle cell disease.[289] All patients who were identified with a stroke were younger than 25 years, the majority had some immunodeficiency (75%), and only a minority presented with a prodromal viral syndrome or a rash (13%).[289] The diagnosis is established with evidence of PVB19 DNA in CSF by PCR.[287]

The complete reference list can be found on the companion Expert Consult website at www.expertconsult.inkling.com.

KEY REFERENCES

1. Jennette JC, Falk RJ, Bacon PA, et al. 2012 Revised International Chapel Hill Consensus Conference nomenclature of vasculitides. Arthritis Rheum 2013;65:1–11.
2. Berlit P. Diagnosis and treatment of cerebral vasculitis. Ther Adv Neurol Disord 2010;3:29–42.
3. Salvarani C, Giannini C, Miller DV, et al. Giant cell arteritis: Involvement of intracranial arteries. Arthritis Rheum 2006;55: 985–9.
4. Salvarani C, Brown RD Jr, Calamia KT, et al. Primary central nervous system vasculitis: Analysis of 101 patients. Ann Neurol 2007;62:442–51.
6. Miller DV, Salvarani C, Hunder GG, et al. Biopsy findings in primary angiitis of the central nervous system. Am J Surg Pathol 2009;33:35–43.
7. Iwase T, Ojika K, Mitake S, et al. Involvement of CD45RO + T lymphocyte infiltration in a patient with primary angiitis of the central nervous system restricted to small vessels. Eur Neurol 2001;45:184–5.
8. Salvarani C, Brown RD Jr, Hunder GG. Adult primary central nervous system vasculitis. Lancet 2012;380:767–77.

11. Salvarani C, Brown RD Jr, Calamia KT, et al. Primary central nervous system vasculitis: Comparison of patients with and without cerebral amyloid angiopathy. Rheumatology 2008;47: 1671–7.
12. Salvarani C, Hunder GG, Morris JM, et al. Abeta-related angiitis: Comparison with CAA without inflammation and primary CNS vasculitis. Neurology 2013;81:1596–603.
21. Calabrese LH, Dodick DW, Schwedt TJ, et al. Narrative review: Reversible cerebral vasoconstriction syndromes. Ann Intern Med 2007;146:34–44.
23. Kuker W, Gaertner S, Nagele T, et al. Vessel wall contrast enhancement: A diagnostic sign of cerebral vasculitis. Cerebrovasc Dis 2008;26:23–9.
24. Mandell DM, Matouk CC, Farb RI, et al. Vessel wall mri to differentiate between reversible cerebral vasoconstriction syndrome and central nervous system vasculitis: Preliminary results. Stroke 2012;43:860–2.
33. Ebinger F, Mannhardt-Laakmann W, Zepp F. Cerebral vasculitis stabilised by methotrexate. Eur J Pediatr 2000; 159:712.
34. Zoller B, Li X, Sundquist J, et al. Risk of subsequent ischemic and hemorrhagic stroke in patients hospitalized for immune-mediated diseases: A nationwide follow-up study from sweden. BMC Neurol 2012;12:41.
35. Gonzalez-Gay MA, Vazquez-Rodriguez TR, Lopez-Diaz MJ, et al. Epidemiology of giant cell arteritis and polymyalgia rheumatica. Arthritis Rheum 2009;61:1454–61.
38. Borchers AT, Gershwin ME. Giant cell arteritis: A review of classification, pathophysiology, geoepidemiology and treatment. Autoimmun Rev 2012;11:A544–54.
39. Katan M, Moon YP, Paik MC, et al. Infectious burden and cognitive function: The Northern Manhattan study. Neurology 2013;80:1209–15.
47. Kang JH, Sheu JJ, Lin HC. Polymyalgia rheumatica and the risk of stroke: A three-year follow-up study. Cerebrovasc Dis 2011;32: 497–503.
56. Mahr A, Saba M, Kambouchner M, et al. Temporal artery biopsy for diagnosing giant cell arteritis: The longer, the better? Ann Rheum Dis 2006;65:826–8.
57. Walvick MD, Walvick MP. Giant cell arteritis: Laboratory predictors of a positive temporal artery biopsy. Ophthalmology 2011;118:1201–4.
58. Schmidt WA, Kraft HE, Vorpahl K, et al. Color duplex ultrasonography in the diagnosis of temporal arteritis. N Engl J Med 1997;337:1336–42.
59. Garcia-Garcia J, Ayo-Martin O, Argandona-Palacios L, et al. Vertebral artery halo sign in patients with stroke: A key clue for the prompt diagnosis of giant cell arteritis. Stroke 2011;42: 3287–90.
60. Meller J, Sahlmann CO, Gurocak O, et al. FDG-PET in patients with fever of unknown origin: The importance of diagnosing large vessel vasculitis. Q J Nucl Med Mol Imaging 2009;53: 51–63.
62. Bley TA, Uhl M, Carew J, et al. Diagnostic value of high-resolution MR imaging in giant cell arteritis. AJNR Am J Neuroradiol 2007;28:1722–7.
63. Narvaez J, Bernad B, Roig-Vilaseca D, et al. Influence of previous corticosteroid therapy on temporal artery biopsy yield in giant cell arteritis. Semin Arthritis Rheum 2007;37:13–19.
64. Mukhtyar C, Guillevin L, Cid MC, et al. Eular recommendations for the management of large vessel vasculitis. Ann Rheum Dis 2009;68:318–23.
65. Mahr AD, Jover JA, Spiera RF, et al. Adjunctive methotrexate for treatment of giant cell arteritis: An individual patient data meta-analysis. Arthritis Rheum 2007;56:2789–97.
67. Nuenninghoff DM, Matteson EL. The role of disease-modifying antirheumatic drugs in the treatment of giant cell arteritis. Clin Experiment Rheumatol 2003;21:S29–34.
68. Yates M, Loke YK, Watts RA, et al. Prednisolone combined with adjunctive immunosuppression is not superior to prednisolone alone in terms of efficacy and safety in giant cell arteritis: Meta-analysis. Clin Rheumatol 2013.
71. Hwang J, Kim SJ, Bang OY, et al. Ischemic stroke in Takayasu's arteritis: Lesion patterns and possible mechanisms. J Clin Neurol 2012;8:109–15.
72. Andrews J, Mason JC. Takayasu's arteritis – recent advances in imaging offer promise. Rheumatology 2007;46:6–15.
73. Desai MY, Stone JH, Foo TK, et al. Delayed contrast-enhanced MRI of the aortic wall in Takayasu's arteritis: Initial experience. AJR Am J Roentgenol 2005;184:1427–31.
76. Clifford A, Hoffman GS. Recent advances in the medical management of Takayasu arteritis: An update on use of biologic therapies. Curr Opin Rheumatol 2013.
78. Saadoun D, Lambert M, Mirault T, et al. Retrospective analysis of surgery versus endovascular intervention in Takayasu arteritis: A multicenter experience. Circulation 2012;125: 813–19.
79. Pagnoux C, Seror R, Henegar C, et al. Clinical features and outcomes in 348 patients with polyarteritis nodosa: A systematic retrospective study of patients diagnosed between 1963 and 2005 and entered into the French Vasculitis Study Group database. Arthritis Rheum 2010;62:616–26.
82. Reichart MD, Bogousslavsky J, Janzer RC. Early lacunar strokes complicating polyarteritis nodosa: Thrombotic microangiopathy. Neurology 2000;54:883–9.
83. Stone JH. Limited versus severe Wegener's granulomatosis: Baseline data on patients in the Wegener's granulomatosis Etanercept trial. Arthritis Rheum 2003;48:2299–309.
86. Suppiah R, Judge A, Batra R, et al. A model to predict cardiovascular events in patients with newly diagnosed Wegener's granulomatosis and microscopic polyangiitis. Arthritis Care Res 2011; 63:588–96.
87. Sinico RA, Di Toma L, Maggiore U, et al. Prevalence and clinical significance of antineutrophil cytoplasmic antibodies in Churg-Strauss syndrome. Arthritis Rheum 2005;52:2926–35.
88. Wolf J, Bergner R, Mutallib S, et al. Neurologic complications of Churg-Strauss syndrome – a prospective monocentric study. Eur J Neurol 2010;17:582–8.
90. Sable-Fourtassou R, Cohen P, Mahr A, et al. Antineutrophil cytoplasmic antibodies and the Churg-Strauss syndrome. Ann Intern Med 2005;143:632–8.
91. Solans R, Bosch JA, Perez-Bocanegra C, et al. Churg-strauss syndrome: Outcome and long-term follow-up of 32 patients. Rheumatology 2001;40:763–71.
92. Schonermarck U, Gross WL, de Groot K. Treatment of ANCA-associated vasculitis. Nat Rev Nephrol 2013.
93. Galossi A, Guarisco R, Bellis L, et al. Extrahepatic manifestations of chronic HCV infection. J Gastrointestin Liver Dis 2007;16: 65–73.
94. Ramos-Casals M, Robles A, Brito-Zeron P, et al. Life-threatening cryoglobulinemia: Clinical and immunological characterization of 29 cases. Semin Arthritis Rheum 2006;36:189–96.
97. Zaidan M, Mariotte E, Galicier L, et al. Vasculitic emergencies in the intensive care unit: A special focus on cryoglobulinemic vasculitis. Ann Intensive Care 2012;2:31.
98. Acharya JN, Pacheco VH. Neurologic complications of hepatitis C. Neurologist 2008;14:151–6.
100. Al-Araji A, Kidd DP. Neuro-Behcet's disease: Epidemiology, clinical characteristics, and management. Lancet Neurol 2009;8: 192–204.
101. Sfikakis PP, Markomichelakis N, Alpsoy E, et al. Anti-TNF therapy in the management of Behcet's disease – review and basis for recommendations. Rheumatology 2007;46:736–41.
102. Barnes CG. Treatment of Behcet's syndrome. Rheumatology 2006;45:245–7.
104. Kampylafka EI, Alexopoulos H, Kosmidis ML, et al. Incidence and prevalence of major central nervous system involvement in systemic lupus erythematosus: A 3-year prospective study of 370 patients. PLoS ONE 2013;8:e55843.
105. Chiu CC, Huang CC, Chan WL, et al. Increased risk of ischemic stroke in patients with systemic lupus erythematosus: A nationwide population-based study. Intern Med 2012;51:17–21.
106. Mok CC, Ho LY, To CH. Annual incidence and standardized incidence ratio of cerebrovascular accidents in patients with systemic lupus erythematosus. Scand J Rheumatol 2009;38: 362–8.
107. Urowitz MB, Gladman D, Ibanez D, et al. Atherosclerotic vascular events in a multinational inception cohort of systemic lupus erythematosus. Arthritis Care Res (Hoboken) 2010;62: 881–7.

108. Mikdashi J, Handwerger B, Langenberg P, et al. Baseline disease activity, hyperlipidemia, and hypertension are predictive factors for ischemic stroke and stroke severity in systemic lupus erythematosus. Stroke 2007;38:281–5.
111. Magder LS, Petri M. Incidence of and risk factors for adverse cardiovascular events among patients with systemic lupus erythematosus. Am J Epidemiol 2012;176:708–19.
112. Maksimowicz-McKinnon K, Magder LS, Petri M. Predictors of carotid atherosclerosis in systemic lupus erythematosus. J Rheumatol 2006;33:2458–63.
113. Devinsky O, Petito CK, Alonso DR. Clinical and neuropathological findings in systemic lupus erythematosus: The role of vasculitis, heart emboli, and thrombotic thrombocytopenic purpura. Ann Neurol 1988;23:380–4.
115. Kumral E, Evyapan D, Keser G, et al. Detection of microembolic signals in patients with neuropsychiatric lupus erythematosus. Eur Neurol 2002;47:131–5.
121. Petri M. Update on anti-phospholipid antibodies in SLE: The Hopkins' lupus cohort. Lupus 2010;19:419–23.
122. Law G, Magder LS, Fang H, et al. Hydroxychloroquine reduces thrombosis (both arterial and venous) in systemic lupus erythematosus, particularly in antiphospholipid positive patients. American College of Rheumatology 76th Annual Meeting 2012.
123. Bertsias GK, Ioannidis JP, Aringer M, et al. Eular recommendations for the management of systemic lupus erythematosus with neuropsychiatric manifestations: Report of a task force of the Eular Standing Committee for Clinical Affairs. Ann Rheum Dis 2010;69:2074–82.
124. Kitas GD, Gabriel SE. Cardiovascular disease in rheumatoid arthritis: State of the art and future perspectives. Ann Rheum Dis 2011;70:8–14.
125. Libby P. Role of inflammation in atherosclerosis associated with rheumatoid arthritis. Am J Med 2008;121:S21–31.
129. Epstein SE, Zhu JH, Najafi AH, et al. Insights into the role of infection in atherogenesis and in plaque rupture. Circulation 2009;119:3133–U3160.
131. Cordato DJ, Djekic S, Taneja SR, et al. Prevalence of positive syphilis serology and meningovascular neurosyphilis in patients admitted with stroke and TIA from a culturally diverse population (2005-09). J Clin Neurosci 2013;20:943–7.
133. Liu LL, Zheng WH, Tong ML, et al. Ischemic stroke as a primary symptom of neurosyphilis among HIV-negative emergency patients. J Neurol Sci 2012;317:35–9.
136. Kayal AK, Goswami M, Das M, et al. Clinical spectrum of neurosyphilis in North East India. Neurol India 2011;59:344–50.
137. Dharmasaroja PA, Dharmasaroja P. Serum and cerebrospinal fluid profiles for syphilis in Thai patients with acute ischaemic stroke. Int J STD AIDS 2012;23:340–5.
138. Workowski KA, Berman S. Sexually transmitted diseases treatment guidelines, 2010. MMWR Recomm Rep 2010;59:1–110.
139. Jay CA. Treatment of neurosyphilis. Curr Treat Options Neurol 2006;8:185–92.
140. Anderson NE, Somaratne J, Mason DF, et al. Neurological and systemic complications of tuberculous meningitis and its treatment at Auckland City Hospital, New Zealand. J Clin Neurosci 2010;17:1114–18.
141. Pasticci MB, Paciaroni M, Floridi P, et al. Stroke in a patient with tuberculous meningitis and HIV infection. Mediterr J Hematol Infect Dis 2013;5:e2013017.
142. Misra UK, Kalita J, Maurya PK. Stroke in tuberculous meningitis. J Neurol Sci 2011;303:22–30.
143. Pasticci MB, Paciaroni M, Floridi P, et al. Stroke in patients with tuberculous meningitis in a low tb endemic country: An increasing medical emergency? New Microbiol 2013;36:193–8.
144. Anuradha HK, Garg RK, Agarwal A, et al. Predictors of stroke in patients of tuberculous meningitis and its effect on the outcome. QJM 2010;103:671–8.
146. Sheu JJ, Chiou HY, Kang JH, et al. Tuberculosis and the risk of ischemic stroke: A 3-year follow-up study. Stroke 2010;41:244–9.
147. Kalita J, Prasad S, Maurya PK, et al. MR angiography in tuberculous meningitis. Acta Radiol 2012;53:324–9.
148. Chan KH, Cheung RT, Lee R, et al. Cerebral infarcts complicating tuberculous meningitis. Cerebrovasc Dis 2005;19:391–5.
149. Nair PP, Kalita J, Kumar S, et al. MRI pattern of infarcts in basal ganglia region in patients with tuberculous meningitis. Neuroradiology 2009;51:221–5.
152. Silva RAE, Araujo SD, Avellar IFDE, et al. Granulomatous amoebic meningoencephalitis in an immunocompetent patient. Arch Neurol-Chicago 2010;67:1516–20.
159. Kaushik RM, Kaushik R, Varma A, et al. *Plasmodium falciparum* malaria presenting with vertebrobasilar stroke. Int J Infect Dis 2009;13:e292–4.
161. Lompo LD, Kamdem FK, Revenco E, et al. *Toxocara canis* cerebral vasculitis revealed by iterative strokes. Rev Neurol-France 2012;168:533–7.
164. Song T, Wang WS, Zhou BR, et al. CT and mR characteristics of cerebral sparganosis. Am J Neuroradiol 2007;28:1700–5.
166. Sarazin M, Caumes E, Cohen A, et al. Multiple microembolic borderzone brain infarctions and endomyocardial fibrosis in idiopathic hypereosinophilic syndrome and in Schistosoma mansoni infestation. J Neurol Neurosur Ps 2004;75:305–7.
167. Wu LQ, Wu MC, Tian DF, et al. Clinical and imaging characteristics of cerebral schistosomiasis. Cell Biochem Biophys 2012;62:289–95.
168. Finsterer J, Auer H. Parasitoses of the human central nervous system. J Helminthol 2013;87:257–70.
170. Carod-Artal FJ, Gascon J. Chagas disease and stroke. Lancet Neurol 2010;9:533–42.
172. Pinto AYD, Valente SA, Valente VD, et al. Acute phase of Chagas disease in the Brazilian Amazon region. Study of 233 cases from Para, Amapa and Maranhao observed between 1988 and 2005. Rev Soc Bras Med Tro 2008;41:602–14.
176. Carod-Artal FJ, Vargas AP, Falcao T. Stroke in asymptomatic Trypanosoma cruzi-infected patients. Cerebrovasc Dis 2011;31:24–8.
177. Jesus PA, Neville I, Cincura C, et al. Stroke history and chagas disease are independent predictors of silent cerebral microembolism in patients with congestive heart failure. Cerebrovasc Dis 2011;31:19–23.
186. Bouldin A, Pinter JD. Resolution of arterial stenosis in a patient with periarterial neurocysticercosis treated with oral prednisone. J Child Neurol 2006;21:1064–7.
194. Castro-Lima H, Raicher I, Lee HW, et al. Neurocysticercosis presenting with stroke. Arq Neuro-Psiquiat 2010;68:146.
195. Agarwal R, Kalita J, Marak RS, et al. Spectrum of fungal infection in a neurology tertiary care center in India. Neurol Sci 2012;33:1305–10.
198. Lee B, Anekthananon T, Poungvarin N, et al. Etiology and risk factors of stroke in HIV-infected patients in Siriraj Hospital: A case-control study. J Med Assoc Thai 2012;95(Suppl. 2):S227–34.
200. Tipping B, de Villiers L, Wainwright H, et al. Stroke in patients with human immunodeficiency virus infection. J Neurol Neurosurg Psychiatry 2007;78:1320–4.
201. Chen SF, Lu CH, Lui CC, et al. Acute/subacute cerebral infarction (ASCI) in HIV-negative adults with cryptococcal meningoencephalitis (CM): A MRI-based follow-up study and a clinical comparison to HIV-negative CM adults without ASCI. BMC Neurol 2011;11:12.
205. Ahsan H, Ajmal F, Saleem MF, et al. Cerebral fungal infection with mycotic aneurysm of basilar artery and subarachnoid haemorrhage. Singapore Med J 2009;50:e22–5.
206. van de Beek D, Patel R, Campeau NG, et al. Insidious sinusitis leading to catastrophic cerebral aspergillosis in transplant recipients. Neurology 2008;70:2411–13.
207. Lee JH, Im SA, Cho B. Renal infarction secondary to invasive aspergillosis in a 5-year-old girl with acute lymphoblastic leukemia. J Pediatr Hematol Oncol 2014;36:e296–8.
210. Charlot M, Pialat JB, Obadia N, et al. Diffusion-weighted imaging in brain aspergillosis. Eur J Neurol 2007;14:912–16.
212. Hurst RW, Judkins A, Bolger W, et al. Mycotic aneurysm and cerebral infarction resulting from fungal sinusitis: Imaging and pathologic correlation. AJNR Am J Neuroradiol 2001;22:858–63.
213. Ueno A, Hamano T, Fujii A, et al. Effects of voriconazole and vascular lesions in invasion of aspergillosis into the central nerve system. Rinsho Shinkeigaku 2009;49:468–73.
220. Alsuhaibani AH, Al-Thubaiti G, Al Badr FB. Optic nerve thickening and infarction as the first evidence of orbital involvement

with mucormycosis. Middle East Afr J Ophthalmol 2012;19: 340–2.

224. Giuliani A, Mettimano M, Viviani D, et al. An uncommon case of systemic mucormycosis associated with spinal cord infarction in a recently diagnosed diabetic. Int J Immunopathol Pharmacol 2010;23:355–8.
225. Koc Z, Koc F, Yerdelen D, et al. Rhino-orbital-cerebral mucormycosis with different cerebral involvements: Infarct, hemorrhage, and ophthalmoplegia. Int J Neurosci 2007;117:1677–90.
227. Dussaule C, Nifle C, Therby A, et al. Teaching neuroimages: Brain mri aspects of isolated cerebral mucormycosis. Neurology 2012;78:e93.
229. Alacacioglu I, Kargi A, Ozcan MA, et al. Fatal disseminated mucormycosis in a patient with mantle cell non-hodgkin's lymphoma: An autopsy case. Braz J Infect Dis 2009;13:238–41.
231. Vinikoor MJ, Napravnik S, Floris-Moore M, et al. Incidence and clinical features of cerebrovascular disease among HIV-infected adults in the southeastern united states. AIDS Res Hum Retroviruses 2013;29:1068–74.
232. Triant VA, Lee H, Hadigan C, et al. Increased acute myocardial infarction rates and cardiovascular risk factors among patients with human immunodeficiency virus disease. J Clin Endocrinol Metab 2007;92:2506–12.
241. Goldstein DA, Timpone J, Cupps TR. HIV-associated intracranial aneurysmal vasculopathy in adults. J Rheumatol 2010;37: 226–33.
243. Gutierrez J, Ortiz G. Hiv/aids patients with hiv vasculopathy and VZV vasculitis: A case series. Clin Neuroradiol 2011;21:145–51.
244. Tipping B, de Villiers L, Candy S, et al. Stroke caused by human immunodeficiency virus-associated intracranial large-vessel aneurysmal vasculopathy. Arch Neurol 2006;63:1640–2.
245. Modi G, Ranchod K, Modi M, et al. Human immunodeficiency virus associated intracranial aneurysms: Report of three adult patients with an overview of the literature. J Neurol Neurosur Ps 2008;79:44–6.
246. Eugenin EA, Morgello S, Klotman ME, et al. Human immunodeficiency virus (HIV) infects human arterial smooth muscle cells in vivo and in vitro: Implications for the pathogenesis of hiv-mediated vascular disease. Am J Pathol 2008;172:1100–11.
247. Gutierrez J, Glenn M, Isaacson RS, et al. Thinning of the arterial media layer as a possible preclinical stage in HIV vasculopathy: A pilot study. Stroke 2012;43:1156–8.
248. Gutierrez J, Elkind MS, Petito C, et al. The contribution of HIV infection to intracranial arterial remodeling: A pilot study. Neuropathology 2012.
249. Gutierrez J, Murray J, Jackson T, et al. HIV-associated brain arterial remodeling is correlated with increased MMP-2 expression: A pilot study. Stroke 2013;44:AWP439.
250. Law MG, Friis-Moller N, El-Sadr WM, et al. The use of the Framingham equation to predict myocardial infarctions in hiv-infected patients: Comparison with observed events in the d:A:D study. HIV Med 2006;7:218–30.
251. Weber R, Ruppik M, Rickenbach M, et al. Decreasing mortality and changing patterns of causes of death in the Swiss HIV cohort study. HIV Med 2013;14:195–207.
252. Ovbiagele B, Nath A. Increasing incidence of ischemic stroke in patients with HIV infection. Neurology 2011;76:444–50.
253. Gutierrez J, Elkind MSV, Marshall RS. Cardiovascular profile and events of us adults 20–49 years with HIV: Results from the nhanes 1999–2008. AIDS Care 2013;1–7.
255. Petoumenos K, Worm S, Reiss P, et al. Rates of cardiovascular disease following smoking cessation in patients with HIV infection: Results from the d:A:D study(*). HIV Med 2011;12: 412–21.
256. Baker JV, Duprez D, Rapkin J, et al. Untreated HIV infection and large and small artery elasticity. J Acquir Immun Defic Syndr 2009;52:25–31.
259. Friis-Moller N, Reiss P, Sabin CA, et al. Class of antiretroviral drugs and the risk of myocardial infarction. N Engl J Med 2007;356:1723–35.
270. Ridker PM, Hennekens CH, Stampfer MJ, et al. Prospective study of herpes simplex virus, cytomegalovirus, and the risk of future myocardial infarction and stroke. Circulation 1998;98:2796–9.
271. Nagel MA, Cohrs RJ, Mahalingam R, et al. The varicella zoster virus vasculopathies: Clinical, CSF, imaging, and virologic features. Neurology 2008;70:853–60.
272. Newsome SD, Nath A. Varicella-zoster virus vasculopathy and central nervous system immune reconstitution inflammatory syndrome with human immunodeficiency virus infection treated with steroids. J Neurovirol 2009;1–4.
273. Ortiz GA, Koch S, Forteza A, et al. Ramsay Hunt syndrome followed by multifocal vasculopathy and posterior circulation strokes. Neurology 2008;70:1049–51.
274. Katchanov J, Siebert E, Klingebiel R, et al. Infectious vasculopathy of intracranial large- and medium-sized vessels in neurological intensive care unit: A clinico-radiological study. Neurocrit Care 2010.
277. Nagel MA, Traktinskiy I, Choe A, et al. Varicella-zoster virus expression in the cerebral arteries of diabetic subjects. Arch Neurol 2012;69:142–4.
280. Nagel MA, Forghani B, Mahalingam R, et al. The value of detecting anti-VZV IGG antibody in CSF to diagnose VZV vasculopathy. Neurology 2007;68:1069–73.
286. Guidi B, Bergonzini P, Crisi G, et al. Case of stroke in a 7-year-old male after parvovirus b19 infection. Pediatr Neurol 2003; 28:69–71.
289. Douvoyiannis M, Litman N, Goldman DL. Neurologic manifestations associated with parvovirus b19 infection. Clin Infect Dis 2009;48:1713–23.

37 Reversible Cerebral Vasoconstriction Syndromes

Aneesh B. Singhal

KEY POINTS

- Reversible Cerebral Vasoconstriction Syndromes (RCVS) are a group of conditions characterized by reversible narrowing and dilatation of the cerebral arteries.
- The mean age is 42 years; age range 10–76 years. The female : male ratio ranges from 2 : 1 to 4 : 1.
- The etiology is unknown. Associated triggers include vasoconstrictive medications, illicit drugs, sexual intercourse, and recent pregnancy, among others.
- Most patients present with sudden, severe "thunderclap" headaches that can recur over a span of 1–4 weeks.
- Approximately one-third to one-half develop visual deficits, weakness, or seizures.
- Despite the often severe and widespread arterial narrowing, the admission brain scan is normal in over 50% of patients. New brain lesions can develop, usually within 8–12 days after onset. Ultimately, around one-third of the brain scans remain normal; the rest show ischemic strokes, convexal (non-aneurysmal) subarachnoid hemorrhages, lobar hemorrhages, and reversible brain edema (alone or in combination).
- Cerebral angiographic abnormalities are dynamic, usually progressing from distal to proximal segments, resulting in a "sausage on a string" appearance of the circle of Willis arteries and their branches. These angiographic abnormalities usually resolve spontaneously within 3 months.
- While some patients can develop new, usually mild neurological deficits in the first few days, the clinical outcome is benign in 95% of patients. Rare patients develop severe irreversible deficits or death from progressive cerebral vasoconstriction.
- There is no proven treatment. Oral calcium-channel blockers are often administered. Empiric glucocorticoid treatment has been associated with poor outcome. Intra-arterial vasodilator therapy has been attempted in fulminant cases, with variable success.
- Recurrence of an episode of reversible cerebral vasoconstriction syndromes (RCVS) is rare.

Reversible cerebral vasoconstriction syndromes (RCVS) are a group of conditions characterized by reversible multifocal narrowing of the cerebral arteries, typically associated with recurrent sudden, severe (thunderclap) headaches and often complicated by ischemic or hemorrhagic strokes.[1,2] A typical case is illustrated in Figure 37-1. Over the past 60 years, this enigmatic reversible angiographic phenomenon has been reported under a variety of names and eponyms, each reflecting the associated clinical setting (Box 37-1) or the presumed pathophysiology – for example, migrainous "vasospasm" or "angiitis";[3,4] thunderclap headache with reversible vasospasm;[5–7] postpartum cerebral angiopathy, angiitis, or vasospasm;[5–7] drug-induced cerebral arteritis or angiopathy;[8,9] Call's or Call-Fleming syndrome:[10,11] central nervous system (CNS) pseudovasculitis;[12] and benign angiopathy of the central nervous system.[13] Only recently has it become apparent that patients with reversible cerebral arterial narrowing have similar clinical, laboratory, imaging, and prognostic features regardless of the associated underlying condition(s).[14–16] The descriptive term *reversible cerebral vasoconstriction syndrome* (RCVS) has been proposed to facilitate the recognition and management of this group of disorders.[1]

HISTORY, EVOLUTION, AND ASSOCIATED CONDITIONS

Stroke was historically attributed to cerebral "vasospasm" for centuries. However, from the 1950s onward, the work of C.M. Fisher and others enumerated pathologic causes of stroke, such as carotid atherosclerosis, lipohyalinosis, and cardioembolism. As a result, "vasospasm" disappeared from the stroke lexicon except in the setting of aneurysmal subarachnoid hemorrhage. Ironically, Dr. Fisher himself was later instrumental in bringing to world attention the phenomenon of reversible segmental cerebral vasoconstriction. In the early 1970s, he described unusual cases of postpartum women with transient neurologic dysfunction associated with reversible cerebral arterial irregularities.[17] One patient was discussed at the first Sâlpetrière Hospital stroke conference in Paris;[18] at the second conference, Rascol and associates[19] presented four similar cases, and the entity became known as "postpartum angiopathy." Over the next decade, similar cases were documented in association with such diverse conditions as pregnancy,[8] migraine,[4,20,21] vasoconstrictive drugs and medications,[8,9] neurosurgical procedures,[22] hypercalcemia,[23] and even unruptured saccular aneurysms.[5] In 1987, Dr. Marie Fleming presented the cases of two patients with transient cerebral arterial narrowing at the Boston Stroke Society meeting held at Massachusetts General Hospital. Dr. Fisher promptly recognized the similarity between her cases and others, and in a collaborative effort reported on 19 patients.[10] Thereafter, some investigators referred to this syndrome as Call's or Call-Fleming syndrome,[24–26] but the use of variable terminology persisted.

Meanwhile, this syndrome was probably being misinterpreted as primary angiitis of the central nervous system (PACNS), an inflammatory condition affecting brain arteries, because of overlapping angiographic as well as clinical features such as headache, seizures, and stroke.[27–29] Calabrese and colleagues[13] recognized that these patients did not exhibit the typical progressive course of PACNS; instead, their angiographic abnormalities reversed promptly and clinical resolution occurred within weeks, even without immunosuppressive therapy. These researchers suspected that the patients had a transient or mild form of PACNS and proposed the term "benign angiopathy of the central nervous system" (BACNS).[13]

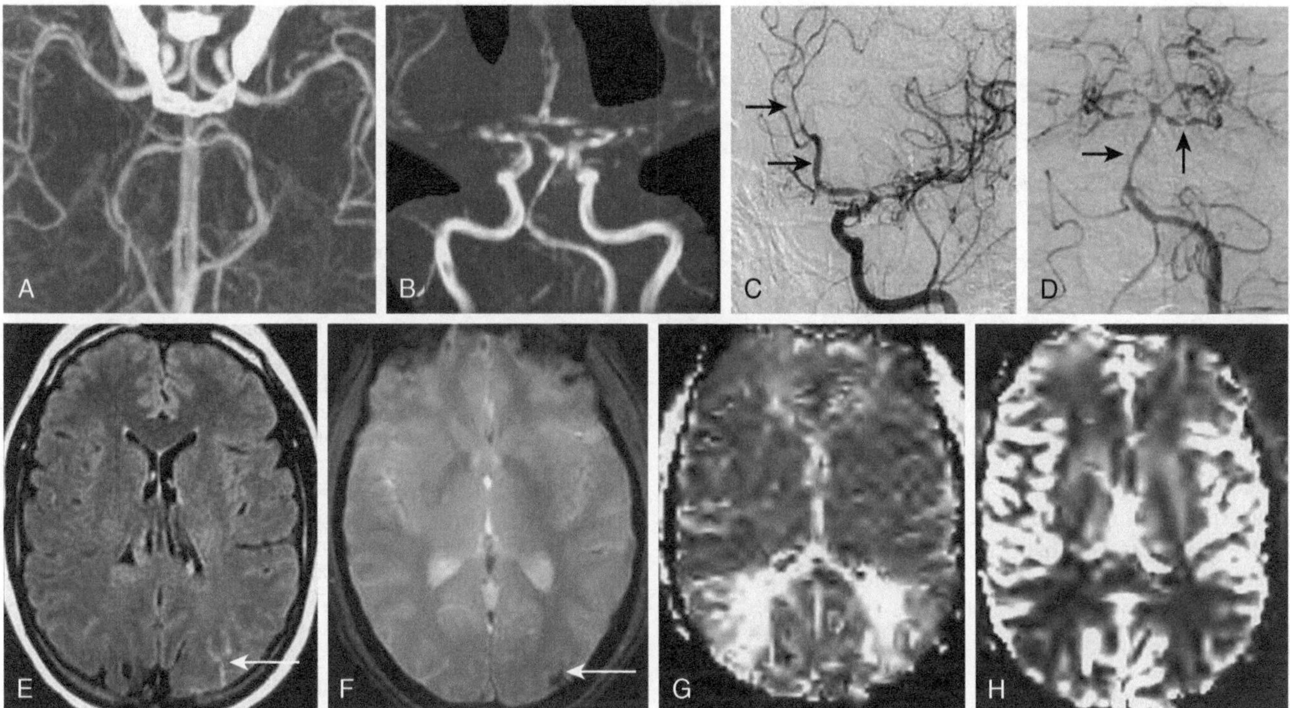

Figure 37-1. Typical case of reversible cerebral vasoconstriction syndrome (RCVS). A 44-year-old woman with prior migraine and depression experienced a sudden, excruciating (thunderclap) headache while exercising. The headache did not resemble her prior migraines and resolved over 30 minutes. Over the next week, three more thunderclap headaches occurred. Blood pressure and neurologic findings were normal. CT angiogram (A), MR angiogram (B), and digital subtraction angiogram (C and D) show segmental narrowing and dilatation of multiple intracerebral arteries. Note the abnormal dilatation followed by abrupt narrowing of the anterior cerebral artery (*arrows*, C), the basilar artery (*horizontal arrow*, D) and the superior cerebellar artery (*vertical arrow*, D). This "sausage on a string" appearance is characteristic of RCVS. Brain MRI showed sulcal hyperintensity in the left occipital lobe on axial fluid-attenuated inversion recovery (FLAIR) images (*arrow*, E), and corresponding sulcal hypointensity on gradient-echo images (*arrow*, F), consistent with cortical surface subarachnoid hemorrhage. Perfusion-weighted MRI showed abnormally increased mean transit time (G) and reduced cerebral blood flow (H) in the "watershed" regions of the bilateral middle and posterior cerebral arteries; fortunately these regions did not progress to infarction. Cerebrospinal fluid examination findings were normal. Results of extensive tests for vasculitis were negative. She was treated with nimodipine. Over the next 2 weeks, her headaches resolved, and follow-up brain imaging showed resolution of the subarachnoid blood and vascular abnormalities.

Calabrese's group subsequently analyzed the clinical characteristics and long-term outcomes of BACNS and concluded that it is consistent with RCVS.[30,31]

Over the past few years, it has become apparent that virtually the same clinicoangiographic syndrome has been reported separately by stroke neurologists, headache specialists, obstetricians, internists, and rheumatologists, each in turn imparting their own biases to nomenclature, theories of pathogenesis, and clinical approach. The proposal and adoption of the broad term RCVS, along with its main clinical and imaging features (Box 37-2), have encouraged relatively large retrospective and prospective studies that have helped characterize the syndrome.[1,2,32–38] The now-routine use of relatively non-invasive angiographic techniques, such as computed tomography angiography (CTA) and magnetic resonance angiography (MRA), combined with the widespread use of illicit drugs such as ecstasy and cocaine and of serotonergic and sympathomimetic medications, makes it likely that vascular neurologists and other specialists will encounter an increasing number of patients with RCVS.

DEMOGRAPHICS AND CLINICAL FEATURES

Once considered rare, RCVS is being reported with increasing frequency, presumably as a result of the widespread use of relatively non-invasive imaging tests such as CT and MRA as well as greater awareness of the syndrome. Cases have been documented from numerous countries including France, the US, Mexico, Canada, Spain, South Africa, China, India, Japan, and Australia. RCVS appears to affect individuals of all races. Most patients are young adults in the age range of 25–50 years, with a mean age of approximately 42 years;[2,33] although children can be affected.[39] There is an impressive female preponderance (2 : 1 to 10 : 1, depending on the case series), even after cases related to pregnancy have been accounted for.

The onset is typically dramatic with a sudden "worst ever" headache that reaches its peak intensity within seconds, often referred to as a "thunderclap headache."[5,40] Screaming, agitation, confusion, and collapse due to the extreme severity of the pain are common. More than 80% of patients experience thunderclap headaches, and the rest have subacute or less severe headaches; the absence of headache at onset is exceptional. The location of the headache could be occipital, vertex, or diffuse. It is usually throbbing and accompanied by nausea, emesis, or photosensitivity, but patients with migraines clearly identify the thunderclap headaches as different from their usual headaches. Severe pain usually subsides within 1–2 hours, although 50–75% of patients report mild baseline headache between acute exacerbations. Thunderclap headaches recur frequently over the ensuing 1–3 weeks, with an average of four recurrences; however, the intensity and frequency diminish over time. Headache remains the only symptom in one-half to three-fourths of patients.

BOX 37-1 Conditions Associated with Reversible Cerebral Vasoconstriction Syndrome

IDIOPATHIC

No identifiable precipitating factor. Associated with headache disorders (migraine, primary thunderclap headache,* benign exertional headache, benign sexual headache, and primary cough headache)

EXPOSURE TO MEDICATIONS, DRUGS, AND BLOOD PRODUCTS

Phenylpropanolamine, pseudoephedrine, amphetamine derivatives,* methergine, bromocriptine, ergotamine tartrate, suma-triptan,* isometheptene, oral contraceptives, lisuride, licorice, khat leaves, selective serotonin reuptake inhibitors (SSRIs),* cocaine, ecstasy, marijuana,* lysergic acid diethylamide (LSD), tacrolimus (FK-506), cyclophosphamide,* erythropoietin,* intravenous immune globulin (IVIG),* red blood cell transfusion*

PREGNANCY AND PUERPERIUM

Early puerperium, late pregnancy, eclampsia,* preeclampsia,* delayed postpartum eclampsia*

MISCELLANEOUS CONDITIONS

Hypercalcemia, porphyria,* thrombotic thrombocytopenic purpura, pheochromocytoma, bronchial carcinoid tumor, unruptured saccular cerebral aneurysm, head trauma, spinal subdural hematoma, postcarotid endarterectomy,* neurosurgical procedures, cervical arterial dissection

*Also associated with the reversible posterior leukoencephalopathy syndrome.

BOX 37-2 Summary of Critical Elements for the Diagnosis of Reversible Cerebral Vasoconstriction Syndromes

1. Transfemoral angiography or indirect (CT or MR) angiography documenting segmental cerebral artery vasoconstriction
2. No evidence for aneurysmal subarachnoid hemorrhage
3. Normal or near-normal cerebrospinal fluid analysis results (total protein content <80 mg/dL, white blood cell count <10/mm^3, normal glucose content)
4. Severe, acute headache, with or without additional neurologic signs and symptoms
5. The diagnosis cannot be confirmed until reversibility of the angiographic abnormalities is documented within 12 weeks after onset or, if death occurs before the follow-up studies are completed, autopsy rules out conditions such as vasculitis, intracranial atherosclerosis, and aneurysmal subarachnoid hemorrhage, which can also manifest as headache and stroke.

Modified from Calabrese LH, Dodick DW, Schwedt TJ, et al: Narrative review: Reversible cerebral vasoconstriction syndromes. *Ann Intern Med* 146:34–44, 2007.

While a preceding history of hypertension is uncommon, the blood pressure can be elevated in the initial stages, either due to underlying pain, eclampsia, or recent exposure to drugs such as cocaine, or as a result of the systemic response to cerebral vasoconstriction. The frequency of other neurologic signs and symptoms varies according to the method of case ascertainment.[1,2,32–38] Generalized tonic-clonic seizures are reported in 0–21% of patients at the time of presentation; however, recurrent seizures are rare. Focal neurologic deficits from ischemic stroke or parenchymal hematoma are reported in 9–63% of patients, the frequency being higher in inpatient series. Visual deficits are common, including scotomas, blurring, hemianopia, and cortical blindness (full or partial Balint's syndrome). Hemiplegia, tremor, ataxia, and aphasia have also been reported. Some patients demonstrate acute transient deficits consistent with transient ischemic attacks, and others have subacute and recurrent positive visual or sensory symptoms mimicking the aura of migraine. Hyper-reflexia is common, similar to the observation in patients with eclampsia, but the basis for hyper-reflexia is not clear since it occurs regardless of the presence of brain lesions. Blood pressure can be normal or elevated from the pain, the disease itself, or the associated condition (e.g., eclampsia). Over the next few weeks, most patients show gradual resolution of visual and other focal neurologic signs or symptoms. Few are left with minor or moderate permanent deficits. Less than 5% experience progressive cerebral arterial vasoconstriction culminating in massive strokes, brain edema, severe morbidity, or death.[41–44] For this reason, it is reasonable to admit patients for observation for the first few days after symptom onset.

LABORATORY FINDINGS

Blood counts, erythrocyte sedimentation rate, serum electrolyte levels, and liver and renal function test results are usually normal. Tests for rheumatoid factor, antinuclear and antinuclear cytoplasmic antibodies, Lyme disease antibodies, and urine vanillylmandelic acid and 5-hydroxyindoleacetic acid are useful to rule out systemic diseases and evaluate for vasoactive tumors (e.g., pheochromocytoma, carcinoid) that have been associated with RCVS. Serum and urine toxicology screens, in addition to a careful medication history, are important to uncover exposure to vasoactive drugs and medications. Cerebrospinal fluid examination findings are normal (protein level less than 60 mg/dL, fewer than five white blood cells per mm^3) in more than 85% of patients;[33] minor abnormalities can result from ischemic or hemorrhagic strokes. There is no role for brain biopsy or temporal artery biopsy other than to rule out cerebral vasculitis when the diagnosis of RCVS cannot be secured within the clinical context, including presentation and associated conditions (see Boxes 37-1, 37-2) and brain imaging and angiographic findings. Distinguishing RCVS from cerebral vasculitis can be challenging and is discussed further later (see "Differential Diagnosis"). Brain and temporal artery biopsies as well as full autopsy in patients who died from progressive vasoconstriction have shown normal arterial histology.[20,26,42] However, in some cases, the interpretation of pathologic samples can be difficult because prolonged severe vasoconstriction can itself induce secondary inflammation.[45]

BRAIN IMAGING

Patients with RCVS typically present to the emergency department for evaluation of thunderclap headaches and appropriately undergo urgent brain and vascular imaging to rule out secondary causes. Between 30% and 70% of patients ultimately diagnosed with RCVS show no parenchymal lesion on initial head CT or brain MRI, despite having widespread vasoconstriction on concomitant cerebral angiography.[2,33,46–48] Brain scans remain normal in 15% of cases reported from in-hospital settings; this number is much higher in emergency department case series. The wide variability in the frequency of abnormal brain imaging findings reflects the wide clinical spectrum, which ranges from isolated headache and normal brain imaging findings (more common), to the more

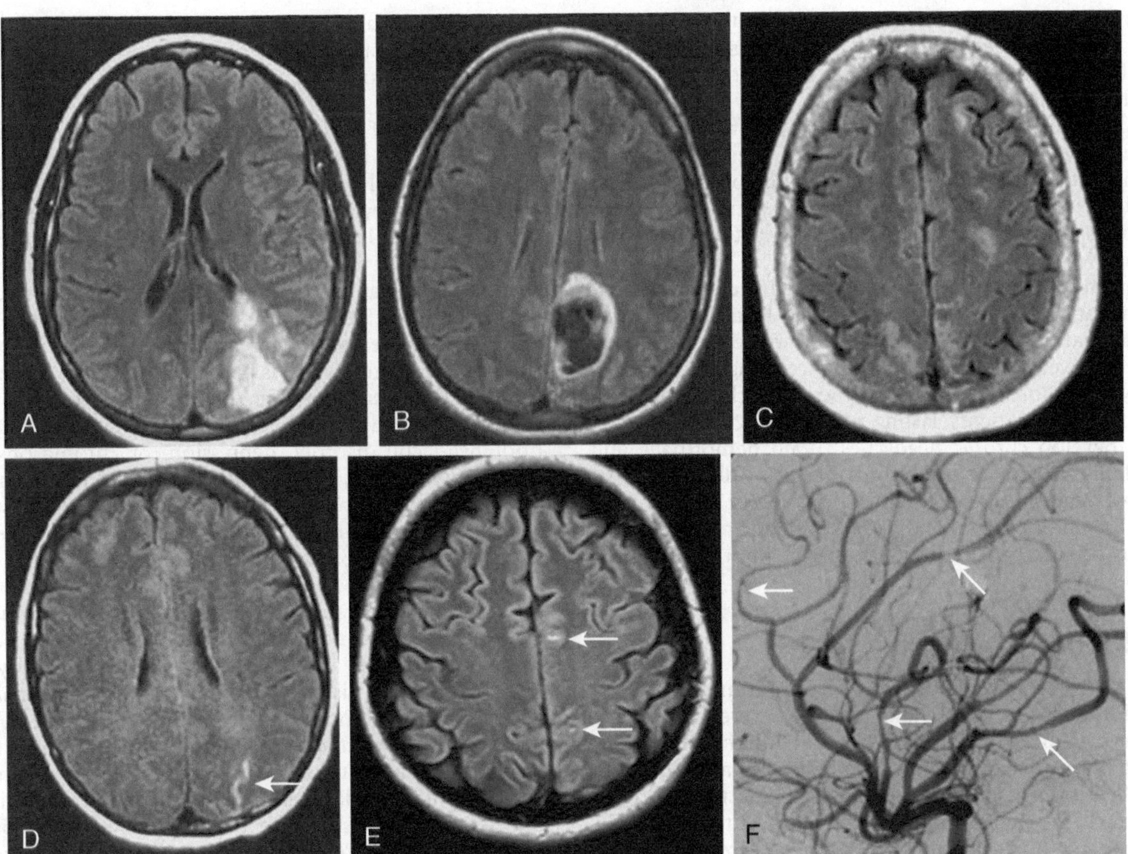

Figure 37-2. Brain MRI findings in reversible cerebral vasoconstriction syndrome (RCVS). A to E, Axial fluid-attenuated inversion recovery (FLAIR) images show the typical brain imaging abnormalities in RCVS, including an ischemic stroke in the watershed distribution of the left middle and posterior cerebral artery (A), parenchymal brain hemorrhage (B), reversible hyperintense lesions (brain edema) in subcortical regions (C), non-aneurysmal cortical surface subarachnoid hemorrhage *(arrow)* overlying the left hemisphere (D), and dilated cortical surface vessels *(arrows)* overlying the left hemisphere (E). However, it is important to note that in many patients with RCVS, no parenchymal lesion is seen on brain MRI. F, Digital subtraction angiogram from a patient with RCVS shows the typical segmental narrowing ("sausaging") of multiple cerebral arteries that usually reverse within weeks. *(From Calabrese LH, Singhal AB: Primary angiitis of the central nervous system (PACNS) and reversible cerebral vasoconstriction syndromes (RCVS). In Stone JH, editor:* A clinician's pearls and myths in rheumatology, *New York, 2010, Springer.)*

pernicious course with multiple strokes, seizures, and permanent neurologic impairment.

Abnormal brain imaging findings can consist of a variety of lesions, either initially or on follow-up studies (Fig. 37-2). Ischemic stroke is the most frequent lesion, followed by cortical surface (non-aneurysmal) subarachnoid hemorrhage, parenchymal hemorrhage, and reversible brain edema.[2,33,46–48] Any combination of lesions can be present. Infarcts are often bilateral and symmetrical and located in arterial "watershed" regions of the cerebral hemispheres. Cerebellar infarcts are also common. Smaller infarcts typically abut the cortical–subcortical junction, and larger infarcts are often wedge-shaped. Perfusion-weighted MRI may show areas of hypoperfusion. Cortical surface hemorrhages are typically minor, restricted to a few sulcal spaces.[49–51] Accumulating data suggest that RCVS is the predominant cause of convexal subarachnoid hemorrhage in individuals below age 60 years.[52–54] Single as well as multiple lobar hemorrhages can occur. Subdural hemorrhage has been reported.[55] It appears that hemorrhages are more common in women and are more frequently associated with medication or drug exposure. Interestingly, some patients with negative initial imaging findings go on to have lobar hemorrhage after their second or third headache exacerbation, reflecting the dynamic nature of this condition. Fluid-attenuated inversion recovery (FLAIR) MRI may show dot or linear hyperintensities within sulcal spaces, which are distinct from subarachnoid hemorrhage, probably reflect slow flow within dilated surface vessels, and may correlate with worse outcome.[56,57] The presence of reversible lesions suggesting transient brain edema in patients with RCVS, and the high frequency of reversible cerebral angiographic abnormalities in patients with the posterior reversible leukoencephalopathy syndrome (PRES), suggests an overlapping pathophysiology between these syndromes.[51,58]

The diagnosis of RCVS can be considered only after documenting cerebral vasoconstriction with transfemoral, CT, or MR angiography. Findings of the first angiogram can be normal if it is performed within 3 to 5 days after symptom onset. In one study, 21% of patients with RCVS had normal findings on initial MRA, and 9% had normal findings on both MRA and transcranial Doppler ultrasonography.[2] The rate of diagnosis can be increased by repeating the angiographic study after a few days; however, the value of repeat testing is limited by the instantly recognizable clinical presentation and the usually benign nature of this condition. Angiographic abnormalities are dynamic, with different segments (usually the more proximal segments) becoming affected over time. Angiography often reveals arterial dissection and unruptured saccular aneurysms,[5,59–61] and in some patients the vasoconstriction can affect the extracranial internal carotid or vertebral artery and rarely, systemic arteries.[62] Patients with typical clinical features have been diagnosed on the basis of elevated blood flow velocities on transcranial Doppler ultrasonography.[63] This non-invasive bedside tool has utility in monitoring the progression of vasoconstriction.[32] However, there is little correlation between ultrasonographic and angiographic findings, and most investigators prefer angiographic studies to establish resolution and confirm the diagnosis. The time course of vasoconstriction is variable, but most patients show resolution within 3 months.

Prospective case series have highlighted the characteristic temporal pattern and relationship of clinical features and arterial abnormalities.[2] Thunderclap headaches recur frequently over the first week, with the last attack occurring an average of 7–8 days after onset.[2] Mild baseline headaches may then persist in 70% of patients, lasting a mean of 22 days;[2,32] some patients develop chronic headaches. Brain hemorrhage and brain edema are early complications, occurring during the first week, whereas ischemic complications occur significantly later, at the end of the second week.[2] Ischemic complications may thus occur when the headaches have improved or even resolved.

DIFFERENTIAL DIAGNOSIS

RCVS is easily recognized upon presentation from the features outlined in Box 37-2. Most patients report severe thunderclap headaches and have benign cerebrospinal fluid findings, characteristic brain imaging features, and vascular abnormalities that resolve over a few weeks. Many patients report trigger factors, such as orgasm, physical exertion, acute stressful or emotional situations, straining, coughing, sneezing, bathing, and swimming. The syndrome is known to occur in certain clinical settings (see Box 37-1). Individually, however, the clinical and imaging features carry a wide range of differential diagnoses.

Thunderclap headaches can signify a variety of ominous conditions, including aneurysmal subarachnoid hemorrhage, parenchymal hemorrhage, cerebral artery dissection, and cerebral venous sinus thrombosis.[40] These conditions are easily excluded with appropriate brain imaging. Patients with negative initial brain scan results are often subjected to a second imaging procedure to exclude these secondary conditions; however, the presence of *recurrent* thunderclap headaches is pathognomonic for RCVS. If imaging findings are negative and the patient does not prove to have vasoconstriction, primary headache disorders such as primary thunderclap headache, primary exertional headache, and orgasmic headache are usually considered.[64] In one study, 39% of patients presenting with thunderclap headache and normal brain MRI findings proved to have vasoconstriction on MRA, and those with and without vasoconstriction had similar clinical features, suggesting that RCVS and primary thunderclap headache belong to the same spectrum of disorders.[47]

Migraine is another consideration because a prior history of migraine is frequently elicited and because abnormal cerebral angiographic results have been documented in migraine.[65,66] Although there may be some overlap, RCVS appears distinct from migraine because, unlike migraine, it rarely (if ever) recurs, the nature of the headache is dissimilar, and the angiographic abnormalities persist for several weeks. Nevertheless, attribution of the severe headache and even the stroke to migraine is a common problem, frequently leading to inappropriate treatment with antimigraine agents such as sumatriptan, which can exacerbate vasoconstriction and stroke.[26,67]

Brain imaging demonstration of infarction or hemorrhage might raise consideration of the broad range of etiologies for stroke in young adults. The presence of thunderclap headache and cerebral vasoconstriction appropriately raises initial concern for a ruptured brain aneurysm.[36] The presence of cortical surface subarachnoid hemorrhage (which occurs in up to 22% of patients with RCVS) adds to the diagnostic dilemma.[36,49,50] However it should be noted that in patients with aneurysmal subarachnoid hemorrhage, cerebral "vasospasm" can be evident within hours and then reappear days or a week or so later. It is restricted to the artery surrounded by blood rather than affecting multiple distant arteries, and cerebral angiography does not reveal the alternating segments of arterial dilatation that give RCVS the characteristic "sausage on a string" appearance. Moreover, subarachnoid hemorrhage from ruptured aneurysms is usually deep-seated, for example, in the Sylvian fissure, rather than restricted to a few cortical sulci as in RCVS. In one study, features such as young age, prior headache disorder, depression, or chronic obstructive pulmonary disease, low Hunt-Hess grade, low Fisher SAH group, and the presence of diffuse, bilateral vasoconstriction, proved to be significant in distinguishing RCVS-associated subarachnoid hemorrhage from other causes of subarachnoid hemorrhage.[36]

Cerebral angiographic abnormalities can raise suspicion for cerebral arteriopathies such as intracranial atherosclerosis, infectious arteritis, vasculitis, and fibromuscular dysplasia. Detailed medical history and laboratory testing usually help distinguish these conditions from RCVS. The one condition that historically has been difficult to exclude is PACNS, because features such as headache, focal deficits, stroke, seizures, and angiographic irregularities are common to both conditions. An understandable presumptive diagnosis of "vasculitis" based on angiographic features alone may lead to the risks of brain biopsy and to the adverse effects of long-term immunosuppressive therapy. Delays of several days before such steps are taken should help distinguish RCVS, in which the initial clinical syndrome is typically more stable and even improving, from PACNS, in which clinical status may be worsening. Dramatic clinical presentations with explosive headaches, normal cerebrospinal fluid findings, and normal brain imaging strongly favor a diagnosis of RCVS. Furthermore, in patients with RCVS, there is often a history of associated cofactors to provide clues to the diagnosis, such as a temporal relationship with childbirth or incriminating drug exposure (see Box 37-1). Imaging clues that strongly favor a diagnosis of RCVS in the appropriate clinical setting are the absence of brain lesions on initial imaging and the presence of cortical surface subarachnoid hemorrhages, lobar hemorrhage, symmetrical "watershed" territory infarctions (usually high parietal), and bilateral edematous lesions.[33,46,48] Angiographic findings of smooth concentric narrowing and dilatation affecting multiple medium-sized intracerebral arteries and their branches ("string of beads" or "sausage on a string" appearance) is characteristic for RCVS, whereas "notched," irregular, and eccentric narrowing, presumably due to arterial inflammation, predicts PACNS.[34] Though rare exceptions exist,[68] the reversibility over days to weeks is the feature that best distinguishes this disorder from PACNS and other arteriopathies. The anxiety of awaiting reversal affects even the most experienced clinical teams.

ETIOLOGY AND PATHOPHYSIOLOGY

The etiology of the prolonged but reversible vasoconstriction, and the relationship between acute headache and vasoconstriction, is not known. Altered cerebral arterial tone due to abnormal vascular receptor activity or sensitivity appears critical; it may result from either a spontaneous or evoked central vascular discharge or a variety of exogenous or endogenous factors, including vasoconstrictive drugs and medications, female reproductive hormones, hypercalcemia, and others (see Box 37-1). The anatomic basis to explain both the vasoconstriction and the headache may be the dense innervation of cerebral blood vessels with sensory afferents from the first division of the trigeminal nerve and dorsal root of C2. At the molecular level, it is reasonable to postulate a role for the numerous immunologic and biochemical factors known to be involved in vasospasm associated with aneurysmal subarachnoid hemorrhage (catecholamines, endothelin-1, serotonin, nitric oxide, prostaglandins).[69] Serotonin is believed to play a central role in RCVS, on the basis of the association of the syndrome with serotonin-enhancing medications and tumors.[24,26,67] Some authorities have speculated that the vasoconstriction is related to transient vasculitis, but findings of histologic studies do not support a role for inflammation.[42]

MANAGEMENT

In the absence of controlled trials, management is guided by observational data and expert opinion. For patients who present with thunderclap headache but have not undergone vascular imaging, empiric therapy is not justified. Once cerebral vasoconstriction has been documented, however, treatment can be considered. The literature is replete with various treatment approaches invariably showing good outcome, probably reflecting strong publication biases. It is important to recognize that clinical and angiographic resolution occurs spontaneously, without any medical intervention, in approximately 90% of patients. However, since up to one-third can develop transient symptoms in the initial few days,[35] and since rare cases can develop a progressive clinical course, it is reasonable to admit patients for observation for the first few days after symptom onset.

Calcium channel blockers such as nimodipine and verapamil,[25] brief courses of glucocorticoids,[70] magnesium sulfate,[71] serotonin antagonists, and dantrolene[72] have been administered in an effort to relieve the vasoconstriction. Data from two prospective case series suggest that nimodipine does not affect the time course of cerebral vasoconstriction.[2,32] However, nimodipine might relieve the number and intensity of headaches, and it has documented effects on the smaller vasculature not easily imaged by angiography. These agents can be discontinued after resolution of symptoms or angiographic abnormalities.

Glucocorticoids are often administered to minimize the risk of delaying treatment in patients who may actually have PACNS, a condition that (as stated above) shares certain features with RCVS and which is believed to be progressive and potentially fatal without prompt immunosuppressive therapy. Unfortunately, many patients remain on glucocorticoids for prolonged durations and incur the risk of serious steroid-related adverse effects. In this author's opinion, empiric glucocorticoid therapy should be avoided for several reasons. First, several recent publications characterizing RCVS and PACNS have made it straightforward to distinguish these conditions in the acute setting.[1,2,73-76] Second, there is little evidence that a therapeutic delay by a few days would increase the risk for worse outcome in PACNS; even with diagnostically challenging cases, the diagnosis usually becomes apparent after a brief period of observation. Finally, glucocorticoids may be associated with worse outcome.[74] Bedside efforts should focus on distinguishing RCVS from PACNS on the basis of the initial clinical and imaging features, and reserve empiric glucocorticoid therapy for the rare patient with a rapidly worsening clinical course while the diagnosis remains uncertain.

Balloon angioplasty and direct intra-arterial administration of nicardipine, papaverine, milrinone, and nimodipine have been used with variable success.[77-79] In patients with RCVS, intra-arterial infusion of vasodilators into a single constricted artery can promptly reverse vasoconstricton in multiple brain arteries, including the contralateral arteries. A similar response has not been observed in RCVS mimics such as PACNS and intracranial atherosclerosis. On this basis, the demonstration of arterial dilatation using intra-arterial vasodilator infusions, has been proposed as a "diagnostic test" for RCVS.[80] In this author's opinion, intra-arterial interventions carry a risk for reperfusion injury and should be reserved for patients exhibiting clear signs of clinical progression,[42] particularly since over 90–95% of RCVS patients have a benign, self-limited syndrome despite the presence of severe angiographic vasoconstriction and ischemic or hemorrhagic brain lesions. Unfortunately, no known clinical or imaging features reliably predict disease progression.

Patients with severe angiographic abnormalities are often admitted to the intensive care unit for neurologic monitoring and blood pressure management. The goals of blood pressure control need careful consideration. Theoretically, pharmacologically induced hypertension can induce further cerebral vasoconstriction or result in brain hemorrhage, and in the setting of cerebral vasoconstriction, even mild hypotension can trigger ischemic stroke.[81] Acute seizures may warrant treatment; however, long-term seizure prophylaxis is probably unnecessary. It is logical to avoid further exposure to any potential precipitating factors, such as marijuana, cocaine, exercise stimulants, amphetamines, and other vasoconstrictive medications which can worsen the clinical course, as well as counsel patients about the possible risk of recurrence with re-exposure. There are no known genetic implications. The pain of RCVS-associated headache is extreme and frequently warrants round-the-clock use of opioid analgesics. Sumatriptan and the ergot derivatives are contraindicated because of their vasoconstrictive actions.[26,67] Patients should be counseled to avoid physical exertion, the Valsalva maneuver, and other known triggers of recurrent headaches for a few weeks. Usual stroke preventive medications, such as antiplatelets, anticoagulants, and cholesterol-lowering agents, are probably not indicated.

OUTCOME AND PROGNOSIS

Most patients with RCVS have complete resolution of headaches and angiographic abnormalities within days to weeks. Less than 15–20% of patients are left with residual deficits from stroke. Progressive vasoconstriction resulting in progressive symptoms[77] or death[41-44] can occur in rare cases. It should be noted that "reversibility" in the term RCVS refers to the dynamic and reversible nature of vasoconstriction; clinical deficits from brain damage might persist, and the vasoconstriction (particularly if severe and prolonged) may not fully reverse in some patients. Recurrence of an "episode" of RCVS is extremely rare.[82] Some patients go on to have intractable chronic migraine-like headaches or depression.

REFERENCES

1. Calabrese LH, Dodick DW, Schwedt TJ, et al. Narrative review: reversible cerebral vasoconstriction syndromes. Ann Intern Med 2007;146:34–44.
2. Ducros A, Boukobza M, Porcher R, et al. The clinical and radiological spectrum of reversible cerebral vasoconstriction syndrome. A prospective series of 67 patients. Brain 2007;130(Pt 12): 3091–101.
3. Serdaru M, Chiras J, Cujas M, et al. Isolated benign cerebral vasculitis or migrainous vasospasm? J Neurol Neurosurg Psychiatry 1984;47:73–6.
4. Jackson M, Lennox G, Jaspan T, et al. Migraine angiitis precipitated by sex headache and leading to watershed infarction. Cephalalgia 1993;13:427–30.

5. Day JW, Raskin NH. Thunderclap headache: symptom of unruptured cerebral aneurysm. Lancet 1986;2:1247–8.
6. Slivka A, Philbrook B. Clinical and angiographic features of thunderclap headache. Headache 1995;35:1–6.
7. Dodick DW, Brown RD Jr, Britton JW, et al. Nonaneurysmal thunderclap headache with diffuse, multifocal, segmental, and reversible vasospasm. Cephalalgia 1999;19:118–23.
8. Henry PY, Larre P, Aupy M, et al. Reversible cerebral arteriopathy associated with the administration of ergot derivatives. Cephalalgia 1984;4:171–8.
9. Raroque HG Jr, Tesfa G, Purdy P. Postpartum cerebral angiopathy. Is there a role for sympathomimetic drugs? Stroke 1993;24: 2108–10.
10. Call GK, Fleming MC, Sealfon S, et al. Reversible cerebral segmental vasoconstriction. Stroke 1988;19:1159–70.
11. Singhal AB, Caviness VS, Begleiter AF, et al. Cerebral vasoconstriction and stroke after use of serotonergic drugs. [see comment]. Neurology 2002;58(1):130–3.
12. Razavi M, Bendixen B, Maley JE, et al. CNS pseudovasculitis in a patient with pheochromocytoma. Neurology 1999;52(5): 1088–90.
13. Calabrese LH, Gragg LA, Furlan AJ. Benign angiopathy: a distinct subset of angiographically defined primary angiitis of the central nervous system. J Rheumatol 1993;20(12):2046–50.
14. Singhal AB. Cerebral vasoconstriction syndromes. Top Stroke Rehabil 2004;11(2):1–6.
15. Singhal AB. Cerebral vasoconstriction without subarachnoid blood: associated conditions, clinical and neuroimaging characteristics. Ann Neurol 2002;S:59–60.
16. Singhal AB, Bernstein RA. Postpartum angiopathy and other cerebral vasoconstriction syndromes. Neurocrit Care 2005;3(1): 91–7.
17. Fisher CM. Cerebral ischemia – less familiar types (review). Clin Neurosurg 1971;18:267–336.
18. Millikan CH, editor. Accidents vasculaires cerebraux chez les femmes agees de 15 a 45 ans. Maladies vasculaires cerebrales I Conference de la Salpetriere. Hospital de la Salpetriere, Paris: J-B Balliere; 1975.
19. Rascol A, Guiraud B, Manelfe C, et al., editors. Accidents vasculaires cerebraux de la grossesse et du post partum. II Conference de la Salpetriere sue les maladies vasculaires cerebrales. Hospital de la Salpetriere, Paris: JB Balliere; 1979.
20. Serdaru M, Chiras J, Cujas M, et al. Isolated benign cerebral vasculitis or migrainous vasospasm? J Neurol Neurosurg Psychiatry 1984;47(1):73–6.
21. Case records of the Massachusetts General Hospital. Weekly clinicopathological exercises. Case 35-1985. Abrupt onset of headache followed by rapidly progressive encephalopathy in a 30-year-old woman. New Eng J Med 1985;313(9):566–75.
22. Suwanwela C, Suwanwela N. Intracranial arterial narrowing and spasm in acute head injury. J Neurosurg 1972;36(3):314–23.
23. Yarnell PR, Caplan LR. Basilar artery narrowing and hyperparathyroidism: illustrative case. Stroke 1986;17(5):1022–4.
24. Noskin O, Jafarimojarrad E, Libman RB, et al. Diffuse cerebral vasoconstriction (Call-Fleming syndrome) and stroke associated with antidepressants. Neurology 2006;67(1):159–60.
25. Nowak DA, Rodiek SO, Henneken S, et al. Reversible segmental cerebral vasoconstriction (Call-Fleming syndrome): are calcium channel inhibitors a potential treatment option? Cephalalgia 2003;23(3):218–22.
26. Singhal AB, Caviness VS, Begleiter AF, et al. Cerebral vasoconstriction and stroke after use of serotonergic drugs. Neurology 2002; 58(1):130–3.
27. Snyder BD, McClelland RR. Isolated benign cerebral vasculitis. Arch Neurol 1978;35(9):612–14.
28. Bettoni L, Juvarra G, Bortone E, et al. Isolated benign cerebral vasculitis. Case report and review. Acta Neurol Belg 1984;84(4): 161–73.
29. van Calenbergh F, van den Bergh V, Wilms G. Benign isolated arteritis of the central nervous system. Clin Neurol Neurosurg 1986;88(4):267–73.
30. Hajj-Ali RA, Furlan A, Abou-Chebel A, et al. Benign angiopathy of the central nervous system: cohort of 16 patients with clinical course and long-term followup. Arthritis Rheum 2002;47(6): 662–9.
31. Hajj-Ali RA, Calabrese LH. Central nervous system vasculitis. Curr Opin Rheumatol 2009;21(1):10–18.
32. Chen SP, Fuh JL, Chang FC, et al. Transcranial color Doppler study for reversible cerebral vasoconstriction syndromes. Ann Neurol 2008;63(6):751–7.
33. Singhal AB, Hajj Ali R, Calabrese LH. Reversible cerebral vasoconstriction syndrome: two-center experience of 139 cases. Bangkok, Thailand: 19th World Congress of Neurology; 2009.
34. Fok JW, Nogueira RG, Singhal AB. Cerebral angiographic features can distinguish reversible cerebral vasoconstriction syndromes from primary angiitis of the CNS. Bangkok, Thailand: 19th World Congress of Neurology; 2009.
35. Katz BS, Fugate JE, Ameriso SF, et al. Clinical worsening in reversible cerebral vasoconstriction syndrome. JAMA Neurol 2014;71(1): 68–73.
36. Muehlschlegel S, Kursun O, Topcuoglu MA, et al. Differentiating reversible cerebral vasoconstriction syndrome with subarachnoid hemorrhage from other causes of subarachnoid hemorrhage. JAMA Neurol 2013;70(10):1254–60.
37. Fugate JE, Ameriso SF, Ortiz G, et al. Variable presentations of postpartum angiopathy. Stroke 2012;43(3):670–6.
38. Chen SP, Fuh JL, Wang SJ, et al. Magnetic resonance angiography in reversible cerebral vasoconstriction syndromes. Ann Neurol 2010;67(5):648–56.
39. Kirton A, Diggle J, Hu W, et al. A pediatric case of reversible segmental cerebral vasoconstriction. Can J Neurol Sci 2006;33(2): 250–3.
40. Schwedt TJ, Matharu MS, Dodick DW. Thunderclap headache. Lancet Neurol 2006;5(7):621–31.
41. Buckle RM, Du Boulay G, Smith B. Death due to cerebral vasospasm. J Neurol Neurosurg Psychiatry 1964;27:440–4.
42. Singhal AB, Kimberly WT, Schaefer PW, et al. Case records of the Massachusetts General Hospital. Case 8-2009. A 36-year-old woman with headache, hypertension, and seizure 2 weeks post partum. N Engl J Med 2009;360(11):1126–37.
43. Williams TL, Lukovits TG, Harris BT, et al. A fatal case of postpartum cerebral angiopathy with literature review. Arch Gynecol Obstet 2007;275(1):67–77.
44. Fugate JE, Wijdicks EF, Parisi JE, et al. Fulminant postpartum cerebral vasoconstriction syndrome. Arch Neurol 2012;69(1): 111–17.
45. Calado S, Vale-Santos J, Lima C, et al. Postpartum cerebral angiopathy: vasospasm, vasculitis or both? Cerebrovasc Dis 2004; 18(4):340–1.
46. Singhal AB, Topcuoglu MA, Caviness VS, et al. Call-Fleming syndrome versus isolated cerebral vasculitis: MRI lesion patterns. Stroke 2003;34:264.
47. Chen SP, Fuh JL, Lirng JF, et al. Recurrent primary thunderclap headache and benign CNS angiopathy: Spectra of the same disorder? Neurology 2006;67(12):2164–9.
48. Singhal AB. Brain hemorrhages in reversible cerebral vasoconstriction syndromes (RCVS). Neurology 2007;68(12 (Suppl. 1)):A221–2.
49. Edlow BL, Kasner SE, Hurst RW, et al. Reversible cerebral vasoconstriction syndrome associated with subarachnoid hemorrhage. Neurocrit Care 2007;7(3):203–10.
50. Moustafa RR, Allen CM, Baron JC. Call-Fleming syndrome associated with subarachnoid haemorrhage: three new cases. J Neurol Neurosurg Psychiatry 2008;79(5):602–5.
51. Singhal AB. Postpartum angiopathy with reversible posterior leukoencephalopathy. Arch Neurol 2004;61(3):411–16.
52. Kumar S, Goddeau RP Jr, Selim MH, et al. Atraumatic convexal subarachnoid hemorrhage: clinical presentation, imaging patterns, and etiologies. Neurology 2010;74(11):893–9.
53. Rico M, Benavente L, Para M, et al. Headache as a crucial symptom in the etiology of convexal subarachnoid hemorrhage. Headache 2014;54(3):545–50.
54. Mathon B, Ducros A, Bresson D, et al. Subarachnoid and intracerebral hemorrhage in young adults: Rare and underdiagnosed. Rev Neurol (Paris) 2014;170(2):110–18.
55. Santos E, Zhang Y, Wilkins A, et al. Reversible cerebral vasoconstriction syndrome presenting with haemorrhage. J Neurol Sci 2009;276(1-2):189–92.
56. Iancu-Gontard D, Oppenheim C, Touze E, et al. Evaluation of hyperintense vessels on FLAIR MRI for the diagnosis of multiple intracerebral arterial stenoses. Stroke 2003;34(8):1886–91.

57. Chen SP, Fuh JL, Lirng JF, et al. Hyperintense vessels on flair imaging in reversible cerebral vasoconstriction syndrome. Cephalalgia 2012;32(4):271–8.
58. Bartynski WS, Boardman JF. Catheter angiography, MR angiography, and MR perfusion in posterior reversible encephalopathy syndrome. AJNR Am J Neuroradiol 2008;29(3):447–55.
59. Arnold M, Camus-Jacqmin M, Stapf C, et al. Postpartum cervicocephalic artery dissection. Stroke 2008;39(8):2377–9.
60. Singhal AB. Thunderclap headache, reversible cerebral arterial vasoconstriction, and unruptured aneurysms. J Neurol Neurosurg Psychiatry 2002;73(1):96, author reply 96–7.
61. Mawet J, Boukobza M, Franc J, et al. Reversible cerebral vasoconstriction syndrome and cervical artery dissection in 20 patients. Neurology 2013;81(9):821–4.
62. Rothrock JF, Walicke P, Swenson MR, et al. Migrainous stroke. Arch Neurol 1988;45(1):63–7.
63. Bogousslavsky J, Despland PA, Regli F, et al. Postpartum cerebral angiopathy: reversible vasoconstriction assessed by transcranial Doppler ultrasounds. Eur Neurol 1989;29(2):102–5.
64. The International Classification of Headache Disorders. ed 2. Cephalalgia 2004;24(Suppl. 1):9–160.
65. Masuzawa T, Shinoda S, Furuse M, et al. Cerebral angiographic changes on serial examination of a patient with migraine. Neuroradiology 1983;24(5):277–81.
66. Sanin LC, Mathew NT. Severe diffuse intracranial vasospasm as a cause of extensive migrainous cerebral infarction.[see comment]. Cephalalgia 1993;13(4):289–92.
67. Meschia JF, Malkoff MD, Biller J. Reversible segmental cerebral arterial vasospasm and cerebral infarction: possible association with excessive use of sumatriptan and Midrin. Arch Neurol 1998; 55(5):712–14.
68. Calado S, Vale-Santos J, Lima C, et al. Postpartum cerebral angiopathy: vasospasm, vasculitis or both? Cerebrovasc Dis 2004; 18(4):340–1.
69. Dietrich HH, Dacey RG Jr. Molecular keys to the problems of cerebral vasospasm. Neurosurgery 2000;46(3):517–30.
70. Hajj-Ali RA, Furlan A, Abou-Chebel A, et al. Benign angiopathy of the central nervous system: cohort of 16 patients with clinical course and long-term followup. Arthritis Rheum 2002;47(6): 662–9.
71. Singhal AB. Postpartum angiopathy with reversible posterior leukoencephalopathy. Arch Neurol 2004;61(3):411–16.
72. Muehlschlegel S, Rordorf G, Bodock M, et al. Dantrolene mediates vasorelaxation in cerebral vasoconstriction: a case series. Neurocrit Care 2009;10(1):116–21.
73. Singhal AB. Diagnostic challenges in RCVS, PACNS, and other cerebral arteriopathies. Cephalalgia 2011;31(10):1067–70.
74. Singhal AB, Hajj-Ali RA, Topcuoglu MA, et al. Reversible cerebral vasoconstriction syndromes: analysis of 139 cases. Arch Neurol 2011;68(8):1005–12.
75. Hajj-Ali RA, Singhal AB, Benseler S, et al. Primary angiitis of the CNS. Lancet Neurol 2011;10(6):561–72.
76. Ducros A. L37. Reversible cerebral vasoconstriction syndrome: distinction from CNS vasculitis. Presse Med 2013;42(4 Pt 2): 602–4.
77. Ringer AJ, Qureshi AI, Kim SH, et al. Angioplasty for cerebral vasospasm from eclampsia. Surg Neurol 2001;56(6):373–8, discussion 8–9.
78. Song JK, Fisher S, Seifert TD, et al. Postpartum cerebral angiopathy: atypical features and treatment with intracranial balloon angioplasty. Neuroradiology 2004;46(12):1022–6.
79. Bouchard M, Verreault S, Gariepy JL, et al. Intra-arterial milrinone for reversible cerebral vasoconstriction syndrome. Headache 2008.
80. Linn J, Fesl G, Ottomeyer C, et al. Intra-arterial application of nimodipine in reversible cerebral vasoconstriction syndrome: A diagnostic tool in select cases? Cephalalgia 2011.
81. Rosenbloom MH, Singhal AB. CT angiography and diffusion-perfusion MR imaging in a patient with ipsilateral reversible cerebral vasoconstriction after carotid endarterectomy. AJNR Am J Neuroradiol 2007;28(5):920–2.
82. Ursell MR, Marras CL, Farb R, et al. Recurrent intracranial hemorrhage due to postpartum cerebral angiopathy: implications for management. Stroke 1998;29(9):1995–8.

38 Hypertensive Encephalopathy

Catherine Lamy, Jean-Louis Mas

KEY POINTS

- Hypertensive encephalopathy is characterized by elevated blood pressure associated with headache, seizures, altered mental status, and visual disturbances.
- Neuroimaging typically reveals a reversible vasogenic edema involving parietooccipital regions.
- Prompt diagnosis is important to avoid unnecessary evaluation and obtain prompt control of blood pressure.
- A similar clinicoradiological syndrome, posterior reversible encephalopathy syndrome (PRES), has been described in numerous medical conditions, including eclampsia and immunosuppressive treatments.

The term *hypertensive encephalopathy* was introduced by Oppenheimer and Fishberg[1] in 1928 to designate a constellation of neurologic symptoms that punctuated the course of severe hypertension. Hypertensive encephalopathy is currently defined as an acute syndrome characterized by elevated blood pressure associated with rapidly progressive signs and symptoms, including headache, seizures, altered mental status, visual disturbances, and other focal or diffuse neurologic signs.[1-3] Neuroimaging typically reveals a reversible vasogenic edema involving parietooccipital regions in a relatively symmetrical pattern.[4-7] Its pathogenesis is still incompletely understood, although it seems to be related to breakthrough of autoregulation, leading to cerebral edema. Recognition is important to avoid unnecessary evaluation and orient treatment toward prompt control of blood pressure. In contrast, when unrecognized, conversion to irreversible cytotoxic edema may occur.

PATHOGENESIS

The brain is protected from extremes of blood pressure by an autoregulation system that ensures constant perfusion over a wide range of systemic pressures (Fig. 38-1). Under normal circumstances, brain vessels possess intrinsic vascular tone. In response to systemic hypotension, cerebral arterioles dilate to maintain adequate perfusion, whereas vessels constrict in response to high pressure.[7,8] The basic mechanism of autoregulation of cerebral blood flow is still controversial. The autoregulatory vessel caliber changes are most likely mediated by an interplay between myogenic and metabolic mechanisms. The endothelium plays a central role in blood pressure homeostasis by secreting relaxing factors such as nitric oxide and vasoconstriction factors (thromboxane A_2 and endothelin). In normotensive individuals, cerebral blood flow remains unchanged between mean blood pressures of approximately 60 mm Hg and 150 mm Hg.[9-11] At pressures above the upper limit of autoregulation, hypertensive encephalopathy may occur. Conversely, when cerebral perfusion pressure decreases below the lower limit of autoregulation, cerebral blood flow decreases and cerebral ischemia occurs. There may be differences between individuals in the degree of hypertension that can give rise to autoregulatory dysfunction leading to encephalopathy as well as differences within a single person over time, depending on comorbid factors. The degree of hypertension required to induce encephalopathy depends on the baseline pressure.[8] Rapidly developing, fluctuating, or intermittent hypertension carries a particular risk for hypertensive encephalopathy. Long-standing hypertension causes a shift of the cerebral blood flow curve to the right, presumably owing to structural changes (vascular hypertrophy and inward remodeling) and diminished responsiveness of resistance vessels. Therefore, sudden elevations to relatively higher blood pressures are required to produce hypertensive encephalopathy in a patient with chronic hypertension than in a normotensive person.[8] In children and young adults, the curve may shift to the left, leaving them more at risk for the development of hypertensive encephalopathy.[2]

Over the previous century, two theories were advanced to explain the pathogenesis of hypertensive encephalopathy. The earlier theory postulated that hypertensive encephalopathy results from intense cerebral autoregulatory vasoconstriction in response to acute hypertension, resulting in decreased cerebral blood flow, ischemia, and subsequent edema involving mainly the borderzone arterial regions.[2,9]

The current popular theory implicates forced vasodilatation of cerebral vessels (autoregulation breakthrough) rather than vasoconstriction as the major component of hypertensive encephalopathy that results in the extravasation of fluid into the interstitium, termed vasogenic edema. In fact, patterns of cerebral blood flow with acute hypertension may be complex with both low-flow and high-flow areas coexisting in adjacent cortical regions. The concept of breakthrough of autoregulation has been initially characterized as a passive phenomenon, as the autoregulatory capacity of vessels is exceeded and the vessels dilate passively. Later evidence suggests that breakthrough of autoregulation may be an active process initiated by calcium-dependent potassium channels. This process generates reactive oxygen species and an active increase in permeability of the blood–brain barrier as well as an increase in vesicular transport, rather than disruption of tight junctions.[12] Abnormalities in vasoactive factors released by the endothelium may contribute to the pathophysiology of hypertensive encephalopathy. Ultimately, loss of endothelial fibrinolytic activity, activation of coagulation and platelets, and degranulation of damaged endothelium may promote further inflammation, thrombosis, and vasoconstriction.[11]

The preferential distribution of white matter lesions in posterior brain regions is recognized but not fully understood. One likely explanation involves the regional heterogeneity of the sympathetic innervation.[13] It is known that anterior cerebral circulation is richly innervated by sympathetic nerves from the superior cervical ganglion, in contrast to the vertebrobasilar vessels, which are relatively devoid of sympathetic innervation.[14] It is possible that sympathetically mediated

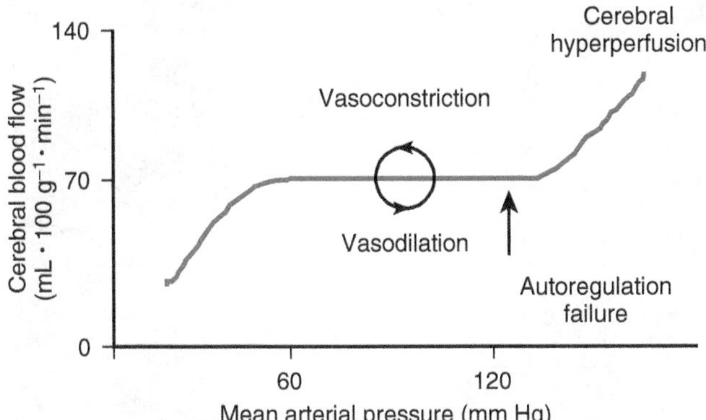

Figure 38-1. Autoregulation of cerebral blood flow

vasoconstriction protects the anterior circulation from overperfusion in acute hypertension.[13]

PATHOLOGIC FEATURES

The neuropathologic findings of hypertensive encephalopathy as shown in autopsy studies[15,16] consist of varying degrees of vascular alterations (fibrinoid necrosis of arterioles, thrombosis of arterioles and capillaries), and of parenchymal lesions (microinfarcts, petechial hemorrhages, cerebral edema). Ring hemorrhage around a thrombosed precapillary constitutes the classic microscopic lesion. If hypertensive encephalopathy develops in a patient with long-standing hypertension, a variety of additional hypertensive cerebrovascular changes may be found, including medial atrophy, hyperplasia, hyalinization, and microaneurysms.

The lesions are most often multiple and bilateral, being most prominent in the deep white matter and at the gray–white junction in the watershed and posterior areas; the brainstem is usually severely affected.[15] They may also be present in the basal ganglia, diencephalon, and cerebral cortex. Their extent and severity vary but are generally correlated with the severity of neurologic manifestations and blood pressure, especially during the terminal stage. Brain swelling, occasionally sufficient to cause herniation of cerebellar tonsils through the foramen magnum, has been documented. The vascular changes are not confined to the brain and may also affect the eyes (retinal hemorrhages, papilledema), kidneys (fibrinoid arteriolar lesions of glomeruli), and other organs.[15] These findings, however, may not be representative of those in surviving patients, instead representing the extreme of a spectrum of abnormalities. A brain biopsy performed in one patient with hypertensive encephalopathy has been reported to demonstrate white matter edema with no evidence of vessel wall damage or infarction, consistent with MRI findings of vasogenic edema; the patient made a full neurologic recovery, and follow-up MRI revealed complete resolution of lesions.[17]

CLINICAL FEATURES

The classic clinical manifestations of hypertensive encephalopathy include severe headache, nausea and vomiting, mental abnormalities including confusion and diminished spontaneity, seizures, and speech and visual disturbances.[2,3,6,15] Alterations in consciousness occur and range in severity from mild somnolence to frank confusion, stupor, or coma, in extreme cases. Temporary restlessness and agitation may alternate with lethargy. The mental functions are slowed; memory and the ability to concentrate are impaired, although severe amnesia is unusual. Abnormalities of visual perception are nearly always detectable. Patients often report blurred vision. Hemianopia, visual neglect, visual hallucinations,[18] and frank cortical blindness may occur. Papilledema may be present with flame-shaped retinal hemorrhages and exudates,[2] but normal ocular fundus findings do not exclude a diagnosis of hypertensive encephalopathy. The tendon reflexes are often brisk, and some patients have weakness and incoordination. Occasionally, focal neurologic signs may be noted. Paraparesis and signs of brainstem or cerebellar dysfunction have been reported.[19,20] Seizures are frequently reported; they can be generalized, tonic-clonic or partial.[6,21,22] Patients may have multiple seizures or status epilepticus.[6,23]

The onset is usually subacute, with symptoms developing over 24 to 48 hours, but may be heralded by a seizure.[21] The electroencephalogram may show focal sharp waves, slowing, or normal findings.[6] Examination of the cerebrospinal fluid in patients with hypertensive encephalopathy has revealed elevated pressure,[3] mild pleocytosis, and elevated protein concentration.[6]

The clinical presentation of hypertensive encephalopathy is often non-specific.[6] The differential diagnosis includes various neurologic conditions, such as stroke, venous thrombosis, and encephalitis, all of which can mimic hypertensive encephalopathy, and transient elevations of blood pressure may be the consequence of cerebral lesions. In cases with sudden onset of neurologic deficits, the clinical presentation may be indistinguishable from bilateral posterior cerebral artery territory infarct.[4] Therefore, patients with hypertension and altered neurologic status represent a difficult diagnosis problem, and hypertensive encephalopathy should remain a diagnosis of exclusion.

NEURORADIOLOGIC FEATURES

Conventional Imaging

The most characteristic imaging pattern in hypertensive encephalopathy is the presence of edema involving the white matter of the posterior portions of both cerebral hemispheres, especially the parietooccipital regions (Fig. 38-2), in a relatively symmetric pattern.[4-7] The calcarine and paramedian occipital lobe structures are usually spared, a feature that could help distinguish hypertensive encephalopathy from bilateral infarction in the posterior cerebral artery territory.[4] Other regions of the brain are also frequently affected, including the frontal and temporal lobes, and cerebellar hemispheres.[24] Although the abnormalities affect primarily the subcortical white matter, the cortex and the basal ganglia may also be involved. A tendency for the milder cases to have a greater involvement of gray than white matter has been reported, suggesting that the edema may originate in the cortex.[25] Lesion confluence may develop as the extent of the edema increases. The basic pattern of hypertensive encephalopathy resembles the brain watershed zones, with the cortex and subcortical and deep white matter involved to varying degrees.[26] Isolated or predominant posterior fossa lesions (Fig. 38-3) are less often reported.[19,27,28] In some rare cases, the posterior fossa lesions are severe enough to cause hydrocephalus.[29-31] Spinal cord involvement has been reported.[20]

The abnormalities are often apparent on CT scan but are best depicted by MRI.[4,6,7] The most commonly observed abnormalities on MRI are punctate or confluent areas of increased foci on proton density and T2-weighted images. Fluid-attenuated inversion recovery (FLAIR) sequences improve the ability to detect subtle peripheral lesions and have showed cortical lesions to be more common than previously thought.[25] Gradient-echo imaging may reveal petechial hemorrhages. Mild or large hematomas and subarachnoid

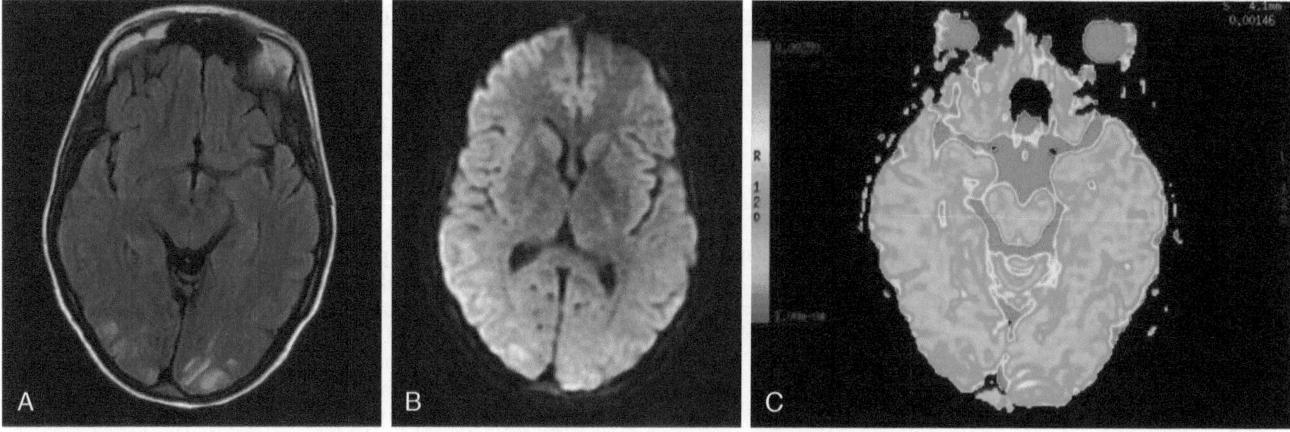

Figure 38-2. Eclampsia in a 28-year-old woman, who had severe headaches, generalized seizures, and blurred vision, and complete clinical recovery after delivery. A, Axial fluid-attenuated inversion recovery (FLAIR) MR image showing bilateral high signal in the occipital regions. B, Diffusion-weighted MR image with normal signal in the occipital regions. C, ADC (apparent diffusion coefficient) MRI map showing increased ADC in the posterior regions.

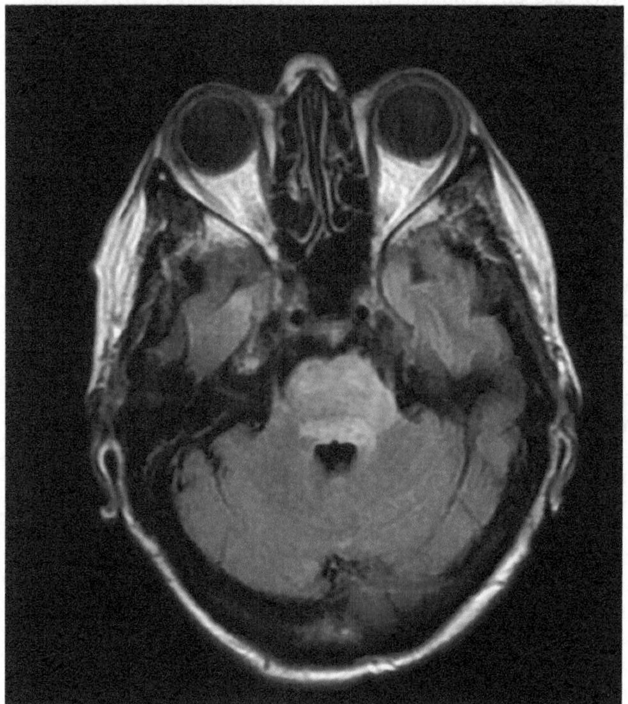

Figure 38-3. Hypertensive encephalopathy in a 52-year-old man. The patient presented with headache, nausea, and unsteady gait. He was drowsy and dysarthric. His blood pressure was 230 mm Hg systolic/150 mm Hg diastolic. This axial fluid-attenuated inversion recovery (FLAIR) MR image shows an extensive increased signal in the brainstem. After blood pressure was controlled, neurologic symptoms improved over days. MRI control 7 weeks later showed complete resolution of abnormalities.

hemorrhage have also been described.[7,32] Signal enhancement, due to disruption of the blood–brain barrier, asymmetric and unilateral lesions have been reported, sometimes making the diagnosis of hypertensive encephalopathy challenging.[25,33]

In most patients, imaging abnormalities are regressive after appropriate therapy, suggesting transient edema rather than true infarction.[4] Follow-up MR studies may be key in the diagnosis because initial differentiation between a reversible and permanent parenchymal lesion is not possible on the basis of conventional MR imaging or CT scan. The ideal timing of repeated brain imaging to document recovery is unclear. Resolution of neuroimaging abnormalities probably occurs in the range of several days to weeks. Recurrent episodes of hypertensive encephalopathy have been occasionally reported.[34]

Other Magnetic Resonance Imaging Sequences

Diffusion-weighted MRI sequences show increased apparent diffusion coefficient (ADC) in the involved brain regions consistent with vasogenic edema in the majority of cases (Fig. 38-2), with a predominant watershed distribution. These areas with increased ADC values may appear hyperintense, hypointense, or isointense on diffusion-weighted imaging (DWI), depending on the amount of the "T2 shine-through" effect. Interpretation of diffusion-weighted MR images alone, without the benefit of quantitative diffusion information, may underestimate the extension of lesions.[35,36] ADC values provide a wealth of prognostic information. Lesions with high ADC values are most often reversible, whereas those with decreased ADC values usually progress to true infarction.[6,35-38] The extent of signal changes on T2-weighted MRI and DWI and of ADC values seem to correlate well with patient outcome and can help guide more aggressive treatment in more severely affected patients.

Both single-photon emission CT[7] and perfusion-weighted MRI[39] have shown preserved or increased perfusion to edematous portions of the brain in patients with hypertensive encephalopathy. These data support the hypothesis that the condition begins with hyperperfusion, resulting in failure of autoregulation and breakthrough accumulation of vasogenic edema. Further perfusion-weighted imaging is needed to clarify the precise evolution of lesions in hypertensive encephalopathy. A few cases of patients with eclampsia examined with proton magnetic resonance spectroscopy imaging have been reported.[40] Widespread metabolic abnormalities, consisting of increased choline and creatinine levels and mildly decreased N-acetylaspartate, occurred in regions with both normal and abnormal MRI appearances. These findings suggest a diffuse metabolic defect, possibly consistent with microglial activation and neuronal dysfunction. Metabolite levels may return to normal.[41] However, an abnormal metabolite ratio may persist[40]

Diffuse vasoconstriction, focal vasoconstriction, vasodilatation, and even string of beads appearance, consistent with

BOX 38-1 Main Causes and Contributing Factors of Posterior Reversible Encephalopathy Syndrome

HYPERTENSIVE ENCEPHALOPATHY

Acute or chronic renal diseases
Vasculitis
- Systemic lupus erythematosus
- Polyarteritis nodosa
- Wegener's

Endocrine disorders
- Pheochromocytoma
- Primary aldosteronism

Porphyria
Thermal injury
Scorpion envenomation
Cocaine or amphetamine abusers
Over-the-counter stimulants
- Phenylpropanolamine
- Hydrochloride
- Ephedrine
- Pseudoephedrine
- Caffeine

ECLAMPSIA

Carotid dissection
Hyperperfusion syndrome
Thrombotic thrombocytopenic purpura
Hemolytic and uremic syndrome
Guillain–Barré syndrome
Triple-H therapy

IMMUNOSUPPRESSIVE DRUGS

- Cyclosporin A
- Tacrolimus
- Sirolimus
- Vincristine
- Cisplatin
- Cytarabine
- L-asparaginase
- Gemcitabine
- Bortezomib
- Bevacizumab
- Intrathecal chemotherapy
- Combination chemotherapy

OTHER DRUGS

- Interferon-α
- TNF-antagonist
- Immunotherapy with interleukin
- Antiretroviral therapy in HIV-infected patients
- Erythropoietin
- Granulocyte stimulating factor
- Intravenous immunoglobulin

OTHER CONDITIONS OR ASSOCIATIONS

Reversible cerebral vasoconstriction syndrome
Infection/sepsis/shock
Blood transfusion
Tumor lysis syndrome
Cholesterol embolism syndrome
Hypomagnesemia
Hypercalcemia
Hypocholesterolemia

vasospasm, have been demonstrated at catheter or MR angiography in patients with eclampsia and preeclampsia.[42–44] Results of follow-up MRA demonstrated reversibility of this vasculopathy.[7]

These imaging features are close to those of reversible cerebral vasoconstriction syndrome (RCVS), which has been associated with various conditions such as the postpartum or exposure to various vasoactive substances.[45] Vasospasm may be a more common finding in hypertensive encephalopathy than previously thought. Small- or medium-sized arterial narrowing might escape detection with magnetic resonance angiography. Timing of vascular imaging might explain that vasospasm escapes detection, since vasoconstriction is not always present at the onset of symptoms, can begin abruptly, fluctuate or resolve within days.[46]

Clinical features such as abrupt onset, severe headaches, confusion, seizures, and visual deficits are common in patients with RCVS and with hypertensive encephalopathy. The topographic features of ischemic strokes that occasionally complicate hypertensive encephalopathy are similar to those of strokes associated with RCVS.[46] Finally, brain lesions consistent with reversible vasogenic edema have been described in patients with RCVS.[45,47]

CAUSES

Hypertensive Encephalopathy

Hypertensive encephalopathy occurs as a result of a sudden, sustained rise in blood pressure, from any cause, sufficient to exceed the upper limit of cerebral blood flow autoregulation. As would be predicted from the physiology of autoregulation (see above), the degree of hypertension required to precipitate encephalopathy depends on the premorbid pressure. Previously normotensive individuals can show signs of encephalopathy at blood pressures as low as 160 mm Hg systolic, 100 mm Hg diastolic (160/100 mm Hg).[11] The condition may occur at any age but is most common in the 2nd to 4th decades of life.

It is estimated that about 1% of patients with hypertension will, at some point, develop a hypertensive crisis (defined as a systolic BP of 180 mmHg or greater or a diastolic BP of 110 mmHg or greater). Hypertensive crisis can be further classified as a hypertensive urgency or hypertensive emergency depending on end-organ involvement including cardiovascular, renal, and neurologic injury (i.e., hypertensive encephalopathy). Hypertensive emergencies represent approximately 25% of hypertensive crises and require immediate BP reduction (not necessarily to normal levels) to prevent or limit target organ damage.[48,49]

Antihypertensive treatment has markedly reduced the incidence of hypertensive encephalopathy in individuals with known hypertension. However, abrupt elevations of blood pressure (characteristically above 220/110 mm Hg) in patients with chronic hypertension who are receiving either no treatment or insufficient treatment or in patients whose treatment has been discontinued may cause hypertensive encephalopathy.

Acute or chronic renal disease (acute glomerulonephritis, renovascular disease, renal infarction,[50] renal failure[51]) is the most common cause (Box 38-1) of hypertensive encephalopathy.[11] Whether the greater tendency toward development of hypertensive encephalopathy in patients with renal hypertension than in those with essential hypertension is related to increased circulating permeability factors or to endothelial damage remains to be determined.

Other clinical situations associated with hypertensive encephalopathy include autoimmune disorders,[22] endocrine disorders (pheochromocytoma[28], primary aldosteronism, Cushing's syndrome, renin-secreting tumors), porphyria,[52] thermal injury,[53] head injuries and central nervous system (CNS) trauma, autonomic hyperactivity (Guillain–Barré syndrome),[54] scorpion envenomation,[55] cocaine or amphetamine abuse,[56] interactions with monoamine oxidase inhibitors (tyramine), triple-H therapy for symptomatic subarachnoid hemorrhage-related vasospasm[57] and use of over-the-counter stimulants[58] (phenylpropanolamine hydrochloride, ephedrine, pseudoephedrine, caffeine).

Eclampsia

Eclampsia has been considered a form of hypertensive encephalopathy on the basis of similarities in clinical, radiologic, and pathologic features.[16,59,60] The fluid accumulation often observed during pregnancy may accentuate the tendency for brain edema to develop. However, several findings suggest that eclampsia is more than hypertensive encephalopathy. There is not always a good correlation between symptoms and signs of eclampsia and level of blood pressure and blood pressure is reported as only minimally elevated in 23% of patients.[61] Several findings suggest that vascular endothelial damage may play a role in preeclampsia/eclampsia.[61,62] Preeclampsia/eclampsia is a multisystem disorder characterized by abnormal vascular response to placentation that is associated with increased systemic vascular resistance, enhanced platelet aggregation, activation of the coagulation system, and endothelial cell dysfunction.[63] Production of placental anti-angiogenic factors, specifically soluble fms-related tyrosine kinase 1 and soluble endoglin, have been shown to be upregulated in preeclampsia. These placental anti-angiogenic factors are released into the maternal circulation; their actions disrupt the maternal endothelium and result in hypertension, proteinuria, and the other systemic manifestations of preeclampsia/eclampsia.[64] Generalized endothelial dysfunction may lead to increased sensitivity to normally circulating pressor agents and impaired synthesis of vasoactive compounds, which may result in vasospasm and reduced organ perfusion; platelet activation with transitory platelet-rich microvascular occlusion; activation of the coagulation cascade, and loss of fluid from the intravascular compartment.[65]

The classic clinical presentation of eclampsia consists of epileptic seizures or coma manifesting during the third trimester or early puerperium in women who already have the preeclamptic symptom triad of edema, proteinuria, and hypertension. However, hypertension or proteinuria may be absent in 10–15% of women who develop HELLP syndrome (hemolysis, elevated liver enzymes, or low platelet counts) and in 38% of those who develop eclampsia.[63] It has been reported that a substantial subset of women diagnosed with late postpartum eclampsia had not been identified as pre-eclamptic before seizure onset. It remained unclear whether this represented a true variant of the clinical presentation of eclampsia or merely reflected decreased caretaker attention towards pre-eclamptic signs in the postpartum period.[66]

A recent systematic study and meta-analysis has shown that women who have had pre-eclampsia have an increased risk of cardiovascular disease, including an almost fourfold increased risk of hypertension and an approximately twofold increased risk of fatal and non-fatal ischemic heart disease, stroke, and venous thromboembolism in later life.[67] The mechanism underlying this association remains to be defined. Whether these long-term observations are due to persistent and subtle endothelial damage as a result of pre-eclampsia remains unknown.[68]

Posterior Reversible Encephalopathy Syndrome

Hinchey and colleagues[4] reported on 15 patients with a reversible syndrome of headaches, altered mental status, seizures, and visual loss, associated with posterior white matter changes on neuroimaging, that they termed reversible posterior leukoencephalopathy syndrome. Four of the 15 reported patients had hypertensive encephalopathy, three had eclampsia, seven were receiving immunosuppressive therapy (cyclosporine or tacrolimus) after transplantation or as treatment for aplastic anemia, and one was receiving interferon-alpha for melanoma. Most of the patients had an abrupt increase in blood pressure, but three of 15 were normotensive. Since the initial description,[4] there has been some controversy about what should be the proper term for this syndrome and whether it truly represents a leukoencephalopathy. Because MRI has shown that lesions can occur in both gray and white matter, a new name, posterior reversible encephalopathy syndrome (PRES), was coined.[27]

Initially reported in adults, PRES has been subsequently described in children.[69] An increasing number of medical conditions associated with PRES have been reported[6,9,70] (Box 38-1). Most are chemotherapeutic agents, immunosuppressive or cytotoxic treatments, or autoimmune diseases.[6,22,70] PRES may be associated with infection and sepsis, particularly in relation to Gram-positive infections.[22,71]

Although most patients with these conditions had moderate-to-severe hypertension, blood pressure levels were usually lower than those typically encountered with pure hypertensive encephalopathy. Hypertension may therefore be the sole cause leading to PRES or may act as a contributory factor.

The correlation between clinical features, location of imaging abnormalities, and causes has not been elucidated.[70] For example, whether predominant cerebellar or brainstem involvement is more frequent in hypertensive encephalopathy than in other causes of PRES remains to be determined.[6,19]

Hyponatremia, hypomagnesemia, hypercalcemia, renal or hepatic dysfunction may also be contributing factors.[4,6,26] Urinary magnesium wasting, due to glomerular or tubular dysfunction, occurs in patients with eclampsia, and in those treated by cyclosporin and tacrolimus. In some cases, symptoms resolved with adequate magnesium replacement.[72] Hypomagnesemia could promote vasoconstriction but the precise mechanism by which it contributes to PRES is unclear. Close serum magnesium level monitoring has been recommended in patients receiving tacrolimus or cyclosporin in order to prevent neurotoxicity.

Immunosuppressive and cytotoxic drugs can damage the blood–brain barrier by various means: direct toxic effects on the vascular endothelium, endothelial dysfunction secondary to the vascular endothelial growth factor inhibition, vasoconstriction caused by release of endothelin, increases in thromboxane and prostacyclin causing microthrombi.[4,9]

The additional role of seizures has been suggested. Seizures can result in elevations of blood pressure, regional hyperperfusion breakdown of the blood–brain barrier and vasogenic edema.

Failure of the autoregulatory capabilities of the cerebral vessels, itself resulting from various mechanisms, including hypertension and endothelial dysfunction, may represent a common pathophysiologic mechanism leading to this syndrome. Immunosuppressive drugs can damage the blood–brain barrier by various means: direct toxic effects on the vascular endothelium, endothelial dysfunction secondary to the vascular endothelial growth factor (VEGF) inhibition, vasoconstriction caused by release of endothelin, and increases in thromboxane and prostacyclin causing microthrombi.[4,26]

Infection, shock, or severe metabolic abnormalities (e.g., hyponatremia, hypomagnesemia, hypercalcemia, renal or hepatic dysfunction) may also be contributing factors.[4,6,26]

TREATMENT

Failure to recognize the syndrome and correct the underlying cause as well as the associated metabolic abnormalities may result in irreversible brain injury. Hypertensive encephalopathy belongs to hypertensive emergencies which are defined as situations that require immediate blood pressure reduction (not necessarily to normal ranges) to prevent or limit target organ damage. As there have been no large clinical trials, treatment of hypertensive encephalopathy is dictated by consensus.[11]

Most experts recommend that mean arterial blood pressure should not be lowered by more than 20% during the first hour, with a target diastolic blood pressure of 100 to 110 mm Hg.[10] If possible, patients should be admitted to an intensive care unit, and the blood pressure lowered under constant monitoring. Intravenous administration of antihypertensive drugs is generally preferred. Excessive falls in pressure must be avoided, particularly in the elderly patient and the patient with preexisting hypertension, because they may precipitate renal, cerebral, or coronary ischemia. Although not evidence-based, the use of anticonvulsants in patients with hypertensive encephalopathy who are having seizures is reasonable.[10,11]

Suitable agents in the management of hypertensive encephalopathy must satisfy a number of criteria, as follows: are usable by intravenous injection, have rapid onset of action, and are easily titrated with a short half-life allowing more flexible use. The drugs proposed include nicardipine, urapidil, labetalol, and sodium nitroprusside.[10,11,73] There is insufficient evidence from randomized controlled trials to determine which drug or drug class is most effective in reducing mortality and morbidity.[74]

Nicardipine is a second-generation calcium channel antagonist. It is an arterial vasodilator with no negative inotropic activity. The onset of action of intravenous nicardipine is 5–15 minutes from administration with the duration of action being 4–6 hours. Nicardipine has been demonstrated to increase coronary blood flow with favorable effect on myocardial oxygen balance. As a result of its rapid onset of action, its ease of use (dosage independent of body weight), and its demonstrated efficacy, nicardipine has become the first-line treatment for hypertensive emergencies.[10,73]

Labetalol has both α-blocking and β-blocking activity, with a recognized value in the majority of hypertensive emergencies except for acute heart failure. The β-blocking effect of labetalol is about one-fifth that of propranolol. The hypotensive effect of labetalol begins within 2–5 minutes, reaching a peak at 5–15 minutes after administration and lasting for about 2–4 hours. It has the advantage of maintaining cardiac output and cerebral and coronary blood flow, and it is associated with good clinical safety, provided that the usual contraindications to β-blockers are observed. Adverse effects include nausea, vomiting, and flushing. Bradycardia, heart block, bronchospasm, and heart failure can also complicate its use.[10,11,73]

Urapidil is a peripheral A1 postsynaptic receptor antagonist as well as a central 5-hydroxytryptamine 1A receptor agonist. Its vasodilatory action is not accompanied by reflex tachycardia or any significant modification of the renin–angiotensin system. Urapidil decreases both cardiac preload and afterload and also induces selective pulmonary and renal vasodilatation. It has a good safety profile; its single contraindication is aortic stenosis.[10] Sodium nitroprusside is a short-acting arterial and venous dilatator that induces a simultaneous reduction in cardiac preload and afterload, making it useful in the treatment of hypertensive crises accompanied by heart failure. It should be given only by continuous intravenous infusion (0.25–2 μg/kg/min). However, several of the following factors limit its use. First, by increasing intracranial pressure, nitroprusside decreases the cerebral flow rate. Second, it is common for blood pressure to be unintentionally below a safe target level during treatment. Third, nitroprusside promotes baroreflex activation, causing tachycardia that can exacerbate acute coronary syndromes and heart failure. Other complications include cyanate or thiocyanate toxicity when the drug is given for a long period (days), especially in patients with hepatic or renal dysfunction. Finally, nitroprusside infusion requires intra-arterial monitoring of blood pressure, which may not otherwise be required. It is now less widely used as first-line treatment because of its adverse effects and the availability of other drugs that are easier to use.[10,11,73]

Other parenteral drugs used for hypertensive emergencies include fenoldopam, a selective postsynaptic dopamine-1 receptor agonist. Reported side effects of fenoldopam include headache, flushing, and increased intraocular pressure. Enalaprilat is an angiotensin-converting enzyme inhibitor available for intravenous administration. Its onset of action is delayed for 15 minutes, and it does not reach peak effect for about 1 hour. The relative slow onset limits its use in hypertensive encephalopathy. In addition, angiotensin-converting enzyme inhibitors should be used cautiously in patients who are hypovolemic or in those with underlying renal artery stenosis, because these drugs can lead to precipitous falls in blood pressure. Intravenous hydralazine is a commonly administered arteriolar vasodilator that is effective for hypertensive emergencies associated with pregnancies. The most common adverse effect of hydralazine administration is unpredictable hypotension.[75] Phentolamine, clonidine, and diazoxide are no longer part of the treatment of hypertensive emergencies.

Clevidipine is a novel promising option for hypertensive emergencies.[73,76] It is a new, third-generation, ultra-short-acting, calcium-channel blocker recently approved for hypertensive crises in the US, Australia, and New Zealand, with the approval in Europe still pending. Clevidipine has a half-life of around 1 minute, a rapid onset and offset of action and its elimination is not being affected by hepatic and renal dysfunction. This agent acts through inhibition of extracellular calcium influx and exerts a selective arteriolar vasodilatory effect, reducing peripheral vascular resistance without affecting venous vascular tone. To this end, clevidipine produces a selective afterload reduction without an effect on preload and, thus, it increases cardiac output with little influence on left ventricular filling pressures. Furthermore, experimental studies have shown that clevidipine maintains splanchnic blood flow and renal perfusion and can protect against ischemia/reperfusion injury in situations of myocardial ischemia. Clevidipine reduces blood pressure by a direct and selective effect on arterioles, thereby reducing afterload without affecting cardiac filling pressures or causing reflex tachycardia. Stroke volume and cardiac output usually increase. Moreover, clevidipine has been shown to protect against ischaemia/reperfusion injury in an animal model of myocardial ischemia, and to maintain renal function and splanchnic blood flow. These unique pharmacodynamic and pharmacokinetic properties enable the use of the drug in critically ill patients and also minimize the risk of prolonged action and overshoot hypotension. The blood-pressure-lowering effects of the drug are rapid and dose-dependent. The intravenous infusion of clevidipine should be initiated at doses of 1–2 mg/h and then uptitrated by doubling every few minute to a maximum infusion rate of 16 mg/h.

The efficacy and safety of clevidipine have been evaluated in Phase I–III clinical studies, including also various patient populations (i.e., patients with essential hypertension, patients with hypertensive emergencies and in the perioperative setting).[73,76–78] In the ACCELERATE trial,[79] a recent multicenter, single-arm study, clevidipine monotherapy seems to be effective and safe for rapid blood pressure reduction in critically ill patients, with intracerebral hemorrhage.

Oral therapy should be instituted before parenteral agents are discontinued. The management of hypertensive encephalopathy also includes early recognition and removal of exacerbating factors such as immunosuppressive drugs.[4]

The only successful treatment for pre-eclampsia is delivery. No definitive preventive strategies have been identified. Magnesium sulfate is indicated to prevent further seizures in women with eclampsia. Magnesium has cerebral vasodilatory effects, alters the expression of endothelin-1 receptors, and reduces the permeability of the blood–brain barrier. These actions are relevant, since regional vasoconstriction, altered cerebral autoregulation with cerebral hyperperfusion, endothelial dysfunction, and breakdown of the blood–brain barrier are central to the pathophysiology of vasogenic edema in patients with eclampsia.[80] The role of prophylactic magnesium sulfate in preeclampsia is less clear. There is also long-standing experience with several suitable antihypertensive drugs. The parenteral antihypertensive drugs most commonly used during pregnancy are labetalol, nicardipine, hydralazine, and urapidil.[10,36,63,80] Angiotensin-converting enzyme inhibitors and angiotensin receptor antagonists are contraindicated in pregnancy because of unacceptable fetal side effects.

Treatment with antiepileptic medications is the standard of care for seizures associated with hypertensive encephalopathy but long-term antiepileptic therapy is not usually necessary.[6]

REFERENCES

1. Oppenheimer BS, Fishberg AM. Hypertensive encephalopathy. Arch Intern Med 1928;41:264–78.
2. Dinsdale HB. Hypertensive encephalopathy. Stroke 1982; 13:717–19.
3. Healton EB, Brust JC, Feinfeld DA, et al. Hypertensive encephalopathy and the neurologic manisfestations of malignant hypertension. Neurology 1982;32:127–32.
4. Hinchey J, Chaves C, Appignani B, et al. A reversible posterior leukoencephalopathy syndrome. N Engl J Med 1996;334: 494–500.
5. Lamy C, Oppenheim C, Meder JF, et al. Neuroimaging in posterior reversible encephalopathy syndrome. J Neuroimaging 2004; 14:89–96.
6. Lee VH, Wijdicks EF, Manno EM, et al. Clinical spectrum of reversible posterior leukoencephalopathy syndrome. Arch Neurol 2008; 65:205–10.
7. Schwartz RB, Jones KM, Kalina P, et al. Hypertensive encephalopathy: findings on CT, MR imaging and SPECT imaging in 14 cases. AJR Am J Roentgenol 1992;159:379–83.
8. Strandgaard S, Paulson OB. Cerebral autoregulation. Stroke 1984;15:415.
9. Bartynski WS. Posterior reversible encephalopathy syndrome, part 2: controversies surrounding pathophysiology of vasogenic edema. AJNR Am J Neuroradiol 2008;29:1043–9.
10. Slama M, Modeliar SS. Hypertension in the intensive care unit. Curr Opin Cardiol 2006;21:279–87.
11. Vaughan CJ, Delanty N. Hypertensive emergencies. Lancet 2000; 356:411–17.
12. Heistad DD. What's new in the cerebral microcirculation? Microcirculation 2001;8:365–75.
13. Beausang-Linder M, Bill A. Cerebral circulation in acute arterial hypertension-protective effect of sympathetic nervous activity. Physiol Scand 1981;111:193–9.
14. Bill A, Linder J. Sympathetic control of cerebral blood flow in acute arterial hypertension. Acta Physiol Scand 1976;96: 114–21.
15. Chester EM, Agamanolis DP, Banker BQ, et al. Hypertensive encephalopathy: a clinicopathologic study of 20 cases. Neurology 1978;28:928–39.
16. Richards A, Graham D, Bullock R. Clinicopathological study of neurological complications due to hypertensive disorders of pregnancy. J Neurol Neurosurg Psychiatry 1988;51:416–21.
17. Schiff D, Lopes MB. Neuropathological correlates of reversible posterior leukoencephalopathy. Neurocrit Care 2005;2:303–5.
18. Tallaksen CM, Kerty E, Bakke S. Visual hallucinations in a case of reversible hypertension-induced brain oedema. Eur J Neurol 1998;5:615–18.
19. Cruz-Flores S, Assis Aquino GF, Leira EC. Brainstem involvement in hypertensive encephalopathy: clinical and radiological findings. Neurology 2004;62:1417–19.
20. Milia A, Moller J, Pilia G, et al. Spinal cord involvement during hypertensive encephalopathy: clinical and radiological findings. J Neurol 2008;255:142–3.
21. Bakshi R, Bates V, Mechtler L, et al. Occipital seizures as the major clinical manifestation of reversible posterior leukoencephalopathy syndrome: magnetic resonance imaging findings. Epilepsia 1998;39:296–9.
22. Fugate JE, Claassen DO, Cloft HJ, et al. Posterior reversible encephalopathy syndrome: associated clinical and radiologic findings. Mayo Clin Proc 2010;85:427–32.
23. Wartenberg KE, Patsalides AD, Yepes M. Transient diffusion-weighted imaging changes in a patient with reversible leukoencephalopathy syndrome. Acta Radiol 2004;45:674–8.
24. Bartynski WS, Boardman JF. Distinct imaging patterns and lesion distribution in posterior reversible encephalopathy syndrome. AJNR Am J Neuroradiol 2007;28:1320–7.
25. Casey SO, Sampaio RC, Michel E, et al. Posterior reversible encephalopathy syndrome: utility of fluid-attenuated inversion recovery MR imaging in the detection of cortical and subcortical lesions. AJNR Am J Neuroradiol 2000;21:1199–206.
26. Bartynski WS. Posterior reversible encephalopathy syndrome, part 1: fundamental imaging and clinical features. AJNR Am J Neuroradiol 2008;29:1036–42.
27. Casey SO, Truwit CL. Pontine reversible edema: a newly recognized imaging variant of hypertensive encephalopathy? AJNR 2000;21:243–5.
28. Sèze Jd, Mastain B, Stojkovic T, et al. Unusual MR findings of the brainstem in arterial hypertension. AJNR 2000;21:391–4.
29. Keyserling HF, Provenzale JM. Atypical imaging findings in a near-fatal case of posterior reversible encephalopathy syndrome in a child. AJR Am J Roentgenol 2007;188:219–21.
30. Lin KL, Hsu WC, Wang HS, et al. Hypertension-induced cerebellar encephalopathy and hydrocephalus in a male. Pediatr Neurol 2006;34:72–5.
31. Wang MC, Escott EJ, Breeze RE. Posterior fossa swelling hydrocephalus resulting from hypertensive encephalopathy: case report and review of the literature. Neurosurgery 1999;44: 1325–7.
32. Weingarten K, Barbut D, Filippi C, et al. Acute hypertensive encephalopathy: Findings on spin-echo and gradient-echo MR imaging. AJR 1994;162:665–70.
33. McKinney AM, Short J, Truwit CL, et al. Posterior reversible encephalopathy syndrome: incidence of atypical regions of involvement and imaging findings. AJR Am J Roentgenol 2007; 189:904–12.
34. Kanazawa M, Sanpei K, Kasuga K. Recurrent hypertensive brainstem encephalopathy. J Neurol Neurosurg Psychiatry 2005; 76:888–90.
35. Covarrubias DJ, Luetmer PH, Campeau NG. Posterior reversible encephalopathy syndrome: prognostic utility of quantitative diffusion-weighted MR images. AJNR Am J Neuroradiol 2002;23: 1038–48.
36. Provenzale JM, Petrella JR, Cruz LCH, et al. Quantitative assessment of diffusion abnormalities in posterior reversible encephalopathy syndrome. AJNR Am J Neuroradiol 2001;22:1455–61.
37. Ay H, Buonanno F, Schaefer P, et al. Posterior leukoencephalopathy without severe hypertension. Utility of diffusion-weighted MRI. Neurology 1998;51:1369–76.
38. Koch S, Rabinstein A, Falcone S, et al. Diffusion-weighted imaging shows cytotoxic and vasogenic edema in eclampsia. AJNR Am J Neuroradiol 2001;22:1068–70.

39. Jones BV, Egelhoff JC, Patterson RJ. Hypertensive encephalopathy in children. Am J Neuroradiol 1997;18:101–6.
40. Sengar AR, Gupta RK, Dhanuka AK, et al. MR imaging, MR angiography, and MR spectroscopy of the brain in eclampsia. AJNR Am J Neuroradiol 1997;18:1485–90.
41. Eichler FS, Wang P, WITYK RJ, et al. Diffuse metabolic abnormalities in reversible posterior leukoencephalopathy syndrome. AJNR Am J Neuroradiol 2002;23:833–7.
42. Bartynski WS, Boardman JF. Catheter angiography, MR angiography, and MR perfusion in posterior reversible encephalopathy syndrome. AJNR Am J Neuroradiol 2008;29:447–55.
43. Trommer B, Homer D, Mikhael M. Cerebral vasospasm and eclampsia. Stroke 1988;19:326–9.
44. Tsukimori K, Ochi H, Yumoto Y, et al. Reversible posterior encephalopathy syndrome followed by MR angiography-documented cerebral vasospasm in preeclampsia-eclampsia: report of 2 cases. Cerebrovasc Dis 2008;25:377–80.
45. Ducros A, Boukobza M, Porcher R, et al. The clinical and radiological spectrum of reversible cerebral vasoconstriction syndrome. A prospective series of 67 patients. Brain 2007;130: 3091–101.
46. Singhal AB. Cerebral vasoconstriction syndromes. Top Stroke Rehabil 2004;11:1–6.
47. Singhal AB. Postpartum angiopathy with reversible posterior leukoencephalopathy. Arch Neurol 2004;61:411–16.
48. Papadopoulos DP, Mourouzis I, Thomopoulos C, et al. Hypertension crisis. Blood Press 2010.
49. Varon J. The diagnosis and treatment of hypertensive crises. Postgrad Med 2009;121:5–13.
50. Christophe JL, Plaen JFD, Goffette P, et al. Severe hypertension and renal infarct. Physiopatholgy and treatment. Nephrologie 1993;14:133–7.
51. Sharer K, Benninger C, Heimann A, et al. Involvement of the central nervous system in renal hypertension. Eur J Pediatr 1993; 152:59–63.
52. Kupferschmidt H, Bont A, Schnorf H, et al. Transient cortical blindness and bioccipital brain lesions in two patients with acute intermittent porphyria. Ann Intern Med 1995;123:598–600.
53. Popp MB, Friedberg DL, MacMillan BG. Clinical characteristics of hypertension in burned children. Ann Surg 1980;191:473–8.
54. Elahi A, Kelkar P, St Louis EK. Posterior reversible encephalopathy syndrome as the initial manifestation of Guillain-Barre Syndrome. Neurocrit Care 2004;1:465–8.
55. Sofer S, Gueron M. Vasodilatation and hypertensive encephalopathy following scorpion envenomation in children. Chest 1990; 97:118–20.
56. Grewal RP, Miller BL. Cocaine-induced hypertensive encephalopathy. Acta Neurol (Napoli) 1991;13:279–81.
57. Wartenberg KE, Parra A. CT and CT-perfusion findings of reversible leukoencephalopathy during triple-H therapy for symptomatic subarachnoid hemorrhage-related vasospasm. J Neuroimaging 2006;16:170–5.
58. Moawad FJ, Hartzell JD, Biega TJ, et al. Transient blindness due to posterior reversible encephalopathy syndrome following ephedra overdose. South Med J 2006;99:511–14.
59. Digre KB, Varner MW, Osborn AG, et al. Cranial magnetic resonance imaging in severe preeclampsia vs eclampsia. Arch Neurol 1993;50:399–406.
60. Manfredi M, Beltramello A, Bongiovanni LG, et al. Eclamptic encephalopathy: imaging and pathogenetic considerations. Acta Neurol Scand 1997;96:277–82.
61. Schwartz RB, Feske SK, Polak JF, et al. Preeclampsia-eclampsia: clinical and neuroradiographic correlates and insights into the pathogenesis of hypertensive encephalopathy. Radiology 2000; 217:371–6.
62. Mas JL, Lamy C. Severe preeclampsia/eclampsia: hypertensive encephalopathy of pregnancy? Cerebrovasc Dis 1998;8:53–8.
63. Sibai B, Dekker G, Kupferminc M. Pre-eclampsia. Lancet 2005; 365:785–99.
64. Wang A, Rana S, Karumanchi SA. Preeclampsia: the role of angiogenic factors in its pathogenesis. Physiology (Bethesda) 2009; 24:147–58.
65. Roberts JM, Redman CWG. Pre-eclampsia: more than pregnancy-induced hypertension. Lancet 1993;34:1447–50.
66. Veltkamp R, Kupsch A, Polasek J, et al. Late onset postpartum eclampsia without pre-eclamptic prodromi: clinical and neuroradiological presentation in two patients. J Neurol Neurosurg Psychiatry 2000;69:824–7.
67. Bellamy L, Casas JP, Hingorani AD, et al. Pre-eclampsia and risk of cardiovascular disease and cancer in later life: systematic review and meta-analysis. BMJ 2007;335:974.
68. Steinberg G, Khankin EV, Karumanchi SA. Angiogenic factors and preeclampsia. Thromb Res 2009;123(Suppl. 2):S93–9.
69. Pavlakis SG, Frank Y, Chusid R. Hypertensive encephalopathy, reversible occipitoparietal encephalopathy or reversible posterior leukoencephalopathy: three names for an old syndrome. J Child Neurol 1999;14:277–81.
70. Hinchey JA. Reversible posterior leukoencephalopathy syndrome: what have we learned in the last 10 years? Arch Neurol 2008;65: 175–6.
71. Bartynski WS, Boardman JF, Zeigler ZR, et al. Posterior reversible encephalopathy syndrome in infection, sepsis, and shock. AJNR Am J Neuroradiol 2006;27:2179–90.
72. Thompson CB, June CH, Sullivan KM, et al. Association between cyclosporin neurotoxicity and hypomagnesaemia. Lancet 1984;2: 1116–20.
73. Varon J. Treatment of acute severe hypertension: current and newer agents. Drugs 2008;68:283–97.
74. Perez MI, Musini VM. Pharmacological interventions for hypertensive emergencies: a Cochrane systematic review. J Hum Hypertens 2008;22:596–607.
75. McCoy S, Baldwin K. Pharmacotherapeutic options for the treatment of preeclampsia. Am J Health Syst Pharm 2009;66: 337–44.
76. Deeks ED, Keating GM, Keam SJ. Clevidipine: a review of its use in the management of acute hypertension. Am J Cardiovasc Drugs 2009;9:117–34.
77. Singla N, Warltier DC, Ghandi SD, et al. Treatment of acute postoperative hypertension in cardiac surgery patients: an efficacy study of clevidipine assessing its postoperative antihypertensive effect in cardiac surgery-2 (ESCAPE-2), a randomized, double-blind, placebo-controlled trial. Anesth Analg 2008;107:59–67.
78. Pollack CV, Varon J, Garrison NA, et al. Clevidipine, an intravenous dihydropyridine calcium channel blocker, is safe and effective for the treatment of patients with acute severe hypertension. Am Emerg Med 2009;53:329–38.
79. Graffagnino C, Bergese S, Love J, et al. Clevidipine rapidly and safely reduces blood pressure in acute intracerebral hemorrhage: the ACCELERATE trial. Cerebrovasc Dis 2013;36:173–80.
80. Duley L, Gulmezoglu AM, Henderson-Smart DJ. Magnesium sulphate and other anticonvulsants for women with pre-eclampsia. Cochrane Database Syst Rev 2003;CD000025.

39 Stroke and Substance Abuse

John C.M. Brust

KEY POINTS

- Stroke in recreational substance users can be an indirect complication, e.g., endocarditis and cardioembolism in parenteral drug users.
- With some drugs, e.g., cocaine, stroke appears to be the result of a direct effect.
- For illicit drugs, epidemiological studies are few, but numerous case reports of stroke temporally associated with drug use in young subjects without other risk factors provide persuasive (albeit inconclusive) evidence for causality.
- For ethanol and tobacco, epidemiological evidence is strong that these agents are major risk factors in a dose-related fashion for ischemic and hemorrhagic stroke.
- Proposed mechanisms for substance-related stroke vary widely and are not mutually exclusive.

Drug dependence is "a state of psychic or physical dependence, or both, on a drug, arising in a person following administration of that drug on a periodic or continuous basis."[1] Drug abuse, on the other hand, refers to the perception that recreational use of a substance is harmful, regardless of whether the substance is taken continuously, periodically, or infrequently, and regardless of whether it is legally available. When alcohol and tobacco are included, millions of Americans are substance abusers, and many of them are at increased risk of stroke, either ischemic or hemorrhagic.[2–5]

OPIATES

The most commonly abused opiate drug is heroin (diacetylmorphine), which is administered by injection, by snorting, or by smoking. Stroke affects heroin users by diverse mechanisms.

Injectors are at risk of infectious endocarditis, which carries risk for both ischemic and hemorrhagic stroke.[6–10] Infarction follows embolic vessel occlusion or, less, often, bacterial or fungal meningitis. Cerebral or subarachnoid hemorrhage usually occurs after rupture of a septic (mycotic) aneurysm,[11–13] which can affect intracranial or cervical arteries.[14,15] Heroin users are also at risk for hemorrhagic stroke secondary to liver failure with deranged clotting and to heroin nephropathy with uremia or malignant hypertension.

In some heroin users the drug itself appears to be more directly causal. Anecdotal reports describe young people without evident stroke risk factors whose ischemic strokes occurred temporally with heroin use. Some had angiographic changes suggestive of vasculitis, and some had immunologic changes suggestive of hypersensitivity.[16–23] Opiate withdrawal symptoms and cerebral infarction were reported in two newborns whose mothers had used codeine during pregnancy.[24] A young man had an intracerebral hemorrhage within minutes of intravenous injection of heroin.[25]

Heroin could cause stroke by a number of possible mechanisms.[26] After heroin overdose, hypoventilation and hypotension can produce permanent brain damage.[27–30] Delayed post-anoxic encephalopathy also occurs.[31] Bilateral globus pallidus infarction is commonly observed at autopsy in heroin users,[32,33] and hemichorea and bilateral ballism are described in heroin users with pallidal infarction on imaging.[16,30,32–34] In some cases an awkward position of the neck during overdose coma might have kinked the carotid artery and further decreased cerebral perfusion.[28] Three days after injecting heroin, a young man developed hemiparesis, and angiography showed reversible bilateral segmental narrowing of the supraclinoid internal carotid, middle cerebral, and anterior cerebral arteries.[35]

Direct toxic injury from either heroin or an adulterant is another possibility. Heroin is often mixed with quinine and lactose or mannitol; other reported adulterants include talc, starch, curry powder, abrasive cleanser, caffeine, and strychnine.[26] Quinine caused amblyopia in a heroin addict[36] and might contribute to acute adverse reactions with pulmonary edema or sudden death after parenteral injection.[37] There is no evidence, however, linking quinine to stroke.

Embolization of foreign material to the brain has not been observed in parenteral heroin users (even though the jugular vein is commonly used, with occasional accidental arterial injection) but has been documented at autopsy in abusers of other opiates.[38,39] Probably because of restricted heroin supply, pentazocine (Talwin) and tripelennamine (Pyribenzamine) ("Ts and Blues") were widely abused in American midwestern cities during the 1970s. Oral tablets were crushed, suspended in water, and injected intravenously, leading to microembolic cerebral infarcts and hemorrhages.[40] Strokes were also reported following injection of paregoric, of pulverized meperidine tablets, and of hydromorphone suppositories.[41–43]

Some heroin-related strokes follow the first injection after weeks or months of abstinence, and laboratory findings sometimes suggest an immunologic cause. Heroin nephropathy may be immunologically mediated;[44] the C3 component of complement is reduced in patients with heroin pulmonary edema; and heroin addicts frequently have hypergammaglobulinemia,[45–48] circulating immune complexes,[41] antibodies to smooth muscle and lymphocyte membranes,[46] false-positive serologic tests,[45] and lymph node hypertrophy.[26] Opium, morphine, codeine, and meperidine, moreover, have caused urticaria, angioneurotic edema, and anaphylaxis.[49] Morphine binding by gamma globulin is reported in addicts[50] and experimental animals.[51]

Relevant to heroin stroke is heroin myelopathy. Acute paraparesis, sensory loss, and urinary retention occur shortly after injection; frequently after a period of abstinence.[52–56] In some patients symptoms are present on awakening from coma. Proprioception and vibratory sense are often preserved relative to loss of spinothalamic sensory modalities, suggesting infarction in the territory of the anterior spinal artery.[57,58] Possible mechanisms include "borderzone" infarction during a period of coma, hypoventilation, and hypotension, as well as hypersensitivity reaction.[59,60] A man using intravenous heroin for the first time in 2 years became comatose and apneic; after he received an opiate antagonist, quadriplegia, anarthria, dysphagia, and sensory loss consistent with a ventral pontine lesion developed over several hours.[61]

AMPHETAMINE AND RELATED AGENTS

During the 1990s methamphetamine became the fastest-growing illegal drug in North America and parts of Europe.[62] Swallowed, injected, snorted, or smoked, methamphetamine is often taken with heroin, and samples contain a variety of pharmacologically active and inactive adulterants.[2] Strokes common to any parenteral drug abuse are encountered. There are also strokes that may be unique to these agents.[63]

In animals and humans amphetamine overdose can cause severe hyperthermia, coagulopathy, and vascular collapse, with brain petechiae and neuronal degeneration.[64-70] Intracranial hemorrhage is often a feature of heat stroke.[71,72] Amphetamine/methamphetamine users are also at risk for intracranial hemorrhage in the absence of hyperpyrexia and disturbed clotting.

Reports of hemorrhagic stroke in abusers of amphetamine or methamphetamine include more than 60 patients, ages 16–60 years.[73-106] Oral, intravenous, nasal, and inhalational routes of administration have been reported. Most were chronic users, but in several patients, stroke followed a first exposure. The dose was usually unknown, but in one case was as low as 80 mg. Except for one instance each of diethylpropion and pseudoephedrine, all the reported patients took amphetamine or methamphetamine; seven also took methylphenidate, LSD, dimethoxymethylamphetamine ("STP"), cocaine, heroin, or barbiturates. Severe headaches usually occurred within minutes of drug use. Blood pressure was elevated in the majority of patients in whom it was recorded, with diastolic pressure as high as 120 mm Hg. Eight patients died. CT variably showed intracerebral hemorrhage (frequently lobar) or subarachnoid hemorrhage. In some patients, angiography revealed irregular narrowing (beading) of distal cerebral arteries, suggesting (but not pathognomonic for) vasculitis. Some of these patients had taken the drug only orally. Vasculitic changes were present at autopsy in three patients (including one whose angiogram showed only an avascular mass). In another patient, a cerebral vascular malformation was seen on both angiography and CT.

Thus, some of these amphetamine/methamphetamine-induced intracranial hemorrhages seem to have been secondary to acute hypertension, some to cerebral vasculitis, and some to a combination of the two; however, in others neither feature was apparent. A case report described cerebral vasculitis at autopsy after methamphetamine-associated intracerebral hemorrhage.[102] Another autopsy report of methamphetamine-associated intracerebral hemorrhage found no evidence of vasculitis.[101] Although acute hypertension secondary to amphetamine could be causal, it might have been a transient result of the stroke in some patients. Conversely, in other patients, fleeting blood pressure elevations could have been missed.

Amphetamine and methamphetamine-associated ischemic strokes have been less frequently reported.[104-113]

Two epidemiologic studies addressed the association of amphetamine/methamphetamine and stroke. In a population-based case-control study of women aged 15–44 years, amphetamine/methamphetamine was a risk factor for combined hemorrhagic and ischemic stroke (odds ratio, 3.8).[114] Some women in that study used both cocaine and amphetamine/methamphetamine, and drug use was based on self-report at a later interview; claims did not always match what was recorded in the medical record, including positive results on urine drug screening. Hospitalized control subjects, moreover, did not undergo drug screening, and if they were even less likely than case patients to report drug use, the risk of stroke might be exaggerated. A case-control study using a cross-sectional design based on more than 3 million patients discharged from Texas hospitals over a 3-year period found that amphetamine/methamphetamine increased the risk of hemorrhagic stroke (odds ratio, 4.95) but not ischemic stroke.[115]

Amphetamine-induced cerebral vasculitis appears to be of more than one type. Necrotizing angiitis, sometimes affecting the nervous system, occurred in 14 Los Angeles polydrug abusers.[116] All but two patients used intravenous methamphetamine, and one used it exclusively. Five patients were asymptomatic; others had, variably, fever, skin rash, pulmonary edema, renal failure, pancreatitis, gastrointestinal hemorrhage, peripheral neuropathy, anemia, leukocytosis, and hemolysis. One patient had "progressive encephalopathy" and, at autopsy, vasculitis affecting pontine arterioles. Another had cerebral and pontine infarction, cerebellar hemorrhage, and vasculitis in the cerebrum, cerebellum, and brainstem. Vessel lesions were considered typical for polyarteritis nodosa and different from hypersensitivity angiitis, which involves small arteries, capillaries, and venules. The authors acknowledged that more than one drug or adulterant could have caused these lesions.[117,118]

Although such brain lesions have been found pathologically in other amphetamine/methamphetamine abusers,[84,104] in some, cerebral arteritis has been presumed on the basis of cerebral angiography,[73,74,78,88,98,119-122] and sometimes the relation to amphetamine abuse has been tenuous. In a report of thalamic infarction following intranasal methamphetamine use, angiography was not performed.[123]

A radiographic study of 19 young drug abusers, most taking intravenous methamphetamine and hospitalized for coma or stroke, revealed widespread segmental constrictions of large and medium-sized cerebral arteries and stenosis or occlusion of many penetrating arterioles (beading).[119] Such a finding could reflect either multiple emboli, vasculitis, or spontaneous segmental vasoconstriction. The same researchers gave rhesus monkeys intravenous methamphetamine, 1.5 mg/kg (considered the lower limit of dosage for most abusers). Cerebral angiography showed an irregularly decreased caliber of small cerebral vessels, and postmortem examination revealed subarachnoid hemorrhage in some animals, with numerous brain petechial hemorrhages, infarcts, edema, microaneurysms, and perivascular white blood cell cuffing.[124,125]

In rats receiving 2 weeks of intravenous methamphetamine, electron microscopy showed that brain capillaries had abnormal "budding" from the luminal walls of endothelial cells and vesicles within the endothelial cell cytoplasm.[125] These changes affected vessels smaller than 100 μm and would, therefore, be missed on angiography. (The vulnerability of small vessels might be related to their separate innervation; large cerebral vessels are innervated by the peripheral sympathetic nervous system, but nerve terminals on smaller arteries appear to be from central noradrenergic neurons.[126])

These lesions are different from those of polyarteritis nodosa, in which elastic arteries, capillaries, and veins are spared. Whether the lesions in methamphetamine users are the result of direct toxicity or hypersensitivity is unclear, nor can the possibility be excluded that the early angiographic findings are secondary to subarachnoid hemorrhage (although beading of distal pial arteries in subarachnoid hemorrhage is rare).[74] Possibly contributing to methamphetamine-related vasculitis is formation of circulating "advanced glycation end products" with pro-inflammatory immunoreactive properties.[127]

In an adolescent amphetamine abuser with mononeuritis multiplex, sural nerve biopsy showed apparent hypersensitivity angiitis of medium and small muscular arteries, arterioles, venules, and veins.[128] The central nervous system, however, was clinically unaffected.

A study using single-photon emission CT (SPECT) found reduced cerebral blood flow in the cingulate cortex of both long-term and short-term abstinent methamphetamine users.[129]

In mice, pretreatment with methamphetamine exacerbated damage after middle cerebral artery ligation.[130]

Amphetamines cause direct myocardial toxicity with contracton band necrosis, and arrhythmia and thrombosis can cause cardioembolic stroke.[131]

Other Related Psychostimulants

Phenylpropanolamine (PPA), an amphetamine-like drug, was marketed in over-the-counter decongestants and diet pills, as well as in drugs made deliberately to resemble amphetamine ("look-alike pills").[132,133] Acute hypertension, severe headache, psychiatric symptoms, seizures, and hemorrhagic stroke were reported in users.[133–144] PPA with caffeine, from a commercial diet preparation, produced subarachnoid hemorrhage in rats receiving it intraperitoneally at several times the recommended dose.[139] Following epidemiological evidence that subjects taking PPA-containing diet pills and decongestants were at increased risk for hemorrhagic stroke, such products were withdrawn from the market.[145–149]

Ephedrine and pseudoephedrine are present in decongestants and bronchodilators. Complications of these agents include headache, tachyarrhythmia, hypertensive emergency, and hemorrhagic and occlusive stroke.[150–158] Rupture of a cerebral vascular malformation occurred in a man who had used pseudoephedrine daily for more than a year.[159] Thunderclap headache and bilateral severe cerebral vasoconstriction in the absence of subarachnoid hemorrhage occurred in a woman soon after taking pseudoephedrine and dextromethorphan.[160]

Seizures, cardiotoxicity (including sudden death), and ischemic and hemorrhagic strokes are reported in users of dietary supplements containing ephedra alkaloids ("ma huang").[161–168] A case-control study found a non-significant trend toward hemorrhagic stroke among users of these products, and in 2003 they were banned in the US.[169]

Other amphetamine-like drugs promoted as diet pills and anecdotally associated with stroke include phendimetrazine,[170] diethylpropion,[82] and fenfluramine,[171–172] and phentermine.[173] After reports of valvular heart disease in users, fenfluramine and dexfenfluramine were removed from the US market.[174]

3,4-Methylenedioxymethamphetamine (MDMA, "ecstasy") and 3,4-methylenedioxyethamphetamine (MDEA) are "designer drugs" with both amphetamine-like and hallucinogen-like properties. Ischemic and hemorrhagic strokes are described in MDMA users as well as in users of MDMA-like designer drugs such as 4-bromo-2,5-dimethoxyphenylethylamine ("2C-B," "Nexus"), 3,4-methylenedioxyamphetamine (MDA), and 4-iodo-2,5-dimethoxyphenylethylamine ("2C-I").[175–194]

A young woman developed bilateral hemiplegia after inadvertent injection of crushed methylphenidate tablets into both carotid arteries.[195] Talc microemboli have been described in the fundi and brains of intravenous methylphenidate abusers.[38,39,196] As with amphetamine/methamphetamine, cerebral "vasculitis" has been presumed on the basis of angiography in some reports of methylphenidate-associated stroke.[197–199] Angiographic and histologic evidence of small-vessel vasculitis was seen in rats and monkeys receiving methlyphenidate.[125]

A cohort study found no increased risk for stroke or myocardial infarction among adult prescription methylphenidate users.[200] A similar cohort study found increased risk (hazard ratio: 3.44) for transient ischemic attack for prescription users of methylphenidate or atomoxetine (a non-stimulant also used to treat attention deficit hyperactivity disorder).[201]

Mycotic subclavian and carotid aneurysms were reported after inadvertent intra-arterial injection of phentermine.[202]

Death has followed parenteral[203] or oral[204] abuse of propylhexedrine from nasal decongestant inhalers; stroke has not yet been reported in such patients, and the cause of death has been uncertain.

Cerebral and retinal infarcts were reported in chronic intranasal abusers of sprays and drops containing the sympathomimetics oxymetazoline and phenoxazoline.[205,206]

Intracerebral hemorrhage occurred in a young man after intravenous self-administration of epinephrine.[207] A normotensive 73-year-old man had a thalamic hemorrhage after repeated heavy use of an epinephrine inhaler.[208]

Khat (*Catha edulis*), a shrub indigenous to East Africa and the Arabian peninsula, contains cathinone, an amphetamine-like psychostimulant.[2] Millions of people in that part of the world chew khat leaves recreationally, and since the 1980s khat use has spread world-wide. Moreover, designer analogues of cathinone have become popular in Europe and North America. Street products containing compounds such as mephedrone, methylone, and 3,4-methyldioxypyrovalerone (MDPV) and sold as "bath salts" are ingested, inhaled, or injected.[209,210] Ischemic stroke and myocardial infarction have been reported in khat chewers.[211–213] A review of 29 case reports of bath salt toxicity identified cardiac arrest and anoxic/ischemic encephalopathy but not ischemic or hemorrhagic stroke.[210]

COCAINE

Before the 1980s cocaine hydrochloride was usually sniffed or, less often, injected. The emergence of smokable alkaloidal "crack" cocaine allowed much larger doses and more prolonged intoxication than with intranasal (and unsmokable) cocaine hydrochloride. An epidemic of crack cocaine use ensued, and with it a flood of reports describing medical complications, including stroke.[214]

Parenteral cocaine users are at risk of stroke related to infection, including endocarditis, AIDS, and hepatitis. They also experience strokes caused directly by the drug itself, whether taken intranasally, intravenously, or intramuscularly or smoked as crack.[215,216] The first report of a cocaine-related stroke, in 1977, described a mildly hypertensive man who, following intramuscular injection of cocaine, developed aphasia and right hemiparesis.[217] The same year, fatal rupture of a cerebral saccular aneurysm occurred in a young man sniffing cocaine.[218] Further cases were not reported until the mid-1980s, but by 2002, more than 600 cases of cocaine-related stroke had been described, about half occlusive and half hemorrhagic.[2,39,219–297] Moreover, as cocaine users have aged, cocaine-related strokes are not uncommon among patients more than 50 years of age.[298–301]

Ischemic strokes have included transient ischemic attacks and infarction of cerebrum, thalamus, brainstem, spinal cord, retina, and peripheral oculomotor nerve.[232,253,302–311] Infarction has occurred in newborns whose mothers used cocaine shortly before delivery[225,312] and in pregnant women.[215,231,253,302] Pontomesencephalic infarction in a cocaine sniffer was associated with extensive destruction of osteocartilaginous structures of the nose, sinuses, and palate.[296] Bilateral hippocampal infarction followed cocaine-induced cardiac arrest.[297] A young crack smoker had middle cerebral artery branch occlusion, cardiomyopathy, and a left atrial thrombus.[272] A 20-year-old with no other risk factors had superior cerebellar artery occlusion 6 months after the last use of cocaine, raising the possibility of delayed effects.[313] A 27-year-old man developed bilateral anterior cerebral artery infarction and paraparesis following cocaine inhalation.[314] A 44-year-old man who abused both cocaine and ethanol developed unilateral putamen infarction and isolated vocal cord paralysis.[315]

In some cases, cerebral infarction was attributed to vasculitis on the basis of angiographic findings;[248] such changes, however, could represent either cocaine-induced cerebral vasoconstriction or vasospasm after undiagnosed subarachnoid hemorrhage.[316] Autopsies usually show histologically normal cerebral vessels,[215,256,267] although in five cases, mild cerebral vasculitis was observed at biopsy or autopsy.[223,236,253,265] In these cases, cerebral angiographic findings were normal. In one report, cocaine-induced vasculitis was diagnosed on the basis of BOLD-MRI cerebrovascular reactivity.[317] In a man with multiple cerebral infarcts, angiography showed "multifocal areas of segmental stenosis and dilatation," yet brain biopsy revealed no evidence of vasculitis.[261]

In a young occasional cocaine sniffer with "heaviness and paresthesias" in the legs and occasional "forgetfulness," MRI revealed multiple periventricular white matter lesions.[290] A young man who had used cocaine "regularly" for 10 years demonstrated progressively impaired cognition; CT revealed patchy areas consistent with infarction, and cerebral angiography showed marked stenosis of the internal carotid and middle cerebral arteries with moyamoya-like collateral vessels.[310] A young woman who had been using crack for 12 years experienced mental deterioration progressing to mutism over several weeks; CT showed diffuse cerebral atrophy, but SPECT showed more focal reductions in perfusion.[318]

MRI studies in asymptomatic long-term cocaine users found abnormal cerebral white matter signals consistent with "subclinical vascular events."[319] In a study of 32 cocaine-dependent subjects, cerebral white matter hyperintensities on MRI were significantly more frequent among cocaine users than among heroin users (odds ratio (OR), 2.54) or normal control subjects (OR, 2.90).[320]

A population-based study of young adults found that cocaine conferred significant risk of "early retinal vascular abnormalities."[321]

Intracerebral or subarachnoid hemorrhage has occurred during or within hours of cocaine use or has shown a less clear temporal relationship.[267,322–324] In some instances there has been other substance use, especially ethanol. Parenchymal hemorrhages have been located in the cerebrum, brainstem, and cerebellum.[267,292,306,307,309,325,326] In a study of 45 patients with cocaine-associated intracerebral hemorrhage (ICH), functional outcome was worse compared to non-users with ICH.[327]

Also described are superior sagittal sinus thrombosis with hemorrhagic venous infarction, mycotic aneurysm rupture, dural arteriovenous fistula, spontaneous spinal epidural hematoma, and bleeding into embolic infarction or glioma.[291,305,328,329] Nearly half the patients with cocaine-associated intracranial hemorrhage who underwent angiography had saccular aneurysms or vascular malformations.

Two studies found cocaine use to predict poor outcome in patients with subarachnoid hemorrhage.[282,330] In another study, 27 of 440 patients with ruptured aneurysms had used cocaine within 72 hours and, although vasospasm was more likely among the cocaine users, there was no difference in clinical outcome.[331] Other studies did not find increased risk for either vasospasm or delayed cerebral ischemia.[332–334] Cerebral hemorrhages have occurred in newborns and postpartum women.[215,244,262]

Autopsies on patients with cocaine-induced intracranial hemorrhage have revealed histologically normal cerebral vessels.[238,322]

A case-control study from Atlanta failed to find any association between crack use and stroke.[335] This unexpected finding was probably related to lack of information regarding acute crack use in more than half of the subjects and controls as well as the fact that nearly half of the controls with information available had used crack, many acutely, raising the possibility that crack users are more likely than non-users to be hospitalized for a variety of reasons. A population-based study of 10,085 young adults identified 33 with non-fatal stroke and concluded that cocaine use was not a risk factor.[336] In that study the diagnosis of stroke was based on physician report, and "lifetime cocaine use" (i.e., use not necessarily associated temporarily with the stroke) was based on patient report.

A case-control study of women aged 15–44 years found that cocaine use was a strong risk factor for stroke (OR, 13.9).[114] A case-control study of men and women aged 18–49 years found that cocaine use within 3 days was a strong risk factor for subarachnoid hemorrhage (OR, 24.97).[303,337]

The mechanisms of cocaine-related stroke are diverse. Notable is the high frequency of underlying aneurysm or vascular malformation in hemorrhagic strokes in cocaine users compared with amphetamine users and, conversely, the frequency of vasculitis in amphetamine users compared with cocaine users.[338] Cocaine hydrochloride is more often associated with hemorrhagic than occlusive stroke, whereas hemorrhagic and occlusive strokes occur with roughly equal frequency in crack users; however, the rising prevalence of stroke following the appearance of crack was probably attributable to wider use and higher dosage rather than to a peculiarity of crack itself.[339]

Cocaine-induced coronary artery vasoconstriction was documented during cardiac catheterization, and cocaine-associated myocardial infarction, cardiac arrhythmia, and cardiomyopathy carry a risk of embolic stroke.[340] More significant, however, is cocaine's effects on systemic and cerebral circulation. Cocaine is a vasoconstrictor both systemically and intracranially.[341–345] Acute hypertension can lead to intracranial hemorrhage, especially in subjects with underlying aneurysms or vascular malformations.[267] Cerebral vasoconstriction probably causes occlusive stroke, and it is possibly significant that cocaine metabolites, which in some long-term users are detectable in urine for weeks, also cause cerebral vasospasm.[346,347] In healthy young cocaine users, intravenous cocaine caused dose-related cerebral vasoconstriction (as detected by magnetic resonance angiography),[348] and Doppler ultrasonography revealed increased cerebrovascular resistance that persisted for at least 1 month during abstinence.[315,349] In one report, CT perfusion imaging led to a diagnosis of vasospasm-related ischemia rather than thromboembolic stroke, and tissue plasminogen activator (rtPA) was withheld.[350] (rtPA appears to be safe in cocaine-associated thromboembolic stroke.[351])

In women, cocaine-induced cerebral vasospasm is hormonally influenced, occurring during the luteal phase of the menstrual cycle but not during the follicular phase.[352] The situation is complex, however, because cerebral and peripheral vessels frequently respond differently to similar stimuli. Either vasoconstriction or vasodilation might occur, depending on whether a study involves in vitro vessel preparations or live animals and whether the animal is rat, rabbit, cat, dog, or pig.[353–358] Cocaine-induced cerebral vasospasm was reportedly most prominent in brain areas rich in dopamine (which has vasoconstrictor effects on intracortical vessels), and the vasospasm was blocked by calcium channel antagonists.[359] In rabbits cocaine-induced cerebral vasospasm was dependent on endothelin-1 release.[360] Cultured canine vascular smooth muscle cells underwent apoptosis when exposed to cocaine.[361]

Active cocaine users have increased platelet aggregation to adenosine diphosphate, and the abnormality improves with abstinence.[362,363] In vitro studies with platelets are conflicting.[364,365] In rabbits, repeated cocaine injections caused arteriosclerotic aortopathy.[366] In a cocaine user with symptoms of coronary artery disease, protein C and antithrombin III levels were depleted but returned to normal, with clearing of symptoms, when use of the drug was discontinued.[367] Long-term cocaine users had increased numbers of circulating endothelial cells and increased levels of markers of endothelial damage,[368] and intravenous administration of cocaine caused erythrocytosis and increased levels of von Willebrand factor.[368,369] Cocaine users are at increased risk for thrombotic thrombocytopenic purpura.[370]

In the presence of ethanol, cocaine is metabolized to cocaethylene, which, more powerfully than cocaine itself, binds to the synaptic dopamine transporter and blocks reuptake.[371] Cocaine and ethanol synergistically depress myocardial contraction,[372] and a study using SPECT found that cerebral perfusion was reduced to a greater degree in subjects who abused both cocaine and ethanol than in those who abused cocaine alone.[373]

Human studies using control subjects suggest that long-term cocaine use produces subtle cognitive impairment,[374–377] but unlike methamphetamine, cocaine does not produce morphologic damage at dopaminergic or serotonergic nerve endings.[378,379] Studies with positron emission tomography (PET) and SPECT in long-term cocaine users found irregularly decreased blood flow in the cerebral cortex; in some of these subjects, CT or MRI findings were normal, and in some (but not all), PET and SPECT abnormalities were associated with deficits on psychometric testing.[380–385] In mice receiving cocaine, ultrahigh-resolution optical coherence tomography demonstrated marked microcirculatory ischemia.[386]

How cocaine affects the fetus is controversial. Perinatal and neonatal strokes - both occlusive and hemorrhagic - may be under-recognized in newborns exposed to cocaine in utero.[283,387] Cerebral blood flow studies during the first few days of life in cocaine-exposed neonates are consistent with persisting vasoconstriction.[388] Some investigators speculate that cocaine-induced vasospasm during the first trimester is responsible for CNS malformations.[243] Others have doubted such causality.[389] Adolescents exposed to cocaine in utero had significantly reduced global cerebral blood flow compared with control subjects.[390]

PHENCYCLIDINE

Phencyclidine (PCP, "angel dust") became a widely abused US street drug in the 1970s; it can be smoked, eaten, or injected. Large doses cause psychosis, myoclonus, nystagmus, seizures, coma, and sometimes fatal respiratory and circulatory collapse.[391] Hypertension can occur both early and late during intoxication.[391–395]

A 13-year-old boy became comatose after taking PCP; admission blood pressure was normal, and he became more alert. Three days later, however, his condition deteriorated, and his blood pressure was 220/130 mm Hg. Autopsy revealed an intracerebral hemorrhage.[393] Other reported complications of PCP intoxication include seizures and hemiparesis in the presence of a probable vascular malformation,[392] subarachnoid hemorrhage,[396] perforation of the basilar artery,[397] amaurosis fugax,[398] and hypertensive encephalopathy.[399]

LYSERGIC ACID DIETHYLAMIDE

In high doses, lysergic acid diethylamide (LSD), an ergot drug, causes severe hypertension, obtundation, and convulsions.[2] In vitro spasm of cerebral vessel strips immersed in LSD-containing solution was prevented or reversed by methysergide.[395] After ingesting LSD capsules, an adolescent boy experienced seizures and, 4 days later, left hemiplegia; carotid angiography showed progressive narrowing of the internal carotid artery from its origin to the siphon, with occlusion at its bifurcation.[400]A young woman demonstrated sudden left hemiplegia a day after oral ingestion of LSD; angiography showed marked constriction of the internal carotid artery at the siphon; 9 days later, the vessel was occluded at that level.[401]

MARIJUANA

Reports of marijuana-related stroke are few, and not all are convincing.[402–405] In some, however, temporal association, young age, and lack of stroke risk factors or other explanation more persuasively implicate cannabis as playing a causal role. As of 2013, more than 60 cannabis-related cases of stroke had been reported. Most were ischemic, including several with transient ischemic attacks, sometimes followed by infarction.[402–438] Only one patient had a hemorrhagic stroke.[421] Several cases involved cerebellar infarction in teenagers.[413,414,423]

In some cases marijuana smoking was accompanied by heavy ethanol consumption. In one of these, MR angiography demonstrated vasospastic narrowing of branches of the left middle and anterior cerebral arteries.[417] Other reports describe cerebral infarction during an episode of coital headache,[418] in an adolescent heterozygous for factor V Leiden mutation,[419] and in a young man receiving cisplatin chemotherapy.[420]

A single report of intracerebral hemorrhage in a cannabis user involved a young woman who took daily buprenorphine for heroin addiction and who had smoked several joints daily for over a decade.[421]

A hospital-based case-control study failed to identify marijuana use as an independent risk factor for stroke.[439] In another study of hospitalized patients, increased risk for ischemic stroke disappeared after adjusting for tobacco use.[440] A population-based study of over 3 million hospital discharges reported an odds ratio of 1.76 (95%CI, 1.15–2.71) for cannabis exposure associated with ischemic stroke.[115]

A number of mechanisms have been proposed for marijuana-related stroke. Cardiovascular effects of cannabis include atrial fibrillation and sinus tachycardia, supine hypertension and orthostatic hypotension, increased cardiac output, and peripheral vasodilation.[423,441–446] The risk of myocardial infarction is increased 4.8-fold in marijuana smokers.[423,447] Decreased cerebral perfusion is greatest in inexperienced compared to experienced users. Cerebral blood volume was increased in marijuana smokers 36 hours after the last dose.[448] Peripheral arteritis resembling Buerger disease is described in heavy marijuana users, but cerebral vasculitis has not been reported.[424]

In both heavy and moderate marijuana users, abstinent for a month, transcranial Doppler sonography demonstrated increased cerebrovascular resistance.[449] Of 48 young patients with ischemic stroke, multifocal intracranial stenosis was associated with cannabis use in ten patients.[425] A 46-year-old cannabis user had recurrent thunderclap headaches with bilateral infarcts in cerebellum, occipital lobe, and frontal lobe; vascular imaging showed multifocal segmental stenosis which resolved on follow-up.[426] The patient with cannabis-associated brain hemorrhage had reversible multifocal intracranial stenosis.[421]

Marijuana is the most widely used illicit drug, and so it is remarkable that so few reports of marijuana-related stroke have appeared. Possible triggering factors include sexual activity and concomitant ethanol ingestion.[418,422,426] Genetic predisposition has been proposed.[427]

Following the discovery of brain endocannabinoid receptors and ligands, dozens of synthetic cannabinoid agonists and antagonists were developed for pharmacological research, and soon synthetic cannabinoids became available as recreational drugs. Collectively termed "spice" and "K2," preparations often contain a mixture of synthetic compounds sprayed onto herbs and aromatic extracts and marketed as "herbal blends" or "incense."[450,451] Spice is now the second most used illicit drug (after marijuana) among American high school seniors.[452] Two healthy young siblings had ischemic stroke shortly after smoking spice.[453]

BARBITURATES

Usually abused orally, barbiturates and other sedatives and tranquilizers can cause cerebral infarction following overdose and diffusely decreased brain perfusion. Patients reported with barbiturate-associated ischemic stroke were taking additional drugs.[199,120]

INHALANTS

Inhalation of vapors to achieve euphoric intoxication is common in the US, especially among children. Substances include aerosols, enamels, paint thinners, lighter fluid, cleaning fluid, glues, cements, gasoline, and anesthetics. Death results from violence, accidents, suffocation, aspiration, or cardiac arrhythmia. Reports of ischemic stroke are few and not readily explained.[454,455] A 43-year-old man had an aneurysmal subarachnoid hemorrhage while watching a pornographic movie and inhaling amyl nitrite.[456]

ALCOHOL

Coronary artery disease and myocardial infarction are less prevalent in people who drink moderate amounts of alcohol than in abstainers.[457,458] Heavy drinkers have an increased risk of coronary artery disease, however, resulting in an increased risk of cardioembolic stroke. Alcohol intoxication and withdrawal are also directly associated with cardiac arrhythmia ("holiday heart"),[459] and thromboembolism is a prominent feature of alcoholic cardiomyopathy.[222] A large body of literature has addressed whether short-term or long-term alcohol use is a risk factor for stroke independent of its cardiac effects or other risk factors.[460–464]

Retrospective studies, most notably from Finland, found an association between recent heavy alcohol use and both ischemic and hemorrhagic strokes.[465–468] The Finnish studies, however, used population prevalence data as a control, and other similarly designed analyses found either no such association[469] or an association only with intracerebral hemorrhage.[470] One study found that the association between alcohol intoxication and stroke disappeared when data were corrected for cigarette smoking.[471,472]

Numerous case-control and cohort studies have addressed the relationship of stroke to chronic alcohol use.[473–523] Contradictory findings are not surprising because studies have differed in endpoints chosen (e.g., total stroke, ischemic stroke, hemorrhagic stroke, or stroke mortality), amount and duration of alcohol consumption, adjustment for other risk factors (especially hypertension and smoking), ethnicity and socioeconomics of populations being studied, and selection of control subjects. Drinkers tend to be over-represented among hospitalized control subjects, which leads to the impression that alcohol is protective against stroke; they tend to be under-represented among community control subjects identified by a questionnaire, which leads to the impression that alcohol is a risk factor for stroke.[500]

In the Northern Manhattan Stroke Study, "moderate" ethanol intake (two drinks daily) protected against ischemic stroke. Protection was questionable for three to five drinks daily, and seven or more drinks increased the risk. There was no difference in benefit or risk between young and older subjects, between men and women, among white, black, and Hispanic people, or among drinkers of wine, beer, and liquor.[524]

In the U.S. Physicians' Health Study, the risk of ischemic stroke was significantly lower in subjects who had more than one drink weekly than in those who drank less. There was no difference in risk reduction between those who had one drink weekly and those who had one or more drinks daily.[525]

In the Framingham Study, when results were stratified according to age, ethanol intake reduced the risk of ischemic stroke only in subjects aged 60–69 years, and when results were stratified according to type of beverage, only wine was protective.[526] Remote but not current drinking of 12 or more grams of ethanol daily increased the risk of ischemic stroke in men but not in women.[527]

In the Cardiovascular Health Study the relative risks of ischemic stroke were 0.85, 0.75, 1.06, and 1.03 for 1, 1–6, 7–13, and 14 or more drinks per week.[528] There were lower risks among drinkers than abstainers in apoE4-negative subjects, but higher risks among drinkers than abstainers in apoE4-positive subjects. The apoE4 allele is associated with lower levels of high-density lipoprotein (HDL) and increased risk of vascular disease.[529] In another report from the Cardiovascular Health Study, red wine was associated with risk reduction in a dose-dependent manner, but other beverages were not.[530]

In a prospective study of more than 60,000 Chinese men, alcohol consumption increased the risk of both ischemic and hemorrhagic stroke in a dose-related fashion.[437] In neither stroke subtype could a protective or J-shaped relationship be found, which was consistent with other studies of Asian subjects.[531]

In 2003 a meta-analysis of 19 cohort studies and 16 case-control studies over a period of two decades found that compared with abstention, consumption of 12–24 g of ethanol per day reduced the risk of ischemic stroke (relative risk (RR), 0.72) but not of hemorrhagic stroke. Consumption of more than 60 g per day increased the risk of both ischemic stroke (RR, 1.69) and hemorrhagic stroke (RR, 2.18). Thus, as with myocardial infarction (and with the possible exception of East Asians), a J-shaped association appears to exist for ethanol consumption and risk of ischemic stroke, whereas a more linear association exists for ethanol consumption and risk of hemorrhagic stroke.[532]

Subsequent studies have found similar associations,[533–538] and a 2010 meta-analysis of 26 studies concluded that low-to-moderate ethanol consumption protects against ischemic stroke whereas higher exposure increases risk; for hemorrhagic stroke any amount of ethanol conferred risk in a dose-dependent fashion.[536] In one study, however, ethanol was not a risk factor for intracerebral and subarachnoid hemorrhage independent of tobacco smoking.[539] Ethanol does not appear to contribute to the formation or size of saccular aneurysms.[540,541] Severity of intracerebral hemorrhage may be greater among heavy drinkers, perhaps related to concomitant liver disease.[542]

A study of American health professionals found that the protective role of moderate ethanol intake in ischemic stroke was insignificant when adjusted for tobacco smoking, optimal weight, and daily exercise.[543] Healthy lifestyle could be relevant to reports of special benefit conferred by wine.

Among drinkers, stroke risk is greatest within an hour of ethanol ingestion.[542] Binge drinking is more harmful than regular daily consumption, especially in hypertensives.[544,545] Binge drinking also aggravates the development of atherosclerosis.[546]

In a French study initial severity of ischemic stroke was significantly greater among "heavy drinkers" (weekly consumption >300 g).[547] On the other hand, in rats with middle cerebral artery occlusion, ethanol given within 4 hours of ischemia reduced infarct volume.[548]

Among men with atrial fibrillation, thromboembolism was greatest among ethanol abstainers and heavy users compared to moderate drinkers.[549]

Studies with duplex ultrasonography and angiography have shown that heavy ethanol consumption raises the risk of carotid artery and aortic atherosclerosis, whereas low ethanol intake has a beneficial effect.[550–552] Similarly, a study using CT found that one to five drinks daily reduced the risk of leukoaraiosis in patients with stroke, whereas heavier alcohol consumption increased the risk.[553] The Japanese Hisayama study found alcohol to be an independent risk factor for "vascular dementia."[554] The U.S. Cardiovascular Health Study found a "U-shaped" relationship between alcohol consumption and MRI white matter abnormalities; one to seven drinks per week was most protective.[555] Other studies describe a similar relationship between moderate ethanol consumption and improved cognitive performance; the degree to which such benefit is related to alcohol's effects on cerebral circulation is uncertain.[556–561] In the Rotterdam Study, alcohol was especially effective in reducing the risk of "vascular dementia."[562]

In 2006 the American Heart Association recommended that men limit their alcohol intake to no more than two drinks per day and that women should limit their intake to no more than one drink per day. One drink was considered either 12 ounces of beer, 4 ounces of wine, or 1.5 ounces of 80-proof spirits (approximately 12.5 g absolute ethanol).[563]

As with coronary artery disease, several mechanisms might explain the association between alcohol and stroke.[564] Alcohol raises blood pressure in the short and long term,[501,503,565–578] perhaps related to increased adrenergic activity and to increased blood levels of cortisol, renin, aldosterone, and vasopressin.[578,579] Corticotropin-releasing hormone is sympathoexcitatory when administered centrally; in healthy subjects, dexamethasone blocked the increased sympathetic discharge and the increased blood pressure induced by intravenous ethanol.[580] The decline in systolic blood pressure seen during the first week after a stroke is greater in heavy drinkers than in light drinkers or abstainers,[581] and with abstinence, blood pressure may become normal.[582] Perhaps related to its protective effects, alcohol lowers blood levels of low-density lipoproteins (LDLs) and elevates levels of HDLs.[583–586]

Alcohol seems preferentially to protect large vessels from atherosclerosis, perhaps accounting for ethnic differences in patterns of protection or risk.[587] The relationship is uncertain, however, because alcohol may not raise blood levels of the more protective HDL-2 subfraction.[588,589] In the Northern Manhattan Stroke Study, the protective effect of moderate alcohol consumption on stroke risk was independent of the HDL cholesterol level.[590] In the Framingham Study, among men with the apoE2 allele, LDL cholesterol was lower in drinkers than in non-drinkers; among those with the apoE4 allele, LDL cholesterol was higher in drinkers.[591] In the Cardiovascular Health Study alcohol intake was associated with decreased total LDL particles, decreased levels of small LDL, HDL, and very-low-density lipoprotein particles, and higher levels of large LDL and medium- and large-sized HDL particles.[592]

Although heavy alcohol consumption is associated with elevated blood glucose levels, mild-to-moderate drinking lowers the risk of developing type 2 diabetes mellitus.[458,593,594]

Alcohol immediately decreases fibrinolytic activity, increases factor VIII level, increases platelet reactivity to adenosine diphosphate (ADP), and shortens bleeding time.[595–600] Ethanol raises endogenous tissue plasminogen activator,[601] reduces plasma fibrinogen levels,[602] increases levels of prostacyclin,[603,604] decreases platelet function,[559,605–609] and stimulates release of endothelin from endothelial cells.[610] In long-term alcoholics, diminished levels of clotting factors, excessive fibrinolysis, and platelet abnormalities appear to be secondary to liver disease.[579,611]

During or after ethanol withdrawal, "rebound thrombocytosis" and platelet hyperaggregability are observed.[612,613] In rats this rebound followed withdrawal from ethanol or white wine but not from red wine.[614] Human subjects with alcoholism undergoing withdrawal had decreased platelet response to activators[615] and decreased levels of tissue-type plasminogen activator inhibitor.[616]

Non-drinkers and heavy drinkers have higher blood levels of C-reactive protein than moderate drinkers, an observation relevant to the probable role of inflammation in atherosclerosis.[617]

Acute alcohol intoxication is accompanied by cerebral vasodilation[618] and blood–brain barrier leakage of albumin,[619] perhaps contributing to the severity of traumatic intracerebral hemorrhage during drinking.[620] Increased cerebral blood flow is also observed during alcohol withdrawal.[621] Compared with non-drinkers, subjects consuming less than one drink per week had increased global cerebral blood flow, whereas in those consuming more than 15 drinks per week cerebral blood flow was decreased.[622] Alcohol-related hemoconcentration may contribute to reduced cerebral blood flow.[579]

In vitro and in vivo studies involving a variety of mammals show ethanol to be a potent vasoconstrictor of brain arteries.[623–630]

Hyperhomocysteinemia is a risk factor for both myocardial ischemia and ischemic stroke, and alcoholics often have elevated blood homocysteine levels secondary to deficiency of folate, pyridoxine, or cobalamin.[631]

Studies suggesting a special protective benefit of wine, especially red wine, have led to speculation that the responsible constituents might be free radical scavengers in the form of polyphenols and flavonoids (e.g., resveratrol), which, by reducing oxidative damage to LDLs, might reduce atherogenesis.[632–637] Ethanol itself, however, is pro-oxidant.[638]

TOBACCO

Epidemiologic studies show smoking to be a major risk factor for coronary artery and peripheral vascular diseases.[639–643] Although a few reports have found no such relationship or have demonstrated only insignificant trends toward higher risk of stroke among smokers,[644–647] most case-control and cohort studies show that smoking does raise the risk of both ischemic and hemorrhagic stroke.[3,337,472,484,496,648–673]

A review in 2000 of 26 epidemiological studies concluded that current smokers have "at least a two-to-four-fold increased risk of stroke compared to nonsmokers or individuals who had quit smoking more than 10 years prior." The risk was sixfold if smokers were compared with non-smokers who had never been exposed to second-hand smoke.[674] Up to half of cryptogenic ischemic strokes in young adults are attributable to cigarette smoking.[675] In women smokers, the risk of ischemic and hemorrhagic stroke is enhanced in those taking oral contraceptives.[676–680] In one report, smoking in hypertensive men and women carried a 15-fold risk for subarachnoid hemorrhage and was a greater risk than hypertension itself.[649] In another report, the treatment of hypertension reduced stroke incidence in non-smokers but not in smokers.[681] Tobacco smoking, hypertension, and high blood cholesterol levels appear to interact synergistically as stroke risk factors.[682] Patients with ischemic stroke who smoke tend to be younger than those who do not.[683]

Stroke risk among smokers is dose-dependent and independent of age, cardiac disease, oral contraceptives, alcohol, and hypertension.[668,684–688] Stroke risk decreases with cessation of smoking,[577,583,689] but a small long-term excess risk persists.[690] Smoking is a risk factor for central retinal artery occlusion as well as for aortic plaque formation.[691,692]

Smokers were not over-represented among 624 consecutive patients with non-arteritic ischemic optic neuropathy.[693] Among smokers, the risk of stroke mortality is reduced in those who smoke cigarettes with lower tar yield.[694] On the other hand, stroke was reported after application of a nicotine patch.[695]

Several studies found that passive as well as active smoking increased stroke risk,[690,696–699] although a meta-analysis of 16 such studies concluded that a causal relationship was "only suggestive."[700] A 2011 meta-analysis of 20 studies found "a strong consistent and dose-dependent association between exposure to second-hand smoke and risk of stroke." No safe lower limit of exposure was identified.[701] A cross-sectional study found second-hand exposure to be an independent risk factor for peripheral arterial disease.[702]

A study from Sweden found that, although smokeless tobacco (oral snuff) did not increase the risk of stroke, it did increase the risk of fatal stroke.[703] A meta-analysis of 11 studies found an increased risk of fatal myocardial infarction and fatal stroke among users of smokeless tobacco products compared to non-users.[704]

A study in 2000 from the UK estimated that an intensive smoking reduction program (as had been adopted but then abandoned in California) would prevent 455 strokes during the year 2000 and 11,304 strokes by 2010.[705]

A European study, noting a decrease in stroke prevalence in Western Europe but a rise in Eastern Europe, attributed the difference to the higher prevalence of tobacco use in Eastern Europe.[706] A study from China estimated that (1) in 1990, 600,000 Chinese deaths (500,000 in men) were attributable to tobacco, (2) by 2000, this figure would rise to 800,000, and (3) of all Chinese males currently younger than 30 years of age, one-third would die prematurely as a consequence of smoking and 5–8% of their deaths would be caused by stroke.[707]

"Smoker's paradox" refers to decreased mortality in smokers compared to non-smokers following acute myocardial infarction. Smoking is also independently associated with reduced mortality following acute ischemic stroke. Proposed mechanisms include "tobacco-induced changes in cerebrovascular vasoreactivity."[708]

In a case-control study, tobacco use was not a risk factor for vascular dementia. A proposed explanation was "survivorship bias."[709]

Several possible mechanisms could underlie tobacco's association with risk of stroke.[710] Smoking aggravates atherosclerosis. In a study of identical twins who were discordant for smoking, carotid plaques were significantly more prominent in the smokers.[711] In other reports, smoking correlated in dose-related fashion with severity of extracranial carotid atherosclerosis.[712,713]

In the Atherosclerosis Risk in Communities Study, current cigarette smoking was associated with a 50% increase in the progression over 3 years of carotid artery atherosclerosis compared with non-smoking; past smoking was associated with a 25% increase, and passive exposure to environmental smoke was associated with a 20% increase.[714] Smoking one cigarette causes transient increases in arterial wall stiffness that increase the likelihood of plaque formation.[715] The reduction in stroke risk with cessation of smoking, however, argues against the possibility that such large-vessel atherosclerosis is paramount.[572,716–718] Carbon monoxide in cigarette smoke reduces blood's oxygen-carrying capacity, and nicotine constricts coronary arteries.[719,720]

An ultrasound study of 1084 asymptomatic subjects found carotid intima-media thickness (C-IMT) highest in smokers, lower in former smokers, and lowest in never smokers. C-IMT was not related to high or low nicotine, tar, or carbon monoxide.[721]

Coronary artery constriction and the greater myocardial oxygen demand induced by cocaine are exacerbated by concomitant tobacco smoking.[722] In animals, nicotine damages endothelium, and increased numbers of circulating endothelial cells are found in smokers.[723,724] Neonates exposed to environmental tobacco smoke already demonstrated endothelial cell damage during the first month of life.[725] Bovine endothelial cells exposed to nicotine demonstrated giant cell formation and cellular vacuolization.[726] Cigarette smoking produces superoxide anions, reduces production and availability of nitric oxide, and increases production and release of endothelin.[727] Tobacco smoke exacerbates inflammation, with overexpression of vascular adhesion molecules and release of pro-inflammatory cytokines.[728] Endothelial dysfunction includes "leaky brain microvessels" and loss of blood–brain barrier integrity.[729]

Smoking immediately raises blood pressure, systolic more than diastolic.[730,731] Whether smoking is a risk factor for chronic hypertension is less clear,[732] although it does accelerate the progression of chronic hypertension to malignant hypertension.[733,734] Smokers become tachycardic, and atrial fibrillation has been observed after chewing nicotine gum.[719]

Smoking activates the coagulant pathway, increases platelet reactivity, and inhibits prostacyclin formation.[716,735–741] It raises blood fibrinogen levels, and polycythemia secondary to smoking increases blood viscosity.[739] In cultures of human brain endothelial cells, nicotine increased production of plasminogen activator inhibitor-1 (PAI-1).[740] In rats, nicotine-induced depletion of tissue plasminogen activator was associated with enhanced focal ischemic brain injury.[742] Increased plasma levels of PAI-1 are found in smokers.[743,744]

The increased risk of subarachnoid hemorrhage in smokers has been blamed on greater elastolytic activity in the serum.[745]

Smokers who receive intravenous thrombolysis for either acute myocardial infarction or acute ischemic stroke have a better early outcome than non-smokers.[746] A proposed mechanism is that increased circulating levels of fibrinogen induced by smoking makes thrombolysis more effective.[747]

The relative contributions of nicotine, tars, and the gaseous constituents of cigarette smoke to cardiovascular disease are uncertain.[748] Transdermal or oral nicotine produces plasma levels of platelet activation products (platelet factor 4 and β-thromboglobulin) and von Willebrand factor that are intermediate between those of smokers and non-smokers.[749]

Although stroke was reported after application of a nicotine patch, a meta-analysis of 35 clinical trials involving the transdermal nicotine patch found no excess incidence of myocardial infarction or stroke.[750] Effects of tobacco smoke and nicotine on cerebral blood flow are complex because nicotine has both direct and indirect effects on cerebral vessels themselves as well as on neuronal nicotinic receptors, and both carbon dioxide and nitric oxide are vasodilators. In volunteers, several puffs on a lighted cigarette during a 5-minute period increased middle cerebral artery flow velocity in all subjects; onset and offset were detected within a few seconds of starting and stopping smoking. The effect was independent of CO_2 autoregulation, and, in fact, smoking suppressed CO_2-induced vasodilation by 56% in men (but by only 5% in women).[751]

Animal studies confirm the complex interplay of thromboxane A2, sympathetic activation, calcium and potassium channels, and nitric oxide in cerebrovascular responses to nicotine.[752–755]

A possible role for inflammation in tobacco's effects on vessels and coagulation factors is suggested by an increased risk of stroke among young female smokers carrying single nucleotide polymorphisms for particular mediators of inflammation.[756]

Progressive multifocal symptoms were observed in four young women who smoked and used oral contraceptives. Cerebral angiography demonstrated moyamoya vessels. Disease progression ceased with discontinuation of oral contraceptives and reduction in smoking.[757] In another series of 39 patients with moyamoya disease, the use of tobacco and oral contraceptives was also over-represented.[758]

An elderly man had syncopal spells whenever he stood up after smoking a cigarette; the spells ceased when he stopped smoking. SPECT showed decreased cerebral perfusion "in the posterior circulation structures" after this patient smoked a cigarette or chewed nicotine gum.[759]

The complete reference list can be found on the companion Expert Consult website at www.expertconsult.inkling.com.

KEY REFERENCES

2. Brust JCM. Neurological aspects of substance abuse. 2nd ed. Newton, MA: Butterworth-Heinemann; 2004.
5. De los Rios F, Kleindorfer DO, Khoury J, et al. Trends in substance abuse preceding stroke among young adults. A population-based study. Stroke 2012;43:3179.
13. Brust JCM, Dickinson PCT, Hughes JEO, et al. The diagnosis and treatment of cerebral mycotic aneurysms. Ann Neurol 1990; 27:238.
16. Brust JCM, Richter RW. Stroke associated with addiction to heroin. J Neurol Neurosurg Psychiatry 1976;39:194.
32. Anderson SN, Skullerud K. Hypoxic/ischemic brain damage, especially pallidal lesions, in heroin addicts. Forensic Sci Int 1999;102:51.
35. Niehaus L, Meyer B-U. Bilateral borderzone brain infarctions in association with heroin abuse. J Neurol Sci 1998;160:180.
56. Sahni V, Garg D, Garg S, et al. Unusual complications of heroin abuse: transverse myelitis, rhabdomyolysis, compartment syndrome, and ARF. Clin Toxicol 2008;46:153.
62. Esse K, Fossati-Bellani M, Traylor A, et al. Epidemic of illicit drug use, mechanisms of action/addiction and stroke as a health hazard. Brain Behav 2011;doi:10.10002/brb3.7.
63. Ho EL, Josephson SA, Lee HS, et al. Cerebrovascular complications of methamphetamine use. Neurocrit Care 2009;10:295.
101. McGee SM, McGee DN, McGee MB. Spontaneous intracerebral hemorrhage related to methamphetamine abuse. Autopsy findings and clinical correlation. Am J Forensic Med Pathol 2004; 25:334.
114. Petitti DB, Sidney S, Quesenberry C, et al. Stroke and cocaine or amphetamine use. Epidemiology 1998;9:596.
115. Westover AN, McBride S, Haley RW. Stroke in young adults who abuse amphetamines or cocaine. A population-based study of hospitalized patients. Arch Gen Psychiatry 2007;64:495.
116. Citron BP, Halpern M, McCarron M, et al. Necrotizing angiitis associated with drug abuse. N Engl J Med 1970;283:1003.
121. DeSilva DA, Wang MC, Lee MP, et al. Amphetamine-associated ischemic stroke: Clinical presentation and proposed pathogenesis. J Stroke Cerebrovasc Dis 2007;16:185.
145. Kernan WN, Viscdi CM, Brass LM, et al. Phenylpropanolamine and the risk of hemorrhagic stroke. N Engl J Med 2000;343:1826.
147. Cantu C, Arauz A, Murillo-Bonilla LM, et al. Stroke associated with sympathomimetics contained in over-the-counter cough and cold drugs. Stroke 2003;34:1667.
150. Bruno A, Nolte KB, Chapin J. Stroke associated with ephedrine use. Neurology 1993;43:1313.
165. Haller CA, Benowitz NL. Adverse cardiovascular and central nervous system events associated with dietary supplements containing ephedra alkaloids. N Engl J Med 2000;343:1833.
169. Morgenstern MD, Viscoli CM, Kernan WN, et al. Use of ephedra-containing products and risk for hemorrhagic stroke. Neurology 2003;60:132.
175. Schifano F, Oyefeso A, Webb L, et al. Review of deaths related to taking ecstasy, England and Wales, 1997–2000. BMJ 2003; 326:80.
187. De Smet K, De Maeseneer M, Talebian YA, et al. Bilateral globus pallidus infarcts in ecstasy use. JBR-BTR 2011;94:93.
190. Lee GYF, Gong GWK, Vrodos N. "Ecstasy"-induced subarachnoid hemorrhage: an under-reported neurological complication? J Clin Neurosci 2003;10:705.
192. Spatt J, Glawar B, Mamoli B. A pure amnestic syndrome after MDMA ("ecstasy") ingestion. J Neurol Neurosurg Psychiatry 1997;62:418.
193. Drees JC, Stone JA, Wu AHB. Morbidity involving the hallucinogenic designer amines MDA and 2C-I. J Forensic Sci 2009;54:1485.
197. Thomalla G, Kucinski T, Weiller C, et al. Cerebral vasculitis following oral methylphenidate intake in an adult: A case report. World J Biol Psychiatry 2006;7:56.
200. Schelleman H, Bilker WB, Kimmel SE, et al. Methylphenidate and risk of serious cardiovascular events in adults. Am J Psychiatry 2012;169:178.
210. Miotto K, Striebel J, Cho AK, et al. Clinical and pharmacological aspects of bath salt use: a review of the literature and case reports. Drug Alcohol Depend 2013;132:1.
211. Kulkarni SV, Mughani YAA, Onbol EHA, et al. Khat and stroke, Ann India Acad Neurol. 2012;15:139.
214. Kaku DA, Lowenstein DH. Emergence of recreational drug abuse as a major risk factor for stroke in young adults. Ann Intern Med 1990;113:821.
215. Levine SR, Brust JCM, Futrell N, et al. Cerebrovascular complications of the use of the "crack" form of alkaloidal cocaine. N Engl J Med 1990;323:699.
298. Silver B, Miller D, Jankowski M, et al. Urine toxicology screening in an urban stroke and TIA population. Neurology 2013;80: 1702.
299. Bhattacharya P, Taraman S, Shankar L, et al. Clinical profiles, complications, and disability in cocaine-related ischemic stroke. J Stroke Cerebrovasc Dis 2011;20:443.
301. Giraldo EA, Yaqi MA, Vaidean GD. A case-control study of stroke risk factors and outcomes in African American stroke patients with and without crack-cocaine abuse. Neurocrit Care 2012; 16:273.
317. Han JS, Mandell DM, Poublanc J, et al. BOLD-MRI cerebrovascular reactivity findings in cocaine-induced cerebral vasculitis. Nat Clin Pract Neurol 2008;4:628.
320. Streeter LIK, Ahn KH, Lee HK, et al. White matter hyperintensities in subjects with cocaine and opiate dependence and healthy comparison subjects. Psychiatry Res 2004;131:135.
327. Martin-Schild S, Albright KC, Hallevi H, et al. Intracerebral hemorrhage in cocaine users. Stroke 2010;41:680.
332. Chang TR, Kowalski RG, Caserta F, et al. Impact of acute cocaine use on aneurysmal subarachnoid hemorrhage. Stroke 2013; 44:1825.
348. Kaufman MJ, Levin JM, Ross MH, et al. Cocaine-induced cerebral vasoconstriction detected in humans with magnetic resonance angiography. JAMA 1998;279:376.
351. Martin-Schild S, Albright KC, Misra V, et al. Intravenous tissue plasminogen activator in patients with cocaine-associated acute ischemic stroke. Stroke 2009;40:3635.

363. Pereira J, Saez CG, Panes O, et al. Platelet activation in chronic cocaine users: effect of short term abstinence. Platelets 2011; 22:596.
369. Hobbs WE, Moore EE, Penkala RA, et al. Cocaine and specific cocaine metabolites induce von Willebrand factor release from endothelial cells in a tissue-specific manner. Stroke 2013; 33:1230.
371. Randell T. Cocaine, alcohol mix in body to form even longer lasting, more lethal drug. JAMA 1992;267:1043.
385. Bolla K, Ernst M, Kiehl K, et al. Prefrontal cortical dysfunction in abstinent cocaine abusers. J Neuropsychiatry Clin Neurosci 2004;16:456.
390. Rao H, Wang J, Gianetta J, et al. Altered resting cerebral blood flow in adolescents with in utero cocaine exposure revealed by perfusion functional MRI. Pediatrics 2007;120:e1245.
396. Besson HA. Intracranial hemorrhage associated with phencyclidine abuse. JAMA 1982;248:585.
401. Lieberman AN, Bloom W, Kishore PS, et al. Carotid artery occlusion following ingestion of LSD. Stroke 1974;5:213.
422. Wolff V, Armspach J-P, Lauer V, et al. Cannabis-related stroke. Myth or reality? Stroke 2013;44:558.
423. Singh NN, Pan Y, Muengtaweeponsa S, et al. Cannabis-related stroke: case series and review of literature. J Stroke Cerebrovasc Dis 2012;21:555.
425. Wolff V, Lauer V, Rouyer O, et al. Cannabis use, ischemic stroke, and multifocal intracranial vasoconstriction: a prospective study in 48 consecutive young patients. Stroke 2011;42:1178.
450. Seely KA, Papoint J, Moran JH, et al. Spice drugs are more than harmless herbal blends: a review of the pharmacology and toxicology of synthetic cannabinoids. Prog Neuropsychopharmacol Biol Psychiatr 2012;39:234.
453. Freeman MJ, Rose DZ, Myers MA, et al. Ischemic stroke following use of synthetic marijuana "spice". Neurology 2013;81:1.
495. Feigin VL, Rinkel GJ, Lowes CM, et al. Risk factors for subarachnoid hemorrhage: An updated systematic review of epidemiological studies. Stroke 2005;36:2773.
516. Camargo CA. Moderate alcohol consumption and stroke: The epidemiologic evidence. Stroke 1989;20:1611.
524. Sacco RL, Elkind M, Baden-Albala B, et al. The protective effect of moderate alcohol consumption on ischemic stroke. JAMA 1999;281:53.
526. Djoussé L, Ellison RC, Beiser A, et al. Alcohol consumption and risk of ischemic stroke: The Framingham Study. Stroke 2002; 33:907.
528. Mukamal KJ, Chung H, Jenny NS, et al. Alcohol use and risk of ischemic stroke among older adults. The Cardiovascular Health Study. Stroke 2005;36:1830.
538. Feigin VL, Rinkel GJE, Lawes CMM, et al. Risk factors for subarachnoid hemorrhage. An updated systematic review of epidemiological studies. Stroke 2005;36:2773.
542. Hillbom M, Saloheimo P, Juvela S. Alcohol consumption, blood pressure, and the risk of stroke. Curr Hypertens Rep 2011;13:208.
543. Chiuve SE, Rexrode KM, Spiegelman D, et al. Primary prevention of stroke by healthy lifestyle. Circulation 2008;118:947.
544. Sundell L, Salomaa V, Vartianen E, et al. Increased stroke risk is related to binge-driking habit. Stroke 2008;39:3179.
546. Rantakomi SH, Laukkamen JA, Kurl S, et al. Binge drinking and the progression of atherosclerosis in middle-aged men: an 11 year follow-up. Athersclerosis 2009;205:266.
590. Elkind SMV, Sciacca R, Boden-Albala B, et al. Moderate alcohol consumption reduces risk of ischemic stroke in the Northern Manhattan Study. Stroke 2006;37:13.
637. Saremi A, Arora R. The cardiovascular implications of alcohol and red wine. Am J Ther 2008;15:265.
668. Shinton R, Beevers G. Meta-analysis of relation between cigarette smoking and stroke. BMJ 1989;298:789.
672. Anderson CS, Feigin V, Bennett D, et al. Active and passive smoking and the risk of subarachnoid hemorrhage: an international population-based case-control study. Stroke 2004;35:633.
673. Koshinen LO, Blomstedt PC. Smoking and non-smoking tobacco as risk factors in subarachnoid hemorrhage. Acta Neurol Scand 2006;114:33.
674. Shah RS, Cole JW. Smoking and stroke: the more you smoke the more you stroke. Expert Rev Cardiovasc Ther 2010;8:917.
685. Bhat VM, Cole JW, Sorkin JD, et al. Dose-response relationship between cigarette smoking and risk of ischemic stroke in young women. Stroke 2008;39:249.
700. Lea PN, Forey BA. Environmental tobacco smoke exposure and risk of stroke in nonsmokers: a review of meta-analysis. Stroke Cerebrovasc Dis 2006;15:190.
702. Lu L, Mackay DF, Pell JP. Association between level of exposure to secondhand smoke and peripheral arterial disease: cross-sectional study of 5686 never smokers. Athersclerosis 2013; 229:273.
704. Boffetta P, Straif K. Use of smokeless tobacco and risk of myocardial infarction and stroke: systematic review with meta-analysis. BMJ 2009;339:b3060. doi:10.1136/bmj.b.3060.
710. Hawkins BT, Brown RC, Davis TP. Smoking and ischemic stroke: A role for nicotine? Trends Pharmacol Sci 2002;23:8.
721. Baldassarre D, Castelnuovo S, Frigerio B, et al. Effects of timing and extent of smoking, type of cigarettes, and concomitant risk factors on the association between smoking and subclinical atherosclerosis. Stroke 2009;40:1991.
727. Rhaman MM, Laher I. Structural and functional alteration of blood vessels caused by cigarette smoking: an overview of molecular mechanisms. Curr Vasc Pharmacol 2007;5:276.
728. Hossain M, Mazzone P, Tierney W, et al. In vitro assessment of tobacco smoke toxicity at the BBB: do antioxidant supplements have a protective role? BMC Neurosci 2011;12:92.
756. Cole JW, Brown DW, Giles WH, et al. Ischemic stroke risk, smoking, and the genetics of inflammation in a biracial population: The Stroke Prevention in Young Women Study. Thromb J 2008;6:11.

40 Moyamoya Disease

Masahiro Yasaka, Takenori Yamaguchi, Jun Ogata

KEY POINTS

- Moyamoya disease is an unusual form of chronic cerebrovascular occlusive disease that is characterized by angiographic findings of bilateral stenosis or occlusion at the terminal portion of the internal carotid artery together with an abnormal vascular network at the base of the brain.
- The major cellular components of the thickened intima formed in arteries of the circle of Willis and the major branches are smooth muscle cells. Migration and proliferation of smooth muscle cells in the intima, induced by unknown mechanisms, may lead to the intimal thickening in association with morphologic and biochemical alteration of extracellular matrix components including elastin, collagen, and other proteoglycans.
- Clinical symptoms and signs are the manifestations of cerebrovascular events secondary to the intracranial vascular lesions, including hemorrhagic stroke, ischemic stroke, transient ischemic attacks (TIAs) and seizure.
- Ischemic events are common in childhood, whereas hemorrhagic strokes are frequently seen in adulthood.
- The largest peak in age distribution is observed in 10–14-year-old patients, with a smaller peak in their 40s.
- Remarkable regional differences in the frequency have been reported. Incidence is high in Japan and large numbers of patients were also reported in Korea and China. The female-to-male ratio is 1.8 : 1.
- Although genetic linkage analysis demonstrated that hereditary factors may be involved in susceptibility to moyamoya disease, etiology has not been fully elucidated yet.
- Ischemic and hemorrhagic lesions can be detected by MRI and CT. Stenotic or occlusive lesions at the distal ends of the internal carotid arteries are demonstrated by MRA. Apparent moyamoya vessels can be visualized as fine unusual vessels on MRA and also as a signal void on the MRI.
- Carotid ultrasonography is useful to evaluate diameter greatly reduced at the proximal portion of the internal carotid artery above the bulbus like a Champagne bottle neck.
- Antiplatelet agents are prescribed to prevent recurrent ischemic attacks, although they have never been tested thoroughly in clinical trials. Surgical revascularization including direct bypass surgery, indirect bypass surgery, and a combination of the two has been performed to give additional collateral flow to the ischemic brain.

Moyamoya disease is an unusual form of chronic cerebrovascular occlusive disease that is characterized by angiographic findings of bilateral stenosis or occlusion at the terminal portion of the internal carotid artery together with an abnormal vascular network at the base of the brain (Fig. 40-1).[1–5] The first report of a patient with this disease was published in 1957 by Takeuchi and Shimizu[6] with the diagnosis of "bilateral hypoplasia of the internal carotid arteries." This patient was a 29-year-old man who had been suffering from visual disturbance and hemiconvulsive seizures since the age of 10 years. Takeuchi and Shimizu[6] considered this arterial occlusion to be congenital hypoplasia that differed from atherosclerosis on the basis of the histologic examination of a branch of the external carotid artery. Since then, similar cases have been reported, mainly among the Japanese, and a variety of names have been applied to the condition – "cerebral juxtabasal telangiectasia" by Sano,[7] "cerebral arterial rete" by Handa and colleagues,[8] "rete mirabile" by Weidner and associates,[9] and "cerebral basal rete mirabile" by Nishimoto and Takeuchi.[10] The terms "spontaneous occlusion of the circle of Willis," used by Kudo,[11] and "moyamoya disease" are now commonly used in the literature. The term *moyamoya disease* was proposed by Suzuki and Takaku,[12] taken from the characteristic angiographic findings of an abnormal vascular network at the base of the brain; the Japanese word *moyamoya*, meaning "vague or hazy puff of smoke," describes its appearance.

Extensive investigations of patients with this characteristic angiographic finding have been conducted over the past 50 years. It is now well known that progression of stenosis or occlusion of the intracranial major arteries, including the distal ends of the internal carotid arteries, is the primary lesion of this disease and that the abnormal vascular network (moyamoya vessels) at the base of the brain is their collateral supply, developed secondary to brain ischemia (see Fig. 40-1).[2,4,5,13] A guideline for the diagnosis of moyamoya disease was established by the Research Committee on Spontaneous Occlusion of the Circle of Willis, organized by the Ministry of Health and Welfare, Japan (MHWJ), and the latest version (1997) was published in Japanese and English.[2,14–16] Because the clinical features, radiologic findings, progress on etiology and pathogenesis, and pathologic findings have been sufficiently described in the previous edition of this textbook and elsewhere,[4,13] we use the present chapter to add new knowledge on ultrasonography, MRI, etc.

GUIDELINE FOR DIAGNOSIS

The guideline for the diagnosis of moyamoya disease developed by the MHWJ's Research Committee on Spontaneous Occlusion of the Circle of Willis (Boxes 40-1, 40-2)[2] has been used not only for patient diagnosis but also for follow-up and further investigation into the etiology and pathogenesis of this unique and mysterious disorder.

Prior to 1995, the guideline stated that cerebral angiography is indispensable to diagnosis in all but the autopsied cases. Because the quality of the images of MRI and MR angiography

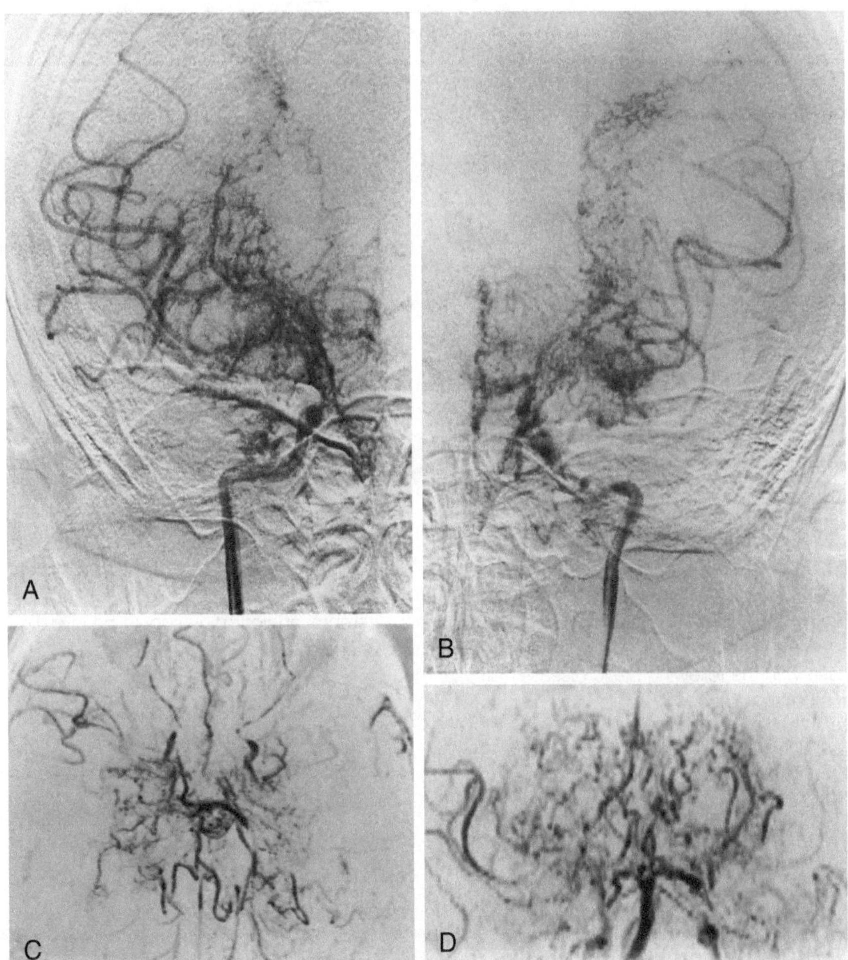

Figure 40-1. Conventional cerebral angiograms (A and B) and MR angiograms (C and D) in a 10-year-old boy with moyamoya disease. Anteroposterior views in conventional angiograms show (A) severe stenosis of the right middle cerebral artery (MCA) and (B) nearly complete occlusion of the left MCA. Well-developed basal moyamoya vessels are also seen. MR angiograms of this patient show findings similar to those observed on conventional angiograms: C, basal view; D, anteroposterior view. *(From Houkin K, Aoki T, Takahashi A, et al: Diagnosis of moyamoya disease with magnetic resonance angiography.* Stroke *25:2159, 1994.)*

(MRA) has improved, the Research Committee concluded in 1995 that the diagnosis can be made without conventional cerebral angiography if MRI and MRA clearly demonstrate all the findings that indicate moyamoya disease.[17–19] The diagnostic criteria applied to the MRI and MRA were added as a supplemented reference in the revision (see Box 40-2).[2] The substitution of non-invasive imaging methods for angiography is helpful for patients, especially children.

This revision also contains the addition of autoimmune disorders to the list of disorders that should be considered in any patient being evaluated for moyamoya disease, to avoid confusing this disease with other disorders in which vascular lesions resembling those of moyamoya disease can form. A correct diagnosis is essential for selecting the optimal plan of treatment.

EPIDEMIOLOGY

The incidence and prevalence of moyamoya disease in the Japanese have been surveyed by collaborative studies in 1984, 1989, and 1994.[20] The prevalence and annual incidence are calculated to be 3.16 and 0.35 per 100,000 population, respectively. Female preponderance has been reported with a female-to-male ratio of 1.8 : 1.[20] The largest peak in age distribution was observed in patients 10 to 14 years old, with a smaller peak in patients in their 40s. The age at onset was younger than 10 years in 47.8% of the patients (childhood moyamoya), although the disease had developed in some patients between the ages of 25 and 49 years (adult-type moyamoya) (Fig. 40-2).

Evidence of familial moyamoya disease has been accumulating in the medical literature.[4,21–23] Family histories of moyamoya disease were found in 10% of patients, and 13 pairs of homozygous twins were reported as having the disease.[20] The contribution of hereditary factors to the occurrence of moyamoya disease is discussed later, in the section on etiology and pathogenesis.

Although regional predilection has never been reported within Japan, there are remarkable regional differences in the frequency of reported moyamoya worldwide.[15,16] After the report by Taveras in 1969,[24] reports of moyamoya disease have been growing among non-Japanese people, including white and black people, although it is rare in white patients.[16,25] None of the races has as high an incidence as the Japanese, but relatively large numbers of patients have been found in Korea[26,27] and China.[28,29]

Korean neurosurgeons performed the first nationwide cooperative survey of moyamoya disease in their country in

BOX 40-1 Diagnostic Guidelines for Spontaneous Occlusion of the Circle of Willis (Moyamoya Disease)

1. Cerebral angiography is indispensable for the diagnosis, and should present at least the following findings:
   a. Stenosis or occlusion at the terminal portion of the internal carotid artery and/or at the proximal portion of the anterior and/or middle cerebral arteries
   b. Abnormal vascular networks seen in the vicinity of the occlusive or stenotic lesions in the arterial phase
   c. These findings should present bilaterally
2. When magnetic resonance imaging (MRI) and magnetic resonance angiography (MRA) clearly demonstrate all the findings described below, conventional cerebral angiography is not mandatory:
   a. Stenosis or occlusion at the terminal portion of the internal carotid artery and at the proximal portion of the anterior and middle cerebral arteries on MRA
   b. An abnormal vascular network in the basal ganglia on MRA. Note: An abnormal vascular network can be diagnosed when more than two apparent flow voids are seen in one side of the basal ganglia on MRI
   c. 2-a and 2-b are seen bilaterally. (Refer to Image Diagnostic Guidelines by MRI and MRA [Box 40-2].)
3. Because the etiology of this disease is unknown, cerebrovascular disease with the following basic diseases or conditions should thus be eliminated:
   a. Arteriosclerosis
   b. Autoimmune disease
   c. Meningitis
   d. Brain neoplasm
   e. Down syndrome
   f. Recklinghausen's disease
   g. Head trauma
   h. Irradiation to the head
   i. Others
4. Instructive pathologic findings:
   a. Intimal thickening and the resulting stenosis or occlusion of the lumen are observed in and around the terminal portion of the internal carotid artery, usually on both sides. Lipid deposit is occasionally seen in thickened intima
   b. Arteries constituting the circle of Willis such as the anterior and middle cerebral and posterior communicating arteries often show stenosis of varying degrees or occlusion associated with fibrocellular thickening of the intima, a waving of the internal elastic lamina, and an attenuation of the media
   c. Numerous small vascular channels (perforators and anastomotic branches) are observed around the circle of Willis
   d. Reticular conglomerates of small vessels are often seen in the pia mater
5. Diagnosis: In reference to 1–4 mentioned above, the diagnostic criteria are classified as follows. Autopsy cases not undergoing cerebral angiography should be investigated separately while referring to 4.
   a. Definite case: One that fulfills either 1 or 2, and 3. In children, however, a case that fulfills 1-a and 1-b (or 2-a and 2-b) on one side and with remarkable stenosis at the terminal portion of the internal carotid artery on the opposite side is also included
   b. A probable case: One that fulfills 1-a and 1-b (or 2-a and 2-b) and 3 (unilateral involvement)

From Fukui M: Guidelines for the diagnosis and treatment of spontaneous occlusion of the circle of Willis ("moyamoya" disease). Research Committee on Spontaneous Occlusion of the Circle of Willis (Moyamoya Disease) of the Ministry of Health and Welfare, Japan. Clin Neurol Neurosurg *99(Suppl 2):S238, 1997.*

BOX 40-2 Image Diagnostic Guidelines for Moyamoya Disease by MRI and MRA

1. When magnetic resonance imaging (MRI) and magnetic resonance angiography (MRA) clearly demonstrate all the findings described below, conventional cerebral angiography is not mandatory:
   a. Stenosis or occlusion at the terminal portion of the intracranial internal carotid artery and at the proximal portion of the anterior and middle cerebral arteries
   b. An abnormal vascular network in the basal ganglia
   c. 1-a and 1-b are seen bilaterally
2. Imaging methods and judgment:
   a. More than a 1.0 tesla magnetic field strength is recommended
   b. There are no restrictions regarding MRA imaging methods
   c. The imaging parameters, such as the magnetic field strength, the imaging methods, and the use of contrast medium, should be clearly documented
   d. An abnormal vascular network can be diagnosed when more than two apparent flow voids are seen on one side of the basal ganglia on MRI
   e. Either an over- or underestimation of the lesion could be made according to the imaging conditions. To avoid a false-positive diagnosis, only definite cases should thus be diagnosed on the MRI and MRA findings
3. Because similar vascular lesions secondary to other disorders are sometimes indistinguishable from this disease in adults, a diagnosis based on MRI and MRA without conventional angiography is thus only recommended in pediatric cases

From Fukui M: Guidelines for the diagnosis and treatment of spontaneous occlusion of the circle of Willis ("moyamoya" disease). Research Committee on Spontaneous Occlusion of the Circle of Willis (Moyamoya Disease) of the Ministry of Health and Welfare, Japan. Clin Neurol Neurosurg *99(Suppl 2):S238, 1997.*

1988, and 289 patients were registered.[26] The reported clinical features of these patients were different from those of Japanese patients, raising questions about whether this heterogeneity suggests racial and regional differences or differences between the criteria used for diagnosis in the two countries. Further analysis by Japanese investigators reclassified the Korean cases into definite, probable, and unlikely cases.[30] The definite cases had similar clinical features and age at onset in both populations. There was a slight female predominance (ratio 1.3 : 1), and the incidence of hemorrhage was higher in females than in males. The incidence of brain infarction and hemorrhage was significantly higher, whereas the rates of transient ischemic

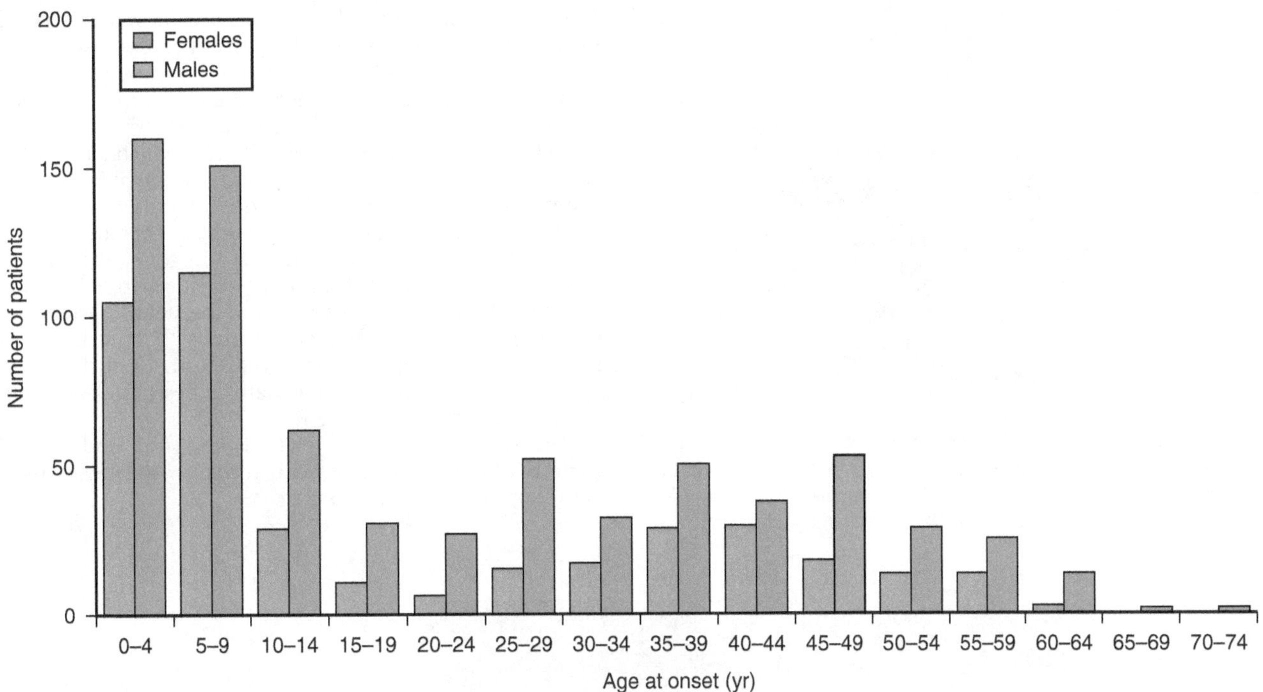

Figure 40-2. Distribution of age at onset and sex of patients with moyamoya disease. *(From Wakai K, Tamakoshi A, Ikezaki K, et al: Epidemiological features of moyamoya disease in Japan: Findings from a nationwide survey.* Clin Neurol Neurosurg *99[Suppl 2]:S1, 1997.)*

attacks and seizures were lower in Korean than in Japanese subjects. The incidence of infarction in children and that of hemorrhage in both children and adults were also statistically higher in Koreans.

Such studies should be undertaken in Western and other Asian countries for clarification of the racial significance and genetic background of this disease.

PATHOLOGY

Pathologic observations of approximately 100 autopsy cases of moyamoya disease revealed various forms of cerebrovascular lesions in the brain, and their macroscopic and microscopic findings have been accumulated.[8,31–38] The lesion observed most commonly at autopsy is intracranial hemorrhage, which is a major cause of death for patients with moyamoya disease.[37] Massive parenchymatous hemorrhage (intracerebral hemorrhage) occurs frequently in the basal ganglia, thalamus, hypothalamus, cerebral peduncle, and midbrain, and often extends and ruptures to the intraventricular spaces.[37] Subarachnoid hemorrhage (SAH) also occurs, but primary SAH caused by rupture of aneurysms seems to be not so frequent as described previously, and many cases appear to be secondary extensions of parenchymatous hemorrhage. In addition, old brain infarction and focal cortical atrophy of the brain are not uncommon findings and are often found in multiples.[37,38] Furthermore, the infarcts are mostly small and localized in the basal ganglia, internal capsule, thalamus, and subcortex. Large arterial territorial infarcts[39] are rare in moyamoya disease, although occlusion of the intracranial major arteries is present. This finding may suggest the function of moyamoya vessels as collateral pathways after arterial occlusion. The frequency and distribution of intracranial hemorrhage and infarction found at autopsy may not be typical of moyamoya disease, as such specimens obtained from the circle of Willis and moyamoya vessels are biased by the unavoidable clinical circumstances related to their deaths. Nevertheless, the histologic and immunohistochemical analyses of the postmortem materials have provided valuable information relating to the pathogenesis of lesion formation in this disease.

The Circle of Willis and the Major Branches

In the guideline for the diagnosis of moyamoya disease, the pathologic findings in the intracranial arteries are included to allow for diagnosis in patients who did not undergo angiography during life (see Box 40-1).[2,3] The histologic appearance of the circle of Willis and the major branches of the patients with moyamoya disease is characteristic, but not specific for this disease.[33,34,38] Therefore, it is not always possible to diagnose moyamoya disease solely on the basis of pathologic findings.

On macroscopic observation, the circle of Willis and the major branches are tapered and narrowed entirely or partially with overgrown and dilated arteries branching from the circle of Willis (Fig. 40-3). The degree of tapering of arteries as well as the network formation of dilated arteries (moyamoya vessels) and their distributions vary from case to case. The distal ends of the internal carotid arteries are affected by severe narrowing or occlusion.

In conventional staining of specimens obtained from the circle of Willis or its major branches with lesion involvement, the arterial lumen is severely narrowed or occluded by fibrocellular intimal thickening (Figs 40-4A, 40-5A).[33,34,36,38] The thickened intima appears to be in a laminated structure with duplication or triplication of internal elastic lamina and a wavy appearance. These features closely resemble the structure noted focally at arterial branching portions in normal controls, the so-called intimal cushion. The outer diameter of the affected artery usually becomes smaller, and the underlying media are markedly attenuated. These histologic features are common to lesions at any site, although the extent of intimal thickening and the distribution in the circle of Willis are variable.

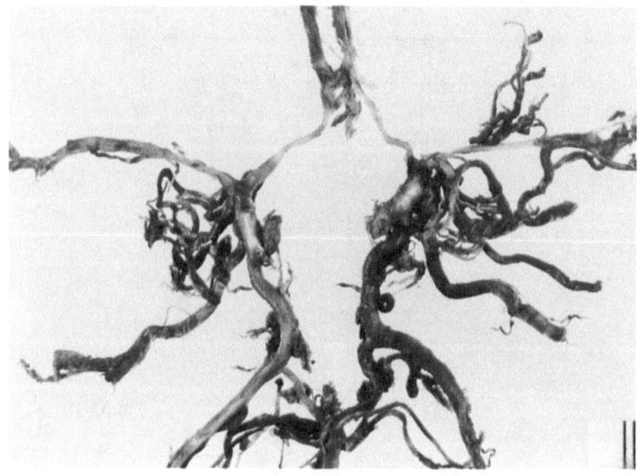

Figure 40-3. Macroscopic appearance of the circle of Willis in a 66-year-old woman with moyamoya disease at autopsy. Tapering of anterior and middle cerebral arteries can be seen bilaterally with network formation of dilated arteries (basal moyamoya vessels).

Immunohistochemical staining demonstrated that the thickened intima is composed mainly of smooth muscle cells (SMCs) (see Fig. 40-5B) that are phenotypically modulated from the contractile type to the synthetic.[36] Some SMCs in the intima were stained positively with the antibody for proliferating cell nuclear antigen (see Fig. 40-5C), which strongly suggests that active SMC proliferation and phenotypic modulation contribute to the formation of fibrocellular intimal thickening of the arteries. Lipid deposition and lipid-containing macrophages (foam cells) have been found in some autopsy cases but are now considered features of atherosclerosis.[3]

Mural thrombi are often found in the stenotic arteries (see Fig. 40-4B), but their frequency varies.[33,34,36,40] Judging from their histologic features, the organization of such thrombi appears to contribute to the pathogenesis of fibrocellular intimal thickening.

Aneurysm formation, a relatively common finding in the circle of Willis in patients with moyamoya disease, and its pathology are summarized later.

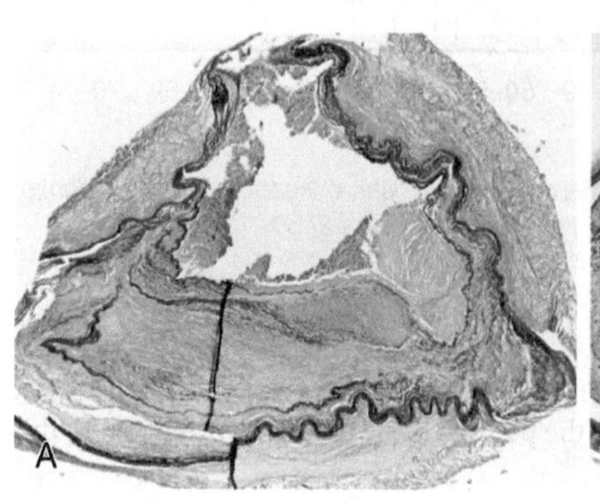

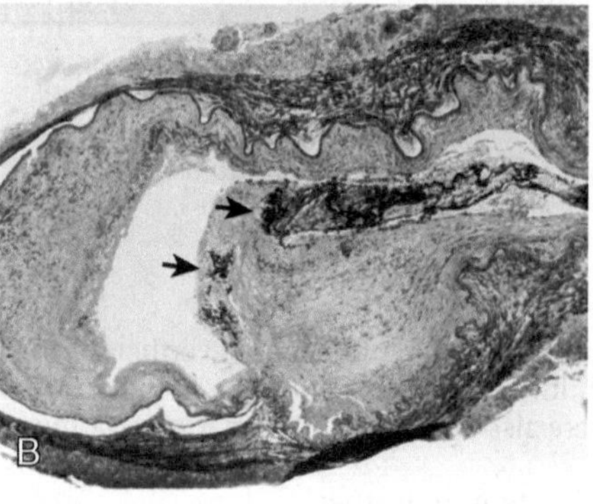

Figure 40-4. Microscopic appearance of the circle of Willis in patients with moyamoya disease at autopsy. A, Intracranial portion of right internal carotid artery of a 60-year-old woman (elastica van Gieson stain). B, Main trunk of the right middle cerebral artery of a 36-year-old man. *Arrows* indicate mural fibrin thrombi with its organization (Mallory's phosphotungstic acid-hematoxylin [PTAH] stain).

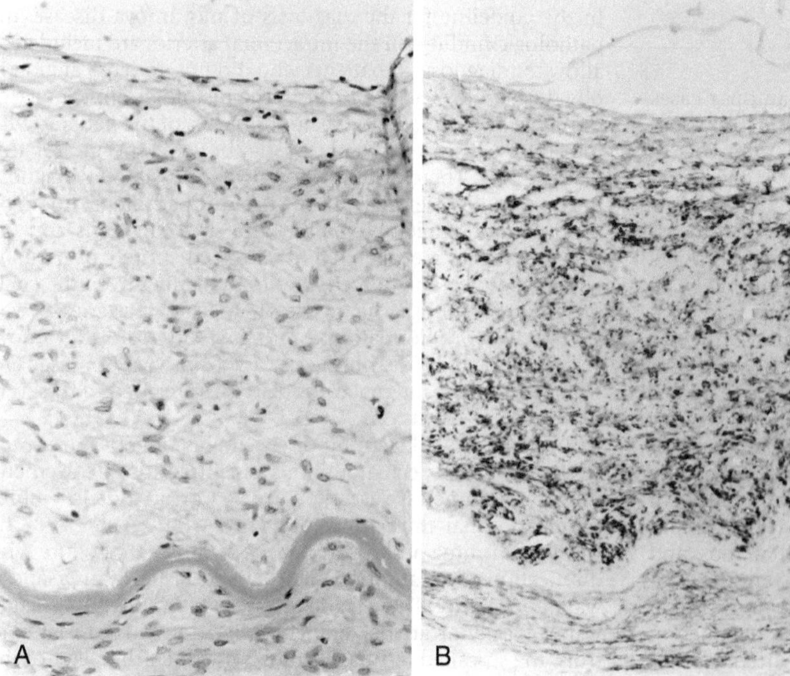

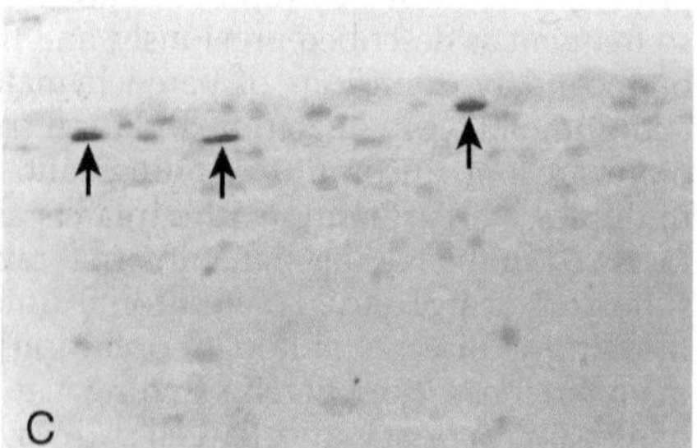

Figure 40-5. Microscopic appearance of the basilar artery of a 14-year-old girl with moyamoya disease at autopsy. A, H&E stain; B, immunohistochemical stain for muscle actin; C, staining for proliferating cell nuclear antigen (PCNA). *Arrows* in C indicate the nuclei stained positively for PCNA. (A and B from *Masuda J, Ogata J, Yutani C: Smooth muscle cell proliferation and localization of macrophages and T-cells in the occlusive intracranial major arteries in moyamoya disease.* Stroke *24:1960, 1993.)*

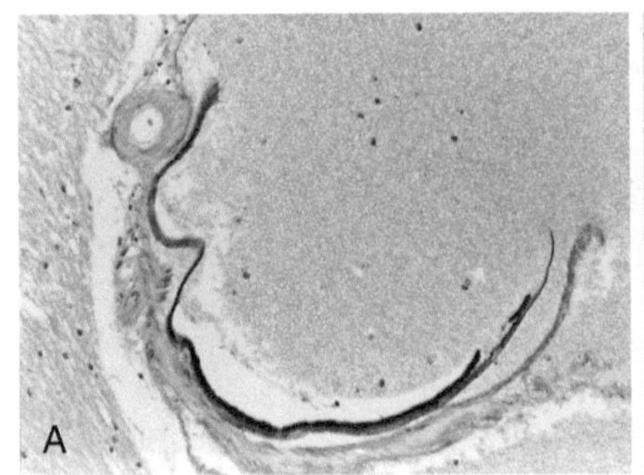

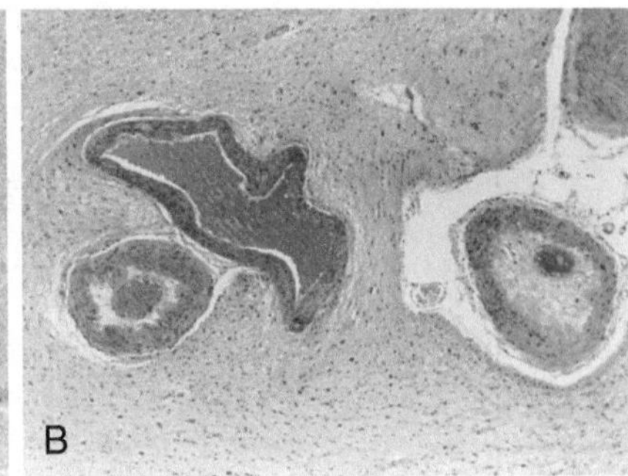

Figure 40-6. Microscopic appearance of the perforating arteries of patients with moyamoya disease at autopsy. A, The artery in the right caudate nucleus of a 60-year-old woman with parenchymatous hemorrhage shows marked dilatation with rupture (elastica van Gieson stain). B, Some of the arteries in the left thalamus of a 39-year-old woman show luminal stenosis due to fibrous and edematous intimal thickening (hematoxylin & eosin stain).

Perforating Arteries (Moyamoya Vessels)

The vascular network at the base of the brain consists of dilated medium-sized or small muscular arteries branching off the circle of Willis, anterior choroidal arteries, intracranial portions of internal carotid arteries, and posterior cerebral arteries. These arteries form complex channels that usually connect to the distal portion of the anterior and middle cerebral arteries. Numerous small dilated and tortuous vessels originating from these channels enter into the base of the brain, corresponding to lenticulostriate and thalamoperforate arteries.

In microscopic observations, these perforating arteries in the brain parenchyma show two patterns of histologic changes: (1) a dilated artery with a relatively thin wall and (2) a thick-walled artery showing luminal stenosis.[37] Dilatation of the arteries is more prominent in young patients. The majority of dilated arteries show fibrosis and marked attenuation of the media with occasional segmentation of the elastic lamina. With hemodynamic stress or aging, the dilated arteries with attenuated walls may predispose to focal protrusion (microaneurysm formation) of the arterial wall, and its rupture is considered one of the mechanisms leading to parenchymatous hemorrhage in patients with moyamoya disease (Fig. 40-6). Fibrinoid necrosis of the perforating arteries in the process of aneurysm formation has been shown in hypertensive parenchymatous hemorrhage, but has never been confirmed pathologically in patients with moyamoya disease.

In contrast, stenotic vessels are less common in young patients.[38] These vessels show concentric thickening of the intima with duplication of the elastic lamina and fibrosis of the tunica media (see Fig. 40-6). Partial dilatation with discontinuity of the elastic lamina and occluding thrombus formation with its organization and recanalization are occasionally found. These histologic changes in the perforating arteries indicate that the arterial obstructive changes in patients with moyamoya disease are not limited to the circle of Willis and its major branches.

Leptomeningeal Vessels

The leptomeningeal anastomoses among the three main cerebral arteries and transdural anastomoses from the external carotid arteries are commonly observed as an abnormal vascular network on cerebral angiograms in patients with moyamoya disease (so-called vault moyamoya).[4,13,41] A histopathologic and morphometric study of the leptomeningeal vessels in autopsied brains with moyamoya disease clarified that such anastomoses are not newly formed vessels, but merely dilated preexisting vessels.[42] Attenuation or disruption of the internal elastic lamina is remarkable in patients with a short history of moyamoya disease, and fibrous intimal thickening is more prominent in patients with a longer history of the disease. These structural adaptations in the vascular walls of the leptomeningeal vessels suggest their participation in the collateral circulation at the cerebral cortical surfaces.

Aneurysm Formation

Intracranial aneurysms are frequently associated with moyamoya disease.[43-46] Intracranial aneurysms are of two types: major artery aneurysms (MAAs) developing from the circle of Willis, and peripheral artery aneurysms (PAAs) located on the moyamoya vessels, choroidal arteries, or any other peripheral arteries serving as collaterals.[43] SAH is caused by rupture of MAAs, whereas parenchymatous hemorrhage or intraventricular hemorrhage is caused by the rupture of PAAs in some cases.

MAAs are commonly found in the arterial complex of the anterior communicating artery - anterior cerebral artery in patients with unilateral moyamoya (probable cases) and in the basilar artery in patients with bilateral moyamoya (Fig. 40-7).[43] MAAs are fourfold higher in unilateral cases than in bilateral cases. Such anatomical distribution of MAAs could be explained if the aneurysms form as a result of increased blood flow through the relatively spared routes of cerebral circulation as the stenotic process progresses. This increased blood flow exerts high pressure on the arterial wall, resulting in aneurysm formation in susceptible places such as branching sites. Histologically, the aneurysmal wall consists of endothelium with adventitial layers and a disappearance of internal elastic lamina and media, which is no different from the walls of saccular aneurysms commonly observed in SAH. Aneurysms formed by dissection of the intima from the media have also been reported in autopsy cases.[47,48]

PAAs are speculated to be responsible for parenchymatous hemorrhage. Two types of aneurysm are reported: saccular (true) aneurysms and pseudoaneurysms, consisting of fibrin and erythrocytes, that might be the result of rupture.[49] The mean size of PAAs is half that of MAAs; PAAs may not be visualized angiographically in many cases. Thus, PAAs detected in angiography may represent only a subset of larger lesions. One-third of angiographically visualized PAAs are reported to disappear spontaneously during the follow-up period; we have reported on the histology of a sclerosed PAA without rupture in an autopsy case[50] and suggested the pathologic processes by which the aneurysms disappear.

Extracranial Cervical Arteries and Systemic Arteries

The luminal stenosis due to fibrocellular intimal thickening in moyamoya disease has been described not only in intracranial arteries but also in extracranial arteries, including carotid arteries, renal arteries, pulmonary arteries, and coronary arteries.[34,51,52] An autopsy of a 7-year-old Japanese girl with moyamoya disease and renovascular hypertension showed

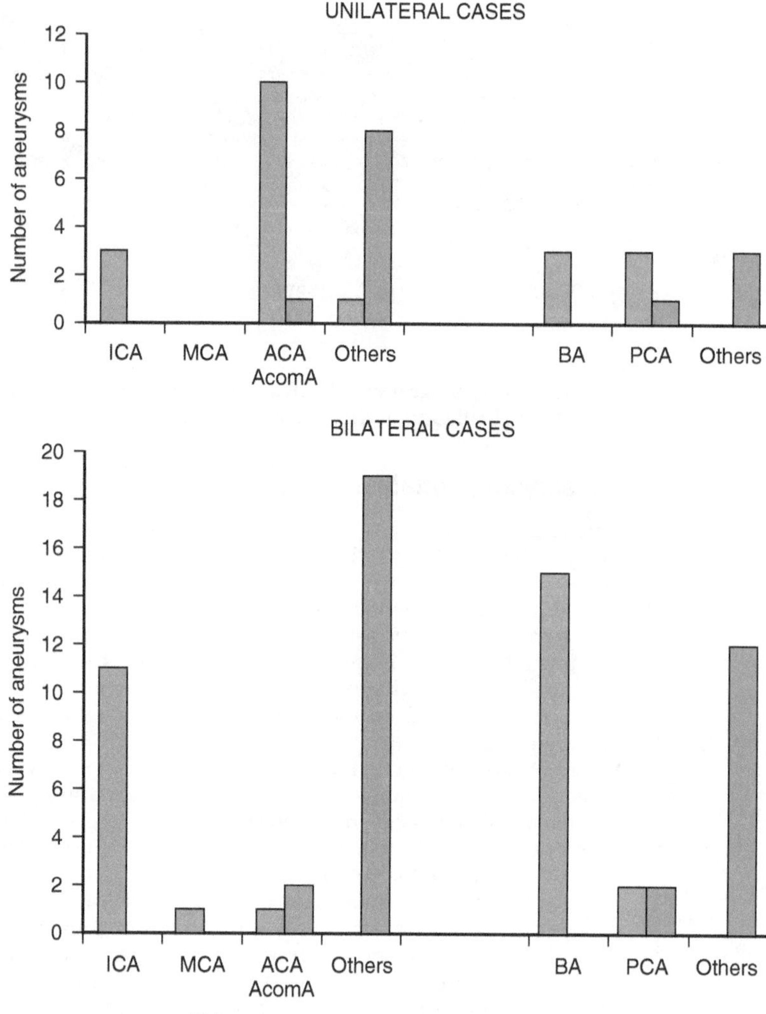

Figure 40-7. Locations of aneurysms in patients with moyamoya disease. ACA, anterior cerebral artery; AcomA, anterior communicating artery; BA, basilar artery; ICA, internal carotid artery; MCA, middle cerebral artery; PCA, posterior cerebral artery. *(Data from Herreman F, Nathal E, Yasui N, et al: Intracranial aneurysm in moyamoya disease: Report of ten cases and review of the literature.* Cerebrovasc Dis *4:329, 1994.)*

systemic involvement of concentric fibrocellular intimal thickening consisting of smooth muscle cells and elastic fibers in intracranial and extracranial carotid, coronary, and renal arteries; their histologic features were similar to those seen in fibromuscular dysplasia (FMD), intimal hyperplasia type. Several other cases of renovascular hypertension associated with moyamoya disease have been reported in the literature,[53–55] many of which show the angiographic or pathologic appearance of FMD. Therefore, it is postulated that the systemic involvement of FMD or FMD-like vascular lesions is present in moyamoya disease, and hypertension may be a result of systemic involvement of the arteries. The intracranial lesions of moyamoya disease might be manifestations of systemic illness, but no pathognomonic changes suggest any specific disease or etiologic factors and the implications of these systemic changes are uncertain at present.

ETIOLOGY AND PATHOGENESIS

There has been serious and continuing debate about whether moyamoya disease is acquired or congenital, and none of the proposed hypotheses for the pathogenesis of this disease has received general agreement.[3,4] Therefore, the cause remains unknown at present. Nevertheless, moyamoya disease is established as a clinical disease entity and the following features are now generally accepted:

1. The progression of stenosis or occlusion of the circle of Willis and the major branches, including distal ends of the internal carotid arteries, is the primary finding in the disease.
2. An abnormal vascular network (moyamoya vessels) at the base of the brain consists of collateral vessels that have formed secondary to brain ischemia.
3. Clinical symptoms and signs are the manifestations of cerebrovascular events secondary to the previously described vascular lesions, including intracranial hemorrhage, infarct, and transient ischemic attacks (TIAs).
4. The major cellular components of the thickened intima formed in arteries of the circle of Willis and the major branches are smooth muscle cells. Migration and proliferation of smooth muscle cells in the intima, induced by unknown mechanisms, may lead to the intimal thickening

in association with morphologic and biochemical alteration of extracellular matrix components including elastin, collagen, and other proteoglycans.

By contrast, the mechanisms responsible for inducing smooth muscle cell proliferation and migration in the arterial intima of patients with the disease are not yet identified. Furthermore, the reason that intimal thickening occurs in only limited arteries, such as the circle of Willis, is unknown. As previously mentioned, hereditary factors have long been suggested to play an important role in the etiology of moyamoya disease, as indicated by the high incidence among Japanese people,[15] occasional familial occurrence,[21] and association with some phenotypes of human leukocyte antigen (HLA)[56] or other congenital diseases, such as sickle cell anemia,[57] von Recklinghausen's disease,[58,59] and Down syndrome.[60,61] In a genetic study of patients in families with moyamoya disease, a multifactorial mode of inheritance was suggested.[62,63] Genetic linkage analysis of the pedigrees of patients with moyamoya disease of familial occurrence has been performed in several institutions. Inoue and coworkers[64,65] demonstrated a possible linkage between moyamoya disease and a region on chromosome 6 where the HLA gene is located. Ikeda and colleagues[66] performed the total genome search and found the possible linkage of markers located on chromosome 3p24.2-p26 in 16 families with moyamoya disease of familial occurrence. Yamauchi and associates,[67] performing a linkage analysis focused on chromosome 17, showed a possible linkage of chromosome 17q25 to familial moyamoya disease. Chromosome 8q23 has been also suggested to have possible linkage to familial moyamoya disease.[68] Recently, several studies identified the ring finger 213 (RNF213) gene as a susceptibility gene for moyamoya disease by the conventional rigorous positional cloning approach, exome analysis, and functional analysis using zebrafish.[69,70] The extensive investigation focusing on the genes contained in, or close to, the candidate regions just described may yield clues for possible hypotheses explaining the pathogenesis of moyamoya disease.

Although hereditary factors may be involved in susceptibility to moyamoya disease, the majority of cases of the disease are sporadic, and the clinical manifestations and disease progression are not congenital. Through the accumulation of patient registrations and analysis of clinical data, acquired factors have been suggested in the occurrence and progression of moyamoya disease. Many hypotheses have been proposed; these include vasculitis with or without an autoimmune mechanism,[12,13,71] infection (virus,[72] anaerobic bacteria such as *Propionibacterium acnes*[73]), thrombosis,[33,34,40] juvenile atherosclerosis,[33,34] cranial trauma,[74] abnormalities of sympathetic nerve endings,[67] and the postirradiation state.[75,76]

As noted in the discussion of pathology, microthrombi are frequently formed in the vasculature of patients with moyamoya disease.[33,34,36,40] Microthrombi appear to contribute to pathogenesis of the fibrocellular intimal thickening through its organization; this hypothesis explains the lamellated structure of the thickened intima of the lesions. If endothelial injury really occurs as the initiation of lesion formation, it is feasible to speculate that smooth muscle cell migration and proliferation in the intima are induced after injury. There has been substantial evidence that endothelial injury provokes phenotypic modulation and proliferation of smooth muscle cells and leads to neointima formation, not only in experimental animals[77-80] but also in patients with angioplasty restenosis.[80,81] In moyamoya disease, however, it is unclear to what extent this process is responsible for lesion formation. Furthermore, microthrombus is a non-specific finding and reveals none of any specific etiologic factors in the endothelial injury.

None of the factors leading to endothelial injury has been identified in moyamoya disease. Ikeda and associates[82] detected loss of the endothelium covering the thickened intima in patients with moyamoya through the use of functional markers (thrombomodulin and von Willebrand factor). In relation to the hypotheses for the mechanisms of arterial injury, prothrombotic abnormalities, including inherited protein S deficiency and antiphospholipid antibodies, have been reported in some patients with moyamoya disease,[83,84] and chronic arteritis due to immunologic reactions may be implicated.[22,85] With cell-type-specific immunohistochemistry, we previously demonstrated the presence of macrophages and T cells in the lesions, especially in the superficial layer of the thickened intima.[36] Such inflammatory cell infiltration observed in patients, however, might be a local reaction to microthrombi or a reflection of systemic inflammation or atherosclerotic changes unrelated to moyamoya disease. Therefore, it is not always easy to separate the histopathologic features of moyamoya disease from those of other pathologic changes, including atherosclerosis and various forms of arteritis.

In addition to the possible migration and proliferation of smooth muscle cells suggested in the genesis of intimal thickening and moyamoya vessel formation, many researchers have focused their attention on the growth factors and cytokines and their receptors, such as basic fibroblast growth factor (b-FGF),[86,87] platelet-derived growth factor (PDGF),[88] transforming growth factor-beta (TGF-β),[89] interleukin-1 (IL-1), prostaglandin E2,[90] and hepatocyte growth factor (HGF).[91,92] Immunohistochemical staining[86,87] and measurements of these proteins in the cerebrospinal fluid[93,94] have been attempted in patients with moyamoya disease. These approaches may help introduce methods of molecular biology and vascular biology, which are now in rapid development in relation to the problem of angioplasty restenosis[79,81] and atherogenesis.[80] Genetic analysis and this work on candidate cytokines and their genes relevant to moyamoya disease may help identify the cause of the disorder.

CLINICAL SYMPTOMS AND SIGNS

Clinical symptoms and signs manifest as a result of the cerebrovascular events that occur in relation to pathologic changes in cerebral arteries in patients with moyamoya disease. Initial symptoms occur abruptly as attacks of cerebrovascular events including TIA, brain infarction, intracranial hemorrhage, and, occasionally, epileptic seizures. Some patients have shown no overt symptoms, and their disease was diagnosed from the angiography performed because of the familial occurrence of the disease.[17]

The MHWJ's Research Committee has defined four clinical types of moyamoya disease according to the initial symptoms and their frequencies in the registered patients accumulated until 1995,[95] as follows:

- Ischemic (63.4%)
- Hemorrhagic (21.6%)
- Epileptic (7.6%)
- Other (7.5%).

The ischemic type dominates in childhood moyamoya, representing 69% of cases in patients younger than 10 years; TIA occurs in 40% and infarction in 29% of patients manifesting a variety of symptoms, including motor paresis, disturbances of consciousness, speech disturbances, and sensory disturbances.[96] The course is sometimes repetitive and progressive and may result in cortical blindness, motor aphasia, or even a vegetative state within several years of onset. The ischemic symptoms are provoked by some conditions involving hyperventilation, such as blowing to play wind instruments, blowing to cool something hot, and crying. They are believed to be induced by decreased cerebral blood flow (CBF) due to diminished $PaCO_2$. Ischemic deterioration is often precipitated by infection of the upper respiratory tract. Mental retardation and low IQ during the long follow-up are other important problems for children; this issue is further discussed in the section on disease progression and prognosis.

The hemorrhagic type is prevalent in adult patients, occurring in 66% of cases of the disease in adults, with predominance in females.[96] Headache, disturbances of consciousness, and motor paresis are frequently encountered in the hemorrhagic type. Events triggering the bleeding are not identified, but hypertension and aging may be suggested as factors. Bleeding occurs often in multiple and repetitive intervals from several days to 10 years, and massive bleeding often leads to death.

Epilepsy was observed in about 5% of all patients, more than 80% of whom were children younger than 10 years old.[96]

LABORATORY FINDINGS

Many groups have attempted to establish a diagnostic laboratory test for moyamoya disease, but none of the tests has proved successful. Some reports, however, showed fragments of data that provided valuable information concerning the etiology and pathogenesis of this disease. Infection by anaerobic bacteria such as *Propionibacterium acnes*,[73] cytomegalovirus, and Epstein–Barr virus,[72] for example, have been examined, with screening for specific antibodies and amplification of viral DNAs with polymerase chain reaction. The reported data suggest positive correlations with moyamoya disease.

Prothrombotic abnormalities have been reported not only in patients with moyamoya disease but also in children with cerebrovascular diseases. Deficiencies of protein S and protein C have been reported in some patients.[83] Anticardiolipin antibody, an autoantibody against phosphatidyl-glycerol, itself a component of cell membrane phospholipid, showed higher percentages in patients with moyamoya disease than in controls.[84,85] These data suggest a possible connection between autoimmune mechanisms and moyamoya disease, because this antibody has been suggested to play an important role in arterial thrombus formation in brain infarction.[85,97]

CLINICAL EXAMINATION

Angiography

The fundamental angiographic finding in moyamoya disease is bilateral stenosis or occlusion at the intracranial portion of the internal carotid arteries together with a retiform arteriolar network (moyamoya vessels) at the base of the brain (see Figs 40-1A, B). The stenotic or occlusive changes often extend along the arteries of the circle of Willis and its main branches. The vertebrobasilar system, however, has rarely been reported to be involved in this disease.[12,13] Formation of leptomeningeal collateral vessels, especially from the branches of the posterior cerebral artery, is frequently noted. Also usually present are transdural anastomoses via the ophthalmic artery, external carotid artery, and vertebral artery.

Suzuki and associates[12,13] divided the progression of moyamoya disease into the following six stages on the basis of angiographic findings, as follows: (1) narrowing of the carotid forks, (2) initial appearance of moyamoya vessels, (3) intensification of moyamoya vessels, (4) minimization of moyamoya vessels, (5) reduction of moyamoya vessels, and (6) disappearance of moyamoya vessels with collateral circulation only from the external carotid arteries. Kitamura and associates[4] confirmed these chronologic changes of angiographic findings in their follow-up patients; that is, as the narrowing of the main arteries advances, the moyamoya vessels increase in number, and they are later reduced when transdural anastomoses develop as disease progresses.

As noted previously, aneurysm formation is commonly seen in moyamoya disease.

Computed Tomography

The features of moyamoya disease on computed tomography (CT) scans vary according to the clinical type. The most striking finding on conventional CT scans is high-density areas (HDAs) in the basal ganglia and thalamus, ventricular system, and subarachnoid spaces of the patients with the hemorrhagic type.[16,98] The HDAs resemble the topography of the hematoma in the internal type of hypertensive intracerebral hemorrhage.

In the ischemic type, CT scans reveal low-density areas (LDAs), which are relatively small and are usually confined to the cerebral cortex and subcortex, along with dilatation of cortical sulci and ventricles. Lacunar infarctions located in the basal ganglia and thalamus are sometimes seen in adults but are rare in children with the disease. Up to 40% of patients with the ischemic type, however, have no abnormalities on a conventional CT scan. Use of a contrast agent often visualizes tortuous and curvilinear vessels in the basal ganglia, which represent moyamoya vessels. The most proximal segments of the anterior and middle cerebral arteries are often poorly opacified.

Magnetic Resonance Imaging and Angiography

Because MRI and MRA are non-invasive techniques that can visualize various pathologic changes of the brain and the arterial tree, they have a big advantage over conventional angiography. MRI can demonstrate small subcortical lesions undetectable on CT. Brain infarctions in patients with moyamoya disease are usually small and located in the subcortex and are often multiple and bilateral. Brain atrophy and slight ventricular dilatation are also seen.[17–19,99] Stenotic or occlusive lesions at the distal ends of the internal carotid arteries can be demonstrated by MRA in most patients with this disease (see Figs 40-1C, D). Apparent moyamoya vessels can be visualized as fine unusual vessels on MRA (see Figs 40-1C, D) and also as a signal void on MRI (Fig. 40-8), particularly in children. Small moyamoya vessels, however, are poorly visualized on both MRI and MRA, particularly in adults.

As described in the guideline for diagnosis of moyamoya disease, the MHWJ's Research Committee has concluded that this disease can be diagnosed without conventional angiography if MRI and MRA visualize the previously described findings bilaterally. To meet this agreement, the guideline was revised in 1995, and the diagnostic criteria on MRI and MRA were supplemented as shown in Box 35-2.[2] MRI and MRA have also been shown to be useful imaging tools for postoperative assessment and longitudinal follow-up of patients with moyamoya disease.[18,100,101] The prevention of rebleeding is important because it clearly worsens outcome (Fig. 40-9).[102] The prevalence of asymptomatic microbleeds (MBs) in patients with moyamoya disease was significantly greater than in healthy individuals.[103] A prospective cohort study using T2*-weighted MRI demonstrated that the presence of microbleeds was a significant predictor for subsequent intracerebral hemorrhage in adult moyamoya disease.[104] The leptomeningeal high signal intensity on fluid-attenuated inversion recovery images in moyamoya disease was called "ivy sign" and indicated decreased cerebral vascular reserve[105,106] (Fig. 40-10).

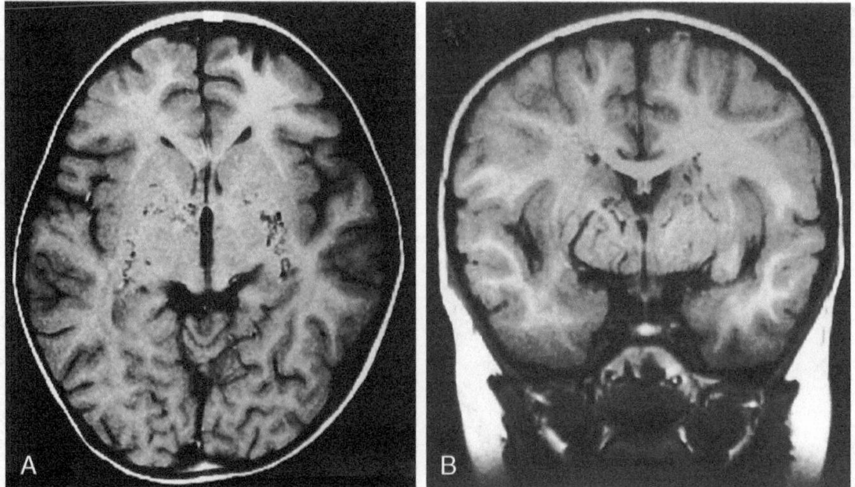

Figure 40-8. Typical MRI appearance of moyamoya vessels. A, Axial image reveals multiple signal voids in the basal ganglia. B, Coronal image shows well-developed basal moyamoya vessels in the bilateral basal ganglia. *(From Houkin K, Aoki T, Takahashi A, et al: Diagnosis of moyamoya disease with magnetic resonance angiography.* Stroke *25:2159, 1994.)*

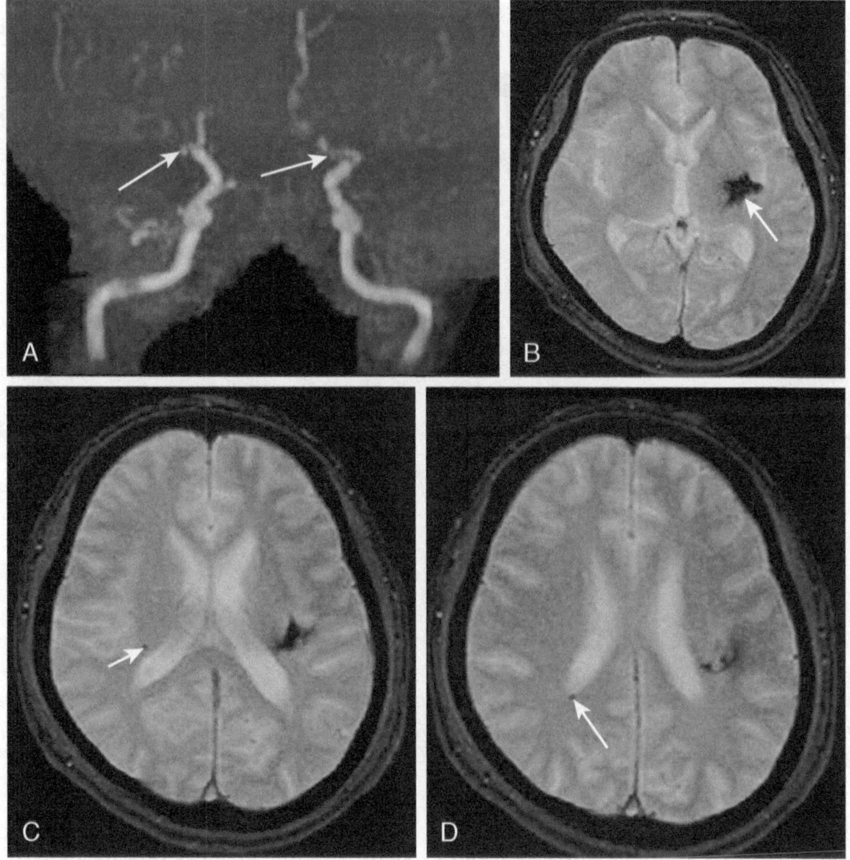

Figure 40-9. MR angiography and MRI in a 52-year-old patient with moyamoya disease. A, MR angiogram demonstrates occlusion or severe stenosis (*arrow*) at the bilateral distal portion of the internal carotid arteries. B to D, T2*-weighted MR images. B shows previous left putaminal hemorrhage (*arrow*). C and D demonstrate multiple microbleeds (*arrows*).

Ultrasonography

Because moyamoya disease is a type of systemic vascular disease, the extracranial internal and external carotid arteries, aorta, pulmonary artery, coronary artery, celiac trunk, and renal artery are reported to be involved, together with intracranial vessels.[107-109] The extracranial carotid artery is observed easily by conventional carotid ultrasonography, and its distal portion is also evaluated by transoral carotid ultrasonography (TOCU).[110-112] An increase in flow velocity in the external carotid artery has been taken as evidence for it functioning as a collateral pathway.[113] Yasaka et al. investigated morphologic features of the extracranial ICA by conventional carotid ultrasonography and TOCU in 19 ICAs in ten patients with

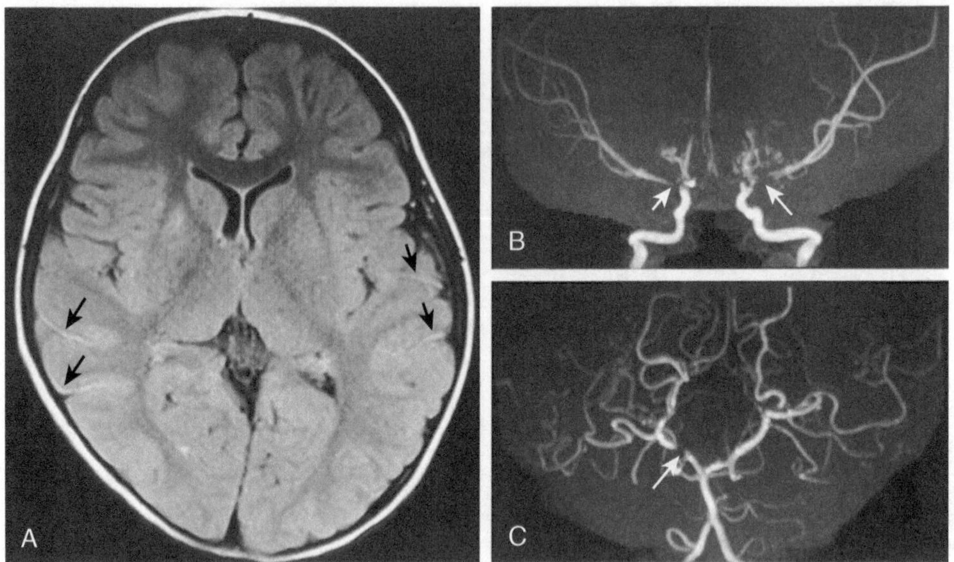

Figure 40-10. MRI-FLAIR and MR angiography in a 5-year-old patient with moyamoya disease, who developed TIA with symptom of right hemiparesis. A, MRI-FLAIR image demonstrates "IVY sign" (*arrows*). B and C show stenosis of distal portion of bilateral internal carotid arteries and their branches (*arrows*) and proximal portion of the right posterior cerebral artery (*arrow*).

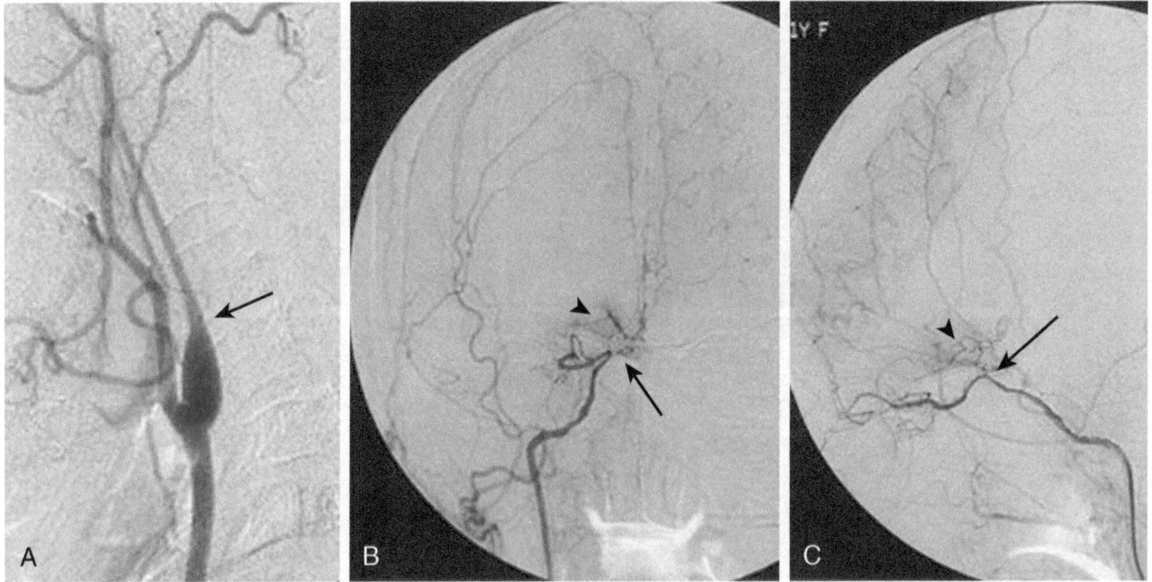

Figure 40-11. Cerebral angiograms in a patient with moyamoya disease. A, Reduction of the diameter of the internal carotid artery (ICA) at its proximal portion (*arrow*). In the anteroposterior (B) and lateral (C) views, *arrows* indicate occlusion of the distal ICA, and *arrowheads* the vascular net at the basal brain. See also Figure 40-12. *(From Yasaka M, Ogata T, Yasumori K, et al: Bottle neck sign of the proximal portion of the internal carotid artery in moyamoya disease.* J Ultrasound Med *25:1547-1552, 2006.)*

moyamoya disease. They described the "champagne bottle neck sign" (diameter greatly reduced at the proximal portion of the ICA above the bulbus like a champagne bottle neck, so as to be less than half of that of the common carotid artery) in 14 ICAs (74%) and "diameter reversal sign" (diameter of the ICA is smaller than that of the external carotid artery) in 16 ICAs (84%) (Figs 40-11, 40-12).[114] These ultrasonographic findings in moyamoya disease may be useful for early detection.[115]

Electroencephalography

Abnormal electroencephalographic (EEG) findings are more frequent in patients with childhood onset of the disease than in adults.[116] Such findings are related to permanent or transient ischemic changes due to a $PaCO_2$ variation that is not specific for moyamoya disease.[4,13] Yoshii and Kudo summarized the EEG findings as: (1) diffuse and bilateral, abnormal, low-voltage or slow waves and spike waves, (2) "buildup" with the appearance of delta waves during hyperventilation, and (3) no effect on photic stimulation.[117]

Other Clinical Examinations

Because the symptoms of the ischemic type and epileptic type of moyamoya disease are caused by impairment of CBF due to arterial stenosis or occlusion, regional CBF and metabolic distribution have been measured by xenon inhalation and

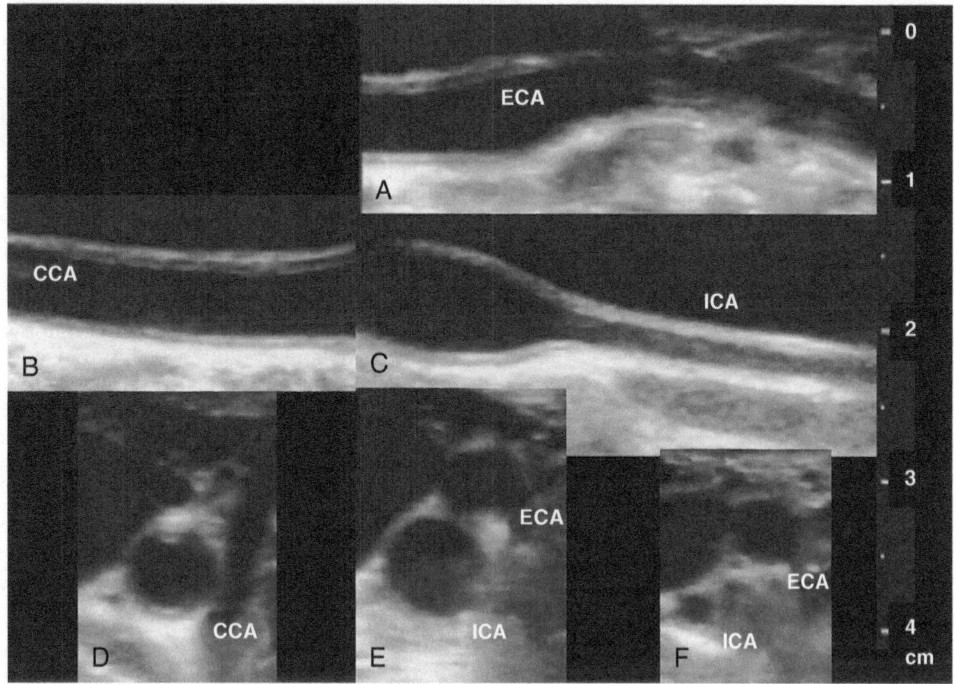

Figure 40-12. A to F, Conventional carotid ultrasonograms demonstrate signs of the "bottle neck" and "diameter reversal" in the same patient as shown in Figure 40-11. CCA, common carotid artery; ECA, external carotid artery; ICA, internal carotid artery. *(From Yasaka M, Ogata T, Yasumori K, et al: Bottle neck sign of the proximal portion of the internal carotid artery in moyamoya disease.* J Ultrasound Med *25:1547-1552, 2006.)*

visualized with CT methods, including stable xenon-enhanced CT, dynamic CT, positron emission computed tomography (PET), and single-photon emission computed tomography (SPECT). Measurements of these physiologic and morphologic parameters have been useful for the follow-up of patients as well as evaluation of medical and surgical treatment and determination of prognosis.[118–124]

DISEASE PROGRESSION AND PROGNOSIS

Disease progression and the prognosis for moyamoya disease differ remarkably between children and adults. In children, angiographic changes progress with time and sometimes rapidly,[125,126] and the formation of abnormal vascular networks at the base of the brain progresses from unilateral to bilateral.[21,126,127] However, the prognosis for activities of daily life (ADLs) and life expectancy in children with moyamoya disease is generally fair, because irreversible ischemic and hemorrhagic complications are rarely encountered. More than 80% of such patients are in good health or in a state of independence, irrespective of treatment received. Nevertheless, many children are reported to be not well accommodated in social or school life because of poor intellectual ability, psychological impairment, and personality changes.[128–132] In general, the earlier the onset of the disease and the longer the period of suffering, the lower the mental function and quality of intelligence.

In adults, however, progression of angiographic changes is uncommon. Prognosis for ADLs and life expectancy, however, is poor because multiple and repetitive intracranial hemorrhages occur in many patients.

TREATMENT

The majority of patients with moyamoya (77%) have been treated surgically by one of several revascularization operations, though some patients with mild or transient symptoms tend to be observed and given conservative treatment.[95] Surgical treatment is more effective than conservative treatment for improving physiologic parameters revealed by regional CBF measurement and PET studies, and is generally believed to have an advantage for a better prognosis.[1,118,133]

Medical Treatment

Vasodilators, antiplatelet agents, antifibrinolytic agents, and fibrinolytic agents are used in patients with moyamoya disease. Other medications, including anticonvulsants and steroids, are used in patients with the epileptic type and in patients with increased intracranial pressure, respectively.[96,98]

Steroids are considered to be effective in certain cases, especially in patients with involuntary movements and during the active phase of recurrent ischemic or hemorrhagic attacks. This effect is presumed to be related to influences of steroids on edema, regional CBF, and vasculitis.

Antiplatelet agents, acetylsalicylic acid, and clopidogrel may also be prescribed to prevent recurrence of ischemic attacks and thrombosis of the circle of Willis and the main branches, which is thought to play an important role in the progression of moyamoya disease. Other drugs, such as vasodilators, antifibrinolytics, and fibrinolytics, are occasionally used for similar purposes. The efficacy of these drugs in patients with moyamoya disease, however, has never been tested thoroughly in clinical trials.

Surgical Treatment

Surgical revascularizations are classified into three categories: direct bypass surgery, indirect bypass surgery, and a combination of the two (Fig. 40-13).[1,134] Surgical revascularization aims to give additional collateral flow to the ischemic brain and thereby to improve regional CBF and prevent or minimize

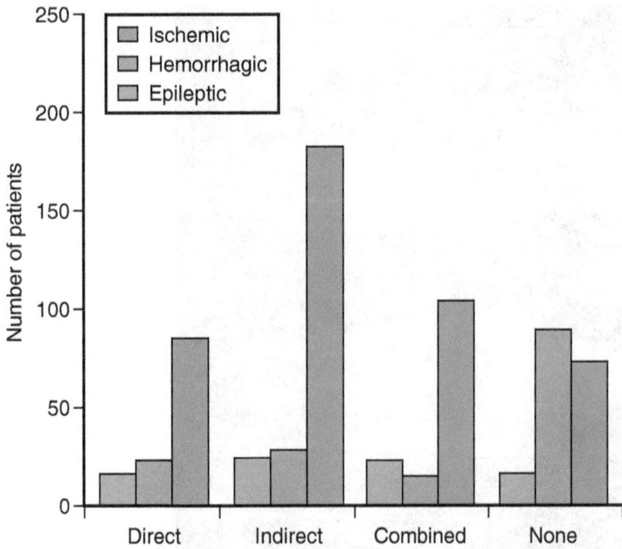

Figure 40-13. Selection of surgical revascularization procedure (x-axis) for patients with moyamoya disease according to type of initial attack. *(Data from Fukui M, Kawano T: Follow-up study of registered cases in 1995. In Fukui M, editor:* Annual report [1995] by the Research Committee on Spontaneous Occlusion of the Circle of Willis [Moyamoya Disease]. *Ministry of Health and Welfare, Tokyo, 1996, p 12.)*

irreversible brain damage. Also, collateral flow through the bypass is expected to have some effects in reducing hemodynamic stress on the moyamoya vessels and eventually to prevent the occurrence of hemorrhagic events. The evacuation of hematoma and ventricular drainage are performed in the acute stage of hemorrhagic complications of moyamoya disease.

Superficial temporal artery–middle cerebral artery (STA-MCA) bypass is a direct revascularization surgery that was pioneered by Yasargil[135] and then applied to moyamoya disease by Karasawa and Kikuchi,[136] and Reichmann and colleagues[137] independently. This direct revascularization surgery seems to achieve a remarkable improvement in CBF and a better prognosis than conservative treatment.[118,138] This technique, however, requires skill in microvascular surgery, and it is not always possible to find a cortical branch suitable for anastomosis. Furthermore, careful intra-operative monitoring of blood pressure and $PaCO_2$ is necessary; otherwise, there is a risk of perioperative ischemic complications.[119]

Indirect revascularizations are surgical procedures that aim to introduce external carotid flow into the internal carotid system via newly developed vascularization through the sutured tissues. Encephaloduroarteriosynangiosis (EDAS)[139] and encephalomyosynangiosis (EMS)[140] are the two representative procedures most commonly used in patients with moyamoya disease. Other operative methods, such as encephaloarteriosynangiosis (EAS), durapexy, and omentum transplantation,[141] also belong to this category. These operations can be performed in patients who do not have a cortical branch suitable for anastomoses, although revascularization is not always sufficient to give a collateral flow sufficient to prevent ischemic symptoms. Therefore, the neurosurgeon often performs a *combination* of direct and indirect revascularization to obtain better collateral flow.[138,142]

These surgical revascularizations are frequently performed in patients with the ischemic type of moyamoya disease (see Fig. 40-9), and the effect of surgery on improvement in regional CBF has been established.[118,119,133,138,143] Further, surgical revascularization seems to be effective for the prevention of ischemic events and for improvement in ADLs and intellectual activity, as long as the surgical procedure is chosen properly and performed successfully.[95,100,132,142] There is controversy as to whether the introduction of collateral flow by revascularization raises the risk of hemorrhagic events[1,144,145]; therefore, bypass surgery is not commonly performed in patients with the hemorrhagic type (see Fig. 40-9).[95,146] Rebleeding has been reported to be lower in patients receiving bypass procedures, but the difference was not significant.[147,148] After surgery, moyamoya vessels actually diminished and often disappeared.[147] To evaluate the effect of bypass surgery on preventing recurrent bleeding, a prospective and randomized multicenter study, the Japan Adult Moyamoya (JAM) Trial, was initiated in January 2001.[149] This trial enrolled 80 patients (surgical, 42; nonsurgical, 38).[150] During the follow up period of 5 years, rebleeding attacks were observed in 5 patients in the surgical group (11.9%) and 12 in the nonsurgical group (31.6%), significantly different in the Kaplan-Meier survival analysis (2.7%/y versus 7.6%/y; $P = 0.042$), suggesting the preventive effect of direct bypass against rebleeding.

CONCLUSION AND FUTURE DIRECTIONS

As a result of the extensive investigation since the first report of this disease in 1957, moyamoya disease is now recognized as a true disease entity all over the world. Angiographic findings and pathophysiologic features of the disorder are well characterized, and the guidelines for diagnosis are also established, including the use of MRI and MRA.[2] Data concerning the epidemiology of the disease as well as the long-term effects of medical and surgical treatment on prognosis have been accumulating and need to be analyzed carefully and accurately.

In regard to the etiology and pathogenesis of this disease, great advances have been achieved, and such data are expected to provide important clues to solve the genesis of this mysterious disorder. Newer techniques, including molecular genetics, cell biology, and experimental pathology, should be applied vigorously. The establishment of an experimental animal model of this disease will be extremely valuable.

REFERENCES

1. Fukui M. Current state of study on moyamoya disease in Japan. Surg Neurol 1997;47:138.
2. Fukui M. Guidelines for the diagnosis and treatment of spontaneous occlusion of the circle of Willis ("moyamoya" disease). Research Committee on Spontaneous Occlusion of the Circle of Willis (Moyamoya Disease) of the Ministry of Health and Welfare, Japan. Clin Neurol Neurosurg 1997;99:S238.
3. Fukui M, Kono S, Sueishi K, et al. Moyamoya disease. Neuropathology 2000;20:S61.
4. Kitamura K, Fukui M, Oka K, et al. Moyamoya disease. In: Toole JF, editor. Handbook of clinical neurology, Vol 11, Vascular diseases, Part III. Amsterdam: Elsevier; 1989. p. 293.
5. Yasaka M, Masuda J, Ogata J, et al. Moyamoya disease. In: Barnett HJM, Mohr JP, Wolf PA, et al., editors. Stroke: Pathophysiology, diagnosis, and management. ed 5. Philadelphia: Elsevier; 2011. p. 815.
6. Takeuchi K, Shimizu K. Hypoplasia of the bilateral internal carotid arteries. No to Shinkei 1957;9:37.
7. Sano K. Cerebral juxta-basal telangiectasia. No to Shinkei 1965;17:748.
8. Handa H, Tani K, Kajikawa H, et al. Clinicopathological study on an adult case with cerebral arterial rete. No to Shinkei 1969;21:181.
9. Weidner W, Hanafee W, Markham C. Intracranial collateral circulation via leptomeningeal and rete mirabile anastomosis. Neurology 1965;15:39.
10. Nishimoto A, Takeuchi S. Abnormal cerebrovascular network related to the internal carotid arteries. J Neurosurg 1968;29:255.

11. Kudo T. Spontaneous occlusion of the circle of Willis: A disease apparently confined to Japanese. Neurology 1968;18:485.
12. Suzuki J, Takaku A. Cerebrovascular "moyamoya disease": A disease showing abnormal net-like vessels in base of brain. Arch Neurol 1969;20:288.
13. Suzuki J, Kodama N. Moyamoya disease: A review. Stroke 1983; 14:104.
14. Ikezaki K, Han DH, Kawano T, et al. A clinical comparison of definite moyamoya disease between South Korea and Japan. Stroke 1997;28:2513.
15. Goto Y, Yonekawa Y. Worldwide distribution of moyamoya disease. Neurol Med Chir (Tokyo) 1992;32:883.
16. Yonekawa Y, Ogata N, Kaku Y, et al. Moyamoya disease in Europe, past and present status. Clin Neurol Neurosurg 1997;99(Suppl. 2):S58.
17. Fukui M, Mizoguchi M, Matsushima T, et al. MR angiography in the families of moyamoya patients. In: Fukui M, editor. Annual report (1994) by research committee of spontaneous occlusion of the circle of Willis (moyamoya disease). Tokyo: Ministry of Health and Welfare; 1995. p. 102.
18. Hasuo K, Mihara F, Matsushima T. MRI and MR angiography in moyamoya disease. J Magn Reson Imaging 1998;8:762.
19. Houkin K, Aoki T, Takahashi A, et al. Diagnosis of moyamoya disease with magnetic resonance angiography. Stroke 1994;25: 2159.
20. Wakai K, Tamakoshi A, Ikezaki K, et al. Epidemiological features of moyamoya disease in Japan: Findings from a nationwide survey. Clin Neurol Neurosurg 1997;99(Suppl. 2):S1.
21. Kitahara T, Ariga N, Yamamura A, et al. Familial occurrence of moyamoya disease: Report of three Japanese families. J Neurol Neurosurg Psychiatry 1979;42:208.
22. Kitahara T, Okumura K, Semba T, et al. Genetic and immunologic analysis of moyamoya disease. J Neurol Neurosurg Psychiatry 1982;45:1048.
23. Yamada H, Nakamura S, Kageyama N. Moyamoya disease in monovular twins. Case report, J Neurosurg 1980;53:109.
24. Taveras JM. Multiple progressive intracranial arterial occlusion: A syndrome of children and young adults. AJR Am J Roentgenol 1969;106:235.
25. Chiu D, Sheden P, Bratina P, et al. Clinical features of moyamoya disease in the United States. Stroke 1998;29:1347.
26. Choi KS. Moyamoya disease in Korea: A cooperative study. In: Suzuki J, editor. Advances in surgery for cerebral stroke. Tokyo: Springer-Verlag; 1988. p. 107.
27. Han DH, Kwon OK, Byun BJ, et al. A co-operative study: Clinical characteristics of 334 Korean patients with moyamoya disease treated at neurosurgical institutes (1976–1994). The Korean Society for Cerebrovascular Disease. Acta Neurochir (Wien) 2000;142:1263.
28. Hung CC, Tu YK, Su CF, et al. Epidemiological study of moyamoya disease in Taiwan. Clin Neurol Neurosurg 1997; 99(Suppl. 2):S23.
29. Matsushima Y, Qian L, Aoyagi M. Comparison of moyamoya disease in Japan and moyamoya disease (or syndrome) in the People's Republic of China. Clin Neurol Neurosurg 1997; 99(Suppl. 2):S19.
30. Ikezaki K, Han DH, Kawano T, et al. Epidemiological survey of moyamoya disease in Korea. Clin Neurol Neurosurg 1997; 99(Suppl. 2):S6.
31. Hanakita J, Kondo A, Ishikawa J, et al. An autopsy case of moyamoya disease. Neurol Surg 1982;10:531.
32. Hirayama A, Kowada M, Fukasawa H, et al. Cerebrovascular moyamoya disease: A case report and review of 12 autopsy cases in Japan. No to Shinkei 1974;26:1215.
33. Hosoda Y, Ikeda E, Hirose S. Histopathological studies on spontaneous occlusion of the circle of Willis (cerebrovascular moyamoya disease). Clin Neurol Neurosurg 1997;99(Suppl. 2):S203.
34. Hosoda Y. Pathology of so-called "spontaneous occlusion of the circle of Willis". Pathol Annu 1984;19:221.
35. Maki Y, Nakata Y. Autopsy of a case with an anomalous hemangioma of the internal carotid artery at the skull base. No to Shinkei 1965;17:764.
36. Masuda J, Ogata J, Yutani C. Smooth muscle cell proliferation and localization of macrophages and T-cell in the occlusive intracranial major arteries in moyamoya disease. Stroke 1960; 24:1993.
37. Oka K, Yamashita M, Sadoshima S, et al. Cerebral hemorrhage in moyamoya disease at autopsy. Virchows Arch 1981;392:247.
38. Yamashita M, Oka K, Tanaka K. Histopathology of the brain vascular network in moyamoya disease. Stroke 1983;14:50.
39. Masuda J, Yutani C, Ogata J, et al. Atheromatous embolism in the brain: A clinicopathologic analysis of 15 autopsy cases. Neurology 1994;44:1231.
40. Yamashita M, Oka K, Tanaka K. Cervico-cephalic arterial thrombi and thromboemboli in moyamoya disease: Possible correlation with progressive intimal thickening in the intracranial major arteries. Stroke 1984;15:264.
41. Kodama N, Fujiwara S, Horie Y, et al. Transdural anastomosis in moyamoya disease: Vault moyamoya. No Shinkei Geka 1980;8: 729.
42. Kono S, Oka K, Sueishi K. Histopathologic and morphometric studies of leptomeningeal vessels in moyamoya disease. Stroke 1990;21:1044.
43. Herreman F, Nathal E, Yasui N, et al. Intracranial aneurysm in moyamoya disease: Report of ten cases and review of the literature. Cerebrovasc Dis 1994;4:329.
44. Kodama N, Suzuki J. Moyamoya disease associated with aneurysm. J Neurosurg 1978;48:565.
45. Konishi Y, Kadowaki C, Hara M, et al. Aneurysms associated with moyamoya disease. Neurosurgery 1985;16:484.
46. Nagamine Y, Takahashi S, Sonobe M. Multiple intracranial aneurysms associated with moyamoya disease. Case report, J Neurosurg 1981;54:673.
47. Pilz P, Hartjes HJ. Fibromuscular dysplasia and multiple dissecting aneurysms of intracranial arteries. A further cause of moyamoya syndrome. Stroke 1976;7:393.
48. Yamashita M, Tanaka K, Matsuo T, et al. Cerebral dissecting aneurysms in patients with moyamoya disease: Report of two cases. J Neurosurg 1983;58:120.
49. Yuasa H, Tokito S, Izumi K, et al. Cerebrovascular moyamoya disease associated with an intracranial pseudoaneurysm. Case report, J Neurosurg 1982;56:131.
50. Ogata J, Masuda J, Nishikawa M, et al. Sclerosed peripheral-artery aneurysm in moyamoya disease. Cerebrovasc Dis 1996;6: 248.
51. Ikeda E. Systemic vascular changes in spontaneous occlusion of the circle of Willis. Stroke 1991;22:1358.
52. Yamashita M, Tanaka K, Kishikawa T, et al. Moyamoya disease associated with renovascular hypertension. Hum Pathol 1984;15: 191.
53. Godin M, Helias A, Tadie M, et al. Moyamoya syndrome and renal artery stenosis. Kidney Int 1978;15:450.
54. Goldberg HJ. Moyamoya associated with peripheral vascular occlusive disease. Arch Dis Child 1974;49:964.
55. Yamano T, Onouchi Z, Shimada M. Moyamoya disease and renal hypertension: A case probably caused by fibromuscular dysplasia. Brain Dev 1974;6:184.
56. Aoyagi M, Ogami K, Matsushima Y, et al. Human leukocyte antigen in patients with moyamoya disease. Stroke 1995;26: 415.
57. Seeler RA, Royal JE, Powe L, et al. Moyamoya disease in children with sickle cell anemia and cerebrovascular occlusion. J Pediatr 1978;93:808.
58. Erickson RP, Wooliscroft J, Allen RJ. Familial occurrence of intracranial arterial occlusive disease (moyamoya) in neurofibromatosis. Clin Genet 1980;18:191.
59. Lamas E, Diez Lobato R, Cabello A, et al. Multiple intracranial arterial occlusions (moyamoya disease) in patients with neurofibromatosis: One case report with autopsy. Acta Neurochir (Wien) 1978;45:133.
60. Mito T, Becker LE. Vascular dysplasia in Down syndrome: A possible relationship to moyamoya disease. Brain Dev 1992;14:248.
61. Nagasaka T, Shiozawa Z, Kobayashi M, et al. Autopsy findings in Down's syndrome with cerebrovascular disorder. Clin Neuropathol 1996;15:145.
62. Fukuyama Y, Kanai N, Osawa M. Clinical genetic analysis on moyamoya disease. In: Yonekawa Y, editor. Annual report (1991) by research committee on spontaneous occlusion of the circle of Willis. Tokyo: Ministry of Health and Welfare; 1992. p. 141.

63. Fukuyama Y, Sugahara N, Osawa M. A genetic study of idiopathic spontaneous multiple occlusion of the circle of Willis. In: Yonekawa Y, editor. Annual Report (1990) by research committee on spontaneous occlusion of the circle of Willis. Tokyo: Ministry of Health and Welfare; 1991. p. 139.
64. Inoue TK, Ikezaki K, Sasazuki T, et al. DNA typing of HLA in the patients with moyamoya disease. Jpn J Hum Genet 1997;42:507.
65. Inoue TK, Ikezaki K, Sasazuki T, et al. Linkage analysis of moyamoya disease on chromosome 6. J Child Neurol 2000;15:179.
66. Ikeda H, Sasaki T, Yoshimoto T, et al. Mapping of a familial moyamoya disease gene to chromosome 3p24.2-p26. Am J Hum Genet 1999;64:533.
67. Yamauchi T, Tada M, Houkin K, et al. Linkage of familial moyamoya disease (spontaneous occlusion of the circle of Willis) to chromosome 17q25. Stroke 2000;31:930.
68. Sakurai K, Horiuchi Y, Ikeda H, et al. A novel susceptibility locus for moyamoya disease on chromosome 8q23. J Hum Genet 2004;49:278.
69. Liu W, Morito D, Takashima S, et al. Identification of RNF213 as a susceptibility gene for moyamoya disease and its possible role in vascular development. PLoS ONE 2011;6:e22542.
70. Kamada F, Aoki Y, Narisawa A, et al. A genome-wide association study identifies RNF213 as the first Moyamoya disease gene. J Hum Genet 2011;56:34.
71. Kasai N, Fujiwara S, Kodama N, et al. The experimental study on causal genesis of moyamoya disease: Correlation with immunological reaction and sympathetic nerve influence for vascular changes. No Shinkei Geka 1982;10:251.
72. Tanigawara T, Yamada H, Sasaki N, et al. Studies on cytomegalovirus and Epstein-Barr virus infection in moyamoya disease. Clin Neurol Neurosurg 1997;99(Suppl. 2):S225.
73. Yamada H, Deguchi K, Tanigawa T, et al. The relationship between moyamoya disease and bacterial infection. Clin Neurol Neurosurg 1997;99(Suppl. 2):S221.
74. Fernandes-Alvares E, Pineda M, Royo C, et al. Moyamoya disease caused by cranial trauma. Brain Dev 1979;1:133.
75. Bitzer M, Topka H. Progressive cerebral occlusive disease after radiation therapy. Stroke 1995;26:131.
76. Rajakulasingam K, Cerullo LJ, Raimondi AJ. Childhood moyamoya syndrome: Postradiation pathogenesis. Childs Brain 1979;5:469.
77. Bai H-Z, Masuda J, Sawa Y, et al. Neointima formation after vascular stent implantation: Spatial and chronological distribution of smooth muscle cell proliferation and phenotypic modulation. Arterioscler Thromb 1994;14:1846.
78. Masuda J, Tanaka K. A new model of cerebral arteriosclerosis induced by intimal injury using a silicone rubber cylinder in rabbits. Lab Invest 1984;51:475.
79. Reidy MA, Fingerle J, Lindner V. Factors controlling the development of arterial lesions after injury. Circulation 1992;86(Suppl. III):1845.
80. Ross R. The pathogenesis of atherosclerosis: A perspective for the 1990s. Nature 1993;362:801.
81. Casscells W. Migration of smooth muscle and endothelial cells: Critical events in restenosis. Circulation 1992;86:723.
82. Ikeda E, Maruyama I, Hosoda Y. Expression of thrombomodulin in patients with spontaneous occlusion of the circle of Willis. Stroke 1993;24:657.
83. Bonduel M, Hepner M, Sciuccati G, et al. Prothrombotic disorders in children with moyamoya syndrome. Stroke 2001;32:1786.
84. Takanashi J, Sugita K, Miyazato S, et al. Antiphospholipid antibody syndrome in childhood strokes. Pediatr Neurol 1995;13:323.
85. Hughes GRV. The antiphospholipid syndrome: Ten years on. Lancet 1993;342:341.
86. Hoshimaru M, Takahashi JA, Kikuchi H, et al. Possible roles of basic fibroblast growth factor in the pathogenesis of moyamoya disease: An immunohistochemical study. J Neurosurg 1991;75:267.
87. Suzui H, Hoshimaru M, Takahashi JA, et al. Immunohistochemical reactions for fibroblast growth factor receptor in arteries of patients with moyamoya disease. Neurosurgery 1994;35:20.
88. Aoyagi M, Fukui N, Sakamoto H, et al. Altered cellular responses to serum mitogens, including platelet-derived growth factor, in cultured smooth muscle cells derived from arteries of patients with moyamoya disease. J Cell Physiol 1991;147:191.
89. Hojo M, Hoshimaru M, Miyamoto S, et al. Role of transforming growth-β1 in the pathogenesis of moyamoya disease. J Neurosurg 1998;89:623.
90. Yamamoto M, Aoyagi M, Fukai N, et al. Increase in prostaglandin E(2) production by interleukin-1β in arterial smooth muscle cells derived from patients with moyamoya disease. Circ Res 1999;85:912.
91. Nanba R, Kuroda S, Ishikawa T, et al. Increased expression of hepatocyte growth factor in cerebrospinal fluid and intracranial artery in moyamoya disease. Stroke 2004;35:2837.
92. Kusaka N, Sugiu K, Tokunaga K, et al. Enhanced brain angiogenesis in chronic cerebral hypoperfusion after administration of plasmid human vascular endothelial growth factor in combination with indirect vasoreconstructive surgery. J Neurosurg 2005;103:882.
93. Takahashi A, Sawamura Y, Houkin K, et al. The cerebrovascular fluid in patients in moyamoya disease contains a high level of basic fibroblast growth factor. Neurosci Lett 1993;160:214.
94. Yoshimoto T, Houkin K, Takahashi A, et al. Angiogenic factors in moyamoya disease. Stroke 1996;27:2160.
95. Fukui M, Kawano T. Follow-up study of registered cases in. In: Fukui M, editor. Annual report (1995) by research committee on spontaneous occlusion of the circle of Willis (moyamoya disease). Tokyo, Japan: Ministry of Health and Welfare; 1995, 1996. p. 12.
96. Handa H, Yonekawa Y, Goto Y, et al. Analysis of the filing data bank of 1500 cases of spontaneous occlusion of the circle of Willis and follow-up study of 200 cases for more than 5 years. In: Handa H, editor. Annual report (1984) by research committee on spontaneous occlusion of the circle of Willis. Tokyo, Japan: Ministry of Health and Welfare; 1985. p. 14.
97. Levine SR, Welch KMA. Cerebrovascular ischemia associated with lupus anticoagulant. Stroke 1987;18:257.
98. Yamaguchi T, Tashiro M, Hasegawa Y. Collective analysis of the patients with spontaneous occlusion of the circle of Willis in Japan, registered from 1977 to 1982. In: Gotoh F, editor. Annual report (1982) by research committee on spontaneous occlusion of the circle of Willis (moyamoya disease). Tokyo, Japan: Ministry of Health and Welfare; 1983. p. 15.
99. Yamada I, Suzuki S, Matsushima Y. Moyamoya disease: Comparison with MR angiography and MR imaging versus conventional angiography. Radiology 1995;196:221.
100. Houkin K, Kuroda S, Nakayama N. Cerebral revascularization for moyamoya disease in children. Neurosurg Clin N Am 2001;12:575.
101. Yamada I, Nakagawa T, Matsushima Y, et al. High-resolution turbo magnetic resonance angiography for diagnosis of moyamoya disease. Stroke 2001;32:1825.
102. Morioka M, Hamada J, Todaka T, et al. High-risk age for rebleeding in patients with hemorrhagic moyamoya disease: long-term follow-up study. Neurosurgery 2003;52:1049.
103. Kikuta K, Takagi Y, Nozaki K, et al. Asymptomatic microbleeds in moyamoya disease: T2*-weighted gradient-echo magnetic resonance imaging study. J Neurosurg 2005;102:470.
104. Kuroda S, Kashiwazaki D, Ishikawa T, et al. Stroke. Incidence, locations, and longitudinal course of silent microbleeds in moyamoya disease: a prospective T2*-weighted MRI study. Stroke 2013;44:516.
105. Maeda M, Tsuchida C. "Ivy sign" on fluid-attenuated inversion-recovery images in childhood moyamoya disease. AJNR Am J Neuroradiol 1999;20:1836.
106. Mori N, Mugikura S, Higano S, et al. The leptomeningeal "ivy sign" on fluid-attenuated inversion recovery MR imaging in Moyamoya disease: a sign of decreased cerebral vascular reserve? AJNR Am J Neuroradiol 2009;30:930.
107. Kaczorowska M, Jozwiak S, Litwin M, et al. Moyamoya disease associated with stenosis of extracranial arteries: a case report and review of the literature. Neurol Neurochir Pol 2005;39:242.
108. Yang SH, Li B, Wang CC, et al. Angiographic study of moyamoya disease and histological study in the external carotid artery system. Clin Neurol Neurosurg 1997;99(Suppl. 2):S61.

109. Hoshimaru M, Kikuchi H. Involvement of the external carotid arteries in moyamoya disease: neuroradiological evaluation of 66 patients. Neurosurgery 1992;31:398.
110. Yasaka M, Kimura K, Otsubo R, et al. Transoral carotid ultrasonography. Stroke 1998;29:1383.
111. Yakushiji Y, Yasaka M, Takada T, et al. Serial transoral carotid ultrasonographic findings in extracranial internal carotid artery dissection. J Ultrasound Med 2005;24:877.
112. Kamouchi M, Kishikawa K, Okada Y, et al. Poststenotic flow and intracranial hemodynamics in patients with carotid stenosis: transoral carotid ultrasonography study. AJNR Am J Neuroradiol 2005;26:76.
113. Takekawa H, Ebata A, Arai M, et al. Usefulness of carotid duplex ultrasonography in a patient with moyamoya disease. No to Shinkei 2003;55:983.
114. Yasaka M, Ogata T, Yasumori K, et al. Bottle neck sign of the proximal portion of the internal carotid artery in moyamoya disease. J Ultrasound Med 2006;25:1547.
115. Yasuda C, Yakusiji Y, Eriguchi M, et al. Usefulness of carotid ultrasonography for the early detection of moyamoya disease. Rinsho Shinkeigaku 2007;47:441.
116. Kodama N, Aoki Y, Hiraga H, et al. Electroencephalographic findings in children with moyamoya disease. Arch Neurol 1979; 36:16.
117. Yoshii N, Kudo T. Electroencephalographical study on occlusion of the Willis arterial ring. Rinsho Shinkeigaku 1968;8:301.
118. Ikezaki K, Matsushima T, Kuwabara Y, et al. Cerebral circulation and oxygen metabolism in childhood moyamoya disease: A perioperative positron emission tomography study. J Neurosurg 1994;81:843.
119. Iwama T, Hashimoto N, Yonekawa Y. The relevance of hemodynamic factors to perioperative ischemic complications in childhood moyamoya disease. Neurosurgery 1996;38:1120.
120. Kuwabara Y, Ichiya Y, Otsuka M, et al. Cerebral hemodynamic changes in the child and adult with moyamoya disease. Stroke 1990;21:272.
121. Kuwabara Y, Ichiya Y, Sasaki M, et al. Cerebral hemodynamics and metabolism in moyamoya disease-a positron emission tomography study. Clin Neurol Neurosurg 1997;99(Suppl. 2):S74.
122. Nariai T, Suzuki R, Hirakawa K, et al. Vascular reserve in chronic cerebral ischemia measured with acetazolamide challenge test: Comparison with positron emission tomography. AJNR Am J Neuroradiol 1995;16:563.
123. Obara K, Fukuuchi Y, Kobari M, et al. Cerebral hemodynamics in patients with moyamoya disease and in patients with atherosclerotic occlusion of the major cerebral arterial trunks. Clin Neurol Neurosurg 1997;99(Suppl. 2):S86.
124. Taki W, Yonekawa Y, Kobayashi A, et al. Cerebral circulation and metabolism in adult's moyamoya disease-PET study. Acta Neurochir (Wien) 1989;100:150.
125. Ezura M, Yoshimoto T, Fujiwara S, et al. Clinical and angiographic follow-up of childhood-onset moyamoya disease. Childs Nerv Syst 1995;11:591.
126. Hirotsune N, Meguro T, Kawada S, et al. Long-term follow-up study of patients with unilateral moyamoya disease. Clin Neurol Neurosurg 1997;99(Suppl. 2):S178.
127. Kawano T, Fukui M, Hashimoto N, et al. Follow-up study of patients with "unilateral" moyamoya disease. Neurol Med Chir (Tokyo) 1994;34:744.
128. Fukuyama Y, Mitsuishi Y, Umezu R. Intellectual prognosis of children with TIA type of spontaneous occlusion of the circle of Willis: With special reference to Wechsler's intelligence test and Benton's visual attention test. In: Handa H, editor. Annual report (1986) of research committee on spontaneous occlusion of the circle of Willis. Tokyo, Japan: Ministry of Health and Welfare; 1987. p. 43.
129. Imaizumi C, Imaizumi T, Osawa M, et al. Serial intelligence test scores in pediatric moyamoya disease. Neuropediatrics 1999;30: 294.
130. Imaizumi T, Hayashi K, Saito K, et al. Long-term outcomes of pediatric moyamoya disease monitored to adulthood. Pediatr Neurol 1998;18:321.
131. Kurokawa T, Tomita S, Ueda K, et al. Prognosis of occlusive disease of circle of Willis (moyamoya disease) in children. Pediatr Neurol 1969;12:288.
132. Matsushima Y, Aoyagi M, Nariai T, et al. Long-term intelligence outcome of post-encephalo-duro-arterio-synangiosis in childhood moyamoya patients. Clin Neurol Neurosurg 1997;99(Suppl. 2):S147.
133. Nakashima H, Meguro T, Kawada S, et al. Long-term results of surgically treated moyamoya disease. Clin Neurol Neurosurg 1997;99(Suppl. 2):S156.
134. Ueki K, Meyer JB. Moyamoya disease: The disorder and surgical treatment. Mayo Clin Proc 1994;69:749.
135. Yasargil MG. Microsurgery applied to neurosurgery. Stuttgart: Thieme; 1969.
136. Karasawa J, Kikuchi H, Furuse S, et al. Treatment of moyamoya disease with STA-MCA anastomosis. J Neurosurg 1978;49: 679.
137. Reichmann O, Anderson RE, Roberts TC, et al. The treatment of intracranial occlusive cerebrovascular disease by STA-cortical MCA anastomosis. In: Handa H, editor. Microneurosurgery. Tokyo: Igaku Shoin; 1975. p. 31.
138. Matsushima T, Inoue T, Suzuki SO, et al. Surgical treatment of moyamoya disease in pediatric patients: Comparison between the results of indirect and direct revascularization procedures. Neurosurgery 1992;31:401.
139. Matsushima Y, Inaba Y. Moyamoya disease in children and its surgical treatment: Introduction of a new surgical procedure and its follow-up angiograms. Childs Brain 1984;11:155.
140. Karasawa J, Kikuchi H, Furuse S. A surgical treatment of moyamoya disease: Encephalomyosynangiosis. Neurol Med Chir (Tokyo) 1977;17:29.
141. Karasawa J, Touhou H, Ohnishi H, et al. Cerebral revascularization using omental transplantation for childhood moyamoya disease. J Neurosurg 1993;79:192.
142. Matsushima T, Inoue TK, Suzuki SO, et al. Surgical techniques and the results of a fronto-temporo-parietal combined indirect bypass procedure for children with moyamoya disease: A comparison with the results of encephalo-duro-arterio-synangiosis alone. Clin Neurol Neurosurg 1997;99(Suppl. 2):S123.
143. Shirane R, Yoshida Y, Takahashi T, et al. Assessment of encephalo-galeo-myo-synangiosis with dural pedicle insertion in childhood moyamoya disease: Characteristics of cerebral blood flow and oxygen metabolism. Clin Neurol Neurosurg 1997;99(Suppl. 2): S79.
144. Aoki N. Cerebrovascular bypass surgery for the treatment of moyamoya disease: Unsatisfactory outcome in the patients presenting with intracranial hemorrhage. Surg Neurol 1993;40:372.
145. Srinivasan J, Britz GW, Newell DW. Cerebral revascularization for moyamoya disease in adults. Neurosurg Clin N Am 2001;12: 585.
146. Ikezaki K, Fukui M, Inamura T, et al. The current status of the treatment for hemorrhagic type moyamoya disease based on a 1995 nationwide survey in Japan. Clin Neurol Neurosurg 1997; 99(Suppl. 2):S183.
147. Houkin K, Kamiyama H, Abe H, et al. Surgical therapy for adult moyamoya disease: Can surgical revascularization prevent the recurrence of intracerebral hemorrhage? Stroke 1996;27:448.
148. Yoshida Y, Yoshimoto T, Shirane R, et al. Clinical course, surgical management, and long-term outcome of moyamoya patients with rebleeding after an episode of intracerebral hemorrhage: An extensive follow-up study. Stroke 1999;30:2272.
149. Miyamoto S. Study on the management of moyamoya disease with hemorrhagic onset. In: Yoshimoto T, editor. Annual report (2000) by research committee on spontaneous occlusion of the circle of Willis. Tokyo, Japan: Ministry of Health, Labor, and Welfare; 2001. p. 61.
150. Miyamoto S, Yoshimoto T, Hashimoto N, et al. Effects of extracranial-intracranial bypass for patients with hemorrhagic moyamoya disease: results of the Japan Adult Moyamoya Trial. Stroke 2014;45:1415.

41 CADASIL: Cerebral Autosomal Dominant Arteriopathy with Subcortical Infarcts and Leukoencephalopathy

Hugues Chabriat, Anne Joutel, Elisabeth Tournier-Lasserve, Marie-Germaine Bousser

KEY POINTS

- CADASIL is a familial small artery disease responsible for migraine with aura, stroke, disability and cognitive decline.
- The disease occurs during midadulthood.
- It is caused by mutations of NOTCH3 gene.

CADASIL (cerebral autosomal dominant arteriopathy with subcortical infarcts and leukoencephalopathy)[1] is an inherited small-artery disease of midadulthood which was identified using both, clinical, MRI, pathological, and genetic tools in the 1990s.[2,3] The disease is due to mutations of the *NOTCH3* gene on chromosome 19,[4] leading to an accumulation of the ectodomain of this receptor within the vascular wall. CADASIL is responsible for subcortical ischemic events and leads progressively to dementia with pseudobulbar palsy. The disease was first reported in European families. Today, CADASIL has been diagnosed in European, American, African and Asiatic pedigrees and reported in all continents. The disease probably remains largely underdiagnosed.

HISTORY

In 1955, Van Bogaert reported two sisters belonging to a family originating from Belgium having a "subcortical encephalopathy of Binswanger's type of rapid course" with onset during midadulthood.[5] Their clinical presentation included dementia, gait disturbances, pseudobulbar palsy, seizures and focal neurological deficits. Two other sisters deceased at age 36 and 43 years after a progressive dementia. The father had a stroke at age 51 and deceased after a myocardial infarct. The pathological examination revealed widespread areas of white-matter rarefaction in the brain associated with multiple small infarcts mainly located in the white-matter and basal ganglia.[5]

In 1977, Sourander and Walinder called "hereditary multi-infarct dementia" a familial condition observed in a Swedish pedigree and characterized by dementia associated with pseudobulbar-palsy occuring 10–15 years after recurrent stroke-like episode.[6] The age of onset was between 29 and 38 years, and age at death varied from 30 to 53. The authors reported brain lesions identical to those observed by Van Bogaert in three cases also caused by a small-vessel disease in the brain. The wall of the small arteries was thickened causing a reduction of their lumen. Atherosclerosis of basal arteries was found only in one family member. In the pedigree, the condition followed an autosomal dominant pattern of transmission. The disease was only recently distinguished from CADASIL.

Up to 1993, several families having a close presentation were reported using numerous eponyms; "chronic familial vascular encephalopathy"[7], "familiäre zerebrale arteriosklerose",[8] "familiäre zerebrale Gefäßerkrankung",[9] "démence sous-corticale familiale avec leucoencéphalopathie artériopathique",[10] "familial disorder with subcortical ischemic strokes, dementia and leukoencephalopathy",[11] "slowly progressive familial dementia with recurrent strokes and white-matter hypodensities on CT-scan".[12]

In 1976, we had a patient who was 50 years old with a clinical history of recurrent lacunar infarcts and who presented with a large and widespread hypodensity of the white matter on CT scan. He had no vascular risk factors. Ten years later, his daughter came to see us with a long history of attacks of migraine with aura, transient ischemic attacks, and a recent minor stroke. Her CT and MRI showed lesions in the white matter identical to those observed in her father. These two observations were the basis of the extensive clinical, MRI and genetic study of the extended family originating from the western part of France called Loire-Atlantique. The data were first presented as "recurrent strokes in a family with diffuse white-matter and muscular lipidosis – a new mitochondrial cytopahy?",[2] then as "autosomal dominant syndrome with stroke-like episodes and leukoencephalopathy"[13] and later as "autosomal dominant leukoencephalopathy and subcortical ischemic strokes".[2] Because of the confusion raised by all these different names, we proposed in 1993 the acronym CADASIL (cerebral autosomal dominant arteriopathy with subcortical infarcts and leukoencephalopathy) to designate this disease and highlight its main characteristics.[2] After genetic analysis in the large family from Loire-Atlantique, the affected gene was located on chromosome 19 in 1993.[1] In 1996, various mutations of the *Notch3* gene were found to be responsible for the disease. Subsequently, CADASIL has been recognized in hundreds of families in all continents. Genetic testing is currently used for diagnosis. The gene identification was also crucial to better understand the pathophysiology of the disease and for the development of transgenic mouse models of the disease.[14]

CLINICAL PRESENTATION

The earliest clinical manifestations of CADASIL are attacks of migraine with aura. Despite their frequency which is four times that of the general population,[15,16] these manifestations are inconstant and observed in 20–30% of symptomatic subjects. In contrast, migraine without aura has the same frequency as the general population. When present, migraine with aura is usually the first symptom, with an average onset of 30 years (range: 6–48 years) and occurs 10 years earlier in women than in men,[17] and possibly in association with a high serum homocysteine level.[18] Most frequently, attacks are typical with visual or sensory aura symptoms, lasting 20–30 minutes, followed by a headache lasting a few hours, but 50% of the patients also have atypical attacks with basilar, hemiplegic or prolonged aura and a few patients have very severe attacks with confusion, fever, meningitis, or coma.[17,19–21] The frequency of attacks is highly variable and trigger factors are the usual migraine ones.[17] Migraine with aura may be the predominant symptom of CADASIL in some families. The frequency of migraine attacks can also largely differ among affected subjects from one attack in life to several attacks per month.[17]

Stroke is the most frequent clinical manifestation of the disease over the lifetime. About two-thirds of symptomatic subjects have had transient ischemic attacks or a completed stroke.[22] These events occur at a mean age of 41 ± 9 years (extreme limits from 20 to 65 years).[15,16,22] Two-thirds of them are classical lacunar syndromes: pure motor stroke, ataxic hemiparesis, pure sensory stroke, sensory motor stroke. Other focal neurologic deficits of abrupt onset are less frequently observed: dysarthria either isolated or associated with motor or sensory deficit, monoparesis, paresthesiae on one limb, isolated ataxia, non-fluent aphasia, hemianopia.[15] The onset of the neurological deficit can be progressive over several hours. Some neurological deficits occur suddenly and are associated with headache. When they are transient, they can mimic attacks of migraine with aura. Ischemic events usually occur in the absence of vascular risk factors. However, they are also observed in some patients with one or several vascular risk factors, most frequently in tobacco users and/or hypertensive subjects. The influence of such factors on the clinical and/or MRI phenotype remains unknown.[4,16]

About 20% of CADASIL patients have a history of severe episodes of mood disturbances. Their frequency is again widely variable between families.[15,23] Some patients have a severe depression of the melancholic type sometimes alternating with typical manic episodes.[15,16,19,24] The location of ischemic lesions in basal ganglia and/or in frontal white matter may play a role in their occurrence.[25,26] Apathy characterized by a lack of motivation associated with a reduction in voluntary behavior, has recently been recognized as a major clinical manifestation present in about 40% of patients, independently from depression.[27]

Dementia is the second most common clinical manifestation of CADASIL. It is reported in one-third of symptomatic patients. The location of cerebral lesions explains the "subcortical" aspect of the cognitive deficit. The neuropsychological deficit of progressive or stepwise course is mainly responsible for attention deficit, apathy, and memory impairment.[10,15,28] Aphasia, apraxia, or agnosia are rare or observed only at the end stage of the disease.[10,12] The cognitive deficit is often subtle, particularly at the onset of the disease, and can be detected using a battery of neuropsychological testing. Tests of executive functions can detect the earliest cognitive alterations before the age of 35.[29] The cognitive decline can occur either suddenly, stepwise or progressively in the total absence of ischemic events, mimicking a degenerative dementia.[15,19] The frequency and severity of cognitive decline can vary among different members of a given family. We recently observed that the severity of white-matter microstructural damage is strongly related to the clinical status in CADASIL.[30] This is in agreement with the correlations observed between the clinical status and the load of infarctions within the white matter[31] and with atrophy.[32] Therefore, the degree of tissue destruction or neuronal loss is crucial for the cognitive status of CADASIL patients. When dementia is present, at a mean age of 60 years, it is observed in the absence of any other clinical manifestations in only 10% of cases. Dementia is always associated with pyramidal signs, pseudobulbar palsy, gait difficulties and/or urinary incontinence.[33] The cognitive and functional decline is usually progressive. The patient becomes bedridden and often dies of pulmonary complications related to dysphagia. Dementia is present in 90% of cases before death which occurs at a median age of 64 years in men, and of 69 years in women.[16]

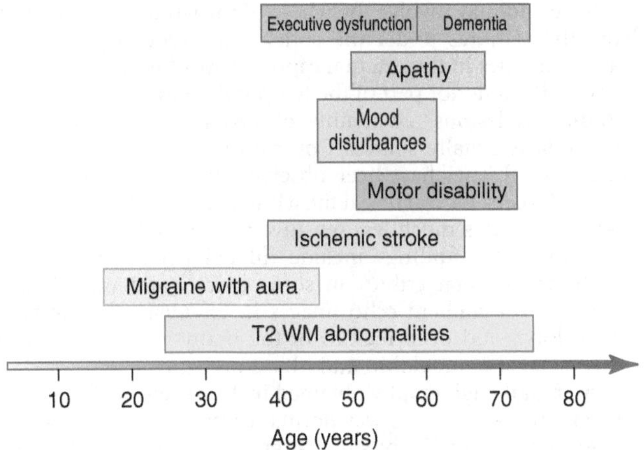

Figure 41-1. Natural history of the main clinical manifestations of CADASIL. *(Modified from Chabriat H, Joutel A, Dichgans M, Tournier-Lasserve E, Bousser MG. CADASIL.* Lancet Neurology *2009;8(7): 643–53.)*

Other neurologic manifestations have occasionally been reported in CADASIL. Focal or generalized seizures have been observed in 6–10% of cases.[15,16] Deafness of acute or rapid onset has been observed in several cases. The lack of cranial nerve palsy, spinal cord disease and of symptoms of muscular origin is noteworthy in CADASIL. The cause of the radiculopathy reported in one case has not been determined.[24]

Finally, the natural history of the disease is summarized in Figure 41-1. CADASIL starts between 20 and 30 years in one-fifth of the patients with attacks of migraine with aura. Ischemic manifestations observed in two-thirds of patients mainly occur during the 4th and 5th decades. Executive dysfunction and apathy are frequent clinical manifestations after age of stroke onset. They are sometimes associated with severe mood disturbances. Dementia mainly occurs during the 6th decade and is found to be nearly constant before death.

No preventive treatment has been evaluated for CADASIL. Because CADASIL is a vascular disorder responsible for cerebral ischemic events, different authors prescribe aspirin for secondary prevention, but its benefit in the disease has not been demonstrated. The occurrence of intracerebral hemorrhage in anecdotal cases suggests that anticoagulant therapy may be dangerous in CADASIL. For migraine, all vasoconstrictive drugs such as ergot derivatives and triptans are not recommended during the course of the disease. And treatment of migraine should be restricted to analgesic agents and nonsteroidal anti-inflammatory drugs.

NEUROIMAGING

MRI is crucial for the diagnosis of CADASIL. It is always abnormal in symptomatic subjects.[2,15,33] In addition, the signal abnormalities can be detected during a presymptomatic period of variable duration. MRI signal abnormalities are observed as early as 20 years of age. After age 35, all subjects having the affected gene have an abnormal MRI.[3,34] The frequency of asymptomatic subjects with abnormal MRI decreases progressively with aging among the gene carriers and becomes very low after 60 years.

T1-weighted MRI shows punctiform or nodular hyposignals in basal ganglia and white matter. T2-weighted images show hypersignals in the same regions often associated with widespread areas of increased signal in the white matter.[29] The severity of MRI signal abnormalities is variable. These lesions dramatically increase with age in affected patients to become diffuse and may involve the whole of the white matter including the U fibres under the cortex. The frequency of signal abnormalities in the external capsule (two-thirds of the cases) and in the anterior part of the temporal lobes is noteworthy.[35] Brainstem lesions are mainly observed in the pons.[30] The medulla is usually spared. Cortical or cerebellar lesions are exceptional. They have been observed in only two cases older than 60 years. CT can reveal the white matter and basal ganglia lesions but it is much less sensitive than MRI.[36]

Other MRI findings include dilated perivascular spaces with typical "etat criblé" in some cases[37] and microbleeds detected on gradient echo images in 25–69% of subjects in both lobar and deep regions of the brain[38,39] related to age, glycosylated hemoglobin and blood pressure.[40]

Cerebral angiography obtained in 14 patients belonging to seven affected families was normal except in one case with a detectable narrowing of small arteries.[15] Worsening of neurological status was reported with high frequency in CADASIL patients after angiography, including possible vasospasm.[41,42] Ultrasound studies and echocardiography are usually normal, although a high frequency of patent foramen ovale (47%) has been reported in an Italian series.[43] CSF examination is usually normal but oligoclonal bands with pleiocytosis have been reported.[36] An isolated increase of complement factor B has been reported in three CADASIL patients.[44] Electromyogram examination is essentially normal. A monoclonal immunoglobulin was detected in the serum of few isolated cases.[13]

PATHOLOGY

Macroscopic examination of the brain shows a diffuse myelin pallor and rarefaction of the hemispheric white matter sparing the U fibres.[2,45] Lesions predominate in the periventricular areas and centrum semi-ovale. They are associated with lacunar infarcts located in the white matter and basal ganglia (lentiform nucleus, thalamus, caudate)[45,46] (Fig. 41-2). The most severe hemispheric lesions are the most profound.[2,10] In the brainstem, the lesions are more marked in the pons and are similar to the pontine rarefaction of myelin of ischemic origin described by Pullicino et al.[47] Microscopic investigations showed that the wall of cerebral and leptomeningeal arterioles is thickened with a significant reduction of the lumen.[2] Such abnormalities can also be detected by leptomeningeal biopsy.[48] Some inconstant features are similar to those reported in patients with hypertensive encephalopathy:[49] duplication and splitting of internal elastic lamina, adventitial hyalinosis and fibrosis, hypertrophy of the media. However, a distinctive feature is the presence of a granular material within the media extending into the adventitia. The PAS-positive staining suggested the presence of glycoproteins; the staining for amyloid substance and elastin are negative.[2,46,50,51] In a single case, these vascular abnormalities were found associated with typical lesions of Alzheimer's disease.[52] Immunohistochemistry does not support the presence of immunoglubulins in the vessel wall. By contrast, the endothelium of the vessels is usually spared. Sometimes, the smooth muscle cells are not detectable and are replaced by collagen fibers.[49] On electron microscopy, the smooth muscle cells appear swollen and often degenerated, some of them with multiple nuclei. There was a granular, electron-dense, osmiophilic material within the media.[45] This material consists of granules of about 10–15 nm of diameter.[49] It is localized close to the cell membrane of the smooth muscle cells where it appears very dense. The smooth muscle cells are separated by large amounts of the unidentified material.

Ruchoux et al. made the crucial observation that the vascular abnormalities observed in the brain were also detectable in other organs.[46,53,54] The granular and osmiophilic material (GOM) surrounding the smooth muscle, cells as seen with electron microscopy is also present in the media of arteries located in the spleen, liver, kidneys, muscle, and skin and also in the wall of carotid and aortic arteries.[46,53] These vascular lesions can also be detected by nerve biopsy.[55] The presence of this material in the skin vessels allows to confirm the intra vitam diagnosis of CADASIL in difficult cases using punch skin biopsies,[56] although the sensitivity and specificity of this method have not yet been completely established.[46,53,57] Skin biopsy immunostaining with a Notch3 monoclonal antibody revealing the accumulation of Notch3 protein in the vessel wall is also another diagnostic tool of high sensitivity (85–95%) and specificity (95–100%).[58,59]

GENETICS

The clinical penetrance of the disease is related to age and is close to 100% after age 50 years. The penetrance based on MRI features reaches 100% at age 35 years. In the absence of a positive familial history, the diagnosis of CADASIL should not be ruled out due to possible de novo mutations of the *Notch3* gene.[60]

CADASIL is caused by stereotyped mutations of the *Notch3* gene. This gene is a 2321-amino-acid protein, it is a transmembrane receptor with an extracellular domain containing 34 EGF repeats (including six cystein residues) and three Lin repeats associated with an intracellular and a transmembrane domain. The stereotyped mis-sense mutations responsible for the disease are within epidermal-growth-factor-like (EGF-like) repeats and only located in the extracellular domain of the Notch3 protein. In 70% of cases, they are located within exons 3 and 4 which encode the first five EGF domains. All mutations in CADASIL lead to an uneven number of cystein residues and presumably alter the function of the receptor.

The Notch3 protein is expressed exclusively in vascular smooth muscle cells.[61] The protein undergoes a proteolytic cleavage leading to an extracellular and a transmembrane fragment. After cleavage, these two fragments form a heterodimer at the cell surface. The ectodomain of the Notch3 receptor accumulates within the vessel wall of affected subjects. It is observed in all vascular smooth mucle cells and in pericytes within all organs (brain, heart, muscles, lungs, skin). An abnormal clearance of the Notch3 ectodomain from the smooth muscle cell surface is presumed to cause this accumulation.[61] Biochemical fractionation of brain samples recently showed that mutant Notch3 extracellular domain (ECD) accumulates in insoluble aggregates in mice and patients with CADASIL. Two functionally important extracellular matrix proteins, tissue inhibitor of metalloproteinases 3 (TIMP3) and vitronectin were found to be sequestered with Notch3(ECD) within the GOM. Experimental data strongly support that aggregation of Notch3 is a central event and enhances the formation of Notch3(ECD)–TIMP3 complex that in turn promotes complex formation including NOTCH3 and VTN. The abnormal recruitment of functionally important extracellular matrix proteins may ultimately cause toxicity by impairing extracellular matrix homeostasis in small vessels.[62]

The identification of the gene of CADASIL was a crucial step to develop a molecular diagnostic test which is now currently used for the positive diagnosis of the disease. Over 95% of mutations in the *NOTCH3* gene are missense mutations. Others are small in-frame deletions or splice-site mutations.[63–67] Remarkably all mutations lead to an odd number of cysteine residues within a given EGFR.[64,68–72] De novo mutations have been reported but their exact frequency is unknown.[60,73] Two homozygous patients have so far been described.[74,75] Genetic testing is the gold standard for the diagnosis of CADASIL. Screening of the 23 exons encoding the 34 EGFR has a 100%

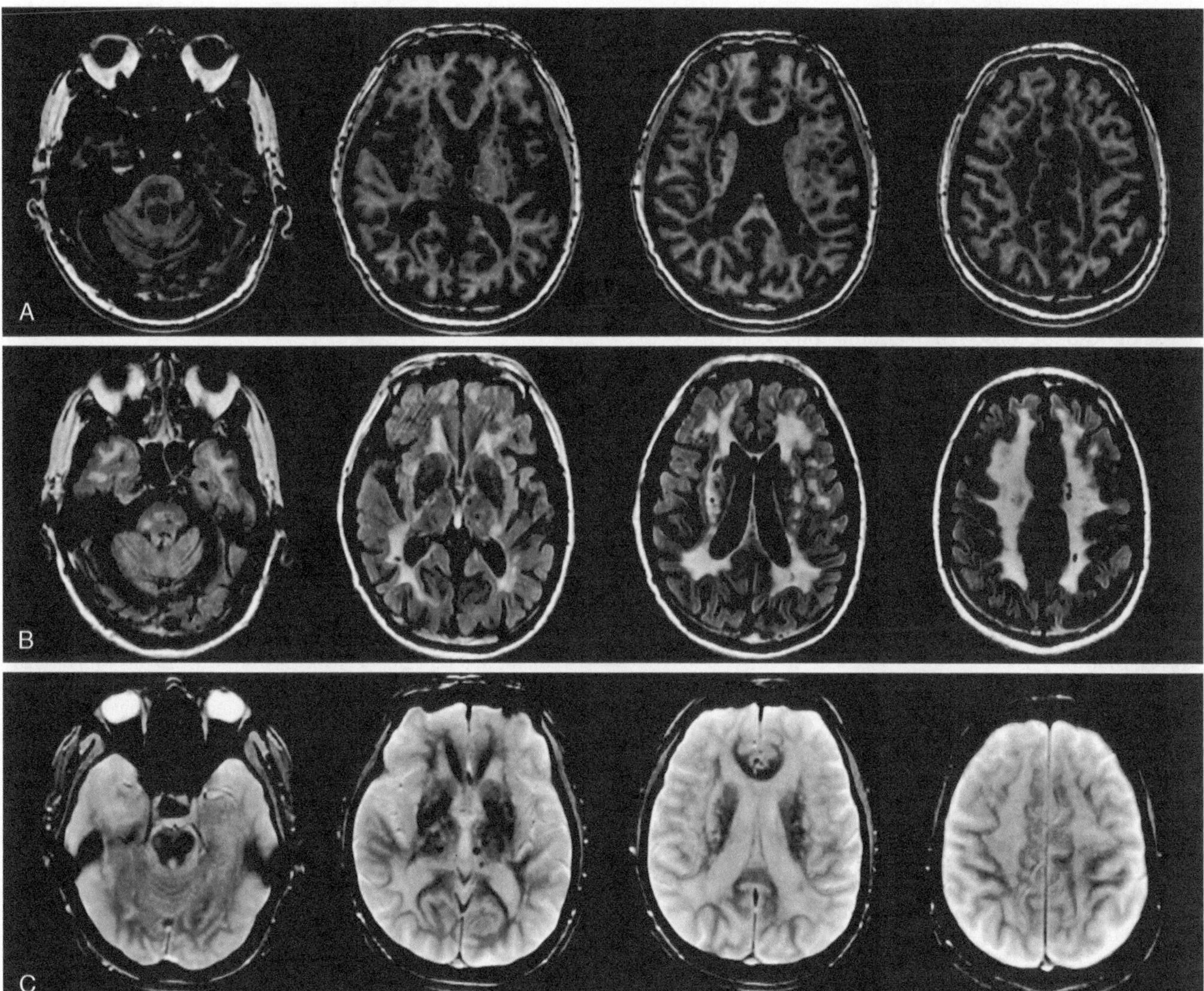

Figure 41-2. MRI aspects in CADASIL. MRI showing (A) on T1-WI lacunar infarcts located in the brainstem (pons), thalamus and lentiform nuclei in a 61-year-old patient with a history of stroke, gait difficulties and cognitive complaints. On FLAIR images (B), the small deep infarcts are detected in association with diffuse and confluent white-matter hyperintensities involving the anterior part of the temporal lobes. On T2* or gradient-echo images (C), microbleeds are visible as small hypointense foci in the thalamus and brainstem. *(Modified from Chabriat H, Joutel A, Dichgans M, Tournier-Lasserve E, Bousser MG. CADASIL.* Lancet Neurology *2009;8(7):643–53.)*

specificity when it detects a mutation leading to an odd number of cysteine residues within an EGFR. Its sensitivity is also close to 100%.[69,71,76]

DIAGNOSIS

The diagnosis of CADASIL should be considered in patients with TIAs or strokes, severe mood disorders, attacks of migraine with aura or dementia, whenever their MRI discloses widespread signal abnormalities in the subcortical white matter and basal ganglia. This association should prompt a genealogical study of the family including all first- and second-degree relatives. Clinical and/or neuroimaging data obtained from these latters are crucial to confirm the hereditary origin of the disease. The diagnosis can be confirmed by genetic testing with or without skin biopsy (see above).

The clinical and MRI presentation of CADASIL is very close to that of Binswanger's disease (BD) but the two conditions differ on three points; in contrast to CADASIL, BD occurs most often in hypertensive patients, is not associated with migraine with aura and is not recognized as an autosomal dominant condition. However, it should be noted that the familial character has not been systematically evaluated in most cases of BD and that, conversely, sporadic mutations of the *Notch3* gene are possible.[60] On MRI, the involvement of the external capsule and anterior white matter of temporal lobes appear more frequent and severe in CADASIL which is useful for differential diagnosis. Some causes of vascular leukoencephalopathies are easy to recognize. Amyloid angiopathies of hereditary origin can present with ischemic strokes and MRI white-matter signal abnormalities but are essentially characterized by recurrent lobar cerebral hemorrhages and the presence of amyloid deposits within the wall of brain vessels.[77,78] The "familial young-onset arteriosclerotic leukoencephalopathy" reported in Japanese pedigrees is an autosomal recessive condition also called CARASIL (cerebral autosomal recessive arteriopathy with subcortical infarcts and leukoencephalopathy), associated with alopecia and skeletal abnormalities, secondary to a thickening of the intima of small cerebral vessels. It is caused by mutations of the HtrA serine protease 1 (*HTRA1*) gene that represses signaling by TGF-beta family members.[79,80] The hereditary leukoencephalopathy described by Lossos et al., a disorder with increased skin collagen content, leads to a progressive dementia and is associated with palmoplantar keratoderma.[81] CADASIL, particularly at onset, can be difficult to differentiate from multiple sclerosis. The autosomal dominant pattern of transmission of the disease, the absence of optic nerve or spinal cord involvement and the symmetrical distribution of white-matter signal abnormalities often associated with basal ganglia infarcts at MRI examination are the most helpful signs to recognize the disease.[63] Also, adrenoleukodystrophy, an X-linked metabolic disorder with accumulation of very-long-chain fatty acids, can be observed in adults but, conversely to CADASIL, it does not involve basal ganglia, the cerebral disease is progressive and associated with spinal cord and peripheral nerve demyelination.

Recently, other ischemic small-vessel diseases with clinical and MRI presentation close to that observed in CADASIL and autosomal dominant transmission but distinct from CADASIL have been identified.[82]

REFERENCES

1. Tournier-Lasserve E, Joutel A, Melki J, et al. Cerebral autosomal dominant arteriopathy with subcortical infarcts and leukoencephalopathy maps to chromosome 19q12. Nat Genet 1993;3:256–9.
2. Baudrimont M, Dubas F, Joutel A, et al. Autosomal dominant leukoencephalopathy and subcortical ischemic stroke. A clinicopathological study. Stroke 1993;24:122–5.
3. Joutel A, Corpechot C, Ducros A, et al. Notch3 mutations in CADASIL, a hereditary adult-onset condition causing stroke and dementia. Nature 1996;383:707–10.
4. Chabriat H, Joutel A, Vahedi K, et al. CADASIL (cerebral autosomal dominant arteriopathy with subcortical infarcts and leukoencephalopathy). J Mal Vasc 1996;21:277–82.
5. Van Bogaert L. Encephalopathie sous-corticale progressive (Binswanger) à évolution rapide chez deux soeurs. Med Hellen 1955;24:961–72.
6. Sourander P, Walinder J. Hereditary multi-infarct dementia. Morphological and clinical studies of a new disease. Acta Neuropathol (Berl) 1977;39:247–54.
7. Stevens DL, Hewlett RH, Brownell B. Chronic familial vascular encephalopathy. Lancet 1977;1:1364–5.
8. Gerhard L. Familiäre zerebrale Arteriosklerose. Zbl Allg Path Bd 1980;124:163.
9. Colmant H. Familiäre zerebrale Gefäberkrankung. Zbl Allg Pathol Bd 1980;124:163.
10. Davous P, Fallet-Bianco C. Familial subcortical dementia with arteriopathic leukoencephalopathy. A clinico-pathological case. Rev Neurol 1991;147:376–84.
11. Mas JL, Dilouya A, De Recondo J. A familial disorder with subcortical ischemic strokes, dementia and leukoencephalopathy. Neurology 1992;42:1015–19.
12. Salvi F, Michelucci R, Plasmati R, et al. Slowly progressive familial dementia with recurrent strokes and white matter hypodensities on CT scan. Ital J Neurol Sci 1992;13(2):135–40.
13. Tournier-Lasserve E, Iba-Zizen MT, Romero N, et al. Autosomal dominant syndrome with strokelike episodes and leukoencephalopathy. Stroke 1991;22(10):1297–302.
14. Brulin-Fardoux P, Godfrain C, Maurage CA, et al. Glycohistochemical characterization of vascular muscle cell destruction in CADASIL subjects by lectins, neoglycoconjugates and galectin-specific antibodies. Neuropathol Appl Neurobiol 2003;29(4): 400–10.
15. Chabriat H, Vahedi K, Iba-Zizen MT, et al. Clinical spectrum of CADASIL: a study of 7 families. Cerebral autosomal dominant arteriopathy with subcortical infarcts and leukoencephalopathy. Lancet 1995;346(8980):934–9.
16. Dichgans M, Mayer M, Uttner I, et al. The phenotypic spectrum of CADASIL: clinical findings in 102 cases. Ann Neurol 1998; 44(5):731–9.
17. Vahedi K, Chabriat H, Levy C, et al. Migraine with aura and brain magnetic resonance imaging abnormalities in patients with CADASIL. Arch Neurol 2004;61(8):1237–40.
18. Singhal S, Bevan S, Barrick T, et al. The influence of genetic and cardiovascular risk factors on the CADASIL phenotype. Brain 2004;127(Pt 9):2031–8.
19. Verin M, Rolland Y, Landgraf F, et al. New phenotype of the cerebral autosomal dominant arteriopathy mapped to chromosome 19: migraine as the prominent clinical feature. J Neurol Neurosurg Psychiatry 1995;59(6):579–85.
20. Schon F, Martin RJ, Prevett M, et al. "CADASIL coma": an underdiagnosed acute encephalopathy. J Neurol Neurosurg Psychiatry 2003;74(2):249–52.
21. Requena I, Indakoetxea B, Lema C, et al. Coma associated with migraine. Rev Neurol 1999;29(11):1048–51.
22. Desmond DW, Moroney JT, Lynch T, et al. The natural history of CADASIL: a pooled analysis of previously published cases. Stroke 1999;30(6):1230–3.
23. Chabriat H, Tournier-Lasserve E, Vahedi K, et al. Autosomal dominant migraine with MRI white-matter abnormalities mapping to the CADASIL locus. Neurology 1995;45(6):1086–91.
24. Ragno M, Tournier-Lasserve E, Fiori MG, et al. An Italian kindred with cerebral autosomal dominant arteriopathy with subcortical infarcts and leukoencephalopathy (CADASIL). Ann Neurol 1995;38(2):231–6.
25. Bhatia K, Marsden C. The behavioural and motor consequences of focal lesions of the basal ganglia in man. Brain 1994;117: 859–76.
26. Aylward ED, Roberts-Willie JV, Barta PE, et al. Basal ganglia volume and white matter hyperintensities in patients with bipolar disorder. Am J Psychiatry 1994;5:687–93.
27. Reyes S, Viswanathan A, Godin O, et al. Apathy: a major symptom in CADASIL. Neurology 2009;72(10):905–10.
28. Davous P, Bequet D. Cadasil–a new model for subcortical dementia. Rev Neurol (Paris) 1995;151(11):634–9.
29. Chabriat H, Levy C, Taillia H, et al. Patterns of MRI lesions in CADASIL. Neurology 1998;51(2):452–7.
30. Chabriat H, Mrissa R, Levy C, et al. Brain stem MRI signal abnormalities in CADASIL. Stroke 1999;30(2):457–9.
31. Viswanathan A, Gschwendtner A, Guichard JP, et al. Lacunar lesions are independently associated with disability and cognitive impairment in CADASIL. Neurology 2007;69(2):172–9.
32. Viswanathan A, Godin O, Jouvent E, et al. Impact of MRI markers in subcortical vascular dementia: a multi-modal analysis in CADASIL. Neurobiol Aging 2010;31(9):1629–36.
33. Bousser MG, Tournier-Lasserve E. Summary of the proceedings of the First International Workshop on CADASIL. Paris, May 19-21, 1993. Stroke 1994;25(3):704–7.
34. Chabriat H, Bousser MG, Pappata S. Cerebral autosomal dominant arteriopathy with subcortical infarcts and leukoencephalopathy: a positron emission tomography study in two affected family members. Stroke 1995;26(9):1729–30.
35. van Den Boom R, Lesnik Oberstein SA, van Duinen SG, et al. Subcortical lacunar lesions: an MR imaging finding in patients with cerebral autosomal dominant arteriopathy with subcortical infarcts and leukoencephalopathy. Radiology 2002;224(3): 791–6.
36. Chabriat H, Joutel A, Vahedi K, et al. CADASIL. Cerebral autosomal dominant arteriopathy with subcortical infarcts and leukoencephalophathy. Rev Neurol 1997;153(6-7):376–85.
37. Cumurciuc R, Guichard JP, Reizine D, et al. Dilation of Virchow-Robin spaces in CADASIL. Eur Neurol 2006;13:187–90.
38. Lesnik Oberstein SA, van den Boom R, van Buchem MA, et al. Cerebral microbleeds in CADASIL. Neurology 2001;57(6): 1066–70.
39. Dichgans M. Cerebral autosomal dominant arteriopathy with subcortical infarcts and leukoencephalopathy: phenotypic and mutational spectrum. J Neurol Sci 2002;203-204:77–80.
40. Viswanathan A, Guichard JP, Gschwendtner A, et al. Blood pressure and haemoglobin A1c are associated with microhaemorrhage in CADASIL: a two-centre cohort study. Brain 2006;129(Pt 9):2375–83.
41. Weller M, Petersen D, Dichgans J, et al. Cerebral angiography complications link CADASIL to familial hemiplegic migraine. Neurology 1996;46:844.

42. Dichgans M, Petersen D. Angiographic complications in CADASIL. Lancet 1997;349(9054):776–7.
43. Zicari E, Tassi R, Stromillo ML, et al. Right-to-left shunt in CADASIL patients: prevalence and correlation with clinical and MRI findings. Stroke 2008;39(7):2155–7.
44. Unlu M, de Lange RP, de Silva R, et al. Detection of complement factor B in the cerebrospinal fluid of patients with cerebral autosomal dominant arteriopathy with subcortical infarcts and leukoencephalopathy disease using two-dimensional gel electrophoresis and mass spectrometry. Neurosci Lett 2000;282(3):149–52.
45. Gutierrez-Molina M, Caminero Rodriguez A, Martinez Garcia C, et al. Small arterial granular degeneration in familial Binswanger's syndrome. Acta Neuropathol (Berl) 1994;87(1):98–105.
46. Ruchoux MM, Guerouaou D, Vandenhaute B, et al. Systemic vascular smooth muscle cell impairment in cerebral autosomal dominant arteriopathy with subcortical infarcts and leukoencephalopathy. Acta Neuropathol (Berl) 1995;89(6):500–12.
47. Pullicino P, Ostow P, Miller L, et al. Pontine ischemic rarefaction. Ann Neurol 1995;37:460–6.
48. Lammie GA, Rakshi J, Rossor MN, et al. Cerebral autosomal dominant arteriopathy with subcortical infarcts and leukoencephalopathy (CADASIL)–confirmation by cerebral biopsy in 2 cases. Clin Neuropathol 1995;14(4):201–6.
49. Zhang WW, Ma KC, Andersen O, et al. The microvascular changes in cases of hereditary multi-infarct disease of the brain. Acta Neuropathol (Berl) 1994;87(3):317–24.
50. Joutel A, Corpechot C, Ducros A, et al. Notch3 mutations in cerebral autosomal dominant arteriopathy with subcortical infarcts and leukoencephalopathy (CADASIL), a mendelian condition causing stroke and vascular dementia. Ann NY Acad Sci 1997;826:213–17.
51. Ruchoux MM, Maurage CA. CADASIL: Cerebral autosomal dominant arteriopathy with subcortical infarcts and leukoencephalopathy. J Neuropathol Exp Neurol 1997;56(9):947–64.
52. Gray F, Robert F, Labrecque R, et al. Autosomal dominant arteriopathic leuko-encephalopathy and Alzheimer's disease. Neuropathol Appl Neurobiol 1994;20(1):22–30.
53. Ruchoux MM, Chabriat H, Bousser MG, et al. Presence of ultrastructural arterial lesions in muscle and skin vessels of patients with CADASIL. Stroke 1994;25(11):2291–2.
54. Lucas C, Pasquier F, Leys D, et al. Cadasil: a new familial disease responsible for cerebral infarction and dementia. Rev Med Interne 1995;16(4):290–2.
55. Schroder JM, Sellhaus B, Jorg J. Identification of the characteristic vascular changes in a sural nerve biopsy of a case with cerebral autosomal dominant arteriopathy with subcortical infarcts and leukoencephalopathy (CADASIL). Acta Neuropathol (Berl) 1995;89(2):116–21.
56. Furby A, Vahedi K, Force M, et al. Differential diagnosis of a vascular leukoencephalopathy within a CADASIL family: use of skin biopsy electron microscopy study and direct genotypic screening. J Neurol 1998;245(11):734–40.
57. Sabbadini G, Francia A, Calandriello L, et al. Cerebral autosomal dominant arteriopathy with subcortical infarcts and leucoencephalopathy (CADASIL). Clinical, neuroimaging, pathological and genetic study of a large Italian family. Brain 1995;118(Pt 1):207–15.
58. Joutel A, Favrole P, Labauge P, et al. Skin biopsy immunostaining with a Notch3 monoclonal antibody for CADASIL diagnosis. Lancet 2001;358(9298):2049–51.
59. Lesnik Oberstein SA, van Duinen SG, van den Boom R, et al. Evaluation of diagnostic NOTCH3 immunostaining in CADASIL. Acta Neuropathol (Berl) 2003;106(2):107–11.
60. Joutel A, Dodick DD, Parisi JE, et al. De novo mutation in the Notch3 gene causing CADASIL. Ann Neurol 2000;47(3):388–91.
61. Joutel A, Andreux F, Gaulis S, et al. The ectodomain of the Notch3 receptor accumulates within the cerebrovasculature of CADASIL patients. J Clin Invest 2000;105(5):597–605.
62. Monet-Lepretre M, Haddad I, Baron-Menguy C, et al. Abnormal recruitment of extracellular matrix proteins by excess Notch-3ECD: a new pathomechanism in CADASIL. Brain 2013;136(Pt 6):1830–45.
63. Auer DP, Putz B, Gossl C, et al. Differential lesion patterns in CADASIL and sporadic subcortical arteriosclerotic encephalopathy: MR imaging study with statistical parametric group comparison. Radiology 2001;218(2):443–51.
64. Dichgans M, Ludwig H, Muller-Hocker J, et al. Small in-frame deletions and missense mutations in CADASIL:3D models predict misfolding of Notch3 EGF-like repeat domains. Eur J Hum Genet 2000;8(4):280–5.
65. Dotti MT, De Stefano N, Bianchi S, et al. A novel NOTCH3 frameshift deletion and mitochondrial abnormalities in a patient with CADASIL. Arch Neurol 2004;61(6):942–5.
66. Chabriat H, Joutel A, Vahedi K, et al. CADASIL (cerebral autosomal dominant arteriopathy with subcortical infarcts and leukoencephalopathy): clinical features and neuroimaging. Bull Acad Natl Med 2000;184(7):1523–31, discussion 1531–3.
67. Holtmannspotter M, Peters N, Opherk C, et al. Diffusion magnetic resonance histograms as a surrogate marker and predictor of disease progression in CADASIL: a two-year follow-up study. Stroke 2005;36(12):2559–65.
68. Bianchi S, Dotti MT, Federico A. Physiology and pathology of notch signalling system. J Cell Physiol 2006;207:300–8.
69. Joutel A, Vahedi K, Corpechot C, et al. Strong clustering and stereotyped nature of Notch3 mutations in CADASIL patients. Lancet 1997;350(9090):1511–15.
70. Joutel A, Chabriat H, Vahedi K, et al. Splice site mutation causing a seven amino acid Notch3 in-frame deletion in CADASIL. Neurology 2000;54(9):1874–5.
71. Peters N, Opherk C, Bergmann T, et al. Spectrum of Mutations in Biopsy-Proven CADASIL: Implications for Diagnostic Strategies. Arch Neurol 2005;62(7):1091–4.
72. Dichgans M, Herzog J, Gasser T. NOTCH3 mutation involving three cysteine residues in a family with typical CADASIL. Neurology 2001;57(9):1714–17.
73. Coto E, Menendez M, Navarro R, et al. A new de novo Notch3 mutation causing CADASIL. Eur J Neurol 2006;13(6):628–31.
74. Tuominen S, Juvonen V, Amberla K, et al. Phenotype of a homozygous CADASIL patient in comparison to 9 age-matched heterozygous patients with the same R133C Notch3 mutation. Stroke 2001;32(8):1767–74.
75. Liem MK, Lesnik Oberstein SA, Vollebregt MJ, et al. Homozygosity for a NOTCH3 mutation in a 65-year-old CADASIL patient with mild symptoms: a family report. J Neurol 2008;255(12):1978–80.
76. Monet M, Domenga V, Lemaire B, et al. The archetypal R90C CADASIL-NOTCH3 mutation retains NOTCH3 function in vivo. Hum Mole Genet 2007;16(8):982–92.
77. Greenberg SM, Vonsattel JP, Stakes JW, et al. The clinical spectrum of cerebral amyloid angiopathy: presentations without lobar hemorrhage. Neurology 1993;43(10):2073–9.
78. Greenberg SM, Vonsattel JP. Diagnosis of cerebral amyloid angiopathy. Sensitivity and specificity of cortical biopsy. Stroke 1997;28(7):1418–22.
79. Razvi SS, Bone I. Single gene disorders causing ischaemic stroke. J Neurol 2006;253(6):685–700.
80. Fukutake T, Hirayama K. Familial young-onset arteriosclerotic leukoencephalopathy with alopecia and lumbago without arterial hypertension. Eur Neurol 1995;35:69–79.
81. Lossos A, Cooperman H, Soffer D, et al. Hereditary leukoencephalopathy and palmoplantar keratoderma: a new disorder with increased skin collagen content. Neurology 1995;45(2):331–7.
82. Verreault S, Joutel A, Riant F, et al. A novel hereditary small vessel disease of the brain. Ann Neurol 2006;59:353–7.

42 Hematologic Disorders and Stroke

Cheryl Bushnell

KEY POINTS

- Patients with hematologic disorders, such as hereditary thrombophilias, are at higher risk for venous thrombosis than ischemic stroke, but these disorders account for a small, but important, percentage of stroke patients.
- The hereditary causes of protein S, C, and antithrombin III deficiencies, in addition to antiphospholipid antibody syndrome, are considered to be very high risk for recurrent thromboembolic events.
- There are no clinical trials to guide secondary prevention in the setting of thrombophilias, and, therefore, the majority of patients are treated with antiplatelet therapy, except in the case of primary antiphospholipid antibody syndrome, in which the general consensus is to treat with adjusted dose warfarin in the range of INRs 2 to 3 because of the high risk of recurrent thromboembolism.
- Myeloproliferative disorders, including polycythemia rubra vera and essential thrombocythemia, are important causes of ischemic stroke, with high risk of morbidity and mortality. Hematology consultation is essential to guide therapy, monitoring for other leukemias, and genetic testing.
- Heparin-induced thrombocytopenia is an important consequence of heparin therapy, and is important to recognize because of the risk of severe thrombosis. HIT type II is the most serious, and requires stopping heparin and switching to alternative anticoagulation with heparinoids or hirudins.
- Sickle cell anemia is associated with stroke primarily in children, but this can continue throughout an affected individual's lifetime. In children, transcranial Doppler studies showing greater than 200 cm/s in the middle cerebral arteries studies can identify those at highest risk of stroke, and therefore guide transfusions for prevention.
- Testing for thrombophilias should be reserved for ischemic stroke patients under age 55 years, with strong family or personal history of venous thrombosis, pregnancy complications, and no clear explanation for the stroke (i.e., vasculopathy, cardioembolic source, or absence of typical risk factors for stroke).

INTRODUCTION

Hemostasis is a complex, highly evolved system involving intricate chemical interactions among soluble clotting factors, blood elements, and vascular tissues all working in concert to stop bleeding when blood vessels are damaged. Coagulation per se is the component of hemostasis that involves the transformation of liquid blood to a solid clot. Practically all ischemic strokes involve activation of hemostasis, sometimes under pathologic circumstances. There are a wide variety of disorders that have been assigned the underlying cause of ischemic stroke, including hereditary and acquired thrombophilias, myeloproliferative disorders, sickle cell anemia, and heparin-induced thrombocytopenia. Although not exhaustive, these disorders are the focus of this chapter because they are the most common and the most important to recognize in the setting of ischemic stroke, especially in young patients.

The formation of a thrombus within an artery is a frequent consequence of vascular endothelial injury, such as happens with rupture of an atherosclerotic plaque or from relative stasis of blood in the fibrillating left atrium or its appendage. Abnormalities in hemostasis that predispose to thrombotic events are referred to as either a "hypercoagulable state" or a "thrombophilia," whereas conditions in which thrombotic events are more prevalent, such as diabetes mellitus, are considered to be a *prothrombotic state;* however, these terms are frequently interchanged. A detailed understanding of the hypercoagulable state hones the mechanistic diagnosis of stroke and may also help define treatment. Some measures of hemostatic function show promise as biomarkers for monitoring the risk of stroke.

PATHOGENESIS OF THROMBOSIS

Vascular Injury

Hemostasis is a complex system of reactions that are normally held in check by a dynamic interplay between the normal blood vessel endothelial surface and regulatory plasma proteins that prevent activation of platelets and the prothrombin pathway.[1] The circulating regulatory plasma proteins include protein C, protein S, antithrombin III (ATIII), tissue factor pathway inhibitor (TFPI), and protein Z.[2,3] On the vascular endothelium, a key protein, thrombomodulin, promotes the activation of protein C. The combination of activated protein C with another endogenous anticoagulant, protein S, results in a complex that can rapidly inactivate activated coagulation factors Va and VIIIa, thereby suppressing thrombin activation (see, for example, Fig. 42-1). Protein S is found in the plasma as both an active (free) and an inactive (C4b-binding protein) form. A member of the coagulation cascade, protein Z, along with protein Z-related protease inhibitor, directly degrades factor Xa.

The vascular endothelium forms another key element in the regulation of hemostasis by expressing a number of regulatory molecules on the endothelial surface. Among these are thrombomodulin and the glycosaminoglycan, heparin, which by binding ATIII, greatly amplifies the ATIII functional ability to rapidly neutralize thrombin and other activated prothrombotic serine proteases, including factors Xa and IXa.[4,5] Healthy vascular endothelium also inhibits platelet adhesion and aggregation by several mechanisms. When the endothelium is stimulated by local injury, inflammation, or other thrombogenic processes, prostacyclin (PGI_2) is released. PGI_2 causes

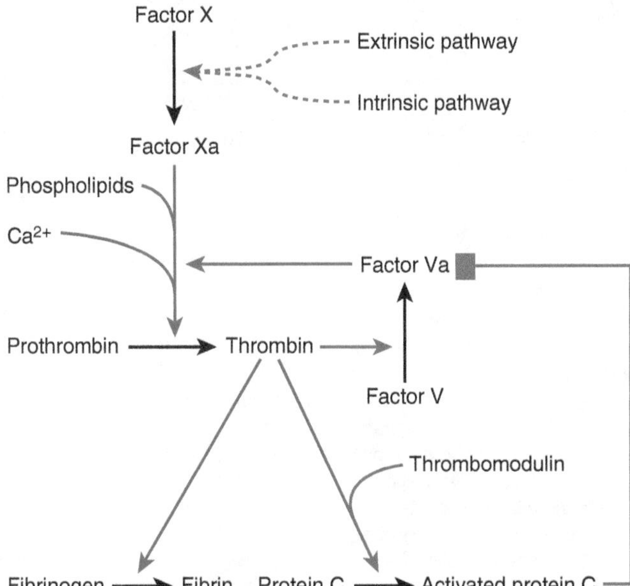

Figure 42-1. Regulation of factor V activity by thrombin and activated protein C. Thrombin activates protein C, which degrades factor V. Factor V Leiden is resistant to inactivation by protein C, which leads to a hypercoagulable state. *(Adapted from Hamedani AG, Cole JW, Mitchell BD, et al: Meta-analysis of factor V Leiden and ischemic stroke in young adults: The importance of case ascertainment.* Stroke *41:1599-1603, 2010.)*

vasodilatation and inhibits platelet plug formation. Vascular endothelium also synthesizes and releases nitric oxide, a potent vasodilator and inhibitor of platelet activation.[6,7] Furthermore, if a clot does begin to form, the vascular endothelium promotes local fibrinolysis via the synthesis and release of tissue plasminogen activator (t-PA).

Although usually a barrier against thrombosis, the normal vascular endothelium becomes a strongly prothrombotic surface when injured.[6] Mediators of inflammation such as interleukin-1, tumor necrosis factor, and immune complexes can induce the endothelium to express tissue factor and other such substances, expose binding sites for clotting factors, and downregulate thrombomodulin expression.[5] With severe injury, endothelial cells may be lost from the vascular surface altogether, thereby exposing thrombogenic subendothelial tissues, as happens with rupture of an atheromatous plaque.[8,9] The brain vascular endothelium also appears to vary in its effectiveness as a barrier against thrombosis because the expression of thrombomodulin within the cerebral circulation varies regionally and is limited in amount compared with systemic vessels.[10–12]

Factor V Leiden, Antithrombin III, Protein C, Protein S, and Protein Z Deficiencies; Prothrombin G20210A Polymorphism; and von Willebrand Factor

Hereditary Deficiencies

Genetic modifications that affect function or concentration of the regulatory coagulation proteins in the hemostatic pathways are associated with an increased risk of stroke. As a general rule the risk is similar for both ischemic stroke and myocardial infarction (MI) in adults, but there are some exceptions. Abnormalities in proteins S, C, and ATIII are associated most strongly with stroke in neonates and young children.[13] Their role in adult stroke is less certain, but recent studies suggest importance in selected populations. For example, the Atherosclerosis Risk in Communities Study (ARIC), reported that the lowest quintile of protein C levels was associated with a 1.5-fold greater risk of ischemic stroke than the highest quintile, and that these levels were most likely associated with non-lacunar stroke subtype.[14]

The presence of factor V Leiden,[15] activated protein C (APC) resistance,[16] and the prothrombin G20210A gene mutation[17] have been associated with stroke in children and young adults. In addition, low levels of protein Z have all been associated with increased risk of stroke.[18] APC resistance, caused by a mutation in factor V (factor V Leiden), which renders factor Va unable to be cleaved by APC, is by far the most common inherited defect associated with venous thrombosis. This mechanism and the related role of thrombin activation and protein C are summarized in Figure 42-1. In white populations, the factor V Leiden defect is present in 5–7% of the normal population and accounts for more than 95% of the total APC resistance. Although APC resistance due to factor V Leiden has a well-recognized association with cerebral venous thrombosis,[15] the relationship to arterial stroke in adults is less certain; currently, the strongest evidence suggests a role in children with stroke.[19] In adult populations such as in the Physicians' Health Study, the presence of factor V Leiden did not increase the risk of stroke or MI,[20] and similar results have been found in some case-control studies;[21] however, in one large study, factor V Leiden was significantly more common in patients with large infarcts (13.6%; $P < 0.025$; confidence interval [CI], 1.16–4.34) than in the stroke-free control subjects (6.5%).[22] Furthermore, a meta-analysis of 18 case-control studies in adults, both young and those older than 50 years, with stroke found inconsistent results with such a heterogeneous mixture of subjects. Among unselected individuals with ischemic stroke, the odds ratio for factor V Leiden was 1.40 (P = NS), whereas the odds ratio associating stroke with factor V Leiden was statistically significant at 2.73 ($P = 0.003$) when individuals who were likely to have a prothrombotic state were specified.[23] In the Genetics of Early Onset Stroke (GEOS) study, there was no significant association between the factor V Leiden mutation and stroke in young men and women vs age-matched controls, and this relationship did not change when the analysis was restricted to strokes of undetermined etiology.[24]

In adults with stroke, the association between inherited deficiencies in protein C, protein S, and ATIII and *arterial* thrombosis is less convincing.[25,26] Case-control and cohort studies provide inconsistent results: some show a positive relationship to stroke while others show a negative relationship. Such discrepancies reflect differences in the selection of subjects to be tested. In a prospective case-control study that initially enrolled subjects with acute MI, it was found on follow-up that individuals with low levels of protein C and/or antithrombin, even if in the low normal range, tended to have an increased risk of recurrent cardiovascular events including stroke (four of the 35 patients with recurrent events).[27]

An increased risk of stroke is also reported with elevated levels of von Willebrand factor (vWF), factor VIIIc, and plasma fibrinogen.[28,29] Unlike the other regulatory proteins that interact with normal vascular endothelial function, vWF comes into play when endothelium is damaged and the factor interacts with platelet activation. The levels of vWF are influenced by inflammation, genetic influences (e.g., ABO blood groups), and a metalloprotease known as "A Disintegrin And Metalloprotease with ThromboSpondin motif (ADAMTS13)."[29] When coupled with inflammation, high levels of vWF triple the relative risk of stroke compared with individuals with low vWF levels. Lip et al.[30] found that constantly elevated vWF levels in persons with chronic atrial fibrillation were associated with an increased likelihood of cardioembolic-related stroke. From a clinical perspective many of these studies emphasize the importance of the role of inflammation as a critical influence on levels and function. When considering the results of measurements obtained during the early phase of stroke, one must keep in mind that levels of these substances can be affected by the extent of the early inflammatory phase response. For example, one study reported that low protein S levels were common in patients hospitalized for any reason,[31] which makes the role of this substance in stroke much more difficult to establish.

A single mutation in the 3′-untranslated region of the prothrombin gene resulting in a G-to-A (glycine-to-alanine) substitution has been associated with familial thrombophilia.[17] Prothrombin, or factor II, is the precursor of thrombin. A vitamin-K-dependent zymogen, this protein is produced by the liver and has a central role in the conversion of fibrinogen to fibrin. Prothrombin also has inhibitory functions that limit the hemostasis process (see Fig. 42-1). Thrombin also has regulatory functions that are important in the pathogenesis of atherosclerosis, such as initiating platelet aggregation and endothelial activation.

Factor II G20210A occurs in about 2.5% of the general population and in 6% of patients with a family history of venous thrombosis.[32] This mutation is seen almost exclusively in white persons; in the presence of traditional vascular risk factors, the addition of factor II G20210A has a synergistic effect on the risk of MI, but results are conflicting.[17] Few studies have investigated the role of factor II G20210A in stroke. A case-control study of consecutive patients with stroke or transient ischemic attack (TIA) found no difference in prevalence of the prothrombin mutation between the patients and control subjects.[21] Another study of 72 young patients with stroke and without traditional vascular risk factors found an increased prevalence in patients compared with control subjects (9.7% of patients had heterozygous mutations vs 2.5% of control subjects; 2.8% of patients had homozygous mutations vs 0% of control subjects).[14] The stroke risk associated with the heterozygous mutation was increased 3.8-fold, either mutation was increased 5.5-fold, and the homozygous mutation was increased 208-fold. From a clinical perspective more studies are needed to clarify the role of this mutation in stroke from either a diagnostic or therapeutic perspective.

Combined Genetic Prothrombotic Factors and Association with Patent Foramen Ovale

In a cohort of young (aged 55 or younger) patients with ischemic stroke and non-stroke controls, genetic polymorphisms for factor V Leiden, G20210A prothrombin, C677T MTHFR, and 4G/5G PAI-1 were evaluated along with other traditional stroke risk factors.[33] The prothrombotic gene mutations were added to provide a genetic sum score, which resulted in an independent association with ischemic stroke in this cohort (odds ratio [OR] 2.31, 95%CI, 1.64–3.25), in addition to decreased HDL cholesterol, hypertension, obesity, and smoking. The authors concluded that these prothrombotic genetic abnormalities act synergistically to increase the risk of ischemic stroke in young patients.[33]

Although patent foramen ovale (PFO) appears to be a conduit for paradoxical embolism in patients with prothrombotic disorders, one study showed that FII G20210A was associated with cryptogenic stroke regardless of the presence of PFO. In addition, there was no increased association with FVL mutation and PFO.[34]

BOX 42-1 Acquired Deficiencies of Antithrombin III and Proteins C and S

- Consumption coagulopathy
- Disseminated intravascular coagulation (shock, sepsis)
- Surgery
- Preeclampsia
- Liver dysfunction
- Acute hepatic failure
- Cirrhosis
- Renal disease
- Nephrotic syndrome
- Hemolytic-uremic syndrome
- Malignancies
- Leukemia (acute promyelocytic leukemia)
- Malnutrition or gastrointestinal loss
- Vascular reconstruction (diabetes, age)
- Protein-calorie deprivation
- Inflammatory bowel disease
- Various medicines (e.g., warfarin)
- Estrogens-progestins
- Heparin
- L-Asparaginase
- Other
- Vasculitis (? systemic lupus erythematosus)
- Infection – neutropenia
- Hemodialysis
- Plasmapheresis

Acquired Deficiencies

Acquired deficiencies of ATIII and proteins C and S are associated with a prothrombotic state and thereby to brain infarction in a variety of special clinical settings, as listed in Box 42-1. Reductions of the anticoagulant proteins have been found in perioperative settings, and in patients with malignancies, hepatic failure, or nephrotic syndrome. Short-term fluctuations of anticoagulant protein levels can also follow plasmapheresis and hemodialysis. In a patient with any of the foregoing conditions who experiences TIA, stroke, or amaurosis fugax, careful evaluation may uncover one of these prothrombotic states.

Association with Prothrombotic States and Hormonal Use. Hormonal contraception (oral contraceptive pills and transdermal patches) have been associated with an increased risk of stroke in young women, but the risk appears to be increased even further in women who also have prothrombotic disorders. The Risk of Arterial Thrombosis in relation to Oral Contraceptives (RATIO) study showed that women with the factor F Leiden and the MTHFR 677T mutation were at increased risk for ischemic stroke, with a suggestion of synergy between the pills and the genetic predisposition since non-users did not have an increased risk.[35]Similarly, women with elevated VWF and ADAMTS13 levels had an increased association with ischemic stroke, but only in OC users.[36] Further research is needed to understand the relationship between these disorders and longitudinal risk of stroke in young women using oral contraceptives, weighing the risks and benefits with pregnancy.

Laboratory Investigation

The decision to order thrombophilia testing for a patient with ischemic stroke is dependent on several important factors, including age younger than 50 years, family or personal history of venous thromboembolism, or thrombosis during pregnancy.[37] Genetic tests are available for factor V Leiden and the prothrombin G20210A polymorphism.[38] For deficiencies of protein C, protein S, and ATIII, the underlying defect may be attributable to several different mutations, and DNA testing is not practical. In general, in situations for which genetic tests are unavailable (or their results would be negative in the case of acquired deficiencies), functional or activity-based assays should be used. Ten percent of defects are in the functional aspect of the molecule and would be missed with antigen assays.[38]

Functional-based assays for protein C are commercially available, but their results may be affected by conditions such as APC resistance and high concentrations of factor VIII and may be difficult to interpret.[39,40] For protein S, a functional assay should be theoretically superior to antigen measurement; however, the distribution of protein S in the plasma is 60% of the whole protein bound to C4b-binding protein, and 40% is free and active as APC cofactor.[41] The most common defect in protein S is a normal total protein S level but decreased levels of free protein S.[42] Therefore, free protein S is likely the best quantitative test.[43] The two types of functional assays for ATIII deficiency are progressive inhibitory activity (performed without heparin) and heparin cofactor activity. The assay using heparin cofactor activity is able to detect all clinically relevant cases of ATIII deficiency. Factor Xa is probably a better target enzyme than thrombin because factor Xa is not affected by the presence of the other main plasma inhibitor of thrombin, heparin cofactor II.[44]

Functional thrombophilia testing should be delayed until 6 months after the event because of the impact of the acute thromboembolic event on the interpretation of the test. Treatment for thromboembolic events with anticoagulation (heparins or warfarin) will also interfere with the test results. Therefore, the recommendations are to wait for at least 2 weeks after discontinuation of anticoagulation prior to testing.[38]

Fibrinolysis

Homeostasis depends on the balance between clot formation and clot degradation, or *fibrinolysis*. Depression of fibrinolytic activity can tip the balance toward thrombosis. The fibrinolytic system is equilibrated between t-PA and its primary inhibitor, plasminogen activator inhibitor type 1 (PAI-1). Either reductions of t-PA or elevations of PAI-1 can inhibit fibrinolysis and predispose to thrombosis.[45]

Fibrinolytic degradation products such as cross-linked D-dimer are increased after stroke,[46–50] and their levels are correlated with infarct size, stroke severity, and subsequent mortality.[51] Prospective population studies have demonstrated the seemingly paradoxical finding that elevations of t-PA antigen are associated with a greater risk of MI and stroke.[17,52,53] Elevations of t-PA antigen are also associated with the severity of carotid atherosclerosis.[54] Elevations of t-PA antigen do not necessarily denote increased fibrinolytic activity, but instead may indicate an ongoing response to atherosclerosis and thrombosis and greater clot formation rather than a more effective fibrinolytic response. Furthermore, t-PA antigen elevation may merely be a marker for ongoing endothelial damage.[55] Genetic evaluation of tPA revealed that only the DD genotype and D allele of this gene were associated with stroke in a Saudi Arabian cohort and that there may be gene–gene interactions with more variants that increase susceptibility of ischemic stroke.[56]

Lipoprotein (a) – or Lp(a) – can inhibit fibrinolysis in vitro and may have a similarly important effect in vivo, and elevated levels of Lp(a) increase the risk of stroke and MI.[57] Lp(a) has substantial homology to plasminogen, the precursor to plasmin.[58] Lp(a) also stimulates the release of PAI-1 from endothelial cells and effectively competes with plasminogen for binding either to fibrin or to the surface of vascular endothelial cells, inhibiting fibrinolysis.[59,60] Lp(a) levels have been found to be high in selected populations with cerebrovascular disease, and most but not all studies have shown Lp(a) elevation to be a potent risk factor for stroke, especially in young patients.[61–66] However, Lp(a) levels do not appear to be associated with stroke characteristics, recurrence, or prognosis.[59,60] Unfortunately, there is no established treatment for increased Lp(a) levels, and management consists of aggressively controlling other risk factors, especially lowering the low-density lipoprotein (LDL) cholesterol level to less than 100 mg/dL.

Myeloproliferative Disorders and Stroke

Patients with myeloproliferative disease (MPD), including polycythemia rubra vera (PV) and essential thrombocythemia (ET), have increases in platelet reactivity and platelet counts as well as large, dysfunctional platelets, which are strongly associated with stroke.[67–69] Thrombosis occurs more frequently in PV and ET than in acute myelocytic leukemia or chronic granulocytic leukemia and is a major cause of morbidity and mortality in patients with these myeloproliferative disorders. Up to 40% of patients with PV or ET experience a thrombotic episode, and the incidence of thrombosis could be as high as 75% per year. Arterial occlusions are more common than venous events,[69–74] and stroke is often the presenting feature of both PV and ET. At the time of diagnosis, 25% of patients with myeloproliferative syndromes manifest atherosclerosis, and 50% of patients have evidence of carotid intimal thickening. Increasing age, elevated hematocrit level, and treatment with phlebotomy in PV all predispose to thromboembolism.

Importantly, in ET, the magnitude of the elevation of the platelet count does not correlate with the risk of thrombosis, since many patients with ischemic stroke have platelet counts lower than 400,000 cell/mm^3. Another risk factor for thrombotic events in patients with ET is the presence of the JAK2 V617F mutation. Patients with this mutation and ET have been found to have lower levels of protein S, and have elevated markers of platelet and endothelial activation (tissue factor, soluble P-selectin, sCD40L, vWF antigen, and soluble thrombomodulin) than those without the mutation.[75]

In addition to pharmacologic antithrombotic measures, lowering of elevated platelet counts should be considered in patients with MPD and a history of thrombosis. Hydroxyurea (e.g., 1 g daily to start) has been shown in a randomized trial to prevent thrombotic complications in patients with essential thrombocytosis.[76,77] A platelet count of 250,000 to 450,000 cells/mm^3 is an appropriate target. The use of anagrelide to lower platelet counts should be considered for cases refractory to hydroxyurea or for patients unable to tolerate the drug.[76]

Heparin-induced Thrombocytopenia

Heparin-induced thrombocytopenia (HIT) is a potentially serious consequence of heparin administration. Type I is a result of a non-immunogenic response to heparin occurring in the first 2 days of therapy, with a transient reduction in platelet count and a gradual return to pre-treatment levels, even if heparin is not discontinued. HIT type II is immune-mediated, less frequent, but more severe than type I. In HIT II, platelet counts are reduced by >30% and occur in delayed fashion. The incidence of HIT is lower in patients receiving low-molecular-weight heparin (LMWH). HIT II happens when antibodies, usually immunoglobulin G (IgG), are produced that bind the heparin–platelet factor 4 (PF4) complex.[78,79] The antibody binding causes further platelet activation that produces more PF4 release, thereby propagating the cycle. An elevation of circulating adhesion molecules (selectins) has also been observed in HIT.[80] Platelet–neutrophil complexes are mediated by P-selectin, which is also important in leukocyte adhesion. This finding supports a role for inflammation in the underlying pathophysiology of HIT. Platelet activation leads to release of platelet microparticles, triggering an activation of the coagulation system.[80] Although platelets are consumed and the counts fall, the syndrome is characterized by vascular occlusive events rather than bleeding. HIT II occurs 6–10 days after heparin exposure and is associated with a significant thrombocytopenia and a high risk of thrombotic events, including stroke.[78,79,81-84] The incidence of HIT II is 1–5%. The risk is higher with higher doses of heparin, but has been described after very low doses such as those used for intravenous line flushes.[85-88]

A 14-year retrospective review found that in patients diagnosed with isolated HIT II the 30-day risk of thrombosis was 53%.[87] Most thromboses were venous. Although platelet counts in HIT may fall to as low as 20,000 cells/mm,[3] hemorrhagic complications are uncommon. HIT is often seen in post-operative settings, perhaps because of the combined influence of surgery-induced inflammation and heparin exposure. Atkinson et al.[82] have emphasized the relationship between HIT and ischemic stroke after carotid endarterectomy. Becker and Miller,[78] reviewing data on 29 patients with HIT II-related stroke from the literature, found that few patients had previous cerebrovascular disease and that most patients either died (25%) or were left disabled after their strokes. HIT has also been associated with cerebral venous thrombosis.[89] Other risk factors for the development of HIT are diabetes, neoplasm, heart failure, infection, antiphospholipid antibodies, and trauma.[90] The diagnosis of HIT is based on a combination of clinical findings and demonstration of heparin-dependent antiplatelet antibodies.[87,91,92]

Prevention of HIT is the best management strategy, and platelet counts should be closely monitored in patients undergoing heparin therapy. Once HIT is recognized, heparin should be promptly discontinued; thrombosis risk is high in these patients, however, so some antithrombotic treatment must be given.[93] Because LMWH will cross-react with anti-heparin antibodies, this agent cannot be used for anticoagulation in patients with HIT.[86] Currently, heparinoids and recombinant hirudins are appropriate treatments in patients with HIT.[94-96] Thrombin inhibitors may also have a role. Many patients need long-term anticoagulation with warfarin; however, this therapy cannot be initiated until platelet counts have normalized because the severe drop in protein C in HIT contraindicates early treatment with warfarin.[94,96]

Antiphospholipid Antibodies

Consisting of a heterogeneous group of immunoglobulins, antiphospholipid antibodies (aPLs) are directed against anionic phospholipids, phospholipid–protein complexes, or phospholipid binding proteins.[97-99] aPL antibodies are produced in a variety of clinical situations and are associated with a hypercoagulable state characterized primarily by thrombosis, thrombocytopenia, and fetal loss. In the 1950s it was noted that some patients with systemic lupus erythematosus (SLE) often had prolonged aPTTs and false-positive results on Venereal Disease Research Laboratory (VDRL) tests,[100] but experienced thrombotic episodes despite the elevation of the aPTT. Among these thrombotic events are a variety of cerebrovascular manifestations.

The lupus anticoagulant (LA) test is a functional assay characterized by prolongation of phospholipid-dependent coagulation, whereas aCL antibodies are identified by immunoassay and target molecular variants of cardiolipin to measure antibody concentration and binding avidity.[97,101,102] Positive results of either test have been independently associated with thrombosis, and their combined presence and repeated positivity amplify the risk of thrombotic complications.[103,104] The preponderance of evidence, however, indicates that the LA test is more specific for patients at risk of thromboembolic events.[101,102] In contrast, the aCL antibody test is a more sensitive assay, but is non-specific, and positive results could also be found in various other individuals, such as those taking certain medications, those with malignancies or infectious diseases, and even in some healthy individuals.[97,101,103]

In 1990, three groups independently recognized that aPL antibodies were not directed against phospholipids alone but rather against a complex of plasma glycoprotein β_2 glycoprotein 1 (β_2GP1) and phospholipid. The cationic plasma glycoprotein β_2GP1, or apolipoprotein H, was noted to be an antigenic target that identifies most but not all aPL antibodies.[102,105,106] Data suggest that endothelial cells have cell surface receptors that attract and bind to β_2GP1, which in turn can attract aPL antibodies, which can lead to endothelial cell activation, increased secretion of proinflammatory cytokines, release of tissue factor, and subsequent initiation of the coagulation cascade.[98,105] One of the most promising aspects of the discovery of β_2GP1 as a target antigen for aPL is that β_2GP1, a minor natural anticoagulant, competes in vitro for available phospholipid surface area needed for assembly of the prothrombinase complex, thereby inhibiting prothrombinase activity. It is thought that only autoimmune aPL antibodies react in vivo with β_2GP1 after binding to phospholipids; therefore, immunoassays for β_2GP1 have been added to the revised criteria for definite antiphospholipid syndrome (APS).[101,102,107] In some studies, the presence of β_2GP1 antibodies rivals the presence of other aPL antibody markers in identifying patients with the highest risk of thrombosis.[108]

The Sapporo diagnostic criteria for APS were revised in 2006 and include the clinical criteria of either vascular thrombosis or pregnancy morbidity as well as the laboratory criteria of aCL antibody, LA, or anti-β_2GP1 antibody on at least two occasions at least 6 weeks apart (Box 42-2).[107] Other clinical manifestations that have been associated with aPLs are livedo reticularis, optic changes, primary adrenal insufficiency, and a variety of neurologic symptoms including movement disorders, epilepsy, and dementia.[99,109-112] The strength of the association between these clinical manifestations and the presence of aPLs is not strong enough for them to be included as diagnostic features.

Antibodies to other negatively charged phospholipids (e.g., phosphatidylserine (aPS), prothrombin (aPT), phosphatidylserine/prothrombin complex (aPS/PT), and phosphatidylethanolamine) are also associated with the classic clinical manifestations of APS. A recent systematic review of case-control studies that summarized data from 38 studies and over 7,000 patients and controls showed that aPT was associated with a 1.8-fold increased odds of thrombosis (OR 1.82, 95%CI, 1.44–2.75).[113] The strongest association with thrombosis, both arterial and/or venous, was aPS/PT, with an OR of 5.11 (95%CI, 4.2–6.3).[113] In a cohort of 158 patients with TIA, anti-PS/PT IgG antibodies (but not other antiphospholipid antibodies) were associated with high risk of stroke/death (OR 15.7, 95%CI, 1.0–125.6), and non-significantly related to the primary composite outcome of stroke or death within 90 days or identification of a high-risk stroke mechanism (OR 4.7, 95%CI, 0.8–29.2).[114]

BOX 42-2 Revised Sapporo Classification Criteria for the Antiphospholipid Syndrome

Antiphospholipid antibody syndrome (APS) is present if at least one of the following clinical criteria and one of the laboratory criteria are met:

CLINICAL CRITERIA

1. Vascular thrombosis: One or more clinical episodes of arterial, venous, or small-vessel thrombosis, in any tissue or organ
2. Pregnancy and morbidity:
   a. One or more unexplained deaths of a morphologically normal fetus at or beyond the tenth week of gestation
   b. One or more premature births of a morphologically normal neonate before the 34th week of gestation
   c. Three or more unexplained consecutive spontaneous abortions before the 10th week of gestation

LABORATORY CRITERIA

1. Lupus anticoagulant (LA) present in plasma, on two or more occasions at least 12 weeks apart
2. Anticardiolipin (aCL) antibody of IgG and/or IgM isotype present in medium or high titer on two or more occasions at least 12 weeks apart
3. Anti-β2 glycoprotein-I antibody of IgG and/or IgM isotype present on two or more occasions at least 12 weeks apart

Adapted from Miyakis S, Lockshin MD, Atsumi T, et al: International consensus statement on an update of the classification criteria for definite antiphospholipid syndrome (APS). *J Thromb Haemost* 4:295–306, 2006.

Individuals with APS but without SLE or other rheumatologic or autoimmune disorders have primary APS (PAPS). Those with APS along with SLE or other collagen vascular diseases have secondary APS.[97,102,115] However, the recent consensus statement on APS advises against using the term *secondary* APS because most of these individuals have SLE and documenting the coexistence of SLE (or another disease) is more advantageous for classification.[107] Turiel et al.[115] found that the main independent risk factors for vascular complications in PAPS patients were previous thrombosis and high IgG aCL titers (>40 GPL units). However, in those with APS and SLE, aPLs impart an increased risk of thrombosis that is at least equal to and may be greater than that observed in PAPS.[116,117] Cerebrovascular ischemia associated with APS generally occurs at a younger age; however, in the absence of clinical complications, the presence of aPLs does not indicate APS, and the role in predicting thrombotic events is controversial.[108,115] The prevalence of aPLs in healthy adults rises with age and is estimated to be as high as 12–50% in healthy elders, depending on the test used for detection.[98] A recent review of aPL prevalence in multiple thrombotic disorders estimated a frequency of 13.5% for stroke, 6% for pregnancy morbidity, 11% for myocardial infarction, and 9.5% for DVT.[118] There are multiple limitations to these estimates given that many of the included studies were published prior to 2000, did not follow the Sapporo criteria for repeat testing, and used lower titer cut-offs than currently recommended.[118] A prospective study, the Antiphospholipid Antibodies, Brain Infarcts, and Cognitive and Motor Decline in Aging (ABICMA) study, is currently underway to determine whether aPLs are truly associated with an increased risk of pathologically proven brain infarcts and outcomes of aging (motor and cognitive function) in community-dwelling older adults enrolled in the Religious Orders Study and the Memory and Aging Project.[119] The investigators will test the significance of four different aPLs: aCL, anti-β2GP1, aPS, lupus anticoagulant in relation to evidence of brain infarction, as well as cognition, and functional status.[119] The mean age at the time of the sample collection for aPL testing was 84 years, so clearly this is not going to answer questions related to testing for patients with APS, but it will provide important longitudinal data for important outcomes related to aging.

One of the largest studies to evaluate the natural history and risk factors for recurrent thrombosis in patients with aPLs comes from the Italian Registry of 360 patients studied prospectively for 4 years.[120] The inclusion criteria were presence of aPLs and availability of the subject for follow-up. aPL assays were performed clinically for a thrombotic event, a coagulation abnormality suggesting the presence of LA, or a disease known to be associated with APS. Treatment was at the discretion of the physician. Over the 4-year period, 34 patients had thrombotic events, including ten strokes and six TIAs. Risk factors for thrombosis in this cohort included an aCL antibody titer greater than 40 GPL units and either a prior thrombotic event or SLE. Other studies have also evaluated the association of APS with recurrent stroke.[120–125] Some,[120,123–127] but not all,[104,122,128] have suggested an association with recurrent thrombosis. Most of these studies are small to medium-sized case series, however, and their results thus cannot be considered conclusive. It is crucial to know whether APS raises the risk of recurrent stroke.

Many case-control studies have shown an association between different types of aPL antibodies and initial stroke,[129–136] but some have not.[137–140] The methodologic differences among studies, such as the type of aPL studied, sample size, and study population, could explain these discrepant results. It is interesting, however, that many of the larger studies found an association between aPLs and incident stroke, whereas the association with recurrent stroke is weaker. The explanation is not clear but may be related to the higher importance of other stroke risk factors in the risk of recurrent stroke, which overshadow the recurrent stroke risk contributed by aPLs.[127]

Few prospective studies have examined the association between aPL and either an initial stroke or MI. However, patients included in these studies would not meet current criteria for APS as these studies were limited to performance of aCL antibody testing performed on only one occasion.[141,142] The first prospective association between aCL and stroke was reported by Brey et al.[130] in a study of the association between aCL and stroke and MI in men enrolled in the Honolulu Heart Program over 20 years. Only the presence of β_2GP1-dependent aCL IgG antibodies was significantly associated with incident ischemic stroke and MI. However, this association was attenuated during the last 5 years of follow-up. The risk factor-adjusted relative odds for men with the presence versus the absence of β_2GP1-dependent aCL of the IgG class was 2.2 at 15 years.

The clinical presentation of stroke and TIA associated with aPLs does not have particular distinguishing features. Both large and small cerebral arterial occlusions in the anterior and posterior circulations as well as venous occlusions are all reported to occur. Although deep lacunar infarctions and isolated white matter signal-enhancing lesions are detected on magnetic resonance imaging (MRI) and large brain infarctions occur, most strokes are relatively small and involve the cortex and subjacent white matter.[121] No single mechanism for stroke associated with aPLs has been established, but a few pathologic reports have demonstrated non-specific microvascular platelet–fibrin plugs, which suggest possible thrombosis in situ. However, cardiac valvular lesions, predominantly left-sided and mitral, often accompany APS and could also be responsible for these lesions.[104,106,143]

Mechanisms underlying the aPL-associated vascular events, in the absence of SLE, are probably multifactorial and include associations of strokes with valvular disease,[104,106] cerebral microemboli,[130,144] thrombosis and endothelial hyperplasia,[98,145,146] antibodies to brain endothelium,[147,148] and adhesion molecule expression.[149] Some aPLs interfere with the vascular endothelial anticoagulant functions, whereas others directly activate endothelial thrombogenic mechanisms. Membranes of circulating white blood cells and platelets have also been implicated as a target for prothrombotic binding of aPLs. The thrombogenicity of aPLs may stem from their targeting of prothrombin on damaged membrane surfaces and their interference with the APC pathway. aPLs can interfere with thrombomodulin-induced protein C activation and also with protein S cofactor function for protein C. The importance of platelet activation in the process is supported by analysis of brain tissue removed from patients with aPL-related stroke, in which small arteries and microvessels are occluded by platelet–fibrin plugs. Single-photon emission computed tomography[150,151] and MRI spectroscopy[152] studies show diffuse damage that is compatible with many of these mechanisms. The thorough evaluation of patients in whom aPL is suspected often requires multiple testing procedures because, unfortunately, no one test can adequately screen a patient for aPLs.[153] An effective initial screen is a sensitive aPTT test and the aCL assay. If results of these evaluations are negative but clinical suspicion remains high, then the following tests should be performed: (1) kaolin clotting time, (2) dilute Russell viper venom time (dRVVT), and (3) lupus inhibitor screen (different aPTT reagents). Antiphosphatidylserine/antiprothrombin (anti-PS/PT) antibodies may be utilized more frequently in the future because they can be tested in patients that are therapeutic on warfarin, whereas the lupus anticoagulant test cannot. The anti-PS/PT test correlated highly with anti-β2-GP1 IgG and IgA, lupus anticoagulant positivity, and predicted a high risk of thrombosis.[154] This test is not currently widely available, however.

One caveat about aPL testing is that levels of aPLs may fall during thrombotic events, so tests may have to be repeated when the patient reaches a steady state.

The largest secondary stroke prevention study was performed by the prospective Antiphospholipid Antibody in Stroke Study (APASS) group. The APASS group, in collaboration with the Warfarin-Aspirin for Recurrent Stroke Study (WARSS) group,[104] was a controlled and blinded study in patients with ischemic stroke who were randomly assigned to receive either aspirin therapy (325 mg/day) or warfarin therapy (target international normalized ratio [INR] range, 1.4 to 2.8). A single aPL determination was performed in each patient at study entry. The rates of recurrent stroke were not found to be statistically different between treatment groups, and there were no differences in major bleeding complication rates. Therefore, aspirin therapy is equivalent to adjusted-dose warfarin for patients with ischemic stroke and positive aPLs, but this is not equivalent to patients with definite APS.[104]

Does targeting a higher INR with warfarin decrease the risk of recurrent events in high-risk APS patients? To address this question, Crowther et al.[126] performed a randomized double-blind trial of 114 patients followed-up for 2.7 years. Recurrent thrombosis including MI, deep venous thrombosis, pulmonary embolism, and stroke, occurred in 3.4% (2/58) of those patients assigned to moderate-intensity warfarin (average INR, 2.3) and in 10.7% (6/56) of those assigned to receive high-intensity warfarin (average INR, 3.3). In addition, 22.4% (13/58) of the moderate-intensity group and 37.5% (21/56) of the high-intensity group discontinued warfarin prematurely because of either thrombosis while receiving therapy or complications; however, there was no difference in bleeding rates between the two groups. These results suggest that high-intensity warfarin therapy with an INR of 3.1 to 4.0 is not more efficacious than moderate-intensity warfarin with an INR of 2.0 to 3.0 for prevention of recurrent thrombosis in patients with aPL antibodies. With the current level of knowledge, however, patients with previous arterial thrombosis and persistent medium-high titers of aCL, LA, or both seem to be at the highest risk of recurrent events. Currently, there is no evidence to support the use of any specific treatment strategies for primary prevention of aPL-associated ischemic stroke.[127]

A small case series showed that in five primary APS patients with thrombotic events refractory to anticoagulation, treatment with IVIG was effective in preventing recurrent thrombosis.[155] For a few patients who experience the catastrophic variant of APS that resembles disseminated intravascular coagulation, the combination of corticosteroids with plasmapheresis and/or intravenous immunoglobulin and possibly immunosuppression has been effective for short-term management.[156–158]

Sneddon's Syndrome

Sneddon's syndrome is an uncommon condition characterized by ischemic stroke and widespread livedo reticularis in the absence of other systemic diseases. Approximately three of four individuals with Sneddon's syndrome have increased levels of aPLs.[159,160] Besides livedo reticularis, some patients with the syndrome experience Raynaud's phenomenon and acrocyanosis. Sneddon's syndrome typically affects young adults and is more common in women than in men and has been linked to tobacco use. Skin biopsies, which are particularly useful for diagnosing aPL-seronegative individuals, show focal epidermal ulceration with chronic inflammatory infiltrates in the dermis, without evidence of vasculitis.[161] Neurologic symptoms associated with Sneddon's syndrome include headaches, vertigo, TIA, retinal artery occlusion, ischemic stroke, and mental deterioration and vascular dementia, presumably from recurrent stroke.[160] However, the presence of aPLs in individuals with Sneddon's syndrome indicates a worse prognosis.[159] Individuals with Sneddon's syndrome are typically younger and have fewer stroke risk factors than most persons with stroke, except that migraine-like headaches and hypertension are common in these individuals. Some individuals with Sneddon's syndrome experience progressive cognitive deterioration leading to dementia, despite having only minor or minimal clinical stroke-like episodes. Such progressive decline can happen even in persons receiving antithrombotic therapy. This clinical course epitomizes the observations of Sneddon[162] and Rebello et al.,[163] who emphasized that stroke in affected individuals often leaves little neurologic deficit but the subjects gradually became demented nonetheless. Unfortunately, except for the possible relationship to high aCL levels and the presence of LA and livedo reticularis, no specific laboratory or clinical finding predicts who will likely develop Sneddon's. Many individuals with Sneddon's syndrome eventually experience complex partial seizures.

What sets Sneddon's apart from other forms of aPL syndromes is not understood. It has been hypothesized that endothelial dysfunction and cell detachment with perivascular inflammation in small arterioles are the initiating events, which are followed by occlusion of the vascular lumen by mononuclear cells, erythrocytes, and fibrin, which leads to a cellular and fibrotic plug. It has yet to be determined whether the vascular occlusive events of Sneddon's syndrome reflect primary endothelial cell dysfunction or an unusual arteriosclerotic-like condition of young adults or result from recurrent thrombotic events in the setting of a hypercoagulable state or possibly from a combination of these conditions.[159]

HOMOCYSTINURIA AND HOMOCYSTINEMIA

The 20-fold or higher increases in plasma homocysteine, homocystine, cysteine–homocysteine, and related mixed disulfides (together termed *homocyst(e)ine* [Hcy]) that typify homocystinuria produce premature atherosclerosis that is frequently complicated by early stroke or other large arterial occlusions.[164] Homocystinuria is a metabolic consequence of one of several inborn errors of metabolism that impair cystathionine β-synthase (CBS) and several other enzyme systems important for methionine metabolism (Fig. 42-2). These are autosomal recessive traits, and persons homozygous for CBS deficiency often develop premature atherosclerosis and thromboembolic complications, including stroke, by age 30 years.[165] The classic phenotype of homocystinuria includes ocular, vascular, skeletal, and nervous system abnormalities. Affected individuals may have a marfanoid habitus, with arm spans greater than body height, setting-sun lenticular dislocations, and cognitive impairment. A malar flush and livedo reticularis are sometimes present, but the phenotypic expression varies considerably; some individuals with homocystinuria exhibit none of these characteristics. About 0.3% to 1.5% of the general population may be heterozygous for CBS deficiency, and the estimated incidence of homocystinuria is approximately 1 in 332,000 live births.[165] In obligate heterozygotes, CBS activity is reduced by 50%, but whether these individuals are at increased risk of stroke is not known.

Dietary folate deficiency raises Hcy levels, and before 1996, almost 90% of Americans did not ingest the minimum 400 μg/day of folate. The U.S. Food and Drug Administration published a regulation that, starting in 1998, all enriched-flour breads, rice, pasta, cornmeal, and other cereal grain products would be required to contain 140 μg of folic acid per 100 g of flour. The goal of this policy was to increase folic acid intake among women of child-bearing potential and reduce the risk of neural tube defects in their children. Since that time, studies evaluating the effect of vitamin supplementation have shown only a modest further reduction in Hcy levels. Thus, the effect of what was once suspected to be a major health problem and potential stroke risk factor may have been lessened by a change in public health policy.[166]

Besides genetic predispositions, many individuals are at risk of hyperhomocysteinemia because of acquired defects in methionine metabolism. As shown in Figure 42-2, decreased CBS activity and reduced remethylation of Hcy may produce hyperhomocysteinemia via abnormalities in folate-, cobalamin-, or betaine-dependent metabolic pathways. Data from case-control studies of healthy subjects as well as subjects with vascular disease indicate that an inverse relationship exists between plasma levels of folate and vitamin B_{12} and plasma concentrations of Hcy.

A mutation in methylenetetrahydrofolate reductase (MTHFR) in the folate pathway has been correlated with an increase in plasma Hcy levels and may possibly be a risk factor for cardiovascular disease.[167] The common thermolabile MTHFR variant results from a C-to-T point mutation at nucleotide C677T (changing alanine to valine), which significantly reduces the enzyme's basal activity.[168] This mutation is prevalent in the population: the frequency of heterozygotes is 40–50% and that of homozygotes is 5–15% in several populations. The presence of the mutation is associated with elevated plasma Hcy levels, but data are currently lacking for support of this mutation as a risk factor for stroke, although the risk may be more significant in children than in adults.[169]

As indicated in Figure 42-2, when an elevation of Hcy is detected, serum folate and vitamin B_{12} levels should also be measured. Lowering homocysteine levels with vitamins has shown no benefits of reducing recurrent vascular events in randomized controlled trials of ischemic stroke patients.[170,171] Although treatment with folate and B vitamins is safe, the current guidelines do not strongly recommend folate supplementation (Class IIb; Level B).[172]

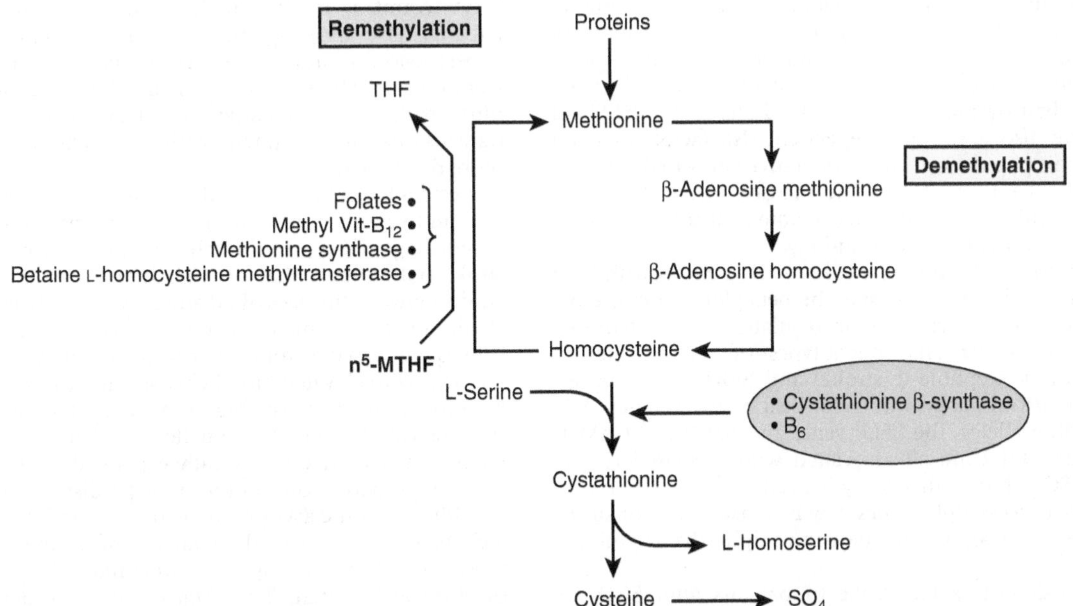

Figure 42-2. Methionine metabolism and homocysteinemia. Plasma homocysteine levels may rise because of genetic or acquired metabolic deficiencies in pathways of methionine metabolism. The principal causes are dysfunction of the cystathionine β-synthase enzyme system for cysteine metabolism and dysfunction of remethylation of the tetrahydrofolate (THF) pathway, and these may occur with folate or vitamin B_{12} deficiencies. See text for details. B_6, vitamin B_6; B_{12}, vitamin B_{12}; n^5-MTHF, methyltetrahydrofolate.

SICKLE CELL DISEASE

A critical single-point mutation that causes the substitution of valine for glutamic acid in the hemoglobin β chain underlies sickle cell anemia (SSA) and its consequent disease, sickle cell disease (SCD). Biochemically, when exposed to acidotic or hypoxemic environments, the hydrophobic valine residue polymerizes, resulting in a gel that changes red cell morphology.[173] The extremely rigid, sickled erythrocyte produces a tremendous increase in blood viscosity that contributes to red blood cell sludging in the microcirculation during sickle crises. Even in the absence of crisis, SSA can cause a progressive occlusive systemic vasculopathy leading to SCD involving many organs, including the brain. This untoward result happens in approximately 30% of individuals with SSA, which suggests that other factors buffer the effects of the HbSS gene. Individuals with SCD are at increased risk of vascular occlusive events, often recurrent, including catastrophic stroke, as well as infarctions of the kidney, lung, bone, skin, and eye. Symptoms usually begin in early childhood, but occasionally, persons with SSA may live into early or middle adulthood before manifesting adverse effects.

The prevalence of sickle trait (HbSA) in black Americans is estimated at about 8.5%; hemoglobin HbSS occurs in up to 0.16%, and the variant HbSC occurs in 0.21%. SCD occurs in approximately 1 in 500 black births in the US,[174] and the incidence of cerebrovascular disease is ten times greater in blacks with SCD than in those without SCD.[175] Roughly 11% of those with SCD develop clinically overt stroke by age 20,[175-177] which peaks at age 10 but increases to 24% overt stroke by age 45.[178] The highest incidence of stroke occurs between the ages of 2 and 9 years, and a second peak occurs after age 20;[178,179] unfortunately, up to two-thirds of individuals with first stroke experience recurrent infarcts.[180] Typically, infarctions include both deep brain and cortical structures, but brainstem, spinal cord, and retinal infarctions as well as dural sinus thrombosis are reported. Pavlakis et al.[181] have emphasized the occurrence of watershed or borderzone infarctions, particularly in territories of the middle cerebral artery. They speculate that a combination of occlusive arteriopathy and perfusion failure produces watershed strokes. Silent infarcts (evidence of ischemic injury by imaging in the absence of clinical history of stroke, but with possible associated cognitive impairment) are also relatively common and increase with age; their overall incidence is 17–22%.[175,176,182,183] Silent infarcts are also a strong independent risk factor for overt stroke in this population. The Cooperative Study of Sickle Cell Disease (CSSCD) found a 14-fold increase in the stroke rate in patients with silent infarction on brain MRI compared with those with normal brain MRI findings.[184]

The susceptibility to ischemic stroke in persons with SCD appears to involve genes outside the beta-globin locus, especially genes that affect immune regulation and inflammation.[176,183] Particular HLA phenotypes of interest include DPB1*0401 (susceptible to stroke) and BPB1*1701 (protective).[183] Transforming growth factor-beta pathway genes, AGT microsatellite alleles, the SELP gene, and SNPs in VCAM-1, IL4R, and ADRB2 are all associated with increased risk of stroke in SCD, but further study is needed.[176,179,185-189] It also appears that excess alpha genes may be a risk factor for stroke in SCD, whereas alpha gene deletion (alpha thalassemia) is protective.[190]

Other risk factors for stroke in patients with SCD are anemia with persistent hemoglobin levels below 7 g/dL, recent or recurrent episodes of chest pain, increased leukocyte count, elevated blood pressure, and the moyamoya phenomenon on brain imaging.[176,180,183,191-193] Parvovirus B19-induced aplasia has also been associated with stroke occurring coincident with the infection, possibly secondary to severely lowered hemoglobin, but the reason for this observation is unclear.[178,194] Chronic hemoglobin desaturation could increase the risk of stroke by perturbing endothelial function and limiting oxygen delivery to the brain. Children with SCD who demonstrate decreased daytime SpO_2 (2–3% absolute difference), which declines over time, appear to be at increased risk of stroke.[195] A useful clinical marker is high middle cerebral artery blood flow velocities, as evidenced by transcranial Doppler (TCD) ultrasonography. Abnormal TCD velocities greater than 200 cm/s were identified in 5–10% of children with SCD and confer a 10% annual risk for developing primary stroke in children.[196] TCD velocities in adults with SCD are lower than in children but are still elevated compared with adult control subjects.[175,197]

As SCD develops, sickled cells adhere to endothelium, contributing to a cascade of acute inflammatory cells and clotting factors resulting in a nidus for thrombus formation and a relative deficiency of nitric oxide that reduces the compensatory vasodilatation and contributes to endothelial expression of cell adhesion molecules and activation of hemostatic pathways, including activation of platelets.[173,198] There is progressive segmental narrowing of the distal internal carotid artery, portions of the circle of Willis, and proximal branches of the major intracranial arteries. Pathologically, this large-vessel arteriopathy demonstrates intimal proliferation and an increase in fibroblasts and smooth muscle cells within the arterial wall. This process is schematized in Figure 42-3. The progressive nature of this occlusive arteriopathy is evidenced by the development of the moyamoya phenomenon in 20–40% of individuals who have had an overt stroke. In addition to disease in large arteries, sickled cells can plug the microcirculation and cerebral veins.[179]

There has been a recent classification of SSA into a viscosity-vaso-occlusion subphenotype (VVO) and a hemolysis-endothelial dysfunction subphenotype (HED).[199] The VVO spectrum is associated with high hemoglobin level and frequent vaso-occlusive pain crises, acute chest syndrome, and osteonecrosis. The HED subphenotype includes patients with high levels of lactate dehydrogenase (LDH) and a high reticulocyte count as markers of hemolysis, and clinically, these patients have stroke (perhaps not definitively), pulmonary hypertension, priapism, and leg ulcers.[199,200] The underlying feature of the HED phenotype is the decreased bioactivity of nitric oxide, and these patients are likely to benefit most from transfusions and treatment with hydroxyurea, described in more detail below.[199]

Besides brain infarctions, these alterations of arterial, capillary, and venous circulation increase the risk of intracerebral hemorrhage (ICH). Although the prevalence of ischemic stroke outnumbers that of ICH, ICH occurs more often in adults between the ages of 20 and 30 years.[173] ICH in SCD can result either from medial necrosis of cerebral arterioles with subsequent vascular rupture or from venous thrombosis that happens with elevated blood viscosity and sludging. The combination of increased cerebral mean arterial blood flow velocities, increased cerebral blood flow, and intracerebral blood volume, which are only partially explained by the underlying anemia, probably contributes to the predisposition to ICH.[201]

Although some asymptomatic persons with SSA may tolerate HbSS of up to 50%, the mainstay of treatment for SCD is repeated exchange transfusion to maintain the concentration of HbSS at less than 30%. Transfusion provides benefit by correcting low oxygen-carrying capacity and improving microvascular perfusion by decreasing the proportion of sickled red cells as well as intravascular hemolysis.[202] The Stroke Prevention Trial in Sickle Cell Anemia (STOP) evaluated the role of repeated red cell transfusion in children with increased stroke

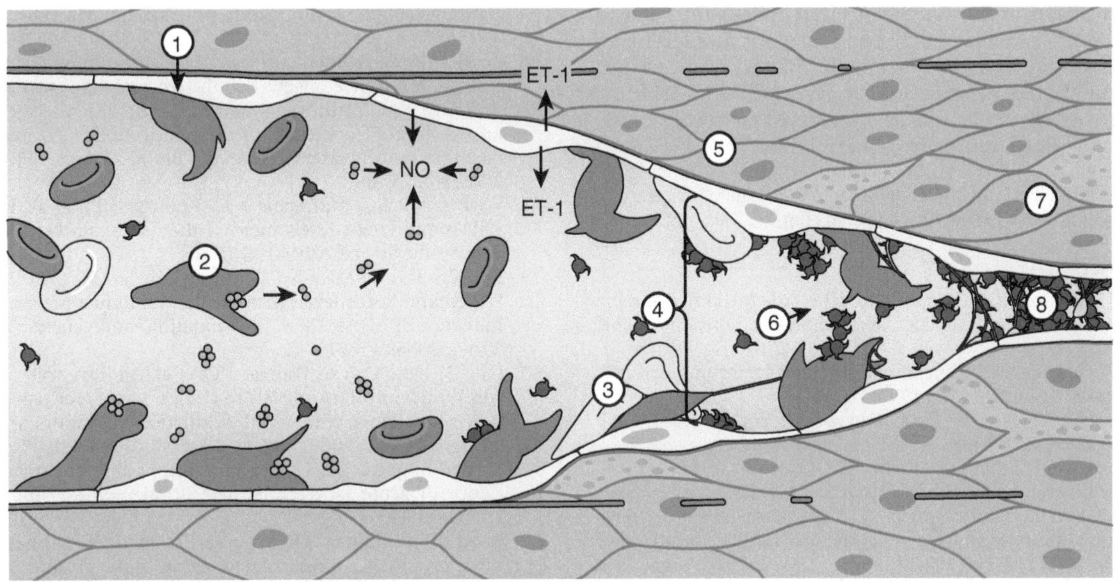

Figure 42-3. Occlusive vasculopathy in sickle cell disease. The sickle erythrocyte adheres to vascular endothelium (1), undergoes hemolysis (2), thereby producing a proinflammatory state with leukocyte adhesion and platelet activation at the vessel wall (3,4,5). These events promote endothelin release and antagonize the effects of nitric oxide (NO) on vascular tone and promote smooth muscle proliferation leading to a progressive occlusive vasculopathy. *(Adapted from Switzer JA, Hess DC, Nichols FT, et al: Pathophysiology and treatment of stroke in sickle-cell disease: Present and future.* Lancet Neurol *5:501-512, 2006.)*

risk and abnormal TCD and showed a decreased incidence of stroke from 10% per year to less than 1% per year[196,202–204] in children maintained with transfusions. Therefore, children with sickle cell disease should have regular screening TCD and undergo transfusion for confirmed TCD velocities greater than 200 cm/s.[196,204] Pegelow et al.[205] also showed that transfusion therapy reduced recurrent silent lesions. Transfusion therapy should be maintained over the long term because discontinuation results in a high rate of reversion to abnormal blood flow velocities on TCD and stroke.[202,203] However, the optimal duration of therapy remains undefined. Scothorn et al.[206] report that, in the 2-year period after an initial stroke, patients with SCD are particularly vulnerable to development of a second stroke but that, after 2 years, those with an antecedent or concurrent medical event at the time of initial stroke have a much lower recurrent stroke risk.

Hematopoietic stem-cell transplantation (HSCT) is the only curative treatment available for SCD and might be more effective than transfusion, specifically for prevention of cerebrovascular disease, but its use has been limited by transplant-related morbidity and mortality. The timing of bone-marrow transplantation is controversial. One would like to perform HSCT before end-stage organ damage occurs yet limit this therapy to patients destined to experience these complications. Therefore, it is generally reserved for those with severe disease, even though those with less severe disease have better outcomes.[207]

Hydroxyurea has decreased the incidence of sickle cell crisis in adults and children with severe disease by increasing hematocrit, inhibiting erythrocyte sickling by increasing HbF, reducing red cell adhesion, and decreasing lactate dehydrogenase and total bilirubin concentrations.[208] It has been shown to provide similar protection as compared with long-term transfusion for decreased TCD velocity and stroke, but the long-term side effects are not known.[177,208] Inhaled nitric oxide and sodium nitrate have also been proposed as potential treatments for SCD because they increase vasodilatation; however, further investigations are needed.[198] For secondary prevention, the currently published guidelines do not specifically recommend antiplatelet or anticoagulant therapy other than for general vascular benefit, as there are no trials performed in the sickle cell population to aid in decision-making.[172]

BOX 42-3 Laboratory Screening Tests for Coagulopathies in Selected Patients*

- Protein C, protein S, and antithrombin III measurements by functional assay
- Free protein S antigen measurement
- Anticardiolipin antibody assay by enzyme-linked immunosorbent assay (ELISA)
- Functional assay for lupus anticoagulant
- Hemoglobin electrophoresis (especially in black people)
- Lipoprotein(a) measurement
- Either factor V Leiden by polymerase chain reaction or functional assay for activated protein C resistance, and prothrombin G20210A mutation

*Patients under age 55 years, with strong family or personal history of venous thrombosis, pregnancy complications, and no clear explanation for the stroke (i.e., vasculopathy, cardioembolic source, or absence of typical risk factors for stroke).

SCREENING OF PATIENTS WITH STROKE FOR COAGULOPATHIES

Besides the usual routine clinical tests for coagulation, the majority of individuals with stroke and TIA do not require an extensive evaluation to look for abnormalities in the hemostatic system or to diagnose a hypercoagulable state.[209,210] The yield of screening is likely to be highest in those who are young, in those with repeated unexplained strokes, and in those with a prior history of thrombosis (particularly venous thrombosis). Patients with unexplained cerebral venous thrombosis (i.e., cortical vein or sagittal sinus thrombosis) should be investigated for hypercoagulable conditions, described in detail in the American Heart Association Scientific Statement.[211] Patients with livedo reticularis and left heart valvular abnormalities and women with a history of spontaneous abortion should be screened for aPL antibodies. Hemoglobin electrophoresis should be considered in young black patients. A suggested approach is summarized in Box 42-3.

The complete reference list can be found on the companion Expert Consult website at www.expertconsult.inkling.com.

KEY REFERENCES

1. Levy JH, Dutton RP, Hemphill JC III, et al. Multidisciplinary approach to the challenge of hemostasis. Anesth Analg 2010;110:354–64.
5. Wu KK, Thiagarajan P. Role of endothelium in thrombosis and hemostasis. Annu Rev Med 1996;47:315.
7. Galley HF, Webster NR. Physiology of the endothelium. Br J Anaesth 2004;93:105–13.
8. Breitenstein A, Tanner FC, Lüscher TF. Tissue factor and cardiovascular disease: Quo vadis? Circ J 2010;74:3–12.
9. Jennings LK. Mechanisms of platelet activation: need for new strategies to protect against platelet-mediated atherothrombosis. Thromb Haemost 2009;102:248–57.
11. Tran ND, Wong VL, Schreiber SS, et al. Regulation of brain capillary endothelial thrombomodulin mRNA expression. Stroke 1996;27:2304.
12. Kwaan HC, Samama MM. The significance of endothelial heterogeneity in thrombosis and hemostasis. Semin Thromb Hemost 2010;36:286–300.
13. Kenet G, Lütkhoff LK, Albisetti M, et al. Impact of thrombophilia on risk of arterial ischemic stroke or cerebral sinovenous thrombosis in neonates and children: A systematic review and meta-analysis of observational studies. Circulation 2010;121: 1838–47.
14. Folsom AR, Ohira T, Yamagishi K, et al. Low protein C and incidence of ischemic stroke and coronary heart disease: The Atherosclerosis Risk in Communities (ARIC) Study. J Thromb Haemost 2009;7:1774–8.
15. Laugesaar R, Kahre T, Kolk A, et al. Factor V Leiden and prothrombin 20210G>A [corrected] mutation and paediatric ischaemic stroke: A case-control study and two meta-analyses. [Erratum appears in Acta Paediatr 2010 Jul;99(7):1112]. Acta Paediatr 2010;99:1168–74.
16. Press RD, Liu XY, Beamer N, et al. Ischemic stroke in the elderly – role of the common factor V mutation causing resistance to activated protein C. Stroke 1996;27:44.
17. Bentley P, Peck G, Smeeth L, et al. Causal relationship of susceptibility genes to ischemic stroke: Comparison to ischemic heart disease and biochemical determinants. PLoS ONE 2010;5(2): e9136.
18. Staton J, Sayer M, Hankey GJ, et al. Protein Z gene polymorphisms, protein Z concentrations, and ischemic stroke. Stroke 2005;36:1123–7.
19. Herak DC, Antolic MR, Krleza JL, et al. Inherited prothrombotic risk factors in children with stroke, transient ischemic attack, or migraine. Pediatrics 2009;123:e653–60.
20. Ridker PM, Vaughan DE, Stampfer MJ, et al. Endogenous tissue-type plasminogen activator and risk of myocardial infarction. Lancet 1993;341:1165.
21. Moskau S, Smolka K, Semmler A, et al. Common genetic coagulation variants are not associated with ischemic stroke in a case-control study. Neurol Res 2010;32:519–22.
22. Szolnoki Z, Somogyvari F, Kondacs A, et al. Evaluation of the roles of the Leiden V mutation and ACE I/D polymorphism in subtypes of ischemic stroke. J Neurol 2001;248:756.
23. Hamedani AG, Cole JW, Mitchell BD, et al. Meta-analysis of factor V Leiden and ischemic stroke in young adults: The importance of case ascertainment. Stroke 2010;41:1599–603.
24. Hamedani AG, Cole JW, Cheng Y, et al. Factor V Leiden and Ischemic Stroke Risk: The Genetics of Early Onset Stroke (GEOS) Study. J Stroke Cerebrovasc Dis 2013;22(4):419–23.
25. Reiner AP, Carty CL, Jenny NS, et al. PROC, PROCR and PROS1 polymorphisms, plasma anticoagulant phenotypes, and risk of cardiovascular disease and mortality in older adults: The Cardiovascular Health Study. J Thromb Haemost 2008;6: 1625–32.
26. de Moerloose P, Boehlen F. Inherited thrombophilia in arterial disease: A selective review. Semin Hematol 2007;44:106–13.
27. Pelkonen KM, Wartiovaara-Kautto U, Nieminen MS, et al. Low normal level of protein C or of antithrombin increases risk for recurrent cardiovascular events. Blood Coagul Fibrinolysis 2005;16:275–80.
28. Wieberdink RG, van Schie MC, Koudstaal PJ, et al. High von Willebrand factor levels increase the risk of stroke: The Rotterdam study. Stroke 2010;41:2151–6.
29. Bongers TN, de Maat MPM, vaan Goor M-LPJ, et al. High von Willebrand factor levels increase the risk of first ischemic stroke. Influence of ADAMTS13, inflammation, and genetic variability. Stroke 2006;37:2672–7.
30. Lip GY, Lane D, Van Walraven C, et al. Additive role of plasma von Willebrand factor levels to clinical factors for risk stratification of patients with atrial fibrillation. [Erratum appears in Stroke 37:2444, 2006]. Stroke 2006;37:2294–300.
31. Mayer SA, Sacco RL, Hurlet-Jensen A, et al. Free protein S deficiency in acute ischemic stroke: A case-control study. Stroke 1993;24:224.
32. Poort SR, Rosendaal FR, Reitsma PH, et al. A common genetic variation in the 3′-untranslated region of the prothrombin gene is associated with elevated plasma prothrombin levels and an increase in venous thrombosis. Blood 1996;88:3698.
33. Supanc V, Sonicki Z, Vukasovic I, et al. The Role of Classic Risk Factors and Prothrombotic Factor Gene Mutations in Ischemic Stroke Risk Development in Young and Middle-Aged Individuals. J Stroke Cerebrovasc Dis [Internet] Available from: <http://www.sciencedirect.com/science/article/pii/S1052305713003996>; [cited 2013 Nov 25.].
34. Favaretto E, Sartori M, Conti E, et al. G1691A factor V and G20210A FII mutations, acute ischemic stroke of unknown cause, and patent foramen ovale. Thromb Res 2012;130(5): 720–4.
35. Slooter AJ, Rosendaal FR, Tanis BC, et al. Prothrombotic conditions, oral contraceptives and the risk of ischemic stroke. J Thromb Haemost 2005;3:1213–17.
36. Andersson HM, Siegerink B, Luken BM, et al. High VWF, low ADAMTS13, and oral contraceptives increase the risk of ischemic stroke and myocardial infarction in young women. Blood 2012;119(6):1555–60.
37. Bushnell C, Goldstein LB. Screening for hypercoagulable syndromes following stroke. Curr Atheroscler Rep 2003;5(4): 291–8.
38. Tripodi A, Mannucci PM. Laboratory investigation of thrombophilia. Clin Chem 2001;47:1597.
39. De Moerloose P, Reber G, Bouviar CA. Spuriously low levels of protein C with Protac activation clotting assay [letter]. Thromb Haemost 1988;59:543.
40. Faioni EM, Franchi F, Asti D, et al. Resistance to activated protein C mimicking dysfunctional protein C: Diagnostic approach. Blood Coagul Fibrinolysis 1996;7:349.
41. Dahlback B. The protein C anticoagulant system: Inherited defects as basis for venous thrombosis. Thromb Res 1995; 77:1.
42. Comp PC, Doray D, Patton D, et al. An abnormal distribution of protein S occurs in functional protein S deficiency. Blood 1986;67:504.
43. Simmonds RE, Ireland H, Lane DA, et al. Clarification of the risk for venous thrombosis associated with hereditary protein S deficiency by investigation of a large kindred with a characterized gene defect. Ann Intern Med 1998;128:8.
45. Juhan-Vague I, Valdier J, Alessi M, et al. Deficient t-PA release and elevated PA inhibitor levels in patients with spontaneous or recurrent deep venous thrombosis. Thromb Haemost 1987; 57:67.
46. Feinberg WM, Bruck DC, Ring ME, et al. Hemostatic markers in acute stroke. Stroke 1989;20:592.
47. Takano K, Yamaguchi T, Uchida K. Markers of a hypercoagulable state following acute ischemic stroke. Stroke 1992;23:194.
48. Tohgi H, Kawashima M, Taa K, et al. Coagulation-fibrinolysis abnormalities in acute and chronic phases of cerebral thrombosis and embolism. Stroke 1990;21:1663.

49. Feinberg WM, Bruck DC. Time course of platelet activation following acute ischemic stroke. J Stroke Cerebrovasc Dis 1991; 1:124.
50. Fisher M, Francis R. Altered coagulation in cerebral ischemia: Platelet, thrombin, and plasmin activity. Arch Neurol 1990;47: 1075.
51. Takano K, Yamaguchi T, Kato H, et al. Activation of coagulation in acute cardioembolic stroke. Stroke 1991;22:12.
52. de Bono D. Significance of raised plasma concentrations of tissue-type plasminogen activator and plasminogen activator inhibitor in patients at risk from ischaemic heart disease. Br Heart J 1994;71:504.
53. Ridker PM. Plasma concentration of endogenous tissue plasminogen activator and the occurrence of future cardiovascular events. J Thromb Thrombolysis 1994;1:35.
54. Salomaa V, Stinson V, Kark JD, et al. Association of fibrinolytic parameters with early atherosclerosis: The ARIC Study. Atherosclerosis Risk in Communities Study. Circulation 1995;91:284.
55. Oates JA, FitzGerald GA, Branch RA, et al. Clinical implications of prostaglandin and thromboxane A_2 formation. N Engl J Med 1988;319:689.
56. Babu MS, Prabha TS, Kaul S, et al. Association of genetic variants of fibrinolytic system with stroke and stroke subtypes. Gene 2012;495(1):76–80.
57. Scott J. Lipoprotein (a): Thrombogenesis linked to atherosclerosis at last? Nature 1989;341:22.
58. McLean JW, Tomlinson JE, Kuang WJ, et al. cDNA sequence of human apolipoprotein (a) is homologous to plasminogen. Nature 1987;330:132.
59. Etingin OR, Hajjar DP, Hajjar KA, et al. Lipoprotein (a) regulates plasminogen activator inhibitor-1 expression in endothelial cells: A potential mechanism in thrombogenesis. J Biol Chem 1991;266:2459.
60. Hajjar KA, Gavish D, Breslow JL, et al. Lipoprotein (a) modulation of endothelial cell surface fibrinolysis and its potential role in atherosclerosis. Nature 1989;339:303.
61. Franceschini G, Cofrancesco E, Safa O, et al. Association of lipoprotein (a) with atherothrombotic events and fibrinolytic variables: A case-control study. Thromb Res 1995;78:227.
62. Jürgens F, Költringer P. Lipoprotein (a) in ischemic cerebrovascular disease: A new approach to the assessment of stroke. Neurology (NY) 1987;37:513.
63. Lassila R, Manninen V. Hypofibrinolysis and increased lipoprotein (a) coincide in stroke. J Lab Clin Med 1995;125:301.
64. Schreiner PJ, Chambless LE, Brown SA, et al. Lipoprotein (a) as a correlate of stroke and transient ischemic attack prevalence in a biracial cohort: The ARIC study. Ann Epidemiol 1994;4:351.
65. Shintani S, Kikuchi S, Hamaguchi H, et al. High serum lipoprotein (a) is an independent risk factor for cerebral infarction. Stroke 1993;24:965.
66. Zenker G, Költringer P, Boné G, et al. Lipoprotein (a) as a strong indicator for cerebrovascular disease. Stroke 1986;17:942.
67. Arboix A, Besses C, Acin P, et al. Ischemic stroke as first manifestation of essential thrombocythemia: Report of six cases. Stroke 1995;26:1463.
68. Jabaily J, Iland HJ, Laszlo J, et al. Neurologic manifestations of essential thrombocythemia. Ann Intern Med 1983;99:513.
69. Alvarez-Larran A, Cervantes F, Bellosillo B, et al. Essential thrombocythemia in young individuals: Frequency and risk factors for vascular events and evolution to myelofibrosis in 126 patients. Leukemia 2007;21:1218.
70. De Stefano V, Za T, Rossi E, et al. Recurrent thrombosis in patients with polycythemia vera and essential thrombocythemia: Incidence, risk factors, and effect of treatments. Haematologica 2008;93:372.
71. Johnson M, Gernsheimer T, Johansen K. Essential thrombocytosis: Underemphasized cause of large-vessel thrombosis. J Vasc Surg 1995;22:443.
72. Murphy S, Peterson P, Iland H, et al. Experience of the Polycythemia Vera Study Group with essential thrombocythemia: A final report on diagnostic criteria, survival, and leukemic transition by treatment. Semin Hematol 1997;34:29.
73. Riuniti O, Barbui T, Finazzi G, et al. Polycythemia vera: The natural history of 1213 patients followed for 20 years. Ann Intern Med 1995;123:656.
74. Vadher BD, Machin SJ, Patterson KG, et al. Life-threatening thrombotic and haemorrhagic problems associated with silent myeloproliferative disorders. Br J Haematol 1993;85:213.
75. Arellano-Rodrigo E, Alvarez-Larrán A, Reverter J-C, et al. Platelet turnover, coagulation factors, and soluble markers of platelet and endothelial activation in essential thrombocythemia: Relationship with thrombosis occurrence and JAK2 V617F allele burden. Am J Hematol 2009;84(2):102–8.
76. Van Genderen PJJ, Mulder PGH, Waleboer M, et al. Prevention and treatment of thrombotic complications in essential thrombocythaemia: Efficacy and safety of aspirin. Br J Haematol 1997;97:179.
77. Harrisnon CN, Campbell PJ, Buck G, et al. Hydroxyurea compared with anagerlide in high-risk essential thrombocythemia. N Engl J Med 2005;353:33.
78. Becker PS, Miller VT. Heparin-induced thrombocytopenia. Stroke 1989;20:1449.
79. Otis SA, Zehnder JL. Heparin-induced thrombocytopenia: Current status and diagnostic challenges. Am J Hematol 2010;85: 700–6.
80. Walenga JM, Jeske WP, Messmore HS. Mechanisms of venous and arterial thrombosis in heparin-induced thrombocytopenia. J Thromb Thrombolysis 2000;10(Suppl.):S13.
81. Ansell J, Deykin D. Heparin-induced thrombocytopenia and recurrent thromboembolism. Am J Hematol 1980;8:325.
82. Atkinson JL, Sundt TM Jr, Kazmier FJ, et al. Heparin-induced thrombocytopenia and thrombosis in ischemic stroke. Mayo Clin Proc 1988;63:353.
83. Bell WR. Heparin-associated thrombocytopenia and thrombosis. J Lab Clin Med 1988;111:600.
84. King DJ, Keltron JG. Heparin-associated thrombocytopenia. Ann Intern Med 1984;100:535.
85. Fabris F, Ahmad S, Cella G, et al. Pathophysiology of heparin-induced thrombocytopenia: Clinical and diagnostic implications: A review. Arch Pathol Lab Med 2000;124:1657.
86. Fabris F, Luzzatto G, Stefani PM, et al. Heparin-induced thrombocytopenia. Haematologica 2000;85:72.
87. Warkentin TE, Kelton JG. Heparin and platelets. Hematol Oncol Clin North Am 1990;4:243.
88. Warkentin TE, Levine MN, Hirsh J, et al. Heparin-induced thrombocytopenia in patients treated with low-molecular-weight heparin or unfractionated heparin. N Engl J Med 1995; 332:1330.
89. Kyritsis AP, Williams EC, Schutta HS. Cerebral venous thrombosis due to heparin-induced thrombocytopenia. Stroke 1990;21: 1503.
90. Goor Y, Goor O, Eldor A. Heparin-induced thrombocytopenia with thrombotic sequelae: A review. Autoimmun Rev 2002; 1:183.
91. Spencer FA. Heparin-induced thrombocytopenia: Patient profiles and clinical manifestations. J Thromb Thrombolysis 2000; 10(Suppl.):S21.
92. Warkentin TE. Heparin-induced thrombocytopenia: A clinicopathological syndrome. Thromb Haemost 1999;82:439.
93. Wallis DE, Workman DL, Lewis BE, et al. Failure of heparin cessation as treatment for heparin-induced thrombocytopenia. Am J Med 1999;106:629.
94. Greinacher A. Treatment of heparin-induced thrombocytopenia. Thromb Haemost 1999;82:457.
95. Lewis BE, Walenga JM, Wallis DE. Anticoagulation with Novastan (argatroban) in patients with heparin-induced thrombocytopenia, and heparin-induced thrombocytopenia and thrombosis syndrome. Semin Thromb Hemost 1997;23:197.
96. Lubenow N, Greinacher A. Management of patients with heparin-induced thrombocytopenia: Focus on recombinant hirudin. J Thromb Thrombolysis 2000;10(Suppl.):S47.
97. Lim W, Crowther MA, Eikelboom JW. Management of antiphospholipid antibody syndrome: A systematic review. JAMA 2006; 295:1050–7.
98. Janardhan V, Wolf PA, Kase CS, et al. Anticardiolipin antibodies and risk of ischemic stroke and transient ischemic attack: The Framingham cohort and offspring study. Stroke 2004;35: 736–41.
99. Lim W, Crowther MA. Antiphospholipid antibodies: A critical review of the literature. Curr Opin Hematol 2007;14:494–9.

101. Caso V, Parnetti L, Panarelli P, et al. Selection of thrombogenetic antiphospholipid antibodies in cerebrovascular disease patients. J Neurol 2003;250:593–7.
102. Galli M, Luciani D, Bertolini G, et al. Lupus anticoagulants are stronger risk factors for thrombosis than anticardiolipin antibodies in the antiphospholipid syndrome: A systematic review of the literature. Blood 2003;101:1827–32.
103. Ruiz-Irastorza G, Hunt BJ, Khamashta MA. A systematic review of secondary thromboprophylaxis in patients with antiphospholipid antibodies. Arthritis Rheum 2007;57:1487–95.
104. Levine SR, Brey RL, Tilley BC, et al. Antiphospholipid antibodies and subsequent thrombo-occlusive events in patients with ischemic stroke. JAMA 2004;35:736–41.
105. Nojima J, Kuratsune H, Suehisa E, et al. Strong correlation between the prevalence of cerebral infarction and the presence of anti-cardiolipin/beta2-glycoprotein I and anti-phosphatidylserine/prothrombin antibodies: Co-existence of these antibodies enhances ADP-induced platelet activation in vitro. Thromb Haemost 2004;91:967–76.
106. Brey RL. Antiphospholipid antibodies in young adults with stroke. J Thromb Thrombolysis 2005;20:105–12.
107. Miyakis S, Lockshin MD, Atsumi T, et al. International consensus statement on an update of the classification criteria for definite antiphospholipid syndrome (APS). J Thromb Haemost 2006;4: 295–306.
108. Ali HY, Abdullah ZA. Anti-beta(2)-glycoprotein I autoantibody expression as a potential biomarker for strokes in patients with anti-phospholipid syndrome. J Immunotoxicol 2008;5:173–7.
109. Suvajac G, Stojanovich L, Milenkovich S. Ocular manifestations in antiphospholipid syndrome. Autoimmun Rev 2007;6: 409–14.
110. Espinosa G, Cervera R, Font J, et al. Adrenal involvement in the antiphospholipid syndrome. Lupus 2003;12:569–72.
111. Arnson Y, Shoenfeld Y, Alon E, et al. The antiphospholipid syndrome as a neurological disease. Semin Arthritis Rheum 2010;40: 97–108.
112. Cavera R, Piette J-C, Font J, et al. Antiphospholipid syndrome. Clinical and immunologic manifestations and patterns of disease expression in a cohort of 1000 patients. Arthritis Rheum 2002;46:1019–27.
113. Sciascia S, Sanna G, Murru V, et al. Anti-prothrombin (aPT) and anti-phosphatidylserine/prothrombin (aPS/PT) antibodies and the risk of thrombosis in the antiphospholipid syndrome. A systematic review. Thromb Haemost 2013;111(2).
114. Mullen MT, Messé SR, Kasner SE, et al. Anti-phosphatidylserine-prothrombin antibodies are associated with outcome in a TIA cohort. Front Stroke 2012;3:137.
115. Turiel M, Sarzi-Puttini P, Peretti R, et al. Thrombotic risk factors in primary antiphospholipid syndrome: A 5-year prospective study. Stroke 2005;36:1490–4.
116. Horbach DA, Oort EV, Donders RC, et al. Lupus anticoagulant is the strongest risk factor for both venous and arterial thrombosis in patients with systemic lupus erythematosus: Comparison between different assays for the detection of antiphospholipid antibodies. Thromb Haemost 1996;76:916.
117. Goldstein R, Moulds JM, Smith CD, et al. MHC studies of the primary antiphospholipid antibody syndrome and of antiphospholipid antibodies in systemic lupus erythematosus. J Rheum 1996;23:1173.
118. Andreoli L, Chighizola CB, Banzato A, et al. Estimated Frequency of Antiphospholipid Antibodies in Patients With Pregnancy Morbidity, Stroke, Myocardial Infarction, and Deep Vein Thrombosis: A Critical Review of the Literature. Arthritis Care Res 2013;65(11):1869–73.
119. Arvanitakis Z, Brey RL, Rand JH, et al. Antiphospholipid Antibodies, Brain Infarcts, and Cognitive and Motor Decline in Aging (ABICMA): Design of a Community-Based, Longitudinal, Clinical-Pathological Study. Neuroepidemiology 2013;40(2):73–84.
120. Finazzi G, Brancaccio V, Moia M, et al. Natural history and risk factors for thrombosis in 360 patients with antiphospholipid antibodies: A four-year prospective study from the Italian registry. Am J Med 1996;100:530.
122. Antiphospholipid Antibody in Stroke Study (APASS) Group. Anticardiolipin antibodies and the risk of recurrent thrombooc-clusive events and death. Neurology 1997;48:91.
123. Levine SR, Salowich-Palm L, Sawaya KL, et al. IgG anticardiolipin antibody titer > 40 GPL and the risk of subsequent thromboocclusive events and death: A prospective cohort study. Stroke 1997;28:1660.
124. Ruiz Irastorza G, Khamashta MA, Hunt BJ, et al. Bleeding and recurrent thrombosis in definite antiphospholipid syndrome: Analysis of a series of 66 patients treated with oral anticoagulation to a target international normalized ratio of 3.5. Arch Intern Med 2002;162:1164.
125. Verro P, Levine SR, Tietjen GE. Cerebrovascular ischemic events with high positive anticardiolipin antibodies. Stroke 1998;29: 2245.
126. Crowther MA, Ginsberg JS, Julian J, et al. A comparison of two intensities of warfarin for the prevention of recurrent thrombosis in patients with the antiphospholipid antibody syndrome. N Engl J Med 2003;349:1133–8.
127. Brey RL. Management of the neurological manifestations of APS – what do the trials tell us? Thromb Res 2004;114:489–99.
128. van Goor MP, Alblas CL, Leebeek FW, et al. Do antiphospholipid antibodies increase the long-term risk of thrombotic complications in young patients with a recent TIA or ischemic stroke? Acta Neurol Scand 2004;109:410–15.
129. Locht H, Wiik A. IgG and IgM isotypes of anti-cardiolipin and anti-beta2-glycoprotein I antibodies reflect different forms of recent thrombo-embolic events. Clin Rheumatol 2006;25: 246–50.
130. Brey RL, Abbott RD, Sharp DS, et al. Beta-2-glycoprotein 1dependent (B2GP1-dep) anticardiolipin antibodies are an independent risk factor for ischemic stroke in the Honolulu Heart Cohort. Stroke 2001;32:1701–6.
131. Brey RL, Stallworth CL, McGlasson DL, et al. Antiphospholipid antibodies and stroke in young women. Stroke 2002;33:2396.
132. Nagaraja D, Christopher R, Manjari T. Anticardiolipin antibodies in ischemic stroke in the young: Indian experience. J Neurol Sci 1997;150:137.
133. Tuhrim S, Rand JH, Wu X, et al. Antiphosphatidylserine antibodies are independently associated with ischemic stroke. Neurology 1999;53:1523–7.
134. Tuhrim S, Rand JH, Wu XX, et al. Elevated anticardiolipin antibody titer is an independent risk factor for stroke in a multiethnic population independent of isotype or degree of positivity. Stroke 1999;30:1561–5.
135. Toschi V, Motta A, et al. High prevalence of antiphosphatidylinositol antibodies in young patients with cerebral ischemia of undetermined cause. Stroke 1998;29:1759–64.
136. Zielinska J, Rygiewicz D, Wierzchowska E, et al. Anticardiolipin antibodies are an independent risk factor for ischemic stroke. Neurol Res 1999;21:653–7.
137. Metz LM, Edworthy S, Mydlarski R, et al. The frequency of phospholipid antibodies in an unselected stroke population. Can J Neurol Sci 1998;25:64.
138. Tanne D, D'Olhaberriague L, Schultz LR, et al. Anticardiolipin antibodies and their associations with cerebrovascular risk factors. Neurology 1999;52:1368–73.
139. Ahmed E, Stegmayr B, Trifunovic J, et al. Anticardiolipin antibodies are not an independent risk factor for stroke. An incident case-referent study nested within the MONICA and Vasterbotten cohort project. Stroke 2000;31:1289–93.
140. Blohorn A, Guegan-Massardier E, Triquenot Y, et al. Antiphospholipid antibodies in the acute phase of cerebral ischemia in young adults: A descriptive study of 139 patients. Cerebrovasc Dis 2002;13:156–62.
141. Ridker PM, Manson JE, Buring JE, et al. Homocysteine and risk of cardiovascular disease among postmenopausal women. JAMA 1999;281:1817.
142. Wu R, Nityanand S, Berglund L, et al. Antibodies against cardiolipin and oxidatively modified LDL in 50-year-old men predict myocardial infarction. Arterioscler Thromb Vasc Biol 1997; 17:3159.
143. Turiel M, Muzzupappa S, Gottardi B, et al. Evaluation of cardiac abnormalities and embolic sources in primary antiphospholipid syndrome by transesophageal echocardiography. Lupus 2000;9: 406–12.
144. Rademacher J, Sohngen D, Specker C, et al. Cerebral microembolism: A disease marker for ischemic cerebrovascular events in

the antiphospholipid syndrome of systemic lupus erythematosus? Acta Neurol Scand 1999;99:356.
145. Chen WH, Kao YF, Lan MY, et al. The increase of blood anticardiolipin antibody depends on the underlying etiology in cerebral ischemia. Clin Appl Thromb Hemost 2006;12: 69–76.
146. Shoenfeld Y, Ziporen L. Lessons from experimental APS models. Lupus 1998;7(Suppl. 2):S158.
147. Katzav A, Shoenfeld Y, Chapman J. The pathogenesis of neural injury in animal models of the antiphospholipid syndrome. Clin Rev Allergy Immunol 2010;38:196–200.
148. Lanir N, Zilberman M, Yron I, et al. Reactivity patterns of antiphospholipid antibodies and endothelial cells: Effect of antiendothelial antibodies on cell migration. J Lab Clin Med 1998;131:548.
149. Kaplanski G, Cacoub P, Farnarier C, et al. Increased soluble vascular cell adhesion molecule 1 concentrations in patients with primary or systemic lupus erythematosus-related antiphospholipid syndrome: Correlations with the severity of thrombosis. Arthritis Rheum 2000;43:55.
150. Hilker R, Thiel A, Geisen C, et al. Cerebral blood flow and glucose metabolism in multi-infarct dementia related to primary antiphospholipid antibody syndrome. Lupus 2000;9:311.
151. Kao CH, Lan JL, Hsieh JF, et al. Evaluation of regional cerebral blood flow with 99mTc-HMPAO in primary antiphospholipid antibody syndrome. J Nucl Med 1999;40:1446.
152. Sabet A, Sibbitt WL, Stidley CA, et al. Neurometabolite markers of cerebral injury in the antiphospholipid antibody syndrome of systemic lupus erythematosus. Stroke 1998;29:2254.
153. Bostom AG, Selhub J, Jacques PF, et al. Power shortage: Clinical trials testing the "homocysteine hypothesis" against a background of folic acid-fortified cereal grain flour. Ann Intern Med 2001;135:133.
154. Akhter E, Shums Z, Norman GL, et al. Utility of Antiphosphatidylserine/Prothrombin and IgA Antiphospholipid Assays in Systemic Lupus Erythematosus. J Rheumatol 2013;40(3):282–6.
155. Sciascia S, Giachino O, Roccatello D. Prevention of thrombosis relapse in antiphospholipid syndrome patients refractory to conventional therapy using intravenous immunoglobulin. Clin Exp Rheumatol 2012;30(3):409–13.
156. Bucciarelli S, Erkan D, Espinosa G, et al. Catastrophic antiphospholipid syndrome: Treatment, prognosis, and the risk of relapse. Clin Rev Allergy Immunol 2009;36:80–4.
157. Uthman I, Shamseddine A, Taher A. The role of therapeutic plasma exchange in the catastrophic antiphospholipid syndrome. Transfus Apher Sci 2005;33:11–17.
158. Ioannou Y, Lambrianides A, Cambridge G, et al. B cell depletion therapy for patients with systemic lupus erythematosus results in a significant drop in anticardiolipin antibody titres. Ann Rheum Dis 2008;67:246–425.
159. Ayoub N, Esposita G, Barete S, et al. Protein Z deficiency in antiphospholipid-negative Sneddon's syndrome. Stroke 2004;35: 1329–32.
160. Boesch SM, Plorer AL, Auer AJ, et al. The natural course of Sneddon syndrome: Clinical and magnetic resonance imaging findings in a prospective six year observation study. J Neurol Neurosurg Psychiatry 2003;74:542–4.
161. Levine SR, Langer SL, Albers JW, et al. Sneddon's syndrome: An antiphospholipid antibody syndrome? Neurology (NY) 1998;38: 798.
162. Sneddon IB. Cerebrovascular lesions and livedo reticularis. Br J Dermatol 1965;77:180.
163. Rebello M, Val JF, Garijo F, et al. Livedo reticularis and cerebrovascular lesions (Sneddon's syndrome). Brain 1983;106:965.
164. Skovby F, Gaustadnes M, Mudd SH. A revisit to the natural history of homocystinuria due to cystathionine beta-synthase deficiency. Mol Genet Metab 2010;99:1–3.
165. Testai FD, Gorelick PB. Inherited metabolic disorders and stroke part 2: Homocystinuria, organic acidurias, and urea cycle disorders. Arch Neurol 2010;67:148–53.
169. Djordjevic V, Stankovic M, Brankovic-Sreckovic V, et al. Prothrombotic Genetic Risk Factors in Stroke A Possible Different Role in Pediatric and Adult Patients. Clin Appl Thromb 2012; 18(6):658–61.
170. B vitamins in patients with recent transient ischaemic attack or stroke in the VITAmins TO Prevent Stroke (VITATOPS) trial: a randomised, double-blind, parallel, placebo-controlled trial. Lancet Neurol 2010;9(9):855–65.
171. Toole JF, Malinow M, Chambless LE, et al. Lowering homocysteine in patients with ischemic stroke to prevent recurrent stroke, myocardial infarction, and death: The vitamin intervention for stroke prevention (visp) randomized controlled trial. JAMA 2004;291(5):565–75.
172. Furie K, Kasner S, Adams R, et al. Guidelines for the prevention of stroke in patients with stroke or transient ischemic attack. A guideline for healthcare professionals from the American Heart Association/American Stroke Association. Stroke 2010;doi: 10.1161/STR.0b013e3181f7d043.
173. Prengler M, Pavlakis SG, Prohovnik I, et al. Sickle cell disease: The neurological complications. Ann Neurology 2002;51:543–52.
174. Wahl S, Quirolo KC. Current issues in blood transfusion for sickle cell disease. Curr Opin Pediatr 2009;21:15–21.
175. Sampaio SG, Vicari P, Figueiredo MS, et al. Brain magnetic resonance imaging abnormalities in adult patients with sickle cell disease. Correlation with transcranial Doppler findings. Stroke 2009;40:2408–12.
176. Hoppe C, Klitz W, Cheng S, et al. Gene interactions and stroke risk in children with sickle cell anemia. Blood 2004;103: 2391–6.
177. Sumoza A, de Bisotti R, Sumoza D, et al. Hydroxyurea (HU) for prevention of recurrent stroke in sickle cell anemia (SCA). Am J Hematol 2002;71:161–5.
178. Wong WY, Powars DR. Overt and incomplete (silent) cerebral infarction in sickle cell anemia: Diagnosis and management. Neuroimaging Clin N Am 2007;17:269–80.
179. Switzer JA, Hess DC, Nichols FT, et al. Pathophysiology and treatment of stroke in sickle-cell disease: Present and future. Lancet Neurol 2006;5:501–12.
180. Dobson SR, Holden KR, Nietert PJ, et al. Moyamoya syndrome in childhood sickle cell disease: A predictive factor for recurrent cerebrovascular events. Blood 2002;99:3144–50.
181. Pavlakis SG, Bello J, Prohovnik I, et al. Brain infarction in sickle cell anemia: magnetic resonance imaging correlates. Ann Neurol 1988;23:125.
182. Steen RG, Emudianughe T, Hankins GM, et al. Brain imaging findings in pediatric patients with sickle cell disease. Radiology 2003;228(1):216–25.
183. Hoppe C, Klitz W, Noble J, et al. Distinct HLA associations by stroke subtype in children with sickle cell anemia. Blood 2003; 101:2865–9.
184. Miller ST, Macklin EA, Pegelow CH, et al. Silent infarction as a risk factor for overt stroke in children with sickle cell anemia: A report from the Cooperative Study of Sickle Cell Disease. J Pediatr 2001;139:385.
185. Sebastiani P, Ramoni MF, Nolan V, et al. Genetic dissection and prognostic modeling of overt stroke in sickle cell anemia. Nat Genet 2005;37:435–40.
186. Hayward P. Genetic model predicts stroke in sickle-cell disease. Lancet Neurol 2005;4:277.
187. Taylor JGVI, Tang DC, Savage SA, et al. Variants in the VCAM1 gene and risk for symptomatic stroke in sickle cell disease. Blood 2002;100:4303–9.
188. Romana M, Diara JP, Doumbo L, et al. Angiotensinogen gene associated polymorphisms and risk of stroke in sickle cell anemia: Additional data supporting an association. Am J Hematol 2004;76:310–11.
189. Tang DC, Prauner R, Lui W, et al. Polymorphisms within the angiotensinogen gene (GT-repeat) and the risk of stroke in pediatric patients with sickle cell disease: A case-control study. Am J Hematol 2001;68:164–9.
190. Sarnaik SA, Ballas SK. Molecular characteristics of pediatric patients with sickle cell anemia and stroke. Am J Hematol 2001;67:179–82.
191. Miller ST, Sleeper LA, Pegelow CH, et al. Prediction of adverse outcomes in children with sickle cell disease. N Engl J Med 2000;342:83–9.
192. Kratovil T, Bulas D, Driscoll MC, et al. Hydroxyurea therapy lowers TCD velocities in children with sickle cell disease. Pediatr Blood Cancer 2006;47:894–900.

193. Strouse JJ, Holbert ML, DeBaun MR, et al. Primary hemorrhagic stroke in children with sickle cell disease is associated with recent transfusion and use of corticosteroids. Pediatrics 2006;118: 1916–24.
194. Wierenga KJ, Serjeant BE, Serjeant GR. Cerebrovascular complications and parvovirus infection in homozygous sickle cell disease. J Pediatr 2001;139:438–42.
195. Quinn CT, Sargent JW. Daytime steady-state haemoglobin desaturation is a risk factor for overt stroke in children with sickle cell anaemia. Br J Haematol 2008;140:336–9.
196. Adams RJ, McKie VC, Hsu L, et al. Prevention of a first stroke by transfusions in children with sickle cell anemia and abnormal results on transcranial Doppler ultrasonography. N Engl J Med 1998;339:5–11.
197. Valadi N, Silva GS, Bowman LS, et al. Transcranial Doppler ultrasonography in adults with sickle cell disease. Neurology 2006;67: 572–4.
198. Kato GJ, Gladwin MT. Evolution of novel small-molecule therapeutics targeting sickle cell vasculopathy. JAMA 2008;300: 2638–46.
199. Kato GJ, Gladwin MT, Steinberg MH. Deconstructing sickle cell disease: Reappraisal of the role of hemolysis in the development of clinical subphenotypes. Blood Rev 2007;21(1):37–47.
200. Kato GJ, McGowan V, Machado RF, et al. Lactate dehydrogenase as a biomarker of hemolysis-associated nitric oxide resistance, priapism, leg ulceration, pulmonary hypertension, and death in patients with sickle cell disease. Blood 2006;107(6):2279–85.
201. Adams RJ, Ohene-Frempong K, Wang W. Sickle cell and the brain. Hematology Am Soc Hematol Educ Program 2001; 31–46.
202. Adams RJ, Brambilla D. Optimizing Primary Stroke Prevention in Sickle Cell Anemia (STOP 2) Trial Investigators: Discontinuing prophylactic transfusions used to prevent stroke in sickle cell disease. N Engl J Med 2005;353:2769–78.
203. Brousse V, Hertz-Pannier L, Consigny Y, et al. Does regular blood transfusion prevent progression of cerebrovascular lesions in children with sickle cell disease? Ann Hematol 2009;88: 785–8.
204. Lee MT, Piomelli S, Granger S, et al. Stroke Prevention Trial in Sickle Cell Anemia (STOP): Extended follow-up and final results. Blood 2006;108:847–52.
205. Pegelow CH, Wang W, Granger S, et al. Silent infarcts in children with sickle cell anemia and abnormal cerebral artery velocity. Arch Neurol 2001;58:2017–21.
206. Scothorn D, Price C, Schwartz D, et al. Risk of recurrent stroke in children with sickle cell disease receiving blood transfusion therapy for at least five years after initial stroke. J Pediatr 2002; 140:348.
207. Bhatia M, Walters MC. Hematopoietic cell transplantation for thalassemia and sickle cell disease: Past, present and future. Bone Marrow Transplant 2008;41:109–17.
208. Zimmerman SA, Schultz WH, Burgett S, et al. Hydroxyurea therapy lowers transcranial Doppler flow velocities in children with sickle cell anemia. Blood 2007;110:1043–7.
209. Bushnell C, Goldstein LB. Screening for hypercoagulable syndromes following stroke. Curr Atheroscler Rep 2003;5: 291–8.
210. Rahemtullah A, Van Cott EM. Hypercoagulation testing in ischemic stroke. Arch Pathol Lab Med 2007;131:890–901.
211. Saposnik G, Barinagarrementeria F, Brown R, et al. Diagnosis and management of cerebral venous thrombosis: A statement for healthcare professionals from the American Heart Association/American Stroke Association. Stroke 2011;42: 1158–92.

43 Migraine and Stroke

Hans-Christoph Diener, Tobias Kurth

KEY POINTS

- Migraine and particularly migraine with aura has been consistently associated with increased risk of ischemic stroke. New evidence also suggest links with hemorrhagic stroke.
- In only few cases migraine directly result in a stroke.
- Treatment of stroke in patients with migraine is generally similar to patients without. However, several acute treatment option to stop a migraine attack are contraindicated after stroke.
- Distinction between migraine aura and a transient ischemic attack can be challenging, particularly among the elderly.

Migraine is a chronic-intermittent headache disorder with episodes of headache that are unilateral or bilateral in location, pulsating in quality, moderate to severe in intensity, and exacerbated by physical activity. Associated symptoms include nausea or vomiting, photophobia, and phonophobia. The prevalence of migraine is 12% to 18% in females and 6% to 8% in males.[1-3] The prevalence of migraine with aura (which includes familial hemiplegic migraine) is lower, around 4%, and about 25% of migraine patients have either migraine with aura or migraine both with and without aura.[4] Aura is, in general, a recurrent visual disorder manifesting in attacks of reversible focal neurologic symptoms that usually develops gradually over 5 to 20 minutes and lasts for less than 60 minutes. Various forms of migraine are recognized, generally classified according to the transient, though sometimes persistent, neurologic deficits that may precede, accompany, or outlast the headache phase. The most accepted current classification was published by the International Headache Society (IHS) in 2013 (Table 43-1).[5]

Migraine with aura of different types, retinal or ocular migraine, ophthalmoplegic migraine, familial hemiplegic migraine, and basilar artery migraine may mimic transient ischemic attack (TIA) or ischemic stroke may be associated with an increased stroke risk. Each may be transient, prolonged, or persistent.[6] When the aura symptoms of a migraine attack persist for more than 24 hours, *migraine-induced stroke* is suspected. The clinical features that often mimic stroke are described next.

CLINICAL FEATURES

The most prevalent migraine syndromes include typical migraine headache without aura of neurologic deficit, and migraine headache associated with aura of neurologic deficit. Visual disturbances account for well over half the transient neurologic manifestations. Most frequently, these consist of positive phenomena such as stars, spark photopsia, complex geometric patterns, and fortification spectra. These positive phenomena may leave in their wake "negative" phenomena such as increasing scotoma and slowly developing hemianopia. The symptoms are characteristically slow in onset and slow in progression, although occasionally the onset is more abrupt, and a migraine headache may be confused with amaurosis fugax.[7] Visual symptoms sometimes progress to visual distortion or misperception, such as micropsia or dysmetropsia. The patterns of symptoms indicate the spread of neurologic dysfunction from the occipital cortex into the contiguous regions of the temporal or parietal lobes.[8-11] It is critical, in making the differential diagnosis from stroke, to establish that the neurologic deficit in aura crosses arterial territories. The second most common symptoms are somatosensory and characteristically hand and lower face (cheiro-oral) in distribution. Less frequently, the symptoms include aphasia, dysarthria, or clumsiness of one limb. Mostly, a slow, marchlike progression of symptoms is characteristic.

CLASSIFICATION

The major problem that faces the clinician is a lack of consistency in the definition of migraine-related stroke in the studies conducted so far. Strict definition of terms is essential for future comprehensive epidemiologic or population-based studies. The following major questions arise:

- Does stroke occur in the course of the migraine attack, causing true migraine-induced cerebral infarction?
- Does migraine cause stroke because other risk factors for stroke are present to interact with the migraine-induced pathogenesis?
- Can stroke present as a migraine syndrome, that is, symptomatic migraine?

Some of the latest developments serve to clarify the association between migraine and stroke. The IHS classification from 1988 has led to improved definitions of migraine and migraine-induced stroke in a more specific comprehensive manner.[12] New techniques of brain imaging have provided new insights into the relationship of the disorders through improvements in diagnosis.

Migrainous cerebral infarction (IHS 1.5.4) is described in the IHS classification as "one or more migraine aura symptoms associated with an ischaemic brain lesion in the appropriate territory demonstrated by neuroimaging".

Diagnostic criteria include:

1. A migraine attack fulfilling criteria B and C.
2. Occurring in a patient with 1.2 migraine with aura and typical of previous attacks except that one or more aura symptoms persists for >60 minutes.
3. Neuroimaging demonstrates ischemic infarction in a relevant area.
4. Not better accounted for by another diagnosis.

Table 43-1 presents an extended classification of stroke in association with migraine or migraine-related stroke. Included in this classification is migrainous cerebral infarction.

TABLE 43-1 Classification of Migraine Subtypes

International Headache Society ICHD—3 Betae	World Health Organization ICD-10NA Code	Diagnosis (and Etiologic ICD-10 Code for Secondary Headache Disorders)
1.	[G43]	Migraine
1.1	[G43.0]	Migraine without aura
1.2	[G43.1]	Migraine with aura
1.2.1	[G43.10]	Migraine with typical aura
1.2.2	[G43.103]	Migraine with brainstem aura
1.2.3.1	[G43.105]	Familial hemiplegic migraine
1.2.3.2	[G43.105]	Sporadic hemiplegic migraine
1.2.6		Basilar-type migraine
1.3	[G43.3]	Chronic migraine
1.4.1	[G43.2]	Status migrainosus
1.4.2	[G43.3]	Persistent aura without infarction
1.4.3	[G43.3]	Migrainous infarction
1.4.4	[G43.3] + [G40.x or G41.x]*	Migraine-aura triggered seizures
1.5	[G43.83]	Probable migraine

Modified slightly from Headache Classification Subcommittee of the International Headache Society: The International Classification of Headache Disorders, 2nd edition. *Cephalalgia* 24(Suppl 1): 1–160, 2004.

ICD-10NA, International Classification of Diseases, 10th revision: Neurological Adaptation; ICHD-II, International Classification of Headache Disorders, 2nd ed.

*The additional code specifies the type of seizure.

Migraine-Induced Stroke

Definition: See previous discussion.

The major problem with the IHS classification is that it does not permit the diagnosis of migraine-induced stroke in patients who have migraine without aura (see previous discussion). Perhaps migraine without aura begins in "silent" brain areas and has the same pathogenesis as migraine with aura. This possibility is indicated by the blood flow measurements reported by Woods and colleagues,[8] who found a decrease of 30–40% in cerebral blood flow (CBF) in the occipital lobe in a woman during an episode of migraine without aura. Migraine-induced stroke might occur in patients without other vascular risk factors.

Coexisting Stroke and Migraine

Definition: A clearly defined clinical stroke syndrome must occur remotely in time from a typical attack of migraine with aura.

Among young individuals, stroke is a rare event, whereas migraine is common. Clearly, the two conditions can coexist without migraine's being a contributive factor to stroke. When the two conditions coexist in the young, the true pathogenesis of stroke may be difficult to elucidate. A comorbidity of stroke risk in migraine sufferers seems apparent from the case-control series reviewed later in this chapter, in which none of the strokes was directly induced by the migraine attack. This finding increases the clinical significance of coincident stroke and should serve to raise clinical consciousness of the need for stroke risk factor awareness in all migraine sufferers.

Stroke with Clinical Features of Migraine

Definition: A structural lesion unrelated to migraine pathogenesis that manifests as clinical features typical of migraine.

Symptomatic Cases

In symptomatic cases, established structural lesions of the central nervous system or cerebral vessels episodically cause symptoms typical of migraine with aura. Such cases should be termed "symptomatic migraine."[13] Migraine-like headache secondary to another disorder (symptomatic migraine) is coded as a secondary headache attributed to that disorder.[5] Cerebral arteriovenous malformations frequently masquerade as migraine with aura.[14] Migraine attacks associated with cerebral autosomal dominant arteriopathy with subcortical infarcts and leukoencephalopathy (CADASIL) also may be symptomatic of the membrane dysfunction associated with this disorder.[15–17] Subarachnoid hemorrhage, venous-sinus thrombosis, and viral meningitis can mimic migraine attacks with or without aura in patients who suffer from migraine or who have a family history of migraine.

Migraine Mimic

In this category, stroke due to acute and progressing structural disease is accompanied by headache and a constellation of progressive neurologic signs and symptoms indistinguishable from those of migraine. This might best be termed a migraine mimic but is also referred to as secondary migraine.[18]

The diagnostic discrimination of a migraine mimic can be most difficult to define in patients with established migraine. Many of the cases described in the literature on the conceptual evolution of migraine-related stroke were likely migraine mimics, the diagnosis being hampered by limitation in investigative tools and uncertainty in the knowledge of migraine pathogenesis.

The issue of spontaneous carotid artery dissection is relevant because patients with migraine are at increased risk for dissections[19–21] and because the occurrence of a dissection as a typical migraine mimic has been reported.[22] Although the mechanism of pain production is not clearly understood, the occurrence of headache is an expected finding, present in 60% of patients[23] and headache is more frequent in vertebral dissection, along with a variable incidence of ischemic complications, a combination that may mimic accompanied migraine. Fisher[24] analyzed 21 selected cases of angiographically documented cervical carotid dissection, observing that almost all patients (19 of 21) had ipsilateral pain in one or more regions of the head, including forehead, orbit, temple, retro-orbit, side of head, and frontal region. In addition, 12 patients had neck pain, usually in the upper neck and localized to a region including the mastoid, the upper carotid, behind or below the angle of the jaw, and along the sternocleidomastoid muscle. The pain was usually severe, often sudden in onset, described equally as steady or throbbing, and occasionally accompanied by alterations in ipsilateral scalp sensation. The duration ranged from several hours to 2 years, with most lasting no longer than 3–4 weeks. About three-fourths of Fisher's patients experienced ischemic complications, and in one-half, the headache preceded the ischemic event by a few hours to 4 days. Other common diagnostic findings were Horner's syndrome, subjective bruit, dysgeusia, and visual scintillations.

Uncertain Classification

Complex or multiple factors: Many migraine-related strokes cannot be categorized with certainty.

EPIDEMIOLOGY

Numerous studies have evaluated the association between migraine and risk of stroke. The vast majority were case-control studies,[25–36] followed by prospective cohort studies,[37–42] a few cross-sectional studies,[43,44] and some studies using data from stroke registries.[45,46] Three retrospective case-control studies found increased risk of ischemic stroke among women younger than 45 years who reported a history of migraine with aura,[28,29,34] with risk estimates ranging from 3.8[29] to 8.4.[34] Two additional case-control studies found an increased risk for migraine sufferers with aura in both genders.[26,32] In only one case-control study, was migraine without aura associated with increased risk of ischemic stroke.[28] The association between migraine and hemorrhagic stroke was evaluated in a case-control study,[47] which found increased risk for those with a family history of migraine (odds ratio [OR] 2.30; 95% confidence interval [CI], 1.35–3.90) and also suggested that there might be an increased risk among participants with migraine without aura (OR 1.84; 95%CI, 0.77–4.39). In another case-control study, the association between migraine and hemorrhagic stroke produced conflicting results, because the association was dependent on the control selection.[25] Results from a prospective cohort study among women indicate that the association between migraine and hemorrhagic stroke is limited to the subgroup of women with MA (relative risk [RR] = 2.25; 95%CI, 1.11–4.54). The risk was stronger for fatal hemorrhagic strokes and appeared to be limited to women aged ≥55 years.[48] A meta-analysis of eight studies involving a total of 1600 hemorrhagic strokes found a pooled adjusted effect of 1.48 (95%CI, 1.16–1.88).[49] When the interaction between migraine and other risk factors for stroke was evaluated, the risk was more than tripled by smoking (OR 10)[28] and quadrupled by oral contraceptive use (ORs 14–17).[29,50] The combination of migraine, oral contraceptives, and smoking further increased the risk.

A meta-analysis of 11 case-control and three cohort studies published up to 2004 suggested that the risk of stroke is increased in individuals with migraine (pooled RR 2.16; 95%CI, 1.89–2.48). In this analysis, the risk was consistent among individuals who had migraine with aura (RR 2.27; 95%CI, 1.61–3.19) and migraine without aura (RR 1.83; 95%CI, 1.06–3.15) and was markedly increased for women taking oral contraceptives (RR 8.72; 95%CI, 5.05–15.05).[51]

Two large-scale prospective cohort studies and one population-based case-control study were published after the meta-analysis. The first used data from the Women's Health Study, which included more than 39,000 apparently healthy women 45 years or older.[36] This study found a 1.7-fold increased risk of ischemic stroke (RR 1.71; 95%CI, 1.11–2.66) for women who reported migraine with aura versus women without migraine. The associated risk was magnified in those women who were 45 to 55 years of age (RR 2.25; 95%CI, 1.30–3.91) and was not seen in the older age group. Migraine without aura was not associated with an increased risk of ischemic stroke.

The second prospective study used data from the Atherosclerosis Risk in Communities Study and included more than 12,000 men and women 55 years and older.[38] The study evaluated the migraine–stroke association in different time windows (i.e., retrospective and prospective). The only strict prospective evaluation (i.e., the migraine assessment preceded the stroke event) showed a 1.8-fold increased risk of ischemic stroke (RR 1.84; 95%CI, 0.89–3.82) in migraine sufferers with aura than in participants without migraine. The fact that the risk estimates did not reach statistical significance may be due to the specific migraine and aura classification used in the study. This study found no further effect modification by age, and the migraine–stroke association persisted after data were controlled for a large number of traditional stroke risk factors. The results of these prospective studies suggest that the migraine–stroke association may not be limited to individuals younger than 45.

The Stroke Prevention in Young Women Study matched 386 women age 15 to 49 years with first ischemic stroke with 614 age- and ethnicity-matched controls.[36] Subjects were classified as having no headache, probable migraine without visual symptoms, or probable migraine with visual symptoms. Compared with women without headache, those who reported probable migraine with visual symptoms had a 1.5-fold higher risk of ischemic stroke (OR 1.5; 95%CI, 1.1–2.0), which was slightly attenuated after control for stroke risk factors. This risk further increased for women who reported a probable migraine frequency of at least 12 per year (OR 2.3; 95%CI, 1.5–3.5) and for those who had begun having migraines during the prior year (OR 6.7; 95%CI, 2.3–19.2). Women with probable migraine without visual symptoms were not at increased risk for ischemic stroke. When effect modification by smoking and oral contraceptive use was considered, the combination of smoking and oral contraceptive use increased the risk of ischemic stroke to sevenfold that in women without probable migraine. The risk in women who did smoke and use oral contraceptives was ten fold that in women without probable migraine who did not smoke and who did not use oral contraceptives.[36]

Furthermore, migraine with aura is associated with silent brain infarcts, as summarized in a recent meta-analyses.[44,52] The CAMERA study from the Netherlands randomly selected patients with migraine with aura (n = 161), patients with migraine without aura (n = 134), and controls (n = 140) who were frequency-matched to cases for age, sex, and place of residence were studied by means of MRI. The investigators found no significant difference between patients with migraine and controls in overall infarct prevalence (8.1% vs 5.0%, respectively). However, patients with migraine had a higher prevalence of silent infarcts in the cerebellar region of the posterior circulation territory than did controls (5.4% vs 0.7%, respectively; $P = 0.02$; adjusted OR, 7.1; 95%CI, 0.9–55). The adjusted OR was 13.7 (95%CI, 1.7–112) for patients with migraine with aura in comparison with that in controls. In patients with migraine with a frequency of attacks of one or more per month, the adjusted OR was 9.3 (95%CI, 1.1–76). The highest risk was in patients with migraine with aura who experienced one attack or more per month (OR, 15.8; 95%CI, 1.8–140).[44]

Because the absolute occurrence of ischemic stroke among migraine sufferers is a rare event, the absolute risks are extremely low. The estimated attributable risk from epidemiologic studies ranges from 18 to 40 additional ischemic stroke cases per 100,000 women per year.[37,51]

Potential Factors Increasing the Risk of Stroke among Patients with Migraine

Oral contraceptives are recognized to increase stroke risk in general and in migraine sufferers and may cause coexisting stroke and migraine. In some instances, however, stroke occurs during the migraine attack, and the medication may have increased the risk of coagulopathy but may not have induced stroke in the absence of the migrainous process. The Collaborative Group for the Study of Stroke in Young Women used a case-control design to evaluate the risk of cerebrovascular disease in users of oral contraceptives.[25] The risk of cerebral thrombosis among women using oral contraceptives was 9.5 times greater than that among non-users. The role of migraine was assessed in both users and nonusers of contraceptives. Among migraine sufferers not exposed to birth control pills, the risk of stroke was equivocal, depending on the control group used for comparison. The use of oral contraceptives in combination with migraine, however, increased the RR for thrombotic stroke from 2.0 to 5.9.

A study from Denmark found a multiplicative relationship between the risk of oral contraceptives and migraine.[31] A smaller French case-control study of women younger than 45 years found an increased risk for ischemic stroke among women who had migraine without aura (OR 3.0; 95%CI, 1.5–5.8). The risk was even greater in women suffering from migraine with aura (OR 6.2; 95%CI, 2.1–18.0).[28] There was a dose–effect relationship between risk of stroke and the dose of estrogen: the OR was 4.8 for pills containing 50 µg of estrogen, 2.7 for 30–40 µg, 1.7 for 20 µg, and 1 µg for progestogen. In none of these cases was the stroke induced by the migraine attack. Use of oral contraceptive in absence of migraine resulted in an OR of 3.5. The combination of oral contraceptive use and migraine resulted in an OR of 13.9 (95%CI, 5.5–35.1). A case-control study from Italy in patients with TIA and stroke studied 308 patients aged 15–44 with either transient ischemic attack or stroke and 591 age- and sex-matched controls from seven university hospitals. A history of migraine was more frequent in patients than in controls, and none of the controls reported the combination of migraine and oral contraceptive use.[32] The latest data on this topic come from the Stroke Prevention in Young Women Study. In this study, the association between risk of stroke and probable migraine with aura was markedly increased in women who used oral contraceptives and smoked, but each factor individually only modestly increased the risk of stroke for women with probable migraine with aura.[36]

An interesting link had been described between migraine and cardiovascular risk factors. The Genetic Epidemiology of Migraine (GEM) study found that compared with controls, migraine sufferers are more likely to smoke and to have a parental history of early myocardial infarction. The study also found that migraine sufferers with aura are more likely to have an unfavorable cholesterol profile and an elevated blood pressure, to report a history of early-onset coronary heart disease or stroke, and to have a twofold greater risk of a high Framingham-risk-score-predicted 10-year risk of coronary heart disease even after adjustments for age were made.[53] Although, as mentioned previously, the risk of ischemic stroke is further increased for women with migraine with aura who smoke, newer data suggest that this association is limited to individuals without cardiovascular risk factors. For example, in the Stroke Prevention in Young Women Study, probable migraine with visual aura was associated with ischemic stroke only among women without hypertension, without diabetes, and without a history of myocardial infarction.[36] These results are complemented by data from the Women's Health Study.[54] The association between active migraine with aura and ischemic stroke was apparent only among women in the lowest Framingham risk score group. Interestingly, the association between migraine with aura and myocardial infarction in this cohort was apparent only among women with migraine with aura with high Framingham risk score. With regard to the individual components of the Framingham risk score, this diametric pattern of association was driven by a particularly increased risk of ischemic stroke among women with active migraine with aura who were young (45 to 49 years) and who had low total cholesterol values. In contrast, women with active migraine with aura who had high total cholesterol values had increased risk for myocardial infarction.[54]

Another interesting interrelationship exists among migraine, vascular disease, and the methylenetetrahydrofolate reductase (*MTHFR*) gene. The TT genotype of this polymorphism impairs enzyme activity, thus elevating homocysteine levels. Some studies have shown that carriers of the TT genotype are more likely to have migraine, in particular migraine with aura.[55] Although data from the Women's Health Study could not confirm this finding,[56] two studies have shown that women with migraine with aura who carry the TT polymorphism are at particular increased risk for ischemic stroke.[56,57]

Taking all these studies together, patients with migraine have an increased stroke risk, although the increase is small if one considers it in absolute numbers. The incidence of stroke caused directly by a migraine attack is low. Additional risk factors for stroke in migraine patients are migraine with aura, smoking, and oral contraceptive use, the last particularly if women also smoke. Further, there is evidence that, with the exception of smoking, a low cardiovascular risk profile further increases the risk of stroke. In addition, specific genetic markers may also increase this risk. There is currently some evidence that migraine increases also the risk of hemorrhagic stroke.

NEUROIMAGING

In a radiologic series of selected migrainous patients with or without focal neurologic deficits, the prevalence of CT scan abnormalities ranged from 34% to 71%. Cala and Mastaglia[58] reported a large series in which they examined 94 patients with a history of "recurrent migrainous headaches," of whom six showed evidence of cerebral infarction. Of these patients, four had fixed visual field defects with mesial occipital low densities. Of the 49 migrainous patients studied, 21 had evidence of low attenuation in the white matter, which was most extensive in the hemisphere on the side of the headache and contralateral to the sensory aura or signs.

Magnetic Resonance Imaging

The diagnosis of migraine-induced stroke has been greatly enhanced by the use of MRI. From the research viewpoint, great interest stemmed from observations of increased white matter lesions in approximately 30% of routinely studied migraine patients compared with healthy controls.[59] Lesions were found in the centrum semiovale and frontal white matter, in some cases extending to deeper structures in the region of the basal ganglia. In some series such findings were more prevalent in patients with the migraine subtypes associated with neurologic aura.[60] Not all case series found a greater incidence than controls, however. Another series found a higher incidence of white matter lesions in patients with migraine as well as in patients with tension-type headache.[61] The mechanisms of these changes remain to be determined. If relevant, they may represent small foci of ischemic infarction of obscure origin, or gliosis.

More important, two MRI studies found an increased prevalence of white matter lesions and silent brain infarcts in women with frequent migraine with aura.[44,52,62] Silent brain infarcts were preferentially observed in the occipital lobes and the posterior fossa. Whether these lesions are predictors of vascular dementia later in life or an increased risk of symptomatic brain infarcts is not yet known. In a population-based study with 760 participants 163 (20.9%) reported a history of severe headache and 116 had migraine, of whom 17 (14.7%) reported aura symptoms. An association was found between any history of severe headache and increasing volume of white matter hyperintensities in MRI.[63] The adjusted odds ratio of being in the highest third for total volume of white matter hyperintensities was 2.0 (95%CI, 1.3–3.1, P for trend 0.002) for participants with any history of severe headache when compared with participants without severe headache being in the lowest third. Migraine with aura was the only headache type strongly associated with volume of deep white matter hyperintensities (highest third OR 12.4,

1.6–99.4, P for trend 0.005) and with brain infarcts (3.4, 1.2–9.3).

Positron Emission Tomography

Weiller and associates[64] found normal cortical blood flow during migraine attacks and after subcutaneous injection of 6 mg sumatriptan.

Headache of Vascular Disease

Not surprisingly, a major difficulty in differential diagnosis is that the symptom of head pain occurs in various forms of acute cerebrovascular disease, including ischemic stroke. The landmark experiments of Ray and Wolff[65] demonstrated that sensitivity to pressure, traction, and faradization occurred in the intracranial internal carotid artery, the first 1–2 cm of the middle cerebral artery stem, the first several centimeters of the anterior cerebral artery just beyond the A2 segment, and the first 1–2 cm of the vertebral, anterior, and posterior inferior cerebellar and pontine arteries. These sensitive structures, when electrically stimulated, provoke pain that is localized to specific areas of the scalp and face.

Fisher's[24,66] clinicopathologic observations extended these findings. A study of the headache syndromes due to ischemic cerebrovascular disease showed that most patients complained of the symptom at the onset of a persisting neurologic deficit, although in some cases headache was premonitory of, or accompanied, TIAs. The headache was usually not throbbing, often localized, and frequently lateralized ipsilateral to the presumed arterial occlusion; it was occasionally severe. Of special interest was the relatively high frequency of headache in posterior cerebral artery territory infarctions compared with that seen in carotid or basilar disease. Headache was the exception in lacunar strokes with pure motor or pure sensory syndromes, and no headaches occurred in any of the 58 patients with transient monocular blindness. Overall, the frequency of headache was 31% in carotid disease and 42% in vertebrobasilar disease. Mitsias and Ramadan[67] have extensively reviewed the literature on this topic up to 1997.

Drug-Induced Migraine-Related Stroke

Migraine-related stroke associated with ergot therapy is appropriately discussed in this category because it is impossible to confidently exclude an interaction of the drug with the migrainous process to induce stroke. Rarely, ergot therapy, even in therapeutic doses, may produce focal and diffuse cerebral dysfunction. The peripheral vascular and central nervous system effects of ergot alkaloids in toxic doses have long been recognized, consisting of gangrene, seizures, encephalopathy, and coma. The mechanism responsible for diffuse cerebral dysfunction is not settled and may be the result of either a direct central nervous system toxic effect or severe cerebral vasoconstriction, although in therapeutic doses ergotamine usually has no effect on CBF. Scattered reports have appeared linking ergotamine use to focal disturbances in the ophthalmic and cerebral circulations, manifested as transient monocular blindness, bilateral papillitis, and sensorimotor deficits.[68–70] Epidemiologic studies show an increased stroke risk with the use of ergots but not of triptans.[71] Since the introduction of triptans, such as sumatriptan, there have also been scattered reports of strokelike events, but so far none that has been persuasive of primary involvement of the drug or can exclude its use in an event that mimics migraine. In most of the reported cases of stroke following injection of 6 mg sumatriptan, the time window between the injection and the stroke ranged from 5 to 329 days.[72] Only one case of sinus thrombosis was reported with the use of sumatriptan.[73] Another case report described spinal cord infarction after use of zolmitriptan.[74]

Angiography

The precipitation of migraine-like signs and symptoms during cerebral angiography is not uncommon and can potentially progress to stroke, although not all observers agree.[75] Angiography performed during migraine carries risk because of potential interaction with the migraine mechanism. Nevertheless, because arteriography can be complicated by stroke in all patients, the true pathogenesis of stroke cannot be attributed with certainty to migraine. In any case, in patients with migraine, CT or MR angiography should be performed when angiography is indicated.

Transient Focal Neurologic Events and Late-onset Migraine Accompaniments

Headache is not an invariable occurrence in migraine. Adding to the potential for diagnostic confusion is the occurrence of isolated migraine auras consisting of visual disturbances or focal deficits not accompanied by typical headache, often termed "migraine sine hemicrania." Charcot identified an incomplete form of ophthalmic migraine as "migraines ophtalmiques frustes" consisting only of "les troubles oculaires."

More controversial has been the entity of accompanied migraine without headache, originally described by Whitty.[76] Fisher[7,77] emphasized that the migrainous syndrome, despite the absence of headache, could be diagnosed on the basis of characteristic clinical features. Since then, painless transient and persistent migraine accompaniments have become more widely recognized.[78] The cause of late-onset migraine accompaniments has not been established. As the name of the syndrome suggests, the clinical features are essentially indistinguishable from those of migraine without headache. Brain imaging and cerebral arteriography do not reveal accountable structural lesions.

Hemorrhage

Cases of intracerebral hemorrhage due to migraine have been reported rarely and have been reviewed.[79] In our view, investigations have failed to establish true migraine-induced hemorrhage, most cases likely being symptomatic migraine or migraine mimics. Epidemiologic studies also showed only a weak association between migraine and cerebral hemorrhage.[37] From the viewpoint of pathogenesis, however, it is not unreasonable that ischemic softening of tissue during true migraine-induced cerebral infarction might become hemorrhagic, so dogmatism must be avoided. Experience with this entity in the context of the current IHS classification is awaited.

Retinal or Ocular Migraine

This group of disorders is designated as uncertain in classification because of limited clinical information; most clinical case reports or series were communicated prior to the development of contemporary, advanced neurologic investigation. Although transient homonymous scintillations or fortification scotoma are well-recognized cortical migrainous phenomena, monocular visual loss due to retinal involvement is less often a manifestation of migraine, although still a differential diagnostic point in the patient presenting with amaurosis fugax. Because both retinal and ciliary circulations may be affected, the term *ocular migraine* is preferred[80] and should be distinguished from the term *ophthalmic migraine*, which refers to any migrainous disturbance of vision, whether ocular or cortical.

MIGRAINE THAT MIMICS STROKE

Hemiplegic Migraine

Liveing,[81] in 1873, first described transient hemiparesis associated with a migraine attack. Whitty[82] classified the disorder into hemiplegic migraine with a family history of migraine with or without aura and familial hemiplegic migraine (FHM), in which attacks occur with stereotypical features in family members, often with severe and long-lasting hemiparesis or other persistent aura symptoms, and an autosomal dominant inheritance pattern.

The IHS classifies "hemiplegic migraine" under "migraine with typical aura" (IHS 1.2.1). FHM is classified as a subgroup of migraine with aura (IHS 1.2.3), and sporadic hemiplegic migraine as 1.2.3.2. The working definition for FHM includes the criteria for migraine with aura (1.2.1,1.2.2) with hemiplegic features that may be prolonged together with at least one first-degree relative with identical attacks. As noted previously, the overall prevalence of migraine with aura is around 4%; this figure includes hemiplegic migraine.

Hemiplegic migraine attacks are characterized by hemiparesis or hemiplegia. The arm and leg are involved in the majority of attacks, often combined with face and hand paresis. Less often, isolated facial and arm paresis occurs. The progression of the motor deficit is slow, with a spreading or marching quality. In most cases symptoms are accompanied by homolateral sensory disturbance, particularly cheiro-oral in distribution, again with a slowly spreading or marching quality. Infrequently, the hemiparesis may alternate from side to side, even during an attack.[83] Visual disturbance, which takes the form of hemianopic loss or typical visual aura, is common. Homolateral or contralateral localization of the visual disturbance is often obscure, however. When dysphasia occurs, it is more often expressive than receptive. The neurologic symptoms last 30 to 60 minutes and are followed by severe pulsating headache that is hemicranial or whole head in distribution. Nausea, vomiting, photophobia, and phonophobia are associated features. In severe cases, the aura can persist throughout the headache phase.

Manifestations of severe hemiplegic migraine attacks include fever, drowsiness, confusion, and coma, all of which can be prolonged from days to weeks.[83] Severe hemiplegic migraine may lead rarely to persistent minor neurologic deficit, in which the cumulative effect of repeated attacks progresses to profound multifocal neurologic deficit, even dementia.

FHM is characterized by the neurologic deficit described previously that is identical in at least one other first-degree relative. There is an autosomal dominant inheritance pattern of the disorder. Other neurologic deficits have been described in association with FHM. Most common is a syndrome of progressive cerebellar disturbance, dysarthria, nystagmus, and ataxia.[83] Retinitis pigmentosa, sensory neural deafness, tremor, dizziness, oculomotor disturbances with nystagmus, ataxia, and coma have also been described.[84,85] These neurologic deficits are present between attacks and are not part of the aura. Hemiplegic migraine attacks also may be part of other familial disorders affecting other systems, for example mitochondrial encephalomyopathy with lactic acidosis, and stroke-like episodes syndrome (MELAS) and CADASIL.[17] Attacks of hemiplegic migraine are less likely to be stereotyped in family members with these conditions, however, because the migraine attack is probably "symptomatic" of the underlying brain disorder.

A breakthrough in establishing the cause of FHM was achieved during the clinical investigation of CADASIL.[86–88] This disease is characterized by recurring small deep infarcts, dementia, and leukoencephalopathy. Some patients also experience recurrent attacks of severe migraine-like headache with aura symptoms that include transient headache and hemiparesis. Joutel and coworkers[89,90] identified the gene locus on chromosome 19. Ophoff and colleagues[91] and Joutel and coworkers[92] have isolated, on chromosome 19p13.1, a gene encoding the alpha$_1$ subunit of a brain-specific voltage-gated P/Q type neuronal calcium channel (CACNL1A4) from patients with FHM. The third gene was identified by Dichgans and associates[93] on chromosome 2q24.

Several missense mutations were also identified.[94–96] The investigators also detected premature stop mutations predicted to disrupt the reading frame of CACNL1A4 in two unrelated patients with episodic ataxia type 2 (EA-2). Thus, FHM and episodic ataxia type 2 can be regarded as allelic channelopathies but of differing molecular mechanism, the former involving a gain-of-function variant of the Ca^{2+} channel subunit, and the latter a decrease in channel density. The results also indicate that different mutations in a single gene may cause phenotypic heterogeneity.[93,97]

Since this report, the same French group identified ten different missense mutations in the *NOTCH3* genes of 14 unrelated families with CADASIL. The Notch genes are intimately involved in intercellular signaling during development. Proteins belonging to the Notch family are transmembrane receptors. Nine of the ten mutations either added or mutated a cysteine residue in one of the epidermal growth factor (EGF)-like repeats, which are to be found in the extracellular domain. It is likely that this mutation strongly affects protein conformation, although how it leads to CADASIL remains to be established. Possibly, however, membrane instability and abnormality of cell signaling could be the underlying basis of the migraine attacks in this disorder. The generalizability of the genetic findings in FHM, one of the rarest subtypes of migraine, to the more prevalent migraine subtypes also remains to be established. It must be noted that cases of non-familial hemiplegic migraine studied by Ophoff and colleagues[91] did not show mutations. Sometimes head trauma can lead to fatal brain edema in patients with FHM.[98]

Migraine with Brainstem Aura

The concept of migraine with brainstem aura, formerly basilar artery migraine (IHS 1.2.2) was first proposed by Bickerstaff.[99,100] The diagnostic criteria are those of migraine with aura, consisting of at least two of the following fully reversible symptoms, but no motor weakness: dysarthria, vertigo, tinnitus, hypacusia, diplopia, visual symptoms present simultaneously in both temporal and nasal fields of both eyes, ataxia, decreased level of consciousness, and simultaneously bilateral paresthesias.

Reviewing a personal series of 300 cases, Bickerstaff[100] noticed 34 patients who experienced attacks that were usually heralded by visual disturbances – either complete visual loss or positive phenomena such as teichopsia so dazzling as to obscure the entire field of vision. Other basilar symptoms followed, including dizziness or vertigo; gait ataxia; dysarthria; tinnitus; bilateral acral, perioral, and lingual numbness; and paresthesias. These symptoms persisted for 2 to 60 minutes, ending abruptly, although the visual loss generally recovered more gradually. After the premonitory phase subsided, a severe throbbing occipital headache supervened and was accompanied by vomiting. The patients recovered completely, and between such attacks, many had episodes of classic migraine. Typically affected were adolescent girls. Attacks were usually infrequent and strongly related to menstruation. In Bickerstaff's series, all but two patients were younger than 23 years, and 26 of the 34 were girls. A clear-cut family history of migraine in close relatives was obtained in 82% of cases.

Lapkin and associates[101] encountered this entity in a younger population, reporting a group of 30 children with a mean age at onset of 7 years (range 7 months to 14 years). The duration of episodes ranged from minutes to many hours; one patient was symptomatic for nearly 3 days. Unlike in the adolescent cases previously described, the most common complaint was vertigo (73%), and visual disturbances occurred in 43% of cases. In children who were more severely affected, pyramidal tract dysfunction was observed as well as cranial nerve abnormalities, including internuclear ophthalmoplegia and facial nerve paresis. A family history of migraine was obtained in 86% of patients. During the follow-up period of 6 months to 3 years, none of the patients showed signs of progressive neurologic dysfunction, although one child was noted to have a permanent oculomotor nerve paralysis.

In the majority of cases of basilar migraine, the aura lasts between 5 and 60 minutes but can extend up to 3 days. Visual symptoms commonly occur first, predominantly in the temporal and nasal fields of vision. The visual disturbance may consist of blurred vision, teichopsia, scintillating scotoma, graying of vision, or total loss of vision. The features may start in one visual field and then spread to become bilateral. Bickerstaff pointed out that when vision is not completely obscured, diplopia might occur, usually as a sixth nerve weakness. Some form of diplopia may occur in up to 16% of cases.[102] Vertigo and gait ataxia are the next most common symptoms, each occurring in 63% of patients in one series.[102] The ataxia can be independent of vertigo. Tinnitus may accompany vertigo. Dysarthria is as common as ataxia and vertigo. Tingling and numbness, in the typical cheiro-oral spreading pattern seen in migraine with aura, occur in more than 60% of cases. This is usually bilateral and symmetric but may alternate sides with a hemidistribution. Occasionally, dysesthesias extend to the trunk. Bilateral motor weakness occurs in more than 50% of cases.

The syndrome of basilar artery migraine was later expanded to include alteration in consciousness. Bickerstaff[99] cited four cases of altered consciousness in detail and recorded a total of eight of 32 patients with previously diagnosed basilar artery migraine. The onset of impaired consciousness occurred in the context of other basilar symptoms with a leisurely onset, not causing the patient to fall or incur self-injury, and was sometimes preceded by a dreamlike state. Ranging from drowsiness to stupor, the altered consciousness was akinetic and usually brief, lasting up to several minutes and not accompanied by rigidity, posturing, tongue biting, urinary incontinence, or changes in the respiratory pattern. As in the usual basilar artery migraine, a throbbing headache occurred on recovery. Laboratory investigations were generally unrevealing, with normal cerebrospinal fluid analysis and electroencephalography results. Lee and Lance[103] encountered seven patients with a similar syndrome of altered consciousness, using the term *migraine stupor*. Unlike the brief episodes observed by Bickerstaff,[99] the duration of stupor in their patients ranged from 2 hours to 5 days. Four patients showed aggressive and hysterical behavior during the attacks, leading to initial psychiatric diagnoses. Although impairment of consciousness in some form is common in basilar artery migraine, it progresses to stupor and prolonged coma. Other forms of altered consciousness are amnesia and syncope. Drop attacks are rare.

Headache occurs in almost all patients with basilar artery migraine. The headache has an occipital location in the majority and a throbbing, pounding quality and is accompanied by severe nausea and vomiting. It is unusual for the headache to be unilateral or localized to the more anterior parts of the cranium. Photophobia and phonophobia occur in one-third to one-half of patients. As with other forms of migraine, the symptoms may occur without headache, but usually in no more than 4% of cases.[102] Seizures have been observed in association with basilar migraine. Electroencephalographic changes without seizures, occurring with attacks of typical basilar artery migraine, also have been described. In all, electroencephalographic abnormalities are detected in less than one-fifth of cases of basilar artery migraine and are mostly independent of any clinical manifestation of the disorder.

Permanent brainstem deficits as a result of basilar artery migraine have been reported rarely. None of Bickerstaff's cases had persisting neurologic disturbances; indeed, he stressed return to complete normality as a criterion for the diagnosis. Among the cases of migraine-associated stroke uncovered in the literature, only four of five have occurred in the vertebrobasilar territory, excluding the posterior cerebral artery. In Connor's presentation[104] of 18 cases of complicated migraine, three patients were considered to have lesions in the brainstem. In no instance did the transient episodes clearly resemble basilar artery migraine, as defined previously. Cerebral infarction specifically affecting the brainstem circulation territory understandably has been offered as evidence for a primary vascular cause of basilar migraine. Skinhoj and Paulson,[105] in studies performed during the migraine aura, found that angiographic findings were normal despite reduction of CBF, except for impaired filling in the top of the basilar artery.[105] Cerebral angiography can itself precipitate migraine aura, however, albeit after a time lag of hours. Nevertheless, the combination of the clinical features plus the arteriographic studies mentioned previously emphasizes a primary vascular alternative for the cause of basilar artery migraine. Cerebrovascular disease is the most serious disorder in the differential diagnosis of basilar artery migraine.

Ischemic stroke in the brainstem and posterior cortical regions, due to either cerebral embolism or thrombosis, manifests as a constellation of neurologic symptoms and signs of brainstem and posterior circulation defects accompanied in approximately one-third of cases by headache. Basilar artery occlusive disease can, therefore, mimic basilar artery migraine. Another basilar artery migraine "mimic" for which migraine patients are at increased risk is vertebral artery dissection.

TIAs involving any part of the vertebrobasilar territory must figure largely in the differential diagnosis, particularly if basilar artery migraine occurs for the first time in later years of life. Certain familial disorders manifest as neurologic deficit in which attacks of hemiplegic or basilar migraine may be part of the symptom complex. This group includes CADASIL, MELAS, and variants of MELAS that are associated with seizures, particularly those occipital in origin.

MECHANISMS

From the preceding review, it should be apparent that migraine can mimic cerebrovascular disorders, especially ischemic stroke, and stroke can mimic migraine. This fact poses diagnostic problems for the clinician that in most cases will be resolved. It is uncertain how much of the past literature on migraine-induced stroke described cerebrovascular disorders that were mistaken for migraine. This statement is made not to criticize these earlier reports but to recognize that they were communicated at a time when diagnostic tools were less well developed and that concepts of migraine mechanisms have changed. How a migraine attack can induce permanent neurologic deficit and brain damage remains to be determined. Perhaps even more intriguing is the question, what constitutes the comorbid increased risk for stroke between attacks? The latter is the most difficult to speculate on because, although comorbid factors may be present (such as increased platelet aggregation), many are uncertain risk factors for stroke. Indeed, when definite risk factors for stroke are present in migraine sufferers, the stroke is attributed to this cause and not to migraine. On the basis of the epidemiologic data described, however, there must be stroke risk factors yet to be identified that are comorbid with migraine.

With regard to the mechanisms whereby stroke is induced during a migraine attack, information provides some limited understanding. The current literature on CBF has been reviewed. To summarize, spreading cortical depression of Leão may induce short-lived increases in CBF, followed by a more profound oligemia. Ischemic foci, however, may occasionally occur during attacks of migraine with aura. Possibly, SD is also associated with depolarization of intrinsic neurons that also supply intraparenchymal resistance microvessels, leading to constriction and a consequent flow reduction below the threshold for K^+ release from the neuron. Increased extracellular K^+ then might precipitate depolarization of contiguous cortical neurons. Alternatively, the decreased extracellular space and brain swelling that accompany spreading cortical depression and possibly migraine could increase microvascular resistance by mechanical compression. Thus, low flow in major intracerebral vessels may be due to increased downstream resistance, not major intracranial arterial vasospasm. Essentially, low CBF and sluggish flow in large intracerebral vessels during the aura of migraine, when combined with factors predisposing to coagulopathy, could lead, although rarely, to intravascular thrombosis and thus migraine-induced cerebral infarction. Release of vasoactive peptides and endothelin, activation of cytokines, and upregulation of adhesion molecules during the neurogenically mediated inflammatory response that may be responsible for headache also may induce intravascular thrombosis. This could explain why migraine-induced stroke usually respects intracranial arterial territories even though the aura involves more widespread brain regions. In addition, frequent aura, if due to spreading depression, could induce cytotoxic cell damage and gliosis based on glutamate release or excess intracellular calcium accumulation. This process could explain persistent neurologic deficit without evidence of ischemic infarction on the basis of selective neuronal necrosis. Increased extracellular K^+, which might precipitate rarely during episodes of migraine, probably relates to variability in the coagulation status, the degree of the neuronal and hemodynamic changes, and the interaction of each during the course of the migraine attack.

MIGRAINE AND PATENT FORAMEN OVALE

Several case-control studies reported a possible link between patent foramen ovale (PFO) and migraine. Del Sette and coworkers[106] compared 44 patients with migraine with aura, 73 patients younger than 50 years with focal cerebral ischemia, with 50 control individuals without cerebrovascular disease and migraine using transcranial Doppler ultrasonography. The prevalence of right-to-left shunt was significantly higher in patients with migraine with aura (41%) and cerebral ischemia (35%) than in controls (8%). Anzola and colleagues[107] performed a case-control study in 113 consecutive patients with migraine with aura, 53 patients with migraine without aura, and 25 age-matched non-migraine individuals. The prevalence of PFO was significantly higher in patients with migraine with aura (48%) than in patients with migraine without aura (23%) and controls (20%). Further studies confirmed by different methods (transcranial Doppler ultrasonography, transesophageal echocardiography) the relationship between PFO and migraine with aura.[108,109] There seems to be a much weaker association of PFO with migraine without aura and other headaches. A meta-analysis from 2013 included 37 studies.[110] The overall pairwise associations between PFO, cryptogenic ischemic stroke and migraine did not suggest a causal role for PFO. Studies with population-based comparators showed weaker associations between migraine with aura and cryptogenic ischemic stroke in younger women (OR 1.4; 95%CI, 0.9–2.0; one study), PFO and ischemic stroke (HR 1.6; 95%CI, 1.0–2.5; two studies; OR 1.3; 95%CI, 0.9–1.9; three studies), or PFO and migraine (OR 1.0; 95%CI, 0.6–1.6; one study). A possible explanation might be that both conditions, migraine with aura and PFO, could be dominantly inherited and share a common genetic background.[111]

Coincident occurrence of two conditions, however, does not necessarily imply a causal relationship. Moreover, it is difficult to imagine how PFO would lead to a migraine attack with aura – a neural event in the occipital cortex caused by spreading depression. Even if small emboli arise from a PFO, they would travel preferentially into the anterior circulation rather than into the posterior cerebral artery.

Should PFOs be closed in patients with migraine? Even if we assume that there is a causal relationship between PFO and migraine, closure of PFO should then result in migraine improvement. To date, only one randomized and controlled prospective trial examining this issue has been performed, in the UK. The Migraine Intervention with STARFlex Technology (MIST) trial recruited patients with frequent migraine with aura that was refractory to preventive treatment (although topiramate and lamotrigine were not used).[112,113] The trial randomly assigned 147 patients to undergo either transcutaneous PFO closure with a STARFlex septal repair implant (NMT Medical, Boston) or a sham procedure. After 6 months, 135 patients had completed the trial. The primary endpoint, cure of migraine, was not significantly different between the two treatment groups. There was a trend for a reduction of migraine frequency in the operated group that was also not significant.[114] The procedure was associated with some serious adverse events – cardiac tamponade, pericardial effusion, retroperitoneal bleed, atrial fibrillation, and chest pain. Adverse events in the sham procedure group included incision site bleed, anemia, nosebleed, and a brainstem stroke.

In a retrospective study, 215 stroke patients with PFO were examined and underwent closure of PFO as a secondary prevention measure.[115] A year later, patients were asked about their migraine frequency before and after PFO closure to determine whether this intervention affected migraine attacks. Patients with a PFO and a history of stroke had higher migraine prevalence (22%) than the general population (10%). In patients with migraine with aura, percutaneous PFO closure reduced the frequency of migraine attacks by 54% (1.2 ± 0.8 vs 0.6 ± 0.8 per month; $P = 0.001$) and in patients with migraine without aura by 62% (1.2 ± 0.7 vs 0.4 ± 0.4 per month; $P = 0.006$). PFO closure did not have a statistically significant effect on headache frequency in patients with non-migraine headaches. Several other retrospective studies found a similar relationship between PFO closure and migraine improvement.[116–121] However, with one exception, all of these studies had major limitations. First, even though migraine improves spontaneously with age, no study had a control group. Second, the high rate of placebo response can reduce the frequency of migraine by up to 70%. Third, after PFO closure, most patients received aspirin, which has a modest migraine prophylactic activity, at least in men.[122,123] Clopidogrel, given as an aspirin alternative, might also reduce migraine frequency.[124,125] Fourth, retrospective collection of headache data is highly unreliable; recall bias has a major influence on the results. Furthermore, the latest study observed that as many patients experience migraine improvement as experience new-onset migraine after PFO closure.[118]

Thus, to date, there is insufficient evidence to support the hypothesis that migraine frequency is improved by PFO closure. PFO closure should not be used for the prophylaxis of migraine.

TABLE 43-2 Treatment of Acute Migraine Attacks in Otherwise Healthy Patients and in Patients With Transient Ischemic Attack (TIA) or Stroke and Patients at Risk for Stroke*

Drug	Dose (mg)	Patients with Migraine without Vascular Risk	Patients with Migraine and with TIA or Stroke
Aspirin	500–1000	+++	+++
Paracetamol, acetaminophen	500–1000	++	++
Nonsteroidal anti-inflammatory drugs		+++	+++
Ergotamine oral	1–2	++	Contraindicated
α-Dihydroergocryptine, intravenous, subcutaneous (SC)		+++	Contraindicated
Sumatriptan	25–100 oral, 6 SC	+++	Contraindicated
Naratriptan	2.5	++	Contraindicated
Rizatriptan	10	+++	Contraindicated
Zolmitriptan	2.5	+++	Contraindicated
Eletriptan	20, 40, 80	+++	Contraindicated
Almotriptan	12.5	+++	Contraindicated
Frovatriptan	2.5	+	Contraindicated
Neuroleptics		+	+

*Number of plus signs indicates efficacy, from low (+) to high (+++), shown in clinical trials.

STROKE PREVENTION IN PATIENTS WITH MIGRAINE

Most patients with TIA or ischemic stroke receive antiplatelet treatment. Aspirin lowers stroke risk[126] and has a weak preventive action in migraine.[123,127] Clopidogrel is more effective than aspirin in the prevention of the combined endpoint of stroke, myocardial infarction, and vascular death[128] and can be given to patients with migraine. In some patients clopidogrel might even improve migraine.[124] The combination of aspirin plus slow-release dipyridamole is more effective than aspirin in stroke prevention.[129] Dipyridamole may lead to headache in the first few days of intake. If it is tolerated over this period, the headache will improve. According to clinical experience, patients who used to suffer from migraine or patients from families with migraine get headache more often with dipyridamole than patients with no history of migraine. Titration of the dosage results in a lower headache incidence and a lower rate of therapy dropout.[130] Anticoagulation in patients with cardio-embolic stroke creates no problems for patients with migraine. This is also true for the new anticoagulants. In patients with significant carotid stenosis angiography, carotid endarterectomy or stenting with angioplasty can induce migraine attacks in people who formerly had migraine or who still suffer from migraine.

Patients with hypertension and migraine should be treated with β-blockers that have shown efficacy in migraine prophylaxis, such as propranolol, metoprolol, bisoprolol, and atenolol.[131] Whether angiotensin-converting enzyme inhibitors such as lisinopril are effective in migraine prophylaxis is under debate.[132] Candesartan was as effective in migraine prevention as propranolol and superior to placebo.[133]

Cholesterol-lowering drugs and antidiabetic treatment do not interfere with migraine or migraine treatment. Women with migraine with aura who suffer from additional diseases like hypertension, diabetes, and obesity and who are smoking should treat these risk factors and should be advised about the risk of oral contraceptives.[134,135]

TABLE 43-3 Drugs for Migraine Prophylaxis in Otherwise Healthy Patients and in Patients with Transient Ischemic Attack or Stroke and Patients at Risk for Stroke*

Drug	Dose (mg)	Patients with Migraine without Vascular Risk	Patients with Migraine and TIA or Stroke
Metoprolol	50–200	+++	+++
Propranolol	40–160	+++	+++
Bisoprolol	5–10	++	++
Flunarizine	5–10	+++	+++
Valproic acid	500–600	+++	+++
Gabapentin	2400	++	++
Topiramate	50–200	+++	+++
Pizotifen	1.5	+	Contraindicated
Methysergide	4–8	++	Contraindicated
Magnesium	500	+	+
α-Dihydroergocryptine	10	+	+
Aspirin	300	+	+

*Plus signs indicate efficacy, from low (+) to high (+++), shown in clinical trials.

TREATMENT OF MIGRAINE ATTACKS IN PATIENTS AT RISK FOR STROKE OR IN PATIENTS WITH TRANSIENT ISCHEMIC ATTACK OR STROKE

Migraine attack treatment with one of the triptans (almotriptan, eletriptan, frovatriptan, naratriptan, rizatriptan, sumatriptan, or zolmitriptan) is contraindicated in patients with TIA or stroke and in patients with multiple vascular risk factors (Table 43-2). The reason is that triptans have a vasoconstrictive action[136–138] and might result in a decrease of already decreased blood flow. For patients with vascular disease, calcitonin-gene-related peptide (CGRP) antagonists are the drugs of choice in the future; these agents have no vasoconstrictive properties.[139] Ergot alkaloids are also contraindicated for the same reason.[138,140] Treatment of acute migraine attacks in patients at high risk for stroke is restricted to analgesic drugs. In some countries aspirin is available as an intravenous (IV) injection for the treatment of acute migraine attack; 1000 mg intravenous aspirin is inferior to 6 mg subcutaneous sumatriptan in terms of efficacy but is better tolerated.[141] Patients with frequent migraine attacks and vascular disease should receive migraine prophylaxis (Table 43-3). Drugs of first choice are β-blockers.[131] They are effective and will also lower increased blood pressure. The later stroke trials indicate that lower blood pressure might even prevent vascular events in patients with normal blood pressure.[142] Flunarizine is not available in all countries but can be given to most patients with vascular disease.[143] The same is true for anticonvulsants.[144,145] Serotonin antagonists such as pizotifen and methysergide[146] are contraindicated in patients at risk for stroke. Aerobic exercise has migraine-preventive action and lowers stroke risk.[147,148]

Patients who suffered cerebral or subarachnoid hemorrhage should not use acetylsalicylic acid to treat migraine attacks or nonsteroidal anti-inflammatory drugs (NSAIDs) for migraine prophylaxis. Triptans are contraindicated to treat headache after subarachnoidal hemorrhage. Valproic acid for migraine prophylaxis should only be used with regular platelet count. Valproic acid can lead to thrombocytopenia.[149] The treatment of the acute phase of cerebral hemorrhage and subarachnoid hemorrhage is the same in patients with or without migraine.

Acknowledgments

HCD is supported by a grant from the German Ministry of Education and Science via the German Headache Consortium. TK is supported by the French Institute of Health and Medical Research (Inserm) and the French National Agency for Research (ANR).

REFERENCES

1. Stewart WF, Lipton RB, Celentano DD, et al. Prevalence of migraine headache in the United States: relation to age, race, income, and other sociodemographic factors. JAMA 1992;267: 64–9.
2. Lipton RB, Stewart WF. Epidemiology and comorbidity of migraine. In: Goadsby PJ, Silberstein SD, editors. Headache. Boston: Butterworth-Heinemann; 1997. p. 75–97.
3. Russel MB, Rasmussen BK, Thornvaldesen P, et al. Prevalence and sex ratio of the subtypes of migraine. Int J Epidemiol 1995; 24:612–18.
4. Rasmussen BK, Olesen J. Migraine with aura and migraine without aura: An epidemiological study. Cephalalgia 1992;12: 221–8.
5. Headache Classification Committee of the International Headache Society. The International Classification of Headache Disorders, 3rd edition (beta version). Cephalalgia 2013;33:629–808.
6. Fisher CM. Late-life migraine accompaniments as a cause of unexplained transient ischemic attacks. Can J Med Sci 1980;7:9.
7. Queiroz AP, Rapaport AM, Weeks RE, et al. Characteristics of migraine visual aura. Headache 1997;37:137–41.
8. Woods RP, Iacoboni M, Mazziotta JC. Bilateral spreading cerebral hypoperfusion during spontaneous migraine headache. N Engl J Med 1994;331:1689–92.
9. Olesen J, Tfelt-Hansen P, Henriksen L, et al. Difference between cerebral blood flow reactions in classic and common migraine. In: Rose FC, editor. Advances in migraine research and therapy. New York: Raven Press; 1982. p. 105–15.
10. Diener H. Positron emission tomography studies in headache. Headache 1997;37:622–5.
11. Cutrer FM, Sorensen AG, Weisskopf RM, et al. Perfusion-weighted imaging defects during spontaneous migrainous aura. Ann Neurol 1998;43:25–31.
12. Headache Classification Committee of the International Headache Society. Classification and diagnostic criteria for headache disorders, cranial neuralgias and facial pain. Cephalalgia 1988; 8:1–93.
13. Olesen J, Friberg L, Olsen TS, et al. Ischaemia-induced (symptomatic) migraine attacks may be more frequent than migraine-induced ischaemic insults. Brain 1993;116:187–202.
14. Silvestrini M, Cupini LM, Calabresi P, et al. Migraine with aura-like syndrome due to arteriovenous malformation: The clinical value of transcranial Doppler in early diagnosis. Cephalalgia 1992;12:115–19.
15. Davous P. CADASIL: a review with proposed diagnostic criteria. Eur J Neurol 1998;5:219–33.
16. Chabriat H, Vahedi K, Iba-Zizen MT, et al. Clinical spectrum of CADASIL: A study of 7 families. Lancet 1995;346:934–9.
17. Dichgans M, Mayer M, Uttner I, et al. The phenotypic spectrum of CADASIL: Clinical findings in 102 cases. Ann Neurol 1998; 44:731–9.
18. Welch KM. Stroke and migraine–the spectrum of cause and effect. Funct Neurol 2003;18(3):121–6.
19. Tzourio C, Benslamia L, Guillon B, et al. Migraine and the risk of cervical artery dissection: A case-control study. Neurology 2002;59:435–7.
20. Metso TM, Tatlisumak T, Debette S, et al. Migraine in cervical artery dissection and ischemic stroke patients. Neurology 2012; 78:1221–8.
21. Rist PM, Diener HC, Kurth T, et al. Migraine, migraine aura, and cervical artery dissection: a systematic review and meta-analysis. Cephalalgia 2011;31:886–96.
22. Ramadan NM, Tietjen GE, Levine SR, et al. Scintillating scotoma associated with internal carotid artery dissection. Neurology 1991;41:1084–7.
23. Sibert PL, Mokri B, Schievink WI. Headache and neck pain in spontaneous internal carotid and vertebral artery dissections. Neurology 1995;45:1517–22.
24. Fisher CM. The headache and pain of spontaneous carotid dissection. Headache 1982;22:60.
25. Collaborative Group for the Study of Stroke in Young Women. Oral contraception and stroke in young women: Associated risk factors. JAMA 1975;231:718–22.
26. Henrich JB, Horwitz RI. A controlled study of ischemic stroke risk in migraine patients. J Clin Epidemiol 1989;42: 773–80.
27. Tzourio C, Iglesias S, Hubert JB, et al. Migraine and risk of ischaemic stroke: A case-control study. BMJ 1993;307:289–92.
28. Tzourio C, Tehindrazanarivelo A, Iglesias S, et al. Case-control study of migraine and risk of ischaemic stroke in young women. BMJ 1995;310:830–3.
29. Chang CL, Donaghy M, Poulter N; World Health Organisation Collaborative Study of Cardiovascular Disease and Steroid Hormone Contraception. Migraine and stroke in young women: Case-control study. BMJ 1999;318:13–18.
30. Marini C, Carolei A, Roberts R, et al. Focal cerebral ischemia in young adults: a collaborative case-control study. The National Research Council Study Group. Neuroepidemiology 1993;12: 70–81.
31. Lidegaard O. Oral contraceptivces, pregnancy and the risk of cerebral thromboembolism: the influence of diabetes, hypertension, migraine and previous thrombotic disease. Br J Obstet Gynaecol 1995;102:153–9.
32. Carolei A, Marini C, DeMatteis G. History of migraine and risk of cerebral ischaemia in young adults. Lancet 1996;347: 1503–6.
33. Haapaniemi H, Hillbom M, Juvela S. Lifestyle-associated risk factors for acute brain infarction among persons of working age. Stroke 1997;28:26–30.
34. Donaghy M, Chang CL, Poulter N, on behalf of the European Collaborators of The World Health Organisation Collaborative Study of Cardiovascular Disease and Steroid Hormone Contraception. Duration, frequency, recency, and type of migraine and the risk of ischaemic stroke in women of childbearing age. J Neurol Neurosurg Psychiatry 2002;73:747–50.
35. Schwaag S, Nabavi DG, Frese A, et al. The association between migraine and juvenile stroke: a case-control study. Headache 2003;43:90–5.
36. MacClellan LR, Giles W, Cole J, et al. Probable migraine with visual aura and risk of ischemic stroke: The stroke prevention in young women study. Stroke 2007;38:2438–45.
37. Kurth T, Slomke MA, Kase CS, et al. Migraine, headache, and the risk of stroke in women: a prospective study. Neurology 2005;64:1020–6.
38. Stang PE, Carson AP, Rose KM, et al. Headache, cerebrovascular symptoms, and stroke: The Atherosclerosis Risk in Communities Study. Neurology 2005;64:1573–7.
39. Buring JE, Hebert P, Romero J, et al. Migraine and subsequent risk of stroke in the Physicians' Health Study. Arch Neurol 1995;52:129–34.
40. Nightingale A, Farmer R. Ischemic stroke in young women: A nested case-control study using the UK General Practice Research Database. Stroke 2004;35:1574–8.
41. Hall G, Brown M, Mo J, et al. Triptans in migraine: The risks of stroke, cardiovascular disease, and death in practice. Neurology 2004;62:563–8.
42. Velentgas P, Cole JA, Mo J, et al. Severe vascular events in migraine patients. Headache 2004;44:642–51.
43. Merikangas KR, Fenton BT, Cheng SH, et al. Association between migraine and stroke in a large-scale epidemiological study of the United States. Arch Neurol 1997;54:362–8.
44. Kruit M, van Buchem M, Hofman P, et al. Migraine as a risk factor for subclinical brain lesions. JAMA 2004;291:427–34.

45. Sochurkova D, Moreau T, Lemesle M, et al. Migraine history and migraine-induced stroke in the Dijon stroke registry. Neuroepidemiology 1999;18:85–91.
46. Milhaud D, Bogousslavsky J, van Melle G, et al. Ischemic stroke and active migraine. Neurology 2001;57:1805–11.
47. Chang CL, Donaghy M, Poulter N. Migraine and stroke in young women: case-control study. The World Health Organisation Collaborative Study of Cardiovascular Disease and Steroid Hormone Contraception. BMJ 1999;318:13–18.
48. Kurth T, Kase CS, Schurks M, et al. Migraine and risk of haemorrhagic stroke in women: prospective cohort study. BMJ 2010; 341:c3659.
49. Sacco S, Ornello R, Ripa P, et al. Migraine and hemorrhagic stroke: a meta-analysis. Stroke 2013;44:3032–8.
50. Tzourio C, Tehindrazanarivelo A, Iglesias S, et al. Case-control study of migraine and risk of ischaemic stroke in young women. BMJ 1995;310:830–3.
51. Etminan M, Takkouche B, Isorna FC, et al. Risk of ischaemic stroke in people with migraine: Systematic review and meta-analysis of observational studies. BMJ 2005;330:63–5.
52. Bashir A, Lipton RB, Ashina S, et al. Migraine and structural changes in the brain: a systematic review and meta-analysis. Neurology 2013;81:1260–8.
53. Scher AI, Terwindt GM, Picavet HS, et al. Cardiovascular risk factors and migraine: the GEM population based study. Neurology 2005;64:614–20.
54. Kurth T, Schürks M, Logroscino G, et al. Migraine, vascular risk, and cardiovascular events in women: Prospective cohort study. BMJ 2008;337:a636.
55. Scher AI, Terwindt GM, Verschuren WM, et al. Migraine and MTHFR C677T genotype in a population-based sample. Ann Neurol 2006;59:372–5.
56. Schurks M, Zee RY, Buring JE, et al. Interrelationships among the MTHFR 677C>T polymorphism, migraine, and cardiovascular disease. Neurology 2008;71:505–13.
57. Pezzini A, Grassi M, Del Zotto E, et al. Migraine mediates the influence of C677T MTHFR genotypes on ischemic stroke risk with a stroke subtype effect. Stroke 2007;38:3145–51.
58. Cala LA, Mastaglia FL. Computerized axial tomography findings in patients with migrainous headaches. BMJ 1976;2:149–50.
59. Igarashi H, Sakai F, Kan S, et al. Magnetic resonance imaging of the brain in patients with migraine. Cephalalgia 1991;11:69–74.
60. Fazekas F, Koch M, Schmidt R, et al. The prevalence of cerebral damage varies with migraine type: A MRI study. Headache 1992;32:287–91.
61. De Benedittis G, Lorenzetti A, Sina C, et al. Magnetic resonance imaging in migraine and tension type headache. Headache 1995;35:264–8.
62. Kruit MC, Launer LJ, Ferrari MD, et al. Brain stem and cerebellar hyperintense lesions in migraine. Stroke 2006;37:1109–12.
63. Kurth T, Mohamed S, Maillard P, et al. Headache, migraine, and structural brain lesions and function: population based Epidemiology of Vascular Ageing-MRI study. BMJ 2011;342:c7357.
64. Weiller C, May A, Limmroth V, et al. Brain stem activation in spontaneous human migraine attacks. Nature Med 1995;1: 658–60.
65. Ray BS, Wolff HG. Experimental studies on headache: Pain-sensitive structures of the head and their significance in headache. Arch Surg 1940;41:813–56.
66. Fisher CM. Headache in cerebrovascular disease. In: Vinken PJ, Bruyn GW, editors. Handbook of clinical neurology. Amsterdam: Elsevier; 1968. p. 124–6.
67. Mitsias P, Ramadan NM. Headache in ischemic cerebrovascular disease. Part I: clinical features. Cephalalgia 1992;12:269–74.
68. Brohult J, Forsberg O, Hellstrom R. Multiple arterial thrombosis after oral contraceptives and ergotamine. Acta Med Scand 1967; 181:453.
69. Merkhoff GC, Poter JM. Ergot intoxication: Historical review and description. Ann Surg 1974;180:773.
70. Senter HJ, Liebermann AN. Cerebral manifestations of ergotism. Report of a case and review of the literature. Stroke 1976; 7:88–92.
71. Wammes-van der Heijden EA, Rahimtoola H, Leufkens HG, et al. Risk of ischemic complications related to the intensity of triptan and ergotamine use. Neurology 2006;67:1128–34.
72. Fox AW. Comparative tolerability of oral 5-HT 1B/1D agonists. Headache 2000;40:521–7.
73. Cavazos JE, Carees JB, Chilukuri VR. Sumatriptan-induced stroke in sagittal sinus thrombosis. Lancet 1994;343:1105–6.
74. Vijayan N, Peacock JH. Spinal cord infarction during use of zolmitriptan: A case report. Headache 2000;40:57–60.
75. Shuaib A, Hachinski C. Migraine and the risks from angiography. Arch Neurol 1988;45:911–12.
76. Whitty CWM. Migraine without headache. Lancet 1967; 2(7510):283.
77. Fisher CM. Migraine accompaniments versus arteriosclerotic ischemia. Trans Am Neuol Assoc 1968;93:211.
78. Wijman CA, Wolf PA, Kase CS, et al. Migrainous visual accompaniments are not rare in late life: The Framingham Study. Stroke 1998;29:1539–43.
79. Caplan L. Intracerebral hemorrhage revisited. Neurology 1988;38:624.
80. Corbett JJ. Neuro-ophthalmic complications of migraine and cluster headaches. Neurol Clin 1983;1:973–95.
81. Liveing E. On megrim, sick-headache, and some allied disorders: a contribution to the pathology of nerve-storms. London: J & A Churchill; 1873.
82. Whittey CWM. Familial hemiplegic migraine. J Neurol Neurosurg Psychiatry 1953;16:172.
83. Ducros A, Denier C, Joutel A, et al. The clinical spectrum of familial hemiplegic migraine associated with mutations in a neuronal calcium channel. N Engl J Med 2001;345:17–24.
84. Elliott MA, Peroutka SJ, Welch S, et al. Familial hemiplegic migraine, nystagmus, and cerebellar atrophy. Ann Neurol 1996; 39:100–6.
85. Vahedi K, Denier C, Ducros A, et al. CACNA1A gene de novo mutation causing hemiplegic migraine, coma and cerebellar atrophy. Neurology 2000;55:1040–2.
86. Hutchinson M, Oriordan J, Javed M, et al. Familial hemiplegic migraine and autosomal dominant arteriopathy with leukoencephalopathy (CADASIL). Ann Neurol 1995;38:817–24.
87. Chabriat H, Vahedi K, Iba-Zizen MT, et al. Clinical spectrum of CADASIL: A study of 7 families. Lancet 1995;346:934–9.
88. Chabriat H, Tournier-Lasserve E, Vahedi K, et al. Autosomal dominant migraine with MRI white-matter abnormalities mapping to the CADASIL locus. Neurology 1995;45:1086–91.
89. Joutel A, Corpechet C, Ducros A, et al. Notch3 mutations in CADASIL, a hereditary adult-onset condition causing stroke and dementia. Nature 1996;383:707–10.
90. Joutel A, Corpechot C, Vayssière C, et al. Characterization of Notch3 mutations in CADASIL patients. Neurology 1997; 48:1729–30.
91. Ophoff RA, Terwindt GM, Vergouwe MN, et al. Familial hemiplegic migraine and episodic ataxia type-2 are caused by mutations in the Ca^{2+} channel gene CACNLA4. Cell 1996;87:543–52.
92. Joutel A, Bousser M, Biousese V, et al. A gene for familial hemiplegic migraine maps to chromosome 19. Nat Genet 1993;5: 40–5.
93. Dichgans M, Freilinger T, Eckstein G, et al. Mutation in the neuronal voltage-gated sodium channel SCN1A in familial hemiplegic migraine. Lancet 2005;366:371–7.
94. Terwindt GM, Ophoff RA, Haan J, et al. Variable clinical expression of mutations in the P/Q-type calcium channel gene in familial hemiplegic migraine. Neurology 1998;50:1105–10.
95. Terwindt GM, Ophoff RA, Haan J, et al. Familial hemiplegic migraine: a clinical comparison of families linked and unlinked to chromosome 19. Cephalalgia 1996;16:153–5.
96. Carrera P, Piatti M, Stenirri S, et al. Genetic heterogeneity in Italian families with familial hemiplegic migraine. Neurology 1999;53:26–32.
97. Battistini S, Stenirri S, Piatti M, et al. A new CACNA1A gene mutation in acetazolamide-responsive familial hemiplegic migraine and ataxia. Neurology 1999;53:38–43.
98. Kors EE, Terwindt GM, Vermeulen FLMG, et al. Delayed cerebral edema and fatal coma after minor head trauma: role of CACNA1A calcium channel subunit gene and relationship with familial hemiplegic migraine. Ann Neurol 2001;49:753–60.
99. Bickerstaff ER. The basilar artery and migraine epilepsy syndrome. Proc R Soc Med 1962;55:167.
100. Bickerstaff ER. Basilar artery migraine. Lancet 1961;1(7211):15.
101. Lapkin ML, French JH, Golden GS. The EEG in childhood basilar artery migraine. Neurology 1977;27:580.
102. Sturzenegger MH, Meienberg O. Basilar artery migraine: a follow-up study of 82 cases. Headache 1985;25:408.

103. Lee CH, Lance JW. Migraine stupor. Headache 1977;17:32.
104. Connor RCR. Complicated migraine. A study of permanent neurological and visual defects caused by migraine. Lancet 1962; 2(7265):1072–5.
105. Skinhoj E, Paulson OB. Regional cerebral blood flow in the internal carotid artery distribution during migraine. BMJ 1969; 3:569–70.
106. Del Sette M, Angeli S, Leandri M, et al. Migraine with aura and right-to-left shunt on transcranial Doppler: a case-control study. Cerebrovasc Dis 1998;8:327–30.
107. Anzola GP, Magoni M, Guindani M, et al. Potential source of cerebral embolism in migraine with aura: a transcranial Doppler study. Neurology 1999;52:1622–5.
108. Schwerzmann M, Nedeltchev K, Lagger F, et al. Prevalence and size of directly detected patent foramen ovale in migraine with aura. Neurology 2005;65:1415–18.
109. Carod-Artal FJ, da Silveira Ribeiro L, Braga H, et al. Prevalence of patent foramen ovale in migraine patients with and without aura compared with stroke patients. A transcranial Doppler study. Cephalalgia 2006;26:934–9.
110. Davis D, Gregson J, Willeit P, et al. Patent foramen ovale, ischemic stroke and migraine: systematic review and stratified meta-analysis of association studies. Neuroepidemiology 2013; 40:56–67.
111. Wilmshurst PT, Pearson MJ, Nightingale S, et al. Inheritance of persistent foramen ovale and atrial septal defects and the relationship to familial migraine with aura. Heart 2004;90:1245–7.
112. Lampl C, Bonelli S, Ransmayr G. Efficacy of topiramate in migraine aura prophylaxis: preliminary results of 12 patients. Headache 2004;44:174–7.
113. Lampl C, Katsarava Z, Diener HC, et al. Lamotrigine reduces migraine aura and migraine attacks in patients with migraine with aura. J Neurol Neurosurg Psychiatry 2005;76:1730–2.
114. Dowson A, Mullen MJ, Peatfield R, et al. Migraine Intervention with STARFlex Technology (MIST) trial: a prospective, multicenter, double-blind, sham-controlled trial to evaluate the effectiveness of patent foramen ovale closure with STARFlex septal repair implant to resolve refractory migraine headache. Circulation 2008;117:1397–404.
115. Schwerzmann M, Wiher S, Nedeltchev K, et al. Percutaneous closure of patent foramen ovale reduces the frequency of migraine attacks. Neurology 2004;62:1399–401.
116. Post M, Thijs V, Herroelen L, et al. Closure of a patent foramen ovale is associated with a decrease in prevalence of migraine. Neurology 2004;62:1439–40.
117. Wilmshurst PT, Nightingale S, Walsh KP, et al. Effect on migraine of closure of cardiac right-to-left shunts to prevent recurrence of decompression illness or stroke or for haemodynamic reasons. Lancet 2000;356(9242):1648–51.
118. Mortelmans K, Post M, Thijs V, et al. The influence of percutaneous atrial septal defect closure on the occurrence of migraine. Eur Heart J 2005;26:1533–7.
119. Reisman M, Christofferson RD, Jesurum J, et al. Migraine headache relief after transcatheter closure of patent foramen ovale. J Am Coll Cardiol 2005;45:493–5.
120. Azarbal B, Tobis J, Suh W, et al. Association of interatrial shunts and migraine headaches: impact of transcatheter closure. J Am Coll Cardiol 2005;45:489–92.
121. Anzola GP, Frisoni GB, Morandi E, et al. Shunt-associated migraine responds favorably to atrial septal repair: a case-control study. Stroke 2006;37:430–4.
122. Buring JE, Peto R, Hennekens CH, et al. Low-dose aspirin for migraine prophylaxis. JAMA 1990;264:1711–13.
123. Diener HC, Hartung E, Chrubasik J, et al. A comparative study of acetylsalicyclic acid and metoprolol for the prophylactic treatment of migraine. A randomised, controlled, double-blind, parallel group phase III study. Cephalalgia 2001;21:140–4.
124. Wilmshurst PT, Nightingale S, Walsh KP, et al. Clopidogrel reduces migraine with aura after transcatheter closure of persistent foramen ovale and atrial septal defects. Heart 2005;91: 1173–5.
125. Sharifi M, Burks J. Efficacy of clopidogrel in the treatment of post-ASD closure migraines. Catheter Cardiovasc Interv 2004; 63:255.
126. Antiplatelet Trialists Collaboration. Collaborative overview of randomised trials of antiplatelet therapy. I: Prevention of death, myocardial infarction, and stroke by prolonged antiplatelet therapy in various categories of patients. BMJ 1994;308:81–106.
127. Bensenor IM, Cook NR, Lee I-M, et al. Low-dose aspirin for migraine prophylaxis in women. Cephalalgia 2001;21:175–83.
128. CAPRIE Steering Committee. A randomised, blinded, trial of clopidogrel versus aspirin in patients at risk of ischaemic events (CAPRIE). Lancet 1996;348:1329–39.
129. Diener HC, Cuhna L, Forbes C, et al. European Stroke Prevention Study 2: Dipyridamole and acetylsalicylic acid in the secondary prevention of stroke. J Neurol Sci 1996;143:1–13.
130. Chang YJ, Ryu SJ, Lee TH. Dose titration to reduce dipyridamole-related headache. Cerebrovasc Dis 2006;22:258–62.
131. Silberstein SD, for the US Headache Consortium. Practice parameter: evidence-based guidelines for migraine headache (an evidence-based review). Report of the Quality Standards Subcommitee of the American Academy of Neurology. Neurology 2000;55:754–63.
132. Schrader H, Stovner LJ, Helde G. Prophylactic treatment of migraine with angiotensin converting enzyme inhibitor (lisinopril): randomised, placebo-controlled, crossover trial. BMJ 2001; 322:19–22.
133. Stovner LJ, Linde M, Gravdahl GB, et al. A comparative study of candesartan versus propranolol for migraine prophylaxis: A randomised, triple-blind, placebo-controlled, double cross-over study. Cephalalgia 2013;34:523–32.
134. Bousser M-G. Migraine, female hormones, and stroke. Cephalalgia 1999;19:75–9.
135. MacGregor A. Gynaecological aspects of migraine. Rev Contemp Pharmacother 2000;11:75–90.
136. Jansen I, Edvinson L, Mortensens A, et al. Sumatriptan is a potent vasoconstrictor in human dural arteries via a 5-HT1-like receptor. Cephalalgia 1992;12:202–5.
137. Longmore J, Hargreaves RJ, Boulanger CM, et al. Comparison ot the vasoconstrictor properties of the 5-HT1D-receptor agonists rizatriptan (MK-462) and sumatriptan in human isolated coronary artery: outcome of two independent studies using different experimental protocols. Funct Neurol 1997;12:3–9.
138. Saxena PR, den Boer MO, Ferrari MD. The pharmacology of antimigrainous drugs. Clin Neuropharm 1992;15:375A–376A.
139. Olesen J, Diener H, Husstedt IW, et al. Calcitonin gene-related peptide (CGRP) receptor antagonist BIBN4096BS is effective in the treatment of migraine attacks. N Engl J Med 2004;350: 1104–10.
140. Saxena VK, De Deyn PP. Ergotamine: its use in the treatment of migraine and its complications. Acta Neurol (Napoli) 1992; 14:140–6.
141. Diener HC, for the ASASUMAMIG Study Group. Efficacy and safety of intravenous acetylsalicylic acid lysinate compared to subcutaneous sumatriptan and parenteral placebo in the acute treatment of migraine. A double-blind, double-dummy, randomized, multicenter, parallel group study. Cephalalgia 1999; 19:581–8.
142. Hansson L, Zanchetti A, Carruthers SG, et al. Effects of intensive blood-pressure lowering and low-dose aspirin in patients with hypertension: principal results of the Hypertension Optimal Treatment (HOT) randomised trial. Lancet 1998;351:1755–62.
143. Diener HC, Peters C, Rudizo M. Ergotamine, flunarizine and sumatriptan do not change cerebral blood flow velocity in normal subjects and migraineurs. J Neurol 1991;238:245–50.
144. Mathew NT, Rapoport A, Saper J, et al. Efficacy of gabapentin in migraine prophylaxis. Headache 2001;41:119–28.
145. Klapper J, on behalf of the Divalproex Sodium in Migraine Prophylaxis Study Group. Divalproex sodium in migraine prophylaxis: a dose-controlled study. Cephalalgia 1997;17: 103–8.
146. Silberstein SD. Methysergide. Cephalalgia 1998;18:421–35.
147. Sacco RL, Gan R, Boden-Albala B, et al. Leisure-time physical activity and ischemic stroke risk - The Northern Manhattan Stroke Study. Stroke 1998;29:380–7.
148. Wannamethee G, Shaper AG. Physical activity and stroke in British middle aged men. BMJ 1992;304:597–601.
149. Vasudev K, Keown P, Gibb I, et al. Hematological effects of valproate in psychiatric patients: what are the risk factors? J Clin Psychopharmacol 2010;30:282–5.

44 Cryptogenic Stroke

Martin O'Donnell, Scott E. Kasner

KEY POINTS

- In a proportion of patients, a defined etiology of ischemic stroke is not identified. These patients are categorized as cryptogenic (unknown cause) ischemic stroke.
- The estimated proportion of ischemic strokes that are cryptogenic varies from 15% to 35%, reflecting the lack of a standardized definition for cryptogenic ischemic stroke, inconsistency of the extent and quality of etiological diagnostic testing, variable type of populations included (e.g., younger versus older), and differences in the attribution of causality to some common findings. The proportion of patients categorized as cryptogenic ischemic stroke also varies by etiological classification scheme.
- Cryptogenic ischemic stroke may comprise three groups: under-classified, under-measured, and truly cryptogenic strokes. Under-classified represents populations where an etiology is present (e.g., carotid disease), but does not fulfill strict criteria for diagnosis (<50%). Under-measured represents a population where diagnostic evaluation is incomplete, especially in those with a high probability of large-vessel disease or atrial fibrillation. True cryptogenic ischemic stroke is defined by a thorough but normal diagnostic evaluation.
- The natural history of recurrent major vascular events in patients with cryptogenic ischemic stroke is strongly associated with population characteristics. In older populations, the risk of recurrent stroke is high, while in younger populations with truly cryptogenic stroke, the risk of recurrent stroke is low.
- Most cryptogenic ischemic strokes have an embolic topology and may be better described as "embolic stroke of undetermined source" (ESUS). The rationale for this new classification is to define a patient population for clinical trials.

Determining the etiology of ischemic stroke is a cornerstone of early evaluation, as it allows tailoring of management strategies to optimally reduce the risk of recurrent stroke in some patients, and provides prognostic information.[1,2] However, in a proportion of patients, the etiology of ischemic stroke is not identified[3] and these are termed cryptogenic or unexplained stroke. The proportion of patients with cryptogenic ischemic stroke depends on the extent and quality of diagnostic evaluation, the age and ethnicity of the population, and which findings are considered etiological (or causal) on diagnostic testing.[4] From a pragmatic management perspective, implications of many common potential etiological findings are uncertain, as evidence-based recommendations for stroke prevention are either generically applied to all ischemic strokes or additionally tailored for selected findings, particularly carotid artery stenosis and atrial fibrillation/flutter.[5] In many cases, patients with cryptogenic stroke have topographical findings that suggest an embolic source of stroke (Fig. 44-1), and/or clinical characteristics that suggest a cardioembolic etiology, but without objective documentation of an established source.[6]

DEFINITIONS

Definition of Cryptogenic Ischemic Stroke

There is no formal consensus definition for cryptogenic stroke, and definitions have varied by the particular scheme used to classify ischemic stroke cause or mechanism (see section on classification schemes below). There is no gold standard for diagnostic criteria.[4] There is, of course, no animal model of cryptogenic stroke pathophysiology, since it is fundamentally unknown. One widely used classification system, designed for the Trial of ORG-10172 for Acute Stroke Treatment (TOAST) trial, defined undetermined stroke as "brain infarction that is not attributable to a source of definite cardioembolism, large artery atherosclerosis, or small artery disease, despite extensive vascular, cardiac and serological evaluation."[7] As such, the definition is framed in negative terms, based on the absence of findings. An alternative proposed definition, based on infarct topography is: "non-lacunar ischemic stroke of unknown etiology but suggestive of embolism despite an exhaustive search for etiologic cause,"[4] the inference being that all non-lacunar ischemic strokes are due to embolism. Based on these considerations, a recent proposal extends the use of infarct topography to categorize such patients as, "embolic stroke of undetermined source" (ESUS).[6] The main rationale for such an approach has been to define this group of patients in a positive manner, to enable a clearer definition for the conduct of randomized controlled trials, with, by extension, implications for clinical practice. Developing a consensus definition for cryptogenic ischemic stroke requires agreement on what is considered to be an extensive or adequate diagnostic evaluation and which findings are considered etiological.

Classification Schemes for Ischemic Stroke Etiological Subtypes

There are a number of classification schemes, which seek to provide an objective and reliable framework for describing ischemic stroke etiology. In general terms, classification schemes include the domains of small-vessel disease, large-vessel atherosclerotic disease, cardiac causes of thromboembolism, unusual causes of stroke, and cryptogenic (also termed unknown, undetermined, or unexplained).[7] The category of cryptogenic stroke often includes multiple groups, including those with unexplained stroke in the setting of extensive testing, stroke due to incomplete or inadequate diagnostic evaluation, and mixed or competing etiologies (e.g., concurrent carotid stenosis and atrial fibrillation). These subgroups within cryptogenic stroke are likely quite different in terms of the risks of future stroke and true underlying pathophysiology.

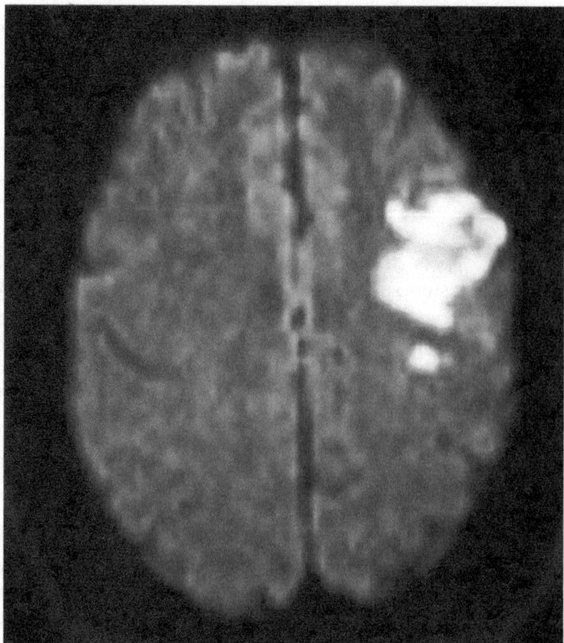

Figure 44-1. Diffusion-weighted MRI showing acute left cortical infarction suggestive of an embolic origin.

The three most prominent classification schemes are summarized below. While overall inter-rater agreement between these classification schemes is good-to-excellent, the proportion of patients classified as "undetermined" varies between schemes, ranging from 26% to 42% in one direct comparison.[8] Each scheme utilizes information on clinical presentation, topographical features on neuroimaging, findings on imaging of large vessels, cardiac rhythm monitoring and imaging of the heart, and results of some serological studies. However, there are differences in use of this information to assign subtypes:

1. *Trial of ORG-10172 in Acute Stroke Treatment (TOAST)* subtype classification system is the most widely used and has been incorporated into routine clinical practice, following initial development for clinical research purposes.[7] The TOAST criteria categorize ischemic stroke into small-vessel occlusion, large-vessel atherosclerosis, cardioembolism, stroke of other determined etiology, and stroke of undetermined etiology. The definition of 'undetermined' etiology includes three circumstances: the diagnostic evaluation is incomplete, no cause is found despite an extensive evaluation, or most likely cause cannot be determined because there is more than one plausible etiology found. Using the TOAST criteria, the inter-rater reliability of diagnosing stroke of undetermined etiology (i.e., cryptogenic stroke) is poor, which presents clinical and research challenges.
2. *The Causative Classification Scheme* (CCS) is a computerized algorithm that provides causative and phenotypic stroke subtypes, categorized as evident, probable, or possible supra-aortic large-vessel disease, cardioaortic embolism, small-vessel occlusion, other uncommon causes, or undetermined. Within the category of undetermined stroke, there is a further subtyping into unknown-cryptogenic embolism, unknown-other cryptogenic, unclassified, and incomplete evaluation.[9] Of the three schemes discussed in this chapter, CCS appears to provide the lowest proportion classified as undetermined (26% versus 39% for TOAST in the North Dublin Stroke Study, n = 381).[8] Inter-rater reliability for this scheme is very good to excellent, because a low proportion of patients are labeled as unclassified, likely due to the use of a heavily probabilistic approach that more commonly assigns an alternative etiology than other classification schemes.
3. *Atherosclerosis, Small-vessel disease, Cardiac causes, Other, and Dissection (ASCOD):* The ASCOD scheme categorizes patients with ischemic stroke into A: atherosclerosis, S: small-vessel disease, C: cardiac source, O: other cause, and D: dissection. The "other" category includes those disorders or findings that are uncommon, and is further subcategorized based on whether the finding is potentially causal, the causal link is uncertain, or the causal link is unlikely but an abnormality is present.[10] The "other" category also includes patients for whom no cause is detected based on best available diagnostic tests and stroke-specific history. There is no specific category for undetermined or cryptogenic stroke, as these are included in the "other" category.

Probabilistic Approach to Etiological Diagnosis

Common to all etiological classification schemes, either stated or implied, is an assessment of probability that a finding is the putative cause of the stroke, through both direct and indirect inferences. First, identification of stroke etiology is usually based on identifying a probable source of thrombosis, rather than direct visualization of thrombus. For example, the presence of atrial fibrillation supports the diagnosis of cardioembolism, but thrombus in the left atrium or its appendage is only observed in a minority of patients.[11] Second, the actual etiological source may not be measured directly. For example, the diagnosis of small-vessel disease is not based on imaging small vessels but based on the assumption that small deep infarcts (<1.5 cm), especially in locations rich in perforator vessels, are probably due to occlusion of small vessels from processes that are inherent to the small vessel. Third, etiologies commonly co-exist, requiring subjective judgment about which is most likely causal. Finally, some classification schemes assign a probability within etiological subcategories, such as the CCS and ASCOD, because potential etiological findings have differing levels of evidence to support a causal role.

EPIDEMIOLOGY AND DIAGNOSIS

Prevalence of Cryptogenic Stroke

The prevalence of cryptogenic ischemic stroke varies among studies, but estimates range from 15% to 35% of consecutive patients (Table 44-1).[6] Between-study comparisons are challenging, and often unreliable because of differences in etiologic classification scheme used, extent and quality of etiological diagnostic testing completed, type of populations included (e.g., younger versus older), and variations in attributing causality to some common findings (e.g., patent foramen ovale). Accordingly, valid inferences from between-study comparisons of temporal trends and regional variations in cryptogenic stroke are often not possible. Similarly, incidence cannot be reliably estimated from combining existing data.

Factors Influencing Prevalence of Cryptogenic Stroke

Population Characteristics

Age of the cohort is an important determinant of the proportion of patients categorized as cryptogenic ischemic stroke. The proportion of patients with cryptogenic stroke is greater in younger cohorts. This is expected since increasing age is an independent risk factor for development of the better characterized stroke etiologies such as small-vessel disease,

TABLE 44-1 Frequency of Cryptogenic Ischemic Stroke Varies According to Study Design, Age, and Diagnostic Criteria for Cryptogenic Stroke

Reference	Study Design	Sample Size	Mean Age (years)	Criteria for Cryptogenic Stroke	Frequency of Cryptogenic Stroke
Besancon Stroke Registry (2000)[63]	Prospective registry	1776	71	Study-specific	18%
Athens Stroke Registry (2000)[64]	Prospective registry of first-ever strokes	885	70	Not specified	21%
German Stroke Data Bank (2001)[65]	Prospective registry	5017	66	Modified TOAST criteria	23%
WARSS (2001)[66]	Randomized trial	2206	63	TOAST criteria	26%
Erlangen Study (2001)[67]	Population-based	583	73	TOAST criteria	32%
Ankara (2002)[68]	Prospective registry	264	66	TOAST criteria	33%
Suwon (2003)[69]	Prospective registry	204	62	TOAST criteria	18%
TULIPS (Japan) (2004)[70]	Prospective registry	831	72	NINDS SDB	23%
Perugia (2006)[71]	Prospective stroke unit	358	NR	TOAST criteria	17%
PRoFESS (2008)[72]	Randomized trial	20,332	66	TOAST criteria	16%
Bern (2008)[73]	Prospective registry	1288	NR	TOAST criteria	39%
Buenos Aires (2010)[74]	Retrospective case series	155	67	TOAST criteria	27%
ASTRAL (2010)[75]	Prospective inpatient registry	1633	73	Modified TOAST criteria	12%
North Dublin (2010)[8]	Population-based registry	381	NR	Causative Classification System	26%
VITATOPS (2010)[76]	Randomized trial	8164	63	Study-specific	14%
PERFORM (2011)[77]	Randomized trial	19,100	67	Study-specific	22%
Mannheim Stroke Center (2012)[78]	Prospective case series	103	69	TOAST criteria	30%
Hebi, China (2012)[79]	Retrospective case series	425	65	TOAST criteria	16%
South Korea (2012)[80]	Prospective hospital-based registry	3278	64	TOAST criteria	21%
Miami/Mexico City (2012)[81]	Prospective registry of Hispanics	671	NR	Modified TOAST criteria	17%
Santiago, Chile (2012)[82]	Prospective stroke unit	380	66	TOAST criteria	20%
Barcelona (2012)[83]	Prospective stroke unit	274	NR	TOAST criteria	32%
Santiago de Compostela (2013)[84]	Prospective case series	1050	NR	TOAST criteria	35%
Bavaria (2013)[85]	Prospective stroke unit	393	62	TOAST criteria	17%

Adapted from Hart RG, Diener H-C, Coutts SB, Easton JD, Granger CB, O'Donnell MJ, Sacco RL, Connolly SJ, for the Cryptogenic Stroke/ESUS International Working Group, with permission.

NR = not reported. TIA = transient ischemic attack. NINDS SDB = National Institute of Neurological Disorders and Stroke Data Bank.

large-vessel atherosclerosis, and atrial fibrillation. Sex has not been identified as an important determinant of cryptogenic stroke prevalence. However, race and ethnicity may be a factor, as a few large epidemiologic studies found that cryptogenic stroke was more common in black and Hispanic stroke patients, and this finding did not appear to be due to differences in use of diagnostic testing among racial groups.[12,13,14] Typical vascular risk factors are associated with identifiable stroke etiologies, and cohorts with greater burdens of such factors, particularly hypertension, tend to have lower proportions of cryptogenic stroke in some studies.[13,15] However, patients with cryptogenic stroke may have an increased prevalence of hypertension compared with stroke-free controls.[16]

Diagnostic Testing

By definition, the prevalence of cryptogenic ischemic stroke depends on the proportion of patients who do not fulfill diagnostic criteria for large, small vessel, cardioembolic and other causes of stroke. Of these, large-vessel disease is most amenable to reliable objective testing, using standardized criteria to detect stenosis >50%. However, the extent and modality of large-vessel imaging will influence the proportion of patients diagnosed with large-vessel disease, and in turn, impact on the proportion labeled cryptogenic. In particular, imaging of both extracranial and intracranial vessels is required to exclude large-vessel disease. This is especially important in populations reported to have a higher prevalence of intracranial stenosis, such as Asians.[17] Modality of vascular imaging is also important, since ultrasound methods have lower sensitivity and positive predictive values than angiographic modalities (MR, CT, or catheter-based angiography),[18,19] and the use of the latter will result in a higher proportion of patients diagnosed with large-vessel disease. The diagnosis of small-vessel disease will depend on modality of neuroimaging, experience and skill-set of the clinician in determining a lacunar clinical syndrome, and extent of diagnostic testing to exclude other causes. MRI, compared to CT, will increase the yield of small infarcts identified, but will also identify patients with multi-territory small infarction suggestive of an embolic mechanism in about 10–15% of patients.[20] Arguably, the etiological subtype most dependent on extent of diagnostic work-up is

TABLE 44-2 Potential Etiological Findings on Cardiac Diagnostic Work-Up (Based on Anticipated Probability of Management Implication)

Cardiac Finding	Risk of Causing Stroke
Atrial fibrillation	Major
Prosthetic mechanical valve	
Intracardiac thrombus	
Atrial myxoma	
Bacterial endocarditis	
Aortic arch atherosclerosis	Moderate
Severe left ventricular dysfunction	
Bioprosthetic valve	
Mitral stenosis	
Spontaneous echocardiographic contrast	
Patent foramen ovale*	Minor/Uncertain
Atrial septal aneurysm	
Mitral valve prolapse	
Mitral annular calcification	
Aortic valve stenosis	
Calcific aortic valve	
Valve strands	

*Suspicion of causality is contextual, and may depend on size and morphology of PFO, age of patients and presence or absence of venous thrombosis.

cardioembolism. A single electrocardiogram (ECG) is less likely to detect atrial fibrillation or flutter than 24 hours of cardiac telemetry.[21] Similarly, more prolonged monitoring of cardiac rhythm will further increase the yield of detection (discussed in detail below). Use of transthoracic echocardiography, or with greater sensitivity, transesophageal echocardiography, will detect a structural cardiac abnormality that may be a potential stroke etiology in about 40% of patients who are considered cryptogenic stroke.[22-29] These findings include aortic arch disease, left ventricular dysfunction, patent foramen ovale, atrial septal aneurysm, spontaneous echocardiographic contrast in the left atrium, among others, but the clinical relevance of each of these findings then needs to be determined as these findings have varying risks of recurrent stroke (see Table 44-2 and Chapter 32 on cardiac diseases).

Association vs Causation

A causal relationship for ischemic stroke has been firmly established for some etiological findings, such as carotid artery stenosis, where prospective studies have consistently reported a significant graded increase in stroke risk with increasing stenosis, and removal of stenosis reduces the risk of recurrent stroke dramatically. However, for other findings, evidence to support a causal relationship is considerably weaker, and is especially an issue when those findings are common. Inclusion of a common risk factor as causal will have a considerable impact on the proportion of patients labeled as cryptogenic. For example, patent foramen ovale occurs in about 25% of the general population, and has been reported to be a risk factor for ischemic stroke, especially in young populations with otherwise unexplained stroke, since PFO has been identified in about 40% of such patients. However, evidence demonstrating it to be a risk factor for recurrent stroke is weak,[30] and closure does not significantly reduce the risk of recurrent stroke (see Chapter 32 for further details). PFO may, therefore, be inconsequential in many stroke patients. Moreover, the size, shape, and shunt proclivity of the PFO may influence whether it is causal, although that also is currently uncertain. Therefore, within a potential etiology such as PFO, there is also a range of findings that impact causal inference. Similarly, additional information, for example documenting deep venous thrombosis, may also influence the clinical impression of whether a PFO is likely to be causally related to stroke.

Proposed Etiologies of Cryptogenic Stroke

As detailed, the category of cryptogenic stroke represents a spectrum of patients who have differing probabilities of underlying causes of ischemic stroke. In many cases, patients have clinical presentations, co-morbidities, and findings on diagnostic testing that support one likely etiology, without fulfilling definitive criteria necessary to formally classify stroke subtype. Ten common risk factors, including hypertension, smoking, hypercholesterolemia, obesity and diabetes, are associated with 90% of the population-attributable risk for stroke[31] and share in the pathophysiology of small vessel, large vessel and cardiac causes of stroke; the key reason for the common co-occurrence of stroke etiologies. Although not considered in etiological classification schemes, such information is routinely engaged in clinical practice. In contrast, many young patients with ischemic stroke have no traditional risk factors for stroke and have an entirely normal etiological diagnostic work-up, resulting in a truly unexplained cause of ischemic stroke. Therefore, within ischemic stroke, there lies a continuum of etiological uncertainty.

We propose the following conceptual framework for understanding the likely mechanisms underlying cryptogenic ischemic stroke, which may be considered in the following headings, under-classified, under-measured, and truly cryptogenic. Exemplary cases of these are described in Table 44-3.

Under-Classified Cryptogenic Stroke. This is stroke that is likely due to an established mechanism but does not fulfill the formal criteria required to include in an etiological category. Such under-classification is most common when the standard definition is based on dichotomization of a continuous parameter. For example, in large-vessel atherosclerotic disease, a stenosis of at least 50% is required to fulfill diagnostic criteria. However, ischemic stroke may result from plaque rupture and other vessel wall characteristics independent of the severity of stenosis. It is likely that there is a continuum of risk over the full range of stenosis.[32,33] In coronary heart disease, for example, there is a lower than expected correlation between degree of stenosis of coronary vessel and future site of myocardial infarction.[34] In large part, the selection of the 50% threshold is because this is the degree of stenosis when the benefits of carotid endarterectomy outweigh the risks in symptomatic patients, not because the risk of stroke abruptly increases when a stenosis reaches the 50% threshold.[35] Moreover, most assessments of stenosis in clinical practice are based on non-invasive testing, not angiography, and measurements are not likely as carefully measured or as precise as in clinical trials. Similarly, the most widely used definition for diagnosing aortic arch disease is atheroma >4 mm,[36] although the association between atheroma thickness and risk of stroke is again more likely continuous than threshold, and there is between-study variation in definition of thickness required to diagnose aortic arch disease. For small deep infarcts, a small-vessel occlusive etiology can only be formally invoked when the infarct is ≤1.5 cm in maximal diameter. As with the above examples, measurement error and individual variability likely render this threshold arbitrary and overly restrictive. Even atrial fibrillation, which could be dichotomously defined as present or absent, is subject to these threshold effects. The duration of atrial fibrillation is likely important,[37] though this is controversial. Some only consider durations of >30 minutes to be considered significant, others select 2 or 6 minutes, while others consider any evidence of atrial fibrillation in patients with other clinical features

TABLE 44-3 Examples of Cryptogenic Stroke Populations

UNDER-CLASSIFIED CRYPTOGENIC STROKE

Case

72-year-old man with prior history of myocardial infarction and peripheral vascular disease is admitted with left hemiparesis and hemineglect. CT of brain reveals right hemispheric cortical-based infarction (4 cm max diameter). CT angiography of carotids reports 40% stenosis bilaterally. Cardiac monitoring and transthoracic echocardiogram are normal. Transesophageal echocardiogram reveals mild atherosclerosis of aortic arch (<4 mm)

Interpretation

Although findings on large-vessel imaging do not comply with definition of large-vessel disease, this patient has multi-bed atherosclerosis, with evidence of large-vessel disease in other vascular beds. Novel approaches to imaging acute thrombosis or unstable plaque in large vessels may clarify these types of cases in the future. Alternative etiologies (e.g., paroxysmal atrial fibrillation) that may co-exist in patients with atherosclerosis should also be considered

UNDER-MEASURED CRYPTOGENIC

Case

62-year-old woman with prior history of hypertension and obesity is admitted with right hemiparesis and global aphasia. CT of brain reveals left hemispheric cortical-based infarction. CT angiography of intra- and extra-cranial vessels is normal. In-hospital cardiac monitoring is normal. Transthoracic echocardiography reveals moderate left ventricular hypertrophy and increased left atrial size. Patient is discharged home, and re-admitted to hospital 3 months later with severe palpitations, and diagnosed with atrial fibrillation, and switched from antiplatelet therapy to oral anticoagulant therapy

Interpretation

Initial presentation supports an embolic etiology, with normal large vessels. Patient has risk factors for atrial fibrillation, namely hypertension and obesity, as well as an enlarged left atrium, which is expected to increase the probability of atrial fibrillation. At the time of initial presentation, patient may be considered embolic stroke of uncertain source (ESUS).[6] The patient transpires to have paroxysmal atrial fibrillation, which was in retrospect the likely cause of her initial stroke

TRUE CRYPTOGENIC STROKE

Case

38-year-old woman with no prior medical history presents with right visual field loss. MRI reveals acute infarction in left occipital cortex and is otherwise normal. She has no traditional risk factors for ischemic stroke, no medical co-morbidities, and no clinical features suggestive of a systemic illness (infection, cancer, chronic inflammation, etc.). There is no family history of premature stroke. Transthoracic and transesophageal echocardiograms are normal. Five-day Holter monitor is normal. CT angio of extracranial and intracranial vessels is normal. MRV: normal. Thrombophilic screen is negative

Interpretation

Initial presentation supports an embolic etiology, and after an extensive work-up, no cause is identified. In these cases, the risk of recurrent stroke is low. Blood pressure and lipids are normal, the role of antihypertensive agents and statins is not known. In general, we recommend chronic antiplatelet therapy for secondary prevention, and adherence with guideline targets for other modifiable risk factors

suggestive of embolic stroke as clinically important, and likely to be etiologic. No specific duration was required in any of the classification schemes described above, leaving the diagnosis and relevance of atrial fibrillation to the inconsistent judgment of the clinician. Other examples include specific thresholds of left ventricular ejection fraction[38] and the mobility of an atrial septal aneurysm.[39] Notably, all of these thresholds were typically developed for research purposes, to enable standardized descriptions of populations in multi-center clinical trials, rather than primarily for routine clinical use, but have nevertheless found their way into clinical practice guidelines and consequently routine care.

Under-Measured Cryptogenic Stroke. This is defined as the failure to identify a known etiology for stroke due to limitations in extent or quality of diagnostic testing. For a number of reasons, there are varying intensities of diagnostic evaluation among patients with ischemic stroke. For example, access to diagnostic testing is a necessity, and this may be limited in settings with reduced resources. In the extreme, there may be no brain or vascular imaging at all. More typically, ultrasound modalities are available, but provide less accurate classification than other technologies. In well-resourced settings, very extensive testing may be performed. Such variability in access to diagnostic testing makes international comparisons of epidemiologic studies almost impossible. In all settings, patients with very severe stroke may undergo limited testing because they are too unstable or may be considered inappropriate if goals of care are palliative, and may ultimately be declared cryptogenic by default.

Decisions on extent of diagnostic testing are not entirely based on availability and access of individual investigations. From a strict evidence-based management perspective, it may be argued that the vast majority of patients with ischemic stroke only require exclusion of atrial fibrillation and significant carotid artery disease, as these are the only common findings where there is definitive evidence from randomized clinical trials that a specific intervention favorably alters the natural history of recurrent stroke, beyond the generic approach to secondary prevention. It is acknowledged that other uncommon etiologies may also have specific management implications, such as infective endocarditis, cerebral vasculitis, and others, but those are uncommon "other" causes and may be suggested by compelling clinical history or features. Thus, a diagnostic strategy based on this reductionist approach will result in a high proportion of patients with an undocumented etiology, in part, due to under-measurement.

Common under-measured etiologies due to insufficient testing include intracranial stenosis, aortic arch disease, and paroxysmal atrial fibrillation. All of these impact prognosis and may have implications for medical therapy,[40-42] most obviously for atrial fibrillation. Rare etiologies often require more extensive testing, but not every consecutive patient needs every test. The identification of those uncommon causes (e.g. infective endocarditis) begins with clinical suspicion.

True Cryptogenic Stroke. This is defined by the true absence of an identified cause after a thorough evaluation. This is the most challenging group of patients to understand. These patients have a very low burden, or the absence of, established vascular risk factors, and an entirely normal extensive etiological work-up, or where findings are confined to questionable etiologies (e.g., small patent foramen ovale) (Table 44-2). In general, these are young patients (<45 years of age), and have embolic patterns of infarction on neuroimaging. As these patients do not have established modifiable risk factors, optimal secondary prevention strategies are uncertain. Conceptually, the mechanism of thromboembolism may be from a temporal collision of transient and perhaps underlying risk factors, supporting a "multiple hit theory." For example, thromboembolism from a deep vein thrombosis has to coincide with left-to-right shunting to cause an ischemic stroke in people with patent foramen ovale. The mechanisms of stroke in the truly cryptogenic stroke population have yet to be elucidated, though unknown thrombophilic, inflammatory, and infectious causes have been speculated. Over the last three decades, there has been a modest increase in the number of

TABLE 44-4 Atrial Fibrillation Detection after Cryptogenic Stroke

	Number of Subjects	Monitoring Method and Duration	Minimum AF Duration	Detection Rate	Predictors of Detecting AF
Tayal 2008[86]	56	Mobile cardiac outpatient telemetry, 21 days	Any	23%	(n/a)
Ziegler 2010[87]	163	Implantable cardiac defibrillator/ pacemaker, 400 days	5 minutes	28%	(n/a)
Gaillard 2010[88]	98	Transtelephonic ECG (patient-triggered), 24 days	30 seconds	9%	>100 PACs 24-hour Holter Non-lacunar anterior circulation acute infarctions
Bhatt 2011[89]	62	Mobile cardiac outpatient telemetry, 28 days	30 seconds	24%	PVC >2 m Stroke >TIA Multiple vs single acute infarctions
Cotter 2013[90]	51	Implantable loop recorder, <229 days	2 minutes	26%	Age Left atrial volume Interatrial block PACs
Miller 2013[91]	156	Mobile cardiac outpatient telemetry, 30 days	Any	17%	Age Female LA diameter PACs Stroke severity
Gladstone 2014[51]	287	Event monitor belt, 30 days	30 seconds	16%	Age>75
Sanna 2014[52]	225	Implantable loop recorder, 180 days	30 seconds	9%	(n/a)

AF = atrial fibrillations, PAC = premature atrial contraction, PVC = premature ventricular contraction, LA = left atrium.

novel etiologies identified for stroke, which has led to the reclassification of those strokes from cryptogenic to "other determined cause." The frequency of these etiologies is low, and they include Fabry's disease,[43] CADASIL,[44] other genetic disorders,[45] and cancer. It is likely that additional rare etiologies will be identified, including more genetic causes, which may be important in specific populations. However, the probability that a common novel potent genetic risk factor exists in the general population of patients with stroke is unlikely based on large population-based studies to date, and the estimated contribution of traditional risk factor for stroke on overall population-attributable risk.[31, 46] Rather, genetic risk factors may have important "main effects" in niche populations, and may modify the risk associated with common risk factors in general populations, which may have important management implications yet to be determined.

Why Cardiac Sources are Suspected to Cause Cryptogenic Strokes

The following considerations have implicated cardiac pathologies to be the most likely source of cryptogenic ischemic stroke. First, findings on imaging small and large vessels are mostly static and most amenable to objective confirmation. Measurement of large-vessel stenosis and infarct size is reliable over time and between readers. In contrast, many cardiac causes of ischemic stroke are dynamic and intermittent, particularly paroxysmal atrial fibrillation and other arrhythmias. Second, infarct topography studies have identified a superficial hemispheric infarct in 62–84% of patients with cryptogenic stroke,[47] a pattern that is also associated with atrial fibrillation.[48,49] Third, TEE has identified numerous potential causative factors and potential novel mechanisms of ischemic stroke (e.g., retrograde flow in aortic arch). Occult atrial fibrillation has been the focus of extensive research recently. Multiple studies have employed a variety of techniques of prolonged cardiac monitoring to detect atrial fibrillation after cryptogenic stroke (Table 44-4). Atrial fibrillation was detected in 3–28% of patients, though the definition of atrial fibrillation varied depending on the minimum duration.[50] Higher yields occurred when any duration (even less than 10 seconds) was considered. Two of these studies were randomized clinical trials.[51,52] The EMBRACE trial compared a 24-hour Holter monitor to 30 days of monitoring with a dry-electrode belt with an event-triggered loop recorder in patients aged 55 years and older with cryptogenic stroke. Using a threshold of at least 30 seconds, atrial fibrillation was detected in only 3% of the 24-hour Holter group vs 16% of the prolonged monitoring group. A total of 10% of patients in the prolonged monitoring group had at least one documented AF episode lasting 2.5 minutes or more, vs 2% in the Holter monitoring group. The device tested in the EMBRACE trial is not commercially available. The CRYSTAL-AF trial compared usual care to an implantable loop recorder and followed subjects for at least 6 months. This trial defined atrial fibrillation if the duration was at least 30 seconds. Atrial fibrillation was detected in 1.4% of patients with routine care and 8.9% with the implantable REVEAL device in the first 6 months, and in 2% vs 12.4% at 12 months, and 3% vs 30% at 36 months. The vast majority (92%) of subjects with atrial fibrillation were documented as having at least one episode of 6 minutes or longer. Other observations support the contention other left atrial potential sources of thrombosis in the absence of atrial fibrillation/flutter contribute to stroke. Other non-specific atrial tachyarrhythmias and increased left atrial volume have also been associated with cryptogenic ischemic stroke and the risk of recurrent stroke.[53]

NATURAL HISTORY OF CRYPTOGENIC ISCHEMIC STROKE

The risk of recurrent ischemic stroke, myocardial infarction, and mortality after cryptogenic ischemic stroke varies among studies and is dependent on the age of the population and burden of co-morbidities. In young patients, mostly with true cryptogenic stroke, including those with patent foramen ovale, the risk of recurrent stroke and major vascular events is low (1–3% per year).[54] This suggests that in most of those with true cryptogenic stroke, the pathogenesis relates to a transient period of increased thromboembolic risk. For example, it may be conjectured that venous thrombosis formation with opportune shunting of patent foramen ovale may be a distinctly rare event, and the probability of occurrence, and therefore recurrence, is low.

In contrast, cryptogenic ischemic stroke in older unselected population has a formidable risk of recurrent stroke and major vascular events (~5–10% per year), comparable with other patients with known causes of stroke.[55] Estimates suggest that the risk of recurrent stroke is lower than in patients with documented large-vessel disease and known atrial fibrillation, but higher than in patients with small-vessel disease. These contrasting natural history data support the contention that cryptogenic stroke is heterogeneous, with higher risk under-classified and under-measured cryptogenic stroke predominating in the older populations and greater proportion of true cryptogenic stroke in the younger, but definitive data are lacking due to inconsistent classification across studies.

MANAGEMENT IMPLICATIONS OF CRYPTOGENIC ISCHEMIC STROKE

Acute Management

Evidence-based interventions that reduce disability or death in patients with acute ischemic stroke appear to be as effective in patients with cryptogenic ischemic stroke, compared to other stroke subtypes, including thrombolysis, aspirin, and stroke unit care.[56–58]

Secondary Prevention

Common to all stroke subtypes, approaches to secondary prevention include lifestyle modification, antihypertensive therapy in those with hypertension, statin therapy in those with dyslipidemia, and antithrombotic therapy. There is no evidence that cryptogenic ischemic stroke should alter the choice of antihypertensive or statin therapy. However, there is emerging debate about the choice of antiplatelet versus anticoagulant therapy.[6] Since there is a high clinical suspicion of cardioembolism in many patients with cryptogenic ischemic stroke, the introduction of oral anticoagulation seems logical, but is, at best, an educated projection. However, since oral anticoagulation is associated with a higher risk of bleeding compared to antiplatelet therapy, convincing evidence of efficacy needs to be demonstrated before it can be recommended in this patient population. The only randomized evaluation of anticoagulation in cryptogenic stroke is the subgroup analysis of the Warfarin-Aspirin Recurrent Stroke Study (WARSS).[59] Among the 2206 patients between 30 and 85 years old with recent (<30 days) ischemic stroke who were randomized to aspirin 325 mg/d or adjusted-dose warfarin (target INR 1.4–2.8, median achieved INR = 1.9), 26% (n=576) were deemed cryptogenic based on the TOAST criteria. For cryptogenic stroke patients, the primary outcome of ischemic stroke or death occurred in 15.0% assigned to warfarin vs 16.5% assigned to aspirin over 2 years (HR 0.92, 95%CI, 0.6–1.4). Among those patients with cryptogenic stroke, 338 had neuroimaging suggesting an embolic pattern, as indicated by a superficial, cortical or cerebellar, large deep, or superficial and deep combined infarct. This strategy effectively eliminated small deep infarcts that were labeled as cryptogenic but were likely due to under-classified small-vessel occlusive disease. In this group with embolic cryptogenic stroke, the 2-year risk of recurrent ischemic stroke or death was 12% with warfarin vs 18% with aspirin (HR=0.66, 95%CI, 0.4–1.2). This analysis is suggestive of both a high risk in this population and a potential benefit of anticoagulation, but is ultimately an underpowered subgroup and is by no means definitive. To date, no clinical trial has been performed to compare antiplatelet therapy to oral anticoagulant therapy in patients with cryptogenic ischemic stroke with an embolic topographic pattern on neuroimaging. However, the emergence of novel oral anticoagulants (NOACs) into clinical practice, and their efficacy and safety in patients with atrial fibrillation, had prompted enthusiasm to complete such trials.[6,60]

CLINICAL AND RESEARCH ISSUES FOR CRYPTOGENIC ISCHEMIC STROKE

Ischemic stroke etiological subtypes have been defined for clinical research. Those definitions were established based on the knowledge and tools available when they were developed. The definition of cryptogenic stroke remains a work in progress, potentially changing every time a new risk factor, disease, or diagnostic test emerges or becomes widely accessible. Clinical researchers need to strive for more detailed characterization of cryptogenic stroke in all studies, particularly distinguishing under-classified, under-measured, and true cryptogenic stroke, as well as the clinical, radiographical, and other features. A number of novel approaches to imaging plaque and acute thrombosis may advance our ability to more precisely characterize ischemic stroke mechanisms.[61,62] Research will always ultimately require specific thresholds and rigid parameters, and these will subsequently be incorporated into clinical practice guidelines. Clinicians need to be aware of this evolution and adapt accordingly, allowing for clinical judgment in the face of some uncertainty. A reasonable approach is to first perform a thorough evaluation to look for high-risk or modifiable stroke etiologies, with emphasis on atrial fibrillation/flutter and carotid stenosis. For under-classified strokes, treat them with aggressive medical therapy. For the true cryptogenic strokes, if all else is unrevealing, the risk of recurrent stroke appears low, but consider evaluation at a stroke center and inclusion in research studies, as novel diseases are yet to be discovered.

REFERENCES

1. Davis SM, Donnan GA. Clinical practice. Secondary prevention after ischemic stroke or transient ischemic attack. N Engl J Med 2012;366:1914–22.
2. Lovett JK, Coull AJ, Rothwell PM. Early risk of recurrence by subtype of ischemic stroke in population-based incidence studies. Neurology 2004;62:569–73.
3. Davis SM, Donnan GA. Clinical practice. Secondary prevention after ischemic stroke or transient ischemic attack. N Engl J Med 2012;366:1914–22.
4. Liberman AL, Prabhakaran S. Cryptogenic stroke: how to define it? How to treat it? Curr Cardiol Rep 2013;15:423.
5. Furie KL, Kasner SE, Adams RJ, et al. Guidelines for the prevention of stroke in patients with stroke or transient ischemic attack: a guideline for healthcare professionals from the american heart association/american stroke association. Stroke 2011; 42:227–76.
6. Hart RG, Diener HC, Coutts SB, et al. Embolic strokes of undetermined source: the case for a new clinical construct. Lancet Neurol 2014;13:429–38.
7. Adams HP Jr, Bendixen BH, Kappelle LJ, et al. Classification of subtype of acute ischemic stroke. Definitions for use in a multicenter clinical trial. TOAST. Trial of Org 10172 in Acute Stroke Treatment. Stroke 1993;24:35–41.
8. Marnane M, Duggan CA, Sheehan OC, et al. Stroke subtype classification to mechanism-specific and undetermined categories by

TOAST, A-S-C-O, and causative classification system: direct comparison in the North Dublin population stroke study. Stroke 2010;41:1579–86.
9. Ay H, Benner T, Arsava EM, et al. A computerized algorithm for etiologic classification of ischemic stroke: the Causative Classification of Stroke System. Stroke 2007;38:2979–84.
10. Amarenco P, Bogousslavsky J, Caplan LR, et al. The ASCOD phenotyping of ischemic stroke (Updated ASCO Phenotyping). Cerebrovasc Dis 2013;36:1–5.
11. Yahia AM, Shaukat AB, Kirmani JF, et al. Treatable potential cardiac sources of embolism in patients with cerebral ischemic events: a selective transesophageal echocardiographic study. South Med J 2004;97(11):1055–9.
12. White H, Boden-Albala B, Wang C, et al. Ischemic stroke subtype incidence among whites, blacks, and Hispanics: the Northern Manhattan Study. Circulation 2005;111(10):1327–31.
13. Zweifler RM, Lyden PD, Taft B, et al. Impact of race and ethnicity on ischemic stroke. The University of California at San Diego Stroke Data Bank. Stroke 1995;26(2):245–8.
14. Woo D, Gebel J, Miller R, et al. Incidence rates of first-ever ischemic stroke subtypes among blacks: a population-based study. Stroke 1999;30(12):2517–22.
15. Schulz UG, Rothwell PM. Differences in vascular risk factors between etiological subtypes of ischemic stroke: importance of population-based studies. Stroke 2003;34(8):2050–9.
16. Karttunen V, Alfthan G, Hiltunen L, et al. Risk factors for cryptogenic ischaemic stroke. Eur J Neurol 2002;9(6):625–32.
17. Kim BJ, Kim JS. Ischemic stroke subtype classification: an Asian viewpoint. J Stroke 2014;16(1):8–17.
18. Feldmann E, Wilterdink JL, Kosinski A, et al. The Stroke Outcomes and Neuroimaging of Intracranial Atherosclerosis (SONIA) trial. Neurology 2007;68(24):2099–106.
19. Nederkoorn PJ, van der Graaf Y, Hunink MG. Duplex ultrasound and magnetic resonance angiography compared with digital subtraction angiography in carotid artery stenosis: a systematic review. Stroke 2003;34(5):1324–32.
20. Wessels T, Rottger C, Jauss M, et al. Identification of embolic stroke patterns by diffusion-weighted MRI in clinically defined lacunar stroke syndromes. Stroke 2005;36(4):757–61.
21. Liao J, Khalid Z, Scallan C, et al. Noninvasive cardiac monitoring for detecting paroxysmal atrial fibrillation or flutter after acute ischemic stroke: a systematic review. Stroke 2007;38(11):2935–40.
22. Albers GW, Comess KA, DeRook FA, et al. Transesophageal echocardiographic findings in stroke subtypes. Stroke 1994; 25(1):23–8.
23. Censori B, Colombo F, Valsecchi MG, et al. Early transoesophageal echocardiography in cryptogenic and lacunar stroke and transient ischaemic attack. J Neurol Neurosurg Psychiatry 1998; 64(5):624–7.
24. Cujec B, Polasek P, Voll C, et al. Transesophageal echocardiography in the detection of potential cardiac source of embolism in stroke patients. Stroke 1991;22(6):727–33.
25. Pearson AC, Labovitz AJ, Tatineni S, et al. Superiority of transesophageal echocardiography in detecting cardiac source of embolism in patients with cerebral ischemia of uncertain etiology. J Am Coll Cardiol 1991;17(1):66–72.
26. Wessler BS, Thaler DE, Ruthazer R, et al. Transesophageal echocardiography in cryptogenic stroke and patent foramen ovale: analysis of putative high-risk features from the risk of paradoxical embolism database. Circ Cardiovasc Imaging 2014;7(1): 125–31.
27. Yahia AM, Shaukat AB, Kirmani JF, et al. Treatable potential cardiac sources of embolism in patients with cerebral ischemic events: a selective transesophageal echocardiographic study. South Med J 2004;97(11):1055–9.
28. Zahuranec DB, Mueller GC, Bach DS, et al. Pilot study of cardiac magnetic resonance imaging for detection of embolic source after ischemic stroke. J Stroke Cerebrovasc Dis 2012;21(8): 794–800.
29. Liebeskind DS, Kosinski AS, Lynn MJ, et al. Noninvasive fractional flow on MRA predicts stroke risk of intracranial stenosis. J Neuroimaging 2014.
30. Almekhlafi MA, Wilton SB, Rabi DM, et al. Recurrent cerebral ischemia in medically treated patent foramen ovale: a meta-analysis. Neurology 2009;73(2):89–97.
31. O'Donnell MJ, Xavier D, Liu L, et al. Risk factors for ischaemic and intracerebral haemorrhagic stroke in 22 countries (the INTERSTROKE study): a case-control study. Lancet 2010;376(9735): 112–23.
32. Mazighi M, Labreuche J, Gongora-Rivera F, et al. Autopsy prevalence of intracranial atherosclerosis in patients with fatal stroke. Stroke 2008;39(4):1142–7.
33. Mazighi M, Labreuche J, Gongora-Rivera F, et al. Autopsy prevalence of proximal extracranial atherosclerosis in patients with fatal stroke. Stroke 2009;40(3):713–18.
34. Giroud D, Li JM, Urban P, et al. Relation of the site of acute myocardial infarction to the most severe coronary arterial stenosis at prior angiography. Am J Cardiol 1992;69(8): 729–32.
35. Barnett HJ, Taylor DW, Eliasziw M, et al. Benefit of carotid endarterectomy in patients with symptomatic moderate or severe stenosis. North American Symptomatic Carotid Endarterectomy Trial Collaborators. N Engl J Med 1998;339(20):1415–25.
36. Amarenco P, Rother J, Michel P, et al. Aortic arch atheroma and the risk of stroke. Curr Atheroscler Rep 2006;8(4):343–6.
37. Boriani G, Diemberger I, Ziacchi M, et al. AF burden is important – fact or fiction? Int J Clin Pract 2014;68(4):444–52.
38. Homma S, Thompson JL, Pullicino PM, et al. Warfarin and aspirin in patients with heart failure and sinus rhythm. N Engl J Med 2012;366(20):1859–69.
39. Kitsios GD, Dahabreh IJ, Abu Dabrh AM, et al. Patent foramen ovale closure and medical treatments for secondary stroke prevention: a systematic review of observational and randomized evidence. Stroke 2012;43(2):422–31.
40. Derdeyn CP, Chimowitz MI, Lynn MJ, et al. Aggressive medical treatment with or without stenting in high-risk patients with intracranial artery stenosis (SAMMPRIS): the final results of a randomised trial. Lancet 2014;383(9914):333–41.
41. Amarenco P, Davis S, Jones EF, et al. Clopidogrel plus aspirin versus warfarin in patients with stroke and aortic arch plaques. Stroke 2014;45(5):1248–57.
42. Aguilar MI, Hart R, Pearce LA. Oral anticoagulants versus antiplatelet therapy for preventing stroke in patients with non-valvular atrial fibrillation and no history of stroke or transient ischemic attacks. Cochrane Database Syst Rev 2007;(3): CD006186.
43. Rolfs A, Bottcher T, Zschiesche M, et al. Prevalence of Fabry disease in patients with cryptogenic stroke: a prospective study. Lancet 2005;366(9499):1794–6.
44. Chabriat H, Joutel A, Dichgans M, et al. Cadasil. Lancet Neurol 2009;8(7):643–53.
45. Zhou Q, Yang D, Ombrello AK, et al. Early-onset stroke and vasculopathy associated with mutations in ADA2. N Engl J Med 2014;370(10):911–20.
46. Traylor M, Farrall M, Holliday EG, et al. Genetic risk factors for ischaemic stroke and its subtypes (the METASTROKE collaboration): a meta-analysis of genome-wide association studies. Lancet Neurol 2012;11(11):951–62.
47. Lamy C, Giannesini C, Zuber M, et al. Clinical and imaging findings in cryptogenic stroke patients with and without patent foramen ovale: the PFO-ASA Study. Atrial Septal Aneurysm. Stroke 2002;33(3):706–11.
48. Evans A, Perez I, Yu G, et al. Should stroke subtype influence anticoagulation decisions to prevent recurrence in stroke patients with atrial fibrillation? Stroke 2001;32(12):2828–32.
49. Miller VT, Rothrock JF, Pearce LA, et al. Ischemic stroke in patients with atrial fibrillation: effect of aspirin according to stroke mechanism. Stroke Prevention in Atrial Fibrillation Investigators. Neurology 1993;43(1):32–6.
50. Kishore A, Vail A, Majid A, et al. Detection of atrial fibrillation after ischemic stroke or transient ischemic attack: a systematic review and meta-analysis. Stroke 2014;45(2):520–6.
51. Gladstone DJ, Sharma M, Spence JD. Cryptogenic stroke and atrial fibrillation. *N Engl J Med* 2014;371(13):1260.
52. Sanna T, Diener HC, Passman RS, et al. Cryptogenic stroke and underlying atrial fibrillation. *N Engl J Med* 2014;370(26): 2478–86.
53. Healey JS, Connolly SJ, Gold MR, et al. Subclinical atrial fibrillation and the risk of stroke. N Engl J Med 2012;366(2): 120–9.

54. Arauz A, Murillo L, Marquez JM, et al. Long-term risk of recurrent stroke in young cryptogenic stroke patients with and without patent foramen ovale. Int J Stroke 2012;7(8):631–4.
55. Homma S, Sacco RL, Di Tullio MR, et al. Effect of medical treatment in stroke patients with patent foramen ovale: patent foramen ovale in Cryptogenic Stroke Study. Circulation 2002;105(22):2625–31.
56. Hsia AW, Sachdev HS, Tomlinson J, et al. Efficacy of IV tissue plasminogen activator in acute stroke: does stroke subtype really matter? Neurology 2003;61(1):71–5.
57. Saposnik G, Hassan KA, Selchen D, et al. Stroke unit care: does ischemic stroke subtype matter? Int J Stroke 2011;6(3):244–50.
58. Lansberg MG, O'Donnell MJ, Khatri P, et al. Antithrombotic and thrombolytic therapy for ischemic stroke: Antithrombotic Therapy and Prevention of Thrombosis, 9th ed: American College of Chest Physicians Evidence-Based Clinical Practice Guidelines. Chest 2012;141(2 Suppl.):e601S–e636S.
59. Sacco RL, Prabhakaran S, Thompson JL, et al. Comparison of warfarin versus aspirin for the prevention of recurrent stroke or death: subgroup analyses from the Warfarin-Aspirin Recurrent Stroke Study. Cerebrovasc Dis 2006;22(1):4–12.
60. Diener HC, Easton JD, Hankey GJ, et al. Novel oral anticoagulants in secondary prevention of stroke. Best Pract Res Clin Haematol 2013;26(2):131–9.
61. Marnane M, Prendeville S, McDonnell C, et al. Plaque inflammation and unstable morphology are associated with early stroke recurrence in symptomatic carotid stenosis. Stroke 2014;45(3):801–6.
62. Fujimoto M, Salamon N, Mayor F, et al. Characterization of arterial thrombus composition by magnetic resonance imaging in a swine stroke model. Stroke 2013;44(5):1463–5.
63. Moulin T, Tatu L, Vuillier F, et al. Role of a stroke data bank in evaluating cerebral infarction subtypes: patterns and outcome of 1,776 consecutive patients from the Besancon stroke registry. Cerebrovasc Dis 2000;10(4):261–71.
64. Vemmos KN, Takis CE, Georgilis K, et al. The Athens stroke registry: results of a five-year hospital-based study. Cerebrovasc Dis 2000;10(2):133–41.
65. Grau AJ, Weimar C, Buggle F, et al. Risk factors, outcome, and treatment in subtypes of ischemic stroke: the German stroke data bank. Stroke 2001;32(11):2559–66.
66. Mohr JP, Thompson JL, Lazar RM, et al. A comparison of warfarin and aspirin for the prevention of recurrent ischemic stroke. N Engl J Med 2001;345(20):1444–51.
67. Kolominsky-Rabas PL, Weber M, Gefeller O, et al. Epidemiology of ischemic stroke subtypes according to TOAST criteria: incidence, recurrence, and long-term survival in ischemic stroke subtypes: a population-based study. Stroke 2001;32(12):2735–40.
68. Murat SM, Erturk O. Ischemic stroke subtypes: risk factors, functional outcome and recurrence. Neurol Sci 2002;22(6):449–54.
69. Bang OY, Lee PH, Joo SY, et al. Frequency and mechanisms of stroke recurrence after cryptogenic stroke. Ann Neurol 2003;54(2):227–34.
70. Soda T, Nakayasu H, Maeda M, et al. Stroke recurrence within the first year following cerebral infarction–Tottori University Lacunar Infarction Prognosis Study (TULIPS). Acta Neurol Scand 2004;110(6):343–9.
71. Acciarresi M, Caso V, Venti M, et al. First-ever stroke and outcome in patients admitted to Perugia Stroke Unit: predictors for death, dependency, and recurrence of stroke within the first three months. Clin Exp Hypertens 2006;28(3–4):287–94.
72. Sacco RL, Diener HC, Yusuf S, et al. Aspirin and extended-release dipyridamole versus clopidogrel for recurrent stroke. N Engl J Med 2008;359(12):1238–51.
73. Nedeltchev K, Wiedmer S, Schwerzmann M, et al. Sex differences in cryptogenic stroke with patent foramen ovale. Am Heart J 2008;156(3):461–5.
74. Sposato LA, Klein FR, Jauregui A, et al. Newly diagnosed atrial fibrillation after acute ischemic stroke and transient ischemic attack: importance of immediate and prolonged continuous cardiac monitoring. J Stroke Cerebrovasc Dis 2012;21(3):210–16.
75. Michel P, Odier C, Rutgers M, et al. The Acute STroke Registry and Analysis of Lausanne (ASTRAL): design and baseline analysis of an ischemic stroke registry including acute multimodal imaging. Stroke 2010;41(11):2491–8.
76. B vitamins in patients with recent transient ischaemic attack or stroke in the VITAmins TO Prevent Stroke (VITATOPS) trial: a randomised, double-blind, parallel, placebo-controlled trial. Lancet Neurol 2010;9(9):855–65.
77. Bousser MG, Amarenco P, Chamorro A, et al. Terutroban versus aspirin in patients with cerebral ischaemic events (PERFORM): a randomised, double-blind, parallel-group trial. Lancet 2011;377(9782):2013–22.
78. Wolf ME, Sauer T, Alonso A, et al. Comparison of the new ASCO classification with the TOAST classification in a population with acute ischemic stroke. J Neurol 2012;259(7):1284–9.
79. Shang W, Liu J. Stroke subtype classification: a comparative study of ASCO and modified TOAST. J Neurol Sci 2012;314(1–2):66–70.
80. Nam HS, Kim HC, Kim YD, et al. Long-term mortality in patients with stroke of undetermined etiology. Stroke 2012;43(11):2948–56.
81. Romano JG, Arauz A, Koch S, et al. Disparities in stroke type and vascular risk factors between 2 Hispanic populations in Miami and Mexico city. J Stroke Cerebrovasc Dis 2013;22(6):828–33.
82. Vallejos J, Jaramillo A, Reyes A, et al. Prognosis of cryptogenic ischemic stroke: a prospective single-center study in Chile. J Stroke Cerebrovasc Dis 2012;21(8):621–8.
83. Santamarina E, Penalba A, Garcia-Berrocoso T, et al. Biomarker level improves the diagnosis of embolic source in ischemic stroke of unknown origin. J Neurol 2012;259(12):2538–45.
84. Rodriguez-Yanez M, Arias-Rivas S, Santamaria-Cadavid M, et al. High pro-BNP levels predict the occurrence of atrial fibrillation after cryptogenic stroke. Neurology 2013;81(5):444–7.
85. Etgen T, Hochreiter M, Mundel M, et al. Insertable cardiac event recorder in detection of atrial fibrillation after cryptogenic stroke: an audit report. Stroke 2013;44(7):2007–9.
86. Tayal AH, Tian M, Kelly KM, et al. Atrial fibrillation detected by mobile cardiac outpatient telemetry in cryptogenic TIA or stroke. Neurology 2008;71(21):1696–701.
87. Ziegler PD, Glotzer TV, Daoud EG, et al. Incidence of newly detected atrial arrhythmias via implantable devices in patients with a history of thromboembolic events. Stroke 2010;41(2):256–60.
88. Gaillard N, Deltour S, Vilotijevic B, et al. Detection of paroxysmal atrial fibrillation with transtelephonic EKG in TIA or stroke patients. Neurology 2010;74(21):1666–70.
89. Bhatt A, Majid A, Razak A, et al. Predictors of occult paroxysmal atrial fibrillation in cryptogenic strokes detected by long-term noninvasive cardiac monitoring. Stroke Res Treat 2011;2011:172074.
90. Cotter PE, Martin PJ, Ring L, et al. Incidence of atrial fibrillation detected by implantable loop recorders in unexplained stroke. Neurology 2013;80(17):1546–50.
91. Miller DJ, Khan MA, Schultz LR, et al. Outpatient cardiac telemetry detects a high rate of atrial fibrillation in cryptogenic stroke. J Neurol Sci 2013;324(1–2):57–61.

45 Cerebral Venous Thrombosis

José M. Ferro, Patrícia Canhão

KEY POINTS

- A high suspicion rate is needed to identify cerebral venous thrombosis (CVT).
- Confirmation of the diagnosis of CVT requires MRI and MR venography or CT and CT venography.
- Prothrombotic screening should be performed in all patients.
- Anticoagulants must be used for almost all patients in the acute phase.
- Hemicraniectomy or local thrombolysis are lifesaving interventions to be performed in selected severe cases.

Cerebral vein and dural sinus thrombosis (CVT) are less frequent than other types of strokes and have a quite different clinical presentation and involve different etiologic investigations. They rarely manifest as a stroke syndrome. The clinical features are rather diverse. CVTs are more challenging to diagnose than other types of stroke. Once considered a rare, often fatal disease related to the puerperium and to infections of the central nervous system (CNS), sinuses, and mastoid,[1] CVT is now recognized with increasing frequency. The apparent rise in the frequency of CVT is related to increasing awareness of its diagnosis among neurologists and emergency physicians and to the use of magnetic resonance imaging (MRI) for the investigation of patients with headache, seizures, and unclear neurologic pictures. Because it can be the initial manifestation of, or can complicate, several systemic conditions, CVT is a disease of interest not only for neurologists but also for neurosurgeons; ear, nose, and throat (ENT) specialists; ophthalmologists; internists; rheumatologists; oncologists; hematologists; and obstetricians.

EPIDEMIOLOGY

There are few epidemiologic studies of CVT that meet the current standards for a good-quality epidemiologic study[2-7] and the true incidence of CVT is probably underestimated. A prevalence of only 1% was found in consecutive autopsies. Autopsy studies are biased because they reflect severe fatal cases of CVT, in particular those associated with intracranial infection. In a nationwide hospital-based series in Portugal, including patients admitted to all neurology services in the country, 91 new cases of CVT were identified, corresponding to an incidence of 0.22/100,000/year.[4] A hospital discharge registry in the US gave an incidence of CVT during pregnancy of 11.6 per 100,000 deliveries.[5] The incidence in the multicenter Canadian registry of CVT in infants and children younger than 18 years was 0.67/100,000.[6] In a recent well-designed cross-sectional study in two provinces in the Netherlands, the overall incidence of CVT was 1.32/100 000/year, but among women between the ages of 31 and 50 years, the incidence was 2.78. These figures are higher than those of the incidence of bacterial meningitis in adults and indicate that the incidence of CVT among adults is probably higher than previously believed.[7]

In hospital-based series, CVT is more common in children than in adults. Among children, CVT is more common in neonates than in older children.[6] In adults, CVT affects patients who are younger than those with other types of strokes, and the incidence apparently decreases in older subjects. In the International Study on Cerebral Vein and Dural Sinus Thrombosis (ISCVT) study, the largest international cohort of CVT patients, the median age was 37 years,[8] with only 8% of the patients older than 65 years. CVT is more common in females than in males (female-to-male ratio 2.9 : 1).[8]

A few studies addressed the chronobiology of CVT. In Portugal, CVTs were more frequent in autumn and winter, raising the hypothesis that upper respiratory infections are the trigger of CVT in prone individuals.[9] However, in Germany, CVTs were more frequent in winter and summer.[10]

VENOUS ANATOMY

Blood of the brain is drained by the cerebral venous system, which consists of the cerebral veins and dural venous sinuses. Cerebral veins encompass the superficial venous system, deep venous system, and posterior fossa veins (Fig. 45-1). Superficial cerebral veins course over the surface of the brain, draining the major part of the cerebral cortex, with the exception of the inner face of temporal and occipital lobes, and a portion of the subjacent white matter. They are variable in number and location. They have no valves and are linked by several anastomoses, allowing the development of collateral circulation in the event of vein or sinus occlusion. Ascending superficial veins are named according to the area of cortex they drain. Anastomotic Trolard and Labbé's veins connect the Sylvian or superficial middle cerebral veins with the superior sagittal sinus and the lateral sinus, respectively.

The deep venous system drains the inferior frontal lobe, most of the deep white matter, the corpus callosum, the basal ganglia, and the upper brainstem. It includes the internal cerebral and basal veins of Rosenthal which join to form the great cerebral vein of Galen, which drains into the straight sinus. The deep venous system is relatively constant compared with the superficial cortical venous system. Posterior fossa veins are variable in their number and course. Three groups of veins may be recognized: superior veins draining into the great vein of Galen, anterior veins draining into the petrosal sinus, and posterior veins draining into the torcular Herophili or the straight or lateral sinuses.

Cerebral veins drain the blood into the dural sinuses, which are endothelium-lined channels without valves and enclosed in the leaves of the dura mater. There are two groups of dural sinuses, superior and inferior. The superior group comprises the superior and inferior sagittal sinus, and the straight, transverse, and sigmoid sinuses (see Fig. 45-1). Superficial veins drain into the superior sagittal and transverse sinuses, and the deep cerebral veins into the straight and transverse sinuses. The confluence of the sinuses (torcular Herophili) results from the junction of superior sagittal,

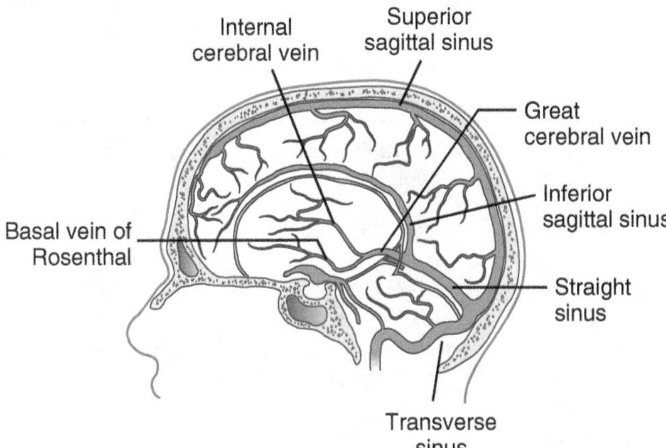

Figure 45-1. Sagittal view of the anatomy of superficial and deep cerebral veins and dural sinuses.

straight, and transverse sinuses and is often asymmetrical. The inferior group drains the basal and medial parts of the undersurface of the brain, the orbits, and the sphenoparietal sinus and collects at the cavernous sinus. Cavernous sinuses connect with the lateral sinuses via superior and inferior petrosal sinuses and with the pterygoid plexus.

Most of the cerebral venous blood flows posteriorly, from the superior sagittal sinus or the straight sinus via the lateral sinuses into the internal jugular veins. A smaller proportion flows to the cavernous sinuses.

There are several anatomic variations of the dural sinuses. The most important are atresia of the anterior part of the superior sagittal sinus; duplication of the superior sagittal sinus, mainly in its posterior part; asymmetry of the transverse sinus with dominance of the right transverse sinus in the majority of cases; and aplasia or hypoplasia of the posteromedial segment of the left transverse sinus. The straight sinus may join the torcular, the right transverse sinus, the left transverse sinus, or all three. Owing to the variability of cerebral veins and anatomic variants of the dural sinus, the angiographic diagnosis of vein or dural sinus thrombosis can be challenging.

PATHOPHYSIOLOGY

Developments in imaging modalities, such as diffusion-weighted MRI (DWI) and perfusion-weighted MRI (PWI), improved our knowledge of the pathophysiology of CVT and established some differences between venous and arterial infarction.[11-20] Nevertheless, data are still conflicting, and the pathogenesis of parenchymal lesions due to venous occlusion remains insufficiently understood. There are few experiments in adequate animal models of CVT.[21] The variability of venous system anatomy makes the understanding of venous flow disturbances and mechanisms of lesions difficult.

At least two different mechanisms may contribute to the clinical features of CVT: the thrombosis of the cerebral veins or dural sinus, leading to cerebral lesions; and the occlusion of the dural sinus, resulting in disturbance of cerebrospinal fluid (CSF) absorption and increased intracranial pressure.

Venous or dural sinus occlusion may have different consequences in the brain: no detectable lesions, focal edema, or hemorrhage. Several mechanisms may be involved, namely vasogenic edema, cytotoxic edema, both vasogenic and cytotoxic edema, and hemorrhage. One of the first consequences of venous occlusion is the increase in venous pressure. At an early stage, the collateral pathways of venous drainage allow for significant compensation, and parenchymal lesions may not develop. Some animal experiments have shown that thrombosis of the cortical veins is required to induce brain lesions, but this may not be the case in human CVT. As venous and capillary pressure rise, dilatation of veins and capillaries ensue, followed by blood-brain barrier disruption with leakage of blood plasma into the interstitial space, resulting in vasogenic edema. This pattern is confirmed by diffusion-weighted MRI, which shows isointensity, hypointensity, or hyperintensity signal abnormality in the affected area without significantly lower apparent diffusion coefficient (ADC) values than in unaffected regions.[11,19] On perfusion-weighted MRI, relative cerebral blood volume (rCBV) and mean transit time (MTT) are increased in affected areas, with preserved relative cerebral blood flow (rCBF).[11,19] Experimental animal data suggest that vasogenic edema occurs earlier in venous stroke than in arterial stroke.[22] At this stage, if collateral pathways are efficacious or recanalization occurs, tissue perfusion may be possible, and swollen brain cells are potentially recoverable.[23] Further increase in intravenous pressure may lead to venous or capillary rupture, causing brain hemorrhage. In addition, elevation of intravenous pressure produces venous congestion, raises intravascular pressure, and lowers cerebral perfusion pressure. Cerebral blood flow may then fall below the penumbra or ischemic threshold, resulting in energetic failure, loss of the Na^+, K^+-ATPase pump activity, and intracellular entry of water, with consequent cytotoxic edema. MRI has confirmed a cytotoxic pattern of edema in patients with CVT, characterized by high signal intensity on DWI and low ADC values.[12,15,17,24] In summary, the pathogenesis of venous lesions is different from that of arterial infarcts. Vasogenic edema predominates, and cytotoxic edema is far less common. After venous occlusion, large areas of the brain may be functionally and metabolically disturbed. Reversibility is very typical of venous lesions, reflected in both favorable clinical recovery and vanishing lesions on neuroimaging.[25]

Besides parenchymal changes, dural sinus thrombosis may impair CSF circulation and cause intracranial hypertension. CSF absorption occurs mainly in the arachnoid villi and granulations (pacchionian bodies) contained in the superior sagittal sinus and other sinuses. Thrombosis of the sinuses leads to increased venous pressure, impaired CSF absorption, and, increased intracranial pressure. This process is more frequent with superior sagittal sinus occlusion, but it may also result from a rise in sinus pressure without thrombosis of the superior sagittal sinus, such as in lateral sinus or jugular vein thrombosis.

ETIOLOGY

A large number of conditions are known to cause or predispose to CVT (Box 45-1). At least one risk factor can be identified in more than 85% of patients with CVT, and multiple risk factors may be found in about half.[8]

The more frequent risk factors are prothrombotic conditions, oral contraceptive use, puerperium or pregnancy states, infection, and malignancy.[8] The patient genetic background most likely determines the inherent individual risk. In the presence of some prothrombotic conditions, patients are at increased risk for developing a CVT when exposed to specific precipitants. Thrombophilic disorders are leading risk factors for CVT (Box 45-2). The most frequent are G20210A prothrombin polymorphism (identified in 6% to 20% of patients with CVT),[26-29] factor V Leiden (10– 24%),[27-33] and anticardiolipin/antiphospholipid antibodies (6– 8%).[8,30] Less often, protein C, protein S, or antithrombin III deficiencies are identified (0–9%).[27-32] A systematic review confirmed the increased risk of CVT in patients with G20210A prothrombin mutation (pooled odds ratio [OR] 5.48; 95% confidence

BOX 45-1 Risk Factors Associated With Cerebral Venous Thrombosis

Prothrombotic condition
- Genetic
- Acquired (e.g., antiphospholipid syndrome)

Infection
- Central nervous system (e.g., abscess, empyema, meningitis)
- Ear, sinus, mouth, face and neck (e.g., otitis, mastoiditis, tonsillitis, stomatitis, sinusitis, skin)
- Systemic infectious disease (e.g., sepsis, endocarditis, tuberculosis, HIV)

Inflammatory disease
- Systemic lupus erythematosus
- Behçet's disease
- Sjögren's syndrome
- Wegener's granulomatosis
- Temporal arteritis
- Thromboangiitis obliterans
- Inflammatory bowel disease
- Sarcoidosis

Malignancy
- Central nervous system (meningioma, metastasis, glomus tumor, medulloblastoma)
- Solid tumor outside the central nervous system
- Hematologic (leukemias, lymphomas)

Hematologic condition
- Anemia
- Sickle cell disease or trait
- Iron deficiency
- Paroxysmal nocturnal hemoglobinuria
- Polycythemia (primary or secondary)
- Thrombocythemia (primary or secondary)

Pregnancy and puerperium

Other disorders
- Dehydration
- Nephrotic syndrome
- Congenital heart disease
- Diabetic ketoacidosis
- Thyroid disease (hyperthyroidism or hypothyroidism)
- Central nervous system disorder
  - Dural fistula
  - Arachnoid cyst

Other precipitants
- Head trauma
- Lumbar puncture, myelography, intrathecal steroids
- Neurosurgical procedures, irradiation
- Jugular catheter occlusion
- Drugs (oral contraceptives, hormone replacement therapy, androgens, medroxyprogesterone acetate, L-asparaginase, cyclosporine, tamoxifen, steroids, lithium, thalidomide, MDMA (3,4-methylenedioxy-methamphetamine), sildenafil)

interval [CI], 3.88–7.74), and in patients with factor V Leiden mutation (pooled OR 2.40; 95%CI, 1.75–3.30).[34] There was heterogeneity in the studies assessing the contribution of methylene tetrahydrofolate reductase/C677T gene homozygoty as a risk factor for CVT,[35] although after iterative analysis controlling for interstudy heterogeneity, it was suggested to be associated with the risk of CVT (pooled OR 2.30; 95% CI, 1.20–4.42).[34] Hyperhomocysteinemia was shown to be associated with increased risk of CVT in a systematic review (pooled OR, 4.07; 95%CI, 2.54–6.52).[36]

The influence of thrombophilia in CVT risk may vary with age. In a meta-analysis on the impact of thrombophilia on first childhood stroke, including CVT, the pooled OR was lower

BOX 45-2 Thrombophilia Conditions Associated with Increased Risk of Cerebral Venous Thrombosis

- Antiphospholipid antibody/anticardiolipin antibody (immunoglobulins G and M)
- Protein S deficiency
- Protein C deficiency
- Antithrombin III deficiency
- G20210A prothrombin gene mutation
- Factor V Leiden mutation
- Hyperhomocysteinemia (may or may not be caused by gene polymorphism TT homozygosity in methylene tetrahydrofolate reductase)
- Homocystinuria
- Increased coagulation factor VIII
- Plasminogen deficiency

than in adults for both factor V Leiden gene variant (OR 2.74; 95%CI, 1.73–4.34) and prothrombin G20210A polymorphism (OR 1.95; 95%CI, 0.93–4.07).[37]

Infective causes of CVT have declined, being responsible for 6–12% in large series of adults.[1,8] In developing countries, systemic and nervous system infections may remain an important cause of CVT (18%).[38] Although uncommon, cavernous sinus thrombosis is caused predominantly by skin infections of the face.

Cancers account for 7.4% of CVT. Of these, 2.2% were associated with CNS malignancy, 3.2% with solid tumors outside the CNS, and 2.9% with hematologic disorders.[8] Sinus or venous thrombosis can result from local compression or invasion by the tumor, can be caused by a hypercoagulable state, or, less commonly, can be associated with local or systemic infections, can be therapy-related, or can be paraneoplastic.[39] Many of the precipitants of CVT are systemic diseases or conditions known to predispose to venous thrombosis in other parts of the body, but others are peculiar to CVT. Among the latter are local causes such as brain tumors or arteriovenous malformations, major or minor head trauma,[40] spontaneous intracranial hypotension,[41] and some invasive procedures (e.g., neurosurgery, jugular catheterization, irradiation, and lumbar puncture with or without drug infusion) (see Box 45-1).

The risk factors of CVT vary throughout life. In the Canadian Pediatric Ischemic Stroke Study Group, a risk factor was identified in 98% of the children.[6] In neonates, acute systemic illness such as perinatal complications and dehydration were frequent, occurring in 84% of patients.[6] Head and neck disorders, mostly infections, and chronic systemic diseases (e.g., connective tissue diseases, hematologic disorders, and cancers) were common in older children. A prothrombotic state was found in 41% of the patients, most often in non-neonates.

The most common risk factor in young women is oral contraceptive use. Two case-control studies have shown an increased risk of CVT in women taking oral contraceptives.[29,31] A meta-analysis showed that the risk of CVT in women taking oral contraceptives was almost six times higher than that of non-users (OR 5.59; 95%CI, 3.95–7.91).[36] The risk for women who use oral contraceptives and carry a prothrombotic defect is higher than that for women without such risk factors.[31] Another frequent setting related to CVT in women is pregnancy and the puerperium,[8,42,43] more common in less developed world regions with higher pregnancy rates.[44] CVT has also been diagnosed in association with the ovarian hyperstimulation syndrome resulting from in vitro fertilization.[45]

Despite extensive examination, no underlying risk factor is found in almost 13% of adult patients with CVT. The cause may be revealed weeks or months after the acute phase. Therefore, it is recommended to monitor the patient and to continue searching for a cause (vasculitis, antiphospholipid syndrome, cancer).

CLINICAL ASPECTS

The clinical presentation of CVT is highly variable.[1] In more than half of patients the onset is subacute, with symptoms increasing in intensity and severity over several days. In one-third of the patients the onset is acute, the full clinical picture being established within 24 hours, but onset is rarely apoplectic. A few cases have a protracted, chronic presentation. A patient with CVT manifesting as multiple transient ischemic attacks (TIAs) has also been reported.[47] Symptoms and signs of CVT can be grouped in three frequent syndromes, as follows: (1) isolated intracranial hypertension syndrome, consisting of headache with or without vomiting, papilledema, and visual troubles,[48] (2) focal syndrome, including focal deficits, seizures, or both, and (3) encephalopathy, with bilateral or multifocal signs, delirium, or dysexecutive or consciousness disturbances.[1,4] Less frequent syndromes include the (4) cavernous sinus syndrome, consisting of orbital pain, oculomotor palsies, proptosis, and chemosis and (5) syndromes of multiple palsies of the lower cranial nerves and subarachnoid haemorrhage, either generalized or localized at a single or few cortical sulci of the hemispheric convexity.[49,50]

Clinical symptoms and signs depend on the (1) gender and (2) age of the patient,[6,46] (3) on the interval from onset to presentation,[51,52] (4) on the presence of parenchymal lesions, (5) on site and number of occluded sinus and veins and (6) the underlying disease, if any. As in the general population, headaches are more frequent in women than in men with CVT. Symptoms of CVT differ in neonates and older children.[6] In neonates, presentation is often non-specific, with seizures in more than half of the babies, respiratory distress syndrome or apnea, poor feeding, lethargy, and hypotonia or hypertonia.[53] Diffuse signs of brain damage, with coma and seizures, are also the main manifestations in younger children. Clinical manifestations in older children, such as headache with or without vomiting, papilledema, sixth nerve palsy, motor deficits, focal or generalized seizures, and disturbances of consciousness, are more similar to the adult presentation.[6,54–56] Elderly patients have a clinical picture distinct from that in younger adults: decreased vigilance and mental symptoms are more common in the elderly, whereas headaches and isolated intracranial hypertension are less common.[46] The clinical picture also depends on the time elapsed from onset to presentation.[58] Patients with more severe clinical features, such as disturbance of consciousness or of mental status, seizures, or motor deficits, tend to present earlier.[52] Isolated intracranial hypertension and papilledema are more frequent in patients with a chronic presentation. As expected, if the admission neuroimaging shows either a hemorrhage or a venous infarct, the clinical picture is more severe. Coma and consciousness disturbances, paresis, aphasia, and seizures are more common in patients with such brain lesions than in subjects without them. Conversely, patients with brain lesions are less likely to present with isolated headache.

Up to 90% of patients with CVT complain of headache, which is the most frequent symptom of CVT and usually the initial one. In 9% of patients in the ISCVT, headache was the only symptom of CVT. As for other secondary headaches, headaches associated with CVT are more frequent in women and young patients. The localization of the headaches has no relationship with the localization of the occluded sinus or of the parenchymal lesions.[57,58] CVT-associated headaches are more severe and of more acute onset than other types of headaches requiring emergency care,[59] with the exception of subarachnoid hemorrhage. Headache is more frequently localized and continuous, with an acute–subacute onset of pain and moderate-to-severe intensity. The most frequent type of headache is the intracranial hypertension variety, a severe, generalized headache worsening with Valsalva's maneuvers and when the patient is lying down. Transient loss of vision can occur in association with spells of more intense headache. In CVT manifesting only as headache, the onset of the latter is usually progressive, and the pain is continuous. Headache is more often unilateral and ipsilateral to the occluded lateral sinus than it is diffuse.[60] A few cases of CVT manifesting only as sudden, explosive headache and neck stiffness,[61,62] mimicking subarachnoid hemorrhage, have been reported. In a minority of patients with headache and stiffness, the CSF is bloody, but in the majority, the headache meets the criteria of the thunderclap type.[63] Migraine with aura has also been reported.[64–66] CVT must also be included as a possible cause of persisting headache after lumbar puncture,[67] in particular if the pattern of headache changes, losing its characteristic postural relief when lying down.

Some patients may complain of visual loss (13% of cases) or are found to have papilledema (28%), a finding more frequent in chronic cases.[51] Severe acute cases of CVT manifest as disturbances of consciousness, ranging from drowsiness to coma (14%), or mental troubles (22%), such as delirium, apathy, or dysexecutive syndrome. Unilateral or, less frequently, bilateral motor deficits, in the form of monoparesis or hemiparesis, are the most common focal deficits (37%). Aphasia can also occur (19%). Fluent aphasia is a manifestation of an occlusion of the left lateral sinus with a posterior temporal lobe lesion. Sensory deficits (5%) and visual field defects are less common. Seizures are more frequent in CVT than in other stroke types. They can be focal (20%) or generalized (30%) and may be complicated by status epilepticus, which can occur rarely from the onset. Seizures are more frequent in patients with brain lesions, motor or sensory deficits, and sagittal sinus and cortical vein thrombosis.[68,69] Cerebellar signs are rare, but can be found in posterior fossa CVT with cerebellar venous infarct or haemorrhage.[70]

The clinical presentation of CVT also varies according to the location of the occluded sinus or vein. In cavernous sinus thrombosis, which is rare and usually has an infectious cause, ocular signs dominate the clinical picture, consisting of headache, orbital pain, chemosis, proptosis, ptosis, diplopia, and oculomotor palsies. Isolated cortical vein thrombosis is probably under-identified, and its diagnosis is difficult to confirm. The diagnostic accuracy is much improved by the use of T2 spin-echo (SE) sequences. Typically, cortical vein thrombosis produces motor or sensory deficits and seizures.[71–74] In occlusion of the sagittal sinus, motor deficits (46%) and focal (35%) and generalized (47%) seizures are frequent, but presentation as an isolated intracranial hypertension syndrome (17%) is infrequent. Bilateral motor deficits are not uncommon (7%). The opposite is found in patients with isolated thrombosis of the lateral sinus, who often at presentation have isolated intracranial hypertension (31–47%), but rarely have paresis (11–15%) or focal (9–12%) or generalized seizures (20–24%). Aphasia is frequent in left transverse sinus occlusion (40%). Multiple cranial nerve palsies (Collet-Sicard syndrome) are a rare manifestation of lateral sinus,[75] jugular, or posterior fossa vein thrombosis. A pulsating tinnitus may be the sole symptom of a jugular vein or lateral sinus thrombosis.[76,77] When the deep cerebral venous system is occluded, the clinical picture is often severe, with coma (67%), mental deficits (87%), and paresis (56%) that can be bilateral (11%).[78-80] In deep CVT, the severity of the clinical picture depends on the extent of the thrombosis in the deep veins and the territory of the involved vessels, the establishment of collaterals, and the duration of the occlusion. Limited thrombosis of the deep venous system can produce relatively mild symptoms without disturbances of consciousness.[81]

DIAGNOSIS

The confirmation of the diagnosis of CVT depends on the demonstration of thrombi in the cerebral veins or sinuses.

Computed Tomography

Computed tomography (CT) is usually the first investigation performed, particularly if patients are evaluated in an emergency setting. CT is useful to rule out other acute or subacute cerebral disorders that CVT may imitate, such as tumor, subdural hematoma, and abscess. CT is normal in up to 30% of cases of CVT, and most of the findings are nonspecific. CT signs are divided into direct and indirect. Direct signs of CVT, present in about one third of cases, correspond to the visualization of thrombus (Fig. 45-2):[1,82] the cord sign (thrombosed cortical or deep vein), the dense triangle sign (visualization of the clot inside the sinus), and the empty delta sign, visible after injection of a contrast agent as a contrast between the non-opacified thrombus inside the sinus and the collateral veins of the sinus wall. Indirect signs are more frequent and include intense contrast enhancement of falx and tentorium, dilated transcerebral veins, small ventricles, localized or diffuse white matter hypodensity without contrast enhancement, and hemorrhagic lesions. Parenchymal abnormalities may occur in 60–80% of cases, and some topographic lesions are suggestive of a specific sinus occlusion: bilateral parasagittal hemispheric lesions, temporooccipital lesions, and bilateral thalamic lesions, which are highly suspicious for thrombosis of the superior sagittal sinus, lateral sinus, and deep venous system, respectively. A small subdural hematoma or convexity subarachnoid hemorrhage may rarely be demonstrated (Fig. 45-3).[61] In serial CT scans, new lesions may appear, and some may disappear ("vanishing infarcts").

CT Venography

Helical CT venography with bolus injection of contrast material provides excellent anatomic detail of venous circulation and can demonstrate filling defects in the dural sinus and cortical veins, sinus wall enhancement, and increased collateral venous drainage (Fig. 45-4).[83,84]

CT venography has several advantages over intra-arterial angiography: it is less invasive and less expensive, and easy to be carried out immediately after brain CT. Visualization of the cavernous sinus, the inferior sagittal sinus, and the basal vein of Rosenthal with multiplanar reformatted images can be superior to that with conventional intra-arterial angiography.[85] There are some advantages of CT/CT venography over MRI in diagnosing CVT: rapid image acquisition, fewer motion artifacts, no contraindication to patients with ferromagnetic devices, and easier to be used in patients with claustrophobia.[84] Furthermore, CT venography is more commonly able to image sinuses or cerebral veins with low flow than is MR venography.[83] Some limitations of CT/CT venography are limited visualization of skull base structures in three-dimensional display, low resolution for small parenchymal

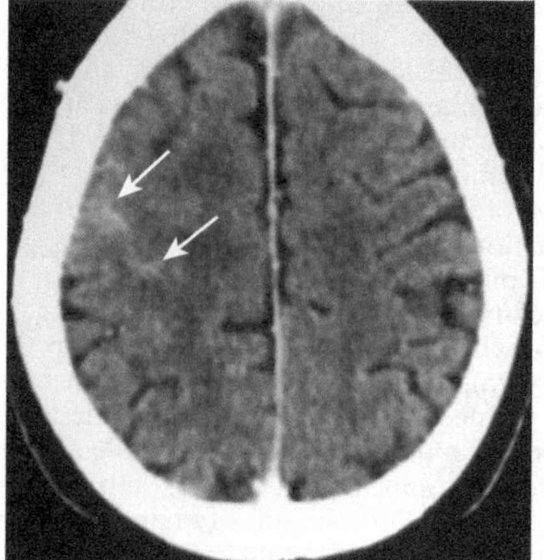

Figure 45-3. Subarachnoid hemorrhage as a manifestation of cerebral venous thrombosis *(arrows)*.

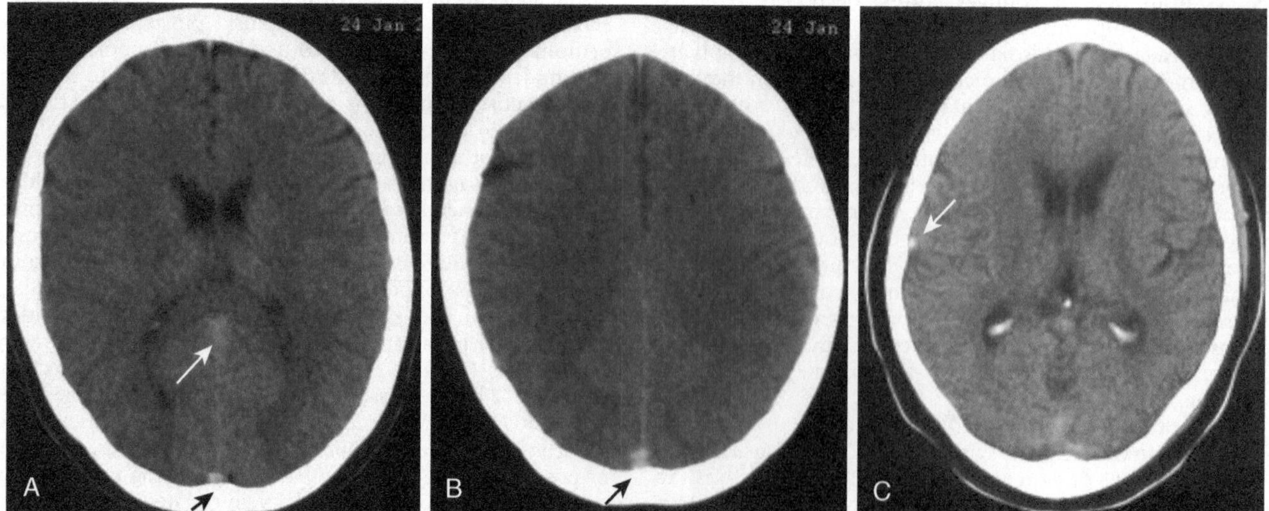

Figure 45-2. Unenhanced CT scans showing direct signs of cerebral thrombosis. A and B, The dense triangle sign – hyperdensities in the torcular Herophili (*A, black arrow*), the straight sinus (A, *white arrow*), and the superior sagittal sinus (B, *arrow*). C, The cord sign *(arrow)*.

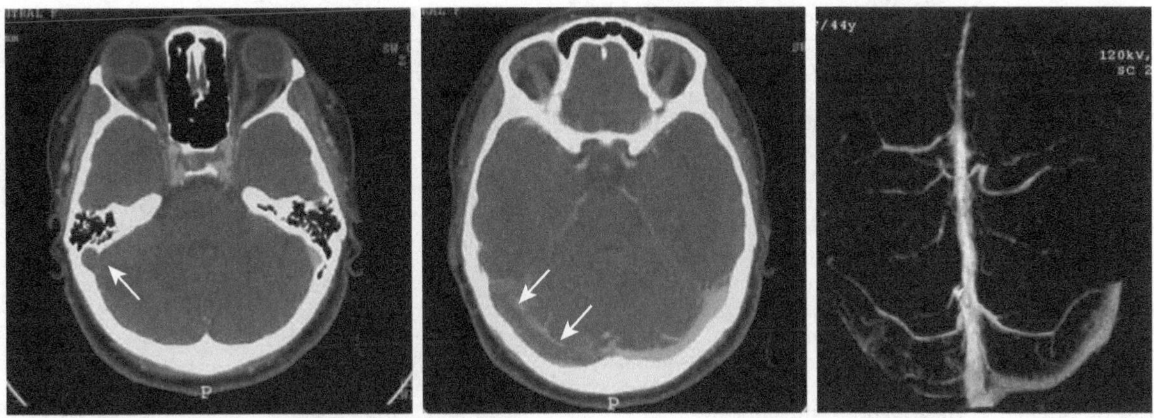

Figure 45-4. CT venograms in a patient with headache showing filling defects in the right lateral sinus *(arrows)*.

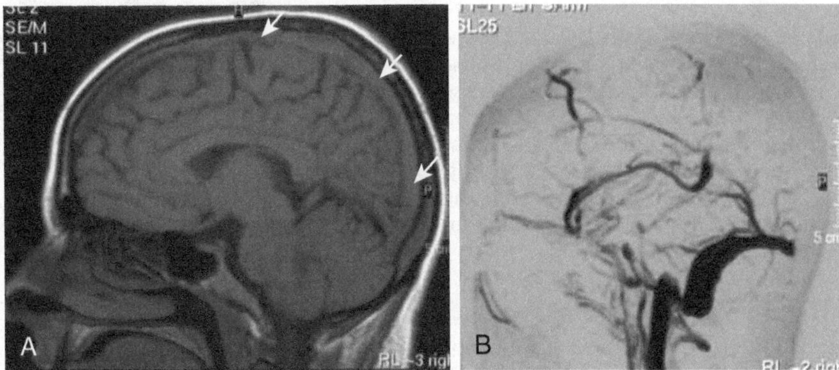

Figure 45-5. A, T1-weighted MR image discloses an isointense signal in the superior sagittal sinus *(arrows)*, corresponding to a thrombus. B, Magnetic resonance venogram showing the corresponding absence of flow.

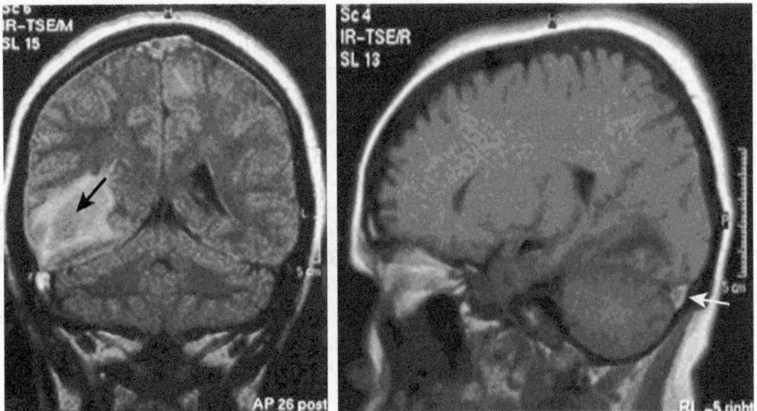

Figure 45-6. Lateral sinus thrombosis demonstrated as a hyperintense signal in T1- and T2-weighted FLAIR (fluid-attenuated inversion recovery) MR images. Concomitant hemorrhagic infarct can be seen *(arrow)*.

abnormalities, poor detection of cortical and deep venous thrombosis, exposure to ionizing radiation, adverse reactions to iodinated contrast medium, and risk of iodinated contrast nephropathy (e.g., in patients with diabetes, renal failure) which may limit its use in pregnant women, children, and patients with renal failure.[84]

Magnetic Resonance Techniques

MRI combined with MR venography is currently the best method to confirm the diagnosis of CVT: it is non-invasive, allows the visualization of the thrombi and the occluded dural sinus or vein, and depicts parenchymal lesions (Figs 45-5, 45-6).[1,79,86] Even so, there are some limitations and diagnostic pitfalls with MR.[87,88] The combination of an abnormal signal in a sinus and a corresponding absence of flow on MR venography support the diagnosis of CVT. Administration of contrast material and application of specific MR sequences and venographic techniques are often required for a confident diagnosis.

Magnetic Resonance Imaging

The signal intensity of the thrombus on T1- and T2-weighted MR images depends on the age of the thrombus: in the first 5 days, the signal is predominantly isointense on T1-weighted images and hypointense on T2-weighted images; after this time, the diagnosis becomes easier because of an increased signal on both T1- and T2-weighted images. After the first month, there is a variable pattern of signal, which may more frequently become isointense or hyperintense on T2-weighted images and hypointense or isointense on T1;[89,90] after gadolinium administration, marked contrast enhancement and flow voids may be observed within the thrombosed sinuses,[90] which could be related to organized thrombus with intrinsic vascularization, slow flow in dural and intrathrombus collateral channels, or recanalization. Echo-planar T2 susceptibility-weighted imaging (T2*SW) sequences improve the diagnosis of CVT, enabling the identification of intraluminal thrombus as a hypointense area. T2*SW sequences are particularly useful in the acute stage of dural sinus thrombosis and in the diagnosis of isolated cortical venous thrombosis.[73,86,91] On diffusion-weighted MRI, hyperintense signals in veins or dural sinus can be observed,[16,92] and may be predictive of a low rate of recanalization.[92]

MRI is also useful in showing parenchymal lesions secondary to venous occlusion: brain swelling, focal or diffuse edema (which is demonstrated as a hypointense or isointense lesion on T1-weighted images and a hyperintense lesion on T2-weighted images), and hemorrhagic lesions, which appear as hyperintense lesions on both MRI sequences. DWI abnormalities consistent with acute infarction may occur, but the degree of DWI findings may be reduced in venous infarction compared with arterial infarction.[11]

MR Venography

Several methods can assess venous or dural sinus flow: unenhanced 2D time-of-flight (TOF) MR venography, 3D TOF MR venography, contrast enhancement MR venography and phase-contrast MR venography.[88] In comparison with TOF MR venography, contrast enhancement MR venography with elliptic centric ordering allows superior depiction of small vessels and dural sinuses.[88,93]

The 2D TOF MR venography is the most commonly used method for the diagnosis of CVT, which typically demonstrates the absence of flow in the thrombosed vessel. MR venography has several limitations and potential pitfalls in the diagnosis of cortical vein thrombosis, of partial sinus occlusion, and distinction between hypoplasia and thrombosis. Other sequences such as T2* gradient echo, susceptibility weighted imaging, and contrast MRI/MRV may help in those situations. T2*gradient-echo sequence or susceptibility-weighted imaging will improve the diagnosis of cortical vein thrombosis. They can also be useful in the case of non-thrombosed hypoplastic sinus, which will not present abnormal low signal in T2*gradient-echo or SW imaging. The thrombosed hypoplastic sinus will have marked enhanced sinus signal and no flow on 2D TOF venography.

Intra-arterial Angiography

At present, intra-arterial angiography is rarely required for diagnosis. It may be performed mainly when the diagnosis of CVT is doubtful, namely, in the rare cases of isolated cortical vein thrombosis or when it is mandatory to exclude a dural arteriovenous fistula or distal aneurysm, such as in the presence of subarachnoid hemorrhage. Typical signs of CVT on angiography are partial or complete lack of filling of veins or sinuses, delayed emptying, dilated collaterals, and the sudden stopping of cortical veins surrounded by dilated and tortuous collateral "corkscrew veins" (Fig. 45-7). Anatomic variations may complicate the interpretation of angiography, such as hypoplasia of the anterior part of the superior sagittal sinus,

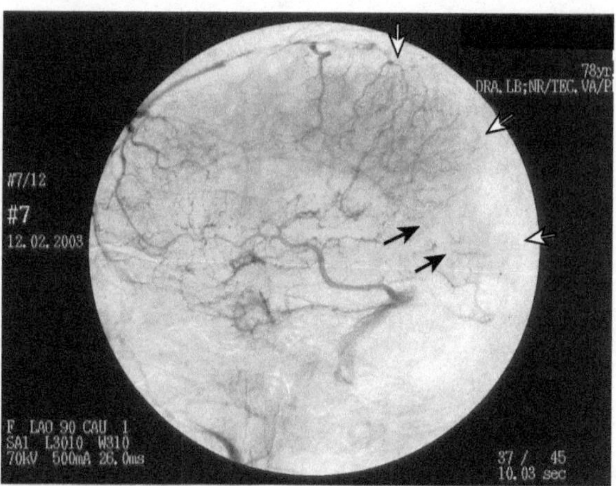

Figure 45-7. Intra-arterial angiogram showing typical signs of cerebral venous thrombosis: lack of filling of part of sagittal sinus *(white arrows)* and of the straight sinus *(black arrows)*; non-filling of the deep venous system; and dilated and tortuous collateral veins.

duplication of the superior sagittal sinus, and hypoplasia or aplasia of the transverse sinuses.[1]

Interobserver Agreement on Neuroimaging Diagnosis of Cerebral Venous Thrombosis

The interobserver agreement on CVT diagnostic imaging is not perfect. The proportion of agreement is 62% for intra-arterial angiography and 94% for MRI plus intra-arterial angiography.[94] A study using MRI and MR venography suggested that the agreement between observers in the diagnosis of the location of CVT varies with the location of sinus or vein thrombosis. It is good or very good for most of the occluded sinus and veins, moderate to very good for the left lateral sinus and jugular vein, and poor to good for the cortical veins.[95]

Transcranial Doppler Ultrasonography

Transcranial Doppler ultrasonography[96,97] and transcranial power or color Doppler imaging, with or without the use of a contrast agent,[98-100] were reported as potential non-invasive techniques for the diagnosis or follow-up of CVT, but more studies are needed to determine the true clinical value of these methods.

D-Dimer Levels

A systematic review examined 14 published studies that had analyzed the value of measuring plasma levels of the fibrin degradation product D-dimer in the diagnosis of 1134 patients with CVT.[101] D-dimer accuracy was good, with a sensitivity of 93.9% (95%CI, 87.5–97.1) and specificity of 89.7% (95%CI, 86.5–92.2). Importantly, potential conditions for false-negative D-dimer results included isolated headache, longer duration of symptoms, and small extent of sinus involvement. Subsequently, a cohort of 71 CVT patients found low levels of D-dimer in 12% of patients. Longer symptom duration was correlated with low D-dimer levels, reinforcing that low levels of D-dimer cannot reliably exclude CVT in patients with subacute or chronic disease.[102]

Although D-dimer may be a useful diagnostic tool of particular clinical presentations of CVT, a normal D-dimer level cannot rule out the diagnosis, and, consequently, measurement of plasma D-dimer level is not a good screening test in patients with suspected CVT.

PROGNOSIS

Several prospective series,[103] and above all the large ISCVT cohort,[8] clarified the contemporary prognosis of patients with acute CVT. The aggregate rate of death or dependency at the end of follow-up in these studies was 15%. In the ISCVT cohort, 79% of patients recovered completely. In a meta-analysis that also included retrospective studies, the overall rate of acute death was 5.6%, that of death at the end of follow-up was 9.4%, and that of complete recovery was 88%.[104] Predictors of poor long-term prognosis derived from the ISCVT cohort were CNS infection, malignancy, deep cerebral venous system thrombosis, hemorrhage on admission CT/MRI, Glasgow Coma Scale score on admission less than 9, mental status disorder, age older than 37 years, and male gender.[8] This predictive model was validated in two independent cohorts.[105] From the model a risk score was derived: 2 points each for malignancy, thrombosis of the deep venous system and coma; 1 point each for mental status disturbance, intracerebral haemorrhage and male gender. A score of ≥3 points indicates a higher risk of unfavourable outcome.[105]

Although patients with CVT often have a favorable prognosis, 4% die during the acute phase. Predictors of mortality at 30 days in the ISCVT cohort were depressed consciousness, mental status disorder, thrombosis of the deep cerebral venous system, right hemispheric hemorrhage, and posterior fossa lesions.[106] The main cause of death in acute CVT is transtentorial herniation secondary to a large hemorrhagic lesion.[106] Other causes of death are herniation due to multiple lesions or to diffuse brain edema, status epilepticus, medical complications, and pulmonary embolism.[107]

Among patients with CVT who have hemorrhagic lesions, 21% are dead or dependent at 6 months.[108] Prognosis is less favorable in patients at both extremes of age. One study found that the prognosis in adults older than 64 years is considerably worse than that in younger patients.[46] Only 47% of elderly patients made a complete recovery, whereas 27% died and 22% were dependent at the end of follow-up. In children, the death, dependency, and late complication rates are also higher than those in adults. The death rate ranges from 2% to 13%,[6,56,109,110] especially in neonates, whose mortality may be as high as 25%.[56] Only 22% of neonates survive free of any impairment.[53] Half of the deaths are a direct consequence of the venous thrombosis.[6] Sequelae of CVT include cognitive and motor impairments, seizures, and symptomatic persistent increased intracranial hypertension. Predictors of unfavorable outcome include coma, seizures, and venous infarcts,[6,56] whereas older age, anticoagulation, and transverse sinus involvement were predictors of good cognitive outcome, although the last item predicted isolated intracranial hypertension syndrome.[110] Women have a better prognosis than men (complete recovery 81% vs 71%), which may relate to gender-specific risk factors (oral contraceptives, pregnancy-puerperium). Women without gender-specific risk factors have an outcome similar to men.[111]

Classically, the clinical course of CVT is unpredictable.[1] Clinical course after admission was prospectively investigated in the ISCVT cohort, with the following conclusions: about one-fourth of the patients deteriorate in status after admission. Neurologic worsening may occur several days after admission and may consist of depressed consciousness, mental state disturbance, new seizures, worsening of a previous symptom or a new focal deficit, increase in headache severity, or visual loss. About one-third of patients whose status deteriorates show new parenchymal lesions on repeat neuroimaging.[112] Deterioration is less frequent but can occur in patients presenting with isolated headache or with isolated intracranial hypertension syndrome.

Patients who survive the acute phase of CVT are at risk for complications; especially further venous thrombotic events, seizures, and headaches. The underlying disease, in particular malignancies, may lead to death in the months or years following CVT. Headaches severe enough to require bed rest or hospital admission afflict 14% of patients with CVT.[8] MRI and MR venography are necessary to exclude recurrent CVT and other intracranial lesions and to document persistent cerebral venous occlusion, partial or complete sinus recanalization, or dural sinus stenosis.

Recurrent CVT is rare and sometimes difficult to document. It is useful for the patient to undergo MRI/MR angiography 3–6 months after CVT to document the extent of recanalization. If new symptoms suggesting recurrence of CVT, such as new headaches or headaches increasing in severity, seizures, or a new focal sign, occur, MRI and MR venography should be performed and the images compared with original images. Other thrombotic events, specifically DVT of the limbs or pelvis and pulmonary embolism, occur in about 5% of patients. In the Mayo Clinic case series of 154 patients with CVT followed for a mean of 36 months, recurrent CVT occurred in 6.5%.[113] In the ISCVT cohort 2.2 % had a recurrent CVT and 4.3% had other thrombotic events. Male gender and polycythemia/thrombocythemia were associated with a higher risk of recurrent venous thrombotic events.[114] Similar rates were found in a series from a thrombosis center, where male gender and severe thrombophilia entailed an increased risk of venous thrombosis.[115] The rate of further venous thrombotic events is similar in children: in a European cohort of 396 children with CVT (median age 5.2 years) followed for a median of 36 months, recurrent venous thrombosis occurred in 22 (6%) children at a median of 6 months, including CVT in 13 children (3%).[109] There were no recurrences of CVT among children younger than 25 months. Absence of administration of anticoagulant therapy before relapse, persistent venous occlusion on repeat venous imaging, and heterozygosity for the prothrombin G20210A mutation[109] were independently associated with recurrent cerebral and systemic venous thrombosis in children.

Seizures may occur in up to 11% of patients. Risk factors for these remote seizures are seizures during the acute phase, a hemorrhagic supratentorial parenchymal lesion, and a motor deficit.[116,117]

Severe visual loss due to intracranial hypertension is very rare.[8,103,118] However, when evaluated by a neuroophthalmologist, a few CVT survivors may be found to have subnormal visual acuity or visual fields as well as esodeviation.[118]

Psychological and cognitive complaints are not uncommon among CVT survivors. About half of the survivors of CVT feel depressed or anxious[119] and demonstrate minor cognitive or language deficits,[120] which may preclude resumption of previous levels of professional activity.[121]

An important practical question is the outcome of future pregnancies in women who have had a CVT. Information to answer this question is available in few studies.[8,43,103,122,123] The large majority (88%) of the pregnancies ended in normal births, the remaining being prematurely terminated by voluntary or spontaneous abortion. The rate of spontaneous abortion was higher than expected. There were no instances of recurrent CVT and only two cases of DVT out of 101 pregnancies.

Recanalization of thrombosed cerebral vein and sinus occurs in 40–90% of patients after CVT, mostly within the first 4 months.[124] This process was confirmed by a systematic review that identified only five small studies evaluating recanalization after CVT. In the pooled population of these studies, recanalization rates at 3 months (84%) and 1 year of follow-up (85%) were nearly identical. Recanalization is more common after thrombosis of the deep cerebral veins and of the cavernous sinuses, and less common in lateral sinus occlusion.[124]

Limited data suggest that recanalization of the occluded sinus is not related to outcome after CVT;[125] in children, however, non-recanalization is associated with higher risk of recurrence.[109] The presence of hyperintensities in the veins or sinus on DWI sequences predicts a low chance of recanalization.[92]

TREATMENT

The treatment of CVT includes (1) antithrombotic treatment, (2) symptomatic treatment of intracranial hypertension, seizures, headache, and visual failure, and (3) etiologic treatment to manage the associated conditions and risk factors, which is beyond the scope of this chapter (Box 45-3). Guidelines for the treatment of cerebral venous and sinus thrombosis were issued by the European Federation of Neurological Societies (EFNS) in 2006[126] and the American Heart Association/American Stroke Association.[127]

The therapeutic priorities in the acute phase are to stabilize the hemodynamic and physiologic parameters, to prevent or reverse cerebral herniation, to stop seizures, and to treat infections or other associated conditions needing urgent management.

Antithrombotic Treatment

The aims of antithrombotic treatment in CVT are (1) to recanalize the occluded sinus or vein, (2) to combat the propagation of the thrombus, namely to the bridging cerebral veins, thus preventing cerebral edema and infarct, (3) to prevent pulmonary embolism,[107] and (4) to treat the underlying prothrombotic state in order to prevent venous thrombosis in other parts of the body and the recurrence of CVT.

Two randomized controlled trials (RCTs) of anticoagulation in acute CVT have been performed in Europe.[128,129] Both have some methodologic problems, namely their modest sample size, selection, and measurement bias. The trial performed by Einhäupl and coworkers[129] compared intravenous (IV) heparin with placebo. This trial showed a significantly better outcome for patients randomly assigned to the heparin arm. The Dutch trial compared subcutaneous (SC) nadroparin with placebo. This trial showed a non-significant difference, but a trend toward superiority of nadroparin over placebo. Two other trials were performed in India, but for these trials, outcome assessment was not blind, and the diagnosis of CVT was confirmed by CT alone.[130,131] Two cases of pulmonary embolism occurred in the placebo groups of the German and Dutch trials. The meta-analysis of the German and Dutch trials showed a relative risk of 0.46 (95%CI, 0.16–1.31) (60% relative risk reduction) of death or dependency after anticoagulant therapy in comparison with placebo.[132]

There is a theoretical safety concern because heparin might cause venous infarcts to become hemorrhagic or might increase bleeding in already existing hemorrhagic lesions. In case series, the risks of intracranial hemorrhage (<5%) and systemic hemorrhage (<2%) were also low, and such hemorrhages did not influence outcome.[133] Anticoagulants are also safe to use in patients with intracranial hemorrhages, either intracerebral or subarachnoid.[126] This finding is in accord with the fact that such intracranial hemorrhages are secondary to venous outflow blockage. Anticoagulant therapy is also safe in children.[134] Both the German and Dutch trials included patients with hemorrhagic infarcts on baseline scans, but there were no intracranial hemorrhagic complications and only one major extracranial bleed. These findings support the choice of full anticoagulation with intravenous heparin or subcutaneous high-dose low-molecular-weight heparin (LMWH) as the initial treatment for nearly all patients with acute or subacute sinus thrombosis. There is a large consensus on the use of heparin or LMWH in acute CVT. For instance, more than 80% of the patients in the ISCVT underwent anticoagulation.[135] The European Federation of Neurological Societies guidelines on the treatment of CVT recommended that patients with CVT but with no contraindications to anticoagulation should be treated either with aPTT-adjusted IV heparin or with body-weight-adjusted LMWH.[126]

Although antiplatelet drugs may be used as alternatives when anticoagulants are contraindicated, there is no evidence,

BOX 45-3 Treatment of Cerebral Venous Thrombosis (CVT): Fundamentals Following European Federation of Neurological Societies Guidelines

ACUTE PHASE

Treatment of the Etiology

Antithrombotic Treatment

Subcutaneous low-molecular-weight heparin or intravenous heparin in therapeutic dosages

In experienced centers, if neurologic worsening occurs despite heparin and the best medical treatment and other causes of deterioration are excluded, local intravenous thrombolysis with/without mechanical thrombectomy is an option

Symptomatic Treatment

Antiepileptics
- In patients with acute seizures and supratentorial lesions
- Consider as an option also for patients with either acute seizures or supratentorial lesions

Intracranial hypertension
- Headache
  - Analgesics
  - Lumbar puncture, if there are no parenchymal lesions; perform before starting anticoagulation
  - Acetazolamide

Impairment of consciousness of herniation
- Osmotic therapy
- Sedation and hyperventilation
- Hemicraniectomy

Threatened vision
- Lumbar puncture, if there are no parenchymal lesions; perform before starting anticoagulation
- Acetazolamide
- Lumboperitoneal shunt
- Optic nerve fenestration

POST-ACUTE PHASE

Treatment of the Etiology

Antithrombotic Treatment

Oral anticoagulants

For 3–6 months if CVT related to a transient risk factor

For 6–12 months if CVT idiopathic or related to "mild" hereditary thrombophilia

For life for recurrent CVT or "severe" hereditary thrombophilia

Symptomatic Treatment

Antiepileptics
- In patients with acute seizures or seizures in the post-acute phase and supratentorial lesions
- Consider as an option also for patients without seizures but with either supratentorial lesions or motor deficits

even from uncontrolled series, regarding the efficacy and safety of antiplatelet agents in CVT.

Thrombolysis

The majority of patients with CVT experience a good outcome, but 4% die during the acute phase of CVT,[106] and the condition of some patients worsens despite anticoagulant therapy. Direct thrombolysis has been used as an alternative treatment in the latter case. Direct thrombolysis aims to dissolve the thrombus by delivering a thrombolytic substance (urokinase or recombinant tissue plasminogen activator [rt-PA]) within the occluded sinus (transverse, superior sagittal, or straight sinus) through an IV catheter. In some cases, mechanical endovascular disruption of the thrombus alone or in combination with chemical thrombolysis has also been used. Endovascular thrombolysis, when successful, can remove the thrombus from the major sinuses within hours. However, this procedure is complicated and expensive. The patient needs anesthesia and intensive care monitoring, and usually the catheter remains in the sinus for hours to days, with repeated applications of the thrombolytic agent and radiologic assessments.

Many case reports or case series describing the use of thrombolytics have been published, suggesting that these agents might be useful and safe, but no RCTs evaluating the efficacy and safety of systemic or local thrombolysis in patients with CVT have yet been completed. In a systematic review of 169 patients treated with local thrombolysis, only 5% died during the acute phase of CVT, and 8% were dependent at discharge.[136] The results of this systematic review suggest a possible benefit of thrombolytics in cases of severe CVT, indicating that the agents may reduce the case fatality rate in critically ill patients. Intracranial hemorrhages were reported in 17% of cases and were associated with clinical deterioration in 5%. Extracranial hemorrhages were reported in 19% of cases and were severe in 2%. A more recent systematic review emphasized the non-negligible incidence of major bleeding (9.8%) complications, including 7.6% of intracranial hemorrhages, 58.3% of which were fatal.[137] Furthermore, there is certainly publication bias in the literature for this issue, with under-reporting of cases with poor outcomes and complications. Treatment and evaluation were non-blinded, leading to bias in evaluating outcomes. In a Dutch series of 20 patients treated with IV local thrombolysis, 12 recovered to independent living, and six died.[138] Local thrombolysis was not useful in patients with large infarcts and impending herniation. These results are worse than those in the previously published literature, but may reflect the prevailing results in clinical practice. Currently, there is no evidence to support the routine use of thrombolysis. Endovascular thrombolysis may be performed in selected centers with expertise in interventional radiology as a therapeutic option in patients with a poor prognosis (e.g., those with thrombosis of the cerebral deep venous system whose condition worsens despite best medical treatment and anticoagulation), provided that other causes of the worsening condition are excluded and treated. A randomized trial to compare endovascular treatment (TO-ACT) is currently ongoing.[139]

Prevention of Thrombotic Events after the Acute Phase

After the acute phase of CVT, recurrence of cerebral venous thrombosis can be detected in 2% to 7% of patients and extracerebral venous thrombosis can occur in up to 5%. To prevent further thrombotic events, anticoagulation with warfarin is recommended. In the Rochester Mayo Clinic series, the likelihood of recurrent venous thrombosis was the same after CVT and lower-extremity DVT. Recurrence of CVT was not influenced by warfarin therapy.[113] In children, non-administration of anticoagulation predicts recurrent CVT or systemic venous thrombosis.[127] The optimal duration of anticoagulation is not known, because it was not addressed in RCTs. Anticoagulation is usually maintained for 3–12 months after acute CVT, aiming at an international normalized ratio (INR) of 2–3. The EFNS and the AHA/ASA guidelines suggest that when CVT is related to a transient risk factor (e.g., pregnancy, infection), anticoagulants may be used for a short period (3 or 3–6 months). In patients with idiopathic CVT or CVT associated with "mild" thrombophilia, the period of anticoagulation must be longer (6 to 12 months). In patients with "combined" or "severe" thrombophilia (e.g., two or more prothrombotic abnormalities; antithrombin, protein C or S deficiencies, antiphospholipid syndrome, cancer), or recurrent venous thrombosis, anticoagulants should be given for life.

Symptomatic Treatment

Treatment of Intracranial Hypertension

In the acute phase, increased intracranial pressure (ICP) due to single or multiple large hemorrhagic lesions, infarcts, or massive brain edema may be fatal by causing transtentorial herniation. General recommendations to control acutely increased ICP include elevating the head of the bed, osmotic diuretics such as mannitol, intensive care unit admission with sedation, hyperventilation to a target $PaCO_2$ of 30 to 35 mm Hg, and ICP monitoring.[126] Although corticosteroids may decrease vasogenic edema, they cannot be recommended routinely to decrease ICP. Steroids may even promote thrombosis. A case-control study failed to demonstrate any benefit of steroids even in patients with parenchymal lesions.[140] In patients with acute CVT who have severe headache with or without papilledema, intracranial hypertension can be reduced and symptoms relieved through a therapeutic lumbar puncture when not contraindicated by parenchymal lesions. In patients with impending herniation due to large unilateral hemispherical lesion, decompressive surgery, either hemicraniectomy or hematoma evacuation, is life-saving and often results in good functional outcome, even in patients with severe clinical conditions.[141–143] In a multicenter registry and systematic review of published cases, 38% recovered completely. Only 16% died and 6% were alive and severely dependent.[141] Shunting alone is not effective in preventing death from brain herniation in acute CVT. Acute obstructive hydrocephalus is rare in acute CVT. Despite shunting half of these patients have a bad outcome.[144]

In patients with chronically increased intracranial pressure, treatment of intracranial hypertension is necessary to improve headache and prevent visual failure. A diagnostic/therapeutic lumbar puncture decreases the CSF pressure and offers headache relief. Although its efficacy is not proven, administration of a diuretic such as acetazolamide or furosemide is a therapeutic option. If severe headaches persist or if visual acuity is decreasing, repeated lumbar punctures, a lumboperitoneal shunt, stenting of a sinus stenosis,[145–147] or fenestration of the optic nerve sheath can be considered.[148,149]

Treatment and Prevention of Seizures

Acute seizures and supratentorial lesions are the risk factors for subsequent early seizures. Patients with seizures or with both risk factors should be prescribed antiepileptic drugs. Prophylactic antiepileptics are not recommended for patients without seizures.[68,126,127]

The long-term risk of remote seizures is approximately 11%.[8,69,116] The risk factors for remote seizures and post-CVT epilepsy are acute seizures, supratentorial hemorrhagic lesions, and motor deficits. Antiepileptics are recommended for patients with seizures in the acute phase of CVT and for those who experience a seizure after the acute phase.[126,127] The optimal duration of antiepileptic treatment is unknown. General recommendations for the selection and withdrawal of antiepileptic drugs can be used as options. Patients with status epilepticus should be treated according to guidelines for this epileptic condition.

CONTRACEPTION AND FUTURE PREGNANCIES

Women of fertile age with past CVT should not become pregnant while taking an oral anticoagulant, because of its teratogenic effects. They should use contraceptive methods other than oral or parenteral contraceptives. Emergency contraception is also contraindicated.[150] Hormonal replacement therapy should also be stopped. CVT and pregnancy and puerperium-related CVT are not contraindications to future pregnancy. Although pregnancy and the puerperium are risk factors for CVT, the risk of complications and of venous thrombotic events during subsequent pregnancy among women who have a history of CVT is low.[8,43,122,123]

There is no indication for termination of pregnancy either in acute CVT during pregnancy or in woman who became pregnant after a CVT. The only exception is if they became pregnant while taking oral anticoagulants.

REFERENCES

1. Bousser MG, Russell RR. Cerebral venous thrombosis. In: Warlow CP, Van Gijn J, editors. Major problems in neurology, vol. 33. London: WB Saunders; 1997.
2. Kalbag RM, Woolf AL. Cerebral venous thrombosis. London: Oxford University Press; 1967.
3. Bienfait HP, van Duinen S, Tans JT. Latent cerebral venous and sinus thrombosis. J Neurol 2003;250:436–9.
4. Ferro JM, Correia M, Pontes C, et al., for the Cerebral Venous Thrombosis Portuguese Collaboration Study Group (VENOPORT). Cerebral venous thrombosis in Portugal 1980–98. Cerebrovasc Dis 2001;11:177–82.
5. Lanska DJ, Kryscio RJ. Risk factors for peripartum and postpartum stroke and intracranial venous thrombosis. Stroke 2000;31:1274–82.
6. deVeber G, Andrew M, Adams C, et al. Canadian Pediatric Ischemic Stroke Study Group: Cerebral sinovenous thrombosis in children. N Engl J Med 2001;345:417–23.
7. Coutinho JM, Zuurbier SM, Aramideh M, et al. The incidence of cerebral venous thrombosis: a cross-sectional study. Stroke 2012;43:3375–7.
8. Ferro JM, Canhão P, Stam J, et al. ISCVT Investigators: Prognosis of cerebral vein and dural sinus thrombosis: Results of the International Study on Cerebral Vein and Dural Sinus Thrombosis (ISCVT). Stroke 2004;35:664–70.
9. Ferro JM, Lopes GC, Rosas MJ, et al. VENOPORT Investigators: Chronobiology of cerebral vein and dural sinus thrombosis. Cerebrovasc Dis 2002;14:265.
10. Stolz E, Klötzsch C, Rahimi A, et al. Seasonal variations in the incidence of cerebral venous thrombosis. Cerebrovasc Dis 2003;16:455–6.
11. Keller E, Flacke S, Urbach H, et al. Diffusion- and perfusion-weighted magnetic resonance imaging in deep cerebral venous thrombosis. Stroke 1999;30:1144–6.
12. Manzione J, Newman GC, Shapiro A, et al. Diffusion- and perfusion-weighted MR imaging of dural sinus thrombosis. AJNR Am J Neuroradiol 2000;21:68–73.
13. Doege CA, Tavakolian R, Kerskens CM, et al. Perfusion and diffusion magnetic resonance imaging in human cerebral venous thrombosis. J Neurol 2001;248:564–71.
14. Ducreux D, Oppenheim C, Vandamme X, et al. Diffusion-weighted imaging patterns of brain damage associated with cerebral venous thrombosis. AJNR Am J Neuroradiol 2001;22:261–8.
15. Forbes KP, Pipe JG, Heiserman JE. Evidence for cytotoxic edema in the pathogenesis of cerebral venous infarction. AJNR Am J Neuroradiol 2001;22:450–5.
16. Lövblad KO, Bassetti C, Schneider J, et al. Diffusion-weighted MR in cerebral venous thrombosis. Cerebrovasc Dis 2001;11:169–76.
17. Peeters E, Stadnik T, Bissay F, et al. Diffusion-weighted MR imaging of an acute venous stroke. AJNR Am J Neuroradiol 2001;22:1949–52.
18. Yoshikawa T, Abe O, Tsuchiya K, et al. Diffusion-weighted magnetic resonance imaging of dural sinus thrombosis. Neuroradiology 2002;44:481–8.
19. Makkat S, Stadnik T, Peeters E, et al. Pathogenesis of venous stroke: Evaluation with diffusion- and perfusion-weighted MRI. J Stroke Cerebrovascular Dis 2003;12:132–6.
20. Mullins ME, Grant PE, Wang B, et al. Parenchymal abnormalities associated with cerebral venous sinus thrombosis: Assessment with diffusion-weighted MR imaging. AJNR Am J Neuroradiol 2004;25:1666–75.
21. Schaller B, Graf R. Cerebral venous infarction: The pathophysiological concept. Cerebrovasc Dis 2004;18:179–88.
22. Gotoh M, Ohmoto T, Kuyama H. Experimental study of venous circulatory disturbance by dural sinus occlusion. Acta Neurochir (Wien) 1993;124:120–6.
23. Frerichs KU, Deckert M, Kempski O, et al. Cerebral sinus and venous thrombosis in rats induces long-term deficits in brain function and morphology: Evidence for a cytotoxic genesis. J Cereb Blood Flow Metab 1994;14:289–300.
24. Rother J, Waggie K, van Bruggen N, et al. Experimental cerebral venous thrombosis: Evaluation using magnetic resonance imaging. J Cereb Blood Flow Metab 1996;16:1353–61.
25. Röttger C, Trittmacher S, Gerriets T, et al. Reversible MR imaging abnormalities following cerebral venous thrombosis. AJNR Am J Neuroradiol 2005;26:607–13.
26. Biousse V, Conard J, Brouzes C. Frequency of 20210 GA mutation in the 3′-untranslated region of the prothrombin gene in 35 cases of cerebral venous thrombosis. Stroke 1998;29:1398–400.
27. Reuner KH, Ruf A, Grau A, et al. Prothrombin gene G20210→A transition is a risk factor for cerebral venous thrombosis. Stroke 1998;29:1765–9.
28. Weih M, Vetter B, Castell S, et al. Hereditary thrombophilia in cerebral venous thrombosis. Cerebrovasc Dis 2000;10:161–2.
29. Martinelli I, Sacchi E, Landi G, et al. High risk of cerebral-vein thrombosis in carriers of prothrombin-gene mutation and in users of oral contraceptives. N Engl J Med 1998;338:1793–7.
30. Deschiens MA, Conard J, Horellou MH, et al. Coagulation studies, factor V Leiden, and anticardiolipin antibodies in 40 cases of cerebral venous thrombosis. Stroke 1996;27:1724–30.
31. de Bruijn SF, Stam J, Koopman MM, et al. Case-control study of risk of cerebral sinus thrombosis in oral contraceptive users and in carriers of hereditary prothrombotic conditions. BMJ 1998;316:589–92.
32. Ludemann P, Nabavi DG, Junker R, et al. Factor V Leiden mutation is a risk factor for cerebral venous thrombosis: A case-control study of 55 patients. Stroke 1998;29:2507–10.
33. Zuber M, Toulon P, Marnet L, et al. Factor V Leiden mutation in cerebral venous thrombosis. Stroke 1996;27:1721–3.
34. Marjot T, Yadav S, Hasan N, et al. Genes associated with adult cerebral venous thrombosis. Stroke 2011;42:913–18.
35. Gouveia LO, Canhão P. Allele 677T MTHFR: Prothrombotic risk factor for cerebral venous thrombosis? A meta-analysis. Cerebrovasc Dis 2008;25:152–3.
36. Dentali F, Crowther M, Ageno W. Thrombophilic abnormalities, oral contraceptives, and the risk of cerebral vein thrombosis: A meta-analysis. Blood 2006;107:2766–73.
37. Kenet G, Lutkhoff LK, Albisetti M, et al. Impact of thrombophilia on risk of arterial ischemic stroke or cerebral sinovenous thrombosis in neonates and children: a systematic review and meta-analysis of observational studies. Circulation 2010;121:1838–47.
38. Khealani BA, Wasay M, Saadah M, et al. Cerebral venous thrombosis: A descriptive multicenter study of patients in Pakistan and Middle East. Stroke 2008;39:2707–11.

39. Grisold W, Oberndorfer S, Struhal W. Stroke and cancer: A review. Acta Neurol Scand 2009;119:1–16.
40. Dalgiç A, Seçer M, Ergüngör F, et al. Dural sinus thrombosis following head injury: Report of two cases and review of the literature. Turk Neurosurg 2008;18:70–7.
41. Savoiardo M, Armenise S, Spagnolo P, et al. Dural sinus thrombosis in spontaneous intracranial hypotension: Hypothesis on possible mechanisms. J Neurol 2006;253:1197–202.
42. Cantu C, Barinagarrementeria F. Cerebral venous thrombosis associated with pregnancy and puerperium; Review of 67 cases. Stroke 1993;24:1880–4.
43. Srinivasan K. Cerebral venous and arterial thrombosis in pregnancy and puerperium: A study of 135 patients. Angiology 1983; 34:731–46.
44. Canhão P, Bousser MG, Barinagarrementeria F, et al. ISCVT Collaborators: Predisposing conditions for cerebral vein thrombosis. J Neurol 2002;249(Suppl. 1):52.
45. Edris F, Kerner CM, Feyles V, et al. Successful management of an extensive intracranial sinus thrombosis in a patient undergoing IVF: Case report and review of the literature. Fertil Steril 2007;88: 705.e9–e14.
46. Ferro JM, Canhão P, Bousser MG, et al. ISCVT Investigators: Cerebral vein and dural sinus thrombosis in elderly patients. Stroke 2005;36:1927–32.
47. Ferro JM, Falcão F, Melo TP, et al. Dural sinus thrombosis mimicking "capsular warning syndrome". J Neurol 2000;247: 802–3.
48. Biousse V, Ameri A, Bousser MG. Isolated intracranial hypertension as the only sign of cerebral venous thrombosis. Neurology 1999;53:1537–42.
49. Oppenheim C, Domigo V, Gauvrit JY, et al. Subarachnoid hemorrhage as the initial presentation of dural sinus thrombosis. AJNR Am J Neuroradiol 2005;26:614–17.
50. Geraldes R, Sousa PR, Fonseca AC, et al. Nontraumatic convexity subarachnoid hemorrhage: different etiologies and outcomes. J Stroke Cerebrovasc Dis 2014;23:e23–30.
51. Ferro JM, Lopes MG, Rosas MJ, et al. VENOPORT Investigators: Delay in hospital admission of patients with cerebral vein and dural sinus thrombosis. Cerebrovasc Dis 2005;19:152–6.
52. Ferro JM, Canhão P, Stam J, et al. ISCVT Investigators: Delay in the diagnosis of cerebral vein and dural sinus thrombosis : Influence on outcome. Stroke 2009;40:3133–8.
53. Fitzgerald KC, Williams LS, Garg BP, et al. Cerebral sinovenous thrombosis in the neonate. Arch Neurol 2006;63:405–9.
54. Lancon JA, Killough KR, Tibbs RE, et al. Spontaneous dural sinus thrombosis in children. Pediatr Neurosurg 1999;30:23–9.
55. Heller C, Heinecke A, Junker R, et al. Childhood Stroke Study Group: Cerebral venous thrombosis in children: A multifactorial origin. Circulation 2003;108:1362–7.
56. Wasay M, Dai AI, Ansari M, et al. Cerebral venous sinus thrombosis in children: A multicenter cohort from the United States. J Child Neurol 2008;23:26–31.
57. Ameri A, Bousser MG. Headache in cerebral venous thrombosis: A study of 110 cases. Cephalalgia 1993;13:110.
58. Lopes MG, Ferro J, Pontes C, et al. for the Venoport Investigators: Headache and cerebral venous thrombosis. Cephalalgia 2000;20: 292.
59. Iurlaro S, Ciccone E, Beghi A, et al. Headache in early diagnosis of cerebral venous thrombosis: Clinical experience in 59 patients. Cerebrovasc Dis 2003;16:109.
60. Cumurciuc R, Crassard I, Sarov M, et al. Headache as the only neurological sign of cerebral venous thrombosis: A series of 17 cases. J Neurol Neurosurg Psychiatry 2005;76:1084–97.
61. Sztajzel R, Coeytaux A, Dehdashti AR, et al. Subarachnoid hemorrhage: A rare presentation of cerebral venous thrombosis. Headache 2001;41:889–92.
62. Oppenheim C, Domingo V, Gauvrit JY, et al. Subarachnoid hemorrhage as the initial presentation of dural sinus thrombosis. Am J Neuroradiol 2005;26:614–17.
63. de Bruijn SF, Stam J, Kappelle LJ, et al. Thunderclap headache as first symptom of cerebral venous sinus thrombosis. Lancet 1996;348:1623–5.
64. Newman DS, Levine SR, Curtis VL, et al. Migraine-like visual phenomena associated with cerebral venous thrombosis. Headache 1989;29:82–5.
65. Martins IP, Sá J, Pereira RC, et al. Cerebral venous thrombosis may mimic migraine with aura. Headache Q 2001;12:121–4.
66. Slooter A, Ramos L, Lapelle L. Migraine-like headache as the presenting symptom of cerebral venous sinus thrombosis. J Neurol 2002;249:775–6.
67. Canhão P, Batista P, Falcão F. Lumbar puncture and dural sinus thrombosis: A causal or casual association? Cerebrovasc Dis 2005;19:53–6.
68. Ferro JM, Canhão P, Bousser MG, et al. Early seizures in cerebral vein and dural sinus thrombosis: Risk factors and role of antiepileptics. Stroke 2008;39:1152–8.
69. Ferro JM, Correia M, Rosas MJ, et al. Cerebral Venous Thrombosis Portuguese Collaborative Study Group (VENOPORT): Seizures in cerebral vein and dural sinus thrombosis. Cerebrovasc Dis 2003;15:78–83.
70. Ruiz-Sandoval JL, Chiquete E, Navarro-Bonnet J, et al. Isolated vein thrombosis of the posterior fossa presenting as localized cerebellar venous infarctions or hemorrhages. Stroke 2010;41: 2358–61.
71. Jacobs K, Moulin T, Bogousslavsky J, et al. The stroke syndrome of cortical vein thrombosis. Neurology 1996;47:376–82.
72. Ahn TB, Roh JK. A case of cortical vein thrombosis with the cord sign. Arch Neurol 2003;60:1314–16.
73. Cakmak S, Hermier M, Montavon A, et al. T2*-weighted MRI in cortical venous thrombosis. Neurology 2004;63:1698.
74. Duncan IC, Fourie PA. Imaging of cerebral isolated cortical vein thrombosis. AJR Am J Roentgenol 2005;184:1317–19.
75. Kuehnen J, Schwartz A, Neff W, et al. Cranial nerve syndrome in thrombosis of the transverse/sigmoid sinuses. Brain 1998;121: 381–8.
76. Utz N, Mull M, Kosinski C, et al. Pulsatile tinnitus of venous origin as a symptom of dural sinus thrombosis. Cerebrovasc Dis 1997;7:150–3.
77. Waldvogel D, Mattle HP, Sturzenegger M, et al. Pulsatile tinnitus—a review of 84 patients. J Neurol 1998;245:137–42.
78. Crawford SC, Digre KB, Palmer CA, et al. Thrombosis of the deep venous drainage of the brain in adults: Analysis of seven cases with review of the literature. Arch Neurol 1995;52: 1101–8.
79. Lafitte F, Boukobza M, Guichard JP, et al. Deep cerebral venous thrombosis: Imaging in eight cases. Neuroradiology 1999;41: 410–18.
80. Lacour JC, Ducrocq X, Anxionnat R, et al. Les thromboses veineuses profondes de l'encéphale de l'adulte: aspects cliniques et approche diagnostique. Rev Neurol (Paris) 2000;156:851–7.
81. Van den Bergh WM, van der Schaaf I, van Gijn J. The spectrum of presentations of venous infarction caused by deep cerebral vein thrombosis. Neurology 2005;65:192–6.
82. Buonanno F, Moody DM, Ball MR, et al. Computed cranial tomographic findings in cerebral sino-venous occlusion. J Comput Assist Tomogr 1978;2:281–90.
83. Ozsvath RR, Casey SO, Lustrin ES, et al. Cerebral venography: Comparison of CT and MR projection venography. AJNR Am J Neuroradiol 1997;169:1699–707.
84. Rodallec MH, Krainik A, Feydy A, et al. Cerebral venous thrombosis and multidetector CT angiography: Tips and tricks. Radiographics 2006;26:S5–18.
85. Wetzel SG, Kirsch E, Stock KW. Cerebral veins: Comparative study of CT venography with intra-arterial digital subtraction angiography. Am J Neuroradiol 1999;20:249–55.
86. Selim M, Fink J, Linfante I, et al. Diagnosis of cerebral venous thrombosis with echo-planar T2*-weighted magnetic resonance imaging. Arch Neurol 2002;59:1021–6.
87. Ayanzen RH, Bird CR, Keller PJ, et al. Cerebral MR venography: Normal anatomy and potential diagnostic pitfalls. AJNR Am J Neuroradiol 2000;21:74–8.
88. Leach JL, Fortuna RB, Jones BV, et al. Imaging of cerebral venous thrombosis: Current techniques, spectrum of findings and diagnostic pitfalls. Radiographics 2006;26:S19–43.
89. Isensee C, Reul J, Thron A. Magnetic resonance imaging of thrombosed dural sinuses. Stroke 1994;25:29–34.
90. Leach JL, Wolujewics M, Strub WM. Partially recanalized chronic dural sinus thrombosis: Findings on MR imaging, time-of-flight MR venography, and contrast-enhancement venography. AJNR Am J Neuroradiol 2007;28:782–9.

91. Idbaih A, Boukobza M, Crassard I, et al. MRI of clot in cerebral venous thrombosis: High diagnostic value of susceptibility-weighted images. Stroke 2006;37:991–5.
92. Favrole P, Guichard JP, Crassard I, et al. Diffusion-weighted imaging of intravascular clots in cerebral venous thrombosis. Stroke 2004;35:99–103.
93. Farb RI, Scott JN, Willinsky RA, et al. Intracranial venous system: Gadolinium-enhanced three-dimensional MR venography with auto-triggered elliptic centric-ordered sequence—initial experience. Radiology 2003;226:203–9.
94. de Bruijn SF, Majoie CB, Koster PA, et al. Interobserver agreement for MR-imaging and conventional angiography in the diagnosis of cerebral venous thrombosis. In: de Bruijn SF, editor. Cerebral venous sinus thrombosis: clinical and epidemiological studies. Thesis Publishers: Amsterdam; 1998. p. 23–33.
95. Ferro JM, Morgado C, Sousa R, et al. Interobserver agreement in the magnetic resonance location of cerebral vein and dural sinus thrombosis. Eur J Neurol 2007;14:353–6.
96. Canhão P, Batista P, Ferro JM. Venous transcranial Doppler in acute dural sinus thrombosis. J Neurol 1998;245:276–9.
97. Valdueza JM, Hoffmann O, Weih M, et al. Monitoring of venous hemodynamics in patients with cerebral venous thrombosis by transcranial Doppler ultrasound. Arch Neurol 1999;56:229–34.
98. Becker G, Bogdahn U, Gehlberg C, et al. Transcranial color-coded real-time sonography of intracranial veins: Normal values of blood flow velocities and findings in superior sagittal sinus thrombosis. J Neuroimaging 1995;5:87–94.
99. Ries S, Steinke W, Neff KW, et al. Echocontrast-enhanced transcranial color-coded sonography for the diagnosis of transverse sinus venous thrombosis. Stroke 1997;28:696–700.
100. Stolz E, Kaps M, Dorndorf W. Assessment of intracranial venous hemodynamics in normal individuals and patients with cerebral venous thrombosis. Stroke 1999;30:70–5.
101. Dentali F, Squizzato A, Marchesi C, et al. D-dimer testing in the diagnosis of cerebral vein thrombosis: a systematic review and a meta-analysis of the literature. J Thromb Haemost 2012;10: 582–9.
102. Hiltunen S, Putaala J, Haapaniemi E, et al. D-dimer and clinico-radiologic features in cerebral venous thrombosis. J Neurol Sci 2013;327:12–14.
103. Ferro JM, Lopes MG, Rosas MJ, et al. Cerebral Venous Thrombosis Portuguese Collaborative Study Group (VENOPORT): Long-term prognosis of cerebral vein and dural sinus thrombosis: Results of the VENOPORT Study. Cerebrovasc Dis 2002;13: 272–8.
104. Dentali F, Gianni M, Crowther MA, et al. Natural history of cerebral vein thrombosis: A systematic review. Blood 2006;108: 1129–34.
105. Ferro JM, Bacelar-Nicolau H, Rodrigues T, et al. ISCVT and VENOPORT investigators: Risk score to predict the outcome of patients with cerebral vein and dural sinus thrombosis. Cerebrovasc Dis 2009;28:39–44.
106. Canhão P, Ferro JM, Lindgren AG, et al. ISCVT Investigators: Causes and predictors of death in cerebral venous thrombosis. Stroke 2005;36:1720–5.
107. Diaz JM, Schiffman JS, Urban ES, et al. Superior sagittal sinus thrombosis and pulmonary embolism: A syndrome rediscovered. Acta Neurol Scand 1992;86:390–6.
108. Girot M, Ferro JM, Canhão P, et al. ISCVT Investigators: Predictors of outcome in patients with cerebral venous thrombosis and intracerebral hemorrhage. Stroke 2007;38:337–42.
109. Kenet G, Kirkham F, Niederstadt T, et al. European Thromboses Study Group: Risk factors for recurrent venous thromboembolism in the European collaborative paediatric database on cerebral venous thrombosis: A multicentre cohort study. Lancet Neurol 2007;6:595–603.
110. Sébire G, Tabarki B, Saunders DE, et al. Cerebral venous sinus thrombosis in children: Risk factors, presentation, diagnosis and outcome. Brain 2005;128:477–89.
111. Coutinho JM, Ferro JM, Canhão P, et al. Cerebral venous and sinus thrombosis in women. Stroke 2009;40:2356–61.
112. Crassard I, Canhão P, Ferro JM, et al. Neurological worsening in the acute phase of cerebral venous thrombosis in ISCVT (International Study on Cerebral Venous Thrombosis). Cerebrovasc Dis 2003;16(Suppl. 4):60.
113. Gosk-Bierska I, Wysokinski W, Brown RD Jr, et al. Cerebral venous sinus thrombosis: Incidence of venous thrombosis recurrence and survival. Neurology 2006;67:814–19.
114. Miranda B, Ferro JM, Canhão P. Venous thromboembolic events after cerebral vein thrombosis. Stroke 2010;41:1901–6.
115. Martinelli I, Bucciarelli P, Passamonti SM. Long-term evaluation of the risk of recurrence after cerebral sinus-venous thrombosis. Circulation 2010;121:2740–6.
116. Ferro JM, Vasconcelos J, Canhão P, et al. Remote seizures in acute cerebral vein and dural sinus thrombosis (CVT): Incidence and associated conditions. Cerebrovasc Dis 2007;23(Suppl. 2):48.
117. Davoudi V, Keyhanian K, Saadatnia M. Risk factors for remote seizure development in patients with cerebral vein and dural sinus thrombosis. Seizure 2014;23:135–9.
118. Purvin VA, Trobe JD, Kosmorsky G. Neuro-ophthalmic features of cerebral venous obstruction. Arch Neurol 1995;52:880–5.
119. Madureira S, Canhão P, Ferro JM. Cognitive and behavioural outcome of patients with cerebral venous thrombosis. Cerebrovasc Dis 2001;11:108.
120. Buccino G, Scoditti U, Patteri I, et al. Neurological and cognitive long-term outcome in patients with cerebral venous sinus thrombosis. Acta Neurol Scand 2003;107:330–5.
121. de Bruijn SF, Budde M, Teunisse S, et al. Long-term outcome of cognition and functional health after cerebral venous sinus thrombosis. Neurology 2000;54:1687–9.
122. Lamy C, Hamon JB, Coste J, et al. Ischemic stroke in young women: Risk of recurrence during subsequent pregnancies. French Study Group on Stroke in Pregnancy. Neurology 2000;55: 274.
123. Mehraein S, Ortwein H, Busch M, et al. Risk of recurrence of cerebral venous and sinus thrombosis during subsequent pregnancy and puerperium. J Neurol Neurosurg Psychiatry 2003;74: 814–16.
124. Baumgartner RW, Studer A, Arnold M, et al. Recanalisation of cerebral venous thrombosis. J Neurol Neurosurg Psychiatry 2003;74:459–61.
125. Strupp M, Covi M, Seelos K, et al. Cerebral venous thrombosis: Correlation between recanalization and clinical outcome—a long-term follow-up of 40 patients. J Neurol 2002;249:1123–4.
126. Einhäupl K, Stam J, Bousser MG, et al. EFNS guideline on the treatment of cerebral venous and sinus thrombosis in adult patients. Eur J Neurol 2010;17:1229–35.
127. Saposnik G, Barinagarrementeria F, Brown RD Jr, et al. Diagnosis and management of cerebral venous thrombosis: a statement for healthcare professionals from the American Heart Association/American Stroke Association. Stroke 2011;42:1158–92.
128. de Bruijn SF, Stam J, Study Group CVST. Randomized, placebo-controlled trial of anticoagulant treatment with low-molecular-weight heparin for cerebral sinus thrombosis. Stroke 1999;30: 484–8.
129. Einhäupl KM, Villringer A, Meister W, et al. Heparin treatment in sinus venous thrombosis. Lancet 1991;338:597–600.
130. Maiti B, Chakrabarti I. Study on cerebral venous thrombosis with special reference to efficacy of heparin. J Neurol Sci 1997; 50:s147.
131. Nagaraja D, Rao B, Taly AB, et al. Randomized controlled trial of heparin in puerperal cerebral venous/sinus thrombosis. Nimhans Journal 1995;13:111–15.
132. Coutinho J, de Bruijn SF, Deveber G, et al. Anticoagulation for cerebral sinus thrombosis. Cochrane Database Syst Rev 2011;(8): CD002005.
133. Wingerchuk DM, Wijdicks EF, Fulgham JR. Cerebral venous thrombosis complicated by hemorrhagic infarction: Factors affecting the initiation and safety of anticoagulation. Cerebrovasc Dis 1998;8:25–30.
134. deVeber G, Chan A, Monagle P, et al. Anticoagulation therapy in pediatric patients with sinovenous thrombosis: A cohort study. Arch Neurol 1998;55:1533–7.
135. Ferro JM, Bousser MG, Barinagarrementeria F, et al. and the ISCVT Collaborators, Variation in management of acute cerebral vein and dural sinus thrombosis. Cerebrovasc Dis 2002;13(Suppl. 3):60.
136. Canhão P, Falcão F, Ferro JM. Thrombolytics for cerebral sinus thrombosis: A systematic review. Cerebrovasc Dis 2003;15: 159–66.

137. Dentali F, Squizzato A, Gianni M, et al. Safety of thrombolysis in cerebral venous thrombosis. A systematic revie of the literature. Thromb Haemost 2010;104:1055–62.
138. Stam J, Majoie BLM, van Delden OM, et al. Endovascular thrombectomy and thrombolysis for severe cerebral sinus thrombosis: A prospective study. Stroke 2008;39:1487–90.
139. Coutinho JM, Ferro JM, Zuurbier SM, et al. Thrombolysis or anticoagulation for cerebral venous thrombosis: rationale and design of TO-ACT trial. Int J Stroke 2013;8:135–40.
140. Canhão P, Cortesão A, Cabral M, et al. for the ISCVT Investigators: Are steroids useful to treat cerebral venous thrombosis? Stroke 2008;39:105–10.
141. Ferro JM, Crassard I, Coutinho JM, et al. Decompressive surgery in cerebovenous thrombosis: a multicenter registry and a systematic review of individual patient data. Stroke 2011;42:2825–31.
142. Rajan Vivakaran TT, Srinivas D, Kulkarni GB, et al. The role of decompressive craniectomy in cerebral venous sinus thrombosis. J Neurosurg 2012;117:738–44.
143. Aaron S, Alexander M, Moorthy RK, et al. Decompressive craniectomy in cerebral venous thrombosis: a single centre experience. J Neurol Neurosurg Psychiatry 2013;84:995–1000.
144. Lobo S, Ferro JM, Barinagarrementeria F, et al. Shunting in acute cerebral venous thrombosis: a systematic review. Cerebrovasc Dis 2013;37(1):38–42.
145. Higgins JN, Owler BK, Cousins C, et al. Venous sinus stenting for refractory benign intracranial hypertension. Lancet 2002;359: 228–30.
146. Owler BK, Parker G, Halmagyi GM, et al. Pseudotumor cerebri syndrome: Venous sinus obstruction and its treatment with stent placement. J Neurosurg 2003;98:1045–55.
147. Tsumoto T, Miyamoto T, Shimizu M, et al. Restenosis of the sigmoid sinus after stenting for treatment of intracranial venous hypertension: Case report. Neuroradiology 2003;45: 911–15.
148. Horton JC, Seiff SR, Pitts LH, et al. Decompression of the optic nerve sheath for vision-threatening papilledema caused by dural sinus occlusion. Neurosurgery 1992;31:203–11.
149. Acheson JF. Optic nerve disorders: Role of canal and nerve sheath decompression surgery. Eye 2004;18:1169–74.
150. Horga A, Santamaria E, Quinlez A, et al. Cerebral venous thrombosis associated with repeated use of emergency contraception. Eur J Neurol 2007;14:e5.

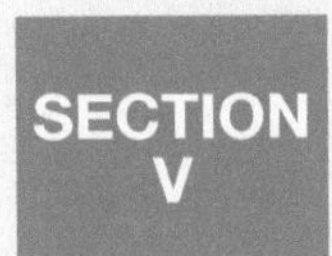

Diagnostic Studies

Gregory W. Albers

As highlighted throughout this textbook, stroke is an enormously heterogeneous condition with a diverse array of etiologies and manifestations. Initial diagnostic imaging results typically provide the first evidence of the size and location of an ischemic or hemorrhagic lesion and frequently reveal clues about the etiology. More focused diagnostic imaging studies can confirm specific pathologies and newer techniques show promise for identifying salvageable tissue, which may guide future therapies. Diagnostic imaging is one of the fastest-moving topics in the field of cerebrovascular disorders and a number of notable advances are highlighted in this section.

The section opens with a chapter on the role of ultrasound, which remains the gold standard for non-invasive real-time monitoring of cerebral blood flow. Ultrasound techniques are used for both diagnostic and therapeutic purposes. For example, recanalization following thrombolytic therapy can be instantaneously detected by transcranial Doppler ultrasonography and high-frequency ultrasound can enhance the efficacy of thrombolysis.

Non-contrast computed tomography remains the initial diagnostic image for the vast majority of patients who present with a clinical syndrome suspicious for stroke. This technique continues to be the only type of brain imaging that is required prior to initiating intravenous thrombolysis. More advanced CT techniques, including CT angiography and CT perfusion, are now playing a fundamental role in most comprehensive stroke centers. The new generation of endovascular therapy trials relies on CT angiography to identify appropriate vessel occlusions prior to endovascular intervention and some of the cutting-edge trials are selecting patients based on CT perfusion evidence of salvageable tissue.

Although accessibility of acute stroke MRI remains primarily limited to specialty centers, new rapidly acquired and processed "stroke MRI" protocols can provide additional data that are not available from CT. Acute restrictions in water proton movement, easily visualized by DWI and ADC maps, provide the most accurate assessment of the volume and location of early ischemic injury. Therefore, especially when combined with MR perfusion techniques, MRI may identify patients who are optimal candidates for acute stroke therapies. MRI is as reliable as CT for identification of acute intracerebral hemorrhage and can be used as the sole imaging modality for evaluating patients with acute stroke. MR angiography and venography are also valuable modalities for evaluation of arterial venous pathology.

This section closes with a chapter on conventional cerebral angiography. This technique remains the gold standard for identification and quantification of specific cerebral arterial and venous pathologies as well as collateral blood flow and also represents the initial phase of all endovascular stroke therapies. Although widespread use of CT angiography and MR angiography has reduced the need for conventional cerebral angiography in many clinical settings, emerging data on the efficacy of endovascular thrombectomy for acute stroke therapy will lead to a substantial increase in demand for conventional angiography studies.

46 Ultrasonography

Michal Haršány, Georgios Tsivgoulis, Andrei V. Alexandrov

Funding:

Supported by European Regional Development Fund – Project FNUSA-ICRC (No. CZ.1.05/1.1.00/02.0123) and by European Social Fund and the State Budget of the Czech Republic – Project Young Talent Incubator II (reg. no. CZ.1.07/2.3.00/20.0117).

KEY POINTS

- Measurement of carotid intima media thickness (IMT) and detection of carotid plaques can reclassify patients at intermediate risk and predict cardiovascular disease (CVD) events.
- Reversed Robin Hood syndrome is diagnosed when the detected blood flow steal is coupled with a deterioration of ≥2 points in NIHSS-score points or recurrence of a neurological deficit.
- For better yield of microembolic signals (MES), power-motion Doppler (PMD) is superior to single-channel transcranial Dopper (TCD).
- TCD yields good-to-excellent results in detecting steno-occlusive intracranial lesions in the setting of acute cerebral ischemia when compared against computed tomography angiography (CTA) or magnetic resonance angiography (MRA).
- Waveform pattern yields more information about thrombus location, hemodynamic significance of occlusion and resistance in the distal vessels compared to velocity difference by itself.
- High-frequency (MHz) ultrasound-enhanced thrombolysis is safe and effective in increasing recanalization and improving functional outcome in patients with acute proximal intracranial occlusions as a potential new therapeutic tool in patients with acute cerebral ischemia.
- Besides the synergistic effect of microbubbles with ultrasound in enhancing gene expression, microbubbles may also be exploited as carriers of therapeutic agents.

INTRODUCTION

Carotid duplex ultrasonography (CDU) and transcranial Doppler ultrasonography (TCD) remain the only non-invasive real-time neuroimaging modalities for the evaluation of characteristics of blood flow in cervical and basal intracerebral vessels that add physiologic information to structural imaging. They have been rapidly evolving from simple diagnostic tools to imaging modalities with a broad spectrum of clinical applications. In acute stroke, they can provide rapid information about vascular stenosis and occlusion, collateral circulation, the hemodynamic status of the cerebral circulation, and real-time monitoring of vasomotor reactivity, embolization and recanalization. Specific applications such as vasomotor reactivity testing, emboli monitoring, and right-to-left shunt detection help clinicians ascertain stroke mechanisms at the bedside, plan and monitor treatment, and determine prognosis. In the neurointensive care unit, TCD is useful for detection and monitoring vasospasm after spontaneous subarachnoid hemorrhage, monitoring waveform changes with increasing intracranial pressure and confirming cerebral circulatory arrest. In this chapter, we discuss the clinical merits and limitations of ultrasound for evaluation of cerebrovascular disease.

APPLIED PRINCIPLES OF ULTRASOUND PHYSICS

Real-time assessment of arterial blood flow started with continuous-wave (CW) Doppler, a technique consisting of two piezo-electric crystals, one emitting ultrasound and another receiving the backscattered signal.[1] Even though this technique displays the Doppler frequency shifts and resulting velocity measurements without an artifact called aliasing, this technique is no longer in routine use since it was supplanted by ultrasound imaging, which will be described below. The main disadvantage of CW is it lacks information about the depth of the signal backscattered, leading to its inability to generate an image beyond a spectral waveform.

In contrast, pulsed-wave (PW) Doppler is based on a single piezoelectric crystal that emits and receives ultrasound. By timing the arrival of the returned echoes, PW technique enables determination of the depth of the insonated structures. In other words, PW determines where the signals came from based on estimation of the time necessary for an ultrasound wave to reach a vessel at a certain depth in the body and for the reflected echoes to return back to the transducer. PW systems need to wait a certain amount of time to register the arrival time of the returned echoes and this poses a limit (relative to CW) of how high the Doppler frequency shift and corresponding velocities can be displayed without an artifact. The advantage is the ability to generate real-time images in addition to spectral waveforms.[2,3]

Ultrasound images are generated using the brightness-modulated (B-mode) technique that determines the amplitude of sequentially arriving returned echoes. The timing of arrival determines the depth at which the returned echoes will be displayed as either white (strong) or dark (weak). The images are encoded in gray-scale. B-mode is used to display carotid and vertebral arteries, and features of their walls, as well as to assess the intracranial structures.

Color-coded Doppler flow imaging (CDFI) depicts blood flow as color images within the gray-scale B-mode display. This modality is useful in recognition of turbulence and disturbed flow patterns with arterial stenoses as well as changes in flow direction. The drawbacks of CDFI include an insufficient ability to display very high or very low blood velocities in high-grade stenotic vessels and tortuous and deep-situated vessels without artifacts.

Power Doppler imaging (PDI) is based on acquisition of Doppler amplitude and, therefore, there is no aliasing. This technique is more angle-independent than CDFI. In this mode, no color change due to blood flow direction is displayed, however, it is sensitive enough to detect blood flow in deep-located, smaller vessels, and lesions with low-flow and slow velocities. Moreover, PDI is useful in assessment of plaque morphology and carotid artery stenosis[4] as it helps to better outline the surface of the plaque and display tortuous residual lumen.

B-flow imaging is a new method that can visualize real-time hemodynamic flow in relation to stationary tissue in B-mode without adding a separate flow signal processing and viewing window. It can display flow changes without aliasing in stenotic lesions in the cervical carotid artery.[5]

Harmonic imaging (HI) is based on detection of a harmonic frequency originating from emitted, or fundamental, frequency. Harmonic frequency is twice the scanning frequency. HI mode can be activated with B-mode scanning in order to improve resolution (this can be called tissue harmonic imaging). Also, HI can be combined with gas-filled ultrasound contrast agents (UCAs) in order to visualize the blood flow within large vessels and the microcircluation. Insonated tissues respond primarily at the fundamental frequency and UCAs increase the generation of harmonic frequencies. HI with UCAs can improve vessel assessment with color flow or power modes. Harmonic imaging permits the receipt of harmonic frequency only and thereby increases signal-to-noise ratio.[6] This technique can be used in brain perfusion studies, distinguishing between arterial occlusion and subtotal stenosis, and in the assessment of vessel wall pathologies.

Doppler velocity spectral display enables analysis of blood-flow velocities with structural and color flow imaging.

Three-dimensional (3D) ultrasonography is a technique that permits conversion of 2D to 3D images in order to better examine extracranial vessels and their wall pathologies.[7-9]

EXTRACRANIAL ULTRASOUND ASSESSMENT

Endothelium-Dependent Flow-Mediated Vasodilatation

Endothelial dysfunction plays an essential role in the pathophysiology of atherosclerosis, it precedes the development of morphological changes and contributes to atherosclerotic lesion development and progression.[10-13] The assessment of endothelium-dependent flow-mediated dilatation (FMD) may be performed with ultrasonography by detection of incremental blood flow changes in the brachial artery if ischemia-induced hyperemia in the distal forearm occurs.[14-16]

Aging is associated with gradual impairment of FMD due to increased oxidative stress.[17] Children with familial hypercholesterolemia and patients with hypercholesterolemia have impaired FMD. However, this association in patients with non-inherited hypercholesterolemia is relatively low. Interestingly, the degree of FMD deterioration correlates with levels of low-density lipoproteins (LDL) and Lp(a) lipoprotein.[18,19] FMD deterioration in young patients was reported in relation to duration of diabetes and LDL levels.[20] Active and passive cigarette smoking are associated with diminished FMD in a dose-dependent manner.[21] Other studies showed a relationship between acute endothelial dysfunction and nicotine levels.[22,23] Furthermore, visceral obesity is associated with endothelial dysfunction.[24]

Intima-media Thickness

Thickening of the two inner layers (intima and media) of the carotid artery wall is regarded as the first morphological sign of atherosclerosis and is also reported to be a marker for systemic atherosclerosis.[25-38] Nevertheless, increased intima-media thickness (IMT) may also occur in other non-atherosclerotic conditions that render intimal hyperplasia or medial hypertrophy. The differentiation between IMT and the non-atherosclerotic entities is often limited and requires subsequent follow-up studies. Basically, the IMT is defined by B-mode ultrasonography as a double-line pattern in which two parallel lines correspond to the lumen–intima and media–adventitia interfaces.[39] Moreover, a pathological study concluded that ultrasonography accurately measures the far-wall IMT[40], i.e., the carotid artery wall located deeper in soft tissues and further away from the transducer surface. Further studies showed good intra-observer and inter-observer reproducibility.[41,42] Regarding the anatomical variability, focal localization of thickening of carotid wall and initial stages of atherosclerotic lesions, several IMT measurement protocols have been developed. Recently, the Mannheim Carotid Intima-Media Thickness and Plaque Consensus released guidance on how to assess IMT. According to this group, carotid examination should include all vessels of the carotid tree and arterial wall segments should be assessed in a longitudinal view, strictly perpendicular to the ultrasound beam, and both walls should be depicted during diastole in order to obtain diameter measurements.[43] Increased common carotid intima-media thickness is a generalized marker of atherosclerosis and is associated with a higher risk of first-ever and recurrent stroke.[44-46] IMT measurements can also help refine cardiovascular risk stratification based on the Framingham score.[45]

Early Carotid Plaque

Plaques are defined according to the Mannheim Consensus as focal structures encroaching into the arterial lumen of at least 0.5 mm or 50% of the surrounding IMT value, or demonstrating a thickness >1.5 mm as measured from intima–lumen interface to the media–adventitia interface.[43] Similarly, a report from the American Society of Echocardiography and the Society of Vascular Medicine and Biology specified carotid plaque as focal wall thickening that is at least 50% greater than that of the surrounding vessel wall or as a focal region with carotid IMT >1.5 mm that protrudes into the lumen and is distinct from the adjacent boundary.[47] Prospective studies have shown a relationship between carotid IMT and increased cardiovascular disease (CVD) risk.[30,32,35,38,45,48-53] Moreover, further studies demonstrated similar or greater predictive power for carotid plaque and CVD risk.[50-52,54-62] According to the ASE report, measurement of carotid IMT and detection of carotid plaques can reclassify patients at intermediate risk and predict CVD events. The most appropriate groups of patients who can benefit from refining CVD risk assessment by measuring carotid IMT and carotid plaque detection are patients, aged 40–70 years without a condition indicating high CVD risk, at intermediate CVD risk (i.e., 6–20% 10-year risk of myocardial infarction or coronary heart disease death using the Framingham risk score); with family history of premature CVD in a first-degree relative; individuals older than 60 years with severe abnormalities in a single risk factor who otherwise would not be candidates for pharmacotherapy; or women younger than 60 years with ≥2 CVD risk factors. This examination is reasonable if the level of the aggressiveness of preventive therapy is uncertain and additional information about the burden of subclinical vascular disease or future CVD risk is needed. Imaging should not be performed if the results would not be expected to alter therapy or in patients with history of CVD.[47,63]

Plaque Features

Ultrasound is the most common imaging method used to study carotid plaque morphology in order to assess the high-risk vulnerable plaques. Pathological changes that occur in carotid plaques were defined by Fisher as:

1. neovascularity
2. calcification
3. intraplaque hemorrhage
4. ulceration
5. thrombosis.[64]

Studies of plaque features are typically focused on echogenicity, surface and ulceration of the lesions. Homogeneous carotid plaques, which are mainly comprised of fibrotic tissue, are imaged by ultrasound with lower intensity of echogenicity, and these plaques are typically stable with rare ulcerations.[65,66] In contrast, heterogeneous plaques consist of matrix deposition, cholesterol accumulation, necrosis, calcification, and intraplaque hemorrhage.[65–67] It has been shown that B-mode imaging can determine carotid plaque features that correlate with histopathologic criteria.[68] Furthermore, ultrasound can assess fibrous cap thickness and is inversely associated with the risk of plaque rupture.[69] These unstable plaques may contribute to the pathophysiology of embolic stroke[70] and account for 15–70% of all ischemic strokes.[71] Among patients with severe carotid stenosis, the degree of stenosis is the most significant predictor of ischemic stroke, however, patients with less than 70% carotid stenosis are not without risk of ischemic stroke due to unstable or vulnerable plaques. Hence, stroke risk assessment based on carotid plaque features may help stratify patients without severe carotid stenosis who have increased risk of ischemic stroke.[58,72] The assessment of carotid plaque features by ultrasound may be diminished by plaque calcification, depending on its extent and the localization of the plaque. Earlier, several studies showed an association between heterogeneous plaques and the occurrence of cerebrovascular events.[73–77] Subsequently, other studies investigating endarterectomy specimens demonstrated a relationship between intraplaque hemorrhage and transient ischemic attacks and stroke.[78–80] However, further studies were unable to support these findings.[81–83] It is still unclear whether ultrasound echogenicity can reliably distinguish symptomatic and asymptomatic carotid plaques. Some studies indicate that heterogeneous plaques are associated with intraplaque hemorrhage and neurologic events, and point out that carotid plaque morphology assessment may be a useful indication of carotid endarterectomy.[84–86] One study suggests an association between intraplaque hemorrhage and high lipid content, and concludes that lipid-rich plaques are more prone to rupture.[87] However these findings were not confirmed in another study that showed little correlation between plaque morphology and histologic specimens.[88] Finally, the study of Hatsukami and colleagues, which evaluated the significance of heterogeneous plaque, showed no differences in the volume of intraplaque hemorrhage, lipid core, necrotic core, or plaque calcification in patients with highly stenotic carotid lesions undergoing endarterectomy, regardless of preoperative symptom status.[89]

B-mode imaging can assess carotid plaque surface with a relatively good differentiation between smooth, irregular, and ulcerative plaque surfaces compared to postmortem carotid artery specimens.[66] However, the accuracy in studies comparing to carotid endarterectomy was poor.[68,88,90,91] Furthermore, B-mode imaging showed only 47% sensitivity for identifying ulcerative plaques.[68] Likewise, B-mode also failed to distinguish between the presence and absence of intimal ulcerations.[92] Detection of carotid plaque ulceration with ultrasonography is influenced by the degree of the stenosis, with increasing sensitivity to 77% in plaques with 50% or less stenosis.[68] Pathophysiologically, it is asserted that plaque ulcerations are prone to thrombosis and thereby cause embolization, however, it is still unclear if, or to what extent, carotid plaque irregularities or ulcerations contribute to the risk of carotid embolic events. This assertion is sustained by a study wherein medically treated symptomatic patients with angiographically confirmed ulcerations had increased risk of stroke.[93] Interestingly, many ulcerations are smooth and thick without signs of thrombosis,[94] however, on the other hand, it should be noted that angiography generally has poor sensitivity and specificity for identification of plaque ulcerations.[68] According to a pathological study, asymptomatic plaques with > 60% stenosis have a higher frequency of plaque hemorrhages, ulcerations, and mural thrombi as well as numerous healed ulcerations and organized thrombi.[95] Similarly, a study comparing asymptomatic and symptomatic carotid endarterectomy plaques found that in each group there occurs complex plaque structure and complications.[81] Consequently, there emerges little difference in plaque structure and surface between patients with symptomatic and asymptomatic carotid plaques. Hence, description of plaque structure and ulcerations appears to be insufficient for prediction of carotid plaque vulnerability and this concurs with guidelines from the American Society of Echocardiography and the Society of Vascular Medicine and Biology.[96]

Another surrogate marker of the plaque vulnerability appears to be intimal neovascularization within the plaque. Histologically, studies demonstrated that the normal vessel intima is without vasculature and vascularization is present in IMT and plaque formations. Moreover, histological studies showed an association between angiogenesis and microvessels in coronary atheroma, and unstable angina and myocardial infarction. Contrast-enhanced ultrasound imaging enables the investigation of the adventitial vasa vasorum.[97–101] Contrast carotid ultrasonography might be useful in identification of microvessels with neoangiogenesis at the base of carotid plaques, and may differentiate symptomatic from asymptomatic plaques.[102]

Carotid Artery Stenosis

For the assessment of carotid stenosis by ultrasound peak systolic velocity (PSV), end-diastolic velocity (EDV) and the systolic internal carotid artery/common carotid artery (ICA/CCA) velocity ratio are essential parameters (Fig. 46-1). All these measurements must be assessed in the prestenotic, stenotic and poststenotic segments of the vessel. Moreover, the degree of carotid stenosis can be investigated by B-mode ultrasound. Likewise, the presence of carotid artery stenosis can be assessed indirectly via the ophthalmic artery.[103,104] In principle, Doppler ultrasonography via the orbital approach enables detection of retrograde collateral blood flow through the ophthalmic anastomosis if there is a severe stenosis or occlusion of the ICA; however, this indirect test is insufficient in up to 20% of cases with hemodynamically significant stenosis. For the assessment of distal carotid stenoses specific types of transducers can be used.

The Society of Radiologists in Ultrasound Consensus Conference issued criteria for assessment of ICA stenosis (Table 46-1). The stratification of carotid stenoses is based on gray-scale and Doppler ultrasound.[105]

CCA occlusion can be manifested either by total occlusion of CCA, ICA and external carotid artery (ECA), or by proximal CCA occlusion with patent ICA and ECA. In the latter scenario, there can be reversed blood flow in the ECA and antegrade flow in the ICA, or vice versa. Reversed ICA flow indicates a competent circle of Willis which is able to compensate for the CCA occlusion and supply the ECA as well as brain vasculature.

Likewise, stenoses in the carotid siphon or in the middle cerebral artery (MCA) may alter flows in the ipsilateral carotid artery. Moreover, the increases in blood flow velocities in the proximal carotid artery may be rendered by intracranial arteriovenous malformations and shunts. Hence, these finding should suspect and lead to further examination to rule out intracranial vascular pathology. At our laboratories, all patients with symptoms of stroke or transient ischemic attack (TIA) undergo both carotid duplex and TCD examinations routinely.

Duplex ultrasonography including B-mode and PW Doppler imaging improves the accuracy of carotid artery sampling with spectral Doppler. Doppler frequency spectrum measures blood flow velocities used to estimate the NASCET range of carotid stenosis. These velocity measurements may be technically difficult if an extensive (>2 cm) plaque calcification is present causing shadowing artifact, thus obscuring the view of the residual lumen.

For the assessment of residual vessel lumen CDFI and PDI are more accurate than B-mode imaging.[106–109] Transverse lumen reduction on CDFI correlates with diameter reduction on carotid stenosis angiography.[109,110] Owing to better visualization of the residual vessel lumen by PDI assessment of local diameter and area reduction of carotid stenosis is carried out more accurately than by CDFI.[111,112] Three-dimensional ultrasound angiography is a precise imaging method for the quantification of carotid artery atherosclerosis.[113,114] Color Doppler flow patterns may render other information in the assessment of the degree in the carotid artery. However, despite these advantages, diameter or area reduction calculations derived from B-mode and flow imaging techniques are not recommended, and velocity criteria and ratios remain the mainstay of grading carotid stenosis with ultrasound. Imaging information is only used to determine:

1. plaque or thrombus presence
2. if the residual lumen is <50% or greater than 50% narrowed by visual inspection
3. if complete occlusion seems to be present with no detectable flow within the lumen.

Carotid Artery Dissection

Ultrasonography may contribute to the diagnosis of carotid artery dissection that can manifest with diverse ultrasound findings. CDFI may present reversed systolic blood flow at the origin of the ICA and absent or minimal diastolic blood flow that concurs with high-resistance bidirectional Doppler signal.[115] In addition, a tapered lumen with a characteristic dural-tail appearance (Fig. 46-2) as well as a floating intimal flap may be shown by B-mode imaging.[116] The true lumen can be oppressed by the false lumen thrombus, and subsequently a low-velocity Doppler waveform can be imaged. The flow direction in a patent false lumen may fluctuate from forward to reversed or bidirectional. The overall flow dynamics hinges on the thrombus presence within the false lumen, the entry and exit flaps in patent false lumen, the flap wall motion, and the extent of the dissection.[117] Some patients may only manifest by a retromandibular high-velocity signal with a finding of a distal cervical carotid artery stenosis.[118]

Within a few weeks to months over two-thirds of patients have successive normalization of ultrasound finding.[119] Moreover, carotid aneurysms may supervene the course of ICA dissection.

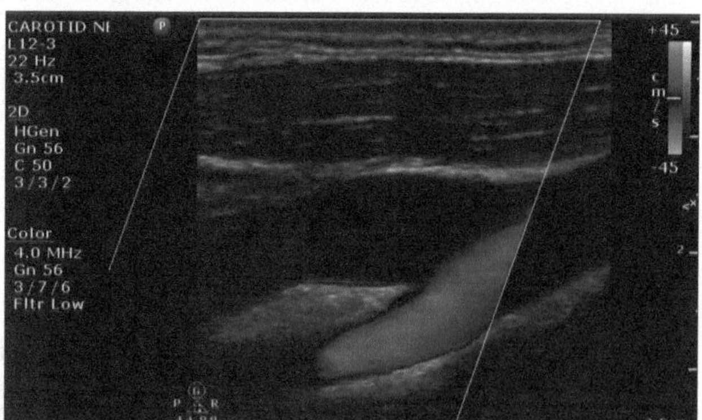

Figure 46-1. Total internal carotid artery (ICA) thrombosis with isoechoic material inside ICA lumen causing complete ICA occlusion.

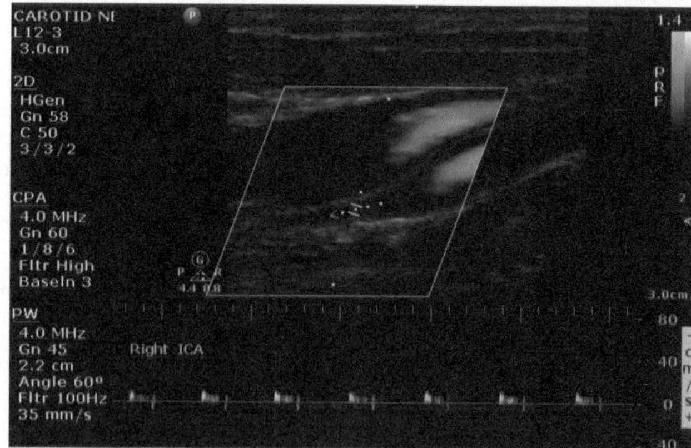

Figure 46-2. Chronic internal carotid artery (ICA) dissection with distal ICA lumen tapering. Spectral interrogation displays the characteristic "thumb sign" appearance.

TABLE 46-1 The Society of Radiologists in Ultrasound Consensus Criteria for Carotid Stenosis[105]

Stenosis Range	ICA PSV	ICA/CCA PSV ratio	ICA EDV	Plaque
Normal	<125 cm/second	<2.0	<40 cm/second	None
<50%	<125 cm/second	<2.0	<40 cm/second	<50% diameter reduction
50–69%	125–230 cm/second	2.0–4.0	40–100 cm/second	≥50% diameter reduction
70–near occlusion	>230 cm/second	>4.0	>100 cm/second	≥50% diameter reduction
Near occlusion	May be low or undetectable	Variable	Variable	Significant, detectable lumen
Occlusion	Undetectable	Not applicable	Not applicable	Significant, no detectable lumen

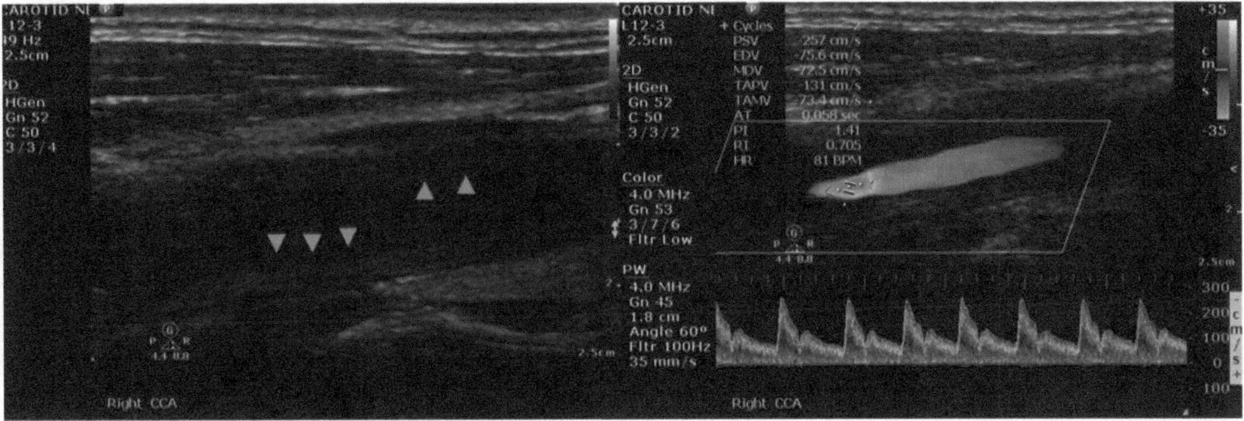

Figure 46-3. Takayasu arteritis with concentric intima-media thickening (arrowheads) in right common carotid artery leading to elevation of peak systolic velocity (257 cm/second) and end diastolic velocity (76 cm/second).

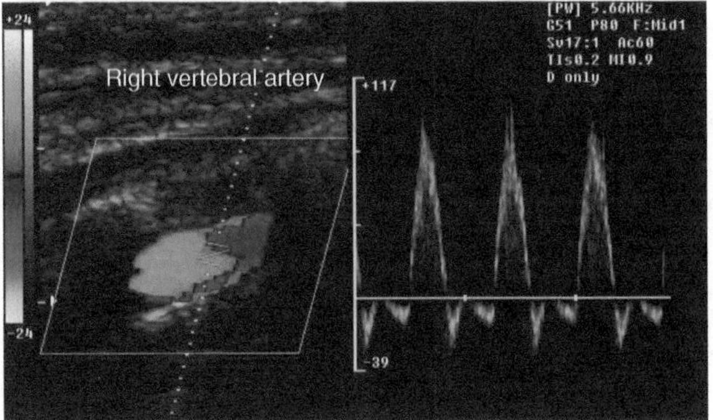

Figure 46-4. Characteristic cervical duplex appearance of subclavian steal syndrome with alternating flow appearance.

Inflammatory Disease of the Carotid Arteries

Takayasu arteritis is associated with concentric increased intima-media thickening on B-mode imaging IMT[120] in proximal cervical vessels (common carotid artery, innominate artery and subclavian artery), which is typically diffusely distributed (Fig. 46-3). Of note, is the fact that 79% of patients have bilateral diffuse increase of IMT. Typically, patients with Takayasu arteritis have affected CCA with sparing of ICA and ECA.[121] Active lesions are significantly thicker than inactive ones, however, hyperechogenicity is present in active as well as inactive stages of the course of Takayasu arteritis.[121] Takayasu arteritis may also lead to subclavian artery stenosis manifesting with subclavian artery syndrome (Fig. 46-4).[122]

Vertebral Artery Stenosis

Extracranial vertebral artery examination by ultrasound is confined to its origin from the subclavian artery, inter-transverse segments between the third and sixth vertebrae, and the atlas loop. Diagnosis and classification of vertebral artery stenosis are more demanding than in the carotid arteries. However, several studies defined PW Doppler criteria to assess vertebral artery stenosis which are comparable to those in diagnosis of carotid artery stenosis.[123–125] For assessment of vertebral arteries it is important to consider the variability of arterial caliber and the presence of numerous collateral pathways which allows supply to the basilar artery even if there is a vertebral occlusion. Flow in the vertebral arteries in over 95% of patients may be quantified by CDFI.[126] This technique also favors recognition of the origin, proximal segment, location of extracranial vertebral stenosis, and the atlas loop.[127] In addition, normal values of flow velocities in the origin, the proximal segment, and the inter-transverse segment have been identified by this imaging method.[128] In order to assess velocities in a vertebral artery it is requisite to know the Doppler values from the contralateral vertebral artery as well as from the carotid arteries, since many abnormalities in the contralateral vertebral artery (e.g., aplasia, hypoplasia, stenosis, and occlusion) or severe stenosis in the carotid arteries may be demonstrated with altered affect blood flow in the vertebral artery. Vertebral artery stenoses are most commonly located in the origin from the subclavian artery, while the atlas loop and the intracranial segment are affected less frequently. Finally, stenoses in the inter-transverse segments are less common.

Vertebral Artery Dissection

Diagnosis of the vertebral artery dissection in the V2 through V4 segments is challenging since there are no defined salient ultrasonographic findings. Dissection of the atlas loop may be demonstrated by absent blood flow, low bidirectional flow, or by low post-stenotic blood flow.[129] The stenotic segment within dissection of the V1 segment may be detected by ultrasound and absent blood flow in the inter-transverse segments may by suspected from vertebral dissection. Moreover, at the same level may be found a localized broadening of a vessel diameter with hemodynamically present stenosis or occlusion.[130,131] Rarely, ultrasound imaging may provide a direct finding of intramural hematoma.[132] Furthermore, ultrasound sensitivity to detect cervical artery dissection is high, however, intramural hematomas may be missed either if they render no hemodynamically significant stenosis or if located outside the arterial segment.[133] For all patients with stenosis or occlusion, ultrasound imaging is a convenient method to follow-up vertebral artery dissection, however, without identification of vertebral artery pseudoaneurysms.[134] In order to assess the length of dissection, transcranial Doppler (TCD) plays a useful role.[135] Clinically, if there is a suspicion on dissection further imaging workup should be performed even if ultrasound results are negative.

TRANSCRANIAL DOPPLER

Introduction

In 1982 Rune Aaslid introduced transcranial Doppler ultrasound.[136] TCD enables a repeatable non-invasive neurovascular evaluation of proximal intracranial arteries at the bedside in real time.

Clinical Indications and Expected Outcomes

TCD is most commonly indicated in patients with ischemic stroke in order to assess intracranial vessel patency, collateral circulation, cerebral vasomotor reactivity/autoregulation, and to detect emboli. In addition, in patients with subarachnoid hemorrhage TCD provides information about the presence and changing degree of vasospasm.

Acute Cerebral Ischemia

TCD can provide the following diagnostic information in the setting of acute cerebral ischemia:[137,138]

- Detect arterial patency, collaterals, emboli, shunts, steal, and cerebral circulatory arrest
- Refine MRA or CTA findings
- Provide real-time physiological monitoring of arterial patency
- Monitor recanalization and detect reocclusion in patients treated with acute reperfusion therapies
- Diagnose a subgroup of patients with acute cerebral ischemia with neurological deterioration caused by a vascular steal phenomenon.

Intracranial Collateralization and Reversed Robin Hood Syndrome

Intracranial collateralization in patients with stenosis or occlusion of the extracranial carotid arteries or intracranial arteries may be assessed by TCD. The main collateral pathways include anterior communicating artery (AComA), posterior communicating artery, reversed flow in ophthalmic artery and in basilar artery, which are open only if there is a change in pressure gradients due to hemodynamically significant stenosis or occlusion. TCD detects the presence and flow direction in collateral pathways that can be a double-edged sword in acute cerebral ischemia. If a pressure gradient is maintained, collaterals can reduce stroke severity, lesion volume and lead to better outcomes. If systemic and local hemodynamic conditions are not maintained, collateral channels can deliver insufficient blood flow and that worsens the ischemia.

Intracranial collaterals detectable by TCD include:

1. anterior communicating artery
2. posterior communicating artery
3. ophthalmic artery
4. flow diversion to branches indicating transcortical collateralization of flow.

The anterior cross-filling via AComA is manifested either by only elevated velocities in the donor anterior cerebral artery (ACA) (suspect A1 stenosis or atresia on the affected side) or by elevated velocities in the donor ACA with stenotic flow at midline depths (distal A1 stenosis, ICA siphon stenosis and cross-filling via AComA) resulting in a reversed A1 segment flow on the affected side.

PComA has a convenient angle of insonation and can be assessed by TCD under abnormal circumstances when there is a detectable blood flow. The blood flow can be directed from either anterior to posterior circulation or vice versa; however, the direction may be deceptive due to the vessel tortuosity or anatomical variations. Moreover, the collateral blood flow via PComA has a systolic flow pattern from donor vessels. The reversed flow in the ophthalmic artery is a pathological finding that implies a severe stenosis or occlusion in the proximal ICA and an incompetent (or incomplete) circle of Willis that is not able to compensate through AComA or PComA.

Intracranial arterial blood flow steal is manifested as paradoxical decreases in flow velocity during episodes of hypercapnia or other vasodilatory stimuli in vessels supplying ischemic areas of the brain at the time of expected velocity increase in non-affected vessels.[139] Reversed Robin Hood syndrome (RRHS) is diagnosed when the detected blood flow steal is coupled by a deterioration of ≥ 2 points in NIHSS-score points or recurrence of a neurological deficit. This neurological deterioration has to be temporarily linked to steal found on TCD and causatively not linked to other known factors that can lead to neurological deterioration, i.e., concurrent changes in blood pressure or arterial patency. Interestingly, in patients with reversed Robin Hood syndrome collateral flow via AComA, PComA and reversed ophthalmic artery occurs more frequently indicating that proximal collaterals can participate in the steal phenomenon.[140]

Vasomotor Reactivity

Determination of vasomotor reactivity with transcranial Doppler has been used to assess intracranial hemodynamics since the 1980s.[141] Most methods were developed using:

1. dose-controlled CO_2 inhalation
2. intravenous injection of Diamox.

Both of these methods have limitations with regard to the need for equipment and potential for complications with intravenous vasoactive drug injection. Therefore, Markus and Harrison[142] introduced a method to quantify the vasomotor reactivity by measuring the MCA velocity response to 30 seconds of breath-holding which is called the breath-holding index (BHI). This method is less reliable since the induced level of CO_2 changes is unknown and it requires patient cooperation. On the other hand, it can be rapidly administered at the bedside.

Patients with asymptomatic severe ICA stenosis and symptomatic occlusion are at higher risk of stroke if their BHI values are under 0.69.[143,144]

Emboli Detection

Ultrasound is able to detect, quantify and localize emboli in real time.[145] Ultrasound is the gold standard technique for emboli detection and its ability has been confirmed in laboratory experiments and animal models.[146] In practice, an emitting frequency of 2 MHz is most commonly used to monitor stroke patients with suspected cardiac, arterial or paradoxical embolization in order to affirm ongoing brain embolization. In addition, ultrasound may be used to monitor patients during carotid and cardiac surgical procedures. Since microemboli have different acoustic properties than blood, they render a transient increase in ultrasound signal named high-intensity transient signals (HITS). Interestingly, most of the detected microembolic signals (MES) by TCD are asymptomatic; however, MES are associated with cognitive decline after cardiac surgery,[147–149] and have also been detected during angiography,[150] carotid endartectomy,[151,152] carotid angioplasty,[153] and open heart surgery.[154] Moreover, detection of MES has also been reported in patients with stroke or TIAs,[155–158] asymptomatic carotid stenosis,[159] intracranial arterial disease,[160] and heart valve prosthesis.[161,162] Interestingly, emboli may cross to the contralateral intracranial vessels through collateral pathways and, moreover, some studies showed more than 10% of MES occurring on the contralateral side to the revascularized carotid artery.[163,164] MES are defined according to the International Hemodynamics Society by the following criteria:[165] duration less than 300 ms, higher intensity usually by 3 dB more than the background blood flow signal, unidirectional signal, and an audible output. For better yield of MES a study showed that PMD is superior to single-channel TCD.[166] Further studies proved this hypothesis, and subsequently criteria for detection of embolic flow pattern on PMD have been developed. Transcranial PMD detected more microbubbles due to greater spatial sampling with insonation of MCA and ACA which resulted in increased yield of MES (Fig. 46-5); however, a post hoc analysis demonstrated ameliorated MES detection when only MCA was assessed.[167] Furthermore, another study compared PMD insonation of submandibular extracranial ICA with standard MCA insonation and ICA insonation was found to be at least as sensitive and specific as the MCA approach in regard of detection of right-to-left shunts (RLS).[168] In addition, due to air microbubble decay and their entry into the ipsilateral ACA this approach appears to be more sensitive for low-volume RLS. Patients with echocardiographically proven RLS had an observed higher microbubble count by this approach. As a consequence, PMD of submandibular extracranial ICA was suggested to be performed in every patient suspected of RLS. Another study comparing PMD TCD with single-gate TCD during PFO closure found out that PMD detected significantly more bubble emboli, and subsequently, a six-level Spencer's Logarithmic Scale (SLS) for the grading of RLS was developed.[169] Grades III–V of SLS showed a high sensitivity and specificity in prediction of a functional PFO, and a higher positive predictive value in detecting large and functional RLS in comparison with the International Consensus Criteria (ICC). Another study compared ICC and SLS criteria and concluded that SLS criteria provide a broader range for grading of shunt conductance and are more specific in the detection of large RLS.[170]

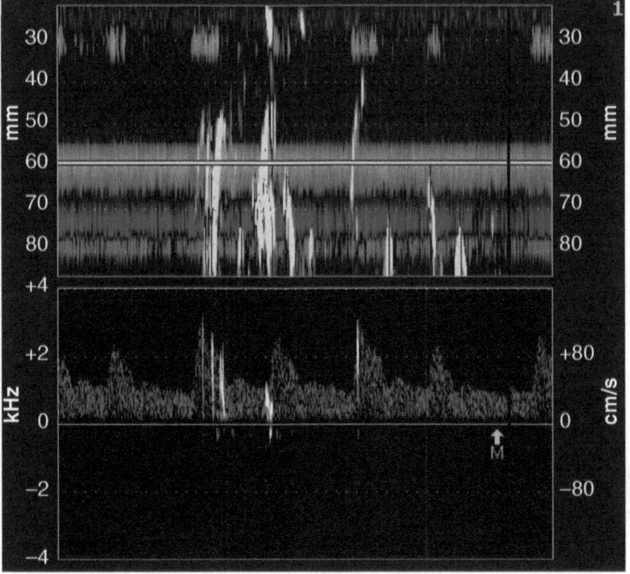

Figure 46-5. Power motion-mode spectrum appearance of microembolic signals.

Intracranial Stenosis

Intracranial stenosis is associated with a higher risk of ischemic stroke and is genetically related to Asian, African, and Hispanic ethnicity.[171–176] However, our recent study indicates that it can also be common in Caucasian acute stroke patients living in the Stroke Belt of the US.[177] The main goal of TCD in patients with ischemic stroke is to detect hemodynamically significant stenosis (≥50%) of intracranial vessels. As a rule for a vessel with straight walls, a 50% diameter reduction doubles the velocity, and a 70% stenosis may quadruple the velocity at the exit of stenosis compared with a prestenotic segment or to the contralateral non-affected side. According to the Warfarin-Aspirin Stroke in Intracranial Disease (WASID) trial, patients with intracranial stenosis at 50% diameter reduction or greater, angiographically confirmed, have significantly higher risk.[178] However, several diagnostic criteria have been developed to identify the hemodynamically significant intracranial stenosis in various intracranial arteries. However, none of them is absolute and it is important to validate the values in each neurosonology laboratory against angiographical findings. A set of proposed TCD mean flow velocity (MFV) criteria that have been developed over the past decade in our neurosonology laboratory are shown in Tables 46-2 and 46-3.

TCDI most reliably detects the proximal MCA stenosis[179] (Fig. 46-6) and it also can detect stenoses in other proximal intracranial arteries.[180] The velocity values measured by TCDI may differ from those on TCD if angle correction is deployed. Of note, only a few angle-corrected criteria are available for TCDI. We therefore recommend using a Doppler carrying frequency of 2 MHz and measuring velocities using zero degree angle with TCDI equipment in order to obtain values closer to TCD and deploying TCD-derived criteria for grading intracranial stenosis. TCD yields good-to-excellent results in detecting steno-occlusive intracranial lesions in the setting of acute cerebral ischemia when compared against CTA or MRA.[181–183]

Cerebral Vasospasm after Subarachnoid Hemorrhage

Cerebral vasospasm is a delayed sustained contraction of the cerebral arteries which may be induced by blood products that remain in contact with the outside of the cerebral vessel after subarachnoid hemorrhage (SAH). Arterial vasospasm is a complication of SAH which becomes symptomatic in more than 25% of patients leading to a delayed ischemic

TABLE 46-2 Normal Depth, Direction, and Mean Flow Velocities at Assumed Zero Degree Angle of Insonation of the Arteries of the Circle of Willis

Artery	Depth (mm, adults)	Direction	Children*	Adults
M2 MCA	30–45	Bidirectional	<170 cm/second	<80 cm/second
M1 MCA	45–65	Towards	<170 cm/second	<80 cm/second
A1 ACA	62–75	Away	<150 cm/second	<80 cm/second
A2 ACA**	45–65	Towards	NA	<80 cm/second
ICA siphon	60–65	Bidirectional	<130 cm/second	<70 cm/second
OA	40–60	Towards	Variable	Variable
PCA	55–70	Bidirectional	<100 cm/second	<60 cm/second
BA	80–100+	Away	<100 cm/second	<60 cm/second
VA	45–80	Away	<80 cm/second	<50 cm/second

*Values are given for children with sickle cell anemia.
**A2 ACA can be found through the frontal windows with TCCD in select patients.[26]

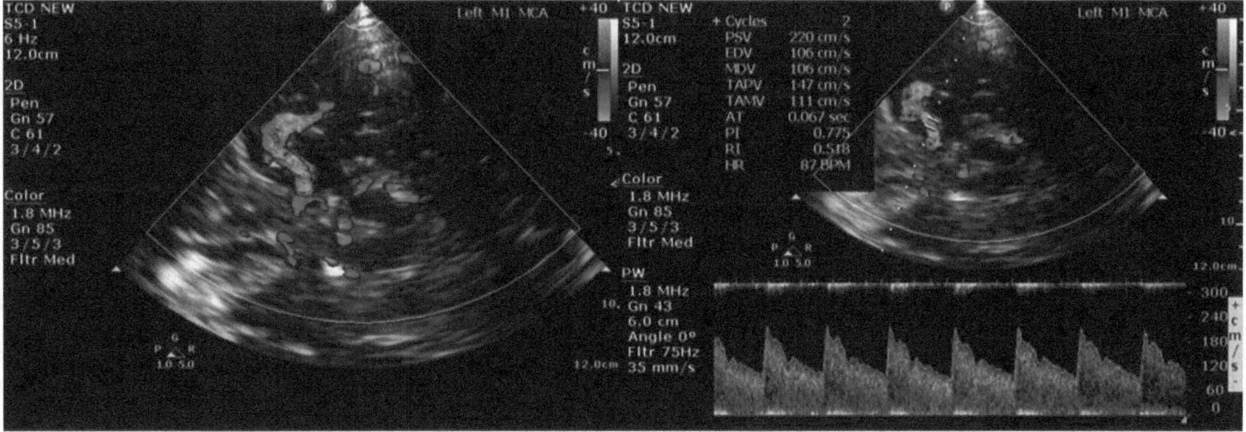

Figure 46-6. Transcranial color-coded duplex appearance of proximal middle cerebral artery (MCA) stenosis with aliasing artifact in color spectrum in proximal MCA (60 mm) and elevated peak systolic velocity (220 cm/second), end diastolic velocity (106 cm/second) and mean flow velocity (144 cm/second).

TABLE 46-3 WASID/SAMMPRIS TCD MFV Criteria[322]

Artery	≥50% stenosis	≥70% stenosis
MCA	MFV >100 cm/second SPR ≥2	MFV >120 cm/second SPR ≥3
VA and BA	MFV >90 cm/second SPR ≥2	MFV >110 cm/second SPR ≥3

SPR: stenotic-to-prestenotic ratio.

deficit.[184–189] Vasospasm occurring after SAH causes narrowing of intracranial arteries, and if there is a severe stenosis (≤1 mm) blood flow decrease with high velocities may be detected. The most common location affected by vasospasm is the MCA, bilateral ACAs, basilar and terminal vertebral artery, or distal branches.[190]

TCD was initially developed with a purpose to non-invasively detect and monitor vasospasm after SAH and it is now a standard method for detection, quantification and monitoring of the severity of vasospasm after SAH and assessment of treatment.[184,191–196] A study showed that vasospasm of MCA is accompanied by an increased velocity above 120 cm/second, whereas velocity is inversely related to arterial diameter and velocities above 200 cm/seconds are predictive of 1 mm or less residual MCA diameter.[197] Furthermore, another study demonstrated a correlation between the changes in velocity on TCD and arterial narrowing measured by angiography, and the best correlation was found in the MCA.[184,197] A ratio between the MFVs (MCA/ICA) can facilitate in differentiation of vasospasm severity and contribution of hyperemia (Table 46-4).[198,199] Moreover, TCD has a relatively poor diagnostic accuracy in the ACA territory which limits this method in a common location of aneurysms.[200]

Finally, there is a need to revise TCD diagnostic criteria for vasospasm (Tables 46-5, 46-6) and make them age-adjusted, and to investigate the effect of new treatment paradigms deployed in the neurointensive care in this setting.

Cerebral Circulatory Arrest

TCD may be used to confirm cerebral circulatory arrest in patients with the suspected clinical diagnosis of brain death.[201,202] Cerebral circulatory arrest is described by TCD as a reverberating flow pattern in both MCA and BA for 30 minutes (Figs 46-7, 46-8). Accuracy in main arteries may yield almost 100% at experienced centers; however, false-positive

TABLE 46-4 Transcranial Doppler Criteria for Grading Proximal MCA Vasospasm

Mean Flow Velocity (cm/second)	MCA/ICA MFV Ratio	Interpretation
<120	≤3	Normal
≥120	3–4	Development of mild spasm and hyperemia
≥120	4–5	Moderate spasm and hyperemia
>120	5–6	Moderate spasm
≥180	6	Moderate-to-severe spasm
≥200	≥6	Severe spasm
>200	4–6	Moderate spasm and hyperemia
>200	3–4	Hyperemia and mild (often residual) spasm
>200	<3	Hyperemia

Note that listed velocity cut-offs are applicable to patients whose baseline MFVs (before vasospasm) were below 60 cm/second.

TABLE 46-5 Sloan's Optimized Criteria for Grading Vasospasm in Intracranial Arteries[184,323]

Artery/ MFV	Possible vasospasm	Probable vasospasm	Definite vasospasm
ICA	>80	>110	>130
ACA	>90	>110	>120
PCA	>60	>80	>90
BA	>70	>90	>100
VA	>60	>80	>90

After hyperemia has been mostly ruled out by the focal velocity increase and by the intracranial artery/extracranial ICA ratio ≥3 except for posterior circulation vessels.

TABLE 46-6 Sviri's Optimized Criteria for Grading Vasospasm in The BA Using Soustiel's Ratio[324,325]

Vasospasm	Soustiel's ratio	BA MFV
BA vasospasm	>2	>70 cm/second
Moderate-to-severe vasospasm	>2.5	>85 cm/second
Severe vasospasm	>3	>85 cm/second

Soustiel's ratio: MFV BA/MFV extracranial VA; VA sampled at the first cervical level, depth 45–55 mm.

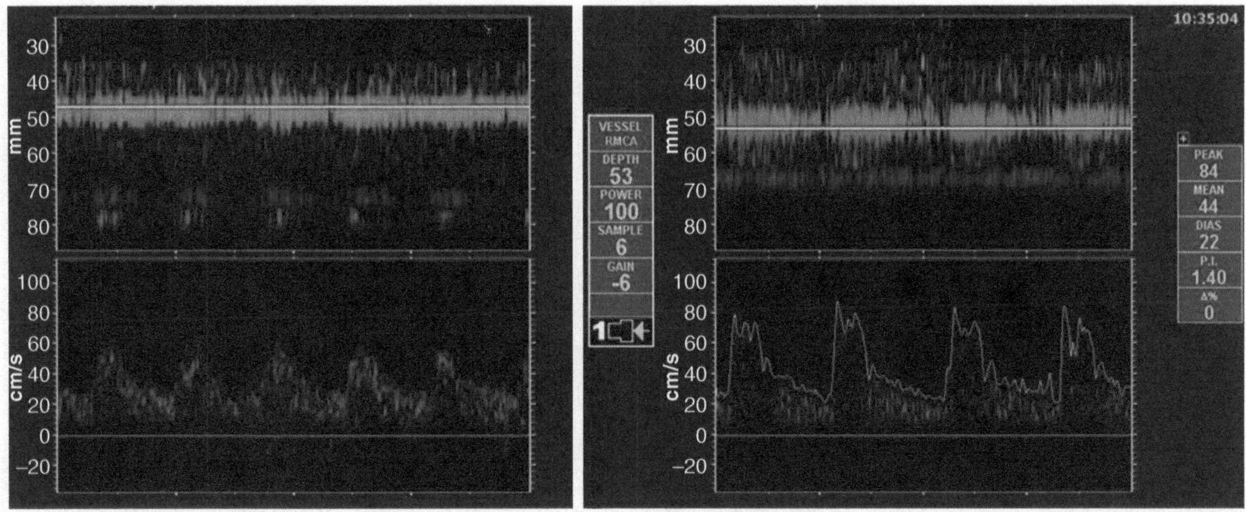

Figure 46-7. Spectral waveform appearance of middle cerebral artery with normal (low flow resistance flow) and increased intracranial pressure (increased flow resistance with pulsatility index of 1.40).

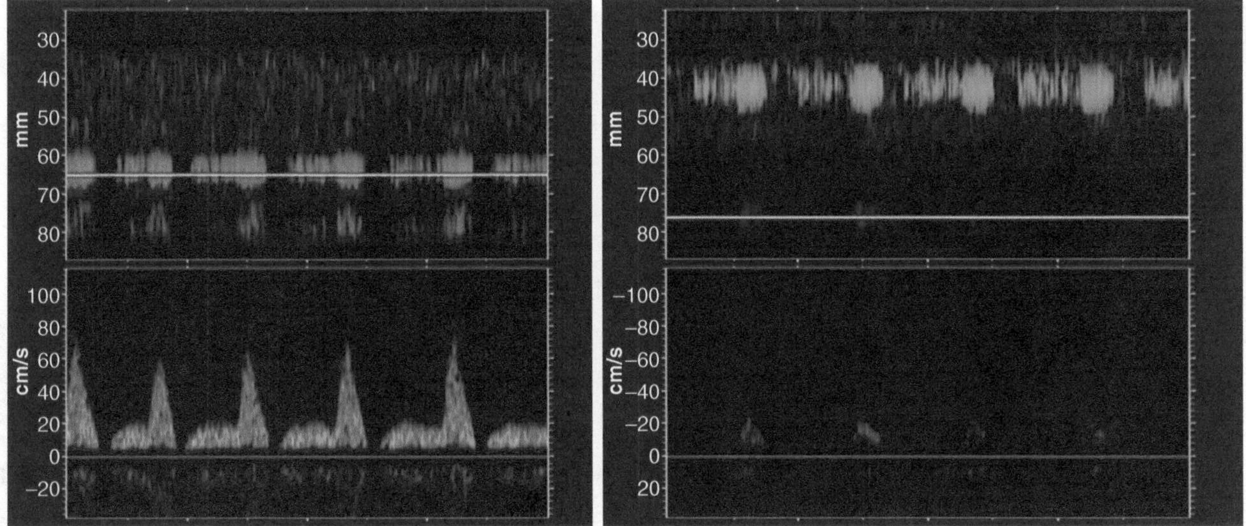

Figure 46-8. Transcranial Doppler waveform appearance of cerebral circulatory arrest.

results may occur and a subsequent nuclear flow scanning may reveal some residual parenchymal blood flow.

Subclavian Steal

Subclavian steal is a hemodynamic condition of reversed flow in one vertebral artery to compensate for a proximal hemodynamic stenosis in the unilateral subclavian artery.[203] TCD may detect various forms of alternating blood flow in one VA at rest or the steal may be augmented by hyperemia cuff test.[123,204,205] Finally, the third-degree subclavian steal syndrome may manifest with complete flow reversal during systole and absent antegrade flow during diastole (Figs 46-9–46-11).

Subclavian steal rarely results in a neurological manifestation and most commonly is an accidental finding indicating widespread atherosclerosis in aortic branches. Under these circumstances it is called subclavian steal phenomenon, otherwise if neurological symptoms from the vertebral-basilar territory are present it is called subclavian steal syndrome. TCD findings of the steal presented at rest include a difference in blood pressure between arms of ≥20 mmHg, systolic flow reversal in the stealing VA, and a low resistance flow in the donor artery. In fact, due to the anatomic differences at the origin of the arteries right to left steal is more common (85%). Nonetheless, dissection of intracranial VA should be involved in the differential diagnosis.

Insufficient Transcranial Bone Windows

Approach through temporal bone window may be impaired by an insufficient signal-to-noise ratio, especially in elderly and female patients. In order to improve the yield of TCD through insufficient temporal approach some echo contrast agents have been introduced. Currently, available are the galactose and palmitinic acid-based Levovist and the perfluorocarbon-based Sonovue or Definity providing improved detection and visualization of intracranial vessels, even in elderly patients.[206] Similarly, Albunex ameliorates visualization of the ICA, MCA and the circle of Willis;[207] however, the effect persists only for a relatively short time. Contrast agents have also improved the quality of examination by transcranial CDFI.[208] Apparently, the use of contrast agents with TCD in acute stroke may be justified by several studies. For

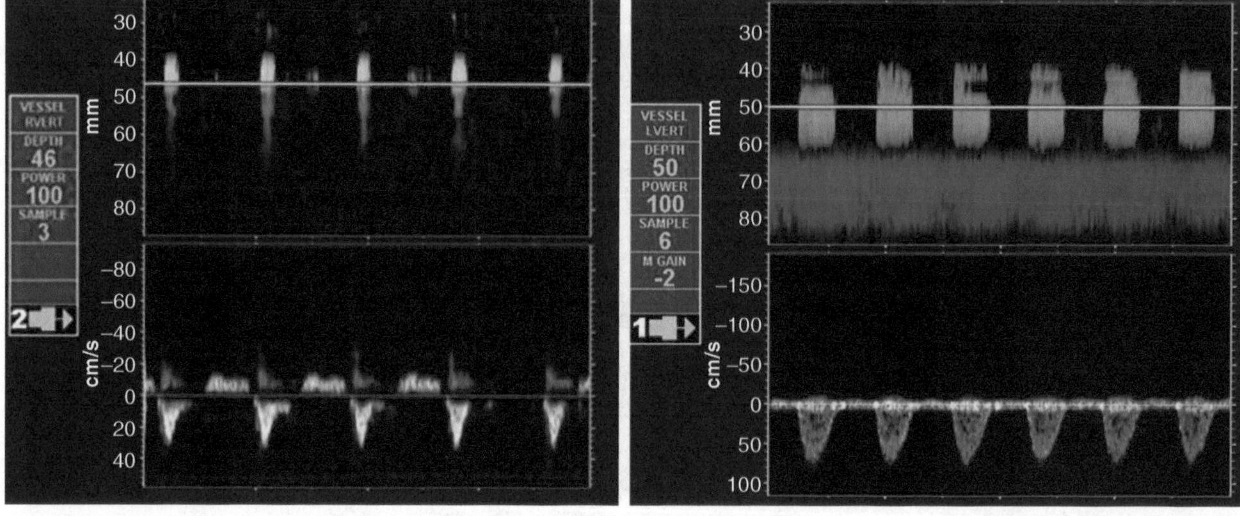

Figure 46-9. Transcranial Dopper waveform appearance of second (alternating flow) and third degree (complete flow reversal) appearance of subclavian steal syndrome.

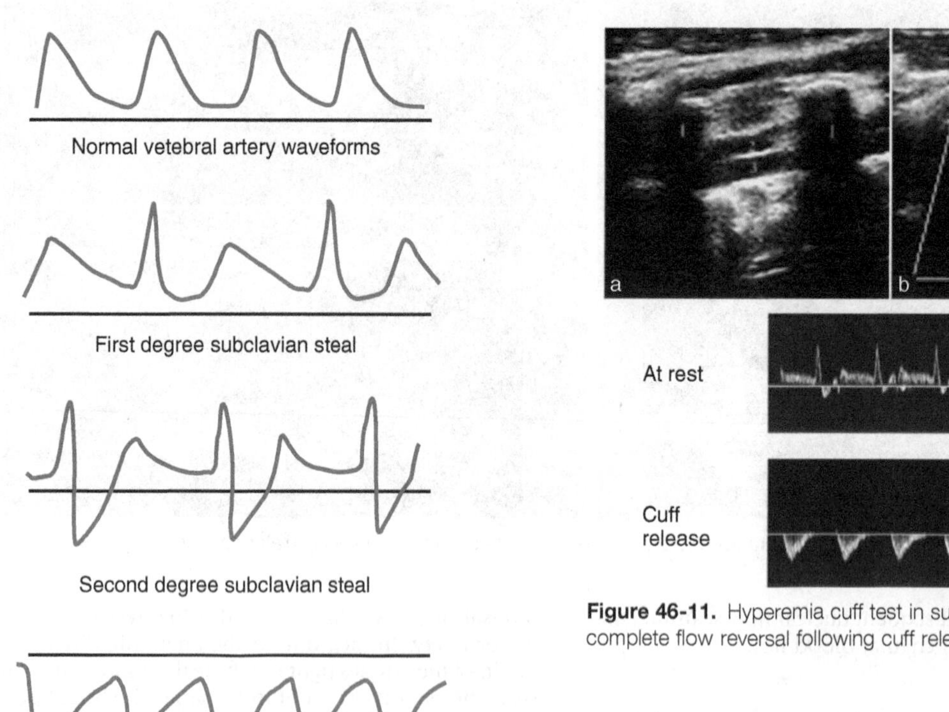

Figure 46-10. Subclavian steal syndrome waveforms.

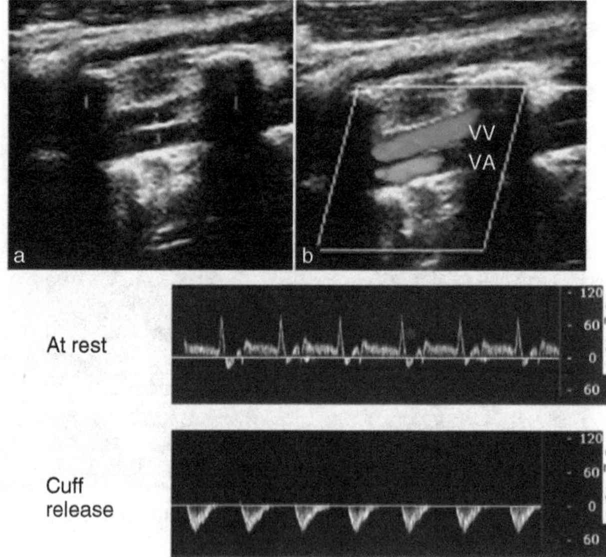

Figure 46-11. Hyperemia cuff test in subclavian steal syndrome with complete flow reversal following cuff release.[321]

instance, findings of transcranial CDFI with contrast agents were conclusive in 66% of patients with ischemic stroke or TIA, and insufficient temporal bone approach.[209] Likewise, in a similar study acute stroke patients with TCD without contrast agents had inadequate results of TCD studies.[210] Patients with poor quality of TCD imaging (i.e., B-mode imaging is not able to visualize intracranial structures and CDFI to depict vessel segments), have little chance of a conclusive contrast study finding.[211] A similar situation was also found in acute ischemic stroke patients.[209]

Echocontrast Studies

Intravenous contrast media are able to increase the echogenicity of blood flow,[212] which has been used in the development of echocontrast-enhancing agents in diagnosis of cerebrovascular diseases. The indications of TCD with contrast agents include insufficient temporal bone window, calcification within internal carotid stenosis, differentiation between internal carotid occlusion and pseudoocclusion, evaluation of intracranial aneurysms and AVMs, and assessment of basilar and intracranial vertebral arteries.

Currently available contrast agents are comprised of microbubbles (3–6 μm) stabilized by surfactants, phospholipids, or partially denatured albumin. The main property of contrast agents is to enhance ultrasound signals by 10 to 30 dB[213] and thereby improve the amplitude of returned signals from blood flow in deeper and smaller vessels.

The first generation of contrast agents was based on air-filled microbubbles. The disadvantage of this generation arises in the fast diffusion of the air from the microbubbles after administration into the body.[214] The properties of the gas in the microbubbles influence the dwell time in the circulation[215] and the back-scattered signal.[216] The second generation of contrast agents introduced less-soluble gases (e.g., perfluorocarbons and sulfur hexafluoride). In addition, echogenic liposomes consist of phospholipid bilayers encapsulating a mixture of liquid and gas. Moreover, this kind of agents may also be exploited due to their better stability in drug delivery.

ULTRASOUND IN STROKE THERAPY

Assessment of Recanalization after Thrombolysis

The diagnosis of an acute intracranial arterial occlusion by TCD is based on flow waveforms and signs of flow diversion, collateralization and embolization. This approach provides a greater yield of abnormal TCD findings that are highly predictive of the presence of a thrombus at acute angiography.[217–219] In fact, more than 75% of acute intracranial occlusions may have some residual flow at presumed thrombus location.[218,219] Thus, waveform pattern yields more information about thrombus location, hemodynamic significance of occlusion and resistance in the distal vessels compared to velocity difference by itself. Hence, there has been introduced the Thrombolysis In Brain Infarction (TIBI) flow grading system to predict success of intracranial thrombolysis and short-term improvement after ischemic stroke.[220] The TIBI residual flow classification consists of six grades (TIBI 0-5) wherein absent and minimal residual flow (TIBI 0-1) (Fig. 46-12) corresponds to persisting occlusion (TIMI 0-1), blunted and dampened flow patterns entail to persisting occlusion with sluggish antegrade flow (TIMI 2), and stenotic and normal waveforms agree with complete recanalization (TIMI 3). Interestingly, in the vertebrobasilar system acute occlusion may manifest with high-resistance reverberating flow both in PMD and spectral display (Fig. 46-13). In addition, an international Consensus On Grading Intracranial Flow obstruction (COGIF) score has been developed to assess recanalization with transcranial color-coded Doppler.[221] The COGIF score encompasses four grades. Herein, no flow pattern (grade 1) represents vessel occlusion, waveforms with low flow (grades 2–3) entail partial recanalization, and established perfusion (grade 4) may correspond to normal flow pattern (4a), stenotic flow waveform (4b), and high flow velocities in hyperperfusion.

Moreover, arterial recanalization may be preceded by detection of MES by TCD at the site of arterial occlusion. TCD is able to detect clusters of MES distal to high-grade M stenosis before spontaneous clinical recovery. Furthermore, there have been detected minimal MCA flow signals followed by MES, increased velocities, and normal flow signals over a period of 2 minutes before complete recanalization.[222]

The yield of TCD in detecting recanalization when compared in real-time with DSA is satisfactory with accuracy parameters >80% for detection of complete recanalization.[223]

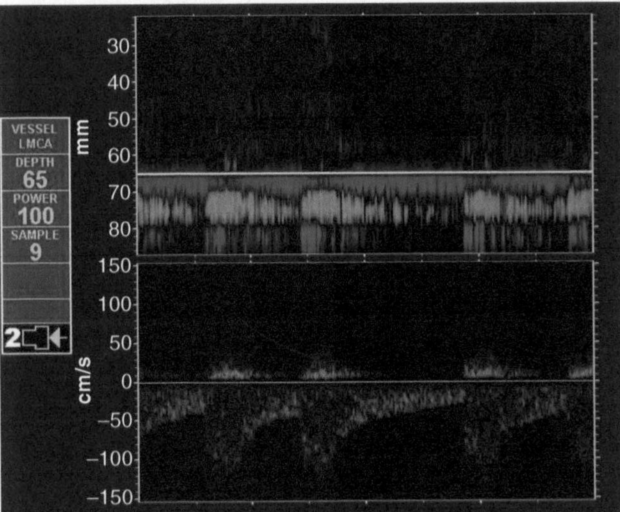

Figure 46-12. Transcranial Dopper waveform of proximal M1 middle cerebral artery occlusion (thrombolysis in brain ischemia residual flow: Grade I) with ipsilateral anterior cerebral artery flow diversion.

Sonothrombolysis

Currently, the only approved treatment option for acute ischemic stroke patients remains intravenous tissue plasminogen activator (tPA) that is administered with the goal of achieving early recanalization.[224] In the absence of vascular imaging, it is assumed that most patients suffering from an acute ischemic stroke have some degree of thrombo-embolic occlusion, and studies showed that shorter symptom onset-to-treatment time results in better functional outcomes.[225] Therefore, amplification of tPA ability to lyse larger clots faster may yield even better functional outcomes after ischemic stroke. According to several studies, a 2-MHz pulsed wave ultrasound enhances thrombolysis.[226–228] Moreover, sonothrombolysis with microbubbles may even further enhance the thrombolytic effect of tPA. Interestingly, ultrasound with microbubbles without tPA have also been used to achieve vessel recanalization.[229]

Ultrasound-enhanced tPA Thrombolysis

Ultrasound delivers mechanical pressure waves to the clot, thus exposing more thrombus surface to circulating drug, an effect called micro-streaming.[139,230–233] Several experimental studies have demonstrated that ultrasound enhance the lytic activity of tPA.[234–242] The effect of ultrasound-enhanced thrombolysis is achieved by improved drug transport, reversible alteration of fibrin structure and increased tPA binding to fibrin.[243–245] Ultrasound frequencies of low KHz range were

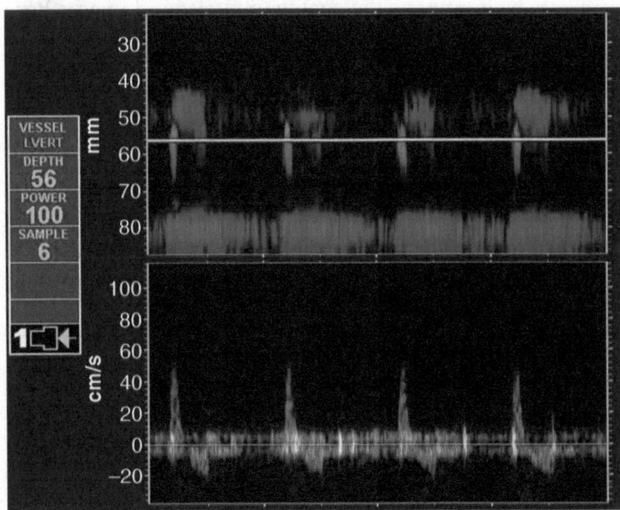

Figure 46-13. Acute vertebral artery occlusion with high-resistance reverberating flow both in power motion-mode and spectral display.

deemed to induce mechanical stretching whereas megahertz frequencies enhance fybrinolysis through enzymatic mechanisms.[236,243,246–248] Kilohertz frequencies penetrate better with less heating, however, adding tPA increases the risk of intracerebral hemorrhage in stroke patients.[249]

In the CLOTBUST trial patients treated by tPA more commonly had early recanalization with early dramatic recovery when being exposed to continuous 2-MHz PW TCD for 2 hours (25% vs 8%). Moreover, more patients tended to recover at 3 months to modified Rankin score 0–1 (42% vs 29%).[250] Briefly, 126 acute ischemic stroke patients in the multicenter randomized CLOTBUST trial with MCA occlusion were given tPA within 3 hours of symptom onset while half of these patients were continuously monitored by 2-MHz PW TCD for 2 hours compared to the rest who were intermittently and briefly assessed by TCD at 30, 60, 90, and 120 minutes in the control group.[250] Ultrasound exposure posed no safety concerns, and the CLOTBUST trial showed the existence of a positive biological effect of a low-power diagnostic-level ultrasound energy that enhanced tPA-induced early recanalization.

Two recent meta-analyses confirmed findings of the CLOTBUST trial and also showed that TCDI might be less effective than conventional TCD.[251,252] Most of the studies used TCD and only a few performed transcranial color-coded sonography (TCCS).[253,254] Of note, is that these studies enrolled patients with M1 MCA occlusions, which resulted in more homogeneous as well as a more severely affected sample of patients. The advantage of TCDI over TCD seems to be in visualization of the occluded intracranial artery and in placement of the sample volume of a PW Doppler ultrasound beam for spectral analysis on the site of occlusion.[206,255,256] Two meta-analyses conducted by our international collaborative group have concluded that high-frequency (MHz) ultrasound-enhanced thrombolysis is safe and effective in increasing recanalization and improving functional outcome in patients with acute proximal intracranial occlusions as a potential new therapeutic tool in patients with acute cerebral ischemia.[251,252] These observations have also been confirmed by a systematic Cochrane review.[257] Finally, sonothrombolysis is now tested in an ongoing multi-national phase III randomized trial (www.clinicaltrials.gov; NCT01098981).

Microbubble-enhanced Thrombolysis

The microbubbles that were originally designed for diagnostic purposes by improving the quality of ultrasound images have also been recently tested to enhance the effect of sonothrombolysis in patients with acute ischemic stroke.[258–262] The microbubbles are administered by intravenous injection and are able to cross the lung capillaries. Subsequently, they are intercepted by an ultrasound beam in the brain arteries, which results in an expansion in size, transient oscillation or complete breakup. During the oscillation, the microspheres transmit mechanical energy momentum from the passing ultrasound wave to the surrounding fluid and structures. At the clot–residual flow interface, interception of an ultrasound beam with the microbubbles ameliorates fibrinolysis with or even without tPA.[258–261] Based on meta-analysis data, sonothrombolysis with microbubbles is safe and there is the same rate of symptomatic intracranial hemorrhage as in sonothrombolysis alone. Moreover, the rate of complete recanalization and favorable functional outcome are as well ameliorated and are substantially greater in microbubble-potentiated sonothrombolysis when compared to systemic thrombolysis alone.[251] Further studies of microbubbles in this setting depend on success of the CLOTBUSTER trial that evaluates an operator-independent therapeutic ultrasound device suitable for deployment of sonothrombolytic treatment in any level of emergency room.

Clot Lysis with Ultrasound and Microbubbles without Thrombolytic Agents

In recent animal model studies, ultrasound with microbubbles alone (sonolysis) was as effective as tPA thrombolysis and as safe with less risk of hemorrhage.[263,264] According to in vitro studies, clot breakup is achieved through a mechanical effect of the microbubbles interfering with the thrombus and their eroding properties in the presence of an ultrasound beam.[265–267] Nonetheless, in vivo models provide a more comprehensive insight, considering interaction such as the endogeneous tPA effect of the ischemic vessel wall or any other endothelial factors emerging during a local ischemia.[268–273]

Historically, success of the combination of ultrasound and microbubbles was demonstrated in a rabbit iliac artery model in 1998.[268] Subsequently, two other studies with albumin microbubbles in thrombosed canine dialysis provided further data.[269,271] Another study using a pig model revealed adequate ultrasound penetration into the center of a human scale head whereas the efficacy of microbubbles with ultrasound remained unaffected.[270] Another study exploited albumin microbubbles labeled by GPIIb/IIIa inhibitor (eptifibatide) to foster microbubble accumulation at the thrombus and thus ameliorated sonothrombolysis.[272] Moreover, microbubbles aimed against human platelets (immunobubbles) have been recently investigated. The immunobubbles contain abciximab which is the ligand for the GPIIb/IIIa receptor expressed by activated platelets. In vitro and in vivo models of acute arterial thrombotic occlusion abciximab immunobubbles ameliorate visualization of human clots, thereby demonstrating the feasibility of using a therapeutic agent for selective targeting in vascular imaging.[274] A subsequent study showed that 2-MHz ultrasound in combination with abciximab immunobubbles induces thrombolysis without lytic agents better than insonation of non-specific immunobubbles.[275]

Sonothrombolysis of Spontaneous Intracranial Hemorrhage

A new clinical application for sonothrombolysis includes patients with intracerebral hemorrhage (ICH). When an external ventricular drainage device is inserted to relieve ICP with intraventricular ICH extension, a small dose of tPA can be injected directly into the clot. To enhance the ability of tPA to dissolve these intraventricular clots faster, a catheter-mounted ultrasound transducer is used to deliver a pulse wave ultrasound in a frequency range close to 2 MHz. Based on the data from MISTIE (Minimally Invasive Surgery plus T-PA for Intracranial hemorrhage Evacuation) and CLEAR (Clot Lysis Evaluating Accelerated Resolution of intraventricular hemorrhage II) trials, rt-PA can be safely administered and may lead to better radiological and functional outcomes in patients with intraventricular hemorrhage (IVH).[276,277] Feasibility of sonothrombolysis deployment in this setting was shown in the SLEUTH (Safety of Lysis with EKOS Ultrasound in the Treatment of intracerebral and intraventricular Hemorrhage) trial.[276]

Brain Perfusion Imaging

Ischemic lesions can be detected by perfusion imaging much earlier than by non-contrast CT. Moreover, this technique enables assessment of the severity of ischemic stroke and differentiates the stroke etiology. The introduction of low mechanical index (MI) real-time perfusion imaging permits the detection of UCAs in the brain microcirculation with minimal or no bubble destruction in comparison to the high MI imaging. Also, this method harbors an improved time resolution of bolus kinetics and obviates the shadowing effect. Furthermore, multiplanar real-time brain imaging can be attained by this method.[278] Nonetheless, the main limitation of the low MI imaging is related to a diminished investigation depth. However, low MI imaging allows depiction of microbubbles flowing through the brain microvasculature and creates dynamic microvascular microbubble maps, which are able to distinguish MCA infarctions. Interestingly, ischemic areas with delayed contrast bolus arrival on perfusion-weighted MRI correlate with a decrease in microbubble refill kinetics. Subsequently, this approach has been used in diagnosis of acute ischemic stroke. Additionally, real-time ultrasound perfusion imaging with analysis of microbubble replenishment showed the ability to properly display ischemic brain tissue in patients with acute ischemic MCA stroke.[279]

Monitoring of Carotid Stenting, Endarterectomy and Endovascular Reperfusion

Surgical treatment of symptomatic carotid artery has become a part of secondary prevention of stroke since clinical trials NASCET and ECST revealed that carotid endarterectomy (CEA) is superior to medical secondary prevention in patients with symptomatic carotid stenosis.[280,281] During carotid intervention neurological deficits may occur as a consequence of perioperative:

1. hypoperfusion
2. thrombosis
3. embolism
4. hyperperfusion.[282]

According to published data peri-procedural stroke rates range between 2% and 10%.[283] Besides symptomatic thromboembolic events, silent subclinical embolism occurs at an even higher rate.[163,284] Monitoring and real-time detection of the emboli by TCD is crucial to prevent, diagnose, and treat procedure-related events.

Carotid artery stenting (CAS) has been approved for clinical use since 2004 and has become an acceptable alternative to CEA. Sometimes carotid interventions are performed without any neurophysiological monitoring, which may markedly affect the ability to respond when complications emerge. In fact, TCD is the only examination to allow the monitoring of intracranial blood flow in real time, thus detecting asymptomatic and symptomatic cerebrovascular events occurring during carotid procedure.[285]

TCD enables assessment of blood flow direction and velocity in the intracranial vessels, thus detecting potential collateral pathways through ophthalmic, anterior and posterior communicating arteries rendered by hemodynamically significant carotid artery stenosis. Assessment of the collateral flow patterns may in fact influence the course of carotid intervention by, e.g., CEA versus CAS, whether or not to place a shunt during CEA, and which embolic protection device to choose during CEA based on the intracerebral flow patterns. Since no arterial clamping is needed, unlike CEA, sudden flow velocity and waveform changes are not generally observed in CAS. However, showers of emboli may be documented during a severe lesion crossing and briefly during stent deployment. One of the indications for choosing CAS over CEA is contralateral ICA occlusion. In fact, acute hypoperfusion is less of a concern in CAS; however, CAS is more commonly associated with hyperperfusion and thromboembolism. TCD monitoring of the ipsilateral MCA during the intervention provides clinicians with useful information if any complications occur. Moreover, TCD may, in the real-time setting, yield hemodynamic information in real time to allow for pertinent procedural adjustments to be made sooner than with any other monitoring method.

Nevertheless, TCD has some limitations including operator-dependence, and suboptimal or absent transtemporal windows that need to be taken into consideration before periprocedural carotid artery interventions. Essentially, TCD is highly operator-dependent and the insufficient skull bone window is also to some extent a limiting factor.

NEW TRENDS IN ULTRASOUND

Molecular Imaging

Molecular imaging is a method that depicts cellular and molecular processes in order to detect and diagnose molecular changes, complex molecular mechanisms, and gene expression present in the course of the disease. Basically, specific contrast agents delineate molecular and genetic markers of the disease and can be combined with targeted ultrasound techniques. Moreover, contrast agents have high echogenicity compared to other structures, and tagging of contrast agents (microbubbles) by specific ligands is a new approach to study vascular occlusions or cerebral injury. In areas of angiogenesis, inflammation, and thrombus an overexpression of adhesion molecules (ICAM-1), and fibrinogen receptor GPIIb/IIIa is frequently observed and can be tracked by tagged contrast agents. Microbubbles targeted to α_v-integrins have been used in imaging of angiogenesis.[286] Similarly, lipid-based perfluorobutane-filled microbubbles tagged by anti-ICAM-1 monoclonal antibodies have been exploited in the study of early stages of atherosclerosis.[287] Furthermore, microbubbles aimed at activated platelets (receptor GPIIb/IIIa) have been introduced for thrombus detection.[274,288,289] To sum up, leukocyte-targeted contrast agents may be used to assess the severity of post-ischemic myocardial inflammation[290] and to detect inflamed plaques.[291]

Contrast ultrasound perfusion imaging and molecular imaging with microbubbles targeted to activated neutrophils, α_5-integrins, or vascular cell adhesion molecule (VCAM-1) has been performed in murine models of vasculogenesis and ischemia-mediated arteriogenesis. Interestingly, targeted imaging demonstrated early signal enhancement for neutrophils, monocyte α_5-integrin, and VCAM-1 at day 2 when blood flow was very low. Hence, the different components of the inflammatory response that participate in vascular development and remodeling can be assessed separately with targeted molecular imaging.[292]

Another study using mice deficient for the LDL-receptor and the Apobec-1 editing peptide (DKO mice) as an age-dependent model of atherosclerosis showed that non-invasive ultrasound molecular imaging of endothelial activation can detect lesion-prone vascular phenotype before the appearance of obstructive atherosclerotic lesions. Ultrasound molecular imaging of the proximal thoracic aorta was performed with contrast agents targeted to P-selectin and VCAM-1 found selective signal enhancement for DKO mice and en face microscopy demonstrated preferential attachment of targeted microbubbles to regions of lesion formation.[293]

The role of inflammation, angiogenesis, and thrombus formation in the pathophysiology of cerebrovascular as well as cardiovascular diseases may be detected by ultrasound molecular imaging. The potential clinical role of this technology will be contingent on further refinement of targeted microbubble chemistry and studies that indicate that the unique diagnostic information from molecular imaging can positively affect patient care.[294]

Opening the Blood–Brain Barrier

Efforts to transport new diagnostic and therapeutic agents to the central nervous system (CNS) are limited by the presence of the blood–brain barrier (BBB). This barrier hinders the transport of small molecules and macromolecular agents that could be beneficial in the treatment and diagnosis of various disorders affecting the CNS. As of today, there have been many attempts to improve the design of new drugs or to develop new delivery methods so as to circumvent the BBB. In this setting ultrasound showed the ability to open the BBB. After application of acoustic energy large molecules and genes are able to cross the plasma membrane of cultured cells.[295] Interestingly, electron microscopy revealed ultrasound-induced porosity in both in vitro and in vivo models.[296] High-intensity focused ultrasound disrupts the BBB in rats by opening capillary endothelial cell tight junctions.[297] Microbubbles may transiently open the BBB at the ultrasound focus without neuronal damage.[298] The presence of microbubbles in the bloodstream can diminish the ultrasound effects to the vasculature and reduce the intensity necessary to open the BBB. Thus, the risk of tissue damage may be lower. Disruption of the BBB has been confirmed in studies with MR contrast imaging at targeted locations[298–300] or with postmortem histological examination.[301]

A study with focused ultrasound attained the delivery of antibodies into the brain. After disruption of the BBB by ultrasound, dopamine D_4 receptor antibody was able to recognize antigen in the murine brain.[299] Furthermore, chemotherapeutic drug doxorubicin was able to cross the BBB using ultrasound with microbubbles.[302] Of note, is that different levels of doxorubicin were detected in the brain by changing the microbubble concentration, which indicates further possibilities for this technique and indicated the need for more studies in this field.

Also, there are other known mechanisms of crossing the BBB after ultrasound exposure including transcytosis, passage through endothelial cell cytoplasmatic openings, opening of tight junctions (TJs), and free passage through injured endothelium.[303] The integrity of TJs in rat brain microvessels after BBB disruption by ultrasound bursts (1.5 MHz) in combination with Optison have been studied.[304] It was concluded that the effect of ultrasound on TJs is transient, lasting less than 4 hours.

Interestingly, reorganization of gap-junctional plaques in neurons and astrocytes may occur at the upper thresholds of acoustic pressure for safe opening of the BBB.[305] In fact, gap junctions are responsible for communication between adjacent cells and for tissue homeostasis. Moreover, it has been observed that ubiquitinylation of proteins in neuronal cells may be increased in BBB disruption by focused ultrasound and contrast agents,[306] which implies that brain molecular stress pathways are involved.

Ultrasound-enhanced Gene Therapy

Ultrasound has a direct effect on gene expression, and acoustically active materials, microbubbles, and gaseous precursor agents have been developed that bind or entrap genetic materials. Moreover, targeting ligands have also been incorporated onto the surface of these agents for cell-specific delivery. The advantage of this new technology is in delivering genes more selectively than other methods and less invasively than direct injection.[307]

Liposomal transfection experiments in cell cultures revealed that exposure to ultrasound for 30 seconds or less at a power level of 0.5 watts/cm^2 resulted in significant increases in gene expression. Thus, relatively low levels of ultrasound energy enhance gene expression from liposomal transfection agents.[308] There is further evidence from a study evaluating the capacity of ultrasound-targeted microbubble destruction to deliver angiogenic genes, improve perfusion, and recruit progenitor cells after a myocardial infarction in mice. The physiologic impact of VEGF and SCF gene delivery was confirmed by increased myocardial recruitment of VEGF receptor 2- and SCF receptor (c-kit)-expressing cells. Consequently, capillary and arteriolar density (Factor VIII and alpha-smooth muscle actin staining), myocardial perfusion, and cardiac function were all enhanced in recipients of VEGF or SCF. Thus, non-invasive ultrasound-targeted microbubble destruction successfully delivered VEGF and SCF genes into the infarcted heart, increased vascular density, and improved myocardial perfusion and ventricular function.[309] Furthermore, the investigators studied repeated delivery of stem-cell-mobilizing genes so as to boost the ability of this therapy to enhance cardiac repair and ventricular function after a myocardial infarction. In conclusion, multiple ultrasound-targeted microbubble destruction treatments enhanced tissue repair, perfusion, and cardiac function.[310] This evidence provides a basis for angiogenesis and recruitment of progenitor cells after ischemic stroke.

Targeted Drug Delivery with Ultrasound

Besides the synergistic effect of microbubbles with ultrasound in enhancing the gene expression, microbubbles may also be exploited as carriers of gene therapeutic agents.[307,311] Thus far, there are different ways that microbubbles may entrap different drugs. Drugs may be incorporated into the membrane or wall-forming materials that stabilize microbubbles. Charged drugs can be stabilized in or onto the surfaces of microbubbles by virtue of electrostatic interactions. Thus, cationic lipid-coated microbubbles can bind DNA that is a polyanion (i.e., negatively charged) and avidly bound to cationic (positively charged) microbubbles. Furthermore, drugs can be incorporated into the interior of microbubbles, i.e., drug- and gas-filled microspheres. Of note, is that the gas lowers the cavitation threshold for the microspheres, thus creating a layer of oil (e.g., triacetin) that stabilizes the outer surface of the bubble. Hydrophobic drugs can then be incorporated into the oil layer. Subsequently, the drugs are released when ultrasound energy cavitates the microbubble. Basically, these methods for making drug-carrying microbubbles are probably most applicable to drugs that are highly active. This is certainly the case for gene-based drugs, in which the amount of gene injected is usually on the order of micrograms or milligrams. Hence, a large volume of bubbles is not required to deliver highly active drugs as would be the case for delivery of genes.[307]

Thus far, there has been evidence from several studies indicating that the entrapment of tissue plasminogen activator into liposomes provides the selective targeting needed to improve the efficacy of the fibrinolytic agent.[312–316] Furthermore, liposomal drug delivery may be targeted by ultrasound, particularly by its cavitational effects and acoustic radiation force.[317] Interestingly, reports from studies combining nanotechnology with microbubbles in drug delivery may be exploited in thrombolytic treatment in the future.[318,319]

A fibrin-specific, liquid perfluorocarbon nanoparticle has been introduced that is surface-modified to deliver the plasminogen activator streptokinase. Targeting of clot-dissolving therapeutics has the potential to decrease the frequency of complications while simultaneously increasing treatment effectiveness, by concentrating the available drug at the desired site and permitting a lower systemic dose. Effective concentrations of targeted streptokinase were orders of magnitude lower than equivalently efficacious levels of free drug. As little as 1% surface targeting of streptokinase nanoparticles produced significant decreases in clot volumes in 1 hour. This new nanoparticle-based thrombolytic agent provides specific and rapid fibrinolysis in vitro and may have a clinical role in early reperfusion during acute ischemic stroke.[320]

The complete reference list can be found on the companion Expert Consult website at www.expertconsult.inkling.com.

KEY REFERENCES

10. Juonala M, Viikari J, Laitinen T, et al. Interrelations between brachial endothelial function and carotid intima-media thickness in young adults – The Cardiovascular Risk in Young Finns Study. Circulation 2004;110:2918–23.
11. Halcox J, Donald A, Ellins E, et al. Endothelial Function Predicts Progression of Carotid Intima-Media Thickness. Circulation 2009;119:1005–12.
13. Kobayashi K, Akishita M, Yu W, et al. Interrelationship between non-invasive measurements of atherosclerosis: flow-mediated dilation of brachial artery, carotid intima-media thickness and pulse wave velocity. Atherosclerosis 2004;173:13–18.
14. Celermajer D, Sorensen K, Gooch V, et al. Noninvasive detection of endothelial dysfunction in children and adults at risk of atherosclerosis. Lancet 1992;340:1111–15.
21. Celermajer DS, Sorensen KE, Georgakopoulos D, et al. Cigarette smoking is associated with dose-related and potentially reversible impairment of endothelium-dependent dilation in healthy young adults. Circulation 1993;88:2149–55.
25. Hennerici M, Meairs S. Imaging arterial wall disease. Cerebrovasc Dis 2000;10(Suppl. 5):9–20.
26. OLeary D, Polak J, Kronmal R, et al. Thickening of the carotid wall – A marker for atherosclerosis in the elderly? Stroke 1996; 27:224–31.
28. Bots M, Hoes A, Koudstaal P, et al. Common carotid intima-media thickness and risk of stroke and myocardial infarction – The Rotterdam Study. Circulation 1997;96:1432–7.
29. O'Leary D, Polak J, Kronmal R, et al. Carotid-artery intima and media thickness as a risk factor for myocardial infarction and stroke in older adults. N Engl J Med 1999;340:14–22.
30. Chambless L, Heiss G, Folsom A, et al. Association of Coronary Heart Disease incidence with carotid arterial wall thickness and major risk factors: The Atherosclerosis Risk in Communities (ARIC) Study, 1987-1993. Am J Epidemiol 1997; 146:483–94.
31. Chambless L, Folsom A, Clegg L, et al. Carotid wall thickness is predictive of incident clinical stroke – The Atherosclerosis Risk in Communities (ARIC) Study. Am J Epidemiol 2000;151: 478–87.
32. Lorenz M, von Kegler S, Steinmetz H, et al. Carotid intima-media thickening indicates a higher vascular risk across a wide age range – Prospective data from the Carotid Atherosclerosis Progression Study (CAPS). Stroke 2006;37:87–92.
33. Salonen J, Salonen R. Ultrasound B-mode imaging in observational studies of atherosclerotic progression. Circulation 1993; 87:56–65.
34. Kitamura A, Iso H, Imano H, et al. Carotid intima-media thickness and plaque characteristics as a risk factor for stroke in Japanese elderly men. Stroke 2004;35:2788–94.
37. Lorenz M, Markus H, Bots M, et al. Prediction of clinical cardiovascular events with carotid intima-media thickness – A systematic review and meta-analysis. Circulation 2007;115:459–67.
41. Riley WA, Barnes RW, Applegate WB, et al. Reproducibility of noninvasive ultrasonic measurement of carotid atherosclerosis. The Asymptomatic Carotid Artery Plaque Study. Stroke 1992;23: 1062–8.
43. Touboul PJ, Hennerici MG, Meairs S, et al. Mannheim carotid intima-media thickness and plaque consensus (2004-2006-2011). An update on behalf of the advisory board of the 3rd, 4th and 5th watching the risk symposia, at the 13th, 15th and 20th European Stroke Conferences, Mannheim, Germany, 2004, Brussels, Belgium, 2006, and Hamburg, Germany, 2011. Cerebrovasc Dis 2012;34:290–6.
44. Grobbee DE, Bots ML. Carotid artery intima-media thickness as an indicator of generalized atherosclerosis. J Intern Med 1994; 236:567–73.
45. O'Leary DH, Polak JF, Kronmal RA, et al. Carotid-artery intima and media thickness as a risk factor for myocardial infarction and stroke in older adults. Cardiovascular Health Study Collaborative Research Group. N Engl J Med 1999;340:14–22.
46. Tsivgoulis G, Vemmos K, Papamichael C, et al. Common carotid artery intima-media thickness and the risk of stroke recurrence. Stroke 2006;37:1913–16.
47. Roman MJ, Naqvi TZ, Gardin JM, et al. Clinical application of noninvasive vascular ultrasound in cardiovascular risk stratification: a report from the American Society of Echocardiography and the Society of Vascular Medicine and Biology. J Am Soc Echocardiogr 2006;19:943–54.
49. Salonen JT, Salonen R. Ultrasound B-mode imaging in observational studies of atherosclerotic progression. Circulation 1993; 87:II56–65.
50. Kitamura A, Iso H, Imano H, et al. Carotid intima-media thickness and plaque characteristics as a risk factor for stroke in Japanese elderly men. Stroke 2004;35:2788–94.
51. van der Meer IM, Bots ML, Hofman A, et al. Predictive value of noninvasive measures of atherosclerosis for incident myocardial infarction: the Rotterdam Study. Circulation 2004;109:1089–94.
52. Lorenz MW, Markus HS, Bots ML, et al. Prediction of clinical cardiovascular events with carotid intima-media thickness: a systematic review and meta-analysis. Circulation 2007;115:459–67.
55. Belcaro G, Nicolaides AN, Ramaswami G, et al. Carotid and femoral ultrasound morphology screening and cardiovascular events in low risk subjects: a 10-year follow-up study (the CAFES-CAVE study(1). Atherosclerosis 2001;156:379–87.
58. Prabhakaran S, Rundek T, Ramas R, et al. Carotid plaque surface irregularity predicts ischemic stroke: the northern Manhattan study. Stroke 2006;37:2696–701.
59. Störk S, van den Beld AW, von Schacky C, et al. Carotid artery plaque burden, stiffness, and mortality risk in elderly men: a prospective, population-based cohort study. Circulation 2004; 110:344–8.
60. Spence JD, Eliasziw M, DiCicco M, et al. Carotid plaque area: a tool for targeting and evaluating vascular preventive therapy. Stroke 2002;33:2916–22.
61. Johnsen SH, Mathiesen EB, Joakimsen O, et al. Carotid atherosclerosis is a stronger predictor of myocardial infarction in women than in men: a 6-year follow-up study of 6226 persons: the Tromsø Study. Stroke 2007;38:2873–80.
62. Rundek T, Arif H, Boden-Albala B, et al. Carotid plaque, a subclinical precursor of vascular events: the Northern Manhattan Study. Neurology 2008;70:1200–7.
63. Roman MJ, Naqvi TZ, Gardin JM, et al. American society of echocardiography report. Clinical application of noninvasive vascular ultrasound in cardiovascular risk stratification: a report from the American Society of Echocardiography and the Society for Vascular Medicine and Biology. Vasc Med 2006;11:201–11.
69. Devuyst G, Karapanayiotides T, Ruchat P, et al. Ultrasound measurement of the fibrous cap in symptomatic and asymptomatic atheromatous carotid plaques. Circulation 2005;111:2776–82.
70. Rundek T. Beyond percent stenosis: carotid plaque surface irregularity and risk of stroke. Int J Stroke. 2007;2:169–71.
71. Foulkes MA, Wolf PA, Price TR, et al. The Stroke Data Bank: design, methods, and baseline characteristics. Stroke 1988; 19:547–54.
72. Mathiesen EB, Bønaa KH, Joakimsen O. Echolucent plaques are associated with high risk of ischemic cerebrovascular events in carotid stenosis: the tromsø study. Circulation 2001;103: 2171–5.
78. Imparato AM, Riles TS, Gorstein F. The carotid bifurcation plaque: pathologic findings associated with cerebral ischemia. Stroke 1979;10:238–45.
83. Lennihan L, Kupsky WJ, Mohr JP, et al. Lack of association between carotid plaque hematoma and ischemic cerebral symptoms. Stroke 1987;18:879–81.
89. Hatsukami TS, Ferguson MS, Beach KW, et al. Carotid plaque morphology and clinical events. Stroke 1997;28:95–100.
92. Bluth EI, McVay LV, Merritt CR, et al. The identification of ulcerative plaque with high resolution duplex carotid scanning. J Ultrasound Med 1988;7:73–6.
93. Eliasziw M, Streifler JY, Fox AJ, et al. Significance of plaque ulceration in symptomatic patients with high-grade carotid stenosis.

North American Symptomatic Carotid Endarterectomy Trial. Stroke 1994;25:304–8.
96. Stein JH, Korcarz CE, Hurst RT, et al. Use of carotid ultrasound to identify subclinical vascular disease and evaluate cardiovascular disease risk: a consensus statement from the American Society of Echocardiography Carotid Intima-Media Thickness Task Force. Endorsed by the Society for Vascular Medicine. J Am Soc Echocardiogr 2008;21:93–111, quiz 89–90.
108. Steinke W, Kloetzsch C, Hennerici M. Variability of flow patterns in the normal carotid bifurcation. Atherosclerosis 1990;84: 121–7.
109. Steinke W, Hennerici M, Rautenberg W, et al. Symptomatic and asymptomatic high-grade carotid stenoses in Doppler color-flow imaging. Neurology 1992;42:131–8.
110. Sitzer M, Fürst G, Fischer H, et al. Between-method correlation in quantifying internal carotid stenosis. Stroke 1993;24:1513–18.
111. Steinke W, Meairs S, Ries S, et al. Sonographic assessment of carotid artery stenosis. Comparison of power Doppler imaging and color Doppler flow imaging. Stroke 1996;27:91–4.
112. Griewing B, Morgenstern C, Driesner F, et al. Cerebrovascular disease assessed by color-flow and power Doppler ultrasonography. Comparison with digital subtraction angiography in internal carotid artery stenosis. Stroke 1996;27:95–100.
115. Hennerici M, Steinke W, Rautenberg W. High-resistance Doppler flow pattern in extracranial carotid dissection. Arch Neurol 1989; 46:670–2.
116. Steinke W, Rautenberg W, Schwartz A, et al. Ultrasonographic diagnosis and monitoring of cervicocephalic arterial dissection. Cerebrovasc Dis 1992;2:195.
118. Sturzenegger M, Mattle HP, Rivoir A, et al. Ultrasound findings in carotid artery dissection: analysis of 43 patients. Neurology 1995;45:691–8.
119. Steinke W, Rautenberg W, Schwartz A, et al. Noninvasive monitoring of internal carotid artery dissection. Stroke 1994;25: 998–1005.
122. Tsivgoulis G, Heliopoulos I, Vadikolias K, et al. Piperidou C. Subclavian steal syndrome secondary to Takayasu arteritis in a young female Caucasian patient. J Neurol Sci 2010;296:110–11.
123. Ackerstaff RG, Hoeneveld H, Slowikowski JM, et al. Ultrasonic duplex scanning in atherosclerotic disease of the innominate, subclavian and vertebral arteries. A comparative study with angiography. Ultrasound Med Biol 1984;10:409–18.
129. Sturzenegger M, Mattle HP, Rivoir A, et al. Ultrasound findings in spontaneous extracranial vertebral artery dissection. Stroke 1993;24:1910–21.
130. Touboul PJ, Mas JL, Bousser MG, et al. Duplex scanning in extracranial vertebral artery dissection. Stroke 1988;19:116–21.
131. Bartels E. Flügel KA. Evaluation of extracranial vertebral artery dissection with duplex color-flow imaging. Stroke 1996;27: 290–5.
136. Aaslid R, Markwalder TM, Nornes H. Noninvasive transcranial Doppler ultrasound recording of flow velocity in basal cerebral arteries. J Neurosurg 1982;57:769–74.
137. Alexandrov AV, Sloan MA, Tegeler CH, et al. Practice standards for transcranial Doppler (TCD) ultrasound. Part II. Clinical indications and expected outcomes. J Neuroimaging 2012;22: 215–24.
138. Tsivgoulis G, Alexandrov AV, Sloan MA. Advances in transcranial Doppler ultrasonography. Curr Neurol Neurosci Rep 2009;9: 46–54.
139. Alexandrov AV, Sharma VK, Lao AY, et al. Reversed Robin Hood syndrome in acute ischemic stroke patients. Stroke 2007;38: 3045–8.
140. Alexandrov AV, Nguyen HT, Rubiera M, et al. Prevalence and risk factors associated with reversed Robin Hood syndrome in acute ischemic stroke. Stroke 2009;40:2738–42.
142. Markus HS, Harrison MJ. Estimation of cerebrovascular reactivity using transcranial Doppler, including the use of breath-holding as the vasodilatory stimulus. Stroke 1992;23:668–73.
143. Silvestrini M, Vernieri F, Pasqualetti P, et al. Impaired cerebral vasoreactivity and risk of stroke in patients with asymptomatic carotid artery stenosis. JAMA 2000;283:2122–7.
144. Vernieri F, Pasqualetti P, Matteis M, et al. Effect of collateral blood flow and cerebral vasomotor reactivity on the outcome of carotid artery occlusion. Stroke 2001;32:1552–8.
146. Russell D, Madden KP, Clark WM, et al. Detection of arterial emboli using Doppler ultrasound in rabbits. Stroke 1991; 22:253–8.
150. Markus H, Loh A, Israel D, et al. Microscopic air embolism during cerebral angiography and strategies for its avoidance. Lancet 1993;341:784–7.
151. Jansen C, Ramos LM, van Heesewijk JP, et al. Impact of microembolism and hemodynamic changes in the brain during carotid endarterectomy. Stroke 1994;25:992–7.
153. Markus HS, Clifton A, Buckenham T, et al. Carotid angioplasty. Detection of embolic signals during and after the procedure. Stroke 1994;25:2403–6.
154. Bunegin L, Wahl D, Albin MS. Detection and volume estimation of embolic air in the middle cerebral artery using transcranial Doppler sonography. Stroke 1994;25:593–600.
155. Siebler M, Sitzer M, Steinmetz H. Detection of intracranial emboli in patients with symptomatic extracranial carotid artery disease. Stroke 1992;23:1652–4.
156. Siebler M, Sitzer M, Rose G, et al. Silent cerebral embolism caused by neurologically symptomatic high-grade carotid stenosis. Event rates before and after carotid endarterectomy. Brain 1993;116:1005–15.
158. Grosset DG, Georgiadis D, Abdullah I, et al. Doppler emboli signals vary according to stroke subtype. Stroke 1994;25: 382–4.
159. Markus HS, Droste DW, Brown MM. Detection of asymptomatic cerebral embolic signals with Doppler ultrasound. Lancet 1994; 343:1011–12.
160. Diehl RR, Sliwka U, Rautenberg W, et al. Evidence for embolization from a posterior cerebral artery thrombus by transcranial Doppler monitoring. Stroke 1993;24:606–8.
161. Georgiadis D, Mallinson A, Grosset DG, et al. Coagulation activity and emboli counts in patients with prosthetic cardiac valves. Stroke 1994;25:1211–14.
165. Basic identification criteria of Doppler microembolic signals. Consensus Committee of the Ninth International Cerebral Hemodynamic Symposium. Stroke 1995;26:1123.
167. Saqqur M, Dean N, Schebel M, et al. Improved detection of microbubble signals using power M-mode Doppler. Stroke 2004;35:e14–17.
170. Lao AY, Sharma VK, Tsivgoulis G, et al. Detection of right-to-left shunts: comparison between the International Consensus and Spencer Logarithmic Scale criteria. J Neuroimaging 2008;18: 402–6.
171. Sacco RL, Kargman DE, Gu Q, et al. Race-ethnicity and determinants of intracranial atherosclerotic cerebral infarction. The Northern Manhattan Stroke Study. Stroke 1995;26:14–20.
172. Wityk RJ, Lehman D, Klag M, et al. Race and sex differences in the distribution of cerebral atherosclerosis. Stroke 1996;27: 1974–80.
173. Wong KS, Huang YN, Gao S, et al. Intracranial stenosis in Chinese patients with acute stroke. Neurology 1998;50: 812–13.
174. Caplan LR, Gorelick PB, Hier DB. Race, sex and occlusive cerebrovascular disease: a review. Stroke 1986;17:648–55.
175. Gorelick PB, Caplan LR, Hier DB, et al. Racial differences in the distribution of anterior circulation occlusive disease. Neurology 1984;34:54–9.
176. Nishimaru K, McHenry LC, Toole JF. Cerebral angiographic and clinical differences in carotid system transient ischemic attacks between American Caucasian and Japanese patients. Stroke 1984;15:56–9.
177. Sands KA, Bavarsad Shahripour R, Tsivgoulis G, et al. Abstract T MP28: High Rate of Symptomatic Intracranial Stenosis (sICS) in Patients Treated with Systemic Thrombolysis at a United States Stroke Belt Tertiary Care Center. Stroke 2014;45: ATMP28–ATMP.
178. Chimowitz MI, Kokkinos J, Strong J, et al. The Warfarin-Aspirin Symptomatic Intracranial Disease Study. Neurology 1995;45: 1488–93.
179. Baumgartner R, Mattle H, Schroth G. Assessment of >= 50% and < 50% intracranial stenoses by transcranial color-coded duplex sonography. Stroke 1999;30:87–92.
180. Bogdahn U, Becker G, Winkler J, et al. Transcranial color-coded real-time sonography in adults. Stroke 1990;21:1680–8.

181. Tsivgoulis G, Sharma VK, Lao AY, et al. Validation of transcranial Doppler with computed tomography angiography in acute cerebral ischemia. Stroke 2007;38:1245–9.
182. Tsivgoulis G, Sharma VK, Hoover SL, et al. Applications and advantages of power motion-mode Doppler in acute posterior circulation cerebral ischemia. Stroke 2008;39:1197–204.
183. Navarro JC, Lao AY, Sharma VK, et al. The accuracy of transcranial Doppler in the diagnosis of middle cerebral artery stenosis. Cerebrovasc Dis 2007;23:325–30.
187. Kistler J, Crowell R, Davis K, et al. The relation of cerebral vasospasm to the extent and location of subarachnoid blood visualized by CT scan – A prospective study. Neurology 1983;33: 424–36.
189. Reynolds A, Shaw C. Bleeding patterns from ruptured intracranial aneurysms – An autopsy series of 205 patients. Surg Neurol 1981;15:232–5.
190. Newell D, Grady M, Eskridge J, et al. Distribution of angiographic vasospasm after subarachnoid hemorrhage – implications for diagnosis by transcranial Doppler ultrasonography. Neurosurgery 1990;27:574–7.
191. Aaslid R, Huber P, Nornes H. Evaluation of cerebrovascular spasm with transcranial Doppler ultrasound. J Neurosurg 1984; 60:37–41.
198. Lindegaard KF, Nornes H, Bakke SJ, et al. Cerebral vasospasm diagnosis by means of angiography and blood velocity measurements. Acta Neurochir (Wien) 1989;100:12–24.
199. Lindegaard KF. The role of transcranial Doppler in the management of patients with subarachnoid haemorrhage – a review. Acta Neurochir Suppl 1999;72:59–71.
200. Lennihan L, Petty GW, Fink ME, et al. Transcranial Doppler detection of anterior cerebral artery vasospasm. J Neurol Neurosurg Psychiatry 1993;56:906–9.
201. Wijdicks EF. The diagnosis of brain death. N Engl J Med 2001; 344:1215–21.
206. Gerriets T, Goertler M, Stolz E, et al. Feasibility and validity of transcranial duplex sonography in patients with acute stroke. J Neurol Neurosurg Psychiatry 2002;73:17–20.
208. Otis S, Rush M, Boyajian R. Contrast-enhanced transcranial imaging. Results of an American phase-two study. Stroke 1995; 26:203–9.
209. Baumgartner RW, Arnold M, Gönner F, et al. Contrast-enhanced transcranial color-coded duplex sonography in ischemic cerebrovascular disease. Stroke 1997;28:2473–8.
210. Nabavi DG, Droste DW, Kemény V, et al. Potential and limitations of echocontrast-enhanced ultrasonography in acute stroke patients: a pilot study. Stroke 1998;29:949–54.
217. Chernyshev OY, Garami Z, Calleja S, et al. Yield and accuracy of urgent combined carotid/transcranial ultrasound testing in acute cerebral ischemia. Stroke 2005;36:32–7.
218. Demchuk AM, Burgin WS, Christou I, et al. Thrombolysis in brain ischemia (TIBI) transcranial Doppler flow grades predict clinical severity, early recovery, and mortality in patients treated with intravenous tissue plasminogen activator. Stroke 2001; 32:89–93.
219. Burgin WS, Malkoff M, Felberg RA, et al. Transcranial doppler ultrasound criteria for recanalization after thrombolysis for middle cerebral artery stroke. Stroke 2000;31:1128–32.
221. Nedelmann M, Stolz E, Gerriets T, et al. Consensus recommendations for transcranial color-coded duplex sonography for the assessment of intracranial arteries in clinical trials on acute stroke. Stroke 2009;40:3238–44.
222. Alexandrov AV, Demchuk AM, Felberg RA, et al. Intracranial clot dissolution is associated with embolic signals on transcranial Doppler. J Neuroimaging 2000;10:27–32.
223. Tsivgoulis G, Ribo M, Rubiera M, et al. Real-time validation of transcranial Doppler criteria in assessing recanalization during intra-arterial procedures for acute ischemic stroke: an international, multicenter study. Stroke 2013;44:394–400.
224. Tissue plasminogen activator for acute ischemic stroke. The National Institute of Neurological Disorders and Stroke rt-PA Stroke Study Group. N Engl J Med 1995;333:1581–7.
225. Lees KR, Bluhmki E, von Kummer R, et al. Time to treatment with intravenous alteplase and outcome in stroke: an updated pooled analysis of ECASS, ATLANTIS, NINDS, and EPITHET trials. Lancet 2010;375:1695–703.
229. Meairs S, Culp W. Microbubbles for thrombolysis of acute ischemic stroke. Cerebrovasc Dis 2009;27(Suppl. 2):55–65.
230. Tsivgoulis G, Alexandrov AV. Ultrasound enhanced thrombolysis: applications in acute cerebral ischemia. J Clin Neurol. 2007; 3:1–8.
231. Tsivgoulis G, Alexandrov AV. Ultrasound-enhanced thrombolysis in acute ischemic stroke: potential, failures, and safety. Neurother 2007;4:420–7.
232. Tsivgoulis G, Culp WC, Alexandrov AV. Ultrasound enhanced thrombolysis in acute arterial ischemia. Ultrasonics 2008;48: 303–11.
233. Tsivgoulis G, Alexandrov A. Ultrasound-enhanced thrombolysis: from bedside to bench. Stroke 2008;39:1404–5.
235. Lauer CG, Burge R, Tang DB, et al. Effect of ultrasound on tissue-type plasminogen activator-induced thrombolysis. Circulation 1992;86:1257–64.
236. Blinc A, Francis CW, Trudnowski JL, et al. Characterization of ultrasound-potentiated fibrinolysis in vitro. Blood 1993;81: 2636–43.
239. Suchkova V, Siddiqi FN, Carstensen EL, et al. Enhancement of fibrinolysis with 40-kHz ultrasound. Circulation 1998;98: 1030–5.
240. Behrens S, Daffertshofer M, Spiegel D, et al. Low-frequency, low-intensity ultrasound accelerates thrombolysis through the skull. Ultrasound Med Biol 1999;25:269–73.
241. Behrens S, Spengos K, Daffertshofer M, et al. Transcranial ultrasound-improved thrombolysis: diagnostic vs. therapeutic ultrasound. Ultrasound Med Biol 2001;27:1683–9.
243. Daffertshofer M, Hennerici M. Ultrasound in the treatment of ischaemic stroke. Lancet Neurol 2003;2:283–90.
244. Polak JF. Ultrasound energy and the dissolution of thrombus. N Engl J Med 2004;351:2154–5.
245. Alexandrov AV. Ultrasound enhanced thrombolysis for stroke. Int J Stroke. 2006;1:26–9.
249. Daffertshofer M, Gass A, Ringleb P, et al. Transcranial low-frequency ultrasound-mediated thrombolysis in brain ischemia: increased risk of hemorrhage with combined ultrasound and tissue plasminogen activator: results of a phase II clinical trial. Stroke 2005;36:1441–6.
250. Alexandrov AV, Molina CA, Grotta JC, et al. Ultrasound-enhanced systemic thrombolysis for acute ischemic stroke. N Engl J Med 2004;351:2170–8.
251. Saqqur M, Tsivgoulis G, Nicoli F, et al. The Role of Sonolysis and Sonothrombolysis in Acute Ischemic Stroke: A Systematic Review and Meta-analysis of Randomized Controlled Trials and Case-Control Studies. J Neuroimaging 2013;doi:10.1111/jon .12026.
252. Tsivgoulis G, Eggers J, Ribo M, et al. Safety and efficacy of ultrasound-enhanced thrombolysis: a comprehensive review and meta-analysis of randomized and nonrandomized studies. Stroke 2010;41:280–7.
253. Eggers J, Seidel G, Koch B, et al. Sonothrombolysis in acute ischemic stroke for patients ineligible for rt-PA. Neurology 2005;64:1052–4.
254. Eggers J, König IR, Koch B, et al. Sonothrombolysis with transcranial color-coded sonography and recombinant tissue-type plasminogen activator in acute middle cerebral artery main stem occlusion: results from a randomized study. Stroke 2008;39: 1470–5.
255. Gerriets T, Postert T, Goertler M, et al. DIAS I: duplex-sonographic assessment of the cerebrovascular status in acute stroke. A useful tool for future stroke trials. Stroke 2000;31:2342–5.
256. Kenton AR, Martin PJ, Abbott RJ, et al. Comparison of transcranial color-coded sonography and magnetic resonance angiography in acute stroke. Stroke 1997;28:1601–6.
257. Ricci S, Dinia L, Del Sette M, et al. Sonothrombolysis for acute ischaemic stroke. Cochrane Database Syst Rev 2012;10:CD008348.
258. Molina CA, Ribo M, Rubiera M, et al. Microbubble administration accelerates clot lysis during continuous 2-MHz ultrasound monitoring in stroke patients treated with intravenous tissue plasminogen activator. Stroke 2006;37:425–9.
261. Sharma VK, Tsivgoulis G, Lao AY, et al. Quantification of microspheres appearance in brain vessels: implications for residual flow velocity measurements, dose calculations, and potential drug delivery. Stroke 2008;39:1476–81.

262. Alexandrov AV. Therapeutic applications of transcranial ultrasound devices. Expert Rev Med Devices 2007;4:1–3.
263. Culp WC, Flores R, Brown AT, et al. Successful microbubble sonothrombolysis without tissue-type plasminogen activator in a rabbit model of acute ischemic stroke. Stroke 2011; 42:2280–5.
272. Culp WC, Porter TR, Lowery J, et al. Intracranial clot lysis with intravenous microbubbles and transcranial ultrasound in swine. Stroke 2004;35:2407–11.
274. Alonso A, Della Martina A, Stroick M, et al. Molecular imaging of human thrombus with novel abciximab immunobubbles and ultrasound. Stroke 2007;38:1508–14.
276. Newell DW, Shah MM, Wilcox R, et al. Minimally invasive evacuation of spontaneous intracerebral hemorrhage using sonothrombolysis. J Neurosurg 2011;115:592–601.
277. Webb AJ, Ullman NL, Mann S, et al. Resolution of intraventricular hemorrhage varies by ventricular region and dose of intraventricular thrombolytic: the Clot Lysis: Evaluating Accelerated Resolution of IVH (CLEAR IVH) program. Stroke 2012; 43:1666–8.
280. Barnett HJ, Taylor DW, Eliasziw M, et al. Benefit of carotid endarterectomy in patients with symptomatic moderate or severe stenosis. North American Symptomatic Carotid Endarterectomy Trial Collaborators. N Engl J Med 1998;339:1415–25.
281. Farrell B, Fraser A, Sandercock P, et al. European Carotid Surgery Trialists' Collaborative Group. Randomised trial of endarterectomy for recently symptomatic carotid stenosis: final results of the MRC European carotid surgery trial (ECST). Lancet 1998;351:1379–87.
282. Spencer MP. Transcranial Doppler monitoring and causes of stroke from carotid endarterectomy. Stroke 1997;28:685–91.
283. Mas JL, Chatellier G, Beyssen B, et al. Endarterectomy versus stenting in patients with symptomatic severe carotid stenosis. N Engl J Med 2006;355:1660–71.
288. Schumann PA, Christiansen JP, Quigley RM, et al. Targeted-microbubble binding selectively to GPIIb IIIa receptors of platelet thrombi. Invest Radiol 2002;37:587–93.
311. Shohet RV, Chen S, Zhou YT, et al. Echocardiographic destruction of albumin microbubbles directs gene delivery to the myocardium. Circulation 2000;101:2554–6.
322. Zhao L, Barlinn K, Sharma VK, et al. Velocity criteria for intracranial stenosis revisited: an international multicenter study of transcranial Doppler and digital subtraction angiography. Stroke 2011;42:3429–34.
323. Sloan MA, Alexandrov AV, Tegeler CH, et al. Assessment: transcranial Doppler ultrasonography: report of the Therapeutics and Technology Assessment Subcommittee of the American Academy of Neurology. Neurology 2004;62:1468–81.
324. Soustiel JF, Shik V, Shreiber R, et al. Basilar vasospasm diagnosis: investigation of a modified "Lindegaard Index" based on imaging studies and blood velocity measurements of the basilar artery. Stroke 2002;33:72–7.
325. Sviri GE, Ghodke B, Britz GW, et al. Transcranial Doppler grading criteria for basilar artery vasospasm. Neurosurgery 2006; 59:360–6, discussion 360–6.

47 Computed Tomography-based Evaluation of Cerebrovascular Disease

Imanuel Dzialowski, Volker Puetz, Marc Parsons, Rüdiger von Kummer

KEY POINTS

- Non-contrast CT is the standard diagnostic modality for acute stroke patients. It reliably differentiates hemorrhagic from ischemic stroke, enables rapid thrombolysis and thereby improves stroke recovery.
- On non-contrast CT, different types of "early ischemic changes" can be found: hypodensity, isolated cortical swelling and hyperdense arteries. Patients with extensive hypodensity do not appear to benefit from thrombolysis, whereas isolated cortical swelling or hyperdense arteries should encourage recanalization therapies.
- CT angiography (CTA) is a fast and reliable tool to diagnose and grade intra- and extracranial occlusive disease. Patients with a large thrombus burden on CTA might benefit from endovascular recanalization.
- In patients with posterior circulation stroke, CTA enables rapid diagnosis of basilar thrombosis.
- CTA improves prediction of irreversible brain tissue injury using a low contrast and window level.
- CTP provides additional information about extent of irreversible brain injury as well as extent of salvageable tissue that is not possible with NCT and CTA.
- Whole-brain CTP can also allow dynamic CTA acquisition which provides valuable insights into collateral flow in acute ischemic stroke.

This chapter studies the clinical efficacy of computed tomography (CT) in patients with acute ischemic or hemorrhagic stroke. We will discuss non-contrast CT (NCT) as well as CT angiography (CTA) and CT perfusion imaging (CTP) for acute stroke. Because of the differing prognosis between anterior and posterior circulation ischemic strokes, we will separately discuss CT imaging for these. In theory, CT, like magnetic resonance imaging (MRI), can be clinically effective in patients with acute stroke on five different levels: (1) technical capacity, (2) diagnostic accuracy, (3) diagnostic impact, (4) therapeutic impact, and (5) patient outcome or prognostic impact.[1]

We will focus on the use of CT in the acute stroke setting. Whenever applicable, we will compare CT with MRI – the other important acute stroke imaging modality discussed in Chapter 48.

NON-CONTRAST COMPUTED TOMOGRAPHY

Feasibility and Technical Capacity

A potential advantage of CT over MRI is its wide availability and excellent feasibility.[2] Even with older-generation scanners a plain CT scan can be performed within minutes. Performing a CTA or CTP requires a spiral CT scanner, the application of contrast media, and processing afterward. Each examination will usually only require an extra 5 minutes' scan time. Recently, CT scanners with up to 320 detector rows that cover a tissue volume of 16 cm thickness have become available.[3] These scanners can examine the whole brain in less than 1 second and can repeatedly image the entire cerebral circulation, allowing time-resolved images of the brain vessels and whole brain CTP.

Downsides of Computed Tomography Imaging

The main downsides of CT brain imaging are radiation and the use of iodinated contrast agents. The radiation dose per CT scan is in the range of 1 to 3 mSv depending on the scanner type. Therefore, repeating a CT to follow-up brain and vessel pathology, and in particular the repetition of CTP, can be problematic. For brain imaging the lenses should be protected. The risk of kidney function failure or thyrotoxic crisis caused by iodinated contrast agents is relatively low, but requires tests of kidney and thyroid gland function. Another disadvantage of unenhanced CT is that automatically measured volumes of pathologic tissue, such as can be performed on CTP or ADC maps, are not available.

Detection of Ischemic Core

Acute brain ischemia below the cerebral blood flow (CBF) threshold of 20–30 mL/100 g/min leads to loss of neurologic function, cell membrane dysfunction with cellular edema (so-called cytotoxic edema), and subsequent shrinkage of the extracellular space. This type of edema is potentially reversible and can be visualized by MRI with diffusion-weighted imaging (DWI). Acute severe brain ischemia with CBF values below 10 mL/100 g/min causes immediate net water uptake into gray matter.[4,5] This so-called ionic edema[6] characterizes brain tissue destined for tissue necrosis, even with early reperfusion.[7] Only this net uptake of water into brain tissue causes a decrease in x-ray attenuation on CT.[4] The decrease in x-ray attenuation is linearly and indirectly correlated to the amount of water uptake. A 1% increase in tissue water causes a decrease of approximately 2 Hounsfield units (HU) in x-ray attenuation that can be detected by the human eye.[8] CT is thus a very specific method for depicting irreversible brain infarction.[9]

Early Signs of Infarction on Non-contract Computed Tomography

Early changes visible on head CT during ischemia are often summarized as "early ischemic changes" (EIC). We should, however, distinguish between at least three different kinds of EIC with different pathophysiologic and diagnostic relevance:

1. Reduced x-ray attenuation of gray matter is the common cause of CT signs such as "loss of the insular or cortical

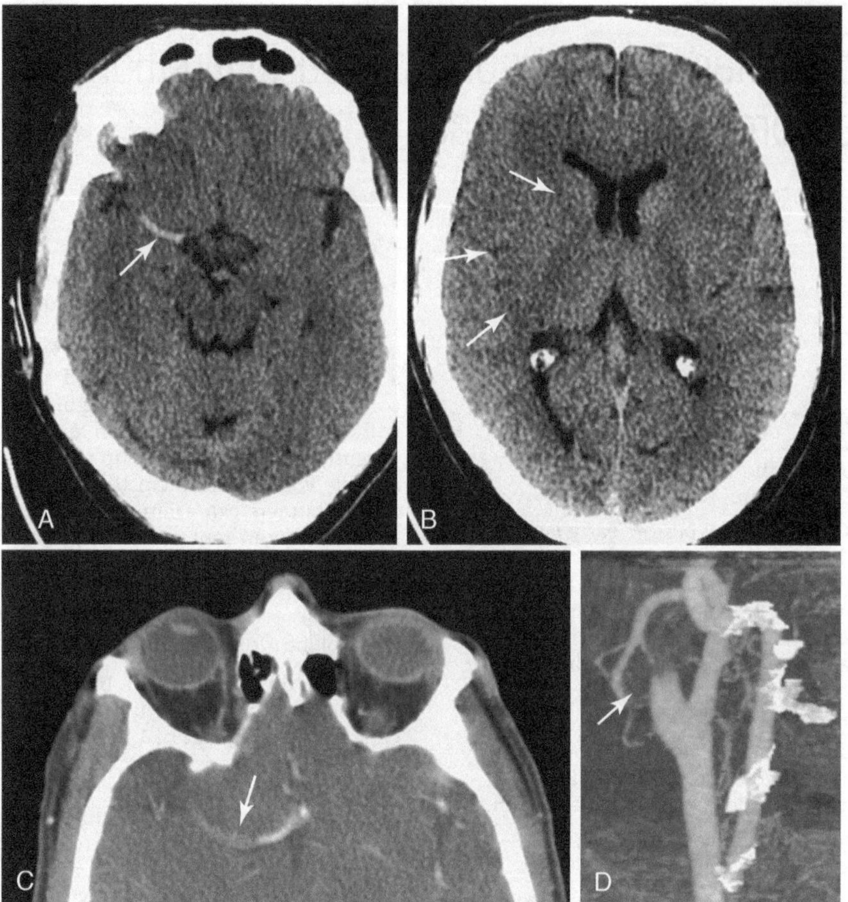

Figure 47-1. Acute middle cerebral artery (MCA) infarction in a patient with occlusion of the internal carotid artery (ICA) and MCA. A, Hyperdense MCA sign *(arrow)* on baseline noncontrast CT (NCT) scan. B, NCT with hypoattenuation of the right lentiform nucleus, head of caudate nucleus, and insula *(arrows)*. C, Intracranial CT angiography (CTA) source image showing right proximal MCA occlusion *(arrow)*. D, Extracranial CTA maximal intensity projection of the right common carotid artery, external carotid artery, and ICA showing proximal ICA occlusion.

ribbon," "obscuration of the lentiform nucleus," reduction in gray matter–white matter contrast, or "hypodensity." These phenomena are all consequences of ionic cerebral edema and thus represent ischemic infarction on CT (Fig. 47-1).

2. Isolated brain tissue swelling without reduced x-ray attenuation (Fig. 47-2): this phenomenon has been extensively studied recently and is likely caused by compensatory vasodilation with an increase of cerebral blood volume (CBV).[10–12] It represents tissue at risk of infarction that might be salvaged with reperfusion, i.e., ischemic penumbra. It was observed in 10–20% of ischemic brain regions.[10] The presence of isolated cortical swelling on CT - even if very extensive - should NOT prevent stroke neurologists from attempting urgent recanalization.
3. The hyperdense artery sign is highly specific for the presence of an intra-arterial thrombus,[13] but its detection depends on the thrombus' hematocrit value, which determines its x-ray attenuation.[14] Recently, it has been shown that accuracy of thrombus detection can be markedly improved using thin-slice (1.25 or 2.5 mm) reconstructions.[15] Using these, thrombus length can be accurately measured. Thrombi with a length of > 8 mm may have no chance to be fully lysed by IV thrombolytics.[16] The term *EIC* should not be used for the hyperdense artery sign because arterial obstruction by an intraluminal thrombus can be fully compensated by collateral flow (see Fig. 47-1A).

Diagnostic Accuracy

In the first 6 hours after ischemic stroke, two of three stroke patients will develop ionic edema that can be detected by NCT.[17] Poor sensitivity of NCT is often blamed for the fact that ischemic (i.e., ionic) edema cannot be diagnosed early in many patients with ischemic stroke. Stroke symptoms occur at CBF reduction to 20–30 mL/100 g/min, which is well above the accepted threshold for ionic edema. We can thus assume that around one-third of ischemic stroke patients have not *yet* developed relevant ionic edema (i.e., no irreversible damage) and may have an excellent prognosis if reperfusion is achieved. X-ray hypoattenuation on early NCT, however, is subtle and hard to detect without training (see Fig. 47-1B). Interrater reliability for ischemic tissue hypoattenuation varies between a kappa value of 0.4 and 0.6.[18] The "sensitivity" of NCT for infarction on follow-up imaging varies between 20% and 87% depending on image quality, experience, and training.[17] Using systematic scores like the Alberta Stroke Program Early CT Score (ASPECTS) facilitates detection of x-ray hypoattenuation and improves reliability and sensitivity.[19] Once a hypoattenuating area has been detected, it is highly predictive of subsequent infarction.[9]

Diagnostic Impact

The diagnostic impact of stroke imaging refers to the proportion of patients in whom the specific diagnosis of stroke type

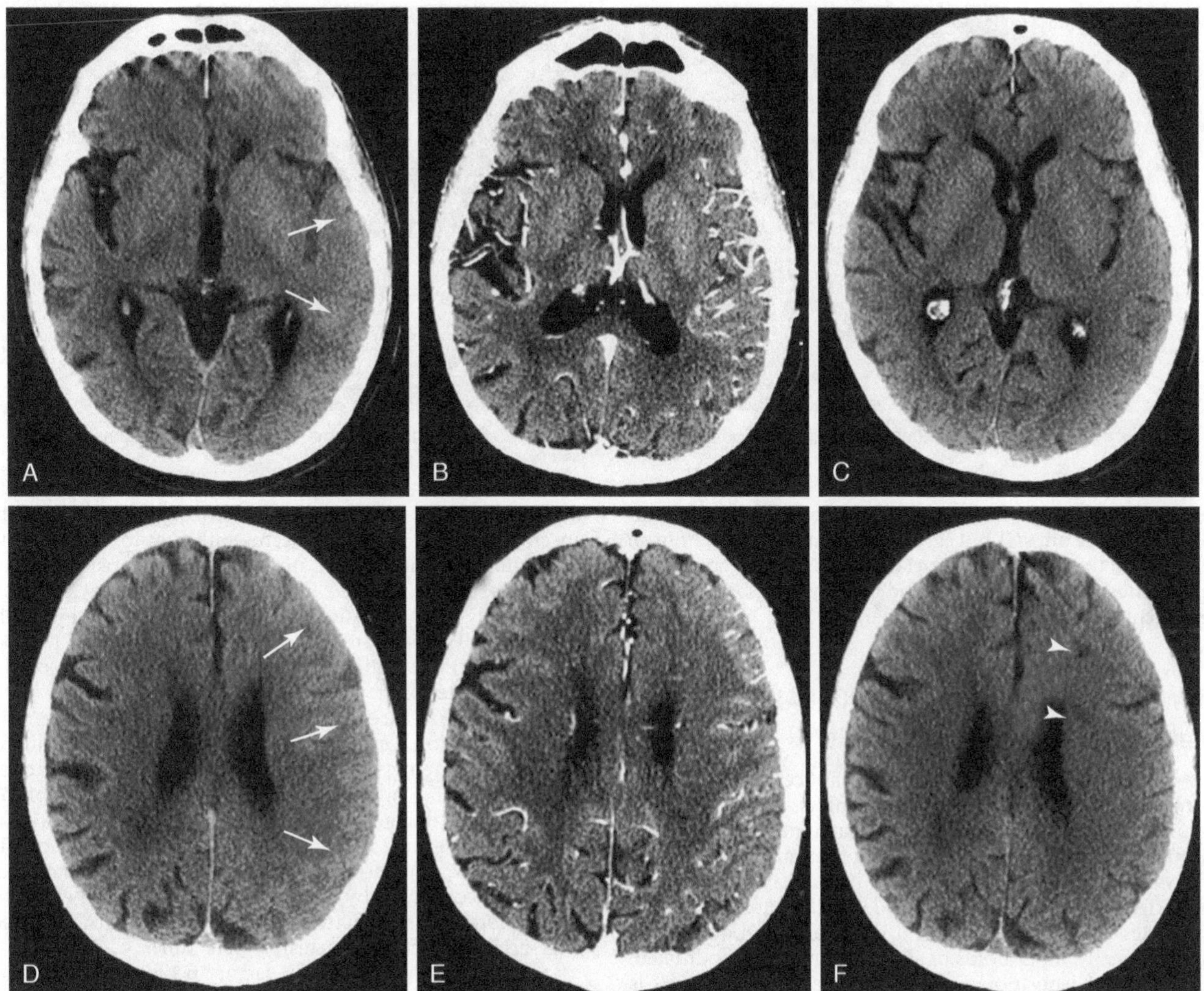

Figure 47-2. A 79-year-old man seen with acute aphasia and right-sided hemiplegia. Baseline noncontrast CT (NCT) shows hemispheric cortical swelling *(arrows)* without hypoattenuation (A, D). CT angiography demonstrates dilated cortical vessels in these regions (B, E). The patient had marked spontaneous clinical improvement. Follow-up NCT (C, F) 3 days later revealed minor infarcts in the internal borderzone *(arrowheads)* and regressive cortical swelling.

relies on imaging. NCT has a huge diagnostic impact simply by differentiating ischemic from hemorrhagic stroke, enabling thrombolysis. In addition, the extent of hypoattenuation on NCT is an important positive predictor of thrombolysis-induced brain hemorrhage, which is the most feared complication of thrombolysis.[20–22] MR DWI is highly sensitive for ischemic brain tissue, even above the CBF level of the penumbra and indicates brain tissue at high risk, if not already irreversibly injured, whereas hypoattenuation on NCT depicts irreversible tissue damage with high specificity. High signal intensity on DWI may allow assessment of ischemic brain patterns and thus the cause of stroke early on and signals an increased early risk of recurrent stroke in patients with transient ischemic attacks (TIAs).[23]

Therapeutic Impact

In acute ischemic stroke, thrombolysis with intravenous (IV) recombinant tissue plasminogen activator (rt-PA) within 4.5 hours of stroke onset can increase the proportion of nondisabled patients by an absolute 11%.[24–26] The National Institute of Neurological Disorders and Stroke (NINDS) rt-PA Study Group was able to prove benefit for thrombolysis simply by using NCT to identify ischemic stroke patients. The European Cooperative Acute Stroke Study (ECASS) investigators used NCT to additionally exclude patients with extended ischemic edema.[24,27,28] These studies show that NCT is sufficient to identify a group of patients in whom IV thrombolytics have a moderate beneficial effect within 4.5 hours of symptom onset.

Prognostic Impact

The impact of CT on the functional outcome of stroke patients is the most important level of clinical efficacy. As shown above, NCT enables thrombolysis in ischemic stroke patients and thereby reduces long-term disability. There is good evidence that patients with extended hypoattenuation (infarction) on NCT have a poorer natural history and less chance to benefit from thrombolysis.[29,21,22]

In summary, brain tissue imaging by NCT ignores the changes above the CBF threshold of irreversible injury, with the exception of brain tissue swelling without hypoattenuation due to compensatory vasodilation. NCT has a rather low sensitivity for identifying brain ischemia but a high specificity for identifying irreversible ischemic injury. One may conclude

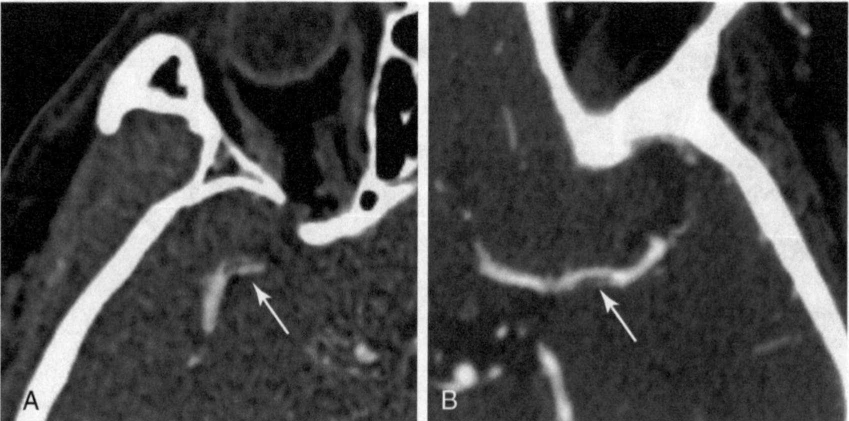

Figure 47-3. Example of intracranial non-occlusive thrombus *(arrows)* in the distal right M1 segment (A) and left M1 segment (B).

that mainly patients who have small volumes of hypoattenuating brain tissue on NCT but severe symptoms will benefit from reperfusion therapy. In fact, several studies have demonstrated that the response to thrombolytic therapy is associated with the extent of hypoattenuation on early CT.[22]

COMPUTED TOMOGRAPHY ANGIOGRAPHY

Feasibility and Technical Capacity

The advent of spiral data acquisition has accelerated CT performance tremendously. With this technique, data acquisition occurs continuously while the gantry table moves the patient through the gantry, so a volume of interest can be scanned in a very short time.

A CTA study of the neck and head usually requires less than 5 minutes' examination time and the application of contrast media. Usually, an IV bolus of about 100 mL of an iodinated, nonionic and isoosmolar or low osmolar contrast agent is given, and image acquisition will be initiated when the contrast reaches the aortic arch or common carotid artery. In our experience, feasibility of CTA is excellent and images are diagnostic in almost every patient. Immediately after data acquisition, CTA source images can be viewed, and large-vessel occlusions can be diagnosed instantaneously (see Fig. 47-1C). Within a few minutes, 3D reformats can be generated, enabling detection of peripheral vessel and other abnormalities (see Fig. 47-1D).

The utility of CTA is tremendous, and it has already replaced conventional catheter angiography in many situations. Recent technical development enables CTA with time-resolution (4D-CTA) and digital subtraction of the bone.

Diagnostic Accuracy

Intracranial Disease

The need for rapid decisions makes CTA an ideal technique in the detection of large-vessel intracranial arterial stenosis or occlusion (see Fig. 47-1). For intracranial atherosclerotic stenosis, non-invasive imaging modalities should identify lesions with high sensitivity and specificity as compared with the gold standard of digital subtraction angiography (DSA).

Compared with MRA, CTA has increased sensitivity (70% vs 98%, respectively) and PPV (65% vs 93%, respectively) for revealing intracranial arterial stenosis.[30] Similar results were found in a recent study, where the sensitivity of CTA to detect 50% or greater intracranial stenosis was 97% and the specificity 99%.[31] Thus, CTA seems sufficient to detect or rule out significant intracranial atherosclerotic stenosis. We have recently used CTA to detect intracranial non-occlusive thrombi (iNOT; Fig. 47-3) in patients seen with acute ischemic stroke and TIAs.[32] These thrombi seem to be rare (2.7% of patients in our study) but indicate stroke patients with increased risk of clinical deterioration during the hospital course.

CTA also has excellent accuracy in detecting intracranial arterial occlusion. Lev et al.[33] studied 44 consecutive patients with acute ischemic stroke who underwent CTA of the circle of Willis within 6 hours of onset of symptoms. A total of 572 vessels were evaluated, and angiographic correlation was available for 224 of these vessels. Sensitivity and specificity of CTA were both 98%, and accuracy was 99%. The results of Lev et al. have been confirmed by a study by Nguyen-Huynh et al.[31] in which both the sensitivity and specificity of CTA to detect large-artery intracranial occlusion were 100%.

As an additional prognostic factor and for the purpose of immediate treatment decisions, the intracranial thrombus extent can be estimated with CTA. Patients' prognoses and responses to therapy can be judged by a ten-point clot burden score (CBS; Fig. 47-4). CBS is a simple measure of the location and extent of intracranial thrombus.[34] Patients with a higher thrombus burden (i.e., lower CBS scores) had higher baseline National Institutes of Health Stroke Scale (NIHSS) scores and more extended infarctions compared with patients with less thrombus burden. Moreover, CBS was an independent predictor of independent functional outcomes and death in this study. These results have been confirmed in a recent study by Tan et al.[35] Their study also demonstrated a correlation of CBS with the perfusion defects on CTP maps and CTA source images and confirmed the hypothesis that a higher thrombus burden is associated with lower recanalization rates with IV thrombolysis.[36]

In summary, CTA is an ideal tool for the rapid and accurate detection of intracranial stenosis and occlusion of major intracranial arteries and may help to differentiate patients who will benefit from specific recanalization techniques.

Extracranial Carotid Artery Disease

Cerebral angiography has been the diagnostic procedure of choice for the quantification of extracranial carotid artery stenosis. Although generally safe, angiography is still associated with a 0.5–5% rate of stroke as a complication when used in routine clinical practice.[37,38] With the advent of ultrafast helical CT imaging, the complication is avoided, and CTA is being used with increasing frequency in the diagnosis of extracranial

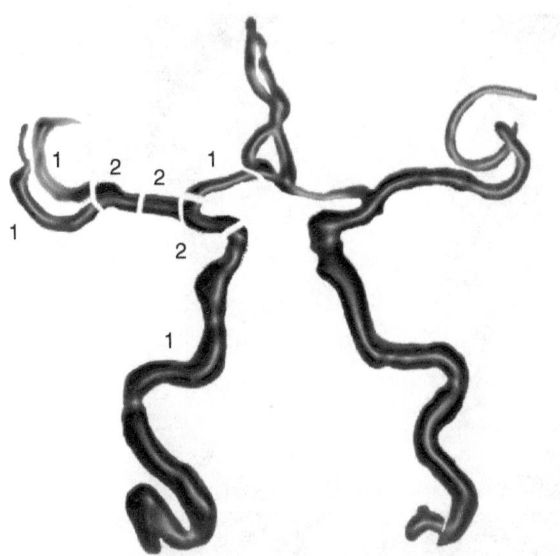

Figure 47-4. A 10-point clot burden score (CBS): 1 or 2 points each (as indicated) are subtracted for absent contrast opacification on CT angiography in the infraclinoid internal carotid artery (ICA) (1), supraclinoid ICA (2), proximal M1 segment (2), distal M1 segment (2), M2 branches (1 each) and A1 segment (1). The CBS score applies only to the symptomatic hemisphere.

carotid artery disease. An example of severe right internal carotid stenosis is depicted in Figure 47-5A, on conventional arteriography, and in Figure 47-5B, on CTA (axial cuts).

Several studies to date have reported excellent agreement between conventional catheter cerebral angiography and CTA. In a comparative study, a strong correlation was found between CTA and angiography ($r = 0.987$; $P < 0.0001$) in 128 carotid bifurcations in 64 patients.[39] CTA has the additional benefit of providing precise information regarding the surrounding vascular and bony anatomy, including arterial wall calcification that is not depicted by DSA or MRA.

In a prospective study, 40 patients (80 carotid arteries) underwent evaluation by CTA, digital DSA, and Doppler ultrasonography.[40] The overall correlation between Doppler ultrasonography and DSA was less robust ($r = 0.808$) than that between CTA and DSA ($r = 0.92$); CTA provided superb correlation in the detection of mild stenosis (0–29%), stenosis greater than 50%, and carotid occlusion and had sensitivities and specificities exceeding 0.90. CTA performed less well in the detection of 70–99% stenosis and had a sensitivity of 0.73 (axial source images) and a PPV of only 0.62 (negative predictive value, 0.95). The relatively poorer degree of discrimination on CTA in this study between moderate (50–69%) and severe (70–99%) stenosis is an important limiting factor to consider in the use of this technology.

Detection of Brain Tissue Infarction

In addition to providing information on the vessel status, CTA may also predict the fate of ischemic brain parenchyma; that is, it improves early detection of ischemic infarction.[41] Viewing the CTA source images at a low contrast and window level (e.g., 40/40 HU) downstream to a large-vessel occlusion, CTA will show an area of diminished tissue contrast enhancement (Figs 47-6, 47-7). This area likely represents severely hypoperfused brain tissue that will be irreversibly damaged without reperfusion. In comparison with NCT, the sensitivity and accuracy in prediction of final infarct extension can be improved.[42,43] The benefit of CTA-SI over NCT is especially evident in the first 3 hours after symptom onset.[44] CTA source images are also closely correlated to MR DWI sequences.

Diagnostic Impact

Within minutes, CTA reliably diagnoses arterial occlusions and stenoses from the aortic arch to the distal intracranial arterial segments. Compared with MRI, CTA is sensitive for calcified plaques and can thus elucidate the underlying stroke etiology in many cases. Patients with MCA occlusion have a lesser chance to benefit from IV thrombolytics if the ipsilateral carotid is obstructed.[45] A systematic study of arterial pathology with CTA may enable more specific treatments of arterial occlusions. In addition, CTA can distinguish patients seen with seizures and postictal paresis (Todd's paralysis) from those with true ischemic hemiparesis and early seizures by demonstrating arterial occlusion.[46]

Therapeutic Impact

The usefulness of CTA for therapeutic decisions has not yet been prospectively studied. There is evidence from secondary analyses of randomized trials that patients with a small core of infarction on NCT (or possibly CTA source images) and an intracranial large-vessel occlusion on CTA might be ideal candidates for recanalization, even beyond the accepted time window. This hypothesis is currently being studied in at least two large, randomized controlled trials.[47]

Many centers use CTA to select acute ischemic stroke patients for intra-arterial interventions. The PROACT II study demonstrated that patients with an MCA occlusion benefit from intra-arterial thrombolysis up to 6 hours after onset.[48] Another approach for patients with known intracranial occlusions is the intravenous–intra-arterial bridging concept. The Interventional Management of Stroke III trial could not show that this strategy is superior to standard IV thrombolysis.[49] In a post-hoc analysis, however, patients with a CTA-proven combined carotid and MCA occlusion at baseline showed a benefit from the bridging approach.[50] Potentially, patients with proximal arterial occlusion (e.g., carotid T occlusion) and/or large thrombus burden may benefit from additional intra-arterial therapy, whereas patients with minor thrombus burden (e.g., MCA M2 branch occlusion) may receive no additional benefit. Estimation of thrombus burden with a CBS could be a simple and readily available tool to help in deciding whether a patient will benefit from aggressive treatment paradigms.

CTA might also be useful for excluding patients without visible arterial occlusion from thrombolysis. Angiographic studies have shown that arterial occlusion cannot be detected in one-third of patients seen within 6 hours of onset.[51]

COMPUTED TOMOGRAPHY PERFUSION IMAGING

Technical Capacity and Feasibility

With the development of helical CT scanning technology, it is now possible to track a bolus of IV contrast material as it passes through the brain. The measurement technique for CBF has its theoretical basis in the central volume principle, which relates CBF (mL/100g/min), CBV (mL/100 g), and mean transit time (MTT; seconds) by the following equation:

$$CBF = \frac{CBV}{MTT}$$

It is assumed that a linear relationship exists between the CT enhancement and the concentration of contrast material

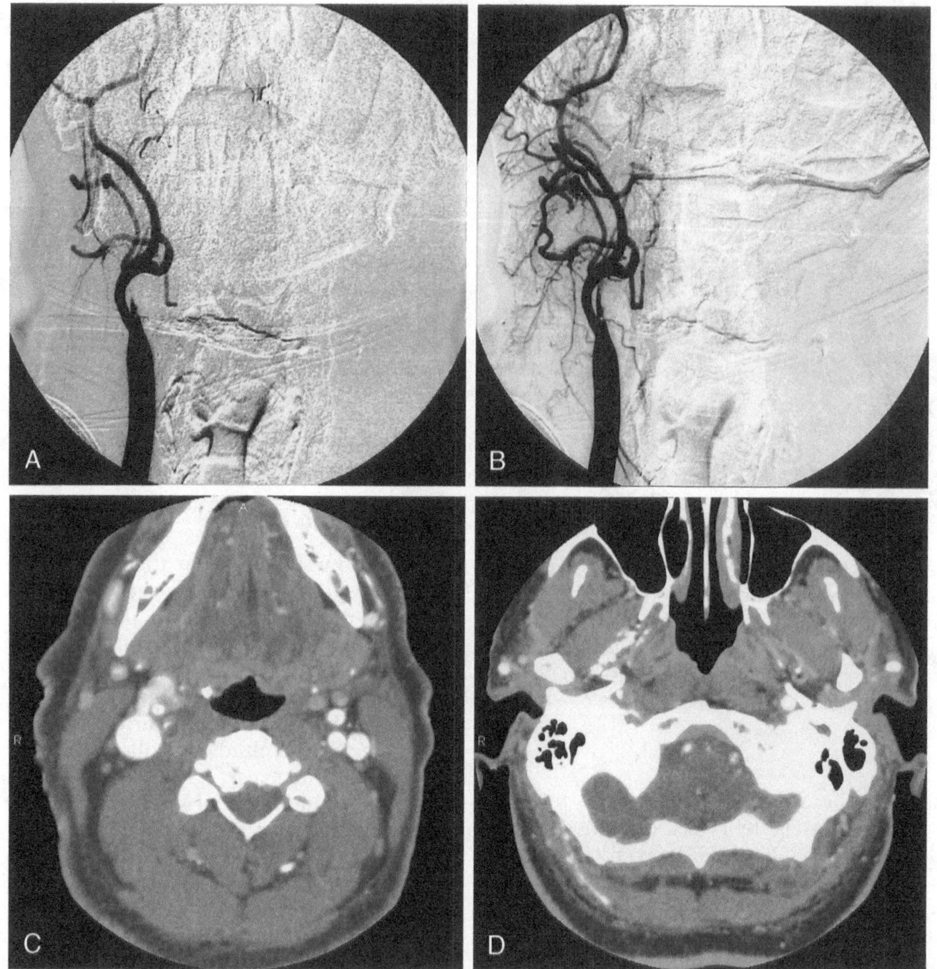

Figure 47-5. Conventional angiographic depiction (A, B) of right internal carotid artery occlusion in a patient seen with an acute ischemic right middle cerebral artery distribution infarction. CT angiography source images (C, D) confirm right ICA occlusion *(arrow)*.

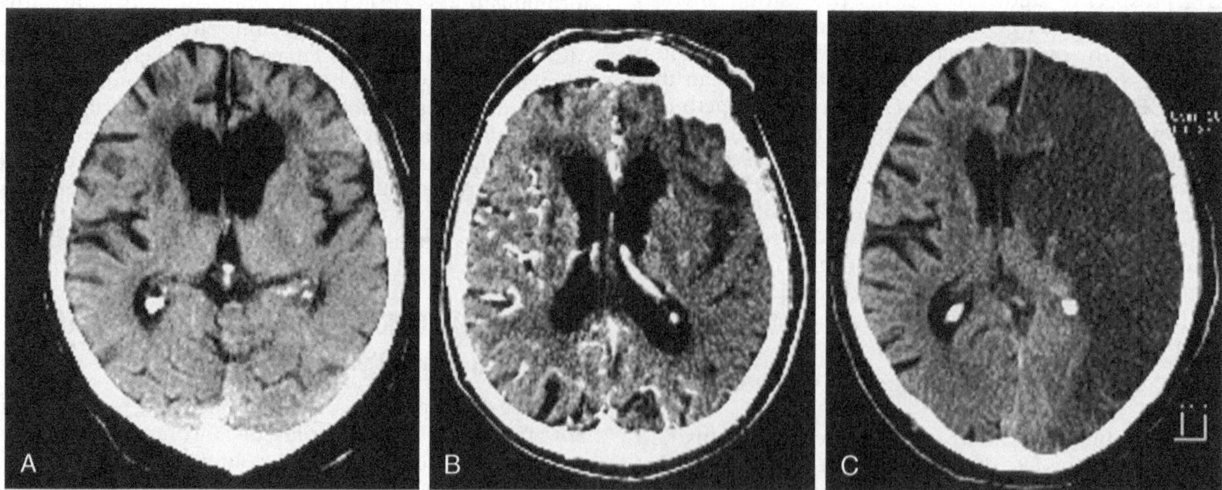

Figure 47-6. Noncontrast CT (NCT) (A) and CT angiography (CTA) source images (B) of a patient 1 hour after acute aphasia and right hemiparesis. NCT shows subtle hypoattenuation of left basal ganglia, insula, and anterior cerebral artery (ACA) territory. CTA clearly shows contrast hypoattenuation in the complete middle cerebral artery and ACA territory caused by an internal carotid artery occlusion. Follow- up CT (C) shows the resulting infarction.

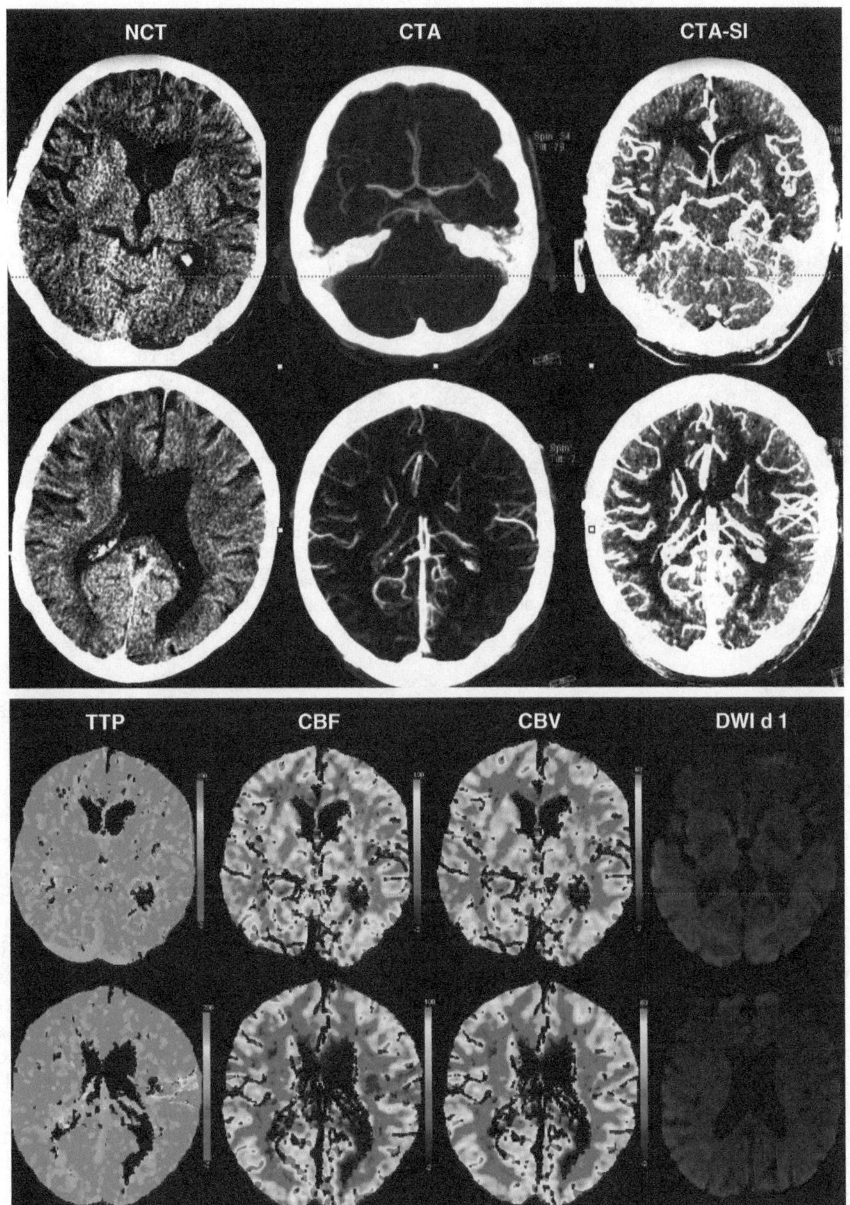

Figure 47-7. Noncontrast CT (NCT), CT angiography (CTA), and CT perfusion imaging (CTA-SI) of an 82-year-old patient 2 hours after aphasia and mild right hemiparesis. NCT and CTA results are normal without evidence of intracranial arterial occlusion *(upper two rows).* Time-to-peak (TTP) and cerebral blood flow (CBF) parameter maps reveal hypoperfusion in the left insula and corona radiata without reduction of cerebral blood volume (CBV, *lower two rows*). After thrombolysis with recombinant tissue plasminogen activator (rt-PA), follow-up MRI-diffusion-weighted imaging (DWI) shows a tiny infarction in the left insula.

within brain tissue and arteries. After IV administration of a bolus of iodinated contrast agent, measurements are made of the arterial enhancement curve, $C_a(t)$, the supplying artery, and the tissue enhancement curve, $Q(t)$, for a region of the central parenchyma. For the calculation of MTT, a mathematical process of deconvolution is applied to the functions $C_a(t)$ and $Q(t)$ to determine an impulse (or residue) function, $R(t)$, which would be the theoretical tissue enhancement curve obtained from a rapidly injected bolus of contrast material. The MTT is calculated from the following formula:

$$\text{MTT} = \frac{\text{area underneath } R(t)}{\text{height of } R(t) \text{ plateau}}$$

CBV is calculated from $Q(t)$ and $C_a(t)$, the two parameters measured directly during the CTP study:

$$\text{CBV} = \frac{\text{area underneath } Q(t)}{\text{area underneath } C_a(t)}$$

In addition to the above perfusion parameters, other measures of perfusion that can be calculated relate to time of contrast transit.[52] These include: (i) time to peak (TTP) = time in seconds from injection to peak enhancement of the tissue time versus contrast concentration curve, (ii) Tmax = time in seconds from onset of contrast arrival to peak height of the residue function, and (iii) delay time (DT) = time in seconds from onset of contrast arrival to peak height of the residue

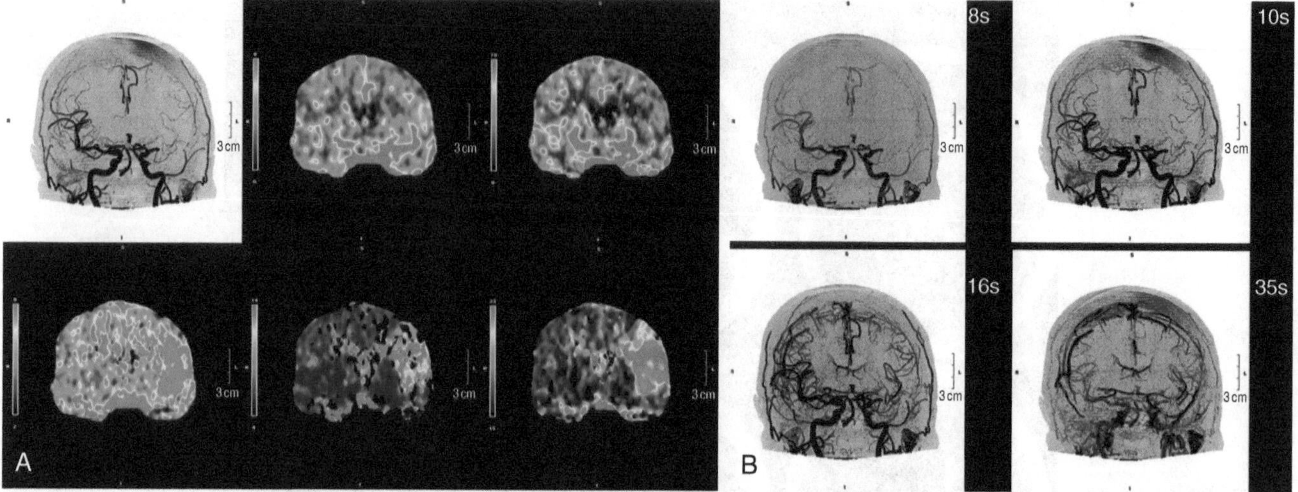

Figure 47-8. Coronal slice from a patient with left MCA occlusion. CTP and CTA acquired simultaneously with 320 detector scanner. A, shows the CTA at a single time-point, as well as various CTP maps: CBV (top middle), CBF, (top right), MTT (bottom left), Delay time (bottom middle), and TTP (bottom right). Note there is a large region of delay/prolonged MTT with relatively preserved CBV suggesting significant tissue at risk. B, shows the dynamic nature of the CTA with four images at different time-points after contrast injection. Note the retrograde flow distal to the left M1 MCA occlusion.

function after a mathematical correction for delay and dispersion of the contrast bolus (Fig. 47-8).[53]

Ischemic stroke represents a hypoperfused vascular territory. On CTP, regions with hypoperfusion are seen as decreased CBF, decreased CBV, prolonged MTT, and prolonged contrast transit measured as TTP, Tmax, or DT. These changes are detectable immediately after stroke onset. Additionally, these perfusion parameters can be used to estimate the ischemic penumbra and the infarct core. Penumbra refers to tissue with hypoperfusion severe enough to cause neuronal dysfunction (and clinical symptoms), but still salvageable if blood supply is restored promptly. Salvage of penumbra correlates with better clinical outcome. Ischemic core, on the other hand, is tissue that is severely hypoperfused and destined to infarct (thus cannot be salvaged by reperfusion). On CTP maps, penumbra can be estimated by delayed MTT/TTP/Tmax/DT and with CBF and CBV that is usually reduced but not below a critical threshold, while infarct core can be delineated as delayed MTT/TTP/Tmax/DT (often more severe delay than penumbra) and with CBV and CBF below critical levels (Fig. 47-9).[53,54]

There is yet no universal consensus as to how one should best define acute ischemia with perfusion CT. Attempts at quantitative validation of this technology in humans through comparison with other techniques, such as xenon-CT, are ongoing.[55] There has been considerable effort to assess the accuracy of perfusion CT in identifying ischemic core and penumbra, mostly by using perfusion thresholds (see next section). One of the points that must be kept in mind when interpreting any studies of perfusion imaging that attempt to distinguish irreversibly injured tissue from salvageable tissue is that depth of perfusion abnormality only provides a probability that tissue might become infarcted (ischemic core) or be salvageable with reperfusion (penumbra). It does not directly tell us about actual tissue viability in the manner that hypodensity on NCT due to ionic edema (i.e., infarction), or even hyperintensity on diffusion-weighted MRI does. Accepting this limitation, the enthusiasm for using CTP and perfusion thresholds as part of a multimodal CT exam in hyperacute stroke relates to the limitations of NCT alone in hyperacute stroke. Firstly, perfusion abnormalities are often seen well before one can see hypodensity on NCT and therefore might provide earlier information about tissue that cannot be salvaged (Fig. 47-10).[11] Thus CTP should be seen as providing complimentary information to NCT.

Although this technique is rapidly evolving, difficulties which interfere with accurate perfusion values include patient motion artifacts, partial averaging effects, and variability in post-processing of the raw perfusion data, which leads in differences in perfusion results across different CT vendor maps.[56] There are many factors that can lead to this variability in perfusion values and may include, depending on choice of post-processing software, drawing regions of interest (ROIs) directly over arterial vessels (which would artefactually increase CBV and CBF values for example), and the site of selection of the arterial input vessel. Further, different CTP acquisition protocols compound this variability in CTP results; a common problem is failure to capture the whole contrast bolus due to insufficient scan duration. This has led to a concerted push for standardization of both the acquisition and post-processing of perfusion imaging.[57]

To date, a further limitation of CTP has been the incomplete coverage of total brain tissue scanned during contrast passage. Depending on the CT manufacturer, only about 2–4 cm (craniocaudal extension) of brain tissue can be covered. This volume is usually placed at the level of the basal ganglia so that perfusion of all major supratentorial vascular territories can be captured. However, new-generation CT scanners with up to 320 detector rows can now provide whole-brain perfusion images.[58] These scanners have the added advantage of providing dynamic CTA acquisition at the same time as CTP acquisition (Fig. 47-8).

Diagnostic Accuracy

Qualitative assessment of CTP parameter maps improves diagnostic accuracy for tissue at risk and irreversibly damaged brain tissue. For example, Lin et al. studied 28 patients with multimodal CT seen with territorial infarction within 3 hours of symptom onset and assessed 280 ASPECTS regions for a relative CBV reduction. They found a 91% sensitivity and 100% specificity for predicting a DWI lesion on follow-up imaging.[52] Parsons et al.[42] showed that CBV best predicts final infarct extent in patients with major reperfusion, whereas CBF

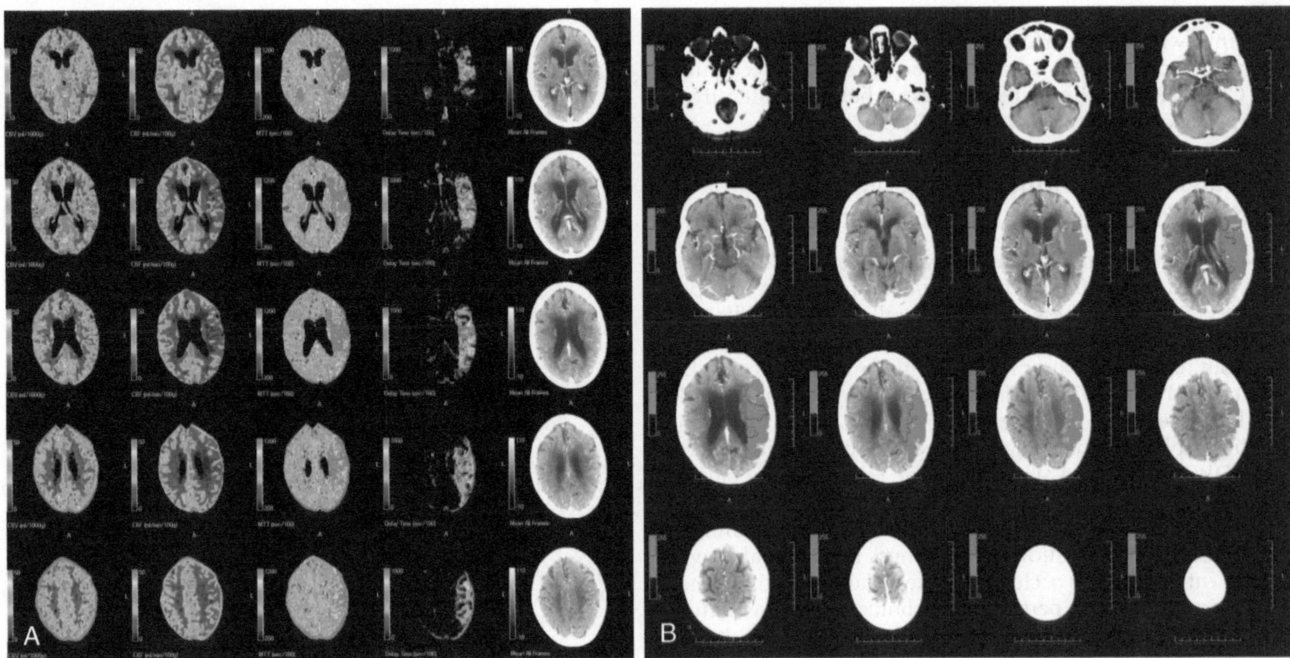

Figure 47-9. Patient imaged at 4 hours after left distal M1 MCA occlusion. A, shows five axial slices of all CTP maps and CTP source image (right). There is a large area of delay (column from right) and MTT prolongation (middle column). This corresponds with reduction in CBF (2nd left column) and preserved CBV (left column). B, shows the core/penumbra maps for all slices based on a delay time threshold (>3 seconds) (shown in green) and a CBF threshold (<30%) (shown in red). The core is small (16 mL) and the penumbra relatively large (64 mL). This is an ideal imaging candidate for acute reperfusion therapy.

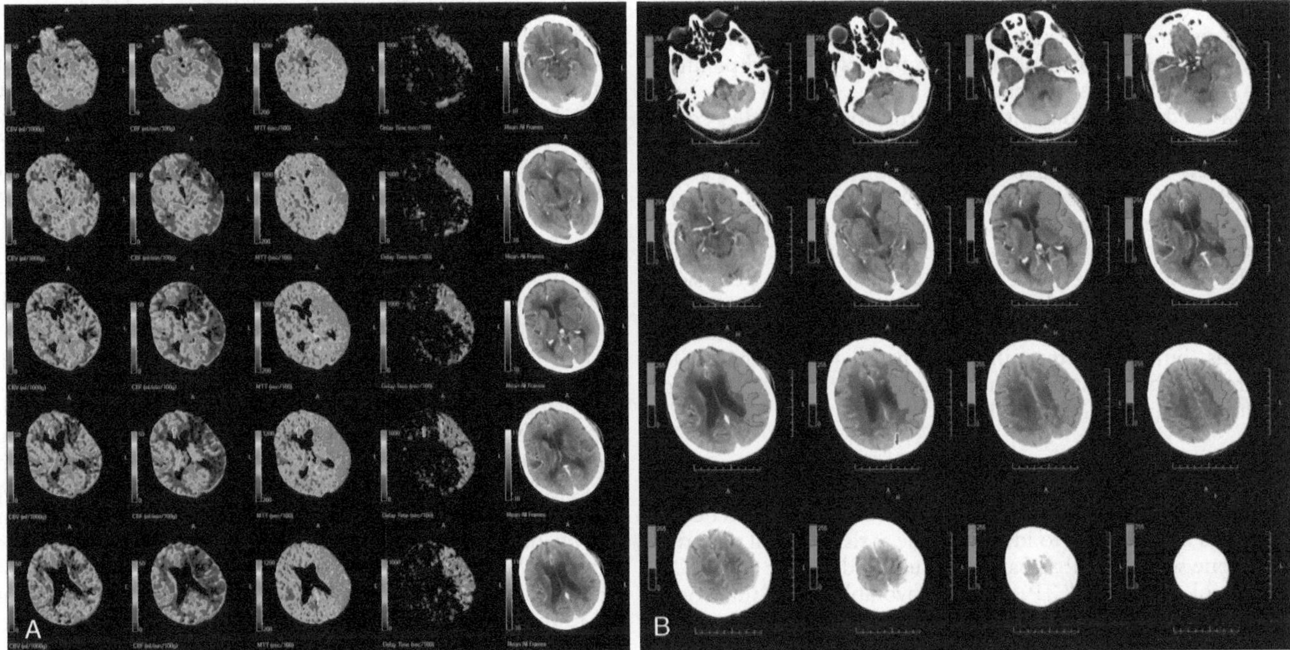

Figure 47-10. Patient imaged at only 2 hours on 320-slice scanner after left M1 MCA occlusion. A, shows five axial slices of all CTP maps and CTP source image (right). There is a large area of severe delay (column from right) and MTT prolongation (middle column). This corresponds with marked reduction in CBF (2nd left column) and CBV (left column). B, shows the core/penumbra maps for all slices based on a delay time threshold (>3 seconds) and a CBF threshold (<30%). The core is more than 100 mL (shown in red). Although there is still some penumbra, reperfusion treatment is futile in such a case as the outcome is already determined.

and MTT were the best predictors of final infarct size in patients without reperfusion. In some patients with MCA branch or other distal intracranial occlusions not recognized on CTA, TTP or MTT parameter maps are helpful in identifying the presence and site of occlusion (Fig. 47-7).

Thresholds and Diffusion-weighted Image and Magnetic Resonance Perfusion

There are many studies, which have assessed the accuracy of CTP in defining ischemic core and penumbra.[59-61] It is important to realize that these studies generally used the follow-up infarct as the reference standard for penumbra in patients without recanalization or reperfusion. For ischemic core, they either used acute DWI performed within a few hours of CTP as the reference, or used the follow-up final infarct in patients with complete recanalization or reperfusion. It is still believed that DWI reversal is a significant issue (although the balance of evidence is now against this).[62] The use of follow-up infarction is also confounded by lack of knowledge of timing of reperfusion/recanalization or by changes in collateral flow in those with persistent occlusion. Others claim, based on anecdotal experience, that perfusion thresholds may vary with time (such that a low CBF region, for example, might still be salvageable with reperfusion at 60 minutes, but not at 180 minutes).[63] These issues would generally impair accuracy of the perfusion thresholds to estimate core and penumbra. Despite that, studies have consistently shown that a CBF threshold below 30–40% (depending on method), as does a CBV threshold below 50–55%, has a high sensitivity and specificity to detect tissue that ultimately infarcts. The data for penumbra are also quite consistent showing delay measures (Tmax >6 seconds, or DT >3 seconds) have the highest sensitivity and specificity. Thus, the "best" group threshold may not necessarily be the most accurate estimate of core and penumbra in an individual patient.

Given the above data, it is not surprising that studies comparing MR perfusion–diffusion mismatch and CT mismatch (between the core and perfusion lesion) show quite good correlations.[64-66] The agreement between modalities appears to be strongest when the Tmax>6 second threshold is used to determine the perfusion lesion for CTP and MR perfusion (MRP). Indeed, the most recent data comparing perfusion lesions across CTP (whole brain coverage) and MRP suggest that there is minimal difference between Tmax perfusion lesions, but with some other parameters (CBF, CBV, MTT) there is a significant difference between CTP and MRP lesion volume at the same threshold.[66]

Diagnostic Impact

CTP facilitates and improves identification of the infarct core and has the potential to identify tissue at risk. Typical patterns that one sees on CTP as part of a multimodal acute stroke CT protocol (NCT/CTA/CTP) are the "favorable" and "unfavorable" mismatch patterns.[52] These are typically seen with proximal intracranial vessel occlusion (especially MCA). In a favorable pattern the ischemic core (CBV or CBF defined) is relatively small and overall perfusion lesion (Tmax/DT) is much larger. Such patients have potential to benefit from acute reperfusion therapy. At the other end of the scale is the patient with a large infarct core, with or without a larger perfusion lesion (unfavorable). These patients may not benefit from reperfusion therapy, indeed, where the core is very large (e.g., greater than 100 mL) reperfusion therapy may be harmful or futile. This has been termed a "malignant mismatch pattern".[67] The adequacy of leptomeningeal collateral flow has a crucial influence on the extent of core and penumbra seen on CTP

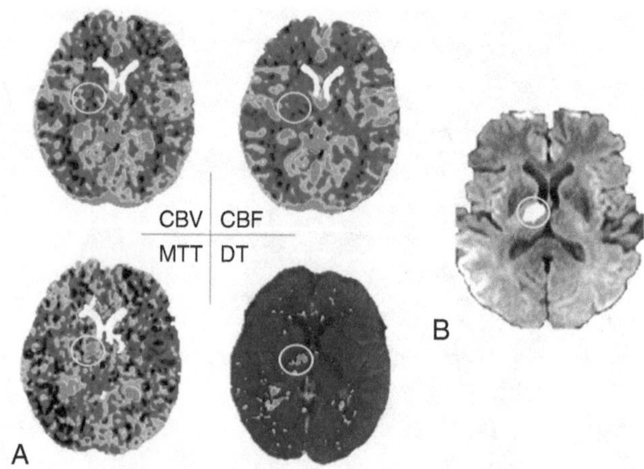

Figure 47-11. Patient imaged with CTP (A) at 2 hours after onset of left hemisensory disturbance. Note prolongation of MTT and delayed-time in right thalamus (yellow circle). However, it is difficult to be sure whether this is a "true" lesion as there are other small areas of prolonged MTT and delayed-time, which are "noise". DWI at 24 hours confirms lacunar infarction in right thalamus.

(and is probably more important than time after onset, at least in the first 3–6 hours).[68]

CTP is relatively limited in detecting small ischemic lesions (Fig. 47-11). In patients with normal NCT, CTA, and CTP findings but persistent neurologic deficit, immediate MR DWI will usually show one or multiple small ischemic lesions. This may be due to limited slice coverage, which can be addressed with whole-brain CTP. In the case of small hemispheric lesions seen on DWI but not on CTP, this might reflect reperfusion. In these cases, one cannot measure infarction with CTP, as CTP (as opposed to DWI) relies on the presence of hypoperfusion. Unfortunately, reperfusion prior to CTP is not well appreciated by many stroke clinicians or radiologists, and may lead to false-negative diagnosis of ischemic lesion on multimodal CT (Fig. 47-12). In such cases it is particularly important to assess the NCT and the source images for subtle hydodensity. If CTP is performed acutely and there is already established hypodensity on CTP source images +/– NCT, the absence of a perfusion abnormality on CTP indicates reperfusion has occurred. Such patients probably do not benefit from reperfusion therapy.

Lacunar stroke, caused by occlusion of small penetrating artery, is smaller than 1.8 ml, or 15 mm in diameter.[69] Thus, the detection of lacunar infarction requires high spatial resolution. Diffusion MR (DWI) meets the requirement, detecting acute lacunar stroke with high sensitivity and specificity, both over 90%.[69,70] Perfusion MR and CTP do not perform well for lesions of this size. Low sensitivity for detection of lacunar lesion has been observed in CTP images with limited slice coverage.[71] Lesions may be outside the slice coverage. Additionally, the CTP data are acquired with slice thickness of 5–10 mm, thus the lacunar lesion may be missed due to partial volume effect (Fig. 47-13).

With newer technology, such as 320-slice CTP, sensitivity of detecting lacunar lesion is increased; 320-slice CTP has whole-brain coverage and thin-slice (0.5–1 mm) acquisition, reducing partial volume effect.

Therapeutic and Prognostic Impact

The role of multimodal CT examination, including CTP, in selection of patients for acute reperfusion therapy needs further study. Firstly, a reliable measure of ischemic core is essential, and non-contrast CT may not always be sufficient

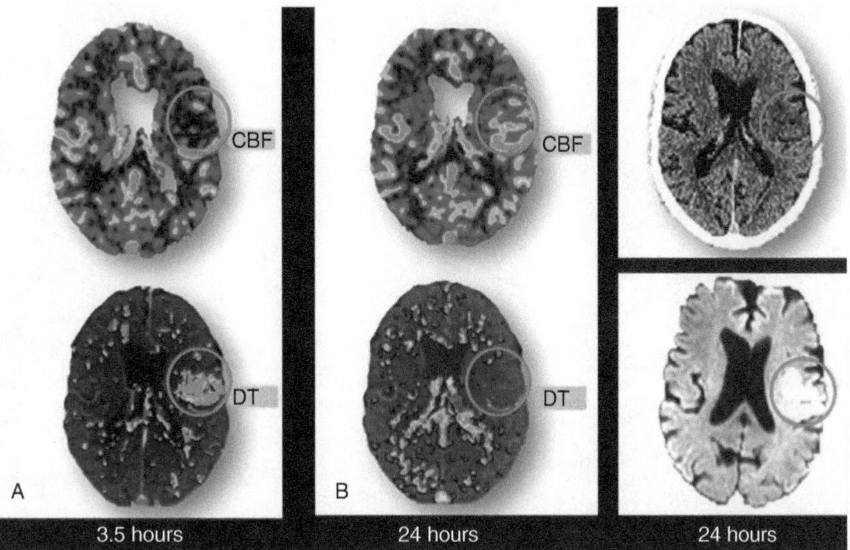

Figure 47-12. CBF and delayed-time maps from a patient at 3.5 hours (left) after M2 MCA occlusion and then at 24 hours (middle) after recanalization of the occlusion. Note that perfusion lesion seen as reduced CBF and delay on the acute maps have disappeared due to reperfusion at 24 hours. Thus, one might mistakenly think there is no infarction unless attention is paid to the NCT at the same time point. DWI on same day confirms infarction. This illustrates that CTP cannot measure the ischemic core after reperfusion.

for this purpose (as it may underestimate "dead brain"). CTP can fulfill this role.[42,60] Second, one must determine where the cutoff point of benefit lies in terms of infarct core volume. Trials such as EXTEND[72] are using a core volume of 70 ml. Finally, an assessment of the tissue at risk and collateral status is also crucial, although there is still not consensus on how best to measure this. Dynamic CT angiography holds promise in measuring collateral status,[73] but CTP can also quantify collateral status and thus has the advantage of avoiding more subjective angiographic grading scales such as American Society of Therapeutic Neuroradiology/Society of Interventional Radiology (SIR) Collateral Flow Grading System (ASITN/SIR) (Fig. 47-13).[74]

When multimodal CT imaging is routinely performed before reperfusion therapy, CTP findings are often used in combination with clinical assessment and NCCT and CTA data to predict likely treatment response and to help make a final decision about reperfusion therapy (Fig. 47-14).[75]

Although level 1 evidence is lacking for CTP to be used in treatment selection, we do now have considerable data that at least help us to predict the likely response to treatment. Patients with a small ischemic core and large areas of salvageable tissue may have a dramatic response to effective reperfusion.[76] Reperfusion of infarcted tissue is futile, and may even be harmful, with data now showing reperfusion of tissue that is severely hypoperfused pre-treatment increases risk of major hemorrhage and edema.[77] On at the other end of the spectrum, patients with small perfusion lesions (particularly without a co-existing occlusion on CTA) may have a very good outcome without reperfusion therapy,[78] likely due to high rates of spontaneous reperfusion.

Prospective trials are currently underway to test the hypothesis that patients with so-called target mismatch on CTP (or MRI) are the ideal candidates for acute reperfusion therapy.[72,79]

POSTERIOR CIRCULATION COMPUTED TOMOGRAPHY IMAGING

Ischemic Stroke

About 20% of cerebrovascular ischemic events involve the posterior circulation.[80] Clinical signs and symptoms are frequently less specific compared with anterior circulation stroke. Isolated transient loss-of-consciousness or dizziness can be misattributed to vertebrobasilar ischemia, whereas many cases of true vertebrobasilar ischemia remain undiagnosed.[81] However, similar to anterior circulation stroke, early diagnosis is crucial for initiating systemic thrombolysis or mechanical revascularization procedures. The relevance of acute brain imaging with CT is to reliably rule out intracranial hemorrhaging and to identify patients with basilar artery occlusion. The latter patients have a devastating prognosis: nearly 80% die or are severely disabled if treated conservatively.[82]

The sensitivity of DWI for identifying final infarction is better than NCT in posterior circulation ischemia.[83] This is relevant in differentiating cerebral ischemic events from other disease entities with similar clinical symptomatology (e.g., basilar migraine or vestibular neuritis). The reliability of CT to detect hypodensity in the posterior circulation is limited by bone and beam hardening artifacts in the posterior fossa. Newer-generation CT scanners with helical scan techniques seem to diminish this limitation[84] but have not been analyzed systematically. The sensitivity for detection of a final infarct in the posterior circulation is improved with CTA source images compared with NCT (Fig. 47-15).[85]

A hyperdense basilar artery sign[86] (see Fig. 47-15) and a hyperdense posterior cerebral artery sign[87] specifically indicate occlusion of these arteries. By application of CTA, vertebrobasilar occlusion can be diagnosed with high sensitivity and specificity.[33] In the study by Lev et al., the diagnostic accuracy of CTA was 96% for vertebral artery occlusion and 100% for basilar artery occlusion. Thus, in a patient with patency of the basilar artery on CTA, the diagnosis of symptomatic basilar artery occlusion can be excluded. In contrast, evidence of basilar artery occlusion on CTA should immediately prompt recanalization strategies. In patients with clinically suspected posterior circulation ischemia, both basilar artery occlusion and vertebral artery occlusion on CTA are predictors of increased risk of mortality and poorer functional outcome.[88]

In contrast to anterior circulation stroke, posterior circulation stroke currently has limited imaging-based selection criteria for identifying patients who may benefit from thrombolysis. Several imaging scores have recently been developed

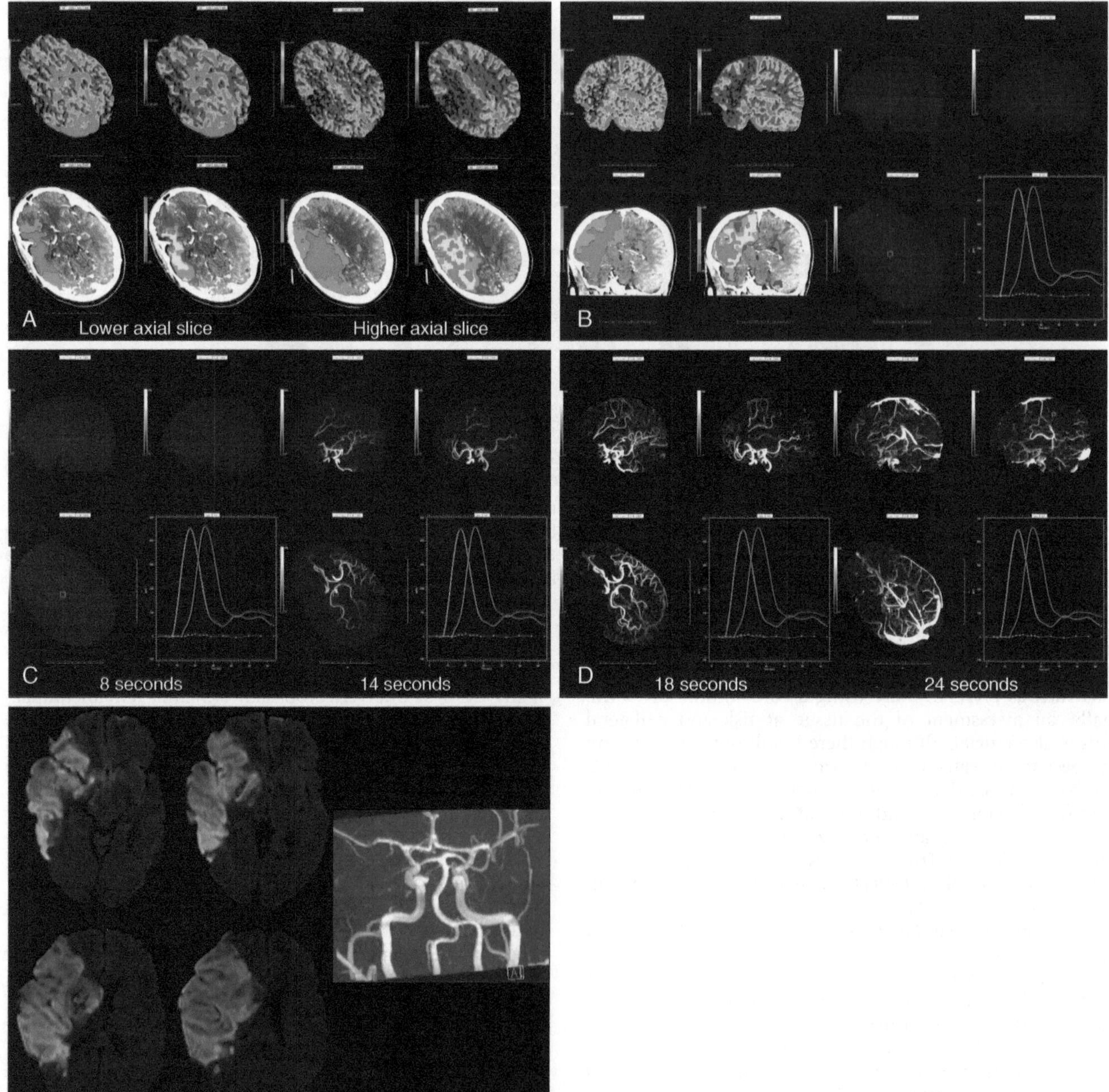

Figure 47-13. Patient (only 47 years old) with whole-brain CTP and dynamic CTA acquired concurrently on 320-slice scanner at 2.5 hours after right M1 MCA occlusion. A, shows two CTP slices with prolonged delayed-time and very low CBV and CBF in much of the MCA territory (with very large core of 190 mL = red on core/penumbra maps). Despite the presence of penumbra of >100 mL this patient has minimal chance of benefit from reperfusion treatment. B, shows a coronal slice. On the right are the pre-contrast arrival CTA axial, coronal and sagittal images. The large core is explained by the patient's very poor collateral flow distal to the occlusion seen in C and D. C, shows the dynamic CTA at 8 and 14 seconds after injection of contrast. D, shows dynamic CTA at 18 and 24 seconds after injection of contrast. The dynamic CTA images show virtually no collateral flow distal to the occlusion. The patient subsequently had IV tPA with M1 recanalization. However, because the patient already had a huge infarct core before treatment he required life-saving hemicraniectomy. E, shows DWI and perfusion MR maps at 72 hours (post-hemicraniectomy) massive MCA infarction despite M1 recanalization. The message is that poor collaterals = very rapid infarction and that attempts at reperfusion therapy may well be futile.

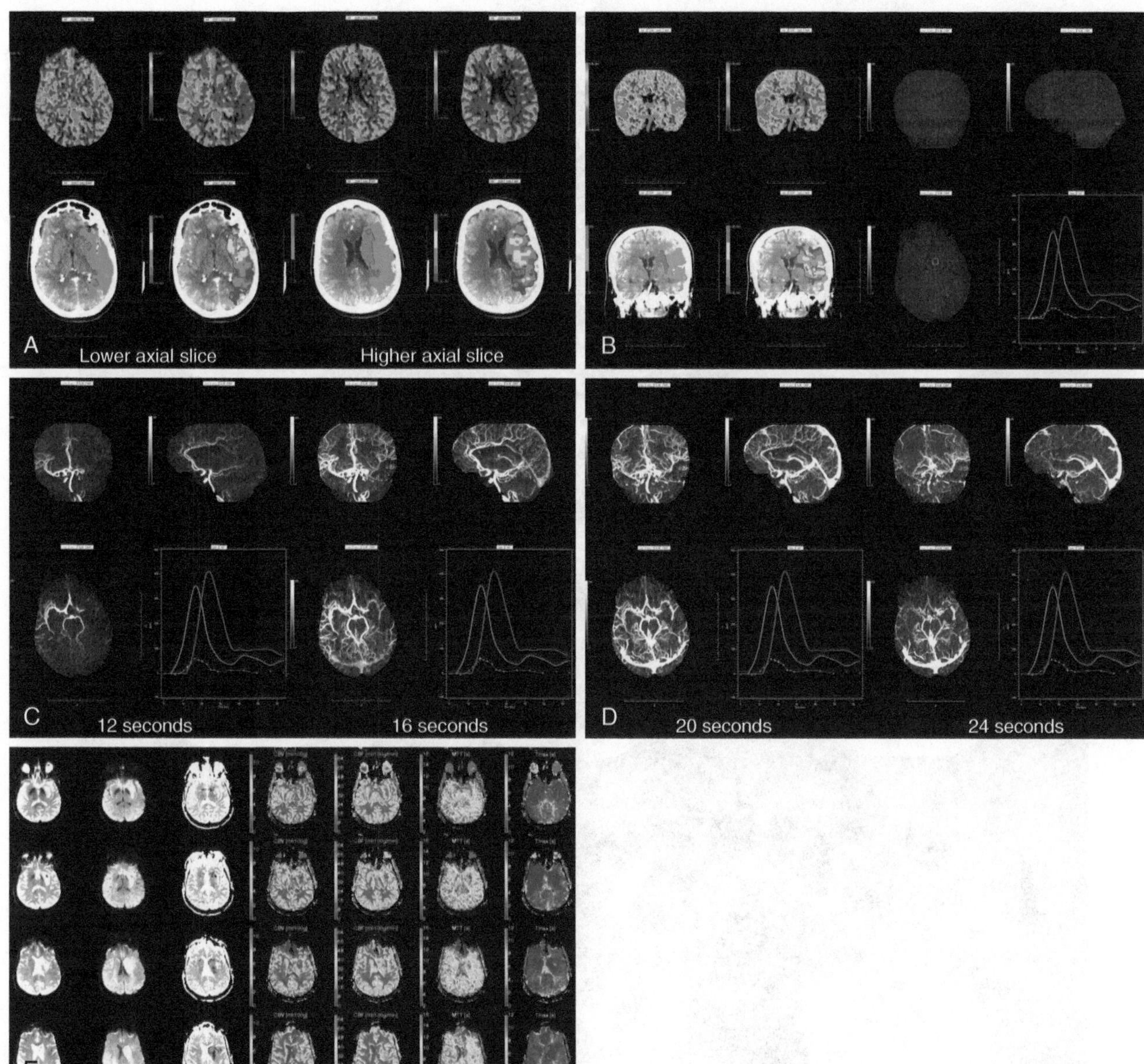

Figure 47-14. Patient with whole-brain CTP and dynamic CTA acquired concurrently on 320-slice scanner at 2 hours after left M1 MCA occlusion. A, shows two CTP slices with prolonged delayed-time and preserved CBV except in striatum where there is ischemic core based on CTP thresholds (red on core/penumbra maps). The patient has considerable tissue to salvage. B, shows a coronal image of CTP maps demonstrating core in deep MCA territory but penumbra in MCA cortex. On the right are the pre-contrast arrival CTA axial, coronal and sagittal images. C, shows the dynamic CTA at 12 and 16 seconds after injection of contrast. D, shows dynamic CTA at 20 and 24 seconds after injection of contrast. The dynamic CTA images show excellent collateral flow distal to the occlusion. The patient subsequently had IV tPA and then mechanical clot retrieval. E, shows DWI and perfusion MR maps at 24 hours showing complete reperfusion with salvage of all of acute penumbra with the infarct on DWI being very similar to that shown on CTP acutely. The message is that good collaterals keep the penumbra viable long enough for reperfusion treatments to work.

to quantify early ischemic changes in the posterior circulation territory to predict functional outcome of patients with basilar artery occlusion.[89–91] Demonstration of small DWI lesions or a diffusion–perfusion mismatch have been proposed for identifying patients with basilar artery occlusion who may potentially benefit from thrombolysis.[89,92] A TTP delay in the posterior cerebral artery territory on CTP parameter maps indicates vertebrobasilar occlusion (Fig. 47-11).[93] The therapeutic and prognostic implications of these techniques for patients with posterior circulation strokes need to be studied.

Quantification of CTA source image hypoattenuation in the posterior circulation with a systematic score, the posterior circulation Acute Stroke Prognosis Early CT Score, identified patients with basilar artery occlusion who were unlikely to have a favorable functional outcome despite recanalization of the basilar artery.[94] In a similar study, CTA source image hypoattenuation in the mesencephalon and pons indicated patients with basilar artery occlusion and poor functional outcomes.[90] Both studies demonstrate that CTA source image hypoattenuation can identify areas with ischemic changes in the posterior circulation, including the brainstem. Moreover, this information has prognostic relevance in patients with basilar artery occlusion. The prognostic value of pc-ASPECTS applied to CTA-SI has been validated in the CTA subgroup of

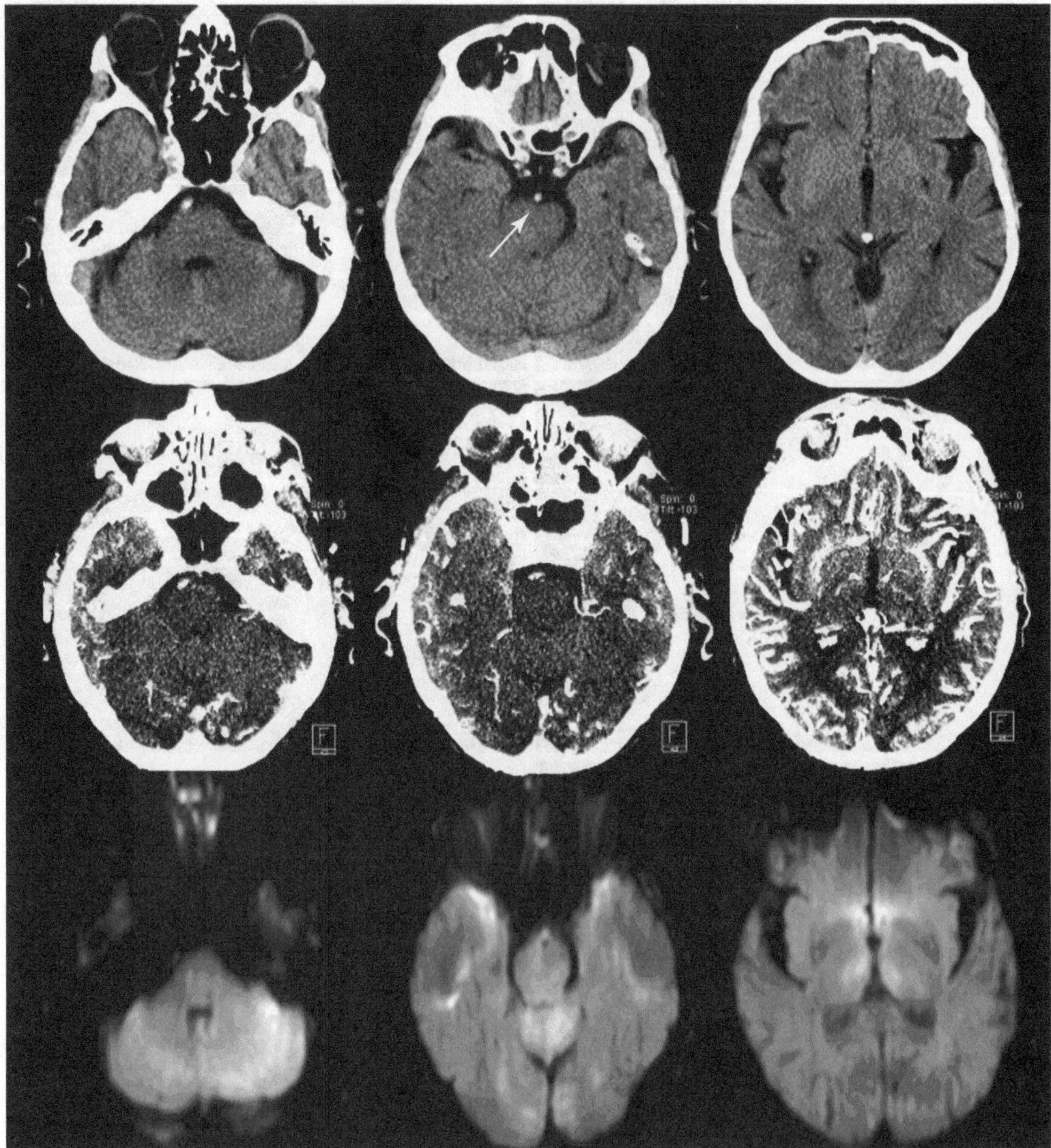

Figure 47-15. Noncontrast CT (NCT) *(upper row)* and CT angiography (CTA) source images *(middle row)* of a patient with acute basilar artery occlusion 3.5 hours and 4.5 hours after symptom onset, respectively. NCT demonstrates hyperdense basilar artery sign *(arrow)* but does not reveal early ischemic changes. CTA source images demonstrate hypoattenuation in all posterior circulation territories (posterior circulation Acute Stroke Prognosis Early CT Score [pc-ASPECTS] = 0). The patient was treated with systemic thrombolysis with alteplase. Diffusion-weighted MRI *(lower row)* performed after thrombolysis (6.5 hours after symptom onset) demonstrates lesions in the same territories (pc-ASPECTS = 0). *(Images courtesy of the Seaman Family MR Research Centre, University of Calgary, Canada.)*

the BASICS registry population.[95] Moreover if applied to CTP, MTT parameter maps were most sensitive for ischemic changes compared with CBF, CBV, and CTA-SI in the CTP-subgroup of the BASICS registry population.[96] Extensive ischemic changes on CBV parameter maps (CBV-pc-ASPECTS of 7 or below) were associated with a fatal outcome in this study (Fig. 47-16).

Currently no study has demonstrated a differential clinical treatment response of imaging scores to IVT or IAT in patients with basilar artery occlusion and, therefore, imaging findings alone should currently not influence immediate treatment decision making in patients with posterior circulation strokes, particularly for those with basilar artery occlusion. However, the extent of ischemic changes on NCCT quantified with the pc-ASPECTS score may identify patients with basilar artery occlusion who have a good functional outcome with IVT regardless of a fixed time-window.[97]

NON-CONTRAST COMPUTED TOMOGRAPHY AND COMPUTED TOMOGRAPHY ANGIOGRAPHY IN ACUTE HEMORRHAGIC STROKE

NCT is the imaging modality of choice in the diagnosis of acute intracerebral hemorrhage. It seems to easily detect the hyperdense (60–80 HU) appearance of a fresh blood clot. Studies on the reliability and validity of this finding, however, have not been performed. The conditions under which intracerebral blood is not hyperdense on CT are not well studied.

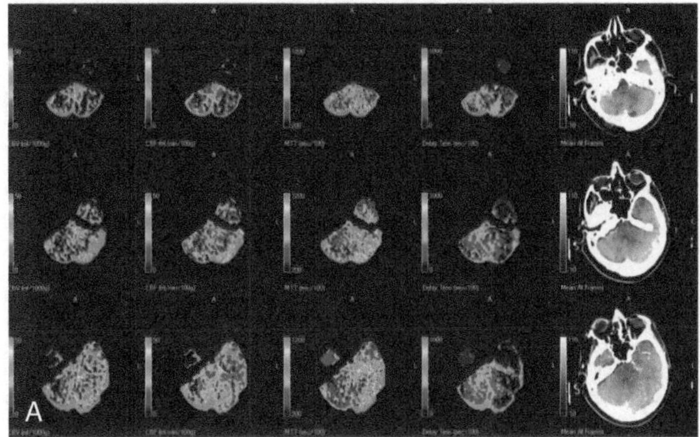
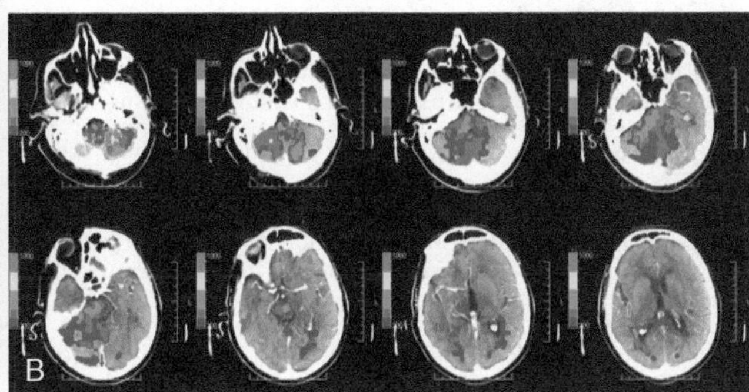

Figure 47-16. A, shows three axial slices of all CTP maps and CTP source image (right) in a patient imaged with whole-brain CTP 2 hours after proximal basilar occlusion. The maps show prolongation of MTT in the pons and medulla as well as in the left cerebellar hemisphere. There also appears to be some delay in the right cerellum. B, shows color-coded delay maps (less severe delay is blue and most severe is red). This confirms there is a bilateral perfusion delay in the brainstem and both cerebellar hemispheres. Note there is also mild perfusion delay in the white matter posterior to the posterior horns of the lateral ventricles (commonly seen in patients with chronic white matter "ischemia").

Low hematocrit levels and impairment of clotting may be possible conditions. CT is as sensitive and specific as MRI in detecting acute intracranial hemorrhage. CT is less sensitive in detecting subacute or old intracerebral hematomas.[98]

The utility of CTA after NCT has been shown in intracerebral hemorrhage to be tremendous and it might replace catheter angiography in the future. Cerebral aneurysms can be diagnosed accurately down to a diameter of 2 mm.[99] Similarly, arteriovenous malformations and venous thrombosis can be diagnosed in many cases.

Approximately 30% of acute hemorrhagic stroke patients show evidence of hematoma growth within the first hours after onset.[100] This increase in hematoma size is a key factor in predicting a poor prognosis for the disease. When CTA source images are used, it is possible to predict hematoma growth early on. The so-called spot sign characterizes a leak of contrast media that is clearly hyperdense in relation to the surrounding hematoma.[101] Wada et al. found the spot sign in 13 of 39 patients (33%) with acute intracerebral hemorrhage within the first 3 hours. The presence of the spot sign was significantly correlated with a poor functional outcome. A large multicenter prospective study has recently shown that the presence of a spot sign at baseline predicts hematoma growth, long-term mortality and functional outcome.[102]

Acknowledgment

We would like to acknowledge Charles A. Jungreis and Steven Goldstein for their work on previous editions of this chapter.

REFERENCES

1. Kent D, Larson E. Disease, level of impact, and quality of research methods; three dimensions of clinical efficacy assessment applied to magnetic resonance imaging. Invest Radiol 1992;27: 245–54.
2. Hand P, Wardlaw J, Rowat A, et al. MR brain imaging in patients with acute stroke – feasibility and patient-related difficulties. J Neurol Neurosurg Psychiatry 2005;76:1525–7.
3. Murayama K, Katada K, Nakane M, et al. Whole-brain perfusion CT performed with a prototype 256-detector row ct system: Initial experience. Radiology 2009;250:202–11.
4. Schuier FJ, Hossmann KA. Experimental brain infarcts in cats. Ii. Ischemic brain edema. Stroke 1980;11:593–601.
5. Todd N, Picozzi P, Crockard A, et al. Reperfusion after cerebral ischemia: Influence of duration of ischemia. Stroke 1986;17: 460–5.
6. Simard JM, Kent TA, Chen M, et al. Brain oedema in focal ischaemia: Molecular pathophysiology and theoretical implications. Lancet Neurol 2007;6:258–68.
7. Dzialowski I, Klotz E, Goericke S, et al. Ischemic brain tissue water content: CT monitoring during middle cerebral artery occlusion and reperfusion in rats. Radiology 2007;243:720–6.
8. Dzialowski I, Weber J, Doerfler A, et al. Brain tissue water uptake after middle cerebral artery occlusion assessed with CT. J Neuroimaging 2004;14:42–8.
9. von Kummer R, Bourquain H, Bastianello S, et al. Early prediction of irreversible brain damage after ischemic stroke by computed tomography. Radiology 2001;219:95–100.
10. Na D, Kim E, Ryoo J, et al. CT sign of brain swelling without concomitant parenchymal hypoattenuation: Comparison with diffusion- and perfusion-weighted MR imaging. Radiology 2005; 235:992–8.
11. Parsons MW, Pepper EM, Bateman GA, et al. Identification of the penumbra and infarct core on hyperacute noncontrast and perfusion CT. Neurology 2007;68:730–6.
12. Butcher KS, Lee SB, Parsons MW, et al. Differential prognosis of isolated cortical swelling and hypoattenuation on CT in acute stroke. Stroke 2007;38:941–7.
13. von Kummer R, Meyding-Lamadé U, Forsting M, et al. Sensitivity and prognostic value of early computed tomography in middle cerebral artery trunk occlusion. AJNR Am J Neuroradiol 1994;15: 9–15.
14. Kirchhof K, Welzel T, Mecke C, et al. Differentiation of white, mixed, and red thrombi: Value of CT in estimation of the prognosis of thrombolysis-phantom study. Radiology 2003;228: 126–30.
15. Riedel CH, Jensen U, Rohr A, et al. Assessment of thrombus in acute middle cerebral artery occlusion using thin-slice nonenhanced computed tomography reconstructions. Stroke 2010;41: 1659–64.
16. Riedel CH, Zimmermann P, Jensen-Kondering U, et al. The importance of size: Successful recanalization by intravenous thrombolysis in acute anterior stroke depends on thrombus length. Stroke 2011;42:1775–7.
17. Wardlaw J, Mielke O. Early signs of brain infarction at CT: Observer reliability and outcome after thrombolytic treatment – systematic review. Radiology 2005;235:444–53.
18. Marks M, Holmgren E, Fox A, et al. Evaluation of early computed tomographic findings in acute ischemic stroke. Stroke 1999;30: 389–92.
19. Barber P, Demchuk A, Zhang J, et al. Validity and reliability of a quantitative computed tomography score in predicting outcome of hyperacute stroke before thrombolytic therapy. Lancet 2000; 355:1670–4.
20. Lansberg MG, Albers GW, Wijman CA. Symptomatic intracerebral hemorrhage following thrombolytic therapy for acute ischemic stroke: A review of the risk factors. Cerebrovasc Dis 2007;24:1–10.
21. Dzialowski I, Hill MD, Coutts SB, et al. Extent of early ischemic changes on computed tomography (CT) before thrombolysis:

Prognostic value of the Alberta Stroke Program early CT score in ECASS II. Stroke 2006;37:973–8.
22. von Kummer R, Allen K, Holle R, et al. Acute stroke: Usefulness of early CT findings before thrombolytic therapy. Radiology 1997;205:327–33.
23. Coutts S, Simon J, Eliasziw M, et al. Triaging transient ischemic attack and minor stroke patients using acute magnetic resonance imaging. Ann Neurol 2005;57:848–54.
24. Hacke W, Kaste M, Bluhmki E, et al. Thrombolysis with alteplase 3 to 4.5 hours after acute ischemic stroke. N Engl J Med 2008; 359:1317–29.
25. Lees KR, Bluhmki E, von Kummer R, et al. Time to treatment with intravenous alteplase and outcome in stroke: An updated pooled analysis of ecass, atlantis, ninds, and epithet trials. Lancet 2010;375:1695–703.
26. [No authors listed]. Tissue plasminogen activator for acute ischemic stroke. The National Institute of Neurological Disorders and Stroke rt-PA Stroke Study Group. N Engl J Med 1995; 333:1581–7.
27. Hacke W, Kaste M, Fieschi C, et al. Intravenous thrombolysis with recombinant tissue plasminogen activator for acute hemispheric stroke. The European Cooperative Acute Stroke Study (ECASS). JAMA 1995;274:1017–25.
28. Hacke W, Kaste M, Fieschi C, et al. Randomised double-blind placebo-controlled trial of thrombolytic therapy with intravenous alteplase in acute ischaemic stroke (ECASS II). Lancet 1998;352:1245–51.
29. Hill MD, Buchan AM. Thrombolysis for acute ischemic stroke: Results of the Canadian Alteplase for Stroke Effectiveness Study. CMAJ 2005;172:1307–12.
30. Bash S, Villablanca JP, Jahan R, et al. Intracranial vascular stenosis and occlusive disease: Evaluation with ct angiography, MR angiography, and digital subtraction angiography. AJNR Am J Neuroradiol 2005;26:1012–21.
31. Nguyen-Huynh MN, Wintermark M, English J, et al. How accurate is CT angiography in evaluating intracranial atherosclerotic disease? Stroke 2008;39:1184–8.
32. Puetz V, Dzialowski I, Coutts SB, et al. Frequency and clinical course of stroke and transient ischemic attack patients with intracranial nonocclusive thrombus on computed tomographic angiography. Stroke 2009;40:193–9.
33. Lev M, Farkas J, Rodriguez V, et al. CT angiography in the rapid triage of patients with hyperacute stroke to intraarterial thrombolysis: Accuracy in the detection of large vessel thrombus. J Comput Assist Tomogr 2001;25:520–8.
34. Puetz V, Dzialowski I, Hill MD, et al. Intracranial thrombus extent predicts clinical outcome, final infarct size and hemorrhagic transformation in ischemic stroke: The clot burden score. Int J Stroke 2008;3:230–6.
35. Tan IY, Demchuk AM, Hopyan J, et al. CT angiography clot burden score and collateral score: Correlation with clinical and radiologic outcomes in acute middle cerebral artery infarct. AJNR Am J Neuroradiol 2009;30:525–31.
36. Lee KY, Han SW, Kim SH, et al. Early recanalization after intravenous administration of recombinant tissue plasminogen activator as assessed by pre- and post-thrombolytic angiography in acute ischemic stroke patients. Stroke 2007;38:192–3.
37. Mamourian A, Drayer BP. Clinically silent infarcts shown by MR after cerebral angiography. AJNR Am J Neuroradiol 1990; 11:1084.
38. Johnston DC, Chapman KM, Goldstein LB. Low rate of complications of cerebral angiography in routine clinical practice. Neurology 2001;57:2012–14.
39. Sameshima T, Futami S, Morita Y, et al. Clinical usefulness of and problems with three-dimensional CT angiography for the evaluation of arteriosclerotic stenosis of the carotid artery: Comparison with conventional angiography, MRA, and ultrasound sonography. Surg Neurol 1999;51:301–8, discussion 308–9.
40. Anderson GB, Ashforth R, Steinke DE, et al. CT angiography for the detection and characterization of carotid artery bifurcation disease. Stroke 2000;31:2168–74.
41. Ezzeddine MA, Lev MH, McDonald CT, et al. CT angiography with whole brain perfused blood volume imaging: Added clinical value in the assessment of acute stroke. Stroke 2002;33: 959–66.
42. Parsons MW, Pepper EM, Chan V, et al. Perfusion computed tomography: Prediction of final infarct extent and stroke outcome. Ann Neurol 2005;58:672–9.
43. Coutts SB, Lev MH, Eliasziw M, et al. Aspects on CTA source images versus unenhanced CT: Added value in predicting final infarct extent and clinical outcome. Stroke 2004;35: 2472–6.
44. Bal S, Bhatia R, Menon BK, et al. Time dependence of reliability of noncontrast computed tomography in comparison to computed tomography angiography source image in acute ischemic stroke. Int J Stroke 2012.
45. Rubiera M, Ribo M, Delgado-Mederos R, et al. Tandem internal carotid artery/middle cerebral artery occlusion. An independent predictor of poor outcome after systemic thrombolysis. Stroke 2006;37:2301–5.
46. Sylaja PN, Dzialowski I, Krol A, et al. Role of CT angiography in thrombolysis decision-making for patients with presumed seizure at stroke onset. Stroke 2006;37:915–17.
47. von Kummer R, Albers GW, Mori E. The Desmoteplase in Acute Ischemic Stroke (DIAS) Clinical Trial Program. Int J Stroke 2012; 7:589–96.
48. Furlan A, Higashida R, Wechsler L, et al. Intra-arterial prourokinase for acute ischemic stroke. JAMA 1999;282:2003–11.
49. Broderick JP, Palesch YY, Demchuk AM, et al. Endovascular therapy after intravenous t-PA versus t-PA alone for stroke. N Engl J Med 2013;368:893–903.
50. Demchuk AM, Goyal M, Yeatts SD, et al. Recanalization and clinical outcome of occlusion sites at baseline CT angiography in the Interventional Management of Stroke III Trial. Radiology 2014;273(1):202–10.
51. Kassem-Moussa H, Graffagnino C. Nonocclusion and spontaneous recanalization rates in acute ischemic stroke: A review of cerebral angiography studies. Arch Neurol 2002;59:1870–3.
52. Lin L, Bivard A, Parsons MW. Perfusion patterns of ischemic stroke on computed tomography perfusion. J Stroke 2013;15: 164–73.
53. Bivard A, Spratt N, Levi C, et al. Perfusion computer tomography: Imaging and clinical validation in acute ischaemic stroke. Brain 2011;134:3408–16.
54. Bivard A, McElduff P, Spratt N, et al. Defining the extent of irreversible brain ischemia using perfusion computed tomography. Cerebrovasc Dis 2011;31:238–45.
55. Wintermark M, Thiran JP, Maeder P, et al. Simultaneous measurement of regional cerebral blood flow by perfusion CT and stable xenon CT: A validation study. AJNR Am J Neuroradiol 2001;22:905–14.
56. Bivard A, Levi C, Spratt N, et al. Perfusion CT in acute stroke: A comprehensive analysis of infarct and penumbra. Radiology 2013;267:543–50.
57. Wintermark M, Warach SJ. Stir, Virtual International Stroke Trials Archive – Imaging I. Acute stroke imaging research roadmap ii and international survey of acute stroke imaging capabilities: We need your help! AJNR Am J Neuroradiol 2013;34:1671.
58. Bivard A, Levi C, Krishnamurthy V, et al. Defining acute ischemic stroke tissue pathophysiology with whole brain CT perfusion. J Neuroradiol 2014;41:307–15.
59. Wintermark M, Flanders A, Velthuis B, et al. Perfusion-CT assessment of infarct core and penumbra: Receiver operating characteristic curve analysis in 130 patients suspected of acute hemispheric stroke. Stroke 2006;37:979–85.
60. Campbell BC, Christensen S, Levi CR, et al. Cerebral blood flow is the optimal CT perfusion parameter for assessing infarct core. Stroke 2011;42:3435–40.
61. Kamalian S, Kamalian S, Maas MB, et al. CT cerebral blood flow maps optimally correlate with admission diffusion-weighted imaging in acute stroke but thresholds vary by postprocessing platform. Stroke 2011;42:1923–8.
62. Campbell BC, Purushotham A, Christensen S, et al. The infarct core is well represented by the acute diffusion lesion: Sustained reversal is infrequent. J Cereb Blood Flow Metab 2012;32:50–6.
63. Gonzalez RG. Low signal, high noise and large uncertainty make CT perfusion unsuitable for acute ischemic stroke patient selection for endovascular therapy. J Neurointerv Surg 2012;4: 242–5.

64. Wintermark M, Meuli R, Browaeys P, et al. Comparison of CT perfusion and angiography and MRI in selecting stroke patients for acute treatment. Neurology 2007;68:694–7.
65. Campbell BC, Christensen S, Levi CR, et al. Comparison of computed tomography perfusion and magnetic resonance imaging perfusion-diffusion mismatch in ischemic stroke. Stroke 2012;43:2648–53.
66. Lin L, Bivard A, Levi CR, et al. Comparison of computed tomographic and magnetic resonance perfusion measurements in acute ischemic stroke: Back-to-back quantitative analysis. Stroke 2014;45:1727–32.
67. Inoue M, Mlynash M, Straka M, et al. Patients with the malignant profile within 3 hours of symptom onset have very poor outcomes after intravenous tissue-type plasminogen activator therapy. Stroke 2012;43:2494–6.
68. Miteff F, Levi CR, Bateman GA, et al. The independent predictive utility of computed tomography angiographic collateral status in acute ischaemic stroke. Brain 2009;132:2231–8.
69. Gerraty RP, Parsons MW, Barber PA, et al. Examining the lacunar hypothesis with diffusion and perfusion magnetic resonance imaging. Stroke 2002;33:2019–24.
70. Gass A, Ay H, Szabo K, et al. Diffusion-weighted MRI for the "small stuff": The details of acute cerebral ischaemia. Lancet Neurol 2004;3:39–45.
71. Campbell BC, Weir L, Desmond PM, et al. CT perfusion improves diagnostic accuracy and confidence in acute ischaemic stroke. J Neurol Neurosurg Psychiatry 2013;84:613–18.
72. Ma H, Parsons MW, Christensen S, et al. A multicentre, randomized, double-blinded, placebo-controlled phase iii study to investigate extending the time for thrombolysis in emergency neurological deficits (extend). Int J Stroke 2012;7:74–80.
73. Menon BK, O'Brien B, Bivard A, et al. Assessment of leptomeningeal collaterals using dynamic ct angiography in patients with acute ischemic stroke. J Cereb Blood Flow Metab 2013;33:365–71.
74. Higashida R, Furlan A, Roberts H, et al. Trial design and reporting standards for intraarterial cerebral thrombolysis for acute ischemic stroke. J Vasc Interv Radiol 2003;14:S493–4.
75. Bivard A, Spratt N, Levi CR, et al. Acute stroke thrombolysis: Time to dispense with the clock and move to tissue-based decision making? Expert Rev Cardiovasc Ther 2011;9:451–61.
76. Parsons M, Spratt N, Bivard A, et al. A randomized trial of tenecteplase versus alteplase for acute ischemic stroke. N Engl J Med 2012;366:1099–107.
77. Yassi N, Parsons MW, Christensen S, et al. Prediction of poststroke hemorrhagic transformation using computed tomography perfusion. Stroke 2013;44:3039–43.
78. Lemmens R, Christensen S, Straka M, et al. Patients with single distal mca perfusion lesions have a high rate of good outcome with or without reperfusion. Int J Stroke 2014;9:156–9.
79. Campbell BC, Mitchell PJ, Yan B, et al. A multicenter, randomized, controlled study to investigate extending the time for thrombolysis in emergency neurological deficits with intra-arterial therapy (extend-ia). Int J Stroke 2014;9:126–32.
80. Savitz SI, Caplan LR. Vertebrobasilar disease. N Engl J Med 2005;352:2618–26.
81. Ferro JM, Pinto AN, Falcao I, et al. Diagnosis of stroke by the nonneurologist. A validation study. Stroke 1998;29:1106–9.
82. Schonewille WJ, Algra A, Serena J, et al. Outcome in patients with basilar artery occlusion treated conventionally. J Neurol Neurosurg Psychiatry 2005;76:1238–41.
83. Muir K, Buchan A, von Kummer R, et al. Imaging of acute stroke. Lancet Neurol 2006;5:755–68.
84. Schulte-Altedorneburg G, Bruckmann H. Imaging techniques in diagnosis of brainstem infarction. Nervenarzt 2006;77:731–43, quiz 744.
85. Puetz V, Khomenko A, Hill MD, et al. Extent of hypoattenuation on CT angiography source images in basilar artery occlusion: Prognostic value in the basilar artery international cooperation study. Stroke 2011;42:3454–9.
86. Vonofakos D, Marcu H, Hacker H. CT diagnosis of basilar artery occlusion. AJNR Am J Neuroradiol 1983;4:525–8.
87. Krings T, Noelchen D, Mull M, et al. The hyperdense posterior cerebral artery sign: A computed tomography marker of acute ischemia in the posterior cerebral artery territory. Stroke 2006;37:399–403.
88. Sylaja PN, Puetz V, Dzialowski I, et al. Prognostic value of CT angiography in patients with suspected vertebrobasilar ischemia. J Neuroimaging 2008;18:46–9.
89. Renard D, Landragin N, Robinson A, et al. MRI-based score for acute basilar artery thrombosis. Cerebrovasc Dis 2008;25:511–16.
90. Schaefer PW, Yoo AJ, Bell D, et al. CT angiography-source image hypoattenuation predicts clinical outcome in posterior circulation strokes treated with intra-arterial therapy. Stroke 2008;39:3107–9.
91. Cho TH, Nighoghossian N, Tahon F, et al. Brain stem diffusion-weighted imaging lesion score: A potential marker of outcome in acute basilar artery occlusion. AJNR Am J Neuroradiol 2009;30:194–8.
92. Ostrem JL, Saver JL, Alger JR, et al. Acute basilar artery occlusion: Diffusion-perfusion mri characterization of tissue salvage in patients receiving intra-arterial stroke therapies. Stroke 2004;35:e30–4.
93. Nagahori T, Hirashima Y, Umemura K, et al. Supratentorial dynamic computed tomography for the diagnosis of vertebrobasilar ischemic stroke. Neurol Med Chir (Tokyo) 2004;44:105–10, discussion 110–1.
94. Puetz V, Sylaja PN, Coutts SB, et al. Extent of hypoattenuation on CT angiography source images predicts functional outcome in patients with basilar artery occlusion. Stroke 2008;39:2485–90.
95. Puetz V, Khomenko A, Hill MD, et al. Extent of hypoattenuation on CT angiography source images in basilar artery occlusion: Prognostic value in the basilar artery international cooperation study. Stroke 2011;42:3454–9.
96. Pallesen LP, Gerber J, Dzialowski I, et al. Diagnostic and prognostic impact of PC-aspects applied to perfusion CT in the basilar artery international cooperation study. J Neuroimaging 2014;2014.
97. Strbian D, Sairanen T, Silvennoinen H, et al. Thrombolysis of basilar artery occlusion: Impact of baseline ischemia and time. Ann Neurol 2013;73:688–94.
98. Kidwell CS, Chalela JA, Saver JL, et al. Comparison of MRI and CT for detection of acute intracerebral hemorrhage. JAMA 2004;292:1823–30.
99. Chen W, Wang J, Xin W, et al. Accuracy of 16-row multislice computed tomographic angiography for assessment of small cerebral aneurysms. Neurosurgery 2008;62:113–21, discussion 121–2.
100. Brott T, Broderick J, Kothari R, et al. Early hemorrhage growth in patients with intracerebral hemorrhage. Stroke 1997;28:1–5.
101. Wada R, Aviv RI, Fox AJ, et al. CT angiography "spot sign" predicts hematoma expansion in acute intracerebral hemorrhage. Stroke 2007;38:1257–62.
102. Demchuk AM, Dowlatshahi D, Rodriguez-Luna D, et al. Prediction of haematoma growth and outcome in patients with intracerebral haemorrhage using the CT-angiography spot sign (predict): A prospective observational study. Lancet Neurol 2012;11:307–14.

48 Magnetic Resonance Imaging of Cerebrovascular Diseases

Maarten G. Lansberg, Max Wintermark, Chelsea S. Kidwell, Steven Warach, Gregory W. Albers

KEY POINTS

- The MRI acute stroke protocol includes T2, FLAIR, GRE, MRA, DWI, and PWI and can be acquired in 15–20 minutes.
- Diffusion-weighted MRI (DWI) is an excellent tool to detect acute cerebral infarcts, and to distinguish these from chronic infarcts, in patients with stroke or TIA.
- MRI has great promise as a tool to select patients who are the optimal candidates for acute stroke therapy.
- MRI is as reliable as CT in the identification of acute intracerebral hemorrhage and can therefore be used as the sole imaging modality for evaluating patients with acute stroke.
- MRI is superior to CT in identifying the underlying cause of intracerebral hemorrhage.
- MR angiography and venography are ideal imaging modalities for evaluation of cerebrovascular pathology such as arterial stenosis or occlusions, dissections, aneurysms, and venous thrombosis.

Nuclear magnetic resonance imaging (MRI) techniques were first employed in the 1940s. The first MR images were obtained in the 1970s. In the 1980s structural MRI emerged as a clinically useful diagnostic modality for stroke and other neurologic disorders.[1–5] In the detection of ischemic stroke lesions MRI is more sensitive than computed tomography (CT), particularly for small infarcts and in sites such as the cerebellum and brainstem and deep white matter.[6–8] In the investigation of ischemic stroke, conventional structural MRI techniques, such as T1-weighted imaging (T1WI), T2-weighted imaging (T2WI), and fluid-attenuated inversion recovery (FLAIR) imaging, reliably detect ischemic parenchymal changes beyond the first 12–24 hours after stroke onset. These methods can be combined with MR angiography (MRA) to non-invasively assess the intracranial and extracranial vasculature. However, within the critical first 3–6 hours, the period of greatest therapeutic opportunity, these methods do not adequately assess the extent and severity of ischemic changes.

The 1990s witnessed the development of diffusion-weighted imaging which is sensitive and specific for delineating irreversibly injured ischemic brain tissue within the first 6 hours from stroke onset.[9,10] Around the same time, contrast-based MR perfusion (MRP) techniques gained popularity to delineate hemodynamic changes.[11,12] These two techniques were recognized for their potential clinical utility in the early detection and investigation of patients with stroke.[13,14] That initial optimism began to bear fruit as further technical developments, most notably echoplanar imaging (EPI),[15] made diffusion and perfusion MRI feasible in routine clinical practice. The detection of hyperacute intraparenchymal hemorrhagic stroke by susceptibility-weighted MRI also has been established as comparable to CT. In combination with MRA, the multimodal stroke MRI examination opened the door for the detection of the site, age, extent, mechanism, and tissue viability of acute stroke lesions in a single imaging study. A number of potential clinical applications have emerged that could allow therapeutic and clinical decisions to be based on the physiologic state of the tissue in addition to clinical assessment. Stroke MRI is applied as a multimodal examination to evaluate the stroke patient for arterial pathology, hemodynamic changes, hyperacute parenchymal injury, subacute and chronic infarct, and evidence of acute or chronic hemorrhage (Fig. 48-1). Beyond its role as an aid in routine clinical diagnosis, the most promising applications of current MRI methodology are as a patient selection tool for experimental and interventional therapies and as a biomarker of therapeutic response in clinical trials.

In this review, we describe the applications of structural and functional MR techniques in cerebrovascular diseases. First, the general MRI principles and pulse sequences are discussed, followed by clinical applications of MRI in the evaluation of patients with TIA, ischemic stroke, intracranial hemorrhage and cerebrovascular pathology. Broader applications of MRI to specific cerebrovascular topics are illustrated in the other chapters of this book. A fuller treatment of the technical topics discussed in this chapter may be found elsewhere.[16,17]

GENERAL PRINCIPLES OF MAGNETIC RESONANCE IMAGING

Routine MR imaging is based on the interaction of radio waves with atomic nuclei (most commonly protons or hydrogen nuclei) in tissue. Hydrogen is present in nearly all of the organs of the body. Protons have a net magnetic moment such that when they are placed in a magnetic field they align with the magnetic field and can be excited by radiofrequency (RF) pulses. Water and fat protons are the most extensively imaged nuclei. Other nuclei can be imaged, such as phosphorus, sodium, and fluorine, but these are much less abundant than hydrogen and have no current clinical application to stroke.

When undergoing an MRI study, the patient is placed in a strong magnetic field. In general, this main magnetic field is always on, so safety precautions around the MRI scanner are essential even when a scan is not being performed. The strength of the magnetic field depends on the specific scanner. In practice, a number of the current clinical MRI are performed at 1.5 Tesla (1.5 T), but lower and higher field strength scanners are also in use. Over the past decade clinical 3T MRI has become commonplace. The next decade may see 7T MRI become a product for routine clinical use.[18] In general, for brain and cerebrovascular imaging, higher field strengths give greater signal-to-noise ratio, which is advantageous for

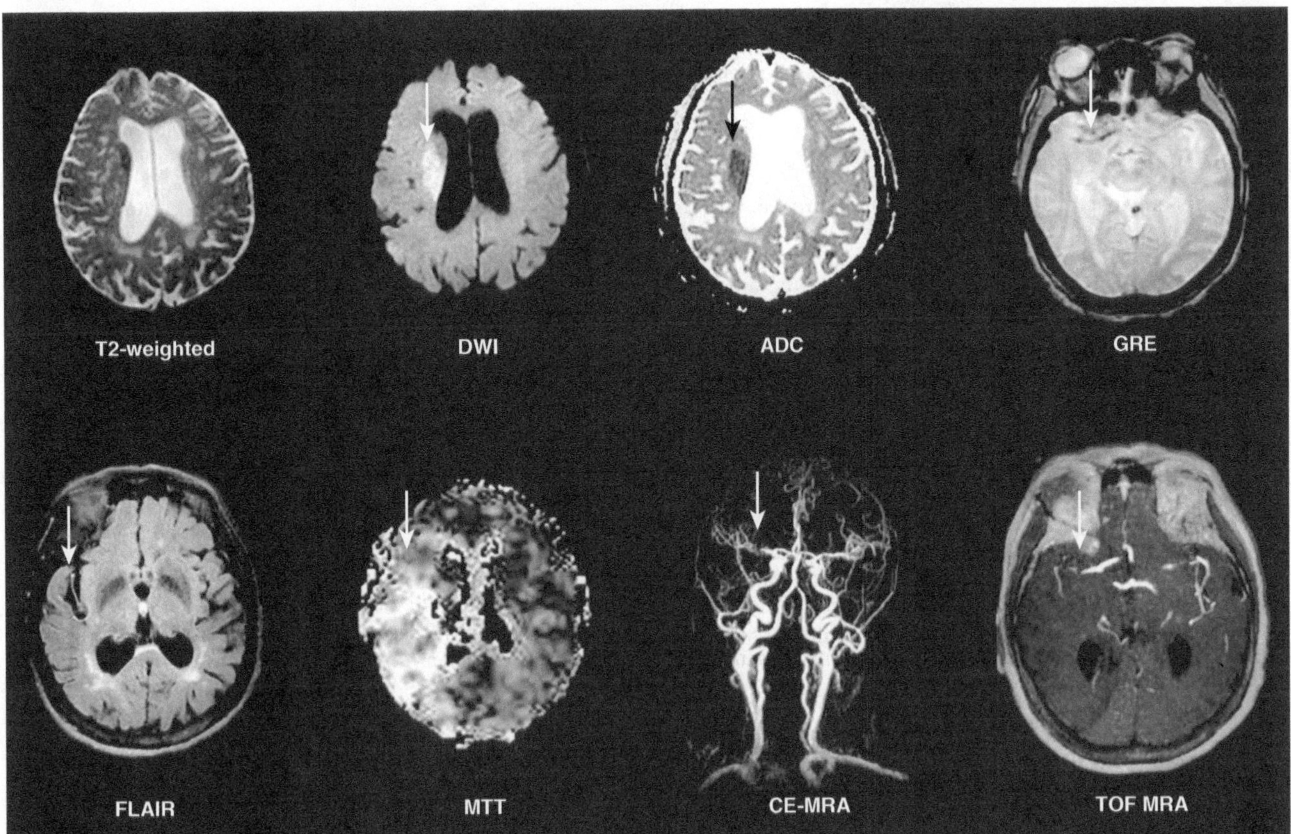

Figure 48-1. Multimodal MRI of acute stroke. *Arrows* point to the sequence-specific acute cerebrovascular pathology. T2-weighted image from the b0 images of the diffusion-weighted imaging (DWI) sequence appears normal. DWI image shows acute ischemic injury as a region of relative hyperintensity. The apparent diffusion coefficient (ADC) is reduced, as is characteristic of hyperacute stroke. The gradient recalled echo (GRE) image illustrates the susceptibility blooming of an acute thrombus *(arrow)*. Fluid-attenuated inversion recovery (FLAIR) image shows hyperintense middle cerebral artery (MCA) distal to the occlusion. The mean transit time (MTT) map of the perfusion-weighted image illustrates delayed perfusion in the right MCA territory. The contrast-enhanced (CE) and time-of-flight (TOF) MR angiograms identify the site of occlusion in the right MCA.

reducing scanning time and improving spatial resolution. Higher field strengths also come with challenges, including those related to susceptibility.

To acquire images, RF pulses are applied at the Larmor frequency of hydrogen, the proton's resonant spin frequency. The energy from the RF pulses is absorbed and then released until the tissue being scanned has reemitted the energy absorbed and undergone relaxation. The *echo time* (TE) is the time the machine waits after the applied RF pulse to receive the RF echo from the patient. The *repetition time* (TR) is the time between RF pulses. The energy released occurs over a short time according to two relaxation constants, known as T1 (longitudinal relaxation constant) and T2 (transverse relaxation constant). Varying the TE and TR enables images of different contrast to be obtained, depending on which of the constants is dominant in the tissue. Spatial localization of the signal source from the tissue is achieved by the superimposition of brief gradient magnetic field pulses.

In the sections below, the most commonly used MR pulse sequences are reviewed. Conventional MRI pulse sequences include T2WI, T1WI, proton density (PD) imaging, and FLAIR imaging. These are of most value in the evaluation of subacute and chronic stroke. The conventional sequences are based on two families of sequences termed spin echo (or fast spin echo) and gradient echo. In the former, the energy is refocused with the use of a series of RF pulses, whereas the latter uses a reversal of the magnetic field gradient to refocus the energy. The gradient echo sequences are most useful for MR angiography and hemorrhage detection. Supplementing the anatomical information obtained from conventional sequences, contemporary MR protocols also include diffusion-weighted imaging (DWI), diffusion kurtosis imaging (DKI), MR perfusion (MRP), and MR-angiography (MRA). These sequences allow a multimodal evaluation of the patient with acute stroke by imaging tissue injury, perfusion, and the vasculature within the short period feasible for an acute stroke evaluation.

T1-Weighted Images

T1WIs are based on the longitudinal relaxation of spins. They are generated primarily from sequences of short TE and short TR; the shorter the TE and TR, the more T1-weighted the image is. On T1WI, the cerebrospinal fluid (CSF) has low signal intensity, whereas fat has high signal intensity. Gray matter appears less intense (darker) than white matter. Ischemic infarcts appear hypointense on T1WI. The T1WI is not an essential part of the multimodal stroke MRI examination but is valuable in specific cases: axial fat-suppressed T1WI of neck soft tissue can identify the intramural thrombus of an arterial dissection.[19]

T2-Weighted Images

T2WIs are based on the transverse relaxation of spins. They are generated from sequences of long TE and long TR. On T2WI, the CSF signal is hyperintense. Gray matter appears less intense (darker) than white matter. Ischemic lesions also appear hyperintense and may be difficult to distinguish from normal CSF spaces, a potential problem for smaller lesions.

Proton Density Images

PD images are generated with long TR and short TE, and the CSF and fat are of similar signal intensity. One advantage of PD imaging is that lesions appear hyperintense relative to CSF, although in practice PD imaging has been supplanted by FLAIR imaging.

Fluid-attenuated Inversion Recovery Images

On FLAIR, an additional RF pulse (inversion pulse) is applied with the purpose of nulling signal from the normal CSF. As applied in routine practice, on T2-weighted FLAIR imaging the CSF signal is nearly fully suppressed and appears dark as in T1WI, but the lesions appear bright, as in T2WI, allowing better visualization of cortical lesions and periventricular lesions. In practice, FLAIR imaging is used in place of PD imaging and often preferred to T2WI, although FLAIR acquisition times are somewhat longer. Some radiologists prefer both FLAIR imaging and T2WI for the comprehensive head MRI examination, because of the diagnostic advantages of the latter for non-cerebrovascular pathologies. Unique features of FLAIR sequences for acute stroke imaging include hyperintensity of extra-axial blood (e.g., subarachnoid hemorrhage [SAH],[20] subdural hematoma, Figs 48-2A, B) and delayed gadolinium enhancement of intrasulcal CSF, indicative of early blood–brain barrier disruption (Fig. 48-2C).[21] FLAIR imaging may also depict hyperintense arterial signal indicative of very slow flow associated with acute occlusions or severe stenosis (Figs 48-1, 48-3)[22-25] A disadvantage of FLAIR imaging is its high sensitivity to pulsation artifacts of CSF that may mimic SAH, for instance in the basilar cisterns.

Diffusion-weighted Imaging

DWI has transformed the diagnosis of ischemic stroke in its earliest stage, from reliance on a mostly clinical inference about the presence, localization, and size of an ischemic lesion, to imaging confirmation of the infarct. This technique is the only brain imaging method to reliably demonstrate ischemic parenchymal impact within the first minutes to hours after onset, well before changes are detectable on CT and T2WI or FLAIR MR images (Figs 48-1, 48-4). DWI detects the self-diffusion of water, which is the mobility of water molecules among other water molecules (brownian

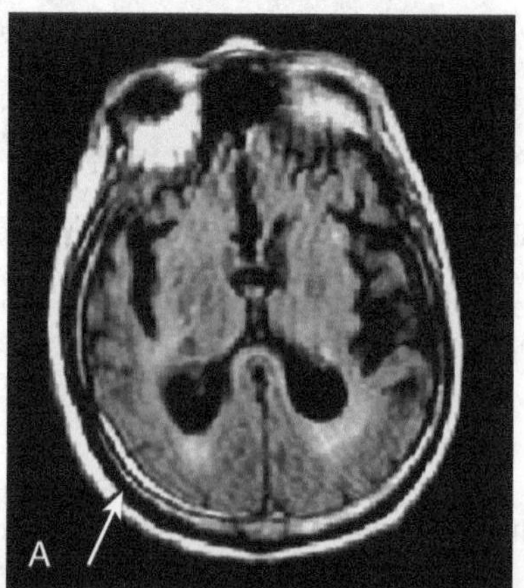

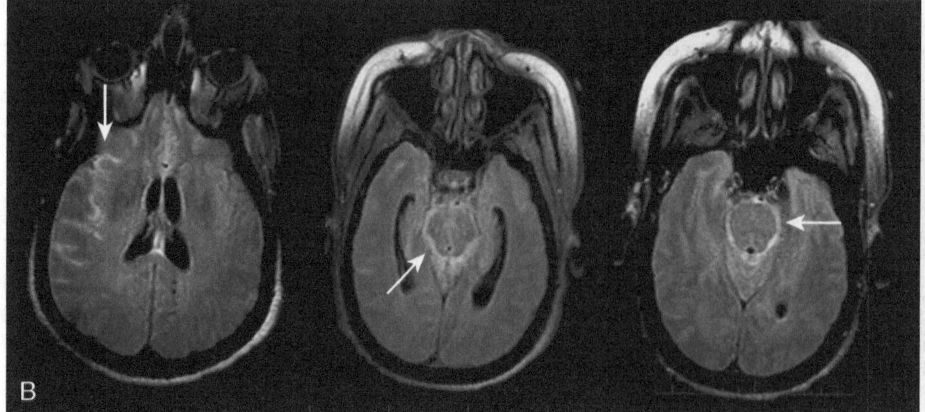

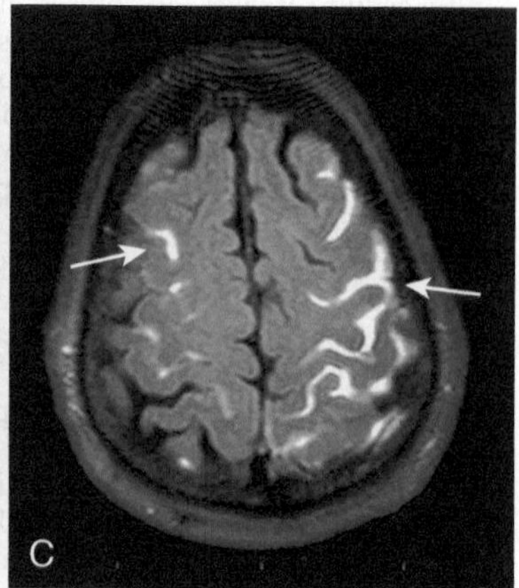

Figure 48-2. Extra-axial hyperintensity on fluid-attenuated inversion recovery (FLAIR). A, An example of a subdural hematoma seen on fluid-attenuated inversion recovery image (FLAIR) *(arrow)*, with clear contrast between the hyperintensity of the blood and the background tissue. This small subdural hematoma was not seen on CT. B, FLAIR images from a 47-year-old man with a subarachnoid hemorrhage. Blood appears hyperintense in the subarachnoid space at multiple levels. C, FLAIR images showing gadolinium enhancement of cerebrospinal fluid in hemispheric sulci *(arrows)* after intravenous tissue-type plasminogen activator (t-PA) treatment. This is the hyperintense acute reperfusion marker (HARM) sign, which indicates early blood–brain barrier disruption in stroke and is associated with reperfusion and increased risk of hemorrhagic transformation. The HARM sign is more likely to be seen following thrombolytic therapy. The main imaging differential is blood, which can be ruled out by gradient recalled echo MRI or CT.

Figure 48-3. Fluid-attenuated inversion recovery (FLAIR) hyperintense vessel sign. *Left,* Hyperintense vessel sign on FLAIR imaging in a patient with a 2-hour-old occlusion of the left internal carotid artery (*arrow*). Note the normal flow void (hypointensity) of the contralateral carotid artery. *Right,* Hyperintense vessel (*arrows*) sign in branches of the right middle cerebral artery territory distal to an occlusion, indicating slow flow in a patient with penumbral flow in that territory.

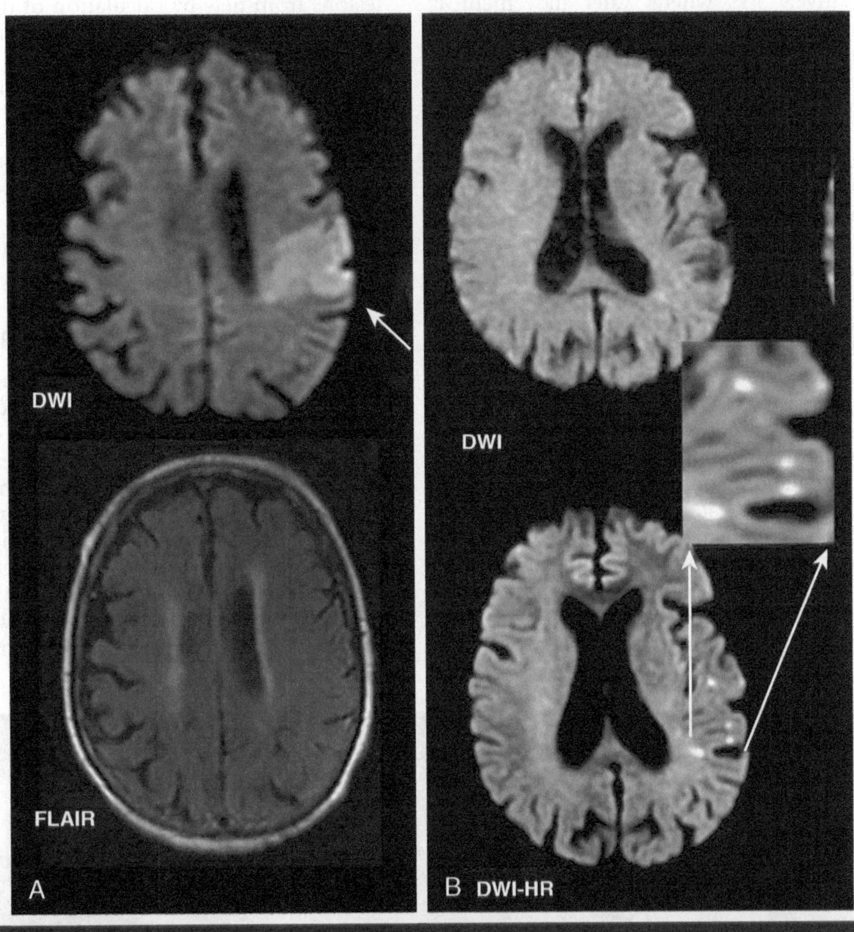

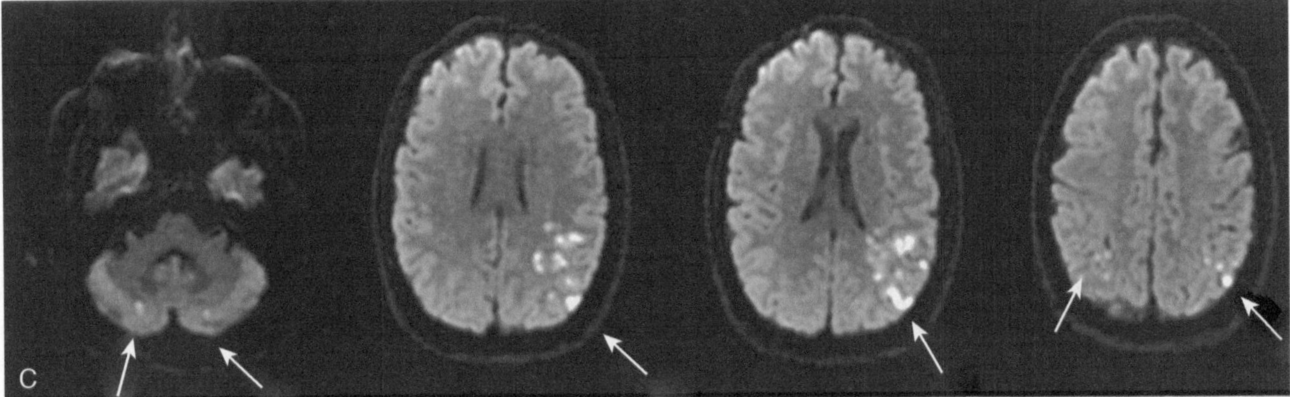

Figure 48-4. Detection of hyperacute ischemic stroke with diffusion-weighted imaging (DWI). A, The characteristic MRI pattern of hyperacute ischemic stroke, which is DWI-positive (*arrow*) and fluid-attenuated inversion recovery (FLAIR)-negative. B, High-resolution DWI (DWI-HR) may reveal punctate acute ischemic lesions not seen on the more typical lower-resolution DWI. The use of DWI-HR may further reduce the probability of false-negative DWI in stroke. C, Acute ischemic lesions (*arrows*) in multiple arterial territories suggestive of cardioembolic mechanism.

motion).[9,26] With use of single-shot echoplanar imaging, whole-brain DWI of stroke can be obtained in a scanning time as short as 2 seconds;[27] in current practice, however, multiple DWI acquisitions are obtained and combined for greater signal-to-noise ratio. The typical DWI pulse sequence actually acquires two sets of images, one with and the other without diffusion weighting. An EPI T2WI sequence is set without diffusion weighting. A bipolar pair of diffusion-sensitizing magnetic field gradient pulses to the T2WI pulse sequence cause a dephasing and then rephasing of the spinning protons in water molecules.[26] Where there has been net displacement of a water molecule (i.e., protons) between application of the two diffusion gradient pulses (on the order of tens of milliseconds), there is a net dephasing and subsequent signal loss in the resulting image. The more the water has moved, the greater the signal loss, so that signal intensity is reduced everywhere but relatively less where water movement is restricted. CSF appears very dark, normal brain appears intermediate, and ischemic brain, where parenchymal diffusion is reduced, appears relatively bright.

DWI is quantitative in that it both measures a physiologic parameter – the apparent diffusion coefficient (ADC) of water in mm^2/second – and can define the acute ischemic lesion volume, which can be used to study ischemic pathophysiology in vivo. The ADC is calculated from the reduction in signal intensity that occurs with diffusion weighting. Thus a DWI pulse sequence usually contains at least two sets of images, one without diffusion weighting, a T2WI, and one with high diffusion weighting. The strength of diffusion weighting is described by a set of pulse sequence features called the b-value, so these two sets of images may be referred to as b0, indicating the T2WI without diffusion weighting, and the b1000, referring to the most commonly used b-value in practice.

DWI measurements also contain geometric information, primarily axonal orientation, because DWI acquires its information in one direction at a time. This anisotropy results in higher signal perpendicular to fiber tracts and lower signal parallel to them. For routine stroke imaging, it is preferable to minimize anisotropy by effectively averaging the diffusion measurements across three orthogonal directions, reducing the hyperintensity not due to ischemia, a potential confounding factor for small ischemic lesion in white matter tracts. These averaged images are often referred to as *isotropic DWI*. Diffusion tensor imaging (DTI)[28,29] is a type of DWI that, rather than eliminate anisotropy, uses this information to determine the direction and integrity of degenerated white matter tracts. There are emerging data suggesting that DTI can be used to assess stroke recovery.[30,31]

In acute cerebral ischemia, the ischemic lesion appears hyperintense (bright) on DWI and hypointense (dark) on an ADC map (see Figs 48-1, 48-4). This appearance reflects cytotoxic edema, and a reduction in the volume and increased tortuosity of the extracellular space. As the ischemic lesion evolves through the phases of cytotoxic edema, vasogenic edema, tissue necrosis, and cavitation, the ADC normalizes and then becomes elevated in the chronic phase of stroke.[32] This feature makes it possible to distinguish old ischemic lesions from new by calculation of the ADC value. As a rule of thumb, DWI hyperintensity without T2WI or FLAIR changes usually implies reduced ADC and can be taken as evidence of acute ischemic impact. Signal hyperintensity on DWI can persist during later stages of stroke (the "T2 shine-through" effect) and cannot by itself be evidence of acute ischemic stroke. In addition, non-ischemic pathologies may be associated with DWI hyperintensity.[33] For these reasons, in patients with suspected ischemic stroke, DWI should always be interpreted with T2WI and FLAIR and ideally with a calculation of the ADC maps.

Magnetic Resonance Perfusion Imaging

Brain perfusion, defined in the broadest sense as some aspect of cerebral circulation, may be studied by various MRI strategies. Two categories of MRI methods, one requiring the injection of contrast agent and the other not, have been used to study abnormal perfusion in human stroke (mainly ischemic) (Fig. 48-5). The first strategy, which is the standard method in clinical practice, is dynamic susceptibility contrast (DSC) imaging, involves a bolus injection of gadolinium and the rapid acquisition of a series of susceptibility-weighted or $T2^*$-weighted images repeated every 1 to 2 seconds through an entire brain volume.[11,12] The intravascular passage of

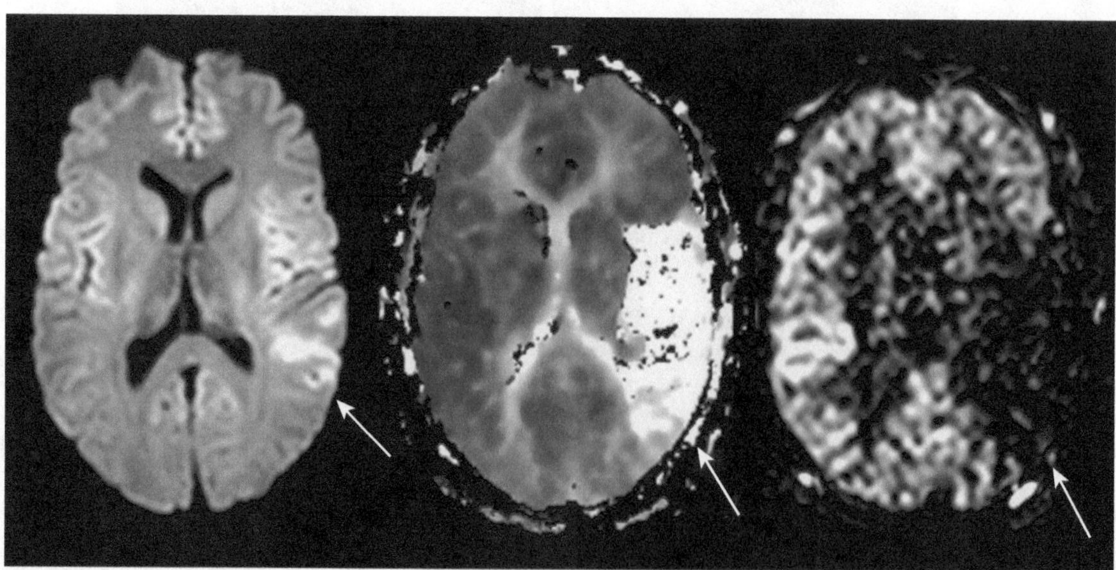

Figure 48-5. MR perfusion imaging. A, Acute ischemic changes in left middle cerebral artery territory on diffusion-weighted imaging (DWI). B, Larger region of ischemia on perfusion mean transit time (MTT) map using the standard dynamic susceptibility contrast (DSC) method. C, MR perfusion without gadolinium is acquired using arterial spin labeling (ASL), showing a comparable perfusion defect on this relative cerebral blood flow map obtained 1 hour 40 minutes after stroke onset. *Arrows* point to regions of abnormality.

gadolinium in sufficiently high concentration distorts the local magnetic field owing to magnetic susceptibility effects, causing dephasing of spins in brain tissue adjacent to the blood vessels and therefore results in signal loss. The amount of signal loss over time in a series of rapidly acquired images has been shown to be proportional to cerebral blood volume (CBV) in healthy brain tissue. The time it takes for the change in signal intensity to reach a maximum is the time to peak (TTP) and is related to the Tmax and mean transit time (MTT) of an idealized bolus of contrast agent. Because cerebral blood flow (CBF) in these intravascular models equals the ratio CBV/MTT, information about cerebral blood flow can potentially be inferred with this technique. In patients with acute stroke, perfusion maps of the relative MTT, Tmax, CBV, and CBF can be generated, permitting visualization of perfusion defects in acute infarcts, tissue reperfusion occurring after recanalization of blood vessels, and hyperperfusion of subacute infarcts that have reperfused. Postprocessing of the MRP images occurs within minutes of image acquisition at the scanner and so the images are rapidly available to the treating physician. The optimal and accurate assessment of these and other perfusion parameters is an area of intense investigation,[34–40] but in clinical practice, the MRP source images and scanner-generated perfusion maps are sufficient to determine the presence or absence of acute focal ischemia. For cases in which patient head movement during MRP acquisition renders the maps inadequate for diagnosis, assessment of the individual source MRP images can be useful, because these EPI source images are virtually unaffected by patient motion.

Because of the recognized toxicity of gadolinium-based contrast agents in patients with renal failure, which is not uncommon in older stroke patients, there has been increased interest in MR perfusion methods that do not require contrast agent administration. The second MR perfusion strategy involves arterial spin labeling (ASL) methods, which use RF inversion pulses to magnetically label spins in the arterial supply to brain regions, using arterial water as an endogenous diffusible tracer.[41–44] It can be applied either as pulsed,[45,46] as continuous labeling,[47] or as a combination of both. In ischemic stroke, ASL appears to give comparable diagnostic information to that from the gadolinium bolus tracking methods (see Fig. 48-5),[48] although the reduced signal-to-noise ratio requires averaging of multiple acquisitions, requiring longer acquisition times, and thus is more vulnerable to motion artifacts. However, the more straightforward quantitative measurement of tissue perfusion with ASL[49,50] is an advantage of this methodology over the bolus tracking method. Innovations have now permitted multiple brain slices to be imaged with ASL,[51] and ASL perfusion methods are available for routine imaging on most MRI scanners.

Magnetic Resonance Angiography

In cerebrovascular diagnosis, MRA with contrast-enhanced (CE) or time-of-flight (TOF) methods are the standard approaches. In CE-MRA, a rapid MR acquisition is timed to a bolus injection of contrast agent over a large field of view, permitting routine imaging of the vasculature from the aortic arch through to the branches of the circle of Willis (see Fig. 48-1). The vascular anatomy is outlined by the blood containing the contrast agent. In TOF MRA, no contrast agent injection is required, and the vascular signal depends on direction and velocity of blood flowing into the plane of imaging. The magnetization of protons in stationary tissue occurs through saturation by repeated low-flip-angle RF pulses, whereas protons in the vessels flowing into the tissue remain unsaturated and appear relatively bright. The data are then postprocessed for an angiographic reconstruction. In practice, inspection of the source images is often necessary to evaluate subtle or ambiguous findings, and most scanners permit scrolling through a reformatted slab of source MRA images for this purpose (see Fig. 48-1). For imaging of the arteries of the circle of Willis, 3D rather than 2D TOF MRA is the most common method of MRA in clinical practice, since it gives superior spatial resolution and is less prone to signal loss from turbulent flow at sites of stenoses. Limitations of TOF MRA are its tendency to overestimate the degree of stenosis (particularly when there is slow or turbulent flow or calcifications) and its insensitivity to collateral sources of flow. Its advantages include greater spatial resolution than CE-MRA for the intracranial circulation and its application to the imaging of the cerebral venous system (MR venography). TOF is an alternative for patients unable to receive gadolinium-based contrast agents. Notwithstanding its tendency to overestimate the degree of stenosis, MRA rivals CT angiography and conventional angiography for the detection of arterial stenoses, occlusions, and dissections.[52–55] The sensitivity of MRA to detect aneurysm after SAH is estimated to be 69–100%, with a specificity of 75–100%.[56] The sensitivity for smaller aneurysms is less.[57]

Susceptibility-weighted Imaging

SWI refers to a family of MRI sequences in which the tissue contrast is based on magnetic susceptibility differences between different tissue types. Magnetic susceptibility is the property of matter that distorts an applied magnetic field. Although often a source of artifacts at the interface of differing tissue types or in the presence of metal, this principle can be used to make pulse sequences sensitive to hemorrhage, to functional changes in blood oxygenation, and to hemodynamic parameters. The conventional GRE pulse sequence (commonly called $T2^*$-weighted images) is sensitive to the susceptibility effects of paramagnetic molecules such as gadolinium-containing contrast agents as well as deoxyhemoglobin and other hemoglobin breakdown products that are present during all stages of intracranial hemorrhage. Single-shot EPI has intrinsic susceptibility weighting, and EPI using a GRE technique, as in MRP, is the most sensitive of all to susceptibility effects in routine clinical practice. A specific variation of GRE, termed simply SWI, measures phase differences and may be more sensitive than conventional GRE in the detection of acute hemorrhage, chronic microbleeds, and cerebral veins.[58–60]

Magnetic Resonance Spectroscopy

MRS allows the non-invasive in vivo assessment of brain chemistry by measuring resonances from important metabolites. Clinical studies of MRS have been performed predominantly on ^1H nuclei (proton MRS), for which there is a relatively favorable signal-to-noise ratio compared with MRS of other nuclei. Although data collection from single voxels (single voxel spectroscopy) is more straightforward, differences between tissue compartments following stroke are more easily appreciated with chemical shift imaging (CSI). In CSI, spectra from multiple voxels within a grid corresponding to one or more slices are displayed. Typically metabolite peaks are presented as a spectrum in the "frequency domain" on a scale expressed in parts per million (ppm), which conventionally runs from right to left. CSI data can also be displayed as a color-coded "map" overlying a structural image, but it should be stressed that analysis of individual spectra is mandatory. Although a large number of metabolites can be detected, particularly in those studies using a short TE, stroke studies have focused on metabolites with large peaks including *N*-acetyl-L-aspartate (NAA) at 2.01 ppm, lactate at 1.33 ppm, and, to a lesser extent, choline at 3.22 ppm and creatine at 3.03 ppm. Values of metabolite peaks can be expressed in relative terms, for example, as a ratio to another metabolite within the same voxel, or to the same metabolite in a voxel in the contralateral hemisphere. Absolute concentrations may be derived by using the signal from water as an internal reference[61] or, less commonly, by using a reference solution placed in the scanner external to the patient. MRS spectroscopy is time-consuming and therefore has limited clinical applications for acute stroke imaging.

CLINICAL APPLICATIONS OF MRI IN PATIENTS WITH CEREBROVASCULAR DISEASE

The objective of multimodal MRI of acute stroke, also referred to as the stroke MRI examination, is to obtain diagnostic information about the acute parenchymal injury, subacute or chronic infarct, arterial pathology, tissue perfusion, and presence of hemorrhage. In this section the clinical application of multimodal MRI in the diagnostic work-up of patients with transient ischemic attacks, ischemic stroke, intracranial hemorrhage, and vascular pathology is discussed. Finally, we describe the utility of MRI as a tool to guide acute stroke therapy.

The full multimodal MR sequences listed in Table 48-1 can be acquired within 15–20 minutes of scanning. All patients must be screened by MRI personnel for safety related to metal or electronic devices. Updated online resources relating to MRI safety are available (e.g., www.mrisafety.com). Approximately, 10–15% of patients suspected of acute stroke are unable to undergo MRI because of contraindications. In 2006, a link between gadolinium-based contrast agents and nephrogenic systemic fibrosis (NSF), a potentially debilitating fibrosing disease of the skin and viscera occurring in patients with chronic kidney disease was recognized. Readers are referred to European and North American guidelines for specific management recommendations.[62,63] In general, caution is recommended when the glomerular filtration rate (GFR) is between 30 and 60 mL/min/1.73 m^2 in the patient with chronic kidney disease, but local hospital policies may differ. Gadolinium should not be used when the GFR is less than 30 mL/min/1.73 m^2 or if the patient is dialysis-dependent. Estimated GFR based on serum creatinine is used to screen patients undergoing MRI for this risk.

TABLE 48-1 MRI Sequences in Acute Stroke

Sequence	Primary Diagnostic Use in Cerebrovascular Disease
Diffusion-weighted imaging (DWI)	Hyperacute acute ischemic lesions Distinguish old lesions from new by apparent diffusion coefficient (ADC) imaging
T2-weighted imaging (T2WI)	Subacute and chronic ischemic lesions Rule out non-cerebrovascular pathology
Fluid-attenuated inversion recovery (FLAIR)	Subacute and chronic ischemic lesions Rule out non-cerebrovascular pathology Hyperintense vessel sign Blood–brain barrier breakdown
Gradient recalled echo (GRE)	Acute intracranial hemorrhage Hemorrhagic transformation Microbleeds Intravascular thrombus
MR angiography (MRA)	Acute arterial occlusion Other arterial lesions: stenosis, dissection, aneurysm MR venogram for sinus and cerebral venous thrombosis
Perfusion-weighted imaging (PWI)	Focal hemodynamic defect Diffusion–perfusion mismatch as marker of ischemic penumbra

Transient Ischemic Attacks

Conventional MRI

Conventional MRI (e.g., T2WI) is more sensitive than CT in identifying both new and preexisting ischemic lesions in patients with transient ischemic attacks (TIAs) (employing the classic definition of TIA as a focal neurologic deficit of vascular etiology that resolves within 24 hours). One of the earliest studies reported that 77% of patients had focal ischemic changes on MRI compared with 32% on CT.[64] In subsequent studies, the percentage of TIA patients with at least one infarct on conventional MRI varies from 46% to 81%, but the majority of lesions do not correlate with symptomatology.[65,66] The percentage of patients with an infarct on MRI in a location that could have accounted for the deficits observed during the TIA varies from 31% to 39% on conventional MRI.[65,67] With conventional MRI it is difficult to determine what proportion of these appropriately localized infarcts occurred at the time of the index TIA and what proportion existed prior to the presenting event. Contrast-enhanced MRI studies can help determine the acuity of the lesion. In series of TIA patients who underwent contrast-enhanced MRI, contrast enhancement of an infarct was observed in 11–39%.[65,65]

Diffusion-weighted MRI

Newer MRI techniques, including diffusion weighting and perfusion have revolutionized the MRI assessment of patients with TIA (Fig. 48-6).[68–75] The high sensitivity and specificity of DWI for detection of acute infarcts has been particularly useful in the work-up of TIA patients. In a pooled analysis of 19 studies, the aggregate rate of DWI positivity was 39%, with frequency ranging from 25% to 67%.[76] In studies that also obtained a follow-up MRI, 56–80% of patients demonstrated a subsequent infarct in the region corresponding to the original DWI abnormality (Fig. 48-7).[68,80]

Several studies have demonstrated that DWI positivity is associated with specific clinical characteristics, including longer symptom duration, motor deficits, aphasia, and large-vessel occlusion demonstrated on MRA.[68,77–79] A study exploring the characteristics of "DWI-negative" patients with TIA, found that patients with brainstem location ischemia or lacunar syndromes were most likely to have a negative initial DWI result and a positive follow-up imaging result.[81]

Identification of DWI-positive lesions in TIA patients is often clinically relevant. For patients who have multiple lesions on T2WI, DWI helps to clarify whether the lesions were related to a recent ischemic event in 31%,[79] and the DWI image alters the physician's opinion regarding vascular localization and probable TIA mechanism in also approximately one-third of patients.[68] It has also been shown that patients with TIA who have abnormalities on DWI scans have a higher risk of recurrent ischemic events than those without such abnormalities.[74,78,82] The presence of a DWI lesion alone or in combination with clinical variables such as the ABCD score (age, blood pressure, type of symptoms and symptom duration) is a strong predictor of 7-day and 3-month stroke risk.[74,83]

MR Perfusion

Several studies have demonstrated that MRP can provide additive value to DWI and in some cases is more sensitive than DWI in detecting acute ischemic changes in patients with TIA.

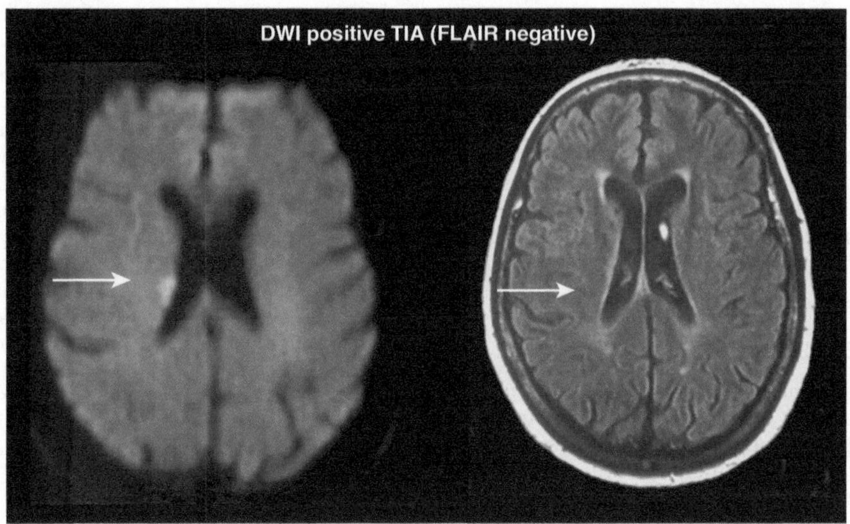

Figure 48-6. Diffusion-weighted imaging (DWI) of a patient with a transient ischemic attack (TIA). MRI findings in a 63-year-old man with a 30-minute episode of left arm weakness, imaged 4 hours after resolution. *Left,* DWI sequence shows right periventricular white matter lesion (*arrow*) not apparent on the fluid-attenuated inversion recovery (FLAIR) sequence (*right, arrow*).

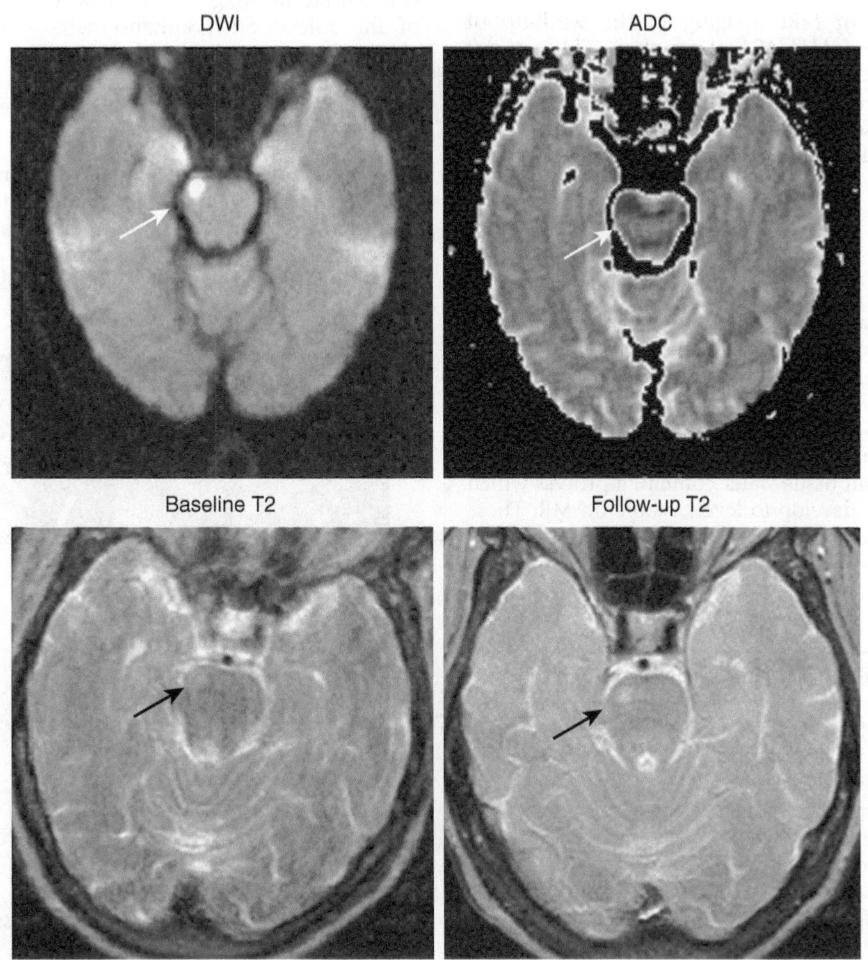

Figure 48-7. Baseline and follow-up MRI in a patient with TIA. An acute ischemic lesion is evident on the baseline MRI as a bright lesion on the DWI sequence (top left) and as a dark lesion on the ADC map (top right), but is inconspicuous on the T2 sequence. Follow-up imaging demonstrates a subsequent infarct in the region corresponding to the original diffusion-weighted imaging (DWI) abnormality. TIA, transient ischemic attack; ADC, apparent diffusion coefficient.

Because MRP is able to detect regions of relative hypoperfusion that do not reach the threshold of tissue bioenergetic compromise required to cause a lesion on DWI, a greater number of patients with modest degrees of ischemia may be detected with MRP.

In series of TIA patients evaluated with MRP within 48 hours of symptom onset, approximately 33% of patients had a perfusion lesion.[73,84] The percentage of patients with a DWI lesion was also approximately 33% and the combined yield of DWI plus MRP was 51%.[73]

Implications of MRI for Transient Ischemic Attack Definition and Clinical Guidelines

TIAs are "brief episodes of neurological dysfunction resulting from focal cerebral ischemia not associated with permanent cerebral infarction."[76] Historically, transient episodes of neurological dysfunction lasting less than 24 hours have been considered TIAs. However, the MRI studies discussed above have shown that 30–50% of patients with short spells sustain permanent injury as evidenced by the presence of acute infarcts. Because of this, a new definition for TIA that includes imaging criteria has been proposed. This defines TIA as "a transient episode of neurological dysfunction caused by focal brain, spinal cord, or retinal ischemia, without acute infarction".[76,85]

Given the utility of MRI imaging in the work-up of patients with TIA, the AHA/ASA states that "TIA patients should undergo neuroimaging evaluation within 24 hours of symptom onset, preferably with magnetic resonance imaging, including diffusion sequences; noninvasive imaging of the cervical vessels should be performed and noninvasive imaging of intracranial vessels is reasonable".[76,85]

Ischemic Stroke

Conventional MRI

The Acute Stroke Stage. Early MRI findings in patients with acute stroke are summarized in Box 48-1. Within the first few hours of ischemia, standard MRI sequences (T1WI, T2WI, and FLAIR) are relatively insensitive to ischemia, showing abnormalities in less than 50% of cases.[84] The earliest changes, seen as increased signal on T2WI and FLAIR sequences, are due to a net increase in overall tissue water content, a process which takes several hours to develop to levels visible on MR. These changes are uncommon prior to 6 hours from onset but can be readily appreciated by 12–24 hours. Although the majority of ischemic lesions are evident on both CT and conventional MRI by 24 hours, standard MRI is superior to CT in identifying lesions earlier as well as lesions that are smaller or in the posterior fossa.[6,7]

Whereas ischemic parenchymal changes are not apparent on conventional sequences in the first few hours, intravascular signs of acute stroke may be apparent. Specific findings include: absence of arterial flow void on T2WI, the hypointense intravascular sign due to acute thrombus on GRE sequences (Figs 48-1, 48-8),[86,87], and intravascular hyperintensity on FLAIR (Figs 48-1, 48-3).[22–25] This hyperintense vessel sign on FLAIR is indicative of slow anterograde flow through an incomplete occlusion, or slow retrograde flow via leptomeningeal collaterals. This finding is associated with large diffusion-perfusion mismatch, but is not predictive of response to thrombolytic therapy.[22,23,88,89] Similarly, after the administration of gadolinium, enhancement of the blood vessels in the area of infarction can be seen on T1WI, indicating slow flow within these vessels.

On FLAIR imaging, CSF signal is suppressed which makes this sequence very sensitive to blood or gadolinium-based contrast agents in the CSF. SAH and subdural hemorrhage can therefore readily be detected on FLAIR. Leakage of gadolinium contrast into the CSF space in stroke patients with early disruption of their blood–brain barrier can be detected on post-contrast FLAIR images. It is characterized by a hyperintensity of the sulci.[21] Such enhancement – termed hyperintense acute reperfusion marker, or HARM – is associated with reperfusion, thrombolytic therapy, an increase in the risk of hemorrhagic transformation, and an increase in plasma matrix metalloproteinase-9[21,90–92] (Fig. 48-2).

The Subacute Stroke Stage. When infarcts evolve their MR characteristics gradually change. Subacute infarcts are characterized by varying amounts of vasogenic edema and sometimes hemorrhagic transformation. Vasogenic edema is maximum between 1 and 6 days but persists to varying degrees

BOX 48-1 Early MRI Findings in Acute Ischemic Stroke

- Hyperintensity on diffusion-weighted imaging, with minimal or no changes on T2-weighted imaging (T2WI) or fluid-attenuated inversion recovery (FLAIR) imaging
- Hypointensity on apparent diffusion coefficient (ADC) imaging
- Hypointense ("blooming") artery sign of acute intravascular thrombus on gradient recalled echo (GRE) imaging
- Arterial occlusion on MR angiography
- Absence of arterial flow-void, indicative of occlusion, on T2WI or FLAIR imaging
- Hyperintense vessel sign, indicative of slow or collateral flow, on FLAIR imaging
- Focal reduction or absence of contrast on dynamic perfusion source images
- Focal reduction or absence of perfusion on perfusion parameter maps

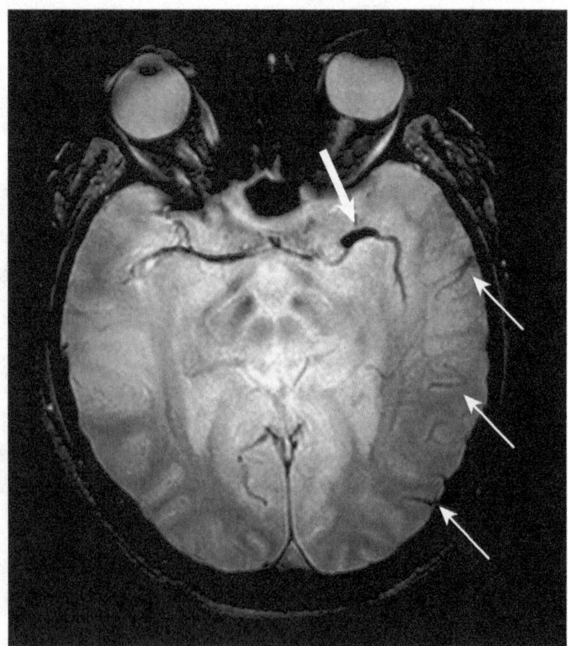

Figure 48-8. The blooming hypointensity of an acute arterial thrombus on gradient recalled echo (GRE) MRI (*large arrow*). The *small arrows* point to dilated veins commonly seen on GRE within the penumbral region, as defined on diffusion–perfusion mismatch (not shown).

for 3 or 4 weeks. This edema appears as a hyperintense signal on T2-weighted and FLAIR images and as hypointense on T1WI. Subacute strokes are also characterized by breakdown of the blood–brain barrier. This breakdown results in gadolinium enhancement. The typical sequence of enhancement of the infarct is that enhancement is uncommon in the first 6 days, is most common between 7 and 30 days and disappears after that but can persist for up to 6 weeks.[93] Two patterns of enhancement have been seen, a slowly progressive form that follows the T2WI changes and then an early form of enhancement which may be associated with better outcome. Occasionally a fogging effect may be seen in this phase or in the acute phase that is postulated to be due to developing hemorrhagic infarction.

The Chronic Stroke Stage. In the chronic stage of stroke the edema that was present in the subacute phase has resolved. At very late time points there may be atrophy and cavity formation. At this stage infarcts appear hyperintense on T2-weighted and FLAIR imaging. On T1WI, infarcts are hypointense and no longer have contrast enhancement. On DWI there is the T2 shine-through pattern and the ADC is elevated. Also at this stage, Wallerian degeneration may be seen as a secondary phenomenon in the white matter tracts.[94]

Ischemic Lesions on MRI in Patients without a Clinical Stroke. Focal hyperintensities in the subcortical white matter demonstrated by T2-weighted or FLAIR images are a common incidental finding in patients undergoing brain MRI for indications other than stroke. They are indicative of chronic microvascular disease. These white matter hyperintensities are an indication of chronic cerebrovascular disease. They are associated with advanced age, history of hypertension, and pathologic changes such as arteriosclerosis, dilated perivascular spaces, and vascular ectasia.[142–145,148–151] These white matter lesions may progress in number and frequency. Their clinical significance in the asymptomatic patient for cognitive decline or risk of stroke, independent of the other coexisting stroke risk factors, is uncertain.

Diffusion-Weighted MRI

DWI allows visualization of regions of ischemia within minutes of symptom onset.[95] DWI lesions follow a relatively consistent pattern of growth during the first 3 days, followed by a subsequent gradual decrease in size.[96–100] The increased (bright) signal on DWI reflects restricted diffusion of water molecules in areas with cytotoxic edema. This can be quantitatively measured on the ADC maps, where darker areas represent decreased diffusion. The increase in signal on DWI may persist for several weeks or longer partially owing to a T2 effect. The average ADC, however, remains reduced for only 4 to 7 days then returns to normal or supranormal levels within 7 to 10 days from ischemia onset.[32,101,102] This feature makes it possible to distinguish old ischemic lesions from new by calculating the ADC. Although the average ADC generally follows this pattern, studies have now clearly demonstrated that marked heterogeneity of the ADC value can occur within the ischemic lesion, even in the hyperacute time window.[103]

Test Characteristics of DWI. DWI has a high degree of sensitivity (88% to 100%) and specificity (95% to 100%) for acute cerebral ischemia, even at very early time points.[104–107] Studies performed in the acute stroke setting have consistently demonstrated marked superiority in accuracy of diagnosis of ischemic change for DWI (95% to 100%) over that for CT (42% to 75%) or standard MRI sequences such as FLAIR (46%).[108–112] A prospective, blinded comparison of DWI with non-contrast CT in a consecutive series of 356 patients referred for emergency assessment of suspected acute stroke proved the superiority of DWI in a broad, representative sample.[113] The sensitivity of DWI for ischemic acute stroke ranged from 73% (within 3 hours after the event) to 92% (more than 12 hours). By contrast, the sensitivity of CT at these times was 12% and 16%, respectively. The specificity of MRI for stroke detection was 92% (at 3 hours) and 97% (more than 12 hours).[113] The superiority of DWI over CT was observed regardless of clinical severity or time from stroke onset to scan. A study comparing DWI lesions with pathologically confirmed infarction at autopsy also demonstrated an overall accuracy of 95%.[114]

Despite the high sensitivity of DWI, false-negative results might occur: Mild or small infarcts, early imaging, and brainstem location are factors associated with false-negative scans, and the false-negative rate is higher when patients have two or more of these factors than when individuals have one or none.[81,113] The reported rate of false-negative results with DWI in consecutive patients assessed for acute stroke was 17% (versus 84% for CT) for the entire sample and 27% (versus 88% for CT) for patients imaged within the first 3 hours.[113] False-positive DWI lesions are rare, but occasionally, DWI hyperintensities may be seen in other cerebral disorders, including status epilepticus, tumors, infections, and Creutzfeldt-Jakob disease. Given the overall excellent test characteristics of DWI for detection of acute infarcts, the 2010 practice guideline of the American Academy of Neurology states that DWI should be performed for the most accurate diagnosis of acute ischemic stroke.[115]

Clinical Utility of DWI. DWI's high sensitivity and specificity for identifying acute infarcts and its ability to distinguish acute from chronic infarcts can provide important diagnostic and prognostic information.[116–119] The neuroanatomic site and the vascular territory of acute infarcts can almost always be demonstrated with DWI. Knowledge about the location of the acute infarcts can provide insight into stroke etiology, because certain lesion patterns are associated with specific stroke subtypes.[120,121] Multiple lesions in the unilateral anterior circulation, and small scattered lesions in one vascular territory, particularly in a watershed distribution, are typically related to large-artery atherosclerosis.[121,122] The presence of multiple acute lesions in different vascular territories in patients who have only one clinically symptomatic acute insult suggests an embolic stroke mechanism. This pattern may be seen in 3–5% of patients.[120] These imaging patterns, together with information obtained from other MRI sequences, such as MRA, might help in the selection of the most appropriate measures for secondary prevention of stroke.

DWI lesion characteristics can also be used to help determine the age of a stroke in patients with unwitnessed onset of stroke, including individuals whose deficits are present on awakening. A DWI lesion without a matching hyperintensity on FLAIR imaging suggests that the stroke occurred within 6 hours. Acute stroke studies are ongoing that use this pattern as a selection criterion for study enrollment.[123–126]

The volume of the baseline DWI lesion provides prognostic information regarding final infarct volume and neurologic and functional outcomes in patients with stroke affecting the anterior circulation but not the posterior circulation[99,127–134] Prognostic accuracy is improved when DWI volume data are combined with clinical variables.[135] The number of acute DWI lesions can also be used prognostically, as the presence of multiple DWI lesions is associated with an increased risk of future ischemic events.[136–138]

MR Perfusion

MR bolus perfusion imaging (MRP) is playing an ever more important role in the initial evaluation of the patient with acute stroke. Perfusion measures that can be derived from this technique include mean transit time (MTT), time to peak (TTP), time to maximum of the residue function (Tmax), cerebral blood volume (CBV), and cerebral blood flow (CBF).[35,38,139,140] Controversy persists regarding which perfusion measure is optimal for identification of critically hypoperfused tissue in the acute stroke setting. The role of perfusion imaging in the assessment of the acute stroke patients is discussed in detail in the section on *MRI-guided acute stroke therapy* at the end of this chapter.

Magnetic Resonance Spectroscopy

MRS provides an opportunity to study brain biochemistry in vivo after stroke. This technique may be used to image the ischemic penumbra, provide prognostic information, and may offer additional imaging endpoints in clinical trials. MRS, however, has a number of limitations. First, even under ideal conditions, signal-to-noise ratio is limited by the low concentration of brain metabolites relative to water. Second, movement of patients during scanning not only may distort spectra and introduce confounding signal from scalp lipid, but also may displace the head from its original position, thereby limiting the spatial sensitivity of the technique. Third, interpretation of metabolite ratios requires an appreciation that all major metabolites may change after stroke and with aging.[141] Finally, MRS is time-consuming and therefore not practical in the acute stroke setting. In the paragraphs below, we describe the expected changes in the major metabolites following stroke that can be measured with MRS.

NAA is considered a marker of neuronal integrity[142] on the basis of its predominantly neuronal localization.[143] NAA values fall after stroke,[144-150] with greater decreases in the center than in the periphery of the infarct.[157,161] The early reduction of NAA can be as much as 20% within an hour[151] and 50% within 6 hours.[152] NAA levels continue to decrease in the first 2 weeks after stroke,[150] and remain chronically low or absent thereafter. Low NAA levels have therefore been implied as a marker of the ischemic core.

The *creatine* peak is influenced by both creatine and phosphocreatine and therefore is considered a marker of energy stores. Reductions in this peak are seen after stroke,[144,145,147,149] but are less dramatic than the reduction in NAA.[146]

Lactate levels are raised within the infarct and manifest as a "doublet" peak at 1.33 ppm, projecting above and below the baseline at long and intermediate TEs, respectively. Lactate production results from anaerobic glycolysis and is generally considered to be undetectable in the healthy brain, although low levels of lactate may be detectable in older healthy adults[153] and in the hemisphere contralateral to stroke lesions.[150] Animal studies of ex vivo and in vivo MRS demonstrate that lactate is present within minutes of ischemia and that lactate levels continue to increase over hours, particularly in the center of the ischemic lesion.[151,152,154] Reperfusion after focal ischemia precipitates a gradual decrease in lactate over days[151,155] but a decline in lactate is also seen in permanent MCA occlusion models.[151] Clinical studies are consistent with these findings. High levels of lactate are present in the infarct of patients imaged in the hyperacute phase.[156,157] Subsequently, lactate levels fall during the first week[145,146] and are undetectable after 2 weeks.[147,150] Measurements after a number of months have shown a second rise in lactate levels,[150] consistent with the presence of inflammatory infiltrate.

Changes in the *choline* peak, which represents total choline levels and is a marker of cell membrane turnover are more variable. Choline levels after stroke can be decreased,[144,149] unchanged,[147] or increased.[145] Although decreases may represent cell loss, it has been postulated that increases may represent myelin damage in infarct regions with a significant proportion of white matter.[148]

Clinical Utility of MR Spectroscopy in Stroke. While MR spectroscopy can theoretically be used to refine the MR definition of "tissue at risk",[156] its clinical applicability in the acute stroke setting is limited because MR spectroscopy is time-consuming. It has been hypothesized that tissue with a raised lactate but normal NAA levels may indicate metabolically compromised yet intact neurons, and therefore the ischemic penumbra (Fig. 48-9).[148] One human MRS study of acute stroke patients confirmed that the MRP–DWI mismatch region has raised lactate levels and normal NAA levels.[156] Another study showed less lactate and more NAA in the ischemic penumbra compared to the ischemic core.[157]

MRS studies also have the potential to provide markers of the efficacy of stroke therapy. This may include the measurement of brain temperature in different tissue compartments,[158,159] assessment of the interplay between ischemia and redox status,[160] or, theoretically, even the demonstration that certain drugs have actually reached the target tissues. In addition, MRS could be used to evaluate the effect of revascularization procedures such as endarterectomy or EC–IC bypass surgery. MRS studies have shown a reduction of NAA, an increase in choline, and sometimes an increase in lactate in the hemisphere ipsilateral to an internal carotid artery stenosis.[161,162] Such changes can be reversed with carotid

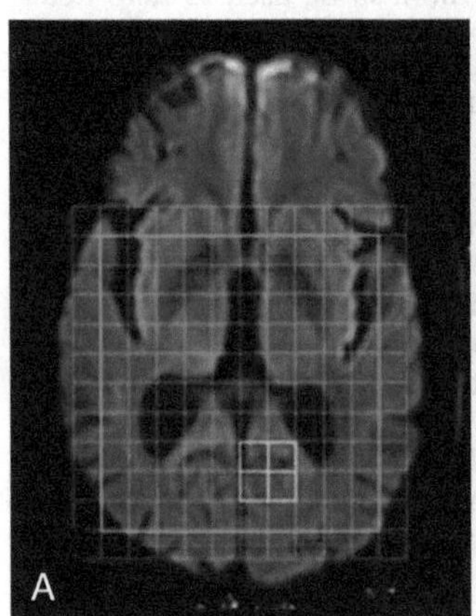

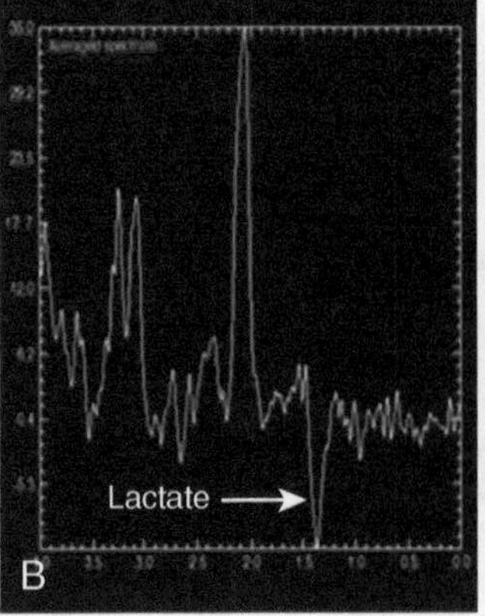

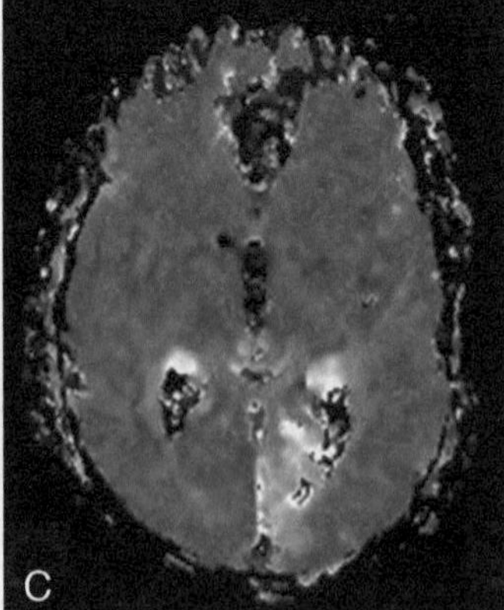

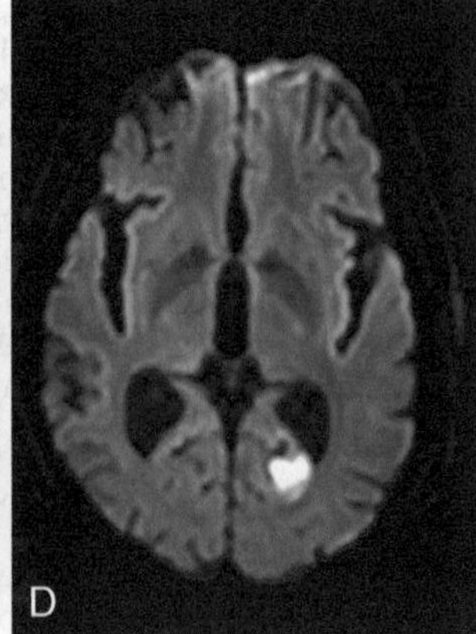

Figure 48-9. Identification of lactate in 2-hour acute stroke in diffusion-negative, perfusion-positive region, preceding the diffusion-weighted imaging (DWI) lesion. A, Baseline DWI with magnetic resonance spectroscopy (MRS) grid overlaid. B, MRS abscissa from highlighted voxels in A, which shows the presence of lactate *(arrow)*. C, Baseline lesion on mean transit time (MTT) map. D, Follow-up DWI demonstrating lesion in region on early lactate peak.

TABLE 48-2 Appearance of Hemorrhage on Various MRI Sequences

Stage	T1-Weighted	T2-Weighted	Fluid-Attenuated Inversion Recovery	Gradient Recalled Echo or T2*
Hyperacute (<12 hour)	Isointense or mildly hyperintense	Hyperintense	Hyperintense	Hypointense rim
Acute (12 hour to 2 days)	Isointense or hypointense	Hypointense	Hypointense	Hypointense rim gradually progressing centrally
Early subacute (2–7 days)	Hyperintense	Hypointense	Hypointense	Hypointense
Late subacute (8 days to 1 month)	Hyperintense	Hyperintense	Hyperintense	Hypointense
Chronic (>1 month to years)	Isointense or hypointense	Hypointense	Hypointense	Slit-like hyperintense or isointense core surrounded by a hypointense rim

endarterectomy, particularly in patients who do not have lactate in the lesion prior to surgery,[161] and in those in whom the postoperative CBV is demonstrably improved.[163] Finally, MRS may play a role in assessing prognosis after stroke, as lactate-to-choline ratios[164] and changes in NAA[165] correlate with clinical outcome.

Intracranial Hemorrhage

Although non-contrast CT has traditionally been considered the gold standard for the assessment of hemorrhage, advances in MRI techniques have provided both improved diagnostic capabilities for detection of intracranial hemorrhage and better understanding of the underlying pathophysiology, etiology, and prognosis of these disorders.

The appearance of blood on various MRI sequences depends on the stage of evolution of the blood breakdown products (Table 48-2).[166] The hemoglobin that is present in freshly extravasated blood exists primarily in the form of oxyhemoglobin, which is non-paramagnetic. However, conversion of intracellular oxyhemoglobin to deoxyhemoglobin likely begins at the periphery of the hematoma almost immediately. Deoxyhemoglobin contains four unpaired electrons, making it highly paramagnetic. Around days 2 or 3, deoxyhemoglobin is converted to methemoglobin, which initially is formed intracellularly then becomes extracellular as the red blood cells lyse. Around day 7, macrophages and phagocytes begin transforming the methemoglobin to hemosiderin and ferritin.

Conventional T1- and T2-weighted MRI sequences are highly sensitive for the detection of subacute and chronic blood, but they are less sensitive to parenchymal hemorrhage less than 6 hours old. Studies now suggest that hyperacute parenchymal blood can be accurately detected using standard or echoplanar imaging T2*-weighted sequences, including gradient recalled echo (GRE) and susceptibility-weighted imaging (SWI).[167–169] Echoplanar T2*-weighted imaging can be performed with a very low acquisition time (seconds), representing a significant advantage in patients with acute intracranial hemorrhage who are unable to cooperate or lie still for extended periods of time.

The hallmark of hyperacute hemorrhage on T2*-weighted sequences is a rim of hypointense signal surrounding an isointense core (Fig. 48-10). Subsequently, in the acute and subacute stages, the hematoma becomes diffusely hypointense, and in the chronic stage, the hematoma appears as a slit-like signal with a hyperintense or isointense core with a rim of hypointensity.

Several large multicenter prospective studies have demonstrated that these MRI sequences are as reliable as CT in the

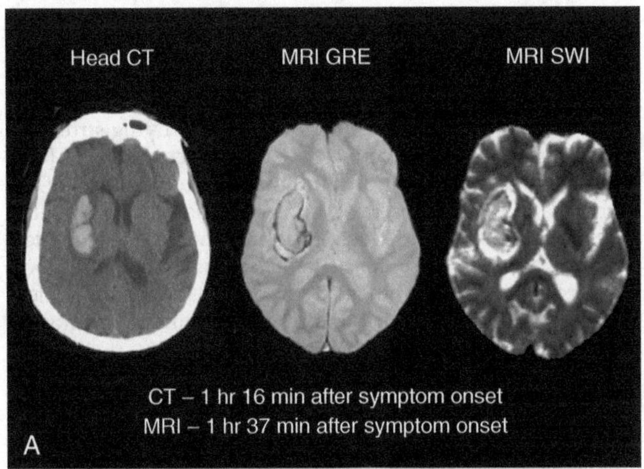

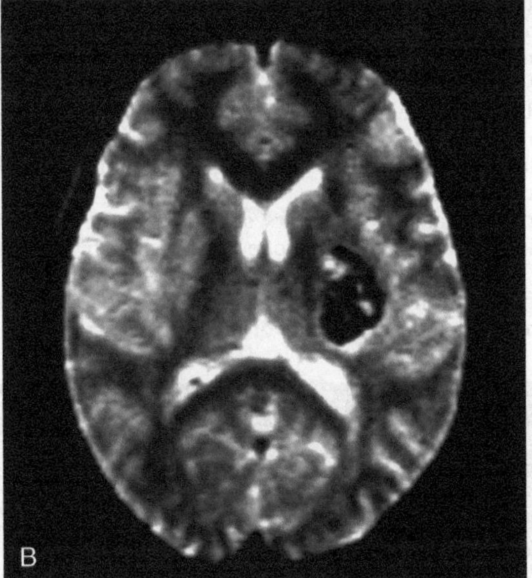

Figure 48-10. A, An example of an acute intraparenchymal hematoma, less than 2 hours from onset, on CT as well as gradient recalled echo (GRE) MRI and MRI using echoplanar imaging (EPI) and susceptibility weighted imaging (SWI). Note on MRI the appearance of a heterogeneous central hypointense periphery of the hematoma, surrounded by the hyperintense rim of edema. B, In a hematoma at a later point, approximately 3 hours from onset in this figure, hypointensity predominates.

identification of acute blood, and superior to CT for detection of chronic blood including microbleeds and chronic hemorrhages.[113,170,171] In some cases, MRI detects hemorrhages that are not evident on CT.[170,172] These findings have allowed MRI to be employed as the sole imaging modality to evaluate patients with acute stroke at capable centers. However, up to 20% of patients with acute stroke may not tolerate or may have contraindications to MRI.[173]

Intraparenchymal Hemorrhage

The most frequent underlying etiologies of adult primary intracerebral hemorrhage (ICH) are hypertension and cerebral amyloid angiopathy (CAA), and MRI findings can often assist in making this determination. Primary ICH associated with hypertension most often occurs in deep brain structures (e.g., putamen, thalamus, cerebellum, and pons), and is often accompanied by deep microbleeds. In contrast, primary ICH occurring in lobar regions, particularly in the elderly, is most commonly related to CAA but may also be associated with hypertension.[174] CAA-related hemorrhage is frequently characterized by a distinct pattern of lobar microbleeds.

MRI is superior to CT in identifying underlying structural lesions that are less frequent causes of parenchymal ICH (e.g., arteriovenous malformations, tumors) and in quantifying the amount and extent of perihematomal edema (fluid attenuated inversion recovery [FLAIR] sequence). A contrast study (highest yield in subacute phase once edema has dissipated and blood been reabsorbed) is indicated in patients without a clear underlying etiology or in hemorrhages occurring in unusual locations.[175]

MRI techniques have provided new insights into the underlying pathophysiology of ICH, specifically the role of ongoing secondary neuronal injury in the perihematomal region. A number of studies (but not all) have demonstrated perihematomal regions of hypoperfusion, bioenergetic compromise, or both.[176,177] These MRI studies have suggested that approximately one-third of patients imaged in the acute phase may have reduced perihematomal ADC values.[176,178,179] Further studies have characterized the evolving time course, with ADC values being low within the first day and then gradually elevated, likely reflecting the evolution of perihematomal edema.

In aggregate, these studies suggest that there may be a subset of patients with a rim of perihematomal hypoperfusion and possibly ischemia in the hyperacute phase. It is likely that this region rapidly disappears in the subacute phase as edema and inflammation evolve.[177,180] The development of edema and toxicity from blood breakdown products are the most significant contributors to ongoing perihematomal injury. MRI studies thus have the potential to monitor the impact of these findings on recovery and in the future may be used as surrogate outcome markers for studies of putative interventions.[181,182]

Recently, a series of studies have reported a high frequency of small acute ischemic lesions visualized on DWI in the acute and subacute periods following the onset of primary ICH. These lesions are remote from the index hemorrhage and have been reported in approximately one-quarter to one-third of patients with primary ICH due to either hypertensive disease or cerebral amyloid angiopathy.[183–188] Several of the studies have found an association with blood pressure reductions or fluctuations in the acute hospital setting[184,188,189] and they have also been associated with the presence of microbleeds, white matter disease, and prior stroke.[185,186,188] Notably, a number of these studies have also found an association between remote ischemic lesions on DWI and poor functional outcome or death following primary ICH.[184,186,190]

Microbleeds

T2*-weighted MRI sequences have the ability to detect clinically silent prior microbleeds, not visualized on CT (Figs 48-11, 48-12). Microbleeds are defined as punctate, homogeneous, rounded, hypointense parenchymal lesions, usually

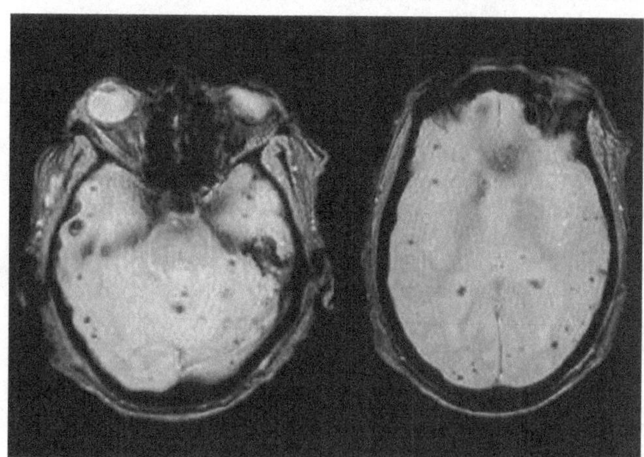

Figure 48-11. Gradient recalled echo MRI sequence demonstrating multiple scattered old microbleeds (punctate hypointensities) from a patient with cerebral amyloid angiopathy.

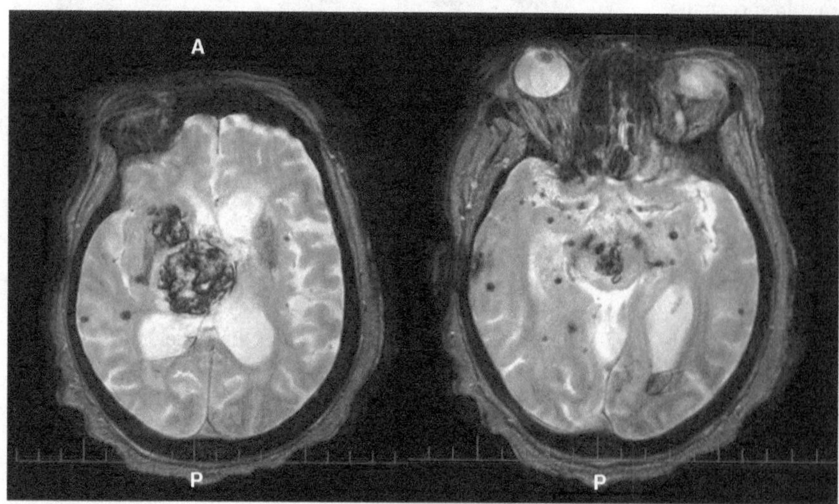

Figure 48-12. Example of GRE from a patient with ICH attributable to hypertensive disease, in whom microbleeds are most commonly found in deep and infratentorial regions.

less than 5–10 mm in size. A number of studies have demonstrated that the pathologic correlate of GRE-visualized microbleeds is a region with hemosiderin-laden macrophages that occurs adjacent to small vessels. These findings are indicative of previous extravasation of blood at the vessel wall.[191] Studies have suggested that the ability to detect microbleeds is greater with higher magnet strength, high-resolution 3D T2*-weighted imaging, and/or the use of susceptibility-weighted imaging sequences compared to standard GRE; however, the clinical relevance of these differences remains unclear.[192–195] A number of standardized approaches and scoring systems have been proposed for quantifying microbleed burden, including automated or semi-automated approaches.[196–200]

MRI evidence of microbleeds is seen in 38–80% of patients with primary ICH, in 21–26% of patients with ischemic stroke, and in 5–6% of asymptomatic individuals.[201–203] In the Rotterdam study of a general elderly population, prevalence of microbleeds increased from 24.4% to 38% over a 3-year interval.[204] Hypertension and/or blood pressure variability, CAA, and advancing age are the most commonly reported risk factors for microbleeds.[205–210] Chronic kidney disease, statin use, antithrombotic use, elevated blood inflammatory markers, and elevated serum uric acids levels have also been reported as independent risk factors for microbleeds.[211–217] In one study, microbleeds have been found to be more prevalent in black patients with primary ICH (74%) than in whites (42%) (P = 0.005).[218] Microbleeds have also been found to occur more commonly in persons with greater white matter and small-vessel disease.[219] Less common risk factors are cerebral autosomal dominant arteriopathy with silent infarcts and leukoaraiosis (CADASIL)[210] moyamoya disease,[220] and SAH where they were associated with the presence of ischemic DWI lesions.[221]

A growing body of evidence indicates that microbleeds represent a marker of a bleeding-prone angiopathy as well as an active, dynamic small-vessel disease process.[222–226] Several case reports and small series suggested that patients with microbleeds may be at increased risk for development of hemorrhage following antithrombotic or thrombolytic therapies. In contrast, two large series did not show an increased risk of hemorrhage in patients treated with intravenous tissue plasminogen activator (t-PA).[227,228] However, in both of these studies, very few patients were included who had a large microbleed burden, thus representing a potentially biased sample. A more recent meta-analysis did report a significant relationship between increasing microbleed burden and symptomatic hemorrhage post thrombolysis.[229] One study found that almost 5% of patients treated with intravenous thrombolysis developed new microbleeds.[230]

The pattern of microbleed topography can provide insights into the underlying risk factors and etiology, particularly in patients with primary ICH. It has been shown that microbleeds are a common occurrence in patients with CAA and most frequently are found in lobar regions (see Fig. 48-11).[205] A pattern of multiple lobar microbleeds in the setting of a lobar ICH is highly suggestive of CAA as the underlying etiology. However, a recent study found that both small-vessel disease and CAA contribute to the pathogenesis of lobar microbleeds.[231] In contrast, in patients with ICH attributable to hypertensive disease, microbleeds are most commonly found in deep and infratentorial regions, although it is likely that hypertension may also contribute to lobar-located microbleeds (see Fig. 48-12).[208] A number of studies have suggested an association between microbleeds and apolipoprotein genotype status, with increased rates in persons with apolipoprotein ε4 and ε4 alleles, particularly in CAA-related lobar microbleeds.[232–234]

The presence of microbleeds and the overall microbleed burden appear to have important prognostic significance. One study demonstrated that the total number of microbleeds predicts risk of future symptomatic hemorrhage in patients with probable CAA.[207] In addition, new microbleeds demonstrated on repeat MRI were found to also predict increased risk of future symptomatic ICH.[235] Several studies have shown a correlation between microbleeds and new vascular events.[206,236,237] In patients with TIA or stroke, microbleeds have been associated with an increased risk of future stroke in general but not symptomatic ICH.[238,239] The presence of prior microbleeds has also been associated with development of new microbleeds both in ischemic disease and ICH. Moreover, microbleed burden and rate of accumulation have been found to predict cognitive decline and poor neurologic or functional outcome in this population, and even vascular death.[240–243] In particular, microbleeds have been found to be associated with executive dysfunction.[244,245] In patients with TIA or stroke, microbleeds have been associated with an increased risk of future stroke in general but not symptomatic ICH.[238,239]

Hemorrhagic Transformation

Hemorrhagic transformation (HT) of an ischemic infarction is a common occurrence, visualized in up to 42% of patients in pathologic series. The MRI evolution of blood breakdown products in HT is similar to that seen with primary ICH (see Table 48-2). However, T2*-weighted MR sequences often demonstrate regions of petechial hemorrhage not visualized with CT or standard MR sequences. Prospective studies, employing serial MRI with gradient echo sequences, are required to clarify the frequency of these findings in various stroke subtypes with and without reperfusion treatments, and their role in antithrombotic treatment decisions. The most commonly used radiologic classification system for rating the type and severity of hemorrhagic transformation was developed for head CT scans and divides hemorrhage into two major categories, hemorrhagic infarct (HI) and parenchymal hematoma (PH), each with two subcategories based on severity.[246] However, it is important to note that the application of this classification system to MRI has not been fully validated. One small study suggested that T2*-weighted GRE was the most reproducible method to categorize HT with excellent reliability for severe parenchymal hematoma category.[247] A modified classification system has also been developed with high rates of interobserver agreement.[248]

MRI information can, however, assist in distinguishing hemorrhagic transformation of an ischemic infarct from a primary hematoma. Most hemorrhagic transformations are smaller than the field of the ischemic infarct as seen on DWI. Primary hematomas also tend to have rounder edges and often have a greater amount of surrounding edema than would be seen in an ischemic stroke. Finally, hematomas frequently do not respect vascular territories.

A growing number of studies have evaluated the clinical and radiologic (including MRI) predictors of HT in the setting of thrombolytic therapy. Contrast agent extravasation visualized on FLAIR, T1-weighted, or T2*-weighted sequences has been identified as an important marker of blood–brain barrier disruption, and therefore a predictor of HT.[218,249–253] Several studies have also suggested that a large baseline DWI lesion, low ADC values, and very low cerebral blood volume are also independent predictors of subsequent symptomatic hemorrhage.[254–258] Some studies,[259] but not all,[260] suggest that early infarct FLAIR hyperintensity is associated with increased rates of hemorrhagic transformation following thrombolysis. Higher rates of HT have been reported in patients treated with intravenous thrombolysis and with enlargement of medullary veins visualized on T2*-weighted sequences.[261] These findings provide potential imaging biomarkers for testing of treatments designed to minimize risk of blood–brain barrier opening and subsequent hemorrhagic transformation.

Subarachnoid Hemorrhage

Later studies have explored the clinical utility of MRI sequences in patients with subarachnoid hemorrhage (SAH). Although standard spin-echo sequences are relatively insensitive to subarachnoid blood, newer sequences, including FLAIR and gradient echo T2* imaging, have been shown to have modest sensitivity, particularly in the subacute phase when the CT result is often negative.[262–264] Subarachnoid blood appears as a region of high signal intensity relative to normal CSF on FLAIR sequences and as a region of hypointensity on gradient echo images. Overall, studies have suggested that FLAIR imaging is as sensitive as CT for acute SAH, but compared with the findings at lumbar puncture, the findings on FLAIR imaging are not definitive in excluding acute SAH.[263,265–267]

Evaluation of patients with SAH and vasospasm is an emerging role for multimodal MRI. Several reports have demonstrated that patients with vasospasm secondary to aneurysmal SAH demonstrate a high rate of DWI lesions, often indicative of silent ischemia.[268,269] In studies employing perfusion imaging, these ischemic lesions were associated with regions of hemodynamic compromise and angiographic evidence of vessel vasospasm.[270–272] Later studies have employed combined diffusion and perfusion imaging to characterize the pathophysiology and evolution of ischemia due to vasospasm.[273,274]

Superficial Siderosis

Superficial siderosis (or hemosiderosis) is defined as hemosiderin deposition within the subpial brain layers due to chronic iron deposition in subarachnoid or CSF spaces that can be visualized on T2*-weighted sequences. It can be caused by or associated with other forms of CNS hemorrhage including SAH, SDH, and primary intraparenchymal hemorrhage or intraventricular hemorrhage. Superficial siderosis is a common finding in cerebral amyloid angiopathy and has been associated with a clinical presentation of transient focal neurological episodes.[275–277] Cortical superficial siderosis in this population may be associated with an increased risk of symptomatic ICH.[278]

Subdural and Epidural Hematomas

Subdural hematomas appear as crescent-shaped lesions adjacent to the brain parenchyma. The MRI appearance depends on the age of the hematoma and the sequences acquired. In the acute stage, subdural hemorrhages appear as hyperintense on FLAIR and T2-weighted sequences. On GRE sequences, they may be isointense or hypointense in the acute stage, on the basis of the stage of blood breakdown products. In the subacute stage, they appear hypointense. In the chronic stage, subdural hematomas appear as either isointense or mixed signals, depending on the degree of blood reabsorption.

Epidural hematomas appear as lentiform (biconvex) extra-axial lesions adjacent to the brain parenchyma. The displaced dura appears as a thin line of low signal intensity between the brain and hematoma. Rapid enlargement may lead to significant midline shift, often associated with herniation. MRI signal intensities usually follow the previously described temporal evolution of intraparenchymal ICH.

Cerebrovascular Pathology

Arterial Stenosis and Occlusion

MRA rivals conventional angiography and CT angiography for the detection of arterial stenoses and occlusions,[52–55,279] but there is a tendency of MRA, especially TOF, to overestimate the degree of stenosis because of dephasing of protons caused by turbulent flow or calcifications at the site of the stenosis. Smaller intracranial vessels are not well visualized with routine applications of MRA, however, ultra-high field MRA at 7 Tesla has shown promising results to reliably visualize small, micro-vessels at a sensitivity approaching that of angiography.[280] A normal screening MRA of the extracranial carotid is reliable to exclude hemodynamically significant stenosis but false-positive results can arise when the degree of carotid stenosis is overestimated. This can occur when the carotid artery is kinked or changes direction abruptly, when assessing stenosis of the distal ICA as it enters the carotid canal (owing to susceptibility artifact between vessel and bone), and when assessing stenosis in the presence of surgical clips. A false-positive occlusion on MRA is usually deducible by the reconstitution of flow distal to the point of signal loss. Sensitivity and specificity for carotid occlusion have been found to be 100% for most studies. In general, if MRA shows no stenosis or a stenosis of less than 70%, no further evaluation is necessary. If MRA shows a stenosis of 70% or more, duplex ultrasonography should be performed. If results of the two studies agree, no further evaluation is suggested,[281,282] and appropriate management can be provided. If MRA and duplex ultrasonography do not agree, then further evaluation with conventional angiography is recommended. A promising new approach is contrast-enhanced MRA of the carotid arteries, in which a more rapid MR acquisition is timed to a bolus injection of contrast agent over a larger field of view in less than 1 minute. This technique compares favorably to conventional angiography for the diagnosis of carotid stenosis.[283–286] The accuracy of contrast-enhanced MRA for the detection of vascular disease of the vertebral artery origins and the aortic arch is being investigated.

Arterial Plaque Morphology

A newer application of vascular imaging with MRI is high spatial resolution multimodal imaging of the carotid plaque to identify the various components, such as lipid deposits, fibrous caps, calcium, and thrombus.[287] Although not yet a routine practice, high-resolution carotid plaque imaging appears promising as a way to document decreased lipid content and plaque stabilization following lipid-lowering therapy[288] and to identify a ruptured fibrous cap associated with a recent history of TIA or stroke.[287] Technical developments in high-resolution MR imaging of MCA stenosis have the potential to yield excellent visualization of intracranial stenosis and atherosclerotic plaque.[289]

Arterial Dissection

The diagnosis of dissection of the internal carotid or vertebral artery can be made with MRI and MRA.[290–293] Findings suggestive of dissection on MRI are increased signal from parts of, or the entire, vessel wall on axial T1-weighted images (with fat suppression) consistent with hematoma (Fig. 48-13), a border of increased signal surrounding the lumen with luminal narrowing, poor or absence of visualization of the vessel, or significant compromise of the vessel lumen by adjacent abnormally increased signal tissue. If a false lumen with an intimal flap is present, it is best appreciated on the T2WI. Vessel abnormalities such as narrowings, aneurysmal dilatation, and a second lumen may be demonstrable by MRA. When a TOF technique is used, MRA may show a normal or simply widened outer contour of the vessel at the site of dissection. This is caused by the addition of signal from the vessel wall due to methemoglobin in the hematoma, and by the high-flow lumen. False-negative MRI/MRA assessments for dissection occur, and CT angiography is recommended if there is a high degree of clinical suspicion and the MR results are negative. Review of the literature indicates that, in general, the positive-predictive and negative-predictive values of MRI combined with MRA were similar to those of CTA for diagnosis of dissection of the carotid and vertebral arteries.[294]

Aneurysms

MRA has a sensitivity of 92–95% for the detection of intracranial aneurysms.[240,241] False-negative and false-positive aneurysms detected on MRA are mainly located at the skull base and middle cerebral artery.[295] The sensitivity of MRA to detect aneurysm after SAH is 69–100%, with a specificity of 75–100%.[56] The sensitivity of this technique for the detection of small aneurysms is lower.[57] Lesions as small as 2–3 mm in diameter have been shown by MRA, and the technique has occasionally demonstrated small aneurysms missed on conventional angiography.[296] However, aneurysms smaller than 5 mm may be missed with MRA. Slow flow and turbulence within small aneurysms may interfere with their detection in up to 27% of cases, leading to limitation in study interpretation.[297] These problems can be partially overcome by using intravenous contrast media. Small aneurysms may be difficult to differentiate from vessel loops because, unlike with conventional angiography, there is no increase in signal at the point of vessel overlap with use of an MIP (maximum intensity projection) algorithm. The use of MRA as a routine screening test for the detection of aneurysms is controversial.[298,299] If aneurysm size is the only factor, the insensitivity to small aneurysms may not be of clinical consequence. The accuracy of MRA in detecting small aneurysms is likely to improve as techniques are further refined.

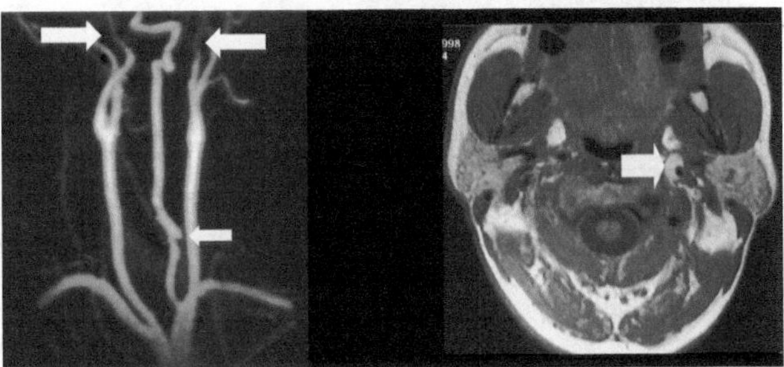

Figure 48-13. MR images from a 48-year-old man with dissections *(arrows)* of bilateral carotid and vertebral arteries. *Left,* Power-injector contrast-enhanced neck MR angiogram shows an intimal flap in the left vertebral artery as well as progressive tapering of the distal internal carotid arteries. *Right,* A T1-weighted axial MR image through the internal carotid artery illustrates the pathognomonic crescent sign of dissection. In this image, the blood within the vessel wall of the right internal carotid artery appears hyperintense.

Venous Thrombosis

Although diagnosis of cerebral venous thrombosis remains a diagnostically challenging entity, advances in MRI have substantially aided in the ability of physicians to perform a rapid, non-invasive, and comprehensive neuroimaging evaluation. The combination of brain MRI with MR venography (MRV) has a sensitivity of up to 95% in detecting cerebral venous sinus thrombosis.[300] Moreover, MRI has provided further insight into the underlying differences in the pathophysiologic processes involved in venous versus arterial infarction. In cerebral venous thrombosis, breakdown of the blood–brain barrier combined with venous congestion leads to a unique combination of coexistent vasogenic and cytotoxic edema, which in turn often leads to frank infarction, hemorrhage, or both. MRI studies are able to visualize venous congestion, venous infarction, and hemorrhage.

Venous hypertension may produce cytotoxic edema, vasogenic edema, or a combination of the two. These changes can be visualized as hyperintensity on T2-weighted or FLAIR images. If venous hypertension is mild, no signal abnormalities may occur. In patients with superior sagittal sinus thromboses, parasagittal lesions are common and may be bilateral. Transverse sinus thrombosis frequently causes posterior temporal lobe lesions, whereas thrombosis of the deep sinus system often causes bithalamic lesions. With contrast agent administration, there may be lesion enhancement in a tumor-like pattern. Hemorrhagic transformation of venous infarction occurs frequently and has the typical MR appearance of hemorrhage based on the stage of the blood breakdown product (see earlier discussion of hemorrhage).

Venous sinus occlusion is usually well demonstrated by MR venography (MRV) (Fig. 48-14), making conventional angiography unnecessary in the majority of cases. MRV has been accepted as the procedure of choice in the diagnosis of sagittal sinus thrombosis.[301,302] Direct findings of cerebral thrombosis by MRV include lack of typical high flow signal from a sinus and direct visualization of thrombus on individual frames of the 2D slices. These must be distinguished from an aplastic or hypoplastic sinus and from the appearance of a sinus after recanalization. Thrombosed veins and/or sinuses may also be

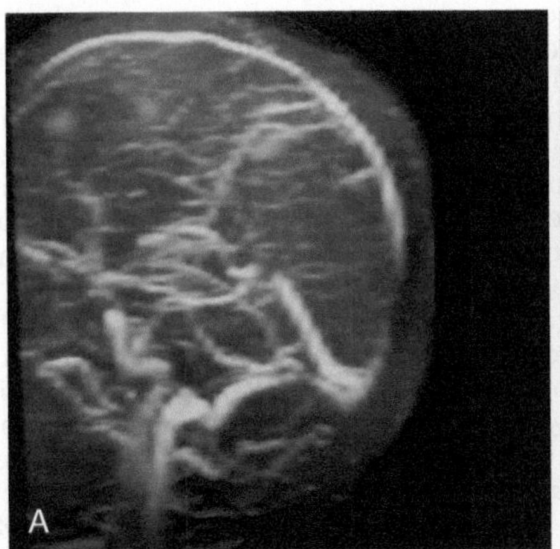

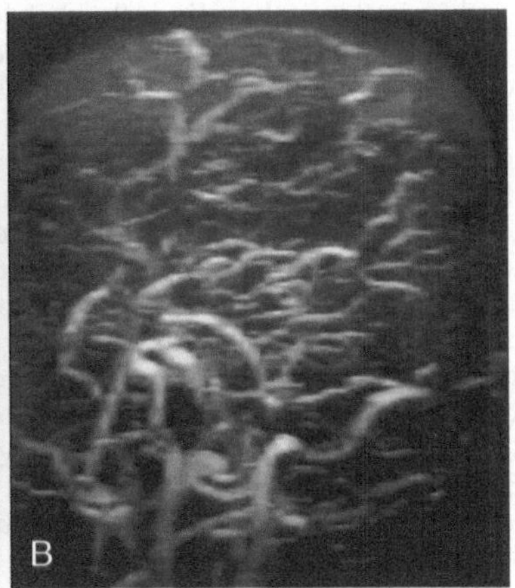

Figure 48-14. A, Normal MR venogram of the brain. B, Straight sinus thrombosis. Note the lack of flow signal in the straight sinus, lateral sinus, vein of Galen, and internal cerebral veins.

visualized on axial gradient echo T2*-weighted sequences with greater conspicuity than standard T1- and T2-weighted scans.[303,304] One group reported that the sensitivity of T2*WI and T1WI sequences to detect clot in the sinuses or veins was estimated at 90% and 71%, respectively, between days 1 and 3.[305] Cerebral veins have a smaller caliber that the cerebral sinuses and there is more variability in terms of their anatomic location. As a result, the cerebral veins are more difficult to visualize on MRV than the cerebral sinuses. However, 97% of thrombosed cortical veins have been detected on T2*SWI, even in the absence of visible occlusion on MRV.

Studies now suggest that the majority of cases of cerebral venous sinus thrombosis can be initially diagnosed by a combination of MRI studies, including T1WI, T2WI, DWI, GRE, FLAIR, MRA, and MRV, and that MRI provides a useful means for follow-up.[306,307] Several reports have begun to elucidate the diffusion–perfusion MR characteristics of venous sinus thrombosis. Abnormal DWI signal intensity may be associated with low ADC values indicative of cytotoxic edema, high ADC values indicative of vasogenic edema, or mixed values indicative of a combination of both vasogenic and cytotoxic edema.[301,308,309] Consequently, MR lesions caused by venous thrombosis are more frequently reversible than those due to arterial ischemia, because of the reversibility of vasogenic edema. Several groups have also demonstrated perfusion imaging abnormalities, including increased MTT[310] and increased CBV.[311]

MRI-Guided Acute Stroke Therapy

The role of MRI in acute stroke management is an area of intense research. The results from MRI-based clinical trials are helping to refine the mismatch concept, and penumbral imaging is a promising tool that has the potential to identify individuals who might benefit from reperfusion therapies at extended time windows.[312–318]

There has been extensive research focused on the optimal MRI criteria to identify the ischemic penumbra. DWI is generally felt to be the gold standard for the ischemic core, but animal studies and case series in humans have shown that a limited volume of the early diffusion abnormalities can be temporarily or permanently reversed with early reperfusion[319–321] (Figs 48-15–48-17). ADC values may predict which portion of the early DWI lesion is most likely to be permanently reversible, and one recent study identified an ADC of ≤620 × 10⁻⁶ mm²/seconds as the optimal threshold for identification of ischemic core (sensitivity 69% and specificity 78%).[322]

Studies that focus on identifying PWI criteria that mark the outer border of the ischemic penumbra (i.e., the border between tissue that is critically hypoperfused and tissue with benign oligemia) have typically optimized perfusion thresholds that predict final infarct size in patients without reperfusion. The underlying rationale for this approach is that, in the absence of reperfusion, the infarct grows to consume the entire penumbra to the benign oligemia border (see Fig. 48-16).[323–326] Because the baseline perfusion lesion identifies tissue that is likely to infarct if vessel recanalization does not occur, its volume correlates well with final infarct volume as well as neurologic and functional outcomes and, in fact, correlates better than the baseline diffusion lesion volume.[128,130,133,327] DEFUSE, Echoplanar Imaging Thrombolysis Evaluation Trial (EPITHET) and DEFUSE 2 used the perfusion parameter Tmax (time to maximum of tissue residue function) and found that a Tmax contrast arrival delay of >4–6 seconds predicts ischemic tissue destined to become infarcted in acute stroke patients who do not experience reperfusion.[328,329] A Tmax threshold of 5–6 seconds has also been shown to approximate penumbral cerebral blood flow values on positron emission tomography.[330]

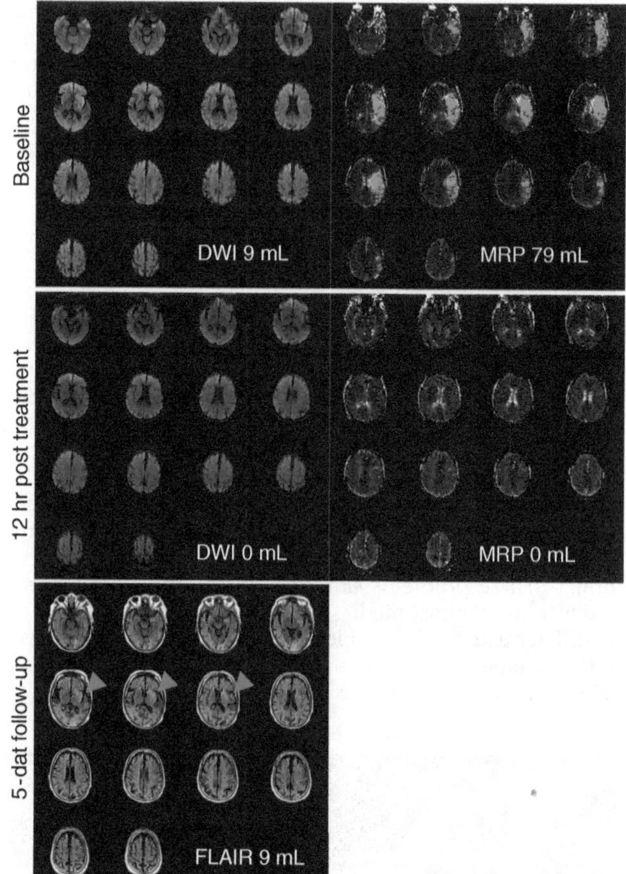

Figure 48-15. The baseline MRI scan (top row) in a patient with a left MCA stroke shows a large mismatch between the diffusion and the perfusion lesion. The diffusion lesion (pink) is segmented based on a ADC threshold <620 × 10^{-6} mm²/second. The perfusion lesion (green) is segmented based on a Tmax>6 second threshold. The patient underwent successful endovascular therapy resulting in complete recanalization of the middle cerebral artery. A follow-up MRI obtained 12 hours after endovascular therapy (middle row) demonstrates complete reperfusion and complete reversal of the initial DWI lesion. The 5-day follow-up MRI (bottom panel) demonstrates an infarct in the location of the baseline DWI lesion which illustrates the transient nature of DWI reversal following endovascular reperfusion.

Serial diffusion/perfusion MR studies have demonstrated that the natural history of diffusion MRI abnormalities is to grow over time, particularly in patients with a large perfusion–diffusion mismatch imaged early after symptom onset.[96,97,99,100,130,331–333] As the diffusion lesion grows, the extend of the mismatch decreases and, as a result, it is less common to see a substantial mismatch when the MRI is obtained later after symptom onset. Nevertheless, a substantial percentage of patients in whom the diffusion lesion grows slowly, still have regions of mismatch 24 hours after symptom onset.[332,334] An altered evolution of infarction can be visualized on serial diffusion and perfusion imaging studies. Inhibition of lesion growth has been demonstrated in patients experiencing reperfusion in comparison with patients with persistent perfusion deficits or vessel occlusions.[335–338] These studies suggest that it is feasible and potentially advantageous to use diffusion–perfusion MRI to select patients for thrombolytic therapy.

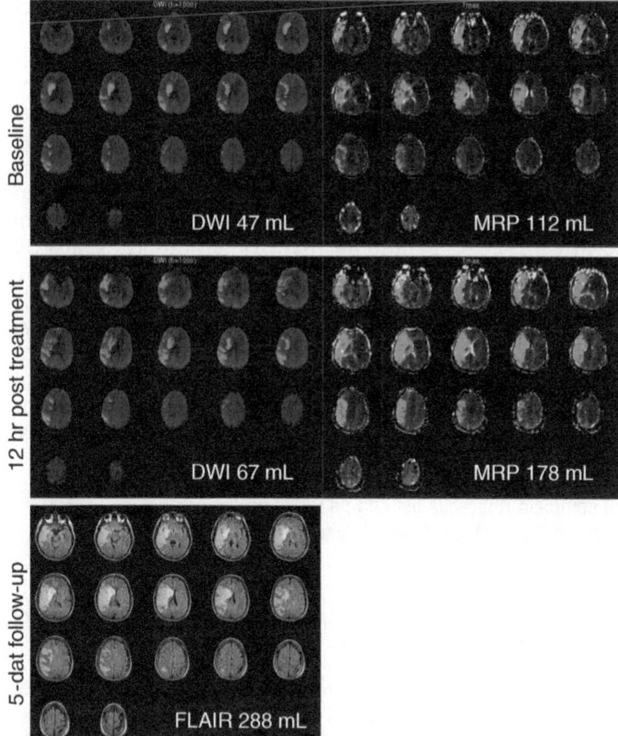

Figure 48-16 The baseline MRI (top row) of a 42-year-old man with a left MCA occlusion shows a moderate-size ischemic core (pink lesion measuring 47 ml on DWI) and a larger territory of critical hypoperfusion (green lesion measuring 112 ml on the MRP [Tmax>6 second] map). Based on these numbers the patient has a MRP–DWI mismatch ratio of 2.4. Endovascular therapy was unsuccessful as evidenced by a persistent perfusion deficit on early follow-up imaging. In the absence of reperfusion, the ischemic core has grown some between baseline (47 ml) and early follow-up (67 ml). At 5-day follow-up there has been further expansion of the infarct into the perfusion lesion.

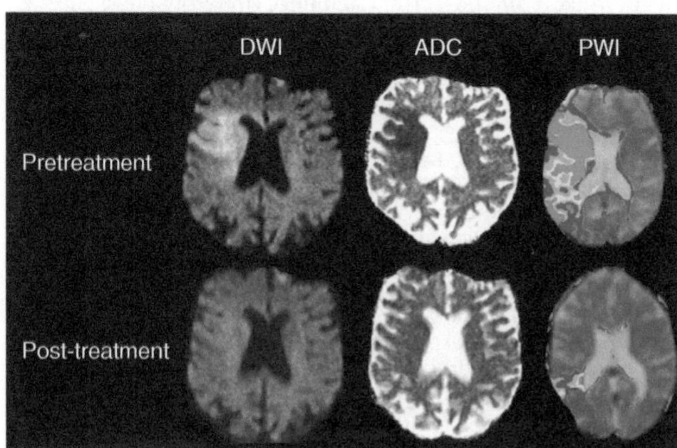

Figure 48-17 Examples of diffusion-weighted (DWI) and perfusion-weighted (PWI) imaging from a patient treated with intra-arterial thrombolytic therapy for a right middle cerebral artery occlusion. *Top row* shows pretreatment images, and *bottom row*, early post-treatment images. Perfusion images are in the form of color-coded maps of the time to peak of the residue function (Tmax) with *red* indicating greatest delay. The intra-arterial treatment resulted in complete recanalization which is evidenced by near-complete reversal of the baseline PWI lesion. There is accompanying complete reversal of the initial DWI and apparent diffusion coefficient (ADC) abnormalities.

The combination of DWI and perfusion imaging allows the identification of several different patterns that appear to have prognostic significance. In about 50% of patients studied within 24 hours of symptom onset, there is a "perfusion–diffusion mismatch" (Fig. 48-16). It has been proposed that patients with a mismatch are the patients who are most likely to respond favorably to reperfusion. In other patients, the DWI lesion is larger than the perfusion lesion (presumably a result of early reperfusion), and in about 10–15%, the DWI and perfusion lesions are of similar size (likely indicating that little or no salvageable tissue is present and operationally defined as a completed infarct). Some patients (about 10%) rapidly develop very large DWI lesions (>70–100 ml) and/or very large and severe perfusion lesions, presumably related to the combination of poor collaterals and a large-vessel occlusion. These patients have been termed "Malignant profile" and appear to have very poor outcomes regardless of early reperfusion.[339,340]

In addition to predicting response to reperfusion, there is a growing body of data suggesting that baseline MRI characteristics may be used to predict risk of hemorrhagic transformation.[222,341] Moreover, follow-up MRI imaging obtained after reperfusion therapy can provide insights into the evolving pathophysiology of human ischemia. The phenomenon of postischemic hyperperfusion has been demonstrated in approximately half of patients undergoing successful vessel recanalization with intra-arterial thrombolysis.[342] Late secondary ischemic injury has been demonstrated on DWI and ADC maps in humans and in animal models, following vessel recanalization.[222] These findings may become important targets for neuroprotective therapy in the future.

The use of MRI signatures to select patients for reperfusion therapy may extend the time window for treatment beyond current standards and improve safety by enabling treatment decisions to be based on individual patient pathophysiology rather than rigid time windows.

Clinical Trials of Intravenous Thrombolysis

Multimodal MRI for acute stroke can now be performed and interpreted rapidly and the additional diagnostic information obtained has the potential to improve both patient selection as well as cost-effectiveness of thrombolytic therapy.[343–348] Several large stroke centers rely on MRI to screen patients for thrombolytic or endovascular therapies and many have contributed to clinical trials evaluating various MR imaging techniques.[349] The Echoplanar Imaging Thrombolytic Evaluation Trial (EPITHET) as well as the Diffusion and Perfusion Imaging Evaluation for Understanding Stroke Evolution (DEFUSE), Desmoteplase in Acute Ischemic Stroke (DIAS), and Dose Escalation of Desmoteplase for Acute Ischemic Stroke (DEDAS) studies showed that in patients with a DWI–MR perfusion mismatch, reperfusion following intravenous thrombolytic therapy was strongly associated with favorable clinical outcomes even in extended time windows.[312–315,350] The DEFUSE study involved stroke patients treated with intravenous alteplase 3 to 6 hours after onset of symptoms. These patients were not selected on the basis of the DWI–MR perfusion mismatch; however, early reperfusion in patients with a mismatch (an MR perfusion lesion of at least 10 mL and ≥20% larger than the DWI lesion) was associated with a favorable clinical outcome, and the benefit of reperfusion appeared to be enhanced in patients with the Target mismatch profile (neither DWI nor MR perfusion with severe delay [Tmax > 8 seconds] exceeded 100 mL). In patients without a mismatch, there was no association between reperfusion and favorable clinical outcomes.[312] In the EPITHET, treatment with intravenous alteplase vs placebo led to attenuation of some measures of infarct volume growth in patients with a mismatch, and similar to DEFUSE, there was a strong association between reperfusion and favorable clinical outcomes in patients with the Target mismatch profile.[313] The trials of desmoteplase (DIAS and DEDAS) enrolled patients in whom a DWI–MR perfusion mismatch was detected 3–9 hours from onset of symptoms. The DIAS and DEDAS studies showed a positive dose–response relationship for desmoteplase on early reperfusion and beneficial clinical effects were seen in patients treated with desmoteplase.[314,315] DIAS-2, a phase 3 study, did not confirm the clinical benefit of desmoteplase;[316] although, in a subgroup analysis, patients with a large mismatch (>60 mL) had more favorable outcomes in the desmoteplase vs placebo group.[351] Results of these late thrombolysis trials are encouraging, but larger clinical trials, such as the ongoing EXTEND study, are required to establish the role of the diffusion–perfusion mismatch in selecting patients for intravenous thrombolysis.[352]

Endovascular Therapy

The role of multimodal MR imaging in selecting patients for endovascular therapy was evaluated in the recently reported MR RESCUE and DEFUSE 2 studies. MR RESCUE was a randomized multi-center study in which patients with a large-vessel anterior circulation stroke were randomized to embolectomy vs standard care within 8 hours of symptom onset.[353] To be eligible for enrollment, multimodal MRI or CT perfusion was required and randomization was stratified based on imaging finding of a "favorable penumbral pattern", defined as infarct core <90 mL and substantial salvageable tissue vs a non-penumbral pattern, defined as large core or small/absent penumbra. MRI was the primary imaging modality employed; however, CT perfusion was also allowed towards the end of the study and was used in about 20% of the patients. To assess salvageable tissue, an automated software program was employed and the penumbral pattern defined based on a voxel-by-voxel algorithm which included measures of the apparent diffusion coefficient, cerebral blood flow, mean transit time, and Tmax for the MRI model.[354] One-hundred and eighteen patients eligible were recruited from 22 North American Stroke Centers between 2004 and 2011. Functional outcomes at 3 months were not different in the embolectomy vs standard care groups, irrespective of penumbral vs non-penumbral pattern. Potential explanations for the failure of this trial to demonstrate benefits of embolectomy include the fact that the median predicted infarct core volume at the time of baseline imaging was large, 60 mL (34.1–107), there was a delay of 2 hours between start of imaging and femoral puncture, and the rate of good reperfusion (TICI 2b/3) achieved in the endovascular group (27%) was low.

DEFUSE 2 was a prospective cohort study in which patients received an MRI scan prior to endovascular therapy.[355] One-hundred and thirty-eight patients were enrolled at nine stroke centers over 3 years. The definition of the Target mismatch pattern was an MR perfusion lesion (Tmax > 6 seconds) that was at least 1.8 times larger than the DWI lesion (defined by an ADC value <600) and the absence of a "Malignant profile" defined as either DWI >70 mL or an MR perfusion lesion with severe delay (Tmax >10 seconds) exceeding 100 mL. The rate of TICI 2b/3 reperfusion obtained in DEFUSE 2 was 46%. DEFUSE 2 demonstrated that patients with a "Target Mismatch" pattern who experienced early reperfusion after endovascular therapy had significantly more favorable clinical outcomes. There was no association between reperfusion and favorable outcomes in the "No Target Mismatch" group. Comparing outcomes in MR RESCUE and DEFUSE 2, it is apparent that the Target mismatch group who underwent endovascular therapy in DEFUSE 2 had more favorable clinical outcomes than the endovascular-treated penumbral group in MR RESCUE (Rankin 0–2 outcomes at 90 days occurred in 46% in DEFUSE 2 vs 21% in MR RESCUE). Among DEFUSE patients who achieved complete reperfusion, Rankin 0–2 outcomes at 90 days were achieved in 75%.[356] The disparities in outcomes between DEFUSE 2 and MR RESCUE may be explained by differences in baseline imaging characteristics as well as reperfusion rates obtained. The estimated infarct core volumes in the MR RESCUE "penumbral pattern" groups (medians 36 and 37 mL) were substantially larger than the "Target Mismatch" group of DEFUSE 2 (13 mL). Of note, the EPITHET trial documented a substantial reduction in favorable clinical outcomes at core volumes >25 mL.[357]

A number of ongoing trials are using a variety of different imaging selection techniques to clarify which imaging patterns will identify patients who are likely to benefit from endovascular therapy.

The complete reference list can be found on the companion Expert Consult website at www.expertconsult.inkling.com.

KEY REFERENCES

1. Bydder GM, Steiner RE, Young IR, et al. Clinical NMR imaging of the brain: 140 cases. AJR Am J Roentgenol 1982;139:215–36.
6. Bryan RN, Levy LM, Whitlow WD, et al. Diagnosis of acute cerebral infarction: Comparison of CT and MR imaging. AJNR Am J Neuroradiol 1991;12:611–20.
9. Le Bihan D, Breton E, Lallemand D, et al. MR imaging of intravoxel incoherent motions: Application to diffusion and perfusion in neurologic disorders. Radiology 1986;161:401–7.
10. Moseley ME, Cohen Y, Mintorovitch J. Early detection of regional cerebral ischemia in cats: Comparison of diffusion- and T2-weighted MRI and spectroscopy. Magn Reson Med 1990;14: 330–46.
12. Rosen BR, Belliveau JW, Buchbinder BR, et al. Contrast agents and cerebral hemodynamics. Magn Reson Med 1991;19:285–92.
14. Warach S, Li W, Ronthal M, et al. Acute cerebral ischemia: Evaluation with dynamic contrast-enhanced MR imaging and MR angiography. Radiology 1992;182:41–7.
16. Edelman R, Hesselink J, Zlatkin M, et al., editors. Clinical magnetic resonance imaging. 3rd ed. Philadelphia, PA: Elsevier; 2006.
17. Davis S, Fisher M, Warach S, editors. Magnetic resonance imaging in stroke. Cambridge, UK: Cambridge University Press; 2003.
18. Duyn JH. Study of brain anatomy with high-field MRI: Recent progress. Magn Reson Imaging 2010;28(8):1210–15.
21. Latour LL, Kang DW, Ezzeddine MA, et al. Early blood-brain barrier disruption in human focal brain ischemia. Ann Neurol 2004;56:468–77.
23. Kamran S, Bates V, Bakshi R, et al. Significance of hyperintense vessels on FLAIR MRI in acute stroke. Neurology 2000;55:265–9.
26. Moseley ME, Kucharczyk J, Mintorovitch J. Diffusion-weighted MR imaging of acute stroke: Correlation with T2-weighted and magnetic susceptibility-enhanced MR imaging in cats. AJNR Am J Neuroradiol 1990;11:423–9.
27. Warach S, Gaa J, Siewert B, et al. Acute human stroke studied by whole brain echo planar diffusion-weighted magnetic resonance imaging. Ann Neurol 1995;37:231–41.
29. Pierpaoli C, Jezzard P, Basser PJ, et al. Diffusion tensor MR imaging of the human brain. Radiology 1996;201:637–48.
30. Liang Z, Zeng J, Zhang C, et al. Progression of pathological changes in the middle cerebellar peduncle by diffusion tensor imaging correlates with lesser motor gains after pontine infarction. Neurorehabil Neural Repair 2009;23:692–8.
32. Lansberg MG, Thijs VN, O'Brien MW. Evolution of apparent diffusion coefficient, diffusion-weighted, and T2-weighted signal intensity of acute stroke. AJNR Am J Neuroradiol 2001;22: 637–44.
35. Smith AM, Grandin CB, Duprez T, et al. Whole brain quantitative CBF, CBV, and MTT measurements using MRI bolus tracking: Implementation and application to data acquired from hyperacute stroke patients. J Magn Reson Imaging 2000;12:400–10.

37. Ostergaard L, Sorensen AG, Kwong KK, et al. High resolution measurement of cerebral blood flow using intravascular tracer bolus passages. Part II: Experimental comparison and preliminary results. Magn Reson Med 1996;36:726–36.
38. Ostergaard L, Johannsen P, Host-Poulsen P, et al. Cerebral blood flow measurements by magnetic resonance imaging bolus tracking: Comparison with [(15)O]H2O positron emission tomography in humans. J Cereb Blood Flow Metab 1998;18: 935–40.
40. Christensen S, Mouridsen K, Wu O, et al. Comparison of 10 perfusion MRI parameters in 97 sub-6-hour stroke patients using voxel-based receiver operating characteristics analysis. Stroke 2009;40:2055–61.
41. Roberts DA, Detre JA, Bolinger L, et al. Quantitative magnetic resonance imaging of human brain perfusion at 1.5 T using steady-state inversion of arterial water. Proc Natl Acad Sci U S A 1994;91:33–7.
48. Siewert B, Schlaug G, Edelman RR, et al. Comparison of EPISTAR and T2*-weighted gadolinium-enhanced perfusion imaging in patients with acute cerebral ischemia. Neurology 1997;48: 673–9.
51. Alsop DC, Detre JA. Multisection cerebral blood flow MR imaging with continuous arterial spin labeling. Radiology 1998;208:410–16.
52. Debrey SM, Yu H, Lynch JK, et al. Diagnostic accuracy of magnetic resonance angiography for internal carotid artery disease: A systematic review and meta-analysis. Stroke 2008;39: 2237–48.
56. Wardlaw JM, White PM. The detection and management of unruptured intracranial aneurysms. Brain 2000;123:205–21.
59. Mittal S, Wu Z, Neelavalli J, et al. Susceptibility-weighted imaging: Technical aspects and clinical applications, part 2. AJNR Am J Neuroradiol 2009;30:232–52.
60. Haacke EM, Mittal S, Wu Z, et al. Susceptibility-weighted imaging: Technical aspects and clinical applications, part 1. AJNR Am J Neuroradiol 2009;30:19–30.
62. Leiner T, Kucharczyk W. NSF prevention in clinical practice: Summary of recommendations and guidelines in the United States, Canada, and Europe. J Magn Reson Imaging 2009;30: 1357–63.
63. Thomsen HS. How to avoid nephrogenic systemic fibrosis: Current guidelines in Europe and the United States. Radiol Clin North Am 2009;47:871–5, vii.
73. Mlynash M, Olivot JM, Tong DC, et al. Yield of combined perfusion and diffusion MR imaging in hemispheric TIA. Neurology 2009;72:1127–33.
74. Calvet D, Touze E, Oppenheim C, et al. DWI lesions and TIA etiology improve the prediction of stroke after TIA. Stroke 2009;40:187–92.
76. Easton JD, Saver JL, Albers GW, et al. Definition and evaluation of transient ischemic attack. A scientific statement for healthcare professionals from the American Heart Association/American Stroke Association Stroke Council; Council on Cardiovascular Surgery and Anesthesia; Council on Cardiovascular Radiology and Intervention; Council on Cardiovascular Nursing; and the Interdisciplinary Council on Peripheral Vascular Disease. Stroke 2009;40:2276–93.
79. Shah SH, Saver JL, Kidwell CS, et al. A multicenter pooled, patient-level data analysis of diffusion-weighted MRI in TIA patients. Stroke 2007;38.
81. Sylaja PN, Coutts SB, Krol A, et al. When to expect negative diffusion-weighted images in stroke and transient ischemic attack. Stroke 2008;39:1898–900.
82. Prabhakaran S, Chong JY, Sacco RL. Impact of abnormal diffusion-weighted imaging results on short-term outcome following transient ischemic attack. Arch Neurol 2007;64:1105–9.
84. Krol AL, Coutts SB, Simon JE, et al. Perfusion MRI abnormalities in speech or motor transient ischemic attack patients. Stroke 2005;36:2487–9.
85. Albers GW, Caplan LR, Easton JD, et al; for the TIA Working Group. Transient ischemic attack: proposal for a new definition. N Engl J Med 2002;347:1713–16.
89. Lee KY, Latour LL, Luby M, et al. Distal hyperintense vessels on FLAIR: An MRI marker for collateral circulation in acute stroke? Neurology 2009;72:1134–9.
91. Warach S, Latour LL. Evidence of reperfusion injury, exacerbated by thrombolytic therapy, in human focal brain ischemia using a novel imaging marker of early blood-brain barrier disruption. Stroke 2004;35(Suppl. 1):2659–61.
93. Crain MR, Yuh WT, Greene GM, et al. Cerebral ischemia: Evaluation with contrast-enhanced MR imaging. AJNR Am J Neuroradiol 1991;12:631–9.
95. Baird AE, Warach S. Magnetic resonance imaging of acute stroke. J Cereb Blood Flow Metab 1998;18:583–609.
96. Warach S, Pettigrew LC, Dashe JF, et al. Effect of citicoline on ischemic lesions as measured by diffusion-weighted magnetic resonance imaging. Citicoline 010 Investigators. Ann Neurol 2000;48:713–22.
97. Baird AE, Benfield A, Schlaug G, et al. Enlargement of human cerebral ischemic lesion volumes measured by diffusion-weighted magnetic resonance imaging. Ann Neurol 1997;41:581–9.
98. Lansberg MG, O'Brien MW, Tong DC, et al. Evolution of cerebral infarct volume assessed by diffusion-weighted magnetic resonance imaging. Arch Neurol 2001;58:613–17.
101. Schlaug G, Siewert B, Benfield A, et al. Time course of the apparent diffusion coefficient (ADC) abnormality in human stroke. Neurology 1997;49:113–19.
107. Gonzalez RG, Schaefer PW, Buonanno FS, et al. Diffusion-weighted MR imaging: Diagnostic accuracy in patients imaged within 6 hours of stroke symptom onset. Radiology 1999;210: 155–62.
110. Lansberg MG, Norbash AM, Marks MP, et al. Advantages of adding diffusion-weighted magnetic resonance imaging to conventional magnetic resonance imaging for evaluating acute stroke. Arch Neurol 2000;57:1311–16.
113. Chalela JA, Kidwell CS, Nentwich LM, et al. Magnetic resonance imaging and computed tomography in emergency assessment of patients with suspected acute stroke: A prospective comparison. Lancet 2007;369:293–8.
115. Schellinger PD, Bryan RN, Caplan LR, et al. Evidence-based guideline: The role of diffusion and perfusion MRI for the diagnosis of acute ischemic stroke: Report of the Therapeutics and Technology Assessment Subcommittee of the American Academy of Neurology. Neurology 2010;75:177–85.
116. Lutsep HL, Albers GW, DeCrespigny A, et al. Clinical utility of diffusion-weighted magnetic resonance imaging in the assessment of ischemic stroke. Ann Neurol 1997;41:574–80.
120. Baird AE, Lovblad KO, Schlaug G, et al. Multiple acute stroke syndrome: Marker of embolic disease? Neurology 2000;54: 674–8.
121. Kang DW, Chalela JA, Ezzeddine MA, et al. Association of ischemic lesion patterns on early diffusion-weighted imaging with TOAST stroke subtypes. Arch Neurol 2003;60:1730–4.
126. Thomalla G, Rossbach P, Rosenkranz M, et al. Negative fluid-attenuated inversion recovery imaging identifies acute ischemic stroke at 3 hours or less. Ann Neurol 2009;65:724–32.
128. Lovblad KO, Baird AE, Schlaug G, et al. Ischemic lesion volumes in acute stroke by diffusion-weighted magnetic resonance imaging correlate with clinical outcome. Ann Neurol 1997;42: 164–70.
132. Thijs VN, Lansberg MG, Beaulieu C, et al. Is early ischemic lesion volume on diffusion-weighted imaging an independent predictor of stroke outcome? A multivariable analysis. Stroke 2000;31: 2597–602.
135. Baird AE, Dambrosia J, Janket S, et al. A three-item scale for the early prediction of stroke recovery. Lancet 2001;357:2095–9.
136. Sylaja PN, Coutts SB, Subramaniam S, et al. Acute ischemic lesions of varying ages predict risk of ischemic events in stroke/TIA patients. Neurology 2007;68:415–19.
137. Kang DW, Latour LL, Chalela JA, et al. Early ischemic lesion recurrence within a week after acute ischemic stroke. Ann Neurol 2003;54:66–74.
139. Ostergaard L, Sorensen AG, Kwong KK, et al. High resolution measurement of cerebral blood flow using intravascular tracer bolus passages. Part II: Experimental comparison and preliminary results. Magn Reson Med 1996;36:726–36.
140. Ostergaard L, Weisskoff RM, Chesler DA, et al. High resolution measurement of cerebral blood flow using intravascular tracer bolus passages. Part I: Mathematical approach and statistical analysis. Magn Reson Med 1996;36:715–25.

141. Haga KK, Khor YP, Farrall A, et al. A systematic review of brain metabolite changes, measured with 1H magnetic resonance spectroscopy, in healthy aging. Neurobiol Aging 2009;30:353–63.
147. Gideon P, Henriksen O, Sperling B, et al. Early time course of *N*-acetylaspartate, creatine and phosphocreatine, and compounds containing choline in the brain after acute stroke. A proton magnetic resonance spectroscopy study. Stroke 1992;23:1566–72.
150. Munoz Maniega S, Cvoro V, Chappell FM, et al. Changes in NAA and Lactate following ischemic stroke. A serial MR spectroscopic imaging study. Neurology 2008;71:7.
155. Allen K, Busza AL, Crockard HA, et al. Acute cerebral ischaemia: Concurrent changes in cerebral blood flow, energy metabolites, pH, and lactate measured with hydrogen clearance and 31P and 1H nuclear magnetic resonance spectroscopy. III. Changes following ischaemia. J Cereb Blood Flow Meta 1988;8:816–21.
156. Nicoli F, Lefur Y, Denis B, et al. Metabolic counterpart of decreased apparent diffusion coefficient during hyperacute ischemic stroke: A brain proton magnetic resonance spectroscopic imaging study. Stroke 2003;34:e82–7.
158. Karaszewski B, Wardlaw JM, Marshall I, et al. Measurement of brain temperature with magnetic resonance spectroscopy in acute ischemic stroke. Ann Neurol 2006;60:438–46.
161. van der Grond J, Balm R, Klijn CJ, et al. Cerebral metabolism of patients with stenosis of the internal carotid artery before and after endarterectomy. J Cereb Blood Flow Metab 1996;16:320–6.
166. Kidwell CS, Wintermark M. Imaging of intracranial haemorrhage. Lancet Neurol 2008;7:256–67.
170. Kidwell CS, Chalela JA, Saver JL, et al. Comparison of MRI and CT for detection of acute intracerebral hemorrhage. JAMA 2004;292:1823–30.
174. Lang EW, Ren Ya Z, Preul C, et al. Stroke pattern interpretation: The variability of hypertensive versus amyloid angiopathy hemorrhage. Cerebrovasc Dis 2001;12:121–30.
175. Broderick J, Connolly S, Feldmann E, et al. Guidelines for the management of spontaneous intracerebral hemorrhage in adults: 2007 update: A guideline from the American Heart Association/American Stroke Association Stroke Council, High Blood Pressure Research Council, and the Quality of Care and Outcomes in Research Interdisciplinary Working Group. Stroke 2007;38:2001–23.
176. Kidwell CS, Saver JL, Mattiello J, et al. Diffusion-perfusion MR evaluation of perihematomal injury in hyperacute intracerebral hemorrhage. Neurology 2001;57:1611–17.
177. Butcher KS, Baird T, MacGregor L, et al. Perihematomal edema in primary intracerebral hemorrhage is plasma derived. Stroke 2004;35:1879–85.
180. Herweh C, Juttler E, Schellinger PD, et al. Evidence against a perihemorrhagic penumbra provided by perfusion computed tomography. Stroke 2007;38:2941–7.
183. Prabhakaran S, Naidech AM. Ischemic brain injury after intracerebral hemorrhage: a critical review. Stroke 2012;43:2258–63.
185. Gregoire SM, Charidimou A, Gadapa N, et al. Acute ischaemic brain lesions in intracerebral haemorrhage: multicentre cross-sectional magnetic resonance imaging study. Brain 2011;134(Pt 8):2376–86.
188. Menon RS, Burgess RE, Wing JJ, et al. Predictors of highly prevalent brain ischemia in intracerebral hemorrhage. Ann Neurol 2012;71:199–205.
191. Fazekas F, Kleinert R, Roob G, et al. Histopathologic analysis of foci of signal loss on gradient-echo T2*-weighted MR images in patients with spontaneous intracerebral hemorrhage: Evidence of microangiopathy-related microbleeds. AJNR Am J Neuroradiol 1999;20:637–42.
193. Goos JD, van der Flier WM, Knol DL, et al. Clinical relevance of improved microbleed detection by susceptibility-weighted magnetic resonance imaging. Stroke 2011;42(7):1894–900.
199. Greenberg SM, Vernooij MW, Cordonnier C, et al. Cerebral microbleeds: a guide to detection and interpretation. Lancet Neurol 2009;8(2):165–74.
204. Poels MM, Ikram MA, van der Lugt A, et al. Incidence of cerebral microbleeds in the general population: the Rotterdam Scan Study. Stroke 2011;42(3):656–61.
219. van Es AC, van der Grond J, de Craen AJ, et al. Risk factors for cerebral microbleeds in the elderly. Cerebrovasc Dis 2008;26(4):397–403.
222. Kidwell CS, Saver JL, Villablanca JP, et al. Magnetic resonance imaging detection of microbleeds before thrombolysis: An emerging application. Stroke 2002;33:95–8.
226. Lee SH, Lee ST, Kim BJ, et al. Dynamic temporal change of cerebral microbleeds: long-term follow-up MRI study. PLoS ONE 2011;6(10):e25930.
228. Fiehler J, Albers GW, Boulanger JM, et al. Bleeding risk analysis in stroke imaging before thromboLysis (BRASIL): Pooled analysis of T2*-weighted magnetic resonance imaging data from 570 patients. Stroke 2007;38:2738–44.
229. Shoamanesh A, Kwok CS, Lim PA, et al. Postthrombolysis intracranial hemorrhage risk of cerebral microbleeds in acute stroke patients: a systematic review and meta-analysis. Int J Stroke 2013;8(5):348–56.
231. Park JH, Seo SW, Kim C, et al. Pathogenesis of cerebral microbleeds: In vivo imaging of amyloid and subcortical ischemic small vessel disease in 226 individuals with cognitive impairment. Ann Neurol 2013;73(5):584–93.
234. Maxwell SS, Jackson CA, Paternoster L, et al. Genetic associations with brain microbleeds: Systematic review and meta-analyses. Neurology 2011;77(2):158–67.
235. Gregoire SM, Brown MM, Kallis C, et al. MRI detection of new microbleeds in patients with ischemic stroke: five-year cohort follow-up study. Stroke 2010;41(1):184–6.
238. Kwa VI, Algra A, Brundel M, et al. Microbleeds as a predictor of intracerebral haemorrhage and ischaemic stroke after a TIA or minor ischaemic stroke: a cohort study. BMJ Open 2013;3(5).
239. Thijs V, Lemmens R, Schoofs C, et al. Microbleeds and the risk of recurrent stroke. Stroke 2010;41(9):2005–9.
250. Bang OY, Buck BH, Saver JL, et al. Prediction of hemorrhagic transformation after recanalization therapy using T2*-permeability magnetic resonance imaging. Ann Neurol 2007;62:170–6.
254. Lansberg MG, Thijs VN, Bammer R, et al. Risk factors of symptomatic intracerebral hemorrhage after tPA therapy for acute stroke. Stroke 2007;38:2275–8.
255. Singer OC, Humpich MC, Fiehler J, et al. Risk for symptomatic intracerebral hemorrhage after thrombolysis assessed by diffusion-weighted magnetic resonance imaging. Ann Neurol 2007.
257. Campbell BC, Christensen S, Parsons MW, et al. Advanced imaging improves prediction of hemorrhage after stroke thrombolysis. Ann Neurol 2013;73:510–19.
259. Kufner A, Galinovic I, Brunecker P, et al. Early infarct FLAIR hyperintensity is associated with increased hemorrhagic transformation after thrombolysis. Eur J Neurol 2013;20(2):281–5.
260. Campbell BC, Costello C, Christensen S, et al. Fluid-attenuated inversion recovery hyperintensity in acute ischemic stroke may not predict hemorrhagic transformation. Cerebrovasc Dis 2011;32(4):401–5.
262. Singer MB, Atlas SW, Drayer BP. Subarachnoid space disease: Diagnosis with fluid-attenuated inversion-recovery MR imaging and comparison with gadolinium-enhanced spin-echo MR imaging—blinded reader study. Radiology 1998;208:417–22.
263. Mitchell P, Wilkinson ID, Hoggard N, et al. Detection of subarachnoid haemorrhage with magnetic resonance imaging. J Neurol Neurosurg Psychiatry 2001;70:205–11.
270. Rordorf G, Koroshetz WJ, Copen WA, et al. Diffusion- and perfusion-weighted imaging in vasospasm after subarachnoid hemorrhage. Stroke 1999;30:599–605.
275. Charidimou A, Peeters A, Fox Z, et al. Spectrum of transient focal neurological episodes in cerebral amyloid angiopathy: multicentre magnetic resonance imaging cohort study and meta-analysis. Stroke 2012;43(9):2324–30.
278. Charidimou A, Peeters AP, Jager R, et al. Cortical superficial siderosis and intracerebral hemorrhage risk in cerebral amyloid angiopathy. Neurology 2013;81(19):1666–73.
280. Kang CK, Park CW, Han JY, et al. Imaging and analysis of lenticulostriate arteries using 7.0-Tesla magnetic resonance angiography. Magn Reson Med 2009;61:136–44.
282. Long A, Lepoutre A, Corbillon E, et al. Critical review of non- or minimally invasive methods (duplex ultrasonography, MR- and

CT-angiography) for evaluating stenosis of the proximal internal carotid artery. Eur J Vasc Endovasc Surg 2002;24:43–52.
286. Randoux B, Marro B, Koskas F, et al. Carotid artery stenosis: Prospective comparison of CT, three-dimensional gadolinium-enhanced MR, and conventional angiography. Radiology 2001;220:179–85.
287. Yuan C, Zhang SX, Polissar NL, et al. Identification of fibrous cap rupture with magnetic resonance imaging is highly associated with recent transient ischemic attack or stroke. Circulation 2002;105:181–5.
288. Zhao XQ, Yuan C, Hatsukami TS, et al. Effects of prolonged intensive lipid-lowering therapy on the characteristics of carotid atherosclerotic plaques in vivo by MRI: A case-control study. Arterioscler Thromb Vasc Biol 2001;21:1623–9.
289. Degnan AJ, Gallagher G, Teng Z, et al. MR angiography and imaging for the evaluation of middle cerebral artery atherosclerotic disease. AJNR Am J Neuroradiol 2012;33:1427–35.
290. Sue DE, Brant-Zawadzki MN, Chance J. Dissection of cranial arteries in the neck: Correlation of MRI and arteriography. Neuroradiology 1992;34:273–8.
294. Provenzale JM, Sarikaya B. Comparison of test performance characteristics of MRI, MR angiography, and CT angiography in the diagnosis of carotid and vertebral artery dissection: a review of the medical literature. AJR Am J Roentgenol 2009;193: 1167–74.
295. Sailer AM, Wagemans BA, Nelemans PJ, et al. Diagnosing Intracranial Aneurysms With MR Angiography: Systematic Review and Meta-Analysis. Stroke 2014;45:119–26.
298. Ronkainen A, Puranen MI, Hernesniemi JA, et al. Intracranial aneurysms: MR angiographic screening in 400 asymptomatic individuals with increased familial risk. Radiology 1995;195: 35–40.
300. Qu H, Yang M. Early imaging characteristics of 62 cases of cerebral venous sinus thrombosis. Exp Ther Med 2013;5:233–6.
302. Yuh WT, Simonson TM, Wang AM, et al. Venous sinus occlusive disease: MR findings. AJNR Am J Neuroradiol 1994;15: 309–16.
307. Bousser MG, Ferro JM. Cerebral venous thrombosis: An update. Lancet Neurol 2007;6:162–70.
309. Ducreux D, Oppenheim C, Vandamme X, et al. Diffusion-weighted imaging patterns of brain damage associated with cerebral venous thrombosis. AJNR Am J Neuroradiol 2001;22: 261–8.
312. Albers GW, Thijs VN, Wechsler L, et al. Magnetic resonance imaging profiles predict clinical response to early reperfusion: The diffusion and perfusion imaging evaluation for understanding stroke evolution (DEFUSE) study. Ann Neurol 2006;60: 508–17.
313. Davis SM, Donnan GA, Parsons MW, et al. Effects of alteplase beyond 3 h after stroke in the Echoplanar Imaging Thrombolytic Evaluation Trial (EPITHET): A placebo-controlled randomised trial. Lancet Neurol 2008;7:299–309.
314. Hacke W, Albers G, Al-Rawi Y, et al. The Desmoteplase in Acute Ischemic Stroke Trial (DIAS): A phase II MRI-based 9-hour window acute stroke thrombolysis trial with intravenous desmoteplase. Stroke 2005;36:66–73.
315. Furlan AJ, Eyding D, Albers GW, et al. Dose Escalation of Desmoteplase for Acute Ischemic Stroke (DEDAS): Evidence of safety and efficacy 3 to 9 hours after stroke onset. Stroke 2006; 37:1227–31.
316. Hacke W, Furlan AJ, Al-Rawi Y, et al. Intravenous desmoteplase in patients with acute ischaemic stroke selected by MRI perfusion-diffusion weighted imaging or perfusion CT (DIAS-2): A prospective, randomised, double-blind, placebo-controlled study. Lancet Neurol 2009;8:141–50.
317. Donnan GA, Baron JC, Ma H, et al. Penumbral selection of patients for trials of acute stroke therapy. Lancet Neurol 2009;8:261–9.
319. Kidwell CS, Saver JL, Mattiello J, et al. Thrombolytic reversal of acute human cerebral ischemic injury shown by diffusion/perfusion magnetic resonance imaging. Ann Neurol 2000;47: 462–9.
322. Purushotham A, Campbell BC, Straka M, et al. Apparent diffusion coefficient threshold for delineation of ischemic core. Int J Stroke 2013.
324. Thijs VN, Adami A, Neumann-Haefelin T, et al. Relationship between severity of MR perfusion deficit and DWI lesion evolution. Neurology 2001;57:1205–11.
325. Rose SE, Chalk JB, Griffin MP, et al. MRI based diffusion and perfusion predictive model to estimate stroke evolution. Magn Reson Imaging 2001;19:1043–53.
329. Wheeler HM, Mlynash M, Inoue M, et al. Early diffusion-weighted imaging and perfusion-weighted imaging lesion volumes forecast final infarct size in defuse 2. Stroke 2013;44: 681–5.
330. Zaro-Weber O, Moeller-Hartmann W, Heiss WD, et al. Maps of time to maximum and time to peak for mismatch definition in clinical stroke studies validated with positron emission tomography. Stroke 2010;41:2817–21.
331. Sorensen AG, Copen WA, Ostergaard L, et al. Hyperacute stroke: Simultaneous measurement of relative cerebral blood volume, relative cerebral blood flow, and mean tissue transit time. Radiology 1999;210:519–27.
334. Darby DG, Barber PA, Gerraty RP, et al. Pathophysiological topography of acute ischemia by combined diffusion-weighted and perfusion MRI. Stroke 1999;30:2043–52.
335. Jansen O, Schellinger P, Fiebach J, et al. Early recanalisation in acute ischaemic stroke saves tissue at risk defined by MRI. Lancet 1999;353:2036–7.
339. Mlynash M, Lansberg MG, De Silva DA, et al. Refining the definition of the malignant profile: Insights from the defuse-epithet pooled data set. Stroke 2011;42:1270–5.
342. Kidwell CS, Saver JL, Mattiello J, et al. Diffusion-perfusion MRI characterization of post-recanalization hyperperfusion in humans. Neurology 2001;57:2015–21.
345. Kohrmann M, Juttler E, Fiebach JB, et al. MRI versus CT-based thrombolysis treatment within and beyond the 3 h time window after stroke onset: A cohort study. Lancet Neurol 2006;5:661–7.
349. Hjort N, Butcher K, Davis SM, et al. Magnetic resonance imaging criteria for thrombolysis in acute cerebral infarct. Stroke 2005;36: 388–97.
350. Lansberg MG, Lee J, Christensen S, et al. Rapid automated patient selection for reperfusion therapy: A pooled analysis of the echoplanar imaging thrombolytic evaluation trial (epithet) and the diffusion and perfusion imaging evaluation for understanding stroke evolution (defuse) study. Stroke 2011;42: 1608–14.
351. Warach S, Al-Rawi Y, Furlan AJ, et al. Refinement of the magnetic resonance diffusion-perfusion mismatch concept for thrombolytic patient selection: Insights from the desmoteplase in acute stroke trials. Stroke 2012;43:2313–18.
352. Ma H, Parsons MW, Christensen S, et al. EXTEND investigators. A multicentre, randomized, double-blinded, placebo-controlled Phase III study to investigate EXtending the time for Thrombolysis in Emergency Neurological Deficits (EXTEND). Int J Stroke 2012;7(1):74–80.
353. Kidwell CS, Jahan R, Gornbein J, et al. A trial of imaging selection and endovascular treatment for ischemic stroke. N Engl J Med 2013;368:914–23.
354. Kidwell CS, Wintermark M, De Silva DA, et al. Multiparametric MRI and CT models of infarct core and favorable penumbral imaging patterns in acute ischemic stroke. Stroke 2013;44: 73–9.
355. Lansberg MG, Straka M, Kemp S, et al. MRI profile and response to endovascular reperfusion after stroke (defuse 2): A prospective cohort study. Lancet Neurol 2012;11:860–7.
356. Inoue M, Mlynash M, Straka M, et al. DEFUSE 1 and 2 Investigators. Clinical outcomes strongly associated with the degree of reperfusion achieved in target mismatch patients: pooled data from the Diffusion and Perfusion Imaging Evaluation for Understanding Stroke Evolution studies. Stroke 2013;44(7):1885–90.
357. Parsons MW, Christensen S, McElduff P, et al. Pretreatment diffusion- and perfusion-mr lesion volumes have a crucial influence on clinical response to stroke thrombolysis. J Cereb Blood Flow Metab 2010;30:1214–25.

49 Cerebral Angiography

Ronald J. Sattenberg, Jason Meckler, Jeffrey L. Saver, Y. Pierre Gobin, David S. Liebeskind

KEY POINTS

- The technique of cerebral angiography emanates from before the advent of non-invasive imaging, yet this approach serves a unique role in the management of patients with cerebrovascular disorders.
- The risks and benefits of cerebral angiography include morbidity due to vascular injury with the advantage of exquisite spatial and temporal resolution to diagnose and treat numerous vascular lesions.
- Common indications include ischemic or hemorrhagic stroke, as well as the underlying or causative vascular lesions.
- Interpretation of cerebral angiography is based on recognition of normal anatomy, collateral flow patterns and pathologic findings.
- Cerebral angiography may be particularly useful in the setting of acute stroke in the young adult or in other potentially elusive diagnoses such as vasculitis.
- Cerebral angiography may simultaneously allow for accurate diagnosis and tailored therapies such as endovascular revascularization for acute stroke or angioplasty/stenting.
- Limitations of cerebral angiography exist, including invasive nature of the procedure, operator-dependent image quality, limited generalizability, and cost.
- Peri-procedural patient care, including monitoring for complications, are unique to this diagnostic modality.

After Egas Moniz invented cerebral angiography in 1927, it became the method of choice for the diagnosis of brain lesions[1,2] until the development of computed tomography (CT) and later magnetic resonance imaging (MRI) limited the indication for catheter angiography to visualize cerebral vessels. CT angiography (CTA) and magnetic resonance angiography (MRA) have demonstrated excellent performance in non-invasively imaging large cervicocerebral vessels, further reducing the need for invasive angiography. Other non-invasive imaging techniques such as duplex ultrasonography and transcranial Doppler ultrasonography provide hemodynamic information that further limits the indications for cerebral angiography. Because of its exquisite spatial and temporal resolution that enables visualization of the smallest vascular lesions and flow patterns, cerebral angiography is still the reference standard for imaging the cervical and cerebral circulation. Moreover, the dramatic expansion of percutaneous treatments for ischemic and hemorrhagic cerebrovascular disease has brought a resurgence in catheter angiography as a necessary prelude and guide to endovascular interventions.[3,4]

TECHNIQUE

Cerebral angiography is increasingly performed by a diverse range of specialists, and this diversity has prompted the publication of qualification requirements for diagnostic and interventional procedures.[5] With miniaturization and other advances in catheter technology and the development of non-ionic contrast agents, cerebral angiography is now usually a straightforward procedure that takes 30–60 minutes to complete. Cerebral angiography is painless and can generally be performed with the use of local anesthesia administered at the groin and no or mild sedation. General anesthesia is required only in patients unable to cooperate or in children. With the use of a closure device[6] such as a collagen plug or percutaneous arterial suture for hemostasis, patients may be ambulatory within 1 hour after the procedure is completed, and anticoagulation need not be halted before the procedure. However, closure devices are only used in a select population of patients. Without closure devices, the patient can usually ambulate within 6 to 8 hours.

Vascular access is most often obtained via the common femoral artery and rarely via the brachial or axillary artery. After arterial puncture, an arterial sheath is placed into the artery. A *sheath* is a short catheter with a diaphragm at its exterior end that allows the passage and manipulation of additional smaller catheters without damaging the femoral artery. Catheterization of the aortic arch and further selective catheterizations are performed with the combined use of a catheter and a guidewire. A plethora of catheters and guidewires is available. Selection of the catheters and guidewires used in a particular patient is based on the patient's vascular anatomy, the diagnostic question to be answered by the procedure, and the preferences of the operator. A hockey-stick-shaped catheter and a guidewire with a simple 45° curve are commonly used, both with hydrophilic coating. For difficult anatomy, other catheter shapes are available. The catheter is continuously flushed with heparinized saline to prevent thrombus formation.

The precise vessels catheterized depend on the indication for the procedure. Sometimes catheterizing only one vessel is all that is required, for instance, for immediate follow-up evaluation after aneurysm clipping. At other times, the bilateral vertebral arteries, bilateral external and internal carotid arteries, and bilateral common carotid arteries all must be catheterized. In many instances, catheterization and angiography of the aortic arch and three to four vessels are necessary. The injection variables employed may alter contrast bolus delivery and have considerable effects on the opacification of downstream arteries, parenchyma, and veins.[7] Standardized technique is therefore important for comparison of angiographic results.

At the very end of the procedure, the common femoral artery sheath is removed, and manual compression is applied at the access site until hemostasis is obtained. Arteriotomy closing devices are now routinely used. These are essentially tools that percutaneously place a suture into or a plug at the puncture site to obtain immediate hemostasis. The indications for the use of a percutaneous closure device vary among institutions. One common approach is not to use these devices for routine angiography, but to reserve their application for patients who are undergoing anticoagulation, who are being treated with thrombolytics, or who have coagulation deficits from other causes.

RISKS

The risks associated with cerebral angiography have declined over the years. Increasing procedural safety is due to many factors, including nonionic contrast agents, new catheters and guidewires that have safer designs and are made of less thrombogenic materials, and digital subtraction angiography.[8,9,10]

The risks associated with cerebral angiography are related to patient age and medical condition, the number of catheter exchanges, the total time for the procedure, and the load of contrast agent.[8,11] Contrast-induced neurotoxicity may elicit neurologic symptoms.[12] Headaches or even transient encephalopathy during angiography have also been documented, although the underlying factors that trigger such events remain unclear.[13–15] Interestingly, some data suggest that the performance of cerebral angiography may directly affect the tone of the vasculature, and vasodilation is the condition most often noted.[16] Increased use of angiography as part of therapeutic interventions and introduction of novel acquisition techniques that may increase radiation exposure also warrant consideration in the future.[17] Cerebral angiography is more risky in the elderly and in patients with particular conditions that predispose to thrombus formation on the catheter (hypercoagulable states) and to vessel dissection and rupture (e.g., Marfan's disease). In the setting of acute ischemic stroke, it has also been suggested that microcatheter injections may predispose to hemorrhagic transformation.[18]

Many studies have been performed to quantify the risks of cerebral angiography.[19] Hankey et al.[20] reviewed several series and found the general risk for permanent neurologic sequelae after cerebral angiography to be 1%. The mortality rate was less than 0.1%. The overall risk for a neurologic complication was about 4%.[20] In a prospective study by Dion et al.,[8] of 1002 cerebral angiography procedures, the rate of permanent neurologic deficit was 0.1% and that of transient deficits was 1.2%. Other studies cite a persistent neurologic deficit rate of 0.3% to 0.5% and a total neurologic complication rate of 0.5–2%.[9] The most recent data suggest angiography complication rates that may be exceedingly low.[19,21,22] Kaufmann et al.[19] reported neurologic complications in 2.63%, including 0.14% with strokes and permanent disability, and a mortality rate of 0.06% in a consecutive series of 19,826 procedures. Fifi et al.[21] reported a complication rate of 0.30% across 3636 diagnostic cerebral angiograms over a 6-year period. Recent studies have also considered operator training or specialty as a factor in complication rates.[23]

Among the potential neurologic complications of cerebral angiography are embolic events and vascular dissections.[24] Transcranial Doppler ultrasonography studies monitoring for microembolic events during diagnostic angiography have shown that, although nonpathogenic air emboli introduced at the time of contrast injection are common, formed element emboli are uncommon.[25] Symptomatic air embolism during angiography may occur in 0.08% of procedures.[26] Carotid or vertebral artery dissections secondary to catheterization depend on operator experience and are less frequent (0.4%) with the newer, safer catheter designs. Although neurologically symptomatic complications from cerebral angiography are rare, clinically silent "complications," diagnosed on diffusion-weighted MRI, are more common, being found in 26% of diagnostic angiography procedures.[27] Covert MRI diffusion lesions are associated with the presence of multiple vascular risk factors, greater difficulty in probing vessels, amount of contrast medium needed, longer fluoroscopy time, and the use of multiple catheters.[27]

One particular concern of cerebral angiography in the setting of recently ruptured cerebral aneurysms is the risk of precipitating rebleeding by injecting contrast agent with an increased pressure head. This risk is extremely low. In a meta-analysis of 415 patients with acute subarachnoid hemorrhage, Cloft et al.[28] found no cases of rebleeding during angiography.

Non-neurologic complications consist of local complications (i.e., hematoma, pseudoaneurysm, and infection[29]), renal failure, contrast agent allergies, and arterial occlusions. Contrast or even heparin during angiography may also cause transient reductions in serum calcium values, possibly due to chelation.[30] In a cooperative study among leading interventional radiologic societies, non-neurologic major complication rates were as follows: renal failure, 0–0.15%; arterial occlusion requiring surgical intervention, 0–0.4%; arteriovenous fistula or pseudoaneurysm, 0.01–0.22%; and hematoma requiring transfusion or evacuation, 0.26–1.5%.[11] Recent use of percutaneous closure devices has demonstrated low rates of complications, although the use of concomitant antithrombotic agents may increase events.[6]

When an allergy to iodine contrast medium is known before procedure initiation, premedication with steroids and antihistamines is usually sufficient to prevent any adverse reactions. In patients with previous severe allergy such as shock, in whom iodine is contraindicated even with premedication, gadolinium-based contrast agents, which are radiopaque as well as paramagnetic, may be used.

ANGIOGRAPHIC CEREBRAL VASCULATURE: NORMAL ANATOMY

To recognize and understand vascular disease, one must first be acquainted with the normal angioarchitecture of the cerebrovascular system and its variants. The three phases of an angiographic imaging sequence – arterial, capillary, and venous – are shown in Figures 49-1–49-3. Each phase has its particular sensitivity for the different pathologic entities. One should be able to recognize common variants, such as persistent fetal anomalies, vascular fenestrations (Fig. 49-4), and collateral pathways.

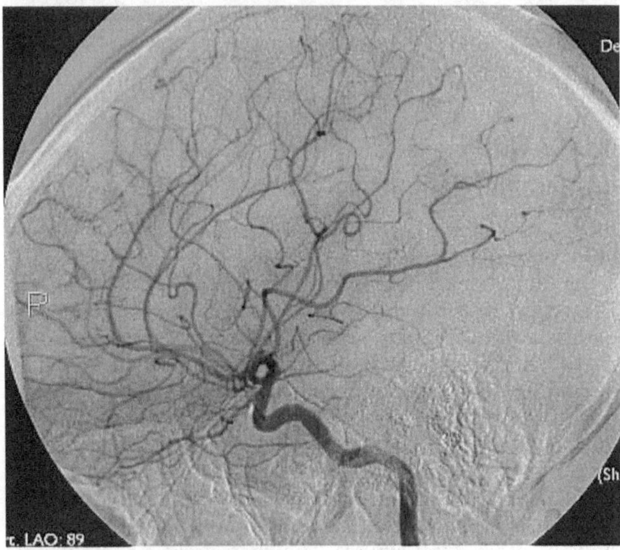

Figure 49-1. Internal carotid artery injection, lateral projection, arterial phase. The arteries are primarily opacified during this phase.

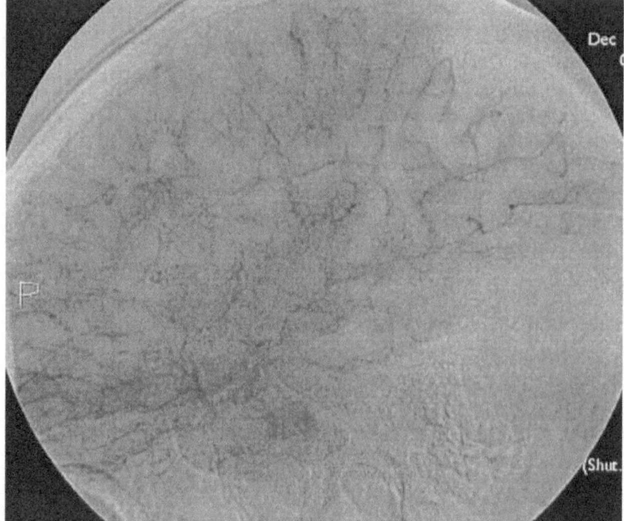

Figure 49-2. Internal carotid artery injection, lateral projection, capillary phase. No significant arterial or venous opacification is noted during this phase.

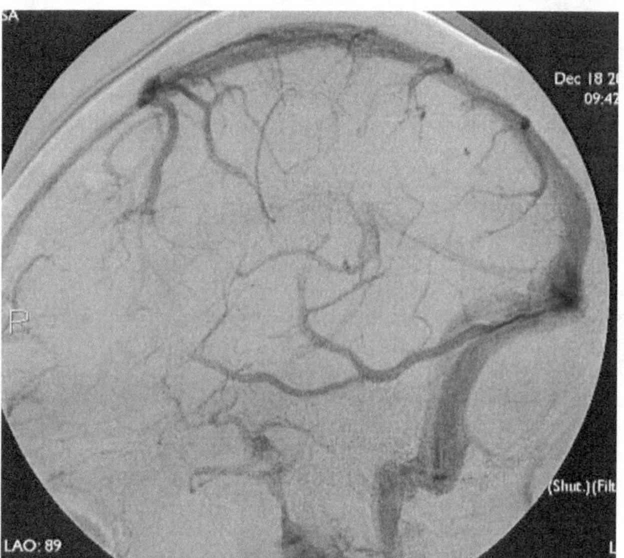

Figure 49-3. Internal carotid artery injection, lateral projection, venous phase. The veins are primarily opacified during this phase.

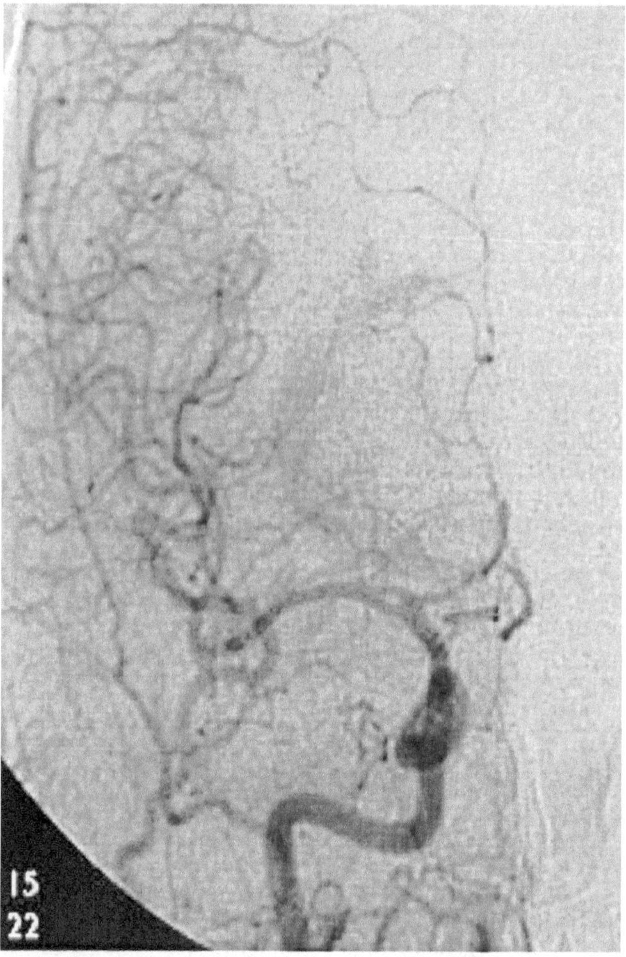

Figure 49-4. Common carotid artery injection, anteroposterior projection. Note the "filling defect" in the M1 segment, just at the carotid bifurcation. This is a fenestration.

INDICATIONS

Intracranial Hemorrhage

Intracranial hemorrhage may be epidural, subdural, subarachnoid, or intraparenchymal.

Epidural hemorrhage is usually secondary to head trauma. The vessels coursing in the epidural space, most notably the middle meningeal artery, are torn and arterial bleeding results. These hemorrhages are often associated with skull fractures. Because epidural hemorrhages are usually of traumatic origin, correlation with the clinical history as well as non-invasive imaging almost invariably identifies the cause, obviating the need for angiographic evaluation.

Subdural hemorrhage (SDH) is secondary to bleeding from the cortical bridging veins that drain into the superior sagittal sinus or other dural sinuses. The characteristic angiographic appearance is a lentiform avascular collection outlined by displaced cortical vessels. The cortical bridging veins are vulnerable to venous hypertension or tearing in the subdural space secondary to trauma. Venous hypertension can be caused by a variety of reasons, including sinus thrombosis and dural arteriovenous fistulas (Fig. 49-5). Uncommonly, a subdural hematoma may result when an intracerebral aneurysm that previously hemorrhaged creates adhesions that direct subsequent hemorrhaging into the subdural compartment. In this situation, an intraparenchymal focus of hemorrhage is also often present, detection of which should raise the suspicion for aneurysmal bleeding. In a subdural hemorrhage, if a dural arteriovenous fistula or aneurysm is suspected, cerebral angiography should be performed. However, if trauma or significant brain parenchyma atrophy is present in an older patient, angiography should be reserved.

Subarachnoid hemorrhage (SAH) has an incidence of 6–8 per 100,000 person-years, and studies suggest that 2–6% of the population have an intracranial aneurysm. In 85% of SAHs, the cause is a ruptured aneurysm, usually a berry aneurysm. Among the other causes of SAH are trauma (in which case a parenchyma focus of contusion or hemorrhage is often seen on imaging), intraparenchymal hemorrhage extending into the ventricular system, cerebral or cervical arteriovenous malformation (AVM) or fistula, venous thrombosis, mycotic aneurysm, non-aneurysmal perimesencephalic hemorrhage, vasculitis, and dissections; some SAHs are cryptogenic.

In less than 5% of AVMs that bleed, the hemorrhage is confined to the subarachnoid space, and no intraparenchymal

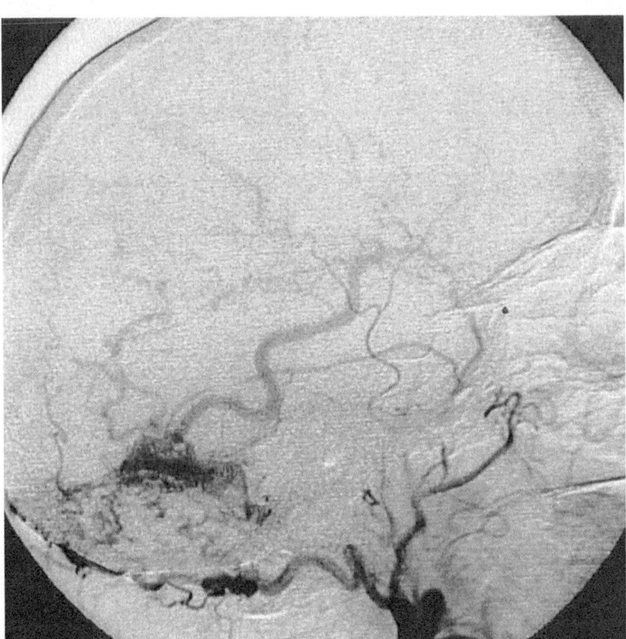

Figure 49-5. External carotid artery injection, lateral projection. There is arterial and early venous opacification with contrast simultaneously. The dural fistula is also opacified.

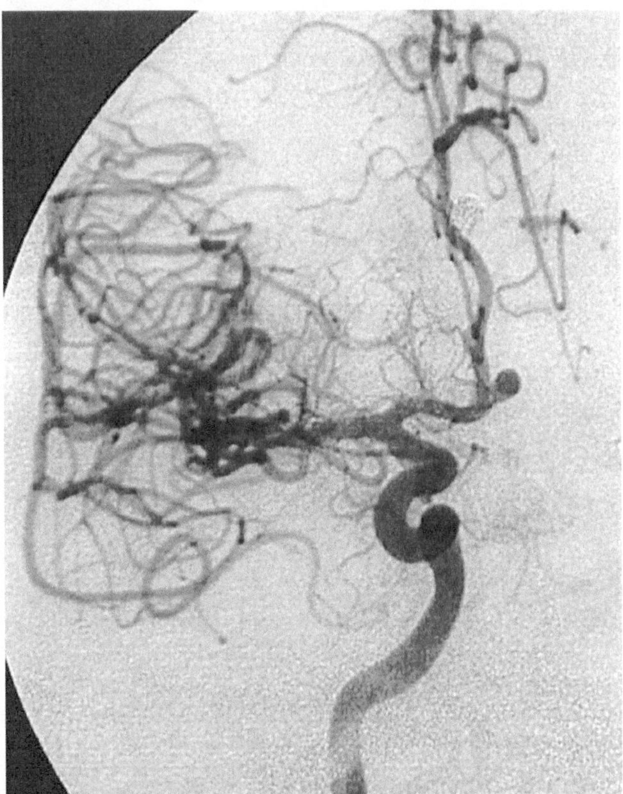

Figure 49-6. Right internal carotid artery injection, frontal projection, demonstrates an anterior communicating artery aneurysm. The aneurysm dome points superomedially.

blood is present. Generally, if the findings of angiography performed in the early phase of a non-traumatic SAH are normal, the procedure should be repeated after 1 week. There are several explanations why an aneurysm may not be detected on angiography; among these are parenchymal hematoma compressing the aneurysm; thrombus in the aneurysm, its neck, or both; perianeurysmal vasospasm; and suboptimal views of the region harboring the aneurysm. The diagnostic yield of a second cerebral angiogram in eight different series was 17%.[31] If findings on the second angiogram are also normal, a third angiographic procedure performed several months later can be of benefit. In one series, aneurysm was detected by a third angiogram in 1 of 14 patients.[31] For a patient in whom a CT scan shows a truly perimesencephalic hemorrhage pattern, the probability that cerebral angiography will reveal a vertebrobasilar aneurysm is 4%.[32] Thus, the diagnosis of perimesencephalic hemorrhage requires normal findings on a cerebral angiogram. In a truly perimesencephalic pattern of SAH, a second angiographic procedure is not necessary if the findings of the first angiogram are normal.[33]

Berry or saccular aneurysms are the most prevalent intracranial aneurysms. They are localized mostly in the anterior circulation (90%) as follows: anterior communicating artery, 40%; middle cerebral artery bifurcation, 30%; intracranial internal carotid artery, 20%; and posterior circulation, 10%. Other cerebral aneurysms are fusiform, traumatic (pseudoaneurysm), mycotic, or dissecting. A selection of aneurysms is illustrated in Figures 49-6–49-18. Cerebral aneurysms have been associated with autosomal dominant polycystic kidney disease and Marfan's syndrome.

Angiography should evaluate the location of the aneurysm, size of the neck and dome (dome–neck ratio), morphology, and relationship to the parent vessel and should show whether the aneurysm incorporates the origin of other vessels. Multiple aneurysms are found in 20% of aneurysmal SAHs, and it may be difficult to identify which aneurysm bled and should be treated first. Three important features indicating the causative aneurysm are (1) the location of the aneurysm in relation to the SAH, (2) the aneurysm shape, because a ruptured aneurysm may be lobulated or have a teat, and (3) the aneurysm size. Active extravasation of contrast material from an aneurysm at the time of angiography is exceptional and indicates intraprocedural rupture. Three-dimensional rotational angiography may be more sensitive for aneurysm detection[34–36]

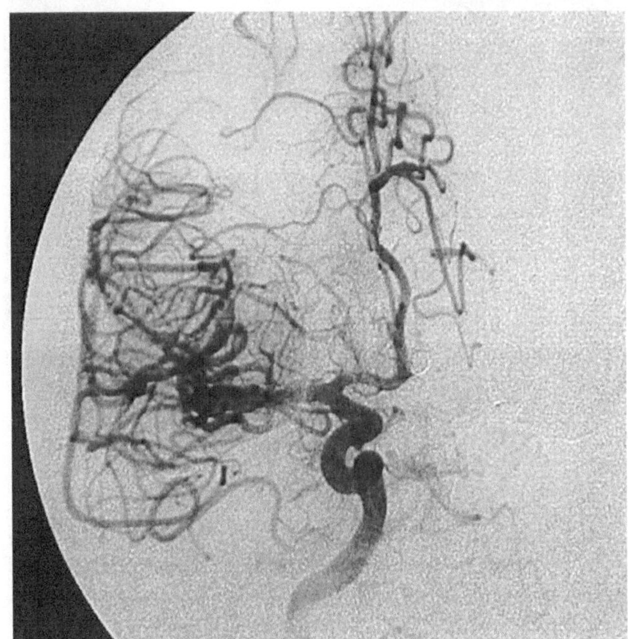

Figure 49-7. Right internal carotid artery injection, anteroposterior projection, after embolization. The anterior communicating artery aneurysm seen previously is no longer opacifying.

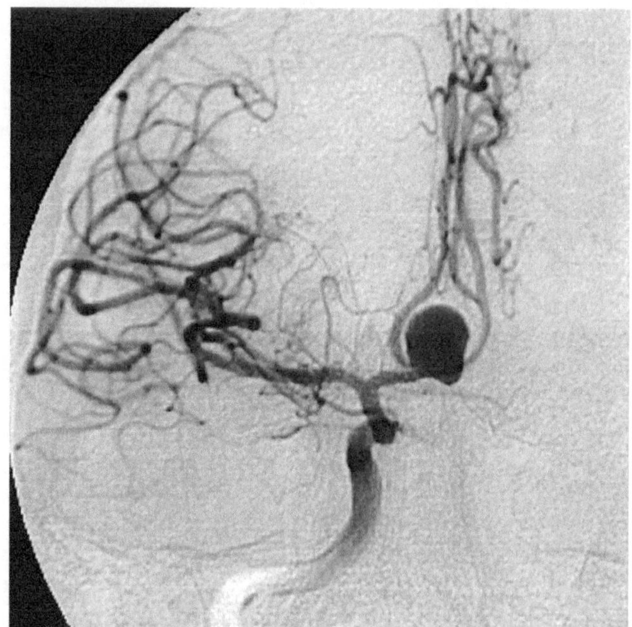

Figure 49-8. Right internal carotid artery injection, frontal view, arterial phase, demonstrating a large anterior communicating artery aneurysm. Notice how the A2 segments of the anterior cerebral artery are splayed by the aneurysm.

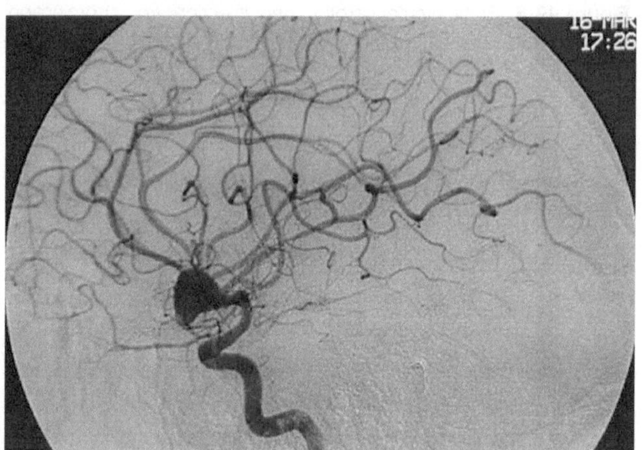

Figure 49-9. Internal carotid artery injection, lateral projection, arterial phase, demonstrating a large anterior communicating artery aneurysm.

yet may still result in a 4.2% rate of angiogram-negative SAH.[37,38] Angiography may also be used for later assessment of arterial status after definitive treatment of an aneurysm, and evidence shows very low complication rates.[39]

Intraparenchymal hemorrhage can be secondary to a variety of pathologic entities, including hypertension (80%), amyloid angiopathy, trauma, hemorrhagic transformation of ischemic stroke, arterial dissection, tumor, sinus thrombosis, AVM, cavernous hemangioma, and saccular aneurysm. About 20% of hemorrhages due to intracranial aneurysms have an intraparenchymal component, especially if a mycotic aneurysm is the cause. If an AVM is suspected on MRI or CT, angiography is required to characterize the lesion, its venous drainage, arterial feeding arteries (feeders), and nidus. The characteristic angiographic appearance of an AVM consists of

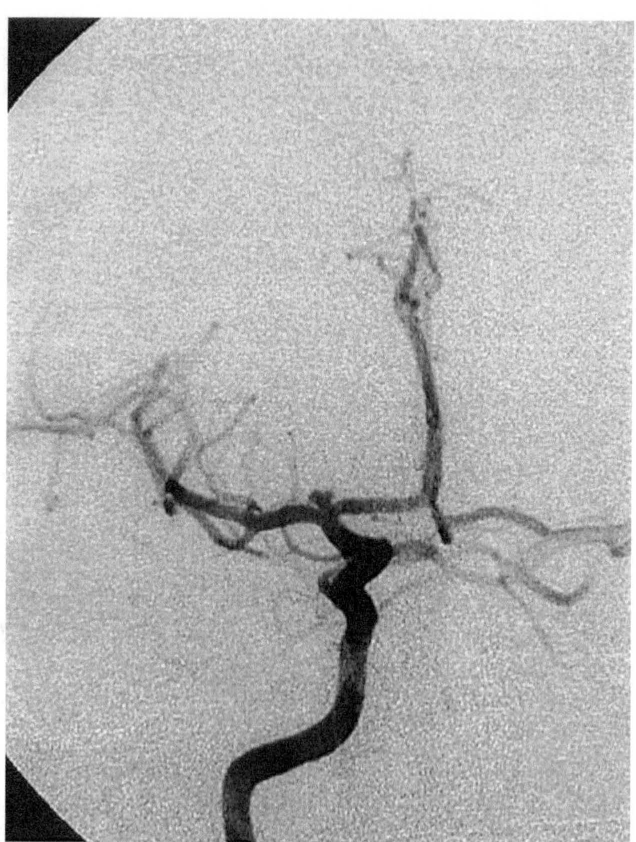

Figure 49-10. Right internal carotid artery injection, anteroposterior projection, arterial phase, demonstrating a carotid bifurcation aneurysm. The aneurysm is bilobed and irregular in contour.

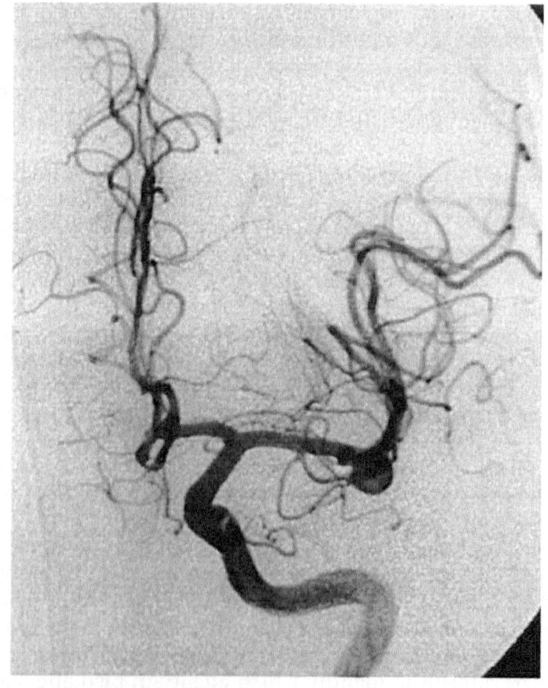

Figure 49-11. Left internal carotid artery injection, frontal projection, arterial phase, demonstrating a middle cerebral artery aneurysm. The aneurysm dome is pointing inferiorly.

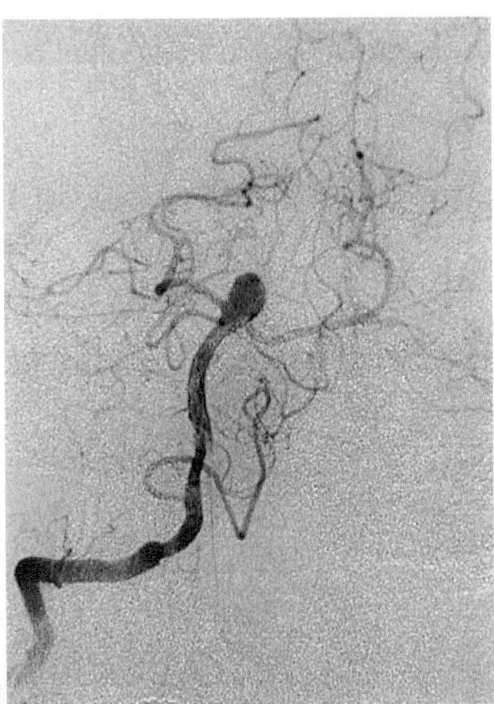

Figure 49-12. Right vertebral artery injection, frontal projection, arterial phase, demonstrating a basilar tip aneurysm.

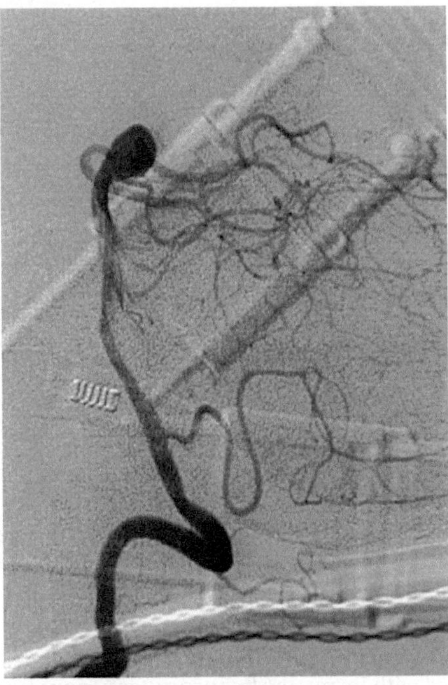

Figure 49-13. Vertebral artery injection, lateral projection, arterial phase, demonstrating a basilar tip aneurysm.

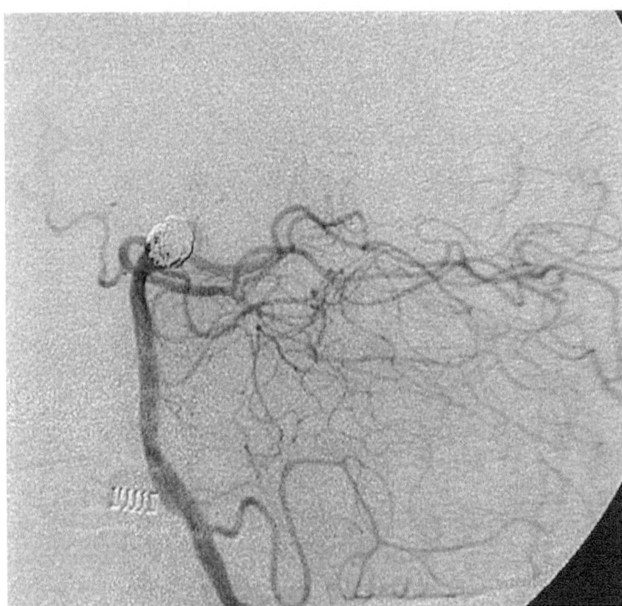

Figure 49-14. Lateral projection, posterior circulation, arterial phase. Status: postembolization; the basilar tip aneurysm is no longer opacifying.

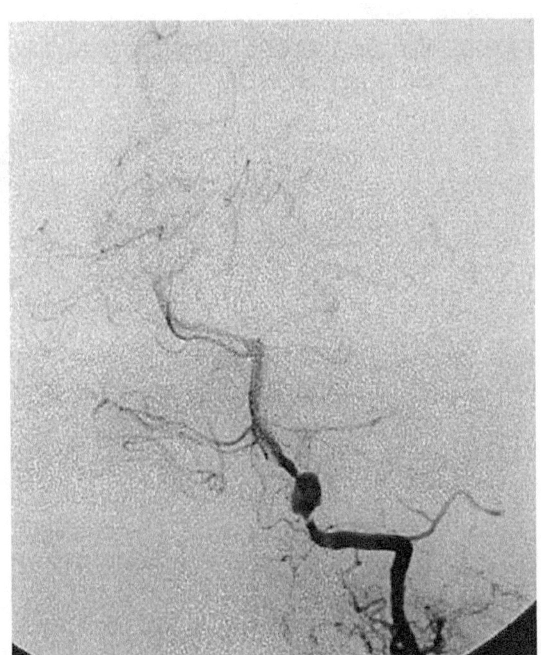

Figure 49-15. Vertebral artery injection, frontal projection, demonstrating a vertebrobasilar aneurysm. Notice how the contrast column rapidly narrows and there is significantly decreased opacification of the vasculature distal to the aneurysm. This is consistent with a dissecting aneurysm.

enlarged arterial feeders, a nidus, and early draining veins (Figs 49-19–49-22).

The association of AVMs and aneurysms on the arterial feeders is well-known and is secondary to the high-flow state through the AVM (see Figs 49-21, 49-22). Furthermore, selection of optimal treatment modalities for AVMs requires knowledge of the detailed angioarchitecture of the lesion. For example, the presence of a lenticulostriate arterial supply to the nidus makes surgery more difficult (see Fig. 49-22).

In general, angiography should be considered in the evaluation of intracranial hemorrhage in (1) any patient younger than 70 years with a lobar hemorrhage and (2) any patient of any age with a deep hemorrhage who does not have a history of hypertension or CT or MRI evidence of small-vessel arteriopathy.

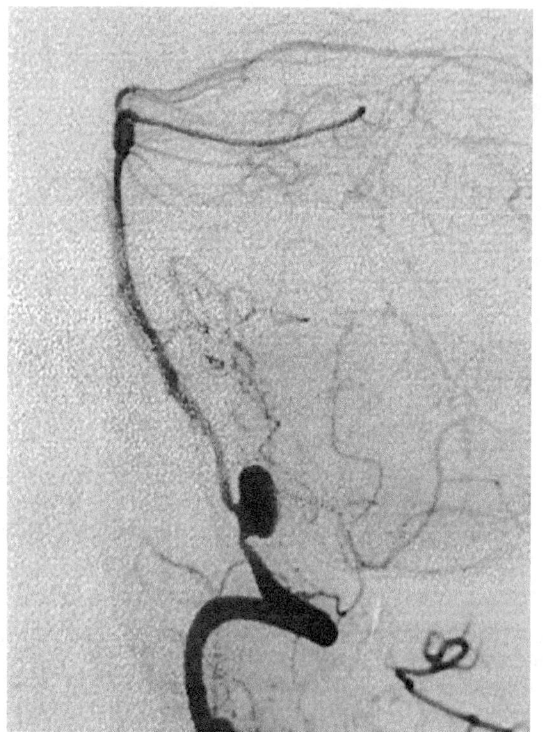

Figure 49-16. Vertebral artery injection, lateral projection, arterial phase, demonstrating a dissecting vertebrobasilar aneurysm.

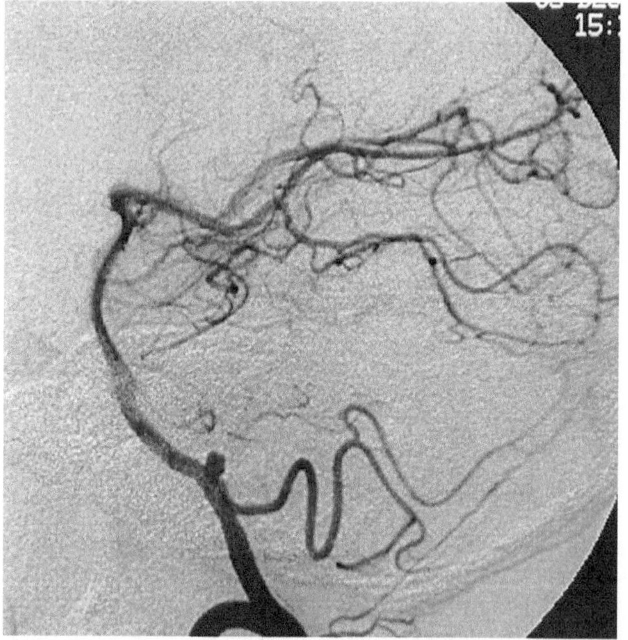

Figure 49-17. Vertebral artery injection, lateral projection, arterial phase, demonstrating a posterior inferior cerebellar artery (PICA) aneurysm.

Ischemia

Cerebral Infarction and Transient Ischemic Attack

Cerebral angiography remains a mainstay in the evaluation of cerebral ischemia in the young (e.g., <45 years), in whom the potential causes are diverse and include entities often best characterized on angiographic studies, including vasculitis and

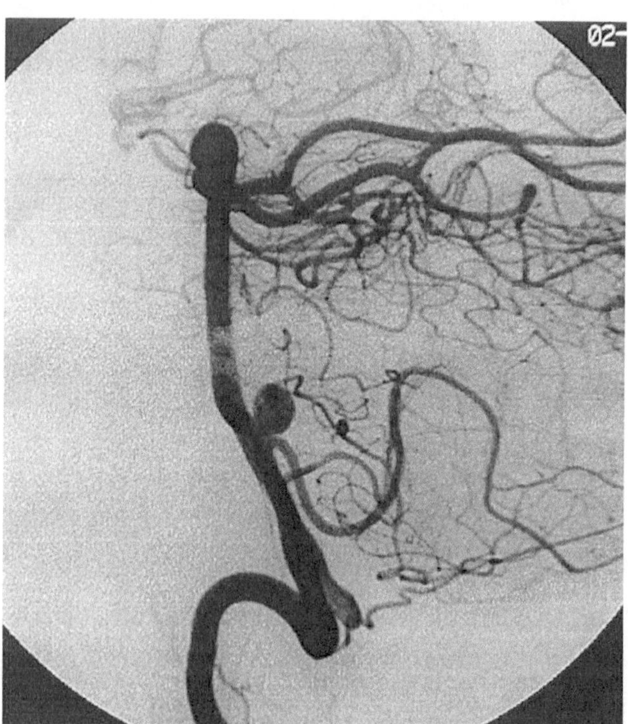

Figure 49-18. Vertebral artery injection, lateral projection, arterial phase, demonstrating both a basilar tip aneurysm and a posterior inferior cerebellar artery aneurysm.

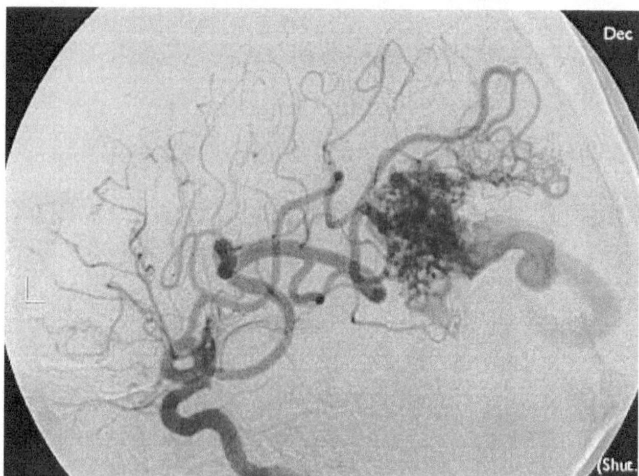

Figure 49-19. Internal carotid artery injection, lateral projection, arterial phase, demonstrating early venous opacification, as well as a nidus, consistent with an arteriovenous malformation.

dissection. Pediatric neuroendovascular procedures are being performed with increasing frequency, for various indications.[40] Even when detailed imaging features of ischemia are evident on multimodal CT or MRI, angiography may still provide further information.[41,42]

Angiography remains fundamentally important in the evaluation of cervical carotid atherosclerosis. The decision of whether to proceed with carotid endarterectomy or carotid stenting depends on the extent of stenosis at the carotid bifurcation. In general, patients with symptomatic carotid disease benefit from surgical intervention if the severity of stenosis on angiography is 50–99%, whereas those with asymptomatic stenosis derive a modest benefit from surgery if the severity of stenosis is 60–99%. The common non-invasive imaging

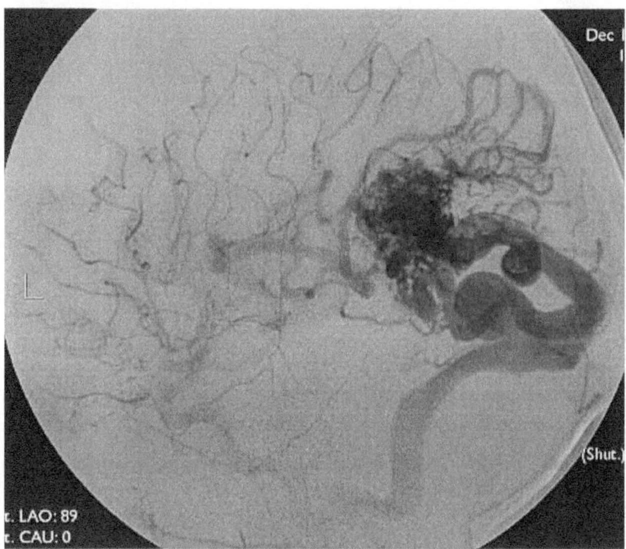

Figure 49-20. Internal carotid artery injection, lateral projection, venous phase, demonstrating the venous phase of an arteriovenous malformation. Note the enlarged vein draining the arteriovenous malformation nidus.

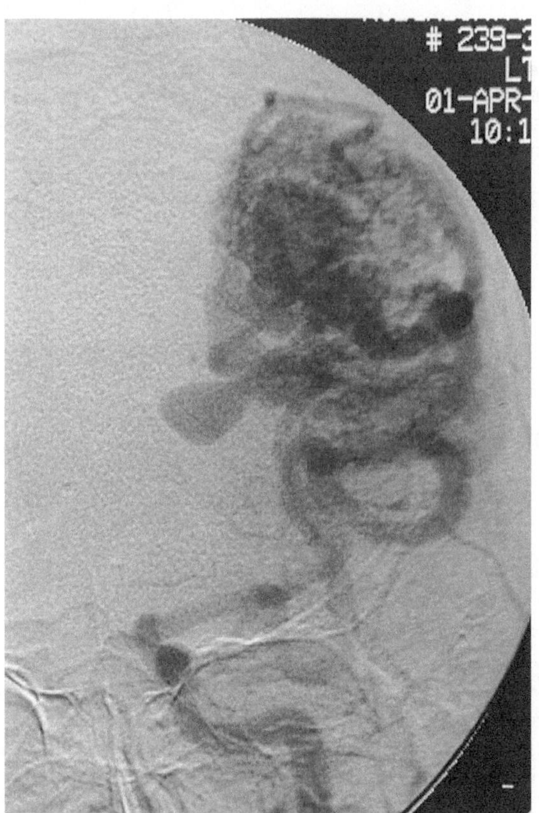

Figure 49-21. Left internal carotid artery injection, anteroposterior projection, arterial phase, demonstrating an enlarged middle cerebral artery vasculature feeding an arteriovenous malformation with an aneurysm whose dome points inferomedially.

modalities, carotid duplex ultrasonography, CTA, and MRA, are generally quite good, but each has intrinsic as well as operator- and reader-dependent limitations. When two non-invasive tests provide congruent results regarding the severity of stenosis, a decision for or against surgery may be made with

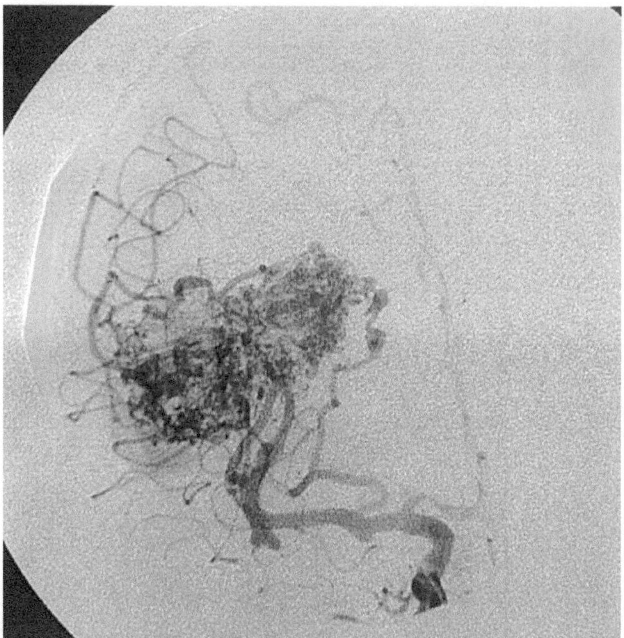

Figure 49-22. Right internal carotid artery injection, frontal projection, arterial phase, demonstrating an arteriovenous malformation being opacified by middle cerebral arterial vessels, as well as a lenticulostriate artery originating from the M1 segment of the middle cerebral artery.

confidence. If non-invasive test results disagree, however, catheter angiography is desirable for definitively characterizing the lesion.

Although both modalities can assess the severity of an internal carotid artery stenosis well, an important advantage of cerebral angiography over standard carotid duplex ultrasonography is that the evaluation of the morphology of a plaque is better accomplished by catheter angiography (Figs 49-23, 49-24). Plaque morphology can be very important because, even if stenosis is not severe, an ulcerated plaque can be the cause of transient ischemic attacks (TIAs) and similarly may be the harbinger of a stroke. Arterial wall imaging with CT or MRI may be another option in the future.

Intracranial atherosclerotic stenosis is one cause of cerebral infarction and TIAs (Figs 49-25, 49-26). For middle cerebral artery atherosclerotic stenosis, a stroke rate of up to 10% annually has been reported. The Warfarin-Aspirin Symptomatic Intracranial Disease (WASID) trial demonstrated that aspirin may be as effective as anticoagulation in this disorder.[43] Particular risk factors, such as severe degree of luminal arterial stenosis, have also been noted and indicate a high risk of recurrent ischemia.[44] Accurate determination of luminal stenosis with angiography is therefore important in risk assessment. The intracranial vasculature can be assessed with CTA, MRA, and transcranial Doppler ultrasonography to some extent; however, these intracranial vessels are smaller in diameter than the internal carotid artery, and the sensitivity and specificity of non-invasive studies for detecting and characterizing intracranial stenoses are not yet as well documented as for cervical stenoses. In fact, the Stroke Outcomes and Neuroimaging of Intracranial Atherosclerosis (SONIA) trial showed prominent discordance in non-invasive angiographic detection rates.[45] Quantifying the severity of intracranial stenosis at angiography requires a different measurement technique from that used for extracranial stenosis – that established by the North American Symptomatic Carotid Endarterectomy Trial (NASCET). Intracranial vessels tend to taper distal to

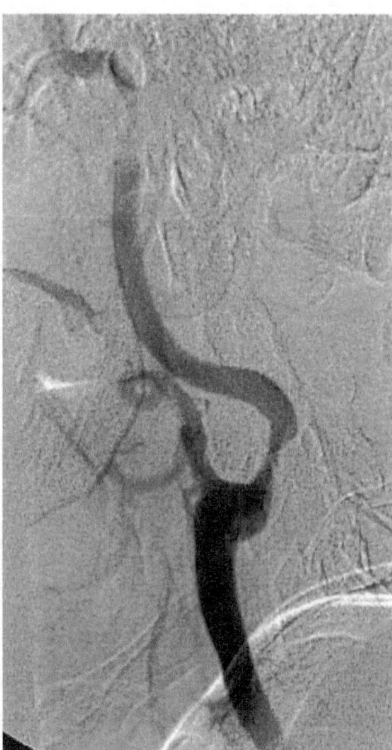

Figure 49-23. Common carotid artery injection, lateral projection, arterial phase, demonstrates an internal carotid artery stenosis just distal to the bifurcation.

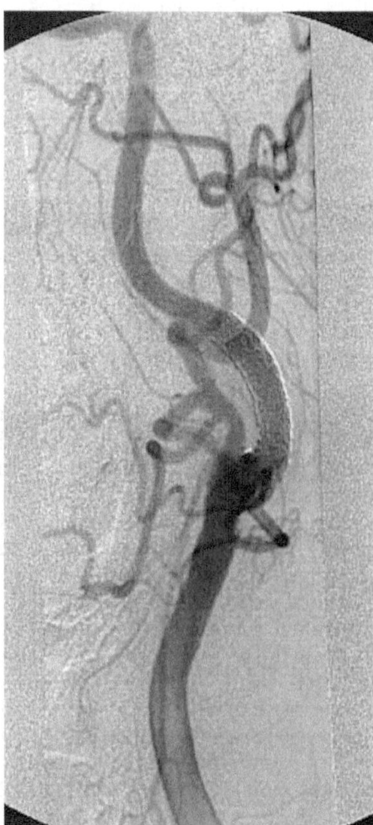

Figure 49-24. Common carotid artery injection, lateral projection, arterial phase, demonstrating internal carotid artery status after angioplasty and stent placement. The stenotic segment is no longer present.

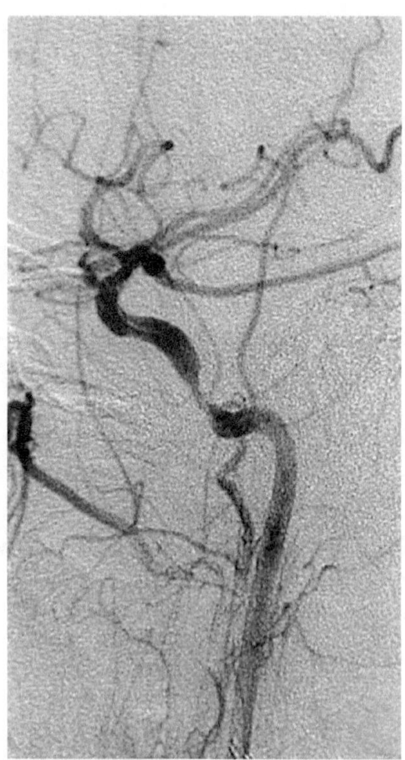

Figure 49-25. Common carotid artery injection, lateral projection, arterial phase, demonstrating a stenosis in the petrous segment of the internal carotid artery. Note that there is also opacification of some of the external carotid artery vasculature.

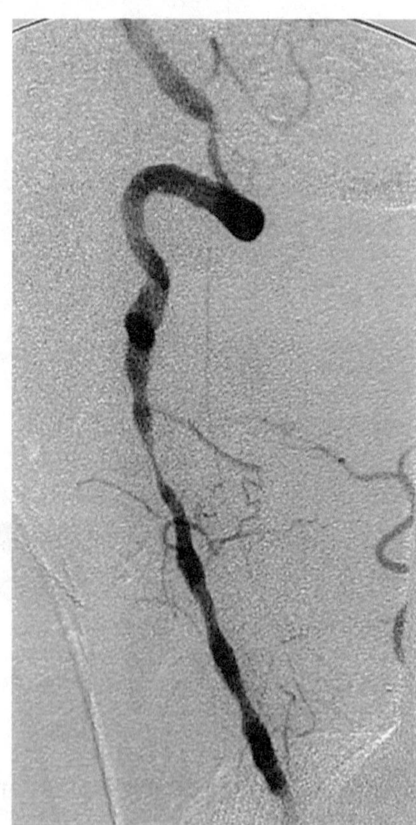

Figure 49-26. Vertebral artery injection, lateral projection, arterial phase. Note the tandem stenoses.

stenoses, leading to possible underestimation of the extent of narrowing if the NASCET method were employed. A standardized measure has been introduced for intracranial stenoses, where percent stenosis = [(1 − (D(stenosis)/D(normal)))] × 100, where D(stenosis) = the diameter of the artery at the site of the most severe stenosis and D(normal) = the diameter of the proximal normal artery.[46]

Acute Ischemia

In approximately 80% of acute ischemic strokes, early angiography demonstrates a large-artery occlusion, either embolic (from arterial origin or cardioembolic) or due to in situ atherothrombosis. Cerebral angiography is indicated as an emergency procedure if intra-arterial thrombolysis or mechanical thrombectomy is being considered. In the last several years, mechanical devices for clot retrieval and aspiration have been cleared by the United States Food and Drug Administration for restoration of cerebral arterial patency in the setting of acute ischemic stroke.[47–51] More recent efforts have expanded revascularization techniques to possibly include stenting of intracranial arteries to restore patency.[52–56]

The cerebral angiographic findings in acute ischemic stroke are varied. One finding is the abrupt cutoff of a vessel (Figs 49-27–49-33). In this situation contrast opacification is noted in the vessel (i.e., artery) up to a specific and definite point, beyond which there is no contrast opacification, hence the appearance of the vessel being abruptly cutoff. If an embolus is the etiology of the acute ischemia, a meniscus sign may be seen. The meniscus sign is created by the intra-arterial contrast medium delineating the edge of the embolus within the vessel. While a large-vessel abrupt cutoff (such as a M1 of the middle cerebral artery) can often be appreciated on both MRA and CTA, small-vessel occlusions may best be appreciated on digital subtraction angiography and may not be appreciated on MRA or CTA. While abrupt vascular cutoff represents total or near-complete vascular occlusion, relative stagnation of contrast in a vessel without being abruptly cutoff may also be seen in acute ischemia, and can represent severe narrowing of the given vessel distally (possibly from atherosclerotic plaque, not totally occlusive embolus, dissection). The clot burden or

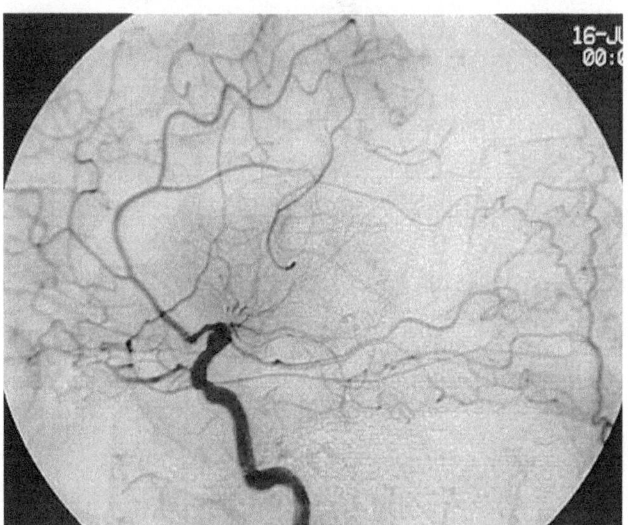

Figure 49-28. Internal carotid artery injection, lateral projection, demonstrating the absence of opacification of the middle cerebral artery vasculature.

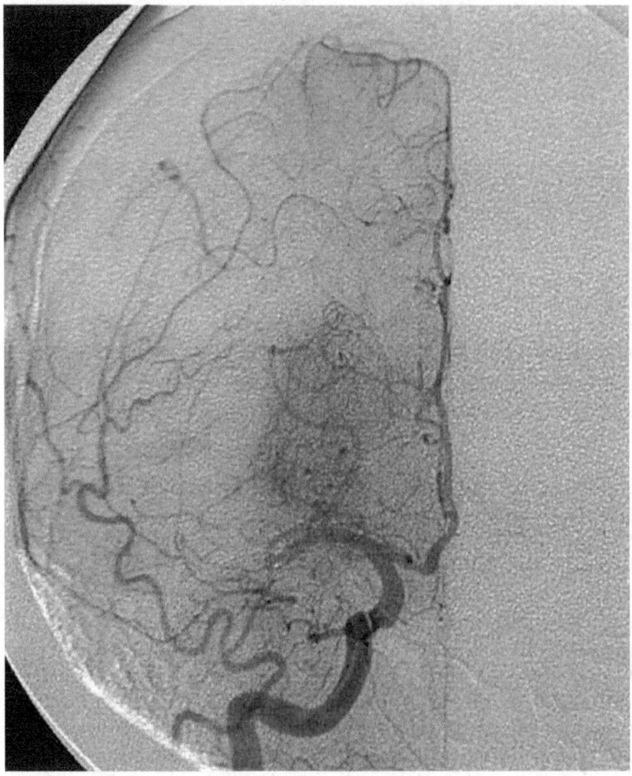

Figure 49-27. Right internal carotid artery injection, frontal projection, demonstrating an abrupt M1 segment "cutoff."

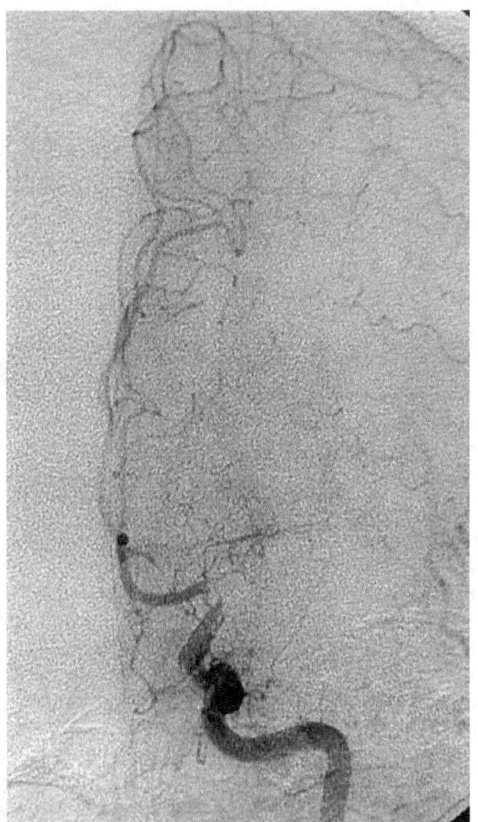

Figure 49-29. Left internal carotid artery injection, frontal projection, demonstrates significant occlusion at the top of the internal carotid artery at its bifurcation. Note that some opacification of the left anterior cerebral artery vasculature is seen.

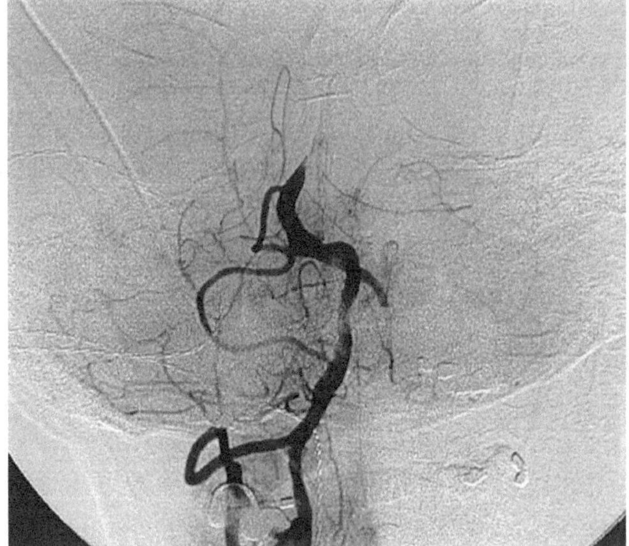

Figure 49-30. This anteroposterior projection of the vertebrobasilar artery demonstrates occlusion of the basilar artery. Notice the parenchymal blush.

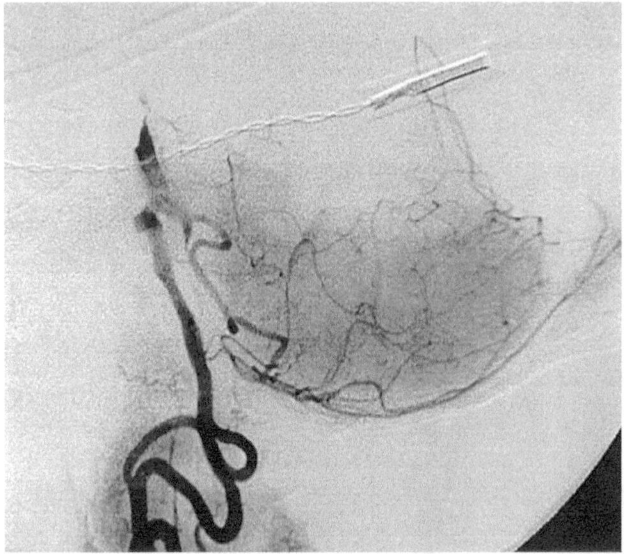

Figure 49-31. Vertebral artery injection, lateral projection, demonstrating an abrupt "cutoff" of the basilar artery opacification.

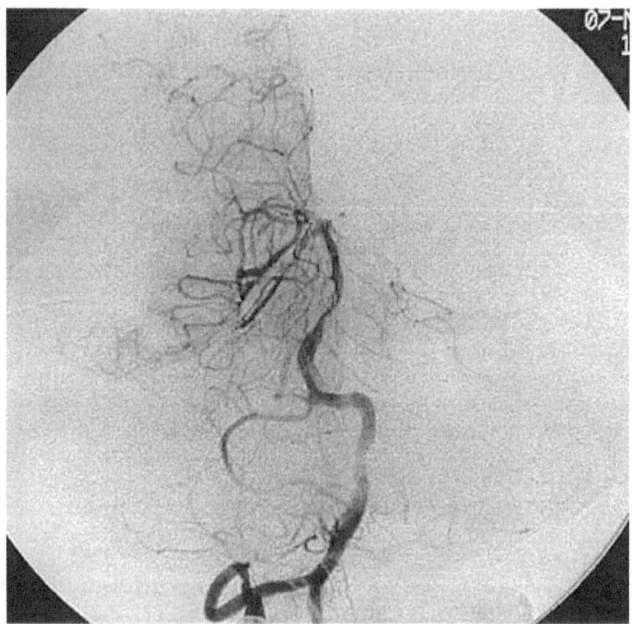

Figure 49-32. Vertebral artery injection, anteroposterior projection, after thrombolysis, demonstrates opacification of the entire basilar artery and the posterior cerebral artery vasculature.

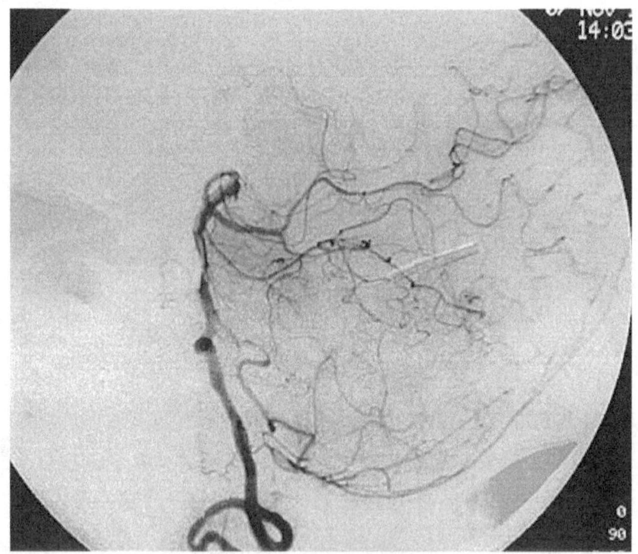

Figure 49-33. Vertebral artery injection, lateral projection, demonstrating basilar artery status after thrombolysis with opacification of the entire basilar artery as well as posterior cerebral artery opacification.

volume of thrombus may also be assessed at angiography, facilitating the planning of revascularization approaches and other potential therapeutic maneuvers.[57] Another possible finding could be a relatively bare area seen in the capillary phase of the examination. This is perhaps the most sensitive angiographic sign of ischemia. This bare area in the capillary phase represents a paucity of blood flow (and hence a paucity of contrast medium) getting to the ischemic tissue, while the adjacent non-ischemic tissues have good or better contrast opacification creating the appearance of the (relatively) bare area in the ischemic tissue. To best appreciate the capillary phase of the angiographic study the intra-arterial contrast should be injected into the catheterized vessel using appropriate technique to evaluate this phase of vascular opacification. Collateralization should be routinely assessed in evaluation of acute stroke because the presence of collateral flow may indicate that the hypoperfused territory has residual blood supply, so irreversible injury may not occur for some time, or throughout the full extent of the territory. Collateralization can take the following forms: (1) flow through the circle of Willis (i.e., through the anterior communicating artery and/or posterior communicating artery). The anterior communicating artery and posterior communicating artery are two of the major arterial collaterals which are amongst the anatomic variants often seen; (2) flow through the external carotid artery through the ophthalmic artery and then to the internal carotid artery, which is another anatomic variant often present, and (3) through leptomeningeal or pial collaterals at the surface of the brain. These leptomeningeal collaterals have the ability to offer flow to ischemic tissues to a variable extent, but can be extensive at times. Collaterals may widely vary across individuals, partly accounting for the marked heterogeneity of stroke outcomes in a given vascular territory. The extent of collateralization or collateral grade has been established as a potent predictor of angiographic and clinical outcomes in acute ischemic stroke and intracranial atherosclerosis. Of note is that cerebral angiography also allows one to appreciate both spatial and temporal extent of collateral perfusion, delineating the capillary blush and collateralization beyond the steno-occlusive lesion. Although gross markers of such findings may be noted on multimodal CT or MRI, cerebral angiography remains the reference standard for collateral flow. In the subacute phase, hours to weeks after ischemic strokes, "luxury perfusion" (hyperperfusion visualized as increased contrast radiodensity) may be seen.

The recent increase in endovascular therapies for revascularization as a treatment for acute ischemic stroke has led to increased investigation of serial angiographic changes that may accompany revascularization of an occluded cerebral artery. Recanalization and re-occlusion may be readily illustrated at angiography.[58] The role of collateral circulation as a key facet of ischemic pathophysiology[59,60] and pivotal determinant of recanalization has been underscored by angiographic analyses in this setting. Revascularization after thrombolysis or thrombectomy has also been the focus of intense investigation as the distinction between recanalization, or restoration of proximal arterial patency, and reperfusion of the downstream territory has become apparent.[61] The use of specific angiographic scales, as well as the inherent advantages or disadvantages of each tool, has become an important area of research because such features of revascularization may have different implications on the neurologic outcome of the stroke patient. Consideration of serial angiographic details, including features of collateral flow, arterial patency, and downstream territorial perfusion, with the use of validated scales and methodology[62] will be important in linking the technical success of endovascular devices with treatment outcomes in clinical trials,[48,50] future registries, and routine clinical practice.

Arteriovenous Malformations

An *arteriovenous malformation* is an abnormal connection between arteries and veins without an intervening capillary, producing a high-flow state with arteriovenous shunting of blood (see Figs 49-19–49-22). These lesions can be associated with headaches, seizures, and other neurologic symptoms. Hemorrhages may be due to nidus vessel rupture, to rupture of an associated aneurysm, or to venous congestion. Associated aneurysms may be in the nidus or on a feeding artery, so-called flow-related aneurysms (see Figs 49-21–49-22). This diagnosis is often made or at least suspected on MRI, MRA, or CTA. Although time-resolved non-invasive angiographic techniques have been refined,[63] cerebral angiography remains necessary for adequately characterizing the arterial feeders and venous drainage and its dynamics, as well as for searching for associated aneurysms.

Some angiographic findings often seen with arteriovenous malformations (AVMs) on cerebral angiography or DSA may include enlarged arteries supplying the AVM, representing their high-flow state. The supplying arteries to the AVM can come from many vascular territories, and for this reason a thorough evaluation should be done to fully evaluate the AVM. The vascular nidus of the AVM, representing a vascular tangle between the arteries and veins may be extensive or at times, not discernible. The classic DSA appearance of an AVM is early draining vein(s), reflecting accelerated arterial to venous transit. This appears as opacification of select venous structures before the "venous phase" of the angiogram for the rest of the tissues. An important aspect of the evaluation of an AVM includes assessment as to where the draining veins go, superficial or deep drainage (e.g., drainage to the superior sagittal sinus or internal cerebral veins). The evaluation of the AVM also needs to evaluate the presence of aneurysms associated with the AVM. There may be aneurysms on the feeding arteries (perhaps related to the high-flow state), draining veins, as well as the AVM nidus itself. Aneurysms will appear as opacification of a vascular outpouching, and can be quite large or alternatively, quite small. During the angiogram it is important to observe the vascular opacification in real time, as a nidus may not be appreciated and an early draining vein may be the only appreciable finding of the AVM. While MRA and CTA may diagnose an AVM, small AVMs may not be appreciated on these non-invasive studies and DSA is far more sensitive. Similarly, DSA better determines the flow characteristics and detailed anatomy of the AVM.

Treatment is based on the characteristics of the AVM and whether it involves neurologically eloquent territory. Among the treatment modalities are endovascular embolization, surgery, and stereotactic radiation surgery. Often, a combination of two or three therapies is required (see Chapter 65).

Cervicocephalic Artery Dissection

Cervicocephalic arterial dissection has many possible causes, including trauma, fibromuscular dysplasia, and other vasculopathies. Dissection can manifest as ischemic stroke and, less often, SAH. The diagnosis of dissection can often be made on MRI, MRA, or CTA. In particular, non-enhanced axial T1-weighted, fat-saturated MR images are sensitive for subacute dissection because the blood in the vessel wall appears as high-signal intensity, contrasting with the flow void in the vessel lumen. Characteristic of dissection on angiography is tapering or narrowing of the vessel, in some cases to a string, or even total occlusion; in other cases, a flap may be visualized. Dissecting aneurysms may also be seen (see Figs 49-15, 49-16). Affected patients are most often managed medically. However, in case of progressing ischemia, an endovascular procedure involving angioplasty and stenting may be beneficial.

Vasculitis

Intracranial vasculitis is suspected when multiple cerebral infarcts are detected in different vascular territories. There are many causes of intracranial vasculitis, both autoimmune and infectious. CT and especially MRI can strongly suggest the diagnosis in conjunction with the clinical history, but a cerebral angiogram is generally required for confirmation. The angiographic findings in intracranial vasculitis range from normal to demonstration of focal concentric narrowings, most prominent in the more distal vasculature. This appearance may mimic the vasospasm of SAH, but the clinical history distinguishes the two entities. Cerebral angiography is important in confirming the diagnosis of vasculitis before a patient is subjected to long-term corticosteroid and cytotoxic therapies with their potential side effects. In rare cases, angiography may be unrevealing because of vasculitic changes primarily situated at more diminutive vessel calibers.[64]

Another benefit of cerebral angiography in suspected vasculitis is that the external carotid artery can be injected as part of the procedure so that a superficial temporal artery biopsy can be planned, if it is indicated to aid in diagnosis.

Takayasu's arteritis involves the proximal segments of the supra-aortic arteries. Its angiographic appearance is shown in Figure 49-34.

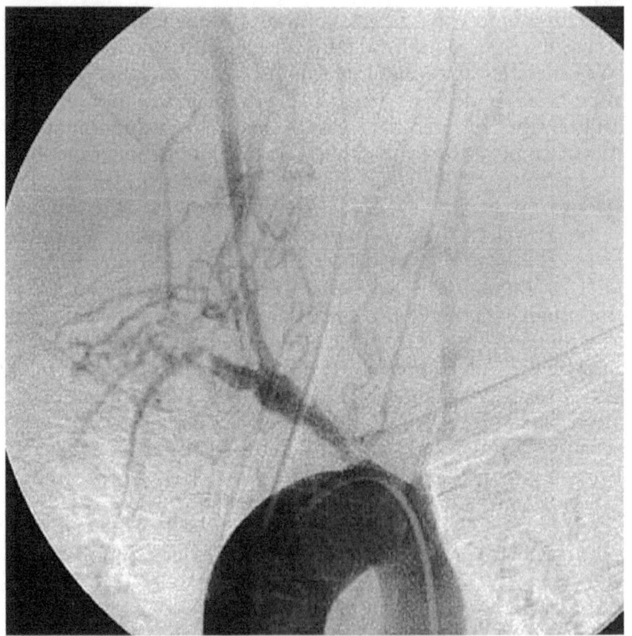

Figure 49-34. Aortic arch injection demonstrating multiple large vessel tandem stenoses in Takayasu's arteritis. Notice how poorly the arch vessels are opacifying secondary to stenoses at vessel origins.

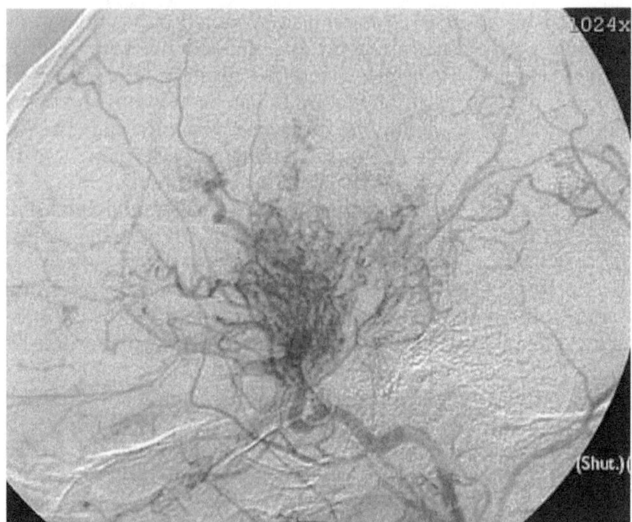

Figure 49-35. Internal carotid artery injection, lateral projection, demonstrating absence of the normal vasculature and a "puff of smoke" appearance to the distribution of opacification.

Fibromuscular Dysplasia

Fibromuscular dysplasia is a vasculopathy of medium-sized arteries, with a prevalence of 0.5–0.7%.[65,66] This entity affects the cervical and intracranial vasculature. Most lesions occur at the C1–C2 level and spare the proximal aspect of the supra-aortic arteries.[65] The diagnosis is often made incidentally on cerebral angiography performed for diagnosis of intracranial aneurysm or dissection, both of which are often associated with fibromuscular dysplasia. The characteristic angiographic finding is alternation of dilated and stenosed regions to give a "string of beads" appearance or, alternatively, a long tubular stenosis.

Moyamoya Syndrome

Moyamoya disease is a condition named for its cerebral angiographic appearance – *moya moya* is the Japanese word for "puff of smoke." The cloudlike collateral networks of vessels in moyamoya disease are multiple small channels formed in response to the chronic occlusive vasculopathy affecting large arteries at the base of the brain, mainly the distal internal carotid artery (see Chapter 35). Moyamoya disease can produce both ischemic and hemorrhagic strokes; cerebral infarcts predominate in children, and hemorrhagic and ischemic events are relatively equally common in adults. Among the pathologic concomitants of this disease are aneurysms and AVMs, which were detected in 11% of patients reported by Chiu et al.[67] Moyamoya syndrome has recently been characterized in reports from Europe and North America, offering insight on this rare disorder.[68,69]

The diagnosis of moyamoya syndrome may be suspected from MRI or MRA findings. Cerebral angiography is required, however, for confirmation, precise anatomic depiction, and study of the external carotid circulation to guide revascularization therapy. The angiographic findings consist of bilateral stenotic occlusive disease in the intracranial internal carotid artery with thin multiple collateral vessels (Fig. 49-35). The angiographic changes occur idiopathically in moyamoya disease but also in response to stenosing vasculopathy from diverse identified causes (moyamoya syndrome), including radiation vasculopathy, Down's syndrome, and early-onset intracranial atherosclerosis.

Cerebral Arterial Vasospasm

Arterial vasospasm of the intracranial arteries after SAH has an associated 15–20% risk of mortality (see Chapter 40).[71] Vasospasm is most common between 3 and 10 days after SAH. It is the principal cause of death and disability once the aneurysm has been secured by clipping or coiling. The diagnosis of vasospasm is generally suspected from clinical findings as well as transcranial Doppler ultrasonography, but confirmation usually requires a cerebral angiogram. Admission angiographic cerebral circulation time may be used to predict subsequent angiographic vasospasm after aneurysmal SAH.[72] Patients with symptomatic vasospasm despite adequate medical management, including hypertensive–hypervolemic therapy, are usually candidates for urgent cerebral angiography and angioplasty (balloon and/or chemical). In a patient with vasospasm, angiography shows narrowing of the vessels in a single or multiple regions. Spasm in the proximal intracranial arteries may be amenable to balloon angioplasty, and more distal spasm may be treated with intra-arterial injection of papaverine or nicardipine.[73]

Cerebral Venous Thrombosis

Cerebral venous thrombosis refers to the occlusion of the cerebral veins or sinuses by thrombus (see Chapter 28). The superior sagittal sinus is affected in 72% of cases, and the lateral sinuses are affected in 70%.[74] Multiple predisposing factors are associated with cerebral venous thrombosis, and a predisposing factor is identified in as many as 80% of cases.[74] Among these factors are intracranial infection, sepsis, brain surgery, tumor, hormonal causes, puerperium, oral contraceptives, hypercoagulable states, and dehydration. The clinical scenario is often one of slow progression of symptoms. Initial symptoms are generally non-specific. A headache is the most common presenting symptom. Additional common symptoms are papilledema, vomiting, seizures, and focal neurologic deficits. CT or MRI findings often suggest the diagnosis.

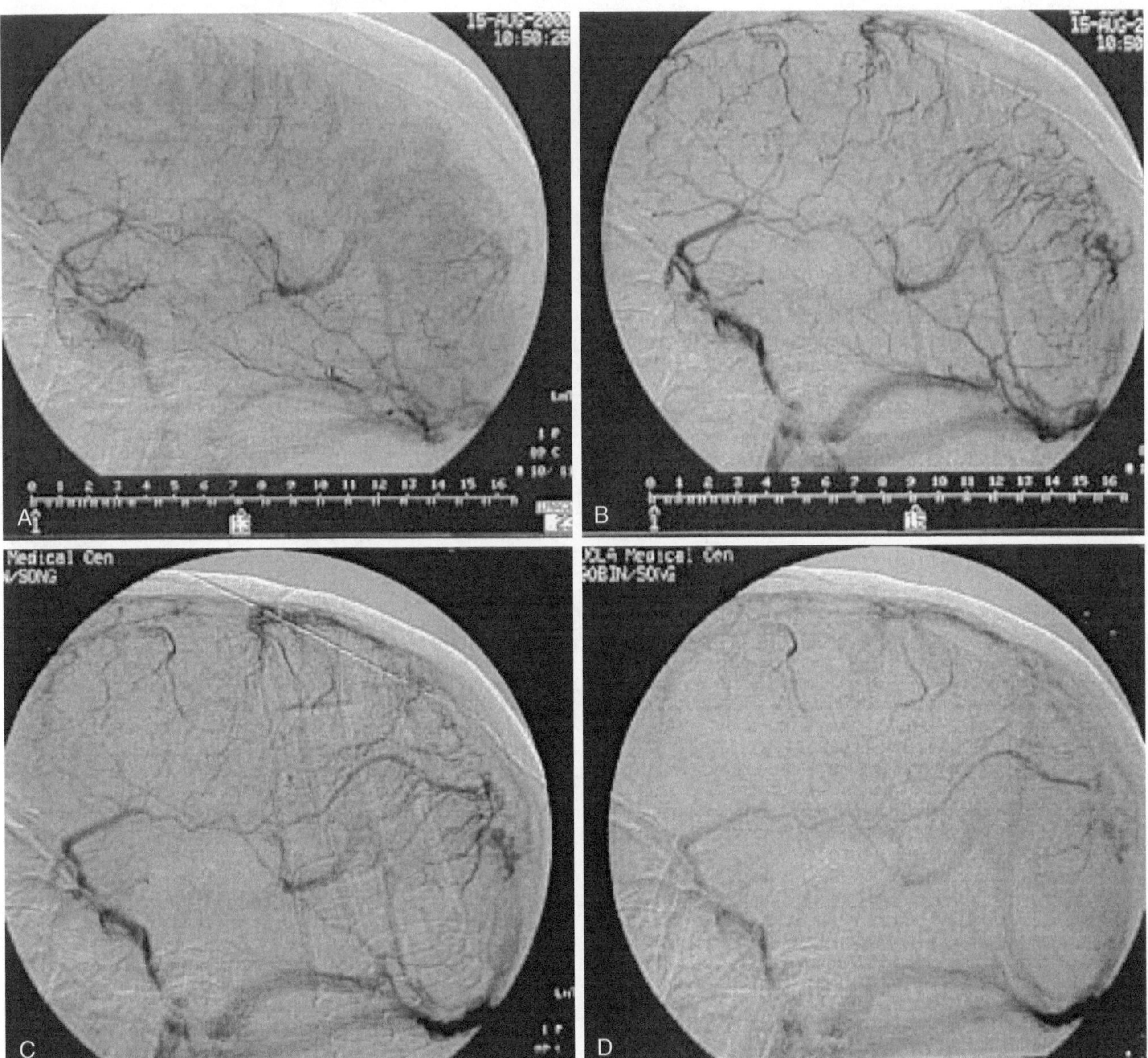

Figure 49-36. A–D, Lateral view of entire venous phase demonstrating no significant opacification of the superior sagittal sinus. (Images are a sequence of the "venous phase" – A being earlier than D.)

The angiographic appearance of cerebral venous thrombosis is characteristically seen in the venous phase of the imaging sequence. There is no (or little) opacification of the thrombosed sinus. A long arterial injection as well as a long imaging time must be used so as to give the venous system an adequate chance to opacify. Anteroposterior (AP), lateral, and oblique views should be obtained. Oblique imaging is very valuable because often the entire sinus cannot be shown on the lateral view, and the anterior and posterior aspects of the sinus overlap on a true AP view. Imaging of superior sagittal sinus thrombosis is shown in Figure 49-36.

Anticoagulation is usually the first treatment attempted for cerebral venous thrombosis. If the patient's symptoms progress or there is no improvement over time, local catheter-guided pharmacologic or mechanical thrombolysis can be considered.

Idiopathic Intracranial Hypertension

Idiopathic intracranial hypertension (IIH) or *pseudotumor cerebri* is an entity clinically characterized by headache, visual changes, pulsatile tinnitus, papilledema, and increased CSF pressure by lumbar puncture. Various etiologies have been hypothesized including arachnoid granulation abnormalities and venous sinus stenosis. Dural venous sinus stenosis has been demonstrated in 30–93% of patients with IIH demonstrated by various imaging techniques including cerebral angiography. Permanent visual loss and optic nerve atrophy are potential long-term sequelae of inadequately or insufficiently treated disease. The mainstay of therapy has been treatment with carbonic anhydrase inhibitors, diuretics or therapeutic lumbar puncture(s). In resistant cases optic nerve sheath fenestration and/or CSF diversion have been utilized. Cerebral angiography has been employed with placement of stents across stenotic vessels with a complication rate of 6% in a combined cohort of 143 patients. Major complications consisted primarily of subdural hematoma. Improvement in headache occurred in 88% and 97% had improvement or resolution of papilledema were reported.[79,80]

Brain Death

The diagnosis of brain death rarely requires a cerebral angiogram. The use of an invasive test for the diagnosis of brain death is regarded as problematic in some countries. If confirmatory laboratory tests are needed to supplement clinical findings, a diagnosis can be established with the use of nuclear medicine, electrophysiology, transcranial Doppler ultrasonography, and other non-invasive methods. Multimodal CT, including CTA and CT perfusion, has recently been studied and holds promise as a potential rapid alternative for diagnosis of brain death.[75–78] For brain death to be diagnosed on cerebral angiography, there should be no contrast opacification of intracranial vessels after injection of contrast agent into the brachiocephalic vasculature. The shutdown of the entire cerebral circulation reflects increased intracranial pressure due to brain swelling.[70]

REFERENCES

1. Wolpert SM. Neuroradiology classics. AJNR Am J Neuroradiol 1999;20:1752–3.
2. Rosenbaum AE, Eldevik OP, Mani JR, et al. In re: Amundsen P. Cerebral angiography via the femoral artery with particular reference to cerebrovascular disease. Acta Neurol Scand 1967; (Suppl 31):115. AJNR Am J Neuroradiol 2001;22:584–9.
3. Jayaraman MV. Cerebral angiography: not yet ready to join the dinosaurs. AJNR Am J Neuroradiol 2013;34:840.
4. Sawiris N, Venizelos A, Ouyang B, et al. Current utility of diagnostic catheter cerebral angiography. J Stroke Cerebrovasc Dis 2014;23:e145–50.
5. Qureshi AI, Abou-Chebl A, Jovin TG. Qualification requirements for performing neurointerventional procedures: A Report of the Practice Guidelines Committee of the American Society of Neuroimaging and the Society of Vascular and Interventional Neurology. J Neuroimaging 2008;18:433–47.
6. Geyik S, Yavuz K, Akgoz A, et al. The safety and efficacy of the Angio-Seal closure device in diagnostic and interventional neuroangiography setting: A single-center experience with 1,443 closures. Neuroradiology 2007;49:739–46.
7. Ahmed AS, Deuerling-Zheng Y, Strother CM, et al. Impact of intra-arterial injection parameters on arterial, capillary, and venous time-concentration curves in a canine model. AJNR Am J Neuroradiol 2009;30:1337–41.
8. Dion JE, Gates PC, Fox AJ, et al. Clinical events following neuroangiography: A prospective study. Stroke 1987;18:997–1004.
9. Leffers AM, Wagner A. Neurologic complications of cerebral angiography. A retrospective study of complication rate and patient risk factors. Acta Radiol 2000;41:204–10.
10. Chohan MO, Sandoval D, Buchan A, et al. Cranial radiation exposure during cerebral catheter angiography. J Neurointerv Surg 2014;6:633–6.
11. Quality improvement guidelines for adult diagnostic neuroangiography: Cooperative study between the ASNR, ASITN, and the SCVIR. American Society of Neuroradiology. American Society of Interventional and Therapeutic Neuroradiology. Society of Cardiovascular and Interventional Radiology. AJNR Am J Neuroradiol 2000;21:146–50.
12. Frontera JA, Pile-Spellman J, Mohr JP. Contrast-induced neurotoxicity and selective cortical injury. Cerebrovasc Dis 2007;24: 148–51.
13. Gil-Gouveia R, Fernandes Sousa R, Lopes L, et al. Headaches during angiography and endovascular procedures. J Neurol 2007; 254:591–6.
14. Gil-Gouveia RS, Sousa RF, Lopes L. Post-angiography headaches. J Headache Pain 2008;9:327–30.
15. Guimaraens L, Vivas E, Fonnegra A, et al. Transient encephalopathy from angiographic contrast: a rare complication in neurointerventional procedures. Cardiovasc Intervent Radiol 2010; 33:383–8.
16. Kochanowicz J, Lewszuk A, Kordecki K. Diagnostic cerebral angiography affects the tonus of the major cerebral arteries. Med Sci Monit 2007;13(Suppl. 1):55–8.
17. Bridcut RR, Murphy E, Workman A. Patient dose from 3D rotational neurovascular studies. Br J Radiol 2007;80:362–6.
18. Khatri P, Broderick JP, Khoury JC. Microcatheter contrast injections during intra-arterial thrombolysis may increase intracranial hemorrhage risk. Stroke 2008;39:3283–7.
19. Kaufmann TJ, Huston J 3rd, Mandrekar JN, et al. Complications of diagnostic cerebral angiography: evaluation of 19,826 consecutive patients. Radiology 2007;243:812–19.
20. Hankey GJ, Warlow CP, Sellar RJ. Cerebral angiographic risk in mild cerebrovascular disease. Stroke 1990;21:209–22.
21. Fifi JT, Meyers PM, Lavine SD, et al. Complications of modern diagnostic cerebral angiography in an academic medical center. J Vasc Interv Radiol 2009;20:442–7.
22. Thiex R, Norbash AM, Frerichs KU. The safety of dedicated-team catheter-based diagnostic cerebral angiography in the era of advanced noninvasive imaging. AJNR Am J Neuroradiol 2010;31: 230–4.
23. Hussain SI, Wolfe TJ, Lynch JR. Diagnostic cerebral angiography: The interventional neurology perspective. J Neuroimaging 2010; 20:251–4.
24. Sato M, Nakai Y, Tsurushima H, et al. Risk factors of ischemic lesions related to cerebral angiography and neuro-interventional procedures. Neurol Med Chir (Tokyo) 2013;53(6):381–7. PubMed PMID:23803616.
25. Gerraty RP, Bowser DN, Infeld B. Microemboli during carotid angiography. Association with stroke risk factors or subsequent magnetic resonance imaging changes? Stroke 1996;27:1543–7.
26. Gupta R, Vora N, Thomas A, et al. Symptomatic cerebral air embolism during neuro-angiographic procedures: Incidence and problem avoidance. Neurocrit Care 2007;7:241–6.
27. Bendszus M, Koltzenburg M, Burger R, et al. Silent embolism in diagnostic cerebral angiography and neurointerventional procedures: A prospective study. Lancet 1999;354:1594–7.
28. Cloft HJ, Joseph GJ, Dion JE. Risk of cerebral angiography in patients with subarachnoid hemorrhage, cerebral aneurysm, and arteriovenous malformation: A meta-analysis. Stroke 1999;30: 317–20.
29. Kelkar PS, Fleming JB, Walters BC, et al. Infection risk in neurointervention and cerebral angiography. Neurosurgery 2013; 72(3):327–31. PubMed PMID:23151621.
30. Hassan AE, Hussain MS, Chowdhury F, et al. Changes in serum calcium levels associated with catheter-based cerebral angiography. J Neuroimaging 2007;17:336–8.
31. van Gijn J, Rinkel GJ. Subarachnoid haemorrhage: Diagnosis, causes and management. Brain 2001;124:249–78.
32. Ruigrok YM, Rinkel GJ, Buskens E. Perimesencephalic hemorrhage and CT angiography: A decision analysis. Stroke 2000;31: 2976–83.
33. Huttner HB, Hartmann M, Kohrmann M, et al. Repeated digital subtraction angiography after perimesencephalic subarachnoid hemorrhage? J Neuroradiol 2006;33:87–9.
34. Pedicelli A, Rollo M, Di Lella GM, et al. 3D rotational angiography for the diagnosis and preoperative assessment of intracranial aneurysms: Preliminary experience. Radiol Med 2007;112: 895–905.
35. van Rooij WJ, Peluso JP, Sluzewski M, et al. Additional value of 3D rotational angiography in angiographically negative aneurysmal subarachnoid hemorrhage: How negative is negative? AJNR Am J Neuroradiol 2008;29:962–6.
36. van Rooij WJ, Sprengers ME, de Gast AN. 3D rotational angiography: The new gold standard in the detection of additional intracranial aneurysms. AJNR Am J Neuroradiol 2008;29: 976–9.
37. Ishihara H, Kato S, Akimura T, et al. Angiogram-negative subarachnoid hemorrhage in the era of three dimensional rotational angiography. J Clin Neurosci 2007;14:252–5.
38. Delgado Almandoz JE, Crandall BM, Fease JL, et al. Diagnostic yield of catheter angiography in patients with subarachnoid

hemorrhage and negative initial noninvasive neurovascular examinations. AJNR Am J Neuroradiol 2013;34:833–9.
39. Ringer AJ, Lanzino G, Veznedaroglu E, et al. Does angiographic surveillance pose a risk in the management of coiled intracranial aneurysms? A multicenter study of 2243 patients. Neurosurgery 2008;63:845–9, discussion 849.
40. Wolfe TJ, Hussain SI, Lynch JR. Pediatric cerebral angiography: Analysis of utilization and findings. Pediatr Neurol 2009;40: 98–101.
41. Liebeskind DS. Location, location, location: Angiography discerns early MR imaging vessel signs due to proximal arterial occlusion and distal collateral flow. AJNR Am J Neuroradiol 2005; 26:2432–3.
42. Sanossian N, Saver JL, Alger JR, et al. Angiography reveals that fluid-attenuated inversion recovery vascular hyperintensities are due to slow flow, not thrombus. AJNR Am J Neuroradiol 2009;30:564–8.
43. Chimowitz MI, Lynn MJ, Howlett-Smith H, et al. Comparison of warfarin and aspirin for symptomatic intracranial arterial stenosis. N Engl J Med 2005;352:1305–16.
44. Kasner SE, Lynn MJ, Chimowitz MI, et al. Warfarin vs aspirin for symptomatic intracranial stenosis: Subgroup analyses from WASID. Neurology 2006;67:1275–8.
45. Feldmann E, Wilterdink JL, Kosinski A, et al. The Stroke Outcomes and Neuroimaging of Intracranial Atherosclerosis (SONIA) trial. Neurology 2007;68:2099–106.
46. Samuels OB, Joseph GJ, Lynn MJ. A standardized method for measuring intracranial arterial stenosis. AJNR Am J Neuroradiol 2000;21:643–6.
47. Gobin YP, Starkman S, Duckwiler GR, et al. MERCI 1: A phase 1 study of mechanical embolus removal in cerebral ischemia. Stroke 2004;35:2848–54.
48. Smith WS, Sung G, Saver J, et al. Mechanical thrombectomy for acute ischemic stroke: Final results of the Multi MERCI trial. Stroke 2008;39:1205–12.
49. Smith WS, Sung G, Starkman S, et al. Safety and efficacy of mechanical embolectomy in acute ischemic stroke: Results of the MERCI trial. Stroke 2005;36:1432–8.
50. The Penumbra Pivotal Stroke Trial: safety and effectiveness of a new generation of mechanical devices for clot removal in intracranial large vessel occlusive disease. Stroke 2009;40:2761–8.
51. Bose A, Henkes H, Alfke K, et al. The Penumbra System: a mechanical device for the treatment of acute stroke due to thromboembolism. AJNR Am J Neuroradiol 2008;29:1409–13.
52. Brekenfeld C, Schroth G, Mattle HP, et al. Stent placement in acute cerebral artery occlusion: Use of a self-expandable intracranial stent for acute stroke treatment. Stroke 2009;40:847–52.
53. Levy EI, Mehta R, Gupta R, et al. Self-expanding stents for recanalization of acute cerebrovascular occlusions. AJNR Am J Neuroradiol 2007;28:816–22.
54. Levy EI, Siddiqui AH, Crumlish A, et al. First Food and Drug Administration-approved prospective trial of primary intracranial stenting for acute stroke: SARIS (stent-assisted recanalization in acute ischemic stroke). Stroke 2009;40:3552–6.
55. Yoo AJ, Simonsen CZ, Prabhakaran S, et al. Refining angiographic biomarkers of revascularization: improving outcome prediction after intra-arterial therapy. Stroke 2013;44:2509–12.
56. Zaidat OO, Yoo AJ, Khatri P, et al. Recommendations on angiographic revascularization grading standards for acute ischemic stroke: a consensus statement. Stroke 2013;44:2650–63.
57. Qureshi AI, Alkawi A, Hussein HM, et al. Angiographic analysis of intravascular thrombus volume in patients with acute ischemic stroke. J Endovasc Ther 2007;14:475–82.
58. Qureshi AI, Hussein HM, Abdelmoula M. Subacute recanalization and reocclusion in patients with acute ischemic stroke following endovascular treatment. Neurocrit Care 2009;10:195–203.
59. Liebeskind DS. Collateral circulation. Stroke 2003;34:2279–84.
60. Liebeskind DS. Collaterals in acute stroke: Beyond the clot. Neuroimaging Clin N Am 2005;15:553–73.
61. Tomsick T. Timi, TIBI, TICI: I came, I saw, I got confused. AJNR Am J Neuroradiol 2007;28:382–4.
62. Higashida RT, Furlan AJ, Roberts H, et al. Trial design and reporting standards for intra-arterial cerebral thrombolysis for acute ischemic stroke. Stroke 2003;34:e109–37.
63. Eddleman CS, Jeong HJ, Hurley MC, et al. 4D radial acquisition contrast-enhanced MR angiography and intracranial arteriovenous malformations: Quickly approaching digital subtraction angiography. Stroke 2009;40:2749–53.
64. Salvarani C, Brown RD Jr, Calamia KT, et al. Angiography-negative primary central nervous system vasculitis: A syndrome involving small cerebral vessels. Medicine (Baltimore) 2008;87: 264–71.
65. Kubis N, Von Langsdorff D, Petitjean C, et al. Thrombotic carotid megabulb: Fibromuscular dysplasia, septae, and ischemic stroke. Neurology 1999;52:883–6.
66. Finsterer J, Strassegger J, Haymerle A, et al. Bilateral stenting of symptomatic and asymptomatic internal carotid artery stenosis due to fibromuscular dysplasia. J Neurol Neurosurg Psychiatry 2000;69:683–6.
67. Chiu D, Shedden P, Bratina P, et al. Clinical features of moyamoya disease in the United States. Stroke 1998;29:1347–51.
68. Kraemer M, Heienbrok W, Berlit P. Moyamoya disease in Europeans. Stroke 2008;39:3193–200.
69. Hallemeier CL, Rich KM, Grubb RL Jr, et al. Clinical features and outcome in North American adults with moyamoya phenomenon. Stroke 2006;37:1490–6.
70. Chakraborty S, Kenny SA, Adas RA. The use of dynamic computed tomographic angiography ancillary to the diagnosis of brain death. Can Assoc Radiol J 2013;64(3):253–7. PubMed PMID: 23149045.
71. Lysakowski C, Walder B, Costanza MC, et al. Transcranial Doppler versus angiography in patients with vasospasm due to a ruptured cerebral aneurysm: A systematic review. Stroke 2001;32: 2292–8.
72. Udoetuk JD, Stiefel MF, Hurst RW. Admission angiographic cerebral circulation time may predict subsequent angiographic vasospasm after aneurysmal subarachnoid hemorrhage. Neurosurgery 2007;61:1152–9, discussion 1159–61.
73. Linfante I, Delgado-Mederos R, Andreone V, et al. Angiographic and hemodynamic effect of high concentration of intra-arterial nicardipine in cerebral vasospasm. Neurosurgery 2008;63:1080–6, discussion 1086–7.
74. Allroggen H, Abbott RJ. Cerebral venous sinus thrombosis. Postgrad Med J 2000;76:12–15.
75. Escudero D, Otero J, Marques L, et al. Diagnosing brain death by CT perfusion and multislice CT angiography. Neurocrit Care 2009;11:261–71.
76. Frampas E, Videcoq M, de Kerviler E, et al. CT angiography for brain death diagnosis. AJNR Am J Neuroradiol 2009;30: 1566–70.
77. Greer DM, Strozyk D, Schwamm LH. False positive CT angiography in brain death. Neurocrit Care 2009;11:272–5.
78. Quesnel C, Fulgencio JP, Adrie C, et al. Limitations of computed tomographic angiography in the diagnosis of brain death. Intensive Care Med 2007;33:2129–35.
79. Puffer RC, Mustafa W, Lanzino G. Venous sinus stenting for idiopathic intracranial hypertension: a review of the literature. J Neurointerv Surg 2013;5:483–6.
80. Fields JD, Javedani PP, Falardeau J, et al. Dural venous sinus angioplasty and stenting for the treatment of idiopathic intracranial hypertension. J Neurointerv Surg 2013;5:62–8.

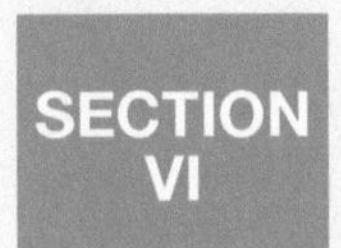

Therapy

PART A Medical Therapy

James C. Grotta

The treatment of acute stroke begins with prehospital management, before the neurologist is even involved, including the extremely important contributions of EMS services, the emergence of stroke centers, the exciting prospect of Mobile Stroke Units, and the role of emergency medicine. Since the chapter by Gensic and Pancioli was written, more data have been published from the Get With the Guidelines consortium suggesting better clinical outcomes with tPA treatment in the first hour after stroke onset compared to later treatment, and additional data from the Berlin group and from Houston and Cleveland in the U.S. that such ultra-early treatment is possible using Mobile Stroke Units. Further studies of the long term benefits and cost of the concept of pre-hospital treatment of stroke are needed and are underway.

The various aspects of intravenous thrombolysis are then covered in detail, including a review of thrombolytic agents, clinical trial data pertaining to benefits and risks, community experience, guidelines, and, finally, practical tips. In response to the publication of important clinical trial experience, endovascular treatment has now been moved to its own separate section. Be sure to read Dr Broderick's introduction for review of the latest studies.

Specialized care in stroke units and intensive care units is addressed with emphasis on the effectiveness and components of each. Details of good ICU care are reviewed with attention to correcting disturbed physiology and treatment of specific stroke syndromes. The possibility of reversing the pathologic cascade of injury at the cellular level is followed by a detailed review of neuroprotective agents, with an eye on how to finally establish the utility of such therapy.

Treatment of specific stroke conditions (e.g., dissection and venous thrombosis) is covered with an emphasis on what is known and where new information is needed, as well as selection of patients for surgical intervention.

The emerging scientific inquiry and evidence surrounding stroke recovery is expanded with chapters on rehabilitation and its outcomes, a new chapter on interventions to improve recovery such as robotics, brain stimulation, and telerehabilitation, and an updated chapter on cell-based treatment.

The topic of secondary prevention begins with a detailed review of platelet physiology in stroke, the mechanism of various antiplatelet agents and choices among them based on clinical trial data, and new antiplatelet strategies. Cardioembolic stroke and its prevention are then covered in detail including discussion of direct thrombin and factor Xa inhibitors, as is treatment to modify important risk factors such as blood pressure and cholesterol and the selection of patients for carotid intervention.

The section concludes with a rewritten review covering important aspects of designing, conducting, and analyzing clinical research studies in stroke prevention and treatment.

SECTION VI Therapy

PART A Medical Therapy

50 Prehospital and Emergency Department Care of the Patient with Acute Stroke

Anna Gensic, Arthur Pancioli

KEY POINTS

- The primary focus of the prehospital and emergency department care of the stroke patient is facilitating rapid diagnosis and initiation of treatment.
- Stroke symptom onset to first medical contact is the largest component of treatment delay in the stroke patient, which may be decreased if patients and family members understand that stroke is a serious and treatable disease process, and activate emergency medical services (EMS) immediately.
- EMS should be dispatched at the highest level of priority for potential stroke patients, to minimize both prehospital and emergency department (ED) delays.
- Patients with a potential stroke should be transported immediately to the nearest stroke center, bypassing non-stroke-certified hospitals if at all feasible.
- EMS should provide advance notification of a potential stroke patient en route to the ED, to allow mobilization of resources prior to the patient's arrival.
- Concurrently with management of the patient's ABCs, rapid neurologic evaluation and intracranial imaging should be performed as rapidly as possible upon arrival.
- Multidisciplinary clinical pathways should be in place to identify and treat potential thrombolysis candidates as rapidly as possible.
- Management of intracranial hemorrhage (ICH) and subarachnoid hemorrhage (SAH) in the ED consists primarily of supportive care and prevention of complications, with little evidence-based guidance for blood pressure management or other medical therapies.

Optimal care of patients with acute stroke depends on rapid recognition of symptoms by the patient or bystanders in the prehospital setting, activation of emergency medical services (EMS), and transport to a hospital capable of delivering state-of-the-art acute stroke care 24 hours a day. Table 50-1 lays out the 2010 advanced cardiac life support stroke chain of survival,[1] which emphasizes the critical importance of prehospital and emergency department (ED) actions in the optimal care of the acute stroke patient. This chapter addresses the roles that prehospital care providers and ED teams play in the evaluation and management of patients with acute stroke.

The EMS community and ED team are vital in the evaluation and management of patients with acute stroke. In 2004, the American Heart Association/American Stroke Association (AHA/ASA) convened a taskforce on the development of stroke systems. That taskforce determined that the approach to care in many systems across the United States was fragmented and that this uneven approach may contribute to stroke morbidity and mortality, and identified the prehospital and ED phases of care as key components within stroke care.[2] Subsequently, an ASA expert panel was convened and issued specific recommendations for optimizing prehospital care of the stroke patient within the larger system of stroke care.[3] These recommendations and potential solutions addressed the specific components necessary for the rapid identification and transportation of stroke patients, facilitating appropriate management and seamless transitions of care. The panel included a recommendation that patients should be transported to the nearest stroke center for evaluation and care if a stroke center is located within a reasonable transport distance and transport time. This recommendation was reiterated in the 2013 AHA/ASA guidelines for the early management of patients with acute ischemic stroke.[4]

This point should be particularly emphasized as it could have implications for regional practices, whereby, as in the case of trauma victims and trauma centers, a closer hospital may be bypassed so that a stroke patient may be better served, evaluated, and treated at a certified stroke center. It may also entail crossing state lines. Given the time-sensitive nature of acute stroke treatment, preexisting systems should facilitate the appropriate prehospital and ED care of stroke patients. Examples of a systematic approach improving care are seen in two subsequent prospective cohort studies that used historical controls, in two different Australian communities; implementation of a prehospital stroke triage protocol that included bypass of non-stroke center hospitals improved thrombolytic

TABLE 50-1 Stroke Chain of Survival

Detection	Patient or bystander recognition of stroke signs and symptoms
Dispatch	Immediate activation of 9-1-1 and priority EMS dispatch
Delivery	Prompt triage and transport to most appropriate stroke hospital and prehospital notification
Door	Immediate ED triage to high-acuity area
Data	Prompt ED evaluation, stroke team activation, laboratory studies, and brain imaging
Decision	Diagnosis and determination of most appropriate therapy; discussion with patient and family
Drug	Administration of appropriate drugs or other interventions
Disposition	Timely admission to stroke unit, intensive care unit, or transfer

administration among stroke patients from 4.7% to 21.4%,[5] and from 7% to 19%,[6] respectively.

THE COURSE OF EVENTS FOR THE ACUTE STROKE PATIENT

Speed and efficiency of initial management, diagnosis, and communication are significant components of the contribution to acute stroke care provided by prehospital and ED teams. The major components in the evaluation and treatment process of patients with acute stroke can be divided into prehospital and ED phases, as follows.

Prehospital Components

1. Recognition of stroke symptoms by the patient or family members
2. First contact with medical care (for example, phoning 911 in the United States)
3. Dispatch of appropriate level of prehospital care providers
4. Prehospital evaluation, management, and transport
5. Prehospital identification of stroke
6. Prehospital notification of pending ED arrival.

Emergency Department

1. ED triage
2. ED evaluation and management
3. Divergence of pathway according to whether stroke is ischemic or hemorrhagic
4. Disposition of patient from the ED.

The single largest component of the delay between symptom onset and definitive therapy exists between symptom onset and arrival at the ED. In a recent evaluation of the Get With The Guidelines–Stroke national database, from 2002 to 2009, only 25.1% of stroke patients arrived to the ED in less than 3 hours after symptom onset, with only an additional 10.7% arriving from 3 to 8 hours after onset.[7] Thus, it is clear that the prehospital times must be decreased if the number of patients eligible for immediate therapy is to be improved.

RECOGNITION OF STROKE SYMPTOMS BY THE PATIENT OR FAMILY MEMBERS

Possibly the largest component in the prehospital delay is failure of the patient or family members to recognize stroke symptoms and act accordingly. In recognition of this, the AHA recently issued a statement that summarizes the issues relating to delayed presentation in acute stroke and offered some suggestions for further study regarding approaches for minimizing prehospital delay.[8] Factors that have been shown to be associated with delay in arrival at the ED are as follows:[9-16]

- The patient (or family member) initially phones the primary care physician instead of the local emergency service phone number.
- The patient lives alone.
- Stroke begins while the patient is asleep.
- Symptoms appear while the patient is at home versus at work.
- The stroke is mild rather than severe.

Similar factors have been associated with pre-hospital delay in numerous international studies on the subject, as well.[17-27]

In addition, stroke often damages the areas of the brain that control either the patient's perception of a problem or the patient's ability to communicate. In a population-based study in Corpus Christi, Texas, only 4.3% of stroke patients who utilized EMS activated EMS themselves.[28] Similar studies have shown that, in all cases of stroke, whether EMS is utilized or not, someone other than the patient makes the decision regarding when and how to seek treatment 66–80% of the time.[18,26]

The major reasons for time-to-treatment delay appear to be the lack of recognition of stroke signs and symptoms and the lack of a proper response. This lack of knowledge of the warning signs of and risk factors in stroke was quantified in a large telephone survey in the greater Cincinnati, Ohio, area in 1995.[29] That survey assessed the level of stroke knowledge within a population whose demographics matched those of patients with acute stroke. Using open-ended questions, the researchers in this study found that only 57% of the respondents were able to name even one warning sign of stroke. Similarly, only 68% could name even one risk factor for stroke. The survey was repeated in 2000 within the same community and with the identical methodology to both reassess the level of stroke knowledge and look for incremental change in the overall level of stroke knowledge in the public.[30] The researchers found an increase in the public knowledge of stroke warning signs, in that 70% of respondents in the 2000 survey were able to name at least one stroke warning sign. Although this survey population had a slightly higher number of respondents who described themselves as having at least "some college," which may account for the increase in knowledge of stroke warning signs, there was no change in the percentage of respondents who could name one risk factor. Other recent studies in the US and in Europe have found that 50–78% of people are able to correctly name at least one warning sign of stroke.[17,26,31]

In recognition of the lack of public knowledge and understanding of stroke warning signs and risk factors, a number of public education campaigns have been launched in hopes of improving community awareness, including the American Stroke Association's Power to End Stroke Campaign, the National Stroke Association's Act FAST campaign, and local projects such as the Beauty Shop Stroke Education Project,[32] the "Hip-hop" Stroke project,[33] and the Kids Identifying and Defeating Stroke project.[34]

Unfortunately, however, a significant portion of the general public still has minimal knowledge and understanding of stroke warning signs and risk factors. Moreover, numerous studies have found that there is strikingly little association between knowledge of stroke symptoms and activation of EMS in the case of a potential or suspected stroke.[17,18,25,35,36] In a 2010 comparison study of two matched counties in Montana, one county was exposed to an intensive 20-week public education campaign involving paid advertisements in multiple mass-media formats. Telephone surveys conducted before and after the intervention period revealed that, while the intervention county showed a significant improvement regarding knowledge of stroke symptoms after the campaign, there was no significant change in the proportion of respondents who would call 911 if they thought that someone was having a stroke.[37]

Similarly, in a nationwide survey of the Czech Republic,[17] knowledge of stroke was relatively good, with 78% of respondents able to name at least one warning sign of stroke, and 60% able to state that stroke is caused by an occlusion of a brain artery. However, even the most typical stroke symptoms of unilateral weakness and speech impairment only prompted 44% of respondents to call 911. Interestingly, however, people who knew that stroke is a serious and treatable disease were about twice as likely to call 911. It appears that the activation of EMS for stroke-like symptoms is not driven primarily by knowledge of those symptoms, but by an understanding of the seriousness and treatability of stroke. In future public awareness campaigns, a focus on the time-dependent nature of the treatment of stroke may be more successful in changing behavior in the community.

FIRST CONTACT WITH MEDICAL CARE

In the US, the EMS system is the point of first medical contact for about half of people having acute stroke.[9,10,13,38] In other countries, reported EMS use for acute stroke varies from 18% to 45%.[18,19,21,23,25,39] Although the symptomatology and presentation of many acute strokes are dramatic enough to lead patients or bystanders toward prompt action, less dramatic presentations often lead to significant delay.

Unfortunately, any action other than the immediate activation of the EMS system via 911 or equivalent will lead to significant delays in treatment. The Second Delay in Accessing Stroke Healthcare study (DASH II) was a prospective multicenter study that enrolled 617 patients with suspected stroke.[40] EMS use was found to be associated with decreased prehospital and in-hospital delays to care. Patients who used EMS had a median prehospital delay time of 2.85 hours compared with 4.03 hours for those who did not use EMS ($P = 0.002$). Those who used EMS had significantly shorter times from symptom onset to arrival, time to seeing an emergency physician, time to computed tomography (CT) scan, and time to being seen by a neurologist.[40] In another study, use of the EMS system shortened time to arrival as well as time to treatment in patients with acute stroke. Patients arriving by ambulance were more likely to arrive earlier (OR for arrival within 3 hours, 3.7) than individuals arriving via other modes of transport and were more likely to be seen by a physician within 15 minutes of arrival (OR, 2.3).[41]

In the Get With the Guidelines-Stroke data set, the two most important predictors of onset-to-arrival times of 60 minutes or less are greater NIHSS score and use of EMS.[42] In a statewide registry in Michigan, stroke patients who arrive by EMS are more than twice as likely to arrive within 2 hours of onset as those who do not.[27] In a registry study of young adults with strokes, ages 15–49, from Detroit, 90% of those who arrived by EMS received some form of therapy for their stroke, versus 10% of those who arrived by other means.[43] Thus, it is clear that the use of the EMS system is one critical link in reducing delay to ED arrival for patients with acute stroke.

DISPATCH OF APPROPRIATE LEVEL OF PREHOSPITAL PROVIDERS

Once the EMS-911 system is activated, EMS dispatchers gather initial information and dispatch prehospital care providers. Thus, the first triage by any form of medical provider occurs on receipt of the 911 call. However, dispatcher recognition of potential strokes varies across EMS systems, with dispatchers identifying 52%,[44] 53%,[45] and 83%[46] of strokes in individual studies. In a retrospective review of San Francisco dispatcher performance for acute stroke or TIA calls, dispatchers were able to identify cases as "cerebrovascular accidents" only 31% of the time.[47] Surprisingly, 51% of callers to 911 used the word *stroke* to describe their emergency, but only 48% of the patients for whom *stroke* was used in the 911 call were categorized by dispatchers as having cerebrovascular accidents.

In the majority of cases in this study (59%), ambulances were dispatched at lower priority than they would have been for an identified stroke.[47] Other studies, too, have shown that dispatcher recognition of stroke symptoms improves patient care from the outset, as dispatchers sent ALS ambulances more frequently (84% vs 73%), offered help and instructions to the caller more frequently, and total transport times were decreased when the dispatcher diagnosed/suspected stroke, than when they did not.[45]

This decision about the level of prehospital provider to dispatch to a possible stroke victim is relatively important. One study indicated that advanced life support (ALS) transport might be better suited to the evaluation and transport of potential stroke victims. In that study, up to 29% of patients with acute ischemic stroke required prehospital interventions for treatable medical conditions, including compromised airway and cardiac instability. The patients transported by basic life support units arrived at the hospital earlier (40 ± 1 minutes) than those transported by ALS units staffed by paramedics (45 ± 1 minutes; $P = 0.004$). However, patients transported by ALS units were seen by a physician sooner after arrival at the ED (10 ± 2 minutes) than those who arrived via basic life support units (20 ± 4 minutes; $P = 0.02$). Thus, although the transport times were similar, the level of care for patients transported by ALS teams was higher. In that community, stroke is treated as a level I emergency equivalent to trauma and myocardial infarction.[48] Not all local EMS networks treat stroke as a level I emergency,[2,3] however, a study from Stockholm, Sweden, showed that, when the Emergency Medical Communications Center increased the priority level for patients with a possible stroke from 2 to 1, this resulted in shorter times throughout the chain of care, both pre-hospital and in-hospital, and ultimately led to an increase in thrombolysis rates from 10% to 24%.[49] Current AHA/ASA guidelines recommend that 911 dispatchers should make suspected stroke a priority dispatch, and transport times should be minimized.[4]

A recent AHA/ASA expert panel recommended that prehospital providers, emergency physicians, and stroke experts should collaborate in the development of EMS training, assessment, treatment, and transportation protocols for stroke.[3] This should facilitate education of local providers and appropriate-level dispatch for possible stroke cases.

PREHOSPITAL EVALUATION AND MANAGEMENT

Upon identification of a potential stroke victim, prehospital care providers must begin stabilization of the patient and measures aimed toward diagnosis (Table 50-2).[4] An assessment of the patient's airway, breathing, and circulation (ABCs) with measurement of vital signs and pulse oximetry must be performed, and abnormalities must be addressed. The initial assessment should proceed with application of a cardiac monitor, measurement of the patient's serum glucose level, initiation of intravenous (IV) access, and application of supplemental oxygen. Notably, these measures should be performed during transport of the patient and, unless resuscitative measures are required, should not delay transport.

TABLE 50-2 Guidelines for Prehospital Management of Stroke

Do ...	Do Not ...
Assess and manage ABCs Initiate cardiac monitoring Establish IV access Treat hypotension Give supplemental oxygen to maintain O_2 saturation > 94% Measure blood glucose level and treat accordingly Determine time of symptom onset or last known normal, and obtain family contact information, preferably a cell phone Triage and rapidly transport patient to the nearest most appropriate stroke hospital Prenotify hospital of pending stroke patient arrival	Initiate interventions for hypertension unless directed by medical command Administer excessive IV fluids Administer dextrose without evidence of hypoglycemia Administer medications by mouth (maintain NPO) Delay transport for prehospital interventions

ABC, airway, breathing, and circulation; IV, intravenous; NPO, nothing by mouth.

TABLE 50-3 The Cincinnati Prehospital Stroke Scale*

Facial Droop	Have patient smile or show teeth
Normal	Both sides move equally
Abnormal	One side does not move as well
Arm Drift	Patient closes eyes and holds both arms out
Normal	Both sides move equally
Abnormal	One side does not move as well
Speech	Have patient say "you can't teach an old dog new tricks."
Normal	Patient uses correct words without slurring
Abnormal	Slurs words, uses inappropriate words, or is unable to speak

*Any one or more abnormal findings is suggestive of acute stroke.

One critical component of the prehospital care provider's assessment is to attempt to establish the exact time of onset of the patient's symptoms, as the time that the patient was last known to be normal is the most important piece of information necessary for potential treatment with fibrinolytic therapy. It is also important for EMS to elicit the history of relevant events surrounding the episode, such as trauma, seizure activity, or migraine headache, as well as salient features of the patient's past medical history, including prior stroke, diabetes mellitus, hypertension, or atrial fibrillation, which would increase the likelihood that the patient's symptoms are caused by a stroke. To facilitate decision-making regarding the use of fibrinolysis, it is exceedingly helpful for EMS to either obtain contact information for family members or witnesses, or even to consider transporting a family member along with the patient.[4]

In addition to stabilization and establishing the time that the patient was last known to be normal, prehospital care providers should pay specific attention to the management of blood pressure, fluid status, and glucose level. Interventions to lower blood pressure should not be attempted in the prehospital setting. The differentiation between acute hemorrhagic and acute ischemic stroke requires neurologic imaging and determines the aggressiveness of blood pressure management once the patient is in the ED.

Hypoglycemia is a potential stroke mimic that must be ruled out or treated. Ideally, hypoglycemia can be diagnosed in the prehospital setting by paramedics and other ALS providers. If hypoglycemia is documented and symptoms of stroke are present, administration of 50% dextrose in water is appropriate. Intramuscular glucagon may be given instead of dextrose if there is difficulty obtaining venous access. The severity of the patient's symptoms, the time of glucose administration, and subsequent changes in the patient's clinical status must be documented by the EMS provider. Administration of glucose to a patient with suspected stroke but without documented hypoglycemia should be avoided because elevations of the serum glucose level have been associated with worse outcomes after ischemic stroke.[50-52]

Given this concern, the prehospital administration of IV fluids to the patient with stroke should also be approached with caution. Dextrose-containing fluids, such as 5% dextrose in water, should be administered only to patients with documented hypoglycemia. For resuscitation needs, isotonic crystalloid is the fluid of choice and should be given as needed to appropriately treat the patient with stroke and associated shock.[4]

PREHOSPITAL IDENTIFICATION OF STROKE

Ideally, prehospital providers should be well versed in acute stroke recognition and should quickly initiate protocols for acute stroke.[53] Two tools, the Los Angeles Prehospital Stroke Screen (LAPSS) and the Cincinnati Prehospital Stroke Scale (CPSS), have emerged for use by prehospital care providers to allow for early stroke recognition and communication with hospital-based teams.

The LAPSS was created to be a stroke recognition tool specifically for prehospital care personnel (Fig. 50-1).[54] It is a one-page instrument that takes less than 3 minutes to perform. The LAPSS consists of four history items, three physical examination items, and a serum glucose test. In a prospective validation study of the LAPSS, paramedics identified acute stroke victims with a sensitivity of 91% and a specificity of 97%.[55]

The CPSS is a three-item neurologic examination that was developed to assist prehospital care providers in identifying patients with stroke who may be candidates for thrombolysis (Table 50-3). The CPSS was derived via the selection of the three most sensitive and specific components of the National Institutes of Health Stroke Scale (NIHSS)[56] – facial palsy, arm weakness, and speech abnormality. When performed by a trained physician, this scale has been shown to be effective in identifying such patients. The CPSS can be taught in approximately 10 minutes and performed in less than 1 minute.

The CPSS has also been shown to identify potential stroke victims accurately when performed by prehospital care providers.[57] Correlation for the total score (number of abnormal items) between prehospital care providers and physicians was excellent. The CPSS is valid in identifying patients with stroke (sensitivity, 66%; specificity, 87%), especially anterior circulation stroke (sensitivity, 88%). In the evaluation study, presence of a single abnormality on the CPSS identified all patients with anterior circulation stroke who would have been candidates for thrombolytic therapy. The addition of a test for ataxia to the CPSS would have identified six of the ten patients with posterior circulation stroke who were not identified in this study. However, ataxia is one of the most poorly reproducible items on the NIHSS and is not included in the CPSS.

Both the LAPSS and the CPSS have been widely utilized in and are accepted tools for the EMS community. The LAPSS has greater overall sensitivity but requires slightly more time to perform. The CPSS is rapidly taught and performed but has a lower sensitivity for posterior circulation stroke.

Los Angeles Prehospital Stroke Screen (LAPSS)

1. Patient Name: ______________ ______________
   Last First
2. Information History from:
   [ ] Patient
   [ ] Family Member ______________ ______________
   [ ] Other Name Phone
3. Last known time patient was at baseline or deficit free and awake: Military Time: ________
   Date: ________

SCREENING CRITERIA:

	Yes	Unknown	No
4. Age > 45	[ ]	[ ]	[ ]
5. History of seizures or epilepsy **absent**	[ ]	[ ]	[ ]
6. Symptom duration **less than** 24 hours	[ ]	[ ]	[ ]
7. At baseline, patient is **not** wheelchair bound or bedridden	[ ]	[ ]	[ ]

	Yes	No
8. Blood glucose between 60 and 400:	[ ]	[ ]

9. Exam: **LOOK FOR OBVIOUS ASYMMETRY**

	Normal	Right	Left
Facial Smile/Grimace:	_	_ Droop	_ Droop
Grip:	_	_ Weak Grip _ No Grip	_ Weak Grip _ No Grip
Arm Strength	_	_ Drifts Down _ Falls Rapidly	_ Drifts Down _ Falls Rapidly

	Yes	No
Based on exam, patient has **only unilateral** (and not bilateral) weakness:	[ ]	[ ]
10. **Items 4,5,6,7,8,9 all YES's (or unknown) LAPSS screening criteria met:**	[ ]	[ ]

11. If LAPSS criteria for stroke met, call receiving hospital with a "code stroke"; if not, then return to the Appropriate Treatment Protocol. (Note: the patient may still be experiencing a stroke even if LAPSS criteria are not met.)

Figure 50-1. The Los Angeles Prehospital Stroke Screen. *(From Kidwell CS, Saver JL, Schubert GB, et al: Design and retrospective analysis of the Los Angeles Prehospital Stroke Screen [LAPSS].* Prehosp Emerg Care *2:267–273, 1998.)*

PREHOSPITAL NOTIFICATION OF PENDING EMERGENCY DEPARTMENT ARRIVAL

The use of EMS or advance hospital notification by EMS providers has been associated with decreased arrival to CT times in the ED and increased likelihood of treatment with thrombolytics.[58-63] Thus, to help diminish the time from symptom onset to definitive therapy for a patient with stroke, prehospital care providers can facilitate rapid delivery of therapy via an advance notification call to the patient's destination hospital. Armed with tools such as the LAPSS or CPSS, prehospital care providers can, with good accuracy, make a presumptive diagnosis of acute stroke and set an ED or "stroke team" into motion via advance notification.

Organizations designed to improve stroke care have formally recognized the importance of EMS in systems such as "stroke centers." In a recommendation for the establishment of primary stroke centers, Alberts et al.[64] state, "It is vital that the EMS system be integrated with the stroke center. The stroke center should be able to communicate effectively with EMS personnel in the out-of-hospital setting during transportation of a patient experiencing an acute stroke. The ED should be able to efficiently receive and triage patients with stroke arriving via EMS. The stroke center staff should support and participate in educational activities involving EMS personnel."

The community of prehospital care providers and the physician leaders in this field are committed to continuous improvement in stroke care and explicitly endorse ongoing efforts to include EMS in the continuum of acute stroke care.[40] To this end, it should be reemphasized that appropriate prehospital stroke triage entails EMS personnel taking the patient to the closest hospital best equipped to fully evaluate and treat the patient's stroke, independent of all other considerations.

THE FUTURE OF PREHOSPITAL CARE

In the future, the prehospital arena of stroke care will almost certainly be of increasing importance. Investigations are underway regarding the use of telemedicine systems in ambulances, to allow for the prehospital confirmation of stroke symptoms by a stroke physician.[65,66] However, these have thus far had poor success, primarily due to telecommunications system dropouts, and technological improvements will be necessary for this to be a feasible option. Hospital systems that have enacted protocols to successfully decrease treatment times and increase thrombolysis rates have generally included, as essential steps in their protocols, accurate prehospital identification of stroke patients, with prenotification of the receiving hospital, and pre-activation of the stroke team, sometimes involving transport directly from the ambulance to immediate neuroimaging.[6,67–69]

The most dramatically successful stroke protocol thus far was enacted in Helsinki over the course of about a decade, and has, in recent years, improved their door-to-needle (DTN) times such that half of their thrombolysis patients are treated within 20 minutes, with an associated ten fold increase in thrombolysis rates.[70] This was accomplished through a series of measures, implemented in a gradual fashion, following the rule of thumb, "Do as much as possible during the transportation of a suspected stroke patient to the ED, and do only what is absolutely necessary for that patient once he or she has arrived to the ED."[71]

Finally, the most striking example of prehospital stroke care thus far is the "mobile stroke unit" (MSU) developed in Germany, which brings a complete diagnostic arsenal and the initiation of treatment to stroke patients in the field. This concept was first proposed in 2003,[72] developed at Saarland University Hospital, and reported its first successful treatments in 2010.[73] The MSU consists of a specialized ambulance equipped with a small, lead-shielded CT scanner, a point-of-care (POC) laboratory, and a telemedicine connection to the hospital, and is staffed with a paramedic, a physician trained in stroke care, and a neuroradiologist.

These resources allow not only for rapid diagnosis and initiation of thrombolysis in the field, when appropriate, but also for rapid diagnosis, initiation of treatment, and appropriate triage of patients who are found not to have acute ischemic strokes, or who are not thrombolysis candidates. For example, a patient found to have an acute intracerebral hemorrhage on CT may have immediate hypertension management initiated in the field, and may be taken directly to the neurosurgical unit, while a patient found to be septic on rapid POC evaluation rather than experiencing an acute ischemic stroke may be transported to a primary hospital for further management rather than a specialized stroke unit.[74] In a randomized controlled trial of MSU care versus standard hospital-based stroke care, use of the MSU was seen to decrease the time from the initial emergency call to therapy decision by about one half, from 76 minutes to 35 minutes.[75] In this trial, of the patients treated with IV thrombolysis, the alarm-to-treatment and onset-to-treatment times were each also decreased by about one half (from 73 to 38 minutes, and from 153 to 72 minutes, respectively).

Although these are the shortest times thus far reported for stroke evaluation and treatment, the study was not powered to detect a concomitant improvement in outcomes, and although the researchers suspect that the initial costs incurred by use of the MSU in the initial phase of stroke management will eventually be outweighed by the cost-savings associated with improved stroke outcomes from more rapid treatment, this has yet to be demonstrated. Moreover, the success of the MSU has been demonstrated in a relatively low-volume, rural environment, and its generalizability as a treatment model has yet to be proven. Currently, the Pre-Hospital Acute Neurological Therapy and Optimization of Medical Care in Stroke Patients (PHANTOM-S) study is engaged in trialing a similar prehospital stroke treatment model, the stroke emergency mobile unit (STEMO), similarly equipped with a CT scanner, POC laboratory, and teleradiological as well as videoconferencing support, in the metropolitan setting of Berlin. The primary outcome to be studied will be the time between activation of EMS and initiation of thrombolysis (alarm to needle time), with secondary endpoints to include treatment rates, functional outcomes, and cost-effectiveness.[76]

EMERGENCY DEPARTMENT TIME DELAYS

Delays in the ED are another barrier to the optimal treatment of patients with acute stroke. Table 50-4 lists the recommendations of the National Institute of Neurological Diseases and Stroke (NINDS)-sponsored National Symposium on Rapid Identification and Treatment of Acute Stroke for time intervals from ED arrival for a patient with suspected stroke.[4,77]

This conference also provided a recommended algorithm for triage and the evaluation of patients with stroke in the ED. Triage of patients, based on stroke severity, available resources, and time from symptom onset, is one way to focus resources appropriately. For example, the patient with a mild or moderate stroke and stable neurologic deficit who presents more than 6 hours after symptom onset should be evaluated promptly, but it is more urgent to treat a patient who is a potential candidate for a thrombolytic agent within a very small time window (e.g., 3 hours).

Opportunities for physicians to intervene exist only for a limited time regardless of whether a patient is having an ischemic or a hemorrhagic stroke. Delays in patient arrival and delivery of care can significantly affect a patient's potential for a good outcome. Accordingly, until the patient is stabilized and imaging is performed, the care of a patient with acute stroke should be kept on a course aimed at early intervention.

Directing acute stroke care toward a rapid, aggressive path of intervention requires a "paradigm shift" from the approach used in the recent past. This shift is similar to the changes in practice mentality for acute myocardial infarction (AMI) that first occurred with the availability of thrombolytic agents and

TABLE 50-4 Guidelines for Rapid Evaluation of the Patient with Acute Stroke

Period Measured	Optimal Time (min)
From ED arrival to emergency physician evaluation	10
From ED arrival to CT scan initiation	25
From ED arrival to CT scan interpretation	45
From ED arrival to initiation of therapy (80% compliance)*	60

CT, computed tomography; ED, emergency department.
*Target should be compliance with these guidelines in at least 80% of cases.

then again with the advent of percutaneous intervention. To optimize the chance of successful treatment, management protocols for patients with stroke similar to those for patients with AMI or trauma must be designed.

EMERGENCY DEPARTMENT TRIAGE

Triage is derived from the French term *trier*, which means to sort or prioritize. This seemingly simple act of setting the patient's priority level via triage is one of the most important aspects of the ED management of an acute stroke. Like the decision a patient or family member makes about whether to call 911, the triage nurse's assignment of a patient with stroke to the critical care arena within an ED rather than to a "non-critical" bed entirely changes the dynamic of the patient's evaluation and treatment. Current AHA/ASA guidelines recommend that patients with suspected stroke be triaged with the same priority as acute myocardial infarction or serious trauma regardless of the severity of their neurological deficits.[4] However, one Australian study demonstrated that, although triage nurses are excellent at identifying patients with acute stroke symptoms, only two-thirds were allocated to an urgent triage category,[78] with patients having loss of coordination as a primary symptom, or who were felt to have improving or resolving symptoms, less likely to be classified as urgent.

Hospital systems seeking to improve the speed and efficiency of evaluation for patients with stroke must involve the ED nursing staff in the effort and must provide education to enable ED triage nurses to assign patients with acute stroke to receive the highest priority of care, regardless of the initial perceived severity of their deficits. It is also useful to give the ED nursing staff clear, concise guidelines for the triage of such patients. Similarly, having a well-understood and easily activated "acute stroke care pathway" with ED orders and a template for documentation can dramatically improve the management of acute stroke.[79,80]

EMERGENCY DEPARTMENT EVALUATION AND MANAGEMENT

Similar to other critically ill patients, the patient with a possible acute stroke must immediately be stabilized. The ABC assessment is primary. Simultaneously, the diagnostic evaluation must be initiated.

Airway

Intubation and mechanical ventilation are the primary mechanism for airway protection in the ED setting. The decision to intubate a patient is based on answering the following three fundamental clinical questions:

1. Is there a failure of airway maintenance or protection?
2. Is there a failure of ventilation or oxygenation?
3. What is the anticipated clinical course?

Airway compromise and the need for intubation may have multiple causes. They include diminished level of consciousness and inability to protect the airway, impairment of oropharyngeal mobility and sensation, and loss of protective reflexes due to ischemic or compressive brainstem dysfunction. A common clinical error in airway assessment and management occurs when a patient is found to be "breathing on his or her own." Although they may be breathing, patients with stroke may be at serious risk of aspiration, at which point airway protection should be considered. Current AHA/ASA guidelines recommend airway support and ventilator assistance for the treatment of the stroke patient with decreased consciousness or bulbar dysfunction that causes compromise of the airway.[4] If a patient cannot adequately maintain oxygen saturation despite supplemental oxygen or cannot properly eliminate carbon dioxide, mechanical ventilation is required. Finally, patients whose status can be expected to deteriorate or who require prolonged procedures such as angiography should be considered for early intubation under controlled circumstances.[81]

BOX 50-1 Rapid Sequence Intubation

Preparation
Preoxygenation
Pretreatment:
- Lidocaine 1.5 mg/kg IV
- Vecuronium 0.01 mg/kg IV
- Fentanyl 3 μg/kg (over 1 minute)

Paralysis with induction:
- Etomidate 0.3 mg/kg IV
- Succinylcholine 1.5 mg/kg IV

Placement – confirm tube placement
Postintubation management

Adapted from Walls R, editor: *Manual of emergency airway management*, Philadelphia, 2000, Lippincott Williams & Wilkins.

Before sedation and intubation, the emergency physician should take a few moments to perform as complete a neurologic examination as is safe for the patient. Once sedation and intubation are achieved, a significant component of the diagnostic and prognostic data is compromised because baseline neurologic data can no longer be obtained. It is therefore critical to record baseline neurologic status before these interventions.

If a patient requires intubation, rapid sequence intubation should be performed (Box 50-1). This process begins with careful preparation of all necessary equipment and medication so as to provide as controlled an environment as possible. The patient should be thoroughly preoxygenated. During intubation, careful consideration must be given to avoiding raising the intracranial pressure (ICP).

The use of the laryngoscope results in significant sympathetic activity and a marked catecholamine discharge. If autoregulation is impaired, the hemodynamic response may result in an increase in ICP. Premedication with IV lidocaine (1.5 mg/kg) may be considered for its purported ability to blunt the hemodynamic response and possibly blunt the rise in ICP that is associated with laryngoscopy. Ideally, the lidocaine should be given at least 3 minutes before intubation. In addition, opiates can be used to decrease the sympathetic response. Fentanyl, given in a dose of 3 μg/kg, is recommended as an adjunct to block the potential hemodynamic response and the potential rise in ICP due to laryngoscopy, if the patient is hemodynamically stable.[82] The patient should next receive a sedative-induction agent. Etomidate, an ultra-short-acting non-barbiturate hypnotic, is a superb induction agent. Given in a dose of 0.3 mg/kg IV, etomidate causes very little alteration in hemodynamics and, therefore, has gained considerable favor in the induction of critically ill patients. Ketamine, although increasingly coming into favor as an induction agent in the emergency department, should be avoided in patients where there is a concern for elevation of ICP, as it directly stimulates the central nervous system, causing increases in cerebral metabolism, cerebral metabolic oxygen demand, and cerebral blood flow. However, there may be an argument for its use in hypotensive patients, as it releases catecholamines, and, therefore, augments heart rate and blood pressure, rather than reducing them.[83]

A defasciculating dose of a non-depolarizing neuromuscular blocking agent should also be part of the premedication before laryngoscopy; an example is vecuronium, 0.01 mg/kg IV. Such an agent is given to blunt the rise in ICP that can occur in relation to the fasciculations that result from the use of a depolarizing neuromuscular blocking agent. Ideally, this dose is given 3 minutes before the use of a depolarizing neuromuscular blocking agent. Neuromuscular blockade should be achieved with a short-acting agent, such as succinylcholine, in a dose of 1.5 to 2 mg/kg IV. Prolonged paralysis is undesirable because of the loss of clinical signs and symptoms. Sedation must be maintained after intubation, however, to avoid agitation and elevation of ICP.

The ED team must be constantly aware that any patient with an altered level of consciousness may have suffered trauma. A careful examination for evidence of injury is required. Cervical spine immobilization is required for all traumatized patients with an altered level of consciousness.

Breathing

Once the airway has been addressed, the patient's respiratory status must be assessed. Stroke patients may also have significant comorbidity, such as congestive heart failure, chronic obstructive pulmonary disease, or cancer. Oxygen delivery and oxygenation should be optimized. Although there is no literature currently supporting the routine use of supplemental oxygen in patients with stroke but without hypoxia,[84] current ASA/AHA guidelines recommend supplemental oxygen as needed to maintain oxygen saturations >94%.[4] Because up to one-third of patients with stroke experience pneumonia within 1 month of the stroke, aspiration pneumonia prevention must begin in the ED. Elevation of the head to 30 degrees, careful pulmonary toilet, and strict avoidance of any oral intake until a formal swallowing evaluation has been performed are imperative.

Circulation

Once a patient has been determined to be capable of protecting the airway or the airway has been secured and adequate ventilation and oxygenation have been established, attention is turned to the cardiovascular status. This assessment should address hypertension, hypotension, and electrocardiographic (ECG) abnormalities.

Hypertension

Hypertension is extremely common in patients with acute stroke and should be treated cautiously, if at all.[4,85,86] The management of hypertension depends on the cause of the stroke.[87] Hypertension in patients with intracranial hemorrhage, presumed aneurysmal subarachnoid hemorrhage (SAH), or other vascular anomalies, in which the hypertension may clearly be detrimental, should be treated more aggressively. Patients with acute ischemic stroke should be treated conservatively.

In patients being considered for thrombolytic therapy, clear guidelines for blood pressure management have been developed. In order to bring pressures below 185/110, to qualify for fibrinolysis, labetalol 10–20 mg IV may be given and repeated once, or a nicardipine drip may be initiated at 5 mg/h, and titrated up by 2.5 mg/h every 5–15 minutes to a maximum of 15 mg/h. Other agents, such as hydralazine or enalaprilat may be considered.[4] Following fibrinolysis, the blood pressure must be maintained at or below 180/105, with similar recommended measures.

Management of hypertension in patients not treated with fibrinolysis is less clear. Several studies have shown a U-shaped relationship between presenting blood pressure and outcomes in patients with ischemic stroke, with worse outcomes at the extremes of hypotension and hypertension.[88] Unfortunately, however, the target blood pressure in this patient population has yet to be defined. Current ASA/AHA guidelines continue to recommend that action to acutely lower blood pressure not be taken in the first 24 hours, unless the blood pressure exceeds 220/120, or there is a concomitant specific medical condition that would benefit from lowering of the blood pressure.[4]

If it is deemed critical to alter a patient's blood pressure, the following principles should guide the choice of agents and approach to the ED management of hypertension. First, short-acting, titratable agents should be used; examples are labetalol, nicardipine, and esmolol. Second, physicians should start with very low doses and titrate the dosage according to desired parameters. Third, physicians should avoid agents that may be harmful; diuretics should be avoided except in the setting of acute and compromising heart failure. Oral medications should be avoided. Also, using more than one medication with different mechanisms of action in the acute setting may be particularly dangerous. The combination of two antihypertensive agents may have a summary effect significantly greater than the presumed individual effects of the two medications at their standard dosing. Finally, the goal should be a relatively slow and modest reduction in blood pressure to avoid a significant diminution in perfusion. For this reason, sodium nitroprusside should be avoided.[87] Additionally, simple bedside maneuvers such as elevation of the head of the bed may help control hypertension by improving cerebral venous drainage.[4,87]

Hypotension

Hypotension can decrease cerebral perfusion pressure and lead to a significant extension of the area of cerebral infarction. During an acute stroke, perfusion of ischemic areas is directly related to the mean arterial pressure, therefore hypotension should be evaluated and aggressively treated. As an initial intervention, putting the patient's head down flat can increase blood pressure and cerebral perfusion and sometimes results in clinical improvement. In addition, hypotension can be treated with IV fluids, inotropic agents, or vasopressors as necessary to maintain perfusion and prevent extension of an infarct. Physicians must search for a cause for a patient's relative hypotension, as this is rare during acute ischemic stroke, and suggests another cause. The emergency physician must be constantly vigilant for other diseases, such as AMI, gastrointestinal bleeding, occult trauma, aortic dissection, and sepsis.

Electrocardiographic Abnormalities

An evaluation of the patient's cardiac rhythm and an ECG are imperative. Cardiac rhythm can be significantly affected by acute stroke or may be the underlying cause of the stroke. Cardiac rhythm disturbances such as atrial fibrillation are a significant risk factor for ischemic stroke. Similarly, acute or subacute myocardial infarction can precipitate either cardiovascular compromise leading to cerebral hypoperfusion or thrombus presenting as cerebrovascular embolism. Finally, acute dissection of the thoracic aorta may involve the carotid and/or vertebral arteries. Patients who have hemodynamic compromise or chest pain at the time of presentation with acute stroke should be evaluated for potential AMI or thoracic aortic dissection. In addition, patients who are mute or who have significant difficulty communicating should be even more aggressively screened for these possibilities. A baseline ECG and a chest radiograph should be considered. Conversely, cardiac rhythm and function can be affected by acute stroke. Hemispheric ischemic strokes that involve the insula and both SAH and intracerebral hemorrhage (ICH) can affect cardiac rhythm. ECG changes such as T-wave inversion occur in 50–75% of patients with acute stroke.[89]

Other Issues

Issues that must be addressed in the ED in addition to stabilization of the airway, breathing, and circulation include hyperglycemia, hyperpyrexia, seizures, and emesis.

Hyperglycemia

Patients with hyperglycemia at the time of the acute stroke have worse outcomes.[51] In the NINDS rt-PA Stroke Trial, a higher admission blood glucose level was associated with lower odds of desirable clinical outcome and a greater likelihood of a symptomatic ICH, regardless of recombinant tissue plasminogen activator (rt-PA) treatment.[50] For this reason, IV fluids should not include glucose, and patients with hyperglycemia should be treated with insulin to achieve euglycemia.

Thus far, only one randomized efficacy trial of hyperglycemia management in acute stroke has been reported: the Glucose Insulin in Stroke Trial (GIST-UK) randomly assigned ischemic and hemorrhagic stroke patients seen within 24 hours of symptom onset who had elevated blood glucose levels at admission to aggressive glucose control versus standard therapy. Unfortunately, the trial was stopped because of slow enrollment, and fewer than half of the 2355 patients it would have taken to detect a 6% mortality difference were ultimately enrolled, showing no difference in clinical outcome between the two treatment groups.[90] Thus, while hyperglycemia should be avoided, it remains unclear whether aggressive early glucose reduction would be beneficial in the setting of acute stroke. Current guidelines recommend treating hyperglycemia to achieve blood glucose levels of 140–180 mg/dL, with close monitoring to prevent hypoglycemia.[4]

Hyperpyrexia

Temperature control is also important. Elevations in brain temperature have been shown to worsen cerebral ischemia and are associated with increases in stroke severity, infarct size, and mortality rates, as well as worse outcomes.[91,92] In a study of 390 patients with acute ischemic stroke, each temperature increase of 1 °C raised the risk of poor outcome by a factor of 2.2.[93] Elevations in temperature have the greatest effect in the first 24 hours after stroke. Hyperthermia is easy to underestimate because brain temperature is higher than core body temperature and varies within regions of the brain.[94] Trials of hypothermia in patients who have experienced cardiac arrest have had encouraging results;[95,96] results of studies of the use of induced hypothermia in acute ischemic stroke have also been encouraging but are not definitive.[97] At this time, fever of any degree, even mild hyperthermia, should be treated with antipyretics (acetaminophen), and its cause should be investigated.

Seizures

Seizures can be a serious complication of acute stroke. They occur in approximately 5% of patients with acute ischemic stroke and may be related to involvement of the cerebral cortex or to very large strokes. The incidence of seizures in patients with ICH is approximately 25%. Seizures occur most commonly in patients with lobar hemorrhages or hemorrhages that extend into the cortex.[98] Seizures or seizure-like episodes occur in approximately 25% of patients with acute SAH.

Current guidelines recommend against the prophylactic use of anticonvulsants in acute ischemic stroke, and recommend that any seizures, which do occur be managed according to established standards for any other seizure activity.[4] Acute seizures are managed with benzodiazepines; if unsuccessful, these agents should be followed with a loading dose of fosphenytoin. Following that, barbiturates or levatiracetam may be considered.[99] Divalproex sodium (Depakote), a commonly used anticonvulsant, should be avoided in the setting of ICH because this agent has an antiplatelet effect, which may be deleterious in hemorrhagic stroke. Continuous electroencephalographic monitoring should be considered in comatose patients or in those with a poor neurologic examination unexplained by the primary stroke, as non-convulsive seizures may be responsible for poor responsiveness. A careful examination by the emergency physician should be undertaken to ensure that poor responsiveness is not due to neurologic posturing that may indicate worsening of a mass lesion or progression of mass effect.

Emesis

Emesis is relatively common in acute hemorrhagic stroke and, because it may increase ICP, may be deleterious. Thus, throughout the ED phase of the patient's care, emesis should be avoided or controlled. Phenothiazine antiemetics such as promethazine (Phenergan) are usually adequate but do carry the theoretical burden of decreasing a patient's seizure threshold and causing sedation. The 5-hydroxytryptamine receptor antagonists (also known as the serotonin antagonists), such as ondansetron, are superior inhibitors of nausea and vomiting; they neither decrease the seizure threshold nor cause sedation. The use of serotonin antagonists should be considered early in acute stroke if emesis occurs and is especially important for hemorrhagic stroke.

Diagnostic Studies

Basic diagnostic studies should be included in the initial evaluation of patients with acute stroke. The AHA recommends an ECG, complete blood count, platelet count, measurements of partial thromboplastin time, prothrombin time, markers of cardiac ischemia, and serum electrolyte levels, and serum glucose level.[4] However, it is recommended that only CT, blood glucose, and oxygen saturation are strictly necessary for thrombolysis, and that fibrinolytic therapy should not be delayed while awaiting the results of other tests, unless there is suspicion of anticoagulation or comorbid disease. Other laboratory studies and imaging, such as hepatic function tests and chest radiography, should be ordered as indicated.

DIVERGENCE OF PATHWAYS BASED ON ISCHEMIC VERSUS HEMORRHAGIC STROKE

Once the initial stabilization and evaluation of a patient with stroke have been accomplished, laboratory and imaging data will lead to a divergence of potential pathways for treatment. First, the clinician is charged with ruling out stroke mimics while proceeding on the course toward rapid institution of stroke management. Second, although there is significant overlap in presentation, the management of acute ischemic stroke differs considerably from that of acute ICH and SAH.

Stroke Mimics

A number of stroke mimics may be encountered in an ED. The most common are hypoglycemia, seizure with postictal paralysis, migraine headaches, a lesion in the brain, systemic infection, trauma, positional vertigo, and metabolic derangements.[100] Because rapid stroke evaluation is labor intensive and costly and because the definitive therapies may carry significant risk, stroke mimics must be ruled out as early as possible in the ED.

Ischemic Stroke

Management

Currently, the optimal therapy for an appropriately selected patient with acute ischemic stroke is the initiation of thrombolysis. The ED's role in the treatment of ischemic stroke with thrombolytics is highly system dependent. The patient with undifferentiated stroke must be kept on the "fast track" toward therapy until either (1) the patient is deemed an appropriate candidate and therapy is offered or (2) the patient is clearly excluded from thrombolytic intervention because of well-defined exclusion criteria.

A number of procedures can ensure that appropriate candidates are considered for therapy in the ED. First, the consistent and reinforced use of the NIHSS confirms and quantifies the extent of the stroke, facilitates discussions about risks and benefits, improves communication among colleagues, and allows for accurate reassessment of progress. Second, a stroke team whose role and availability are clearly defined has been shown to be one of the essential elements in optimizing rapid stroke treatment. Ideally, ED faculty would be members of this team.[61] Third, an agreed-on clinical pathway should be developed and implemented by the institution along with emergency physicians and nurses, the stroke team, laboratory services, radiology services, and hospital administration; this pathway should be initiated in the ED.

Each hospital should develop a treatment plan for patients with acute stroke that reflects its abilities and limitations.[61] Hospitals without brain imaging facilities should never treat patients with a thrombolytic agent. Hospitals with easy access to brain imaging facilities, radiologic expertise, and an experienced physician should be able to treat appropriately identified patients with IV alteplase. However, in a hospital without an active intensive care unit or neurosurgical expertise, it is probably best that patients treated with alteplase be transferred immediately after treatment has begun to a hospital with these capabilities. Additionally, AHA/ASA guidelines now support the implementation of telestroke consultation, in conjunction with stroke education and training for healthcare providers in order the increase the use of rtPA at community hospitals that would otherwise not have access to adequate onsite stroke expertise.[4]

Prevention of Complications

The ED team may initiate critical preventive measures in the care of patients with acute stroke. Ideally, the measures would be initiated via the predefined stroke treatment pathway. They include not giving the patient anything by mouth, initiating a consultation for a formal swallowing study, and beginning prophylaxis against deep venous thrombosis in patients not receiving thrombolytics. Because urosepsis is a significant risk, use of Foley catheters should be avoided whenever possible.[101] Finally, it cannot be overemphasized that the initiation of a stroke treatment pathway in the ED will help ensure complete and consistent care throughout a patient's hospitalization.

Special Consideration: Transient Ischemic Attacks

TIAs have been previously clinically defined as "temporary focal brain or retinal deficits caused by vascular disease that clear completely in less than 24 hours."[102] Neurovascular experts now adhere to a tissue-based definition of TIA as "a brief episode of neurologic dysfunction caused by focal brain ischemia, with clinical symptoms typically lasting less than 1 hour and without evidence of accompanying infarction on brain imaging."[103] This newer definition should help clinicians avoid labeling mild strokes as TIAs.

TIAs are common and represent a significant warning of ischemic stroke.[104] On the basis of estimates of stroke incidence, approximately 300,000 TIAs occur each year in the United States.[105,106] In one study, one in 15 individuals older than 65 years reported a history of TIA.[107] Labeled by some clinicians as "unstable angina of the brain," this disease and its significance are becoming increasingly well understood.

Identification of TIAs in the ED is a complex and difficult task. TIAs often manifest as vague complaints that can be difficult to discern, especially in the patient without a classic medical history for the disease. Another problem is the fact that, in the majority of cases of true TIA, the symptoms have abated by the time the patient is evaluated by an emergency physician. In addition, the differential diagnosis of TIAs is extensive; it includes syncope, seizure and/or Todd's paralysis, hypoglycemia, complicated migraines, multiple sclerosis, neuromuscular disorders, SAH, Bell's palsy, neoplasm, hemorrhagic stroke, functional disorders, and vertigo. These factors combine to make the identification of TIAs difficult. It is important for the ED physician to realize that a TIA is the final common pathway of a number of disease processes and is not necessarily an entity unto itself. For that reason, the history and physical examination are of paramount importance in the diagnosis of the source of the TIA. Careful questioning of paramedics, family, friends, and other possible witnesses is usually required.

The role of the ED in the care of the patient with a suspected TIA has three primary components. The first is identification of the possibility of TIA and initiation of a rapid and aggressive evaluation for causes, which is a process aimed at reducing stroke risk. The second is prevention of ischemic stroke via the institution of antiplatelet or antithrombotic agents. Third is the disposition of the patient, with a strong emphasis on admission to the hospital so that monitoring and completion of the evaluation can be facilitated. Nonrandomized studies suggest that urgent preventive intervention may reduce subsequent stroke risk in patients with TIAs.[108,109]

Hemorrhagic Stroke

Intracerebral Hemorrhage

ED management for patients with ICH consists of standard resuscitative techniques such as airway management and hemodynamic monitoring for stability. Blood pressure control is the primary therapeutic goal of the emergency physician for patients with dramatic hypertension in the setting of ICH. Hypertension is theoretically thought to contribute to hematoma expansion, peri-hematomal edema, and rebleeding, although a clear association has not been proven.[110]

The exact parameters for blood pressure control remain unproven. There has historically been concern that intensive efforts at blood pressure control could lead to worsening neurological outcomes secondary to decreased cerebral perfusion of a postulated "peri-hematomal penumbra".[111] The INTERACT[112] and ATACH[113] pilot studies both previously demonstrated the safety of intensive blood pressure management in the acute phase of ICH, and the more recent ICH ADAPT[111] study used CT perfusion imaging to show that aggressive lowering of systolic blood pressure (SBP), with goals of <150 mmHg, does not lead to decreased perfusion about the hematoma. Most recently, the INTERACT2 study[114] randomly assigned patients within 6 hours of a spontaneous ICH to either intensive blood pressure management (goal SBP <140) or guideline-recommended treatment (goal SBP <180), using agents of the physician's choosing. The primary outcome was defined as death or major disability at 90 days, which was noted in 52% of the intensive treatment cohort, compared to 55.6% of the guideline-recommended treatment group, which was not statistically significant. The difference in hematoma growth between the two groups in the 24 hours after baseline was also not significant (relative difference 1.4%, P=0.27). However, a prespecified ordinal analysis of the modified Rankin scores showed significantly lower scores among the intensive treatment group (OR for greater disability, 0.87; 95% CI, 0.77–1.00; $P = 0.04$). The ATACH-II study is forthcoming, which will eventually present more homogenous data, in that nicardapine will be the only intervention used.

On the basis of these data, it appears that intensive blood pressure management in acute ICH is safe, even when instituted rapidly to goals of SBP <140, and may offer some benefit in functional outcome, although this effect thus far seems smaller than would have been expected.[115] Current AHA/ASA guidelines recommend aggressive reduction of BP with IV agents if SBP is >200 or MAP is >150 mmHg, a modest reduction of BP to a goal of 160/90 or MAP of 110 if SBP is >180 and there is no evidence of increased ICP, and monitoring of ICP with reduction of BP to maintain a cerebral perfusion pressure ≥60 mmHg if SBP is >180 and there is concern for elevated ICP. Additionally, these most recent guidelines assert that, in patients presenting with a SBP of 150–220 mmHg, acute lowering of SBP to 140 mmHg is probably safe.[110]

Because nitroprusside, verapamil, and hydralazine are all cerebral vasodilators, these agents may be suboptimal and should be avoided in the setting of presumed increased intracerebral pressure associated with intracerebral hematomas. Additional choices for blood pressure control in the setting of ICH are labetalol, nicardipine, and esmolol.[87] Management of elevated ICP may be initiated in the ED. In the setting of an acute herniation syndrome, hyperventilation can be instituted. This measure immediately lowers cerebral blood flow and thereby decreases ICP. Hyperventilation should not be instituted for patients other than those with impending herniation syndrome, however, because of a theoretical concern that the perihematoma regions will suffer significant ischemia due to the decrease in intracerebral blood flow. Hypertonic saline and mannitol can also be used but should be reserved for the patient with herniation syndrome or with a hematoma so large that herniation can be expected.

The ED team must remain vigilant for rapid changes in the neurologic status of patients with ICH. For many years, it was believed that ICH occurred over a brief time and that growth in hemorrhage volume was arrested very shortly after ictus. Brott et al.,[116] however, found that substantial growth in the volume of hematomas occurred in 26% of patients within the first hour after baseline CT. In addition, growth occurred in 12% of patients between 1 hour and 20 hours after baseline CT. Thus, 38% of patients had substantial growth (greater than one-third of the volume) in the first 20 hours after baseline CT scanning. These results reveal a significant potential for a decline in a patient's neurologic status while the patient remains in the ED, and the treatment team must maintain a constant watch to be able to respond appropriately to such a change. Patients who are seen early, those with prior antiplatelet use, and those with large baseline ICHs or any intraventricular hemorrhage on the initial CT are particularly susceptible to hematoma expansion.[117]

Special Consideration: Anticoagulant-Associated Intracerebral Hemorrhage

In ICH patients with coagulopathy due to concomitant medical conditions or medications, specific therapies may be available depending on the primary process. Recent estimates suggest that one in every five cases of ICH occur in patients receiving warfarin.[118–120] In these patients, current options for correcting the coagulopathy include administration of vitamin K, fresh frozen plasma (FFP), prothrombin complex concentrates (PCC), and rFVIIa. Vitamin K should be administered because it addresses the effects of warfarin, and is necessary for long-term reversal, but its onset of activity is far beyond the early time window when it would have an impact on limiting hematoma expansion. Some concerns are frequently raised about anaphylactic reactions after IV administration of vitamin K. The emergency physician and others caring for patients with life-threatening bleeding receiving anticoagulation should be aware that a retrospective analysis of the experience at the Mayo Clinic over 5 years found the incidence of anaphylactoid reaction from IV vitamin K to be three in 10,000 administrations, similar to that for *all* penicillins.[121] Thus, vitamin K may be as safely administered as other medications that are routinely used in medical practice. A slow infusion over an hour may be preferred to a bolus infusion.

Patients with elevated international normalized ratio (INR, >1.3) due to warfarin have also historically been treated with FFP. Time to initiation of FFP infusion has been found to be highly predictive of normalization of INR at 24 hours in warfarin-associated hemorrhages.[122] ICH patients receiving anticoagulation have a higher mortality rate than patients not receiving anticoagulation, and higher INR levels in patients receiving anticoagulation have been associated with worse outcomes.[123] Given the life-threatening impact of anticoagulant-associated ICH, 10–12 mL/kg of FFP have been recommended, rapidly administered to correct the coagulopathy. Hospitals without the ability to care for patients with warfarin-associated ICH should administer both vitamin K and FFP before the transfer of patients to tertiary care centers, if possible. Delaying this critical intervention may allow for further hematoma expansion and associated worse outcomes.

Although FFP has been the accepted urgent reversal agent for many years, increased attention has been brought to the use of PCCs for this purpose. PCCs require much smaller volume infusions than FFP and are thought to act more rapidly in reversing anticoagulation from warfarin than FFP and, as such, may result in less hematoma expansion in the setting of ICH.[124–127] These products do have an increased risk of thromboembolic events,[125,126] although this risk appears relatively low.[127] As such, although the lack of large, well-controlled, randomized trials are acknowledged, current AHA/ASA guidelines state that PCCs are reasonable to consider as an alternative to FFP in oral-anticoagulant associated ICHs with elevated INR.[110] The use of rFVIIa for warfarin-associated ICH has also been evaluated. In a study of seven patients with warfarin-associated ICH, 15–90 μg/kg of rFVIIa was given in addition to standard therapy (FFP and vitamin K).[128] Rapid normalization of INR occurred, but rebound increased INR developed, and full doses of FFP and vitamin K were still required. The rebound phenomenon presumably occurred as a result of the short half-life of rFVIIa (2.6 hours). Another study compared 13 patients with warfarin-associated ICH treated with rFVIIa plus vitamin K and FFP to 15 patients treated with vitamin K and FFP alone.[129] A fourfold faster decrease in INR was found in the rFVIIa treated group compared with the standard therapy group.

Although rFVIIa is able to rapidly normalize INR, it does not replenish all of the vitamin-K-dependent clotting factors, and therefore may not restore thrombin generation as well as FFP or PCCs.[110] A 2008 American Society of Hematology evidence-based review recommended against the routine use of rFVIIa in acute warfarin reversal, primarily based on a lack of good-quality clinical studies of efficacy.[130] Therefore, although this may be a potential therapy for warfarin-associated ICH, larger prospective studies are needed, and current AHA/ASA guidelines recommend against the use of rFVIIa as a sole agent for oral anticoagulant reversal in ICH.[110]

Patients who develop an ICH while receiving heparin therapy should be treated promptly with protamine sulfate to reverse the effects of heparinization. For every 100 units of continuous heparin infusion per hour, 1 mg of protamine may be given. The same dose may be administered to patients who received a bolus of heparin.

Whether use of antiplatelet agents at the time of a spontaneous ICH is associated with increased hematoma expansion and worsened neurologic outcome is unclear, as several studies have had conflicting results.[131] Moreover, the literature regarding the effectiveness of reversal of antiplatelet medication effects is equivocal.[131] Various protocols have been proposed involving platelet transfusion, with or without the addition of desmopressin (DDAVP), but no randomized studies are thus far available regarding their effectiveness or outcomes. Current AHA/ASA guidelines describe platelet transfusions in ICH patients with a history of antiplatelet use as "investigational".[110]

Patients with underlying coagulopathies due to comorbidities such as liver disease, essential thrombocytopenia, hemophilia, and von Willebrand's disease should be treated with the appropriate replacement product, which addresses the underlying condition. Failure to initiate these therapies specifically aimed at limiting hematoma expansion may expose patients to further bleeding and clinical deterioration.

Subarachnoid Hemorrhage

The most critical issue in the ED management of acute SAH is making the diagnosis. The diagnosis is not difficult in the setting of catastrophic SAH; nevertheless, hidden within the myriad patients with headaches who are seen at an ED are those few individuals with SAH whose symptoms are limited to a headache. Such patients have the best prognosis if the diagnosis is made, but also the greatest likelihood that the diagnosis will be missed.

Patients with acute cephalgia account for approximately 1.2% of the more than 100 million ED encounters per year in the US.[132] On the basis of this statistic, more than 1 million patients per year seen at an ED are evaluated for acute headaches. Buried within that group are approximately 30,000 patients with aneurysmal SAH, of whom only 48% are seen with symptoms that would lead to their assignment to Hunt and Hess category 1 or 2.[133] Thus, patients with aneurysmal SAH who are assigned to Hunt and Hess category 1 or 2 at presentation represent approximately 1% of ED headache evaluations. It is exactly those patients in whom great vigilance is required to maximize their potential for a favorable outcome.

In the ED, the diagnosis is based on clinical suspicion followed by a non-contrast-enhanced head CT scan; if CT does not yield a diagnosis, lumbar puncture is performed. There is continued debate in the emergency medicine literature regarding the need to perform lumbar puncture in all patients to rule out SAH if findings on head CT scanning performed with a third- or fourth-generation scanner are negative for SAH.[134-140] The latest generation CT scanners are extremely sensitive for detection of SAH, with overall sensitivities reported at 93–97.8%.[138,140,141] Several studies have now reported a 100% sensitivity of third-generation CT scanners for the detection of SAH within 6 hours of headache onset.[138,140,142] However, given the severe morbidity and mortality associated with a missed diagnosis of SAH, the standard evaluation for patients with the sudden onset of a severe (often termed *thunderclap*) headache remains imaging, followed by lumbar puncture when imaging findings are normal, as recommended by the most recent AHA/ASA guidelines.[143]

Specific ED management of patients with non-traumatic SAH revolves around the basics of resuscitation and stabilization as well as management of the frequent complications of acute SAH. First, consultation with a neurosurgeon is required as soon as this diagnosis is made. Second, as with any potentially critically ill ED patient, the ED physician must begin with the ABCs of treatment. Patients with SAH frequently are seen with, or progress to, obtundation. Endotracheal intubation of obtunded patients protects them from aspiration caused by depressed airway protective reflexes and allows for hyperventilation, if required.

There is general agreement that acute hypertension should be controlled after acute SAH until the aneurysm has been secured, although clear parameters for blood pressure management have not been defined.[143] Although it is based on limited evidence, the current recommendation is to maintain SBP <160 mmHg in patients with an unsecured aneurysm.[88,143] When medications are required for blood pressure control, the clinician should use only agents that can be titrated rapidly. Patients receiving vasoactive agents require invasive arterial line monitoring because labile blood pressure is common in acute SAH.[87]

Pulmonary Edema, Cardiac Events, Electrocardiography, Dysrhythmias

Left ventricular dysfunction occurs in an estimated 22% of SAH patients[144] and is predicted by elevations in cardiac troponin I and abnormal ECG findings. Although reversible, this left ventricular dysfunction predisposes a sizeable proportion of SAH patients to pulmonary edema, hypotension, and cardiac arrhythmias. The mechanisms responsible for these derangements in SAH are poorly understood, but it is postulated to be due to increased ICP resulting in a catecholamine surge. ED treatment measures should prevent further complications. The ED team should monitor cardiac activity, oximetry, automated blood pressure measurements, and end-tidal carbon dioxide and should avoid excessive or inadequate hyperventilation. The head of the patient's bed should be elevated to 30° so that intracranial venous drainage can occur.

If the patient manifests evidence of herniation, a number of interventions should be started. The patient should receive osmotic agents, such as mannitol or hypertonic saline, and hyperventilation should be initiated or maintained.

DISPOSITION FROM THE EMERGENCY DEPARTMENT

Patients with hemorrhagic stroke or large ischemic stroke and all patients receiving rt-PA for an acute ischemic stroke should be admitted to a dedicated neuroscience intensive care unit, if available, or the stroke care unit or general intensive care unit. Of note, special attention should be given to patients with posterior circulation strokes, as they may benefit from a high level of monitoring. In particular space-occupying edema can develop in 17–54% of patients with cerebellar infarction, essentially creating a mass lesion in the posterior fossa, which can lead to brainstem compression and obstructive hydrocephalus.[145,146] Development of this edema peaks in days 2–4 after infarction,[146] and can lead to progressive neurologic deterioration. Of patients who progress to coma, 85% die without surgical intervention; however, with craniectomy, about half will have good outcomes.[145] As a result, patients with cerebellar infarctions, even those who are alert and clinically stable, should ideally be managed in a stroke center with a neurologic intensive care unit, where close clinical monitoring, rapid neuroimaging, and neurosurgical interventions are rapidly available.[145,146]

Patients with smaller ischemic strokes who are deemed unlikely to be at risk of clinically significant cerebral edema would ideally be assigned to a monitored bed in a dedicated stroke unit. Because dedicated stroke units do not exist in many facilities, predesignated monitored beds should be assigned to where the acute stroke care pathway is well understood. Hospitals without the required capabilities should have a prearranged transfer agreement with a facility that can meet these requirements. It is rare for a patient with stroke to be discharged from the ED to other than an inpatient bed.

One area of considerable importance to the ED team is disposition of the patient with a suspected TIA. The disposition of the patient with a neurologic emergency such as TIA should be no different from that of any other patient with critical status and is in many ways analogous to that of the patient with unstable angina. Nonetheless, patients with neurologic emergencies commonly are not admitted and do not receive the urgent evaluation that data suggest they need to prevent recurrence or evolution of their medical problems. The disposition of an ED patient with a suspected TIA requires great care. TIAs represent a significant warning of potentially impending stroke.

When considering disposition of such a patient, the emergency physician must keep in mind the short-term prognosis after a suspected TIA. In an early incidence study from Rochester, Minnesota, investigators found a 10% incidence of ischemic stroke in the 3 months after a TIA.[147] In a study of 1707 patients evaluated for TIA in EDs, 10.5% experienced a stroke within 90 days of diagnosis, 2.6% were hospitalized for cardiac events, and 1.4% died of causes other than stroke.[148] This risk of stroke was more than 50 times that expected in a cohort of similar age.[104,105] Half of the strokes occurred within 2 days of the TIAs.[148] A 2008 cross-sectional study of mostly community hospitals across 11 states in the US found that 53% of patients with TIAs were admitted to the hospital.[149] Another study over a 10-year period found that 54% of patients with TIAs were admitted from the ED and the admission rate did not change over the 10 years. The strongest predictors of hospital admission were location in the northeast region of the US and the performance of a head CT in the ED.[150]

Non-randomized studies suggest that urgent preventive intervention may reduce subsequent stroke risk in patients with TIAs.[107,108] Thus, the emergency physician should initiate the evaluation of a TIA patient beyond a baseline CT, when possible. The physician should also initiate or advance the patient's antiplatelet therapy. Then, the patient's care can be turned over to a primary care provider or neurologist for continuation of the observation and completion of the necessary evaluation.

The basis for admission is the rapid evaluation of these TIA patients for the cause of disease. While recently published risk stratification scores such as the $ABCD^2$ score hold promise in terms of deriving a tool that may guide emergency physicians in identifying high-risk patients,[151] it should be noted that all patients seen in the ED in the derivation and validation cohorts were admitted to the hospital. Other patients were seen in outpatient settings. Thus, the ED TIA patient population likely represents a high-risk group that warrants more aggressive evaluation and intervention. One possible solution for these patients is an observation unit with clinical protocols for diagnostic testing (e.g., carotid duplex ultrasonography and echocardiography) and rapid disposition with risk factor modification and follow-up. These protocols have yet to be implemented on a national, scale but do hold promise for the treatment of TIA and other diseases.

It is critical that the emergency physician consider the literature that highlights the significant potential morbidity that TIA heralds. It is becoming clear that initial therapeutic intervention, thorough evaluation, initial testing, and admission with subsequent testing must be undertaken to prevent devastating harm to this group of patients. Because half of TIA patients are discharged home from the ED, this change is truly a paradigm shift for many practitioners and consultants.[149,150] Current AHA/ASA guidelines recommend that it is reasonable to admit patients to the hospital for a TIA if they present within 72 hours of the event, and if any of the following criteria are present:

1. ABCD2 score ≥3
2. ABCD2 score of 0 to 2 and uncertainty that diagnostic workup can be completed within 2 days as an outpatient
3. ABCD2 score of 0 to 2 and other evidence that indicates the patient's event was caused by focal ischemia.

CONCLUSION

The care of a patient with an acute stroke should exist as a continuum from access to prehospital care through definitive therapies. Prehospital care providers are critical players in the pursuit of optimal care for acute stroke. As the point of first medical contact for many stroke victims, they serve as the first opportunity for identification of stroke and for the initiation of the cascade of events that must occur to optimize a patient's chance for recovery. The prehospital arena has been shown to be the part of a patient's care in which the greatest delays between symptom onset and definitive therapy occur. It is within this arena that symptom recognition and a decision to act based on symptom recognition make the difference between potential eligibility for acute therapy and automatic exclusion based on time. The fact that "all care begins prehospital" for the patient with acute stroke must not be lost on researchers and treating physicians. Improvements in public education, prehospital care provider education, protocol development, triage and communication, and destination selection can mean the difference between the implementation of advanced therapies and a lost opportunity.

The ED is the next critical point in the care of a patient with stroke. In the ED, stabilization and a carefully coordinated evaluation, in concert with appropriate subspecialists, optimizes the patient's chance of receiving the most appropriate definitive therapy in the shortest time. This process involves significant preplanning with the establishment of clear delineation of responsibilities and a well-designed stroke care pathway. Thus, a major focus in the initial management of acute ischemic stroke revolves around well-orchestrated coordination of patient care to ensure that physician evaluation and diagnostic testing are performed very quickly. During this "golden hour of stroke," however, there remain multiple patient care issues for the clinician.[152]

Such system building, with the emphasis on prehospital and ED teams, represents a new paradigm in acute stroke care and will serve to create opportunities for patients to receive optimal therapies in an efficient manner.

REFERENCES

1. Jauch EC, Cucchiara B, Adeoye O, et al. Part 11: adult stroke: 2010 American Heart Association guidelines for cardiopulmonary resuscitation and emergency cardiovascular care. Circulation 2010;122:S818–28.
2. Schwamm LH, Pancioli A, Acker JE 3rd, et al. Recommendations for the establishment of stroke systems of care: recommendations from the American Stroke Association's Task Force on the Development of Stroke Systems. Circulation 2005;111: 1078–91.
3. Acker JE 3rd, Pancioli AM, Crocco TJ, et al. Implementation strategies for emergency medical services within stroke systems of care: a policy statement from the American Heart Association/ American Stroke Association Expert Panel on Emergency Medical Services Systems and the Stroke Council. Stroke 2007;38: 3097–115.
4. Jauch EC, Saver JL, Adams HP Jr, et al., on behalf of the American Heart Association Stroke Council; Council on Cardiovascular Nursing; Council on Peripheral Vascular Disease; Council on Clinical Cardiology. Guidelines for the early management of patients with acute ischemic stroke. Stroke 2013;44:870–947.
5. Quain DA, Parsons MW, Loudfoot AR, et al. Improving access to acute stroke therapies: A controlled trial of organised prehospital and emergency care. Med J Aust 2008;189:429–33.
6. O'Brien W, Crimmins D, Donaldson W, et al. FASTER (Face, Arm, Speech, Time, Emergency Response): Experience of Central Coast Stroke Services implementation of a pre-hospital notification system for expedient management of acute stroke. J Clin Neurosci 2012;19:241–5.
7. Tong D, Reeves MJ, Hernandez AF, et al. Times from symptom onset to hospital arrival in the Get With The Guidelines-Stroke Program 2002 to 2009. Stroke 2012;43:1912–17.
8. Moser DK, Kimble LP, Alberts MJ, et al. Reducing delay in seeking treatment by patients with acute coronary syndrome and stroke. Circulation 2006;114:168–82.
9. Barsan W, Brott T, Broderick J, et al. Time of hospital presentation in patients with acute ischemic stroke. Arch Intern Med 1993;153:2558–61.
10. Adeoye O, Lindsell C, Broderick J, et al. Emergency medical services use by stroke patients: A population based study. Am J Emerg Med 2009;27:141–5.
11. Anderson N, Broad J, Bonita R. Delays in hospital admission and investigation in acute stroke. BMJ 1995;311:162.
12. Fogelholm R, Murros K, Rissanen A, et al. Factors delaying hospital admission after acute stroke. Stroke 1996;27:398–400.
13. Rosamond DW, Gorton RA, Hinn AR, et al. Rapid response to stroke symptoms: The delay in accessing stroke healthcare (DASH) study. Acad Emerg Med 1998;5:45–51.
14. Ferro J, Melo T, Oliveria V, et al. An analysis of the admission delay of acute strokes. Cerebrovasc Dis 1994;4:71–5.
15. Jorgensen H, Nakauama H, Reith J, et al. Factors delaying hospital admission in acute stroke. Neurology 1996;47:383–7.
16. Derex L, Adeleine P, Nighoghossian N. Factors influencing early admission in a French stroke unit. Stroke 2002;33:153–9.
17. Mikulik R, Bunt L, Hrdlicka D, et al. Calling 911 in Response to Stroke: A Nationwide Study Assessing Definitive Individual Behavior. Stroke 2008;39:1844–9.
18. Geffner D, Soriano C, Perez T, et al. Delay in seeking treatment by patients with stroke: Who decides, where they go, and how long it takes. Clin Neurol Neurosurg 2012;114:21–5.
19. Chen NC, Hsieh MJ, Tang SC, et al. Factors associated with use of emergency medical services in patients with acute stroke. Am J Emerg Med 2013;31:788–91.
20. Fang J, Yan W, Jiang GX, et al. Time interval between stroke onset and hospital arrival in acute ischemic stroke patients in Shanghai, China. Clin Neurol Neurosurg 2011;113:85–8.
21. Jin H, Zhu S, Wei JW, et al. Factors associated with prehospital delays in the presentation of acute stroke in urban China. Stroke 2012;43:362–70.
22. Kim HJ, Ahn JH, Kim SH, et al. Factors associated with prehospital delay for acute stroke in Ulsan, Korea. J Emer Med 2011; 41:59–63.
23. Kuster GW, Alves MB, Neto MC, et al. Determinants of emergency medical services use in a Brazilian population with acute ischemic stroke. J Stroke Cerebrovas Dis 2013;22:244–9.
24. Hagiwara Y, Imai T, Yamada K, et al. Impact of life and family background on delayed presentation to hospital in acute stroke. J Stroke Cerebrovas Dis 2014;23:625–9.
25. Faiz KW, Sundseth A, Thommessen B, et al. Factors related to decision delay in acute stroke. J Cerebrovasc Dis 2014;23: 534–9.
26. Zerwic J, Hwang SY. Tucco L: Interpretation of symptoms and delay in seeking treatment by patients who have had a stroke: Exploratory study. Heart Lung 2007;36:25–34.
27. Gargano JW, Webner S, Reeves M. Presenting symptoms and onset-to-arrival time in patients with acute stroke and transient ischemic attack. J Stroke Cerebrovas Dis 2011;20: 494–502.
28. Wein TH, Staub L, Felberg R, et al. Activation of emergency medical services for acute stroke in a nonurban population: The T.L.L. Temple Foundation Stroke Project. Stroke 2000;31: 1925–8.
29. Pancioli A, Broderick J, Kothari R, et al. Public perception of stroke warning signs and potential risk factors. JAMA 1998;279: 1288–92.
30. Schneider A, Pancioli A, Khoury J, et al. Trends in community knowledge of the warning signs and risk factors for stroke. JAMA 2003;289:343–6.
31. Neau JP, Ingrand P, Godeneche G. Awareness within the French population concerning stroke signs, symptoms, and risk factors. Clin Neurol Neurosurg 2009;111:659–64.
32. Kleindorfer D, Miller R, Sailor-Smith S, et al. The challenges of community-based research: the beauty shop stroke education project. Stroke 2008;39:2331–5.
33. Williams O, Noble JM. "Hip-hop" stroke: a stroke educational program for elementary school children living in a high-risk community. Stroke 2008;39:2809–16.
34. Morgenstern LB, Gonzales NR, Maddox KE, et al. A randomized, controlled trial to teach middle school children to recognize stroke and call 911: the Kids Identifying and Defeating Stroke project. Stroke 2007;38:2972–8.
35. Kleindorfer D, Lindsell CJ, Moomaw CJ, et al. Which stroke symptoms prompt a 911 call? A population-based study. Am J Emerg Med 2010;28:607–12.
36. Fussman C, Rafferty AP, Lyon-Callo S, et al. Lack of association between stroke symptom knowledge and intent to call 911: a population-based study. Stroke 2010;41:1501–7.
37. Fogle CC, Oser CS, McNamara MJ, et al. Impact of media on community awareness of stroke warning signs: a comparison study. J Stroke Cerebrovas Dis 2010;19:370–5.
38. Govindarajan P, Gonzales R, Maselli JH, et al. Regional differences in emergency medical services use for patients with acute stroke (findings from the National Hospital Ambulatory Medical Care Survey Emergency Department Data File). J Cerebrovas Dis 2013;22:e257–63.
39. Mosley I, Nicol M, Donnan G, et al. The impact of ambulance practice on acute stroke care. Stroke 2007;38:2765–70.
40. Schroeder EB, Rosamond WD, Morris DL, et al. Determinants of use of emergency medical services in a population with stroke symptoms: The Second Delay in Accessing Stroke Healthcare (DASH II) Study. Stroke 2000;31:2591–6.
41. Lacy C, Suh D-C, Bueno M, et al. Delay in presentation and evaluation for acute stroke. Stroke Time Registry for Outcomes Knowledge and Epidemiology (STROKE). Stroke 2001;32: 63–9.
42. Saver JL, Smith EE, Fonarow GC, et al. The "golden hour" and acute brain ischemia: presenting features and lytic therapy in >30,000 patients arriving within 60 minutes of stroke onset. Stroke 2010;41:1431–9.
43. Nagaraja N, Bhattacharya P, Norris G, et al. Arrival by ambulance is associated with acute stroke intervention in young adults. J Neurol Sci 2012;316:168–9.
44. Kothari R, Barsan WG, Brott T, et al. Frequency and accuracy of prehospital diagnosis of acute stroke. Stroke 1995;26:937–41.
45. Caceres JA, Adil MM, Jadhav V, et al. Diagnosis of stroke by emergency medical dispatchers and its impact on the prehospital care of patients. J Cerebrovas Dis 2013;(Epub ahead of print).
46. Ramanujam P, Castillo E, Patel E, et al. Prehospital transport time intervals for acute stroke patients. J Emer Med 2009;37: 40–5.

47. Porteous G, Corry M, Smith W. Emergency medical services dispatcher identification of stroke and transient ischemic attack. Prehosp Emerg Care 1999;3:211–16.
48. Kothari R, Barsan WG, Brott T, et al. Frequency and accuracy of prehospital diagnosis of acute stroke. Stroke 1995;26(6):937–41.
49. Berglund A, Svensson L, Sjostrand C, et al. Higher prehospital priority level of stroke improves thrombolysis frequency and time to stroke unit: The Hyper Acute STroke Alarm (HASTA) Study. Stroke 2012;43:2666–70.
50. Bruno A, Levine SR, Frankel M, et al. Relation between admission glucose level and outcome in the NINDS rt-PA Stroke Trial. Stroke 2002;59:669–74.
51. Wass C, Lanier W. Glucose modulation of ischemic brain injury: Review and clinical recommendations. Mayo Clin Proc 1996;71: 801–12.
52. Bruno A, Biller J, Adams HP Jr, et al. Acute blood glucose level and outcome from ischemic stroke. Neurology 1999;52:280–4.
53. Zachariah B, Van Cott C, Dunford J. Dispatch life support and the acute stroke patient: Making the right call. In: Marler J, Winters-Jones P, Emr M, editors. Proceedings of a National Symposium on Rapid Identification and Treatment of Acute Stroke. Bethesda, Md: The National Institute of Neurological Disorders and Stroke; 1997. p. 29–33.
54. Kidwell CS, Saver JL, Schubert GB, et al. Design and retrospective analysis of the Los Angeles Prehospital Stroke Screen (LAPSS). Prehosp Emerg Care 1998;2:267–73.
55. Kidwell CS, Starkman S, Eckstein M, et al. Identifying stroke in the fields. Prospective validation of the Los Angeles Prehospital Stroke Screen (LAPSS). Stroke 2000;31:71–6.
56. Kothari R, Hall K, Brott T, et al. Early stroke recognition: Developing an out-of-hospital NIH Stroke Scale. Acad Emerg Med 1997;4:986–90.
57. Kothari R, Pancioli A, Liu T, et al. Cincinnati Prehospital Stroke Scale: Reproducibility and validity. Ann Emerg Med 1999;33: 373–8.
58. Abdullah AR, Smith EE, Biddinger PD, et al. Advance hospital notification by EMS in acute stroke is associated with shorter door-to-computed tomography time and increased likelihood of administration of tissue-plasminogen activator. Prehosp Emerg Care 2008;12:426–31.
59. California acute stroke pilot registry (CASPR) investigators. Prioritizing interventions to improve rates of thrombolysis for ischemic stroke. Neurology 2005;64:654–9.
60. Rossnagel K, Jungehulsing GJ, Nolte CH, et al. Out-of-hospital delays in patients with acute stroke. Ann Emerg Med 2004;44: 476–83.
61. Sahni R. Acute stroke: Implications for prehospital care. National Association of EMS Physicians Standards and Clinical Practice Committee. Prehosp Emerg Care 2000;4:270–2.
62. Patel MD, Rose KM, O'Brien EC, et al. Prehospital Notification by Emergency Medical Services Reduces Delays in Stroke Evaluation: Findings From the North Carolina Stroke Care Collaborative. Stroke 2011;42:2263–8.
63. McKinney JS, Mylavarapu K, Lane J, et al. Hospital prenotification of stroke patients by emergency medical services improves stroke time targets. J Stroke Cerebrovas Dis 2013;22:113–18.
64. Alberts MJ, Hademenos G, Latchaw RE, et al. Recommendations for the establishment of primary stroke centers. JAMA 2000;283: 3102–9.
65. Bergrath S, Reich A, Rossaint R, et al. Feasibility of prehospital teleconsultation in acute stroke – a pilot study in clinical routine. PLoS ONE 2012;7:e36796.
66. Liman TG, Winter B, Waldschmidt C, et al. Telestroke ambulances in prehospital stroke management: concept and feasibility study. Stroke 2012;43:2086–90.
67. Puolakka T, Vayrynen T, Happola O, et al. Sequential analysis of pretreatment delays in stroke thrombolysis. Acad Emerg Med 2010;17:965–9.
68. Dalloz MA, Bottin L, Muresan IP, et al. Thrombolysis rate and impact of a stroke code: A French hospital experience and a systematic review. J Neurol Sci 2012;314:120–5.
69. Joux J, Olindo S, Girard-Claudon A, et al. Prehospital medicalization increases thrombolysis rate in acute ischemic stroke. A French stroke unit experience. Clin Neurol Neurosurg 2013;115: 1583–5.
70. Meretoja A, Strbian D, Mustanoja S, et al. Reducing in-hospital delay to 20 minutes in stroke thrombolysis. Neurology 2012;79: 306–13.
71. Meretoja A, Kaste M. Pre- and in-hospital intersection of stroke care. Ann N Y Acad Sci 2012;1268:145–51.
72. Fassbender K, Walter S, Liu Y, et al. "Mobile stroke unit" for hyperacute stroke treatment. Stroke 2003;34:e44.
73. Walter S, Kostpopoulos P, Haass A, et al. Bringing the hospital to the patient: first treatment of stroke patients at the emergency site. PLoS ONE 2010;5:e13758.
74. Kostpopoulos P, Walter S, Haass A, et al. Mobile stroke unit for diagnosis-based triage of persons with suspected stroke. Neurology 2012;78:1849–52.
75. Walter S, Kostpopoulos P, Haass A, et al. Diagnosis and treatment of patients with stroke in a mobile stroke unit versus in hospital: a randomised controlled trial. Lancet Neurol 2012;11: 397–404.
76. Ebinger M, Rozanski M, Waldschmidt C, et al. PHANTOM-S: the prehospital acute neurological therapy and optimization of medical care in stroke patients – study. Int J Stroke 2012;7: 348–53.
77. Bock B. Response system for patients presenting with acute ischemic stroke. In: Marler J, Winters-Jones P, Emr M, editors. Proceedings of a National Symposium on Rapid Identification and Treatment of Acute Stroke. Bethesda, Md: The National Institute of Neurological Disorders and Stroke; 1997. p. 55–7.
78. Mosley I, Morphet J, Innes K, et al. Triage assessments and the activation of rapid care protocols for acute stroke patients. Aus Emerg Nurs J 2013;16:4–9.
79. Baraff L, Lee TJ, Kader S, et al. Effect of a practice guideline on the process of emergency department care of falls in elder patients. Acad Emerg Med 1999;6:1216–23.
80. Bonnono C, Criddle LM, Lutsep H, et al. Emergi-paths and stroke teams: An emergency department approach to acute ischemic stroke. J Neurosci Nurs 2000;32:298–305.
81. Walls R. The decision to intubate. In: Walls R, editor. Manual of Emergency Airway Management. Philadelphia: Lippincott Williams & Wilkins; 2000. p. 3–7.
82. Jagoda AS, Bruns JJ. Increased intracranial pressure. In: Walls R, editor. Manual of Emergency Airway Management. 2nd ed. Philadelphia: Lippincott Williams & Wilkins; 2004. p. 262–9.
83. Schneider RE, Caro DA. Sedative and induction agents. In: Walls R, editor. Manual of Emergency Airway Management. 2nd ed. Philadelphia: Lippincott Williams & Wilkins; 2004. p. 262–9.
84. Pancioli AM, Bullard MJ, Grulee ME, et al. Supplemental oxygen use in ischemic stroke patients: Does utilization correspond to need for oxygen therapy? Arch Intern Med 2002;162:49–52.
85. Lisk D, Grotta JC, Lamki LM, et al. Should hypertension be treated after acute stroke? A randomized controlled trial using single photon emission computed tomography. Arch Neurol 1993;50:855–62.
86. Powers W. Acute hypertension after stroke: The scientific basis for treatment decisions. Neurology 1993;43:461–7.
87. Pancioli AM. Hypertension management in neurologic emergencies. Ann Emerg Med 2008;51(3S):524–7.
88. Grise EM, Adeoye O. Blood pressure control for acute ischemic and hemorrhagic stroke. Curr Opin Crit Care 2012;18:132–8.
89. Dimant J, Grob D. Electrocardiographic changes and myocardial damage in patients with acute cerebrovascular accidents. Stroke 1977;8:448–55.
90. Gray CS, Hildreth AJ, Sandercock PA, et al. Glucose-potassium-insulin infusions in the management of post-stroke hyperglycaemia: The UK Glucose Insulin in Stroke Trial (GIST-UK). Lancet Neurol 2007;6:397–406.
91. Azzimondi G, Bassein L, Nonino F, et al. Fever in acute stroke worsens prognosis. A prospective study. Stroke 1995;26: 2040–3.
92. Hajat C, Hajat S, Sharma P. Effects of post-stroke pyrexia on stroke outcome: A meta-analysis of studies in patients. Stroke 2000;31:410–14.
93. Reith J, Jorgensen H, Pedersen PM, et al. Body temperature in acute stroke: Relation to stroke severity, infarct size, mortality, and outcome. Lancet 1996;347:422–5.

94. Schwab S, Spranger M, Aschoff A, et al. Brain temperature monitoring and modulation in patients with severe MCA infarction. Neurology 1997;48:762–7.
95. Bernard S, Gray TW, Buist MD, et al. Treatment of comatose survivors of out-of-hospital cardiac arrest with induced hypothermia. N Engl J Med 2002;346:557–63.
96. The Hypothermia After Cardiac Arrest Study Group. Mild therapeutic hypothermia to improve the neurologic outcome after cardiac arrest. N Engl J Med 2002;346:549–56.
97. Schwab S, Georgiadis D, Berrouschot J, et al. Feasibility and safety of moderate hypothermia after massive hemispheric infarction. Stroke 2001;32:2033–5.
98. Vespa PM, O'Phelan K, Shah M, et al. Acute seizures after intracerebral hemorrhage: A factor in progressive midline shift and outcome. Neurology 2003;60:1441–6.
99. Brophy GM, Bell R, Claassen J, et al. Guidelines for the evaluation and management of status epilepticus. Neurocrit Care 2012;17:3–23.
100. Libman R, Wirkowski E, Alvir J, et al. Conditions that mimic stroke in the emergency department: Implications for acute stroke trials. Arch Neurol 1995;52:1119–22.
101. Roth EJ, Lovell L, Harvey RL, et al. Incidence of and risk factors for medical complications during stroke rehabilitation. Stroke 2001;32:523–9.
102. The Study Group on TIA Criteria and Detection. XI. Transient focal cerebral ischemia: Epidemiologic and clinical aspects. Stroke 1974;5:277–84.
103. Albers GW, Caplan LR, Easter JD, et al. Transient ischemic attack – proposal for a new definition. N Engl J Med 2002;347: 1713–16.
104. Brown RJ, Petty GW, O'Fallon WM, et al. Incidence of transient ischemic attack in Rochester, Minnesota, 1985-1989. Stroke 1998;29:2109–13.
105. Broderick J, Brott T, Kothari R, et al. The Greater Cincinnati/ Northern Kentucky Stroke Study: Preliminary first-ever total incidence rates of stroke among blacks. Stroke 1998;29:415–21.
106. Williams G, Jiang JG, Matchar DB, et al. Incidence and occurrence of total (first-ever and recurrent) stroke. Stroke 1999;30: 2523–8.
107. Rothwell PM, Giles MF, Chandratheva A, et al. Early use of Existing Preventive Strategies for Stroke (EXPRESS) study. Lancet 2007;370:1432–42.
108. Lavallee PC, Meseguer E, Abboud H, et al. A transient ischaemic attack clinic with round-the-clock access (SOS-TIA): Feasibility and effects. Lancet Neurol 2007;6:953–60.
109. National Stroke Association. TIA/Mini Strokes: Public Knowledge and Experience – Roper Starch Worldwide Survey. Roper Starch Worldwide. Englewood, Colo: National Stroke Association; 2000. p. 55.
110. Morgenstern LB, Hemphill JC, Anderson C, et al., on behalf of the American Heart Association Stroke Council and Council on Cardiovascular Nursing. Guidelines for the management of spontaneous intracerebral hemorrhage. Stroke 2010;41: 2108–29.
111. Butcher KS, Jeerakathil T, Hill M, et al. The Intracerebral Hemorrhage Acutely Decreasing Arterial Pressure Trial. Stroke 2013;44: 620–6.
112. Anderson CS, Huang Y, Wang JG, et al. Intensive blood pressure reduction in acute cerebral hemorrhage trial (INTERACT): A randomised pilot trial. Lancet Neurol 2008;7:391–9.
113. Antihypertensive Treatment of Acute Cerebral Hemorrhage (ATACH) investigators. Antihypertensive treatment of acute cerebral hemorrhage. Crit Care Med 2010;38:637–48.
114. Anderson CS, Heeley E, Huang Y, et al. Rapid blood-pressure lowering in patients with acute intracerebral hemorrhage. N Engl J Med 2013;368:2355–65.
115. Hill MD, Muir KW. INTERACT-2, Should blood pressure be aggressively lowered acutely after intracerebral hemorrhage? Stroke 2013;44:2951–2.
116. Brott T, Broderick J, Kothari R, et al. Early hemorrhage growth in patients with intracerebral hemorrhage. Stroke 1997;28: 1–5.
117. Broderick JP, Diringer MN, Hill MD, et al. Determinants of intracerebral hemorrhage growth: an exploratory analysis. Stroke 2007;38:1072–5.
118. Hart RG, Tonarelli SB, Pearce LA. Avoiding central nervous system bleeding during antithrombotic therapy: Recent data and ideas. Stroke 2005;36:1588–93.
119. Flaherty ML, Kissela B, Woo D, et al. The increasing incidence of anticoagulant-associated intracerebral hemorrhage. Neurology 2007;68:116–21.
120. Cabral KP, Fraser GL, Duprey J, et al. Prothrombin complex concentrates to reverse warfarin-induced coagulopathy in patients with intracranial bleeding. Clin Neurol Neurosurg 2013;115:770–4.
121. Reigert-Johnson DL, Volcheck GW. The incidence of anaphylaxis following intravenous phytonadione (vitamin K[1]): a 5-year retrospective review. Ann Allergy Asthma Immunol 2002;89: 400–6.
122. Goldstein JN, Thomas SH, Frontiero V, et al. Timing of fresh frozen plasma administration and rapid correction of coagulopathy in warfarin-related intracerebral hemorrhage. Stroke 2006;37:151–5.
123. Rosand J, Eckman MH, Knudsen KA, et al. The effect of warfarin and intensity of anticoagulation on outcome after intracerebral hemorrhage. Arch Intern Med 2004;164:880–4.
124. Huttner HB, Schellinger PD, Hartmann M, et al. Hematoma growth and outcome in treated neurocritical care patients with intracerebral hemorrhage related to oral anticoagulant therapy: Comparison of acute treatment strategies using vitamin K, fresh frozen plasma, and prothrombin complex concentrates. Stroke 2006;37:1465–70.
125. Makris M, Greaves M, Phillips WS, et al. Emergency oral anticoagulant reversal: The relative efficacy of infusions of fresh frozen plasma and clotting factor concentrate on correction of the coagulopathy. Thromb Haemost 1997;77:477–80.
126. Lankiewicz MW, Hays J, Friedman KD, et al. Urgent reversal of warfarin with prothrombin complex concentrate. J Thromb Haemost 2006;4:967–70.
127. Leissinger CA, Blatt PM, Hoots WK, et al. Role of prothrombin complex concentrates in reversing warfarin anticoagulation: A review of the literature. Am J Hematol 2008;83:137–43.
128. Freeman WD, Brott TG, Barrett KM, et al. Recombinant factor VIIa for rapid reversal of warfarin anticoagulation in acute intracranial hemorrhage. Mayo Clin Proc 2004;79:1495–500.
129. Brody DL, Aiyagari V, Shackleford AM, et al. Use of recombinant factor VIIa in patients with warfarin-associated intracranial hemorrhage. Neurocrit Care 2005;2:263–7.
130. Rosovsky RP, Crowther MA. What is the evidence for the off-label use of recombinant factor viia (rFVIIa) in the acute reversal of warfarin? Hematology Am Soc Hematol Educ Program 2008; 2008:36–8.
131. Campbell PG, Sen A, Yadla S, et al. Emergency reversal of antiplatelet agents in patients presenting with an intracranial hemorrhage: a clinical review. World Neurosurg 2010;74: 279–85.
132. Morgenstern L, Huber JC, Luna-Gonzales H, et al. Headache in the emergency department. Headache 2001;41:537–41.
133. Whisnant JP, Sacco SE, O'Fallon WF, et al. Referral bias in aneurysmal subarachnoid hemorrhage. J Neurosurg 1993;78: 726–32.
134. Sidman R, Connolly E, Lemke T. Subarachnoid hemorrhage diagnosis: Lumbar puncture is still needed when the computed tomography scan is normal. Acad Emerg Med 1996;3:827–31.
135. Edlow JA, Wyer PC. How good is a negative cranial computed tomographic scan result in excluding subarachnoid hemorrhage? Ann Emerg Med 2000;36:507–17.
136. Prosser RL Jr, Edlow JA, Wyer PC. Feedback: Computed tomography for subarachnoid hemorrhage. Ann Emerg Med 2001;37: 679–80.
137. McCormack RF, Hutson A. Can computed tomography angiography of the brain replace lumbar puncture in the evaluation of acute-onset headache after a negative computed tomography scan? Acad Emerg Med 2010;17:444–51.
138. Gee C, Dawson M, Bledsoe J, et al. Sensitivity of newer-generation computed tomography scanners for subarachnoid hemorrhage: a Bayesian analysis. J Emerg Med 2012;43:13–18.
139. Farzad A, Radin B, Oh JS, et al. Emergency diagnosis of subarachnoid hemorrhage: an evidence-based debate. J Emerg Med 2013;44:1045–53.

140. Stewart H, Reuben A, McDonald J. LP or not LP, that is the question: gold standard, or unnecessary procedure in subarachnoid haemorrhage? Emerg Med J June 11, 2013;(Published online first).
141. Perry J, Stiell I, Silvotti M, et al. Sensitivity of computed tomography performed within six hours of onset of headache for diagnosis of subarachnoid haemorrhage: prospective cohort study. BMJ 2011;343:d4277.
142. Backes D, Rinkel GJE, Kemperman H, et al. Time-dependent test characteristics of head computed tomography in patients suspected of nontraumatic subarachnoid hemorrhage. Stroke 2012; 43:2115–19.
143. Connolly ES, Rabinstein AA, Carhuapoma JR, et al., on behalf of the American Heart Association Stroke Council, Council on Cardiovascular Radiology and Intervention, Council on Cardiovascular Nursing, Council on Cardiovascular Surgery and Anesthesia, and Council on Clinical Cardiology. Guidelines for the Management of Aneurysmal Subarachnoid Hemorrhage. Stroke 2012;43:1711–37.
144. Naidech AM, Kreiter KT, Janjua N, et al. Cardiac troponin elevation, cardiovascular morbidity, and outcome after subarachnoid hemorrhage. Circulation 2005;112:2851–6.
145. Edlow JA, Newman-Toker DE, Savitz SI. Diagnosis and initial management of cerebellar infarction. Lancet Neurol 2008;7: 951–64.
146. Neugebauer H, Witsch J, Zweckberger K, et al. Space-occupying cerebellar infarction: complications, treatment, and outcome. Neurosurg Focus 2013;34:E8.
147. Whisnant J, Matsumoto N, Elveback L. Transient cerebral ischemic attacks in a community – Rochester, Minnesota, 1955 through 1969. Mayo Clin Proc 1973;48:194–8.
148. Johnston S, Gress DR, Browner WS, et al. Short-term prognosis after emergency-department diagnosis of transient ischemic attack. JAMA 2000;284:2901–6.
149. Coben JH, Owens PL, Steiner CA, et al. Hospital and demographic influences on the disposition of transient ischemic attack. Acad Emerg Med 2008;15:171–6.
150. Edlow JA, Kim S, Pelletier AJ, et al. National study on emergency department visits for transient ischemic attack, 1992-2001. Acad Emerg Med 2006;13:666–72.
151. Johnston SC, Rothwell PM, Nguyen-Huynh MN, et al. Validation and refinement of scores to predict very early stroke risk after transient ischaemic attack. Lancet 2007;369:283–92.
152. Thurman J, Jauch EC. Emergency department management of acute ischemic stroke. Emerg Med Clin North Am 2002;20: 609–30.

51 Intravenous Thrombolysis

Wendy Brown, Patrick D. Lyden

KEY POINTS

- Intravenous rt-PA remains the most commonly used therapy that is effective and safe for acute ischemic stroke.
- Pivotal trials in the 1990s demonstrated the effect of rt-PA; subsequent trials have confirmed the initial results and extended the evidence of benefit to include key subgroups such as the very old or patients with very mild strokes.
- Intravenous thrombolytic therapy is cost-effective, and like childhood vaccinations, actually provides a net cost saving to the healthcare system.
- The benefits of intravenous thrombolysis could be improved upon. Newer thrombolytic agents may prove safer and more effective. Combination treatment with intra-arterial intervention appears promising and of proven benefit.
- The original protocol for using intravenous rt-PA must be followed scrupulously to obtain the safety and benefit seen in the trials. The selection criteria, however, may be safely ignored in some special cases and in experienced centers.

Thrombolysis offers the simplest and most direct treatment for thrombotic disorders, including ischemic strokes. Plasminogen activators produce clinical improvement in patients with coronary artery thrombosis, peripheral vascular disease, venous thrombosis, pulmonary embolism, and acute ischemic stroke. According to the pivotal National Institutes of Neurological Disorders and Stroke (NINDS) study, intravenous (IV) tissue plasminogen activator (t-PA) improved the clinical outcome of all types of ischemic stroke (i.e., large-artery, embolic, and small-vessel or lacunar strokes) if treatment began within 3 hours of the onset of symptoms.[1] Consequently, the U.S. Food and Drug Administration (FDA) approved recombinant t-PA (rt-PA) for the treatment of acute ischemic strokes within 3 hours of onset, excluding all patients with intracranial hemorrhage (ICH).

To date, other IV agents have proved useful, but none is yet approved by the FDA for treatment of ischemic stroke. In this chapter we review the historical background of thrombolytic therapy in preclinical and clinical trials, summarize the different agents in previous as well as current use, and discuss the management protocol for thrombolytic treatment in patients with stroke.

THROMBOSIS AND THROMBOLYSIS

Thrombosis involves the processes of endothelial injury, platelet adherence and aggregation, and thrombin generation. Thrombin plays a major role in clot formation; it is responsible for cleaving fibrinogen to fibrin, which forms the clot matrix. Thrombin also activates factor XIII, which accomplishes interfibrin cross-linking. Figure 51-1 illustrates the coagulation cascade.[2] In a process involving platelet membrane receptors and phospholipids, thrombin is generated locally by the extrinsic and intrinsic pathways. Factors V and XIII interact with specific platelet membrane phospholipids to facilitate activation of factor X to factor Xa and the conversion of prothrombin to thrombin on the platelet surface. Platelet-bound thrombin-modified factor V (factor Va) serves as a high-affinity platelet receptor for factor Xa, which accelerates the rate of thrombin generation. The relative platelet–fibrin composition of a specific thrombus depends on regional blood flow or shear stress. At arterial flow rates, thrombi are predominantly platelet-rich, whereas at lower venous flow rates, activation of coagulation predominates. The efficacy of thrombolysis perhaps depends on the relative fibrin content and fibrin cross-linking, the latter possibly determined by the age of the thrombus. Theoretically, therefore, plasminogen activators may act less well on fibrin-poor clots, but such distinctions have not been observed clinically.

In addition to both endothelial-cell-derived antithrombotic characteristics and circulating anticoagulants (activated protein C and protein S), thrombus growth is limited by the endogenous thrombolytic system, in which plasmin plays a central role. One effect of endogenous thrombolysis is continuous remodeling of the thrombus. This effect results from the preferential conversion of plasminogen to plasmin on the thrombus surface, where fibrin binds t-PA in proximity to its substrate plasminogen, accelerating plasmin formation. Plasminogen activation may also occur on cells that express plasminogen receptors and produce plasminogen activators, such as endothelial and polymorphonuclear cells. If sufficient quantities of plasminogen activators are produced or administered, plasminogen can be activated in plasma, where it cleaves circulating fibrinogen and fibrin to produce fibrin split products.

The naturally circulating plasminogen activators, t-PA and single-chain urokinase-type PA (scu-PA), catalyze plasmin formation from plasminogen. In the circulation, plasmin rapidly binds to its inhibitor, α_2-antiplasmin, and is inactivated. Endogenous fibrinolysis is modulated by several inhibitors of plasmin and plasminogen activators. The half-life of plasmin in the circulation is estimated to be approximately 0.1 second. α_2-Antiplasmin is the primary inhibitor

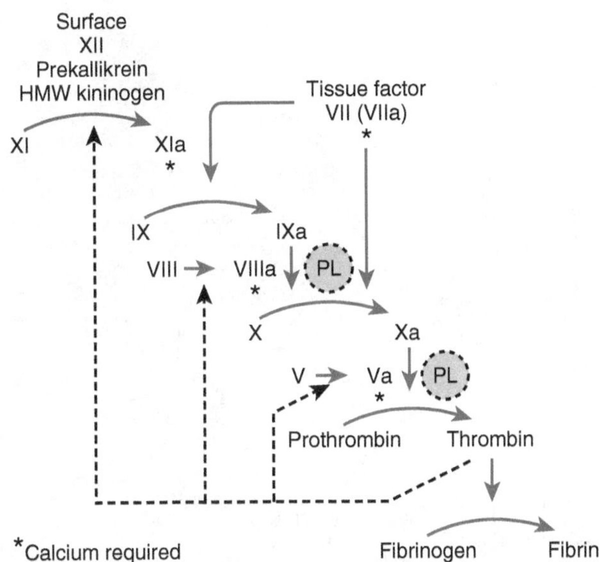

Figure 51-1. Coagulation cascade. The different factors of the coagulation system are portrayed. The cascade culminates in the conversion of prothrombin to thrombin. The *dashed lines* show the autocatalytic action of thrombin. PL, Phospholipids. *(From Douglas S: Coagulation history.* Br J Haematol *107:22–32, 1999.)*

of fibrinolysis through plasmin inhibition by binding to excessive plasmin. Thrombospondin interferes with the t-PA-mediated, fibrin-associated activation of plasminogen. Contact activation inhibitors and C1 inhibitor have indirect effects on thrombolysis.

A competitive inhibitor of plasminogen is histidine-rich glycoprotein (HRG). In addition to inhibitors of plasmin, there are specific plasminogen activator inhibitors that decrease the activity of t-PA, scu-PA, and urokinase (UK) plasminogen activator (u-PA). Both plasma t-PA and u-PA are inhibited by plasminogen activator inhibitor-1 (PAI-1), which is derived from platelets and endothelial cells. The potential risk for thrombosis reflects the relative concentrations of circulating PAI-1 and the endogenous plasminogen activators t-PA and u-PA. In addition, other plasminogen activator inhibitors are derived from different tissues. Within the thrombus, however, plasmin is protected from this inhibitor and t-PA is also relatively protected from circulating plasma inhibitors. This is why plasmin and t-PA can achieve their fibrinolytic effect better within the clot than in serum and also why clot lysis can be achieved with a relatively low risk of bleeding when these agents are used. Plasminogen activation is enhanced further by the complex formed by t-PA, fibrin, and plasminogen. The complex increases the clot-selective fibrinolytic activity of t-PA. Fibrinolysis occurs predominantly within the thrombus and at its surface. Lysis of thrombus is augmented by contributions from local blood flow. During thrombus consolidation, plasminogen bound to fibrin and to platelets allows local release of plasmin. Within the circulation, plasmin cleaves the fibrinogen to different fragments, which incorporate into the fibrin and cause destabilization of its network, therefore allowing further degradation.

All thrombolytic agents in current use are obligate plasminogen activators that act on fibrin and thrombin. Current thrombolytic agents are either endogenous plasminogen activators, which are involved in physiologic fibrinolysis, or exogenous plasminogen activators, which are not.

Endogenous Plasminogen Activators

Tissue-Type Plasminogen Activator

Tissue-type plasminogen activator is a single-chain, 70-kilodalton (kDa), glycosylated serine protease. It has four domains: finger or F domain, growth factor or E domain, two kringle regions (K1 and K2), and a serine protease domain. The COOH-terminal serine protease domain has the active site for the cleavage of plasminogen. The two kringle domains of t-PA (Fig. 51-2) are similar to the kringle domains on plasminogen. The finger domain residues and the K2 domain residues are responsible for fibrin affinity. The single t-PA chain is converted to the double-chain t-PA form by plasmin cleavage of the arginine (position 275)–isoleucine (position 276) bond. Both the single- and double-chain forms are enzymatically active and have fibrin-selective properties. The plasma half-life of the single- and double-chain forms is 3–8 minutes. Tissue-type plasminogen is secreted by endothelial cells, neurons, astrocytes, and microglia. It is cleared by the liver. It is considered to be fibrin-dependent because of favorable activation of plasminogen in association with fibrin. Exercise and certain vasoactive substances, such as desmopressin, raise t-PA levels. Heparin and heparan sulfate increase t-PA activity. Recombinant DNA techniques are used to produce rt-PA for commercial use in both single-chain (alteplase) and double-chain (dulteplase) forms. Figure 51-2 illustrates the amino acid sequence of t-PA.[3]

Urokinase

Urokinase plasminogen activator and its precursor scu-PA, or pro-UK, are glycoproteins. Urokinase is synthesized by endothelial, renal, and malignant cells. The single-chain pro-UK possesses fibrin-selective plasmin-generating activity. Pro-UK has been synthesized by recombinant techniques to be used as an exogenous agent. Removal of the amino acid lysine at position 158 from scu-PA by plasmin produces the high-molecular-weight (HMW) double-chain u-PA (54 kDa) linked by the disulfide bridge; further cleavage produces the low-molecular-weight (LMW) u-PA (31 kDa). Both LMW and HMW forms are enzymatically active. HMW u-PA activates plasminogen to plasmin directly. The half-life of the two forms is 9–12 minutes. Pro-UK has been studied in patients with stroke but has not been approved for clinical use.

Novel Plasminogen Activators

Different mutant forms of t-PA and u-PA have been developed through alteration of the original amino acid sequences by point mutations and deletions. These changes alter the specificity and stability of the molecules. A good example is TNK-t-PA (tenecteplase), a mutant form of t-PA with delayed clearance and a longer half-life than t-PA. In patients with myocardial infarction (MI), TNK has a half-life of 17 ± 7 minutes, as compared with 3.5 ± 1.4 minutes for alteplase.[4] TNK has higher fibrin selectivity and greater resistance to plasminogen-activator inhibitor with enhanced lytic activity on the thrombus and induces earlier reperfusion than t-PA. The name TNK is derived from the fact that the molecule is produced through alteration of the amino acid sequence at the T, N, and K domains of t-PA, as portrayed in Figure 51-3, resulting in the improved characteristics already described.[5]

TNK was shown to be effective for the treatment of coronary thrombosis. The Assessment of the Safety and Efficacy of New Thrombolytic Trial–study 1 (ASSENT-1) evaluated the safety of TNK in 3325 patients with MI. The ICH rates were 0.7% with the 30-mg dose and 0.6% with the 40-mg dose of TNK, which are similar to rates for t-PA in previous MI trials.

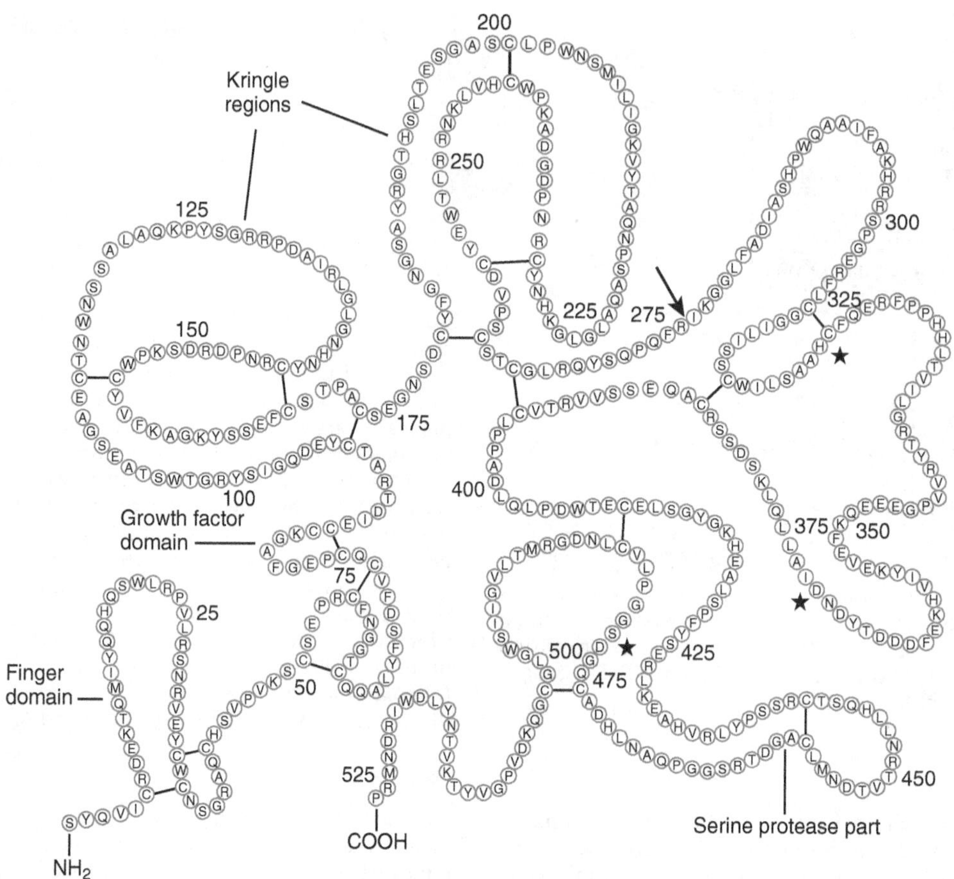

Figure 51-2. Schematic representation of the amino acid sequence of t-PA. The amino acids are represented by their letter symbols. *Black bars* indicate the disulfide bonds. The active site residues histidine-322, asparagine-371, and serine-478 are indicated with an *asterisk*. The *arrow* indicates the plasmin cleavage site for conversion of single-chain to double chain t-PA. *(From Collen D: Fibrin-selective thrombolytic therapy for acute myocardial infarction.* Circulation *93:857–865, 1996.)*

The rate of serious bleeding complications requiring transfusions was 1.4% for TNK compared with 7% for t-PA (statistically significant difference with the lesser bleeding rates in the TNK group).[6] In ASSENT-2, 16,949 patients with acute MI were assigned to receive either a single-bolus dose of TNK or a 30-minute infusion of t-PA. All patients also received heparin and aspirin. The ICH rates were statistically similar in the two groups (0.93% in the TNK group and 0.94% in the t-PA group). There was a slightly but statistically significantly lower rate of major bleeding requiring transfusion with TNK (4.25% for the TNK group versus 5.49% for the t-PA group; $P = 0.0003$). The ASSENT-2 investigators concluded that TNK, which has higher fibrin specificity than t-PA and can be given as a single bolus, is associated with a lesser overall systemic bleeding rate but a similar ICH rate when given to patients with acute MI.[7]

After these successes with coronary thrombosis, it was natural to pursue an indication for cerebral thrombosis. A dose-finding study showed safety in acute stroke patients treated with TNK. Twenty-five patients were enrolled into each tier, and the study included four TNK dose tiers. Patients were followed-up at 24 hours, at discharge, and at 3 months. Symptomatic ICHs within 36 hours of treatment did not occur in the first two tiers, but *asymptomatic* ICH occurred in 8% and 32% in the first two tiers, respectively. Clinical systemic bleeding that did not require treatment occurred in 16% and 40% in the first two tiers, respectively.[8] Two hemorrhages occurred at the highest dose tier after 13 patients were enrolled, prompting a halt to the trial.[9] A phase 2 study of the best two doses of TNK was organized and funded, but unfortunately the FDA imposed an additional two tiers. As a result, enrollment in the trial proceeded poorly, but a summary of the data collected was published.[9] In 2012, Parsons et al. published a trial comparing tenceteplase to aleplase.[10] This was an open-label trial in which 75 patients were randomized to receive alteplase at 0.9 mg/kg, tenecteplase at 0.1 mg/kg or tenecteplase at 0.25 mg/kg. Patients had to have a perfusion lesion at least 20% greater than the core infarct on CT perfusion imaging as well as an associated vessel occlusion on CT angiogram. The two tenecteplase groups together had a higher reperfusion rate on imaging at 24 hours (79.3% in the tenecteplase group versus 55.4 in the aletplase group; $P = 0.004$). Patients treated with tenecteplase were more likely to improve on the NIH score at 24 hours (8% in the tenecteplase group vs 3% in the alteplase group at 8%, $P < 0.001$). Seventy-two percent of the patients treated with the higher dose of tenecteplase versus 40% of the patients treated with alteplase had minimal or no deficit at 90 days ($P = 0.02$). There was no difference in symptomatic intracranial hemorrhage rate or death between patients treated with either dose of tenecteplase and those treated with alteplase. Thus, although TNK appears to be more effective than rt-PA and to have fewer complications, a definitive, adequately powered trial remains ongoing.

Microplasmin

A recombinant form of human microplasminogen has recently been investigated. Whereas t-PA is a specific proteolytic

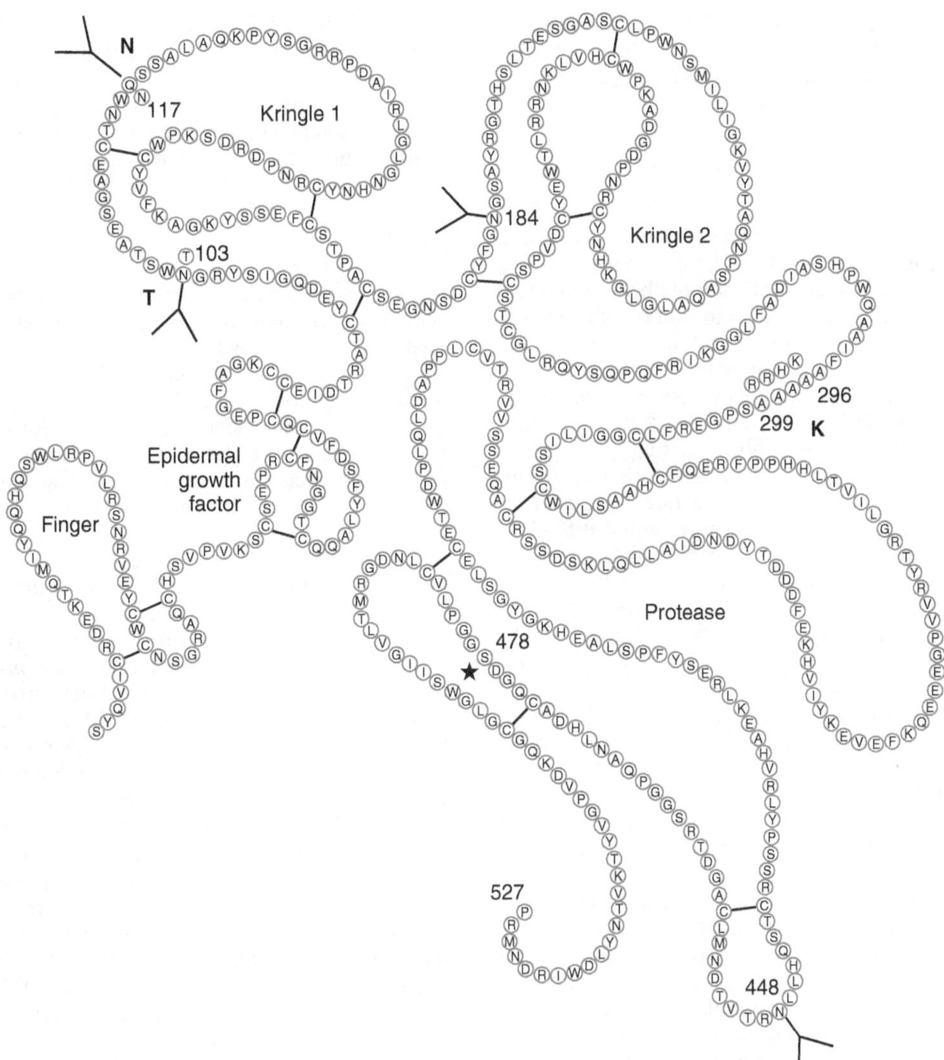

Figure 51-3. The structure of the mutant form of t-PA called TNK-t-PA. This name is given to this compound because of substitution at the T site (asparagine for threonine at position 103), N site (glutamine for asparagine at position 117), and K site (replacing one lysine, one histidine, and two arginines with four alanines at positions 296 through 299) of the original t-PA molecule. The t-PA and TNK structures have the following domains: finger domain, epidermal growth factor domain, the two kringle structures, as well as the serine protease domain. Glycosylation sites are marked by a *Y*. The *star* marks the serine site where plasminogen activation occurs. There are *short lines* that show the bridging between the different loops of the molecule. The amino acid substitutions enhance the selectivity and increase the half-life of the molecule, as fully explained in the text. *(From Benedict CR, Refino CF, Keyt BA, et al: New variant of human tissue plasminogen activator [TPA] with enhanced efficacy and a lower incidence of bleeding compared with recombinant human TPA.* Circulation *92:3032–3040, 1995.)*

enzyme that converts the inactive proenzyme plasminogen to plasmin, microplasmin is a truncated form of plasmin, which, in recent years, has been tested in rodent models of ischemic stroke for safety and neuroprotective properties. It has been shown that in mice with inactivation of genes encoding α_2-antiplasmin, this inactivation significantly reduced infarct size after ischemia, which suggests that there may be some neuroprotective properties inherent in the molecule.[11] Microplasmin reacts with α_2-antiplasmin and neutralizes it. Microplasmin was tested in two rabbit clot embolic stroke models, both small and large, with escalating weight-based dosing. Microplasmin improved behavioral rating scores 60 minutes after embolization without increasing hemorrhagic conversion. There have been no human studies up to now; however, this seems to be a promising new agent for further study.

Exogenous Plasminogen Activators

Exogenous plasminogen activators are produced or extracted from non-human sources. Pharmacologic quantities of endogenous plasminogen activators produced by recombinant techniques, such as rt-PA, or produced through different mutations in the original physiologic plasminogen activator molecules, such as TNK, have already been discussed.

Streptokinase

Streptokinase (SK) is a single-chain polypeptide derived from group C β-hemolytic streptococci. SK combines with plasminogen, and the complex activates circulating plasminogen to plasmin and undergoes conversion to SK–plasmin itself. This complex is not inhibited by α_2-antiplasmin, but SK activity can be eliminated by the presence of SK-neutralizing antibodies produced after previous infection with streptococci. The kinetics of SK elimination are complex, consisting of an initial half-life of 4 minutes and a second half-life of 30 minutes.

Plasminogen Activators Derived from Saliva of *Desmodus rotundus*

The recombinant plasminogen activators that are identical to the ones derived from the saliva of the vampire bat (*Desmodus rotundus*) include an alpha form that is more fibrin-dependent than t-PA. Its half-life is also longer than that of t-PA. Experimental studies have shown that the recombinant alpha-1 form and the bat plasminogen activator may be superior to t-PA in sustaining recanalization and may cause less fibrinogenolysis.[12] The Desmoteplase in Acute Ischemic Stroke Study (DIAS) was a dose-finding randomized, phase 2 trial designed to evaluate the safety and efficacy of IV desmoteplase.[13] This study selected patients between 3 and 9 hours after stroke onset based on mismatch of perfusion-weighted/diffusion-weighted MRI. Eligible patients had a National Institutes of Health Stroke Scale (NIHSS) score between 4 and 20 and MRI evidence of perfusion/diffusion mismatch. The perfusion/diffusion mismatch is considered to be reflective of the "ischemic penumbra," which is potentially salvageable tissue. Fixed doses of desmoteplase were evaluated, but the evaluation was terminated early due to the excessive rate of symptomatic ICH, defined as a four-point or more worsening of the NIHSS with CT-confirmed ICH. Subsequently, the lower weight-adjusted doses were investigated in 57 patients. A significantly higher rate of reperfusion was observed with desmoteplase compared with placebo ($P = 0.0012$). Early reperfusion was found to correlate favorably with clinical outcome assessed by the NIHSS, modified Rankin scale, and Barthel Index (BI) at 90 days ($P = 0.0028$).

The Dose Escalation of Desmoteplase in Acute Stroke (DEDAS) study accompanied the DIAS study to further define the safety and efficacy of IV desmoteplase in patients with perfusion/diffusion mismatch 3–9 hours after stroke onset.[14] DEDAS was a randomized, placebo-controlled, body-weight-adjusted dose-escalation study. Included were patients with an NIHSS score of 4 through 20 with a perfusion/diffusion mismatch on MRI. The primary safety end point was symptomatic ICH defined as in the DIAS study. The study randomly assigned 37 patients: 14 received an IV bolus of 90 μg/kg of desmoteplase over 1 to 2 minutes, and 15 received 125 μg/kg. As was seen in the DIAS trial, reperfusion was found to correlate with a good clinical outcome at 90 days compared with those without reperfusion ($P = 0.003$). Also, no symptomatic ICHs were observed.

Subsequently, DIAS 2, a prospective, randomized, double-blind, placebo-controlled study was completed to confirm the results of the DIAS/DEDAS studies and to further evaluate the safety and efficacy of desmoteplase.[15] Patients were included if they had an NIHSS score between 4 and 24 and onset of symptoms within 3 to 9 hours, as well as a perfusion/diffusion mismatch on MRI of 20%. Perfusion CT was also allowed depending on site experience. There was no statistically significant difference in clinical outcome between the 90 μg/kg or 125 μg/kg of desmoteplase or placebo. Symptomatic ICH, defined as in DIAS, was observed in 4% of patients in the desmoteplase groups. Questions have been raised, however, regarding the reproducibility of the perfusion studies in DIAS 2, which allowed site investigators to use an "eyeball" method (i.e., non-quantitative) measurement of mismatch. Post-hoc data analysis suggested that there may have been important overestimation and underestimation of mismatch in DIAS 2 (personal communication, Greg Albers, MD). Desmoteplase will be studied again in DIAS 3 and DIAS 4, trials organized to find a positive effect of desmoteplase on clinical outcomes without the use of mismatch selection criteria from imaging. Instead, patients will be selected if imaging documents a large-artery occlusion and the absence of large areas of infarcted brain (hypodensity on CT imaging).

Ancrod

Ancrod is a purified fraction of venom from the Malaysian pit viper (*Calloselasma rhodostoma*) and induces rapid defibrinogenation in humans by splitting fibrinopeptide A from fibrinogen.[16] This agent has been the target for acute ischemic stroke since the 1980s.[17,18] Ancrod is given as a continuous infusion for up to 72 hours, and fibrinogen levels are checked before treatment and at designated intervals during and after treatment to determine the activity. Ancrod's effects on plasma fibrinogen levels can be measured. The dosing strategy is to maintain a target fibrinogen level throughout the 5 to 7 days of dosing.[19]

The North American Stroke Treatment with Ancrod Trial (STAT) was a randomized clinical trial that enrolled patients within 3 hours of stroke onset with pretreatment blood pressures maintained at 185 mm Hg systolic/105 mm Hg diastolic or less.[20] The patients received IV ancrod or placebo continuously for 72 hours, then intermittently for 2 days so that a target fibrinogen level could be obtained, which was based on their pretreatment fibrinogen level. This study was found to increase the proportion of patients with ischemic stroke who had a favorable functional status, as measured by a BI score of 95 or greater at 90 days. This study showed significant efficacy ($P = 0.041$), and similar mortality rates were seen between ancrod treatment and placebo. Significantly more asymptomatic ICHs were also found in the ancrod group than in the placebo group at rates similar to those found in the NINDS t-PA trial. Following this study was the European Stroke Treatment with Ancrod Trial (ESTAT), which administered treatment within 6 hours of acute stroke onset.[21] ESTAT was a randomized, double-blind placebo-controlled, phase 3 trial of 1222 patients randomly assigned to ancrod or placebo. Unlike the STAT study, treatment was started within 6 hours of symptom onset and blood pressure was allowed to be 220/120 mm Hg or less. As in the STAT study, pretreatment fibrinogen levels were measured, and infusions were adjusted to maintain a prespecified target fibrinogen range. The time to treatment was more than 3 hours in 43% of the ancrod-treated group and in 42% of the placebo-treated group. Functional outcome at 3 months, as measured by a BI score greater than 95 or return to prestroke values, was similar in the ancrod and placebo groups. Symptomatic ICH occurred significantly more often in patients given ancrod compared with those given placebo ($P = 0.007$).

A pivotal phase 3 trial was organized to confirm whether ancrod significantly altered the outcome after stroke in a large cohort of patients. The dose was carefully titrated to fibrinogen. Unfortunately, the trial was halted after an interim analysis for futility, which suggests that ancrod does not benefit patients with acute stroke.[22]

PRECLINICAL STUDIES OF THROMBOLYSIS FOR ACUTE STROKE

Considerable preclinical development showed that thrombolysis might be an effective stroke therapy. After recombinant technology was developed to produce large quantities of t-PA, animal studies could be conducted to show that t-PA, administered immediately after experimental embolic occlusion, caused reperfusion with significantly less neurologic damage. This development helped overcome the negative experience of early human use that accumulated before modern imaging techniques.

As early as 1963, Meyer et al. studied embolic stroke models in cats and monkeys and administered IV or intra-arterial bovine or human plasmin; this treatment resulted in clot lysis without higher rates of hemorrhagic infarction.[23] In 1986, del Zoppo et al. demonstrated in baboons that after 3 hours of reversible balloon inflation compressing the middle cerebral artery (MCA), intracarotid administration of UK improved neurologic function and reduced infarct size without an increase in the rate of ICH detectable by CT.[24] In 1985, Zivin et al. documented that t-PA could substantially improve neurologic function after embolization with artificially made clots.[25] These studies together strongly suggested that thrombolysis, by restoring blood flow soon after stroke onset, could prevent neurologic deficits.

Preclinical trials also yielded insights into the potential risks of thrombolysis. In 1986, del Zoppo et al. studied t-PA-induced hemorrhagic transformation of ischemic baboon brains within 3.5 hours of MCA occlusion followed by 30 minutes of reperfusion.[24] There was no significant difference in incidence or volume of infarct-related hemorrhage between any of the t-PA groups and the control group. In 1987, Slivka and Pulsinelli investigated the hemorrhagic potential of both t-PA and SK given 24 hours after experimental strokes in rabbits as well as that of SK given 1 hour after experimental stroke.[26] These investigators found that the thrombolytic agents increased the risk of ICH unless they were given early after the insult. In 1989, Lyden et al. found no difference in the frequency of hemorrhagic transformation in the ischemic brains of rabbits whether t-PA was administered 10 minutes, 8 hours, or even 24 hours after cerebral embolism.[27] In 1991, Clark et al. demonstrated that aspirin and t-PA act synergistically to cause intracranial bleeding in the rabbit embolism model.[28]

To learn whether hemorrhagic risk was associated with thrombolytic agents in general or with a particular agent specifically, Lyden et al. compared t-PA, SK, and saline given after embolic stroke in rabbits.[29] SK, but not t-PA, was associated with a significant increase in ICH rate and size. Table 51-1 demonstrates those results. It should be noted that there was no clear dose–response effect for hemorrhages, and the doses used were comparable to those used for cardiac disease in humans. Only the rabbits in which t-PA achieved thrombolysis had twice the frequency of ICH than those given placebo, which suggests that reperfusion might be the basis for the higher rate of hemorrhagic transformation.

In summary, preclinical studies suggested that t-PA had reliably opened cerebral arteries in embolic experimental models. Considerable benefit was achieved if thrombolysis occurred early after occlusion onset. Hemorrhages occurred after thrombolysis and seemed to be related to the particular agent used, and SK carried a greater risk than t-PA.

CLINICAL STUDIES OF THROMBOLYSIS FOR ACUTE STROKE

The clinical development of thrombolysis for stroke proceeded logically from preclinical testing. Early experiments benefited from preclinical data and emphasized several factors: agent, dose, timing, and concomitant management. We review first human-use studies that documented thrombolysis in humans after administration of thrombolytic agents.

Dose-ranging studies yielded important data about the dose of t-PA to use in pivotal trials; the efficacy of the agents seemed to be counterbalanced by hemorrhages at higher doses. Large placebo-controlled trials confirmed the efficacy and hazards of these agents as well as observations from preclinical studies that SK was more hazardous. Finally, after regulatory approval of t-PA for treatment of acute stroke, open-label studies confirmed the findings of the definitive trials and showed that IV thrombolysis is feasible and efficacious in a variety of settings. Data from experimental cerebral ischemia studies pointed to the need to treat acute stroke within a few hours, and this observation also proved true in human trials.

Feasibility Studies

Results of early attempts to achieve thrombolysis for acute ischemic stroke were discouraging, especially in studies conducted without the benefit of brain CT to exclude hemorrhage; in these preliminary trials, patients were enrolled within significantly longer time windows than currently approved. In 1965, Meyer et al. studied 73 patients with acute progressive strokes; the treatment group received SK plus anticoagulation, and the control group received anticoagulation only. There was a higher incidence of death in the treatment group, and better clinical improvement in the control group.[30]

In 1976, Fletcher et al. studied 31 patients with acute ischemic stroke who were treated with one of three different doses of IV UK; treatment was given within 36 hours of symptom onset.[31] The study concluded that UK could be

TABLE 51-1 Rates of Intracranial Hemorrhage and Thrombolysis in Rabbits with Embolic Strokes after Administration of t-PA as Compared with Streptokinase and Saline*

				Hemorrhage		*Thrombolysis*	
Treatment	**Dose**	**Time (min)**	***n***	***n***	**%**	***n***	**%**
Saline		†	48	12	25	17	35
t-PA	3 mg/kg	90	16	5	31	9	56
t-PA	5 mg/kg	90	22	3	14	15	68
t-PA	10 mg/kg	90	11	4	36	10	91†
SK	30,000 units/kg	5	11	6	55	5	45
SK	30,000 units/kg	90	17	11	65‡	14	82†
SK	30,000 units/kg	300	12	10	83‡	10	83†

ICH, Intracranial hemorrhage; SK, streptokinase; Time, time after embolization that treatment was initiated; t-PA, tissue-type plasminogen activator.
*Results of t-PA treatment at 5 minutes and 4, 8, and 24 hours are contained in Douglas 1999[2] and Collen 1996[3].
†Saline-treated control rabbits were treated 5, 90, or 300 minutes after embolization.
‡$P < 0.05$ different from saline by chi-squared test.
From Lyden PD, Madden KP, Clark WA, et al. Comparison of cerebral hemorrhage rates following tissue plasminogen activator or streptokinase treatment for embolic strokes in rabbits. *Stroke* 21:981–983, 1990.

administered to patients in doses that achieve substantial thrombolysis without producing other than mild coagulation deficits; this study could not address the efficacy of the treatment, however, because the number of patients was too low. The mortality rate was 16%, and there was no placebo group for comparison. On the basis of these two studies, which were widely discussed, IV thrombolysis for stroke was abandoned pending better agents and better selection procedures.

After the efficacy and safety of t-PA were proved in animal models, thrombolysis was pursued again in acute clinical stroke trials. In 1992, del Zoppo et al. studied 139 patients with acute ischemic stroke who received different doses of IV t-PA within 8 hours of stroke onset.[32] An angiogram confirmed occlusion of an extracranial or intracranial arterial cerebral blood supply in all patients. Exclusion criteria included a minor deficit, a transient ischemic attack (TIA), a clinically large stroke with a combination of hemiplegia, impaired consciousness, and forced gaze deviation, blood pressure higher than 200 mm Hg systolic, 120 mm Hg diastolic, and radiologic (CT) evidence of bleeding or radiologic evidence of significant mass effect or midline shift. Patients with early CT hypoattenuation changes were not excluded from the study. Primary endpoints were angiographic recanalization and ICH with neurologic deterioration. This landmark study re-established the clinical promise of thrombolysis; 40% of all patients experienced recanalization of occluded arteries. Intriguingly, there was no relation between dose and recanalization, but patients with distal (i.e., smaller) clots showed higher recanalization rates. The frequency of all hemorrhages was 30.8%, although symptomatic hemorrhages occurred in 9.6% of all patients. The mortality rate during hospitalization was 12.5%. There was no increase in hemorrhages with doses comparable to those used to achieve coronary reperfusion, although it could not be assumed that the safe and effective dose for acute coronary events would be the perfect dose for acute stroke treatment. Therefore, the effective and safe dose for stroke treatment was yet to be determined.

In 1992, the first in a series of government-sponsored trials appeared. In a dose-finding trial sponsored by the NINDS, 74 patients with acute ischemic stroke received escalating doses of t-PA (0.35–1.08 mg/kg) within the time window of 90 minutes. Intracranial hematomas did not occur in any of the 58 patients who received doses of 0.85 mg/kg or less. Intracranial hematomas occurred with higher doses. Hemorrhages associated with neurologic deterioration (symptomatic hemorrhages) occurred in three of the 74 patients, although such hemorrhages did not occur at t-PA doses of less than 0.95 mg/kg. Major improvement, manifesting as a significant improvement in the NIHSS score, occurred at 2 hours in 30% of the patients and at 24 hours in 46% of patients. Major neurologic improvement was not related to the dose of t-PA. The investigators concluded that the highest safe dose of t-PA was probably less than 0.95 mg/kg, but it is important to keep in mind that this conclusion was based on only three symptomatic hemorrhages occurring in a total experience of 74 patients. The distinct possibility remains that a higher dose could, in fact, prove to be safe and more efficacious.[33]

In 1992, Haley et al studied 20 patients with acute ischemic stroke in another dose-escalating trial in which t-PA treatment was given between 91 and 180 minutes after stroke onset.[34] The risks of symptomatic ICH were 10% overall and 17% with the two higher dosage levels (the three doses used were 0.6 mg/kg, 0.85 mg/kg, and 0.95 mg/kg). Three patients (15%) improved by 4 points on the NIHSS at 24 hours.

Mori et al. conducted a trial in Japan in which either 6 million or 12 million units of IV t-PA or placebo was administered within 6 hours of stroke onset.[35] Using angiograms before and after thrombolysis, these investigators confirmed that t-PA increased the rate of MCA recanalization. Of considerable importance is the fact that functional outcome measured by the BI score was also significantly improved by thrombolysis. Like the del Zoppo trial, this trial established unequivocally that IV thrombolytics could open occluded cerebral vessels. Further, and perhaps even more important, the trial results suggested that angiographic confirmation of cerebral vessel occlusion might not be essential before IV thrombolysis.

In 1993, in the "bridging trial," a forerunner of the definitive NINDS study, Haley et al. studied 27 patients who received 0.85 mg/kg of IV t-PA or placebo within 3 hours of stroke onset.[36] This was a randomized, double-blinded, placebo-controlled study. Despite the small sample size, there was suggestion of early neurologic improvement (at 24 hours) in the patients treated with t-PA. In the treatment arm in which therapy was given up to 90 minutes after stroke onset, six of the 10 patients who received t-PA improved by 4 or more points on the NIHSS, compared with one of the 10 patients given placebo. In the treatment arm in which therapy was given between 91 and 180 minutes after stroke onset, two patients in the t-PA group and two patients from the placebo subgroups improved by 4 or more points on the NIHSS at 24 hours. The results of the bridging trial anticipated those of the larger NINDS study in a surprising number of respects. Nevertheless, large, rigorous, placebo-controlled, randomized trials were needed to confirm any beneficial effects afforded by IV thrombolytic agents.

Large, Randomized, Multicenter, Placebo-Controlled Trials

ECASS

Published in 1995, the European Cooperative Acute Stroke Study (ECASS) included 620 patients treated with 1.1 mg/kg of IV t-PA or placebo within 6 hours of stroke onset.[37] The trial showed no significant efficacy in the intent-to-treat primary analysis. On exclusion of patients with protocol violations (109 patients, 17.4%), a target population of 511 patients was selected for further analysis. Protocol violations consisted of inclusion of patients with large strokes (i.e., hypodensity of greater than one-third of the MCA territory on CT), concurrent use of anticoagulants or volume expanders, detection of hemorrhage on baseline CT, uncontrolled hypertension, and lack of complete follow-up. The first hypothesis in this study was that there would be a 15-point difference in the BI between the two groups in the study, favoring the t-PA treatment group. The second hypothesis was that there would be a difference on the modified Rankin Scale (mRS) score in favor of the t-PA group.

In the target population, there was a 1-point difference in the mRS score between the two groups ($P = 0.035$) in favor of the t-PA group. There was no statistically significant difference in ICH rates between the groups, but there was an increase in frequency of large parenchymal hemorrhages in the t-PA group and an increase in frequency of hemorrhagic infarcts in the placebo group. There was no statistically significant difference in mortality rates at 30 days. Although ECASS failed to show a benefit (the hypothesis was not proved), subsequent analyses showed a significant treatment effect. In particular, on post hoc reanalysis of ECASS with the use of NINDS global end-point statistics, a statistically significant treatment effect was detected in the intent-to-treat group.[38] This finding suggests that ECASS might have shown a beneficial effect of thrombolytic agents in stroke even though one cannot definitely reach that conclusion from a post hoc analysis. Furthermore, when the patients treated within 3 hours were examined

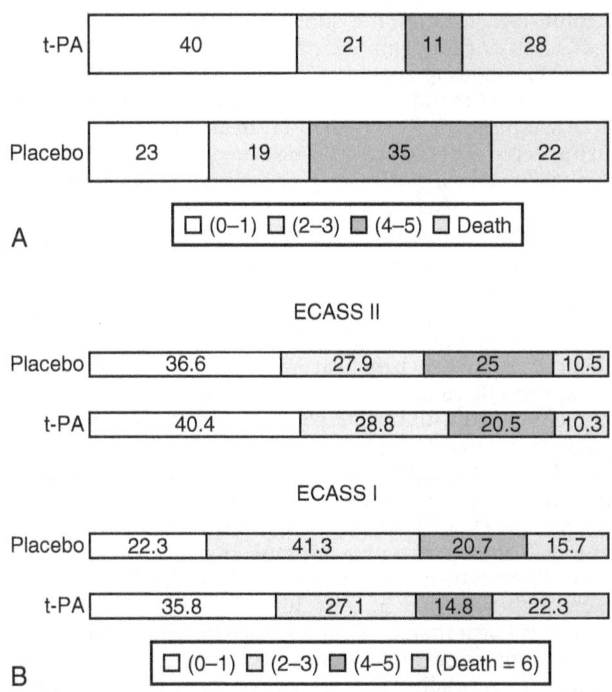

Figure 51-4. A, Intention to treat subpopulation (n = 87, t-PA = 49, placebo = 38) in the ECASS-I patients who received treatment within 3 hours, using the same analysis method implemented previously in NINDS: global odds ratio is 2.3 (0.9, 5.3), *P* = 0.07. The results are not statistically significant because of the small number of patients within 3 hours. B, Patient outcome by modified Rankin scale (mRS) in ECASS-I and ECASS-II. Both ECASS-I and ECASS-II were positive for the endpoint of mRS ≤ 2 (no disability to slight disability). Each *bar* shows the percent of patients with that grade. Grade 0: asymptomatic patients. Grade 1: no significant disability despite symptoms; patient is able to carry out all usual activities and duties. Grade 2: slight disability; the patient is unable to carry out all previous activities but able to look after his or her affairs without assistance. Grade 3: moderate disability with the requirement of some help but with preservation of the ability to walk without assistance. Grade 4: moderately severe disability with inability to walk without assistance and inability to attend to one's own bodily needs without assistance. Grade 5: severe disability; the patient is bedridden, incontinent, and requires constant nursing care and attention. Grade 6: death.

separately (38 given placebo, 49 given t-PA), a non-statistically significant treatment effect (Fig. 51-4A) was demonstrated by the same statistical analysis methods used in the NINDS study (global odds ratio [OR], 2.3; *P* = 0.07).[39] The ECASS post hoc analyses suggested that an independent 3-hour trial might show a benefit for thrombolytic agents.

The NINDS Studies

In December 1995, the NINDS study was published; it was a randomized, placebo-controlled, multicenter trial that showed the efficacy of t-PA in treating acute ischemic strokes within 3 hours of onset.[1] This NINDS study differed from ECASS in several respects besides the dose of t-PA and time to treatment. Most importantly, NINDS protocol required that the blood pressure had to be controlled to below 185 mm Hg systolic, 95 mm Hg diastolic. Box 51-1 summarizes the inclusion and exclusion criteria of the NINDS study.

The NINDS study had two parts with identical protocol but different endpoints. Part 1 tested whether t-PA showed clinical activity, as indicated by a statistically significant difference on the primary endpoint, chosen arbitrarily to be either an improvement of 4 or more points on the NIHSS or complete resolution of the neurologic deficit within 24 hours. Part 2 used a global test statistic to assess clinical outcome after 3 months, based on scores on the BI, mRS, Glasgow Outcome Scale (GOS), and NIHSS. Part 1 enrolled 291 patients (144 in the t-PA group and 147 in the placebo group), and part 2 enrolled 333 patients (168 patients in the t-PA group and 165 patients in the placebo group). In part 1, on the primary endpoint, the number of patients improving by 4 or more points on the NIHSS at 24 hours was 67 (47%) in the t-PA group and 57 (39%) in the placebo group (not statistically significant, with a P value of 0.21). Subsequent analysis showed that any other cutoff improvement in the 24-hour NIHSS score, such as 5 or more points, would have yielded a statistically significant difference between the two groups (Fig. 51-5).[40]

In part 2 of the NINDS, benefit was observed on all four primary efficacy measures (i.e., NIHSS, BI, mRS, and GOS scores) at 3 months from onset of stroke. Figure 51-6 demonstrates the increase in proportion of patients with good clinical outcomes in the t-PA group compared with the placebo group as measured by these scales. Patients treated with t-PA were 30–50% more likely to have minimal or no disability at 3 months, depending on the outcome measure. For example, the percentage of patients with an mRS score of 1 or less at 3 months was 39% in the t-PA group versus 26% in the placebo group (statistically significant difference in favor of t-PA). Symptomatic ICH occurred in 6.4% of patients who received

BOX 51-1 Inclusion and Exclusion Criteria of the NINDS Study*

INCLUSION CRITERIA OF NINDS

Ischemic stroke of defined onset <3 hours
Deficit measurable on NIHSS
Baseline CT of the brain without evidence of hemorrhage

EXCLUSION CRITERIA OF NINDS

A prior stroke within the last 3 months PTP
Major surgery within the last 14 days PTP
Serious head trauma within the last 3 months PTP
History of ICH
Systolic BP >185 mm Hg or diastolic BP >110 mm Hg or if aggressive treatment was required to lower the BP to below these limits
Rapidly improving or minor symptoms
Symptoms suggestive of SAH
Gastrointestinal bleeding or urinary tract hemorrhage within 3 weeks PTP
Arterial puncture at a noncompressible site within the last 7 days PTP
Seizure at the onset of symptoms
Anticoagulants or heparin within 48 hours before stroke onset or elevated PTT or elevated PT >15 sec
Platelet count <100,000/mL
Blood glucose <50 mg/dL or above 400 mg/dL

BP, Blood pressure; CT, computed tomography; ICH, intracranial hemorrhage; NIHSS, National Institutes of Health Stroke Scale; NINDS, National Institute of Neurological Disorders and Stroke; PT, prothrombin time; PTP, prior to presentation; PTT, partial thromboplastin time; SAH, subarachnoid hemorrhage.
*Tissue plasminogen activator for acute ischemic stroke.
Tissue plasminogen activator for acute ischemic stroke. The National Institute of Neurological Disorders and Stroke rt-PA Stroke Study Group. *N Engl J Med* 333:1581–1587, 1995.

treatment but only in 0.6% of patients who received placebo. Mortality rates at 3 months were not statistically different between the two groups, being 17% in the t-PA group and 21% in the placebo group.[1] Thus, despite an increased risk of hemorrhage, the mortality rate was not affected, and IV t-PA provided considerable benefit and improved outcomes, as depicted in Figure 51-7. Furthermore, the NINDS data analysis showed that t-PA treatment resulted in a more favorable outcome regardless of the subtype of stroke (small-vessel, large-vessel, or cardioembolic stroke) diagnosed at baseline.[1]

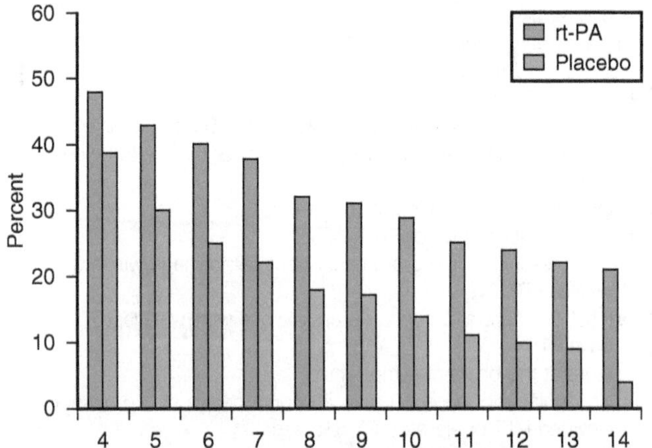

Figure 51-5. The percentage of patients within each improvement category of National Institutes of Health Stroke Scale (NIHSS) at 24 hours in Part 1 of National Institute of Neurological and Communicable Diseases and Stroke (NINDS) study. The improvement in NIHSS score at 24 hours was significantly better in the t-PA treated group as compared with placebo ($P < 0.05$) in each of the categories of improvement in the NIHSS score, except for a drop of NIHSS of ≥4 points (chosen as the primary endpoint of Part I of NINDS). Therefore, had the primary endpoint been chosen to be a drop in NIHSS at 24 hours ≥ any number other than 4, Part 1 would have shown a statistically significant benefit of t-PA at 24 hours.

Further subgroup analysis of the NINDS data showed that the only variables independently associated with an increased risk of symptomatic ICH in the t-PA-treated patients were the baseline severity of the stroke as measured by the NIHSS, brain edema defined by hypodensity on baseline CT, and mass effect on baseline CT (before treatment).[41] These factors did not interact with treatment, however, which suggests that such factors might not be predictive in excluding patients from treatment.

Subsequent prespecified analyses of the NINDS database with the use of a global statistical method showed sustained, statistically significant benefit at 6-month and 1-year follow-up points: the OR values for a favorable outcome in the t-PA group compared with the placebo group were 1.7 with a 95% confidence interval (CI) of 1.3 to 2.3 at 6 months and 1.7 with a 95% CI of 1.2 to 2.3 at 1 year.[42] At 1 year, the range of absolute increase in the percentage of patients with a favorable outcome was 11–13%, and the range of relative increase in the percentage of patients with a favorable outcome was 32– 46% for the three outcome scales (mRS, BI, and GOS). Patients treated with t-PA were at least 30% more likely to be independent at 1 year than those given placebo. Importantly, favorable outcomes were not accompanied by an increase in severe disability or mortality. The proportion of patients surviving between 3 months and 12 months after stroke was consistently higher in the t-PA group than in the placebo group. However, there was no statistically significant difference in mortality at 6 months and 1 year. After adjustment for those variables, treatment with t-PA still offered better outcomes.

As was the case for the 3-month follow-up data, there was no evidence of interaction between the subtype of stroke at baseline and treatment, meaning that all stroke subtypes (large-vessel, small-vessel, and embolic) benefitted from t-PA. Moreover, there was no significant difference in the incidence of recurrent stroke between the t-PA and placebo groups at 1 year.[42] Furthermore, another analysis of the NINDS data

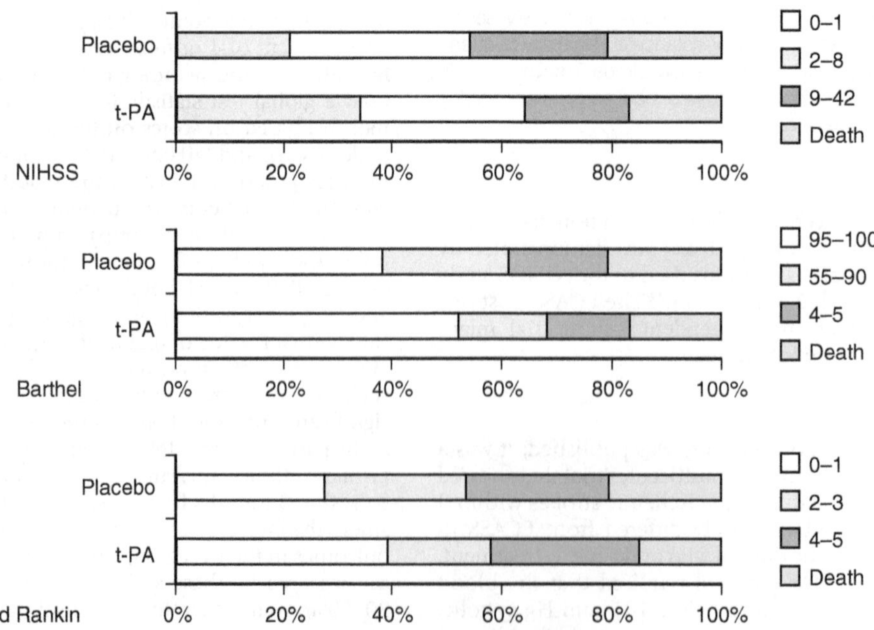

Figure 51-6. Statistically significant improvement on all primary outcome measures at 3 months in National Institute of Neurological and Communicable Diseases and Stroke (NINDS) study, Part 2. National Institutes of Health Stroke Scale (NIHSS), Barthel Index, and modified Rankin Scale (mRS) at 3 months are depicted here, and there is a statistically significant improvement in the t-PA treated patients as compared with placebo in each of these categories as well as in the Glasgow Outcome Scale (GOS), which is not shown here.

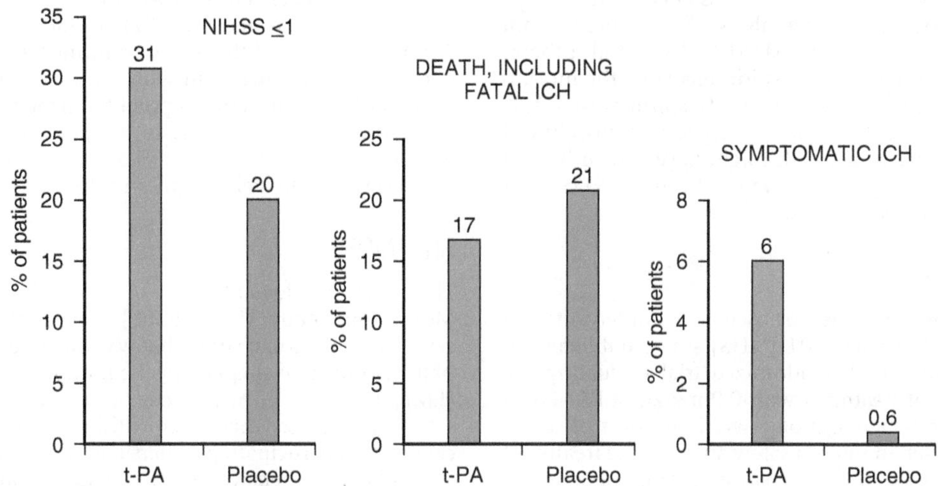

Figure 51-7. Benefit and risk of t-PA in National Institute of Neurological and Communicable Diseases and Stroke (NINDS) for Acute Stroke Trial: Benefit from t-PA is shown as a statistically significant higher percent of patients with National Institutes of Health Stroke Scale (NIHSS) score of 0–1 in the t-PA group as compared with placebo. Risk is depicted as a statistically significant increase in symptomatic intracranial hemorrhage (ICH) at 36 hours that is attributable to t-PA treatment. Despite that risk, there is no significant difference in mortality between the t-PA and placebo groups at 3 months.

addressed finding the binary measures that predicted effectiveness of t-PA during the first 3 months. Measures using NIHSS and mRS scores of 1 or less were the most sensitive discriminators of effectiveness of t-PA in the NINDS study. The best measure was NIHSS score of 2 or less at 24 hours. High-quality analysis of the volume of brain infarction as measured by CT was not as sensitive in detecting a treatment effect as the clinical scale measures.[43]

ECASS II

ECASS II was a multicenter double-blind, randomized trial of 800 patients with acute stroke who received either 0.9 mg/kg t-PA (409 patients) or placebo (391 patients) within 6 hours of stroke onset.[44] Exclusion criteria were similar to those for the NINDS, with the addition of evidence of early infarction changes on CT greater than one-third of the MCA territory, coma or stupor, and hemiplegia with fixed eye deviation. The use of anticoagulants and antiplatelet agents was prohibited for the first 24 hours after random assignment of patients to treatment.

There were 72 protocol violations (17%), 34 in the t-PA group and 38 in the placebo group; the majority resulted from failure to abide by the CT criteria. There was no statistically significant difference in the proportion of favorable outcomes (mRS score 0 to 1 at day 90) between the two groups; favorable outcomes occurred in 40.3% of the t-PA group and in 36.6% of the placebo group ($P \geq 0.05$). A post hoc analysis of the 90-day mRS score, classifying each patient as either functionally independent (mRS score, ≤2) or dependent (mRS score, >2), found a statistically significant difference between the two groups in favor of t-PA (54.3% in the t-PA group versus 46.0% in the placebo group with an 8.3% absolute difference; $P = 0.024$). The incidence of symptomatic ICH was higher in the t-PA group (8.8%) than in the placebo group (3.4%). Figure 51-4B shows the mRS scores for the t-PA and placebo groups at 90 days in both ECASS-1 and ECASS-2.

Streptokinase Trials

Three clinical trials attempted to investigate the benefits and risks of SK treatment in acute stroke. These trials were all terminated prematurely because of complications. The Multicentre Acute Stroke Trial in Europe (MAST-E) was a double-blind, placebo-controlled, randomized study of SK published in 1996.[45] Patients with acute MCA strokes presenting within 6 hours of onset received either 1.5 million units of IV SK or placebo. There was no difference in the primary outcome measures (death and severe disability and mRS score ≥ 3 at 6 months after treatment). In-hospital death and symptomatic ICH occurred more often in the SK group. The use of anticoagulants or antiplatelet agents was allowed: 65% of patients given SK and 75% of patients given placebo received heparin concomitantly with thrombolysis, and 20% of patients in each group also received aspirin. At 6 months, the mortality rate was higher in the SK group ($P = 0.06$). There was a trend toward less severe disability with SK and a significantly shorter rehabilitation or nursing home stay ($P = 0.003$). This study found no evident benefit from SK treatment.

The Multicentre Acute Stroke Trial in Italy (MAST-I), published in 1995, was a randomized controlled trial that studied patients who received IV SK, SK plus aspirin, aspirin alone, or placebo within 6 hours of stroke onset.[46] Anticoagulants were to be avoided in this trial, except for limited doses of subcutaneous heparin for prophylaxis of deep venous thrombosis. There was no proved benefit in any therapy group. Symptomatic hemorrhages were more common in the SK groups than in the placebo and aspirin-only groups. Aspirin plus SK therapy was associated with a statistically significant increase in early mortality compared with placebo.

In the Australian Streptokinase (ASK) study, 340 patients were randomly assigned to receive either placebo or SK intravenously within 4 hours of stroke onset.[47] The study had to be suspended because of poorer outcomes in the SK group. There was no relationship between the dose of SK and the risk of hemorrhage. The hematoma rate was 9.6% in the SK group and 0% in the placebo group for patients who received treatment within 3 hours of stroke onset. The SK group had higher mortality, worse clinical outcome, and increased ICH rates. Hypotension was an adverse event that occurred in the SK-treated patients. Subsequent analysis comparing the 70 patients treated within 3 hours and the 270 patients treated after 3 hours of stroke onset found that earlier treatment was associated with better outcomes than was later treatment.[48]

A further multivariate meta-analysis of all patients from previous SK studies (MAST-E, MAST-I, ASK, and others) showed that concomitant use of aspirin increased the mortality in SK-treated patients (17% without aspirin versus 91% with aspirin treatment, $P = 0.005$).[49] There remains clinical uncertainty, therefore, whether SK might have shown benefit if tested with the same protocol as used in the NINDS rt-PA trial. This issue remains unsolved.

The ATLANTIS Study

The Alteplase Thrombolysis for Acute Noninterventional Therapy in Ischemic Stroke (ATLANTIS) study, published in 1999, was a double-blind, randomized trial evaluating the efficacy and safety of treatment with 0.9 mg/kg of IV t-PA in patients with acute ischemic strokes within 6 hours of stroke onset (part A).[50] After an interim safety analysis, the treatment window was changed to 5 hours (part B) because of concerns about safety in patients treated between 5 and 6 hours of onset. The trial ended prematurely in 1998 on the basis of analysis that the treatment was unlikely to be beneficial. In the final analysis of part B, the median time to treatment was 4.5 hours; a minority of patients received treatment within 3 hours. There was no difference in the primary endpoint, that is, in the percentage of patients with an NIHSS score of ≤1 at 90 days. The symptomatic ICH rate, however, was greater in the t-PA group.

Albers et al. retrospectively evaluated data for the ATLANTIS patients who had received t-PA or placebo within the 3-hour time window.[51] The primary endpoint was the percentage of patients who had complete recovery, as determined by an NIHSS score of ≤1 at 90 days after treatment. The total number of patients was 61: 38 in the placebo arm and 23 in the t-PA arm. The patients receiving t-PA were significantly more likely to have a favorable outcome, defined as an NIHSS score of ≤1 ($P = 0.01$); 60.9% of the t-PA group had an NIHSS score of ≤1 at 3 months versus only 26.3% in the placebo group, with an absolute difference of 34.6% (OR, 4.4; $P < 0.01$). The symptomatic ICH rate was 13% in the t-PA group versus 0% in the placebo group (statistically significant difference; $P = 0.05$). There was a trend toward higher mortality in the t-PA group that did not reach statistical significance.

Pooled Analysis of NINDS, ECASS II, and ATLANTIS

Despite its proven effectiveness in treating acute ischemic strokes, alteplase is still only given to a minority of patients with acute ischemic strokes, primarily because of the short time window in which it is currently being used. In 2004, the investigators of the ATLANTIS, ECASS II, and NINDS studies performed a pooled analysis of six randomized controlled trials of alteplase given up to 6 hours to determine the effect of time to treatment on functional outcome.[52] A total of 2775 patients were included from the NINDS trials, the ECASS trials and the ATLANTIS trials. The median onset to treatment was 243 minutes. The study confirmed a clear association between time to treatment and meaningful recovery. As the time interval to treatment increased, the odds of a favorable outcome (defined as an mRS of <2) decreased ($P < 0.005$). The odds ratios were 2.8 (95%CI, 1.8–4.5) for 0–90 minutes, 1.6 (1.1–2.2) for 91–180 minutes, 1.4 (1.1–1.9) for 180–270 minutes, and 1.2 (0.9–1.5) for 271–360 minutes. Symptomatic ICH occurred in 5.9% of patients treated with alteplase compared with 1.1% of placebo-treated patients ($P < 0.0001$). An association was found between ICH and treatment with alteplase as well as age but not with time to treatment. The hazard ratio for death adjusted for baseline NIHSS was not significantly different from 1.0 for patients treated within 270 minutes but exceeded 1.0 for patients treated from 271 to 360 minutes (1.0; 1.02–2.07). The results of this study confirmed a strong association between time to treatment with alteplase and treatment efficacy, but it also suggested a potential benefit beyond 3 hours. The most important finding in the pooled analysis, however, was a confirmation that the odds of favorable outcome declined with every minute delay from symptom onset.

SITS-MOST

The Safe Implementation of Thrombolysis in Stroke-Monitoring Study (SITS-MOST) was a prospective, multicenter, observational study that was initiated as a requirement of the approval of alteplase by the European Medicines Agency (EMEA) in 2002.[53] The purpose of the trial was to confirm the safety of alteplase when given within 3 hours in routine clinical practice. Participating centers had to have routine monitoring and comprehensive care for all stroke patients. Safety and functional outcomes were compared with pooled results from the NINDS, ECASS I and II, and the ATLANTIS trials for patients treated within 3 hours. Between 2002 and 2006, 6483 patients received alteplase. At 7 days, the rate of symptomatic hemorrhage was 7.3% (468/6438) compared with 8.6% (40/465) in the pooled randomized analysis. In the SITS-MOST, 54.8% of patients had good functional outcomes (defined as an mRS of 0 to 2) compared with 49% in the pooled analysis. While SITS-MOST confirmed the safety of alteplase in routine clinical practice, it should be noted that the study did not include patients older than 80 years or with an NIHSS score of 25 or higher.

Additional analysis of SITS-MOST data suggested that new centers, that is, those that began thrombolytic programs for the first time, could deliver thrombolytic therapy as safely as more experienced centers. This finding, although counterintuitive, suggests that centers without active programs can design and initiate teams to deliver thrombolytic therapy to stroke patients with good safety and efficacy.

SITS-ISTR

The SITS (Safe Implementation of Treatments in Stroke) is an interactive database of unselected patients treated with thrombolysis for acute strokes in more than 700 clinical centers in 35 countries. The SITS-ISTR study was a retrospective study of 664 patients registered with the SITS-ISTR between 2002 and 2007 who were treated with alteplase between 3 and 4.5 hours after symptom onset.[54] The rates of functional independence (defined as an mRS of 0 to 2) and symptomatic ICH were compared with patients registered in the SITS-ISTR who were treated within 3 hours. Differences between the treatment groups suggested a possible selection bias because patients treated between 3 and 4.5 hours were younger (65 years compared with 68 years, $P < 0.0001$), had a lower median NIHSS score (11 versus 12, $P < 0.0001$), and were more likely to be treated in experienced stroke centers. There was no difference between groups in rate of functional independence (58% vs 56.3%) or symptomatic ICH (2.2% vs 1.6%). The authors concluded that alteplase can be safely given at 4 to 4.5 hours but acknowledged the need for a randomized controlled study to confirm their findings.

ECASS III

In 2002, the EMEA approved alteplase with two requirements. The first request was for the implementation of an observational study, which resulted in the SITS-MOST study. The second was for a randomized trial in which the time window was extended beyond 3 hours.

The ECASS III trial was a randomized controlled, double-blind trial of 821 patients with acute ischemic stroke who received either 0.9 mg/kg of alteplase (418) intravenously or placebo (403) at 3–4.5 hours after symptom onset.[55] Patients with a history of diabetes and a previous stroke and an NIHSS score of more than 25 were excluded. Treatment groups were generally well-matched, but patients treated beyond 3 hours had a significantly higher mean NIHSS compared with the alteplase group (11.6 versus 10.7, $P = 0.03$). The average time to treatment was 3 hours and 59 minutes in the alteplase group and 3 hours and 58 minutes in the placebo group. Of the patients in the alteplase group, 52% had a favorable outcome (defined as an mRS of ≤1) compared with 45.2% in the placebo group ($P < 0.04$). The difference remained significant even after adjustment for the baseline NIHSS score (OR, 1.42; 95%CI, 1.02 to 1.98, $P = 0.04$). The rate of symptomatic ICH was 2.4% in the alteplase group compared with 0.3% in the placebo group ($P = 0.008$).

Some critics argue that the use of the mRS changed significantly between the ECASS II and the ECASS III trials and that the unusually high response rate in the placebo group reflects this secular trend. Others, however, noted the fact that the ECASS III resembled the NINDS trial in important respects – other than the age and severity limits – and that the statistically significant result confirms the original NINDS trial of rt-PA for acute stroke.[56]

On the basis of this study, the European Stroke Organization modified its guidelines to include patients with symptom onset up to 4.5 hours, and other countries are expected to follow. The critical point, however, is that increasing the time window for thrombolysis should increase the number of acute strokes that can be treated with alteplase, not provide a reason to delay treatment. While the ECASS III study shows that alteplase is still effective when given after 3 hours, early treatment is essential because its benefit is time-dependent.

After the ECASS-3 was published, a metanalysis done by Lansberg et al. was performed in 2009 to further assess the treatment effect of intravenous thrombolysis within the 3–4.5 hour time window.[57] This meta-analysis included patients from the ECASS-1, ECASS-2, ECASS-3 and ATLANTIS trials that were treated with t-PA between 3 and 4.5 hours from time of onset. Compared to placebo, patients treated with t-PA were more likely to have good functional outcome at 90 days based on the Global Outcome Measure (OR 1.31; 95%CI, 1.10 to 1.56; $P = 0.002$) and Modified Rankin Scale (OR 1.31; 95%CI, 1.07–1.59; $P = 0.008$). There was no significant difference in mortality. Because patients in the ECASS-1 received a higher dose of tPA of 1.1 mg/kg, a separate meta-analysis was performed using only the other three trials that used a tPA dose of 0.9 mg/kg. Patients that received tPA still were more likely to have a favorable outcome with no difference in mortality with an OR of 1.27 on the Global Outcome Measure ($P = 0.001$) and 1.28 on the Modified Rankin Scale ($P = 0.03$). This study added further evidence that intravenous thrombolysis at 3–4.5 hours can improve functional outcome without an increase in mortality.

IST-3

Published in 2012, the Third International Stroke Trial (IST-3) was an multicenter, randomized open-label trial in which 3035 patients were randomized to receive intravenous t-PA (1515 patients) or standard care (1520 patients).[58–60] Patients were eligible based on the uncertainty principle meaning the use of intravenous thrombolysis was thought to be promising, but not necessarily proven. Over 53% of the patients were therefore over the age of 80. In the first 7 days, t-PA was associated with a higher rate of intracerebral hemorrhage and mortality. Symptomatic intracerebral hemorrhage occurred in 7% of the t-PA group and 1% in the control group, and the mortality rate at 7 days was 11% in the t-PA group versus 7% in the control group. However, between 7 days and 6 months, there were fewer deaths in the t-PA group, so by the end 6 months, there was no significant difference in mortality between groups (27% in both groups). Functional outcome was measured with the Oxford Handicap Score. At 6 months, there was no significant difference in disability with 37% patients in the t-PA group versus 35% in the control group alive and independent. This study therefore showed that despite the early adverse events with t-PA, thrombolysis within 6 hours improved functional outcomes at 6 months.

A follow-up study to the IST-3 was published in 2013 to assess the long-term effects of t-PA at 18 months.[61] The primary outcome measure was a score based on the EuroQol instrument which is a self-reported questionnaire on health. At 18 months, treatment with thrombolysis was associated with a significantly higher self-reported health on the EuroQol Instrument ($P = 0.019$). Thirty-five percent in the t-PA group verses 31.4% in the control group were more likely to be independent based on the Oxford Handicap Scale for an OR of 1.28 (95%CI, 1.03–1.57; $P = 0.024$). Patients over 80 in particular that were treated with t-PA were more likely to be alive and independent based the Oxford Handicap Score compared to their controls ($P = 0.032$). There was no significant difference in mortality between groups. This study, therefore, showed sustained benefits in IV alteplase at 18 months.

Following the IST-3, Wardlaw et al. published meta-analysis in 2012 that included 7012 patients from 12 randomized trials of t-PA given within 12 hours of onset.[62] At follow-up, 46.3% of patients treated with t-PA versus 42.1% of the control patients had a Modified Rankin score of 0–1 with an OR of 1.17 (95%CI, 1.06–1.29; $P = 0.001$). The benefit of t-PA was greatest in patients treated within 3 hours of onset with 40.7% of patients treated with t-PA having a modified Rankin score of 0–2 versus 31.7% of control patients, for a OR of 1.53 (95%CI, 1.26–1.86; $P < 0.0001$). The number of deaths at 7 days was increased in patients treated with t-PA (8.9% in patients treated with t-PA versus 6.4% patients treated with placebo, $P = 0.0003$). Symptomatic hemorrhage occurred in 7.7% of patients treated with t-PA versus 1.8% patients treated with placebo ($P < 0.001$). However, at follow-up, there was no significant difference in mortality. The benefit of t-PA was shown to extend to patients over the age of 80, particularly when treated early.

COMMUNITY EXPERIENCE OF THROMBOLYSIS FOR ACUTE STROKE

On the basis of the results of the two NINDS studies and the post hoc analysis of the ECASS trials, the FDA approved t-PA as treatment for acute ischemic stroke in June 1996. Almost immediately, critics suggested that somehow the trials had been conducted only in specialized stroke centers and therefore the results could not be generalized to the larger stroke population. Despite the fact that the NINDS study included more patients randomly assigned for treatment at community medical centers than in academic centers, a need existed to demonstrate efficacy in community experience. Several such observational studies have now appeared, and the results nearly uniformly confirm those of the ECASS and NINDS studies. If the NINDS protocol is not followed, however, lower response rates and higher hemorrhage rates can be observed.

In 1998, Chiu et al.[63] published the first *Houston* community experience, which evaluated 30 patients with acute ischemic stroke who were treated with IV t-PA between December 1995 and December 1996 at a dose of 0.9 mg/kg. The rate of symptomatic ICH was 7%, and the rate of fatal ICH was 3%. On follow-up in December 1996, 37% of patients had recovered to fully independent function (BI, 95–100), and 30% of patients had no disability (mRS score, 0–1). The 3-month mortality rate was 20% (compared with 17% in the corresponding NINDS group). Three patients were treated outside the 3-hour window. This study concluded that t-PA therapy is a feasible, safe, and effective treatment for acute ischemic stroke in one academic and three community medical centers. There was no difference in any outcome or safety measure between the two types of medical centers.

The results of the *STARS* (Standard Treatment with Alteplase to Reverse Stroke) study were published in March 2000.[64] Albers et al. looked at 389 consecutive patients with stroke enrolled between February 1997 and December 1998 from different academic and community hospitals in the US. Those patients were seen with acute ischemic stroke within 3 hours of onset. The median NIHSS score was 13. Protocol violations occurred in 127 patients (32.6%). The violations were anticoagulant use, treatment outside the recommended period, and non-adherence to blood pressure guidelines. The measure of recovery was mRS score at 30 days after t-PA treatment; the mRS score was ≤1 in 35% of patients and ≤2 (independence) in 43% of patients. Symptomatic ICH occurred in 3.3% of patients, and asymptomatic ICH occurred in 8.2%. This study showed favorable clinical outcomes with t-PA treatment and a relatively low rate of symptomatic hemorrhage, comparable with that of the NINDS studies.

In April 2001, Barber et al. published the *Calgary* experience, in which 2165 consecutive patients with acute stroke in Calgary, Canada, treated between October 1996 and December 1999 were studied. Of these patients, 1168 (53.9%) were given a diagnosis of ischemic stroke. Hemorrhagic stroke was diagnosed in 31.8%, and TIAs were diagnosed in 13.9%. Of the 1168 patients with ischemic stroke, 73.1% were excluded from the study because of delayed presentation. Causes for delay included uncertain time of onset (24.2%), waiting to see whether the deficit would improve (29%), transfer from another hospital (8.9%), and poor accessibility to the treating hospital (patient's home a long distance from the treating hospital or transfer of patients from an outlying hospital) (5.7%). Of the 1168 patients with ischemic stroke, 314 patients (27%) were admitted to the hospital within 3 hours of onset, and 84 of the 314 (26.7%) received IV t-PA. Exclusion of the rest of the patients seen within the 3-hour window was due to different reasons: 13.1% had mild strokes, 18.2% showed clinical improvement, 13.6% had other protocol exclusions, 8.9% experienced ED referral delay, and 8.3% had significant morbidity. At 3 months, 54% of the patients included in the study had an mRS score ≤ 2. The symptomatic ICH rate was 7.1%. Only 4.7% of all patients seen during the study period were treated with t-PA; the majority of t-PA treatment exclusions were related to a delay in presentation. Of those patients whose strokes were considered too mild to be treated or who showed rapid improvement, 32% either remained dependent on hospital discharge or died during hospital admission. This finding implied that one-third of the patients who were excluded because of minimal deficits or dramatic improvement had poor outcomes, which raises the question of whether such patients should also be treated.[65]

In an article published in December 2001, Grotta et al. described their own *Houston* community experience with t-PA treatment in patients with acute ischemic stroke between January 1996 and June 2000.[66] The design was a prospective inception cohort registry of patients seen by the stroke team at the University of Texas–Houston Medical School and three community hospitals in addition to a retrospective medical record review of all patients treated with t-PA within the same 4-year period. A total of 269 patients were treated, representing 15% of all patients who were seen with acute ischemic stroke during the study period. The mean door-to-needle time was 70 minutes, and 28% of patients were treated within 2 hours of onset. The symptomatic ICH rate was 4.5%. Protocol violations occurred in 13% of all treated patients, and patients with protocol violations had an ICH rate of 15%. The mean NIHSS score was 14.4 ± 6.1 before treatment, 10 ± 8 at 24 hours, and 7 ± 7 on discharge. The in-hospital mortality rate was 15%. These investigators concluded that IV t-PA could be given in up to 15% of patients with acute ischemic stroke with a low risk of intracerebral bleeding; they also concluded that successful experience with such treatment depends not only on the experience and organization of the treating team, but also on following the treatment protocol.[72]

In May 2002, the final results of the Canadian Activase for Stroke Effectiveness Study (CASES) were published.[67] A total of 1099 stroke patients who were treated with IV t-PA were enrolled between February 1999 and June 2001. The median baseline NIHSS score was 15 (range, 2 to 40). On follow-up evaluation at 90 days after the stroke, 30% of those patients had minimal or no residual neurologic deficit, and 46% were independent (mRS, 0 to 2). The ICH rate was 4.6%. Protocol violations occurred in 15%. Predictors of outcome were baseline NIHSS, baseline ASPECT score (evaluates the radiologic changes of stroke on brain CT), patient age, atrial fibrillation, and the patient's baseline serum sugar level. Predictors of ICH were mean arterial blood pressure as well as baseline serum glucose level. The CASES group concluded that IV alteplase (Activase) is safe and efficacious in Canada.

The *Lyon* trial was a phase 2 trial of thrombolysis using a protocol that was very different from that of the NINDS study: the t-PA dose was 0.8 mg/kg; 10% of the dose was given as an IV bolus, and the remaining 90% was given as IV drip over 1 hour after that.[68] The time window for t-PA administration was 7 hours after stroke; the majority of patients received the t-PA within 3–6 hours. Heparin or LMW heparin was also given. The rate of good outcome (mRS score, ≤1) at 5 years was 37.4%. The mortality rate was 23.9%. The rate of good outcomes (mRS score, 0 and 1) was 35% at 3 months. The rate of parenchymal anatomic hematoma within 7 days was 9%, and that of symptomatic hematomas was 5.5%. Mortality at 3 months occurred in 11.5%. Independent predictive factors of poor outcomes appeared to be structured hypodensity on Day 1 CT, hyperdense MCA sign, internal carotid thrombosis, gray-white matter indistinction, no IV heparin within 24 hours or after 24 hours, the use of LMW heparin, and the use of mannitol.

GUIDELINES FOR INTRAVENOUS THROMBOLYSIS IN ACUTE STROKE

Given the relationship between adverse events and protocol violations, it is important to understand the NINDS protocol for the use of t-PA in acute stroke. The study was originally intended to be a phase 2B confirmatory dose-finding and safety study, not a definitive phase 3 protocol, but because it proved efficacy, no further phase 3 trial was pursued. Therefore, the protocol contains some idiosyncrasies that were never intended to be included in the FDA package insert.

Treatment Protocol

Patients should be seen within the 3-hour window of stroke onset.[69,70] Thrombolysis should not be implemented unless (1) the stroke diagnosis is established by a physician with expertise in stroke and (2) brain CT is assessed by a physician with expertise in reading this imaging study. A total dose of 0.9 mg/kg of recombinant t-PA is given, not to exceed a maximal dose of 90 mg. The first 10% of the dose is given as an IV bolus, and the rest of the dose (90%) is given as an IV drip over the following hour. A list of inclusion and exclusion criteria is used to determine whether a patient should be given t-PA. These criteria were defined by the NINDS study (see Box 51-1) and were adopted nearly verbatim by the FDA, even though they were not intended for clinical use. At this time, it is important to follow these guidelines, but the physician's judgment is required in individual cases.

Expedited Treatment Protocol

Although studies are now beginning to show that alteplase may be safely given beyond the 3-hour window, the chance of a favorable outcome diminishes with time; thus treatment should still be rendered as soon as possible. In 2006, Sattin et al. demonstrated that alteplase could be safely given using an expedited protocol with a benchmark onset-to-treatment time of less than 2 hours.[71] This protocol avoids delays pending coagulation studies or platelet count, unless clinically indicated, and allows no delays pending a formal CT interpretation by a radiologist. Between July 2003 and June 2005, 781 patients were evaluated for acute stroke with the use of this protocol, and 103 patients (13.2%) received t-PA. Of those patients treated with alteplase, 49 (47.6%) were treated within 2 hours of symptom onset. The overall rate of symptomatic hemorrhage in the group treated in less than 2 hours was two of 49 (4.1%), which was not significantly different from the rate of 6.4% in the NINDS trial ($P = 0.42$) or from the group treated between 2 and 3 hours, who had a rate of two of 54 (3.7%). While this study demonstrated that an expedited protocol is feasible and appears safe, it reflects the experience in only one institution; thus its generalization to other centers cannot be made.

Although it is important to follow the guidelines, a physician's judgment is required in individual cases, especially in those cases in which the safety of thrombolysis is not known. Many physicians may also decide to administer alteplase in extreme situations in which the benefits seem to outweigh the risks, despite a contraindication. As experience with alteplase increases, it is likely that there will be more circumstances in which patients are deliberately or inadvertently given alteplase in "off-label" situations. In 2007, Aleu et al. performed a literature review that identified 273 patients who received off-labeled IV or intra-arterial t-PA for acute ischemic stroke.[72] Hemorrhagic complications occurred in a total of 36 patients; 19 of 273 patients (6.95%) had a symptomatic ICH and 17 of 273 (6.22%) had extracranial hemorrhages.

Tong et al. have promoted a reduced set of rt-PA selection criteria known as SMART.[73] Initial safety and efficacy experience appears promising, although none of these streamlined selection criteria have been approved by the US FDA.

Patients are excluded for any of the exclusion criteria; we consider some of the more important criteria in the following discussion.

Use of Oral Anticoagulants, Prothrombin Time Longer than 15 Seconds, or International Normalized Ratio 1.7 or Greater

This criterion is obviously needed to exclude patients receiving anticoagulation therapy. In the original trial, any patient was excluded who had consumed any oral warfarin (Coumadin) in the previous day, no matter what the prothrombin time might be at the time of the stroke.[1] The final package insert was written in such a way, however, as to allow thrombolysis even if the patient has taken warfarin recently; the criterion is only that the international normalized ratio (INR) be less than 1.7. The physician confronted with this situation must use judgment and must proceed thoughtfully; however, generally, we recommend thrombolytic treatment if the INR is below the stated limit even if the patient has taken warfarin before the stroke occurred. In routine practice, physicians *should not wait* for INR results before beginning the rt-PA bolus, unless some clinical clue suggests that the patient may have below-normal coagulation status. On the other hand, there may be residual risk in patients with low INR who have recently taken warfarin.[74] Experience with other anti-coagulants that are not vitamin-K antagonists is too preliminary to provide any guidance.[75]

Use of Heparin in the Last 24 Hours with a Prolonged Partial Thromboplastin Time

This is an absolute contraindication, given the potential risk of hemorrhaging. We are aware of anecdotal cases in which heparin was reversed with protamine, and t-PA was given after the partial thromboplastin time was recorded as normal. Because this approach has never been studied for safety, we cannot recommend it and do not use it routinely in our own practice. We are also aware of many cases in which reocclusion occurs after successful thrombolysis; preliminary data using serial transcranial ultrasonography has indicated that the reocclusion rate may be as high as 27%.[76] Certainly, after coronary thrombolysis, heparin is required to maintain vessel patency. We believe that further study on this point is warranted.

Platelet Count Less than 100,000 cells/mm^3

The limit of 100,000 cells/mm^3 for the platelet count is arbitrary and was chosen by the NINDS investigators on the basis of limited review of literature and consultation with hematologists. No one knows, however, how many functioning platelets are needed to protect a patient from hemorrhaging during thrombolysis. The physician should exercise caution and judgment; in some situations, it may be wise to treat a patient with a platelet count below the limit.

Prior Stroke within the Last 3 Months

The time limit on prior stroke was set somewhat arbitrarily at 3 months, and no mention is made of severity. For example, does a minor motor lacune with signs lasting 3 days and resolving completely contraindicate thrombolytic therapy for 3 months? The physician must use considerable judgment in individual cases and consider the following questions:

- How mild was the prior stroke?
- Did it resolve completely or partially?
- How long ago was the prior stroke?
- What is the potential for bleeding into the prior stroke if thrombolysis is used today?

There may be situations in which the benefit of treating the current stroke outweighs the risk due to recent, resolved minor stroke.

Head Trauma within the Last 3 Months

The considerations applying to this exclusion criterion are similar to those mentioned for prior stroke. The guidelines do not mention severity. The critical question for the clinician is as follows: how likely is the previous head trauma to predispose the patient to bleeding if thrombolysis is given now? The benefit of thrombolysis for the current event may outweigh the potential risks of bleeding after minor head trauma in the previous 3 months.

Major Surgery within the Last 14 Days

This contraindication is generally absolute, although we often consult with the surgeon who performed the surgery before making the decision. Often the devastation of the current stroke outweighs any harm that could be caused by rebleeding at the operative site. An individual exception to this exclusion rule could be considered in rare cases after careful consideration and discussion with the patient or family or both regarding the risks of hemorrhage.

Pretreatment Systolic Blood Pressure Greater than 185 mm Hg or Diastolic Blood Pressure Greater than 110 mm Hg

This exclusion criterion is absolute. If gentle antihypertensive therapy, such as 10–20 mg of IV labetalol, or an infusion of 5 mg/h nicardipine does not bring the blood pressure under the limits, no thrombolytic agents should be used. Hypertension at the time of thrombolysis has been shown to predict hemorrhagic transformation. On the other hand, the careful physician should be aware that most patients with stroke have elevated blood pressure on arrival at the ED. The first blood pressure values obtained by paramedics or the triage nurse must not be used to exclude the patient from t-PA therapy. The patient should be allowed to acclimate to the ED for a few minutes; often, the blood pressure declines spontaneously. The patient who exhibits persistent hypertension despite the passage of time and gentle antihypertensive therapy should always be excluded from t-PA treatment.

Rapidly Improving Neurologic Signs

This exclusion criterion causes considerable discomfort for most physicians because stroke symptoms wax and wane over the first few hours. To qualify as rapidly improving, the symptoms must improve monotonically and dramatically. Patients whose deficits oscillate from severe to mild or who show only slight improvement should be treated. Generally, patients with TIA have complete resolution of symptoms within 1 or 2 hours. Patients who show only slight improvement over the first hour should be treated. The risk of ICH associated with thrombolytic treatment in a patient with TIA appears to be extremely low.[77] In an observational study by Odzemir et al. 13 patients with marked clinical fluctuations defined as an increase or decrease on the NIHSS of 4 points were treated with alteplase.[78] Only one patient had an asymptomatic hemorrhage, and all patients had a favorable functional outcome.

Isolated Mild Neurologic Deficits

Patients with isolated mild neurologic deficits, such as isolated ataxia, isolated hemisensory loss, or isolated dysarthria, tend to recover completely with little residual effect. This criterion assumes a careful neurologic examination and a search for symptoms that could easily be overlooked, such as quadrantanopsia, hemispatial neglect, and mild expressive aphasia. The only patients who should be excluded from t-PA therapy are those with pure sensory or isolated ataxic symptoms. Also, individual judgment must be used; an isolated, mild expressive aphasia could end the career of a patient who speaks for a living. We routinely consider treating mild aphasia if the patient works in an occupation such as teaching, television broadcasting, or therapy. Likewise, an isolated hemianopsia could end some careers, such as truck or taxi driving, and treatment could be considered. Mild symptoms other than pure dysarthria or sensory deficit are associated with adverse outcomes. As mentioned earlier, of the patients studied by Barber et al. whose deficits were considered mild or were rapidly improving, 32% were dependent at hospital discharge or died during hospital admission.[65] Therefore, unless the symptoms are truly isolated to a purely sensory deficit or dysarthria, the patient should be treated. This study was confirmed by Smith et al.: of all stroke patients arriving at one institution within 3 hours, 34% were not given thrombolytic therapy because of mild deficits; of these, 27% had poor functional outcomes.[79]

Prior or Current Intracerebral Hemorrhage

This contraindication is relative: if the patient has ever had an ICH, thrombolysis should not be used if the cause was such that thrombolytic therapy is likely to promote rebleeding. Individual exceptions may be considered if the bleeding was due to some nonrecurring condition, such as remote history of post-traumatic subdural hematoma that is proven to be resolved.

Blood Glucose Level Less than 50 mg/dL or Greater than 400 mg/dL

Hypoglycemia should be treated with glucose replacement; the deficit will most likely resolve, but if it does not, then thrombolysis could be considered. Hypoglycemia mimics stroke in 1.7% of cases.[80] On the other hand, incidental hypoglycemia could accompany a stroke and should not exclude the patient from therapy if the neurologic deficit persists despite blood glucose correction. Hyperglycemia is associated with increased hemorrhage risk and very low rates of successful outcome. Again, if insulin therapy brings the glucose value down to an acceptable level, it would theoretically be permissible to treat with t-PA. This approach has not been studied, however, and cannot be recommended in routine practice.

Seizure at the Onset of Stroke

The purpose of this exclusion is to ensure that post-ictal paralysis is not mistaken for stroke. In actual practice, some patients with stroke do suffer tonic or clonic jerks, which witnesses may report to paramedics or the physicians as seizures. Generally, post-ictal paralysis occurs in a patient with a known seizure disorder who has a typical tonic–clonic convulsion. Physicians must sort out from witnesses what actually occurred and whether the movements were tonic–clonic. There is probably little risk, however, in giving a thrombolytic to a patient with no stroke and post-ictal paralysis; one could argue for erring on the side of treatment, reasoning that failure to treat the patient with true ischemic stroke could result in much greater harm.

Gastrointestinal or Genitourinary Bleeding

Excluding patients with gastrointestinal or genitourinary bleeding from thrombolytic therapy is necessary because thrombolysis could activate bleeding from sources in the gastrointestinal or genitourinary tract. On the other hand, many patients consider blood loss inconsequential compared with the devastating effects of stroke. It is important to consider the nature of the bleeding, how recently it occurred, and how difficult it might be to control if it were to recur. Women with active menstruation and menometrorrhagia have been successfully and safely treated with t-PA for acute stroke, after consultation with the gynecologist, because an urgent uterine artery embolization or ligation could easily be performed to halt uncontrollable bleeding.[81] Giving such therapy to a patient with colonic polyposis or diverticulosis, however, could result in bleeding that would be far less easily controlled. Considerable physician judgment is required in this setting, and full discussion with the patient or family or both about the potential risks and benefits is essential.

Recent Myocardial Infarction

This is an absolute contraindication because of the possibility of pericardial rupture and tamponade. No specific time limit is specified, but *recent* is generally considered to be on the order of weeks. As with other exclusion criteria, one must consider the size of the myocardial infarct, the treatment given, and the current status of the patient in assessing the potential risk of cardiac rupture in a specific case.

Additional Treatment Considerations

Thrombolytic treatment should not be given unless ancillary care and the facility to handle bleeding complications are present, best provided in an intensive care unit setting. We are aware of many stroke units and "step-down" care units that are perfectly appropriate for monitoring patients after thrombolysis. Vital signs and neurologic examinations (neurochecks) are required for monitoring the patient for blood loss (causing hypotension), hypertension above the post-treatment limits, neurologic deterioration (suggesting hemorrhage or reocclusion), and other complications of stroke.

Risks and benefits of thrombolytic treatment should be explained to the family, and consent should be obtained. Consent can be waived if the patient is not fit to give it and no family member is available. We recommend, however, that if any deviation from the protocol is contemplated, full consent from the family be obtained before it is initiated.

Early Computed Tomography Findings Are Not Contraindications to Treatment

In 1997, von Kummer et al. analyzed the ECASS data and concluded that the clinical severity of stroke could be associated with hemorrhagic infarction and that the risk of hemorrhagic infarction might be increased when early CT changes indicating hypoattenuation and mass effect are detected.[82] It was clear that hemorrhaging and death occurred more frequently in patients with early ischemic changes constituting more than one-third of the MCA territory. They also concluded that rising age and treatment with t-PA were related to the risk of increased parenchymal hemorrhaging. However, the analysis was post hoc and, therefore, should have served to generate hypotheses, not guide patient care. Furthermore, the finding was not statistically significant, even in the first report. Unfortunately, the logical caveats expressed by these investigators in their report went unheeded, and the result has been widely applied as a common reason not to treat patients who would otherwise qualify.

In a retrospective analysis, the NINDS group looked at early ischemic changes (EICs) on baseline CT scans and tried to correlate them with outcome, CT lesion volume at 3 months, development of symptomatic ICH, and negative or positive interaction with t-PA treatment.[83] The EICs based on von Kummer's original report were (1) loss of distinction between gray matter and white matter, (2) hypodensity or hypoattenuation on baseline CT, or (3) compression of cerebrospinal fluid spaces (sulcal effacement). The hyperdense MCA sign was not included. Overall, EICs were present in 35% of the patients given placebo and in 28% of the patients given t-PA (similar in the two groups; $P = 0.09$). There was a strong association between stroke severity as measured by the NIHSS and the incidence of EICs; after correction for the NIHSS variable, however, there was no proven interaction between t-PA treatment and EIC. In other words, there was no higher risk associated with t-PA treatment when EICs were present on baseline CT. The patients given t-PA seemed to have a better outcome regardless of whether they had EICs. The findings are summarized in Figure 51-8. The investigators in this study concluded that the presence of EICs should not be contraindications in the decision for t-PA treatment if the patient otherwise meets eligibility criteria. They also commented that the analysis of the ECASS data and conclusions about EICs prohibiting treatment should have been established after correction for the variable of stroke severity. Gilligan et al. published similar results arising from the reanalysis of the ASK trial in 2002.[84] The authors found that predictors of major hemorrhage were SK treatment and elevated systolic blood pressure before treatment (>165 mm Hg); however, EICs less than one-third or more than one-third of MCA territory were not associated with major hemorrhaging.

In an attempt to reconcile the two positions and the contradiction between the analyses of the two studies (ECASS and NINDS), we may argue that the implication of ischemic changes in more than one-third of the MCA territory on early CT might be different beyond 3 hours (ECASS) than they would be within 3 hours (NINDS). In the latter case, a substantial portion of the remaining two-thirds of the MCA territory might be hypoperfused, but still salvageable, if lysis of the clot is successful, which might result in a clinical benefit to offset the risk of bleeding. Beyond 3 hours, however, a smaller ischemic area might still be penumbral and have less of a hypothetical volumetric mismatch between the hypoperfused area and the irreversibly injured area.

It appears, therefore, that the CT findings should be used with caution in selecting patients for thrombolytic therapy. Certainly, a hemorrhage contraindicates therapy. Areas of marked hypodensity, suggesting that the stroke is more than 3 hours old, should give the physician pause. Mild EIC such as sulcal effacement, loss of gray–white matter distinction, or loss of the so-called insular ribbon sign, no matter how large a portion of the MCA territory is involved, should not necessarily contraindicate therapy if the patient otherwise qualifies for treatment. Presence of the so-called hyperdense MCA sign, or hyperdense dot sign, should not be regarded as a contraindication to therapy either, although the prospects for a good outcome are very low in this setting, regardless of the type of treatment.[85,86] Figure 51-9 demonstrates the CT of a 40-year-old man with the different CT signs mentioned and EICs at baseline and 24 hours after thrombolysis.

Considerable research is ongoing to find imaging variables that may guide selection of treatment. It is probably true that many patients with remaining salvageable brain tissue are deprived of useful treatment if physicians strictly adhere to the 3-hour time limit. Similarly, it is clear that many patients do not have salvageable brain tissue even earlier than 3 hours after stroke onset. There remains a need for a truly reliable, rapid, and widely available imaging method that will indicate when brain tissue becomes irretrievably damaged. Many techniques, such as magnetic resonance imaging (MRI) diffusion and perfusion techniques have been proposed and are under intense evaluation. To date, however, no imaging modality has proved better for selection of patients for particular therapies than existing published clinical criteria.

Effect of Time to Thrombolytic Treatment

Thrombolytic therapy should be administered within 3 hours from time of onset, as discussed before, but a 2000 analysis of the NINDS study data showed that the benefit of treatment was higher when t-PA was given earlier in this time window.[87] This analysis showed that patients treated within 90 minutes

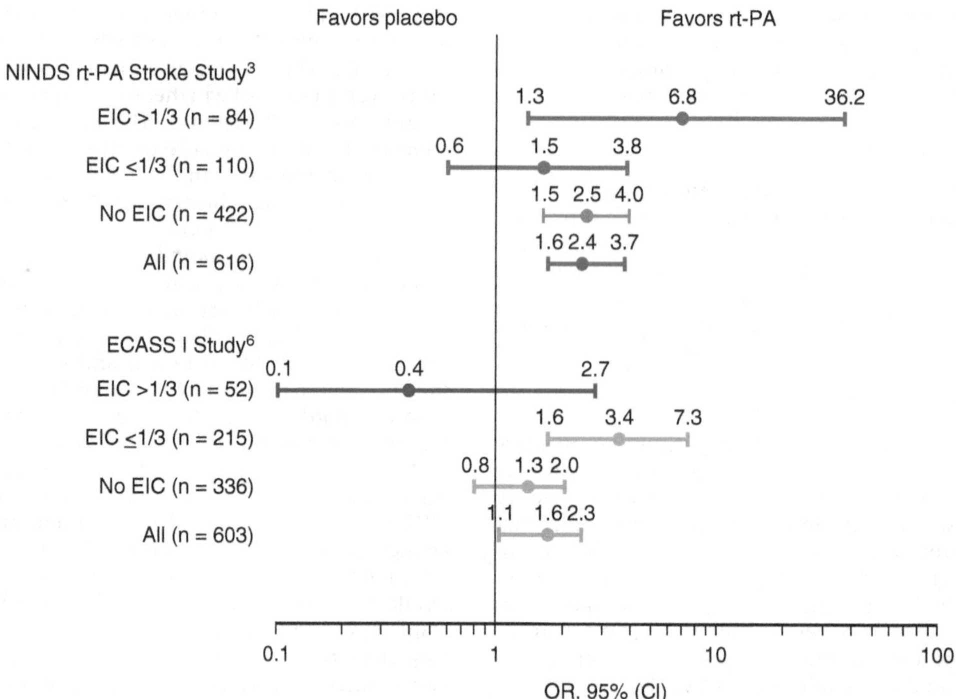

Figure 51-8. Early ischemic changes (EIC) are not contraindications for t-PA treatment. The odds ratio from ECASS for patients with EIC of more than one third of the middle cerebral artery vascular territory shows that there was no statistical difference in bad outcome between the t-PA and placebo groups in the presence of these early ischemic changes but that there was benefit with t-PA treatment in the NINDS for Acute Stroke Trial even in the presence of these early ischemic changes. *(From Patel S, Levine S, Tilley B, et al: Lack of clinical significance of early ischemic changes on computed tomography in acute stroke.* JAMA *286:2830–2838, 2001.)*

of stroke onset had greater odds of improvement at 24 hours and a higher favorable 3-month outcome than patients treated between 91 and 180 minutes after onset. The time of treatment within 3 hours had no effect on the ICH rate. Therefore, the earliest possible treatment is recommended, not for fear of ICH, but because of decreased benefit with later treatment. Figure 51-10 shows that the OR for a favorable outcome approaches 1 as the time to treatment approaches 3 hours (the benefit of t-PA is greater than that of placebo if the OR is greater than 1, as depicted in the graph). This effect of time has been confirmed in the pooled analyses described above.[52,88]

Generalized Efficacy of t-Pa for Acute Stroke

A post hoc analysis of the NINDS data was conducted to try to establish whether any factors might have had negative interactions with t-PA treatment or, in other words, to identify any pretreatment patient information that significantly affected the patient's response to t-PA treatment.[89] The investigators included 27 baseline variables to check for possible interaction with t-PA treatment. These variables were age, race, sex, cigarette smoking, alcohol abuse, diabetes mellitus, hypertension, baseline NIHSS score, percentage of correct t-PA dose received, history of atherosclerosis, history of atrial fibrillation, history of other cardiac disease, prior stroke, aspirin administration, baseline stroke subtype, early CT findings, presence or absence of thrombus, weight, admission and baseline mean arterial blood pressure, admission and baseline systolic as well as admission and baseline diastolic blood pressure, centers of treatment, time from stroke onset to treatment, and admission temperature. This analysis also tested interactions among these factors and among confounding variables. Independent of t-PA therapy, outcome was related to age by deficit or age by NIHSS score, diabetes, age by blood pressure interaction, and early CT findings. These factors and their interactions altered the patient's long-term outcome, but did not alter the likelihood of a favorable response to t-PA treatment; the efficacy of t-PA as shown by the NINDS data were generalized to all subgroups. The investigators concluded that treatment for patients with acute stroke should be selected according to the NINDS guidelines and that further subselection is not supported.

Recanalization and Arterial Reocclusion after t-Pa Treatment

Early studies by del Zoppo et al. and Mori et al., as described earlier, showed that IV t-PA could recanalize the cerebral vessels on angiograms.[32,35] Further data have been published to support their conclusions. In 2002, Alexandrov et al. published the results of a series of 60 consecutively treated patients with occlusion of the M1 or M2 segment of the MCA who received t-PA (bolus followed by IV infusion) and were monitored by transcranial Doppler ultrasonography for 2 hours after t-PA treatment.[76] The median prebolus NIHSS score was 16, and the median time to administration of the bolus was 120 minutes; 58% of patients received the t-PA within the first 2 hours. Recanalization was complete in 30% (18 patients), partial in 48% (29 patients), and null in 22% (13 patients). Early reocclusion occurred in 34% of patients given t-PA who experienced any initial recanalization, accounting for two-thirds of deteriorations after improvement. Note that reocclusion occurred more often in patients with earlier and partial recanalization, along with secondary neurologic deterioration and higher in-hospital mortality. Nevertheless, patients with reocclusion had better long-term outcomes than patients without any early recanalization.

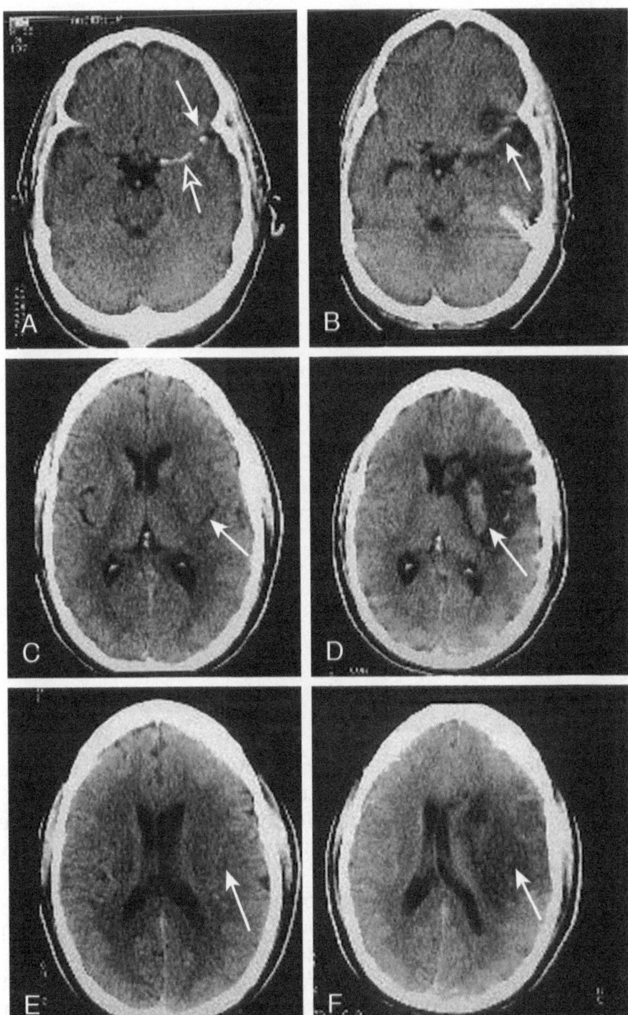

Figure 51-9. Early ischemic changes (EICs) on CT are not contraindications for thrombolysis. This is the brain CT of a 40-year-old man with acute left hemispheric stroke on presentation (A, C, and E) and 48 hours after thrombolysis (B, D, and F). A, A linear hyperdense middle cerebral artery (MCA) sign *(open head white arrow)* and a hyperdense dot MCA sign *(closed head white arrow)*, on presentation. B, The hyperdense MCA sign 48 hours later. C, Portrays loss of the left insular ribbon as one of the early ischemic changes. D, Portrays an island of relative hyperdensity within the stroke bed that might be either hemorrhagic transformation or an island of spared nonischemic brain tissue within the ischemic bed at 24 hours after thrombolysis. E, Portrays ischemic-related hypodense changes in the MCA territory on presentation. F, Portrays progression of the hypodense ischemic changes at 48 hours.

BOX 51-2 Emergency Management of Arterial Hypertension for Patients Receiving Thrombolytic Treatment for Acute Ischemic Stroke

Indication that patient is eligible for treatment with intravenous rt-PA or other acute reperfusion intervention:

Blood pressure level

Systolic >185 mm Hg or diastolic >110 mm Hg

- Labetalol 10 to 20 mg IV over 1 to 2 minutes, may repeat ×1; or
- Nitropaste 1 to 2 inches; or
- Nicardipine infusion, 5 mg/h, titrate up by 0.25 mg/h at 5- to 15-minute intervals, maximum dose 15 mg/h; when desired blood pressure attained, reduce to 3 mg/h

If blood pressure does not decline and remains >185/110 mm Hg, do not administer rt-PA.

MANAGEMENT OF BLOOD PRESSURE DURING AND AFTER TREATMENT WITH RT-PA OR OTHER ACUTE REPERFUSION INTERVENTION

Monitor blood pressure every 15 minutes during treatment and then for another 2 hours, then every 30 minutes for 6 hours, and then every hour for 16 hours:

Blood pressure level

Systolic 180 to 230 mm Hg or diastolic 105 to 120 mm Hg

- Labetalol 10 mg IV over 1 to 2 minutes, may repeat every 10 to 20 minutes, maximum dose of 300 mg; or
- Labetalol 10 mg IV followed by an infusion at 2 to 8 mg/min

Systolic >230 mm Hg or diastolic 121 to 140 mm Hg

- Labetalol 10 mg IV over 1 to 2 minutes, may repeat every 10 to 20 minutes, maximum dose of 300 mg; or
- Labetalol 10 mg IV followed by an infusion at 2 to 8 mg/min; or
- Nicardipine infusion, 5 mg/h, titrate up to desired effect by increasing 2.5 mg/h every 5 minutes to maximum of 15 mg/h

If blood pressure not controlled, consider sodium nitroprusside.

From Adams HP Jr, del Zoppo G, Alberts M, et al: Guidelines for the early management of adults with ischemic stroke. *Stroke* 38: 1655–1711, 2007.

Management During and After Thrombolytic Treatment

As mentioned before, the patient should be admitted to a skilled care unit, such as an intensive care unit or a stroke care unit that provides close observation, careful cardiovascular monitoring, and frequent neurologic evaluations. Blood pressure should be monitored and controlled carefully during the treatment and the following 24 hours. An excessively high blood pressure might predispose the patient to bleeding intracranially, whereas low blood pressure might worsen cerebral ischemia. According to American Heart Association recommendations, blood pressure should be monitored every 15 minutes for 2 hours from the start of t-PA infusion, then every 30 minutes for 6 hours, then every 60 minutes over the rest of the 24 hours after initiation of t-PA treatment.[70]

The protocol for blood pressure treatment after thrombolysis is listed in Box 51-2. Recommended drugs listed in the table were selected because of their rapid onset of action and their predictable effects with a low potential for overshooting. Note that in the NINDS study, these medications were used, in addition to other medications such as IV nicardipine, hydralazine, sublingual nifedipine, and sustained-release or topical nitroglycerin.[90] Furthermore, although abrupt substantial declines in mean arterial pressure have been shown to reduce cerebral flow, the threshold below which it is unsafe to lower mean arterial pressure is unknown. The blood pressure eligibility criteria that were applied are similar to those used in the t-PA dose-finding trial. The blood pressure management algorithm was used because of the low incidence of symptomatic hemorrhaging in the pilot study and recognition of the potential link between high blood pressure and ICH.

Post hoc analyses of data from the NINDS study have shown that, after randomization but not before, blood

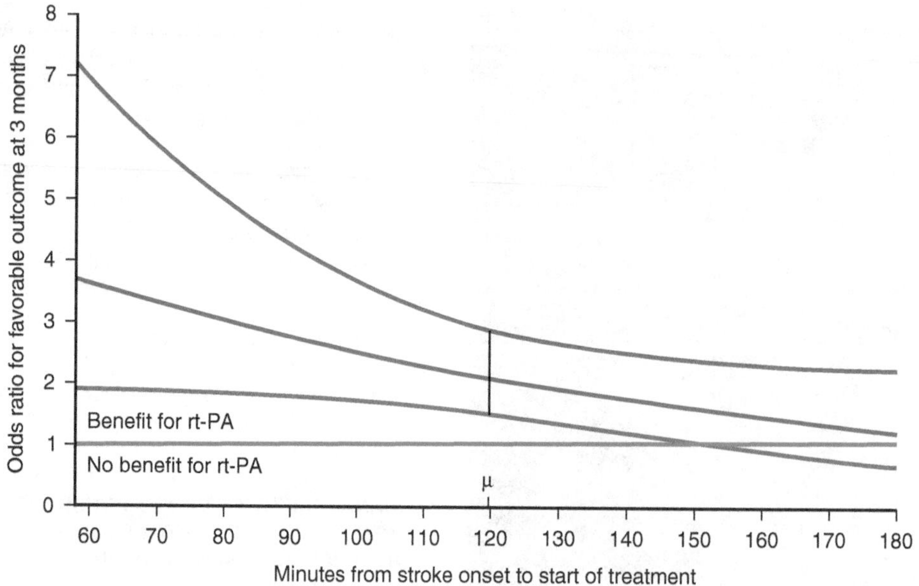

Figure 51-10. Time to treatment effect: This figure shows that t-PA benefit disappears as the time from onset to t-PA treatment approaches 3 hours. *(From Marler J, Tilley B, Lu M, et al: Early stroke treatment associated with better outcome: The NINDS rt-PA Stroke Study.* Neurology *55:1649–1655, 2000.)*

pressure treatment was associated with a less favorable 3-month outcome in the t-PA group. However, because of the non-randomized use of antihypertensive therapy and the many post hoc comparisons leading to statistical errors, the significance of this observation was unclear, and the importance of controlling blood pressure after thrombolysis still holds because of the possible association of ICH with high blood pressure.[91]

Central lines and arterial puncture should be restricted in the first 24 hours after thrombolytic treatment. However, the physician should be aware that the serum half-life of t-PA is very short, and after 20 minutes, there is very little systemic thrombolytic activity. Therefore, if clinical circumstances require a central line or triple-lumen catheter for monitoring of cardiopulmonary pressures, such a line could be safely established an hour or more after thrombolysis was complete. Urinary tract instrumentation (placement of a Foley catheter) should be avoided during infusion of t-PA and at least 30 minutes after the infusion ends. Placement of a nasogastric tube should be avoided during the first 24 hours after initiation of treatment; as with central lines and arterial puncture, we routinely insert this catheter earlier if required by patient circumstances.

For 36 hours after thrombolysis, hemorrhagic complications of t-PA are the major worry; these can be intracranial or extracranial hemorrhages. If bleeding is suspected, then a blood specimen is collected for measurement of hemoglobin level, hematocrit, partial thromboplastin time, prothrombin time, INR, platelet count, and fibrinogen level. Blood should be typed and cross-matched when the need for transfusion arises. Arterial or venous sites should be compressed if they are the bleeding source.

If major life-threatening bleeding occurs, including ICH, gastrointestinal bleeding, and retroperitoneal bleeding, thrombolytic treatment should be stopped if it is still going. Urgent CT of the brain should be obtained for suspected ICH. Neurosurgical consultation for possible surgical intervention should also be obtained. Surgery should not be performed, however, unless the fibrinolytic state is corrected; such a correction usually requires both cryoprecipitate and fresh frozen plasma to overcome clotting factor deficiencies induced by the t-PA. The presence of immediate neurosurgical treatment, however, is not a mandatory element of using rt-PA for acute ischemic stroke because the efficacy of early surgery has never been established.

For major extracranial hemorrhages, the appropriate emergency imaging techniques should be performed, along with surgical consultations and interventions when appropriate. For 24 hours after IV t-PA treatment, patients should not receive aspirin, heparin, warfarin, or other antithrombotic or antiplatelet drugs. As mentioned elsewhere, however, reocclusion may be a considerable problem after thrombolysis, and we are concerned that further studies of post-thrombolytic anticoagulation are lacking.

Predictors of Good Outcome with Thrombolytic Treatment

In a 2001 article, Demchuk et al. analyzed data collected from 1205 patients treated in different centers in Germany, the United States, and Canada with IV t-PA as per NINDS protocol.[92] A good outcome was defined as an mRS score of 0 to 1, and a poor outcome was an mRS score greater than 1. The independent predictors of good outcome in patients treated with IV t-PA, in relative order of decreasing magnitude, were milder baseline stroke severity, no history of diabetes mellitus, normal CT scan result, normal pretreatment blood glucose level, and normal pretreatment blood pressure. Confounding was observed among the variables: history of diabetes, CT scan appearance, baseline serum glucose level, and blood pressure (baseline mean arterial pressure), suggesting important relationships among these variables. Symptomatic ICH was associated with a poor outcome. The known risk factors for poor outcome in untreated patients, such as age and stroke mechanism, were not associated with outcome in this cohort study.

Risks of Thrombolysis

Plasminogen activators raise the risk of ICH by altering the framework of the platelet plug and by changing vascular permeability as well as the integrity of the vascular basal lamina at the site of injury; the latter two effects contribute to dissolution of the blood–brain barrier. Therefore, there is an increased risk of brain edema and ICH. As mentioned before, subgroup analysis of the NINDS data showed that the only variables that were independently associated with an increased risk of symptomatic ICH were baseline stroke severity as measured by NIHSS, the amount of edema defined by acute hypodensity, and mass effect on CT before treatment (baseline CT).[41]

Reperfusion injury is another hypothetical risk. It has been shown that reperfusion is associated with a secondary wave of glutamate and other neurotransmitter release, which results in calcium influx and excitotoxicity. Restoration of blood flow might allow synthesis of damaging proteins and other cytokines as well as a supply of oxygen to ischemic areas, providing a substrate for peroxidation of lipids and formation of free radicals. Moreover, thrombolysis might allow the clot to break and cause secondary embolization to a distal vascular distribution.

Cost-Effectiveness of Thrombolysis

The cost-effectiveness of t-PA was demonstrated in 1998, in a study that used certain assumptions about stroke costs and outcomes based on data from the literature and from the NINDS study.[93] Even though it shortened the stay at the hospital, t-PA therapy increased the hospital cost for each additional patient who was discharged home rather than to a nursing home or in-patient rehabilitation center. On the other hand, t-PA reduced the costs of nursing home care and rehabilitation. The overall effect on both acute and long-term care costs (90% certainty) to the healthcare system is a net decrease of more than $4,000,000 for every 1000 patients treated.[93] These results have been confirmed in other trials.[94,95]

COMBINATION TREATMENT

Combining thrombolysis with other treatment regimens has not proved to be beneficial so far in clinical studies. Previous studies have combined anticoagulants with fibrinolysis. In the MAST-E study, 65% of the patients received SK and 75% of the placebo group also received heparin.[45] There was no evidence of statistically significant benefit, and the study was terminated early because of increased ICH in the SK group. It is recommended that no anticoagulants be given within 24 hours of t-PA treatment. Previous studies have shown that SK with antiplatelet treatment (aspirin) is associated with a higher risk of ICH compared with SK alone or aspirin alone (MAST-I).[46] Clinical studies have not tested t-PA in combination with aspirin. Experimental models, however, have shown that t-PA with heparin is safe and did not increase the rate of ICH.[28] A small group of patients (n = 30) received a combination of t-PA and heparin in a feasibility study described by von Kummer et al.; these researchers concluded that when the combination treatment was given within 6 hours of stroke onset, the incidence of fatal ICH occurred in 9% of patients, whereas asymptomatic hemorrhagic infarction occurred in 28%.[96] Reperfusion occurred in 34% of patients 90 minutes after initiation of thrombolysis and in 53% within 12 to 24 hours of thrombolysis initiation. Good clinical outcomes correlated with reperfusion ($P < 0.05$). Recent data suggest that the direct thrombin inhibitors may directly and powerfully protect the neurovascular unit, apart from any anti-coagulant effect.[97,98] An initial pilot safety study that used argatroban to raise the PTT to 1.5x control confirmed safety and no increased risk of hemorrhage due to the combination of rt-PA and an anticoagulant.[99] Future randomized controlled studies are needed to determine whether this or other antithrombotic strategies combined with IV t-PA are better than thrombolysis alone, weighing the benefits and risks involved.

Neuroprotective agents in combination with thrombolysis have been tested in experimental models and in clinical studies. Studies showed benefit in animals receiving neuroprotective agents within a short time window after the cerebrovascular occlusion. For example, in 1991, Zivin and Mazzarella used MK-801, a glutamate antagonist, followed by thrombolysis with t-PA and proved that such a combination was more effective than t-PA alone in reducing neurologic damage after stroke.[100] MK-801 had no effect when used alone in the same stroke model. Neuroprotective agents can reduce the side effects of thrombolysis because they enhance the integrity of the vascular endothelium and protect ischemic brain tissue from the hypothetical reperfusion injury discussed earlier.[101]

Several clinical studies combined thrombolysis with neuroprotective agents. However, two very large studies failed to show benefit, putting a pall on such studies for the past several years.[102] In a series of large, well-designed trials, combinations of a free radical scavenger, NXY-059, failed to provide benefit beyond that provided by intravenous rt-PA.[103–105] Of considerable interest, a moderately size large trial (n = 1699) showed benefit on the primary outcome ($P = 0.038$) as well as on post-hoc measures such as reduced rates of intracerebral hemorrhage when NXY-059 was given after rt-PA but within 6 hours of stroke onset.[105] A confirmatory study included 3306 patients and was powered to detect a 7% absolute treatment effect, also using a 6-hour treatment window. The study showed no benefit favoring the neuroprotectant.[103] A pooled analysis of both studies confirmed the absence of effect on any measures of efficacy or safety.[106] Future studies combining neuroprotective agents with thrombolysis should be pursued, keeping in mind that the neuroprotective agent should be administered earlier, and maybe earlier than the thrombolytic treatment, in light of animal models that show benefit only with very early administration of neuroprotective agents.[107] Similarly, new approaches to pre-clinical qualification of putative neuroprotectants will be needed.[108,109]

Hypothermia in combination with thrombolysis is under investigation. Future studies will evaluate whether hypothermia might prolong the time window of thrombolysis so that benefit might be achieved from t-PA given in combination with induced hypothermia even later than 3 hours after stroke onset.[110] Initial experience shows that hypothermia can be combined safely with thrombolysis; pivotal trials are being organized.[111] Intra-arterial thrombolysis in combination with IV thrombolysis is discussed in Chapter 62.

CONCLUSION

Thrombolysis with the use of IV t-PA is safe and improves the outcome of patients with stroke, despite a higher risk of ICH (but no increased risk of mortality). The emphasis should be on (1) treating the patient as early as possible, (2) excluding ICH on CT before treatment, and (3) controlling hypertension before and after treatment. A specialized unit setting is ideal for monitoring the patient. Treatment with anticoagulants and antiplatelet agents are forbidden within the first 24 hours after thrombolysis, according to the NINDS protocol. Newer generation thrombolytic agents are currently under study for acute stroke treatment and, because they are more clot-selective, may show a greater rate of lysis with a lower risk of bleeding. It is hoped that future clinical studies using combination treatments of IV thrombolysis with intra-arterial lytics or mechanical clot disruption, antithrombotic therapy, or neuroprotective agents within a short time window might build on the positive results obtained so far with t-PA.

REFERENCES

1. The National Institute of Neurological Disorders and Stroke rt-PA Stroke Study Group. Tissue plasminogen activator for acute ischemic stroke. N Engl J Med 1995;333:1581–7.
2. Douglas S. Coagulation history. Br J Haematol 1999;107:22.
3. Collen D. Fibrin-selective thrombolytic therapy for acute myocardial infarction. Circulation 1996;93:857.
4. Benedict CR, Refino CJ, Keyt BA, et al. New variant of human tissue plasminogen activator (TPA) with enhanced efficacy and lower incidence of bleeding compared with recombinant human TPA. Circulation 1995;92:3032.
5. Stewart RJ, Fredenburgh JC, Leslie BA, et al. Identification of the mechanism responsible for the increased fibrin specificity of TNK-tissue plasminogen activator relative to tissue plasminogen activator. J Biol Chem 2000;275:10112–20.
6. Van de Werf F, Cannon C, Luyten A, et al. Safety assessment of single-bolus administration of TNK tissue-plasminogen activator in acute myocardial infarction: the ASSENT-1 trial. Am Heart J 2000;137:786.
7. Van de Werf F, Barron HV, Armstrong PW, et al. Incidence and predictors of bleeding events after fibrinolytic therapy with fibrin-specific agents. Eur Heart J 2001;22:2253.
8. Haley EC Jr, Lyden PD, Johnston KC, et al. A pilot dose-escalation safety study of tenecteplase in acute ischemic stroke. Stroke 2005;36:607–12.
9. Haley EC Jr, Thompson JL, Grotta JC, et al. Phase IIB/III trial of tenecteplase in acute ischemic stroke: results of a prematurely terminated randomized clinical trial. Stroke 2010;41:707–11.
10. Parsons M, Spratt N, Bivard A, et al. A randomized trial of tenecteplase versus alteplase for acute ischemic stroke. N Engl J Med 2012;366:1099–107.
11. Lapchak PA, Araujo DM, Pakola S, et al. Microplasmin: a novel thrombolytic that improves behavioral outcome after embolic strokes in rabbits. Stroke 2002;33(9):2279. PubMed PMID: 5907.
12. Witt W, Baldus B, Bringmann P, et al. Thrombolytic properties of *Desmodus rotundus* (vampire bat) salivary plasminogen activator in experimental pulmonary embolism in rats. Blood 1992;79(5):1213–17. PubMed PMID: 1536947.
13. Hacke W, Albers G, Al-Rawi Y, et al. The Desmoteplase in Acute Ischemic Stroke Trial (DIAS): a phase II MRI-based 9-hour window acute stroke thrombolysis trial with intravenous desmoteplase. Stroke 2005;36(1):66–73. PubMed PMID: 15569863.
14. Furlan AJ, Eyding D, Albers GW, et al. Dose Escalation of Desmoteplase for Acute Ischemic Stroke (DEDAS): evidence of safety and efficacy 3 to 9 hours after stroke onset. Stroke 2006;37(5):1227–31. PubMed PMID: 16574922.
15. Hacke W, Furlan AJ, Al-Rawi Y, et al. Intravenous desmoteplase in patients with acute ischaemic stroke selected by MRI perfusion-diffusion weighted imaging or perfusion CT (DIAS-2): a prospective, randomised, double-blind, placebo-controlled study. Lancet Neurol 2009;8(2):141–50. PubMed PMID: 19097942.
16. Bell WR, Pitney WR, Goodwin JF. Therapeutic defibrination in the treatment of thrombotic disease. Lancet 1968;1(7541):490–3. PubMed PMID: 4170831.
17. Hossmann V, Heiss WD, Bewermeyer H, et al. Controlled trial of ancrod in ischemic stroke. Arch Neurol 1983;40:803. PubMed PMID: 2186.
18. Olinger CP, Brott TG, Barsan WG, et al. Use of ancrod on acute or progressing ischemic cerebral infarction. Ann Emerg Med 1988;17:1208. PubMed PMID: 2183.
19. Levy DE, Trammel J, Wasiewski WW. Ancrod Stroke Program Study T. Ancrod for acute ischemic stroke: a new dosing regimen derived from analysis of prior ancrod stroke studies. J Stroke Cerebrovasc Dis 2009;18(1):23–7. PubMed PMID: 19110140.
20. Sherman DG, Atkinson RP, Chippendale T, et al. Intravenous Ancrod for Treatment for Acute Ischemic Stroke. JAMA 2000; 283(18):2395. PubMed PMID: 4025.
21. Hennerici MG, Kay R, Bogousslavsky J, et al. Intravenous ancrod for acute ischaemic stroke in the European Stroke Treatment with Ancrod Trial: a randomised controlled trial. Lancet 2006;368(9550):1871–8. PubMed PMID: 17126719.
22. Levy DE, del Zoppo GJ, Demaerschalk BM, et al. Ancrod in acute ischemic stroke: results of 500 subjects beginning treatment within 6 hours of stroke onset in the ancrod stroke program. Stroke 2009;40(12):3796–803. PubMed PMID: 19875736.
23. Meyer JS, Gilroy J, Barnhart ME, et al. Therapeutic thrombolysis in cerebral thromboembolism. In: Siekert RG, Whisnant JP, editors. Cerebral Vascular Diseases. Philadelphia: Grune & Stratton; 1963. p. 160.
24. del Zoppo G, Copeland BR, Waltz TA, et al. The beneficial effect of intracarotid urokinase on acute stroke in a baboon model. Stroke 1986;17:638. PubMed PMID: 84.
25. Zivin JA, Fisher M, DeGirolami U, et al. Tissue plasminogen activator reduces neurological damage after cerebral embolism. Science 1985;230:1289. PubMed PMID: 85.
26. Slivka A, Pulsinelli WA. Hemorrhagic complications of thrombolytic therapy in experimental stroke. Stroke 1987;18:1148. PubMed PMID: 87.
27. Lyden PD, Zivin JA, Clark WA, et al. Tissue plasminogen activator mediated thrombolysis of cerebral emboli and its effect on hemorrhagic infarction in rabbits. Neurology 1989;39:703. PubMed PMID: 539.
28. Clark WM, Madden KP, Lyden PD, et al. Cerebral hemorrhagic risk of aspirin or heparin therapy with thrombolytic treatment in rabbits. Stroke 1991;22:872. PubMed PMID: 770.
29. Lyden PD, Madden KP, Clark WA, et al. Comparison of cerebral hemorrhage rates following tissue plasminogen activator or streptokinase treatment for embolic stroke in rabbits. Stroke 1990;21:981. PubMed PMID: 546.
30. Meyer JS, Gilroy J, Barnhart ME, et al. Therapeutic thrombolysis in cerebral thromboembolism: Randomized evaluation of intravenous streptokinase. Cerebral Vascular Diseases, Fourth Princeton Conference. New York: Grune and Stratton; 1965. p. 200.
31. Fletcher AP, Alkjaersig N, Lewis M, et al. A pilot study of urokinase therapy in cerebral infarction. Stroke 1976;7:135. PubMed PMID: 81.
32. del Zoppo G, Poeck K, Pessin MS, et al. Recombinant tissue plasminogen activator in acute thrombotic and embolic stroke. Ann Neurol 1992;32:78. PubMed PMID: 960.
33. Brott TG, Haley EC Jr, Levy DE, et al. Urgent therapy for stroke: Part 1. Pilot study of tissue plasminogen activator administered within 90 minutes. Stroke 1992;23:632. PubMed PMID: 954.
34. Haley EC Jr, Levy DE, Brott TG, et al. Urgent therapy for stroke. Part II. Pilot study of tissue plasminogen activator administered 91–180 minutes from onset. Stroke 1992;23:641. PubMed PMID: 2012.
35. Mori E, Yoneda Y, Tabuchi M, et al. Intravenous recombinant tissue plasminogen activator in acute carotid artery territory stroke. Neurology 1992;42:976. PubMed PMID: 946.
36. Haley EC, Brott TG, Sheppard GL, et al. Pilot randomized trial of tissue plasminogen activator in acute ischemic stroke. Stroke 1993;24:1000. PubMed PMID: 1921.
37. Hacke W, Kaste M, Fieschi C, et al. Intravenous thrombolysis with recombinant tissue plasminogen activator for acute hemispheric stroke: The European Cooperative Stroke Study (ECASS). JAMA 1995;274(13):1017. PubMed PMID: 2595.
38. Hacke W, Bluhmki E, Steiner T, et al. Dichotomized efficacy end points and global end-point analysis applied to the ECASS intention-to-treat data set. Stroke 1998;29:2073. PubMed PMID: 3206.
39. Steiner T, Bluhmki E, Kaste M, et al. The ECASS 3-Hour Cohort. Cerebrovasc Dis 1998;8:198. PubMed PMID: 3227.
40. Haley EC Jr, Lewandowski C, Tilley BC. Group Nr-PSS. Myths Regarding the NINDS rt-PA Stroke Trial: Setting the Record Straight. Ann Emerg Med 1997;30(5):676. PubMed PMID: 2739.
41. The NINDS rt-PA for Stroke Study Group. Intracerebral hemorrhage after intravenous t-PA therapy for ischemic stroke. Stroke 1997;28:2109. PubMed PMID: 2838.
42. Kwiatkowski TG, Libman RB, Frankel M, et al. Effects of tissue plasminogen activator for acute ischemic stroke at one year. N Engl J Med 1999;340:1781. PubMed PMID: 3576.
43. Broderick J, Lu M, Kothari R, et al. Finding the most powerful measures of the effectiveness of tissue plasminogen activator in the NINDS stroke trial. Stroke 2000;31(10):2335. PubMed PMID: 4271.
44. Hacke W, Kaste M, Fieschi C, et al. Randomised double-blind placebo-controlled trial of thrombolytic therapy with

intravenous alteplase in acute ischaemic stroke (ECASS II). Lancet 1998;352:1245. PubMed PMID: 3175.
45. The Multicenter Acute Stroke Trial – Europe Study Group. Thrombolytic therapy with streptokinase in acute ischemic stroke. N Engl J Med 1996;335(3):145–50. PubMed PMID: 8657211.
46. Multicentre Acute Stroke Trial – Italy (MAST-I) Group. Randomised controlled trial of streptokinase, aspirin, and combination of both in treatment of acute ischaemic stroke. Lancet 1995;346(8989):1509–14. PubMed PMID: 7491044.
47. Donnan GA, Davis SM, Chambers BR, et al. Streptokinase for acute ischemic stroke with relationship to time of administration: Australian Streptokinase (ASK) Trial Study Group. JAMA 1996;276(12):961–6. PubMed PMID: 8805730.
48. Donnan GA, Davis SM, Chambers BR, et al. ASK Trial: unfavourable outcome if treated more than three hours after onset. Cerebrovasc Dis 1995;5:225. PubMed PMID: 2325.
49. Cornu C, Boutitie F, Candelise L, et al. Streptokinase in acute ischemic stroke: an individual patient data meta-analysis: The thrombolysis in acute stroke pooling project. Stroke 2000;31(7):1555. PubMed PMID: 5005.
50. Clark WM, Wissman S, Albers GW, et al. Recombinant tissue-type plasminogen activator (Alteplase) for ischemic stroke 3 to 5 hours after symptom onset. The ATLANTIS Study: a randomized controlled trial. Alteplase Thrombolysis for Acute Noninterventional Therapy in Ischemic Stroke. JAMA 1999; 282(21):2019–26. PubMed PMID: 10591384.
51. Albers GW, Clark W, Madden K, et al. ATLANTIS Trial – results for patients treated within 3 hours of stroke onset. Stroke 2002;33:493. PubMed PMID: 5000.
52. Hacke W, Donnan G, Fieschi C, et al. Association of outcome with early stroke treatment: pooled analysis of ATLANTIS, ECASS, and NINDS rt-PA stroke trials. Lancet 2004;363(9411):768. PubMed PMID: 5760.
53. Wahlgren N, Ahmed N, Davalos A, et al. Thrombolysis with alteplase for acute ischaemic stroke in the Safe Implementation of Thrombolysis in Stroke-Monitoring Study (SITS-MOST): an observational study. Lancet 2007;369(9558):275–82. PubMed PMID: 17258667.
54. Wahlgren N, Ahmed N, Davalos A, et al. Thrombolysis with alteplase 3–4.5 h after acute ischaemic stroke (SITS-ISTR): an observational study. Lancet 2008;372(9646):1303–9. [Epub 2008/09/16]; PubMed PMID: 18790527. eng.
55. Hacke W, Kaste M, Bluhmki E, et al. Thrombolysis with alteplase 3 to 4.5 hours after acute ischemic stroke. N Engl J Med 2008; 359(13):1317–29. PubMed PMID: 18815396.
56. Lyden P. Thrombolytic therapy for acute stroke – not a moment to lose. N Engl J Med 2008;359(13):1393–5. PubMed PMID: 18815401.
57. Lansberg MG, Bluhmki E, Thijs VN. Efficacy and safety of tissue plasminogen activator 3 to 4.5 hours after acute ischemic stroke: a metaanalysis. Stroke 2009;40(7):2438–41. PubMed PMID: 19478213, Pubmed Central PMCID: 2725521.
58. Sandercock P, Lindley R, Wardlaw J, et al. Third international stroke trial (IST-3) of thrombolysis for acute ischaemic stroke. Trials 2008;9:37. [Epub 2008/06/19]; PubMed PMID: 18559104, Pubmed Central PMCID: 2442584. eng.
59. Sandercock P, Wardlaw JM, Lindley RI, et al. The benefits and harms of intravenous thrombolysis with recombinant tissue plasminogen activator within 6 h of acute ischaemic stroke (the third international stroke trial [IST-3]): a randomised controlled trial. Lancet 2012;379(9834):2352–63. PubMed PMID: 22632908, Pubmed Central PMCID: 3386495.
60. Sandercock P, Lindley R, Wardlaw J, et al. Update on the third international stroke trial (IST-3) of thrombolysis for acute ischaemic stroke and baseline features of the 3035 patients recruited. Trials 2011;12(1):[Epub November 30, 2011]; Pubmed Central PMCID: PMC3286387.
61. IST-3 collaborative group. Effect of thrombolysis with alteplase within 6 h of acute ischaemic stroke on long-term outcomes (the third International Stroke Trial [IST-3]): 18-month follow-up of a randomised controlled trial. Lancet Neurol 2013;12(8):768–76. PubMed PMID: 23791822, Pubmed Central PMCID: 3854835.
62. Wardlaw JM, Murray V, Berge E, et al. Recombinant tissue plasminogen activator for acute ischaemic stroke: an updated systematic review and meta-analysis. Lancet 2012;379(9834):2364–72. PubMed PMID: 22632907, Pubmed Central PMCID: 3386494.
63. Chiu D, Krieger D, Villar-Cordova C, et al. Intravenous tissue plasminogen activator for acute ischemic stroke feasibility, safety, and efficacy in the first year of clinical practice. Stroke 1998;29:18. PubMed PMID: 2741.
64. Albers GW, Bates V, Clark W, et al. Intravenous tissue-type plasminogen activator for treatment of acute stroke: The Standard Treatment with Alteplase to Reverse Stroke (STARS) Study (STARS). JAMA 2000;283:1145. PubMed PMID: 4000.
65. Barber PA, Zhang J, Demchuk A, et al. Why are stroke patients excluded from TPA therapy? Neurology 2001;56:1015. PubMed PMID: 4827.
66. Grotta J, Burgin WS, El-Mitwalli A, et al. Intravenous tissue-type plasminogen activator therapy for ischemic stroke. Arch Neurol 2001;58(12):2009. PubMed PMID: 4933.
67. Hill MD, Buchan A, Investigators C. The Canadian Activase for Stroke Effectiveness Study (CASES): final results. Stroke 2002;33(1):359. PubMed PMID: 5002.
68. Trouillas P, Nighoghosian N, Derex L, et al. Final Results of the Lyon rtPA Protocol (200 cases): Effect of intravenous rtPA within 7 hours without radiological and clinical exclusions in carotid territory acute cerebral infarcts. Stroke 2006;37:556–61.
69. Adams HP Jr, del Zoppo G, Alberts MJ, et al. Guidelines for the early management of adults with ischemic stroke: a guideline from the American Heart Association/American Stroke Association Stroke Council, Clinical Cardiology Council, Cardiovascular Radiology and Intervention Council, and the Atherosclerotic Peripheral Vascular Disease and Quality of Care Outcomes in Research Interdisciplinary Working Groups: the American Academy of Neurology affirms the value of this guideline as an educational tool for neurologists. Stroke 2007;38(5):1655–711. PubMed PMID: 17431204.
70. Jauch EC, Saver JL, Adams HP Jr, et al. Guidelines for the early management of patients with acute ischemic stroke: a guideline for healthcare professionals from the American Heart Association/American Stroke Association. Stroke 2013;44(3):870–947. PubMed PMID: 23370205.
71. Sattin JA, Olson SE, Liu L, et al. An expedited code stroke protocol is feasible and safe. Stroke 2006;37(12):2935–9. PubMed PMID: 17095736.
72. Aleu A, Mellado P, Lichy C, et al. Hemorrhagic complications after off-label thrombolysis for ischemic stroke. Stroke 2007; 38(2):417–22. PubMed PMID: 17185641.
73. Tong D. Are all IV thrombolysis exclusion criteria necessary?: Being SMART about evidence-based medicine. Neurology 2011; 76(21):1780–1. [Epub 2011/04/15]; PubMed PMID: 21490320. eng.
74. Ruecker M, Matosevic B, Willeit P, et al. Subtherapeutic warfarin therapy entails an increased bleeding risk after stroke thrombolysis. Neurology 2012;79(1):31–8. [Epub 2012/06/01]; PubMed PMID: 22649217. eng.
75. Hart RG, Pogue J, Eikelboom JW. Direct-Acting Oral Anticoagulants: The Brain Gets a Break. JAMA Neurol 2013;PubMed PMID: 24166449.
76. Alexandrov AV, Grotta JC. Arterial reocclusion in stroke patients treated with intravenous tissue plasminogen activator. Neurology 2002;59:862. PubMed PMID: 5129.
77. Lyden P, Lu M, Kwiatkowski TG, et al. Thrombolysis in patients with transient neurologic deficits. Neurology 2001;57:2125. PubMed PMID: 4991.
78. Ozdemir O, Beletsky V, Chan R, et al. Thrombolysis in patients with marked clinical fluctuations in neurologic status due to cerebral ischemia. Arch Neurol 2008;65(8):1041–3. PubMed PMID: 18695054.
79. Smith EE, Abdullah AR, Petkovska I, et al. Poor outcomes in patients who do not receive intravenous tissue plasminogen activator because of mild or improving ischemic stroke. Stroke 2005;36(11):2497–9. PubMed PMID: 16210552.
80. Hemmen TM, Meyer BC, Hayes KA, et al. Identification of "Stroke Mimics" among 411 Code Strokes at the UCSD Stroke Center from September 1998 to March 2001. Stroke 2002; 33(1):385. PubMed PMID: 5034.

81. Wein TH, Hickenbottom SL, Morgenstern LB, et al. Safety of tissue plasminogen activator for acute stroke in menstruating women. Stroke 2002;2002(33):2506. PubMed PMID: 5137.
82. von Kummer R, Allen KL, Holle R, et al. Acute Stroke: usefulness of early CT findings before thrombolytic therapy. Radiology 1997;205:327. PubMed PMID: 4642.
83. Patel SC, Levine SR, Tilley BC, et al. Lack of clinical significance of early ischemic changes on computed tomography in acute stroke. JAMA 2001;286(22):2830–8. [Epub 2001/12/12]; PubMed PMID: 11735758. eng.
84. Gilligan. Early CT changes do not predict parenchymal hemorrhage following streptokinase therapy in acute stroke. Stroke 2000;31(11):2887. PubMed PMID: 5016.
85. Tomsick TA, Brott TG, Chambers AA, et al. Hyperdense middle cerebral artery sign on CT: Efficacy in detecting middle cerebral artery thrombosis. AJNR 1990;11:473. PubMed PMID: 884.
86. Barber P, Demchuk A, Hudon ME, et al. Hyperdense Sylvian Fissure MCA "DOT" Sign. Stroke 2001;32:84. PubMed PMID: 4399.
87. Marler JR, Tilley BC, Lu M, et al. Early stroke treatment associated with better outcome: the NINDS rt-PA stroke study. Neurology 2000;55(11):1649–55. PubMed PMID: 11113218.
88. Lees KR, Bluhmki E, von Kummer R, et al. Time to treatment with intravenous alteplase and outcome in stroke: an updated pooled analysis of ECASS, ATLANTIS, NINDS, and EPITHET trials. Lancet 2010;375(9727):1695–703. [Epub 2010/05/18]; PubMed PMID: 20472172. eng.
89. NINDS rt-PA Stroke Study Group. Generalized Efficacy of t-PA for Acute Stroke. Stroke 1997;28:2119. PubMed PMID: 2837.
90. Brott T, Lu M, Kothari R, et al. Hypertension and its treatment in the NINDS rt-PA stroke trial. Stroke 1998;29:1504. PubMed PMID: 3238.
91. Brott T, Broderick J, Kothari R, et al. Early hemorrhage growth in patients with intracerebral hemorrhage. Stroke 1997;28:1. PubMed PMID: 2661.
92. Demchuck AM, Tanne D, Hill MD, et al. Predictors of Good Outcome After Intavenous tPA for Acute Ischemic Stroke. Neurology 2001;57(3):474. PubMed PMID: 4916.
93. Fagan SC, Morgenstern LB, Petitta A, et al. Cost-effectiveness of tissue plasminogen activator for acute ischemic stroke. Neurology 1998;50:883. PubMed PMID: 2918.
94. Demaerschalk BM, Yip TR. Economic benefit of increasing utilization of intravenous tissue plasminogen activator for acute ischemic stroke in the United States. Stroke 2005;36(11):2500–3. PubMed PMID: 16224087.
95. Sandercock P, Berge E, Dennis M, et al. Cost-effectiveness of thrombolysis with recombinant tissue plasminogen activator for acute ischemic stroke assessed by a model based on UK NHS costs. Stroke 2004;35(6):1490. PubMed PMID: 5744.
96. von Kummer R, Hacke W. Safety and efficacy of intravenous tissue plasminogen activator and heparin in acute middle cerebral artery stroke. Stroke 1992;23:646. PubMed PMID: 956.
97. Chen B, Friedman B, Whitney MA, et al. Thrombin activity associated with neuronal damage during acute focal ischemia. J Neurosci 2012;32(22):7622–31. [Epub 2012/06/01]; PubMed PMID: 22649241, Pubmed Central PMCID: 3383068. eng.
98. Chen B, Cheng Q, Yang K, et al. Thrombin mediates severe neurovascular injury during ischemia. Stroke 2010;41(10):2348–52. PubMed PMID: 20705928.
99. Barreto AD, Alexandrov AV, Lyden P, et al. The argatroban and tissue-type plasminogen activator stroke study: final results of a pilot safety study. Stroke 2012;43(3):770–5. [Epub 2012/01/10]; PubMed PMID: 22223235, Pubmed Central PMCID: 3289043. eng.
100. Zivin JA, Mazzarella V. Tissue plasminogen activator plus glutamate antagonist improves outcome after embolic stroke. Arch Neurol 1991;48(12):1235–8. PubMed PMID: 1688257.
101. Wang Y, Zhang Z, Chow N, et al. An activated protein C analog with reduced anticoagulant activity extends the therapeutic window of tissue plasminogen activator for ischemic stroke in rodents. Stroke 2012;43(9):2444–9. [Epub 2012/07/20]; PubMed PMID: 22811462, Pubmed Central PMCID: 3429704. eng.
102. O'Collins VE, Macleod MR, Donnan GA, et al. 1,026 Experimental treatments in acute stroke. Ann Neurol 2006;59(3): 467–77.
103. Shuaib A, Lees KR, Lyden P, et al. NXY-059 for the treatment of acute ischemic stroke. N Engl J Med 2007;357(6):562–71. PubMed PMID: 17687131.
104. Lyden PD, Shuaib A, Lees KR, et al. Safety and tolerability of NXY-059 for acute intracerebral hemorrhage: the CHANT Trial. Stroke 2007;38(8):2262–9. [Epub 2007/06/16]; PubMed PMID: 17569876. eng.
105. Lees KR, Zivin JA, Ashwood T, et al. NXY-059 for acute ischemic stroke. N Engl J Med 2006;354(6):588–600. PubMed PMID: 16467546.
106. Diener HC, Lees KR, Lyden P, et al. NXY-059 for the treatment of acute stroke: pooled analysis of the SAINT I and II Trials. Stroke 2008;39(6):1751–8. PubMed PMID: 18369171.
107. Grotta J. Neuroprotection is unlikely to be effective in humans using current trial designs. Stroke 2001;33:306. PubMed PMID: 5228.
108. Lapchak PA, Zhang JH, Noble-Haeusslein LJ. RIGOR Guidelines: Escalating STAIR and STEPS for Effective Translational Research. Transl Stroke Res 2013;4(3):279–85. PubMed PMID: 23658596, Pubmed Central PMCID: 3644408.
109. O'Collins VE, Macleod MR, Cox SF, et al. Preclinical drug evaluation for combination therapy in acute stroke using systematic review, meta-analysis, and subsequent experimental testing. J Cereb Blood Flow Metab 2011;31(3):962–75. [Epub 2010/10/28]; PubMed PMID: 20978519, Pubmed Central PMCID: 3063631. eng.
110. Hemmen TM, Raman R, Guluma KZ, et al. Intravenous thrombolysis plus hypothermia for acute treatment of ischemic stroke (ICTuS-L): final results. Stroke 2010;41(10):2265–70. [Epub 2010/08/21]; PubMed PMID: 20724711, Pubmed Central PMCID: 2947593. eng.
111. Lyden PD, Hemmen TM, Grotta J, et al. Endovascular therapeutic hypothermia for acute ischemic stroke: ICTuS 2/3 protocol. Int J Stroke 2013;PubMed PMID: 24206528.

52 Antithrombotic Therapy for Treatment of Acute Ischemic Stroke

Harold P. Adams Jr., Patricia H. Davis

KEY POINTS

- Aspirin therapy (initial dose of 325 mg and subsequently 81 mg a day) should be initiated in acute stroke patients within 24 to 48 hours. Patients receiving thrombolytic therapy should delay treatment until after 24 hours.
- Full-dose anticoagulation in acute ischemic stroke patients does not improve stroke outcomes or reduce the risk of recurrent stroke but increases the risk of intracerebral hemorrhage.
- While some subgroups may benefit from anticoagulation, including patients with arterial dissection, aortic arch atheroma, or active cancer, no data are currently available to support this therapy. Trials comparing antiplatelet therapy to anticoagulation are underway.
- In immobilized patients following stroke, deep vein thrombosis prophylaxis should be started early using LMW heparin, heparin, or intermittent compression stockings. The duration of therapy is unclear.
- Oral anticoagulants for long-term prevention of recurrent ischemic stroke in patients with cardioembolism should be initiated but the timing of starting treatment is unclear and the size of the ischemic stroke should be considered in this decision. The new oral anticoagulants are associated with a lower risk of intracerebral hemorrhage but have a more rapid onset of action than vitamin K antagonists. These medications have not been tested in patients with acute stroke.
- Dual antiplatelet therapy with aspirin and clopidogrel loading following TIA or minor stroke is being tested and it was safe and effective in an Asian population.
- Combined antithrombotic therapy (argatroban and eptifibatide) with intravenous thrombolytic therapy is being tested for safety and appears promising.

Because most ischemic strokes are secondary to arterial thromboembolism, antithrombotic agents (i.e., anticoagulants and antiplatelet agents) are a mainstay of medical treatment to prevent ischemic stroke. The utility of these medications in long-term management to prevent stroke or recurrent stroke is well established.[1–4] Oral anticoagulants including vitamin K antagonists (VKA) and new oral anticoagulants (NOAC) are of confirmed usefulness in the prevention of cardioembolic stroke among patients with high-risk heart diseases, including most patients with atrial fibrillation including those with prior stroke or transient ischemic attack.[5–7] Antiplatelet agents are the standard medical therapy for lowering the risk of stroke among patients with arterial diseases, including those patients with either intracranial or extracranial atherosclerosis.[3] Because of their established efficacy in long-term care and because most strokes are secondary to formation of clots, there continues to be considerable interest in the emergency use of either anticoagulant or antiplatelet agents in the setting of acute stroke. A number of antithrombotic agents can be considered (Table 52-1). These agents may be used as the primary intervention or as an adjunct to other measures aimed at restoring perfusion to the brain. The rationale for these medications includes halting the propagation of an intra-arterial thrombus, forestalling early recurrent embolization, and maintaining collateral flow to the area of ischemia. In addition, their adjunctive use after mechanical or pharmacologic thrombolysis centers on preventing rethrombosis or reocclusion after recanalization. In particular, intravenously administered antiplatelet agents are given in conjunction with emergency angioplasty and stenting or following thrombolytic therapy.[8] Antithrombotic agents also are a potential therapy for those patients with stroke who are bedridden and have an increased risk of deep vein thrombosis (DVT) and pulmonary embolism (PE), which add to the morbidity and potential mortality of the neurologic event. The antithrombotic medications are used both to prevent and to treat these thromboembolic events. Recent guidelines address the use of antithrombotic agents for treatment of acute ischemic stroke.[1,3,4] Several reviews have also discussed the role of antithrombotic therapy in ischemic stroke.[2,9–12]

PHARMACOLOGY

Heparin, Low-Molecular-Weight Heparins, and Danaparoid

Heparin, low-molecular-weight (LMW) heparins, and *danaparoid* have been used for more than 60 years. Heparin is a mixture of glycosaminoglycans that is usually obtained from porcine or bovine sources. Its molecular weight ranges from 5000 to 30,000 daltons (d).[13] Because of the high risk of local bleeding at the injection site, heparin is given either subcutaneously or intravenously, not intramuscularly. The antithrombotic effects of heparin are immediate if it is given intravenously in a bolus dose followed by a continuous intravenous infusion.

Heparin binds to plasma proteins, platelet-derived proteins, and endothelial cells. Differences in levels of those proteins might explain variations in clinical responses to heparin among patients. Heparin binds to and alters the conformation of antithrombin, which in turn increases the ability of antithrombin to inactivate thrombin, activated factor X (factor Xa), and activated factor IX (factor IXa). Heparin binds to the amino terminus of the molecule site of antithrombin, which leads to a conformational change in the antithrombin. This change increases the ability of antithrombin to inactivate thrombin by a ratio of 1000 to 4000 times. Heparin does not directly affect either thrombin or factor Xa already

TABLE 52-1 Antithrombotic Agents that May be Used in the Management of Patients with Acute Ischemic Stroke

Anticoagulants	Benefit (Level of Evidence)	Increased Risk of ICH
GLYCOSAMINOGLYCANS		
Heparin	Low-dose – DVT prevention (IA)	Yes
Low-molecular-weight heparins	Low-dose DVT prevention (IA)	Yes
Danaparoid	No	Yes
DIRECT THROMBIN INHIBITORS		
Argatroban	IIIB	Yes
Dabigatran	Prevention in AF(1A)	
XA INHIBITORS		
Fondaparinux	NT	
Rivaroxaban, apixaban	Prevention in AF (1A)	
ANTIPLATELET AGENTS		
Aspirin (ASA)	Yes (1A)	Yes (low)
Clopidogrel	No data	Uncertain
Dipyridamole	No data	
Cilostazol	Stroke prevention (1A)	No
Vorapaxar	No	Yes
Terutroban	Not compared to ASA	No
GLYCOPROTEIN IIb/IIIa RECEPTOR BLOCKERS		
Abciximab	No	Yes
Eptifibatide (Integrilin)	Uncertain	No
Tirofiban	Not compared to ASA	No

DVT, deep vein thrombosis; AF, atrial fibrillation.
For more details refer 'AHA Evidence box index' in the FM.

incorporated in a formed thrombus; thus, it does not have thrombolytic effects. The ratio of inhibition of activated thrombin to factor Xa is 1:1. Heparin also prevents fibrin formation through its inhibition of thrombin-induced activation of platelets and factors V and VIII. It does not affect factor Xa already bound to platelets. Heparin also inactivates thrombin through heparin cofactor II, which is an action that occurs at high concentrations and is independent from its effects on antithrombin. In addition, the high-molecular-weight components of heparin can alter endothelial modulation of clotting factors and interact with platelet factor 4 (PF4). The binding of heparin to von Willebrand factor (vWF) also affects platelet function.[13]

Heparin also binds to macrophages and endothelial cells. This binding, which is saturable, relates to the rapid clearance of heparin from the circulation. Heparin has a narrow therapeutic window; differences between safe but effective doses and dangerous levels are small. There is a strong association between the risks of serious bleeding with increases in the dose of heparin. Some patients are relatively resistant to the actions of heparin (heparin resistance). This response may be secondary to a deficiency of antithrombin, increased heparin clearance or to an elevation of heparin-binding proteins, including fibrinogen, factor VIII, or PF4.[13] Heparin does not cross the placenta.

The activated partial thromboplastin time (aPTT) is the most widely used test to monitor the biologic (antithrombotic) effects of heparin. This test measures responses to heparin-induced inhibition of thrombin, factor Xa, and factor IXa. The optimal level of anticoagulation is uncertain but is assumed to be approximately 1.5 times control values. The aPTT test has a number of serious limitations. Variability in reagents between institutions may lead to spurious aPTT results.[14] Patients with the lupus anticoagulant–antiphospholipid antibody syndrome often have falsely elevated aPTT values; in this situation, monitoring heparin therapy with this test may be problematic and alternative ways to assess heparin's activity include measuring inhibition of factor Xa or measuring heparin levels via neutralization with protamine sulfate. The usual therapeutic level of heparin is inhibition of factor Xa to 0.3 to 0.7 U/mL.

Most high-risk patients receive 5000 units of heparin two to three times a day for prevention of DVT. A different regimen is often given to patients with acute thrombotic events. The usual daily dose is approximately 24,000 to 30,000 units to maintain a therapeutic antithrombotic effect. Traditionally, a bolus of heparin (usually 5000 units) is given to start treatment; thereafter, heparin is given as a continuous intravenous infusion. Initially, the aPTT value is markedly prolonged, so follow-up assessments are usually delayed until 6 hours after the initiation of therapy. The patient's weight is an important variable that affects biologic responses to heparin. As a result, weight-based nomograms are now used to administer heparin. Current guidelines now recommend a nomogram, such as that included in Box 52-1, for initiation of heparin treatment and subsequent adjustments in doses in response to levels of anticoagulation.[13]

Heparin also has subtle anti-inflammatory actions that may differ from its effects on coagulation factors.[15] In addition, heparin may have effects on major neurotransmitters of the brain. The interactions of these effects and the potential utility of heparin for treatment of patients with acute brain ischemia are not obvious.

Because of the many limitations of unfractionated (traditional) heparin, other parenterally administered, rapidly acting anticoagulants have been developed.[13] The leading alternatives are the LMW heparins and danaparoid. These medications have a weak effect on thrombin and selective antithrombotic actions on factor Xa. The LMW heparins weigh approximately 1000 to 10,000 d. The reduction into low-weight compounds leads to lessened binding to platelets, proteins, endothelial cells, and macrophages. This probably explains the longer duration of effect and the relatively predictable responses to the use of the LMW heparins.

The LMW heparins and danaparoid have a reduced effect on thrombin function compared with unfractionated heparin but more selective inhibition of factor Xa. The ratio for thrombin and factor Xa is approximately 1:2 to 1:4. Because

BOX 52-1 Weight-Based Regimen for Administration of Unfractionated Heparin

INITIAL DOSAGE REGIMEN

80 units/kg intravenous bolus
Followed by 18 units/kg/hour
Check aPTT in 6 hours

ADJUSTMENT OF DOSAGE

aPTT level of <35 second (approximately 1.2 × control)
- Administer another 50 units/kg bolus
- Increase infusion to 22 units/kg/hour (increase 4 units/hour)

aPTT level of 35–45 second (approximately 1.2 to 1.5 × control)
- Administer another 40 units/kg bolus
- Increase infusion to 20 units/kg/hour (increase 2 units/hour)

aPTT level of 46 to 70 second (approximately 1.5 to 2.3 × control)
- Continue infusion at 18 units/kg/hour

aPTT level of 71 to 90 second (approximately 2.3 to 3 × control)
- Decrease infusion to 16 units/kg/hour (decrease 2 units/hour)

aPTT level of >90 second (approximately 3 × control)
- Halt infusion for 1 hour
- Restart infusion at 16 units/kg/hour
- Decrease infusion to 15 units/kg/hour (decrease 3 units/hour)

aPTT, activated partial thromboplastin time.

these agents do not affect thrombin activity except in very high concentrations, assessment of the responses by the use of the aPTT is unreliable. Rather, measuring inhibition of factor Xa tests the antithrombotic effects of these medications. The desired levels are 0.3–0.7 U/mL. Because these agents are excreted renally, the level of anticoagulation may be high among patients with renal failure.[13] Clinical trials have demonstrated that neonates and infants need a relatively higher dose of the LMW heparins than do older children or adults to achieve targeted levels for inhibition of factor Xa.[16]

Although the LMW heparins and danaparoid may be given intravenously, most clinical studies have focused on subcutaneously administered regimens using a weight-based nomogram, particularly in the scenario of preventing DVT. The responses to specific LMW heparins generally are similar, but the specific pharmacologic effects differ; thus, these agents should be evaluated individually. In particular, the ratio of antithrombin activity to antifactor Xa activity varies among the several compounds. Danaparoid is no longer available in the US.

Another group of parenteral anticoagulants that inhibit factor Xa, mediated via antithrombin but do not interact with PF4, are the pentasaccarides (*fondaparinux, idraparinux, idrabiotaparinux*). They are renally excreted and may be safe for patients with heparin-induced thrombocytopenia (HIT). Fondaparinux is used for prophylaxis and treatment of venous thromboembolism (VTE) as an alternative to LMW heparins. Idraparinux has a longer half-life and was tested for stroke prevention in atrial fibrillation (AMADEUS trial) but the study was terminated because of excess bleeding, as was a trial of idrabiotaparinux (BOREALIS-AF) which was terminated by the manufacturer for commercial reasons.[17]

Other Anticoagulants

Because of the lag between the initiation of therapy with VKA and an antithrombotic response, these agents are not used as an intervention for treatment of an acute ischemic stroke. In addition, these medications may have an initial and transient prothrombotic effect through their initial inhibition of the actions of proteins C and S, which limit their applicability. However, oral agents with direct or indirect inhibition of activated factors Xa have a more rapid onset of action. These agents include *rivaroxaban, apixaban,* and *edoxaban*.[18] Rivaroxaban is effective in preventing and treating VTE.[19,20] There are three double-blind trials which tested Xa inhibitors for stroke prevention in atrial fibrillation; these are ARISTOTLE and AVERROES (apixaban), and ROCKET-AF (rivaroxaban). Both showed similar efficacy in preventing stroke compared to VKA and are approved by the U.S. Food and Drug Administration (FDA) for this indication. An ongoing study, ENGAGE-AF TIMI 48 is testing edoxaban at two different doses for stroke prevention in patients with atrial fibrillation.[21] Otamixaban is a parenteral Xa inhibitor with a short half-life which is being studied in acute coronary syndrome (ACS).[17]

Direct thrombin inhibitors may affect unbound thrombin and don't require antithrombin, resulting in a more reliable antithrombotic effect than unfractionated heparin. These agents also do not affect platelet function and do not interact with PF4 so are suitable for patients with or at risk of HIT. They may be bivalent like the agent *Hirudin* - originally derived from the salivary gland of the medicinal leech - which is now available with the use of recombinant technology (*lepirudin, desirudin*).[17] It is a potent and irreversible inhibitor of thrombin function. The anticoagulant activity of hirudin is monitored by the aPTT. Antihirudin antibodies may develop within 5 days of treatment in 40–70% of patients treated with lepirudin. These antibodies may increase drug potency or cause anaphylaxis with re-exposure. Desirudin and lepirudin have been used in the treatment of patients with ACS, but they have not been used to treat patients with stroke. Leptirudin is no longer available. *Bivalirudin* (*hirulog*) another direct thrombin inhibitor which is reversible has been used to treat patients undergoing percutaneous coronary interventions (PCI), particularly in those patients at risk of HIT. There is a lower risk of bleeding compared to heparin.

Argatroban is a univalent selective thrombin inhibitor that competitively acts at the active site of thrombin; it has an immediate antithrombotic effect. Argatroban is metabolized by the liver and has a short half-life (approximately 50 minutes); thus, anticoagulation may be initiated or terminated more rapidly than with either unfractionated heparin or the LMW heparins.[22] It also is monitored by the aPTT. It is approved for treatment of HIT and is being tested as an adjunctive for thrombolytic therapy in stroke patients.[23]

Dabigatran is an oral direct thrombin inhibitor that was as effective as warfarin in preventing thromboembolism with less risk of bleeding when administered at a lower dose. At a higher dose, it was more effective than warfarin in preventing stroke and systemic embolism but had a similar rate of bleeding and is FDA-approved for stroke prevention.[24]

Aptamers are small RNA or DNA oligonucleotides that bind target molecules through high-affinity interactions. The advantage of these molecules is that they can be inactivated rapidly by a complementary antidote aptamer.[25] Pegnivacogin is a RNA aptamer that blocks factors IX and Xa and can be rapidly reversed by a complementary RNA aptamer, anivamersen. It is being tested in patients with ACS.[17]

Antiplatelet Agents

Antiplatelet agents target different receptors to prevent platelet aggregation (Fig. 52-1). *Aspirin* irreversibly blocks the cyclooxygenase (COX) activity of prostaglandin (PG) H synthase 1 (COX-1) and 2 (COX-2) by acetylation of a serine residue of the COX channel.[26] Aspirin's actions on platelet COX-1 are

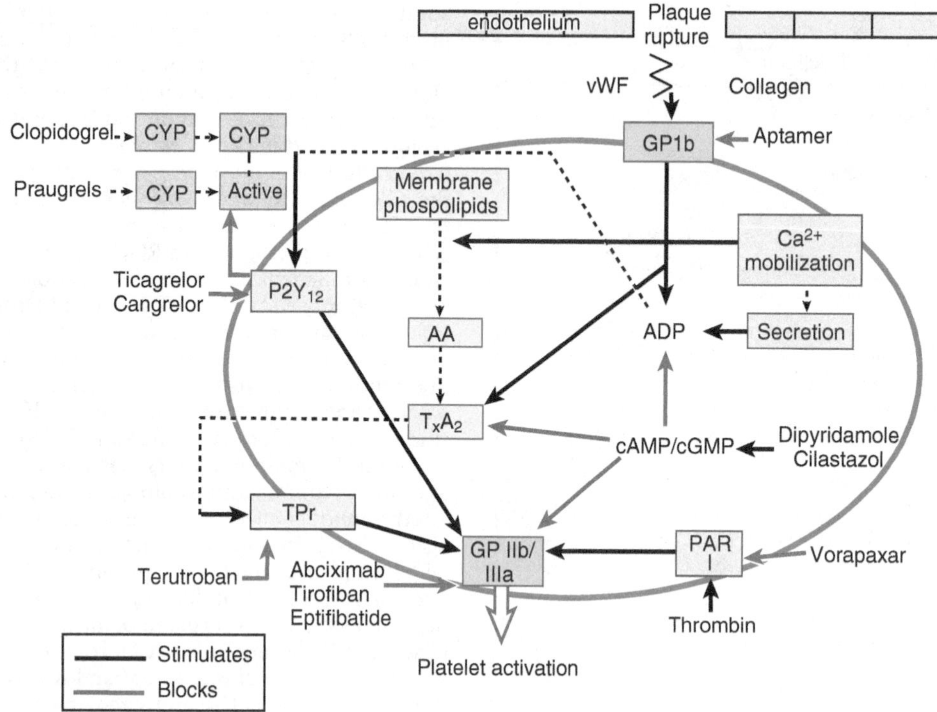

Figure 52-1. Mechanisms of action of antiplatelet therapy.The figure shows the site of action of antiplatelet medications to block platelet aggregation.[41,62] vWF = von Willebrand factor, CYP = cytochrome P 450 enzymes, COX-1 = cyclooxygenase-1, CAMP/cGMP = cyclic adenosine monophosphate/cyclic guanosine monophosphate, ADP = adenosine diphosphate, TxA2 = thromboxane A2, AA = arachadonic acid.

approximately 170-fold more potent than on monocyte COX-2.[27] It produces a permanent defect of thromboxane-A_2-dependent platelet function that induces platelet aggregation and causes vasoconstriction. Aspirin also alters endothelial production of prostacyclin, an agent that inhibits platelet aggregation and prevents vasoconstriction. The potentially prothrombotic effects of prostacyclin inhibition appear to be less relevant clinically because the endothelial cells may regenerate new COX unlike the anuclear platelet, in which COX inhibition is irreversible.[27]

The antithrombotic actions of aspirin occur over a broad range of doses. Aspirin is readily absorbed, so peak plasma levels are reached within 30–40 minutes. The portal circulation is the point of contact with platelets with aspirin which has a half-life of 15–20 minutes.[28] Enteric coating of the tablet does delay absorption with peak levels at 3–4 hours. There is not a lower risk of gastrointestinal (GI) bleeding with this formulation suggesting that it is the systemic effect of aspirin to inhibit the production of prostaglandins responsible for gastric protection that cause GI side-effects.[28,29] The risk of GI bleeding is directly related to the dose of aspirin.[26,30] A single dose of 100 mg of aspirin has an almost immediate effect on platelet aggregation. Lower doses of aspirin (<100 mg) may take longer than 24 hours to achieve maximal suppression of COX. Subsequently, lower daily doses are able to maintain the antiplatelet effects. Current guidelines recommend low-dose aspirin for secondary prevention of stroke or coronary events.[1,31] Thus, the minimum initial dose of aspirin appears to be at least 160 mg; that is the dose used in the Chinese Acute Stroke Trial.[32] Most non-steroidal anti-inflammatory drugs (NSAIDs) reversibly bind COX receptors with a stronger affinity than aspirin so that these receptors are occupied when aspirin is exposed to platelets in the portal circulation if NSAIDs are taken prior to aspirin.[33] Guidelines recommend taking NSAIDs 30 minutes after aspirin or at least 8 hours before aspirin.[31] Other potential antiplatelet actions may be the result of platelet activation by neutrophils, which is mediated by nitric oxide, and enhancement of the production of nitric oxide by endothelial cells.[27] The utility of aspirin as a neuroprotective agent for use in acute stroke is not established, but there is evidence that strokes may be less severe among patients who have previously used aspirin and infarct volume may be reduced.[34–36] There have been concerns that patients may develop resistance to aspirin and that higher doses of the medication may be needed to achieve antiplatelet effects.[26,29,33] Reasons for aspirin treatment failure include non-compliance, high platelet turnover due to an inflammatory process such as atherosclerosis, interaction with medication such as NSAIDs' alternative pathway of platelet activation, tachyphylaxis with reduced effect of aspirin with prolonged use, and genetic polymorphisms with the first three reasons probably the most important contributory causes.[29] There is no evidence that switching to an alternative antiplatelet agent decreases the risk of stroke.[33]

Terutroban is a selective thromboxane-prostaglandin receptor antagonist. A clinical trial comparing it to aspirin in stroke prevention (PERFORM) was stopped prematurely because of futility and an increased risk of minor bleeding.[37]

Dipyridamole and *cilostazol* block the actions of phosphodiesterase resulting in decreased reuptake of adenosine and elevated levels of cAMP and gAMP.[26] These agents prolong platelet survival, reduce inflammation, scavenge free radicals and produce vasodilation. Bioavailability of dipyridamole is low unless it is combined with tartaric acid to provide an acid environment for absorption in the extended-release formulation.[38] The interval from initiation of treatment with extended-release dipyridamole to the achievement of antiplatelet effects may be too slow to make this medication useful to treat acute ischemic stroke, although in combination with aspirin, it is effective in preventing recurrent stroke.[39] Cilostazol has only been investigated for the secondary prevention of stroke. In a meta-analysis, cilostazol was more effective than aspirin in preventing recurrent stroke, myocardial infarction (MI) or vascular death (relative ratio [RR] 0.72, 95% confidence interval [CI], 057–0.89) and had a lower risk of hemorrhage.[40]

The thienopyridines, *ticlopidine, clopidogrel, prasugrel, ticagrelor, elinogrel* and *cangrelor,* inhibit platelet aggregation induced by adenosine diphosphate by blocking the platelet receptor P2Y12, which interacts with fibrinogen.[41] The ability of clopidogrel to limit platelet aggregation occurs in a dose-dependent manner. The inhibition of platelet function starts within 2 hours of a 600 mg loading dose of clopidogrel and is irreversible. Inhibition of platelet aggregation is greater with a 600 mg loading dose than a 300 mg dose but a trial of the 600 mg loading dose followed by double-dose clopidogrel (150 mg) did not show any additional benefit in preventing recurrent vascular events compared to a 300 mg loading dose and 75 mg dose in patients with ACS. The risk of stent thrombosis in those patients undergoing PCI was lower with the high-dose regime.[42] Clopidogrel is a prodrug that requires a two-step activation process by the cytochrome P-450 (CYP) isoenzymes. Inhibition of these enzymes, particularly CYP2C19, by other drugs such as fluoxetine or by competition for the catalytic site on CYP2C19 by proton pump inhibitors (PPIs) can lead to interindividual variability in platelet aggregation.[43] However, in one randomized study of co-administration of clopidogrel and omeprazole in patients with ACS, there was more than 50% reduction of GI bleeding with PPI use and no increased risk of vascular events.[44] While PPIs decrease the efficacy of platelet inhibition by clopidogrel in vitro, there are conflicting data about whether co-administration of PPIs with clopidogrel increases the risk of thrombotic events and guidelines suggest selective use of PPIs in patients at high risk of GI bleeding.[31,45] There are also genetic variations that affect the antiplatelet response to clopidogrel. Carriers of specific alleles of CYP2C19 and CYP3A4 had less response to clopidogrel but there are conflicting results about these genotypes conferring a higher risk of recurrent vascular events after MI.[46,47] In a small Asian study, these genotypes were associated with a worse outcome after acute ischemic stroke.[48] There are significant ethnic differences in the frequency of these alleles, with 65% of East Asians and 35% of Western populations having a loss of function allelle.[49] Smoking increases the clinical benefit of clopidogrel by inducing the activity of CYP1A2, another isoenzyme which activates clopdiogrel.[50] The clinical usefulness of genotyping patients or performing tests of platelet inhibition to select the appropriate antiplatelet agent or to adjust the dose is being assessed.[51] Prasugrel has a tenfold to 100-fold greater and irreversible inhibition of platelet aggregation than either clopidogrel or ticlopidine. Prasugrel also has more rapid effects on platelet function. It is also a prodrug but requires only one-step activation by CYP enzymes and is not affected by genetic variability of these isoenzymes. Prasugrel was approved for the treatment of patients with ACS because there was a significant reduction in ischemic events when it was compared with clopidogrel.[52] However, it is contraindicated in patients with prior stroke or TIA because of an increased risk of ICH (2.3% vs 0%).[52] Ticagrelor, unlike clopidogrel and prasugrel, binds reversibly to the P2Y12 receptor and has a half-life of 7–8 hours. It is not a prodrug, has a rapid onset of action, and is more potent than clopidogrel. It is more effective than clopidogrel in preventing vascular death, MI, or stroke among patients with ACS, (PLATO trial).[53] It should be used with low-dose aspirin (<100 mg) as efficacy is improved.[54] A subgroup analysis of patients with prior stroke or TIA which comprised 6.2% of randomized patients showed similar benefit in preventing thrombotic events and no increased risk of ICH (0.9% vs 0.7%).[55] However, caution is recommended in treating patients with prior stroke or TIA with ticagrelor.[56] Ticagrelor is not approved for treatment of patients with a prior history of ICH. Of interest, a secondary prevention trial in ACS patients (PEGASUS) will compare ticagrelor to aspirin, but patients with stroke or TIA are excluded so further data will not be available about safety in these patients.[56] Cangrelor is an intravenous adenosine triphosphate analogue that reversibly binds to the P2Y12 platelet receptor. It has a half-life of 3–6 minutes, and the antiplatelet effect is gone within 60 minutes after the infusion is stopped. In a meta-analysis of the CHAMPION trials, cangrelor significantly reduced death, MI, revascularization, and stent thrombosis among 24,910 patients with ACS compared to clopidogrel. There was no increased risk of severe or moderate bleeding (0.2%) compared to clopidogrel but only 5% of the enrolled patients had a history of TIA or stroke.[57] Elinogrel is an oral or intravenous reversible P2Y12 receptor blocker which was tested in patients with ACS but the manufacturer suspended production.[58]

The glycoprotein (integrin) IIb/IIIa receptor antagonists are potent blockers of platelet aggregation by affecting the binding of fibrinogen to the platelets.[28] These agents do not affect platelet adhesion, but they do limit formation of a clot.[28] *Abciximab* is a monoclonal chimeric murine-human antibody that blocks the receptor. A bolus dose of abciximab may block more than 80% of the platelet receptors and maintain antiplatelet effects for several hours.[28] Platelet function is inhibited within 2 hours of administration of a bolus dose. The usual loading dose of abciximab is 0.25 mg/kg, and the maintenance infusion is 0.125 mcg/kg/min (maximum, 10 mcg/min). Platelet function recovers within 48 hours following an infusion lasting 12 hours.[28] The antiplatelet effects of abciximab are potentiated by the concomitant administration of aspirin.[59] Abciximab also may have some effect on the formation of thrombin. Abciximab in conjunction with other antithrombotic medications has been used to treat patients with ACS, including those undergoing PCI.

Tirofiban is a non-peptide derivative of tyrosine. It selectively and reversibly blocks the glycoprotein IIb/IIIa receptor. Marked inhibition of platelet aggregation and prolongation of the bleeding time occur within 5 minutes of the start of an intravenous infusion of the medication. Platelet function is normal within 2–6 hours after the infusion is halted.[28] Tirofiban is used to treat ACS.

Eptifibatide is a heptapeptide that has high affinity and specificity for the glycoprotein IIb/IIIa receptor. It also affects integrin-mediated binding of the smooth muscle cells to thrombospondin and prothrombin. After administration of a bolus dose followed by an intravenous infusion, platelet aggregation is diminished markedly within 15 minutes. Eptifibatide also affects thrombin generation and markedly prolongs the bleeding time. Platelet function returns to normal within 4 hours after withdrawal of the drug. The agent is used to treat patients' ACS and is the most widely used of the IIb/IIIa receptor antagonists. The usual dose is 180 mcg/kg (maximum, 22.6 mg) given over 1–2 minutes followed by a continuous infusion of 2 mcg/kg/min (maximum dose, 15 mg/h). All the IIb/IIIa receptor antagonists can cause an immune-mediated thrombocytopenia.[27]

Thrombin mediates platelet activation via an interaction with the protease-activated receptor 1 (PAR-1) on the platelet. Vorapaxar is a competitive and selective inhibitor of the PAR-1 receptor without affecting the production of fibrin by thrombin. The (TRA 2°P)-TIMI 50 trial was a double-blind, placebo-controlled trial that tested the addition of vorapaxar to standard therapy in patients with MI, peripheral vascular disease, or stroke. The trial was halted prematurely for the subgroup of patients with prior TIA or stroke because of an associated increased risk of intracerebral hemorrhage (ICH.)[60]

Novel antiplatelet are being developed that target the interaction between vWF and the platelet receptor glycoprotein 1b.

TABLE 52-2 Rates of Symptomatic Intracranial Hemorrhage and Serious Extracranial Hemorrhage with Antithrombotic Treatment of Acute Ischemic Stroke

		Intracranial Hemorrhage		Extracranial Hemorrhage	
Trial	**Agent**	**n**	**%**	**n**	**%**
UNFRACTIONATED HEPARIN					
Chamorro	Heparin	8/83	9.6	–	
Camerlingo	Heparin	2/45	4.4	0/45	0
IST	LD heparin	16/2429	0.7	10/2429	0.4
	HD heparin	43/2426	1.8	33/2426	1.4
Camerlingo	Heparin	13/208	6.2	6/208	2.9
RAPID	Heparin	2/32	6.3		
LMW HEPARINS OR DANAPAROID					
FISS	LD nadroparin	0/100	0	4/100	4.0
	HD nadroparin	0/101	0	6/101	5.9
TOAST	Danaparoid	19/638	2.9	25/638	3.9
FISS-bis	LD nadroparin	10/271	3.7		–
	HD nadroparin	15/245	6.1		–
HAEST	Dalteparin	6/224	2.7	13/224	5.8
TOPAS	Certoparin	2/99	2.0	1/99	1.0
	Certoparin	1/102	0.9	0	0
	Certoparin	2/103	1.9	0	0
	Certoparin	4/100	4.0	5/100	5.0
TAIST	LD tinzaparin	3/507	0.6	2/507	0.4
	HD tinzaparin	7/486	1.4	4/486	0.8
Fiss-tris	Nadroparin	1/180	0.5	25/180	14.0
ANTIPLATELET AGENTS					
MAST	Aspirin	3/153	1.9	–	
IST	Aspirin	87/9720	0.9	109/9720	1.1
CAST	Aspirin	115/10,335	1.1	86/10,335	0.8
HAEST	Aspirin	4/225	1.8	4/225	1.8
TAIST	Aspirin	1/491	0.2	2/491	0.4
FISS-tris	Aspirin	5/173	2.8	10/173	5.7
Abciximab	Abciximab	0/54	0	0/54	0
AbESTT	Abciximab	8/195	4.1	3/195	1.5
AbESTT-II	Abciximab	23/397	5.8	24/394	6.1

Abciximab, Abciximab in Ischemic Stroke Study; AbESTT, Abciximab Emergent Stroke Treatment Trial; CAST, Chinese Acute Stroke Trial; FISS, Fraxiparin in Stroke Study; HAEST, Heparin in Acute Embolic Stroke Trial; IST, International Stroke Trial; LD, low-dose; HD, high-dose; LMW, low-molecular-weight; MAST, Multicentre Acute Stroke Trial – Italy; RAPID, Rapid Anticoagulation Prevents Ischemic Damage study; TAIST, Tinzaparin in Acute Ischemic Stroke; TOAST, Trial of Org 10172 in Acute Stroke Treatment; TOPAS, Therapy of Patients with Acute Stroke.

An aptamer (ARC1779) was tested in a small pilot study of patients undergoing carotid endarterectomy and showed reduced embolic signals.[61] A nanobody has also been developed against vWF.[62]

SAFETY OF EMERGENCY ANTITHROMBOTIC TREATMENT FOR PATIENTS WITH ACUTE ISCHEMIC STROKE

Physicians are concerned about the safety of emergency administration of antithrombotic medications in the treatment of patients with acute ischemic stroke. Intracranial hemorrhage, including hemorrhagic transformation of the infarction, is a potential complication of any therapy aimed at restoring or improving perfusion to the brain. Bleeding complications also may occur in other locations in the body. In addition, some of the antithrombotic agents also may be associated with nonhemorrhagic complications.

Heparin

In a 2008 meta-analysis, Sandercock et al.[63] found that heparin is associated with an increased risk of bleeding. Data on the safety of heparin are shown in Table 52-2. Two doses of subcutaneously administered heparin were tested in the International Stroke Trial. Intracranial bleeding was diagnosed in 16 of 2429 patients (0.7%) given the lower dose and in 43 of 2426 patients (1.8%) receiving the higher dose.[64] In a subgroup of patients with atrial fibrillation, the rates of hemorrhage were 1.3% and 2.8% for the lower and higher doses of heparin.[65] The risk of bleeding with heparin is generally associated with the level of anticoagulation and the dose of medication. A significantly increased risk of bleeding has also been observed with low-dose anticoagulation used for prophylaxis of VTE in several recent meta-analyses.[66–68] Lederle et al.[68] found that heparin prophylaxis in acute stroke patients was associated with an increased major bleeding risk (OR, 1.66; 95%CI, 1.20–2.28) which was an absolute increased risk of six events per 1,000 people treated.

Non-neurologic hemorrhages also may complicate heparin; in one study of heparin for evolving stroke, ten of 69 patients had bleeding complications; most were non-neurologic.[106] In the International Stroke Trial, extracranial hemorrhage was diagnosed in 33 of 2426 patients (1.4%) given the higher dose of heparin and in ten of 2429 patients (0.4%) receiving low-dose heparin.[64] The most common locations for serious bleeding are the gastrointestinal tract, urinary system, retroperitoneal space, and joints.

Heparin should be discontinued if a patient experiences severe bleeding. Protamine sulfate also may be administered. The calculated dosage of protamine is based on the assumption that heparin has a half-life of approximately 60 minutes and that the dosage of the antidote corresponds to the amount of heparin given in the previous 90 minutes.[69]

Approximately 1 mg of protamine sulfate negates the effects of 100 units of heparin. Intravenous protamine sulfate should be infused slowly (over at least 10 minutes) because it can induce hypotension. Anaphylaxis may also complicate administration of protamine.[69]

Thrombocytopenia is a potential complication of treatment with heparin. Ramirez-Lassepas et al.[70] found a greater than 40% decline in platelet count among 21 of 137 patients with stroke who were treated with heparin; most were asymptomatic. A more severe, autoimmune-mediated thrombocytopenia (HIT) associated with antibodies to anti-PF4/heparin complex may appear 5–15 days after heparin is started. Prior use of heparin may sensitize a patient, and a second exposure may induce a severe thrombocytopenia within hours. The autoimmune reaction is not related to the dose of heparin. The diagnosis of HIT is based on an unexplained drop in the platelet count of at least 50% or skin lesions at sites of heparin injection and the presence of anti-PF4/heparin complex antibodies. The secondary white clot syndrome may lead to myocardial or cerebral ischemia. A study of acute ischemic stroke patients treated with heparin found a 1.7% incidence of definite HIT.[71] Ischemic stroke patients receiving heparin should have platelet counts checked every 2 to 3 days from days 4 to 14 (or until heparin is stopped).[72] Patients with HIT with thrombosis should be treated with lepirudin or argatroban. Further studies are needed to assess the role of fondaparinux in HIT.[72]

Low-Molecular-Weight Heparins and Danaparoid

Bleeding is the most likely potential complication of treatment with an LMW heparin or danaparoid. Because of a more predictable dose–response relationship, the risk of bleeding appears to be less with these agents than with unfractionated heparin. The long duration of their pharmacologic actions is a potential disadvantage if serious bleeding does happen. There is no effective antidote but current guidelines recommend treatment with protamine.[13]

The safety of these agents in patients with acute ischemic stroke has been evaluated in several clinical trials (see Table 52-2). Most of the trials have tested subcutaneous administration. A trial performed in Hong Kong found no increase in the risk of intracranial or extracranial hemorrhage with the administration of nadroparin.[73] However, a second trial of nadroparin found a significantly increased risk of serious bleeding.[74] In a study comparing aspirin or dalteparin in patients with atrial fibrillation and recent stroke, symptomatic intracranial hemorrhage was diagnosed in 2.7% of the patients given the LMW heparin and in 1.8% of patients receiving aspirin.[75] Extracranial hemorrhage also was more common among the patients treated with dalteparin. A German trial tested four doses of certoparin; the risks of symptomatic intracranial or extracranial bleeding were the greatest among the group that received the highest dose of the medication.[76] In a trial that tested two doses of tinzaparin in comparison with aspirin, the risks for symptomatic intracranial hemorrhage were 0.2% for aspirin, 0.6% for low-dose tinzaparin, and 1.4% for the highest dose of tinzaparin.[77] Wong et al.[78] compared the utility of aspirin or a LMW heparin, nadroparin, in patients with recent stroke associated with large-artery occlusive disease. The rates of hemorrhagic transformation of the infarction and severe adverse events were similar in both treatment groups.

One trial tested the intravenous administration of danaparoid in treatment of patients with acute ischemic stroke.[79] The medication was given with a bolus followed by a continuous intravenous infusion, and subsequent treatment was adjusted according to levels of inhibition of factor Xa. Enrollment of patients with more than a moderately severe stroke (as indicated by a National Institutes of Health Stroke Scale [NIHSS] score of 15 or greater) was halted because of an unacceptably high rate of symptomatic intracranial hemorrhage. Overall, symptomatic hemorrhage occurred in six of 628 patients given placebo (0.9%) and in 19 of 638 patients treated with danaparoid (2.9%). A meta-analysis of the randomized trials of anticoagulants among patients with cardioembolism concluded that early administration of anticoagulants is associated with a significant increase in the risk of symptomatic ICH (2.5% vs 0.7%; OR, 2.89; 95%CI, 1.19–7.01).[80]

A clinical trial compared the utility of enoxaparin or unfractionated heparin in preventing DVT after stroke.[81] The trial, which involved entry within 48 hours after stroke, demonstrated no difference in neurologic outcomes in the two groups.[82] Symptomatic ICH occurred in 0.69% of the heparin group and 0.46% of the enoxaparin group.[82] Another clinical trial compared the utility of certoparin or unfractionated heparin in preventing VTE among patients treated within 24 hours of stroke.[83] The rates of major bleeding complications were 1.1% with certoparin and 1.8% with heparin. A systematic review that compared aspirin or LMW heparin after stroke found that the anticoagulant was associated with a significant increase in major extracranial hemorrhage.[84] Among patients treated within 24 hours, symptomatic ICH was significantly more common among patients treated with LMW heparin. In a prospective cohort of 215 children with acute ischemic stroke, full-dose anticoagulation was associated with a 4% risk of symptomatic ICH.[85]

Thrombocytopenia is a potential complication of treatment with the LMW heparins and danaparoid, but the risk of this complication is lower than with unfractionated heparin.[13] Because of the potential for cross-reactivity, patients who have HIT probably should not receive the LMW heparins.

Other Anticoagulant Agents

The other rapidly acting antithrombotic agents have not been extensively, tested in the setting of acute ischemic stroke. LaMonte et al.[22] performed a multicenter trial that enrolled 171 patients within 12 hours of stroke; two different doses of argatroban were tested. The primary outcome of this safety trial was symptomatic intracranial hemorrhage; it occurred in 5.1% of 59 subjects treated with the larger dose of argatroban, 3.4% of 58 subjects in the lower dose group, and in none of the 52 subjects in the control group. Argatroban was administered as an adjunct to standard full-dose t-PA to 65 patients with middle cerebral artery occlusions in a safety study. Significant ICH occurred in 6.2%.[23] A further phase 2 trial of this combination is in progress (ARTSS-2).[86]

New Oral Anticoagulants

The new oral anticoagulants (NOACs) including dabigatran, apixaban, and rivaroxaban are associated with a reduced risk of intracranial hemorrhage compared to VKA. In a meta-analysis, the OR of ICH was 0.49 (95%CI, 0.36–0.65).[87] A Cochrane review found a reduced risk of ICH with oral factor Xa inhibitors (OR, 0.56; 95%CI, 045–0.64).[5] The reasons for the lower risk may be a factor VII sparing effect with NOACs and the fact that these agents do not decrease the substrates required to produce thrombin.[88] No trials in acute ischemic stroke are available.

Antiplatelet Agents

The safety of administration of aspirin started within 48 hours of onset of stroke was explored in two large trials, and the medication was compared with LMW heparin in other clinical trials.[32,64,75,77,78] In the Chinese Acute Stroke Trial, bleeding events developed in 115 of 10,335 patients (1.1%) who received aspirin within 48 hours of onset of stroke.[32] In the International Stroke Trial, hemorrhages were reported in 87 of the 9720 patients treated with aspirin (0.9%).[64] The risk was lower among those patients who received aspirin without concomitant heparin; only 26 of 4858 patients had bleeding (0.5%). Two trials comparing aspirin or LMW heparin reported less bleeding with aspirin, but a more recent trial did not find any difference in hemorrhagic complications.[75,77] While the likelihood of serious ICH is relatively low with aspirin, there is some associated risk from the early use of the medication after stroke.

There are limited data about the safety of clopidogrel loading in patients with acute ischemic stroke.[89] A retrospective study of 55 acute ischemic stroke patients loaded with clopidogrel compared to 55 patients who did not receive this therapy showed no difference in serious bleeding events.

The greater potency of platelet inhibition of prasugrel compared with clopidogrel is associated with a higher risk of serious bleeding. In a trial of patients with ACS, those with a history of TIA or stroke had a risk of intracranial hemorrhage of 2.3% for prasugrel versus 0% for clopidogrel ($P = 0.02$). Prior stroke or TIA is a contraindication to using prasugrel in ACS.[45] In a meta-analysis of the CHAMPION trials, there was no increase in severe or moderate bleeding but there was an increase in minor bleeding with cangrelor.[57] An increased risk of dyspnea has been noted in reversible P2Y12 receptor inhibitors (ticagrelor, elinogrel, and cangrelor) is postulated to be due to an acute autoimmune lung injury.[90]

The parenterally administered glycoprotein IIb/IIIa receptor blockers have been given in patients with acute ischemic stroke. The experience is greatest with abciximab, which has been tested in a series of clinical trials. A dose escalation study of abciximab reported no hemorrhages among 54 subjects; no dosage relationship was found.[91] A dose confirmation study reported seven cases of symptomatic ICH among 195 subjects administered abciximab compared with two cases in 199 subjects treated with placebo.[92] An international trial testing abciximab given within 6 hours after stroke was halted prematurely after 808 patients were enrolled; symptomatic intracranial hemorrhages were more common among those treated with abciximab than among those assigned to receive placebo.[93] A subgroup of patients treated within 3 hours of awakening with a stroke had a high rate of bleeding with abciximab.[94] In a series of 24 patients with neurologic deterioration after a subcortical infarct, infusion of eptifibatide was not associated with any ICH.[95] A safety study of 260 patients with moderate ischemic stroke received intravenous tirofiban or placebo (SaTIS trial). There was no significant difference in ICH between the two groups.[96] Based on a systemic review, Ciccone et al. concluded that the glycoprotein IIb/IIIa receptor blockers were associated with non-significant increases in symptomatic intracranial hemorrhages or major extracranial hemorrhages.[97]

Combined Antithrombotic and Fibrinolytic Therapy

A trial found that early administration of aspirin added to streptokinase was associated with high risk of ICH.[98] A trial of 300 mg of intravenous aspirin following thrombolytic therapy was halted early because of an excessive rate of symptomatic ICH (4.3% vs 1.6%, $P = 0.04$) and no benefit on outcomes.[99] A retrospective analysis of 139 patients receiving oral aspirin less than 24 hours after thrombolytic therapy compared to those receiving aspirin after 24 hours did not demonstrate higher rate of bleeding.[100]

Qureshi et al.[101] reported one symptomatic intracranial hemorrhage among 20 patients receiving abciximab in addition to reteplase. The same group reported two asymptomatic hemorrhages among 20 patients who were treated with eptifibatide and reteplase.[102] In 13 patients with middle cerebral artery occlusion, half-dose intravenous t-PA combined with abciximab caused only one symptomatic ICH. However, in one case series, an 18% symptomatic ICH rate (9/51 cases) was observed using abciximab in neurovascular procedures and the authors suggested that the shorter-acting agents (eptifibatide and tirofiban) may be preferable to abciximab to reduce the risk of bleeding.[103] In the ReoPro and Retavase to treat Acute Stroke study (ROSIE/ROSIE-CT), an open-label dose-escalation study, the safety of abciximab combined with a thrombolytic agent is being tested (http://www.clinicaltrials.gov/ct2/show/NCT00046293?term=ReoPro&rank=4). In the CLEAR-ER trial, eptifibatide was given in combination with low-dose intravenous t-PA within 3 hours after the onset of acute ischemic stroke and compared with standard-dose intravenous t-PA. Of 126 enrolled subjects, 101 received combination therapy with a symptomatic ICH rate of 2% compared to 12% with standard dose t-PA therapy.[8] A further phase 2 study (CLEAR-FDR) is comparing standard dose t-PA with and without IV eptifibatide (http://www.clinicaltrials.gov/ct2/show/NCT01977456?term=Eptifibatide+Rt-PA+in+stroke&rank=3).

Heparin also has been given in conjunction with thrombolytic agents. Studies of intra-arterially administered prourokinase involved the use of heparin as a concomitant therapy.[104,105] The risk of bleeding approached 10% and was increased with the larger of the two doses of heparin. The lower dose heparin protocol has been used in subsequent trials of intra-arterial thrombolytic therapy and in the Interventional Management of Stroke III (IMSIII) trial, the risk of symptomatic ICH was 6.2%, in the endovascular group which was not different than those receiving intravenous thrombolytic therapy alone.[106]

Dual Oral Antiplatelet Therapy

Longer-term administration of the combination of aspirin and clopidogrel in comparison with monotherapy with either aspirin or clopidogrel alone is associated with higher rates of bleeding with the combination.[107] The MATCH trial enrolled only patients with ischemic cerebrovascular disease and life-threatening and major bleeding were significantly increased with combination therapy.[108] In the ACTIVE-A trial, patients with atrial fibrillation received either the combination of aspirin and clopidogrel with an associated 2.0% per year risk of major bleeding or aspirin alone with a 1.3% per year risk ($P < 0.001$).[109] In the Secondary Prevention of Small Subcortical Strokes (SPS3) trial that enrolled patients with small vessel disease, there was a statistically significant increase in major bleeding with combined long-term aspirin and clopidogrel therapy (2.1%/year vs 1.1%/year, $P < 0.001$) and a non-significant increase in ICH (0.42%/year vs 0.28%/year, $P = 0.21$). However, double antiplatelet therapy was not started until 14 days after the ictus.[110] A meta-analysis of patients receiving dual antiplatelet therapy for more than a year showed no benefit in stroke prevention and dual therapy compared to clopidogrel alone showed an elevated risk of ICH (relative ratio [RR], 1.46; 95%CI, 1.17–1.82).[107] Shorter duration of dual antiplatelet therapy seems to have a lower risk of hemorrhage. In the medical treatment group included in a trial testing endovascular therapy in patients with symptomatic intracranial stenosis (SAMMPRIS trial), combined therapy with aspirin and clopidogrel was started within 30 days after onset of symptoms and continued for 90 days. There was a low risk of ICH (0.4%) but there was no single antiplatelet group for comparison.[111] In a Chinese population, a trial (Clopidogrel in High-Risk Patients with Acute Non-disabling Cerebrovascular Events (CHANCE)) testing a loading dose of 300 mg of clopidogrel combined with aspirin within 24 hours after TIA or minor stroke and continued for 3 weeks followed by aspirin alone compared to aspirin only did not demonstrate an increased risk of ICH (0.3% in both groups at 3 months) or moderate-to-severe bleeding, but there was a non-significant increase in minor bleeding.[112] It is uncertain whether these results will also apply to other ethnic groups as there is a higher prevalence of intracranial stenosis and CYP2C19 in Asian populations. One study found a higher risk of bleeding with combined aspirin and clopidogrel therapy in patients not previously treated with aspirin compared to those already taking aspirin.[113] A trial of initiation of dual therapy with aspirin and dipyridamole within 24 hours after TIA or stroke showed no increased risk of hemorrhage compared to waiting a week to start dual therapy. A meta-analysis of 9,012 patients who were treated within 3 days with dual antiplatelet therapy compared to single antiplatelet agents after a non-cardioembolic stroke or TIA showed a non-significantly increased risk of major bleeding (RR, 1.35; 95%CI, 0.70–2.59).[114,115]

CONCLUSIONS

Clinical trials confirm that both anticoagulants and antiplatelet agents are associated with a risk of serious bleeding complications. The likelihood for either major extracranial or symptomatic intracranial hemorrhage appears to be greatest with unfractionated heparin, the LMW heparins, argatroban, and danaparoid. Bleeding side effects also appear to be greater with the glycoprotein IIb/IIIa receptor blockers than with aspirin. The new thienopyridines appear to have increased risk of ICH in patients with prior stroke or TIA (prasugrel) or uncertain risk (ticagrelor and cangrelor). There are insufficient data to determine the safety of using loading doses of clopidogrel in acute ischemic stroke but while dual antiplatelet therapy appears to be associated with increased risk of hemorrhage in long-term use, it may be safe if used for a short duration after a minor stroke. Further trials are investigating this combination.

Although the risk of bleeding is relatively low with anticoagulants, it is high enough to mandate that strong evidence for efficacy is needed to justify their use. The LMW heparins do not appear to be either more dangerous or safer than unfractionated heparin. The likelihood of hemorrhage with heparin or LMW heparins is associated with the severity of neurologic impairments or the size of stroke on the initial brain imaging study. Patients with more severe strokes (NIHSS score >15) and those with a large area of hypodensity on CT probably should not be treated with either unfractionated heparin or one of the LMW heparins. The NOACs are associated with lower risk of intracranial bleeding than warfarin but have not been tested in acute ischemic stroke.

Starting aspirin within 48 hours after stroke is accompanied by a relatively low rate of symptomatic bleeding. The safety of a combination of either an anticoagulant or antiplatelet agent with a thrombolytic agent has not been established. Current guidelines recommend delaying the start of these medications until at least 24 hours after intravenous treatment with t-PA.[1] Besides intracranial bleeding, physicians should be alert to non-neurologic hemorrhagic complications after the use of an anticoagulant or antiplatelet agent. Patients with active bleeding or other illnesses that are associated with a high chance of serious bleeding (e.g., recent surgery or recent trauma) may be well-served by not receiving these medications. Immune-mediated side-effects such as thrombocytopenia or dyspnea should be kept in mind when antithrombotic medications are administered to patients with acute ischemic stroke.

EFFICACY OF TREATMENT OF ACUTE ISCHEMIC STROKE

The primary goal of acute anticoagulation has been to limit brain injury and improve neurologic outcome by halting neurologic worsening and preventing early recurrent thromboembolism. In the past, some subgroups of patients with stroke, such as those with cardioembolism, large artery atherosclerosis, or arterial dissection have been preferentially treated with urgent anticoagulation.

Unfractionated Heparin

In a very large trial that enrolled approximately 20,000 participants, investigators of the International Stroke Trial tested two doses of subcutaneously administered heparin against placebo (Tables 52-2–52-5).[64] Within 48 hours of onset of stroke, subjects were assigned treatment with either 5000 units (low dose) or 12,500 units (high dose) of heparin twice a day. Some subjects also received aspirin. The trial has limitations in design. For a sizable number of patients enrolled in the trial, baseline brain imaging studies were not performed beforehand to exclude primary hemorrhages. Both the treating physicians and the subjects were aware of the treatment allocation; this information may have biased the physicians' and subjects' reporting of adverse experiences. No monitoring of the level of anticoagulation and no adjustment of doses of heparin were included. The trial demonstrated a modest decline in the frequency of recurrent stroke within the first 14 days with the use of heparin. No reduction in mortality or an improvement in the rate of favorable outcomes was seen. As a result, the trial found no net benefit from treatment with heparin. In addition, no net benefit from treatment with heparin was noted among the subgroup of patients who had atrial fibrillation.

Despite the publication of the results of the International Stroke Trial, interest persisted in the potential usefulness of heparin for treatment of patients with recent stroke. In a small multicenter clinical trial, Chamorro et al.[116] tested intravenously administered heparin with adjustments in dosage in response to aPTT. The trial was halted prematurely when only 67 subjects were enrolled because of slow enrollment. Not surprisingly, outcomes between the two treatment groups were not different. In a single-center, placebo-controlled study, Camerlingo et al.[117] enrolled 418 subjects in a clinical trial that tested intravenous heparin administered within 3 hours of onset of stroke. Favorable outcomes were found in 38.9% of 208 subjects given heparin and in 28.6% of 210 subjects in the control group. There was a higher rate of symptomatic ICH in the heparin group (6.2% vs 1.4%). A meta-analysis performed by Sandercock et al.[118] could not confirm the efficacy of heparin for improving outcomes after stroke or lowering the risk of recurrent embolization. Guidelines from the US and Europe do not recommend full-dose anticoagulation in the treatment of acute ischemic stroke.[1,3,4] Two studies have shown a temporal decline in the use of full-dose heparin in acute stroke patients. In Sweden, the rate declined from 7.5% to 1.6% between 2001 and 2008 and in Germany, it declined from 24.5% to 6% between 2001 and 2006.[119,120]

TABLE 52-3 Rates of Early Recurrent Stroke after Antithrombotic Therapy for Acute Ischemic Stroke

		Treatment		Comparison Group		
Trial	**Agent**	***n***	**%**	***Type***	***n***	**%**
UNFRACTIONATED HEPARIN						
IST	LD heparin	78/2429	1.6	Control	214/4859	2.2
	HD heparin	86/2426	1.8			
IST – AF	Heparin	44/1557	2.8	Control	79/1612	4.9
LMW HEPARINS AND DANAPAROID						
FISS	LD nadroparin	2/101	1.9	Placebo	5/105	4.7
	HD nadroparin	1/102	1			
TOAST	Danaparoid	7/638	1.1	Placebo	7/628	1.1
TOAST – CE	Danaparoid	0/143	0	Placebo	2/123	1.6
HAEST	Dalteparin	19/224	8.5	Aspirin	17/225	7.5
TOPAS	Certoparin	3/99	3.0			
	Certoparin	3/102	2.9			
	Certoparin	4/103	3.9			
	Certoparin	3/100	3.0			
TAIST	LD tinzaparin	24/507	4.7	Aspirin	15/491	3.1
	HD tinzaparin	16/486	3.3			
TAIST – CE	Tinzaparin	4/256	1.6	Aspirin	2/112	1.8
Fiss-tris	Nadroparin	8/180	4.0	Aspirin	8/173	5.0
ANTIPLATELET AGENTS						
MAST	Aspirin	1/153	0.6	Control	0/156	0
IST	Aspirin	275/9719	2.8	Control	368/9714	3.8
CAST	Aspirin	220/10,335	2.1	Placebo	258/10,320	2.5
HAEST	Aspirin	17/225	7.5	Dalteparin	19/224	8.5
TAIST	Aspirin	15/491	3.2	Tinzaparin	40/993	4.0
FISS-tris	Aspirin	8/173	5.0	Nadroparin	8/180	4.0
Abciximab	Abciximab	1/54	2.0	Placebo	1/20	5.0
AbESTT	Abciximab	7/195	3.9	Placebo	8/199	3.9
AbESTT-II	Abciximab	12/403	2.9	Placebo	7/398	1.7

Abciximab, Abciximab in Ischemic Stroke Study; AbESTT, Abciximab Emergent Stroke Treatment Trial; AF, atrial fibrillation; CAST, Chinese Acute Stroke Trial; CE, cardioembolic; FISS, Fraxiparin in Stroke Study; HAEST, Heparin in Acute Embolic Stroke Trial; IST, International Stroke Trial; LD, low-dose; HD, high-dose; LMW, low-molecular-weight; MAST, Multicentre Acute Stroke Trial – Italy; TAIST, Tinzaparin in Acute Ischemic Stroke; TOAST, Trial of Org 10172 in Acute Stroke Treatment; TOPAS, Therapy of Patients with Acute Stroke.

TABLE 52-4 Rates of Neurologic Worsening after Treatment of Acute Ischemic Stroke

		Treatment		Comparison Group		
Trial	**Agent**	***n***	**%**	***Type***	***n***	**%**
UNFRACTIONATED HEPARIN						
Rödén-Jüllig	Heparin		30	Control		33
RAPID	Heparin	8/32	25	Aspirin	7/35	20
LMW HEPARINS AND DANAPAROID						
TOAST	Danaparoid	63/635	10	Placebo	62/633	9.9
HAEST	Dalteparin	24/224	10.7	Aspirin	17/225	7.6
TAIST	LD tinzaparin	55/508	11.4	Aspirin	58/491	11.9
	HD tinzaparin	58/486	11.9			
Wong	Nadroparin	10/180	6	Aspirin	8/173	5
ANTIPLATELET AGENTS						
MAST	Aspirin	18/153	11.8	Control	21/156	13.4
IST	Aspirin	567/4858	11.7	Control	604/4859	12.4
CAST	Aspirin	545/10,335	5.3	Placebo	614/10,320	5.9
HAEST	Aspirin	17/225	7.6	Dalteparin	24/224	10.7
TAIST	Aspirin	58/491	11.9	Tinzaparin	116/993	11.7
RAPID	Aspirin	7/35	20.0	Heparin	8/32	25.0
FISS-tris	Aspirin	8/173	5.0	Nadroparin	10/180	6.0
Abciximab	Abciximab	6/54	11.0	Placebo	3/20	15.0
AbESTT	Abciximab	14/195	7.1	Placebo	24/199	12.0
AbESTT-II	Abciximab	35/403	8.6	Placebo	45/398	11.3

Abciximab, Abciximab in Ischemic Stroke Study; AbESTT, Abciximab Emergent Stroke Treatment Trial; AF, atrial fibrillation; CAST, Chinese Acute Stroke Trial; CE, cardioembolic; FISS, Fraxiparin in Stroke Study; HAEST, Heparin in Acute Embolic Stroke Trial; HD, high-dose; IST, International Stroke Trial; LD, low-dose; LMW, low-molecular-weight; MAST, Multicentre Acute Stroke Trial – Italy; TAIST, Tinzaparin in Acute Ischemic Stroke; TOAST, Trial of Org 10172 in Acute Stroke Treatment; TOPAS, Therapy of Patients with Acute Stroke.

TABLE 52-5 Rates of Favorable Outcomes after Antithrombotic Treatment of Acute Ischemic Stroke

Trial	Agent	Treatment *n*	%	Comparison Group Type	*n*	%
UNFRACTIONATED HEPARIN						
IST	LD heparin	1776/4860	36.5	Control	3852/9718	36.9
	HD heparin	1802/4856	37.1			
Camerlingo	Heparin	81/208	38.9	Control	60/210	28.6
RAPID	Heparin	13/32	40.6	Aspirin	19/35	54.3
LMW HEPARINS AND DANAPAROID						
FISS	LD nadroparin	48/101	47.5	Placebo	37/105	35.2
	HD nadroparin	57/102	55.8			
TOAST	Danaparoid	482/641	75.2	Placebo	467/634	73.6
FISS-bis	LD nadroparin	155/271	57.2	Placebo	142/250	56.8
	HD nadroparin	145/245	59.2			
HAEST	Dalteparin	76/224	33.9	Aspirin	79/225	35.1
TOPAS	Certoparin	37/96	38.5			
	Certoparin	38/97	39.2			
	Certoparin	36/98	36.7			
	Certoparin	42/96	43.7			
TAIST	LD tinzaparin	188/507	38.3	Aspirin	206/491	42.5
	HD tinzaparin	181/486	38.4			
FISS-tris	Nadroparin	131/180	72.7	Aspirin	119/173	68.9
ANTIPLATELET AGENTS						
MAST	Aspirin	59/153	38.6	Control	50/156	32.1
IST	Aspirin	1860/4858	38.3	Control	1795/4859	36.9
CAST	Aspirin	7182/10335	69.5	Placebo	7054/10321	68.3
HAEST	Aspirin	79/225	35.1	Dalteparin	76/224	33.9
TAIST	Aspirin	206/491	42.5	Tinzaparin	369/993	38.3
FISS-tris	Aspirin	119/173	68.9	Nadroparin	131/180	72.7
Abciximab	Abciximab	24/54	44.0	Placebo	8/20	40.0
AbESTT	Abciximab	97/200	48.5	Placebo	80/200	40.0
AbESTT-II	Abciximab	154/403	38.2	Placebo	167/398	41.9

Abciximab, Abciximab in Ischemic Stroke Study; AbESTT, Abciximab Emergent Stroke Treatment Trial; CAST, Chinese Acute Stroke Trial; FISS, Fraxiparin in Stroke Study; HAEST, Heparin in Acute Embolic Stroke Trial; HD, high-dose; IST, International Stroke Trial; LD, low-dose; LMW, low-molecular-weight; MAST, Multicentre Acute Stroke Trial – Italy; RAPID, Rapid Anticoagulation Prevents Ischemic Damage study; TAIST, Tinzaparin in Acute Ischemic Stroke; TOAST, Trial of Org 10172 in Acute Stroke Treatment; TOPAS, Therapy of Patients with Acute Stroke.

Low-Molecular-Weight Heparins and Danaparoid

Several trials tested subcutaneously administered LMW heparins (see Tables 52-2–52-5). Two dosages of nadroparin (4100 anti-factor Xa units daily or 4100 anti-factor Xa units twice daily) were tested in a placebo-controlled trial performed by Kay et al.[73] Medications were started within 48 hours of stroke and continued for 10 days. Recurrent strokes occurred more frequently in the subjects receiving placebo than in either group that received nadroparin. At an assessment performed 6 months after stroke, excellent outcomes were significantly more common among the subjects who received the larger dose of nadroparin than among those who received placebo. A second trial of nadroparin tested two doses of nadroparin against placebo. The medications were administered within 24 hours of onset of stroke, but no monitoring or dose adjustments were included. No improvement in outcomes was noted.[74]

A Norwegian trial tested dalteparin or aspirin in preventing early recurrent stroke or improving outcomes among patients with atrial fibrillation who had strokes.[75] Dalteparin was given subcutaneously for 10 days. Recurrent strokes occurred in 8.5% of 224 subjects treated with dalteparin and in 7.5% of 225 subjects receiving aspirin. No differences in the rates of favorable outcomes were found. German investigators evaluated four doses of subcutaneously administered certoparin (3000 U/day, 3000 U/twice a day, 5000 U/twice a day, or 8000 U/twice a day) in a study that enrolled approximately 400 subjects. Therapy was initiated within 12 hours of stroke. No differences in the rates of recurrent stroke or favorable outcomes were seen among the groups.[76] In a three-arm treatment trial, two doses of tinzaparin (100 anti-factor Xa U/kg or 175 anti-factor Xa U/kg) were compared with aspirin (300 mg/day).[77] Treatment was started within 48 hours of stroke. No reduction in mortality or improvement in the rate of favorable outcome was seen with either dose of tinzaparin.

Intravenously administered danaparoid was compared with placebo in a randomized trial that enrolled approximately 1300 subjects.[79] Patients were enrolled within 24 hours of onset of stroke. Treatment was initiated with a bolus dose and maintained with a continuous infusion for 7 days. Infusion rates were adjusted in response to levels of inhibition of factor Xa. A weight-based regimen also was used. No differences were noted between the two treatment groups in the rates of neurologic worsening or early recurrent stroke. No reduction in the rate of early recurrent embolism among those patients with presumed cardioembolic stroke was noted between the two treatment groups. Although a trend in favor of treatment with danaparoid was detected during the first 7 days, no difference in outcomes was found at 3 months. Patients with stroke secondary to large artery atherosclerosis (primarily stenosis or occlusion of the internal carotid artery) seemed to benefit from treatment.[121] This response was not replicated in the trial of tinzaparin described previously.[77] In a meta-analysis of the trials of LMW heparins and danaparoid, Bath et al.[122] could not establish efficacy of these agents in any group of patients with acute ischemic stroke. Subsequently, Wong et al.[78] tested nadroparin (3800 anti-factor Xa U twice daily) or aspirin (160 mg daily) in 603 subjects. Enrollment was within 48 hours of onset of stroke; 353 subjects had evidence of large artery occlusive disease demonstrated by vascular imaging. Almost all the subjects had primarily intracranial stenoses. Favorable outcomes were similar in the two treatment groups. In an exploratory subgroup analysis, the authors suggested there may be benefit in patients over the age of 68 years, those not taking antiplatelet therapy and in patients with posterior circulation stenosis.[123] Another trial looked at the utility of early anticoagulation in treatment of patients with atrial fibrillation as identified by clinical variables or laboratory findings of D-dimer, prothrombin fragments (1 + 2), soluble fibrin monomer, or C-reactive protein. Dalteparin (100 U/kg twice a day) or aspirin (160 mg/day) was administered, and outcomes at 3 months were compared. No improvement in outcomes with administration of dalteparin was found.[124] A meta-analysis of LMW heparin versus aspirin for acute ischemic stroke showed no difference in outcomes.[125]

No clinical trials have tested NOACs in acute ischemic stroke. A Chinese trial (Apixiban Versus Dual-antiplatelet Therapy (Clopidogrel and Aspirin) in High-risk Patients with Acute Non-disabling Cerebrovascular Events (ADANCE) is testing apixiban (http://www.clinicaltrials.gov/ct2/show/NCT01924325?term=ADANCE&rank=1).

There are no clinical trials comparing anticoagulation to antiplatelet therapy in children. Findings from a large international registry of 661 children with acute ischemic stroke showed that 27% received anticoagulant therapy alone, 28% received antiplatelet therapy and 16% received combined anticoagulants and antiplatelet agents. Anticoagulants were more frequently used with a diagnosis of cardiac disease or arterial dissection.[126]

In a meta-analysis of the trials testing unfractionated heparin or LMW heparins in acute stroke patient, there was no difference in death or disability.[66] When the analysis was restricted to patients with cardioembolic stroke, Paciaroni et al.[80] found that the medications were associated with a non-significant reduction in recurrent stroke within 7 to 14 days (3.0% vs 4.9%; OR, 0.68; 95%CI, 0.44–1.06; $P = 0.09$). No major difference in disability or death at follow-up was seen (73.5% vs 73.8%; OR, 1.01; 95%CI, 0.82–1.24; $P = 0.9$). Whiteley et al.[127] evaluated individual patient data from 22,655 patients treated with anticoagulants compared to aspirin and could not find a subgroup that benefited from anticoagulation, including those at higher risk of thrombotic events. Risk factors for thrombotic events included advanced age, increased neurological impairments, or atrial fibrillation but these same risk factors also increased the risk of hemorrhage.

Antiplatelet Agents

Aspirin has been examined in several clinical trials (see Tables 52-2–52-5). Aspirin often has been the reference agent for trials testing LMW heparins. In general, aspirin was as effective as the anticoagulant in preventing recurrent stroke, in achieving favorable outcomes, and in preventing mortality.

In the International Stroke Trial, aspirin (300 mg daily) was given alone to 4858 subjects and in conjunction with heparin to another 4861 subjects.[32] Recurrent stroke was diagnosed in 156 (3.2%) of the subjects who received only aspirin and in 119 (2.4%) of the subjects who were given both aspirin and heparin. The reduction in recurrent events was statistically significant. The rates of recurrent stroke among patients treated with aspirin alone and with heparin, in comparison with the rates in those not taking aspirin are shown in Table 52-4. The rates of death or disability were modestly reduced in patients who were treated with either aspirin or the combination of heparin and aspirin, but the differences were not significant. In the randomized Chinese Acute Stroke Trial, which enrolled more than 20,000 subjects, aspirin (160 mg/day) was compared with placebo.[32] Therapy was started within 48 hours of stroke and continued for 28 days. The long interval from onset of stroke and the long treatment period are sources of concern; in particular, the long treatment period during which the control group received placebo overlaps with the time that many physicians would consider that long-term stroke preventive medications should have been started. Aspirin reduced the risk of recurrent stroke: rates of stroke were 2.1% (220/10,335) in the aspirin group and 2.5% (258/10,320) in the placebo group. The trial found a modest decline in mortality and disability with aspirin (30.5% vs 31.6% for placebo). The investigators of the CAST and International Stroke Trials had prespecified an analysis of combined data; the results found a significant reduction in the prevention of recurrent strokes (7 per 1000), and a benefit was seen in all subgroups of patients for improving outcomes.

The FASTER trial enrolled 392 patients with TIA or minor stroke, and all patients received aspirin in addition to either a 300-mg loading dose of clopidogrel or placebo and simvastatin versus placebo in a factorial design. The trial was stopped early because of difficulty recruiting patients due to the widespread use of statins, but the risk of recurrent stroke within 90 days was 7.1% in the clopidogrel group and 10.8% on placebo (RR, 0.7; 95%CI, 0.3–1.2).[128] In the CHANCE trial, the risk of recurrent stroke at 3 months was lower in the clopidogrel/aspirin group compared to aspirin alone (8.2% vs 11.7%, hazard ratio [HR], 0.68; 95%CI, 0.57–0.81; $P < 0.001$).[112] A large trial (Platelet-Oriented Inhibition in New TIA and minor ischemic stroke [POINT] trial) is testing a loading dose of 600 mg of clopidogrel vs placebo in addition to aspirin started within 12 hours in patients with minor stroke or high-risk TIA and continued for 90 days.[129] A second trial (TARDIS), the combination of aspirin, dipyridamole and clopidogrel will be compared to aspirin and dipyridamole within 48 hours after TIA or stroke. A third study (COMPRESS) is assessing the effect of combined aspirin and clopidogrel vs aspirin alone within 48 hours after acute ischemic stroke on the occurrence of new diffusion weighted imaging (DWI) lesions on MRI at 30 days.[130] Early treatment during the front-loaded high-risk period for recurrent stroke may be beneficial.

A pilot dose-escalation study of abciximab found that the medication might improve outcomes among patients treated within 24 hours of stroke.[91] A second dose-confirmation, randomized, double-blinded, placebo-controlled study tested the efficacy of abciximab when started within 6 hours of onset of stroke.[92] Abciximab was given in a 0.25 mg/kg bolus followed by a 12-hour infusion of 0.125 μg/kg/min (maximum, 10 μg/min). The trial, which enrolled 400 patients, showed a non-significant shift in favorable outcomes at 3 months (OR, 1.20; 95%CI, 0.84–1.70; $P = 0.33$). The benefit was strongest among patients treated within 5 hours of onset of stroke. The results of this trial prompted the Abciximab in Emergent Stroke Treatment Trial-II, which enrolled subjects into three groups: those enrolled within 5 hours of stroke onset, 5–6 hours after stroke, or within 3 hours of awakening with a stroke.[93] The trial was halted prematurely when an interim analysis did not demonstrate a favorable risk–benefit ratio. A small trial of tirofiban compared with aspirin within 6 hours of the onset of acute ischemic stroke was halted early because of no difference between the two groups.[131]

Conclusions

Preventing Early Recurrent Stroke

The data from clinical trials provide conflicting evidence as to whether early administration of antithrombotic agents is effective in lowering the risk of early recurrent stroke. On the basis of the information collected from several of the larger trials, the risk of early recurrent stroke is much lower than was assumed previously.[32,64,79] A reasonable estimate is that approximately 2% of patients have recurrent stroke within 1 week of the stroke. By 2 weeks, the rate probably increases to between 3% and 4%. Although the risk of recurrent stroke is higher in patients with presumed cardioembolic stroke, the rates are approximately 2% to 8% in the first 7–14 days.[64,65,75,79] However, although the risk of early recurrent stroke is not high, the likelihood of a poorer neurologic outcome after a second event is considerable.

Because the overall risk of early recurrent embolization is relatively low, demonstration of the efficacy of emergency anticoagulation in lessening that risk will be difficult. Some trials have not specifically evaluated the utility of anticoagulants in preventing early recurrent stroke, and others have not demonstrated that unfractionated heparin, LMW heparins, or danaparoid are effective. At present, early anticoagulation is not efficacious in preventing early recurrent stroke, including presumed cardioembolic stroke. There has been no subgroup of stroke patients identified who have been judged as having a very high risk of recurrent stroke and who might benefit from emergency anticoagulation.

Results of the large trials of aspirin are somewhat conflicting. Although aspirin lowered the risk of early recurrences, the benefit from aspirin was reduced when the aggregate of hemorrhagic and ischemic stroke was evaluated.[32,64] In trials of LMW heparin, aspirin was administered as the control medication. In the trial conducted by Berge et al.,[75] the rate of recurrent embolic stroke among patients with atrial fibrillation was slightly lower among the patients treated with aspirin than among those receiving dalteparin. Overall, the results suggest that aspirin, started within 48 hours of stroke, may produce a modest reduction in the risk of early recurrent stroke. Aspirin should not be started in lieu of other effective treatments for acute stroke, such as t-PA. Aspirin should not be started sooner than 24 hours after the administration of t-PA.[1]

Halting Neurologic Worsening

Neurologic worsening (stroke-in-evolution) is associated with a greater likelihood of poor outcomes; thus, preventing this deterioration should be a primary focus of acute stroke care.[132] As a result, antithrombotic agents often are prescribed to patients who are judged to be at risk of neurologic decline. Prediction of those patients who will deteriorate cannot be made with certainty.[133] Neurologic decline seems to be more common with strokes in the vertebrobasilar circulation than in the carotid circulation.[134] Patients with multilobar or large brainstem strokes are at high risk of neurologic worsening. At the other end of the spectrum, 20–30% of patients with lacunar stroke progress in the days after onset.[135] In addition, neurologic worsening may be secondary to a number of medical or neurologic complications of stroke that are not ameliorated by antithrombotic medications including brain edema, hydrocephalus, seizures, electrolyte disturbances, and infections.[136–138] None of these conditions may be successfully treated with antithrombotic agents.

A small Swedish placebo-controlled, randomized, double-blind trial tested the usefulness of aspirin (325 mg/day) in preventing progressing stroke.[139] Patients who had taken an antiplatelet agent within 72 hours before the stroke were excluded. The medication was started within 48 hours of stroke. At 5 days, progression of neurologic impairments was found in 15.9% of the 220 subjects treated with aspirin and in 16.7% of the subjects assigned placebo. Rödén-Jüllig and Britton[140] compared outcomes among 314 patients not receiving heparin with those in 907 patients treated with anticoagulants. Progression of neurologic deficits was noted in 28% of patients who did not receive heparin and in 21% of those who did, and the investigators concluded that heparin did not improve outcomes or halt neurologic worsening. The addition of cilostazol to antithrombotic therapy was not beneficial in preventing stroke progression in a Japanese study.[141,142] It also was not effective in a study of acute strokes in the lenticulostriate artery territory.[143] There have been several cases reports of clopidogrel loading showing benefit in patients with capsular warning syndromes.[144–146]

Clinical trials that have examined the impact of anticoagulants or antiplatelet agents on halting neurologic worsening have reported neutral results.[15,32,64,75,78,79,92,116,140] Overall, the trials report that the frequency of neurologic deterioration within the first 7–10 days after stroke was approximately 10% regardless of whether the patient received antithrombotic therapy. Overall, the data suggest that the effect of antithrombotic therapy in halting neurologic deterioration after stroke is likely to be small.

Improving Neurologic Outcomes

Overall, the data from the clinical trials of unfractionated heparin, LMW heparins, and danaparoid are similar. The trials do not show a net long-term benefit from initiation of anticoagulant therapy within the first 12–48 hours after stroke.[64,76–79,116] There is no evidence that anticoagulants are more effective in any subgroup of patients, including those with cardioembolic events or large artery atherosclerosis. The data about argatroban are too limited to determine its effectiveness.

Most of the information about the utility of antiplatelet agents comes from two large trials testing aspirin.[32,64] Although there are marked differences in the rates of favorable outcomes between the two trials, the aggregate data suggest that starting aspirin within 48 hours of onset of stroke is associated with a modest improvement in the rate of favorable outcomes. Several of the trials of anticoagulants included aspirin as part of the control management; these studies show that aspirin is at least equal to the anticoagulants.[75,77,78] An international trial of abciximab did not demonstrate a benefit in improving neurologic outcomes.[131]

At present, there is no evidence that antithrombotic therapy improves outcome after acute ischemic stroke.

PREVENTION OF DEEP VEIN THROMBOSIS

DVT and PE are important causes of morbidity and mortality after stroke. Bedridden patients with a paralyzed lower extremity have the greatest risk of these complications. Approximately 5–25% of deaths after stroke are due to PE, and most of these vascular events occur more than 1 week after stroke. Institution of measures to prevent DVT is a quality indicator for inpatient management of patients with recent stroke. In a retrospective database analysis from the US, 1% of patients had symptomatic VTE during hospitalization or within 30 days after discharge. Only 46% received prophylaxis for VTE while hospitalized.[147] In a study of the Get-With-Guidelines-Stroke population, the risk of clinically diagnosed VTE was 3% and 95% of patients received prophylaxis, likely this high percentage is related to the selection of this population.[148] Several measures can prevent DVT including early mobilization, low-dose anticoagulation, and intermittent compression stockings.[149] Elastic compression stockings are not effective and increase the risk of skin complications.[150,151] Antithrombotic agents are the principal medical therapy for prevention or treatment of DVT in the US. A large international trial compared unfractionated heparin and enoxaparin in 1762 subjects with recent ischemic stroke and found no difference in risk of bleeding but a lower rate of VTE in the enoxaparin group.[81,81] A meta-analysis found a reduction in DVT, but non-significant results for PE or mortality with anticoagulant therapy.[66] Greenage et al.[67] argued that the increase in ICH outweighed the benefit in prevention of PE and recommended against the routine use of low-dose anticoagulation in stroke patients. The American Stroke Association recommends the subcutaneous administration of low-dose anticoagulants for the treatment of immobilized stroke patients to prevent DVT.[1] The American College of Physicians recommends pharmacological prophylaxis with heparin or LMW heparin unless the assessed risk for bleeding outweighed the benefits.[152] British guidelines do not recommend prophylactic low-dose anticoagulation in acute stroke patients because of increased risk of hemorrhage. (http://guidance.nice.org.uk/CG92). External pneumatic calf compression devices reduced the risk of proximal vein or symptomatic DVT compared to no device (8.5% vs 12.1%, OR, 0.65; 95%CI, 0.51–0.84) in a large clinical trial (Clots in Legs or Stockings [CLOTS] 3).[149] About 30% of patients also received heparin but this was balanced between the two groups. The value of combined mechanical and anticoagulant therapy is uncertain in acute stroke patients although a synergistic effect has been noted in hospitalized patients.[153] Another controversial issue is the duration of VTE prophylaxis in acute stroke patients. In the Extended Prophylaxis for Venous ThromboEmbolism in Acutely Ill Medical Patients With Prolonged Immobilization (EXCLAIM) trial, a benefit of extended prophylaxis with enoxaparin for 28 days compared to 10 days in reducing VTE was seen in acute stroke patients. This was balanced by an increased risk of major bleeding.[19] Similarly, extended VTE prophylaxis with rivaroxaban in patients hospitalized with an acute medical illness was compared to a standard period of treatment and there was an increased risk of major bleeding (4.1% vs 1.7%; $P < 0.001$) as well as a decreased risk of VTE (4.4% vs 5.7%; $P = 0.02$).[154]

Aspirin provides some protection against VTE. It is an alternative to treatment with anticoagulants but has not been directly compared with anticoagulation. Placement of a filter in the inferior vena cava (Greenfield filter) prevents life-threatening PE in patients who cannot receive antithrombotic agents.[155] Treatment of PE includes LMW heparin, heparin, or fondaprinux.[20]

OTHER INDICATIONS

With the initiation of therapy, warfarin lowers the levels of the antithrombotic factors, proteins C and S, before its effects on prothrombin are detected. Thus, a transient hypercoagulable state might occur during the first days of starting warfarin. The complication of a pro-thrombotic state with secondary ischemic events is most commonly detected among patients who have an inherited or acquired deficiency of protein C or protein S. Because of the concern about this risk, physicians may prescribe a brief course of heparin or an LMW heparin during the initiation of treatment with warfarin. In a retrospective review of 204 patients with cardioembolic stroke, those who were treated with warfarin and bridged with heparin or enoxaparin had an increased risk of serious bleeding compared with those treated with warfarin without bridging.[156] In another study, the outcome with bridging therapy was the same as without bridging except there was a longer hospital stay.[157] If oral anticoagulants are to be prescribed to prevent recurrent stroke, several steps should be taken to increase the safety of their use. If the medications are to be started 24 hours after treatment with t-PA, a brain imaging study should be performed to exclude bleeding before starting the anticoagulants. Anticoagulation should be delayed several days if a brain imaging study shows a multilobar infarction, hemorrhagic transformation of the infarction, or if the patient has severe neurologic impairments. Current guidelines recommend that these agents not be started within 24 hours after treatment with t-PA but beyond that, the timing of initiation of anticoagulation after an infarction has not been established. NOACs have a faster onset on action than VKA and this should be considered when initiating this therapy.

Anticoagulation has been recommended for treatment of patients with stroke secondary to extracranial arterial dissection. A Cochrane review in 2010[158] and a meta-analysis in 2013 that included more than 1,991 patients did not show any difference in efficacy or complications between antiplatelet and anticoagulant therapy in preventing stroke, TIA, or death.[159] A non-randomized study of 298 consecutive patients with spontaneous dissection of the cervical carotid artery also showed no difference in efficacy.[160] Most studies have demonstrated a low rate of recurrent stroke of less than 3% at 3 months.[159] One non-randomized study showed a 10.7% risk of recurrent stroke at 1 year which was 2% in those treated with aspirin and 16.7% in those receiving anticoagulants (RR, 0.11; 95%CI, 0.02–0.69).[161] The Cervical Artery Dissection in Stroke Study (CADISS) is a randomized controlled trial in which antiplatelet therapy is being compared with anticoagulation with heparin followed by warfarin in patients with cervical artery dissection. A feasibility phase has enrolled 250 subjects to determine the necessary sample size and to see if an adequate number of patients can be recruited.[162]

An increased risk of recurrent stroke is seen in patients with aortic atheroma, particularly with thickness of at least 4 mm compared to those without aortic atherosclerosis (6.6% vs 2.2% in 1 year).[163] A trial of combined aspirin and clopidogrel therapy is being compared to warfarin therapy in the Aortic Arch Related Cerebral Hazard Trial (ARCH).[164] Patients with active cancer and ischemic stroke have elevated D-dimer levels and a higher prevalence of embolic signals on transcranial Doppler studies which is postulated to be due to a hypercoagulable state.[165–167] A randomized safety trial of full-dose enoxaparin versus aspirin in active cancer patients with acute ischemic stroke is in progress (http://www.clinicaltrials.gov/ct2/show/NCT01763606?term=stroke+and+cancer&rank=2).

Patients with acute stroke with a non-occlusive intraluminal thrombus have a high-risk of complications when treated with carotid endarterectomy or endovascular treatment. A case series of 18 patients received intravenous heparin with no occurrence of intracranial hemorrhage.[168]

Patients with acute ischemic heart disease often receive anticoagulants, antiplatelet agents, or both as part of the treatment regimen to limit the cardiac injury. These agents are administered as adjuncts to pharmacologic or mechanical thrombolysis. A similar strategy may be important in treating acute brain ischemia. Concomitant administration of an anticoagulant or antiplatelet agent might limit the occurrence of reocclusion. The concern is whether the addition of the antithrombotic medications would increase the risk of serious intracranial bleeding. Heparin and glycoprotein IIb/IIIa receptor blockers have been used as periprocedural adjunctive therapy in conjunction with angipoplasty and stenting or intra-arterial thrombolytic agents.[169] One study used low-pressure angioplasty supplemented with eptifibatide.[170] The authors concluded that the regimen was successful in achieving recanalization and in preventing reocclusion. Qureshi et al.[102] found that eptifibatide within 24 hours of treatment with thrombolytic therapy may help prevent subsequent neurologic worsening. Eckert et al.[171] found that the addition of abciximab to t-PA and endovascular interventions was associated with improved degrees of recanalization and neurologic outcomes in patients with acute vertebrobasilar occlusion. In another study, 20 patients with acute basilar artery occlusion treated with abciximab and intra-arterial t-PA, there was a poor outcome despite a high recanalization rate.[172] Nahab et al. provide recommendations about the dosing of adjunctive antithrombotic therapy used with endovascular procedures.[169] At present, there are no conclusive data about safety or efficacy of adjunctive periprocedural antithrombotic therapy.

CURRENT STATUS OF ANTITHROMBOTIC THERAPY

The many clinical trials performed in the last 10 to 15 years provide no support for the emergency administration of a rapidly acting anticoagulant for treatment of a patient with an acute ischemic stroke. These medications are associated with a small but statistically significant risk of ICH or other serious bleeding. The risk of hemorrhage is less than that attributed to emergency administration of thrombolytic medications, but the anticoagulants have not been found to improve neurologic outcomes, halt neurologic worsening, or forestall early recurrent stroke. Because of the lack of efficacy, the use of potentially risky medications is problematic. There does not appear to be any proven subgroup with clear evidence of benefit. Ongoing trials are testing anticoagulants compared to antiplatelet agents in patients with arterial dissection, aortic atherosclerosis and active cancer. There is also a need for clinical trials in children.

Low-dose anticoagulation has been recommended in North American guidelines for immobilized patients with acute ischemic stroke to reduce the risk of DVT. LMW heparins may be superior to heparin but both are associated with a small increased risk of ICH.[3] Intermittent compression stockings have also been proven to prevent VTE.[149] There is not a direct comparison of these two therapies and they may be synergistic.

Early administration of aspirin modestly reduces the frequency of recurrent events and improves outcomes. Aspirin's utility in the emergency management of stroke (within the first hours) is not clear. The use of aspirin should not be regarded as equal to thrombolytic therapy in improving outcomes after stroke. Still, starting aspirin within the first 48 hours after stroke seems prudent. There appear to be no particular limitations for starting aspirin with regard to the severity of stroke as determined by clinical and brain imaging findings. Aspirin should not be given within 24 hours after treatment with t-PA. Currently, the glycoprotein IIb/IIIa receptor blockers should not be prescribed to patients with ischemic stroke. Adjunctive therapy after intravenous thrombolysis with argatroban or eptifibatide is being tested. Short duration combined antiplatelet therapy with clopidogrel and aspirin after TIA or minor stroke is also under investigation.

FUTURE OF ANTITHROMBOTIC THERAPY

Ideally, an antithrombotic agent used for acute ischemic stroke treatment will have a rapid onset of action and can rapidly be reversed in the event of major bleeding. Rapid reversal could be accomplished by an agent with a short half-life or an antidote. Future possibilities include aptamers with their complementary reversal agents or intravenous PY12 inhibitors with a short half-life. Newer oral anticoagulants have not been tested but their slower onset of action and lack of an antidote detracts from their potential usefulness.

The future role of antiplatelet agents and anticoagulants in the management of patients with acute ischemic stroke might be as a component in multimodality therapy. The adjunctive use of antithrombotic medications may maintain the efficacy of pharmacologic or mechanical thrombolysis. The use of these medications might lower the risk of bleeding because the dose of the thrombolytic agents may be reduced. Hopefully, future clinical trials will test the safety and efficacy of new antithrombotic agents as well as multimodality thrombolytic and antithrombotic therapy for treatment of patients with acute ischemic stroke.

The complete reference list can be found on the companion Expert Consult website at www.expertconsult.inkling.com.

KEY REFERENCES

1. Jauch EC, Saver JL, Adams HP Jr, et al., American Heart Association Stroke Council, Council on Cardiovascular Nursing, Council on Peripheral Vascular Disease, Council on Clinical Cardiology. Guidelines for the early management of patients with acute ischemic stroke: A guideline for healthcare professionals from the American Heart Association/American Stroke Association. Stroke 2013;44:870–947.
3. Lansberg MG, O'Donnell MJ, Khatri P, et al., American College of Chest Physicians. Antithrombotic and thrombolytic therapy for ischemic stroke: Antithrombotic therapy and prevention of thrombosis, ed 9. American College of Chest Physicians evidence-based clinical practice guidelines. Chest 2012;141: e601S–636S.
4. European Stroke Organisation Executive Committee. Guidelines for management of ischaemic stroke and transient ischaemic attack 2008. Cerebrovasc Dis 2008;25:457–507.
5. Bruins Slot KM, Berge E. Factor Xa inhibitors versus vitamin k antagonists for preventing cerebral or systemic embolism in patients with atrial fibrillation. Cochrane Database Syst Rev 2013;(8):CD008980.
6. Cove CL, Hylek EM. An updated review of target-specific oral anticoagulants used in stroke prevention in atrial fibrillation, venous thromboembolic disease, and acute coronary syndromes. J Am Heart Assoc 2013;2:e000136.
7. Hankey GJ, Patel MR, Stevens SR, et al., ROCKET-AF Steering Committee and Investigators. Rivaroxaban compared with warfarin in patients with atrial fibrillation and previous stroke or transient ischaemic attack: A subgroup analysis of ROCKET-AF. Lancet Neurol 2012;11:315–22.
8. Pancioli AM, Adeoye O, Schmit PA, et al., CLEAR-ER Investigators. Combined approach to lysis utilizing eptifibatide and recombinant tissue plasminogen activator in acute ischemic stroke-enhanced regimen stroke trial. Stroke 2013;44:2381–7.
9. Pudusseri A, Shameem R, Spyropoulos AC. A new paradigm shift in antithrombotic therapy. Front Pharmacol 2013;4:133.
10. Kraft P, De Meyer SF, Kleinschnitz C. Next-generation antithrombotics in ischemic stroke: Preclinical perspective on 'bleeding-free antithrombosis'. J Cereb Blood Flow Metab 2012;32: 1831–40.
11. Bansal S, Sangha KS, Khatri P. Drug treatment of acute ischemic stroke. Am J Cardiovasc Drugs 2013;13:57–69.
12. Weber R, Brenck J, Diener HC. Antiplatelet therapy in cerebrovascular disorders. Handb Exp Pharmacol 2012;519–46.
13. Garcia DA, Baglin TP, Weitz JI, et al., American College of Chest Physicians. Parenteral anticoagulants: Antithrombotic therapy and prevention of thrombosis, ed 9. American College of Chest Physicians evidence-based clinical practice guidelines. Chest 2012;141:e24S–43S.
14. Hankey GJ, Eikelboom JW. Antithrombotic drugs for patients with ischaemic stroke and transient ischaemic attack to prevent recurrent major vascular events. Lancet Neurol 2010;9:273–84.
15. Chamorro A. Role of inflammation in stroke and atherothrombosis. Cerebrovasc Dis 2004;17:1–5.
16. Nowak-Gottl U, Bidlingmaier C, Krumpel A, et al. Pharmacokinetics, efficacy, and safety of LMWHs in venous thrombosis and stroke in neonates, infants and children. Br J Pharmacol 2008;153:1120–7.
17. van Es N, Bleker SM, Buller HR, et al. New developments in parenteral anticoagulation for arterial and venous thromboembolism. Best Pract Res Clin Haematol 2013;26:203–13.

18. Ageno W, Gallus AS, Wittkowsky A, et al., American College of Chest Physicians. Oral anticoagulant therapy: Antithrombotic therapy and prevention of thrombosis, 9th ed: American College of Chest Physicians evidence-based clinical practice guidelines. Chest 2012;141:e44S–88S.
19. Turpie AG, Hull RD, Schellong SM, et al., EXCLAIM Investigators. Venous thromboembolism risk in ischemic stroke patients receiving extended-duration enoxaparin prophylaxis: Results from the EXCLAIM study. Stroke 2013;44:249–51.
21. Ruff CT, Giugliano RP, Antman EM, et al. Evaluation of the novel factor xa inhibitor edoxaban compared with warfarin in patients with atrial fibrillation: Design and rationale for the Effective Anticoagulation with Factor Xa Next GEneration in Atrial Fibrillation-Thrombolysis In Myocardial Infarction study 48 (ENGAGE AF-TIMI 48). Am Heart J 2010;160:635–41.
22. LaMonte MP, Nash ML, Wang DZ, et al., ARGIS-1 Investigators. Argatroban anticoagulation in patients with acute ischemic stroke (ARGIS-1): A randomized, placebo-controlled safety study. Stroke 2004;35:1677–82.
23. Barreto AD, Alexandrov AV, Lyden P, et al. The Argatroban and Tissue-type Plasminogen Activator Stroke Study: Final results of a pilot safety study. Stroke 2012;43:770–5.
24. Connolly SJ, Ezekowitz MD, Yusuf S, et al., RE-LY Steering Committee and Investigators. Dabigatran versus warfarin in patients with atrial fibrillation. N Engl J Med 2009;361:1139–51.
25. De Meyer SF, Stoll G, Wagner DD, et al. Von Willebrand Factor: An emerging target in stroke therapy. Stroke 2012;43: 599–606.
26. Eikelboom JW, Hirsh J, Spencer FA, et al. Antiplatelet drugs: Antithrombotic therapy and prevention of thrombosis, ed 9. American College of Chest Physicians evidence-based clinical practice guidelines. Chest 2012;141:e89S–119S.
27. Awtry EH, Loscalzo J. Aspirin. Circulation 2000;101:1206–18.
28. Kalra K, Franzese CJ, Gesheff MG, et al. Pharmacology of antiplatelet agents. Curr Atheroscler Rep 2013;15:371.
29. Floyd CN, Ferro A. Mechanisms of aspirin resistance. Pharmacol Ther 2014 Jan;14(1):69–78.
31. Anderson JL, Adams CD, Antman EM, et al., American College of Cardiology Foundation/American Heart Association Task Force on Practice Guidelines. 2012 ACCF/AHA focused update incorporated into the ACCF/AHA 2007 guidelines for the management of patients with unstable angina/non-st-elevation myocardial infarction: A report of the American College of Cardiology Foundation/American Heart Association Task Force on Practice Guidelines. Circulation 2013;127:e663–828.
32. CAST (Chinese Acute Stroke Trial) Collaborative Group. Randomised placebo-controlled trial of early aspirin use in 20,000 patients with acute ischaemic stroke. CAST. Lancet 1997;349: 1641–9.
33. Thomson RM, Anderson DC. Aspirin and clopidogrel for prevention of ischemic stroke. Curr Neurol Neurosci Rep 2013; 13:327.
35. Wilterdink JL, Bendixen B, Adams HP Jr, et al. Effect of prior aspirin use on stroke severity in the Trial of Org 10172 in Acute Stroke Treatment (TOAST). Stroke 2001;32:2836–40.
37. Bousser MG, Amarenco P, Chamorro A, et al., Investigators PS. Terutroban versus aspirin in patients with cerebral ischaemic events (PERFORM): A randomised, double-blind, parallel-group trial. Lancet 2011;377:2013–22.
38. Eisert WG. Dipyridamole in antithrombotic treatment. Adv Cardiol 2012;47:78–86.
39. Sacco RL, Diener HC, Yusuf S, et al., PRoFESS Study Group. Aspirin and extended-release dipyridamole versus clopidogrel for recurrent stroke. N Engl J Med 2008;359:1238–51.
40. Dinicolantonio JJ, Lavie CJ, Fares H, et al. Meta-analysis of cilostazol versus aspirin for the secondary prevention of stroke. Am J Cardiol 2013;112:1230–4.
41. Chua D, Nishi C. New antiplatelet agents for cardiovascular disease. CMAJ 2013;185:1405–11.
42. Mehta SR, Bassand JP, Chrolavicius S, et al., CURRET-OASIS 7 Investigators. Dose comparisons of clopidogrel and aspirin in acute coronary syndromes. N Engl J Med 2010;363:930–42.
44. Bhatt DL, Cryer BL, Contant CF, et al., COGENT Investigators. Clopidogrel with or without omeprazole in coronary artery disease. N Engl J Med 2010;363:1909–17.
45. Tanguay JF, Bell AD, Ackman ML, et al. Focused 2012 update of the Canadian Cardiovascular Society Guidelines for the Use of Antiplatelet Therapy. Can J Cardiol 2013;29:1334–45.
46. Holmes MV, Perel P, Shah T, et al. Cyp2c19 genotype, clopidogrel metabolism, platelet function, and cardiovascular events: A systematic review and meta-analysis. JAMA 2011;306:2704–14.
48. Jia DM, Chen ZB, Zhang MJ, et al. Cyp2c19 polymorphisms and antiplatelet effects of clopidogrel in acute ischemic stroke in China. Stroke 2013;44:1717–19.
49. Man M, Farmen M, Dumaual C, et al. Genetic variation in metabolizing enzyme and transporter genes: Comprehensive assessment in 3 major East Asian subpopulations with comparison to Caucasians and Africans. J Clin Pharmacol 2010;50: 929–40.
50. Gurbel PA, Nolin TD, Tantry US. Clopidogrel efficacy and cigarette smoking status. JAMA 2012;307:2495–6.
51. Society for Cardiovascular Angiography and Interventions, Society of Thoracic Surgeons Writing Committee Members, Holmes DR Jr, Dehmer GJ, Kaul S, et al. ACCF/AHA clopidogrel clinical alert: Approaches to the FDA "boxed warning": A report of the American College of Cardiology Foundation Task Force on Clinical Expert Consensus Documents and the American Heart Association. Circulation 2010;122:537–57.
52. Wiviott SD, Braunwald E, McCabe CH, et al., TRITON-TIMI 38 Investigators. Prasugrel versus clopidogrel in patients with acute coronary syndromes. N Engl J Med 2007;357:2001–15.
53. Wallentin L, Becker RC, Budaj A, et al., PLATO Investigators. Ticagrelor versus clopidogrel in patients with acute coronary syndromes. N Engl J Med 2009;361:1045–57.
54. Mahaffey KW, Wojdyla DM, Carroll K, et al., PLATO Investigators. Ticagrelor compared with clopidogrel by geographic region in the platelet inhibition and patient outcomes (PLATO) trial. Circulation 2011;124:544–54.
55. James SK, Storey RF, Khurmi NS, et al., PLATO Study Group. Ticagrelor versus clopidogrel in patients with acute coronary syndromes and a history of stroke or transient ischemic attack. Circulation 2012;125:2914–21.
57. Steg PG, Bhatt DL, Hamm CW, et al., for the CHAMPION Investigators. Effect of cangrelor on periprocedural outcomes in percutaneous coronary interventions: A pooled analysis of patient-level data. Lancet 2013;382:1981–92.
59. Schneider DJ, Baumann PQ, Holmes MB, et al. Time and dose dependent augmentation of inhibitory effects of abciximab by aspirin. Thromb Haemost 2001;85:309–13.
60. Morrow DA, Alberts MJ, Mohr JP, et al., Thrombin Receptor Antagonist in Secondary Prevention of Atherothrombotic Ischemic Events TIMI 50 Steering Committee and Investigators. Efficacy and safety of vorapaxar in patients with prior ischemic stroke. Stroke 2013;44:691–8.
61. Markus HS, McCollum C, Imray C, et al. The von Willebrand inhibitor ARC1779 reduces cerebral embolization after carotid endarterectomy: A randomized trial. Stroke 2011;42: 2149–53.
63. Sandercock PA, Counsell C, Gubitz GJ, et al. Antiplatelet therapy for acute ischaemic stroke. Cochrane Database Syst Rev 2008; (16):CD000029.
64. Internal Stroke Trial Collaborative Group. The International Stroke Trial (IST): A randomised trial of aspirin, subcutaneous heparin, both, or neither among 19435 patients with acute ischaemic stroke. Lancet 1997;349:1569–81.
65. Saxena R, Lewis S, Berge E, et al. Risk of early death and recurrent stroke and effect of heparin in 3169 patients with acute ischemic stroke and atrial fibrillation in the International Stroke Trial. Stroke 2001;32:2333–7.
66. Sandercock PA, Counsell C, Tseng MC. Low-molecular-weight heparins or heparinoids versus standard unfractionated heparin for acute ischaemic stroke. Cochrane Database Syst Rev 2008;CD000119.
67. Geeganage CM, Sprigg N, Bath MW, et al. Balance of symptomatic pulmonary embolism and symptomatic intracerebral hemorrhage with low-dose anticoagulation in recent ischemic stroke: A systematic review and meta-analysis of randomized controlled trials. J Stroke Cerebrovasc Dis 2013;22:1018–27.
68. Lederle FA, Zylla D, MacDonald R, et al. Venous thromboembolism prophylaxis in hospitalized medical patients and those with

stroke: A background review for an American College of Physicians Clinical Practice Guideline. Ann Intern Med 2011;155: 602–15.

70. Ramirez-Lassepas M, Cipolle RJ, Rodvold KA, et al. Heparin-induced thrombocytopenia in patients with cerebrovascular ischemic disease. Neurology 1984;34:736–40.
71. Kawano H, Yamamoto H, Miyata S, et al. Prospective multicentre cohort study of heparin-induced thrombocytopenia in acute ischaemic stroke patients. Br J Haematol 2011;154:378–86.
72. Linkins LA, Dans AL, Moores LK, et al., American College of Chest Physicians. Treatment and prevention of heparin-induced thrombocytopenia: Antithrombotic therapy and prevention of thrombosis, ed 9. American College of Chest Physicians evidence-based clinical practice guidelines. Chest 2012;141: e495S–530S.
73. Kay R, Wong KS, Yu YL, et al. Low-molecular-weight heparin for the treatment of acute ischemic stroke. N Engl J Med 1995;333: 1588–93.
74. Hommel M. Fraxiparin in ischemic stroke study (fiss-bis). Cerebrovasc Dis 1998;8:63–8.
75. Berge E, Abdelnoor M, Nakstad PH, et al. Low molecular-weight heparin versus aspirin in patients with acute ischaemic stroke and atrial fibrillation: A double-blind randomised study. HAEST study group. Heparin in Acute Embolic Stroke Trial. Lancet 2000;355:1205–10.
76. Diener HC, Ringelstein EB, von Kummer R, et al. Treatment of acute ischemic stroke with the low-molecular-weight heparin certoparin: Results of the TOPAS trial. Therapy of Patients with Acute Stroke (TOPAS) investigators. Stroke 2001;32:22–9.
77. Bath PM, Lindenstrom E, Boysen G, et al. Tinzaparin in acute ischaemic stroke (TAIST): A randomised aspirin-controlled trial. Lancet 2001;358:702–10.
78. Wong KS, Chen C, Ng PW, et al., FISS-tris Investigators. Low-molecular-weight heparin compared with aspirin for the treatment of acute ischemic stroke in Asian patients with large artery occlusive disease: A randomised study. Lancet Neurol 2007;6: 407–13.
79. The Publications Committee for the Trial of Org 10172 in Acute Stroke Treatment (TOAST) Investigators. Low molecular weight heparinoid, org 10172 (danaparoid), and outcome after acute ischemic stroke: A randomized controlled trial. JAMA 1998;279: 1265–72.
81. Sherman DG, Albers GW, Bladin C, et al., Investigators P. The efficacy and safety of enoxaparin versus unfractionated heparin for the prevention of venous thromboembolism after acute ischaemic stroke (PREVAIL study): An open-label randomised comparison. Lancet 2007;369:1347–55.
82. Kase CS, Albers GW, Bladin C, et al., PREVAIL Investigators. Neurological outcomes in patients with ischemic stroke receiving enoxaparin or heparin for venous thromboembolism prophylaxis: Subanalysis of the Prevention of VTE after Acute Ischemic stroke with LMWH (PREVAIL) Study. Stroke 2009;40: 3532–40.
83. Diener HC, Ringelstein EB, von Kummer R, et al., PROTECT Trial Group. Prophylaxis of thrombotic and embolic events in acute ischemic stroke with the low-molecular-weight heparin certoparin: Results of the PROTECT trial. Stroke 2006;37:139–44.
85. Schechter T, Kirton A, Laughlin S, et al. Safety of anticoagulants in children with arterial ischemic stroke. Blood 2012;119: 949–56.
86. Khatri P, Mono ML. Combining antithrombotic and fibrinolytic agents: Can it be done? Stroke 2013;44:1489–91.
87. Chatterjee S, Sardar P, Biondi-Zoccai G, et al. New oral anticoagulants and the risk of intracranial hemorrhage: Traditional and Bayesian meta-analysis and mixed treatment comparison of randomized trials of new oral anticoagulants in atrial fibrillation. JAMA Neurol 2013;70:1486–90.
88. Hart RG, Pogue J, Eikelboom JW. Direct-acting oral anticoagulants: The brain gets a break. JAMA Neurol 2013;70:1483–4.
89. Leung LY, Albright KC, Boehme AK, et al. Short-term bleeding events observed with clopidogrel loading in acute ischemic stroke patients. J Stroke Cerebrovasc Dis 2013;22:1184–9.
91. Abciximab in Ischemic Stroke Investigators. Abciximab in acute ischemic stroke. A randomized, double-blind, placebo-controlled, dose-escalation study. Stroke 2000;31:601–9.
92. Abciximab Emergent Stroke Treatment Trial Investigators. Emergency administration of abciximab for treatment of patients with acute ischemic stroke: Results of a randomized phase 2 trial. Stroke 2005;36:880–90.
93. Adams HP Jr, Effron MB, Torner J, et al., AbESTT-II Investigators. Emergency administration of abciximab for treatment of patients with acute ischemic stroke: Results of an international phase iii trial: Abciximab in Emergency Treatment of Stroke Trial (ABESTT-II). Stroke 2008;39:87–99.
94. Adams HP Jr, Leira EC, Torner JC, et al., for the AbESTT II Investigators. Treating patients with 'wake-up' stroke: The experience of the AbESTT-II Trial. Stroke 2008;39:3277–82.
95. Martin-Schild S, Shaltoni H, Abraham AT, et al. Safety of eptifibatide for subcortical stroke progression. Cerebrovasc Dis 2009;28:595–600.
96. Siebler M, Hennerici MG, Schneider D, et al. Safety of tirofiban in acute ischemic stroke: The SATIS trial. Stroke 2011;42: 2388–92.
98. Ciccone A, Motto C, Aritzu E, et al. Negative interaction of aspirin and streptokinase in acute ischemic stroke: Further analysis of the Multicenter Acute Stroke Trial-Italy. Cerebrovasc Dis 2000;10:61–4.
99. Zinkstok SM, Roos YB, ARTIS Investigators. Early administration of aspirin in patients treated with alteplase for acute ischemic stroke: A randomised controlled trial. Lancet 2012;380:731–7.
100. Amaro S, Llull L, Urra X, et al. Risks and benefits of early antithrombotic therapy after thrombolytic treatment in patients with acute stroke. PLoS ONE 2013;8:e71132.
101. Qureshi AI, Harris-Lane P, Kirmani JF, et al. Intra-arterial reteplase and intravenous abciximab in patients with acute ischemic stroke: An open-label, dose-ranging, phase I study. Neurosurgery 2006;59:789–96.
102. Qureshi AI, Hussein HM, Janjua N, et al. Postprocedure intravenous eptifibatide following intra-arterial reteplase in patients with acute ischemic stroke. J Neuroimaging 2008;18: 50–5.
103. Walsh RD, Barrett KM, Aguilar MI, et al. Intracranial hemorrhage following neuroendovascular procedures with abciximab is associated with high mortality: A multicenter series. Neurocrit Care 2011;15:85–95.
104. Furlan A, Higashida R, Wechsler L, et al. Intra-arterial prourokinase for acute ischemic stroke. The PROACT II Study: A randomized controlled trial. Prolyse in acute cerebral thromboembolism. JAMA 1999;282:2003–11.
105. del Zoppo GJ, Higashida RT, Furlan AJ, et al. Proact: A Phase II randomized trial of recombinant pro-urokinase by direct arterial delivery in acute middle cerebral artery stroke. PROACT investigators. Prolyse in acute cerebral thromboembolism. Stroke 1998;29:4–11.
106. Broderick JP, Palesch YY, Demchuk AM, et al., Interventional Management of Stroke III Investigators. Endovascular therapy after intravenous t-pa versus t-pa alone for stroke. N Engl J Med 2013;368:893–903.
107. Lee M, Saver JL, Hong KS, et al. Risk-benefit profile of long-term dual- versus single-antiplatelet therapy among patients with ischemic stroke: A systematic review and meta-analysis. Ann Intern Med 2013;159:463–70.
108. Diener HC, Bogousslavsky J, Brass LM, et al., MATCH Investigators. Aspirin and clopidogrel compared with clopidogrel alone after recent ischaemic stroke or transient ischaemic attack in high-risk patients (MATCH): Randomised, double-blind, placebo-controlled trial. Lancet 2004;364:331–7.
109. Connolly SJ, Pogue J, Hart RG, et al., ACTIVE Investigators. Effect of clopidogrel added to aspirin in patients with atrial fibrillation. N Engl J Med 2009;360:2066–78.
110. Benavente OR, Hart RG, McClure LA, et al., SPS Investigators. Effects of clopidogrel added to aspirin in patients with recent lacunar stroke. N Engl J Med 2012;367:817–25.
111. Chimowitz MI, Lynn MJ, Derdeyn CP, et al., SAMMPRIS Trial Investigators. Stenting versus aggressive medical therapy for intracranial arterial stenosis. N Engl J Med 2011;365: 993–1003.
112. Wang Y, Wang Y, Zhao X, et al., CHANCE Investigators. Clopidogrel with aspirin in acute minor stroke or transient ischemic attack. N Engl J Med 2013;369:11–19.

113. Geraghty OC, Kennedy J, Chandratheva A, et al. Preliminary evidence of a high risk of bleeding on aspirin plus clopidogrel in aspirin-naive patients in the acute phase after tia or minor ischaemic stroke. Cerebrovasc Dis 2010;29:460–7.
114. Wong KS, Wang Y, Leng X, et al. Early dual versus mono antiplatelet therapy for acute non-cardioembolic ischemic stroke or transient ischemic attack: An updated systematic review and meta-analysis. Circulation 2013;128:1656–66.
115. Geeganage CM, Diener HC, Algra A, et al., Acute Antiplatelet Stroke Trialists Collaboration. Dual or mono antiplatelet therapy for patients with acute ischemic stroke or transient ischemic attack: Systematic review and meta-analysis of randomized controlled trials. Stroke 2012;43:1058–66.
116. Chamorro A, Busse O, Obach V, et al., RAPID Investigators. The Rapid Anticoagulation Prevents Ischemic Damage Study in acute stroke–final results from the writing committee. Cerebrovasc Dis 2005;19:402–4.
117. Camerlingo M, Salvi P, Belloni G, et al. Intravenous heparin started within the first 3 hours after onset of symptoms as a treatment for acute nonlacunar hemispheric cerebral infarctions. Stroke 2005;36:2415–20.
118. Sandercock PA, van den Belt AG, Lindley RI, et al. Antithrombotic therapy in acute ischaemic stroke: An overview of the completed randomised trials. J Neurol Neurosurg Psychiatry 1993;56:17–25.
119. Eriksson M, Stecksen A, Glader EL, et al., Riks-Stroke Collaboration. Discarding heparins as treatment for progressive stroke in Sweden 2001 to 2008. Stroke 2010;41:2552–8.
121. Adams HP Jr, Bendixen BH, Leira E, et al. Antithrombotic treatment of ischemic stroke among patients with occlusion or severe stenosis of the internal carotid artery: A report of the Trial of Org 10172 in Acute Stroke Treatment (TOAST). Neurology 1999;53:122–5.
122. Bath PM, Iddenden R, Bath FJ. Low-molecular-weight heparins and heparinoids in acute ischemic stroke : A meta-analysis of randomized controlled trials. Stroke 2000;31:1770–8.
123. Wang QS, Chen C, Chen XY, et al. Low-molecular-weight heparin versus aspirin for acute ischemic stroke with large artery occlusive disease: Subgroup analyses from the Fraxiparin In Stroke Study for the treatment of ischemic stroke (FISS-tris) study. Stroke 2012;43:346–9.
124. O'Donnell MJ, Berge E, Sandset PM. Are there patients with acute ischemic stroke and atrial fibrillation that benefit from low molecular weight heparin? Stroke 2006;37:452–5.
126. Goldenberg NA, Bernard TJ, Fullerton HJ, et al., International Pediatric Stroke Study Group. Antithrombotic treatments, outcomes, and prognostic factors in acute childhood-onset arterial ischaemic stroke: A multicentre, observational, cohort study. Lancet Neurol 2009;8:1120–7.
127. Whiteley WN, Adams HP Jr, Bath PM, et al. Targeted use of heparin, heparinoids, or low-molecular-weight heparin to improve outcome after acute ischaemic stroke: An individual patient data meta-analysis of randomised controlled trials. Lancet Neurol 2013;12:539–45.
128. Kennedy J, Hill MD, Ryckborst KJ, et al., FASTER Investigators. Fast Assessment of Stroke and Transient ischaemic attack to prevent Early Recurrence (FASTER): A randomised controlled pilot trial. Lancet Neurol 2007;6:961–9.
129. Johnston SC, Easton JD, Farrant M, et al. Platelet-Oriented Inhibition in New TIA and Minor Ischemic Stroke (POINT) Trial: Rationale and design. Int J Stroke 2013;8:479–83.
131. Torgano G, Zecca B, Monzani V, et al. Effect of intravenous tirofiban and aspirin in reducing short-term and long-term neurologic deficit in patients with ischemic stroke: A double-blind randomized trial. Cerebrovasc Dis 2010;29:275–81.
132. Britton M, Roden A. Progression of stroke after arrival at hospital. Stroke 1985;16:629–32.
133. Tei H, Uchiyama S, Ohara K, et al. Deteriorating ischemic stroke in 4 clinical categories classified by the oxfordshire community stroke project. Stroke 2000;31:2049–54.
134. Yamamoto H, Bogousslavsky J, van Melle G. Different predictors of neurological worsening in different causes of stroke. Arch Neurol 1998;55:481–6.
135. Del Bene A, Palumbo V, Lamassa M, et al. Progressive lacunar stroke: Review of mechanisms, prognostic features, and putative treatments. Int J Stroke 2012;7:321–9.
136. Thanvi B, Treadwell S, Robinson T. Early neurological deterioration in acute ischaemic stroke: Predictors, mechanisms and management. Postgrad Med J 2008;84:412–17.
137. Ali LK, Saver JL. The ischemic stroke patient who worsens: New assessment and management approaches. Rev Neurol Dis 2007;4:85–91.
138. Balami JS, Chen RL, Grunwald IQ, et al. Neurological complications of acute ischaemic stroke. Lancet Neurol 2011;10:357–71.
139. Roden-Jullig A, Britton M, Malmkvist K, et al. Aspirin in the prevention of progressing stroke: A randomized controlled study. J Intern Med 2003;254:584–90.
140. Roden-Jullig A, Britton M. Effectiveness of heparin treatment for progressing ischemic stroke: Before and after study. J Intern Med 2000;248:287–91.
141. Cook CD, Hainsworth M. Tuberculosis of the conjunctiva occurring in association with a neighbouring lupus vulgaris lesion. Br J Ophthalmol 1990;74:315–16.
142. Shimizu H, Tominaga T, Ogawa A, et al., Tohoku Acute Stroke Progressing Stroke Study Group. Cilostazol for the prevention of acute progressing stroke: A multicenter, randomized controlled trial. J Stroke Cerebrovasc Dis 2013;22:449–56.
143. Kondo R, Matsumoto Y, Furui E, et al. Effect of cilostazol in the treatment of acute ischemic stroke in the lenticulostriate artery territory. Eur Neurol 2013;69:122–8.
144. Kawano H, Nakajima M, Inatomi Y, et al. Loading dose of clopidogrel in combination with other antithrombotic therapy for capsular warning syndrome. J Stroke Cerebrovasc Dis 2013;23: 1265–6.
145. Fahey CD, Alberts MJ, Bernstein RA. Oral clopidogrel load in aspirin-resistant capsular warning syndrome. Neurocrit Care 2005;2:183–4.
146. Asil T, Ir N, Karaduman F, et al. Combined antithrombotic treatment with aspirin and clopidogrel for patients with capsular warning syndrome: A case report. Neurologist 2012;18: 68–9.
147. Amin AN, Lin J, Thompson S, et al. Rate of deep-vein thrombosis and pulmonary embolism during the care continuum in patients with acute ischemic stroke in the United States. BMC Neurol 2013;13:17.
148. Douds GL, Hellkamp AS, Olson DM, et al. Venous thromboembolism in the Get With the Guidelines-stroke acute ischemic stroke population: Incidence and patterns of prophylaxis. J Stroke Cerebrovasc Dis 2014;23:123–9.
149. Dennis M, Sandercock P, Reid J, et al., CLOTS (Clots in Legs Or sTockings after Stroke) Trials Collaboration. Effectiveness of intermittent pneumatic compression in reduction of risk of deep vein thrombosis in patients who have had a stroke (CLOTS 3): A multicentre randomised controlled trial. Lancet 2013;382: 516–24.
150. Jain P, Ward E, Nevatte T, et al. Incidence of venous thromboembolism in the wake of the clots in legs or stockings after stroke (CLOTS) study. Stroke 2013;44:2910–12.
151. Dennis M, Sandercock P, Reid J, et al., Collaboration CT. The effect of graduated compression stockings on long-term outcomes after stroke: The CLOTS trials 1 and 2. Stroke 2013;44: 1075–9.
152. Qaseem A, Chou R, Humphrey LL, et al., Clinical Guidelines Committee of the American College of Physicians. Venous thromboembolism prophylaxis in hospitalized patients: A clinical practice guideline from the American College of Physicians. Ann Intern Med 2011;155:625–32.
153. Ho KM, Tan JA. Stratified meta-analysis of intermittent pneumatic compression of the lower limbs to prevent venous thromboembolism in hospitalized patients. Circulation 2013;128: 1003–20.
154. Cohen AT, Spiro TE, Buller HR, et al., MAGELLAN Investigators. Rivaroxaban for thromboprophylaxis in acutely ill medical patients. N Engl J Med 2013;368:513–23.
155. Somarouthu B, Yeddula K, Wicky S, et al. Long-term safety and effectiveness of inferior vena cava filters in patients with stroke. J Neurointerv Surg 2011;3:141–6.
157. Audebert HJ, Schenk B, Tietz V, et al. Initiation of oral anticoagulation after acute ischaemic stroke or transient ischaemic attack: Timing and complications of overlapping heparin or conventional treatment. Cerebrovasc Dis 2008;26:171–7.

158. Lyrer P, Engelter S. Antithrombotic drugs for carotid artery dissection. Cochrane Database Syst Rev 2010;CD000255.
159. Sarikaya H, da Costa BR, Baumgartner RW, et al. Antiplatelets versus anticoagulants for the treatment of cervical artery dissection: Bayesian meta-analysis. PLoS ONE 2013;8: e72697.
160. Georgiadis D, Arnold M, von Buedingen HC, et al. Aspirin vs anticoagulation in carotid artery dissection: A study of 298 patients. Neurology 2009;72:1810–15.
161. Weimar C, Kraywinkel K, Hagemeister C, et al., German Stroke Study Collaboration. Recurrent stroke after cervical artery dissection. J Neurol Neurosurg Psychiatry 2010;81:869–73.
162. Kennedy F, Lanfranconi S, Hicks C, et al., CADISS Investigators. Antiplatelets vs anticoagulation for dissection: CADISS nonrandomized arm and meta-analysis. Neurology 2012;79:686–9.
163. Guidoux C, Mazighi M, Lavallee P, et al. Aortic arch atheroma in transient ischemic attack patients. Atherosclerosis 2013;231: 124–8.
164. Zavala JA, Amarrenco P, Davis SM, et al. Aortic arch atheroma. Int J Stroke 2006;1:74–80.
165. Schwarzbach CJ, Schaefer A, Ebert A, et al. Stroke and cancer: The importance of cancer-associated hypercoagulation as a possible stroke etiology. Stroke 2012;43:3029–34.
167. Kim SJ, Park JH, Lee MJ, et al. Clues to occult cancer in patients with ischemic stroke. PLoS ONE 2012;7:e44959.
168. Mokin M, Kass-Hout T, Kass-Hout O, et al. Intravenous heparin for the treatment of intraluminal thrombus in patients with acute ischemic stroke: A case series. J Neurointerv Surg 2013;5: 144–50.
169. Nahab F, Kass-Hout T, Shaltoni HM. Periprocedural antithrombotic strategies in acute ischemic stroke interventional therapy. Neurology 2012;79:S174–81.
170. Nogueira RG, Schwamm LH, Buonanno FS, et al. Low-pressure balloon angioplasty with adjuvant pharmacological therapy in patients with acute ischemic stroke caused by intracranial arterial occlusions. Neuroradiol 2008;50:331–40.
172. Barlinn K, Becker U, Puetz V, et al. Combined treatment with intravenous abciximab and intraarterial tpa yields high recanalization rate in patients with acute basilar artery occlusion. J Neuroimaging 2012;22:167–71.

53 General Stroke Management and Stroke Units

Turgut Tatlisumak, Risto O. Roine

KEY POINTS

- All stroke patients should be admitted to hospitals that offer 24/7 specialized stroke care with access to stroke unit care.
- Multiprofessional stroke unit care reduces significantly death, dependency, and long-term institutional care independent of patients' age and gender or subtype and severity of stroke.
- Each stroke patient should undergo a full investigation including clinical, laboratory, and imaging examinations that ascertain diagnosis, subtype, etiology, mechanisms, as well as risk factors of stroke.
- Prevention, early diagnosis, and aggressive treatment of medical complications are essential, as well as early prevention of recurrence and timely rehabilitation.
- Incorporating research, teaching, and stroke registry activity to patient care as well as implementation of quality measures are the key for success.

INTRODUCTION

Only few acute treatments have been shown to improve the outcome of stroke. Whereas most acute treatments could only be given to limited numbers of patients, stroke unit care has the advantage of being applicable to almost all stroke patients. This chapter characterizes stroke unit care, including all aspects of general stroke management that can optimally be delivered in stroke units. There is strong evidence that treatment of patients with stroke in dedicated stroke units significantly results in lower rates of death, dependency, and the need for institutional care than treatment in general medical wards. The acute stroke unit is a key element in the critical care pathway and the chain of recovery of a patient with stroke after emergency care in the emergency department. Early recognition of stroke in the field, rapid transfer to a fully equipped stroke center, stat neurological evaluation including brain imaging and laboratory testing, as well as delivery of acute treatments such as intravenous thrombolysis for eligible patients, access to interventional procedures and intensive care unit are discussed in other chapters. This chapter will cover the stroke care after the patient has received acute treatments and transferred to a stroke unit although we are aware that some centers has the practice of admitting stroke patients directly to stroke units and giving acute treatments in the same facility.

STROKE UNIT CARE

Following numerous trials on efficacy of stroke unit care in various stroke patient populations in several countries, The Stroke Unit Trialists' Collaboration verified these results and demonstrated that organized care in stroke units reduced the rates of death or institutional care and death or dependency.[1] The most recent review of this working group, including 28 randomized controlled trials involving almost 6000 participants, compared stroke unit care with alternative services.[2] Stroke unit care reduced significantly the risk of death (odds ratio [OR], 0.76; confidence interval [CI], 0.66–0.88), death or dependency (OR, 0.80; CI, 0.67–0.97), and death or institutional care (OR, 0.76; CI, 0.67–0.86) without prolonging length of stay in a hospital or institution in up to 1-year follow-up.[2] These benefits were independent of patient age, sex, initial stroke severity or stroke type (ischemic or hemorrhagic), and appeared to be better in stroke units based in a discrete ward.[2] Patients with more severe strokes and those with hemorrhagic stroke seemed to benefit even more.[2] Furthermore, these results sustained at 5-year follow-up time points when available. The authors, thus, concluded that stroke patients who received organized inpatient care in a stroke unit were more likely to be alive, independent, and living at home 1 year after the stroke.[2]

The target population of stroke unit covers ischemic stroke (IS), intracerebral hemorrhage (ICH), intraventricular hemorrhage (IVH), transient ischemic attack (TIA), cerebral venous thrombosis (CVT), and subarachnoidal hemorrhage (SAH) patients. Patients with cerebral vasculitides or reversible cerebral vasoconstriction syndrome are best treated in a stroke unit even if they do not have parenchymal lesions.

Stroke Unit Design

The observed benefits are apparent for a wide variety of stroke services, including stroke centers, acute stroke units, combined acute and rehabilitation stroke units, rehabilitation stroke units admitting patients after a delay of 1 or 2 weeks, and mobile stroke teams.

A *stroke center* consists of a comprehensive stroke service that offers the infrastructure to bring patients as quickly as possible to the stroke center. It provides immediate diagnosis and treatment, as well as early rehabilitation, and refers patients to the appropriate further treatment, rehabilitation, and secondary prevention. A stroke center offers 24-hour availability of laboratory, radiological, neurosurgical, and cardiologic services (Box 53-1). Stroke centers need a large catchment area, and most often, they are part of a large teaching hospital located in a metropolitan area. A primary stroke center (PSC) has the necessary staffing, infrastructure, and programs to stabilize and treat most acute stroke patients.[3] A comprehensive stroke center (CSC) is defined as a facility or system with the necessary personnel, infrastructure, expertise,

BOX 53-1 Requirements for Acute Stroke Units

MINIMUM REQUIREMENTS FOR STROKE CENTERS

Written protocols for diagnostic and treatment guidelines and operational procedures for medical and nursing staff
Availability of CT 24 hours a day
Availability of blood tests 24 hours a day, including immediate availability of coagulation parameters
Availability of neurosonographic investigations 24 hours a day (color-coded duplex ultrasonography of extracranial vessels and transcranial Doppler ultrasonography of intracranial vessels)
Continuous or frequent monitoring of blood pressure, levels of blood gases and blood glucose, and body temperature
Continuous ECG monitoring and availability of ECG within 24 hours
Close cooperation of neurologists, internists, neuroradiologists, and neurosurgeons in evaluation and treatment
Trained nursing staff specialized in acute care of stroke
Early rehabilitation, including physical therapy, speech therapy, neuropsychology, and occupational therapy
Established network of rehabilitation facilities

ADDITIONAL FACILITIES RECOMMENDED IN ACUTE STROKE UNITS

Diffusion and perfusion MRI and MRA
CT angiography and perfusion CT
Transesophageal echocardiography
Cerebral angiography

CT, Computed tomography; ECG, electrocardiography; MRA, magnetic resonance angiography; MRI, magnetic resonance imaging.
Modified from Kaste M, Skyhoj Olsen T, Orgogozo J-M, et al for the European Stroke Initiative (EUSI) Executive Committee: Organization of stroke care: Education, stroke units and rehabilitation. Cerebrovasc Dis *10(Suppl 3):1–11, 2000.*

and programs to diagnose and treat stroke patients who require a high intensity of medical and surgical care, specialized tests or interventional therapies.[4] A CSC may act as a resource center for other facilities in their region and as an educational resource for other hospitals and health care professionals in a region. Furthermore, a CSC can provide telestroke support to remote hospitals.

Organized stroke unit care incorporates three basic and mandatory features: (1) it provides a disease-specific service in a geographically defined area of a hospital ward and is exclusively dedicated to the management of patients with stroke and TIA. Such units can be organized in a variety of medical departments: neurology, internal medicine, geriatric medicine, and rehabilitation medicine. (2) It has a multidisciplinary team (physician, nurse, physiotherapist, occupational therapist, speech therapist, neuropsychologist, and social-worker) with a special interest, training, and expertise in stroke, educational programs for the staff, and involvement of caregivers. (3) A comprehensive system for stroke care forms the infrastructure that is around the clock admission (24/7 principle), rapid clinical, radiological, and laboratory evaluation of stroke patients (diagnostic work-up), delivery of acute treatments, monitoring facility, access to various procedures and intensive care, prevention and treatment of complications, early mobilization and rehabilitation, risk factor mapping, as well as in-house written guidelines for stroke care.

Although there is universal agreement that stroke units are dedicated exclusively to stroke patients; not much evidence-based data exist on the essential components that should be present in different types of stroke units. In a survey among European stroke experts the levels of care were defined.[5] According to experts, all facilities considered necessary should be available in CSCs (Box 53-2), and research and teaching should also be important parts of the activity. In PSCs, all stroke patients should receive the highest level of care except for a few specific investigations or treatments requiring resources and expertise available only in tertiary hospitals (see Box 53-2). The third level should include the minimum level of care considered necessary by the experts for any hospital ward (AHW) treating stroke patients (see Box 53-2). The eight components considered absolutely necessary by more than 75% of experts for both CSCs and PSCs were a multidisciplinary team, stroke-trained nurses, brain CT available 24 hours a day 7 days a week (24/7), CT priority for stroke patients, extracranial Doppler sonography, automated electrocardiographic monitoring, IV recombinant tissue plasminogen activator (rt-PA) protocol available 24/7, and an in-house emergency department. Eleven other components in the fields of vascular surgery, neurosurgery, interventional radiology, and clinical research were considered to be necessary in CSCs by more than 75% of the experts.[5] Only eight components – brain CT 24/7, CT priority for stroke patients, in-house emergency department with dedicated staff, stroke care roadmap for patient admission, stroke pathway, prevention program, and collaboration with outside rehabilitation center – were considered important for AHW, but not absolutely necessary by more than 50% of the experts.[5] This classification is close to that of the Brain Attack Coalition[3,4] and the German and Swiss models,[6–8] although it does not closely relate to stroke units included in the Cochrane systematic review.[2]

Availability of Stroke Unit Care

The first Pan-European Consensus Meeting on Stroke Management recommended that by the year 2005 all patients in Europe with acute stroke should have access to care in specialized stroke units or from stroke teams. This ambitious goal was not reached, but in Sweden the majority of stroke patients (up to 80%) are already treated in stroke units, according to the Swedish national quality assessment register for stroke care, Riks-Stroke.[9] The Norwegian Board of Health has recommended that all hospitals treating stroke patients should have stroke units. In Germany, stroke patients are treated nationwide in stroke units.

The second Pan-European Consensus Meeting on Stroke Management stated that all stroke patients should have access to a continuum of care from organized stroke units in the acute stage to appropriate rehabilitation and secondary prevention by 2015.[10] The random survey of European hospitals admitting stroke patients revealed that only 14% of stroke patients are treated in CSCs and PSCs, 44% are treated in AHWs, and 42% of acute stroke patients are admitted to hospitals that do not have the minimum facilities for acute stroke care as specified by the European Stroke Organisation (ESO).[11] Only in Finland, Luxembourg, Sweden, and the Netherlands did most hospitals of the survey have appropriate level of care.[11] Accordingly, in Europe there is still a long way to go until the goals specified in the Helsingborg Declaration of 2006 are met.

Because stroke incidence is increasing more rapidly in low-income than high-income countries, the burden of stroke is increasing more rapidly in poorer than in richer communities.[12,13] An analysis limited to randomized trials of stroke unit care in middle- and low-income countries favored strongly the use of stroke unit care.[13] Although stroke unit care is clearly cost-effective,[14] it has been challenging to establish adequately equipped stroke units even in high-income countries.[11]

BOX 53-2 Components Considered Essential* for Stroke Care

CSC
Stroke-trained physician (24/7)
Interventional neuroradiologist on call
Neurosurgeon on call
Multidisciplinary team
CEA vascular surgeon
Stroke-trained nurses
Emergency department staff
Physician expert in carotid ultrasonology
Physician expert in echocardiography
Social worker
Physician trained in rehabilitation
Speech therapy start within 2 days
Physiotherapy start within 2 days
Brain CT scan 24/7
CT priority for stroke patients
MRI (T_1, T_2, T_2*- weighted, FLAIR) 24/7
Diffusion-weighted MRI
Extracranial Doppler sonography 24/7
Extracranial duplex sonography 24/7
TCD 24/7
CT angiography 24/7
Magnetic resonance angiography 24/7
Transfemoral cerebral angiography 24/7
Transthoracic echocardiography
Transesophageal echocardiography
Automated ECG monitoring (bedside)
Automated monitoring of pulse oximetry
Automated monitoring of BP
Automated monitoring of breathing
Monitoring of temperature
Intravenous rt-PA protocols 24/7
Intra-arterial thrombolysis 24/7
Respiratory support
Surgery for hematoma
Carotid surgery
Angioplasty and stenting
Hemicraniectomy
Ventricular drainage
Surgery for hematoma
Emergency department (in-house)
Stroke outpatient clinic
Multidisciplinary ICU
Inpatient rehabilitation (in-house)
Outpatient rehabilitation available
Collaboration with outside rehabilitation center
Anticoagulation clinic
Stroke faculty
Stroke care map for patient admission
Stroke database
Intravenous rt-PA protocols
Community stroke awareness program
Prevention program
Stroke pathways
Clinical research
Research grants
Drug research
Stroke clinical fellowship
Stroke study coordinator
Stroke research unit

PSC
Neurologist on call
Neurologist on staff
Stroke-trained physician (24/7)
Diagnostic radiologist on call
Multidisciplinary team
Stroke-trained nurses
Emergency department staff
Physician expert in carotid ultrasonology
Social worker
Speech therapy starts within 2 days
Physiotherapy starts within 2 days
Brain CT scan 24/7
CT priority for stroke patients
Extracranial Doppler sonography
Extracranial duplex sonography
Transthoracic echocardiography
Transesophageal echocardiography
Automated ECG monitoring at bedside
Automated monitoring of pulse oximetry
Automated monitoring of blood pressure
Automated monitoring of breathing
Monitoring of temperature
Intravenous rt-PA protocols 24/7
Emergency department (in-house)
Stroke outpatient clinic
Multidisciplinary ICU
Inpatient rehabilitation (in-house)
Outpatient rehabilitation available
Collaboration with outside rehabilitation center
Stroke care map for patient admission
Intravenous rt-PA protocols
Community stroke awareness program
Prevention program
Stroke pathways

AHW
Emergency department staff
Brain CT scan 24/7
CT priority for stroke patients
Emergency department (in-house)
Collaboration with outside rehabilitation center
Stroke care map for patient admission
Prevention program
Stroke pathways

*Considered absolutely necessary by more than 50% of the experts.

CSC, comprehensive stroke center; PSC, primary stroke center; AHW, Any hospital ward; CEA, carotid endarterectomy; BP, blood pressure; CT, computed tomography; MRI, magnetic resonance imaging; FLAIR, fluid-attenuated inversion recovery; TCD, transcranial Doppler; ECG, electrocardiographic; ICU, intensive care unit; rt-PA, recombinant tissue plasminogen activator.

From Leys D, Ringelstein EB, Kaste M, Hacke W; European Stroke Initiative Executive Committee: The main components of stroke unit care: Results of a European expert survey. Cerebrovasc Dis 23:344–352, 2007.

BOX 53-3 Main Goals in the Acute Stroke Unit

1. Reassess the patient medically and neurologically
2. Ascertain definite diagnosis and rule out other diseases
3. Establish stroke subtype, mechanisms, and etiology
4. Deliver hyperacute/acute treatments
5. Achieve and maintain vital functions within or close to physiological ranges (homeostasis)
6. Prevent, diagnose, and treat complications
7. Detect risk factors and start preventive measures for avoiding recurrences
8. Start early rehabilitation and make mid-/long-term plans
9. Recruit as many patients as possible to scientific projects including randomized controlled trials
10. When hope is lost, remember organ donation

BOX 53-4 Stroke Mimics

Epidural hematoma	Hypoglycemia
Subdural hematoma	Hyponatremia
Traumatic brain hemorrhage	Toxic and metabolic disorders
Brain tumor	Syncope
Multiple sclerosis	Sepsis
Encephalitis	Psychogenic
Abscess and cyst	Peripheral nerve diseases (rare)
Seizure and postictal state	Other rare conditions
Migraine with aura	
Transient global amnesia	

Therefore, it will likely be even more challenging to spread stroke units in low-income countries.

A number of quality indicators for a stroke unit has been set by the AHA[15] and ESO[16] aiming at improving quality of care and allow for benchmarking between performances of different stroke centers. Further, establishing local and national stroke registries is strongly recommended. Quality indicators include a wide range of activities including quick patient evaluation, imaging, delivery of acute treatments, initiation of various preventive measures, and rehabilitation. Stroke unit certification programs have been initiated in several countries and similar efforts are under way elsewhere.

GENERAL STROKE MANAGEMENT

The main goals of stroke care in a stroke unit are shown in Box 53-3. Every patient with acute stroke, even with mild symptoms or with stable vital functions, must be recognized as an urgently ill medical patient. Even transitory, rapidly resolving, or fluctuating symptoms may be associated with complete acute occlusion of a major artery in patients with excellent collateral circulation. If the artery is not recanalized, the situation is likely to lead to expansion of the brain infarction and worsening of the patient's clinical status over several hours. In some cases, hemodynamic ischemia may accentuate the symptoms, if the patient is dehydrated, hypotensive, or is immediately mobilized without knowledge of the state of recanalization.

The decision where to treat the patient depends on local resources and the level of care and monitoring at the stroke unit; some stroke units do have intensive care facilities, such as continuous arterial blood pressure (BP) monitoring, central venous catheters, mechanical ventilators, and continuous positive airway pressure (CPAP) ventilation. The vital functions of a patient with stroke are stable if (1) the patient has a secure airway and ventilatory function, (2) BP is not extremely high or low, (3) the cardiac rhythm is hemodynamically sufficient, and (4) unstable coronary ischemia is not present. Endotracheal intubation is indicated for patients with reduced consciousness (generally when Glasgow Coma Scale is ≤7 points), and controlled ventilation is needed for patients with spontaneous hypoventilation.

REASSESS THE PATIENT MEDICALLY AND NEUROLOGICALLY

A quick evaluation of the patient upon arrival to the stroke unit ascertains any deteriorations as the patients are most vulnerable during the earliest hours and days of their stroke. All stroke patients should undergo a stroke severity measurement (preferably with NIHSS) and Glasgow Coma Scale. At the same time, necessary diagnostic tests, rehabilitation evaluations, and preventative measures can be ordered. Patient and family history may be collected in more detail at this point. Patients and relatives can briefly be informed of the situation and the next steps. If the patient's condition worsened, the cause must be quickly detected and corrected.

ASCERTAIN DEFINITE DIAGNOSIS AND RULE OUT OTHER DISEASES

Stroke mimics (Box 53-4) are conditions where a non-stroke cause of the patient's symptoms and signs is erroneously interpreted as a stroke.[17,18] Patients presenting with stroke mimics are usually younger, are more often females, and have more often vertebrobasilar-territory-like symptoms.[19] Most stroke mimics can be diagnosed with appropriate imaging and laboratory studies as well as using clinical skills. However, a few per cent of thrombolysis-treated patients are harboring a stroke mimic. Fortunately, serious complications following thrombolysis in stroke mimic patients are rare.[19] Strokes with atypical presentations that clinically appear to be caused by another disease are called chameleons.[18,20] Among them are movement disorders (e.g., acute hemiballismus, limb-shaking TIAs), syncopes, hypertensive crises, systemic infections, and altered mental status (psychosis, delirium confusional states, and agitation). In some cases of chameleons, establishing the correct diagnosis will take time and time window for acute treatments will usually be over. However, only rarely are they suitable candidates for thrombolysis.

Imaging is the cornerstone of stroke diagnostics. Early imaging with CT upon arrival will help in establishing a definite diagnosis in majority of ischemic stroke patients and almost all hemorrhagic stroke patients. Structural abnormalities mimicking a stroke, such as tumors, can be grossly diagnosed by CT, especially if combined with contrast imaging. When MRI is used at the emergency room, only few ischemic stroke patients will not demonstrate an acute ischemic lesion. MRI is superior to CT in diagnosing stroke mimics. Metabolic disorders mimicking stroke can usually be diagnosed with simple and quick blood tests. Patients who are considered candidates for acute therapies such as thrombolysis and thrombectomy should follow the institutional short-cut imaging guidelines. In other cases, a comprehensive diagnostic imaging protocol with "one-stop" principle with a versatile sequence package of MRI and MRA is preferable.

ESTABLISH STROKE SUBTYPE, MECHANISMS, AND ETIOLOGY

Brain imaging reliably distinguishes between ischemic and hemorrhagic strokes and gives hints on their mechanisms. Ancillary tests and clinical data help in identifying stroke mechanisms in ischemic stroke (e.g., hypoperfusion, embolic, artery-to-artery embolism from atherosclerotic plaques, dissections), presence of underlying structural causes in ICH patients, or presence of aneurysm(s) in SAH.

Etiologic stroke classification is an integral part of individual patient care and stroke research. The benefits of precise etiologic classification are manifold: (1) it necessitates a systematic comprehensive search for pathologies, mechanisms, and risk factors underlying stroke, (2) guides treatment choices and risk factor management, (3) helps estimating outcomes and recurrence rates, (4) allows for correct statistics and epidemiological studies, (5) helps recording correct diagnosis in discharge notes (using ICD-codes where possible), (6) sometimes leads to extending diagnostic studies to family members (e.g., in mitochondrial disease), (7) detects correct patients for ongoing or future studies, (8) serves for developing new diagnostic tests and biomarkers, and (9) allows clear-cut phenotype descriptions that may help in phenotype–genotype analyses for detecting potentially underlying genetic factors. Etiologic studies change patient management, e.g., by prescribing anticoagulant agents in most cardioembolic strokes and in some other occasions (antiphospholipid syndromes, lupus erythematosus, etc.) and antiplatelet agents in majority of patients. In amyloid angiopathy associated with ICH, vice versa, antiplatelets should be avoided. In patients with intracranial stenosis and with ischemic stroke due to hypoperfusion, aggressive antihypertensive treatment may be avoided. Patients with moyamoya are universally operated on with various techniques of extracranial–intracranial anastomosis. Detecting and treating risk factors have shown significant benefits in reducing the burden of future strokes.

There are several classification systems for ischemic stroke such as Trial of Org 10172 in Acute Stroke Treatment (TOAST),[21] Causative Classification System (CSS),[22] and ASCOD (A for atherosclerosis; S for small-vessel disease, C for cardiac pathology, O for other causes, and D for dissection),[23] TOAST being the most commonly used. SAH is usually classified simply into aneurysmal and non-aneurysmal that determines interventive treatments and recurrence risks. Instead, there is a shortage of classification systems in ICH, reflecting the difficulty of developing one. Recently published SMASH-U (S=structural, M=medication-related, A=amyloid angiopathy-caused, S = systemic disease-related, H = hypertensive, U = undetermined) may provide a useful tool as it is also a prognostic classification system,[24] but needs to be validated in large independent patient cohorts.

DELIVER HYPERACUTE/ACUTE TREATMENTS

Recanalization

In ischemic stroke patients who received or not received early IV and intra-arterial thrombolysis as well as mechanical thrombectomy, one critical step is to ascertain recanalization and in case of deterioration whether this is due to reocclusion, hemorrhage, or other cause. Rapid and significant improvement in severity of the stroke symptoms and signs is a robust marker of recanalization. Additionally, imaging brings more definite answers: the intraluminal thrombus is often visible as a hyperdensity on the initial CT scan, showing as the characteristic dense media sign but also as the dense posterior, anterior, or basilar artery sign. In borderline cases, the CT diagnosis can be difficult, and persistent arterial occlusion can be suspected only because of calcified atherosclerotic arteries. If the dense artery sign matches the perfusion defect in perfusion CT images, the artery has not recanalized. CT angiography, if available, will provide the final answer. Magnetic resonance angiography (MRA) is also sensitive but is more time-consuming and is not always readily available to diagnose lack of blood flow in the artery. The dynamic recanalization process calls for more feasible methods that can be repeated at the bedside or used in continuous monitoring mode, such as the transcranial Doppler (TCD) ultrasonography. A new thrombolysis in brain ischemia (TIBI) classification, analogous to the angiographic thrombolysis in myocardial ischemia (TIMI) classification to measure residual flow and recanalization of cardiac vessels, has been developed for noninvasive monitoring of intracranial vessel residual flow signals with TCD ultrasonography.[25] TIBI classification as determined by emergency TCD ultrasonography correlated with initial stroke severity, clinical recovery, and mortality in patients with stroke who were treated with IV t-PA, and a flow-grade improvement has been found to correlate with clinical improvement.[25,26] If reocclusion has occurred or no reperfusion has been achieved, further interventions must be considered.

Unstable Cerebral Ischemia and Progressing Stroke

The unstable phase of cerebral ischemia generally extends up to the point that recanalization is complete and, in some cases, beyond, depending on the status of the cerebrovascular tree and the overall cardiopulmonary condition of the patient. The unstable phase is characterized by both persisting arterial occlusion and fluctuating symptoms due to reduced perfusion or embolization of the thrombus that may or may not be accentuated if the blood pressure falls or as the patient is mobilized.[27]

Progressing stroke is an old concept, originated before the era of modern imaging technology. Transition of the penumbral area into infarction over time has been demonstrated by several perfusion methods, including perfusion-weighted magnetic resonance imaging (PWI). Deterioration of the clinical condition of the patient has many potential reasons (Box 53-5); however, only few are directly related to the thrombus itself.[28] Because of the heterogeneous nature of progressing stroke, it should not be used for research or clinical decision-making unless the diagnosis is based on visualization of clot material, recanalization, or mismatch patterns on imaging. Treatment of progressing symptoms can be successful only if the pathophysiologic mechanism or multiple mechanisms behind the deterioration have been clarified. The main reasons for progressing stroke include most of the acute complications (Box 53-6), which can be prevented in well-organized stroke unit care and, if they do occur, can be treated.

Malignant middle cerebral artery infarction requires close monitoring and timely intervention with urgent decompressive craniectomy which is often life-saving and leads to significantly better and reasonable long-term outcomes.[29] Similarly, complicated cerebral venous thrombosis patients as well as intracerebral hemorrhage patients might benefit from decompressive craniectomy, but evidence is yet scarce.

ACHIEVE AND MAINTAIN VITAL FUNCTIONS WITHIN OR CLOSE TO PHYSIOLOGICAL RANGES (HOMEOSTASIS)

The clinical condition of the patient with acute stroke should be stabilized already in the emergency department. For

BOX 53-5 Reasons for Deterioration in Acute Ischemic Stroke

SYSTEMIC CAUSES

Dehydration
Arterial hypotension
Extreme degrees of arterial hypertension
Increased body temperature, fever
Hyperglycemia
Hypoventilation, CO_2 retention
Hypoxia
Aspiration and pneumonia
Sepsis, infection
Pulmonary embolism
Myocardial ischemia
Cardiac arrhythmias
Congestive heart failure
Neurogenic pulmonary edema
Hypoglycemia
Epileptic seizure activity
Hyponatremia and other disturbances of electrolyte balance
Overhydration
Thiamine deficiency
Organic delirium
Psychiatric factors

CAUSES RELATED TO ARTERIAL OCCLUSION OR CEREBRAL INFARCT

Re-embolization
Progressing thrombosis
Reocclusion
Infarct edema
Increased intracranial pressure and reduced perfusion pressure
Compartmental brain herniation
Hemorrhagic transformation
Decreasing collateral flow
Reduced perfusion due to multiple stenosing arterial lesions
Extension of the infarct core
Extension of the penumbral area

BOX 53-6 Complications of Ischemic Stroke

Medical Complications	Neurological Complications
Chest infections	Brain edema and herniation
Urinary tract infections	Stroke progression
Fever	Recurrent stroke
Pain	Dysphagia and aspiration
Pressure sores	Hydrocephalus
Falls and fractures	Symptomatic hemorrhagic transformation
Fluid and electrolyte imbalance	Seizures and epilepsy
Deep vein thrombosis/ pulmonary embolism	Delirium or confusion
Myocardial infarction and angina pectoris	Fatigue
Congestive heart failure	Depression
Cardiac arrest/arrhythmias	Apathy
Gastrointestinal bleeds	Hiccups
Incontinence	Central post-stroke pain
Sepsis	Sleep disorders
Pulmonary edema	Movement disorders (chorea, athetosis, etc.)
Respiratory failure	Malnutrition
Hypo- or hyperglycemia	

a patient in whom airway, breathing, or cardiovascular function (the ABCs) is compromised, intensive care facilities are used until the clinical situation is stable.

One monitored stroke unit bed is required for each 100 stroke admissions as the average stay on monitoring is 72 hours.[16] Close monitoring of the acute stroke patient is essential for detecting any deteriorations and timely diagnosis of a number of life-threatening conditions. Further, one or several days of cardiac monitoring may disclose acute myocardial infarctions as well as previously undiagnosed atrial fibrillations disclosing the etiology. Close monitoring in a stroke unit includes 24/7 presence of a nurse within the same observation room with direct visual contact, frequent automated measurements of blood pressure (continuous on-line measurement with intra-arterial line in selected patients), continuous EKG, pulse, respiratory rate, and oxygen saturation monitoring on a large and visible monitor preferably with continuous recording on a hard disk, and blood sugar measurements a few times a day. If a temperature-probe urinary catheter is inserted, core temperature can be monitored on line, otherwise can be frequently measured by various methods. Stroke patients should not be fed orally for 24 hours and afterwards until swallowing is tested and considered safe.

Fluid and Electrolyte Balance

Almost all patients with stroke are somewhat dehydrated on admission, and dehydration is associated with less favorable outcomes. Several reasons may account for dehydration after acute stroke – unconsciousness, swallowing, communication, and cognitive problems as well as immobility, infection, diuretic therapy, hyperthermia, and restlessness. In the prehospital care setting, one of the first things to be done for a patient with stroke is to establish an IV line with Ringer's solution or physiologic saline; rehydration will continue at the stroke unit. IV fluid therapy is virtually always needed, and no patient with stroke should be deprived of it during the early phase. The fluid balance during the first 24 hours after stroke should be more or less positive, depending on the level of dehydration on admission, which can be assessed by a measurement of hematocrit and osmolality. Because both volume depletion and volume overloading should be avoided, the fluid balance of a patient with acute stroke must be closely monitored, especially during the unstable phase.

Body Temperature

Body temperature is commonly elevated to above 37.5 °C in the early phase of stroke which may be a marker of stroke severity, may reflect infectious complications, or may be an independent prognostic factor adversely affecting morbidity and mortality.[30] There is compelling evidence that even mild hyperthermia has a clear-cut, clinically significant deleterious effect in acute stroke and may lead to expanding infarct, edema, hemorrhage, and increased ICP. A landmark work by Reith et al. is the largest retrospective study showing that admission body temperature is highly correlated with initial stroke severity and infarct size as well as with poor outcome and mortality.[30] These researchers found that the relative risk of poor outcome increased by a factor of 2.2 per each 1 °C rise in body temperature. Furthermore, this relationship was independent of stroke severity, and the presence of infection was not independently predictive of poor outcome. Similarly, fever occurs in 40% of patients after ICH and is independently associated with poor outcome and increased mortality, especially in patients with IVH.[31] Fever is common and usually central in origin in SAH patients, and independently associated with higher mortality[32,33] and worse outcomes in survivors,[32,34] clearly related to the amount of extravasated blood and presence of IVH.[32] Improved functional outcomes with control of fever have been reported.[35]

Normothermia should be aimed in acute stroke patients because of deleterious effects of hyperthermia and fever. Many stroke units combat fever aggressively, and routine administration of paracetamol or acetaminophen is common; for acetaminophen, a mean reduction of 0.4 °C for 24 hours compared with placebo has been demonstrated. Physical cooling methods are effective in most patients. Emerging pivotal hypothermia trials will address whether hypothermia is beneficial in the acute phase in ischemic or hemorrhagic stroke patients or possibly in some subgroups. Recent works indicated that mild-to-moderate hypothermia can be achieved in wake stroke patients when anti-shivering medications are used[36] whereas deep hypothermia necessitates general anesthesia and intensive care unit admission.

Blood Glucose

Hypoglycemia is extremely rare in stroke patients. Approximately half of patients with acute stroke are hyperglycemic on admission even in the absence of previously diagnosed diabetes. Hyperglycemia has various effects that lead to increased infarct size and hemorrhagic transformation in experimental reperfusion models.[37]

An elevated blood glucose level leads to a 12-fold increase in the rate of hemorrhagic complications with intra-arterial thrombolysis, as reported by the second Prolyse in Acute Cerebral Thromboembolism Trial (PROACT II) investigators.[38] Hyperglycemia enhances hemorrhagic transformation in ischemic stroke patients with[39–41] and without intravenous thrombolysis.[42]

Admission hyperglycemia is associated with increased infarct size.[43] The strong and consistent association between admission hyperglycemia and poor prognosis after stroke observed in non-diabetic patients suggests that glucose level is an important risk factor for morbidity and mortality after stroke.[44] After ischemic stroke, even a mildly elevated admission blood glucose level of 110 to 126 mg/dL (6.1 to 7.0 mmol/L) was associated with an increased risk of 30-day mortality in non-diabetic patients only (relative risk, [RR], 3.28; 95% confidence interval [CI], 2.32–4.64). In non-diabetic stroke survivors, mild acute hyperglycemia seems to be associated with in-hospital mortality and a higher risk of poor functional recovery.[44] Very strict blood glucose control (80 to 110 mg/dL [4.4 to 6.1 mmol/L]) has significantly reduced the early mortality rate of patients admitted to a surgical intensive care unit by 42% (95%CI, 22–62%).[45]

What are the clinical implications of these data? No glucose-containing solutions should be given to patients with ischemic stroke, especially during the first few days. Blood glucose levels exceeding 144 mg/dL (8 mmol/L) are to be treated with small doses of rapidly acting subcutaneous insulin or, in resistant cases, IV insulin infusion. In SAH patients undergoing cerebral aneurysm surgery, intraoperative hyperglycemia has been associated with long-term decline in cognition and gross neurological function.[46] Therefore, prevention of intraoperative hyperglycemia during aneurysm surgery is probably indicated.[47] In ICH patients, increased admission serum glucose levels are associated with larger hematoma size, hematoma expansion, poor outcomes and increased mortality rates in both diabetic and non-diabetic patients.[48] Therefore, a similar treatment approach is justified.

Blood Pressure

A transient elevation of arterial BP is the rule at the onset of stroke, occurring in 70–80% of the patients with higher BP values in hemorrhagic stroke patients.[49,50] It has been attributed to a number of factors, such as catecholamine secretion in response to stress, neuroendocrine factors, alcohol abuse, increased cardiac output, pain, urinary retention, and topographic presentation of the lesion.[51] The BP usually declines during the first few days. Although the general recommendation has been not to treat a moderate elevation in BP during the first few days, the issue is not entirely settled. Extreme BP is certainly detrimental and requires aggressive treatment. However, ideal BP levels are not determined and may differ in individual patients.

Acute hypertension should be controlled in SAH patients until aneurysm obliteration.[47] The magnitude of blood pressure control to reduce the risk of rebleeding in aneurysmal SAH patients has not been established, but a decrease in systolic blood pressure to < 160 mmHg is reasonable.[47]

According to the current recommendations of the American Heart Association (AHA), BP values exceeding 220 mm Hg systolic and/or 120 mm Hg diastolic in all ischemic stroke patients and over 180/105 mmHg in patients receiving thrombolysis are reasonable to lower preferably with intravenous antihypertensive medications and start long-term antihypertensive treatment after the first day of the stroke onset.[52]

Vasodilators typically cause a severe ischemic steal phenomenon and should be avoided, except when strongly indicated as, for example, in myocardial ischemia. The drugs of choice for emergency IV antihypertensive treatment are (1) labetalol in IV boluses of 10 mg, which can be repeated as necessary, or as a continuous infusion at 30 to 60 mg/h and (2) enalapril in repeated boluses of 1 mg every 15 to 30 minutes. Nicardipine can be used with a starting dose of 2 to 5 mg/h as a continuous infusion (or nimodipine, 1 to 2 mg/h); one must keep in mind, however, that calcium entry blockers can lead to steal of blood flow from ischemic to healthy regions of the brain and that the effect of a sharp drop in BP can be harmful. The use of peroral nifedipine is strongly discouraged. In resistant cases, sodium nitroprusside can be considered, although this agent carries the risk of severe compromise of cerebral perfusion with a sudden drop of BP, reflex tachycardia, and myocardial ischemia. Either IV nimodipine or IV nitroglycerin effectively treats elevated BP when there is a special indication, such as SAH or myocardial ischemia, for the use of either of these drugs.

The recent INTERACT-2 study results indicate that aggressive lowering of BP is safe in acute setting of ICH, and is probably beneficial, although the main result of this study remained statistically insignificant.[53] Hypotension is rare in acute ischemic stroke, found in 0.6% of the patients in one large study.[54] The brain is vulnerable to arterial hypotension during acute ischemic stroke with reportedly poor outcomes in these patients.[54] The cause of hypotension should be found and corrected. Intravenous volume expanders and vasopressor agents are empirically used.

PREVENT, DIAGNOSE, AND TREAT COMPLICATIONS

Stroke patients are particularly prone to both medical and neurological complications (Box 53-6). They may stem from the brain injury itself, but also from co-existing diseases (e.g., diabetes, hypertension, and heart disease), immobilization, and medications. Whereas complications increase mortality and morbidity as well as the length of hospital stays, successful prevention, early recognition, and early-initiated aggressive treatment of a wide range of complications improve patient outcomes and reduce costs. Stroke unit care is able to reduce stroke progression/recurrence, infections, complications, and bedsores.[52] Most serious complications occur early (within days) and are more common in patients with advanced age, severe strokes, and premorbidities. Probably, one-fourth to one-half of total deaths in ischemic stroke patients is caused by complications. Majority of stroke patients develop one or more complications.[48,52,55,56] Further, complications are likely underdiagnosed, underreported, and undertreated.

Brain Edema and Elevated Intracranial Pressure

Patients with large hemispheric infarcts, large intracerebral hematomas, or profuse subarachnoid bleeding, are at risk of development of cerebral edema followed by mass effect, herniation, and death. Patients with large cerebellar infarcts and hematomas associated with secondary edema may develop hydrocephalus through obliteration of the IVth ventricle and secondary hydrocephalus, brainstem compression, and both descending (transforaminal) and ascending (transtentorial) herniation. The clinical picture is that of a progressive decline in level of consciousness, sighing, and vomiting, followed by decorticate or decerebrate posturing and pupillary dilatation as the herniation proceeds. Close monitoring of neurological status and serial CT scans are the diagnostic method of choice for guiding interventions.

Ischemic brain edema develops during the first 24–48 hours after ischemic infarcts. In younger patients, brain edema with elevated ICP may become a major complication, potentially leading to herniation and death.[57] Such patients usually show a rapid decline in consciousness and demonstrate the signs of herniation 2–4 days after onset of symptoms. Brain edema involving the gray and white matter surrounding the infarcted tissue could be seen within 24 hours, reached its maximum on days 3–5, and then subsided completely within 2 weeks. A malignant MCA infarct typically caused by an embolic occlusion of either the distal ICA or the proximal MCA trunk has been defined as a space-occupying infarct of at least the total MCA territory, with signs of an increasing space-occupying effect on serial CT scans with a midline shift of more than 10 mm at the septum pellucidum level.[58,59] The outcome is often fatal, and a mortality rate of up to 80% has been reported for standard care. Decompressive hemicraniectomy is now the treatment of choice and level I class A recommendation for these patients if younger than 60 years of age.[29] Decompressive craniectomy reduces mortality significantly in older patients, too, but the majority of additional survivors will have substantial disability.[60] Craniectomy window must be large enough to allow additional space for the swollen brain tissue and reinstitute microcirculation. Generally speaking, older patients may stand brain edema better because general brain atrophy offers larger available space within the cranium. Whether craniectomy is beneficial in ICH and selected cerebral venous thrombosis patients is a matter of great interest.

Basic management of elevated ICP after stroke usually consists of (1) placement of the patient in a semi-sitting position with elevation of the head and upper trunk to approximately 30° degrees without turning the head to extreme lateral positions, (2) avoidance of noxious stimuli, (3) pain relief, and (4) a low normal body temperature (36–37°C). Osmotherapy with 10% glycerol (250 mL of 10% glycerol over 60 minutes every 6 hours), 15% mannitol (100–200 mL every 4–6 hours), dexametasone, hypertonic saline (up to 5% or more), and others are widely used for dismal brain edema in patients with ischemic or hemorrhagic strokes without solid scientific evidence.

Hemorrhagic Transformation

Hemorrhagic transformation of the infarct occurs in 30–40% of cases and is often asymptomatic. Symptomatic hemorrhagic transformation equaling to parenchymal hemorrhage occurs more commonly following intravenous (6%) or intra-arterial (7%) thrombolysis, mechanical thrombectomy (8.5%),[61] and more often in patients with cardiogenic embolism, carotid artery dissections, and large infarcts.[62] Symptomatic hemorrhagic transformation, especially when leading to solid hematomas, worsens patient outcomes and highly increases mortality.[41,63] Bed rest and avoidance of antithrombotic agents for the first 24 hours and treatment of hypertension, hyperglycemia, and fever may decrease the risk of hemorrhagic transformation.

Seizures

Partial (focal) and secondarily generalized seizures may occur as part of presenting symptoms (onset seizures), early during the course of stroke (within 1 week, early seizures), or later (late seizures). The frequency of seizures following an ischemic or hemorrhagic stroke is around 10%, being more common in SAH.[64,65] But, seizures are most common in CVT patients (40%). Late recurrent seizures (i.e., epilepsy) develop in 2.5–10% of stroke patients. Status epilepticus in the early phase is rare in stroke patients; non-convulsive status epilepticus may be seen in hemorrhagic stroke patients[66] and is likely associated with poor outcomes.[66]

Monitoring with electroencephalography (EEG) may be useful in some cases, but routine EEG monitoring is not recommended. Non-convulsive seizure activity in EEG is much more common than clinically detected seizures, and is associated with worse outcome. Single seizures and status epilepticus should be treated according to general guidelines. Despite lack of evidence, it is common practice to treat recurrent early seizures with anticonvulsants for a few months. CVT patients presenting with any seizure or having parenchymal lesions even without a clinical seizure are usually treated with anticonvulsant drugs for 3–6 months. Stroke patients with no seizures do not need prophylactic anticonvulsant treatment. Otherwise late recurrent seizures need long-term anticonvulsant treatment.

Recurrent Stroke

Early recurrent stroke is common following an ischemic stroke and TIA. The risk is around 10% within 1 week, an additional 2–4% within 1 month, and approximately 5% per year afterwards following a TIA.[56] Older age, presence of multiple risk factors, atrial fibrillation, and severe carotid artery stenosis all increase the risk of forthcoming ischemic strokes.

ICH patients with underlying lesions will benefit from early surgery before rebleeding occurs. Recurrence of ICH occurs in 2.1–3.7% per patient-year.[67,68] Lobar location likely representing cerebral amyloid angiopathy is a significant predictor of ICH recurrence. Treating hypertension and avoiding antithrombotic agents in amyloid angiopathy-related ICH are beneficial.

If a ruptured aneurysm is left untreated, one-third of the patients who recover from the initial hemorrhage will die because of recurrent bleeding within 6 months after SAH.[69,70] When a ruptured cerebral aneurysm was obliterated with either clipping or coiling, rebleeding during 1 year follow-up was extremely unlikely.[71]

Early recurrence led clinical deterioration in 11.3% of 1964 ischemic stroke patients and 4.5% of 8291 transient ischemic attack or minor stroke patients.[72] Early recurrent ischemia is clearly associated with worse outcomes. Data indicate that early mobilization and management of physiological variables within or close to normal range improve outcomes and reduce recurrent strokes. Early initiation of secondary preventive measures in full extent including life habit changes and early surgery for significant carotid artery stenosis may prevent most recurrent ischemic strokes, even up to 80%.

Delirium

Delirium, an acute decline in attention and cognition, with a fluctuating course in orientation, memory, thought, and behavior, is common in acute stroke patients and increases with advancing age.[73] Delirium has been reported in up to half of stroke patients (10–48%), most commonly during the first week of hospitalization.[74] Delirium is associated with a five-fold increased risk of mortality and morbidity (threefold risk of being discharged to a long-term care institution), longer stay in hospital, loss of independence, and increased costs.[73] Further, patients with delirium might injure themselves or hospital staff. Restlessness, confusion, and aggressiveness typically start or worsen through the night. Recent studies suggest that delirium persists much longer than previously believed.

The pathophysiology of delirium remains poorly understood. Electroencephalography often shows diffuse slowing of background activity, consistent with widespread cortical dysfunction.[75] Brain injury itself, as well as factors such as advanced age, underlying cognitive or mental disorder, intensive care, surgical interventions, poor vision or hearing, severe illness, pain, fever, infections, hypoxia, polypharmacy, abstinence, dehydration, immobility, and various medications may ignite delirium. Several neurotransmitter systems may be involved, among them, most evidence point to an imbalance between the cholinergic (relative deficiency of acetylcholine) and dopaminergic (relative excess of dopamine) systems.

Delirium presents in three different forms: hyperactive (marked by agitation and vigilance), hypoactive (marked by lethargy with a decreased level of motor activity and is difficult to recognize), and in a mixed form. Hyperactive delirium has the best prognosis. Most stroke patients present with the hyperactive form. Facial inexpressiveness, motor retardation, speech retardation, a decrease in reactivity, perplexity, and mental slowness are typical in hypoactive delirium, whereas logorrhea, motor hyperactivity, aggressiveness, stereotyped activities, hyper-reaction, and delusions are closely associated with the hyperactive type.[76]

Usage of delirium assessment methods such as the Confusion Assessment Method (CAM)[77] or the Delirium Rating Scale (DRS)[78] improves quick recognition of delirium with a reasonably high accuracy. Adaptations of the CAM include the CAM-ICU for non-verbal ventilated patients (or aphasic stroke patients), adaptations for emergency room and nursing home settings. The diagnostic algorithm of CAM has four components: acute onset and fluctuating course, inattention, disorganized thinking, and altered level of consciousness.

Identification of patients at risk, early recognition and prevention, elimination of precipitating factors, general supportive measures, arranging an optimal environment and nursing care, sedation with medication, using restraints only in extreme situations, and reassurance of family members are the main management elements for delirium. In a randomized trial, early mobilization, adequate hydration, ensuring good communication (replace missing eyeglasses or hearing aids), and preventing sleep deprivation were found effective in preventing delirium leading to a one-third reduction in delirium rates.[79] Underlying causes need to be corrected when feasible. Haloperidol in small, but frequently repeated, doses is the first-line treatment.[73] Anticholinergic drugs must be avoided. Atypical antipsychotics and benzodiazepines can be used as second-line drugs. Benzodiazepins are useful if delirium is caused by or associated with withdrawal of alcohol or sedative drugs. Parenteral thiamine substitution is started on admission for all patients at risk of delirium. Restraints should be reserved for patients with extreme agitation and aggression who are at risk of hurting themselves or others.

Depression

Depression affects approximately one-third of patients early after stroke and interferes with recovery.[80,81] Other neuropsychiatric problems such as anxiety, fatigue, and apathy are approximately equally common and may present together with or without depression. Only one small-sized (n = 128) population-based study recruited controls to allow estimates of the relative risks of depression after stroke.[82] The prevalence of depression in stroke survivors was twice that found in controls.[82]

Depression starts shortly after stroke and is a chronic relapsing disease with a similar incidence along several years after stroke.[80] Stroke severity, disability, cognitive impairment, lack of social support, and anxiety (most studies excluded patients with prestroke depression) are the consistent predictors of post-stroke depression.[80,81] A clear correlation between lesion location and depression could not be demonstrated. Post-stroke depression is likely underdiagnosed and undertreated. In addition to clinical evaluation, a number of interviewer-administered or self-completed depression screening instruments exist, and some of them (The Center of Epidemiological Studies-Depression Scale, Hamilton Depression Rating Scale, and Patient Health Questionnaire-9 Scale) were found to be modestly useful for case-finding in stroke patients.[83] Stroke Aphasic Depression Questionnaire[84] or The Depression Intensity Scale Circles[85] can be used in stroke patients with communication problems. However, all these scales are only supplementary to clinical bedside judgment.

A Cochrane review[86] and a meta-analysis[87] showed that use of antidepressant agents at various doses and length of time periods in post-stroke depression was beneficial. When started, antidepressants should be continued for long periods, e.g., 6 months. Indeed, new antidepressants are shown to have positive effects on brain recovery and plasticity in animal models of stroke that reignited the interest on antidepressants in stroke research. A recent small randomized controlled multicenter trial in non-depressed ischemic stroke patients showed a clear benefit in terms of functional outcomes in fluoxetine-treated patients.[88] Thus, antidepressants may potentially have dual benefits given that these results can be replicated in large randomized future trials. While selective serotonin reuptake inhibitors are widely used to treat depression in stroke patients, exposure to these agents is reported to be associated with a slightly increased risk of intracranial hemorrhages; yet, given the rarity of the event, absolute risks are likely to be very low.[89] Further, a causal relationship between exposure to selective serotonin reuptake inhibitors and increased risk of ICH has not been established. Several randomized trials with fluoxetine in stroke patients are under progress and hopefully will report on potential benefits on stroke recovery and whether its use is associated with increased risk for ICH or other serious adverse events.

Electrolyte Disorders

Hyponatremia, frequently associated with diabetes and chronic renal failure and an independent predictor of long-term mortality, was found in over 10% of ischemic stroke patients upon admission.[90] Similarly, hypopotassemia was found in 20% of acute stroke patients during admission and was associated with poor outcomes.[91] Severe electrolyte disorders require correction and close monitoring. Sometimes complex electrolyte disturbances ensue, as seen in such cases with low intake of salt or, very rarely, preexisting syndrome of inappropriate antidiuretic hormone (SIADH). The occurrence of SIADH is exceptional after stroke and hyponatremia and volume depletion are usually caused by the cerebral salt wasting syndrome (CSWS). CSWS is produced by excessive secretion of natriuretic peptides leading to hyponatremia from excessive natriuresis, which may provoke volume contraction.[92] In these cases, the conventional recommendation to restrict fluids for correcting hyponatremia is risky and may even prove fatal; instead, volume and sodium loading must be performed. As a rule, fluid restriction is virtually never indicated in acute stroke. In very severe stroke with compression or destruction of the hypothalamus, lack of antidiuretic hormone may lead to diabetes insipidus, which must be treated with vasopressin.

Cardiovascular Complications

Cardiac arrhythmias and myocardial ischemia secondary to stroke are very common. A systematic review of 39 studies reported a risk of 2% for myocardial infarction in patients with TIA and strokes.[93] Even in young ischemic stroke patients, cardiac death was the dominant cause of death in long-term follow-up.[94] Patients with stroke frequently harbor some degree of coronary disease which may be yet undiagnosed. Within 3 months of ischemic stroke, 19% suffered from serious cardiac events and 4% died from cardiac reasons in the placebo arm analysis of a VISTA-registered multicenter trial patients' registry.[95] Which high-risk patients should be further investigated for coronary heart disease at their post-stroke phase is not clear. A recent grading system (PRECORIS Score) in TIA and ischemic stroke patients was reported to identify moderately well the subpopulation of patients with occult severe coronary artery stenosis.[96] A large single-center study showed that 4.1% of consecutive ICH patients had ≥1 acute in-hospital cardiac complications, most often acute heart failure that required treatment.[97] Similarly, after SAH, 4.3% experienced a cardiac arrhythmia in one study of 580 patients, with no other cardiac outcomes analyzed.[98] Acute heart failure in subacute period was reported to range between 2% and 11% after all strokes.[99]

Significant alterations in the ST segments and the T waves on an electrocardiogram (ECG) may appear in the early phase, representing true myocardial ischemia, sometimes in the absence of coronary disease. Cardiac enzymes may be elevated in stroke, more commonly in severe stroke, including stroke due to ICH or SAH. Distinguishing true myocardial ischemia from stroke-related neurally induced myocardial damage may be difficult as no clear-cut threshold level has been established to reliably distinguish between cardiac and neural mechanisms for increased myocardial enzyme concentrations. The routine treatment for this phenomenon, which depends mainly on excess circulating catecholamines, is beta-blocker or alpha and beta-blocker therapy. Beta-blockers are routinely administered to protect the myocardium, especially in severe strokes. One must, however, abide by any pre-existing and acute contraindications to this therapeutic modality, such as bronchoconstriction, congestive heart failure, severe bradycardia, and disturbances of atrioventricular or intraventricular conduction (i.e., prolonged PQ or QT interval).

An initial ECG should be performed on admission in every stroke patient followed by continuous ECG monitoring in a stroke unit. Cardiac enzyme levels are routinely monitored for 24 hours or for several days in unstable patients. Etiologic studies, including echocardiography and invasive cardiologic evaluation, are an essential part of the diagnostic work-up for many patients with stroke.

Takotsubo syndrome (apical ballooning cardiomyopathy, broken heart syndrome) is a stress-induced non-ischemic cardiomyopathy characterized by sudden weakening of the myocardial muscle function and leading to acute cardiac failure. Cardiac ultrasound studies demonstrate that the apical and mid-segments of the myocardium do not contract. Limited reports indicate a frequency of 1.2% in both ischemic stroke and SAH,[100-103] female dominance, and possible insular damage.[103]

Respiratory Failure

In acute ischemic stroke, early changes in ventilatory drive and early respiratory disturbances due to reduced consciousness are rare. However, patients with complete MCA infarct, large supratentorial ICH, severe SAH, or brainstem stroke may have early ventilatory problems. Continuous monitoring of oxygen saturation and frequent arterial blood gas measurements are necessary in unstable patients. Supplemental oxygen, usually 2–4 L/min via nasal tube or a mask, should be used in the emergency and unstable phases. Temporary CPAP ventilation is sometimes necessary for refractory pulmonary edema. CPAP can also be used for severe obstructive sleep apnea, which is commonly diagnosed in acute stroke patients. Studies showed feasibility of this approach, but efficacy has not been demonstrated.

If intubation is indicated, it should be preplanned and performed by an experienced anesthesiologist because CBF can be compromised during the procedure; such compromise may also provoke unwanted autonomic reflexes and BP changes, thereby precipitating intracranial shifts or bleeding. The following findings are sufficient indications for intubation:

- Unconsciousness (Glasgow Coma Scale [GCS] score ≤ 7)
- Inability to swallow or clear secretions from the mouth
- Absence of cough and gag reflexes
- Severe stridor.

A patient with stroke should undergo intubation only if the possibility for independent recovery is present; that is, intubation should not be used only to prolong the terminal phase. However, early withdrawal of care decisions must be avoided and patients should be intubated during the first few days if prognosis is not deemed to be completely hopeless. Intubated stroke patients have well over 50% mortality, but pessimistic approaches leading to rather easy withholding of active treatments likely increase mortality.

Pneumonia

In a recent meta-analysis comprising 87 studies and 137,817 patients, the overall infection rate was 30% among stroke patients, the most common infections being pneumonia and urinary tract infections.[104] In a multicenter cohort study with 8251 patients, pneumonia increased 30-day mortality by 2.2 times and 1-year mortality by three times.[105] One of the most important risks in the early phase after stroke is aspiration pneumonia. Dysphagia increases the risk of pneumonia threefold, rising to 11-fold in patients with confirmed aspiration.[106] Bacterial pneumonia accounts for 15–25% of stroke-related deaths and triples the mortality rates. Aspiration is commonly found in patients with reduced consciousness as well as in patients with impaired gag reflexes or swallowing disturbances, which occur in patients with severe stroke, who are initially unconscious or vomiting, or who lay for hours after stroke before being found and brought for treatment are assumed to have aspirated, implicating the need for antibiotics covering both the aerobic and anaerobic pathogens of aspiration pneumonia. Delay in initiation of antibiotics may worsen the outcome.

Nasogastric feeding is helpful in preventing aspiration pneumonia, although it does not completely abolish the risk. Other reasons for pneumonia are poor cough (hypostatic pneumonia) and immobilization. Frequent changes of the patient's position in bed and pulmonary physical therapy may prevent this type of pneumonia. Oral care and dental hygiene may also reduce pneumonia risk. Preventive antibiotic therapy decreased the rate of infections in stroke patients, however, did not ameliorate mortality figures.[107] Until ongoing trials bring definite data, routine prophylactic antibiotic treatment in stroke patients is not recommended.

Urinary Tract Infection

Urinary tract infection (UTI) is one of the most common medical complications of stroke occurring in up to one-fourth of patients[108] and is usually caused by *Escherichia coli*. Patients with stroke are particularly prone to developing UTI due to immunosuppression, bladder dysfunction, and use of urinary tract catheters. Diagnosis of UTI in stroke patients within 2 days of stroke onset is unusual as most UTIs develop after hospital admission as a nosocomial infection.[109] The majority of hospital-acquired UTIs are associated with the use of indwelling catheters. In the general medical population, the risk of UTI is 3–10% per day of catheterization.[110] Catheter-associated UTI may be caused by contamination from personnel's hands and equipment (exogenous) or from nearby (meatal, rectal, or vaginal) colonization of bacteria. Closed-drainage catheterization systems prevent intraluminal migration of bacteria from external sources into the urinary bladder, however, a biofilm of bacteria develops on the surface of the catheters already one day after catheterization followed by colonization and migration of pathogens up in the urinary tract.[110] Risk of UTI after stroke is increased in older patients, in females, with functional dependence, severe strokes, poor cognitive function, and catheterization.

There are almost no high-quality data on the frequency, type, duration, and indications for urinary catheter use in stroke patients, mainly because of poor documentation and that the topic has received little attention. Probably one-fourth of all hospital catheterizations are unnecessary and inappropriate reasons for catheterizations include monitoring urine output without a critical need, incontinence, and nursing convenience.[108] Appropriate reasons for catheterization include acute urinary retention or obstruction, need for accurate measurements of urinary output in critically ill patients, and in patients requiring prolonged immobilization. Urinary retention and incontinence are common in the early phase after stroke. Some patients already have micturition and continence problems before stroke. A small study carried out in stroke patients in three teaching hospitals showed that no catheterization policy or standard continence assessment was utilized and documentation was often lacking, reflecting that the topic did not receive much attention.[111]

Dysuria is a strong marker or UTI, however, most stroke patients do not report dysuria (high specificity, but low sensitivity). Once urinary infection is detected, appropriate antibiotics should be started. Urine cultures are helpful in diagnosis and guiding appropriate antibiotic selection. However, prophylactic antibiotics are not recommended. Acidification may reduce the risk of infection, whereas intermittent catheterization has not been shown to do so. New approaches include antiseptic-coated catheters, antibiotic-impregnated catheters, and condom catheters in male patients, but more evidence is needed. Educational interventions[112] and computer-based order entry approaches[113] reduced catheter use and catheter-associated UTI rates in non-stroke patient populations.

Dysphagia and Malnutrition

Dysphagia commonly occurs in stroke patients, initially affecting 27–64% of them[114] and increasing risk for aspiration, pneumonia, and malnutrition. Half of these patients will recover within 2 weeks as spontaneous improvement is common, but at least one in six patients will still have swallowing problems 1 month after stroke.[114] There is good evidence that early identification and management of dysphagia reduce the occurrence of pneumonia. Thus, swallowing tests should be an integral part of acute stroke unit treatment protocols. Swallowing screening should be quick and minimally invasive bedside test that includes dysphagia risk identification (abnormality in the oropharyngeal swallowing system) along with risk for aspiration (subglottic penetration of food or liquid). These tests include the Water-Swallowing-Test (WST) with 50 mL of aqua, the Multiple-Consistency-Test or Gugging Swallowing Screen (GUSS) and the Swallowing-Provocation-Test (SPT) with 0.4 mL of aqua to nasopharynx. The videofluoroscopic barium swallowing test (VFSS) has been the gold standard for many years, but may soon be replaced by FEES (Flexible Endoscopic Evaluation of Swallowing). FEES is more sensitive than VFSS in detecting residuals, penetration and aspiration.

Diagnostic procedures of dysphagia as well as interventions for treating dysphagia are often administered by speech and language therapists (SLTs). Modification of fluid and food consistencies, postural techniques, swallowing exercises, as well as thermal or electrical stimulation of oral and pharyngeal structures, transcranial direct current stimulation (TDCS) and transcranial magnetic stimulation (TMS) and even acupuncture have all been used for this purpose. However, none of these approaches is currently evidence-based.[114] Ongoing randomized trials are soon expected to shed some light on this issue.

Pre-existing malnutrition is common in elderly patients amounting to 8–28% in stroke patients on hospital admission. Stroke itself is a catabolic state. However, caloric need may not be increased in acute stroke patients as they have reduced mobility. Indirect calorimetric studies on days 7–90 after stroke revealed that caloric need was only 10% higher than predicted by the Harris-Benedict equation, but energy needs did not differ by stroke subtypes.[115] Initial (admission) body weight and weekly weight measurements may help in estimating nutritional needs and energy insufficiency. A general recommendation for protein intake is 1.0 to 1.5 g per kilogram of body weight. Malnutrition was found in 6–60% of stroke patients and presence of dysphagia increased the risk of malnutrition 2.5-fold.[116] Malnutrition is associated with increased mortality, length of hospital stay and costs, poor functional status and poor outcome after rehabilitation. Dysphagia, depression, apathy, and loss of appetite all contribute to malnutrition following stroke.

There are insufficient data on the effects of swallowing therapies, feeding, and nutritional and fluid supplementation on functional outcome in patients with stroke.[114] It is common practice to avoid oral feeding in stroke patients for 24 hours or until swallowing is tested. Patients with swallowing difficulties will require nasogastric tubing (NGT) if the need for feeding is expected to be short (e.g., 1 week). Patients with complete or near-complete pharyngeal region paresis will likely require long-term feeding and may be suitable candidates for insertion of percutaneous endoscopic gastrostomy (PEG). However, it is unclear whether PEG is superior to NGT in patients with acute to subacute stroke, the ideal time to start feeding following stroke onset, and the ideal time to insert PEG if indicated. The insertion of both PEG and NGT may give rise to complications. NGT is uncomfortable for the patients and disoriented patients frequently pull their NGT. Intravenous feeding of dysphagic stroke patients should be limited to cases with enteral failure.

Pulmonary Embolism and Deep Vein Thrombosis

Pulmonary embolism (PE) accounts for 10% of deaths after stroke, being a major concern, especially in patients with severe lower limb paresis. In an old literature review, DVT was found in as high as 50% of stroke patients within the first 2 weeks without thromboprophylaxis.[117] A prospective study that used MRI for direct thrombus imaging detected venous thrombus in legs or pelvis in 40% and a PE in 12% of patients with ischemic stroke who were on aspirin and graded compression stockings 3 weeks of stroke onset.[118] The risk of DVT and PE can be reduced by early mobilization and by the use of low-molecular-weight heparin. Although an increase in the rate of hemorrhagic complications is expected, nevertheless, prophylaxis with subcutaneous anticoagulants every 12 hours, is recommended for bedridden patients with stroke until mobilization. Tachypnea, pain, and oxygen desaturation may be signs of PE or pneumonia. Most fatal PEs occur between 2 and 4 weeks after a stroke. The lower extremities should be examined daily to detect signs of DVT, which can be excluded by venous ultrasonography. Most DVTs are asymptomatic and thus not clinically detectable. Physical therapy and the use of support or pump stockings are suggested as an alternative to low-molecular-weight heparin.

Management of DVT and PE is more complicated in patients with hemorrhagic stroke as the risk of thromboembolism must be balanced against the risk of rebleeding. A recent multicenter prospective randomized trial recruited 2876 acute stroke patients (13% hemorrhagic strokes) within 3 days of admission in 94 UK-based centers. The patients received either intermittent pneumatic compression or no intervention. Thromboprophylaxis was given according to investigators' own preference and was similarly given to both groups. DVTs were reduced significantly (12.1% vs 8.5%), but mortality and proven PE rates were only non-significantly lower in the treatment arm.[119] Treatment effect was stronger in hemorrhagic stroke patients. This approach may prove beneficial in stroke patients, especially when thromboprophylaxis is associated with a significant risk of serious bleeding.

Decubitus Ulcer

Decubitus ulcers (or pressure sores), once a major problem in bedridden patients, have become a rarity in western hospitals as preventive measures such as early mobilization, frequent repositioning of patients by turning to other side every 2 hours, good skin care, use of special decubitus mattresses and padded heel booths have become routine measures. It is easier to prevent decubitus ulcers than treating them once they appeared. In bedridden patients, sacrum, buttocks, heels, and ankles should be examined frequently. If the decubitus ulcer does not respond to conservative treatment, antibiotic therapy for several days may be justified, before definitive surgical debridement.

Complications Specific to Intracerebral Hemorrhage

Complications specific to ICH include hematoma expansion, perihematomal edema leading to increased intracranial pressure, and intraventricular extension of hemorrhage with hydrocephalus. These complications are associated with early neurological deterioration and increased mortality. Early neurological deterioration was found in one-third of ICH patients within 48 hours of disease of onset, the period when half of the deaths in ICH patients occurred.[48] Hematoma expansion is usually defined as an increase in hematoma volume by 33% or an absolute change of >6 mL on repeat CT imaging, occurs in up to 40% of ICH patients. Large hematoma volume on presentation, presence of spot sign, early arrival to ER, heterogeneity of hematoma density, and prior use of anticoagulation are important predictors of hematoma expansion. Bed rest, pain control, reversal of anticoagulation, and aggressive reduction of arterial blood pressure are universally recommended to avoid or minimize hematoma expansion. Perihematomal edema develops early, increasing over days, reaching its maximum between 1 and 2 weeks after bleeding.[48] Edema volume might even exceed the hematoma volume leading to mass effects with tissue shifts, increased intracranial pressure, obstructive hydrocephalus, and herniation. Head positioning by slight elevation, fever and pain control, and bed rest are universally recommended. Anti-edema treatments are widely used despite lack of scientific evidence. Surgical interventions should be considered in critical patients. Intraventicular hemorrhage is found in 40% of all ICH patients, although IVH alone without ICH is rare. Presence of IVH in ICH patients doubles mortality and halves good functional outcome in survivors compared to ICH patients without IVH.[48] Up to half of IVH patients will develop hydrocephalus caused by obstruction of the third and the fourth ventricles. External ventricular drainage and lumbar drainage are often used in critical patients.

Complications Specific to Subarachnoidal Hemorrhage

Hydrocephalus, cerebral vasospasm leading to delayed cerebral ischemia, and recurrent bleeding are serious complications underlying SAH. Early rebleeding occurs in one-third of conservatively-treated aneurysmal SAH patients within 6 months.[69] The risk of rebleeding is maximal in the first hours, with reported rates between 4% and 13.6% within the first 24 hours.[47] Therefore, aneurysm clipping or coiling should be performed as early as possible aiming at complete obliteration of the aneurysm. Absolute bed rest, pain control, and avoiding constipation are crucial measures until clipping or coiling of ruptured aneurysms.[120] Hydrocephalus occurs in at least 20% of patients during the acute phase and in about 10% during the chronic phase after SAH.[121] Hydrocephalus may be asymptomatic in up to one-third of these patients, and half of the patients with initial hydrocephalus and impairment of consciousness improve spontaneously within 24 hours.[121] External ventricular drainage for obstructive and lumbar drainage for communicating hydrocephalus are frequently used despite risks of rebleeding and infection.[122,123] Widespread cerebral vasospasm is found in 30% of aneurysmal SAH patients usually during the 4–10 days resolving gradually over 21 days after the initial bleeding, but leads to ischemic deficits in about half of them.[124] A Cochrane review, including 16 trials with 3361 patients with SAH, found a clear benefit of calcium antagonists for death and dependence.[125] Therefore, a standard regimen is oral nimodipine 60 mg every 4 hours for 3 weeks in all patients with a ruptured aneurysmal SAH.

DETECT RISK FACTORS AND START PREVENTIVE MEASURES FOR AVOIDING RECURRENCES

Secondary prevention should start as early as possible or on admission to the stroke unit at the latest. Aspirin should be given early after ischemic stroke if thrombolysis is not administered or 24 hours after thrombolysis. Early mobilization of stable patients is strongly recommended. Adequate secondary prevention of stroke may reduce the risk of recurrent stroke substantially even by 80%.[126] Anticoagulation alone in patients with atrial fibrillation reduces ischemic stroke recurrence by about two-thirds and antiplatelets in non-cardioembolic ischemic stroke approximately by one-fourth. Carotid endarterectomy, when indicated, must be performed early. All risk factors must be systematically searched and treated.

Home measurements of arterial blood pressure, blood sugar, and international normalized ratio are widely available and reliable. A major challenge is patient compliance in regular use of medications, but even more challenging is changing lifestyle habits and maintaining the improved lifestyles (cessation of smoking, alcohol abuse and illicit drug use, increased exercising, weight-control, implementing a diet rich in vegetables, salt restriction). These measures are effective in all stroke subtypes. So far, there is little evidence that long-term nursing staff-facilitated close follow-ups would improve maintaining secondary prevention.

START EARLY REHABILITATION

Following a stroke, approximately 50–70% of survivors will regain functional independence; however, 15–30% of patients will remain with serious permanent disabilities.[15] Early initiation of rehabilitation improves long-term recovery and may reduce mortality rates through decreased complications and recurrences.[127] Any patient with stroke should be mobilized as soon as considered safe by the treating physician. There are a number of situations in which mobilization is believed to carry a risk. Thrombolysis and thrombectomy are followed by immobilization for 24 hours. Hemodynamically unstable patients should be kept in bed until becoming stable. Patients with ICH require bed rest for at least 24 hours because of high risk of additional bleeding. Unstable cardiopulmonary status, coronary ischemia, and pulmonary embolism are typical contraindications to mobilization of a stroke patient, but respiratory insufficiency is usually not because the ventilatory function commonly improves with sitting and upright positions.

Most stroke patients will require various combinations of physiotherapy, occupational therapy, speech therapy, and neuropsychologic assessment. Working-aged patients should be investigated more thoroughly for ascertaining their working abilities and limitations. Majority of stroke patients will survive, but greatest health effects are the long-term consequences of stroke that can be diminished by early-initiated multidisciplinary rehabilitation. Recovery is a complex process including restitution, substitution, and compensation. Engaging the patient and the family is crucial as rehabilitation outcomes are strongly associated with patient motivation. Enhancing social coping and promoting integration into the community are better achieved by involving family members.

Stroke unit staff should make mid- and long-term plans including transfer to a rehabilitation unit, supported discharge, home care, and outpatient rehabilitation. Further, the length of sick leave, ability to drive, and other medicolegal issues need to be solved during the stroke unit care. Social workers are in key roles in most of these aspects. Stroke units should introduce novel rehabilitation methodologies such as constraint-induced movement therapies or robotics and work closely with regional rehabilitation facilities. Stroke units should have clear-cut contracts with regional health care providers that ensure timely transfer of patients to institutional or outpatient rehabilitation, discharge with home support, and continuum of secondary preventive measures.

Advanced age, neglect, depression, stroke severity, comorbidities, cognitive disorders, and lack of social support network are factors known to impair recovery. However, it is often difficult to estimate early which patients will regain their independence and make their way back home. Therefore, all but clearly hopeless patients should be treated actively and offered rehabilitation until a decision on the activity level of further rehabilitation can be reached. Stroke unit staff should have regular weekly meetings where each patient is discussed by the multidisciplinary team. Stroke information leaflets targeted to patients and relatives as well as nurse-led information sessions regularly organized in the stroke unit are well-received and highly appreciated by patients and relatives.

RECRUIT AS MANY PATIENTS AS POSSIBLE TO SCIENTIFIC PROJECTS INCLUDING RANDOMIZED CONTROLLED TRIALS

Progress in stroke care requires active research work along with high-quality education. All dedicated and prestigious stroke centers have enormous research output. Different stroke centers have different research profiles depending on their own interest and local conditions. Nevertheless, each stroke research center must ascertain that they have an active long-standing plan on scientific activities. There is clear evidence that patients involved with clinical research have better outcomes than those not involved in such research.[128] National networking such as the Canadian Stroke Network (www.canadianstrokenetwork.ca) help in improving routine patient care, promotes research, and may facilitate fund-raising. Multinational networks may even be more productive and are more competitive in terms of funding opportunities and having large sample sizes. Stroke unit lead should be well-connected nationally and internationally.

WHEN HOPE IS LOST, REMEMBER ORGAN DONATION

Despite the pleasing reduction in mortality rates during the last decades in all, but most prominently among ischemic stroke patients, a substantial portion of stroke patients will decease.[129] In SAH, 12% of all patients die before reaching medical attention[130] and over 40% within 1 month.[129] In ICH patients, 1-month mortality is approximately 40%.[129] Among ischemic stroke patients, early mortality is frequent in large MCA infarcts and basilar occlusion patients and is equal to 11% within 1 month.[129] All stroke patients, except some extreme cases, should be treated actively during the first few days including intensive unit-level care.[131] Do not resuscitate and withdrawal of care decisions should not be done hastily and when done should preferably by senior stroke physicians after meticulous consideration. Early do-not-resuscitate decisions may have an independent impact on mortality and lead to a self-fulfilling prophecy in individual patients.[132] These decisions must be written and described clearly and well-communicated to nursing staff and relatives of the patient. Unfortunately, most international guidelines on stroke care do not explicitly deal with do-not-resuscitate or withdrawal of care decisions.

Approximately 80% of organ donations are from patients with acute brain catastrophes leading to brain death[133] and over half come from stroke patients SAH being the dominant source. Currently, there are few absolute contraindications for donorship. Absolute contraindications are mainly transmissible diseases and target organ failure. Corneas are eligible for transplantation after death, whereas internal organs are eligible after brain death in hemodynamically stable patients without severe ongoing infections. Age is no longer an absolute contraindication. Organ donorship must be considered in all hopeless stroke patients. Stroke unit and neurointensive care physicians and nursing staff should be educated for transplantation matters periodically, a simple and concise transplantation folder as well as a contact person (transplantation coordinator) should be available at all times. By improving care pathways and awareness within institutions, the number of organ donations from brain death ICH patients could significantly increase.[134]

Further, how and where terminal care for hopeless patients should be arranged is a crucial question. If possible, terminal care should be given in the same department in a single room if it is judged that it is likely that the patient will decease within a few days.

CONCLUSIONS

Stroke unit care is highly evidence-based medicine. Stroke unit care is cost-effective and reduces the likelihood of death, disability, and the need for long-term institutional care. These benefits are not restricted to any special group of patients. All stroke patients who were independent before their index stroke, regardless of age, sex, severity or subtype of stroke, benefit from stroke unit care. The beneficial effect is long-standing for up to 5–10 years. Acute stroke care should take place in stroke units. Therefore, all stroke patients should be admitted to hospitals where acute treatments can be delivered on-site immediately on a 24/7 basis, except that if a patient's condition requires otherwise (e.g., intensive care unit or if explicitly clear that withdrawal of care is well-founded). Specialized stroke unit care possesses a number of interventions such as quick and thorough diagnostic work-up, maintenance of vital parameters, early prevention, recognition, and treatment of complications, introduction of early mobilization and full-scale rehabilitation leading to more favorable outcomes. Stroke units should also invest on continuous education and research activities.

REFERENCES

1. Stroke. Unit Trialists' Collaboration. Organised inpatient (stroke unit) care for stroke. Cochrane Database Syst Rev 2007;(4): CD000197.
2. Stroke Unit Trialists' Collaboration. Organised inpatient (stroke unit) care for stroke. Cochrane Database Syst Rev 2013;(9): CD000197.
3. Alberts MJ, Hademenos G, Latchaw RE, et al. Recommendations for the establishment of primary stroke centers. Brain Attack Coalition. JAMA 2000;283:3102–9.
4. Alberts MJ, Latchaw RE, Selman WR, et al. Recommendations for comprehensive stroke centers: A consensus statement from the Brain Attack Coalition. Stroke 2005;36:1597–616.
5. Leys D, Ringelstein EB, Kaste M, et al. The main components of stroke unit care: Results of a European expert survey. Cerebrovasc Dis 2007;23:344–52.
6. Ringelstein EB, Berlit P, Busse O, et al. Konzept der überregionalen und regionalen Schlaganfallversorgung in Deutschland. Fortschreibung der Empfehlungen der Kommission 1.06 "Stroke Units und akute Schlaganfalltherapie" der Deutschen Gesellschaft für Neurologie. Akt Neurol 2000;27:101–3.
7. Ringelstein EB, Grond M, Busse O. Time is brain – Competence is brain. Further development of a European stroke unit concept. Nervenarzt 2005;76:1024–7.
8. Engelter S, Lyrer P. Stroke Units in der Schweiz: Bedarfsanalyse, Richtlinien und Anforderungsprofil. Schweiz Medical Forum 2004;4:200–3.
9. Asplund K, Hulter Asberg K, Norrving B, et al. Riks-stroke – a Swedish national quality register for stroke care. Cerebrovasc Dis 2003;15(Suppl. 1):5–7.
10. Kjellstrom T, Norrving B, Shatchkute A. Helsingborg Declaration 2006 on European stroke strategies. Cerebrovasc Dis 2007;23: 231–41.
11. Leys D, Ringelstein EB, Kaste M, et al., Executive Committee of the European Stroke Initiative. Facilities available in European hospitals treating stroke patients. Stroke 2007;38:2985–91.
12. Johnston SC, Mendis S, Mathers CD. Global variation in stroke burden and mortality: estimates from monitoring, surveillance, and modelling. Lancet Neurol 2009;8:345–54.
13. Langhorne P, de Villiers L, Pandian JD. Applicability of stroke-unit care to low-income and middle-income countries. Lancet Neurol 2012;11:341–8.
14. Launois R, Giroud M, Megnigbeto AC, et al. Estimating the cost-effectiveness of stroke units in France compared with conventional care. Stroke 2004;35:770–5.
15. Schwamm LH, Pancioli A, Acker JE 3rd, et al. Recommendations for the establishment of stroke systems of care: recommendations from the American Stroke Association's Task Force on the Development of Stroke Systems. Stroke 2005;36: 690–703.
16. Ringelstein EB, Chamorro A, Kaste M, et al. European Stroke Organisation recommendations to establish a stroke unit and stroke center. Stroke 2013;44:828–40.
17. Libman RB, Wirkowski E, Alvir J, et al. Conditions that mimic stroke in the emergency department. Implications for acute stroke trials. Arch Neurol 1995;52:1119–22.
18. Huff JS. Stroke mimics and chameleons. Emerg Med Clin North Am 2002;20:583–95.
19. Zinkstok SM, Engelter ST, Gensicke H, et al. Safety of thrombolysis in stroke mimics: results from a multicenter cohort study. Stroke 2013;44:1080–4.
20. Dupre CM, Libman R, Dupre SI, et al. Stroke chameleons. J Stroke Cerebrovasc Dis 2014;23:374–8.
21. Adams HP Jr, Bendixen BH, Kappelle LJ, et al. Classification of subtype of acute ischemic stroke. Definitions for use in a multicenter clinical trial. TOAST. Trial of Org 10172 in Acute Stroke Treatment. Stroke 1993;24:35–41.
22. Ay H, Furie KL, Singhal A, et al. An evidence-based causative classification system for acute ischemic stroke. Ann Neurol 2005;58:688–97.
23. Amarenco P, Bogousslavsky J, Caplan LR, et al. The ASCOD phenotyping of ischemic stroke (Updated ASCO Phenotyping). Cerebrovasc Dis 2013;36:1–5.
24. Meretoja A, Strbian D, Putaala J, et al. SMASH-U: a proposal for etiologic classification of intracerebral hemorrhage. Stroke 2012; 43:2592–7.
25. Demchuk AM, Scott Burgin W, Christou I, et al. Thrombolysis in Brain Ischemia (TIBI) transcranial Doppler flow grades predict clinical severity, early recovery, and mortality in patients treated with intravenous tissue plasminogen activator. Stroke 2001;32: 89–93.
26. Burgin WS, Malkoff M, Felberg RA, et al. Transcranial doppler ultrasound criteria for recanalization after thrombolysis for middle cerebral artery stroke. Stroke 2000;31:1128–32.
27. Alexandrov AV, Felberg RA, Demchuk AM, et al. Deterioration following spontaneous improvement: Sonographic findings in patients with acutely resolving symptoms of cerebral ischemia. Stroke 2000;31:915–19.
28. Jansen O, Schellinger P, Fiebach J, et al. Early recanalisation in acute ischaemic stroke saves tissue at risk defined by MRI. Lancet 1999;353:2036–7.
29. Vahedi K, Hofmeijer J, Juettler E, et al. Early decompressive surgery in malignant infarction of the middle cerebral artery: a pooled analysis of three randomised controlled trials. Lancet Neurol 2007;6:215–22.
30. Reith J, Jørgensen HS, Pedersen PM, et al. Body temperature in acute stroke: Relation to stroke severity, infarct size, mortality, and outcome. Lancet 1996;347:422–5.
31. Schwarz S, Hafner K, Aschoff A, et al. Incidence and prognostic significance of fever following intracerebral hemorrhage. Neurology 2000;54:354–61.
32. Dorhout Mees SM, Luitse MJ, van den Bergh WM, et al. Fever after aneurysmal subarachnoid hemorrhage: relation with extent of hydrocephalus and amount of extravasated blood. Stroke 2008;39:2141–3.
33. Zhang G, Zhang JH, Qin X. Fever increased in-hospital mortality after subarachnoid hemorrhage. Acta Neurochir Suppl 2011;110: 239–43.
34. Fernandez A, Schmidt JM, Claassen J, et al. Fever after subarachnoid hemorrhage: risk factors and impact on outcome. Neurology 2007;68:1013–19.

35. Badjatia N, Fernandez L, Schmidt JM, et al. Impact of induced normothermia on outcome after subarachnoid hemorrhage: a case-control study. Neurosurgery 2010;66:696–700, discussion 700–1.
36. Piironen K, Tiainen M, Mustanoja S, et al. Mild hypothermia after intravenous thrombolysis in patients with acute stroke: a randomized controlled trial. Stroke 2014;45:486–91.
37. Kawai N, Keep RF, Betz AL. Hyperglycemia and the vascular effects of cerebral ischemia. Stroke 1997;28:149–54.
38. Kase CS, Furlan AJ, Wechsler LR. Symptomatic intracranial hemorrhage after intraarterial thrombolysis with recombinant prourokinase in acute ischemic stroke. Neurology 2000;54: A260–1.
39. Demchuk AM, Morgenstern LB, Krieger DW, et al. Serum glucose level and diabetes predict tissue plasminogen activator-related intracerebral hemorrhage in acute ischemic stroke. Stroke 1999; 30:34–9.
40. Strbian D, Engelter S, Michel P, et al. Symptomatic intracranial hemorrhage after stroke thrombolysis: the SEDAN score. Ann Neurol 2012;71:634–41.
41. Whiteley WN, Slot KB, Fernandes P, et al. Risk factors for intracranial hemorrhage in acute ischemic stroke patients treated with recombinant tissue plasminogen activator: a systematic review and meta-analysis of 55 studies. Stroke 2012;43:2904–9.
42. Paciaroni M, Agnelli G, Caso V, et al. Acute hyperglycemia and early hemorrhagic transformation in ischemic stroke. Cerebrovasc Dis 2009;28:119–23.
43. Toni D, De Michele M, Fiorelli M, et al. Influence of hyperglycaemia on infarct size and clinical outcome of acute ischemic stroke patients with intracranial arterial occlusion. J Neurol Sci 1994;123:129–33.
44. Capes SE, Hunt D, Malmberg K, et al. Stress hyperglycemia and prognosis of stroke in nondiabetic and diabetic patients: A systematic overview. Stroke 2001;32:2426–32.
45. Van Den Berghe G, Wouters P, Weekers F, et al. Intensive insulin therapy in critically ill patients. New Engl J Med 2001;345: 1359–67.
46. Pasternak JJ, McGregor DG, Schroeder DR, et al. Hyperglycemia in patients undergoing cerebral aneurysm surgery: its association with long-term gross neurologic and neuropsychological function. Mayo Clin Proc 2008;83:406–17.
47. Connolly ES Jr, Rabinstein AA, Carhuapoma JR, et al. Guidelines for the management of aneurysmal subarachnoid hemorrhage: a guideline for healthcare professionals from the American Heart Association/american Stroke Association. Stroke 2012;43: 1711–37.
48. Balami JS, Buchan AM. Complications of intracerebral haemorrhage. Lancet Neurol 2012;11:101–18.
49. Qureshi AI, Ezzeddine MA, Nasar A, et al. Prevalence of elevated blood pressure in 563,704 adult patients with stroke presenting to the ED in the United States. Am J Emerg Med 2007;25: 32–8.
50. Qureshi AI. Acute hypertensive response in patients with stroke: pathophysiology and management. Circulation 2008;118: 176–87.
51. Carlberg B, Asplund K, Hagg E. Factors influencing admission blood pressure levels in patients with acute stroke. Stroke 1991;22:527–30.
52. Jauch EC, Saver JL, Adams HP Jr, et al. Guidelines for the early management of patients with acute ischemic stroke: a guideline for healthcare professionals from the American Heart Association/ American Stroke Association. Stroke 2013;44:870–947.
53. Anderson CS, Heeley E, Huang Y, et al. Rapid Blood-Pressure Lowering in Patients with Acute Intracerebral Hemorrhage. N Engl J Med 2013;368:2355–65.
54. Ahmed N, Wahlgren N, Brainin M, et al. Relationship of blood pressure, antihypertensive therapy, and outcome in ischemic stroke treated with intravenous thrombolysis: retrospective analysis from Safe Implementation of Thrombolysis in Stroke-International Stroke Thrombolysis Register (SITS-ISTR). Stroke 2009;40:2442–9.
55. Kumar S, Selim MH, Caplan LR. Medical complications after stroke. Lancet Neurol 2010;9:105–18.
56. Balami JS, Chen RL, Grunwald IQ, et al. Neurological complications of acute ischaemic stroke. Lancet Neurol 2011;10:357–71.
57. Hacke W, Schwab S, Horn M, et al. 'Malignant' middle cerebral artery territory infarction: Clinical course and prognostic signs. Arch Neurol 1996;53:309–15.
58. Rieke K, Schwab S, Krieger D, et al. Decompressive surgery in space-occupying hemispheric infarction: Results of an open, prospective trial. Crit Care Med 1995;23:1576–87.
59. Krieger DW, Demchuk AM, Kasner SE, et al. Early clinical and radiological predictors of fatal brain swelling in ischemic stroke. Stroke 1999;30:287–92.
60. Juttler E, Unterberg A, Woitzik J, et al. Hemicraniectomy in older patients with extensive middle-cerebral-artery stroke. N Engl J Med 2014;370:1091–100.
61. Nogueira RG, Gupta R, Jovin TG, et al. Predictors and clinical relevance of hemorrhagic transformation after endovascular therapy for anterior circulation large vessel occlusion strokes: a multicenter retrospective analysis of 1122 patients. J Neurointerv Surg 2014;7(1):16–21.
62. Mustanoja S, Haapaniemi E, Putaala J, et al. Haemorrhagic transformation of ischaemic stroke in young adults. Int J Stroke 2014;9(Supple A100):85–92.
63. Strbian D, Sairanen T, Meretoja A, et al. Patient outcomes from symptomatic intracerebral hemorrhage after stroke thrombolysis. Neurology 2011;77:341–8.
64. Butzkueven H, Evans AH, Pitman A, et al. Onset seizures independently predict poor outcome after subarachnoid hemorrhage. Neurology 2000;55:1315–20.
65. Lin CL, Dumont AS, Lieu AS, et al. Characterization of perioperative seizures and epilepsy following aneurysmal subarachnoid hemorrhage. J Neurosurg 2003;99:978–85.
66. Dennis LJ, Claassen J, Hirsch LJ, et al. Nonconvulsive status epilepticus after subarachnoid hemorrhage. Neurosurgery 2002;51:1136–43, discussion 1144.
67. Bailey RD, Hart RG, Benavente O, et al. Recurrent brain hemorrhage is more frequent than ischemic stroke after intracranial hemorrhage. Neurology 2001;56:773–7.
68. Viswanathan A, Rakich SM, Engel C, et al. Antiplatelet use after intracerebral hemorrhage. Neurology 2006;66:206–9.
69. Pakarinen S. Incidence, aetiology, and prognosis of primary subarachnoid haemorrhage. A study based on 589 cases diagnosed in a defined urban population during a defined period. Acta Neurol Scand 1967;43(Suppl. 29):1–28.
70. Phillips LH 2nd, Whisnant JP, O'Fallon WM, et al. The unchanging pattern of subarachnoid hemorrhage in a community. Neurology 1980;30:1034–40.
71. Molyneux A, Kerr R, Stratton I, et al. International Subarachnoid Aneurysm Trial (ISAT) of neurosurgical clipping versus endovascular coiling in 2143 patients with ruptured intracranial aneurysms: a randomised trial. Lancet 2002;360:1267–74.
72. Ferrari J, Knoflach M, Kiechl S, et al. Early clinical worsening in patients with TIA or minor stroke: the Austrian Stroke Unit Registry. Neurology 2010;74:136–41.
73. Inouye SK. Delirium in older persons. N Engl J Med 2006;354: 1157–65.
74. Shi Q, Presutti R, Selchen D, et al. Delirium in acute stroke: a systematic review and meta-analysis. Stroke 2012;43: 645–9.
75. Jacobson S, Jerrier H. EEG in delirium. Semin Clin Neuropsychiatry 2000;5:86–92.
76. Camus V, Gonthier R, Dubos G, et al. Etiologic and outcome profiles in hypoactive and hyperactive subtypes of delirium. J Geriatr Psychiatry Neurol 2000;13:38–42.
77. Inouye SK, van Dyck CH, Alessi CA, et al. Clarifying confusion: the confusion assessment method. A new method for detection of delirium. Ann Intern Med 1990;113:941–8.
78. Trzepacz PT, Baker RW, Greenhouse J. A symptom rating scale for delirium. Psychiatry Res 1988;23:89–97.
79. Inouye SK, Bogardus ST Jr, Charpentier PA, et al. A multicomponent intervention to prevent delirium in hospitalized older patients. N Engl J Med 1999;340:669–76.
80. Ayerbe L, Ayis S, Crichton S, et al. The natural history of depression up to 15 years after stroke: the South London Stroke Register. Stroke 2013;44:1105–10.
81. Hackett ML, Anderson CS. Predictors of depression after stroke: a systematic review of observational studies. Stroke 2005;36: 2296–301.

82. House A, Dennis M, Mogridge L, et al. Mood disorders in the year after first stroke. Br J Psychiatry 1991;158:83–92.
83. Meader N, Moe-Byrne T, Llewellyn A, et al. Screening for post-stroke major depression: a meta-analysis of diagnostic validity studies. J Neurol Neurosurg Psychiatry 2014;85:198–206.
84. Benaim C, Cailly B, Perennou D, et al. Validation of the aphasic depression rating scale. Stroke 2004;35:1692–6.
85. Turner-Stokes L, Kalmus M, Hirani D, et al. The Depression Intensity Scale Circles (DISCs): a first evaluation of a simple assessment tool for depression in the context of brain injury. J Neurol Neurosurg Psychiatry 2005;76:1273–8.
86. Hackett ML, Anderson CS, House A, et al. Interventions for treating depression after stroke. Cochrane Database Syst Rev 2008;(4):CD003437.
87. Chen Y, Patel NC, Guo JJ, et al. Antidepressant prophylaxis for poststroke depression: a meta-analysis. Int Clin Psychopharmacol 2007;22:159–66.
88. Chollet F, Tardy J, Albucher JF, et al. Fluoxetine for motor recovery after acute ischaemic stroke (FLAME): a randomised placebo-controlled trial. Lancet Neurol 2011;10:123–30.
89. Hackam DG, Mrkobrada M. Selective serotonin reuptake inhibitors and brain hemorrhage: a meta-analysis. Neurology 2012;79: 1862–5.
90. Huang WY, Weng WC, Peng TI, et al. Association of hyponatremia in acute stroke stage with three-year mortality in patients with first-ever ischemic stroke. Cerebrovasc Dis 2012;34:55–62.
91. Gariballa SE, Robinson TG, Fotherby MD. Hypokalemia and potassium excretion in stroke patients. J Am Geriatr Soc 1997;45:1454–8.
92. Rahman M, Friedman WA. Hyponatremia in neurosurgical patients: clinical guidelines development. Neurosurgery 2009;65: 925–35, discussion 935–6.
93. Touze E, Varenne O, Chatellier G, et al. Risk of myocardial infarction and vascular death after transient ischemic attack and ischemic stroke: a systematic review and meta-analysis. Stroke 2005;36:2748–55.
94. Putaala J, Curtze S, Hiltunen S, et al. Causes of death and predictors of 5-year mortality in young adults after first-ever ischemic stroke: the Helsinki Young Stroke Registry. Stroke 2009;40: 2698–703.
95. Prosser J, MacGregor L, Lees KR, et al. Predictors of early cardiac morbidity and mortality after ischemic stroke. Stroke 2007;38:2295–302.
96. Calvet D, Song D, Yoo J, et al. Predicting Asymptomatic Coronary Artery Diseasein Patients With Ischemic Stroke and Transient Ischemic Attack: The PRECORIS Score. Stroke 2014;45: 82–6.
97. Putaala J, Lehto M, Meretoja A, et al. In-hospital cardiac complications after intracerebral hemorrhage. Int J Stroke 2014;9: 741–6.
98. Frontera JA, Parra A, Shimbo D, et al. Cardiac arrhythmias after subarachnoid hemorrhage: risk factors and impact on outcome. Cerebrovasc Dis 2008;26:71–8.
99. Roth EJ, Lovell L, Harvey RL, et al. Incidence of and risk factors for medical complications during stroke rehabilitation. Stroke 2001;32:523–9.
100. Lee VH, Connolly HM, Fulgham JR, et al. Tako-tsubo cardiomyopathy in aneurysmal subarachnoid hemorrhage: an underappreciated ventricular dysfunction. J Neurosurg 2006;105: 264–70.
101. Yoshimura S, Toyoda K, Ohara T, et al. Takotsubo cardiomyopathy in acute ischemic stroke. Ann Neurol 2008;64:547–54.
102. Kilbourn KJ, Levy S, Staff I, et al. Clinical characteristics and outcomes of neurogenic stress cadiomyopathy in aneurysmal subarachnoid hemorrhage. Clin Neurol Neurosurg 2013;115: 909–14.
103. Porto I, Della Bona R, Leo A, et al. Stress cardiomyopathy (takotsubo) triggered by nervous system diseases: a systematic review of the reported cases. Int J Cardiol 2013;167:2441–8.
104. Westendorp WF, Nederkoorn PJ, Vermeij JD, et al. Post-stroke infection: a systematic review and meta-analysis. BMC Neurol 2011;11:110-2377-11-110.
105. Finlayson O, Kapral M, Hall R, et al. Risk factors, inpatient care, and outcomes of pneumonia after ischemic stroke. Neurology 2011;77:1338–45.
106. Martino R, Foley N, Bhogal S, et al. Dysphagia after stroke: incidence, diagnosis, and pulmonary complications. Stroke 2005;36: 2756–63.
107. Chamorro A, Horcajada JP, Obach V, et al. The Early Systemic Prophylaxis of Infection After Stroke study: a randomized clinical trial. Stroke 2005;36:1495–500.
108. Poisson SN, Johnston SC, Josephson SA. Urinary tract infections complicating stroke: mechanisms, consequences, and possible solutions. Stroke 2010;41:e180–4.
109. Stott DJ, Falconer A, Miller H, et al. Urinary tract infection after stroke. QJM 2009;102:243–9.
110. Maki DG, Tambyah PA. Engineering out the risk for infection with urinary catheters. Emerg Infect Dis 2001;7:342–7.
111. Cowey E, Smith LN, Booth J, et al. Urinary catheterization in acute stroke: clinical realities. A mixed methods study. Clin Rehabil 2012;26:470–9.
112. Gokula RM, Smith MA, Hickner J. Emergency room staff education and use of a urinary catheter indication sheet improves appropriate use of foley catheters. Am J Infect Control 2007;35: 589–93.
113. Topal J, Conklin S, Camp K, et al. Prevention of nosocomial catheter-associated urinary tract infections through computerized feedback to physicians and a nurse-directed protocol. Am J Med Qual 2005;20:121–6.
114. Geeganage C, Beavan J, Ellender S, et al. Interventions for dysphagia and nutritional support in acute and subacute stroke. Cochrane Database Syst Rev 2012;(10):CD000323.
115. Finestone HM, Greene-Finestone LS, Foley NC, et al. Measuring longitudinally the metabolic demands of stroke patients: resting energy expenditure is not elevated. Stroke 2003;34:502–7.
116. Foley NC, Martin RE, Salter KL, et al. A review of the relationship between dysphagia and malnutrition following stroke. J Rehabil Med 2009;41:707–13.
117. Brandstater ME, Roth EJ, Siebens HC. Venous thromboembolism in stroke: literature review and implications for clinical practice. Arch Phys Med Rehabil 1992;73:S379–91.
118. Kelly J, Rudd A, Lewis RR, et al. Venous thromboembolism after acute ischemic stroke: a prospective study using magnetic resonance direct thrombus imaging. Stroke 2004;35:2320–5.
119. CLOTS (Clots in Legs Or sTockings after Stroke) Trials Collaboration. Effectiveness of intermittent pneumatic compression in reduction of risk of deep vein thrombosis in patients who have had a stroke (CLOTS 3): a multicentre randomised controlled trial. Lancet 2013;382:516–24.
120. Steiner T, Juvela S, Unterberg A, et al. European Stroke Organization guidelines for the management of intracranial aneurysms and subarachnoid haemorrhage. Cerebrovasc Dis 2013;35: 93–112.
121. Heros RC. Acute hydrocephalus after subarachnoid hemorrhage. Stroke 1989;20:715–17.
122. Bota DP, Lefranc F, Vilallobos HR, et al. Ventriculostomy-related infections in critically ill patients: a 6-year experience. J Neurosurg 2005;103:468–72.
123. Huttner HB, Schwab S, Bardutzky J. Lumbar drainage for communicating hydrocephalus after ICH with ventricular hemorrhage. Neurocrit Care 2006;5:193–6.
124. Vergouwen MD, Vermeulen M, van Gijn J, et al. Definition of delayed cerebral ischemia after aneurysmal subarachnoid hemorrhage as an outcome event in clinical trials and observational studies: proposal of a multidisciplinary research group. Stroke 2010;41:2391–5.
125. Dorhout Mees SM, Rinkel GJ, Feigin VL, et al. Calcium antagonists for aneurysmal subarachnoid haemorrhage. Cochrane Database Syst Rev 2007;(3):CD000277.
126. Rantanen K, Tatlisumak T. Secondary prevention of ischemic stroke. Curr Drug Targets 2004;5:457–72.
127. Diserens K, Moreira T, Hirt L, et al. Early mobilization out of bed after ischaemic stroke reduces severe complications but not cerebral blood flow: a randomized controlled pilot trial. Clin Rehabil 2012;26:451–9.
128. Concato J, Shah N, Horwitz RI. Randomized, controlled trials, observational studies, and the hierarchy of research designs. N Engl J Med 2000;342:1887–92.
129. Lackland DT, Roccella EJ, Deutsch AF, et al. Factors influencing the decline in stroke mortality: a statement from the American

Heart Association/American Stroke Association. Stroke 2014;45:315–53.

130. Huang J, van Gelder JM. The probability of sudden death from rupture of intracranial aneurysms: a meta-analysis. Neurosurgery 2002;51:1101–5, discussion 1105–7.

131. Morgenstern LB, Hemphill JC 3rd, Anderson C, et al. Guidelines for the management of spontaneous intracerebral hemorrhage: a guideline for healthcare professionals from the American Heart Association/American Stroke Association. Stroke 2010;41:2108–29.

132. Silvennoinen K, Meretoja A, Strbian D, et al. Do-not-resuscitate (DNR) orders in patients with intracerebral hemorrhage. Int J Stroke 2014;9:53–8.

133. Salih MA, Harvey I, Frankel S, et al. Potential availability of cadaver organs for transplantation. BMJ 1991;302:1053–5.

134. Sairanen T, Koivisto A, Koivusalo AM, et al. Lost potential of kidney and liver donors amongst deceased intracerebral hemorrhage patients. Eur J Neurol 2014;21:153–9.

54 Critical Care of the Patient with Acute Stroke

Marek Sykora, Silvia Schönenberger, Julian Bösel

KEY POINTS

- Mechanical ventilation and sedation in acute stroke
- Brain edema and increased intracranial pressure
- Blood pressure and blood glucose management
- Targeting hematoma growth
- Neuromonitoring
- Hypothermia.
- Large Middle Cerebral Artery Stroke
- Basilar Artery Occlusion
- Large Cerebellar Infarction
- Medical Treatment of Intracerebral hemorrhage
- Cerebral Venous Thrombosis

GENERAL PRINCIPLES OF NEUROLOGIC CRITICAL CARE

Initial Assessment of Patients with Stroke

Initial clinical assessment of patients with severe stroke should concentrate on the following issues:

1. Vital functions (pulmonary function, heart rate, blood pressure)
2. Neurologic symptoms, severity of neurologic deficit based on validated stroke scales
3. Time of symptom onset, potential eligibility for specific treatment options
4. Blood sampling for electrolytes, full blood count, and coagulation studies.

One should always bear in mind that most emergency measures depend on the cause of the stroke (ischemic versus hemorrhagic). Thus, it is vital that appropriate neuroimaging studies not be unnecessarily delayed. Additionally, caution is warranted to avoid measures that have the potential to interfere with further treatment options (for example, insertion of a central venous line in a patient eligible for thrombolysis).

Ancillary Tests

Diagnostic studies and their indication in stroke patients are discussed in detail elsewhere in this book. As a general rule, the need for further diagnostics has to be weighted carefully against the potential risk that in-house transportations bear for the critically ill. These procedures usually require disconnection from the ventilator to a transportable ventilator or those suitable for the use in MRI scanners, which may not be tolerated easily by patients with severe pulmonary dysfuntion. Moreover, monitoring is not as good as on the intensive care unit and the options for intervention during critcal situations may be limited. Before transportation of a critically ill patient, one should always question the therapeutic consequences that are likely to be drawn from the results. If there are no consequences, one should resign from the procedure. Diagnostic procedures that do not require transportation of the patient should be preferred. Optimal neuro-monitoring as will be described later in the chapter may help to reduce the need for imaging scans.

If a diagnostic or therapeutic procedure requiring transportation of the patient cannot be avoided, careful preparation is obligatory. The physician has to decide about the medications that may be discontinued and the adequate monitoring that has to be taken along; catheters need to be fixed properly; extraventricular drainages should be closed during transportation to avoid overdrainage. Emergency medication should be taken along and unnecessary delays should be avoided. Deeper sedation frequently becomes necessary for transportation and to allow acquisition of diagnostic studies of acceptable quality. One should bear in mind, however, that the clinical evaluation of the patient may be markedly limited therafter; short-acting sedatives should be preferred. All patients with severe stroke have to be accompanied by a physician or trained physician-extender during all diagnostic procedures.

Clinical Examinations

Neuro-intensive care patients should have a complete clinical examination at least three times per day. Because of analogo-sedation, the neurological exam frequently is restricted to evaluation of pupillary and brainstem reflexes, motor reaction upon painful stimuli, reflex status and pathologic reflexes. Particularly, signs of raised intracranial pressure (ICP) and transtentorial hernation such as sequential loss of brainstem reflexes have to be recognized immediately. New motor deficts or pathologic reflexes may indicate enlargement of infarction or vasospasm in subarachnoid hemorrhage (SAH) patients. Changes in ventilator settings as the need to switch from assisted ventilation to fully controlled mechanical ventilaton under stable levels of sedation may indicate loss of brainstem function. Auscultation of heart and lung, palpation and auscultation of the abomen and careful inspection of the patient (edema, signs of dehydration, skin lesions, wounds) complete the clinical exam. Additionally, ventilator settings, blood gas analyses, laboratory parameters, temperature, urine excretion and central venous pressure have to be reviewed regularly by the attending physicians.

Pulmonary Function and Mechanical Ventilation

Maintenance of adequate oxygenation is essential in patients with acute stroke and hypoxia could be deleterious for the ischemic penumbra. Avoidance of hypercapnia is of equal importance, as it potentially leads to vasodilation in the cerebral arterioles supplying healthy brain tissue, thereby reducing blood supply to the lesion site, where cerebral vessels are already maximally dilated under resting conditions. The need to secure the airway and mechanically ventilate a patient with severe stroke may be one of the main reasons, if not the main one, to transfer this patient from the stroke unit to the neurointensive care unit (NICU). Several publications in the 90s have suggested that cerebrovascular patients requiring mechanical ventilation have a very bad prognosis and questioned its usefulness[1–6] while other studies indicated that a considerable part of these, even long-term ventilated, patients may have a good outcome. [7,8] Of note, mechanical ventilation in these studies was almost invariably an indicator of illness severity only and less often looked at with regard to the details of its application. Today, with evidence from several studies that treatment on specialized NICUs improves outcome, with more treatment options for cerebrovascular patients, as well as advances in ventilation techniques, the only justifications to withold these live-saving procedures from neurocritical stroke patients appears to be obvious futility or the patient's explicit will. Since the further course and eventual outcome are often unclear in the acute phase of the disease, the physician in charge should initiate airway management and ventilation without delay. Although standard, basic principles of airway and ventilation management from the general ICU can mostly be applied to the NICU patient as well, the NICU stroke patient merits some more specific considerations.

There are distinct neurologic disease-related causes of respiratory failure to be aware of. All sorts of severe cerebraovascular compromise of the central nervous system, i.e., supra- and infratentorial acute ischemic (AIS) or hemorrhagic stroke, SAH or cerebral venous and sinus thrombosis (CVST) and their sequelae, such as hydrocephalus and/or increased ICP, can cause respiratory failure. The complex connections between the central respiratory centers, i.e., the cortex and the autonomic centers in pons and medulla, as well as their connections to the phrenic nerve and the upper motor neurons can be affected on every level. This does not necessarily (only) result in loss of respiratory drive or respiratory rhythm, but also might cause loss of protective airway reflexes and airway patency, and thus impair ventilation. Major reasons for intubation and ventilation in stroke patients are decline in level of consciousness, loss in glossopharyngeal muscle tone, or loss of protective reflexes and dysphagia with consequently impending or occurred aspiration (Box 54-1). Specific patterns of pathologic breathing (e.g. Cheyne-Stokes, Cluster, Biot) have been suggested for topographic diagnosis of lesion levels. However, the correlation seems to be less consistent in clinical reality.

During the course of the disease, however, respiratory function can be further compromised by the development of various pathologic conditions, including hypoventilation-associated atelectasis or pneumonia due to immobilization, decreased level of consciousness, epileptic seizures, critical illness polyneuropathy, and stroke-related immunosuppression. The percentage of unselected patients with stroke who have to undergo mechanical ventilation has been reported as 10%.[6] Significant differences in rate of mechanical ventilation have been found to be related to the cause of stroke; Mayer and associates reported that 5% of patients with ischemic stroke, 26% of patients with intracerebral hemorrhage (ICH), and 47% of patients with SAH underwent mechanical ventilation,[6] whereas Gujjar and colleagues found rates of 6% for ischemic stroke and 30% for ICH.[9] In 54 out of 218 patients with AIS who needed mechanical ventilation, Berrouschot et al. found that 90% had to be ventilated for neurological deterioration and 10% for cardiopupmonary compromise.[2] Intubation of stroke patient has hardly been investigated[10, 11] with regard to the timing and technique itself. Clinical signs of impending respiratory failure are tachypnea exceeding 35 breaths per minute, dyspnea with use of accessory muscles, sweating and paradoxical breathing. Transcutaneous pulse oximetry for assessing arterial saturation of oxygen ($SatO_2$) constitutes the minimal requirement for monitoring of pulmonary function. Enhanced intermittent arterial blood sampling for blood gas analysis is recommended in suspected respiratory compromise. Intubation should be undertaken as soon as clinical signs of pulmonary dysfunction or aspiration risk are present or $SatO_2$ drops below 90% despite O_2-application via face mask, PaO_2 values drop below 60 mmHg, $PaCO_2$ values exceed 60 mmHg, or both (Box 54-2). The principles of non-invasive airway support by head positioning, airway clearing and application of nasal prongs or an oronasal mask for O_2 insufflation, and possibly the insertion of oro/nasopharyngeal airways, apply to almost all stroke patients with respiratory deterioration in the beginning and might be followed by intubation later. For patients with less severe stroke these non-invasive measures might suffice and be followed by non-invasive ventilation (i.e., BiPAP). It has to be confirmed regularly, however, whether these patients are still awake, cooperative, not respiratorily exhausted and have not lost their airway protective reflexes or developed other indications for intubation. Otherwise rapid initiation of the latter is warranted.

Orotracheal intubation is the approach of first choice because it enables the use of larger-diameter tubes, avoids the tube contamination that occurs during passage of oronasal tubes, and is associated with a lower prevalence of maxillary sinusitis.[12,13] Intubation almost always involves an episode of hypotension or at least variance in blood pressure. This can be detrimental in cerebrovascular disease in case of impaired cerebral autoregulation and subsequent decreased cerebral perfusion pressure (CPP). Hypotension during pharmacological induction for intubation is more common in patients with more severe underlying disease, a baseline MAP < 70 mmHg, age > 50 years and with use of propofol or increasing doses of fentanyl as inductor drugs.[14] Therefore, the less vascular-active etomidate might be more appropriate for

BOX 54-1 Mechanisms of Central Respiratory Failure

IMPAIRED RESPIRATORY DRIVE

Lesions to pons or medulla
Brainstem compression by raised intracranial ICP/herniation
Neurotransmitter imbalance/diffuse brain dysfunction
Sympathetic overdrive

IMPAIRED AIRWAY AND VENTILATORY CONTROL

Lesions to brainstem swallowing centers, dysphagia, loss of glossopharyngeal muscle tone
Lesions to reticular formation/bilateral thalami/large hemispheric lesions/hydrocephalus with subsequent coma and loss of protective airway reflexes
Vomiting, dysphagia, aspiration
Neurogenic pulmonary edema

IMPAIRED VENTILATION MECHANICS

High (above C3–C5) spinal ischemia, reducing ventilatory force to accessory neck muscles

BOX 54-2 Indications for Mechanical Ventilation

PO_2 < 70 mm Hg despite O_2 administration via nasal probe or facial mask
PCO_2 > 60 mm Hg (except for patients with chronic obstructive airway disease and chronically elevated CO_2)
Vital capacity <500–600 mL
Clinical signs of respiratory failure (tachypnea, use of accessory muscles)
Severe respiratory acidosis
Airway protection (gag and swallowing reflexes absent, level of consciousness decreased)

induction in cerebrovascular patients, it can be accompanied by fasciculations that should not be taken for seizures. Ketamine as an alternative induction agent was suggested to be associated with increases in ICP, but this was not confirmed in several studies that followed, in fact, in many of these studies it was shown to decrease ICP. Contrary to other sedatives, ketamine does not have depressing but activating circulatory effects. It can thus cause tachycardia and hypertension and should not be used in patients already in the upper ranges of these parameters. The concept of rapid sequence induction commonly used in non-fasting patients, involves the rapidly acting muscular blocker succinylcholine for excellent intubation conditions (i.e., glottis wide open). The depolarizing succinylcholine has been reported to induce small, but at times (e.g., in traumatic brain injury (TBI)) relevant ICP increases and can cause rhabdomyolysis and hyperkalemia in patients with seizures or post-immobilization. As the non-depolarizing muscular blocker rocuronium has been found only little inferior (i.e., comparable) to succinylcholine in a recent Cochrane analysis of almost 40 good-quality studies on the subject,[15] we prefer rocuronium for rapid sequence induction (RSI) in neurocritically ill stroke patients or avoid muscular blockers at all. Any drugs used for intubation should preferably be short-acting. Continuous infusion of sedatives and analgesics is warranted for the duration of mechanical ventilation. Further details on sedation and analgesia are given in the next section of this chapter.

A group of stroke patients increasingly often intubated in the first hours of their disease is that with acute ischemic large vessel stroke recieving endovascular revascularization. Most interventionalists prefer to have these patients intubated and put on general aesthesia for several (unproven) technical and safety reasons.[16] A few retrospective studies, however, have suggested that it is more beneficial not to intubate these patients (instead conscious sedation), as the intubated state was associated with more complications and higher mortality,[17-19] possibly owing to time delay, hypotension, and inadvertent hyperventilation with subsequent detrimental vasoconstriction in the penumbra.

Optimal ventilation management in stroke patients has not been clarified. The choice of ventilation modes and parameter settings should follow general principles. The following table (Box 54-3) contains suggestions for initial ventilator settings that have to be adjusted according to the clinical state and blood gas analysis results in the further course.

Oxygenation is the main goal of mechanical ventilation to provide the essential brain nutrient besides glucose. It is important to aim for tissue oxygenation and not for arbitrary levels of oxygen in the blood, however. Toxic levels of oxygen ($FiO_2 > 0.6$) in patients that are not hypoxemic should be avoided. Not only is there ample evidence that hyperoxia is associated with tissue damage resulating from free oxygen radical formation, lipid peroxidation and other mechanisms. It might also impede brain perfusion by a not completely understood process called hyperoxia-related cerebral vasoconstriction that may counterbalance and thus abolish the gain in blood oxygenation or might theoretically even lead to secondary ischemia.[20,21] It thus seems reasonable to aim for normoxemia but not more. Improving oxygenation is not limited to increasing FiO_2 or aggressiveness of ventilation, but can also be achieved by reducing cerebral oxygen demand by reducing work of breathing, treating infections and fever, fight agitation, delirium, and shivering, use anticonvulsants in seizures and/or employ certain sedatives that reduce the cerebral metabolic rate of oxygen ($CMRO_2$). Normocarbia may be an even more impoartant aim to strive for in the NICU patient, as $PaCO_2$ plays such a prominent role to influence cerebral blood flow (CBF) via pH changes in both directions, as long as cerebral autoregulation is intact (which is often not the case in brain-lesioned patients but difficult to determine). Both hypercarbia, with subsequent fall in pH, cerebral vasodilation, increase in CBF, and rise in ICP, and hypocarbia, with subsequent rise in pH, cerebral vasoconstriction, and decrease in CBF, increase the risk of secondary ischemia. This might be detrimental, depending on the extent and duration of the derangement, the specific neurological disease and the stage it is at (acute vs subacute). Changes in $PaCO_2$ may have very different implications for an SAH patient with vasopasm than for an AIS patient with brain edema. The concept of lung-protective ventilation with permissive hypercarbia as part of treating acute respiratory distress syndrome (ARDS) may be problematic in brain-injured patients and neuromonitoring should be installed if this is performed. Hyperventilation may be used transiently to induce hypocarbia and high pH to bring down raised ICP rapidly. However, if applied chronically or prophylactically, it may be associated with higher morbidity and mortality in TBI patients[22,23] or with cerebral ischemia in SAH and ICH patients.[24] The application of increased positive end-expiratory pressure (PEEP) might theoretically cause raised intrathoracic pressure with subsequently reduced venous return from the brain and thus increased ICP. Alternatively or additionally, reduced cardiac output and reduced mean arterial pressure (MAP) (see above, in itself potentially detrimentral via reduced CPP) can lead to raised ICP indirectly via reductions on CBF and brain oxygenation. However, the individual patient's ICP reaction to raised PEEP seems to vary greatly, possibly according to their lung and ventricular compliance, those with normal or poor pulmonary compliance seem not to show relevant ICP crises (TBI and SAH[25]). In patients with NICU-dependent stroke, raised PEEP did not transduce into significant ICP changes (but reductions in MAP and thus CPP).[26] Also, PEEP can be absolutely necessary to achieve adequate oxygenation which is the primary prerequisite for brain integrity and should not be subordinated to potential changes in ICP. Furthermore, no increase in mortality has been linked to the use of PEEP in brain-injured patients so far. In essence, higher PEEP should not be withheld from NICU stroke patients that are in need of improved oxygenation. However, neuromonitoring should be installed in these patients to detect changes in ICP and thus CPP and be able to take measures to achieve a reasonable compromise, as by raising MAP.

Changing the I:E ratio to 1:1 or even higher to improve oxygenation has also been thought to reduce venous return from the brain and raise ICP. Studies in ventilated patients with ischemic stroke, intracerebral hemorrhage and TBI have not confirmed this.[27-29] Pre-existing pulmonary disorders such as chronic obstructive pulmonary disease (COPD), pneumonia or the development of ARDS may require more invasive ventilator settings. Lung-protective strategies comprise the application of low tidal volume, low inspiratory pressure and sufficiently high PEEP levels[30] and should be applied in stroke

BOX 54-3 Initial Ventilator Settings

FiO_2 <0.6
Vt 6 ml/kg of ideal (=predicted) body weight (IBW):
IBW male = 50 + (2.3 × (height in inches − 60))
IBW female = 45.5 + (2.3 × (height in inches − 60))
RR < 35/min
PEEP 5–7 cmH_2O
P plat <30 cmH_2O
I:E 1:2

patients as well, although data suggest that this is neglected when compared to other ventilated NICU patients.[31]

Theoretically, higher PEEP levels result in higher intrathoracic pressure and reduced venous return and thereby may promote an increased ICP. Moreover, the PEEP could affect cerebral perfusion pressure (CPP) by lowering MAP. In a recent study in SAH patients, stepwise elevation of PEEP to 20 cmH_2O (14.7 mmHg) resulted in an increase in central venous pressure and a significant decrease of MAP and regional cerebral blood flow.[32] However, reduction of cerebral blood flow depended on mean arterial pressure changes as a result of disturbed cerebrovascular autoregulation and normalization of MAP restored regional cerebral blood flow to baseline values. Likewise, PEEP levels up to 12 mmHg did not increase ICP in patients with acute stroke.[26] Equally, it was shown that alterations of the I:E ratio from 1:2 to 1:1 do not influence ICP or CPP, and could therefore be readily applied in patients with acute stroke.[27] In summary, PEEP application seems to be safe; provided that MAP is maintained. However, monitoring of MAP, ICP and CPP is desirable.

Weaning from the ventilator should not be delayed in NICU stroke patients, even if they are still comatose. The best method of weaning, i.e., continuous vs discontinuous, is unclear (as in general ICU patients). Discontinuous weaning methods, however, involve successive spontaneous breathing trials and thus wake-up trials. These have been found to be associated with a release of stress hormones[33] and rises in ICP in brain-injured patients, particularly those with a higher ICP from the outset.[34] In a small randomized pilot study in ventilated patients with severe stroke, patients weaned by a gradual weaning method employing the ASV mode had a shorter duration of ventilation (Teismann, Dziewas, et al. Poster ANIM 2013).

Extubation can only be considered in patients that are respiratorily re-constituted and are cardiocirculatorily stable. A central problem, however, is that classical extubation criteria involve having an awake and cooperative patient, something rarely encountered in the NICU where patients might present with aphasia, anarthria, apraxia, agitation, delirium or reduced level of consciousness, depending on their brain lesion. Classical extubation criteria (see above) have failed to predict extubation failures in NICU patients, which occur far more often than in non-neurological ICU patients, at a rate of 15–35% in patients with cerebrovascular brain lesions.[35-37] However, to delay extubation in NICU patients for not meeting classical extubation criteria, especially the one regarding consciousness, leads to complications, such as more ventilator-associated pneumonias (VAPs) and prolonged ICU-length of stay (LOS), while earlier or later extubated patents do not seem to differ with regard to the re-intubation rate.[38] Coma should not be the only reason to withhold weaning or extubation from these patients. Rather, particular attention should be paid to presence of dysphagia, which is much more frequent in the NICU population.[39] Endoscopic swallowing tests that do not necessarily involve cooperation from the patient have been successfully applied in stroke patients and might help to guide the extubation decision in other NICU patients.[40]

While 10–15% of ICU patients receive a tracheostomy during their stay, this rate is about 35% in NICU patients.[41] This may reflect the fact that neurological ICU patients often are not compromised with regard to their pulmonary function, but rather to their capacity to protect the airway and handle secretions. The question of the optimal time to tracheostomize patients with severe stroke has hardly been studied.[42] A retrospective study suggested that among ICU patients, the neurological/neurosurgical ones were those fastest to be weaned from the ventilator.[43] Two retrospective studies investigated predictors of tracheostomy need in ICH and found ganglionic location, hematoma volume, hydrocephalus, midline-shift, GCS and presence of COPD as predictors.[44,45] The optimal time point for tracheostomy was restrospectively investigated in cerebrovascular patients,[8,46] the studies suggesting that duration of ventilation and ICU-LOS was reduced in patients recieving earlier tracheostomy. This could not be confirmed in the only prospective randomized trial on early tracheostomy (up to day 3 vs days 7–14 from intubation) in ventilated NICU stroke patients.[47] However, the study showed that early tracheostomy is safe, feasible and reduces sedative demand.

Until the potential benefits of early tracheostomy in NICU patients are clarified in larger prospective trials, it is probably reasonable to proceed to tracheostomy as part of a weaning protocol if extubation trials failed or were deemed not feasible, i.e., the patient appears to require mechanical ventilation for more than 1 week.

Sedation and Analgesia

All patients treated in the ICU are exposed to various stress factors, including anxiety, unfamiliar auditory and visual stimuli, awareness of severe illness, and sleep disturbances, and stroke patients are no exception. Medical conditions such as pain, respiratory insufficiency, cardiovascular impairment, and sepsis constitute further stress factors; the most important of these might be mechanical ventilation via an orotracheal tube. However, invasive therapeutic or diagnostic procedures can be equally stressful and are often not feasible without proper analgesia and sedation. Inadequate sedation and analgesia can cause agitation and combativeness, which results in greater metabolic rate and oxygen consumption, potentially further endangering the ischemic penumbra. General goals of analgesia and sedation are freedom from pain, anxiety and agitation. In stroke patients requiring NICU treatment, some more specific goals have to be added, these comprise preservation of CPP, reduction of ICP, compensation of disturbed autoregulation, avoidance of seizures, the option of neurological examination and the prevention of prolonged coma and delirium, the latter of which brain-injured NICU patients are particularly prone to. Risks of sedation and analgesia are circulatory compromise, immunosuppression, GIT-disorders, deep vein thrombosis and pulmonary embolism, critical illness neuropathy and myopathy, prolonged coma and delirium. Therefore the daily goal must be to reduce or even discontinue sedation, if the cerebral lesion allows this. It is important not to use sedatives to treat conditions that have to be treated more specifically in other ways, such as pain, seizures, fever, infections, or psychological disorders.

Sedation in the general ICU has undergone changes during the last decade. These include the overall reduction of sedative dosing to achieve a less deep sedation, the emphasis on analgesia, the employment of protocols and sedation scores, and the implimentation of "drug holidays" and daily "wake-up trials". These measures have hardly been studied in NICU patients but still deserve to be considered. A patient-directed, protocol-based sedation has led to benefits such as reduced ICU-length of stay, duration of ventilation and even mortality in general ICU patients.[48-50] The implementation of analgesia-based sedation protocols (only using sedatives as add-on if necessary) as part of this individualized form of treatment has been studied in 215 NICU patients, many of which had suffered SAH,[51] and in 162 NICU patients (again involving many SAH patients),[52] and reduced sedative need/increased pain-free days as well as equal feasibility/better neurological judgability had been found, respectively. Modern analgesia and sedation involves scores that have, again, hardly been validated in NICU patients. The previously widespread RAMSAY score has shown weaknesses in several more recent studies and has largely been substituted by the well-validated Richmond Agitation Sedation Score (RASS)[53] and the Sedation-Agitation Scale (SAS).[54] RASS and SAS were found useful at least in two small studies in NICU patients.[52,55] Analgesia has been assessed by the nociception coma scale (NCS) to differentiate between minimal vegetative state and minimal cognitive state in comatose post-NICU patients.[56] Although overall backed-up by a very weak base of evidence, we think that RASS, SAS and NCS are feasible and probably useful to guide sedation and analgesia in NICU stroke patients as well. Finally, daily wake-up trials are a matter of controversy with regard to NICU patients. Studies on this question in NICU patients (including SAH) have reported increases in ICP[34] and the release of stress hormones[33] and other safety concerns.[57] Also, a recent study in 413 general ICU patients has not confirmed the benefits that were suggested by previous studies.[58] In essence, we recommend that a wake-up trial be carried out in sedated stroke patients after the acute management is completed and if the brain lesion allows this, but to refrain from further such trials if there is physiological derangement and rather choose a gradual reduction of sedation over time or early tracheostomy.

Benzodiazepines are the most frequently administered drugs for long-term sedation in the ICU. Their mechanism is facilitating the action at the GABA-receptor. They vary in their potency, onset of duration and action, distribution and metabolism, including presence or absence of active metabolites. Advantages are good titrability, only weak circulatory side effects, anxiolysis, anticonvulsive effect and the option to antagonise. Patient-specific factors, such as age, prior alcohol abuse and concomitant drug therapy, affect the intensity and duration of benzodiazepine activity. Especially older patients exhibit a slower clearance of benzodiazepines. Accumulation of benzodiazepines and their active metabolites, especially under continuous infusion, may produce prolonged oversedation, tolerance, withdrawal syndrome and delirium. Midazolam is a benzodiazepine with a rapid onset and short duration with single doses (elimination half time 1.5–2.5 hours). However, accumulation and prolonged sedative effects commonly are observed after long-term sedation with midazolam, especially in the elderly, in obese patients and those with low albumin levels or renal insufficiency. Yet, the use of the benzodiazepine antagonist flumazenil is problematic after prolonged therapy because of the risk of inducing withdrawl syndromes and seizures.

Propofol is an intravenous, general anesthetic agent with rapid onset and short duration of sedation, even after longer infusion. Its mechanism of action is unclear. Advantages are the very good titrability, short action, ICP-reducing and anticonvulsive potential. Common adverse effects include severe hypotension and bradycardia. Prolonged administration of high doses of propofol has been associated with lactic acidosis and hypertriglycidemia, since the agent comes in a phospholipid emulsion (1.1 kcal/mL). There have been reported incidents of the life-threatening rhabdomyelitic propofol-infusion syndrome (PRIS), mostly in children, that is probably not a major problem in the adult NICU, if recommendations on dosing and duration are being followed.

Studies comparing the effects of propofol and midazolam have reported a reliable, safe, and controllable sedation for both agents.[60–64] The main observed differences were: (1) a higher incidence of arterial hypotension in patients receiving propofoland, and (2) a faster recovery in patients treated with propofol, also resulting in faster weaning. The use of midazolam infusion for treatment of refractory status epilepticus is well established; case reports suggest that propofol also possesses therapeutic potential for patients with this condition.[65] Additionally, initial comparisons have described no differences in antiepileptic properties between the two agents.[66]

Ketamine has strong analgetic effects and induces a dissociative anesthesia, besides being an NMDAR-antagonist. Due to its psychomimetic effect, potentially leading to nightmares and hallucinations, it should preferably be combined with other sedative agents, although the enantiomere S-ketamine does seem to be associated with "bad trips" often. Ketamine possesses sympathomimetic properties leading to higher cardiac output and bronchodilation, which is in contrast to all other sedatives and makes it particularly interesting for stroke patients depending on circulatory stability. The use of ketamine has been debated and its use is controversial in neurologic intensive care patients because of its putative effect on ICP. However, recent studies suggest that it can be administered safely in patients with elevated ICP, if the patient is under sedation (propofol or midazolam) and $PaCO_2$ is maintained by controlled mechanical ventilation.[67,68]

There are several substances that do not have the sedative potency on their own to sufficiently address the needs of cerebrovascular NICU patients in the acute phase of their disease, but can be used very well as an add-on or in the later de-escalative phase. Among these are alpha-2-agonists that "shield" the patient from stress rather than deeply sedate him. In the US and many other countries, dexmedetomidine is in fairly widespread use in the ICU and the NICU. This very specific alpha-2-agonist has an analgetic component and has been shown to cause less delirium, shorter ventilation times and benefits in sepsis compared to conventional sedatives used in the general ICU population. Its use in NICU patients has only been investigated in one small study, which reported no severe side effects but a lack of sedative power.[69] Dexmedetomidine is now approved in Europe as well, but is contraindicated there for patients with acute cerebrovascular disease for (questionable) fear of interference with cerebral autoregulation. Clonidine is another central α-agonist that is less specific and potent than dexmedetomidine, but can be recommended for light sedation, as add-on therapy to reduce dose-requirements of sedatives, and to treat drug-withdrawal syndromes in the ICU, although it is only approved as an antihypertensive. Side effects of both agents include bradycardia and hypotension. Other drugs to be used as add-ons or for very specific situations are barbiturates for (transient!) reduction of ICP and treating super-refractary status epilepticus, neuroleptics for hallucinations, or morphine (histaminergic sedative component) for palliative or stressful tachypneic situations. A special group of sedatives are the volatile (inhalative) anesthetics isoflurane and sevoflurane. These can now be used outside the operating room (OR) for long-term sedation in the ICU via a miniature vaporizer (Anesthetic Conserving Device, AnaConDaTM, Sedana Medical, Sweden, not available in the US) that can be connected to any respirator. Potential advantages of these substances are very good titrability, little accumulation, anticonvulsive and analgetic components, and potential neuro/cardio/pulmoprotective effects.[70,71] Disadvantages are side effects, such as hypotension and bradycardia, CO_2 accumulation via an enlarged dead space, and a potentially ICP-raising effect via cerebral vasodilation. Volatile anesthetics have just started to be investigated in stroke NICU patients. Two small prospective observational studies in mixed cerebrovascular[72] and SAH patients[73] have been partially encouraging, but further research is necessary to show whether volatile sedation constitutes more benefit than risk for the stroke NICU patient.

It must be stressed that sedation is never a substitute for adequate analgesia. Almost every patient in an ICU experiences pain at some point; the treatment of choice depends on the cause and severity of the pain. Non-opioids (paracetamol [acetaminophen], salicylate, or non-steroidal agents [indometacin, ibuprofen, diclofenac]) may be adequate in some cases. Still, most patients require opioids for satisfactory pain control.

Three substances from this group frequently applied are fentanyl, sufentanil and the ultra-short-acting remifentanil. Fentanyl possesses an approximately 150 times higher analgesic potency than morphine. The maximal effect is already reached 5 minutes after intravenous infusion. However, fentanyl accumulates in fatty tissue and has an elimination half-time of up to 4 hours. Its redistribution can cause significant rebound effects after its discontinuation, and even respiratory depression. Fentanyl is applied as a continuous intravenous infusion, at doses ranging between 0.05 and 0.3 mg/h, usually combined with midazolam or propofol.

Sufentanil (not available on the US market) has an analgesic potency approximately 1000 higher than morphine. Its context-sensitive half-life is significantly shorter than that of fentanyl during continuous infusion (elimination half-time about 1 hour), making it the agent of choice in many neurological intensive care units. Moreover, it is reported to provide better patient comfort with less respiratory depression than fentanyl.[74] Sufentanil has an additional sedative effect, which reduces the required dose of sedatives. It is applied as continuous intravenous infusion at rates of 0.5–0.75 μg/kg/hour.

Remifentanil (not available on the US market) is an ultra-short-acting opioid, increasingly used today in neuroanesthesia and neurointensive care. It has the shortest elimination half-time, the smallest volume of distribution and the highest clearance rate of all opioids. Its context-sensitive half-life remains stable even after long-term continuous infusion (elimination half-time 6–14 minutes). These characteristics make Remifentanil attractive for neurological ICU patients where regular clinical evaluation of the neurological status is desirable. Analgesia-based sedation with Remifentanil permitted significantly faster and more predictable awakening for neurological assessment.[52,75]

A frequent complication in long-term treatment with opioids is gastrointestinal hypomotility leading to pharmacologically induced sub-ileus. Prophylactic application of laxative agents may be considered. Although good cardiovascular properties were reported under fentanyl and sufentanil, hypotension and bradycardia may occur, especially when large doses are rapidly administered intravenously. Studies on the effects of remifentanil on ICP have suggested that infusion of the drug usually decreases ICP with minimal changes in CPP.[75] However, the exact effect of sufentanil, fentanyl and remifentanil on cerebral hemodynamics remains uncertain.[76–79]

Fluid and Electrolyte Balance

Fluid and electrolyte disturbances are common findings in ICU patients. They may be due to: (1) sympathetic responses to ischemic or hemorrhagic neuronal injury, (2) unbalanced fluid and electrolyte substitution (calculation of daily fluid requirement; see Table 54-1), (3) unbalanced nutritional regimen, or (4) administration of diuretics and other drugs (particularly osmotherapeutics). Sympathetic nervous system stimulation reduces renal blood flow, thus activating the renin-angiotensin system and increasing the secretion of aldosterone, an effect that in turn causes sodium retention and kaliuresis. Antidiuretic hormone (ADH) secretion may also be affected by central nervous system lesions, resulting in sodium and water retention and decreased urine output (syndrome of inappropriate antidiuretic hormone secretion [SIADH]) or in diabetes insipidus. Finally, release of brain derived natriuretic peptide (BNP) has been associated to cerebral salt waste syndrome (CSWS, see below).

TABLE 54-1 Assessment of Daily Fluid Requirement

Basal Requirement	30 mL Per kg Body Weight
+ Urinary output	Urine volume over last 24 hours
+ Stool water	Approximately 100 mL/day (more in diarrhea)
+ Insensible loss	Approximately 800 mL/day (spontaneously breathing patient) Approximately 400 mL/day (mechanically ventilated patient) Fever correction: add 500 mL per 1°C > 37°C

Fluid disturbances can be assessed by: (1) clinical observation, (2) evaluation of fluid intake and output, (3) measurement of CVP via a central venous line or pulscontour continous cardiac output analysis (PiCCO), and (4) measurements of serum osmolarity, urine osmolarity, and serum sodium concentration. Sodium, the main electrolyte of the extracellular fluid, accounts for more than 90% of its osmolarity. There is a close relationship between sodium and water shifts. Sodium concentrations and the hydration state of the patient provide the required information for diagnosis and the treatment of fluid imbalances. Isotonic volume depletion is the most common abnormality encountered. The treatment of choice is enteral or IV administration of isotonic fluids. Careful fluid balancing and monitoring of the CVP are warranted to allow determination of the amount of fluids needed. In patients with concomitant left ventricular failure, chest radiograph, echocardiography, or PiCCO analysis should be used to avoid potentially deleterious fluid overload.

For hypernatremic or hyponatremic states, the therapeutic regimen depends on the hydration state of the patient. Hyponatremia is the most common electrolyte disturbance in the NICU. Rapidly developing and severe hyponatremia <110 mmol/L may lead to generalized seizures, coma and brain edema. The differential diagnosis includes SIADH versus cerebral salt wasting syndrome (CSWS). The correct and early diagnosis is important, because the recommended fluid management is exactly opposite in the two conditions. While SIADH is caused by excessive secretion of antidiuretic hormone (ADH) leading to water retention, hypervolemia and secondary diuresis and natriuresis, CSWS is associated with the release of brain natriuretic factor, resulting in diuresis, natriuresis and concomitant hypovolemia. Therefore, treatment of SIADH is based on water restriction while in contrast treatment of CSWS requires fluid and sodium administration. Differential diagnosis between both syndromes requires correct estimation of hydration state, measurement of urine volume, serum and urine osmolality and the ratio of both, and urine sodium concentration. However, it remains still controversial whether both syndromes are separate entities or rather different manifestations of a common pathophysiologic origin. Some studies claim that hyponatremia more frequently should be attributed to CSWS rather than SIADH[80–82] while other studies entirely doubt the concept of CSWS.[83,84]

In the setting of a central diabetes insipidus, SC or IV administration of 2–5 units of aqueous vasopressin or 1–5 μg of its analog, desmopressin (DDAVP), effectively reduces water diuresis. Further details concerning fluid management are provided in textbooks of clinical medicine.

Nutrition

Nutrition in hospitalized patients with acute stroke is an often overlooked, though significant issue. Davalos and coworkers reported protein-energy malnutrition in 16.3% of 104 patients admitted with acute stroke, and in 26.4% and 35% of the same population after the first and second weeks in hospital, respectively; additionally, malnutrition was identified as an independent predictor of poor outcome.[85] Similar results were reported by Gariballa and associates; they assessed 96 patients with acute stroke upon admission and after 2 weeks, and 51 of them again at 4 weeks.[86] They found that nutritional status deteriorated significantly during the study period. Serum albumin concentrations showed a significant association with infective complications and were an independent predictor of death at 3 months. Davalos and coworkers postulated a hypercatabolic state due to stress reaction or a neuroendocrine response to injury that modified the carbohydrate metabolism as a possible explanation for the observed malnutrition.[85] The demonstrated prognostic significance of malnutrition in patient outcome highlights the importance of an adequate caloric and protein supply in patients with acute stroke. Rough estimates for basal energy expenditure (BEE) are 25 kcal/kg/day for adults between 20 and 30 years, 22.5 kcal/kg/day for adults between 30 and 70 years and 20 kcal/kg/day for those older than 70. A closer estimation is provided by the formula of Harris and Benedict (BEE (men) = 66.5 + 13.75 × weight (kg) + 5 × height (cm) − 6.8 × age (years); BEE (women) = 655 + 9.6 × weight (kg)+ 1.8 × height (cm) − 4.7 × age (years)).

For nutritional support of the critically ill, partly contradictory guidelines exist[87-89] since there is little evidence from randomized controlled trials on the issue. Consideration of some basic pathopyhsiological mechanisms may be helpful to guide therapy. Typically, different metabolic stages can be distinguished during critical illness. An initial phase of reduced metabolism that has been found predominantly in trauma patients is followed by a catabolic stage. In this stage, acute-phase proteins are synthesized and regulation of metabolism underlies stress hormones such as epinephrine, cortisol and glucagon. Metabolism thereby becomes detached from substrate intake; independently from the external supply of glucose, gluconeogenesis in the liver is triggered and cells of organs such as the musle develop insuline resistance in order to ensure substrate supply of the brain. This phase is then followed by an anabolic stage with a high-energy expenditure that in contrast to the previous phase is reactive to external energy supply.

A meta-analysis has shown that parenteral hyperalimentaion may increase complications and mortality rates in critically ill patients.[90] An uncontrolled observational study of ICU patients found that moderate caloric intake (33–65% of recommended caloric intake target of 25 kcal/kg/day; approximately 9–18 kcal/kg per day) was associated with better outcomes than higher levels of caloric intake.[91] Other studies have provided evidence for the negative effect of hyperglycemia on the survival of critically ill patients.[92] However, the fact that energy expenditure and reactivity to external supply of substrates varies during the different phases of critical illness renders the use of fixed formulas problematic. Current guidelines state that substituted energy during acute critical illness should not exceed 25–30 kcal/kg/day, and in the acute phase 15–20 kcal/kg/day are sufficient. Afterwards, energy supply should be augmented slowly to ~ 1.2 times (~1.5 times for patients with malnutrition) of the actual energy turnover. Therefore, nutritional concepts may constantly change during the intensive care stay: while during acute sepsis hyperalimentation and hyperglycemia should be avoided, a patient that is to be weaned from the respirator should be provided with an adequate energy supply. It is important to note, that while hyperalimentation may be harmful, at the same time nutritional support offering an adequate caloric input should not be delayed in critical care patients. Delaying initiation of nutritional support exposes the patients to energy deficits that cannot be compensated for later on. Essential amino acids, fatty acids, and vitamins are already included in standard parenteral and enteral feeding preparations. Protein requirements in critically ill patients may be higher (1.2–1.5 g per kg body weight) than in non-stressed, healthy persons (0.8 g per kg body weight).

Concepts now suggest that enteral rather than parenteral nutrition should be pursued in ICU. If possible, oral feeding should be allowed. However, supplemental nutritional support is required in most patients treated in a neurocritical care unit because of depressed levels of consciousness, impaired swallowing function, or mechanical ventilation. For nutritional support, enteral nutrition with a nasogastric tube is the approach of first choice. Patients who are bound to require long-term enteral nutritional support may be considered for percutaneous endoscopic gastrostomy (PEG), which is better tolerated and causes fewer local complications. The enteral route has several advantages, including simpler application, lower risk of infection, utilization of the normal physiologic functions of digestion and absorption, maintenance of the intestinal mucosa, and lower cost. Intestinal function and motility must be regularly monitored (bowel sounds, aspiration of gastric residuals) and, if necessary, supported by a stimulant such as metoclopramide. Gastric retention enhances the risk of regurgitation and pulmonary aspiration. If motility is still not restored, postpyloric feeding (endoscopically placed nasoduodenal or nasojejunal probe) or parenteral nutrition should be considered. Another common complication of enteral feeding is diarrhea, which occurs as a result of the hyperosmolar electrolyte solutions or of quick build-up of enteral feeding after an extended period of fasting or parenteral nutrition.

Additional parenteral nutrition is indicated when enteral feeding does not cover nutritional requirements. A peripheral venous line is adequate for short-term parenteral nutrition, provided that the osmolarity of the infused solutions does not exceed approximately 1000 mOsm/kg. Long-term parenteral nutrition, meeting the patients' full caloric and protein requirements without giving an excess fluid volume, requires hyperosmolar formulas of up to 1800 mOsm/kg. These are very irritating to the venous endothelium and thus must be administered via central venous lines (see earlier discussion). Complications of parenteral feeding thereby include the risks associated with the necessity of a central catheter.

Nutritonal support should be carefully monitored. This includes assessment of blood glucose levels at least every 4 hours, daily assessment of blood urea (daily increase <30 mg/dl) and measurement of triglyceride levels at least twice per week (<400 mg/dl). Hyperglycemia often requires continuous insulin infusion. In case insulin requirements exceed 6 IE per hour, external glucose supply should be lowered. Further monitoring of nutritional therapy includes regular assessment of albumin, electrolytes, phosphate and liver enzymes. Liver-function abnormalities, with mild-to-moderate elevations of serum liver enzyme activity and bilirubin, are also very common, but usually benign and self-limiting.

Blood Pressure Control

A variety of drugs can be used for treatment of acute arterial hypertension (Table 54-2). Continuous infusion of intravenous drugs with a short half-life time provides optimal therapeutic control. Modes of action and potential influence on ICP and CBF of the intravenous antihypertensive agents most commonly used in intensive care are described in this section. Specific aspects of managing blood pressure according to

TABLE 54-2 Antihypertensives Commonly Used in Patients Treated in Neurocritical Care Units

Drug	Dose	Onset of Action	Duration of Action	Comments
ADRENERGIC INHIBITORS				
Labetalol	20–80 mg bolus every 10 minutes, up to 300 mg; 0.5–2.0 mg/minute infusion	5–10 minutes	3–6 hours	Indicated in ischemic and hemorrhagic stroke; contraindicated in acute heart failure
Esmolol	250–500 μg/kg/minute bolus then 50–100 μg/kg/min infusion	1–2 minutes	10–30 minutes	Indicated in stroke and aortic dissection; contraindicated in bradycardia, atrioventricular block, heart failure, and bronchospasm
Urapidil	1.25–2.5 mg bolus; 5–40 mg/hour infusion	3–5 minutes	4–6 hours	Indicated in most hypertensive emergencies including stroke; avoid in coronary ischemia
VASODILATORS				
Nitroprusside	0.2–10 μg/kg/minute as infusion	Within seconds	2–5 minutes	Indicated in most hypertensive emergencies, including stroke, when diastolic blood pressure >140 mm Hg; contraindicated in high intracranial pressure
Nicardipine	5–15 mg/hour infusion	5–10 minutes	0.5–4 hours	Indicated in stroke; contraindicated in acute heart failure, coronary ischemia, and aortic stenosis
Enalapril	1.25–5 mg every 6 hours	15–30 minutes	6–12 hours	Indicated in acute left ventricular failure; avoid in acute myocardial infarction and hypotension
Hydralazine	10–20 mg bolus	10–20 minutes	1–4 hours	Indicated in eclampsia; avoid in tachycardia and coronary ischemia
Fenoldopam	0.1–0.3 μg/kg/minute infusion	<5 minutes	30 minutes	Indicated in most hypertensive emergencies, including stroke; avoid in glaucoma, tachycardia, and portal hypertension
DIURETIC				
Furosemide	20–40 mg bolus	2–5 minutes	2–3 hours	Avoid in hypokalemia, eclampsia, and pheochromocytoma

Adapted from Steiner T, Kaste M, Forsting M, et al: Recommendations for the management of intracranial haemorrhage – part I: Spontaneous intracerebral haemorrhage. The European Stroke Initiative Writing Committee and the Writing Committee for the EUSI Executive Committee. Cerebrovasc Dis *22:294–316, 2006.*

cause of stroke and individual findings are covered later in the chapter.

Peripheral Vasodilators

Vasodilators cause relaxation of arterial and venous smooth muscle cells. This effect is accompanied by baroreceptor-mediated tachycardia. These agents are also active in the cerebral vasculature, increasing CBF and ICP. In patients with acute stroke, cerebral vessels supplying the affected brain region are already maximally dilated. Thus, use of vasodilators can result in vasodilation of the vessels supplying unaffected brain regions, causing a redistribution of CBF (steal phenomenon) and potentially aggravating ischemic injury. Although this pathophysiologic concept has not been demonstrated in clinical studies, most institutions refrain from using vasodilators in patients with acute stroke.

The most commonly used vasodilators are nitroprusside, nitroglycerin, and hydralazine. Nitroprusside and nitroglycerin, which have a fast onset and short duration of action, should be administered as continuous intravenous infusions. The main limitation of nitroprusside is the risk of cyanide intoxication, particularly in association with doses exceeding 18 μg/kg/hour or used longer than 48-72 hours. Nitroglycerin has been shown to dilate large cerebral arteries.[93] Rogers and colleagues demonstrated significant ICP increases in association with the decrease in arterial blood pressure in a cat model.[94] Cottrell and associates reported similar findings in five anesthetized patients.[95] Thus, the use of nitroglycerin is not indicated in patients with intracranial hypertension. Hydralazine has a slower onset of action, although its effect after intravenous bolus administration lasts for approximately 4 hours. Like nitroprusside and nitroglycerin, Hydralazine is best administered as a continuous intravenous infusion. Studies on head-injured patients showed that hydralazine administration is associated with increases in ICP.[96,97] To date, no clinical studies have examined the effect of hydralazine in patients with acute stroke.

Anti-Adrenergic Agents

Urapidil (not available on the US market) is an alpha$_1$ receptor antagonist that has both a peripheral effect and a central effect. Owing to its central effect, administration of urapidil is not associated with tachycardia. Animal studies demonstrated that urapidil does not influence ICP when applied as a continuous intravenous infusion.[98,99] Results of bolus administration were not unanimous; one study described an ICP increase in cats with experimental cerebral cold lesions,[99] and the other described no ICP effects in dogs with intracranial hypertension.[98] Still, loss of cerebral autoregulation and significant decrease in cerebral perfusion pressure were reported.[100] A clinical study in eight patients undergoing craniotomy for intracerebral tumor showed that the decrease in systemic arterial blood pressure due to urapidil does not influence ICP.[101]

Clonidine stimulates alpha$_2$-adrenergic inhibitory neurons in the medulla, thus reducing sympathetic nervous system outflow. This reduction leads to decreases in arterial blood pressure, heart rate, and cardiac output. Clonidine also has sedative and analgesic properties.[102,103] It can be administered orally, subcutaneously, and as an intravenous infusion. Acute withdrawal results in rebound hypertension. The effects of clonidine on CBF remain unclear. Greene and coworkers used clonidine in 13 patients with severe hypertension. Goal blood pressure was reached in 12 patients; a significant increase in CBF (>10%) occurred in five patients, and a significant decrease in 4.[104] The magnitude of CBF changes depended on the initial values, patients with initially low CBF experiencing an increase, and those with initially high CBF, a decrease. Asgeirsson and colleagues found no effect of clonidine on CBF and ICP in six patients with severe head injuries.[105] Kanawati and associates observed a significant reduction in CBF after administration of clonidine; because this effect could not be reproduced with use of a structural analogue of clonidine that does not cross the blood–brain barrier, these investigators suggested that the CBF response of clonidine is mediated by central mechanisms rather than by alterations in CPP.[106] Favre and coworkers observed significant changes in MAP and CPP in 12 patients who received clonidine during the preinduction period, while ICP remained unchanged.[107] Ter Minassian and associates also observed significant decreases in MAP and CPP after intravenous administration of clonidine; in contrast to the previous study, clonidine also resulted in a transient increase in ICP in three subjects.[108] Thus, although thoroughly studied, the effects of clonidine on CBF remain unclear. The effect of clonidine on the cerebrovascular CO_2 response is also a matter of debate, with two studies reporting a reduced response[107,109] and another an increased response.[110]

Propranolol is a non-selective β-antagonist. Its administration results in decreases in blood pressure, heart rate, and cardiac output. No effect of propranolol on ICP was observed after oral administration in patients with intracerebral hemorrhage[111] or in patients with head injury.[101] Equally, no effect on CBF was noted in 31 hypertensive patients after long-term propranolol therapy.[112] Because this agent can be administered either orally or by slow intravenous injection, it cannot be used for long-term control of hypertension in the ICU.

Labetalol is a mixed α- and β-antagonist. It can lower MAP by reducing systemic vascular resistance while preventing reflex tachycardia through the additional β-blockade. Labetalol can be administered as a continuous intravenous infusion, a feature that augments its applicability in ICU. This agent appears to have no effect on ICP in experimental studies using animal models[113,114] or in clinical studies in hypertensive patients.[115] Orlowski and associates observed a slight but statistically significant ICP reduction in patients treated with nitroprusside alone compared with patients treated either with labetalol or with a combination of labetalol and nitroprusside.[116] As with other agents in this category, studies examining the effectiveness of labetalol in patients with acute stroke are lacking.

Calcium Channel Blockers

Calcium channel blockers cause vasodilation (more pronounced in arteries than in veins) and a decrease in heart rate, myocardial contractility, and conduction at the atrioventricular node. These effects can lead to myocardial depression, atrioventricular block, bradycardia, heart failure, and even cardiac arrest. Nifedipine and nicardipine are the most commonly used calcium channel blockers.

Nifedipine was shown to produce a discrete but statistically significant elevation in ICP when given intravenously to cats with normal baseline ICP; this increase, however, was larger in the presence of intracranial hypertension.[117] Similar results were reported by Anger and colleagues in a further animal study; Wusten and associates observed significant increase in ICP after administration of nifedipine but found that administration of urapidil did not influence ICP.[118,119] Likewise Tateishi and coworkers reported a significant ICP increase, ranging from 1 to 10 mmHg, in ten patients with head trauma or cerebrovascular disease.[120] Bertel and associates compared oral nifedipine with placebo in 25 hypertensive patients who did not have intracranial disease.[121] They observed significant reductions in MAP with nifedipine; however, in this study, nifedipine administration resulted in CBF elevation in four out of five patients in whom CBF was evaluated. Current stroke guidelines do not recommend the sublingual administration of nifedipine because of a prolonged effect and the potential for a precipitous decline in blood pressure.[122]

Nicardipine is a potent vasodilator that also affects cerebral blood vessels. Its effect on CBF remains unclear. Sakabe and associates observed significant postischemic rises in CBF in both nicardipine-treated and control animals; CBF significantly decreased in the control group but remained unchanged in the nicardipine-treated group.[123] Kittaka and colleagues observed no CBF changes with administration of nicardipine after an ischemic insult in rats;[124] in contrast, in an animal model without intracranial disease, Tanaka and coworkers saw CBF increases after administration of the agent.[125] Interestingly, Sakabe and colleagues observed no improvement in neurologic outcome in treated animals,[123] but Kittaka and colleagues reported with treatment significant decreases in neuron-specific enolase and in infarction and edema volume, which were associated with an improved neurologic outcome.[124] After topical application of nicardipine during extracranial-to-intracranial bypass procedures, Gaab and associates observed a marked dilation in the small cortical arteries; a nicardipine infusion, however, was associated with an increase in cerebral Po_2.[126] Akopov and colleagues could demonstrate no consistent pattern in regional (r) global CBF changes in 75 hypertensive patients with symptoms of chronic ischemic cerebrovascular disorders.[127] Abe and coworkers, however, reported a moderate increase in local CBF after administration of nicardipine.[128]

Halpern and coworkers compared the efficacy and safety of intravenous nicardipine versus sodium nitroprusside in the treatment of postoperative hypertension.[129] In that study including 137 patients, intravenous nicardipine controlled hypertension more rapidly than sodium nitroprusside (14 minutes ± 1 versus 30 minutes ± 3.5) and the total number of dose changes required was lower with nicardipine. Other studies came to similar results.[130,131]

Lisk and associates examined the effect of nicardipine, captopril, or clonidine in hypertensive patients with acute ischemic stroke (treated within 72 hours of onset).[132] Nicardipine administration resulted in the most marked drop in MAP. A total of four patients demonstrated an MAP decrease greater than 16%, which was associated with sustained or decreased CBF. Three of these four patients were treated with nicardipine. Administration of nicardipine also appears to increase ICP; Nishikawa and associates observed significant rises in cerebrospinal fluid (CSF) pressure (approximately 5 mmHg), which were associated with significant decreases in MAP and CPP in 17 patients without intracranial disease.[133] Interestingly, this effect was not influenced by the dose administered (0.1–0.3 mg/kg).

Angiotensin-Converting Enzyme Inhibitors

Various angiotensin-converting enzyme (ACE) inhibitors have been developed. Of those, enalapril is the only agent currently available for intravenous administration and therefore also the one relevant for use in neurocritical care units. Enalapril apparently has no effect on CBF in patients without intracranial disease or in patients with a unilateral stenosis of the internal carotid artery greater than 70%.[134,135] Kobayashi and associates observed a mean 8% CBF increase in patients with chronic cerebral infarction.[136] These findings, together with its insignificant side effects, suggest that enalapril is an attractive alternative for treatment of arterial hypertension in patients with acute stroke. An important contraindication is stenosis of the renal artery. One and one-quarter milligrammes are administered intravenously over 5 minutes. Continuous application is possible, a dose of 10 mg/day should not be exceeded.

Maintenance or Elevation of Arterial Blood Pressure

Maintenance of adequate cerebral perfusion is essential for patients with acute brain injury. Patients with arterial hypotension should initially be assessed clinically, and underlying conditions (for example, arrhythmia or hypovolemia) treated accordingly, before catecholamines are administered. One should note that cardiac failure due to acute myocardial ischemia is a common cause of acute hypotension that should be excluded before other measures are initiated. Other frequent causes of severe hypertension include hypovolemia, sepsis or iatrogenic induced hypotension due to sedation or excessive application of anti-hypertensive agents. Crystalloid or colloid fluids should be applied and fluid homeostasis maintained through precise evaluation of fluid intake and output. The target value of CVP lies between 8 and 12 cm H_2O. In prolonged, severe hypotonia, PiCCO-monitoring may provide useful parameters to guide cardio-circulatory treatment. Catecholamines are administered after adequate optimization of volume status in order to enhance cardiac output and optimize systemic peripheral resistance. All catecholamines augment cardiac oxygen consumption and a proarrhythmogenic. No studies have yet compared the efficacy or side effects of various catecholamines in patients with acute stroke, so no definitive recommendations are possible. Norepinephrine (noradrenaline) is a strong vasopressor and the drug of choice in order to augment peripheral systemic resistance, for example during septic shock. Dobutamine is administered to enhance cardiac output. Epinephrine (adrenaline) is the catecholamine of choice for cardio-vascular resuscitation. Specific therapeutic concepts utilizing induced arterial hypertension are discussed later in the chapter.

Invasive Monitoring Procedures

Central Venous Line

Venous access can be achieved by catheterizing a peripheral vein. Although several veins can be used, one must bear in mind that antecubital veins are not appropriate in awake and mobile patients because of discomfort and the risk of thrombosis; risk of thrombosis also prohibits the use of pedal veins, except for immobile bedridden patients. Central venous lines should be used: (1) if no peripheral venous access can be obtained, (2) for administration of drugs that irritate peripheral veins or can cause tissue necrosis after extravasation, and (3) in unstable patients requiring several intravenous lines for drug administration.

The femoral, internal jugular, external jugular, and subclavian veins can be used for central venous access. Each approach has its own advantages and disadvantages. It is important to note that cannulation of the internal jugular vein should be avoided in patients with, or in danger of potential development of, intracranial hypertension, because of possible impairment of cerebral venous drainage. Puncture of the internal carotid artery may occur, but the incidence of pneumothorax is quite low. Cannulation of the subclavian vein bears an increased risk of pneumothorax; on the other hand, this vein does not collapse and can, therefore, be used in cases of shock or hypovolemia. Although cannulation of the femoral vein is relatively easy, this approach should be used only as a last resort, mainly because of the risk of infection. The position of all central venous lines, except for those inserted in the femoral vein, should be verified on a chest radiograph before they are used.

Pulse Contour Analysis

Pulse contour analysis has replaced the use of pulmonary artery catheters for monitoring of cardiac output in many intensive care units. It has the advantage of being less invasive than the pulmonary artery catheter, diminishing the risk of severe complications; in patients who already have a central line, the system only requires an additional central artery catheter. The PiCCO (pulse contour cardiac output system) uses transpulmonary thermodilution and pulse contour analysis to calculate cardiac output, stroke volume variation, intrathoracic blood volume, and extravascular lung water. Thereby, cardiac function can be monitored continuously and volume status can be better estimated than by the use of the unreliable CVP alone. There have been some initial reports on the use of pulse contour analysis to direct hypertensive and hypervolemic therapy in patients with vasospasm[137] and more studies are to follow. A valuable, completely non-invasive alternative for hemodynamic monitoring is transthoracal echocardiography.

Invasive Monitoring of Arterial Blood Pressure

The main indications for peripheral arterial cannulation are continuous direct blood-pressure measurement and access for blood sampling, particularly in patients whose peripheral veins are inadequate for repeated blood sampling. The radial artery is most commonly used. The pulse of the ulnar artery should be confirmed as palpable before cannulation of the radial artery is attempted. Alternatively, evaluation of the ulnar artery can be performed with Doppler ultrasonography.

Invasive Monitoring of Intracranial Pressure

ICP monitoring is essential in patients at risk for ICP increase during the course of their disease, particularly comatose or sedated patients, in whom clinical assessment is not feasible. ICP monitoring reduces the need for neuroradiologic examinations and allows evaluation of the effectiveness of diverse therapeutic approaches. From ICP and MAP, CPP is calculated as follows: CPP = MAP − ICP. ICP monitoring is routinely performed unilaterally; tissue shifts in the contralateral hemisphere are, therefore, detected with a certain temporal latency. However, ICP transducers are mostly inserted in the affected hemisphere, so that ICP increases are readily recognized. The majority of studies on neuromonitoring has been performed in traumatic brain injury (TBI) patients. Data from stroke patients are very scarce. Recommendations for neuromonitoring in stroke patients are therefore approximated from the TBI data including the thresholds for target ICP and CPP. The evidence for the clinical relevance of ICP monitoring *in general* remains controversial. A recent study by Chestnut compared in 324 traumatic brain injury patients treated according two specific protocols: one including invasive ICP-monitoring and other based on clinical and imaging examinations. The primary outcome was a composite of survival time, impaired consciousness, and functional status at 3 months and 6 months and neuropsychological status at 6 months. There was no significant difference in the primary outcome between the groups. Six-month mortality was 39% in the pressure-monitoring group and 41% in the imaging–clinical examination group (P = 0.60). The median length of stay in the ICU was similar in the two groups (12 days in the pressure-monitoring group and 9 days in the imaging–clinical examination group; P = 0.25), although the number of days of brain-specific treatments (e.g., administration of hyperosmolar fluids and the use of hyperventilation) in the ICU was higher in the imaging–clinical examination group than in the pressure-monitoring group (4.8 vs 3.4, $P = 0.002$). The distribution of serious adverse events was similar in the two groups. Thus, for patients with severe TBI, care focused on maintaining monitored intracranial pressure at 20 mm Hg or less was not shown to be superior to care based on imaging and clinical examination. However, several studies found increased ICP to be associated with increased mortality and poor outcome and thus highlight indirectly the intuitive meaningfulness of ICP-monitoring in brain injured patients.[138,139] Moreover, ICP monitoring allows fewer neuroimaging transports which are potentially harmful to the neurocritically ill patient as well as targeted antiedema therapy.

Currently, monitoring can be performed with intraventricular, intraparenchymatous, or epidural catheters as well as subarachnoid bolts.

Intraventricular Catheters. Intraventricular catheters (IVCs) possess the highest accuracy and still are the reference standard for ICP monitoring. First introduced in 1953, they continue to constitute an attractive option for ICP monitoring, because they also allow CSF drainage. An IVC is mostly introduced through a skin incision and burr hole over the posterior frontal lobe of the non-dominant hemisphere, and forwarded for 5–8 cm, until CSF is encountered. A three-way stopcock allows CSF drainage. The amount of CSF drained can be regulated by adjustment of the height of the reservoir. The external acoustic meatus usually serves as reference point for estimating reservoir height. Simultaneous performance of ICP monitoring and CSF drainage is a common mistake; the ICP measured under these conditions equals the atmospheric pressure. Thus, drainage must be temporarily interrupted to achieve an accurate measurement. The accuracy of the measured ICP can be compromised by accumulation of blood clots, debris, or air in the lumen of an IVC.

The major complication of IVCs is infection, the actual incidence of which varies widely among the different studies (0–22%),[140–142] probably largely due to the various definitions for ventriculostomy-related infections. A recent large series was reported by Bota and associates,[142] who analyzed clinical, laboratory and microbiological data of 638 critically ill patients in whom an external ventriculostomy catheter was placed; incidence rate of ventriculitis was 9%. This is in line with data from a review by Lozier and colleagues[143] who found a 8.8% incidence of positive CSF cultures. They proposed definition criteria for five categories of CSF infections in patients who underwent ventriculostomy ranging from contamination, colonization, suspected infection, ventriculostomy-related infection and ventriculitis. According to those criteria, it requires progressively declining glucose CSF level, increasing CSF protein and pleocytosis and at least one positive CSF culture without clinical symptoms other than fever to diagnose ventriculostomy-related infection. Patients with ventriculitis should additionally have clinical signs of meningitis including nuchal rigidity. However, the value of CSF glucose, CSF protein and standard laboratory parameters, such as peripheral leukocyte count, has been doubted by other authors.[144,145] New approaches include assessment of intrathecal interleukin-6 levels, but need to be evaluated in larger patient series.[146]

Several factors in the risk of IVC-associated infection remain unclear, including: (1) the potential influence of the duration of intraventricular catheterization and (2) the usefulness of prophylactic antibiotic treatment. In a prospective study of 172 consecutive neurosurgical patients, Mayhall and coworkers identified ventricular catheterization for longer than 5 days as a risk factor for infection (ventriculitis or meningitis).[141] Previous ventriculostomy, however, did not raise the risk of infection with subsequent procedures. These researchers thus concluded that an IVC should remain in place for up to 5 days, after which the catheter should be removed and re-inserted at a different site. These results were challenged by Holloway and associates, who did not observe significant differences in infection rates between patients in whom catheters were replaced prior to 5 days and those whose catheters remained in place for longer periods; these results suggest that catheter exchange is not beneficial.[140] In this context, it must be noted that even the association between duration of IVC and infection still is not unequivocally documented and remains a matter of debate. In their review, Lozier and associates found that extended duration of ventriculostomy is correlated with an increasing risk for infections during the first 10 days of catheterization. Likewise, Bota et al. found a peak at day 9, followed by a rapid decrease after day 10. Other risk factors for ventriculostomy related infections were intraventricular hemorrhage, subarachnoid hemorrhage, cranial fracture with CSF leak systemic infections and catheter irrigation.[143]

Prophylactic use of antibiotics was reported as beneficial by some investigators,[147,148] but not by others.[149,150] According to a 1999 survey, 72% of centers do use antibiotics (mainly cephalosporins and semisynthetic penicillins) in patients with IVCs.[150] This issue remains unclear and should be addressed in a randomized controlled trial. Currently we do not use prophylactic antibiotic treatment.

Friedmann and Vries reported that percutaneous tunneling of the IVC reduces the infection rate; they encountered no infections after 100 consecutive procedures in 66 patients, with a mean drainage duration of 6.2 days.[151] This finding was later confirmed by Khanna and associates, who reported no infection during the first 16 days after IVC insertion in a series of 100 consecutive procedures; the overall infection incidence in their patients was quite low (4% for an average IVC duration of 18.3 days).[152]

Parenchymal or subdural bleeding along the insertion site constitutes a further complication of IVC. Its incidence, however, is negligibly low.

Prior to removal of the IVC, it is vital to acquire some information about the CSF absorption. For this purpose, catheter drainage should be discontinued for 24 hours, and ICP values closely monitored. Provided that ICP values do not increase by more than 15–20 mmHg during this period, removal of the catheter can be regarded as safe. The quantity of drained CSF is a further indicator for the patency of CSF absorption and the necessity of external drainage; CSF drainage less than 250 mL/day with the reservoir hanging 20 cm above the external acoustic meatus indicates an adequate CSF absorption.

Epidural Catheters. Epidural ICP monitoring is the least invasive approach, in which bleeding complications or infections are extremely rare. Unfortunately, this method is also the most vulnerable to artifacts, and the results are, therefore, not reproducible. Kosteljanetz and associates examined the efficacy of epidural catheters in 35 neurosurgical patients.[153] Satisfactory catheter function was noted in approximately two-thirds of cases. In seven patients, ICP was simultaneously monitored with IVCs and epidural catheters; differences in measured ICP values of up to 25 mmHg were noted. The researchers thus concluded that epidural catheters do not constitute an appropriate method for ICP monitoring. Bruder and colleagues reported similar findings; they observed no agreement between epidural and intraparenchymatous ICP values.[154]

Intraparenchymal Microtransducers. Catheter-tip intraparenchymal ICP measurement is a popular alternative to the ventricular catheter. Parenchymal ICP probes are likely to cause less damage to brain tissue and are associated with low infection rates. On the other hand, problems regarding zero-drift and robustness have been reported in various laboratory and clinical studies.[155-159] There are different techniques of pressure transduction including: (1) fiberoptic, (2) piezo-electric, or (3) pneumatic systems.

Fiberoptic systems are based on a device sensing changes in light reflection off a pressure-sensitive diaphragm. They have been shown to have a relatively good zero-drift and sensitivity stability. Good long-term zero drift properties are crucial. Although devices provide an electrical calibration for calibration of external monitors, their recordings cannot be corrected for inherent zero-drift of the catheter once it is placed, their pressure output being dependent on zero drift of the sensor. *Piezo-electric* systems based on silicon chips seem to be more robust than fiberoptic transducers.[160] The *Spiegelberg ICP monitoring* system is an example for a special pneumatic catheter-transducer system. ICP is measured by a catheter that has an air pouch balloon situated at the top. The pressure within the internal air pouch balloon is equivalent to the surrounding pressure and is transduced by an external strain gauge transducer. This design allows an automatic *in-vivo* zeroing of the ICP system.

The current guidelines for the brain trauma state that with regard to current technology, the ventricular catheter connected to an external strain gauge is the most accurate, low cost, and reliable method of monitoring ICP. ICP transduction via fiberoptic or catheter-tip micro strain gauge devices placed in ventricular catheters provide similar benefits but at higher costs. Other devices such as subarachnoid, subdural or epidural monitors are less accurate.

Multimodality Brain Monitoring

The rationale for multimodality monitoring in large ischemic stroke is the protection of healthy brain tissue adjacent to the infarcted area or in the contralateral hemisphere that may become affected due to the expanding brain edema. In patients with intracranial hemorrhage, brain monitoring is applied to recognize secondary brain injury caused by re-bleeding, by the space-occupying effects of the hematoma and the surrounding edema or to detect vasospasm in SAH. Thus, the main goals of multimodality brain monitoring are: (1) to detect deterioration before irreversible secondary brain injury develops,[161,162,163-165,166] (2) to monitor the effect of therapeutic measures,[167-169] and (3) to predict outcome.[170,171] The benefit of extensive brain monitoring in terms of clinical outcome has yet to be determined. In an early series, ICP monitoring in patients with malignant MCA infarction predicted clinical outcome, but was not helpful in guiding long-term treatment of increased ICP.[172] Moreover, the authors stated that in most cases, clinical signs of hernation preceded ICP increase. However, all patients in the series were treated conservatively and in none, elevation of ICP triggered decompressive surgery. With the advent and evaluation of new therapeutic strategies, brain monitoring becomes increasingly meaningful. Multimodality brain monitoring in addition to ICP and CPP, includes measurement of brain tissue oxygen pressure ($PtiO_2$), cerebral microdialysis, measurement of cerebral blood flow and eventually continuous EEG monitoring.

$PtiO_2$ is measured by a microprobe that is usually placed within the frontal white matter or the region of interest such as the penumbra of an infarct or adjacent to a hematoma. Depending on the catheter, brain temperature, pH, tissue partial pressure of oxygen and carbon dioxide and ICP can be measured simultaneously. The measured tissue surface is approximately 17 mm^2. The measured values depend on localization of the catheter: oxygen levels are highest in areas with dense populations of neurons as the cortex and lowest in the white matter. Most of the experience was gained in patients with traumatic brain injury or subarchnoid hemorrhage so far. However, we routinely use $PtiO_2$- monitoring in the indications listed above supplementary to ICP and CPP measurement. Normal values are 20 mm Hg in the white and 35–45 mm Hg in the gray matter.

Cerebral microdialysis likewise requires the placement of a small catheter (~ 0.65 mm diameter) within the brain tissue. It allows analysis of various substances derived from the extracellular space in brain tissue such as glucose and its metabolites lactate and pyruvate, the neurotransmitter glutamate, and glycerol that is set free from membrane phospholipes during neuronal cell decay. Additionally, post-hoc analyses using high performance liquid chromatography can be performed. Under aerobic conditions, glucose will be metabolized to pyruvate and adenosine triphosphate; in contrast, during hypoxia, the endproduct will be lactate instead. Thus, the lactate/pyruvate ratio is a sensitive indicator of lack of oxygen or ischemia. Another sensitive parameter to detect ischemia is glutamate, moderately high levels indicating ischemia in a reversible state while excessively high levels and a concomitant increase in glycerol indicate an irreversible loss of neurons. These changes in the extracellular milieu often precede elevations of ICP or manifestation of new neurological deficits.

Cerebral blood flow can be estimated by a variety of techniques including transcranial Doppler ultrasonography (TCD), xenon-CT, single photon emission CT (SPECT), oxygen-15-positron emission tomography (PET), perfusion CT and perfusion weighted MRI. Except TCD, these methods do not offer the possibility of continuous monitoring. Placement of a thermal diffusion probe offers the possibility to continuously assess regional cerebral perfusion based on the tissue's ability to dissipate heat. Other systems measure ICP and changes in CBF by laser Doppler flowmetry.

Continuous EEG (cEEG) monitoring in the ICU setting usually was used to detect (non-convulsive) seizures, to monitor burst-suppression during barbiturate therapy, to assess levels of sedation, or to predict outcome.[173] With the advent of digital EEG and quantitative EEG analysis, EEG monitoring has become more user-friendly. Recent reports have shown the value of cEEG monitoring and quantitative EEG analysis to predict vasospasm in SAH patients,[174,175] to detect hypoperfusion or predict outcome in malignant MCA stroke.[176,177]

Treatment of Raised Intracranial Pressure

The main goal of ICP treatment is to minimize or, if possible, eliminate secondary ischemic insults and mechanical damage caused by shifts and local compression of brain tissue. The focus has hereby changed from the initially proposed regimen, which was purely ICP-oriented, to a regimen aiming at maintaining CPP. Sustained CPP drops can result in hypoperfusion of the ischemic brain regions, because the supplying arterioles are maximally dilated and cerebral autoregulation is impaired (Figs 54-1, 54-2).

Basic Measures

Although the optimal blood pressure in patients with intracranial hypertension remains unknown, it is important to avoid sustained hypotensive episodes encompassing the risk of further ischemic brain injury, especially in patients with disturbed autoregulation. We usually maintain CPP above

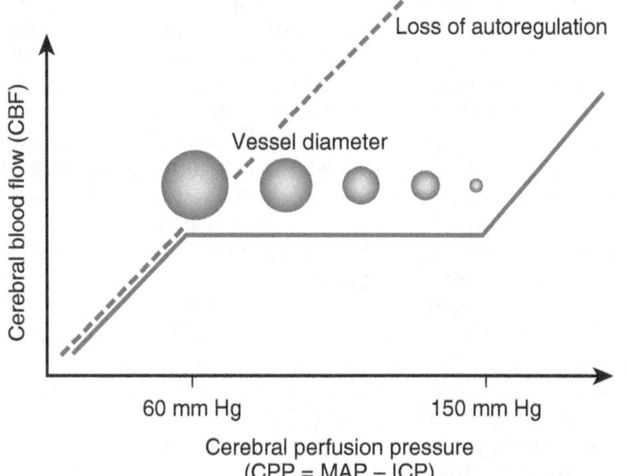

Figure 54-1. Autoregulation of cerebral blood flow (CBF). The cerebral vascular bed is capable of maintaining a constant CBF from a mean arterial blood pressure of 60–150 mm Hg. This phenomenon of "autoregulation" is achieved through either a reduction (vasodilation) or an increase (vasoconstriction) of arterial resistances when the cerebral perfusion pressure (CPP) decreases or increases. If the autoregulation is impaired (dotted line), the CBF passively changes with the CPP. ICP, intracranial pressure.

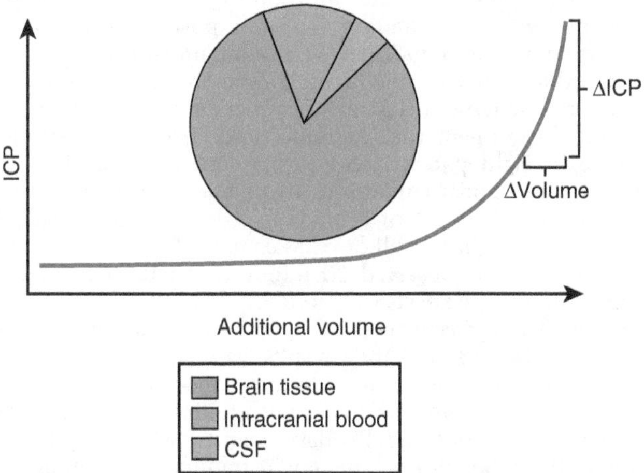

Figure 54-2. Cerebral compliance. An increase of edematous brain tissue requires a compensatory decrease of the other two physiologic compartments contained in the skull, intravascular blood and cerebrospinal fluid (CSF). After the failure of these very limited compensatory mechanisms, the ICP rapidly rises, and even a small increase in the intracranial volume (Δvolume) may substantially raise the intracranial pressure (ΔICP). However, in this situation, even a small reduction in brain edema can dramatically lower the ICP.

60–70 mm Hg. In patients with traumatic brain injury, continuous assessment of autoregulatory parameters was used in order to calculate optimal CPP.[178] In a cohort of 114 head-injured patients, Steiner and colleagues could show that outcome at 6 months correlated with the difference between CPP and CPPopt. However, data on optimal CPP levels and their association to outome in stroke patients are lacking.

Avoidance of hypovolemia is the simplest way to maintain blood pressure; in patients with a central line, CVP should be kept above 8 mm Hg. Crystalloid solutions, colloid solutions, and blood products can be used, in the order given. In patients with decreased peripheral resistance, vasopressors can be necessary; dopamine and epinephrine are the drugs of first choice. Dobutamine is the drug of choice when arterial hypotension is presumed to be caused by decreased cardiac output.

Keeping the patient's head elevated 15–30° increases cerebral venous and CSF outflow, and could thus contribute to an ICP reduction. On the other hand, such a position compromises venous return to the heart, possibly decreasing arterial pressure. Ropper and colleagues examined the influence of body position on ICP in 19 patients in ICU;[179] ICP was lowest when the head was raised to 60° in 10 patients and with the head horizontal in two patients; ICP remained unchanged in both positions in five patients. Rosner and Coley examined the effect of various head positions (0–50°, in steps of 10°) on ICP and CPP. An average ICP decrease of 1 mm Hg was noted for each step, but was associated with a reduction in CPP of 2–3 mm Hg;[180] CPP was not beneficially affected by any degree of head elevation and was maximal in the horizontal position. Feldman and coworkers observed no significant changes in CPP with elevation of the patient's head from horizontal to 30°, and ICP was significantly reduced.[181] Similar results were reported by Meixensberger and associates, who also found that brain tissue oxygen pressure remained unaffected by the body position.[182] Moraine and colleagues, however, observed no ICP changes when the patient's head was elevated from horizontal to 30°; ICP values did drop, however, when the head was further elevated to 45°.[183] At the same time, CBF gradually decreased with head elevation from horizontal to 45°, a change that these investigators attributed mainly to changes in arteriovenous pressure gradients.

It must be noted that all of the studies just summarized examined patients with severe head injury. In a study in 18 patients with acute stroke, ICP, MAP, and CPP values were compared when head position was changed from horizontal to 30° of elevation. A mild but statistically significant reduction in ICP was evident; it was accompanied by a reduction in MAP of a much higher magnitude, so this maneuver mildly reduced ICP at the expense of a CPP reduction.[184] Like Ropper and colleagues, they observed different behaviors of the monitored parameters among the patients studied.[179] We thus suggest that optimal head positioning be decided on an individual basis, rather than routine positioning of all patients with 30° head elevation, as is currently practiced in most ICUs.

Specific Treatment

Osmotherapy. Osmotherapeutic agents are hypertonic solutions of low molecular weight that increase serum osmolarity, thus creating an osmotic gradient between blood and brain tissue. An intact blood–brain barrier is essential for this osmotic gradient. Migration of osmotic substances through the damaged blood–brain barrier can reverse the osmotic gradient and aggravate brain edema (rebound effect). This result was demonstrated by Kaufmann and Cardoso, in 23 cats with a cortical cold injury and vasogenic edemav,[185] and by Garcia-Sola and associates in a goat model in which inflation of an epidural balloon was used to produce intracranial hypertension.[186] Furthermore, volume reduction is more pronounced in the healthy hemisphere; this could potentially increase the pressure gradient between the two hemispheres and facilitate displacement and herniation of brain tissue. It must be noted, however, that such an increase in the pressure gradient constitutes a pathophysiologic model, which has not been substantiated in any animal or clinical studies. The few available data in humans are inconsistent.[187–189]

Mannitol is the most commonly used osmotherapeutic agent. In addition to drawing water from interstitial and intercellular spaces it may improve rheologic properties of blood.

Initially, mannitol leads to an increased intravascular volume, resulting in reduction of hematocrit and higher MAP levels. Provided intact autoregulation, a concomitant increase in cerebral perfusion pressure leads to cerebral vasoconstriction that is followed by a reduction of cerebral blood volume and finally ICP.

Its effectiveness was demonstrated in several studies examining patients with head injury.[190-192] Pollay and coworkers also described a synergistic effect of mannitol and furosemide in reducing ICP, related to preferential excretion of water through the renal distal tubule, which sustains the osmotic gradient, and potentially also to reduced production of CSF.[193] Although a large body of animal studies has investigated the effects of mannitol on cerebral ischemia and edema formation, only a few clinical trials have investigated the use of mannitol in stroke patients. Most experimental studies found beneficial effects of mannitol regarding edema formation, lowering of ICP and infarct volume.[194,195] However, enhanced brain swelling and midline shift after repetitive doses of mannitol have been reported.[185] Bereczki and associates analyzed the case fatality with respect to mannitol treatment in 805 stroke patients. They could not find any association between mannitol use and better prognosis at 30 days and 1 year after stroke. Depending on the factors included in the logistic regression models, mannitol either did not have a significant effect on case fatality or was associated with an adverse outcome.

In their recent Cochrane analysis, Bereczki and associates evaluated the evidence for the effectiveness of mannitol in patients with acute ischemic and hemorrhagic stroke.[196,197] They identified a total of three randomized studies, comparing the effect of mannitol with placebo or open control in patients with ischemic stroke or non-traumatic intracerebral hemorrhage. Based on these three trials (including 21 and 128 patients with ICH, and 77 patients with ischemic stroke), neither beneficial nor harmful effects could be proved. Thus, the use of mannitol in patients with acute stroke is based solely on the results of experimental studies or studies in patients with head trauma.

However, these trials were not designed to investigate efficacy of reducing edema formation in malignant, space-occupying ischemic stroke. In this special setting, some case series have described effective lowering of ICP by using mannitol. In ten of 14 episodes, single doses of 40 g mannitol in eight patients with hemispheric stroke and massive brain edema did effectively lower elevated ICP for up to 4 hours.[198] Likewise, in another observational study, mannitol effectively reduced ICP, associated with a concomitant increase in CPP and brain tissue oxygen pressure in the ipsi- and contralateral hemisphere.[199] Effects on long-term outcome have not been investigated, but the data suggest that mannitol can be efficiently employed to manage an acute ICP crisis and to bridge the time until further interventions, such as hemicraniectomy, can be initiated.

The sugar glycerol is another frequently used osmotic agent. Theoretically, the risk of a rebound phenomenon is lower compared to mannitol, since glycerol can be metabolized by the brain. As with mannitol, the occurrence of a rebound phenomenon remains controversial.[200] Biestro and colleagues compared the effectiveness of mannitol and glycerol for decreasing ICP, using a modified therapeutic intensity level to compare the two approaches.[201] Although both agents were effective at reducing ICP, the duration of this effect was longer for glycerol, leading these investigators to suggest that glycerol should best be used as basic treatment and that a bolus of mannitol should be applied to counteract sudden increases in ICP. A recent Cochrane review identified 10 randomized studies including a total of mannitol-treated 482 patients compared to 463 control patients.[202] Despite a small favorable effect of glycerol treatment on short-term survival, results have to be interpreted cautiously due to the relatively small number of patients, and the fact that most of the trials were performed in the pre-CT era. Moreover, there was no evidence of benefit in long-term survival or functional outcome. Focusing on intensive-care treatment, it has to be noted that only a few patients had their stroke confirmed by CT scan and only one study had clinical signs of brain edema as inclusion criterion. There is no randomized clinical trial addressing the effect of glycerol on outcome in patients with massive brain edema secondary to hemispheric infarction.

Theoretically, 40% sorbit solutions can be applied as well. However, they have two major drawbacks: (1) they are metabolized through the liver, and thus cannot be used in patients with liver dysfunction, and (2) they are contraindicated in patients with fructose intolerance. For this reason, we refrain from their routine use.

The effectiveness of hypertonic saline solutions in the treatment of intracranial hypertension after head trauma has been documented in several studies.[203,204] Gemma and colleagues observed a comparable ICP decrease after the administration of 7.5% hypertonic saline or 20% mannitol in 50 patients during elective supratentorial procedures.[205] In a similar study, Schwarz and associates compared the effects of a combination of hypertonic saline–hydroxyethyl starch (HS-HES) and of mannitol; both substances were effective in reducing ICP.[198] In contrast, Qureshi and coworkers reported a favorable trend toward ICP reduction after infusion of 3% saline/acetate in patients with head trauma (n=8) or postoperative edema (n=6), but not in patients with nontraumatic intracranial hemorrhage (n=8) or ischemic stroke (n=6).[206] This result could not be reproduced, however, in a later study conducted in our department that examined the effect of hypertonic saline in eight patients with stroke and increased ICP, in whom the standard mannitol treatment showed no effect; treatment with 75 mL of 10% saline over 15 minutes resulted in an ICP reduction in all cases. Maximal ICP decrease (mean, 9.9 mmHg) was observed 20 minutes after the end of the infusion. No side effects were noted.[207] Thus, few studies have examined the effectiveness of hypertonic saline in patients with acute stroke, and their results, as described previously, were not unanimous. The optimum concentration of hypertonic saline remains controversial, multiple concentrations ranging from 3% to 23.4% have been tested with different application schedules in patients with traumatic brain injury.[208] Severe side effects of hypertonic saline solutions include severe hypernatremia, congestive heart failure and pulmonary edema.

Given the results already summarized, no evidence-based recommendation can be made on the use of osmotic agents in stroke. Regardless of the therapeutic regimen, it is vital to monitor serum electrolyte levels and osmolarity closely (at least twice daily) while osmotic agents are used. We initially use mannitol (100 mL of a 20% mannitol solution) for control of intracranial hypertension. This is given as bolus infusion (over 15 minutes), preferably through a central line. Because the half-life of mannitol is short (approximately 1 hour), several administrations (4 to 6 per day) are necessary. In predisposed patients, a cumulative dose of 300 g may already be nephrotoxic and induce tubular necrosis. Therefore, mannitol accumulation in the serum has to be monitored. This can be done by simultaneous calculation and measurement of serum osmolality.[209] Usually, both values should be identical. If mannitol accumulates, an osmolar gap will occur with serum osmololity exceeding the calculated osmolality. We aim for a target serum osmolarity of 320 mOsm/L, avoiding higher values in an effort to minimize the risk of acute tubular necrosis and because of the previously cited risk of rebound effect.

We often combine mannitol with furosemide in an attempt to increase the osmotic gradient. If mannitol therapy is not sufficient for ICP control, we use HS-HES, a hypertonic saline, or both.

Tromethamine. Tromethamine (Tham) has been shown to decrease ICP in animal models.[210] It acts by entering the CSF compartment, reducing cerebral acidosis, and causing vasoconstriction, thus reducing ICP. A prospective randomized clinical trial in 149 patients with severe head injury who received either Tham or placebo for 5 days demonstrated that the use of Tham was associated with: (1) a significantly lower incidence of ICP values exceeding 20 mmHg during the first two treatment days and (2) a significantly lower number of patients with barbiturate coma requiring treatment.[211] Nevertheless, no difference in outcome for the two groups was observed at 3, 6, or 12 months.

Tham should always be infused via a central line, because extravasation leads to severe tissue necrosis. Initially, the effectiveness of Tham should be assessed by infusing 1 mmol/kg in 100 mL of 5% glucose over 45 minutes. Continuous Tham infusion should be initiated only if the first application leads to an ICP reduction by approximately 10–15 mm Hg. The dose is adapted so as to achieve and then maintain blood pH between 7.5 and 7.55.

Hyperventilation. Hyperventilation results in reduction in arterial pressure of carbon dioxide ($PaCO_2$), which causes vasoconstriction, thus reducing CBF, cerebral blood volume, and, subsequently, ICP. This effect usually occurs within minutes of initiation of hyperventilation. It must be noted that metabolic autoregulation is not intact in ischemic brain regions, where brain arterioles are maximally dilated. Vasoconstriction is therefore limited to vessels supplying unaffected brain tissue, a feature that could theoretically lead to redistribution of CBF (reverse steal phenomenon). Michenfelder and Milde examining the effect of hypocapnia in a primate model of acute ischemic stroke, found no differences in mortality or level of neurologic function, although they did note a tendency toward smaller infarct volumes.[212] The applicability of hyperventilation is limited by the following major factors: (1) cerebral vasoconstriction can result in cerebral ischemia and (2) the induced elevation of CSF pH is compensated by the choroid plexus within hours, in contrast to the much slower compensation of blood pH, which can require several days. This latter finding implies that the effect of hyperventilation lasts for only a few hours, after which cerebral vessels regain their normal diameter. Termination of hyperventilation at this stage results in an increase of $PaCO_2$ in both blood and CSF, which in turn causes cerebral vasodilation, potentially leading to a rebound effect on ICP. In a randomized trial, Muizelaar and associates examined the effects of hyperventilation alone, hyperventilation plus Tham, and normoventilation (control) in 113 patients with severe head injury, who were divided into two subgroups according to the initial motor score.[23] These investigators observed a significantly worse outcome at 3 and 6 months after injury in patients with severe motor scores who were treated with hyperventilation alone. They also demonstrated that hyperventilation alone, in contrast to hyperventilation plus Tham, could not sustain CSF alkalinization. A variety of clinical studies on head injury suggested deleterious effects of hyperventilation on cerebral oxygenation[213,214] and metabolism.[215]

Hyperventilation is a treatment option for short interventions, to counteract sudden ICP elevations. Under these conditions, the risk of rebound is minimal. Hyperventilation is easily induced through an approximate 10% increase in tidal volume, target levels are 30–35 mm Hg arterial PCO_2. However, with regard to the large body of evidence indicating possible deleterious effects of hyperventilation on cerebral oxygenation, metabolism and blood flow, and the lack of any beneficial effect on outcome, long-term hyperventilation cannot be recommended in stroke patients.[216]

Barbiturates. The main effects of barbiturates are decreases in cerebral metabolism and CBF; the mechanism of these changes is unclear, although an enhancement of the binding of gamma-aminobutyric acid (GABA) to its receptor and a direct effect on vascular tone have been postulated.[217] The effect of barbiturates on ICP appears to be less uniform than that of other agents. ICP reductions were observed in 11 of 15 patients with non-traumatic lesions by Woodcock and associates;[218] in 14 of 21 patients with neurosurgical trauma by Lee and colleagues; [219] in 50 of 60 patients with acute ischemic stroke by Schwab and coworkers;[220] and in 57 of 67 patients with severe head injuries by Cormio and associates,[221] who found that ICP values were reduced, but remained higher than 20 mm Hg in 27 of 67 patients. Schwartz and colleagues found no differences in efficacy between barbiturate coma and mannitol in reducing ICP in 95 patients with head injury.[222] Only 5 of 60 (8%) patients treated with barbiturates survived in the study reported by Schwab and coworkers.[220] Sustained ICP control was only achieved in the five survivors. It must be noted, however, that barbiturates were mostly used as the last line of treatment, after failure of other treatment options; thus, outcome in some patients treated with barbiturates may already have been predetermined by the extent of brain lesions. In another series comprising 21 patients with elevated ICP after large MCA infarction, ICP was temporarily decreased in every case by barbiturate treatment, but this effect was associated with a reduction in cerebral oxygen pressure and reduced CPP.[199]

Because of several potential and partially severe side effects of barbiturate coma (marked arterial hypotension, myocardial damage, electrolyte disturbances, impairment of liver function, predisposition to infection), this treatment should only be used as a therapy of last resort, accompanied by invasive monitoring of arterial blood pressure and frequent evaluations of serum electrolyte and liver enzyme levels. Barbiturates should be infused slowly over a separate venous line. Thiopental is the barbiturate used most often in the neurocritical care unit. It is advisable to apply a bolus injection of 100 mg of thiopental initially and to proceed with further applications only if a marked ICP reduction is observed. The barbiturate effect is monitored on the basis of the appearance of a burst-suppression pattern on electroencephalography (EEG). Serum levels of barbiturates are not reliable.

Glucocorticoids. Qizilbash and associates[176] have reviewed the use of corticosteroids for acute stroke. Seven trials involving 453 patients were chosen for analysis; the follow-up period varied between 1 and 12 months, and only one study utilized CT to exclude hemorrhagic stroke.[223] The reviewers concluded that corticosteroid treatment did not influence mortality at 1 year or improve functional outcome in survivors. Reported adverse effects included gastrointestinal hemorrhage, infection, and hyperglycemia. A clinical study of corticosteroid therapy in 93 patients with supratentorial intracranial hemorrhage found no evidence of a beneficial effect, and the rates of complications already mentioned were significantly increased.[224] Obviously, the possibility that inclusion of patients with hemorrhagic infarcts may have influenced the results of early studies cannot be ruled out. Thus, it is possible that a subgroup of patients with ischemic stroke (particularly those with large infarcts and vasogenic edema) could potentially benefit from corticosteroid treatment. At the same time, the adverse effects observed in these early trials discourage conducting further research in this area.

Hemicraniectomy. As early as 1901, Kocher suggested performing decompressive surgery in order to alleviate intracranial hypertension.[225] Decompressive surgery is based on purely mechanical considerations. The vector of brain extension is reverted into the newly created compensatory spaces so as to relieve the pressure on the midline structures. The rationale of removing a part of the neurocranium is simply to create space for the expanding brain. This ideally normalizes the intracranial pressure and reduces ventricular compression and midline shift. Cerebral blood flow can also be restored, thus increasing tissue oxygen supply. In this way, secondary damage to the surrounding healthy tissue may be avoided.

Most studies on decompressive surgery have been performed in the context of malignant infarction of the middle cerebral artery and traumatic brain injury. Occasionally, hemicraniectomy was carried out in patients with venous sinus thrombosis, subarachnoid hemorrhage, or brain infections. Several stroke animal models provide evidence that decompressive surgery improves cerebral perfusion and reduces the volume of infarction.[226-228] Likewise, in animal models of traumatic brain injury it could be shown that decompression significantly reduced secondary brain damage.[229] Recently, there has been a strong body of evidence showing that decompressive surgery effectively lowers ICP, as well as mortality, and improves outcome in large ischemic stroke[230-233] This is discussed approach in detail in another chapter.

Hypothermia. Normal body temperature is 37 °C, with a significant diurnal variation of 0.6 °C. Body core temperature can be measured at varying sites; the shell temperatures are measured either sublingually, axillary, or on the skin. Core temperatures reflect tympanic membrane, esophageal, rectal, bladder, and intravasal temperature measurements. Hypothermia is defined as mild (33 °C), moderate (29–33 °C), or deep (29 °C).

With a drop in core body temperature, the systemic oxygen demand lessens. Correspondingly, decreases in carbon dioxide production, plasma potassium levels, and carbohydrate metabolism are observed. Several studies have demonstrated a neuroprotective effect of moderate hypothermia in animal models of focal cerebral ischemia.[234-236] Potential underlying neuroprotective mechanisms include decrease in excitatory amino acid levels,[237,238] stabilization of the blood–brain barrier and cell membranes,[239,240] and a downregulation of cerebral metabolism.[241] Additionally, alteration of CBF during hypothermia may contribute to its neuroprotective effects.[241]

Deep hypothermia has routinely been used during open heart surgery and also occasionally for cerebral protection during neurosurgical operations. Although initial clinical studies in patients with brain injury suggested a potential clinical benefit of moderate hypothermia.[242,243] these results could not be confirmed in a later multicenter trial.[244] Yet, moderate hypothermia appears to improve outcomes in patients with coma after resuscitation from out-of-hospital cardiac arrest.[245,246] Application of moderate hypothermia for ischemic and hemorrhagic stroke is detailed later in this chapter.

Antiepileptic Therapy

Reported frequencies for epileptic seizures in acute stroke range from 2% to 23%, depending on study design, diagnostic criteria, duration of follow-up, study population and the extent of monitoring. Incidence seems to be higher in hemorrhagic stroke.[247] In ICH, lobar location and small hemorrhages seem to be associated with the occurrence of seizures within 24 hours after ictus.[248] Seizures are usually partial, secondary generalization may occur. Recent reports focus on the occurrence of non-convulsive seizures. Vespa and co-workers, performed continuous EEG monitoring on 109 patients with acute ischemic or hemorrhagic stroke.[247] Electrographic seizures occurred in 28% of patients with ICH compared to 6% of patients with ischemic stroke. The risk for recurrent seizures after stroke in the acute phase is unclear, estimates range from 20% to 80%.[249] History of alcohol abuse increased the risk of status epilepticus in ICH patients.[248] Data from MRI studies suggest that prolonged seizures may be associated with formation of cerebral edema, which could potentially increase ICP.[179-182] The same holds true for seizure-related cerebral vasodilation, and increases in oxygen and substrate demand can aggravate cerebral ischemia. In the study by Vespa and colleagues, posthemorrhagic non-convulsive seizures were associated with a significant increase in midline shift.[247]

Few data are available on the utility of prophylactic application of antiepileptic drugs after stroke. Prophylactic administration of antiepileptic drugs is therefore not recommended in current guidelines for the management of ischemic or hemorrhagic stroke. An exception may be patients with lobar hemorrhages.[250] In a small prospective study, prophylactic use of antiepileptic treatment in patients with lobar hemorrhage led to a reduction in seizures.[248] We administer antiepileptics only in patients who experience seizures. Epileptic seizures should be treated initially with intravenous benzodiazepines, followed by phenytoin (18–20 mg/kg) if unsuccessful. In the case of refractory status epilepticus please refer to current guidelines, for example provided by the European Federation of Neurological Societies (http://www.efns.org).

Prevention of Deep Vein Thrombosis and Pulmonary Embolism

Early in-hospital mortality in acute stoke patients has been attributed not only to neurological deterioration caused by brain edema, recurrent ischemia or hemorrhage growth, but also to secondary medical complications, such as aspiration pneumonia, cardiac complication, sepsis and pulmonary embolism.[251-253] The incidence of pulmonary embolism after acute stroke shows a large variation between studies.[254] Incidences between 0% and 46% in post-mortem studies have been reported. A study by Widjicks and associates found that pulmonary embolism was associated with sudden death in 50% of the cases;[255] in the other cases, clinical diagnosis was based on the occurrence of sudden dyspnea, pleuritic pain or tachycardia. Studies applying MR direct thrombus imaging have reported high incidences of deep vein thrombosis (DVT) (17.7%) in hemiplegic stroke patients having received aspirin and compression stockings.[256]

The risk of DVT and pulmonary embolism can be reduced by hydration and early mobilization, although the latter is not an option for many intensive care unit patients. Compression stockings have been found effective in surgical patients, however, their efficacy after stroke remains unproven.[257] Studies in ischemic stroke patients have shown that administration of low-molecular-weight heparin (LMWH) reduced the incidence of DVT and pulmonary embolism without increasing the risk of intracerebral hemorrhage.[254,258,259] Current guidelines therefore recommend the use of low-dose subcutaneous heparin or LMWHs for patients with ischmemic stroke at high risk for DVT or pulmonary embolism.[122] Because of the fear of triggering re-bleeding in hemorrhagic stroke patients, thrombembolism prophylaxis is frequently withheld during the first days after ICH or administered at half of the normal dose in patients at high risk for DVT. The intermittent use of pneumatic compression devices has recently been recommended.[250] In a small randomized trial, Boeer and associates have compared early versus late application of low-dose subcutaneous heparin in patients with hemorrhagic stroke. The group of patients where prophylaxis was started on the second day after ICH onset had a significant reduction of pulmonary embolism compared to patients who had treatment initiated on day 4 and 10 after ictus. No overall increase of rebleeding was observed in any of the groups. Therefore, it has been recommended that in neurologically stable patients low-dose heparin can be started on the second day after onset of ICH.[260] Other guidelines recommend starting after day 3 and 4.[261] Monitoring of PTT or anti-factor Xa have been recommended.

Recently, a large multicenter parallel group randomized trial confirmed robustly the effects of intermittent pneumatic compression (IPC) stockings to reduce the risk of DVT in patients immobilized after ischemic and hemorrhagic stroke. The primary outcome (DVT in the proximal veins detected on a screening ultrasound or any symptomatic DVT within 30 days of randomisation) occurred in 122 (8.5%) of 1438 patients allocated IPC and 174 (12.1%) of 1438 patients allocated no IPC; an absolute risk reduction of 3.6% (95%CI, 1.4–5.8). Use of prophylactic-dose heparin or LMWH after randomization was very similar between treatment groups (17% both groups). The authors concluded that IPC is an effective method of reducing the risk of DVT and possibly improving survival in a wide variety of patients who are immobile after stroke.[262]

A special issue arises in patients on vasopressors. A small study has investigated bioavailability of subcutaneous LMWH in ICU patients on vasopressors. Those on vasopressors had lower plasma concentrations of factor-Xa activity than ICU patients without vasopressors or postoperative controls and might therefore be insufficiently protected from venous thrombembolism. This could be caused by impaired perfusion of subcutaneous tissue due to pharmacologically induced adrenergic vasoconstriction. These results suggest that ICU patients on vasopressors may need a different mode of administration to attain adequate thrombosis prophylaxis.[263]

Management of Blood Glucose

Post-stroke hyperglycemia is a common finding and occurs in around 43–68% of patients.[264] Several large clinical trials have found an association between post-stroke hyperglycemia and higher mortality and poor functional outcome.[264–267] Suggested mechanisms include tissue acidosis secondary to anaerobic glykolysis, lactic acidosis and free radical production.[268,269] Others argue that hyperglycemia may be part of a stroke-related stress response and reflect the seriousness of the event itself.[270]

Furthermore, in a study including critically ill surgical patients, van den Berghe and colleagues had shown that intensive insulin therapy in order to maintain blood glucose levels between 80 and 110 mg/dl lowered in-hospital mortality from 10.9% to 7.2%.[92] This was achieved mostly by reducing deaths from multi-organ failure with a proven septic focus. However, in a follow-up study by the same group in medical ICU patients, intensive insulin therapy had no beneficial effects on survival rates, but was associated with five- to sixfold increase in hypoglycemic events.[271] Despite these conflicting results, intensive insulin therapy had been widely advocated, especially in patients with severe sepsis.[272] This procedure was now challenged by the results of a large trial on intensive insulin therapy in severe sepis.[273] The trial had to be stopped prematurely for safety reasons. The rate of severe hypoglycemia was higher in the intensive insulin-therapy group than in the conventional group (17% vs 4.1%), as was the rate of serious adverse events (10.9% vs 5.2%). Moreover, a larger randomized trial comparing conventional and intensive glycemic control (target 80–110 mg/dl) in general ICU patients (NICE-SUGER trial) showed increased mortality in the arm with intensive glycemic control.[274,275] A recent microdialysis study in patients with severe brain injury demonstrated that tight glycemic control might be associated with increased prevalence of brain metabolic crises defined as glucose <0.7 mmol/L and lactate/pyruvate ratio >40, which was in turn associated with increased mortality.[276]

Likewise, so far the largest randomized trial of blood glucose management in stroke patients found no difference between mortality and functional outcome in patients with mild-to-moderate glucose elevations (median 137 mg/dl) that were not treated with insulin and those with intensive insulin therapy targeted at achieving blood glucose levels between 72 and 126 mg/dl.[277] Therefore, current guidelines do not recommend the routine use of insulin infusion in stroke patients with moderate hyperglycemia and refer to the common practice of lowering blood glucose to levels of >180 mg/dl.[122,278]

Temperature Management

In experimental stroke, hyperthermia was associated with increased infarct size and poor outcome.[279,280] A retrospective study of patients with supratentorial ICH found a high incidence of fever, especially in patients with ventricular hemorrhage. The duration of fever was associated with poor outcome and appeared to be an independent prognostic factor.[281] Research in experimental cerebral ischemia revealed a variety of possible mechanisms by which hyperthermia contributes to a worse outcome. These include enhanced release of neurotransmitters, exaggerated oxygen radical production, more extensive blood–brain barrier breakdown, increased numbers of potentially damaging ischemic depolarizations in the focal ischemic penumbra and impaired recovery of energy metabolism, enhanced inhibition of protein kinases and worsening of cytoskeletal proteolysis.[282] The basic pathophysiological principles probably also apply to ICH patients. A raise in body temperature should prompt a search for an infectious focus and treatment should aim to maintain body temperature below 37.5 °C. A frequently used agent is acetaminophen or paracetamol; external cooling with cooling blankets may work well. Some centers employ an intravenous cooling catheter to maintain body temperature at the desired level. The theoretical benefits of hypothermia have been discussed previously in this chapter.

SPECIFIC TREATMENT OF VARIOUS STROKE SYNDROMES

Large Middle Cerebral Artery Stroke

The clinical course of severe infarction of the MCA (malignant MCA syndrome) or of infarction of the MCA plus the anterior cerebral artery (ACA) and/or the posterior cerebral artery (PCA), that is treated with medical therapy alone follows a predictable pattern in most patients.[283,284] Within the first few hours after onset of symptoms, patients with large supratentorial infarcts are typically fully awake, although some may show mild drowsiness. Bilateral motor signs, coma, posturing, and pupillary abnormalities are usually not observed in the very early phase of large supratentorial infarcts. Neurologic deterioration occurs during the first 24 hours in most patients with large supratentorial infarcts, corresponding to the development of brain edema, see Figure 54-3. Such patients lose consciousness to varying degrees from drowsiness to coma. Pupillary enlargement and loss of pupillary reactivity – initially occurring only on the side of the infarction and later bilaterally – nausea, vomiting, posturing, and abnormal breathing patterns are signs of secondary brainstem dysfunction due to impending herniation. If ICP is being monitored,

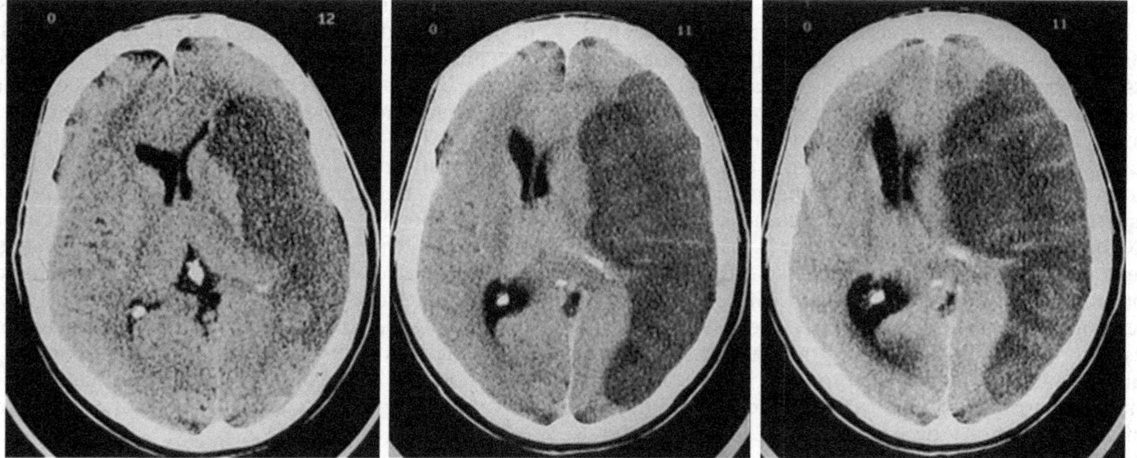

Figure 54-3. Left to right, Course of edema formation in complete infarction of the middle cerebral artery.

it is typically only moderately elevated (20 mm Hg), at the first onset of deterioration. ICP values subsequently rise over the next 24–48 hours. Elevated ICP is a reliable prognostic sign, and an ICP exceeding 30 mm Hg is usually associated with a fatal course.[172]

Most patients demonstrating neurologic deterioration within the first few hours after stroke onset eventually die. Various predictors for deterioration and poor clinical outcome have been identified. Regarding vascular disease, distal internal carotid artery (ICA) occlusion almost uniformly indicates fatal outcome. Proximal occlusion of the MCA stem is also an unfavorable radiologic finding, typically leading to a complete MCA infarction, including the basal ganglia, which are often spared in patients with a more distal MCA occlusion. It seems plausible that the extent of the infarcted area closely correlates with mortality. Complete MCA plus ACA infarcts and infarcts involving the complete hemisphere are usually lethal. Rapid onset of neurologic deterioration with loss of consciousness during the first 6 hours indicates an aggressive course of the disease and is associated with a high mortality.[283] The extent of brain edema depends largely on the size and location of the infarct, but also shows substantial individual variability. As a general rule, young and middle-aged patients have less compensation capacity for space-occupying intracranial lesions than older patients with cerebral atrophy.

A large hemispheric infarct must be recognized in the emergency department as a life-threatening condition that requires prompt and massive intervention. After stabilization of the airway, breathing, and circulation, the initial diagnostic evaluation and transfer of the patient to a neurocritical care unit should not be delayed. If indicated, early reperfusion therapies can be initiated in the emergency department. Venous access, continuous monitoring of blood pressure, electrocardiography (ECG), and pulse oxygenation are part of routine intensive care measures. Continuous ECG monitoring is especially important because neurogenic cardiac arrhythmias are commonly observed, particularly in patients with large infarcts of the right hemisphere. Although respiratory problems are uncommon upon presentation, their frequency sharply rises within the first 24 hours, reflecting increasing brain edema and brainstem dysfunction. Most patients with large infarcts require ventilatory support. To achieve sufficient cerebral oxygenation, oxygen should be insufflated via a face mask to achieve arterial Po_2 values greater than 90 mm Hg. Indications for intubation and mechanical ventilation were discussed earlier in the chapter.

Hemicraniectomy

The most effective treatment of malignant middle cerebral artery syndrome is decompressive surgery, which is discussed in a separate chapter.

Moderate Hypothermia

As already discussed previously in this chapter, hypothermia: (1) theoretically offers neuroprotective effects and (2) may help to control ICP. Since patients with acute stroke were rarely treated with hypothermia within the first 12 hours after symptom onset, neuroprotection has been barely considered in case studies on hypothermia in ischemic stroke. Those studies rather have focused on the effect of hypothermia regarding reduction of brain edema and control of ICP.

The first clinical trial on the effect of moderate hypothermia (33 °C) in patients with severe MCA infarction was reported by Schwab and colleagues in 1998.[285] Hypothermia was induced at a mean of 14 hours after symptom onset and maintained for 72 hours. Mortality was 44%, and survivors had a favourable outcome, with a mean Barthel index of 70, even though all patients had met the criteria for diagnosis of a "malignant" MCA infarction. Although hypothermia significantly reduced ICP, a secondary rise in ICP, occasionally exceeding initial ICP levels and requiring additional treatment with osmotherapeutics, was observed upon rewarming. The rewarming period constitutes a critical phase, because metabolic needs potentially outstrip oxygen delivery. This ICP rebound after rewarming might be due to a hypermetabolic response after induced hypothermia, which has already been described after cardiopulmonary bypass surgery. Schwab and colleagues[286] reported similar results in a multicenter observational study of 50 prospective patients with cerebral infarction involving at least the complete MCA territory who were treated with moderate hypothermia (33 °C). Overall mortality was 38%; 8% of patients died during hypothermia, 30% during rewarming owing to uncontrollable ICP increase. Median neurologic outcome were National Institute of Health Stroke Scale score (NIHSS) of 28, and median modified Rankin Scale score of (mRS) of 2.9, at 4 weeks and at 3 months after stroke, respectively. Krieger et al. reported initial results in 10 patients with acute ischemic stroke (NIHSS, 19.8 ± 3.3) who were treated with moderate hypothermia (32 °C) after thrombolysis.[287] Mortality was 33%, and the mean mRS at 3 months was 3.1 ± 2.3.

Hypothermia affects virtually every organ system. Ventricular ectopy and fibrillation limit the extent of hypothermia, but these effects are known to occur only at temperatures below 30 °C. Pneumonia was the only severe side effect of moderate hypothermia in the first study reported by Schwab and colleagues.285 The complications of moderate hypothermia most commonly described in the later multicenter trial were thrombocytopenia (70%), bradycardia (62%), and pneumonia (48%).[286] Four patients (8%) died during hypothermia, because of severe coagulopathy, cardiac failure, or uncontrollable intracranial hypertension. Complications in the 10 patients studied by Krieger and associates were bradycardia (n=5), ventricular ectopy (n=3), hypotension (n=3), melena (n=2), fever after rewarming (n=3), and infection (n=4). Also, four patients with chronic atrial fibrillation experienced a rapid ventricular rate, and three patients had myocardial infarctions during hypothermia.[287]

Initially, surface cooling with cooling blankets, alcohol applied to exposed skin, or application of ice bags to groin, axilla, and neck were used to induce hypothermia. This approach, however, requires intensive effort from the medical and nursing staff for induction as well as for maintenance of the target temperature and steering of temperature is not easy. Modern techniques like endovascular cooling[288] use a central line with a single infusion lumen and another lumen that ends in three balloons located at the distal end of the catheter. The balloons are perfused with a sterile solution of normal saline via a closed-loop tubing system. The tubing is connected to a mobile temperature management device placed at the patient's bedside. The device consists of a water bath with adjustable temperature; a pump circulates the saline solution through the water bath. The catheter is inserted into the femoral vein and advanced to the inferior vena cava. Initial results of this approach were promising, as target temperature was reached after 3 ±1 hours (range, 2–4.5 hours) and deviations from the target temperature were minimal (>0.2 °C or >0.3 °C during 21% or 10% of the time, respectively).[288] Surface cooling has also been considerably advanced. Several devices are available that use cooling pads attached to the patient perfused with cold fluid from a mobile unit that allows good steering of the temperature. Additionally, many methods for inducing hypothermia (ice-cold saline, cooling pads, cooling helmets, nasal cavity tubing, etc.) do emerge. Data are not sufficient to clarify the favorable device and technique of cooling the stroke patient, yet. Particularly, the advantages of endovascular over surface cooling have still not convincingly been demonstrated.

Hemicraniectomy has certainly to be regarded as the therapy of choice in space-occupying MCA infarction, but still leaves a considerable number of patients substantially disabled, and it was questioned whether hypothermia could be an alternative or even an adjunct to hemicraniectomy.

In one study, a total of 36 patients with severe acute ischemic stroke were treated with hemicraniectomy (n=17) or moderate hypothermia (n=19). Age, baseline NIHSS score, sex, cranial computed tomography (CCT) findings, level of consciousness, and time to treatment were similar in the two groups. Mortality was 12% for hemicraniectomy and 47% for moderate hypothermia; one patient treated with moderate hypothermia died of treatment complications (sepsis) and three on ICP crises that occurred during re-warming. The researchers concluded that in patients with acute ischemic stroke, hemicraniectomy is associated with lower rates of both mortality and complications than moderate hypothermia.[289]

In one small trial Els et al. have investigated additional benefits of hypothermia by randomizing 25 patients with large MCA-infarcts either to hemicraniectomy alone or to the combination of hemicraniectomy and mild hypothermia (35 °C) for 48 hours.[290] They observed a tendency to lower mortality in the combination group (mortality 8% after 6 months) and concluded the safety and feasibility thereof. Currently, a larger randomized controlled trial investigates the same question.[291]

New clinical applications for hypothermia may also focus on the early neuro-protective effect rather than the potential to decrease brain edema and ICP. As mentioned above, the studies so far conducted on hypothermia in ischemic stroke did not focus on neuron-protection. Promising data derive from two studies including patients after cardiac arrest.[245,246] The positive results of these studies lead to inclusion of hypothermia into current guidelines for resuscitation. However, limiting factors for large-scale clinical application of early hypothermia for neuroprotection in acute ischemic stroke include the question about the required depth of hypothermia and thereby its feasibility in awake patients. Until now hypothermia was restricted to intubated and sedated patients, but new monocentric and multicentric trials are beginning to investigate hypothermia in awake stroke patients as well. The use of hypothermia in ischemic stroke, although principally promising, still remains experimental and no evidence-based recommendation can currently be given.

Blood Pressure Management

Blood pressure management is a critical issue in the treatment of acute stroke. Both, hyper- and hypotension can be associated with poor outcome after stroke.[292] Theoretical reasons to lower blood pressure in the acute phase are decreasing the risk of severe hemorrhagic transformation, especially after thrombolysis, to prevent further cardiovascular damage and eventually to diminish the formation of brain edema. On the other hand, it is feared that aggressive reduction of blood pressure may negatively affect cerebral perfusion, especially in the penumbra and thereby enlarge ischemic damage of the brain. Furthermore, it has to be kept in mind that in a majority of patients, blood pressure spontaneously declines during the first hours after stroke. The additional effect of sedative medication may enhance this effect in intensive care patients. A systematic review on blood-pressure management in acute stroke has failed to provide evidence that active management of blood pressure influences patient outcomes.[293] In the absence of conclusive, evidence-based data, current guidelines recommend to cautiously initiate treatment when systolic or diastolic blood pressure exceeds 220 mm Hg and 120 mm Hg respectively, or in the presence of other medical factors that may require lowering of blood pressure, such as cardiac insufficiency, myocardial infarction, aortic dissection or pulmonary edema.[249,278] Lower thresholds apply for patients after intravenous or intra-arterial thrombolysis. Special caution is required in patients with hemodynamic causes for stroke. No specific antihypertensive agent can be recommended (please see previous section of this chapter). However, intravenous application is preferable for better controlability. The use of sublingual administration of nifedipine is discouraged because of the potential for a prolonged and precipitous effect. A randomized controlled trial (CHHIPS) investigated blood pressure lowering in the acute phase of ischemic and hemorrhagic stroke initiated at the level SBP >160 mm Hg within 36 hours of symptom onset. The primary outcome – death or dependency at 2 weeks – occurred in 61% (69) of the active and 59% (35) of the placebo group (RR, 1.03; 95%CI, 0.80–1.33; $P = 0.82$). There was no evidence of early neurological deterioration with active treatment (RR, 1.22; 0.33–4.54; $P = 0.76$) despite the significantly greater fall in SBP within the first 24 hours in this group compared with placebo (21 [17–25] mm Hg vs 11 [5–17] mm Hg; $P = 0.004$). No increase in serious adverse events was reported with active treatment (RR, 0.91; 0.69–1.12; $P = 0.50$), but 3-month mortality was halved (9.7% vs 20.3%; HR, 0.40; 95%CI, 0.2–1.0; $P = 0.05$). However, in view of the small sample size, results have to be regarded as preliminary.[294] More recent large randomized studies (SCAST, CATIS), however, failed to show any outcome benefit of early blood pressure lowering, the evidence for which, if anything, suggested a harmful effect.[295,296]

Acute Basilar Artery Occlusion

Occlusion of the basilar artery (BAO) is the cause of the most desolate strokes and associated with a grave prognosis; early studies reported a mortality rate up to and in excess of 90%.[297–299] Without treatment the chances for survival or independent outcome are negligible. Survival mainly depends on immediate recanalization.[300,301] The clinical presentation includes sudden onset of severe motor and bulbar symptoms such as tetraplegia, ophthalmoplegia and dysarthria, combined with reduced consciousness. Up to 60% of affected patients have prodromal symptoms. They are predominantly non-specific, such as nausea, tinnitus, hearing loss, and vertigo.[302,303] A gradual or stuttering course may occur as well. The prospective multicenter BASICS registry by Schoenwille et al. compared an antithrombotic treatment (AT) (n = 183) with primary intravenous thrombolysis (IVT) including subsequent intra-arterial thrombolysis (n = 121) and intra-arterial therapy (IAT) (n = 288) in patients with basilar artery occlusion.[304,305] In a direct comparison of IAT with IVT, patients with a mild-to-moderate deficit had a higher risk of a poor outcome when treated with IAT whereas patients with a severe deficit had similar outcomes when treated with either IAT or IVT. Results for AT compared to IVT were similar for patients with mild-to-moderate deficits, but individuals with severe deficits had a better outcome in the IVT group compared to patients of the AT collective. Although IAT was associated with a slightly higher recanalization rate (72%) compared to IVT (67%), survival rates, when related to the severity of pre-existing symptoms, were equal. Four-hundred and two (68%) of 592 analyzed patients had a poor clinical outcome at 1-month follow-up and 214 (36%) patients died. The authors thus draw two main conclusions: first the efficacy of treatment strategies depends primarily on the severity of stroke. Outcome of patients with a mild-to-moderate deficit was poorer if treated with IAT rather than with IVT. When analyzing all assessed patients authors found out that the chances of recanalization, and hence a favorable outcome, were slightly higher after IAT. Hence, secondly, the chance of a favorable response to therapy will probably decrease in the course of time, so that the initiation of IVT should not be delayed while waiting for IAT. Therefore, centers that have a 24-hour interventional neuroradiology should employ intra-arterial thrombolysis. Moreover, the intra-arterial approach offers mechanical options like PTA, stenting or catheter devices for thrombus extraction.[306] However, centers without a interventional neuroradiologist should not delay treatment and immediately start intravenous thrombolysis.[307] Eckert et al.[308] and Nagel et al. [301] have both performed studies assessing outcomes in patients treated initially with an intravenous bolus, then infusion of a glycoprotein IIb/IIIa receptor antagonist abciximab followed by IAT including tPA and, where appropriate, angioplasty with or without stenting for underlying atherothrombotic lesions. Both studies demonstrated improved rates of recanalization in the bridging groups as well as an improved survival rate compared to IAT alone (58–62% vs 25–32%). Also rates of favorable outcome (mRS score 0–3) were higher in the bridging groups (35% vs 12.5–17%). The rationale for applying anti-platelet agents and/or immediate PTA/stenting is to prevent reocclusion. Reocclusion rates of 17% have been reported during intra-arterial thrombolysis.[309] Reocclusion may be a reason why in the BASICS registry, discussed above, there was no significant benefit of intra-arterial thrombolysis regarding survival rates despite significantly higher recanalization rates.

There is no established time-window for recanalization therapy in basilar artery occlusion; however, aggressive treatment more than 12 hours after onset of symptoms or in patients already presenting with complete loss of brainstem reflexes seems not to be justified.

A current prospective, monocenter study by Strbian et al. evaluated the impact of extensive baseline ischemia on functional outcome after BAO thrombolysis.[310] In this investigation 184 patients were analyzed and IVT was given to 175 (95.1%) patients, 97% of them received accompanying AT with full-dose heparin. A mechanical recanalization was applied in 13 (7.1%) patients and an endovascular procedure was performed only when systemic thrombolysis with rtPA was contraindicated. The study protocol advises thrombolysis up to 12 hours in case of sudden massive onset. In contrast, for patients with clinical aggravation, the time window was 48 hours from onset. The extent of baseline ischemia was evaluated with the posterior circulation Acute Stroke Prognosis Early CT score (pc-ASPECTS). In the analysis 132 of 184 (72%) patients had pc-ASPECTS ≥8. The majority (96%) of patients with baseline pc-ASPECTS <8 had a poor 3-month outcome, and 94% were observed in those with confirmed recanalization (51.5%). In contrast, half of patients with pc-ASPECTS ≥8 and successful recanalization (73.2%) achieved good outcome. In these patients, onset-treatment-time (OTT) was associated with poor outcome neither as a continuous nor as a categorical variable. When analyzing all assessed patients authors found out that pc-ASPECTS <8 was independently associated with poor outcome. The authors thus draw one main conclusion: in the absence of extensive baseline ischemia, recanalization of BAO up to 48 hours, independent of time to treatment, can produce good outcomes in 50% of patients.

Our routine emergency protocol for patients with reduced consciousness and suspected acute basilar occlusion includes immediate magnetic resonance imaging (MRI) with MR-angiography (MRA). If MRA confirms the clinical diagnosis, a bridging intravenous thrombolysis therapy with rtPA is started and the patient is immediately transferred to angiography. If no immediate angiographic recanalization can be achieved the application of the remaining dose of intravenous or intra-arterial rtPA combined with intravenous application of the platelet glycoprotein IIb/IIIa antagonist tirofiban is being considered according to strict indications. Due to a reduction of consciousness, most patients arrive already intubated and mechanically ventilated at the emergency room. Patients who are still awake are intubated for the procedure, short-acting sedatives such as propofol and remifentanil are preferable for immediate neurological assessment following the procedure in order to estimate prognosis. Post-angiographic radiological assessment includes CT or MRI to exclude intracerebral hemorrhage. All patients with acute basilar artery occlusion are transferred to an intensive care unit.

Cerebellar Infarction

Cerebellar infarction accounts for 1.9–10.5% of cases in clinicopathologic series of patients with cerebral infarctions. Neurologic deterioration occurs as a result of a growing mass effect of the infarcted cerebellum in the posterior fossa. Therefore, patients with signs of increased pressure in the posterior fossa on CCT scan should be carefully monitored in a neurocritical care unit. One must always bear in mind that deterioration in such a patient can occur within minutes, although the clinical condition prior to this can appear to be stable or even improving. Although there seems to be a maximum of deterioration of consciousness around the third day within ictus,[311] deterioration can occur anytime within the first 2 weeks after onset of a cerebellar infarct and may be delayed compared with that in supratentorial stroke, indicating the need for prolonged monitoring in conservatively treated patients with cerebellar infarcts.

No controlled study has yet assessed the efficacy of decompressive surgery for cerebellar infarctions. Nevertheless, this is an important issue, because increasing mass effect of the infarcted cerebellum in the posterior fossa can lead to clinical deterioration and brainstem compression. Identifying patients with cerebellar infarctions who are bound to experience intracranial hypertension is not always straightforward; prognostic factors include underlying size of the infarction, hemorrhagic transformation, and poor collateral blood flow. Neurologic deterioration can also be caused by occlusive hydrocephalus or progression of concurrent brainstem infarction. Close clinical monitoring and frequent CT scanning to estimate the severity of obstructive hydrocephalus are mandatory. In patients with fast decline of consciousness, decompressive surgery of the posterior fossa – with or without removal of infarcted cerebellar tissue – is significantly better than ventriculostomy.[312,313] Ventriculostomy alone may be a temporary measure, but great care must be taken in such a procedure because it may promote ascending herniation. Recently, Neugebauer et al. reviewed all available studies and series on patients with space-occupying cerebellar infarction including 750 patients altogether. Albeit therapeutically heteregenous, the analysis showed that conservative treatment alone is associated with a high mortality rate of 42.9%, increasing to a rate as high as 85% in those patients who progress to coma. Surgical treatment was associated with much higher survival rates: 81.6% for patients treated with EVD alone, 76.8% for those treated with SDC alone, and 77.5% for those treated with both EVD and SDC. Despite the general belief that the clinical outcome of patients with space-occupying cerebellar stroke who have undergone successful life-saving surgery is usually good irrespective of other prognostic factors, this issue has to be regarded with caution. Two studies including 108 patients treated with different strategies reported a low long-term survival rate of 60%. Twenty-seven percent of survivors showed a favorable outcome (mRS score 0–1) and 38% showed an independent outcome (mRS score 0–2). Age and the presence of brainstem infarction were identified as independent prognostic factors. Interestingly, insertion of an external ventricular drain, either alone or in combination with decompressive craniectomy, seemed to have no effect on survival or outcome. These results indicate very heterogeneous outcome results, with 40% of patients dying and a considerable number of patients left with severe neurological deficits.[314,315] However, surgical decompression of posterior fossa remains the life-saving procedure and first-line treatment of choice in space-occupying cerebellar infarction.

Spontaneous Intracerebral Hemorrhage

ICH accounts for 10–17% of all strokes.[260] In retrospective studies, mortality within the first month was between 35% and 52%; only 20% of patients regained functional independence by 6 months. Volume of ICH, Glasgow Coma Scale on admission, age >80 years, infratentorial origin of ICH and presence of intraventricular blood have been identified as independent predictors of 30-day mortality.[316] However, implementation of do-not-resuscitate-orders in ICH patients may have lead to self-fulfilling prophecies and to a pessimistic overestimation of prognosis in ICH. Of importance, is that it has been shown that treatment within specialized neurological intensive care units can decrease the mortality rate to 28–38% compared to a rate of 25–83% in patients treated in general intensive care units.[317] Moreover, during recent years, there has been a large increase in clinical trials of ICH, providing hope for new and effective treatments. Since more than half of ICH patients require intubation and mechanical ventilation,[9] the neurointensivist has to know these options to be able to make meaningful therapeutic decisions in time.

Three pathophysiological concepts are considered of high importance for intensive care treatment of ICH patients and have been the target of recent studies. First, ICH is a dynamic process; in about one-third of patients substantial hematoma enlargement occurs within the first 24 hours[318] and in up to 70% of patients who have CT scanning performed within 3 hours after onset of symptoms.[319] Although it remains unclear whether this is due to re-bleeding or continuous bleeding, hemorrhage growth has been shown to be an independent determinant of mortality and functional outcome after ICH.[319] Each 1 ml growth of hematoma has been associated with a 7% increased risk of death or disability.[319,320] Thus, attenuation of hematoma growth is a major therapeutic strategy. Second, a low-density region develops frequently surrounding the hematoma. Thrombin and several serum proteins were suggested to trigger an inflammatory reaction in the perihematomal zone.[321–323] Additionally, Sansing and colleagues have proposed that interaction of thrombin with factors released from activated platelets at the site of hemorrhage increases vascular permeability, thereby contributing to the development of edema.[324] Parallel to ICH enlargement, perihematomal edema seems to grow during the first 24 hours.[325] Furthermore, significant, delayed edema growth can occur up to 2 weeks after ictus. The prognostic and pathophysiological significance of brain edema in ICH remains controversial. Edema volume has not been independently associated with worse outcome, but was associated with increased mass effect and neurological deterioration.[326] On the other hand, another group has found an association between early edema size relative to hemorrhage volume and good outcome.[327] Third, 36–50% of ICH patients have additional intraventricular hemorrhage. Intraventricular blood volume was significantly associated with mortality at 30 days. Concomitant hydrocephalus was identified as independent predictor of early mortality.[328]

Therapeutic strategies of ICH, therefore, must be targeted primarily to stop hematoma enlargement and to prevent deleterious consequences of mass effect evoked by the hemorrhage itself and the surrounding edema. Development of hydrocephalus has to be monitored and adequate measures such as placement of an extraventricular drain have to be carried out in time.

Medical Treatment of Intracerebral Hemorrhage

Recombinant Activated Factor VII. Considering aforementioned prognostic significance, hematoma expansion seems an ideal therapeutic target. Thus the use of haemostatic agents has been tried in ICH and SAH with various agents including tranexamic acid, ε-aminocaproic acid and aprotinin with disappointing results. Recombinant activated factor VII (rFVIIa) was originally developed for patients with hemophilia and was applied to stop intracerebral bleeding in these patients. rFVIIa acts locally at the sites of tissue injury and vascular wall disruption by binding to tissue factor. It thus generates small amounts of thrombin sufficient to activate platelets. At higher doses, rFVIIa directly activates factor X on the surface of activated platelets, leading to a thrombin burst and acceleration of coagulation. Following two small prospective, randomized dose-escalating phase-IIa trials, a larger phase-II trial was performed including 399 patients with spontaneous ICH. Patients were randomized to treatment with 40, 80 or 160 µg/kg rFVIIa within 4 hours of ictus. Compared to placebo, treatment with rFVIIa limited hematoma expansion, decreased mortality and improved 3-month clinical outcome; a 5% increase in arterial thromboembolic events was found within the group receiving the highest dose. The results lead to initiation of a larger phase III trial[329] that included 841 patients within 3 hours of ICH onset; patients with a GCS <5 were excluded. Two-hundred and sixty-eight patients were randomized to placebo, 276 patients had 20 µg/kg rFVIIa and 297 patients had 80 ug/kg rFVIIa within 4 hours of stroke. At 24 hours, treatment with 80 µg/kg significantly reduced hemorrhage growth as compared with placebo (26% vs 11%), corresponding to a moderate but statistically significant reduction of 3.8 mL in the growth in volume as compared to placebo. Total final lesion volumes at 72 hours were similar in the three groups. There was no significant difference regarding survival or functional outcome between the three groups. The overall frequency of thromboembolic serious adverse events was similar in the three groups; however, arterial events were significantly more frequent in the 80 µg group compared to the placebo group. The investigators point out imbalances between groups with a higher rate of intraventricular extension in the treatment group; moreover, they mainly attribute the disappointing results to the fact that the placebo group had a much more favorable outcome compared to the placebo group of the previous phase IIa trial (mortality 19% vs 29%; mRS 5 and 6, 24% vs 45%). However, other recent studies on neuron-protective treatment in ICH found comparably lower mortality rates.[330,331] Thus, outcomes of ICH may have improved due to advances in neurointensive care. Post-hoc analysis of the FAST trial suggests specific subgroups that may benefit from rFVIIa treatment. Patients under 70 years of age, with ICH volumes less than 60 ml and IVH less than 5 mL treated within 2.5 hours may have improved outcome when treated with rFVIIa (OR for poor outcome 0.28, 95%CI, 0.08–1.06).[332] Another promising approach to the selection patients for rFVIIa treatment may be the identification of patients at high-risk for hematoma growth by using the spot-sign. Spot-sign, contrast extravasation into the hematoma, has been repeatedly shown to be a very strong predictor of hematoma growth. The ongoing STOP-IT trial is investigating this issue. This randomized, prospective, controlled study includes ICH patients within 6 hours of onset and compares rFVIIa versus placebo for patients with ICH and positive spot-sign on the CT-angiography.

Blood Pressure Management

Severe hypertension is commonly observed in patients with acute ICH. Current guidelines recommend maintaining systolic blood pressure at <180 mmHg and diastolic blood pressure at <105 mm Hg. MAP should not exceed 130–120 mmHg.[260,261] The importance of selecting a target blood pressure on the basis of individual patient factors, such as baseline blood pressure, history of hypertension, presumed cause of hemorrhage, age and elevated ICP, was outlined.

Two main pathophysiological considerations have to be weighed against one another. The rationale for lowering blood pressure is to avoid hemorrhagic expansion, which is especially important for hemorrhages caused by aneurysms or arteriovenous malformations. On the other hand, aggressive lowering of blood pressure bears the theoretical risk of inducing ischemia in the edematous region adjacent to the hemorrhage. Studies underlining and mitigating the importance of both principles have been published so far. Several questions remain unresolved: (1) Does hypertension promote hemorrhage growth? Or is it rather a bystander effect of hematoma enlargement? Does reduction of blood pressure result in better patient outcome? (2) Is autoregulation impaired in ICH? If so, does overaggressive treatment of blood pressure decrease CPP and thereby worsen brain injury and finally patient outcome? What are the mechanisms involved?

A randomized pilot trial (INTERACT) investigated intensive BP reduction in acute ICH.[320] Patients with spontaneous ICH were included within 6 hours of onset and randomly assigned to early intensive lowering of BP with target systolic BP of 140 mm Hg (n=203) or standard-based management (n=201) with target systolic BP of 180 mmHg. Mean BP in the first hour was 153 mm Hg in the intensive group vs 167 mm Hg in the guideline group. Within the first 24 hours, BP was 146 mm Hg vs 157 mmHg. At 24 hours, mean proportional hematoma growth was 36.3% in the guideline group vs 13.7% in the intensive group. The mean absolute difference in hematoma volume between both groups was 1.7 mL at 24 hours. This pilot study established the safety of decreasing BP acutely after ICH by absence of significant adverse events or increased mortality and showed a trend toward reduced hematoma growth. Another randomized, controlled trial (ATACH) confirmed the feasibility and safety of BP lowering in ICH using IV nicardipine. Systolic BP reduction to 110–140 mm Hg in the first 24 hours was well tolerated and associated with a trend towards reduced hematoma expansion and neurological deterioration.[13] Recently, the results of the INTERACT-2 trial have been published. Within 6 hours after ICH onset, 2839 patients were randomized to intensive treatment to lower their blood pressure (with a target systolic level of <140 mm Hg within 1 hour) or guideline-recommended treatment (with a target systolic level of <180 mm Hg). The primary outcome was death or major disability (mRS 3–6). Seven-hundred and nineteen of 1382 participants (52%) receiving intensive treatment, as compared with 785 of 1412 (55.6%) receiving guideline-recommended treatment, had a primary outcome event (OR with intensive treatment, 0.87; 95%CI, 0.75–1.01; $P = 0.06$). The ordinal analysis showed significantly lower modified Rankin scores with intensive treatment (OR for greater disability, 0.87; 95%CI, 0.77–1.00; $P = 0.04$). Mortality with 11.9% in the group receiving intensive treatment and 12% in the group receiving guideline-recommended treatment was unchanged. Non-fatal serious adverse events occurred in 23.3% and 23.6% of the patients in the two groups, respectively.

Interestingly, the outcome effect seemed not to be associated with the attenuation of hemorrhage growth. The mean hematoma volumes were 15.7 ± 15.7 mL and 15.1 ± 14.9 mL in the two groups, respectively, at baseline and 18.2 ± 19.1 mL and 20.6 ± 24.9 mL, respectively, at 24 hours The difference in hematoma growth between the groups in the 24 hours after baseline was not significant (relative difference, 4.5%; [95%CI, – 3.1–12.7; $P = 0.27$], and absolute difference, 1.4 ml [95%CI, – 0.6–3.4; $P = 0.18$]). Summarized, acute lowering of the systolic BP to 140 mm Hg seems to be reasonable, safe and might improve outcome in ICH. Results from this trial will probably be considered in future guidelines.

Although prospective studies in animals and humans have challenged the concept of major ischemia in the perihematomal edema,[113,333] human MRI and SPECT data indicate the existence of a rim of tissue at risk for secondary ischemia in large hematomas with elevated ICP.[334,335] Yet, more recent MRI and CT studies again have dispelled this concept.[336,337] Few data are available to date with respect to autoregulation in ICH. In a human PET study, Powers and colleagues have found that reduction in MAP by 15% (mean 142 ± 10 to 119 ± 11 mm Hg) did not result in CBF reduction.[333] In an earlier SPECT study Kuwata and collegues reported that autoregulation in the perihematomal zone seemed to be preserved in the acute phase; however, global CBF significantly dropped in both hemispheres after reducing MAP > 20%.[338] It may be relevant to consider that stroke patients frequently suffer from chronic hypertension and their brain autoregulatory curve may be shifted to the right. While in normal individuals, CBF remains constant for MAP levels between 50 and 120 mm Hg, patients with chronic hypertension can be at risk for critical hypoperfusion at MAP levels that would be tolerated by normal individuals. The same holds true for patients with elevated ICP. Mainly based on data from patients with traumatic brain injury and one study in ICH patients, current guidelines recommend a preservation of a CPP > 60 mm Hg.[339,340] However, as discussed previously in this chapter, further research is to be done in the field with respect to recent studies claiming optimal CPP may differ between patients and should be determined aided by autoregulatory-based parameters.[178]

Appropriate agents for blood-pressure management have been discussed earlier in this chapter.

Coagulation and Reversal of Anticoagulation

Early assessment and correction of the coagulation status of a patient with ICH are particularly important, because it may affect both the progression of cerebral bleeding and the incidence of early re-bleeding. A therapeutic dilemma arises in patients with anticoagulant-associated ICH and an underlying condition associated with a high risk of recurrent embolism. Between 0.3% and 0.6% of patients on warfarin anticoagulation suffer from ICH, risk factors including age, intensity of anti-coagulation and leukoaraiosis. However, the annual risk of 5–10% of a thromboembolic complication without anticoagulation in patients with prosthetic valves can be translated as a 2-week risk of 0.2–0.4% that should be weighted against a rather high risk of early re-bleeding.[260,341]

Patients with a prolonged activated partial thromboplastin time because of heparin therapy should be treated with protamine sulfate, 1 mg/100 IU of heparin, adjusted to the time since last heparin use (30–60 minutes, 0.5–0.75 mg/IU; 60–120 minutes, 0.375–0.5 mg/IU; >120 minutes, 0.25–0.375 mg/IU, according to Broderick et al.[261]). The total dose should not exceed 50 mg and the infusion rate should be below 5 mg/minute; eventually PCC or FFP may be added. LMWH are increasingly employed for anti-coagulation in clinical practice. However, there is no uniformly effective or specific antidote to reverse bleeding complications. Protamine sulfate only partially antagonizes the anticoagulant effects of LMWH. PCC have proven more efficient.[342]

A prolonged prothrombin time due to phenprocoumon or warfarin therapy should be reversed with intravenous prothrombin complex concentrates (PCC), fresh frozen plasma (FFP), or both. Dosages and composition of factors of PCC largely vary between products and details should be obtained from the manufacturer. For FFP, the following approximation can be applied: 10 mL/kg will reduce an INR of 4.2–2.4, an INR of 3.0–2.1 or an INR of 2.4–1.8; reducing an INR of 4.2–1.4 would therefore require 40 mL/kg.[260] Treatment must be combined with vitamin K_1 (1–2 × 5–10 mg IV), since half-lives of phenoprocoumon (7 days) and warfarin (24 hours) exceed that of vitamin-K-dependent factors. Currently, there are no randomized clinical trials comparing PCC and FFP. However, PCC seems to reverse anticoagulation faster than FFP. In one retrospective study with 55 patients the use of PCC as compared to FFP showed faster effect and reduced hematoma growth.[343] The use of FFP may require infusion of relatively large volumes of plasma. The necessary time for infusion may give place to hematoma enlargement and can lead to volume overload, at worst provoking heart failure. Moreover, the concentration of factors varies between different batches, making the degree of effectiveness somewhat unpredictable.[261] PCC concentrates can correct coagulopathy faster with smaller volumes, at the price of a higher risk for thromboembolic complications. Repeated measurements of coagulation status are necessary; INR should be reevaluated 15 minutes after application of PCC. The ongoing randomized comparison between PCC and FFP in OAT-related ICH (INCH trial) has been designed to resolve these questions.[344]

The efficacy of novel direct oral anticoagulants (NOAC) dagibratran (factor II-inhibitor), apixaban and rivaroxaban (factor Xa-inhibitors) for stroke prevention in non-valvular atrial fibrilation has been demostrated in three non-inferiority trials against warfarin.[345–347] The rate of ICH in all three studies was significantly lower as compared to warfarin (0.2–0.5% vs 0.7–0.8%). The substantial issue in NOAC-related hemorrhages is the fact that routine hemocoagulation tests (Quick, PTT) are not sufficient to detect and measure the anticoagulatory activity of these drugs and that at present no specific antidote is known. Existing tests for dagibatran – the ecarin clotting time (ECT), thrombin time (TT) and the Hemoclot-test, for rivaroxaban and apixaban – the anti-factor Xa-levels, are mostly not available for the clinical routine. In NOAC-related intracranial hemorrhages, off-label PCC, factor VIIa or FFP administration may be tried.[348,349] However, no data on reversal of DOAC in patients with intracranial hemorrhage has been published so far.

Re-initiation of anticoagulation primarily concerns patients with a high risk of cardiogenic embolism associated with mechanical heart valves or atrial fibrillation. Current guidelines have summarized the available data as follows: in 114 patients from three clinical series, antagonizing anticoagulation with FFP and discontinuation of warfarin for a mean of 7–10 days was associated with embolism in 5% of patients. Re-bleeding upon reinstitution of anticoagulation between day 7 and 10 occurred in one patient (0.8%). Seven additional clinical series including 78 patients used PCC for reversal of anticoagulation, resulting in 5% of thromboembolic events; hematoma expansion occurred in 6%.[261] These limited data suggest that reversal of anticoagulation with FFP or PCC seems to be safe in patients with high risk for cardioembolic events; re-initiation of warfarin appears to be safe within the 14 days.

Antiplatelet Agents and Platelet Transfusions

Studies of the effects of prior antiplatelet agents, including aspirin, clopidogrel or both, on ICH hematoma growth, mortality and outcome produced conflicting results. In the CHANT study, reported antiplatelet agent use was not associated with hematoma expansion or clinical outcome.[350] A meta-analysis of cohort studies, however, showed slight increased mortality, but not worse functional outcome in ICH patients on antiplatelets. Non-randomized studies on platelet transfusion in ICH patients on antiplatelet agents failed to show any mortality or outcome benefits. Unfortunately, there was no standardization of the platelets dose or timing of transfusion,which may be of the utmost importance.[351] Identification of reduced platelet activity and early administration may be crucial for patient selection and the hemostatic effects. Two recent studies suggested smaller hemorrhage growth and potential outcome benefits with this setting.[352,353] In general, the utility and safety of platelet transfusions in ICH patients with a normal platelet count is not adequately known and cannot be recommended at this point.[250]

Intraventricular Hemorrhage and Hydrocephalus

One differentiates between primary and secondary intraventricular hemorrhage. Primary intraventricular hemorrhage (IVHs) constitutes a distinct entity; it originates from intraventricular structures as the choroid plexus. Symptoms are similar to those of SAH (severe headache of acute onset, neck stiffness, depressed level of consciousness), although motor deficit usually is either absent or minimal. Prognosis is more benign than that of secondary IVH.[354] Secondary IVH occurs in up to 40% of all patients with ICH and in up to 20% of all patients with SAH. There is strong evidence that IVH contributes to mortality after cerebral hemorrhage. Retrospective studies identified the presence and amount of intraventricular blood, time to clearance of the ventricles and development of hydrocephalus as independent predictors of poor outcome.[328,355] Hydrocephalus due to IVH develops via two different pathomechanisms. In the acute phase, obstruction of the third and fourth ventricle results in obstructive hydrocephalus. Later, malresorptive hydrocephalus may occur due to loss of function of pacchionian granulations. Typically, decline in the level of consciousness is the major symptom of a developing hydrocephalus. External ventricular drainage (EVD) is the treatment of choice which lowers the ICP immediately. Typically, the EVD is placed ipsilateral on the side of the hemorrhage. In case of occlusion of the foramina of Monroi, bilateral placement of an EVD may become necessary. The drainage has to be continued until the ventricular clot has dissolved, and CSF circulation normalized. Although a life-saving procedure, placement of a ventricular drainage does not affect the clot resolution or the incidence of communicating hydrocephalus. Therefore, intraventricular thrombolysis was proposed as an effective measure to hasten the resolution of the intraventricular blood clot, reduce the duration of extraventricular drainage, decrease the severity and incidence of communicating hydrocephalus, and reduce IVH-associated mortality. Clinical experience with this approach has grown over the last years.[356–358] The use of urokinase or streptokinase has been widely replaced by administration of rtPA, dosages varying between 4 mg and 20 mg.[359] At the moment, one prospective study on intraventricular thrombolysis with rtPA is ongoing (CLEARIII). This study was preceeded by two randomized pilot dose-finding studies employing 1 mg rtPA every 8 hours until clearing of the third and fourth ventricle or a cumulative dose of 8 mg, showing an acceptable safety profile and good resolution rates.[356,360]

Complications that may counteract the advantages of intraventricular thrombolysis are secondary hemorrhage and EVD infection. Therefore, vascular malformations should be ruled out with either CT angiography (CTA) or conventional angiography before intraventricular lysis is initiated (Fig. 54-4).

A promising approach to shorten the need for EVD is placement of a lumbar drainage. In a retrospective series including 55 patients with ICH, Huttner and colleagues investigated the effect of the placement of a lumbar drainage on duration of need for an EVD.[361] Placement of the lumbar drainage was performed in patients with persistent hydrocephalus after complete clearing of the third and fourth ventricles. In these cases, a communication between the inner and outer CSF spaces was assumed and lumbar drainage was performed with clamped EVD. EVD was only reopened when ICP increased. As soon as clamping of the EVD was tolerated for at least 24 hours without increase in ICP and no enlargement of the ventricles was observed in the CT scan, the EVD was removed. After that, the lumbar drainage was clamped every other day and hydrocephalus was monitored by CT scan. If no hydrocephalus reoccurred, the lumbar drainage was removed. After five futile attempts of clamping the lumbar drainage, a VP-shunt was placed. In this small series, placement of a lumbar drainage shortened the duration of required EVD and the frequency of a VP-shunt was reduced. The authors do not report an increased risk for axial herniation or infection.

Hypothermia

Hyperthermia in acute stroke is associated with poor outcome and increased mortality. High incidences of fever were reported in a retrospective study including ICH patients, especially for patients with ventricular hemorrhage; the duration of fever was associated with poor outcome.[281] Possible mechanisms by which hyperthermia affects outcome include release of neurotransmitters, oxygen radical production, blood–brain barrier breakdown, increase of ischemic depolarizations and impaired recovery of energy metabolism, inhibition of protein kinases and propagation of cytoskeletal proteolysis.[282] A raise in body temperature should prompt a search for an infectious focus and treatment should aim to maintain body temperature below 37.5 °C. A frequently used agent is paracetamol; external cooling with cooling blankets may be more effective. Some centres employ intravascular cooling catheters. However, outcome effects of temperature control are unproven. A recent small pilot study using historical controls showed that mild hypothermia is feasible in ICH and may reduce perihematomal edema.[362]

General management

The treatment of SAH is covered in Chapter 29.

Cerebral Venous Thrombosis

Cerebral venous and sinus thrombosis (CVST) constitutes less than 0.5–1% of all strokes and occurs predominantly in young female adults.[363] In general, 75% of patients diagnosed with CVST have a favorable clinical outcome, but 3–15% of patients die in the acute phase, in the majority of cases due to cerebral herniation caused by edema, infarctions and parenchymal hemorrhages.[364,365] Four percent of CVST takes a severe (sometimes called "malignant") course.[366] The diverse clinical presentation oftentimes obscures diagnosis, thus leading to a delayed initiation of therapeutical measures. Typical clinical symptoms of CVST are constitutional symptoms such as cephalgia, seizures, change of personality or disturbance of consciousness up to paralysis.

The optimal management of CVST is presently unclear and data on therapeutic strategies, apart from the guideline-recommended[365,367] anticoagulation with heparin, are still scarce and mainly based on case-series. A prospective cohort study of Coutinho et al. compared patients who received LMWH (n = 119) with patients who received unfractionated heparin (UFH) (n = 302) as anticoagulation treatment of cerebral venous thrombosis.[368] The analysis of this investigation showed that the frequency of new intracranial hemorrhages was increased among UFH (10% vs. 16%) and suggests a better efficacy and safety of LMWH over UFH.

Invasive therapeutical techniques such as endovascular thrombectomy and decompressive surgery are gaining attention, the latter having been shown to improve survival and functional outcome after malignant MCA infarction.[233] Their potential benefits in complicated CVST are uncertain, as prospective trials do not exist and evidence is limited to retrospective registries[365] or anecdotal reports.[369–375] These suggest that decompressive hemicraniectomy (HC) oftentimes results in good functional outcomes in CVST patients with impeding transtentorial herniation.[373,376] More persuading data regarding decompressive HC in CVST come from a recent investigation by Ferro et al.[365] This multicenter registry and review of

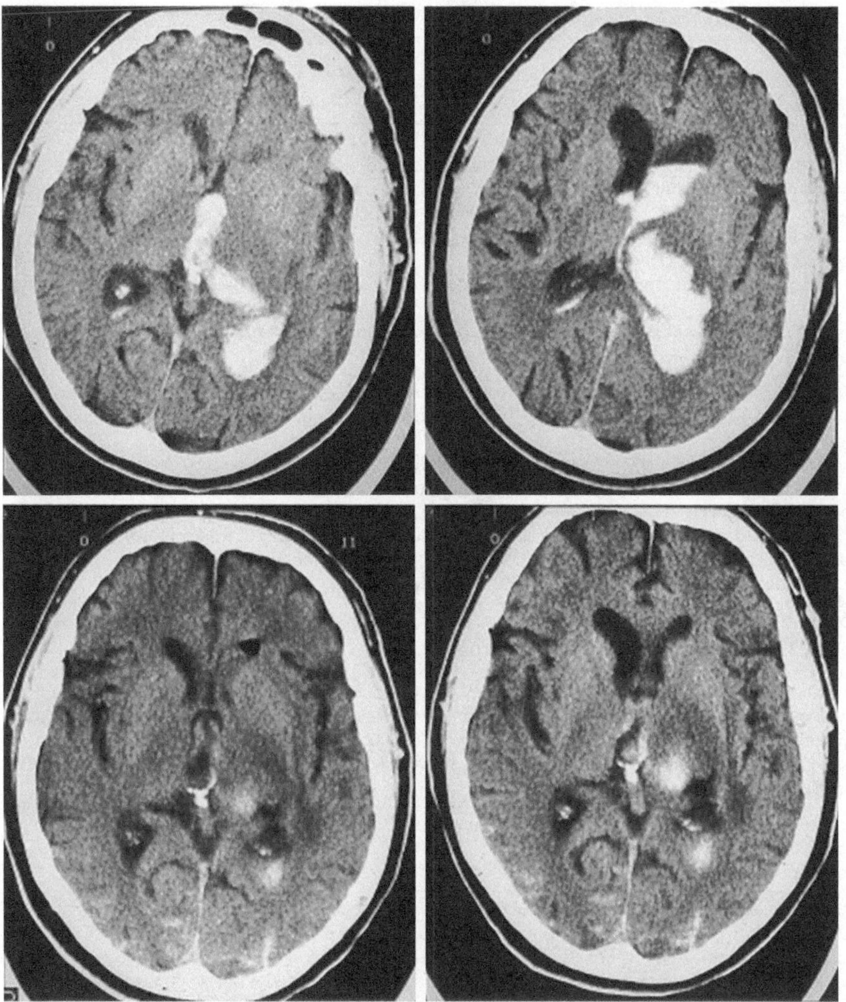

Figure 54-4. Intraventricular thrombolysis after basal ganglia hemorrhage with intraventricular bleeding. Time course of therapy with recombinant tissue-plasminogen activator (rt-PA) for thrombolysis of intraventricular blood. Top row, before treatment; bottom row, after treatment.

literature shows that good functional outcome was related to decompressive surgery, even in patients with poor neurological status. In this study the majority of the registered patients (n = 38) had a severe condition with early signs of transtentorial herniation: 65.8% of patients were comatose before surgery and 52% had dilated fixed pupils. Decompressive surgery was performed in 60.5% of patients, hematoma evacuation was performed in 18.4%, and 21.1% of patients underwent both types of surgery. The authors thus draw two main conclusions: firstly HC was lifesaving in patients with large parenchymal lesions causing herniation. Secondly, even in patients with severe clinical conditions HC often resulted in good functional outcome. A subsequent prospective registry study on an invasive interdisciplinary therapeutic approach to severe CVST (International Study on Dural Sinus and Cerebral Vein Thrombosis II (ISCVT II)) has already been initiated by Ferro et al., but results are still outstanding.

Few reports showed that EVT and thrombolysis can be performed successfully, but authors emphasize that this therapeutical approach is a last resort for selected and severe cases.[374,377] A study by Stam et al. investigated EVT and thrombolysis as a treatment option for patients with poor prognosis. The analysis showed that patients with severe CSVT did not benefit from the sole application of this method.[378] A subsequent prospective registry study on an endovascular therapeutic approach to severe CVST (thrombolysis or anticoagulation for cerebral venous thrombosis: rationale and design of the TO-ACT trial) has already been initiated by Coutinho et al. At present, efficacy of endovascular thrombolysis on its own remains without proof of evidence.

Conservative neurocritical care treatment of severe CVST involves anticoagulation management, intubation and ventilation, airway management, treatment of seizures, temperature control and ICP-management. With regard to the latter, osmotherapy has been controversial in CVST.[367,379]

CONCLUSION

Significant developments in the field of intensive care treatment have led to improved care and outcome for critically ill stroke patients. Robust evidence suggests that treatment in a specialized stroke units or neurological intensive care units is associated with more favorable outcome as compared to general ICU wards.[317,380] Therefore patients with acute stroke ideally should be treated in such units including standardized care, neuromonitoring, with neurosurgeons and neuroradiologists in reach, and development of these structures are strongly encouraged. Despite the fact that for the basic therapeutic questions such as optimal blood pressure management, osmotherapy or hypothermia, reversal and re-initialization of anticoagulation, etc., there still is insufficient evidence, neurocritical care of stroke as a complex of specialized measures in a dedicated unit seems to be more effective than general multidisciplinary critical care.

TABLE 54-3 Selected Conclusions/Recommendations

Aspect/ Stroke Type	Conclusion/Recommendation	Class of Recommendation	Level of Evidence
General Management			
Initial assessment of acute stroke	Clinical, monitoring and blood test assessment should not add up to more than 30 minutes to be able to provide imaging and, in AIS, recanalizing therapy within 60 minutes. It should involve the use of severity scores of (such as NIHSS, HuntHess/WFNS, ICH score, as adequate)	I	A
	Laboratory tests on hematology, coagulation, and biochemistry are recommended, and assessment of blood glucose is compulsory	I	B
	Echocardiographic monitoring should be initiated and maintained for at least the first 24 hours from stroke onset	I	B
	Realization of adequate imaging in acute stroke is paramount and must not be unnecessarily delayed	I	A
Airway and ventilation	In AIS (and probably in other stroke types as well), normoxemia (SpO_2>94%) should be aimed for	I	C
	In AIS (and probably in other stroke types as well), non-hypoxic patients should not receive supplementary oxygen	III	B
	Airway support (if adequate, by intubation) and ventilatory assistance should be provided without delay in stroke patients with respiratory failure, a decline in level of consciousness, bulbar dysfunction, and loss of protective reflexes	I	C
	Due to a high incidence of dysphagia and disturbed vigilance in ventilated patients with severe stroke, extubation failure is frequent and classical ICU extubation criteria not reliable	IIa	B
	(Early) tracheostomy in stroke patients is safe and feasible	IIb	B
Nutrition and GIT	Swallowing should be assessed by clinical and/or endoscopic swallowing tests and detection of dysphagia lead to nasogastric tube placement	I	B
	Nasogastric tubes can be used for feeding for 2–3 weeks after stroke onset, before placement of a percutaneous endoscopic gastrostomy tube may be considered	IIa	B
	Energy expenditure and caloric demand of sedated and ventilated stroke patients can be estimated using the Harris-Benedict equation	IIb	C
	Enteral should be preferred over parenteral feeding, the routine use of nutritional supplements is not of proven benefit	III	C
Infection	Infections (such as pneumonias or UTIs) should be screened for and detection leads to adequate antibiotic treatment without delay	I	A
	The use of prophylactic antibiotics in stroke patients has not been proven beneficial	III	B
DVT-prophylaxis	Immobilized patients with severe stroke should have intermittent compression for prevention of DVT	I	B
	Additional use of low-dose unfractionated or low-molecular-weight heparin should be considered in stroke patients for DVT prophylaxis, but withheld for 24 hours after SAH and ICH, following securing the aneurysm in SAH and demonstrating hematoma stability in ICH	I(AIS), IIb	A(AIS),B
Blood glucose	Aiming for intermediate levels of blood glucose (140–180 mg/dL) appears feasible and advisable in stroke. Both hyperglycemia exceeding 180 mg/dL and hypoglycemia (<80 mg/dL) should be avoided and treated	I	B
Temperature	Fever is detrimental in stroke, its sources should be screened for and, if accessible (such as infections), be treated	I	A
	Normothermia should be aimed for by active fever-lowering measures, although the benefit thereof remains to be confirmed	IIa	C
	Active hypothermia may lead to complications and its benefits are not established in stroke	III	C
Seizures	Manifest seizures and status epilepticus must be treated rapidly by adequate antiepileptics	I	A
	In patients with a changed mental status and electrographic seizure correlates on EEG should be treated with antiepileptics	I	C
	There is no sufficiently proven benefit of prophylactic antiepileptics in stroke, but may be considered in the immediate posthemorrhagic period of SAH	IIa	B
Monitoring	Patients with severe stroke should be managed on a dedicated neurocritical care unit and receive continuous basic systemic (such as ECG, BP, SaO_2, PaO_2, $PaCO_2$, CVP, fluid status, etc.)	I	B
	Enhanced hemodynamic monitoring (such as by volumetric devices, pulmonary artery catheter or TEE) may be advisable in certain settings (e.g., SAH with vasospasm), but the benefit thereof needs to be further investigated	IIb	C
	Enhanced neuromonitoring (such as by ICP, $PbtO_2$, cont. EEG, etc.) may be advisable in analog-sedated patients with severe stroke prone to brain edema, ICP increases, and secondary brain damage, but the benefits thereof need to be further investigated	IIb	C

TABLE 54-3 Selected Conclusions/Recommendations—cont'd

Aspect/ Stroke Type	Conclusion/Recommendation	Class of Recommendation, Level of Evidence	
Specific Management			
AIS	Elevated blood pressure should be lowered to <185/110 mmHg if the patient is to receive thrombolysis and maintained at this level for the following 24 hours	I	B
	Outside of thrombolysis, elevated blood pressure should be left untreated, and only be lowered if it exceeds >220/120 mmHg	I	C
	Potential side effects of thrombolysis, such as ICH, systemic bleeding, or angioedema need to be anticipated. Prompt cessation of thrombolysis, diagnostic tests and specific treatment have to follow in case these are observed	I	B
	If IAT is selected, intubation and general anesthesia are advisable in posterior circulation stroke, and/or if the patient is comatose, agitated or has vomited. In all other patients, conscious sedation without intubation may possibly be advantageous	IIb	C
	Urgent or early anticoagulation, therapeutic heparin or early antiplatelets other than aspirin (or aspirin/ clopidogrel after stent placement) are not well established and should be avoided	III	B-C
	Re-initiation of oral anticoagulation in patients at risk of cardioembolism (e.g., with AF or heart valve) has to be judged individually depending on size of infarction and risk of embolism. Re-initiation between 2 and 4 weeks appears reasonable	IIa	C
	In patients with large hemispheric stroke prone to massive brain edema, decompressive surgery within 48 hours reduces mortality and morbidity and hence should be considered	I	B
	In patients with space-occupying cerebellar stroke prone to hydrocephalus and brain stem compression, placement of an EVD and suboccipital decompressive trepanation may be life-saving and improve outcome, and should hence be considered	IIa	C
ICH	In patients with elevated SBP > 200 (or MAP >150) mmHg, aggressive BP lowering, and in those with SBP >180 (or MAP >130) mmHg, modest BP lowering, respectively, should be considered (target 160/90 mmHg), ideally under ICP/CPP monitoring to keep CPP >60 mmHg. In patients with SBP between 150 and 220 mmHg, aggressive BP lowering to 140 mmHg is probably safe	IIa	B
	Patients with severe coagulation deficiency or severe thrombocytopenia should receive appropriate factor replacement therapy or platelets, respectively	I	C
	Patients whose INR is elevated due to OAC, should have their OAC withheld, be given vitamin K (if they were in warfarin) and PCC or FFP to normalize coagulation	I	C
	PCC may have fewer complications than FFP and are reasonable to be considered as an alternative, though an outcome benefit has not been shown. Coagulation tests for NOACs may not be available and basic coagulation tests may not be reliable for excluding ongoing activity	IIa	B
	rFVIIa does not replace all clotting factors, and although the INR may be lowered, clotting may not be restored in vivo; therefore rFVIIa is not routinely recommended as a sole agent for OAC reversal in ICH	III	C
	Although rFVIIa can limit secondary hematoma expansion in non-coagulation ICH patients, there is no proven clinical benefit and an increase in thromboembolic events, hence it is not recommended in unselected patients	III	A
	In IVH and hydrocephalus leading to decline in level of consciousness, external ventricular drainage is reasonable	IIa	B
	Although intraventricular administration of rtPA via the EVD to speed drainage in IVH seems to have a low complication rate, its efficacy is uncertain and the treatment is considered experimental, at present	IIb	B
	The benefits of surgery for clot removal, either by open craniotomy or minimal invasive techniques, are uncertain for most ICH patients	IIb	B, C
	Surgical clot removal may be considered in selected patients, e.g., those with ongoing mid-line shift and progressive clinical worsening, those with cerebellar hemorrhage leading to brainstem compression and hydrocephalus, and those with superficial lobar clots >30 mL	I, IIb	B
	Current methods of prognostication are probably biased by failure to account for the influence of withdrawal of support and early DNR orders. Aggressive full care early after ICH onset and postponement of new DNR orders until at least the second full day of hospitalization is probably recommended in most ICH patients who had no preexisting DNR orders	IIa	B
CVST	Basic treatment of CVST should contain antithrombotic therapy by either unfractionated heparin or low-molecular-weight heparinoids, even if congestive ICH is present	IIa	B
	Hemicraniectomy should be considered early in severe CVST with brain edema, space-occupying ICH and/or ICP increase. This should probably not include ICH evacuation	IIa	C

Abbreviations: NIHSS, National Institutes of Health Stroke Scale; WFNS, World Federation of Neurosurgeons Scale; ICH, intracerebral hemorrhage; AIS, acute ischemic stroke; SpO_2; pulse oxiymetry arterial oxygen saturation; ICU; intensive care unit; GIT; gastrointestinal tract; UTI; urinary tract infection; DVT; deep vein thrombosis; SAH, subarachnoid hemorrhage; EEG, electroencephalography; ECG; electrocardiography; BP, blood pressure; PaO_2, partial arterial pressure of oxygen; $PaCO_2$, partial arterial pressure of carbon dioxide; CVP, central venous pressure; TEE, transesophageal echocardiography; ICP, intracranial pressure; $PbtO_2$, brain tissue tension of oxygen; IAT, intra-arterial thrombolysis; EVD, external ventricular drain; SBP, systolic blood pressure; MAP, mean arterial pressure; CPP, cerebral perfusion pressure; INR, international normalized ratio; (N)OAC, (new) oral anticoagulants; PCC, prothrombin complex concentrates; FFP, fresh-frozen plasma; rFVIIa, recombinant factor VIIa; IVH, intraventricular hemorrhage; rtPA, recombinant tissue-type plasminogen activator; DNR, do-not-rescuscitate; aSAH, aneurysmal SAH; CT, computed tomography; MRI, magnetic resonance tomography; CSF, cerebrospinal fluid; CVST, cerebral venous and sinus thrombosis.

Classification of recommendations and levels of evidence are based on the AHA categories.

These selected conclusions/recommendations are corresponding to some relevant parts of the chapter and based on current evidence and guidelines, in part they are adapted from: Jauch, E.C., et al., Guidelines for the early management of patients with acute ischemic stroke: a guideline for healthcare professionals from the American Heart Association/American Stroke Association. *Stroke, 2013. 44(3): p. 870–947; Morgenstern, L.B., et al.,* Guidelines for the management of spontaneous intracerebral hemorrhage: a guideline for healthcare professionals from the American Heart Association/American Stroke Association. *Stroke, 2010. 41(9): p. 2108–29; Connolly, E.S., Jr., et al.,* Guidelines for the management of aneurysmal subarachnoid hemorrhage: a guideline for healthcare professionals from the American Heart Association/American Stroke Association. *Stroke, 2012. 43(6): p. 1711–37.*

For more details refer to 'AHA Evidence box index' in the FM.

The complete reference list can be found on the companion Expert Consult website at www.expertconsult.inkling.com.

KEY REFERENCES

2. Berrouschot J, Rössler A, Köster J, et al. Mechanical ventilation in patients with hemispheric ischemic stroke. Crit Care Med 2000;28:2956–61.
4. Wijdicks EF, Scott JP. Causes and outcome of mechanical ventilation in patients with hemispheric ischemic stroke. Mayo Clin Proc 1997;72:210–13.
5. el-Ad B, Bornstein NM, Fuchs P, et al. Mechanical ventilation in stroke patients – is it worthwhile? Neurology 1996;47:657–9.
7. Roch A, Michelet P, Jullien AC, et al. Long-term outcome in intensive care unit survivors after mechanical ventilation for intracerebral hemorrhage. Crit Care Med 2003;31:2651–6.
9. Gujjar AR, Deibert E, Manno EM, et al. Mechanical ventilation for ischemic stroke and intracerebral hemorrhage: indications, timing, and outcome. Neurology 1998;51:447–51.
11. Bushnell CD, Phillips-Bute BG, Laskowitz DT, et al. Survival and outcome after endotracheal intubation for acute stroke. Neurology 1999;52(7):1374–81.
12. Holzapfel L, Chevret S, Madinier G, et al. Influence of long-term oro- or nasotracheal intubation on nosocomial maxillary sinusitis and pneumonia: results of a prospective, randomized, clinical trial. Crit Care Med 1993;21(8):1132–8.
15. Perry J, Lee J, Wells G. Rocuronium versus succinylcholine for rapid sequence induction intubation. Cochrane Database Syst Rev 2003;(1):CD002788.
17. Abou-Chebl A, Lin R, Hussain MS, et al. Conscious sedation versus general anesthesia during endovascular therapy for acute anterior circulation stroke: preliminary results from a retrospective, multicenter study. Stroke 2010;41(6):1175–9.
18. Jumaa MA, Zhang F, Ruiz-Ares G, et al. Comparison of safety and clinical and radiographic outcomes in endovascular acute stroke therapy for proximal middle cerebral artery occlusion with intubation and general anesthesia versus the nonintubated state. Stroke 2010;41(6):1180–4.
19. Davis MJ, Menon BK, Baghirzada LB, et al. Anesthetic management and outcome in patients during endovascular therapy for acute stroke. Anesthesiology 2012;116(2):396–405.
20. Iscoe S, Fisher JA. Hyperoxia-induced hypocapnia: an underappreciated risk. Chest 2005;128(1):430–3.
21. Johnston AJ, Steiner LA, Gupta AK, et al. Cerebral oxygen vasoreactivity and cerebral tissue oxygen reactivity. Br J Anaesth 2003; 90(6):774–86.
22. Coles JP, Minhas PS, Fryer TD, et al. Effect of hyperventilation on cerebral blood flow in traumatic head injury: clinical relevance and monitoring correlates. Crit Care Med 2002;30(9): 1950–9.
26. Georgiadis D, Schwarz S, Baumgartner RW, et al. Influence of positive end-expiratory pressure on intracranial pressure and cerebral perfusion pressure in patients with acute stroke. Stroke 2001;32(9):2088–92.
31. Pelosi P, Ferguson ND, Frutos-Vivar F, et al. Management and outcome of mechanically ventilated neurologic patients. Crit Care Med 2011;39(6):1482–92.
33. Skoglund K, Enblad P, Hillered L, et al. The neurological wake-up test increases stress hormone levels in patients with severe traumatic brain injury. Crit Care Med 2012;40(1):216–22.
46. Qureshi AI, Suarez JI, Parekh PD, et al. Prediction and timing of tracheostomy in patients with infratentorial lesions requiring mechanical ventilatory support. Crit Care Med 2000;28(5): 1383–7.
50. Sessler CN, Varney K. Patient-focused sedation and analgesia in the ICU. Chest 2008;133(2):552–65.
53. Sessler CN, Gosnell MS, Grap MJ, et al. The Richmond Agitation-Sedation Scale: validity and reliability in adult intensive care unit patients. Am J Respir Crit Care Med 2002;166(10): 1338–44.
54. Riker RR, Picard JT, Fraser GL. Prospective evaluation of the Sedation-Agitation Scale for adult critically ill patients. Crit Care Med 1999;27(7):1325–9.
55. Deogaonkar A, Gupta R, DeGeorgia M, et al. Bispectral Index monitoring correlates with sedation scales in brain-injured patients. Crit Care Med 2004;32(12):2403–6.
58. Mehta S, Burry L, Cook D, et al. Daily sedation interruption in mechanically ventilated critically ill patients cared for with a sedation protocol: a randomized controlled trial. JAMA 2012; 308(19):1985–92.
60. Aitkenhead AR, Pepperman ML, Willatts SM, et al. Comparison of propofol and midazolam for sedation in critically ill patients. Lancet 1989;2(8665):704–9.
61. Barrientos-Vega R, Mar Sánchez-Soria M, Morales-García C, et al. Prolonged sedation of critically ill patients with midazolam or propofol: impact on weaning and costs. Crit Care Med 1997; 25(1):33–40.
62. Chamorro C, de Latorre FJ, Montero A, et al. Comparative study of propofol versus midazolam in the sedation of critically ill patients: results of a prospective, randomized, multicenter trial. Crit Care Med 1996;24(6):932–9.
63. Shafer A. Complications of sedation with midazolam in the intensive care unit and a comparison with other sedative regimens. Crit Care Med 1998;26(5):947–56.
67. Bourgoin A, Albanèse J, Wereszczynski N, et al. Safety of sedation with ketamine in severe head injury patients: comparison with sufentanil. Crit Care Med 2003;31(3):711–17.
68. Albanese J, Arnaud S, Rey M, et al. Ketamine decreases intracranial pressure and electroencephalographic activity in traumatic brain injury patients during propofol sedation. Anesthesiology 1997;87(6):1328–34.
70. Kitano H, Kirsch JR, Hurn PD, et al. Inhalational anesthetics as neuroprotectants or chemical preconditioning agents in ischemic brain. J Cereb Blood Flow Metab 2007;27(6):1108–28.
79. Werner C, Kochs E, Bause H, et al. Effects of sufentanil on cerebral hemodynamics and intracranial pressure in patients with brain injury. Anesthesiology 1995;83(4):721–6.
85. Davalos A, Ricart W, Gonzalez-Huix F, et al. Effect of malnutrition after acute stroke on clinical outcome. Stroke 1996;27(6): 1028–32.
90. Heyland DK, MacDonald S, Keefe L, et al. Total parenteral nutrition in the critically ill patient: a meta-analysis. JAMA 1998; 280(23):2013–19.
91. Krishnan JA, Parce PB, Martinez A, et al. Caloric intake in medical ICU patients: consistency of care with guidelines and relationship to clinical outcomes. Chest 2003;124(1): 297–305.
92. van den Berghe G, Wouters P, Weekers F, et al. Intensive insulin therapy in the critically ill patients. N Engl J Med 2001;345(19): 1359–67.
93. Kistler JP, Vielma JD, Davis KR, et al. Effects of nitroglycerin on the diameter of intracranial and extracranial arteries in monkeys. Arch Neurol 1982;39(10):631–4.
98. Puchstein C, Van Aken H, Anger C, et al. Influence of urapidil on intracranial pressure and intracranial compliance in dogs. Br J Anaesth 1983;55(5):443–8.
103. Hall JE, Uhrich TD, Ebert TJ. Sedative, analgesic and cognitive effects of clonidine infusions in humans. Br J Anaesth 2001; 86(1):5–11.
106. Kanawati IS, Yaksh TL, Anderson RE, et al. Effects of clonidine on cerebral blood flow and the response to arterial CO_2. J Cereb Blood Flow Metab 1986;6(3):358–65.
108. ter Minassian A, Beydon L, Decq P, et al. Changes in cerebral hemodynamics after a single dose of clonidine in severely head-injured patients. Anesth Analg 1997;84(1):127–32.
110. Lee HW, Caldwell JE, Dodson B, et al. The effect of clonidine on cerebral blood flow velocity, carbon dioxide cerebral vasoreactivity, and response to increased arterial pressure in human volunteers. Anesthesiology 1997;87(3):553–8.
113. Qureshi AI, Wilson DA, Hanley DF, et al. Pharmacologic reduction of mean arterial pressure does not adversely affect regional cerebral blood flow and intracranial pressure in experimental intracerebral hemorrhage. Crit Care Med 1999;27(5): 965–71.
123. Sakabe T, Nagai I, Ishikawa T, et al. Nicardipine increases cerebral blood flow but does not improve neurologic recovery in a canine model of complete cerebral ischemia. J Cereb Blood Flow Metab 1986;6(6):684–90.

129. Halpern NA, Goldberg M, Neely C, et al. Postoperative hypertension: a multicenter, prospective, randomized comparison between intravenous nicardipine and sodium nitroprusside. Crit Care Med 1992;20(12):1637–43.
132. Lisk DR, Grotta JC, Lamki LM, et al. Should hypertension be treated after acute stroke? A randomized controlled trial using single photon emission computed tomography. Arch Neurol 1993;50(8):855–62.
141. Mayhall CG, Archer NH, Lamb VA, et al. Ventriculostomy-related infections. A prospective epidemiologic study. N Engl J Med 1984;310(9):553–9.
161. Berger C, Annecke A, Aschoff A, et al. Neurochemical monitoring of fatal middle cerebral artery infarction. Stroke 1999;30(2): 460–3.
170. Dohmen C, Bosche B, Graf R, et al. Identification and clinical impact of impaired cerebrovascular autoregulation in patients with malignant middle cerebral artery infarction. Stroke 2007; 38(1):56–61.
171. Dohmen C, Bosche B, Graf R, et al. Prediction of malignant course in MCA infarction by PET and microdialysis. Stroke 2003; 34(9):2152–8.
172. Schwab S, Aschoff A, Spranger M, et al. The value of intracranial pressure monitoring in acute hemispheric stroke. Neurology 1996;47(2):393–8.
178. Steiner LA, Czosnyka M, Piechnik SK, et al. Continuous monitoring of cerebrovascular pressure reactivity allows determination of optimal cerebral perfusion pressure in patients with traumatic brain injury. Crit Care Med 2002;30(4):733–8.
184. Schwarz S, Georgiadis D, Aschoff A, et al. Effects of body position on intracranial pressure and cerebral perfusion in patients with large hemispheric stroke. Stroke 2002;33(2):497–501.
188. Manno EM, Adams RE, Derdeyn CP, et al. The effects of mannitol on cerebral edema after large hemispheric cerebral infarct. Neurology 1999;52(3):583–7.
189. Videen TO, Zazulia AR, Manno EM, et al. Mannitol bolus preferentially shrinks non-infarcted brain in patients with ischemic stroke. Neurology 2001;57(11):2120–2.
195. Paczynski RP, He YY, Diringer MN, et al. Multiple-dose mannitol reduces brain water content in a rat model of cortical infarction. Stroke 1997;28(7):1437–43, discussion 1444.
196. Bereczki D, Fekete I, Prado GF, et al. Mannitol for acute stroke. Cochrane Database Syst Rev 2007;(3):CD001153.
197. Bereczki D, Mihálka L, Szatmári S, et al. Mannitol use in acute stroke: case fatility at 30 days and 1 year. Stroke 2003;34: 1730–5.
198. Schwarz S, Schwab S, Bertram M, et al. Effects of hypertonic saline hydroxyethyl starch solution and mannitol in patients with increased intracranial pressure after stroke. Stroke 1998; 29(8):1550–5.
202. Righetti E, Celani MG, Cantisani T, et al. Glycerol for acute stroke. Cochrane Database Syst Rev 2004;(2):CD000096.
206. Qureshi AI, Suarez JI. Use of hypertonic saline solutions in treatment of cerebral edema and intracranial hypertension. Crit Care Med 2000;28(9):3301–13.
207. Schwarz S, Georgiadis D, Aschoff A, et al. Effects of hypertonic (10%) saline in patients with raised intracranial pressure after stroke. Stroke 2002;33(1):136–40.
215. Marion DW, Puccio A, Wisniewski SR, et al. Effect of hyperventilation on extracellular concentrations of glutamate, lactate, pyruvate, and local cerebral blood flow in patients with severe traumatic brain injury. Crit Care Med 2002;30(12): 2619–25.
223. Qizilbash N, Lewington SL, Lopez-Arrieta JM. Corticosteroids for acute ischaemic stroke. Cochrane Database Syst Rev 2002;(2): CD000064.
224. Poungvarin N, Bhoopat W, Viriyavejakul A, et al. Effects of dexamethasone in primary supratentorial intracerebral hemorrhage. N Engl J Med 1987;316(20):1229–33.
228. Forsting M, Reith W, Schäbitz WR, et al. Decompressive craniectomy for cerebral infarction. An experimental study in rats. Stroke 1995;26(2):259–64.
232. Juttler E, Schwab S, Schmiedek P, et al., DESTINY Study Group. Decompressive Surgery for the Treatment of Malignant Infarction of the Middle Cerebral Artery (DESTINY): a randomized, controlled trial. Stroke 2007;38(9):2518–25.
233. Vahedi K, Hofmeijer J, Juettler E, et al., DECIMAL, DESTINY, and HAMLET investigators. Early decompressive surgery in malignant infarction of the middle cerebral artery: a pooled analysis of three randomised controlled trials. Lancet Neurol 2007;6(3): 215–22.
234. Colbourne F, Corbett D, Zhao Z, et al. Prolonged but delayed postischemic hypothermia: a long-term outcome study in the rat middle cerebral artery occlusion model. J Cereb Blood Flow Metab 2000;20(12):1702–8.
237. Nakashima K, Todd MM. Effects of hypothermia on the rate of excitatory amino acid release after ischemic depolarization. Stroke 1996;27(5):913–18.
240. Karibe H, Zarow GJ, Graham SH, et al. Mild intraischemic hypothermia reduces postischemic hyperperfusion, delayed postischemic hypoperfusion, blood-brain barrier disruption, brain edema, and neuronal damage volume after temporary focal cerebral ischemia in rats. J Cereb Blood Flow Metab 1994;14(4): 620–7.
244. Clifton GL, Miller ER, Choi SC, et al. Lack of effect of induction of hypothermia after acute brain injury. N Engl J Med 2001; 344(8):556–63.
245. Hypothermia after Cardiac Arrest Study Group. Mild therapeutic hypothermia to improve the neurologic outcome after cardiac arrest. N Engl J Med 2002;346(8):549–56.
246. Bernard SA, Gray TW, Buist MD, et al. Treatment of comatose survivors of out-of-hospital cardiac arrest with induced hypothermia. N Engl J Med 2002;346(8):557–63.
247. Vespa PM, O'Phelan K, Shah M, et al. Acute seizures after intracerebral hemorrhage: a factor in progressive midline shift and outcome. Neurology 2003;60(9):1441–6.
249. Adams HP Jr, del Zoppo G, Alberts MJ, et al., American Heart Association/American Stroke Association Stroke Council; American Heart Association/American Stroke Association Clinical Cardiology Council; American Heart Association/American Stroke Association Cardiovascular Radiology and Intervention Council; Atherosclerotic Peripheral Vascular Disease Working Group; Quality of Care Outcomes in Research Interdisciplinary Working Group. Guidelines for the early management of adults with ischemic stroke: a guideline from the American Heart Association/American Stroke Association Stroke Council, Clinical Cardiology Council, Cardiovascular Radiology and Intervention Council, and the Atherosclerotic Peripheral Vascular Disease and Quality of Care Outcomes in Research Interdisciplinary Working Groups: The American Academy of Neurology affirms the value of this guideline as an educational tool for neurologists. Circulation 2007;115(20):e478–534.
251. Johnston KC, Li JY, Lyden PD, et al. Medical and neurological complications of ischemic stroke: experience from the RANTTAS trial. RANTTAS Investigators. Stroke 1998;29(2):447–53.
253. Langhorne P, Stott DJ, Robertson L, et al. Medical complications after stroke: a multicenter study. Stroke 2000;31(6):1223–9.
256. Kelly J, Rudd A, Lewis RR, et al. Venous thromboembolism after acute ischemic stroke: a prospective study using magnetic resonance direct thrombus imaging. Stroke 2004;35(10):2320–5.
257. Mazzone C, Chiodo GF, Sandercock P, et al. Physical methods for preventing deep vein thrombosis in stroke. Cochrane Database Syst Rev 2004;(4):CD001922.
258. Diener HC, Ringelstein EB, von Kummer R, et al. Prophylaxis of thrombotic and embolic events in acute ischemic stroke with the low-molecular-weight heparin certoparin: results of the PROTECT Trial. Stroke 2006;37(1):139–44.
259. Sherman DG, Albers GW, Bladin C, et al. PREVAIL Investigators The efficacy and safety of enoxaparin versus unfractionated heparin for the prevention of venous thromboembolism after acute ischaemic stroke (PREVAIL Study): an open-label randomised comparison. Lancet 2007;369(9570):1347–55.
261. Broderick J, Connolly S, Feldmann E, et al., American Heart Association/American Stroke Association Stroke Council; American Heart Association/American Stroke Association High Blood Pressure Research Council; Quality of Care and Outcomes in Research Interdisciplinary Working Group. Guidelines for the management of spontaneous intracerebral hemorrhage in adults: 2007 update: a guideline from the American Heart Association/American Stroke Association Stroke Council, High Blood Pressure Research Council, and the Quality of Care and

Outcomes in Research Interdisciplinary Working Group. Circulation 2007;116(16):e391–413.
262. Dennis M, Sandercock P, Reid J, et al. Effectiveness of intermittent pneumatic compression in reduction of risk of deep vein thrombosis in patients who have had a stroke (CLOTS 3): a multicentre randomised controlled trial. Lancet 2013;382(9891):516–24.
263. Dorffler-Melly J, de Jonge E, Pont AC, et al. Bioavailability of subcutaneous low-molecular-weight heparin to patients on vasopressors. Lancet 2002;359(9309):849–50.
264. Capes SE, Hunt D, Malmberg K, et al. Stress hyperglycemia and prognosis of stroke in nondiabetic and diabetic patients: a systematic overview. Stroke 2001;32(10):2426–32.
265. Scott JF, Robinson GM, French JM, et al. Prevalence of admission hyperglycaemia across clinical subtypes of acute stroke. Lancet 1999;353(9150):376–7.
268. Lindsberg PJ, Roine RO. Hyperglycemia in acute stroke. Stroke 2004;35(2):363–4.
269. Parsons MW, Barber PA, Desmond PM, et al. Acute hyperglycemia adversely affects stroke outcome: a magnetic resonance imaging and spectroscopy study. Ann Neurol 2002;52(1):20–8.
270. Candelise L, Landi G, Orazio EN, et al. Prognostic significance of hyperglycemia in acute stroke. Arch Neurol 1985;42(7):661–3.
271. Van den Berghe G, Wilmer A, Hermans G, et al. Intensive insulin therapy in the medical ICU. N Engl J Med 2006;354(5):449–61.
272. Dellinger RP, Carlet JM, Masur H, et al., Surviving Sepsis Campaign Management Guidelines Committee. Surviving Sepsis Campaign guidelines for management of severe sepsis and septic shock. Crit Care Med 2004;32(3):858–73.
273. Brunkhorst FM, Engel C, Bloos F, et al., German Competence Network Sepsis (SepNet). Intensive insulin therapy and pentastarch resuscitation in severe sepsis. N Engl J Med 2008;358(2):125–39.
274. Finfer S, Chittock DR, Su SY, et al., NICE-SUGAR Study Investigators. Intensive versus conventional glucose control in critically ill patients. N Engl J Med 2009;360(13):1283–97.
275. Finfer S, Liu B, Chittock DR, et al., NICE-SUGAR Study Investigators. Hypoglycemia and risk of death in critically ill patients. N Engl J Med 2012;367(12):1108–18.
276. Oddo M, Schmidt JM, Carrera E, et al. Impact of tight glycemic control on cerebral glucose metabolism after severe brain injury: a microdialysis study. Crit Care Med 2008;36(12):3233–8.
277. Gray CS, Hildreth AJ, Sandercock PA, et al. Glucose-potassium-insulin infusions in the management of post-stroke hyperglycaemia: the UK Glucose Insulin in Stroke Trial (GIST-UK). Lancet Neurol 2007;6(5):397–406.
280. Takagi K. Body temperature in acute stroke. Stroke 2002;33(9):2154–5, author reply 2154–5.
281. Schwarz S, Häfner K, Aschoff A, et al. Incidence and prognostic significance of fever following intracerebral hemorrhage. Neurology 2000;54(2):354–61.
283. Hacke W, Schwab S, Horn M, et al. Malignant' middle cerebral artery territory infarction: clinical course and prognostic signs. Arch Neurol 1996;53(4):309–15.
285. Schwab S, Schwarz S, Spranger M, et al. Moderate hypothermia in the treatment of patients with severe middle cerebral artery infarction. Stroke 1998;29(12):2461–6.
286. Schwab S, Georgiadis D, Berrouschot J, et al. Feasibility and safety of moderate hypothermia after massive hemispheric infarction. Stroke 2001;32(9):2033–5.
287. Krieger DW, De Georgia MA, Abou-Chebl A, et al. Cooling for acute ischemic brain damage (cool aid): an open pilot study of induced hypothermia in acute ischemic stroke. Stroke 2001;32(8):1847–54.
288. Georgiadis D, Schwarz S, Kollmar R, et al. Endovascular cooling for moderate hypothermia in patients with acute stroke: first results of a novel approach. Stroke 2001;32(11):2550–3.
289. Georgiadis D, Schwarz S, Aschoff A, et al. Hemicraniectomy and moderate hypothermia in patients with severe ischemic stroke. Stroke 2002;33(6):1584–8.
292. Castillo J, Leira R, García MM, et al. Blood pressure decrease during the acute phase of ischemic stroke is associated with brain injury and poor stroke outcome. Stroke 2004;35(2):520–6.
293. Blood pressure in Acute Stroke Collaboration (BASC). Interventions for deliberately altering blood pressure in acute stroke. Cochrane Database Syst Rev 2001;(3):CD000039.
294. Potter JF, Robinson TG, Ford GA, et al. Controlling hypertension and hypotension immediately post-stroke (CHHIPS): a randomised, placebo-controlled, double-blind pilot trial. Lancet Neurol 2009;8(1):48–56.
295. Sandset EC, Bath PM, Boysen G, et al., SCAST Study Group. The angiotensin-receptor blocker candesartan for treatment of acute stroke (SCAST): a randomised, placebo-controlled, double-blind trial. Lancet 2011;377(9767):741–50.
296. He J, Zhang Y, Xu T, et al., CATIS Investigators. Effects of immediate blood pressure reduction on death and major disability in patients with acute ischemic stroke: The CATIS Randomized Clinical Trial. JAMA 2014;311:479–89.
297. Archer CR, Horenstein S. Basilar artery occlusion: clinical and radiological correlation. Stroke 1977;8(3):383–90.
298. Castaigne P, Lhermitte F, Gautier JC, et al. Arterial occlusions in the vertebro-basilar system. A study of 44 patients with post-mortem data. Brain 1973;96(1):133–54.
299. Fields WS, Ratinov G, Weibel J, et al. Survival following basilar artery occlusion. Arch Neurol 1966;15(5):463–71.
300. Hacke W, Zeumer H, Ferbert A, et al. Intra-arterial thrombolytic therapy improves outcome in patients with acute vertebrobasilar occlusive disease. Stroke 1988;19(10):1216–22.
301. Nagel S, Schellinger PD, Hartmann M, et al. Therapy of acute basilar artery occlusion: intraarterial thrombolysis alone vs bridging therapy. Stroke 2009;40(1):140–6.
302. Ferbert A, Bruckmann H, Drummen R. Clinical features of proven basilar artery occlusion. Stroke 1990;21(8):1135–42.
304. Mattle HP, Arnold M, Lindsberg PJ, et al. Basilar artery occlusion. Lancet Neurol 2011;10(11):1002–14.
305. Schonewille WJ, Wijman CA, Michel P, et al. Treatment and outcomes of acute basilar artery occlusion in the Basilar Artery International Cooperation Study (BASICS): a prospective registry study. Lancet Neurol 2009;8(8):724–30.
306. Gobin YP, Starkman S, Duckwiler GR, et al. MERCI 1: a phase 1 study of Mechanical Embolus Removal in Cerebral Ischemia. Stroke 2004;35(12):2848–54.
308. Eckert B, Koch C, Thomalla G, et al. Aggressive therapy with intravenous abciximab and intra-arterial rtPA and additional PTA/stenting improves clinical outcome in acute vertebrobasilar occlusion: combined local fibrinolysis and intravenous abciximab in acute vertebrobasilar stroke treatment (FAST): results of a multicenter study. Stroke 2005;36(6):1160–5.
310. Strbian D, Sairanen T, Silvennoinen H, et al. Thrombolysis of basilar artery occlusion: impact of baseline ischemia and time. Ann Neurol 2013;73(6):688–94.
312. Chen HJ, Lee TC, Wei CP. Treatment of cerebellar infarction by decompressive suboccipital craniectomy. Stroke 1992;23(7):957–61.
313. Heros RC. Surgical treatment of cerebellar infarction. Stroke 1992;23(7):937–8.
314. Juttler E, Schweickert S, Ringleb PA, et al. Long-term outcome after surgical treatment for space-occupying cerebellar infarction: experience in 56 patients. Stroke 2009;40(9):3060–6.
315. Pfefferkorn T, Eppinger U, Linn J, et al. Long-term outcome after suboccipital decompressive craniectomy for malignant cerebellar infarction. Stroke 2009;40(9):3045–50.
316. Hemphill JC 3rd, Bonovich DC, Besmertis L, et al. The ICH score: a simple, reliable grading scale for intracerebral hemorrhage. Stroke 2001;32(4):891–7.
317. Diringer MN, Edwards DF. Admission to a neurologic/neurosurgical intensive care unit is associated with reduced mortality rate after intracerebral hemorrhage. Crit Care Med 2001;29(3):635–40.
318. Brott T, Broderick J, Kothari R, et al. Early hemorrhage growth in patients with intracerebral hemorrhage. Stroke 1997;28(1):1–5.
319. Davis SM, Broderick J, Hennerici M, et al., Recombinant Activated Factor VII Intracerebral Hemorrhage Trial Investigators. Hematoma growth is a determinant of mortality and poor outcome after intracerebral hemorrhage. Neurology 2006;66(8):1175–81.
320. Anderson CS, Huang Y, Wang JG, et al. Intensive blood pressure reduction in acute cerebral haemorrhage trial (INTERACT): a randomised pilot trial. Lancet Neurol 2008;7(5):391–9.

328. Diringer MN, Edwards DF, Zazulia AR. Hydrocephalus: a previously unrecognized predictor of poor outcome from supratentorial intracerebral hemorrhage. Stroke 1998;29(7):1352–7.
329. Mayer SA, Brun NC, Begtrup K, et al. Efficacy and safety of recombinant activated factor VII for acute intracerebral hemorrhage. N Engl J Med 2008;358(20):2127–37.
332. Mayer SA, Davis SM, Skolnick BE, et al., FAST trial investigators. Can a subset of intracerebral hemorrhage patients benefit from hemostatic therapy with recombinant activated factor VII? Stroke 2009;40(3):833–40.
333. Powers WJ, Zazulia AR, Videen TO, et al. Autoregulation of cerebral blood flow surrounding acute (6 to 22 hours) intracerebral hemorrhage. Neurology 2001;57(1):18–24.
334. Kidwell CS, Zazulia AR, Videen TO, et al. Diffusion-perfusion MR evaluation of perihematomal injury in hyperacute intracerebral hemorrhage. Neurology 2001;57(9):1611–17.
336. Schellinger PD, Fiebach JB, Hoffmann K, et al. Stroke MRI in intracerebral hemorrhage: is there a perihemorrhagic penumbra? Stroke 2003;34(7):1674–9.
340. Robertson CS, Valadka AB, Hannay HJ, et al. Prevention of secondary ischemic insults after severe head injury. Crit Care Med 1999;27(10):2086–95.
341. Flibotte JJ, Hagan N, O'Donnell J, et al. Warfarin, hematoma expansion, and outcome of intracerebral hemorrhage. Neurology 2004;63(6):1059–64.
345. Connolly SJ, Ezekowitz MD, Yusuf S, et al., RE-LY Steering Committee and Investigators. Dabigatran versus warfarin in patients with atrial fibrillation. N Engl J Med 2009;361(12):1139–51.
346. Patel MR, Mahaffey KW, Garg J, et al., ROCKET AF Investigators. Rivaroxaban versus warfarin in nonvalvular atrial fibrillation. N Engl J Med 2011;365(10):883–91.
347. Granger CB, Alexander JH, McMurray JJ, et al., ARISTOTLE Committees and Investigators. Apixaban versus warfarin in patients with atrial fibrillation. N Engl J Med 2011;365(11):981–92.
354. Butler AB, Partain RA, Netsky MG. Primary intraventricular hemorrhage. A mild and remediable form. Neurology 1972;22(7): 675–87.
355. Tuhrim S, Horowitz DR, Sacher M, et al. Volume of ventricular blood is an important determinant of outcome in supratentorial intracerebral hemorrhage. Crit Care Med 1999;27(3):617–21.
360. Naff N, Williams MA, Keyl PM, et al. Low-dose recombinant tissue-type plasminogen activator enhances clot resolution in brain hemorrhage: the intraventricular hemorrhage thrombolysis trial. Stroke 2011;42(11):3009–16.
364. Ferro JM, Canhão P, Stam J, et al., ISCVT Investigators. Prognosis of cerebral vein and dural sinus thrombosis: results of the International Study on Cerebral Vein and Dural Sinus Thrombosis (ISCVT). Stroke 2004;35(3):664–70.
365. Saposnik G, Barinagarrementeria F, Brown RD Jr, et al., American Heart Association Stroke Council and the Council on Epidemiology and Prevention. Diagnosis and management of cerebral venous thrombosis: a statement for healthcare professionals from the American Heart Association/American Stroke Association. Stroke 2011;42(4):1158–92.
368. Coutinho JM, Ferro JM, Canhão P, et al. Unfractionated or low-molecular weight heparin for the treatment of cerebral venous thrombosis. Stroke 2010;41(11):2575–80.
372. Coutinho JM, Majoie CB, Coert BA, et al. Decompressive hemicraniectomy in cerebral sinus thrombosis: consecutive case series and review of the literature. Stroke 2009;40(6):2233–5.
376. Theaudin M, Crassard I, Bresson D, et al. Should decompressive surgery be performed in malignant cerebral venous thrombosis?: a series of 12 patients. Stroke 2010;41(4):727–31.
378. Stam J, Majoie CB, van Delden OM, et al. Endovascular thrombectomy and thrombolysis for severe cerebral sinus thrombosis: a prospective study. Stroke 2008;39(5):1487–90.

55 Pharmacologic Modification of Acute Cerebral Ischemia

Nicole R. Gonzales, James C. Grotta

KEY POINTS

- The ideal cytoprotective agent should be low in cost and complexity to allow access in emergency settings of variable sophistication.
- Cerebral ischemia is a process providing the potential to modify the process both during and after the event to affect outcome.
- Challenges in translation of clinical trials in acute ischemic stroke include standardization of stroke physiology, sample size estimation, optimal time to treatment, coupling cytoprotection with reperfusion, dose, and selecting the appropriate outcome measures.
- Clinical trial design needs to undergo a paradigm shift to minimize the known problems in demonstrating cytoprotection.
- Despite the inability to demonstrate clinical cytoprotection after stroke to date, human studies of hypothermia after cardiac arrest suggest that meaningful cytoprotection after stroke may still be achievable.

Pharmacologic therapy of acute ischemic stroke (AIS) promises the opportunity to reduce brain injury and hence disability in a large proportion of patients with stroke. Treatments are needed that can be proven effective for important clinical outcomes in well-designed clinical trials. Optimally, these treatments should be low in morbidity, cost, and complexity so that they can be quickly and widely used in emergency settings of variable sophistication, as are common in the care of most patients with stroke worldwide.

BACKGROUND: PRECLINICAL AND CLINICAL CYTOPROTECTION

The Definition and Role of Cytoprotection

Pharmacologic therapy of ischemic stroke can be split into broad groups on the basis of the sequence and location of physiologic events thought to occur on occlusion of a cerebral artery, although as in most complex biological systems, these events overlap both temporally and spatially. In some instances, the opportunity for "pretreatment" exists. Ischemic preconditioning, in which a noxious stimulus is given below the threshold of damage, can induce protection when a subsequent deleterious event occurs. The mechanisms of ischemic preconditioning are the focus of ongoing study and important mediators such as Toll-like receptors (TLRs)[1] and astrocyte-mediated mechanisms may play a role.[2] There is mounting evidence that the genomic response to the ischemic cascade can be reprogrammed,[1] thus introducing the concept of prophylactic ischemic stroke therapy in high-risk patients (e.g., those undergoing endovascular or surgical procedures with periprocedural risk of ischemic stroke).

The next group of therapies targets the events occurring within the artery lumen by reversing the arterial occlusion and restoring perfusion to damaged brain tissue. The prototypes of such therapy are thrombolytics, fibrinolytics, and anticoagulants. Reversing arterial occlusion has been the area of greatest clinical success to date in stroke treatment. Other therapies targeting later events will probably have much less impact on outcome than fast removal of the offending arterial occlusion, and it is even possible that further improvement in treatment cannot be achieved unless it is also accompanied by reperfusion of the damaged tissue. Much can be learned from the preclinical and clinical development of these "reperfusion" drugs, and the lessons will be brought into this chapter. However, such therapy is discussed in detail in other chapters and so is not specifically addressed further here.

A third, broad category of pharmacotherapy for stroke targets the consequences of arterial occlusion on the blood vessel wall, neuron, glia, and neuronal environment. Although often labeled *neuroprotection,* this approach to therapy actually has a wide variety of targets, many of which are non-neuronal, so a more appropriate term would be *cytoprotection*. Common to this approach is the effort to improve outcome by preventing progression to cellular death of tissue initially damaged by the ischemic event. Although unlikely to salvage irreversibly damaged cells, such therapies may "modify" the biologic perturbations induced at the cellular level in brain tissue whose fate still hangs in the balance. This type of pharmacotherapy is the subject of the present chapter.

A final category of stroke pharmacotherapy aims to augment recovery of brain function by targeting events during the restorative phase occurring after tissue damage is complete. This therapy is the subject of another chapter.

The concept of cytoprotection relies on the principle that delayed cellular injury occurs after ischemia. Neurons suffer irreversible damage after only a few minutes of complete cessation of blood flow. Such a condition might exist during cardiac arrest. In most instances of acute focal brain ischemia, however, if a state of zero blood flow occurs, it would only be in the core of the ischemic region. The larger surrounding penumbral area receives reduced blood flow, which causes loss of normal function that may lead to permanent cellular damage if uncorrected, but allows for recovery if blood flow is restored by either clot lysis or collateral flow.

Because ischemia is clearly a process and not an instantaneous event, there is potential both for modifying the process after the clinical ictus and for altering the final outcome. It is equally apparent from experimental models that if cytoprotective treatments are to succeed, they must be instituted within a few minutes after the onset of ischemia. Previous clinical trials may have failed because such treatment was delayed and was therefore unlikely to render a benefit.

The concept of cytoprotection is not new in the clinical domain. It has been known for years that hypothermia reduces ischemic neuronal injury. Accidental hypothermia can protect a drowning victim from otherwise fatal hypoxic-ischemic brain damage. Animal models of both global and focal ischemia confirm the beneficial effects of hypothermia. The benefit of hypothermia in treating global cerebral ischemic injury after cardiac arrest has also been dramatically demonstrated in humans. The importance of this result cannot be overemphasized because it is the first proof that experimental brain cytoprotection, which can be demonstrated so readily in the laboratory, can be translated into human benefit.

Targets of Cytoprotection: The Ischemic Cascade

A major accomplishment of in vivo and in vitro model systems of cerebral ischemia is an understanding of the *ischemic cascade*. The details of the physiologic events that constitute the brain's response to injury and this cascade are discussed in detail in other chapters. Each step of this cascade might be a potential target for therapeutic intervention. Several variables exist that may affect the pathobiology of the ischemic cascade and, consequently, the severity of injury; the most important are the depth of blood flow reduction, its duration before reperfusion occurs, its distribution (i.e., global or focal), comorbidities (e.g., diabetes or hypertension), and the adequacy of reperfusion, if one assumes that reperfusion occurs. However, many of the events that have been described seem to follow in a fairly predictable order.

Preclinical Stroke Models

The development of reproducible, relatively simple animal models mimicking cerebral ischemia in humans subsequently led to numerous preclinical studies testing the efficacy of cytoprotective therapies that targeted each of the steps of the ischemic cascade. Although the general nature of the cerebral damage produced by ischemia is the same among species, the severity and other features may differ not only between species but also among various strains and within strains, depending on age, sex, and size. To maintain reproducibility of results of such studies, investigators must pay careful attention to the choice of anesthetic as well as to physiologic variables which must be carefully controlled both during and after ischemia. The standardization of physiologic variables is an important difference between animal stroke models and human stroke, the latter being characterized by great variability in severity and other phenotypic features. Broadly, the models can be divided into those of global forebrain ischemia, which reflect the type of cerebral injury incurred with cardiac arrest, and focal ischemia, similar to what occurs with ischemic stroke in humans. Many permutations of these models exist.

Preclinical Testing of Cytoprotective Therapies

The disturbing reality is that despite the substantial positive effect of cytoprotective drugs in animal stroke models – except for hypothermia after cardiac arrest – results of all clinical trials of this approach to stroke treatment have been neutral (no effect) or negative (harmful). Before we discuss this conundrum, we deal with several general themes that have proved useful in achieving positive results with cytoprotective therapies in preclinical models. Careful attention to these issues will be important in achieving positive results with neuroprotective drugs, either in the laboratory or at the bedside.

The Need for Careful Physiologic Monitoring

Core temperature, blood glucose concentration, pH, oxygenation, blood pressure, and cerebral blood flow and collateral circulation all have important effects on outcome after ischemia. If these variables are not controlled in the laboratory, variability in stroke severity occurs and consistent results are not detected. For instance, if cerebral blood flow is not monitored during an experiment in which the MCA is occluded, animals in two comparison treatment groups may have different levels of ischemic insult; thus differences in outcome may be due to these imbalances rather than to the therapy that is being tested. Minor differences in the location or number of vessels occluded or in the level of blood pressure can have major effects on the depth and distribution of cerebral hypoperfusion. As another example, some drugs, such as the glutamate antagonists, can lower brain temperature. Unless this effect is monitored, positive results occurring from the neuroprotective properties of hypothermia may be attributed to the drug instead.

Penumbra as Target

Because cytoprotective therapies are aimed at interrupting the ischemic cascade in tissue that is not yet dead, most logically they should be tested in animal models of focal cerebral ischemia in which there is a relatively extensive ischemic penumbra. *Penumbra* can be operationally defined as tissue that has been exposed to a reduction in perfusion shy of the threshold leading to immediate destruction but that would not survive without reperfusion or cytoprotective intervention.[3,4] Such regions of "penumbral level" hypoperfusion are most often seen in MCA occlusion models with rather extensive cortical involvement and in which the damage is of a moderate nature, more typical of reversible occlusion models. Penumbra is also time-related; it gradually disappears over minutes to hours after arterial occlusion to become incorporated into the irreversibly damaged "core," or areas that spontaneously improve their perfusion and function ("benign oligemia"). It is likely that both in the laboratory and at the bedside, strokes with extensive penumbral tissue are the most likely to respond to cytoprotection and vice versa; that is, strokes with irreversible damage are the least likely. The current challenge is reliable determination of penumbra. The hope is that the ischemic penumbra can be imaged as a surrogate marker of reversible versus irreversible injury. So far, this surrogate marker remains elusive.

Reperfusion Injury

There is considerable debate regarding whether reperfusion itself has damaging effects. Certainly, if there is disruption of the blood–brain barrier, reperfusion can be associated with cerebral edema and hemorrhage. However, even in the absence of such gross abnormalities, reperfusion after a period of occlusion long enough to produce cellular injury may result in increased production of free radicals, gene expression, and inflammatory events that may augment cellular damage.

Downstream Targets

Many of the initial events in the ischemic cascade, such as release of glutamate and increase in intracellular calcium, occur almost instantaneously, and their effect might not be dampened by a cytoprotective agent even if it is started as early as 1 or 2 hours after the onset of ischemia. Later events in the cascade, such as production of NO and free radicals, inflammatory cytokines, transcription factors, and caspases may be more effectively targeted by post ischemic cytoprotective therapies.

Multimodality Therapy

An understanding of the ischemic cascade has enabled us to design cytoprotective therapy aimed at each of these steps.

This has led to the emerging concept that multimodality therapy may be necessary to maximize a therapeutic attack on AIS. A therapy targeting only one of these processes is unlikely to result in a therapeutic "home run." A multimodality approach to neuroprotection will probably be more effective clinically than the use of a single agent. The negative or neutral results of clinical trials of drugs targeting specific neurotransmitter pathways (see later), despite their efficacy in animal models, suggest that, to detect a signal of clinical efficacy, we need a more potent intervention that might be achieved only by simultaneously targeting multiple pathways. However, such clinical studies will be complex and more difficult to design and carry out. The dosing, benefit, and interactions of the various candidate combinations must be worked out in animal models before this approach can be taken at the bedside.

Early Pharmacologic Intervention May Influence Functional Recovery

Brain plasticity and functional recovery depend on the contributions of synaptogenesis, dendritic arborization, trophic factors, and progenitor cells. The timing and amount of these reparative processes may be influenced by neurotransmitter function, inflammation, and gene expression that all occur earlier and that may be the targets of neuroprotective pharmacotherapy.

The outcome in rodent stroke models used to test neuroprotective drugs is usually measured by histologic quantification of infarct volume within the first few days after stroke onset. These measures may miss an additional positive effect of the drug on recovery or an inhibitory effect on reparative processes. Evaluation of behavioral outcome during the weeks after stroke may provide a more accurate picture of the effect of a neuroprotective agent on the complex interaction of acute injury and delayed recovery.

Relevance of Animal Models

Much has been written about the failure of benefit in clinical trials of neuroprotective drugs despite the positive results of the same drugs in animal models.[5,6] Such discordance has raised the question of whether the animal models of stroke, particularly rodent models, reflect what is occurring in human stroke. Indeed, the juvenile lissencephalic rodent brain used in most laboratory studies may not respond to ischemic injury or to a neuroprotective drug the same way as an elderly gyrencephalic human brain. However, data correlating thresholds of both the depth and duration of perfusion needed to produce irreversible damage have been similar in rodents and humans,[7,8] such that the positive results of thrombolytic trials in patients with stroke were predicted by data from animal models. Therefore, although biological differences between rodent and human brain certainly exist, it is likely that the discrepancy between results of clinical and laboratory testing of neuroprotective drugs rests more on differences between the way we have tested drugs in the laboratory and how we have designed the clinical trials to test them at the bedside.

This principle has been demonstrated in a review of preclinical neuroprotection studies that compared the experimental efficacy of interventions that have been taken forward to clinical trials with that of drugs that have only been tested in the laboratory.[9] There was no evidence that drugs used clinically were more effective experimentally than those tested only in animal models. The results of this review highlight the importance of the quality of trial design in the preclinical stages of development because it provides the foundation for translational clinical trials. Even the most well-designed clinical trials are doomed to failure if the premise on which they are based is not solid.

Stroke Therapy Academic Industry Roundtables (STAIR) are consensus conferences on translational stroke research and have addressed how to reconcile our laboratory and clinical studies to achieve successful translation of laboratory results.[6,10,11] Some of the conferences' recommendations for making our laboratory studies more reliable were as follows:

1. Evaluate most drugs in both permanent and transient models of ischemia.
2. Provide an adequate dose–response curve.
3. Determine the therapeutic index between efficacy and toxicity; a narrow index would indicate less clinical utility.
4. Explore the time window of benefit.
5. Perform studies with blinded assessment of outcome and with careful monitoring of potentially confounding physiologic variables.
6. Measure outcome both histologically and functionally and both immediately and at later points.
7. Ensure that preclinical studies follow the intent-to-treat model of clinical trials – animals should not be excluded from the analysis just because they are "data outliers" and so on.
8. Before proceeding to clinical trials, a drug should be seen to have positive results consistently in multiple laboratories and with multiple models. Comparison of magnitude of benefit with positive controls may be useful for determining relative efficacy.
9. Test novel first-in-class drugs in gyrencephalic species.

In the following discussion, we describe some of the important things we need to do in the future design of clinical trials to achieve the success realized in the laboratory.

Important Issues to Clarify in Design of Future Clinical Trials

Standardization of Stroke

Along with time to treatment, the biggest discrepancy between laboratory and clinical trials has been in the area of standardized stroke physiology, severity, type, location, perfusion, and reversibility. We have already emphasized that controlling physiologic variables is important in detecting a therapeutic effect in laboratory stroke models. This control is more difficult to achieve in patients who have a wide variety of underlying illness such as pulmonary disease (hypoxia), cardiac disease (hypotension, reduced cardiac output), diabetes (elevated blood glucose and lactate levels), advanced age and associated atherosclerosis (reduced collateral circulation), and infection (fever). Distribution of such underlying conditions that are known to influence outcome must be balanced among the treatment groups in any clinical trial.

The single most important determinant of stroke outcome is stroke severity, as reflected in the clinical deficit.[12] This deficit can be quantified with various stroke scales. It is critical that the distribution and level of stroke severity be comparable in the treatment groups of any stroke trial. Most patients with very minor deficits recover spontaneously, and those with very severe deficits often do not survive. Patients at these extremes of the clinical spectrum therefore only provide "noise" in the analysis because their data are least likely to show a difference between an effective treatment and the control group. Most trials now use the baseline stroke scale to exclude patients with the most minor or severe strokes and to ensure that the treated groups are well balanced in the critical variable of stroke severity. However, there is debate about what the thresholds should be.

The presence of reversible damage, or penumbra, is likely to be important as well, in terms of a treatment target.

Numerous studies have attempted to define the imaging signature of penumbral tissue.[13-20] To date, however, the appropriate imaging thresholds for distinguishing either penumbra from benign oligemia or irreversibly from reversibly injured core tissue are still uncertain. Though this imaging tool may be useful for subgroup analysis or stratification, it is not yet justifiable for patient selection.[21]

Such issues of stroke standardization and selection of the optimal set of patients for a pivotal efficacy trial should be worked out in multiphasic phase 2 studies before embarking on a large phase 3 efficacy trial.

Sample Size

As will become apparent in the discussion of the individual clinical trials that have been conducted, most have been insufficiently powered to detect small clinical benefits. If one considers that t-PA given within 3 hours of stroke onset produced an absolute difference of 12–15% in good outcome in a trial of roughly 300 patients,[22] then a trial of a cytoprotective drug, which would most likely produce substantially less effect than t-PA, would have to be much larger to reach significance. Later efficacy trials, such as the Glycine Antagonist (gavestinel) in Neuroprotection (GAIN International) study,[23] the Intravenous Magnesium Efficacy in Acute Stroke trial (IMAGES),[24] and Stroke - Acute Ischemic NXY Treatment (SAINT)[25] were powered to detect a 5% difference in outcome, which is a treatment effect that is more realistic to expect.

Time

Perhaps the biggest deficiency of clinical trials to date has been the substantial delay in starting treatment compared with animal studies. The calcium antagonist and glutamate antagonist trials are excellent examples (see later). In the laboratory, these drugs work only if started within an hour or so of the onset of ischemia, presumably because they are targeting events that occur immediately on the interruption of blood flow. The clinical trials testing these compounds, however, enrolled patients 6–12 hours after stroke onset. There are many reasons for designing trials to allow delayed therapy; mainly, they include the difficulty in accruing large numbers of patients into trials within 1–3 hours of onset and marketing pressures dictating that treating so few patients would not be profitable. However, these are practical and not biological reasons, and our negative experiences to date tell us that we must pay more attention to the biology of the disease to be successful. The clinical trial, therefore, should reflect the time window determined in preclinical studies. It is possible to treat patients more rapidly after stroke onset, as evidenced by the successful National Institute of Neurological Diseases and Stroke (NINDS) t-PA trial (treatment given within 90–180 minutes)[22] and later studies temporally linking use of t-PA within 3 hours and random assignment to therapy with the cytoprotective agent.[26] Even more aggressive have been efforts to train paramedics to recognize stroke with sufficient accuracy to allow field administration of the first dose of the cytoprotective drug.[27]

Coupling Cytoprotection with Reperfusion

Besides the practical issue of delivering drug faster, there are other theoretical advantages of coupling cytoprotection with the use of t-PA or other reperfusion strategies. Logically, it would allow greater penetration of the cytoprotective agent into the target tissue than if the arterial occlusion remained untreated. Furthermore, as already discussed, one of the consequences of reperfusion might be a second wave of pathologic events leading to "reperfusion injury" that might be advantageously targeted by the cytoprotective agent.

Dose

It will become apparent in the discussion to follow that several cytoprotective drugs have been taken through clinical trial progression from phase 1 to large phase 3 efficacy trials even though side effects limited the doses that were given so that blood levels of drug analogous to those that had been protective in animals were never achieved in humans.

More Sensitive Outcome Measures

Animal stroke models most often rely on histologic outcome, whereas clinical trials in humans are based on functional performance. Which measure is more sensitive? More important, which is more important to patients? Clearly, patients are more interested in what they can do functionally regardless of what an MR image or CT scan shows.

Another question concerns the best functional outcome measure to use. This issue is still uncertain because no one measurement reflects the total clinical condition of the patient. Any scale that is used to measure outcome must be validated as reflecting a true deficit in function, its entire range and distribution in patients with stroke must be understood, and its reliability through repeated measurements and among different examiners must be established.

CLINICAL CYTOPROTECTIVE THERAPY TRIALS

To date, many cytoprotective drugs have reached the stage of pivotal phase 3 efficacy trials in patients with acute stroke (Table 55-1). Unfortunately, throughout the neuroprotective literature, the phrase "failure to demonstrate efficacy" is a common thread in the many trials with neutral or negative results despite the largely encouraging results yielded by preclinical studies. The reasons for this discrepancy are multiple and have been discussed in the preceding paragraphs. Many of the later trials have addressed deficiencies of the previous ones with more rigorous trial design, including more specific patient selection criteria (ensuring homogeneity of stroke location and severity), stratified randomization algorithms (time-to-treatment), narrowed therapeutic window, and pharmacokinetic monitoring. Current trials have also incorporated biological surrogate markers of toxicity and outcome, such as serum drug levels and neuroimaging. Lastly, multimodal therapies and coupled cytoprotection–reperfusion strategies are being investigated to optimize tissue salvage. In the remainder of this chapter, we focus on individual therapeutic strategies and, sometimes, provide the historical rationale for pursuing a particular agent. We emphasize what has been learned from these trials in terms of both trial design and the biological effect (or lack thereof) of these agents.

Calcium Antagonists

The first practical pharmacologic agents to be clinically evaluated for cytoprotection in stroke were the calcium channel antagonists. There are several classes of calcium channels that play a role in brain ischemia. The presynaptic voltage-activated N-type calcium channels are largely restricted to neurons and regulate neurotransmitter release. The ubiquitous voltage-gated L-type calcium channels trigger excitation–contraction coupling in smooth muscle and regulate vasomotor tone. These L-type calcium channels are sensitive to the dihydropyridine compounds, of which nimodipine and nicardipine are examples. Calcium influx through NMDA receptor-mediated

TABLE 55-1 Past and Current Cytoprotective Clinical Trials

Drug	Phase	Latest Extent of Time Window (h)	Adequate Power*	Adequate Dose	Dose-Limiting Adverse Effects	Results*	Classification of Recommendation, Level of Evidence
CALCIUM ANTAGONISTS							
Nimodipine	3	6–48	+	?	Hypotension	Neutral	III, A
Nicardipine	2	12		?	Hypotension	Neutral	III, C
GLUTAMATE ANTAGONISTS							
Selfotel	3	6–12	+	No	Neuropsychological	Negative	III, A
Dextrorphan	2	48		Yes	Neuropsychological	Neutral	III, B
Aptiganel (Cerestat)	3	6–24	+	Yes	Hypertension	Negative	III, B
AR-R15696AR	2	12		Yes	Neuropsychological	Neutral	III, B
MAGNESIUM							
IMAGES	3	12	+	Yes	No	Neutral	III, A
FAST-MAG	3	2	+	Yes	No	Neutral	
AMPA ANTAGONISTS							
YM872	2b	3–6	+	?	?	Neutral	III, A
ZK200775	2	24		?	Sedation	Negative	III, B
INDIRECT GLUTAMATE MODULATORS							
Eliprodil	3	?	?	?	?	Negative	III, B
Gavestinel	3	6	+	Yes	No	Neutral	III, A
Sipatrigine	2	12		?	Neuropsychological	Negative	III, B
Fosphenytoin	2/3	4	+	?	No	Neutral	III, B
BMS-204352	3	6	+	?	No	Neutral	III, B
Lifarizine	2	?		?	Hypotension	Neutral	III, B
Lubeluzole	3	4-8	+	No	Cardiac	Neutral	III, A
OTHER NEUROTRANSMITTER MODULATORS							
Trazodone	2	?	?	?	?	Neutral	III, B
Repinotan	3	6	+	Yes	?	Negative	III, B
ONO-2506	2/3	6	+	?	?	?	III, B
OPIOID ANTAGONISTS							
Naloxone	2	8–60		?	No	Neutral	III, B
Nalmefene	3	6	+	?	No	Neutral	III, B
GABA AGONISTS							
Clomethiazole	3	12	+	Yes	Sedation	Neutral	III, A
Diazepam	3	12	+	?	?	Neutral	III, B
FREE RADICAL SCAVENGERS							
Tirilazad	3	6	+	?	No	Negative	III, A
Ebselen	3	48	+	?	?	?	III, B
Edaravone	3	72			No	Positive	IIb, B
NXY-059	3	6	+	Yes	No	Neutral	III, A
ANTI-INFLAMMATORY AGENTS							
Enlimomab	3	6	+	Yes	Fever	Negative	III, B
LeukArrest	3	12		?	?	Neutral	III, B
Interferon-β	1	24		?	?	?	III, B
UK-279276	2	6		?			III, B
Minocycline	2	24		?	?		III, B
Lovastatin	1	24				NA	III, B
FK-506	2	12		?	?	?	III, B
Steroids	2	48		?	Infection	Negative	III, B

TABLE 55-1 Past and Current Cytoprotective Clinical Trials—cont'd

Drug	Phase	Latest Extent of Time Window (h)	Adequate Power*	Adequate Dose	Dose-Limiting Adverse Effects	Results*	Classification of Recommendation, Level of Evidence
Membrane Stabilizers, Trophic Factor							
Glyburide	1	10			No	NA	III, B
GM1	3	72	+	?	No	Neutral	III, A
Cerebrolysin	2	12-24		?	No	Neutral	III, B
Citicoline	3	24	+	?	No	Neutral	III, A
Albumin	3	5		Yes		Neutral	III, B
EPO	3	6		?	?	Negative	III, B
bFGF	2/3	6	+	?	Hypotension	Negative	III, B
G-CSF	2	9	?	?		Negative	III, B
Hypothermia	1	5-24		Yes	Pneumonia, arrhythmia, hypotension	NA	III, B
Caffeinol	2	4		Yes	No	NA	III, B
Oxygen							
DCLHb	2	18		?	Hypertensive nephropathy	Negative	III, B
HBO	2/3	24		?	?	Neutral	III, B
NBO	2	9	?	?		Negative	III, B

AMPA, α-amino-3-hydroxy-5-methyl-4-isoxazole proprionic acid; bFGF, basic fibroblast growth factor; DCLHb, diaspirin-cross-linked hemoglobin; EPO, erythropoietin; FAST-MAG, Field Administration of Stroke Therapy – Magnesium Trial; GABA, γ-aminobutyric acid; GM1, genetic marker (monosialoganglioside); G-CSF, granulocyte colony-stimulating factor; HBO, hyperbaric oxygen; NBO, normobaric oxygen; IMAGES, Intravenous Magnesium Efficacy in Acute Stroke study; NA, not applicable.
*Relevant only to phase 2b or 3 efficacy trial.

channels is both ligand- and voltage-dependent. Other classes of calcium channels have distinct activation or inactivation characteristics or resemble L-type channels but are insensitive to dihydropyridines. Many calcium channel antagonists have been reported to preferentially antagonize the cerebral vascular smooth muscle and have a high affinity for calcium channels in the inactivated state, such as those found in the depolarized environment of the ischemic penumbra.[28] This selective interaction may be beneficial for the neuroprotectant potential of these agents.

The calcium channel antagonist that has undergone the most extensive investigation in stroke is *nimodipine*. The cytoprotective effect of nimodipine results from its ability to block calcium influx and prevent the excessive accumulation of intracellular calcium that initiates the final common pathway to cell death. Nimodipine has been studied in clinical trials of subarachnoid hemorrhage, head injury, and cardiac arrest, as well as acute focal ischemia.[29]

Oral nimodipine has been investigated in ischemic stroke in at least 29 randomized placebo-controlled trials. A few of the earlier studies found a significant difference in mortality and neurologic function in favor of nimodipine therapy; however, subsequent larger studies and a later meta-analysis failed to replicate this benefit.[30,31] Several studies have actually shown a better outcome in the placebo-treated patients, which is a finding attributed to hypotension induced by both oral and intravenous (IV) administration of the drug.[32]

The most extensive meta-analysis of 22 calcium antagonist trials, studying more than 6800 patients, did not demonstrate any beneficial effect of treatment, even in subgroups receiving early treatment (within 12 hours of stroke onset) (Fig. 55-1).[30] In addition, meta-analysis limited to the "good-quality" trials showed a statistically significant negative effect of calcium antagonists. A similar analysis of "poor-" and "moderate-quality" trials found that calcium antagonists exerted no effect on outcome. In fact, the results of this meta-analysis prompted the premature termination of the Very Early Nimodipine Use in Stroke (VENUS) trial, which was designed to determine the efficacy of nimodipine administered within 6 hours of stroke onset.[33] The interim analysis of 454 patients showed no effect of nimodipine; within the ischemic stroke subgroup, however, an increase in poor outcome at 3 months was found in the nimodipine-treated patients (relative risk [RR], 1.4; 95% confidence interval [CI], 1.0–2.1).

In summary, given the weight of the evidence, calcium channel antagonists cannot be considered generally effective in improving the outcome of ischemic stroke and may even cause a worsened outcome. The lack of effect, or the presence of detrimental effect, may be due to the hypotension caused by blocking of the vascular smooth muscle cells. Blockade of L-type calcium channels in the setting of maximal vasodilation and impaired autoregulation within the ischemic region may cause relative hypotension and a steal phenomenon with shunting of blood flow to non-ischemic regions, thereby further decreasing perfusion to the penumbra.[34] Another plausible explanation for the failure of calcium channel antagonists to show efficacy is that neurotransmitter release is a proximal event in the excitotoxic cascade with immediate effects; therefore, any delay in administration of the drug precludes its theoretical efficacy in preventing cell necrosis. Delayed or prolonged use of L-type calcium antagonists may actually induce apoptotic cell death because modest increases in calcium inhibit apoptosis.[35] This mechanism may overcome other protective actions of these agents. Ultra-early antagonism of other receptor subtypes, such as the N-type, may be more beneficial in penumbral preservation through inhibition

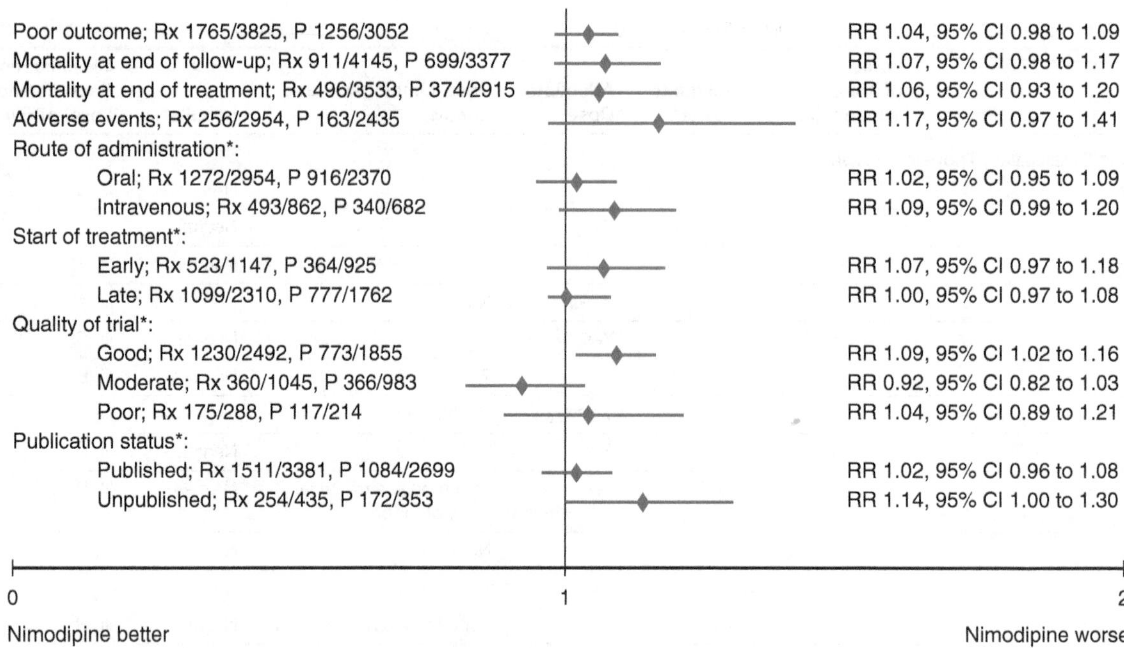

Figure 55-1. Results from meta-analyses comparing nimodipine to placebo in acute ischemic stroke. 0, Nimodipine better; 2, nimodipine worse; CI, confidence intervals; P, placebo group; RR, relative risk; Rx, treatment group; *, assessment of analyses indicated poor outcome. *(Adapted from Horn J, Limburg M: Calcium antagonists for ischemic stroke: A systematic review.* Stroke *32:570, 2001.)*

of neurotransmitter release without undesired hypotension. Such agents have demonstrated cytoprotection in animal models, but they have not been extensively studied in humans because of poor blood–brain barrier permeability of these peptides.[36] Critical review of these studies highlights the importance of beginning treatment as quickly as possible, that is, within a few hours of injury as opposed to the 24- or 48-hour treatment window allowed in some studies. The importance of adequate sample size necessary to demonstrate modest benefit is also underscored.[37]

Glutamate Antagonists

NMDA receptor antagonists were the first class of therapeutic agents for acute stroke to proceed from development in the laboratory to testing in humans that employed modern principles of clinical trial design, of which the most important was relatively early treatment. The potential utility of NMDA antagonists in stroke was first recognized when it was observed that a hypoxic or ischemic insult results in elevation of brain levels of the excitatory neurotransmitter glutamate. The excitotoxic theory of ischemic brain injury implicates glutamate as a pivotal mediator of cell death via ligand-gated receptors (NMDA and AMPA receptors), as reviewed in previous chapters.

The complex structure of the NMDA receptor provides multiple sites for therapeutic inhibition. Competitive NMDA antagonists bind directly to the glutamate site of the NMDA receptor to inhibit the action of glutamate. Non-competitive antagonists block the NMDA-associated ion channel in a use-dependent manner. Other sites on the NMDA receptor susceptible to antagonism are the glycine site and the polyamine site. Prototypes of these competitive and non-competitive NMDA antagonists have been studied in phase 3 clinical trials for the treatment of stroke.

CGS19755 (*selfotel*) is a competitive NMDA receptor antagonist that limits neuronal damage in animal stroke models.[38–40] Phase 2 studies of selfotel revealed that the dosing regimen was limited by dose-related neuropsychiatric adverse events including hallucinations, agitation, confusion, dysarthria, ataxia, delirium, paranoia, and somnolence. Phase 3 parallel studies in the United States and Europe were suspended because of an unfavorable efficacy-to-toxicity ratio.[41] The proportion of patients with neurologic progression or decreased arousal was higher in the selfotel group, as were both 8- and 30-day mortality rates. There was no difference between selfotel and placebo in the primary endpoint of functional independence, even when stroke subtype subgroup analysis was performed.

We may conclude from these trials that selfotel is not efficacious as a cytoprotectant and may potentially exert a neurotoxic effect in patients with severe stroke. The selfotel trials exhibit an important principle of cytoprotectant failure – the narrow therapeutic index. Animal models determined that a plasma selfotel level of 40 μg/mL was cytoprotective. However, the highest tolerated level in human patients with stroke was only half of this target cytoprotective concentration (21 μg/mL), and even these "subtherapeutic" levels produced marked neurologic and psychiatric effects.[42]

The non-competitive NMDA antagonist CNS1102 (aptiganel, *Cerestat*) was evaluated in a nested phase 2–phase 3 study comparing low-dose (3-mg bolus then 0.5 mg/h; total 9 mg) and high-dose (5-mg bolus then 0.75 mg/h; total 14 mg) aptiganel regimens with placebo.[43] Patients with AIS were randomly assigned to one of three treatment arms within 6 hours of symptom onset. There were no criteria for stroke severity or syndrome, and no stratified randomization procedure was used to enforce recruitment of patients within a 3-hour window. Phase 3 enrollment was terminated early when analysis of the phase 2 data revealed an increase in mortality within the aptiganel cohort. Analysis of available phase 3 data (628 patients) showed no difference in 90-day outcome, as measured by mRS, among the three groups. The difference in 90-day mortality was not significant, but mortality at 120 days was marginally increased in the high-dose group. On the basis of this evidence, aptiganel is not efficacious when given within 6 hours of onset of stroke and may be harmful at higher doses.

Magnesium (Mg^{2+}) is theoretically an ideal neuroprotectant because of its diverse mechanisms of action, low cost, ease of administration, wide therapeutic index, good blood–brain barrier permeability, and established safety profile. Mg^{2+} ions endogenously function as a physiologic voltage-dependent block of the NMDA receptor ion channel and inhibitor of ischemia-induced glutamate release.[44] In addition to these antiexcitotoxic actions, Mg^{2+} antagonizes voltage-gated calcium (Ca^{2+}) channels of all types, promotes vasodilation, enhances mitochondrial buffering of calcium overloading, prevents depletion of ATP, and inhibits the inflammatory response and calcium-mediated activation of intracellular enzymes.[44–46]

Pilot studies demonstrated the safety and tolerability of IV Mg^{2+} in patients with AIS.[45,47] The hypotension or hyperglycemia that was experienced in some preclinical evaluations of $MgCl$[48] did not prove to be an issue in clinical evaluation. The majority of reported adverse events was the expected complication of the initial stroke and did not differ from those reported in patients given placebo. A systematic review of four phase 2 clinical trials disclosed a non-significant, 8% absolute reduction in the combined endpoint of death or functional dependence.[24]

The IMAGES Study Group conducted a large phase 3 trial of $MgSO_4$ administered within 12 hours of onset designed to detect a 5.5% absolute difference in death or dependence.[49] A total of 2589 patients were randomly assigned within 12 hours of acute stroke to receive either $MgSO_4$ intravenously or placebo. The primary outcome was a global endpoint statistic expressed as the common odds ratio for death or disability at day 90. The efficacy dataset included 2386 patients. The primary outcome was not improved by magnesium (odds ratio [OR], 0.95; 95% CI, 0.80–1.13, $P = 0.59$).

One of the greatest impediments to translating experimental efficacy to a clinical reality is the delay in administration of potentially cytoprotective therapies. More recent trials of magnesium administration have been designed to specifically address this issue. The Field Administration of Stroke Therapy – Magnesium (FAST-MAG) pilot study was an open-label evaluation of the safety and feasibility of paramedic-initiated magnesium therapy to patients with stroke identified in the field.[27] The average time to treatment was only 29 minutes from symptom onset, which is the shortest onset-to-treatment interval reported to date. More than two-thirds of patients had a good functional outcome.

The Field Administration of Stroke Therapy – Magnesium Phase 3 Clinical Trial, a phase 3 multicenter, randomized, placebo-controlled trial to evaluate the efficacy of field-administered, hyperacute Mg^{2+} therapy (given within 2 hours of stroke onset) recently completed enrollment. Because patients were identified by paramedics before neuroimaging, both ischemic (73%) and hemorrhagic strokes (23%) were included. The study enrolled 1700 subjects (843 placebo, 857 magnesium). The median interval from "last known well" to the start of the study agent was 45 minutes. Treatment was initiated within 1 hour of onset in 74% and between 1 and 2 hours in 25%. Analysis was based on time-to-treatment stratification. The primary endpoint, the shift in the distribution of functional outcomes on the mRS–global disability at 90 days, was not different between the two groups.[50]

In summary, although preclinical studies of competitive and non-competitive NMDA antagonists suggest that they can effectively protect penumbral regions, results of clinical studies have thus far been disappointing. Trial design, lacking forced time-to-treatment stratification and patient selection criteria for stroke homogeneity, may have contributed to these results. As with calcium antagonists, achieving neuroprotection by blocking glutamate-induced damage means interrupting events that are triggered almost immediately after the onset of ischemia; thus the time to treatment from onset must be brief. This small time window, seen in all animal studies, was ignored in all clinical trials of these drugs except for the FAST-MAG trial.

Even more important, the negative clinical results with NMDA antagonists may be attributed to the dose-limiting phencyclidine-like side effects, which prevent achievement of therapeutic drug levels in brain tissue. An understanding of the clinically apparent neurotoxicity of NMDA antagonists involves a condition described as "NMDA receptor hypofunction." NMDA antagonists have been shown to induce large vacuoles within the adult rodent brain that may signify irreversible damage.[51,52] Molecular experiments have demonstrated that an indirect complex network disturbance is responsible for the NMDA receptor hypofunction. Blockade of NMDA receptors on subcortical inhibitory neurons leads to disinhibition of glutamatergic and cholinergic cortical projections.[53] This disinhibited state, coupled with simultaneous stimulation of non-NMDA glutamate receptors, may lead to enhanced neurotoxicity. Concurrent administration of GABAergic or α-adrenergic agents appears to diminish the excitotoxic damage.[54] Finally, a model of immature rodents demonstrates that administration of NMDA antagonists during the period of synaptogenesis triggers diffuse apoptotic degeneration throughout the brain.[55]

These complex interactions indicate the potential problems with using drugs that target specific neurotransmitter function. Attempts have been made to develop strategies inhibiting glutamate-induced damage while avoiding the toxicity profile of direct NMDA receptor antagonism. Several agents with such properties have been tested in phase 2 and 3 trials, including polyamine site blockers, glycine antagonists, AMPA receptor antagonists, presynaptic glutamate release inhibitors, ion channel blockers, and GABA agonists. These agents are discussed individually in the following sections.

Agents Acting Indirectly on Glutamate

GV150526 (*gavestinel*) is a glycine site antagonist at the NMDA receptor complex.

Two large phase 3 randomized, placebo-controlled, double-blind trials failed to demonstrate the efficacy of gavestinel despite statistical power adequate to detect even small differences. The GAIN Americas trial randomly assigned 1367 patients to treatment or placebo within 6 hours of stroke onset, and concomitant treatment with IV t-PA was allowed in eligible patients.[56] Patients were stratified at randomization by age and initial stroke severity. Mean NIHSS score was 12 and median time to treatment was 5.2 hours. No significant difference in mortality rate or 3-month outcome was found between the gavestinel and placebo groups.

The GAIN International trial recruited 1804 patients within 6 hours of stroke onset and used the same dosing regimen and stratified randomization schema as the GAIN Americas trial.[23] The primary efficacy measure, survival combined with 3-month BI, was analyzed only in the ischemic stroke population (721 patients given gavestinel; 734 given placebo). Secondary endpoints were BI, NIHSS score, mRS, death within 3 months, and global statistical test of combined neurologic status at 3 months. In comparison with placebo, gavestinel had no effect on primary or secondary outcome measures when baseline NIHSS score and age were included as covariates. Minor adverse events (transient increase in liver function values and phlebitis) were seen more commonly in the gavestinel group, but no significant differences were found in rates of serious adverse events.

The neutral results of the large gavestinel trials are disconcerting for several reasons. First, the clinical testing closely mimicked the experimental models that had exhibited neuroprotection even after 6 hours of ischemia. Second, these trials incorporated an adequate number of patients to exclude a clinically significant benefit of gavestinel, which is a point that has been used to criticize previous trials. Third, these trials appropriately stratified patients according to baseline stroke severity and age, which are factors that may otherwise cause imbalances within treatment and placebo groups, thereby confounding results. Fourth, "supratherapeutic" levels of the neuroprotective agent were achieved with only minimal and tolerable side effects. Therefore, unlike with other modulators of glutamate activity, doses of gavestinel were not limited by intolerability of "therapeutic" doses.

The reason for the neutral results for gavestinel clinical trials remains to be identified. It is possible that the time window to effectively antagonize glutamate is simply less than 6 hours and that the neuroprotective benefit of infarct size reduction in animals does not translate into improved functional outcome measured in clinical trials. Just as likely, however, is that expectations for gavestinel were overinflated because only positive preclinical results were published (it is common for negative results in animal studies to go unreported). Mild beneficial effects were seen only in carefully standardized stroke models that do not reflect the heterogeneity of patients with stroke, in whom more robust efficacy would be needed to achieve clinical significance.

Blockade of glutamate-activated AMPA receptors represents another target of cytoprotection with several advantages over NMDA receptor antagonism. AMPA receptors are co-localized with NMDA receptors on cortical neurons but are also present on oligodendrocytes in the white matter.[57] These receptors are more permeable to sodium and mediate fast synaptic transmission and depolarization, thereby facilitating activation of NMDA receptors. Favorable attributes of AMPA antagonism include potential preservation of both cortical and subcortical regions as well as reduction of secondary activation of NMDA receptor and voltage-gated calcium channels. One promising AMPA antagonist, *YM872*, exhibits high-affinity competitive activity at the AMPA receptor as well as low affinity for the NMDA receptor, the glycine site on the NMDA receptor, and the kainite receptor.

Enrollment was terminated prematurely in two concurrent YM872 clinical trials,[58,59] the AMPA Receptor Antagonist Treatment in Ischemic Stroke (ARTIST) trials, on the basis of an interim futility analysis. These multicenter, randomized, double-blind, placebo-controlled trials were designed to "fill in the gaps" left by past neuroprotection trials: combination of reperfusion and neuroprotection strategies and the use of a biological marker of efficacy. The ARTIST+ trial compared the efficacy of YM872 plus t-PA with that of placebo plus t-PA. Patients with acute hemispheric ischemic stroke and a moderate-to-severe deficit treated with standard protocol t-PA were eligible. The planned enrollment was 600 patients, and more than 400 patients were enrolled. YM872 administration was started before the end of t-PA infusion and continued for 24 hours. Primary efficacy-outcome measures included neurologic function and disability scales.

The second trial, ARTIST MRI, evaluated the safety and potential efficacy of YM872 administered to patients with stroke within 6 hours of onset and used MRI as a surrogate marker of outcome. Baseline ischemic lesion volume on DWI was compared with final lesion volume on T2-weighted imaging with fluid-attenuated inversion recovery (FLAIR) to detect the effect of YM872 on lesion growth. The abandonment of these very well-designed trials is disappointing. Further investigation of YM872 is not planned at this time.

Another approach to the biological monitoring of neurotherapeutics is highlighted in a stroke trial investigating another AMPA antagonist, *ZK200775*.[60] This dose-finding trial utilized serum concentrations of S-100B and neuron-specific enolase as peripheral markers of glial and neuronal injury, respectively. The study found a significant worsening in the mean NIHSS score 48 hours after the start of treatment in the highest dose group (525 mg/48 hours). This neurologic deterioration was associated with a higher than expected elevation in serum S-100B levels in a multiple regression analysis controlling for stroke severity. There was no significant increase in neuron-specific enolase. Although these data suggest glial rather than neuronal damage, the oligodendrocytes are critical for neuronal homeostasis, and glial damage may contribute to neuronal dysfunction. These results provide corroborative evidence of the potential toxicity of glutamate antagonists suggested by the clinically apparent dose-related toxicity observed in previous trials. Such markers may be useful surrogate markers of cytoprotection and toxicity in future trials.

Inhibitors of glutamate release are a heterogeneous group of agents, including anticonvulsants and antidepressants. The proposed mechanism of action for these drugs is ion channel blockade. While some of these treatments have been shown to reduce infarct volume in preclinical models, the cytoprotective effect is present only when administered at the onset of ischemia.[61–63] When these drugs were evaluated clinically, sipatrigine was limited by intolerable neuropsychiatric side effects[64] and phase 2–3 evaluation of IV fosphenytoin was terminated prematurely after interim analysis showed no difference between placebo and fosphenytoin in any of the functional or disability outcomes.[65]

A calcium-sensitive, maxi-K potassium channel opener, *BMS-204352 (MaxiPost)*, causes neuronal hyperpolarization, decreased calcium influx, and glutamate release.[66] A phase 3 trial, the Potassium-Channel Opening Stroke Trial (POST) of 1978 patients with moderate-tosevere cortical strokes (NIHSS score, 6 to 20) treated within 6 hours of onset failed to show any significant beneficial effect compared with placebo.[65]

Lubeluzole is a benzothiazole compound that has emerged as a neuroprotective agent in animal models of focal ischemia.[67–69] There are several putative mechanisms by which lubeluzole protects the penumbral region. First, lubeluzole normalizes neuronal activity in the peri-infarct region by inhibiting glutamate release possibly via blockade of non-L-type calcium channels.[70] Additionally, blockade of sodium channels and taurine release by lubeluzole suggests that it may reduce osmoregulatory stress in the peri-infarct zone.[71] Finally, lubeluzole down-regulates the glutamate-induced NOS pathway and diminishes NO-related neurotoxicity.[72]

A phase 3 randomized, multicenter, double-blind, placebo-controlled trials adopted a low-dose regimen to test the efficacy of lubeluzole in patients with AIS. The low-dose regimen was selected partly due to concern for cardiac toxicity with a higher dose regimen. However, it is essential to note that the low-dose regimen produced a mean plasma concentration that was below the minimal neuroprotective level established in animals.[73]

Three large-scale, multicenter, double-blind, placebo-controlled, randomized, phase 3 trials of low-dose lubeluzole in patients with stroke have produced conflicting results. The European and Australian trial randomly assigned 725 patients to treatment within 6 hours of onset and demonstrated similar overall mortality rates, rates of adverse events, and clinical outcomes in all placebo- and lubeluzole-treated patients.[74] However, an unplanned post hoc analysis found that lubeluzole treatment decreased mortality among patients with mild-to-moderate stroke as measured by the Clinical Global Impression rating. The North American trial involved 721 patients treated within 6 hours of onset of moderate to severe hemispheric stroke (NIHSS score, >7).[75] The mean time to treatment was 4.7 hours. The primary outcome measure, mortality at 12 weeks, was not significantly different between groups; however, the extent of functional recovery (BI score) and disability (mRS) at 3 months significantly favored lubeluzole over placebo after the data were controlled for appropriate covariates. The odds of favorable outcome were 38% higher with lubeluzole according to the global test statistic. This study also confirmed the safety of the low-dose regimen, reporting no significant differences in cardiac-related complications or adverse events.

The third trial evaluating the efficacy of low-dose lubeluzole randomly assigned to treatment a total of 1786 patients who were stratified according to time to treatment (0 to 6 hours and 6 to 8 hours).[76] During the trial, a target stroke population (core stroke group) was defined on the basis of results of a meta-analysis identifying patients who might benefit from treatment. The core stroke group consisted of patients with ischemic stroke, excluding patients 75 years or older with severe strokes, who were treated within 6 hours. Only the core stroke group was used in the primary efficacy analyses. Lubeluzole had no significant effect on mortality or 12-week functional status in the core stroke group. Similar neutral results were found in the non-target population, including all patients treated within 6–8 hours of onset and patients 75 years or older with severe stroke. The most commonly reported adverse experiences were fever, constipation, and headache. Lubeluzole-treated patients experienced more cardiac events, including atrial fibrillation and QT interval prolongation, but this higher rate was not associated with increased mortality.

Finally, lubeluzole was the first potentially neuroprotective agent to be evaluated in a dedicated combination trial with t-PA. Patients who qualified for and received IV t-PA within 3 hours of symptom onset were randomly allocated 1 : 1 to receive either lubeluzole or placebo.[77] The lubeluzole infusion was started before the end of the 1-hour t-PA infusion. Eighty-nine patients were enrolled before the trial was terminated early because of negative results of the previously described concurrent lubeluzole phase 3 trial. In the enrolled patients (45% of the planned population), t-PA and the study drug were administered at a mean of 2.5 and 3.2 hours from symptom onset, respectively. There were no significant differences in rates of death, intracerebral hemorrhage, or serious adverse events or in functional outcomes (BI) between the lubeluzole and placebo groups. These results demonstrate the safety and feasibility of linking ultra-early neuroprotection with thrombolysis; however, the premature stoppage of enrollment led to a study with insufficient power to detect efficacy.

A systematic review of five randomized trials, involving a total of 3510 patients, found no evidence that lubeluzole given at any dose reduced the odds of death or dependency at the end of follow-up (OR, 1.03; 95% CI, 0.91–1.19).[78] At any given dose, however, lubeluzole was associated with a significant excess of cardiac conduction disorders.

There are several reasons that the lubeluzole trials may have failed to show efficacy. As with many other agents, the time from stroke onset to drug administration is most likely too long to meaningfully inhibit glutamate release and action. Although an extended 6-hour time window for efficacious treatment has been reported, other animal models have failed to replicate the efficacy of lubeluzole initiated more than 30 minutes after ischemia. The discrepancy in results between the North American and European trials may be in part due to time to drug initiation. In the North American trial, the mean interval was 4.7 hours. Although a similar mean is not reported by the European trial, more than 80% of patients were treated after 4 hours, which may potentially have led to lessened efficacy. Also, dose-limiting side effects, primarily cardiac, led to a narrow therapeutic index with resultant serum drug levels below the minimum neuroprotective level reported in animal studies. Although the combination trial of lubeluzole and t-PA required treatment within 4 hours, its early termination yielded a small sample size and a study with insufficient power to detect efficacy.

Other Neurotransmitter Modulators

Serotonin agonists may exert cytoprotection via several actions at presynaptic and postsynaptic 5-hydroxytryptamine-1A (5-HT_{1A}) receptors. Primarily, activation of this receptor causes neuronal membrane hyperpolarization by opening G-protein-coupled potassium channels.[79] Activation of presynaptic serotonin receptors may lead to a reduction in glutamate release.[80] Lastly, these agents may inhibit apoptosis.[81]

The neuroprotective efficacy, safety, and tolerability of *repinotan* (*BAY x 3702*), a serotonin agonist of the 5-HT_{1A} subtype, has been evaluated. The results of a double-blind, placebo-controlled phase 3 efficacy trial comparing repinotan to placebo in patients with moderate-to-severe stroke (NIHSS scores, 8 to 23) within 6 hours of symptom onset failed to demonstrate a clinical benefit with repinotan.[82]

ONO-2506 is a neurotransmitter modulator. Its proposed mechanism of action is modulation of glutamate transporter uptake capacity and expression of GABA receptors.[83] A safety and efficacy study of ONO-2506, which recruited patients with stroke within 6 hours of onset of a radiographically confirmed cortical infarct, was terminated; however, details have not been published.[65]

Although no overall treatment effect was observed in phase 2 evaluation, a subgroup analysis suggested that nalmefene may confer a beneficial effect in young patients (<70 years old).[84] On the basis of phase 2 data, a phase 3 trial was designed to study the safety and efficacy of 60 mg of nalmefene.[85] A total of 368 patients were randomly assigned to undergo treatment within 6 hours of stroke onset. The study found no significant treatment effect on 3-month outcome with any of the planned analyses, including secondary analyses in young patients and thrombolytic-treated patients.

There are several potential explanations for the neutral results of the opioid antagonist trials. As with other upstream modulators of excitotoxicity, delayed treatment may not confer neuroprotection because the pivotal steps in the cascade have already occurred by the time of treatment. Also, the trial design did not enforce recruitment of adequate numbers of patients to the subgroups most likely to derive benefit (e.g., young patients, patients with moderate-to-severe deficits, and patients eligible for thrombolytic treatment), which resulted in insufficient power. Last, no pharmacokinetic studies were performed so the adequacy of dosage is unknown.

Enhancement of GABA-induced inhibition may be a useful target of cytoprotection. *Clomethiazole* is a GABA agonist that theoretically prevents damage due to excessive excitatory neurotransmitters by enhancing inhibition at the $GABA_A$ receptor level.[86] Activation of the GABA receptor increases chloride conductance and membrane hyperpolarization, thereby depressing neuronal depolarization and excitability.[87]

The Clomethiazole Acute Stroke Study (CLASS) evaluated clomethiazole in a randomized, placebo-controlled fashion in patients with hemispheric ischemic stroke with moderate to severe deficit who were treated within 12 hours of onset.[88] Efficacy analysis of 1353 patients revealed a non-significant 1.2% difference favoring clomethiazole in achievement of functional independence as assessed by BI. Sedation, the most common adverse event, led to withdrawal of treatment in 15.6% of patients. Subgroup analyses found a significant beneficial effect of clomethiazole in two overlapping groups:

patients with severe baseline neurologic deficit and those classified as having a total anterior circulation stroke. An interaction between stroke syndrome classification and treatment was identified. In patients with total anterior circulation strokes, 40.8% of clomethiazole-treated patients reached relative functional independence compared with 29.8% of placebo-treated patients, which suggests that patients with the largest strokes may have a larger penumbra that may be salvaged by cytoprotective therapy.

The Clomethiazole Acute Stroke Study in Ischemic Stroke (CLASS-I) was designed to test the hypothesis generated by the previous CLASS trial, which was that clomethiazole is effective in patients with large ischemic anterior circulation strokes.[89] Patients with ischemic stroke who showed evidence of higher cortical dysfunction plus visual field and motor deficits were randomly assigned within 12 hours of onset to receive either placebo or clomethiazole. There was no evidence of drug efficacy on any of the outcome variables, including NIHSS score, BI, mRS, and 30-day lesion volume.

The absence of treatment effect occurred despite adequate trial design, appropriate patient selection, and adequate plasma drug concentrations. As with other trials, the lack of efficacy is most likely due to either the prolonged treatment time window or the inadequate prediction of human pharmacokinetics based on rodent data.

In summary, a large number of drugs that target glutamate and other neurotransmitter functions have shown efficacy in preclinical studies but not in clinical trials. A major factor has been side effects that limit dose, but even in studies that have achieved therapeutic dose ranges and that have been sufficiently powered, such as the GAIN and CLASS trials, results have been neutral or negative. There is a recurrent theme in preclinical studies of benefit being seen when treatment is administered very early after ischemia. In subsequent clinical trials, however, a much larger treatment window was allowed. Currently, the best remaining hope for this strategy is with clinical trials which require a very rapid time to treatment.[90]

Free Radical Scavengers, Adhesion Molecule Blockers, Steroids, and Other Anti-inflammatory Strategies

Reactive oxygen intermediates play a role in ischemic tissue damage and represent another target for cytoprotection. Free radical scavengers affect a late stage of the ischemic process. *Tirilazad mesylate* is a 21-aminosteroid free radical scavenger and potent membrane lipid peroxidation inhibitor that has shown neuroprotective promise in focal ischemia and subarachnoid hemorrhage models.[91,92] This agent protects the microvascular endothelium and maintains intact blood–brain barrier and cerebral autoregulatory mechanisms. Unfortunately, its penetration into the brain parenchyma is limited, possibly leading to unsatisfactory efficacy in stroke, as demonstrated by clinical trials to date.[93] However, a newer group of antioxidants, pyrrolopyrimidines, with significantly improved blood–brain barrier penetrance, have demonstrated successful neuroprotection in focal ischemia with a postischemic treatment window of 4 hours.[93]

A phase 3 randomized trial of Tirilazad therapy started within 6 hours of stroke onset was terminated prematurely after a preplanned interim analysis of 660 patients determined the futility of continued enrollment.[94] No significant difference was found in the proportion of patients demonstrating a favorable outcome because of tirilazad treatment administered at a median of 4.3 hours. The lack of drug efficacy in this trial was, in part, ascribed to inadequate dosing, especially in women. A second tirilazad trial was designed using higher dosing regimens.[95] This trial was discontinued prematurely after safety concerns were raised in a concurrent European trial, despite trends toward reduced rates of mortality and dependence in both men and women. A systematic review of six randomized controlled trials involving more than 1700 patients included previously unpublished data from two large European trials with negative results.[96] This review found that tirilazad actually increases rates of death and disability by one-fifth.

Whether tirilazad not only exhibits a lack of neuroprotection but also induces worsening within specific populations of patients with stroke is still unclear. Potential reasons for these conclusions include controversial results of preclinical studies,[97] delay in drug administration (>75% of patients were treated >3 hours after stroke onset), thrombophlebitis causing a systemic inflammatory state, and inadequate blood–brain barrier permeability. Finally, it is possible that generation of free radicals plays a positive role in the recovery of patients with stroke.

Ebselen is another type (selenoorganic) of antioxidant that potentially inhibits lipid peroxidation through multiple mechanisms. These mechanisms include inhibition of lipoxygenase within the arachidonate cascade, blocked production of superoxide anions by activated leukocytes,[98] inhibition of inducible NOS,[99] and glutathione-like inhibition of membrane lipid peroxidation.[100]

A single randomized efficacy trial has shown that early treatment with ebselen improved outcome after AIS.[101] Ebselen was administered orally to patients within 48 hours of ischemic stroke onset (mean time to treatment, 29.7 hours). There was no significant difference in mortality. Intention-to-treat analysis demonstrated that ebselen therapy achieved a significantly better outcome at 1 month, but only a trend to improvement was observed at 3 months. Although the ebselen group contained slightly more patients with mild impairment than the placebo group, the difference was not significant, and the efficacy of ebselen was also demonstrated in patients with moderate to severe deficits. Ebselen treatment given within 24 hours significantly improved the likelihood of good recovery on the Glasgow Outcome Scale compared with placebo (42% vs 22%; $P = 0.038$), whereas treatment after 24 hours led to no significant differences between the groups. The ebselen-treated patients were marginally more likely to report adverse events, but the incidence was not significantly different from that in the placebo group. On the basis of the results of this adequately powered trial, ebselen is believed to be safe and possibly efficacious. A multicenter phase 3 ebselen trial was completed in 2002 with a total of 394 patients; however, the results have not been reported.[65] These studies were submitted for registration for use in cerebral ischemia to the Japanese regulatory authority; however, the drug was not approved for use since reviewers considered that the efficacy was insufficient.[102]

Free radicals are produced during ischemia and reperfusion and contribute to the neuronal injury after stroke. Edaravone (MCI-186) is a free radical scavenger whose mechanism of neuroprotection includes inhibition of endothelial cell injury, delayed neuronal death, and prevention of edema after ischemia.[103,104] A Japanese multicenter randomized clinical trial of edaravone was published in 2003. Patients were randomly assigned to edaravone or placebo within 72 hours after symptom onset. A significant improvement in functional outcome on the mRS at 3 months was noted in the edaravone group ($P = 0.0382$).[105] Edaravone has been approved in Japan since 2001 as a neuroprotective agent for treatment of acute cerebral infarct within 24 hours after symptom onset.[104] A Cochrane Review including three trials with 496 participants reported that edaravone appeared to increase the proportion of patients with marked neurological improvement compared with control (risk ratio (RR), 1.99; 95%CI, 1.60–2.49).[106] A phase 2 randomized controlled safety study in Europe demonstrated safety and tolerability of a new formulation and dose regimen of edaravone with plasma concentrations which reached prespecified target levels. This information will allow a more practical treatment regimen for additional trials.[107]

Several nitrone free radical-trapping agents (spin-trap agents) have demonstrated neuroprotection in rodent models of both transient and permanent focal ischemia.[108,109] *NXY-059* (disodium 4-((*tert*-butylimino) methyl) benzene-1,3-disulfonate *N*-oxide) is a nitrone-based compound that has free radical-trapping properties.

The SAINT I study[110] was a randomized, double-blind, placebo-controlled trial involving 1722 patients with AIS who were randomly assigned to receive a 72-hour infusion of placebo or IV NXY-059 within 6 hours after the onset of the stroke. The primary outcome was mRS at 90 days. All patients received standard of care, including IV rt-PA, when indicated.

Approximately 96% of the patients assigned to NXY-059 achieved plasma concentrations of NXY-059 greater than 150 μmol/L. Analysis for the primary outcome was positive. Among the 1699 subjects included in the efficacy analysis, NXY-059 significantly improved the overall distribution of scores on the mRS compared with placebo ($P = 0.038$). The OR for improvement across all categories of the scale was 1.20 (95% CI, 1.01–1.42). Rates of adverse events and mortality were similar in the two groups. Although the effect on disability was moderate, it was believed to be consistent with a neuroprotective action. Additional support for the suggestion that NXY-059 was neuroprotective was a biological signal from post hoc analysis, which revealed that treatment with NXY-059 significantly reduced the incidence of intracranial hemorrhage among patients in whom alteplase was also used.[111]

As expected, these findings generated much excitement, and confirmation of these results was planned in SAINT II. Based on the results of SAINT I, the SAINT II protocol was modified to include an increase in the sample size from 1700 to 3200 patients, which would provide at least 80% power to detect an OR of 1.2 (across all cutoff points of the mRS), which was seen in SAINT I. In addition, a revised approach to analysis of the NIHSS score and a prospective analysis of intracerebral hemorrhage were planned.[25] The efficacy analysis was based on 3195 patients (1588 in the NXY-059 group and 1607 in the placebo group). Mortality and adverse event rates were similar in the two groups. The distribution of scores on the mRS did not differ between the NXY-059 and placebo groups ($P = 0.33$; OR, 0.94; 95%CI, 0.83–1.06). Analysis of categorized scores on the mRS confirmed the lack of benefit: the OR for trichotomization into mRS scores of 0–1 vs 2–3 vs 4–6 was 0.92 (95%CI, 0.80–1.06). There was no evidence of efficacy for any of the secondary endpoints. Alteplase was administered to 44% of patients in both groups; however, there was no difference in the frequency of symptomatic or asymptomatic hemorrhage between treatment groups. The authors concluded that NXY-059 is ineffective for the treatment of AIS within 6 hours after the onset of symptoms. Lastly, a pooled analysis of the SAINT trials confirmed neutral results, not only in the overall population, but also in important prespecified subgroups, such as those treated early after stroke or those who were offered alteplase.[112]

The SAINT II investigators considered whether the conflicting results of the two trials might be related to the higher rate of alteplase use in SAINT II. However, no evidence of an interaction between alteplase use and the effect of NXY-059 was found in either trial.[25] Although NXY-059 was tested rigorously in the preclinical setting relative to other neuroprotective agents, in retrospect, investigators identified red flags in the preclinical stages including lack of benefit across animal models and concerns with timing of administration.[113] The results from SAINT II are disappointing, but they highlight many opportunities for improvement in both preclinical testing of neuroprotective agents and in clinical trial design.

Complex inflammatory processes mediate ischemic- and reperfusion-related brain injury, representing an ideal downstream target for cytoprotection. Modulation of cytokines, inflammatory-related enzymes (NOS), endothelial leukocyte interactions, leukocyte activation, and gene transcription factors have been investigated in experimental models and a few clinical trials.

Enlimomab is a murine monoclonal anti-ICAM-1 antibody that has undergone phase 3 testing in patients with stroke. A phase 3 trial compared the efficacy of enlimomab with placebo in 625 patients with ischemic stroke who received treatment within 6 hours of symptom onset.[114] The target serum drug level was achieved in 96.6% of patients after the first dose, and adequate trough levels were maintained throughout the duration of treatment. Enlimomab treatment was associated with worse disability and greater mortality rates than was placebo. This negative treatment effect was evident by day 5 of treatment and was confirmed with adjustments for age and stroke severity. The hazard of death averaged over the first 90 days was 43% higher in enlimomab-treated patients than in placebo-treated patients.

There are several possible explanations for the negative effect of enlimomab. First, enlimomab is a different type of antibody from that used in experimental models. Murine anti-ICAM antibody may have led to up-regulation of endogenous adhesion molecules and precipitated a paradoxical inflammatory response. It has been shown that all enlimomab-treated patients develop anti-mouse antibodies.[115] An experimental model was subsequently designed to mimic the clinical trial that had negative results. First, administration of this murine antibody to rats was shown to lead to production of host humoral responses against the protein, consisting of the activation of complement, neutrophils, and the microvascular system.[116] Second, no preclinical model delayed treatment for 6 hours or administered the drug for 5 consecutive days as in the clinical trial. Most important, animal studies showed no treatment benefit in permanent ischemia models. Only a minority of patients (4–24%) had spontaneous reperfusion; hence most enrolled patients were not comparable with transient ischemia models, which were associated with treatment benefit. Therefore, the rational approach to future immunomodulatory therapies would be development of a humanized anti-adhesion molecule strategy with a revised (shorter) dosage regimen coupled with thrombolysis.

To this end, a humanized immunoglobulin (Ig) G1 antibody against human CD18 (*Hu23F2G* or rovelizumab, *LeukArrest*) was developed to block leukocyte infiltration while avoiding the complications of enlimomab due to sensitization. A phase 3 trial enrolled patients within 12 hours of stroke onset, allowed concomitant use of t-PA, and employed a reduced frequency of dosing schema compared with enlimomab. The three groups received either a single dose at enrollment, the first dose at enrollment and a second dose 60 hours later, or placebo. The phase 3 trial of rovelizumab was terminated after interim futility analysis determined that treatment was unlikely to confer significant benefit if the trial were continued.[117] To date, the data from this trial remain unpublished.

The immunomodulator, interferon-β (IFN-β), has been evaluated in a small number of preclinical trials. Its well-known side effect profile in patients with multiple sclerosis provides the opportunity to move forward more quickly in clinical trials of acute stroke. While the exact mechanism by which IFN-β provides neuroprotection is not clear, potential mechanisms include a reduction in neutrophil infiltration, decreased blood–brain barrier disruption,[118] and promotion of cell survival factors possibly mediated by NF-κB activation.[119] The preclinical data in AIS, however, are limited and conflicting.[120–122] A randomized controlled dose-escalation phase 1 trial of IFN-β1a administered within 24 hours of symptom onset has been completed.[65] Five dose cohorts of five patients (4 : 1 active:placebo) were studied at 11 μg, 22 μg, 44 μg, 66 μg, and 88 μg administered daily for 7 days. The results have not been published.

Leukocyte activation is another event in the inflammatory process that may be interrupted. A recombinant protein inhibitor of CD11b/CD18 receptor (*UK-279276*) blocks neutrophil activation and has shown neuroprotection in animal models of focal ischemia.[123] The Acute Stroke Therapy by Inhibition of Neutrophils (ASTIN) study was an adaptive phase 2 dose-response finding, proof-of-concept study to establish whether UK-279276 improves recovery in AIS. The investigators utilized a Bayesian sequential design with real-time efficacy data capture and continuous reassessment of the dose response using a double-blind, randomized, adaptive allocation to 1 of 15 doses (dose range, 10–120 mg) or placebo and early termination for efficacy or futility. The primary endpoint was change from baseline to day 90 on the Scandinavian Stroke Scale. Nine hundred sixty-six acute stroke patients (887 ischemic, 204 cotreated with IV t-PA) were treated within 6 hours of symptom onset. There was no treatment effect for UK-279276, and the trial was stopped early for futility. The authors concluded that UK-279276 was well-tolerated and without serious side effects, but that it did not improve recovery in patients with AIS. The adaptive design facilitated early termination for futility.[124]

Promising new strategies are developing to target other "downstream" events of the ischemic–excitotoxic cascade: the calcium-dependent enzymatic reactions mediating necrotic and apoptotic cell death. Theoretically, because these processes occur "later" in the cascade, the therapeutic time window may be longer. Several important enzymes have been characterized as potential targets of neuroprotection.[125–130] However, the inability of these large protein compounds to cross the blood–brain barrier has limited clinical development.

Minocycline, a semisynthetic second-generation drug of the tetracycline group, is a safe and readily available compound that exerts anti-inflammatory effects such as inhibition of microglial activation[131] and production of other inflammatory mediators.[132] Furthermore, minocycline may inhibit the activity of matrix metalloproteinases (MMPs) and diminish permeability of the blood–brain barrier. The neuroprotective efficacy of minocycline has been demonstrated in animal models even when delayed up to 4 hours,[132] has been shown to be as neuroprotective as hypothermia,[133] and may extend the t-PA treatment time window in ischemic stroke models.[134] Minocycline appears to be an ideal neuroprotective candidate on the basis of its established safety profile, good central nervous system (CNS) penetration, wide availability, and inexpensive cost. Interestingly, the possibility of a gender-related response to treatment, with no reduction in infarct size in female rodents, has been reported[135] and highlights an important trial design aspect that may need to be taken into account in future studies.

The results of an open-label, evaluator-blinded study of 152 patients has been reported.[136] Minocycline at a dosage of 200 mg was administered orally for 5 days within 6–24 hours after onset of stroke. The primary outcome measure was change in NIHSS score from baseline to day 90 in the minocycline group compared with placebo. Seventy-four patients received minocycline, and 77 received placebo. NIHSS, mRS, and BI scores were all significantly improved in minocycline-treated patients. Rates of adverse events and hemorrhagic transformation did not differ by treatment group. The trial did have some limitations, including the pseudorandomized design and open-label treatment. In addition, the placebo group did unusually poorly in this particular trial. Nonetheless, these findings support the preclinical data, which suggested a potential benefit of minocycline in AIS.

Two clinical trials of minocycline in patients with AIS were terminated early, one for futility[137] and the other was not able to meet enrollment requirements.[138] The Minocycline to Improve Neurologic Outcome (MINOS) trial, evaluated four different IV doses (between 3 and 10 mg/kg) of minocycline for safety and tolerance in patients with AIS. Results demonstrate that doses between 3 and 10 mg/kg daily for 3 days is safe and achieved concentrations that have been shown to be neuroprotective in experimental models.[139] An efficacy trial was suggested, but none is currently registered as of the time of this update.

Corticosteroids, theoretically, may interrupt the inflammatory cascade that occurs during stroke. Although corticosteroids substantially reduce stroke size in experimental models, trials using various routes of administration, dosage, and duration of treatment with *dexamethasone* have failed to demonstrate a beneficial effect of steroids.[140,141] A systematic review of published randomized trials comparing steroids with placebo given within 48 hours of onset concluded that there is insufficient evidence to justify corticosteroid use after ischemic stroke.[142] The substantial delay from stroke onset to drug administration is a possible culprit in the negative results. Additionally, the detrimental side effects of corticosteroids may be mediated by the transcriptional genomic activities of steroids, thereby limiting their clinical utility.[143]

A growing interest in studying the pleiotropic effects of the 3-hydroxy-3-methylglutaryl coenzyme A (HMG CoA) reductase inhibitors (*"statins"*) has uncovered a potential neuroprotective effect. The possible mechanisms of neuroprotection include improved endothelial function, increased endothelial NOS activity, antioxidant effects, promotion of neovascularization, and anti-inflammatory properties.

The Neuroprotection with Statin Therapy for Acute Recovery Trial (NeuSTART) was the first clinical trial evaluating the use of lovastatin in the early stage of stroke.[144] NeuSTART was a phase 1B dose-escalation and dose-finding study in which ischemic stroke patients were treated with increasing doses of lovastatin within 24 hours of symptom onset. The primary safety outcomes were the occurrence of myotoxicity or hepatotoxicity. A total of 33 patients were enrolled, receiving between 1 and 8 mg/kg. No clinical liver disease or myopathy elevations occurred. NeuSTART identified 8 mg/kg/day for 3 days as the maximum tolerated dose of lovastatin to carry forward in future efficacy trials.[145]

Human serum albumin is a multifunctional protein with neuroprotective properties in experimental models of focal ischemia even when administered up to 4 hours after induction of reversible ischemia.[146] Several mechanisms have been speculated for its neuroprotective capacity, including inhibition of lipid peroxidation (antioxidant), maintenance of microvascular integrity, inhibition of endothelial cell apoptosis,[147] hemodilution, and mobilization of the free fatty acids required for restoration of damaged neurons.[148] Although non-albumin hemodilution trials have not demonstrated a benefit, these were designed to test efficacy of hemodilution, not cytoprotection per se.

The promising preliminary results from the Albumin in Acute Stroke (ALIAS) Pilot Trial led to a multicenter, randomized, placebo-controlled efficacy trial of albumin in AIS. The ALIAS-Part 2 Trial was a phase 3 trial in which human serum albumin, at a dose of 2 g/kg, administered IV over 2 hours was compared with placebo isovolumic normal saline in patients with AIS. The major change in ALIAS-Part 2 was that infusion of the study drug began within 5 hours of stroke onset. Patients received standard of care including concurrent treatment with IV or intra-arterial thrombolysis, when appropriate. The primary endpoint was favorable outcome at 90, defined as either a modified Rankin scale (mRS) score of 0 or 1 or NIHSS score of 0 or 1, or both. Estimated enrollment was 1100 patients; however, the study was stopped early for futility after 841 patients were enrolled. The primary outcome did not differ between patients in the albumin group and those in the saline group (186 [44%] vs 185 [44%]; RR 0·96; 95%CI 0.84–1.10, adjusted for baseline NIHSS score and thrombolysis stratum). Mild-to-moderate pulmonary edema and symptomatic intracranial hemorrhage were more common in patients given albumin. Although the rate of favorable outcome in patients given albumin remained consistent at 44–45% over the course of the trial, the cumulative rate of favorable outcome in patients given saline rose steadily from 31% to 44%.[149] Several reasons were postulated to explain the neutral results including treatment window to 5 hours, differences in preclinical models demonstrating the neuroprotective benefit of albumin compared to the clinical scenario and possible improvement in general stroke care over the 3.5 years of enrollment.[149] The latter being particularly important since organized stroke unit care has been shown to improve outcomes.[150]

Membrane "Stabilizers" and Trophic Factors

SUR1, while best known for its role in the formation of K_{ATP} channels, has recently been associated with a non-selective cation channel, the NC(Ca-ATP) channel, in ischemic astrocytes, which is regulated by SUR1. NC(Ca-ATP) is opened by depletion of ATP and, when opened, leads to cytotoxic edema and cell necrosis.[151] This channel is upregulated in neurons, astrocytes, and capillary endothelial cells after CNS ischemia or injury. The SUR1 antagonist, glibenclamide, has been shown to have a significant benefit across multiple ischemic stroke models with a large window for treatment opportunity (4–6 hours after ischemic insult).[152]

The Glyburide Advantage in Malignant Edema and Stroke Pilot (GAMES-PILOT) study was a prospective study of 10 patients with DWI lesion volumes of 82–210 cm^3 treated with RP-1127 (glyburide for injection) to determine the feasibility of recruiting and treating patients with severe stroke within 10 hours of symptom onset.[153] A dose of 3 mg/d was well tolerated and additional evaluation is planned. The Glyburide Advantage in Malignant Edema and Stroke-Remedy Pharmaceuticals (GAMES-RP) is a phase 2 randomized, prospective, double blind study evaluating the efficacy of RP-1127 compared to placebo in subjects with a severe anterior circulation ischemic stroke who are likely to develop malignant edema. Primary outcome is day 90 mRS ≤4 without the need for decompressive craniectomy.[154] This innovative study is ongoing and results are eagerly awaited.

The monosialoganglioside *GM-1* is thought to limit excitotoxicity and facilitate nerve repair and regrowth. In a study of 792 patients with acute stroke, there was a non-significant trend toward greater recovery in patients treated for 3 weeks with GM-1 than in those given placebo.[155] Post hoc analysis showed a statistically significant difference in neurologic outcome favoring GM-1 in the subgroup of patients treated within 4 hours. There was no difference in mortality rates, and the drug had no significant side effects. A Cochrane meta-analysis reported that there is not enough evidence to conclude that gangliosides are beneficial in acute stroke. In addition, caution was warranted due to sporadic cases of Guillain-Barré syndrome after ganglioside therapy.[156]

Cerebrolysin is a compound consisting of free amino acids and biologically active small peptides that are products of the enzymatic breakdown of lipid free brain products. Experimental models have demonstrated neuroprotection, although the mechanism of action is unclear.[157] The results of a placebo-controlled, double-blind clinical trial enrolling 119 patients with acute ischemic hemispheric stroke randomized to a combined treatment with alteplase plus cerebrolysin or placebo administered 1 hour after thrombolytic treatment starting within 3 hours after onset of symptoms were recently reported. The combination of tpa with cerebrolysin was safe, but did not demonstrate improved outcomes at 90 days.[158] The study was powered to detect a difference of 20% which is probably unrealistic for a neuroprotective agent, as mentioned previously.

Energy failure and activation of phospholipases during ischemia lead to breakdown of cellular membranes and, ultimately, to neuronal death. *Cytidine-5'-diphosphocholine (citicoline)*, the rate-limiting intermediate in the biosynthesis of phosphatidylcholine, is incorporated into the membrane of injured neurons and may prevent membrane breakdown into free-radical-generating lipid byproducts. Citicoline has exhibited a neuroprotective effect in a variety of CNS injury models, including focal ischemia.[159] However, the neuroprotective capacity is modest and is lost if treatment is started beyond 3 hours after onset of injury.[160] Despite the extensive work performed with experimental models, the exact mechanism of action of citicoline remains elusive. However, it is believed to be due to increased phosphatidylcholine synthesis and inhibition of phospholipase A_2 within the injured brain. During ischemia, the choline supply is limited, and membrane phospholipids are hydrolyzed to provide a source of choline for neurotransmitter synthesis. This autocannibalism ultimately leads to death of cholinergic neurons.[160] Additionally, there is evidence that citicoline reduces expression of procaspases and other proteins involved in apoptotic cell death after focal ischemia.[161]

A pooled analysis of oral citicoline clinical trials in AIS reported that[162] 3-month recovery (composite NIHSS score <1, mRS score <1, BI value >95) was achieved in 25.2% of citicoline-treated patients compared with 20.2% of placebo-treated patients. The largest difference in recovery was seen in patients treated with the highest dose (2000 mg) of citicoline.

The Citicoline in the treatment of acute ischemic stroke: an international, randomized, multicenter, placebo-controlled study (ICTUS trial) began enrollment in 2006 to confirm the efficacy findings noted in the pooled analysis. The study enrolled 2298 of a planned 2600 patients (1148 assigned to citicoline and 1150 to placebo) with moderate-to-severe anterior circulation stroke within 24 hours of symptom onset. The primary outcome measure was total recovery at 3 months, based on a global test analysis including the NIHSS, mRS, and BI. The trial was stopped for futility at the third interim analysis on the basis of complete data from 2078 patients. The final randomized analysis was based on data for 2298 patients. Global recovery was similar in both groups (OR, 1.03; 95%CI, 0.86–1.25; $P = 0.364$). Again, several reasons for the discrepancy between the meta-analysis results and ICTUS were outlined by the authors including the 10-year difference in time during which the management of stroke patients has improved, older patients with more severe strokes and an increase in the use of IV tpa in ICTUS.[163]

Erythropoietin (EPO) is a mediator of the physiologic response to hypoxia via activation of the EPO receptor, a member of the cytokine receptor superfamily. Both astrocytes and neurons produce EPO in response to hypoxia, and this glycoprotein has been demonstrated to cross the blood–brain barrier.[164] The overall result of EPO receptor activation is cell proliferation, inhibition of apoptosis, and erythroblast differentiation.[165] EPO may also provide antioxidant activity and resistance to glutamate toxicity.[166,167] An initial safety and subsequent proof-of-concept study showed that intravenously administered EPO is safe and able to enter the brain in patients with stroke. In addition, treatment with EPO was associated with an improvement in clinical outcomes at 1 month.[168] A phase 2/3 randomized controlled trial that enrolled 522 patients within 6 hours of symptom onset evaluated the effect of a 3-day high-dose, IV EPO treatment on functional outcome (BI) at 90 days. Greater than 60% of patients received tPA. There was no difference in the primary outcome or any of the other outcome parameters between groups. An overall death rate of 16.4% in the EPO and 9% in the placebo group (OR, 1.98; 95%CI, 1.16–3.38; $P = 0.01$) without any particular mechanism of death unexpected after stroke was reported, raising safety concerns, particularly in patients receiving thrombolysis.

Because of the potential of EPO to stimulate production of red blood cells and to promote blood coagulation, a modified version of EPO, Lu AA24493 or carbamylated erythropoietin (CEPO), has been developed and studied in a phase 1 trial. A subsequent study further evaluating safety and pharmacokinetics has been completed but results have not been reported.[169]

Trophic factors are emerging as potential cytoprotective agents, although their role may be more important in the recovery phase. *bFGF* (*trafermin [Fiblast]*) is a polypeptide that is trophic for brain neurons, glia, and endothelial cells and may prevent downregulation of antiapoptotic proteins such as Bcl-2.[170]

A double-blind, placebo-controlled clinical trial compared two doses of bFGF (5 mg or 10 mg) with placebo.[171] Patients with acute, moderate to severe stroke (NIHSS score >6) were randomly assigned within 6 hours of onset to receive a single 24-hour infusion of either bFGF or placebo. An interim efficacy analysis predicted only a nominal chance of significant benefit, and the trial was terminated after enrollment of 286 of the 900 patients planned. A non-significant trend for favorable outcome was seen in the low-dose group, whereas a non-significant disadvantage was seen in the high-dose group. Post hoc analysis further suggested efficacy of the low-dose regimen. Dose-dependent adverse events included leukocytosis and relative hypotension. An unpublished, multicenter, controlled phase 2/3 trial of bFGF was halted after interim analysis revealed a significant higher mortality rate in patients treated with this agent.

Granulocyte colony-stimulating factor (G-CSF) is a colony-stimulating factor hormone. It is a glycoprotein, growth factor, or cytokine produced by a number of different tissues to stimulate the bone marrow to produce granulocytes and stem cells. In acute stroke, G-CSF has been shown to be neuroprotective, antiapoptotic, and anti-inflammatory. In chronic stroke, G-CSF improves neurologic function weeks after stroke, induces neurogenesis, and enhances plasticity and stem cell mobilization from bone marrow. A phase 2 randomized, double-blind, placebo-controlled trial evaluating the safety and tolerability of AX 200 (G-CSF) compared with placebo in patients with acute stroke within 12 hours of symptom onset was completed in 2007. Patients with MCA infarct confirmed by MRI were randomly assigned on a 1:2 basis to receive either placebo or one of four different escalating doses of AX 200 (30, 90, 135, 180 μg/kg total) as an IV infusion.[65,110] A total of 44 patients were recruited. Thromboembolic complications (stroke and heart attack) were similar between G-CSF and placebo (7/30 versus 4/14, respectively) and serious adverse events were evenly distributed between groups.[172] Based on these findings, AXIS 2 (AX200 for the Treatment of Ischemic Stroke – A Multinational, Multicenter, Randomized, Double-blind, Placebo-Controlled phase 2 trial) evaluated a dose of 135 μg/kg administered IV over 72 hours against placebo in 328 patients. Primary and secondary end points were the mRS score and NIHSS score at day 90, respectively. G-CSF did not provide any significant benefit with respect to either clinical outcome or imaging biomarkers.[173]

Many of the novel neuroprotectants, especially trophic factors and anti-inflammatory agents, exist as peptides unable to cross the blood–brain barrier. Animal models have demonstrated enhancement of delivery and neuroprotection when protein agents are conjugated to a delivery vector. Such enhanced delivery mechanisms include (1) reformulation of the neurotherapeutic protein by conjugation and biotinylation and (2) creation of a fusion protein linked to transduction domains. Enhanced drug delivery systems have several benefits. First, obviously, they may enable delivery of neurotherapeutic agents that otherwise do not have access to the brain. Second, neuroprotection may be achieved at lower systemic doses, thereby allowing administration of agents that previously had dose-limiting side effects. Last, conjugation of an agent to blood–brain barrier delivery vectors may decrease its distribution to peripheral organs.

Hypothermia

The neuroprotective action of mild to moderate (29°C to 35°C) systemic hypothermia has been demonstrated in numerous animal models of global and focal cerebral ischemia.[174–179] The many hypothesized mechanisms for this protection include restoration of neurotransmitter balance,[180,181] reduction in cerebral metabolism,[182] preservation of the blood–brain barrier,[177] inhibition of apoptosis,[183] and attenuation of the inflammatory response.[184,185] Perhaps the consistent and robust benefit of hypothermia in multiple laboratories and animal models is due to the fact that it works through multiple pathways, all conspiring to have a greater effect than more precisely targeted therapies. Many of the clinically relevant questions regarding hypothermia have been addressed with varying degrees of success in animal studies: optimal mechanism of induction, target temperature, therapeutic time window, duration of treatment, rewarming, safety, reduction of shivering threshold, and persistence of benefit.

Several general principles have emerged from the extensive work investigating the cerebroprotective effects of hypothermia.[176] First, hypothermia applied during the ischemic period (intra-ischemic) is more protective than hypothermia applied after reperfusion (post-ischemic). Second, the efficacy of post-ischemic hypothermia depends on the interval between onset of ischemia and induction of hypothermia, achievement of target temperature, and duration of treatment. Third, hypothermia is more efficacious for global ischemia–reperfusion than for focal ischemia and more efficacious for transient focal ischemia than for permanent focal ischemia, which suggests that hypothermia may be most beneficial when coupled with thrombolysis and recanalization.

Two large trials have conclusively established the neuroprotective effects and safety of hypothermia after cardiac arrest.[186,187] These studies are the first proof of principle that neuroprotection can be realized in humans.

The Cooling for Acute Ischemic Brain Damage (COOL-AID) study group completed two clinical trials of hypothermia in AIS in patients with severe MCA infarcts. The first study used surface cooling,[188] and the second used endovascular cooling.[189] Hypothermia (target, 31 °C to 33 °C) was achieved with surface cooling within 5 hours after onset (after IV t-PA) or within 8 hours (after endovascular thrombolysis). Both trials demonstrated feasibility but were not powered to answer questions regarding safety and efficacy.

The Intravascular Cooling in the Treatment of Stroke-Longer t-PA Window (ICTuS-L) was a phase 1 trial originally designed to establish the safety of endovascular cooling combined with t-PA. In addition, by enrolling patients treated with t-PA from 3 to 6 hours after onset, extension of the therapeutic time window for thrombolysis using hypothermia would also be evaluated. There were a total of six treatment groups: patients who were seen within 3 hours received t-PA with or without hypothermia (groups 1 and 2) and patients who were seen within 3–6 hours of symptom onset randomly assigned to hypothermia plus t-PA, hypothermia alone, t-PA alone, or no treatment assignment (standard of care) comprised groups 3 through 6. ICTuS-L utilized an aggressive antishivering regimen, including buspirone and meperidine. ICTuS-L began in 2003; however, in 2008 both SITS-ISTR and ECASS 3 showed that IV thrombolysis was effective in patients treated between 3 and 4.5 hours after symptom onset. At this point, the investigators elected to close the ICTuS-L study early for analysis. As of December 2008, 59 patients were enrolled in ICTuS-L: 28 patients were randomly assigned to hypothermia and 30 patients were randomly assigned to normothermia. Overall, the rate of serious adverse events between those who received t-PA and those who did not were equivalent. Pneumonia occurred more frequently in the hypothermia patients than in the normothermia patients (7/28 versus 2/30, $P < 0.05$). This led to a protocol change to decrease the risk of pneumonia. The rates of intracranial hemorrhage, including both asymptomatic and symptomatic, were comparable in the two groups at 48 hours (33% hypothermia, 25% normothermia). There appeared to be no other safety concerns besides pneumonia, specifically, no increased risk of deep vein thrombosis due to the endovascular catheter; no liver, renal or hematologic concerns; and no coagulopathy.

The ICTuS-L trial confirmed that hypothermia, using an endovascular catheter, can be safely combined with thrombolytic therapy and that an aggressive antishivering protocol is feasible in awake stroke patients. ICTuS 2/3 is an on-going prospective, multisite phase 2/3 pivotal efficacy trial of thrombolysis combined with hypothermia in awake patients with moderately severe MCA distribution strokes. This trial will investigate the clinical efficacy of hypothermia, further delineate safety in combination with thrombolysis, and confirm that the changes to the treatment protocol successfully limit the occurrence of pneumonia. The target population in phase 2 will include 450 assessable patients and in phase 3 will include 1600 assessable patients diagnosed with AIS. IV infusion of cooled saline will be added to the hypothermia protocol and will be followed by catheter placement for endovascular hypothermia therapy as soon as possible. Patients will receive hypothermia therapy to 33 °C for 24 hours followed by 12 hours of controlled rewarming to 36.5 °C (normothermia). Each subject will be followed up for 90 days after the onset of their stroke.

Hypothermia remains one of the most potent neuroprotective agents yet studied. The use of a treatment protocol that obviates the need for intubation makes this early treatment more relevant for practical clinical use. Future studies will investigate the effect of hypothermia on clinical outcome, the safety of combination with thrombolysis, and the potential for utilization with other neuroprotective modalities as discussed next.

Caffeinol

A novel combination of caffeine and ethanol (*caffeinol*) has demonstrated more robust neuroprotection than many other experimental and clinically relevant agents tested in the laboratory.[190] When used individually, caffeine had no effect, and ethanol actually increased infarct volume. The protective mechanism of the combination remains largely unknown but may be due to the synergistic effect of caffeine and ethanol on the excitatory–inhibitory balance between neurotransmitter systems. Adenosine and NMDA receptor antagonism and GABA enhancement are hypothesized to be mechanistically involved in this neurochemical action.

An open-label, dose-escalation pilot study of caffeine and ethanol in patients with AIS identified the optimal dose resulting in plasma levels comparable with those producing therapeutic effect in animals (caffeine, 5 to 10 μg/mL; ethanol, 30 to 50 mg/dL) and that is clinically tolerated by patients without any significant adverse effects.[191]

Combining caffeinol with hypothermia to 35 °C conferred greater neuroprotection in a transient focal ischemia model than either caffeinol or hypothermia alone. A second clinical trial designed to establish the feasibility and safety of administering both caffeinol and mild systemic hypothermia to patients with AIS who had been treated with IV t-PA within 5 hours of symptom onset has been completed.[192] Twenty patients with AIS were treated with caffeinol (8 to 9 mg/kg caffeine + 0.4 g/kg IV ethanol over 2 hours, started within 4 hours after symptom onset) and hypothermia (started within 5 hours of symptom onset and continued for 24 hours followed by 12 hours of rewarming). IV t-PA was given to eligible patients. Meperidine and buspirone were used to suppress shivering. All patients received caffeinol, and most reached target blood levels. Cooling was attempted in 18 patients via endovascular (n = 8) or surface (n = 10) approaches. Thirteen patients reached the target temperature; average time from symptom onset was 9 hours and 43 minutes. Three patients died: one from symptomatic hemorrhage, one from malignant cerebral edema, and one from unrelated medical complications. No adverse events were attributed to caffeinol. At this point, the details of feasibility have been identified, and a prospective placebo-controlled randomized study is needed to further assess safety and to test the efficacy of caffeinol, hypothermia, or both.

Blood Substitutes and Oxygen Delivery

Compounds derived from human hemoglobin have a dual property: they may be neuroprotective through improvement in tissue oxygenation and may also augment perfusion because of their low viscosity. Several cell-free hemoglobin solutions are under clinical evaluation, but development has been cautious because of concerns about potential allergic and infectious complications as well as nephrotoxicity. *Diaspirin-cross-linked hemoglobin* (*DCLHb*) is human hemoglobin derived from banked red blood cells, heat treated, and cross-linked to diaspirin to prevent dissociation. Its oxygen affinity is similar to that of blood. Probably because hemoglobin binds endothelial NO, it has a slight pressor effect. The drug may be particularly effective in maintaining flow and oxygenation in the core of the infarct, thereby maintaining it in a "penumbral" state until definitive reperfusion by spontaneous or therapeutic thrombolysis occurs.

A multicenter, randomized, single-blind phase 2 safety and dose-finding trial randomly assigned 85 patients to receive either DCLHb or saline.[193] Patients who had AIS in the anterior circulation and were identified within 18 hours of onset of symptoms were enrolled. DCLHb caused a rapid rise in mean arterial blood pressure. The pressor effect was not accompanied by complications or excessive need for antihypertensive treatment. More serious adverse events and deaths occurred in DCLHb-treated patients than in control patients.

Normobaric hyperoxia (NBO) confers cortical protection when administered within 30 minutes of ischemia in rodents.[194] Practically, NBO therapy is easier to deliver than hyperbaric oxygen (HBO) therapy. Because of its simplicity, low cost, and safety, NBO may be initiated by first responders in the field. A phase 2 randomized controlled trial which enrolled 85 patients to compare the safety and efficacy of treating AIS patients with NBO (within 9 hours of symptom onset) to standard medical treatment was terminated due to an imbalance in deaths favoring the control arm. Deaths were not attributed to treatment.[195]

HBO treatment presumably increases oxygen delivery to the ischemic penumbra, thereby prolonging the functional activity of this potentially salvageable tissue. Administration of 100% oxygen at greater than atmospheric ambient pressure increases the amount of oxygen physically dissolved in blood. Although the majority of animal models demonstrate a beneficial effect of HBO therapy on outcome and infarct volume,[196–200] others do not,[201–203] and controversy prevails regarding the neuroprotective potential of this modality in both clinical and experimental focal ischemia. Increased free radical generation and lipid peroxidation is a theoretical risk of HBO therapy that may counteract its neuroprotective mechanisms of action. Human experience with ischemic stroke and HBO treatment yields similar conflicting results.[204,205]

CONCLUSION

In light of recent several clinical trials of cytoprotection demonstrating neutral results, it is becoming increasingly more challenging to encourage continued clinical research in neuroprotection in the same traditional fashion as has been done over the past decade. Past clinical trials are ridden with recurrent problems that dampen any possible treatment effect.

Despite these disappointing results, the search for cytoprotective therapy should not be abandoned; rather, clinical trial design needs to undergo a paradigm shift to minimize the known problems in demonstrating cytoprotection. Conducting pre-hospital treatment has its barriers, but should continue to be pursued. Efforts to take the emergency department to the patient with mobile stroke units[206] are currently underway in Germany with plans to begin in the US in 2014. Before valuable resources are committed to more, large, phase 3 studies, clinical researchers and funding agencies must come to a consensus about how to carry out future trials. Important issues to address include solid preclinical data, targeted patient populations, shorter time windows for treatment and adaptive trial design. Any preclinical agent that seems promising should first show robust benefit in careful and thorough preclinical testing in multiple laboratories and models with clinically realistic treatment delay. It may be necessary to demonstrate a convincing proof of concept in a more targeted population such as patients who will undergo cardiac procedures where the opportunity for pretreatment exists. A review of randomized clinical trials evaluating pharmacological perioperative brain neuroprotection reports the use of atorvastatin and magnesium sulfate was associated with a lower incidence of new postoperative neurological deficit.[207] Indeed, these types of studies are already being conducted.[208]

Encouraging signals have been detected in human studies of hypothermia after cardiac arrest, suggesting that clinically meaningful cytoprotection after stroke may still be achievable despite >10 years of trials of various agents that have largely failed to demonstrate it. A change in the way we approach clinical trials will be necessary before a successful cytoprotective agent is shown to improve outcomes.

The complete reference list can be found on the companion Expert Consult website at www.expertconsult.inkling.com.

KEY REFERENCES

2. Trendelenburg G, Dirnagl U. Neuroprotective role of astrocytes in cerebral ischemia: focus on ischemic preconditioning. Glia 2005;50:307–20.
3. Hossmann KA. Viability thresholds and the penumbra of focal ischemia. Ann Neurol 1994;36:557–65.
4. Ginsberg M. Neuroprotection in brain ischemia: An update. Neuroscientist 1995;1(95):164.
5. Grotta JC. The current status of neuronal protective therapy: Why have all neuronal protective drugs worked in animals but none so far in stroke patients? Cerebrovasc Dis 1994;4:115–20.
6. Fisher M, Ratan R. New perspectives on developing acute stroke therapy. Ann Neurol [Review] 2003;53:10–20.
8. Kaplan B, Brint S, Tanabe J, et al. Temporal thresholds for neocortical infarction in rats subjected to reversible focal cerebral ischemia. Stroke [Research Support, U.S. Gov't, P.H.S.] 1991;22: 1032–9.
9. O'Collins VE, Macleod MR, Donnan GA, et al. 1,026 experimental treatments in acute stroke. Ann Neurol 2006;59:467–77.
10. Stroke Therapy Academic Industry Roundtable (STAIR). Recommendations for standards regarding preclinical neuroprotective and restorative drug development. Stroke 1999;30: 2752–8.
11. Stroke Therapy Academic Industry Roundtable II (STAIR-II). Recommendations for clinical trial evaluation of acute stroke therapies. Stroke 2001;32(7):1598–606.
12. Adams HP Jr, Davis PH, Leira EC, et al. Baseline NIH Stroke Scale score strongly predicts outcome after stroke: A report of the Trial of Org 10172 in Acute Stroke Treatment (TOAST). Neurology [Clinical Trial Comparative Study Multicenter Study Randomized Controlled Trial Research Support, U.S. Gov't, P.H.S.] 1999;53(1):126–31.
13. Heiss WD, Graf R, Lottgen J, et al. Repeat positron emission tomographic studies in transient middle cerebral artery occlusion in cats: residual perfusion and efficacy of postischemic reperfusion. J Cereb Blood Flow Metab 1997;17(4):388–400.
14. Baron JC. Mapping the ischaemic penumbra with PET: implications for acute stroke treatment. Cerebrovasc Dis 1999;9(4): 193–201.
15. Marchal G, Beaudouin V, Rioux P, et al. Prolonged persistence of substantial volumes of potentially viable brain tissue after stroke: a correlative PET-CT study with voxel-based data analysis. Stroke [Research Support, Non-U.S. Gov't] 1996;27(4): 599–606.
16. Neumann-Haefelin T, Moseley ME, Albers GW. New magnetic resonance imaging methods for cerebrovascular disease: emerging clinical applications. Ann Neurol [Research Support, Non-U.S. Gov't Review] 2000;47(5):559–70.
17. Schellinger PD, Fiebach JB, Jansen O, et al. Stroke magnetic resonance imaging within 6 hours after onset of hyperacute cerebral ischemia. Ann Neurol 2001;49(4):460–9.
18. Schlaug G, Benfield A, Baird AE, et al. The ischemic penumbra: operationally defined by diffusion and perfusion MRI. Neurology [Research Support, Non-U.S. Gov't Research Support, U.S. Gov't, P.H.S.] 1999;53(7):1528–37.
19. Li F, Silva MD, Liu KF, et al. Secondary decline in apparent diffusion coefficient and neurological outcomes after a short period of focal brain ischemia in rats. Ann Neurol [Research Support, Non-U.S. Gov't] 2000;48(2):236–44.
20. Kidwell CS, Saver JL, Mattiello J, et al. Thrombolytic reversal of acute human cerebral ischemic injury shown by diffusion/ perfusion magnetic resonance imaging. Ann Neurol [Clinical Trial Research Support, Non-U.S. Gov't] 2000;47(4):462–9.
21. Tymianski M. Novel approaches to neuroprotection trials in acute ischemic stroke. Stroke [Research Support, Non-U.S. Gov't] 2013;44(10):2942–50.

22. Tissue plasminogen activator for acute ischemic stroke. The National Institute of Neurological Disorders and Stroke rt-PA Stroke Study Group. N Engl J Med 1995;333(24):1581–7.
23. Lees KR, Asplund K, Carolei A, et al. Glycine antagonist (gavestinel) in neuroprotection (GAIN International) in patients with acute stroke: a randomised controlled trial. GAIN International Investigators. Lancet 2000;355(9219):1949–54.
24. Muir KW. Magnesium for neuroprotection in ischaemic stroke: rationale for use and evidence of effectiveness. CNS Drugs 2001;15(12):921–30.
25. Shuaib A, Lees KR, Lyden P, et al. NXY-059 for the treatment of acute ischemic stroke. N Engl J Med 2007;357(6):562–71.
27. Saver JL, Kidwell CS, Leary M, et al. The Field Administration of Stroke Therapy-Magnesium: A study of prehospital neuroprotective therapy. Abstract presented at the Ongoing Clinical Trials Session, 26th International Stroke Conference. 2001.
29. Grotta JC. Clinical aspects of the use of calcium antagonists in cerebrovascular disease. Clin Neuropharmacol 1991;14(5): 373–90.
30. Horn J, de Haan RJ, Vermeulen M, et al. Nimodipine in animal model experiments of focal cerebral ischemia: a systematic review. Stroke 2001;32(10):2433–8.
31. Clinical trial of nimodipine in acute ischemic stroke. The American Nimodipine Study Group. Stroke 1992;23(1):3–8.
32. Wahlgren N, MacMahon D, De Keyser J, et al. Intravenous Nimodipine West European Stroke Trial (INWEST of nimodipine in the treatment of acute ischemic stroke. The INWEST Study Group. Cerebrovasc Dis 1994;4:204.
33. Horn J, de Haan RJ, Vermeulen M, et al. Very Early Nimodipine Use in Stroke (VENUS): a randomized, double-blind, placebo-controlled trial. Stroke 2001;32(2):461–5.
35. Koh JY, Cotman CW. Programmed cell death: its possible contribution to neurotoxicity mediated by calcium channel antagonists. Brain Res 1992;587(2):233–40.
37. Ginsberg MD. Neuroprotection for ischemic stroke: Past, present and future. Neuropharmacology 2008;55(3):363–89.
38. Grotta JC, Picone CM, Ostrow PT, et al. CGS-19755, a competitive NMDA receptor antagonist, reduces calcium-calmodulin binding and improves outcome after global cerebral ischemia. Ann Neurol 1990;27(6):612–19.
39. Simon R, Shiraishi K. N-methyl-D-aspartate antagonist reduces stroke size and regional glucose metabolism. Ann Neurol 1990; 27(6):606–11.
41. Davis SM, Lees KR, Albers GW, et al. Selfotel in acute ischemic stroke : possible neurotoxic effects of an NMDA antagonist. Stroke 2000;31(2):347–54.
43. Albers GW, Goldstein LB, Hall D, et al. Aptiganel hydrochloride in acute ischemic stroke: a randomized controlled trial. JAMA 2001;286(21):2673–82.
45. Muir KW, Lees KR. A randomized, double-blind, placebo-controlled pilot trial of intravenous magnesium sulfate in acute stroke. Stroke 1995;26(7):1183–8.
46. Weglicki WB, Phillips TM. Pathobiology of magnesium deficiency: a cytokine/neurogenic inflammation hypothesis. Am J Physiol 1992;263(3 Pt 2):R734–7.
47. Muir KW, Lees KR. Dose optimization of intravenous magnesium sulfate after acute stroke. Stroke 1998;29(5):918–23.
49. Muir KW, Lees KR, Ford I, et al. Magnesium for acute stroke (Intravenous Magnesium Efficacy in Stroke trial): randomised controlled trial. Lancet 2004;363(9407):439–45.
53. Farber NB, Kim SH, Dikranian K, et al. Receptor mechanisms and circuitry underlying NMDA antagonist neurotoxicity. Mol Psychiatry 2002;7(1):32–43.
56. Sacco RL, DeRosa JT, Haley EC Jr, et al. Glycine antagonist in neuroprotection for patients with acute stroke: GAIN Americas: a randomized controlled trial. JAMA 2001;285(13): 1719–28.
57. Akins PT, Atkinson RP. Glutamate AMPA receptor antagonist treatment for ischaemic stroke. Curr Med Res Opin 2002;18(Suppl. 2):s9–13.
58. Inc AP. A Study to Evaluate the Effects of YM872 on Brain Function and Disability When Administered in Combination With Alteplase (Tissue Plasminogen Activator). Available from: <http://clinicaltrials.gov/ct2/show/NCT00044057>; 2006 [updated March 31, 2006; cited 2013 December 1].
59. Inc AP. A Study to Evaluate the Effects of YM872 on Stroke Lesion Volume in Acute Stroke Patients. Available from: <http://clinicaltrials.gov/show/NCT00044070>; 2006 [updated March 31, 2006; cited 2013 December 1].
60. Elting JW, Sulter GA, Kaste M, et al. AMPA antagonist ZK200775 in patients with acute ischemic stroke: possible glial cell toxicity detected by monitoring of S-100B serum levels. Stroke [Clinical Trial Clinical Trial, Phase II Multicenter Study Randomized Controlled Trial Research Support, Non-U.S. Gov't] 2002;33(12): 2813–18.
64. Muir KW, Holzapfel L, Lees KR. Phase II clinical trial of sipatrigine (619C89) by continuous infusion in acute stroke. Cerebrovasc Dis 2000;10(6):431–6.
67. De Ryck M, Keersmaekers R, Clincke G, et al. Lubeluzole, a novel benzothiazole, protects neurologic function after cerebral thrombotic stroke in rats: An apparent stereospecific effect abstract. Soc Neurosci Abstr 1994;20:185.
68. Aronowski J, Strong R, Grotta JC. Treatment of experimental focal ischemia in rats with lubeluzole. Neuropharmacology 1996;35(6):689–93.
69. De Ryck M, Verhoye M, Van der Linden AM. Diffusion-weighted MRI of infarct growth in a rat photochemical stroke model: effect of lubeluzole. Neuropharmacology 2000;39(4):691–702.
74. Diener HC. Multinational randomised controlled trial of lubeluzole in acute ischaemic stroke. European and Australian Lubeluzole Ischaemic Stroke Study Group. Cerebrovasc Dis 1998; 8(3):172–81.
75. Grotta J. Lubeluzole treatment of acute ischemic stroke. The US and Canadian Lubeluzole Ischemic Stroke Study Group. Stroke 1997;28(12):2338–46.
76. Diener HC, Cortens M, Ford G, et al. Lubeluzole in acute ischemic stroke treatment: A double-blind study with an 8-hour inclusion window comparing a 10-mg daily dose of lubeluzole with placebo. Stroke 2000;31(11):2543–51.
77. Grotta J. Combination Therapy Stroke Trial: recombinant tissue-type plasminogen activator with/without lubeluzole. Cerebrovasc Dis 2001;12(3):258–63.
78. Gandolfo C, Sandercock P, Conti M. Lubeluzole for acute ischaemic stroke. Cochrane Database Syst Rev 2002;(1):CD001924.
79. Davies MF, Deisz RA, Prince DA, et al. Two distinct effects of 5-hydroxytryptamine on single cortical neurons. Brain Res 1987;423(1–2):347–52.
81. Schaper C, Zhu Y, Kouklei M, et al. Stimulation of 5-HT(1A) receptors reduces apoptosis after transient forebrain ischemia in the rat. Brain Res 2000;883(1):41–50.
82. Teal P, Davis S, Hacke W, et al. A randomized, double-blind, placebo-controlled trial to evaluate the efficacy, safety, tolerability, and pharmacokinetic/pharmacodynamic effects of a targeted exposure of intravenous repinotan in patients with acute ischemic stroke: modified Randomized Exposure Controlled Trial (mRECT). Stroke [Clinical Trial, Phase II Comparative Study Controlled Clinical Trial Multicenter Study Randomized Controlled Trial Research Support, Non-U.S. Gov't] 2009;40(11): 3518–25.
83. Pettigrew LC, Kasner SE, Albers GW, et al. Safety and tolerability of arundic acid in acute ischemic stroke. J Neurol Sci 2006;251(1–2):50–6.
84. Clark W, Ertag W, Orecchio E, et al. Cervene in acute ischemic stroke: Results of a double-blind, placebo-controlled, dose-comparison study. J Stroke Cerebrovasc Dis 1999;8(4):224–30.
85. Clark WM, Raps EC, Tong DC, et al. Cervene (Nalmefene) in acute ischemic stroke: final results of a phase III efficacy study. The Cervene Stroke Study Investigators. Stroke 2000;31(6):1234–9.
86. Green AR, Hainsworth AH, Jackson DM. GABA potentiation: a logical pharmacological approach for the treatment of acute ischaemic stroke. Neuropharmacology 2000;39(9):1483–94.
88. Wahlgren NG, Ranasinha KW, Rosolacci T, et al. Clomethiazole acute stroke study (CLASS): results of a randomized, controlled trial of clomethiazole versus placebo in 1360 acute stroke patients. Stroke 1999;30(1):21–8.
89. Lyden P, Shuaib A, Ng K, et al. Clomethiazole Acute Stroke Study in ischemic stroke (CLASS-I): final results. Stroke 2002;33(1): 122–8.
90. Saver JE, Ekstein M, Stratton S, et al., editors. Poster Presentation: The Field Administration of Stroke Therapy – Magnesium

(FAST-MAG) Phase 3 Clinical Trial. International Stroke Conference. San Diego, CA: The American Heart Association; 2009.
94. A randomized trial of tirilazad mesylate in patients with acute stroke (RANTTAS). The RANTTAS Investigators. Stroke 1996; 27(9):1453–8.
95. Haley EC Jr. High-dose tirilazad for acute stroke (RANTTAS II). RANTTAS II Investigators. Stroke 1998;29(6):1256–7.
96. Tirilazad mesylate in acute ischemic stroke: A systematic review. Tirilazad International Steering Committee. Stroke 2000;31(9): 2257–65.
97. Beck T, Bielenberg GW. Failure of the lipid peroxidation inhibitor U74006F to improve neurological outcome after transient forebrain ischemia in the rat. Brain Res 1990;532:336.
99. Hattori R, Inoue R, Sase K, et al. Preferential inhibition of inducible nitric oxide synthase by ebselen. Eur J Pharmacol 1994; 267(2):R1–2.
101. Yamaguchi T, Sano K, Takakura K, et al. Ebselen in acute ischemic stroke: a placebo-controlled, double-blind clinical trial. Ebselen Study Group. Stroke 1998;29(1):12–17.
103. Watanabe T, Yuki S, Egawa M, et al. Protective effects of MCI-186 on cerebral ischemia: possible involvement of free radical scavenging and antioxidant actions. J Pharmacol Exp Ther 1994; 268(3):1597–604.
104. Yoshida H, Yanai H, Namiki Y, et al. Neuroprotective effects of edaravone: a novel free radical scavenger in cerebrovascular injury. CNS Drug Rev 2006;12(1):9–20.
105. Effect of a novel free radical scavenger, edaravone (MCI-186), on acute brain infarction. Randomized, placebo-controlled, double-blind study at multicenters. Cerebrovasc Dis 2003;15(3): 222–9.
106. Feng S, Yang Q, Liu M, et al. Edaravone for acute ischaemic stroke. Cochrane Database Syst Rev [Meta-Analysis Review] 2011;(12):CD007230.
107. Kaste M, Murayama S, Ford GA, et al. Safety, tolerability and pharmacokinetics of MCI-186 in patients with acute ischemic stroke: new formulation and dosing regimen. Cerebrovasc Dis 2013;36(3):196–204.
108. Zhao Z, Cheng M, Maples KR, et al. NXY-059, a novel free radical trapping compound, reduces cortical infarction after permanent focal cerebral ischemia in the rat. Brain Res 2001;909(1–2): 46–50.
109. Sydserff SG, Borelli AR, Green AR, et al. Effect of NXY-059 on infarct volume after transient or permanent middle cerebral artery occlusion in the rat; studies on dose, plasma concentration and therapeutic time window. Br J Pharmacol 2002;135(1): 103–12.
110. Lees KR, Zivin JA, Ashwood T, et al. NXY-059 for acute ischemic stroke. N Engl J Med 2006;354(6):588–600.
111. Lees KR, Davalos A, Davis SM, et al. Additional outcomes and subgroup analyses of NXY-059 for acute ischemic stroke in the SAINT I trial. Stroke 2006;37(12):2970–8.
112. Diener HC, Lees KR, Lyden P, et al. NXY-059 for the treatment of acute stroke: pooled analysis of the SAINT I and II Trials. Stroke 2008;39(6):1751–8.
114. Use of anti-ICAM-1 therapy in ischemic stroke: results of the Enlimomab Acute Stroke Trial. Neurology 2001;57(8): 1428–34.
115. Schneider D, Berrouschot J, Brandt T, et al. Safety, pharmacokinetics and biological activity of enlimomab (anti-ICAM-1 antibody): an open-label, dose escalation study in patients hospitalized for acute stroke. Eur Neurol 1998;40(2):78–83.
116. Furuya K, Takeda H, Azhar S, et al. Examination of several potential mechanisms for the negative outcome in a clinical stroke trial of enlimomab, a murine anti-human intercellular adhesion molecule-1 antibody: a bedside-to-bench study. Stroke 2001; 32(11):2665–74.
117. Becker KJ. Anti-leukocyte antibodies: LeukArrest (Hu23F2G) and Enlimomab (R6.5) in acute stroke. Curr Med Res Opin [Research Support, U.S. Gov't, P.H.S.] 2002;(18 Suppl. 2):s18–22.
118. Veldhuis WB, Floris S, van der Meide PH, et al. Interferon-beta prevents cytokine-induced neutrophil infiltration and attenuates blood-brain barrier disruption. J Cereb Blood Flow Metab 2003; 23(9):1060–9.
120. Veldhuis WB, Derksen JW, Floris S, et al. Interferon-beta blocks infiltration of inflammatory cells and reduces infarct volume after ischemic stroke in the rat. J Cereb Blood Flow Metab 2003;23(9):1029–39.
122. Maier CM, Yu F, Nishi T, et al. Interferon-beta fails to protect in a model of transient focal stroke. Stroke 2006;37(4):1116–19.
123. Jiang N, Chopp M, Chahwala S. Neutrophil inhibitory factor treatment of focal cerebral ischemia in the rat. Brain Res 1998; 788(1–2):25–34.
124. Krams M, Lees KR, Hacke W, et al. Acute Stroke Therapy by Inhibition of Neutrophils (ASTIN): an adaptive dose-response study of UK-279,276 in acute ischemic stroke. Stroke 2003; 34(11):2543–8.
125. Manabat C, Han BH, Wendland M, et al. Reperfusion differentially induces caspase-3 activation in ischemic core and penumbra after stroke in immature brain. Stroke 2003;34(1):207–13.
131. Yenari MA, Xu L, Tang XN, et al. Microglia potentiate damage to blood-brain barrier constituents: improvement by minocycline in vivo and in vitro. Stroke 2006;37(4):1087–93.
132. Yrjanheikki J, Tikka T, Keinanen R, et al. A tetracycline derivative, minocycline, reduces inflammation and protects against focal cerebral ischemia with a wide therapeutic window. Proc Natl Acad Sci U S A 1999;96(23):13496–500.
133. Nagel S, Su Y, Horstmann S, et al. Minocycline and hypothermia for reperfusion injury after focal cerebral ischemia in the rat: effects on BBB breakdown and MMP expression in the acute and subacute phase. Brain Res 2008;1188:198–206.
134. Murata Y, Rosell A, Scannevin RH, et al. Extension of the thrombolytic time window with minocycline in experimental stroke. Stroke 2008;39(12):3372–7.
135. Li J, McCullough LD. Sex differences in minocycline-induced neuroprotection after experimental stroke. J Cereb Blood Flow Metab 2009;29(4):670–4.
136. Lampl Y, Boaz M, Gilad R, et al. Minocycline treatment in acute stroke: an open-label, evaluator-blinded study. Neurology 2007; 69(14):1404–10.
139. Fagan SC, Waller JL, Nichols FT, et al. Minocycline to improve neurologic outcome in stroke (MINOS): a dose-finding study. Stroke [Research Support, N.I.H., Extramural Research Support, Non-U.S. Gov't] 2010;41(10):2283–7.
140. Mulley G, Wilcox RG, Mitchell JR. Dexamethasone in acute stroke. Br Med J 1978;2(6143):994–6.
141. Norris JW, Hachinski VC. High dose steroid treatment in cerebral infarction. Br Med J (Clin Res Ed) 1986;292(6512):21–3.
142. Qizilbash N, Lewington SL, Lopez-Arrieta JM. Corticosteroids for acute ischaemic stroke. Cochrane Database Syst Rev 2000;(2):CD000064.
144. Elkind MS, Sacco RL, MacArthur RB, et al. The Neuroprotection with Statin Therapy for Acute Recovery Trial (NeuSTART): an adaptive design phase I dose-escalation study of high-dose lovastatin in acute ischemic stroke. Int J Stroke 2008;3(3): 210–18.
145. Elkind MS, Sacco RL, Macarthur RB, et al. High-dose lovastatin for acute ischemic stroke: results of the phase I dose escalation neuroprotection with statin therapy for acute recovery trial (NeuSTART). Cerebrovasc Dis [Clinical Trial, Phase I Multicenter Study Research Support, N.I.H., Extramural] 2009;28(3): 266–75.
146. Belayev L, Liu Y, Zhao W, et al. Human albumin therapy of acute ischemic stroke: marked neuroprotective efficacy at moderate doses and with a broad therapeutic window. Stroke 2001;32(2): 553–60.
148. Rodriguez de Turco EB, Belayev L, Liu Y, et al. Systemic fatty acid responses to transient focal cerebral ischemia: influence of neuroprotectant therapy with human albumin. J Neurochem 2002; 83(3):515–24.
149. Ginsberg MD, Palesch YY, Hill MD, et al. High-dose albumin treatment for acute ischaemic stroke (ALIAS) part 2: a randomised, double-blind, phase 3, placebo-controlled trial. Lancet Neurol [Research Support, N.I.H., Extramural Research Support, Non-U.S. Gov't] 2013;12(11):1049–58.
151. Simard JM, Chen M, Tarasov KV, et al. Newly expressed SUR1-regulated NC(Ca-ATP) channel mediates cerebral edema after ischemic stroke. Nat Med 2006;12(4):433–40.
153. Sheth KN, Kimberly WT, Elm JJ, et al. Pilot study of intravenous glyburide in patients with a large ischemic stroke. Stroke 2013.

154. Remedy Pharmaceuticals I. Glyburide Advantage in Malignant Edema and Stroke – Remedy Pharmaceuticals (GAMES-RP). Available from: <http://clinicaltrials.gov/ct2/show/NCT01794182>; 2013 [updated November 18, 2013; cited 2013 December 2].
155. Lenzi GL, Grigoletto F, Gent M, et al. Early treatment of stroke with monosialoganglioside GM-1. Efficacy and safety results of the Early Stroke Trial. Stroke 1994;25(8):1552–8.
156. Candelise L, Ciccone A. Gangliosides for acute ischaemic stroke. Cochrane Database Syst Rev 2001;(4):CD000094.
157. Schwab M, Antonow-Schlorke I, Zwiener U, et al. Brain-derived peptides reduce the size of cerebral infarction and loss of MAP2 immunoreactivity after focal ischemia in rats. J Neural Transm Suppl 1998;53:299–311.
158. Lang W, Stadler CH, Poljakovic Z, et al. A prospective, randomized, placebo-controlled, double-blind trial about safety and efficacy of combined treatment with alteplase (rt-PA) and Cerebrolysin in acute ischaemic hemispheric stroke. Int J Stroke [Randomized Controlled Trial] 2013;8(2):95–104.
161. Krupinski J, Ferrer I, Barrachina M, et al. CDP-choline reduces pro-caspase and cleaved caspase-3 expression, nuclear DNA fragmentation, and specific PARP-cleaved products of caspase activation following middle cerebral artery occlusion in the rat. Neuropharmacology 2002;42(6):846–54.
162. Davalos A, Castillo J, Alvarez-Sabin J, et al. Oral citicoline in acute ischemic stroke: an individual patient data pooling analysis of clinical trials. Stroke 2002;33(12):2850–7.
163. Dávalos A, Alvarez-Sabín J, Castillo J, et al. Citicoline in the treatment of acute ischaemic stroke: an international, randomised, multicentre, placebo-controlled study (ICTUS trial). Lancet 2012;380(9839):349–57.
165. Siren AL, Ehrenreich H. Erythropoietin – a novel concept for neuroprotection. Eur Arch Psychiatry Clin Neurosci 2001; 251(4):179–84.
166. Sakanaka M, Wen TC, Matsuda S, et al. In vivo evidence that erythropoietin protects neurons from ischemic damage. Proc Natl Acad Sci U S A 1998;95(8):4635–40.
167. Morishita E, Masuda S, Nagao M, et al. Erythropoietin receptor is expressed in rat hippocampal and cerebral cortical neurons, and erythropoietin prevents in vitro glutamate-induced neuronal death. Neuroscience 1997;76(1):105–16.
168. Ehrenreich H, Hasselblatt M, Dembowski C, et al. Erythropoietin therapy for acute stroke is both safe and beneficial. Mol Med 2002;8(8):495–505.
170. Ay I, Sugimori H, Finklestein SP. Intravenous basic fibroblast growth factor (bFGF) decreases DNA fragmentation and prevents downregulation of Bcl-2 expression in the ischemic brain following middle cerebral artery occlusion in rats. Brain Res Mol Brain Res 2001;87(1):71–80.
171. Bogousslavsky J, Victor SJ, Salinas EO, et al. Fiblast (trafermin) in acute stroke: results of the European-Australian phase II/III safety and efficacy trial. Cerebrovasc Dis 2002;14(3–4): 239–51.
173. Ringelstein EB, Thijs V, Norrving B, et al. Granulocyte colony-stimulating factor in patients with acute ischemic stroke: results of the AX200 for Ischemic Stroke trial. Stroke [Research Support, Non-U.S. Gov't] 2013;44(10):2681–7.
174. Buchan A, Pulsinelli WA. Hypothermia but not the N-methyl-D-aspartate antagonist, MK-801, attenuates neuronal damage in gerbils subjected to transient global ischemia. J Neurosci [Research Support, Non-U.S. Gov't Research Support, U.S. Gov't, P.H.S.] 1990;10(1):311–16.
176. Barone FC, Feuerstein GZ, White RF. Brain cooling during transient focal ischemia provides complete neuroprotection. Neurosci Biobehav Rev [Review] 1997;21(1):31–44.
177. Maier CM, Ahern K, Cheng ML, et al. Optimal depth and duration of mild hypothermia in a focal model of transient cerebral ischemia: effects on neurologic outcome, infarct size, apoptosis, and inflammation. Stroke 1998;29(10):2171–80.
178. Corbett D, Hamilton M, Colbourne F. Persistent neuroprotection with prolonged postischemic hypothermia in adult rats subjected to transient middle cerebral artery occlusion. Exp Neurol 2000;163(1):200–6.
180. Nakashima K, Todd MM. Effects of hypothermia on the rate of excitatory amino acid release after ischemic depolarization. Stroke 1996;27(5):913–18.
181. Koizumi H, Fujisawa H, Ito H, et al. Effects of mild hypothermia on cerebral blood flow-independent changes in cortical extracellular levels of amino acids following contusion trauma in the rat. Brain Res 1997;747(2):304–12.
182. Sick TJ, Xu G, Perez-Pinzon MA. Mild hypothermia improves recovery of cortical extracellular potassium ion activity and excitability after middle cerebral artery occlusion in the rat. Stroke 1999;30(11):2416–21, discussion 2422.
183. Babu PP, Yoshida Y, Su M, et al. Immunohistochemical expression of Bcl-2, Bax and cytochrome c following focal cerebral ischemia and effect of hypothermia in rat. Neurosci Lett 2000; 291:196.
184. Ishikawa M, Sekizuka E, Sato S, et al. Effects of moderate hypothermia on leukocyte-endothelium interaction in the rat pial microvasculature after transient middle cerebral artery occlusion. Stroke 1999;30(8):1679–86.
185. Inamasu J, Suga S, Sato S, et al. Post-ischemic hypothermia delayed neutrophil accumulation and microglial activation following transient focal ischemia in rats. J Neuroimmunol 2000;109(2):66–74.
186. Bernard SA, Gray TW, Buist MD, et al. Treatment of comatose survivors of out-of-hospital cardiac arrest with induced hypothermia. Clinical Trial Comparative Study Randomized Controlled Trial. N Engl J Med 2002;346(8):557–63.
187. Mild therapeutic hypothermia to improve the neurologic outcome after cardiac arrest. N Engl J Med 2002;346(8): 549–56.
188. Krieger DW, De Georgia MA, Abou-Chebl A, et al. Cooling for acute ischemic brain damage (cool aid): an open pilot study of induced hypothermia in acute ischemic stroke. Stroke 2001; 32(8):1847–54.
189. De Georgia MA, Krieger DW, Abou-Chebl A, et al. Cooling for Acute Ischemic Brain Damage (COOL AID): a feasibility trial of endovascular cooling. Neurology 2004;63(2):312–17.
190. Strong R, Grotta JC, Aronowski J. Combination of low dose ethanol and caffeine protects brain from damage produced by focal ischemia in rats. Neuropharmacology 2000;39(3): 515–22.
191. Piriyawat P, Labiche LA, Burgin WS, et al. Pilot dose-escalation study of caffeine plus ethanol (caffeinol) in acute ischemic stroke. Stroke 2003;34(5):1242–5.
192. Martin-Schild S, Hallevi H, Shaltoni H, et al. Combined neuroprotective modalities coupled with thrombolysis in acute ischemic stroke: a pilot study of caffeinol and mild hypothermia. J Stroke Cerebrovasc Dis 2009;18(2):86–96.
193. Saxena R, Wijnhoud AD, Carton H, et al. Controlled safety study of a hemoglobin-based oxygen carrier, DCLHb, in acute ischemic stroke. Stroke 1999;30(5):993–6.
194. Singhal AB, Dijkhuizen RM, Rosen BR, et al. Normobaric hyperoxia reduces MRI diffusion abnormalities and infarct size in experimental stroke. Neurology 2002;58(6):945–52.
198. Veltkamp R, Warner DS, Domoki F, et al. Hyperbaric oxygen decreases infarct size and behavioral deficit after transient focal cerebral ischemia in rats. Brain Res 2000;853(1): 68–73.
199. Chang CF, Niu KC, Hoffer BJ, et al. Hyperbaric oxygen therapy for treatment of postischemic stroke in adult rats. Exp Neurol 2000;166(2):298–306.
200. Sunami K, Takeda Y, Hashimoto M, et al. Hyperbaric oxygen reduces infarct volume in rats by increasing oxygen supply to the ischemic periphery. Crit Care Med 2000;28(8):2831–6.
202. Roos JA, Jackson-Friedman C, Lyden P. Effects of hyperbaric oxygen on neurologic outcome for cerebral ischemia in rats. Acad Emerg Med 1998;5(1):18–24.
203. Hjelde A, Hjelstuen M, Haraldseth O, et al. Hyperbaric oxygen and neutrophil accumulation/tissue damage during permanent focal cerebral ischaemia in rats. Eur J Appl Physiol 2002;86(5): 401–5.
204. Anderson DC, Bottini AG, Jagiella WM, et al. A pilot study of hyperbaric oxygen in the treatment of human stroke. Stroke [Clinical Trial Comparative Study Randomized Controlled Trial Research Support, Non-U.S. Gov't] 1991;22(9):1137–42.
205. Nighoghossian N, Trouillas P, Adeleine P, et al. Hyperbaric oxygen in the treatment of acute ischemic stroke. A double-blind pilot study. Stroke 1995;26(8):1369–72.

206. Walter S, Kostopoulos P, Haass A, et al. Diagnosis and treatment of patients with stroke in a mobile stroke unit versus in hospital: a randomised controlled trial. Lancet Neurol [Comparative Study Randomized Controlled Trial Research Support, Non-U.S. Gov't] 2012;11(5):397–404.

208. Messe SR, McGarvey ML, Bavaria JE, et al. A pilot study of darbepoetin alfa for prophylactic neuroprotection in aortic surgery. Neurocrit Care [Clinical Trial, Phase II Research Support, Non-U.S. Gov't] 2013;18(1):75–80.

56 Treatment of "Other" Stroke Etiologies

Scott E. Kasner, Brett L. Cucchiara

KEY POINTS

- There are a variety of specific but relatively uncommon causes of stroke, many of which have unique treatment implications.
- For most uncommon causes of stroke, there are few data from randomized trials, and treatment is based largely on clinical experience.
- Uncommon causes of stroke are more common in the young and in those without traditional vascular risk factors.
- Inflammatory and non-inflammatory vasculopathies, hematologic disorders, migraine-related stroke, mitochondrial disease, and cerebral vein thrombosis represent the major categories reviewed in this chapter.

The relatively uncommon or "other determined causes" of stroke often require therapeutic approaches that are distinct from the strategies employed for the more typical atherothromboembolic, cardioembolic, and small vessel occlusive stroke. These unusual stroke etiologies are myriad, but can be broadly classified as vascular, hematologic, and miscellaneous diseases (Boxes 56-1–56-3). The clinical manifestations, pathophysiology, and diagnostic considerations for these disorders are discussed elsewhere in this text, while this chapter will address the unique issues of treatment of those disorders for which specific therapies have been proposed. Because of the relative rarity of these stroke etiologies, most of the putative treatments have not been subjected to randomized clinical trials and are supported by limited data from observational or descriptive studies.

VASCULAR DISORDERS

The extracranial and intracranial arteries are susceptible to a diverse set of non-atherosclerotic disorders that may cause stroke (see Box 56-1). In young stroke victims, these nonatherosclerotic vasculopathies are particularly overrepresented, accounting for approximately 20–30% of strokes.[1-4] These disorders can be further classified as inflammatory and non-inflammatory.

Non-inflammatory Vasculopathies

Arterial Dissection[5,6]

Dissection of the internal carotid artery and vertebral artery may occur as a result of significant head and neck trauma, but may also occur spontaneously or after a trivial injury. A number of underlying connective tissue disorders appear to be risk factors for spontaneous dissection, including fibromuscular dysplasia (FMD), Marfan's syndrome, Ehlers–Danlos syndrome (Type IV), osteogenesis imperfecta, and other genetic conditions in which collagen is abnormally formed.[7-11] At present, none of these underlying conditions are amenable to specific treatment, although several of these conditions may be associated with systemic abnormalities warranting monitoring and in some cases intervention. Further, identification of conditions such as Ehlers–Danlos is relevant as endovascular procedures are extremely high risk in this population and should generally be avoided.

Ischemic stroke may result from either extracranial or intracranial dissection. However, intracranial dissection may also produce subarachnoid hemorrhage and will be discussed separately below. The clinical manifestations of extracranial carotid and vertebral artery dissection are distinct, but their treatment appears to be identical.

In the first 3 hours after the onset of acute ischemic stroke, thrombolytic therapy must be considered[12] regardless of whether dissection is suggested by the patient's history or examination. While intravenous tissue plasminogen activator (t-PA) is contraindicated in patients with a known history of recent major systemic trauma, spontaneous dissection is not easily diagnosed during the critical time window. There is a theoretical risk of causing increased hemorrhage into the vessel wall. However, there have been no reports to substantiate the theoretical risk. To the contrary, multiple case series have demonstrated no dissection-specific complications related to IV tPA and have found outcomes with tPA comparable to patients with more typical stroke etiologies.[13,14] In the time window beyond 4.5 hours, intravenous tPA is no longer a viable option, but intra-arterial thrombolysis is a potential treatment[15] that has been used successfully for stroke due to dissection.[16-20] In these cases, the catheter tip is placed in the distal thrombus beyond the site of the dissection, thus minimizing the exposure of the torn intima to the thrombolytic agent. Emergent endovascular therapy using angioplasty and stenting with or without thrombolysis has also been reported in cases with high-risk large vessel occlusions or demonstrable penumbral tissue defined by diffusion–perfusion MRI and fluctuating or progressive symptoms.[21-24]

The optimal strategy for prevention of stroke in patients with arterial dissection is controversial. Options include anticoagulation, antiplatelet therapy, angioplasty with or without stenting, surgery, or conservative observation without specific medical or surgical therapy. As stroke related to dissection may be a result of thromboembolism or hemodynamic compromise, treatment should be directed at the mechanism by which the dissection caused the stroke. Thromboembolism seems to be the dominant mechanism,[25] and microembolic signals are detectable with transcranial Doppler monitoring in about half of patients.[26] Historically, early anticoagulation with heparin or low-molecular-weight heparin (LMWH) has been widely recommended at the time of diagnosis,[27-30] particularly because the risk of stroke appears to be greatest in the first few days after the initial vascular injury.[31-33] As with

BOX 56-1 Unusual Vasculopathies

NON-INFLAMMATORY VASCULOPATHIES

Dissection
Fibromuscular dysplasia
Vasospasm after subarachnoid hemorrhage
Reversible cerebral vasoconstriction syndromes
Radiation-induced vasculopathy
Moyamoya disease
Hereditary disorders
  Homocystinuria, Fabry disease, CADASIL

INFLAMMATORY VASCULOPATHIES

Isolated angiitis of the central nervous system
Temporal (giant cell) arteritis
Collagen vascular diseases
  Polyarteritis nodosa, Churg–Strauss angiitis, systemic lupus erythematosus, Wegener's granulomatosis, Henoch-Schönlein purpura, rheumatoid arthritis, cryoglobulinemia, Takayasu disease
Infectious arteriopathy
  Syphilis, tuberculosis, bacterial and fungal infections, varicella-zoster virus, human immunodeficiency virus
Toxin-related arteriopathy
  Amphetamines, cocaine, phenylpropanolamine, LSD, heroin
Neoplasm-related arteriopathy

CADASIL, cerebral autosomal dominant arteriopathy with subcortical infarcts and leukoencephalopathy; LSD, lysergic acid diethylamide.

BOX 56-2 Hematologic Causes of Stroke

DISORDERS OF COAGULATION

Hereditary disorders
  Factor V Leiden mutation, prothrombin G20210A mutation, protein C deficiency, protein S deficiency, antithrombin III deficiency, other factor deficiencies
Acquired disorders
  Disseminated intravascular coagulation
  Antiphospholipid antibody syndrome
  Factor excess, deficiency, or dysfunction
    Dysfibrinogenemia, nephrotic syndrome, liver disease, pregnancy, paroxysmal nocturnal hemoglobinuria, iatrogenic causes

RED CELL DISORDERS

Hemoglobinopathies
  Sickle cell disease, hemoglobin SC disease
Polycythemia rubra vera

PLATELET DISORDERS

Essential thrombocytosis
Sticky platelet syndrome

BOX 56-3 Miscellaneous Unusual Causes of Stroke

Migraine-related stroke
Mitochondrial encephalopathy, lactic acidosis, and strokelike episodes (MELAS)
Atypical embolism
  Fat embolism, tumor embolism, air embolism, cholesterol embolism
Cerebral venous thrombosis

thrombolysis, it has been proposed that immediate anticoagulation of an acute dissection could cause worsening hemorrhage into the vessel wall, but this has never been proven to occur. A Cochrane database systematic review and pooled analysis of 1285 patients with carotid dissection in 36 studies (all of which were observational studies) reported a non-significant trend towards greater risk of death or disability with antiplatelet compared to anticoagulant therapy (odds ratio [OR], 1.77; 95%CI, 0.98–3.22, $P = 0.06$).[5] Recurrent stroke was not significantly different between anticoagulant and antiplatelet treated groups (1.87% with anticoagulation vs 2% with antiplatelet therapy). These data must be considered severely limited given the non-randomized nature of the included studies. Interpretation of these data is also complicated by the extreme variability in stroke rates reported across the larger observational studies, ranging from 0.3% to 10%.[6,34–36] The Cervical Artery Dissection in Stroke Study (CADISS)[37] was a pilot trial that randomized 250 subjects to either antiplatelet or anticoagulant therapy within 7 days of symptom onset. At 3 month follow-up, ipsilateral ischemic stroke occurred in 3 of 126 subjects in the antiplatelet group compared to 1 of 124 subjects in the anticoagulant group, but there was 1 subarachnoid hemorrhage with hydrocephalus in the anticoagulant group, yielding no net effect. All events occurred within the first 2 weeks after randomization. In both this trial and in the observational studies, most recurrent strokes occurred early after symptom onset, such that the choice of antithrombotic therapy may be influenced by the time from initial symptoms to presentation.

Dissections usually heal over time, and patients are commonly maintained on antithrombotic therapy for at least 3 months. The 3 month duration of therapy is arbitrary, and some authors suggest that imaging studies be repeated to confirm recanalization of the dissected vessel prior to a change in therapy.[32,38] Patients with complete vascular healing and those with complete and persistent occlusions on follow-up imaging appear to be at relatively low risk and prolonged anticoagulation, if employed initially, is not necessary. Prolonged anticoagulation may be warranted for dissections with residual luminal irregularities and stenosis, but even these irregular vessels are believed to eventually pose a low risk, so anticoagulation beyond 12 months is seldom inicated. There are no reliable data to indicate whether prolonged or indefinite antiplatelet therapy should be used beyond the first few months; the perceived risk of recurrent dissection may be taken into consideration when making this decision. A dissecting aneurysm (often erroneously referred to as "pseudoaneurysm") may occur in 5–40% of patients with dissection.[29,39–44] These have been thought to represent a potential source of thromboembolism and to pose a risk of arterial rupture. Consequently, aggressive treatments such as ligation of the parent artery, bypass procedures, and stenting have been advocated.[45–50] However, long-term observational data have demonstrated a very low risk of complications related to these aneurysms, arguing against aggressive intervention. The three case series that have been reported included a total of 89 patients with 109 aneurysms, with average follow-up ranging from 3 to 6.5 years. No cases of aneurysm rupture were identified, and there were only three recurrent cerebral ischemic events, none of which was clearly related to the aneurysm.[44,51,52] Most of these patients were treated with either early anticoagulation for a few months followed by long-term antiplatelet therapy or antiplatelet therapy alone.

While most ischemic strokes due to dissection are a result of early thromboembolic phenomena, a minority appear to be due to hemodynamic compromise.[53,54] The prognosis may be worse in these cases, and revascularization procedures such as stenting or surgery have occasionally been proposed in this setting, although prospective studies do not currently exist.[53,55,56] Routine treatment of clinically asymptomatic persistent stenosis following dissection is probably not warranted given that procedural risk seems to outweigh the long-term risk of stroke with medical management.[57]

Intracranial dissection may result in either ischemic stroke or subarachnoid hemorrhage. In the setting of subarachnoid hemorrhage, anticoagulation is contraindicated and patients should be medically managed as with aneurysmal subarachnoid hemorrhage. In the setting of ischemic stroke, the same treatment principles likely apply as for extracranial dissection, but this has not been studied. Caution and vigilance is certainly warranted since hemorrhage may be catastrophic. It has been proposed that intracranial dissections that cause ischemia could be treated with surgical extracranial-to-intracranial arterial bypass[58] in order to avoid anticoagulation, but again data regarding this approach are completely lacking. At least one report of acute extracranial-to-intracranial arterial bypass surgery following intra-arterial thrombolysis in a patient with intracranial carotid dissection has been reported.[59]

Some dissections are believed to occur without producing any symptoms and therefore are presumed to remain completely unrecognized. Therefore, it is possible that some dissections have a benign prognosis and do not require therapy. Unfortunately, there is no reliable method to identify these low-risk patients at present and observation without any therapy cannot be recommended.

Patients who have had cervicocerebral arterial dissections should probably avoid activities that may cause sudden rotation or extension of the neck. However, no reliable data exist to define the limits of activity for these patients. There is no apparent reason to manage their physical therapy differently during rehabilitation after stroke because of the dissection.

Fibromuscular Dysplasia

Fibromuscular dysplasia (FMD) is a non-inflammatory arteriopathy that predominantly affects the extracranial cephalic, renal, splanchnic, and iliac arteries. About one-third of patients with FMD also harbor intracranial berry aneurysms. FMD is frequently an incidental finding on conventional angiography, but is occasionally associated with stroke. When FMD is implicated as a cause of ischemic stroke, it is usually by way of a poorly characterized predisposition toward arterial dissection, although local atherosclerosis and local in-situ thrombosis have been described.[60-67] Hypertension is extremely common in patients with FMD and must be aggressively controlled in order to prevent the development of cardiovascular and cerebrovascular atherosclerotic disease. An evaluation of the renal arteries is indicated to identify FMD causing renal artery stenosis and secondary hypertension, which may be effectively treated with renal artery angioplasty in many cases.[68]

Acute treatment of stroke attributed to FMD has not been reported. As with dissection, FMD is often not diagnosed in the hyperacute period. There is no current evidence to suggest a differential response to thrombolytic therapy in patients with FMD.

Prevention of stroke and treatment of FMD are largely unknown since there is a paucity of information about its natural history, though it is often believed to be benign. In a series of 79 patients with FMD, only one elderly patient had a stroke in the territory of the affected artery, and it occurred 18 years after the initial diagnosis.[64] Two other elderly patients had strokes in regions that were unrelated to the affected vessel, about 4 and 11 years after diagnosis. All three of these patients were on no treatment, while no strokes or TIAs occurred among patients treated with antithrombotic medications. Thus, even without therapy, the risk of stroke related to FMD appears to be relatively low, and may be particularly minimal in younger patients in whom FMD is an often incidental finding. Nevertheless, antithrombotic strategies should be considered since they appear to further ameliorate the risk, most importantly among patients with FMD and stroke without an alternative etiology. In most cases, antiplatelet therapy is generally preferable to anticoagulation since the annual risk of stroke (approximately 1–2%) appears to be less than the bleeding risk attributable to anticoagulation.[69-71] However, anticoagulation should be carefully considered as a short-term therapy for patients with dissections (as described in the above section).

Surgical and endovascular treatment has been advocated for patients with FMD causing symptomatic focal carotid artery stenosis. Since FMD is often associated with atherosclerosis, patients with accessible symptomatic carotid artery stenosis which appears atherosclerotic should probably be managed as if the FMD were an incidental anomaly.[72] In the absence of concomitant atherosclerosis, surgical intraluminal dilatation of the FMD-related stenosis has been attempted with mixed results.[60,65,73-78] Perioperative morbidity is estimated at 3–6% and may negate any potential benefit compared to medical therapy alone or no therapy at all. Angioplasty and/or stenting of FMD has also been successfully performed in a number of cases and is increasingly used, although the efficacy of this approach in stroke prevention has not been formally assessed.[79-87] Surgical considerations for FMD-associated intracranial aneurysms are likely to be similar to those for all intracranial aneurysms.

Vasospasm after Subarachnoid Hemorrhage

Among survivors of aneurysmal subarachnoid hemorrhage (SAH), symptomatic vasospasm is a leading cause of morbidity and mortality. Although vasospasm resembles a dynamic constrictive process, there is evidence that it is largely a proliferative arteriopathy. Compromise of the vascular lumen may lead to impaired cerebral autoregulation and ultimately to ischemia. This non-atherosclerotic vasculopathy and its treatment are discussed extensively elsewhere in the text and will not be reiterated here.

Reversible Cerebral Vasoconstriction Syndromes

Reversible cerebral vasoconstriction syndromes (RCVS) encompass several interrelated disorders associated with dysregulation of cerebral vascular tone, leading to vasoconstriction of medium and large arteries.[88] Patients often present with thunderclap headache, and SAH, intracerebral hemorrhage, or ischemic stroke may occur. A number of vasoactive drugs have been identified as possible precipitants of RCVS (Box 56-4).[89-100] A detailed history with attention to these agents should be taken and their use, if present, permanently

BOX 56-4 Drugs Associated with Reversible Cerebral Vasoconstriction Syndrome

SYMPATHOMIMETIC DRUGS

Phenylpropanolamine, pseudoephedrine, amphetamine and amphetamine derivatives, cocaine, ephedra-containing herbal supplements, isometheptene

SEROTONERGIC DRUGS

Serotonin selective reuptake inhibitors, sumatriptan, ergotamine

MISCELLANEOUS

Bromocriptine, lisuride, tacrolimus, cyclophosphamide, erythropoietin, intravenous immune globulin, licorice discontinued. Rarely, RCVS occur secondary to underlying conditions, including pheochromocytoma, carcinoid tumors, hypercalcemia, porphyria, or following vascular or neurosurgical procedures.[88] Such conditions should be identified and specific treatment implemented as appropriate.

Optimal treatment for RCVS is uncertain given the lack of any controlled therapeutic trials. Spontaneous recovery without intervention is probably common.[101] Treatment with calcium channel blockers, particularly nimodipine and verapamil, has been proposed based on anecdotal evidence and the possibly comparable role of calcium channel blockers in treating vasospasm following aneurysmal SAH.[101–105] If used, care should be taken in patients with extensive segmental vascular narrowing to avoid decreased cerebral perfusion and subsequent ischemia. Intra-arterial administration of calcium channel blockers has been used in patients with RCVS and severe progressive neurologic deterioration with reports of improvement.[106,107] A short course of high-dose steroids has also been suggested as a possible therapy based on efficacy in experimentally induced vasoconstriction, although one retrospective case series of 139 patients with RCVS suggested that steroids might be associated with worse outcomes.[101,105,108] Magnesium sulfate is often used in patients with RCVS in the post-partum period given parallels with the central nervous system involvement seen with eclampsia.[109]

Follow-up imaging to confirm resolution of vasoconstriction is generally warranted in order to determine the duration of treatment. Transcranial Doppler may be used as a noninvasive modality for monitoring and follow-up, and is particularly useful if elevated blood flow velocities are present initially.[110–112]

Radiation-induced Vasculopathy

Radiotherapy for cancers of the head and neck often leads to delayed toxicity to the nervous system. Cerebral necrosis is the predominant result, but vascular endothelial damage is believed to be a critical component of its pathogenesis.[113,114] In addition, larger vessels are often affected by fibrosis and accelerated atherosclerosis at atypical locations.[115–118] The extracranial carotid and vertebral arteries, intracranial vessels of the circle of Willis, and the microvasculature may all be affected, depending on the field and dose of radiation.[119] Microvascular disease tends to be particularly insidious and progressive. Anticoagulation with heparin and warfarin was reported to be beneficial in a small series of patients with radiation-induced nervous system disease,[113] but has not been replicated and the risk-to-benefit ratio is unknown. The role of antiplatelet therapy and statins has not been studied. For large vessel disease, angioplasty with or without stenting, and carotid endarterectomy have been reported to be viable treatment options for some patients.[120–124] The endovascular approach may be preferable for radiation-induced carotid disease because local scarring and soft-tissue injury from radiation often makes the surgical field for endarterectomy less manageable. However, a meta-analysis of 27 non-randomized studies comprising 533 patients comparing CEA to CAS in the setting of previous cervical radiation found no difference in perioperative stroke between the two approaches, and a lower rate of long-term cerebrovascular events in those patients treated with CEA.[125] These data should be interpreted with caution given the observational, non-randomized nature of the included studies. The risk of late restenosis appears to be substantial in patients with radiation vasculopathy treated with CAS, ranging from 10 to 40%.[125]) For patients with radiation-induced intracranial disease, encephaloduroarteriomyosynangiosis combined with superficial temporal artery to middle cerebral artery (STA-MCA) bypass has been reported.[126]

Moyamoya Disease

Moyamoya disease is a rare idiopathic arteriopathy in which there is progressive stenosis and occlusion of the terminal portions of the internal carotid arteries and formation of an anomalous vascular network at the base of the brain. A similar vascular pattern may occur with systemic diseases including severe atherosclerosis, hemoglobinopathies, prothrombotic disorders, radiation therapy, head trauma, and inflammatory or infectious diseases, and is often labeled as "quasi-moyamoya" or moyamoya syndrome rather than moyamoya disease.[127,128] Patients with moyamoya disease are prone to ischemic stroke, intracerebral hemorrhage, and aneurysm formation with subsequent subarachnoid hemorrhage. Ischemic complications tend to predominate in children, while hemorrhage is more typical of moyamoya in adults, but this pattern is not constant. Epilepsy is also common in moyamoya, occurring in about 5% of all patients,[129,130] and usually relates to the underlying cerebrovascular disease. Medical and surgical treatments exist for moyamoya disease, but their rigorous assessment has been limited by the rarity of the disease. Management of concurrent vascular risk factors, such as hypertension or smoking, is recommended to prevent additional vascular injury. Further, in quasi-moyamoya, treatment should target the underlying disorder when possible.

Ischemic stroke in moyamoya should initially be treated with supportive measures as with other ischemic strokes. Hyperacute therapy with intravenous tPA has not been assessed in this setting, and discretion with this approach is advised because of the propensity for intracerebral hemorrhage in moyamoya. Antiplatelet therapies are frequently used to prevent recurrent cerebral thromboembolic events, both acutely and chronically, although this approach has not been formally evaluated in this population. Further, there is no specific information about the choice of antiplatelet agent, although dipyridamole has a vasodilatory effect that is conjectured to offer a potential but untested benefit. Anticoagulation with warfarin also has not been studied, but because of the risk of intracerebral hemorrhage, it should probably be used with caution in moyamoya.

Other vasodilators, calcium channel antagonists in particular, are believed to improve transient ischemic symptoms in moyamoya, and may also offer modest prevention against stroke. Corticosteroids are also believed to useful in some patients, notably when there is evidence of cerebral edema or vascular inflammation. However, there are considerable data that argue against the use of steroids for more typical causes of ischemic stroke[131–135] that make this approach somewhat dubious. Further, inflammation does not appear to play a major role in the pathophysiology of moyamoya, again arguing against the empiric use of steroids.

Medical management of intracerebral hemorrhage due to moyamoya is similar to that due to the more common causes, and is again principally supportive. As with hypertensive hemorrhage, surgical evacuation is controversial,[136,137] and may offer limited benefit since the intraparenchymal hemorrhages of moyamoya tend to be deep. Management of subarachnoid hemorrhage due to rupture of a moyamoya-related aneurysm is also similar to the management of more generic aneurysms. However, the surgical issues are quite distinct, since the abnormal network of moyamoya vessels is extremely susceptible to manipulation. Moreover, the aneurysms tend to be in unusual locations or in the posterior circulation, thereby complicating the approach. Endovascular techniques have limited utility in dealing with aneurysms of the anterior circulation since the occlusion of the terminal internal carotid artery renders them inaccessible. Vasospasm after subarachnoid hemorrhage may contribute substantially to morbidity and mortality in moyamoya, particularly since cerebral perfusion is already impaired. Early detection of vasospasm is therefore critical, yet non-invasive diagnosis with transcranial Doppler ultrasound may be unreliable because of the obliteration of the major intracranial cerebral vessels. When suspected, the diagnosis of vasospasm should be pursued with angiography and aggressively treated as outlined above, although the utility of HHH therapy or nimodipine in this setting is unknown.

There are some patients with moyamoya for whom the disease is relatively benign, limited to mild, transient symptoms, and conservative medical therapy may suffice.[138] However, in the majority of patients, these medical therapies offer very limited efficacy, and more aggressive surgical therapies should be considered. Occasionally, moyamoya is discovered incidentally in asymptomatic patients. A small observational study of 40 such patients in Japan found a 3.2% annual stroke risk among 34 non-surgically treated patients, and no subsequent stroke among six surgically treated patients, suggesting a possible benefit for aggressive surgical therapies even in patients without symptoms.[139]

Surgical revascularization procedures have two key goals: (1) improving regional cerebral blood flow to prevent ischemic complications, and (2) alleviating the pressure and/or flow through deep moyamoya collateral vessels, thus reducing the risk of hemorrhage. Direct bypass (such as superficial temporal artery to middle cerebral artery anastamosis), indirect bypass (such as encephaloduroarteriosynangiosis and encephaloduroarteriomyosynangiosis), or a combination of both have been described as effective treatments in a number of series and small uncontrolled studies,[140–148] but their roles have never been studied in a randomized clinical trial. Several case reports of angioplasty and stenting for early moyamoya have been published; the success of this approach appears to be variable and durability uncertain.[149–152] These surgical techniques and their proposed importance in moyamoya are described in detail elsewhere in this text.

Hyperhomocyst(e)inemia and Homocystinuria

Elevated levels of the amino acid homocyst(e)ine appear to cause endothelial injury and proliferation of vascular smooth muscle cells, thereby leading to premature atherosclerosis.[153,154] In addition, homocyst(e)ine may interfere with endogenous anticoagulant mechanisms, resulting in a prothrombotic state.[155,156] Homocyst(e)ine levels can be reduced with folic acid, pyridoxine (vitamin B_6), and cyanocobalamin (vitamin B_{12}) supplementation.

Homocystinuria is a rare autosomal recessive disease caused by a genetic deficiency of cystathionine synthase. This defect leads to high blood levels of homocysteine and excretion of homocysteine in the urine, and is associated with a number of clinical symptoms including vascular disease and thromboembolic events. Most patients develop clinical symptoms during early childhood, though vascular events often occur in early adulthood. Treatment is aimed at normalizing homocysteine levels through vitamin B6, B12, and folate supplementation. For patients who do not respond to vitamin supplementation, a methionine-restricted, cystine-supplemented diet is added to vitamin therapy. Betaine has also been used as an adjunctive therapy.[157] A multicenter observational study demonstrated a substantial reduction in vascular events in patients with homocystinuria treated with aggressive homocysteine lowering therapy compared to historical controls.[158]

In contrast to the specific situation of homocystinuria, the role of vitamin supplementation in patients with modest hyperhomocyst(e)inemia and vascular disease is much less clear. While hyperhomocyst(e)inemia appears to be independently associated with risk of ischemic stroke, it is uncertain whether this is a cause or effect of vascular disease.[153,154] Controlled trials of homocysteine lowering therapy have shown some beneficial effects on surrogate indicators of vascular function, however, these indicators may not directly correlate with clinical vascular events.[159,160] Two large randomized trials assessing the role of vitamin therapy in preventing recurrent vascular events following stroke, the Vitamins in Stroke Prevention (VISP) study, and the Vitamins to Prevent Stroke Study (VITATOPS), have been completed. The VISP trial randomized 3680 patients with stroke to either high-dose (daily doses of 25 mg B6, 0.4 mg B12, 2.5 mg folic acid) or low-dose (200 μg B6, 6 μg B12, 20 μg folic acid) vitamin supplementation.[161] There was a mean reduction in homocysteine levels of 2 μmol/L, but no therapeutic benefit was seen on any vascular endpoint. A subgroup analysis of the VISP trial focused on the patients theoretically most likely to benefit from treatment.[162] In this analysis, patients with low and very high B12 levels at baseline were excluded in an attempt to eliminate patients with B12 malabsorption (low levels) and those receiving B12 supplementation outside of the study (very high levels). In the remaining 2155 patients, a 21% relative reduction in the composite endpoint of stroke, coronary event, or death was demonstrated ($P = 0.05$) with high-dose compared to low-dose vitamin supplementation.

VITATOPS randomized 8164 patients with stroke/TIA to either placebo or vitamin supplementation (daily doses of 25 mg B6, 500 μg B12, 2 mg folic acid).[163] Over a median follow-up period of 3.4 years, the primary endpoint of stroke, MI, or vascular death occurred in 15.1% of patients in the vitamin arm compared to 16.6% in the placebo arm (relative ratio [RR] 0.91; 95%CI, 0.82–1.00; $P = 0.05$). Vitamin therapy was associated with a reduction in stroke (RR 0.92) and vascular death (RR 0.86), but not myocardial infarction (RR 1.03). No adverse events were seen with vitamin therapy. Several large randomized controlled trials have assessed the role of vitamin therapy in patients with known coronary artery disease or other vascular disease, but have not focused specifically on patients with prior stroke. These trials have uniformly failed to show benefit to homocysteine lowering therapy.[164–166] A meta-analysis evaluating the role of homocysteine lowering therapy in reducing stroke demonstrated a modest reduction in overall stroke events associated with vitamin supplementation (RR, 0.93; 95%CI, 0.86–1.00; $P = 0.04$). Benefit seemed to be greatest in populations with low antiplatelet use and without widespread cereal folic acid fortification. Based on the totality of the current data, it remains uncertain whether vitamin supplementation for prevention of stroke in patients with elevated homocysteine is beneficial (outside the specific context of homocystinuria); if real, it is likely that any benefit is small.

Fabry Disease

Fabry disease is a rare X-linked inherited deficiency of the lysosomal enzyme alpha-galactosidase, which causes lipid deposition in the vascular endothelium and results in progressive vasculopathy of the brain, heart, skin, and kidneys.[167] Cerebral arteriopathy usually becomes clinically event in young men by the 4th decade, and occasionally in older women.[168] The intracranial vertebrobasilar system is often dolichoectatic and may be the proximate source of ischemic stroke, although cardiogenic embolism and progressive small vessel occlusive disease with deep infarctions are also observed.[167,169,170] In young stroke victims, Fabry disease may underdiagnosed. A pooled analysis of nine studies with 8302 patients suggested that Fabry disease may explain about 1% of

TABLE 56-1 Immunosuppressive Drugs Used in the Treatment of Inflammatory Vasculopathies

Drug	Indications	Dosing Regimens	Adverse Effects	LOE
Prednisone or methylprednisolone	IACNS GCA CVD-related ? Infection-related ? Toxin-related ? Neoplasm-related	*Induction:* 0.5–2 mg/kg/day orally or: up to 1000 mg/day IV for acute or severe cases *Taper:* as tolerated over 3–12 months *Maintenance:* 5–10 mg/day orally	Infections, cushingoid features, adrenal insufficiency, behavioral/mood changes, osteopenia, diabetes mellitus, many others	IIa, C IIa, C IIa, C IIb, C IIb, C IIb, C
Cyclophosphamide	IACNS CVD-related	*Induction:* 1–2 mg/kg/day orally or: 750 mg/m² BSA IV monthly for acute, severe cases *Taper:* as tolerated over 3–12 months *Maintenance*: lowest dose without recurrent symptoms; consider switch to azathioprine	Bone marrow suppression, infections, malignancy, nausea/vomiting, alopecia, hemorrhagic cystitis, diarrhea, rash	IIa, C IIb,C
Azathioprine*	IACNS GCA CVD-related	*Induction*: not used as induction therapy *Maintenance*: start 1 mg/kg/day orally; increase by 0.5 mg/kg/day every 4 weeks to max. 2.5 mg/kg/day	Bone marrow suppression, infections, hepatotoxicity, nausea/vomiting, diarrhea	IIa, C IIa, C IIa, C
Methotrexate†	GCA CVD-related	*Induction and maintenance:* 10 mg/day orally	Bone marrow suppression, hepatotoxicity, nephrotoxicity, nausea/vomiting, fatigue, fever/chills	IIb, A IIb, C

BSA, Body surface area; CVD, collagen vascular disorder; GCA, giant cell (temporal) arteritis; IACNS, isolated angiitis of the central nervous system; IV, intravenous.
*Used as an alternative to cyclophosphamide.
†Used in conjunction with corticosteroids.
For more details refer to "Evidence box index" in the FM.

stroke in the young, and 3–5% of cryptogenic strokes in this population.[171]

Antiplatelet agents are believed to be useful in preventing ischemic events related to existing vascular disease,[172] but the disease itself was untreatable until recombinant alpha-galactosidase became available as an intravenous infusion. Enzyme replacement therapy has been shown to have beneficial effects on surrogate outcome measures. In a randomized controlled trial in 58 patients with Fabry disease, alpha-galactosidase was given intravenously every other week for 20 weeks.[173] Only 31% of patients in the treated group developed new microvascular endothelial lipid deposits after 20 weeks, compared with 100% of the patients in the placebo group ($P < 0.001$). In addition, after 6 months of open-label therapy provided to all subjects, all patients in the former placebo group and 98% of patients in the former recombinant alpha-galactosidase A group had clearance of microvascular endothelial deposits. Enzyme replacement therapy has been shown to have a favorable effect on cerebral blood flow.[174] However, despite these findings, the benefit of enzyme therapy on clinical outcomes remains uncertain, with small randomized trials offering no convincing evidence of a reduction in stroke or cardiac events, and observational data suggesting a substantial risk of stroke despite therapy.[175-181] The major adverse effects of recombinant alpha-galactosidase infusions are fever and rigors, which may occur in 25–50% of treated patients, but may be minimized with slow infusion rates and premedication with acetaminophen and hydroxyzine.

Inflammatory Vasculopathies

Cerebrovascular disease may rarely occur as a result of derangement of cell-mediated and antibody-mediated immune responses. The vasculitides are a heterogeneous group of disorders in which inflammation of the blood vessels causes vascular narrowing, occlusion, or necrosis, which may result in cerebral ischemia, infarction, or hemorrhage.[182] Vasculitis may be a primary process (isolated angiitis of the central nervous system) or may occur secondary to an identifiable systemic inflammatory disorder, infection, toxin, or neoplasm. Immunosuppression appears to be the key element of treatment (Table 56-1).

Isolated Angiitis of the Central Nervous System

Isolated angiitis of the central nervous system (IACNS) affects only the brain and spinal cord, and there is a complete absence of any systemic manifestation of the disease. Symptoms of IACNS may include headache, seizure, stroke, and multifocal encephalopathy. In the early descriptions of this disease, the prognosis was uniformly poor, but immunotherapy may alter the course of the disease. Clinical and angiographic improvement has been attributed to corticosteroids and cyclophosphamide, but because of the profound rarity of IACNS, randomized clinical trials have not been performed. In a review of the literature and description of eight additional cases, Calabrese and Mallek[183] observed that nearly all untreated patients died or were persistently dependent, whereas four of 13 treated with steroids and ten of 13 treated with both steroids and cyclophosphamide improved. In a series of 101 patients from the Mayo Clinic, 34 of 42 patients (81%) treated initially with prednisone alone had a favorable response, compared with 38 of 47 patients (81%) treated with cyclophosphamide (most of whom also received treatment with steroids).[184] The median duration of treatment was approximately 10 months with both steroids and cyclophosphamide. Relapse leading to a change in therapy occurred in 26 of 101 patients (26%). In contrast, others[185,186] have found that corticosteroids alone offered a transient effect at best, and that combination therapy with cyclophosphamide was required for a clinical benefit. The appropriate dosage for both medications is unclear and varies among centers. For induction therapy, prednisone or prednisolone 1–2 mg/kg per day is recommended at the time of diagnosis; tapering should occur over 3–12 months to a minimal dose of 5–10 mg per day. Some centers initiate steroid treatment with intravenous pulse steroids, such as methylprednisolone 1 g daily for 1–6 days.[184] Cyclophosphamide can be administered orally at 1–2 mg/kg per day or intravenously with 3–6 monthly pulses of 750 mg per m^2 of body surface area or 15 mg/kg.[182,187] Intravenous cyclophosphamide may be safer than oral cyclophosphamide; in both formulations the most serious toxicity relates to infection, cancer (particularly of the bladder), and infertility.[188] Patients may be followed with serial neurological examination, neuropsychiatric testing, cerebrospinal fluid examination, and/or MRI at 3–6-month intervals. Serial angiography is seldom necessary. If remission or stabilization occurs, then cyclophosphamide may be gradually weaned over several months. Long-term steroid sparing agents may be considered for maintenance of remission, including azathioprine 1–2 mg/kg per day, methotrexate 20–25 mg/week, or mycophenolate 1–2 g per day.[188] These therapeutic regimens have only been evaluated for relatively brief terms of a few years, and their longer term efficacy has not been described. Longer-term therapy seems to be required for patients who relapse. One study of 12 patients found a high relapse rate in patients with predominantly small vessel involvement, whereas no patients with middle-sized vessel involvement relapsed, suggesting that patients with small vessel vasculitis may require longer term or more aggressive treatment.[189] On the other hand, some evidence indicates that subjects with predominantly small vessel vasculitis manifested by prominent leptomeningeal enhancement on MRI with normal cerebral angiography may have a more benign course with a good response to steroids alone.[188,190] Titration of medication doses is somewhat empiric in response to each individual patient's clinical response. Patients taking cyclophosphamide or azathioprine require careful monitoring of the leukocyte count for evidence of bone marrow suppression. In addition, oral fluid intake must be increased to minimize the risk of hemorrhagic cystitis. Antiemetics may be needed to manage nausea, particularly with intravenous pulse cyclophosphamide. Finally, patients must be monitored and treated for steroid-induced diabetes mellitus and should receive prophylaxis against pneumocystis infection (trimethoprim 80 mg and sulfamethoxazole 400 mg daily) and osteoporosis (vitamin D 800 IU and calcium 1200 mg daily; for patients at very high risk of fracture, bisphosphonates may be considered as well).

Other immunomodulatory approaches, including other chemotherapeutic agents, plasma exchange, intravenous immunoglobulin, and tumor necrosis factor blockers have not been studied in IACNS beyond individual case reports. Similarly, the role of antithrombotic medication in IACNS has not been evaluated.

Amyloid Angiitis and Cerebral Amyloid Angiopathy-Related Inflammation

Amyloid angiitis and cerebral amyloid angiopathy-related inflammation represent distinct but related entities with a transmural, often granulomatous, vasculitis in the former and perivascular inflammation in the latter, both occurring in and around vessels containing amyloid-B deposits.[191–193] Given the small number of reported cases, evidence for various treatment strategies is largely anecdotal, but in general treatment is similar to that for isolated CNS angiitis. However, it does appear that many patients will respond rapidly and completely to steroids alone, although relapse may occur frequently. In one small series of 12 patients, relapse occurred in three patients over about 3 years of follow-up.[194]

Temporal (Giant Cell) Arteritis

Temporal (giant cell) arteritis is a systemic inflammatory vasculopathy that should be considered in any stroke patient older than 50 years.[195] Treatment decisions are often necessary before confirmation of the diagnosis. When the diagnosis is suspected, a unilateral temporal artery biopsy should be performed. Corticosteroids, the mainstay of therapy, can be initiated prior to the biopsy and will not affect the results if performed within approximately 10–14 days.[195,196] For patients presenting with acute visual loss, immediate treatment with high-dose (up to 1000 mg daily) intravenous methylprednisolone for 3–5 days has been advocated by some authors,[197,198] although others have suggested that intravenous steroid pulses offer no benefit compared with oral therapy, but carry greater expense and risk.[199,200] Chevalet et al. performed a randomized clinical trial of 164 patients with uncomplicated temporal arteritis comparing three dosing regimens: 240 mg intravenous pulse of methylprednisolone (IVMP) followed by 0.7 mg/kg/day oral prednisone (group 1), or 0.7 mg/kg/day oral prednisone without an IV pulse (group 2), or 240 mg IVMP followed by 0.5 mg/kg/day oral prednisone (group 3).[201] Steroid doses were then tapered starting at 6 months after therapy. At 1 year, there were no significant differences among the three groups with regard to clinical symptoms, laboratory parameters, or steroid-related side effects. In contrast, Mazlumzadeh et al. performed a randomized clinical trial in 27 patients with temporal arteritis comparing a 3-day course of IVMP (15 mg/kg per day) to placebo. All patients were also treated with 40 mg/day of prednisone. Patients randomized to IVMP were able to taper steroids more rapidly and had a higher frequency of sustained remission after stopping steroid treatment.[202] Further, Chan et al. performed a retrospective cohort study of 100 patients with acute visual loss due to giant cell arteritis and found that there was an increased likelihood of improved vision in the group treated with intravenous steroids (40%) compared with those who received oral steroids (13%).[203] Based on these data, the role of intravenous steroids remains somewhat uncertain, and some authors recommend using high-dose intravenous steroids only for those patients whose clinical condition progresses in the face of oral steroids.[204,205]

Regardless of whether intravenous steroids are used, maintenance therapy with daily oral prednisone, starting at 40–80 mg daily (0.5–1.0 mg/kg),[206] should be initiated; eventual gradual tapering should then occur. The goal of maintenance therapy is to prevent subsequent ischemic events, and the taper should likely be adjusted according to the patient's clinical response and ESR and C-reactive protein levels. There is great controversy over the duration of therapy and the rapidity of the taper. However, in a cohort study involving 90 patients, the timing of cessation of therapy had no effect on the risk of recurrent symptoms.[207] A reasonable approach is treatment for 4 weeks until clinical signs and symptoms have resolved and the ESR and C-reactive protein levels have normalized, then reduction of the steroid dose gradually every 1–2 weeks by 10% or less of the total daily dose.[208] If symptoms recur or there is an increase in ESR or C-reactive protein levels during the taper, the prednisone dose should be increased by 20–40 mg per day for 2–3 weeks, then the taper can be resumed. Careful attention should be given to steroid side effects such as diabetes, hypertension, osteoporosis, avascular necrosis of the hip, cataracts, and gastrointestinal bleeding. Calcium (1200 mg/day) and vitamin D (800 IU/day) supplementation is recommended.[208] Bisphosphonates may be appropriate for patients with reduced bone-mineral density. In the setting of concurrent aspirin therapy, the use of a proton-pump inhibitor to protect gastric mucosa should be considered.

Experience with other immunosuppressive agents for temporal arteritis is limited. Methotrexate has been studied in three randomized controlled trials, and an individual patient data meta-analysis of the 161 patients in these trials has been published.[209] All patients were treated with steroids initially. Adjunctive methotrexate significantly lowered the risk of first and second relapse. The estimated numbers needed to treat were 3.6 to prevent a first relapse, and 4.7 to prevent a second relapse. The overall incidence of adverse events, including typical steroid side effects, did not differ between the methotrexate and placebo arms. It, therefore, appears reasonable to consider the use of adjunctive methotrexate to reduce the risk of relapse, but it does not appear that methotrexate is effective at reducing the incidence of steroid side effects. Azathioprine was shown to reduce the required dose of corticosteroids in a randomized trial involving 31 patients with temporal arteritis and/or polymyalgia rheumatica.[210] Based on these limited data, the role of azathioprine remains poorly defined, but it may be reasonable to consider if a steroid-sparing agent is required and methotrexate is not tolerated. Cyclosporine A offered no benefit over steroids alone in a small open trial.[211] The tumor necrosis factor-alpha inhibitor infliximab has been tested in a randomized trial of 44 patients with temporal arteritis and was found to be ineffective and associated with a higher rate of infection.[212] A small randomized trail of 17 patients compared etanercept to placebo and reported a reduction in steroid use in the etanercept group with no increase in adverse events.[213]

In patients with stroke related to temporal arteritis, it seems logical to use antiplatelet therapy to reduce the risk of recurrent vascular events, although this has not been subject to randomized trials. Two small observational studies do support a significant reduction in ischemic events in patients with temporal arteritis treated with antithrombotic therapy.[214,215]

Cerebral Vasculitis Related to Collagen Vascular Disorders

Systemic vasculitides include polyarteritis nodosa (PAN), Sjögren's disease, Churg–Strauss angiitis, Wegener's granulomatosis, Henoch–Schönlein purpura, cryoglobulinemia, systemic lupus erythematosus, scleroderma, and rheumatoid arthritis, each of which is characterized by the pattern of involvement of other organ systems.[216–228] Neurologic involvement is variable in each of these disorders and is typically less prominent than the other features, but may be the initial manifestation in some cases. Further, neurological symptoms when present, are rarely due to cerebral vasculitis or cerebritis, but rather are more frequently related to cardiac emboli (such as nonbacterial thrombotic endocarditis), hypercoagulable states (such as antiphospholipid antibody syndrome), or atherosclerosis (as a result of renovascular hypertension or steroid-induced diabetes mellitus).[229,230] Treatment of the cerebral component is, in general, dictated by the treatment of the systemic disease and often includes corticosteroids and other immunosuppressant agents.[216,231] When the diagnosis of concomitant cerebral vasculitis exists and persists despite treatment of the systemic process, then more aggressive treatment, such as that for IACNS may be warranted, but again data to support this approach are lacking.

Cerebral Vasculitis Related to Infection

Among the secondary causes of vasculitis, infectious etiologies include meningovascular syphilis, tuberculous meningitis, other bacterial (*Streptococcus pneumoniae, Neisseria*) meningitis, fungal (*Aspergillus, Candida, Coccidioides, Cryptococcus, Histoplasma,* and *Mucor*) meningoencephalitides, neurocysticercosis, varicella-zoster virus (VZV) encephalitis, human immunodeficiency virus (HIV), and hepatitis C virus.[232–265] Specifically directed antimicrobial therapy is advisable for each of these disorders and may improve the vasculopathic angiographic findings,[238] although this approach may not necessarily improve the clinical course.[266,267] Immunosuppressive regimens are often used in patients with persisting vasculopathy,[238,266,268] although the efficacy of this approach is unproven. The role of antiplatelet agents, anticoagulation, and thrombolysis in infection-related vasculopathy is also uncertain, and caution is advised since there may be a necrotizing component of the vasculitis as well as dysfunction of the blood–brain barrier, thereby increasing the risk of intracerebral hemorrhage.[269]

Cerebral Vasculitis Related to Toxins

Toxins implicated in cerebral vasculitis include cocaine, amphetamines, heroin, lysergic acid diethylamide (LSD), and inhaled volatile solvents (glue sniffing), although these may result in a process more like vasospasm after subarachnoid hemorrhage than a true inflammatory vasculitis.[270–275] Other sympathomimetic agents, including ephedrine and phenylpropanolamine, may have similar effects.[276–278] In the setting of acute ischemic stroke associated with drug use (cocaine, in particular), there is evidence to suggest that a combination of vasospasm and superimposed thrombosis may occur.[279] In such cases, thrombolysis may be a reasonable therapeutic option in the first few hours, whereas antiplatelet therapy may be appropriate later in the course.[280]

No specific therapy has been shown to improve the vasculopathy, but the offending agent should certainly be removed.[275] Patients should be closely monitored and treated for symptoms of drug withdrawal. As many abusers of illicit drugs also abuse alcohol, a low threshold should exist for initiating benzodiazepines for symptoms or signs of alcohol withdrawal.

Ideal therapy for ongoing vasculitis among users of methamphetamine has not been identified, in part because the pathogenesis of the vasculitis is unclear. Steroid therapy has been used in some patients on a short-term basis, but there is little evidence to suggest this is beneficial.[275] Calcium channel blockers have been advocated for the treatment of cocaine users with vasospasm/vasculitis, but no formal data exist regarding efficacy.

Long-term secondary stroke prevention strategies should include cessation of the identified abused drug. Antiplatelet therapy is probably indicated for patients with ischemic stroke, although there are limited data specifically applicable to stroke in the setting of drug abuse.

Cerebral Vasculitis Related to Neoplasms

Arteriopathies may rarely complicate the course of systemic neoplasms. The small and middle-sized intracranial arteries may be affected by carcinomatous or lymphomatous meningitis, as well as intravascular lymphomatosis. The prognosis is quite poor in these cases. Steroids, palliative chemotherapy, and radiation therapy may offer some transient benefit for the inflammatory vasculopathy, although in some cases this approach led to acute worsening of symptoms.[281–284]

HEMATOLOGIC DISORDERS

Ischemic stroke may be associated with a number of hereditary and acquired prothrombotic states, including abnormalities of red cell or platelet function, coagulation factors, or endogenous fibrinolysis (see Box 56-2). These disorders are uncommon, but are over represented among young stroke victims and should be considered when no alternative etiology is identified.[1,2,285,286]

Prothrombotic Disorders

Defects of the Coagulation System

The factor V Leiden, prothrombin G20210A, and methylenetetrahydrofolate reductase (MTHFR) C677T gene mutations have been associated with a hypercoagulable state, particularly with regard to venous thrombosis. Meta-analysis of published studies suggests that the relationship between these genetic variants and arterial events such as ischemic stroke is relatively modest but possibly stronger in younger patients.[287,288] Stroke is also associated with inherited deficiencies of protein C, protein S, and antithrombin III, which are far less common but are probably associated with a higher risk of recurrent thrombotic events; acquired deficiencies may also occur because these factors may be depleted in nephrotic syndrome, hepatic disease, and pregnancy. Prothrombotic tendencies are also found in association with oral contraceptive use, systemic inflammatory disorders, and malignancies. Hyperhomocyst(e)-inemia may also predispose to thrombosis, as already described.

In the hyperacute setting of ischemic stroke, these underlying inherited or acquired disorders may not be recognized and patients may be treated with standard thrombolytic or antithrombotic therapy.[289] Chronic anticoagulation is often recommended for secondary prevention among stroke survivors with a confirmed prothrombotic state, although this remains controversial and guidelines suggest that either antiplatelet or anticoagulant therapy may be considered.[290,291] Those rare patients with known protein C or protein S deficiencies should not be initially treated with warfarin unless heparin is given concurrently because there is a small risk of inducing a transient hypercoagulable state.[292] Given the modest association of the factor V, prothrombin G20210A, and MTHFR C677T gene mutations with arterial events, it is probably reasonable to use antiplatelet therapy for secondary stroke prevention in these patients unless multiple thrombotic events have occurred.

Antiphospholipid Antibody Syndrome

Antiphospholipid antibodies (aPLs) may occur with systemic disorders or may occur in isolation; they appear to be an independent risk factor for both arterial and venous thromboembolism in some but not all studies, as their presence may be confounded by other disorders or medications.[293-302] The mechanism by which aPLs may lead to thrombosis is uncertain, but they appear to interfere with endogenous anticoagulants, protein C, and platelet homeostasis. aPLs are relatively common, occurring in up to 10% of the normal population.[303,304] It is important to distinguish between the mere presence of aPLs and the aPL syndrome, which is characterized by the occurrence of vascular thrombosis and medium to high-titer aPLs or a positive lupus anticoagulant on two separate measurements at least 12 weeks apart.[305]

In the acute setting, tPA has been used for stroke due to aPL syndrome.[289] However, assessment of the eligibility of such patients for thrombolysis may be obscured if the partial thromboplastin time (PTT) is spuriously elevated due to the presence of aPL. Elevated PTT is an exclusion criterion for the use of intravenous tPA only if the patient has received heparin or has a known predisposition to bleed (such as a factor deficiency).[306] This is not the case with aPL, so patients with falsely elevated PTT due to aPL should still be considered as candidates for thrombolysis. Anti-tPA antibodies have been identified in patients with aPL syndrome[307] which might, theoretically, attenuate the potential effect of thrombolysis, but the clinical significance of this is unknown.

Preventative strategies for patients who have had stroke or other thromboembolic events include antithrombotic and immunomodulatory therapies. The prospective Antiphospholipid Antibody Stroke Study (APASS) specifically addressed the role of aPL in a large population of patients with noncardioembolic stroke as part of the Warfarin versus Aspirin for Recurrent Stroke Study (WARSS).[308] In APASS, 1770 patients had testing for aPL before the initiation of antithrombotic therapy, and 41% were classified as aPL positive.[309] During 2 years of follow-up, there was no difference in the incidence of thrombo-occlusive events between patients with and without aPL. Further, there was no difference in the risk of these events between those treated with warfarin or aspirin. Several important limitations of this study should be noted. First, patients enrolled in WARSS/APASS were, for the most part, older (mean age 62 years) with typical atherosclerotic risk factors and mostly lacunar stroke. Second, aPLs were measured only on a single occasion; therefore, it is unknown what proportion of patients would have met criteria for aPL syndrome. Third, the vast majority of aPL positive patients had low-to-medium titer antibodies (only 0.2% of patients had high-titer positive IgG anticardiolipin antibodies). The results of APASS do emphasize that older patients with typical atherosclerotic risk factors, a single thrombotic event, and positive aPL at a single measurement should be managed with antiplatelet therapy alone. These findings should not be extrapolated, however, to patients who meet criteria for aPL syndrome.

In a retrospective study of 147 patients with aPL syndrome, recurrent thromboembolic events occurred in 101 patients during a median follow-up period of 6 years.[310] The relative risk of recurrence was dramatically and significantly lower in patients treated with warfarin to maintain the international normalized ratio (INR) ≥ 3.0, compared with those treated with aspirin or with lower levels of anticoagulation. Corticosteroids, azathioprine, and cyclophosphamide had no significant effect on thrombotic events in this study. Similarly, a later study with 61 patients followed for a median of 77 months showed that warfarin significantly reduced the risk of recurrence by about 75% when the prothrombin ratio (patient versus control) was maintained between 1.5 and 2.0.[311] Aspirin was no better than observation without treatment, and prednisone was associated with a possible increased risk of thrombotic episodes. More recently, two randomized controlled trials enrolling 114 and 109 patients, respectively, compared high-intensity warfarin (goal INR 3.0 to 4.0 or 4.5) to moderate intensity warfarin (goal INR 2.0 to 3.0) in aPL syndrome.[312,313] Both studies found no benefit and more bleeding complications with higher-intensity warfarin. On the basis of these data, it is recommended that patients with aPL syndrome who are treated with warfarin should have a goal INR of 2.0 to 3.0. In contrast to other immunosuppressant drugs, there is some evidence to suggest a possible benefit for hydroxychloroquine in aPL, particularly in those patients with systemic lupus erythematosus.[314] Its use may be reasonable in those with aPL and recurrent thrombotic events despite therapeutic anticoagulation, or in those with coexistent systemic lupus erythematosus.

Catastrophic antiphospholipid antibody syndrome refers to the rare but dramatic occurrence of thrombotic events involving multiple organ systems over a short period of time (generally <7 days) in patients with aPLs. This condition is associated with a poor prognosis, and aggressive treatment is required. Given the rarity of the condition, treatment recommendations are based entirely on clinical experience.[315] Intravenous heparin should be started immediately and administered for 7–10 days before conversion to oral anticoagulation. High-dose steroids are recommended to attenuate cytokine release from widespread tissue necrosis. Plasmapheresis and/or intravenous immunoglobulin is used in an attempt to modulate the pathogenic aPLs. If progression occurs despite these interventions, then more aggressive immunosuppression with cyclophosphamide or rituximab should be considered.[316]

Disseminated Intravascular Coagulation

Disseminated intravascular coagulation (DIC) is caused by disequilibrium of the coagulation system that usually occurs in the context of malignancy, sepsis, surgical/obstetrical complications, or trauma. Fibrin and platelet thrombi form in the microcirculation and obstruct tissue perfusion.[317] Simultaneously, free platelets are depleted and fibrin degradation products are formed, which results in a systemic lytic state. Both ischemic stroke and intracerebral hemorrhage may occur in DIC.[317–319]

Treatment should be directed primarily toward correcting the underlying or precipitating disorder, if possible. When ischemic thromboembolic events are the prevailing process, anticoagulation with heparin or LMWH is reasonable though unproven; LMWH may be preferred to unfractionated heparin (UFH) based on one small randomized trial.[320–323] Prophylactic doses of either LMWH or UFH to prevent venous thromboembolism should be used in patients not treated will full dose anticoagulation and who are not actively bleeding. Thrombolysis is likely contraindicated in patients with ischemic stroke due to DIC because of low platelet counts, depleted coagulation factors, and the increased risk of hemorrhage, although this remains speculative given the lack of clinical data.

After the acute thrombotic event, if the underlying disorder cannot be treated, long-term prophylactic therapy should be considered for chronic DIC. Chronic DIC does not typically respond well to oral anticoagulation with warfarin, so parenteral heparin or LMWH is preferred.[320,321]

When intracerebral or systemic hemorrhage is the predominant event, bleeding should be controlled by replacement of depleted clotting factors and platelets. Fresh frozen plasma may be used in patients with prolonged PT/PTT or decreased fibrinogen levels; cryoprecipitate may be used in the setting of active bleeding with persistent decreased fibrinogen levels after FFP administration.[324] Antithrombotic therapy should be avoided. In patients with DIC and bleeding refractory to conventional therapy, recombinant factor VIIa and prothrombin complex concentrates have been suggested as possible additional therapeutic options.[324,325]

Sickle Cell Disease

Sickle cell disease rarely has stroke as its presenting symptom, but stroke may occur in 10–20% of patients with the disorder.[326,327] Sickle trait alone may also be rarely associated with stroke, particularly in the setting of severe dehydration or hypoxia. Sickle cell disease causes a progressive nonatherosclerotic large vessel arteriopathy that, in the extreme, may evolve into a quasi-moyamoya pattern.[328,329] Increased blood viscosity during a sickle crisis may impair perfusion and infarction may also occur due to direct occlusion of the microvasculature by cellular aggregates. The co-existing anemia may cause compensatory arteriolar vasodilatation and increase cerebral blood flow, which may in turn increase the risk of intracerebral hemorrhage.[330]

Early treatment of stroke due to sickle cell disease consists of emergent simple blood transfusion or exchange transfusion to reduce the proportion of sickle hemoglobin (HbS) to less than 30%, although this approach is based on consensus rather than evidence.[331] Generic supportive measures are indicated in the acute setting, aiming for normovolemia, normothermia, and normoglycemia. Thrombolytic therapy for acute ischemic stroke may be associated with an increased risk of intracerebral hemorrhage, however formal studies to evaluate this have not been performed and there is no definite reason to withhold this treatment option from patients who otherwise meet standard eligibility criteria.[331] At least one case study of successful thrombolysis for cerebral venous sinus thrombosis in sickle cell disease has been reported.[332] Extracranial carotid occlusion, in some cases consistent with arterial dissection, may cause stroke in patients with sickle cell disease, and there may be benefit to early antithrombotic therapy with antiplatelet or anticoagulant therapy in such cases.[333]

Transfusion therapy is better characterized as a strategy for prevention of stroke in sickle cell disease. The Stroke Prevention Trial in Sickle Cell Anemia (STOP) was a randomized clinical trial that tested whether long-term transfusion therapy could reduce the risk of stroke in 130 high-risk children with the disease.[334] Participants were identified as being at high risk if transcranial Doppler ultrasonography (TCD) revealed velocities exceeding 200 cm/second in the intracranial internal carotid artery or the middle cerebral artery. Transfusions were performed to maintain the hemoglobin S (HbS) concentration at less than 30% of the total hemoglobin. Only one of 63 children treated with transfusion therapy developed a stroke, compared with 11 of 67 who received standard care ($P < 0.001$). The study was terminated prematurely because of the overwhelming benefit, a 92% reduction in the risk of stroke. Transfusion is strongly recommended as first-line, primary prevention in children at high risk based on this study, and may be advisable as secondary prevention in children and adults who have already had cerebrovascular events. The optimal concentration of HbS for long-term secondary prevention is controversial, ranging from 30% to 60%.[335–337] The optimal duration of transfusion therapy was assessed in the Optimizing Stroke Prevention in Sickle Cell Anemia (STOP 2) trial.[338] This trial enrolled 79 patients with sickle cell disease, no history of stroke, elevated TCD velocities, and who had undergone at least 30 months of transfusion therapy with normalization of their TCD velocities. Patients were randomly assigned to continued transfusion therapy versus discontinuation of transfusion therapy. In the 41 patients who stopped transfusion therapy, 14 developed recurrent high-risk TCD velocities and two experienced a stroke. The 38 patients who continued transfusion therapy had neither of these endpoints. Furthermore, silent brain lesions consistent with infarction on MRI were present at study end in 8% of patients in the continued transfusion group compared to 28% of those who stopped transfusion therapy ($P = 0.03$).[339]

As short-term or prophylactic therapy, transfusions can be performed as either simple transfusions or exchange transfusions. Simple transfusions are straightforward transfusions of packed red blood cells to reduce the relative proportion of HbS. The number of required units of blood is based on the patient's pre-transfusion levels of HbS and total hematocrit and an estimate of the total circulating blood volume. The short-term risks of simple transfusion are volume overload and hyperviscosity; therefore, it is most suited for patients who are already severely anemic, volume depleted, or both. Exchange transfusions allow for reduction in the HbS level without increasing the hematocrit. This can be performed manually or automatically with apheresis equipment, and both approaches involve removal of about 2 units (about 1 L) of blood with replacement of about 4 units of packed red blood cells and normal saline, depending on the initial HbS level and the patient's size. Over the long term, exchange transfusions may be better tolerated than simple transfusions and pose a lower risk of iron toxicity, but are more expensive and require exposure to more units of blood. Blood-borne infections are infrequent, but their risk increases with chronic transfusion therapy. With either approach, transfusions are also associated with alloimmunization, but this may be minimized with the use of red blood cells that are phenotypically matched for specific antigens (Kell blood group and Rh antigens C and E).[340] In a retrospective review of patients treated with transfusion therapy for secondary stroke prevention, eight of 14 (57%) of those treated with initial simple transfusion had recurrent stroke, compared to eight of 38 (21%) of those treated with exchange transfusion.[341] These data must be interpreted cautiously given the non-randomized nature of the observations.

Hydroxyurea is a chemotherapeutic agent that appears to increase the concentration of fetal hemoglobin and improve red blood cell survival.[342] It has also been shown to increase cerebral oxygenation as measured by near-infrared spectroscopy.[343] Several studies have shown that treatment with hydroxyurea lowers TCD flow velocities, suggesting a possible benefit in stroke prevention.[344–346] In a double-blinded clinical trial, 299 patients with frequent painful sickle crises (without a history of stroke) were randomly assigned to receive either hydroxyurea or placebo, and were followed for a mean of 21 months.[347] Hydroxyurea was given at an initial dose of 15 mg/kg per day, and increased by 5 mg/kg per day every 12 weeks, unless bone marrow suppression (neutrophil count <2000/mm^3, platelet count <80,000/mm^3, or hemoglobin <4.5 g/dL) occurred. If marrow depression occurred, treatment was stopped until blood counts recovered and was then resumed at a lower dose. The maximum dose in the study was 35 mg/kg per day. Painful crises occurred at a median rate of 2.5 times per year in treated patients compared with 4.5 times per year among those given placebo ($P < 0.001$). Time between crises was also extended by hydroxyurea therapy. The study was too small to address the effect of treatment on the risk of stroke, although the findings are encouraging because the mechanism by which painful crises occur is likely similar to the pathogenesis of stroke. In one long-term prospective observational study of patients with sickle cell syndromes (sickle cell disease and thalassemia), treatment with hydroxyurea was associated with a lower rate of fatal stroke compared to those not treated with hydroxyurea (2% versus 5%).[348] The benefit of hydroxyurea seen in older children and adults appears to extend to very young children as well.[349] One small prospective study in 35 children with a history of stroke suggested that hydroxyurea plus phlebotomy might be as effective as chronic transfusion therapy and iron chelation for long-term recurrent stroke prevention.[350] However, in a multicenter randomized trial comparing these two strategies for secondary stroke prevention, none of the 66 patients assigned transfusion and chelation had recurrent stroke compared to seven of 67 assigned hydroxyurea plus phlebotomy.[351] Therefore, while hydroxyurea is beneficial for patients with sickle cell disease it does not appear to be a substitute for transfusion therapy in those with a history of stroke. The major side effect of hydroxyurea is reversible, dose-related bone marrow suppression.

Quasi-moyamoya disease resulting from sickle cell disease should presumably be managed in a manner similar to that for true moyamoya disease, as already described.[352–355] Bone-marrow or hematopoietic stem-cell transplantation may be considered for patients with high-risk sickle cell disease and may reduce the risk of recurrent stroke, although this remains controversial.[356–358]

MISCELLANEOUS DISORDERS

Migraine-related Stroke

Epidemiologic evidence demonstrates that patients with migraine, particularly migraine with aura, have an increased risk of stroke.[359] The relationship between migraine and stroke is complex and probably bidirectional. Cortical spreading depression, a slowly spreading wave of cortical depolarization associated with a brief, transient increase in cerebral blood flow followed by a more prolonged period of relative hypoperfusion, appears to underlie the aura in migraine, and may be present in migraine without aura as well.[360,361] Multiple shared mechanisms may trigger both cerebral ischemia and cortical spreading depression, including microemboli, impaired endothelial function, and coagulation abnormalities.[362–368] Cerebral ischemia itself may trigger cortical spreading depression, and once triggered, the relative hypoperfusion produced by cortical spreading depression may potentially lead to, or exacerbate, ischemia. Disentangling the relative contributions of these various factors in an individual patient is probably impractical. Given this, in conjunction with a lack of data specific to treatment of stroke or prevention of recurrent stroke in the setting of concurrent migraine, it seems reasonable to use thrombolytic and antithrombotic medications as would be used in stroke due to more typical causes.

Cerebral vasoconstrictive medications used for abortive migraine therapy, including ergots and triptans, should be avoided because of the concern that they may further reduce cerebral blood flow to the ischemic territory or precipitate a recurrent event.[369–372] Whether migraine prophylaxis might reduce the risk of recurrent stroke is unknown. Oral calcium channel antagonists including verapamil or amlodipine are widely used in this setting; however, evidence for this approach is lacking. Smoking cessation and aggressive treatment of traditional vascular risk factors are warranted in all patients with migraine, particularly those who have experienced stroke. Furthermore, given epidemiological evidence suggesting a roughly eightfold increase in stroke risk in patients with migraine taking oral contraceptive agents, these should be discontinued after migraine-related stroke and alternative contraceptive strategies employed.[373,374]

Mitochondrial Encephalopathy, Lactic Acidosis, and Stroke-Like Episodes

Inherited abnormalities in the mitochondrial respiratory chain complexes may lead to the syndrome of mitochondrial encephalopathy, lactic acidosis, and stroke-like episodes (MELAS). Stroke is usually attributed to a metabolic energy failure, rather than a vascular mechanism, although there may be altered function of the smooth muscle cells in the microvasculature.[375] While no specific therapy has been proven effective, a number of potential therapies have been suggested. Supportive care is appropriate for all patients and includes the removal of offending systemic conditions which might exacerbate mitochondrial dysfunction, such as hypoxemia, acidosis, and infection. Medications which may worsen mitochondrial function should be avoided, including barbiturates, valproic acid, statins, aminoglycosides, and linezolid amongst others (Box 56-5).[376,377] Administration of agents that alter mitochondrial metabolism has been used to limit the production of excess lactic acid. The drug used most often, coenzyme Q10, has been shown to reduce abnormally elevated ratios of lactate to pyruvate,[378] although its clinical effect is uncertain. A randomized, blinded cross-over trial in 30 subjects comparing treatment for 60 days with coenzyme Q10 at a dose of 1200 mg daily to placebo showed minor effects on aerobic exercise capacity and post-exercise rise in lactate production, but no significant change in other clinical variables.[379] An early, smaller trial suggested a possible benefit in muscle strength with coenzyme Q10 supplementation.[380] Coenzyme Q is well-tolerated without significant side effects, such that empiric use is reasonable in patients with MELAS. Sodium dichloroacetate also appears to reduce lactate and pyruvate, and early reports

BOX 56-5 Medications Potentially Associated with Worsening of Mitochondrial Function

Valproic acid
Antiretrovirals
Aminoglycosides
Linezolid
Statins
Metformin
Propofol
Volatile anesthetics
Bupivicaine

suggested a possible clinical benefit.[381] However, a small randomized controlled trial involving 30 patients comparing dichloroacetate to placebo demonstrated unacceptable peripheral nerve toxicity associated with this agent without evidence of clinical benefit.[382] Several reports have suggested a role for l-arginine in the treatment of patients with MELAS, possibly mediated by improvements in endothelial dysfunction and tissue perfusion.[383–385] In one study of 24 patients with MELAS, intravenous infusion of L-arginine seemed to attenuate the neurologic symptoms occurring during acute stroke-like episodes, and long-term oral L-arginine supplementation appeared to decrease the frequency and severity of subsequent episodes.[386] Given the lack of a comparator placebo group, these observations must be interpreted cautiously. Other agents that have been reported in isolated case reports to be potentially beneficial include high dose corticosteroids, idebenone and vitamins K3 (menadiol sodium diphosphate), C, riboflavin, niacin, thiamine, and pyridoxine.[387–391]

Cerebral Venous Thrombosis

Cerebral venous thrombosis (CVT) is a rare but important cause of stroke for which specific therapy is available. Etiologic treatment is a principal consideration. CVT related to an infectious etiology, seen most commonly in children with otitis, sinusitis, tonsillitis, or pharyngitis, requires early administration of appropriate antibiotics. In adults, most cases are not related to infection but systemic processes often are implicated.[392] A number of infrequent but potentially treatable causes of CVT include severe dehydration, malignancy, myeloproliferative disorders, hypercoagulable states, and inflammatory bowel disease, all of which require treatment of the systemic disorder. Many adult cases are associated with pregnancy and the puerperium and are more readily treated after the delivery of the child. Oral contraceptive agents have also been implicated as risk factors and should be discontinued.[374,393,394] The cause remains unknown in about 20% of cases.[395]

Symptomatic management of CVT should include attention to the treatment of seizures, metabolic derangements, cerebral edema, and elevated intracranial pressure, as dictated by the clinical situation. Seizures usually respond to standard anticonvulsant agents. Cerebral edema may be medically treated with mannitol, glycerol, acetazolamide, dextran, barbiturates, or corticosteroids, although there is considerable debate about the relative advantages of each.[395–397] Osmotherapy with mannitol or glycerol in repeated boluses may be particularly useful in dealing with abrupt elevations of intracranial pressure, particularly while more specific thrombolytic or antithrombotic medications are being initiated. Acetazolamide tends to be most useful in patients with relatively mild symptoms but is unlikely to offer great benefit in patients with severe cerebral edema. Corticosteroids have no proven role in CVT and may increase the risk of systemic infection. Barbiturates are problematic because they obscure the neurologic examination and may cause significant hypotension. In very severe cases, consideration may be given to lumbar puncture, shunting, or surgical decompression.[392] Decompressive craniectomy has been reported in cases with clinical signs of impending or active herniation, and many patients have had surprisingly good outcomes at long-term follow-up.[398–400] These invasive approaches may, however, limit the use of antithrombotic or thrombolytic treatments that are more likely to relieve the venous hypertension and the resultant cerebral edema. On the other hand, in one series of four patients undergoing decompressive craniectomy, half-dose heparin was restarted 12 hours post-operatively, and full-dose heparin was resumed at 24 hours, without bleeding complications.[399]

Therapeutic options for dealing with the thrombosis itself include anticoagulation, pharmacologic thrombolysis, mechanical devices for clot removal, or conservative observation. The role of anticoagulation in the treatment of CVT is rooted in a long history of controversy. Anticoagulation prevents further thrombus formation, thereby preventing the development of venous infarctions, both bland and hemorrhagic. However, in patients with hemorrhagic venous infarction due to CVT, anticoagulation may pose a risk of increased intracerebral bleeding. Some authors favor anticoagulation with heparin only in patients without radiologic and cerebrospinal fluid evidence of hemorrhage, while others favor a more aggressive stance and recommend heparin even in patients with documented hemorrhagic infarctions. CVT is one of the few uncommon causes of stroke that has been subjected to randomized controlled clinical trials. Einhaupl and colleagues[401] planned to study 60 patients with CVT, randomly assigning them to receive either intravenous heparin (adjusted to a PTT of 80–100 seconds) or placebo saline infusion. The study was halted prematurely after only 20 patients were enrolled because of the dramatic and statistically significant benefit of heparin. At 3 months after treatment, eight of the 10 heparin-treated patients had complete recovery and the remaining two had slight residual deficits. In contrast, only one patient in the placebo group had complete recovery, six had residual deficits, and three died ($P < 0.01$). Moreover, the benefit of heparin was demonstrable after only 3 days of treatment. Einhaupl et al. also performed a retrospective analysis to evaluate the role of heparin in CVT with hemorrhagic venous infarction, and found that, of 43 patients, the mortality rates were 15% among patients treated with heparin and 69% among those not treated with heparin. A clinical trial of nadroparin, a LMWH, was performed in 60 patients with CVT. The results were less dramatic than with unfractionated heparin, with a non-significant reduction in poor outcomes: 13% of the treated group and 21% in the placebo group. There were no new symptomatic intracerebral hemorrhages associated with nadroparin.[402] Taken together, these two trials suggest an absolute reduction in the risk of death or dependency of 13% (95%CI, 30−–3%).[403] It remains uncertain whether efficacy differs between UFH and LMWH, although one small randomized trial and one prospective observational study suggested better outcomes with LMWH.[404,405] Based on these results, acute anticoagulation is recommended for the majority of patients with CVT, even in the presence of hemorrhagic infarction.[406] Reflecting this, in the International Study on Cerebral Vein and Dural Sinus Thrombosis (ISCVT), a multicenter, prospective, observational study, more than 80% of patients were treated with immediate anticoagulation.[407]

Thrombolysis offers the possibility of a more aggressive intervention than heparin, but its role remains poorly defined. Intravenous thrombolytic therapy for CVT has been reported to be of value in a few case series, but data are limited.[408,409] Local infusion of urokinase or tPA into dural sinus thrombosis has been more widely used, although no controlled trials have been published.[410] In most reported series of local thrombolysis, relatively low doses of thrombolytic agent are administered (tPA, 1–2 mg/h) as a continuous infusion. Mechanical thrombolysis, in particular with the use of rheolytic thrombectomy (Angiojet catheter), has been increasingly reported, typically in conjunction with pharmacologic thrombolysis.[411–416] Most series have also treated patients concurrently with intravenous heparin as already described. In a non-randomized comparison of 40 patients with superior sagittal sinus thrombosis, 16 of 20 patients (80%) treated with local urokinase returned to normal compared with only nine of 20 (45%) treated with heparin ($P = 0.019$), even though patients in the thrombolysis group had more severe deficits before treatment.[417] A systematic review of 72 studies reporting 169 patients treated with pharmacologic thrombolysis, including roughly 30% with hemorrhagic infarcts, found a relatively low rate of bleeding complications (5% intracerebral hemorrhage with neurologic deterioration, 2% extracranial hemorrhage requiring transfusion), and good outcomes were achieved in most patients. However, a prospective case series of 20 patients treated with pharmacologic and mechanical thrombolysis, 70% of whom had hemorrhagic infarction, found a much higher risk of symptomatic hemorrhage (25%), raising the possibility of publication bias in prior case reports.[418] Given the apparent efficacy of heparin in most cases, thrombolytic therapy should probably be reserved for patients who decline despite adequate anticoagulation, patients who rapidly deteriorate owing to extensive thrombosis in multiple venous sinuses, and possibly patients with thrombosis of the deep venous system given the worse prognosis associated with this location.[407,419,420] A randomized trial comparing endovascular therapy to standard anticoagulation in CVT patients with a high probability of poor outcome is underway.[421]

After early treatment with intravenous heparin and/or thrombolytics, oral anticoagulation with warfarin is typically used for ongoing therapy, although the ideal duration of therapy has not been established. A standard recommendation is to continue warfarin for 3–6 months in those with a transient provoking factor and for 6–12 months in those with unprovoked CVT.[406] Some experts recommend MRI and MR venography to determine whether flow is reestablished to help inform the decision about when to discontinue anticoagulation, although this strategy may be complicated by the fact that many subjects have permanently abnormal MR venography following CVT. Life-long anticoagulation therapy may be indicated for patients with an underlying persistent high-risk thrombophilia or in those with prior venous thromboembolism.[406,422] In women with CVT related to pregnancy or the puerperium, many experts advocate prophylactic anticoagulation during future pregnancies.[395] If the CVT developed during a prior pregnancy, then subcutaneous LMWH is often recommended during the next pregnancy and for up to 8 weeks postpartum. If the prior CVT was a puerperal event, then anticoagulation is solely used for 4 to 8 weeks after delivery.

The complete reference list can be found on the companion Expert Consult website at www.expertconsult.inkling.com.

KEY REFERENCES

5. Lyrer P, Engelter S. Antithrombotic drugs for carotid artery dissection. Cochrane Database Syst Rev 2010;(6):CD000255.
6. Weimar C, Kraywinkel K, Hagemeister C, et al. Recurrent stroke after cervical artery dissection. J Neurol Neurosurg Psychiatry 2010;81:869–73.
13. Zinkstok SM, Vergouwen MDI, Engelter ST, et al. Safety and functional outcome of thrombolysis in dissection-related ischemic stroke: a meta-analysis of individual patient data. Stroke 2011;42:2515–20.
14. Fuentes B, Masjuan J, de Leciñana MA, et al. Benefits of intravenous thrombolysis in acute ischemic stroke related to extra cranial internal carotid dissection. Dream or reality? Int J Stroke 2012;7:7–13.
18. Gomez CR, May AK, Terry JB, et al. Endovascular therapy of traumatic injuries of the extracranial cerebral arteries. Crit Care Clin 1999;15:789–809.
26. Molina CA, Alvarez-Sabin J, Schonewille W, et al. Cerebral microembolism in acute spontaneous internal carotid artery dissection. Neurology 2000;55(11):1738–40.
34. Georgiadis D, Arnold M, von Buedingen HC, et al. Aspirin vs anticoagulation in carotid artery dissection: a study of 298 patients. Neurology 2009;72:1810–15.
35. Touzé E, Gauvrit J-Y, Moulin T, et al. Risk of stroke and recurrent dissection after a cervical artery dissection: a multicenter study. Neurology 2003;61:1347–51.
36. Kennedy F, Lanfranconi S, Hicks C, et al. Antiplatelets vs anticoagulation for dissection: CADISS nonrandomized arm and meta-analysis. Neurology 2012;79:686–9.
37. The CADISS Trial Investigators. Antiplatelet therapy vs. anticoagulation in cervical artery dissection: the Cervical Artery Dissection in Stroke Study (CADISS), a randomised trial. Lancet Neurol 2015;14:361–367.
44. Benninger DH, Gandjour J, Georgiadis D, et al. Benign long-term outcome of conservatively treated cervical aneurysms due to carotid dissection. Neurology 2007;69(5):486–7.
51. Guillon B, Brunereau L, Biousse V, et al. Long-term follow-up of aneurysms developed during extracranial internal carotid artery dissection. Neurology 1999;53(1):117–22.
52. Touze E, Randoux B, Meary E, et al. Aneurysmal forms of cervical artery dissection: associated factors and outcome. Stroke 2001;32(2):418–23.
64. Corrin LS, Sandok BA, Houser OW. Cerebral ischemic events in patients with carotid artery fibromuscular dysplasia. Arch Neurol 1981;38(10):616–18.
75. Stewart MT, Moritz MW, Smith RB 3rd, et al. The natural history of carotid fibromuscular dysplasia. J Vasc Surg 1986;3(2):305–10.
88. Calabrese LH, Dodick DW, Schwedt TJ, et al. Narrative review: reversible cerebral vasoconstriction syndromes. Ann Intern Med 2007;146(1):34–44.
101. Singhal AB, Hajj-Ali Ra, Topcuoglu Ma, et al. Reversible cerebral vasoconstriction syndromes: analysis of 139 cases. Arch Neurol 2011;68:1005–12.
105. Hajj-Ali RA, Furlan A, Abou-Chebel A, et al. Benign angiopathy of the central nervous system: cohort of 16 patients with clinical course and long-term followup. Arthritis Rheum 2002;47(6):662–9.
106. Ioannidis I, Nasis N, Agianniotaki E, et al. Reversible cerebral vasoconstriction syndrome: treatment with multiple sessions of intra-arterial nimodipine and angioplasty. Interv Neuroradiol 2012;18:297–302.
107. Wilder M, Digre KB, French KF, et al. Repetitive use of intra-arterial verapamil in the treatment of reversible cerebral vasoconstriction syndrome. J Clin Neurosci 2012;19:174–6.
108. Chen D, Nishizawa S, Yokota N, et al. High-dose methylprednisolone prevents vasospasm after subarachnoid hemorrhage through inhibition of protein kinase C activation. Neurol Res 2002;24(2):215–22.
113. Glantz MJ, Burger PC, Friedman AH, et al. Treatment of radiation-induced nervous system injury with heparin and warfarin. Neurology 1994;44(11):2020–7.
119. Campen CJ, Kranick SM, Kasner SE, et al. Cranial irradiation increases risk of stroke in pediatric brain tumor survivors. Stroke 2012;43(11):3035–40.
124. Harrod-Kim P, Kadkhodayan Y, Derdeyn CP, et al. Outcomes of carotid angioplasty and stenting for radiation-associated stenosis. AJNR 2005;26(7):1781–8.
125. Fokkema M, den Hartog AG, Bots ML, et al. Stenting versus surgery in patients with carotid stenosis after previous cervical radiation therapy: systematic review and meta-analysis. Stroke 2012;43:793–801.

128. Bonduel M, Hepner M, Sciuccati G, et al. Prothrombotic disorders in children with moyamoya syndrome. Stroke 2001;32(8): 1786–92.
139. Kuroda S, Hashimoto N, Yoshimoto T, et al. Radiological findings, clinical course, and outcome in asymptomatic moyamoya disease: results of multicenter survey in Japan. Stroke 2007;38(5): 1430–5.
140. Houkin K, Ishikawa T, Yoshimoto T, et al. Direct and indirect revascularization for moyamoya disease surgical techniques and peri-operative complications. Clin Neurol Neurosurg 1997; 99(Suppl. 2):S142–5.
144. Kawaguchi S, Okuno S, Sakaki T. Effect of direct arterial bypass on the prevention of future stroke in patients with the hemorrhagic variety of moyamoya disease. J Neurosurg 2000;93(3): 397–401.
149. Rodriguez GJ, Kirmani JF, Ezzeddine MA, et al. Primary percutaneous transluminal angioplasty for early moyamoya disease. J Neuroimaging 2007;17(1):48–53.
150. Drazin D, Calayag M, Gifford E, et al. Endovascular treatment for moyamoya disease in a Caucasian twin with angioplasty and Wingspan stent. Clin Neurol Neurosurg 2009;111:913–17.
151. El-Hakam LM, Volpi J, Mawad M, et al. Angioplasty for acute stroke with pediatric moyamoya syndrome. J Child Neurol 2010;25:1278–83.
152. Khan N, Dodd R, Marks MP, et al. Failure of primary percutaneous angioplasty and stenting in the prevention of ischemia in Moyamoya angiopathy. Cerebrovasc Dis 2011;31:147–53.
158. Yap S, Boers GH, Wilcken B, et al. Vascular outcome in patients with homocystinuria due to cystathionine beta-synthase deficiency treated chronically: a multicenter observational study. Arterioscler Thromb Vasc Biol 2001;21(12):2080–5.
160. Hackam DG, Peterson JC, Spence JD. What level of plasma homocyst(e)ine should be treated? Effects of vitamin therapy on progression of carotid atherosclerosis in patients with homocyst(e)ine levels above and below 14 micromol/L. Am J Hypertens 2000;13(1 Pt 1):105–10.
161. Toole JF, Malinow MR, Chambless LE, et al. Lowering homocysteine in patients with ischemic stroke to prevent recurrent stroke, myocardial infarction, and death: the Vitamin Intervention for Stroke Prevention (VISP) randomized controlled trial. JAMA 2004;291(5):565–75.
162. Spence JD, Bang H, Chambless LE, et al. Vitamin Intervention For Stroke Prevention trial: an efficacy analysis. Stroke 2005; 36(11):2404–9.
163. The VITATOPS Trial Study Group. B vitamins in patients with recent transient ischaemic attack or stroke in the VITAmins TO Prevent Stroke (VITATOPS) trial: a randomised, double-blind, parallel, placebo-controlled trial. Lancet Neurol 2010;9(9): 855–65.
164. Ebbing M, Bleie O, Ueland PM, et al. Mortality and cardiovascular events in patients treated with homocysteine-lowering B vitamins after coronary angiography: a randomized controlled trial. JAMA 2008;300(7):795–804.
165. Bonaa KH, Njolstad I, Ueland PM, et al. Homocysteine Lowering and Cardiovascular Events after Acute Myocardial Infarction. N Engl J Med 2006;354(15):1578–88.
166. The Heart Outcomes Prevention Evaluation I. Homocysteine lowering with folic acid and B vitamins in vascular disease. N Engl J Med 2006;354(15):1567–77.
170. Frustaci A, Chimenti C, Ricci R, et al. Improvement in cardiac function in the cardiac variant of Fabry's disease with galactose-infusion therapy. N Engl J Med 2001;345(1):25–32.
171. Shi Q, Chen J, Pongmoragot J, et al. Prevalence of Fabry Disease in Stroke Patients-A Systematic Review and Meta-analysis. J Stroke Cerebrovasc Dis 2014;23(5):985–92.
172. Rolfs A, Bottcher T, Zschiesche M, et al. Prevalence of Fabry disease in patients with cryptogenic stroke: a prospective study. Lancet 2005;366(9499):1794–6.
173. Eng CM, Guffon N, Wilcox WR, et al. Safety and efficacy of recombinant human alpha-galactosidase A - replacement therapy in Fabry's disease. N Engl J Med 2001;345(1):9–16.
174. Moore DF, Scott LT, Gladwin MT, et al. Regional cerebral hyperperfusion and nitric oxide pathway dysregulation in Fabry disease: reversal by enzyme replacement therapy. Circulation 2001;104(13):1506–12.
175. Banikazemi M, Bultas J, Waldek S, et al. Agalsidase-beta therapy for advanced Fabry disease: a randomized trial. Ann Intern Med 2007;146(2):77–86.
179. El Dib RP, Nascimento P, Pastores GM. Enzyme replacement therapy for Anderson-Fabry disease. Cochrane Database Syst Rev 2013;(2):CD006663.
180. Wilcox WR, Banikazemi M, Guffon N, et al. Long-term safety and efficacy of enzyme replacement therapy for Fabry disease. Am J Hum Genet 2004;75(1):65–74.
181. Weidemann F, Niemann M, Stork S, et al. Long-term outcome of enzyme-replacement therapy in advanced Fabry disease: evidence for disease progression towards serious complications. J Intern Med 2013;274(4):331–41.
184. Salvarani C, Brown RD Jr, Calamia KT, et al. Primary central nervous system vasculitis: analysis of 101 patients. Ann Neurol 2007;62(5):442–51.
188. Salvarani C, Brown RD, Hunder GG. Adult primary central nervous system vasculitis. Lancet 2012;380:767–77.
190. Salvarani C, Brown RD, Calamia KT, et al. Primary central nervous system vasculitis with prominent leptomeningeal enhancement: a subset with a benign outcome. Arthritis Rheum 2008;58:595–603.
191. Salvarani C, Hunder GG, Morris JM, et al. Aβ-related angiitis: Comparison with CAA without inflammation and primary CNS vasculitis. Neurology 2013;81:1596–603.
192. Eng Ja, Frosch MP, Choi K, et al. Clinical manifestations of cerebral amyloid angiopathy-related inflammation. Ann Neurol 2004;55:250–6.
193. Salvarani C, Brown RD, Calamia KT, et al. Primary central nervous system vasculitis: comparison of patients with and without cerebral amyloid angiopathy. Rheumatol 2008;47:1671–7.
194. Kinnecom C, Lev MH, Wendell L, et al. Course of cerebral amyloid angiopathy-related inflammation. Neurology 2007;68: 1411–16.
201. Chevalet P, Barrier JH, Pottier P, et al. A randomized, multicenter, controlled trial using intravenous pulses of methylprednisolone in the initial treatment of simple forms of giant cell arteritis: a one year followup study of 164 patients. J Rheumatol 2000;27(6):1484–91.
202. Mazlumzadeh M, Hunder GG, Easley KA, et al. Treatment of giant cell arteritis using induction therapy with high-dose glucocorticoids: a double-blind, placebo-controlled, randomized prospective clinical trial. Arthritis Rheum 2006;54(10):3310–18.
204. Staunton H, Stafford F, Leader M, et al. Deterioration of giant cell arteritis with corticosteroid therapy. Arch Neurol 2000;57(4): 581–4.
206. Nesher G, Rubinow A, Sonnenblick M. Efficacy and adverse effects of different corticosteroid dose regimens in temporal arteritis: a retrospective study. Clin Exp Rheumatol 1997;15(3): 303–6.
208. Salvarani C, Cantini F, Hunder GG. Polymyalgia rheumatica and giant-cell arteritis. Lancet 2008;372(9634):234–45.
209. Mahr AD, Jover JA, Spiera RF, et al. Adjunctive methotrexate for treatment of giant cell arteritis: an individual patient data meta-analysis. Arthritis Rheum 2007;56(8):2789–97.
212. Hoffman GS, Cid MC, Rendt-Zagar KE, et al. Infliximab for maintenance of glucocorticosteroid-induced remission of giant cell arteritis: a randomized trial. Ann Intern Med 2007;146(9): 621–30.
213. Martínez-Taboada VM, Rodríguez-Valverde V, Carreño L, et al. A double-blind placebo controlled trial of etanercept in patients with giant cell arteritis and corticosteroid side effects. Ann Rheum Dis 2008;67:625–30.
214. Lee MS, Smith SD, Galor A, et al. Antiplatelet and anticoagulant therapy in patients with giant cell arteritis. Arthritis Rheum 2006;54(10):3306–9.
215. Nesher G, Berkun Y, Mates M, et al. Low-dose aspirin and prevention of cranial ischemic complications in giant cell arteritis. Arthritis Rheum 2004;50(4):1332–7.
231. Jayne D. Evidence-based treatment of systemic vasculitis. Rheumatology 2000;39(6):585–95.
239. Picard O, Brunereau L, Pelosse B, et al. Cerebral infarction associated with vasculitis due to varicella zoster virus in patients infected with the human immunodeficiency virus. Biomed Pharmacother 1997;51(10):449–54.

251. Weststrate W, Hijdra A, de Gans J. Brain infarcts in adults with bacterial meningitis. Lancet 1996;347(8998):399.
252. Azuma T, Matsubara T, Shima Y, et al. Neurosteroids in cerebrospinal fluid in neurologic disorders. J Neurol Sci 1993;120(1): 87–92.
256. Goel A, Pandya SK, Satoskar AR. Whither short-course chemotherapy for tuberculous meningitis? Neurosurgery 1990;27(3): 418–21.
265. Casato M, Saadoun D, Marchetti A, et al. Central nervous system involvement in hepatitis C virus cryoglobulinemia vasculitis: a multicenter case-control study using magnetic resonance imaging and neuropsychological tests. J Rheumatol 2005;32(3): 484–8.
269. Reynard CA, Calain P, Pizzolato GP, et al. Severe acute myocardial infarction during a staphylococcal septicemia with meningoencephalitis. A possible contraindication to thrombolytic treatment. Int Care Med 1992;18(4):247–9.
272. Sloan MA, Kittner SJ, Feeser BR, et al. Illicit drug-associated ischemic stroke in the Baltimore-Washington Young Stroke Study. Neurology 1998;50(6):1688–93.
273. Aggarwal SK, Williams V, Levine SR, et al. Cocaine-associated intracranial hemorrhage: absence of vasculitis in 14 cases. Neurology 1996;46(6):1741–3.
274. Brust JC. Vasculitis owing to substance abuse. Neurol Clin 1997;15(4):945–57.
275. Calabrese LH, Duna GF. Drug-induced vasculitis. Curr Opin Rheumatol 1996;8(1):34–40.
276. Mourand I, Ducrocq X, Lacour JC, et al. Acute reversible cerebral arteritis associated with parenteral ephedrine use. Cerebrovasc Dis 1999;9(6):355–7.
277. Kernan WN, Viscoli CM, Brass LM, et al. Phenylpropanolamine and the risk of hemorrhagic stroke. N Engl J Med 2000;343(25): 1826–32.
278. Bruno A, Nolte KB, Chapin J. Stroke associated with ephedrine use. Neurology 1993;43(7):1313–16.
279. Konzen JP, Levine SR, Garcia JH. Vasospasm and thrombus formation as possible mechanisms of stroke related to alkaloidal cocaine. Stroke 1995;26(6):1114–18.
284. Calamia KT, Miller A, Shuster EA, et al. Intravascular lymphomatosis. A report of ten patients with central nervous system involvement and a review of the disease process. Adv Exp Med Biol 1999;455:249–65.
289. Julkunen H, Hedman C, Kauppi M. Thrombolysis for acute ischemic stroke in the primary antiphospholipid syndrome. J Rheumatol 1997;24(1):181–3.
292. Sallah S, Abdallah JM, Gagnon GA. Recurrent warfarin-induced skin necrosis in kindreds with protein S deficiency. Haemostasis 1998;28(1):25–30.
305. Miyakis S, Lockshin MD, Atsumi T, et al. International consensus statement on an update of the classification criteria for definite antiphospholipid syndrome (APS). JTH 2006;4:295–306.
308. Mohr JP, Thompson JLP, Lazar RM, et al. A Comparison of Warfarin and Aspirin for the Prevention of Recurrent Ischemic Stroke. N Engl J Med 2001;345:1444–51.
309. Investigators A. Antiphospholipid antibodies and subsequent thrombo-occlusive events in patients with ischemic stroke. JAMA 2004;291(5):576–84.
310. Khamashta MA, Cuadrado MJ, Mujic F, et al. The management of thrombosis in the antiphospholipid-antibody syndrome. N Engl J Med 1995;332(15):993–7.
312. Crowther MA, Ginsberg JS, Julian J, et al. A comparison of two intensities of warfarin for the prevention of recurrent thrombosis in patients with the antiphospholipid antibody syndrome. N Engl J Med 2003;349(12):1133–8.
313. Finazzi G, Marchioli R, Brancaccio V, et al. A randomized clinical trial of high-intensity warfarin vs. conventional antithrombotic therapy for the prevention of recurrent thrombosis in patients with the antiphospholipid syndrome (WAPS). J Thromb Haemost 2005;3(5):848–53.
314. Ruiz-Irastorza G, Ramos-Casals M, Brito-Zeron P, et al. Clinical efficacy and side effects of antimalarials in systemic lupus erythematosus: a systematic review. Ann Rheum Dis 2010;69(1): 20–8.
315. Asherson RA, Cervera R, de Groot PG, et al. Catastrophic antiphospholipid syndrome: international consensus statement on classification criteria and treatment guidelines. Lupus 2003; 12(7):530–4.
319. Schwartzman RJ, Hill JB. Neurologic complications of disseminated intravascular coagulation. Neurology 1982;32(8):791–7.
320. de Jonge E, Levi M, Stoutenbeek CP, et al. Current drug treatment strategies for disseminated intravascular coagulation. Drugs 1998;55(6):767–77.
323. Sakuragawa N, Hasegawa H, Maki M, et al. Clinical evaluation of low-molecular-weight heparin (FR-860) on disseminated intravascular coagulation (DIC) – a multicenter co-operative double-blind trial in comparison with heparin. Thromb Res 1993;72:475–500.
324. Wada H, Thachil J, Di Nisio M, et al. Guidance for diagnosis and treatment of DIC from harmonization of the recommendations from three guidelines. JTH 2013;761–7.
325. Franchini M, Manzato F, Salvagno GL, et al. Potential role of recombinant activated factor VII for the treatment of severe bleeding associated with disseminated intravascular coagulation: a systematic review. Blood Coagul Fibrinolysis 2007;18(7): 589–93.
331. Adams RJ. Stroke prevention and treatment in sickle cell disease. Arch Neurol 2001;58(4):565–8.
332. Sidani CA, Ballourah W, El Dassouki M, et al. Venous sinus thrombosis leading to stroke in a patient with sickle cell disease on hydroxyurea and high hemoglobin levels: Treatment with thrombolysis. Am J Hematol 2008.
333. Telfer PT, Evanson J, Butler P, et al. Cervical carotid artery disease in sickle cell anemia: clinical and radiological features. Blood 2011;118:6192–9.
334. Adams RJ, McKie VC, Hsu L, et al. Prevention of a first stroke by transfusions in children with sickle cell anemia and abnormal results on transcranial Doppler ultrasonography. N Engl J Med 1998;339(1):5–11.
335. Cohen AR, Martin MB, Silber JH, et al. A modified transfusion program for prevention of stroke in sickle cell disease. Blood 1992;79(7):1657–61.
338. Adams RJ, Brambilla D. Discontinuing prophylactic transfusions used to prevent stroke in sickle cell disease. N Engl J Med 2005;353(26):2769–78.
339. Abboud MR, Yim E, Musallam KM, et al. Discontinuing prophylactic transfusions increases the risk of silent brain infarction in children with sickle cell disease: data from STOP II. Blood 2011;118:894–8.
341. Hulbert ML, Scothorn DJ, Panepinto JA, et al. Exchange blood transfusion compared with simple transfusion for first overt stroke is associated with a lower risk of subsequent stroke: a retrospective cohort study of 137 children with sickle cell anemia. J Pediatr 2006;149(5):710–12.
344. Zimmerman SA, Schultz WH, Burgett S, et al. Hydroxyurea therapy lowers transcranial Doppler flow velocities in children with sickle cell anemia. Blood 2007;110(3):1043–7.
345. Gulbis B, Haberman D, Dufour D, et al. Hydroxyurea for sickle cell disease in children and for prevention of cerebrovascular events: the Belgian experience. Blood 2005;105(7):2685–90.
346. Kratovil T, Bulas D, Driscoll MC, et al. Hydroxyurea therapy lowers TCD velocities in children with sickle cell disease. Pediatr Blood Cancer 2006;47(7):894–900.
347. Charache S, Terrin ML, Moore RD, et al. Effect of hydroxyurea on the frequency of painful crises in sickle cell anemia. Investigators of the Multicenter Study of Hydroxyurea in Sickle Cell Anemia. N Engl J Med 1995;332(20):1317–22.
348. Voskaridou E, Christoulas D, Bilalis A, et al. The effect of prolonged administration of hydroxyurea on morbidity and mortality in adult patients with sickle cell syndromes: results of a 17-year, single-center trial (LaSHS). Blood 2010;115:2354–63.
349. Wang WC, Ware RE, Miller ST, et al. Hydroxycarbamide in very young children with sickle-cell anaemia: a multicentre, randomised, controlled trial (BABY HUG). Lancet 2011;377: 1663–72.
350. Ware RE, Zimmerman SA, Sylvestre PB, et al. Prevention of secondary stroke and resolution of transfusional iron overload in children with sickle cell anemia using hydroxyurea and phlebotomy. J Pediatr 2004;145(3):346–52.
351. Ware RE, Helms RW. Stroke With Transfusions Changing to Hydroxyurea (SWiTCH). Blood 2012;119:3925–32.

355. Hankinson TC, Bohman LE, Heyer G, et al. Surgical treatment of moyamoya syndrome in patients with sickle cell anemia: outcome following encephaloduroarteriosynangiosis. J Neurosurg Pediatr 2008;1(3):211–16.
356. Walters MC, Storb R, Patience M, et al. Impact of bone marrow transplantation for symptomatic sickle cell disease: an interim report. Multicenter investigation of bone marrow transplantation for sickle cell disease. Blood 2000;95(6):1918–24.
357. Woodard P, Helton KJ, Khan RB, et al. Brain parenchymal damage after haematopoietic stem cell transplantation for severe sickle cell disease. Br J Haematol 2005;129(4):550–2.
358. Walters MC, Hardy K, Edwards S, et al. Pulmonary, gonadal, and central nervous system status after bone marrow transplantation for sickle cell disease. Biol Blood Marrow Transplant 2010;16: 263–72.
359. Spector JT, Kahn SR, Jones MR, et al. Migraine headache and ischemic stroke risk: an updated meta-analysis. Am J Med 2010; 123:612–24.
362. Dalkara T, Nozari A, Moskowitz Ma. Migraine aura pathophysiology: the role of blood vessels and microembolisation. Lancet Neurol 2010;9:309–17.
364. Hering-Hanit R, Friedman Z, Schlesinger I, et al. Evidence for activation of the coagulation system in migraine with aura. Cephalalgia 2001;21(2):137–9.
365. Lassen LH, Ashina M, Christiansen I, et al. Nitric oxide synthase inhibition in migraine. Lancet 1997;349(9049):401–2.
366. Zeller JA, Frahm K, Baron R, et al. Platelet-leukocyte interaction and platelet activation in migraine: a link to ischemic stroke? J Neurol Neurosurg Psychiatry 2004;75(7):984–7.
367. Tietjen GE, Al-Qasmi MM, Athanas K, et al. Increased von Willebrand factor in migraine. Neurology 2001;57(2):334–6.
368. Schwerzmann M, Nedeltchev K, Meier B. Patent foramen ovale closure: A new therapy for migraine. Catheter Cardiovasc Interv 2007;69(2):277–84.
369. Meschia JF, Malkoff MD, Biller J. Reversible segmental cerebral arterial vasospasm and cerebral infarction: possible association with excessive use of sumatriptan and Midrin. Arch Neurol 1998;55(5):712–14.
373. Etminan M, Takkouche B, Isorna FC, et al. Risk of ischaemic stroke in people with migraine: systematic review and meta-analysis of observational studies. BMJ 2005;330(7482):63.
374. Gillum LA, Mamidipudi SK, Johnston SC. Ischemic stroke risk with oral contraceptives: A meta-analysis. JAMA 2000;284(1): 72–8.
376. Parikh S, Saneto R, Falk MJ, et al. A modern approach to the treatment of mitochondrial disease. Curr Treat Options Neurol 2009;11:414–30.
377. Cope TE, McFarland R, Schaefer A. Rapid-onset, linezolid-induced lactic acidosis in MELAS. Mitochondrion 2011;11: 992–3.
379. Glover EI, Martin J, Maher A, et al. A randomized trial of coenzyme Q10 in mitochondrial disorders. Muscle Nerve 2010;42: 739–48.
380. Chen RS, Huang CC, Chu NS. Coenzyme Q10 treatment in mitochondrial encephalomyopathies. Short-term double-blind, crossover study. Eur Neurol 1997;37:212–18.
384. Kubota M, Sakakihara Y, Mori M, et al. Beneficial effect of L-arginine for stroke-like episode in MELAS. Brain Dev 2004; 26(7):481–3, discussion 0.
385. Koga Y, Akita Y, Junko N, et al. Endothelial dysfunction in MELAS improved by l-arginine supplementation. Neurology 2006;66(11):1766–9.
386. Koga Y, Akita Y, Nishioka J, et al. L-arginine improves the symptoms of strokelike episodes in MELAS. Neurology 2005;64(4): 710–12.
387. Walcott BP, Edlow BL, Xia Z, et al. Steroid responsive A3243G mutation MELAS: clinical and radiographic evidence for regional hyperperfusion leading to neuronal loss. Neurologist 2012;18: 159–70.
400. Ferro JM, Crassard I, Coutinho JM, et al. Decompressive surgery in cerebrovenous thrombosis: a multicenter registry and a systematic review of individual patient data. Stroke 2011;42(10): 2825–31.
401. Einhaupl KM, Villringer A, Meister W, et al. Heparin treatment in sinus venous thrombosis. Lancet 1991;338:597–600.
402. de Bruijn SFTM, Stam J, for the Cerebral Venous Sinus Thrombosis Study Group. Randomized, placebo-controlled trial of anticoagulant treatment with low-molecular-weight heparin for cerebral sinus thrombosis. Stroke 1999;30:484–8.
403. Coutinho J, de Bruijn SF, Deveber G, et al. Anticoagulation for cerebral venous sinus thrombosis. Cochrane Database Syst Rev 2011;CD002005.
404. Coutinho JM, Ferro JM, Canhão P, et al. Unfractionated or low-molecular weight heparin for the treatment of cerebral venous thrombosis. Stroke 2010;41:2575–80.
405. Misra UK, Kalita J, Chandra S, et al. Low molecular weight heparin versus unfractionated heparin in cerebral venous sinus thrombosis: a randomized controlled trial. Eur J Neurol 2012;19: 1030–6.
406. Saposnik G, Barinagarrementeria F, Brown RD, et al. Diagnosis and management of cerebral venous thrombosis: a statement for healthcare professionals from the American Heart Association/ American Stroke Association. Stroke 2011;42:1158–92.
407. Ferro JM, Canhao P, Stam J, et al. for the II. Prognosis of cerebral vein and dural sinus thrombosis: results of the International Study on Cerebral Vein and Dural Sinus Thrombosis (ISCVT). Stroke 2004;35(3):664–70.
410. Canhao P, Falcao F, Ferro JM. Thrombolytics for cerebral sinus thrombosis: a systematic review. Cerebrovasc Dis 2003;15(3): 159–66.
412. Zhang A, Collinson RL, Hurst RW, et al. Rheolytic thrombectomy for cerebral sinus thrombosis. Neurocrit Care 2008;9(1): 17–26.
417. Wasay M, Bakshi R, Kojan S, et al. Nonrandomized comparison of local urokinase thrombolysis versus systemic heparin anticoagulation for superior sagittal sinus thrombosis. Stroke 2001; 32(10):2310–17.
418. Stam J, Majoie CBLM, van Delden OM, et al. Endovascular thrombectomy and thrombolysis for severe cerebral sinus thrombosis: a prospective study. Stroke 2008;39(5):1487–90.
421. Coutinho JM, Ferro JM, Zuurbier SM, et al. Thrombolysis or anticoagulation for cerebral venous thrombosis: rationale and design of the TO-ACT trial. Int J Stroke 2013;8:135–40.

57 Medical Therapy of Intracerebral and Intraventricular Hemorrhage

Darin B. Zahuranec, Lewis B. Morgenstern

KEY POINTS

- Patients with ICH should be cared for in specialized units with a focus on monitoring for deterioration and avoiding medical complications such as fever, hyper- or hypoglycemia, and deep vein thrombosis.
- Blood pressure lowering after ICH to a target systolic blood pressure (SBP) of 140–160 mmHg is probably safe and may improve outcome, though caution is advised for very elevated blood pressure (e.g. SBP > 220 mmHg) or if elevated intracranial pressure is suspected.
- Prevention of early hematoma expansion is likely an important treatment target, though optimal methods to identify and treat those at highest risk remain active areas of investigation.
- Indications for craniotomy and hematoma removal remain uncertain for most cases of supratentorial ICH, though minimally invasive surgical treatments are a promising area of investigation. For cerebellar hemorrhage with mass effect or hydrocephalus, surgical hematoma evacuation can be lifesaving.
- Outcome prediction after ICH may be confounded by very frequent limitations in life-sustaining treatments. Clinicians should be cautious of early limitations in the supportive treatment provided and work to ensure that the goals of treatment are in line with patient and family values and treatment preferences.

Blood frightens people. Although acute hemorrhage is white rather than red on a CT scan, it usually prompts an emergency department physician to rapidly call a tertiary referral center to transfer the patient. The physician accepting the call at the referral center is frequently left wondering what the referral center can do for the patient that the local community hospital cannot. The good news is that, although we still have no "magic bullet" to treat intracerebral and intraventricular hemorrhage, intensive therapy is likely to reduce mortality and improve outcome. Surgery remains controversial, and many therapies can be provided at any hospital with a good intensive care unit and neurologic or neurosurgical expertise.

In this chapter, we discuss medical therapy of spontaneous intracerebral hemorrhage (ICH) and intraventricular hemorrhage (IVH) in adults. Epidemiology, clinical presentation, imaging, and surgical treatment are covered elsewhere in this book. Care for ICH or IVH begins in the community with prompt recognition, transport, and triage of the patient with acute stroke. In the emergency department, after a *stat* head CT scan determines that a spontaneous cerebral hemorrhage has occurred and a search for the cause begins, therapy commences with blood pressure control and assessment of cerebral edema. A watchful eye for hydrocephalus and complications are critical. Early rehabilitation and avoiding malnutrition are important.

We begin with emergency department management of the patient with acute ICH or IVH and follow it with a discussion of the utility of specialized wards for patients with ICH or IVH and the importance of intensive medical therapies. We then consider edema, hydrocephalus, and ventricular drainage procedures; instillation of thrombolytic medication is considered in this section. Next we discuss hematoma expansion and the steps to prevent this serious complication. Consideration then is given to patient selection for surgical interventions. Finally, we deal with circumstances special to anticoagulant-associated cerebral hemorrhage and predictors of outcome. Primary IVH is rare.[1] One study found that primary IVH accounted for only 3% of all cases of IVH.[2] We therefore discuss ICH and IVH as one entity. When recommendations in this chapter cite the American Heart Association/American Stroke Association (AHA/ASA) ICH Guidelines, the classification and level of evidence are noted.[3] Full explanations of evidence classifications are listed in the front matter of the text.

EMERGENCY DEPARTMENT MANAGEMENT

Box 57-1 reviews the first steps in the care of patients with ICH or IVH. Initial concerns should focus on the ABCs of emergency therapy. The patient who has brainstem injury or reduced consciousness may have compromise of airway or breathing. These complications are treated with airway management (with adequate cervical spine protection for those in whom trauma is suspected) and intubation, as discussed in Chapter 54. Patients who have been immobile for long periods before they are brought to the emergency department may have rhabdomyolysis and renal failure; these possibilities should be kept in mind.

THE IMPORTANCE OF INTENSIVE MEDICAL THERAPIES

Stroke Units and Intensive Care Units

Patients with ICH or IVH should be cared for in specialized units where personnel are familiar with both intensive care procedures and neurologic injury (Class I, Level B).[3] At the minimum, this statement implies training of nurses to perform frequent neurologic examinations and to promptly recognize deterioration so that rescue therapies can be instituted to halt worsening. At many institutions, this implies that ICH patients should be in an intensive care unit (ICU), though some ICH patients without respiratory compromise or elevated intracranial pressure may be able to be cared for in specialized stroke units as long as access to higher levels of care is immediately available. Support for providing care in specialized hospital areas comes from the data on stroke units,[4–6] and some evidence suggests stroke units may be more beneficial for ICH compared with other stroke types.[7] Considering studies specific to ICH, Ronning et al.[8] randomly assigned 121 patients with ICH to care in an acute stroke unit or a general medical ward, demonstrating a reduction in 30-day mortality (39% in stroke unit compared with 63% in the general medical

BOX 57-1 Emergency Department Considerations for Suspected Intracerebral Hemorrhage (ICH)

1. Secure airway, breathing, and circulation
2. Check for history of recent head trauma, hypertension, tumor, arteriovenous malformation (AVM), aneurysm, antithrombotic medication use, clotting disorder, or chemotherapy
3. Order *stat* head CT scan
4. Collect and send specimens for complete blood count, prothrombin time (INR), partial thromboplastin time, chemistry panel, and urine drug screen
5. Insert intravenous and Foley bladder catheters
6. If CT confirms ICH and increased ICP is not suspected: reduce blood pressure to systolic blood pressure of 140–160 mm Hg if initial systolic blood pressure is ≤220 mmHg. If initial systolic blood pressure is >220 mmHg, reduce blood pressure by no more than 15–20%
7. Obtain neurologic and neurosurgical consultations
8. Suspect aneurysm or AVM if CT shows subarachnoid hemorrhage or hemorrhage in an atypical location or if the patient is not known to have hypertension
9. Watch the patient closely for signs of deterioration; repeat CT if deterioration occurs
10. Treat fever and hyperglycemia or hypoglycemia

BOX 57-2 Representative Standard Orders for Patients Admitted to an Intensive Care Unit or Stroke Unit with Cerebral Hemorrhage

Admit to Intensive Care Unit/Stroke Unit
Diagnosis: intracerebral hemorrhage
Condition: critical
Vital signs: q1h with neurologic checks and pulse oximetry
Activity: bed rest; have patient up with therapists after 24 hours if stable
Call physician if: temp >38.0° C (obtain chest x-ray, urinalysis and urine culture, blood culture × 2, and give acetaminophen, 1g q6h, and cooling blanket to keep temp <38.0° C); systolic blood pressure >160 mm Hg; finger-stick glucose q6h, call if glucose >150 or <70 mg/dL for sliding scale; pulse <60, >120 bpm; respirations <8, >24 min; change in National Institutes of Health Stroke Scale score of ≥2 points
Diet: NPO until swallow screen or cleared by speech pathologist
Allergies: ?
Lab tests: electrolytes, blood chemistry, blood counts including platelets, coagulation profile
IV fluids: normal saline at 80 mL/hour
Pneumatic compression stockings; may add heparin 5000 U SC q8–12 hours after 1–4 days
Ventilator settings as needed
Consult physical, occupational and speech therapy

ward group). The decision to assign patients to a neurologic intensive care unit (ICU) rather than a general ICU is also supported by an observational study demonstrating that patients who were *not* in a neurologic ICU had a higher odds ratio (OR) for mortality, of 3.4 (95% confidence interval [CI], 1.7–7.6).[9] Patients in ICUs that had a full-time intensivist on staff had lower odds of death (OR, 0.39; 95%CI, 0.2–0.7). Specialized units not only provide rescue treatment for patients with worsening neurologic signs, but also can help prevent complications and avoid conditions that are toxic to damaged neurons. Representative standard orders are shown in Box 57-2.

The decision to transfer a patient with ICH to a tertiary care center versus keep them at a local presenting hospital is complex. Despite the expected benefits of care in specialized units, some studies have suggested a worse outcome in patients transferred to tertiary centers,[10] though this finding is not consistent across studies,[11] and these analyses are almost certainly confounded by unmeasured severity of illness. Hospitals that lack the capability to provide all available diagnostic and surgical procedures for ICH patients should work with their regional tertiary centers to develop protocols for which patients may be cared for locally and which should be transferred, taking into consideration patient factors, local hospital capabilities, geography, and family preferences.

Fever

Fever is an independent predictor of poor outcome in ICH.[12] Routine prophylactic administration of acetaminophen to all stroke patients has not been found to improve outcome,[13] but there is good evidence that patients with stroke do worse if they have fever.[14,15] In patients with elevated temperatures, an infectious source should be sought assiduously. Prompt use of acetaminophen and of mechanical cooling devices (blankets) is advocated with a goal of normothermia.

Hyperglycemia

Elevated serum glucose concentration is associated with poor outcome in ICH,[16] though it remains uncertain to what degree hyperglycemia is a cause of poor outcome versus a marker of severity of brain injury. Elevated serum glucose level may also predispose to secondary ICH after intravenous recombinant tissue-type plasminogen activator (rt-PA) for ischemic stroke.[17] Efforts to control glucose in stroke patients with an insulin drip have not proved useful to date,[18] though additional studies are ongoing. The injured brain is particularly sensitive to deleterious effect from hypoglycemia, and intensive insulin protocols targeting normoglycemia (e.g. <~110mg/dL) have been found to increase the risk of hypoglycemia in neurocritical patients.[19] No specific targets for glucose can be recommended based on existing evidence, though frequent monitoring of blood glucose is recommended to avoid extremes of both hyper- and hypoglycemia (Class I, Level C).[3]

Hypertension

Although lowering the blood pressure in acute hemorrhage holds the theoretical promise of preventing enlargement of the hematoma, many researchers have worried that perihematomal ischemia may be worsened. Evidence now suggests that this concern is a moot point. Experimental laboratory data in dogs first showed that lowering mean arterial pressure (MAP) within normal limits of cerebral autoregulation did not detrimentally affect regional cerebral blood flow or intracranial pressure (ICP).[20] Positron emission tomography (PET) also fails to demonstrate tissue hypoxia surrounding cerebral hematomas in humans.[21] Powers et al.[22] performed a controlled trial of blood pressure reduction in acute patients with ICH and measured perihematomal and global cerebral blood flow; neither declined.

The pilot Intensive Blood Pressure Reduction in Acute Cerebral Haemorrhage Trial (INTERACT) was carried out primarily in China and demonstrated that blood pressure could be lowered in the acute setting with relative safety in comparison with a control group.[23] The pivotal INTERACT2 trial also demonstrated safety and a trend to improved outcome. The study randomized 2839 patients, 68% from China, who had a primary ICH within 6 hours of randomization. The intensive treatment arm (goal SBP < 140 mmHg) had a 3.6% decreased chance of death or disability (52% vs 55.6%) compared with the guideline concordant treatment arm (goal SBP < 180 mmHg; OR, 0.87; 95%CI, 0.75–1.01; $P = 0.06$). Treating physicians chose the blood-pressure-lowering agent to use. Mortality and safety did not differ between the treatment groups.[24] The antihypertensive treatment of intracerebral hemorrhage (ATACH) group reported a 60-person dose-finding pilot trial using IV nicardipine to lower blood pressure in acute ICH. Outcomes were generally better than expected at all doses.[25] The ATACH-II study is a large multinational randomized control trial whose results will help the interpretation of the INTERACT2 trial.[26] Of some concern is the observation that many patients with ICH have positive diffusion signal on brain MRI in locations away from the hemorrhage. One study of 118 ICH patients found that 22.9% had positive diffusion signal reflecting acute ischemia during the first month after ICH. The overwhelming majority of these diffusion changes were small and asymptomatic, though blood pressure lowering was associated with these abnormalities.[27] The AHA/ASA Guidelines currently available at the time of writing this chapter[3] were written prior to the results of INTERACT2 and therefore we wait for the new guidelines to define blood pressure management in ICH. However, it appears that acutely lowering SBP to a target of 140 mmHg is probably safe if the initial SBP is ≤ 220 mmHg.

When ICP is elevated, it takes higher MAPs to drive cerebral perfusion pressure. Choice of antihypertensive agent may be important.[28] Intravenous labetalol[29] or nicardipine may provide smooth onset of action and allow physicians to control blood pressure in patients without cardiac contraindications to these agents. Labetalol is begun as 10–20 mg intravenous (IV) push over 1–2 minutes. Doses can be increased up to 40–80 mg every 10 minutes, or a continuous infusion starting at 2 mg/minute can be used if needed. The maximum dose is 300 mg/day. Nicardipine infusions are begun at 5 mg/hour. The dose can be increased by 2.5 mg/hour every 10 minutes if needed. The maximum dose is 15 mg/hour. Nitrates theoretically may worsen cerebral edema owing to their vasodilatory properties and should probably be avoided, given the other available agents.

Deep Vein Thrombosis

Prevention of deep vein thrombosis (DVT) is critical, though prevention efforts must be balanced against the risks of early hematoma expansion. Mechanical prophylaxis with thigh-high intermittent pneumatic compression stockings reduced the risk of DVT, with a trend toward reduced mortality in a prospective randomized trial of mixed ischemic stroke and ICH.[30] Graduated compression stockings have traditionally been considered another option for mechanical prophylaxis, though recent randomized trials of their effectiveness in stroke have shown mixed results. The CLOTS 1 study suggested that thigh-high compression stockings were ineffective at preventing DVT when compared with no treatment,[31] while a subsequent study suggested that thigh-high stockings were superior to below-knee stockings for prevention of proximal DVT.[32] Interpretation of these apparently disparate findings is challenging, as evidenced by mixed recommendations from several organizations on the use of graduated compression stockings.[33,34] Based on these studies, ICH patients with reduced mobility should be immediately fitted with pneumatic compression stockings (Class I, Level B) though the utility of graduated compression stockings is less certain. After documentation of cessation of intracranial bleeding, subcutaneous heparin can be added 1–4 days from onset (Class IIb, Level B).[3] While studies of ischemic stroke have suggested possible benefits of enoxaparin over subcutaneous unfractionated heparin,[35] ICH patients were not included in this study and, therefore, we use subcutaneous unfractionated heparin in patients with ICH.

Steroids

Two randomized trials have examined the role of steroids in ICH.[36,37] Both failed to demonstrate a benefit for steroids in patients with ICH. In fact, in one study,[36] patients who were treated with steroids had more infectious complications than those who were not.

Anticonvulsants

Early seizures are common after ICH, occurring in about 3–17% of patients.[38] However, no prospective randomized trials support the use of prophylactic anticonvulsants after ICH,[39,40] and observational studies suggest that preventative anticonvulsants may be associated with harm.[41,42] Prophylactic anticonvulsants are not recommended (Class III, Level B), though a low threshold should be maintained to order EEG monitoring to assess for non-convulsive seizures in patients with unexplained alteration of consciousness (Class IIa, Level B).[3,38] If a seizure does occur, we administer a loading dose with IV fosphenytoin 10–20 mg phenytoin equivalents/kg, followed by maintenance phenytoin 4–7 mg/kg daily. Levetiracetam 500–1500 mg twice daily can be considered if drug-drug interactions are an issue.

Other Therapies

Issues of airway management and of mechanical ventilation are addressed in Chapter 54. Critically ill patients should be monitored for infection, and appropriate antibiotics should be instituted if necessary. Frequent change of positioning reduces pressure sores. Gastrointestinal hemorrhage is one potential complication in the high stress of an ICU stay, though the utility of medical prophylaxis with acid-reducing agents remains uncertain. A meta-analysis of randomized trials suggested that prophylactic use of histamine (H_2) blockers may not be necessary if early (within 48 hours) enteral nutrition is used.[43] Early rehabilitation is advisable, but has not been well studied (Class IIa, Level B).[3] Avoidance of sedation except for treatment of elevated ICP allows the patient to more actively participate in rehabilitation and any neurologic changes to be observed and managed.

PREVENTION OF HEMATOMA EXPANSION

Evidence now suggests that much of the morbidity and mortality in ICH stems from early hematoma expansion. The first report of the regrowth of cerebral hematomas came from Fujii et al.[44] They observed that of their 419 patients with ICH who presented within 24 hours of symptom onset, hematoma growth was observed in 14% when imaging was repeated within 24 hours of admission. Liver disease, an irregularly shaped hematoma on CT, and coagulation abnormalities were also associated with hematoma expansion. Kazui et al.[45] reported that 36% of 74 patients who underwent imaging within 3 hours had hematoma expansion on later imaging studies. Even after 6 hours, 17% had enlargement of hematoma, but none expanded after 24 hours.

In another study, Brott et al.[46] performed head CT in patients with ICH upon emergency department presentation, 1 hour later, and 20 hours later. These researchers found that 26% of the 103 study subjects experienced a greater than 33%

enlargement of hemorrhage volume within 1 hour of hospital arrival. Another 12% of the remaining patients experienced expansion between the 1-hour and 20-hour CT scans. It seems that hematoma growth happens early, in the majority of cases within the first minutes to hours of the initial bleed. Patients who have coagulation disorders or a hepatic predisposition for coagulation deficits are at greater risk, and may have expansion of hematoma later than patients with normal coagulation.[47] The roles of blood pressure and glucose are also potential factors.

Two trials investigated the effect of recombinant factor VIIa (rfVIIa), which is used in bleeding disorders such as hemophilia, on the prevention of hematoma expansion in acute ICH. The first was a dose-finding, phase 2b, randomized, controlled trial of 399 patients.[48] The group that received rfVIIa had significantly less hematoma growth, severe disability and mortality than the placebo group. There was a trend to increased thromboembolic complications in the rfVIIa -treated groups. The absolute reduction in hemorrhage growth was quite small (4.5 mL). Unfortunately, the pivotal, phase 3 trial showed absolutely no difference in functional outcome or mortality between rfVIIa-treated and placebo-treated patients, and there was a higher rate of arterial thromboembolic events in rfVIIa-treated patients.[49] The AHA/ASA Guidelines state clearly that rfVIIa should not be used in unselected patients (Class III, Level A).[3] At this time the only indications for use of rfVIIa approved by the U.S. Food and Drug Administration (FDA) are bleeding prophylaxis and bleeding treatment in known factor deficiencies.

One possible way to determine whether hemostasis has occurred is through CT with contrast imaging. Becker et al.[50] found that extravasation of contrast material in patients with ICH suggested that the hemorrhage was still growing. Extravasation of contrast material can also be demonstrated on MRI, with the same correlation with hematoma expansion.[51] CT angiography (CTA) is perhaps the easiest acute vascular imaging test to obtain, and continuous bleeding on CTA has been labeled the "spot sign."[52] This finding suggests that patients with imaging evidence of continued bleeding may be candidates for local or systemic therapies to promote clotting, and trials to evaluate this possibility are under way.

The coagulation factors related to the occurrence and growth of hemorrhage remain unknown. Finding specific therapies to intervene in the acute period requires an understanding of the natural phenomena in patients with ICH. One study found that normal systemic hemostatic activation does not occur unless the cerebral hematoma extends into the ventricular system or subarachnoid space.[53] Platelet transfusions have not shown mortality or functional outcome benefit in the limited studies performed to date,[54] though additional studies of platelet transfusion are ongoing. AHA/ASA Guidelines suggest that the usefulness of platelet transfusions is considered unclear and their use is investigational (Class IIb Level of Evidence B).[3]

MANAGEMENT OF CEREBRAL EDEMA, HYDROCEPHALUS, AND INTRAVENTRICULAR HEMORRHAGE

Significant causes of mortality in ICH or IVH are cerebral edema and hydrocephalus. There are therapies for these conditions, and their results are mixed, as discussed here.

Cerebral Edema

Cerebral edema is a well-recognized complication of ICH. Whether the edema is due to an acute space-occupying lesion or the toxic effects of blood is unknown. An intriguing finding is that patients with thrombolysis-related ICH have far less cerebral edema than patients with spontaneous ICH,[55] suggesting that something in the clotting process may be directly responsible for development of cerebral edema. Mass effect and midline shift maximize around 48 hours after symptom onset and, perhaps, during a second peak 2–3 weeks after hemorrhage.[56] Despite the success of antiedema therapies in controlling ICP in animal models,[57] the therapeutic value of these agents has not been borne out in human studies. Two randomized trials of therapy for cerebral edema in patients with ICH have been performed. The first randomized 216 patients to intravenous glycerol or placebo.[58] There was no difference in 6-month mortality rates or functional outcomes between the two groups. A similar trial of hemodilution in ICH compared with the best medical therapy failed to demonstrate an advantage for hemodilution treatment.[59] A link between iron deposition, cerebral edema, and neuronal injury in ICH has been elucidated.[60,61] A pilot trial of iron chelation with deferoxamine in acute ICH demonstrated safety and tolerability,[62] and a larger-scale study is underway.[63] Animal models have also suggested that agonists of peroxisome proliferator-activated receptor gamma may be able to enhance hematoma resolution and reduce secondary injury after ICH, and preliminary human studies of pioglitazone are underway.[64,65]

Hydrocephalus and Intraventricular Hemorrhage

Hydrocephalus is an independent predictor of poor outcome from ICH or IVH.[66,67] It can occur because of obstruction of cerebrospinal fluid (CSF) flow in patients with ventricular clot or communicating hydrocephalus from a variety of causes. The treatment is placement of a ventriculostomy for external drainage of CSF and blood in the ventricular system as well as measurement of ICP. Ventricular drain should be considered for patients with hydrocephalus and decreased consciousness (Class IIa, Level B) or for those with extensive intraventricular hemorrhage, GCS ≤8, or transtentorial herniation (Class IIb, Level C).[3] The drain is usually set at 15 cm above the ear to facilitate drainage. The risk of infection rises with time, so a ventricular fluid specimen can be collected every other day for analysis to monitor cell count, differential cell counts, and glucose and protein levels as well as for bacterial culture. The drain should remain in place until the pressure returns to normal (<20 cm H_2O).

Often, when ventricular blood is copious, hydrocephalus becomes chronic, and the patient is drain-dependent. Conversion of the ventriculostomy to an internalized shunt must be timed properly. If the externalized shunt is internalized when too much blood still remains, there is the danger of blockage of the shunt by clotting. Waiting too long, however, raises the risk of ventriculitis. In general, when the CSF visually clears of blood and the CSF protein level has decreased toward the normal range, it is time to consider a shunt in a patient who cannot maintain a normal ICP after a trial of 7–10 days.

Observational studies suggest that external CSF drainage is associated with a 25% lower risk of death and poorer outcome than conservative treatment.[68] Unfortunately, no trials have been conducted to guide our management of hydrocephalus. Certainly, hydrocephalus is a treatable condition that leads to reductions in consciousness and therefore makes patients look more severely impaired. This appearance may lead to early withdrawal of life-sustaining treatments and the missed opportunity to intervene and help patients with ICH.[69]

An intriguing possibility for IVH is lysis of the clot in the ventricular system to improve hydrocephalus and accelerate reabsorption of blood products. A meta-analysis of observational and small randomized studies suggested a substantial reduction in mortality with intraventricular fibrinolysis using urokinase or tPA when compared to external ventricular drainage alone (pooled OR, 0.32; 95%CI, 0.19–0.52).[70] The favorable findings from these studies have prompted a larger trial of ventricular clot lysis that is currently under way, the Clot Lysis Evaluation of Accelerated Resolution of Intraventricular Hemorrhage (CLEAR-III) trial[71] though existing guidelines still cite this treatment as investigational (Class IIb, Level B).[3]

Intracranial Pressure Considerations

Cerebral edema and hydrocephalus are two causes of increased ICP. ICP must be maintained below 20 cm H_2O. To accomplish this goal, evaluation of the underlying cause of the elevation in ICP should proceed. If it is not possible to remove the underlying cause (e.g., surgical removal of the hematoma), management of elevated ICP, as discussed in detail in Chapter 54, is suggested.

Two experimental therapies may hold promise in the future for the management of cerebral edema and increased ICP. Hypothermia dramatically lowers ICP in animal models. Studies show impressive results of hypothermia in the form of improved neurologic outcome in patients who have experienced cardiac arrest.[72,73] One potential side effect of hypothermia is coagulopathy, so studies must be performed before this therapy can be advocated for ICH. The other therapy is hemicraniectomy and duraplasty. This treatment involves removing a large portion of the skull and making a broad incision in the dura to allow the brain to swell without added tissue pressure inside the enclosed skull cavity. Decompressive hemicraniectomy has been shown to be life-saving in malignant hemispheric ischemic stroke.[74] A series of small nonrandomized studies have suggested possible benefit for selected ICH patients, though no large randomized trials have been performed.[75]

SELECTION OF PATIENTS FOR SURGERY

Several small studies and two large studies have investigated surgical treatment of ICH. The best reported benefits for hematoma evacuation come from surgical removal of thrombolytic-related ICH. In an observational study, patients treated with surgery had a 65% 30-day survival, compared with a 35% survival for patients treated medically ($P <$ 0.001).[76] For patients with spontaneous hemorrhage, it seems that operating long after symptom onset does not improve outcome. The goals of early surgery are to reduce mortality and to improve functional outcome.[77] One randomized study of 20 patients treated within 24 hours of symptom onset found a non-significant trend toward better outcome in those treated medically.[78]

In a randomized trial of 34 patients undergoing either medical treatment or surgery within 12 hours of symptom onset for spontaneous supratentorial ICH, mortality was found to be 24% in the medical group and 19% in the surgical group (the difference was not statistically significant).[79] Functional outcome was unchanged. When these researchers added another surgical arm to the study, involving operation within 4 hours of symptom onset, they found that early post-operative rebleeding was a problem.[80] Figure 57-1 shows examples of a successful clot evacuation and an evacuation complicated by post-operative hematoma reaccumulation. Clearly, residual hematoma volume is directly related to poor outcome,[79] suggesting that if early surgery could be performed with good hemostasis, the procedure might be of benefit. Achieving hemostasis is probably related in part to the compulsiveness of the surgeon in identifying bleeding of microvessels and to careful coagulation.[81,82]

The international Surgical Trial for Intracerebral Hemorrhage (iSTICH) was a herculean effort using a randomized, controlled design to determine whether surgical clot removal was safe and effective.[83] The study found no difference in patients treated surgically and those receiving the best medical treatment. The study had several factors that may have diminished its ability to demonstrate a surgical benefit. Inclusion in the study and randomization to treatment occurred only in patients whom the surgeon was uncertain if they would benefit from surgery, rather than all eligible subjects. There were many crossovers between treatment arms, and, perhaps most problematic, operations occurred very late (24 hours) post ictus. In a subgroup analysis of iSTICH, patients with hematomas within 1 cm of the brain surface did better with surgery than with medical treatment. A second iSTICH, focusing on these superficial hematomas was completed and found no benefit in this subgroup either.[84] However, frequent crossovers and late surgery in many patients were also concerns in this second study. Despite the negative results of the iSTICH studies and other studies, there still may be a group of ICH patients who benefit from surgery, though determining who these individuals are remains a challenge.

Earlier attempts at synthesizing the evidence to determine the relative value of surgery in spontaneous supratentorial ICH usually concluded that the evidence was insufficient to allow any conclusions to be drawn.[85,86] A meta-analysis using original patient data found that early surgery (<8 hours) from symptom onset, moderate hematoma volume (20 to 50 cc), mild-to-moderate impairment (Glasgow Coma Scores between 9 and 12), and middle-age patients (50 and 69 years) were significantly associated with improved outcome with surgical hematoma evacuation.[87] Many clinicians consider clinical deterioration due to mass effect to be an indication for surgery, though this has not been formally addressed in randomized trials.

In the last version of the AHA/ASA ICH Guidelines, the usefulness of surgery was considered uncertain for most ICH patients (Class IIb; Level of Evidence: C).[3] Stereotactic and endoscopic approaches allow less disruption of tissue than open craniotomy for deep hemorrhages, but may not be able to remove enough hematoma volume in a timely manner (Class IIb, Level B). Stereotactic approaches coupled with local thrombolysis may be promising, but remain unproven (Class IIb, Level B).[3] The Minimally-Invasive Surgery Plus rtPA for Intracerebral Hemorrhage Evacuation (MISTIE) trial reported a beneficial effect on edema formation[88] using this combined approach. A pivotal trial is ongoing.[89]

For patients with infratentorial hemorrhage, the indications for surgery are different. Patients with cerebellar hemorrhage may experience brainstem compression syndromes quickly at any time within the first 3 weeks after the event. Surgical evacuation of the hematoma is therefore recommended for those with brainstem compression, neurological deterioration, or hydrocephalus from ventricular obstruction (Class I, Level B).[3] Patients recover well if the procedure is carried out at the earliest threat of brainstem compression, before frank herniation occurs.[90]

SPECIAL CONSIDERATIONS IN ANTICOAGULANT-RELATED INTRACRANIAL HEMORRHAGE

Warfarin-related ICH has higher mortality than non-warfarin-related ICH, likely due to both a higher initial hemorrhage volume and a greater risk of early hematoma expansion.[47,91,92] Ensuring that the bleeding has stopped is imperative. Vitamin K should be administered urgently (though it takes time to

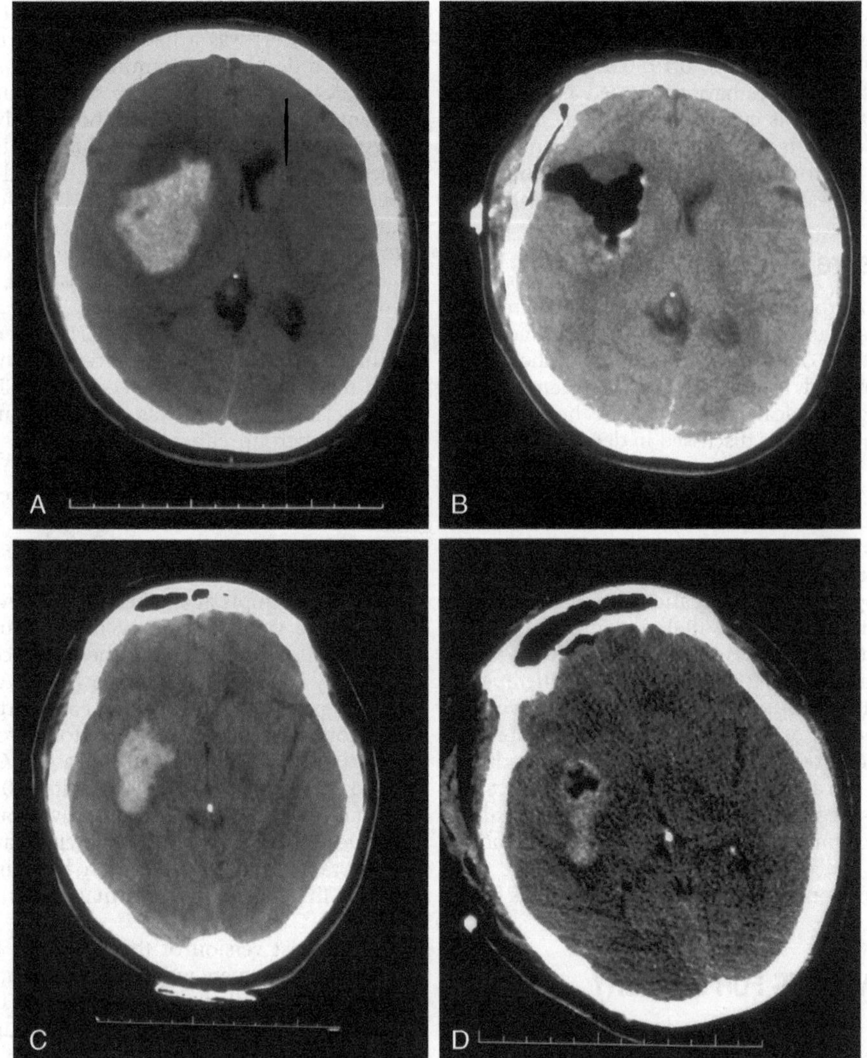

Figure 57-1. Surgical clot removal by craniotomy for intracranial hemorrhage within 4 hours of symptom onset in two patients. Baseline CT scan (A) and 24-hour post-operative CT scan (B) of the head of a patient in whom clot evacuation was successful. Dark areas in the hematoma cavity represent absorbable gelatin sponge (Gelfoam) and air, which subsequently were reabsorbed. Baseline CT scan (C) and 24-hour post-operative CT scan (D) of the head of a patient in whom hematoma regrowth occurred after clot evacuation.

work), and vitamin-K-dependent clotting factors should be repleted (Class I, Level C).[3] However, the best method for repletion of clotting factors remains uncertain. Fresh-frozen plasma (FFP) has been the traditional "gold standard" for warfarin reversal. However, prothrombin complex concentrate (PCC) has theoretical advantages of lower volume of infusion and no need for blood-type matching, though the risk of thrombotic complications may be higher. Non-randomized studies have suggested possible faster normalization of INR with PCC, though results on mortality have been mixed.[93-95] A prospective randomized study comparing PCC to FFP for treatment of major warfarin-related bleeding demonstrated that PCC was not inferior to FFP in terms of INR correction with a similar safety profile, though only 12% of patients in this study had ICH.[96] Specific studies of PCC versus FFP in ICH are ongoing.[97]

Recently, several novel oral anticoagulants (NOAC) have been approved for use in the treatment of atrial fibrillation or venous thromboembolism. Dabigatran, apixiban, and rivoroxaban have all been tested against warfarin in non-inferiority trials for treatment of atrial fibrillation.[98-100] All three of the NOACs have been found to have a lower risk of intracranial hemorrhage than warfarin. This lower risk of hemorrhage has to be balanced against the fact that methods to accurately monitor or reverse the anticoagulant effect of these medications are still under development. Despite the lack of a dedicated reversal agent, the risk of fatal or life-threatening bleeding appears to be lower with NOACs when compared with warfarin,[100-102] suggesting that theoretical concerns about lack of a reversal agent do not translate to excess mortality. There is no evidence to guide treatment for patients who sustain an ICH while on a NOAC, though blood pressure lowering is reasonable to potentially lower the risk of hematoma expansion.[103] Activated charcoal could be considered if the dose was given recently, and some authors have suggested use of PCC due to ease of administration,[103] though no randomized trials are available. Until more data are available, emergent consultation with hematology and pharmacy is probably indicated to individualize a reversal plan for each patient.

RESTARTING ANTITHROMBOTIC MEDICATIONS AFTER INTRACEREBRAL HEMORRHAGE

Determining whether to use antithrombotic medication (antiplatelet or anticoagulant therapy) after initial ICH is an important concern, because many patients with ICH are also at risk for ischemic stroke and myocardial infarction.[104] In general, for patients with a prior ICH, the risk of recurrent ICH is higher than the risk of recurrent ischemic stroke, particularly for the case of lobar hemorrhage, which has double the risk of recurrence when compared with non-lobar hemorrhage.[105] Therefore, most patients with ICH should probably have antithrombotic medications withheld in the future. However, the relative risk of ischemic vascular events versus recurrent hemorrhage likely varies considerably across individual patients, and some patients may be at very high risk of recurrent ischemic events. The presence of cerebral microbleeds may help to stratify the risk of recurrent ICH,[106] though precise thresholds for the number and location of microbleeds that would indicate that antithrombotic therapy is either safe or contraindicated have not been well established.

This issue is particularly challenging for patients at the highest risk of ischemic stroke, as is the case for mechanical heart valves or atrial fibrillation. NOACs may be a theoretically attractive option to consider for patients with atrial fibrillation and prior ICH, based on the lower risk of ICH compared to warfarin seen in clinical trials.[98–100] However, since patients with prior ICH were excluded from these studies it is not known if the lower risk of ICH extends to those with a known prior intracranial hemorrhage. A decision analysis of patients with non-valvular atrial fibrillation and ICH suggested that only those at lower risk of recurrent hemorrhage (e.g., deep ICH) who were at especially high risk for ischemic stroke should receive anticoagulation after an ICH.[107] Patients who restart anticoagulation after ICH are at a non-trivial risk of recurrent ICH, though withholding anticoagulation is associated with risk of thromboembolic events.[108–110] If anticoagulation is to be restarted after ICH, the optimal timing for resumption of anticoagulation is unknown. One observational study suggested that restarting warfarin between 10 and 30 weeks after ICH may optimally balance risks of recurrent ICH and thromboembolic events.[109] However, this decision of whether and when to restart anticoagulation remains a clinical judgment that should be individualized based on balancing the patient's estimated risks of hemorrhagic and ischemic events.

PREDICTORS OF OUTCOME AND WITHDRAWAL OF LIFE SUSTAINING TREATMENTS

Many researchers have developed prognostic models to help stratify the risk of death or disability after ICH. While the precise elements included in various prognostic models vary, common predictors in most models include age, level of clinical impairment (e.g., Glasgow Coma Scale or NIH Stroke Scale), and hematoma volume.[111–114] It is important to note that all of these prognostic models describe what happens on average to a group of patients, and they are not necessarily able to predict the future for any one individual.

Becker et al.[115] considered the role of withdrawal of life-sustaining treatments in patients with ICH. They found that the level of medical support was the most important predictor of outcome and that withdrawal of life support is likely to bias outcome data and lead to self-fulfilling prophecies. None of the commonly used ICH prognostic models have accounted for the intensity of treatment provided, leaving the existing models open to bias from these decisions made by physicians and families.[116,117] Therefore, it is difficult to know the true outcome of ICH if all available supportive treatments were offered.

Early do-not resuscitate orders (DNR) are very common after ICH, with about 25–35% of ICH patients having a DNR order written within the first day of admission.[118,119] Hemphill et al.[119] found that hospitals that use do not resuscitate (DNR) orders more frequently have worse ICH outcomes, even when data are controlled for individual patient factors. The AHA/ASA Guidelines suggest that clinicians not make new "do not resuscitate" orders for patients with ICH within the first 24 hours (Class IIa, Level B).[3] This recommendation reflects the true uncertainty we have regarding ICH outcome. Better methods are needed to help physicians and families work together to make decisions regarding the appropriate level of medical support to provide to patients with ICH. Measures of quality of life after ICH are important barometers of recovery and should guide future clinical trial results.[120]

CONCLUSIONS

Although ICH is a devastating disease, intensive medical therapy can make a large difference in outcome. Much of the therapy is "supportive," but it is also intensive and must be started urgently. A nihilistic approach to the care of patients with ICH is quickly dissipating. When life support is limited, recovery is all but impossible. Future studies of surgery, neuroprotection, and strategies to prevent hematoma expansion will likely revolutionize ICH therapy.

In the interim, meticulous attention to medical treatment and avoidance of complications of the patient with ICH is warranted. Control of blood pressure, treatment of fever, and glucose regulation are important. Patients with ICH or IVH should be cared for in specialized units with well-trained personnel. Early feeding and rehabilitation are also important. Prevention of complications such as pneumonia, ventriculitis, and deep vein thrombosis are necessary. Compulsive attention to these intensive medical therapies is of great value for the patient with ICH.

Acknowledgment

The authors would like to thank Dr. Venkatakrishna Rajajee for his review and comments on this chapter.

REFERENCES

1. Marti-Fabregas J, Piles S, Guardia E, et al. Spontaneous primary intraventricular hemorrhage: clinical data, etiology and outcome. J Neurol 1999;246:287–91.
2. Darby DG, Donnan GA, Saling MA, et al. Primary intraventricular hemorrhage: clinical and neuropsychological findings in a prospective stroke series. Neurology 1988;38:68–75.
3. Morgenstern LB, Hemphill JC 3rd, Anderson C, et al. Guidelines for the management of spontaneous intracerebral hemorrhage: a guideline for healthcare professionals from the American Heart Association/American Stroke Association. Stroke 2010;41:2108–29.
4. Langhorne P, Dennis M. Stroke units: an evidence based approach. London: BMJ Publishing Group; 1998.
5. Ronning OM, Guldvog B. Stroke units versus general medical wards, I: twelve- and eighteen-month survival: a randomized, controlled trial. Stroke 1998;29:58–62.
6. Ronning OM, Guldvog B. Stroke unit versus general medical wards, II: neurological deficits and activities of daily living: a quasi-randomized controlled trial. Stroke 1998;29:586–90.
7. Terent A, Asplund K, Farahmand B, et al. Stroke unit care revisited: who benefits the most? A cohort study of 105,043 patients in Riks-Stroke, the Swedish Stroke Register. J Neurol Neurosurg Psychiatry 2009;80:881–7.
8. Ronning OM, Guldvog B, Stavem K. The benefit of an acute stroke unit in patients with intracranial haemorrhage: a controlled trial. J Neurol Neurosurg Psychiatry 2001;70:631–4.

9. Diringer MN, Edwards DF. Admission to a neurologic/neurosurgical intensive care unit is associated with reduced mortality rate after intracerebral hemorrhage. Crit Care Med 2001;29:635–40.
10. Rincon F, Morino T, Behrens D, et al. Association between out-of-hospital emergency department transfer and poor hospital outcome in critically ill stroke patients. J Crit Care 2011;26:620–5.
11. Adeoye O, Haverbusch M, Woo D, et al. Is ED disposition associated with intracerebral hemorrhage mortality? Am J Emerg Med 2011;29(4):391–5.
12. Schwarz S, Hafner K, Aschoff A, et al. Incidence and prognostic significance of fever following intracerebral hemorrhage. Neurology 2000;54(2):354–61.
13. den Hertog HM, van der Worp HB, van Gemert HM, et al. The Paracetamol (Acetaminophen) In Stroke (PAIS) trial: a multicentre, randomised, placebo-controlled, phase III trial. Lancet Neurol 2009;8(5):434–40.
14. Azzimondi G, Bassein L, Nonino F, et al. Fever in acute stroke worsens prognosis. A prospective study. Stroke 1995;26(11): 2040–3.
15. Reith J, Jorgensen HS, Pedersen PM, et al. Body temperature in acute stroke: relation to stroke severity, infarct size, mortality, and outcome. Lancet 1996;347(8999):422–5.
16. Passero S, Ciacci G, Ulivelli M. The influence of diabetes and hyperglycemia on clinical course after intracerebral hemorrhage. Neurology 2003;61(10):1351–6.
17. Demchuk AM, Morgenstern LB, Krieger DW, et al. Serum glucose level and diabetes predict tissue plasminogen activator-related intracerebral hemorrhage in acute ischemic stroke. Stroke 1999; 30(1):34–9.
18. Gray CS, Hildreth AJ, Sandercock PA, et al. Glucose-potassium-insulin infusions in the management of post-stroke hyperglycaemia: the UK Glucose Insulin in Stroke Trial (GIST-UK). Lancet Neurol 2007;6(5):397–406.
19. Tiemessen CA, Hoedemaekers CW, van Iersel FM, et al. Intensive insulin therapy increases the risk of hypoglycemia in neurocritical care patients. J Neurosurg Anesthesiol 2011;23(3): 206–14.
20. Qureshi AI, Wilson DA, Hanley DF, et al. Pharmacologic reduction of mean arterial pressure does not adversely affect regional cerebral blood flow and intracranial pressure in experimental intracerebral hemorrhage. Crit Care Med 1999;27(5):965–71.
21. Hirano T, Read SJ, Abbott DF, et al. No evidence of hypoxic tissue on 18F-fluoromisonidazole PET after intracerebral hemorrhage. Neurology 1999;53(9):2179–82.
22. Powers WJ, Zazulia AR, Videen TO, et al. Autoregulation of cerebral blood flow surrounding acute (6 to 22 hours) intracerebral hemorrhage. Neurology 2001;57(1):18–24.
23. Anderson CS, Huang Y, Wang JG, et al. Intensive blood pressure reduction in acute cerebral haemorrhage trial (INTERACT): a randomised pilot trial. Lancet Neurol 2008;7(5):391–9.
24. Anderson CS, Heeley E, Huang Y, et al. Rapid blood-pressure lowering in patients with acute intracerebral hemorrhage. N Engl J Med 2013;368(25):2355–65.
25. Antihypertensive Treatment of Acute Cerebral Hemorrhage (ATACH) investigators. Antihypertensive treatment of acute cerebral hemorrhage. Crit Care Med 2010;38(2):637–48.
26. Qureshi AI, Palesch YY. Antihypertensive Treatment of Acute Cerebral Hemorrhage (ATACH) II: design, methods, and rationale. Neurocrit Care 2011;15:559–76.
27. Prabhakaran S, Gupta R, Ouyang B, et al. Acute brain infarcts after spontaneous intracerebral hemorrhage: a diffusion-weighted imaging study. Stroke 2010;41(1):89–94.
28. Kuroda K, Kuwata N, Sato N, et al. Changes in cerebral blood flow accompanied with reduction of blood pressure treatment in patients with hypertensive intracerebral hemorrhages. Neurol Res 1997;19(2):169–73.
29. Patel RV, Kertland HR, Jahns BE, et al. Labetalol: response and safety in critically ill hemorrhagic stroke patients. Ann Pharmacother 1993;27(2):180–1.
30. Dennis M, Sandercock P, Reid J, et al. Effectiveness of intermittent pneumatic compression in reduction of risk of deep vein thrombosis in patients who have had a stroke (CLOTS 3): a multicentre randomised controlled trial. Lancet 2013;382(9891):516–24.
31. Dennis M, Sandercock PA, Reid J, et al. Effectiveness of thigh-length graduated compression stockings to reduce the risk of deep vein thrombosis after stroke (CLOTS trial 1): a multicentre, randomised controlled trial. Lancet 2009;373(9679): 1958–65.
32. CLOTS (Clots in Legs Or sTockings after Stroke) Trial Collaboration. Thigh-length versus below-knee stockings for deep venous thrombosis prophylaxis after stroke: a randomized trial. Ann Intern Med 2010;153(9):553–62.
33. Kahn SR, Lim W, Dunn AS, et al. Prevention of VTE in nonsurgical patients: Antithrombotic Therapy and Prevention of Thrombosis, 9th ed: American College of Chest Physicians Evidence-Based Clinical Practice Guidelines. Chest 2012;141(2 Suppl.):e195S–226S.
34. Qaseem A, Chou R, Humphrey LL, et al. Venous thromboembolism prophylaxis in hospitalized patients: a clinical practice guideline from the American College of Physicians. Ann Intern Med 2011;155(9):625–32.
35. Sherman DG, Albers GW, Bladin C, et al. The efficacy and safety of enoxaparin versus unfractionated heparin for the prevention of venous thromboembolism after acute ischaemic stroke (PREVAIL Study): an open-label randomised comparison. Lancet 2007;369(9570):1347–55.
36. Poungvarin N, Bhoopat W, Viriyavejakul A, et al. Effects of dexamethasone in primary supratentorial intracerebral hemorrhage. New Eng J Med 1987;316(20):1229–33.
37. Tellez H, Bauer RB. Dexamethasone as treatment in cerebrovascular disease. 1. A controlled study in intracerebral hemorrhage. Stroke 1973;4(4):541–6.
38. Claassen J, Taccone FS, Horn P, et al. Recommendations on the use of EEG monitoring in critically ill patients: consensus statement from the neurointensive care section of the ESICM. Intensive Care Med 2013;39(8):1337–51.
39. Sykes L, Wood E, Kwan J. Antiepileptic drugs for the primary and secondary prevention of seizures after stroke. Cochrane Database Syst Rev 2014;(1):CD005398.
40. Gilad R, Boaz M, Dabby R, et al. Are post intracerebral hemorrhage seizures prevented by anti-epileptic treatment? Epilepsy Res 2011;95(3):227–31. [Epub 2011/06/03. eng]; PubMed PMID: 21632213.
41. Naidech AM, Garg RK, Liebling S, et al. Anticonvulsant use and outcomes after intracerebral hemorrhage. Stroke 2009;40(12): 3810–15.
42. Messe SR, Sansing LH, Cucchiara BL, et al. Prophylactic antiepileptic drug use is associated with poor outcome following ICH. Neurocrit Care 2009;11(1):38–44.
43. Marik PE, Vasu T, Hirani A, et al. Stress ulcer prophylaxis in the new millennium: a systematic review and meta-analysis. Crit Care Med 2010;38(11):2222–8.
44. Fujii Y, Tanaka R, Takeuchi S, et al. Hematoma enlargement in spontaneous intracerebral hemorrhage. J Neurosurg 1994;80(1): 51–7.
45. Kazui S, Naritomi H, Yamamoto H, et al. Enlargement of spontaneous intracerebral hemorrhage. Incidence and time course. Stroke 1996;27(10):1783–7.
46. Brott T, Broderick J, Kothari R, et al. Early hemorrhage growth in patients with intracerebral hemorrhage. Stroke 1997;28(1): 1–5.
47. Flibotte JJ, Hagan N, O'Donnell J, et al. Warfarin, hematoma expansion, and outcome of intracerebral hemorrhage. Neurology 2004;63(6):1059–64.
48. Mayer SA, Brun NC, Begtrup K, et al. Recombinant activated factor VII for acute intracerebral hemorrhage. N Engl J Med 2005;352(8):777–85.
49. Mayer SA, Brun NC, Begtrup K, et al. Efficacy and safety of recombinant activated factor VII for acute intracerebral hemorrhage. N Engl J Med 2008;358(20):2127–37.
50. Becker KJ, Baxter AB, Bybee HM, et al. Extravasation of radiographic contrast is an independent predictor of death in primary intracerebral hemorrhage. Stroke 1999;30(10): 2025–32.
51. Murai Y, Ikeda Y, Teramoto A, et al. Magnetic resonance imaging-documented extravasation as an indicator of acute hypertensive intracerebral hemorrhage. J Neurosurg 1998;88(4):650–5.
52. Boulouis G, Dumas A, Betensky RA, et al. Anatomic pattern of intracerebral hemorrhage expansion: relation to ct angiography spot sign and hematoma center. Stroke 2014;45:1154–6.

53. Fujii Y, Takeuchi S, Harada A, et al. Hemostatic activation in spontaneous intracerebral hemorrhage. Stroke 2001;32(4):883–90.
54. Martin M, Conlon LW. Does platelet transfusion improve outcomes in patients with spontaneous or traumatic intracerebral hemorrhage? Ann Emerg Med 2013;61(1):58–61.
55. Gebel JM, Brott TG, Sila CA, et al. Decreased perihematomal edema in thrombolysis-related intracerebral hemorrhage compared with spontaneous intracerebral hemorrhage. Stroke 2000; 31(3):596–600.
56. Zazulia AR, Diringer MN, Derdeyn CP, et al. Progression of mass effect after intracerebral hemorrhage. Stroke 1999;30(6): 1167–73.
57. Qureshi AI, Wilson DA, Traystman RJ. Treatment of elevated intracranial pressure in experimental intracerebral hemorrhage: comparison between mannitol and hypertonic saline. Neurosurgery 1999;44(5):1055–63.
58. Yu YL, Kumana CR, Lauder IJ, et al. Treatment of acute cerebral hemorrhage with intravenous glycerol. A double-blind, placebo-controlled, randomized trial. Stroke 1992;23(7):967–71.
59. Italian Acute Stroke Study Group. Haemodilution in acute stroke: results of the Italian haemodilution trial. Lancet 1988; 1(8581):318–21.
60. Huang FP, Xi G, Keep RF, et al. Brain edema after experimental intracerebral hemorrhage: role of hemoglobin degradation products. J Neurosurg 2002;96(2):287–93.
61. Nakamura T, Keep RF, Hua Y, et al. Deferoxamine-induced attenuation of brain edema and neurological deficits in a rat model of intracerebral hemorrhage. Neurosurg Focus 2003;15(4): ECP4.
62. Selim M, Yeatts S, Goldstein JN, et al. Safety and tolerability of deferoxamine mesylate in patients with acute intracerebral hemorrhage. Stroke 2011;42(11):3067–74.
63. Yeatts SD, Palesch YY, Moy CS, et al. High dose deferoxamine in intracerebral hemorrhage (HI-DEF) trial: rationale, design, and methods. Neurocrit Care 2013;19(2):257–66.
64. Gonzales NR, Shah J, Sangha N, et al. Design of a prospective, dose-escalation study evaluating the Safety of Pioglitazone for Hematoma Resolution in Intracerebral Hemorrhage (SHRINC). Int J Stroke 2013;8(5):388–96.
65. Zhao X, Sun G, Zhang J, et al. Hematoma resolution as a target for intracerebral hemorrhage treatment: role for peroxisome proliferator-activated receptor gamma in microglia/macrophages. Ann Neurol 2007;61(4):352–62.
66. Diringer MN, Edwards DF, Zazulia AR. Hydrocephalus: a previously unrecognized predictor of poor outcome from supratentorial intracerebral hemorrhage. Stroke 1998;29(7):1352–7.
67. Phan TG, Koh M, Vierkant RA, et al. Hydrocephalus is a determinant of early mortality in putaminal hemorrhage. Stroke 2000;31(9):2157–62.
68. Nieuwkamp DJ, de Gans K, Rinkel GJ, et al. Treatment and outcome of severe intraventricular extension in patients with subarachnoid or intracerebral hemorrhage: a systematic review of the literature. J Neurol 2000;247(2):117–21.
69. Zahuranec DB, Gonzales NR, Brown DL, et al. Presentation of intracerebral haemorrhage in a community. J Neurol Neurosurg Psychiatry 2006;77(3):340–4.
70. Gaberel T, Magheru C, Parienti JJ, et al. Intraventricular fibrinolysis versus external ventricular drainage alone in intraventricular hemorrhage: a meta-analysis. Stroke 2011;42(10):2776–81.
71. Ziai WC, Tuhrim S, Lane K, et al. A multicenter, randomized, double-blinded, placebo-controlled phase III study of Clot Lysis Evaluation of Accelerated Resolution of Intraventricular Hemorrhage (CLEAR III). Int J Stroke 2014;9:536–942.
72. Hypothermia after Cardiac Arrest Study Group. Mild therapeutic hypothermia to improve the neurologic outcome after cardiac arrest. N Engl J Med 2002;346(8):549–56.
73. Bernard SA, Gray TW, Buist MD, et al. Treatment of comatose survivors of out-of-hospital cardiac arrest with induced hypothermia. N Engl J Med 2002;346(8):557–63.
74. Vahedi K, Hofmeijer J, Juettler E, et al. Early decompressive surgery in malignant infarction of the middle cerebral artery: a pooled analysis of three randomised controlled trials. Lancet Neurol 2007;6(3):215–22. [Epub 2007/02/17. eng]; PubMed PMID: 17303527.
75. Takeuchi S, Wada K, Nagatani K, et al. Decompressive hemicraniectomy for spontaneous intracerebral hemorrhage. Neurosurg Focus 2013;34(5):E5.
76. Mahaffey KW, Granger CB, Sloan MA, et al. Neurosurgical evacuation of intracranial hemorrhage after thrombolytic therapy for acute myocardial infarction: experience from the GUSTO-I trial. Global Utilization of Streptokinase and tissue-plasminogen activator (tPA) for Occluded Coronary Arteries. Am Heart J 1999; 138(3 Pt 1):493–9.
77. Fujitsu K, Muramoto M, Ikeda Y, et al. Indications for surgical treatment of putaminal hemorrhage. Comparative study based on serial CT and time-course analysis. J Neurosurg 1990;73(4): 518–25.
78. Zuccarello M, Brott T, Derex L, et al. Early surgical treatment for supratentorial intracerebral hemorrhage: a randomized feasibility study. Stroke 1999;30(9):1833–9.
79. Morgenstern LB, Frankowski RF, Shedden P, et al. Surgical treatment for intracerebral hemorrhage (STICH): a single-center, randomized clinical trial. Neurology 1998;51(5):1359–63.
80. Morgenstern LB, Demchuk AM, Kim DH, et al. Rebleeding leads to poor outcome in ultra-early craniotomy for intracerebral hemorrhage. Neurology 2001;56(10):1294–9.
81. Kaneko M, Koba T, Yokoyama T. Early surgical treatment for hypertensive intracerebral hemorrhage. J Neurosurg 1977;46(5): 579–83.
82. Kaneko M, Tanaka K, Shimada T, et al. Long-term evaluation of ultra-early operation for hypertensive intracerebral hemorrhage in 100 cases. J Neurosurg 1983;58(6):838–42.
83. Mendelow AD, Gregson BA, Fernandes HM, et al. Early surgery versus initial conservative treatment in patients with spontaneous supratentorial intracerebral haematomas in the International Surgical Trial in Intracerebral Haemorrhage (STICH): a randomised trial. Lancet 2005;365(9457):387–97.
84. Mendelow AD, Gregson BA, Rowan EN, et al. Early surgery versus initial conservative treatment in patients with spontaneous supratentorial lobar intracerebral haematomas (STICH II): a randomised trial. Lancet 2013;382(9890):397–408.
85. Hankey GJ, Hon C. Surgery for primary intracerebral hemorrhage: is it safe and effective? A systematic review of case series and randomized trials. Stroke 1997;28(11):2126–32.
86. Prasad K, Browman G, Srivastava A, et al. Surgery in primary supratentorial intracerebral hematoma: a meta-analysis of randomized trials. Acta Neurol Scand 1997;95(2):103–10.
87. Gregson BA, Broderick JP, Auer LM, et al. Individual patient data subgroup meta-analysis of surgery for spontaneous supratentorial intracerebral hemorrhage. Stroke 2012;43(6): 1496–504.
88. Mould WA, Carhuapoma JR, Muschelli J, et al. Minimally invasive surgery plus recombinant tissue-type plasminogen activator for intracerebral hemorrhage evacuation decreases perihematomal edema. Stroke 2013;44(3):627–34.
89. MISTIE-II Clinical Trial [March 16, 2013]. Available from: http://braininjuryoutcomes.com/mistie-about.
90. Montes JM, Wong JH, Fayad PB, et al. Stereotactic computed tomographic-guided aspiration and thrombolysis of intracerebral hematoma: protocol and preliminary experience. Stroke 2000;31(4):834–40.
91. Rosand J, Eckman MH, Knudsen KA, et al. The effect of warfarin and intensity of anticoagulation on outcome of intracerebral hemorrhage. Arch Intern Med 2004;164(8):880–4.
92. Cucchiara B, Messe S, Sansing L, et al. Hematoma growth in oral anticoagulant related intracerebral hemorrhage. Stroke 2008;39(11):2993–6. [Epub 2008/08/16. eng]; PubMed PMID: 18703803.
93. Majeed A, Meijer K, Larrazabal R, et al. Mortality in vitamin K antagonist-related intracerebral bleeding treated with plasma or 4-factor prothrombin complex concentrate. Thromb Haemost 2014;111(2):233–9.
94. Hanger HC, Geddes JA, Wilkinson TJ, et al. Warfarin-related intracerebral haemorrhage: better outcomes when reversal includes prothrombin complex concentrates. Intern Med J 2013;43(3):308–16.
95. Dowlatshahi D, Butcher KS, Asdaghi N, et al. Poor prognosis in warfarin-associated intracranial hemorrhage despite anticoagulation reversal. Stroke 2012;43(7):1812–17.

57

96. Sarode R, Milling TJ Jr, Refaai MA, et al. Efficacy and safety of a 4-factor prothrombin complex concentrate in patients on vitamin K antagonists presenting with major bleeding: a randomized, plasma-controlled, phase IIIb study. Circulation 2013; 128(11):1234–43.
97. Steiner T, Freiberger A, Griebe M, et al. International normalised ratio normalisation in patients with coumarin-related intracranial haemorrhages–the INCH trial: a randomised controlled multicentre trial to compare safety and preliminary efficacy of fresh frozen plasma and prothrombin complex–study design and protocol. Int J Stroke 2011;6(3):271–7.
98. Patel MR, Mahaffey KW, Garg J, et al. Rivaroxaban versus warfarin in nonvalvular atrial fibrillation. N Engl J Med 2011;365(10): 883–91.
99. Granger CB, Alexander JH, McMurray JJ, et al. Apixaban versus warfarin in patients with atrial fibrillation. N Engl J Med 2011; 365(11):981–92.
100. Connolly SJ, Ezekowitz MD, Yusuf S, et al. Dabigatran versus warfarin in patients with atrial fibrillation. N Engl J Med 2009; 361(12):1139–51.
101. Wasserlauf G, Grandi SM, Filion KB, et al. Meta-analysis of rivaroxaban and bleeding risk. Am J Cardiol 2013;112(3):454–60.
102. Halvorsen S, Atar D, Yang H, et al. Efficacy and safety of apixaban compared with warfarin according to age for stroke prevention in atrial fibrillation: observations from the ARISTOTLE trial. Eur Heart J 2014;35:1864–72.
103. Steiner T, Bohm M, Dichgans M, et al. Recommendations for the emergency management of complications associated with the new direct oral anticoagulants (DOACs), apixaban, dabigatran and rivaroxaban. Clin Res Cardiol 2013;102(6):399–412.
104. Vermeer SE, Algra A, Franke CL, et al. Long-term prognosis after recovery from primary intracerebral hemorrhage. Neurology 2002;59(2):205–9.
105. Bailey RD, Hart RG, Benavente O, et al. Recurrent brain hemorrhage is more frequent than ischemic stroke after intracranial hemorrhage. Neurology 2001;56:773–7.
106. Biffi A, Halpin A, Towfighi A, et al. Aspirin and recurrent intracerebral hemorrhage in cerebral amyloid angiopathy. Neurology 2010;75(8):693–8.
107. Eckman MH, Rosand J, Knudsen KA, et al. Can patients be anticoagulated after intracerebral hemorrhage? A decision analysis. Stroke 2003;34(7):1710–16.
108. Poli D, Antonucci E, Dentali F, et al. Recurrence of ICH after resumption of anticoagulation with VK antagonists: CHIRONE Study. Neurology 2014.
109. Majeed A, Kim YK, Roberts RS, et al. Optimal timing of resumption of warfarin after intracranial hemorrhage. Stroke 2010; 41(12):2860–6.
110. Claassen DO, Kazemi N, Zubkov AY, et al. Restarting anticoagulation therapy after warfarin-associated intracerebral hemorrhage. Arch Neurol 2008;65(10):1313–18.
111. Broderick JP, Brott TG, Duldner JE, et al. Volume of intracerebral hemorrhage. A powerful and easy-to-use predictor of 30-day mortality. Stroke 1993;24(7):987–93.
112. Hemphill JC 3rd, Bonovich DC, Besmertis L, et al. The ICH score: a simple, reliable grading scale for intracerebral hemorrhage. Stroke 2001;32(4):891–7.
113. Rost NS, Smith EE, Chang Y, et al. Prediction of functional outcome in patients with primary intracerebral hemorrhage: the FUNC score. Stroke 2008;39(8):2304–9.
114. Weimar C, Benemann J, Diener HC. Development and validation of the Essen Intracerebral Haemorrhage Score. J Neurol Neurosurg Psychiatry 2006;77(5):601–5.
115. Becker KJ, Baxter AB, Cohen WA, et al. Withdrawal of support in intracerebral hemorrhage may lead to self-fulfilling prophecies. Neurology 2001;56(6):766–72.
116. Creutzfeldt CJ, Becker KJ, Weinstein JR, et al. Do-not-attempt-resuscitation orders and prognostic models for intraparenchymal hemorrhage. Crit Care Med 2011;39(1):158–62.
117. Zahuranec DB, Morgenstern LB, Sanchez BN, et al. Do-not-resuscitate orders and predictive models after intracerebral hemorrhage. Neurology 2010;75(7):626–33.
118. Zahuranec DB, Brown DL, Lisabeth LD, et al. Early care limitations independently predict mortality after intracerebral hemorrhage. Neurology 2007;68(20):1651–7.
119. Hemphill JC 3rd, Newman J, Zhao S, et al. Hospital usage of early do-not-resuscitate orders and outcome after intracerebral hemorrhage. Stroke 2004;35(5):1130–4.
120. Hamedani AG, Wells CK, Brass LM, et al. A quality-of-life instrument for young hemorrhagic stroke patients. Stroke 2001;32(3): 687–95.

58 Rehabilitation and Recovery of the Patient with Stroke

Bruce H. Dobkin

KEY POINTS

- Neurologic rehabilitation strategies draw upon basic mechanisms of learning and memory.
- The reacquisition of skills depends on experience- and training-induced synaptic reorganization, as well as behavioral compensation.
- Many preventable and reversible medical complications may impede progress toward lessening impairments, disabilities, and a return to more normal participation in daily life.
- Focused, progressive, task-related, intensive practice clearly improves outcomes for cognitive, language, and motor skills.
- Whereas most of the major improvements in walking and self-care occur within the first 3–4 months after stroke, further gains in speed, endurance, accuracy, and strength can be accomplished with additional practice of desired motor skills and exercise at any time after stroke.

The rehabilitation of the patient with stroke aims to lessen physical and cognitive impairments, increase functional independence, lessen the burden of care provided by significant others, reintegrate the patient into the family and community, and restore the patient's health-related quality of life. Rehabilitation differs from usual neurologic care in that its long-term goal is to lessen disability and to give patients the opportunity to participate in their typical roles and activities. Strategies for neurologic rehabilitation draw heavily from the neuroscientific bases for learning and training-induced neuroplasticity. Increasingly, information gleaned from the molecular, physiologic, genetic, cellular, and neural network signaling cascades post stroke are providing insights into what may promote and what may limit neural adaptations for recovery.

Physicians who consider the management of stroke a "done deal" beyond the first few days after a disabling brain injury are abandoning their obligation to provide best patient care. Along with offering interventions to prevent another stroke, stroke neurologists and other clinicians who treat acute stroke ought to be familiar with the short-term and long-term interventions that may prevent complications of immobility, reduce impairments and disabilities, and improve quality of life for their patients. Specialized scales to assess these aspects of recovery are described in Chapter 21.

MECHANISMS FOR GAINS

A decrease in impairments and disabilities over the first 3–6 months after a stroke is often called *spontaneous recovery*. Resolution of edema, heme, ion fluxes, cell and axon physiologic dysfunction, and diaschisis from transsynaptic and neurotransmitter dysfunction may lead to *restitutive* intrinsic biologic activity that augments gains in the first month or so. Rehabilitation interventions may aim for *substitutive* extrinsic drives to manipulate biologic activity.[1] The multilevel effects of activity-dependent plasticity associated with practice and skills learning have become increasingly clear from molecular, electrophysiologic, and morphologic studies in recovering animals as well as from functional neuroimaging studies in humans.[2,3] Patients make gains by experience-driven or training-induced changes within partially spared pathways, within flexible neuronal assemblies that represent movements, sensation, and cognition, and within multiple representational maps in parallel, distributed networks. In recent years, new modalities to facilitate or modulate these pathways in combination with skills practice have come into clinical trials, including repetitive transcranial magnetic stimulation (TMS) or transcranial direct cortical stimulation (tDCS), drugs that may act on targets for learning and memory, and drugs, vectors and cellular interventions for neuromodulation and tissue repair.

Rehabilitation approaches also emphasize *compensatory strategies* for impairments and disabilities. Patients are trained to substitute a latent skill, learn a new way to accomplish a goal, alter the environment to make a task easier, or change their expectations about performing a particular task. Most compensatory approaches require learning, and gains may be reflected in experience-dependent plasticity.

The optimal duration and intensity of training are uncertain for human rehabilitation strategies. More intensive, task-oriented practice seems to enhance learning and performance.[4] Most patients, however, receive no more than a few months of formal inpatient and outpatient retraining. *Intensive rehabilitation* often amounts to less than 20 hours of engagement in physical, occupational, or speech therapy across many tasks. This modest amount of practice may be far less than what is needed to, say, regain the ability to walk at a speed that permits community activities or to improve word-finding skills.

ASSESSING IMPAIRMENT, DISABILITY, ACTIVITY, AND QUALITY OF LIFE

Outcome measurements that are unique to stroke rehabilitation emphasize ordinal scales that reflect changes in self-care and community-related activities and burden of caregiving. The Barthel Index (BI) and the Functional Independence Measure (FIM) are commonly used for the semi-quantification of the level of independence in activities of daily living (ADLs). On admission to inpatient rehabilitation, the majority of patients have a moderate level of disability, with a BI of 40–60 or a total FIM score of 40–80 with a mean of 60 (Table 58-1). These scales do not reflect fine motor function, the quality and time of execution of a skill, or whether an affected upper extremity is used to carry it out. Patients who score 100 on the

TABLE 58-1 Metrics for First Admission for Inpatient Stroke Rehabilitation Based on National Results (419,823 Patients) Reported by the Uniform Data System for Medical Rehabilitation (Accessed 09/16/13)

Functional Independence Measure subscores (0–7 per item)	At Admission	At Discharge
Self-care (6 items; max 42)	20.0	30.4
Sphincter (2 items)	7.7	10.2
Mobility (3 items)	8.3	13.8
Locomotion (2 items)	3.7	8.1
Communication (2 items)	8.9	10.9
Social cognition (3 items)	12.0	15.3
Total	60.6	88.7
PATIENT CHARACTERISTICS		
Age (years)	70	
Onset (days)	12	
Stay (days)		13.5
LIVING SITE (%)		
Community		78
Long-term care		7.1
Acute care		9.6

(FIM scale: 1 = total assistance, 4 = minimal contact help, 7 = completely independent.)

BI or more than 60 on the motor subscore of the FIM are usually continent and can feed, bathe, and dress themselves; get up out of bed and chairs; ambulate household distances; and ascend and descend stairs. A maximum score does not imply that they can cook, keep house, live alone, and meet the public, but they usually get along without attendant care. A BI of less than 60 at hospital discharge predicts a level of dependence that makes discharge to home less likely.

A general relationship exists between motor impairment and disability scores. The Fugl-Meyer Assessment of Sensorimotor Recovery tests for selective versus synergistic movements and is often used in trials for rehabilitation interventions and is particularly useful for assessing the upper extremity and thus dividing patients into groups of mild, moderate, and severe. The NIHSS score also describes the severity of impairment observed during inpatient stroke rehabilitation, but it is less sensitive to changes beyond 3 months in relationship to gains in ADLs.

Health-related quality of life (QOL), which includes a patient's perception of physical functioning as well as mental, psychosocial, and emotional state, has been measured most often with the Sickness Index Profile and the Medical Outcomes Study Short Form-36. Caregiver strain may be another dimension of QOL for the patient and family.[9,10] The Stroke Impact Scale (SIS) is a self-report measure with 64 items (a short form includes 16) that assess eight domains and covers strength, hand function, ADLs, instrumental ADLs, mobility, communication, memory, emotion, thinking, and participation. Its reliability, validity, responsiveness, and clinically meaningful changes are well described,[5] but self-reports may over- and under-state ground truth. The Neuro-QOL includes many additional instruments.[6]

Organization of Services

Patients who are at a supervised or minimally assisted level of self-care are usually discharged from the acute hospital setting to the home with either home health or outpatient therapy.[7] By the end of the first 2 weeks after a stroke, from 12% to 20% of patients in the US are referred for inpatient rehabilitation. These patients must need ongoing supervision by physicians and nurses, have enough stamina to participate in rehabilitation therapies for at least 3 hours a day, and have adequate psychosocial supports, so the rehabilitation team can anticipate discharge to the home or to a board-and-care facility. Further criteria include adequate motivation and cognition for learning. Patients who do not meet these criteria may receive therapies in a skilled nursing facility.

Although the issue is difficult to study formally, the literature suggests that the earlier the initiation of an inpatient rehabilitation program (within 20 days of onset of stroke, compared with 20–60 days in subjects with similar levels of disability), the better the outcomes. Length of stay in inpatient rehabilitation is determined during weekly conferences in which the team reassesses the patient's progress toward reasonable functional goals. In the US, the average stay has gradually fallen to about 14 days compared to 20 days early in this century. Patients often need appropriate durable medical equipment, such as a lightweight wheelchair, a cane, an ankle-foot-orthosis (AFO), and a tub bench, along with follow-up medical and disability-oriented community care.

The milieu of a dedicated stroke unit that provides rehabilitation or of a dedicated rehabilitation unit appears to improve outcomes, partly from the focus on prevention of medical complications related to immobility, on retraining functional activities, on family training, on the intensity of retraining skills, on early recognition of mood disorders, and on organizing outpatient follow-up.[8] An intention-to-treat randomized trial with 250 subjects showed that rehabilitation on an inpatient unit after a brief stay in an acute stroke unit or general medical ward produced better outcomes in moderate to severely disabled patients (BI < 50) than rehabilitation treatment in the community.[9]

Community mobility, cooking and cleaning skills, leisure activities, social isolation, and support for caregivers often continue to be problematic for 2-year survivors of a stroke. The clinician should ask about instrumental ADLs and mobility during chronic care. A short added pulse of therapy focused on training specific skills such as walking and using the affected arm, may improve what has been practiced, given the gains noted in most randomized clinical trials (RCTs) of interventions carried out beyond 1 year after stroke.

REHABILITATION-RELATED MEDICAL COMPLICATIONS

During inpatient rehabilitation, about one-third of patients have a urinary tract infection, urinary retention, musculoskeletal pain, or depression. Up to 20% fall, experience a rash, or need continuous management of blood pressure, hydration, nutrition, or glucose levels. About 10% have a transient toxic-metabolic encephalopathy, pneumonia, cardiac arrhythmias, pressure sores, or thrombophlebitis. Up to 5% have a pulmonary embolus, seizures, gastrointestinal bleeding, heart failure, or other medical complications. Beyond inpatient care, bowel and bladder dysfunction, pain-induced spasticity, and other complications require ongoing vigilance.

Bladder Dysfunction

Urinary incontinence occurs in up to 60% of patients in the first week after a stroke, but the rate tends to decline to less than 25% at hospital discharge without a specific medical treatment.[42] Across studies, about 18% of those who were incontinent at 6 weeks after stroke are still so at 1 year. Urinary tract infections develop in about 40% of patients during acute stroke and rehabilitation care. Persistent lack of bladder control is often secondary to an unstable detrusor muscle or to detrusor-sphincter dyssynergia.[43]

TABLE 58-2 Pharmacologic Manipulation of Bladder Dysfunction

Medication and Dosage	Indication	Mechanism of Action
Bethanechol, 25 mg bid to 50 mg qid	Facilitate emptying	Increase detrusor contraction
Prazosin, 1 mg bid to 2 mg tid	Decrease outlet obstruction	Alpha blockade of external sphincter to decrease tone
Tamsulosin, 0.4 mg qd	Prostatic hypertrophy	
Oxybutinin, 2.5 mg hs to 5 mg qid	Urge incontinence	Relax detrusor; increase internal sphincter tone
Tolterodine, 2 mg bid	Frequency	
Imipramine, 25–50 mg hs	Urge incontinence Enuresis	Increase internal sphincter tone; decrease detrusor contractions

Evidence for all interventions: IIa, B.
For more details refer to "Evidence box index" in the FM.

In patients with retention of urine volumes greater than 250 mL, intermittent bladder catheterization with a clean technique probably lessens the risk of an infection, although there is little evidence for this claim. Perineal cleanliness should lessen the risk of infection by fecal contamination. Most patients with incontinence after a hemispheric stroke either have a small bladder and are unable to suppress the micturition reflex or become aware of filling too late to void in a urinal, commode, or toilet. Scheduled voiding is one good approach. Urodynamic testing, usually not performed as an inpatient, may point to an abnormality of urine filling and storage, bladder emptying, or a combination of both, making the choice of medication more rational (Table 58-2). Use of an anticholinergic agent such as 5 mg of oxybutynin before sleep may allow greater filling and less urgency or incontinence overnight. Medications may reduce outlet obstruction in men, but prostate surgery may be indicated for a stable outpatient.

Musculoskeletal and Central Pain

Pain is common after a stroke and can limit participation in therapy. Central pain may become a major source of disability, especially after a thalamoparietal stroke, but affects fewer than 5%. Some patients only need assurance that the pain or dysesthesia does not represent a serious complication or a warning signal of another stroke.

Shoulder pain in the hemiparetic arm develops in 5–50% of patients in different studies. Pain exacerbates hypertonicity and may trigger flexor and extensor spasms and dystonic postures. Physical modalities, analgesics, anti-inflammatory agents, and an occasional local anesthetic or steroid injection reduce most sources of musculo-ligamentous pain. A sling for the shoulder or an orthotic to hold the wrist and fingers in extension may also prevent further complications.

Burning or hypersensitivity from central pain may respond to gabapentin, carbamazepine, lamotrigine, tricyclic antidepressants, pregabalin, baclofen, and other medications, based on small RCTs.

Depression

Depression was diagnosed in the community-based Framingham Study in 47% of 6-month stroke survivors, but was simultaneously diagnosed in 25% of age- and sex-matched controls. In a population-based cohort of Swedish patients with stroke whose mean age was 73 years, the prevalence of major depression was 25% at hospital discharge, 30% at 3 months after stroke, 16% at 1 year, 19% at 2 years, and 29% at 3 years.[10] By 3 months after stroke, greater dependence in ADLs and social isolation have been associated with depression. Premorbid depression was a strong risk factor for major depression after stroke. The symptoms that lead to a treatment trial during rehabilitation tend to be lack of motivation and carryover of therapies from day to day, feelings of fatigue and lack of energy, hopelessness, and poor sleep with recurrent negative thoughts, which seem to limit progress.

Counseling during rehabilitation may lessen the risk for depression, especially when directed toward concerns that patients have about becoming a burden on others. A meta-analysis of 52 rather small trials of one of several selective serotonin reuptake inhibitors (fluoxetine, sertraline, citalopram and others) suggested a modest benefit, compared to no treatment, on dependence, disability, impairment, anxiety, and depression at any time after stroke. Side effects were not significant. The results were quite heterogeneous and larger trials were recommended.[11] Tricyclic antidepressants at 10–25 mg in the evening may lessen insomnia and depression, but their anticholinergic effects may have a negative impact. Methylphenidate at a dose of 5–10 mg bid during daytime sometimes has a rapid onset of effect on mood and attention, especially in the elderly. Exercise in subacute and chronic stroke seems to lessen depression during the period of trying to build strength and endurance at an intensity of at least 30 min 3–5 days a week.[12]

Fatigue

The symptom of fatigue after hemiparetic stroke is described by 20–40% of community dwellers. Although a bit vague in meaning, fatigue includes sluggishness, easy tiring, low energy, lack of motivation, impaired endurance, and sleepiness. The source may be a mood disorder or psychological and physical manifestations of disability, medications, cardiovascular fitness, and disease. Symptoms may also arise from fatigability, meaning diminishing strength that follows repetitive movements, leading to greater weakness superimposed on underlying paresis, as well as from deconditioning. Interventions that have had modest success include SSRI antidepressants or stimulants such as methylphenidate and modafinal, ruling out a sleep disorder, conditioning and strengthening exercises, and scheduled rest periods after scheduled physical activity.

Dysphagia

Swallowing disorders may cause malnutrition, dehydration, and aspiration pneumonia. The stroke and any associated toxic-metabolic encephalopathy may combine to cause lethargy, inattention, poor judgment, and impaired control or sensitivity of the tongue and cheek. These problems often impair the oral stage of swallowing. Patients cannot form a bolus; food is pocketed in the cheek; the swallowing reflex may be delayed; and the bolus slides over the base of the tongue and collects in the valleculae and hypopharynx. In addition, patients may take too much food or liquid in a bolus, which then enters the airway before triggering a swallow reflex. Slow oral intake, a cough or wet voice after swallowing, and a rising blood urea nitrogen level point to the potential for clinical complications of dysphagia.

A videofluoroscopic modified barium swallow (MBS) study provides the best information about the safety and efficacy of the stages of swallowing. An MBS study performed with less than a teaspoonful of thin barium, the same of thickened barium, and a test of swallowing with a barium-coated piece of cookie help document problems at the oral, pharyngeal, and esophageal stages. The therapist can simultaneously assess the effect of changes in head and neck position on deglutition. During inpatient rehabilitation, an abnormal MBS study result reveals the greater risk for pneumonia in aspirators compared to non-aspirators. Nasogastric feeding tubes and gastrostomies do not appreciably lessen the risk of aspiration, probably because of gastric reflux, aspiration of oral secretions, and errors in tube placement.

Therapies include compensatory head repositioning such as flexing or turning to one side, tongue and sucking exercises, double swallowing, and supraglottic and dry coughing. If dysphagia persists near the time of discharge from inpatient rehabilitation, a gastrostomy or gastrojejunostomy tube is a comfortable portal for nutrition. Recovery from dysphagia may be associated with a greater motor representation for the pharyngeal muscles in the uninjured hemisphere that evolves over time and with practice in swallowing. With this in mind, pilot studies of TMS during swallowing are proceeding.

Sexual Dysfunction

After stroke, sexual desire may persist, but many men and women who had been sexually active experience sexual dysfunction. Premorbid problems from diabetes, medications, vascular disease, and psychogenic causes can be exacerbated by new neural dysfunction, decreased mobility, pain, and polypharmacy. Counseling and education with patient and spouse help. Sildenafil and related drugs, if angina is not present, and prostheses for men can assist in the treatment of erectile dysfunction.

Sleep Disorders

During rehabilitation, insomnia, sleep apnea, and excessive daytime sleepiness can interfere with attention and perhaps with learning. Medications, pain, anxiety, depression, and chronically poor sleep habits contribute to sleep deficits. Reversed sleep–wake cycles are common in the first days of inpatient rehabilitation. Pharyngeal muscle weakness and impairment of neural control of the nasopharyngeal and pharyngolaryngeal muscles due to a stroke contribute to the risk for new onset of obstructive apnea. The number of oxygen desaturation events and the oximetry measures during sleep-disordered breathing correlate with poorer functional recovery scores at 1 and 12 months after stroke.

Insomnia during the first week or two of rehabilitation can be managed with short-acting hypnotic agents such as temazepam and zolpidem, night-time non-narcotic analgesics, and careful positioning in bed. Nocturia more than two times that awakens the patient can be diminished by avoiding liquid intake after dinner and using medications that lessen activation of the bladder detrusor muscle. Melatonin may help correct a reversed day–night sleep cycle. As an outpatient, polysomnography and consideration of continuous positive airway pressure may be necessary.

Spasticity

A number of still ill-defined mechanisms after stroke alter neural membrane properties and morphologically and physiologically reorganize spinal circuits, leading to hypertonicity, clonus, spasms, and contractures. However, the paresis, slowness, and fatigability that accompany an upper motor neuron (UMN) syndrome are usually more serious contributors to impairment and disability than hypertonicity. The difficulty in quantifying spasticity and measuring a functional consequence has made research and drug testing difficult. The Modified Ashworth Scale is most often used, but the scoring is little more than an extension of the clinical examination of resistance to passive movement. Also, the properties of joints, ligaments, tendons, and muscles change with paresis after a UMN injury and contribute to the alteration in resistance to joint stretch.

Small trials of modest resistance exercises have not revealed a risk of inducing an increase in tone. Indeed, clonus and spasms often diminish with weight bearing on the leg or arm. Excessive resistance exercises, however, that only flex the arm, as in performing curls, or that only extend the leg may drive flexor or extensor postures, respectively, and produce a dystonic arm or leg.

Pathologically increased muscle tone in patients with hemiplegia can usually be managed by aiming to maintain the normal length of the muscle and soft tissue across a joint and by helping patients avoid abnormal flexor and extensor patterns at rest and during movement. Spasticity should be treated more aggressively when it interferes with nursing care and perineal hygiene or contributes to contractures and pressure sores.

No studies offer convincing evidence of benefits for the motor control of functional movements from use of systemic antispasticity medications after a stroke, but range of motion, pain, and flexor postures of the arm or hand may improve. Dantrolene, baclofen, a benzodiazepine such as clonazepam, and tizanidine can be tried for a few weeks to test their utility. Intramuscular injection of botulinum toxin may reduce local features of spasticity for about 3 months, especially flexor postures of the arm and hand and equinovarus foot positioning. These agents may improve the Modified Ashworth Scale score, but they rarely improve the torque around a joint or actual usage of the limb.[13] Injections should be followed by physical or occupational therapy to try to maintain range of motion. Tendon lengthening of the hamstrings, Achilles, and toe or finger and wrist flexors is an occasional consideration to improve range of motion.

OVERVIEW OF PRACTICES

Do neurologic rehabilitation therapies improve outcomes? One may better ask whether specific interventions for clearly defined impairments and disabilities really work. Newer RCTs discussed below point to many cognitive and physical interventions that clearly improve outcomes compared to no focused, progressive retraining intervention.[14] The robustness of the broad range of physical interventions varies greatly, in part related to the limitations of clinical trials in stroke rehabilitation.[15]

Cognitive Rehabilitation

Disabilities arise from aphasia and hemineglect as well as from faltering attention, visuoperception, memory, and executive functions. Lesions within the frontal-subcortical circuit that include the caudate, basal ganglia, or thalamus may lead to deafferentation of the dorsolateral prefrontal cortex and impair working memory, judgment, problem-solving skills, and creative thought. Neuropsychological tests help define these problems. A modest number of RCTs have suggested efficacy of specific interventions for aphasia, apraxia, and visuospatial rehabilitation.[16]

Memory Disorders

Encoding and retrieving new information is essential during rehabilitation. Up to 30% of all stroke survivors, however, have a disturbance in memory. Community-based studies report dementia in 15–30% of patients after stroke within 3 months to 1 year and in 33% within 5 years.[17] Cognitive remediation for memory disorders aims to train compensatory strategies such as rehearsal, visual imagery, semantic elaboration, and memory aids such as notebooks, diary calendars, and electronic message devices. In general, patients with stroke have good procedural or motor learning abilities. Donepezil and galantamine may improve aspects of memory and cognitive functioning in some patients with vascular dementia.[18,19]

Visuospatial and Attentional Disorders

Visual neglect is found in up to one-third of patients with moderate disability after a new stroke. Patients with anosognosia, visual neglect, tactile extinction, motor impersistence, or auditory neglect at 10 days after stroke have the lowest BI value 1 year later. Recovery is most rapid within the first 2 weeks, regardless of the side of the stroke, and visual neglect improves by 3 months in most patients. Many still have more subtle impairments that are found by formal tests.

Treatments for left hemi-inattention aim to engage attention to the left, disengage attention to the right, shift spatial coordinates to the left, and increase arousal. Well-described behavioral interventions for visuospatial retraining have been employed to improve attention to the left.[20] The techniques include a stimulus such as a red ribbon on the left to anchor attention followed by a gradual withdrawal of left-sided spatial cues, work on sensory awareness to physical stimuli on the left, prism lenses to shift the center of focus,[21] and tasks to aid spatial organization. Computer-based visual scanning training to increase saccadic eye movements into the field, scanning combined with trunk rotation, self-cuing by movement of the left arm, or a warning tone to increase spatial awareness have improved scores on tests of left hemi-space awareness. Some of these techniques may be better than conventional occupational therapy.[22] These interventions do not necessarily improve left hemi-attention during ADLs. Rotigotine, a dopamine agonist, did improve outcomes in a small RCT.[23]

Speech and Language Therapies

The Copenhagen Stroke Study reported that 38% of 881 patients were aphasic on admission and 20% were rated as severe on the Scandinavian Stroke Scale (SSS).[24] Nearly half of the patients with severe aphasia died early after stroke onset, and half of those with mild aphasia recovered by 1 week. Only 18% of community survivors were still aphasic at the time of acute and rehabilitation hospital discharges. Ninety-five percent of subjects with mild aphasia reached their best level of recovery by 2 weeks, those with a moderate aphasia by 6 weeks, and those with severe aphasia by 10 weeks. Only 8% of the severely aphasic patients fully recovered according to the scoring system by 6 months. Social communication was not measured. This natural history does not imply that aphasic patients cannot improve in aspects of comprehension and expression for months, even years, after stroke onset.

Interventions

For the aphasic patient, speech therapists attempt to find ways to circumvent or compensate for impairments in the comprehension and expression of language. Interventions are mostly specific to a syndrome (Chapter 24). Visual and verbal cuing techniques include picture matching and sentence completion tasks. Frequent repetition and positive reinforcement are used as the patient approaches the desired responses. A large variety of approaches for particular language and linguistic impairments have evolved.[24] Melodic intonation therapy for non-fluent aphasics who have good comprehension, for example, may enhance expression. Audio-visual speech stimuli may increase speech fluency in Broca's aphasics.[25]

The intensity and specificity of practice may be most important in testing the efficacy of a particular therapy. One well-designed study employed a picture card game in which a group of aphasic subjects were prompted to request and provide cards of depicted objects from their hands of cards. The results suggest that behaviorally relevant mass practice for at least 3 hours a day for 10 days that also constrains the use of non-verbal communication, and reinforces appropriate responses within a group setting, could improve comprehension and naming skills more effectively than less intensive and formalized therapy.[21] Computer software offers other forms of practice. Numerous mobile apps are also available for smartphones and tablets. Small trials have also tried rTMS and tDCS protocols to lessen dysnomia.

Clinical trials in modest numbers of patients with amphetamine, piracetam, and cholinergic, and dopaminergic agents and memantine,[26] plus language training, have suggested modest efficacy for particular aphasic syndromes and language impairments (Chapter 24).

MOTOR REHABILITATION

Mobility Training

Sensorimotor impairments and disabilities in mobility and other ADLs are managed by at least four general approaches:

1. Task-oriented retraining that emphasizes motor learning by progressive, repetitive practice of challenging tasks that increasingly shape whole-limb movements and are relevant to the patient.
2. Sensory facilitation and techniques to limit spasticity and develop synergistic movements drawn from therapy schools such as Bobath, especially in the face of severe impairments.
3. Compensatory training to adapt to disability and enable participation when sensorimotor control is limited.
4. Exercise and selective muscle group strengthening, along with fitness training.

Natural History for Walking Gains

In the Copenhagen Stroke Study,[27] at discharge after acute and rehabilitative care, 22% of survivors could not walk, 14% walked with assistance, and 64% walked independently. About 80% of those who were initially non-walkers reached their best walking function within 6 weeks, and 95% within 11 weeks. Of patients who initially walked with physical assistance, 80% reached best function within 3 weeks, and 95% within 5 weeks. Independent walking was achieved by 34% of the survivors who had been dependent and by 60% of those who initially required assistance. Recovery of ambulation correlated directly with residual leg strength. In general, patients who can flex the hip and extend the hemiparetic lower leg against gravity will be able to ambulate without human assistance. Figure 58-1 shows recovery data according to impairment group for one cohort of patients.

Interventions

Therapy is initiated as soon as feasible. Range of motion in the plegic leg is maintained with positioning, ankle splints, and slow rhythmic rotation and stretch of all joints several

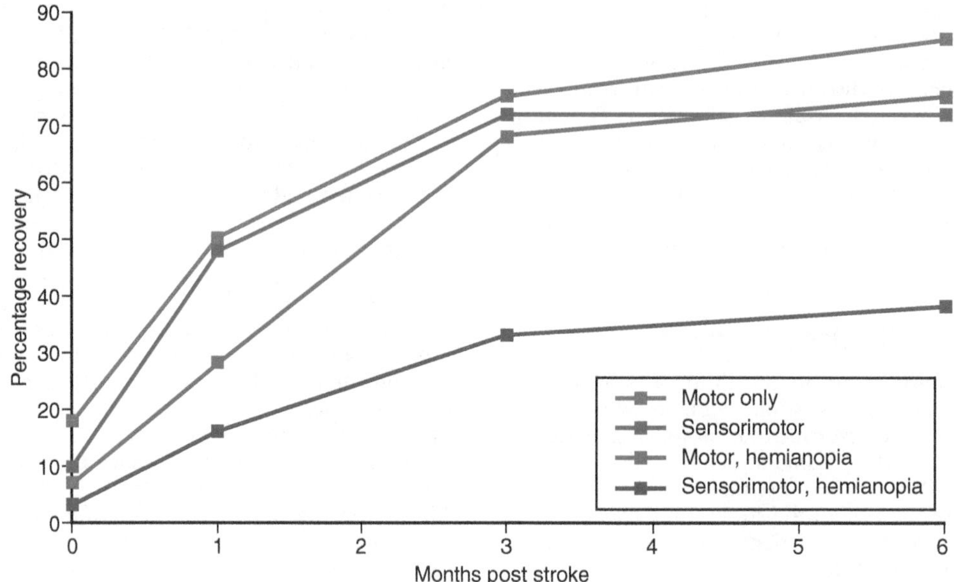

Figure 58-1. Recovery of walking in patients grouped by impairments at onset of stroke.[63]

times a day, along with weight bearing as soon as possible. These exercises also help prevent excessive hypertonicity. Patient and family are taught to assist. Head and trunk stability and reaching and grasping with the affected upper extremity start early to enable head and trunk control for transfers and standing. Flexion at the hip, knee, and ankle are encouraged by mat exercises. Elicitation of muscle synergies is where the Bobath technique is especially useful. Once the patient has adequate endurance and stability to stand in the parallel bars or at a hemibar with the therapist's help to control the paretic leg, gait training begins. The therapist concentrates on the most prominent deviations from normal during the gait cycle, such as circumduction of the hip, pelvic drop, hyperextension or flexor give-way of the knee, inadequate dorsiflexion of the ankle, and toe clawing. The physical therapist also encourages heel strike at initial stance, greater weight bearing on the paretic leg, push-off at the end of stance, at least 5–10° of hip extension in late stance, and a longer step length. Concentration on timing of loading the mid-stance leg with simultaneous initiation of the swing phase of the other leg can help engrain more symmetrical stepping and better toe clearance of the hemiplegic leg.

The hemiparetic patient who cannot control ankle movement, whose foot tends to turn over during gait, or who lacks enough knee control to prevent the knee from snapping back is fitted with a polypropylene AFO. Inpatient therapy for gait progresses away from the parallel bars to increasing distances walked with an assistive device such as a quad cane, then to stair climbing and outdoor ambulation on uneven surfaces.

Progress in the development of lightweight, lower-extremity exoskeletons with actuators that can manipulate the affected leg to control the knee and flex the hip, knee, or ankle are now available for paraplegia and may come into use for serious hemiplegia with hemisensory loss. No trials of commercially available devices (e.g., ReWalk and Ekso bilateral leg exoskeletons) are available.

Task-related Training

Treadmill walking is considered as a task-oriented approach for ambulation. Body-weight-supported treadmill training (BWSTT) allows a therapist to employ different levels of weight support to gradually load the affected leg and practice stepping at a variety of treadmill speeds. The step pattern is assisted with physical and verbal cues to optimize the temporal, kinematic, and kinetic parameters of the step cycle. The opportunity to better control sensory input may improve the timing and increase the activation of residual descending locomotor outputs on spinal motor pools. Trials that included small numbers of subjects suggested that BWSTT may be superior to usual care or no intervention in subacute and chronically slow walkers, but well-designed RCTs show no differences in outcomes compared to an equal amount of either walking-related therapy or supervised home-based therapy that focuses on balance and strengthening.[4] In addition, treadmill training with weight support that is assisted by a robotic device for stepping appears equal to the same intensity of more conventional over-ground training.[28] No clinically important differences for walking speed, distance, or physical functioning have been found with these seemingly task-related locomotor training strategies,[29] although meta-analyses may find possible benefit for some outcomes in some subgroups, such as initiation early vs late after onset or highly vs less impaired.[15,30,31] However, these improvements are not clinically robust. Perhaps the training environs of a treadmill and robotic stepper differ from over-ground practice or do not enable motor learning as well as was once thought, or there is a limit as to how much improvement can be expected based on, for example, residual neural networks that represent walking.

Another multicenter trial during inpatient stroke rehabilitation found that simply giving patients and their therapists feedback about how fast the person walked 10 m each day, without any other specific intervention, led to improved walking speed at discharge by 24%.[32] Thus, positive feedback about performance may be a critical motivating drive for gains. Peroneal nerve stimulation may improve foot clearance and may modestly improve walking speed, but RCTs reveal no greater improvements than obtained from wearing an AFO.[33] Rhythmic practice of stepping entrained by the temporal elements of music may also improve walking speed and the symmetry of both stance and swing phases of gait.[34] Studies aimed at improving balance and gait with virtual reality and exercise games have shown only modest, if any, benefit so far, but the strategy is still evolving.

Strengthening and Fitness Exercise

Selective bilateral muscle strengthening and exercise to improve physical fitness are central to rehabilitation, both early and late after stroke.[35,36] Up to 85% of stroke survivors are deconditioned, in part because they are far more sedentary than age-matched peers who are not hemiparetic.[37] Being sedentary also leads to a potential non-use myopathy that can weaken even the non-hemiparetic leg. A statin-induced myopathy may also induce weakness that can be appreciated by a careful examination. Strengthening of the hip and knee muscles can be achieved with resistance exercises against weights, elastic bands, in the pool, and on a stationary recumbent bike. Reconditioning by aerobic exercise is feasible in those with enough motor control to bicycle or walk on a treadmill.[38] The clinician should encourage patients to continuously increase the duration and distance of daily walking (and thus walking speed) under safe conditions, both to improve mobility and fitness, and to reduce risk factors for recurrent stroke.

UPPER EXTREMITY AND SELF-CARE SKILLS

ADL tasks are emphasized by therapists during inpatient rehabilitation. Community and leisure activities are addressed during outpatient therapy. Outcomes for prospective studies of patients undergoing rehabilitation, as well as for the overall population of patients admitted for acute care after a first stroke, suggest that 60–70% of patients recover the ability to manage basic ADLs, although the majority do not return to their premorbid level of socialization.

Natural History

Using the BI and SSS, the Copenhagen Study graded recovery before and after acute and rehabilitative inpatient stays and at 6 months. Within the same facility, all patients who needed rehabilitation received services for an average stay of 35 days (S.D. 41). By then, 11% had severe impairment, 11% had moderate impairment, and 78% had mild or no deficits. At the same time, 20% had severe, 8% moderate, and 26% mild disability, and 46% had no disability. ADL scores plateaued by 9 weeks in patients with initially mild strokes, within 13 weeks in those with moderate strokes, within 17 weeks in those with severe strokes, and within 20 weeks in those with most severe stroke. For patients initially admitted to a US rehabilitation inpatient program, 65% achieved a BI of more than 95 by 15 weeks if they had only motor deficits and by 26 weeks with sensorimotor loss, but only 10% of those with sensorimotor and hemianoptic deficits scored that high by 18–30 weeks.[39] However, 100% of patients with motor loss achieved a BI higher than 60 by 14 weeks, 75% of those with SM deficits by 23 weeks, and 60% of those with SMH loss by 29 weeks.

Functional recovery of the upper extremity was assessed in the Copenhagen Stroke Study with the use of BI subscores for feeding and grooming for the affected arm. Within 9 weeks, 95% of patients achieved their best function. With mild paresis, this was accomplished by 6 weeks after stroke onset. In those with severe paresis, best function was achieved by 11 weeks. The ability to shrug or abduct the affected shoulder within the first few weeks after stroke may predict outcomes better than synergistic hand function. Patients who have no movement of the hand or proximal muscles by several weeks after onset of the stroke most often do not recover independent feeding and dressing with that hand.[40] Patients who have some voluntary finger and wrist extension within the first few weeks may show improvement in hand coordination for practiced tasks for 12 months or more.

General Interventions

Occupational therapy to improve upper-extremity function first puts an emphasis on visually and manually patterning the patient through parts of a task and then through the entire task with frequent positive feedback. Synergistic movements, which may represent both fractionation and merging of cortical and spinal motor modules,[41] are elicited and, if necessary, inhibited. Techniques that conserve energy and promote independence in dressing, grooming, bathing, and toileting involve relearning how to carry out the task with compensation when using the unaffected arm and adaptive strategies with the affected arm. If needed, the therapist also provides an arm sling or electrical stimulation if shoulder subluxation or pain arises, a compression glove to reduce hand edema if elevation and massage fail to do so, and static and dynamic splints to maintain wrist and finger position in extension. Assistive devices may be needed at home, such as grab bars, rails, ramps, environmental controls, and architectural changes such as widening a doorway to allow wheelchair access.

Task-Oriented Approaches

Failed early attempts to use the affected limb may suppress subsequent use. Forced use of the affected arm and gradual shaping of a variety of functional movements may increase the incorporation of the affected arm into daily activities. This approach was developed as constraint-induced movement therapy (CIMT), which has been the focus of many clinical trials at various stages of rehabilitation.[42,43]

A randomized trial of CIMT in subjects who, at 3–9 months after their stroke were able to extend several fingers and the wrist at least 10°, revealed significantly better outcomes compared to no intervention.[43,44] The intervention involved 6 hours of daily supervised upper extremity therapy plus a mitten on the unaffected hand throughout the day for 2 weeks. Other trials suggest that less time in formal therapy and less restraint may be as effective.[45]

Robotic and other mechanical assistive training devices have led to modest improvements in the performance of reaching, usually in the plane of practice or across the joints most used.[46,47] Trials that do not augment the amount of practice time generally produce negative results for gains in arm function.[48] Not unlike robotic steppers, rehabilitation via upper-extremity electromechanical devices may require additional strategies to promote an iterative process of skills learning with practice on and off the device.

Other Training

EMG-triggered neuromuscular stimulation feedback produces modest gains in wrist extensor strength. Studies give both positive and negative results for functional electrical stimulation to prevent or reduce shoulder pain related to subluxation after hemiplegia. Commercial orthotic devices placed across the wrist and designed to electrically stimulate surface muscles for a grasp or pincer movement can improve use of the paretic hand if adequate shoulder–elbow movement is present.[49] Acupuncture has not improved motor function or performance of ADLs.[50]

Virtual reality systems that augment feedback about the position of the hand in space represent a potentially powerful form of practice, offering feedback such as knowledge of performance and of results using parameters such as velocity, trajectory, and accuracy of the reaching movement.[51,52] Bimanual upper extremity practice with coupling of movements,[53] mental practice of actions that precedes attempted limb function, and mirror therapy, in which the hemiparetic arm appears to move, show some promise in some patients,[54] but one progressive practice paradigm tends to be equal to another.[55] The optimal style, daily intensity, and overall duration of training and the best outcome measures, in terms of sensitivity to change and relevance to useful movements, are a work in progress for all interventions.

Repetitive TMS and tDCS have enabled modest improvements in small trials for arm or hand function, when the participants had no more than mild-to-moderate loss of motor control.[56] The combination of non-invasive cortical stimulation with simultaneous robotic therapy to maximize Hebbian plasticity for skills learning has been minimally encouraging, so far.[57] Overall, the evidence for the effectiveness of rTMS and tDCS for lessening impairment and disability is modest to date.[58,59] Optimized protocols need to be tested in a properly powered RCT.[60]

Pharmacotherapy

In small, randomized trials, amphetamine, methylphenidate, levodopa, and fluoxetine have shown modest levels of success for improving strength or motor control, but the trials did not necessarily improve ADLs. No differences in gains were found, however, in an adequately powered trial when upper-extremity therapy was provided to chronic, moderately hemiparetic patients randomly assigned to receive ropinirole, a dopamine agonist.

Amphetamine has received the most acclaim. Side effects of amphetamine, when using 10 mg every other morning, have been minimal; most trials have probably used exclusion criteria that were too strict. Best, if modest, improvements were achieved when physical therapy relevant to the outcome measure was combined with the drug.[61]

Clinicians may consider 2-week, N-of-1 trials of pharmacologic adjuncts to enhance motor gains. Such an approach may be worthwhile in patients with some sensorimotor function who are undergoing active rehabilitation and in whom motor control lags and limits gains in walking or use of the upper extremity. To date, the most promising medication to start is fluoxetine, 20 mg daily beginning within the first week after stroke.[62]

CONCLUSIONS

The milieu and focus on functional gains provided by an inpatient rehabilitation team lead to better outcomes than those achieved by general medical care and less organized services. Patients may improve by spontaneous processes at first, but important gains are likely related to intrinsic biologic mechanisms that are driven by external stimuli, especially formal, progressive practice. Progressively difficult or complex task-oriented practice and problem-solving with reinforcement paradigms may be a critical element for successful motor and cognitive retraining. Practice must be relevant to the subject, frequent, and of adequate duration, but these parameters are a work in progress.

To improve motor performance, practice should engage the patient and aim to improve selective movements, motor control, skill, strength, endurance for an activity, and generalized fitness. This approach to training may lead to synaptic and morphologic changes associated with activity-dependent plasticity at the levels of the spinal cord, brainstem, and cerebral hemispheres. Certain pharmacologic interventions may help drive experience-induced learning and neural adaptations for specific tasks, but clinical trials to date offer only modest support for this theory. Biological interventions such as cellular therapies and dendritic and axonal regeneration show some promise in animal models (Chapter 60). These rewiring and neuromodulation strategies will require relevant rehabilitation interventions to produce clinical efficacy. The physician with expertise in neurorehabilitation can help therapists develop training paradigms drawn from an integration of basic neuroscience, cognitive neuroscience, clinical neuromedicine, clinical research study designs, and outcomes research.

REFERENCES

1. Dobkin B. The clinical science of neurologic rehabilitation. New York: Oxford University Press; 2003.
2. Carmichael ST. Themes and strategies for studying the biology of stroke recovery in the poststroke epoch. Stroke 2008;39:1380–8.
3. Buma F, Lindeman E, Ramsey N, et al. Functional neuroimaging studies of early upper limb recovery after stroke: A systematic review. Neurorehabil Neural Repair 2010;24:589–608.
4. Duncan P, Sullivan K, Behrman A, et al. Body-weight-supported treadmill rehabilitation program after stroke. N Engl J Med 2011;364:2026–36.
5. Lin K, Fu T, Wu C, et al. Minimal detectable change and clinically important difference of the Stroke Impact Scale in stroke patients. Neurorehabil Neural Repair 2010;24:486–92.
6. Cella D, Lai J, Nowinski C, et al. Neuro-QOL: Brief measures of health-related quality of life for clinical research in neurology. Neurology 2012;78:1860–7.
7. Dobkin B. Rehabilitation after stroke. New Engl J Med 2005;352:1677–84.
8. Langhorne P, Taylor G, Murray G, et al. Early supported discharge services for stroke patients: a meta-analysis of individual patients' data. Lancet 2005;365:501–6.
9. Ronning OM, Guldvog B. Outcome of subacute stroke rehabilitation: a randomized controlled trial. Stroke 1998;29:779–84.
10. Astrom M, Adolfsson R, Asplund K. Major depression in stroke patients: a 3-year longitudinal study. Stroke 1993;24:976–82.
11. Mead G, Hsieh C, Lee R, et al. Selective serotonin reuptake inhibitors (SSRIs) for stroke recovery. Cochrane Database Syst Rev 2012;(11):CD009286.
12. Eng J, Reime B. Exercise for depressive symptoms in stroke patients: a systematic review. Clin Rehabil 2014;doi:10.1177/0269215514523631; [epub Feb 17].
13. Foley N, Pereira S, Salter K, et al. Treatment with botulinum toxin improves upper-extremity function post stroke: a systematic review and meta-analysis. Arch Phys Med Rehabil 2013;94:977–89.
14. Langhorne P, Bernhardt J, Kwakkel G. Stroke rehabilitation. Lancet 2011;377:1693–702.
15. Veerbeek J, van Wegen E, van Peppen R, et al. What is the evidence for physical therapy poststroke? A systematic review and meta-analysis. PLoS ONE 2014;9:e87987.
16. Cicerone K, Langenbahn D, Braden C, et al. Evidence-based cognitive rehabilitation: updated review of the literature from 2003 through 2008. Arch Phys Med Rehabil 2011;92:519–30.
17. Desmond D, Moroney J, Paik M, et al. Frequency and clinical determinants of dementia after ischemic stroke. Neurology 2000;54:1124–31.
18. Roman GC, Wilkinson DG, Doody RS, et al. Donepezil in vascular dementia: combined analysis of two large-scale clinical trials. Dement Geriatr Cogn Disord 2005;20:338–44.
19. Birks J, Craig D. Galantamine for vascular cognitive impairment. Cochrane Database Syst Rev 2006;(4):CD004746.
20. Gordon W, Diller L, Lieberman A, et al. Perceptual remediation in patients with right brain damage: A comprehensive program. Arch Phys Med Rehabil 1985;66:353–9.
21. Mizuno K, Tsuji T, Takebayashi T, et al. Prism adaptation therapy enhances rehabilitation of stroke patients with unilateral spatial neglect. Neurorehabil Neural Repair 2011;25:711–20.
22. Modden C, Behrens M, Damke I, et al. A randomized controlled trial comparing 2 interventions for visual field loss with standard occupational therapy during inpatient stroke rehabilitation. Neurorehabil Neural Repair 2012;26:463–9.
23. Gorgoraptis N, Mah Y, Machner B, et al. The effects of the dopamine agonist rotigotine on hemispatial neglect following stroke. Brain 2012;135:2478–91.
24. Pedersen P, Jorgensen H, Nakayama H, et al. Aphasia in acute stroke: Incidence, determinants, and recovery. Ann Neurol 1995;38:659–66.

25. Frikriksson J, Hubbard H, Hudspeth S, et al. Speech entrainment enables patients with Broca's aphasia to produce fluent speech. Brain 2012;135:3815–29.
26. Berthier M, Green C, Lara J, et al. Memantine and constraint-induced aphasia therapy in chronic poststroke aphasia. Ann Neurol 2009;65:577–85.
27. Jorgensen HS, Nakayama H, Raaschou HO, et al. Outcome and time course of recovery in stroke. Part II: Time course of recovery. The Copenhagen Stroke Study. Arch Phys Med Rehabil 1995;76: 406–12.
28. Hidler J, Nichols D, Pelliccio M, et al. Multicenter randomized clinical trial evaluating the effectiveness of the Lokomat in subacute stroke. Neurorehabil Neural Repair 2009;23: 5–13.
29. Dobkin B, Duncan P. Should body weight-supported treadmill training and robotic-assistive steppers for locomotor training trot back to the starting gate? Neurorehabil Neural Repair 2012;26: 308–17.
30. Mehrholz J, Elsner B, Werner C, et al. Electromechanical-assisted training for walking after stroke: Updated evidence. Cochrane Database Syst Rev 2013;(7):CD006185.
31. Mehrholz J, Pohl M, Elsner B. Treadmill training and body weight support for walking after stroke. Cochrane Database Syst Rev 2014;(1):CD002840.
32. Dobkin B, Plummer-D'Amato P, Elashoff R, et al. International randomized clinical trial, Stroke Inpatient Rehabilitation With Reinforcement of Walking Speed (SIRROWS) improves outcomes. Neurorehabil Neural Repair 2010;24:235–42.
33. Sheffler L, Taylor P, Gunzler D, et al. Randomized controlled trial of surface peroneal nerve stimulation for motor relearning in lower limb hemiparesis. Arch Phys Med Rehabil 2013;94: 1007–14.
34. Thaut M, Leins A, Rice R, et al. Rhythmic auditory stimulation improves gait more than NDT/Bobath training in near-ambulatory patients early poststroke: a single-blind, randomized trial. Neurorehabil Neural Repair 2007;21:455–9.
35. Brazzelli M, Saunders D, Greig C, et al. Physical fitness training for stroke patients. Cochrane Database Syst Rev 2011;(11): CD003316.
36. Stoller O, de Bruin E, Knols R, et al. Effects of cardiovascular exercise early after stroke: systematic review and meta-analysis. BMC Neurol 2012;12:45.
37. Rand D, Eng JJ, Tang PF, et al. How active are people with stroke? Use of accelerometers to assess physical activity. Stroke 2009;40: 163–8.
38. Globus C, Becker C, Cerny J, et al. Chronic stroke survivors benefit from high-intensity aerobic treadmill exercise. Neurorehabil Neural Repair 2012;26:85–95.
39. Reding MJ, Potes E. Rehabilitation outcome following initial unilateral hemispheric stroke. Life table analysis approach. Stroke 1988;19:1354–8.
40. Houwink A, Nijland R, Geurts A, et al. Functional recovery of the paretic upper limb after stroke: who regains hand capacity? Arch Phys Med Rehabil 2013;94:839–44.
41. Cheung V, Turolla A, Agostini M, et al. Muscle synergy patterns as physiological markers of motor cortical damage. Proc Natl Acad Sci 2012;109:14652–6.
42. Dromerick A, Edwards D, Hahn M. Does the application of constraint-induced movement therapy during acute rehabilitation reduce arm impairment after ischemic stroke? Stroke 2000; 31:2984–8.
43. Wolf SL, Winstein CJ, Miller JP, et al. Effect of constraint-induced movement therapy on upper extremity function 3 to 9 months after stroke: the EXCITE randomized clinical trial. JAMA 2006; 296:2095–104.
44. Wolf SL, Winstein CJ, Miller JP, et al. Retention of upper limb function in stroke survivors who have received constraint-induced movement therapy: the EXCITE randomised trial. Lancet Neurol 2008;7:33–40.
45. Smania N, Goandolfi M, Paolucci S, et al. Reduced intensity modified constraint-induced movement therapy versus conventional therapy for upper extremity rehabilitation after stroke. Neurorehabil Neural Repair 2012;26:1035–45.
46. Volpe BT, Lynch D, Rykman-Berland A, et al. Intensive sensorimotor arm training mediated by therapist or robot improves hemiparesis in patients with chronic stroke. Neurorehabil Neural Repair 2008;22:305–10.
47. Lo A, Guarino P, Richards L, et al. Robot-assisted therapy for long-term upper-limb impairment after stroke. N Engl J Med 2010;362: 1772–83.
48. Mehrholz J, Hadrich A, Platz T, et al. Electromechanical and robot-assisted arm training for improving generic activities of daily living, arm function, and arm muscle strength after stroke. Cochrane Database Syst Rev 2012;(6):CD006876.
49. Alon G, Levitt AF, McCarthy PA. Functional electrical stimulation enhancement of upper extremity functional recovery during stroke rehabilitation: a pilot study. Neurorehabil Neural Repair 2007;21:207–15.
50. Kong J, Lee M, Shin B, et al. Acupuncture for functional recovery after stroke: a systematic review. CMAJ 2010;182:1723–9.
51. Subramanian S, Lourenco C, Chilingaryan G, et al. Arm recovery using a virtual reality intervention in chronic stroke. Neurorehabil Neural Repair 2012;27:13–23.
52. Saposnik G, Levin M. Virtual reality in stroke rehabilitation: a meta-analysis. Stroke 2011;42:1380–6.
53. Luft A, McCombe-Waller S, Whitall J, et al. Repetitive bilateral arm training and motor cortedx activation in chronic stroke. JAMA 2004;292:1853–61.
54. Thieme H, Mehrholz J, Pohl M, et al. Mirror therapy for improving motor function after stroke. Cochrane Database Syst Rev 2012;(3):CD008449.
55. van Delden A, Peper C, Niehuys K, et al. Unilateral versus bilateral upper limb training after stroke: the upper limb training after stroke clinical trial. Stroke 2013;44:2613–16.
56. Lindenberg R, Renga V, Zhu L, et al. Bihemispheric brain stimulation facilitates motor recovery in chronic stroke patients. Neurology 2010;75:2176–84.
57. Hesse S, Waldner A, Mehrholz J, et al. Combined transcranial direct current stimulation and robot-assisted arm training in subacute stroke patients. Neurorehabil Neural Repair 2011;25: 838–46.
58. Hao Z, Wang D, Zeng Y, et al. Repetitive transcranial magnetic stimulation for improving function after stroke. Cochrane Database Syst Rev 2013;(5):CD008862.
59. Elsner B, Kugler J, Pohl M, et al. Transcranial direct current stimulation for activities after stroke. Cochrane Database Syst Rev 2013;(11):CD009645.
60. Adeyemo B, Simis M, Macea D, et al. Systematic review of parameters of stimulation, clinical trial design characteristics, and motor outcomes in non-invasive brain stimulation in stroke. Front Psychiatry 2012;3:88.
61. Schuster C, Maunz G, Lutz K, et al. Dexamphetamine improves upper extremity outcome during rehabilitation after stroke. Neurorehabil Neural Repair 2011;25:749–55.
62. Chollet F, Tardy J, Albucher J, et al. Fluoxetine for motor recovery after acute ischemic stroke (FLAME): a randomised placebo-controlled trial. Lancet Neurol 2011;10:123–30.
63. Patel A, Duncan P, Lai S, et al. The relation between impairments and functional outcomes poststroke. Arch Phys Med Rehabil 2000;81:1357–63.

59 Interventions to Improve Recovery after Stroke

Steven C. Cramer

KEY POINTS

- Neural repair is a therapeutic strategy that is separate from acute stroke strategies such as reperfusion and neuroprotection, and has distinct biological targets, time windows for therapeutic efficacy, and issues to address in clinical trial design.
- Many classes of therapy are under study to improve stroke recovery including small molecules, growth factors, monoclonal antibodies, stem cells, robotic devices, brain stimulation, activity-based therapies, telerehabilitation, and cognitive-based strategies.
- Some repair-based therapies are introduced within days of stroke onset, in an attempt to amplify innate repair mechanisms, while other therapies are offered to patients from months to years after stroke onset, where the goal is to stimulate new forms of neural repair.
- Restorative therapies improve behavioral outcomes on the basis of experience-dependent brain plasticity – a drug may galvanize the brain for repair, but behavioral reinforcement is also needed to achieve maximal gains. This is an important difference as compared to neuroprotective, reperfusion, and preventative stroke therapies, where the patient generally does not need to engage in any particular behavioral regimen to derive treatment benefit.
- Several positive late-phase clinical trials of restorative therapies have been published, e.g., for activity-based therapies and for small molecules such as serotonergic drugs.

BIOLOGY OF STROKE RECOVERY SUGGESTS THERAPEUTICS TARGETS

A new stroke sets numerous biological pathways into motion. These include the ischemic cascade acutely, immunological events that evolve from pro-inflammatory systemic immunosuppression,[1] and later a sequence of restorative events that support tissue repair and that also represent potential targets to improve stroke recovery.

Animal studies indicate that an experimental stroke results in an ordered change in expression of numerous genes. Numerous growth-related events are seen, such as growth factor release, increased levels of growth inhibitors such as Nogo and MAG, capillary growth, axonal sprouting, synaptogenesis, glial cell activation, and changes in cortical excitability. These changes are seen both near and distant from injury, and generally peak during the initial weeks post-stroke.[2–6]

Studies of stroke recovery mechanisms in humans, informed by non-invasive neuroimaging and neurophysiological methods, are overall concordant with preclinical findings.[7] In parallel with behavioral improvement, cortical maps undergo reorganization.[8–10] compensatory changes in brain function and brain networks[11–13] arise, often bilaterally,[14–17] and are associated with changes in brain structure.[18,19] Uninjured areas that are normally connected to the infarct region as part of a distributed network may show depressed function, a process known as diaschisis,[20,21] resolution of which may be linked with behavioral improvement. These restorative events represent potential therapeutic targets to promote brain repair.

NEURAL REPAIR IS DISTINCT FROM NEUROPROTECTION

A clear distinction must be made between therapeutic targets related to neuroprotection and those related to repair. These are parallel treatment strategies that have temporally distinct targets – a neuroprotective therapy is initiated from minutes to hours after stroke onset to salvage threatened tissue, while a repair therapy is typically introduced days after stroke onset or later. Brain repair aims to improve function by restoring normal patterns of brain structure and function, e.g., regaining voluntary control of arm reaching; this is distinguished from compensation, which aims to improve function by substituting new patterns, e.g, teaching a patient to reach by swinging his torso to propel a paretic arm.[22]

Many classes of restorative therapy are under study, using many different strategies.[6,23–27] These are listed in Box 59-1, which emphasizes interventions that have reached the point of human trials. Some repair-based therapies are introduced within days, or perhaps weeks, of stroke onset in an attempt to amplify innate repair mechanisms. For some restorative therapies, a critical period exists, whereby introduction within a specific time window provides a therapeutic benefit that is lost when treatment is delayed.[28–30] This is one of the many parallels between stroke recovery and normal brain development.[7,31] Other repair-based therapies are less limited by a time window and that may be offered to patients in the chronic phase, from months to years after stroke onset. Advantages of this approach include availability of a large enrollment pool and a stable baseline that is helpful to interpret treatment effects.

DRUGS

Many types of drugs have been studied in relation to stroke recovery, particularly small molecules, which may have advantages in terms of transport through the blood–brain barrier[32] or availability as repurposing of an approved drug. Many of the small molecules studied for neural repair target a specific brain neurotransmitter system.

Monoaminergic drugs have been most frequently studied. An early focus was on amphetamine,[33] which acts on multiple monoaminergic targets. Initial human experience in small studies was favorable,[34,35] but the Subacute Therapy with Amphetamine and Rehabilitation for Stroke (STARS) study was not. This was a randomized, double-blind, placebo-controlled trial that did not demonstrate a drug benefit.[36]

BOX 59-1 Therapies Studied to Improve Recovery after Stroke

- Drugs, including small molecules such as amphetamine, dopamine agonists, SSRIs such as fluoxetine, and many others
- Traditional and alternative medicines such as traditional Chinese medicines
- Growth factors such as G-CSF, erythropoietin, and BDNF
- Monoclonal antibodies such as those targeting MAG or Nogo-A
- Stem cell therapies
- Robotic devices
- Brain stimulation methods such as transcranial magnetic stimulation and transcranial direct current stimulation
- Other device-based approaches such as a brain–computer interface
- Rehabilitation therapies such as constraint-induced movement therapy, gait training, and other forms of activity-based therapies
- Telerehabilitation
- Cognitive-based therapies using approaches such as mental imagery, motor observation, mirror visual feedback, and enriched environment

These authors examined 5 weeks of twice-weekly amphetamine vs. placebo in 71 patients enrolled 5–10 days post-stroke. The drug was safe but did not improve the primary outcome, motor recovery over 3 months using the arm/leg Fugl-Meyer motor score.[36] Strengths of this study include use of a single therapist to administer all physiotherapy, and use of a single examiner to assess study outcomes, which reduces variance and increases study power. The treatment protocol was not directly translated from preclinical findings, which might theoretically help define the optimal dose, timing, and frequency of amphetamine to promote stroke recovery.

Dopamine is a monoaminergic catecholamine neurotransmitter important to key brain functions that include learning, plasticity, reward, motivation, and movement.[37] Drugs increasing dopaminergic neurotransmission may improve learning and plasticity in healthy subjects.[38] A randomized, double-blind, placebo-controlled study was consistent with these results, finding 100 mg L-dopa/day, given as Sinemet and combined with physical therapy, to be significantly better than placebo on the primary endpoint, motor status by the Rivermead Motor Assessment after 3 weeks.[39] These authors randomized 53 patients within 6 months of stroke onset to 3 weeks of daily L-dopa or placebo coupled with physiotherapy. Dopaminergic drugs have the potential advantage that measures of genetic variability may help predict inter-subject differences in treatment response.[40] This study awaits replication. Smaller studies using other dopamine agonists have been largely negative, for example, a placebo-controlled, double-blind study of 33 patients 1–12 months post-stroke did not find a difference between a 9-week course of ropinirole+physiotherapy compared to placebo+physiotherapy on gait velocity.[41] Small studies hint at the potential for noradrenergic drugs.[42–44]

Serotonin is another monoaminergic neurotransmitter of interest. Recent reports suggest that increasing serotonin neurotransmission improves stroke recovery. Robinson et al.[45] performed a multisite randomized controlled trial for prevention of depression among 176 non-depressed patients enrolled within 3 months of stroke onset. Patients randomized to the placebo arm were significantly ($P < 0.001$) more likely to reach the primary outcome, development of major or minor depression, compared to patients in either of the two active study arms, the selective serotonin reuptake inhibitor (SSRI) escitalopram or problem-solving therapy. One analysis of a subgroup of these patients found that cognitive outcomes at 12 months were significantly better among those randomized to escitalopram, independent of depression, while a separate subgroup analysis found a lower incidence of generalized anxiety disorder with escitalopram or problem-solving therapy.[46]

The Fluoxetine for Motor Recovery After Acute Ischemic Stroke (FLAME) study[47] was a double-blind, placebo-controlled trial that enrolled non-depressed hemiplegic/hemiparetic patients within 10 days of ischemic stroke onset. Patients were randomized to 3 months of oral fluoxetine (20 mg/day) or placebo. Patients randomized to fluoxetine showed significantly greater gains on the primary endpoint, change in the arm/leg Fugl-Meyer motor score to day 90 ($P = 0.003$), a remarkable 9.7 point difference on this 100-point scale. Measures of genetic variability may inform likelihood of response to a serotonergic drug.[48,49]

Drugs that modulate neurotransmission in acetylcholinergic pathways have received limited study in relation to neural repair. Luria found cholinergic drugs useful for enhancing recovery after brain injury.[50] Studies in rodents[51] and primates[52] with experimental stroke support this, but data from human subjects with stroke are sparse.[53]

Many other small molecules are under study as restorative agents, including inosine;[54] niacin,[55,56] HMG-CoA reductase inhibitors,[57] sigma-1 receptor agonists,[58] BDNF ligands,[59] and drugs targeting extracelluar matrix such as chondroitinase ABC.[60] Sildenafil[61,62] has a time window of at least 7 days and has been tested in human subjects recovering from stroke.[63] An extended-release formulation of the potassium channel blocker 4-aminopyridine has been approved by the U.S. FDA to improve walking ability in patients with multiple sclerosis,[64] and is now being studied after stroke.[65] A randomized, placebo-controlled trial of citicoline initiated within 24 hours of stroke onset was stopped for futility.[66]

TRADITIONAL AND ALTERNATIVE MEDICINES

These medicines have also been suggested as potentially useful for improving outcome after stroke. This reflects a number of factors, including cultural mores, availability of herbal remedies, dietary supplements, patterns of regulatory oversight of nutraceuticals, and patient frustration – treatments based on alternative medicine attract interest whenever symptoms persistent after using approved therapies. Alternative medicines may be drug-based or device-based such as acupuncture and acupressure. Few traditional and alternative medicines have undergone formal evaluation. One exception is the Chinese Medicine Neuroaid Efficacy on Stroke recovery (CHIMES) study,[67] a multicenter, double-blind, placebo-controlled clinical trial that randomized 1,100 patients to 3 months of Neuroaid vs placebo, provided in the form of three daily doses of four oral capsules each. Neuroaid is a traditional Chinese medicine containing extracts of nine herbal and five animal components. Patients started therapy within 72 hours of stroke onset. No difference between treatment arms was seen in the primary outcome measure, shift in the modified Rankin Scale at 3 months.

BIOLOGICAL PRODUCTS

Growth Factors

These are normally produced by the body as signaling molecules, e.g., for development, learning, and brain plasticity.

Brain levels of many growth factors increase after stroke.[68] These play a critical role in neural repair through mechanisms that include angiogenesis, reduced apoptosis, stem cell proliferation, and immunomodulation.[69] Preclinical studies suggest that administration of certain exogenous growth factors, e.g., brain-derived neurotrophic factor (BDNF), improves stroke recovery[70] when introduced within days of stroke onset.

Human studies of growth factors to date have focused on hematopoietic factors, some of which have extensive human experience. Granulocyte-colony stimulating factor (G-CSF) showed favorable preclinical findings. The AX200 for Ischemic Stroke (AXIS) study[71] found G-CSF given within 12 hours of stroke to be safe, feasible, and well-tolerated in 44 patients; these good safety results were echoed by a separate study of 60 patients.[72] The AXIS-2 study[73] compared the middle G-CSF dose from the AXIS study (135 ug/kg) with placebo in 328 patients <9 hours post-stroke using a multicenter, randomized, placebo-controlled design. G-CSF was not different from placebo on the primary endpoint, modified Rankin Scale score at day 90.

Preclinical studies suggest that systemically administered erythropoietin may enter the brain and improve outcome when introduced with a delay such as 24 hours post-stroke.[74] Other studies found favorable effects of sequential growth factor administration, giving epidermal growth factor[75] or beta-human chorionic gonadotropin (hCG)[76] followed by erythropoietin, beginning 1–7 days after stroke, possibly by increasing neural stem cell levels. This approach was directly translated to humans in the beta-hCG+erythropoietin in acute stroke (BETAS) study, a single-dose, multisite, open-label, non-controlled safety trial that gave three hCG doses beginning 1–2 days post-stroke followed by three erythropoietin doses beginning 7–8 days after stroke. No safety concerns were identified.[77] The safety of erythropoietin was also found in a randomized placebo-controlled study of 167 patients who received two doses of erythropoietin vs placebo beginning 48 hours post-stroke.[78]

The BETAS study was followed by the REGENESIS study.[79] This was intended to be a randomized, placebo-controlled, double-blind proof of concept study of sequential hCG and erythropoietin using the BETAS study treatment schedule. This trial was put on hold by regulatory authorities due to concerns related to an acute stroke neuroprotective trial[80] that initiated erythropoietin <6 hours after stroke onset, even though the REGENESIS trial initiated erythropoietin 7–8 days post-stroke. Subsequently, the REGENESIS trial was modified to be a dose-ranging safety study and due to financial constraints largely moved to India. Enrollment was terminated by the sponsor early after 96 enrollees. Treatment groups did not differ in safety or in the primary endpoint, NIHSS score change to day 90.

Delivering growth factors to brain targets presents challenges. Alternate approaches under study include intranasal or intracerebral delivery, a Trojan horse strategy involving conjugation of a growth factor with a molecule that can cross the blood–brain barrier, delivery via gene-modified stem cells, and development of small ligands.[81–83]

Monoclonal Antibody

A monoclonal antibody modulates activity within a targeted signaling pathway by binding to a specific target such as a receptor or cell surface marker. Axonal growth occurs in the peripheral nervous system.[84] In the CNS, however, inhibitory molecules such as myelin-associated glycoprotein (MAG) and Nogo-A, result in the lack of a permissive growth environment; furthermore, levels of these molecules increase after stroke.[4,85] A monoclonal antibody can be used to neutralize these inhibitory CNS signals and promote axon growth after injury. A recent study randomized 42 patients with stroke to placebo vs one of three doses of intravenous GSK249320, a humanized IgG1 monoclonal antibody to MAG that has a disabled Fc region. Each patient received two infusions, the first being 24–72 hours after stroke onset and the second being 9 days later. No safety concerns were identified,[86] and a phase II proof-of-concept study is ongoing.

Stem Cells

Numerous cell-based therapies are under study to improve stroke recovery.[87,88] Examples include transformed tumor cells, adult stem cells such as mesenchymal stromal cells, umbilical cord cells, placental cells, fetal stem cells, embryonic stem cells, and induced pluripotent cells. Cells can be autologous, allogeneic, or xenogeneic; introduced with a bioscaffold; cultured using conditions such as hypoxia or an enriched medium; contain modified genes; and can be introduced through various routes including intracerebral, intra-arterial, and intravenous. Few human studies of stem cells after stroke have been published. These are reviewed elsewhere in this volume.

Cellular therapies may introduce complexities that are uncommon to other therapeutic classes. As these are living cells, potency and identity could change over time or after storage and so must be confirmed prior to release.[89] Some stem cells persist for months or years after administration, requiring extended assessment of their long-term fate - 10 years for the first embryonic stem cell trial approved by the U.S. FDA.[90] Some patients and scientists have ethical concerns with use of certain cells.[91]

DEVICE-BASED THERAPIES

A robot is a mechanical device, guided by a computer, that senses or moves within its environment.[92,93] Many robotic devices have been designed.[93–95] Robotic devices have potential advantages such as consistent output, programmability, utility for gaming applications, ability to precisely measure patient behavior, and the potential for an improved therapist : patient ratio.[96]

Clinical experience with robotic devices has been variable but generally favorable. Generalization is difficult due to major differences between studies such as in the robot, population studied, treatment protocol, and mode of robotic assistance.[92,93,95,97] One of the largest stroke recovery trials of a robotic device[98] recruited 127 patients an average of 4.6 years post-stroke among whom baseline motor deficits were severe. Using a multi-center, controlled randomized design, enrollees were randomized to robot-assisted upper-extremity rehabilitation, which employed high-intensity, repetitive proximal and distal arm movements (36 1-hour sessions over 12 weeks); a dose-matched and intensity-matched comparison therapy using conventional rehabilitation methods; or to usual care. No significant difference was seen in the primary endpoint, change in arm motor FM score to 12 weeks, though robot-assisted therapy appeared favorable in secondary analyses to 36 weeks.

Robotic therapies are being studied for many other applications, including lower extremity deficits; pediatric populations;[99] activities limitations (disability);[100] sensory deficits;[101] and as an outcome measure.[102] Challenges for robotic therapy include identifying optimal populations and protocols, attention to human issues such as fatigue, consideration of object affordance and ecology, and identifying optimal types of assistance.[92–95,103] Patient acceptance of these devices as a treatment option must be considered, although one stroke study found that most patients, after being exposed to both conventional and robotic therapy, preferred the robot.[103]

BRAIN STIMULATION

The brain is an electrical organ and so modulation of brain function can be achieved via electromagnetic approaches. Brain stimulation, in the form of electroconvulsive therapy, is more effective than all other forms of treatment and remains the gold standard for treating depression.[104] Many types of brain stimulation have been examined to improve outcome after stroke. Surgical approaches have been studied, including a phase III trial that did not find a benefit;[105] most investigation has focused on non-invasive approaches.

Transcranial magnetic stimulation (TMS) provides focal brain stimulation. The key innovation of TMS was to excite cerebral cortex by passing a magnetic pulse rather than electrical current through the skull. An insulated stimulator coil is placed onto the scalp, which issues a magnetic pulse that induces action potentials in neurons of underlying cortex. A single TMS pulse over motor cortex produces a brief contralateral muscle twitch. TMS over most other cortical areas transiently disrupts behavioral output of the stimulated regions. Neurophysiological measures using single-pulse TMS may be useful to stratify patients after stroke.[106,107]

Delivery of TMS in other modes may affect cortical function and could have therapeutic value. Repetitive TMS (rTMS) involves delivery of multiple TMS pulses. At low frequencies (e.g., 1 Hz), the effect is generally decreased cortical excitability, of potential interest if overactivity within a particular cortical region is seen as an impediment to stroke recovery.[108,109] High-frequency rTMS (e.g., 5–20 Hz) can increase cortical excitability, which carries potential risks; specific guidelines must be followed to insure safety.[110]

Use of rTMS within recommended parameters after stroke is safe[111] and may improve selected behaviors.[112] A recent Cochrane review concluded that current evidence does not support routine use of rTMS to improve function after stroke, possibly due to heterogeneity between trials and small sample sizes.[111] Another factor may be that grouping together disparate stroke studies can complicate stroke recovery meta-analyses; consistent with this, a meta-analysis of rTMS studies that focused on arm motor recovery did identify a significant benefit.[113] As with many restorative therapies, challenges include identifying target populations, patterns of injury most likely to benefit, ideal treatment protocols including optimal rTMS Hz, best brain target(s), best time post-stroke, and best approaches to behavioral reinforcement.[114]

TRANSCRANIAL DIRECT CURRENT STIMULATION

Transcranial direct current stimulation (tDCS) passes current through the scalp, skull, and meninges in order to stimulate the brain, generally undetectably. A small electric current (1–2 mA) is delivered to the scalp by a battery-driven device connected to two saline-soaked surface electrodes. The current is not sufficient to generate action potentials but instead alters neuronal resting membrane potentials. Like rTMS, tDCS can alter cortical excitability, with anodal tDCS generally increasing cortical excitability and cathodal tDCS decreasing it.[112,115] In patients with stroke, tDCS has been found safe, and a number of studies suggest the potential to improve certain behaviors.[112,116] A recent Cochrane review combining wide-ranging tDCS studies noted that evidence was limited for the effectiveness of tDCS for improving function after stroke.[117] As with rMTS, a meta-analysis of studies focused on arm motor recovery did find significant benefit of tDCS.[118]

OTHER DEVICES

A brain–computer interface (BCI) is a computer-based system that acquires brain signals, analyzes them, and translates them into commands that are relayed to an output device to carry out a desired action. In this way, a BCI bypasses the region of stroke injury by recording signals directly from intact brain regions and then delivering that signal, or a derivative, to an effector that can modify the environment.[119,120] Some BCI systems are invasive, e.g., implanting electrodes directly into the brain to decode neural signals to control movement of a robotic arm.[121] Less invasive approaches use techniques such as scalp EEG to record brain signals, but the precision of this information is reduced; one such approach captures event-related peri-Rolandic mu rhythms as subjects make a selection or decision, e.g., to begin movement, and this triggers a device such as a neuromotor prosthesis or functional electrical stimulation.[122,123]

Numerous other devices have been proposed as useful to improve outcome and function after stroke. These span a wide range of complexity, and include resistance splints, neuroprosthetics, functional electrical stimulation, motorized orthotic devices for specific joints, and novel computer interfaces.

REHABILITATION AND OTHER ACTIVITY-BASED THERAPIES

Rehabilitation therapy is generally standard of care following a stroke. Strong evidence exists that interdisciplinary rehabilitation, which includes activity-based therapies, provided subacutely after stroke, is associated with reduced death and dependency.[124] Activity-based therapies achieve their effects by promoting brain plasticity. Substantial evidence indicates that greater amount and duration of activity-based therapy after stroke are associated with improved outcome.[125–128] The same is true for greater intensity of therapy.[125,129,130] Effects are also increased when therapy is challenging, motivating, and interesting.[131–134] Results extend to patients in the subacute or chronic phase after stroke.[135,136]

Activity-based interventions are important to brain repair after stroke for at least two reasons: first as a stand-alone therapy, and second as an adjuvant therapy for many pharmacological and biological therapies. Whether there are differences across the various schools of post-stroke rehabilitation remains uncertain.[137] A potential advantage of activity-based therapies is that regulatory concerns may be reduced as compared to many biological products or devices.

Constraint-induced movement therapy (CIMT) is a form of activity-based therapy that focuses on overcoming learned disuse of a stroke-affected hand to improve motor function and has been found useful in selected subpopulations of patients with unilateral hemiparesis.[138] With CIMT, the non-affected hand is restrained while the affected hand undergoes a very intense course of therapy. The long-term efficacy of CIMT for patients with moderate arm motor deficits was supported by the "Extremity Constraint Induced Therapy Evaluation" (EXCITE) study,[139] a prospective, single-blind, randomized, multisite clinical trial that enrolled 222 patients with stroke 3–9 months prior and moderate arm motor deficits. Subjects were randomized to customary care or 2 weeks of CIMT, 6 hours/day. Significant results were found for both primary endpoints, Wolf Motor Function Test (52% reduction in time to complete its tasks) and Motor Activity Log (76–77% increase in quantity and quality of affected arm use) at 1 year. Gains were persistent at 2 years.[140] The limitations of the EXCITE trial include that intensive therapy was compared to a non-active intervention; also, the fraction of patients with stroke eligible for this intervention is uncertain. However

EXCITE is a positive Phase III clinical trial targeting stroke recovery. Simplified forms of CIMT may also be useful,[141] and the overall approach has been extended to other domains such as language.[142,143]

The Very Early Constraint Induced Movement during Stroke Rehabilitation (VECTORS) trial[144] was a single-site, single-blind, controlled clinical trial that randomized patients with moderate-to-severe motor deficits to 2 weeks of study intervention in place of occupational therapy (OT) during their post-acute inpatient rehabilitation admission. Patients were randomized to standard CIMT, high-intensity CIMT, or a control treatment that mimicked usual OT. Patients averaged 10 days post-stroke at enrollment. The primary endpoint, change in arm motor function to 90 days after stroke onset, was significantly different across groups. To the authors' surprise, subjects in the high-intensity CIMT group showed significantly *less* gains vs the other two groups. VECTORS suggests that more therapy is not always better, and emphasizes that activity-based interventions also benefit from dose-finding studies. VECTORS also underscores the value of including a dose-matched control group in an activity-based trial. Finally, CIMT was as effective as a similar dose of conventional therapy for reducing arm motor impairment and disability, echoing that in at least some cases, the dose of activity-based therapy may be more important than particulars of treatment content.[137]

The Locomotor Experience Applied Post-Stroke (LEAPS) trial[145] targeted post-stroke gait, an endpoint of high interest because it is commonly affected by stroke, ranked as the top priority by hemiplegic patients,[146] and though a measure of impairment (loss of body function and structure) it is directly linked to quality of life[147] and social participation.[148] At time of randomization 2 months post-stroke, enrollees were <2 months post-stroke and had leg weakness plus gait velocity < 0.8 m/second. Enrollees were randomized to 36 sessions of 90 minutes duration of either body-weight support treadmill training (BWSTT) starting 2 months post-stroke, BWSTT starting 6 months post-stroke, or home exercises starting 2 months post-stroke. The primary outcome, the proportion of patients who at 1 year post-stroke improved functional walking ability, was found in 52% of enrollees, with no significant difference between treatment groups. LEAPS provides evidence that months after stroke onset, when standard of care is no longer providing physical therapy, the functional status of many patients can, nonetheless, be improved by a therapeutic intervention. A strength of the study design was the use of active control groups that were matched in intensity of intervention. LEAPS is one of a growing number of studies that relies upon modality-specific endpoints, an approach that may be of particular value for restorative therapies.[64,149,150] LEAPS also used sliding dichotomous outcomes, with different criteria used to define success across various strata of baseline patient deficits, an approach that can be expected to attract increased attention over time.[151,152]

Unfortunately, many patients do not receive high-dose/intensity therapy in clinical practice.[153-157] For example, in one recent U.S. study, patients receiving inpatient stroke rehabilitation received on average only 23 functional arm repetitions per treatment session.[153]

TELEREHABILITATION

This may be a useful approach to increasing the quantity and intensity of stroke rehabilitation. Telerehabilitation has been defined as "the delivery of rehabilitation services via information and communication technologies," and encompasses services that include assessment, prevention, treatment, education, and counseling.[158]

Increasing evidence supports the potential of a telerehabilitation approach for reducing neurological deficits.[159-165] A major component of this may be derived from promoting patient participation in health care via the use of games,[166-170] which can motivate patients to engage in enjoyable play behavior that involves useful therapy-related movements.[171,172] Recent reviews have criticized the quality of published stroke telerehabilitation studies but noted high levels of user satisfaction.[173-176]

COGNITIVE-BASED THERAPIES

Humans are cognitive creatures and so the potential exists to enhance outcomes by focusing on cognitive skills. It has long been known that athletes who mentally practice a motor skill improve performance, from tasks ranging from dart throwing to badminton serving to golf.[177] Consistent with this, increasing evidence suggests that mental imagery has value for improving some outcomes after stroke.[178] Other therapies, building on the neurobiology of mirror neuron systems, have focused on motor observation.[179] Other cognitive strategies include those focused on music,[155] mirror visual feedback to overcome hemi-inattention,[180] computerized delivery of stimuli target activity in selected neural circuits,[181] real-time neural feedback,[182-184] and techniques focused on virtual reality and augmented reality.[44,185] Animal studies have long demonstrated that an enriched environment has favorable effects on the brain and behavior in the healthy state[186] and after stroke;[187,188] comparable studies in humans are needed.[189]

ISSUES RELATED TO THE DESIGN OF RESTORATIVE CLINICAL TRIALS AFTER STROKE

Many of the larger stroke recovery studies to date have provided useful insights (Table 59-1). Key questions remain for many classes of restorative intervention. What is the optimal time for safe and effective initiation? What is the best frequency of duration of therapy? Indeed, for some therapies, a single dose may be effective,[190-192] whereas, for others, repeated exposures are emphasized as necessary.[55,61,75,193,194] How will the target population be defined? Emerging studies are paying increasing attention to these questions.

An issue important to stroke recovery trials is that neural repair occurs on the basis of experience-dependent plasticity. This issue is generally not considered in acute stroke therapies – the patient need not engage in any particular behavioral regimen to enable tPA effectiveness – but it is central to promoting recovery after stroke. The issue was well described in the landmark study by Feeney et al.,[33] who found that in rodents with an experimental stroke, amphetamine therapy improved motor outcome, but only if drug dosing was paired with training. Subsequent studies have confirmed this principle across many other classes of post-stroke restorative therapy.[195-199] This is an additional analogy with normal development, where the brain is galvanized for learning and plasticity, but must be shaped by experience to achieve maximal behavioural gains.

For some restorative therapies, use of a modality-specific outcome measure may be important to capturing treatment effects.[149] A treatment that improves outcome by promoting neuroplasticity might have maximum effect in a brain network that has sustained subtotal injury, but show no effect in a network that has been obliterated by stroke. A restorative drug given to a patient with dense aphasia but moderate hemiparesis might provide useful gains in motor function, but not in language function; a motor scale would have superior granularity for measuring this treatment effect as compared to a global scale.

TABLE 59-1 Lessons from Recent Key Stroke Recovery Trials

Study	n	Time Post-Stroke	Treatment Arms	Main Finding	Key Lessons for Restorative Stroke Trials
Robinson et al.[45]	176	<3 months	[1] Escitalopram [2] Problem-solving therapy [3] Placebo	[1] and [2] > [3] to prevent depression at 12 months	Concerns include the need to control amount of interaction with study personnel, and the low incidence of primary endpoint
FLAME[47]	118	5–10 days	[1] 20 mg/day fluoxetine [2] placebo	[1] > [2] in Fugl-Meyer score change to day 90	No measurement of outside therapy from baseline to day 90
LEAPS[145]	408	2 months	[1] BWSTT at 2 months post-stroke [2] BWSTT at 6 months post-stroke [3] Home exercise at 2 months post-stroke	Functional walking ability improved after 1 year in 52% of subjects, but no difference between groups	Use of active control groups matched in treatment intensity, and use of sliding dichotomous outcomes, are strengths. Absence of a "no therapy" group, useful for some analyses, is a potential concern
Lo et al.[98]	127	>6 months	[1] Robot therapy [2] Non-robotic therapy [3] Usual care	No difference in Fugl-Meyer score after 12 weeks	Enrolled patients with very severe baseline deficits, among whom treatment gains are often limited
EXCITE[139]	222	3–9 months	[1] Constraint-induced movement therapy [2] Usual care	After 12 months, [1] > [2] in Wolf Motor Function Test and Motor Activity Log	Treatment arms were not matched in intensity, difficult to ascertain if findings are due to differences in treatment content or treatment intensity
Everest[105]	164	>4 months	[1] Epidural cortical stimulation +physiotherapy [2] Physiotherapy alone	No difference in proportion of patients with both ≥4.5 point Fugl-Meyer score and ≥0.21 Arm Motor Ability Test score increase 4 weeks post-therapy	Need to match neurological features of trial enrollees with features present in preclinical studies[217]
STARS[36]	71	5–10 days	[1] Amphetamine + physiotherapy [2] Placebo + physiotherapy	No difference between groups	Uncertain basis for choosing drug dose and schedule. Use of a single examiner and use of a single therapist reduced study variance and increased power

Restorative trials often must address the issue of therapy provided to patients outside of study procedures, which could complicate interpretation of clinical trial results. Occupational therapy, physical therapy, and speech therapy can influence recovery. These will, therefore, be provided as standard of care to most patients enrolled in a stroke recovery clinical trial, and in a variable manner across treatment sites.[200] For example, in the LEAPS trial,[145] where functional walking ability was the primary endpoint, 81.9% of enrollees received physical therapy outside of study procedures (an average of 25 such sessions). Several options for addressing this issue have been suggested, including limiting outside therapy,[144] though patients might be non-compliant and this could slow recruitment; measuring the amount of outside therapy, to be used as a covariate in data analysis;[41] and restricting enrollment to healthcare systems where such therapy is relatively standardized.[23]

An issue of concern to stroke recovery trials also shared by acute stroke trials is that many treatments are time-sensitive. Indeed, some therapies have a bimodal effect over time, e.g., GABA agonists or NMDA receptor blockers can be favorable if administered in the early hours after stroke,[201,202] but deleterious if initiated days later;[203–205] the reverse may be true for VEGF,[206] AMPA receptor signaling,[207] matrix metalloproteinases,[208] and immune modulators.[209,210]

Patient stratification is another issue common to many types of stroke trial, including restorative trials. Many different measures can affect stroke recovery and response to restorative therapies, such as injury location and size,[211,212] genotype,[213] differences in brain function,[214] and level of depression.[215,216] Such measures may be of pivotal value for defining the stroke subpopulation that is most likely to benefit from a given therapy.[217]

The complete reference list can be found on the companion Expert Consult website at www.expertconsult.inkling.com. 

KEY REFERENCES

1. Iadecola C, Anrather J. The immunology of stroke: from mechanisms to translation. Nat Med 2011;17:796–808.
2. Wieloch T, Nikolich K. Mechanisms of neural plasticity following brain injury. Curr Opin Neurobiol 2006;16:258–64.
3. Nudo RJ. Neural bases of recovery after brain injury. J Commun Disord 2011;44:515–20.
4. Li S, Carmichael ST. Growth-associated gene and protein expression in the region of axonal sprouting in the aged brain after stroke. Neurobiol Dis 2006;23(2):362–73.
6. Zhang ZG, Chopp M. Neurorestorative therapies for stroke: underlying mechanisms and translation to the clinic. Lancet Neurol 2009;8:491–500.
7. Cramer S, Chopp M. Recovery recapitulates ontogeny. Trends Neurosci 2000;23:265–71.
8. Cramer S, Moore C, Finklestein S, et al. A pilot study of somatotopic mapping after cortical infarct. Stroke 2000;31:668–71.
9. Cramer S, Crafton K. Somatotopy and movement representation sites following cortical stroke. Exp Brain Res 2006;168: 25–32.

10. Rosen H, Petersen S, Linenweber M, et al. Neural correlates of recovery from aphasia after damage to left inferior frontal cortex. Neurology 2000;55:1883–94.
11. Sharma N, Baron JC, Rowe JB. Motor imagery after stroke: relating outcome to motor network connectivity. Ann Neurol 2009;66(5):604–16.
12. Grefkes C, Nowak DA, Eickhoff SB, et al. Cortical connectivity after subcortical stroke assessed with functional magnetic resonance imaging. Ann Neurol 2008;63(2):236–46.
13. Carter AR, Astafiev SV, Lang CE, et al. Resting interhemispheric functional magnetic resonance imaging connectivity predicts performance after stroke. Ann Neurol 2010;67(3):365–75.
14. Chollet F, DiPiero V, Wise R, et al. The functional anatomy of motor recovery after stroke in humans: A study with positron emission tomography. Ann Neurol 1991;29:63–71.
15. Weiller C, Chollet F, Friston K, et al. Functional reorganization of the brain in recovery from striatocapsular infarction in man. Ann Neurol 1992;31:463–72.
16. Weiller C, Isensee C, Rijntjes M, et al. Recovery from Wernicke's aphasia: a positron emission tomographic study. Ann Neurol 1995;37(6):723–32.
17. Cramer S, Nelles G, Benson R, et al. A functional MRI study of subjects recovered from hemiparetic stroke. Stroke 1997;28(12): 2518–27.
18. Gauthier LV, Taub E, Mark VW, et al. Atrophy of spared gray matter tissue predicts poorer motor recovery and rehabilitation response in chronic stroke. Stroke 2012;43(2):453–7.
19. Schaechter JD, Moore CI, Connell BD, et al. Structural and functional plasticity in the somatosensory cortex of chronic stroke patients. Brain 2006;129(Pt 10):2722–33.
21. Carmichael ST, Tatsukawa K, Katsman D, et al. Evolution of diaschisis in a focal stroke model. Stroke 2004;35(3):758–63.
22. Levin MF, Kleim JA, Wolf SL. What do motor "recovery" and "compensation" mean in patients following stroke? Neurorehabil Neural Repair 2009;23(4):313–19.
23. Cramer SC. Repairing the human brain after stroke. II. Restorative therapies. Ann Neurol 2008;63(5):549–60.
26. Langhorne P, Bernhardt J, Kwakkel G. Stroke rehabilitation. Lancet 2011;377(9778):1693–702.
27. Dobkin BH, Dorsch A. New evidence for therapies in stroke rehabilitation. Curr Atheroscler Rep 2013;15(6):331.
28. Biernaskie J, Chernenko G, Corbett D. Efficacy of rehabilitative experience declines with time after focal ischemic brain injury. J Neurosci 2004;24(5):1245–54.
29. Ren J, Kaplan P, Charette M, et al. Time window of intracisternal osteogenic protein-1 in enhancing functional recovery after stroke. Neuropharmacology 2000;39(5):860–5.
30. Clarkson AN, Huang BS, Macisaac SE, et al. Reducing excessive GABA-mediated tonic inhibition promotes functional recovery after stroke. Nature 2010;468:305–9.
31. Cramer SC, Sur M, Dobkin BH, et al. Harnessing neuroplasticity for clinical applications. Brain 2011;134(Pt 6):1591–609.
32. Pardridge WM. Drug transport across the blood-brain barrier. J Cereb Blood Flow Metab 2012;32(11):1959–72.
33. Feeney D, Gonzalez A, Law W. Amphetamine, Halperidol, and experience interact to affect the rate of recovery after motor cortex injury. Science 1982;217:855–7.
36. Gladstone DJ, Danells CJ, Armesto A, et al. Physiotherapy coupled with dextroamphetamine for rehabilitation after hemiparetic stroke: a randomized, double-blind, placebo-controlled trial. Stroke 2006;37(1):179–85.
38. Floel A, Cohen LG. Recovery of function in humans: cortical stimulation and pharmacological treatments after stroke. Neurobiol Dis 2010;37(2):243–51.
39. Scheidtmann K, Fries W, Muller F, et al. Effect of levodopa in combination with physiotherapy on functional motor recovery after stroke: a prospective, randomised, double-blind study. Lancet 2001;358:787–90.
40. Pearson-Fuhrhop KM, Minton B, Acevedo D, et al. Genetic variation in the human brain dopamine system influences motor learning and its modulation by L-dopa. PLoS ONE 2013;8(4): e61197.
41. Cramer SC, Dobkin BH, Noser EA, et al. Randomized, placebo-controlled, double-blind study of ropinirole in chronic stroke. Stroke 2009;40(9):3034–8.
42. Small SL, Llano DA. Biological approaches to aphasia treatment. Curr Neurol Neurosci Rep 2009;9(6):443–50.
43. Wang LE, Fink GR, Diekhoff S, et al. Noradrenergic enhancement improves motor network connectivity in stroke patients. Ann Neurol 2011;69(2):375–88.
45. Robinson RG, Jorge RE, Moser DJ, et al. Escitalopram and problem-solving therapy for prevention of poststroke depression: a randomized controlled trial. JAMA 2008;299(20): 2391–400.
47. Chollet F, Tardy J, Albucher JF, et al. Fluoxetine for motor recovery after acute ischaemic stroke (FLAME): a randomised placebo-controlled trial. Lancet Neurol 2011;10(2):123–30.
49. Kohen R, Cain KC, Buzaitis A, et al. Response to psychosocial treatment in poststroke depression is associated with serotonin transporter polymorphisms. Stroke 2011;42(7):2068–70.
52. Ramanathan D, Tuszynski MH, Conner JM. The basal forebrain cholinergic system is required specifically for behaviorally mediated cortical map plasticity. J Neurosci 2009;29(18): 5992–6000.
53. Berthier ML, Green C, Higueras C, et al. A randomized, placebo-controlled study of donepezil in poststroke aphasia. Neurology 2006;67(9):1687–9.
54. Zai L, Ferrari C, Subbaiah S, et al. Inosine alters gene expression and axonal projections in neurons contralateral to a cortical infarct and improves skilled use of the impaired limb. J Neurosci 2009;29(25):8187–97.
56. Yan T, Chopp M, Ye X, et al. Niaspan increases axonal remodeling after stroke in type 1 diabetes rats. Neurobiol Dis 2012; 46(1):157–64.
57. Karki K, Knight RA, Han Y, et al. Simvastatin and atorvastatin improve neurological outcome after experimental intracerebral hemorrhage. Stroke 2009;40(10):3384–9.
58. Ruscher K, Shamloo M, Rickhag M, et al. The sigma-1 receptor enhances brain plasticity and functional recovery after experimental stroke. Brain 2011;134:732–46.
59. Han J, Pollak J, Yang T, et al. Delayed administration of a small molecule tropomyosin-related kinase B ligand promotes recovery after hypoxic-ischemic stroke. Stroke 2012;43(7):1918–24.
60. Soleman S, Yip PK, Duricki DA, et al. Delayed treatment with chondroitinase ABC promotes sensorimotor recovery and plasticity after stroke in aged rats. Brain 2012;135:1210–23.
61. Zhang R, Wang Y, Zhang L, et al. Sildenafil (Viagra) induces neurogenesis and promotes functional recovery after stroke in rats. Stroke 2002;33(11):2675–80.
63. Silver B, McCarthy S, Lu M, et al. Sildenafil treatment of subacute ischemic stroke: a safety study at 25-mg daily for 2 weeks. J Stroke Cerebrovasc Dis 2009;18(5):381–3.
65. Iaci JF, Parry TJ, Huang Z, et al. Dalfampridine improves sensorimotor function in rats with chronic deficits after middle cerebral artery occlusion. Stroke 2013;44(7):1942–50.
66. Davalos A, Alvarez-Sabin J, Castillo J, et al. Citicoline in the treatment of acute ischaemic stroke: an international, randomised, multicentre, placebo-controlled study (ICTUS trial). Lancet 2012;380(9839):349–57.
67. Chen CL, Young SH, Gan HH, et al. Chinese medicine neuroaid efficacy on stroke recovery: a double-blind, placebo-controlled, randomized study. Stroke 2013;44(8):2093–100.
70. Ren JM, Finklestein SP. Growth factor treatment of stroke. Curr Drug Targets CNS Neurol Disord 2005;4(2):121–5.
71. Schabitz WR, Laage R, Vogt G, et al. AXIS: a trial of intravenous granulocyte colony-stimulating factor in acute ischemic stroke. Stroke 2010;41(11):2545–51.
73. Ringelstein EB, Thijs V, Norrving B, et al. Granulocyte colony-stimulating factor in patients with acute ischemic stroke: results of the AX200 for Ischemic Stroke trial. Stroke 2013;44(10): 2681–7.
75. Kolb B, Morshead C, Gonzalez C, et al. Growth factor-stimulated generation of new cortical tissue and functional recovery after stroke damage to the motor cortex of rats. J Cereb Blood Flow Metab 2007;27(5):983–97.
76. Belayev L, Khoutorova L, Zhao KL, et al. A novel neurotrophic therapeutic strategy for experimental stroke. Brain Res 2009;1280: 117–23.
77. Cramer SC, Fitzpatrick C, Warren M, et al. The beta-hCG+erythropoietin in acute stroke (BETAS) study: a 3-center,

single-dose, open-label, noncontrolled, phase IIa safety trial. Stroke 2010;41(5):927–31.
79. Cramer SC, Hill MD. Human choriogonadotropin and epoetin alfa in acute ischemic stroke patients (REGENESIS-LED trial). Int J Stroke 2014;9(3):321–7.
80. Ehrenreich H, Weissenborn K, Prange H, et al. Recombinant human erythropoietin in the treatment of acute ischemic stroke. Stroke 2009;40(12):e647–56.
82. Zhang Y, Pardridge WM. Conjugation of brain-derived neurotrophic factor to a blood-brain barrier drug targeting system enables neuroprotection in regional brain ischemia following intravenous injection of the neurotrophin. Brain Res 2001; 889(1–2):49–56.
83. Yasuhara T, Borlongan C, Date I. Ex vivo gene therapy: transplantation of neurotrophic factor-secreting cells for cerebral ischemia. Front Biosci 2006;11:760–75.
85. Cheatwood JL, Emerick AJ, Schwab ME, et al. Nogo-A expression after focal ischemic stroke in the adult rat. Stroke 2008;39(7): 2091–8.
86. Cramer SC, Abila B, Scott NE, et al. Safety, pharmacokinetics, and pharmacodynamics of escalating repeat doses of GSK249320 in patients with stroke. Stroke 2013;44(5):1337–42.
87. Lindvall O, Kokaia Z. Stem cell research in stroke: how far from the clinic? Stroke 2011;42(8):2369–75.
88. Savitz SI, Cramer SC, Wechsler L. Stem cells as an emerging paradigm in stroke 3: enhancing the development of clinical trials. Stroke 2014;45(2):634–9.
90. Chapman AR, Scala CC. Evaluating the first-in-human clinical trial of a human embryonic stem cell-based therapy. Kennedy Inst Ethics J 2012;22(3):243–61.
91. Hyun I. The bioethics of stem cell research and therapy. J Clin Invest 2010;120(1):71–5.
92. Reinkensmeyer DJ. Robotic approaches to stroke recovery. In: Cramer SC, Nudo RJ, editors. Brain repair after stroke. Cambridge, UK: Cambridge University Press; 2010. p. 195–205.
93. Volpe BT, Huerta PT, Zipse JL, et al. Robotic devices as therapeutic and diagnostic tools for stroke recovery. Arch Neurol 2009;66(9):1086–90.
95. Reinkensmeyer D, Emken J, Cramer S. Robotics, motor learning, and neurologic recovery. Annu Rev Biomed Eng 2004;6: 497–525.
96. Cramer SC. Brain repair after stroke. N Engl J Med 2010;362(19): 1827–9.
98. Lo AC, Guarino PD, Richards LG, et al. Robot-assisted therapy for long-term upper-limb impairment after stroke. N Engl J Med 2010;362(19):1772–83.
99. Fasoli SE, Ladenheim B, Mast J, et al. New horizons for robot-assisted therapy in pediatrics. Am J Phys Med Rehabil 2012;91(11 Suppl. 3):S280–9.
101. Semrau JA, Herter TM, Scott SH, et al. Robotic identification of kinesthetic deficits after stroke. Stroke 2013;44(12):3414–21.
103. Reinkensmeyer DJ, Wolbrecht ET, Chan V, et al. Comparison of three-dimensional, assist-as-needed robotic arm/hand movement training provided with Pneu-WREX to conventional tabletop therapy after chronic stroke. Am J Phys Med Rehabil 2012; 91(11 Suppl. 3):S232–41.
104. American Psychiatric Association. Practice guideline for the treatment of patients with major depressive disorder. ed 3. Arlington, VA: American Psychiatric Association; 2010.
105. Levy R, Benson R, Winstein C, et al., editors. Cortical stimulation for upper-extremity hemiparesis from ischemic stroke: everest study primary endpoint results. New Orleans, LA: International Stroke Conference; 2008.
106. Hoyer EH, Celnik PA. Understanding and enhancing motor recovery after stroke using transcranial magnetic stimulation. Restor Neurol Neurosci 2011;29(6):395–409.
107. Talelli P, Greenwood RJ, Rothwell JC. Arm function after stroke: Neurophysiological correlates and recovery mechanisms assessed by transcranial magnetic stimulation. Clin Neurophysiol 2006; 117(8):1641–59.
108. Naeser MA, Martin PI, Nicholas M, et al. Improved picture naming in chronic aphasia after TMS to part of right Broca's area: an open-protocol study. Brain Lang 2005;93(1):95–105.
110. Rossi S, Hallett M, Rossini PM, et al. Safety, ethical considerations, and application guidelines for the use of transcranial magnetic stimulation in clinical practice and research. Clin Neurophysiol 2009;120(12):2008–39.
111. Hao Z, Wang D, Zeng Y, et al. Repetitive transcranial magnetic stimulation for improving function after stroke. Cochrane Database Syst Rev 2013;(5):CD008862.
112. Shah PP, Szaflarski JP, Allendorfer J, et al. Induction of neuroplasticity and recovery in post-stroke aphasia by non-invasive brain stimulation. Front Hum Neurosci 2013;7:888.
113. Hsu WY, Cheng CH, Liao KK, et al. Effects of repetitive transcranial magnetic stimulation on motor functions in patients with stroke: a meta-analysis. Stroke 2012;43(7):1849–57.
114. Castel-Lacanal E, Tarri M, Loubinoux I, et al. Transcranial magnetic stimulation in brain injury. Ann Fr Anesth Reanim 2014;33(2):83–7.
115. Nitsche MA, Paulus W. Transcranial direct current stimulation – update 2011. Restor Neurol Neurosci 2011;29(6):463–92.
116. Lindenberg R, Renga V, Zhu LL, et al. Bihemispheric brain stimulation facilitates motor recovery in chronic stroke patients. Neurology 2010;75(24):2176–84.
117. Elsner B, Kugler J, Pohl M, et al. Transcranial direct current stimulation (tDCS) for improving function and activities of daily living in patients after stroke. Cochrane Database Syst Rev 2013;(11):CD009645.
118. Butler AJ, Shuster M, O'Hara E, et al. A meta-analysis of the efficacy of anodal transcranial direct current stimulation for upper limb motor recovery in stroke survivors. J Hand Ther 2013;26(2):162–70, quiz 171.
119. Ifft PJ, Shokur S, Li Z, et al. A brain-machine interface enables bimanual arm movements in monkeys. Sci Transl Med 2013; 5(210):210ra154.
120. Shih JJ, Krusienski DJ, Wolpaw JR. Brain-computer interfaces in medicine. Mayo Clin Proc 2012;87(3):268–79.
121. Hochberg LR, Bacher D, Jarosiewicz B, et al. Reach and grasp by people with tetraplegia using a neurally controlled robotic arm. Nature 2012;485(7398):372–5.
122. Do AH, Wang PT, King CE, et al. Brain-computer interface controlled functional electrical stimulation device for foot drop due to stroke. Conf Proc IEEE Eng Med Biol Soc 2012;2012:6414–17.
125. Kwakkel G, Wagenaar R, Twisk J, et al. Intensity of leg and arm training after primary middle-cerebral-artery stroke: a randomised trial. Lancet 1999;354(9174):191–6.
127. Kwakkel G, van Peppen R, Wagenaar RC, et al. Effects of augmented exercise therapy time after stroke: a meta-analysis. Stroke 2004;35(11):2529–39.
128. Outpatient Service Trialists. Rehabilitation therapy services for stroke patients living at home: systematic review of randomised trials. Lancet 2004;363:352–6.
129. Bhogal S, Teasell R, Speechley M. Intensity of aphasia therapy, impact on recovery. Stroke 2003;34(4):987–93.
131. Woldag H, Hummelsheim H. Evidence-based physiotherapeutic concepts for improving arm and hand function in stroke patients: a review. J Neurol 2002;249(5):518–28.
133. Kleim JA, Jones TA. Principles of experience-dependent neural plasticity: implications for rehabilitation after brain damage. J Speech Lang Hear Res 2008;51(1):S225–39.
135. Kerr AL, Cheng SY, Jones TA. Experience-dependent neural plasticity in the adult damaged brain. J Commun Disord 2011; 44(5):538–48.
136. Pollock A, Baer G, Campbell P, et al. Physical rehabilitation approaches for the recovery of function and mobility following stroke. Cochrane Database Syst Rev 2014;(4):CD001920.
138. Taub E, Uswatte G, Mark VW, et al. The learned nonuse phenomenon: implications for rehabilitation. Euro Medicophys 2006; 42(3):241–56.
139. Wolf SL, Winstein CJ, Miller JP, et al. Effect of constraint-induced movement therapy on upper extremity function 3 to 9 months after stroke: the EXCITE randomized clinical trial. JAMA 2006; 296(17):2095–104.
141. Page SJ, Levine P. Back from the brink: electromyography-triggered stimulation combined with modified constraint-induced movement therapy in chronic stroke. Arch Phys Med Rehabil 2006;87(1):27–31.
143. Berthier ML, Pulvermuller F. Neuroscience insights improve neurorehabilitation of poststroke aphasia. Nat Rev Neurol 2011;7(2): 86–97.

144. Dromerick AW, Lang CE, Birkenmeier RL, et al. Very Early Constraint-Induced Movement during Stroke Rehabilitation (VECTORS): A single-center RCT. Neurology 2009;73(3):195-201.
145. Duncan PW, Sullivan KJ, Behrman AL, et al. Body-weight-supported treadmill rehabilitation after stroke. N Engl J Med 2011;364(21):2026-36.
148. Perry J, Garrett M, Gronley J, et al. Classification of walking handicap in the stroke population. Stroke 1995;26(6):982-9.
149. Cramer SC, Koroshetz WJ, Finklestein SP. The case for modality-specific outcome measures in clinical trials of stroke recovery-promoting agents. Stroke 2007;38(4):1393-5.
151. Bath PM, Lees KR, Schellinger PD, et al. Statistical analysis of the primary outcome in acute stroke trials. Stroke 2012;43(4): 1171-8.
153. Lang CE, Macdonald JR, Reisman DS, et al. Observation of amounts of movement practice provided during stroke rehabilitation. Arch Phys Med Rehabil 2009;90(10):1692-8.
164. Deutsch JE, Lewis JA, Burdea G. Technical and patient performance using a virtual reality-integrated telerehabilitation system: preliminary finding. IEEE Trans Neural Syst Rehabil Eng 2007; 15(1):30-5.
166. Baranowski T, Buday R, Thompson DI, et al. Playing for real: video games and stories for health-related behavior change. Am J Prev Med 2008;34(1):74-82.
168. Hansen MM. Versatile, immersive, creative and dynamic virtual 3-D healthcare learning environments: a review of the literature. J Med Internet Res 2008;10(3):e26.
170. Thompson D, Baranowski T, Buday R, et al. Serious video games for health how behavioral science guided the development of a serious video game. Simul Gaming 2010;41(4):587-606.
173. Johansson T, Wild C. Telerehabilitation in stroke care–a systematic review. J Telemed Telecare 2011;17(1):1-6.
174. Saposnik G, Levin M. Virtual reality in stroke rehabilitation: a meta-analysis and implications for clinicians. Stroke 2011;42(5): 1380-6.
177. Feltz D, Landers D. The effects of mental practice on motor skill learning and performance: A meta-analysis. J Sport Psychol 1983;5:25-57.
178. Kho AY, Liu KP, Chung RC. Meta-analysis on the effect of mental imagery on motor recovery of the hemiplegic upper extremity function. Aust Occup Ther J 2014;61(2):38-48.
179. Small SL, Buccino G, Solodkin A. The mirror neuron system and treatment of stroke. Dev Psychobiol 2010;54(3):293-310.
180. Ramachandran VS, Altschuler EL. The use of visual feedback, in particular mirror visual feedback, in restoring brain function. Brain 2009;132(Pt 7):1693-710.
181. Dodakian L, Sharp K, See J, et al. Targeted engagement of a dorsal premotor circuit in the treatment of post-stroke paresis. Neurorehabilitation 2013;33(1):13-24.
182. Berman BD, Horovitz SG, Venkataraman G, et al. Self-modulation of primary motor cortex activity with motor and motor imagery tasks using real-time fMRI-based neurofeedback. Neuroimage 2012;59(2):917-25.
184. Sulzer J, Haller S, Scharnowski F, et al. Real-time fMRI neurofeedback: progress and challenges. Neuroimage 2013;76:386-99.
185. Hondori H, Khademi M, McKenzie A, et al. Utility of augmented reality in relation to virtual reality in stroke rehabilitation. Stroke 2014;45:ATMP43.
186. Bennett E, Rosenzweig M, Diamond M. Rat brain: effects of environmental enrichment on wet and dry weights. Science 1969;163(869):825-6.
187. Johansson B. Brain plasticity and stroke rehabilitation. The Willis lecture. Stroke 2000;31(1):223-30.
188. Janssen H, Bernhardt J, Collier JM, et al. An enriched environment improves sensorimotor function post-ischemic stroke. Neurorehabil Neural Repair 2010;24(9):802-13.
190. Kawamata T, Ren J, Chan T, et al. Intracisternal osteogenic protein-1 enhances functional recovery following focal stroke. Neuroreport 1998;9(7):1441-5.
191. Kawamata T, Dietrich W, Schallert T, et al. Intracisternal basic fibroblast growth factor (bFGF) enhances functional recovery and upregulates the expression of a molecular marker of neuronal sprouting following focal cerebral infarction. Proc Natl Acad Sci 1997;94:8179-84.
192. Shen LH, Li Y, Chen J, et al. Therapeutic benefit of bone marrow stromal cells administered 1 month after stroke. J Cereb Blood Flow Metab 2007;27:6-13.
193. Stroemer R, Kent T, Hulsebosch C. Enhanced neocortical neural sprouting, synaptogenesis, and behavioral recovery with D-amphetamine therapy after neocortical infarction in rats. Stroke 1998;29(11):2381-95.
194. Chen J, Zhang C, Jiang H, et al. Atorvastatin induction of VEGF and BDNF promotes brain plasticity after stroke in mice. J Cereb Blood Flow Metab 2005;25(2):281-90.
195. Fang PC, Barbay S, Plautz EJ, et al. Combination of NEP 1-40 treatment and motor training enhances behavioral recovery after a focal cortical infarct in rats. Stroke 2010;41(3):544-9.
196. Starkey ML, Schwab ME. Anti-Nogo-A and training: Can one plus one equal three? Exper Neurol 2012;235:53-61.
198. Adkins-Muir D, Jones T. Cortical electrical stimulation combined with rehabilitative training: enhanced functional recovery and dendritic plasticity following focal cortical ischemia in rats. Neurol Res 2003;25(8):780-8.
200. Freburger JK, Holmes GM, Ku LJ, et al. Disparities in postacute rehabilitation care for stroke: an analysis of the state inpatient databases. Arch Phys Med Rehabil 2011;92(8):1220-9.
202. Ovbiagele B, Kidwell CS, Starkman S, et al. Neuroprotective agents for the treatment of acute ischemic stroke. Curr Neurol Neurosci Rep 2003;3(1):9-20.
203. Kozlowski D, Jones T, Schallert T. Pruning of dendrites and restoration of function after brain damage: Role of the NMDA receptor. Restor Neurol Neurosci 1994;7:119-26.
204. Wahlgren N, Martinsson L. New concepts for drug therapy after stroke. Can we enhance recovery? Cerebrovasc Dis (Basel, Switzerland) 1998;8(Suppl. 5):33-8.
207. Clarkson AN, Overman JJ, Zhong S, et al. AMPA receptor-induced local brain-derived neurotrophic factor signaling mediates motor recovery after stroke. J Neurosci 2011;31(10): 3766-75.
209. Allan SM, Rothwell NJ. Inflammation in central nervous system injury. Philos Trans R Soc Lond B Biol Sci 2003;358(1438): 1669-77.
210. Lucas SM, Rothwell NJ, Gibson RM. The role of inflammation in CNS injury and disease. Br J Pharmacol 2006;147(Suppl. 1):S232-40.
211. Stinear CM, Barber PA, Smale PR, et al. Functional potential in chronic stroke patients depends on corticospinal tract integrity. Brain 2007;130(Pt 1):170-80.
212. Riley JD, Le V, Der-Yeghiaian L, et al. Anatomy of stroke injury predicts gains from therapy. Stroke 2011;42(2):421-6.
213. Siironen J, Juvela S, Kanarek K, et al. The Met allele of the BDNF Val66Met polymorphism predicts poor outcome among survivors of aneurysmal subarachnoid hemorrhage. Stroke 2007;38(10):2858-60.
214. Cramer SC, Parrish TB, Levy RM, et al. Predicting functional gains in a stroke trial. Stroke 2007;38(7):2108-14.
215. Lai SM, Duncan PW, Keighley J, et al. Depressive symptoms and independence in BADL and IADL. J Rehabil Res Dev 2002; 39(5):589-96.
217. Nouri S, Cramer SC. Anatomy and physiology predict response to motor cortex stimulation after stroke. Neurology 2011;77: 1076-83.

60 Enhancing Stroke Recovery with Cellular Therapies

Sean I. Savitz, Kaushik Parsha

KEY POINTS

- Over the past decade, cell therapies have attracted intense interest in their use as a potential treatment in a multitude of neurological disorders including stroke. A large number of pre-clinical studies have provided important information on the mechanisms, efficacy, and potential clinical application of cell therapies to enhance recovery after stroke.
- Cell therapies have been obtained from a variety of sources ranging from embryos to adults, and from various tissues, such as the brain, bone marrow, adipose, etc.
- Increasing evidence points towards paracrine and immunomodulatory mechanisms of action for many different types of cell therapies rather than tissue replacement and restoration of severed connections. The principal mediators of benefit may be a range of biological factors secreted by cell therapies including microparticles.
- Multiple clinical trials have been initiated world-wide, to assess the safety profiles of cell therapies in patients with acute, subacute, and chronic stroke. These trials have involved different delivery routes including intravenous, intra-arterial, and intracerebral injections. Few clinical trials have been reported yet that involve randomized placebo controlled designs.
- Further work is needed to understand mechanisms of action, address translational barriers, and develop and apply clinically relevant imaging modalities to track labeled cells in patients.

WHAT ARE CELL THERAPIES?

Cell therapy refers to cellular material with biological activities that cause a desired effect either in vitro or in vivo. For over 15 years, an expanding number and variety of cell types, prepared for exogenous administration, have been discovered with therapeutic activity demonstrated in animal models of neurological disorders.[1,2] Cell therapies as a potential treatment for neurological disease began in the 1990s as a transplantation source for certain neurodegenerative disorders. The first clinical trials were conducted to graft fetal tissues in patients with Parkinson's disease.[3] Some of the transplanted patients showed sustained improvement over time and no longer required dopaminergic medications. The results were preliminary but served as a proof of principle that grafting cellular tissue might effectively treat a neurological disorder. Since then, the field of cell therapy evolved in a completely different direction when it was found that the bone marrow and umbilical cord contain various different types of cells that reduce injury and promote recovery in a range of animal models of stroke, traumatic brain injury, multiple sclerosis, and neurodegenerative disorders. Some of these cell therapies possess the properties of bona fide stem cells while others are heterogeneous collections of progenitor, immature, and/or mature cell types. The mechanisms underlying how these types of cell therapies enhance stroke recovery are completely different than cell transplantation and need to be understood within the context of their intended use.

MECHANISMS, RATIONALE, AND TEMPORAL WINDOWS

Rather than serving as a source of cell replacement, almost all types of cell therapies at the present time are under development for stroke because they release biological factors that modulate other endogenous host cells within the brain and/or other organs. Many types of cell therapies release growth factors and cytokines involved in brain repair, immunomodulation, and cell survival[1,4–6] (Fig. 60-1). Some types of cell therapies release biologically active microparticles such as exosomes that by themselves are much smaller in size than cells, can circulate through the body and possibly directly enter into the brain[7,8] (Fig. 60-2). Therefore, there may be a biological rationale to apply certain types of cell therapies with systemic administration. The timing of when to administer cell therapies very much would depend upon the intended targets and there is extensive evidence that the acute to subacute stages of ischemic stroke may be an important window to consider clinical applications. In the days to weeks after stroke, there is a brisk inflammatory response involving multiple, interconnected processes both within the brain and in the periphery. During this same time period, there is a cascade of molecular signaling events leading to angiogenesis, neurogenesis, and axonal sprouting.[9] Furthermore, neuroplasticity occurs at the molecular and cellular levels within the peri-infarct zone and areas remote from the infarct. Certain types of cell therapies modulate the inflammatory response and/or may facilitate and amplify many of the repair mechanisms operating during this time period. The temporal window for cell therapies during this subacute to chronic period of stroke is not well-defined and likely depends on the intended targets, cell type, and delivery route (Fig. 60-3).

In the chronic period of stroke, months after symptom onset, the potential therapeutic applications of cell therapies are also being studied in several different ways (see Fig. 60-3). The route of delivery has principally involved a stereotactic intracranial administration, with the intent of placing therapeutic cells in the infarct area or around the infarct. In fact, in the 1990s, there were preliminary clinical trials studying intracranial delivery of neural cells in patients with chronic stroke,[10,11] studies that were designed in the wake of fetal transplantation approaches for patients with Parkinson disease. The goal of these pilot trials was to graft neural cells in the

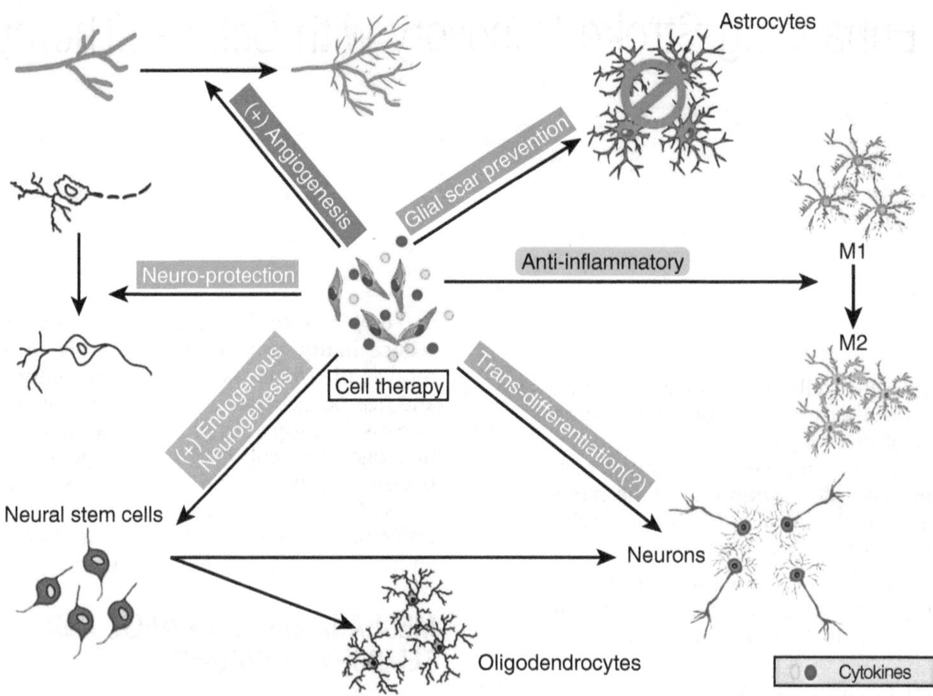

Figure 60-1. Cell therapy – mechanisms of action in stroke. Several mechanisms by which various types of cell therapies may improve recovery after stroke. Different types of cell therapies release biological factors that directly influence local endogenous repair responses, promote neuroprotection, and modulate the inflammatory/immune response. Some types of cell therapies may activate endogenous cells to release biological factors that promote repair and protection. *Illustration by Suhas Bajgur and Kaushik Parsha.*

infarct cavity, but current intracranial clinical studies have been designed with a different intention to implant cells to stimulate local endogenous repair pathways. The current cell therapy platforms principally involve direct injections of (1) modified marrow stromal cells (sponsored by San Bio) and (2) feta-derived neural fetal cells (ReNeuron and Neuralstem).

It is important to point out from the beginning of this chapter that the concept of grafting cells to restore lost neural circuitry is still in an early stage of preclinical development for any neurological disorder.[12] There are several biological and logical challenges and barriers to consider for stroke that are well covered in recent reviews,[12] but there are some promising preclinical studies.[13]

DIFFERENT CELL TYPES AND THEIR CATEGORIZATION

Among the various types of cell therapies, there are different kinds of cells that fall into the categories of embryonic, fetal, birth-related, and adult cell types, all of which are under development as potential new treatments for stroke (Fig. 60-4). A growing body of extensive animal data suggests that cell therapies derived from a range of tissues improve neurological outcome in rodent models of stroke. Among the most studied, the investigation of adult-derived cell therapies has surged during the past 10 years, when it was discovered that the bone marrow harbored mesenchymal stromal cells, hematopoietic stem cells, and other cell types that exert therapeutic effects in rodent stroke models, even when administered by intravenous delivery.[14] Subsequently, a range of either purified cell types or mixed cell types from bone marrow, umbilical cord, adipose, and other tissues have been shown to improve neurological outcome in rodents and other animals with stroke.[15-17]

DELIVERY ROUTES

In addition to a wide variety of cell types, there are several delivery routes under consideration for cell delivery. The intravenous route is a preferred approach because of the ease of administration and most effective means if the intent is to circulate cells throughout the body. For example, the intent for some cell therapy platforms in the acute to subacute stage of stroke is for cells to target the immune response after stroke. Umbilical cord cells, for example, and bone-marrow-derived multipotent adult progenitor cells (MAPCs) may exert their main therapeutic effects in models of stroke and TBI by targeting the spleen. If the spleen and other immune-related organs are the main targets of certain cell therapies, an IV delivery route may be optimal. Furthermore, over 10 years of research have consistently shown that IV administration of MSCs improves neurological outcome after stroke[18] and other acute neurological disorders while it remains contentious if these cells enter the CNS in any significant numbers.[19-21] Others have even shown, for example, that umbilical cells do not need to enter the brain to exert therapeutic effects.[22] Both MSCs and umbilical cord cells may enhance recovery because of the factors that they release into the circulation suggesting that their products are the critical mediators of their effects and not the cells (see Fig. 60-2). All of these studies support the IV delivery route as the most preferred approach for several types of cell therapy platforms.[23]

The endovascular route is also being explored by several investigators because intra-arterial (IA) delivery (1) selectively targets cells to an area of injury within the brain, (2) delivers

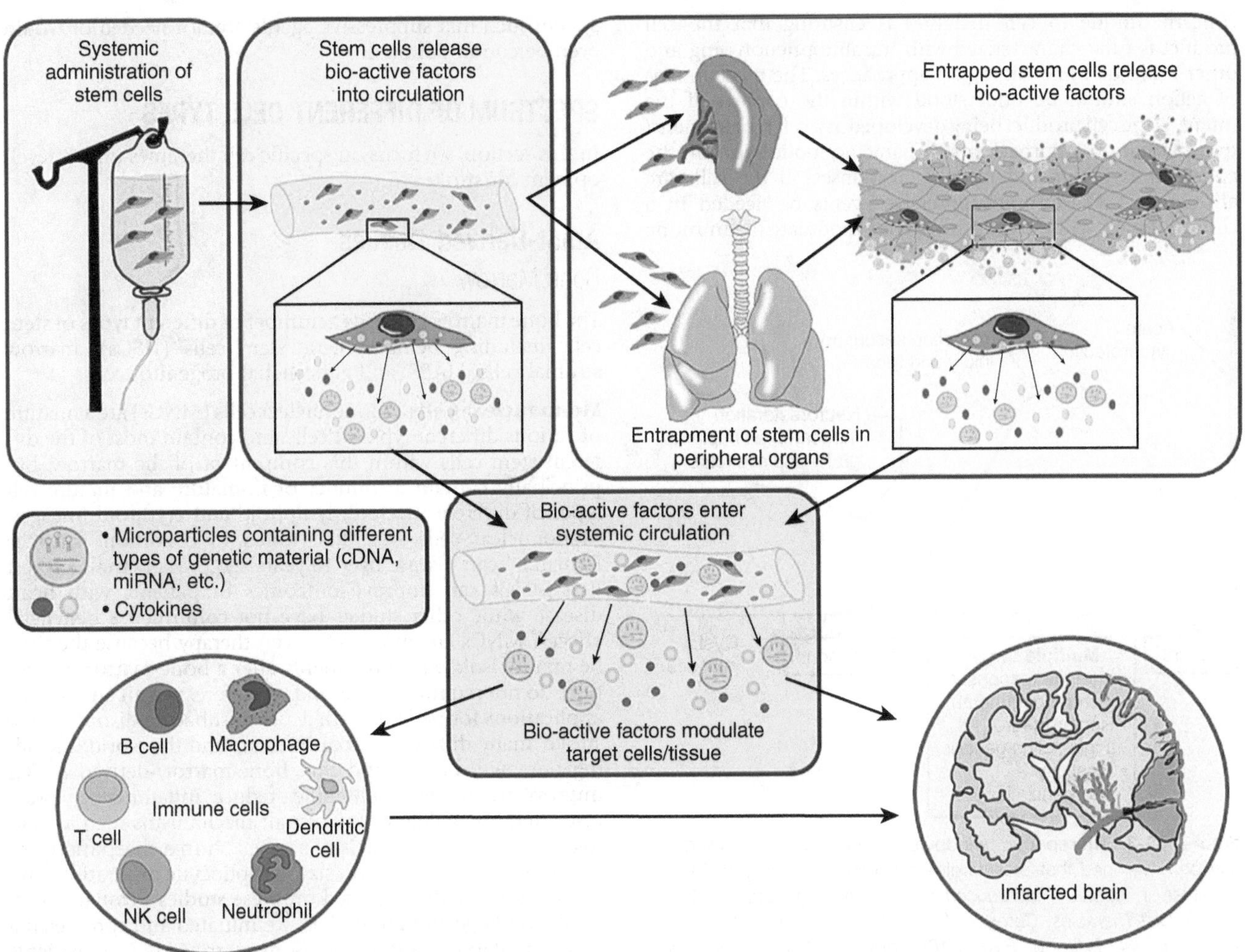

Figure 60-2. Cell therapies – paracrine action – release of microparticles/exosomes and cytokines. Potential mechanisms of how systemic administration of certain types of cell therapies may promote brain repair. Within the peripheral circulation and when entrapped in peripheral organs (lungs and spleen), some types of cell therapies may release bioactive factors such as microparticles. Microparticles containing different types of genetic material can directly alter immune cells and possibly even cross the blood–brain barrier and directly influence parenchymal cells in the brain. *Illustration by Suhas Bajgur and Kaushik Parsha.*

a more concentrated number of cells at a lower dose to the brain, and (3) bypasses the entrapment of cells in peripheral organs. Overall, it is theorized that IA could lead to better control of cell delivery and cover a greater surface area within the brain at a lower dose compared to any other delivery route. However, IA delivery will lead to cell migration into the systemic circulation and other organs once they pass through the CNS. Our studies indicate that for smaller-sized cells, IA does not lead to a greater effect on various different biological endpoints compared with IV.[24] There are also clear risks that need to be addressed with the IA route. IA delivery of larger-sized cells can lead to microvascular plugging and focal reductions in cerebral blood flow, leading to ischemic injury. This risk depends on cell size, number of cells injected, the adhesiveness of the cells, the target arteries involved, and the infusion rate.[25–27]

In contrast to systemic delivery routes, stereotactic injection ensures placement of cells in a focal area and is a preferred route for such cell types where migration outside of the CNS may be unwanted. There are various opinions as to whether intracranial delivery is a preferred approach and is superior to systemic delivery. Decisions on which approaches require an understanding of intended effects with planned trajectories and placement of cells, the cell types involved, a demonstration that intracranial delivery leads to a clear superior effect compared with systemic delivery, and clear safety data that the cells do not cause tumors or cause neurological worsening. There are other routes of delivery under investigation including intrathecal delivery and intranasal delivery.

STEPS GUIDELINES FOR TRANSLATION FROM BENCH TO CLINICAL

Recognizing the tremendous potential of cell therapies to become a new future treatment for stroke, investigators from academia convened with industry leaders and members of the federal government in a meeting called the STEPS (Stem cells as an Emerging Paradigm for Stroke) conference. The principal goal was to discuss how to successfully translate cell therapies from animal studies to clinical trials. The meeting followed the format of the STAIR conferences and set forth a series of guidelines for anyone interested in developing cell therapies for stroke.[28–31] These conferences have stressed the importance of defining doses, therapeutic time window, optimal delivery route, and biocompatibility of delivery devices. Of special concern unique to cell therapies is ensuring that the cell product is fully characterized with immunophenotyping and other molecular and biological approaches. The mechanisms of action should be understood within the context of the intent. Is the cell product being developed as a cell replacement/transplantation approach or a paracine/modulator of the endogenous repair and immune responses? If the cells are allogeneic, will immunosuppressive agents be needed in a clinical trial or will the cells themselves modulate the immune system such that suppressive agents are not needed or would even be contraindicated.

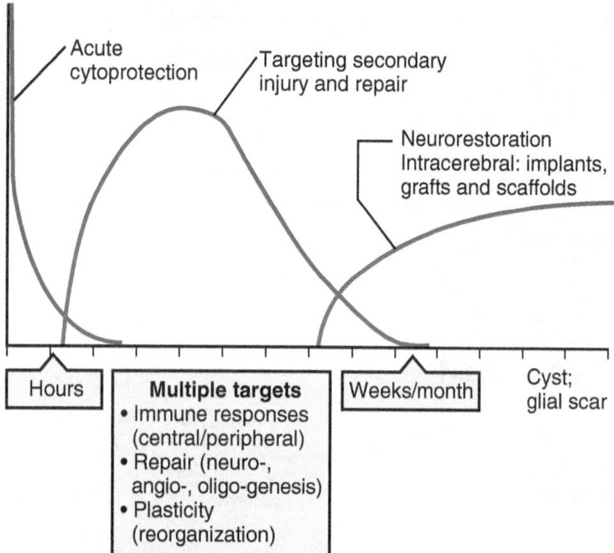

Figure 60-3. Therapeutic windows. Various temporal windows can be envisioned that provide different mechanistic targets for cell therapies in stroke. *(Reproduced with permission from Savitz SI; Stroke; Cell Therapies: Careful Translation From Animals to Patients; 2013; Vol 44: Issue 6: S107–S109;Copyright © American Heart Association, Inc.)*

SPECTRUM OF DIFFERENT CELL TYPES

In this section, we focus on specific cell therapies under development for stroke.

Adult-Derived Tissues

Bone Marrow

The bone marrow contains a number of different types of stem cells including hematopoietic stem cells (HSCs), marrow stromal cells, MAPS, and endothelial progenitor cells.

Mononuclear Cells. Mononuclear cells (MNCs) are a mixture of various different types of cells and contain most of the different stem cells within this component of the marrow, but principally contain a number of immature and mature cell types of different myeloid, lymphoid and erythroid lineages. Mononuclear cells were first tested in conditions such as ischemic heart disease over 10 years ago.[32] Many trials suggest that MNCs can improve outcomes in patients with heart disease while other studies have not confirmed a beneficial effect.[33] MNCs are an attractive cell therapy because they can be rapidly isolated from patients after a bone-marrow aspiration, do not require culture, and, therefore, permit autologous applications for patients with acute to subacute disorders. For stroke, many different laboratories around the world, including our own, have found that bone-marrow-derived MNCs improve neurological outcome, reduce inflammatory processes, and upregulate various repair mechanisms such as neurogenesis in rodent models of stroke.[34–37] In a sheep model of stroke, MNCs reduce lesion size, lymphocytic infiltration, and axonal degeneration.[38] Based on these studies involving both small and large animal models, we initiated and completed a phase I trial testing autologous bone marrow MNCs in patients with acute ischemic stroke.[39] There have been several other

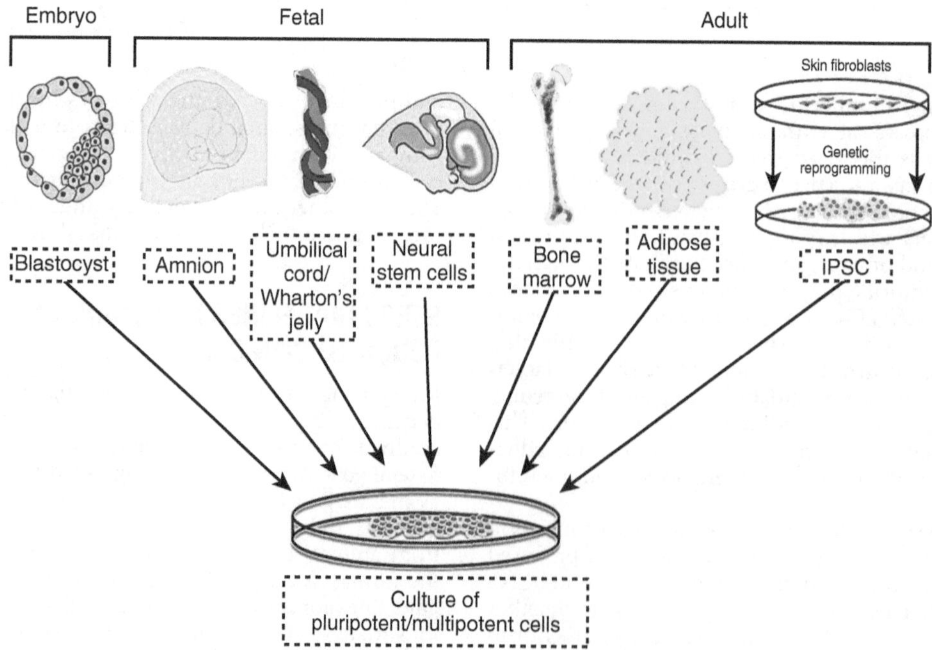

Figure 60-4. Stem cells – sources. Cell therapies have been isolated and cultured from a variety of sources for their use as a therapeutic modality in experimental studies of ischemic stroke and other neurological disorders. *Illustration by Suhas Bajgur and Kaushik Parsha.*

small clinical trials testing MNCs in patients with subacute and chronic stroke.[40,41]

Mesenchymal Stem Cells. Within MNCs lies a more specific population of mesenchymal cells residing in the stromal compartment of the marrow that have been termed marrow stromal cells. These cells are fibroblast-like cells that adhere to plastic and are thus easily isolated in culture. They display morphologic and functional heterogeneity, possibly related to variations in tissue source and culture protocols. Marrow stromal cells are an example of mesenchymal stem cells (MSCs) that can be isolated from a range of tissues, exert a number of therapeutic effects in a range of medical disorders, and are identified based on the expression of CD105, CD73, CD90 markers, along with lack of CD45, CD34, CD14 markers. MSCs display low immunogenicity and powerful immunomodulatory activity, supporting host tolerance toward MSCs as an allogeneic off-the-shelf product.[42,43] A large body of work has been conducted demonstrating that MSCs, when delivered with intracerebral, intravenous, or intracarotid approaches, enhance recovery from stroke in animal models.[44] Three excellent reviews have recently been published describing the various studies around the world on the therapeutic efficacy of MSCs in animal stroke models.[45–47] MSCs have been shown to reduce neurologic deficits even when administered at 30 days after stroke and exert benefit in a range of species from mice to rat, to stroke and even primates in stroke models. A meta-analysis of several published studies shows a large effect size for MSCs in pre-clinical models.[18] MSCs require passage in cell culture and may exert different biological properties depending on the cell passage.

Multipotent Adult Progenitor Cells. The bone marrow also contains stem cells that may be more primitive than MSCs displaying pluripotent, regenerative properties.[48] In 2001, Reyes et al.[49] described the isolation from the bone marrow of multipotent adult progenitor cells, which expressed embryonic stem cell markers and demonstrated broad differentiation capability, including epithelial, endothelial, neural, myogenic, hematopoietic, osteogenic, hepatogenic, chondrogenic, and adipogenic lineages. MAPCs share similar features with MSCs with respect to strong immunomodulatory properties, but also have distinct phenotypes separate from those of MSC and also elaborate different gene and protein expression patterns from MSCs.[50] In the rat stroke model, stereotactic or intravenous injections of MAPCs (termed Multistem by Athersys) up to 1 week after ischemic injury lead to significant improvement in motor outcomes compared with saline and cyclosporine-A-treated control animals.[51] In these studies, there was no evidence that MAPCs differentiate into neurons.

Adipose. Studies also suggest that adipose tissue contains pluripotent stromal cell. Stem cell density may be 500–1000 times more than bone marrow. Primary cultures of adipose tissue are a heterogeneous collection of hematopoietic cells, pericytes, endothelial cells, and smooth muscle cells. Several passages in cultures yield stromal cells that exhibit cell-surface markers consistent with mesenchymal stem cells.[52,53] Stromal cells can be cultured from human liposuction adipose tissue and are therefore being investigated as a potential therapy for stroke.[54–57]

Dental Stem Cells. The dental pulp represents another source of stem cells that show similarities with other stem cells in the nervous system and that can differentiate into different neural cell types. Intracerebral injection of dental pulp stem cells improves functional recovery in a rodent stroke model through paracrine mechanisms similar to other types of cell therapies.[17,58] Dental pulp cells stimulate endogenous neurogenesis and vasculogenesis.[59]

Birth-Derived Tissues

Umbilical Cord Blood Cells. Cord blood contains an enriched fraction of progenitor cells, but also several other different cell types including erythrocytes and platelets. A number of animal studies have been conducted evaluating the therapeutic benefits of umbilical cord blood cells (UCBCs) in the treatment of acute ischemic stroke.[15,60,61] The studies can be divided based on the type of cells investigated:

1. UCB MNCs – The mononuclear fraction comprising all the leukocytes (excluding the granulocytes) and the various types of stem and progenitor cells (HSCs, MSCs and EPCs).
2. UCB MSCs – The stromal cells obtained from the cord blood or the cord itself (Wharton's Jelly) by a process of culture in media.[62]
3. Enriched UCB populations – Cell populations obtained by selection of a specific subset of progenitor cells from the MNC fraction such as CD 34+ or CD 133+ cells[63]

Most initial studies exploring the use of UCBCs in cerebral ischemia employed the MNC fraction of the cord blood while more recently, studies have investigated MSCs or other specific sub-populations such as CD 34+ or CD 133+ cells.[64,65] An overwhelming majority of the studies have shown a beneficial effect of the administration of UCBC neurological behavior. However, there have been a few studies reporting no beneficial effects of UCBCs in the stroke model.[66] Similar to bone marrow, it is not clear which sub-population of cells is optimal that would maximize positive outcome and that mechanisms of benefit might involve a complex interaction of the various cell types with the host environment represented by the host blood/immune cells as well as the cells of the injured brain. Nevertheless, certain sub-populations of the cord blood cells are being shown to be critical in their beneficial effects after stroke.[67]

Many of the initial reports showed engraftment of the administered cells in the injured regions of the stroked brain. Subsequent work showed that the number of cells in the brain can be low relative to number of cells administered and that cellular replacement cannot account for the extent of the benefit observed.[22] Similar perhaps to bone marrow cells, UCBCs modulate the inflammatory response after stroke at peripheral and central levels. Studies have also shown UCBCs migrate to the spleen and thereby alter circulating inflammatory responses.[68,69] In addition to their anti-inflammatory effects, UCBCs have been shown to increase angiogenesis as well as enhance neurogenesis in the peri-infarct zone. These cells also have neuroprotective effects which help in rescuing the neuronal populations around the infarcted zone. Current evidence suggests that the beneficial effects shown by the cells are a result of the secretory/paracrine actions.[70] The cells have been shown to release cytokines and factors that suppress inflammation and enhance neuroprotection and angiogenesis.[71]

In considering a clinical trial, a number of translational issues have been addressed. Positive outcomes have been shown when the UCBCs are administered at doses ranging from 2×10^5 to 5×10^7 with one study suggesting that the threshold dose of cells is 10^6 cells.[61] A study investigating the efficacy of single vs multiple IV UCB MSC administrations concluded that multiple dosages were not superior to a one-time administration of the cells.[72] The literature indicates that the ideal post-stroke time for the administration of UCBCs is not known, but most studies report favorable behavioral outcome when the cells are administered between 24 and 72 hours.[73,74] One study even suggests that favorable outcome can be achieved when umbilical-derived cells are administered up to 30 days after stroke.[75]

When it became increasingly shown that HUBCs improve outcome in models of hypoxic-ischemic encephalopathy, the most logical clinical application for these cells has been an intravenous autologous infusion for neonates with HIE.[76,77] We await large clinical trials to test the efficacy of this approach in HIE.

Placenta. **Human placenta-derived adherent cells** (PDAC) are a mesenchymal-like cell population derived from normal human placental tissue. IV administration improves outcome in several animal studies and the mechanisms appear very similar to bone marrow and umbilical cord cells.[78,79]

Fetal-Derived

Embryonic. Studies have indicated that injection of embryonic stem cells (ESCs) to the side of the brain contralateral to a stroke leads to ESC migration to the ischemic lesion. However, it has clearly been shown that the injection of predifferentiated ESCs in the rodent stroke model leads to teratocarcinomas.[80] Therefore, the use of predifferentiated ESCs as a therapy for stroke is not an option at present.

Neural Stem Cells. Neural stem cells (NSCs) are a group of ectodermal progenitor cells, which can differentiate into committed neural sub-types, such as neurons, astrocytes, or oligodendrocytes. The identification of neurogenesis in specific areas of the adult brain, the sub-ventricular zone bordering the lateral ventricles[81–83] and the sub-granular zone of the dentate gyrus,[84,85] has stimulated rich and intense investigations to study the biology and potential applications of neural stem cells (NSCs). NSCs contribute to the production of neuroblasts, which may play a part in adult learning and memory as well the process of cell repair and replenishment after brain pathologies, including stroke. NSCs, therefore, as natural precursors of the different neural cell types, have been considered very attractive candidates for use as therapeutic agents in disorders of the nervous system, such as ischemic stroke. NSCs can be sourced from the ectodermal cells of the embryonic inner cell mass as well as the fetal brain. Indeed, most of the initial work investigating NSCs as agents of cellular therapy employed embryonic and fetal brain tissue. Additionally, neural stem cells have also been derived from induced pluripotent stem cells obtained from adult fibroblasts and these cells are being closely studied due to their dual advantages of being autologous as well as being clear of ethical issues.[86]

Over the last two decades, NSCs have been tested extensively in animal models of ischemic stroke and have shown encouraging results leading to the initiation of early human clinical trials. NSCs are seen as highly promising agents of cellular therapy as they are natural precursors of the cells they are intended to repair or replace. NSCs carry the advantage of being native to the affected region, thereby having the potential for greater survival, engraftment, and ability to modulate the local environment. The NSCs that have been studied in animal stroke models can be categorized into the following four types: (a) embryonic stem cell derived NSC (ESC-NSC),[87,88] (b) cultured fetal neural stem cell,[89–91] or, (c) induced pleuripotent stem cell derived neural stem cell (iPSC-NSC).[13,92] Some of the NSCs tested have been genetically modified for better control of growth, production, and scalability for clinical trials.[93]

Most studies administer NSCs stereotactically via intracerebral delivery. In comparing different delivery routes among IA, ICV, and IC, one study showed that the NSCs migrated to the cortex by all routes of administration.[94] Although various studies report engraftment and survival of some injected cells, the principal mechanisms of action are likely still paracrine effects. NSCs interact with many of the cell types of the neurovascular unit, which may lead to an enhanced expression of various growth factors such as NGF, BDNF, CNTF, and GDNF,[95,96] which play a role in their immune-modulatory and neuroprotective effects. Some types of NSCs attenuate brain inflammation, modulate microglia activation, and limit demyelination.[96] Over the past few years, it has even been shown that transplanted NSCs induce endogenous neurogenesis[89] and promote white matter repair and re-modeling likely via paracrine effects.[97] Intravenous administration of NSCs may also enhance recovery, at least in part, through their direct effects on the peripheral immune response.[98] Still, many investigators are aiming to use NSCs for brain cell replacement.[13]

Amniotic Cells. The amniotic membrane (AM) is an avascular tissue that forms the innermost layer of the fetal membranes and has been shown to be a source of multi-potential cells.[99–101] It has been shown that many types of amnion-derived cells possess stem-cell characteristics[102–105] and immunomodulatory properties.[106,107] The amnion-derived cells have, therefore, been tested in stroke models in which they similarly reduce motor deficits and improve behavioral outcomes through mechanisms that likely overlap with paracrine effects of other cell therapies.[108,109]

Inducible Pluripotent Stem Cells. In its own category we discuss inducible pluripotent stem cells (iPS). Recent technological advancements have now made it possible to reprogram somatic cells such that they behave similar to an embryonic stem cell and have been termed inducible pluripotent stem cells (iPS). The prototypical example that launched this area of regenerative medicine is the pioneering work of Yamanaka, who converted skin fibroblasts to iPS cells.[110] Converting somatic cells to pluripotent cells is a major revolution in the stem cell field. While the applications of iPS cells could one day lead to generating various different autologous brain cells that might be needed to treated the injured brain, at this point in time, there is much concern about potential tumorigenicity and immunogenicity associated with iPS.[111,112] iPS cells by themselves when injected into the brain after stroke can cause tumors.[113] However, neural cells derived from iPS have been shown to enhance recovery in stroke animal models either by paracrine effects or even possibly by host integration.[114–116]

CLINICAL TRIALS

Overview

The majority of clinical trials testing cell therapies in stroke have been early-phase pilot studies testing autologous bone-marrow-derived cells.

Bone-Marrow Mononuclear Cell Studies

Based upon extensive animal studies,[2] we conducted a phase I trial of autologous bone marrow MNCs in patients 24–72 hours after acute ischemic stroke. All patients underwent a limited bone-marrow aspiration followed by an intravenous re-infusion of separated MNCs. The study design followed from published data on MNCs in animal stroke models. The patients underwent bone-marrow aspiration under conscious sedation and received their own MNCs by intravenous infusion within 3–6 hours of cell separation in a good manufacturing production (GMP) facility. Safety results on the first ten patients were published in 2011 and after the subsequent enrolment of an additional 15 patients, the study was stopped because there were no severe adverse events definitely related to the study.[39] Investigators in Brazil have also been conducting clinical trials of BM-MNCs but with an intra-arterial delivery either by injection into the carotid or middle cerebral artery. They began their investigations in patients several months after stroke. After finding that this approach with intra-arterial delivery was safe in more chronic patients, they recently reported safety in a 20-patient study in which intra-arterial MNCs were delivered in the 3–7-day period after stroke.[117] Using technetium labeling and SPECT, they have also found that MNCs do migrate to the brain within hours after infusion. Investigators in Spain also conducted a small ten-patient study of intra-arterially delivered MNCs in patients 5–9 days after stroke and found that the intervention was safe and feasible.[41] Finally, in India, several small studies have reported on the safety of IV administration of autologous BM-MNCs in patients 7–30 days[40] after stroke as well as in cases of chronic ischemic stroke.[118]

Marrow Stromal Cell Studies

The more homogeneous stem cell population, marrow stromal cells have also undergone safety testing in stroke patients. All of the published clinical studies have been conducted in patients with chronic stroke, led by investigators in Asia, and involve the application of autologous patient-derived bone marrow cells. The first pilot study was completed in South Korea as an open label clinical trial in which the investigators harvested bone marrow from patients with an MCA infarct, isolated and purified the MSCs in fetal bovine serum, and re-injected the cells with an intravenous administration.[119] Five patients received 5 million autologous MSCs at 4–5 weeks after stroke and another 5 million cells at 7–9 weeks after stroke. No adverse effects were reported up to 1 year later. This study was followed by a subsequent publication describing the same patients with longer-term follow-up and enrollment of more patients, totaling 16 study patients and 36 controls.[120] There was blinded randomization to the two groups along with blinded outcome assessments. The control patients did not receive any additional interventions aside from standard of care. There were no statistical differences in adverse events or mortality between the two groups. In Japan, 12 patients were administered one infusion IV of their own MSCs anywhere from 36 to 133 days after stroke.[121] Distinguishing this trial from the Korean studies, the MSCs were grown with the patient's own serum. There was also variability in the dose of MSCs 0.6×10^8 to 1.6×10^8 cells per patient. No study-related adverse events were reported within the prior 3–12 months. Finally, in India, 12 patients who had had a stroke 3–12 months beforehand, were divided into two groups; six patients serving as controls while the other six received IV autologous MSCs.[122] There were no significant differences clinically between the two groups up to 24 weeks after enrollment. Larger, randomized trials are now underway in various countries to determine if autologous bone-marrow-derived MSCs improve outcome in stroke.

Collectively, the trials thus far illustrate the safety and feasibility of preparing autologous MSCs from patients with stroke, but the time required to grow the cells before injection does not allow for applications in the acute or subacute period after stroke. There is very limited work on the therapeutic efficacy of MSCs at such late time points, raising the question as to whether autologous MSCs will be a practical option or whether such cells need to be used at earlier passages in culture. The cell passage and the specific cell culture conditions, including the use of serum, likely will have an impact on the potential efficacy of MSCs in various neurologic disorders. These issues need to be considered in the planning of future clinical trials in stroke.

Aldehyde Dehydrogenase Bright Cells. Stem cells can also be isolated from the bone marrow by the expression of enzymes. For example, cell populations that express high levels of aldehyde dehydrogenase which are termed aldehyde dehydrogenase bright ($ALDH^{br}$) cells participate in tissue repair, contain hematopoietic, endothelial, and mesenchymal progenitor cells, and can be readily isolated by flow cytometry from a patient's bone marrow, permitting autologous applications.[123,124] $ALDH^{br}$ cell populations have also been sorted from human cord blood, mobilized peripheral blood, and skeletal muscle. Intracarotid infusion of $ALDH^{br}$ cells reduces neurological deficits in an animal stroke model (unpublished data). The mechanism of these cells is likely very similar to other types of cell therapies by releasing a variety of cytokines.[125] Autologous bone-marrow-derived $ALDH^{br}$ cells are safe to administer by transendocardial injection in patients with chronic heart failure and by intramuscular injection in critical limb ischemia.[126,127] Based upon animal model studies and safety shown in other clinical conditions, Cytomedix sponsored a clinical trial testing the intracarotid injection of $ALDH^{br}$ cells in patients with middle cerebral artery (MCA) ischemic stroke. The clinical trial was a phase I/II double-blind safety and efficacy study in which patients 11–17 days after symptoms were randomized to the study intervention or sham control. The intervention group underwent a bone-marrow harvest followed 2 days later by distal carotid injection $ALDH^{br}$ cells. The sham group underwent a simulated harvest and a simulated angiography. To preserve blinding of endpoints, two groups of blinded and unblinded teams were needed. After enrollment of 48 patients, a resizing analysis determined that there was no difference in the primary endpoint on the mRS. It was determined that $ALDH^{br}$ cells can be safely harvested from the bone marrow and delivered via ipsilateral intracarotid injection in the subacute phase of stroke. This trial was the most advanced study to date to test the intra-arterial delivery of autologous stem cells in stroke patients.

Allogeneic Multistem Trial. Multistem cells are MAPC derived from bone marrow, which have been shown to modulate immune responses, protect cells from injury, and promote repair in various disorders, even by intravenous administration. Owned by Athersys, Multistem cells have shown much potential to treat a range of medical conditions and are under clinical development for ischemic heart disease, Crohn's disease, and graft vs host disease. In animal models, Multistem enhances recovery after stroke by reducing inflammatory responses emanating from the spleen.[128,129] Based on results from animal studies, Athersys went forward to test Multistem in patients 24–48 hours after acute stroke. This is the first trial to test an allogeneic stem cell product, by intravenous administration, in patients with acute ischemic stroke. The trial began first as a dose escalation study in which it was found that 1.2 billion cells could safely be administered without causing serious adverse events. The trial is now in phase II in which 120 patients from various sites in the US and UK are being randomized 1:1 either to receive Multistem or vehicle IV. The primary efficacy endpoint is a dichotomized outcome on the mRS.

Clinical Trials Testing Intracerebral Administration of Stem Cells. In the past few years, cell therapy platforms have emerged to bring forward new stem cell treatments by intracranial administration in patients with chronic stroke. ReNeuron has been developing an immortalized neural stem cell called CTX0E03, which is a cell line derived from fetal brain tissue, infected with c-mycERTAM.[93] Intracerebra injection of CTX0E03 after stroke reduces neurologic deficits in rodent models.[130] Based on these animal studies, ReNeuron conducted the PISCES study (Pilot Investigation of Stem Cells in Stroke), a phase I dose escalation study to test the safety of stereotactic implantation of a single administration of CTX0E03. Among 11 patients enrolled at least 6 months after their stroke, all had disabling deficits with a median NIHSS of 7 (at least 2 points for hemiparesis). In long-term follow-up data at 12 months in all patients, there were no cell-related or immunological adverse events reported. Adverse events were related to the implantation procedure or co-morbidities. At 12 months, the median NIHSS had decreased by 3 points and there were also sustained reductions in spasticity in most of the patients compared to their pre-treatment baseline. A phase II single arm study is now underway for patients with stable upper limb paresis, treated between 8 and 12 weeks after their stroke, a time window chosen to optimize the potential treatment window for this cell type.

San Bio has also conducted in the US a phase I/IIA dose escalation safety trial in 18 patients testing the implantation of genetically modified marrow stromal cells. SB623 cells are marrow stromal cells transfected with a Notch1 intracellular domain (NICD)-expressing plasmid and have been shown to promote functional improvement in rodent models of stroke.[131] SB623 cells resemble MSCs with respect to morphology and cell surface markers and transfection with NICD enhances some of the immunomodulatory and pro-angiogenic properties of MSCs compared with their parental MSC counterparts. For the clinical trial, allogeneic bone marrow cells prepared from healthy donors were implanted to the regions adjacent to the infarct. Patients were 7–36 months post stroke and had fixed motor deficits prior to transplantation.

CLINICAL DEVELOPMENT OF EARLY- AND LATER-STAGE TESTING OF CELL THERAPIES

To facilitate successful translation of cell therapies from the bench to the bedside, the STEPS conference re-convened for a second meeting (STEPS 2). The major focus of STEPS 2[30] was to provide guidelines on early-stage clinical trials primarily focused on testing safety and obtaining potential signals of efficacy. Because a few different types of cell therapies are being, or have been, cleared through initial safety trials, larger more advanced trials have already begun. Designing phase IIB and even phase III trials for cell therapies involves several complicated decisions. The STEPS 3 conference, therefore,[31] focused on the design of clinical trials testing cell therapies in later stages of testing. Six areas were covered on patient selection, time window for enrollment, trial endpoints, biomarkers of activity, concurrent rehabilitation therapy, and the application of cell therapies in chronic stroke.

FUTURE DIRECTIONS

As some types of cell therapies advance to later stages of clinical testing and new types of cell therapies enter clinical testing, there are several key areas that need to be addressed to advance the field:

1. Labeling cells and imaging biodistribution: a critical question in the application of cell therapies is tracking where the cells migrate after administration into the body. Various imaging technologies are available for animal studies;[132,133] however, there are only a few studies in stroke patients. Most of the studies in patients were conducted by investigators in Brazil who used SPECT to study the biodistribution of bone marrow mononuclear cells radiolabeled with ^{99m}Tc.[134–136] In these studies, a small number of systemically administered cells migrate to the injured brain, but larger numbers travel to peripheral organs such as the lungs, liver, and spleen. These studies raise hope that imaging can be safely applied to monitor cell therapies in stroke patients in the future.
2. Surrogates of activity: a major gap in developing therapies for stroke recovery has been a lack of validated biomarkers. Newer technologies have emerged that may provide biochemical or imaging data indicative of restorative events. In the next several years, we hope to see major advancements in this area to understand the biological effects of cell therapies in stroke patients.
3. Combinations with other modalities: because cell therapies are being applied to promote stroke recovery, it will likely become increasingly more important to assess their effects in combination with other therapeutic modalities under investigation to promote stroke recovery. How cell therapies might affect or be affected by novel rehabilitation paradigms that go beyond usual rehab care (e.g., more intensive motor training) is unknown. Similarly, how cell therapies will affect or interact with the application of non-invasive brain stimulation or other emerging approaches that involve robotics or pharmacological approaches will require formal studies, some of which can be explored in animal models before attempting investigations in patients.

REFERENCES

1. Lunn JS, Sakowski SA, Hur J, et al. Stem cell technology for neurodegenerative diseases. Ann Neurol 2011;70:353–61.
2. Savitz SI. Cell therapies: careful translation from animals to patients. Stroke 2013;44:S107–9.
3. Freed CR, Breeze RE, Rosenberg NL, et al. Survival of implanted fetal dopamine cells and neurologic improvement 12 to 46 months after transplantation for Parkinson's disease. N Engl J Med 1992;327:1549–55.
4. Caplan AI, Dennis JE. Mesenchymal stem cells as trophic mediators. J Cell Biochem 2006;98:1076–84.
5. Crigler L, Robey RC, Asawachaicharn A, et al. Human mesenchymal stem cell subpopulations express a variety of neuro-regulatory molecules and promote neuronal cell survival and neuritogenesis. Exp Neurol 2006;198:54–64.
6. Lindvall O, Kokaia Z. Stem cells in human neurodegenerative disorders – time for clinical translation? J Clin Invest 2010;120:29–40.
7. Xin H, Li Y, Cui Y, et al. Systemic administration of exosomes released from mesenchymal stromal cells promote functional recovery and neurovascular plasticity after stroke in rats. J Cereb Blood Flow Metab 2013;33:1711–15.
8. Xin H, Li Y, Liu Z, et al. MiR-133b promotes neural plasticity and functional recovery after treatment of stroke with multipotent mesenchymal stromal cells in rats via transfer of exosome-enriched extracellular particles. Stem Cells 2013;31:2737–46.
9. Carmichael ST. Themes and strategies for studying the biology of stroke recovery in the poststroke epoch. Stroke 2008;39:1380–8.
10. Kondziolka D, Steinberg GK, Wechsler L, et al. Neurotransplantation for patients with subcortical motor stroke: a phase 2 randomized trial. J Neurosurg 2005;103:38–45.
11. Savitz SI, Dinsmore J, Wu J, et al. Neurotransplantation of fetal porcine cells in patients with basal ganglia infarcts: a preliminary safety and feasibility study. Cerebrovasc Dis 2005;20:101–7.
12. Dihne M, Hartung HP, Seitz RJ. Restoring neuronal function after stroke by cell replacement: anatomic and functional considerations. Stroke 2011;42:2342–50.
13. Oki K, Tatarishvili J, Wood J, et al. Human-induced pluripotent stem cells form functional neurons and improve recovery after grafting in stroke-damaged brain. Stem Cells 2012;30:1120–33.
14. Schwarting S, Litwak S, Hao W, et al. Hematopoietic stem cells reduce postischemic inflammation and ameliorate ischemic brain injury. Stroke 2008;3910:2867–75.
15. Chen J, Sanberg PR, Li Y, et al. Intravenous administration of human umbilical cord blood reduces behavioral deficits after stroke in rats. Stroke 2001;32:2682–8.
16. Gutierrez-Fernandez M, Rodriguez-Frutos B, Otero-Ortega L, et al. Adipose tissue-derived stem cells in stroke treatment: from bench to bedside. Discov Med 2013;16:37–43.
17. Leong WK, Henshall TL, Arthur A, et al. Human adult dental pulp stem cells enhance poststroke functional recovery through non-neural replacement mechanisms. Stem Cells Transl Med 2012;1:177–87.
18. Vu Q, Xie K, Eckert M, et al. Meta-analysis of preclinical studies of mesenchymal stromal cells for ischemic stroke. Neurology 2014;82:1277–86.
19. Honma T, Honmou O, Iihoshi S, et al. Intravenous infusion of immortalized human mesenchymal stem cells protects against

injury in a cerebral ischemia model in adult rat. Exp Neurol 2006;199(1):56–66.
20. Zangi L, Margalit R, Reich-Zeliger S, et al. Direct imaging of immune rejection and memory induction by allogeneic mesenchymal stromal cells. Stem Cells 2009;27:2865–74.
21. Chopp M, Li Y, Zhang ZG. Mechanisms underlying improved recovery of neurological function after stroke in the rodent after treatment with neurorestorative cell-based therapies. Stroke 2009;40:S143–5.
22. Borlongan CV, Hadman M, Sanberg CD, et al. Central nervous system entry of peripherally injected umbilical cord blood cells is not required for neuroprotection in stroke. Stroke 2004; 35:2385–9.
23. Willing AE, Shahaduzzaman M. Delivery routes for cell therapy in stroke. In: Jolkkonen J, Walczak P, editors. Cell-based Therapies in Stroke. NY, USA: Springer; 2013. p. 15–28.
24. Yang B, Migliati E, Parsha K, et al. Intra-arterial delivery is not superior to intravenous delivery of autologous bone marrow mononuclear cells in acute ischemic stroke. Stroke 2013;44: 3463–72.
25. Janowski M, Lyczek A, Engels C, et al. Cell size and velocity of injection are major determinants of the safety of intracarotid stem cell transplantation. J Cereb Blood Flow Metab 2013;33: 921–7.
26. Walczak P, Zhang J, Gilad AA, et al. Dual-modality monitoring of targeted intraarterial delivery of mesenchymal stem cells after transient ischemia. Stroke 2008;39:1569–74.
27. Li L, Jiang Q, Ding G, et al. Effects of administration route on migration and distribution of neural progenitor cells transplanted into rats with focal cerebral ischemia, an MRI study. J Cereb Blood Flow Metab 2010;30:653–62.
28. Stroke Therapy Academic Industry Roundtable (STAIR). Recommendations for standards regarding preclinical neuroprotective and restorative drug development. Stroke 1999;30:2752–8.
29. Stem Cell Therapies as an Emerging Paradigm in Stroke Participants. Stem Cell Therapies as an Emerging Paradigm in Stroke (STEPS): bridging basic and clinical science for cellular and neurogenic factor therapy in treating stroke. Stroke 2009;40: 510–15.
30. Savitz SI, Chopp M, Deans R, et al. Stem Cell Therapy as an Emerging Paradigm for Stroke (STEPS) II. Stroke 2011;42: 825–9.
31. Savitz SI, Cramer SC, Wechsler L, et al. Stem cells as an emerging paradigm in stroke 3: enhancing the development of clinical trials. Stroke 2014;45:634–9.
32. Strauer BE, Brehm M, Zeus T, et al. Repair of infarcted myocardium by autologous intracoronary mononuclear bone marrow cell transplantation in humans. Circulation 2002;106:1913–18.
33. Jeevanantham V, Butler M, Saad A, et al. Adult bone marrow cell therapy improves survival and induces long-term improvement in cardiac parameters: a systematic review and meta-analysis. Circulation 2012;126:551–68.
34. Wang J, Yu L, Jiang C, et al. Bone marrow mononuclear cells exert long-term neuroprotection in a rat model of ischemic stroke by promoting arteriogenesis and angiogenesis. Brain Behav Immun 2013;34:56–66.
35. Franco EC, Cardoso MM, Gouveia A, et al. Modulation of microglial activation enhances neuroprotection and functional recovery derived from bone marrow mononuclear cell transplantation after cortical ischemia. Neurosci Res 2012;73:122–32.
36. Brenneman M, Sharma S, Harting M, et al. Autologous bone marrow mononuclear cells enhance recovery after acute ischemic stroke in young and middle-aged rats. J Cereb Blood Flow Metab 2010;30:140–9.
37. Giraldi-Guimardes A, Rezende-Lima M, Bruno FP, et al. Treatment with bone marrow mononuclear cells induces functional recovery and decreases neurodegeneration after sensorimotor cortical ischemia in rats. Brain Res 2009;1266:108–20.
38. Boltze J, Nitzsche B, Geiger KD, et al. Histopathological Investigation of Different MCAO Modalities and Impact of Autologous Bone Marrow Mononuclear Cell Administration in an Ovine Stroke Model. Transl Stroke Res 2011;2:279–93.
39. Savitz SI, Misra V, Kasam M, et al. Intravenous autologous bone marrow mononuclear cells for ischemic stroke. Ann Neurol 2011;70:59–69.
40. Prasad K, Mohanty S, Bhatia R, et al. Autologous intravenous bone marrow mononuclear cell therapy for patients with subacute ischaemic stroke: a pilot study. Indian J Med Res 2012; 136:221–8.
41. Moniche F, Gonzalez A, Gonzalez-Marcos JR, et al. Intra-arterial bone marrow mononuclear cells in ischemic stroke: a pilot clinical trial. Stroke 2012;43:2242–4.
42. Le Blanc K, Pittenger M. Mesenchymal stem cells: progress toward promise. Cytotherapy 2005;7:36–45.
43. Barry FP, Murphy JM, English K, et al. Immunogenicity of adult mesenchymal stem cells: lessons from the fetal allograft. Stem Cells Dev 2005;14:252–65.
44. Li Y, Chopp M. Marrow stromal cell transplantation in stroke and traumatic brain injury. Neurosci Lett 2009;456:120–3.
45. Eckert MA, Vu Q, Xie K, et al. Evidence for high translational potential of mesenchymal stromal cell therapy to improve recovery from ischemic stroke. J Cereb Blood Flow Metab 2013;33: 1322–34.
46. Honmou O, Onodera R, Sasaki M, et al. Mesenchymal stem cells: therapeutic outlook for stroke. Trends Mol Med 2012;18:292–7.
47. Doeppner TR, Hermann DM. Mesenchymal stem cells in the treatment of ischemic stroke: progress and possibilities. Stem Cells Cloning 2010;3:157–63.
48. Jiang Y, Jahagirdar BN, Reinhardt RL, et al. Pluripotency of mesenchymal stem cells derived from adult marrow. Nature 2002; 418:41–9.
49. Reyes M, Lund T, Lenvik T, et al. Purification and ex vivo expansion of postnatal human marrow mesodermal progenitor cells. Blood 2001;98:2615–25.
50. Anjos-Afonso F, Bonnet D. Nonhematopoietic/endothelial SSEA-1+ cells define the most primitive progenitors in the adult murine bone marrow mesenchymal compartment. Blood 2007; 109:1298–306.
51. Mays RW, Borlongan CV, Yashuhara T, et al. Development of an allogeneic adherent stem cell therapy for treatment of ischemic stroke. J Exper Stroke Transpl Med 2010;3:34–46.
52. Gronthos S, Franklin DM, Leddy HA, et al. Surface protein characterization of human adipose tissue-derived stromal cells. J Cell Physiol 2001;189:54–63.
53. Tallone T, Realini C, Bohmler A, et al. Adult human adipose tissue contains several types of multipotent cells. J Cardiovasc Transl Res 2011;4:200–10.
54. Leu S, Lin YC, Yuen CM, et al. Adipose-derived mesenchymal stem cells markedly attenuate brain infarct size and improve neurological function in rats. J Transl Med 2010;8:63.
55. Gutierrez-Fernandez M, Rodriguez-Frutos B, Ramos-Cejudo J, et al. Effects of intravenous administration of allogenic bone marrow- and adipose tissue-derived mesenchymal stem cells on functional recovery and brain repair markers in experimental ischemic stroke. Stem Cell Res Ther 2013;4:11.
56. Kang SK, Lee DH, Bae YC, et al. Improvement of neurological deficits by intracerebral transplantation of human adipose tissue-derived stromal cells after cerebral ischemia in rats. Exp Neurol 2003;183:355–66.
57. Jiang W, Liang G, Li X, et al. Intracarotid transplantation of autologous adipose-derived mesenchymal stem cells significantly improves neurological deficits in rats after MCAo. J Mater Sci Mater Med 2014;25:1357–66.
58. Yalvac ME, Rizvanov AA, Kilic E, et al. Potential role of dental stem cells in the cellular therapy of cerebral ischemia. Curr Pharm Des 2009;15:3908–16.
59. Sugiyama M, Iohara K, Wakita H, et al. Dental pulp-derived CD31(−)/CD146(−) side population stem/progenitor cells enhance recovery of focal cerebral ischemia in rats. Tissue Eng Part A 2011;17:1303–11.
60. Willing AE, Lixian J, Milliken M, et al. Intravenous versus intrastriatal cord blood administration in a rodent model of stroke. J Neurosci Res 2003;73:296–307.
61. Vendrame M, Cassady J, Newcomb J, et al. Infusion of human umbilical cord blood cells in a rat model of stroke dose-dependently rescues behavioral deficits and reduces infarct volume. Stroke 2004;3510:2390–5.
62. Erices A, Conget P, Minguell JJ. Mesenchymal progenitor cells in human umbilical cord blood. Br J Haematol 2000;109: 235–42.

63. Boltze J, Reich DM, Hau S, et al. Assessment of neuroprotective effects of human umbilical cord blood mononuclear cell subpopulations in vitro and in vivo. Cell Transplant 2012;21:723–37.
64. Nystedt J, Makinen S, Laine J, et al. Human cord blood CD34+ cells and behavioral recovery following focal cerebral ischemia in rats. Acta Neurobiol Exp (Wars) 2006;66:293–300.
65. Iskander A, Knight RA, Zhang ZG, et al. Intravenous administration of human umbilical cord blood-derived AC133+ endothelial progenitor cells in rat stroke model reduces infarct volume: magnetic resonance imaging and histological findings. Stem Cells Transl Med 2013;2:703–14.
66. Makinen S, Kekarainen T, Nystedt J, et al. Human umbilical cord blood cells do not improve sensorimotor or cognitive outcome following transient middle cerebral artery occlusion in rats. Brain Res 2006;1123:207–15.
67. Womble TA, Green S, Shahaduzzaman M, et al. Monocytes are essential for the neuroprotective effect of human cord blood cells following middle cerebral artery occlusion in rat. Mol Cell Neurosci 2014;59:76–84.
68. Vendrame M, Gemma C, Pennypacker KR, et al. Cord blood rescues stroke-induced changes in splenocyte phenotype and function. Exp Neurol 2006;199:191–200.
69. Golden JE, Shahaduzzaman M, Wabnitz A, et al. Human umbilical cord blood cells alter blood and spleen cell populations after stroke. Transl Stroke Res 2012;3:491–9.
70. Newman MB, Willing AE, Manresa JJ, et al. Cytokines produced by cultured human umbilical cord blood (HUCB) cells: implications for brain repair. Exp Neurol 2006;199:201–8.
71. Vendrame M, Gemma C, de Mesquita D, et al. Anti-inflammatory effects of human cord blood cells in a rat model of stroke. Stem Cells Dev 2005;14:595–604.
72. Shehadah A, Chen J, Kramer B, et al. Efficacy of single and multiple injections of human umbilical tissue-derived cells following experimental stroke in rats. PLoS ONE 2013;8:e54083.
73. Boltze J, Schmidt UR, Reich DM, et al. Determination of the therapeutic time window for human umbilical cord blood mononuclear cell transplantation following experimental stroke in rats. Cell Transplant 2012;21:1199–211.
74. Newcomb JD, Ajmo CT Jr, Sanberg CD, et al. Timing of cord blood treatment after experimental stroke determines therapeutic efficacy. Cell Transplant 2006;15:213–23.
75. Zhang L, Li Y, Zhang C, et al. Delayed administration of human umbilical tissue-derived cells improved neurological functional recovery in a rodent model of focal ischemia. Stroke 2011;42:1437–44.
76. Carroll J. Human cord blood for the hypoxic-ischemic neonate. Pediatr Res 2012;71:459–63.
77. Verina T, Fatemi A, Johnston MV, et al. Pluripotent possibilities: human umbilical cord blood cell treatment after neonatal brain injury. Pediatr Neurol 2013;48:346–54.
78. Shehadah A, Chen J, Pal A, et al. Human placenta-derived adherent cell treatment of experimental stroke promotes functional recovery after stroke in young adult and older rats. PLoS ONE 2014;9:e86621.
79. Chen J, Shehadah A, Pal A, et al. Neuroprotective effect of human placenta-derived cell treatment of stroke in rats. Cell Transplant 2013;22:871–9.
80. Erdo F, Buhrle C, Blunk J, et al. Host-dependent tumorigenesis of embryonic stem cell transplantation in experimental stroke. J Cereb Blood Flow Metab 2003;23:780–5.
81. Lledo PM, Alonso M, Grubb MS. Adult neurogenesis and functional plasticity in neuronal circuits. Nat Rev Neurosci 2006;7:179–93.
82. Doetsch F, Caille I, Lim DA, et al. Subventricular zone astrocytes are neural stem cells in the adult mammalian brain. Cell 1999;97:703–16.
83. Gage FH. Mammalian neural stem cells. Science 2000;287:1433–8.
84. Ming GL, Song H. Adult neurogenesis in the mammalian central nervous system. Annu Rev Neurosci 2005;28:223–50.
85. Eriksson PS, Perfilieva E, Bjork-Eriksson T, et al. Neurogenesis in the adult human hippocampus. Nat Med 1998;4:1313–17.
86. Chang DJ, Lee N, Park IH, et al. Therapeutic potential of human induced pluripotent stem cells in experimental stroke. Cell Transplant 2013;22:1427–40.
87. Chang DJ, Oh SH, Lee N, et al. Contralaterally transplanted human embryonic stem cell-derived neural precursor cells (ENStem-A) migrate and improve brain functions in stroke-damaged rats. Exp Mol Med 2013;45:e53.
88. Tang Y, Wang J, Lin X, et al. Neural stem cell protects aged rat brain from ischemia-reperfusion injury through neurogenesis and angiogenesis. J Cereb Blood Flow Metab 2014;34:1138–47.
89. Mine Y, Tatarishvili J, Oki K, et al. Grafted human neural stem cells enhance several steps of endogenous neurogenesis and improve behavioral recovery after middle cerebral artery occlusion in rats. Neurobiol Dis 2013;52:191–203.
90. Andres RH, Horie N, Slikker W, et al. Human neural stem cells enhance structural plasticity and axonal transport in the ischaemic brain. Brain 2011;134:1777–89.
91. Darsalia V, Kallur T, Kokaia Z. Survival, migration and neuronal differentiation of human fetal striatal and cortical neural stem cells grafted in stroke-damaged rat striatum. Eur J Neurosci 2007;26:605–14.
92. Yuan T, Liao W, Feng NH, et al. Human induced pluripotent stem cell-derived neural stem cells survive, migrate, differentiate, and improve neurologic function in a rat model of middle cerebral artery occlusion. Stem Cell Res Ther 2013;4:73.
93. Thomas RJ, Hope AD, Hourd P, et al. Automated, serum-free production of CTX0E03: a therapeutic clinical grade human neural stem cell line. Biotechnol Lett 2009;31:1167–72.
94. Jin K, Sun Y, Xie L, et al. Comparison of ischemia-directed migration of neural precursor cells after intrastriatal, intraventricular, or intravenous transplantation in the rat. Neurobiol Dis 2005;18:366–74.
95. Liu YP, Lang BT, Baskaya MK, et al. The potential of neural stem cells to repair stroke-induced brain damage. Acta Neuropathol 2009;117:469–80.
96. Martino G, Pluchino S. The therapeutic potential of neural stem cells. Nat Rev Neurosci 2006;7:395–406.
97. Andres RH, Horie N, Slikker W, et al. Human neural stem cells enhance structural plasticity and axonal transport in the ischaemic brain. Brain 2011;134:1777–89.
98. Lee ST, Chu K, Jung KH, et al. Anti-inflammatory mechanism of intravascular neural stem cell transplantation in haemorrhagic stroke. Brain 2008;131:616–29.
99. Soncini M, Vertua E, Gibelli L, et al. Isolation and characterization of mesenchymal cells from human fetal membranes. J Tissue Eng Regen Med 2007;1:296–305.
100. Antonucci I, Stuppia L, Kaneko Y, et al. Amniotic fluid as a rich source of mesenchymal stromal cells for transplantation therapy. Cell Transplant 2011;20:789–95.
101. Yu SJ, Soncini M, Kaneko Y, et al. Amnion: a potent graft source for cell therapy in stroke. Cell Transplant 2009;18:111–18.
102. Miki T, Strom SC. Amnion-derived pluripotent/multipotent stem cells. Stem Cell Rev 2006;2:133–42.
103. Alviano F, Fossati V, Marchionni C, et al. Term Amniotic membrane is a high throughput source for multipotent Mesenchymal Stem Cells with the ability to differentiate into endothelial cells in vitro. BMC Dev Biol 2007;7:11.
104. Miki T, Lehmann T, Cai H, et al. Stem cell characteristics of amniotic epithelial cells. Stem Cells 2005;23:1549–59.
105. Ilancheran S, Michalska A, Peh G, et al. Stem cells derived from human fetal membranes display multilineage differentiation potential. Biol Reprod 2007;77:577–88.
106. Wolbank S, Peterbauer A, Fahrner M, et al. Dose-dependent immunomodulatory effect of human stem cells from amniotic membrane: a comparison with human mesenchymal stem cells from adipose tissue. Tissue Eng 2007;13:1173–83.
107. Kang JW, Koo HC, Hwang SY, et al. Immunomodulatory effects of human amniotic membrane-derived mesenchymal stem cells. J Vet Sci 2012;13:23–31.
108. Tajiri N, Acosta S, Glover LE, et al. Intravenous grafts of amniotic fluid-derived stem cells induce endogenous cell proliferation and attenuate behavioral deficits in ischemic stroke rats. PLoS ONE 2012;7:e43779.
109. Liu T, Wu J, Huang Q, et al. Human amniotic epithelial cells ameliorate behavioral dysfunction and reduce infarct size in the

rat middle cerebral artery occlusion model. Shock 2008;29: 603–11.

110. Takahashi K, Yamanaka S. Induction of pluripotent stem cells from mouse embryonic and adult fibroblast cultures by defined factors. Cell 2006;126:663–76.
111. Liu J. Induced pluripotent stem cell-derived neural stem cells: new hope for stroke? Stem Cell Res Ther 2013;4:115.
112. Pluchino S, Peruzzotti-Jametti L. Rewiring the ischaemic brain with human-induced pluripotent stem cell-derived cortical neurons. Brain 2013;136:3525–7.
113. Kawai H, Yamashita T, Ohta Y, et al. Tridermal tumorigenesis of induced pluripotent stem cells transplanted in ischemic brain. J Cereb Blood Flow Metab 2010;30:1487–93.
114. Yuan T, Liao W, Feng NH, et al. Human induced pluripotent stem cell-derived neural stem cells survive, migrate, differentiate, and improve neurologic function in a rat model of middle cerebral artery occlusion. Stem Cell Res Ther 2013;4:73.
115. Tornero D, Wattananit S, Gronning Madsen M, et al. Human induced pluripotent stem cell-derived cortical neurons integrate in stroke-injured cortex and improve functional recovery. Brain 2013;136:3561–77.
116. Tatarishvili J, Oki K, Monni E, et al. Human induced pluripotent stem cells improve recovery in stroke-injured aged rats. Restor Neurol Neurosci 2014;32:547–58.
117. Friedrich MA, Martins MP, Araujo MD, et al. Intra-arterial infusion of autologous bone marrow mononuclear cells in patients with moderate to severe middle cerebral artery acute ischemic stroke. Cell Transplant 2012;21:S13–21.
118. Bhasin A, Srivastava M, Bhatia R, et al. Autologous intravenous mononuclear stem cell therapy in chronic ischemic stroke. J Stem Cells Regen Med 2012;8:181–9.
119. Bang OY, Lee JS, Lee PH, et al. Autologous mesenchymal stem cell transplantation in stroke patients. Ann Neurol 2005;57: 874–82.
120. Lee JS, Hong JM, Moon GJ, et al. A long-term follow-up study of intravenous autologous mesenchymal stem cell transplantation in patients with ischemic stroke. Stem Cells 2010;28: 1099–106.
121. Honmou O, Houkin K, Matsunaga T, et al. Intravenous administration of auto serum-expanded autologous mesenchymal stem cells in stroke. Brain 2011;134(Pt 6):1790–807.
122. Bhasin A, Srivastava MV, Kumaran SS, et al. Autologous mesenchymal stem cells in chronic stroke. Cerebrovasc Dis Extra 2011;1:93–104.
123. Armstrong L, Stojkovic M, Dimmick I, et al. Phenotypic characterization of murine primitive hematopoietic progenitor cells isolated on basis of aldehyde dehydrogenase activity. Stem Cells 2004;22:1142–51.
124. Keller LH. Bone marrow-derived aldehyde dehydrogenase-bright stem and progenitor cells for ischemic repair. Congest Heart Fail 2009;15:202–6.
125. Balber AE. Concise review: aldehyde dehydrogenase bright stem and progenitor cell populations from normal tissues: characteristics, activities, and emerging uses in regenerative medicine. Stem Cells 2011;29:570–5.
126. Perin EC, Silva GV, Zheng Y, et al. Randomized, double-blind pilot study of transendocardial injection of autologous aldehyde dehydrogenase-bright stem cells in patients with ischemic heart failure. Am Heart J 2012;163:415–21, 421.e1.
127. Perin EC, Silva G, Gahremanpour A, et al. A randomized, controlled study of autologous therapy with bone marrow-derived aldehyde dehydrogenase bright cells in patients with critical limb ischemia. Catheter Cardiovasc Interv 2011;78:1060–7.
128. Yang B, Hamilton J, Strong R, et al. Abstract 78: Human multipotential bone marrow stem cells exert immunomodulatory effects, prevent splenic contraction, and enhance functional recovery in a rodent model of ischemic stroke. Stroke 2011;42:e67.
129. Yang B, Schaar K, Hamilton J, et al. Abstract 198: The spleen is a pivotal target of functional recovery after treatment with multistem for acute ischemic stroke. Stroke 2012;43:A198.
130. Smith EJ, Stroemer RP, Gorenkova N, et al. Implantation site and lesion topology determine efficacy of a human neural stem cell line in a rat model of chronic stroke. Stem Cells 2012;30: 785–96.
131. Yasuhara T, Matsukawa N, Hara K, et al. Notch-induced rat and human bone marrow stromal cell grafts reduce ischemic cell loss and ameliorate behavioral deficits in chronic stroke animals. Stem Cells Dev 2009;18:1501–14.
132. Adamczak J, Hoehn M. In vivo imaging of cell transplants in experimental ischemia. Prog Brain Res 2012;201:55–78.
133. Tennstaedt A, Aswendt M, Adamczak J, et al. Noninvasive multimodal imaging of stem cell transplants in the brain using bioluminescence imaging and magnetic resonance imaging. Methods Mol Biol 2013;1052:153–66.
134. Barbosa da Fonseca LM, Gutfilen B, Rosado de Castro PH, et al. Migration and homing of bone-marrow mononuclear cells in chronic ischemic stroke after intra-arterial injection. Exp Neurol 2010;221:122–8.
135. Rosado-de-Castro PH, Schmidt Fda R, Battistella V, et al. Biodistribution of bone marrow mononuclear cells after intra-arterial or intravenous transplantation in subacute stroke patients. Regen Med 2013;8:145–55.
136. Barbosa da Fonseca LM, Battistella V, de Freitas GR, et al. Early tissue distribution of bone marrow mononuclear cells after intra-arterial delivery in a patient with chronic stroke. Circulation 2009;120:539–41.

61 Antiplatelet Therapy for Secondary Prevention of Stroke

Thalia S. Field, Mar Castellanos, Babette B. Weksler, Oscar R. Benavente

KEY POINTS

- Antiplatelet agents are the gold standard for secondary prevention of non-cardioembolic stroke.
- The combination of aspirin plus clopidogrel should not be used for long-term secondary stroke prevention.
- Aspirin, aspirin plus dypidiridamole or clopidogrel are accepted therapeutic alternatives.
- For prevention of early stroke prevention, it is possible that the combination of aspirin and clopidogrel is effective; however, this needs to be confirmed by results of the ongoing POINT trial.
- For patients with atrial fibrillation unable to receive anticoagulation, aspirin plus clopidogrel confers protection in reducing stroke, however with a significant increase in the risk of major hemorrhages.

Stroke is the second-leading cause of death worldwide, after ischemic heart disease, and is the sixth leading cause of adult disability-adjusted life-years worldwide.[1] The predominant mechanisms for ischemic stroke are cardioembolic, thromboembolic, and small-vessel disease. The rest are due to unusual mechanisms or are classified as cryptogenic.

Cerebral ischemia tends to recur after a primary episode of either transient ischemic attack (TIA) or stroke. Most commonly, cerebral ischemia is caused by thromboemboli that form on damaged vascular surfaces of extracranial or intracerebral arteries. Local activation of platelets on the walls of diseased arteries initiates thrombus formation under conditions of high flow typical of arteries because activated platelets not only clump together but also directly catalyze thrombin generation. These thrombi are classically considered "white clots"; that is, they are composed mainly of platelets plus some fibrin. These platelet-rich thrombi that form on atherosclerotic plaques may either occlude small arterioles directly or embolize into intracerebral end arteries, producing vascular occlusion that results in neurologic dysfunction.

Because platelet activation is causally linked to episodes of cerebral arterial ischemia, therapies that diminish or block the early steps in hemostasis that are platelet-dependent are used in patients with TIAs or stroke to prevent further episodes of cerebral ischemia.

Stroke prevention can be considered under the rubrics of primary prevention and secondary prevention, this can be divided into: (a) early and (b) late. Risk-factor management is of the utmost importance in primary prevention of stroke - control of hypertension, for example, is associated with a 30–40% reduction in stroke - although antiplatelet use may have a role in primary prevention in certain populations.

However, despite the use of a variety of antithrombotic therapies for secondary prevention of stroke, risk reduction has been disappointing; it has been only about 15–20% in most large clinical trials.[2,3] Increasing the intensity of treatment, either antiplatelet therapy or anticoagulation (or both together), has the important adverse effect of increasing intracerebral and systemic hemorrhage and negates the net therapeutic benefit. The success of antiplatelet drugs in reducing the recurrence of ischemic stroke further incorporates the fact that bleeding is less common during antiplatelet therapy than during anticoagulant therapy.

In contrast to arterial thrombi, venous thrombi form under conditions involving vascular stasis, consist mainly of fibrin and erythrocytes, and are much less dependent on platelet activation. Venous thrombosis, including cerebral venous thrombosis, is thus better prevented by anticoagulation than by antiplatelet therapy.[4] This is also true for cardioembolic strokes associated with atrial fibrillation (AF). However, the distinctions between factors contributing to arterial versus venous thrombi are far from absolute. Both platelet-dependent phases and coagulation-factor-dependent phases of hemostasis intermingle to a considerable extent, for example, because of the prominent role played by platelets in catalyzing thrombin generation.

Moreover, combining antiplatelet and anticoagulant agents in the search for more powerful effects during long-term, secondary prevention of cerebral ischemia has been notably unsuccessful because an unacceptably high incidence of intracerebral and extracranial bleeding ensues when the drug combinations are used at doses that effectively block both platelet function and blood coagulation.[4]

PLATELET PHYSIOLOGY IN THE PLANNING OF ANTIPLATELET THERAPY

The evidence is clear that persons at increased risk of stroke have excessively active platelets and that even normal platelet activation in the setting of arterial disease imparts thromboembolic risk. This provides the pathophysiologic basis for antiplatelet therapy in the secondary reduction of stroke risk. To understand the rationale for using particular antiplatelet drugs, it is important first to consider how platelets regulate normal hemostasis. Hemostasis is defined as the appropriate physiologic response to vascular injury that provides prompt control of blood loss. In contrast, thrombosis is excessive or inappropriate blood clotting. Platelet hemostatic function needs then to be contrasted with platelet prothrombotic function, that is, how platelets promote inappropriate formation of blood clots in the setting of arterial vascular disease. Because platelets interact with the blood vessel wall in both hemostasis and thrombosis, the status of the arterial endothelial lining is an important determinant of platelet behavior. Normal vascular endothelium is non-thrombogenic and prevents platelet interactions with it and with other platelets or leukocytes by multiple mechanisms including secretion

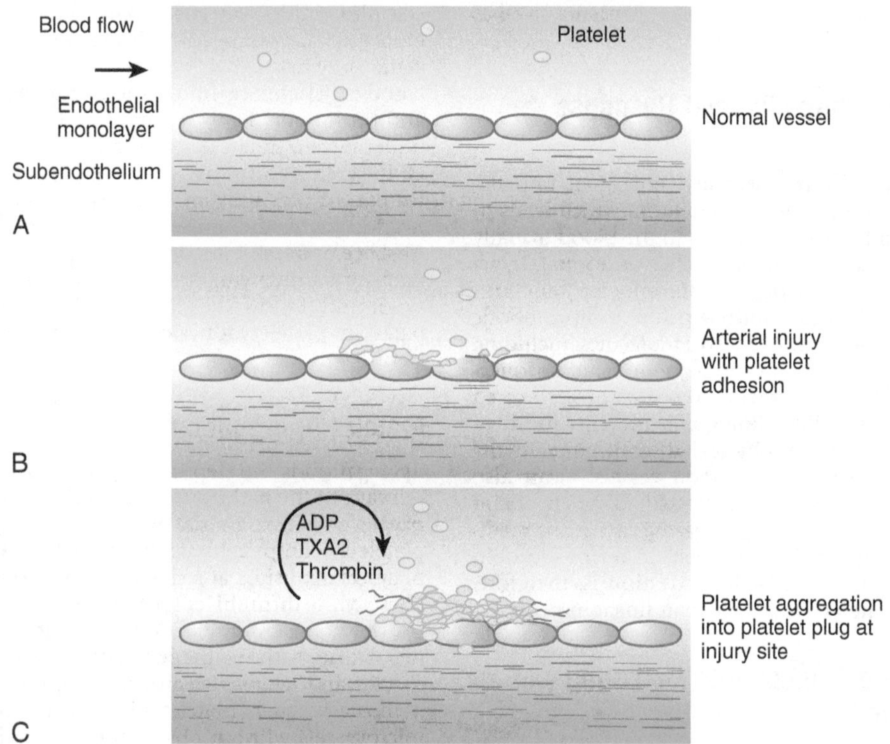

Figure 61-1. Platelets and primary hemostatic plug formation. Sequence of events in primary hemostasis after arterial injury. A, Blood flow over normal arterial endothelium. No interaction of platelets with the vascular wall. B, Immediately after injury that disrupts the arterial endothelium, platelets adhere to the subendothelium exposed at the injury site, forming a platelet monolayer, change shape, spread out, and begin to release vasoactive substances. C, Within a few minutes, activated platelets aggregate on the first layer of spread platelets, clumping together and releasing vasoactive mediators such as adenosine diphosphate (ADP) and thromboxane A_2 (TXA_2), and catalyze generation of thrombin so that fibrin strands (designated by *wavy lines*) form and stabilize the platelet plug.

of prostaglandins and nitric oxide, surface expression of anticoagulant heparan sulfate and adenosine-diphosphate (ADP)-metabolizing enzymes, and facilitation of smooth, non-turbulent blood flow.

Normal Functions of Platelets in Hemostasis

Normal platelets circulate for about 7–10 days after being released from megakaryocytes in the bone marrow, even though they lack nuclei and are almost incapable of protein synthesis. The youngest platelets are the most hemostatically active. The relatively long life of platelets in the blood has permitted effective, once-daily dosing with several antiplatelet drugs. Circulating platelets do not normally interact with one another, with other blood cells, or with the surface of the normal vascular endothelium. If a blood vessel is injured and endothelial continuity is broken; however, platelets undergo, within seconds, a rapid series of coordinated activation changes that quickly leads to a hemostatic platelet plug. This primary hemostatic plug prevents bleeding at the injury site without blocking blood flow through the vessel (Fig. 61-1).

These activation steps start with adhesion of single platelets to the damaged vessel wall, in which the platelets change in shape from flat, unreactive disks to "spiny spheres" that spread out over the surface. Next is aggregation, in which additional platelets join into masses or clumps on top of the original spread layer of platelets, blocking blood loss. During this process, the now activated platelets release vasoactive substances from storage granules, including adhesive glycoproteins, procoagulants, agonists for platelet activation, enzymes, and inflammatory mediators (Table 61-1). Moreover, once platelets are activated, vasoactive lipids, such as thromboxane A_2 (TXA_2) and leukotrienes, are rapidly synthesized and released. Many of these substances either recruit other platelets or produce vascular contraction, which are functions that help stop bleeding promptly at the injury site. Most importantly, the surface membranes of activated platelets catalyze thrombin generation with great efficiency, such that activated platelets serve to initiate, augment, and localize fibrin

TABLE 61-1 Platelet-Derived Vasoactive Mediators

Dense granule contents	Adenosine diphosphate, adenosine triphosphate, Ca^{2+}, serotonin
Alpha granule contents	Adhesive proteins: fibronectin, fibrinogen, thrombospondin, vitronectin
	Coagulation factors: von Willebrand factor, factor V, factor X
	Growth factors: fibroblast growth factor, platelet-derived growth factor, transforming growth factor-β
	Membrane proteins: P-selectin, amyloid precursor protein
	Others: albumin, immunoglobulin G, antibacterial proteins, platelet inhibitor activator-1
Lysosomes	Acid hydrolases, neutral proteases, elastase, complement-activating enzymes, heparitinase
Peroxisomes	Catalase
Lipid mediators (not preformed)	Prostaglandin endoperoxides, thromboxane A_2, prostaglandin D_2, 12-hydroxyeicosatetraenoic acid, isoprostanes

formation, further amplifying thrombotic potential as well as participating in clot stabilization.

Participants in the Initial Platelet Response to Vascular Injury

In both hemostasis and thrombosis, the major signal for platelet activation is a local injury to endothelium, which leads to exposure of prothrombotic components to the blood, usually localized in the subendothelial matrix. Whereas normal, intact endothelium displays numerous antithrombotic functions and repels platelets, subendothelium is rich in prothrombotic substances such as collagen and adhesive molecules, including von Willebrand factor (vWF), thrombospondin, and fibronectin. In addition, subtle endothelial dysfunction produced by turbulent blood flow, hyperlipidemia, inflammation, or atherosclerosis – without any physical discontinuity in the endothelial monolayer lining the blood vessels – can also activate platelets. Moreover, once activated, platelets themselves recruit additional platelets by releasing vasoactive mediators and catalyzing thrombin formation; in turn, thrombin is a potent platelet activator. Platelet activation is, therefore, an exponential and interactive, rather than linear, process.

Platelet Membrane Components Mediating Platelet Activation

Platelet activation involves changes in both the morphologic and biochemical state of the platelet membrane, including conformational changes in adhesion receptors, binding of adhesive proteins, mobilization of intracellular granule contents, interactions with the cytoskeleton, initiation of signaling, and platelet–platelet interaction. Glycoprotein (GP) platelet adhesion receptors mediate attachment of platelets to substrate proteins. Adhesion receptors that are important for normal hemostasis, thus representing potential therapeutic targets for thrombosis prevention, include the following: GPIa, a collagen receptor; GPIb, a receptor for vWF; the GPIIb/IIIa complex, a major receptor for fibrinogen, fibronectin, and vWF; GPIV, a thrombospondin receptor, required for irreversible platelet activation; glycoproteins V and IX; and $\alpha_v\beta_3$, a receptor for vitronectin, fibrinogen, and fibronectin. These receptors are all functional on resting platelets except for GPIIb/IIIa, which requires platelet activation to undergo the conformational change that permits this complex to bind fibrinogen.

Many of the adhesive glycoproteins that are ligands for these receptors share the peptide sequence RGD (R, arginine; G, glycine; D, aspartic acid), which is directly involved in cell–cell adhesion.

Platelet Adhesion

Adhesion of platelets to other platelets, to the subendothelium exposed by vascular injury, or to activated endothelium is the first major step in the platelet activation sequence. Platelet adhesion is mediated by a complex of GPIb–V–IX, which binds to matrix vWF at high shear rates and is also a binding site for thrombin, thus acting to amplify platelet responses to thrombin.[5,6] GPIb–V–IX is mainly involved in platelet activation resulting from abnormal shear stress, such as is found in arteries narrowed by atherosclerosis. Changes in conformation of the GPIbα component of the complex or of vWF can induce interaction between these two molecules. Binding of vWF to collagen induces small conformational changes in vWF that permit its binding to GPIb. Furthermore, binding of vWF to GPIb causes redistribution of the GPIb–V–IX glycoprotein complex within platelets, linking the complex to the cytoskeleton and activating phosphorylating enzymes that regulate actin polymerization and the activation of the GPIIb/IIIa complex. Therefore, inhibition of platelet adhesion should be antithrombotic. Peptides that block GPIb–V–IX function are under development as novel antiplatelet drugs. Activation of GPIb–V–IX in a thromboxane-independent manner accounts for part of the "resistance" to aspirin that is observed in connection with the presence of atherosclerotic risk factors. Absence or dysfunction of GPIb is characteristic of a rare platelet disorder involving soft-tissue bleeding, the Bernard-Soulier syndrome. At low shear, the GPIIb/IIIa complex also participates in platelet adhesion to surfaces through binding of fibrinogen.

Platelet Aggregation

Aggregation is the step in the platelet activation process most relevant to the pathogenesis of occlusive vascular events in an oxygen-sensitive arterial bed. During aggregation, activated platelets clump together atop an initial, adherent layer of platelets deposited at a site of injury or diseased vascular wall. These white thrombi, composed mainly of platelets and fibrin, may be transient or may become stabilized by further fibrin deposition, forming the nidus of bulkier clots in which erythrocytes and leukocytes also become trapped. During normal hemostasis, such platelet plugs halt bleeding from injured microvessels without obstructing blood flow, but in diseased vessels (e.g., in atherosclerosis or vasculitis or after irradiation), excessive platelet plug formation can occlude cerebral vasculature, producing TIA or stroke.

Platelet Membrane Receptors in Aggregation

The most important membrane receptor for aggregation is the integrin GPIIb/IIIa, a bimolecular membrane complex unique to platelets and megakaryocytes. Platelet aggregation by all known pathways depends on conformational changes in GPIIb/IIIa induced by platelet agonists.[7,8] Three main physiologic pathways independently triggered by different ligands can activate the GPIIb/IIIa complex; one pathway is activated by arachidonic acid leading to TXA_2 formation, the second by ADP, and the third by thrombin (Fig. 61-2).[9–11] All of these signaling pathways converge in a final common mechanism to produce a conformational change in GPIIb/IIIa that exposes a high-affinity fibrinogen binding site. The activated GPIIb/IIIa complex thus markedly increases fibrinogen binding, becomes associated with cytoskeletal proteins and signaling kinases (e.g., pp60[c-src]), forms receptor clusters, and becomes phosphorylated. All of these functions favor platelet–platelet interactions. Both outside–inside signaling (e.g., agonist-driven) and inside–outside signaling (i.e., kinase/phosphatase-driven) are involved in this activation process.

Because the final common pathway for platelet activation requires the GPIIb/IIIa complex, therapeutic blockade of the complex inhibits all further platelet activation. In contrast, drugs that inhibit only one of the three pathways, such as aspirin inhibition of the thromboxane pathway or clopidogrel inhibition of the ADP pathway, do not prevent GPIIb/IIIa activation. Drugs that directly block the functions of the GPIIb/IIIa complex thus have profound inhibitory effects on platelet function and are currently used to treat acute cardiac ischemia. Development of the monoclonal antibody abciximab (ReoPro), of peptides such as eptifibatide (Integrilin), and of peptidomimetics such as tirofiban (Aggrastat), which inhibit GPIIb/IIIa function when administered intravenously, has permitted highly successful antiplatelet therapy in acute cardiac interventions. Used over a short interval in

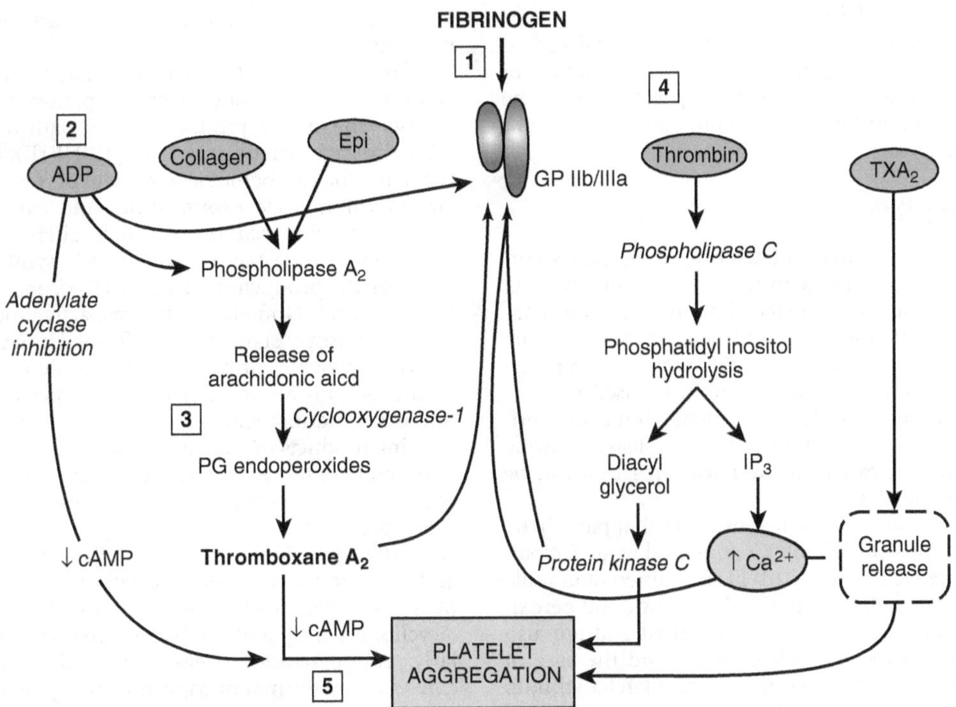

Figure 61-2. Platelet activation pathways and their inhibition. Specific, seven-transmembrane-spanning, G-protein-linked receptors on the platelet surface (depicted as *ellipses*) are activated by binding of their specific ligands and initiate different pathways for platelet activation, which converge on the conformational activation of the glycoprotein (GP) IIb/IIIa receptor complex to increase fibrinogen binding. These pathways lead to activation of the arachidonic acid pathway, hydrolysis of phosphatidyl inositol, increase in intraplatelet calcium ion (Ca^{2+}) concentration, release of vasoactive substances from platelet granules, synthesis of vasoactive lipids, and platelet aggregation. Mechanisms of inhibition of specific activation mechanisms by antiplatelet drugs (numbers in boxes) are (1) blocking of GPIIb/IIIa function and therefore blocking of fibrinogen binding and platelet aggregation; (2) blocking of the adenosine diphosphate (ADP) receptor; (3) inhibition of cyclooxygenase-interrupting arachidonic acid metabolism and prevention of the production of thromboxane A_2 (TXA_2); (4) blocking of thrombin action and thrombin receptor activation; (5) maintenance of high intraplatelet cyclic adenosine monophosphate (cAMP), which prevents platelet aggregation. Not depicted is inhibition of thromboxane A_2 synthase or thromboxane A_2 receptor function because drugs with these activities have not been clinically useful. *Epi*, Epinephrine; *IP_3*, inositol 1,4,5-triphosphate; *PG*, prostaglandin.

combination with heparin and aspirin, these GPIIb/IIIa inhibitors prevent early thrombosis and deter vascular reocclusion after coronary angioplasty and stent placement. Unfortunately, the use of oral GPIIb/IIIa inhibitors for long-term prevention of cardiac thrombosis has been unsuccessful to date in numerous clinical trials, in which administration of such agents has been accompanied by higher rates of thrombosis or bleeding. A single clinical trial testing the safety of abciximab in treatment of acute stroke has been published (see later). Indeed, the Blockage of the Glycoprotein IIb/IIIa Receptor to Avoid Vascular Occlusion (BRAVO) study of lotrafiban (an oral GPIIb/IIIa inhibitor) and heparin for prevention of cardiovascular and cerebrovascular events, initiated in 2000, had to be discontinued because of excess occurrences of thrombosis.

Multiple Independent Pathways to Aggregation

Each of the three independent biochemical pathways of platelet aggregation provides a separate potential for therapeutic intervention. One major pathway involves metabolism of arachidonic acid, which is released from membrane phospholipids during platelet activation (see Fig. 61-2, center left). This pathway is sensitive to aspirin and other non-steroidal anti-inflammatory drugs (NSAIDs). Receptor engagement by various platelet agonists activates phospholipase C to cleave membrane-bound phosphatidyl inositol to inositol 1,4,5-triphosphate (IP_3) and diacylglycerol. IP_3 in turn releases stored calcium ions, permitting activation of platelet phospholipase A_2, which releases esterified arachidonic acid from membrane phospholipids. The enzyme cyclooxygenase-1 in platelets rapidly converts the released arachidonic acid to prostaglandin endoperoxides that are isomerized to thromboxane A_2 (TXA_2), a potent platelet agonist and vasoconstrictor. The TXA_2 diffuses from the platelets and binds to its specific seven-transmembrane receptor on the platelet surface, signaling further activation of phospholipase C. Concomitantly, the liberated diacylglycerol activates protein kinase C, which translocates to the platelet plasma membrane and triggers activation of GPIIb/IIIa, exposing its fibrinogen binding site, thereby permitting platelet aggregation and secretion of platelet granule contents (see Fig. 61-2, right side). Aspirin, which irreversibly binds to cyclooxygenase-1, blocks the formation of TXA_2 for the entire life span of circulating platelets because platelets are incapable of synthesizing new cyclooxygenase protein.

Platelets that cannot produce TXA_2 can still be activated via the ADP-dependent and thrombin-dependent activation pathways. Platelet aggregation can be initiated via two interacting ADP receptors by ADP that is released by platelets or derived from extraplatelet sources such as red blood cells, even in the presence of aspirin.[10,11] Thrombin acts on several specific protease-activated membrane receptors (PARs) that signal the activation of phospholipase C and irreversible platelet aggregation and the release reaction that is independent of arachidonic acid metabolism.[9] Similarly, platelet activation by the phosphorylcholine-derivative platelet-activating factor (PAF), which is produced by leukocytes or by disturbed endothelial cells, is also aspirin-insensitive. The existence of these separate pathways for platelet aggregation may be regarded as representing fail-safe or redundant mechanisms to avoid hemorrhages.

Platelet Release Reaction

Release of vasoactive contents of platelet storage granules normally accompanies platelet activation, augments platelet aggregation, and accelerates localized clot formation, vasoconstriction, and the initiation of wound healing. Not only are preformed glycoprotein mediators, ADP, vasoactive amines, growth factors, calcium ions, and serotonin released into the blood or displayed on the surface membrane, but also short-lived lipid mediators are synthesized and released during platelet activation. The extent of the release reaction can be modulated by antiplatelet drugs.

Several types of granules rich in substances that participate in blood coagulation, cell–cell interactions, and wound repair are present in platelets (see Table 61-1). The different granule types – dense granules, alpha granules, lysosomes, and peroxisomes – can be morphologically distinguished and are also functionally characterized by their contents and the ease of release of their contents. For example, weak platelet stimuli, such as ADP, adenosine triphosphate (ATP), serotonin, and calcium – all of which participate in potentiating irreversible platelet aggregation – release the contents of the dense granules. By contrast, strong stimuli are required for release of alpha granule contents: fibrinogen, fibronectin, vWF, platelet-derived growth factor (PDGF), epidermal growth factor (EGF), transforming growth factor-β (TGF-β), platelet factor-4 (PF-4) and β-thromboglobulin. Alpha granules also contain albumin, immunoglobulins, antibacterial proteins, and a complement inhibitor. The membrane of the alpha granules contains P-selectin and the amyloid precursor protein; on platelet activation, P-selectin is transferred to the surface of the platelets, where it mediates cell–cell interactions with leukocytes and plays an important role in inflammatory reactions. Platelet lysosomes, the last granule type to be released, contain acid hydrolases, neutral proteases, elastase, enzymes that activate complement, and a heparitinase. Peroxisomes contain catalase.

In general, release of components of both dense bodies and alpha granules usually accompanies platelet aggregation, but may also occur from platelets that are adherent to damaged endothelium or subendothelium, even without formation of platelet aggregates.

Platelet Synthesis of Vasoactive Lipid Mediators

In contrast to the release of preformed proteins or amines from platelet granules, vasoactive lipid mediators are not stored by platelets, but instead are rapidly synthesized and released on platelet activation. Most of these lipids are oxygenated metabolites of arachidonic acid, which is mobilized from membrane phospholipids when agonists interact with platelet membrane receptors. The released arachidonate is the substrate for several different metabolic pathways producing eicosanoids and hydroxylated fatty acids. TXA_2 is the major platelet product of arachidonic acid metabolism by the eicosanoid pathway, and its synthesis occurs very rapidly – within seconds – on platelet activation. G-protein linked, seven membrane-spanning receptors for TXA_2 are present on platelets, leukocytes, and vascular cells.[12] These receptors bind TXA_2 and also its endoperoxide precursors, which have similar vasoconstrictor properties. Signal transduction via TXA_2 receptors initiates platelet activation and causes vasoconstriction.

Platelets also synthesize hydroxylated fatty acids from arachidonate via a separate enzymatic pathway involving lipoxygenase. The major product of this pathway in platelets is 12-hydroxyeicosatetraenoic acid (12-HETE), an inflammatory mediator that is chemotactic for leukocytes, stimulates vascular smooth muscle proliferation, and can be converted to additional inflammatory mediators, di-HETEs, by leukocytes. In contrast to the rapid burst of TXA_2 synthesis by activated platelets, the production of 12-HETE occurs continuously over a long period. Non-enzymatic, vasoactive metabolites of arachidonate, isoprostanes are also formed by oxidation; they can inactivate vascular or platelet nitric oxide (NO).

Interactions among different cell types can produce additional arachidonic acid products via transcellular metabolism, yielding products that are not made by a single cell type alone. Thus, platelet-released arachidonic acid can be converted into other vasoactive products by leukocytes or endothelial cells in close proximity. As mentioned previously, leukocytes can convert 12-HETE into various di-HETEs that have chemotactic and inflammatory properties. Endothelial cells can convert platelet-derived arachidonic acid or endoperoxide into prostacyclin, an antiplatelet substance that is a vasodilator. Similarly, endoperoxides released by endothelial cells can be converted by normal or aspirin-treated platelets into TXA_2.

How Platelet Activation Promotes Blood Coagulation

Platelets responding to strong agonists such as collagen, TXA_2, and thrombin accelerate both primary hemostatic plug formation and catalysis of blood coagulation, efficiently localized on the surface of the activated platelets. By providing specific sites, receptors, procoagulant factors, and lipid cofactors for the assembly of the key complexes of procoagulant enzymes, the activated platelet surface markedly accelerates the rate of localized thrombin generation, increasing by more than 200,000-fold the reaction rate in the fluid phase. Furthermore, activated platelets themselves contribute coagulation factors such as factor V and factor X released from their granules into a local clot as well as antifibrinolytic factors such as plasminogen activator inhibitor-1 (PAI-1). Because thrombin is a strong stimulus for platelet activation, the release reaction, and TXA_2 formation, the initial production of trace amounts of thrombin at the site of vascular injury directly stimulates further platelet activation and promotes coagulation. Microparticles shed from activated platelets also catalyze thrombin generation. Platelets additionally participate in clot stabilization by releasing the fibrin cross-linking protein factor XIII and by supporting clot retraction.

Platelet Participation in Fibrinolysis and Thrombolysis

During fibrinolysis, blood clots are dissolved by the protease plasmin, which cleaves insoluble fibrin. Platelets both promote and inhibit fibrinolysis, and the products of fibrinolysis can affect platelet function.[13] Activated platelet surfaces favor fibrinolysis by localizing plasminogen and promoting its activation. Thus, platelets bind plasminogen and plasminogen activators (both urokinase and tissue-type activators) via the GPIIb/IIIa complex. Thrombospondin released from platelet granules and then displayed on the platelet surface also binds plasminogen and enhances the activation of bound plasminogen. Because plasmin is more efficiently formed on a surface than in the fluid phase, activated platelets provide an alternative surface for promoting fibrinolysis. Platelet-bound plasminogen, therefore, is more readily activated by either tissue plasminogen activator or streptokinase than is free plasminogen, which suggests a mechanism by which platelets can enhance local fibrinolysis. In turn, plasmin at low concentrations enhances and at high concentrations depresses platelet activation.[14]

Platelets also contain and secrete two fibrinolytic antagonists, PAI-1 and α_2-antiplasmin. The net effects of these different platelet activities are that platelet-rich thrombi resist fibrinolysis and thrombolysis and that platelets become activated during therapeutic thrombolysis.[15]

Physiologic Mechanisms That Limit Platelet Activation

For clinical practice, the coexistence of multiple pathways mediating platelet activation means that drugs inhibiting only one pathway - for example, aspirin inhibiting cyclooxygenase, thus blocking TXA_2 formation - only partially block platelet activation. The existence of multiple pathways of platelet activation thus protects against hemorrhage, but permits thrombosis. Several natural mechanisms exist in normal blood vessels to limit the extent of platelet activation. These mechanisms are also vasodilatory. They are (1) plasma ADPase enzymes and endothelial ectoADPases that metabolize ADP to adenosine, a vasodilator and inhibitor of platelet activation, (2) prostacyclin, the vasodilator metabolite of arachidonic acid released by endothelial cells, which stimulates platelet adenylate cyclase, raising intraplatelet cyclic adenosine monophosphate (cAMP) levels, blocking calcium release, and inhibiting platelet aggregation and secretion, and (3) NO produced by endothelial cells, platelets, and monocytes via NO synthases.[16,17]

NO stimulates platelet guanylate cyclase and raises levels of cyclic guanosine monophosphate (cGMP), thus inhibiting platelet activation. It also relaxes vascular smooth muscle via stimulation of cGMP in the vessel wall. NO is formed from L-arginine, an amino acid that has been shown to inhibit platelet aggregation. In arterial vascular disease, it is clear that NO-mediated mechanisms are diminished. At present, development of soluble ADPases and stimulators of NO synthase or NO donors as clinical antithrombotic agents is being actively pursued, but such drugs have not yet entered the clinical trial phase of development.

Platelet Activation as a Link between Hemostasis and Inflammation

Activated platelets recruit leukocytes to sites of vascular injury, setting up an inflammatory response that assists in repair of damaged tissue after hemostasis but promotes atherosclerotic progression in vascular disease. Numerous substances released from platelets are directly chemotactic for neutrophils (12-HETE), monocytes (PF-4, PDGF), or both. Platelet proteases release chemotactic complement fragment C5a from plasma C5 and potentiate C3 activation, enhancing leukocyte function. Platelet P-selectin translocated to the surface membrane of activated platelets mediates interactions between platelets and leukocytes, including initial leukocyte rolling on vascular endothelium, and P-selectin also augments leukocyte activation. Activated platelets remain coated with P-selectin, which permits long-lasting inflammatory effects in the vicinity of platelet plugs, whereas display of P-selectin on activated endothelium is a transient phenomenon. Activation of endothelium, however, induces platelet thrombus formation.[18]

Adhesive proteins released by platelets promote inflammation as well as hemostasis; therefore, they contribute to thrombosis. Circulating levels of vWF, fibrinogen, thrombospondin, and PDGF rise during inflammation and are chronically elevated in patients with occlusive vascular disease. The growth factors released by aggregating platelets are chemotactic for leukocytes, smooth muscle cells, and endothelial cells and, during wound healing, stimulate cell division of smooth muscle cells and fibroblasts. Among these factors is TGF-β. Platelets are a major source of circulating TGF-β, which is released on their activation. TGF-β stimulates the synthesis of matrix proteins, a component of atherosclerotic lesions. Because these growth factors can also be released by single platelets adhering to an abnormal vascular wall, they can stimulate excessive proliferative responses in the vessel wall that favor both restenosis after revascularization and progression of atherosclerosis. Platelets are rich in cholesterol, which is also released during platelet activation and can be incorporated into the arterial wall. Therefore, antiplatelet therapy that depresses release of platelet granule contents has potential anti-atherosclerotic as well as direct antithrombotic value.

PLATELET FUNCTION IN PATIENTS AT RISK OF OCCLUSIVE STROKE

Factors Contributing to Platelet Hyperactivity

Patients at risk of occlusive stroke often have activated platelets.[19,20] Their platelet hyperreactivity most likely reflects the interactions between platelets and an abnormal vascular surface. Most frequently atherosclerosis, but also vasculitis, infection, trauma, or congenital anomaly may lead to vascular endothelial dysfunction. Stroke risk factors such as hypertension, hypercholesterolemia, smoking, diabetes mellitus, and inflammation contribute both to increased platelet reactivity and to abnormal endothelial behavior with consequently higher risk of arterial thrombosis.[21] In addition, turbulent blood flow that accompanies atherosclerotic or hypertensive arterial changes (e.g., endothelial dysfunction, stiff vascular wall, atherosclerotic plaque, or altered pressure gradients) further contributes to increased platelet reactivity in the absence of actual breaches in the endothelium. High levels of platelet activation markers have been associated with carotid artery wall thickening.

Plasma factors may also contribute to increased platelet reactivity in stroke-prone patients. The higher levels of circulating catecholamines associated with advancing age and with stress contribute to platelet reactivity. Catecholamines are weak direct platelet agonists but augment platelet aggregation by other agonists, oppose the effects of natural antiplatelet factors such as prostacyclin and NO, and offset some of the antiplatelet efficacy of aspirin. A circadian rhythm in acute myocardial infarction (MI), stroke, and sudden death has been observed in which the peak incidence is seen in the early morning, soon after patients awaken.[22,23] Platelet aggregability is highest soon after waking and correlates with elevations in plasma catecholamines and free fatty acids.[23] A diminution in the morning excess of cardiovascular events in patients who take aspirin points to platelet involvement in the process.

In clinical settings marked by stress, in which catecholamine levels are increased, plasma fibrinogen and vWF–factor VIII are also elevated, which contributes to platelet activation.[27] Elevated plasma fibrinogen by itself is an independent risk factor for stroke and is known to increase platelet aggregability.[24] Recent infection may also contribute to the risk of recurrent cerebral ischemia.[25] In the elderly, a seasonal rise in stroke incidence during the winter months may reflect a higher incidence of infection.[26,27]

Role of Platelet Count

High platelet counts may but do not necessarily represent a stroke risk factor. In situations in which platelet turnover is continually enhanced, a compensatory increase in megakaryocyte size may result in release of platelets that are "younger," larger, and more hemostatically active than usual. Young platelets have been found to be larger than average, to produce more prothrombotic factors, and to aggregate in response to lower concentrations of agonists. Large platelets are a risk factor for death and recurrent vascular events after MI.[32] Platelet volume is greater in patients with acute stroke than in age- and sex-matched control subjects, and the high platelet volume may persist for months.[28]

In myeloproliferative diseases, platelets are often very large, and platelet mass is increased even more than platelet count; platelet numbers, therefore, underestimate total platelet mass. The greater platelet mass probably contributes to the higher thrombotic risk observed in these diseases. High platelet counts in a setting of myeloproliferative disease are associated with increased risk of thrombosis, including cerebral thrombosis, and lowering the platelet count with chemotherapy appears to reduce the risk of both stroke and thrombosis in these diseases.[34] Low-dose aspirin therapy also decreases stroke risk in patients with myeloproliferative diseases, especially if the platelet count has been normalized. In contrast, secondary thrombocytosis that accompanies inflammation or follows splenectomy, for example, is not usually associated with a higher risk of thrombosis or stroke.

Chronic Changes in Platelet Reactivity

The question of whether greater platelet reactivity in patients with stroke merely reflects the body's inflammatory response to tissue damage is, however, clearly answered with a no. Increases in platelet activation not only may follow an acute stroke for many months but also may be chronically present before an episode of cerebral ischemia. In adults, increased platelet aggregability after atherosclerotic stroke has been demonstrated to continue for at least 3–9 months after the acute event in 60% of patients; this time extends well beyond that required for resolution of the acute inflammatory changes typical of cerebral tissue damage.[21] Similar changes in platelet aggregability are not observed after stroke caused by cardiac emboli, even though brain tissue damage may be extensive. A long-term increase in platelet aggregation after acute cerebral ischemia correlates with a poorer outcome. In some unusual circumstances, oxidative stress has been correlated with chronic platelet activation. In familial stroke, infants seen with stroke can be shown to have a chronic platelet hyperreactivity that is not blocked by NO; such infants lack the plasma enzyme glutathione peroxidase and, therefore, have low blood antioxidant potential that counters the protective effect of NO on platelets.[29] In most cases of adult ischemic stroke, however, no such simple correlation between oxidative stress and platelet hyperreactivity can be made.

The pathologic consequences of greater platelet reactivity in stroke-prone patient clearly show that more is not better. In normal arteries, hemostasis rapidly controls bleeding, and the damaged area is soon precisely repaired, whereas in a diseased arterial bed, even this normal hemostatic response may have the unwanted consequences of arterial thrombosis. This dysequilibrium between hemostasis and thrombosis appears to be particularly true in vessels vulnerable to even temporary occlusion, such as the end arteries of the brain. Furthermore, normal platelet contributions to wound repair can similarly be detrimental in stroke-prone patients, in whom platelet-derived mediators promote excessive vascular cell proliferation that accelerates intimal hyperplasia and vascular narrowing.[21,30]

ANTIPLATELET DRUGS AND PREVENTION OF STROKE

The sequential steps in platelet activation are sensitive to different pharmacologic interventions. Antiplatelet drugs that mainly affect platelet aggregation and mediator release tend to block platelet-initiated thrombosis without much depression of hemostasis and, therefore, involve a smaller chance of hemorrhagic complications. On the other hand, antiplatelet drugs that block platelet adhesion, the initial step in platelet activation at a vascular surface, or the GPIIb/IIIa complex and, thus, all aggregation pathways, are highly effective in preventing thrombosis; thus far, however, they continue to impose an unacceptable risk of bleeding, particularly in the brain. Only direct inhibitors of thrombin, factor Xa, or both block the capacity of platelets to catalyze thrombin generation. Such agents might pose a major bleeding risk with long-term use in secondary prevention of cerebral ischemia and have not been tested for prevention of non-cardioembolic stroke.

Antiplatelet drugs in current use for secondary prevention of stroke include aspirin, clopidogrel, dipyridamole, and various combinations of these agents (Table 61-2). In clinical settings in which platelets are not major factors in the production of vasoocclusive arterial emboli, anticoagulation is an effective form of secondary prevention of stroke. The foremost of settings is cardioembolic stroke associated with nonvalvular AF and valvular heart disease. Other important causes of stroke that are relatively independent of platelets are cholesterol emboli released from ulcerated atherosclerotic plaques, patent foramen ovale, fibrin-rich emboli from intracardiac mural thrombus, "bland" cardiac valve vegetations in inflammatory disease, thalassemia, and sickle cell disease;[31-37] these causes together represent about 15% of cerebral ischemic episodes. Even in some of these settings, antiplatelet agents may have a role in stroke prevention if anticoagulation alone does not suffice or if the patient also has atherosclerotic risk factors for stroke.

Aspirin

Mechanism of the Antiplatelet Effect of Aspirin

Aspirin has long been known to prolong bleeding time. That the lengthened bleeding time involves decreased platelet aggregation was first demonstrated in the 1960s. In 1971, aspirin was first shown to affect platelet function by irreversible acetylation and thus inactivation of the platelet enzyme cyclooxygenase-1 (prostaglandin endoperoxide synthase-1), thus preventing the addition of molecular oxygen to arachidonic acid to form prostaglandin endoperoxides G_2 and H_2 and blocking downstream formation of TXA_2 from endoperoxides.[38-40] Because platelets do not synthesize proteins, platelet functions that depend on TXA_2 activity are inhibited for the life span of the platelet. The separate peroxidase function of cyclooxygenase, not involved in eicosanoid synthesis, remains unaffected by aspirin. Very small doses of aspirin rapidly (within minutes) block platelet cyclooxygenase in vivo.[41] Certain peculiarities of platelet kinetics favor the profound and long-lasting effect of aspirin. Platelets circulate for 7–10 days, but once exposed to aspirin, they are permanently unable to produce TXA_2. Because only about 10% of circulating platelets are replaced each day by new platelets released from bone-marrow megakaryocytes, a single daily dose of aspirin produces virtually complete inhibition of platelet cyclooxygenase. Therefore, high, persistent blood

TABLE 61-2 Actions of Antiplatelet Drugs

Activity	Effect on Platelets	Drug
Inhibition of membrane GPIb receptor	Block GPI-V-IX function, prevent adhesion and aggregation	S-nitroso-AR545C*
Inhibition of membrane GPIIb/IIIa receptor	Prevent bending of fibrinogen Prevent platelet–platelet interaction	Abciximab RGD peptide analogues Disintegrins
Inhibition of membrane ADP $P2Y_{12}$ receptor	Prevent binding of ADP Prevent ADP-mediated aggregation Decrease GPIIb/IIIa activation	Ticlopidine, clopidogrel AR-C69931 MX†
Inhibition of membrane ADP $P2Y_1$ receptor	Prevent binding of ADP Prevent calcium mobilization	Adenosine 3′-phosphate, 5′-phosphosulfate†
Catabolism of ADP	Prevent ADP-mediated aggregation Foster disaggregation	Soluble recombinant CD39*
Inhibition of cyclooxygenase-1	Prevent TXA_2 generation Inhibit arachidonic-acid-mediated platelet aggregation and secretion	Aspirin (irreversible effect) NSAIDs (competitive effect)
Stimulate adenylate cyclase	Raise platelet cAMP, preventing aggregation and secretion	Epoprostenol, Iloprost Fish oils, ω3 fatty acids*
Inhibition of phophodiesterase	Maintain elevated cAMP once raised	Dipyridamole Methylxanthines*
Stimulate guanylate cyclase	Raise platelet CGMP, preventing aggregation and secretion	NO, NO donors (e.g., *S*-nitrosoglutathione, nitroglycerin)
Inhibit calcium flux	Prevent calcium mobilization Decrease aggregation and secretion	Ca^{2+} channel blockers* Local anesthetics* Beta-blockers*
Inhibit thrombin generation or action	Inhibit aggregation and secretion Inhibit procoagulant activity	Heparins, hirudin Antithrombin peptides†

ADP, Adenosine diphosphate; Ca^{2+}, calcium ion; cGMP, cyclic guanosine monophosphate; NO, nitric oxide; NSAID, non-steroidal anti-inflammatory drug; TXA_2, thromboxane A_2.
*Weak or adjunctive effect.
†Under development.

levels of aspirin are not required for the inhibitory effect on platelet function, even in patients with cerebral ischemia.

In contrast to platelets, other cells in vascular endothelium, cells in kidney or lung epithelium, and monocytes are capable of rapid resynthesis of cyclooxygenase. The inhibitory effect of aspirin on eicosanoid synthesis in cells other than platelets is, therefore, much briefer. Moreover, these other tissues also synthesize cyclooxygenase-2, a related isoform inducible by inflammatory stimuli and cytokines. Platelets neither contain nor synthesize cyclooxygenase-2. Cyclooxygenase-2 is also inhibited by aspirin, but because of its rapid resynthesis in many cell types (i.e., monocytes, vascular endothelium, and smooth muscle), net eicosanoid production by these cells is less durably inhibited by aspirin.[42] In terms of the vascular bed, once-daily dosage with aspirin selectively inhibits platelet function, usually without impairing production of vasoprotective prostaglandins such as prostacyclin and prostaglandin (PG) E_2 by the blood vessel wall.

Pharmacokinetics

After oral administration, aspirin is rapidly absorbed from the stomach and upper small intestine, reaching a peak plasma level 30 minutes after a single dose. It is rapidly deacetylated in the liver to salicylate. Although salicylate has little or no antiplatelet efficacy, it does have independent anti-inflammatory effects through modulation of NFκB-regulated genes. By 3 hours after oral ingestion of aspirin, the plasma acetylsalicylate level is negligible. However, because aspirin exposure inactivates platelet cyclooxygenase within minutes, even a brief exposure of circulating platelets to aspirin produces full inactivation of cyclooxygenase and depresses platelet function. Intravenous aspirin works even faster.[43]

As little as 1 mg aspirin taken orally per hour – a dose completely deacetylated on first pass through the liver – fully inhibits platelet cyclooxygenase within about 12 hours because platelets traveling through the portal circulation encounter sufficient newly absorbed aspirin to inhibit their cyclooxygenase.[44] In clinical studies, an initial dose of 162 mg fully blocks platelet cyclooxygenase in an adult, and 81 mg/day (one pediatric aspirin tablet) maintains full inhibition.[45] As little as 30 mg taken once daily for several days builds to the same net effect within 1 week, because the antiplatelet effects of aspirin are cumulative over time.[46,51] Effects of enteric-coated aspirin are similar to those of plain aspirin, except for a slightly slower onset of action.[47]

Dose–Response Effects

Antiplatelet effects of aspirin usually maximize at 81 to 325 mg/day, and higher doses do not inhibit platelet function any further.[41] Only in persons with a very rapid rate of platelet turnover are higher or more frequent doses needed for full effect (see later). TXA_2 synthesis must be decreased by 95% for full inhibitory effects of aspirin on platelet function to be achieved.[44] Aspirin was approved by the U.S. Food and Drug Administration (FDA) in 1980 for the prevention of TIAs and stroke and in 1985 for the prevention of unstable angina and secondary prevention of MI; the recommended dosage is 50–325 mg/day.

At these doses, the bleeding time lengthens to about double the baseline time in at least 60% of individuals;

larger doses of aspirin do not prolong bleeding time further. Indeed, very high doses may slightly shorten the bleeding time because of inhibition of vascular cyclooxygenase. Prolongation of bleeding time by aspirin correlates poorly with either gastric irritation or gastrointestinal bleeding. After aspirin is stopped, bleeding time returns to normal within 1–2 days regardless of the dose administered. Concomitant alcohol ingestion can further lengthen aspirin-induced prolongation of bleeding time and slows recovery; this factor may contribute to the incidence of gastrointestinal bleeding in aspirin users.

Once aspirin is stopped, platelet aggregation and TXA_2 formation return to normal levels within 7–10 days, and linear kinetics after a 1- to 2-day lag likely reflects the acetylation of megakaryocyte cyclooxygenase, resulting in release of aspirin-impaired platelets during the first 2 days. In patients at major risk of stroke, such as those with high-grade carotid stenosis, doses of aspirin up to 1300 mg/day have been tried, but the data obtained do not show greater clinical efficacy of doses higher than 325 mg (see later).[48–50]

NSAIDs inhibit platelet cyclooxygenase in a reversible, competitive manner, so their antiplatelet effects all depend on maintenance of a high blood level of drug. Therefore, their duration of antiplatelet activity is relatively brief. However, the coadministration of an NSAID, such as ibuprofen or naproxen, with low-dose aspirin can decrease the irreversible effects of aspirin on platelet cyclooxygenase by competition and may impair the antiplatelet efficacy of aspirin.[51]

In contrast, the "coxib" cyclooxygenase-2 inhibitors do not block the ability of aspirin to acetylate platelet cyclooxygenase-1 and so do not diminish the antiplatelet effects of aspirin. No definitive data are currently available on the incidence of cardiovascular events and stroke, in particular, in patients taking both aspirin and cyclooxygenase-2 inhibitors, although patients taking only the latter have been reported in some studies to have a higher incidence of MI; more information is clearly needed.

Range and Limits of Aspirin Effects on Platelet Function

The effects of aspirin on platelet activation all result from cyclooxygenase inhibition. These effects include blocking of TXA_2 production, complete inhibition of arachidonate-induced platelet aggregation, a decreased release reaction that is reflected in diminished and slowed platelet responses to collagen and epinephrine, and reduced platelet aggregation to low-dose ADP. In contrast, aspirin does not affect platelet adhesion, prolong the shortened platelet life span, decrease secretion of vascular growth factors from platelets, or block thrombin-induced platelet activation. Because TXA_2, the major eicosanoid produced by blood platelets, is a strong stimulus for platelet aggregation and release and a powerful vasoconstrictor, all of the aspirin-induced changes in platelet activation previously listed are related to blocking of the TXA_2 pathway of platelet activation.

Because thrombin affects platelets in a cyclooxygenase-independent manner, activation of platelets by thrombin is not inhibited by aspirin. Even so, use of aspirin (325–500 mg/day) has been reported to reduce platelet-dependent thrombin generation in vitro and in vivo.[52] The inhibitory effect of aspirin on thrombin generation is weaker in hypercholesterolemic patients, who are known to have a hypercoagulable state and who often show enhanced platelet TXA_2 generation. It is postulated that the antithrombinogenic effect of aspirin may involve acetylation of platelet membrane proteins, but the mechanism is not yet clear. The clinical relevance of aspirin-induced impairment of thrombin generation remains to be assessed.

Aspirin has little or no effect on the lipoxygenase pathway of arachidonic acid metabolism; thus, 12-HETE production by platelets is not altered. Production of epoxyeicosatrienoic acids and isoprostanes, which are formed non-enzymatically, is also unaltered by aspirin.

Aspirin Resistance

In spite of the well-reported efficacy of aspirin in the secondary prevention of cardiovascular disease,[2,3] recurrent vascular events are not uncommon in patients prescribed aspirin. The recurrence of coronary heart disease, stroke, and peripheral vascular disease syndromes under prescription of a regular therapeutic dose of aspirin defines what is known as clinical aspirin resistance or aspirin treatment failure. This may or may not be accompanied by biochemical aspirin resistance, a phenomenon of persistent platelet activation, measured by platelet function tests, despite prescription of a regular therapeutic dose of aspirin.[53] Whereas the incidence of aspirin resistance by the clinical definition has been estimated at 12.9% with a range from 10.9% to 17.3% depending on the dosage, the estimated incidence of biochemical resistance ranges from as little as 5.2% to as much as 60% depending on the studied population and the platelet function assay used.[54] A few studies have attempted to quantify both clinical and pharmacologic resistance, but the reported data are hampered by internal and external validity concerns including small sample sizes, lack of agreement between different platelet function tests, different dose regimens and non-adherence, and insufficient information about measurement stability over time. Moreover, none of the available platelet aggregation assays have convincingly been shown to predict clinical events, and the results between different assays have also been discordant. At present, no standardized definition or test can be used to quantify either type of aspirin resistance. However, it is clear that there is individual biochemical variability in the response to aspirin administration, which may be responsible for treatment failures and secondary vascular clinical events. Research into the mechanisms involved in the aspirin resistance phenomenon is necessary for development of more accurate platelet function tests and correlation of their results with clinical event occurrence.

Measurement of Aspirin Effects on Platelets. Because platelet activation leads to a change in platelet shape and aggregation as well as the release of different platelet constituents, the examination of these changes and/or the analysis in blood and urine of the metabolic products of platelets is the basis for determining the degree of platelet function,[55,56] which can be evaluated by different in vivo and in vitro tests.

In vivo ***Tests***

1. Measurement of TXA_2 pathway end products. The analysis of TXA_2 metabolites, which include serum thromboxane B_2 and urinary 11-dehydrothromboxane B_2, has been used to determine aspirin resistance. However, these tests seem to reflect the contribution of monocyte/macrophages to TXA_2 synthesis as well as the cyclooxygenase-2 linked pathway of arachidonic acid, but not specifically platelet activity. The levels of 11-dehydrothromboxane B_2 in urine are highly dependent on the renal function, and ex vivo platelet activation during blood sample collection, storage, and processing may also interfere with the results of these tests.[57–59].
2. Expression of P-selectin on platelet membranes. P-selectin moves to the plasma membrane when platelets are activated and degranulated; thus increased P-selectin expression on the platelet surface is indicative of platelet activation. However, selectins are also expressed on all blood cell types, which is a fact that results in conflicting

data when this marker is used to assess aspirin efficacy.[60] In addition, testing is not easy because it requires expensive equipment and carefully controlled test conditions.[61]

3. Analysis of soluble P-selectin in plasma. Plasma levels of P-selectin increase as a result of platelet activation; thus, this marker may be useful in determining platelet status.[48,61] The test is simple to perform, but relatively expensive. Moreover, because of its stability, the sample can be stored for long periods. However, the same concerns regarding the validity of the expression of P-selectin on platelet membranes as a marker of platelet activation also apply for the analysis of P-selectin in plasma.

In vitro Tests

1. Optical platelet aggregation tests. These tests measure optical changes in plasma caused by platelet aggregation induced by the addition of various substrates, including arachidonic acid, ADP, collagen, epinephrine (adrenaline), and thrombin, in the absence of erythrocytes and blood flow. The induction of platelet aggregation results in a decrease in the turbidity of the solution as the platelets crosslink and clump together. The amount of platelet aggregation is directly related to the amount of light that is allowed to be transmitted through the solution. Aspirin almost completely inhibits platelet aggregation induced by arachidonic acid and collagen, but aggregation in response to ADP and epinephrine is only partially inhibited. Moreover, platelet aggregation is sensitive to changes in temperature and pH and so must be carried out within hours of sample collection. In addition, these tests do not correlate well with other indicators of platelet function. Finally, although these tests have been the most widely used to date, the technical difficulties of the tests, which require a specialized laboratory setting, make them unsuitable for routine clinical practice.[55,62,63]
2. PFA-100 (Dade-Behring Inc.). The PFA-100 is a whole blood, point-of-care, platelet aggregometer that functions by aspirating a blood sample through a capillary tube at a high shear rate and through a small slit aperture that is cut into a membrane coated with either collagen-epinephrine or collagen-ADP platelet agonists.[64,65] Given that measurement is performed in the presence of erythrocytes and at a high shear rate, it can be considered more clinically relevant than platelet aggregometry, which is conducted in the absence of erythrocytes and blood flow. The time for a platelet plug to occlude the slit aperture, reported in seconds as the closure time, is inversely related to platelet activity. A closure time value of 193 seconds is considered normal and a closure time of more than 300 seconds is considered as non-closure.[64,65] This test is easy to perform, requires only a small volume of blood (800 μL), is quick, and has good sensitivity and reproducibility. However, the PFA-100 test is quite expensive, depends on plasma vWF and hematocrit levels, and testing must be done within 4 hours of blood collection.
3. VerifyNow Aspirin Assay (Accumetrics Inc.). Another point-of-care, easy-to-use, and rapid test for measuring platelet-induced aggregation is the VerifyNow Aspirin Assay (formerly called the Ultegra Rapid Platelet Function Analyzer). Unlike the PFA-100, VerifyNow is designed only to detect platelet dysfunction as the result of exposure to antiplatelet agents, including aspirin, clopidogrel, and glycoprotein IIb/IIIa inhibitors. The VerifyNow Aspirin Assay originally used a proprietary platelet agonist consisting of metallic cations and propyl gallate, but this has recently been substituted by an arachidonic acid agonist (Accumetrics Inc, VerifyNow Aspirin Assay package insert, San Diego, Calif; 2004). Platelet aggregation detection is based on the agglutination of platelets on fibrinogen-coated beads detected by an optical turbidimetric method. Platelet inhibition measured by the VerifyNow Aspirin Assay in response to single-dose aspirin has correlated well with measurements by the PFA-100 (r^2 = 0.73–0.86) and with traditional optical platelet aggregation (r^2 = 0.902).[66] Platelet responsiveness is expressed in aspirin response units (ARU) with a cutoff for aspirin resistance at 550 ARU. The most important limitation of this test relates to its diagnostic criteria because these were set in comparison with optical aggregation in response to adrenaline after only a single 325-mg dose of aspirin.[59]

Mechanisms of Aspirin Resistance. Several factors have been mentioned and investigated as related to aspirin resistance, but so far, the exact mechanism responsible for this phenomenon is not known.

A reduction in the bioavailability secondary to lack of adherence to the treatment, low dosage of aspirin, or concurrent intake of NSAIDs such as ibuprofen, naproxen, and indomethacin, which appear to antagonize the antiplatelet effects of aspirin by blocking its union to the cyclooxygenase-1 binding site, may explain the lack of efficacy of the drug in some cases. In fact, it has been reported that about 10% of outpatients who are prescribed aspirin or ticlopidine are non-compliant with their medication and showed a decreased inhibition of platelet aggregation on repeated testing.[67,68]

The activation of platelet function by the stimulation of alternative pathways that are not blocked by aspirin such as red-cell-induced platelet activation, stimulation of collagen, ADP, epinephrine, and thrombin receptors on platelets, and the biosynthesis of thromboxane by pathways not inhibited by aspirin has also been mentioned as a possible cause of aspirin non-responsiveness.[69]

The existence of comorbid conditions increasing vascular risk such as smoking habit, hyperlipidemia, ischemic heart disease, prosthetic heart valves, or arteritis also explain the recurrence of stroke in patients taking aspirin. In one large study, 5.7% of patients consecutively admitted for ischemic stroke were classified as aspirin non-responders as they had been taking aspirin at the time of stroke. Pertinent characteristics of these patients included significant hyperlipidemia, ischemic heart disease, and lower dose of aspirin, which suggests that individuals with greater risk factors for occlusive vascular disease might benefit less from aspirin.[70]

Moreover, some patients seem to develop aspirin resistance over time. In a study including poststroke patients prescribed aspirin who were repeatedly tested at 6-month intervals to observe the effect of aspirin on platelet aggregation,[71] 75% of 306 patients were found to have a maximum effect and 25% a partial effect of aspirin at the initial testing, but on repeated testing, only 33% continued to show good inhibition. Increasing the aspirin dose restored maximum inhibition in about two-thirds of those who had experienced a reduced effect, but this improvement was only temporary. Patients were reminded to take aspirin on the day of testing, but neither compliance with dosing nor lipid status was directly assessed in this study. Overall, about 8% of patients showed aspirin resistance, even at 1300 mg/day. Interestingly, eight patients experienced a stroke during follow-up, all of whom had previously been classified as having aspirin resistance during at least one study visit.

Finally, genetic factors also seem to be involved in aspirin resistance. Several single nucleotide polymorphisms that have been linked to changes in platelet function and thrombosis, including a polymorphism on the cyclooxygenase-1 gene, overexpression of cyclooxygenase-2 mRNA on platelets and endothelial cells, the platelet alloantigen A1/A2 of the gene encoding glycoprotein IIIa, and the homozygous 807T (873A) polymorphism allied with increased density of platelet glycoprotein Ia/IIa collagen-receptor gene, may contribute to aspirin resistance and increased risk of vascular events.[72] However, the effect of these polymorphisms on the antithrombotic effects of aspirin is only based on measurements of platelet function; thus, studies are needed to characterize the prevalence of these polymorphisms fully and, especially, to elucidate whether their presence can influence clinical outcomes.

Aspirin Resistance and Stroke Recurrence. Data regarding the percentage recurrence of ischemic stroke in patients treated with aspirin are scarce. Grotemeyer et al.[73] studied the prevalence of aspirin resistance in 174 poststroke patients treated with 1500 mg of aspirin daily, who were followed up for a period of 2 years. Twenty-nine of the 174 patients had major vascular events: 16 patients (9.2%) had MI, and 13 (7.5%) had a second stroke. The authors specified that, of the 29 patients with major events, only 4.4% (five of 114) belonged to the aspirin responder group as compared with 40% (24 of 60) of the secondary aspirin non-responder group ($P < 0.0001$). However, no specific data as to the prevalence of the different major vascular events in the group of responders vs non-responders were supplied.

As has been mentioned earlier, in Bornstein et al.,[70] 129 of 2231 consecutive patients (5.7%) admitted over a 4-year period with ischemic stroke were found to have had a recurrent ischemic stroke while already taking aspirin. The authors found that the average period until stroke was longer for patients taking higher aspirin doses and suggested that doses of 500 mg daily or more should be used in secondary stroke prevention. Moreover, comparison of patients resistant to aspirin with a control group matched for age, sex, date of first ischemic stroke, and aspirin dose demonstrated that these patients more often had statistically significant hyperlipidemia and ischemic heart disease, which confirms the importance of adequate control of vascular risk factors related to stroke, regardless of aspirin intake. Eikelboom et al.[58] analyzed the levels of 11-dehydrothromboxane B_2 in urine from 488 patients with MI, stroke, or cardiovascular death during a period of 5 years. Whereas baseline urinary concentrations of 11-dehydrothromboxane B_2 were significantly higher in patients with MI and in those who died of a cardiovascular cause, the levels were not significantly different between case patients who subsequently had a stroke and their matched control group. The adjusted odds for the composite outcome of MI, stroke, or cardiovascular death increased with each increasing quartile of baseline urinary 11-dehydrothromboxane B_2 concentrations, and patients in the highest quartile had a risk 1.8-fold higher than those in the lowest quartile. A similar association was seen with MI and cardiovascular death, but not for stroke. Andersen et al.[74] analyzed aspirin resistance using the PFA-100 system in a total of 202 patients with acute MI who were randomly assigned to aspirin 160 mg/day (n = 71), aspirin 75 mg/day together with warfarin (international normalized ratio [INR], 2.0 to 2.5) (n = 58), or warfarin alone (INR, 2.8 to 4.2) (n = 73). Although the authors reported a higher incidence of vascular events, including MI, stroke, and revascularization procedures, over a period of 4 years in the group of patients with aspirin resistance, the results were not statistically significant. Data about the separate prevalence of stroke recurrence in the group with aspirin resistance were not supplied in the article. Using the same system to evaluate platelet function, Grundmann et al.[75] reported that 12 of 35 patients (34%) who had a stroke recurrence had evidence of aspirin resistance, whereas none of the patients without further cerebrovascular events had evidence of biochemical aspirin resistance. Gum et al.[76] used platelet aggregation to analyze platelet function in a group of 326 prospective stable cardiovascular patients receiving aspirin 325 mg/day for at least 7 days and followed them up for a mean of 679 days. Clinical endpoints included the composite of death, MI, or cerebrovascular accident. Of the patients studied, 17 (5.2%) were classified as having aspirin resistance by optical aggregation and 309 (94.8%) were classified as aspirin sensitive. During follow-up, aspirin resistance was associated with an increased risk of death, MI, or stroke compared with patients who were aspirin sensitive (24% versus 10%; hazard ratio [HR], 3.12; 95% confidence interval [CI], 1.10–8.90; $P = 0.03$). However, despite there being a consistent trend, the association between aspirin resistance and individual clinical events including stroke did not reach statistical significance (12% aspirin-resistant versus 1% aspirin-sensitive, $P = 0.09$).

Recently, a post-hoc analysis form the Secondary Prevention of Small Subcortical Strokes (SPS3) trial,[77] showed that the addition of clopidogrel to aspirin in patients who had lacunar stroke while taking aspirin did not result in reduction of vascular events when compared to those that continued only on aspirin after randomization. The risk of recurrent stroke was 3.1%/year on dual antiplatelet vs 3.3%/year only on aspirin (HR 0.91; 95%CI, 0.59–1.38), however there was a significant increased on major systemic bleeding on those allocated to dual antiplatelet therapy (HR 2.7; 95%CI, 1.1–6.9).[78]

In spite of these data, the association between aspirin resistance and stroke recurrence as well as other cardiovascular events still remains uncertain. Comparison between studies is difficult because of differences in the platelet function tests used and the studied populations.

Therapeutic Management of Aspirin Resistance. Because aspirin resistance seems to be a multifactorial phenomenon, different factors need to be addressed when clinical vascular events occur in patients already being treated with this drug. Therapeutic compliance as well as the adequate control of vascular risk factors related to cerebrovascular events may increase the efficacy of aspirin administration.[70,71] However, the decision to increase aspirin dosage has to be considered individually. In fact, it has recently been reported that, in patients with diabetes mellitus, a high dosage of aspirin seems to be neither effective nor safe.[79]

The association between different antiplatelet drugs appears to be the best therapeutic approach in case of aspirin resistance. In fact, patients with aspirin resistance have been shown to have increased platelet sensitivity to ADP as well as increased plasma levels of this agonist. Moreover, those patients with a very low sensitivity to the effect of aspirin on the arachidonic acid pathway appear to be highly sensitive to the $P2Y_{12}$ platelet ADP receptor antagonist clopidogrel,[80] which suggests that the association of both drugs might have a greater effect on platelet action. In an attempt to clarify this question, several clinical trials have tested the efficacy of combining aspirin and clopidogrel in the secondary prevention of stroke.[81,82] However, some recent data seem to demonstrate the existence of clopidogrel resistance[83] and even a dual aspirin–clopidogrel resistance.[84-86] although this deserves further investigation. The combination of different dosages of aspirin and 400 mg extended-release dipyridamole (ERDP) daily has been found to be more effective than aspirin alone in the secondary prevention of stroke.[87,88] However, the combination of 25 mg aspirin and 200 mg ERDP twice a day has been reported to be equally effective as 75 mg clopidogrel daily in secondary stroke prevention. The design and results of these clinical trials are discussed in another section of this chapter.

Finally, the administration of new antiaggregants that modify platelet aggregation by a different mechanism than aspirin can be an alternative for patients who have a recurrent stroke while receiving aspirin.

Aspirin Toxicity

Gastrointestinal irritation and bleeding, well-known side effects of aspirin, can cause major or fatal bleeding, partly through a direct irritant action and partly through blocking the production of protective prostaglandins in the gastric mucosa. Risk increases with dose and duration of use.[2,3,44] Reexamination of the occurrence of hemorrhagic stroke, the major central nervous system toxicity of aspirin as an antithrombotic agent, in a meta-analysis of more than 55,000 subjects enrolled in 16 clinical trials of secondary prevention of vascular events showed that aspirin use gave an absolute risk reduction per 10,000 persons of 137 MIs and 39 ischemic strokes, which was offset by an absolute risk increase of 12 hemorrhagic strokes.[89] These were all statistically significant effects (in each case, $P < 0.001$). The risk of hemorrhagic stroke did not depend on aspirin dose. Thus, in this later, more focused analysis, as in the analysis by the Antiplatelet Trialists' Collaboration,[2,3] a real increase in hemorrhagic stroke was clearly observed in patients taking aspirin; this adverse effect was considerably less, however, than the decreases in both MI and ischemic stroke seen when patients with extensive vascular disease took aspirin prophylactically.

Clopidogrel, a Thienopyridine Inhibitor of ADP-Mediated Platelet Activation

Mechanism of Action

Thienopyridine drugs, specifically ticlopidine (Ticlid) and a closely related compound, clopidogrel (Plavix, Iscover), have been clinically tested as antiplatelet agents that are chemically and functionally unrelated to prior classes of antiplatelet drugs.[90] These drugs block the binding of ADP to one specific type of purinergic receptor on platelets ($P2Y_{12}$) and therefore inhibit ADP-mediated platelet activation and G_i protein association with platelet membranes.[11] Thienopyridines, therefore, prevent the activation of GPIIb/IIIa, the fibrinogen receptor, to its high-affinity form, but do not inhibit ADP-induced calcium flux or changes in platelet shape. Ticlopidine and clopidogrel have similar antiplatelet effects but differ in potency and pharmacokinetics.[90]

Bleeding time is prolonged much more by thienopyridines than by aspirin, and the prolongation is dose-dependent.[90] When ticlopidine or clopidogrel is given together with aspirin, the effects on bleeding time are additive. The prolongation of bleeding time due to thienopyridines can be reversed by the administration of corticosteroids, although the antiplatelet effects are not reversed. In emergency situations - for example, when urgent surgery is required in a patient taking a thienopyridine - the prolongation of bleeding time can be reversed quickly by desmopressin or by a bolus dose of dexamethasone (20 mg). Clopidogrel is more potent, can be rapidly effective, and is safer than ticlopidine; thus, it is rapidly taking the place of ticlopidine in clinical practice.

In addition to decreasing binding of ADP and fibrinogen to platelet membranes, thienopyridines decrease platelet adhesion to artificial surfaces, reduce platelet deposition on atheromatous plaque,[91] and restore abnormally short platelet survival toward normal. In contrast, they do not affect platelet arachidonic acid metabolism or decrease TXA_2 synthesis. Thienopyridines also reduce plasma fibrinogen levels and blood viscosity and enhance red cell deformability, which suggests possibly beneficial rheologic properties.[90] They can oppose the action of several vasoconstrictors, such as endothelin and TXA_2, presumably by acting on vascular purinergic receptors.[92] In many different experimental thrombosis systems, these drugs have been shown to reduce thrombosis and improve outcomes regardless of whether platelets are important in the pathogenesis of the thrombosis. There is no gender or age difference in response to the drugs.

Pharmacokinetics and Dosing

Clopidogrel is administered orally at 75 mg/day. Clopidogrel blocks ADP-mediated platelet activation processes in vivo; however, it is a prodrug inactive in vitro, which indicates that its antiplatelet activity depends on drug metabolites. The prodrug is activated by hepatic metabolism. Clopidogrel is converted to active metabolites on first pass through the liver and, therefore, develops antiplatelet efficacy within a few hours when a loading dose (300 mg) is used. The antiplatelet effects last for up to 1 week after administration is stopped because its effect on circulating platelets is not reversible and active metabolites are slowly cleared.

Clopidogrel Resistance

The concept of clopidogrel resistance has emerged as a possible explanation for the continued occurrence of ischemic events despite the adequate dosage of the antiplatelet agent and proper compliance. *Resistance* is the term used to reflect failure to inhibit platelet function in vitro, and failure of therapy reflects patients who have recurrent events while receiving therapy. The prevalence of clopidogrel non-response in different populations has been described as being between 4% and 30%. The reason for the response variability among different studies depends on the technique used to evaluate platelet aggregation. In addition, the definition of non-responders is not standardized or validated.[93,94]

The potential mechanisms of clopidogrel resistance are multiple and can be divided into two main groups: (1) extrinsic mechanisms, that is, drug interactions involving CYP3A4, and (2) intrinsic mechanisms, that is, polymorphisms of $P2Y_{12}$ receptor and CYP3As.

Regarding drug interactions, any medication that interacts with (either inhibiting or increasing) CYP3A4 can potentially block the conversion of clopidogrel into its active metabolite. Among these drugs, statins, except pravastatin, might interfere with clopidogrel metabolism. Also, the antiplatelet activity has been shown to be reduced in persons receiving omeprazole, which is a CYP2C19 inhibitor. However, other studies have not confirmed this observation.

Recently, several reports indicate that certain polymorphisms in the hepatic cytochrome P450 system are associated with an excess of vascular events. Patients who are carriers of a loss-of-function of CYP2C19 allele (including the *2 and *3 alleles) might have a reduced rate in the conversion to an active metabolite, thus resulting in decreased inhibition of platelets. Compared with non-carriers, carriers of loss-of-function alleles showed a significant increase in the risk of major vascular events.[95,96] However, these data were obtained only from clopidogrel-treated patients. Despite the potential limitations of these data, the FDA issued a black box warning about the potential reduced effectiveness of clopidogrel in patients who are carriers of two loss-of-function alleles (poor metabolizers) and has suggested that these patients receive a higher dose of clopidogrel or other antiplatelet agent. A recent analysis of data among 5059 patients with acute coronary syndromes or AF showed that the response to clopidogrel compared with placebo was consistent, irrespective of CYP2C19 loss-of-function carrier status.[97] Therefore, it is possible that loss-of-function variants do not directly alter the efficacy and safety of clopidogrel. Consequently, clopidogrel should be used regardless of the carrier status until further studies can elucidate this paradox.

Currently, the management of clopidogrel resistance is a challenge, and there are no standardized guidelines. Until new data are available, it seems prudent to avoid interactions of drugs with a well-known effect on hepatic cytochrome P450 that might affect the metabolism of clopidogrel.

Antiplatelet Agents in Primary Prevention of Stroke

The role of aspirin versus control for primary prevention of stroke, MI, or vascular death has been studied in six major trials – the British Doctors Study (BDS),[98] US Physicians Study (PHT), Thrombosis Prevention Trial (TPT),[99] Hypertension Optimal Treatment Study (HOT),[100] Primary Prevention Project (PPP) , and Women's Health Study (WHS)[101] – and in meta-analyses.[3,102] No other antiplatelet agent has been widely investigated for primary prevention of cerebrovascular disease.

In meta-analyses by the Antithrombotic Trialists' Collaboration (ATTC), the trials, which followed up 95,000 patients and accounted for 660,000 patient-years, showed a 12% reduction in overall events with a small but significant benefit in favor of aspirin. There were 0.51% events per year vs 0.57% in the control group (rate ratio [RR], 0.88; 95%CI, 0.82–0.94). The authors attributed this effect largely to a 23% reduction in non-fatal MI with 0.18% events per year vs 0.23% in the control group (RR, 0.77; 95%CI, 0.67–0.89). There was no significant benefit in reduction of vascular death, with 0.19% events per year in both groups (RR, 0.97; 95%CI, 0.87–1.09). Subgroup analysis revealed no benefit in the aspirin group for primary stroke prevention, with 0.20% events per year versus 0.21% in the control group (RR, 0.95; 95%CI, 0.85–1.06). There was no significant difference when these events were subdivided into fatal and non-fatal stroke or ischemic and hemorrhagic stroke. Major extracranial bleeding was increased in the aspirin group (0.10% vs 0.07% per year; RR, 1.54; 95% CI, 1.30–1.82; $P < 0.0001$).[3]

In Women

Three of the six trials included women: PPP, HOT, and WHS. WHS, with 39,876 subjects, accounted for 74% of female subjects. The results in WHS showed no benefit in the aspirin group for primary prevention of fatal or non-fatal MI with 198 events versus 193 events in the control group (RR, 1.02; 95%CI, 0.67–0.97). Aspirin did, however, confer a significant protective benefit against stroke with a 17% reduction in events, that is, a total of 221 events versus 266 in the control group (RR, 0.83; 95%CI, 0.69–0.99; $P = 0.04$). Rates of ischemic stroke showed a greater reduction in the aspirin group with 170 events versus 266 in the control group (RR, 0.76; 95%CI, 0.63–0.93; $P = 0.009$), but the benefit was reduced by a non-significant increase in hemorrhagic stroke, with 51 versus 41 events (RR, 1.24; 95%CI, 0.82–1.87; $P = 0.31$).[101]

Patients aged 65 or older comprised 10% of the study population but experienced 30% of events. Analysis of this subgroup found a significant reduction in MI, ischemic stroke, and vascular death in the intervention group that was counterbalanced by an increase in gastrointestinal bleeding requiring transfusion.

In Diabetic Patients

Diabetic patients experience MI and cerebral ischemia at a rate of two to five times that of their age-and sex-matched counterparts. The role of aspirin in primary prevention in this susceptible patient group has been investigated in independent prospective trials, in subgroup analyses of other primary prevention trials, and in meta-analysis.

The Prevention of Progression of Arterial Disease and Diabetes (POPADAD) trial, a prospective population-based trial of antiplatelet agents in diabetic patients to prevent stroke and other vascular death, found no benefit for aspirin in the primary prevention of vascular events. A total of 1276 patients with type 1 or type 2 diabetes and asymptomatic peripheral vascular disease as determined by an ankle-brachial index of 0.99 or less were randomly assigned to aspirin or placebo and antioxidant or placebo in a 2 × 2 fashion. Over 6.7 years of follow-up, there was no significant difference in the number of primary vascular events between groups, with 116 in the aspirin group and 117 in the control group (HR, 0.98; 95%CI, 0.76–1.26). There was no significant benefit seen in the stroke subgroup, nor was there a difference seen when patients were subdivided by gender or by age older than or younger than 60.[103]

The Japanese Primary Prevention of Atherosclerosis with Aspirin for Diabetes (JPAD) trial enrolled 2539 diabetic patients without a history of atherosclerotic disease. Patients were randomly assigned to daily aspirin (81 to 100 mg), and the median follow-up was 4.37 years. With respect to the primary endpoints of MI, stroke, and peripheral vascular disease, there was no significant difference between groups (13.6 events/1000 patient-years in the aspirin group versus 17.0 in control group; HR, 0.80; $P = 0.16$). There was no significant difference in the rates of fatal and non-fatal ischemic stroke, nor was there a significant difference in composite rates of major bleeding.[104]

The rates of vascular events for both JPAD and POPADAD were much lower than predicted, which is an effect that the authors of POPADAD suggested may have been due to statin use. The ongoing Aspirin and Simvastatin Combination for Cardiovascular Events Prevention Trial in Diabetes (ACCEPT-D), which aims to enroll more than 5000 patients, may further clarify the role of aspirin versus placebo for primary prevention in diabetic patients taking daily simvastatin.[105]

Prevention of Early Stroke Recurrence

Aspirin given within 48 hours after an ischemic stroke has been documented to decrease stroke recurrence in two very large studies, the Chinese Acute Stroke Trial (CAST, 20,655 patients)[106] and the International Stroke Trial (IST, 19,435 patients).[107] In the CAST, patients were randomly assigned to receive either 160 mg/day aspirin or placebo starting within 48 hours of the stroke (in some, as early as 6 hours) and continuing for 4 weeks. Death or recurrent nonfatal stroke occurred in 5.3% of aspirin-treated patients and in 5.9% of patients receiving placebo, which translates into a significant absolute risk reduction (0.68%; $2P = 0.03$) – in other words, a decrease of seven strokes per 1000 patients treated. The absolute risk reduction for ischemic stroke (0.47%; $2P = 0.01$) was offset by a small excess of hemorrhagic strokes (0.21%; $2P > 0.1$), that is, 2 per 1000 patients treated.[106]

The IST examined the safety and efficacy of 300 mg/day aspirin, subcutaneous unfractionated heparin, or both drugs together in preventing recurrent stroke; treatment was started within 48 hours of the first ischemic event and continued for 14 days. Aspirin therapy in the IST led to an absolute reduction of 1.1% ($2P < 0.001$) for recurrent ischemic strokes without an increase in the risk of hemorrhagic stroke, although the risk of other bleeding rose significantly. Heparin use significantly increased the risk of hemorrhagic stroke or fatal extracranial bleeding, and although it did reduce the risk of recurrent ischemic stroke, this benefit was negated by an equal increase in hemorrhagic stroke. Functional status at 6 months was not altered by early poststroke use of aspirin in either CAST or IST.

A later analysis combined data from both CAST and IST to evaluate the effects of early aspirin use after ischemic stroke on the balance between reduced risk of recurrent ischemic stroke and risk of hemorrhagic stroke.[108] Among all treated subgroups examined, the absolute risk reduction of about seven recurrent ischemic strokes per 1000 was similar (1.6% recurrent strokes with aspirin vs 2.3% without aspirin; $2P < 0.01$), and the benefit from early aspirin treatment did not vary with respect to patient age or sex, level of consciousness, computed tomographic (CT) findings, blood pressure, stroke subtype, prognostic category, or concomitant heparin use. Neither AF nor treatment assignment without a prior CT scan (which occurred in 9000 patients, or 22%) altered the net benefit of aspirin treatment. The risk reduction for those taking aspirin was similar regardless of whether they also received heparin. Overall, there was an absolute decrease of four deaths per 1000 without further stroke, and the increase in hemorrhagic stroke averaged about two per 1000. In aspirin-treated patients, there was a 1.0% rate of hemorrhagic stroke or hemorrhagic transformation, whereas the placebo group had a rate of 0.8% ($2P = 0.07$). Extracranial bleeding that required transfusion was significantly more common in patients receiving aspirin, especially in those also receiving heparin (1.8% of those taking aspirin plus heparin versus 0.9% of those taking aspirin alone; excess bleeding occurred in nine per 1000 treated; $2P = 0.0001$). Most of the cases of hemorrhage were non-fatal. Indeed, among 800 patients inadvertently randomly assigned to receive aspirin after a hemorrhagic stroke, there was no evidence of net hazard, including further stroke and death. The conclusions of this meta-analysis of the CAST and IST data are that low-dose aspirin started early after an acute ischemic stroke produces a definite reduction of recurrent ischemic stroke that is of net benefit to a wide range of patients. Of particular interest is that the benefit was also observed in patients who started aspirin therapy without a prior CT scan, who might have been expected to have a higher incidence of intracranial bleeding. Patients of both sexes, older patients, patients with AF, and hypertensive patients all benefited. It was also concluded that the reduction of further stroke or death from early aspirin use within 1 month of the first event compared favorably with the monthly benefits previously reported for long-term antiplatelet therapy.

In the Fast Assessment of Stroke and TIA to prevent Early Recurrence (FASTER) trial, patients with minor stroke or TIA were given antiplatelet therapy within 24 hours of symptom onset. All patients enrolled received 81 mg of aspirin daily for the study duration, and patients received a loading dose of 162 mg if they were naive to aspirin before study enrollment. They were then randomly assigned to receive either placebo or a 300-mg clopidogrel loading dose immediately followed by 75 mg clopidogrel daily or to receive placebo or 40 mg simvastatin immediately followed by 40 mg daily in the evening. The primary endpoint of the study was total stroke (ischemic and hemorrhagic) within 90 days. Although the trial was prematurely terminated because of failure to recruit patients at the prespecified minimum enrollment rate, which was caused by a generalized use of statins in cardiovascular prevention, the results of this pilot study showed a reduction in stroke recurrence in patients who had received clopidogrel together with aspirin. In fact, 7.1% of patients treated with clopidogrel had a stroke within 90 days compared with 10.8% of patients in the placebo group (RR, 0.7; 95%CI, 0.3–1.2; absolute risk reduction −3.8%; 95%CI, −9.4 to 1.9; $P = 0.19$). Despite the increased rate of bleeding complications with clopidogrel, the authors concluded that in patients with minor stroke or TIA the addition of this drug to aspirin within 24 hours of onset might reduce the risk of stroke recurrence. The data come from a pilot study and thus cannot be taken as proof of clinical utility, but they do provide strong support for undertaking a large clinical trial.

Recently, the Clopidogrel in High-Risk Patients with Acute Nondisabling Cerebrovascular Events (CHANCE) trial randomized 5170 patients in China within 24 h after onset of minor stroke or high-risk TIA to combination therapy with clopidogrel and aspirin (clopidogrel loading dose of 300 mg, then 75 mg per day for 90 days plus ASA 75 mg daily for the first 21 days) or ASA + placebo (75 mg per day for 90 days). The primary outcome (ischemic and hemorrhagic stroke) during 90 days was reduced from 11.7% in those on ASA alone to 8.2% in dual antiplatelet group (HR 0.68; 95%CI, 0.57-0.81; $P < 0.001$). There were no differences in the rates of systemic or intracranial bleeding between treatment groups.[109] Implementation of optimal secondary prevention strategies and post-stroke care in China and in the CHANCE population may differ from Western norms. Differences in proportions of stroke subtype, or other genetic, environmental, or undetermined factors may affect the benefit–risk ratio of combination antiplatelet therapy in other ongoing trials, thus whether results similar to that in CHANCE will be replicated has yet to be determined. However, the results of CHANCE are consistent with prior studies conducted in different populations.[110]

The ongoing National Institutes of Health-National Institute of Neurological Diseases and Stroke (NIH-NINDS)-sponsored Platelet-Oriented Inhibition in New TIA and Minor Ischemic Stroke (POINT) Trial (NCT00991029) plans to enroll 5840 patients with minor stroke (NIH Stroke Scale < 3) or high-risk TIA (as determined by a simple clinical score of age, blood pressure, clinical features, symptom duration, and diabetes [ABCD2] > 4). This study may further clarify the benefit of short-term combined antiplatelet therapy. Patients receiving 50–325 mg aspirin daily are being randomly assigned within 12 hours of symptom onset to a 600-mg clopidogrel loading dose, then 75 mg daily, or placebo. The primary outcome is a composite of ischemic stroke, MI, or vascular death at 90 days. The trial started enrollment in early 2010 and is anticipated to be completed by 2017, currently 2298 patients have been enrolled.[111]

Antiplatelet Agents in Secondary Prevention of Noncardioembolic Stroke

Antiplatelets in Comparison with Warfarin

To date, large trials have failed to show the superiority of warfarin over aspirin in secondary prevention of noncardioembolic stroke. Various INR targets have been investigated; the specific indication of intracranial stenosis has been studied, and the indication for high-risk aortic atheroma is currently under investigation.

The Stroke Prevention in Reversible Ischemia Trial (SPIRIT) compared 30 mg daily aspirin against high-target dose-adjusted warfarin (INR target, 3.0 to 4.5) in an open randomized trial. Over 14 months, 1316 patients were enrolled. Because of a high rate of hemorrhagic complications in the warfarin group, the study was terminated early: hemorrhagic events increased by a factor of 1.46 (95%CI, 0.96–2.13) for every increase in INR of 0.5. Major systemic and intracranial hemorrhage rates were 8.1% in the warfarin group and 1.0% in the aspirin group (HR, 9.3; 95%CI, 4.0–22). There was no significant difference between groups (4.1% in both groups; HR, 1.03; 95%CI, 0.6–1.75) in the number of ischemic events, including vascular death, nonfatal ischemic stroke, and nonfatal MI.[112]

More conservative INR targets have also failed to show a benefit for warfarin. The Warfarin–Aspirin Recurrent Stroke Study (WARSS), which compared dose-adjusted warfarin with an INR target of 1.4 to 2.8 with 325 mg daily aspirin in 2206 patients without a cardioembolic source, peri-operative stroke, or carotid stenosis requiring operative intervention, found no significant difference between death or recurrent stroke or major hemorrhage in the two groups. The daily INR remained within the target range for 70.7% of patients; 16.3% of INR values were subtherapeutic.[113]

Warfarin with an INR target of 2.0 to 3.0 was compared with 30 to 325 mg daily aspirin in the European and Australasian Stroke Prevention in Reversible Ischemia Trial (ESPRIT). In a separate arm, aspirin was compared with or without 200 mg twice daily dipyridamole. Treatment was randomized but open; outcome event assessment was blinded. A total of 1068 patients with stroke or TIA were enrolled within 6 months of their index event. After combination antiplatelet therapy was found to be more effective than aspirin monotherapy, the warfarin versus aspirin monotherapy arm was terminated early. Patients were within the INR target 70% of the time, and the median INR was 2.57. There was no significant difference found in the rate of primary outcomes of nonfatal stroke, MI, vascular death, or major bleeding in the aspirin group as compared with warfarin, with an 18% event rate in the aspirin group and a 19% event rate in the warfarin group (HR, 1.02; 95%CI, 0.77–1.35). There was a nonsignificant trend toward a lower rate of ischemic stroke in the warfarin group (7.6% vs 10.0%; HR, 0.76; 95%CI, 0.51–1.15), which was counterbalanced by a significantly higher rate of major bleeding in this group (8.4% vs 3.4%; HR, 2.56; 95%CI, 1.48–4.43). In post-hoc analysis, there were no significant differences between the combination antiplatelet group and the warfarin group (HR, 1.31; 95%CI, 0.98–1.75).[114]

The Warfarin-Aspirin Symptomatic Intracranial Disease (WASID) trial compared high-dose daily aspirin (1300 mg) with dose-adjusted warfarin with an INR target of 2.0–3.0 for secondary stroke prevention in 569 patients with intracranial stenosis of 50–99%. There was no significant difference in the recurrent stroke rate: 22.1% recurrence rate over 1.8 years of follow-up in the aspirin group and 21.8% in the warfarin group (HR, 1.04; 95%CI, 0.73–1.48). Enrollment was stopped early because of high rates of adverse events in the patients receiving warfarin, including death (4.3% in the aspirin group versus 9.7% in the warfarin group; HR, 0.46; 95%CI, 0.23–0.90; *P* = 0.02), major hemorrhage (3.2% vs 8.3%; HR, 0.39; 95%CI, 0.18–0.84; *P* = 0.01), and MI and sudden death (2.9 vs 7.3%; HR, 0.40; 95%CI, 0.18–0.91; *P* = 0.02). Warfarin patients were within the target range 63% of the time.[33]

The ARCH trial randomized patients with recent stroke, TIA or peripheral embolism and aortic atheroma ≥4 mm in thickness and no other identified source of embolus to combination aspirin (75–150 mg/d) and clopidogrel (75 mg/d) versus dose-adjusted warfarin (target INR 2-3).[32] The trial, which used a PROBE (prospective, open-label, blinded-endpoint) design, enrolled 349 subjects, was stopped early due to slow recruitment. After a median follow-up of 3.4 years (range 1–8), there was no significant difference in recurrence of the primary composite endpoint of ischemic stroke, myocardial infarction, vascular death, peripheral embolism or intracerebral hemorrhage between groups (7.6% antiplatelet vs 11.3% warfarin, adjusted HR, 0.76; 95%CI, 0.36–1.61). There was no difference in rates of recurrent ischemic stroke alone (6.4% vs 5.1%). There were four major hemorrhages (including two non-fatal intracranial hemorrhages) with dual antiplatelet and six (including one fatal intracranial hemorrhage) in the warfarin group. The study was unable to include a single-antiplatelet arm due to budget constraints. It remains uncertain as to which antithrombotic strategy is ideal for patients with this stroke mechanism.

Antiplatelets as Monotherapy and in Combination for Secondary Stroke Prevention

Commonly utilized antiplatelet drugs are aspirin, dipyridamole, and clopidogrel. Aspirin is an irreversible inhibitor of cyclooxygenase-1, which in turn inhibits the formation of TXA_2. Dipyridamole increases cAMP by inhibiting platelet phosphodiesterase E5. Clopidogrel is a thienopyridine $P2Y_{12}$-ADP receptor blocker.

Several large trials comparing alternative antiplatelet therapies have demonstrated a modest benefit in favor of clopidogrel or combination aspirin and dipyridamole over aspirin for long-term secondary stroke prevention. In direct comparison, combination aspirin and dipyridamole failed to demonstrate non-inferiority to clopidogrel, mainly because of problems with tolerability. The minimal benefits of the alternatives over aspirin in addition to their higher cost and tolerability issues allows aspirin to remain the most commonly prescribed first-line antiplatelet for secondary prevention. Combination aspirin and clopidogrel has not proven to be superior to aspirin monotherapy for secondary prevention, but is still under investigation for specific indications including subcortical stroke and for short-term secondary prevention immediately after the index event.

Aspirin. In meta-analysis by the ATTC, aspirin was associated with a 23% reduction in the combined events of stroke, MI, and vascular death. Aspirin was associated with a 22% reduction in stroke in secondary prevention trials (2.08% vs 2.54% per year; RR, 0.78; 0.61–0.99, *P* = 0.002). There was a nonsignificant increase in hemorrhagic stroke in the aspirin group.

Aspirin has been shown to be effective in secondary prevention of ischemic events in doses from 30 to 1300 mg daily.[2,3,46,115] Higher doses cause an increased rate of gastrointestinal upset, peptic ulcer disease, and gastrointestinal bleeding.

Aspirin plus Dipyridamole. The European Stroke Prevention Study (ESPS)-2 randomly assigned patients with ischemic stroke or TIA into one of four groups with twice-daily dosing within 3 months after their index event: placebo, 25 mg aspirin, 200 mg ERDP, or combination aspirin and dipyridamole (aspirin-ERDP, same dose and formulation). A total of 6602 patients were followed up for 2 years. The stroke rate in the placebo group was 15.8%. Both aspirin and dipyridamole were independently associated with a reduced rate of stroke (12.9%: odds ratio [OR], 0.79; 95%CI, 0.65–0.97; 13.2%: OR, 0.81; 95%CI, 0.67–0.99, respectively); the effect was most marked in the combination group (9.9%: OR, 0.59; 95%CI, 0.48–0.73), with a 23% relative risk reduction and 3% absolute risk reduction in stroke between the aspirin monotherapy and the combination group over 2 years of follow-up.[87]

Aspirin monotherapy was compared with aspirin-ERDP in the ESPRIT trial, the results of which echoed that of ESPS-2. A separate arm, already discussed, examined warfarin for secondary prevention. Patients were randomly assigned to 30–325 mg aspirin daily with or without 200 mg ERDP twice daily within 6 months of stroke or TIA. A total of 2739 patients were followed up over a mean of 3.5 years. The median aspirin dose was 75 mg, although 44% took 30 mg. There were major ischemic events (vascular death, nonfatal ischemic stroke, and non-fatal MI) in 12.6% of the aspirin group and in 10.3% of the combination group. The absolute risk reduction of major ischemic events was 7% in the combination group (aspirin: HR, 0.81; 95% CI, 0.65–1.01; aspirin-ERDP: HR, 0.88; 95%CI, 0.69–1.02). There was no significant difference in the rates of major bleeding between the two groups (RR, 1.03; 95% CI, 0.84–1.25), although a larger proportion (34%) of the combination group discontinued therapy, mostly because of headaches.[88]

Clopidogrel. The Clopidogrel versus Aspirin in Patients at Risk of Ischemic Events (CAPRIE) trial investigated the effects of clopidogrel. A total of 19,185 patients with a history of stroke, MI, or peripheral vascular disease were randomly assigned to 75 mg daily clopidogrel or 325 mg aspirin. Over a mean follow-up of 1.91 years, the annual rate of non-fatal stroke, non-fatal MI, and vascular death was 5.83% in the aspirin group and 5.32% in the clopidogrel group (relative risk reduction [RRR], 0.087; 95%CI, 0.003–0.165; $P = 0.043$). In the stroke subgroup, however, this trend was not significant. The annual rate of vascular events was 7.71% in the aspirin group and 7.15% in the clopidogrel group (RRR, 0.073; 95%CI, −0.057–0.187; P = 0.26). There was no significant difference in major hemorrhage rates between groups.[116]

Aspirin plus Dipyridamole vs Clopidogrel. Before the Prevention Regimen for Effectively Avoiding Second Strokes (PRoFESS) trial, a study designed to test the non-inferiority of aspirin-ERDP against clopidogrel for secondary stroke prevention, the only means of comparing the efficacy of the two regimens was through the indirect comparison of their performance in previous trials against aspirin. In a 2 × 2 factorial double-blinded trial, 20,332 patients were randomly assigned to 75 mg daily clopidogrel or 25 to 200 mg twice-daily aspirin-ERDP in combination with telmisartan or placebo. The mean follow-up was 2.5 years. Recurrent stroke occurred in 9% of patients in the aspirin-ERDP group and in 8.8% of the clopidogrel group (HR, 1.01; 95%CI, 0.92–1.11). Stroke, MI, and vascular death occurred at 13.1% (HR, 0.99; 95%CI, 0.92–1.07; RRR, 1%; 95%CI, 7–8%). Major hemorrhage rates, including intracranial hemorrhage, were higher in the aspirin-ERDP group (HR, 1.15; 95%CI, 1.00–1.32). Rates of discontinuation were higher with aspirin-EDRP than with clopidogrel (29.1% vs 22.6%; 6.5% difference; 95%CI, 5.3–7.7%), most often because of headache[117] (Table 61-3).

Antiplatelet Agents in Secondary Prevention of Cardioembolic Stroke

Oral anticoagulants remain the treatment of choice for secondary prevention of cardioembolic stroke. Antiplatelet therapy, however, provides an alternative when oral anticoagulation is contraindicated or when patient choice or compliance limits choice of therapy.

The superiority of warfarin over combination antiplatelet therapy for stroke prevention in non-valvular AF has been shown in several trials and in meta-analyses. A meta-analysis of 29 trials incorporating 28,044 patients found a 64% reduction in stroke in the warfarin group as compared with 22% (95%CI, 0.49–0.74) in the antiplatelet groups (95%CI, 0.06–0.35) for a relative risk reduction of 39% (95%CI, 0.22–0.52). The Atrial Fibrillation Clopidogrel Trial with Irbesartan for Prevention of Vascular Events (ACTIVE)-W trial, which compared warfarin to combination aspirin-clopidogrel in 6706 patients, was terminated early because of a clear benefit in the warfarin group, who had a 3.93% annual event rate versus 5.60% in the control group (RR, 1.44; 95%CI, 1.18–1.76; $P =$ 0.0003).[118]

The ACTIVE-A trial enrolled patients with cardioembolic stroke deemed unsuitable for warfarin therapy because of risk of bleeding, physician's judgment, or patient preference. The effects of combination aspirin and clopidogrel versus aspirin and placebo on secondary stroke prevention were compared in 7554 patients over a mean follow-up of 3.6 years. The majority of patients had no history of cerebrovascular disease; 13.2% of patients in the clopidogrel group and 13% of control patients had a history of stroke or TIA. The clopidogrel group experienced major vascular events at a rate of 6.8% per year, as compared with 7.6% per year in the control group (RR, 0.89; 95%CI, 0.81–0.98). The risk reduction was largely due to a significant reduction of ischemic strokes, with rates of 1.9% vs 2.8% per year in the clopidogrel and control groups, respectively (RR, 0.68; 95%CI, 0.57–0.80). This therapeutic

TABLE 61-3 Recent Randomized Clinical Trials Testing Antiplatelet Agents for Secondary Stroke Prevention

Study	Year of Completion	Sample Size	Intervention	Results
ESPS-2	1996	6602	ASA 25 mg bid vs ERDP 200 mg bid vs ASA–ERDP 25/200 mg bid vs placebo	ASA–ERDP vs placebo: 24% RRR ASA–ERDP vs ASA: 13% RRR Primary outcome: stroke/death
CAPRIE	1996	19,185	ASA 325 mg vs clopidogrel 75 mg	Clopidogrel vs ASA: 9% RRR Primary outcome: stroke/MI/vascular death
MATCH	2004	7599	Clopidogrel 75 mg vs ASA + clopidogrel	Non-significant difference Primary outcome: stroke/MI/vascular death
ESPRIT	2006	2739	ASA 30–325 mg vs. ASA/ERDP 30–325/200 mg bid	ASA + EDRP vs ASA: 20% HR Primary outcome: vascular death, stroke, major bleeding
CHARISMA	2006	15,603	ASA 75–162 mg vs ASA + clopidogrel 75 mg qd	No significant diference Primary outcome: MI, stroke, vascular death
PRoFESS	2008	20,332	ASA–ERDP 25–200 mg bid vs clopidogrel 75 mg	No significant difference Primary outcome: stroke

ASA, Acetylsalicylic acid; bid, twice a day; CAPRIE, Clopidogrel versus Aspirin in Patients at Risk of Ischaemic Events [trial]; CHARISMA, Clopidogrel for High Atherothrombotic Risk and Ischemic Stabilization, Management, and Avoidance; ERDP, extended-release dipyridamole; ESPRIT, European and Australasian Stroke Prevention in Reversible Ischemia Trial; ESPS, European Stroke Prevention Study; HR, hazard ratio; MATCH, Management of Atherothrombosis with Clopidogrel in High-Risk Patients with Recent Transient Ischaemic Attack or Ischaemic Stroke; MI, myocardial infarction; PRoFESS, Prevention Regimen for Effectively Avoiding Second Strokes; qd, every day; RRR, relative risk reduction.

benefit, however, was greatly reduced by rates of systemic and intracranial hemorrhages. Annual rates of any major bleeding in the clopidogrel and control groups, respectively, were 2% vs 1.3% (RR, 1.57; 95%CI, 1.29–1.92), and rates of intracranial bleeding were 0.4% vs 0.2% (RR, 1.87; 95%CI, 1.19–2.94).[119]

COMBINATIONS OF ANTIPLATELET AGENTS

Aspirin and Thienopyridines

Given that aspirin and the thienopyridines have quite different modes of action, there has been considerable interest in combining these drugs to improve antiplatelet activity. In particular, there has recently been a significant increase in the simultaneous use of aspirin and clopidogrel. However, completed studies in which aspirin and clopidogrel have been combined are few and mainly concern acute cardiac procedures rather than stroke prevention.

Ischemic Strokes

Favorable results of combination aspirin-clopidogrel for prevention of vascular events in patients with percutaneous coronary intervention in the PCI-CURE and TRITON-TIMI 38 trials and acute MI in the CURE and CREDO trials prompted an interest in investigating this combination in other types of vascular disease.

Clopidogrel (75 mg daily) and placebo vs aspirin-clopidogrel (75/75 mg daily) were compared in the Management of Atherothrombosis with Clopidogrel in High-Risk Patients with Recent Transient Ischaemic Attack or Ischaemic Stroke (MATCH) trial. A total of 7599 patients with previous stroke or TIA and at least one other vascular risk factor were randomly assigned and followed up for 18 months. Nearly one-third were randomly assigned more than 1 month after their index event. There was no significant difference in the two groups with regard to all ischemic strokes (11% in both groups; RRR, 0.066; 95%CI, −0.07–0.185; $P = 0.324$), nor was there a difference in the combined endpoints of non-fatal stroke, non-fatal MI, or vascular death (12% in both groups; RRR, 0.059; 95% CI, −0.071–0.173; $P = 0.360$). The rates of major and life-threatening bleeding (1.3% versus 2.6%; AR increase, 1.3%; 95%CI, 0.6–1.9) were significantly increased in the aspirin-clopidogrel group, although there was no increase in rates of mortality.[82]

The Clopidogrel for High Atherothrombotic Risk and Ischemic Stabilization, Management, and Avoidance (CHARISMA) trial randomly assigned 15,603 patients with a history of vascular disease or multiple vascular risk factors to daily aspirin (75–162 mg) and placebo or combination aspirin-clopidogrel (75 mg to 162/75 mg). Over the 5 years before enrollment, 27% of patients had a history of stroke and 10% of patients had a history of TIA. Rates of MI, stroke, or vascular death were 7.3% in the control group and 6.8% in the aspirin-clopidogrel group (RR, 0.93; 95%CI, 0.83–1.05; $P = 0.22$). There was a non-significant trend toward a reduction in ischemic events in the subgroup with previous stroke (HR, 0.13, 95%CI). There was a non-significant reduction in non-fatal ischemic stroke (2.1% control, 1.7% clopidogrel; RR, 0.81; 95%CI, 0.64–1.02; $P = 0.07$) and a significant reduction in all non-fatal stroke in the clopidogrel group (2.4% control, 1.9% clopidogrel; RR, 0.79; 95%CI, 0.64–0.98; $P = 0.03$). Dual antiplatelet therapy was associated with a non-significant increase in severe and fatal bleeding and a significant increase in moderate bleeding (1.3% control, 2.1% clopidogrel; RR, 1.62; 95%CI, 1.27–2.08; $P < 0.001$). In the asymptomatic subgroup, there was an unanticipated increase in ischemic events and vascular death in addition to the significant increase in severe bleeding in this group. The phenomenon is yet to be fully explained. Proposed explanations have included a higher proportion of diabetic patients in this group and a theoretical risk of platelet hyperaggregability with medication non-compliance.[120]

The Secondary Prevention of Small Subcortical Strokes (SPS3) trial randomized 3020 patients with recent lacunar stroke (verified by MRI) to ASA 325 mg per day + placebo or to ASA + clopidogrel 75 mg daily. The primary outcome was any recurrent stroke (ischemic and hemorrhagic). After a mean follow-up of 3.4 years, the risk of stroke was not reduced with combination therapy (2.5% per year vs 2.7% per year) (HR 0.92; 95%CI 0.72–1.16). The risk of major hemorrhage and all-cause mortality was increased with dual antiplatelet therapy (HR 1.97; 95%CI, 1.41–2.71; $P < 0.001$) and (HR 1.52; 95%CI, 1.14–2.04; $P < 0.004$) respectively. The cause for the excess in mortality has not been elucidated.[77, 121]

In the SAMMPRIS trial patients with symptomatic stenosis ≥70% of a major intracranial artery were randomized to percutaneous stenting versus best medical therapy, consisting of 90 days of combination aspirin plus clopidogrel followed by aspirin alone, and aggressive management of blood pressure, hypercholesterolemia, and lifestyle modification.[122] Though there was a reduction in events in the medical management group, whether the use of dual antiplatelet therapy contributed significantly to the decreased event rate is unclear given that there was no single-platelet medical comparison group. The role for dual antiplatelet therapy for symptomatic intracranial stenosis thus remains uncertain.

Based on the results of the MATCH, CHARISMA and SPS3 trials, the combination of aspirin-clopidogrel should not be routinely indicated for long-term secondary stroke prevention.

Carotid Endarterectomy and Carotid Artery Stenting

On the basis of the results of the Aspirin and Carotid Endarterectomy (ACE) trial,[49] it is recommended that patients undergoing carotid endarterectomy receive 81–325 mg aspirin. Recent data suggest that dual antiplatelet therapy in the preoperative phase of patients undergoing this procedure may be more effective in the reduction of vascular events than aspirin alone. In a study including 100 patients randomly assigned to receive aspirin and concomitant clopidogrel or placebo before carotid endarterectomy, the association of clopidogrel and aspirin reduced the platelet response to ADP by 8.8% while conferring a tenfold decrease in the RR of those patients having more than 20 emboli in the post-operative period. Moreover, this reduction in risk occurred without a significant increase in the risk of bleeding complications.[123] More recently, Markus et al. have also reported that combination clopidogrel-aspirin therapy is more effective than aspirin alone in reducing asymptomatic embolization in patients with a recent diagnosis of symptomatic carotid stenosis.[124] Dual antiplatelet therapy was reported to reduce the number of microembolic signals (MES) (R, 39.8%; 95%CI, 13.8–58.0; $P = 0.0046$) as well as the frequency of MES per hour both at day 2 (RRR, 61.6%; 95%CI, 34.9–77.4; $P = 0.0005$) and day 7 (R, 61.4%; 95%CI, 31.6–78.2; $P = 0.0013$) of randomization. Moreover, the frequency of stroke and TIA was also lower in the group receiving clopidogrel-aspirin: there were four recurrent strokes and seven TIAs in the monotherapy group compared with no stroke and four TIAs in the dual-therapy group.

With respect to the efficacy of associating thienopyridines and aspirin in patients undergoing carotid artery stenting (CAS), dual antiplatelet therapy also seems to be associated with lower rates of ischemic events. In a study by Bhatt et al., results with clopidogrel-aspirin in 139 consecutive patients undergoing this procedure at a single center were compared with those in 23 similar patients who received ticlopidine-aspirin.[120] The cumulative 30-day rate of death, stroke, TIA, or MI was 5.6% in patients who received an ADP antagonist (clopidogrel or ticlopidine) and aspirin. There were no cases of stent thrombosis in patients who were treated with clopidogrel/ticlopidine and aspirin, but one of five patients who did not receive an ADP antagonist did develop in-stent thrombosis. Dual antiplatelet therapy did not increase the incidence of bleeding events. When the association of ticlopidine or clopidogrel with aspirin was compared, the 30-day rate of death, stroke, TIA, or MI was significantly higher in patients receiving clopidogrel-aspirin than in those receiving ticlopidine-aspirin (4.3% vs 13%; $P = 0.01$). Although these data might suggest that the use of clopidogrel-aspirin in patients with CAS is associated with a low rate of ischemic events and that clopidogrel might be better than ticlopidine in this high-risk group, these are the results of a small, unblinded study, so caution is important. Dalainas et al.[125] reported the results of a study comparing two groups of 50 patients each undergoing CAS who were randomly assigned to receive heparin for 24 hours together with 325 mg of aspirin or 250 mg ticlopidine twice a day together with 325 mg of aspirin. Neurologic complications were significantly more frequent at day 30 in the group with heparin (16% vs 2%, $P < 0.05$); there were no significant differences in the rates of bleeding complications or thrombosis/occlusion between the two groups of treatment.

Similar to the recommendation in patients undergoing percutaneous coronary intervention, the presented data support the administration of dual antiplatelet therapy for patients undergoing CAS. With regard to the duration of dual antiplatelet therapy, it seems that, beyond the periprocedural period, the prolongation of this therapy might also be beneficial in patients undergoing CAS,[126] although additional studies are necessary to determine the optimal duration.

OTHER ANTIPLATELET AGENTS

Current data suggest that triflusal, cilostazol, and terutrobran have shown equal efficacy to aspirin. A meta-analysis of five trials comparing 325 mg aspirin daily with triflusal for secondary prevention of stroke and TIA (four trials, 2944 patients; follow-up, 6–47 months) or MI (one trial, 2275 patients; follow-up, 35 days) showed no significant difference in the number of serious vascular events (OR, 1.04; 95%CI, 0.87–1.23). Triflusal had a lower risk of major (OR for aspirin, 2.34; 95%CI, 1.58–3.46) and minor hemorrhage (OR for aspirin, 1.60; 95%CI, 1.31–1.95), but more non-hemorrhagic adverse gastrointestinal events than aspirin (OR for aspirin, 0.84; 95%CI, 0.75–0.95).[127]

Cilostazol was compared against aspirin in CSPS-2, a Japanese randomized, blinded non-inferiority trial for secondary prevention in 2757 patients with recent stroke. Patients aged 20–79 with an infarct within the last 26 weeks (31% randomized ≤28 days after onset) were assigned to cilostazol 100 mg bid vs aspirin 81 mg bid. Over a mean 29 months (SD 16) of follow-up, there was a significantly lower rate of all recurrent stroke (2.8% vs 3.7%; HR ,0.74; 95%CI, 0.56–0.98), the primary endpoint, in the cilostazol group. There were also fewer major hemorrhages in the cilostazol group as compared with aspirin (0.77%/year vs 1.78; HR, 0.46 (0.30–0.71); 8 vs 27 intracerebral hemorrhages, $P = 0.026$), though there was a significantly higher rate of side effects (headache, diarrhea, palpitations, dizziness, tachycardia) and side effects resulting in discontinuation of medication with cilostazol.[128]

The PERFORM trial randomized 19120 participants within 3 months after an ischemic stroke (90% of participants) or 8 days of a transient ischemic attack (10%) to terutroban 30 mg daily vs aspirin 100 mg daily in a randomized, double-blinded design.[129] The primary endpoint was a composite of recurrent ischemic stroke, myocardial infarction or vascular death (excluding hemorrhage). Over a mean 28.3 months (SD 7.7), there was no difference in the recurrence of the primary endpoint (11% in both groups; HR, 1.02; 95%CI, 0.94–1.12) or recurrent ischemic stroke (12% in each group; HR, 1.02; 95%CI, 0.92–1.13) between groups. There was no excess in major hemorrhagic complications between groups (2% in each group; HR, 1.01; 95%CI, 0.83–1.22) or intracranial hemorrhage (2% vs 1%; HR, 1.2; 95%CI, 0.94–1.53), though there was a small but significant excess in minor bleeding in the terutroban group (12% vs 11%; HR, 1.11; 95%CI, 1.02–1.11). The authors concluded that terutroban did not meet criteria for non-inferiority.[129]

In the PLATO trial, 18624 patients with an acute coronary syndrome (ST or non-ST-elevation myocardial infarction) were randomized to ticagrelor (180 mg load followed by 90 mg bid) versus clopidogrel (300–600 mg loading dose followed by 75 mg daily) within 24 hours of symptom onset. The primary end point at 1 year, a composite of vascular death, myocardial infarction and stroke, occurred in 9.8% of patients on ticagrelor vs 11.7% on clopidogrel (HR, 0.84; 95%CI, 0.77–0.92; $P < 0.001$). There was no difference between groups with regards to occurrence of stroke (1.5% vs 1.3%; HR, 1.2; 95%CI, 0.91–1.52). There were no differences overall with respect to major bleeding, though ticagrelor was associated with a non-significant excess of intracranial bleeding (all intracranial bleeding 0.3% vs 0.2%; HR, 1.87 (0.98–3.58); $P = 0.06$; ICH 0.2% vs 0.1%; $P = 0.1$).[130]

The effectiveness of ticagrelor versus aspirin monotherapy for prevention of early recurrence after transient ischemic attack/minor stroke is currently being investigated in the SOCRATES trial. The SOCRATES study (clinicaltrials.gov identifier NCT01994720) is an ongoing international, randomized, blinded trial sponsored by AstraZeneca examining the efficacy of ticagrelor (180 mg loading dose followed by 90 mg bid) vs aspirin (300 mg loading followed by 100 mg daily) for early prevention of major vascular events (composite of stroke, myocardial infarction and death within 90 days) in patients randomized within 24 hours of minor stroke or transient ischemic attack (http://www.clinicaltrials.gov/show/NCT01994720).

Interaction of Antiplatelet Agents and NSAIDs. Nonsteroidal anti-inflammatory drugs (NSAIDs) are one of the most commonly used medications worldwide.[131,132] Patients receiving both antiplatelet medication and NSAIDs may require prophylactic anti-ulcer therapy, including a proton pump inhibitor, misoprostol, or both, to prevent gastropathy if they are at increased risk for toxicity.

Guidelines from the American College of Gastroenterologists identified patients on aspirin therapy as high-risk for gastrointestinal toxicity from NSAIDs if they were over the age of 65, were on high-dose NSAIDs, or had a previous history of GI ulcers.[133] High-risk patients should be considered for prophylactic therapy with proton-pump inhibitors, misoprostol, or both.[134] The optimal treatment strategy with respect to drug choice or dosage is unknown. The use of H2 receptor antagonists[134] or enteric-coated aspirin has not been shown to protect against gastrointestinal bleeding.[135-137] Patients who are positive for H. pylori should be treated prior to initiating NSAID therapy.

ANTIPLATELET AND CEREBRAL MICROBLEEDS

Although the benefit of antiplatelet agents for the secondary prevention of stroke has been clearly demonstrated, it is also good evidence for the increased risk of hemorrhagic complications related to the administration of antiaggregants. Cerebral microbleeds (CMB) are deposits of hemosiderin in the brain that are identified in T2*-weighted gradient-echo magnetic resonance imaging (MRI) sequences because they are residues of small hemorrhages. They are currently regarded as evidence of small artery disease because they are associated with leukoaraiosis and frequently observed in patients with recurrent ischemic and hemorrhagic strokes. Moreover, previous use of antithrombotic drugs has been found to be an independent factor for the presence of CMB.[138]

Because of the increased risk of hemorrhagic side effects including intracranial hemorrhage (ICH), considerable debate has occurred about the possible increased risk of ICH in patients with CMB who are also receiving antiplatelet therapy. CMB prevalence rates are more than 10 times higher among patients with spontaneous ICH. There is some evidence for a topographic association of lobar and non-lobar ICH with the distribution of CMB, which suggests that CMB and ICH share an etiologic basis; that is, CMB represents indicators of imminent ICH. Two prospective studies with baseline and follow-up T2*-weighted MRI have reported data about the significance of CMBs for the future development of ICH. In the study of Fan et al.,[139] 121 patients with acute ischemic stroke were followed up for a mean of 27 months. Among them, 36% were found to have CMBs, and five patients developed ICH during the follow-up period (all taking antithrombotic medication). Four of the five patients had CMBs at the baseline MRI study, and in two cases the ICH was located at the same sites where the CMBs had been found. Greenberg et al.[140] studied 94 consecutive survivors of primary lobar ICH who had been studied with gradient-echo MRI sequences. Seventeen of 34 patients who had a second MRI after a stroke-free interval of 15.6 months were found to have new CMBs, and the authors found that these were associated with an increased risk of subsequent symptomatic ICH (3-year cumulative risk: 19%, 42%, and 67% for subjects with 0, 1 to 3, or ≥4 CMBs; $P = 0.02$). A case-control study by Wong et al.[110] investigated whether asymptomatic CMBs were a risk factor for ICH among aspirin users in a Chinese population. Twenty-one patients with ICH and 21 controls with no ICH were compared. CMBs were present in 19 patients (90%) with ICH, whereas only seven patients (33%) in the control group were found to have CMBs ($P < 0.001$). Moreover, the number of CMBs was also significantly higher in the group of patients with ICH (mean number of CMBs, 13 versus 0.2; $P < 0.001$). On the other hand, patients with CMBs also have a higher risk of recurrent ischemic stroke,[141] which might be decreased by the use of antiplatelets; thus, larger studies are needed to confirm these data. Despite the increased risk of ICH in patients with CMBs treated with antiplatelet agents,[142] recommendations about the use of antithrombotic therapy based on the detection of CMBs are not currently justified.

CONCLUSIONS

Effective primary prevention of stroke depends chiefly on risk factor management. However, based on the current data, aspirin can be considered for primary prevention in women older than 65 years who are at a risk of ischemic events that exceeds their risk of intracranial or extracranial hemorrhage. Aspirin has not been shown to be of significant benefit in primary prevention of stroke in men or in diabetic patients.[143,144]

Antiplatelet drugs are the current gold standard for secondary prevention of non-cardioembolic stroke. There is no current indication for anticoagulants in secondary prevention of atherothrombotic stroke. Aspirin (50 to 325 mg/day) is commonly used given its lower cost, although clopidogrel and aspirin-ERDP are also acceptable options. Clopidogrel is better tolerated than aspirin and offers greater benefit in non-cerebrovascular events. Aspirin-ERDP is superior to aspirin alone in preventing stroke recurrence; however, it may be more poorly tolerated than aspirin-clopidogrel. There is no current indication for long-term combination of aspirin-ERDP plus clopidogrel or aspirin-clopidogrel use in atherothrombotic or lacunar stroke,[145] the use of combination aspirin-clopidogrel in caucasians is under investigation for short-term use. Tests for resistance to aspirin and clopidogrel are not standardized, and their results are not yet validated. Therefore, selection of an antiplatelet agent should not be based on the results of these tests neither on the presence of CMBs on MRI.

Aspirin-clopidogrel confers additional protection over aspirin alone in patients with non-valvular AF who are not suitable for anticoagulation.[145,146]

REFERENCES

1. Donnan GA, Fisher M, Macleod M, et al. Stroke. Lancet 2008; 371:1612–23.
2. Antithrombotic Trialists C. Collaborative meta-analysis of randomised trials of antiplatelet therapy for prevention of death, myocardial infarction, and stroke in high risk patients. BMJ 2002;324:71–86.
3. Antithrombotic Trialists C, Baigent C, Blackwell L, et al. Aspirin in the primary and secondary prevention of vascular disease: collaborative meta-analysis of individual participant data from randomised trials. Lancet 2009;373:1849–60.
4. Hankey GJ. Secondary stroke prevention. Lancet Neurol 2014; 13:178–94.
5. Andrews RK, Shen Y, Gardiner EE, et al. The glycoprotein Ib-IX-V complex in platelet adhesion and signaling. Thromb Haemost 1999;82:357–64.
6. Fitzgerald DJ. Vascular biology of thrombosis: the role of platelet-vessel wall adhesion. Neurology 2001;57:S1–4.
7. Plow EF, Cierniewski CS, Xiao Z, et al. AlphaIIbbeta3 and its antagonism at the new millennium. Thromb Haemost 2001;86: 34–40.
8. Shattil SJ, Brass LF. Induction of the fibrinogen receptor on human platelets by intracellular mediators. J Biol Chem 1987; 262:992–1000.
9. Coughlin SR. Thrombin signalling and protease-activated receptors. Nature 2000;407:258–64.
10. Gachet C. ADP receptors of platelets and their inhibition. Thromb Haemost 2001;86:222–32.
11. Hollopeter G, Jantzen HM, Vincent D, et al. Identification of the platelet ADP receptor targeted by antithrombotic drugs. Nature 2001;409(6817):202–7.
12. Shen RF, Tai HH. Thromboxanes: synthase and receptors. J Biomed Sci 1998;5(3):153–72.
13. Hajjar KA. Cellular receptors in the regulation of plasmin generation. Thromb Haemost 1995;74(1):294–301.
14. Schafer AI, Adelman B. Plasmin inhibition of platelet function and of arachidonic acid metabolism. J Clin Invest 1985;75(2): 456–61.
15. Fitzgerald DJ, Wright F, FitzGerald GA. Increased thromboxane biosynthesis during coronary thrombolysis. Evidence that platelet activation and thromboxane A2 modulate the response to tissue-type plasminogen activator in vivo. Circ Res 1989;65(1):83–94.
16. Loscalzo J. Nitric oxide insufficiency, platelet activation, and arterial thrombosis. Circ Res 2001;88(8):756–62.
17. Marcus A, Broekman M, Drosopoulos J, et al. Thromboregulation by endothelial cells: significance for occlusive vascular diseases. Arterioscler Thromb Vasc Biol 2001;21(2):178–82.
18. Zwaginga JJ, Sixma JJ, de Groot PG. Activation of endothelial cells induces platelet thrombus formation on their matrix. Studies of new in vitro thrombosis model with low molecular weight heparin as anticoagulant. Arteriosclerosis 1990;10(1):49–61.
19. Feinberg WM, Erickson LP, Bruck D, et al. Hemostatic markers in acute ischemic stroke. Association with stroke type, severity, and outcome. Stroke 1996;27(8):1296–300.
20. Uchiyama S, Yamazaki M, Hara Y, et al. Alterations of platelet, coagulation, and fibrinolysis markers in patients with acute ischemic stroke. Semin Thromb Hemost 1997;23(6):535–41.

21. Folsom AR, Rosamond WD, Shahar E, et al. Prospective study of markers of hemostatic function with risk of ischemic stroke. The Atherosclerosis Risk in Communities (ARIC) Study Investigators. Circulation 1999;100(7):736–42.
22. Marler JR, Price TR, Clark GL, et al. Morning increase in onset of ischemic stroke. Stroke 1989;20(4):473–6.
23. Tofler GH, Brezinski D, Schafer AI, et al. Concurrent morning increase in platelet aggregability and the risk of myocardial infarction and sudden cardiac death. N Engl J Med 1987;316(24):1514–18.
24. Ernst E, Resch KL. Fibrinogen as a cardiovascular risk factor: a meta-analysis and review of the literature. Ann Intern Med 1993;118(12):956–63.
25. Becher H, Grau A, Steindorf K, et al. Previous infection and other risk factors for acute cerebrovascular ischaemia: attributable risks and the characterisation of high risk groups. J Epidemiol Biostat 2000;5(5):277–83.
26. Grau AJ, Buggle F, Becher H, et al. Recent bacterial and viral infection is a risk factor for cerebrovascular ischemia: clinical and biochemical studies. Neurology 1998;50(1):196–203.
27. Woodhouse PR, Khaw KT, Plummer M, et al. Seasonal variations of plasma fibrinogen and factor VII activity in the elderly: winter infections and death from cardiovascular disease. Lancet 1994;343(8895):435–9.
28. O'Malley T, Langhorne P, Elton RA, et al. Platelet size in stroke patients. Stroke 1995;26(6):995–9.
29. Kenet G, Freedman J, Shenkman B, et al. Plasma glutathione peroxidase deficiency and platelet insensitivity to nitric oxide in children with familial stroke. Arterioscler Thromb Vasc Biol 1999;19(8):2017–23.
30. Knapp HR, Reilly IA, Alessandrini P, et al. In vivo indexes of platelet and vascular function during fish-oil administration in patients with atherosclerosis. N Engl J Med 1986;314(15):937–42.
31. Amarenco P, Cohen A, Tzourio C, et al. Atherosclerotic disease of the aortic arch and the risk of ischemic stroke. N Engl J Med 1994;331(22):1474–9.
32. Amarenco P, Davis S, Jones EF, et al. Clopidogrel plus aspirin versus warfarin in patients with stroke and aortic arch plaques. Stroke 2014;45(5):1248–57.
33. Chimowitz MI, Lynn MJ, Howlett-Smith H, et al. Comparison of warfarin and aspirin for symptomatic intracranial arterial stenosis. N Engl J Med 2005;352(13):1305–16.
34. Choudhury A, Chung I, Blann AD, et al. Platelet surface CD62P and CD63, mean platelet volume, and soluble/platelet P-selectin as indexes of platelet function in atrial fibrillation: a comparison of "healthy control subjects" and "disease control subjects" in sinus rhythm. J Am Coll Cardiol 2007;49(19):1957–64.
35. Gunning AJ, Pickering GW, Robb-Smith AH, et al. Mural Thrombosis of the Internal Carotid Artery and Subsequent Embolism. Q J Med 1964;33:155–95.
36. Hart RG, Diener HC, Coutts SB, et al. Embolic strokes of undetermined source: the case for a new clinical construct. Lancet Neurol 2014;13(4):429–38.
37. Orgera MA, O'Malley PG, Taylor AJ. Secondary prevention of cerebral ischemia in patent foramen ovale: systematic review and meta-analysis. South Med J 2001;94(7):699–703.
38. Roth GJ, Stanford N, Majerus PW. Acetylation of prostaglandin synthase by aspirin. Proc Natl Acad Sci U S A 1975;72(8):3073–6.
39. Smith JB, Willis AL. Aspirin selectively inhibits prostaglandin production in human platelets. Nat New Biol 1971;231(25):235–7.
40. Vane JR. Inhibition of prostaglandin synthesis as a mechanism of action for aspirin-like drugs. Nat New Biol 1971;231(25):232–5.
41. Patrono C, Roth GJ. Aspirin in ischemic cerebrovascular disease. How strong is the case for a different dosing regimen? Stroke 1996;27(4):756–60.
42. Weksler BB, Tack-Goldman K, Subramanian VA, et al. Cumulative inhibitory effect of low-dose aspirin on vascular prostacyclin and platelet thromboxane production in patients with atherosclerosis. Circulation 1985;71(2):332–40.
43. Goertler M, Baeumer M, Kross R, et al. Rapid decline of cerebral microemboli of arterial origin after intravenous acetylsalicylic acid. Stroke 1999;30(1):66–9.
44. Patrono C, Coller B, Dalen JE, et al. Platelet-active drugs: the relationships among dose, effectiveness, and side effects. Chest 1998;114(5 Suppl.):470S–88S.
45. Kyrle PA, Eichler HG, Jager U, et al. Inhibition of prostacyclin and thromboxane A2 generation by low-dose aspirin at the site of plug formation in man in vivo. Circulation 1987;75(5):1025–9.
46. The Dutch TIA Trial Study Group. A comparison of two doses of aspirin (30 mg vs. 283 mg a day) in patients after a transient ischemic attack or minor ischemic stroke. N Engl J Med 1991;325(18):1261–6.
47. Ali M, McDonald JW, Thiessen JJ, et al. Plasma acetylsalicylate and salicylate and platelet cyclooxygenase activity following plain and enteric-coated aspirin. Stroke 1980;11(1):9–13.
48. O'Connor CM, Gurbel PA, Serebruany VL. Usefulness of soluble and surface-bound P-selectin in detecting heightened platelet activity in patients with congestive heart failure. Am J Cardiol 1999;83(9):1345–9.
49. Taylor DW, Barnett HJ, Haynes RB, et al. Low-dose and high-dose acetylsalicylic acid for patients undergoing carotid endarterectomy: a randomised controlled trial. ASA and Carotid Endarterectomy (ACE) Trial Collaborators. Lancet 1999;353(9171):2179–84.
50. Tohgi H, Takahashi H, Chiba K, et al. Coagulation-fibrinolysis system in poststroke patients receiving antiplatelet medication. Stroke 1993;24(6):801–4.
51. Catella-Lawson F, Reilly MP, Kapoor SC, et al. Cyclooxygenase inhibitors and the antiplatelet effects of aspirin. N Engl J Med 2001;345(25):1809–17.
52. Szczeklik A, Krzanowski M, Gora P, et al. Antiplatelet drugs and generation of thrombin in clotting blood. Blood 1992;80(8):2006–11.
53. Sanderson S, Emery J, Baglin T, et al. Narrative review: aspirin resistance and its clinical implications. Ann Intern Med 2005;142(5):370–80.
54. Mueller MR, Salat A, Stangl P, et al. Variable platelet response to low-dose ASA and the risk of limb deterioration in patients submitted to peripheral arterial angioplasty. Thromb Haemost 1997;78(3):1003–7.
55. Kamath S, Blann AD, Lip GY. Platelet activation: assessment and quantification. Eur Heart J 2001;22(17):1561–71.
56. Kottke-Marchant K, Corcoran G. The laboratory diagnosis of platelet disorders. Arch Pathol Lab Med 2002;126(2):133–46.
57. Bruno A, McConnell JP, Cohen SN, et al. Serial urinary 11-dehydrothromboxane B2, aspirin dose, and vascular events in blacks after recent cerebral infarction. Stroke 2004;35(3):727–30.
58. Eikelboom JW, Hirsh J, Weitz JI, et al. Aspirin-resistant thromboxane biosynthesis and the risk of myocardial infarction, stroke, or cardiovascular death in patients at high risk for cardiovascular events. Circulation 2002;105(14):1650–5.
59. Gasparyan AY, Watson T, Lip GY. The role of aspirin in cardiovascular prevention: implications of aspirin resistance. J Am Coll Cardiol 2008;51(19):1829–43.
60. Nadar S, Blann AD, Lip GY. Effects of aspirin on intra-platelet vascular endothelial growth factor, angiopoietin-1, and p-selectin levels in hypertensive patients. Am J Hypertens 2006;19(9):970–7, discussion 8.
61. Serebruany VL, Kereiakes DJ, Dalesandro MR, et al. The flow cytometer model markedly affects measurement of ex vivo whole blood platelet-bound P-selectin expression in patients with chest pain: are we comparing apples with oranges. Thromb Res 1999;96(1):51–6.
62. De Gaetano G, Cerletti C. Aspirin resistance: a revival of platelet aggregation tests? J Thromb Haemost 2003;1(9):2048–50.
63. Yardumian DA, Mackie IJ, Machin SJ. Laboratory investigation of platelet function: a review of methodology. J Clin Pathol 1986;39(7):701–12.
64. Jilma B. Platelet function analyzer (PFA-100): a tool to quantify congenital or acquired platelet dysfunction. J Lab Clin Med 2001;138(3):152–63.
65. Kundu SK, Heilmann EJ, Sio R, et al. Description of an in vitro platelet function analyzer–PFA-100. Semin Thromb Hemost 1995;21(Suppl. 2):106–12.
66. Malinin A, Spergling M, Muhlestein B, et al. Assessing aspirin responsiveness in subjects with multiple risk factors for vascular

disease with a rapid platelet function analyzer. Blood Coagul Fibrinolysis 2004;15(4):295–301.
67. Komiya T, Kudo M, Urabe T, et al. Compliance with antiplatelet therapy in patients with ischemic cerebrovascular disease. Assessment by platelet aggregation testing. Stroke 1994;25(12): 2337–42.
68. Sappok T, Faulstich A, Stuckert E, et al. Compliance with secondary prevention of ischemic stroke: a prospective evaluation. Stroke 2001;32(8):1884–9.
69. Hankey GJ, Eikelboom JW. Aspirin resistance. BMJ 2004; 328(7438):477–9.
70. Bornstein NM, Karepov VG, Aronovich BD, et al. Failure of aspirin treatment after stroke. Stroke 1994;25(2):275–7.
71. Helgason CM, Bolin KM, Hoff JA, et al. Development of aspirin resistance in persons with previous ischemic stroke. Stroke 1994;25(12):2331–6.
72. Cambria-Kiely JA, Gandhi PJ. Aspirin resistance and genetic polymorphisms. J Thromb Thrombolysis 2002;14(1):51–8.
73. Grotemeyer KH, Scharafinski HW, Husstedt IW. Two-year follow-up of aspirin responder and aspirin non responder. A pilot-study including 180 post-stroke patients. Thromb Res 1993;71(5):397–403.
74. Andersen K, Hurlen M, Arnesen H, et al. Aspirin non-responsiveness as measured by PFA-100 in patients with coronary artery disease. Thromb Res 2002;108(1):37–42.
75. Grundmann K, Jaschonek K, Kleine B, et al. Aspirin non-responder status in patients with recurrent cerebral ischemic attacks. J Neurol 2003;250(1):63–6.
76. Gum PA, Kottke-Marchant K, Welsh PA, et al. A prospective, blinded determination of the natural history of aspirin resistance among stable patients with cardiovascular disease. J Am Coll Cardiol 2003;41(6):961–5.
77. Investigators SPS, Benavente OR, Hart RG, et al. Effects of clopidogrel added to aspirin in patients with recent lacunar stroke. N Engl J Med 2012;367(9):817–25.
78. Cote R, Zhang Y, Hart RG, et al. ASA failure: does the combination ASA/clopidogrel confer better long-term vascular protection? Neurology 2014;82(5):382–9.
79. Campbell CL, Smyth S, Montalescot G, et al. Aspirin dose for the prevention of cardiovascular disease: a systematic review. JAMA 2007;297(18):2018–24.
80. Eikelboom JW, Hankey GJ, Thom J, et al. Enhanced antiplatelet effect of clopidogrel in patients whose platelets are least inhibited by aspirin: a randomized crossover trial. J Thromb Haemost 2005;3(12):2649–55.
81. Bhatt DL, Fox KA, Hacke W, et al. Clopidogrel and aspirin versus aspirin alone for the prevention of atherothrombotic events. N Engl J Med 2006;354(16):1706–17.
82. Diener HC, Bogousslavsky J, Brass LM, et al. Management of atherothrombosis with clopidogrel in high-risk patients with recent transient ischaemic attack or ischaemic stroke (MATCH): study design and baseline data. Cerebrovasc Dis 2004;17(2–3): 253–61.
83. Snoep JD, Hovens MM, Eikenboom JC, et al. Clopidogrel non-responsiveness in patients undergoing percutaneous coronary intervention with stenting: a systematic review and meta-analysis. Am Heart J 2007;154(2):221–31.
84. Lev N, Melamed E, Offen D. Proteasomal inhibition hypersensitizes differentiated neuroblastoma cells to oxidative damage. Neurosci Lett 2006;399(1–2):27–32.
85. Michos ED, Ardehali R, Blumenthal RS, et al. Aspirin and clopidogrel resistance. Mayo Clin Proc 2006;81(4):518–26.
86. Wang TH, Bhatt DL, Topol EJ. Aspirin and clopidogrel resistance: an emerging clinical entity. Eur Heart J 2006;27(6):647–54.
87. Diener HC, Cunha L, Forbes C, et al. European Stroke Prevention Study. 2. Dipyridamole and acetylsalicylic acid in the secondary prevention of stroke. J Neurol Sci 1996;143(1–2): 1–13.
88. Group ES, Halkes PH, van Gijn J, et al. Aspirin plus dipyridamole versus aspirin alone after cerebral ischaemia of arterial origin (ESPRIT): randomised controlled trial. Lancet 2006; 367(9523):1665–73.
89. He J, Whelton PK, Vu B, et al. Aspirin and risk of hemorrhagic stroke: a meta-analysis of randomized controlled trials. JAMA 1998;280(22):1930–5.
90. Sharis PJ, Cannon CP, Loscalzo J. The antiplatelet effects of ticlopidine and clopidogrel. Ann Intern Med 1998;129(5): 394–405.
91. Isaka Y, Kimura K, Etani H, et al. Effect of aspirin and ticlopidine on platelet deposition in carotid atherosclerosis: assessment by indium-111 platelet scintigraphy. Stroke 1986;17(6):1215–20.
92. Yang LH, Hoppensteadt D, Fareed J. Modulation of vasoconstriction by clopidogrel and ticlopidine. Thromb Res 1998;92(2): 83–9.
93. Nguyen TA, Diodati JG, Pharand C. Resistance to clopidogrel: a review of the evidence. J Am Coll Cardiol 2005;45(8): 1157–64.
94. Sugunaraj JP, Palaniswamy C, Selvaraj DR, et al. Clopidogrel resistance. Am J Therapeut 2010;17(2):210–15.
95. Collet JP, Hulot JS, Pena A, et al. Cytochrome P450 2C19 polymorphism in young patients treated with clopidogrel after myocardial infarction: a cohort study. Lancet 2009;373(9660): 309–17.
96. Shuldiner AR, O'Connell JR, Bliden KP, et al. Association of cytochrome P450 2C19 genotype with the antiplatelet effect and clinical efficacy of clopidogrel therapy. JAMA 2009;302(8): 849–57.
97. Pare G, Mehta SR, Yusuf S, et al. Effects of CYP2C19 genotype on outcomes of clopidogrel treatment. N Engl J Med 2010; 363(18):1704–14.
98. Peto R, Gray R, Collins R, et al. Randomised trial of prophylactic daily aspirin in British male doctors. Br Med J (Clin Res Ed) 1988;296(6618):313–16.
99. The Medical Research Council's General Practice Research Framework. Thrombosis prevention trial: randomised trial of low-intensity oral anticoagulation with warfarin and low-dose aspirin in the primary prevention of ischaemic heart disease in men at increased risk. Lancet 1998;351(9098):233–41.
100. Hansson L, Zanchetti A, Carruthers SG, et al. Effects of intensive blood-pressure lowering and low-dose aspirin in patients with hypertension: principal results of the Hypertension Optimal Treatment (HOT) randomised trial. HOT Study Group. Lancet 1998;351(9118):1755–62.
101. Ridker PM, Cook NR, Lee IM, et al. A randomized trial of low-dose aspirin in the primary prevention of cardiovascular disease in women. N Engl J Med 2005;352(13):1293–304.
102. Eidelman RS, Hebert PR, Weisman SM, et al. An update on aspirin in the primary prevention of cardiovascular disease. Arch Intern Med 2003;163(17):2006–10.
103. Belch J, MacCuish A, Campbell I, et al. The prevention of progression of arterial disease and diabetes (POPADAD) trial: factorial randomised placebo controlled trial of aspirin and antioxidants in patients with diabetes and asymptomatic peripheral arterial disease. BMJ 2008;337:a1840.
104. Ogawa H, Nakayama M, Morimoto T, et al. Low-dose aspirin for primary prevention of atherosclerotic events in patients with type 2 diabetes: a randomized controlled trial. JAMA 2008; 300(18):2134–41.
105. De Berardis G, Sacco M, Evangelista V, et al. Aspirin and Simvastatin Combination for Cardiovascular Events Prevention Trial in Diabetes (ACCEPT-D): design of a randomized study of the efficacy of low-dose aspirin in the prevention of cardiovascular events in subjects with diabetes mellitus treated with statins. Trials 2007;8:21.
106. CAST (Chinese Acute Stroke Trial) Collaborative Group. CAST: randomised placebo-controlled trial of early aspirin use in 20,000 patients with acute ischaemic stroke. Lancet 1997; 349(9066):1641–9.
107. International Stroke Trial Collaborative Group. The International Stroke Trial (IST): a randomised trial of aspirin, subcutaneous heparin, both, or neither among 19435 patients with acute ischaemic stroke. Lancet 1997;349(9065):1569–81.
108. Chen ZM, Sandercock P, Pan HC, et al. Indications for early aspirin use in acute ischemic stroke: A combined analysis of 40 000 randomized patients from the chinese acute stroke trial and the international stroke trial. On behalf of the CAST and IST collaborative groups. Stroke 2000;31(6):1240–9.
109. Wang Y, Wang Y, Zhao X, et al. Clopidogrel with aspirin in acute minor stroke or transient ischemic attack. N Engl J Med 2013; 369(1):11–19.

110. Wong KS, Wang Y, Leng X, et al. Early dual versus mono antiplatelet therapy for acute non-cardioembolic ischemic stroke or transient ischemic attack: an updated systematic review and meta-analysis. Circulation 2013;128(15):1656–66.
111. Johnston SC, Easton JD, Farrant M, et al. Platelet-oriented inhibition in new TIA and minor ischemic stroke (POINT) trial: rationale and design. Int J Stroke 2013;8(6):479–83.
112. The Stroke Prevention in Reversible Ischemia Trial (SPIRIT) Study Group. A randomized trial of anticoagulants versus aspirin after cerebral ischemia of presumed arterial origin. Ann Neurol 1997;42(6):857–65.
113. Mohr JP, Thompson JL, Lazar RM, et al. A comparison of warfarin and aspirin for the prevention of recurrent ischemic stroke. N Engl J Med 2001;345(20):1444–51.
114. Group ES, Halkes PH, van Gijn J, et al. Medium intensity oral anticoagulants versus aspirin after cerebral ischaemia of arterial origin (ESPRIT): a randomised controlled trial. Lancet Neurol 2007;6(2):115–24.
115. The SALT Collaborative Group. Swedish Aspirin Low-Dose Trial (SALT) of 75 mg aspirin as secondary prophylaxis after cerebrovascular ischaemic events. Lancet 1991;338(8779):1345–9.
116. Committee CS, CAPRIE Steering Committee. A randomised, blinded, trial of clopidogrel versus aspirin in patients at risk of ischaemic events (CAPRIE). Lancet 1996;348(9038):1329–39.
117. Sacco RL, Diener HC, Yusuf S, et al. Aspirin and extended-release dipyridamole versus clopidogrel for recurrent stroke. N Engl J Med 2008;359(12):1238–51.
118. Investigators AWGotA, Connolly S, Pogue J, et al. Clopidogrel plus aspirin versus oral anticoagulation for atrial fibrillation in the Atrial fibrillation Clopidogrel Trial with Irbesartan for prevention of Vascular Events (ACTIVE W): a randomised controlled trial. Lancet 2006;367(9526):1903–12.
119. Investigators A, Connolly SJ, Pogue J, et al. Effect of clopidogrel added to aspirin in patients with atrial fibrillation. N Engl J Med 2009;360(20):2066–78.
120. Bhatt DL, Kapadia SR, Bajzer CT, et al. Dual antiplatelet therapy with clopidogrel and aspirin after carotid artery stenting. J Invasive Cardiol 2001;13(12):767–71.
121. Sharma M, Pearce LA, Benavente OR, et al. Predictors of Mortality in Patients With Lacunar Stroke in the Secondary Prevention of Small Subcortical Strokes Trial. Stroke 2014.
122. Chimowitz MI, Lynn MJ, Derdeyn CP, et al. Stenting versus aggressive medical therapy for intracranial arterial stenosis. N Engl J Med 2011;365(11):993–1003.
123. Payne DA, Jones CI, Hayes PD, et al. Beneficial effects of clopidogrel combined with aspirin in reducing cerebral emboli in patients undergoing carotid endarterectomy. Circulation 2004; 109(12):1476–81.
124. Markus HS, Droste DW, Kaps M, et al. Dual antiplatelet therapy with clopidogrel and aspirin in symptomatic carotid stenosis evaluated using doppler embolic signal detection: the Clopidogrel and Aspirin for Reduction of Emboli in Symptomatic Carotid Stenosis (CARESS) trial. Circulation 2005;111(17):2233–40.
125. Dalainas I, Nano G, Bianchi P, et al. Dual antiplatelet regime versus acetyl-acetic acid for carotid artery stenting. Cardiovasc Intervent Radiol 2006;29(4):519–21.
126. Hirsh J, Bhatt DL. Comparative benefits of clopidogrel and aspirin in high-risk patient populations: lessons from the CAPRIE and CURE studies. Arch Intern Med 2004;164(19): 2106–10.
127. Matias-Guiu J, Ferro JM, Alvarez-Sabin J, et al. Comparison of triflusal and aspirin for prevention of vascular events in patients after cerebral infarction: the TACIP Study: a randomized, double-blind, multicenter trial. Stroke 2003;34(4):840–8.
128. Shinohara Y, Katayama Y, Uchiyama S, et al. Cilostazol for prevention of secondary stroke (CSPS 2): an aspirin-controlled, double-blind, randomised non-inferiority trial. Lancet Neurol 2010;9(10):959–68.
129. Bousser MG, Amarenco P, Chamorro A, et al. Terutroban versus aspirin in patients with cerebral ischaemic events (PERFORM): a randomised, double-blind, parallel-group trial. Lancet 2011; 377(9782):2013–22.
130. Kohli P, Wallentin L, Reyes E, et al. Reduction in first and recurrent cardiovascular events with ticagrelor compared with clopidogrel in the PLATO Study. Circulation 2013;127(6):673–80.
131. Laine L. Approaches to nonsteroidal anti-inflammatory drug use in the high-risk patient. Gastroenterology 2001;120(3): 594–606.
132. Singh G. Gastrointestinal complications of prescription and over-the-counter nonsteroidal anti-inflammatory drugs: a view from the ARAMIS database. Arthritis, Rheumatism, and Aging Medical Information System. Am J Therapeut 2000;7(2): 115–21.
133. Lanza FL, Chan FK, Quigley EM, et al. Guidelines for prevention of NSAID-related ulcer complications. Am J Gastroenterol 2009; 104(3):728–38.
134. Koch M, Dezi A, Ferrario F, et al. Prevention of nonsteroidal anti-inflammatory drug-induced gastrointestinal mucosal injury. A meta-analysis of randomized controlled clinical trials. Arch Intern Med 1996;156(20):2321–32.
135. Hawthorne AB, Mahida YR, Cole AT, et al. Aspirin-induced gastric mucosal damage: prevention by enteric-coating and relation to prostaglandin synthesis. Br J Clin Pharmacol 1991; 32(1):77–83.
136. Kelly JP, Kaufman DW, Jurgelon JM, et al. Risk of aspirin-associated major upper-gastrointestinal bleeding with enteric-coated or buffered product. Lancet 1996;348(9039):1413–16.
137. Petroski D. Endoscopic comparison of three aspirin preparations and placebo. ClinTherapeutics 1993;15(2):314–20.
138. Haley KE, Greenberg SM, Gurol ME. Cerebral microbleeds and macrobleeds: should they influence our recommendations for antithrombotic therapies? Curr Cardiol Rep 2013;15(12):425.
139. Fan YH, Zhang L, Lam WW, et al. Cerebral microbleeds as a risk factor for subsequent intracerebral hemorrhages among patients with acute ischemic stroke. Stroke 2003;34(10):2459–62.
140. Greenberg SM, Eng JA, Ning M, et al. Hemorrhage burden predicts recurrent intracerebral hemorrhage after lobar hemorrhage. Stroke 2004;35(6):1415–20.
141. Imaizumi T, Horita Y, Chiba M, et al. Dot-like hemosiderin spots on gradient echo T2*-weighted magnetic resonance imaging are associated with past history of small vessel disease in patients with intracerebral hemorrhage. J Neuroimag 2004;14(3): 251–7.
142. Lovelock CE, Cordonnier C, Naka H, et al. Antithrombotic drug use, cerebral microbleeds, and intracerebral hemorrhage: a systematic review of published and unpublished studies. Stroke 2010;41(6):1222–8.
143. Bushnell C, McCullough LD, Awad IA, et al. Guidelines for the prevention of stroke in women: a statement for healthcare professionals from the American Heart Association/American Stroke Association. Stroke 2014;45(5):1545–88.
144. Goldstein LB, Bushnell CD, Adams RJ, et al. Guidelines for the primary prevention of stroke: a guideline for healthcare professionals from the American Heart Association/American Stroke Association. Stroke 2011;42(2):517–84.
145. Kernan WN, Ovbiagele B, Black HR, et al. Guidelines for the prevention of stroke in patients with stroke and transient ischemic attack: a guideline for healthcare professionals from the American Heart Association/American Stroke Association. Stroke 2014;45(7):2160–236.
146. Furie KL, Goldstein LB, Albers GW, et al. Oral antithrombotic agents for the prevention of stroke in nonvalvular atrial fibrillation: a science advisory for healthcare professionals from the American Heart Association/American Stroke Association. Stroke 2012;43(12):3442–53.

62 Secondary Prevention of Cardioembolic Stroke

Karen Furie, Muhib Khan

KEY POINTS

- Cardioembolic stroke is a major etiology accounting for one-fifth of all ischemic strokes.
- Recent advances in technology have enabled us to monitor heart rhythm remotely and detect paroxysmal atrial fibrillation.
- Newer risk stratification scores like CHADS2-Vasc and HAS-BLED have been developed to predict ischemic stroke due to atrial fibrillation as well as bleeding risk on anticoagulation.
- Rheumatic mitral valve disease has the highest risk of ischemic stroke of all native valvular heart disease.
- CLOSURE, RESPECT, and PC trials have shown that device closure of patent foramen ovale (PFO) is not superior to medical therapy in preventing recurrent stroke.
- Newer oral anticoagulants have shown equal or superior efficacy to warfarin in preventing ischemic stroke in non-valvular atrial fibrillation expanding treatment options for this patient population.
- Intracerebral hemorrhage due to anticoagulant therapy has higher morbidity and mortality needing further research in this particular area.

Cardioembolic stroke is a major stroke subtype accounting for one-fifth of all ischemic strokes.[1,2] Advanced imaging technology has enabled us to easily identify potential cardiac sources of emboli. Since, the underlying cardiac condition is often evident before stroke occurs and antithrombotic therapies are notably effective, cardiogenic emboli to the brain are among the most preventable causes of stroke.

With a thorough cardiac evaluation, a potential source of cardiogenic emboli can be identified in at least 30% of all patients with ischemic stroke.[3,4] However, potential cardioembolic sources often coexist with other cardiovascular disease risk factors.[5–7] During the past two decades, new and better non-invasive cardiac imaging became available; therefore, new potential cardioembolic sources have been recognized. This situation is reflected in the increased frequency of cardioembolic stroke over time. Aggregate data from stroke registries conducted between 1988 and 1994 show mean frequency of cardioembolic stroke to be 20% (range, 17–28%).[1,6,8–11] Data from later stroke registries (1995–2001) showed a higher mean prevalence of cardioembolic stroke, 25% (range 16–38%).[12–16]

Cardioembolic stroke is caused by a variety of cardiac disorders, each with a unique natural history and a variable response to antithrombotic therapy (Fig. 62-1). The embolic material originating from the heart and proximal aorta can be quite diverse. The thrombi may be composed of varying proportions of platelets and fibrin, cholesterol fragments, tumor particles, or bacterial clusters. The natural history and response to antithrombotic therapy of each of these conditions are unique, and, consequently, each source of cardioembolic stroke should be considered separately. Thus cardioembolic stroke is not a single disease; it is a syndrome with diverse causes (see Fig. 62-1).

The incidence of ischemic stroke associated with cardioembolic sources varies greatly. Cardioembolic sources of stroke can be divided according to their stroke risk potential as "major-risk sources," for which the risk for stroke is well established, or "minor-risk sources," for which the risk for stroke has been incompletely established (Table 62-1). The major-risk cardioembolic sources carry a substantial annual risk of emboli and a high risk of recurrence, and usually, antithrombotic therapy is warranted for stroke prevention. Conversely, the so-called minor sources of emboli can cause stroke but have a low or uncertain risk of embolism and are more often coincidental than causal; therefore, antithrombotic therapy is usually reserved for selected cases.

ATRIAL FIBRILLATION

Atrial fibrillation (AF) is the most common cardiac arrhythmia, affecting 0.7–0.9% of the general population of the US (2.5 million people).[17,18] Its prevalence increases with age, being present in about 5% of persons at age 65 years and in 10% at age 80 years. AF is equally distributed in men and women, and the mean age of individuals affected is about 75 years (Fig. 62-2).[17,18]

The first-detected episode can proceed along different pathways. It can be self-limited without any recurrence, in which case it is termed "lone AF." It can adopt a recurrence pattern with intervening sinus rhythm termed as "paroxysmal AF." If it persists for 7 days, it is termed "persistent." These forms of AF are proposed by American College of Cardiology (ACC)/American Heart Association (AHA)/European Society of Cardiology (ESC).[19] It is important to note that the AF duration and its persistence can evolve over time either due to ongoing pathophysiological process or treatment. AF can be further divided into valvular vs non-valvular AF. Valvular AF is defined as AF secondary to structural heart disease involving the valves, commonly the mitral valve. Non-valvular AF is defined as AF without evidence of structural valvular heart disease preferably screened by an echocardiogram.[19]

Non-valvular AF is the etiology in 25% of all ischemic strokes.[6,20,21] Older age is a major risk and AF is the diagnosed etiology in more than one-third of patients older than 70 years with ischemic stroke.[22] The risk of ischemic stroke increases fivefold (from 1–5% per year) in elderly patients (mean age, 70 years) with non-valvular AF, and about 18-fold in patients with AF and rheumatic mitral stenosis.[23] AF accounts for about one-half of presumed cardioembolic strokes. Patients with AF are typically older and have large middle cerebral artery strokes associated with a high mortality rate during the first 30 days (Table 62-2).[24,25]

Stroke associated with AF is attributed to embolism of thrombus from the left atrium (LA), the pathogenesis of which is complex.[26] Thrombus most frequently forms in the left atrial appendage (LAA).[27] This thrombus is a result of stasis, endothelial dysfunction and a hypercoagulable state. Stasis results from the decreased emptying of the LAA due to loss of organized mechanical contraction during the cardiac cycle, as evidenced by the reduced LAA flow velocities.[28] Moreover, AF seems to promote a hypercoaguable state and has been associated with biochemical markers of coagulation and platelet activation.[29]

However, AF alone may not be enough to promote thrombi formation. Other factors may also contribute, because associated cardiovascular disease and age appear to influence the stroke risk in AF and, hence, also to influence the formation of atrial appendage thrombi. This variable risk is reflected by the wide range of stroke risk in patients with AF ("lone AF") a phenomenon not observed with other "high-risk" conditions. Temporal variation in factors that influence thrombus formation may explain the intermittency of embolism in different patients with AF and even within each patient. Embolic events are intermittent in AF, sometimes separated by years. A balance between the formation and inhibition of clot is likely present in the atrial appendage of such patients. This balance is influenced by atrial size, appendage flow velocities, and coagulation factors. Therefore, the type and intensity of antithrombotic therapy needed to inhibit appendage thrombi may differ among patients with AF and over time for the same patient. In summary, complex electrophysiological and thromboembolic processes lead to embolic events in AF.

The overall incidence of ischemic stroke among people with AF is about 5% per year. The rate of stroke varies widely, however, ranging from 0.5% per year in young patients with "lone AF" to 12% per year in those with prior transient ischemia attack (TIA) or stroke. This variation depends on coexisting cardiovascular disorders.[26,30,31] Therefore, identification of subgroups of patients with AF with relatively high vs low absolute rates of stroke is important for selecting prophylactic antithrombotic therapy.[22] Different scores have been developed and validated to predict this risk in an individual.

The CHADS2 score is widely used as the most reliable scheme of stratification that allows the separation of AF

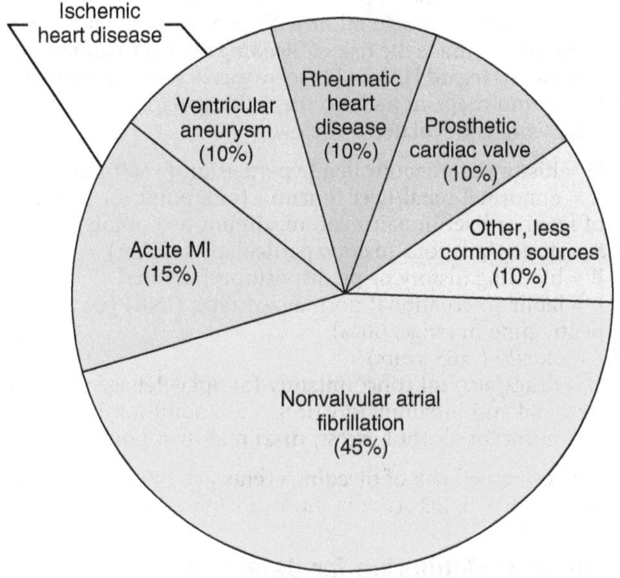

Figure 62-1. Sources of cardioembolic stroke. MI, myocardial infarction.

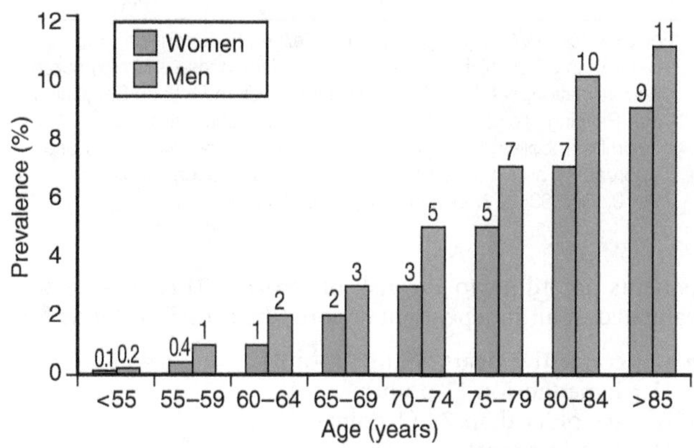

Figure 62-2. Prevalence of atrial fibrillation stratified by age and sex.

TABLE 62-1 Cardioembolic Sources by Location

	Atrial	Valvular	Ventricular
Major-Risk Sources	Atrial fibrillation	Mitral stenosis	Left ventricular thrombus (mobile or protruding)
	Left atrial thrombus	Prosthetic cardiac valves	Recent anterior wall myocardial infarction
	Left atrial myxoma	Infective endocarditis calcification	Non-ischemic dilated cardiomyopathy
	Sustained atrial flutter	Marantic endocarditis	
Minor-Risk Sources	Patent foramen ovale	Mitral valve prolapse	Left ventricular regional wall abnormalities
	Atrial septal aneurysm	Calcific aortic stenosis	Congestive heart failure
		Mitral annular	Akinetic ventricular wall segment
		Giant Lambl's excrescences	
		Fibroelastoma	

TABLE 62-2 Stroke Risk in Relation to Atrial Fibrillation*

Study	Mean Age (years)	Stroke Rate %/year AF	Stroke Rate %/year Non-AF	Increased Relative Risk
Framingham (USA) (Wolf, 1991)[23]	70	4.1	0.7	× 6
Shibata (Japan) (Nakayama, 1997)[23a]	65	5.0	0.9	× 6
Reykjavik (Iceland) (Onundarson, 1987)[23b]	52	1.6	0.2	× 7

*Data from epidemiologic studies.

TABLE 62-3 CHADS2 Score for Risk Stratification of Stroke

$CHADS_2$ Score*	Risk	Stroke Rate (%/year)
0	Low	0.5
1	Low	1.5
2	Moderate	2.5
3	High	5
4	High	6
5-6	Very high	7

*For CHADS2 (congestive heart failure, hypertension, age older than 75 year, diabetes mellitus) score and validation, see Gage BF, Waterman AD, Shannon W, Boechler M, Rich MW, Radford MJ. Validation of clinical classification schemes for predicting stroke: Results from the national registry of atrial fibrillation. *JAMA* 2001;285:2864–2870. Level of Evidence Class I.

TABLE 62-4 CHA2DS2-VASc Score for Risk Stratification of Stroke

$CHADS_2$ Score*	Risk	Stroke Rate (%/year)
0	Low	0
1	Low	1.3
2	Moderate	2.2
3	Moderate	3.2
4	High	4
5	High	6.7
6	Very High	9.8
7	Very High	9.6
8	High	6.7
9	Very High	15.2

*For CHA2DS2-VASc (congestive heart failure, hypertension, age older than 65 yr, diabetes mellitus, vascular disease and sex) score and validation, see Lip GY, Nieuwlaat R, Pisters R, Lane DA, Crijns HJ. Refining clinical risk stratification for predicting stroke and thromboembolism in atrial fibrillation using a novel risk factor-based approach: The Euro Heart Survey on atrial fibrillation. *Chest.* 2010;137:263–272. Level of Evidence Class IIa.

patients according to the risk of stroke.[32] This scheme was validated in an independent cohort. The acronym stands for:

- C = congestive heart failure (1point)
- H = hypertension (1 point)
- A = age older than 75 (1 point)
- D = DM (1 point)
- S2 = history of stroke or transient ischemic attack (TIA) (2 points).

In a large validation cohort the estimated risk of stroke per year based on CHADS2 score is shown in Table 62-3. A limitation of the CHADS2 score applies to secondary prevention in patients with prior stroke or TIA and no other risk factors.[32] Therefore, recently CHA2DS2-VASc index was developed to further refine the risk calculation of CHADS2 by including additional variables of Vascular Disease, Age > 65 and female gender.[33,34]

The score is calculated as below:

- C = congestive heart failure (1 point)
- H = hypertension (1 point)
- A2 = age older than 75 (2 point)
- D = DM (1 point)
- S2 = history of stroke or transient ischemic attack (TIA) (2 points)
- V = vascular disease (previous myocardial infarction, peripheral artery disease, aortic plaque) (1 point)
- Age = 65–74 (1 point)
- Sex = female (1 point).

The estimated risk of stroke per year based on CHA2DS2-VASc score is shown in Table 62-4.[33,34]

TABLE 62-5 HAS-BLED Score for Bleeding Risk on Anticoagulation[36]

HAS-BLED Score*	Bleeding Risk (% per 100 patient-years
0	1.2
1	2.8
2	3.6
3	6.0
4	9.5
5	7.4

*For HAS-BLED (Hypertension, abnormal renal/liver function, stroke, bleeding history or predisposition, labile international normalized ratio, elderly, drugs/alcohol concomitantly) score and validation see Pisters R, Lane DA, Nieuwlaat R, de Vos CB, Crijns HJ, Lip GY. A novel user-friendly score (HAS-BLED) to assess 1-year risk of major bleeding in patients with atrial fibrillation: The Euro Heart Survey. *Chest.* 2010;138:1093–1100. Level of Evidence Class IIb.

The short-term risk of stroke recurrence after an acute stroke in patients with AF is about 5% in 2 weeks which is a value much lower than previously considered.[35]

The goal of anticoagulation is to prevent ischemic events but also to minimize the risk of bleeding related to anticoagulation. In this regard HAS-BLED score was developed to predict risk of hemorrhage in patients on anticoagulation.

The score is calculated as below:

- H = history of uncontrolled hypertension (>160 mm Hg)
- A = abnormal renal/liver function (one point for presence of renal or liver impairment, maximum two points)
- S = stroke (previous history, particularly lacunar)
- B = bleeding history or predisposition (anemia)
- L = labile international normalized ratio (INR) (i.e., therapeutic time in range, 60%)
- E = elderly (>65 years)
- D = drugs/alcohol concomitantly (antiplatelet agents, non-steroidal anti-inflammatory drugs; one point for drugs plus one point for alcohol excess, maximum two points).

The estimated risk of bleeding events per 100 patient-years based on HAS-BLED score is shown in Table 62-5.[36,37]

Long-term Monitoring for Detection of Atrial Fibrillation

The risk of stroke recurrence as highlighted above makes it imperative to diagnose AF promptly to provide effective stroke prevention therapy. Paroxysmal AF (PAF) is a major hindrance in achieving this goal and has been suggested as a cause for cryptogenic strokes.[38] Brief asymptomatic PAF events may remain undetected by traditional methods of screening. Recent technological advances have made it possible to perform long-term invasive and non-invasive cardiac rhythm monitoring up to months or even years after a stroke.[39] The diagnostic yield of these monitoring strategies is high (an average of 11.5%; 95% confidence interval [CI], 8.9–14.3%) and enables detection of AF in large number of cryptogenic stroke patients.[39–42] The currently underway CRYSTAL-AF study is investigating the value of longer-term monitoring with an implantable loop recorder in patients with cryptogenic stroke.[43] Moreover, IMPACT study is also evaluating the impact of therapeutic intervention implied after detection of these events which is the final goal of any diagnostic evaluation in secondary stroke prevention.[44]

Stroke Prevention in Atrial Fibrillation

The efficacy of antithrombotic therapies to prevent stroke in non-valvular AF has been well established by randomized clinical trials. An aggregate analysis showed that anticoagulation with warfarin reduces ischemic stroke by 64% in comparison with the rate in untreated patients, and an efficacy analysis indicated an even greater benefit. Warfarin was effective in preventing disabling stroke by 59% and non-disabling stroke by 61%. The absolute risk reduction in all strokes by the use of warfarin was 2.7% per year for primary prevention (NNT for 1 year to prevent one stroke = 37) and 8.4% per year for secondary prevention (NNT = 12).[45] When only ischemic strokes were considered, adjusted-dose warfarin was associated with a 67% relative risk reduction (RRR) (95%CI, 54–77%). In addition, the increase in rate of major bleeding among elderly patients with AF undergoing anticoagulation in these trials was only 0.3–2.0% per year with a target international normalized ratio (INR) of 1.5–4.0. The risk of major hemorrhage in elderly patients with AF who are taking oral anticoagulants seems to be related to the intensity of anticoagulation, patient age, and fluctuation in INR.[46]

The efficacy of aspirin, with doses ranging from 50 to 1300 mg per day, for stroke prevention in patients with AF has been tested in eight trials that included 4876 participants. Comparing aspirin alone with placebo or no treatment, aspirin was associated with a 19% reduction in incidence of stroke (95%CI, 1–35%). For primary prevention, there was an absolute risk reduction of 0.8% per year (NNT = 125) and for secondary prevention trials a reduction of 2.5% per year (NNT = 40). When only ischemic strokes are considered, aspirin results in a 21% reduction in strokes (95%CI, 1–38%). When all antiplatelet agents are considered, stroke was reduced by 22% (95%CI, 6–35%).[45]

Eight trials compared warfarin and other vitamin K antagonists with various dosages of aspirin, other antiplatelet agents in three trials and aspirin combined with low-fixed-dose warfarin in two trials. For the 11 trials that compared adjusted-dose warfarin with antiplatelet therapy alone, warfarin was associated with a 37% reduction in strokes (95%CI, 23–48%).[45] In the Atrial fibrillation Clopidogrel Trial with Irbesartan for prevention of Vascular Events (ACTIVE-W), anticoagulation therapy was superior to the combination clopidogrel plus aspirin (RRR, 40%; 95%CI, 18–56%).[47] The risk of intracranial hemorrhage with adjusted-dose warfarin was double that with aspirin. The absolute risk increase, however, was small (0.2% per year).[45]

Unquestionably, warfarin is highly efficacious for preventing stroke in patients with AF and relatively safe for selected patients. Aspirin offers less benefit, possibly by decreasing non-cardioembolic strokes in these patients. The choice of antithrombotic prophylaxis is based on the risk stratification (see Tables 62-3 and 62-4). Long-term anticoagulation cannot be recommended for all unselected patients with AF, because most of them would not experience strokes even if untreated. Patients with AF with a relatively low risk of subsequent stroke would not substantially benefit from the use of warfarin, because the absolute risk reduction would be small (RRR, 1% per year). In these patients, anticoagulation may not be warranted. On the contrary, patients with AF who have a high risk for ischemic stroke (higher than 7%) because of a history of hypertension, prior TIA or stroke, or ventricular dysfunction would have a significantly lower stroke rate if they received anticoagulation.[48]

High-risk patients who are good candidates for anticoagulation realize remarkable benefit from warfarin. For high-risk patients 75 years or younger, a target INR of 2.5 (range, 2.0–3.0) is effective and safe; for those older than 75 years, choosing a slightly lower target (INR 2.0–2.5), with the hope of minimizing bleeding complications, appears appropriate. Patients younger than 60 years with "lone AF" may not require long-term anticoagulation, and because their intrinsic risk for stroke is small, aspirin may be sufficient.

Paroxysmal atrial fibrillation (PAF), with underlying causes similar to those in sustained or constant AF, constitutes between 25% and 60% of all cases of AF.[49] Epidemiologic data have suggested that the risk of stroke for patients with PAF is intermediate between those of patients with constant AF and patients with sinus rhythm. However, when data are controlled for stroke risk factors, PAF involves a stroke risk similar to that of constant AF.[50] The risk–benefit ratio for antithrombotic therapy in patients with PAF has not been evaluated in clinical trials. Therefore, the recommendations are based on indirect data from AF trials, so the approach to patients with PAF should be the same as that to patients with sustained AF.[49]

Warfarin Combined with Antiplatelet Agents

The risks and benefits of combination of an oral anticoagulant and an antiplatelet agent compared with an oral anticoagulant alone for secondary prevention of cardioembolic stroke have not been clearly established. Turpie et al. studied young patients with prosthetic valves and showed a significant reduction of embolic events in those assigned to combination therapy and no significant increase in the incidence of ICH (seven patients vs three patients, respectively).[51] However, in view of the occurrence of only a few events and the patients' ages, these results cannot be generalized to different groups of patients (i.e., elderly with established cerebrovascular disease).

Recent meta-analyses comparing warfarin plus antiplatelet with warfarin alone in different populations found that the addition of antiplatelets to warfarin significantly increased the risk of ICH specially in elderly populations and risk–benefit ratio of combination therapy was higher for elderly patients with prior ischemic strokes than that for young patients with prosthetic valvular disease.[52,53] This becomes a major issue in patients who undergo coronary artery stenting and require dual-antiplatelet therapy for drug-eluting stents and also have indication for anticoagulation due to atrial fibrillation. WOEST trial addressed this particular dilemma and found that the risk of bleeding complications is highest with triple therapy and recommended using clopidogrel for warfarin in patients with coronary stents and need for anticoagulation.[54]

NEW ANTITHROMBOTIC AGENTS

Although warfarin is highly efficacious in preventing systemic emboli in AF patients, its use is restricted by the narrow therapeutic window, multiple drug interactions, and the need for permanent INR monitoring.[55] Consequently, owing to the inherent limitations for the use of oral anticoagulants in patients with AF, there is a need to develop and test novel antithrombotic agents with a much safer profile and wider therapeutic window than warfarin.

Recently three new oral anticoagulants dabigatran, rivaroxaban and apixaban have been approved by FDA for use in non-valvular atrial fibrillation patients[48,56] (Table 62-6).

Dabigatran

Dabigatran etexilate is an oral pro-drug that is converted to dabigatran, a direct, competitive inhibitor of factor IIa (thrombin). The Randomized Evaluation of Long-Term Anticoagulation Therapy (RE-LY) compared open-label warfarin with two fixed, blinded doses of dabigatran (110 mg or 150 mg twice daily) in patients with AF and at least one additional stroke risk factor (previous stroke or TIA, left ventricular ejection fraction <40%, New York Heart Association heart

TABLE 62-6 Novel Anticoagulant Agents for Prevention of Stroke in Atrial Fibrillation

Drug	Target	Dosing	Onset (h)	Half-Life (h)	Antidote
Apixaban	Factor Xa	Twice a day	3	12	No
Rivaroxaban	Factor Xa	Once a day	3	9	No
Dabigatran	Thrombin	Twice a day	1-2	12-17	No

failure classification of II or higher, age ≥75 years, or age 65-74 years plus diabetes mellitus, hypertension, or coronary artery disease). The primary outcome was stroke or systemic embolism; secondary outcomes included stroke, systemic embolism, and death. The primary safety outcome was major hemorrhage. A net clinical benefit was defined as an unweighted composite of stroke, systemic embolism, pulmonary embolism, MI, death, or major hemorrhage.[57]

For the primary outcome of stroke or systemic embolism, both dabigatran 110 mg twice daily (1.53% per year) and dabigatran 150 mg twice daily (1.11% per year) were non-inferior to warfarin (1.69% per year); dabigatran 150 mg twice daily was also superior to warfarin (RR, 0.66; 95%CI, 0.53-0.82). Compared with warfarin, the risk of hemorrhagic stroke was lower with both dabigatran 110 mg twice daily (RR, 0.31; 95%CI, 0.17-0.56) and dabigatran 150 mg twice daily (RR, 0.26; 95%CI, 0.14-0.49).

Major bleeding in RE-LY was lower with dabigatran 110 mg twice daily (2.71% per year; RR, 0.80; 95%CI, 0.69-0.93), but similar for dabigatran 150 mg twice daily (3.11% per year; RR, 0.93; 95%CI, 0.81-1.07) compared with warfarin (3.36% per year).[58] The rate of gastrointestinal bleeding was higher with dabigatran 150 mg twice daily (1.51% per year) than with warfarin (1.02% per year) or dabigatran 110 mg twice daily (1.12% per year; $P < 0.05$).[58] Rates of life-threatening and intracranial bleeding, respectively, were higher with warfarin (1.80% and 0.74%) than with either dabigatran 110 mg twice daily (1.22% and 0.23%) or dabigatran 150 mg twice daily (1.45% and 0.30%).[57]

It is interesting to note that Food and Drug Administration (FDA) only approved the 150 mg twice daily dose and the 75 mg twice daily regimen for patients with low creatinine clearance (15-30 mL/min). This decision raised comment in the medical community, since the 110 mg twice daily dose was approved both in Canada and Europe.[58] Moreover, the 110 mg twice daily dose showed better safety profile in terms of bleeding events, as mentioned earlier.[57] The 75 mg twice daily dose was approved only on pharmacokinetic and pharmacodynamics modeling.[48] FDA responded to this concern by highlighting the superiority of the 150 mg twice daily dose over warfarin, assuming normal renal function.[59]

Measuring the anticoagulant effect of dabigatran is difficult. Activated partial thromboplastin time, endogenous thrombin potential lag time, thrombin time, and ecarin clotting time can be used.[60] Ecarin clotting time is a clinical assay which can be used to measure the thrombin activity and subsequently is affected by thrombin inhibitors.[60]

Activated recombinant factor VIIa or purified factor replacement products have been proposed for reversal of dabigatran.[61] Emergency dialysis for rapid reversal of the antithrombotic effect has been recommended.[61] However, there are limited data and there is no widespread consensus on the reversal techniques at this point.[62,63]

Rivaroxaban

Rivaroxaban is a direct factor Xa inhibitor. The Rivaroxaban vs Warfarin in Non valvular Atrial Fibrillation (ROCKET AF) Trial was a double-blind non inferiority trial in randomized patients with non-valvular AF who were at moderate-to-high risk of stroke to rivaroxaban (20 mg/d) or warfarin.[64] The primary end point was the composite of ischemic and hemorrhagic stroke and systemic embolism.

In the rivaroxaban group 1.7% of subjects per year reached the primary end point as compared to 2.2% per year in the warfarin group (HR, 0.79; 95%CI, 0.66-0.96; $P < 0.001$ for non-inferiority). The primary safety end point was a composite of major and non-major clinically relevant bleeding. Primary safety end point occurred in 14.9% of patients per year in the rivaroxaban group and 14.5% in the warfarin group (HR, 1.03; 95%CI, 0.96-1.11; $P = 0.44$). Lower rates of intracranial hemorrhage (0.5% vs 0.7%; $P = 0.02$) and fatal bleeding (0.2% vs 0.5%; $P = 0.003$) occurred in the rivaroxaban group than in the warfarin group.[64]

J-ROCKET AF (Japanese Rivaroxaban Once daily oral direct factor Xa inhibition Compared with vitamin K antagonism for prevention of stroke and Embolism Trial in Atrial Fibrillation) was a prospective, randomized, double-blind phase 3 study in Japanese subjects with AF.[65] This study evaluated the safety of rivaroxaban 15 mg once daily (10 mg daily in patients with moderate renal impairment) vs dose-adjusted warfarin. The primary safety end point in J-ROCKET was the time to first major or non-major clinically relevant bleeding event in both the rivaroxaban and warfarin arms. There were 11 vs 22 bleeding events in the rivaroxaban and warfarin arms, respectively (1.26 vs 2.61 events per 100 patients per year; HR, 0.48; 95%CI, 0.23-1.00).[65]

The effect of rivaroxaban can be measured through prothrombin time, endogenous thrombin potential and anti-thrombin activity.[66] Thrombelastography can also be used to detect the activity of thrombin inhibitors for emergent decisions such as intravenous thrombolysis in acute stroke patients.[67] Prothrombin complex concentrate has been reported to reverse the effect of rivaroxaban.[62] Caution is advised regarding these reversal strategies as their clinical efficacy hasn't been adequately evaluated.

Apixaban

Apixaban is a direct and competitive factor Xa inhibitor. The Apixaban Versus Acetylsalicylic Acid to Prevent Strokes in Atrial Fibrillation Patients Who Have Failed or Are Unsuitable for Vitamin K Antagonist Treatment (AVERROES) trial was a randomized, double-blind trial comparing the efficacy and safety of apixaban to aspirin in patients with non-valvular AF who were unsuitable for vitamin K antagonist therapy primarily on the basis of physician judgment or patient preference.[68]

The dose tested was 5 mg twice daily (94%) or 2.5 mg twice daily (6%). The dose of aspirin was 81 mg (64%), 162 mg (27%), 243 mg (2%), or 324 mg (7%) at the discretion of the investigator. The study was terminated when an interim analysis found that apixaban was superior to aspirin for prevention of stroke or systemic embolism (1.6% per year vs 3.7% per year; HR, 0.45; 95%CI, 0.32-0.62) with a similar rate of major bleeding (1.4% per year vs 1.2% per year; HR, 1.13; 95%CI, 0.74-1.75). Apixaban was superior to aspirin in preventing a disabling or fatal stroke (1% per year vs 2.3% per year; HR, 0.43; 95%CI 0.28-0.65). The net clinical benefit, a composite outcome of stroke, systemic embolism, MI, death of a vascular cause or major bleeding, supported apixaban as being superior to aspirin (5.3% per year vs 7.2% per year; HR, 0.74; 95%CI, 0.6–0.9).[68]

The ARISTOTLE trial was a phase 3 randomized trial comparing apixaban to warfarin for the prevention of stroke (ischemic or hemorrhagic) or systemic embolization among patients with AF or atrial flutter.[69] The doses tested were 5 mg twice daily as well as 2.5 mg twice daily. Warfarin dose was adjusted to achieve a therapeutic INR of 2.0–3.0. Additionally, patients in both groups were permitted to receive up to 162 mg of aspirin daily if clinically indicated.

In the apixaban group 1.27% of the patients experienced the primary outcome of stroke or systemic embolization compared with 1.60% of warfarin group (HR, 0.79; 95%CI, 0.66–0.95). Both non inferiority ($P < 0.001$) and superiority ($P = 0.01$) of apixaban were demonstrated.[69] There was significant reduction in hemorrhagic stroke (49% reduction) compared with ischemic or uncertain types of stroke (8% reduction). Secondary end points of death (3.52% vs 3.94%; HR, 0.89; 95%CI, 0.80–0.99; $P = 0.047$) and major bleeding (2.13% vs 3.09%; HR, 0.69; 95%CI, 0.60–0.80; $P < 0.001$) favored apixaban.[69]

Comparison of New Oral Anticoagulants

There is no direct comparison between the anticoagulants. However, some features distinguish these new oral anticoagulants from each other.

The rate of myocardial infarction appears to be slightly higher with dabigatran than with warfarin.[70] Moreover, gastrointestinal bleeding was higher with both dabigatran and rivaroxaban than with warfarin.[57,64] Apixaban use was not associated with higher gastrointestinal bleeding as compared to warfarin.[69] Dabigatran (150 mg twice daily) reduced both the rates of hemorrhagic and ischemic stroke compared with warfarin.[57] Apixaban, in addition to reduction of hemorrhagic and ischemic stroke also reduced major systemic bleeding.[69]

Patients who are non-compliant with warfarin should not be switched to the new agents because missed doses of these short-acting anticoagulants have the potential to be more detrimental than missed doses of warfarin, which has a half-life of several days.[71] Patients who prefer once-daily drugs, or are poorly compliant with twice-daily dosing regimens, can be prescribed rivaroxaban. Patients with hepatic dysfunction should not be given the new anticoagulants because all three agents undergo some degree of hepatic metabolism.

It has been theorized that the reversal of AF and maintenance of sinus rhythm might reduce the risk of stroke. The Atrial Fibrillation Follow-up Investigation of Rhythm Management (AFFIRM) study compared the outcomes of patients with AF randomly assigned to treatment with a rhythm-control strategy and with a rate-control strategy.[72] One objective of this study was to describe any differences in stroke occurrence in the two groups. The AFFIRM study was designed to compare mortality rates of patients managed with rate control only and those managed with rhythm control utilizing cardioversion and pharmacologic efforts along with anticoagulation. The rate-control and rhythm-control groups did not differ significantly in the primary endpoint, that is, mortality ($P = 0.078$).[72] At 5 years, 94% of patients in both treatment arms remained free of ischemic stroke.[73] Treatment assignment had no significant effect on the occurrence of ischemic stroke.

CARDIOMYOPATHIES

A cardiomyopathy is the second most common cause of cardiogenic stroke after AF, with a threefold increase in relative risk.[74]

The ejection fraction (EF) is a reliable measurement of left ventricular function, with the normal value between 50% and 70%. A decline in EF produces an elevated left ventricular filling pressure and a drop in stroke volume with a consequent reduction of systemic blood flow. The reduced stroke volume creates relative stasis within the left ventricle that promotes thrombus formation and an increased risk of thromboembolic events. Cardiomyopathies can be dilated or hypertrophic. Dilated cardiomyopathy is present if the diastolic dimension of the left ventricle becomes enlarged and hypertrophic when wall thickness is increased.

In patients with CHF who are treated with aspirin or warfarin, the aggregate stroke risk per year has been found to be between 1% and 4%.[75,76] The stroke rate was inversely proportional to the EF in two studies.[75,77] In the Survival And Ventricular Enlargement trial (SAVE) trial, patients with EF of 32% had a stroke rate of 1% per year; with an EF of 28% or less, the rate increased up to 2% per year. This translates into an 18% increment in the risk of stroke for every 5% decline in EF.[77]

Ventricular thrombus formation occurs in about 30–50% of patients with dilated cardiomyopathy.[78] The underlying mechanism for thrombus formation in patients with dilated cardiomyopathy is probably complex and multifactorial, including mechanical factors such as low velocity in the left ventricle and activation of hemostatic factors.[79,80] The intracavitary flow velocity is chronically reduced in these patients; therefore the risk of thrombus formation is constant.

The Study of Left Ventricular Dysfunction (SOLVD) clarified the relation between embolic stroke risk and worsening ventricular function.[75] In SOLVD, warfarin and aspirin were associated with a lower rate of death or hospitalization for heart failure than aspirin, but only warfarin reduced death from worsening heart failure. Although embolic stroke risk when left ventricular EF declines below 28% is double that for a value of 35%, patients with the lower values also benefit from aspirin alone (56% RRR in SAVE trial[77]) and without the bleeding complications.

The Warfarin and Aspirin Therapy in Chronic Heart Failure (WATCH) trial compared aspirin 160 mg/day, clopidogrel 75 mg/day, and warfarin (INR 2.5–3.0) in patients with poor LV function.[81] The primary composite outcome of time to first occurrence of death, non-fatal myocardial infarction, or non-fatal stroke was not significantly different between the groups ($P = 0.57$).[81] Although the rate of nonfatal ischemic strokes was lower in the Warfarin group than aspirin, this benefit was offset by higher bleeding complications in the Warfarin group.[81]

The Warfarin vs Aspirin in patients with Reduced Cardiac Ejection Fraction (WARCEF) trial was a randomized, double-blind, multicenter trial studying the efficacy of warfarin (INR, 2.5–3.0; target, 2.75) vs aspirin (325 mg per day) in all-cause mortality and stroke (both ischemic and hemorrhagic) in patients with left ventricular EF of 35% or less.[82] The rates of the primary outcome were not significantly different between the two groups ($P = 0.40$).[82]

In the light of these trials oral anticoagulation (INR intensity, 2.0–3.0) in patient with severe heart failure should be reserved for those with AF and previous episodes of thromboembolism (systemic or pulmonary embolism), or documented left ventricular thrombus. However, certain high-risk patients with stroke and imaging suggestive of cardioembolism may be considered for anticoagulation but such decisions should be made on an individual basis with extensive discussion with the patient about the risk and benefit of such an approach.

MYOCARDIAL INFARCTION

The stroke rate in survivors of MI is about 1–2% per year. The risk of stroke is particularly high during the first 3 months after MI.[83,84]

The use of long-term anticoagulants after MI is associated with a 75% risk reduction in the incidence of stroke; however, this value represents an absolute risk reduction of only 1% per year. At the same time, anticoagulation (INR, 2.5–4.5) has an associated tenfold higher risk of intracerebral hemorrhage (ICH), or 0.4% per year. In addition, ICHs have a higher mortality and are more disabling than ischemic strokes.[85] In summary, we would need to treat 1000 unselected MI survivors to prevent approximately ten strokes per year, and of those 1000 patients treated, four would suffer a disabling or fatal ICH; therefore, the net benefit is minimal. Aspirin reduces the incidence of stroke in patients with prior MI, with an RRR of 30%, but a very small absolute risk reduction (less than 0.5%). Because of such small net benefit, oral anticoagulation cannot be routinely recommended to prevent stroke in unselected MI survivors.

There are, however, specific subsets of patients with prior MI who are at higher risk of ischemic stroke and benefit from anticoagulation. Patients suffering anterior wall MI have a higher risk for stroke than patients with MI in other locations.[86] The presence of left ventricular thrombi after MI is associated with a much higher incidence of embolic stroke (approximately 5–10% over the following 6 to 12 months).[87] Left ventricular mural thrombus occurs in 20% of all MIs and up to 40% of anterior infarctions involving the apex. Formation of mural thrombi is almost exclusively limited to mural infarctions.[88]

The risk of thromboembolism is greatest in the first week after infarction.[89] The presence of thrombus mobility, proximity to a hypokinetic segment, and protrusion appear to raise the risk of embolism.[90] Additional risk factors predisposing to thrombus formation are EF less than 35%, apical dyskinesia, and anterior infarction.[90] In short, when ventricular thrombus is present, anticoagulants reduce the stroke risk by 60%. Therefore, anticoagulation therapy is indicated for 3–6 months after detection of ventricular thrombi. Chronic thrombi (more than 6 months old) have less emboligenic potential, so anticoagulation after this period would be reasonable only for a patient in whom a thrombus is mobile or protruding.[91]

The presence of AF in MI survivors markedly raises the risk for embolic stroke.[92] Therefore, anticoagulation is routinely recommended in this situation. Patients who experience anterior wall myocardial infarction and are found to have ventricular wall thrombus should receive warfarin therapy, aiming for an INR ranging from 2 to 3, for up to 6 months. Prolonged anticoagulation decreased stroke risk up to 40% over 3 years in the Anticoagulants in the Secondary Prevention of Events in Coronary Thrombosis (ASPECT) trial, although major bleeding complications were increased.[93] Therefore, aspirin should be used after 6 months.

In summary, oral anticoagulation (INR, 2.5–4.8) to prevent stroke does not substantially benefit unselected patients with acute MI. Patients with prior MI and AF or acute left ventricular thrombi are at higher risk of embolic stroke; anticoagulation (INR, 2.0–3.0) is routinely recommended for stroke prevention in these patients. On the basis of the available evidence, oral anticoagulation in the patient with left ventricular thrombus should be administered for at least 6 months; the patient should then be reassessed for the presence and characteristics of left ventricular thrombi by means of echocardiography.

VALVULAR HEART DISEASE

Before the use of surgical replacement of heart valves, valvular disease, especially rheumatic mitral valve disease, was associated with a very high risk of systemic emboli. Now almost all the patients with congenital or acquired valvular disease undergo surgical implantation of prosthetic heart valves. Hence, for most patients with valvular heart disease, the requirement for antithrombotic therapy depends on the thromboembolic risk associated with valve replacement. Data on antithrombotic therapy in patients with native valvular disease is limited, and all published recommendations are based on clinical experience.

Lambl's excrescence (GLE) and valvular strands consists of valvular abnormalities that have a frond-like appearance and a stalk-like attachment that arises mostly from left-sided valvular surfaces (aortic more than mitral) and are of unclear cause (neoplastic, hamartomatous, or reparative).[94] Embolic risk is difficult to quantify for GLE but appears directly proportional to size and mobility. Medical therapy is typically an antiplatelet agent first, and if recurrent cerebral ischemic events occur, anticoagulation or surgical resection is considered for large (more than 1 cm), mobile lesions.[95,96]

Rheumatic Mitral Valve Disease

Of all native valvular diseases, rheumatic mitral valve disease carries the highest risk of systemic emboli. The incidence of systemic emboli ranges from 2% to 5% per year.[97] In short, it can be assumed that a patient with rheumatic mitral valve disease has at least one chance in five of having a symptomatic systemic embolus during his or her life.[97] Mitral stenosis carries a higher risk of embolization than mitral regurgitation, and the presence of AF increases the risk of embolism by about sevenfold.[97] In addition, the risk of systemic emboli in patients with rheumatic heart disease increases with age and is higher in those with associated low EF.[97] After a first episode of embolization, recurrent emboli occur in 30–65% of patients; more than half of recurrences are seen during the first year, most during the first 6 months.[97]

Although long-term anticoagulation was never examined in randomized trials in this population, observational studies have established the effectiveness of this intervention in reducing systemic emboli. In view of these data, all patients with rheumatic mitral valve disease and AF should be treated with long-term anticoagulation if possible. Patients with rheumatic heart disease and prior ischemic stroke should also receive anticoagulation in view of the high recurrence rate.[97] The recommended intensity of anticoagulation is a target INR of 2.5. If recurrent embolism occurs despite adequate anticoagulation, the target INR should be increased to 3.0 or aspirin, 81 mg per day, should be added.

PROSTHETIC CARDIAC VALVES

Systemic embolism is a serious threat in patients who have undergone heart valve replacement. The rate of embolism is high in patients with mechanical prosthetic cardiac valves, being 2% per year even in those with proper anticoagulation.[98] Embolism occurs at estimated rates of 0.5% per year with prosthetic aortic valves, 1% per year with mitral valves, and 1.5% per year for both.[98] Embolism is more frequent with valves in the mitral position, with multiple valves, and with caged-ball valves. Atrial stasis, a risk factor for thrombogenicity, is influenced by valve type and position, coexistent AF, and ventricular pacemakers. AF and enlargement of the left atrium are more common in patients with mitral valve disease.[98]

Permanent anticoagulation is generally recommended to prevent embolic stroke and valve thrombosis with all mechanical prosthetic valves. In addition, anticoagulation is also recommended for bioprosthetic valves in the mitral position in the first 3 months post-operatively. Aspirin can replace anticoagulation after 3 months provided that the patient doesn't have AF, enlarged (more than 55 mm) left atrium, ventricular pacemakers, or evidence of atrial thrombi or prior thromboembolism.[99] Anticoagulation may not be required for bioprosthetic valves in the aortic position in patients with sinus rhythm because the stroke rate is relatively low.[99]

In the past, the intensity of anticoagulation for mechanical valves was a target INR between 3.0 and 4.5. Now it is believed that a lower intensity (INR, 2.0–3.0) for aortic mechanical valves and (INR 2.5–3.5) for mitral mechanical valves would be as effective.[99] Adding an antiplatelet agent such as aspirin to warfarin further reduces embolism risk in mitral mechanical valves; however, this therapeutic strategy may raise the risk of bleeding (mostly minor bleeds when aspirin is added).[99]

The success of antithrombotic therapy in primary stroke prevention in patients with prosthetic valves is influenced by the type of prosthesis, factors associated with left atrial stasis, underlying cardiovascular disease, and tolerability of antithrombotic therapies. The optimal or appropriate intensity of anticoagulation and the decision to use additional antiplatelet agents in individual patients depend on the presence of some of the previously mentioned risk factors and the valve type.

The current recommendations are as follows: Oral anticoagulation with a target INR between 2 and 3 should be used in all patients with mechanical prosthetic valves (St. Jude Medical bileaflet valve or Medtronic ball tilting disk mechanical valve) in the aortic position and with sinus rhythm. For patients with tilting disk valves and bileaflet mechanical valves in the mitral position, the intensity of anticoagulation is a target INR of 2.5 to 3.5. Addition of antiplatelet (low dose aspirin) therapy to both the aortic and mitral mechanical valves is recommended if the bleeding risk is low.[99]

In patients with full anticoagulation, the incidence of stroke is about 1% per year and most of the emboli are minor, leaving mild residual deficits.[99] When stroke occurs in patients receiving anticoagulation, transesophageal echocardiography (TEE) should usually be performed to search for infective valve vegetations, thrombi, spontaneous echodensities, and atrial thrombi.[100] Anticoagulation may be increased if embolism from the left atrium is suspected, but adding an antiplatelet agent might be useful if the stroke is attributed to cerebrovascular disease or valve-related thrombi.[99]

In patients at high risk of thromboembolism, the interruption of anticoagulant therapy before invasive procedures often presents a challenge to clinicians. It is recommended that warfarin therapy be stopped approximately 5 days before surgery, allowing the INR to return to a normal level. Full-dose LMW heparin is begun as the INR falls (about 2 days before surgery). The LMW heparin can be stopped about 6 hours before surgery and restarted between 8 and 12 hours after the procedure.[101]

NON-BACTERIAL THROMBOTIC ENDOCARDITIS

Non-bacterial thrombotic endocarditis (NBTE) or marantic endocarditis is a non-infectious process affecting normal or degenerative cardiac valves that is due to fibrin thrombi deposits in patients with hypercoagulable states associated with adenocarcinomas of the lung, colon, or pancreas that produce mucin.[99,102] Patients with NBTE may present with arterial and venous thromboembolism and disseminated intravascular coagulation. Heparin, but not warfarin, has been associated with benefit[99,102] as well as treatment of the underlying neoplastic disorder.

Libman-Sacks endocarditis is a non-infectious valvular abnormality associated with autoimmune disorders such as systemic lupus erythematosus and the antiphospholipid antibody syndrome.[103] The choice of antiplatelet or anticoagulation doesn't affect the progression of these lesions.[103] Aspirin is recommended for primary prevention and warfarin should be reserved for patients who experience an ischemic stroke in presence of these valvular lesions.[104]

INFECTIOUS ENDOCARDITIS

Infectious seeding of heart valves or endocarditis prior to the advent of antibiotics was associated with a very high cerebral embolic rate (70–90%), which decreased (12–40%) with the advent of antibiotics.[105,106] Specific antibiotic therapy for endocarditis remains the first-line treatment on the basis of blood culture results, whereas anticoagulation remains controversial or contraindicated[105–107] given the early rates of cerebral hemorrhage and the fact that anticoagulation does not reduce the incidence of embolism in native valve endocarditis. Patients with mechanical prosthetic valves, however, may be at higher risk if anticoagulation is discontinued.[108] Controversy remains about the duration and intensity of anticoagulation in patients with prosthetic valve endocarditis, given the risk of embolism vs intracranial hemorrhage.[107] Prosthetic endocarditis also may embolize to the brain, where an infected microscopic nidus (especially when there is *Staphylococcus aureus*) or microaneurysm prone to cerebral hemorrhage may develop. The patient with prosthetic valve endocarditis may be thought of as an anticoagulation dilemma because the ischemic stroke risk must be balanced against cerebral hemorrhagic risk. We recommend careful consideration of the patient's valve type and location and presence or absence of AF to weigh the ischemic and hemorrhagic risks. For example, if the patient had a large ischemic stroke from endocarditis, anticoagulation becomes higher risk for brain hemorrhage and may need to be delayed or not administered at all.[107] Moreover, intracranial vascular imaging is helpful in risk stratification since it can reveal occult mycotic aneurysms at high risk of rupture.[109,110] An attempt should be made to treat these aneurysms before anticoagulation is considered.[107]

Early surgery was historically reserved for heart failure, uncontrolled infection and prevention of recurrent embolic events.[111] Recently there has been an increase in early elective surgery with improved outcomes particularly related to systemic embolization.[112] This approach needs to be validated in a larger randomized controlled trial before it becomes the standard of care.

CARDIAC TUMORS

Primary cardiac tumors are rare (less than 0.2% in unselected autopsy series) and the majority of them benign (50% myxomas and papillary fibroelastoma) but associated with a high frequency of embolic events. Myxomas commonly occur in the left atrium and arise from the interatrial septum. They may embolize to the systemic circulation, particularly to the brain, when tumor pieces break off or there is secondary thrombus formation. TEE is invaluable in defining tumor location, size, and morphology. To prevent embolization, surgical resection of the tumor is recommended in all cases of myxoma.[113,114]

Papillary fibroelastomas are benign tumors that tend to originate on cardiac valves in single or multiple masses. Embolic events are typically the first clinical manifestation, because they are present on highly mobile valve leaflets. The embolic mechanism is the same as myxomas, being tumor fragmentation or secondary thrombus generation. Surgical resection is also indicated for fibroelastomas.[115]

Metastatic tumors to the heart are 20–40 times more frequent than primary cardiac tumors, which are rare (e.g., angiosarcoma, rhabdomyosarcoma).[116] Cerebral embolization can occur from these tumors as well. Surgical treatment can be offered but depends on the underlying tumor type and prognosis.[116]

PATENT FORAMEN OVALE

The high frequency of patent foramen ovale (PFO) is in part the result of advances that have been made in cardiac imaging techniques. PFO has been associated with stroke in several case-control studies, particularly in young individuals without an alternative recognized cause of stroke. PFO is a potential conduit for paradoxical embolism.[117-119] However, its relationship to stroke, its prognosis, and the therapeutic implications are not clearly established. Precordial contrast echocardiography detects some interatrial shunting in about 18% of normal controls[120] especially during early systole or Valsalva maneuver–provoking activities such as coughing.[121] The fossa ovalis and the size of PFO can be directly visualized by TEE, considered the diagnostic "gold standard".[122] Transcranial Doppler (TCD) ultrasonography can detect injected microbubbles that bypass the pulmonary capillaries and enter the cerebral circulation, an observation that correlates well with the TEE evidence of PFO in the majority of patients.[123] The size of the PFO patency varies from 1 to 9 mm at autopsy.[124] The volume of shunting depends on the size of the PFO and the difference in atrial pressures.

Several studies have now shown that the prevalence of PFO in young adults with TIA or ischemic stroke has increased (about 40%; range 32–48%)[125] especially among those with cryptogenic ischemic stroke, in whom the prevalence in some series exceeds 50%.[125] The wide range of PFO prevalence may reflect in part the interobserver variability in the diagnosis of septal abnormalities. Hence, the frequency of PFO is increased twofold to threefold among young adults with cerebral ischemia, and PFO is clearly associated with cryptogenic stroke in young adults, who are less likely to have traditional risk factors for stroke. In older patients with stroke, the prevalence of PFO is lower, probably because its importance as an independent risk factor is offset by the higher prevalence of other stroke mechanisms.[126] PFO is significantly associated with ischemic stroke usually in patients younger than 55 years.[127] Because PFO is also common in normal subjects, it is important to characterize the cases associated with stroke. Therefore, it is possible that patients with PFO plus atrial septal aneurysm (ASA) constitute a subgroup of patients at increased risk of stroke.[128] An ASA is a sustained 15-mm segmental bowing of the interatrial septal membrane in the fossa ovalis of at least 11–15 mm beyond the plane of the interatrial septum or may be a phasic excursion to either side of the same distance.[128] Therefore, an ASA may be the substrate for *in-situ* thrombus to form, which later passes through the PFO (right-to left-sided circulation).

The mechanism of PFO-associated stroke is thought to be due to paradoxical embolism in many patients. Paradoxical embolism occurs when embolic material originating in the venous system or right heart chambers migrates into the systemic circulation through vascular shunts that bypass the pulmonary vasculature. However, this mechanism has been well documented in only a few cases, in which the embolus was seen in its passage through a PFO. A venous source of thromboembolism is rarely found in patients with stroke and PFO.[129,130] The failure to document a venous source does not rule out paradoxical emboli, because in many cases, deep venous thrombosis in the pelvis or legs is under-recognized.[129,130] Another potential mechanism for stroke is direct embolization from thrombi formed locally within the PFO or in an associated ASA.[130] In a prospective study of 503 patients with stroke, PFO or PFO-ASA was detected in 34% and 14% of the patients classified with cryptogenic stroke by Trial of Org 10172 in Acute Stroke Treatment (TOAST) criteria vs 12% and 4%, respectively, with stroke of known type ($P < 0.001$).[131] The study also compared 131 younger patients (less than 55 years) with 372 older patients (more than 55 years) and found that the PFO-ASA combination was more strongly associated with cryptogenic stroke in younger ($P < 0.049$) and older ($P < 0.001$) patients than with known stroke subtype.

In addition to the unclear mechanism of stroke in patients with PFO, the risk of recurrent stroke remains unsettled owing to the lack of prospective data. Studies have reported stroke recurrence between 1% and 2% in patients with PFO.[132,133] A prospective study of 581 patients with cryptogenic stroke treated with aspirin reported that at 4 years, the risk of recurrent stroke was 2% in those with PFO (n = 216), 15% in those with both PFO and ASA (n = 51), and 4% in those with neither. Only 10 patients in the study had ASA alone, and no recurrence was seen in this group. In this study, only the presence of both abnormalities was associated with a significant risk of stroke (relative risk [RR] 4; 95%CI, 1–12). PFO alone, regardless of its size, did not influence the risk of stroke.[134]

Results of the Patent Foramen Ovale in Cryptogenic Stroke Study (PICSS), a substudy of the Warfarin-Aspirin Recurrent Stroke Study (WARSS), were reported in 2002. The 630 patients first underwent TEE, which documented PFO in 34%, and then were randomly assigned to receive either warfarin (INR, 2.0) or aspirin. The stroke rates were similar for the two interventions, and the presence of PFO did not alter the event rate when associated with all or cryptogenic strokes. There was no benefit to using warfarin in patients with large PFO or in those with PFO and ASA (12% of the total).[125]

It is sensible to speculate that closure of PFO by surgical or device-mediated procedures would prevent stroke recurrence in patients with paradoxical emboli. Three major clinical trials have been published since 2012: CLOSURE I, RESPECT, and PC comparing the efficacy of medical therapy vs device closure of PFO.[135-137] CLOSURE I trial used STARFLEX device while RESPECT and PC trials sued AMPLATZER device. There was no significant difference in outcomes between the two approaches in these trials.[135-137] One of the major reasons for no significant difference being found between the two treatment groups was the low risk of recurrence in this subset of population.[135-137] The current data therefore do not support routine device closure of PFO to prevent recurrent stroke. Closure can be considered in young patients with recurrent cryptogenic stroke, deep venous thrombosis or hypercoagulable state, but such decisions should be extensively discussed with patients in light of the known risk and questionable benefits of such an approach.

In short, the role of PFO as a cause of stroke is still unsettled; therefore, the optimal treatment remains undetermined. On the basis of current evidence, every patient with stroke and PFO should receive antiplatelet therapy. In addition, if there is evidence of deep venous thrombosis, pulmonary embolism, hypercoagulable state or recurrent stroke, the use of long-term anticoagulation seems appropriate.

AORTIC ARCH DISEASE

An overlooked but a potentially serious source of embolic stroke is the aortic arch.[138] Aortic embolic events may be misclassified as cryptogenic unless adequate transesophageal echocardiography of the aorta is performed. Patients with ascending aorta or proximal arch plaques of 4 mm thickness are up to seven times more likely to have cerebral infarction than controls (14.4% vs 2%; $P < 0.001$).[138,139] For non-mobile aortic plaque, statin therapy may be protective in preventing stroke,[140] whereas uncertainty remains about the optimal antithrombotic therapy, aspirin or warfarin.[140]

ACUTE ANTICOAGULANT AGENTS

Heparin, Low-Molecular-Weight Heparin, and Heparinoids

Heparin is the most commonly used parenteral anticoagulant. Unfractionated heparin is derived from bovine lung or porcine gut tissue. A glycosaminoglycan of varying molecular weight, heparin binds to antithrombin III to inactivate factors IIa and Xa.[141] Its major anticoagulant effect comes from a unique pentasaccharide with high-affinity binding to antithrombin. Unfractionated heparin is quite heterogeneous, containing saccharides ranging in molecular weight from 5000 to 30,000 daltons. Only about one-third of the unfractionated heparin molecules have anticoagulant activity. This heterogeneity is one of the reasons for the variability in the anticoagulant effect of heparin administration among individuals.

The most common side effect of heparin administration is bleeding. Other complications are thrombocytopenia, osteoporosis, skin necrosis, alopecia, hypersensitivity reactions, and hypoaldosteronism. Thrombocytopenia is somewhat more common with heparin derived from bovine lung than from porcine gut. The thrombocytopenia is thought to occur because of the binding of immunoglobulin (Ig) G to heparin. Thrombocytopenia occurs in between 0.3% (in prophylactic use) and 2.4% (with higher therapeutic doses) of treated patients.

Low-molecular-weight heparin (LMWH) represents a fragment of a standard heparin with lower molecular weight, higher bioavailability, longer half-life, and more predictable anticoagulant effects. LMWH is said to cause fewer bleeding complications and fewer interactions with platelets, but this issue remains somewhat controversial. Heparinoids are analogues of heparin that inhibit factor Xa, have a longer half-life than unfractionated heparin, and cause fewer bleeding complications. LMWH is as effective as, if not more effective than, unfractionated heparin, has the advantage of being given in fixed subcutaneous doses, and does not require monitoring or dose adjustment.[141]

Patients who are not candidates for heparin or heparnoids due to heparin-induced thrombocytopenia (HIT) can benefit from new-generation intravenous anticoagulants.[142] Argatroban and bivalirudin are approved for the treatment of heparin-induced thrombocytopenia. Direct thrombin inhibitors cause a dose-dependent increase in the activated partial-thromboplastin time, which allows for simple monitoring. Argatroban is a synthetic direct thrombin inhibitor derived from the amino acid L-arginine that reversibly binds to the active site of thrombin, inhibiting its catalytic activity. The standard regimen is an intravenous infusion of 2 µg per kilogram of body weight per minute.[143] Bivalirudin is a hirudin analogue that binds to both the active and fibrin-binding sites of circulating and clot-bound thrombin. It is administered intravenously by continuous infusion. A regimen of 0.15 mg per kilogram per hour, adjusted for the activated partial-thromboplastin time, has been suggested.[144]

INTRACEREBRAL HEMORRHAGE ASSOCIATED WITH ANTICOAGULATION

ICH is the most serious complication of anticoagulant therapy because of its high associated mortality. Anticoagulation with INR targets between 2.5 and 4.5 increases the risk of ICH 7 to 10 times[145,146] representing an absolute rate of 1% per year in stroke-prone patients.[46] The mortality related to oral anticoagulants in patients with ICH exceeds 50%. The cerebellum is frequently involved, and simultaneous ICHs at multiple sites can occur, particularly with excessive anticoagulation. One of the unique features of intracerebral hematomas related to anticoagulation is that they can continue to enlarge for 12–24 hours; therefore, anticoagulation should be reversed immediately, even in patients with minimal deficits and small hematomas. ICH-related anticoagulation is usually managed by the following approaches:

- Cessation of anticoagulation therapy
- Administration of vitamin K; the INR is not affected for several hours, and the dose should not exceed 10 mg because higher doses lead to refractoriness to further anticoagulant therapy for days
- Administration of plasma derivatives containing vitamin-K-dependent clotting factors, such as fresh frozen plasma (FFP), cryoprecipitates and prothrombin complex concentrates (PCC).

FFP reverses anticoagulation immediately, but it has the disadvantage of requiring a large infusion to correct the INR, which could be a problem in patients with poor cardiac function. Factor concentrates (factor II, VII, IX, and X) are an alternative for patients who cannot tolerate large volume of fluids but should not be used in patients with liver failure.

The hemostatic agent recombinant activated factor VII (rFVIIa) has been used for the management of hemorrhages in the central nervous system associated with anticoagulation. In the phase 2B randomized controlled trial, Mayer et al. and the Novo Nordisk investigators studied the effect of recombinant factor VIIa (rFVIIa) on early hematoma growth.[147] Three hundred and ninety-nine patients with acute ICH were randomly assigned to placebo or to 40 µg/kg, 80 µg/kg, or 160 µg/kg of rFVIIa within 1 hour after a baseline CT scan. The primary outcome of the study was to assess hematoma growth at 24 hours. A dose-dependent effect on reducing hematoma growth was noticed, with a mean increase of 29%, 16%, 14%, and 11% in the placebo, 40 µg/kg, 80 µg/kg, and 160 µg/kg groups, respectively ($P = 0.01$). The modified Rankin Scale (mRS) performed at 90 days found 69% of placebo-treated patients dead or severely disabled (mRS = 4 to 6), compared with 49–55% for the rFVIIa-treated patients ($P = 0.004$). Mortality at 90 days was 29% for placebo-treated patients, compared with 18% for rFVIIa-treated patients. Thromboembolic events (MI or ischemic stroke) occurred in 7% of rFVIIa-treated patients, compared with 2% of placebo-treated patients ($P = 0.12$).[147]

To address safety and to find an optimal dose, Novo Nordisk and the NovoSeven Investigators completed the phase 3 Factor Seven for Acute Hemorrhagic Stroke (FAST) study in the United States and Europe, which involved 821 patients randomly assigned to receive placebo or 20 µg/kg or 80 µg/kg of rFVIIa.[148] The investigators reported reduced growth of the hematoma and a safety profile similar to results of the phase 2B study. However, the FAST study failed to confirm that rFVIIa given within 4 hours of onset improves survival or functional outcome in ICH and has not gained a U.S. Food and Drug Administration (FDA) label indication for that purpose.[148] In summary, with the available evidence, the use of rFVIIa for the management of ICH is not indicated outside clinical trials. It remains an off-label indication for this agent.

Prothrombin complex concentrate has been shown recently to be effective in warfarin reversal. Effective hemostasis was achieved in 72.4% of patients receiving PCC vs 65.4% receiving plasma. Rapid international normalized ratio reduction was achieved in 62.2% of patients receiving PCC vs 9.6% receiving plasma. The safety profile (adverse events, serious adverse events, thromboembolic events, and deaths) was similar between groups; 66 of 103 (PCC group), and 71 of 109 (plasma group) patients experienced ≥1 adverse event.[149,150]

Well-established risk factors for ICH in patients who have been receiving anticoagulants include advanced age (particularly more than 75 years), hypertension, prior ischemic stroke[151] and intensity of anticoagulation (perhaps also fluctuations in the level of anticoagulation).[152] The significance of high INR levels in influencing the development of ICH was demonstrated in an observational study and in the Stroke Prevention in Reversible Ischemia Trial (SPIRIT) study. In this study, the absolute rate of ICH was 3% per year in patients receiving anticoagulation, particularly those with INR values exceeding 4.0.[153,154]

White matter abnormalities, identified by neuroimaging studies in patients with established cerebrovascular disease, were found to be an independent risk factor for ICH associated with anticoagulation.[155,156] Small hemosiderin deposits (indicative of asymptomatic "microbleeds") are frequently detected by gradient echo MRI in patients with stroke, particularly those with small vessel disease (i.e., lacunar stroke, primary ICH, and white matter abnormalities).[157] It is likely that the presence of microbleeds predisposes to ICH in patients taking anticoagulants.[158-160] Currently, the presence of white matter abnormalities or microbleeds does not preclude the use of anticoagulants; more data are needed to stratify the risk of ICH on the basis of MRI findings. A prospective inception cohort study (CROMIS-2) is underway in UK to answer to address this issue (www.ucl.ac.uk/cromis-2).[160]

Cerebral amyloid angiography (CAA) is characterized by deposition of congophilic amyloid beta protein in cortical and leptomeningeal vessels. ICH associated with CAA is typically seen in an older individual after the age of 55 (predominantly more than 80 years), lobar, often multiple, with a tendency to be located in the posterior half of brain, and prone to recurrence.[160] It is a well-established risk factor for non-coagulopathic ICH, and this information might also apply to WICH.[160]

ANTICOAGULATION IN ACUTE CARDIOEMBOLIC STROKE

Hemorrhagic transformation is defined as the presence of petechiae or confluent petechial hemorrhage confined to the ischemic zone. It is a relatively common consequence of developing cerebral infarction, being present in about 15% of all ischemic strokes and up to 30% of cardioembolic strokes.[161-163] The proposed mechanism for hemorrhagic transformation is the distal migration or lysis of an embolus resulting in reperfusion of the ischemic tissue, which can become hemorrhagic depending on the extent of the ischemic vascular injury.

Detection of hemorrhagic transformation depends on the neuroimaging technique used. MRI with T2-weighted sequences as well as diffusion- and perfusion-weighted imaging has higher sensitivity than CT for early detection of hemorrhagic transformation.[164,165] A prospective MRI study that imaged patients 3 weeks after cardioembolic stroke reported a 60% incidence of hemorrhagic transformation.[162] Autopsy series showed hemorrhagic transformation in even higher numbers (50–70%) of patients undergoing anticoagulation.[166] The great majority of hemorrhagic transformations are asymptomatic in patients not receiving anticoagulants.

The visualization of hemorrhagic transformation in a patient with ischemic stroke is important in that it may provide guidance as to the possible underlying mechanism of stroke (i.e., cardioembolic) and may influence the selection of antithrombotic therapy. Because of the high incidence of secondary hemorrhagic transformation in patients with cardioembolic stroke, early anticoagulation is potentially risky. At present, it is impossible to formulate firm guidelines for anticoagulation in acute cardioembolic stroke because of a paucity of adequate data. The risk–benefit ratio of early anticoagulation is influenced by the specific cardioembolic source of the stroke as well as the size of the infarct.

In the past, the risk of early recurrent stroke or systemic embolism after a recent cardioembolic stroke in untreated patients was estimated to be around 10% during the first week and to be especially high during the first 5 or 6 days after an acute cardioembolic stroke.[167] However these data were not supported by later studies, in which the risk of recurrent stroke within the first 14 days of stroke in patients with AF was between 5% and 8% without anticoagulation.[35]

Pooled data from case-series and one small controlled trial suggest that heparin reduces early stroke recurrence by about 70% in patients with cardioembolic stroke. However, the higher risk of symptomatic ICH in patients in whom anticoagulation is begun early offsets the benefit conveyed by the therapy.[168] It has been shown that these patients can be safely bridged with aspirin until the target INR is achieved.[169]

The relationship between anticoagulants and clinically significant delayed hemorrhage is controversial. The occurrence and timing of asymptomatic hemorrhagic transformation do not seem to be affected by anticoagulation;[170] however, the magnitude and likelihood of associated clinical deterioration are augmented.[170] The incidence of symptomatic hemorrhagic transformation in patients receiving early anticoagulation varies widely (from 1% to 25%).[171]

Patients with a large infarct, excessive anticoagulation, and detection of hemorrhagic infarction on initial CT scan are at higher risk for symptomatic hemorrhagic transformation. Small case-series have advocated the use of anticoagulants even in patients with early CT visualization of hemorrhagic infarction.[172] It appears that hemorrhagic infarction may not be an absolute contraindication to anticoagulation, especially in individual patients who are at high risk of recurrent embolism. Given the lack of prospective studies and the relatively small number of patients in these case-series, however, early anticoagulation in hemorrhagic infarction cannot be routinely recommended without assessment of the risk of recurrent stroke. Delaying the start of anticoagulation for 1–2 weeks after detection of hemorrhagic infarction may be prudent.

For patients at relatively low risk of early stroke recurrence, including those with non-valvular AF or recent MI without associated ventricular thrombi, deferring anticoagulation for several weeks may reduce the risk of hemorrhagic deterioration, particularly for patients with moderate-to-large infarcts or uncontrolled hypertension. Initiation of anticoagulation with oral warfarin (without the use of heparin) is an alternative for these patients. Thus, the "typical" patient with ischemic stroke and AF is unlikely to benefit from initiation of anticoagulation within the first day or two, especially if the stroke is large. In the interest of management efficiency, some physicians initiate oral anticoagulation within the first day or two, assuming that therapeutic and, therefore, dangerous levels of anticoagulation will not be achieved for a few days, when the period of increased risk for symptomatic hemorrhage has past. Since there are no specific studies to address this issue, individualized care is recommended. Presence of blood products on imaging, larger infarct size, mass effect, contrast enhancement on neuroimaging indicating disruption of blood–brain barrier and leukoariaosis may be taken into consideration when deciding about anticoagulation since these factors have been associated with hemorrhagic transformation.[173,174] Moreover, newer oral anticoagulants are therapeutic immediately, in contrast to warfarin, which takes days to weeks to achieve a therapeutic effect. This should also be considered when starting treatment in these patients. Bridging is not recommended when newer oral anticoagulants are started. It has been proposed that even in the presence of hemorrhagic transformation initiation of anticoagulation does not lead to adverse outcomes but we advise caution in such an approach because of the small number of patients studied.[175] Some patients with AF might benefit from early anticoagulation because their recurrent stroke risk is increased – for example, the patient with documented thrombi in the left atrium. The randomized clinical trials that included patients with AF have not studied this subgroup and other potentially important subgroups to establish with certainty whether atrial thrombi or other predictors might identify a subpopulation at sufficiently increased risk of early stroke recurrence to justify prompt initiation of anticoagulation.[35]

For patients at high risk of recurrent embolization (i.e., mechanical prosthetic valve, intracardiac thrombus, AF with valvular disease or CHF), early anticoagulation is recommended, particularly if there are no associated risk factors for brain hemorrhage. Intravenous boluses of heparin and excessive anticoagulation should be avoided.

The value of antiplatelet agents and low-dose subcutaneous heparin in this setting has not been systematically assessed. Both could be alternatives to intravenous heparin, particularly in patients at low risk of early recurrent stroke (e.g., non-valvular AF).

Patients with prosthetic valves who are in full anticoagulation at the time of stroke represent a management challenge. Reversing anticoagulation should be considered in patients with large infarcts or with infarcts already visible on early CT scan (less than 6–12 hours). Anticoagulation is not indicated for embolic stroke secondary to infective endocarditis of native valves.

RESUMPTION OF ANTICOAGULATION IN THE PRESENCE OF INTRACEREBRAL HEMORRHAGE

The risk of ICH in the general population ranges from 0.5% to 2% per year. In patients undergoing anticoagulation, the risk of hemorrhage is about 10 times higher.[176] However, the risk of cerebral emboli in patients with major cardioembolic sources (e.g., left ventricular thrombi, prosthetic valve disease) who are without the protection offered by anticoagulation is high. Therefore, it is essential to estimate the risks and benefits of anticoagulation in this particular group of patients. So far, data are insufficient for firm recommendations to be made in these situations. Results of several small series and retrospective studies have suggested that, when absolutely necessary, resumption of oral anticoagulation after 1 or 2 weeks is associated with a low short-term risk of embolism and no major complications, worsening, or recurrence of ICH.[177,178]

The use of intravenous heparin or continuation of oral anticoagulant therapy in a patient who has ICH or a cerebral infarct with hemorrhagic transformation and a high-risk embolic source is less clear and continues to be a challenge for physicians. There are no large, prospective trials addressing the issue of when to restart anticoagulation after warfarin-associated ICH. The literature ranges from recommendations to withhold warfarin anticoagulation for 4–6 weeks[177] or 1–2 weeks[179] to the use of intravenous heparin immediately after the INR is corrected to normal.[180] The risk of thromboembolism (underlying indication to use anticoagulation) and the risk of recurrent ICH (i.e., lobar vs deep location of the initial ICH vs hemorrhagic infarct) are key factors to be considered.

When to initiate anticoagulation and whether to continue anticoagulant therapy in patients with ICH remain controversial, and it is unlikely that these important issues will be settled by a large study.[181] In view of the lack of evidence, we recommend that each case be assessed individually through balancing of the risks and benefits of the intervention.

SUMMARY

Emboli arising from the heart account for at least 20% of ischemic strokes. Cardiac sources of emboli are being detected with increasing ease with modern echocardiography and long-term cardiac rhythm monitoring. The common clinical dilemma is whether the detection of one of the "minor" cardiac sources of emboli bears any responsibility for causing a stroke in a given patient. Long-term oral anticoagulation is highly effective in preventing recurrent stroke in patients with "major" cardiac abnormalities, including AF, in patients who have received prosthetic cardiac valves and in patients with intracardiac thrombi due to MI or cardiomyopathy. In the near future, likely novel antithrombotic agents with superior safety and efficacy profile will replace warfarin as alternative agents to prevent cardioembolic stroke.

Definitions of Classes and Levels of Evidence Used

Class I: Conditions for which there is evidence for and/or general agreement that the procedure or treatment is useful and effective

Class II: Conditions for which there is conflicting evidence and/or a divergence of opinion about the usefulness/efficacy of a procedure or treatment

Class IIa: The weight of evidence or opinion is in favor of the procedure or treatment

Class IIb: Usefulness/efficacy is less well established by evidence or opinion

Class III: Conditions for which there is evidence and/or general agreement that the procedure or treatment is not useful/effective and in some cases may be harmful

THERAPEUTIC RECOMMENDATIONS

Level of Evidence A: Data derived from multiple randomized clinical trials or meta-analyses

Level of Evidence B: Data derived from a single randomized trial or non-randomized studies

Level of Evidence C: Consensus opinion of experts, case studies, or standard of care

Adapted from Furie et al.[48]

For more details refer to "Evidence box index" in the FM.

The complete reference list can be found on the companion Expert Consult website at www.expertconsult.inkling.com.

KEY REFERENCES

1. Foulkes MA, Wolf PA, Price TR, et al. The stroke data bank: Design, methods, and baseline characteristics. Stroke 1988;19: 547–54.
2. [No authors listed]. Cardiogenic brain embolism. The second report of the cerebral embolism task force. Arch Neurol 1989;46: 727–43.
4. Albers GW, Comess KA, DeRook FA, et al. Transesophageal echocardiographic findings in stroke subtypes. Stroke 1994;25: 23–8.
12. Arboix A, Vericat MC, Pujades R, et al. Cardioembolic infarction in the Sagrat Cor-Alianza Hospital of Barcelona stroke Registry. Acta Neurol Scand 1997;96:407–12.
13. Vemmos KN, Bots ML, Tsibouris PK, et al. Stroke incidence and case fatality in Southern Greece: The Arcadia Stroke Registry. Stroke 1999;30:363–70.

14. Vemmos KN, Takis CE, Georgilis K, et al. The Athens Stroke Registry: Results of a five-year hospital-based study. Cerebrovasc Dis 2000;10:133–41.
15. Lee BI, Nam HS, Heo JH, et al. Yonsei Stroke Registry. Analysis of 1,000 patients with acute cerebral infarctions. Cerebrovasc Dis 2001;12:145–51.
16. Grau AJ, Weimar C, Buggle F, et al. Risk factors, outcome, and treatment in subtypes of ischemic stroke: The German Stroke Data Bank. Stroke 2001;32:2559–66.
18. Go AS, Hylek EM, Phillips KA, et al. Prevalence of diagnosed atrial fibrillation in adults: National implications for rhythm management and stroke prevention: The anticoagulation and risk factors in atrial fibrillation (atria) study. JAMA 2001;285: 2370–5.
19. Fuster V, Ryden LE, Cannom DS, et al. 2011 ACCF/AHA/HRS focused updates incorporated into the ACC/AHA/ESC 2006 guidelines for the management of patients with atrial fibrillation: A report of the American College of Cardiology Foundation/ American Heart Association Task Force on Practice Guidelines. Circulation 2011;123:e269–367.
24. Saxena R, Lewis S, Berge E, et al. Risk of early death and recurrent stroke and effect of heparin in 3169 patients with acute ischemic stroke and atrial fibrillation in the international stroke trial. Stroke 2001;32:2333–7.
32. Gage BF, Waterman AD, Shannon W, et al. Validation of clinical classification schemes for predicting stroke: Results from the national registry of atrial fibrillation. JAMA 2001;285: 2864–70.
33. Lip GY, Nieuwlaat R, Pisters R, et al. Refining clinical risk stratification for predicting stroke and thromboembolism in atrial fibrillation using a novel risk factor-based approach: The Euro Heart Survey on atrial fibrillation. Chest 2010;137:263–72.
34. Lip GY, Frison L, Halperin JL, et al. Identifying patients at high risk for stroke despite anticoagulation: A comparison of contemporary stroke risk stratification schemes in an anticoagulated atrial fibrillation cohort. Stroke 2010;41:2731–8.
35. Hart RG, Palacio S, Pearce LA. Atrial fibrillation, stroke, and acute antithrombotic therapy: Analysis of randomized clinical trials. Stroke 2002;33:2722–7.
36. Pisters R, Lane DA, Nieuwlaat R, et al. A novel user-friendly score (HAS-BLED) to assess 1-year risk of major bleeding in patients with atrial fibrillation: The Euro Heart Survey. Chest 2010;138: 1093–100.
37. Lip GY, Frison L, Halperin JL, et al. Comparative validation of a novel risk score for predicting bleeding risk in anticoagulated patients with atrial fibrillation: The HAS-BLED (hypertension, abnormal renal/liver function, stroke, bleeding history or predisposition, labile INR, elderly, drugs/alcohol concomitantly) score. J Am Coll Cardiol 2011;57:173–80.
38. Seet RC, Friedman PA, Rabinstein AA. Prolonged rhythm monitoring for the detection of occult paroxysmal atrial fibrillation in ischemic stroke of unknown cause. Circulation 2011;124: 477–86.
39. Kishore A, Vail A, Majid A, et al. Detection of atrial fibrillation after ischemic stroke or transient ischemic attack: A systematic review and meta-analysis. Stroke 2014.
40. Ritter MA, Kochhauser S, Duning T, et al. Occult atrial fibrillation in cryptogenic stroke: Detection by 7-day electrocardiogram versus implantable cardiac monitors. Stroke 2013;44:1449–52.
41. Etgen T, Hochreiter M, Mundel M, et al. Insertable cardiac event recorder in detection of atrial fibrillation after cryptogenic stroke: An audit report. Stroke 2013;44:2007–9.
42. Flint AC, Banki NM, Ren X, et al. Detection of paroxysmal atrial fibrillation by 30-day event monitoring in cryptogenic ischemic stroke: The stroke and monitoring for PAF in real time (SMART) registry. Stroke 2012;43:2788–90.
43. Sinha AM, Diener HC, Morillo CA, et al. Cryptogenic stroke and underlying atrial fibrillation (CRYSTAL AF): Design and rationale. Am Heart J 2010;160:36–41 e31.
44. Ip J, Waldo AL, Lip GY, et al. Multicenter randomized study of anticoagulation guided by remote rhythm monitoring in patients with implantable cardioverter-defibrillator and CRT-D devices: Rationale, design, and clinical characteristics of the initially enrolled cohort the impact study. Am Heart J 2009;158:364–70, e361.
45. Hart RG, Pearce LA, Aguilar MI. Meta-analysis: Antithrombotic therapy to prevent stroke in patients who have nonvalvular atrial fibrillation. Ann Intern Med 2007;146:857–67.
46. Hart RG, Boop BS, Anderson DC. Oral anticoagulants and intracranial hemorrhage. Facts and hypotheses. Stroke 1995;26: 1471–7.
47. Investigators AWGotA, Connolly S, Pogue J, Hart R, et al. Clopidogrel plus aspirin versus oral anticoagulation for atrial fibrillation in the atrial fibrillation clopidogrel trial with irbesartan for prevention of vascular events (ACTIVE W): A randomised controlled trial. Lancet 2006;367:1903–12.
48. Furie KL, Goldstein LB, Albers GW, et al. Oral antithrombotic agents for the prevention of stroke in nonvalvular atrial fibrillation: A science advisory for healthcare professionals from the American Heart Association/American Stroke Association. Stroke 2012;43:3442–53.
49. Lip GY, Hee FL. Paroxysmal atrial fibrillation. QJM 2001;94: 665–78.
50. Hart RG, Pearce LA, Rothbart RM, et al. Stroke with intermittent atrial fibrillation: Incidence and predictors during aspirin therapy. Stroke Prevention in Atrial Fibrillation Investigators. J Am Coll Cardiol 2000;35:183–7.
52. Dentali F, Douketis JD, Lim W, et al. Combined aspirin-oral anticoagulant therapy compared with oral anticoagulant therapy alone among patients at risk for cardiovascular disease: A meta-analysis of randomized trials. Arch Intern Med 2007;167: 117–24.
53. Johnson SG, Rogers K, Delate T, et al. Outcomes associated with combined antiplatelet and anticoagulant therapy. Chest 2008; 133:948–54.
54. Dewilde WJ, Oirbans T, Verheugt FW, et al. Use of clopidogrel with or without aspirin in patients taking oral anticoagulant therapy and undergoing percutaneous coronary intervention: An open-label, randomised, controlled trial. Lancet 2013;381:1107–15.
55. Sobieraj-Teague M, O'Donnell M, Eikelboom J. New anticoagulants for atrial fibrillation. Semin Thromb Hemost 2009;35: 515–24.
56. Alberts MJ, Eikelboom JW, Hankey GJ. Antithrombotic therapy for stroke prevention in non-valvular atrial fibrillation. Lancet Neurol 2012;11:1066–81.
57. Connolly SJ, Ezekowitz MD, Yusuf S, et al. Dabigatran versus warfarin in patients with atrial fibrillation. New Engl J Med 2009;361:1139–51.
58. Kowey PR, Naccarelli GV. The food and drug administration decision not to approve the 110 mg dose of dabigatran: Give us a way out. Am J Med 2012;125:732.
59. Beasley BN, Unger EF, Temple R. Anticoagulant options – why the FDA approved a higher but not a lower dose of dabigatran. New Engl J Med 2011;364:1788–90.
60. van Ryn J, Stangier J, Haertter S, et al. Dabigatran etexilate – a novel, reversible, oral direct thrombin inhibitor: Interpretation of coagulation assays and reversal of anticoagulant activity. Thromb Heamost 2010;103:1116–27.
61. Cotton BA, McCarthy JJ, Holcomb JB. Acutely injured patients on dabigatran. New Engl J Med 2011;365:2039–40.
62. Eerenberg ES, Kamphuisen PW, Sijpkens MK, et al. Reversal of rivaroxaban and dabigatran by prothrombin complex concentrate: A randomized, placebo-controlled, crossover study in healthy subjects. Circulation 2011;124:1573–9.
63. Weitz JI, Quinlan DJ, Eikelboom JW. Periprocedural management and approach to bleeding in patients taking dabigatran. Circulation 2012;126:2428–32.
64. Patel MR, Mahaffey KW, Garg J, et al. Rivaroxaban versus warfarin in nonvalvular atrial fibrillation. New Engl J Med 2011;365: 883–91.
65. Hori M, Matsumoto M, Tanahashi N, et al. Rivaroxaban vs. Warfarin in Japanese patients with atrial fibrillation – the J-ROCKET AF study. Circ J 2012;76:2104–11.
66. Steiner T, Bohm M, Dichgans M, et al. Recommendations for the emergency management of complications associated with the new direct oral anticoagulants (DOACS), apixaban, dabigatran and rivaroxaban. Clin Res Cardiol 2013;102:399–412.
67. Bowry R, Fraser S, Archeval-Lao JM, et al. Thrombelastography detects the anticoagulant effect of rivaroxaban in patients with stroke. Stroke 2014;45:880–3.

68. Connolly SJ, Eikelboom J, Joyner C, et al. Apixaban in patients with atrial fibrillation. New Engl J Med 2011;364:806–17.
69. Granger CB, Alexander JH, McMurray JJ, et al. Apixaban versus warfarin in patients with atrial fibrillation. New Engl J Med 2011; 365:981–92.
70. Hohnloser SH, Oldgren J, Yang S, et al. Myocardial ischemic events in patients with atrial fibrillation treated with dabigatran or warfarin in the RE-LY (randomized evaluation of long-term anticoagulation therapy) trial. Circulation 2012;125: 669–76.
71. Weitz JI, Gross PL. New oral anticoagulants: Which one should my patient use? Hematology Am Soc Hematol Educ Program 2012;2012:536–40.
72. Wyse DG, Waldo AL, DiMarco JP, et al. A comparison of rate control and rhythm control in patients with atrial fibrillation. New Engl J Med 2002;347:1825–33.
73. Sherman DG, Kim SG, Boop BS, et al. Occurrence and characteristics of stroke events in the atrial fibrillation follow-up investigation of sinus rhythm management (AFFIRM) study. Arch Intern Med 2005;165:1185–91.
77. Loh E, Sutton MS, Wun CC, et al. Ventricular dysfunction and the risk of stroke after myocardial infarction. New Engl J Med 1997;336:251–7.
80. Maze SS, Kotler MN, Parry WR. Flow characteristics in the dilated left ventricle with thrombus: Qualitative and quantitative Doppler analysis. J Am Coll Cardiol 1989;13:873–81.
81. Massie BM, Collins JF, Ammon SE, et al. Randomized trial of warfarin, aspirin, and clopidogrel in patients with chronic heart failure: The warfarin and antiplatelet therapy in chronic heart failure (WATCH) trial. Circulation 2009;119:1616–24.
82. Homma S, Thompson JL, Pullicino PM, et al. Warfarin and aspirin in patients with heart failure and sinus rhythm. New Engl J Med 2012;366:1859–69.
83. Dexter DD Jr, Whisnant JP, Connolly DC, et al. The association of stroke and coronary heart disease: A population study. Mayo Clin Proc 1987;62:1077–83.
84. Tanne D, Goldbourt U, Zion M, et al. Frequency and prognosis of stroke/TIA among 4808 survivors of acute myocardial infarction. The Sprint Study Group. Stroke 1993;24:1490–5.
85. The Stroke Prevention in Atrial Fibrillation Investigators. Bleeding during antithrombotic therapy in patients with atrial fibrillation. Arch Intern Med 1996;156:409–16.
86. Bodenheimer MM, Sauer D, Shareef B, et al. Relation between myocardial infarct location and stroke. J Am Coll Cardiol 1994;24:61–6.
87. Keren A, Goldberg S, Gottlieb S, et al. Natural history of left ventricular thrombi: Their appearance and resolution in the posthospitalization period of acute myocardial infarction. J Am Coll Cardiol 1990;15:790–800.
88. Friedman MJ, Carlson K, Marcus FI, et al. Clinical correlations in patients with acute myocardial infarction and left ventricular thrombus detected by two-dimensional echocardiography. Am J Med 1982;72:894–8.
89. Mooe T, Eriksson P, Stegmayr B. Ischemic stroke after acute myocardial infarction. A population-based study. Stroke 1997;28:762–7.
90. Mooe T, Teien D, Karp K, et al. Long term follow up of patients with anterior myocardial infarction complicated by left ventricular thrombus in the thrombolytic era. Heart 1996;75:252–6.
93. Anticoagulants in the secondary prevention of events in coronary thrombosis (ASPECT) research group. Effect of long-term oral anticoagulant treatment on mortality and cardiovascular morbidity after myocardial infarction. Lancet 1994;343: 499–503.
94. Roldan CA, Shively BK, Crawford MH. Valve excrescences: Prevalence, evolution and risk for cardioembolism. J Am Coll Cardiol 1997;30:1308–14.
95. Cohen A, Tzourio C, Chauvel C, et al. Mitral valve strands and the risk of ischemic stroke in elderly patients. The French Study of Aortic Plaques in Stroke (FAPS) investigators. Stroke 1997;28: 1574–8.
96. Aziz F, Baciewicz FA Jr. Lambl's excrescences: Review and recommendations. Tex Heart Inst J 2007;34:366–8.
97. Salem DN, Daudelin HD, Levine HJ, et al. Antithrombotic therapy in valvular heart disease. Chest 2001;119:207S–219S.
98. Cannegieter SC, Rosendaal FR, Wintzen AR, et al. Optimal oral anticoagulant therapy in patients with mechanical heart valves. New Engl J Med 1995;333:11–17.
99. Whitlock RP, Sun JC, Fremes SE, et al., American College of Chest P. Antithrombotic and thrombolytic therapy for valvular disease: Antithrombotic therapy and prevention of thrombosis, 9th ed: American College of Chest Physicians Evidence-based Clinical Practice Guidelines. Chest 2012;141:e576S–600S.
100. Scott PJ, Essop R, Wharton GA, et al. Left atrial clot in patients with mitral prostheses: Increased rate of detection after recent systemic embolism. Int J Cardiol 1991;33:141–8.
101. Douketis JD, Spyropoulos AC, Spencer FA, et al. Perioperative management of antithrombotic therapy: Antithrombotic therapy and prevention of thrombosis, 9th ed: American College of Chest Physicians Evidence-based Clinical Practice Guidelines. Chest 2012;141:e326S–350S.
102. Katsouli A, Massad MG. Current issues in the diagnosis and management of blood culture-negative infective and non-infective endocarditis. Ann Thorac Surg 2013;95:1467–74.
103. Roldan CA, Sibbitt WL Jr, Qualls CR, et al. Libman-sacks endocarditis and embolic cerebrovascular disease. JACC Cardiovasc Imaging 2013;6:973–83.
104. Lockshin M, Tenedios F, Petri M, et al. Cardiac disease in the antiphospholipid syndrome: Recommendations for treatment. Committee consensus report. Lupus 2003;12:518–23.
105. Hart RG, Foster JW, Luther MF, et al. Stroke in infective endocarditis. Stroke 1990;21:695–700.
106. Davenport J, Hart RG. Prosthetic valve endocarditis 1976–1987. Antibiotics, anticoagulation, and stroke. Stroke 1990;21: 993–9.
107. Molina CA, Selim MH. Anticoagulation in patients with stroke with infective endocarditis: The sword of Damocles. Stroke 2011; 42:1799–800.
108. Yau JW, Lee P, Wilson A, et al. Prosthetic valve endocarditis: What is the evidence for anticoagulant therapy? Intern Med J 2011;41:795–7.
109. Okazaki S, Yoshioka D, Sakaguchi M, et al. Acute ischemic brain lesions in infective endocarditis: Incidence, related factors, and postoperative outcome. Cerebrovasc Dis 2013;35:155–62.
110. Goulenok T, Klein I, Mazighi M, et al. Infective endocarditis with symptomatic cerebral complications: Contribution of cerebral magnetic resonance imaging. Cerebrovasc Dis 2013;35: 327–36.
111. Hoen B, Duval X. Clinical practice. Infective endocarditis. New Engl J Med 2013;368:1425–33.
112. Kang DH, Kim YJ, Kim SH, et al. Early surgery versus conventional treatment for infective endocarditis. New Engl J Med 2012; 366:2466–73.
113. Bhan A, Mehrotra R, Choudhary SK, et al. Surgical experience with intracardiac myxomas: Long-term follow-up. Ann Thorac Surg 1998;66:810–13.
114. Garatti A, Nano G, Canziani A, et al. Surgical excision of cardiac myxomas: Twenty years experience at a single institution. Ann Thorac Surg 2012;93:825–31.
115. Gowda RM, Khan IA, Nair CK, et al. Cardiac papillary fibroelastoma: A comprehensive analysis of 725 cases. Am Heart J 2003; 146:404–10.
116. Amano J, Nakayama J, Yoshimura Y, et al. Clinical classification of cardiovascular tumors and tumor-like lesions, and its incidences. Gen Thorac Cardiovasc Surg 2013;61:435–47.
117. Di Tullio M, Sacco RL, Gopal A, et al. Patent foramen ovale as a risk factor for cryptogenic stroke. Ann Intern Med 1992;117: 461–5.
118. Cabanes L, Mas JL, Cohen A, et al. Atrial septal aneurysm and patent foramen ovale as risk factors for cryptogenic stroke in patients less than 55 years of age. A study using transesophageal echocardiography. Stroke 1993;24:1865–73.
119. Lechat P, Mas JL, Lascault G, et al. Prevalence of patent foramen ovale in patients with stroke. New Engl J Med 1988;318: 1148–52.
120. Hausmann D, Mugge A, Daniel WG. Identification of patent foramen ovale permitting paradoxic embolism. J Am Coll Cardiol 1995;26:1030–8.
121. Lynch JJ, Schuchard GH, Gross CM, et al. Prevalence of right-to-left atrial shunting in a healthy population: Detection by valsalva

maneuver contrast echocardiography. Am J Cardiol 1984;53: 1478–80.
123. Jauss M, Kaps M, Keberle M, et al. A comparison of transesophageal echocardiography and transcranial Doppler sonography with contrast medium for detection of patent foramen ovale. Stroke 1994;25:1265–7.
124. Hagen PT, Scholz DG, Edwards WD. Incidence and size of patent foramen ovale during the first 10 decades of life: An autopsy study of 965 normal hearts. Mayo Clin Proc 1984;59: 17–20.
125. Homma S, Sacco RL, Di Tullio MR, et al., Investigators PFOiCSS. Effect of medical treatment in stroke patients with patent foramen ovale: Patent foramen ovale in cryptogenic stroke study. Circulation 2002;105:2625–31.
126. Jones EF, Calafiore P, Donnan GA, et al. Evidence that patent foramen ovale is not a risk factor for cerebral ischemia in the elderly. Am J Cardiol 1994;74:596–9.
127. Alsheikh-Ali AA, Thaler DE, Kent DM. Patent foramen ovale in cryptogenic stroke: Incidental or pathogenic? Stroke 2009;40: 2349–55.
128. Lee JY, Song JK, Song JM, et al. Association between anatomic features of atrial septal abnormalities obtained by omni-plane transesophageal echocardiography and stroke recurrence in cryptogenic stroke patients with patent foramen ovale. Am J Cardiol 2010;106:129–34.
129. Lamy C, Giannesini C, Zuber M, et al. Clinical and imaging findings in cryptogenic stroke patients with and without patent foramen ovale: The PFO-ASA study. Atrial septal aneurysm. Stroke 2002;33:706–11.
130. Cramer SC, Rordorf G, Maki JH, et al. Increased pelvic vein thrombi in cryptogenic stroke: Results of the Paradoxical Emboli from Large Veins in Ischemic Stroke (PELVIS) Study. Stroke 2004;35:46–50.
131. Handke M, Harloff A, Olschewski M, et al. Patent foramen ovale and cryptogenic stroke in older patients. New Engl J Med 2007;357:2262–8.
133. Mas JL, Zuber M. Recurrent cerebrovascular events in patients with patent foramen ovale, atrial septal aneurysm, or both and cryptogenic stroke or transient ischemic attack. French Study Group on Patent Foramen Ovale and Atrial Septal Aneurysm. Am Heart J 1995;130:1083–8.
135. Furlan AJ, Reisman M, Massaro J, et al. Closure or medical therapy for cryptogenic stroke with patent foramen ovale. New Engl J Med 2012;366:991–9.
136. Carroll JD, Saver JL, Thaler DE, et al. Closure of patent foramen ovale versus medical therapy after cryptogenic stroke. New Engl J Med 2013;368:1092–100.
137. Meier B, Kalesan B, Mattle HP, et al. Percutaneous closure of patent foramen ovale in cryptogenic embolism. New Engl J Med 2013;368:1083–91.
138. Amarenco P, Cohen A, Tzourio C, et al. Atherosclerotic disease of the aortic arch and the risk of ischemic stroke. New Engl J Med 1994;331:1474–9.
139. The French Study of Aortic Plaques in Stroke Group. Atherosclerotic disease of the aortic arch as a risk factor for recurrent ischemic stroke. New Engl J Med 1996;334:1216–21.
140. Tunick PA, Nayar AC, Goodkin GM, et al. Effect of treatment on the incidence of stroke and other emboli in 519 patients with severe thoracic aortic plaque. Am J Cardiol 2002;90:1320–5.
141. Hirsh J, Anand SS, Halperin JL, et al. Guide to anticoagulant therapy: Heparin: A statement for healthcare professionals from the American Heart Association. Circulation 2001;103: 2994–3018.
142. Kelton JG, Arnold DM, Bates SM. Nonheparin anticoagulants for heparin-induced thrombocytopenia. New Engl J Med 2013;368: 737–44.
143. Lewis BE, Wallis DE, Berkowitz SD, et al. Argatroban anticoagulant therapy in patients with heparin-induced thrombocytopenia. Circulation 2001;103:1838–43.
144. Kiser TH, Burch JC, Klem PM, et al. Safety, efficacy, and dosing requirements of bivalirudin in patients with heparin-induced thrombocytopenia. Pharmacotherapy 2008;28:1115–24.
145. Fogelholm R, Eskola K, Kiminkinen T, et al. Anticoagulant treatment as a risk factor for primary intracerebral haemorrhage. J Neurol Neurosurg Psychiatry 1992;55:1121–4.
146. Franke CL, de Jonge J, van Swieten JC, et al. Intracerebral hematomas during anticoagulant treatment. Stroke 1990;21: 726–30.
147. Mayer SA, Brun NC, Begtrup K, et al. Recombinant activated factor VII for acute intracerebral hemorrhage. New Engl J Med 2005;352:777–85.
148. Mayer SA, Brun NC, Begtrup K, et al. Efficacy and safety of recombinant activated factor VII for acute intracerebral hemorrhage. New Engl J Med 2008;358:2127–37.
149. Woo CH, Patel N, Conell C, et al. Rapid warfarin reversal in the setting of intracranial hemorrhage: A comparison of plasma, recombinant activated factor VII, and prothrombin complex concentrate. World Neurosurg 2014;81:110–15.
150. Sarode R, Milling TJ Jr, Refaai MA, et al. Efficacy and safety of a 4-factor prothrombin complex concentrate in patients on vitamin K antagonists presenting with major bleeding: A randomized, plasma-controlled, phase IIIb study. Circulation 2013;128:1234–43.
151. Torn M, Algra A, Rosendaal FR. Oral anticoagulation for cerebral ischemia of arterial origin: High initial bleeding risk. Neurology 2001;57:1993–9.
152. Hylek EM, Singer DE. Risk factors for intracranial hemorrhage in outpatients taking warfarin. Ann Intern Med 1994;120: 897–902.
153. The Stroke Prevention in Reversible Ischemia Trial (SPIRIT) Study Group. A randomized trial of anticoagulants versus aspirin after cerebral ischemia of presumed arterial origin. Ann Neurol 1997;42:857–65.
154. Hylek EM, Skates SJ, Sheehan MA, et al. An analysis of the lowest effective intensity of prophylactic anticoagulation for patients with nonrheumatic atrial fibrillation. New Engl J Med 1996;335: 540–6.
155. Smith EE, Rosand J, Knudsen KA, et al. Leukoaraiosis is associated with warfarin-related hemorrhage following ischemic stroke. Neurology 2002;59:193–7.
156. Gorter JW. Major bleeding during anticoagulation after cerebral ischemia: Patterns and risk factors. Stroke Prevention in Reversible Ischemia Trial (SPIRIT). European Atrial Fibrillation Trial (EAFT) study groups. Neurology 1999;53:1319–27.
157. Kato H, Izumiyama M, Izumiyama K, et al. Silent cerebral microbleeds on T2*-weighted MRI: Correlation with stroke subtype, stroke recurrence, and leukoaraiosis. Stroke 2002;33: 1536–40.
158. Charidimou A, Kakar P, Fox Z, et al. Cerebral microbleeds and the risk of intracerebral haemorrhage after thrombolysis for acute ischaemic stroke: Systematic review and meta-analysis. J Neurol Neurosurg Psychiatry 2013;84:277–80.
159. Charidimou A, Werring DJ. The dilemma of atrial fibrillation in intracerebral haemorrhage: How to balance the risks of ischaemia and bleeding. Eur J Neurol 2014;21:549–51.
160. Kakar P, Charidimou A, Werring DJ. Cerebral microbleeds: A new dilemma in stroke medicine. JRSM Cardiovasc Dis 2012;1: 2048004012474754.
161. Hart RG, Easton JD. Hemorrhagic infarcts. Stroke 1986;17: 586–9.
162. Hornig CR, Bauer T, Simon C, et al. Hemorrhagic transformation in cardioembolic cerebral infarction. Stroke 1993;24: 465–8.
163. Molina CA, Montaner J, Abilleira S, et al. Timing of spontaneous recanalization and risk of hemorrhagic transformation in acute cardioembolic stroke. Stroke 2001;32:1079–84.
164. Nighoghossian N, Hermier M, Berthezene Y, et al. Early diagnosis of hemorrhagic transformation: Diffusion/perfusion-weighted MRI versus CT scan. Cerebrovasc Dis 2001;11:151–6.
165. Hermier M, Nighoghossian N, Derex L, et al. MRI of acute post-ischemic cerebral hemorrhage in stroke patients: Diagnosis with T2*-weighted gradient-echo sequences. Neuroradiology 2001;43: 809–15.
166. Okada Y, Yamaguchi T, Minematsu K, et al. Hemorrhagic transformation in cerebral embolism. Stroke 1989;20:598–603.
167. Cerebral Embolism Study Group. Immediate anticoagulation of embolic stroke: Brain hemorrhage and management options. Stroke 1984;15:779–89.
168. Sandercock P. Full heparin anticoagulation should not be used in acute ischemic stroke. Stroke 2003;34:231–2.

169. Hallevi H, Albright KC, Martin-Schild S, et al. Anticoagulation after cardioembolic stroke: To bridge or not to bridge? Arch Neurol 2008;65:1169–73.
170. Cerebral Embolism Study Group. Cardioembolic stroke, early anticoagulation, and brain hemorrhage. Arch Intern Med 1987; 147:636–40.
171. Chamorro A, Vila N, Saiz A, et al. Early anticoagulation after large cerebral embolic infarction: A safety study. Neurology 1995;45:861–5.
172. Pessin MS, Estol CJ, Lafranchise F, et al. Safety of anticoagulation after hemorrhagic infarction. Neurology 1993;43:1298–303.
173. Paciaroni M, Agnelli G, Corea F, et al. Early hemorrhagic transformation of brain infarction: Rate, predictive factors, and influence on clinical outcome: Results of a prospective multicenter study. Stroke 2008;39:2249–56.
174. Jickling GC, Liu D, Stamova B, et al. Hemorrhagic transformation after ischemic stroke in animals and humans. J Cereb Blood Flow Metab 2014;34:185–99.
175. Kim JT, Heo SH, Park MS, et al. Use of antithrombotics after hemorrhagic transformation in acute ischemic stroke. PLoS ONE 2014;9:e89798.
176. Gebel JM, Broderick JP. Intracerebral hemorrhage. Neurol Clin 2000;18:419–38.
177. Crawley F, Bevan D, Wren D. Management of intracranial bleeding associated with anticoagulation: Balancing the risk of further bleeding against thromboembolism from prosthetic heart valves. J Neurol Neurosurg Psychiatry 2000;69:396–8.
178. Hacke W. The dilemma of reinstituting anticoagulation for patients with cardioembolic sources and intracranial hemorrhage: How wide is the strait between Skylla and Karybdis? Arch Neurol 2000;57:1682–4.
179. Phan TG, Koh M, Wijdicks EF. Safety of discontinuation of anticoagulation in patients with intracranial hemorrhage at high thromboembolic risk. Arch Neurol 2000;57:1710–13.
180. Bertram M, Bonsanto M, Hacke W, et al. Managing the therapeutic dilemma: Patients with spontaneous intracerebral hemorrhage and urgent need for anticoagulation. J Neurol 2000;247: 209–14.
181. Aguilar MI, Hart RG, Kase CS, et al. Treatment of warfarin-associated intracerebral hemorrhage: Literature review and expert opinion. Mayo Clin Proc 2007;82:82–92.

63 Conduct of Stroke-Related Clinical Trials

Adriana Pérez, Barbara C. Tilley

KEY POINTS

- A trial can be conducted only when there is equipoise.
- Phase 2 trials are under-utilized in stroke research and can reduce the number of ineffective treatments taken to phase 3.
- Common single outcome measures are the NIH stroke scale and modified Rankin scale.
- Properly planned adaptive designs can allow midcourse modifications to the study design while maintaining validity and integrity of study data.
- No single approach to data analysis and sample size estimation fits all trials. Choices depend on the hypothesized distribution of outcomes and questions of interest.
- Bath et al. provide four examples of hypothesized benefits that may require differing power calculations and analytic plans: (i) a neuroprotective effect - mild benefit experienced across all ranges of stroke severity, (ii) an early recanalization effect - a substantial benefit experienced across all ranges of stroke severity, (iii) a late recanalization effect - a benefit experienced across all ranges of stroke severity but with limited ability to attain fully normal outcome, and (iv) benefits clustered at unexpected health state transitions.
- Where possible meta-analyses should use pooled-per-patient data.
- Regulations, guidelines, and ethical considerations for the conduct of stroke clinical trials are international.
- Exception from consent (EFIC) may be useful in emergent stroke research.

Drawing from the general literature on the conduct of clinical trials, this chapter addresses the design, analytical, data management, ethical, and regulatory issues relevant to stroke prevention and therapeutic clinical trials. A clinical trial is defined as "an experiment in which a group of individuals is given an intervention and subsequent outcome measures are taken. Results of the intervention are compared to individuals not given the intervention."[1]

WHEN CAN A STROKE-RELATED TRIAL BE CONDUCTED?

Ethical conduct of a randomized clinical trial requires equipoise, a point in time when the treatment is acceptable to administer to humans but uncertainty remains about treatment outcome. If there is a consensus of potential participants or clinicians that a treatment or procedure is beneficial (or harmful), randomization becomes impractical and possibly unethical, For example, rt-PA cannot be withheld from eligible patients in the first 3 hours after stroke onset[2] and other studies suggested the window should extend to 4.5 hours[3] precluding use of a placebo group in eligible patients. Ethical considerations preclude a trial of the stroke-related risk factor, cigarette smoking, where non-smoking participants are randomly assigned to smoking or non-smoking as an intervention.

TYPES OF PREVENTION TRIALS

Primary prevention trials evaluate interventions in participants who have never had a stroke. Pure primary prevention trials are rare, as most prevention trials include some participants with previous stroke, transient ischemic attack (TIA), or both. A prevention trial also may be a trial with a primary outcome such as cardiovascular disease, and stroke as a secondary outcome. A landmark stroke prevention trial, the Carotid Revascularization Endarterectomy Versus Stenting Trial (CREST) comparing stenting versus carotid endarterectomy for carotid disease included both patients with and without a previous stroke.[4]

Secondary prevention trials evaluate interventions only in participants who have previously had a TIA or stroke. The Warfarin and Aspirin Recurrent Stroke Study (WARSS), comparing warfarin and aspirin in participants with a previous stroke,[5] and the Vitamins To Prevent Stroke (VITATOPS) trial of multivitamin therapy[6] in patients with a recent TIA or ischemic stroke are examples of secondary prevention trials.

THERAPEUTIC TRIALS

Therapeutic stroke trials are generally directed at reducing post-stroke-related disability or mortality. The International Surgical Trial (IST) in Intracranial Hemorrhage assessed the use of a surgical procedure to reduce mortality from spontaneous intracranial hemorrhage.[7] The National Institute of Neurological Disorders and Stroke (NINDS) studies of recombinant tissue-type plasminogen activator (rt-PA)[2] and the more recent European Cooperative Acute Stroke Study III (ECASS III)[3] were designed to reduce post-stroke disability with mortality classified as the most severe disability. A cluster randomized controlled trial of a structured training program for caregivers of inpatients after stroke (TRACS) was designed to reduce post-stroke disability as measured by ability to do activities of daily living and to reduce caregiver burden and cost.[8,9]

THE THREE PHASES OF CLINICAL TRIALS

Although the nomenclature and definition of the phases are, in general, not standardized, the three phases are phase 1 (dose finding and safety), phase 2 (determination of futility, feasibility, and safety), and phase 3 (efficacy or effectiveness). In the development of therapies for stroke, these phases are often not distinct. Phases 1 and 2 or phases 2 and 3 may be combined. After an agent receives approval from the U.S. Food and Drug Administration (FDA) for marketing, phase 4 (post-marketing surveillance) may be conducted, particularly if such a phase is a condition of FDA approval. Phase 4 studies assess long-term effects of the new treatment, monitor subsequent adverse reactions, and can be used for cost-effectiveness assessment and marketing purposes.

Phase 1

Phase 1 studies establish a safe dose in humans with an acceptable level of toxicity, establish a route of administration, and determine the clinical pharmacology. In studies of cancer chemotherapy, the intent of a phase 1 trial is to discover the maximum tolerated dose (MTD) on the premise that the maximum benefit (efficacy) would be observed with the highest tolerable dose. The occurrence of toxicity that is unacceptable is termed dose-limiting toxicity (DLT). Hence, the MTD is determined by the absence of a DLT, with the MTD being one dose level below a DLT.

In stroke, there is no consensus regarding the need to escalate the dose to the MTD. The level of escalation chosen for a phase 1 study would be treatment specific. Another ambiguity in phase 1 studies for stroke is the definition of DLT. Oncology clinical trials use standard definitions for the varying levels of toxicity. Stroke has no such guidelines. A phase 1 study funded by NINDS aimed to establish the MTD of human serum albumin as a neuroprotective agent for participants with recent ischemic stroke.[10] A Safety Evaluation Committee of neurologists and cardiologists evaluated participants' records at each dose level according to pre-specified guidelines to determine whether severe and serious adverse events occurred during the 72 hours after ictus. The existence of DLT was determined by a consensus after each member of the committee reviewed the charts of all the participants at each dose level.

The choice of the initial phase 1 dose is based either on animal experiments for a drug that has never been used in humans or on previous studies in humans for an existing drug. The common approach starts from one-tenth of the dose that causes 10% mortality in the rodents (LD_{10}). The dose is increased by a smaller percentage each time, often using a modified Fibonacci scheme. Continual reassessment methods (CRMs) as an alternative design for a phase 1 study can use either the frequentist or Bayesian methods. Information gathered in the trial from a previous increase in dose is used to estimate the probability of DLT at the next dose level. Simulation studies show that the MTD may be reached sooner with some CRM methods than with the Fibonacci method putting fewer participants at risk from higher doses.[11]

Phase 2

Phase 2 studies have been underutilized in stroke. New therapies often are studied in phase 1 trials and then studied in underpowered phase 3 trials, sometimes called phase 2B studies. Phase 2 studies do not seek to draw definitive conclusions about the treatment effectiveness but seek evidence to justify proceeding to a phase 3 study. Phase 2 studies primarily rule out clearly ineffective treatments, that is, assess futility, and also assess side effects, toxicity, logistics of treatment administration, and project trial costs.[12,13] In phase 2 stroke prevention trials, a surrogate outcome such as a risk factor reduction may be used as the primary outcome when the outcome for a future phase 3 study, new stroke or death, would take years to ascertain. Therapeutic phase 2 and phase 3 stroke trials generally use the same outcome measures taken at 3 months; no surrogate is required.

Using a one-sided test and inflated type-I-error level phase 2 studies require smaller sample sizes, less time and fewer resources than phase 2B studies. Single-arm phase 2 studies using historical data as a reference have the advantage of requiring even smaller sample sizes than a controlled study with the same error and effect size parameters. A critical assumption of a single-arm design is that the course of the disease has not changed over time, that historical controls are an accurate representation of current patients and that the same outcome measure is collected in the same way. In the NINDS trial, a common source of historical data, the modified Rankin was used,[14] not the stroke-related Rankin[15] and the NIH Stroke Scale (NIHSS) was collected under the instructions "score what you see".[16] Newer trials changed the instructions for the Rankin and/or the NIHSS to make the measures more specific to the current stroke. If there is uncertainty about the validity of historical controls, a comparison group must be included but the single-sided hypothesis and an inflated type-I-error level would still lead to a reduction in sample size over a phase 2B design.[12,17] A completed phase 2 stroke treatment trial of combined intravenous and intra-arterial t-PA[18] with historical controls was determined to be worthwhile and moved forward to phase 3.[19,20]

Phase 2 studies may also be used to choose a dose from among a set of tolerable doses or to select the "best" among a set of treatments.[21] In a study of amyotrophic lateral sclerosis (ALS), investigators combined a dose selection study with a phase 2 futility study,[22] a design that may be applicable to dose finding studies in stroke. Bayesian dose-finding studies may also be applicable depending on agreement regarding the level of prior knowledge, whether outcomes can be assessed rapidly, and investigators' ability to reduce bias.[23,24]

A phase 2 design is especially attractive when availability of participants is limited in relation to the rate of development of new treatments. A successful phase 2 study does not guarantee a successful phase 3 trial.[25,26] Nevertheless, using a phase 2 design can reduce the number of futile phase 3 studies and can provide an overall reduction in the long-term cost of trials.[12,13,27]

Phase 3

In a randomized phase 3 clinical trial, whether preventive or therapeutic, each participant is randomly assigned to an intervention or control (placebo, usual care, best medical treatment for the condition, etc.). A well-designed, well-executed, randomized, concurrently controlled phase 3 clinical trial is the ultimate proof (or lack thereof) of the strength of association between the treatment and a clinical effect.[1]

It may be of interest to show that a treatment is as beneficial as another current treatment, given that the new treatment has fewer side effects or lower cost. Studies to demonstrate the equivalence or non-inferiority of one therapy to another require specialized approaches to design and analysis.[28,29]

OUTCOME MEASURES

All clinical trials should begin with a clear definition of the question to be studied and of the expected outcomes. Most primary and secondary prevention trials often use new stroke occurrence or stroke-related mortality, requiring extended follow-up over several years to observe a sufficient number of events.

Prevention trials must obtain sufficient information to define new stroke occurrence and, where applicable, stroke-related mortality, at a cost low enough to allow the trial to be conducted. In planning a new trial, investigators can draw on the experience of other large prevention trials. Investigators in the Asymptomatic Carotid Atherosclerosis Study (ACAS), for example, devised a symptom-based questionnaire and algorithm for detecting TIAs and other neurologic illness,[30] but recommend that positive results be confirmed by neurologic evaluation. Reported stroke events are generally verified and categorized into stroke subtypes by a central events committee, blinded to treatment assignment. Adjudication and classification of stroke events is costly and time-consuming. Classifying deaths as stroke-related adds another level of complexity.

Acute stroke therapeutic trials use some measure of 3 month post-stroke recovery as the outcome measure rather than a long-term mortality or new-stroke outcome. Common measures are the NIH Stroke Scale (NIHSS)[31] and modified Rankin scale,[14] in which participants who have died are given the worst score. There is no consensus on the best single outcome and the amount of difference to be detected is treatment-dependent. It is clear that no one outcome measures all aspects of recovery after stroke. In the NINDS rt-PA Stroke Study, investigators classified participants as having a favorable (minimal or no disability) or unfavorable outcome using four outcome measures, the modified Rankin Scale (mRS),[14] Barthel Index,[32] NIHSS score,[31] and the Glasgow Outcome Scale.[33] The four outcomes were combined to form a single global outcome measure.[2,34] If a trial is planned to use a new outcome measure or to use an existing outcome measure in a new population, the measure should be validated in patients similar to possible trial participants before it is used in the trial.[35,36] In some recent trials a "stroke-related" modified Rankin is being used instead of a traditional modified Rankin, but there is limited information on validation of this outcome[15] and few comparisons between the modified Rankin and the stroke-related modified Rankin.

INCLUSION AND EXCLUSION CRITERIA FOR PHASE 3

Inclusion and exclusion criteria define the trial population to be studied. Investigators may wish to give a treatment its "best chance to succeed" by excluding participants hypothesized not to "do well," such as those who are older or have high NIHSS scores, subtle computerized tomography (CT) findings, or certain stroke subtypes. If one suspects that patients *with* a risk factor will have a *poorer* outcome with treatment than with placebo and patients *without* a risk factor would have a *better* outcome with treatment than with placebo, a *treatment–risk factor interaction* is implied. If no interaction with treatment is expected – patients with the risk factor are expected to do worse than those without it, *regardless* of treatment assignment – there is not a strong rationale to exclude these participants.

The more restrictive the criteria for entry into the trial, the less generalizable are the results. Trials that exclude potential participants with specific stroke subtypes or include participants only from large specialty clinics may not provide data applicable to patients seen in the general practice of neurology. If the treatment appears efficacious, a wider range of patients than used in the trial may receive the treatment without knowing the true benefit. Overly restrictive entry criteria may limit enrollment of older adults and minority populations more likely to have comorbidities and most in need of the new approaches to stroke prevention or therapy. Potential participants at higher risk of unfavorable outcomes are also potential "responders" to treatment.

Table 63-1 shows published data from the NINDS t-PA Stroke Study.[5] The percentage of participants with a favorable outcome decreased with age and with increasing NIHSS score, but the t-PA-treated group had a higher percentage of favorable outcomes in 14 of the 16 age-by-NIHSS subgroups. In the oldest patients with the highest NIHSS scores, there were no

TABLE 63-1 Proportion of 3-Month Favorable Outcomes by Baseline NIHSS Score, Age, and Treatment Group*

	% Patients with Favorable Outcome	
Variable	***t-PA***	***Placebo***
AGE ≤60 YEAR		
Baseline NIHSS Score		
0–9 (n = 46)	59	42
10–14 (n = 35)	38	18
5–20 (n = 49)	41	27
>20 (n = 26)	22	12
AGE 61–68 YEAR		
NIHSS Score		
0–9 (n = 44)	60	37
10–14 (n = 28)	25	25
15–20 (n = 39)	0	25
>20 (n = 30)	7	0
AGE 69–75 YEAR		
NIHSS Score		
0–9 (n = 41)	50	54
10–14 (n = 45)	39	27
15–20 (n = 40)	26	0
>20 (n = 35)	8	0
AGE >75 YEAR		
NIHSS Score		
0–9 (n = 46)	67	36
10–14 (n = 28)	27	15
15–20 (n = 43)	23	6
>20 (n = 49)	0	0

*Favorable outcome: NIHSS score of 0 or 1 at 3 months. The categories for age and baseline NIHSS represent quartiles of the range of each variable.

NIHSS: National Institutes of Health Stroke Scale.

t-PA: tissue-type plasminogen activator.

Data from the NINDS t-PA Study Group. Generalized efficacy of t-PA for acute stroke: subgroup analysis of the NINDS t-PA Stroke Trial. Stroke 1997;28:2119–2125 (Table 3 adapted here).[87]

favorable binary outcomes indicating limited or no disability in either treatment group, but only 74% of the t-PA-treated patients, versus 86% of the placebo-treated patients, experienced severe disability or death.

To minimize problems with missing data, consider excluding potential participants with characteristics that might prevent the participants from completing the study or from complying with the study medication. Stroke trials thus may exclude patients at imminent risk of death such as those with terminal cancer.

RANDOMIZATION

Randomization is the method of allocating participants to the different treatment arms of a randomized clinical trial. Simple randomization is similar to flipping an unbiased coin and using heads or tails to assign a participant to one of two treatment arms. Using alternating assignment of participants to treatment or control as they come in to a study is not a random assignment. To ensure randomness, a random number generator, available in many statistical sample size and/or analysis packages, is generally used to conduct the randomization. Unfortunately, simple randomization may, by chance, result in imbalances in risk factors associated with outcome.[1]

Stratification during randomization helps to balance factors associated with treatment outcome, e.g., the baseline NIHSS score, age, clinical site, and/or other baseline variables. Participants are stratified before randomization into specific subgroups and then randomly assigned to treatment arms within each subgroup. Stratification helps to ensure that one group does not inadvertently have an advantage over another. Stratification can also improve the precision of the statistical analysis but stratifying variables must be included in the primary trial analysis.[1]

There is a rapid increase in the number of subgroups as the number of variables used for stratification increases. In a trial stratified on time from stroke onset (early, late), clinical center (eight locations), NIHSS score (three levels), and age (three levels), there would be 144 subgroups. Given a large number of subgroups and a small sample size, participants could be unequally assigned to treatment groups within strata, inducing an overall imbalance in the treatment arms and a decrease in precision. A complex randomization scheme may also lead to more errors in the randomization.

Most treatment trials and prevention trials have sufficient sample size to make stratification unnecessary except on one or two influential variables. There is little gain in statistical precision once the number of participants per group exceeds 50. The greatest stratification gains come from trials with 20 or fewer participants per treatment arm.[37] If the overall sample size is small and there is concern that stratification by site may lead to serious imbalances in treatment groups, a validated clinical index that takes into account several variables can be used, although this type of index is less available for stroke patients. Another option is *minimization,* a statistical approach to balancing the treatment arms to the extent possible after each participant's entry criteria are ascertained.[38]

Blocking forces the proportion in each of the two treatment arms within strata to be fixed through time, usually at 0.5; that is, blocking provides balance on unknown temporal variables. A block size of four in a trial with equal randomization to the two treatment arms would imply that after every four participants are randomly assigned within a block there would be two participants in each treatment arm. The selected block size should be large enough to make it difficult for an investigator to guess the next treatment assignment or the block size can be randomly chosen from a range of block sizes to make it more difficult to detect the end of a block. In either case, the blocking criteria are not shared with investigators before the end of the trial.[1]

Blinding or *masking* reduces bias in the assessment of the trial outcome measures. In a single-blind study, either the participant or the investigator is blinded to the treatment assignment until the end of the trial. In the more common double-blind study, neither the participant nor the investigator knows the treatment assignment. Bias in classifying a participant as having a new stroke or stroke-related death or assigning a Rankin score could be introduced if the rater assessing the outcomes in an unblinded trial knows the treatment assignment. Even when a rater does not introduce bias, results of an unblinded trial can be considered questionable by an external reviewer. If a trial cannot be blinded (e.g., surgery versus medical care), using someone not present at the time of treatment to assess outcome or using an independent adjudicator can reduce bias. When the outcome is overall mortality, it is more difficult to introduce bias given the same effort is made to determine the outcome in all treatment arms.

In the WARSS,[5] periodic dose adjustments were needed for many participants receiving warfarin. To maintain the blind, the coordinating center fabricated clinically plausible values for participants in the aspirin-placebo treatment arm mimicking the frequency and direction of change in the warfarin-treated group. The laboratory sent messages to investigators mandating a change in placebo dose for some randomly chosen patients.

RECRUITMENT

Planning helps ensure timely recruitment, especially in acute stroke therapy trials where time from admission to treatment must be minimized. In the NINDS t-PA Stroke Study, using methods of total quality improvement investigators flowcharted the process in each emergency department and engaged those involved in the process (CT technicians, laboratory technicians, nurses, pharmacists, neurologists, emergency department physicians and staff) in determining how to enroll patients more quickly.[39] Another important aspect of recruiting is community engagement where community is broadly defined. In acute stroke trials, presentations to the community generally have a low yield, but communication remains important to create a climate of trust and is required if exception from informed consents (EFIC) is used (see ethics section). For acute stroke treatment trials presentations to community emergency medical services help to facilitate prompt arrival of prospective trial participants at participating emergency departments.[40]

For prevention trials, especially those conducted in groups of participants who are not acutely ill, community presentations may substantially increase recruitment and help increase trust among minority groups that may be unwilling to participate in prevention trials. A 2000 survey of minority community members in San Francisco identified altruism and tangible factors associated with willingness to participate in research.[41] There is a growing literature on recruitment of minority participants to non-emergent clinical trials, but few randomized trials have been conducted to assess or compare recruitment strategies.

ADHERENCE TO TREATMENT AND TRIAL FOLLOW-UP

Treatment adherence is increased by simplifying study procedures, case report forms and demands on participants, gathering sufficient information to enable close contact with participants after enrollment, and by providing the patient, family, or both with sufficient information about the trial and its requirements before randomization. Conducting a "run-in" period in long-term stroke prevention trials that mimics the study before randomization may eliminate "non-compliers" before they are entered into the trial, but trial results may also be less generalizable. A run-in period would not be possible in therapeutic trials for acute stroke, where time to treatment must be minimized.

In both stroke prevention and therapeutic trials at all phases, all participants should be encouraged to return for a final trial visit even if they no longer take study medications or participate in other aspects of the intervention, to reduce missing outcome data. For an acute stroke trial with a one-time dose, the possibility of drop-out from therapy is minimal, but completeness of follow-up remains essential to trial integrity.

Measuring Adherence to Treatment

If treatment is an educational intervention to reduce stroke risk factors or an exercise rehabilitation program, a participant's adherence to the regimen should be estimated with process measures (e.g., number of sessions attended) or by changes in knowledge, attitudes, and beliefs. If laboratory tests are applicable, reliable, and affordable, the most accurate assessment of medication compliance may be measurement of blood, saliva, or urine levels of the drug. When, a non-compliant participant takes medication just before a clinic visit, a laboratory measurement may not reflect the true level of adherence. Some trials use pill counts of returned medication or count the number of times a pill container was opened by means of an often expensive miniaturized electronic device in the lid of the pill bottle. Latter methods are only estimates, subject to under- and over-counting, and can be expensive. Morisky et al.[42] suggest posing a brief set of questions as a better measure of compliance than a pill count. The usefulness of these four questions in stroke trials needs validation, although the approach has been validated in trials of Parkinson's disease treatments.[27] Counts of missed visits, missed forms, and missed items on forms are also useful in monitoring adherence to treatment.

DATA ANALYSES

Intent-to-Treat

A guiding principle in clinical trials is the use of intent-to-treat (ITT) analysis. When an ITT analysis is used, all participants undergoing randomization are included in the primary analysis, as randomized whether or not they withdraw or deviate from the protocol. In a surgical trial, under an ITT analysis, all participants randomly assigned to surgery would be analyzed in the surgical group, and all participants assigned to medical care would be analyzed in the medical care group regardless of treatment actually received. ITT is used to reduce the introduction of bias that can interfere with the interpretation of study results.

The terms "completer analysis," "on-treatment analysis," and "analyzable population" are generally used to describe a situation in which participants who stop treatment, did not adhere to protocol, or have incomplete follow-up are excluded. These secondary analyses are useful in addition to ITT analyses and if results agree with the analyses of the full trial data set, the interpretation is clear. If results do not agree, emphasis should be placed on the ITT analysis.

When some ineligible participants are expected to be enrolled, the trial sample size could be increased (see section on sample size). If it is necessary to randomly assign participants to treatment before an entry criterion is ascertained and a high proportion of patients will not be eligible, it may be necessary to redefine the ITT population. For example, if the treatment is expected to be effective for only patients with an uncommon genotype and the treatment must be administered in an emergency situation before the genotype can be ascertained, the number of ineligibles will far outnumber the number of eligible participants and can add noise, obscuring treatment differences. Under the following conditions: (a) eligibility is determined from data collected prior to treatment, (b) eligibility is determined by someone blinded to treatment assignment, and (c) eligibility can be ascertained before outcomes are known. ITT analyses may include only the eligible participants.[43] This design would need pre-approval by the FDA and/or funding agency, where applicable. Missing values in the ITT population are handled as described in the section on missing data.

General approaches to analysis are summarized in standard texts on clinical trials.[1] Standard approaches, such as analyses of time to new stroke or death, can be useful in prevention trials, in which the outcome is binary (yes/no; each participant either survived stroke-free or had a new stroke or died). When the outcome of a therapeutic trial is recovery from stroke, trials are usually designed with a set of correlated outcome measures. Interpretation of a set of outcomes with respect to an overall effect of treatment is difficult, particularly if some outcomes show different degrees of effect. Additionally, having multiple outcome measures generally requires adjustment for multiple comparisons.[44] For this reason some investigators choose a single primary outcome, usually the modified Rankin Scale (mRS) even though the single outcome does not represent the multiple dimensions of recovery. Others use a more powerful global test for multiple outcomes.

Global Tests

A composite outcome can be constructed identifying the results in a subject as a failure if any one of the set of primary outcomes occur.[45] In stroke, a composite outcome could be new stroke or stroke-related death. Composite outcomes are most commonly used in cardiovascular disease. Another approach is the use of a global statistical test,[34,46] such, as in the NINDS t-PA Stroke Trial.[2] Trial investigators dichotomized each outcome measures into minimal or no disability (success/failure) to address the question of interest. Dichotomization also solves the statistical issue of the J-shaped distributions as described under *Sample Size*. When the outcome measures are dichotomous (binary), the global test is reported as odds ratios or can be converted to relative risks. Relative risks for the individual outcomes provide an interpretation of the global test outcome.[47] A combination of continuous and binary outcome measures can be combined into a single outcome using a summed rank approach and tested with a traditional t-test or analysis of variance.[34]

Shift Analysis of the mRS

The modified Rankin Scale (mRS) is the most commonly used outcome measure in stroke trials.[14,15,48] The mRS is an ordered scale coded from 0 (no symptoms at all) through 5 (severe disability) 6 (death).[14] Traditionally, stroke trials collapsed the mRS into two groups, for example scores of 0 to 1 were defined as positive (treatment success) versus scores 2 to 6 were defined as negative (treatment failure) or using other dichotomies. Recent approaches analyze this ordinal scale using a shift analysis based on the Cochran-Mantel-Haenszel test in a particular form known as the van Elteren's test or using an extension of the Wilcoxon rank sum test, or using ordered logistic regression.[48–50] If adjustment for more than one covariate is required ordered logistic is preferred. Two simulation studies compared the dichotomous analysis versus ordinal versus continuous statistical approaches, one using data from acute stroke trials (the optimizing analysis of stroke trials collaboration-OAST)[49] and another using data from traumatic brain injury IMPACT).[51] Results from simulations indicate that ordinal approaches (shift analysis) are more efficient among 16 statistical tests compared except under some situations. Saver and Gornbein[52] proposed four treatment pattern profiles in stroke randomized clinical trials: (i) a neuroprotective effect – mild benefit experienced across all ranges of stroke severity, (ii) an early recanalization effect – a substantial benefit experienced across all ranges of stroke severity, (iii) a late recanalization effect – a benefit experienced across all ranges of stroke severity but with limited ability to attain fully normal outcome, and (iv) benefits clustered at unexpected health state transitions. They found the shift analysis more efficient for patterns (i) and (iv), and dichotomization of the mRS more efficient for patterns (ii) and (iii). The NINDS trial[2] was similar to pattern profile (ii).

Clustering

Special analytic issues arise in the analyses of clustered data in the presence of correlation or association among participants. Examples include clinical trials where the unit of randomization is a physician's practice or an emergency department rather than a patient and there are multiple subjects enrolled in the same treatment arm within those units of randomization (i.e., the INSTINCT trial[53]). Under the assumption that patients in the provider's practice or clinical site are more like one another than like patients in different practices or sites a positive correlation is implied. A variance unadjusted for clustering underestimates the true variance in the trial potentially leading to falsely rejecting the null hypothesis and a false claim of treatment benefit. Analytical techniques accounting for clustering should be implemented in cluster randomized trials.[28]

Analysis of Covariance

Unless most participants in one treatment arm of a study have the risk factor and most participants in the other arm do not have the risk factor, it is possible to adjust statistically for imbalances between treatment groups by including the risk factor in a model testing for a treatment effect. If the imbalance in the risk factor explains away the treatment benefit, the benefit has been artificially enhanced by the imbalance. If a benefit of treatment remains or is enhanced after adjustment for the risk factor, the imbalance was not artificially inflating the treatment benefit. One danger in such post hoc analyses is that many variables may be tested in an attempt to bring out a positive treatment outcome, making the end result less credible. Investigators can avoid this "data dredging" by prespecifying the variables to be included as covariates.[54]

The odds ratio for a favorable outcome in the second NINDS rt-PA Stroke Study (part II) was 1.7 (95% confidence interval [CI], 1.2–2.6), adjusting for pre-specified stratification variables. Post hoc analyses of covariance were also conducted with adjustment for the three variables (age, weight, and aspirin use before stroke) imbalanced ($P < 0.05$) between the two treatment groups at randomization. These post hoc analyses suggested an even greater benefit of t-PA (odds ratio [OR] for a favorable outcome 2.0; 95%CI, 1.3–3.1).[2]

Multiple Comparisons

An argument has been made[55] that if the comparisons represent separate questions (i.e., assessment of the impact of the intervention on two or three different outcomes), each comparison can be considered a separate experiment with no need for adjustment of the type-I-error level (alpha). When an overall hypothesis and a subgroup hypothesis are being tested (e.g., all patients with stroke and patients with severe NIHSS status at baseline), spending some type-I-error level on this overall comparison (i.e., 0.04) and less on the subgroups is another approach.[56] If a global test is used and the comparison is statistically significant, the components of the global test can be tested individually at the 0.05 level. When all possible pairwise comparisons are to be made among a series of treatments, a more stringent adjustment of the type-I-error level for multiple comparisons may be required. Hockberg's correction,[44] a step-down approach, is an example and is less conservative than the traditional Bonferroni approach, which uses the type-I-error level divided by the number of comparisons.

Subgroup Analyses and Interaction

After the completion of a trial, multiple analyses are often performed to determine whether there are subgroups in which the treatment might have been beneficial or harmful. To avoid bias, subgroups should be "proper" – that is, defined by characteristics measured at baseline – before treatment. In the NINDS rt-PA Stroke Study, each participant's stroke subtype was determined 7–10 days after stroke based on CT scans taken 24 hours after thrombolytic treatment and clinical data collected at baseline. The rt-PA could affect the 24-hour CT findings through both its clot-busting properties and its potential hemorrhagic side effects. The grouping of patients by this post-randomization classification of stroke subtype would not constitute a "proper" subgroup.

The more subgroups examined, the more likely the analyses will lead to a type-I-error, i.e., detecting a difference by chance alone. To protect against bias and a type-I-error, the subgroups should be predefined, a priori, based on a clearly justified rationale, and pre-specified in the protocol before the start of the trial. A priori subgroups are less subject to bias than subgroups defined after study results are known (post hoc). Adjusting analyses for multiple comparisons can reduce power with the reduction depending on the number of subgroups. Additionally, to protect against bias and inflated type-I-error levels, particularly in the testing of post hoc hypotheses, a more stringent approach is to require a significant treatment interaction before subgroup analyses are conducted. An interaction between treatment and the subgrouping variable may be present if either (1) the treatment is harmful in one subgroup, but beneficial in another, or (2) the magnitude of treatment benefit differs among subgroups.[57] Generally, interactions are tested at the 0.1 rather than 0.05 type-I-error level as most studies are not designed with sufficient power to test for interactions effects.

Meade and Brennan[58] conducted subgroup analyses of patients in a thrombosis prevention trial with emphasis on detecting subgroups who might derive the most benefit in terms of stroke prevention. The investigators presented analyses with tests of interactions suggesting that participants who had baseline systolic blood pressures of 145 mm Hg and higher and were receiving aspirin therapy were at a higher risk of stroke than those with similar blood pressure levels who were receiving placebo, whereas participants with lower blood pressures experienced a protective effect (*P* value for the interaction, 0.006). The time-treatment interaction in the NINDS tPA Stroke Trial[59] (Fig. 63-1) provides another example of a treatment by covariate interaction.

MISSING DATA

Of particular concern in clinical trials is the biased use of only those participants for whom there is complete outcome data. Bias may arise because the participants who provided data may have a better response to treatment than those who did not, even those in the placebo group. Therefore, a subgroup of fully compliant participants ("completers") is not a random sample of the original sample. Patterns of missing data (i.e., rate, time to withdrawal, and reason for withdrawal) may differ among treatment groups, adding more bias, particularly if the amount of missing data differs among treatment groups. If a substantial proportion of primary outcome data (e.g., >20%) is unobserved the integrity and quality of the entire study could be in question, regardless of the statistical approach to handle the missing data. When data are missing, a variety of statistical methods may be used to perform an ITT analysis.[45,60,61] There are two patterns of missing data in longitudinal clinical trials: intermittent (e.g., due to some missed clinic visits) and monotone (e.g., due to participant withdrawal or loss to follow-up). Missing data have been classified as follows:

- *Missing completely at random (MCAR):* Data that are missing because of an event, circumstances, or measure completely independent of the outcome of interest or other participant-specific measures collected in the study. For example, the participant moved out of the country and the NIHSS could not be ascertained.

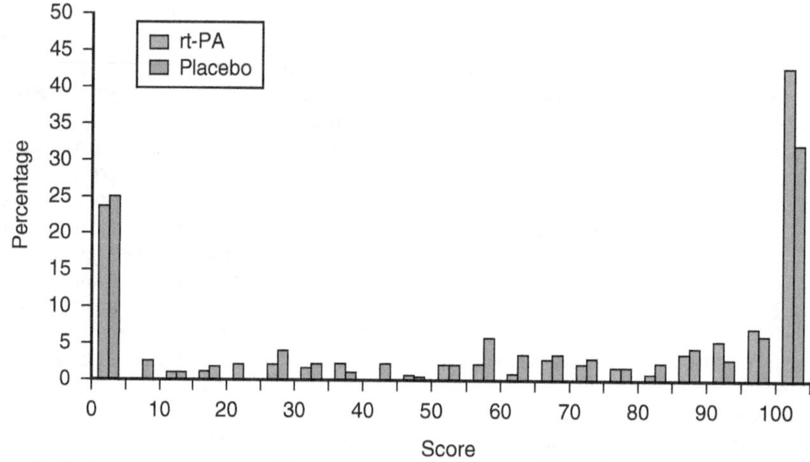

Figure 63-1. Graph of model estimating odds ratio (OR) for favorable outcome at 3 months in patients treated with recombinant tissue-type plasminogen activator (rt-PA) and in those given placebo by onset-to-treatment time (OTT) with 95% confidence intervals, after adjustment for the baseline National Institutes of Health Stroke Scale (NIHSS) score. OR >1 indicates greater odds that rt-PA-treated patients will have a favorable outcome at 3 months than the placebo-treated patients. Range of OTT was 58–180 minutes with a mean (μ) of 119.7 minutes. *(Adapted from Marler JR, Tilley BC, Lu M, et al: Early stroke treatment associated with better outcome.* Neurology *55:1649–1655, 2000.)*[59]

- *Missing at random (MAR):* Data that are missing because of an event, circumstances, or measure independent of the outcome of interest but related to another participant-specific measure. If the 3-month NIHSS score is missing because the participant was feeling depressed and did not wish to make the clinic visit, it is MAR (depression is not measured by NIHSS score).
- *Missing not at random (MNAR or non-ignorable):* The data are missing because of the unobserved outcome of interest. If the 3-month NIHSS score is missing because the participant's neurologic condition, measured by the NIHSS score deteriorated to the extent that the participant was unable to travel to the clinic, the missing data are non-ignorable.

Statistically, MCAR and MAR data are not problematic and standard statistical methods can be applied with minimal or no bias because the missing data are considered a representative sample of the observed data.[60] If more than a minimal amount of data are missing, this approach leads to reduction in statistical power.

For statistical analysis with MAR data, a multiple imputation method is recommended before analysis, because the method adds some uncertainty (variability) to the imputed value, allowing for more appropriate variance estimation.[62] Repeated measures analysis or survival analyses can be conducted with MAR data without imputing, if all other assumptions are met. Non-ignorable missing (MNAR) data are more problematic and conducting sensitivity analyses under several model assumptions is recommended.[60,61] In clinical trials in which an event such as death or recurrent stroke is the primary outcome and are MNAR, using an approach to analysis that assumes MAR and censors participants when they are lost to follow-up can introduce bias. Thus, approaches to multiple imputation specifically for survival data have been developed.[63] Ordinal data have been modeled including a score for treatment failure/death. For drop-outs approaches to handling missing data depend on why the data are missing, as described above.[64] When the reason for the primary outcome being missing is unknown, the most conservative approach is either to assume it is MNAR, or to use a worst-case outcome.

In the WARSS,[5] the primary outcome (recurrent ischemic stroke or death from any cause) for 2173 of the 2206 participants was assessed at the end of the trial. For the remaining 33, a pre-specified stratified imputation procedure was used that was specific to different types of loss to follow-up and assumptions.[5] A senior clinician, blinded to treatment assignments, classified the participants with missing outcomes into three categories and the following decisions were made:

1. Endpoint eminent; an endpoint was assumed to have occurred at the time the participant was lost to follow-up (n = 1) (MNAR).
2. Data missing for reason unrelated to study (e.g., participant moved to Puerto Rico with daughter); participant was censored at the date of loss to follow-up (i.e., participant's outcome was considered unknown after the date specified, and participant does not contribute information after that point in time) (n = 20) (MAR or MCAR).
3. Data missing for a reason possibly related to study (MNAR). For example, a TIA occurred then a participant was lost to follow-up. For this type of participants, methods of multiple imputation were used to impute a value for time to outcome, taking into account baseline covariates (n = 12). Of the 12 participants for whom multiple imputation was used, a primary outcome was imputed for two, and an event-free follow-up imputed for ten.[65] However, a sensitivity analysis was not reported.

ADAPTIVE DESIGNS

General Concepts

In an adaptive design, accumulating data are used to make midcourse modifications to the study design while maintaining validity and integrity of study data. Adaptive designs can involve concurrent changes during the course of the trial, such as changes in the eligibility criteria, length of study follow-up, study outcomes, or in sample size. Designs have been developed to take trials seamlessly from phase 2 to phase 3 using participants from phase 2, to augment the sample size for phase 3, or to take trials from phase 1 to phase 2 such as applied in ischemic stroke.[66] Adaptive designs can allow early termination in the face of strong evidence of efficacy or futility (see section on interim analysis). Potential adaptive design changes must be pre-specified in the protocol for the trial. An FDA guidance document describes approaches to reduce the

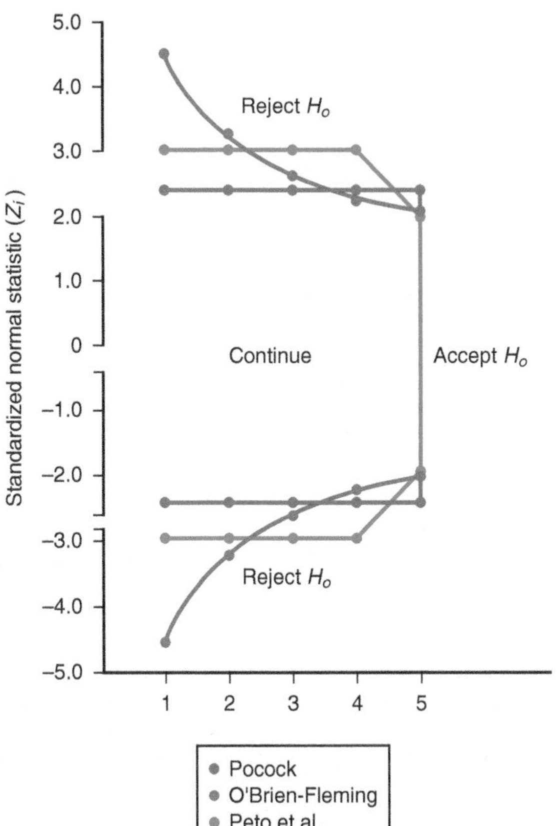

Figure 63-2. Guidelines for stopping a clinical trial. *(Adapted from Friedman LM, Furberg CD, DeMets DL:* Fundamentals of clinical trials, *ed 3, New York, 1998, Springer-Verlag.)*[1]

chance that an adaptive design will diminish the credibility of the trial.[67] In general, changes to the design should not be made where differences have been observed to date in outcome measures.

Interim Analysis

Most stroke trial participants are enrolled sequentially and followed longitudinally. Interim analyses conducted during the trial help to ensure participant safety. Stopping a trial early because of overwhelming evidence of the efficacy means controls have earlier access to an efficacious treatment and spend less time receiving an ineffective treatment; in addition it prevents the wasting of resources. If a pharmaceutical is being tested, time to approval may be shortened. Interim analyses allow the investigators and statisticians to evaluate assumptions made in the trial design regarding participant accrual rate and the parameters used for sample size estimation, and consideration of adaptive designs.

Figure 63-2 provides three examples of guidelines for stopping a trial.[1] Peto et al.[68] and O'Brien and Fleming[69] use more conservative guidelines early in their studies, leading to final type-I-error level for testing close to the planned overall type-I-error level (0.05). Pocock[70] uses a less conservative guideline. The final comparison would be at a type-I-error level much less than 0.05, and potentially less acceptable to investigators.

If all participants are quickly entered into the trial by the time the first or the second interim analysis is to be conducted, further interim analyses may be unnecessary. The Interventional Management of Stroke Study, a phase 2 trial with a planned sample size of 80 enrolled 10 patients per month. Enrollment was completed in 8 months, making planned interim analyses unnecessary.[18]

Stochastic curtailment originated in the quality control field for manufacturing, in which an entire batch of products would be rejected if a certain number of defective items were found; if that number was reached, the rest of the batch was not inspected. In clinical trials, stochastic curtailment determines whether proceeding further with the study would be unlikely to provide a statistically significant result. These analyses are completed separately from analyses of efficacy, and often implemented using a B-statistic[71] or Bayesian rules, derived from subjective prior information. Bayesian approaches have been used more frequently in cancer therapy trials than in trials of stroke prevention and therapy. Interim analyses, formal or informal, should be fully described in the study protocol.

SAMPLE SIZE

There are many commercial user friendly software packages,[72-74] and free shareware such as that developed by Vanderbilt University[75] employing various methods for sample size calculation. Using a sample size program requires choosing to use a one-tailed or two-tailed test and determining the type-I-error level or the power for the study.

One-Tailed or Two-Tailed Tests

A one-tailed test requires a smaller sample size to achieve the same effect with the same power. In phase 2 a one-sided test may be used to reduce sample size. In phase 3 investigators generally design the trial to learn whether the treatment group has an outcome better *or worse* than that of the control group, requiring a two-sided test. An exception, the EC/IC Bypass Study[76] investigators designed the trial using a one-tailed test to compare surgery with best medical care. Investigators assumed that if the trial indicated that surgery was no better than best medical care, surgery would not be recommended in the future due to its cost.

Power and Type I Error Level

In large multicenter phase 3 stroke trials, *power* (1 minus beta, the chance of missing a true difference if such a difference exists) is usually set high, 90% or greater, to allow interpretation of a negative result or lack of a treatment effect. If the investigators will accept a greater chance of missing a true difference if it exists, power can be as low as 80% (i.e., a 20% chance of missing the hypothesized treatment effect). The type-I-error level (chance of calling an ineffective treatment effective) is usually 0.05, but if multiple groups are being compared, the type-I-error level may be set to a smaller value. In a phase 2 study the tolerated type-I-error is often much larger (0.15 or 0.2), but power is usually set to 85% knowing a treatment will be tested further in phase 3 if the futility hypothesis cannot be rejected.[12]

Sample Size Based on Stroke Outcome Distributions

Applying these methods to clinical trials in stroke requires consideration of the expected distribution of stroke outcomes. In therapeutic stroke trials, outcome measures are often measured as a continuum or as ordinal categories to increase the power of the test and reduce the required sample size.[15,77] When considering the four outcomes pattern profiles for *shift analysis* as described in the section on Analysis, above, the smallest sample sizes are required when using mRS as a

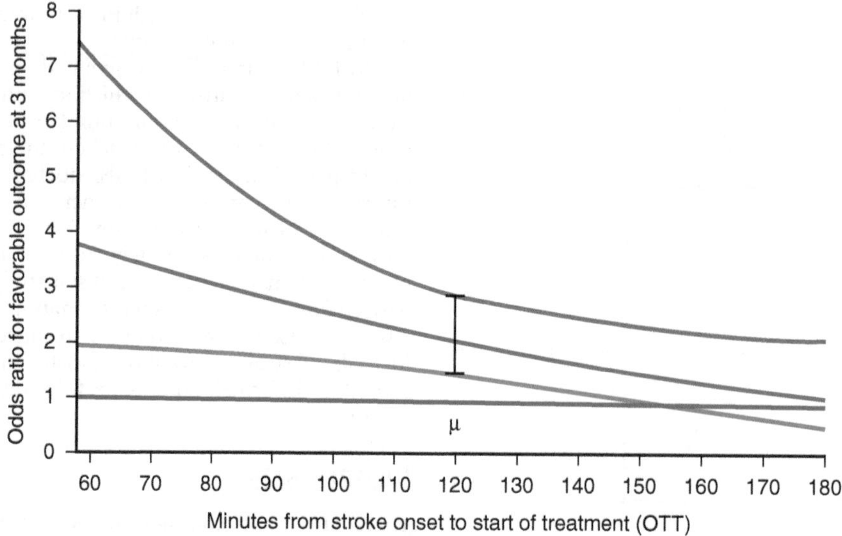

Figure 63-3. Distribution of the Barthel Index. *(Data from Tissue plasminogen activator for acute ischemic stroke. National Institute of Neurological Disorders and Stroke [NINDS] rt-PA Stroke Study Group.* N Engl J Med *333:1581–1587, 1995.)*[2]

continuum for pattern profiles (i) and (iv). If using dichotomization of the mRS then pattern profiles (ii) and (iii) require the smallest sample sizes.[77]

If the outcome distribution takes on a J- or U-shape, the gain from using a continuum is unclear. Figure 63-3 shows an example using the Barthel Index.[78] This J- or U-shaped distribution does not lend itself to transformation into a distribution that is less skewed or more normally distributed. Power can be increased and sample size decreased by dichotomizing J- or U-shaped distribution into success or failure and choosing a value or cut point in the distribution, depending on the question of interest before the start of the study.[77,78]

Sample size for Equivalence or Non-inferiority

When the probability of missing a true difference is high and when the power is low, negative study results are difficult to interpret. The detectable difference is usually chosen to be smaller than for phase 3 efficacy trials. Many software packages include sample size estimation for equivalence studies or non-inferiority studies.[72-74] A large number of drop-outs could lead to a spurious conclusion of non-inferiority or equivalence.[29]

Adjusting the Sample Size for Drop-Outs and Drop-Ins

Drop-outs (patients who are stopping the study therapy) and drop-ins (patients changing over to a study treatment different from their original assignment) must be considered when calculating the sample size. Inflating the sample size by the proportion expected to drop-out or drop-in may underestimate the size needed. The formula $1/(1\text{-R})^2$, where R is the drop-out or drop-in rate or a combination of the two, enlarges the sample size appropriately.[1]

META-ANALYSES AND POOLED ANALYSES

Meta-analysis refers to the statistical combination of results from two or more individual studies.[79] When individual studies are randomized clinical trials a meta-analysis compares the effects of the same or very similar interventions and estimates the overall direction, size, consistency studies.[80] Depending on the validity of assumptions, meta-analyses may provide misleading information. In early meta-analyses streptokinase and rt-PA studies were pooled, but later studies of rt-PA suggested that not all thrombolytics had the same effect.[81] Pooled analyses are meta-analysis of individual data.[82,83] Where the included trials share treatment and design characteristics, the meta-analysis may provide stronger evidence than a simple randomized clinical trial, in part by reducing publication bias if published and unpublished trials are included. Pooled analyses of individual patients are preferred over meta-analysis because there is a decrease in the variability caused by random error providing more precise estimates of effects.[84] Pooled analysis requires close cooperation among many investigators, both a benefit, as new collaborations emerge, and a challenge. Limitations include the cost associated with standardization of the data, the time required, and inability to remove systematic study-related biases.

Protocol and Manual of Procedures

A trial has two key documents, the protocol and the manual of procedures. Both are essential to trial management. The *protocol* provides a blueprint for the trial. The institutional review board and, when necessary, the FDA reviews and approve the protocol, as well as any changes. Protocols should be kept as simple, reflecting the primary aspects of study design with procedures being documented in the *manual of procedures (MOP)*. The MOP contains study instruments (i.e., forms for data collection), detailed instructions for completing study, case report forms, and other instructions for data collection, follow-up, laboratory procedures, and so on. The MOP documents responses to questions raised by investigators conducting the trial in the field so that answers to the same question are consistent over time. The protocol and MOP provide sufficient detail to allow someone who has not been participating in the trial to replicate the trial in another setting.

Training

An important aspect of quality assurance is training of the people collecting data for the trial. Some trials have developed video training and testing programs for stroke outcomes such as the modified Rankin and NIHSS scales.[16] To maintain consistency of NIHSS measurement over time, investigators are often recertified over the course of the trial.

REGULATIONS AND GUIDELINES

Federal and International Regulations

In the US, the two main federal agencies responsible for regulation of stroke-related clinical trials are the U.S. Department of Health and Human Services (DHHS) and the FDA. Federal regulations apply to all clinical investigations and to studies involving FDA-regulated products. Additional regulations and policies (such as the Good Clinical Practice formulated by the International Conference of Harmonisation of Technical Requirements for Registration of Pharmaceuticals for Human Use,[85] those of the U.S. Department of Veterans Affairs and the Joint Commission on Accreditation of Health Care Organizations) may also apply, depending on the source of funding or the purpose of the investigation. Federal regulations govern all clinical trials that are funded by federal money or are conducted in institutions that (1) receive federal money, (2) have federal project-wide assurances, or (3) conduct studies of investigational drugs with human participants. Any clinical trial of drugs, biological products, or medical devices involving interstate shipping or marketing requires prior submission to and approval from the FDA.

Ethics and the Protection of Human Subjects

In clinical trials of stroke therapies the informed consent process may be difficult when a stroke trial requires emergent therapy. In 1996, criteria to waive the informed consent requirement were established for research in emergency settings, exception to informed consent (EFIC). Under EFIC an experimental intervention can be given when the participant cannot provide informed consent because of a life-threatening medical condition and the absence of a legally authorized representative (LAR). The FDA provides detained guidelines on the use of EFIC.[86]

REFERENCES

1. Friedman LM, Furberg CD, DeMets DL. Fundamentals of clinical trials. New York: Springer; 2010.
2. The National Institute of Neurological Disorders and Stroke rt-PA Stroke Study Group. Tissue plasminogen activator for acute ischemic stroke. N Engl J Med 1995;333:1581–7.
3. Hacke W, Kaste M, Bluhmki E, et al. Thrombolysis with alteplase 3 to 4.5 hours after acute ischemic stroke. N Engl J Med 2008;359:1317–29.
4. Brott TG, Hobson RW, Howard G, et al. Stenting versus endarterectomy for treatment of carotid-artery stenosis. N Engl J Med 2010;363:11–23.
5. Mohr JP, Thompson JL, Lazar RM, et al. A comparison of warfarin and aspirin for the prevention of recurrent ischemic stroke. N Engl J Med 2001;345:1444–51.
6. The VITATOPS (Vitamins to Prevent Stroke) Trial: rationale and design of an international, large, simple, randomised trial of homocysteine-lowering multivitamin therapy in patients with recent transient ischaemic attack or stroke. Cerebrovasc Dis 2002; 13:120–6.
7. Little KM, Alexander MJ. Medical versus surgical therapy for spontaneous intracranial hemorrhage. Neurosurg Clin N Am 2002;13: 339–47.
8. Forster A, Young J, Nixon J, et al. A cluster randomized controlled trial of a structured training programme for caregivers of inpatients after stroke (TRACS). Int J Stroke 2012;7:94–9.
9. Forster A, Dickerson J, Young J, et al. A structured training programme for caregivers of inpatients after stroke (TRACS): a cluster randomised controlled trial and cost-effectiveness analysis. Lancet 2013;382:2069–76.
10. Ginsberg MD, Hill MD, Palesch YY, et al. The ALIAS Pilot Trial: a dose-escalation and safety study of albumin therapy for acute ischemic stroke – I: Physiological responses and safety results. Stroke 2006;37:2100–6.
11. Garrett-Mayer E. The continual reassessment method for dose-finding studies: a tutorial. Clin Trials 2006;3:57–71.
12. Palesch YY, Tilley BC, Sackett DL, et al. Applying a phase II futility study design to therapeutic stroke trials. Stroke 2005;36: 2410–14.
13. Tilley BC, Palesch YY, Kieburtz K, et al. Optimizing the ongoing search for new treatments for Parkinson disease: using futility designs. Neurology 2006;66:628–33.
14. Rankin J. Cerebral vascular accidents in patients over the age of 60. II. Prognosis. Scott Med J 1957;2:200–15.
15. Lees KR, Bath PM, Schellinger PD, et al. Contemporary outcome measures in acute stroke research: choice of primary outcome measure. Stroke 2012;43(4):1163–70.
16. National Stroke Association. The National Stroke Association NIH Stroke Scale (NIHSS) Certification Services. NIH Stroke Scale; Available from: <http://www.stroke.org/site/PageServer?pagename=NIHSS>; 2014 [cited 1-29-2014].
17. Tilley BC, Galpern WR. Screening potential therapies: lessons learned from new paradigms used in Parkinson disease. Stroke 2007;38(2 Suppl.):800–3.
18. IMS Study Investigators. Combined intravenous and intra-arterial recanalization for acute ischemic stroke: the Interventional Management of Stroke Study. Stroke 2004;35(4):904–11.
19. Khatri P, Hill MD, Palesch YY, et al. Methodology of the Interventional Management of Stroke III Trial. Int J Stroke 2008;3(2): 130–7.
20. Zaidat OO, Lazzaro MA, Gupta R, et al. Interventional Management of Stroke III trial: establishing the foundation. J Neurointerv Surg 2012;4(4):235–7.
21. Bechhofer RE, Santner TJ, Goldsman DM. Design and Analysis of Experiments for Statistical Selection, Screening and Multiple Comparisons. New York: John Wiley & Sons; 1995.
22. Levy G, Kaufmann P, Buchsbaum R, et al. A two-stage design for a phase II clinical trial of coenzyme Q10 in ALS. Neurology 2006;66(5):660–3.
23. Grieve AP, Krams M. ASTIN: a Bayesian adaptive dose-response trial in acute stroke. Clin Trials 2005;2(4):340–51.
24. Berry DA. Bayesian clinical trials. Nat Rev Drug Discov 2006;5(1): 27–36.
25. Broderick JP, Palesch YY, Demchuk AM, et al. Endovascular therapy after intravenous t-PA versus t-PA alone for stroke. N Engl J Med 2013;368(10):893–903.
26. Ginsberg MD, Palesch YY, Hill MD, et al. High-dose albumin treatment for acute ischaemic stroke (ALIAS) Part 2: a randomised, double-blind, phase 3, placebo-controlled trial. Lancet Neurol 2013;12(11):1049–58.
27. Elm JJ, Kamp C, Tilley BC, et al. Self-reported adherence versus pill count in Parkinson's disease: the NET-PD experience. Mov Disord 2007;22(6):822–7.
28. Campbell MK, Piaggio G, Elbourne DR, et al. Consort 2010 statement: extension to cluster randomised trials. BMJ 2012;345:e5661.
29. D'Agostino RB Sr, Campbell M, Greenhouse J. Non-inferiority trials: continued advancements in concepts and methodology (special papers for the 25th Anniversary of Statistics in Medicine 25(7). Stat Med 2006;25(7):1097–9.
30. Karanjia PN, Nelson JJ, Lefkowitz DS, et al. Validation of the ACAS TIA/stroke algorithm. Neurology 1997;48(2):346–51.
31. Brott T, Adams HP Jr, Olinger CP, et al. Measurements of acute cerebral infarction: a clinical examination scale. Stroke 1989;20(7): 864–70.
32. Mahoney FI, Barthel DW. Functional Evaluation: The Barthel Index. Md State Med J 1965;14:61–5.
33. Jennett B, Bond M. Assessment of outcome after severe brain damage: A Practical Scale. Lancet 1975;305(7905):480–4.
34. Tilley B, Huang P, O'Brien PC. Global Assessment Variables. In: D'Agostino R, Sullivan L, Massaro J, editors. Wiley Encyclopedia of Clinical Trials. New York: John Wiley & Sons, Inc.; 2007.
35. Hantson L. Neurological scales in assessment of stroke. In: Grotta J, Miller LP, Buchan AM, editors. Ischemic Stroke: Recent Advances in Understanding Stroke Therapy. Southborough, MA: International Business Communications; 1985. p. 42–54.

36. Lyden PD, Hantson L. Assessment scales for the evaluation of stroke patients. J Stroke Cerebrovasc Dis 1998;7(2):113–27.
37. Grizzle JE. A note on stratifying versus complete random assignment in clinical trials. Control Clin Trials 1982;3(4):365–8.
38. Scott NW, McPherson GC, Ramsay CR, et al. The method of minimization for allocation to clinical trials. A review. Control Clin Trials 2002;23(6):662–74.
39. Tilley BC, Lyden PD, Brott TG, et al. Total quality improvement method for reduction of delays between emergency department admission and treatment of acute ischemic stroke. The National Institute of Neurological Disorders and Stroke rt-PA Stroke Study Group. Arch Neurol 1997;54(12):1466–74.
40. The National Institute of Neurological Disorders and Stroke (NINDS) rt-PA Stroke Study Group. A systems approach to immediate evaluation and management of hyperacute stroke-Experience at eight centers and implications for community practice and patient care. Stroke 1997;28(8):1530–40.
41. Napoles-Springer AM, Grumbach K, Alexander M, et al. Clinical research with older African Americans and Latinos: perspectives from the community. Res Aging 2000;22(6):668–91.
42. Morisky DE, Green LW, Levine DM. Concurrent and predictive validity of a self-reported measure of medication adherence. Med Care 1986;24(1):67–74.
43. Gillings D, Koch G. The application of the principle of intention-to-treat to the analysis of clinical trials. Drug Inf J 1991;25(3): 411–24.
44. Hochberg Y. A sharper Bonferroni procedure for multiple tests of significance. Biometrika 1988;75(4):800–2.
45. O'Brien PC, Tilley BC, Dyck PJ. Composite Endpoints in Clinical Trials. In: Wiley Encyclopedia of Clinical Trials. New York: John Wiley & Sons, Inc.; 2007.
46. Tilley BC. Contemporary outcome measures in acute stroke research: choice of primary outcome measure and statistical analysis of the primary outcome in acute stroke trials. Stroke 2012;43(4):935–7.
47. Lu M, Tilley BC. Use of odds ratio or relative risk to measure a treatment effect in clinical trials with multiple correlated binary outcomes: data from the NINDS t-PA stroke trial. Stat Med 2001;20(13):1891–901.
48. Bath PM, Lees KR, Schellinger PD, et al. Statistical analysis of the primary outcome in acute stroke trials. Stroke 2012;43(4): 1171–8.
49. Bath PM, Gray LJ, Collier T, et al. Can we improve the statistical analysis of stroke trials? Statistical reanalysis of functional outcomes in stroke trials. Optimising Analysis of Stroke Trials (OAST) Collaboration. Stroke 2007;38(6):1911–15.
50. Savitz SI, Lew R, Bluhmki E, et al. Shift analysis versus dichotomization of the modified Rankin scale outcome scores in the NINDS and ECASS-II trials. Stroke 2007;38(12):3205–12.
51. McHugh GS, Butcher I, Steyerberg EW, et al. A simulation study evaluating approaches to the analysis of ordinal outcome data in randomized controlled trials in traumatic brain injury: results from the IMPACT Project. Clin Trials 2010;7(1):44–57.
52. Saver JL, Gornbein J. Treatment effects for which shift or binary analyses are advantageous in acute stroke trials. Neurology 2009; 72(15):1310–15.
53. Scott PA, Meurer WJ, Frederiksen SM, et al. A multilevel intervention to increase community hospital use of alteplase for acute stroke (INSTINCT): a cluster-randomised controlled trial. Lancet Neurol 2013;12(2):139–48.
54. Koch GG, Davis SM, Anderson RL. Methodological advances and plans for improving regulatory success for confirmatory studies. Stat Med 1998;17(15-16):1675–90.
55. O'Brien PC. The appropriateness of analysis of variance and multiple-comparison procedures. Biometrics 1983;39(3): 787–94.
56. Moye LA. Alpha calculus in clinical trials: considerations and commentary for the new millennium. Stat Med 2000;19(6): 767–79.
57. Yusuf S, Wittes J, Probstfield J, et al. Analysis and interpretation of treatment effects in subgroups of patients in randomized clinical trials. JAMA 1991;266(1):93–8.
58. Meade TW, Brennan PJ. Determination of who may derive most benefit from aspirin in primary prevention: subgroup results from a randomised controlled trial. BMJ 2000;321(7252):13–17.
59. Marler JR, Tilley BC, Lu M, et al. Early stroke treatment associated with better outcome: the NINDS rt-PA stroke study. Neurology 2000;55(11):1649–55.
60. Molenberghs G, Kenward MG. Missing Data in Clinical Studies. Hoboken, NJ: John Wiley & Sons, Ltd.; 2007.
61. Molenberghs G, Thijs H, Jansen I, et al. Analyzing incomplete longitudinal clinical trial data. Biostatistics 2004;5(3):445–64.
62. Schafer JL. Multiple imputation: a primer. Stat Methods Med Res 1999;8(1):3–15.
63. Taylor JM, Murray S, Hsu CH. Survival estimation and testing via multiple imputation. Stat Probab Lett 2002;58(3):221–32.
64. Li N, Elashoff RM, Li G, et al. Joint modeling of longitudinal ordinal data and competing risks survival times and analysis of the NINDS rt-PA stroke trial. Stat Med 2010;29(5):546–57.
65. Thompson JMG, Taylor S, Hsu CH. Statistical Considerations in the WARSS Collaboration. Presented to American Heart Association Stroke Meeting. San Antonio: 2002.
66. Thall PF, Cook JD. Dose-finding based on efficacy-toxicity trade-offs. Biometrics 2004;60(3):684–93.
67. U.S. Department of Health and Human Services. Food and Drug Administration. Center for Drug Evaluation and Research. Center for Biologics Evaluation and Research. Guidance for Industry. Adaptive Design Clinical Trials for Drugs and Biologics; Available from: http://www.fda.gov/downloads/Drugs/.../Guidances/ucm201790.pdf>; 2010 [cited 1-31-2014].
68. Peto R, Pike MC, Armitage P, et al. Design and analysis of randomized clinical trials requiring prolonged observation of each patient. I. Introduction and design. Br J Cancer 1976;34(6): 585–612.
69. O'Brien PC, Fleming TR. A multiple testing procedure for clinical trials. Biometrics 1979;35(3):549–56.
70. Pocock SJ. Group sequential methods in the design and analysis of clinical trials. Biometrika 1977;64:191–9.
71. Lan KK, Wittes J. The B-value: a tool for monitoring data. Biometrics 1988;44(2):579–85.
72. Elashoff JD. NQuery Advisor + nTerim® 2.0. Boston, MA: Statistical Solutions Ltd.; 2012. <http://www.statistical-solutions-software.com/nquery-advisor-nterim/>.
73. PASS 13. Power Analysis and Sample Size Software. 2013. <http://www.ncss.com/software/pass/>.
74. Ruiz A, Morillo LE. Epidemiologia Clínica, Investigación Clínica aplicada. In: Pérez A, Rodríguez N, Gil JFA, et al., editors. Tamaño de la Muestra. Programa sistematizado para el calculo del tamaño de la muestra y el poder en diseños de investigación. [A computer program to estimate the required sample size and power in clinical research]. V 1.1. Editorial Medica Panamericana. Register at Colombian Government Ministry: Book 13, Volume 7, Item 063. Bogotá, Colombia: Panamerican Health Organization/World Health Organization; 2001. <http://paltex.paho.org/bookdetail.asp?bookId=ECR01>.
75. Dupont WD, Plummer WD. PS: Power and Sample size Calculation 3.0.43. 2011. <http://biostat.mc.vanderbilt.edu/wiki/Main/PowerSampleSize>.
76. The International Cooperative Study of Extracranial/Intracranial Arterial Anastomosis (EC/IC Bypass Study): methodology and entry characteristics. The EC/IC Bypass Study Group. Stroke 1985;16(3):397–406.
77. Saver JL, Gornbein J. Treatment effects for which shift or binary analyses are advantageous in acute stroke trials. Neurology 2009;72(15):1310–15.
78. Lesaffre E, Scheys I, Frohlich J, et al. Calculation of power and sample size with bounded outcome scores. Stat Med 1993;12(11): 1063–78.
79. Glass GV. Primary, secondary, and meta analysis of research. Educ Res 1976;5(10):3–8.
80. Higgins JPT, Green S, editors. Cochrane Handbook for Systematic Reviews of Interventions. Version 5.0.1. The Cochrane Collaboration; Available from: <www.cochrane-handbook.org>; 2008, [cited 1-10-2014].
81. Wardlaw JM, Warlow CP, Counsell C. Systematic review of evidence on thrombolytic therapy for acute ischaemic stroke. Lancet 1997;350(9078):607–14.
82. Diener HC, Lees KR, Lyden P, et al. NXY-059 for the treatment of acute stroke: pooled analysis of the SAINT I and II Trials. Stroke 2008;39(6):1751–8.

83. Stroke Thrombolysis Trialists' Collaborative Group. Details of a prospective protocol for a collaborative meta-analysis of individual participant data from all randomized trials of intravenous rt-PA vs. control: statistical analysis plan for the Stroke Thrombolysis Trialists' Collaborative meta-analysis. Int J Stroke 2013; 8(4):278–83.
84. Emberson J, Lees KR, Lyden P, et al. Impact of treatment delay, age and stroke severity on the effects of intravenous thrombolysis with alteplase in acute ischaemic stroke: an individual patient data meta-analysis of randomised trials. Lancet In press;2014.
85. International Conference of Harmonisation. Guidance for Industry. E6. Good Clinical Practice: Consolidated Guidance. U.S. Food and Drug Administration. U.S.Department of Health and Human Services; Available from: <http://www.fda.gov/downloads/Drugs/GuidanceComplianceRegulatoryInformation/Guidances/UCM073122.pdf>; 1996, [cited 1-24-2014.].
86. U.S. Department of Health and Human Services. Food and Drug Administration. Office of Good Clinical Practice. Center for Drug Evaluation and Research. Center for Biologics Evaluation and Research. Center for Devices and Radiological Health. Guidance for Institutional Review Boards, Clinical Investigators, and Sponsors. Exception from Informed Consent Requirements for Emergency Research. Available from: <http://www.fda.gov/downloads/regulatoryinformation/guidances/ucm249673.pdf>; 2013, [cited 1-31-2014.].
87. The NINDS t-PA StrokeStudy Group. Generalized efficacy of t-PA for acute stroke – Subgroup analysis of the NINDS t-PA Stroke Trial. Stroke 1997;28(11):2119–25.

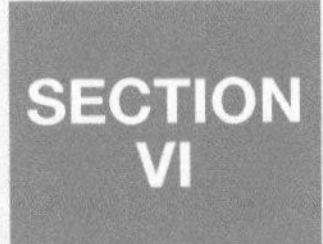

SECTION VI Therapy

PART B Interventional Therapy

Joseph P. Broderick

There are times in medicine when change happens gradually and other times when it happens almost all at once. In late 2014 and early 2015, after the chapters for this section of the book were finalized, positive results from several endovascular therapy trials were either presented or published. The trials employed several design features that differed from previous trials, including demonstration of intracranial occlusion, faster treatment, and use of the latest stent-retriever technology. The results of these studies are summarized in the Table and Figure.

First, the Multicenter Randomized Clinical Trial of Endovascular Treatment for Acute Ischemic Stroke in the Netherlands (MR CLEAN) Trial investigators reported that patients with large artery occlusions treated with endovascular therapy up to 6 hours from stroke onset, after standard therapy, had significantly better functional outcomes at 90 days. There was no difference in mortality rates or symptomatic intracranial hemorrhage rates as compared to standard therapy alone.[1]

Standard therapy included prior IV t-PA in 89% of 267 control subjects and stent-retrievers were used in 82% of 233 subjects randomized to endovascular therapy. The point estimates for endovascular therapy as compared to standard therapy were similar in patients with both moderate and severe baseline NIHSS scores, patients 80 years or older and younger, and those randomized earlier or later. Only the point estimate for patients with a baseline ASPECTS CT score of 0–4 showed no difference between the two treatment groups. The overall safety of endovascular therapy as compared to standard therapy was similar. The authors did report embolization into new arterial territories in 8.6% of endovascular patients, with an accompanying increase in the percentage of patients with new cerebral infarctions in areas outside of the original infarct region, as compared to subjects treated with standard therapy alone.

The population of patients included in MR CLEAN must be understood in order to interpret the significance of the findings. First, the median time to treatment with IV t-PA in both groups was less than 90 minutes from symptom onset; the fastest time to IV t-PA treatment in a trial since the original NINDS t-PA Stroke Trial.[2] The investigators should be congratulated for such an accomplishment. However, there was a substantial delay from start of IV t-PA treatment to randomization, which occurred at a median time of 204 minutes from symptom onset, and to groin puncture, which occurred at a median time of 260 minutes. Although it is not discussed in the primary manuscript, this substantial time delay occurred in many patients because of transport of patients from initial hospitals, where they were treated with IV t-PA, to tertiary centers, where endovascular therapy could be done, or in delays in the arrival of interventional teams. The authors also note that the CT angiography demonstrating the large artery occlusion was carried out in almost all patients after t-PA was started. Randomization required agreement of the stroke neurologist and the interventionalist about whether the patient should be randomized and occurred several hours, on average, after start of t-PA. Patients who had a large artery occlusion prior to IV t-PA and who had an excellent response to t-PA during this several hour period, or who developed advanced CT changes, probably would have been excluded from the trial. Thus, this trial has features of a "failed t-PA" trial rather than a trial where randomization occurred within minutes after onset of t-PA administration. This is reflected in the very low percentage of patients with a modified Rankin score (mRS) of 0–2 (good functional outcome) at 90 days in the standard (mostly IV t-PA) group (19%) and even in the endovascular group (33%).

The Endovascular Treatment for Small Core and Anterior Circulation Proximal Occlusion With Emphasis on Minimizing CT to Recanalization Times (ESCAPE) Trial also crossed a stopping boundary for efficacy in favor of endovascular therapy in late fall of 2014.[3] This trial focused on minimizing the time from hospital arrival to start of endovascular therapy by requiring groin puncture within 1 hour of imaging. This resulted in the fastest onset to treatment time of all the studies, suggesting an effective strategy for speeding endovascular therapy in practice. The time window for this trial was up to 12 hours from onset, thereby allowing "wake up" and t-PA ineligible patients, although 72% of endovascular patients were treated with t-PA (median 110–125 minutes since last seen normal). All subjects had to have documentation of an ASPECT score >5 on pretreatment CT, and the trial excluded patients with poor collaterals at CT angiography or severely decreased perfusion on CT perfusion.

The Extending the Time for Thrombolysis in Emergency Neurologic Deficits – Intra-Arterial (EXTEND IA) Trial also announced that it had stopped and had met its goal for efficacy using a combination primary endpoint of reperfusion at 24 hours and improvement on the NIHSS at 3 days.[4] Patients who received IV t-PA within 4.5 hours of stroke onset were treated out to 6 hours with endovascular therapy. EXTEND IA was the only one of the recent studies that selected patients on the basis of perfusion-core mismatch on MRI or CT perfusion imaging. While the population of patients included into ESCAPE and MR CLEAN overlapped with EXTEND IA, undoubtedly some patients who would have qualified for randomization in the trials based only on non-contrast CT criteria were excluded from EXTEND IA based on imaging. The percent of endovascular patients achieving TICI 2b3 flow and good outcome (mRS) were very high in this study (86% and 71% respectively), which might also reflect the strict imaging criteria for inclusion.

Solitaire With the Intention for Thrombectomy as Primary Endovascular Treatment Trial (SWIFT PRIME)[5] was stopped after enrolling 196 patients, just shy of a planned interim analysis at 200 patients. Patients were selected based either on mismatch imaging as in EXTEND IA, or on measurement of ischemic core on non-contrast CT using ASPECTS as in ESCAPE. Virtually all the patients in this trial were treated with t-PA, had distal ICA or M1 occlusions, and were treated with the Solitaire stent-retriever. SWIFT PRIME achieved the highest

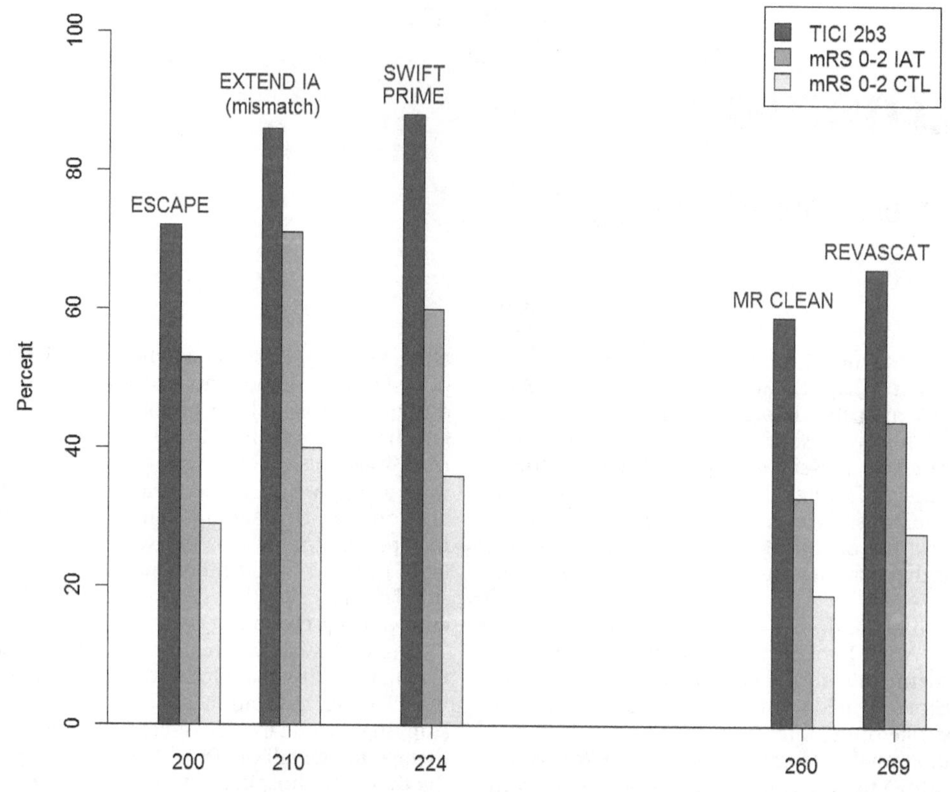

Figure Relationship of percentage of patients achieving thrombolysis in cerebral infarction grade 2b or 3 (TICI2b3) flow and patients achieving modified Rankin Scale (mRS) of 0–2 in intervention (intra-arterial thrombectomy [IAT]) and control (CTL) groups (y axis) vs minutes from last seen normal to groin puncture for each of the five published studies (x axis). The exact time to achieving maximal reperfusion is not available from published data for all studies, but where available is proportionate to time to groin puncture. Note the following: (1) the percentage of patients achieving good outcome is strikingly proportionate to the percentage of patients achieving TICI2b3 flow. (2) There is a consistent difference between the IAT and CTL groups in the percent achieving mRS 0 to 2 across all studies with the difference diminishing with increased time from last seen normal to groin puncture. (3) The percentage of patients achieving good outcome is roughly proportionate to the time from last seen normal to groin puncture (earlier groin puncture=higher proportion good outcome) with the exception being the EXTEND IA study, which was the only study to use advanced imaging for patient selection suggesting its use to identify responsive patients at delayed time intervals. ESCAPE indicates Endovascular Treatment for Small Core and Anterior Circulation Proximal Occlusion With Emphasis on Minimizing CT to Recanalization Times; EXTEND IA, Extending the Time for Thrombolysis in Emergency Neurological Deficits – Intra-Arterial; MR CLEAN, Multicenter Randomized Clinical Trial of Endovascular Treatment for Acute Ischemic Stroke in the Netherlands; SWIFT PRIME, Solitaire With the Intention for Thrombectomy as Primary Endovascular Treatment Trial; and REVASCAT, Randomized Trial of Revascularization With the Solitaire FR Device Versus Best Medical Therapy in the Treatment of Acute Stroke Due to Anterior Circulation Large Vessel Occlusion Presenting Within Eight Hours of Symptom Onset. *(From Grotta and Hacke. Stroke Neurologist's Perspective on the New Endovascular Trials. Stroke. 2015;46:1447–52. DOI: 10.1161/STROKEAHA.115.008384.)*

rate of TICI 2b3 reperfusion of all the studies 88% with corresponding high rates of mRS 0–2 in endovascular subjects (60%) as compared to subjects treated with t-PA alone (36%).

The Randomized Trial of Revascularization With the Solitaire FR Device Versus Best Medical Therapy in the Treatment of Acute Stroke Due to Anterior Circulation Large Vessel Occlusion Presenting Within Eight Hours of Symptom Onset (REVASCAT)[6] was stopped after an interim analysis of the first 206 patients. It allowed endovascular treatment out to 8 hours; though, on average groin, puncture occurred at 269 minutes. mRS 0–2 outcomes at 90 days in subjects treated with endovascular therapy (44%) were markedly better than outcomes in t-PA treated subjects (28%).

Other randomized trials that have been halted and presented at national meetings, but not yet published include Trial and Cost Effectiveness Evaluation of Intra-Arterial Thrombectomy in Acute Ischemic Stroke (THRACE)[7] and Assess the Penumbra System in the Treatment of Acute Stroke (THERAPY).[8] THRACE included basilar thrombosis and allowed a variety of older and newer devices, and THERAPY tested only the Penumbra device and required the presence of a clot >8 mm.

The point of all of these endovascular trials is that we have taken the next step beyond IV t-PA alone for acute therapy of those patients with acute ischemic stroke who harbor large arterial occlusions not likely to respond to IV t-PA alone. This advance has taken about 20 years since the publication of the original NINDS t-PA Stroke Trial. Despite this gap in time, the results of these studies are consistent with previous experience. For instance, the outcomes in the t-PA alone arms of these trials are similar to outcomes in previous t-PA studies treating similar patients within the same time frame. The IV t-PA group of the IMS III trial with a large artery occlusion prior to IV t-PA had 38.5% of patients reaching an mRS of 0–2 at 90 days, similar to SWIFT PRIME and EXTEND IA.[9] Also, prospective analyses of the 12-month outcomes in IMS III, demonstrated a significant benefit in favor of endovascular therapy for those with NIHSS ≥ 20 at baseline.[10] The recent studies were more

TABLE Summary of Data From the Five Published Trials

Trial N IAT+/CTL	NIHSS Range		t-PA	TICI 2B/3	LSN to Groin Median	mRS 0–2 @90d		Symptomatic ICH		Device Complications (No. of events)	Mortality	
	CTL	*IAT+*				*CTL*	*IAT+*	*CTL*	*IAT+*		*CTL*	*IAT+*
MR CLEAN [1] 500 233/267	18 14–21	17 14–22	90%	59%	260	19%	33%	6.4%	7.7%	Distal Embolization (13)	22%	21%
ESCAPE [3] 315 165/150	17 12–20	16 13–20	76%	72%	200	29%	53%	2.7%	3.6%	Vessel Perforation (1)	19%	10%
EXTEND IA [4] 70 35/35	13 9–19	17 13–20	100%	86%	210	40%	71%	6%	0%	Vessel Perforation (1) Distal Embolization (2)	20%	9%
SWIFT PRIME [5] 196 98/98	17 13–19	17 13–20	100%	88%	224	36%	60%	3%	0%	Subarachnoid Hemorrhage (4)	12%	9%
REVASCAT[6] 206 103/103	17 12–19	17 14–20	73%	66%	269	28%	44%	1.9%	1.9%	Vessel Perforation (5) Distal Embolization (5)	16%	18%

CTL indicates control group; IAT+, intra-arterial thrombectomy on top of standard treatment including t-PA; LSN, time (minutes) from last seen normal to groin puncture in IAT+ group; mRS 0–2 at 90 d, modified Rankin Scale of 0–2 at 90 days after randomization; NIHSS, baseline National Institutes of Health Stroke Scale; t-PA, patients in trial treated with recombinant tissue-type plasminogen activator; Symptomatic ICH (SITS), symptomatic intracerebral hemorrhage based on safe implementation of treatments in stroke criteria; and TICI 2b/3, patients in IAT+ group achieving thrombolysis in cerebral infarction grade 2b or 3 reperfusion.

From Grotta and Hacke. Stroke Neurologist's Perspective on the New Endovascular Trials. Stroke. 2015;46:1447–52. DOI: 10.1161/STROKEAHA.115.008384.

alike than different in their design and patients studied (see Table and Figure – documentation of intracranial occlusion – mostly distal ICA and M1, relatively normal pre-treatment non-contrast CT despite high NIHSS scores, IV t-PA treatment in the vast majority of patients, and rapid treatment in experienced endovascular centers with therapy begun within 6 hours of last seen normal using the latest stent-retrievers). We estimate that approximately 20–30% of patients who qualify for IV t-PA may fit into the group which benefitted from endovascular therapy in these trials, though the exact proportion remains to be determined since screening logs from most of these studies have not been reported. Roughly the same magnitude of benefit was seen in all studies, with the shortest delays to endovascular treatment associated with better results, and there was total absence of any signal of increased risk of mortality or bleeding. Although the investigators in all the trials were unblinded to treatment, the consistent and robust difference in favor of the intervention groups in each of these studies (number needed to treat approximately 4 for one additional good outcome) is reassuring that the benefit of endovascular intervention for the subpopulation of patients included in these trials is real.

These studies leave no doubt that rapid and sustained reperfusion will remain the primary treatment for acute ischemic stroke going forward, as it is for acute myocardial infarction.

Yet, many questions remain unanswered: (1) Beyond what time window, and using what imaging and clinical criteria, does endovascular therapy no longer provide benefit? (2) Can we improve endovascular therapy by limiting distal embolization by better devices and by better distal reperfusion using additional medications? (3) Can we provide better sustained *medical* reperfusion than with IV t-PA alone since only a minority of acute stroke patients who qualify for IV t-PA will be candidates for rapid endovascular therapy? (4) Can we safely speed the administration of IV t-PA or prove the efficacy of neuroprotection in the prehospital and early hospital setting to increase the likelihood that reperfusion will provide benefit? (5) Can endovascular therapy without use of prior IV t-PA be as effective as endovascular therapy following IV t-PA in the IV t-PA time window, and for which patients? (6) Can we limit symptomatic hemorrhagic transformation related to reperfusion? (7) What are the biologic limits for reperfusion therapy – those patients whose focal ischemia is so profound that even reperfusion within 30–60 minutes provides no benefit?

Finally, clinical scientific advances are only as impactful as the implementation of these advances in regional healthcare systems. It took more than 10 years from the publication of the NINDS t-PA Stroke Trial before IV t-PA became widely accepted and implemented. This development required changes in hospital reimbursement, institution of primary stroke centers, and education of physicians and the community. Our next primary challenge for endovascular therapy is not so much new trials, but how to implement this scientific advance in regional communities using a triage system that gets the largest number of patients to the right therapy at the right time and which is also cost-effective for our national health systems. Such a triage system should not lead to a proliferation of centers which intermittently use endovascular therapy for financial considerations and market share, but don't have the required "soup to nuts" of comprehensive stroke centers. Endovascular therapy should be carried out at hospitals with highly organized and trained stroke teams, well-defined and implemented processes of stroke care, highly trained cerebrovascular interventionalists, superb neurocritical care, and careful monitoring of outcomes. The trauma model is probably the best approach for healthcare systems to learn from going forward, but the details of how to get there will require new research, regional organization of EMS services, and political skill. Such changes in stroke triage will almost certainly have an impact on the treatment of intracerebral and subarachnoid hemorrhage as well, and recent treatment advances in patients with these stroke subtypes also point to the importance of comprehensive stroke centers for the management of patients with severe stroke of any type.

The stroke community has lots of work to do and it will be fascinating to revisit the progress that we will make by the time the next edition of this book is written. Let's keep stroke patients and their families in clear focus as we implement new changes in the delivery of stroke care in our health systems.

REFERENCES

1. Berkhemer OA, Fransen PS, Beumer D, et al. A randomized trial of intraarterial treatment for acute ischemic stroke. N Engl J Med 2015;372:11–20.
2. NINDS rt-PA Stroke Study Group. Tissue plasminogen activator for acute ischemic stroke. N Engl J Med 1995;333:1581–7.
3. Goyal M, Demchuk AM, Menon BK, et al. Randomized assessment of rapid endovascular treatment of ischemic stroke. N Engl J Med 2015;372:1019–30.
4. Campbell BCV, Mitchell PJ, Kleinig TJ, et al. Endovascular therapy for ischemic stroke with perfusion-imaging selection. N Engl J Med 2015;372:1009–18.
5. Saver JS, Goyal M, Bonafe A, et al. Stent-retriever thrombectomy after intravenous t-PA vs. t-PA alone in stroke [publish online ahead of print April 17, 2015]. N Engl J Med doi:10.1056/NEJMoa1415061.
6. Jovin TG, Chamorro A, Cobo E, et al. Thrombectomy within 8 hours after symptom onset in ischemic stroke [published online ahead of print April 17, 2015]. N Engl J Med doi:10.1056/NEJMoa1503780.
7. ClinicalTrials.gov identifier: NCT01062698.
8. ClinicalTrials.gov Identifier: NCT01429359.
9. Demchuk AM, Goyal M, Yeatts SD, et al. Recanalization and clinical outcome of occlusion sites at baseline CT angiography in the Interventional Management of Stroke III trial. Radiology 2014; 273:202–10.
10. Palesch YY, Yeatts SD, Tomsick TA, et al. Interventional Management of Stroke III Investigators. Twelve-Month Clinical and Quality-of-Life Outcomes in the Interventional Management of Stroke III Trial. Stroke 2015;46:1321–7.

64 Endovascular Therapy of Extracranial and Intracranial Occlusive Disease

Maxim Mokin, Elad I. Levy

KEY POINTS

- The Carotid Revascularization Endarterectomy versus Stenting Trial (CREST) demonstrated higher risk of stroke with carotid angioplasty and stenting (CAS) and higher risk of myocardial infarction with carotid endarterectomy (CEA).
- Age, sex, lesion morphology, lesion location, and aortic arch anatomy influence outcomes after CAS.
- Embolic protection devices improve the safety profile of carotid stenting and have become the standard of care in both investigational trials and routine clinical practice.
- In most patients with symptomatic stenosis, when CAS is indicated, it should be performed within the first 2 weeks of the original neurologic event.
- Endovascular therapy of extracranial vertebral artery stenosis is typically performed in patients with symptoms refractory to medical therapy.
- The Stenting and Aggressive Medical Management for Preventing Recurrent stroke in Intracranial Stenosis (SAMMPRIS) trial showed a higher rate of perioperative complications in patients with symptomatic intracranial stenosis treated with intracranial angioplasty and stenting than medical therapy alone.

Endovascular treatment of extracranial carotid artery disease with angioplasty and stenting has been best studied in patients with carotid artery stenosis at the bifurcation area, which is the most common location of such atherosclerotic lesions.[1] Data gathered from multiple registries and trials provide ample data on the safety and efficacy of carotid angioplasty and stenting (CAS) in patients with both symptomatic (qualifying event of stroke or transient ischemic attack [TIA] attributed to the stenotic lesion that occurred within the previous 6 months) and asymptomatic (qualifying event that occurred beyond the 6-month period or incidental discovery) carotid disease. Endovascular treatment of carotid stenosis has evolved over the last decade. The introduction of new stent and embolic protection technologies and advanced non-invasive imaging of plaque characteristics has resulted in improved safety profiles and lower perioperative complications rates.[2]

In contrast to CAS, catheter-based revascularization of extracranial vertebral artery atherosclerotic disease is less understood and is typically reserved for symptomatic patients in whom medical therapy is a failure. Because far less extracranial vertebral revascularization procedures are performed (compared with CAS procedures), no devices exist that are specifically designed for this purpose.

Intracranial stenting was originally considered a safe and effective alternative to medical therapy for patients with severe intracranial stenosis in whom the stroke risk was estimated to be as high as 20% per year.[3,4] However, direct comparison of intracranial stenting with best medical management demonstrated a significantly higher than expected rate of adverse events with intracranial stenting and a much lower than anticipated rate of stroke in the medical management group.[5] It has yet to be determined whether alternative endovascular treatments, such as submaximal angioplasty, will play a role in the management of patients with symptomatic intracranial stenosis.[5]

In this chapter, we present the current status of catheter-based approaches to the treatment of extracranial and intracranial occlusive disease. We review available data demonstrating indications, safety, and efficacy of such treatments, and also discuss new technological developments of this rapidly evolving field.

CAROTID ARTERY STENOSIS

Carotid angioplasty and stenting is an increasingly utilized minimally invasive endovascular treatment alternative to open surgical repair (carotid endarterectomy [CEA]) in patients with both symptomatic and asymptomatic carotid artery stenosis. A review of the 1998–2008 Nationwide Inpatient Sample demonstrated an increase in the percentage of patients undergoing CAS from 3% to 13%.[6] A correlation between utilization of CAS and publication of randomized trial results was found; an increasing number of CAS procedures followed the publication of CAS-favorable data in 2004 (after publication of the Stenting and Angioplasty with Protection in Patients at High Risk for Endarterectomy [SAPPHIRE] trial[7]) whereas the publication of CEA-favorable studies (Endarterectomy versus Stenting in Patients with Symptomatic Severe Carotid Stenosis [EVA-3S][8] and Stent-Protected Angioplasty versus Carotid Endarterectomy [SPACE][9] in 2006) was followed by a decrease in the number of CAS revascularization procedures. Because the results of the Carotid Revascularization Endarterectomy versus Stenting Trial (CREST) were not available until 2010,[10] the impact of this landmark trial on clinical practice has yet to be determined.

Carotid Stenosis and Stroke Risk

The efficacy of carotid revascularization in reducing the risk of ischemic stroke was first demonstrated by comparison of CEA to medical therapy alone. In the North American Symptomatic Carotid Endarterectomy Trial (NASCET), the greatest benefit of surgical revascularization was seen in patients with severe

TABLE 64-1 High-risk Features for Carotid Endarterectomy

Feature	Explanation
High or low lesion	High lesion extends above the second cervical vertebra (C2); low lesion is near the clavicle. Increased risk for CN injury (most commonly CN VII, X, XII)
History of radiation or previous surgery to the neck	Challenging surgical access
Lesion previously treated with CEA	Challenging surgical access
"Hostile" or immobile neck	Unable to rotate or extend neck due to arthritis or severe obesity. Challenging surgical access
Contralateral carotid occlusion	Unable to tolerate clamping of treated carotid artery
Tandem intracranial lesion, such as high-grade intracranial stenosis	Unable to treat with open surgical approach
Physiological features, examples: severe COPD, congestive heart failure classes III–IV, recent MI, ejection fraction <30%	Increased risk of peri-operative cardiac and pulmonary complications

CN, cranial nerve; COPD, chronic obstructive pulmonary disease; MI, myocardial infarction.

TABLE 64-2 American Heart Association/American Stroke Association Guidelines for Endovascular Treatment of Patients with Extracranial Carotid Disease

Guideline	Classification of Recommendation, Level of Evidence
CAS is considered an alternative to CEA in patients with ≥50% symptomatic carotid stenosis within 6 months of qualifying event (stroke or TIA)	I, B
CAS within 2 weeks of qualifying event, rather than delaying intervention, is reasonable in cases of symptomatic ICA stenosis	IIa, B
Selection of asymptomatic patients for CAS should be guided by an assessment of comorbid conditions and life expectancy	I, C
Dual antiplatelet therapy is recommended for a minimum of 30 days after CAS	I, C
Use of embolic protection devices can be beneficial during CAS to reduce risk of stroke	IIa, C
Non-invasive imaging after CAS is reasonable at 1 month, 6 months, and annually	IIa, C
Repeat angioplasty or stenting is reasonable with rapidly progressive restenosis that indicates a threat of complete carotid occlusion	IIa, C

CAS, carotid angioplasty and stenting; ICA, intenal carotid artery, TIA, transient ischemic attack.
Adapted from Brott TG et al. Circulation *2011; 124:e54–130.*[16]
For more details refer to "Evidence box index" in the FM.

(70–99%) stenosis, with an absolute reduction of 17% in the risk of ipsilateral stroke at 2 years.[11] A moderate benefit of CEA was demonstrated in patients with stenosis on the order of 50–69% (rates of ipsilateral stroke of 15.7% among patients treated surgically and 22% among those treated medically over a 5-year period).[12] There was no benefit of surgery in patients with less than 50% symptomatic stenosis.

The benefit of CEA in asymptomatic carotid stenosis was assessed in another randomized trial, the Asymptomatic Carotid Atherosclerosis Study (ACAS).[13] The trial included 1662 patients with asymptomatic carotid artery stenosis of 60% or more who were randomized to CEA or medical management with an antiplatelet agent and stroke risk factor modification. The 5-year risk for stroke or death was 5.1% for surgical patients and 11% for patients treated medically.

Several anatomical and physiological features are associated with a higher risk of peri-operative complication (including stroke and myocardial infarction [MI]) for patients undergoing CEA (Table 64-1). Anatomical features include the presence of contralateral carotid occlusion, history of previous CEA or radiation to the neck, hostile neck, and extremely low or high anatomical location of the lesion, making CEA technically challenging.[12,14,15] Physiological features include severe medical and surgical comorbidities[12,15] that make a minimally invasive CAS a safer alternative. CAS was first performed exclusively in patients who were considered "high risk" for CEA. Once the data from randomized trials demonstrated clinical equipoise between the two revascularization approaches, the popularity and utilization of CAS in clinical practice increased. Reviewed and discussed below are the results of pivotal randomized trials comparing safety and outcomes of carotid revascularization with CAS and CEA. Table 64-2 provides a summary of evidence that supports the role of CAS in the treatment of patients with extracranial carotid disease.[16]

Randomized Trials of Carotid Angioplasty and Stenting versus Carotid Endarterectomy

The Carotid Revascularization Endarterectomy versus Stenting Trial (CREST) is considered a landmark trial that compared outcomes associated with open surgical versus endovascular treatment of carotid atherosclerotic disease (symptomatic patients with >50% and asymptomatic patients with >60% stenosis).[10] This randomized, controlled trial with blinded end-point adjudication conducted at 108 centers in the US and nine in Canada had a rigorous certification process; all participating operators had to undergo evaluation of their carotid stenting experience and participation in hands-on training.[17] The study committee evaluated 427 applicants for participation in the trial, and only 224 interventionists were selected to participate in the randomized phase. Such a demanding process ensured that every selected operator was qualified to perform either CEA or CAS and emphasized the value of operator experience to avoid criticism seen with previously published trials. For example, in the EVA-3S trial,[8] surgeons had to have performed at least 25 CEA procedures in the year before enrollment, whereas substantially less CAS procedure exposure was required – only five interventions were required for an interventionist to join the trial. The participation of operators with limited CAS training and experience in the EVA-3S trial was subsequently criticized as a potential factor explaining the unusually high peri-operative complication risk in the CAS arm of this trial (the 30-day risk of stroke or death was 9.6% with CAS).[17]

Among the 2,522 patients enrolled in CREST, no significant difference was found in the estimated 4-year rates of primary end points (stroke, MI, or death from any cause during the peri-procedural period or any ipsilateral stroke within 4 years) between the stenting and endarterectomy groups (7.2% and 6.8%, respectively; P = 0.51).[10] In the peri-operative period, both procedures were associated with similar mortality rates (0.7% with CAS versus 0.3% with CEA, P = 0.18). The risk of stroke was higher with CAS (4.1% vs 2.3% with CEA, P = 0.01), and the risk of MI was higher with CEA (2.3% vs 1.1% with CAS, P = 0.03).

A subsequent analysis of the CREST data showed that most strokes were minor (defined as National Institutes of Health Stroke Scale [NIHSS] score ≤8, which was the score in 81% of all strokes in CREST) with the median NIHSS score of 2.[18] An important observation came from a breakdown of the distribution of strokes relative to the time of the interventions; most strokes associated with CAS occurred on the day of the procedure (29 events with CAS vs nine with CEA). Beyond day 0, there was no longer a significant difference in stroke rates between the two procedures. Major strokes were infrequent and occurred in 0.6% of all patients, mostly several days after the procedure (median, 3 days from the date of the procedure). These events included intracranial hemorrhages that were potentially related to hyperperfusion syndrome.

A strong relationship between patient age and stroke risk was shown in CREST.[10] The hazard ratio for the primary end point indicated safety and efficacy of CAS at a younger age and CEA at an older age. At the age of approximately 70 years, both procedures were equally safe. A more detailed analysis of the CREST data on the impact of age in CAS-treated patients confirmed an increased risk for stroke with CAS at an older age.[19] The risk of stroke with CEA remained relatively unchanged at both young and older ages. Such a relationship between age and stroke risk with CAS and CEA was true for both symptomatic and asymptomatic patients.

The influence of age on outcomes of carotid revascularization was addressed in a meta-analysis of three other major randomized trials - EVA-3S, SPACE, and the International Carotid Stenting Study (ICSS).[20] Analysis of outcome data from 3433 patients with symptomatic carotid stenosis identified age as a strong predictor of primary outcome events (stroke and death) in patients treated with CAS. According to the intention-to-treat analysis, in patients younger than 70 years, the estimated 6-month risk of primary outcome events was similar with both types of treatment (5.8% with CAS and 5.7% with CEA); whereas in older patients, the risk doubled with stenting (12% vs 5.9% with CEA).

Nevertheless, the theory that there is an association between age and risk of stroke from CAS is controversial. Other studies have suggested that perioperative stroke risk is increased secondary to unfavorable arch anatomy, such as types II, III, and bovine arch (left common carotid and brachiocephalic arteries with a common origin), which is more commonly seen in the elderly.[21,22] In a carefully selected group of elderly patients, including octogenarians, CAS can be performed with a low complication rate.[21,22] Age is often considered a high-risk feature for CEA.[23] However, similar to CAS, in a highly selected group of elderly patients without major cardiovascular comorbidities, CEA can be performed with a safety profile comparable to that for younger patients.[24]

The influence of gender on outcomes in patients undergoing CAS is another area of ongoing research and is not well understood. In the CREST design, a recruitment goal of 40% women was set to provide data on treatment differences between male and female gender and primary end points (stroke, MI, or death).[10] When the trial was completed, 35% of randomized patients were women. No influence of gender on 4-year rates of primary outcomes from CAS and CEA were seen, based on a pre-specified analysis.[10] Further subgroup analysis showed that women had higher rates of peri-procedural events with CAS than with CEA (6.8% vs 4.3%, P= 0.047) but men did not.[25] The difference was mostly driven by a higher rate of stroke in women during the peri-procedural period (5.5% with CAS compared to 3.7% with CEA, P = 0.013). Although a meta-analysis of other randomized trials of CEA vs CAS did not confirm the influence of gender on short-term outcomes,[20] CREST data emphasize the need for further investigation.

The Stent-Protected Angioplasty versus Carotid Endarterectomy (SPACE) trial was a multicenter European randomized trial of CEA vs CAS that evaluated 1183 patients with ≥50% symptomatic stenosis (per NASCET criteria[11]) between 2001 and 2006.[9] The 30-day rates of ipsilateral ischemic or hemorrhagic stroke or death were 6.8% with CAS and 6.3% with CEA (P-value for non-inferiority, 0.09). The 2-year follow-up results demonstrated similar rates of ipsilateral ischemic stroke and any stroke or death for both treatment groups.[26]

Recurrent stenosis of ≥70% documented by carotid Doppler imaging was more frequent in the CAS group than the CEA group (intention-to-treat life-table estimate of 10.7% vs 4.6%, P = 0.0009).[26] Restenosis was most common in the first 6 months after treatment (52% of all restenosis cases after CAS or CEA). Of 54 total cases of restenosis following CAS during the 2-year period, only two led to neurological symptoms.

A subanalysis of the SPACE data indicated a higher complication rate (ipsilateral stroke or death) with increased age in the CAS group but not in the CEA group (P = 0.001 and P = 0.534, respectively).[27] Similar to the CREST findings, a crossover at the age of 68 years showed the greatest separation between high- and low-risk populations of CAS-treated patients. Analogous to the CREST data, the CEA group in SPACE showed a homogeneous distribution of complication rates across different age groups.

Endarterectomy versus Stenting in Patients with Symptomatic Severe Carotid Stenosis

The EVA-3S trial was conducted to compare CAS with CEA in patients with symptomatic carotid stenosis of 60% or more.[8] After the enrollment of 527 patients, the trial was stopped for safety reasons because of the increased 30-day risk of stroke or death in the CAS group (9.6% vs 3.9% with CEA, P = 0.01).

The trial was started in 2000 and initially did not mandate the use of embolic protection devices with carotid stenting. In 2003, the trial safety committee recommended stopping unprotected CAS because of the associated significant increase of stroke, which was 3.9 times higher than that of protected CAS.[28] Upon completion of the EVA-3S study, a subsequent analysis confirmed the value of cerebral protection devices in reducing peri-operative complications.[29] Significant reduction in stroke or death rates was seen within 24 hours, as well as within 30 days in "protected" stenting cases. Proximal and distal protection devices demonstrated equal safety profiles.

Embolic Protection Devices

The utilization of embolic protection devices was very limited in early trials that evaluated safety and efficacy of CAS. As discussed earlier in this chapter, with accumulated evidence of an improved safety profile of carotid stenting when using such

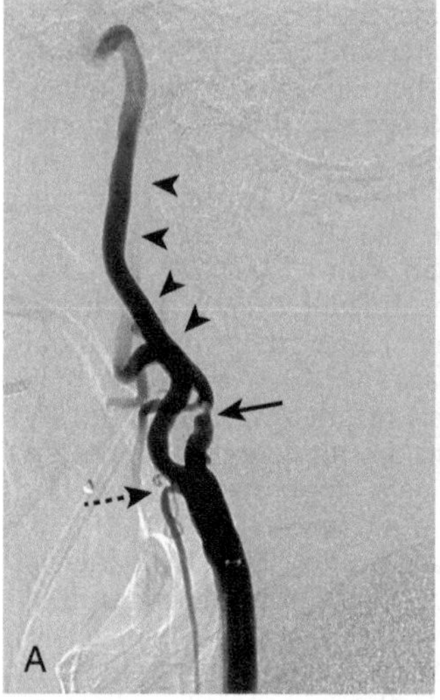

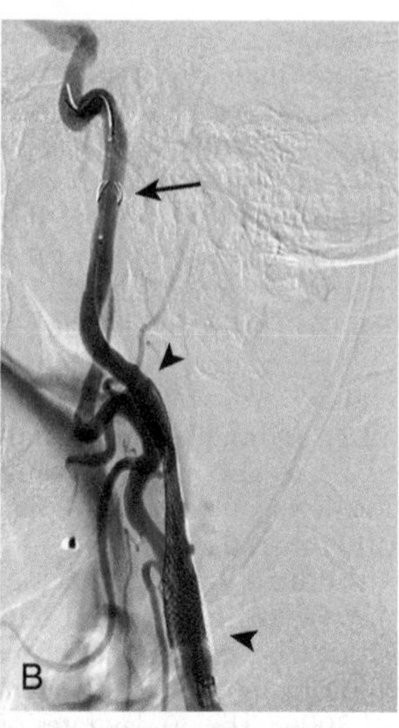

Figure 64-1. Example of distal embolic protection for carotid angioplasty and stenting. A, Diagnostic digital subtraction angiogram, lateral view, showing a focal high-grade stenosis at the origin of the internal carotid artery (ICA) (*arrow*). Note the rather straight course of the cervical ICA (*arrowheads*), allowing easy deployment of the distal filter. Although no disease exists within the proximal external carotid artery, the very early takeoff of the superior thyroid artery (*dashed arrow*) might interfere with obtaining complete flow arrest if a proximal protection device is used. This case is best managed with a distal filter. B, Intraoperative digital subtraction angiogram shows a filter basket successfully deployed within the distal cervical ICA (*arrow*). No lucency is seen within the filter basket, suggesting lack of any significant embolic debris. A closed-cell stent is successfully deployed (*arrowheads* indicate the proximal and distal ends of the stent).

devices, embolic protection has become the standard of care in both investigational trials and routine clinical practice.

Evidence in support of cerebral protection devices comes from two major systematic reviews of studies comparing "unprotected" CAS with the use of various protection devices. The review by Kastrup et al.[30] was based on the analysis of 3433 carotid stenting procedures and demonstrated a threefold increased risk of any stroke or death from CAS without protection compared with protected CAS. In a more recent systematic analysis that included a total of 23,461 stenting procedures, a benefit of protected CAS was confirmed in both symptomatic and asymptomatic patients.[31]

The two main types of embolic protection devices include distal filters (so-called "distal protection") and flow-cessation or flow-reversal devices ("proximal protection"). Distal filters are positioned beyond the lesion, higher in the internal carotid artery, and act as an umbrella by capturing plaque debris that can be released during angioplasty and stenting (Fig. 64-1). Distal filters are manufactured by several companies and vary in pore size and deployment mechanisms, but all share the same basic design. These devices allow continuous cerebral perfusion during the stenting procedure and are easy to use. Their limitations include incomplete apposition to the vessel wall, allowing some debris to escape the filter basket and cause embolic complications, and difficulty in deployment and capture in cases of tortuous internal carotid arteries (Fig. 64-2).

Proximal protection devices create cessation or reversal of blood flow by the introduction and inflation of two balloons – one in the external carotid artery and the second in the common carotid artery (Fig. 64-3), thus not allowing any plaque debris to circulate towards the brain. Because blood flow through the internal carotid artery is arrested for the duration of the procedure, some patients without adequate collateral supply via the contralateral carotid artery or posterior circulation might develop ischemia and not tolerate the procedure. For example, in one registry that evaluated the Mo.Ma proximal protection device (Invatec, Roncadelle, Italy),

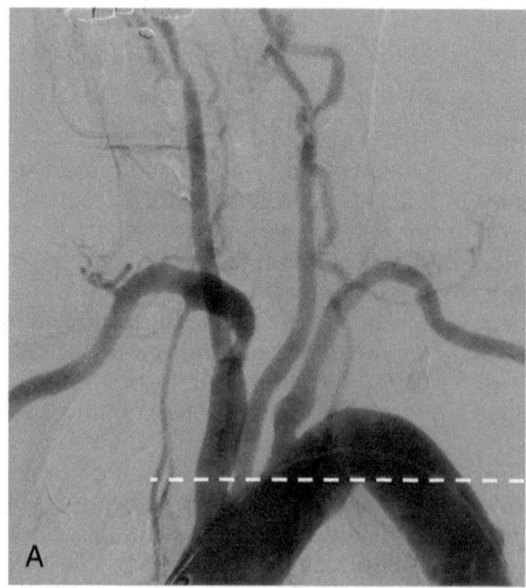

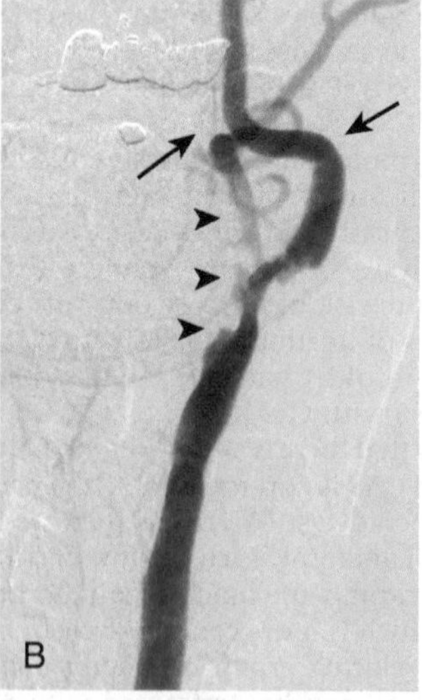

Figure 64-2. Challenging anatomy for carotid angioplasty and stenting in a patient with symptomatic carotid stenosis. A, Diagnostic digital subtraction angiogram, aortic arch run, anteroposterior (AP) view demonstrates type III arch (innominate and left common carotid artery origins are below the inferior margin of the aortic arch, as indicated by the *dashed line*) suggesting technically difficult access for transfemoral carotid artery stenting and high risk for perioperative complications. B, Diagnostic digital subtraction angiogram, AP view, left common carotid artery injection shows an extensive ulcerated plaque causing more than 50% stenosis. Two 90° turns within the cervical left internal carotid artery (*arrows*) make the use of a distal embolic protection device (filter) challenging. A combination of a hypoplastic external carotid artery and extensive plaque ulceration starting at the distal common carotid artery (*arrowheads*) precludes the use of proximal embolic protection devices. This case is best managed with CEA.

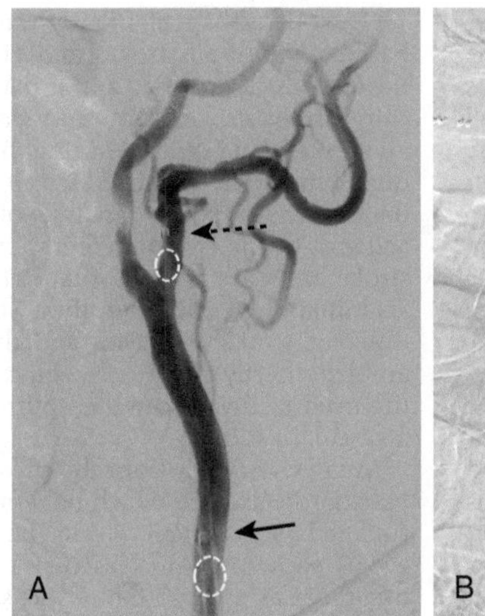

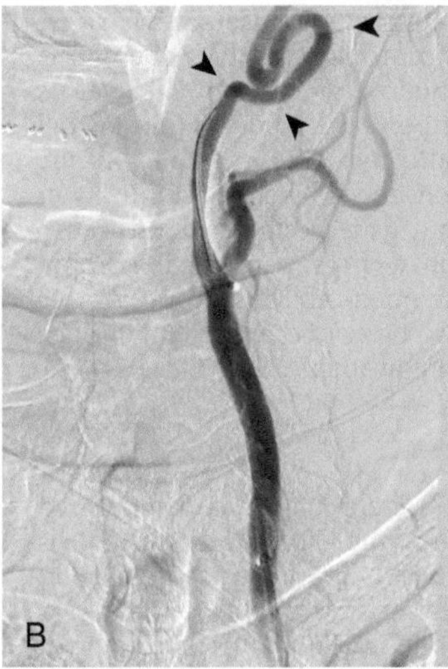

Figure 64-3. Example of proximal embolic protection for carotid angioplasty and stenting. A, Diagnostic digital subtraction angiogram, anteroposterior view, showing near occlusion of the ICA. The Mo.Ma flow arrest device (Invatec, Roncadelle, Italy) is brought into the common carotid artery with the distal balloon marker located in the proximal external carotid artery (*dashed arrow*) and the proximal balloon marker in the common carotid artery (*arrow*). Blood flow is blocked once both balloons are inflated (actual inflation not shown, *dashed circles* used for schematic illustration). B, Once flow arrest is achieved, a stent is brought over the delivery wire (seen inside the stent) and unsheathed. Note the extremely tortuous course of the distal cervical ICA (*arrowheads*), making the use of a distal filter impossible. Also, the use of a distal filter in a case of near-occlusion would increase the risk for plaque rupture while passing the filter through the "unprotected" lesion.

8% of patients developed transient intolerance to flow cessation and required intermittent balloon deflation or alternative cerebral protection devices.[32]

Studies suggest that proximal protection might be more effective than filters in preventing embolic complications during CAS.[33-35] In those studies, embolic load to the brain measured with diffusion-weighted magnetic resonance (MR) imaging or transcranial Doppler imaging was used as a primary end point. Although the rate of clinical events was similar for the two types of protection, given the potential association between cerebral embolization during cardiac interventions and cognitive deficits,[36] further studies are needed to evaluate optimal approaches to embolic protection during CAS.

An alternative approach to transfemoral CAS includes direct transcervical access via a direct carotid artery puncture or a small cut-down. Such an approach circumvents catheterization of the aortic arch and proximal common carotid artery in cases of challenging proximal anatomy and eliminates the risk of the embolic events that happen during this maneuver. An analysis of 12 studies reporting the combined results of 739 CAS procedures with transcervical access showed an impressive 96% technical success rate and a low complication rate.[37] The incidences of stroke, MI, and death were 1.1%, 0.1%, and 0.4%, respectively.

When selecting the type of embolic protection device for CAS, several factors should be considered (Table 64-3). A hypoplastic or stenotic origin of the external carotid artery can interfere with placement of the distal balloon, thereby precluding the use of a proximal protection device. Severe tortuosity of the cervical carotid artery distal to the lesion might interfere with deployment and landing of a distal filter. Severe plaque ulceration and irregularity can be too challenging for the navigation of a distal filter, increasing risk for plaque rupture. Finally, a type II or III arch can be more suitable for direct transcervical access.

TABLE 64-3 High-risk Features for CAS

Feature	Explanation
Type II or III arch, bovine arch, ostial stenosis	Challenging access, increased risk of peri-operative stroke
Tortuosity of the lesion, vessel kinking	Poor stent opposition
History of gastrointestinal hemorrhage	Increased risk for hemorrhagic complications with dual antiplatelet therapy
Allergy to stent materials	Permanent stent placement will trigger allergic reaction with intimal hyperplasia causing in-stent stenosis
Severe contrast material allergy	Increased risk of peri-operative complications

CAS, carotid angioplasty and stenting.

Stents

Self-expanding stents for CAS include two main types: open-cell and closed-cell designs. Open-cell stents have incomplete connections between the stent struts that increase the stent's flexibility, and they can be used in vessel segments with extensive carotid bifurcation angulation or tortuosity. Their free-cell area coverage is larger than that of a closed-cell stent; therefore, theoretically, there is a higher risk of embolic debris release into the circulation, especially when treating plaques with so-called "unstable" features (such as intraplaque hemorrhage and/or ulcerated plaque surface) with open-cell stents. A closed-cell stent design implies a complete connection between all stent struts and provides a small free-cell area.

Data in support of closed-cell versus open-cell design and the risk of peri-procedural neurologic complications are controversial. A review of data from 1684 consecutive patients at ten European centers who underwent CAS with either closed-cell or open-cell stents failed to show an advantage of a specific stent-cell design.[38] An analysis of outcome data from the SPACE trial, which only included patients with symptomatic stenosis, showed a significantly lower rate of ipsilateral stroke or ipsilateral stroke death in patients treated with a closed-cell stent (5.6% vs 11% open-cell stent, $P = 0.029$).[39] Such analyses should be interpreted with caution, because several other factors (such as protected or unprotected CAS, type of embolic protection device, and distribution of symptomatic versus asymptomatic lesions) are all powerful confounding factors and can influence clinical outcomes. For example, in the SPACE trial, embolic protection devices were not utilized in the majority of cases in which a closed-cell stent was used.[39] Conversely, cerebral protection devices were used in more than half of the patients in the open-cell stent group. At this time, trials that compare the two types of carotid stent designs in a randomized fashion are not available.

Restenosis Rates

Restenosis rates following CAS were evaluated and compared to CEA in a secondary analysis of the CREST data (restenosis was defined as ≥70% diameter-reducing stenosis by Doppler ultrasonography).[40] The rates were similar during the 2-year follow-up period after CEA and CAS (Kaplan-Meier rates of 6.3 and 6.0%, respectively). Female sex, diabetes, and dyslipidemia predicted an increased rate of restenosis, irrespective of intervention type or symptomatic status. Interestingly, there was a higher rate of restenosis seen in smokers after CEA but not after CAS. However, this observation was not supported in another study, which demonstrated an increased risk of restenosis post-CAS in smokers.[41] Previous cervical radiation therapy, multiple stent deployments, and increased length of the stenotic lesion are additional risk factors for restenosis.[42,43] Such groups of patients might benefit from closer monitoring for restenosis with non-invasive imaging, which typically includes carotid Doppler ultrasonography.

Balloon angioplasty alone for carotid stenosis is no longer performed in clinical practice or trials due to high restenosis rates and concern for release of unprotected plaque debris into the circulation, which was demonstrated in earlier studies. For example, in the Carotid and Vertebral Artery Transluminal Angioplasty Study (CAVATAS), which was a randomized trial of endovascular versus surgical treatment conducted between 1992 and 1997, most patients in the endovascular arm were treated with balloon angioplasty alone (76% of patients vs 24% treated with a stent).[44] In this study, a significantly lower risk for restenosis in patients treated with a stent than angioplasty alone was observed.[41] The cumulative 1-year incidence of ≥70% restenosis was 13% with a stent and 25% with angioplasty alone. At the 5-year follow-up review, the incidence of restenosis was 17% and 36%, respectively.

Direct comparison of restenosis rates between different trials should be done with caution. The definition of restenosis used in clinical trials is most commonly based on carotid Doppler velocity thresholds, which can vary significantly. A more detailed discussion of this issue can be found in the analysis of restenosis rates of the CREST.[40]

Timing of Revascularization in Symptomatic Stenosis

Current guidelines recommend revascularization of symptomatic carotid stenosis within 2 weeks of the qualifying clinical event.[16] The benefit of early CEA was shown in a pooled analysis of the European Carotid Surgery Trial (ECST) and NASCET in which the relationship between timing of surgical intervention and reduction of stroke risk was investigated.[45] CEA performed within 2 weeks of the original neurologic event resulted in 30% reduction in absolute risk of stroke, whereas delaying CEA by more than 4 weeks weakened the stroke-risk-reduction effect by nearly one-third. The optimal timing of performing CAS is not well understood and is understudied.

The Oxford Vascular Study was a prospective, population-based study of all strokes and TIAs in 91,105 individuals in the UK, which provided ample data on the risks and identifiers of recurrent stroke.[46] The study indicated that almost half of all strokes that occurred during the 30-day period following a qualifying event happened within the first 24 hours. Another dataset from a pooled analysis of observational studies with active outcome ascertainment showed a staggering 10% risk of stroke at 2 days after an initial TIA and 13% at 30 days after an initial TIA.[47] Although these studies include patients with different stroke etiologies and thus the findings cannot be applied directly to patients with carotid stenosis, they indicate the need to investigate the optimal time window for carotid revascularization.

Analysis of data from the prospectively collected Swedish Vascular Registry in which patients received ultra-urgent CEA (defined as treatment within the first 2 days of a qualifying event) showed an increased risk of adverse events, whereas treatment as early as day 3 was safe (comparable to average risk). Ultra-early CAS treatment performed within the first 2 days might have a safety profile similar to procedures performed during the later period; however, studies that support this conclusion are limited by heterogeneity and small size of patient population and should be interpreted with caution.[48–50] For example, the study by Setacci et al.[48] only included patients with TIA or minor strokes, whereas Zaidat et al.[50] also included patients with moderate-to-severe stroke and fluctuating neurological symptoms in their analysis.

EXTRACRANIAL VERTEBRAL ARTERY STENOSIS

Unlike the endovascular treatment of carotid artery stenosis, which has been the subject of multiple investigations and trials, the epidemiology, risks, and treatment strategies of extracranial vertebral artery disease are much less understood. Symptoms of posterior circulation ischemia can often be misinterpreted for peripheral vertigo or cardiac disease, leading to under-recognition and misdiagnosis.[51–53] Imaging of extracranial vertebral stenosis is more challenging than of the anterior circulation due to the smaller size, asymmetry and tortuous course of the posterior circulation.[54]

The anatomy of the vertebral artery is often described by dividing it into four distinct segments (V1–V4). The V1 segment is the most proximal segment, starting from the origin of the vertebral artery and ending at the entrance into the transverse vertebral foramen, whereas V4 is the most distal segment that joints the contralateral vertebral artery to form the vertebrobasilar junction. The V1 segment and, specifically, the vertebral artery origin (ostium), is the most common site for atherosclerotic occlusive disease.[55,56]

Studies estimating the long-term survival and natural history of vertebral artery origin stenosis indicate a high risk of stroke or death associated with this type of lesion. Thompson et al.[57] observed a 5-year survival rate for symptomatic patients who had presented with a stroke and were found to have ostial lesions of 67% compared to a rate of 89% in matched control subjects (patients with a stroke but no ostial lesions on angiography). Similar results were found in a study conducted by Moufarrij et al.,[58] in which the 5-year survival rate was 60% compared to 87% in a matched control population. Table 64-4 provides a summary of evidence in support of the role of endovascular interventions in patients with extracranial vertebral artery disease.

A pooled analysis of data from individual patients presenting with posterior circulation ischemic symptoms, who underwent MR angiography or computed tomographic angiography for the diagnosis of vertebral stenosis from two recent prospective studies (Oxford Vascular Study and St. George's Study), was recently published.[59] The 90-day risk of stroke was 16% in patients with extracranial vertebral stenosis vs 7% in those without.

Angioplasty and Stenting

Endovascular therapy of extracranial vertebral artery stenosis is typically performed in patients with symptoms refractory to medical therapy. No consensus currently exists on the severity of stenosis that warrants endovascular intervention. To this day, no randomized trial has evaluated adequately whether endovascular therapy is superior to medical therapy in patients with symptomatic extracranial vertebral disease.

The aforementioned CAVATAS was a mixed trial that included patients with carotid and vertebral stenoses. The disproportionate number of patients with carotid disease (n = 504) compared with those with vertebral stenosis (n = 16) limits the interpretation and generalizability of the trial data.[44,60] The randomized vertebral artery cases included extracranial stenosis in 15 patients and intracranial stenosis in one patient. The trial failed to show any benefit of endovascular treatment over medical therapy. It is important to consider that of eight patients allocated to the endovascular group, only two were treated with stents, whereas the six other patients were treated with balloon angioplasty alone. Primary angioplasty of extracranial vertebral stenosis is no longer considered the standard of modern clinical practice, due to its high restenosis rate and the risk of dissection.[61–63]

TABLE 64-4 American Heart Association/American Stroke Association Guidelines for Selection and Treatment of Patients with Extracranial Vertebral Artery Disease

Guideline	Classification of Recommendation, Level of Evidence
In patients with posterior circulation ischemia who may be candidates for revascularization, catheter-based angiography can be useful to define vertebral artery pathology	IIa, C
In patients who are status post vertebral artery revascularization, serial non-invasive imaging is reasonable at 1 month 6 months, and annually	IIa, C

Adapter from Brott TG et al. Circulation *2011; 124:e54–130.*[16]
For more details refer to "Evidence box index" in the FM.

A recent systematic review evaluated the safety and durability of endovascular treatment of symptomatic extracranial vertebral artery stenosis.[64] Cumulative data from 993 patients (98.7% treated with stenting and 1.3% with angioplasty alone) demonstrated a very low rate of perioperative neurologic events – 1.1% for stroke and 0.8% for TIA within 30 days of the intervention. The overall technical success rate (defined as residual stenosis <20%) was achieved in 99.3% of cases – a very impressive result for an interventional procedure. The majority of treated lesions were located at the vertebral artery origin (72%). Within a 21-month follow-up period, the rate of vertebrobasilar stroke was 1.3% and 6.5% for a TIA. The review demonstrated a lower rate of restenosis with drug-eluting stents (11.2%) than with bare-metal stents (30%).

Both transfemoral and transbrachial approaches can be used for vertebral stenting (Fig. 64-4). Owing to the small size of the vertebral artery, distal embolic protection devices (filters) are typically not used. Severe tortuosity or extensive calcifications of the proximal vertebral artery can make accurate landing and deployment of the stent more challenging. Currently, there are no endovascular devices designed specifically for vertebral stenosis treatment. Instead, stents and angioplasty balloons approved for cardiac or peripheral interventions are most commonly used.

INTRACRANIAL ATHEROSCLEROSIS

With advances in non-invasive intracranial imaging, intracranial atherosclerotic disease (ICAD) is becoming more recognized in clinical practice. ICAD is most commonly diagnosed in Hispanic, African-American, and Asian patient populations.[65–67] The frequency of large-artery intracranial occlusive disease in patients with stroke is estimated to be as high as 50% in certain Asian populations, and this disorder is likely the most common cause of stroke worldwide.[67,68]

The Warfarin versus Aspirin for Symptomatic Intracranial Disease (WASID) trial was a landmark study that established

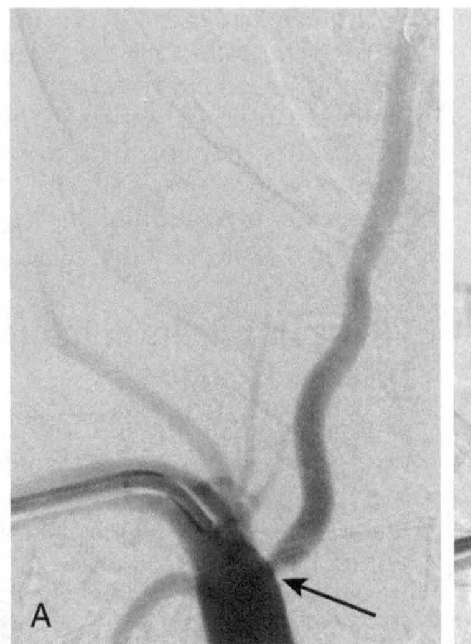

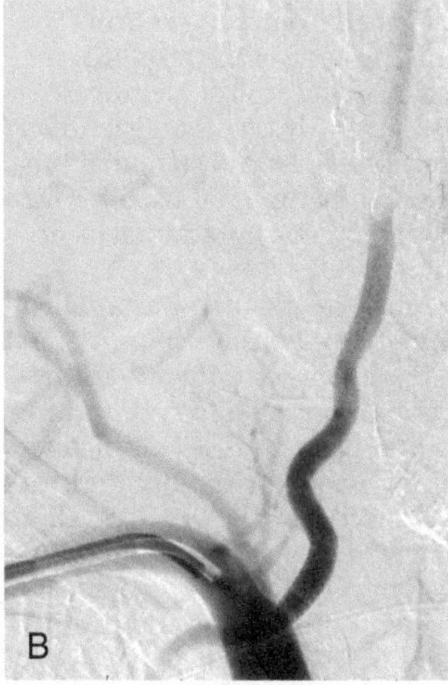

Figure 64-4. Vertebral artery origin stenting. A, Diagnostic digital subtraction angiogram via a transbrachial approach, anteroposterior view, right subclavian artery injection, showing severe stenosis of the right vertebral artery origin (*arrow*) in a patient with a recent posterior circulation stroke and a hypoplastic contralateral vertebral artery (not shown). B, Following placement of a balloon-mounted stent, there is complete resolution of the vertebral artery origin stenosis.

the superiority of an antiplatelet agent (aspirin) over an anticoagulant (warfarin) in the treatment of symptomatic ICAD.[69] Treatment with warfarin was found to be associated with a significantly higher rate of adverse events and without any added benefit over aspirin in preventing a secondary stroke or death. Importantly, the trial's pre-specified analysis helped identify patients with the highest risk for stroke in the territory of the stenotic artery and established a foundation for the stenting trial of ICAD, which will be discussed later in this chapter.

The WASID trial enrolled patients who had had a qualifying event (stroke or TIA) within 3 months of randomization that was attributed to 50–99% stenosis of a major intracranial artery (both anterior and posterior circulation included), which was confirmed with angiography. Patients with concurrent extracranial carotid stenosis were excluded from the trial. The key finding was that stenosis severity correlated with subsequent stroke risk; stenosis ≥70% resulted in a higher risk of stroke in the territory of the stenotic artery than stenosis <70%. Another important finding was identifying the optimal time window for intervention; patients randomized early (≤17 days) after the qualifying event were at highest risk to experience recurrent ischemic symptoms. ICAD location was not associated with increased risk of stroke.

Stenting and Aggressive Medical Management for Preventing Recurrent Stroke in Intracranial Stenosis Study

With the goal of targeting the population of patients at highest risk for recurrent stroke, the SAMMPRIS study enrolled patients with a recent TIA or non-disabling stroke with angiographically verified 70–99% stenosis of a major intracranial artery.[5,70] Study patients were randomized to receive medical management alone versus endovascular treatment with intracranial angioplasty and stenting. The hypothesis was that angioplasty and stenting combined with aggressive medical management would add benefit in preventing primary end points (stroke or death) during the 2-year follow-up period, which was estimated at 24.7% in the medical arm and 16.1% in the angioplasty/stenting arm.

On the basis of WASID data analysis, best medical management alone was estimated to produce a 15% relative-risk reduction for primary events, whereas an even higher relative-risk reduction of 35% was anticipated from intervention. The 35% reduction was estimated on the basis of the results of the prospective multicenter Wingspan stent (Stryker Neurovascular, Fremont, California, USA; formerly Boston Scientific, Natick, Massachusetts, USA) registry (the type of stent that was used in SAMMPRIS).[4] In the registry, stenting was used for the treatment of severe (70–99%) symptomatic intracranial stenosis and demonstrated promising results.

In SAMMPRIS, an aggressive medical regimen was applied that consisted of management of low-density lipoprotein-cholesterol with a statin, blood pressure control with antihypertensive agents, and programs for smoking cessation, weight-loss, and life-style modifications.[5,70] The antiplatelet regimen included aspirin, 325 mg daily, for the duration of the study; and clopidogrel, 75 mg daily, for 90 days after enrollment. Such a dual antiplatelet regimen ensured identical medical management of both arms, because the two agents were required for 90 days in patients undergoing intracranial stenting to prevent in-stent thrombosis.

To qualify for participation in the SAMMPRIS trial, neurointerventionists were required to submit at least 20 previous cases of intracranial angioplasty and stenting to the trial committee for review of procedural outcomes. According to the trial protocol, the intervention consisted of gradual, slow inflation of the Gateway angioplasty balloon (Stryker Neurovascular) for predilatation of the lesion. Once the balloon was fully deflated and removed, the Wingspan self-expanding intracranial stent was centered within the lesion for deployment. If significant residual stenosis was seen after deployment of the stent, post-stenting balloon angioplasty was performed.

The trial was designed with an estimated enrollment of 382 patients in each of the two arms in order to demonstrate superiority of endovascular intervention over medical management alone. However, on the basis of recommendations made by the study's safety committee, enrollment of patients into SAMMPRIS was stopped after a significantly higher rate of stroke and death was seen in patients undergoing angioplasty and stenting. Analysis of 451 patients who underwent randomization between 2008 and 2011 revealed 30-day rates of stroke or death of 14.7% in the stenting group and 5.8% in the medical-management group (P = 0.002).[5] The rate of primary end-point events remained significantly higher for the angioplasty and stenting group than the medical group throughout the entire follow-up period of the study (medical group duration of follow-up, 32 months): 12.6% vs 19.7% at year 1, 14.1% vs 20.6% at year 2, and 14.9% vs 23.9% at year 3.[71]

Lessons from Stenting and Aggressive Medical Management for Preventing Recurrent Stroke in Intracranial Stenosis Study

The majority of strokes in the angioplasty and stenting arm occurred within the first 24 hours of the intervention, prompting detailed analysis of the types and mechanisms of peri-procedural stroke complications after endovascular treatment for symptomatic ICAD.[72] Review of catheter angiography records and post-procedural MR imaging showed that local perforator ischemic stroke was the most frequent type of peri-procedural stroke (likely secondary to displaced plaque debris, the so-called "snow-plowing" effect), whereas distal symptomatic embolic stroke was uncommon. Other common types of stroke were intraparenchymal (possibly secondary to reperfusion hemorrhage) and subarachnoid hemorrhages (from wire perforation).

Criticism of the SAMMPRIS trial included the effect of operator experience on the unexpectedly high rate of peri-procedural events in the angioplasty and stenting group, drawing an analogy with the EVA-3S carotid stenting trial, which we discussed earlier in this chapter.[73] However, analysis of operator training background and experience with the Gateway and Wingspan devices failed to demonstrate any link between peri-procedural stroke rate and individual operator and site experience.[74]

Future Directions of Intracranial Atherosclerotic Disease Treatment

Although the SAMMPRIS trial clearly demonstrated superiority of aggressive risk factor management plus antiplatelet therapy over intracranial stenting in patients with symptomatic high-grade ICAD, the question remains regarding optimal treatment of those patients who develop recurrent stroke symptoms despite best medical management. The reported 5.8% risk of stroke and death at 30 days and 12.6% at 1 year are alarming.

Submaximal angioplasty alone (without stenting) has emerged as an alternative to intracranial stenting (Fig. 64-5). Theoretical benefits include limited intimal injury and

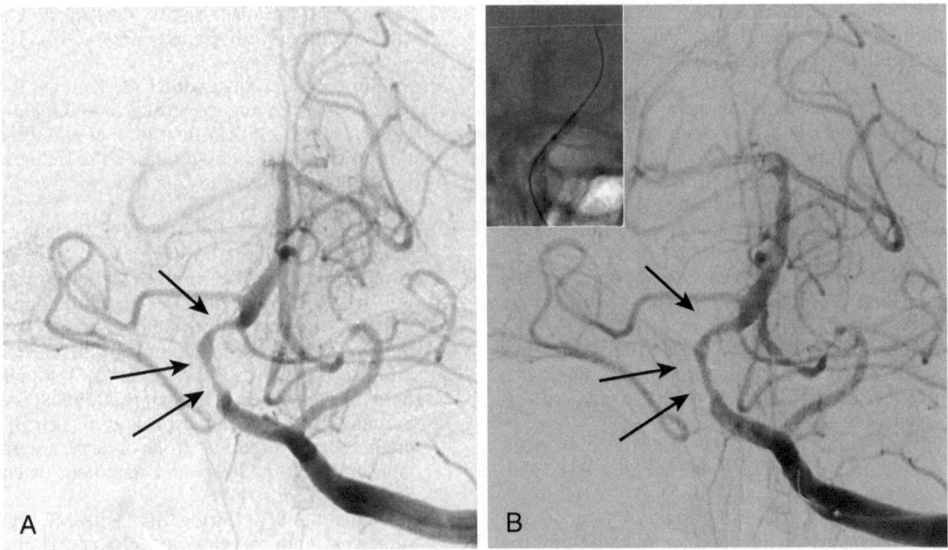

Figure 64-5. Submaximal angioplasty for intracranial atherosclerotic disease. A, Diagnostic digital subtraction angiogram, AP view, left vertebral artery injection, displaying severe stenosis of the vertebrobasilar junction (*arrows*) in a patient with recurrent brainstem strokes while placed on a dual antiplatelet regimen. B, Gentle submaximal angioplasty with a balloon sized to 50% of the diameter of the basilar artery resulted in only moderate improvement in the degree of stenosis (*arrows*). Insert shows the inflated angioplasty balloon delivered over the microwire. Because flow is proportional to the fourth power of the (vessel) radius (Poiseuille's law), even modest improvement in the degree of stenosis results in greatly augmented blood flow.

reduced risk of reperfusion hemorrhage, because the goal of submaximal angioplasty is partial restoration (only) of the original vessel diameter. Even achieving partial recanalization with an undersized balloon results in a significant augmentation of blood flow, because flow is proportional to the fourth power of the (vessel) radius (Poiseuille's law). Studies suggest that this technique has an improved safety profile over intracranial stenting, with the 30-day risk of perioperative stroke of approximately 5%.[75,76] However, direct comparison of submaximal angioplasty to best medical management is lacking. Further research into the role of noninvasive imaging for identification of patients at higher risk for stroke and the roles of medical therapy and intra-arterial interventions is needed.

REFERENCES

1. Fisher CM, Gre I, Okabe N, et al. Atherosclerosis of the carotid and vertebral arteries – extracranial and intracranial. J Neuropathol Exp Neurol 1965;24:455–76.
2. Siddiqui AH, Natarajan SK, Hopkins LN, et al. Carotid artery stenting for primary and secondary stroke prevention. World Neurosurg 2011;76:S40–59.
3. Kasner SE, Chimowitz MI, Lynn MJ, et al. Predictors of ischemic stroke in the territory of a symptomatic intracranial arterial stenosis. Circulation 2006;113:555–63.
4. Zaidat OO, Klucznik R, Alexander MJ, et al. The NIH registry on use of the Wingspan stent for symptomatic 70–99% intracranial arterial stenosis. Neurology 2008;70:1518–24.
5. Chimowitz MI, Lynn MJ, Derdeyn CP, et al. Stenting versus aggressive medical therapy for intracranial arterial stenosis. N Engl J Med 2011;365:993–1003.
6. Dumont TM, Rughani AI. National trends in carotid artery revascularization surgery. J Neurosurg 2012;116:1251–7.
7. Yadav JS, Wholey MH, Kuntz RE, et al. Protected carotid-artery stenting versus endarterectomy in high-risk patients. N Engl J Med 2004;351:1493–501.
8. Mas JL, Chatellier G, Beyssen B, et al. Endarterectomy versus stenting in patients with symptomatic severe carotid stenosis. N Engl J Med 2006;355:1660–71.
9. Ringleb PA, Allenberg J, Bruckmann H, et al. 30 day results from the SPACE trial of stent-protected angioplasty versus carotid endarterectomy in symptomatic patients: a randomised non-inferiority trial. Lancet 2006;368:1239–47.
10. Brott TG, Hobson RW 2nd, Howard G, et al. Stenting versus endarterectomy for treatment of carotid-artery stenosis. N Engl J Med 2010;363:11–23.
11. North American Symptomatic Carotid Endarterectomy Trial Collaborators. Beneficial effect of carotid endarterectomy in symptomatic patients with high-grade carotid stenosis. N Engl J Med 1991;325:445–53.
12. Barnett HJ, Taylor DW, Eliasziw M, et al. Benefit of carotid endarterectomy in patients with symptomatic moderate or severe stenosis. North American Symptomatic Carotid Endarterectomy Trial Collaborators. N Engl J Med 1998;339:1415–25.
13. Executive Committee for the Asymptomatic Carotid Atherosclerosis Study. Endarterectomy for asymptomatic carotid artery stenosis. JAMA 1995;273:1421–8.
14. Gasecki AP, Eliasziw M, Ferguson GG, et al. Long-term prognosis and effect of endarterectomy in patients with symptomatic severe carotid stenosis and contralateral carotid stenosis or occlusion: results from NASCET. North American Symptomatic Carotid Endarterectomy Trial (NASCET) Group. J Neurosurg 1995;83:778–82.
15. Young B, Moore WS, Robertson JT, et al. An analysis of perioperative surgical mortality and morbidity in the asymptomatic carotid atherosclerosis study. Stroke 1996;27:2216–24.
16. Brott TG, Halperin JL, Abbara S, et al. ASA/ACCF/AHA/AANN/AANS/ACR/ASNR/CNS/SAIP/SCAI/SIR/SNIS/SVM/SVS guideline on the management of patients with extracranial carotid and vertebral artery disease. A report of the American College of Cardiology Foundation/American Heart Association Task Force on Practice Guidelines, and the American Stroke Association, American Association of Neuroscience Nurses, American Association of Neurological Surgeons, American College of Radiology, American Society of Neuroradiology, Congress of Neurological Surgeons, Society of Atherosclerosis Imaging and Prevention, Society for Cardiovascular Angiography and Interventions, Society of Interventional Radiology, Society of NeuroInterventional Surgery, Society for Vascular Medicine, and Society for Vascular Surgery. Circulation 2011;124:e54–130.
17. Hopkins LN, Roubin GS, Chakhtoura EY, et al. The Carotid Revascularization Endarterectomy versus Stenting Trial: credentialing of interventionalists and final results of lead-in phase. J Stroke Cerebrovasc Dis 2010;19:153–62.

18. Hill MD, Brooks W, Mackey A, et al. Stroke after carotid stenting and endarterectomy in the Carotid Revascularization Endarterectomy versus Stenting Trial (CREST). Circulation 2012;126:3054–61.
19. Voeks JH, Howard G, Roubin GS, et al. Age and outcomes after carotid stenting and endarterectomy: the carotid revascularization endarterectomy versus stenting trial. Stroke 2011;42:3484–90.
20. Bonati LH, Dobson J, Algra A, et al. Short-term outcome after stenting versus endarterectomy for symptomatic carotid stenosis: a preplanned meta-analysis of individual patient data. Lancet 2010;376:1062–73.
21. Setacci C, Chisci E, Setacci F, et al. Siena carotid artery stenting score: a risk modelling study for individual patients. Stroke 2010;41:1259–65.
22. Dumont TM, Mokin M, Wach MM, et al. Understanding risk factors for perioperative ischemic events with carotid stenting: is patient age over 80 years or is unfavorable arch anatomy to blame? J Neurointerv Surg 2014;6:219–24.
23. Kazmers A, Perkins AJ, Huber TS, et al. Carotid surgery in octogenarians in Veterans Affairs medical centers. J Surg Res 1999;81:87–90.
24. Debing E, Van den Brande P. Carotid endarterectomy in the elderly: are the patient characteristics, the early outcome, and the predictors the same as those in younger patients? Surg Neurol 2007;67:467–71.
25. Howard VJ, Lutsep HL, Mackey A, et al. Influence of sex on outcomes of stenting versus endarterectomy: a subgroup analysis of the Carotid Revascularization Endarterectomy versus Stenting Trial (CREST). Lancet Neurol 2011;10:530–7.
26. Eckstein HH, Ringleb P, Allenberg JR, et al. Results of the Stent-Protected Angioplasty versus Carotid Endarterectomy (SPACE) study to treat symptomatic stenoses at 2 years: a multinational, prospective, randomised trial. Lancet Neurol 2008;7:893–902.
27. Stingele R, Berger J, Alfke K, et al. Clinical and angiographic risk factors for stroke and death within 30 days after carotid endarterectomy and stent-protected angioplasty: a subanalysis of the SPACE study. Lancet Neurol 2008;7:216–22.
28. Mas JL, Chatellier G, Beyssen B, et al. Carotid angioplasty and stenting with and without cerebral protection: clinical alert from the Endarterectomy Versus Angioplasty in Patients With Symptomatic Severe Carotid Stenosis (EVA-3S) trial. Stroke 2004;35:e18–20.
29. Naggara O, Touze E, Beyssen B, et al. Anatomical and technical factors associated with stroke or death during carotid angioplasty and stenting: results from the endarterectomy versus angioplasty in patients with symptomatic severe carotid stenosis (EVA-3S) trial and systematic review. Stroke 2011;42:380–8.
30. Kastrup A, Groschel K, Krapf H, et al. Early outcome of carotid angioplasty and stenting with and without cerebral protection devices: a systematic review of the literature. Stroke 2003;34:813–19.
31. Garg N, Karagiorgos N, Pisimisis GT, et al. Cerebral protection devices reduce periprocedural strokes during carotid angioplasty and stenting: a systematic review of the current literature. J Endovasc Ther 2009;16:412–27.
32. Reimers B, Sievert H, Schuler GC, et al. Proximal endovascular flow blockage for cerebral protection during carotid artery stenting: results from a prospective multicenter registry. J Endovasc Ther 2005;12:156–65.
33. Montorsi P, Caputi L, Galli S, et al. Microembolization during carotid artery stenting in patients with high-risk, lipid-rich plaque. A randomized trial of proximal versus distal cerebral protection. J Am Coll Cardiol 2011;58:1656–63.
34. Bijuklic K, Wandler A, Hazizi F, et al. The PROFI study (Prevention of Cerebral Embolization by Proximal Balloon Occlusion Compared to Filter Protection During Carotid Artery Stenting): a prospective randomized trial. J Am Coll Cardiol 2012;59:1383–9.
35. Schmidt A, Diederich KW, Scheinert S, et al. Effect of two different neuroprotection systems on microembolization during carotid artery stenting. J Am Coll Cardiol 2004;44:1966–9.
36. Pugsley W, Klinger L, Paschalis C, et al. The impact of microemboli during cardiopulmonary bypass on neuropsychological functioning. Stroke 1994;25:1393–9.
37. Sfyroeras GS, Moulakakis KG, Markatis F, et al. Results of carotid artery stenting with transcervical access. J Vasc Surg 2013;58:1402–7.
38. Schillinger M, Gschwendtner M, Reimers B, et al. Does carotid stent cell design matter? Stroke 2008;39:905–9.
39. Jansen O, Fiehler J, Hartmann M, et al. Protection or nonprotection in carotid stent angioplasty: the influence of interventional techniques on outcome data from the SPACE Trial. Stroke 2009;40:841–6.
40. Lal BK, Beach KW, Roubin GS, et al. Restenosis after carotid artery stenting and endarterectomy: a secondary analysis of CREST, a randomised controlled trial. Lancet Neurol 2012;11:755–63.
41. Bonati LH, Ederle J, McCabe DJ, et al. Long-term risk of carotid restenosis in patients randomly assigned to endovascular treatment or endarterectomy in the Carotid and Vertebral Artery Transluminal Angioplasty Study (CAVATAS): long-term follow-up of a randomised trial. Lancet Neurol 2009;8:908–17.
42. Bonati LH, Ederle J, Dobson J, et al. Length of carotid stenosis predicts peri-procedural stroke or death and restenosis in patients randomized to endovascular treatment or endarterectomy. Int J Stroke 2014;9:297–305.
43. Fokkema M, den Hartog AG, Bots ML, et al. Stenting versus surgery in patients with carotid stenosis after previous cervical radiation therapy: systematic review and meta-analysis. Stroke 2012;43:793–801.
44. CAVATAS Investigators. Endovascular versus surgical treatment in patients with carotid stenosis in the Carotid and Vertebral Artery Transluminal Angioplasty Study (CAVATAS): a randomised trial. Lancet 2001;357:1729–37.
45. Rothwell PM, Eliasziw M, Gutnikov SA, et al. Endarterectomy for symptomatic carotid stenosis in relation to clinical subgroups and timing of surgery. Lancet 2004;363:915–24.
46. Chandratheva A, Mehta Z, Geraghty OC, et al. Population-based study of risk and predictors of stroke in the first few hours after a TIA. Neurology 2009;72:1941–7.
47. Wu CM, McLaughlin K, Lorenzetti DL, et al. Early risk of stroke after transient ischemic attack: a systematic review and meta-analysis. Arch Intern Med 2007;167:2417–22.
48. Setacci C, de Donato G, Chisci E, et al. Carotid artery stenting in recently symptomatic patients: a single center experience. Ann Vasc Surg 2010;24:474–9.
49. Wach MM, Dumont TM, Mokin M, et al. Early carotid angioplasty and stenting may offer non-inferior treatment for symptomatic cases of carotid artery stenosis. J Neurointerv Surg 2014;6:276–80.
50. Zaidat OO, Alexander MJ, Suarez JI, et al. Early carotid artery stenting and angioplasty in patients with acute ischemic stroke. Neurosurgery 2004;55:1237–43.
51. Caplan LR. Cerebellar infarcts: key features. Rev Neurol Dis 2005;2:51–60.
52. Gomez CR, Cruz-Flores S, Malkoff MD, et al. Isolated vertigo as a manifestation of vertebrobasilar ischemia. Neurology 1996;47:94–7.
53. Choi KD, Lee H, Kim JS. Vertigo in brainstem and cerebellar strokes. Curr Opin Neurol 2013;26:90–5.
54. Khan S, Cloud GC, Kerry S, et al. Imaging of vertebral artery stenosis: a systematic review. J Neurol Neurosurg Psychiatry 2007;78:1218–25.
55. Hass WK, Fields WS, North RR, et al. Joint study of extracranial arterial occlusion. II. Arteriography, techniques, sites, and complications. JAMA 1968;203:961–8.
56. Wityk RJ, Chang HM, Rosengart A, et al. Proximal extracranial vertebral artery disease in the New England Medical Center Posterior Circulation Registry. Arch Neurol 1998;55:470–8.
57. Thompson MC, Issa MA, Lazzaro MA, et al. The natural history of vertebral artery origin stenosis. J Stroke Cerebrovasc Dis 2014;23:e1–4.
58. Moufarrij NA, Little JR, Furlan AJ, et al. Vertebral artery stenosis: long-term follow-up. Stroke 1984;15:260–3.
59. Gulli G, Marquardt L, Rothwell PM, et al. Stroke risk after posterior circulation stroke/transient ischemic attack and its relationship to site of vertebrobasilar stenosis: pooled data analysis from prospective studies. Stroke 2013;44:598–604.
60. Coward LJ, McCabe DJ, Ederle J, et al. Long-term outcome after angioplasty and stenting for symptomatic vertebral artery stenosis

compared with medical treatment in the Carotid And Vertebral Artery Transluminal Angioplasty Study (CAVATAS): a randomized trial. Stroke 2007;38:1526–30.

61. Cloud GC, Crawley F, Clifton A, et al. Vertebral artery origin angioplasty and primary stenting: safety and restenosis rates in a prospective series. J Neurol Neurosurg Psychiatry 2003;74: 586–90.
62. Motarjeme A, Keifer JW, Zuska AJ. Percutaneous transluminal angioplasty of the vertebral arteries. Radiology 1981;139: 715–17.
63. Chastain HD 2nd, Campbell MS, Iyer S, et al. Extracranial vertebral artery stent placement: in-hospital and follow-up results. J Neurosurg 1999;91:547–52.
64. Stayman AN, Nogueira RG, Gupta R. A systematic review of stenting and angioplasty of symptomatic extracranial vertebral artery stenosis. Stroke 2011;42:2212–16.
65. Rincon F, Sacco RL, Kranwinkel G, et al. Incidence and risk factors of intracranial atherosclerotic stroke: the Northern Manhattan Stroke Study. Cerebrovasc Dis 2009;28:65–71.
66. Feldmann E, Daneault N, Kwan E, et al. Chinese-white differences in the distribution of occlusive cerebrovascular disease. Neurology 1990;40:1541–5.
67. De Silva DA, Woon FP, Lee MP, et al. South Asian patients with ischemic stroke: intracranial large arteries are the predominant site of disease. Stroke 2007;38:2592–4.
68. Wong LK. Global burden of intracranial atherosclerosis. Int J Stroke 2006;1:158–9.
69. Chimowitz MI, Lynn MJ, Howlett-Smith H, et al. Comparison of warfarin and aspirin for symptomatic intracranial arterial stenosis. N Engl J Med 2005;352:1305–16.
70. Chimowitz MI, Lynn MJ, Turan TN, et al. Design of the stenting and aggressive medical management for preventing recurrent stroke in intracranial stenosis trial. J Stroke Cerebrovasc Dis 2011;20:357–68.
71. Derdeyn CP, Chimowitz MI, Lynn MJ, et al. Aggressive medical treatment with or without stenting in high-risk patients with intracranial artery stenosis (SAMMPRIS): the final results of a randomised trial. Lancet epub 2013.
72. Derdeyn CP, Fiorella D, Lynn MJ, et al. Mechanisms of stroke after intracranial angioplasty and stenting in the SAMMPRIS trial. Neurosurgery 2013;72:777–95.
73. Alexander MJ. Intracranial stenting for intracranial atherosclerotic disease: still much to learn. J Neurointerv Surg 2012;4:85–6.
74. Derdeyn CP, Fiorella D, Lynn MJ, et al. Impact of operator and site experience on outcomes after angioplasty and stenting in the SAMMPRIS trial. J Neurointerv Surg epub 2013;5:528–33.
75. Dumont TM, Kan P, Snyder KV, et al. Revisiting angioplasty without stenting for symptomatic intracranial atherosclerotic stenosis after the stenting and aggressive medical management for preventing recurrent stroke in intracranial stenosis (SAMMPRIS) study. Neurosurgery 2012;71:1103–10.
76. Marks MP, Wojak JC, Al-Ali F, et al. Angioplasty for symptomatic intracranial stenosis: clinical outcome. Stroke 2006;37:1016–20.

65 Endovascular Treatment of Acute Ischemic Stroke

Reza Jahan, Jeffrey L. Saver

KEY POINTS

- Endovascular recanalization strategies for acute ischemic stroke include intra-arterial fibrinolysis, aspiration devices, and retrieval devices.
- Compared with intravenous fibrinolysis, endovascular interventions have higher recanalization rates, but longer time-to-therapy start.
- Randomized trials of early-generation neurothombectomy devices did not demonstrate superiority to standard medical care, but had modest recanalization rates and late onset to treatment times.
- Randomized trials demonstrated that newer devices, the stent retrievers, have improved recanalization rates, reduced hemorrhage, and improved functional outcomes.
- The new recanalization devices combined with systems improvements to shorten door-to-recanalization time and improved patient selection (proximal occlusions with substantial penumbra), hold great promise.

INTRODUCTION

In ischemic stroke, an acute arterial occlusion rapidly produces a core of infarcted brain tissue surrounded by hypoxic, but potentially salvageable, tissue, i.e., the ischemic penumbra.[1-3] Penumbral tissue is viable due to collateral blood flow and the time to irreversible injury is largely dependent on the degree of collateral flow. The goal of recanalization therapy is rapid restoration of blood flow and preservation of the ischemic penumbra.[4,5] Intravenous (IV) recombinant tissue plasminogen activator (tPA) is a recanalization agent approved by the Food and Drug Administration (FDA) for the treatment of acute ischemic stroke within 3 hours of symptom onset.[6] However, IV tPA achieves reperfusion in only 30–50% of large-artery occlusion, in part because of the low concentration of lytic agent arriving at the target thrombus.[5]

Given the limitations of systemic thrombolysis for cervicocerebral reperfusion, intense efforts have been directed at developing endovascular reperfusion treatments. Early strategies focused on the intra-arterial (IA) delivery of thrombolytic drugs and primary angioplasty.[7-9] For the last decade, since the 2004 approval of the Merci coil retriever,[10,11] the greatest focus has been on neurothrombectomy devices. Subsequent technical innovations led to the development of novel, more effective strategies to remove blood clots from cerebral vessels and FDA approval of additional devices including the penumbra aspiration catheters and subsequently the stent retrievers.[12-14] In this chapter we present a comprehensive review of clinical trials and discuss the current status of endovascular treatment in acute ischemic stroke.

INTRA-ARTERIAL THROMBOLYSIS

Intra-arterial (IA) thrombolysis was first reported by Zeumer et al. in 1983 where five patients with vertebrobasilar occlusion were treated with local IA fibrinolysis.[15] Subsequently, Zeumer et al. reported treating two patients with ICA occlusions with urokinase.[16] Both patients had clinical improvement. Following that a large number of case series were published.[17-30] Neurologic improvement was variable in these studies with minimal or no neurologic deficit reported in 15–75% of patients. In review of these studies several factors were identified contributing to this wide variation in reported outcome: (1) the grading system used for assessing outcome; (2) dose of thrombolytic agent used; (3) differences in baseline patient demographics, i.e., age, baseline neurologic status; (4) site of arterial occlusion. In these studies, the time from onset to treatment was for the most part within 6 hours in the anterior circulation. Substantial recanalization was seen on the average in approximately 40% of patients and at least partial recanalization in 35%.[17-30] These rates of recanalization were higher than those reported in IV thrombolysis,[31-33] reflecting the greater concentration of lytic agent delivered to the occlusion site.

As initially the majority of experience with IA thrombolysis was based on retrospective studies, no definite conclusions could be drawn with respect to efficacy or safety of IA thrombolysis. Only randomized trials can answer questions regarding the safety and efficacy of IA therapy. Three large, multicenter trials have been performed in IA thrombolysis: Prolyse in Acute Cerebral Thromboembolism Trial (PROACT), PROACT II and the Japanese Middle Cerebral Artery Embolism Local Fibrinolytic Intervention Trial (MELT).[7,8,34]

PROACT I

PROACT I[34] was designed to evaluate the safety and efficacy of IA administration of pro-urokinase in patients with acute ischemic stroke. The study consisted of a uniform population of stroke patients presenting within 6 hours of symptom onset with middle cerebral artery (MCA) M1 or M2 occlusion. This subgroup of patients was expected to have similar clinical presentations and anticipated outcomes. A placebo group was included to evaluate the safety aspects of the angiographic and interventional procedures and to provide a basis for assessment of recanalization by the thrombolytic drug. Mechanical disruption of clot was not allowed in this trial. The grading system used to assess recanalization was the Thrombolysis in Myocardial Infarction (TIMI) classification. This is scored as TIMI 0 – complete occlusion, TIMI 1 – minimal reperfusion, TIMI 2 – partial recanalization, TIMI 3 – complete recanalization. Forty patients were randomized at a median 5.5 hours from symptom onset with 26 receiving pro-urokinase and 14

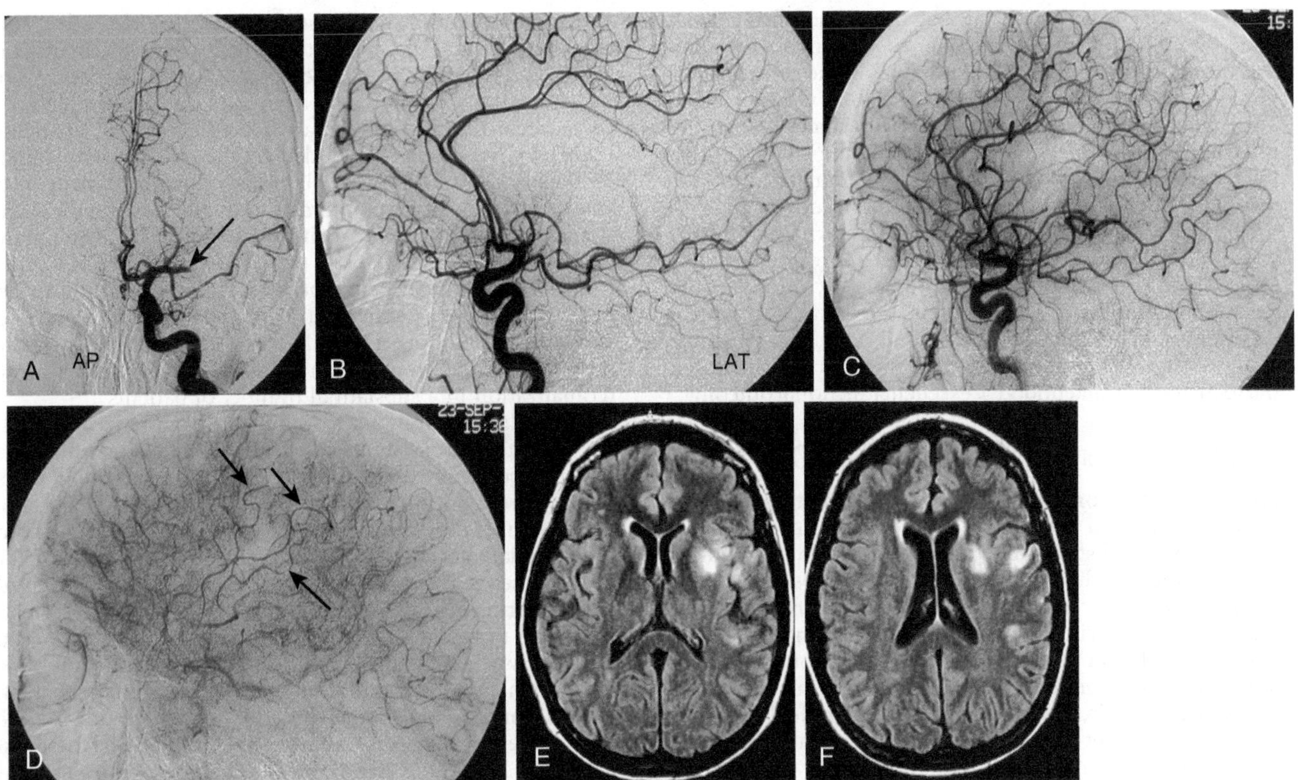

Figure 65-1. Anteroposterior (A) and lateral (B) views of the internal carotid artery injection showing occlusion of the proximal left middle cerebral artery (arrow in A). Lateral views of the internal carotid artery injection following intra-arterial thrombolysis show recanalization of the majority of the middle cerebral artery branches (C) with exception of a few vessels that fill well via retrograde collaterals (arrows in D) in the late arterial phase of the angiogram (D). Magnetic resonance images of the brain 7 days post procedure (E,F) show only a few FLAIR hyperintense lesions with the majority of the middle cerebral artery territory spared.

placebo. Partial or complete recanalization was seen in 15 of 26 (57.7%) patients treated with pro-urokinase and in two of 14 (14.3%) placebo patients. Symptomatic hemorrhage occurred in four of 26 (15.4%) treated patients and in one of 14 (7.1%) placebo patients (*P*-value non-significant). The number of patients was too small to show statistical significance in clinical outcome. The 90-day mortality was 26.9% in the pro-urokinase group and 42.9% in the placebo group (*P*-value non-significant).

PROACT II

Based on the encouraging findings of PROACT I, the PROACT II[7] trial was designed as a larger, pivotal trial with study entry criteria identical to PROACT I. The primary outcome was the ability to live independently at 3 months after the stroke. Of the 180 patients enrolled, 121 received IA pro-urokinase and low-dose IV heparin, and 59 received low-dose IV heparin. At completion of infusion, 66% of patients receiving pro-urokinase had complete or partial recanalization compared to 18% in the heparin only group ($P < 0.001$). Excellent neurological outcome was attained by 40% of the patients treated with pro-urokinase as compared to 25% in the heparin-only group ($P = 0.04$). Symptomatic ICH within 24 hours of treatment was seen in 10% of patients undergoing thrombolysis compared to 2% in the heparin group ($P = 0.06$). There was no significant difference in the 90-day mortality, which was 25% for the treated group, and 27% for the placebo patients. Despite the increased frequency of early hemorrhage, patients receiving IA pro-urokinase exhibited improved clinical outcome at 90 days.

Although PROACT II was a positive trial, it did not lead to regulatory approval of pro-urokinase for acute ischemic stroke, as the FDA typically requires two positive trials for new drug registration and the sponsor did not pursue a confirmatory study. While there are no drugs specifically approved for intra-arterial infusion in acute ischemic stroke, agents approved for other indications can be used off-label for this purpose. In most centers, t-PA is used for intra-arterial thrombolysis (Fig. 65-1).

MELT

The Japanese MELT study was organized to determine the safety and clinical efficacy of intra-arterial infusion of urokinase (UK) in patients with stroke within 6 hours of onset. The patient population was similar to that of the PROACT studies where patients with ischemic stroke presenting within 6 hours of onset and displaying angiographic occlusions of the M1 or M2 portion of the middle cerebral artery were randomized to the UK or control groups. Clinical outcome was assessed by the modified Rankin Scale (mRS), National Institutes of Health Stroke Scale (NIHSS), and Barthel Index (BI). The primary outcome was percentage of patients achieving independent status defined as mRS of 0-2. Following approval of IV rt-PA in Japan, the Independent Monitoring Committee recommended stopping the trial. At that time, a total of 114 patients had undergone randomization, 57 patients in each group. The primary end point of independent outcome at 90 days was somewhat more frequent in the UK group than in the control group (49.1% and 38.6%; OR, 1.54; 95%CI, 0.73–3.23), but did not reach statistical significance ($P = 0.35$).

However, excellent functional outcome (modified Rankin Scale 0 to 1) at 90 days, a preplanned secondary end point, was more frequent in the UK group than in the control group (42.1% and 22.8%; $P = 0.045$; OR, 2.46; 95%CI, 1.09–5.54). There were significantly more patients with National Institutes of Health Stroke Scale 0 or 1 at 90 days in the UK group than the control group ($P = 0.02$). The 90-day cumulative mortality was 5.3% in the UK group and 3.5% in the control group ($P = 1.00$), and symptomatic intracranial hemorrhage within 24 hours of treatment occurred in 9% and 2%, respectively ($P = 0.21$). The investigators and editorialists concluded that despite the trial being aborted prematurely and the primary end point not reaching statistical significance, the secondary analyses suggest that intra-arterial fibrinolysis has the potential to increase the likelihood of excellent functional outcome.[35]

Intra-arterial Thrombolysis in the Posterior Circulation

Posterior circulation stroke differs in several respects from ischemic stroke in the carotid distribution. Reports of the natural history of stroke due to basilar occlusion or bilateral vertebral artery occlusion show a dismal prognosis, with mortality of 70–80%.[36–40] Furthermore, the evolution of clinical signs in posterior circulation stroke differs from those in the anterior circulation. In the anterior circulation onset of symptoms is often concomitant with abrupt occlusion of the vessel. In the posterior circulation there may be a gradual evolution of symptoms rather than a sudden major clinical deficit.[36,41,42] This causes difficulty in accurately defining the time of symptom onset and hence assessing time limits for re-establishing perfusion. In addition, patients with posterior circulation infarcts have a high frequency of severe intracranial large-artery disease.[43,44] Intracranial atherosclerosis with in situ supervening thrombosis occurs more commonly in posterior circulation than anterior circulation strokes (Fig. 65-2). Consequently, fibrinolytic agents may clear only one component of the occlusive lesion, leaving a high potential for re-thrombosis.[15,23,27] Given the potentially slower, stuttering progression of posterior circulation infarcts and the reduced risk of hemorrhagic transformation because of the smaller volume of tissue at risk, intra-arterial thrombolysis therapy beyond 6 hours may be of greater benefit and safety in the posterior than anterior circulation. Reported series have included patients up to 24 hours after symptom onset.[15,17,27,45,46]

A non-randomized pilot study evaluating the safety and efficacy of IA urokinase in patients with posterior circulation stroke was reported by Mitchell et al.[47] Sixteen patients were treated within 24 hours of symptom onset. Complete or partial recanalization was initially achieved in 13 of 16 patients (82%). Of these, two re-occluded within 24 hours with a final recanalization rate of 69%. Six-month functional status was assessed by a neurologist blinded to the degree of recanalization with a good outcome defined as equal to, or greater than, 60 on the Barthel Index 11 (69%) patients survived, nine (56%) with a good outcome while two (13%) were left severely disabled. Recanalization correlated with improved survival. The authors conclude that IA thrombolysis in the posterior circulation is safe and feasible, capable of achieving recanalization in a substantial number of patients.

Following this initial pilot study, the randomized Australian Urokinase Stroke study was mounted.[48] Patients with acute ischemic posterior circulation stroke between 18 and 85 years of age were randomized to receive IA urokinase or placebo. All patients were anticoagulated acutely (5,000 IU heparin intra-arterially followed by IV heparinization to a target APTT of 60–80 seconds for a minimum of 2 days) and then received oral warfarin to a target INR of 1.5–2.5 for 6 months. Treatment had to be initiated within 24 hours after stroke onset. The trial was terminated in June 2003 on account of slow recruitment and the withdrawal of urokinase from the market. Sixteen patients were recruited prior to termination of the study. The investigators reported the results for these 16 patients.[48] Analyzing the primary outcome, seven of eight patients in the anticoagulation arm and four of eight patients in the urokinase arm were dead or disabled at 6 months (odds ratio [OR], 0.14; 95% confidence interval [CI], 0.02–1.43; $P = 0.28$). The protocol specified a subgroup analysis according to time to treatment. Of eight patients treated within 12 hours of symptom onset, five received urokinase while three did not. Disability-free survival was 2/5 for urokinase patients and 1/3 for those who received anticoagulation alone (OR, 1.3; 95%CI, 0.07–26.6). Of eight patients treated between 12 and 24 hours after symptom onset, three received urokinase and five did not; disability-free survival was 2/3 for urokinase patients and 0/5 for those who received anticoagulation alone (OR, 0.05; 95%CI, 0.0–1.9). Among survivors, the median mRS was one in the treatment group compared with three in the control group. There were eight deaths; four in each group. There was

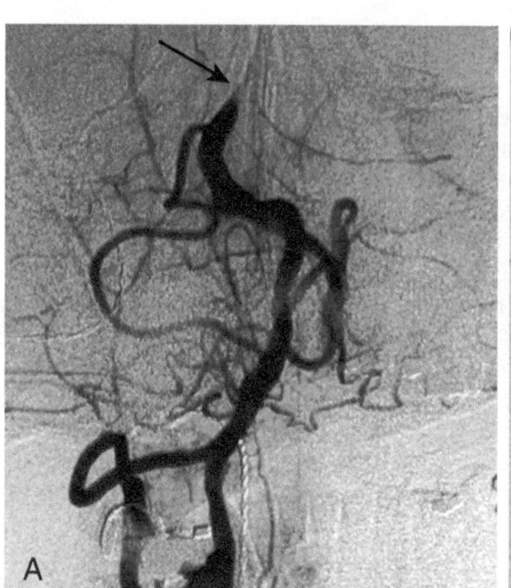

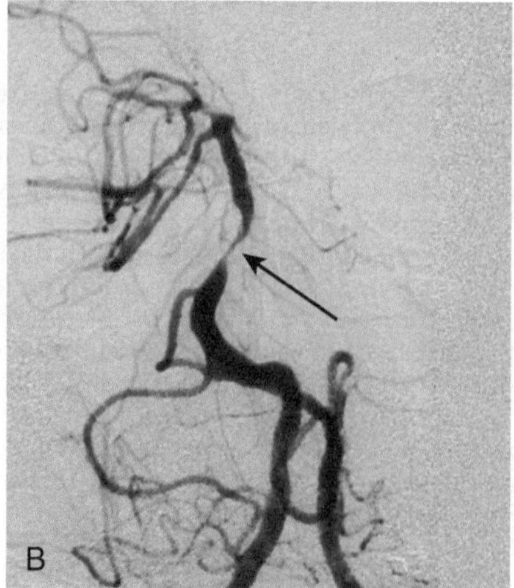

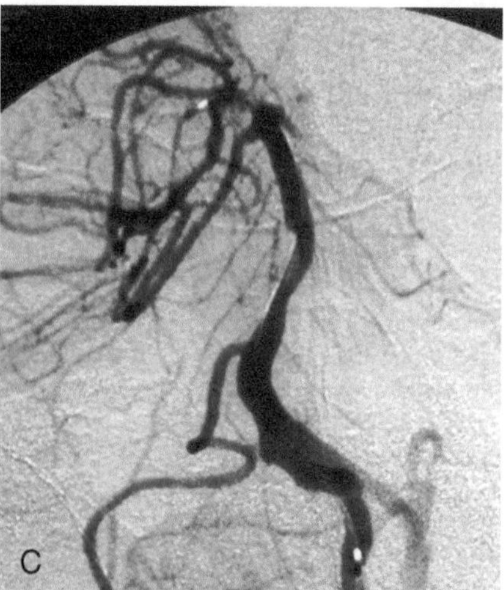

Figure 65-2. Anteroposterior view of the right vertebral artery injection (A) shows occlusion of the mid basilar artery (arrow in A). Following infusion of thrombolytic drug (B), a small channel is recanalized (arrow in B) and an underlying stenosis of the mid basilar artery is appreciated. Angioplasty is performed with significant reopening of the stenotic vessel (C).

one asymptomatic cerebral hemorrhage in the urokinase group and none in the anticoagulation group.

While this small trial does not provide definitive evidence for management of patients with acute posterior circulation stroke, it may provide useful information for the design of future studies. Although patients treated within or beyond 12 hours seemed to benefit from IA thrombolysis, none of the patients in the anticoagulation arm did well if treated beyond 12 hours. Therefore, the potential for benefit of IA thrombolytic treatment does not appear to be restricted to those treated within 12 hours, and future studies should consider including treatment between 12 and 24 hours after the ictus. In summary, the natural history of vetebrobasilar stroke is severe. Neurointerventional therapy with thrombolysis may be life-saving in this patient population. The time limit to IA lytic treatment has not been established and may be greater than 12 hours. Given the high morbidity and mortality in this population, endovascular intervention can be considered in patients with vertebrobasilar stroke.

COMBINED INTRAVENOUS AND INTRA-ARTERIAL TREATMENT

One major disadvantage of endovascular recanalization therapies is delay to treatment initiation. Compared with intravenous thrombolysis, which can be started immediately after initial brain imaging, endovascular therapy requires the neurointerventional team be gathered, the angiography suite prepared to perform the endovascular procedure, a groin be shaved, the access sheath be placed, and the catheter be navigated to the target clot before intervention can begin.[49] Such delays can limit effectiveness of IA therapy. Randomized IV trials and large practice registries have shown that effectiveness of treatment is strongly dependent on the time to start of therapy.[50,51] The greatest benefit has been shown to be in patients treated within 90 minutes. Interest thus developed in combining the advantages of IV and endovascular therapy, beginning with combined intravenous and intra-arterial delivery of pharmacology thrombolysis. The advantage of IV thrombolytic therapy includes its ease and rapidity of administration and wide availability in many hospitals. The advantages of IA thrombolytic therapy include the higher recanalization rates and titrated dosing where repeat angiography during delivery of the thrombolytic allows the physician to deliver only as much drug as is necessary to re-open the occlusion. This can potentially lead to lower dose of thrombolytic and hence reduced chance of bleeding. In addition, although most hospitals are equipped to deliver IV drug, they do not have trained physicians or equipment necessary to deliver IA therapy. With this combined IV/IA approach the IV drug can be started at any hospital and if necessary the patient is transferred to another hospital where IA thrombolysis is available.

This concept of combined therapy was first explored in the Emergency Management of Stroke (EMS) study.[52] In this study, a strategy of combined IV and IA tPA was compared with a strategy of pure IA tPA. In the combined arm, IV tPA was initiated without delay but at a lower than standard dose, allowing the remaining portion of the usual tPA dose to be given intra-arterially. This was a double-blind randomized study with a total of 35 patients enrolled within 3 hours of symptom onset. Of these 17 were randomized to receive IV tPA at a dose of 0.6 mg/kg (maximum dose 60 mg) with 18 patients in the second arm of the study receiving IV placebo. All 35 patients then underwent immediate angiography. If no clot was visualized, the angiogram was stopped at that point. If a clot was visualized, then IA treatment with tPA was initiated with 20 mg of the drug given over 2 hours or until recanalization had been achieved.

The study showed higher recanalization rates in the combined IV/IA group vs the placebo/IA group (55% vs 10% full recanalization). The numbers of symptomatic hemorrhage in the two groups were similar. The investigators concluded that the combined approach was feasible, reasonably safe, and worthy of further study.

This combined IV/IA thrombolysis strategy was evaluated further in the first Interventional Management of Stroke (IMS) trial.[53] Patients with NIHSS greater than 10 within 3 hours of symptom onset were offered treatment with IV rt-PA at 0.6 mg/kg followed by neuroangiography. This included both patients with anterior and posterior circulation stroke. If an arterial occlusive lesion was present, up to 22 mg IA rt-PA was infused over 2 hours. Outcomes were compared to the historical experience of the placebo and treated groups in the two NINDS tPA trials. The 80 subjects recruited in the study had a median NIHSS score of 18. The median time to initiation of IV therapy was 140 minutes and to initiation of IA thrombolysis was 212 minutes. This demonstrates the potential advantage of the combined approach, with the IV treatment able to be started 72 minutes earlier than the IA delivery. Symptomatic intracranial bleeding was seen in 6.3% of the cases in IMS vs 1.0% of the NINDS placebo and 6.6% of the NINDS tPA group. Despite the higher incidence of bleeding in IMS compared to NINDS placebo, mortality was nominally lower, although not statistically significant, at 3 months in the IMS patients vs NINDS placebo (16% vs 24%). Good outcome was seen in 28% of the IMS patients and 15% of the NINDS placebo patients (OR, 2.51; 95%CI, 1.21–5.18).

Upon completion of the IMS I trial, the investigators had planned a large phase 3 trial comparing IV tPA to combined IV/IA tPA. However, the completion of IMS I 1.5 years earlier than expected presented an opportunity to accrue more data and to explore new microcatheter technology for the combined IV/IA approach. IMS II was, therefore, designed to evaluate the safety and effectiveness of the combined IV/IA approach using the investigational EKOS catheter tip ultrasound infusion system.[54] The EKOS System consists of an 0.014-inch micro-infusion catheter consisting of an end-hole infusion lumen with an ultrasound element at the distal tip. This system uses low-energy ultrasound to alter reversibly the structure of the thrombus and facilitate access of the thrombolytic agent to potentially accelerate thrombolysis. Intra-arterial infusion with a standard microcatheter was also allowed.

The median dose of IV rt-PA administered to IMS II subjects was 46.4 mg and the median dose of IA rt-PA was 12 mg. The total median dose of rt-PA for IMS II subjects (56 mg) was significantly less than the total dose of 67.5 mg administered to subjects in the two NINDS tPA stroke trials and similar to the total median dose administered to IMS I subjects (59.95 mg). This lower total rt-PA dose for IMS I and II again points out the advantage of combined treatment where the IA dose can be tailored to recanalization thus leading to less total dose of lytic administered.

The 3-month mortality of 16% (13/81) for IMS II was identical to IMS I and not significantly different than mortality in the two NINDS tPA stroke trials (21% for NINDS tPA group and 24% for NINDS placebo).[6] The 90-day mortality of IMS II and IMS I subjects (16%) was lower than mortality of subjects in PROACT II (27%)[7] despite similar rates of reperfusion after completion of IA therapy. The lower mortality in IMS I and II subjects most likely relates to earlier recanalization because IMS II subjects had IV tPA initiated within a median time of 2 hours and 20 minutes as compared with median time to randomization of 4.7 hours in the PROACT II Trial. This illustrates the advantage of a combined IV/IA approach in which IV tPA can be started as quickly as possible while preparations for IA therapy, either at the same hospital ("mothership" strategy) or a tertiary hospital ("drip and ship" strategy), are underway.

One of the objectives of IMS II was to evaluate whether recanalization could be accelerated with the EKOS system as compared with IA delivery of tPA using a standard microcatheter. The observed modest differences did not reach statistical significance. Complete recanalization of the primary occlusive lesion with any distal flow by 60 minutes was achieved in 41.4% (12 of 29) of IMS II subjects treated with IA rt-PA plus the final generation EKOS catheter compared with 30.4% (seven of 23) in IMS I subjects ($P = 0.41$) treated with a standard microcatheter. From the standpoint of reperfusion of the entire vascular territory of an occluded vessel, the EKOS catheter performed similarly to the standard microcatheter in IMS I. Overall, all IMS II subjects treated with IA rt-PA via the latest generation EKOS catheter had a 62% rate of partial or better reperfusion (Thrombolysis in Cerebral Infarction, TICI, 2a or higher) after completion of the intra-arterial procedure as compared with 56.8% of IMS I subjects (P =not significant).[55]

The rates of symptomatic ICH in IMS II subjects were slightly but non-significantly higher than IMS I and the NINDS tPA stroke trials. There was a trend toward better outcomes (mRS 0–1) in IMS II subjects as compared with tPA-treated subjects in the NINDS tPA stroke trials.

Based on the favorable clinical outcome signals in IMS I and II, the IMS III trial was performed as a pivotal randomized controlled study comparing standard IV tPA to the combined IV and IA approach.[56] The trial randomly assigned eligible patients who had received intravenous rt-PA within 3 hours after symptom onset to receive additional endovascular therapy or intravenous rt-PA alone, in a 2:1 ratio. Permitted endovascular therapies included IA tPA via microcatheter, IA tPA via the EKOS ultrasound catheter, neurothrombectomy with the Merci coil retriever and, late in the course of the trial, aspiration with the Penumbra System or neurothrombectomy with stent retrievers. The primary outcome measure was a modified Rankin Scale (mRS) global disability score of 2 or less at 90 days. Following randomization of 656 patients (434 patients to endovascular therapy and 222 to intravenous tPA alone), the data and safety monitoring board recommended stopping enrollment as a predefined boundary for futility had been crossed. The proportion of participants with a mRS of 2 or less at 90 days did not differ significantly according to treatment arm (40.8% with endovascular therapy and 38.7% with intravenous tPA; absolute adjusted difference, 1.5 percentage points; 95%CI, −6.1–9.1, with adjustment for the National Institutes of Health Stroke Scale [NIHSS] score [8–19, indicating moderately severe stroke, or ≥20, indicating severe stroke]). In addition, there were no significant differences for the predefined subgroups of patients with an NIHSS score of 20 or higher (6.8 percentage points; 95%CI, −4.4–18.1) and those with a score of 19 or lower (−1.0 percentage point; 95%CI, −10.8–8.8). Findings in the endovascular-therapy and intravenous tPA groups were similar for mortality at 90 days (19.1% and 21.6%, respectively; $P = 0.52$) and the proportion of patients with symptomatic intracerebral hemorrhage within 30 hours after initiation of t-PA (6.2% and 5.9%, respectively; $P = 0.83$). The trial thus showed no significant difference in functional independence with endovascular therapy after intravenous t-PA, as compared with intravenous t-PA alone. Of note, there was no difference in safety outcomes between the two groups.

Several aspects of the trial deserve further discussion. Endovascular recanalization technology evolved substantially during the years after trial launch. By the end of the trial, a new generation of stent retriever devices were available that have substantially better recanalization efficacy, safety, and clinical outcomes than earlier catheter-based reperfusion techniques.[13,14] Although newer interventions were incorporated in IMS III as they became available, at study end the tested endovascular interventions consisted largely early generation technology, including of IA thrombolysis with the EKOS or standard microcatheter (160 of 334 interventions), the Merci coil retriever (95 of 334 interventions), and the Penumbra aspiration system (54 of 334). Overall, early generation endovascular interventions constituted at least 94% of the endovascular interventions in the study. Stent retrievers were used in only a small number of patients (five patients treated with Solitaire device) in the IMS III trial before the study was halted because of futility.

The IMS III study enrolled majority of patients without vascular imaging to confirm large vessel occlusion. Of 656 patients enrolled, only 306 (47%) had CT angiogram (CTA) or MR angiogram (MRA). Not surprisingly, 80 of 423 patients (19%) who underwent angiography had no visible occlusion treatable by endovascular means. These patients without a large vessel occlusion and no endovascular intervention received two-thirds the standard therapeutic dose of IV tPA while similar patients in the IV treatment only group received full-dose tPA. These patients with angiographically occult or distal small vessel occlusions typically do well with standard IV tPA. The inclusion of these patients without large vessel occlusion may have obscured the benefits of endovascular therapy.

Patient selection in the study was based on clinical diagnosis of major ischemic stroke as defined by the NIHSS and imaging was mainly used only to rule out intracranial bleed and presence of a definite large area of hypodensity suggestive of a completed infarct. There was no other selection based on imaging and approximately 42% of patients enrolled in the endovascular arm had an Alberta Stroke Program Early CT scores (ASPECTS) of ≤7. Lower ASPECTS scores correlate with poor functional outcomes and inclusion of such patients may have further diluted the benefit of endovascular therapy in this population.

One very important lesson learned from the IMS trials is that the link between reperfusion and outcome rapidly diminishes with increasing time from the onset of symptoms to reperfusion. In both the IMS I and II trials, a 30-minute delay was associated with a 10% decrease in the probability of functional independence (defined as a modified Rankin score of 0, 1, or 2).[57,58] In IMS III the time to endovascular treatment was 32 minutes longer than in the IMS I trial, which was a smaller, phase 2, single-group study conducted at 17 sites. In IMS III, the time from IV tPA bolus to first IA lytic infusion or device deployment was 126 minutes and from endovascular therapy initiation to reperfusion was another 85 minutes.[59] This delay to treatment in IMS III may have been another important reason for the lack of clinical benefit in the study. In IMS III, increased time to reperfusion was associated with decreased likelihood of an independent functional outcome, with the relative risk declining by 12% for every 30 minute reperfusion delay.[60]

MECHANICAL STRATEGIES

Coil/Stent Retrievers and Thrombus Aspiration

Interventions for acute cerebral ischemia have followed, more slowly, the evolution of interventions of acute myocardial ischemia, with the iterative development of mechanical techniques superior in recanalization efficacy to IV or IA thrombolysis alone.[61,62] Diverse strategies have been explored. The

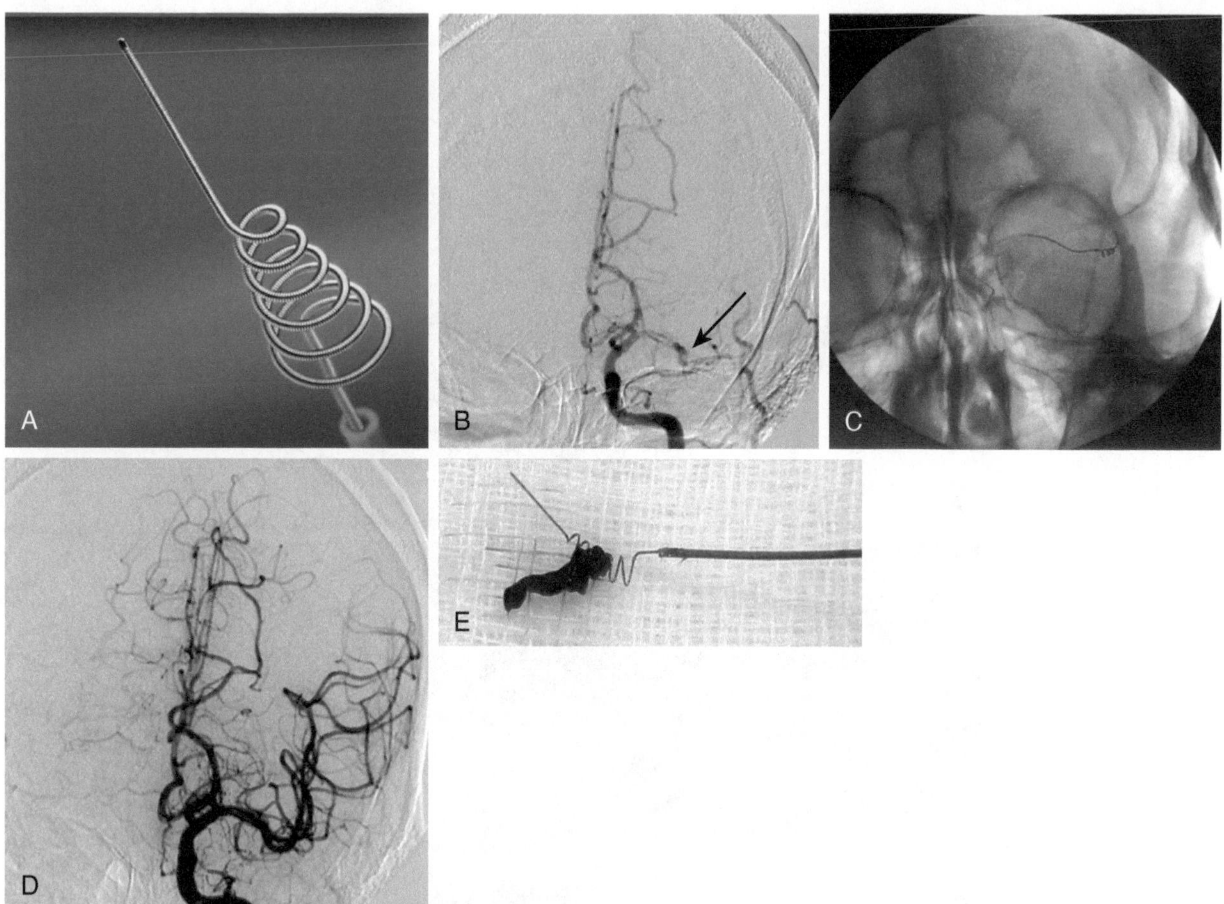

Figure 65-3. Image of the Merci X5 device (A). Anteroposterior view of the left common carotid artery injection (B) showing occlusion of the proximal middle cerebral artery (arrow in B). Unsubtracted anteroposterior view of the skull (C) showing the X5 device deployed in the left middle cerebral artery. Final angiogram post procedure (D) showing recanalization of the vessel with clot captured in the device (E).

use of acute angioplasty with or without stenting and in reopening of cerebral vessels has been reported.[9,63] However, a potential disadvantage of this strategy is forcing the clot into the deep penetrating arteries with worsening ischemia and the potential risk of rupturing the blood vessel. Other strategies included delivering energy to fragment the clot with the utilization of ultrasound and laser devices. The first successful mechanical strategy for ischemic stroke was the Merci device (Concentric Medical, Mountain view, California).[64,65] The initial design of the Merci retriever was a tapered wire with five helical loops of decreasing diameter from 2.8 mm to 1.1 mm at its distal end. The retriever is placed through the microcatheter and as it exits the microcatheter the helical loops begin to reshape in order to snare the clot in the occluded vessel. The clot is then pulled back to the carotid vessel in the neck and aspirated out through the guide catheter.

Two large, non-randomized studies were completed evaluating the Merci retriever.[10,11,66] The MERCI Trial[10] was a non-randomized trial evaluating the early generation coil retrievers of devices, the X5 and X6 devices (Fig. 65-3), in patients with acute ischemic stroke presenting within 8 hours of symptom onset. The trial recruited 141 patients all of whom were treated with the device. The rate of substantial recanalization was 48% and, when coupled with IA thrombolytic drugs, recanalization rates of 60% were reported. Clinically significant procedural complications occurred in ten of 141 (7.1%) patients. Symptomatic intracranial hemorrhages were observed in 11 of 141 (7.8%) patients. Good neurological outcomes (mRS ≤2) were more frequent at 90 days in patients with successful recanalization compared with patients with unsuccessful recanalization (46% vs 10%; relative risk [RR], 4.4; 95%CI, 2.1 to 9.3; $P < 0.0001$), and mortality was less (32% vs 54%; RR, 0.59; 95%CI, 0.39 0.89; $P = 0.01$). Based on this data, the FDA cleared the Merci retriever as a tool for the removal of thrombi in patients experiencing ischemic stroke.

Following the successful MERCI trial, the Multi-MERCI trial[11] was initiated to evaluate the newer generation of merci devices, the L-series. The major difference between the L-series and the X-series was in design of the helical loops (Fig. 65-4). The L-series has five helical loops all of which are of the same diameter rather than tapered helical loops as in the X-series. Multi MERCI was similar in design to the Merci trial. It was a multicenter, prospective, single-arm trial of thrombectomy in patients with large vessel stroke treated within 8 hours of symptom onset. Patients with persistent large vessel occlusion after IV tissue plasminogen activator treatment were included. Primary outcome was recanalization of the target vessel. One hundred and sixty-four patients received thrombectomy and 131 were initially treated with the L5 retriever. Treatment with the L5 retriever resulted in successful recanalization in 75 of 131 (57.3%) treatable vessels and in 91 of 131 (69.5%) after adjunctive therapy (IA tPA plus mechanical thrombectomy). Overall, favorable clinical outcomes (mRS 0 to 2) occurred in 36% and mortality was 34%; both outcomes were significantly related to vascular recanalization. Symptomatic intracerebral hemorrhage occurred in 16 patients (9.8%). Clinically significant procedural complications occurred in nine (5.5%) patients.

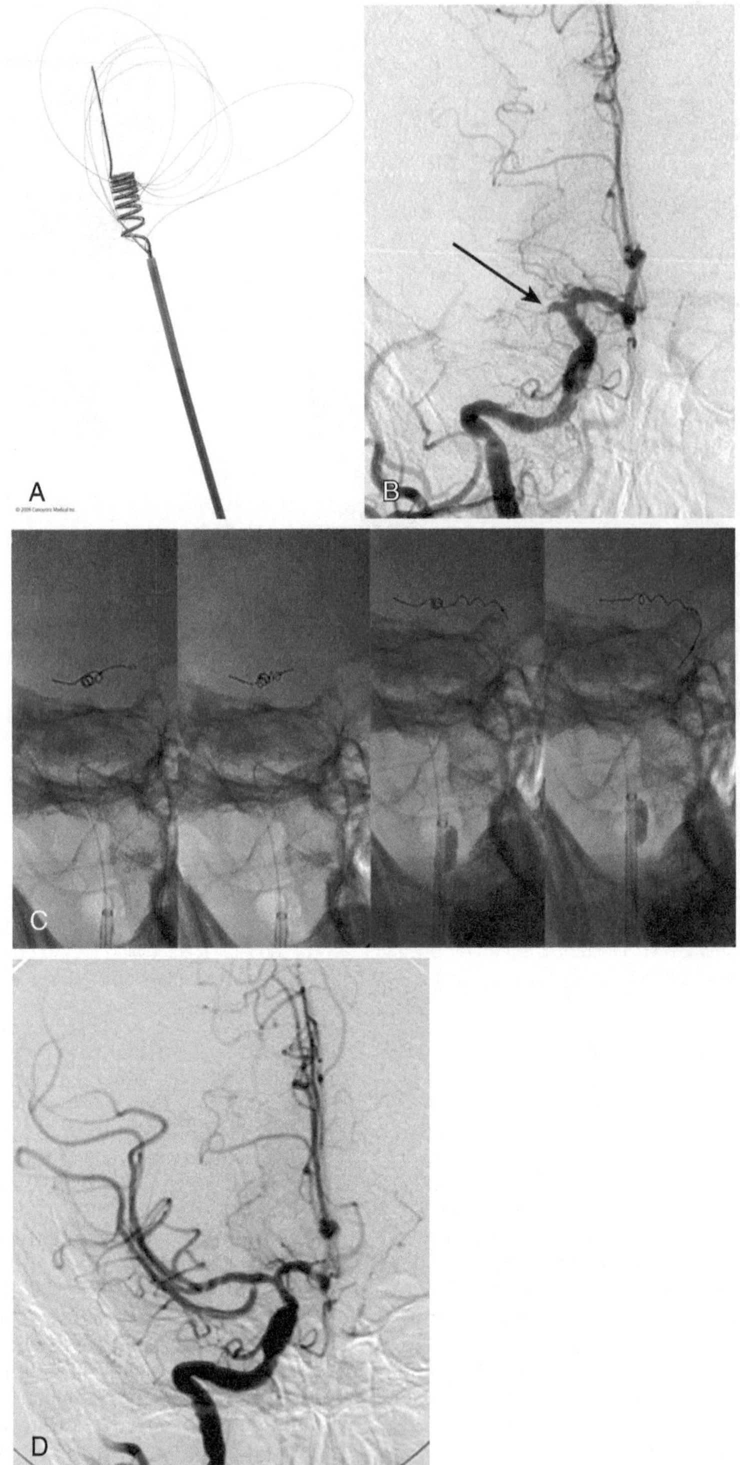

Figure 65-4. Image of the L5 device (A). Anteroposterior view of the right common carotid artery injection (B) showing occlusion of the proximal middle cerebral artery (arrow in B). Unsubtracted images of the L5 device (C) as it is being withdrawn to remove the captured clot within the device with final angiogram (D) showing successful recanalization of the vessel.

Compared to the MERCI trial, higher rates of recanalization were seen with the newer L-5 thrombectomy device compared with first-generation X-series devices, but these differences did not achieve statistical significance. Mortality trended lower compared to the MERCI trial and the proportion of good clinical outcomes trended higher, consistent with better recanalization in the Multi-MERCI trial.

The recanalization rates and good outcomes (69.5% and 36%, respectively) in the Multi-MERCI trial are comparable to the treated group of the PROACT II trial[7] where 66% had successful recanalization and 40% had a good outcome at 3 months. In addition, symptomatic intracerebral hemorrhage was similar with 9.8% in the Multi-MERCI and 10% in the PROACT II trial.

Although the results of the MERCI and Multi-MERCI trials were encouraging, there was much controversy regarding approval of this device based on studies using historical controls rather than based on randomized trials.[67–69]

Aspiration Thrombectomy

In 2009 a new mechanical device, the Penumbra System, was approved by the FDA for clot removal in acute ischemic stroke patients.[70] The Penumbra System (Penumbra, Alameda, California) removes the thrombus primarily by aspiration. It consists of three main components: a reperfusion catheter, a separator, and a vacuum pump. For aspiration, the reperfusion catheter is used in parallel with the separator and an aspiration source to separate the thrombus and aspirate it from the occluded vessel. The initial safety and effectiveness study was carried out enrolling subjects with acute ischemic stroke presenting within 8 hours of symptom onset.[70] Twenty-three subjects were enrolled, and 21 target vessels were treated. All treated vessels (100%) were successfully revascularized. At 30-day follow-up, nine subjects (45%) had a 4-point or more NIHSS improvement or a mRS of 2 or less. The all-cause mortality rate was 45% (nine of 20).

Following the initial safety study, the pivotal study was carried out for the penumbra system.[12] This was a prospective, multicenter, single-arm study, where 125 patients with neurological deficits as defined by a NIHSS score of eight or greater, presenting within 8 hours of symptom onset, and an angiographic occlusion of a treatable large intracranial vessel were enrolled. Patients who presented within 3 hours from symptom onset had to be ineligible or refractory to recombinant tissue plasminogen activator therapy. Post-procedure, 81.6% of the treated vessels were at least minimally reperfused to TIMI 2 to 3. A total of 35 patients (28%) were found to have intracranial hemorrhage on 24-hour CT of which 14 (11.2%) were symptomatic. All-cause mortality was 32.8% at 90 days with 25% of the patients achieving a modified Rankin Scale score of 2 or less.

The reported reperfusion rates in the penumbra pivotal study were higher than all prior studies, but the favorable clinical outcomes was lower than that in the MERCI, Multi-MERCI, and IMS trials. The investigators suggested that this discrepancy between recanalization rates and clinical outcomes was due to differences in the time from stroke onset to start of therapy.[71, 72] All subjects in the IMS I and II Trials had treatment with IV rt-PA begun within 3 hours and had the best reported overall outcomes at 90 days. PROACT II, in which subjects were randomized within 6 hours, had the next best functional outcome and in the MERCI, Multi-MERCI, and Penumbra Trials, despite good recanalization rates, subjects had the lowest proportions of good outcomes with the longest time windows from stroke onset to initiation of therapy.

A further explanation was provided by the review of the parenchymal imaging data in the trial. The baseline ASPECTS score of the patients in the study was reviewed and correlated with outcome. Of 125 patients in the trial, 85 for whom imaging data was readily available were included in this study. Median baseline NIHSS score was 18 (range, 8–34) and median baseline ASPECTS score was 6 (range, 0–10); 81.2% of patients in this cohort achieved recanalization (TIMI, 2–3) and (27.7%) achieved good clinical outcome. Good clinical outcome was significantly greater in the >7 group (n = 31) when compared to the ≤7 group (n = 54) (RR, 3.3; 95%CI, 1.6–6.8). No patient with an ASPECTS score <4 (n = 28) had good clinical outcome. Thus patients with favorable baseline CT scan (ASPECTS >7) have better clinical outcomes with an effect size of 35% and inclusion of significant proportion of patients with unfavorable CT scans, may have obscured the benefit of recanalization in this study.

Finally, the study was criticized for not specifying how they measured the primary trial outcome, angiographic revascularization.[73] The core laboratory in the trial used the TIMI scale to assess revascularization; however, no explanation is provided as to how they applied the TIMI scale to their cerebral angiograms. Many different operationalized versions of the TIMI scale have been described[74] and without further clarification it is difficult to determine whether the reported higher recanalization rate in the Penumbra Trial is an artifact of different angiographic scoring methods or a genuine difference in device technical efficacy. Revascularization rates have since become more comparable across studies with the widespread adoption of scales designed specifically for the cerebral circulation, including the Thrombolysis in Cerebral Infarction (TICI) and the Arterial Occlusive Lesion (AOL) scales.[75]

Stent Retrievers

The stent retriever class of devices was developed to improve upon earlier generation thrombectomy devices by offering immediate flow restoration upon device deployment, more effective capture and clearance of the target thrombus, less fragmentation and embolism of thrombi, and reduced trauma to the vessel wall.[76,77] The first stent retriever device approved by the FDA was the Solitaire FR Revascularization Device (Covidien Neurovascular, Irvine, California), based on the SWIFT randomized trial (Fig. 65-5).[14,78] In SWIFT, the safety and efficacy of the Solitaire FR stent retriever were compared with the Merci coil retriever. This was a randomized, blinded outcome observer, parallel-group trial undertaken at 21 centers in the US and France. Patients with an acute ischemic stroke presenting within 8 hours of symptom onset and with large intracranial artery occlusions were randomized to receive thrombectomy with either the Solitaire FR or the Merci device. The primary endpoint was successful revascularization (core lab assessed) defined as TIMI 2 or 3 flow in all treatable vessels without symptomatic intracranial hemorrhage (SICH). Up to three passes of the assigned device were allowed to achieve revascularization after which the thrombectomy procedure would be deemed a failure and rescue therapy with an FDA approved device would be allowed. Following randomization of 113 patients (58 Solitaire, 55 Merci) a pre-specified efficacy stopping rule was reached resulting in early termination of the trial. The primary efficacy outcome was achieved more often in Solitaire vs Merci patients, 60.7% vs 24.1% (difference 36.6% [18.5% to 53.4%], OR, 4.87; 95%CI, 2.14 to 11.10; non-inferiority $P < 0.0001$; superiority $P = 0.0001$). More patients had good 3 month neurologic outcome (mRS ≤ 2 or equal to the prestroke mRS if prestroke mRS was higher than 2, or NIHSS score improvement of 10 points or more) with Solitaire than Merci, 58.2% vs 33.3% (24.9% [5.5% to 42.9%], OR, 2.78, 95%CI, 1.25–6.22; non-inferiority $P = 0.0001$; superiority $P = 0.02$). Mortality was reduced with Solitaire, 17.2% vs 38.2% (difference −20.9% [−38.6% to −2.7%], OR, 0.34; 95%CI, 0.14–0.81; non-inferiority $P = 0.0001$; superiority $P = 0.02$). Thus in conclusion the Solitaire Flow Restoration device was deemed superior to the Merci Retriever in achieving successful recanalization free of symptomatic intracranial hemorrhage, and was associated with reduced mortality and increased good neurologic outcome.

Several aspects of the trial deserve further mention. SWIFT was the first acute ischemic stroke trial to conduct a direct, randomized comparison of one endovascular recanalization technique to another. Prior studies leading to clearance of devices for neurovascular thrombectomy have been single arm studies with only historical controls[10–12] SWIFT employed the

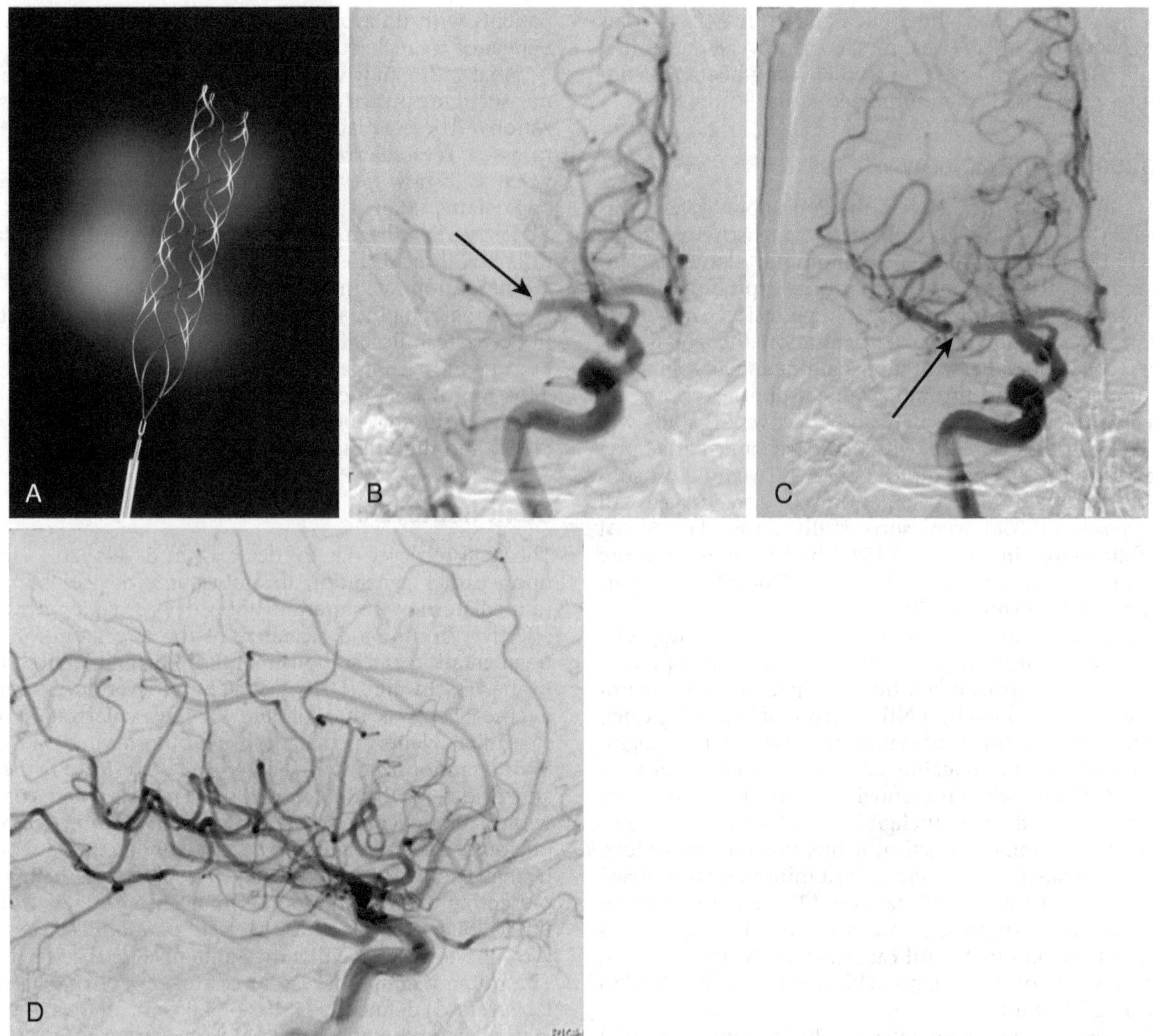

Figure 65-5. Image of the Solitaire FR device (A). Angiogram of the right common carotid artery (B) showing occlusion of the proximal middle cerebral artery (arrow in B). With the device deployed (C), the clot is compressed (arrow in C) and antegrade flow is reestablished immediately. Following clot extraction with the device, angiogram shows successful recanalization (D).

most stringent version of the TIMI scale, requiring revascularization to be achieved in all treatable vessels, not just the most proximal target vessel. This is the same definition that was used in the Merci and MultiMerci trials, however, unlike those studies, the SWIFT revascularization was assessed by a blinded central core laboratory, rather than unblinded site investigators. This likely accounts for the lower reported rates of partial or better recanalization in the primary SWIFT analysis for both devices compared with prior studies. In fact, site assessed revascularization rates were published in the SWIFT study and compared to the core laboratory assessments. For Solitaire, the SWIFT core lab-determined successful recanalization rate of 69% was less than the reported rates of 88–92% in open series,[79–83] but the site-determined rate of 83% is not dissimilar from prior reports. Similarly, for Merci, the Core-Lab determined successful recanalization rate of 30% is less than the partial recanalization rates of 48–55% observed in prior multicenter series,[10,11] but the site-determined rate of 48% is in the same range.

The primary outcome measure in SWIFT, namely, successful recanalization with no symptomatic hemorrhage, was selected at the request of regulatory authorities and was novel in neurovascular reperfusion trials. Previous trials such as the MERCI, Multi-MERCI and the Penumbra Pivotal trial,[10–12] have used successful recanalization as the sole component of the primary efficacy endpoint. The type of combined efficacy outcome as was used in SWIFT has been termed a metric of "unqualified success".[84] Measures of unqualified success assess treatment efficacy adjusted for treatment-induced adverse effects in a single metric. The differences on this primary endpoint in SWIFT were driven by both components, but with a larger contribution from the substantially greater recanalization efficacy of Solitaire vs Merci.

The second stent retrieval device to achieve FDA approval in the US was the Trevo Retriever (Stryker Neurovascular, Mountain View, California). This device was evaluated in a randomized trial and the comparator device was also the Merci Retrieval system.[13] This was an open-label randomized controlled trial at 26 sites in the USA and one in Spain. Adults aged 18–85 years with angiographically confirmed large vessel occlusion ischemic strokes and NIHSS scores of 8–29 within 8 hours of symptom onset were randomly assigned to thrombectomy with Trevo or Merci device. The primary efficacy endpoint, assessed by an unmasked core laboratory, was thrombolysis in cerebral infarction (TICI) scores of 2 or greater reperfusion with the assigned device alone. The study randomized 88 patients to the Trevo Retriever group and 90 patients to Merci Retriever group. Overall safety profiles were similar with the two devices. Time to revascularization was much the same in both groups and the median number of passes with the assigned study device was 2 (IQR 1–3) in the Trevo group (mean 2.4 [SD 1.4]) and 2 (1–3) in the Merci group (2.5 [1.2]). A perfusion channel was noted angiographically in 72% of patients in the Trevo group immediately after device deployment. Good neurologic outcome (mRS 0-2) was seen in 34/85 (40%) in the Trevo group and 19/87 (22%) in the Merci group (*P* value, 0.013; OR, 2.39; 95%CI, 1.16–4.95).

RANDOMIZED TRIALS WITH MEDICAL CONTROL ARMS

By 2012, more than two decades after the first development of endovascular recanalization therapy, endovascular treatment for acute stroke appeared highly promising but, except for the PROACT II study, its clinical effectiveness was yet to be demonstrated in randomized trials with non-interventional control arms. The non-randomized trials carried out for FDA device clearance did not provide adequate data to address the clinical effectiveness of these devices. The discrepancy between recanalization rates and good clinical outcome further complicates the matter as all these studies had recanalization as the primary outcome measure and despite high reported recanalization rates did not demonstrate high rates of good clinical outcome. For example, subjects in the MERCI trial had an overall TIMI 2–3 reperfusion rate of 48% with overall mortality rate at 90 days 44%, and only 28% had a good functional outcome (mRS 0–2). The subsequent Multi-MERCI Trial demonstrated an overall TIMI 2–3 rate of 69% with 90 day mortality of 34%, and 36% of subjects had a Rankin Scale score of 0–2. Results from the non-randomized Penumbra Trial were similar with reported reperfusion rates higher than all prior studies, but the rate of Rankin Scale score of 0–2 at 90 days was lower than the rates in the MERCI and Multi-MERCI. Ultimately the safety and effectiveness of these devices can only be demonstrated in a randomized clinical trial where the clinical outcomes are compared to best medical therapy.

In 2013, the first three major randomized trials of neurothrombectomy devices versus non-interventional control treatment were reported, and all showed disappointingly neutral results. In the early time window, two studies, the IMS III study and SYNTHESIS Expansion trial[56,85] evaluated the benefit of endovascular therapy versus IV tPA. The IMS III study has already been discussed. The SYNTHESIS Expansion trial is discussed below.

The investigators in the SYNTHESIS Expansion trial randomly assigned 362 patients presenting within 4.5 hours of ictus to endovascular therapy (intra-arterial thrombolysis with recombinant tissue plasminogen activator [rt-PA], mechanical clot disruption or retrieval, or a combination of these approaches) or standard dose intravenous rt-PA. The endovascular therapy had to be initiated as soon as possible after randomization and within 6 hours of onset. The primary outcome measure was survival without disability (defined as mRS of 0–1) at 3 months. A total of 181 patients were assigned to receive endovascular therapy, and 181 intravenous t-PA with median time from stroke onset to the start of treatment 3.75 hours for endovascular therapy and 2.75 hours for intravenous t-PA ($P < 0.001$). At 3 months, 55 patients (30.4%) in the endovascular-therapy group and 63 (34.8%) in the intravenous t-PA group were alive without disability (odds ratio adjusted for age, sex, stroke severity, and atrial fibrillation status at baseline, 0.71; 95%CI, 0.44–1.14; $P = 0.16$). Fatal or non-fatal symptomatic intracranial hemorrhage within 7 days occurred in 6% of the patients in each group, and there were no significant differences between groups in the rates of other serious adverse events or the case fatality rate. Thus, the results of this trial indicate that endovascular therapy alone is not superior to standard treatment with intravenous tPA alone.

The SYNTHESIS trial achieved a more rapid imaging to groin puncture time than contemporaneous trials, an important requisite when comparing a pure endovascular strategy to a pure IV tPA strategy. However, some other aspects of study performance may have reduced the opportunity to test optimum endovascular intervention. Of the 181 patients assigned to endovascular treatment, 16 did not receive the treatment (six because of clinical improvement, three because of absence of an intracranial occlusive lesion, three because of dissection, one because of an unknown bleeding diathesis, one because of a groin hematoma, one because of the delayed availability of the interventionist and one procedure was aborted owing to equipment breakdown). Among the 165 patients who received endovascular treatment, interventions were almost entirely early generation, including IA tPA in 109, Merci coil retriever in five, and penumbra aspiration in nine. Stent retrievers were used only in 23 patients (13.9%). The maximum dose of IA rt-PA that was allowed was 0.9 mg/kg (maximum dose 90 mg) to be delivered over 1 hour, which appears to be a rather high dose for local infusion with a microcatheter. The median IA rt-PA dose delivered was 40 mg (IQR 20–50).

Furthermore, just as in IMS III, it has been stated that SYNTHESIS did not target the optimal patient population for endovascular therapy.[86] Experience from previous trials suggests that benefit from endovascular intervention is dependent on several factors including presence of large target vessel occlusion with large target salvageable tissue and fast and effective reperfusion. However, only 30% (109/362) of SYNTHESIS patients underwent CT angiography. Moreover, it is likely that a significant proportion of the SYNTHESIS patients lacked a proximal arterial occlusion as reflected in the low median NIHSS in SYNTHESIS which was only 13 (SWIFT:18; Trevo 2:19) with 36% (129/362) of patients having NIHSS ≤10.

While SYNTHESIS failed to demonstrate superiority of early generation endovascular recanalization therapy to iV tPA alone, it did indicate the two strategies yield roughly equivalent outcomes. This observation has important implications for the treatment of acute ischemic stroke within 3 hours of onset in patients who are ineligible for IV tPA, for example because of active anticoagulation therapy or recent major thoracoabdominal surgery. The SYNTHESIS results indicate these patients likely will be benefitted by active endovascular recanalization therapy, compared with supportive care alone.

In contrast to IMS III and SYNTHESIS, the Mechanical Retrieval and Recanalization of Stroke Clots Using Embolectomy (MR RESCUE) trial recruited patients in the later time window from 3 to 8 hours post symptom onset.[87] Entry criteria included patients ineligible for IV tPA and also patients who had failed to recanalize after IV tPA administration. The primary aim of the study was to assess whether imaging can identify patients who are most likely to benefit from therapies for acute ischemic stroke and whether endovascular thrombectomy improves clinical outcomes in such patients. The investigators randomly assigned patients with large vessel, anterior-circulation strokes presenting within 8 hours of symptom onset to undergo mechanical embolectomy (with the Merci Retriever or Penumbra System) or receive standard care. All patients underwent pre-procedure computed tomography (CT) or magnetic resonance imaging (MRI) of the brain and randomization was stratified according to whether the patient had a favorable penumbral pattern (substantial salvageable tissue and small infarct core) or a non-penumbral pattern (large core or small or absent penumbra). There were thus four groups of patients: (1) penumbral pattern/

embolectomy (n = 34); (2) penumbral pattern/standard care (n = 34); (3) non-penumbral pattern/embolectomy (n = 30); and (4) non-penumbral pattern/standard care (n = 20). Outcomes were assessed by comparing the distribution of Rankin scores in each group at 90-days. Among 118 eligible patients, the mean age was 65.5 years, the mean time to enrollment was 5.5 hours, and 58% had a favorable penumbral pattern. Core laboratory assessed any reperfusion (TICI 2a-3) in the embolectomy group was achieved in 67% of the patients. Ninety-day mortality was 21%, and the rate of symptomatic intracranial hemorrhage was 4%; neither rate differed across groups. In the primary analysis of scores on the 90-day mRS, there was no interaction between the pretreatment imaging pattern and treatment assignment ($P = 0.14$). Among all patients, mean scores on the mRS did not differ between embolectomy and standard care (3.9 vs 3.9; $P = 0.99$). Embolectomy was not superior to standard care in patients with either a favorable penumbral pattern (mean score, 3.9 vs 3.4; $P = 0.23$) or a non-penumbral pattern (mean score, 4.0 vs 4.4; $P = 0.32$). Thus, a favorable penumbral pattern on neuroimaging did not identify patients who would differentially benefit from endovascular therapy for acute ischemic stroke, nor was embolectomy shown to be superior to standard care.

Several drawbacks of the MR-RESCUE trial have been noted. As in SYNTHESIS and IMS III, first-generation thrombectomy devices were used with the majority of patients being treated with the Merci retriever. It is now clear that recanalization efficacy is limited with first-generation devices relative to second-generation thrombectomy devices. Also, the use of two different imaging modalities (CT and MR) to evaluate penumbra further complicates the findings in this study. The acquisition and processing of the images may have led to delays in treatment with relatively long times to groin puncture (onset to groin puncture, mean = 6.2 hours) and this potentially played a role in the overall disappointing clinical outcomes in the trial.

Latest Randomized Trial Results

For a review of the latest trials published after the completion of this chapter, please see the section introduction by Dr Broderick (Section VI, Part B: Interventional Therapy).

CONCLUSIONS

The first 25 years of acute endovascular recanalization therapy for acute ischemic stroke have been marked by technical innovation and progress, resulting in improving reperfusion rates, reduced hemorrhagic complications, and better clinical outcomes. While randomized trials of early generation endovascular interventions did not demonstrate superiority to standard medical care, a paradigm shift has occurred with advent of stent retriever technology. Stroke physicians for the first time can offer patients a highly effective recanalization intervention, achieving substantial reperfusion in 80–90% of patients. If the new generation devices can be paired with systems improvements to shorten door to clot time,[88] there is every reason to expect randomized trials of current treatment approaches may demonstrate their efficacy,[89] and a new era in endovascular reperfusion therapy for acute cerebral ischemia will commence.

REFERENCES

1. Astrup J, Siesjo B, Symon L. Thresholds in cerebral ischemia-the ischemic penumbra. Stroke 1981;12:723–5.
2. Kidwell CS, Alger JR, Saver JL. Beyond mismatch: Evolving paradigms in imaging the ischemic penumbra with multimodal magnetic resonance imaging. Stroke 2003;34:2729–35.
3. Fisher M, Albers GW. Advanced imaging to extend the therapeutic time window of acute ischemic stroke. Ann Neurol 2013; 73:4–9.
4. Fisher M, Ratan R. New perspectives on developing acute stroke therapy. Ann Neurol 2003;53:10–20.
5. Saver JL. Improving reperfusion therapy for acute ischaemic stroke. J Thromb Haemost 2011;9:333–43.
6. The National Institute of Neurological Disorders and Stroke rt-PA Stroke Study Group. Tissue plasminogen activator for acute ischemic stroke. N Engl J Med 1995;333:1581–7.
7. Furlan A, Higashida R, Wechsler L, et al. Intra-arterial prourokinase for acute ischemic stroke. The PROACT II study: A randomized controlled trial. Prolyse in acute cerebral thromboembolism [see comment]. JAMA 1999;282:2003–11.
8. Ogawa A, Mori E, Minematsu K, et al. Randomized trial of intraarterial infusion of urokinase within 6 hours of middle cerebral artery stroke: The middle cerebral artery embolism local fibrinolytic intervention trial (MELT) Japan. Stroke 2007;38: 2633–9.
9. Rha JH, Saver JL. The impact of recanalization on ischemic stroke outcome: A meta-analysis. Stroke 2007;38:967–73.
10. Smith WS, Sung G, Starkman S, et al. Safety and efficacy of mechanical embolectomy in acute ischemic stroke: Results of the merci trial. Stroke 2005;36:1432–8.
11. Smith WS, Sung G, Saver J, et al. Mechanical thrombectomy for acute ischemic stroke: Final results of the multi merci trial. Stroke 2008;39:1205–12.
12. Penumbra Pivotal Stroke Trial Investigators. The penumbra pivotal stroke trial: Safety and effectiveness of a new generation of mechanical devices for clot removal in intracranial large vessel occlusive disease. Stroke 2009;40:2761–8.
13. Nogueira RG, Lutsep HL, Gupta R, et al. Trevo versus merci retrievers for thrombectomy revascularisation of large vessel occlusions in acute ischaemic stroke (TREVO 2): A randomised trial. Lancet 2012;380:1231–40.
14. Saver JL, Jahan R, Levy EI, et al. Solitaire flow restoration device versus the merci retriever in patients with acute ischaemic stroke (swift): A randomised, parallel-group, non-inferiority trial. Lancet 2012;380:1241–9.
15. Zeumer H, Hacke W, Ringelstein EF. Local intraarterial thrombolysis in vertebrobasilar thromboembolic disease. AJNR 1983;4:401–4.
16. Zeumer H, Hundgen R, Ferbert A, et al. Local intraarterial fibrinolytic therapy in inaccessible internal carotid occlusion. Neuroradiology 1984;26:315–17.
17. Zeumer H, Freitag HJ, Zanella F, et al. Local intra-arterial fibrinolytic therapy in patients with stroke: Urokinase versus recombinant tissue plasminogen activator (r-tPA). Neuroradiology 1993;35:159–62.
18. Jansen O, von Kummer R, Forsting M, et al. Thrombolytic therapy in acute occlusion of the intracranial internal carotid artery bifurcation. AJNR 1995;16:1977–86.
19. Theron J, Courtheoux P, Casasco A, et al. Local intraarterial fibrinolysis in the carotid territory. AJNR 1989;10:753–65.
20. Barr JD, Mathis JM, Wildenhain SL, et al. Acute stroke intervention with intraarterial urokinase infusion. J Vasc Interv Radiol 1994;5:705–13.
21. del Zoppo GJ, Ferbert A, Otis S, et al. Local intra-arterial fibrinolytic therapy in acute carotid territory stroke. A pilot study. Stroke 1988;19:307–13.
22. Mori E, Tabuchi M, Yoshida T, et al. Intracarotid urokinase with thromboembolic occlusion of the middle cerebral artery. Stroke 1988;19:802–12.
23. Hacke W, Zeumer H, Ferbert A, et al. Intraarterial therapy improves outcome in patients with acute vertebrobasilar disease. Stroke 1988;19:1216–22.
24. Ezura M, Kagawa S. Selective and superselective infusion of urokinase for embolic stroke. Surg Neurol 1992;38:353–8.
25. Barnwell SL, Clark WM, Nguyen TT, et al. Safety and efficacy of delayed intraarterial urokinase therapy with mechanical clot disruption for thromboembolic stroke. AJNR Am J Neuroradiol 1994;15:1817–22.
26. Brandt T, von Kummer R, Müller-Küppers M, et al. Thrombolytic therapy of acute basilar artery occlusion. Variables affecting recanalization and outcome. Stroke 1996;27:875–81.

27. Becker KJ, Monsein LH, Ulatowski J, et al. Intraarterial thrombolysis in vertebrobasilar occlusion. AJNR Am J Neuroradiol 1996;17:255–62.
28. Ueda T, Sakaki S, Kumon Y, et al. Multivariable analysis of predictive factors related to outcome at 6 months after intra-arterial thrombolysis for acute ischemic stroke. Stroke 1999;30:2360–5.
29. Jahan R, Duckwiler GR, Kidwell CS, et al. Intraarterial thrombolysis for treatment of acute stroke: Experience in 26 patients with long-term follow-up [see comments]. AJNR Am J Neuroradiol 1999;20:1291–9.
30. Suarez JI, Sunshine JL, Tarr R, et al. Predictors of clinical improvement, angiographic recanalization, and intracranial hemorrhage after intra-arterial thrombolysis for acute ischemic stroke. Stroke 1999;30:2094–100.
31. Yamaguchi T, Hayakawa T, Kiuchi H. Intravenous tissue plasminogen activator ameliorates the outcome of hyperacute embolic stroke. Cerebrovasc Dis 1993;3:269–72.
32. Wolpert SM, Bruckmann H, Greenlee R, et al., Group. r-PASS. Neuroradiologic evaluation of patients with acute stroke treated with recombinant tissue plasminogen activator. AJNR 1993;14:3–13.
33. Mori E, Yoneda Y, Tabuchi M, et al. Intravenous recombinant tissue plasminogen activator in acute carotid artery territory stroke [see comments]. Neurology 1992;42:976–82.
34. del ZG, Higashida RT, Furlan AJ, et al. Proact: A phase ii randomized trial of recombinant pro-urokinase by direct arterial delivery in acute middle cerebral artery stroke. Proact investigators. Prolyse in acute cerebral thromboembolism. Stroke 1998; 29:4–11.
35. Saver JL. Intra-arterial fibrinolysis for acute ischemic stroke: The message of melt. Stroke 2007;38:2627–8.
36. Zeumer H, Freitag HJ, Grzyska U, et al. Local intraarterial fibrinolysis in acute vertebrobasilar occlusion. Technical developments and recent results. Neuroradiology 1989;31:336–40.
37. Rosa A, Gautier J. Thrombolytic agents in cerebral infarctions. Rev Neurol 1991;147:99–110.
38. Kubic C, Adams R. Occlusion of the basilar artery: A clinical and pathological study. Brain 1946;69:73–121.
39. Archer CR, Horenstein S. Basilar artery occlusion: Clinical and radiological correlation. Stroke 1977;8:383–90.
40. Caplan LR, Wityk RJ, Glass TA, et al. New England Medical Center Posterior Circulation Registry. Ann Neurol 2004;56:389–98.
41. Ferbert A, Bruckmann H, Drummen R. Clinical features of proven basilar artery occlusion. Stroke 1990;21:1135–42.
42. Searls DE, Pazdera L, Korbel E, et al. Symptoms and signs of posterior circulation ischemia in the New England Medical Center Posterior Circulation Registry. Arch Neurol 2012;69:346–51.
43. Bogousslavsky J, Regli F, Maeder P, et al. The etiology of posterior circulation infarcts: A prospective study using magnetic resonance imaging and magnetic resonance angiography. Neurology 1993;43:1528–33.
44. Caplan L, Wityk R, Pazdera L, et al. New England Medical Center Posterior Circulation Stroke Registry II. Vascular lesions. J Clin Neurol 2005;1:31–49.
45. Ostrem JL, Saver JL, Alger JR, et al. Acute basilar artery occlusion: Diffusion-perfusion MRI characterization of tissue salvage in patients receiving intra-arterial stroke therapies. Stroke 2004;35:e30–4.
46. Barlinn K, Becker U, Puetz V, et al. Combined treatment with intravenous abciximab and intraarterial tpa yields high recanalization rate in patients with acute basilar artery occlusion. J Neuroimaging 2012;22:167–71.
47. Mitchell PJ, Gerraty RP, Donnan GA, et al. Thrombolysis in the vertebrobasilar circulation: The australian urokinase stroke trial – a pilot study. Cerebrovascular Diseases 1997;7:94–9.
48. Macleod MR, Davis SM, Mitchell PJ, et al. Results of a multicentre, randomised controlled trial of intra-arterial urokinase in the treatment of acute posterior circulation ischaemic stroke. Cerebrovasc Dis 2005;20:12–17.
49. Goyal M, Almekhlafi MA, Fan L, et al. Evaluation of interval times from onset to reperfusion in patients undergoing endovascular therapy in the interventional management of stroke iii trial. Circulation 2014;130:265–72.
50. Lees KR, Bluhmki E, von Kummer R, et al. Time to treatment with intravenous alteplase and outcome in stroke: An updated pooled analysis of ECASS, ATLANTIS, NINDS, and EPITHET trials. Lancet 2010;375:1695–703.
51. Saver JL, Fonarow GC, Smith EE, et al. Time to treatment with intravenous tissue plasminogen activator and outcome from acute ischemic stroke. JAMA 2013;309:2480–8.
52. Lewandowski CA, Frankel M, Tomsick TA, et al. Combined intravenous and intra-arterial r-tpa versus intra-arterial therapy of acute ischemic stroke: Emergency management of stroke (ems) bridging trial. Stroke 1999;30:2598–605.
53. IMS Study Investigators. Combined intravenous and intra-arterial recanalization for acute ischemic stroke: The interventional management of stroke study. Stroke 2004;35:904–11.
54. IMS II Trial Investigators. The interventional management of stroke (IMS) II study. Stroke 2007;38:2127–35.
55. Tomsick T, Broderick J, Carrozella J, et al., Investigators ftIMoSI. Revascularization results in the interventional management of stroke ii trial. Am J Neuroradiol 2008;29:582–7.
56. Broderick JP, Palesch YY, Demchuk AM, et al. Interventional Management of Stroke IIII. Endovascular therapy after intravenous t-PA versus t-PA alone for stroke. N Engl J Med 2013;368:893–903.
57. Khatri P, Abruzzo T, Yeatts SD, et al. Good clinical outcome after ischemic stroke with successful revascularization is time-dependent. Neurology 2009;73:1066–72.
58. Mazighi M, Serfaty JM, Labreuche J, et al., Investigators R. Comparison of intravenous alteplase with a combined intravenous-endovascular approach in patients with stroke and confirmed arterial occlusion (recanalise study): A prospective cohort study. Lancet Neurol 2009;8:802–9.
59. Goyal M, Almekhlafi MA, Fan L, et al. Evaluation of interval times from onset to reperfusion in patients undergoing endovascular therapy in the interventional management of stroke iii trial. Circulation 2014;130:265–72.
60. Khatri P, Yeatts SD, Mazighi M, et al. Time to angiographic reperfusion and clinical outcome after acute ischaemic stroke: An analysis of data from the interventional management of stroke (IMS III) phase 3 trial. Lancet Neurol 2014;13:567–74.
61. Weaver WD, Simes RJ, Betriu A, et al. Comparison of primary coronary angioplasty and intravenous thrombolytic therapy for acute myocardial infarction: A quantitative review [see comments] [published erratum appears in JAMA 1998 Jun 17;279(23):1876]. JAMA 1997;278:2093–8.
62. Patel RD, Saver JL. Evolution of reperfusion therapies for acute brain and acute myocardial ischemia: A systematic, comparative analysis. Stroke 2013;44:94–8.
63. Levy EI, Rahman M, Khalessi AA, et al. Midterm clinical and angiographic follow-up for the first food and drug administration-approved prospective, single-arm trial of primary stenting for stroke: Saris (stent-assisted recanalization for acute ischemic stroke). Neurosurgery 2011;69:915–20, discussion 920.
64. Martinez H, Zoarski GH, Obuchowski AM, et al. Mechanical thrombectomy of the internal carotid artery and middle cerebral arteries for acute stroke by using the retriever device. AJNR Am J Neuroradiol 2004;25:1812–15.
65. Gobin YP, Starkman S, Duckwiler GR, et al. Merci 1: A phase 1 study of mechanical embolus removal in cerebral ischemia. Stroke 2004;35:2848–54.
66. Smith WS. Safety of mechanical thrombectomy and intravenous tissue plasminogen activator in acute ischemic stroke. Results of the multi mechanical embolus removal in cerebral ischemia (MERCI) trial, part i. AJNR Am J Neuroradiol 2006;27:1177–82.
67. Saver JL. Does the merci retriever work? For. Stroke 2006;37:1340–1, discussion 1342–3.
68. Wechsler LR. Does the MERCI retriever work? Against. Stroke 2006;37:1341–2, discussion 1342–3.
69. Becker KJ, Brott TG. Approval of the MERCI clot retriever: A critical view. Stroke 2005;36:400–3.
70. Bose A, Henkes H, Alfke K, et al. The penumbra system: A mechanical device for the treatment of acute stroke due to thromboembolism. AJNR Am J Neuroradiol 2008;29:1409–13.
71. Broderick JP. Endovascular therapy for acute ischemic stroke. Stroke 2008.

72. Goyal M, Menon BK, Coutts SB, et al., Penumbra Pivotal Stroke Trial Investigators CSP, the Seaman MRRC. Effect of baseline CT scan appearance and time to recanalization on clinical outcomes in endovascular thrombectomy of acute ischemic strokes. Stroke 2011;42:93–7.
73. Saver JL, Liebeskind DS, Nogueira RG, et al. Need to clarify thrombolysis in myocardial ischemia (TIMI) scale scoring method in the penumbra pivotal stroke trial. Stroke 2010;41: e115–16.
74. Soares BP, Chien JD, Wintermark M. MR and CT monitoring of recanalization, reperfusion, and penumbra salvage: Everything that recanalizes does not necessarily reperfuse! Stroke 2009; 40:S24–7.
75. Zaidat OO, Yoo AJ, Khatri P, et al. Recommendations on angiographic revascularization grading standards for acute ischemic stroke: A consensus statement. Stroke 2013;44:2650–63.
76. Jahan R. Solitaire flow-restoration device for treatment of acute ischemic stroke: Safety and recanalization efficacy study in a swine vessel occlusion model. AJNR Am J Neuroradiol 2010;31: 1938–43.
77. Nogueira RG, Levy EI, Gounis M, et al. The trevo device: Preclinical data of a novel stroke thrombectomy device in two different animal models of arterial thrombo-occlusive disease. J Neurointerv Surg 2012;4:295–300.
78. Saver JL, Jahan R, Levy EI, et al., the ST. Solitaire with the intention for thrombectomy (swift) trial: Design of a randomized, controlled, multicenter study comparing the solitaire flow restoration device and the merci retriever in acute ischaemic stroke. Int J Stroke 2012.
79. Castano C, Dorado L, Guerrero C, et al. Mechanical thrombectomy with the solitaire AB device in large artery occlusions of the anterior circulation: A pilot study. Stroke 2010;41:1836–40.
80. Machi P, Costalat V, Lobotesis K, et al. Solitaire FR thrombectomy system: Immediate results in 56 consecutive acute ischemic stroke patients. J Neurointerv Surg 2012;4:62–6.
81. Miteff F, Faulder KC, Goh AC, et al. Mechanical thrombectomy with a self-expanding retrievable intracranial stent (solitaire AB): Experience in 26 patients with acute cerebral artery occlusion. AJNR Am J Neuroradiol 2011;32:1078–81.
82. Mpotsaris A, Bussmeyer M, Loehr C, et al. Mechanical thrombectomy in severe acute stroke: Preliminary results of the solitaire stent. J Neurol Neurosurg Psychiatry 2012;83:117–18.
83. Roth C, Papanagiotou P, Behnke S, et al. Stent-assisted mechanical recanalization for treatment of acute intracerebral artery occlusions. Stroke 2010;41:2559–67.
84. Mancini GB, Schulzer M. Reporting risks and benefits of therapy by use of the concepts of unqualified success and unmitigated failure: Applications to highly cited trials in cardiovascular medicine. Circulation 1999;99:377–83.
85. Ciccone A, Valvassori L, Nichelatti M, et al., Investigators SE. Endovascular treatment for acute ischemic stroke. N Engl J Med 2013;368:904–13.
86. Nogueira RG, Gupta R, Davalos A. IMS-iii and synthesis expansion trials of endovascular therapy in acute ischemic stroke: How can we improve? Stroke 2013;44:3272–4.
87. Kidwell CS, Jahan R, Saver JL. Endovascular treatment for acute ischemic stroke. N Engl J Med 2013;368:2434–5.
88. Almekhlafi MA, Eesa M, Menon BK, et al. Ultrashort imaging to reperfusion time interval arrests core expansion in endovascular therapy for acute ischemic stroke. J Neurointerv Surg 2013;5(Suppl. 1):i58–61.
89. Saver JL, Jovin TG, Smith WS, et al. Stroke treatment academic industry roundtable: Research priorities in the assessment of neurothrombectomy devices. Stroke 2013;44:3596–601.

66 Endovascular Treatment of Cerebral Aneurysms

Ajay K. Wakhloo, Matthew J. Gounis, Francesco Massari, Ajit S. Puri

KEY POINTS

- Historical review of endovascular treatment (EVT) for aneurysms.
- Safety and efficacy of coil embolization as compared with surgical clipping for ruptured aneurysms.
- Controversies over management of unruptured aneurysms.
- Added value of balloon-assisted coiling for complex aneurysms.
- Stenting improves durability of coiling.
- Introduction of flow diversion to cure aneurysms.
- Understanding and management of peri- and post-operative risks associated with EVT.

HISTORICAL OVERVIEW

The field of neurointerventional surgery has emerged in recent decades to provide safe and effective options for the treatment of intracranial aneurysms. The primary goal of aneurysm treatment, regardless of the means, is to prevent rupture or re-rupture and ameliorate mass effect in some cases of large and giant aneurysms. Before endovascular techniques were developed, craniotomy with clipping was the only definitive treatment for both ruptured and unruptured aneurysms. However, improvements in imaging and medical device technologies have expanded the role of endovascular approaches to intracranial aneurysms, especially for high-risk surgical patients.

The first endovascular intracranial aneurysm occlusion was attempted in 1964 by Luessenhop and Velasquez.[1] Though technically unsuccessful, this ground-breaking procedure provided a fundamental shift in the approach for treating intracranial disease. Contemporaries of Lussenhop and Velasquez investigated other technologies for aneurysm occlusion such as metallic[2] and electric current thrombosis.[3,4] However, the work of Fedor Serbinenko in Cold War-era Soviet Russia revolutionized this new field. Inspired by the sight of tethered helium balloons at a 1959 May Day celebration in Moscow's Red Square,[5] Serbinenko pioneered the development of the first flow-guided intralumenal balloon catheter.[6] Not long after he performed the first therapeutic vessel occlusion in 1970, Serbinenko used a detachable balloon catheter to embolize an intracranial aneurysm.[7]

Widespread news of Serbinenko's innovations at the Burdenko Neurosurgery Institute reached the West in 1974 when he summarized his experiences in English in the *Journal of Neurosurgery*.[8] Serbinenko's techniques immediately attracted curious minds from around the world. Among the pilgrims was Gerard Debrun, the French neuroradiologist who developed a latex balloon occlusion device.[9] The detachable balloon method of aneurysm embolization underwent a period of growth over the next 15 years by numerous investigators.[10-12] However, detachable balloon embolization was not without complications. For example, a detached balloon could act as a ball valve within an aneurysm sac, leading to rapid aneurysm refilling and rupture. Furthermore, the balloons would not appropriately appose to the aneurysm boundaries or would rupture/deflate resulting in dislodgement, distal non-target embolization and suboptimal aneurysm occlusion.

The detachable platinum coil, introduced in 1989, was developed to overcome the deficiencies of detachable balloons and represented another fundamental shift in the neurointerventional treatment of intracranial aneurysms. When tightly packed into the aneurysmal sac, the coil mass prevented blood flow into the aneurysm, initiating intra-aneurysmal clotting.[13,14] Within days of coil embolization, macrophages and fibroblasts infiltrated the dome of the aneurysm as endothelial cells began to proliferate across the neck. The long-term histopathological results showed that coil embolization promoted a vascularized fibrous connective tissue scar within the aneurysm dome and complete endothelialization of the neck.[15-17] Early experience with platinum coils revealed that they were difficult to control and deployment of the coil within the aneurysm sac was unreliable. However, in 1991, Guido Guglielmi published two pivotal articles describing a novel electrolytic coil detachment technique from a stainless steel wire.[18,19] Initial use of Guglielmi Detachable Coils (GDC) in 15 patients demonstrated excellent aneurysm occlusion (70–100%).[19] Periprocedural complications were limited to a single case of transient aphasia. The first multicenter trial of GDC treatment in 43 posterior circulation aneurysms showed a 7% combined morbidity and mortality, notably better than the 20% combined rate reported for similarly sized detachable balloon studies.[20,21]

ENDOVASCULAR TREATMENT OF RUPTURED ANEURYSMS: EVIDENCE

Without treatment, patients with aneurysmal subarachnoid hemorrhage (SAH) have a 19% risk of rebleeding within 2 weeks[22] and a greater than 3% annual risk thereafter.[23] Thus, isolating the aneurysm (i.e., the rupture site) from the circulation is the primary goal of treatment. Although endovascular embolization techniques found widespread use in the early 1990s, there was a lack of data comparing surgery to intervention. The International Subarachnoid Aneurysm Trial (ISAT) was the first large-scale, prospective, randomized trial to compare the safety and efficacy of endovascular coiling to surgical clipping for the treatment of ruptured aneurysms.[24] The primary end-points of this international study were dependency and death at 1 year following treatment. Patient enrollment began in 1994, and was stopped in 2002 after 2143 patients were randomized because of a significantly

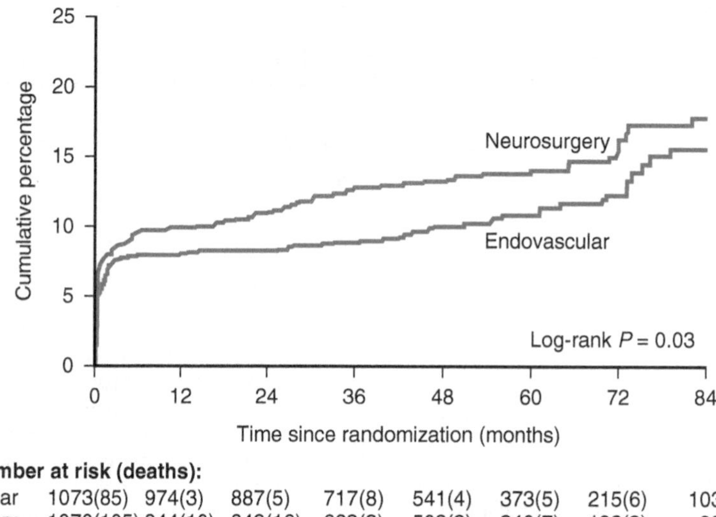

Figure 66-1. Kaplan-Meier graph of cumulative mortality from the surgical and endovascular cohorts of the International Subarachnoid Aneurysm Trial up to 7 years. *(With permission from Molyneux AJ, Kerr RS, Yu LM, Clarke M, Sneade M, Yarnold JA, et al. International subarachnoid aneurysm trial (ISAT) of neurosurgical clipping versus endovascular coiling in 2143 patients with ruptured intracranial aneurysms: a randomised comparison of effects on survival, dependency, seizures, rebleeding, subgroups, and aneurysm occlusion.* Lancet *2005;366(9488):809–17.)*

lower risk of death and disability in the endovascular group (22.6% relative risk reduction, 6.9% absolute risk reduction). One year after treatment, the absolute risk reduction improved to 7.4% in the endovascular group compared to the clipping group, and the survival advantage continued for 7 years (Fig. 66-1).[25] At the time, a criticism of the ISAT trial was the paucity of centers from the United States that participated. To address this perceived limitation, one of the premiere cerebrovascular neurosurgery centers in the country randomized ruptured aneurysms to receive either neurosurgical clipping or endovascular treatment in the Barrow Ruptured Aneurysm Trial.[26] Of the 403 patients screened for the protocol, 358 were randomized and treated. After one-year, there was a 10% absolute reduction in the rate of death or permanent disability in favor of the endovascular arm as compared to microsurgical clipping. The report of the 3-year results continued to show a benefit for those patients receiving coil embolization.[27]

The ISAT trial demonstrated that coil embolization had a superior safety profile compared to surgical clipping for the treatment of ruptured aneurysms (Fig. 66-2). However, questions remained about the durability of aneurysm occlusion, specifically, the efficacy of coils in preventing long-term rebleeding. Previous studies have demonstrated that angiographic follow-up is necessary after aneurysm treatment with detachable coils.[28–30] Although there has been no widely accepted standard for defining recanalization, recanalization rates of aneurysms treated with detachable coils ranged from 4% to 60%, depending on aneurysm size, neck width and location.[29,30] Recanalization may be associated with an increased risk of rebleeding in patients treated either endovascularly or surgically. The Cerebral Aneurysm Rerupture After Treatment (CARAT) study[31,32] was an ambidirectional cohort study designed to compare rebleeding rates in 1001 patients with aneurysm rupture treated either with coil embolization or surgical clipping with an average of 3.6 years of follow-up. The total risk of rerupture after the initial treatment of coiling and clipping were 3.4% and 1.3%, respectively.[32] The rebleeding rate as a function of time from both treatments was reported to be 2.2% in the first year, 0.2% in the second year, and 0% thereafter. These findings were similar to those of the ISAT trial, which found an annual risk of re-rupture 1 year after treatment of 0.21% in the coiling group and 0.03% in the clipping group, respectively.[25,33] In both the ISAT and CARAT, most rebleeds occurred in the first month after treatment. The latest ISAT analysis reports that with more than 8000 person-years of follow-up, aneurysms treated in the coiling and clipping arms rebled at a rate of 1.3% and 0.3% after the first year (treatment received, P = 0.023).[34] Although late rebleeding rate has been shown to be higher in the endovascular treatment arm as compared to surgery, the ISAT investigators concluded the risk remains low and similar to that of SAH from either an existing or newly formed aneurysm. Long-term rebleeding rates were even lower in an impressive single center experience of coil embolization of intracranial, berry aneurysms with 1810 patient-years of follow-up.[35] This extensive experience from a Parisian hospital demonstrated that coiled aneurysms have a risk of early re-bleeding in 0.94%, and only one case of late aneurysmal re-bleed was observed (0.21%).

Subsequent analysis by the CARAT investigators showed that the degree of initial aneurysm occlusion was the strongest predictor of re-bleeding. Aneurysms that were completely occluded had a 1.1% risk of re-bleeding, while the rebleeding risk was 17.6% for aneurysms with only partial initial occlusion.[32] While total obliteration was achieved in significantly more patients that underwent clipping (92% compared to 39% with coiling), there were no cases of rerupture following early retreatment if deemed necessary. It should also be noted, that retreatment of a previously embolized aneurysm is accompanied by low morbidity and mortality of 1.1% and 0%, respectively.[35]

Although there is consensus that surveillance imaging of endovascularly treated aneurysms is mandatory, the precise timing and imaging modalities vary depending on local practices and rupture status of the aneurysm.[36] Generally, catheter angiography is recommended as standard of care at 6 and 18 months following endovascular repair;[36] however, MR angiography is an attractive alternative with specificity and sensitivity approaching 90% for the detection of a residual aneurysm neck.[37] At our institution, catheter angiography following the treatment of ruptured aneurysms is performed at 3–6 and 12 months, and if there is no evidence of aneurysm filling, 3, 5, and 10 years thereafter. Notably, treated dissecting aneurysms

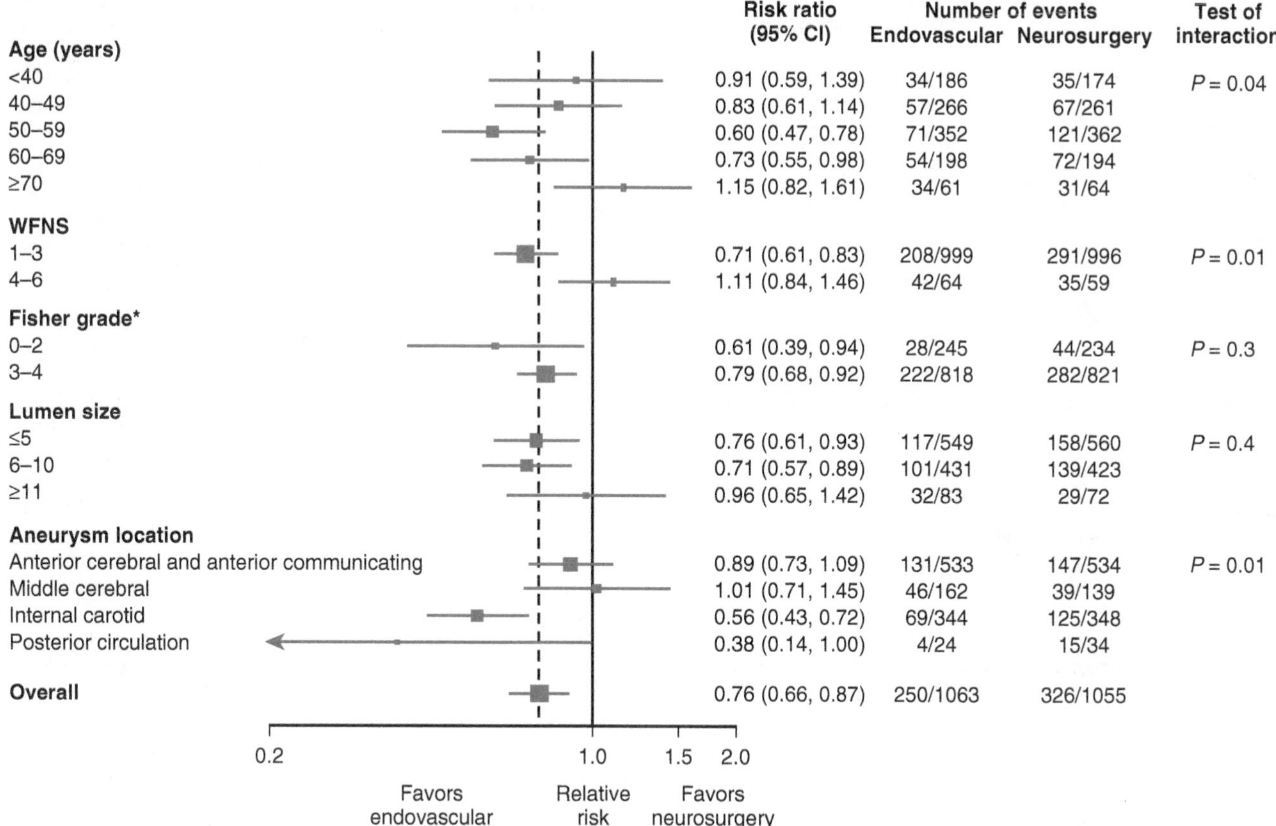

Risk ratio (95% CI)
Number of events
Endovascular
Neurosurgery
Test of interaction
Age (years)
<40 0.91 (0.59, 1.39) 34/186 35/174 P = 0.04
40–49 0.83 (0.61, 1.14) 57/266 67/261
50–59 0.60 (0.47, 0.78) 71/352 121/362
60–69 0.73 (0.55, 0.98) 54/198 72/194
≥70 1.15 (0.82, 1.61) 34/61 31/64
WFNS
1–3 0.71 (0.61, 0.83) 208/999 291/996 P = 0.01
4–6 1.11 (0.84, 1.46) 42/64 35/59
Fisher grade*
0–2 0.61 (0.39, 0.94) 28/245 44/234 P = 0.3
3–4 0.79 (0.68, 0.92) 222/818 282/821
Lumen size
≤5 0.76 (0.61, 0.93) 117/549 158/560 P = 0.4
6–10 0.71 (0.57, 0.89) 101/431 139/423
≥11 0.96 (0.65, 1.42) 32/83 29/72
Aneurysm location
Anterior cerebral and anterior communicating 0.89 (0.73, 1.09) 131/533 147/534 P = 0.01
Middle cerebral 1.01 (0.71, 1.45) 46/162 39/139
Internal carotid 0.56 (0.43, 0.72) 69/344 125/348
Posterior circulation 0.38 (0.14, 1.00) 4/24 15/34
Overall 0.76 (0.66, 0.87) 250/1063 326/1055
0.2
1.0
1.5
2.0
Favors endovascular
Relative risk
Favors neurosurgery
* Fisher grade is a measure of the amount and location of blood on the CT scan.

Figure 66-2. Subgroup analysis from the International Subarachnoid Aneurysm Trial showing the odds ratios of death or dependency after 1 year for the surgical versus endovascular treatment of ruptured brain aneurysms. *(With permission from Molyneux AJ, Kerr RS, Yu LM, Clarke M, Sneade M, Yarnold JA, et al. International subarachnoid aneurysm trial (ISAT) of neurosurgical clipping versus endovascular coiling in 2143 patients with ruptured intracranial aneurysms: a randomised comparison of effects on survival, dependency, seizures, rebleeding, subgroups, and aneurysm occlusion.* Lancet *2005;366(9488):809–17.)*

should be imaged within 3 months of treatment due to the increased risk of aneurysm growth or recanalization and early rerupture.[38] Long-term follow-up of treated aneurysms is controversial since late recurrence or rebleeding is rare,[39] but documented cases of late rebleeding are associated with poor outcomes and perhaps justify continued surveillance.[40] Importantly, imaging is not only necessary for the surveillance of the treated aneurysm, but also to assess formation of de novo aneurysms which may occur in up to 8% of patients during long-term follow-up.[41]

These long-term data on the endovascular treatment of ruptured brain aneurysms confirm that the risk of rebleeding from the treated aneurysms is extremely low and the patients have a good clinical outcome as compared with surgical clipping. However, the recanalization rates and expansion of endovascular treatment (EVT) to otherwise only surgically approachable or non-treatable aneurysms have been the impetus for continuous technological developments to improve treatment durability and to find a cure for the disease. These technologies will be discussed in subsequent sections.

ENDOVASCULAR TREATMENT OF UNRUPTURED ANEURYSMS: EVIDENCE

The management of asymptomatic unruptured aneurysms remains controversial.[42–44] Based primarily on natural history data compiled by the International Study on Unruptured Intracranial Aneurysms (ISUIA) investigators,[45,46] clinical decisions usually take into account the patient's age, aneurysm size and location, patient preferences, and the skills of local neurosurgeons and neuroendovascular interventionalists.[47] Increased rupture risk is also reported for patients with a family history of intracranial aneurysms and a clinical history of smoking and/or hypertension.[48] The ISUIA study was designed with both a retrospective (1449 patients) and prospective arms (4060 patients). The primary objective for the retrospective arm was to compare the natural history of unruptured aneurysms in patients with and without a history of SAH, in an attempt to determine the risk of rupture and treatment options. The prospective arm sought to determine morbidity and mortality rates for patients undergoing treatment for unruptured aneurysms. Mean duration of follow-up was 8.3 years. The authors concluded that in patients without a history of SAH, aneurysms ≤7 mm in size were extremely unlikely to rupture with a rupture risk of 0.05% per year (Fig. 66-3). Patients with aneurysms similar in size and location, but with a history of SAH, were 11 times more likely to rupture (0.5% per year). Aneurysm size was an important predictor of rupture in patients without a history of SAH, with large (relative risk, 11.6) and giant (relative risk, 59) aneurysms at higher risk of rupture. Posterior circulation (vertebrobasilar) and basilar apex aneurysms were also at higher risk of rupture, having a relative risk of 13.6 and 13.8, respectively. In the endovascular cohort, 2% and 5% of patients suffered

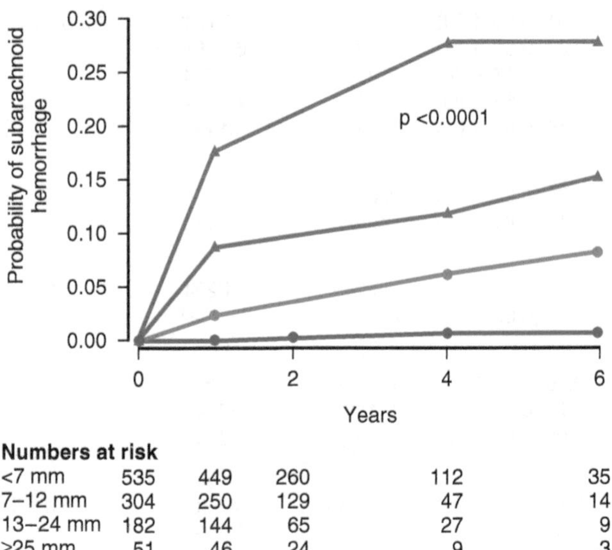

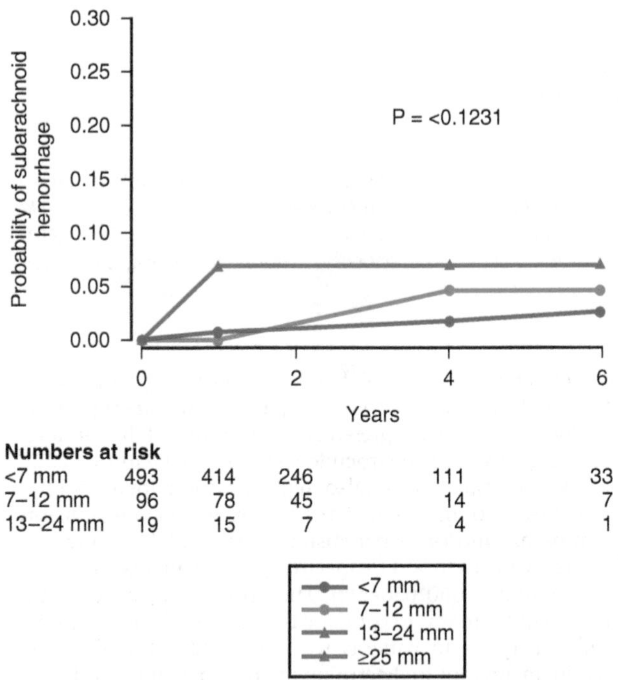

Figure 66-3. Probability of subarachnoid hemorrhage as a function of size separated by previous history of subarachnoid hemorrhage from the International Study of Unruptured Intracranial Aneurysms. The giant aneurysm group is excluded in the analysis of patients with previous subarachnoid hemorrhage due to small sample size. *(With permission from Wiebers DO, Whisnant JP, Huston J, 3rd, et al. Unruptured intracranial aneurysms: natural history, clinical outcome, and risks of surgical and endovascular treatment. Lancet. 2003;362(9378): 103-10.)*

hemorrhage and cerebral infarction, respectively, during the procedure. Complete obliteration of the aneurysm was achieved in 55% of the aneurysm, with a partial occlusion in 24%, and no occlusion in 18%. In 3% of the endovascular cases, the status of aneurysm obliteration was not reported. Rupture of the aneurysm during surgical clipping was observed in 6% of the patients, intracranial hemorrhage and cerebral infarction was seen in 4% and 11% of the patients, respectively. The total morbidity and mortality in the surgical arm at 1 year was 10.1% and 12.6% in patients with and without history of SAH, respectively. In the endovascular cohort, the 1 year morbidity and mortality rates were 7.1% and 9.8% in patients with and without history of SAH, respectively. Overall rates of cognitive impairment 1 year following endovascular or surgical treatment was 3.5% or 5.7%, respectively.

Not long after the ISUIA study was published in 1998, the Stroke Council of the American Heart Association adopted "Recommendations for the management of patients with unruptured intracranial aneurysms."[49] The recommendations were criticized because ISUIA patients were not a good representation of the general population,[50] patient follow-up was limited compared to other large-scale studies of unruptured intracranial aneurysms,[51,52] and anterior circulation aneurysms were under-represented. Since patients with unruptured intracranial aneurysms have never been the subjects of a randomized trial, the Trial on Endovascular Aneurysm Management (TEAM) began enrolling patients with unruptured intracranial aneurysms to compare the combined morbidity and mortality of endovascular treatment with conservative management over a projected 10-year period of follow-up.[53] Unfortunately, the low enrollment rate in the TEAM trial led to its announced cancellation at the 2009 Congress of the World Federation of Interventional and Therapeutic Neuroradiology. More recently, the Unruptured Cerebral Aneurysm Study (UCAS) from Japan that included 6697 aneurysms, confirmed the increased risk of aneurysm rupture as a function of size, with a significant increase in rupture risk beyond 7 mm.[54] Additionally, the UCAS investigators reported increased rupture risk for anterior or posterior communicating artery locations as well as irregular protrusions or blebs from the aneurysm sac.

Particularly controversial is the management of small unruptured intracranial aneurysms, which ISUIA shows have a relatively benign natural history that may not be improved with treatment; however, more recent studies on the natural history and endovascular treatment outcomes in small unruptured aneurysms prove valuable.[55-57] Importantly, advances in endovascular technology that have become available since the ISUIA trial was conducted allow for high rates of complete occlusion and cure of small unruptured aneurysms with a low risk of morbidity and mortality. Six hundred forty-nine patients with a total of 1100 aneurysms were treated endovascularly in 27 Canadian and French neurointerventional centers (Analysis of Treatment by Endovascular approach of Nonruptured Aneurysms, ATENA).[55] Aneurysms were treated with coils alone in 54.5% of the cases, and in 37.3% and 7.8% of the cases a temporary balloon-assistance or stenting was required, respectively. Endovascular treatment failed in 4.3% of the cases. Thromboembolic complications were encountered in 7.1%, intra-operative rupture occurred in 2.6%, and device-related problems were observed in 2.9% of the procedures. Adverse events associated with transient or permanent neurological deficit or deaths were encountered in 5.4% of the cases. Thirty-day morbidity and mortality rates were 1.7% and 1.4%, respectively. The relatively benign natural history of small unruptured intracranial aneurysms along with accurate assessments of the risk–benefit ratio of treating these lesions must be evaluated on a case-by-case basis between a multidisciplinary team of cerebrovascular specialists and the patient. Importantly, modifiable risk factors (reviewed by Andreasen et al.),[58] in particular smoking cessation and control of hypertension, should be aggressively managed with or without subsequent treatment. In cases of small unruptured aneurysms that are under observation, serial non-invasive imaging is necessary at regular intervals to assess morphological changes or growth that may indicate treatment.[59,60]

Key developments in the area of unruptured aneurysms involve the identification of the rupture risk of these lesions. Aneurysm wall inflammation has been correlated with ruptured aneurysms.[61] A more comprehensive understanding of aneurysm wall biology is providing clues as to the progression of an unruptured aneurysm to rupture. Similar to vulnerable plaque, inflammation is central to a vascular remodeling process that may lead to rupture[62] – essentially engendering the concept of a "vulnerable aneurysm." Identifying cellular and molecular mechanisms of human intracranial aneurysm rupture (reviewed in[63]) holds promise for improved decision making regarding the benefit of treatment weighed against the quantitated risk of aneurysm rupture. Human aneurysm specimens were recently analyzed for the presence of myeloperoxidase, an oxidoreductase secreted primarily by neutrophils. It was found that the presence of this inflammatory marker was significantly correlated with the Population, Hypertension, Age, Size of Aneurysm, Earlier Subarachnoid Hemorrhage From Another Aneurysm and Site of Aneurysm (PHASES) model of 5-year aneurysm rupture risk.[62] It has been recently reported that oxidative stress may be the cause of programmed cell death that is predominant in ruptured vs unruptured human aneurysms.[64,65]

Building on previous work with human aneurysm tissue that identified the association of mural cell loss with rupture, a rat model was developed in which an allogeneic arterial graft was decellularized prior to its anastomosis to the aorta of the experimental animal.[66] Nearly half of these decellularized aneurysms grew and three ultimately ruptured during the observation period, whereas control aneurysms remained stable. Pathological analysis demonstrated that thrombus formation within the decellularized aneurysm could not organize, thereby leading to recanalization, inflammation, wall degeneration and ultimately rupture. Similar conclusions regarding the role of incomplete thrombosis and subsequent inflammatory cell infiltration into the aneurysm wall with marked degeneration were confirmed in a swine venous pouch aneurysm model.[67] Ultimately, thorough understanding of aneurysm pathophysiology may enable diagnostic imaging approaches to identify those at risk of rupture[68,69] or eligible for pharmacological treatment for stabilization of these lesions.[70,71]

Due to the advances in cost-effective computational resources, computational fluid dynamic (CFD) analysis of intra-aneurysmal hemodynamics dominates much of the research on aneurysm treatment[72–80] and potential rupture mechanisms.[81–89] The debate about how to implement the information from CFD into clinical workflow remains active.[90–93] Numerous modeling assumptions have been investigated to determine the accuracy of the patient-specific simulations.[94] Studies on the generation of the virtual model,[95–97] the importance of the inlet/outlet boundary conditions,[98,99] and the relevance of the Newtonian fluid assumption[100] serve to refine the technique for eventual clinical utility. A recent high-quality CFD analysis on untreated, unruptured small aneurysms was recently published.[101] Four of the aneurysms followed progressed to rupture, and each case had five controls matched by location and size. There were no significant differences in commonly used parameters such as the aspect ratio, wall shear stress (mean, maximum or minimum), and pressure loss coefficient between the aneurysms that ruptured versus controls. The investigators found a novel parameter, the wall shear stress cumulative distribution function that predicted pending rupture with a sensitivity and specificity of 0.9 and 0.93, respectively. Although this is a small cohort, these results are quite promising. Ultimately, combining detailed biomechanical analysis with information on wall-biology and genetics may serve to develop fluid-solid-growth models that predict the evolution of brain aneurysms.[102]

TECHNIQUES OF ENDOVASCULAR ANEURYSM TREATMENT

The vast majority of aneurysms that were treated endovascularly in the above described clinical trials were performed with the first generation of embolic coils. These coils, the Guglielmi Detachable Coil (GDC), are made of a platinum alloy and have a 2D helical shape. Technological advancements have dramatically improved endovascular treatment of aneurysms in a relatively short span of time. New tools have facilitated access to the lesions, including microcatheters that allow the safe embolization of the aneurysm sac with high rates of complete occlusion. Wide-neck aneurysms can now be addressed via the endovascular approach with the use of adjunctive devices such as temporary occlusion balloons and neurovascular stents. Developments in imaging including flat panel detectors with high spatial and contrast resolution, 3D reconstruction angiography,[103] radiation dose reduction algorithms[104] and cone beam computed tomography[105–107] offer enhanced visualization of the aneurysm morphology and the medical devices deployed endovascularly. The cumulative effects of these advancements, many of which have occurred in the last 5 years, have not yet been captured in large randomized controlled studies with long-term follow-up. Trials to investigate the impact of various new technologies are ongoing and to date we rely on single center studies to demonstrate the positive clinical impact.

Coiling

As noted briefly in the previous section, the major shortcoming of the original 2D GDC bare platinum coils is compaction and aneurysmal recanalization that ranges between 21% and 34% of the cases. Recanalization and regrowth is even higher in subsets of aneurysms including those that are large or have wide necks,[29,30] have large direct blood-flow impingement,[108] or have a large amount of intra-aneurysmal clot. With progressively improving technology, the safety profile of bare platinum coils is acceptable with an approximately 2% mortality and a 4–5% morbidity. Negative outcomes are mostly related to thromboembolic complications and intraoperative rupture.[55,109] In larger series technical success of aneurysm coiling reaches 96.9% and 94% for ruptured and unruptured aneurysms, respectively. The procedural mortality is reported to be 1.4% and 1.7% for ruptured and unruptured aneurysms, respectively, while the morbidity rates are 8.6% and 7.7% for ruptured and unruptured aneurysms, respectively.[28,110]

In addition to thromboembolic complications, intraoperative rupture accounts for major morbidity and mortality.[110,111] In two large multicenter series the rates of thromboembolic complications and intra-operative rupture associated with coiling were reported in 7.3% and 2%, respectively.[110] For both types of complications, no clinical worsening was observed in approximately half the cases, but the mortality rate was higher after intra-operative rupture (16.7%) than thromboembolic complications (4.1%). In ruptured aneurysms, the rates of thromboembolic complications and intraoperative rupture were higher: 13.3% and 3.7%, respectively.[111] Because thromboembolism is the most common complication of aneurysm coiling, operators have adapted perioperative use of intravenous heparin for anticoagulation and aspirin as an antiplatelet agent for unruptured and in some instances for ruptured aneurysms as well.[112]

Early experience showed two main challenges for aneurysm coiling: (1) some aneurysms were not easy to treat because of their shape (large and giant aneurysms, fusiform aneurysms, wide-neck aneurysms, aneurysms with unfavorable size relationship between aneurysm dome, neck, and parent artery). This led to the development of new techniques and technologies, including balloon-assisted coiling (known as the remodeling technique), aneurysm coiling supported by stenting, and more recently, the introduction of flow diversion/disruption. (2) The durability of aneurysm coil embolization was not achieved in all aneurysms.[29,113] A systematic review of a large number of studies showed that aneurysm recanalization and regrowth occurred in 20.8% of the cases, requiring retreatment in 10.3%.[114] Several factors were identified as being associated with an increased risk for recanalization and regrowth, including recent rupture, high blood pressure, smoking, aneurysm diameter and neck size, and quality of immediate post-operative aneurysm occlusion associated with coil packing density.[115-122] To reduce the recanalization rate, a second generation of bare platinum coils was introduced to the endovascular armament that provided a 3D shape of the coils that were more appropriate to the native aneurysm morphology. These improved coils made it possible to maintain a high structural integrity, yet permitted a high and homogenous packing density throughout the aneurysmal sac. Surface-modified coils, including polyglycolic-lactic acid coils and Hydrocoils (Microvention, Tustin, CA), were developed, but their evaluation in large multicenter series showed that they were not more efficacious than bare platinum coils.[123-125] The clinical significance of aneurysm recanalization and regrowth is not very well known, although the CARAT study showed that the degree of aneurysm occlusion after the initial treatment was a strong predictor of the risk of subsequent rupture in patients presenting initially with an SAH.[32] Because aneurysm recanalization can occur, anatomic follow-up with digital subtraction angiography or MR imaging is mandatory (Fig. 66-4A–E).[32,126-129] A recently published trial comparing a polyglycolic/polylactic acid biopolymer-modified coils (Matrix^2) with bare platinum coils, showed non-inferiority of the modified coils regarding safety profile and technical success.[130] However, there were no significant differences in recurrence rates between the coils (14.6% with bare metal coils vs 13.3% with Matrix^2, $P = 0.76$, log-rank test).

Balloon-Assisted Coiling

Several authors have described the use of temporary balloons to enable coil embolization of wide-neck aneurysms and prevent coil herniation or migration into the parent artery.[131,132] The operator first places a non-detachable, super compliant balloon within the parent vessel in front of the aneurysm neck. Subsequently, a microcatheter is then navigated into the aneurysm for coil deployment. During coiling, the balloon is temporarily inflated allowing a proper deployment of each coil within the aneurysm pouch (Fig. 66-5A–F).[133] To allow brain perfusion and limit occlusion time, the balloon is generally deflated within 2 minutes and re-inflated as needed to continue coiling or for deployment of subsequent coils. The time the balloon is left inflated also depends on the collateral flow, branches coming off the balloon inflation site and the region of the brain being treated. In more complex aneurysms, especially in, or adjacent to, bifurcations, such as middle cerebral or anterior communicating artery aneurysms, the approach can resemble artistic work. Several techniques have been carved out, including the use of two balloons or the use of various-shaped balloons. Following embolization, the balloon is deflated and removed from the cerebrovascular system. Optimal anti-coagulation is recommended for balloon remodeling to prevent thromboembolic complications during flow arrest/disruption. The purpose of balloon-assisted coiling (BAC) was to address a subgroup of wide-neck aneurysms in the pre-stent era. However, more recently, balloons were found to be useful in EVT of ruptured and unruptured aneurysms at high-risk for intra-operative rupture.[134] In the event of an iatrogenic rupture, the balloon is readily available at the site and can be inflated immediately. The indication expansion for ruptured and unruptured aneurysms has led to an increased use of balloons during the past years and is now reported to be used in nearly in half of the cases.[135]

A single-center, retrospective series using BAC for ruptured and unruptured aneurysms reported thromboembolic events and intra-operative aneurysm rupture in 9.8% and 4.0% of patients, respectively, while in the same study thromboembolic complications and ruptures with coiling alone were observed in 2.2% and 0.8%, respectively.[136] However, a recently published and well-designed multicenter study on the use BAC for unruptured (Analysis of Treatment by Endovascular approach of Non-ruptured Aneurysms [ATENA]) and ruptured aneurysms (Clinical and Anatomical Results in the Treatment of Ruptured Intracranial Aneurysms [CLARITY])[137,138] showed acceptable peri-operative risks with the technique. In unruptured aneurysms, the rate of thromboembolic events associated with BAC was similar to coiling alone (5.4% vs 6.2%). In the unruptured study, the intra-operative rupture rate was slightly higher with BAC as compared with coiling alone (3.2% vs 2.2%) resulting in a treatment morbidity of 2.3% and 2.2% in the BAC and coiling group, respectively. In addition there was, although not significant, a higher mortality of 1.4% associated with BAC as compared to 0.9% in the coiling group. The data for the ruptured aneurysm series did not show any major differences between the two approaches. The rate of thromboembolic events was 11.3% for BAC and 12.7% for coiling alone. Intra-operative rupture was seen in 4.4% for both modalities. Morbidity and mortality in the BAC group was seen in 2.5% and 1.3% of treated subjects, respectively. Similarly, morbidity and mortality with coiling alone was reported in 3.9% and 1.2%, respectively. Despite more complex aneurysm morphology in the BAC group, both safety and efficacy profiles for both ruptured and unruptured aneurysm treatment are comparable between BAC or coiling alone.

Stent-assisted Coiling

The original concept of using stents for coiling goes back nearly 20 years when pushable coils were used for treatment of aneurysms[139] and was thought to prevent coil herniation in-to the parent artery. Stent-assisted coiling (SAC) also overcame the limitation of EVT in some complex aneurysms, including wide-neck aneurysms with a very small dome-neck ratio, large and giant aneurysms, and fusiform aneurysms (Fig. 66-6A–G).[38,140-144]

For a long period of time only stiffer coronary stents and delivery systems were available to access the challenging cerebrovascular system. Based on early encouraging clinical observations, several medical device manufacturers engineered neurovascular-specific, later FDA approved stents that over the past decade have found their broad application in the clinical realm.

Beyond challenges with access, introduction of stenting for aneurysms posed a new hematological concern. Unlike coils, stents are implanted in the parent artery and used to bridge

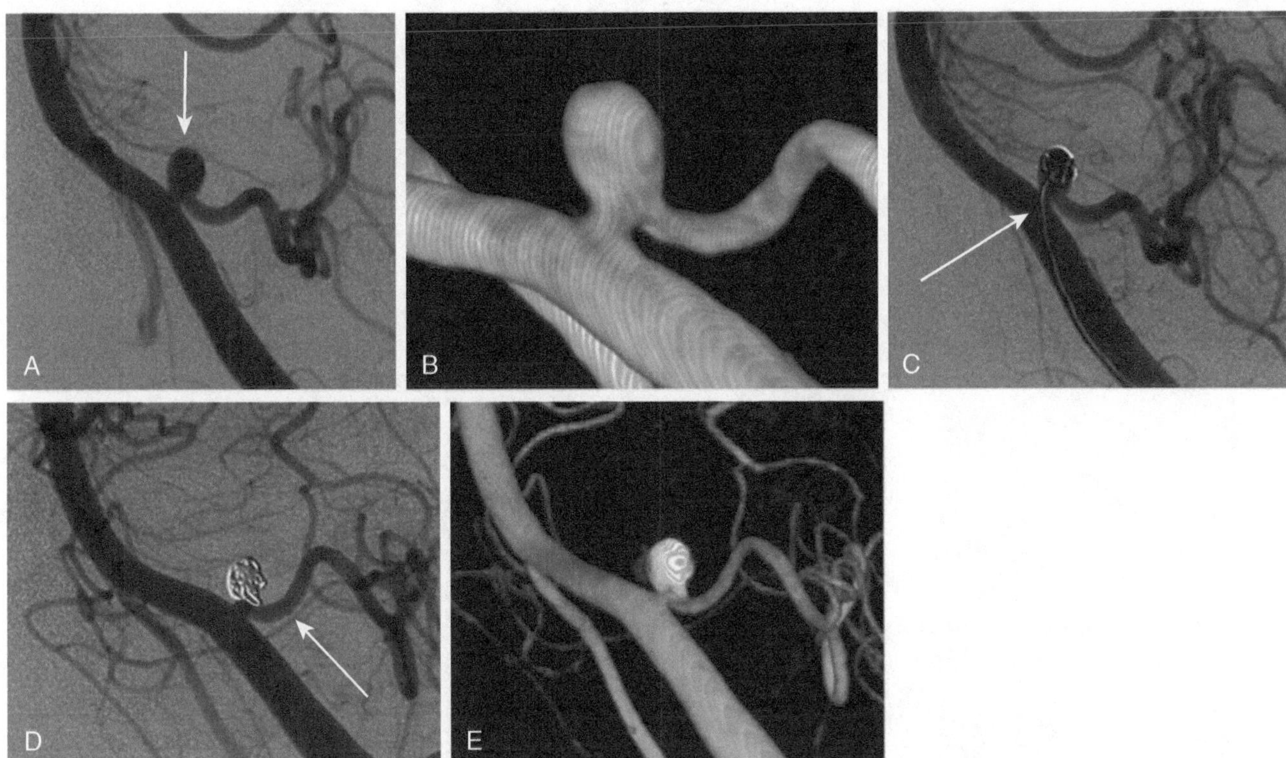

Figure 66-4. A, Lateral view angiogram shows a posterior inferior cerebellar artery (PICA) aneurysm (arrow). B, 3D angiogram shows detailed aneurysm architecture and PICA involvement. C, Coils being placed through a microcatheter for embolization (arrow). D, Post-operative follow-up angiogram shows a complete aneurysm occlusion and patent PICA (arrow). E, Two-year 3D follow-up angiogram shows stable aneurysm occlusion and patent PICA.

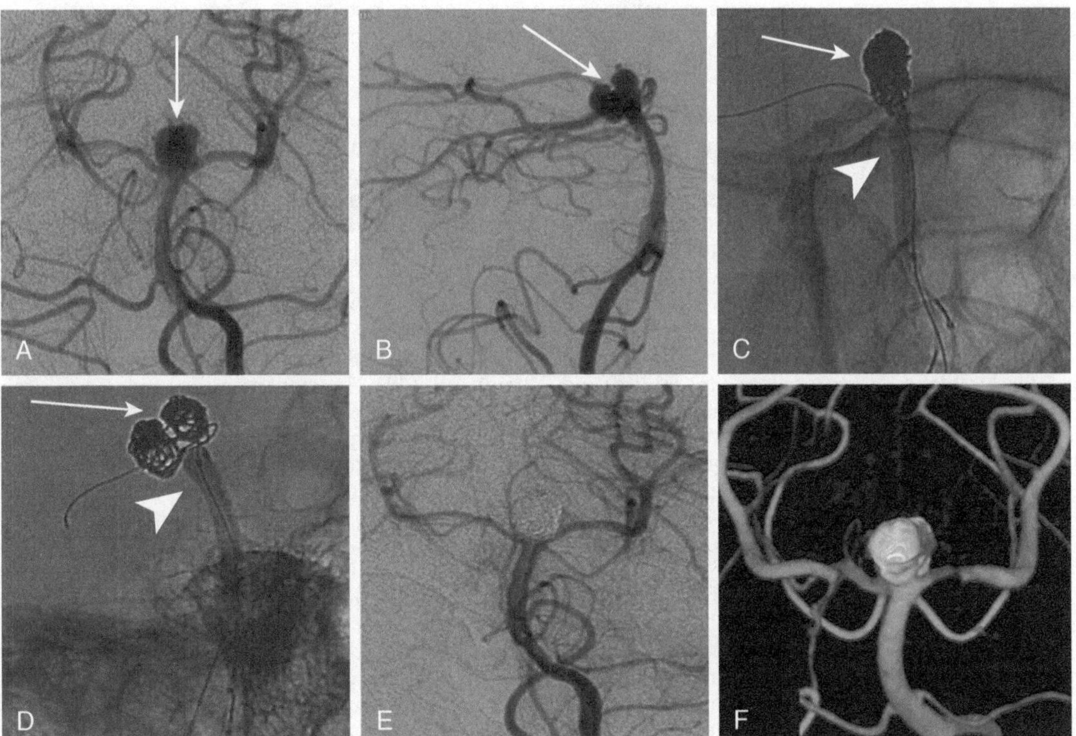

Figure 66-5. A and B, Frontal and lateral view left vertebral artery angiograms show a ruptured wide-neck bilobed and septated basilar artery bifurcation aneurysm (arrows). C and D, A super-compliant temporary balloon (arrowhead) is inflated in the parent artery during placement of coils (arrow) to prevent coil herniation in to the basilar artery. The balloon is deflated and removed at the end of the procedure. E, Follow-up frontal angiogram before removal of the coil delivery microcatheter shows a complete aneurysm occlusion. F, 6-month 3D follow-up angiogram shows stable and complete occlusion of the aneurysm.

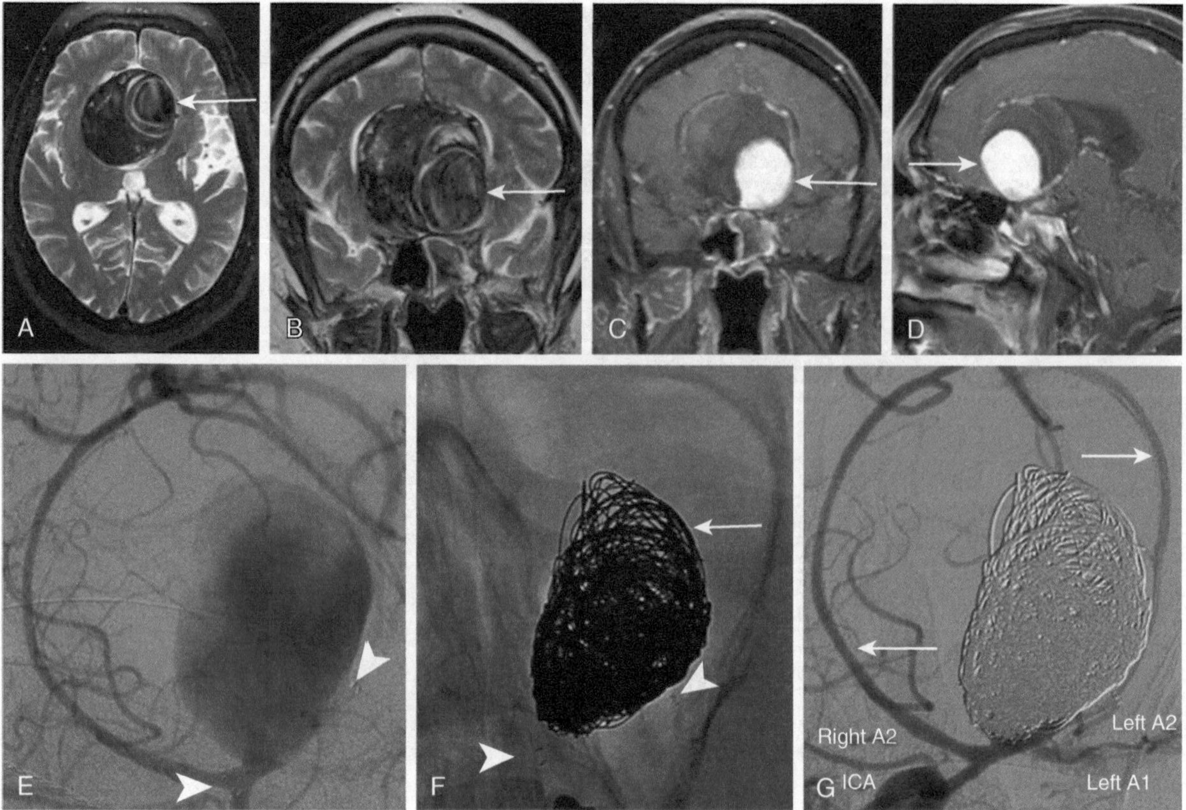

Figure 66-6. A and B, MRI axial and coronal T2-weighted images depicting a partially thrombosed 6.5 cm anterior communicating artery aneurysm with flow-related artifacts centered in the left anterior–inferior portion of the aneurysm (arrows). C and D, MRI coronal and sagittal post-contrast T1-weighted images confirm the presence of a left anterior–inferior patent aneurysm part (arrows). E, Frontal view right internal carotid artery angiogram shows a partially thrombosed giant anterior communicating artery aneurysm with a significant mass effect and stretching of both A2 segments. F, Stenting (arrowheads) across the anterior communicating artery in to the left A2 and coiling (arrow). G, Final follow-up angiogram shows a complete aneurysm occlusion, with preserved antegrade flow in A2 segment of both anterior cerebral arteries (arrows).

the aneurysm neck. Thus, to prevent an implant thrombosis or thromboembolism they require a peri-operative and post-operative antiplatelet treatment. Most operators additionally prescribe an antiplatelet regimen that includes both aspirin and clopidogrel. Subsequently, the use of SAC for ruptured aneurysms may complicate management, especially if the placement of an extraventricular drainage (EVD) or surgical intervention in the acute peri-SAH phase is indispensable. However, with the experience gained during recent years, stenting has been used in selected cases of ruptured aneurysms. Importantly, higher postprocedural morbidity and mortality as compared with unruptured aneurysms still remains a concern.

Beyond expansion of EVT to more complex aneurysms, stent placement has been shown to reduce aneurysm recanalization. This encouraged increased use of SAC. There are several prospective and retrospective single- and multi-center case series that have evaluated safety and efficacy of SAC. However, no prospective randomized clinical trials have been published comparing standard coiling or BAC with SAC. In a recently published large retrospective single-center series of 1137 patients with 1325 aneurysms, 216 aneurysms (16.3%) were treated with stents.[145] Based on architectural features and location, the coiling subgroup was not comparable with the SAC population. Although not significant, SAC was associated with higher rates of permanent neurological complications (7.4%) as compared with coiling (3.8%; $P = 0.644$). Procedure-related mortality in the SAC and coiling group was 4.6% and 1.2% respectively ($P = 0.006$). Follow-up, available in approximately 50% of the patients, showed angiographic recurrence in 33.5% of the coiling group as compared with 14.9% in the stenting group ($P < 0.0001$).

A recently published meta-analysis on SAC showed an overall complication rate of 19% and a mortality of 2.1%.[146] Thromboembolic events and hemorrhage were encountered in 10% and 2.2%, respectively while technical complications were seen in 9% of the treated cases. A complete aneurysm occlusion was observed in 45% of aneurysms following SAC. Unlike coiling, SAC showed a higher rate of progressive occlusion to 61%. In stent-stenosis and stent occlusion were observed in 3.5% and 0.6% of cases, respectively.

Other larger published series[147,148] have reported procedure-related complications of nearly 15% with permanent neurological sequelae in approximately 5% of treated patients. Minor and major recanalization was seen in nearly 20% of treated patients.

A recently completed study on SAC found that risk factors for higher periprocedural complications and morbidity at follow-up were associated with underlying coronary heart disease and neck size of the target aneurysm.[149]

With growing experience, SAC is increasingly used in ruptured aneurysms.[150] Although a high degree of technical success is achieved, authors have reported a significant increase in intracranial hemorrhage (up to 11%) and thromboembolic events (up to 6%)[151] as well as a high mortality of nearly 20%. Two larger multicenter studies confirm these findings.[152,153] The authors reported death in 3.5% of treated patients (16% for all patients with SAH and 1.5% for electively treated patients). Periprocedural or delayed thromboembolic events were observed in 4.4% of patients.[152] In the population with angiographic follow-up, a complete occlusion was observed in 59% and retreatment was required in 8.3% of patients. In-stent stenosis was seen in 3.4% of patients.

In summary, SAC has enabled the treatment of more complex aneurysms with lower rate of recanalization and retreatment. However, increased peri-procedural risk of hemorrhagic and thromboembolic events as well as increased morbidity during follow-up, especially in ruptured aneurysms, warrant a careful selection of patients. No data are available comparing safety and efficacy of SAC with BAC or coiling alone.

Flow Diversion

Prior to the FDA approval of the GDC coil, researchers were already exploring the concept of flow diversion for the treatment of brain aneurysms.[139,154–157] Essentially, the concept incorporates two phenomena, namely, the disruption of the fluid momentum transfer into the aneurysm sac and the scaffold that produces a remodeling effect of the vascular wall. The embodiment today of this concept is low-porosity braided stents (Figs. 66-6, 66-7 and 66-8). In the last edition of this chapter, we concluded that the next decade of development would usher in an era of vascular reconstruction of the diseased segment with this technology. We were, perhaps, too conservative, as this technology is currently presenting a paradigm shift in the endovascular treatment of brain aneurysms.

The first multi-center, single-arm clinical trial, Pipeline for Uncoilable or Failed Aneurysms (PUFS) trial,[158] established the safety and efficacy of the flow diversion concept for human aneurysms. In this study, 108 patients from ten centers were enrolled having an aneurysm that measured at least 10 mm and a neck of at least 4 mm. The location of the aneurysm was restricted to the internal carotid artery, from the petrous segment to the superior hypophyseal artery. Patients with a history of SAH within 60 days or surgery within 42 days from the time of enrollment were excluded. Patients with recurrence following coil embolization or surgical clip placement could be enrolled, as long as no other stent devices were present in the target vessel. Failed implantation of the Pipeline embolization device occurred in a single patient within the study, giving a high rate of technical success (99.1%). The mean aneurysm size in the trial was 18.2 mm, and 6 month follow-up angiography showed that 73.6% of aneurysms were completely occluded without major stenosis of the parent artery or use of adjunctive coils. Major ipsilateral stroke or neurological death occurred in 5.6% of the patients. For aneurysms that had follow-up at 1 year, 86.8% were completely obliterated. Progressive aneurysm occlusion and cure has been reported with a second generation device, the Surpass flow diverter, which has similar porosity of the Pipeline but augmented pore density.[159] This exciting finding shows that unlike coil embolization, where coil compaction leads to aneurysm recurrence over time, there is a progressive thrombosis and healing of the aneurysm following flow diversion treatment. Even more compelling is that this progressive healing was predicted in preclinical studies.[160,161] The next generation technology with substantially improved pore-density (increase in the number of wires braided into the device that have smaller diameter) has shown that using a single device can produce aneurysm occlusion rates at 6 months that exceed 90%.[162]

However, the PUFS trial was very limited in aneurysms that could be included, and nearly half of aneurysms enrolled originated from the petrous and cavernous segments. There are numerous single-center reports of using the Pipeline Embolization Device (eV3 Neurovascular, Irvine CA) outside of the original indication to treat smaller aneurysms located more distally or in the posterior circulation. Several recently published meta-analysis of EVT in more than 1000 intracranial aneurysms treated with flow diversion confirm the efficacy of the device with occlusion rates as high as 76%.[163,164] However, the complication rates were higher than the PUFS trial, with procedure-related morbidity and mortality of 5–10% and 4%, respectively. Morbidity and mortality with the Silk device are reported to be higher with up to 15% and 8%, respectively.[165–167] Generally, adverse clinical events with current flow diversion technology is similar to stent-assisted coil embolization but with higher rates of treatment cure.[159]

Specifically, the complications included post-operative SAH, intraparenchymal hemorrhage (IPH), and perforator infarctions (3% in each category). Beyond the immediate post-operative period but less than 30 days following treatment, the rate of SAH, IPH and ischemia/ischemic stroke was 3%, 3% and 5%, respectively. After 30 days, there was a slight decrease in the rates of SAH, IPH and ischemic stroke (2%, 2% and 3% of the patients, respectively). Perforator occlusions were more common in flow diverter implants of the posterior circulation as compared with those in the anterior circulation. Ischemic stroke was encountered in 6% of the patients.[163]

As we learn more from the clinical experience with flow diversion, certain complications have emerged that include: (1) parenchymal bleeds that occur shortly after implant and are ipsilateral, distal to the device, and (2) acute or delayed aneurysm rupture (reviewed in[168]). Albeit rare (~1%),[158,169–172] the latter complication is devastating since in patients with dual-antiplatelet therapy this complication is often fatal. The mechanism for aneurysm rupture following flow diversion remains unclear. Several explanations have been proposed. Notably, this particular complication is typically only seen in large aneurysms (>10 mm). Given the higher overall risk of rupture from these aneurysms,[54] this observation may well be the result of the natural history of the lesion combined with a given "latency" period required for aneurysm obliteration. Notably, this has been reported with SAC embolization as well.[150] Others have proposed a mechanism that involves rapid yet incomplete thrombosis of the aneurysm that subsequently leads to inflammatory changes in the aneurysm wall that in the unsecured aneurysm can lead to weakening followed by rupture.[61,169,173] Some have proposed abnormal hemodynamics in the aneurysm from the devices causing jets or local pressure increases;[174,175] however, at this time more research is required to fully understand this complication. To prevent this complication, some prefer to sub-totally occlude large aneurysms with coils prior to using flow diversion; however, currently it is not possible to determine if this strategy has a superior safety profile.

Ipsilateral, distal IPH is another concerning complication that may have be seen in as many as 8.5% of the cases.[176] Again, this complication can be quite serious in patients under dual-antiplatelet therapy, and difficult to manage as surgical decompression is often necessary. Again, mechanisms of these delayed ipsilateral bleedings remains unclear and do not correlate with size of the aneurysm or location. One compelling explanation is thromboembolic distal infarction that converts to hemorrhage. There have been autopsy studies that have shown intravascular amorphous foreign materials that likely represent materials from the hydrophilic lining of some medical devices.[177] In one case of this report, the material was extracted from the intracranial parenchymal hematoma evacuation, showing that these materials can lead to hemorrhagic infarction. Recent autopsies performed subsequent to delayed, ipsilateral IPH following Pipeline flow diversion treatment

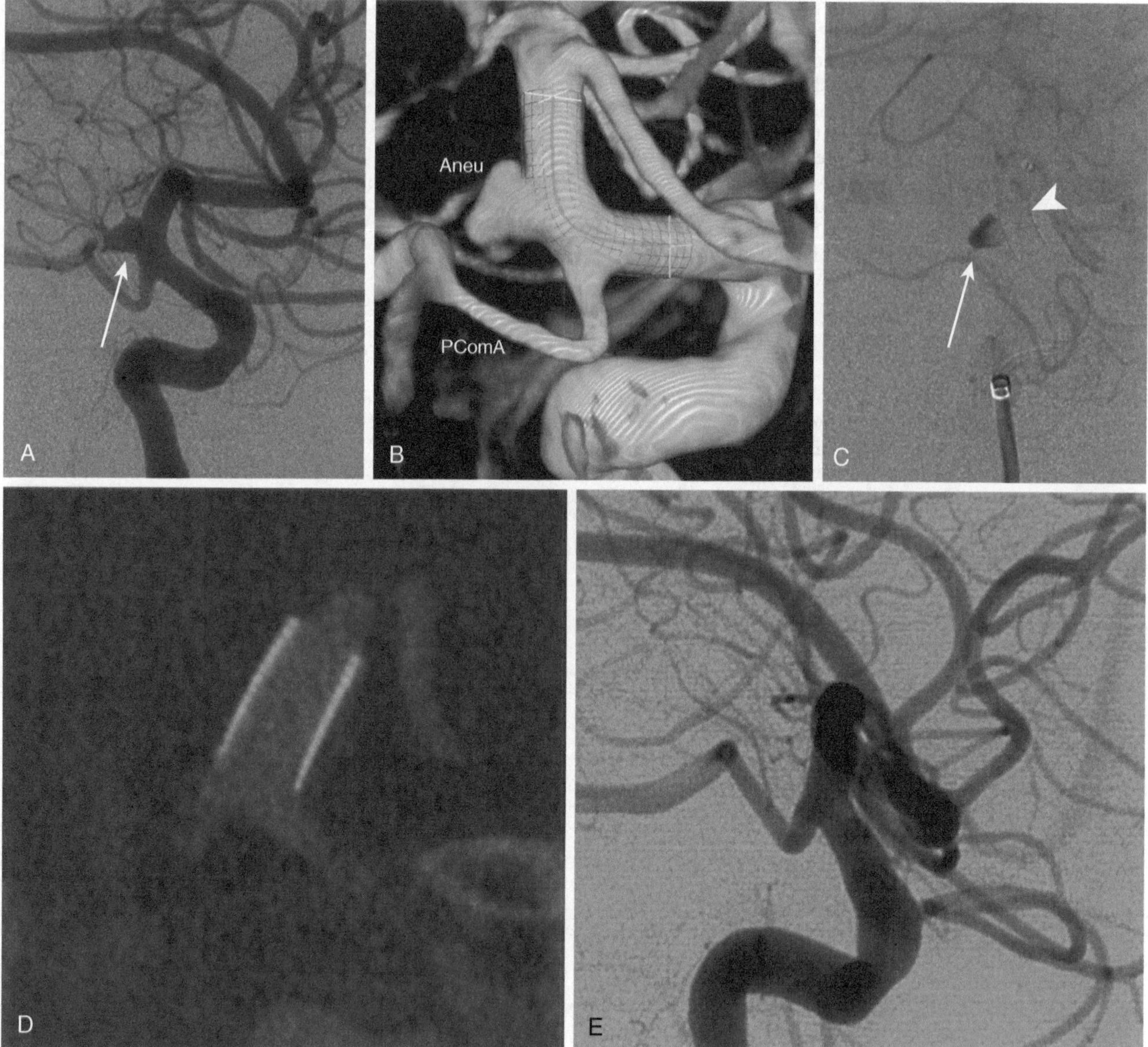

Figure 66-7. A, Lateral view left internal carotid artery angiogram shows an unruptured wide-neck small left anterior choroidal artery aneurysm (arrow). B, 3D view shows the aneurysm and virtual placement of a flow diverter for pre-procedural planning. C, Follow-up angiogram after flow diverter placement (arrowhead) shows contrast stagnation (arrow). D, Cone-beam CT with contrast and E, conventional angiogram at 1-year show complete aneurysm occlusion with preservation of anterior choroidal artery. Note, no major intimal hyperplasia is seen.

revealed in all cases polyvinylpyrrolidone (a material used in hydrophilic coatings for interventional devices) emboli.[178]

Rapid progress towards understanding these complications of flow diversion will ultimately produce technology and methods for their prevention. The efficacy of parent vessel remodeling is very encouraging, and likely will revolutionize the manner in which aneurysms are treated.

A new class of flow diverters that include placement of a fine mesh *within* the aneurysmal sac are undergoing preclinical[179] and preliminary clinical evaluation.[180] This technology is similar to the flow diverter, with the exception that the device is placed within the aneurysm sac rather than within the parent vessel. This strategy does not require dual antiplatelet therapy, which offers a significant advantage over an implant positioned in the parent vessel - particularly for the treatment of ruptured aneurysms. However, evaluation of the technology is still required as there are concerns regarding incomplete occlusion of the aneurysm particularly at the neck and the requirement for larger bore microcatheters for delivering the larger sizes of these devices. Also, it is not clear at this juncture if these devices can be used to treat a wide-class of aneurysms since they may not necessarily conform to the boundaries of irregularly shaped aneurysms.

The rate of rupture per aneurysm per year varies from 1.07% to 6.94% and 10.61% to 126.97% for large and giant aneurysms, respectively.[54] Rupture entails significant rates of morbidity and mortality. Analysis of nearly 1000 aneurysms treated by the Pipeline embolization device shows mortality of 2.2%, stroke/transient ischemic attack rate of 3.9% and risk of hemorrhagic complications of 3.4%; comparable to stent-assisted coil embolization.[181] Presently, this technology is indicated for high-risk (large and giant, wide-neck) intracranial aneurysms of the internal carotid artery; however, a number of trials are ongoing to expand the indication of flow diversion for smaller aneurysms, aneurysms of the posterior circulation, and aneurysms distal to the circle of Willis. These trial data

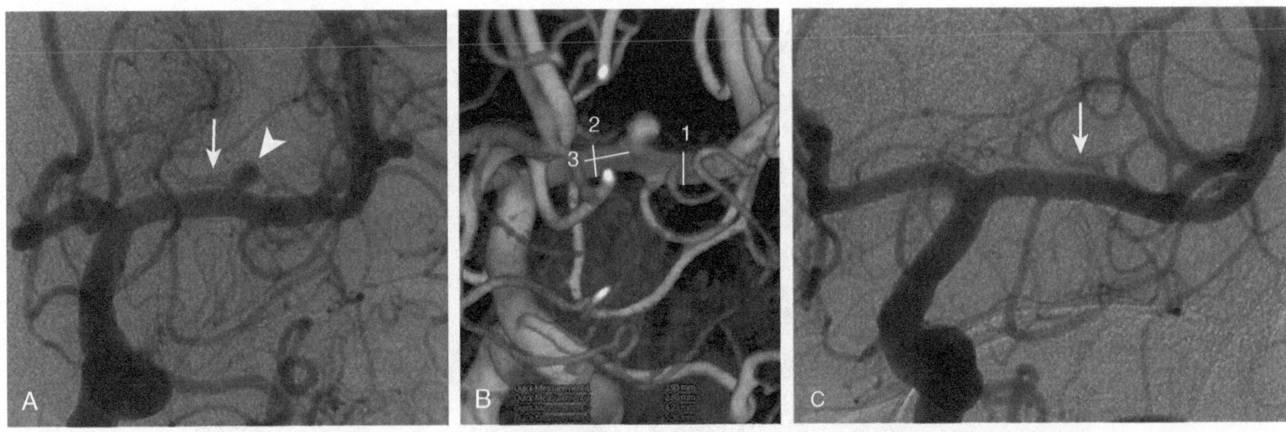

Figure 66-8. A, Frontal view left internal carotid artery angiogram shows an unruptured aneurysm originating from M1 segment of middle cerebral artery (arrowhead) and involving a large lateral lenticulostriate artery (arrow). B, 3D view shows the aneurysm with measurements of proximal and distal parent artery diameter for selection of a flow diverter. C, 6-month follow-up angiogram after treatment shows cure of the aneurysm and preserved patency of lateral lenticulostriate arteries (arrow).

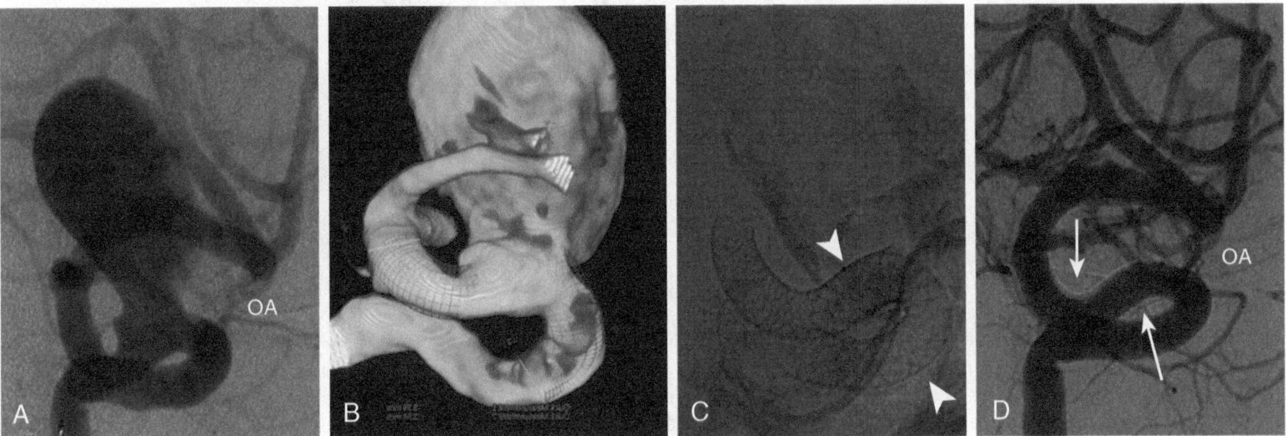

Figure 66-9. A, Right internal carotid artery angiogram of a large partially thrombosed and calcified paraclinoid aneurysm. B, 3D view shows the aneurysm and superimposed virtual placement of a flow diverter for pre-procedural planning. C, Treatment with two telescoping flow diverters (arrowheads). D, 6-month follow-up angiogram shows complete aneurysm obliteration and some mild intimal hyperplasia (arrows). OA, ophthalmic artery.

will provide endovascular specialists and patients with the best practices and indications for flow diverter utilization.

Liquid Embolics

An early technique in the endosaccular embolization of a cerebral aneurysm was performed using cyanoacrylate via needle puncture into the aneurysm dome under direct visualization.[182] It was believed that a liquid which can deform under shear forces can easily conform to the boundaries of the aneurysm and achieve total occlusion. Subsequent polymerization or precipitation of the liquid then led to its solidification. However, even from this early experience, the threats of distal emboli generated by fragmentation of the embolus and parent artery occlusion were identified. Due to this limitation, liquid embolics for the treatment of saccular aneurysms of the large arteries were largely abandoned with the exploration of detachable balloons and later detachable coils. It is important to note that aneurysms associated with arteriovenous malformations and distal traumatic or mycotic aneurysms are often treated via liquid embolic agents with excellent results. One agent, ethylene-vinyl alcohol (Onyx, eV3 Neurovascular, Irvine, CA), was evaluated clinically in the Cerebral Aneurysm Multicenter European Onyx (CAMEO) Trial.[183] CAMEO was a prospective, non-randomized, multicenter study to investigate the safety and efficacy of Onyx for the treatment of brain aneurysms. The study reported results in 97 patients with 100 aneurysms. Permanent neurologic morbidity or death related to the procedure or material was 10%. In 9.3% of patients, parent vessel occlusion occurred, which was asymptomatic in five cases. Modifications of Onyx and ancillary devices used to inject the embolic into unruptured wide-necked aneurysms of the internal carotid artery were investigated in a small series of patients at a single center.[184] The rate of parent artery occlusion or stenosis was 13.6% of the patients after a mean follow-up of 13 months. More recently, larger single center series have shown low rates of recanalization (4.6–12.5% after a minimum of 6 months and up to 5 years) and permanent morbidity in 7.2% and 8.3%.[185,186] Mortality rates in these reports were 2.9% and 3.2%. In both series, a small percentage of the cases involved ruptured aneurysms (6% and 14%), and thus morbidity and mortality of patients treated with liquid embolics do not appear to compare favorably against endovascular coil embolization in unruptured aneurysms. A randomized controlled multicenter clinical trial comparing the safety and efficacy of Onyx liquid embolic against the standard of care procedure, coil embolization, is needed to determine the long-term viability of this procedure. The key challenge with all liquid occlusive

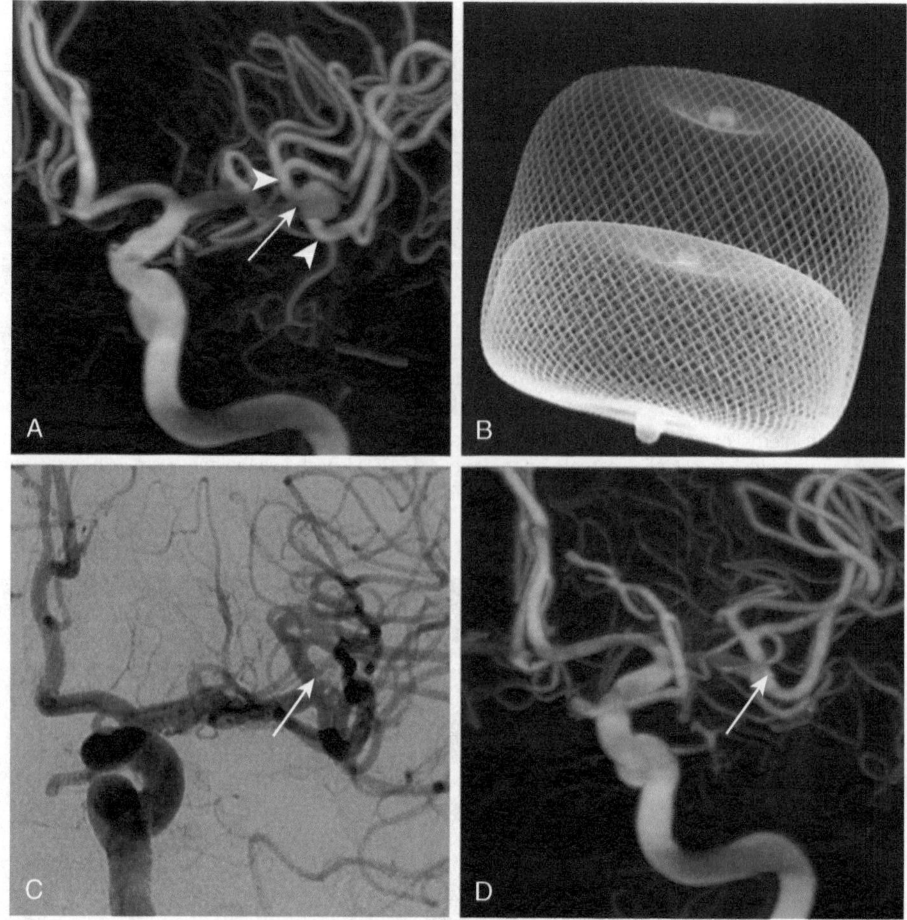

Figure 66-10. A, Unruptured left middle cerebral artery wide-neck bifurcation aneurysm (arrow) and involvement of both M2 divisions (arrowheads). B, Image of a WEB device prior to implantation. C, Follow-up angiogram after intrasaccular placement of the WEB shows no contrast filling of the aneurysms sac and residual opacification of the neck (arrow). D, One-year follow-up angiogram shows complete occlusion of the aneurysm (arrow). *(With permission from Pierot and Wakhloo, Stroke 2013.)*

agents is to maintain material stability within the aneurysm sac during injection which is necessary to prevent embolic complications or obliteration of adjacent perforating arteries secondary to leakage of the embolic material.

PERIPROCEDURAL MANAGEMENT OF PATIENTS UNDERGOING ENDOVASCULAR ANEURYSM TREATMENT

Preprocedural management of patients undergoing elective endovascular treatment for an unruptured intracranial aneurysm differs from that of a patient with emergent aneurysmal SAH. Therefore, the two conditions will be addressed separately.

Preprocedural Management: Unruptured Aneurysms

Patients undergoing elective endovascular embolization of an unruptured intracranial aneurysm require a complete history, physical examination and diagnostic angiography for planning of the intervention. Digital subtraction angiography (DSA) is the traditional gold standard diagnostic test for assessment of intracranial aneurysms.[187,188] Newer technology, such as 3D rotational angiography (3DRA), allows for more elegant pre-procedural planning especially in anatomically challenging areas such as the middle cerebral artery bifurcation and in small aneurysms (≤3 mm) that may be missed on DSA.[189]

A multidisciplinary approach involving neurosurgery, neurology and neurointerventional surgeons is recommended for each case (ruptured or unruptured aneurysm). Aneurysm size, location, and morphology are factors to consider when planning the approach. When endovascular treatment is agreed upon, it is critical to have access to a variety of technology, including various microcatheters, coil sizes and shapes, adjunctive devices such as compliant balloons and neurovascular stents. Wide-neck (neck >4 mm, dome to neck ratio of <2) or fusiform aneurysms often require the use of adjunctive therapies, such as stents. The American Heart Association recommends that dual antiplatelet therapy commence before and continued after stenting in coronary artery disease to lower the risk of acute in-stent thrombosis and delayed thrombotic complications and re-stenosis.[190] There is, however, no consensus recommendation in cerebrovascular stenting, where the re-stenosis rates in intracranial atherosclerosis is reportedly higher.[191,192] One study found that of 55 patients taking clopidogrel after cerebrovascular stent placement, 28 patients (52%) were clopidogrel-resistant.[193] Only 4.2% of patients in the same cohort were aspirin-resistant.[193] In the near future, point-of-care tests of platelet function may be feasible so that antiplatelet regimens may be appropriately modified in antiplatelet-resistant patients or one could use the newer anti-platelet agents that don't have limitations of clopidogrel.[194] However, SAC of aneurysms, which rarely involves local atherosclerosis, poses a different challenge regarding dual-antiplatelet therapy. Although no specific guidelines of dual antiplatelet therapy for aneurysm stenting currently exist, most practitioners have adopted the treatment regimen from the coronary stenting literature. All cases, regardless of the use of stent-supported coil embolization, require anticoagulation with heparin to maintain an activated clotting time (ACT) between 250 and 400 seconds. This is accomplished by an intravenous bolus of heparin followed by continuous administration of maintenance doses and ACT monitoring. Furthermore, all endovascular surgeries are performed under general anesthesia for patients' comfort and to prevent complications associated with patient motion. Regardless of the use of adjunctive devices, it has been shown that patients pre-treated with oral anti-platelet drugs have a lower incidence of periprocedural thromboembolic events, but consequently a higher rate of intracerebral hemorrhage.[195] Currently, there is no standard of practice regarding the use of antiplatelet therapy prior to embolization of unruptured aneurysms.

Adverse reactions to contrast agents, although rare, may be life-threatening. To reduce the risk of allergic contrast media reaction and contrast-induced nephrotoxicity, use of low- or iso-osmolar contrast media is supported.[196,197] Furthermore, there is evidence to support pre-treatment with corticosteroids[198,199] and antihistamines[200] in patients with suspected or documented history of allergic reaction to contrast media. Despite its relatively low incidence (0.03 cases per 1000 patients per year),[201] prophylaxis against contrast-induced nephropathy, especially for patients with elevated serum creatinine levels, is necessary.[197] Pre-procedural hydration with isotonic saline (100 mL per hour for up to 24 hours prior) is the pretreatment of choice. Administration of acetylcysteine or sodium bicarbonate 48 hours before coiling may also be beneficial in high-risk patients. In patients taking metformin, the drug should be stopped 24 hours prior to coiling and remain discontinued up to 48 hours after the procedure to minimize the risk of lactic acidosis.[202]

Preprocedural Management: Ruptured Aneurysms

Eighty percent of non-traumatic SAH cases occur secondary to intracranial aneurysm rupture.[203] Nearly half of all patients will die within the first 30 days[204] and a 46% of survivors will suffer long-term disability.[205] Therefore, a rapid neurological assessment using the World Federation of Neurological Surgeons SAH grade[206] and Hunt and Hess scale[207] is essential. A non-contrast CT of the head is the first imaging test to confirm the presence and assess the degree[208] of subarachnoid blood. All patients with confirmed SAH should be transferred to a center with dedicated neurological critical care services.[209,210] More than only Airway (Airway, Breathing, Circulation (ABC's)), but off course the Airway is especially important in neurologically impaired patients.[211] Once SAH confirmed, a four-vessel DSA (with 3DRA if available) is indicated, during which definitive aneurysm treatment may be performed.[212] CT angiography, readily available in most centers, is becoming first-line diagnostic imaging of choice for aneurysm screening in SAH and for further therapeutic management.[213] Although currently debated, if intracranial stent placement in the emergent setting is indicated, a loading dose of aspirin (325 mg) and clopidogrel (300 mg) can be administered through a nasogastric tube, or abciximab can be administered intravenously. Since, however, an increased risk of intracerebral hemorrhage is seen, a ventriculostomy should be considered prior to antiplatelet therapy with Clopidogrel.[214] Decompressive craniotomy in case of a large intracerebral hematoma associated with an aneurysm rupture may be considered pre- or postprocedural.

Intraprocedural Management

Endovascular aneurysm treatment requires the careful positioning of microwires and microcatheters into the cerebral blood vessels. Therefore, patients should be maintained under general anesthesia with endotracheal intubation to eliminate any movement thus ensuring accurate imaging and catheter placement.[215] The anesthesiologist can also maintain controlled access over the airway and hemodynamics. Angiogram should be obtained under apnea to reduce motion artifact.

Thromboembolic complications, including major and minor stroke and transient ischemic attack, occur in between 2.5% and 28% of all patients undergoing aneurysm coiling[109,216] and this is why doing coiling, stenting, flow-diverting in patients with small unruptured aneurysms doesn't make great sense, except for subgroups with higher risk. Thrombi may form on the surface of catheters and coils, be dislodged from the aneurysm sac during coiling, or occur at sites of catheter-induced vessel injury.[217] In a meta-analysis of 1547 patients from 23 studies treated with GDCs, the majority of thromboembolic complications occurred intra-operatively.[218] Therefore, intra-procedural therapy with a weight-based dosing schedule of heparin[219] is recommended, with baseline activated clotting time (ACT) measured prior to catheter insertion. In the setting of aneurysmal SAH, heparin can be started following placement of the first coil.[220,221] This reduces the risk of devastating rebleeding if the coil should pierce through the aneurysm rupture site. Intra-procedural ACT should be measured at regular intervals (generally hourly) during the procedure and heparin dosing can be titrated to a target ACT of 250 seconds.

Post-procedural Management

Post-procedural use of heparin is controversial and generally not recommended.[218] Aspirin therapy is indicated following coiling for 4 weeks, after which endothelialization of the devices is expected.[222] Thromboembolic complications are very rare after 4 weeks,[218] even if endothelialization is incomplete.[223] For stent-assisted coiling, dual antiplatelet therapy is recommended for 3–6 months for the prevention of in-stent stenosis. At some centers, life-long single anti-platelet therapy with aspirin is advocated.

Pre- and intra-procedural use of heparin and antiplatelets emphasizes the importance of hemostasis at the access site to prevent hematoma formation. A recent meta-analysis of 4000 patients in 30 trials who underwent percutaneous coronary interventions demonstrated that arterial puncture closure devices appear to reduce time to hemostasis, but there is no evidence that these devices reduce complication rates or length of hospital stay compared to traditional manual compression.[224] To aid effectiveness of manual compression, new glycosaminoglycan-containing matrices have been shown to improve hemostasis in animal models.[225]

Upon hemostasis, controlled extubation should take place in the angiography suite prior to monitored patient transfer to the intensive care unit. If needed, a cone beam CT can be obtained with the newer angiography equipment if acute hydrocephalous necessitating ventriculostomy is suspected. This technology is also useful to evaluate size and location of hematoma in the case of an intra-procedural aneurysm rupture potentially requiring an emergency decompression. Neurologic examinations are critical in the immediate post-procedural period, as abnormal findings may indicate the need for emergent re-intervention.

MANAGEMENT OF PERIPROCEDURAL COMPLICATIONS DURING ENDOVASCULAR ANEURYSM TREATMENT

As with all endovascular approaches, intraoperative complications involve aneurysm or arterial rupture (perforation), non-extravasating damage to the vascular wall (dissection, thrombosis), and cessation of antegrade blood flow (embolus). Unfortunately, the tortuous and fragile cerebrovasculature accentuates the risk of these complications and at the same time, the brain is the most unforgiving organ when these complications arise. Hence, the need for highly trained and dedicated endovascular interventionalists who specialize in this procedure must be amply emphasized; specialists who are capable of both preventing complications and know how best to manage them when they occur. Two-decades of experience in the endovascular coil embolization of aneurysms have offered valuable techniques and devices to manage these complications in situ, thereby minimizing adverse clinical events.

Thromboembolic Complications

In the absence of Class I evidence of a superior anti-platelet regimen for both ruptured and unruptured aneurysms, thromboembolic complications during endovascular aneurysm embolization remain the most common with a frequency of 2.4–5.2%.[28,30] The sources of emboli are platelet aggregation in response to catheters, devices, intimal damage, and intra-aneurysmal clot dislodgement. Late thromboembolisms might result from discontinuation of anti-platelet therapy in stent-assisted embolization cases or herniation of coils into the parent artery. Recently, the safety and efficacy of intra-operative selective administration of abciximab has been demonstrated.[226,227] In addition, stents can be used in the event of coil herniation to trap the extra-aneurysmal coil against the vessel wall.[228]

There are a variety of retrieval systems now available when devices, such as embolic coils, compromise the parent artery (examples in[229,230]). These snares and microforceps are navigated through microcatheters and may be employed to remove foreign bodies. Additionally, devices are now becoming available for mechanical thrombectomy to extract clot that does not respond to lytics.[231]

Perforation

Perforation and subsequent hemorrhage caused by the endovascular devices is more common in patients presenting with SAH (4.1%) than those with unruptured aneurysms (0.5%) (meta-analysis in.[232] Resulting morbidity and mortality from intra-operative perforation was 1.8% and 0.2%, respectively. Most aneurysm perforations today do not produce clinical adverse outcomes primarily due to the aggressive and rapid response by experienced interventionalists that include: (1) reversal of anticoagulation, (2) use of temporary occlusion balloon to tamponade the bleed site or leaving the perforating instrument in place if surgical repair is needed, and (3) continuation of coil embolization to secure the perforation. Continuous improvements in coil technology have led to reduced incidence of periprocedural aneurysm perforations.

SUMMARY

In summary, several endovascular approaches are now available for the treatment of intracranial aneurysms, including standard coiling, BAC, SAC, and flow diversion. Ruptured aneurysms have to be treated on an emergency base to avoid rebleeding and minimize further complications associated with SAH like vasospasm and hydrocephalus. Treatment of ruptured aneurysms remains coiling (standard of care) or BAC. Because antiplatelet medication is needed for SAC and flow diversion, these approaches should be used in ruptured aneurysms only if not treatable with standard coiling, BAC or clipping. Indications for treatment of unruptured aneurysms are still discussed on a case-by-case basis, taking into account clinical presentation, age of the patient, comorbidities as well as aneurysm location and size. For small aneurysms with a small neck, treatment with standard coiling or BAC is probably appropriate, and SAC as well as FDs have probably limited value unless aneurysms are prone to recurrence. For large and giant, fusiform, and wide-neck aneurysms, because of the potentially high rate of recanalization, a more sophisticated approach probably has to be used, including SAC, and flow diversion. Progress in imaging and device manufacturing is providing more sophisticated tools that have expanded EVT to aneurysms that were previously neither surgically or endovascularly treatable. Randomized trials will be necessary to evaluate the safety and efficacy of various emerging new technologies for aneurysm treatment.

The complete reference list can be found on the companion Expert Consult website at www.expertconsult.com.

KEY REFERENCES

1. Luessenhop AJ, Velasquez AC. Observations on the tolerance of the intracranial arteries to catheterization. J Neurosurg 1964;21:85–91.
2. Alksne JF. Stereotactic thrombosis of intracranial aneurysms using a magnetic probe. Confin Neurol 1969;31:95–8.
3. Mullan S, Beckman F, Vailati G, et al. An experimental approach to the problem of cerebral aneurysm. J Neurosurg 1964;21:838–45.
4. Mullan S, Raimondi AJ, Dobben G, et al. Electrically induced thrombosis in intracranial aneurysms. J Neurosurg 1965;22:539–47.
5. Teitelbaum GP, Larsen DW, Zelman V, et al. A tribute to Dr. Fedor A. Serbinenko, founder of endovascular neurosurgery. Neurosurgery 2000;46:462–9.
6. Serbinenko FA. Catheterization and occlusion of major cerebral vessels and prospects for the development of vascular neurosurgery. Vopr Neirokhir 1971;35:17–27.
7. Serbinenko FA. Balloon occlusion of saccular aneurysms of the cerebral arteries. Vopr Neirokhir 1974;4:8–15.
8. Serbinenko FA. Balloon catheterization and occlusion of major cerebral vessels. J Neurosurg 1974;41:125–45.
9. Debrun G, Coscas G. Treatment of carotido-cavernous fistulas and intracavernous aneurysms by means of a balloon catheter, which can be inflated and enlarged. Bull Soc Ophtalmol Fr 1975;75:857–64.
10. Higashida RT, Halbach VV, Barnwell SL, et al. Treatment of intracranial aneurysms with preservation of the parent vessel: results of percutaneous balloon embolization in 84 patients. AJNR Am J Neuroradiol 1990;11:633–40.
11. Debrun G, Lacour P, Caron JP, et al. Detachable balloon and calibrated-leak balloon techniques in the treatment of cerebral vascular lesions. J Neurosurg 1978;49(5):635–49.
12. Romodanov AP, Shcheglov VI. Endovascular method of excluding from the circulation saccular cerebral arterial aneurysms, leaving intact vessels patient. Acta Neurochir Suppl (Wien) 1979;28(1):312–15.
13. Bavinzski G, Talazoglu V, Killer M, et al. Gross and microscopic histopathological findings in aneurysms of the human brain treated with Guglielmi detachable coils. J Neurosurg 1999;91:284–93.
18. Guglielmi G, Viñuela F, Sepetka I, et al. Electrothrombosis of saccular aneurysms via endovascular approach. Part 1: Electrochemical basis, technique, and experimental results. J Neurosurg 1991;75(1):1–7.

19. Guglielmi G, Viñuela F, Dion J, et al. Electrothrombosis of saccular aneurysms via endovascular approach. Part 2: Preliminary clinical experience. J Neurosurg 1991;75(1):8–14.
20. Higashida RT, Halbach VV, Dowd C, et al. Endovascular detachable balloon embolization therapy of cavernous carotid artery aneurysms: results in 87 cases. J Neurosurg 1990;72(6): 857–63.
22. Kassell NF, Torner JC. Aneurysmal rebleeding: a preliminary report from the Cooperative Aneurysm Study. Neurosurgery 1983;13(5):479–81.
24. Molyneux A, Kerr R, Stratton I, et al. International Subarachnoid Aneurysm Trial (ISAT) of neurosurgical clipping versus endovascular coiling in 2143 patients with ruptured intracranial aneurysms: a randomised trial. Lancet 2002;360(9342):1267–74.
25. Molyneux AJ, Kerr RS, Yu LM, et al. International subarachnoid aneurysm trial (ISAT) of neurosurgical clipping versus endovascular coiling in 2143 patients with ruptured intracranial aneurysms: a randomised comparison of effects on survival, dependency, seizures, rebleeding, subgroups, and aneurysm occlusion. Lancet 2005;366(9488):809–17.
28. Gallas S, Pasco A, Cottier JP, et al. A multicenter study of 705 ruptured intracranial aneurysms treated with Guglielmi detachable coils. AJNR Am J Neuroradiol 2005;26(7):1723–31.
29. Raymond J, Guilbert F, Weill A, et al. Long-term angiographic recurrences after selective endovascular treatment of aneurysms with detachable coils. Stroke 2003;34(6):1398–403.
30. Murayama Y, Nien YL, Duckwiler G, et al. Guglielmi detachable coil embolization of cerebral aneurysms: 11 years' experience. J Neurosurg 2003;98(5):959–66.
31. CARAT Investigators. Rates of delayed rebleeding from intracranial aneurysms are low after surgical and endovascular treatment. Stroke 2006;37(6):1437–42.
32. Johnston SC, Dowd CF, Higashida RT, et al. Predictors of rehemorrhage after treatment of ruptured intracranial aneurysms: the Cerebral Aneurysm Rerupture After Treatment (CARAT) study. Stroke 2008;39(1):120–5.
34. Molyneux A, Kerr R, Birks J, et al. Risk of recurrent subarachnoid haemorrhage, death, or dependence and standardised mortality ratios after clipping or coiling of an intracranial aneurysm in the International Subarachnoid Aneurysm Trial (ISAT): long-term follow-up. Lancet Neurol 2009;8:427–33.
35. Holmin S, Krings T, Ozanne A, et al. Intradural saccular aneurysms treated by Guglielmi detachable bare coils at a single institution between 1993 and 2005: clinical long-term follow-up for a total of 1810 patient-years in relation to morphological treatment results. Stroke 2008;39(8):2288–97.
36. Meyers PM, Schumacher HC, Higashida RT, et al. Reporting standards for endovascular repair of saccular intracranial cerebral aneurysms. AJNR Am J Neuroradiol 2010;31:E12–24.
38. Wakhloo AK, Mandell J, Gounis MJ, et al. Stent-assisted reconstructive endovascular repair of cranial fusiform atherosclerotic and dissecting aneurysms: long-term clinical and angiographic follow-up. Stroke 2008;39(12):3288–96.
39. Ferns SP, Sprengers ME, van Rooij WJ, et al. Late reopening of adequately coiled intracranial aneurysms: frequency and risk factors in 400 patients with 440 aneurysms. Stroke 2011;42(5): 1331–7.
40. Willinsky RA, Peltz J, da Costa L, et al. Clinical and angiographic follow-up of ruptured intracranial aneurysms treated with endovascular embolization. AJNR Am J Neuroradiol 2009;30(5): 1035–40.
41. Tsutsumi K, Ueki K, Morita A, et al. Risk of aneurysm recurrence in patients with clipped cerebral aneurysms: results of long-term follow-up angiography. Stroke 2001;32(5):1191–4.
45. International Study of Unruptured Intracranial Aneurysms Investigators. Unruptured intracranial aneurysms – risk of rupture and risks of surgical intervention. N Engl J Med 1998; 339(24):1725–33.
46. Wiebers DO, Whisnant JP, Huston J 3rd, et al. Unruptured intracranial aneurysms: natural history, clinical outcome, and risks of surgical and endovascular treatment. Lancet 2003; 362(9378):103–10.
48. Broderick JP, Brown RD Jr, Sauerbeck L, et al. Greater rupture risk for familial as compared to sporadic unruptured intracranial aneurysms. Stroke 2009;40(6):1952–7.
49. Bederson JB, Awad IA, Wiebers DO, et al. Recommendations for the management of patients with unruptured intracranial aneurysms: A Statement for healthcare professionals from the Stroke Council of the American Heart Association. Stroke 2000;31(11): 2742–50.
52. Juvela S, Porras M, Poussa K. Natural history of unruptured intracranial aneurysms: probability of and risk factors for aneurysm rupture. J Neurosurg 2000;93(3):379–87.
54. The UCAS Japan Investigators. The natural course of unruptured cerebral aneurysms in a Japanese cohort. New Engl J Med 2012;366(26):2474–82.
55. Pierot L, Spelle L, Vitry F, ATENA Investigators. Immediate clinical outcome of patients harboring unruptured intracranial aneurysms treated by endovascular approach: results of the ATENA study. Stroke 2008;39(9):2497–504.
56. Ishibashi T, Murayama Y, Urashima M, et al. Unruptured intracranial aneurysms: incidence of rupture and risk factors. Stroke 2009;40(1):313–16.
57. Im S, Han M, Kwon O, et al. Endovascular coil embolization of 435 small asymptomatic unruptured intracranial aneurysms: procedural morbidity and patient outcome. AJNR Am J Neuroradiol 2009;30(1):79–84.
58. Andreasen TH, Bartek J Jr, Andresen M, et al. Modifiable risk factors for aneurysmal subarachnoid hemorrhage. Stroke 2013; 44(12):3607–12.
59. Villablanca JP, Duckwiler GR, Jahan R, et al. Natural history of asymptomatic unruptured cerebral aneurysms evaluated at CT angiography: growth and rupture incidence and correlation with epidemiologic risk factors. Radiology 2013;269(1):258–65.
60. Burns JD, Huston J 3rd, Layton KF, et al. Intracranial aneurysm enlargement on serial magnetic resonance angiography: frequency and risk factors. Stroke 2009;40(2):406–11.
61. Frösen J, Piippo A, Paetau A, et al. Remodeling of saccular cerebral artery aneurysm wall is associated with rupture; histological analysis of 24 unruptured and 42 ruptured cases. Stroke 2004;35:2287–93.
62. Gounis MJ, Vedantham S, Weaver JP, et al. Myeloperoxidase in human intracranial aneurysms: Preliminary evidence. Stroke 2014;45(5):1474–7.
64. Frösen J, Tulamo R, Heikura T, et al. Lipid accumulation, lipid oxidation, and low plasma levels of acquired antibodies against oxidized lipids associate with degeneration and rupture of the intracranial aneurysm wall. Acta Neuropathol Commun 2013;1(1):71.
65. Laaksamo E, Tulamo R, Liiman A, et al. Oxidative stress is associated with cell death, wall degradation, and increased risk of rupture of the intracranial aneurysm wall. Neurosurgery 2013;72(1):109–17.
66. Marbacher S, Marjamaa J, Bradacova K, et al. Loss of mural cells leads to wall degeneration, aneurysm growth, and eventual rupture in a rat aneurysm model. Stroke 2014;45(1):248–54.
67. Raymond J, Darsaut TE, Kotowski M, et al. Thrombosis heralding aneurysmal rupture: an exploration of potential mechanisms in a novel giant swine aneurysm model. AJNR Am J Neuroradiol 2013;34(2):346–53.
68. DeLeo MJ 3rd, Gounis MJ, Hong B, et al. Carotid artery brain aneurysm model: in vivo molecular enzyme-specific MR imaging of active inflammation in a pilot study. Radiology 2009;252(3): 696–703.
83. Cebral JR, Raschi M. Suggested connections between risk factors of intracranial aneurysms: a review. Ann Biomed Eng 2013;41(7): 1366–83.
92. Robertson AM, Watton PN. Computational fluid dynamics in aneurysm research: critical reflections, future directions. AJNR Am J Neuroradiol 2012;33(6):992–5.
94. Valen-Sendstad K, Steinman DA. Mind the gap: impact of computational fluid dynamics solution strategy on prediction of intracranial aneurysm hemodynamics and rupture status indicators. AJNR Am J Neuroradiol 2014;35(3):536–43.
101. Pereira VM, Brina O, Bijlenga P, et al. Wall shear stress distribution of small aneurysms prone to rupture: A case-control study. Stroke 2014;45(1):261–4.
102. Di Achille P, Humphrey JD. Toward large-scale computational fluid-solid-growth models of intracranial aneurysms. Yale J Biol Med 2012;85(2):217–28.

103. Tanoue S, Kiyosue H, Kenai H, et al. Three-dimensional reconstructed images after rotational angiography in the evaluation of intracranial aneurysms: surgical correlation. Neurosurgery 2000; 47(4):866–71.
104. Soderman M, Holmin S, Andersson T, et al. Image noise reduction algorithm for digital subtraction angiography: clinical results. Radiology 2013;269(2):553–60.
105. Patel NV, Gounis MJ, Wakhloo AK, et al. Contrast-enhanced angiographic cone-beam CT of cerebrovascular stents: experimental optimization and clinical application. AJNR Am J Neuroradiol 2011;32(1):137–44.
106. Struffert T, Deuerling-Zheng Y, Engelhorn T, et al. Monitoring of balloon test occlusion of the internal carotid artery by parametric color coding and perfusion imaging within the angiosuite: first results. Clin Neuroradiol 2013;23(4):285–92.
107. Pereira VM, Bonnefous O, Ouared R, et al. A DSA-based method using contrast-motion estimation for the assessment of the intra-aneurysmal flow changes induced by flow-diverter stents. AJNR Am J Neuroradiol 2013;34(4):808–15.
109. Viñuela F, Duckwiler G, Mawad ME. Guglielmi detachable coil embolization of acute intracranial aneurysm: perioperative anatomical and clinical outcome in 403 patients. J Neurosurg 1997; 86(3):475–82.
110. Gallas S, Drouineau J, Gabrillargues J, et al. Feasibility, procedural morbidity and mortality, and long-term follow-up of endovascular treatment of 321 unruptured aneurysms. AJNR Am J Neuroradiol 2008;29(1):63–8.
111. Cognard C, Pierot L, Anxionnat R, et al. Results of embolization used as the first treatment choice in a consecutive nonselected population of ruptured aneurysms: clinical results of the Clarity GDC study. Neurosurgery 2011;69(4):837–41, discussion 42.
113. Cognard C, Weill A, Sprelle L, et al. Long-term angiographic follow-up of 169 intracranial berry aneurysms occluded with detachable coils. Radiology 1999;212(2):348–56.
114. Ferns SP, Sprengers ME, van Rooij WJ, et al. Coiling of intracranial aneurysms: a systematic review on initial occlusion and reopening and retreatment rates. Stroke 2009;40(8):e523–9.
115. Hope JK, Byrne JV, Molyneux AJ. Factors influencing successful angiographic occlusion of aneurysms treated by coil embolization. AJNR Am J Neuroradiol 1999;20(3):391–9.
121. Willinsky RA, Peltz J, da Costa L, et al. Clinical and angiographic follow-up of ruptured intracranial aneurysms treated with endovascular embolization. AJNR Am J Neuroradiol 2009;30(5): 1035–40.
123. Pierot L, Cognard C, Ricolfi F, et al. Mid-term anatomic results after endovascular treatment of ruptured intracranial aneurysms with Guglielmi detachable coils and Matrix coils: analysis of the CLARITY series. AJNR Am J Neuroradiol 2012;33(3):469–73.
124. Fiorella D, Albuquerque FC, McDougall CG. Durability of aneurysm embolization with Matrix detachable coils. Neurosurgery 2006;58(1):51–9.
125. White PM, Lewis SC, Gholkar A, et al. Hydrogel-coated coils versus bare platinum coils for the endovascular treatment of intracranial aneurysms (HELPS): a randomised controlled trial. Lancet 2011;377(9778):1655–62.
126. Buhk J-H, Kallenberg K, Mohr A, et al. Evaluation of angiographic computed tomography in the follow-up after endovascular treatment of cerebral aneurysms—a comparative study with DSA and TOF-MRA. Eur Radiol 2009;19(2):430–6.
130. McDougall CG, Johnston SC, Gholkar A, et al. Bioactive versus Bare Platinum Coils in the Treatment of Intracranial Aneurysms: The MAPS (Matrix and Platinum Science) Trial. AJNR Am J Neuroradiol 2014;35(5):935–42.
131. Moret J, Cognard C, Weill A, et al. Reconstruction technic in the treatment of wide-neck intracranial aneurysms. Long-term angiographic and clinical results. Apropos of 56 cases. J Neuroradiol 1997;24(1):30–44.
132. Mericle RA, Wakhloo AK, Rodriguez R, et al. Temporary balloon protection as an adjunct to endosaccular coiling of wide-necked cerebral aneurysms: technical note. Neurosurgery 1997;41(4): 975–8.
133. Pierot L, Cognard C, Spelle L, et al. Safety and efficacy of balloon remodeling technique during endovascular treatment of intracranial aneurysms: critical review of the literature. AJNR Am J Neuroradiol 2012;33(1):12–15.
134. Santillan A, Gobin YP, Greenberg ED, et al. Intraprocedural aneurysmal rupture during coil embolization of brain aneurysms: role of balloon-assisted coiling. AJNR Am J Neuroradiol 2012;33(10):2017–21.
137. Pierot L, Spelle L, Leclerc X, et al. Endovascular treatment of unruptured intracranial aneurysms: comparison of safety of remodeling technique and standard treatment with coils. Radiology 2009;251(3):846–55.
138. Pierot L, Cognard C, Anxionnat R, et al. Remodeling technique for endovascular treatment of ruptured intracranial aneurysms had a higher rate of adequate postoperative occlusion than did conventional coil embolization with comparable safety. Radiology 2011;258(2):546–53.
139. Wakhloo AK, Schellhammer F, de Vries J, et al. Self-expanding and balloon-expandable stents in the treatment of carotid aneurysms: an experimental study in a canine model. AJNR Am J Neuroradiol 1994;15(3):493–502.
140. Wakhloo AK, Lanzino G, Lieber BB, et al. Stents for intracranial aneurysms: the beginning of a new endovascular era? Neurosurgery 1998;43(2):377–9.
141. Mericle RA, Lanzino G, Wakhloo AK, et al. Stenting and secondary coiling of internal carotid artery aneurysm: technical case report. Neurosurgery 1998;43:1229–34.
142. Lanzino G, Wakhloo AK, Fessler RD, et al. Efficacy and current limitations of intravascular stents for intracranial carotid, vertebral, and basilar artery aneurysms. J Neurosurg 1999;91(4): 538–46.
143. Lylyk P, Ceratto R, Hurvitz D, et al. Treatment of a vertebral dissecting aneurysm with stents and coils: a case report. Neurosurgery 1998;43(2):385–8.
144. Lylyk P, Cohen JE, Ceratto R, et al. Endovascular reconstruction of intracranial arteries by stent placement and combined techniques. J Neurosurg 2002;97(6):1306–13.
145. Piotin M, Blanc R, Spelle L, et al. Stent-assisted coiling of intracranial aneurysms: clinical and angiographic results in 216 consecutive aneurysms. Stroke 2010;41(1):110–15.
146. Shapiro M, Becske T, Sahlein D, et al. Stent-supported aneurysm coiling: a literature survey of treatment and follow-up. AJNR Am J Neuroradiol 2012;33(1):159–63.
148. Gao X, Liang G, Li Z, et al. Complications and adverse events associated with Neuroform stent-assisted coiling of wide-neck intracranial aneurysms. Neurol Res 2011;33(8): 841–52.
149. Hetts SW, Turk A, English JD, et al. Stent-Assisted Coiling versus Coiling Alone in Unruptured Intracranial Aneurysms in the Matrix and Platinum Science Trial: Safety, efficacy, and mid-term outcomes. AJNR Am J Neuroradiol 2014;35(4): 698–705.
150. Wakhloo AK, Linfante I, Silva CF, et al. Closed-cell stent for coil embolization of intracranial aneurysms: clinical and angiographic results. AJNR Am J Neuroradiol 2012;33(9): 1651–6.
151. Bodily KD, Cloft HJ, Lanzino G, et al. Stent-assisted coiling in acutely ruptured intracranial aneurysms: a qualitative, systematic review of the literature. AJNR Am J Neuroradiol 2011;32(7): 1232–6.
152. Fargen KM, Hoh BL, Welch BG, et al. Long-term results of enterprise stent-assisted coiling of cerebral aneurysms. Neurosurgery 2012;71(2):239–44, discussion 44.
153. Gentric JC, Biondi A, Piotin M, et al. Safety and efficacy of neuroform for treatment of intracranial aneurysms: a prospective, consecutive, French multicentric study. AJNR Am J Neuroradiol 2013;34(6):1203–8.
154. Wakhloo AK, Tio FO, Lieber BB, et al. Self-expanding nitinol stents in canine vertebral arteries: hemodynamics and tissue response. AJNR Am J Neuroradiol 1995;16(5):1043–51.
155. Lieber BB, Gounis MJ. The physics of endoluminal stenting in the treatment of cerebrovascular aneurysms. Neurol Res 2002; 24(Suppl. 1):S33–42.
156. Geremia G, Bakon M, Brennecke L, et al. Experimental arteriovenous fistulas: treatment with porous metallic stents. AJNR Am J Neuroradiol 1995;16(10):1965–73.
157. Turjman F, Acevedo G, Moll T, et al. Treatment of experimental carotid aneurysms by endoprosthesis implantation: preliminary report. Neurol Res 1993;15(3):181–4.

158. Becske T, Kallmes DF, Saatci I, et al. Pipeline for uncoilable or failed aneurysms: results from a multicenter clinical trial. Radiology 2013;267(3):858–68.
159. Wakhloo AK, Lylyk P, de Vries J, et al. Surpass Flow Diverter in the Treatment of Intracranial Aneurysms: A Prospective Multicenter Study. AJNR Am J Neuroradiol 2015;36(1):98–107.
160. Sadasivan C, Cesar L, Seong J, et al. An original flow diversion device for the treatment of intracranial aneurysms: evaluation in the rabbit elastase-induced model. Stroke 2009; 40(3):952–8.
161. Kallmes DF, Ding YH, Dai D, et al. A new endoluminal, flow-disrupting device for treatment of saccular aneurysms. Stroke 2007;38(8):2346–52.
162. De Vries J, Boogaarts J, Van Norden A, et al. New generation of flow diverter (Surpass) for unruptured intracranial aneurysms: a prospective single-center study in 37 patients. Stroke 2013;44(6): 1567–77.
163. Brinjikji W, Murad MH, Lanzino G, et al. Endovascular treatment of intracranial aneurysms with flow diverters: a meta-analysis. Stroke 2013;44(2):442–7.
164. Arrese I, Sarabia R, Pintado R, et al. Flow-diverter devices for intracranial aneurysms: systematic review and meta-analysis. Neurosurgery 2013;73(2):193–9, discussion 9–200.
165. Byrne JV, Beltechi R, Yarnold JA, et al. Early experience in the treatment of intra-cranial aneurysms by endovascular flow diversion: a multicentre prospective study. PLoS ONE 2010;5: e12492.
168. Wakhloo AK, Gounis MJ. Revolution in aneurysm treatment: flow diversion to cure aneurysms -a paradigm shift. Neurosurgery 2014;61(Suppl. 1):111–20.
169. Kulcsár Z, Houdart E, Bonafé A, et al. Intra-aneurysmal thrombosis as a possible cause of delayed aneurysm rupture after flow-diversion treatment. AJNR Am J Neuroradiol 2011;32: 20–5.
170. Turowski B, Macht S, Kulcsar Z, et al. Early fatal hemorrhage after endovascular cerebral aneurysm treatment with a flow diverter (SILK-Stent): do we need to rethink our concepts? Neuroradiology 2011;53(1):37–41.
171. Cebral JR, Mut F, Raschi M, et al. Aneurysm rupture following treatment with flow-diverting stents: computational hemodynamics analysis of treatment. AJNR Am J Neuroradiol 2011;32: 27–33.
172. Berge J, Tourdias T, Moreau JF, et al. Perianeurysmal brain inflammation after flow-diversion treatment. AJNR Am J Neuroradiol 2011;32(10):1930–4.
173. Tulamo R, Frösen J, Hernesniemi J, et al. Inflammatory changes in the aneurysm wall: a review. J Neurointerv Surg 2010;2(2): 120–30.
174. Chow M, McDougall C, O'Kelly C, et al. Delayed spontaneous rupture of a posterior inferior cerebellar artery aneurysm following treatment with flow diversion: a clinicopathologic study. AJNR Am J Neuroradiol 2012;33:E46–51.
175. Wakhloo AK, Lieber BB. Changes of intra-aneurysmal pressure during coiling. AJNR Am J Neuroradiol 2006;27:471–2.
176. Cruz JP, Chow M, O'Kelly C, et al. Delayed ipsilateral parenchymal hemorrhage following flow diversion for the treatment of anterior circulation aneurysms. AJNR Am J Neuroradiol 2012; 33(4):603–8.
177. Mehta RI, Mehta RI, Solis OE, et al. Hydrophilic polymer emboli: an under-recognized iatrogenic cause of ischemia and infarct. Mod Pathol 2010;23(7):921–30.
178. Hu YC, Deshmukh VR, Albuquerque FC, et al. Histopathological assessment of fatal ipsilateral intraparenchymal hemorrhages after the treatment of supraclinoid aneurysms with the Pipeline Embolization Device. J Neurosurg 2014;120(2):365–74.
179. Kwon SC, Ding YH, Dai D, et al. Preliminary results of the Luna aneurysm embolization system in a rabbit model: a new intrasaccular aneurysm occlusion device. AJNR Am J Neuroradiol 2011;32(3):602–6.
180. Lubicz B, Klisch J, Gauvrit JY, et al. WEB-DL endovascular treatment of wide-neck bifurcation aneurysms: short- and midterm results in a European study. AJNR Am J Neuroradiol 2014;35(3): 432–8.
184. Weber W, Siekmann R, Kis B, et al. Treatment and follow-up of 22 unruptured wide-necked intracranial aneurysms of the internal carotid artery with Onyx HD 500. AJNR Am J Neuroradiol 2005;26:1909–15.
185. Piske RL, Kanashiro LH, Paschoal E, et al. Evaluation of Onyx HD-500 embolic system in the treatment of 84 wide-neck intracranial aneurysms. Neurosurgery 2009;64(5):E865–75.
189. van Rooij WJ, Sprengers ME, de Gast AN, et al. 3D rotational angiography: the new gold standard in the detection of additional intracranial aneurysms. AJNR Am J Neuroradiol 2008; 29(5):976–9.
190. Smith SC Jr, Feldman TE, Hirshfeld JW Jr, et al. ACC/AHA/SCAI 2005 guideline update for percutaneous coronary intervention: a report of the American College of Cardiology/American Heart Association Task Force on Practice Guidelines (ACC/AHA/SCAI Writing Committee to Update 2001 Guidelines for Percutaneous Coronary Intervention). Circulation 2006;113(7): e166–286.
191. Fiorella D, Levy EI, Turk AS, et al. US multicenter experience with the wingspan stent system for the treatment of intracranial atheromatous disease: periprocedural results. Stroke 2007;38(3): 881–7.
192. Henkes H, Miloslavski E, Lowens S, et al. Treatment of intracranial atherosclerotic stenoses with balloon dilatation and self-expanding stent deployment (WingSpan). Neuroradiology 2005;47(3):222–8.
193. Prabhakaran S, Wells KR, Lee VH, et al. Prevalence and risk factors for aspirin and clopidogrel resistance in cerebrovascular stenting. AJNR Am J Neuroradiol 2008;29(2):281–5.
194. Lee DH, Arat A, Morsi H, et al. Dual antiplatelet therapy monitoring for neurointerventional procedures using a point-of-care platelet function test: a single-center experience. AJNR Am J Neuroradiol 2008;29(7):1389–94.
195. Yamada NK, Cross DT I, Pilgram TK, et al. Effect of antiplatelet therapy on thromboembolic complications of elective coil embolization of cerebral aneurysms. AJNR Am J Neuroradiol 2007;28:1778–82.
197. Thomsen HS, Morcos SK. Contrast media and metformin: guidelines to diminish the risk of lactic acidosis in non-insulin-dependent diabetics after administration of contrast media. ESUR Contrast Media Safety Committee. Eur Radiol 1999;9(4): 738–40.
203. van Gijn J, Rinkel GJ. Subarachnoid haemorrhage: diagnosis, causes and management. Brain 2001;124(Pt 2):249–78.
204. Johnston SC, Selvin S, Gress DR. The burden, trends, and demographics of mortality from subarachnoid hemorrhage. Neurology 1998;50(5):1413–18.
205. Mayer S, Kreiter K. Quality of life after subarachnoid hemorrhage. J Neurosurg 2002;97(3):741–2, author reply 2.
207. Hunt WE, Hess RM. Surgical risk as related to time of intervention in the repair of intracranial aneurysms. J Neurosurg 1968; 28(1):14–20.
208. Claassen J, Bernardini GL, Kreiter K, et al. Effect of cisternal and ventricular blood on risk of delayed cerebral ischemia after subarachnoid hemorrhage: the Fisher scale revisited. Stroke 2001; 32(9):2012–20.
211. Suarez JI, Tarr RW, Selman WR. Aneurysmal subarachnoid hemorrhage. N Engl J Med 2006;354(4):387–96.
212. McKinney AM, Palmer CS, Truwit CL, et al. Detection of aneurysms by 64-section multidetector CT angiography in patients acutely suspected of having an intracranial aneurysm and comparison with digital subtraction and 3D rotational angiography. AJNR Am J Neuroradiol 2008;29(3):594–602.
213. Romijn M, Gratama van Andel HA, van Walderveen MA, et al. Diagnostic accuracy of CT angiography with matched mask bone elimination for detection of intracranial aneurysms: comparison with digital subtraction angiography and 3D rotational angiography. AJNR Am J Neuroradiol 2008;29(1):134–9.
214. Tumialán LM, Zhang YJ, Cawley CM, et al. Intracranial hemorrhage associated with stent-assisted coil embolization of cerebral aneurysms: a cautionary report. J Neurosurg 2008;108(6):1122–9.
215. Varma MK, Price K, Jayakrishnan V, et al. Anaesthetic considerations for interventional neuroradiology. Br J Anaesth 2007;99(1): 75–85.
216. Pelz DM, Lownie SP, Fox AJ. Thromboembolic events associated with the treatment of cerebral aneurysms with Guglielmi detachable coils. AJNR Am J Neuroradiol 1998;19(8):1541–7.

217. Qureshi AI, Luft AR, Sharma M, et al. Prevention and treatment of thromboembolic and ischemic complications associated with endovascular procedures: Part I–Pathophysiological and pharmacological features. Neurosurgery 2000;46(6):1344–59.
218. Qureshi AI, Luft AR, Sharma M, et al. Prevention and treatment of thromboembolic and ischemic complications associated with endovascular procedures: Part II–Clinical aspects and recommendations. Neurosurgery 2000;46(6):1360–75.
220. Raymond J, Roy D. Safety and efficacy of endovascular treatment of acutely ruptured aneurysms. Neurosurgery 1997;41(6):1235–45, discussion 45–6.
222. Van Belle E, Maillard L, Tio FO, et al. Accelerated endothelialization by local delivery of recombinant human vascular endothelial growth factor reduces in-stent intimal formation. Biochem Biophys Res Commun 1997;235(2):311–16.
223. Ferns GA, Stewart-Lee AL, Anggard EE. Arterial response to mechanical injury: balloon catheter de-endothelialization. Atherosclerosis 1992;92(2–3):89–104.
228. Fessler RD, Ringer AJ, Qureshi AI, et al. Intracranial stent placement to trap an extruded coil during endovascular aneurysm treatment: technical note. Neurosurgery 2000;46(1):248–51.
230. Wakhloo AK, Gounis MJ. Retrievable closed cell intracranial stent for foreign body and clot removal. Neurosurgery 2007; 62(5 Suppl. 2):ONS390–3.
231. Smith WS, Sung G, Saver J, et al. Mechanical thrombectomy for acute ischemic stroke: final results of the Multi MERCI trial. Stroke 2008;39(4):1205–12.

67 Interventional Therapy of Brain and Spinal Arteriovenous Malformations

Timo Krings, Sasikhan Geibprasert, Karel Ter Brugge

KEY POINTS

- Brain arteriovenous malformation may present with hemorrhagic and non-hemorrhagic symptoms.
- Hemorrhagic presentation of a brain arteriovenous malformation is a major risk factor for subsequent hemorrhage. While rarely complete, endovascular treatment options can be part of a combined treatment plan.
- Endovascular treatment may be particularly suited to the acute setting in order to obliterate the point of rupture of an arteriovenous malformation (AVM).
- Treatment risks of unruptured brain AVMs have to be carefully weighed against the natural history of these lesions taking into consideration angioarchitecture, pathomechanical considerations, age of the patient and imaging findings.
- Spinal vascular malformations are rare, and little is known about their natural history.
- Similar to brain AVMs, previous hemorrhage appears to be a risk factor for subsequent hemorrhage.
- Endovascular treatment, even partially, appears to lower the risk of repeat hemorrhage in the larger published series.
- Endovascular treatment of spinal AVMs in asymptomatic patients is controversial discussed.

One of the basic principles in medicine is that the understanding of a disease should precede its treatment. Unfortunately, in the case of brain and spinal pial arteriovenous malformations (AVMs), too little is known as yet about their etiology, pathophysiology, and natural history for guidelines about their treatment to be given with confidence. The numerous different classification schemes that should aid in the understanding of arteriovenous (AV) shunts testify to this lack of knowledge. To additionally complicate matters, advances in diagnostic tools for pretreatment risk assessment as well as continuously improved treatment modalities (catheterization and embolization materials) are likely to further change the way we will manage these vascular malformations. Finally, the skills and experience of the physician performing the endovascular treatment will have a more profound impact on the patient's outcome than any of the aforementioned issues.

We subdivide this chapter into two sections, the first one dealing with the brain, the second one with the spine, and we confine ourselves to the discussion of endovascular treatments of the pial AVMs only, leaving the dural (spinal and cranial) AV shunts for a different chapter. In each subdivision, we describe briefly the classification that we use as an aid in understanding the disease, bearing in mind that this classification may be different from those used by other writers.

BRAIN ARTERIOVENOUS MALFORMATIONS

Classification of Vascular Malformations in General

When considering endovascular treatment of AVMs, a classification of pial brain AVMs that is based on the size, the pattern of venous drainage, and the eloquence of the portions of brain adjacent to the AVM is of limited use for three reasons. First, such a classification cannot predict the natural history of a specific AVM for an individual patient; second, it does not anticipate the risk of treating brain AVMs by endovascular techniques; and third, it does not enhance our understanding of this disease.

Concerning the last, a classification that is based on the etiology of vascular malformations may be a more useful approach to assess vascular malformations in general, of which the AVMs are but a subgroup. This etiologic classification takes into account the target, the timing, and the nature of the triggering event. Because arteries and veins are already differentiated early during vasculogenesis, the target of a triggering event may vary according to its location along the vessel tree: from the arterial side to the arterial-capillary, the venous junction venules, veins, sinuses, and lymphatics.[1] The second determinant is the timing, or when the trigger hits its target: an early hit during vasculogenesis (such as a germinal mutation) affects more cells and leads to a metamerically arranged defect, whereas a late hit (such as a somatic mutation that occurs late during the fetal life or even postnatally) has a more focal impact (such as failed localized remodeling during vascular renewal).[2] Finally, the nature of the triggering event – intrinsic (i.e., genetic vs extrinsic), environmental, traumatic, or infectious – adds another level of complexity to this schematic approach of classifying brain vascular malformations.[3] Although there is likely to be a continuous spectrum of vascular diseases rather than clear-cut disease entities, the scheme that is based on the previously mentioned assumptions may help to discern vascular malformations from an etiologic standpoint.

Classification of Pial Brain Arteriovenous Malformations

The main focus of this chapter is on the endovascular treatment of the shunting lesions. Although the previously mentioned classification may be helpful to broadly categorize vascular lesions, the most often encountered shunting lesions, i.e., the pial brain AVMs, deserve further subclassification because the presented classification is too crude to predict the natural history of a specific AVM for an individual patient and is unable to anticipate the endovascular treatment risk.

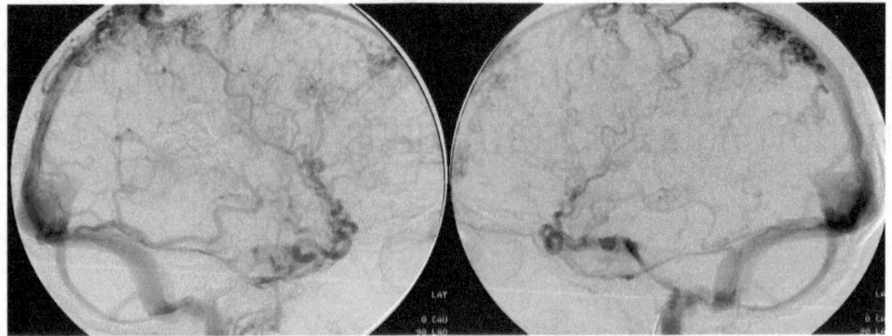

Figure 67-1. Left and right internal carotid artery injection in the venous phase of an angiogram demonstrates the classic "pseudophlebitic" aspect of enlarged and tortuous pial veins, which is a sign of long-standing venous congestion that may go along with epilepsy, headaches, cognitive decline, and focal neurologic deficits.

Natural History

A classification that is able to predict natural history has to distinguish first those AVMs that have bled from those that have not bled, which in most instances is possible through the review of the clinical history. In asymptomatic patients, T2-weighted gradient-echo MRI sequences, which are highly susceptible to depicting signs of old hemorrhage, may assist the identification of those exceedingly rare cases in which a subclinical hemorrhage may have happened.

The future risk of bleeding from a brain AVM has been the subject of many studies. In 1983, Graf et al.[4] published their results concerning the risk for future hemorrhage, which was calculated to be 37% in 20 years for unruptured AVMs and 47% for ruptured AVMs. Crawford et al.[5] found similar 20-year cumulative risks of hemorrhage (33% for unruptured and 51% for ruptured AVMs); however, they added that older age was a major risk factor, with patients older than 60 years harboring a risk for rupture of 90% in 9 years. Both studies demonstrated an annual average risk for hemorrhage of approximately 2%, which was confirmed in the study by Brown et al.[6] in 1988, who investigated unruptured AVMs only. These investigators added that the risks for permanent morbidity and mortality following a hemorrhage of a brain AVM were 29% and 23%, respectively. Ondra et al.[7] in 1990 calculated a slightly higher risk of 5% per year for unruptured brain AVMs with a mortality risk of 1% per year (i.e., 25% for all hemorrhages) and a morbidity of 2.7% per year (more than 50% for all hemorrhages). In a prospective series published by Mast et al.[8] in 1997, the yearly risk of hemorrhage for previously ruptured brain AVMs was calculated as 17% per year, whereas in unruptured AVMs, the risk of hemorrhage was 2% per year. These researchers found male gender, deep vein drainage, and previous hemorrhages to be the major determinants for future hemorrhages.

Pathomechanical Classification

Although there is little discussion about the necessity of treating ruptured pial AVMs because of their larger rebleeding risk. Unruptured pial AVMs have to be further subdivided to identify those patients in whom therapy is indicated, that is, in whom the risk of treatment is lower than the natural history risk. In our practice, we try to classify these "unruptured" AVMs first according to their *pathomechanism* in relation to the angioarchitecture. Owing to their *high-flow shunt,* fistulous pial AVM , especially when present in childhood, can lead to psychomotor developmental retardation and cardiac insufficiency and, when present later in life, to dementia, and, therefore, they merit treatment.[9] Endovascular treatment should be aimed in these cases to reduce the AV shunt. **Venous congestion** (Fig. 67-1) that can be due to a high input (fistulous lesions) or a reduced outflow (secondary stenosis of the outflow pattern) may go along with a cognitive decline or epilepsy, and we would propose treatment in these cases, with the same aim as stated previously.[10] Even if signs of venous congestion are not present, a long pial course of the draining vein may indicate that *venous drainage restriction* is present over a large area, increasing the risk of venous congestion and subsequent epilepsy. Conversely, a short vein that drains almost directly into a dural sinus is unlikely to interfere with the normal pial drainage. If a patient were to have epilepsy in this kind of angioarchitecture, MRI should be scrutinized for signs of *perinidal gliosis.* In the former case (epileptic patient harboring an AVM with a long pial draining vein) endovascular treatment is warranted to reduce the interference with the normal pial drainage and is likely to reduce seizure frequency or severity, but in the latter case (epilepsy following perinidal gliosis), endovascular therapies are unlikely to change the seizure frequency or severity, and we would suggest abstention from an endovascular treatment. *Mass effect* is a rare pathomechanism that may result from large venous ectasias or the nidus proper compressing critical structures and may lead to epilepsy, neurologic deficits, and even hydrocephalus.[11] *Arterial steal* has been associated with clinical findings, such as migraine and focal neurologic symptoms, that most often are transitory in nature.[12] With the advent of new imaging modalities such as functional MRI and perfusion MRI, it has now become possible to demonstrate whether the symptoms of a patient can be attributed to a true steal that can be treated by endovascular means, with the aim of reducing the shunt if the symptoms are disabling (Fig. 67-2).

Angioarchitectonic Classification

As outlined previously, the first step in non-ruptured AVMs is to evaluate whether the specific symptoms of an individual patient can be related to the AVM. Second, one has to evaluate whether the pathomechanism responsible for the symptoms can be treated by endovascular means (as also described previously) (Table 67-1). The third step consists, in our practice, of evaluating the angioarchitecture of the AVM to determine whether endovascular therapies are suitable for a specific brain AVM and whether there are any focal weak points within the AVM of an asymptomatic patient.

The basic principle of the concept of "targeted embolization" of brain AVMs is the hypothesis that specific angioarchitectonic features of a pial brain AVM can be regarded as *focal "weak points"* that may predispose to hemorrhage.[13-15] Although not proven by randomized prospective trials, this principle has

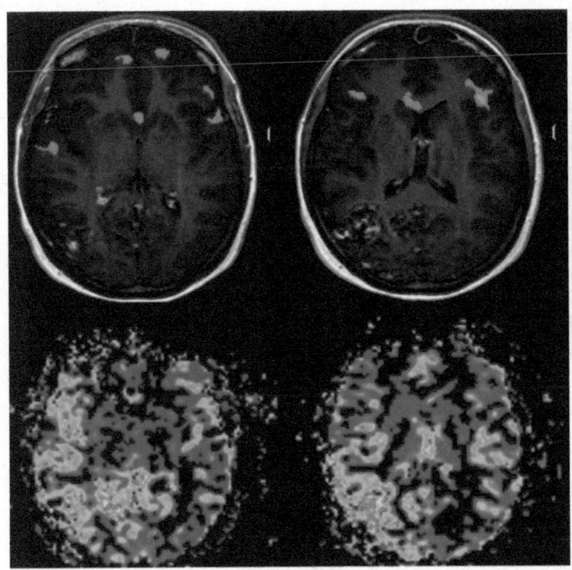

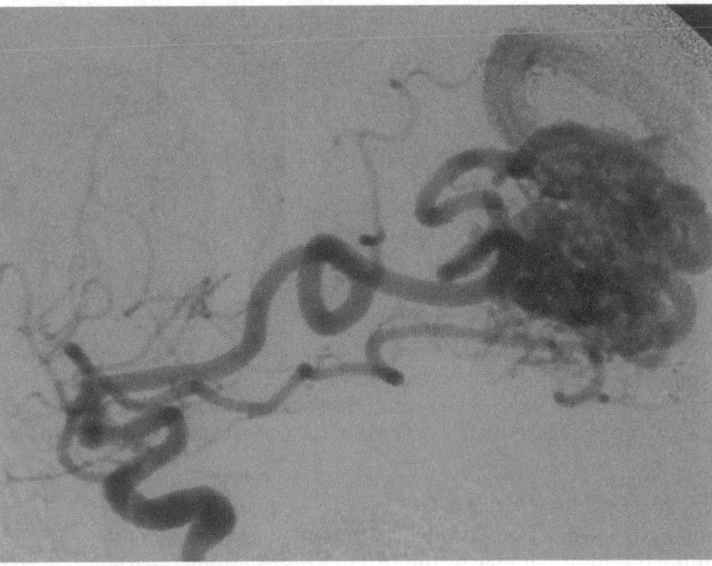

Figure 67-2. The patient complained of repetitive speech arrests without other neurologic signs or symptoms, leading to the discovery of the right parietal arteriovenous malformation (AVM). Functional MRI demonstrates bilateral representation of speech areas. Perfusion MRI was able to show an increased mean transit time in areas remote from the AVM that, however, were active during speech production. Thus the symptoms of the patient could be attributed to the arterial steal effect of the AVM.

TABLE 67-1 Pathomechanical Classification of Brain Arteriovenous Malformations

Clinical Findings	Angiographic Sign	Additional Imaging Diagnostics	Primary Pathophysiology	Treatment Rationale
Neurologic deficits	Perinidal high flow and associated extranidal (remote) hypoperfusion	Perfusion-weighted MRI, (extranidal hypoperfusion), functional MRI (detection of eloquent tissues)	Steal	Reduce shunting volume
	Venous ectasias/pouches close to eloquent brain	MRI (compression, focal edema?), functional MRI (detection of eloquent tissues)	Mass effect	Remove mass effect
Headaches	Occipital high-flow arteriovenous malformation	Perfusion-weighted MRI (extranidal occipital hypoperfusion)	Steal	Reduce shunting volume
	Large draining veins	MRI: hydrocephalus with draining veins close to the aqueduct or interventricular foramen	Mass effect	Decrease size of draining vein
	Pseudophlebitic aspect in venous phase, prolonged venous phase	MRI: edema	Venous congestion	Reduce shunt
Epilepsy	Long-standing high-flow shunts, pseudophlebitic aspect in venous phase	CT: calcifications	Venous congestion	Reduce shunt
	Unspecific	MRI: perinidal gliosis	Gliosis	Surgical removal
	Long pial course of draining vein	Unspecific	Venous restriction	Reduce shunt
Cardiac insufficiency	High-flow shunts	MRI/CT: large venous pouches	Right-to-left shunt	Reduce shunt
Psychomotor developmental retardation	High-flow shunts, pseudophlebitic aspect in venous phase, reduced outflow	MRI: melting brain? CT: calcifications	Venous congestion in not fully matured brain	Reduce shunt
Dementia	Pseudophlebitic aspect in venous phase	MRI: edema	Venous congestion	Reduce shunt

been used in our practice over more than 20 years, and we were able to show an improved outcome on follow-up in comparison with the natural history.[16] These angioarchitectonic weak points are: (1) intranidal aneurysms and venous ectasias,[17] and (2) venous stenosis.[14] The first to state that specific angioarchitectonic features present in brain AVMs make them more prone to future hemorrhage were Brown et al.[6] in 1988, who found that the annual risk of future hemorrhage was 3% in brain AVMs alone, and 7% per year in brain AVMs with associated aneurysms. Meisel et al.[16] found that among 662 patients with brain AVMs, 305 patients had associated aneurysms, and there was a significant increase in rebleed episodes in brain AVMs harboring intranidal aneurysms ($P < 0.002$).[17] In the Toronto series of 759 brain AVMs, associated

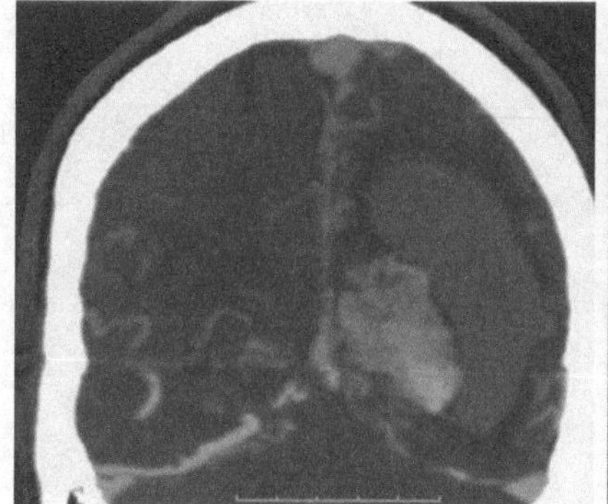
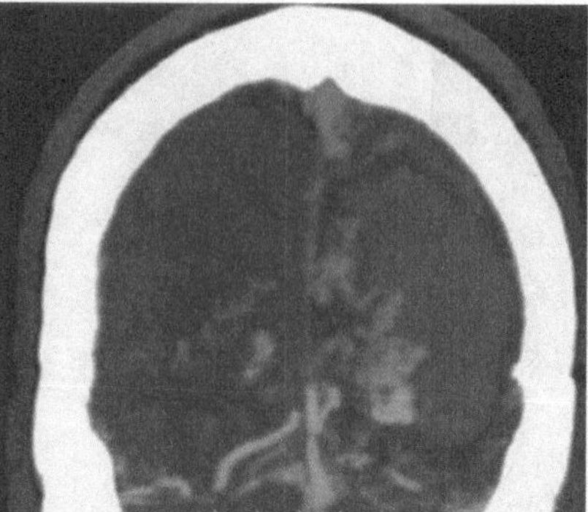
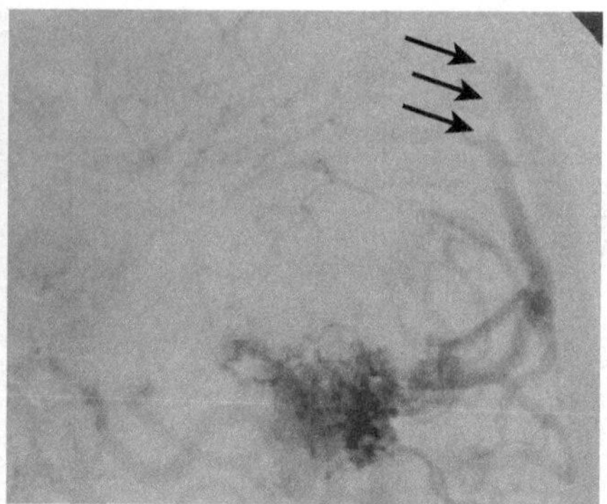

Figure 67-3. The pathomechanism of this ruptured arteriovenous malformation is presumably due to the stenosis of the major venous outlet *(right, arrows)* that led to an increased pressure within the nidus proper. If endovascular therapy is contemplated in cases like these, extreme caution has to be taken that no embolic material penetrates to the venous side.

aneurysms were significantly (P = 0.015) associated with future bleeding.[18] It may be difficult to discern intranidal arterial aneurysms from intranidal venous ectasias, which is why these two angioarchitectonic specificities are grouped as one entity in most series. Venous stenoses, on the other hand, are a separate angiographic weak point and are often seen in ruptured AVMs (Fig. 67-3). The nature of the venous stenosis is not completely understood; most likely high-flow vessel wall changes, failure in remodeling, or an increased vessel wall response to the shear stress induced by the arterialization may be put forward as potential reasons. A stenotic venous outlet will lead to an imbalance of pressure in various compartments of the AVM, which may induce subsequent rupture of the AVM. The compartment that is drained by the stenotic vessel should be scrutinized for contrast agent stagnation, and if endovascular therapy is contemplated, extreme caution has to be undertaken not to push liquid embolic agent toward the already stenosed vein, as doing so may have catastrophic results. In addition to these two angioarchitectonic risk factors, there are also other factors that may lead to an increased risk of hemorrhage. These are: deep venous drainage only, elder age, and male gender.[19]

BOX 67-1 Features Important for a Treatment-Based Classification of Brain Arteriovenous Malformations Employing Endovascular Techniques

ARTERY

Flow-related aneurysms
Number of feeders
Type of feeder (direct vs en passage)

NIDUS

Number of compartments
Intranidal aneurysms
Fistulous vs nidal

VEINS

Stenoses
Number of draining veins per compartment

Angioarchitectonics Related to Endovascular Therapies

Before treatment of an AVM is contemplated, angiography must be scrutinized for the following points: the nature and number of the feeding arteries, the presence or absence of flow-related aneurysms, the number of separate compartments of the malformation, any arterial or venous ectasias near or within the malformation, and the nature of the venous drainage (Box 67-1). On the arterial side, flow-related aneurysms (discussed in greater detail later) are typically present on branching points of the major feeding arteries. They classically resolve following treatment of the AVM and are due to vascular remodeling after increased shear stress.[20] Although such aneurysms are not a contraindication to endovascular treatment, the neurointerventionalist should take special care, because flow-directed catheters are prone to enter the aneurysm rather than the distal vessels. Concerning the arterial side of the AVM, both the number and the nature of the feeding arteries need to be assessed because they determine whether endovascular approaches will make sense. An AVM with a large number of only slightly dilated feeders will make an endovascular therapy more challenging than an AVM with a single large feeder (Fig. 67-4).[21]

Concerning the nature of the feeding artery, there are two basic types of feeding arteries. *Direct arterial feeders* end in the AVM; *indirect arterial feeders* supply the normal cortex and also supply the AVM "en passage" via small vessels that arise from the normal artery (Fig. 67-5). The nature of arterial feeders may be misdiagnosed because of a high-flow AV fistula that attracts all of the contrast agent, leaving the en passage arterial branch invisible. Although direct feeders are safe targets for endovascular therapy, the en passage feeder may carry the risk of inadvertent arterial glue migration to distal healthy vessels. In this regard, the "security margin" of the catheter position has to be briefly discussed. Liquid embolic agents may reflux at the end of the injection. Depending on the agent, the microcatheter, the injection technique, and the skills of the operator, this reflux may be as far as 1 cm proximal to the tip of the catheter. A safe deposition of liquid embolic agent is therefore possible only if the catheter tip is distal enough to any vessel that supplies normal brain tissue. In case of an en passage feeder, this may not be the case, especially if the catheter is only hooked into the feeding artery and so will jump backward because of the jet effect of injecting a liquid embolic agent. Intranidal arterial aneurysms and venous varices that indicate weak points must also be recognized as well as the number of compartments and their nature (nidal versus fistulous). Finally, on the venous side of the AVM, the number of draining veins per compartment (the more the better for endovascular treatment if venous migration should occur), a possible drainage into the deep vein system (higher risk for hemorrhage, more difficult surgical treatment), and stenosis that restricts venous outflow have to be identified to enable

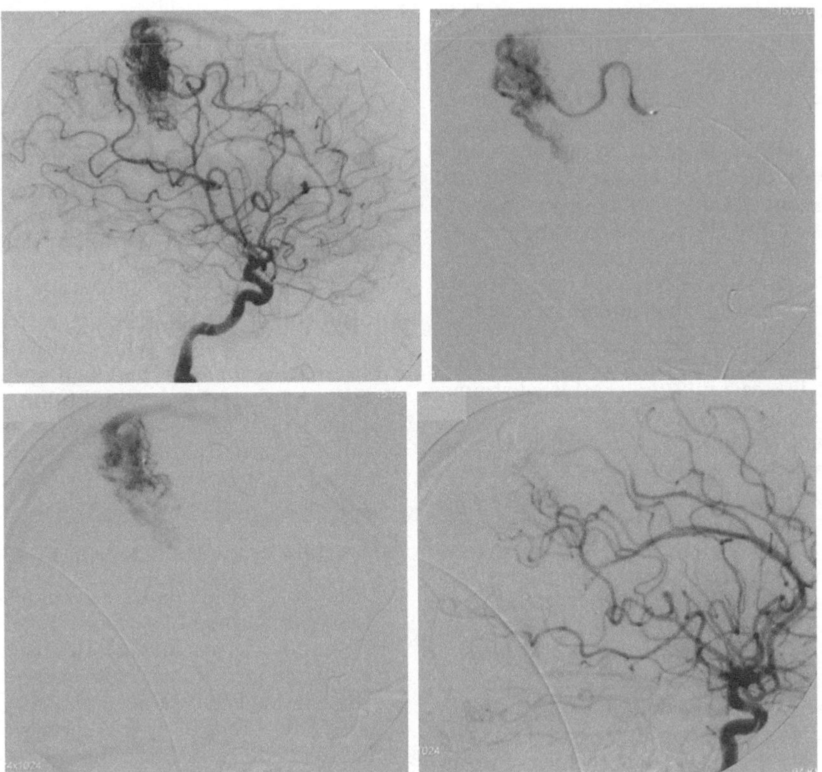

Figure 67-4. Single-feeder arteriovenous malformations (AVMs) are easier to embolize with a higher chance of a complete cure than multiple-feeder AVMs. In this single-compartment AVM, the microcatheter is brought to an intranidal position, where a histoacryl deposition was able to completely occlude the AVM.

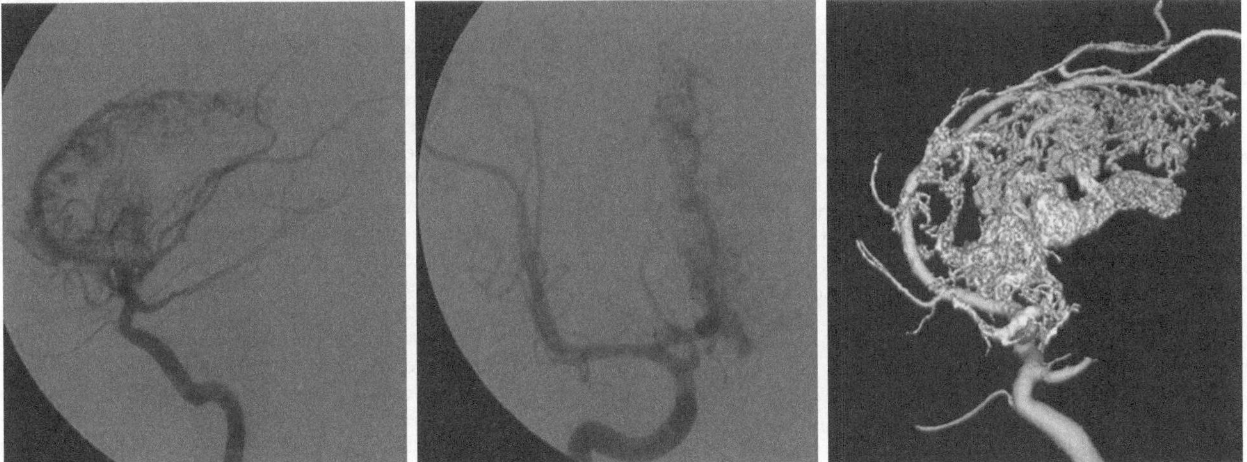

Figure 67-5. Whereas the feeder in Figure 64.8 was of the terminal or "direct" type, the feeder type of this pericallosal arteriovenous malformation is of the "indirect" or "en passage" type. These "en passage" feeders may carry the risk of inadvertent arterial glue migration to distal healthy vessels.

full determination of the risk of a specific AVM. At present, this information can be obtained only by conventional digital subtraction angiography that, in our practice, still must precede any treatment decision in AVMs.

Concepts of Treatment

There is general consensus for treatment of ruptured brain arteriovenous malformations since the major risk factor for future bleeding from a brain AVM is an initial hemorrhagic presentation. However, interventional treatment of unruptured AVMs has been controversial The uncertainty regarding whether interventional or medical therapy was the most effective treatment for patients with unruptured AMVs lead to a prospective multicenter randomized controlled trial of unruptured brain AVMs (ARUBA). This trial aimed to determine whether invasive treatment of unruptured bAVMs provides any significant long-term benefit over medical management. ARUBA showed that after a mean follow-up of 33 months, the event rate (time to stroke or death) in the intervention group was more than three times higher than in the medical management group. This analysis included data from 224 participants enrolled at 39 sites world-wide. The trial's primary endpoint was the composite of death or stroke, defined as "any new focal neurological deficit, seizure, or new-onset headache" associated with imaging findings, while one may argue that a modified Rankin score could have been a clinically more meaningful endpoint. In addition, whether or not the difference in outcomes holds true at longer endpoints cannot be answered by the trial, although the trial was stopped early because of superior outcomes in the medical arm. The rather low recruitment rate (a total of 226 patients were recruited in 39 centers over a period of 7 years) and an inclusion rate per center of only 63% also raise question of selection bias for the patients included and reported upon in the study. Thus it is not clear whether the results of this study are generalizable to all patients with unruptured AVM, but the ARUBA data must be considered strongly in future decision-making for these patients.

A complete cure of a pial brain AVM by endovascular means is possible in approximately 20% of all AVMs irrespective of their angioarchitecture.[22–24] Those AVMs that are favorable to a complete endovascular cure are the small, single-feeder, single-compartment AVMs that have a direct feeding artery. Because such AVMs are also good candidates for both radiosurgery and open neurosurgery, a tailored team approach for each specific AVM in each individual patient, respecting also the patient's wishes and the peculiarities of the clinical presentation, must be taken. In most instances, endovascular therapies are used to diminish the size of an AVM prior to radiotherapy or surgery, to secure focal weak points in the acute and subacute stages of ruptured AVMs and in unruptured AVMs for which radiosurgery is contemplated, or to exclude those compartments of an AVM that may be difficult to reach during surgery (see also the discussion of indications and contraindications). It has to be stressed at this point that, once a therapy of an AVM is contemplated, a pathway to its complete exclusion has to be agreed upon by the treatment team, which should include radiosurgeons, vascular neurosurgeons, neurologists, and neurointerventionalists. It does not make sense, in our opinion, to partially treat an AVM without a strategy on how to handle a possible residual of the AVM.

Once endovascular therapy is decided upon, we proceed with a predefined goal, which may mean a partial, targeted embolization. Such rationale is based on the outcomes in a series of more than 600 patients with AVMs that were partially embolized and showed a significant decrease in hemorrhage episodes in comparison with the conservatively treated series reported in the literature.[16] The yearly hemorrhage incidence rate of patients before partial treatment was 0.062 (95% confidence interval [CI], 0.03–0.11). The observed annual rate after the start of this regimen was 0.02 (95%CI, 0.012–0.030).[16] Given the previously mentioned considerations concerning focal weak points, we think that these numbers reflect the benefit of selectively excluding specific weak compartments of an AVM and thereby providing early protection while the patient is scheduled for radiotherapy (the effects of which take more time, but the results of which concerning complete obliteration are better). In these instances the goal is to secure the AVM during its time to complete occlusion. In other instances the goal may be to exclude those compartments that will be difficult to reach prior to surgery or to diminish the size of the AVM prior to radiosurgery. In the latter instance, compartments in the periphery of the AVM have to be targeted, whereas in the former instance, the neurosurgeon has to point out the target of the neurointerventionalist. Because in combined therapies (endovascular + radiotherapy; endovascular + surgery), the relative risks of each procedure are cumulative, embolization only makes sense if a goal is predefined prior to therapy. In most instances, this goal should be reached during a maximum of two or three endovascular sessions.

Specific Treatment Considerations

Flow-Related Arterial Aneurysms

Redekop et al.[25] reported that there was no difference in the rate of hemorrhagic occurrence during follow-up between the overall population of patients with brain AVMs without aneurysms and those with proximal-flow-related aneurysms. Likewise, in our experience, proximal-flow-related aneurysms are almost never the site of bleeding. Therefore, there is no evidence that treatment of a non-ruptured proximal aneurysm associated with an AVM is needed; and we perform treatment of the AVM before a treatment of the proximal aneurysm (only if the latter is still persistent). We have never observed rupture of a proximal aneurysm following embolization of the related contribution to the AVM. As already pointed out, during endovascular treatment of brain AVMs with associated flow-related aneurysms, great caution is needed to avoid entering and rupturing the flow-related aneurysm with the microcatheter.

Fistulous Arteriovenous Malformations

Although most AVMs have fistulous and glomerular (plexiform) compartments, a specific subset of purely fistulous pial AV shunts, the pial single-hole macrofistulas, deserve special consideration. They are often present in children and should raise the suspicion of an underlying genetic disease such as hereditary hemorrhagic telangiectasia (HHT).[26] HHT is inherited as an autosomal dominant trait with varying penetrance and expressivity. Cerebral pial AV fistulas in HHT are macrofistulas with a high fistula volume and are of the single-hole type. The feeding arteries drain directly into a massively enlarged venous pouch, and often there is only a single feeding artery. Signs of venous congestion are typically present because of venous overload and are responsible for the patients' symptoms. Associated angiographic abnormalities include venous ectasias, venous stenoses, pial reflux, venous ischemia, calcifications, and associated arterial aneurysms. Patients are typically younger than 16 years, but the disease has a propensity for appearing in early infancy; in our series all patients but two were younger than 6 years.[9] Localization of the AVF is either cortical supratentorial or infratentorial, and deep locations are exceptional. Presenting symptoms are intracerebral hemorrhage in the majority of patients; macrocrania, bruit, cognitive deficits, cardiac insufficiency, epilepsy, tonsillar prolapse, and hydrocephalus may also be present.

In our practice, treatment consists of superselective embolization to obliterate the fistulous area by pushing the glue via the artery into the venous pouch to establish a mushroom-shaped cast that occludes the single-hole fistula. Alternatively, coils may be used to selectively occlude the fistulous site. Because a major problem of glue embolization is the uncontrollable propagation of glue into veins with secondary venous occlusion and hemorrhage, we try to minimize this risk in these macrofistulas by using undiluted glue with tantalum powder at a position close to the venous pouch with the catheter tip pointed against the vessel wall.[9] In selected patients flow reduction with coils may be used prior to glue embolization.

Cerebral Proliferative Angiopathy

We have introduced the term cerebral proliferative angiopathy (CPA) to distinguish a specific entity that differs from "classic" pial AVMs in its angiomorphology, histology, presumed pathomechanism, epidemiology, natural history, and clinical presentation.[27]

From an angiomorphologic standpoint, the salient features of CPA, which help discern it from "classic" brain AVMs, are the absence of dominant feeders or flow-related aneurysms, the presence of proximal stenoses of feeding arteries, the extensive transdural supply to both healthy and pathologic tissues, the large size (which might be lobar or even hemispheric), the presence of capillary angioectasia, and the only moderately enlarged veins (compared with the size of the nidus) (Fig. 67-6). Moreover, this special entity of false brain AVM can be suspected when brain tissue is seen on MRI to be intermingled between the vascular spaces. Perfusion MRI indicates an increased blood volume within the nidus with a longer mean transit time (MTT), indicative of capillary and venous ectasias, and an area of hypoperfusion that could be seen throughout the affected hemisphere. This differs from the features of classic brain AVMs, in which the mean transit time is decreased owing to AV shunts and the perinidal areas are not as severely hypoperfused as in CPA. This hypoperfusion trigger might then cause angiogenesis. Whereas transdural supply following iatrogenic ischemia is a normal response to an abnormal demand, the transdural supply in CPA is an abnormal response to an abnormal demand. On histopathology, CPA is characterized by normal brain parenchyma interspersed with the abnormal vascular channels. Brain tissue within the "nidus" of the CPA is, therefore, functional, similar to brain tissue found in between the abnormal vascular channels present in capillary telangiectasias. Patients (typically, young females) usually do not present with an acute neurologic deficit or hemorrhage, but more commonly with epileptic manifestations, headaches, and progressive neurologic deficits. There is a high rate of stroke-like symptoms, transient ischemic attacks (TIAs), and neurologic defects not owing to a hemorrhage that suit the assumption that CPA is a disease related to ischemia rather than hemorrhage. Embolization of these malformations carries an extremely high risk of neurologic deficits, because normal brain tissue is very likely to be embolized owing to the specific histopathology described. We do not recommend endovascular therapy for this condition. Because one of the major pathomechanisms of this disease is ischemia (which in itself is probably multifactorial owing to incompetent angiogenesis, "steal" phenomena, arterial stenosis, and capillary wall involvement), a therapy that enhances cortical blood supply (such as placement of calvarial burr holes) may be adopted.[27]

Cerebrofacial Arteriovenous Metameric Syndromes

The association of AVMs of the brain, the orbit (retinal and/or retrobulbar lesions), and the maxillofacial region was originally named after Bonnet-Dechaume-Blanc and Wyburn-Mason. A potential explanation for this striking association is that neural crest and mesodermal cells originating from a given transverse (metameric) level of the embryo finally occupy the same territory in the head and that these embryonic tissues are regionalized in various areas devoted to providing blood vessels to specific regions of the face and brain. Because these fate maps have shown a striking similarity to the distribution of vascular malformations in the previously mentioned diseases, the term cerebrofacial AV metameric syndrome (CAMS) has been coined, reflecting the putative underlying disorder. Depending on the involved structures, different CAMSs can be differentiated: CAMS 1 is a midline prosencephalic (olfactory) group with involvement of the hypothalamus, corpus callosum, hypophysis, and nose (Fig. 67-7); CAMS 2 is a lateral prosencephalic (optic) group with involvement of the optic nerve, retina, parietotemporooccipital lobes, thalamus, and maxilla; and CAMS 3 is a rhombencephalic (otic) group, with involvement of the cerebellum, pons, petrous bone, and mandible. CAMS 3 is located in a strategic position on the crossroad between the complex cephalic segmental arrangements and the relatively simplified spinal metamers and it may ,therefore, bear transitional characteristics. A more extensive insult will lead to overlapping territories, producing a complete prosencephalic phenotype (CAMS 1+2) or bilateral involvement. The insult producing the underlying lesion would have to develop before the migration occurs and thus before the fourth week of development.[2] The disease spectrum may be incomplete either because some cells are spared or because they have not been triggered to reveal the disease, leading to cases without retinal involvement, cerebral involvement, or facial involvement. Retinal AVM is often the earliest manifestation of a CAMS and it is interesting to note, that in some cases, follow-up showed secondary expression of the full syndrome.

Considered metameric lesions, CAMSs most commonly include intracranial AVMs. Certain angioarchitectural features differentiate cerebral AVMs in CAMS from "classic" AVMs. The AVM nidus in CAMS is a cluster of small vessels with intervening normal brain tissue, some degree of angiogenesis, and a rather small shunting volume. Transdural arterial supply can be present. Progressive enlargement of these cerebral AVMs is one of the special observations in CAMS, suggesting that AVMs in CAMS are not static processes within the segment that carry the embryonic defect. Multifocality is another typical aspect of CAMS AVMs. Despite the common occurrence of cerebral AVMs in CAMS, they are usually clinically silent or asymptomatic at the time of discovery. They rarely manifest as acute neurologic symptoms caused by intracerebral or subarachnoid hemorrhage; rather, they give rise to progressive neurologic deterioration without evidence of intracranial bleeding, most likely owing to a progression in size. About 25% of patients with CAMS-associated AVMs bleed during the course of their disease. Therapeutic management of the cerebral AVMs is particularly challenging. We suggest targeted embolization in an attempt to exclude weak angioarchitectural aspects or to reduce the AV shunt in the least eloquent areas in symptomatic patients who are clinically significantly affected. Brain AVMs associated with CAMS tend to be difficult to cure because of their size, location, and evolving natural history.[2]

Indications for and Contraindications to Endovascular Therapies

With the previously described precautions and considerations in mind, in our practice, we see the following indications for endovascular therapies in ruptured brain AVMs: (1) ruptured brain AVMs in the hyperacute stage when contrast stagnation in a vessel pouch (pseudoaneurysm) is demonstrated during angiography, because this suggests a false sac with a potential rebleeding risk; (2) ruptured brain AVM in the subacute stage, with intranidal aneurysms; (3) surgically unfavorable ruptured AVM in the subacute stage when venous stenosis is present; and (4) surgically unfavorable ruptured AVM in elderly patients with deep vein drainage.

For unruptured AVMs, a more conservative approach appears indicated given the results of the ARUBA trial for AVMs that were similar to those included in the trial, bearing in mind that there was an under-representation of AVMs of the fistulous type, that no pediatric patients and few "symptomatic" AVMs were included and that presence of identifiable risk factors was not reported in the treated patient population. Thus, despite the results of the ARUBA trial, we see the following potential indications for endovascular therapies in our practice in unruptured brain AVMs: (1) pial macrofistulas at any age, to reduce venous congestion, especially for the maturing brain; (2) unruptured but symptomatic AVMs with

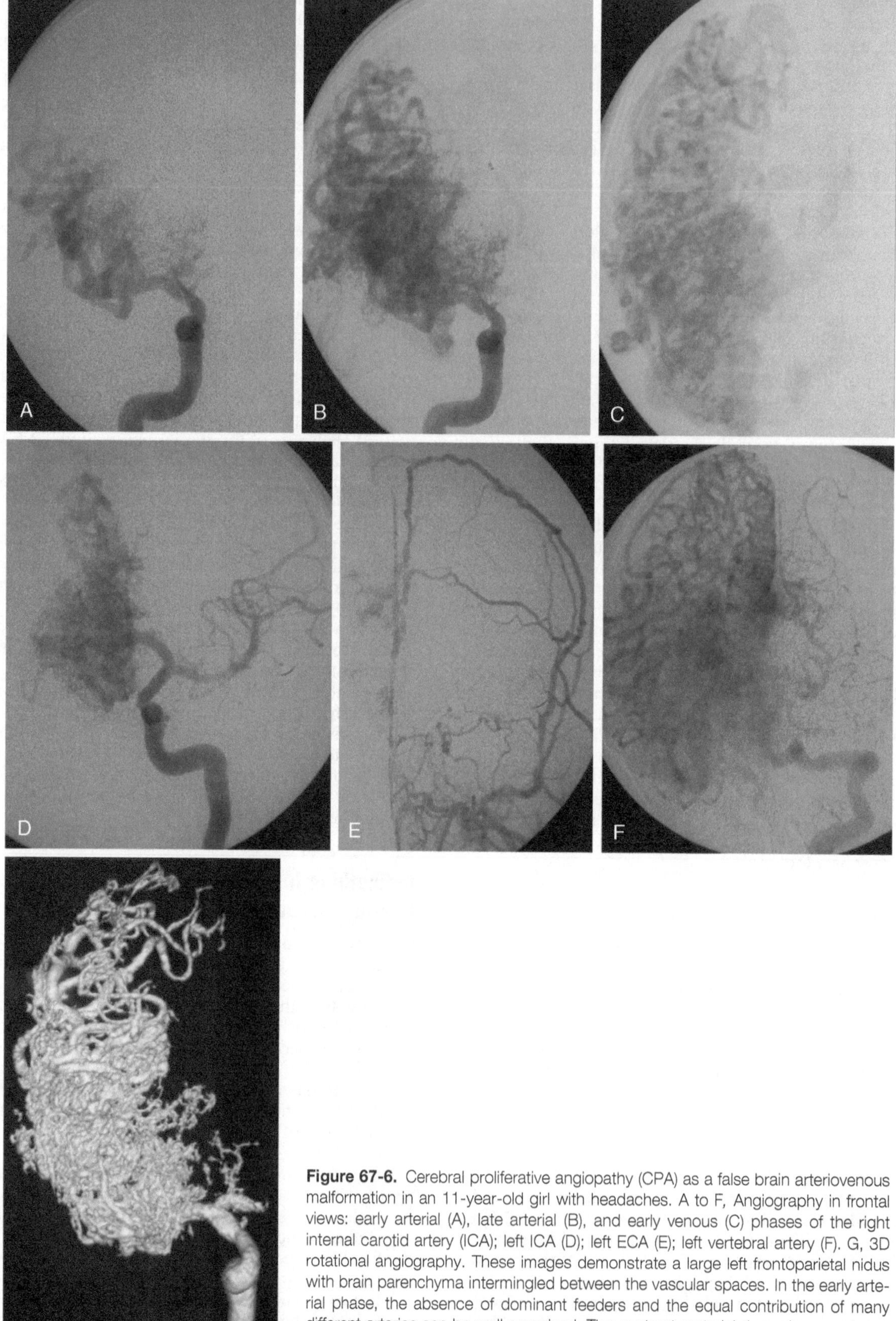

Figure 67-6. Cerebral proliferative angiopathy (CPA) as a false brain arteriovenous malformation in an 11-year-old girl with headaches. A to F, Angiography in frontal views: early arterial (A), late arterial (B), and early venous (C) phases of the right internal carotid artery (ICA); left ICA (D); left ECA (E); left vertebral artery (F). G, 3D rotational angiography. These images demonstrate a large left frontoparietal nidus with brain parenchyma intermingled between the vascular spaces. In the early arterial phase, the absence of dominant feeders and the equal contribution of many different arteries can be well perceived. The contrast material dynamics reveal persistence of contrast material in the malformation and hardly any early venous drainage. The transdural supply testifies to the proliferative component of the disease, whereas injection into the vertebral artery demonstrates diffuse neoangiogenesis in other cortical areas.

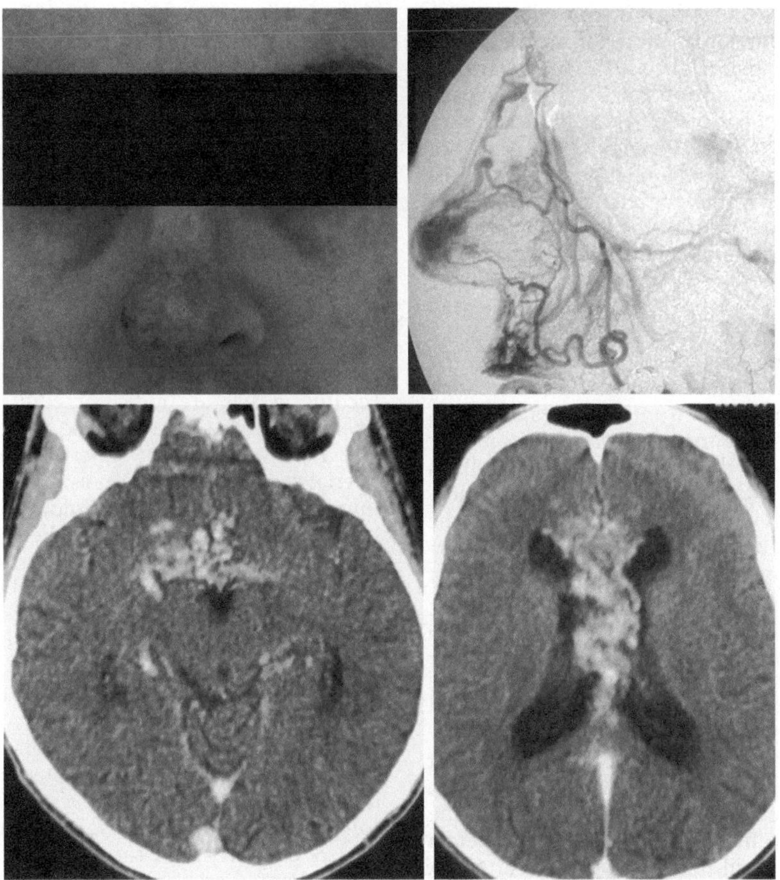

Figure 67-7. Cerebrofacial arteriovenous metameric syndrome type 1 (CAMS 1): Midline or olfactory type with arteriovenous malformation along the nose, hypothalamus, and corpus callosum.

symptoms that are attributable to an endovascularly reachable angioarchitectonic target (mass effect of venous pouches, venous congestion with neurological symptoms are refractory seizures); and (3) surgically unfavorable AVMs with angioarchitectonic risk factors (large intranidal outpouchings/aneurysms, significant venous outflow obstructions, perilesional edema), especially when other risk factors for future hemorrhage are present (male gender, deep vein drainage). Unfortunately, in the ARUBA trial no subgroup analysis was reported, or will ever be reportable as this study is already statistically underpowered given the low recruitment rate. Unfortunately, this study is based on the presumption that all unruptured brain AVMs behave in the same way, irrespective of size, location, age, anatomy, venous drainage, associated aneurysms, perilesional edema, etc. To generalize from this study to ALL patients with unruptured brain AVMs would, therefore, be only acceptable if, indeed, ALL patients from a participating center were included in the study. On the other hand, especially in the light of the ARUBA trial we do not see an indication, for treatment in elderly, asymptomatic patients without angioarchitectonic risks.

In our view, there are no true "contraindications" to endovascular therapies; in other words, any AVM can be partially treated by embolization. There are many AVMs, however, in which partial treatment does not make sense. This is particularly true for small unruptured AVMs with no angioarchitectonic risk factors. Finally, the following angioarchitectonic features should make interventional neuroradiologists cautious about endovascular therapy and to consider alternate treatment strategies: en passage feeder, flow-related aneurysms, and diffuse nidus-type AVM.

SPINAL ARTERIOVENOUS MALFORMATIONS

A classification for spinal AVMs that is based on the same characteristics outlined for brain AVMs is difficult to establish, because of the rarity of the spinal lesions. As in cerebral vascular malformations, there are purely arterial diseases (aneurysms, dissections), AV diseases (i.e., AVMs) and purely venous diseases (cavernomas). In addition, a differentiation between focal (i.e., single spinal AVMs) and metameric diseases can be made, with the latter being similar to the previously mentioned CAM syndromes.[2] Finally, hereditary diseases (such as HHT with its associated spinal neurovascular phenotypes) can be differentiated from non-hereditary lesions.[26] However, for the sake of a treatment-based classification, we use a classification scheme in this chapter that is based on the angioarchitecture in addition to the various pathomechanisms. For an understanding of the rationale for these classifications, it is essential to briefly review the essentials of spinal cord vascularization.

Spinal Cord Vascularization

Segmental arteries supply the spine, including the vertebral bodies, paraspinal muscles, dura, nerve roots, and the spinal cord with blood. Radicular arteries are the first branches of the dorsal division of the segmental arteries. The bony spine is supplied by anterior and posterior central arteries that arise directly from the segmental and radicular arteries. A spinal radicular branch supplying the dura and the nerve root as a radiculomeningeal artery is present at each segment. From these radicular arteries, radiculomedullary and/or radiculopial arteries might branch, following the anterior or posterior nerve roots to reach the anterior or posterior surface of the cord where they form the anterior or posterior spinal arterial systems. In the adult patient, not all lumbar or intercostal arteries have a radiculomedullary feeder and their location for a given patient is not predictable.[28] The anterior and posterior spinal arteries constitute a superficial longitudinal anastomosing system. The anterior spinal artery travels along the anterior sulcus and typically originates from the two vertebral arteries, while the typically paired posterolateral spinal arteries originate from the preatlantal part of the vertebral artery or from the posteroinferior cerebellar artery (PICA). These three arterial systems run from the cervical-medullary junction to the conus medullaris, but are not capable of supplying the entire spinal cord. Instead, they are reinforced by radiculomedullary and radiculopial arteries that derive from various (and unpredictable!) segmental levels. The most known of the anterior radiculomedullary arteries is the artery radiculomedullaris magna (i.e., the Adamkiewicz artery). The anterior radiculomedullary arteries branch in a very typical way to reach the spinal cord. The ascending branch continues along the direction of the radicular artery in the midline of the anterior surface. The descending branch, being the larger one at thoracolumbar levels, forms a hairpin curve as soon as it reaches the midline at the entrance of the anterior fissure.

The intrinsic network of the spinal cord arteries can be divided into central or sulcal arteries from the anterior spinal artery that supply the gray matter and the central part of the cord on one side or the other.[29] The radiculopial network that is derived from the posterolateral spinal arteries supplies via the rami perforantes of the vasa corona the periphery of the spinal cord (i.e., the white matter). The vasa corona gets a small anterolateral supply from the anterior spinal artery. A multitude of anastomoses is present at the spine and spinal cord: extradural interconnections between segmental arteries can compensate for a proximal occlusion of a radicular artery, whereas intradurally, both the anterior and posterior spinal arteries represent a system of longitudinal anastomoses that is reinforced from different levels. Moreover, both the posterior and anterior arterial systems are interconnected at the level of the conus via the "basket" anastomosis and via transverse anastomoses of the intrinsic arteries that interconnect by the pial network of the vasa corona. The venous drainage of the cord is via radially symmetrical intrinsic spinal cord veins and small superficial pial veins that open into the superficial longitudinal median anastomosing spinal cord veins, both anterior and posterior to the spinal cord.[30] They may use the nerve roots to reach the epidural plexus and the extraspinal veins and plexus with a reflux-impeding mechanism within the dura mater.[31]

Angiomorphologic Classification

Spinal AV shunting lesions can be differentiated like those of the brain, that is, grossly into those that are supplied by dural (or radiculomeningeal) arteries, that do *not* serve to supply the brain (or spinal cord) under normal circumstances, and those shunting lesions that are supplied by arteries that under normal circumstances also supply the brain or spinal cord (i.e., pial AVMs). Because spinal dural AV fistulas (i.e., those shunting lesions that are supplied by radiculomeningeal arteries) are discussed in a different chapter in this book, we focus here only on those pial AV shunts of the spinal cord that are supplied by cord-supplying radiculopial or radiculomedullary arteries.[28]

According to their nidus, these spinal pial AVMs are either glomerular or fistulous in nature, and, although the fistulous pial AVMs can be further differentiated into macrofistulas with high fistula volume and microfistulas with small fistula volume, the glomerular (nidus-type of plexiform) AVMs may be further separated into the focal and the diffuse ones. Because the location of the AVM itself (i.e., intramedullary versus perimedullary) depends on the supplying vessel (with AVMs being supplied exclusively by the radiculopial arteries and typically perimedullary in location), we do not use this angiographic feature to further subclassify spinal AVMs.

Fistulous Arteriovenous Malformations

Fistulous AVMs (which in some classifications have been called AVMs of the perimedullary fistula type or intradural AV fistulas) are direct AV shunts located superficially on the spinal cord that only rarely possess intramedullary compartments. Feeding vessels are radiculomedullary arteries, radiculopial arteries, or both (differentiating them from the dural AV fistulas). Draining veins are superficial perimedullary veins. The arterialized blood may even ascend via the foramen magnum into the posterior fossa. Fistulous AVMs can be subdivided into two types according to their feeding vessel size, the volume of the shunt, and the drainage pattern. Microfistulas are small AVMs in which neither the feeding artery nor the draining vein are markedly dilated and the shunt volume is low. Macrofistulas harbor multiple massively dilated arterial feeders and a large shunt volume. These latter fistulas are typically encountered in HHT. Spinal cord AV fistula in HHT is characterized as an intradural AV malformation with a macrofistula and high fistula volume; the fistula drains directly into a massively enlarged venous pouch that can be easily identified on MRI.[26] Feeding vessels might be either the dorsolateral or the anterior spinal arteries or both. Multiple feeders conjoin at the same space into the draining venous pouch. Venous ectasias, stenosis, and pial reflux are present in all patients with these fistulas.

Glomerular Arteriovenous Malformations

The *focal type* of glomerular AVM is confined to the spinal cord. It is fed by radiculomedullary and radiculopial (spinal cord feeding) arteries and drained by spinal cord veins. The shunt flow is high but typically not as high as in macrofistulous AVMs. Glomerular AVMs, which are sometimes called plexiform or nidus-type AVMs, are the most often encountered spinal cord AVM, with a nidus resembling closely those of a brain AVM. This type of malformation usually has an intramedullary location, but superficial nidus compartments can also reach the subarachnoid space. Because of the many anastomoses between the anterior and posterior arterial feeding system of the spines, these AVMs typically have multiple artery supply from both the posterior and anterior system. Drainage is into dilated spinal cord veins (Fig. 67-8).

The *diffuse type* of glomerular AVMs is not confined to the spinal cord and, in correlation to its cerebral counterpart, has, therefore, been called spinal AV metameric syndrome (SAMS; previously called Cobb's syndrome or spinal AVM of the juvenile type). SAMS affects the whole myelomere, so affected patients typically present with multiple shunts of the spinal cord, the nerve root, bone, paraspinal, subcutaneous, and skin tissues that share the same myelomere. SAMS can be further subdivided depending on the affected myelomere from 1 to 31.

Pathophysiologic Classification

As in brain AVMs, a classification of spinal AVMs based on their pathomechanisms and clinical presentations is possible. The major pathophysiologic mechanisms in spinal cord AVMs are venous congestion and hemorrhage.[32] Only rarely,

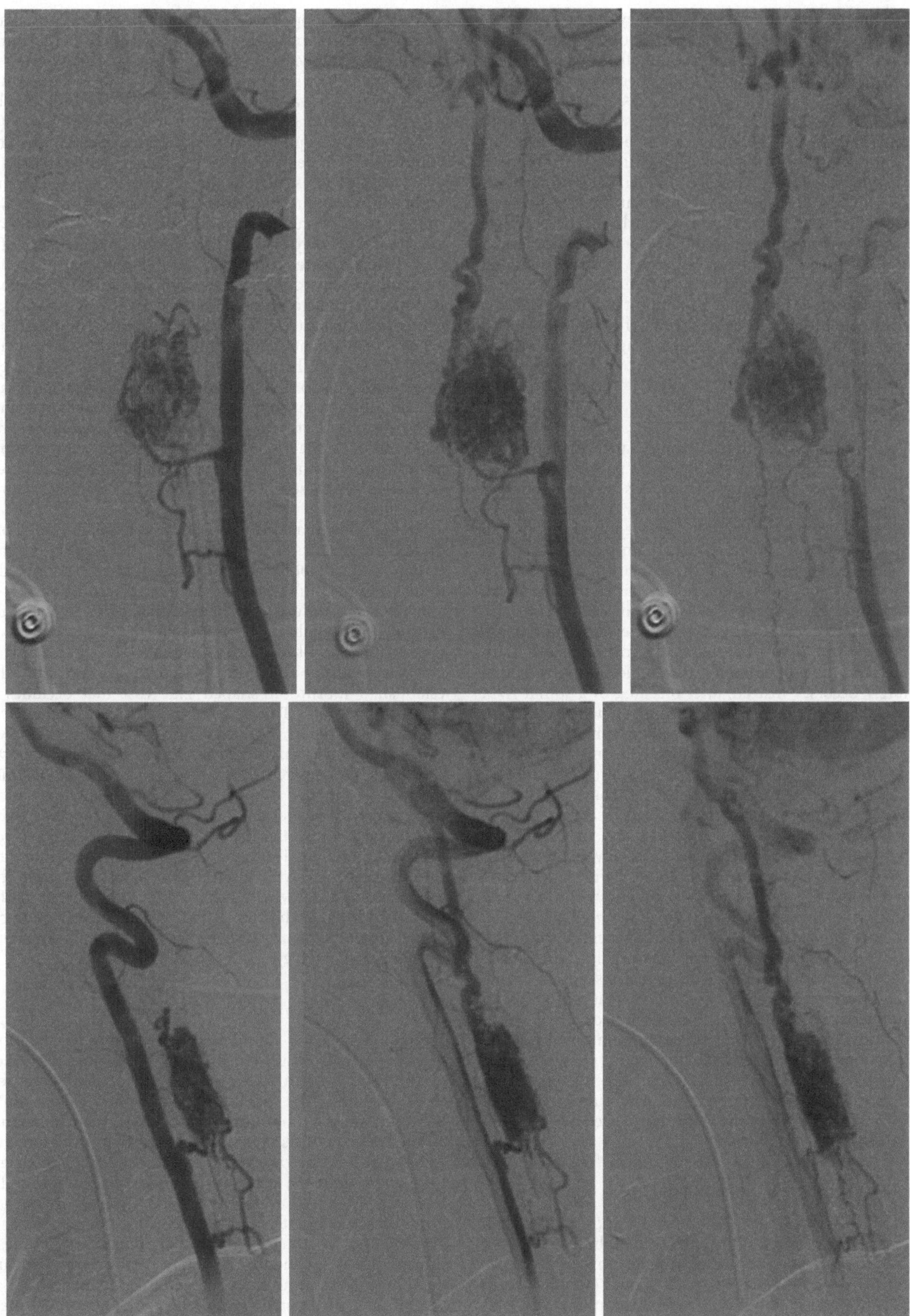

Figure 67-8. Glomerular or nidus-type arteriovenous malformation (AVM). Early arterial to early venous arteriogram phases in anteroposterior views in the *upper row* and the lateral views in the *lower row* demonstrate multiple feeders to an intramedullary AVM that consists of a nidus or glomus of pathologic vessels instead of a single fistula.

space-occupying effects or arterial steal may be present. Acute symptoms may be related to a spontaneous thrombosis of a vein. If the AVM does not manifest initially as acute hemorrhage, symptomatology may be non-specific. Patients may complain about hypesthesia or paresthesia, weakness, and diffuse back and muscle pain. Progressive sensorimotor symptoms can develop slowly or worsen acutely followed by some improvements over time. Glomerular AVMs tend to become symptomatic in younger children and adolescents, whereas fistulous AVMs become symptomatic in young adults, the latter presenting often with a subarachnoid hemorrhage because of the frequent perimedullary location. Glomerular AVMs can become symptomatic by means of venous congestion alone, intraparenchymal hemorrhage, and/or subarachnoid hemorrhage. Macrofistulas manifest as hematomyelia with acute tetraplegia/paresis in the majority of cases; spinal subarachnoid hemorrhage and venous congestion can also be encountered.[33]

Concepts of Treatment

The therapeutic approach to an asymptomatic AVM is difficult since data concerning the spontaneous prognosis are not available; however, in symptomatic AVMs therapy improves the prognosis of the patient as indicated by the Bicetre series[34] and by our own recent results.[35] In fact, we found that overall rebleed rate after presentation with hemorrhage was 7 in 145.5 patient-years (4.8%/yr), if the lesion was not treated; 3 in 102 patient-years (2.9%/yr) following partial treatment and 0 in 47.5 patient-years (0%) following complete treatment.[35] There are some fundamental differences between brain AVMs and spinal AVMs. First, a hyperacute treatment is rarely indicated because, in our opinion, acute rebleeding of a spinal AVM rarely occurs.[36] Instead, after bleeding of a spinal AVM has occurred, we typically wait for approximately 6 weeks for potential vasospasm to resolve or the hemorrhage to absorb. Second, although brain AVMs have to be completely treated to avoid the risk of rebleeding, this seems not to be the case with spinal AVMs, for which partial treatment appears to be sufficient to dramatically improve the prognosis, especially in those cases in which a complete eradication of the AVM is likely to produce neurologic deficits. Especially in unruptured spinal AVMs that have become symptomatic with venous congestion rather than hemorrhage,[37] the goal has to be to reduce the shunting volume rather than to make an "angiographically nice" picture that carries a high risk of treatment-related morbidity.[34] Third, because of the low flow in some glomerular AVMs, endovascular therapies with particles seem to have a better and more stable result, if venous stagnation (with subsequent venous thrombosis of the outlet) occurs. Fourth, in our opinion, there is no role for radiosurgery in spinal vascular malformations, and the endovascular route should be the modality of choice in most instances. Surgery remains an option especially when the endovascular route is too long (which may be the case for AV fistulas located at the filum terminale).

Fistulous Arteriovenous Malformations

In fistulous AVMs, the aim is to obliterate the point of fistulization. A secure way to reach this goal is to embolize the most proximal venous segment together with the most distal arterial segment. This can be done with either liquid embolic agents or coils. Although the choice of embolization material is of minor importance and merely depends on the interventionalist's preference, the most important (and most difficult) part is to know where the artery stops and where the vein starts. A proximal occlusion of the artery will lead to collateral filling and secondary reopening due to the vast network of anastomoses and may carry the risk of inadvertent occlusion of spinal cord supply. A pure venous occlusion that leaves the fistula open may, on the other hand, result in hemorrhage. The transition between artery and vein may be indicated by a venous aneurysm (which is often the site of rupture) (Fig. 67-9), a large venous pouch (as typically present in the large-volume single-hole fistulas), or a slight change in caliber (Fig. 67-10). A 3D reconstruction of the angiogram is in our opinion particularly helpful to define this fistulous point.[38] Great caution must be taken in identifying the normal spinal cord arteries (which may be difficult to demonstrate because of the flow being directed primarily into the fistula). Therefore, before therapy is contemplated, complete spinal angiography is done to evaluate potential collaterals to the anterior and posterior spinal arteries. When therapy with a liquid embolic agent is contemplated, the point of security has to be defined because reflux of the embolic agent may occur (especially in small fistulas). Too short a distance between the microcatheter tip and the adjacent anterior spinal arterial system may, therefore, carry a large risk for the patient. In addition, a too proximal position of the microcatheter tip may prevent the embolic agent from reaching the vein, resulting in a proximal arterial occlusion.[39] In these cases, we rather opt for surgical treatment of the fistula.[40]

In high-flow macrofistulas (which may be indicative of an underlying genetic disease such as HHT), a technique similar to that for single-hole brain AV fistulas has to be adopted. In these types of fistulous AVMs the dilated feeding vessels will allow for superselective catheterization close to the fistula. Closure with highly concentrated glue is, therefore, possible with the aim to obliterate the fistulous area by pushing the glue via the distal artery into the proximal venous pouch to establish a mushroom-shaped glue cast that occludes the single-hole fistula. This is preferably done via a posterior spinal arterial feeder, with occlusion of the fistula being verified during injection of the other feeders. One important caution has to be kept in mind in this kind of treatment, though. Because the volume of the venous pouch is typically large and may further enlarge following thrombosis (which will happen within the first 24 hours after occlusion), compression of the spinal cord may occur. Such rare evolution may need to be treated with surgical decompression. Given these assumptions, a stepwise approach with reduction of the flow (and subsequently the size of the venous pouch) using coils at the site of the fistula in several sessions may be an alternative treatment strategy.

Glomerular Arteriovenous Malformations

In glomerular AVMs, liquid embolic agents can be employed to obliterate the nidus, but even partial embolization seems to improve the natural history of the patient, because in most instances, the pathophysiologic mechanism can be identified prior to the procedure, leading to an individually tailored therapeutic strategy. In most instances of glomerular AVMs that have become symptomatic with a hemorrhage, a focal weak point can be identified and targeted for embolization (Fig. 67-11).[34] On the other hand, in cases in which the symptoms can be attributed to the venous congestion, the aim will be to reduce the shunt as much as possible. As in fistulous AVMs, the first step is to perform complete angiography to determine the collaterals, the main feeders, and the number of different and/or overlapping compartments. Three-dimensional reconstructions will be helpful to demonstrate focal weak points. With the anatomic characteristics of spinal cord vessels taken into consideration, the safest vessels via which an embolization can be performed are the

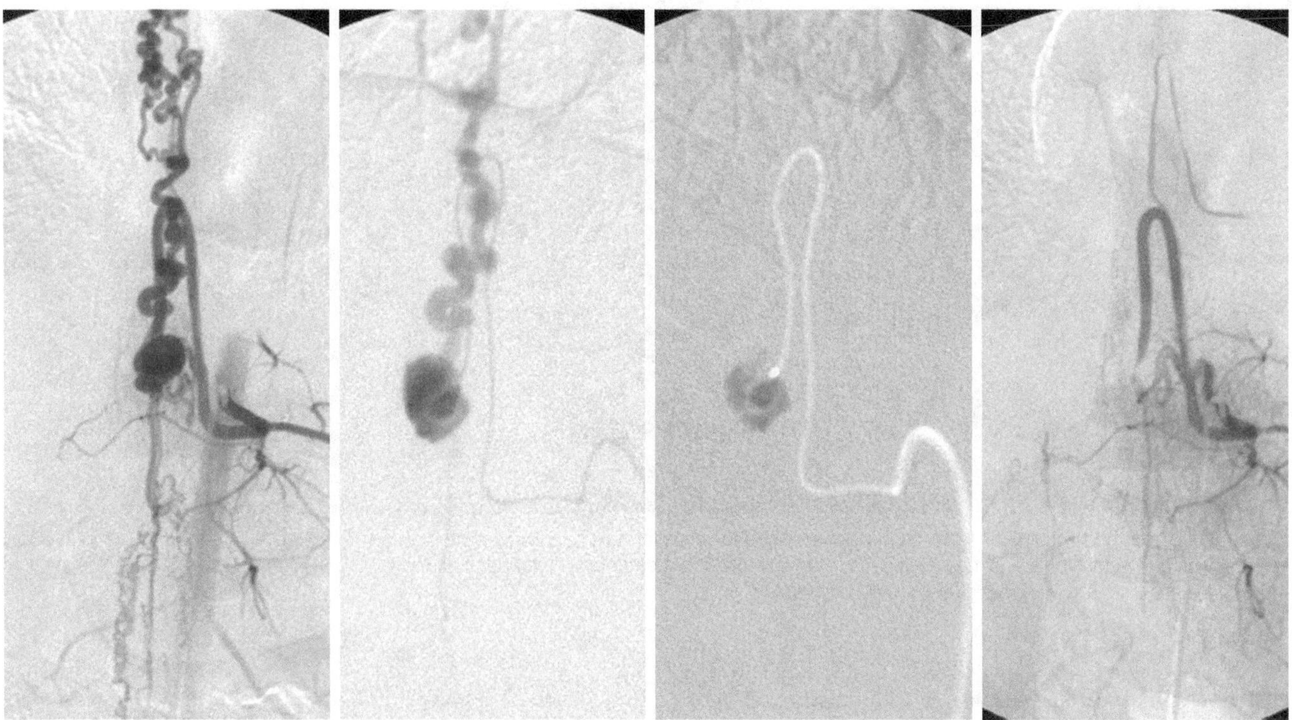

Figure 67-9. This fistulous arteriovenous malformation was characterized by a venous pouch at the transition from the anterior spinal artery to the vein. After selective microcatheterization and glue deposition, the fistula could be completely obliterated with preservation of the anterior spinal artery.

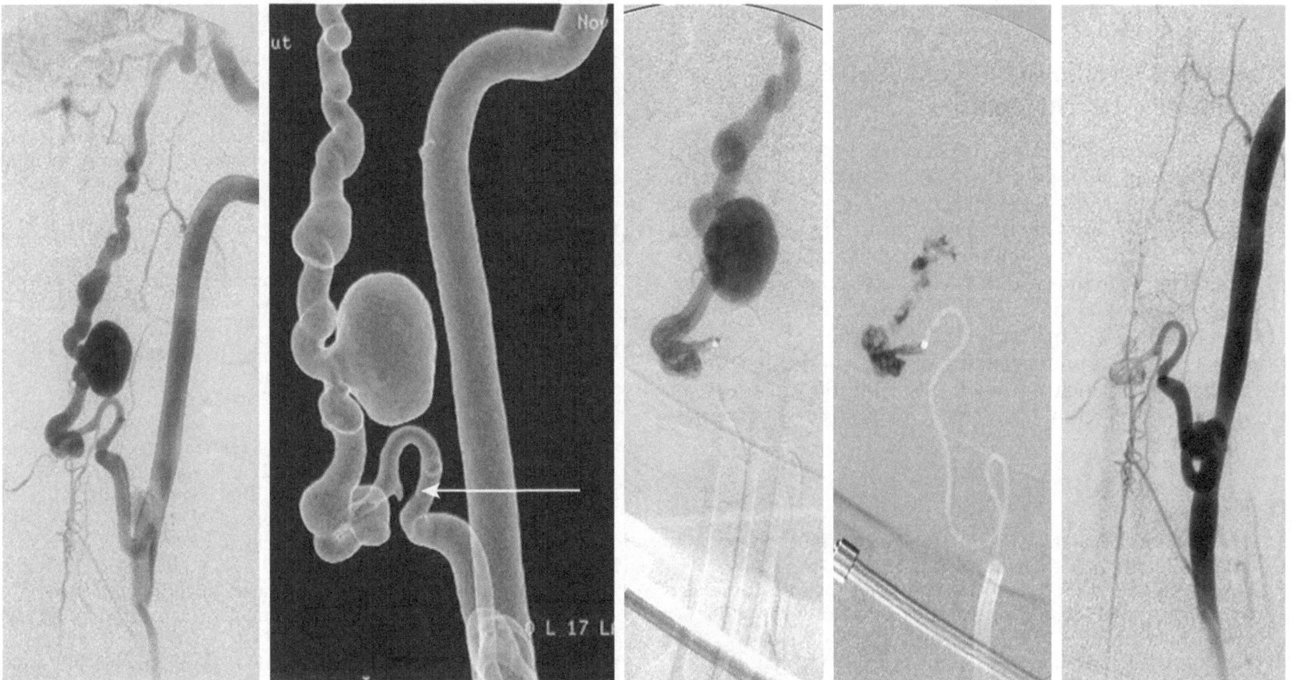

Figure 67-10. Treatment of a microfistula with glue. In this patient, the transition between artery and vein is depicted by the sudden onset of increase in diameter. In addition, the 3D reconstruction demonstrates the further course of the normal anterior spinal artery network *(arrow)*, thereby demonstrating the security margin and the aim of treatment.

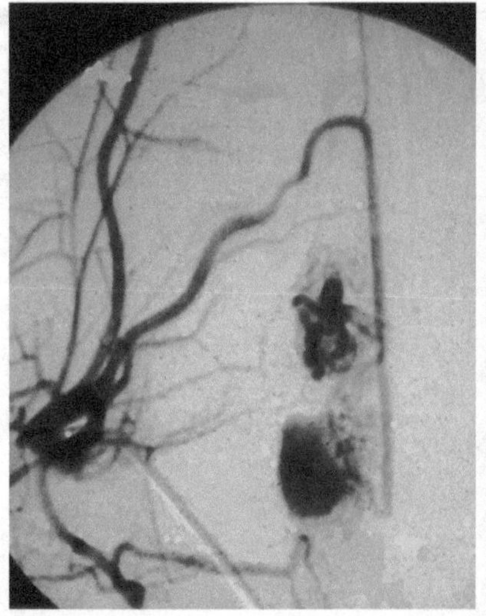
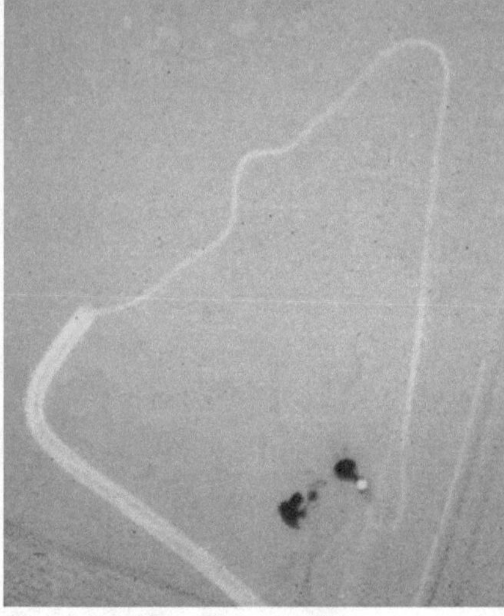
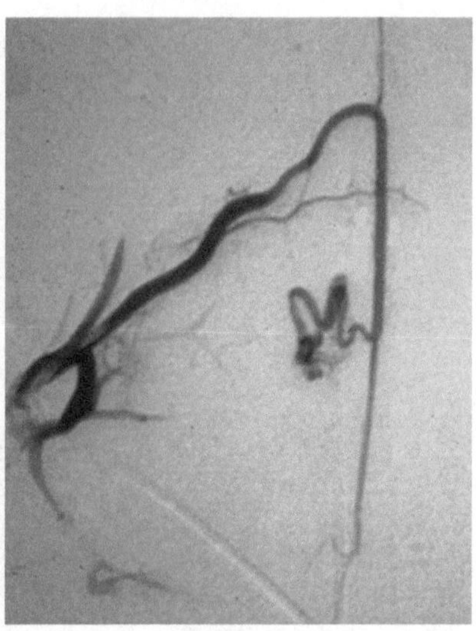

Figure 67-11. In the lower part of this glomerular arteriovenous malformation, a large false aneurysm can be identified with contrast agent stagnation in the venous phase of the arteriogram. After superselective catheterization and glue deposition, the site of bleeding could be secured with preservation of the remainder of the spinal cord vessels.

posterior spinal ones.[41] Because of the vast anastomotic network, compartments belonging to the anterior spinal artery axis can often be reached by the posterior spinal system as well. In diffuse angiomas (SAMS or juvenile angiomas, Cobb's syndrome), a complete obliteration or resection is almost never possible.[42] In these cases, we again adopt the strategy of a partially targeted embolization to reduce shunting zones and to obliterate potential focal weak points.

Indications for and Contraindications to Endovascular Therapies

As stated in the beginning of this section, a therapy of spinal AVMs improves the prognosis in symptomatic patients, whereas in asymptomatic patients, its use has not been proven. Endovascular therapies are definitely the first line of treatment and should be tailored to the specific individual pathomechanisms and angioarchitectonics. We perceive contraindications to endovascular therapy only in those cases in which a safe catheter position cannot be achieved. The term "safe," however, implies a profound understanding of the angioarchitecture of the spinal cord, which is why, in our opinion, treatment of these rare diseases should be carried out exclusively in specialized centers.

REFERENCES

1. Lasjaunias P. Segmental identity and vulnerability in cerebral arteries. Intervent Neuroradiol 2000;6:113–24.
2. Krings T, Geibprasert S, Luo CB, et al. Segmental neurovascular syndromes in children. Neuroimaging Clin North Am 2007;17: 245–58.
3. Lasjaunias PL, Berenstein A, terBrugge K. Clinical vascular anatomy and variations. Surgical Neuroangiography, vol. 1. Berlin: Springer; 2001.
4. Graf CJ, Perret GE, Torner JC. Bleeding from cerebral arteriovenous malformations as part of their natural history. J Neurosurg 1983;58:331–7.
5. Crawford PM, West CR, Chadwick DW, et al. Arteriovenous malformations of the brain: Natural history in unoperated patients. J Neurol Neurosurg Psychiatry 1986;49:1–10.
6. Brown RD Jr, Wiebers DO, Forbes G, et al. The natural history of unruptured intracranial arteriovenous malformations. J Neurosurg 1988;68:352–7.
7. Ondra SL, Troupp H, George ED, et al. The natural history of symptomatic arteriovenous malformations of the brain: A 24-year follow-up assessment. J Neurosurg 1990;73:387–91.
8. Mast H, Young WL, Koennecke HC, et al. Risk of spontaneous haemorrhage after diagnosis of cerebral arteriovenous malformation. Lancet 1997;350:1065–8.
9. Krings T, Chng SM, Ozanne A, et al. Hereditary hemorrhagic telangiectasia in children: Endovascular treatment of neurovascular malformations: Results in 31 patients. Neuroradiology 2005;47: 946–54.
10. Alvarez H, Garcia Monaco R, Rodesch G, et al. Vein of Galen aneurysmal malformations. Neuroimaging Clin N Am 2007;17: 189–206.
11. Geibprasert S, Pereira V, Krings T, et al. Hydrocephalus in unruptured brain arteriovenous malformations: Pathomechanical considerations, therapeutic implications and clinical course. J Neurosurg 2009;110:500–7.
12. Monteiro JM, Rosas MJ, Correia AP, et al. Migraine and intracranial vascular malformations. Headache 1993;33:563–5.
13. Alexander MJ, Tolbert ME. Targeting cerebral arteriovenous malformations for minimally invasive therapy. Neurosurgery 2006;59:S178–83, discussion S173–83.
14. Hademenos GJ, Massoud TF. Risk of intracranial arteriovenous malformation rupture due to venous drainage impairment. A theoretical analysis. Stroke 1996;27:1072–83.
15. Mansmann U, Meisel J, Brock M, et al. Factors associated with intracranial hemorrhage in cases of cerebral arteriovenous malformation. Neurosurgery 2000;46:272–9, discussion 279–81.
16. Meisel HJ, Mansmann U, Alvarez H, et al. Effect of partial targeted N-butyl-cyano-acrylate embolization in brain AVM. Acta Neurochir (Wien) 2002;144:879–87, discussion 888.
17. Meisel HJ, Mansmann U, Alvarez H, et al. Cerebral arteriovenous malformations and associated aneurysms: Analysis of 305 cases from a series of 662 patients. Neurosurgery 2000;46: 793–800.
18. Stefani MA, Porter PJ, terBrugge KG, et al. Angioarchitectural factors present in brain arteriovenous malformations associated with hemorrhagic presentation. Stroke 2002;33:920–4.
19. Hofmeister C, Stapf C, Hartmann A, et al. Demographic, morphological, and clinical characteristics of 1289 patients with brain arteriovenous malformation. Stroke 2000;31:1307–10.
20. Krings T, Geibprasert S, Pereira V, et al. Aneurysms. In: Naidich T, editor. Neuroradiology of the brain and spine. New York: Elsevier; 2008.
21. Willinsky R, TerBrugge K, Montanera W, et al. Micro-arteriovenous malformations of the brain: Superselective angiography in diagnosis and treatment. AJNR Am J Neuroradiol 1992;13:325–30.

22. Richling B, Killer M. Endovascular management of patients with cerebral arteriovenous malformations. Neurosurg Clin North Am 2000;11:123–45, ix.
23. Valavanis A, Yasargil MG. The endovascular treatment of brain arteriovenous malformations. Adv Tech Stand Neurosurg 1998; 24:131–214.
24. Yu SC, Chan MS, Lam JM, et al. Complete obliteration of intracranial arteriovenous malformation with endovascular cyanoacrylate embolization: Initial success and rate of permanent cure. AJNR Am J Neuroradiol 2004;25:1139–43.
25. Redekop G, TerBrugge K, Montanera W, et al. Arterial aneurysms associated with cerebral arteriovenous malformations: Classification, incidence, and risk of hemorrhage. J Neurosurg 1998;89: 539–46.
26. Krings T, Ozanne A, Chng SM, et al. Neurovascular phenotypes in hereditary haemorrhagic telangiectasia patients according to age. Review of 50 consecutive patients aged 1 day-60 years. Neuroradiology 2005;47:711–20.
27. Lasjaunias PL, Landrieu P, Rodesch G, et al. Cerebral proliferative angiopathy: Clinical and angiographic description of an entity different from cerebral AVMs. Stroke 2008;39:878–85.
28. Krings T, Mull M, Gilsbach JM, et al. Spinal vascular malformations. Eur Radiol 2005;15:267–78.
29. Thron A. Vascular anatomy of the spinal cord: Neuroradiological investigations and clinical syndromes. Berlin and New York: Springer; 1988.
30. Krings T, Lasjaunias PL, Hans FJ, et al. Imaging in spinal vascular disease. Neuroimaging Clin North Am 2007;17:57–72.
31. Krings T, Mull M, Bostroem A, et al. Spinal epidural arteriovenous fistula with perimedullary drainage. Case report and pathomechanical considerations. J Neurosurg Spine 2006;5:353–8.
32. Rodesch G, Hurth M, Alvarez H, et al. Angio-architecture of spinal cord arteriovenous shunts at presentation. Clinical correlations in adults and children. The Bicetre experience on 155 consecutive patients seen between 1981–1999. Acta Neurochir (Wien) 2004;146:217–26.
33. Ozanne A, Krings T, Facon D, et al. MR diffusion tensor imaging and fiber tracking in spinal cord arteriovenous malformations: A preliminary study. AJNR Am J Neuroradiol 2007;28:1271–9.
34. Rodesch G, Hurth M, Alvarez H, et al. Spinal cord intradural arteriovenous fistulae: Anatomic, clinical, and therapeutic considerations in a series of 32 consecutive patients seen between 1981 and 2000 with emphasis on endovascular therapy. Neurosurgery 2005;57:973–83.
35. Lee YJ, Terbrugge KG, Saliou G, et al. Clinical Features and Outcomes of Spinal Cord Arteriovenous Malformations: Comparison between Nidus and Fistulous-types. Stroke 2014;45(9):2606–12.
36. Kataoka H, Miyamoto S, Nagata I, et al. Venous congestion is a major cause of neurological deterioration in spinal arteriovenous malformations. Neurosurgery 2001;48:1224–9, discussion 1229–30.
37. Rodesch G, Hurth M, Alvarez H, et al. Embolization of spinal cord arteriovenous shunts: Morphological and clinical follow-up and results—review of 69 consecutive cases. Neurosurgery 2003; 53:40–9.
38. Prestigiacomo CJ, Niimi Y, Setton A, et al. Three-dimensional rotational spinal angiography in the evaluation and treatment of vascular malformations. AJNR Am J Neuroradiol 2003;24: 1429–35.
39. Mourier KL, Gobin YP, George B, et al. Intradural perimedullary arteriovenous fistulae: Results of surgical and endovascular treatment in a series of 35 cases. Neurosurgery 1993;32:885–91, discussion 891.
40. Huffmann BC, Spetzger U, Reinges M, et al. Treatment strategies and results in spinal vascular malformations. Neurol Med Chir (Tokyo) 1998;38(Suppl.):231–7.
41. Niimi Y, Berenstein A. Endovascular treatment of spinal vascular malformations. Neurosurg Clin North Am 1999;10:47–71.
42. Spetzler RF, Zabramski JM, Flom RA. Management of juvenile spinal AVMs by embolization and operative excision. Case report. J Neurosurg 1989;70:628–32.

68 Dural Arteriovenous Malformations

Javed Khader Eliyas, Issam A. Awad

KEY POINTS

- Dural arteriovenous malformation (DAVM) consists of pathological shunting within the dural leaflet, with secondary involvement of the cerebral venous circulation.
- The vast majority of these lesions are acquired in nature; with possible causes including trauma, surgery, dural venous thrombosis and hypercoagulability.
- They are often supplied by branches of external carotid circulation and occur in close proximity to dural venous sinuses.
- Venous drainage can be into the dural venous sinuses or the leptomeningeal/cortical vessels or both.
- Retrograde leptomeningeal drainage portends more aggressive behavior, including hemorrhage, focal neurologic deficits, and seizures. There is high risk of rebleeding from DAVMs that have hemorrhaged previously.
- Treatment options include transarterial or transvenous embolization, microsurgical resection and disconnection, and stereotactic radiosurgery.
- Selection of specific treatment modality or combinations of it depends on symptom presentation, lesion location, and the presence or absence of leptomeningeal venous drainage.

INTRODUCTION

Arteriovenous malformations affecting the central nervous system include a number of pathologic entities, all characterized by abnormal arteriovenous shunting. The most prevalent cerebral arteriovenous malformations consist of a nidus of arteriovenous shunting within brain parenchyma, supplied by the intracranial anterior and posterior circulation and lacking a normal capillary bed. Pial fistulas are characterized by a direct, high-flow shunt from a pial artery to an enlarged vein or varix. In contrast, dural arteriovenous malformations (DAVMs) are comprised of arteriovenous shunts within the dural leaflet, fed predominately by pachymeningeal arteries and located near a major venous sinus.[1]

Historically DAVMs have been a confusing entity. This is in part due to multiple names given to them by different groups and the difficulty in separating the primary abnormality, dural arteriovenous shunting, from other secondary changes. Some believe that DAVMs should be more appropriately named dural arteriovenous shunts, dural arteriovenous fistulas, or dural arteriovenous fistulous malformations.[2] The DAVMs are distinguished from other intracranial vascular lesions by their nidus of arteriovenous shunting, housed wholly within the leaflets of the dura mater (Fig. 68-1). They are typically located adjacent to a major dural sinus and their arterial supply originates from dural (meningeal) arteries, pachymeningeal branches of cerebral arteries, and transsosseous dural branches of scalp arteries. Venous drainage occurs through an adjacent dural sinus and/or other dural and leptomeningeal venous channels. While their etiology is controversial, the vast majority of DAVMs appear to be acquired lesions.[3] DAVMs may remain asymptomatic, or can manifest a wide range of symptoms including headache, tinnitus, bruit, cranial neuropathy, seizures, dementia, intracranial hypertension or focal neurologic deficits from venous congestion.[4–8] They may also present with life-threatening intracranial hemorrhage.[9] While it remains difficult to prognosticate, for a given lesion, the location (i.e., cavernous sinus, anterior cranial fossa or tentorial incisura) and pattern of venous drainage (i.e., sinus versus retrograde leptomeningeal venous drainage) clearly influence clinical presentation.[10–12] Lesions that present with hemorrhage are commonly associated with a significantly increased risk for additional morbidity and mortality. While many unruptured DAVMs are best treated expectantly, there are features which identify high-risk lesions and these may be definitively treated using a careful selection of endovascular, surgical and/or radiosurgical techniques.

CLINICAL PRESENTATION

DAVMs comprise 10–15% of cranial vascular malformations; 6% of supratentorial and 35% of infratentorial vascular lesions are dural fistulas.[13] Typical presentation is between 30 and 50 years of age with a female preponderance, but hemorrhage is more common in males.[14] Lesions are often located in proximity to the major sinuses (50% transverse-sigmoid, 15% cavernous, 10% tentorial, 8% superior sagittal). A few DAVMs present early in life, and are thus thought to be congenital. These are usually associated with complex congenital anomalies, rare phakomatoses, or a vein of Galen malformation – a special form of DAVM.[1] In these cases, there is often gross malformation of dural sinuses with atresia of venous outflow in the region of dura mater involved with the DAVM. The vast majority of DAVMs present later in life and are assumed to be acquired.[15,16] Known or suspected etiologic factors include trauma, infection, hypercoagulable state, and neoplasm. The most important aspect of these etiologic factors may be a shared propensity toward sinus thrombosis with a secondary alteration in venous hemodynamics (restricted outflow and venous hypertension) and development of overt shunting within arteriovenous connections that had involuted during development. Arteriovenous shunting is then thought to promote recruitment of pachymeningeal supply from dural, cerebral and scalp arteries, into the pathologic dural leaflets. Eventually, the pathology progresses to involve changes on the venous side of the circulation (including retrograde leptomeningeal venous reflux of arterialized blood).

Clinical manifestations of DAVMs are highly variable and related to the lesion location, arterial supply, and venous drainage. These range from minor symptoms to catastrophic intracranial hemorrhage. Symptoms can be sudden or slowly progressive. The more benign symptoms of pain, tinnitus, or bruit are related to arteriovenous shunting and vascular

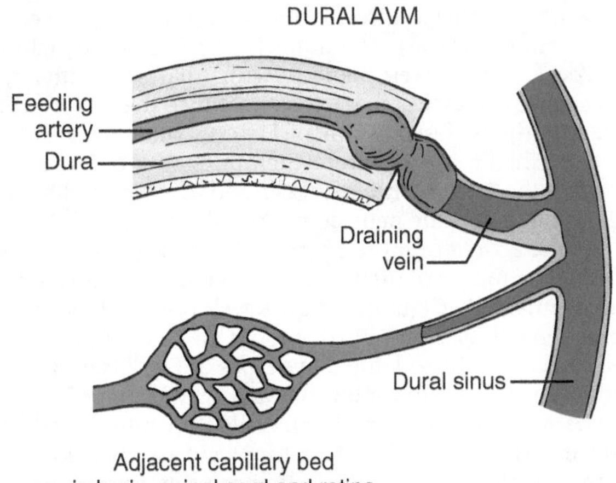

Figure 68-1. Dural arteriovenous malformation (DAVM) schematic. DAVM is comprised of arteriovenous shunts within the dural leaflet, typically supplied predominately by pachymeningeal arteries and located near a major venous sinus. Retrograde leptomeningeal venous drainage is associated with a high risk of hemorrhage.

congestion in the affected dural leaflets and/or adjacent venous sinus. Serious neurological sequelae from DAVMs are associated with retrograde leptomeningeal venous drainage (RLVD).[17] Venous hypertension may cause a myriad of related focal neurologic deficits or seizures (non-hemorrhagic neurologic deficit-NHND), depending on the region of the brain affected.[18–20] Arterialized leptomeningeal veins may become frankly variceal and are prone to hemorrhage. Hemorrhage may also occur within congested brain tissue, again a result of RLVD.

Neuro-ophthalmic manifestations of DAVMs include visual and gaze abnormalities caused by venous hypertension, as well as orbital or ocular venous hypertension with resulting orbital crowding, venous stasis retinopathy and glaucoma. Some cranial DAVMs may present with symptoms of increased intracranial pressure (ICP), including papilledema.[7,21] Headaches associated with DAVMs are multifactorial, often referred from regions of dural congestion, and/or as a result of elevated ICP.

DAVMs may also result in altered cerebrospinal (CSF) hydrodynamics.[6] Dilated venous structures may act as mass lesions, obstructing CSF circulation to cause hydrocephalus. Additionally dural venous hypertension may result in decreased absorption of CSF with secondary intracranial hypertension and papilledema. This phenomenon appears to be more common with high-flow lesions draining into large dural venous sinuses, in the setting of concomitant dural sinus outflow obstruction. Lesions at the anterior cranial fossa or the tentorial incisura rarely drain into a patent dural venous sinus and are more frequently associated with RLVD. They are more likely to cause serious clinical sequelae from RLVD, including focal neurologic deficits and hemorrhage. Hemorrhage in DAVMs has not been reported in the absence of RLVD in any published case, with carefully documented diagnostic studies. Hemorrhage from DAVMs is often associated with rupture of arterialized venous structures in the leptomeningeal circulation. The prognosis of a first hemorrhage from DAVMs is ominous, and is associated with a greater than 30% mortality or serious disability.[22] Hemorrhage from DAVMs in anticoagulated patients can sometimes be fatal.

PATHOPHYSIOLOGY AND LESION EVOLUTION

DAVMs are usually acquired and the exact nature of lesion genesis is frequently unknown.[15,16] It is thought to result from altered angiogenesis within the dura following an inciting event such as thrombosis, trauma, surgery, or chronic infection. It is hypothesized that an initial event precipitates venous sinus thrombosis that leads to opening up of occult arteriovenous vascular channels in the vicinity of the affected sinus. Cases of angiographically proven dural sinus thrombosis in which DAVMs subsequently developed in relation to the obstructed sinus have been documented. Initial microshunts then proliferate, helped by venous hypertension, maturing into clinically significant arteriovenous fistulae. The degree of progression or involution determines the significance of the abnormality. DAVMs cause decreased regional cerebral blood flow in cortical regions where there is RLVD, and this positively predicts the development of hemorrhage, focal neurologic deficits, and/or seizures.[23]

The development of DAVMs following trauma and surgery is well known.[24,25] They have also been reported in association with chronic infection, vascular diseases and tumors, all considered to be related to hypercoagulable state.[26] Many cases of DAVM have no clear etiologic trigger. They may be identified at anatomical sites distinct from the presumed inciting event. It is inferred that development of a DAVM in these diverse settings would probably require a common mechanism, as well as a possible anatomic or genetic predisposition.[27,28] Recent experimental work suggests that the diverse clinical associations of DAVM may be explained by the development of venous obstruction and hypertension with aberrant angiogenesis.[29] This has been confirmed clinically by the reports of fistulas in patients with antithrombin III deficiency or prothrombin gene defects, which render them hypercoagulable.[30,31]

An established DAVM may follow one of several unpredictable natural courses. Some lesions remain asymptomatic or maintain stable clinical symptomatology and angiographic features over many years. Others undergo spontaneous regression, involution and resolution with stabilization or improvement of symptoms.[11,32–34] DAVMs in the region of the cavernous sinus are particularly prone to this phenomenon, with as many as 40% of reported cases having undergone spontaneous involution. In contrast, some DAVMs may demonstrate an increase in size from either arterial or venous enlargement.[1,17] Pachymeningeal arterial feeders may be progressively recruited with enlargement of the nidus. The mechanism behind this recruitment of arterial feeders from numerous sources has not been elucidated. This results in hypertrophy of dural arteries and the re-emergence of involuted embryonic arteries that may not normally be visible in the adult dura mater. In some DAVMs there is also progression of pathology on the venous side. Progressive arterialization of the pathologic dural leaflets results in hypertension in adjacent leptomeningeal venous channels leading to RLVD. Under arterialized pressures, these channels may become tortuous and eventually varicose or aneurysmal, with hemorrhage as the unfortunate result in some patients. In DAVMs that present with intracranial hemorrhage and have retrograde cortical venous drainage, there is a 35% risk of rebleeding within the first 2 weeks.[35]

DIAGNOSTIC IMAGING

Catheter cerebral angiography is the most sensitive and specific diagnostic study for defining DAVMs.[36] In cases of suspected DAVM, the study should include injection of bilateral internal carotid, vertebral and external carotid arteries, as middle meningeal and occipital arteries are principal feeders in many lesions. In cases of suspected clival or foramen magnum region DAVMs, aortic arch injections may reveal additional ascending muscular or pharyngeal arterial feeders. Imaging should capture the very early arterial phase and continue late into the venous phase. Digital subtraction, magnification techniques and the occasional use of superselective angiography greatly enhance the diagnostic potential of angiography. Cerebral angiography provides the spatial diagnostic and dynamic flow information to identify arterial feeders and define in detail the pattern of flow and venous drainage of the DAVM. This information is essential for prognostication and therapeutic decision making.

Other imaging tests may reveal indirect evidence of a DAVM. Imaging with computed tomography (CT) or magnetic resonance (MR) is often performed as part of the initial investigation for presenting neurological symptoms. These studies may reveal thickening of a region of dura mater, tortuosities of leptomeningeal venous drainage or secondary changes reflective of venous hypertension in brain parenchyma. More recently, magnetic resonance angiography (MRA) has been used to detect and follow DAVMs.[37] To maximize the sensitivity of MR, the radiologist should be alerted to the high index of clinical suspicion. At present, these adjuvant diagnostic studies are incapable of totally excluding the presence of a DAVM, and they do not define relevant features of the lesion well enough for prognostic and therapeutic considerations. However, MR imaging and MRA may be used to screen patients with a low clinical suspicion of a DAVM and to follow specific features of DAVMs (i.e., development or enlargement of leptomeningeal venous channels and resolution of venous hypertension), after baseline correlation with angiography. In the setting of strong clinical suspicion, a negative CT or MR should not be used to exclude a DAVM.

LESION CLASSIFICATION

Classification of DAVMs, aimed at prognostication and guiding therapeutic intervention, has evolved over time. Some schemes emphasize the anatomic location (e.g., transverse-sigmoid DAVM, cavernous DAVM, sagittal sinus DAVM) while others focus on drainage pattern. Classification based on location helps define the associated clinical syndrome, but does not fully convey prognostic information or the need and feasibility of therapeutic interventions. Subsequent classifications have incorporated information from diagnostic angiography[38–40] (Table 68-1). The correlation of lesion location, angiographic features and symptoms leads to a clear understanding of clinical behavior, more reliable prognostication, and better planning of therapeutic interventions.

One of the most well-recognized classification schemes specific to DAVMs is that developed by Djindjian et al.[41] This system categorizes a lesion into one of four types: type I DAVMs are characterized by normal antegrade drainage into a venous sinus or meningeal vein; type II lesions drain into a sinus, with reflux into adjacent sinuses or cortical veins; type III DAVMs drain directly into cortical veins with resultant retrograde flow into the cerebral venous compartment; type IV DAVMs have drainage directly into a venous pouch (venous lake or venous ectasia). The authors of the study concluded that type I DAVMs were benign, with each sequential type having more aggressive characteristics. Since the introduction of the Djindjian classification of DAVMs, other studies have been published in the literature attempting to correlate certain features of the DAVM with the likelihood of associated hemorrhage or other specific neurologic complications.[9,12,17,42]

With the advent of more effective endovascular therapeutic techniques, a means of predicting lesion risk and management options emerged. Cognard et al. developed a classification system derived as a modified version of that published by Djindjian et al.[38] They defined five types of DAVMs exclusively based on the pattern of venous outflow. As such, type I DAVMs were characterized by normal antegrade flow into the affected dural sinus (Fig. 68-2). Type II lesions were associated with an abnormal direction of venous drainage within the affected dural sinus (Fig. 68-3). These lesions could be further categorized into three subtypes: type IIa, lesions with retrograde flow exclusively into the sinus or sinuses; type IIb, lesions with retrograde venous drainage into the cortical veins only; and type II a + b, lesions with retrograde drainage into sinuses and cortical veins. Type III DAVMs drained directly into a cortical vein or veins without venous ectasia (Fig. 68-4), whereas type IV DAVMs had drainage into cortical veins with venous ectasia greater than 5 mm in diameter and three times larger than the diameter of the draining vein (Fig. 68-5). A DAVM was considered to be type V when drainage was into spinal perimedullary veins (Fig. 68-6). Correlation with their clinical data yielded the following conclusions: type I DAVMs are considered benign, and treatment is usually not necessary, except possibly for palliation of symptoms; type IIa lesions are best treated with arterial embolization; type IIb and IIa + b lesions usually require both transarterial and transvenous embolization for effective obliteration. For lesions of types III through V, transarterial and occasionally transvenous embolization aimed at complete occlusion of the fistula is necessary and usually will need to be combined with surgical techniques in eliminating the dangerous cortical venous drainage.

Borden et al. proposed a classification system emphasizing venous anatomy.[39,40] This system is appealing in its simplicity, with only three categories. Type I dural AVMs drain directly into dural venous sinuses or pachymeningeal veins. Type II malformations drain into dural sinuses or pachymeningeal veins, but also have retrograde drainage into subarachnoid (leptomeningeal) veins. Type III malformations drain solely into subarachnoid (leptomeningeal) veins and do not have dural sinus or meningeal venous drainage. The prognostic validity of both the Cognard and Borden classification systems were confirmed in 102 intracranial DAVMs in 98 patients.[42]

Current knowledge about natural history of DAVMs with RLVD has dichotomized these categories.[22,43] In a series of 85

TABLE 68-1 Classification of Dural Arteriovenous Malformations

Type	Djindjian	Cognard	Borden
I	Normal antegrade flow into dural sinus	Normal antegrade flow into dural sinus	Drains directly into venous sinus or meningeal vein
II	Drainage into venous sinus with reflux into adjacent sinus or cortical vein	a. Retrograde flow into sinus b. Retrograde filling of cortical veins only c. Retrograde drainage into sinus and cortical veins	Drains into dural sinus or meningeal veins with retrograde drainage into subarachnoid veins
III	Drainage into cortical veins with retrograde flow	Direct drainage into cortical veins with retrograde flow	Drains into subarachnoid veins without dural sinus or meningeal involvement
IV	Drainage into venous pouch (lake)	Direct drainage into cortical veins with venous ectasia >5 mm and 3x larger than diameter of draining vein	
V		Drainage to spinal perimedullary veins	

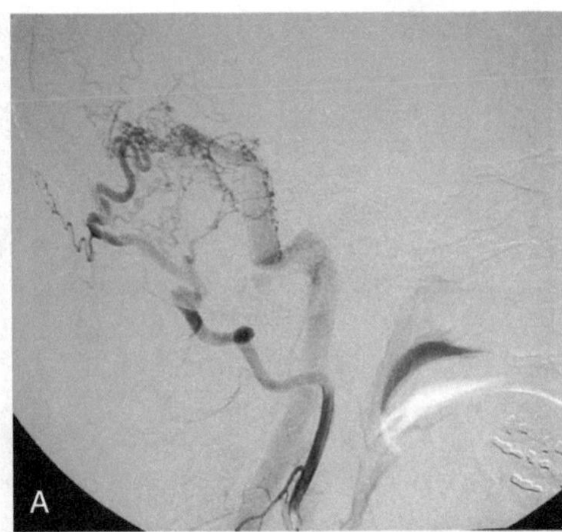

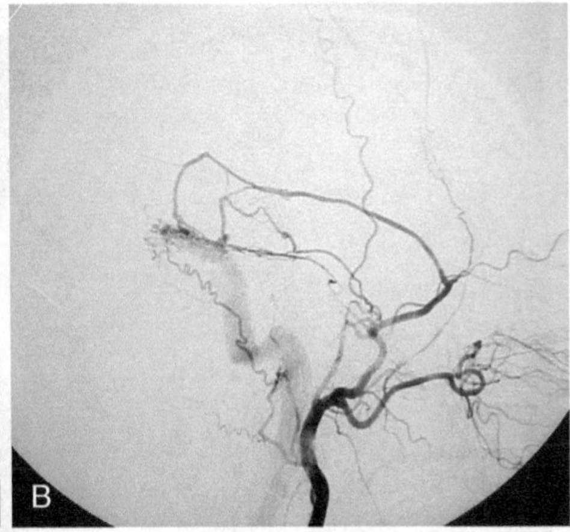

Figure 68-2. Cognard Type I dural arteriovenous malformation: 35-year-old female with new onset bruit behind right ear. Past medical history was notable for head trauma 13 years prior requiring hospitalization. A, Selective injection of right occipital artery (lateral view). There is arterio-venous shunting via numerous small fistula from distal arterial branches to transverse sinus. Venous flow remains antegrade making this a "benign" lesion. B, Selective right external trunk injection (lateral view). Additional fistulae from middle meningeal and posterior auricular arteries.

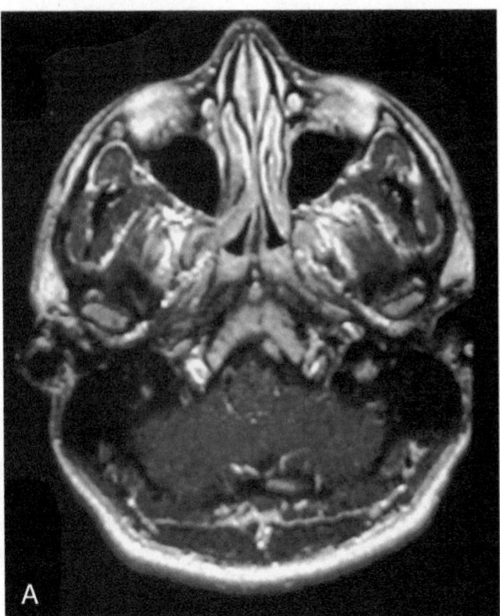

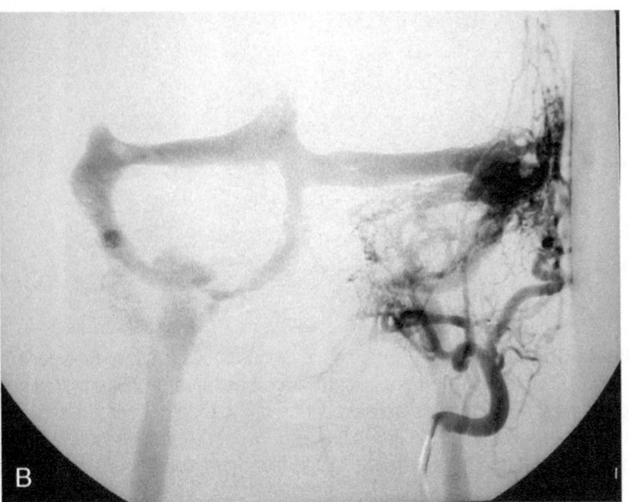

Figure 68-3. Cognard Type II dural arteriovenous malformation: 22-year-old male with new onset of seizures. No past history of head trauma. A, Post contrast T1 axial MR demonstrates increased vascularity along posterior/inferior aspect of cerebellum. B, Left external carotid injection (frontal view). There is prompt venous opacification during the arterial phase. There is retrograde filling of the contralateral sinus across the midline. Contribution is primarily from middle meningeal and posterior auricular branches.

patients with Borden type II and III fistulas, Soderman et al. found the annual risk of hemorrhage in the 32 patients who presented with hemorrhage was 7.4%; while for the remaining 53 who presented without hemorrhage, the risk was only 1.5%.[22] This suggests a higher risk of hemorrhage in patients who have RLVD and have already bled. Gross et al. reported a 10% annual hemorrhage risk and 20% risk of further non-hemorrhagic symptoms in Borden Type II and Type III lesions that presented with non-hemorrhagic symptoms, while those that presented with hemorrhage had a 46% annual hemorrhage risk.[44] Similar results were also noticed by Strom et al., compelling them to conclude that DAVMs with asymptomatic RLVD may have less aggressive behavior than previously thought.[43] Accordingly Zipfel et al. proposed subdividing Borden Type II and Type III into asymptomatic and symptomatic lesions, for more accurate prognostication.[45] This does not imply that lesions with asymptomatic RLVD are benign, but rather portend lesser urgency for intervention as compared to DAVMS with prior hemorrhage or focal neurologic symptoms.

INDICATIONS FOR TREATMENT

Treatment is most often undertaken with the aim of eliminating RLVD, to prevent (further) hemorrhage or (progressive) neurologic deficits. Or it may be considered to alleviate neuro-opthalmic manifestations (including glaucoma, venous stasis retinopathy, ophthalmoplegia, papilledema) and other flow-related symptoms (including disabling pulsatile bruit, tinnitus, or pain). Lesion obliteration can often accomplish both aims, but may not always be possible or justified, hence the occasional selection of palliative interventions. Close

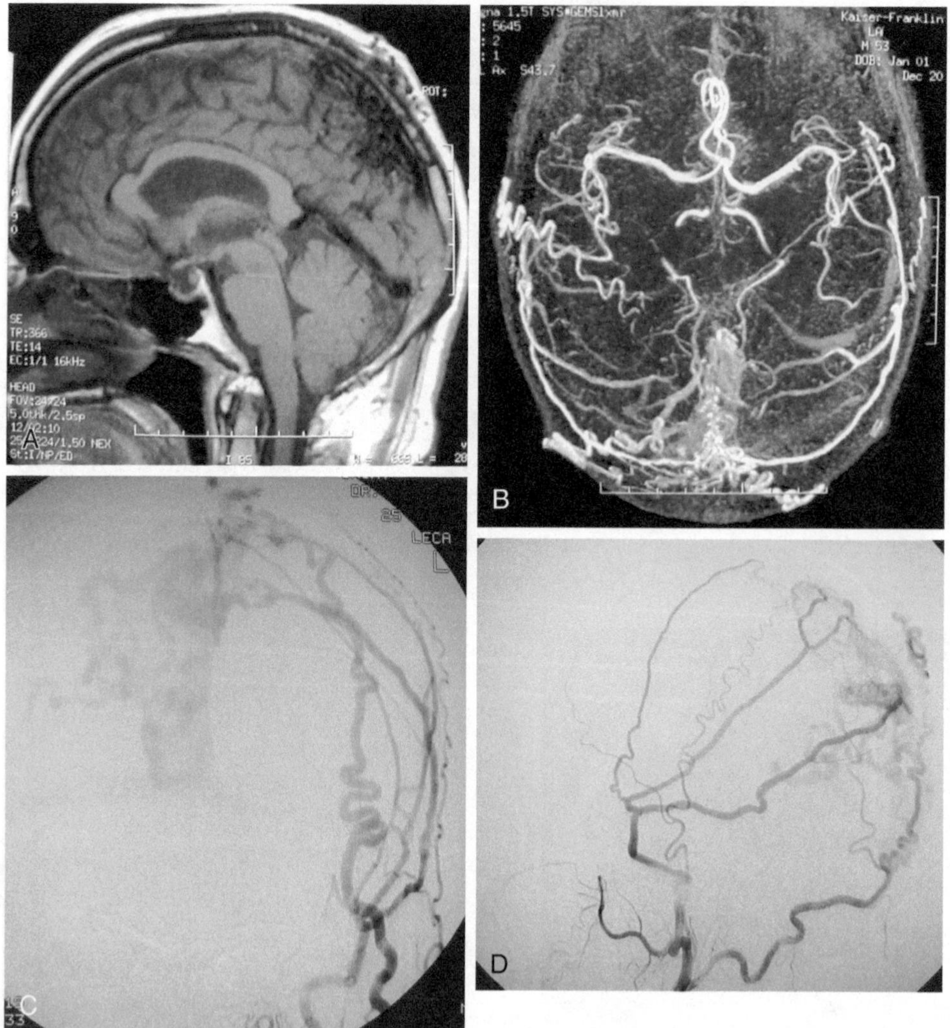

Figure 68-4. Cognard Type III dural arteriovenous malformation: 54-year-old male with new-onset seizure. Patient also noted pulsatile mass on his scalp. A, Sagittal T1 non-contrast MR demonstrates prominent flow voids in the parietal occipital area representing dilated cortical veins. B, Collapsed view MRA. Innumerable branches of the external carotid arteries (bilateral) converge near midline adjacent to sagittal sinus. C and D, Left external carotid injections (frontal, oblique views). Arteriovenous shunting noted with prominent cortical veins to right of midline, and early opacification of right transverse sinus. Contribution from superficial temporal, middle meningeal and occipital arteries.

surveillance of DAVMs is needed in the absence of documented obliteration since a palliated or benign lesion may later progress and develop aggressive features.

The Borden and other classifications emphasize the primary determinant of prospective aggressive neurologic course as the presence of leptomeningeal venous drainage. This sole feature is also the primary determinant of whether therapeutic interventions, with their associated risks, are justifiable. Lesions without significant symptoms and no RLVD can be observed clinically with serial imaging to look for any development of aggressive features.[44,46] In follow-up of 68 patients with Borden Type I or IIa fistula, Satomi and colleagues found only one that developed hemorrhage and by then this patient's lesion had developed RLVD.[46] Lesions with RLVD warrant treatment and cases presenting with clinical symptoms require more urgent intervention.[22,35] Because the clinical presentation and natural history of DAVMs are highly variable, treatment should be individualized based on many factors, including patient age and comorbidities, severity of clinical symptoms and the risk of the proposed treatment.[47]

TREATMENT OPTIONS

There are many patients with non-aggressive lesions who are best managed with symptom palliation. This may include reassurance and counseling, biofeedback and possibly jugular massage.[48] The latter should be used with caution in the elderly who might have coexisting carotid disease or may be vulnerable to vasovagal syncope. Patients with dull aching pain or bothersome pulsatile tinnitus may benefit from non-steroidal anti-inflammatory agents, carbamazepine for tic-like pain or short courses of corticosteroids, which may be particularly effective for retro-orbital discomfort. Patients with DAVMs and tic douloureux should not be treated by percutaneous methods involving puncture of the foramen ovale, since it may result in catastrophic hemorrhage. Once it is decided that a patient with a particular DAVM will benefit from intervention, careful consideration of the available options is required. This includes evaluation of surgery, endovascular techniques, and radiosurgery, alone or in combination, as possible treatment options. Multidisciplinary management

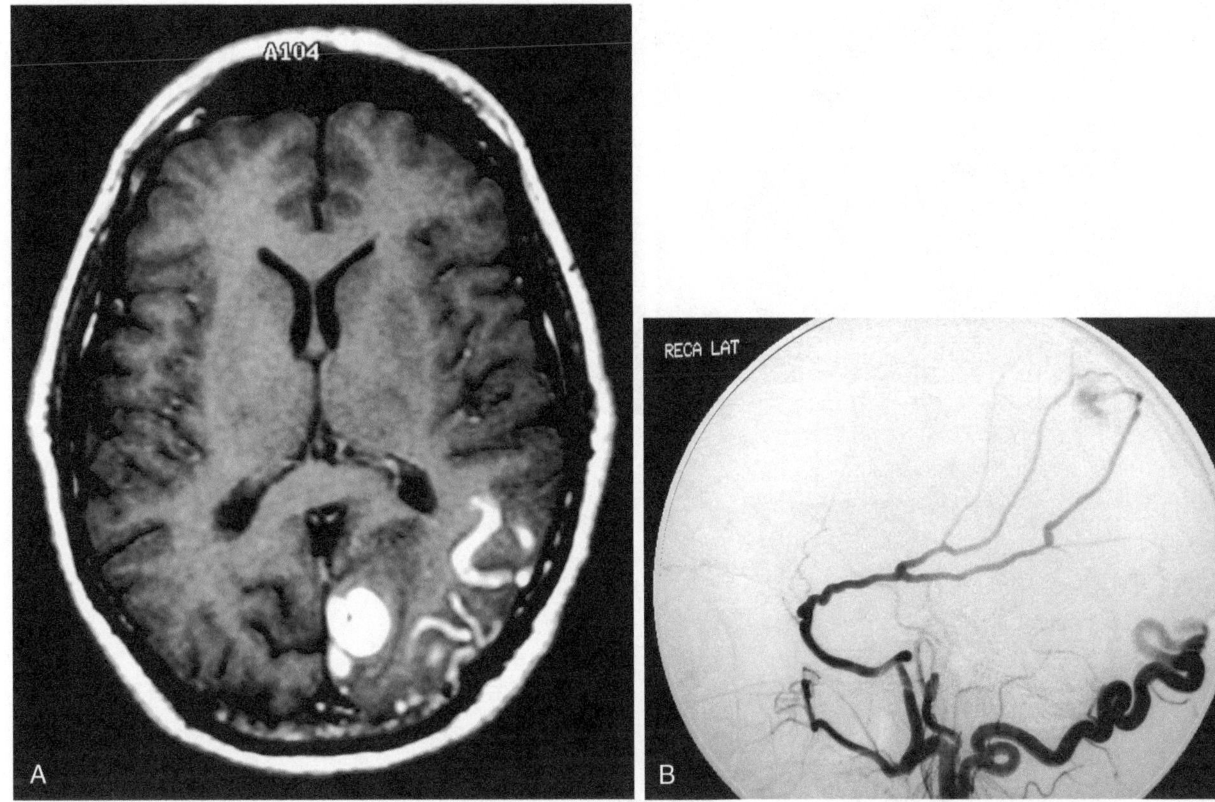

Figure 68-5. Cognard Type IV dural arteriovenous malformation: 57-year-old male who was noted by his family to have personality changes. Patient related intermittent visual changes. A, Axial T1 MR demonstrates prominent cortical veins. High signal represents slow flow status. Note venous varix (pouch) posteriorly adjacent to falx. B, Right external carotid injection (early, late arterial phase). Markedly dilated middle meningeal and occipital arteries. There is early venous opacification with dilated venous varix.

helps define treatment objectives and ensures that the most effective and least risky interventions are chosen, alone or in combination.

Endovascular Techniques

A variety of endovascular techniques are applicable to DAVMs. Unlike the more common brain arteriovenous malformations, DAVMs can be accessed through trans-arterial, trans-venous approaches and sometimes in combined fashion. The presence of small but multiple arterial feeders from external and internal carotid and vertebral artery territories may limit the effectiveness of transarterial embolization toward angiographic cure, unless the fistulous communications are penetrated with embolic material, casting them toward the venous side of the lesion.[49,50,51]

Transarterial embolization has been widely used in the treatment of DAVMs.[1,52,53] The use of flow-guided catheters increased experience with particle, glue and liquid embolic materials and the control of polymerization time has greatly improved the safety and efficacy of this technique.[49,54,55,56] Angiographic cure or significant improvement with transarterial embolization can be accomplished in as many as 70% of DAVMs.[57,58] However, transarterial embolization alone may not succeed in totally eliminating and curing many DAVM, due to multiplicity of feeders and latent recruitment of new feeding arteries following treatment when some fistulous venous channels are left untouched. It may, nevertheless, be quite useful in palliating symptoms and in preparing lesions for curative surgical disconnection.[59-61] Also, palliative transarterial embolization may be useful in conjunction with radiosurgery to the pathologic leaflet, combining the effects toward lesional cure.[56,62]

Arterial embolization may give a false sense of security that the lesion was "treated" while the DAVM may progress to acquire more aggressive features, including leptomeningeal venous drainage (even in the absence of recurrent symptoms). DAVMs that are followed expectantly or treated palliatively should be monitored closely with serial diagnostic studies to watch for the development of RLVD, which may occur without change in clinical symptoms. Non-invasive imaging methods including MRI and MRA may be used for interval studies; although these modalities may miss subtle development of leptomeningeal venous drainage, which may be clinically catastrophic. Depending on the clinical situation and the particular lesion, serial MR studies may be performed on a yearly basis, with formal angiography every few years, or sooner if symptoms change or if there is a suggestion of new leptomeningeal venous drainage on MRI. Even lesions apparently cured with liquid embolic agents have been shown to recanalize (Fig. 68-7), including potentially catastrophic bleeding.[63] Hence, even apparently obliterated lesions with transarterial embolization should be followed with late confirmatory angiogram, after a few months, to confirm effective cure.

Transvenous endovascular obliteration of DAVMs has been used with good results.[64-66] This modality aims at the thrombosis of the venous side of the lesion, often obliterating adjacent dural venous sinus. Occluding the venous side of DAVMs is usually well tolerated if the pathologic dural sinus is arterialized and does not serve as a site of drainage of cerebrovenous circulation (Fig. 68-8). The pathologic dural segment is often associated with harmful RLVD and these

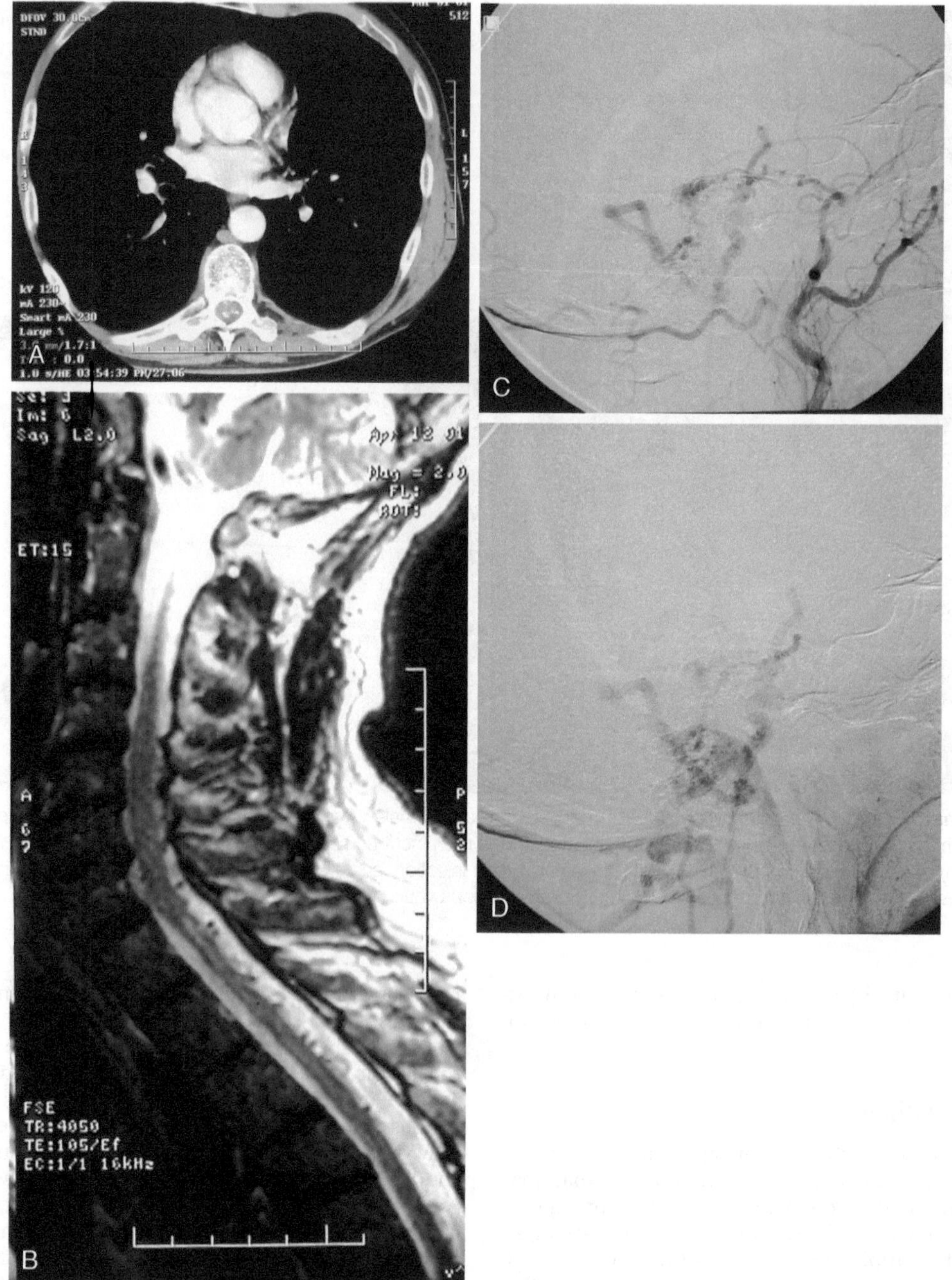

Figure 68-6. Cognard Type V dural arteriovenous malformation: 59-year-old female with multisystem disease including chronic obstructive pulmonary disease. She had unexplained progressive difficulty with ambulation. Chest CT was obtained for pulmonary evaluation. A, Post-contrast CT chest (axial view). There is incidentally noted abnormal vascular enhancement within the spinal canal. B, Sagittal T2 MR image of the cervical spine. Prominent flow voids are seen dorsal to the spinal cord. These represent prominent venous channels. C and D, Left external carotid injection (lateral view). There is early opacification of venous outflow toward spinal perimedullary veins (C: early image; D: delayed image).

channels are secondarily obliterated with thrombosis of the venous side of DAVMs. Transvenous obliteration is particularly effective in the treatment of cavernous sinus DAVMs (access through the inferior petrosal sinus) though in some cases additional transarterial embolization may be necessary.[57] In one series of 28 patients with cavernous sinus lesions, 25 had durable cure with tranvenous coiling through inferior petrosal sinus.[67] In some cases, access to cavernous sinus may be achieved through endovascular or open access of the superior ophthalmic veins.[68,69]

Transvenous obliteration has also been used for transverse-sigmoid sinus DAVMs, and may be substantially safer than open surgical approaches to these lesions.[70] It is important to confirm the retrograde nature of vein of Labbe flow, as occluding a tranverse-sigmoid sinus receiving flow from this vital vein will be detrimental.[50] However, there may be no accessible transvenous route for many DAVMs, including tentorial incisura DAVMs and anterior cranial fossa DAVMs, which frequently behave aggressively. Transvenous obliteration may occasionally be performed after open surgical exposure, through puncture of the dural venous sinus or the arterialized venous varix and the injection of coils or glue.[71] Rarely, transvenous occlusion may result in propagating venous thrombosis or altered hemodynamic patterns with paradoxical clinical

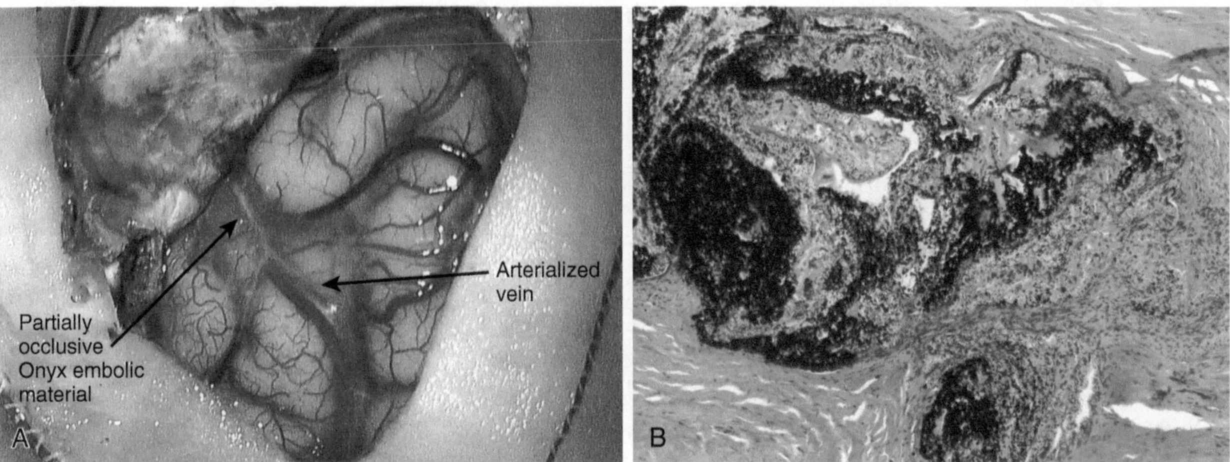

Figure 68-7. Recurrent dural arteriovenous malformation (DAVM) after transarterial embolization. A, Middle-aged man with a history of prior malignancy presented with left temporal intracerebral hemorrhage. A DAVM involving the middle meningeal artery and cortical vein (RLVD) was identified, and readily obliterated by Onyx embolization. This included verification of "casting of the venous side" of the fistula, and absent filling of DAVM on extracranial and intracranial and selective angiographic injections. He did well clinically, except for the development of focal seizures, which responded to medical therapy. At routine follow-up angiography, the DAVM had recurred, including arteriovenous shunting into the cortical vein (RLVD). At surgery, the arterialized cortical vein (arrow) was disconnected, and the DAVM dural leaflet was resected. B, Histopathology of the resected dural leaflet revealed reconstituted vascular channels around the cast of Onyx embolic material (black).

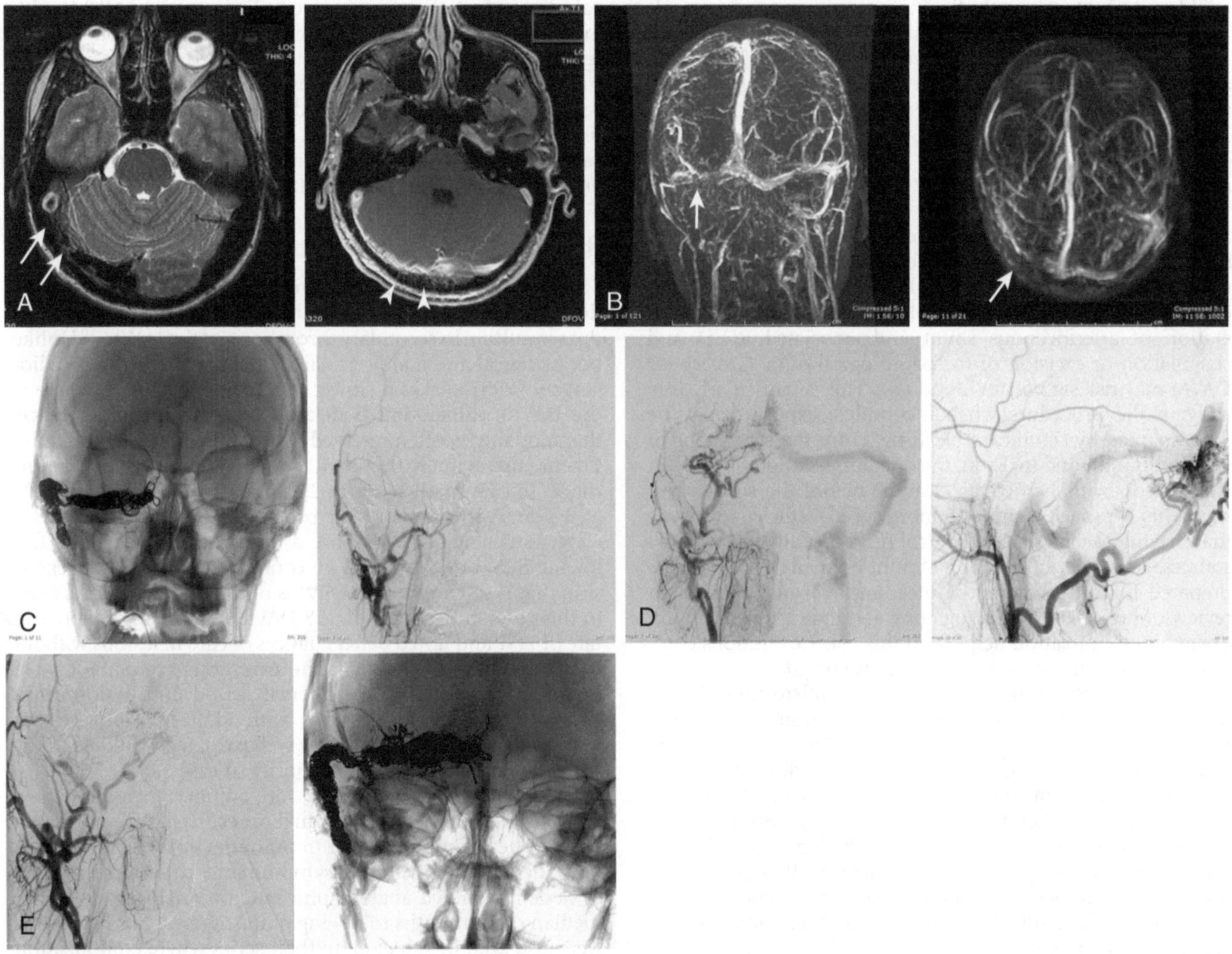

Figure 68-8. Recurrent dural arteriovenous malformation after transvenous coiling. A 29-year-old woman presented with progressive headaches and visual difficulty. A, Axial T2 *(left)* shows abnormal flow void in right transverse and sigmoid sinus *(arrows)*. Postcontrast T1 *(right)* shows abnormal enhancement along the margin of the right transverse sinus *(arrowheads)* indicating the site of fistulous connections. B, Magnetic resonance venogram (MRV) shows lack of normal flow signal in the right transverse sinus, and prominent vasculature adjacent to the sinus *(arrows)*. C, Transvenous approach for treatment. Conventional coil packing of the right transverse/sigmoid sinus with platinum coils *(left)*. External carotid angiogram *(right)* confirms obliteration of shunting. D, Follow-up angiogram at 6 months reveals recurrent fistulas with brisk arterial supply from the right occipital artery (selective right external injection). E, Right external carotid angiogram after transarterial embolization of occipital artery with Onyx *(left)*. Spot film *(right)* reveals density of coils in transverse/sigmoid sinus and Onyx within arterial feeders from the occipital artery.

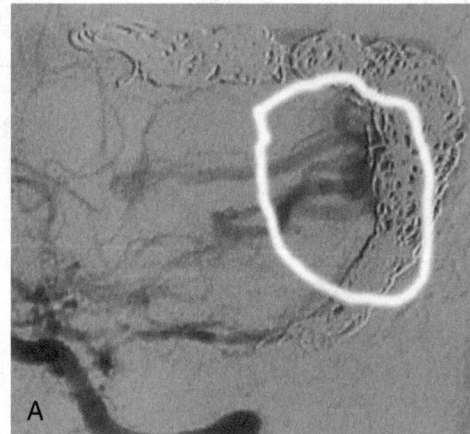

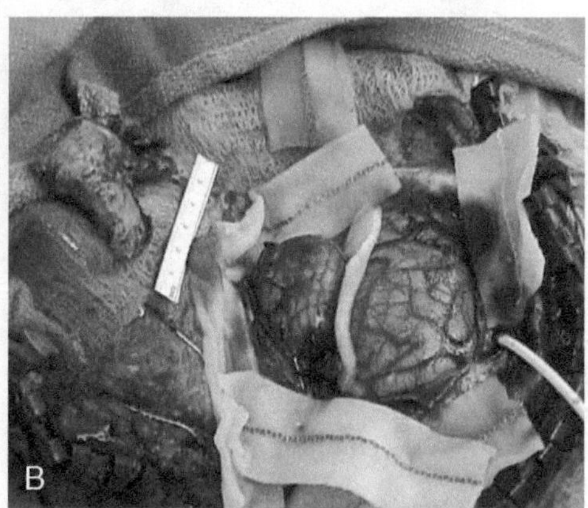

Figure 68-9. Surgical treatment of recurrent dural arteriovenous malformation (DAVM): A, 48-year-old male whose symptoms recurred 2 years following endovascular treatment of his DAVM. The angiogram demonstrates reconstitution of arteriovenous channels within the walls of the previously occluded sinus. B, Surgical excision of the segment of occluded sinus with disconnection of associated arterialized leptomeningeal veins resulted in cure.

deterioration or hemorrhage. Occasionally, a DAVM can recur adjacent to endovascularly occluded venous sinus, and this could represent reconstitution of arteriovenous channels within the walls of the occluded sinus (Fig. 68-8), or recanalization of organized thrombus within the sinus. These cases are amenable to surgical excision of the segment of occluded sinus and disconnection of associated arterialized leptomeningeal veins (Fig. 68-9).

Microsurgical Treatment

Specific situations requiring surgical intervention include persistent RLVD or DAVM recurrence after endovascular therapy or lesions without safe endovascular access. The goals of surgical treatment of DAVMs include physical interruption or obliteration of arteriovenous shunt and associated RLVD and coagulation or excision of the pathological dura. Surgery for DAVM may risk significant blood loss. This is particularly true early in the procedure when incomplete exposure may be accompanied by significant bleeding. From the early steps of skin infiltration and incision, the operation should proceed in small steps, with hemostatic control before the subsequent step. This approach is, indeed, more speedy, efficient and safe than having to take time to control brisk bleeding from many sources. As a rule, no incision should be made unless one is prepared to control potential bleeding from it. A thorough review of pre-operative angiography and judicious use of preoperative embolization helps limit this risk. Continuous communication with the anesthesia team is critical.

Meticulous attention to hemostasis and microsurgical technique is imperative throughout the procedure.[54] Following identification, resection of the abnormal dura is aided by the irrigating bipolar. Small permanent vascular clips in tandem, alternated with dural transection may be useful. Temporary aneurysm clips are helpful in decision making prior to coagulation and sectioning of variceal veins, which may significantly impact adjacent cortical venous circulation. It is sometimes possible to identify discrete arteriovenous connections whose occlusion significantly decreases surrounding subarachnoid venous engorgement.

Direct puncture of large varices with intra-operative placement of obliterating coils has been used successfully.[71] A combination of coils and glue after obtaining access by craniotomy and direct sinus puncture has also been reported.[72] Resection of the dural sinus can be accomplished without the risk of venous infarction if the resected segment is arterialized and collateral channels are well developed.[73] In some cases, surgical clipping of the draining vein close to the DAVM, with extensive dural coagulation rather than resection may be preferred.[74] Utilization of presigmoid skull base exposures has made many inaccessible petrosal and sigmoid lesions currently accessible.[75] Image-guided frameless navigation is useful for flap design and localization of DAVMs or associated cortical venous drainage. Intra-operative angiography helps to ensure complete resection in difficult cases.

Radiosurgical Treatment

The goal of radiosurgical treatment is sclerosis and obliteration of arteriovenous connections within the pathological dura, resulting in secondary thrombosis of the DAVM.[76] Unlike both surgical and endovascular modalities, stereotactic radiosurgery (SRS) evokes a slower therapeutic response, whereby the DAVM obliteration is delayed by many months. Hence, this modality is often reserved for lesions that do not require urgent cure, namely those without RLVD or previous hemorrhage. In one small series of 22 patients cure rates were 51% at 3 years with Kaplan-Meir projection of 80% at 5 years.[77] Cavernous sinus DAVMs have a higher obliteration rate following SRS, but this could be confounded by natural regression that is so common in DAVMs of this region.[77] Gross et al. in their literature review of 558 DAVMs found an obliteration rate of 71% and noted better chances of cure in lesions without RLVD and those located in the cavernous region.[78] Risk of hemorrhage persists in the interval period until lesion obliteration, particularly in lesions with RLVD.[78,79] Flow-related DAVM symptoms are frequently well palliated by radiosurgery (tinnitus, chemosis), in the majority of cases.[77,80]

Radiosurgery also serves as an adjunct, especially post embolization, if there is a residual or recurrent disease. In one series, when combined with transarterial embolization, 95% of patients demonstrated symptomatic improvement and 87% demonstrated angiographic cure on angiography after a median of 12 months following radiosurgery.[81] Similar results were also seen by Oh et al. in their series where embolization combined with SRS, reporting an DAVM cure rate of 83%.[62] Radiosurgery alone can be effective when the DAVM is not amenable to embolization, but the time course for symptomatic improvement is longer. DAVMs of the transverse-sigmoid sinuses treated with a similar strategy yielded a symptom

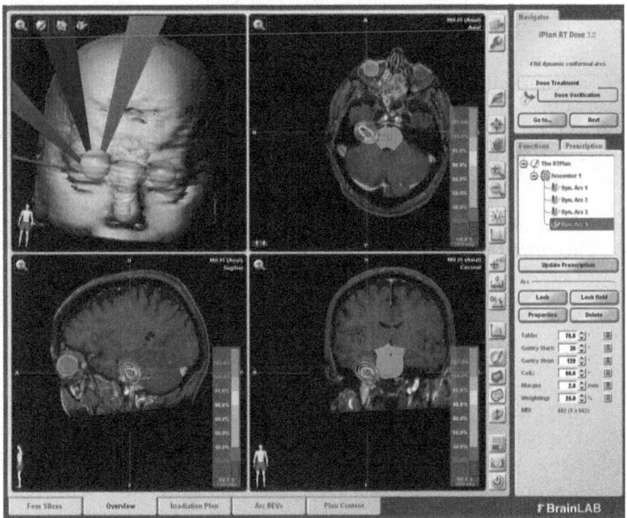

Figure 68-10. Radiosurgery for dural arteriovenous malformation (DAVM). Radiosurgical targeting of a petrous apex DAVM, presenting with disabling tinnitus and pulsatile bruit, but without retrograde leptomeningeal venous drainage. The target was defined to include the pathologic dural leaflet at the petrous apex, and dosimetry was 16 Gy to the 90% isodose line at the target margin. Symptoms gradually resolved after 6 months of treatment, and lesion obliteration was confirmed by angiography after 2 years.

resolution or significant improvement in 96% of patients and total or near-total obliteration in 65% of follow up angiography at a mean of 21 months following radiosurgery.[60] Complications such as hemorrhage, proptosis, worsening chemosis, hearing loss, NHND and cranial nerve palsies can occur after SRS, but are infrequent and often transient.[82,83] Other complications of radiosurgery, including radionecrosis in adjacent brain, may lead to seizures or focal neurologic deficits many months or years after treatment, even long after the DAVM has been successfully obliterated. While the ideal treatment parameters and ultimate role of radiosurgery continue to evolve, it has an established role in the multimodality treatment of DAVMs (Fig. 68-10).

COMPREHENSIVE MANAGEMENT STRATEGY

A DAVM may be discovered on routine imaging studies for associated symptoms, or performed for other indications. Incidental lesions must be carefully assessed for features predisposing to aggressive clinical behavior. Complete angiographic evaluation is indicated in every case of suspected DAVM unless the patient is a poor candidate for therapeutic intervention. Lesions should be evaluated specifically for the presence of RLVD and for any variceal or aneurysmal changes in the venous circulation. In the absence of these features, the lesion should be followed expectantly. There is no evidence to justify the risks of prophylactic interventions for asymptomatic DAVMs that are not associated with RLVD. Expectant follow-up of these lesions can involve serial MR imaging for any evidence of development of leptomeningeal venous dilations, while digital subtraction angiography may be reserved for new, or a change in, symptoms, or to clarify a suspected change on non-invasive imaging. Angiographic re-examination of the lesion every few years should be considered, especially for DAVMs at the anterior cranial fossa or the tentorial incisura, which very commonly develop RLVD, although lesions in all locations may develop this unfavorable feature.

Definitive prophylactic treatment should be considered for asymptomatic and incidentally discovered DAVMs with RLVD and must aim at complete lesion obliteration, including the elimination of RLVD. The specific location of the lesion, classification, type of symptoms and patient fitness should dictate the choice of intervention either alone or in combination. If treatment does not succeed at totally eliminating RLVD, further definitive therapy or very close follow-up of the lesion is indicated. Not all cases of dural sinus thrombosis are associated with DAVMs and invasive angiography may not be needed in such a setting unless clinical symptoms or signs (such as an audible bruit or pulsatile tinnitus) and/or features of MRI (prominent pachymeningeal arteries or venous channels around occluded sinus) suggest an associated fistula. As many cases of sinus thrombosis are treated with anticoagulation, there should be a high index of suspicion in this regard and formal catheter angiography should be performed in cases where the above-mentioned peculiarities are present. If a DAVM with RLVD is detected anticoagulation should be withheld and prompt intervention considered to obliterate the DAVM, or at least eliminate, associated RLVD. It is our belief that anticoagulation is contraindicated in the setting of DAVMs with leptomeningeal venous drainage.

There is no controversy in recommending a definitive intervention for DAVMs that have already behaved aggressively. Nevertheless, the morbidity of a first hemorrhage with DAVMs is substantial, and many patients do not survive or recover to a condition suitable for therapeutic intervention. There are numerous documented cases of progression of focal neurological symptoms resulting in death or major disability unless the DAVM is obliterated. It is our recommendation that lesions that have hemorrhaged or that cause focal neurological symptoms due to parenchymal venous hypertension be considered for urgent and definitive treatment. Palliative therapy is not sufficient in this setting.

Lesions that present with pain or pulsatile tinnitus are evaluated and treated in the same way as incidental lesions. Non-specific measures aimed at the symptoms are usually sufficient in the absence of RLVD. Some cases with bothersome symptoms interfering with patient's life but without RLVD may be considered for palliative treatment (to decrease flow and control intolerable pain or bruit or to treat progressive glaucoma and other sequels of cavernous sinus DAVM). Obviously the choice of treatment must be accompanied by a clear articulation of inherent risk of individual therapeutic modality and its justification. Treatment risk varies with different procedures; open microsurgery carries the highest general risk while endovascular techniques are less risky. These risks need to be weighed in each individual case independently with respect to specific location and features of the lesion, general fitness of the patient and other indications of intervention. Rarely is definitive treatment indicated solely for pain or pulsatile tinnitus. We do not believe that the risk of definitive treatment is justified in such DAVMs if they do not exhibit RLVD. Lesions associated with ophthalmoplegia need to be evaluated on a case-by-case basis. Frequently, painful ophthalmoplegia will resolve spontaneously, and many such lesions involute after angiography. In other cases, ophthalmoplegia may be progressive or associated with retinopathy and visual loss. In such situations, treatment of the associated DAVM is essential. Palliative treatment may be sufficient to stabilize visual symptoms. Again, a radical cure of the DAVM should not be pursued at any risk, and is generally not warranted unless symptoms are truly debilitating or the DAVM is associated with RLVD.

Lesions associated with intracranial hypertension and papilledema require special consideration. Palliation or definitive cure of the DAVM frequently (but not always) results in reversal of papilledema and stabilization of visual symptoms. In other instances, the risks of definitively treating the DAVM may not be justified. Intracranial hypertension may be treated by lumboperitoneal shunting. Ventriculoperitoneal shunting may not be possible in view of small cerebral ventricles, and may be dangerous in the setting of arterialized cortical or subependymal veins. Optic nerve sheath decompression has also been used in cases of progressive papilledema and inoperable DAVMs. Cerebrospinal fluid diversion or optic nerve sheath decompression may be combined with transarterial embolization and/or radiosurgery in the management of some lesions. Transvenous occlusion is rarely possible in this setting, as it may further compromise intracranial venous outflow.

In summary, clinical symptoms other than hemorrhage and neurological deficits rarely warrant radical treatment of a DAVM, unless the lesion is particularly accessible or is associated with features predisposing to subsequent aggressive clinical behavior. Patient reassurance, symptomatic treatment, or lesion palliation are frequently sufficient. In DAVMs with features predisposing to an aggressive clinical course, a more definitive treatment strategy should be adopted. It is obvious that the myriad of clinical manifestations of DAVMs and the wide spectrum of possible angiographic and pathophysiologic scenarios call for highly individualized management strategies. Diagnostic investigation should be thorough so as to identify DAVMs with features predisposing to aggressive clinical behavior. Treatment strategies should include a highly individualized choice of modalities from the available armamentarium of symptomatic treatment, lesion palliation, transarterial and/or transvenous endovascular therapy, open surgical invention, and radiosurgery. The treatment of DAVMs should preferably be entrusted to multidisciplinary teams with expertise in the recognition and management of these lesions, and with experience in a variety of treatment options and approaches. Finally, one should not lose sight of potential risk factors predisposing to the development of DAVMs. Often, a DAVM is the first clinical sign of occult malignancy, or hypercoagulable state. A vigilant stance and screening for these potential conditions is warranted, in addition to addressing the DAVM proper.

SUMMARY

Much has been learned in recent years about the pathoanatomy, pathophysiology, natural history, and therapeutic options for DAVMs. A better understanding of these lesions has allowed precise diagnosis, and a realistic assessment of features predisposing to an aggressive clinical course. Treatment is not only guided toward the palliation of clinical symptoms but also toward prevention of future sequelae. The therapeutic armamentarium includes a number of options with varying risk and effectiveness in individual lesions. Embolization, either transarterial or transvenous, microsurgical therapy and radiosurgery can be used alone or in various combinations as required for individual clinical scenarios.

REFERENCES

1. Lasjaunias P, Lopez-Ibor L, Abanou A, et al. Radiological anatomy of the vascularization of cranial dural arteriovenous malformations. Anat Clin 1984;6:87–99.
2. Awad IA, Barrow DL, editors. Dural arteriovenous malformations. Park Ridge, Illinois: American Association of Neurological Surgeons; 1993. p. xi–xii.
3. Lasjaunias P, Berenstein A. Surgical neuroangiography II: endovascular treatment of craniofacial lesions. New York: Springer-Verlag; 1987.
4. Aminoff MJ, Kendall BE. Asymptomatic dural vascular anomalies. Br J Radiol 1973;46:662–7.
5. Fermand M, Reizine D, Melki JP, et al. Long term follow-up of 43 pure dural arteriovenous fistulae (AVF) of the lateral sinus. Neuroradiology 1987;29:348–53.
6. Gelwan MJ, Choi IS, Berenstein A, et al. Dural arteriovenous malformations and papilledema. Neurosurgery 1988;22:1079–84.
7. Chimowitz MI, Little JR, Awad IA, et al. Intracranial hypertension associated with unruptured cerebral arteriovenous malformations. Ann Neurol 1990;27:474–9.
8. Hurst RW, Bagley LJ, Galetta S, et al. Dementia resulting from dural arteriovenous fistulas: the pathologic findings of venous hypertensive encephalopathy. AJNR Am J Neuroradiol 1998;19: 1267–73.
9. Malik GM, Pearce JE, Ausman JI, et al. Dural arteriovenous malformations and intracranial hemorrhage. Neurosurgery 1984;15: 332–9.
10. Barnwell SL, Halbach VV, Dowd CF, et al. A variant of arteriovenous fistulas within the wall of dural sinuses. Results of combined surgical and endovascular therapy. J Neurosurg 1991;74: 199–204.
11. Bitoh S, Sakaki S. Spontaneous cure of dural arteriovenous malformation in the posterior fossa. Surg Neurol 1979;12(2): 111–14.
12. Lasjaunias P, Chiu M, ter Brugge K, et al. Neurological manifestations of intracranial dural arteriovenous malformations. J Neurosurg 1986;64(5):724–30.
13. Chaichana KL, Coon AL, Tamargo RJ, et al. Dural arteriovenous fistulas: epidemiology and clinical presentation. Neurosurg Clin N Am 2012;23(1):7–13.
14. Singh V, Smith WS, Lawton MT, et al. Risk factors for hemorrhagic presentation in patients with dural arteriovenous fistulae. Neurosurgery 2008;62(3):628–35, discussion 628–35.
15. Chaudhary MY, Sachdev VP, Cho SH, et al. Dural arteriovenous malformation of the major venous sinuses: an acquired lesion. AJNR Am J Neuroradiol 1982;3(1):13–19.
16. Houser OW, Campbell JK, Campbell RJ, et al. Arteriovenous malformation affecting the transverse dural venous sinus–an acquired lesion. Mayo Clin Proc 1979;54(10):651–61.
17. Awad IA, Little JR, Akarawi WP, et al. Intracranial dural arteriovenous malformations: factors predisposing to an aggressive neurological course. J Neurosurg 1990;72(6):839–50.
18. Kim MS, Oh CW, Han DH, et al. Intraosseous dural arteriovenous fistula of the skull base associated with hearing loss. Case report. J Neurosurg 2002;96(5):952–5.
19. Rizzo M, Bosch EP, Gross CE. Trigeminal sensory neuropathy due to dural external carotid cavernous sinus fistula. Neurology 1982;32(1):89–91.
20. Willinsky R, Goyal M, terBrugge K, et al. Tortuous, engorged pial veins in intracranial dural arteriovenous fistulas: correlations with presentation, location, and MR findings in 122 patients. AJNR Am J Neuroradiol 1999;20(6):1031–6.
21. Cognard C, Casasco A, Toevi M, et al. Dural arteriovenous fistulas as a cause of intracranial hypertension due to impairment of cranial venous outflow. J Neurol Neurosurg Psychiatry 1998; 65(3):308–16.
22. Soderman M, Pavic L, Edner G, et al. Natural history of dural arteriovenous shunts. Stroke 2008;39(6):1735–9.
23. Iwama T, Hashimoto N, Takagi Y, et al. Hemodynamic and metabolic disturbances in patients with intracranial dural arteriovenous fistulas: positron emission tomography evaluation before and after treatment. J Neurosurg 1997;86(5):806–11.
24. Ishikawa T, Houkin K, Tokuda K, et al. Development of anterior cranial fossa dural arteriovenous malformation following head trauma. Case report. J Neurosurg 1997;86(2):291–3.
25. Nabors MW, Azzam CJ, Albanna FJ, et al. Delayed postoperative dural arteriovenous malformations. Report of two cases. J Neurosurg 1987;66(5):768–72.
26. Yokota M, Tani E, Maeda Y, et al. Meningioma in sigmoid sinus groove associated with dural arteriovenous malformation: case report. Neurosurgery 1993;33(2):316–19, discussion 319.
27. Yassari R, Jahromi B, Macdonald R. Dural arteriovenous fistula after craniotomy for pilocytic astrocytoma in a patient with protein S deficiency. Surg Neurol 2002;58(1):59–64, discussion 64.
28. Singh V, Meyers PM, Halbach VH, et al. Dural arteriovenous fistula associated with prothrombin gene mutation. J Neuroimaging 2001;11(3):319–21.

29. Lawton MT, Jacobowitz R, Spetzler RF. Redefined role of angiogenesis in the pathogenesis of dural arteriovenous malformations. J Neurosurg 1997;87(2):267–74.
30. Saito A, Takahashi N, Furuno Y, et al. Multiple isolated sinus dural arteriovenous fistulas associated with antithrombin III deficiency – case report. Neurol Med Chir (Tokyo) 2008;48(10): 455–9.
31. Orina JN, Daniels DJ, Lanzino G. Familial intracranial dural arteriovenous fistulas. Neurosurgery 2013;72(2):E310–13, discussion E313.
32. Magidson MA, Weinberg PE. Spontaneous closure of a dural arteriovenous malformation. Surg Neurol 1976;6(2):107–10.
33. Olutola PS, Eliam M, Molot M, et al. Spontaneous regression of a dural arteriovenous malformation. Neurosurgery 1983;12(6): 687–90.
34. Hansen JH, Sogaard I. Spontaneous regression of an extra- and intracranial arteriovenous malformation. Case report. J Neurosurg 1976;45(3):338–41.
35. Duffau H, Lopes M, Janosevic V, et al. Early rebleeding from intracranial dural arteriovenous fistulas: report of 20 cases and review of the literature. J Neurosurg 1999;90(1):78–84.
36. Hu WY, TerBrugge KG. The role of angiography in the evaluation of vascular and neoplastic disease in the external carotid artery circulation. Neuroimaging Clin N Am 1996;6(3):625–44.
37. Ikawa F, Uozumi T, Kiya K, et al. Diagnosis of carotid-cavernous fistulas with magnetic resonance angiography – demonstrating the draining veins utilizing 3-D time-of-flight and 3-D phase-contrast techniques. Neurosurg Rev 1996;19(1):7–12.
38. Cognard C, Gobin YP, Pierot L, et al. Cerebral dural arteriovenous fistulas: clinical and angiographic correlation with a revised classification of venous drainage. Radiology 1995;194(3):671–80.
39. Borden JA, Wu JK, Shucart WA. A proposed classification for spinal and cranial dural arteriovenous fistulous malformations and implications for treatment. J Neurosurg 1995;82(2): 166–79.
40. Borden JA, Wu JK, Shucart WA. Correction: dural arteriovenous fistulous malformations. J Neurosurg 1995;82(4):705–6.
41. Djindjian R, Merland JJ, Theron J, editors. Superselective arteriography of the external carotid artery. New York: Springer-Verlag; 1977.
42. Davies MA, TerBrugge K, Willinsky R, et al. The validity of classification for the clinical presentation of intracranial dural arteriovenous fistulas. J Neurosurg 1996;85(5):830–7.
43. Strom RG, Botros JA, Refai D, et al. Cranial dural arteriovenous fistulae: asymptomatic cortical venous drainage portends less aggressive clinical course. Neurosurgery 2009;64(2):241–7, discussion 247–8.
44. Gross BA, Du R. The natural history of cerebral dural arteriovenous fistulae. Neurosurgery 2012;71(3):594–602, discussion 602–3.
45. Zipfel GJ, Shah MN, Refai D, et al. Cranial dural arteriovenous fistulas: modification of angiographic classification scales based on new natural history data. Neurosurg Focus 2009;26(5):E14.
46. Satomi J, van Dijk JM, Terbrugge KG, et al. Benign cranial dural arteriovenous fistulas: outcome of conservative management based on the natural history of the lesion. J Neurosurg 2002;97(4): 767–70.
47. van Dijk JM, terBrugge KG, Willinsky RA, et al. Clinical course of cranial dural arteriovenous fistulas with long-term persistent cortical venous reflux. Stroke 2002;33(5):1233–6.
48. Halbach VV, Higashida RT, Hieshima GB, et al. Dural fistulas involving the cavernous sinus: results of treatment in 30 patients. Radiology 1987;163(2):437–42.
49. Rabinov JD, Yoo AJ, Ogilvy CS, et al. ONYX versus n-BCA for embolization of cranial dural arteriovenous fistulas. J Neurointerv Surg 2012.
50. Radvany MG, Gregg L. Endovascular treatment of cranial arteriovenous malformations and dural arteriovenous fistulas. Neurosurg Clin N Am 2012;23(1):123–31.
51. Andreou A, Ioannidis I, Nasis N. Transarterial balloon-assisted glue embolization of high-flow arteriovenous fistulas. Neuroradiology 2008;50(3):267–72.
52. Hardy RW, Costin JA, Weinstein M, et al. External carotid cavernous fistula treated by transfemoral embolization. Surg Neurol 1978;9(4):255–6.
53. Vinuela FV, Debrun GM, Fox AJ, et al. Detachable calibrated-leak balloon for superselective angiography and embolization of dural arteriovenous malformations. J Neurosurg 1983;58(6):817–23.
54. Liu JK, Dogan A, Ellegala DB, et al. The role of surgery for high-grade intracranial dural arteriovenous fistulas: importance of obliteration of venous outflow. J Neurosurg 2009;110(5): 913–20.
55. Nesbit GM, Barnwell SL. The use of electrolytically detachable coils in treating high-flow arteriovenous fistulas. AJNR Am J Neuroradiol 1998;19(8):1565–9.
56. Hu YC, Newman CB, Dashti SR, et al. Cranial dural arteriovenous fistula: transarterial Onyx embolization experience and technical nuances. J Neurointerv Surg 2011;3(1):5–13.
57. Cha KC, Yeon JY, Kim GH, et al. Clinical and angiographic results of patients with dural arteriovenous fistula. J Clin Neurosci 2013; 20(4):536–42.
58. Lv X, Jiang C, Li Y, et al. Embolization of intracranial dural arteriovenous fistulas with Onyx-18. Eur J Radiol 2010;73(3): 664–71.
59. Goto K, Sidipratomo P, Ogata N, et al. Combining endovascular and neurosurgical treatments of high-risk dural arteriovenous fistulas in the lateral sinus and the confluence of the sinuses. J Neurosurg 1999;90(2):289–99.
60. Friedman JA, Pollock BE, Nichols DA, et al. Results of combined stereotactic radiosurgery and transarterial embolization for dural arteriovenous fistulas of the transverse and sigmoid sinuses. J Neurosurg 2001;94(6):886–91.
61. Collice M, D'Aliberti G, Arena O, et al. Surgical treatment of intracranial dural arteriovenous fistulae: role of venous drainage. Neurosurgery 2000;47(1):56–66, discussion 66–7.
62. Oh JT, Chung SY, Lanzino G, et al. Intracranial dural arteriovenous fistulas: clinical characteristics and management based on location and hemodynamics. J Cerebrovasc Endovasc Neurosurg 2012;14(3):192–202.
63. Adamczyk P, Amar AP, Mack WJ, et al. Recurrence of "cured" dural arteriovenous fistulas after Onyx embolization. Neurosurg Focus 2012;32(5):E12.
64. Halbach VV, Higashida RT, Hieshima GB, et al. Transvenous embolization of dural fistulas involving the cavernous sinus. AJNR Am J Neuroradiol 1989;10(2):377–83.
65. Roy D, Raymond J. The role of transvenous embolization in the treatment of intracranial dural arteriovenous fistulas. Neurosurgery 1997;40(6):1133–41, discussion 1141–4.
66. Lv X, Jiang C, Li Y, et al. Percutaneous transvenous packing of cavernous sinus with Onyx for cavernous dural arteriovenous fistula. Eur J Radiol 2009;71(2):356–62.
67. He HW, Jiang CH, Wu ZX, et al. Transvenous embolization of cavernous dural arteriovenous fistula: report of 28 cases. Chin Med J (Engl) 2007;120(24):2229–32.
68. Yu Sc, Fau – Cheng HKM, Cheng HK, et al. Transvenous embolization of dural carotid-cavernous fistulae with transfacial catheterization through the superior ophthalmic vein. Neurosurgery 2007;60:1032–7.
69. Klisch J, Huppertz HJ, Spetzger U, et al. Transvenous treatment of carotid cavernous and dural arteriovenous fistulae: results for 31 patients and review of the literature. Neurosurgery 2003;53: 836–56.
70. Wong GK, Poon WS, Yu SC, et al. Transvenous embolization for dural transverse sinus fistulas with occluded sigmoid sinus. Acta Neurochir (Wien) 2007;149:929–35.
71. Endo S, Kuwayama N, Takaku A, et al. Direct packing of the isolated sinus in patients with dural arteriovenous fistulas of the transverse-sigmoid sinus. J Neurosurg 1998;88(3):449–56.
72. Houdart E, Saint-Maurice JP, Chapot R, et al. Transcranial approach for venous embolization of dural arteriovenous fistulas. J Neurosurg 2002;97(2):280–6.
73. Sundt TM Jr, Piepgras DG. The surgical approach to arteriovenous malformations of the lateral and sigmoid dural sinuses. J Neurosurg 1983;59(1):32–9.
74. Hoh BL, Choudhri TF, Connolly ES Jr, et al. Surgical management of high-grade intracranial dural arteriovenous fistulas: leptomeningeal venous disruption without nidus excision. Neurosurgery 1998;42(4):796–804, discussion 804–5.
75. Kattner KA, Roth TC, Giannotta SL. Cranial base approaches for the surgical treatment of aggressive posterior fossa dural

arteriovenous fistulae with leptomeningeal drainage: report of four technical cases. Neurosurgery 2002;50(5):1156–60, discussion 1160–1.
76. See AP, Raza S, Tamargo RJ, et al. Stereotactic radiosurgery of cranial arteriovenous malformations and dural arteriovenous fistulas. Neurosurg Clin N Am 2012;23(1):133–46.
77. Hanakita S, Koga T, Shin M, et al. Role of Gamma Knife surgery in the treatment of intracranial dural arteriovenous fistulas. J Neurosurg 2012;117(Suppl.):158–63.
78. Gross BA, Ropper AE, Popp AJ, et al. Stereotactic radiosurgery for cerebral dural arteriovenous fistulas. Neurosurg Focus 2012; 32(5):E18.
79. Cifarelli CP, Kaptain G, Yen CP, et al. Gamma knife radiosurgery for dural arteriovenous fistulas. Neurosurgery 2010;67(5):1230–5, discussion 1235.
80. Pan DH, Chung WY, Guo WY, et al. Stereotactic radiosurgery for the treatment of dural arteriovenous fistulas involving the transverse-sigmoid sinus. J Neurosurg 2002;96(5):823–9.
81. Pollock BE, Nichols DA, Garrity JA, et al. Stereotactic radiosurgery and particulate embolization for cavernous sinus dural arteriovenous fistulae. Neurosurgery 1999;45(3):459–66, discussion 466–7.
82. Yang HC, Kano H, Kondziolka D, et al. Stereotactic radiosurgery with or without embolization for intracranial dural arteriovenous fistulas. Neurosurgery 2010;67(5):1276–83, discussion 1284–5.
83. Wu HM, Pan DH, Chung WY, et al. Gamma Knife surgery for the management of intracranial dural arteriovenous fistulas. J Neurosurg 2006;105(Suppl.):43–51.

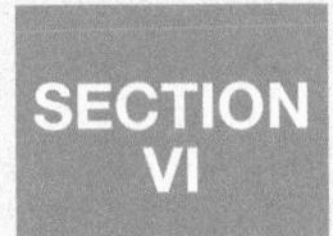

Therapy

PART C Surgical Therapy

A. David Mendelow

The role of cerebrovascular surgery for stroke is rapidly evolving and, therefore, neurosurgeons have to adapt to these changes accordingly. In some countries, neurosurgeons have taken on the tasks of interventional neuroradiologists while in others the two specialties have remained separate. As a result of these changes, there is a decrease in the number of craniotomies for aneurysms, arteriovenous malformations (AVMs), fistulae and bypasses. This will inevitably lead to a "de-skilling" of the neurosurgery workforce. To adjust to this, patients requiring open neurovascular operative procedures and those trainees needing to learn such operative techniques will have to be concentrated in fewer and larger centers.

The chapter on aneurysm surgery by Dannenbaum and colleagues reflects this with accurate details of the precise operative approaches to different ruptured and unruptured aneurysms. The arguments about whether to treat or not and whether to use endovascular approaches or not are not discussed in this chapter in great detail. Suffice it to say that if it is considered better to treat an aneurysm, then usually the endovascular approach will be the one to choose while surgery is reserved for those cases where coiling cannot be undertaken or where technical considerations make them less safe. Such decisions are usually taken by multidisciplinary teams in large centers: in the UK, these larger centers are now using the endovascular approach in more than 90% of cases.

Intraventricular thrombolysis/fibrinolysis or "topical thrombolysis" is a promising therapy that may convert intraventricular hemorrhage (IVH), a condition with a poor prognosis, into one with much more favorable outcomes. J M Findlay refers to the CLEAR III trial that has now completed recruitment of 500 patients with IVH. The results should be known in early 2016 after all the 12-month outcomes are available and analysis has been completed. Although all the prior trials and studies have suggested that IVH is best treated with this form of topical thrombolysis; the CLEAR III trial should provide the class I evidence that is required to set a standard of care. A similar form of topical thrombolysis is being evaluated for intracerebral hemorrhage (ICH) in the MISTIE III trial, which has now recruited its first 100 patients out of the target of 500. This is summarized in the chapter that I have written with Dr Barbara Gregson (statistician) about surgery for ICH.

Spontaneous supratentorial ICH in patients whose Glasgow Coma Scale (GCS) is between 9 and 12 is best treated with early surgery (within 48 hours) according to the meta-analysis that Dr. Gregson has provided. This meta-analysis includes the STICH and STICH II trials where these sub-group analyses were prespecified. It also makes intuitive sense because operating on patients with a GCS of 13 to 15 subjects them to the risks of craniotomy whereas with a policy of watching and waiting, unnecessary craniotomy is avoided, minimizing the risk of the intervention in those patients in whom consciousness is preserved. On the other hand, patients in coma (GCS of 8 or less) have been shown consistently to have worse outcomes with surgery. This use of craniotomy as the surgical intervention also differs from the minimum intervention technique that is used in the MISTIE trials, which may also prove to be more effective in deep-seated hematomas. Cerebellar hematomas are also considered in this chapter but no randomized controlled trials are available. The problem with cerebellar hemorrhage is that it causes obstructive hydrocephalus that has to be treated (often urgently) in its own right. An algorithm is provided that divides patients into the same three levels of consciousness that are intuitive with supratentorial hematomas: those in coma from the outset have poor outcomes, while those that are fully conscious (GCS 13 to 15) can be watched, anticipating the development of hydrocephalus, and those in between (GCS 9 to 12) requiring earlier intervention.

In the chapter by Russin and Spetzler regarding the Surgical Management of Cranial and Spinal Arteriovenous Malformations the Spetzler Martin Grading system and its modifications are discussed. Grade IV and V lesions are less likely to be treated surgically unless there are recurrent hemorrhages. The ARUBA trial of treatment compared to no treatment for unruptured AVMs is discussed critically. ARUBA is not perfect but the best available prospective evidence and it is consistent with the idea that asymptomatic AVMs in older subjects are best treated conservatively. It would, therefore, appear to be better not to treat unruptured AVMs unless they are small, non-eloquent and the patient is young with a long life expectancy. Spinal AVMs are discussed in relation to their location.

Cerebral cavernous malformations (CCMs) have a benign natural history and their pathology and genetic types are now much better understood. Surgery is effective but not usually necessary unless the lesion is in a critical area or has manifested itself with frequent and recurrent hemorrhage. Cerebral venous malformations seldom require surgery. The efficacy of image-guided radiosurgery for these lesions is questioned. El Tecle et al. point out that selected brainstem CCMs can be removed microsurgically with excellent results.

Braca III et al. provide the class I evidence that carotid endarterectomy (CEA) remains the best treatment for tight symptomatic and asymptomatic internal carotid artery stenosis. They describe the many trials that have been conducted over the years and show that CEA is superior to medical treatment alone in preventing ipsilateral stroke. They present a balanced view and meta-analysis that confirms that CEA is superior to stenting for most symptomatic patients. Whether or not CEA remains superior to stenting for asymptomatic patients will not be known until the Asymptomatic Carotid Stenosis Trial (ACST) II has been completed; to date nearly 2000 patients have been randomized but it will be some years before the results of ACST II are known. CEA and stenting are also being evaluated against modern-day intensive medical management in the Carotid Revascularization and Medical Management for Asymptomatic Carotid Stenosis Trial (CREST-2) which is actually two studies of carotid revascularization and intensive medical management versus medical management alone in patients with asymptomatic high-grade carotid stenosis. One trial will randomize patients in a 1:1 ratio to endarterectomy versus no endarterectomy and another will randomize patients in a 1:1 ratio to carotid stenting with embolic protection versus no stenting.

Newell, Vilella and Powers summarize the two main ExtraCranial IntraCranial (ECIC) arterial bypass trials and conclude that the procedure does not reduce subsequent stroke in patients presenting with ischemic symptoms and carotid occlusion with hemodynamic impairment. ECIC bypass is still frequently used to treat patients with moyamoya who have cerebral ischemia, although controlled trials regarding its efficacy for stroke prevention are lacking. ECIC bypass is also still used to augment blood flow to prevent cerebral ischemia with planned vessel occlusion for complex aneurysms or skull base tumors.

Juetler et al. describe the evidence from four relatively small randomized controlled trials for decompressive craniectomy for middle cerebral artery infarction. There is undoubtedly a survival advantage with the procedure, but the very high cost per quality adjusted life year (QALY) must be considered in justifying disabled survival for patients with this type of stroke. At over $100,000 per QALY this procedure, which appears to produce for the most part an increase in Rankin 4 outcomes, is difficult to justify on either an economic or quality of life basis in all but the most affluent societies in our world today. The use of "life-saving" craniotomy for ischemic and hemorrhagic stroke deserves further investigation with the goal of improving the functional state of the survivor and improving our knowledge of costs and benefits.

In conclusion, while endovascular techniques are displacing open surgery in many branches of vascular neurosurgery, CEA appears to remain the best option for tight carotid stenosis. ECIC bypass is still used for patients with moyamoya and when large-vessel occlusion is undertaken. Aneurysm surgery is still needed when endovascular therapy is not possible. The role for surgery in patients with ICH has been partially defined in the 15 trials that have been published to date, but strong class I evidence demonstrating long-term functional improvement is awaited from the CLEAR III and MISTIE III trials before standards of care can be set; hopefully within the next 2–4 years. Rapid evolution in the field of stroke surgery demands rapid adaptation by vascular neurosurgeons who, in the future, will need to be concentrated in fewer and larger centers to maintain excellence.

Acknowledgments

Thanks to Professor D. H. Hanley, Dr. M. Davis, Dr. J. Grotta and Professor R. P. Sengupta for their editorial advice and assistance with this overview.

69 Surgery of Anterior and Posterior Aneurysms

Mark J. Dannenbaum, Matthew R. Fusco, Christopher S. Ogilvy, A. David Mendelow, Arthur L. Day

KEY POINTS

- Endovascular technical methods have advanced the scope for aneurysm treatment, but not all aneurysms can be treated by endovascular means. It is necessary for surgeons, therefore, to continue with the mastery of operative aneurysm treatments and approaches.
- Most intracranial aneurysms occur at arterial branch points; the most common anterior circulation aneurysm locations are the middle cerebral artery bifurcation, anterior communicating artery complex, and the posterior communicating artery while the most common posterior circulation aneurysm location is the basilar apex.
- The majority of anterior circulation aneurysms can be reached through a standard pterional craniotomy with varying degrees of Sylvian fissure splitting. Minimal access techniques via the supra-orbital subfrontal approach allow access to the middle cerebral artery and its aneurysms. Ophthalmic and proximal internal carotid artery (ICA) aneurysms may often require adjunctive cervical carotid exposure and anterior clinoidectomy for complete aneurysm visualization and clipping.
- Distal anterior cerebral artery aneurysms (i.e., pericallosal or callosal-marginal artery aneurysms) are best approached through an interhemispheric approach and thus are the only anterior circulation aneurysms not reachable through a pterional approach.
- Basilar apex bifurcation aneurysms can be reached through multiple surgical corridors; the pterional/trans-Sylvian, anterior subtemporal, or fronto-polar approaches. Choice of which surgical corridor is most appropriate is dictated by surrounding anatomy, particularly the level of the posterior clinoidal processes in relation to the basilar bifurcation.
- Vertebral artery and proximal posterior inferior artery aneurysms are best approached through a far lateral suboccipital craniotomy.

The circle of Willis can be divided into anterior and posterior portions, branches of which supply different regions of the brain (Fig. 69-1). The anterior portion, also known as the anterior circulation, supplies the majority of the cerebrum, and includes the internal carotid artery (ICA), its branches, and its termination into the anterior and middle cerebral arteries. The posterior circulation includes the vertebral and basilar arteries and their branches that supply the brainstem, cerebellum, and occipital lobes via the posterior cerebral arteries.

Aneurysm development typically occurs at points of hemodynamic stress where a bend in the vessel and a branch site coincide.[1] Most intracranial aneurysms are saccular, in that they project from a bifurcation site as a "sac" or pouch in a direction that flow would have continued had a branch point and vessel curve not been present. Saccular aneurysms arise at predictable sites along a vessel (where the branches are), and are usually amenable to clipping or coiling without compromise of the branches and flow around it. In contrast, non-saccular or fusiform aneurysms are generally the result of an arterial dissection, with or without arteriosclerosis, infection, or trauma. This type occurs much more frequently in the vertebrobasilar system than in the anterior circulation. Since the entire vessel circumference is involved in the pathology, these are not usually amenable to simple clipping or coiling strategies. For the purposes herein, this chapter will primarily address saccular aneurysms and their surgical management.

ANTERIOR CIRCULATION (Fig. 69-2)

Currently, the treatment for anterior circulation aneurysms at most centers is divided between open and closed methods. Following subarachnoid hemorrhage, the microvasculature is likely to be more sensitive to microsurgical manipulation required for successful aneurysm obliteration, and the effects of vasospasm may be potentiated. In the unruptured state, however, surgery is especially effective and accurate in completely obliterating most lesions, while endovascular approaches are associated with a significant rate of recanalization or incomplete obliteration (Fig. 69-3). Acute cranial nerve deficits, including visual loss or oculomotor nerve palsies, respond rapidly to surgical decompression. Other lesions still cannot be effectively treated endovascularly without adding stents, a methodology which requires preliminary antiplatelet drugs including Plavix which can raise the bleeding risks associated with ventricular drainage in subarachnoid hemorrhage patients. Others are difficult for endovascular therapy either because of restricted vascular access or because the shape, size, or other anatomic considerations of the aneurysm are not ideal for such methodology.

In such circumstances, microsurgical management is warranted, particularly when performed by surgeons experienced in pterional and skull base approaches. The specifics of this "work-horse" approach for anterior circulation aneurysms, the pterional craniotomy, are demonstrated in Figure 69-4.

Internal Carotid Artery

The subarachnoid portion of the ICA can be divided into four regions which generate aneurysms, including the ophthalmic, communicating, and choroidal segments, as well as the terminal carotid bifurcation. Each region has an

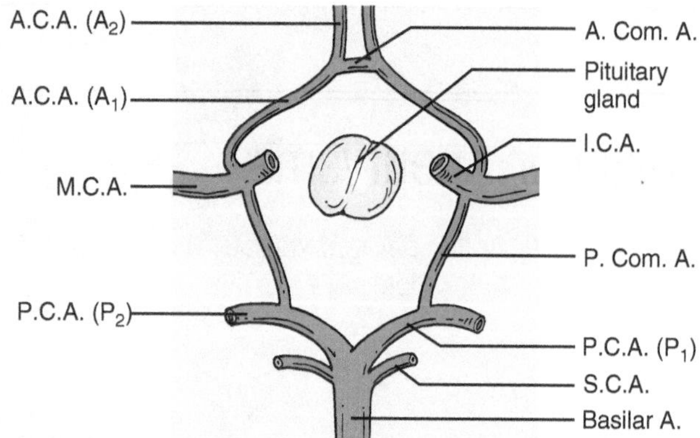

Figure 69-1. The circle of Willis: anterior and posterior circulations.

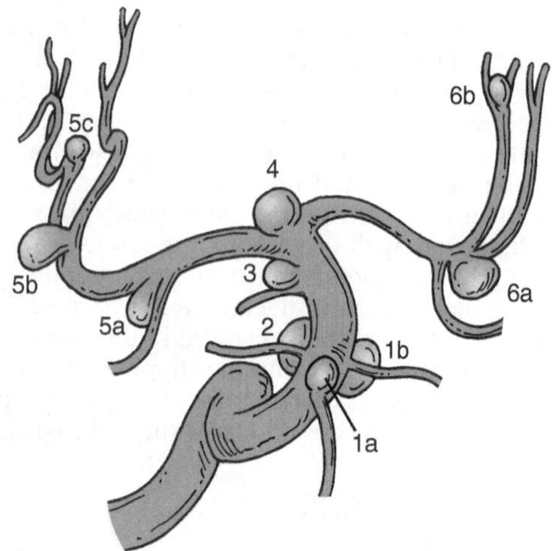

Figure 69-2. Common locations of anterior circulation aneurysms and standard nomenclature. 1a, Opththalmic artery aneurysm. 1b, Superior Hypophyseal artery aneurysm. 2, Posterior communicating artery aneurysm. 3, Anterior choroidal artery aneurysm. 4, ICA bifurcation aneuryusm. 5a, Anterior Temporal artery aneurysm. 5b, Typical MCA bifurcation aneurysm. 5c, M2 segment aneurysm. 6a, Anterior communicating artery aneurysm. 6b, Distal ACA aneurysm (pericallosal/callosomarginal junction).

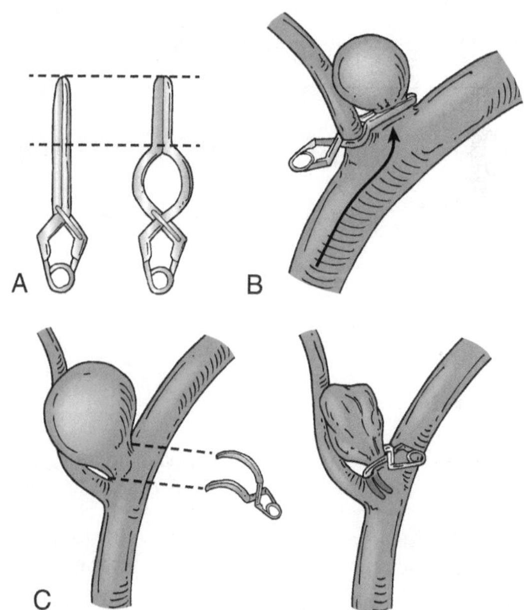

Figure 69-3. Aneurysm clips, general technique. A, Straight and "fenestrated" clips; B, fenestrated clip encircling branch to secure aneurysm neck; C, gently curved clip applied to aneurysm neck, followed by puncture and collapse of the sac; note that the neck of the aneurysm is completely separated from the aneurysm dome, making the risk of regrowth extremely low when applied as illustrated.

origination and intimate association with named ICA branches or perforators.

Ophthalmic Segment Aneurysms (Fig. 69-5)

Anatomy and Terminology. The ophthalmic segment (OphSeg) is typically the longest subarachnoid segment of the ICA, beginning at the dural ring (DR) where the artery penetrates the dura to enter the subarachnoid space, and ending at the origin of the posterior communicating artery. The OphSeg has two major branches, both of which typically originate just above the dural ring. The first, largest, and best known is the ophthalmic artery (OphArt), which provides the majority of blood supply to the ipsilateral optic nerve. It typically arises from the dorsal or dorso-medial surface of the ICA at its first posterior bend, immediately beneath the lateral aspect of the overlying optic nerve. Several perforating vessels also arise from this segment, the largest of which is called the superior hypophyseal artery (SupHypArt). These perforators supply the dura around the cavernous sinus, the superior aspect of the pituitary gland and stalk, and the optic nerves and chiasm. They typically arise from the medial or ventro-medial surface of the OphSeg, usually along the second, medial-to-lateral bend of the ICA prior to the posterior communicating artery origin.

OphSeg aneurysms are divided herein into three types, depending primarily on an association of the aneurysm neck with the arterial branches of the segment:

1. OphArt aneurysms arise from the ICA just distal to the origin of the OphArt, and initially project dorsally or dorso-medially towards the optic nerve.
2. SupHypArt aneurysms have no association with the OphArt, and instead incorporate the medial perforating branches in their origins. Small SupHypArt aneurysms usually arise from the inferior medial surface of the ICA and expand towards the sella dura within a small subarachnoid diverticulum called the carotid cave. Because this medial space is limited, enlarging lesions will eventually expand superomedially above the diaphragma sella into the suprasellar space.
3. Dorsal variant aneurysms are uncommon, and arise from the dorsal aspect of the ICA well distal to and separate from the OphArt origin. Unrelated to any arterial branch point, some are the result of hemodynamic vectors produced by a sharp angulation within the OphSeg. Others appear as "blisters" on the dorsal carotid surface that bleed when small and expand quickly as a fusiform-shaped lesion externally, reflecting a genesis likely representing a dissection.

Clinical and Radiographic Features. Most OphSeg aneurysms arise in women, and their incidence is greatly underestimated because most remain asymptomatic. The low frequency of OphSeg lesions presenting with bleeding when small is probably explained by their reinforcement by adjacent structures such as the overlying optic nerve or parasellar dura.

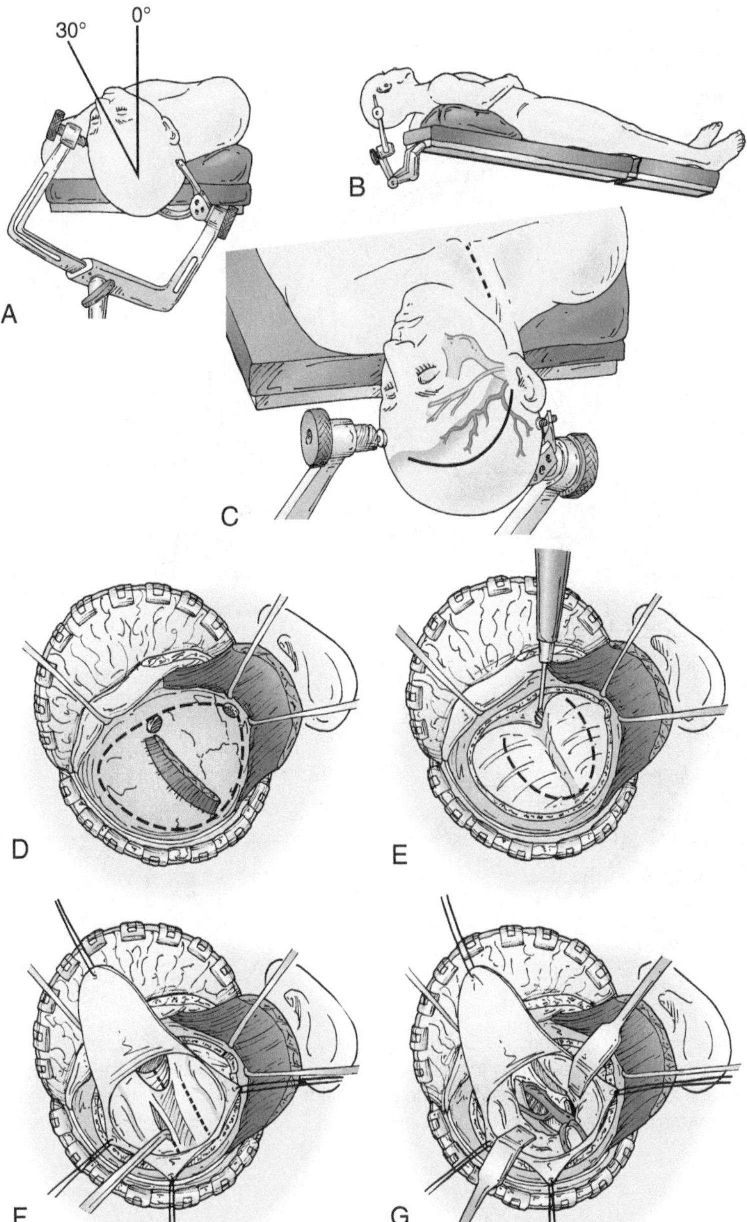

Figure 69-4. Pterional approach: operative position, skull fixation, scalp incision, skull base exposure. A, After the incision is outlined, the scalp is fixated in a three-pronged radiolucent skull clamp, positioned so that the surgical field and the position of the surgeon's hands are not obstructed by the superior-most pins on each side. A femoral catheter is placed beforehand for complex aneurysms; for simpler lesions, the groin is left unimpeded. The head is placed slightly higher than the level of the heart and turned the appropriate degree to place the operative field into the ideal position. The vertex of the skull is dropped slightly to allow gravitational distraction of the frontal and temporal lobes. Evoked potential electrodes are applied in almost all cases, both to monitor ischemic changes during the procedure and to regulate the amount of barbiturates needed to achieve burst suppression should temporary intraoperative arteriogram become necessary (B) clipping will be required (C). The scalp incision (solid line) extends from the midline to the zygoma, and is gently curved to stay approximately 1 cm behind the hairline. The cervical carotid bifurcation region is marked (dotted line), prepped, and draped into the field in cases where a need for proximal control is anticipated (D). Temporalis muscle incision: Interfascial technique for enhanced skull base exposure. The scalp is reflected anteriorly independent of the temporalis muscle, which is detached and retracted posteriorly and inferiorly. The skull base, orbital roof, and sphenoidal compartment of the deep Sylvian fissure can now be seen more easily with less brain retraction (E). The sphenoid ridge and bony indentations of the orbital roof are removed to produce a smooth flat sphenoid surface down to the superior orbital fissure. The dura is incised in a semi-circle (dotted line) based on the sphenoid ridge (F). The Sylvian fissure is generally opened from lateral-to-medial, on the frontal side of the superficial Sylvian veins, with a round arachnoid knife. When the brain is excessively tight, the frontal lobe may be gently retracted to open the carotid and interpeduncular cisterns (short dotted line). For typical bifurcation middle cerebral aneurysms, a superior temporal gyrus approach may be useful (long dotted line), especially when associated with a temporal lobe clot (G). At the end of a broad fissure splitting, the entire course of the internal carotid and middle cerebral arteries can be inspected from the anterior clinoid process to just beyond the genu. Whenever possible, the veins of the Sylvian fissure and sphenoparietal sinus are preserved to minimize venous congestion.

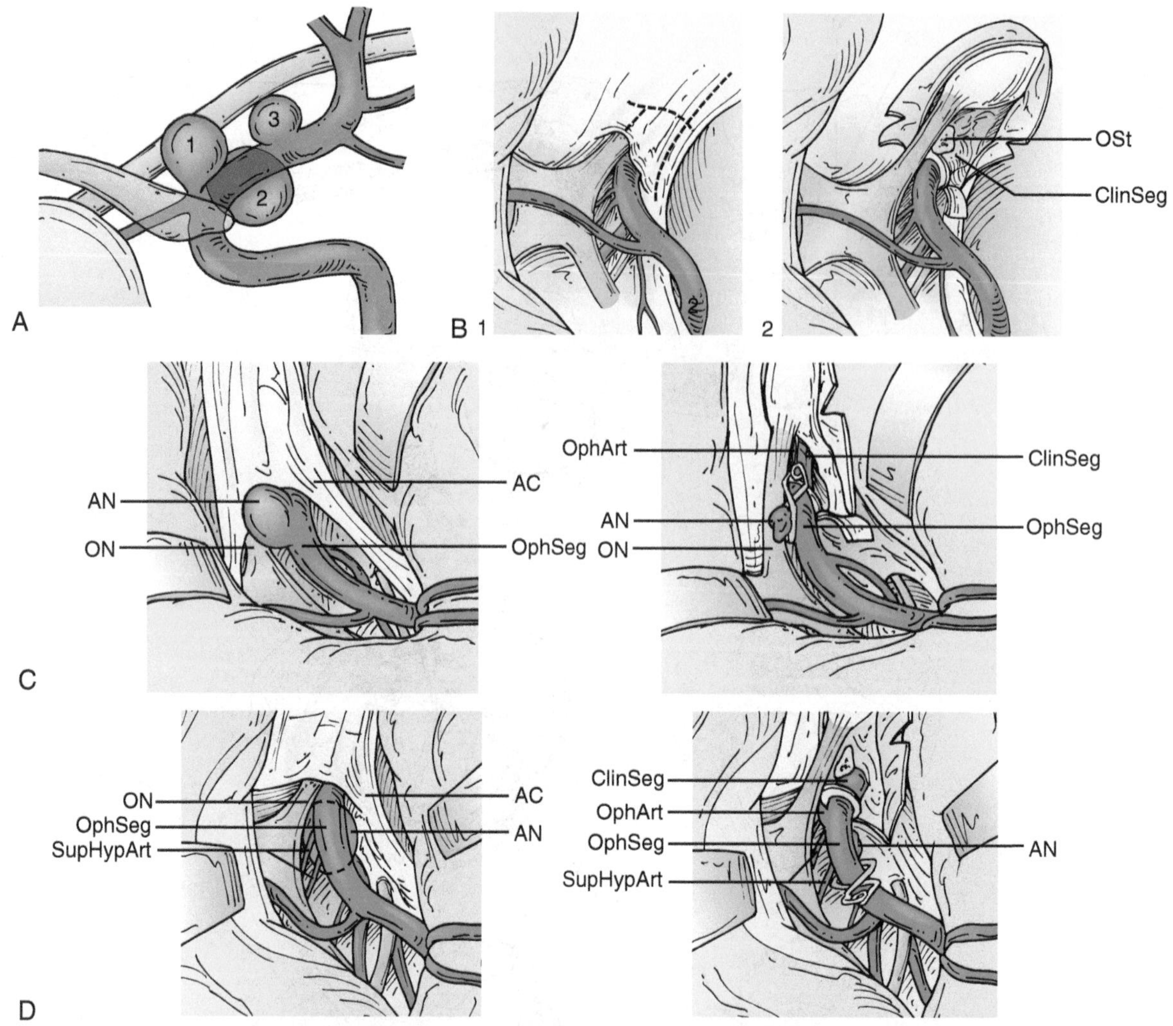

Figure 69-5. Ophthalmic segment aneurysms. A, Types: 1. Ophthalmic artery; 2. Superior hypophyseal; 3. Dorsal variant. B, Anterior clinoid removal; 1. The dotted lines mark the dural incision overlying the clinoid and include a limb to section the falciform ligament to untether the optic nerve; 2. Drilling down the optic strut (OSt) allows isolation of the clinoid segment (ClinSeg) of the internal carotid artery, which may be used for proximal control as necessary. C, Ophthalmic artery aneurysm; operative views. D, Superior hypophyseal artery aneurysm; operative views.

When symptomatic other than headaches, the clinical presentation includes roughly equal proportions between visual symptoms and hemorrhage. Visual loss is most commonly observed in giant lesions (greater than 2.5 cm in external diameter). Smaller lesions may produce acute blindness if they rupture directly into the overlying optic nerve. Visual loss from OphArt aneurysms is produced by the lesion's elevation of the lateral portion of the optic nerve superiorly and medially against the sharp edge of the falciform ligament. Initially, a unilateral ipsilateral inferior nasal field is produced. As the lesion grows, the entire nasal field is affected, followed by a superior temporal field loss in the contralateral eye. SupHypArt aneurysms produce visual field deficits are more closely akin to those seen with pituitary tumors, with the accompanying pressure more directed towards the chiasm.

Small OphSeg aneurysms are frequently not well seen on computerized tomographic (CT) scans, due to their close approximation to the skull base. Magnetic resonance imaging (MRI) can identify these lesions more easily, but the curves of the carotid artery in this region may still create some diagnostic uncertainty. Cerebral arteriography remains the definitive diagnostic test. OphArt aneurysms are easiest to diagnose on the lateral view, as they arise just distal to the OphArt and project superiorly above the plane of the ICA. Enlargement will be evident by a "closing" of the carotid siphon as the overlying optic nerves inhibit superior expansion. SupHypArt aneurysms arise proximal to the posterior communicating artery and project medially or inferomedially seemingly towards or into the cavernous sinus. Enlargement will tend to "open" the siphon and displace the ICA superiorly and laterally.

Surgical Approaches. With proper exposure and a firm understanding of parasellar and vascular anatomy, most OphSeg lesions are clippable with low risks to the brain or visual apparatus. Carotid ligation should be considered a secondary alternative, as the risks of stroke are high from parent vessel sacrifice, the visual system is not as effectively decompressed, and complete thrombosis of the aneurysm is not assured. Endovascular treatments with coils, stents and flow-diversion devices are increasingly being applied to these lesions. Although less invasive, these techniques do not effectively decompress the visual system when it is failing, and have a substantial recanalization rate compared to clipping.

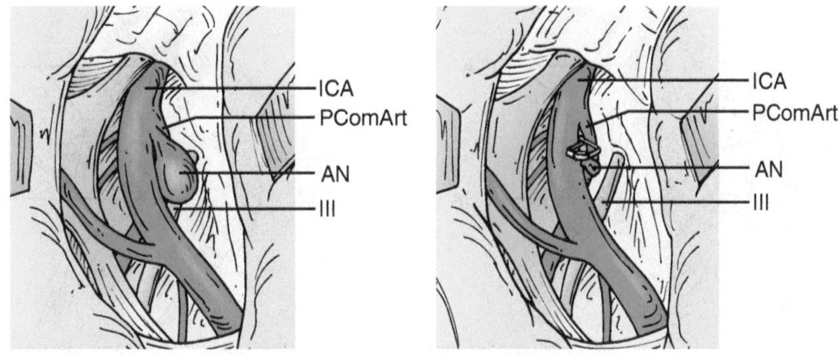

Figure 69-6. Communicating segment aneurysms: operative views before and after clipping.

Excellent visualization of the ICA, its branches, and the dural folds are mandatory for surgically treating lesions in this segment, and cervical carotid exposure for proximal control is often useful. An extensive skull base exposure, including removal of the anterior clinoid process (ACP) is sometimes necessary for safe and accurate clipping, especially for larger lesions.

Because some optic nerve displacement is usually necessary to visualize the proximal neck, the falciform ligament should be sectioned before the aneurysm is manipulated. Once the ACP is removed down to the optic strut, a gentle curved or side-angled clip, closed down parallel to the course of the ICA will secure the neck of OphArt aneurysms, followed by lesion collapse to decompress the visual system. SupHypArt aneurysms are usually best obliterated with fenestrated clips whose blades pass over and then run parallel to the ICA, spanning the distance between the posterior communicating artery and the DR.[2] The posterior communicating artery, anterior choroidal, and of course the SupHypArt must be identified and spared from the clip. "Dorsal" carotid artery blister aneurysms are extremely dangerous if clipped while carrying pulsatile flow, and are best handled surgically by temporarily trapping the affected segment followed by clip-wrapping to support the diffusely weakened wall.

Communicating Segment (Posterior Communicating Artery) Aneurysms (Fig. 69-6)

Anatomy and Terminology. The communicating segment of the ICA begins with the take-off of the posterior communicating artery (PComArt) and ends at the origin of the anterior choroidal artery. Due to its short length, only one aneurysm develops from this segment, traditionally termed a PComArt aneurysm. The hemodynamic stresses from flow through this segment create a potential aneurysm site that projects in two directions, one that points posteriorly and slightly inferiorly medial to the incisural edge, and the other that points laterally towards and into the uncus.

Clinical and Radiographic Features. PComArt aneurysms classically represent the most common type of symptomatic ICA aneurysm in adults, and are the most common specific type of symptomatic aneurysm found in females. These lesions frequently present when small (less than 1 cm), producing retro-orbital headaches, oculomotor nerve deficits invariably involving the pupil (posterior-inferior projecting), or subarachnoid hemorrhage.[3] This aneurysm and other distal ICA lesions have a higher risk of rupture than OphSeg aneurysms when small, as their walls and fundus are not secondarily reinforced by adjacent dural structures or overlying visual system. Visual loss from optic tract compression is rare, and cranial neuropathies other than oculomotor nerve dysfunction do not occur.

Surgical Approaches. The operative position and extent of bone removal to expose this lesion are similar to that required for anterior choroidal, ICA bifurcation, and proximal middle cerebral artery aneurysms. The Sylvian fissure is split from lateral-to-medial until the entire course of the ICA and M1 segment of the middle cerebral artery is delineated. Opening of the Sylvian fissure must be done with caution in laterally projecting cases, so as to avoid avulsion of the fundus from its temporal lobe attachments. With the posteriorly projecting type, part of the neck may be obscured by the basal dura of the tentorial incisura, especially when the OphSeg is shortened, or when the anterior clinoid process is elongated. The clinoid may have to be partially removed to secure adequate exposure and proximal control of the ICA. PComArt aneurysms always arise distal to the origin of the PComArt. With care, the PComArt can be gently dissected away from the anterior wall of the aneurysm. The clip should be advanced just beyond the PComArt origin, without compromising its patency or that of the anterior thalamoperforators, ICA perforators, or anterior choroidal artery. After the clip is properly situated, the aneurysm is sometimes punctured and the membrane of Liliequist opened widely to display and free up any tethering or compromise of the PComArt, its accompanying thalamoperforating vessels, and the oculomotor nerve.

Choroidal Segment (Anterior Choroidal Artery) Aneurysms

Anatomy and Terminology. The choroidal segment (ChorSeg) of the ICA begins with the take-off of the anterior choroidal artery (AChorArt), and ends at the base of the terminal carotid bifurcation into the anterior and middle cerebral arteries. This short segment lies superior and slightly lateral to the communicating segment, and has similar hemodynamic vectors. The single named branch from this segment, the AChorArt, typically arises several mm distal and lateral to the PComArt. The artery initially swings laterally and then posteriorly following the optic tract, often giving off branches or a separate trunk to the uncus and portions of the amygdala and anterior hippocampus. The main trunk continues posteriorly, inferior to the optic tract, and its major flow enters the choroidal fissure to supply the choroid plexus. Variability in size is considerable, and it often continues beyond the choroidal fissure to supply small portions of the basal ganglia, thalamus, internal capsule and brainstem. The artery is duplicated in up to 30% of cases.

Clinical and Radiographic Features. This aneurysm type is often difficult to distinguish radiographically from the

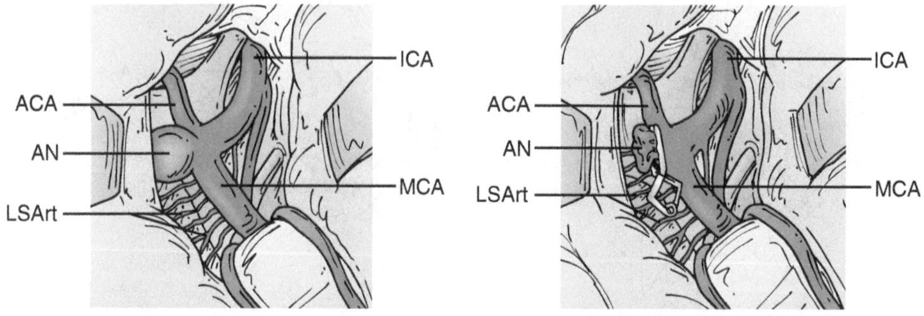

Figure 69-7. Internal carotid artery bifurcation aneurysms: operative views before and after clipping.

PComArt variety, and surgical confirmation is required in many instances. Because the ChorSeg is more lateral and distal than the communicating segment, however, AChorArt aneurysms invariably lie above the tentorium, away from the oculomotor nerve, and palsy of this nerve is much less common. The typical AChorArt aneurysm has an intimate relationship with the mesial temporal lobe, and is not infrequently buried within the uncus, in a fashion quite similar to the lateral variant PComArt aneurysm.

Surgical Approaches. The surgical approach to AChorArt aneurysms is identical to that of PComArt aneurysms for both the temporalis muscle incision, the size of the craniotomy, the degree of basal bone removal, and the method of Sylvian fissure splitting. Aneurysms associated with the AChorArt are usually small and thin walled, accounting for 3–5% of all intracranial saccular aneurysms. During the initial exposure, the surgeon must remember the aneurysm's possible adherence to the temporal lobe, and direct the approach more frontally until this relationship can be visually clarified. A small amount of sub-pial resection of the uncus surrounding the aneurysm's attachment may facilitate completion of the fissure splitting and subarachnoid cistern dissection. Once proximal control is obtained, the number and course of the AChorArt(ies) must be ascertained and separated from the aneurysm neck. Unlike the PComArt, this artery is vital and often unforgiving, and temporary clipping with flow interruption is not well tolerated. This artery must be spared from the clip, as its loss can result in a ganglionic or brainstem infarct often accompanied by a severe neurologic deficit (hemiparesis, hemianesthesia, and hemianopsia).

Internal Carotid Artery Bifurcation Aneurysms (Fig. 69-7)

Anatomy and Terminology. ICA bifurcation aneurysms arise at the distal end of the artery, and project as a direct extension of the terminal carotid flow towards and into the anterior perforated substance. Depending on the tortuosity of the vessel at this site, these aneurysms may point anterior-superiorly, directly superiorly, or posterior-superiorly, and may also be based more towards the anterior cerebral artery medially or the middle cerebral artery laterally. The lenticulostriate perforators, usually arising independent of the aneurysm neck, are invariably displaced posteriorly and are frequently adherent to the posterior wall of the expanding sac.

Clinical and Radiographic Features. Carotid bifurcation aneurysms account for about 3–5% of all saccular intracranial aneurysms, the majority of which present with hemorrhage. This site accounts for nearly 50% of saccular lesions identified in childhood. There is a high incidence of hemiplegia associated with hemorrhage in this location, and the pattern of intracerebral hematoma can closely resemble that seen with hypertensive medial ganglionic bleeds.

Surgical Approaches. The craniotomy and basal bone removal for ICA bifurcation aneurysms is quite similar to that required for PComArt and AChorArt aneurysms. The interfascial temporalis muscle incision, however, is preferable for these lesions to minimize the amount of retraction needed to see this region well. The Sylvian fissure is split from medial-to-lateral, carefully staying on the anterior–inferior surface of the middle cerebral artery until the carotid is encountered to avoid disturbance of the aneurysm. The basal cisterns should be broadly opened to obtain proximal control (ideally just distal to the AChorArt) and to further relieve any tension on the brain. The anterior cerebral and middle cerebral arteries should then be dissected several millimeters distal to the aneurysm origin to allow temporary clips on these trunks if needed. Finally, the aneurysm base is gradually approached from both sides until its neck is completely clarified and separated from the posteriorly displaced lenticulostriate vessels. The recurrent artery of Heubner frequently runs from medially-to-laterally with these perforators on the back surface of the aneurysm, and the AChorArt is also nearby, running from anterior-to-posterior behind the lesion's base. A straight or gentle curved clip is most ideal, placed parallel to the axis of the anterior cerebral – middle cerebral plane while the perforators are gently displaced posteriorly.

Anterior Cerebral Artery (Fig. 69-8)

The anterior cerebral artery (ACA) gives rise to two common types of aneurysms: the anterior communicating type and the distal (pericallosal) lesion.

Anterior Communicating Artery Aneurysms

Anatomy and Terminology. The proximal ACA (A1 segment) begins at the terminal ICA bifurcation, proceeds medially and somewhat anteriorly above the optic chiasm and nerves to the interhemispheric fissure, and ends where it joins its contralateral counterpart at the anterior communicating artery (AComArt). Inequality in the sizes of the two A1 segments occurs in approximately 40% of unselected cases (with severe hypoplasia or aplasia in 5%), and in 85% of patients harboring an AComArt aneurysm. Several small perforators arise from the A1 segment that supply the fornix, optic chiasm, anterior hypothalamus, anterior limb of the internal capsule and other septal region structures.

The AComArt usually exists as a single channel, but variations such as duplications, triplications, fenestrations, etc., are encountered in up to 25% of cases. AComArt aneurysms usually arise as a direct extension of a dominant A1 segment that delivers blood to both distal ACAs, with the aneurysm

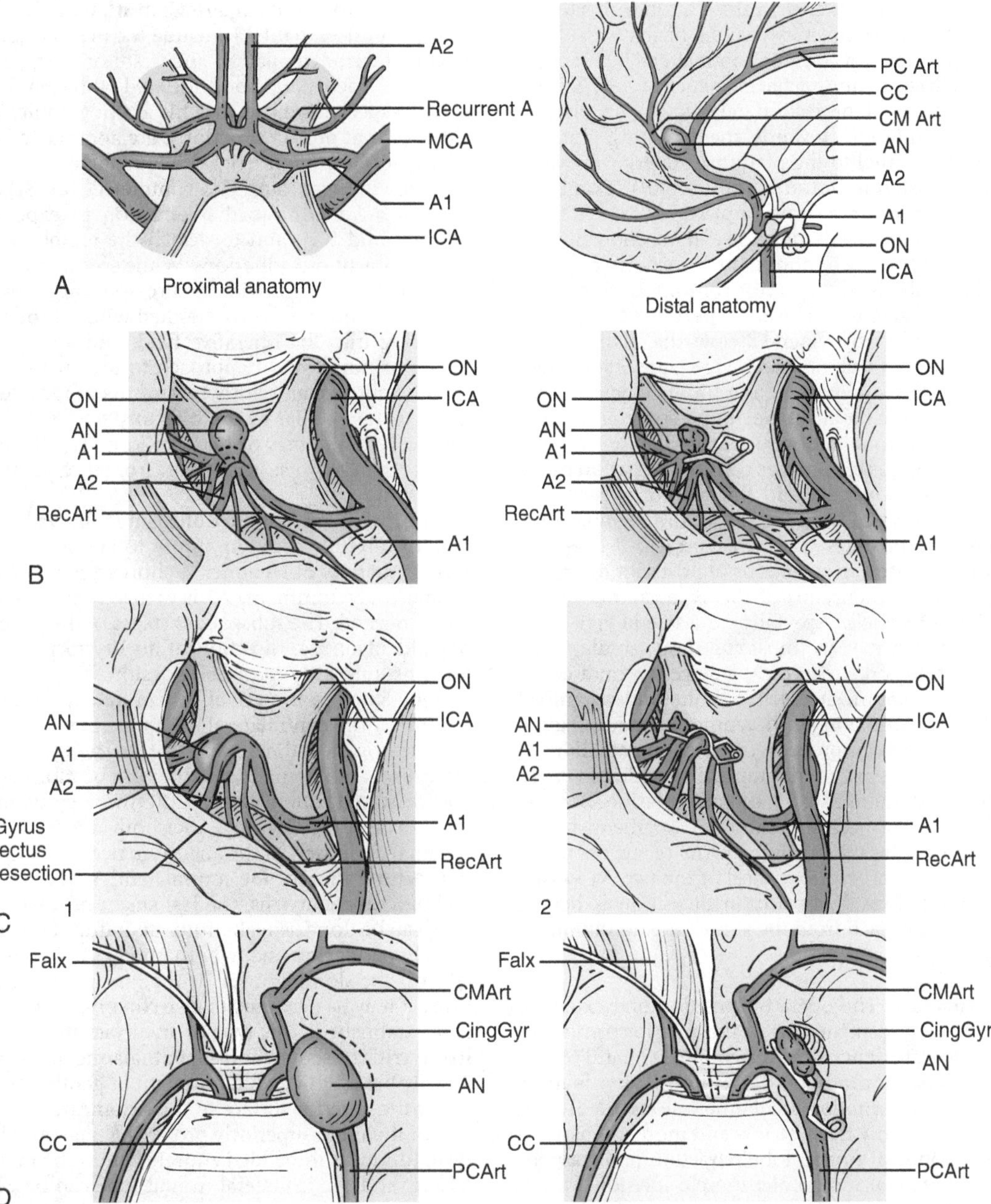

Figure 69-8. Anterior cerebral artery aneurysms. A, Anatomy; B, anterior communicating artery aneurysm: operative view of anterior–inferior projecting lesion before and after clipping. C, Anterior communicating artery aneurysm: operative view of superior projecting lesion before and after clipping. D, Distal anterior cerebral artery aneurysms: operative view before and after clipping.

attributed to the increased hemodynamic stress placed on the communicating channel, and the direction of aneurysm projection determined by the angle that the dominant A1 approaches the communicating region. The posterior–superior surface of the AComArt typically gives rise to at least one perforator supplying the anterior hypothalamic region.

The distal (A2) ACA begins at the AComArt and runs within the interhemispheric fissure to supply the medial third of the cerebral hemispheres and the corpus callosum. In most cases, the A2 segments are equal in size, and each supplies only the ipsilateral hemisphere. Common variations in this pattern and their incidence include an unpaired (azygous) A2 - also known as the "arteria termatica" (2% of cases), and a median callosal artery or third A2 (10% of cases). The first branch of the distal ACA is usually the recurrent artery of Heubner, which typically originates from the lateral surface of A2 just beyond the AComArt and proceeds laterally, paralleling the course of the ipsilateral A1, to supply anterior portions of the caudate, putamen, globus pallidus, and internal capsule.

Clinical and Radiographic Features. AComArt aneurysms represent the single most common saccular aneurysm type identified in adult clinical series, and account for 40–50% of those found in males. Most lesions are identified following subarachnoid hemorrhage; on rare occasions, they reach giant proportions and cause compression of the visual system. Following severe subarachnoid hemorrhage, these lesions are particularly prone to develop electrolyte imbalances (hyponatremia), and dropping serum sodium is invariably a reflection of hypothalamic ischemia caused by vasospasm.

Most AComArt aneurysms arise in association with a dominant A1 segment, and as direct extensions of that vessel, are often somewhat directed towards the contralateral hemisphere (see Fig. 69-2). These aneurysms have been classified, according to their direction of projection relative to the planum sphenoidale, into inferior (towards the planum), anterior (towards the nose parallel to the planum), superior (towards the vertex), and posterior (towards the occiput). Combinations of these projections are commonplace.

A simplistic system that is quite useful in choosing the direction of surgical approach (dominant A1 vs non-dominant hemisphere) basically divides anterior communicating artery aneurysms into two categories. The first type, those that project anteriorly and/or inferiorly, extend below the plane of the ascending A2 vessels (as seen on lateral view), are often adherent to the top of the visual system, and produce hemorrhage patterns confined to the basal subarachnoid space or contralateral inferior frontal lobe and gyrus rectus (Fig. 69-2). The inferior projection of this type makes early visualization of the contralateral A1 more difficult, and this type of aneurysm is invariably best approached from the side of the dominant A1.

The second type includes those that project between or behind the two A2 vessels in a superior or posterior direction. Visualization of small aneurysms of this type can be limited by the overlying A2 vessels, especially on a lateral view. This lesion, in our experience, is the most common saccular anterior circulation aneurysm site to escape detection on a good-quality initial arteriogram. Detailed oblique and magnified films with 3D reconstruction of the communicating region, with and without cross-compression of the contralateral internal carotid artery, or repeat arteriography in suspicious cases, may be required to demonstrate the offending lesion. Because this type of aneurysm projects more into the interhemispheric fissure and is hidden by the overlying gyrus rectus on initial frontal lobe elevation, proximal control of the two A1 vessels is easily obtained before the aneurysm dissection is begun, making a surgical approach from the side of the dominant A1 less advantageous.

Surgical Approaches. The operative position and extent of bone removal to expose aneurysms of the anterior communicating artery region are delineated in Figures 69-8A and 69-8B. Because the aneurysm location and direction of view is more anterior than for other anterior circulation lesions, the frontal portion of the craniotomy must be low and more extensive to minimize the amount of frontal lobe retraction necessary for exposure. An interfascial temporalis muscle incision further facilitates a low sub-frontal angle of approach.

The decision for the laterality of approach is based on the presence or absence of A1 dominance, the direction of projection of the aneurysm fundus, and the presence or absence of a significant intraparenchymal hematoma or other anterior circulation aneurysm. Approaching an AComArt aneurysm from the side of the dominant A1 is both technically easier and safer, especially when the aneurysm is pointing somewhat inferiorly towards the contralateral optic nerve. The surgeon enters the region of the aneurysm in control of the dominant A1, and encounters the aneurysm at its base, with the fundus (and site of rupture) pointing towards the contralateral side. If such cases are approached from the non-dominant A1 side, the aneurysm's adhesions to the visual system may be disrupted during elevation of the frontal lobe, and may limit access to the contralateral A1 should temporary clipping be necessary.

These technical advantages more than compensate for any perceived increased risks associated with dominant hemisphere (left-sided) approaches, especially when a skull-base style of exposure minimizes frontal lobe retraction. Indications to approach an AComArt aneurysm from the side of the non-dominant A1 include the presence of another ipsilateral anterior circulation aneurysm or a large hematoma on that side. Aneurysms not associated with significant A1 asymmetry, especially those that fill arteriographically from both sides, or that project superiorly, are approached from the side of the non-dominant (right) hemisphere.

Once the craniotomy is completed, the Sylvian fissure is split in a lateral-to-medial direction to expose the middle cerebral and ICA, and to detach the temporal lobe from its Sylvian arachnoid adhesions. While seemingly superfluous for this aneurysm type, wide fissure splitting allows the frontal lobe to be independently elevated without the temporal lobe crowding into the operative field, and also permits a more posterior trajectory of approach to the aneurysm base rather than from more anteriorly towards its fundus. Removal of the gyrus rectus medial to the olfactory tract will often facilitate the dissection. It may be better to lose a small amount of gyrus rectus than to use excessive frontal and temporal lobe retraction.

The ipsilateral A1 is identified and followed to the AComArt region, carefully avoiding injury to any perforators or to the recurrent artery of Heubner. A short segment of the ipsilateral (and usually dominant) A1 is prepared to receive a temporary clip if needed. The subsequent stages of dissection then differ, dependent on the direction of aneurysm projection. For the anterior–inferiorly projecting lesion, the aneurysm fundus may be stuck to the visual system, making visualization and control of the contralateral A1 hazardous. The two A2 vessels and the origins of their branches (especially the recurrent arteries) are less problematic, and they can be more easily identified and dissected, often with a little more gyrus rectus removal adjacent to the AComArt. After both A2s have been clarified, the final dissection of the aneurysm neck is completed, including identification of the contralateral A1. For very thin-walled or bulbous aneurysms, the last stages of dissection and clipping can be done using barbiturate-induced burst suppression, mild hypertension and hypothermia (33 °C), and a temporary clip on the dominant A1. If the aneurysm prematurely ruptures, it may be necessary to also clip other vessels until control is re-established. This type of aneurysm usually projects away from critical septal and hypothalamic perforators, and is usually best clipped with a straight or gentle curved clip paralleling the anterior surface of the AComArt.

For the more superiorly projecting type of lesion, the aneurysm fundus is imbedded entirely within the interhemispheric fissure, and the ipsilateral frontal lobe can be gently elevated and detached from the visual system with much more safety. The contralateral A1 is easily seen, and both A1s are prepared to receive a temporary clip as required. The region of the AComArt is clarified, and a subpial resection of the gyrus rectus (about 1 cm) allows visualization of the ipsilateral A2 and its branches. The contralateral A2 is the problematic vessel, usually being obstructed from view by the intervening aneurysm. After both A1s and the ipsilateral A2 (and Heubner's) are ascertained, the final neck dissection is begun, using the same methods of cerebral protection as outlined previously.

This type of aneurysm has a much more intimate association with the septal area perforators, and is often best managed with a short fenestrated clip that encircles the ipsilateral A2 and parallels the posterior and superior surface of the AComArt, carefully avoiding compromise of the contralateral A2 and penetrating vessels. At the completion of apparently satisfactory clipping, the aneurysm should be punctured and collapsed, and all branches carefully inspected for patency, including both A1s, A2s, recurrent arteries of Heubner, perforators, and the AComArt itself.

Many surgeons take the opportunity to perform a 3rd ventriculostomy by opening the lamina terminalis because it is easily visualized during the proper dissection of an anterior communicating artery aneurysm. This allows drainage of CSF from the 3rd ventricle into the chiasmatic cisterns thus avoiding post-operative hydrocephalus.

Distal Anterior Cerebral Artery Aneurysms

Anatomy and Terminology. In the typical situation, two distal anterior cerebral arteries (also known as the A2, post-communicating, or pericallosal arteries) initially run dorsally and then arch posteriorly within the midline pericallosal sulcus deep within the interhemispheric fissure, parallel and closely applied to the genu and body of the corpus callosum. The callosomarginal artery typically arises from the pericallosal artery near the genu and runs within the cingulate sulcus, giving off several major cortical branches to the mesial cerebral hemisphere.

Clinical and Radiographic Features. Distal anterior cerebral aneurysms (DACAs) account for 2–4% of all intracranial aneurysms. Almost all are saccular, but those that originate near the falx cerebri may be traumatic, and those that arise distal to the pericallosal-callosomarginal bifurcation may have infectious origins. The typical distal ACA aneurysm presents with subarachnoid hemorrhage, usually confined to the interhemispheric fissure distal to the AComArt region, but occasionally extending into the cingulate gyrus or subdural space. Most arise from the pericallosal artery, usually at the branching point between the pericallosal and callosomarginal arteries. Less commonly, distal aneurysms will arise at the bifurcation of an azygos A2 segment where it divides to form two pericallosal arteries.

Surgical Approaches. The operative position, scalp incision, and craniotomy flap for the typical DACA aneurysm is shown in Figure 69-8D. In most instances, the bone flap should extend well anterior to the coronal suture to allow dissection of the pericallosal artery around the genu of the corpus callosum. The posterior limit of the flap should be placed so that the surgeon can enter the interhemispheric fissure (sparing as many veins as possible) and identify the pericallosal artery distal to the aneurysm without the retraction disturbing the aneurysm. The pericallosal artery is then followed anteriorly until the aneurysm is encountered, proximal control is obtained, and the aneurysm clipped. Intra-operative navigation is a useful adjuvant to direct the surgeon to the intended spot.

Middle Cerebral Artery Aneurysms (Fig. 69-9)

Anatomy and Terminology. The middle cerebral artery (MCA) begins at the terminal bifurcation of the ICA, and supplies the lateral two-thirds of the cerebral hemisphere centered around the Sylvian fissure. The vessel initially runs laterally, paralleling the sphenoid ridge, within the sphenoidal compartment of the deep Sylvian fissure. At the level of the limen insulae, it makes an abrupt turn (genu) posteriorly and superiorly to enter the insular compartment of the deep fissure. The MCA can be divided into four segments, including: (1) M1 – that segment between the carotid bifurcation and the genu, (2) M2 – those segments that run over the deep insular surface, (3) M3 – the segments that traverse the opercular surface of the Sylvian fissure to reach the cortical surface, and (4) M4 – cortical branches. The M1 segment typically divides into two trunks just proximal to the genu, creating a long pre-bifurcation (main trunk) and short post-bifurcation portion (superior and inferior trunks). The pre-bifurcation segment gives rise to lenticulostriate vessels from its posterior superior surface, and often contributes an early or anterior temporal branch off its anterior inferior surface. Recurrent lateral lenticulostriate branches occasionally originate from the post-bifurcation M1 segment or from proximal portions of the M2 trunks.

Approximately 20% of all clinically significant saccular intracranial aneurysms originate from the MCA. These lesions may be divided into three types: (1) proximal, (2) typical bifurcation, and (3) distal. The majority are typical bifurcation aneurysms that originate as a direct extension of the main trunk to project laterally, anteriorly, and slightly inferiorly between and beyond its two branches and the genu towards the temporal lobe (see Fig. 69-9). A smaller number originate proximal to the genu, and include lesions associated with the main trunk-anterior temporal artery bifurcation, a shortened pre-bifurcation M1 portion (with correspondingly long post-bifurcation trunks straddling the aneurysm), or a lenticulostriate origin. A few arise distally, usually from a delayed bifurcation of the main trunk beyond the genu, or from a second or third order bifurcation thereafter. Whenever distal lesions arise significantly beyond the genu, an infectious or traumatic etiology should at least be considered.

Clinical and Radiographic Features. Unruptured MCA aneurysms are generally asymptomatic, although when larger they may occasionally present with temporal lobe seizures or intra-aneurysmal thrombosis and embolism. Rupture and subarachnoid hemorrhage usually result in a syndrome indistinguishable from that seen with aneurysms at other sites. Certain clinical characteristics, however, favor a middle cerebral origin of the bleed, including a unilateral temporal region headache or a focal neurologic deficit including dysphasia or weakness of the contralateral arm or face. These focal signs and symptoms are presumably related to the tendency of typical bifurcation MCA aneurysms to project into the temporal lobe, resulting in a higher incidence of intracerebral hemorrhage (30–50%) than with saccular intracranial aneurysms at other locations.

The common hemorrhage patterns for proximal, typical bifurcation, and distal middle cerebral aneurysms are different. In an acutely deteriorating patient with a classically located temporal lobe clot, computerized tomographic scanning may be the only study required prior to emergent surgical intervention. The arteriogram should be carefully inspected for the aneurysm's position relative to the genu and for its direction of projection, as subtle differences may alter the choice of temporalis muscle incisions and the method of Sylvian fissure dissection.

Surgical Approaches. Most MCA aneurysms are best approached via a pterional craniotomy, with slight bone flap alterations to broaden the length of Sylvian fissure exposure. The initial scalp incision should ideally preserve the dominant branch of the superficial temporal artery for its potential future use as a bypass donor vessel. The aneurysm may thereafter be exposed by three basic methods, including: (1) transcortical (through the superior temporal gyrus), (2) medial-to-lateral trans-Sylvian (opening the Sylvian fissure medially at the internal carotid artery and following the main trunk laterally until the aneurysm is encountered), and (3) lateral-to-medial trans-Sylvian (opening the fissure laterally and following an M2 trunk proximally to the aneurysm). Regardless of the method chosen, the Sylvian and sphenoparietal veins should be preserved whenever possible to minimize venous congestion and swelling in the frontal and temporal operculum.

The superior temporal gyrus approach requires little brain retraction and can be performed quite rapidly, making it

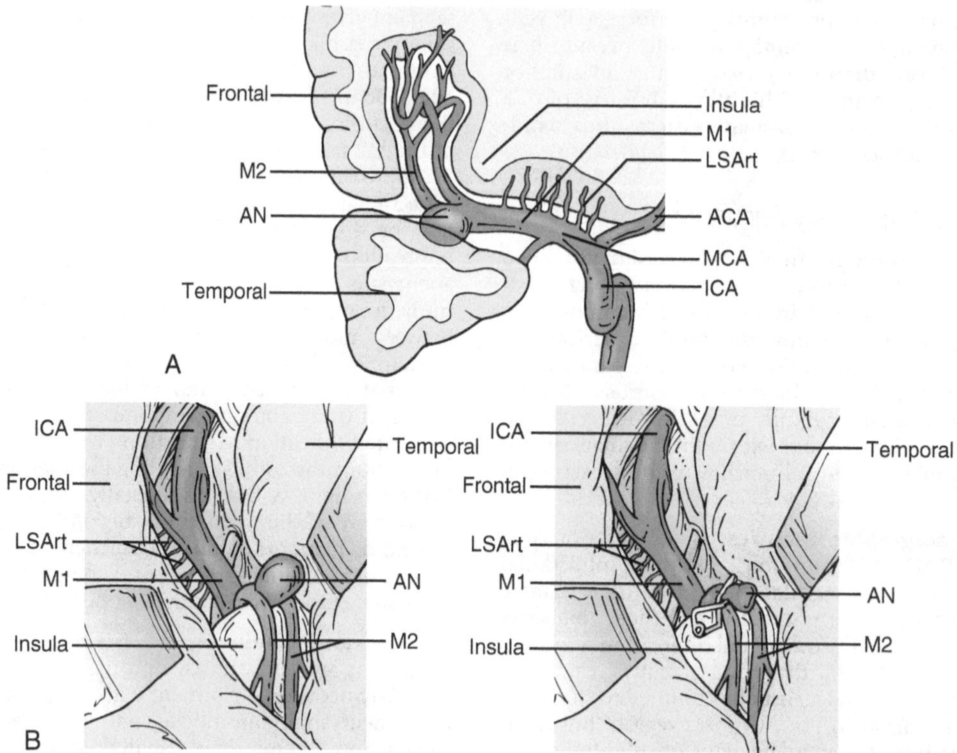

Figure 69-9. Middle cerebral artery bifurcation aneurysms. A, Frontal view: typical bifurcation (schematic). The aneurysm arises at the terminal end of the M1 segment, and continues laterally towards and often into the temporal lobe. The M2 branches, beginning at the genu, sharply angle posteriorly and superiorly to enter the insular compartment of the Sylvian fissure. B, Operative views before and after clipping.

especially useful for typical bifurcation aneurysms with significant temporal lobe hematomas. When the brain is tight, the hematoma should be entered early and evacuated peripherally with gentle suction, taking care not to disturb the clot adjacent to the aneurysm. Once the brain has been decompressed, the Sylvian fissure should be entered, and the anatomy further clarified from within the subarachnoid space. Disadvantages to a transcortical approach include the production of trauma to otherwise normal temporal lobe structures (which may increase the risk of post-operative epilepsy) and premature disturbance of the clot adjacent to the aneurysm (which may precipitate rebleeding). This approach is contraindicated for proximal aneurysms and for distal lesions projecting into more posterior portions of the temporal lobe (i.e., Heschl's gyrus).

The trans-Sylvian fissure methods are more aesthetically appealing as they respect the brain's natural pial barriers. The medial-to-lateral Sylvian fissure splitting approach has the advantage of proximal M1 control before the aneurysm comes into view, while the lateral-to-medial trans-Sylvian approach requires less retraction and reduces the risks of perforator vessel injury. In general, the senior author prefers the lateral-to-medial approach in most instances. For typical bifurcation middle cerebral aneurysms, the Sylvian fissure is entered slightly more posteriorly (3–4 cm behind the sphenoid ridge) than for other aneurysms. Once an M2 branch is encountered, it is followed proximally on the side opposite the aneurysm's projection (i.e., if the aneurysm is projecting temporally, the trunk is followed on the frontal lobe side) until the genu and bifurcation are encountered. Once proximal control is established, the fissure can be more broadly opened as needed to obtain good exposure without undue retraction. The subarachnoid plane between the frontal and temporal lobes may be difficult to preserve, especially in younger patients or in hemorrhage cases, and if lost during the dissection, it is far better to veer inferiorly towards the superior temporal gyrus rather than risk injury to the frontal lobe operculum, especially in the dominant hemisphere.

The type of temporalis muscle incision and the methods of Sylvian fissure dissection vary according to the clinical and radiographic features of the individual aneurysm. Once the fissure is widely opened, typical bifurcation lesions are usually best controlled with a curved or straight clip running parallel to the axis between the two exiting trunks. The aneurysm neck is often bulbous and arteriosclerotic at this location, making "perfect" clip placement difficult in some instances. Most of the lenticulostriate vessels exit prior to the aneurysm origin, but some arise more distally, and in their recurrent course, they may be adherent to the aneurysm and inadvertently included in the clip. After the lesion is satisfactorily secured, it should be punctured and collapsed, and the dissection continued until all significant Sylvian and intracerebral clot is removed. The safe passage of all nearby vessels must be visually ascertained, using intraoperative arteriography in questionable cases.

Proximal MCA aneurysms are somewhat buried beneath the insula, and have a much more intimate association with the lenticulostriate vessel origins, making exposure and clipping more difficult. Temporary clipping under barbiturate and mild hypothermic protection is particularly useful for these aneurysms, as premature rupture risks disastrous perforator injury. Clips of excessive length are particularly hazardous in this region, and all perforators must be spared from the blades. Any neurologic deficit appearing immediately after the operation cannot be attributed to delayed cerebral vasospasm, and if unexplained by intraoperative events, should prompt a re-exploration to inspect for a clipped or kinked perforator.

Distal MCA aneurysms generally lie entirely within the insular compartment of the Sylvian fissure, with little or no association with the lenticulostriate vessels. In this position, the aneurysm will often have a projection that is more superiorly oriented, making any intracerebral hemorrhage more likely be in the frontal lobe than those that originate from the typical bifurcation site (which invariably produces a temporal lobe hematoma). When exposing these lesions, care must be taken to notice which trunk harbors the aneurysm, staying on the "safe" side of the fissure away from the aneurysm until proximal control is obtained.

The "eyebrow" approach has been used successfully by some surgeons for small MCA aneurysms and is safe in good grade patients or with unruptured aneurysms. The craniotomy is subfrontal and should be about 2.5cm long and 1.5 cm high, placed right on the floor of the orbital roof. There are several essential pre-requisites to these minimal access craniotomies: a lumbar drain should be inserted with induction and opened when the skin is incised along the partially shaved upper half of the lateral two-thirds of the eyebrow. Image guidance allows a rapid and safe approach to the aneurysm. Skeletal fixation is needed both for the image guidance and for attachment of retractors. Narrow clip applicators of a bayonet design avoid obstructing the narrow visual field. A wide range of angled and curved clips is needed because of the limited maneuverability of the applicator. The small bone flap is fixed in place with small plates and screws. Various fillers and putty can be used to achieve a smooth and natural bone contour when closing.[4-6]

The hemorrhage from MCA aneurysms is frequently confined to the ipsilateral hemisphere, and the risks of generalized secondary events following the bleed may be reduced compared to more centrally located lesions. The incidence of hydrocephalus and the need for ventricular drainage and later shunting appear lower, presumably because the basal cisterns are less often filled with fresh clot and the contralateral convexity can still conduct and absorb cerebrospinal fluid. Vasospasm is more often confined to the ipsilateral hemisphere, and the incidence of electrolyte disturbances (i.e., hyponatremia) appears reduced, especially when compared to AComArt aneurysms. The surgical approaches to MCA aneurysms require the least brain retraction, and when this fact is combined with the increased facility by which vasospasm affecting the MCA can be treated (with papaverine or angioplasty), early surgery should probably be performed in all good grade patients. Early intervention should also at least be considered in poorer grade patients who are younger or harbor large hematomas, especially if diagnosed soon after the bleeding.

POSTERIOR CIRCULATION

Posterior circulation aneurysms, which include the vertebral and basilar arteries and their branches, are less common than their anterior circulation counterparts, accounting for approximately 15% of all intracranial aneurysms.[7] They most commonly occur in the upper basilar artery at the basilar apex, followed by those of the vertebral–posterior inferior cerebellar artery regions. As a group, posterior circulation aneurysms appear to have a significantly higher rate of rupture when small (<1 cm) than those arising in the anterior circulation.[8]

Currently, the primary means of treatment for the majority of posterior circulation aneurysms at most centers is via an endovascular route. Following subarachnoid hemorrhage, the posterior fossa contents and vasculature are often more sensitive to the microsurgical manipulation required for successful aneurysm obliteration. When this sensitivity is combined with the increased technical difficulty often required, the peri-operative course and postoperative outcomes are more frequently suboptimal in comparison with those of endovascular treatments. In the non-ruptured aneurysm, such heightened sensitivity is not as problematic. Many cannot be treated by current endovascular methodology, either because of restricted vascular access or because the shape, size, or other anatomic considerations of the aneurysm are not ideal for such methodology. In such circumstances, microsurgical management is warranted, particularly when performed by surgeons experienced in posterior fossa and skull base approaches.[9-14]

Basilar Artery

The basilar artery (BA) can be divided into two regions which generate aneurysms: the apex and the trunk formed by the union of the two vertebral arteries.

Basilar Apex Aneurysms (Fig. 69-10)

Anatomy and Terminology. The basilar apex region refers to the terminal basilar bifurcation, including the origins and proximal portions of the posterior cerebral (PCA) and superior cerebellar (SCA) arteries. The terminal basilar bifurcation is most often located at the level of the pontomesencephalic junction, within 1 cm of the dorsum sella in most patients. The upper 5 mm of the BA is a source of multiple perforators that generally arise from the posterior and lateral aspects of the parent vessel. Most of these perforators enter the midbrain or pons near the midline; other lateral circumferential branches terminate in the lateral pons, peduncle, and posterior perforated substance. Perforating vessels that arise from the superior and posterior aspects of the P1 segment (that portion of the PCA from the BA bifurcation to the PComArt origin) are termed the posterior thalamoperforators, and they supply the interpeduncular fossa, mamillary bodies, cerebral peduncle, and posterior mesencephalon. Those that arise from the PComArt are termed the anterior thalamoperforators, and they supply the thalamus, posterior limb of the internal capsule, hypothalamus, subthalamus, substantia nigra, red nucleus, and the oculomotor and trochlear nuclei.[15]

Clinical and Radiographic Features. Saccular aneurysms in the basilar apex region, those that arise within the interpeduncular cistern, originate from the terminal basilar bifurcation,

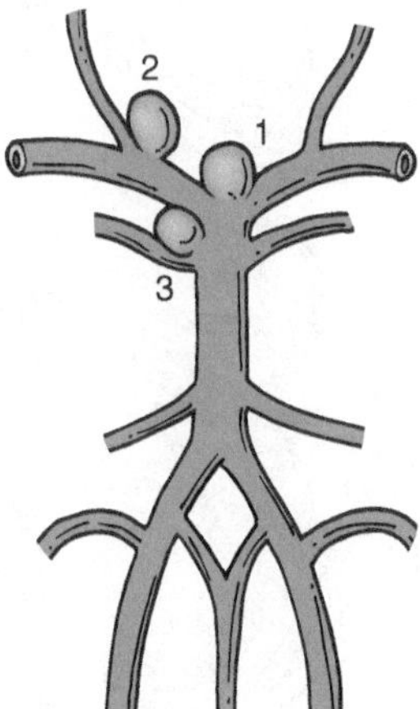

Figure 69-10. Posterior circulation: types of basilar apex saccular aneurysms. 1, Basilar Apex Aneurysm; 2, P1 segment Posterior Cerebral Artery Aneurysm (PCA); 3, Superior Cerebellar Artery Aneurysm.

the posterior cerebral artery–superior cerebellar (PCA-SCA) junction, and the distal P1 segment where it joins the PComArt.

Surgical Approaches. The main problem with basilar tip aneurysms is the lack of proximal control if the aneurysm ruptures during the dissection. The three major surgical approaches to the basilar apex are as follows: (1) trans-Sylvian (frontotemporal or pterional), (2) anterior subtemporal, and (3) temporopolar (Fig. 69-11). Each route has advantages and disadvantages, with no one approach being applicable for every aneurysm. Aneurysm projection and level of origin affects the choice of routes. Most BA apex aneurysms project superiorly. When the aneurysm projects posteriorly, a purely trans-Sylvian approach is difficult, because the posterior–inferior aspect of the aneurysm neck and any posteriorly located perforating arteries are obstructed from view by the BA. Similarly, anteriorly projecting aneurysms are often adherent to the dorsum sellae, and a trans-Sylvian route risks premature aneurysm rupture before the dissection is completed. For most solitary basilar apex aneurysms, a right-sided approach is favored, with any brain retraction confined to the non-dominant frontal and/or temporal lobes. A left-sided approach is preferable in patients presenting with a left CN III palsy or right hemiparesis, coexistent basilar and left-sided anterior circulation aneurysms, and lateral orientation of the BA aneurysm toward the left side.

Trans-Sylvian (Frontotemporal or Pterional) Approach. The pterional or trans-Sylvian approach to the upper BA (Fig. 69-12), first advocated by Yasargil et al.,[16] was applied to lesions at this site because the basilar bifurcation usually lies within 1–2 cm to the intracranial ICA. Wide incision in the membrane of Lilliequist provides visualization of the BA apex and the origins of the SCA and PCA. Advantages of this approach are its general familiarity to most neurosurgeons,

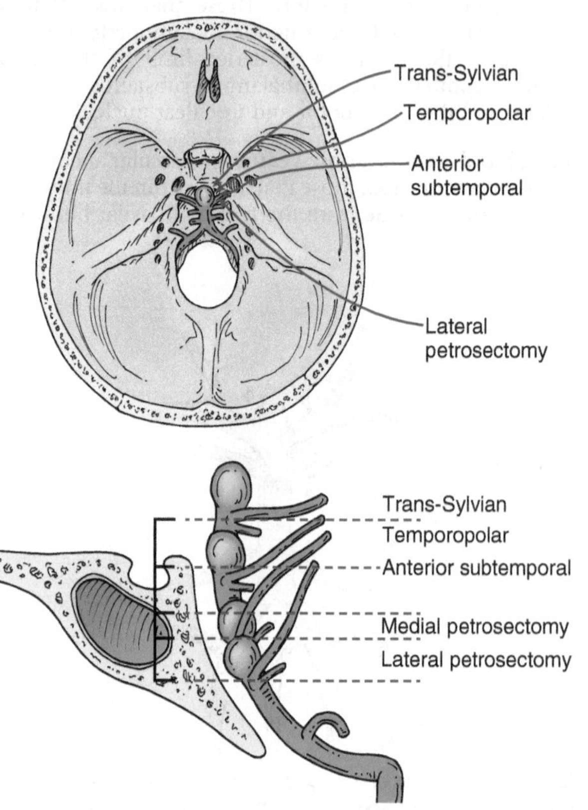

Figure 69-11. Surgical approaches to basilar apex.

minimal temporal lobe retraction, and less manipulation and injury to the oculomotor nerves. This approach also allows concurrent anterior circulation aneurysms to be clipped during the same procedure. The operative field is deeper and narrower, however, and visualization may be further impeded by the posterior clinoid process or the ICA, its branches, or perforators. Other disadvantages include a limited space and direction for final clip application, and greater difficulty in placing a proximal temporary clip, particularly with low-lying bifurcations, where proximal clipping may in fact not be possible at all.

The scalp, temporalis muscle and fascia are reflected using the same interfascial technique as for anterior circulation lesions. The Sylvian fissure is opened in a lateral-to-medial direction, beginning approximately 2–3 cm posterior to the sphenoid ridge on the frontal lobe side of the Sylvian veins. The basal cisterns surrounding the ICA and optic nerves are opened to further relax and broaden the operative exposure. When the procedure is completed, the frontal and temporal lobes fall away from the sphenoid ridge and orbital roof. A broad view of basal structures is provided, without sacrifice of the sphenoparietal veins.

The usual best interval of access to the basilar apex is between the ICA and oculomotor nerve – the carotid-oculomotor interval. The PComArt is identified and followed to and through Lilliequist's membrane to the ipsilateral P1/P2 junction. The oculomotor nerve (cranial nerve III) and SCA are identified and dissected free, creating enough space to allow the anterior–inferior margin of the P1 segment to be followed proximally. Once the P1 origin is reached, the aneurysm neck becomes visible. The BA apex is now carefully exposed, including the origin of the contralateral P1 and a site for a temporary clip below the SCA origins where there are no perforators. The base of the aneurysm is then dissected, with careful delineation of the relationship of the perforators to the aneurysm. Each perforator must be completely free and excluded from the clip.

The "transcavernous-transellar" modification as described by Dolenc et al.[17] was designed to overcome the two major limitations of the standard trans-Sylvian route. In this modification, the posterior lateral orbital wall and roof are removed; both the optic canal and superior orbital fissure are unroofed, and the anterior clinoid process is removed extradurally. The dural ring around the ICA is incised in a circumferential manner, allowing medial mobilization of the ICA and optic nerve. The dura forming the lateral wall of the cavernous sinus is incised, allowing the oculomotor nerve to be mobilized and retracted laterally. If the bifurcation is low, the posterior clinoid process can be removed for increased exposure.

Anterior Subtemporal Approach. The lateral subtemporal approach devised by Drake[18,19] once represented the mainstay of surgical management of BA apex aneurysms. Although initially accompanied by a high incidence of temporal lobe contusion or hematoma, subsequent modification to the anterior subtemporal approach now permits the temporal lobe to be gently elevated with a low incidence of damage to the temporal lobe or its venous structures[20] (Fig. 69-13). The main advantage of this approach is that the BA apex and aneurysm are viewed from a lateral direction, allowing for easier identification and manipulation of the posterior perforators. This direction of approach also allows the clip to be placed parallel to the plane of aneurysm origin from the parent vessels, a substantial advantage especially for bulbous or broad-based aneurysms. In addition, the working space for dissection and clip application is larger and the working distance more superficial than with the trans-Sylvian route. The main disadvantages are the higher incidence of postoperative CN III deficits,

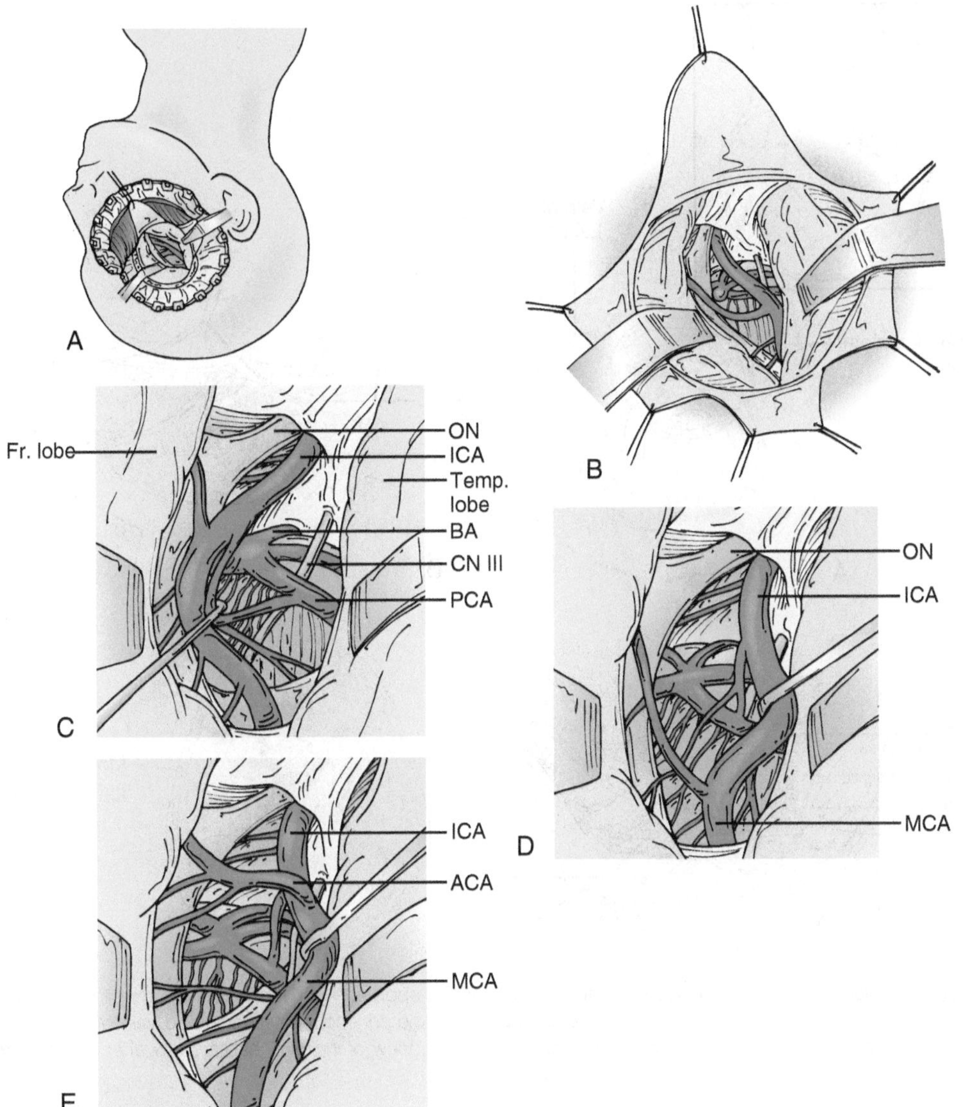

Figure 69-12. Terminal basilar bifurcation aneurysms: trans-Sylvian approach. A, Fronto-temporal pterional craniotomy. B, Sylvian fissure broadly split. C, The carotid-oculomotor interval, posterior to the internal carotid artery. D, The optico-carotid interval, medial to the internal carotid artery. E, Above the terminal internal carotid artery bifurcation.

the inability to clip most concurrent anterior circulation aneurysms, increased difficulty in visualizing the contralateral perforators, and the risk of temporal lobe injury.

The scalp incision is similar to that used in the trans-Sylvian approach, but extends more posteriorly over the ear and posterior temporal bone. A muscle-splitting incision mobilizes the temporalis muscle anteriorly. A temporal craniotomy is performed anteriorly to the temporal pole and inferiorly down to the floor of the middle fossa to expose the anterior and middle portions of the temporal lobe. The superior half of the zygomatic arch is drilled away to further minimize the amount of brain retraction needed to gain a subtemporal view of the incisura.

Gentle retraction, combined with patience and CSF drainage to allow for adequate brain relaxation, is critical to prevent temporal lobe injury. Care is taken to preserve the vein of Labbé and the sphenoparietal sinus to facilitate temporal lobe venous drainage and minimize postoperative brain swelling. The surgical route is obliquely *oriented* across the anterior floor of the middle fossa. When the incisura is reached, the tentorium is incised posterior to the entry point of the trochlear nerve (CN IV), sectioned parallel and posterior to the superior petrosal sinus, and reflected until the SCA is exposed coursing in the ambient cistern. The resultant space allows visualization of a 2-cm interval of the anterior superior brainstem and BA centered at the level of the posterior clinoid process. The anterior–inferior margins of the ipsilateral PCA and SCA are dissected and followed to their origins from the BA. The width of the aneurysm between the two PCA origins is estimated, a critical step because a fenestrated clip encircling the ipsilateral PCA is usually used and must not reach or compromise contralateral perforators.

Visualization of low-lying BA apex or upper basilar trunk aneurysms is hindered by the bony and dural attachments of the posterior clinoid process, clivus, and petrous apex.[16,18,21,22] Extradural resection of the medial petrous apex combined with the anterior subtemporal approach[23-25] creates an exposure that provides access to an additional 1–1.5 cm of the BA over that provided by the anterior subtemporal approach alone.

When the basilar bifurcation is particularly high, the temporalis muscle can limit the desired inferior to superior

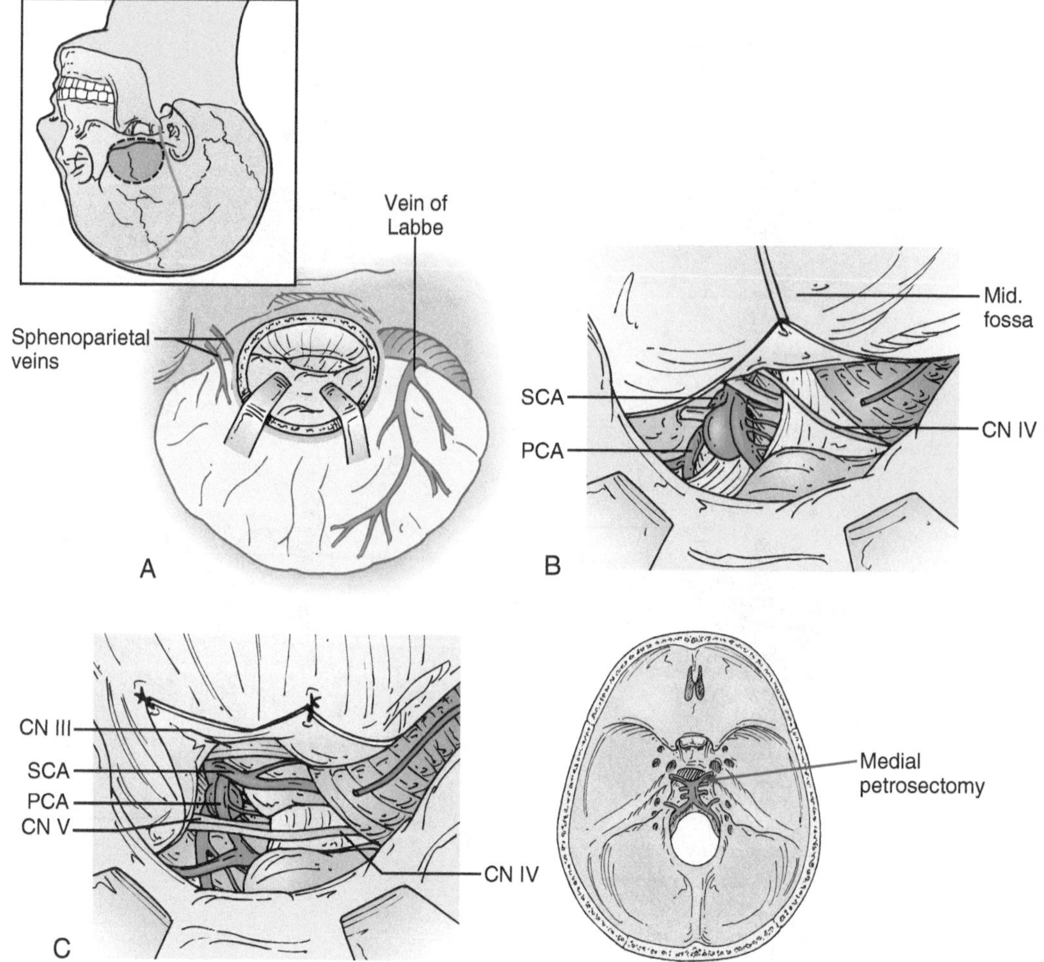

Figure 69-13. Terminal basilar bifurcation aneurysms: anterior subtemporal approach (A). Temporal lobe mobilization: the anterior and middle portions of the temporal lobe are slowly elevated in a gentle arch between the sphenoparietal veins and vein of Labbe to expose the anterior incisura. B, View of incisura, basilar apex after tentorial section, retraction. C, View of incisura, basilar apex after medial petrosectomy.

microscope trajectory. In such cases, the zygomatic arch can be removed, allowing the temporalis to be reflected inferiorly to facilitate a more superior view into the incisura without further temporal lobe retraction.[26]

Temporopolar Approach (Fig. 69-14). The temporopolar or pretemporal route is in many ways a combination of the pterional trans-Sylvian and anterior subtemporal approaches. First mentioned by Drake[18,19] as a "half and half" exposure, it was also described by Sano[26] who coined the term "temporopolar," and Sundt[27] who called it a modified pterional (anterior temporal) approach. Like the trans-Sylvian approach, the temporopolar approach begins with a pterional craniotomy but includes more inferior and anterior temporal bone removal. After wide splitting of the Sylvian fissure, the bridging veins to the sphenoparietal sinus are coagulated and sectioned, the temporal tip is gently retracted posteriorly and laterally to provide a view of the incisura.

The major advantage of this approach is that posterior retraction of the temporal pole, particularly when accompanied by splitting of the Sylvian fissure, produces less temporal lobe swelling than that encountered via the traditional subtemporal approach.[20,28] Like the subtemporal route, a lateral view can be obtained for dissection of the posterior aneurysm wall, but the more anterior view also aids in the visualization of the contralateral P1 segment and the dissection of the opposing aneurysm neck. In addition, concurrent anterior circulation aneurysms can be clipped. The working space is significantly larger than with the pterional trans-Sylvian route. A disadvantage is that the large veins at the temporal pole must be sacrificed, and this maneuver is not always well-tolerated.

The scalp incision is the same as for a trans-Sylvian approach, with interfascial dissection of the temporalis fascia allowing posteroinferior reflection of the temporalis muscle. A larger pterional craniotomy is made that extends more posteriorly and inferiorly into the temporal bone. When the basilar bifurcation is particularly high, a frontoorbitozygomatic craniotomy or zygomatic arch removal can be used to facilitate a desired inferior to superior microscope trajectory.[21,26] Extradural resection of the sphenoid greater and lesser wings, both above and below the superior orbital fissure down to the base of the anterior clinoid process, can further reduce the extent of temporal lobe retraction and subsequent venous congestion.[23,29]

Distal Posterior Cerebral Artery and Superior Cerebral Artery Aneurysms. Aneurysms involving distal portions of SCA and PCA are much less commonly encountered than those arising at or near the basilar apex. Most represent fusiform dissections, flow-related aneurysms associated with arteriovenous malformations (SCA), or mycotic lesions associated with subacute bacterial endocarditis. Parent vessel sacrifice is

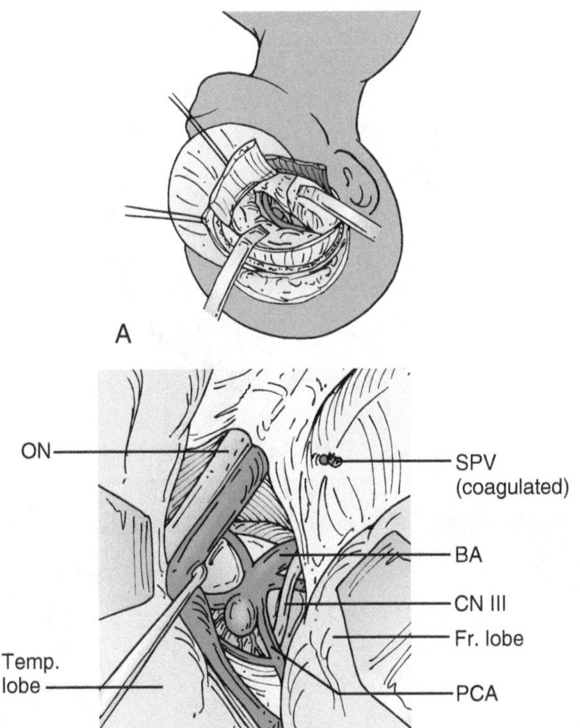

Figure 69-14. Terminal basilar bifurcation aneurysms: temporopolar approach (also referred to as the pre-temporal or "half and half" approach). A, Fronto-temporal pterional craniotomy has been performed and the Sylvian fissure broadly split. B, The sphenoparietal vein is coagulated to allow posterior and lateral retraction of the temporal pole. The basilar apex is approached posterior to the internal carotid artery (retracted with suction).

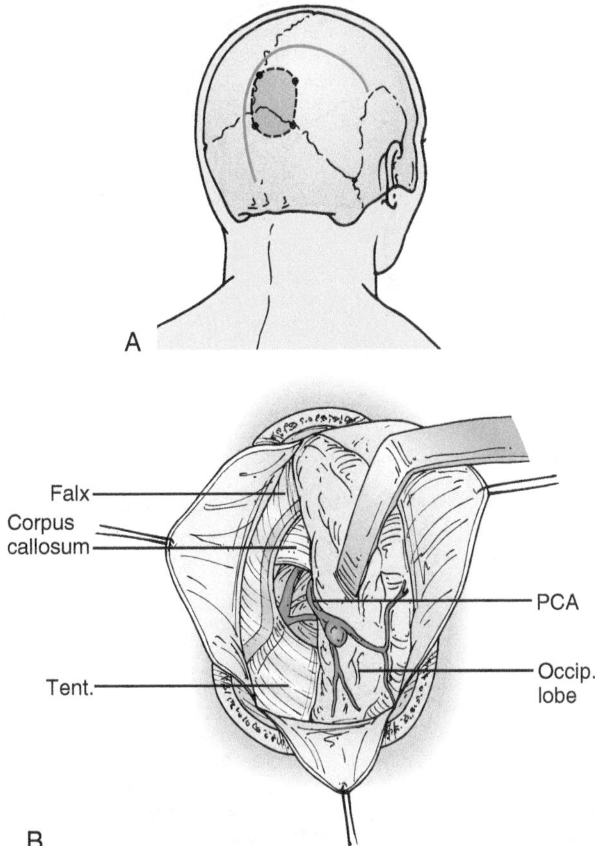

Figure 69-15. Distal posterior cerebral artery aneurysm: posterior interhemispheric approach. A, The scalp incision and bone removal allow exposure of the occipital lobe along the superior sagittal and transverse sinuses. The occipital pole is retracted laterally and superiorly to expose the tentorium. The posterior cerebral artery enters the calcarine sulcus just posterior to the splenium of the corpus callosum. This vessel may be followed distally or traced proximally to the posterior–lateral surface of the mesencephalon, until the aneurysm is encountered (B). PCA, posterior cerebral artery; Occip. Lobe, occipital lobe; Tent, tentorium.

often required, as the entering and exiting vessels arise at opposite ends of the aneurysm. Endovascular sacrifice often requires sacrifice of the parent vessel proximal to the aneurysm, and that segment may harbor important perforators. Clipping, however, offers the advantage of accurate obliteration of the parent vessel right at the aneurysm origin, allowing the perforators to be spared more easily.

The exact surgical approach taken to these lesions depends on the segment and cisternal location of the aneurysm. Many distal SCA or PCA aneurysms in the anterior portions of the ambient cistern can be approached through an anterior subtemporal route (see previous description), with the tentorium being split over a longer interval to provide the necessary posterior exposure. When a PCA aneurysm lies further back in this cistern toward the quadrigeminal cistern, an occipital posterior interhemispheric route can provide a very effective exposure (Fig. 69-15). Very distal SCA aneurysms posterior to the trigeminal nerve exit from the pons can also be approached through a superior-lateral suboccipital craniectomy, similar to that used for microvascular decompression for trigeminal neuralgia (Fig. 69-16).

A mid-PCA segment lesion is most difficult to expose surgically, as its position lies superior to the undersurface of the temporal lobe, making this approach untenable without resection of the parahippocampal gyrus. Furthermore, elevation of the posterior temporal lobe is difficult without injury of the vein of Labbé, a hazardous maneuver often accompanied by temporal lobe venous infarction or hemorrhage. In such situations, a transtemporal (through the inferior temporal gyrus) transventricular (through the temporal horn) approach, followed by splitting of the choroidal fissure, exposes this vessel segment.

Basilar Trunk Aneurysms

Aneurysms of the basilar trunk are very uncommon and are defined anatomically as arising between the vertebrobasilar junction and the SCA. Most commonly they arise at the origin of the anterior inferior cerebellar artery (AICA), in close association with the sixth cranial nerve. Surgical approaches to these lesions may include the anterior subtemporal approach combined with a medial petrosectomy, or a far lateral suboccipital craniectomy with superior and lateral extension as described in the next section. A lateral petrosal presigmoid approach with or without venous sinus sacrifice may be considered in some circumstances, but the operating space and view are usually quite limiting.

Vertebral Artery

The vertebral artery (VA) can be divided into three regions which generate aneurysms: the VA trunk independent of the posterior inferior cerebellar artery (PICA), the VA–PICA junction, and peripheral portions of PICA.

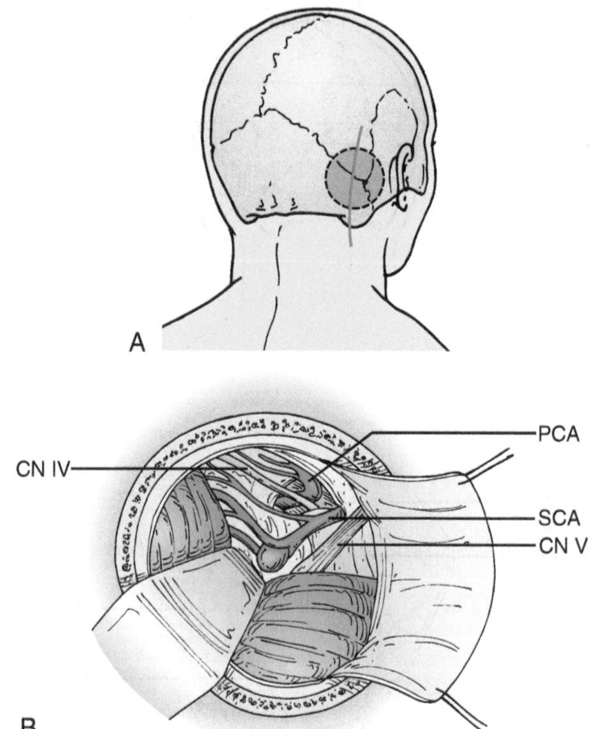

Figure 69-16. Distal superior cerebellar artery aneurysm: lateral supracerebellar approach. A, The scalp incision and bone removal allow exposure of the superior and lateral cerebellar surface along the transverse and sigmoid sinuses. B, The cerebellum is retracted medially and inferiorly, following the tentorial insertion into the petrous apex, until the superior cerebellar artery is identified adjacent to the trigeminal nerve.

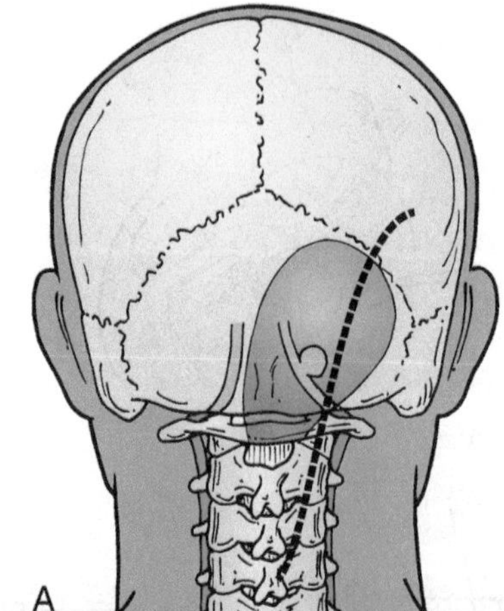

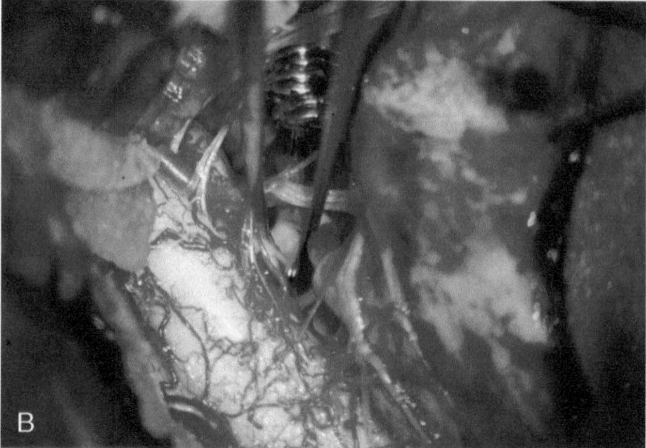

Figure 69-17. Posterior inferior cerebellar artery aneurysm (PICA): far lateral suboccipital approach. A, The incision starts in a vertical paramedian plane centered midway between the midline and the mastoid process and curved at each end to facilitate a broader view, especially laterally and inferiorly. The ipsilateral bony rim of the foramen magnum and posterior arch of C1 are removed, including an aggressive resection of the medial occipital condyle to facilitate access to the anterolateral foramen magnum and brainstem. B, After the dura is opened and cisterna magna drained, the ipsilateral cerebellar tonsil is superiorly and medially displaced so as to expose the lower cranial nerves, the vertebral artery dural entry site (between forceps), and the PICA origin within the field. Note clips on PICA aneurysm between the cranial nerves.

Vertebral Artery Trunk and Vetebral Artery–Posterior Inferior Cerebral Artery Aneurysms

Anatomy and Terminology. The VAs enter the dura at the foramen magnum laterally and then course superiorly and medially, ventral to the brainstem, to merge at the pontomedullary junction into the BA. The PICA is its principal named branch, and it usually originates from the intracranial portion of the VA approximately 1 cm above the foramen magnum and 1 cm proximal to the vertebrobasilar junction. The PICA has the most complex and variable course of the cerebellar arteries, however, and its origin may vary from below the foramen magnum to the vertebrobasilar junction.

Clinical and Radiographic Features. Those aneurysms that occur at the VA independent of the PICA origin are nearly always dissections, and are most often best treated with ipsilateral VA sacrifice and some additional method to preserve PICA flow. VA–PICA junction aneurysms, however, are typically saccular and can be clipped or coiled without PICA compromise.

Surgical Approaches. Most VA and VA–PICA junction aneurysms are best approached with a far lateral suboccipital craniotomy combined with removal of the arch of C1 (Fig. 69-17). The patient is positioned in the three-quarters-prone lateral decubitus position, a head position that provides a wide exposure of the cervicomedullary junction and facilitates visualization of the entire intracranial course of the proximal VA with little or no need for brainstem retraction. The incision generally starts in a vertical paramedian plane centered midway between the midline and the mastoid process. To facilitate a broader view laterally and inferiorly, the incision is curved laterally at its superior end, and medially at its inferior end, in an elongated "S" configuration. The craniotomy exposes the ipsilateral sigmoid sinus laterally and should extend to the midline inferiorly. The ipsilateral bony rim of the foramen magnum and posterior arch of C1 should be removed, including an aggressive resection of the medial occipital condyle to facilitate access to the anterolateral margin of the foramen magnum and brainstem.[30]

After the dura is opened and cisterna magna drained, the arachnoid boundaries of the ipsilateral cerebellar tonsil are dissected to allow superior and medial displacement, so as to expose the lower cranial nerves, the VA dural entry site, and the PICA origin within the field. The VA is followed on its lateral and superior surface superiorly until the PICA origin is visualized, often obscured by branches of the hypoglossal nerve.

After completely defining the aneurysm neck, a clip placed parallel with the VA axis, sometimes using a fenestration clip to encircle the origin of PICA, will effectively eliminate the offending lesion.

For vertebrobasilar junction (VBJ) aneurysms, the positioning, scalp, and bony exposure are the same as those used for the far lateral suboccipital approach. After the VA is dissected distal to the PICA origin, the space between the ninth, tenth, and eleventh cranial nerves and the seventh and eighth nerves is more aggressively expanded to provide visualization of the vertebrobasilar junction.

Peripheral Posterior Inferior Cerebral Artery Aneurysms

Anatomy and Terminology. The PICA can be divided into five segments and two loops, on the basis of its relationship to the medulla oblongata and the cerebellum.

The segments and their distal limits are: (1) anterior medullary, extending from the origin of the PICA at the VA to the inferior olivary prominence, (2) lateral medullary, extending to the origins of the ninth, 10th, and 11th cranial nerves, (3) tonsillomedullary, extending to the level of the tonsillar midportion (includes the caudal loop), (4) telovelotonsillar, extending to the cortical surface of the cerebellum (includes the cranial loop), and (5) cortical, extending to the cerebellar vermis and hemisphere.

Clinical and Radiographic Features. This surgical anatomic classification scheme is a critical concept for surgical planning and in deciding whether the PICA can be potentially sacrificed. The proximal segments (anterior and lateral medullary) invariably contribute brainstem perforators. A transitional (tonsillomedullary) segment may or may not contribute perforating vessels to the brainstem. Distal segments (telovelotonsillar and cortical) can be sacrificed without effects on the brainstem blood supply.

Surgical Approaches. Proximal peripheral PICA aneurysms are best approached with a far lateral suboccipital craniotomy combined with removal of the arch of C1. For distal PICA aneurysms that arise behind the brainstem, a standard midline suboccipital craniotomy and C1 arch removal are usually sufficient. For those aneurysms located beneath the tonsil, where mobilization of this structure may be associated with risk of premature rupture, a subpial tonsillar resection may be used to gain exposure. When applicable, direct clip placement across the neck of the aneurysm is performed.

During treatment, the proximal portions of PICA must be preserved. Whenever its origin is potentially compromised by direct clipping, a more proximal VA sacrifice or some type of flow augmentation procedure should be considered. Additional techniques include aneurysm resection with end-to-end anastomosis or placement of an interposition superficial temporal artery or occipital artery graft or proximal PICA obliteration combined with flow reversal by either distal PICA–PICA or occipital artery–PICA anastomosis.

Many peripheral PICA aneurysms involve dissections that cannot be safely reconstructed without sacrifice of the vessel. Even if no brainstem perforators are at risk, a large cerebellar infarction is a possibility, which should be prevented if possible with distal flow augmentation. Approximately 20% of peripheral PICA aneurysms are flow-related lesions found in tandem with a more peripheral vermian AVM. In such circumstances, the AVM can often be treated simultaneously by a widening of the surgical exposure.[31]

REFERENCES

1. Bor ASE, Velthuis BK, Majoie CB, et al. Configuration of intracranial arteries and development of aneurysms: a follow-up study. Neurology 2008;70:700–5.
2. Dolenc VV. A combined epi- and subdural direct approach to carotid-ophthalmic artery aneurysms. J Neurosurg 1985;62: 667–72.
3. Pikus HJ, Heros RC. Surgical treatment of internal carotid and posterior communicating artery aneurysms. Neurosurg Clin N Am 1998;9:785–95.
4. Reisch R, Perneczky A. Ten-year experience with the supraorbital subfrontal approach through an eyebrow skin incision. Neurosurgery 2005;57:242–53.
5. Brydon HL, Akil H, Ushewokunze S, et al. Supraorbital microcraniotomy for acute aneurysmal subarachnoid haemorrhage: results of first 50 cases. Br J Neurosurg 2008;22:40–5.
6. Mitchell P, Vindlacheruvu RR, Mahmood K, et al. Supraorbital eyebrow minicraniotomy for anterior circulation aneurysms. Surg Neurol 2005;63:47–51.
7. Fox J. Intracranial aneurysms. New York: Springer-Verlag; 1983.
8. Wermer MJH, van der Schaaf IC, Algra A, et al. Risk of rupture of unruptured intracranial aneurysms in relation to patient and aneurysm characteristics: an updated meta-analysis. Stroke 2007;38:1404–10.
9. Sanai N, Tarapore P, Lee AC, et al. The current role of microsurgery for posterior circulation aneurysms: a selective approach in the endovascular era. Neurosurgery 2008;62:1236–49, discussion 1249–53.
10. Krisht AF, Krayenbühl N, Sercl D, et al. Results of microsurgical clipping of 50 high complexity basilar apex aneurysms. Neurosurgery 2007;60:242–50, discussion 250–2.
11. Bendok BR, Getch CC, Parkinson R, et al. Extended lateral transsylvian approach for basilar bifurcation aneurysms. Neurosurgery 2004;55:174–8, discussion 178.
12. Gonzalez LF, Amin-Hanjani S, Bambakidis NC, et al. Skull base approaches to the basilar artery. Neurosurg Focus 2005;19:E3.
13. Lozier AP, Kim GH, Sciacca RR, et al. Microsurgical treatment of basilar apex aneurysms: perioperative and long-term clinical outcome. Neurosurgery 2004;54:286–96, discussion 296–9.
14. Krisht AF, Kadri PAS. Surgical clipping of complex basilar apex aneurysms: a strategy for successful outcome using the pretemporal transzygomatic transcavernous approach. Neurosurgery 2005; 56:261–73, discussion 261–73.
15. Wascher T, Spetzler R. Sacular aneurysms of the basilar bifurcation. In: Carter L, Spetzler R, editors. Neurovascular surgery. New York: McGraw Hill; 1996. p. 729–55.
16. Yasargil MG, Antic J, Laciga R, et al. Microsurgical pterional approach to aneurysms of the basilar bifurcation. Surg Neurol 1976;6:83–91.
17. Dolenc VV, Skrap M, Sustersic J, et al. A transcavernous-transsellar approach to the basilar tip aneurysms. Br J Neurosurg 1987;1: 251–9.
18. Drake CG. Bleeding aneurysms of the basilar artery. Direct surgical management in four cases. 1961. Can J Neurol Sci 1999;26: 335–40.
19. Drake CG. Gordon Murray lecture. Evolution of intracranial aneurysm surgery. Can J Surg 1984;27:549–55.
20. Heros RC, Lee SH. The combined pterional/anterior temporal approach for aneurysms of the upper basilar complex: technical report. Neurosurgery 1993;33:244–50, discussion 250–1.
21. Al-Mefty O. Supraorbital-pterional approach to skull base lesions. Neurosurgery 1987;21:474–7.
22. Malis LI. The petrosal approach. Clin Neurosurg 1991;37: 528–40.
23. Day JD, Fukushima T, Giannotta SL. Microanatomical study of the extradural middle fossa approach to the petroclival and posterior cavernous sinus region: description of the rhomboid construct. Neurosurgery 1994;34:1009–16, discussion 1016.
24. Kawase T, Shiobara R, Toya S. Anterior transpetrosal-transtentorial approach for sphenopetroclival meningiomas: surgical method and results in 10 patients. Neurosurgery 1991;28:869–75, discussion 875–6.
25. MacDonald JD, Antonelli P, Day AL. The anterior subtemporal, medial transpetrosal approach to the upper basilar artery and ponto-mesencephalic junction. Neurosurgery 1998;43:84–9.

26. Sano K, Shiokawa Y. The temporo-polar approach to basilar artery aneurysms with or without zygomatic arch translocation. Acta Neurochir (Wien) 1994;130:14–19.
27. Sundt T. Surgical techniques for saccular and giant intracranial aneurysms. Baltimore: Williams & Wilkins; 1990.
28. Al-Mefty O, Fox JL, Smith RR. Petrosal approach for petroclival meningiomas. Neurosurgery 1988;22:510–17.
29. Day JD, Giannotta SL, Fukushima T. Extradural temporopolar approach to lesions of the upper basilar artery and infrachiasmatic region. J Neurosurg 1994;81:230–5.
30. Heros RC. Lateral suboccipital approach for vertebral and vertebrobasilar artery lesions. J Neurosurg 1986;64:559–62.
31. Samson D, Batjer H: Intracranial aneurysm surgery - Techniques. Mount Kisco: Futura; 1990.

70 Surgery for Intracerebral Hemorrhage

A. David Mendelow, Barbara A. Gregson

Evidence Classifications

Class IIa, Level of Evidence A: Meta-analysis shows that early surgery improves the outcome for patients with spontaneous supratentorial intracerebral hemorrhage.

Class IIa, Level of Evidence A: Meta-analysis indicates that the greatest benefit from surgery is when the patient has a GCS of 9–12.

Class IIb, Level of Evidence B: Post hoc meta-analysis indicates that an even greater benefit occurs with early surgery when the GCS is 9–13.

Class IIb, Level of Evidence B: These generalizations do not apply to intracerebral hemorrhage from aneurysms, arteriovenous malformations, or tumors because they were excluded from most of the trials.

Class IIa, Level of Evidence A: Early surgery reduces mortality without an increase in the vegetative state or lower severe disability.

Class IIa, Level of Evidence A: Independent patient data meta-analysis confirms that surgery reduced the morbidity and mortality in patients with spontaneous intracerebral hematomas and particularly with lobar hematomas.

Class IIa, Level of Evidence B: Aneurysmal intracerebral hemorrhage is better treated with surgery for the clot as well as securing the aneurysm.

For more details refer to the AHA Evidence-based Classifications on Page xvii.

KEY POINTS

- For patients with spontaneous supratentorial intracerebral hemorrhage (ICH), early surgery is a good option particularly if the level of consciousness on the Glasgow Coma Scale is between 9 and 13 at the outset.
- There is no evidence to support early surgery if the patient presents in coma or if the conscious level is well preserved at the outset.
- Most neurosurgeons would undertake surgery if the patient's level of consciousness starts to deteriorate; especially if it is initially good.
- Intracerebral hemorrhage associated with an aneurysm is best treated surgically.

The key to understanding the therapeutic potential in intracerebral hemorrhage (ICH) lies in understanding those aspects of the etiology, pathophysiology, and consequences of ICH that surgery can influence. The etiologic factors to consider are the so-called ictohemorrhagic lesions that may require simultaneous treatment to prevent recurrence of the hemorrhage (Box 70-1). The specific aspects of pathophysiology that require consideration are clot expansion and the existence of a "penumbra" of functionally impaired but potentially viable tissue around the clot. Of the many consequences of ICH, hydrocephalus is the one that requires the most rapid and repeated attention. The therapeutic initiatives can be medical, surgical, or both, and there is an important interaction between them, particularly with regard to peri-procedural care. There is no doubt that the incidence of intracerebral hemorrhage continues to rise because of (1) the more common use of antiplatelet therapy for the primary and secondary prevention of atherosclerosis, (2) the increasing use of anticoagulation, particularly in the elderly population, and (3) the more frequent use of thrombolysis for both myocardial[1] infarction and ischemic stroke, particularly since the Third International Stroke Trial (IST 3) has now extended the time window to 6 hours.[2] It has been estimated that between 1% and 2% of the population is now undergoing anticoagulant therapy.[3] Surgical decision-making, therefore, must often take place against a background of disturbed coagulation, with careful consideration of the etiology, pathophysiology, and their consequences in the individual patient.

There are considerable controversies about the prevention of rebleeding as well as the medical management and surgical treatment of this condition. Surgical indications vary in different countries of the world, with high rates of surgical evacuation for spontaneous ICH found in some centers, and low rates in others.[4] The main controversy is about whether or not to evacuate supratentorial ICH; the randomized International Surgical Trials in Intracerebral Haemorrhage (STICH I and STICH II) involved 1634 patients from 35 countries worldwide, but at 6 months there was no overall benefit of early surgery over initial conservative treatment [5,6] There was, however, a trend toward better outcomes for early surgery in patients with superficial lobar hematomas, particularly if operated upon early (randomization <21 hours and surgery within 12 hours of randomization) and with a GCS of 9–12. A general trend of better outcomes with surgery is reported in the second edition of the *Cochrane Database of Systemic Reviews* article on surgery for ICH.[7] This finding, coupled with further meta-analysis of other trials, has strengthened the hypothesis that early craniotomy for such superficial clots will improve outcome. Controversies also relate to cerebellar hemorrhage, treatment of the underlying cause (arteriovenous malformation [AVM] or aneurysm), and initial medical treatment. Cerebellar hemorrhage is a special case because of its more frequent progression to hydrocephalus.

Although the International Subarachnoid Aneurysm Trial (ISAT) examined outcomes related to endovascular versus microsurgical treatment of ruptured cerebral aneurysms,[8,9] the trial did not specifically set out to evaluate endovascular coiling in the context of ICH. Nor has it resolved the issue of the durability of endovascular coiling, particularly in young people who would otherwise have a long life expectancy.[10] Similar uncertainty surrounds the efficacy of treatment for unruptured aneurysms in relation to subarachnoid hemorrhage and ICH.[11,12]

BOX 70-1 Causes of Intracerebal Hemorrhage

Idiopathic
Hypertension
Amyloid angiopathy
Cerebral aneurysms
Cerebral arteriovenous malformations
Cerebral arteriovenous fistulas
Cavernous malformations
Brain tumors (primary and secondary)
Anticoagulants/antiplatelet agents/tissue-type plasminogen activator
Recreational drugs
Unrecognized trauma
Post-operatively (remote and cerebellar)
Post-infarction (hemorrhagic conversion)
Hereditary hemorrhagic telangiectasia
Blood dyscrasias (e.g., hemophilia, leukemia)

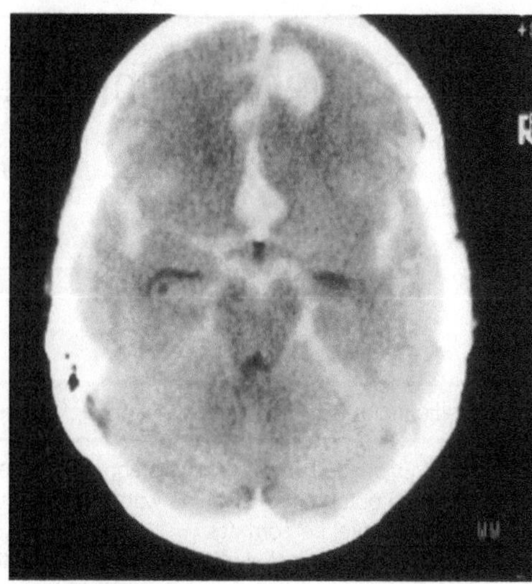

Figure 70-1. CT scan showing interhemispheric hematoma from a ruptured anterior communicating artery aneurysm.

All clinicians who deal with such patients must know the natural history of unruptured aneurysms and must keep up to date with ongoing studies, such as the International Study of Unruptured Intracranial Aneurysms (ISUIA), as the sequential reports appear.[11,12] From these studies, it has now become clear that the critical size is 6 mm; for aneurysms larger than this threshold, the risk of hemorrhage rises toward 1% for each year of future life.

Such ictohemorrhagic lesions play an important role in determining treatment of the ICH itself.[13] For example, Heiskanen et al.[14] showed that surgical evacuation of ICH due to an aneurysm was much more effective than conservative treatment. For this reason, management of aneurysmal ICH must be considered separately. Investigation of the ICH must therefore include imaging that elucidates the causes and consequences of ICH. A discussion about the nature and timing of such imaging in relation to surgical decision-making follows.

IMAGING IN THE DIAGNOSIS OF INTRACEREBRAL HEMORRHAGE

The difficulty of differentiating ischemic stroke from ICH is well known. Although the sudden onset of severe headache, coma, or epilepsy is more likely to be due to ICH, urgent imaging is essential to avoid the danger of using thrombolytic therapy in a patient with an ICH. CT is perfectly adequate for diagnosing ICH, although MRI is similarly diagnostic in the acute phase. MRI has the advantage of defining underlying ictohemorrhagic lesions better without the need for intravenous contrast agents. Because of the dynamic nature of the pathophysiology and consequences of ICH, repeated imaging must be tailored to the clinical status of the patient; hydrocephalus may develop or progress rapidly over just a few hours, so that monitoring of these patients in a critical care area is essential.

Computed Tomography

In the acute phase, spontaneous ICH is easy to recognize on CT as a high-density mass. Subsequently, the area around the ICH develops low-density changes as a result of brain edema. The volume of the hematoma can be calculated with the use of the approximation of the volume of an ellipse, from the following equation described by Broderick et al.:[15]

$$\frac{4}{3}\pi r^3 = \frac{A \times B \times C}{2}$$

where r is the radius, and A, B, and C are the diameters in three planes.

The volume of the hematoma determines the outcome, larger hematomas having a much poorer prognosis than smaller hematomas.[16] Now that CT is performed more frequently in patients with ischemic stroke, a greater number of patients with ICH will be discovered. This trend should help differentiate these two completely different disorders that have, in the past, often been wrongly lumped together as "stroke."

Sites of Hemorrhage

Lesions at certain sites are more likely to be associated with aneurysmal ICH, such as interhemispheric and Sylvian fissures (Figs 70-1, 70-2). The classic hypertensive ICH occurs in the basal ganglia, whereas lobar hematomas are more likely with amyloid angiopathy. Imaging may also demonstrate evidence of underlying tumor or trauma. Adjacent or remote calcification may also give an indication that there is an underlying cerebral AVM or tumor. Contrast-enhanced imaging and angiography may display aneurysms or cerebral AVMs. Cerebellar hematomas can produce non-communicating obstructive hydrocephalus, which may need urgent treatment in its own right.

Magnetic Resonance Imaging

MRI easily differentiates ischemic stroke from ICH. However, the MRI appearances will change as the time from ictus increases (Table 70-1). MRI with diffusion-weighted imaging (DWI) also displays the development of brain edema. The change in DWI appearance that occurs sequentially following an ICH may provide further insight into the pathophysiology of the penumbra.[1] There is no doubt that MRI is being undertaken at the primary investigation in more and more patients with stroke.

Angiography

Some surgeons prefer to obtain an angiogram routinely before undertaking surgery. This step is taken to prevent the unexpected discovery of an otherwise difficult-to-treat AVM. Similarly, for the patient in whom an aneurysm is suspected, most neurosurgeons would recommend angiography to display the aneurysm. CT and MR angiography have now become acceptable alternatives to intra-arterial angiography.

Blood Flow Mapping with Single-Photon Emission CT and Positron Emission Tomography

Single-photon emission CT (SPECT) using technetium hexamethyl-propyleneamineoxime (HM-PAO) has been shown to display a penumbra of functionally impaired, but potentially recoverable, tissue around an ICH. Through the use of the difference-based region-growing (DBRG) method, the penumbra has been objectively identified in patients with supratentorial ICH.[17] Similarly, positron emission tomography (PET) has been used to identify a penumbra around ICH,[18,19] although this issue remains controversial. Clinical[20,21] and experimental studies[22,23] have indicated that the reduced perfusion in the perihematoma region may not be severe enough to induce ischemia and may be secondary to hypometabolism. The importance of demonstrating a penumbra around an ICH is the recognition of the potential for reversal of the oligemic process by either pharmacologic or surgical means. An understanding of this issue is, therefore, essential to appreciating the possible role for surgery in a particular case; the next section, therefore, focuses on this important controversy.

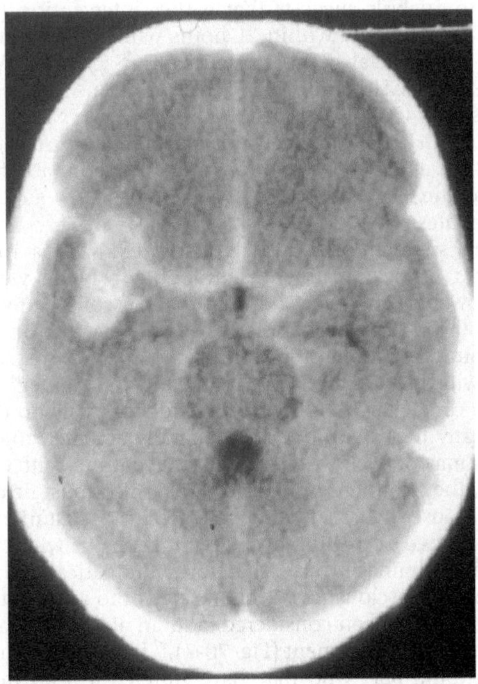

Figure 70-2. CT scan showing intracerebral and subarachnoid hemorrhage from a ruptured middle cerebral artery aneurysm.

PATHOPHYSIOLOGY OF THE PENUMBRA

Controversy, therefore, exists as to whether or not there is a penumbra around an ICH.[17,19,23–26] The importance of the issue is that if a penumbra does exist, there is the potential for medical or surgical intervention to minimize the brain damage in the area surrounding the ICH. Histologic studies have unequivocally established that there is ischemic neuronal damage in the tissue around the ICH. Later studies, using KU80 and fractin antibody stains, have shown that there is apoptosis in the tissue around an ICH (Fig. 70-3). This finding implies that some cells have undergone programmed cell death (apoptosis) and that these cells, having initially survived, may be potential targets for urgent therapeutic intervention.[27]

The first experimental evidence of a large penumbra around an ICH came from experiments in rats in which blood was introduced into the caudate nucleus under arterial pressure (Fig. 70-4).[28,29] Carbon C-14–iodoantipyrene autoradiography demonstrated a large ischemic area (Fig. 70-5). Similarly, in a study using an inflatable and deflatable microballoon (50 μL), deflation of the microballoon 2 hours after inflation produced a much smaller infarct than when the balloon was left inflated for a full 2 hours.[30] These experimental studies provide a background for clinical studies, which have also revealed a penumbra in some patients with ICH. Reduced cerebral blood flow (CBF) has also been demonstrated around ICH in patients by means of dynamic CT perfusion techniques.[19,31] Other clinical studies using MRI and positron emission tomography have similarly demonstrated a penumbra.[17–19]

By contrast, some clinical studies have not shown a penumbra.[32–34] It may well be that a penumbra is present in some patients with ICH, but not in others. Therefore, the patient with a penumbra is likely to benefit from surgical

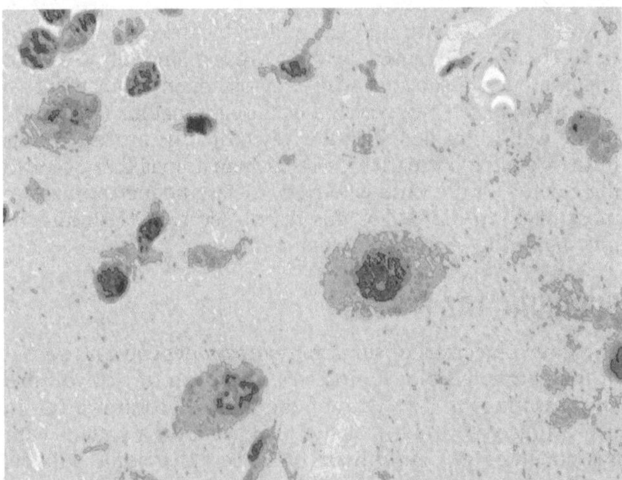

Figure 70-3. Photomicrograph of brain around an intracerebral hemorrhage stained with KU80 antibody to show evidence of apoptosis. (This finding indicates programmed cell death and therefore supports the concept of a penumbra.)

TABLE 70-1 MRI Characteristics of Hemorrhage

Time from Ictus	Clinical Phase	Appearance on T1-Weighted Images	Appearance on T2-Weighted Images	Hemoglobin State
Immediate	Hyperacute	Isointense	Bright	Intracellular oxyhemoglobin
6 hour	Acute	Isointense	Dark	Intracellular deoxyhemoglobin
6–48 hour	Early subacute	Bright	Dark	Extracellular deoxyhemoglobin
2 week	Late subacute	Bright	Bright	Extracellular methemoglobin
>3 week	Chronic	Dark	Dark	Hemosiderin

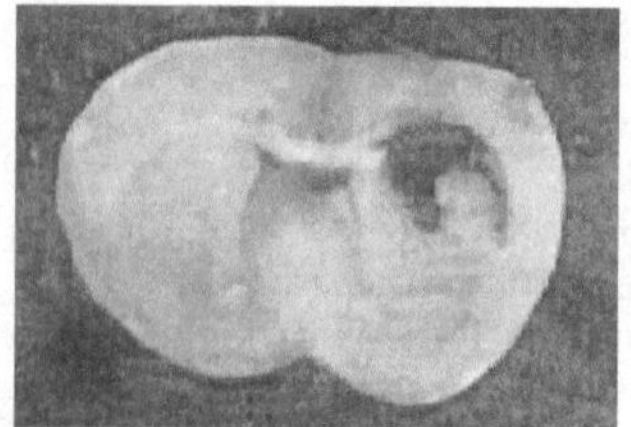

Figure 70-4. Section of rat brain showing caudate intracerebral hemorrhage.

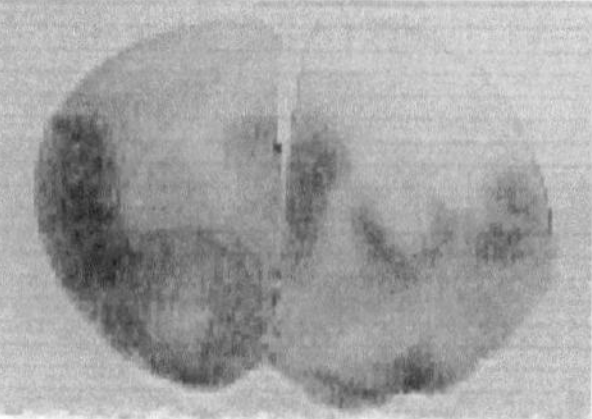

Figure 70-5. Carbon C autoradiograph showing large perfusion defect around caudate intracerebral hemorrhage.

decompression; if such patients could be identified, selective surgery could be applied. Kanno et al.[35] have shown that the use of hyperbaric oxygen leads to an improvement in the clinical condition of some patients. Microdialysis has also found elevated lactate pyruvate ratios in the penumbra.[16] Heiss[36] has clearly shown that a penumbra does exist in some patients. Also, with time, the penumbra changes and perihematoma edema progresses, adversely affecting outcome.[37,38] As discussed previously, if a penumbra can be identified, surgery is more likely to be beneficial if undertaken rapidly, before permanent secondary processes take place. Such secondary processes include release of cytokines and interleukins as well as the products of the clot itself, including fibrin and metalloproteins. As these inflammatory chemicals are produced, secondary vasogenic brain edema increases, and swelling leads to further brain shift and elevated intracranial pressure (ICP).

Underlying Pathology

In some patients with ICH, the underlying disease (e.g., tumor or cerebral AVM) causes the hemorrhage. Similarly, amyloid angiopathy is associated with amyloid deposits in the area around small cerebral vessels. It is thought that the weakening in the wall associated with this vasculopathic process results in the classic lobar parietooccipital hematomas that occur in the elderly. Of the various tumors, metastatic melanomas are most likely to bleed. For this reason, every ICH should be investigated to exclude underlying disease.

SURGICAL TREATMENT

The three objectives of surgical treatment depend on reversal of the pathophysiologic processes, reduction of clot volume, and lowering of ICP. One of the greatest controversies in neurosurgery is whether or not to operate on a patient with a supratentorial ICH. Although it is clear that some patients need surgery and that others do not, there is an area of uncertainty between these extremes. For example, a young patient with ICH in the non-dominant hemisphere who is initially conscious and talking, but who subsequently deteriorates with a lobar ICH would undoubtedly warrant surgical treatment. By contrast, an elderly dependent patient with a large ICH in the dominant hemisphere and extending into the thalamus who is in coma from the outset has such a poor prognosis that surgery would not be considered. Surgery would also not be considered for the patient with a very small volume ICH who has a minimal focal deficit with no disturbance of consciousness, particularly if the clot is deep-seated. It is, therefore, clear that some patients would not undergo surgery because they are too well and others would not undergo surgery because their prospects are hopeless. These two negative aspects in relation to surgery have resulted in confusion about the indications, particularly because there are some patients, as in the example already given, who would clearly benefit. It is the patients between these extremes for whom uncertainty about performing surgery exists.

Prospective Randomized Controlled Trials and Observational Studies

Class I Evidence

In the original review about surgical treatment for ICH reported by Prasad et al.,[39,40] four prospective randomized trials were cited. In a subsequent meta-analysis, Fernandes et al.[41] summarized seven prospective randomized controlled trials. However an individual patient data meta-analysis[42] which was updated with the STICH II results[6] (see Fig. 70-6A) showed benefit with early surgery (Fig. 70-6A). The SICHPA trial of stereotactic aspiration failed to demonstrate improved outcome from thrombolytically assisted aspiration.[43] However the MISTIE II trial has demonstrated benefits from catheter aspiration after TPA.[44] The second edition of the *Cochrane Database of Systematic Reviews* article on surgery for ICH has now indicated that there is substantial evidence in favor of surgical intervention for ICH.[7] The second Surgical Trial in Intracerebral Haemorrhage (STICH II) was published in 2013, and the final results of this trial did not show an overall benefit from early surgery with spontaneous supratentorial ICH with lobar haematomas and no IVH.[6] However, the prespecified subgroup analysis suggests that earlier intervention (admission to neurosurgery within 21 hours with surgery within 12 hours) is beneficial if the presenting GCS is 9–12. A meta-analysis of STICH I and STICH II also confirms this benefit in patients with GCS 9–13 (Fig. 70-6B).

The STICH trial has been misinterpreted by many, and a subsequent analysis of operation and admission rates for ICH in Newcastle, UK, has shown that there has been a reduction in these rates.[45]

When supratentorial ICH is associated with a ruptured aneurysm, surgical treatment is undoubtedly better, yielding a much lower mortality (27%) than that for conservative treatment (80%).[14] The probability of sudden death from a ruptured intracranial aneurysm has been subject to a systematic review with meta-analysis by Huang and van Gelder.[46]

With cerebellar ICH, no class I evidence exists on the efficacy of any treatment, but it is generally accepted that these patients may do well with surgical intervention. With cerebellar ICH, the treatment of hydrocephalus also must be considered, because hydrocephalus may lead to disturbance of consciousness. Correction of the hydrocephalus with external ventricular drainage may, therefore, dramatically improve the level of consciousness. Whether or not to remove the cerebellar ICH has been considered, and an algorithm has been offered for its management (Fig. 70-7).[47] In some patients with supratentorial ICH who may have suffered a head injury, it may be difficult to know whether or not the lesion is traumatic or spontaneous. One small trial has been conducted to ascertain whether surgical treatment should be undertaken in patients with traumatic ICH. It is clear that patients with traumatic ICH (TICH) differ from patients with spontaneous ICH (SICH), and these differences have been characterized by Siddique and colleagues.[48] By and large, patients with traumatic ICH have better outcomes, perhaps because as a group they are younger than patients with spontaneous ICH. The prospective randomized controlled trial of patients with traumatic ICH (Surgical Treatment of Traumatic Intracerebral Haemorrhage [STITCH]) has demonstrated reduced mortality with early surgery.[49]

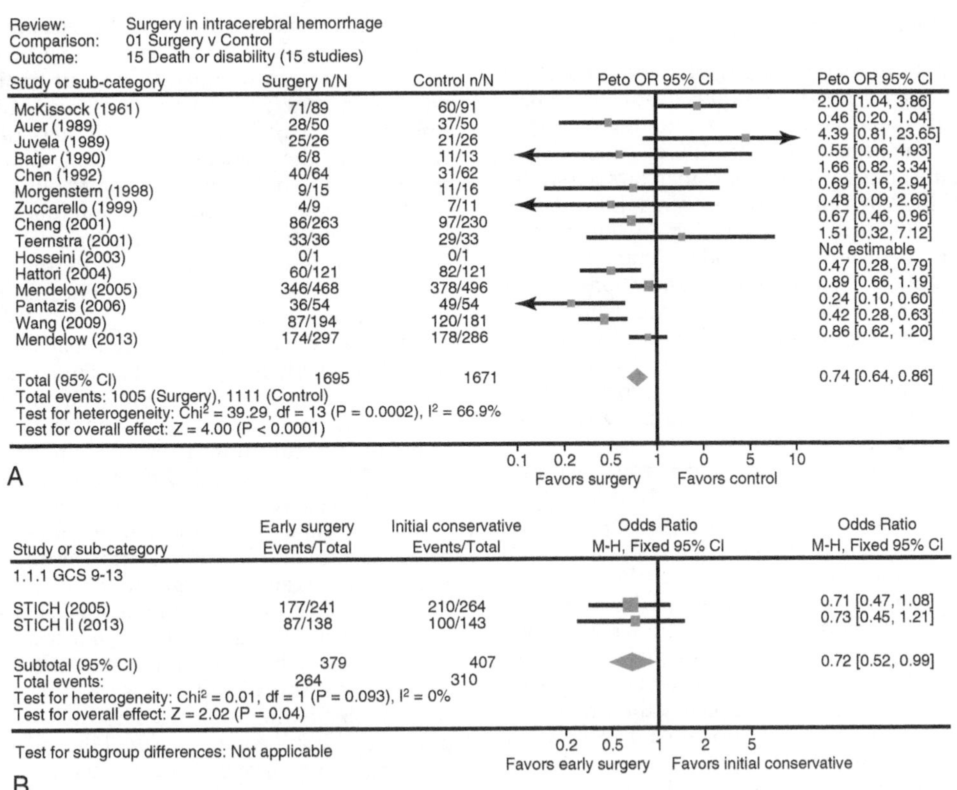

Figure 70-6. A, Meta-analysis of 15 randomized controlled trials of the effect of surgery after a supratentorial spontaneous intracerebral hemorrhage, with death and disability combined. *(From Mendelow AD, et al: Early surgery versus initial conservative treatment in patients with spontaneous supratentorial lobar intracerebral haematomas (STICH II): A randomised trial,* Lancet *382:397–408, 2013.)* B, Meta-analysis of prognosis-based outcome for patients with GCS of 9–13 at randomization in the STICH and STICH II trials.

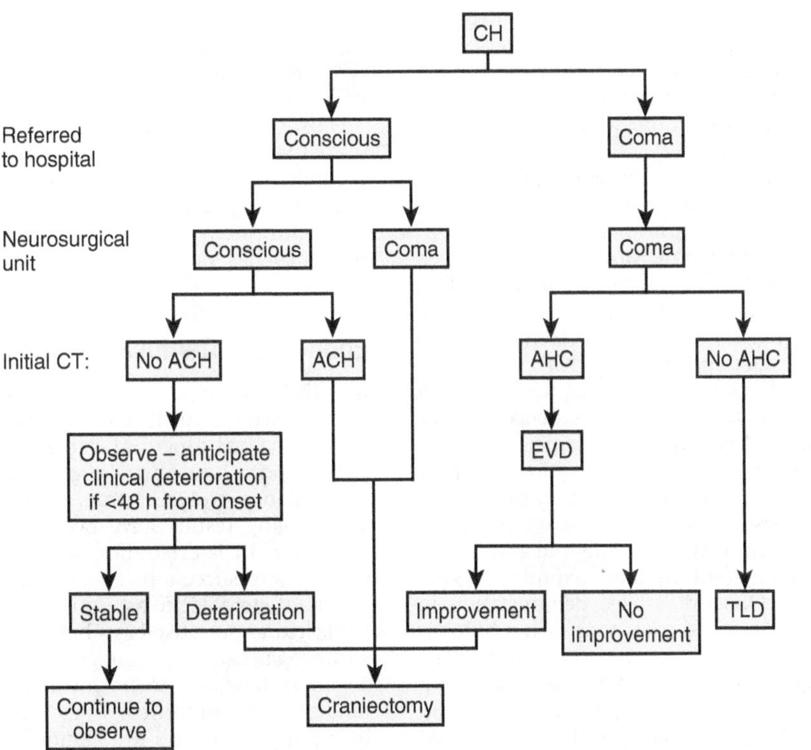

Figure 70-7. Recommendations for neurosurgical management of cerebellar hematomas. ACH, acute hydrocephalus; CH, cerebellar hemorrhage; EVD, external ventricular drainage; TLD, treatment-limiting decision. *(Redrawn from Mathew P, et al: Neurosurgical management of cerebellar hematoma and infarct.* J Neurol Neurosurg Psychiatry *59:287–292, 1995.)*

Class II and Class III Evidence

Many observational studies (yielding class II and class III evidence) have been performed to examine treatment of ICH. Retrospective studies that either compare results of surgery and non-operative management or are "pure" surgical series without controls are numerous, and more than 60 such studies were reported in 2002 by Fernandes.[16] In general, the reports of "new" surgical techniques are encouraging. Such techniques include the well-established and standard craniotomy,[50–53] stereotaxic aspiration,[54–56] and ultrasonic aspirations.[57] Fernandes[16] also summarized the class II evidence, which came from 32 papers comparing medical and surgical treatments prospectively but in a non-randomized way. The results of these studies were mixed, with some finding better results from surgery,[58] some finding no difference,[59] and others finding surgery worse.[60]

In the largest series to date, Kanaya and Kuroda[61] reported on more than 7000 patients in the Japanese ICH register; these investigators found that patients with deep coma and very large ICHs fared badly with surgical treatment. Craniotomy was better for hematomas larger than 50 mL, whereas aspiration was better for smaller clots. Other studies have similarly concluded that surgical results in patients with large hematomas were poor, particularly because the patients were selected for surgery on the basis of their comatose state and large hematomas. It is possible to draw completely the wrong conclusion from results of these observational studies, however, because they were non-randomized studies in which the less severely affected patients underwent medical treatment[50] and the most severely affected with a poor prognosis underwent surgery.

Craniotomy

The majority of neurosurgeons around the world still favor craniotomy for the evacuation of a hematoma. Generally, surgeons are more inclined to operate if the ICH is in the non-dominant hemisphere, if the patient's condition deteriorates, and if the clot is lobar and near the surface.[62] If the clot is lobar and polar, especially in the non-dominant hemisphere, surgery is easier and a larger internal decompression is possible with less risk to neurologic function.

Some surgeons prefer a large craniotomy because it leaves open the option of external decompression for swelling. Although this technique is gaining favor in traumatic ICH[63] and with larger infarcts from ischemic stroke, it has not been formally evaluated in randomized controlled trials in ICH. There are no ongoing or planned trials of external decompression for spontaneous supratentorial ICH at present; the technique is, therefore, unproven in patients with ICH. In a review of the subject of external decompression for ICH, Mitchell et al.[64] concluded that there was insufficient evidence to make any recommendation about decompressive craniectomy.

For a craniotomy, the patient is usually positioned supine with the head rotated, but in elderly patients with osteoarthritic necks, the lateral position may be preferred, especially if the clot is occipital as often occurs with amyloid angiopathy in the elderly. A large bolus of intravenous mannitol is given preoperatively; Cruz and Okuchi[64,65] have demonstrated in prospective randomized controlled trials that such a bolus is effective, although these studies have been called into question.[67] A craniotomy is made over the hematoma, with avoidance of eloquent areas of the brain such as the motor strip and speech areas of the cortex. The exact position is facilitated with the use of image guidance.

If the dura is very tight after administration of mannitol, repositioning, and correction of any other problem such as high central venous pressure or hypercapnia, the clot should initially be gently aspirated with a large-bore-type cannula so that the dura can be opened without trauma to the cortex, which may otherwise herniate alarmingly through the durotomy. Removal of even a few milliliters of clot by cannula may move the patient's condition down the pressure–volume curve. It is better to correct all of these problems at the earliest opportunity to minimize the oligemia or ischemia which would otherwise persist in any penumbra surrounding the hematoma. In theory, the sooner reperfusion is restored, the smaller the volume of ultimate ischemic damage is likely to be.

Once the dura is open, the clot may be visible or the flattened pale overlying gyri may be obvious. If not, image guidance or ultrasonography may prove helpful. A cortical window that avoids arteries and major venous structures is created, rather than a cortical incision. The window avoids or reduces the need for retraction; and for access through non-eloquent cortex, damage is less with a cortical window.

Once located, the clot is entered and easily removed with gentle suction and irrigation, with Hartman's solution rather than saline because it more closely resembles cerebrospinal fluid. Use of the operating microscope, which allows access to all parts of the hematoma through a relatively small cortical window, is highly recommended. Self-retaining retractors facilitate access to all parts of the cavity. Hemostasis is secured with bipolar diathermy. Hemostatic materials can be used, but only after the surgeon has ensured that all arterial and venous bleeding points have been coagulated.

Usually, the brain will have become slack, and the dura can be closed and the bone flap replaced. If the brain is very swollen, however, leaving the dura open with removal of the bone flap is an option. Alternatively, the bone flap can be left riding with the dura open, and the non-eloquent cortex covered with a hemostatic material. If the clot has ruptured into the ventricle, it is reasonable practice to leave an external ventricular drain in situ; the drain either can be used to drain cerebrospinal fluid post-operatively or can be connected to a pressure transducer and opened to drainage only if the ICP rises or the CPP drops below an acceptable threshold (e.g., below a CPP of 65 mm Hg in an adult or 55 mm Hg in a child).[68]

Post-operative neurologic monitoring must be continued until the patient shows signs of recovery of consciousness, because the post-operative rebleeding rate is high. In some units, post-operative CT scanning, ICP monitoring, or both are routine, but the benefit of either of these critical care measures has not yet been formally confirmed in clinical trials.

Endoscopic Removal of Hematoma

In 1989, Auer et al.[69] showed, in a single-center prospective randomized controlled trial, that endoscopic removal of hematoma was superior to medical treatment. Other observational reports have also favored endoscopy, and with stereotactic guidance and real-time ultrasonographic imaging, very encouraging results have been obtained with smaller clots (<30 mL). In later studies, such techniques have been tried with greater success in larger hematomas. Variations on the theme of stereotactic aspiration abound.[70,71] In some reports the laser has been used as a hemostatic tool through the endoscope, again with encouraging results. All these technologic advances have yet to be formally evaluated in prospective randomized controlled trials, although such techniques, including ultrasound dissolution of the clot, are planned in the evaluation that is to become part of the Minimally Invasive Surgery plus t-PA for Intracerebral Hemorrhage Evacuation (MISTIE III) trial.[72]

Ultrasonic Aspiration

Hondo et al.[57] have reported success with a stereotactic aspiration of supratentorial ICH using an ultrasonic aspirator. Studies of this procedure are observational, and the method has not yet been subjected to prospective randomized controlled trials. Similarly Newell et al. have reported sonothrombolysis for ICH.[73]

Intracavity Thrombolysis

Teernstra et al. undertook a small prospective randomized controlled trial in patients with supratentorial ICH; the investigators introduced urokinase into the cavity of the ICH and, after a specified period, aspirated the contents. This small prospective randomized controlled trial was stopped early; results showed no benefit in terms of mortality,[43] although there was a possible benefit in data from a small number of patients analyzed with multivariate analysis.[74] In some patients, in whom ICH has ruptured into the ventricle, external ventricular drainage (EVD) in conjunction with topical thrombolysis[75] may be useful. These techniques are now being evaluated in prospective randomized controlled trials. The results of the phase 2 trials of intracavity (MISTIE[76]) and intraventricular (Clot Lysis: Evaluating Accelerated Resolution of Intraventricular Hemorrhage [CLEAR IVH][77]) thrombolysis are very encouraging, with low morbidity and mortality reported.[78] Observational studies have highlighted the otherwise poor prognoses in these patients.[79]

TREATMENT OF INTRACEREBRAL HEMORRHAGE ASSOCIATED WITH SPECIFIC LESIONS

Aneurysmal Intracerebral Hemorrhage

Heiskanen et al.[14] showed in a prospective randomized controlled trial that the mortality was significantly lower for surgical removal of aneurysmal ICH than for medical treatment. For this reason, it is recommended that for the patient in whom an ICH is associated with aneurysmal rupture, the clot should be removed and the aneurysm should be clipped. Niemann et al.[80] reported that endovascular coiling associated with surgical removal of the hematoma is also an option.[81] However, the reporting of good results with endovascular coiling for ICH is anecdotal, and care should be taken in extrapolating these endovascular therapy results to patients with aneurysmal ICH rather than subarachnoid hemorrhage. Also, if the clot is to be removed surgically, clipping the aneurysm at the same time is convenient and efficient, rather than delaying the evacuation to perform the endovascular procedure. Furthermore, removal of the ICH normalizes the ICP, so the need for operative retraction is lessened and access to the aneurysm is facilitated.

Arteriovenous Malformation

Any ICH may be associated with an AVM. If such a lesion is demonstrated, care should be taken in removing the ICH because uncontrollable bleeding from the AVM may be encountered if the anatomy was not clearly defined preoperatively. If the ICH is being treated conservatively and there is an associated AVM, many surgeons prefer to deal with the AVM within 6–8 weeks of the ICH, because surgical planes lead easily to the AVM, which is often better visualized within the wall of the ICH. The options for treatment of the underlying AVM are endovascular obliteration, surgical excision, stereotaxic radiosurgery, and a combination of these treatment modalities.[82]

If the ICH is being removed in an urgent procedure, surgical excision of the AVM through the same craniotomy is clearly the preferred method of treatment, provided that it is technically possible and the appropriate inaccessible feeders have been occluded first by endovascular means if time permits. It is not necessary to embolize feeders that are on the surface and that are easily accessible at craniotomy, because they can simply be occluded as the dura is opened. Embolization can usually be achieved if the primary ICH was small and was initially treated conservatively, because the planned surgery at 6–8 weeks can be preceded by embolization. The problem occurs when it is deemed necessary to operate on the ICH as an emergency before embolization can be accomplished; in that case, the only option may be to use intra-operative hypotension *after* the ICH has been decompressed, so as to avoid compromising CPP. After removal of the ICH, the brain should have become slack, with an ICP equal to atmospheric pressure, so that the CPP approximates the blood pressure. Under such circumstances with the dura open, a mean blood pressure of about 60 mm Hg (i.e., a CPP of also about 60 mm Hg mean) would be well tolerated in a previously normotensive individual until the AVM has been excised and hemostasis properly secured.

Cerebellar Hemorrhage

A major difference between supratentorial ICH and cerebellar hemorrhage is the delayed onset of obstructive hydrocephalus that occurs with the latter, often necessitating emergency ventriculostomy. Cerebellar hemorrhage may occur at any site in the cerebellum, but lateral cerebellar hemisphere lesions are more common than midline (vermian) lesions. Clinically, such lesions are more likely to cause ataxia, nystagmus, and varying degrees of brainstem signs with the subsequent onset of a deteriorating level of consciousness owing to hydrocephalus.

Serial CT scans may be required to document increasing ventriculomegaly (Fig. 70-8). Cerebellar hemorrhages respond well to surgery, but the effect of hydrocephalus must be considered separately. There are no randomized controlled trials on which to base management decisions. However, Mathew et al.[83] have proposed an algorithm for management that is sensible and easy to use (see Fig. 70-7). As with supratentorial ICH, underlying causes of cerebellar hemorrhage should be sought and treated.

With rapid treatment, the outcome of cerebellar hemorrhage with appropriate management of hydrocephalus may be surprisingly good.[83–92] In fact, patients with short-term brainstem compression causing absence of brainstem reflexes may make a gratifying and full neurologic recovery. Nevertheless, one should not underestimate the morbidity and mortality associated with posterior fossa surgery, which carries a high complication rate compared with ventricular drainage for hydrocephalus, which is relatively straightforward. The counter-argument is that very poor outcomes result from an overly conservative approach.[83,93] Indeed, conservative management is condemned by some clinicians, although the series on which arguments are based may have included large hematomas diagnosed in the pre-CT era.[94,95] As with supratentorial ICH surgery is considered when the GCS is 9–12 (see Fig. 70-7).

PROGNOSIS AND FOLLOW-UP

In general, many studies using multivariate analyses of cases of cerebral ICH have shown that patients in deep coma, with advancing age, or with very large hematomas tend to do poorly. Kanaya and Kuroda[61] analyzed more than 7000 patients

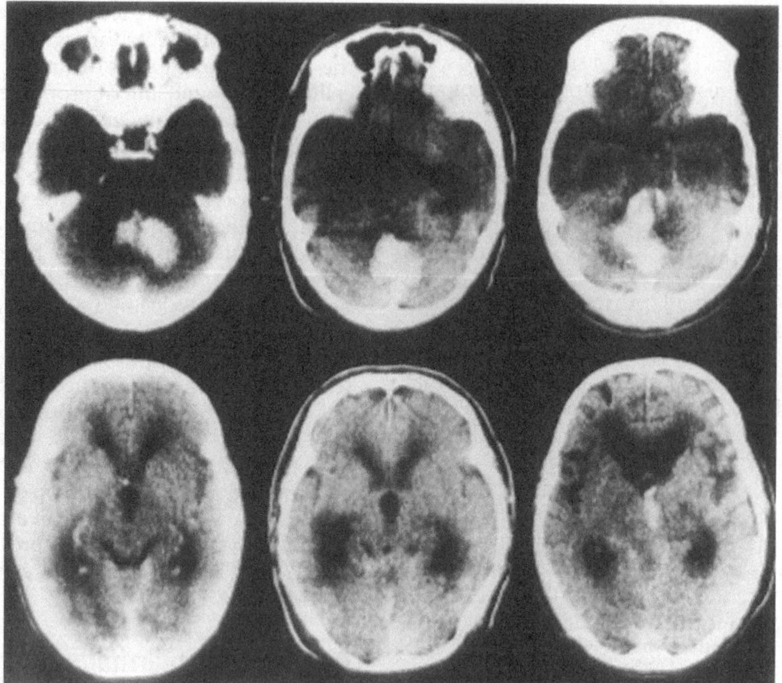

Figure 70-8. CT scans showing cerebellar intracerebral hemorrhage with hydrocephalus.

from Japan and classified them into five groups. They recommended that no surgery should be undertaken in patients in groups IVb and V (patients in coma and patients with herniation).

Our own studies at Newcastle-upon-Tyne have confirmed that elderly patients in coma with large hematomas fare poorly. We treated 440 patients with spontaneous supratentorial ICHs between May 1993 and August 1999. Of these, only 24% had favorable scores on the Glasgow Outcome Scale (GOS). Multivariate analysis of patients in the prospectively collected database (including patients not in the International Surgical Trial of Intracerebral Hemorrhage) has confirmed these findings (Table 70-2). These adverse prognostic factors have been confirmed in the later, prospectively collected studies and trials.[5,96,97]

Epilepsy

Patients with ICH may present with epilepsy for the first time, and epilepsy may be the cause of sudden unexplained death.[98] Faught et al.[99] reported that in patients with ICH, seizure incidence was more common with cortical lobar hemorrhage than with basal ganglia or subcortical hemorrhage and that no epilepsy was found if the bleed was thalamic. Chronic epilepsy after ICH has been reported in 2.5–25% of patients.[100–102] The role of surgery in reducing subsequent seizure frequency after ICH is unknown.

Risk of Rebleeding

Most hematomas enlarge in the first few hours, whatever the cause of the initial bleed, but delayed rebleeding or continued oozing is more likely to occur with a structural vascular cause, such as an aneurysm or AVM, or with an underlying tumor. Emergency angiography is, therefore, necessary if a vascular lesion is suspected. After clot evacuation, delayed angiography should be considered to eliminate an AVM. This step must not be forgotten in a patient who makes a reasonable recovery, because the results of a second hemorrhage are often worse than those of the first.

Assessment of Dependence and Disability

Unfortunately, the quality of life in survivors of ICH is often poor. Most neurosurgeons prefer to use the GOS to quantitate functional outcome. As assessed with this scale, good recovery occurs in only 5% of patients, with 10% moderately disabled (independent) and 40% remaining severely disabled (dependent).[48] Other analyses have employed the Rankin and Barthel scales; very few patients become independent according to ratings on these scales.

The GOS was originally developed by Jennett and Bond[103] for use in head injury studies. "Severe disability" was used for patients who were dependent on daily support because of mental disability, physical disability, or both. Patients with "moderate disability" could travel by public transport and could work in a sheltered environment, could shop independently, and were, therefore, independent as far as daily life was concerned. Moderately disabled patients could have residual disabilities such as hemiparesis, dysphasia, memory deficits, or personality changes, but this category did not include patients who were able only to care for themselves in their own homes; such patients were described instead as being severely disabled. "Good recovery" implied a resumption of normal life, including the capacity to return to work, to leisure, and family relationships. To compare groups treated in different ways, the scale may be dichotomized into unfavorable outcome (dead, vegetative, or severely disabled) and favorable outcome (moderate disability or good recovery).

With time, the GOS has been used more and more frequently to measure outcome in patients with conditions other than head injury, including stroke, aneurysmal subarachnoid hemorrhage, and spontaneous ICH. The use of this scale in such patient groups must take into account the differences in age, health, and social independence before the event and, hence, the potential for recovery. For many elderly patients, it

TABLE 70-2 Logistic Regression Analysis of Independent Predictors of Outcome From 440 Newcastle Patients With Intracerebral Hemorrhage in the Prospectively Collected Database*

			95% Confidence Interval	
	P	**Odds Ratio**	**Lower Value**	**Upper Value**
Age	<0.0001	0.9493	0.9277	0.9715
Verbal Glasgow Coma Scale score	0.0013	1.4697	1.1630	1.8574
Location: basal ganglia or lobar	<0.0001	7.0618	3.3713	14.7922
Hematoma volume <20 mL compared with >40 mL	<0.0001	7.9539	3.3807	18.7132
Hematoma volume 20–40 mL compared with >40 mL	0.0035	3.6871	1.5344	8.8598
Basal cisterns (open)	0.0251	12.2821	1.3685	110.2258

*December 1993–August 1999.

From Siddique MS: Intracerebral hemorrhage: The global magnitude of the problem and the scientific basis for intervention in the acute phase, Newcastle upon Tyne, UK, 2007, Newcastle University.

is clear that independence *within* the home should be regarded as a favorable outcome, but this independence might not include the ability to use public transportation or to shop independently. For patients with ICH, traditional classification to an outcome of severe disability would apply to three-quarters of the group, but the category would vary widely from people who were able to look after themselves all day within their own homes to those who were bedridden and needed total care. The GOS should, therefore, be modified for use in patients with stroke and ICH to take into account these widely differing abilities.

The extended GOS (GOS-E) provides a finer classification of outcome because it subdivides each of the categories into upper and lower levels of disability.[104] It is clear that patients with ICH who are admitted to the hospital in coma very rarely achieve a good recovery or moderate disability whatever treatment they receive, whereas those with ICH and an admission Glasgow Coma Scale score of 14 or 15 may achieve these outcome levels (Fig. 70-9). Thus, a single dichotomous outcome division, uniform for the whole patient group, is less sensitive than measures that take into account the severity of the condition at the outset and the varying potential for improvement in individual patients. A sliding-scale dichotomy has, therefore, been proposed,[96] with the breakpoints between moderate disability and severe disability for the groups with the best prognoses and between upper and lower severe disability for the groups with the worst prognoses.

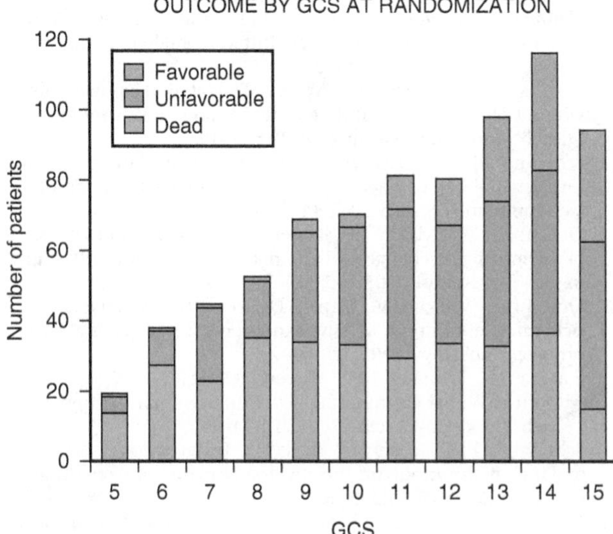

Figure 70-9. Outcome plotted against Glasgow Coma Scale (GCS) score in relation to random assignment to treatment for patients in the Surgical Trial in Intracerebral Hemorrhage (STICH).

REFERENCES

1. Davis S. DWI and perfusion MRI. In: Abstracts of the 6th World Stroke Congress and Xth International Symposium on Thrombolysis and Acute Stroke Therapy. September 24–27, 2008 Vienna, Austria and September 21–23, 2008, Budapest, Hungary. Int Stroke J 2008;3(Suppl. 1):2–474.
2. The IST-3 collaborative group. The benefits and harms of intravenous thrombolysis with recombinant tissue plasminogen activator within 6 h of acute ischaemic stroke (the third international stroke trial [IST-3]): a randomized controlled trial. Lancet 2012; 379:2352–63.
3. Sudlow M, Thomson R, Thwaites B, et al. Prevalence of atrial fibrillation and eligibility for anticoagulants in the community. Lancet 1998;352:1167–71.
4. Gregson BA, Mendelow AD. International variations in surgical practice for spontaneous intracerebral hemorrhage. Stroke 2003; 34:2593–7.
5. Mendelow AD, Gregson BA, Fernandes HM, et al. Early surgery versus initial conservative treatment in patients with spontaneous supratentorial intracerebral haematomas in the International Surgical Trial in Intracerebral Haemorrhage (STICH): A randomised trial. Lancet 2005;365:387–97.
6. Mendelow AD, Gregson BA, Rowan EN, et al. Early surgery versus initial conservative treatment in patients with spontaneous supratentorial lobar intracerebral haematomas (STICH II): A randomised trial. Lancet 2013;382:397–408.
7. Prasad K, Mendelow AD, Gregson BA. Surgery for primary supratentorial intracerebral haemorrhage. Cochrane Database Syst Rev 2008;(4):CD000200.
8. Molyneux A, Kerr R, Stratton I, et al. International Subarachnoid Aneurysm Trial (ISAT) of neurosurgical clipping versus endovascular coiling in 2143 patients with ruptured intracranial aneurysms: A randomised trial. Lancet 2002;360:1267–74.
9. Molyneux A, Kerr R, Sandercock P, et al. International Subarachnoid Aneurysm Trial (ISAT) Collaborative Group: Long term results of ISAT. In: Abstracts of the 6th World Stroke Congress and Xth International Symposium on Thrombolysis and Acute Stroke Therapy. September 24–27, 2008 Vienna, Austria and September 21–23, 2008, Budapest, Hungary. Int Stroke J 2008; 3(Suppl. 1):2–474.
10. Mitchell P, Kerr R, Mendelow AD, et al. Could late rebleeding overturn the superiority of cranial aneurysm coil embolization over clip ligation seen in the International Subarachnoid Aneurysm Trial? J Neurosurg 2008;108:437–42.
11. Brown RDJ. The natural history of unruptured intracranial aneurysms: Prospective data from the International Study of Unruptured Intracranial Aneurysms. In: Abstracts of the 11th European

Stroke Conference. Geneva, Switzerland, May 29–June 1, 2002. Cerebrovasc Dis 2002;(Suppl. 3):O146.
12. Wiebers DO, Piepgras DG, Brown RD Jr, et al. Unruptured aneurysms. J Neurosurg 2002;96:50–1, discussion 58–60.
13. Mitchell P, Mitra D, Gregson BA, et al. Prevention of intracerebral hemorrhage. Curr Drug Targets 2007;8:832–8.
14. Heiskanen O, Poranen A, Kuurne T, et al. Acute surgery for intracerebral haematomas caused by rupture of an intracranial arterial aneurysm. A prospective randomized study. Acta Neurochir (Wien) 1988;90:81–93.
15. Broderick JP, Brott TG, Duldner JE, et al. Volume of intracerebral hemorrhage: a powerful and easy-to-use predictor of 30-day mortality. Stroke 1993;24:987–93.
16. Fernandes HF. MD thesis [MD]. Newcastle upon Tyne, UK: Newcastle University; 2002.
17. Siddique MS, Fernandes HM, Wooldridge TD, et al. Reversible ischemia around intracerebral hemorrhage: A single-photon emission computerized tomography study. J Neurosurg 2002;96: 736–41.
18. Heiss W-D, Beil C, Pawlik G, et al. Nontraumatic intracerebral haematoma versus ischaemic stroke. Regional pattern of glucose metabolism. J Cereb Blood Flow Metab 1985;5:S5–6.
19. Uemura K, Shishido F, Higano S, et al. Positron emission tomography in patients with a primary intracerebral hematoma. Acta Radiol Suppl 1986;369:426–8.
20. Zazulia AR, Diringer MN, Videen TO, et al. Hypoperfusion without ischemia surrounding acute intracerebral hemorrhage. J Cereb Blood Flow Metab 2001;21:804–10.
21. Schellinger PD, Fiebach JB, Hoffmann K, et al. Stroke MRI in intracerebral hemorrhage: Is there a perihemorrhagic penumbra [see comment]? Stroke 2003;34:1674–9.
22. Orakcioglu B, Fiebach JB, Steiner T, et al. Evolution of early perihemorrhagic changes – ischemia vs. edema: An MRI study in rats. Exp Neurol 2005;193:369–76.
23. Qureshi AI, Wilson DA, Hanley DF, et al. No evidence for an ischemic penumbra in massive experimental intracerebral hemorrhage. Neurology 1999;52:266–72.
24. Zazulia AR, Diringer MN, Videen TO, et al. Hypoperfusion without ischemia surrounding acute intracerebral hemorrhage. J Cereb Blood Flow Metab 2001;21:804–10.
25. Schellinger PD, Fiebach JB, Hacke W. Imaging-based decision making in thrombolytic therapy for ischemic stroke: Present status. Stroke 2003;34:575–83.
26. Orakcioglu B, Fiebach JB, Steiner T, et al. Evolution of early perihemorrhagic changes – ischemia vs. edema: An MRI study in rats. Exp Neurol 2005;193:369–76.
27. Siddique MS. Intracerebral hemorrhage: The global magnitude of the problem and the scientific basis for intervention in the acute phase [MD thesis]. Newcastle upon Tyne, UK: Newcastle University; 2007.
28. Mendelow AD, Bullock R, Teasdale GM, et al. Intracranial haemorrhage induced at arterial pressure in the rat: Part 2. Short term changes in local cerebral blood flow measured by autoradiography. Neurol Res 1984;6:189–93.
29. Bullock R, Mendelow AD, Teasdale GM, et al. Intracranial haemorrhage induced at arterial pressure in the rat: Part 1. Description of technique, ICP changes and neurological findings. Neurol Res 1984;6:184–8.
30. Kingman TA, Mendelow AD, Graham DI, et al. Experimental intracerebral mass – time-related effects on local cerebral bloodflow. J Neurosurg 1987;67:732–8.
31. Rosand J, Eskey C, Chang Y, et al. Dynamic single-section CT demonstrates reduced cerebral blood flow in acute intracerebral hemorrhage. Cerebrovasc Dis 2002;14:214–20.
32. Powers WJ, Zazulia AR, Videen TO, et al. Autoregulation of cerebral blood flow surrounding acute (6 to 22 hours) intracerebral hemorrhage. Neurology 2001;57:18–24.
33. Videen TO, Dunford-Shore JE, Diringer MN, et al. Correction for partial volume effects in regional blood flow measurements adjacent to hematomas in humans with intracerebral hemorrhage: Implementation and validation. J Comput Assist Tomogr 1999;23:248–56.
34. Zazulia AR, Diringer MN, Derdeyn CP, et al. Progression of mass effect after intracerebral hemorrhage. Stroke 1999;30: 1167–73.
35. Kanno T, Nonomura K. Hyperbaric oxygen therapy to determine the surgical indication of moderate hypertensive intracerebral hemorrhage. Minim Invas Neurosurg 1996;39:56–9.
36. Heiss WD. Ischemic penumbra: Evidence from functional imaging in man. J Cereb Blood Flow Metab 2000;20: 1276–93.
37. Gebel JM Jr, Jauch EC, Brott TG, et al. Natural history of perihematomal edema in patients with hyperacute spontaneous intracerebral hemorrhage. Stroke 2002;33:2631–5.
38. Gebel JM Jr, Jauch EC, Brott TG, et al. Relative edema volume is a predictor of outcome in patients with hyperacute spontaneous intracerebral hemorrhage. Stroke 2002;33:2636–41.
39. Prasad K, Browman G, Srivastava A, et al. Surgery in primary supratentorial intracerebral hematoma: A meta-analysis of randomized trials. Acta Neurol Scand 1997;95:103–10.
40. Prasad K, Shrivastava A. Surgery for primary supratentorial intracerebral haemorrhage. Cochrane Database Syst Rev 1999; (4):CD000200.
41. Fernandes HM, Gregson B, Siddique MS, et al. Surgery in intracerebral hemorrhage – the uncertainty continues. Stroke 2000; 31:2511–16.
42. Gregson BA, Broderick JP, Auer LM, et al. Individual patient data subgroup meta-analysis of surgery for spontaneous supratentorial intracerebral haemorrhage. Stroke 2012;43:1496–504.
43. Teernstra O, Evers S, Lodder J, et al. Stereotactic treatment of intracerebral hematoma by means of plasminogen activator. A multicentre randomized controlled trial (SICHPA). Stroke 2003;34:968–74.
44. Mould WA, Carhuapoma JR, Muschelli J, et al. Minimally invasive surgery plus recombinant tissue-type plasminogen activator for intracerebral hemorrhage evacuation decreases perihematomal edema. Stroke 2013;44:627–34.
45. Kirkman M, Gregson B, Mahattanakal W, et al. The effect of the STICH trial on management of intracerebral haemorrhage in Newcastle. Br J Neurosurg 2008;22:739–46, discussion 747.
46. Huang J, van Gelder JM. The probability of sudden death from rupture of intracranial aneurysms: A meta-analysis. Neurosurgery 2002;51:1101–7.
47. Mathew P, Teasdale G, Bannan A, et al. Neurosurgical management of cerebellar haematoma and infarct. J Neurol Neurosurg Psychiatry 1995;59:287–92.
48. Siddique MS, Gregson BA, Fernandes HM, et al. Comparative study of traumatic and spontaneous intracerebral hemorrhage. J Neurosurg 2002;96:86–9.
49. Mendelow DA, Gregson BA, Rowan EN, et al. Results from the first randomized controlled trial of surgery for traumatic intracerebral haemorrhage [STITCH(TRAUMA)]. J Neurotrauma 2014; 31:A-30.
50. Chen X, Yang H, Cheng Z. The comparative study of medical and surgical treatment of hypertensive intracerebral haemorrhage. Acta Acad Med Shanghai 1992;19:237–40.
51. Chen B, Hou D. Surgical treatment of hypertensive intracerebral hemorrhage. Chin Med J (Engl) 1981;94:723–8.
52. McKissock W, Richardson A, Taylor J. Primary intracerebral haemorrhage; a controlled trial of surgical and conservative treatment in 180 unselected cases. Lancet 1961;2:221–6.
53. Pia HW. The surgical treatment of intracerebral and intraventricular haematomas. Acta Neurochir 1972;27:149.
54. Lui ZH, Kang HQ, Chen XH, et al. Evacuation of hypertensive intracerebral hematoma by a stereotactic technique. Stereotact Funct Neurosurg 1990;54:451–2.
55. Niizuma H, Shimizu Y, Yonemitsu T, et al. Results of stereotactic aspiration in 175 cases of putaminal haemorrhage. Neurosurgery 1989;24:814–19.
56. Mohadjer M. Computed tomographic-stereotactic evacuation and fibrinolysis of spontaneous intracerebral haematomas. In: Lorenz R, Klinger M, Brock M, editors. Advances in Neurosurgery. Berlin: Springer-Verlag; 1993. p. 47–51.
57. Hondo H, Uno M, Sasaki K, et al. Computed tomography controlled aspiration surgery for hypertensive intracerebral hemorrhage. Experience of more than 400 cases. Stereotact Funct Neurosurg 1990;54:432–7.
58. Kanaya H, Yukawa H, Itoh Z, et al. A neurological grading for patients with hypertensive intracerebral hemorrhage and a classification for hematoma location of computer tomography. In:

7th conference of surgical treatment of stroke; 1978. Japan; 1978. p. 265–70.

59. Kanno T, Sano H, Shinomiya Y, et al. Role of surgery in hypertensive intracerebral hematoma. A comparative study of 305 nonsurgical and 154 surgical cases. J Neurosurg 1984;61: 1091–9.
60. Coraddu M, Floris F, Nurchi GC, et al. Considerations about the surgical indication of the spontaneous cerebral haematomas. J Neurosurg Sci 1990;34:35–9.
61. Kanaya H, Kuroda K. Development in neurosurgical approaches to hypertensive intracerebral haemorrhage in Japan. In: Kaufman HH, editor. Intracerebral Hematomas. New York: Raven Press; 1992. p. 197–209.
62. Fernandes HM, Mendelow AD. Spontaneous intracerebral haemorrhage: A surgical dilemma. Br J Neurosurg 1999;13: 389–94.
63. Taylor ABW, Rosenfeld J, Shann F, et al. A randomized trial of very early decompressive craniectomy in children with traumatic brain injury and sustained intracranial hypertension. Childs Nerv Syst 2001;17:154–62.
64. Mitchell P, Gregson BA, Vindlacheruvu R, et al. Surgical options in ICH including decompressive craniectomy. J Neurol Sci 2007; 261:89–98.
65. Cruz J, Minoja G, Okuchi K. Improving clinical outcomes from acute subdural hematomas with the emergency preoperative administration of high doses of mannitol: A randomized trial. Neurosurgery 2001;49:864–71.
66. Cruz J, Minoja G, Okuchi K. Major clinical and physiological benefits of early high doses of mannitol for intraparenchymal temporal lobe hemorrhages with abnormal pupillary widening: A randomized trial. Neurosurgery 2002;51:628–37, discussion 637–8.
67. Roberts I, Smith R, Evans S. Doubts over head injury studies. BMJ 2007;334:392–4.
68. Chambers IR, Treadwell L, Mendelow AD. The determination of threshold levels of cerebral perfusion pressure and intracranial pressure in severe head injury using receiver operator characteristic curves: An observational study on 291 patients. J Neurosurg 2001;94:412–16.
69. Auer LM, Deinsberger W, Niederkorn K, et al. Endoscopic surgery versus medical treatment for spontaneous intracerebral hematoma: A randomized study. J Neurosurg 1989;70:530–5.
70. Marquardt G, Wolff R, Sager A, et al. Manual stereotactic aspiration of spontaneous deep-seated intracerebral hematomas in non-comatose patients. Br J Neurosurg 2001;15:126–31.
71. Marquardt G, Wolff R, Sager A, et al. Subacute stereotactic aspiration of heamatomas within the basal ganglia reduces occurrence of complications in the course of haemorrhagic stroke in non-comatose patients. Cerebrovasc Dis 2003;15:252–7.
72. <http://braininjuryoutcomes.com/mistie-iii-about>; [Accessed 5 March 2014.].
73. Newell DW, Shah MM, Wilcox R, et al. Minimally invasive evacuation of spontaneous intracerebral hemorrhage using sonothrombolysis. J Neurosurg 2011;115:592–601.
74. Teernstra OPM, Blaauw G. SICHPA: Stereotactic Treatment of Intracerebral Hematoma by Means of a Plasminogen Activator: A multicentre randomised controlled trial. In: 12th World Congress of Neurosurgery; 2001. Sydney; 2001.
75. Naff NJ, Hanley DF, Keyl PM, et al. Intraventricular thrombolysis speeds blood clot resolution: Results of a pilot, prospective, randomized, double-blind, controlled trial. Neurosurgery 2004; 54:577–83, discussion 583–4.
76. <http://braininjuryoutcomes.com/mistie-about>; [Accessed 5 March 2014.].
77. <http://braininjuryoutcomes.com/clear-about>; [Accessed 5 March 2014.].
78. Hanley D. Update of Clinical Trials: CLEAR, MISTIE & STICH. In: European Association of Neurosurgery Societies (EANS); 2007. Glasgow; 2007.
79. Arene NU, Fernandes HM, Wilson S, et al. Intraventricular haemorrhage from spontaneous intracerebral haemorrhage and aneurysmal rupture. Acta Neurochirg Suppl 1998;79:134–8.
80. Niemann DB, Wills AD, Maartens NF, et al. Treatment of intracerebral hematomas caused by aneurysm rupture: coil placement followed by clot evacuation. J Neurosurgery 2003;99:843–7.
81. Molyneux AKR, Stratton I, Sandercock P, et al. International Subarachnoid Aneurysm Trial (ISAT) Collaborative Group: International Subarachnoid Aneurysm Trial (ISAT) of neurosurgical clipping versus endovascular coiling in 2143 patients with ruptured intracranial aneurysms: A randomised trial. Lancet 2002;360(9342):1267–74.
82. Nataraj A, Mohamed MB, Gholkar A, et al. Multimodality treatment of cerebral arteriovenous malformations. World Neurosurg 2014;82:149–59.
83. Mathew P, Teasdale G, Bannan A, et al. Neurosurgical management of cerebellar haematoma and infarct. J Neurol Neurosurg Psychiatry 1995;59:287–92.
84. Auer LM, Auer T, Sayama I. Indications for surgical treatment of cerebellar haemorrhage and infarction. Acta Neurochir 1986;79: 74–9.
85. Donauer E, Loew F, Faubert C, et al. Prognostic factors in the treatment of cerebellar haemorrhage. Acta Neurochir 1994;131: 59–66.
86. Dunne JW, Chakera T, Kermode S. Cerebellar haemorrhage: Diagnosis and treatment: A study of 75 consecutive cases. Q J Med 1987;64:739–54.
87. Firsching R, Huber M, Frowein RA. Cerebellar haemorrhage: Management and prognosis. Neurosurg Rev 1991;14:191–4.
88. Gerritsen van der Hoop R, Vermeulen N, van Gijn J. Cerebellar haemorrhage: diagnosis and treatment. Surg Neurol 1988;29: 6–10.
89. Heros RC. Cerebellar haemorrhage and infarction. Stroke 1982;29:6–10.
90. Koziarski A, Frankiewicz E. Medical and surgical treatment of intracerebellar haematomas. Acta Neurochir 1991;110:24–8.
91. Lui T, Fairholm DJ, Shu T, et al. Surgical treatment of spontaneous cerebellar hemorrhage. Surg Neurol 1985;23:555–8.
92. Waidhauser E, Hamburger C. Marguth F: Neurosurgical management of cerebellar haemorrhage. Neurosurg Rev 1990;13: 211–17.
93. Ott KH, Kase CS, Ojemann RG, et al. Cerebellar hemorrhage: Diagnosis and treatment. A review of 56 cases. Arch Neurol 1974;31:160–7.
94. Brennan RW, Bergland RM. Acute cerebellar haemorrhage. Analysis of clinical findings and outcome in 12 cases. Neurology 1977;27:527–32.
95. Fisher CM, Picard EH, Polak A, et al. Acute hypertensive cerebellar haemorrhage: Diagnosis and surgical treatment. J Nerv Ment Dis 1965;140:38–57.
96. Mendelow AD, Teasdale GM, Barer D, et al. Outcome assignment in the International Surgical Trial of Intracerebral Haemorrhage. Acta Neurochir (Wien) 2003;145:679–81, discussion 681.
97. Hemphill JC 3rd, Bonovich DC, Besmertis L, et al. The ICH score: A simple, reliable grading scale for intracerebral hemorrhage. Stroke 2001;32:891–7.
98. Black M, Graham D. Sudden unexplained death in adults caused by intracranial pathology. J Clin Pathol 2002;55:44–50.
99. Faught E, Peters D, Bartolucci A, et al. Seizures after primary intracerebral hemorrhage. Neurology 1989;39:1089–93.
100. Lancman M, Golimstok A, Norscini J, et al. Risk factors for developing seizures after a stroke. Epilepsia 1993;34:141–3.
101. Sung CY, Chu NS. Epileptic seizures in intracerebral haemorrhage. J Neurol Neurosurg Psychiatry 1989;52:1273–6.
102. Arboix X, García-Eroles L, Massons JB, et al. Predictive factors of early seizures after cerebrovascular disease. Stroke 1997;28: 1590–4.
103. Jennett B, Bond M. Assessment of outcome after severe brain damage: A practical scale. Lancet 1975;1:480–4.
104. Wilson JT, Pettigrew LE, Teasdale GM. Structured interviews for the Glasgow Outcome Scale and the extended Glasgow Outcome Scale: Guidelines for their use. J Neurotrauma 1998;15(8): 573–85.

71 Intraventricular Hemorrhage

J. Max Findlay

KEY POINTS

- The commonest causes of spontaneous intraventricular hemorrhage (IVH) are hypertensive parenchymal hemorrhages (occurring in at least one-third of these patients), saccular aneurysms (most commonly the anterior communicating artery location, and fourth ventricle hemorrhage especially suggestive of a posterior circulation location), and arteriovenous malformations.
- IVH is an independent and important clinical problem that adversely impacts outcome when clots distend the ventricular system, compress adjacent brain, obstruct cerebrospinal fluid and contribute to elevated intracranial pressure (ICP).
- Vascular imaging is recommended for any patient with IVH with no clear cause based on history and CT scanning, and especially for those patients 45 years of age or younger.
- The standard treatment for significant IVH (i.e., associated hydrocephalus) is external ventricular drainage (EVD). Intraventricular fibrinolyis or thrombolysis (IVT), using an enzyme such as rt-PA administered through an external drainage catheter, appears to accelerate IVH clearance, maintain catheter patency and facilitate ICP control in patients with severe IVHs.
- It is not currently known whether IVT in addition to EVD independently improves long-term clinical outcome in any patient group, but it is a subject of continued study especially in patients with IVH associated with ICH due to hypertensive arteriolar degeneration.

Bleeding directly into the ventricles from a source or lesion that is in contact with, or is part of, a ventricular wall, such as a vascular malformation or neoplasm is classified as primary intraventricular hemorrhage (IVH). This type of IVH without an associated intracerebral hematoma is rare, accounting for only about 3% of all spontaneous intracerebral hemorrhages (ICHs).[1] Usually IVH is secondary either to intracerebral bleeding that dissects through brain parenchyma to reach a ventricle or to bleeding into the subarachnoid space that spreads into the ventricles through the fourth ventricular foramina. Primary or secondary IVHs can fill one or more ventricles and, when of sufficient volume and density, can result in formed ventricular blood clots, or hematocephalus. Blood that refluxes into the ventricles from the subarachnoid space often remains unclotted and settles in dependent parts of the ventricular system. Although the presence of IVH per se does not always correlate with neurologic condition or prognosis, IVH is an independent and important clinical problem when clots distend the ventricular system, compress adjacent brain, or obstruct cerebrospinal fluid (CSF) flow to cause hydrocephalus and elevated intracranial pressure (ICP).

There are many causes of spontaneous IVH, but the most common are hypertensive ICH, saccular aneurysms, and arteriovenous malformations (AVMs).[2-8] IVH resulting from germinal matrix hemorrhage in the newborn and traumatic IVH are not discussed in this chapter.

PRIMARY INTRAVENTRICULAR HEMORRHAGE

Spontaneous IVH with no evidence of associated ICH is most often due either to a vascular malformation that contacts the ependyma of one of the ventricular chambers or to an intraventricular or periventricular neoplasm. There have been rare reports of primary IVH due to ruptured intraventricular aneurysms, which arise from distal lenticulostriate or choroidal arteries that reach the ventricular lining or choroid plexus.[9] Aneurysms have been reported on penetrating arteries enlarged by moyamoya disease.[10-12] In many cases, no cause of primary IVH can be established, although in these instances bleeding may be from rupture of arterioles located in the immediate periventricular region that have been weakened by chronic hypertension. Past the 8th decade of life primary IVH carries a particularly poor prognosis, with an over 50% early mortality rate.[13] Primary IVH can be due to any type of bleeding disorder, including anticoagulation[8] and fibrinolytic treatment.[14,15]

The most common brain neoplasms that bleed spontaneously are malignant astrocytomas and melanoma metastases. Less common tumors to cause primary IVH are ependymoma,[16] subependymoma,[17] choroid plexus papilloma,[18] intraventricular meningioma,[19,20] pituitary tumors that erode through the floor of the third ventricle,[21] neurocytoma,[22] granular cell tumor,[23] metastasis,[24] and craniopharyngioma. It is probable that any cause of spontaneous ICH can be responsible for direct bleeding into the ventricles.

HYPERTENSIVE BRAIN HEMORRHAGE AND INTRAVENTRICULAR HEMORRHAGE

Spontaneous hypertensive ICHs are associated with secondary IVH in one-third to one-half of patients.[25] The most significant risk factor for this arteriopathy, which most commonly affects the lenticulostriate and thalamoperforating arterioles, is chronic arterial hypertension; other risk factors are moderate-to-heavy alcohol intake and anticoagulant treatment.[26] IVH most often complicates thalamic, caudate, or putaminal bleeding that decompresses into the lateral or third ventricles (Fig. 71-1). Not surprisingly, IVH in this setting has been associated with larger parenchymal hematomas, midline shift of brain structures, and worse clinical outcome.[27-30] Patients with spontaneous and deep intracerebral hemorrhages complicated by both IVH and hydrocephalus have a particularly bad prognosis,[31-33] although the associated ICH size probably has the greatest influence on clinical outcome.[34] After spontaneous ICH the list of factors consistently associated with death are as follows: increasing age, decreasing level

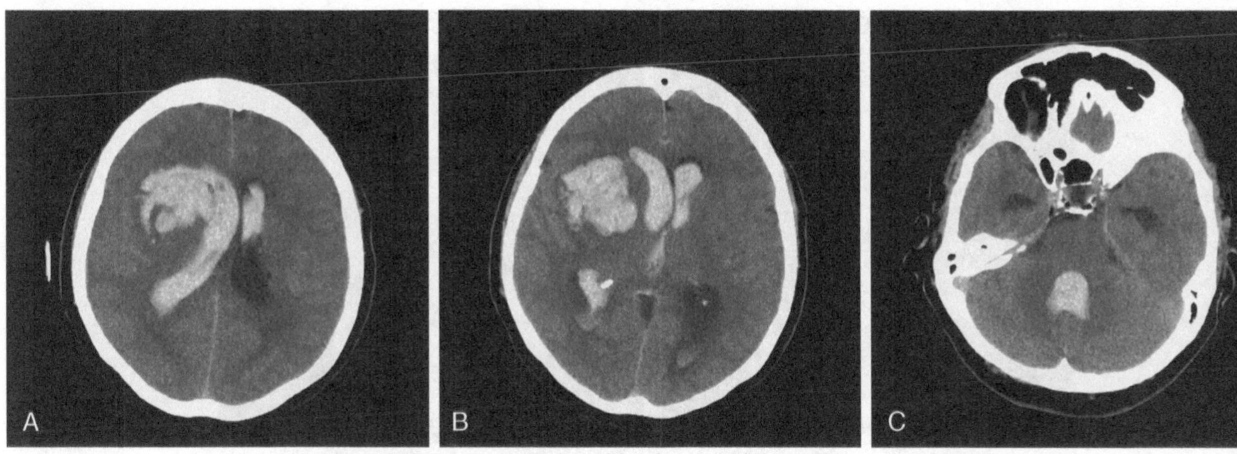

Figure 71-1. A 71-year-old woman presented obtunded and paralyzed on the left side of her body from a right lentiform intracerebral hemorrhage that extended into the ventricular system. See Figure 71-4 for follow-up.

of consciousness, increasing ICH volume, presence of IVH and either a deep or infratentorial (cerebellar and brainstem) ICH location.[35]

ANEURYSMAL INTRAVENTRICULAR HEMORRHAGE

Up to 45% of patients suffering cerebral aneurysm rupture show IVH on their initial CT scan.[36] Patients with IVH in this setting more commonly have a history of hypertension, diabetes, and coronary artery disease, are generally in poorer neurological condition than those without IVH, and the presence of IVH strongly and independently predicts a worse prognosis.[36,37] Not surprisingly, patients with higher volume IVHs are the most likely to do poorly.[38] Clinical deterioration is seen more often in ruptured aneurysm patients with associated IVH, and they have a higher incidence of symptomatic vasospasm.[36] The presence of IVH has been added to the commonly used Fisher scale of subarachnoid hemorrhage severity to predict vasospasm occurrence.[39] However not all analyses have found that IVH is associated with delayed cerebral ischemia or infarction.[38] Aneurysmal IVH is associated with a higher (up to 50%) chance of requiring a ventriculoperitoneal shunt.[40–42]

Aneurysm rupture can cause IVH through several different mechanisms.[43] Blood can reflux into the ventricular system from an aneurysm in any location, but disproportionate or isolated fourth ventricular hemorrhage in association with SAH is especially suggestive of a posterior circulation aneurysm situated closer to the fourth ventricular foramina. Up to one-half of posterior inferior cerebellar artery (PICA) aneurysm ruptures have an accompanying IVH,[44] and indeed on a case-by-case analysis aneurysms located in the posterior circulation more commonly cause IVH than those found in the anterior circulation.[36]

Sudden death from aneurysmal SAH is commonly associated with IVH, and in some patients the mechanism may be acute fourth ventricular dilatation causing brainstem compression.[45,46]

Aneurysms also cause IVH when forceful hemorrhage dissects through intervening brain parenchyma to reach the ventricular system. This occurrence is most commonly seen with anterior communicating artery aneurysms.[47] Accounting for roughly one-third of saccular cerebral aneurysms and with a 25% incidence of associated IVH, anterior communicating artery aneurysms are the single most common type overall to cause IVH (Fig. 71-2). Blood can break directly through the lamina terminalis into the third ventricle or can pass superiorly beneath the rostrum of the corpus callosum to dissect through the septum pellucidum into the lateral ventricles. Frontal hemorrhages resulting from anterior communicating or middle cerebral artery aneurysms can spread into the anterior horn of the lateral ventricles. Parenchymal clots from middle cerebral aneurysms can also rupture into the body or the temporal horn of the lateral ventricles. Internal carotid artery aneurysms, at the origin of either the posterior communicating or the anterior choroidal arteries can rupture into the temporal horn of the lateral ventricles. Basilar apex aneurysms can rupture directly through the hypothalamus to reach the third ventricle, usually with serious clinical consequences.

In large patient series, IVH along with aneurysm rupture is associated with higher intracranial pressures[48] and, as already emphasized, worse clinical outcome.[49]

VASCULAR MALFORMATIONS AND INTRAVENTRICULAR HEMORRHAGE

Cerebral AVMs that are in contact with the ventricular wall and hemorrhage often bleed into the ventricles, and are usually associated with deep cerebral venous drainage (Fig. 71-3). In one prospective AVM database, 16% of first AVM hemorrhages were primarily intraventricular and 31% were combined intracerebral and intraventricular hemorrhages.[50] Periventricular cavernous malformations and dural arteriovenous fistulas with transcerebral venous drainage are less common, but can also cause IVH.

NATURAL CLEARANCE OF INTRAVENTRICULAR HEMORRHAGE

Normally the CSF contains little fibrinolytic activity, although fibrinolysis becomes detectable after bleeding into the CSF. As in plasma, the principal fibrinolytic enzyme in the CSF is plasmin, carried into the ventricles in its precursor form, plasminogen, as a normal blood constituent. It is converted to its active form by tissue-type plasminogen activator (t-PA). Tissue-type plasminogen activator is released from the endothelium of small vessels in the meninges and ependyma, and leukocytes and platelets within the ventricular thrombi are additional sources of plasminogen activator enzymes. These various activators diffuse into clot, bind to fibrin, and activate plasminogen incorporated into the coagulum. The degree of fibrinolytic activity in "activated" CSF is meager

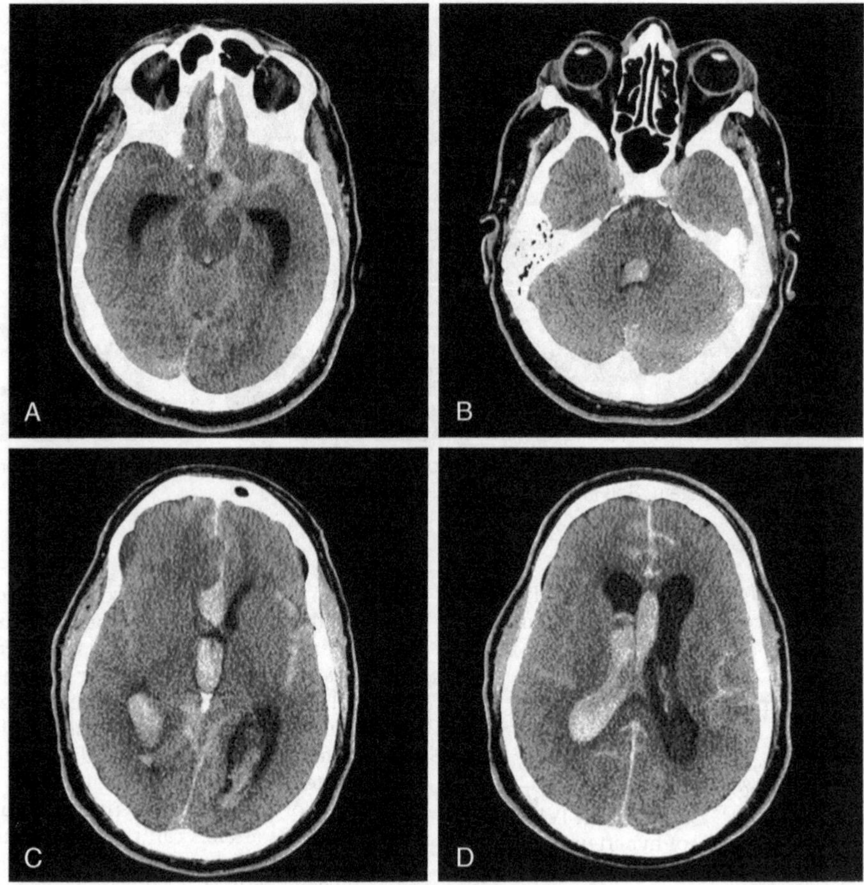

Figure 71-2. A 57-year-old man suffered recurrent hemorrhage from an anterior communicating artery aneurysm resulting in widespread IVH and hydrocephalus (A–D). See Figure 71-5 for follow-up.

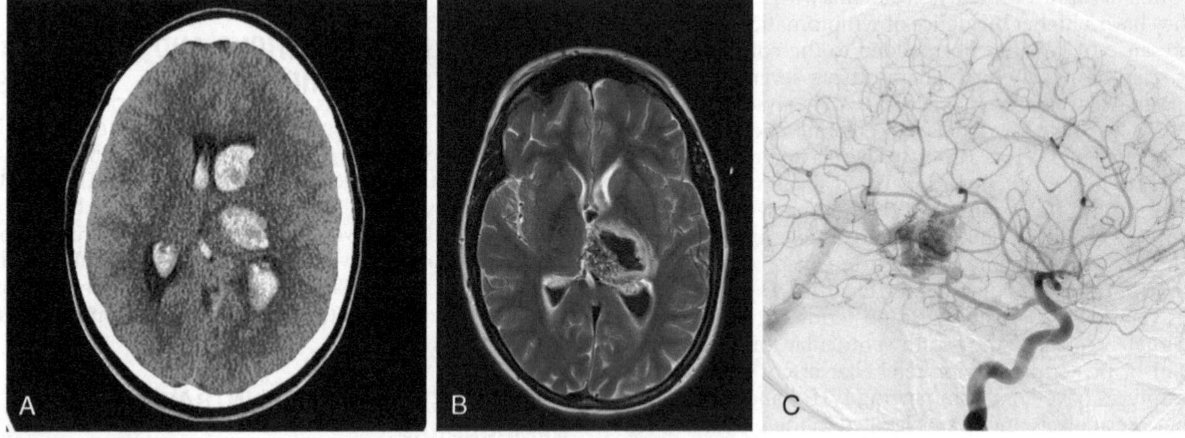

Figure 71-3. A 25-year-old woman presented obtunded with right hemiparesis after spontaneous bleeding from a left thalamic (pulvinar) arteriovenous malformation (AVM) with secondary intraventricular hemorrhage (A, CT scan; B, MRI; C, cerebral angiogram). She had Parinaud's syndrome (conjugate down gaze with paralysis of upgaze – "setting-sun sign", abnormal papillary responses and convergence–retraction nystagmus), but all of her symptoms and signs resolved within 4 months and she was then treated with stereotactic radiosurgery for her AVM. At the time of this writing she is less than 12 months from hemorrhage.

relative to plasma, but is proportional to the volume of blood clot volume. It is also balanced by the presence of inhibitors also released into the CSF by inflamed leptomeninges.[51] Changes in CSF coagulation and fibrinolysis have been studied in the context of SAH and are probably similar to changes following IVH.[52]

The resolution of intraventricular blood clot appears to follow first-order kinetics, such that the daily percentage rate of clot breakdown and clot half-life is constant and the absolute amount of clot broken down per day rises with increasing IVH volume.[53] The clearance of erythrocytes from CSF is accomplished by several mechanisms. The first is hemolysis, which commences within hours and reaches a plateau 2–10 days after IVH, depending on the size of the hemorrhage. Another is phagocytosis by macrophages, which occurs both in the leptomeninges irritated by blood and in arachnoid granulations engorged with erythrocytes.

CLINICAL FEATURES

Spontaneous and primary IVH manifests as sudden headache, vomiting, and sometimes altered mental status.[5,54] A generalized seizure may occur, but without any significant associated ICH, focal signs are generally absent. Symptoms from even a large IVH can sometimes be surprisingly minimal, provided that the ventricles have not become distended and ICP remains within normal limits. The total volume of CSF in adults is approximately 150 mL, and the normal ventricular volume is only 20–30 mL. Acute fourth ventricular distension after aneurysm or AVM rupture causing brainstem compression is associated with rapid and advanced neurologic deterioration and with sudden death.

With secondary IVH, presenting symptoms are usually due to the associated ICH or SAH, and the nature and magnitude of the symptoms and signs correspond to the location and size of the hemorrhage.

Symptomatic vasospasm of the anterior and middle cerebral arteries after an AVM-related IVH has been described,[55,56] but the complication is exceptional after hemorrhage restricted to the ventricles. Delayed-onset cerebral vasospasm after aneurysm rupture depends on thick blood clots deposited in the basal subarachnoid cisterns and left in prolonged contact with the adventitial surfaces of arteries. The presence of thick subarachnoid hematomas along with blood clots also in both lateral ventricles may predict an especially high risk of delayed cerebral ischemia after aneurysm rupture.[57]

Non-communicating hydrocephalus can occur acutely after IVH if clots obstruct CSF drainage within the ventricular system, and communicating hydrocephalus may develop more gradually or even in a delayed fashion because of obstruction and then scarring of the arachnoid granulations from blood elements carried to them by CSF flow. The risk of hydrocephalus correlates with the severity of IVH and is greater if there is blood in the third or fourth ventricles or if there is associated SAH. In spontaneous supratentorial ICH, secondary IVH correlates with the presence of acute hydrocephalus and poor outcome.[58] Acute hydrocephalus is seen in roughly 15% of patients with ruptured aneurysms, and its presence is also significantly related to the presence of IVH.[59]

DIAGNOSIS

IVH is diagnosed with CT, and scoring systems have been devised to quantify the extent of IVH seen on CT scan (Table 71-1). Clinical condition and prognosis are more closely related to ventricular distension, associated parenchymal damage, and the underlying cause of bleeding.

TABLE 71-1 Grading System for Severity of Intraventricular Hemorrhage*

Score	Criterion
1	Less than half of ventricle filled with blood
2	More than half of ventricle filled with blood
3	Ventricle filled and distended with blood

*Third ventricle, fourth ventricle, and each lateral ventricle are scored separately. All the scores are then summed (maximum total score = 12).

Supplied by J. Max Findlay.

If CT scanning shows IVH secondary to a deep thalamic or ganglionic parenchymal hemorrhage in an adult, and especially an older person, a small vessel cause can usually be assumed, and further investigation is not mandatory. Similarly, if the primary hemorrhage is lobar and is strongly suspected on clinical grounds to be related to a bleeding disorder, amyloid angiopathy, or conversion of a cardioembolic infarction, angiography is again unwarranted. If, after these considerations, the underlying cause of IVH remains uncertain, angiography, MRI, or both are indicated, especially if thrombolytic therapy (discussed in the next section) is being considered. Vascular imaging is recommended for any patient with primary IVH of no apparent cause and for any patient younger than 45 years who has an IVH.[6,54,60] In a 2008 review, nearly 60% of patients with primary IVH had positive angiographic findings of a bleeding source, and the two most common causes of primary IVH were AVMs and aneurysms.[54]

TREATMENT

Management is directed at any identified underlying cause of IVH (e.g., aneurysm repair, AVM or tumor excision, blood pressure control, correction of bleeding disorder) and external ventricular drainage to relieve any associated hydrocephalus and help manage raised ICP. Surgical evacuation through a frontal corticotomy of lateral ventricles packed with blood clot after aneurysm rupture was judged not to be useful,[61] but there has been a report of successful fourth ventricle decompression.[62] Surgery for IVH decompression is not generally recommended.

A regular problem with ventriculostomy for IVH is catheter occlusion with blood clot, necessitating irrigation or replacement of the catheter. With obstruction of the foramen of Monro, bilateral ventricular drainage tubes are sometimes necessary. Infection becomes a risk among patients with IVH in whom prolonged drainage is required.[63] In addition, ventricular drainage alone has a limited ability to relieve cerebral compression due to intraventricular blood clots themselves. It has been suggested that pressure exerted on the ventricular walls by hematoma could compromise local microcirculation and blood flow[64] and decaying blood clots may cause secondary neuronal injury due to an inflammatory reaction in the adjacent subependymal tissues.[65] The clinical significance of these latter two phenomena is uncertain.

Intraventricular clot breakdown using fibrinolytic enzymes showed promise in animal models of IVH, speeding clearance of ventricular clots, restoring ventricular size, preventing hydrocephalus, and reducing CSF outflow resistance.[66–70] Reports and case series of intraventricular thrombolysis (IVT) or fibrinolysis (IVF) in human patients followed, consisting of either injections or infusions of urokinase or recombinant tissue plasminogen activator (rt-PA) through external ventricular drainage catheters for IVH resulting from aneurysm and AVM rupture, chronic hypertensive arteriolar disease, ventricular catheter insertion, trauma, and germinal matrix hemorrhage in the newborn.[71–82] Although the type, dose, and duration of fibrinolytic treatment varied, these preliminary studies indicated that IVT accelerated IVH clearance and seemed to have an acceptable risk profile. One case series of mostly aneurysm patients also suggested rt-PA clearance of IVH helped control elevated ICP, especially in younger patients with little intracranial compliance or those in poor neurologic condition due to severe bleeding.[73]

Smaller clinical trials have compared IVT with external ventricular drainage alone (Table 71-2). All indicated that IVT is effective in accelerating intraventricular clot clearance without a large risk of causing new or repeated hemorrhages.[81,83–89] Several reviews have reached the same conclusions[90,91] as did

TABLE 71-2 Comparison Studies of Intraventricular Fibrinolysis with External Ventricular Drainage Versus External Ventricular Drainage Alone

Study, Population, Year	No. Patients	Cause of IVH	Fibrinolytic Agent	Main Study Results
Coplin et al.,[75] single center, 1998	40 (22 received IVF)	Hypertensive ICH in most	Urokinase	IVF resulted in faster clot clearance, lower mortality rate, trend to better outcomes
Naff et al.,[73] multi-center, 2000	20 (16 received IVF, eight randomized)	Hypertensive ICH in most	Urokinase	IVF was associated with better 30-day survival than predicted
Findlay and Jacka,[76] single center, 2004	30 (21 received IVF)	Aneurysm rupture	rt-PA	IVF resulted in more rapid ventricular opening, fewer EVD replacements
Naff et al.,[77] multi-center, 2004	12 (7 randomized to IVF)	Hypertensive ICH	Urokinase	Randomization to IVF (and female gender) favorably affected clot resolution rate
Varelas et al.,[78] single center, 2005	20 (10 received IVF)	Aneurysm rupture	rt-PA	IVF resulted in faster clot clearance, trend to decreased need for shunt placement, better outcome
Torres et al.,[79] single center, 2008	28 (14 received IVF)	Hypertensive ICH	Urokinase	IVF resulted in faster clot clearance, fewer catheter obstructions, improved outcome
Huttner et al.,[80] single center, 2008	135 (27 received IVF)	Hypertensive ICH	rt-PA	IVF hastened clot clearance, reduced the need for repeated EVD exchanges and permanent shunting, but did not influence long-term outcome
Bartek et al.,[9] single center 2011	9	Hypertensive ICH in six, aneurysm rupture in three	Urokinase	IVF resulted in rapid clot clearance, fewer shunt placements
King et al.[92] single center 2011	16 (seven received IVF)	Hypertensive ICH	Urokinase	IVF resulted in increased rate of IVH resolution, no adverse events

EVD, external ventricular drainage; ICH, intracerebral hemorrhage; IVF, intraventricular fibrinolysis; IVH, intraventricular hemorrhage; rt-PA, recombinant tissue-type plasminogen activator.

a small placebo-controlled pilot study using urokinase in patients with spontaneous IVH.[92]

In North America urokinase has been replaced by rt-PA for routine clinical use and is the agent used in the multicenter CLEAR IVH trials (Clot Lysis: Evaluating Accelerated Resolution of Intraventricular Hemorrhage (CLEAR IVH). Phase II of CLEAR IVH examined patients with small spontaneous supratentorial ICHs (≤30 mL) associated with massive intraventricular bleeding.[93] Patients with underlying aneurysms, vascular malformations, tumors or coagulopathies were not included. All 48 patients enrolled had external ventricular drainage and were randomized to receive either 3 mg/3 mL of rt-PA or 3 mL of normal saline injected via the EVD every 12 hours until CT evidence of clot resolution was sufficient to remove the catheter. The addition of thrombolysis was associated with significantly faster clot clearance and a shorter duration of external drainage, but also more intracranial rebleeding, either at the primary hemorrhage site or along the catheter tract. The risk of catheter tract hemorrhage could be related in part to catheter placement with tip fenestrations being located within brain parenchyma after EVD insertion, allowing rt-PA injection into brain tissue.[94] CLEAR III is currently underway (January 2014), using the same protocol in the same patient population as in CLEAR II with clinical outcome at 180 days as the primary outcome measure.[95] This study hopes to determine whether IVT has an impact on clinical outcome, clot reduction, and bleeding events in patients with spontaneous (primarily hypertensive) ICH with extension in the ventricles resulting in ventricular obstruction.

On the basis of current evidence, IVT can be considered for patients with large IVHs that expand and occlude the ventricular system, but without large parenchymal hematomas or clinical conditions that strongly predict unfavorable outcome regardless of the IVH. Fibrinolytic treatment is not likely to be helpful in patients with extensive deep or dominant brain destruction, those with severely elevated ICP, or those with rapidly failing brainstem activity. IVT has been proven useful in maintaining EVD patency, speeding IVH resolution and normalization of ventricular size, and there is some evidence that it assists in ICP control in some patients. It is not known if IVT reduces the need for subsequent ventriculoperitoneal shunting or if it has a favorable effect on long-term outcome.

Our treatment protocol is to begin treatment after CT confirmation of results of uncomplicated surgery for aneurysm or AVM repair (if applicable) and satisfactory placement of a ventricular drain catheter with the fenestrated tip clearly within the lateral ventricular chamber (best seen with on the CT scan "bone window"). It is not necessary to place the EVD on the side of the dominant ventricular clot for effective clot resolution.[96] A 2- to 4-mg (1 mg/mL) dose of rt-PA is given slowly through the ventricular catheter with frequent checks of ICP to ensure that it does not reach dangerous levels, which would compromise cerebral perfusion pressure. It is sometimes possible to facilitate the rt-PA injection by first aspirating and discarding the same volume of CSF from the ventricles. If the patient tolerates only a portion of the 4-mg dose, the remainder can be given 1 hour later. Care must be taken to ensure that the volume of rt-PA dosage exceeds the CSF-filled tubing "dead" space between injection port and ventricle to ensure that the rt-PA reaches the ventricles.

Following rt-PA injection the ventricular drain is closed for 1 hour and is then opened to drain against a pressure gradient of 1–2 cm (above the level of the external auditory canal) for 1 hour. The drain is then opened and closed during alternating hours for the next 24 hours. CT scanning is performed daily for the first several days, and additional rt-PA can be given if necessary, the goal being to open ventricular pathways, restore normal ventricular size, reduce intracranial hypertension, and maintain catheter patency (Figs 71-4, 71-5). Midline ventricles (third and fourth) clear

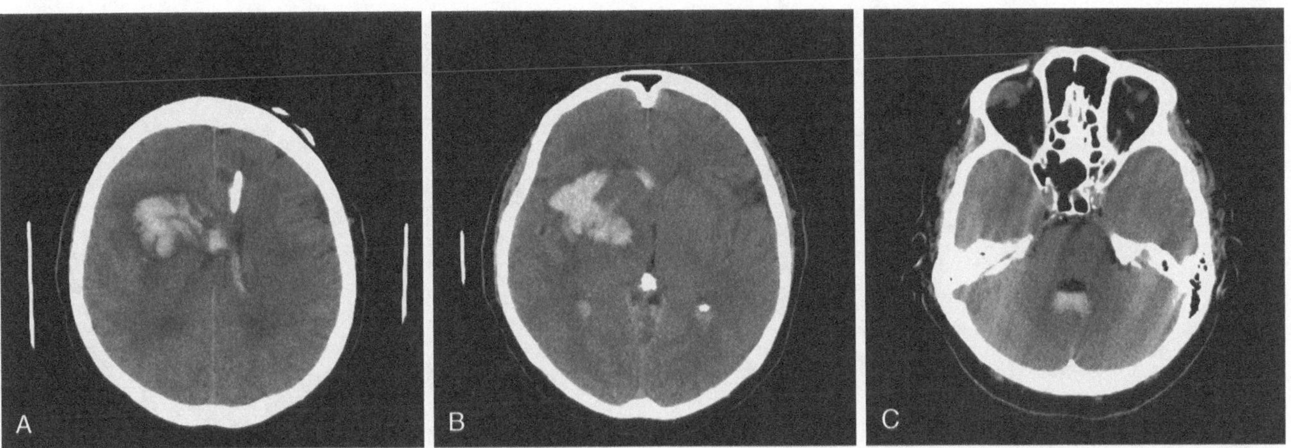

Figure 71-4. Following 2 consecutive days of intraventricular fibrinolysis (rt-PA, 4 mg per day via the external ventricular drain), a 71-year-old woman with a right-sided lentiform hemorrhage with intraventricular extension (see Fig. 71-1) had considerable clot clearance from the ventricular system. A ventriculoperitoneal shunt was not required. She recovered to her baseline cognition but had a permanent left hemiparesis that prevented her from ambulation.

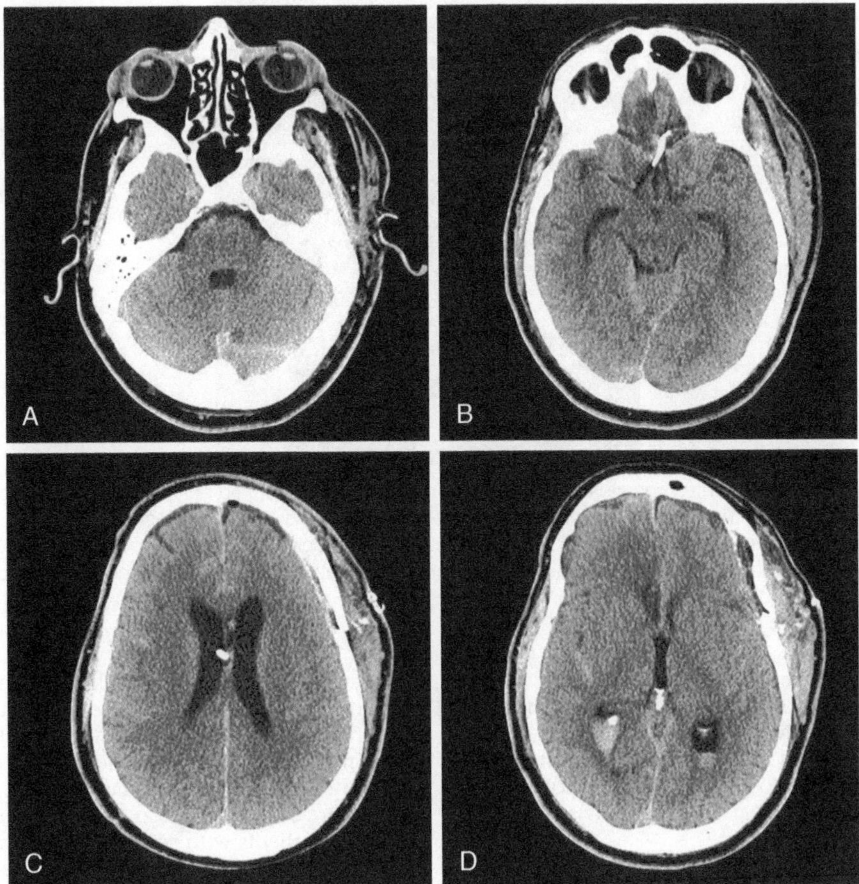

Figure 71-5. Following aneurysm clipping in this 57-year-old man (see Fig. 71-2), 4 mg/4 mL rt-PA was administered via an external ventricular drain over 2 consecutive days, resulting in good clot resolution (A–D). A ventriculoperitoneal shunt was inserted 16 days later. The patient made a good recovery.

most rapidly and the posterolateral (gravity dependent) ventricles last.[97] Subependymal clots are often unresponsive to IVT. Complete clearance of clot settled in dependent parts of the lateral ventricles is not necessary.

We have administered IVF after endovascular coiling of ruptured aneurysms without subsequent bleeding complications (see Fig. 71-6), a therapeutic maneuver reported by others in several patients.[98,99] Interference of aneurysm thrombosis in the coil mass by the administration of rt-PA and the potential risk of aneurysm rebleeding remains a concern. Risks and potential benefits must be taken into account under these circumstances. All of the patients described in the literature who had aneurysm coiling followed by IVF had high-grade aneurysm ruptures with massive IVH, and one of our own

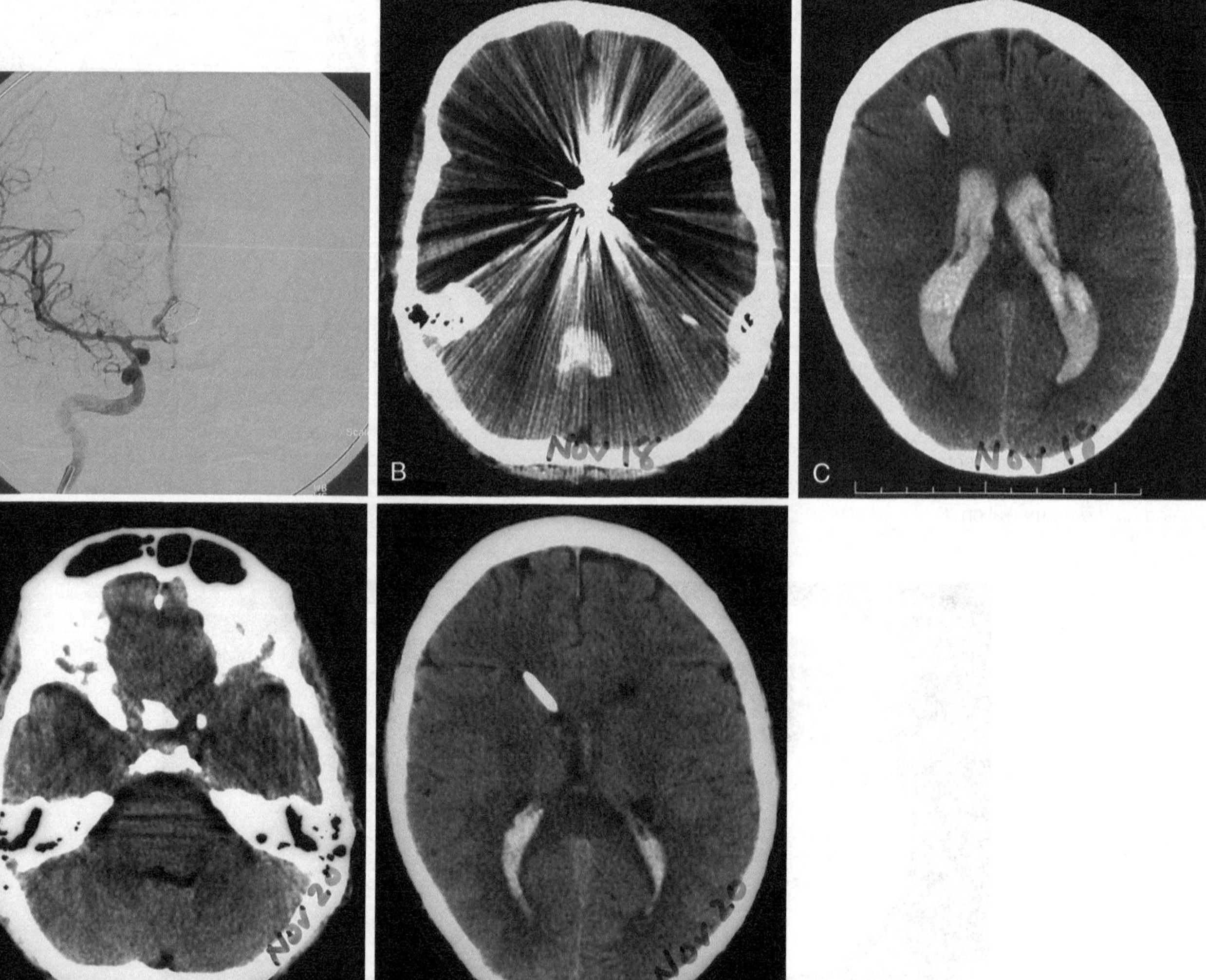

Figure 71-6. A 56-year-old man presented comatose after a sudden collapse. A, A ruptured anterior communicating artery was treated with endovascular coiling. (The patient had a second, small, right middle cerebral artery aneurysm that was not treated.) B and C, CT scanning the next day showed a persistent panventricular hemorrhage that was treated with a single dose of 4 mg of rt-PA via the ventriculostomy catheter. (See text for protocol details.) D and E, CT scans performed 2 days later demonstrate considerable clearance of ventricular clots, and the patient went on to make a good clinical recovery.

patients went on to die from severe subarachnoid hemorrhage; another made a good recovery. Several examples of rt-PA treatment are shown in (Fig. 71-3).

Although "rescue" IVT has been reported in several patients with massive IVHs secondary to ruptured periventricular AVMs prior to their obliteration,[100] great caution is advisable in this rare circumstance.

PROGNOSIS

The presence of IVH does not necessarily portend a poor prognosis in every patient, as was once thought. Even quite large primary IVHs can be associated with a good clinical condition and good outcome.[101,102] However, secondary IVHs associated with severe subarachnoid hemorrhage, centrally destructive ICHs or anticoagulant treatment are associated with poorer neurologic condition on presentation and a worse outcome.[103–105] Massive IVH that produces fourth ventricular distension and periventricular cerebral compression is an especially ominous sign associated with early death.[44]

Patients with large IVHs who survive hemorrhage without vital brain destruction are potential candidates for IVT. Intraventricular thrombolysis/fibrinolysis helps maintain ventriculostomy blockage with blood clot, promotes rapid IVH clearance, and, we believe, facilitates ICP management, all of which are of great practical help in the intensive care management of patients with severe IVH. IVT can result in EVD tract and other hemorrhages especially when the catheter is not placed correctly. It is not currently known whether IVT by itself improves long-term clinical outcome, but this is a subject of ongoing study. As discussed, the CLEAR III trial currently underway will hopefully provide important guidance for IVH secondary to hypertensive arteriolar degeneration and ICH.

REFERENCES

1. Darby DG, Donnan GA, Saling MA, et al. Primary intraventricular hemorrhage: Clinical and neuropsychological findings in a prospective stroke series. Neurology 1988;38:68–75.
2. Pia HW. The surgical treatment of intracerebral and intraventricular haematomas. Acta Neurochir 1972;27:149–64.

3. Little JR, Blomquist GA Jr, Ethier R. Intraventricular hemorrhage in adults. Surg Neurol 1977;8:143–9.
4. Donauer E, Reif J, Al-Khalaf E, et al. Intraventricular haemorrhage caused by aneurysms and angiomas. Acta Neurochir 1993;122:23–31.
5. Angelopoulos M, Gupta SR. Azat KB. Primary intraventricular hemorrhage in adults: Clinical features, risk factors, and outcome. Surg Neurol 1995;44:433–6.
6. Chang DS, Lin CL, Howng SL. Primary intraventricular hemorrhage in adult—an analysis of 24 cases. Kao Hsiung I Hsueh Ko Hsueh Tsa Chih 1998;14:633–8.
7. Marti-Fabregas J, Piles S, Guardia E, et al. Spontaneous primary intraventricular hemorrhage: Clinical data, etiology and outcome. J Neurol 1999;246:287–91.
8. Taheri SA, Wani MA, Lewko J. Uncommon causes of intraventricular hemorrhage. Clin Neurol Neurosurg 1990;92-3:195–202.
9. Bergsneider M, Grazee JG, DeSalles AA. Thalamostriate artery aneurysm within the third ventricle. J Neurosurg 1994;81: 463–5.
10. Hamada J, Hashimoto N. Tskukahara T. Moyamoya disease with repeated intraventricular hemorrhage due to aneurysm rupture. J Neurosurg 1994;80:328–31.
11. Newman P, Al-Menar A. Intraventricular hemorrhage in pregnancy due to moyamoya disease. J Neurol Neurosurg Psychiatry 1998;64:686.
12. Larrazabal R, Pelz D, Findlay JM. Endovascular treatment of a lenticulostriate artery aneurysm with *N*-butyl cyanoacrylate. Can J Neurol Sci 2001;28:256–9.
13. Arboix A, Garcia-Eroles L, Viscens A, et al. Spontaneous primary intraventricular hemorrhage: clinical features and early outcome. ISRN Neurology 2012, Article ID 498303, 7 pages.
14. Szabo K, Sommer A, Gass A, et al. Rapid resorption of intraventricular hemorrhage after thrombolytic therapy of ischemic stroke. Cerebrovasc Dis 2001;12:144.
15. Gebel JL, Sila CA, Sloan MA, et al. Thrombolysis-related intracranial hemorrhage: A radiographic analysis of 244 cases from the GUSTO-1 trial with clinical correlation. Stroke 1998;29: 563–9.
16. Toffol GJ, Biller J, Adams HP Jr. Nontraumatic intracerebral hemorrhage in young adults. Arch Neurol 1987;44:483–5.
17. Lindboe CF, Stolt-Nielsen A, Dale LG. Hemorrhage in a highly vascularized subependymoma of the septum pellucidum: Case report. Neurosurg 1992;31:741–5.
18. Matsushima M, Yamamoto T, Motomochi M, et al. Papilloma and venous angioma of the choroid plexus causing primary intraventricular hemorrhage. J Neurosurg 1973;39:666–70.
19. Lang I, Jackson A, Strang FA. Intraventricular hemorrhage caused by intraventricular meningioma: CT appearance. AJNR Am J Neuroradiol 1995;6:1378–81.
20. Murai Y, Yoshida D, Ikeda Y, et al. Spontaneous intraventricular hemorrhage caused by lateral ventricular meningioma—case report. Neurol Med Chir (Tokyo) 1996;36:586–9.
21. Challa VR, Richards F II, Davis CH Jr. Intraventricular hemorrhage from pituitary apoplexy. Surg Neurol 1981;16:360–1.
22. Okamura A, Goto S, Sato K, et al. Central neurocytoma with hemorrhagic onset. Surg Neurol 1995;43:252–5.
23. Graziani N, Dufour H, Figarella-Branger D, et al. Suprasellar granular-cell tumor, presenting with intraventricular haemorrhage. Br J Neurosurg 1995;9:97–102.
24. Mandybur TI. Intracranial hemorrhage caused by metastatic tumors. Neurology 1977;27:650–5.
25. Young WB, Lee KP, Pessin MS. Prognostic significance of ventricular blood in supratentorial hemorrhage: A volumetric study. Neurology 1990;40:616–19.
26. Juvela S, Hillbom M, Palomäki H. Risk factors for spontaneous intracerebral hemorrhage. Stroke 1995;26:1558–64.
27. Broderick JP, Brott TG, Duldner JE, et al. Volume of intracerebral hemorrhage: A powerful and easy-to-use predictor of 30-day mortality. Stroke 1993;24:987–93.
28. Ruscalleda J, Peiró A. Prognostic factors in intraparenchymatous hematoma with ventricular hemorrhage. Neuroradiology 1986; 28:34–7.
29. Hallevi H, Albright KC, Aronowski J, et al. Intraventricular hemorrhage: Anatomic relationships and clinical implications. Neurology 2008;70:848–52.
30. Hanley DF. Intraventricular hemorrhage severity factor and treatment target in spontaneous intracerebral hemorrhage. Stroke 2009;40:1533–8.
31. Phan TG, Koh M, Vierkant RA, et al. Hydrocephalus is a determinant of early mortality in putaminal hemorrhage. Stroke 2000;31:2157–62.
32. Liliang PC, Liang CL, Lu CH, et al. Hypertensive caudate hemorrhage prognostic predictor, outcome, and role of external ventricular drainage. Stroke 2001;32:1195–200.
33. Bhattathiri PS, Gregson B, Prasad KS, et al. Intraventricular hemorrhage and hydrocephalus after spontaneous intracerebral hemorrhage: Results from the STICH trial. Acta Neurochir Suppl 2006;96:65–8.
34. Huttner HB, Kohrmann M, Berger C, et al. Influence of intraventricular hemorrhage and occlusive hydrocephalus on the long-term outcome of treated patients with basal ganglia hemorrhage: A case-control study. J Neurosurg 2006;105:412–17.
35. Poon MT, Fonville AF, Al-Shahi SR. Long-term prognosis after intracerebral hemorrhage: a systematic review and meta-analysis. J Neurol Neurosurg Psychiatry 2013;doi:10.1136/jnnp-2013-306476.
36. Rosen D, MacDonald RL, Huo D, et al. Intraventricular hemorrhage from ruptured aneurysm: clinical characteristics, complications and outcomes in a large, prospective, multicentre study population. J Neurosurg 2007;107:261–5.
37. Findlay JM. Intraventricular hemorrhage. Neurosurg Q 2000;10: 182–95.
38. Kramer AH, Mikolaenko I, Deis N, et al. Intraventricular hemorrhage volume predicts poor outcomes but not delayed ischemic neurological deficits among patients with ruptured cerebral aneurysms. Neurosurgery 2010;67:1044–53.
39. Claassen J, Bernardini GL, Kreiter K, et al. Effect of cisternal and ventricular blood on risk of delayed cerebral ischemia after subarachnoid hemorrhage: the Fisher scale revisited. Stroke 2001;32:2012–20.
40. Vale FL, Bradley EL, Fisher WS III. The relationship of subarachnoid hemorrhage and the need for postoperative shunting. J Neurosurg 1997;86:462–6.
41. Graff-Radford NR, Torner J, Adams HP Jr, et al. Factors associated with hydrocephalus after subarachnoid hemorrhage. Arch Neurol 1989;46:744–52.
42. de Oliveira JG, Beck J, Setzer M, et al. Risk of shunt-dependent hydrocephalus after occlusion of ruptured intracranial aneurysms by surgical clipping or endovascular coiling: A single-institution series and meta-analysis. Neurosurgery 2007;61:924–34.
43. Inagawa T, Hirano A. Ruptured intracranial aneurysms: An autopsy study of 133 patients. Surg Neurol 1990;33:117–23.
44. Ruelle A, Cavazzani P, Andrioli G. Extracranial posterior inferior cerebellar artery aneurysm causing isolated intraventricular hemorrhage: A case report. Neurosurgery 1988;23:774–7.
45. Schievink WI, Wijdicks EFM, Parisi JE, et al. Sudden death from aneurysmal subarachnoid hemorrhage. Neurology 1995;45: 871–4.
46. Shapiro SA, Campbell RL, Scully T. Hemorrhagic dilation of the fourth ventricle: An ominous predictor. J Neurosurg 1994;80:805–9.
47. Mohr G, Ferguson G, Khan M, et al. Intraventricular hemorrhage from ruptured aneurysm: Retrospective analysis of 91 cases. J Neurosurg 1983;58:482–7.
48. Heuer GG, Smith MJ, Elliott JP, et al. Relationship between intracranial pressure and other clinical variables in patients with aneurysmal subarachnoid hemorrhage. J Neurosurg 2004;101:408–16.
49. Rosengart AJ, Schultheiss KE, Tolentino J, et al. Prognostic factors for outcome in patients with aneurysmal subarachnoid hemorrhage. Stroke 2007;38:2315–21.
50. Hartmann A, Mast H, Mohr JP, et al. Morbidity of intracranial hemorrhage in patients with cerebral arteriovenous malformation. Stroke 1998;29:931–4.
51. Findlay JM, Weir BKA, Kanamaru K, et al. Intrathecal fibrinolytic therapy after subarachnoid hemorrhage: Dosage study in a primate model and review of the literature. Can J Neurol Sci 1989;16:28–40.
52. Ikeda K, Asakura H, Futami K, et al. Coagulative and fibrinolytic activation in cerebrospinal fluid and plasma after subarachnoid hemorrhage. Neurosurgery 1997;41:344–50.

53. Naff NJ, Williams MA, Rigamonti D, et al. Blood clot resolution in human cerebrospinal fluid: Evidence of first-order kinetics. Neurosurgery 2001;49:614–21.
54. Flint AC, Roebken A, Singh V. Primary intraventricular hemorrhage: yield of diagnostic angiography and clinical outcome. Neurocrit Care 2008;8:330–6.
55. Yanaka K, Hyodo A, Tsuchida Y, et al. Symptomatic cerebral vasospasm after intraventricular hemorrhage from ruptured arteriovenous malformation. Surg Neurol 1992;38:63–7.
56. Maeda K, Kurita H, Nakamura T, et al. Occurrence of severe vasospasm following intraventricular hemorrhage from an arteriovenous malformation: Report of two cases. J Neurosurg 1997;87:436–9.
57. Classen J, Bernardini GL, Kreiter K, et al. Effect of cisternal and ventricular blood on risk of delayed cerebral ischemia after subarachnoid hemorrhage: The Fisher Scale revisited. Stroke 2001;32:2012–20.
58. Diringer MN, Edwards DF, Zazulia AR. Hydrocephalus: A previously unrecognized predictor of poor outcome from supratentorial intracerebral hemorrhage. Stroke 1998;29:1352–7.
59. Mohr G, Ferguson G, Khan M, et al. Intraventricular hemorrhage from ruptured aneurysm: Retrospective analysis of 91 cases. J Neurosurg 1983;58:482–7.
60. Graeb DA, Robertson WD, Lapointe JS, et al. Computed tomographic diagnosis of intraventricular hemorrhage. Radiology 1982;143:91–6.
61. Shimoda M, Oda S, Shibata M, et al. Results of early surgical evacuation of packed intraventricular hemorrhage from aneurysm rupture in patients with poor-grade subarachnoid hemorrhage. J Neurosurg 1999;91:408–14.
62. Lagares A, Putman CM, Ogilvy CS. Posterior fossa decompression and clot evacuation for fourth ventricle hemorrhage after aneurysmal rupture: Case report. Neurosurgery 2001;49:208–11.
63. Mayhall CG, Archer NH, Lamb VA, et al. Ventriculostomy-related infections: A prospective epidemiologic study. N Engl J Med 1984;310:553–9.
64. Young WB, Lee KP, Pessin MS, et al. Prognostic significance of ventricular blood in supratentorial hemorrhage: a volumetric study. Neurology 1990;40(4):616–19.
65. Lee KR, Betz AL, Kim S, et al. The role of the coagulation cascade in brain edema formation after intracerebral hemorrhage. Acta Neurochir (Wien) 1996;138(4):396–400.
66. Pang D, Sclabassi RJ, Horton JA. Lysis of intraventricular blood clot with urokinase in a canine model: Part 1: Canine intraventricular blood cast model. Neurosurgery 1986;19:540–6.
67. Pang D, Sclabassi RJ, Horton JA. Lysis of intraventricular blood clot with urokinase in a canine model: Part 2: In vivo safety study of intraventricular urokinase. Neurosurgery 1986;19:547–52.
68. Mayfrank L, Kissler J, Raoofi R, et al. Ventricular dilatation in experimental intraventricular hemorrhage in pigs: Characterization of cerebrospinal fluid dynamics and the effects of fibrinolytic treatment. Stroke 1997;28:141–8.
69. Brinker T, Seifert V, Stolke D. Effect of intrathecal fibrinolysis on cerebrospinal fluid absorption after experimental subarachnoid hemorrhage. J Neurosurg 1991;74:789–93.
70. Brinker T, Seifert V, Dietz H. Subacute hydrocephalus after experimental subarachnoid hemorrhage: Its prevention by intrathecal fibrinolysis with recombinant tissue plasminogen activator. Neurosurgery 1992;31:306–12.
71. Shen PH, Matsuoka Y, Kawajiri K, et al. Treatment of intraventricular hemorrhage using urokinase. Neurol Med Chir (Tokyo) 1990;30:329–33.
72. Todo T, Usui M, Takakura K. Treatment of severe intraventricular hemorrhage by intraventricular infusion of urokinase. J Neurosurg 1991;74:81–6.
73. Findlay JM, Grace MGA, Weir BKA. Treatment of intraventricular hemorrhage with tissue plasminogen activator. Neurosurgery 1993;32:941–7.
74. Findlay JM, Weir BKA, Stollery DE. Lysis of intraventricular hematoma with tissue plasminogen activator. J Neurosurg 1991;74:803–7.
75. Mayfrank L, Lippitz B, Groth M, et al. Effect of recombinant tissue plasminogen activator on clot lysis and ventricular dilatation in the treatment of severe intraventricular hemorrhage. Acta Neurochir 1993;122:32–8.
76. Rhode V, Schaller C, Hassler WE. Intraventricular recombinant tissue plasminogen activator for lysis of intraventricular haemorrhage. J Neurol Neurosurg Psychiatry 1995;58:447–51.
77. Akdemir H, Selcuklu A, Pasaoglu A, et al. Treatment of severe intraventricular hemorrhage by intraventricular infusion of urokinase. Neurosurg Rev 1995;18:95–100.
78. Rainov NG, Burkert WL. Urokinase infusion for severe intraventricular haemorrhage. Acta Neurochir 1995;134:55–9.
79. Grabb PA. Traumatic intraventricular hemorrhage treated with intraventricular recombinant-tissue plasminogen activator: Technical case report. Neurosurgery 1998;43:966–9.
80. Goh KY, Poon WS. Recombinant tissue plasminogen activator for the treatment of spontaneous adult intraventricular hemorrhage. Surg Neurol 1998;50:526–31.
81. Naff NJ, Carhuapoma JR, Williams MA, et al. Treatment of intraventricular hemorrhage with urokinase: Effects on 30-day survival. Stroke 2000;31:841–7.
82. Haines SJ, Lapointe M. Fibrinolytic agents in the management of post hemorrhagic hydrocephalus in preterm infants: The evidence. Childs Nerv Syst 1999;15:226–34.
83. Coplin WD, Vinas FC, Agris JM, et al. A cohort study of the safety and feasibility of intraventricular urokinase for nonaneurysmal spontaneous intraventricular hemorrhage. Stroke 1998;29(8):1573–9.
84. Findlay JM, Jacka MJ. Cohort study of intraventricular thrombolysis with recombinant tissue plasminogen activator for aneurysmal intraventricular hemorrhage. Neurosurgery 2004;55(3):532–7.
85. Naff NJ, Hanley DF, Keyl PM, et al. Intraventricular thrombolysis speeds blood clot resolution: Results of a pilot, prospective, randomized, double-blind, controlled trial. Neurosurgery 2004;54(3):577–84.
86. Varelas PN, Rickert KL, Cusick J, et al. Intraventricular hemorrhage after aneurysmal subarachnoid hemorrhage: Pilot study of treatment with intraventricular tissue plasminogen activator. Neurosurgery 2005;56(2):205–13.
87. Torres A, Plans G, Martino J, et al. Fibrinolytic therapy in spontaneous intraventricular haemorrhage: Efficacy and safety of the treatment. Br J Neurosurg 2008;22(2):269–74.
88. Huttner HB, Tognoni E, Bardutzky J, et al. Influence of intraventricular fibrinolytic therapy with rt-PA on the long-term outcome of treated patients with spontaneous basal ganglia hemorrhage: A case-control study. Eur J Neurol 2008;15(4):342–9.
89. Bartek J, Hansen-Schwartz J, Bergdal O, et al. Alteplase (rtPA) treatment of intraventricular hematoma (IVH): safety of an efficient methodological approach for rapid clot removal. Acta Neurochir Suppl 2011;111:409–13.
90. Nieuwkamp DJ, de Gans K, Rinkel GJE, et al. Treatment and outcome of severe intraventricular extension in patients with subarachnoid hemorrhage: A systematic review of the literature. J Neurol 2000;247:117–21.
91. Engelhard HH, Andrews CO, Slavin KV, et al. Current management of intraventricular hemorrhage. Surg Neurol 2003;60:15–21.
92. King NK, Lai JL, Tan LB, et al. A randomized, placebo-controlled pilot study of patients with spontaneous intraventricular hemorrhage treated with intraventricular thrombolysis. J Clin Neurosci 2012;19(7):961–4.
93. Naff N, Williams MA, Keyl PM, et al. Low-dose recombinant tissue-type plasminogen activator enhances clot resolution in brain hemorrhage: the intraventricular hemorrhage thrombolysis trial. Stroke 2011;42:3009–16.
94. Jackson DA, Patel AV, Darracott RM, et al. Safety of intraventricular hemorrhage (IVH) thrombolysis based on CT localization of external ventricular drain (EVD) fenestrations and analysis of EVD tract hemorrhage. Neurocrit Care 2013;19(1):103–10.
95. Ziai WC, Tuhrim S, Lane K, et al. A multicenter, randomized, double-blinded, placebo-controlled phase III study of Clot Lysis Evaluation of Accelerated Resolution of Intraventricular Hemorrhage (CLEAR III). Int J Stroke 2014;9:536–42.
96. Jaffe J, Melnychuk E, Muschelli J, et al. Ventricular catheter location and the clearance of intraventricular hemorrhage. Neurosurgery 2012;70(5):1258–63.
97. Webb AJ, Ullman NL, Mann S, et al. Resolution of intraventricular hemorrhage varies by ventricular region and dose of

intraventricular thrombolytic: the Clot Lysis: Evaluating Accelerated Resolution if IVH (CLEAR IVH) program. Stroke 2012;43(6): 1666–8.

98. Azmi-Ghadimi H, Heary RF, Farkas JE, et al. Use of intraventricular tissue plasminogen activator and Guglielmi detachable coiling for the acute treatment of casted ventricles from cerebral aneurysm hemorrhage: Two technical case reports. Neurosurgery 2002;50:421–4.
99. Hall B, Parker D Jr, Carhuapoma JR. Thrombolysis for intraventricular hemorrhage after endovascular aneurysmal coiling. Neurocrit Care 2005;3:153–6.
100. Jorens PG, Menovsky TM, Voormolen MH, et al. Intraventricular thrombolysis for massive intraventricular hemorrhage due to periventricular arteriovenous malformations: no absolute contraindications as rescue therapy prior to surgical repair or embolization? Clin Neurol Neurosurg 2009;111(6):544–50.
101. Verma A, Maheshwari MC, Bhargava S. Spontaneous intraventricular haemorrhage. J Neurol 1987;234:233–6.
102. Roos YB, Hasan D, Vermeulen M. Outcome in patients with large intraventricular haemorrhages: A volumetric study. J Neurol Neurosurg Psychiatry 1995;58:622–4.
103. De Weerd AW. The prognosis of intraventricular hemorrhage. J Neurol 1979;222:45–51.
104. Juvela S. Risk factors for impaired outcome after spontaneous intracerebral hemorrhage. Arch Neurol 1995;52:1193–2000.
105. Sjoblom L, Hårdemark HG, Lindgren A, et al. Management of prognostic features of intracerebral hemorrhage during anticoagulant therapy: A Swedish multicenter study. Stroke 2001;32: 2567–74.

72 Surgical Management of Cranial and Spinal Arteriovenous Malformations

Jonathan Russin, Robert F. Spetzler

KEY POINTS

- Review of the natural history and presentation of cerebral arteriovenous malformations (AVMs).
- Surgical indications and morbidity/mortality of surgical intervention for cerebral AVMs.
- Technical nuances for the microsurgical resection of cerebral and spinal AVMs.
- Review and discussion of the impact of the ARUBA trial.
- Classification and treatment recommendations for spinal AVMs.

CEREBRAL ARTERIOVENOUS MALFORMATIONS

Introduction

Cerebral arteriovenous malformations (AVMs) are vascular lesions consisting of tangled anastomoses of blood vessels in which arteriovenous shunting occurs. The majority of AVMs are sporadic; however, they can occur in patients with diagnosed hereditary disorders as well as in familial forms.[1,2] Cerebral AVMs account for between 1% and 2% of all strokes, and for the majority of hemorrhagic strokes in children and young adults.[3-6] The incidence of cerebral AVMs has been approximated as 1 per 100,000 persons per year in unselected populations, with a prevalence of approximately 18 per 100,000 persons.[4,7-9] The annual hemorrhage rate for cerebral AVMs is 3%, with an initial rate of approximately 2% and a re-rupture rate of 4.5%. Re-hemorrhage rates in the first year after presentation with rupture have been reported to be between 6% and 15%.[10] Hemorrhage is the most common presentation and occurs in approximately 50% of cases.[10,11]

The surgical management of cerebral AVMs is undertaken with the goal of complete obliteration of the nidus of the AVM. Although feeding arteries and draining veins are relevant when discussing risks and treatment options, the surgical cure of an AVM is dependent only on the elimination of the arteriovenous shunting. Management strategies for these lesions range from observation to extirpation. The benefits of intervention must be carefully measured against the risks when considering treatment. Validated surgical risk stratification tools exist for cerebral AVMs, and their application is critical for appropriate decision making.[12-14] Modern therapies include stereotactic radiosurgery, endovascular occlusion, and microsurgery. Combinations of these interventions have also proved to be valuable in the treatment of more complex cerebral AVMs.

Pathogenesis

Although the exact pathogenesis of cerebral AVMs is unknown, they are believed to be of embryologic or fetal origin. However, these are not static lesions and multiple studies have identified abnormal expression of angiogenic factors within cerebral AVMs.[15-17] In addition, cases of de novo cerebral AVM formation have been published and serve to further cloud the discussion of the etiology of these lesions.[18] Inheritable genetic mutations on chromosomes 9 and 12 are responsible for hereditary hemorrhagic telangiectasia (HHT). The genes encoded by these mutations are glycoproteins associated with transforming growth factor-β (TGF-β) and are involved in angiogenesis.[19] Clinically, HHT is characterized by telangiectasia and AVMs of almost any organ, but predominantly of the lungs, liver, and brain. Familial cerebral AVMs have also been identified and high-density single nucleotide polymorphism array analysis has been used to try to identify candidate genes.[2] The role of inflammatory cytokines has also been investigated and may be associated with cerebral AVM hemorrhage.[20]

Presentation

The majority of patients with cerebral AVMs (52%) present with hemorrhage.[10] These hemorrhages typically result in acute onset of a severe headache and can include loss of consciousness, nausea, vomiting, neurologic deficit, and seizure. Patients with cerebral AVMs may also present with epilepsy, headaches, focal progressive neurologic deficits, or, in newborns, congestive heart failure.[4] Symptoms from unruptured AVMs can be produced from mass effect, inflammation, altered hemodynamics (steal phenomenon), or recruitment of dilated perinidal capillary networks.[6] Advances in neuroimaging techniques, such as improved image resolution, have allowed for greater detection and evaluation of cerebral AVMs. Due to widening availability of computed tomography (CT), magnetic resonance imaging (MRI), and magnetic resonance angiography (MRA), a greater number of AVMs are now being incidentally discovered.[7] Given the breadth of presentations for these lesions, it is crucial to identify which patients will benefit from intervention versus conservative management.

Natural History

The most severe consequences of cerebral AVMs occur with intracranial hemorrhage. The risk of mortality and morbidity is 10% and 30–50%, respectively, with each episode of AVM-related hemorrhage.[21] Individuals with AVMs who have not had complete obliteration of the nidus are subject to a lifelong risk of hemorrhagic stroke. Significant efforts have been undertaken in an attempt to characterize the long-term overall risk of hemorrhage in patients with untreated AVMs. Most studies report annual rates of intracranial hemorrhage for patients with AVMs to be approximately 2–4% per year; however, wide ranges have been reported between 2% and 32.6%.[22-26] The most recent systematic review and meta-analysis published an annual hemorrhage rate for cerebral AVMs of 3%. The rate of initial rupture was approximately 2%, with a re-rupture rate of 4.5%. Re-hemorrhage rates in the first year

TABLE 72-1 Cerebral Arteriovenous Malformation Risk Factors for Hemorrhage*

Significance	Variable
Statistically significant	Prior hemorrhage Deep AVM location Exclusively deep venous drainage Associated aneurysms
Trending toward but NOT statistically significant	Any deep venous drainage Female sex
Not significant	Small AVM size (<3 cm) Older age

AVM, arteriovenous malformation.
*Data from Gross BA, Du R, Natural history of cerebral arteriovenous malformations: meta-analysis. *J Neurosurg*. 2013;118:437–443.

TABLE 72-2 Spetzler-Martin Grading System for Cerebral Arteriovenous Malformations*

AVM	Score
Size	
<3 cm	1
3–6 cm	2
>6 cm	3
Location	
Non-eloquent	0
Eloquent†	1
Venous drainage	
Superficial only	0
Any deep	1

AVM, arteriovenous malformation.
*Modified from Spetzler RF, Martin NA. A proposed grading system for arteriovenous malformations. *J Neurosurg* 1986;65:476–483.
†Sensorimotor, motor, or visual cortex; hypothalamus; thalamus; internal capsule; brainstem; cerebellar peduncles; or cerebellar nuclei.

after presentation with rupture were reported to be between 6% and 15%.[10] However, the risk of hemorrhage for each AVM is variable and depends on multiple factors, including location, morphology, and angioarchitectural characteristics of the lesion.

In the past numerous variables have been associated with an increased risk of hemorrhage. These include deep or infratentorial AVM location, periventricular location, deep venous drainage, small AVM size, impaired venous drainage, a single draining vein, intranidal aneurysm, multiple aneurysms, elevated feeding artery pressure, and posterior circulation blood supply.[21,27–34] A current meta-analysis of the literature found that prior hemorrhage, deep AVM location, exclusively deep venous drainage, and associated aneurysms were statistically significant risk factors for hemorrhage (Table 72-1). Female sex and the presence of any deep venous drainage showed a trend toward an increased risk of hemorrhage but were not statistically significant. Contrary to prior published studies, there was no increased risk associated with small AVM size (<3 cm) or older age.[10]

Surgical Morbidity and Mortality

Many different variables have been associated with surgical risk but the most pervasive tool for risk stratification is the Spetzler-Martin grading system.[12] Both retrospective and prospective studies have validated the Spetzler-Martin grading system as a clinically applicable and reliable classification system.[35–39] The original grading system classifies cerebral AVMs based on size, eloquent location, and deep venous drainage (Table 72-2). The Spetzler-Martin grades range from grade I to grade V, and as the grade increases so does the surgical risk. Favorable outcomes for patients with Spetzler-Martin grade I lesions have been reported to range from 92% to 100%.[12,35,36] Patients with grade II AVMs achieve a good or an excellent outcome in approximately 95% of cases.[12,35] Large variability exists for Spetzler-Martin grade III lesions, with good or excellent outcomes in 68–96% of patients.[35,36] Spetzler-Martin grade IV and V AVMs are reported to have good or excellent outcomes in 71–75% and 50–70%, respectively.[12,35–37,40] Based on the wide variability in surgical outcomes for patients with grade III lesions, attempts have been made to subclassify these lesions with the hopes of better defining surgical risk. The first subclassification consisted of grade IIIA, which was all AVMs greater than 6 cm in non-eloquent cortex without deep venous drainage, and grade IIIB, which was all other traditional Spetzler-Martin grade III lesions. This modified classification scheme reported fair or bad outcomes in 4.5% of grade IIIA and 30% of grade IIIB AVMs.[41] These results prompted the authors to recommend microsurgical resection or embolization followed by microsurgical resection for grade IIIA and radiosurgery for grade IIIB lesions. A second modification of the Spetzler-Martin grade III AVM category favored deconstructing each combination of AVMs within the grade. The risk of a new neurologic deficit or death due to surgical resection was 2.9% for S1V1E1 (S = size, V = venous drainage, and E = eloquence), 7.1% for S2V1E0, and 14.8% for S2V0E1 Spetzler-Martin grade III AVMs.[42] Despite including a consecutive series of 174 AVMs, the author did not treat any S3V0E0 AVMs in the study.

Spetzler and Ponce published the most recent revision of the Spetzler-Martin classification system, recommending the distillation of the grades into three classes.[13] Class A consists of all Spetzler-Martin grade I and II lesions, class B is all Spetzler-Martin grade III AVMs, and class C includes Spetzler-Martin grade IV and V malformations (Fig. 72-1). Microsurgical resection is recommended for all class A AVMs, and preoperative embolization is discussed as a treatment option but not recommended based on the current risk profile for endovascular treatment. Surgical morbidity for class A AVMs has been reported to be from approximately 1% to 2.5%, which tends to decrease with longer follow-up.[12,13,35,43] Class B AVMs represent a heterogenous group, as evidenced by prior attempts at subclassification. An individualized approach to intervention for class B lesions is highlighted by the authors, who recommend consideration of multimodality therapy. Patients with class C AVMs have surgical morbidity and mortality rates that range from 20% to 30% under the best circumstances.[12,35] Conservative management is recommended for class C AVMs with few exceptions. In cases of repeated hemorrhage or progressive neurologic deficit, treatment may be considered. Aneurysms associated with class C AVMs should also be considered for microsurgical or endovascular treatment.

Additions have also been made to the Spetzler-Martin grading scale in attempts to improve predictive accuracy. Lawton et al. published a large series of microsurgically treated AVMs and compared the predictive accuracy of the Spetzler-Martin grading scale to a supplementary scale.[44] The supplementary scale included the patient's age, diffuseness of the AVM, presence of deep perforating artery supply, and whether the patient presented with a rupture or not. The authors concluded that their supplementary scale is a better predictor of neurologic outcomes after microsurgical treatment of cerebral AVMs. However, the supplementary scale does not translate to the bedside as well as the Spetzler-Martin grading system due to its increased complexity. In addition, the subjective interpretation of diffuseness lends itself to problems with

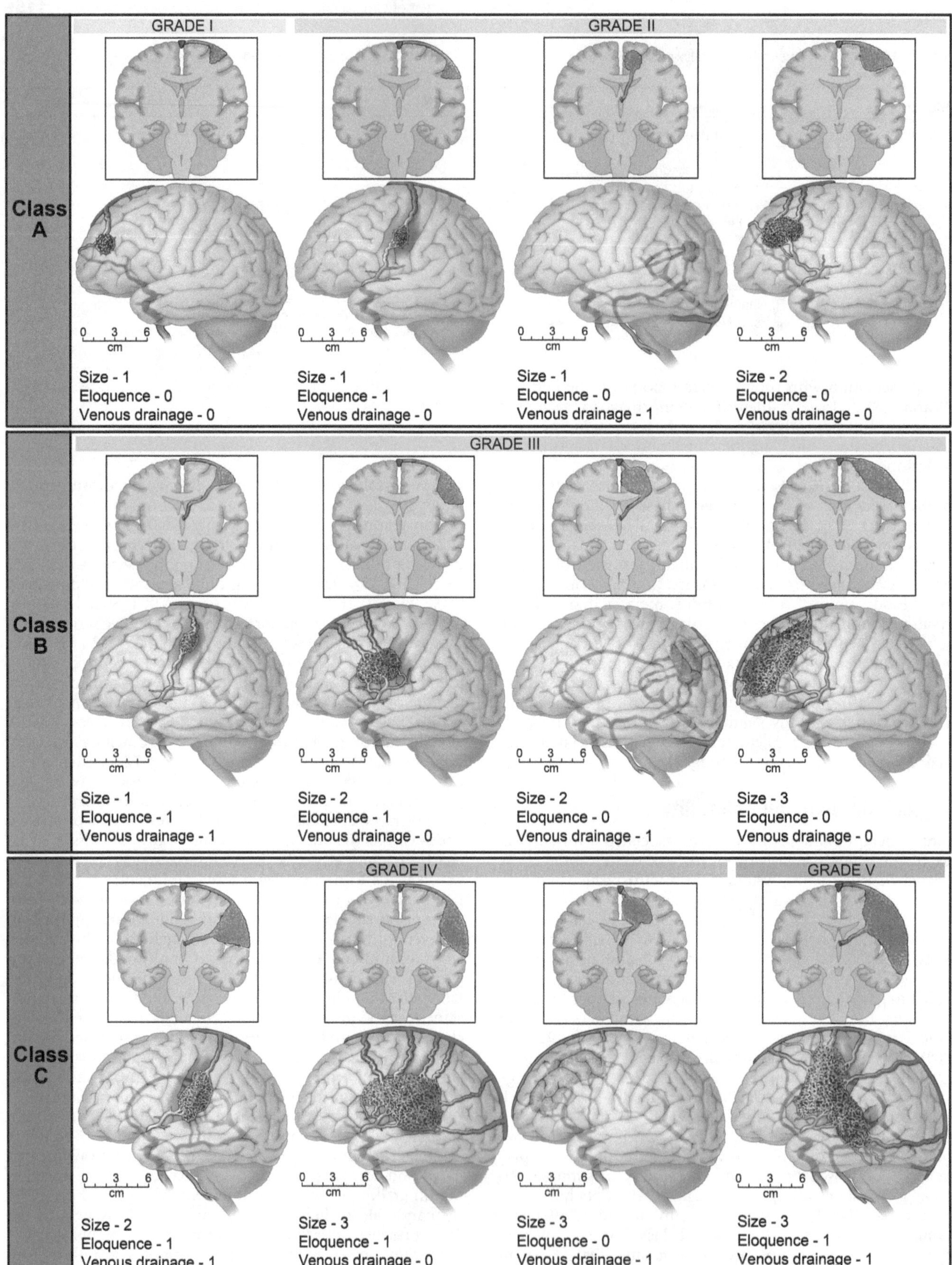

Figure 72-1. Diagrammatic representation of the combinations of graded variables (size, eloquence, and venous drainage) for each class of arteriovenous malformation (AVM). The Spetzler-Martin grading system assigns a score of 1 for small AVMs (<3 cm), 2 for medium (3–6 cm), and 3 for large (>6 cm). The eloquence of adjacent brain is scored as either non-eloquent (0) or eloquent (1). The venous drainage is scored as superficial only (0) or including drainage to the deep cerebral veins (1). Scores for each feature are totaled to determine the grade. In this system class A includes Spetzler-Martin grades I and II; class B includes grade III; and class C includes grades IV and V. *(Modified from Spetzler RF, Martin NA. A proposed grading system for arteriovenous malformations. J Neurosurg 1986;65:476–483, with permission from the American Association of Neurological Surgeons.)*

interobserver reliability. Although the supplementary grading system has not yet found popularity in the clinical setting, it highlights some of the shortcomings of the Spetzler-Martin grading system and the importance of clinical experience when dealing with these complex pathologies.

Surgical Indications and Timing

Combining the patient's demographics, neurologic examination, social history, angioarchitectural features of the AVM, and presentation allows the formulation of a risk–benefit profile for treatment. Comparing the best natural history data with the patient's surgical risk allows the surgeon to provide individual recommendations. However, in general the current indication for therapy based on the above-reviewed surgical morbidity and mortality data is microsurgical resection for class A AVMs. Class B AVMs should be strongly considered for treatment, with special attention to the potential use of multimodality therapy, particularly if patients present with a hemorrhage. At this time class C AVMs should be observed and intervention should be considered only for management of associated aneurysms in cases of serial hemorrhages or progressive neurologic decline.

The initiation of treatment for AVMs is dependent on their presentation. Ruptured AVMs can result in acute intracranial emergencies. In general, it is preferable to manage the intracranial hypertension without having to extirpate the AVM in the acute setting. In most cases medical management, external ventricular drainage, partial clot evacuation, and/or decompressive craniectomy are sufficient to control intracranial pressure. The exception to the rule is when an AVM is well visualized on preoperative imaging, with arterial feeders and venous drainage identifiable, and easily accessible during emergency surgery with the appropriate instrumentation available. In those rare situations, it is reasonable to consider resection of the AVM at the time of emergency intervention. However, the benefits of delayed intervention after hemorrhage make emergency AVM resection the exception rather than the rule.

Delaying resection of a cerebral AVM after hemorrhage allows for a complete preoperative evaluation of the patient. Most emergency interventions are based on rapidly acquired CT scans of the brain, which are insufficient to accurately delineate the angioarchitecture of vascular malformations. CT angiography (CTA) is becoming more available and provides a static image that can help identify an AVM in the setting of acute intracranial hemorrhage. However, CTA does not allow the surgeon to determine the flow through the AVM, which veins are draining the AVM, or whether small deep perforating arteries are involved. A complete four-vessel cerebral angiogram is necessary to appropriately evaluate an AVM for treatment. Delaying the AVM resection after hemorrhage allows for the proper and complete evaluation of the patient and the malformation. In addition, delayed management allows the intracranial hemorrhage to liquefy, frequently leaving a cavity adjacent to the AVM. This corridor to the lesion provides access without having to manipulate a fresh clot. The patient is also allowed time to recover in order to better assess neurologic function prior to intervention. It is the custom of the senior author (R.F.S.) to wait approximately 2 weeks after hemorrhage before performing any microsurgical intervention. Such interventions should take place within the first 3 months of the ictus because the better access provided by the clot cavity will be lost after this time interval.

Patients presenting with unruptured cerebral AVMs should generally be managed electively. Complete preoperative evaluation and education are important for successful outcomes. Functional imaging should be applied when considering treatment for an eloquent-area AVM. Relocation of eloquent function away from cerebral AVMs has been documented and these data can influence treatment recommendations.[45] Multidisciplinary review of class B AVMs is important for the best clinical outcomes, given the recommendations for multimodality therapy. Microsurgical, endovascular, and radiosurgical expert opinions are necessary for a complete assessment. The ARUBA (A Randomized trial of Unruptured Brain Arteriovenous malformations) trial[46] has provided data that call into question the wisdom of intervention in patients with unruptured AVMs unless the patient has a long life expectancy and a low risk from intervention. A detailed discussion of the ARUBA trial is set out below.

Microsurgical Resection

Access to feeding arteries and draining veins tends to dictate the approach for AVM resection. Exposure should attempt to maximize access without unnecessary exposure of cortical structures. Whenever possible, extensive arachnoid dissection around the AVM should be performed prior to beginning to resect the lesion (Fig. 72-2). This facilitates the identification of feeding arteries as they enter the nidus, as well as en passage vessels that must be preserved. Intraoperative indocyanine green angiography can be used to help clarify the anatomy of the malformation (Fig. 72-3). Once the anatomy of the AVM is correlated with preoperative imaging, the feeding vessels to the AVM can be coagulated and divided. Dissection is best executed parallel to the direction of feeding arteries. Cortical feeding vessels can frequently be fragile and may hemorrhage with bipolar cautery, resulting in retraction and risking intracerebral hemorrhage. These vessels are sometimes best managed with clip application. Once the arterial supply to the nidus has been eliminated, the draining vein is frequently deflated and no longer arterialized. Again, indocyanine green angiography can be repeated to confirm that the vein no longer fills ahead of other cortical veins. The venous outflow is the last connection to the nidus that is coagulated and divided prior to removal of the malformation. After removal of the AVM, induced hypertension can help identify any at-risk areas within the resection bed.

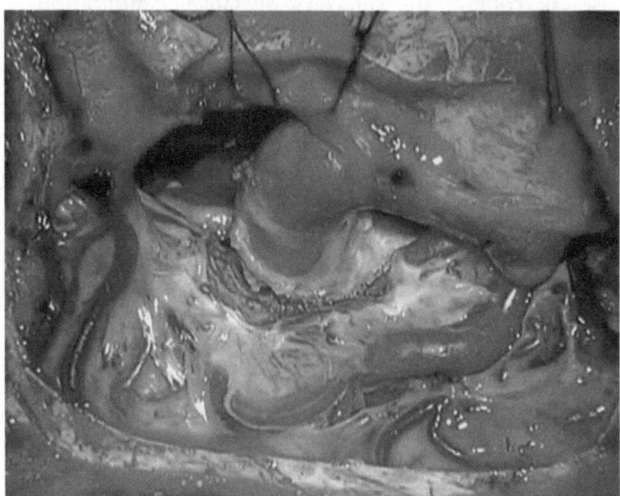

Figure 72-2. Intraoperative microscopic view of a parafalcine arteriovenous malformation during arachnoid dissection. A large dilated arterialized vein is prominent as it drains into the superior sagittal sinus. Feeding arteries from the middle cerebral circulation are appreciated on the cerebral convexity. *(Used with permission from Barrow Neurological Institute, Phoenix, Arizona).*

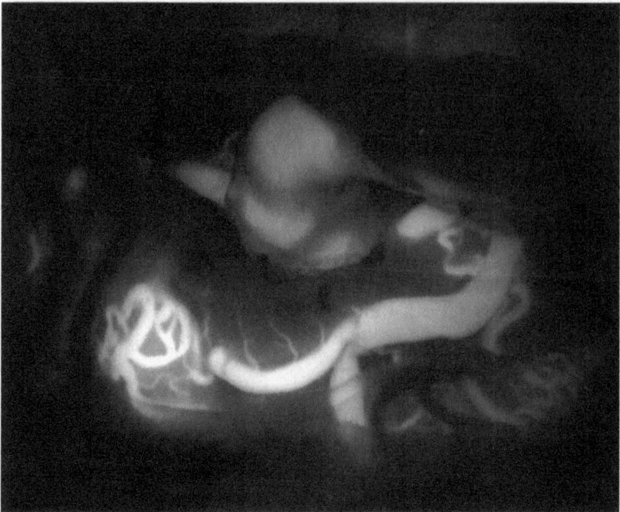

Figure 72-3. Intraoperative indocyanine green angiogram of the arteriovenous malformation (AVM) shown in Figure 72-2. The AVM draining vein obviously fills with contrast out of phase compared to other veins in the field. Arteries feeding the nidus of the AVM are appreciated in the interhemispheric fissure. *(Used with permission from Barrow Neurological Institute, Phoenix, Arizona).*

The resection of AVMs from eloquent cortex forces the surgeon to adhere closely to the coils of the nidus. When lesions are resected from non-eloquent cortex, it is favorable to leave a small layer of cortex between the nidus and the dissection plane. This facilitates the identification of feeding arteries and allows for safer manipulation of the nidus itself. Intraoperative navigation can assist in maintaining a tight adherence to the nidus despite the remaining cortical cleft.

When the AVM nidus extends into the interhemispheric fissure, sylvian fissure, or basal cisterns, the risk of iatrogenic injury to an en passage vessel increases. Special attention must be paid to the anatomy of the nidus, and exhaustive dissection prior to vessel sacrifice is necessary to prevent complications. Intraoperative angiography can be especially helpful in these cases to confirm the surgeon's operative identification of anatomy and to evaluate obliteration of the malformation.

Deep Hemispheric Arteriovenous Malformations

Classically, AVMs of the deep white matter have been considered to harbor too high a risk of morbidity and mortality to warrant consideration for surgical resection. Recent literature has challenged conventional thinking by achieving better than expected results for surgical treatment of basal ganglia, thalamic AVMs, and insular AVMs.[47] Patient selection is particularly critical for this subset of AVMs, and best results are seen in young patients who present with a hemorrhage and have a small, compact nidus. These lesions are reportedly best evaluated using the supplementary grading system discussed above. Although size is included in the Spetzler-Martin grading scale, the other three important features of deep AVMs, when considering resection, are in the supplementary system.[44] For patients harboring deep AVMs that do not meet surgical criteria, a conservative approach versus multimodality therapy should be considered. Unfortunately, the complication rate with radiosurgical treatment for these lesions tends to be higher than that for other locations.[48-50] In addition, the deep feeding arteries that typically supply these lesions make them unfavorable for embolization.

Arteriovenous Malformations of the Posterior Fossa

Posterior fossa AVMs were initially thought to have a more malignant natural history than their supratentorial counterparts. However, autopsy data have shown that a significant portion of posterior fossa AVMs remain asymptomatic, suggesting that there may not be a significant difference between the two groups.[51] It is accepted that patients with these lesions more frequently present with hemorrhage compared to patients with supratentorial AVMs.[4,32,52-54] Malformations of the posterior fossa are generally placed into one of three categories for the purpose of surgical decision making. The AVM is either in the cerebellum, in the brainstem, or in both locations. Class A or B malformations in the cerebellum should be considered for treatment. Class C lesions should be observed unless these patients present with recurrent hemorrhages or progressive neurologic decline. Brainstem AVMs can be subdivided into those that have pial representation and those that do not. Those with surface representation can be considered for surgical resection and those without should be observed or treated with fractionated radiosurgery. Lesions located in the cerebellum and brainstem can be observed, treated with surgical resection, or partially resected from the cerebellum, with the residual component treated with fractionated radiosurgery. In general, posterior fossa AVMs require special attention be paid to the vascular anatomy involved in the lesion. Decisions about intervention for those malformations involving the brainstem must be made individually, with attention to anatomic white matter tracts and potential deficits. Although these are challenging lesions, the current literature indicates that favorable clinical outcomes can be achieved in approximately 70–80% of surgically treated cases.[52,53,55,56]

Cerebral Aneurysms Associated with Arteriovenous Malformations

The incidence of cerebral aneurysms associated with AVMs ranges from approximately 3% to 60% and has been reported to average 10%.[27,57-59] The risk of hemorrhage in AVMs harboring cerebral aneurysms is believed to be higher than in those without.[60,61] It is unclear whether this is related to the presence of the aneurysms or to the angioarchitecture of the AVMs resulting in high-flow conditions that predispose the lesions to a higher risk of hemorrhage. Intranidal aneurysms are treated in conjunction with the AVM. Aneurysms on the direct feeding arteries of the AVM typically regress with treatment of the AVM. Proximal aneurysms on the circle of Willis are less likely to regress and frequently require management and follow-up independent of the AVM.[61] When an unruptured AVM with a direct feeding artery aneurysm is being managed conservatively, the aneurysm should be managed independently. Management options include observation, palliative embolization, and endovascular or surgical obliteration. When patients with AVMs with circle of Willis or direct feeding artery aneurysms present with hemorrhage, the first step is to try to determine whether the hemorrhage was from the AVM or the aneurysm. Aneurysm rupture tends to result in predominantly subarachnoid hemorrhage while AVM rupture is more classically intraparenchymal. If it is determined that the aneurysm has hemorrhaged, then it should be managed primarily and the AVM can be addressed at the same time, if accessible, or in a delayed fashion. The reverse is true if the AVM is determined to be the cause of the rupture. If no determination can be made regarding the source of the hemorrhage, then both lesions should be treated, with priority given to treating the aneurysm secondary to the higher risk of re-rupture.

Multimodality Treatment of Arteriovenous Malformations

Consideration of multiple interventions for the treatment of an AVM requires assessment of the additive risk of the interventions. Class A or Spetzler-Martin grade I and II AVMs have very good outcomes with microsurgical resection, and multimodality therapy is not currently recommended for these lesions. Class B or Spetzler-Martin grade III lesions should be considered for multimodality treatment. Obliteration rates above 80% have been achieved using multimodality therapy for class B AVMs. Higher morbidity rates seem to be related to increasing size of class B lesions rather than the presence of deep drainage or eloquence.[42,43,62] Minor neurologic deficits have been reported in 14–29%, major deficits in 5–6% and mortality rates of 0–1% of class III AVMs treated with multimodal therapy.[62,63] When intervention is considered for class C lesions, a multimodality approach should be considered as well. Reported cure rates with multimodality therapy for Spetzler-Martin grade IV lesions (80%) is significantly better than those for grade V lesions (50%).[64] Since partial treatment does not provide any significant protection from future hemorrhage, the comparatively low obliteration rate of Spetzler-Martin grade V lesions needs to be considered prior to offering intervention.

Arteriovenous Malformation Management during Pregnancy

Despite conflicting reports, the general belief at this time is that there is no significant increase in risk of hemorrhage from a cerebral AVM during pregnancy.[65–67] Given that some literature reports higher rates of hemorrhage, it is reasonable to consider AVM treatment prior to pregnancy. Those lesions that are incidentally diagnosed during pregnancy should generally be observed until after childbirth and then reevaluated for possible treatment. Hemorrhage rates have not been reported to be higher with vaginal delivery compared to cesarean section.[65,68,69] Patients with AVMs who present with hemorrhage during pregnancy should be considered for treatment. There is concern that the re-hemorrhage rate of AVMs is increased during pregnancy and this should be a consideration when debating intervention.[66,70] An obstetric consultation should be obtained early when managing an AVM in a pregnant patient.

Perioperative Management

All patients being considered for treatment should be evaluated by an internist prior to intervention. Blood pressure should be maintained intraoperatively at approximately the baseline. Diuretics, antiepileptics, and corticosteroids can be used at the discretion of the surgeon. Induced hypertension after resection can help to identify any at-risk areas of the resection cavity. Care should be taken to prevent spikes in blood pressure during extubation. Postoperative blood pressure should be strictly maintained in a normotensive range for 24 hours. Prophylaxis for deep vein thrombosis can be initiated 24 hours after surgery. Intraoperative or postoperative angiography should be obtained to confirm complete resection of the AVM.

The ARUBA Trial

The ARUBA trial was a prospective, multicenter, parallel design, randomized, controlled trial that was intended to compare intervention versus medical management for unruptured AVMs.[46] Eligible patients were 18 years of age or older with no prior hemorrhage or intervention and AVMs that were deemed to be suitable for complete obliteration. Of the 1740 patients screened, 726 were deemed eligible. Of those 726 eligible patients, 323 refused to enroll and 177 patients had their management decision made by the treating team outside of the randomization process. Only seven (3%) patients dropped out of the trial. The primary outcome measure was death or symptomatic stroke and the secondary outcome was clinical impairment, defined as ≥2 on the modified Rankin Scale. The authors initially planned to enroll 800 patients for an 87.5% power to detect a 40% reduction in risk for symptomatic stroke or death. Due to low numbers of patients enrolled in the study, the goal sample size was reduced to 400 patients for an 80% power to detect a 46% reduction in risk. However, due to recommendations of an independent data safety monitoring committee, the study ultimately stopped enrolling patients after randomizing 226 patients between April 2007 and April 2013. Of those 226 patients, 114 were randomized to intervention and 109 to medical management. At the time of analysis, 53 of the treatment patients had not completed therapy and 20 had not initiated therapy. Seven patients randomized to medical management ultimately crossed over to the intervention arm, although no hemorrhages were identified in these patients. Interventional therapy included any neurosurgical, endovascular, or radiotherapy procedure (single or multiple) deemed appropriate by local ARUBA investigators to achieve complete AVM obliteration. In the intervention group, 5 were treated with neurosurgical procedures, 30 with embolization, 31 with radiotherapy, and 28 with multimodality therapy. The average follow-up was 33 months and was balanced between the intervention and medical management arms. The primary endpoint was achieved in 35 (30.7%) of the 114 patients randomized to treatment and in 11 (10.1%) of the 109 patients in the medical management arm. The secondary outcome was achieved in 24 (46.2%) of the patients receiving intervention and in 8 (15.1%) of the medically managed patients at 30 months. At 36 months the secondary outcome was achieved in 17 (38.6%) of the treatment patients and in 6 (14%) of the patients in the medical group. The authors concluded that medical management is superior to intervention in preventing death or stroke in patients with unruptured AVMs followed for 33 months.[46]

The authors of the ARUBA trial aimed to address a valid question and their efforts are to be commended. However, the study design and execution have serious flaws that undermine the validity of their conclusions. To start, the authors fail to explain why such a large number of eligible patients, who did not refuse enrollment, were not randomized. Of the 726 eligible patients, 323 refused and 226 were enrolled. The other 177 patients were managed outside of the randomization process. There is no discussion regarding the characteristics of these patients, their lesions, or why they were not included.

The length of follow-up is the most obvious pitfall of this analysis. The 33-month follow-up for a disease with a lifelong risk of stroke and hemorrhage is clearly inadequate to make conclusions. The authors' proposed follow-up of 5 years is also comparatively short. Treatment of AVMs compresses the risk associated with these lesions. It may require more than the planned follow-up period to demonstrate the benefit of eradicating these lesions.

Additionally, the study design lacks any standardization of the treatment arm. A recent large meta-analysis of treated AVMs published obliteration rates of 96% for surgical resection, 38% for stereotactic radiosurgery, and 13% for embolization.[71] The neurosurgical literature supports these findings, and the current recommendation, based on pooled analysis, is for surgical resection as the primary therapy for Spetzler-Martin grades I and II AVMs.[13] Without further detail regarding the treatment arm, it remains difficult to resolve why only five patients received surgical resection alone when 76 patients in the treatment arm had grade I or II AVMs.

The authors also provide no discussion regarding the treatment details of the radiotherapy and embolization groups. What type of radiotherapy was used and with what doses? Was serial or single embolization performed and why? Serial embolization certainly increases the risk of adverse events compared to single therapeutic options. Additionally, embolization is generally not considered a curative procedure, as evidenced by the previously mentioned obliteration rate of 13%, and it is mainly used in combination therapies. It is concerning that 30 of the treatment patients were managed with embolization alone.

There is reference to evaluation of lesion eradication by cerebral angiography within the methods section. However, the authors do not include data regarding eradication in the article. The temporal relationship between treatment and achievement of primary and secondary outcomes is important when considering radiotherapy or serial embolization. Radiotherapy has a significantly delayed therapeutic effect. Serial embolization will not provide therapeutic effect until complete eradication is achieved. Any events in the treatment arm that occur prior to eradication should be noted by the authors.

Given the lack of information and heterogeneity regarding therapies, it is impossible to understand what the treatment arm represents. That said, it is unclear what the authors are concluding medical management is superior to. It seems imprudent to conclude superiority of medical management for AVMs when the treatment arm provides therapies that are seemingly well below the current standard of care for eradication. It is apparent from the prior discussion that many of the treatments provided in the ARUBA trial deviated severely from what is widely accepted as the standard of care for these lesions.

In summary, the ARUBA trial is the first randomized controlled trial attempting to evaluate intervention versus medical management for unruptured AVMs. Unfortunately, shortcomings in study design and execution, as well as a relative lack of information regarding the treatment arm and the enrollment process, invalidate the authors' conclusions. Indeed, the fact that in the medically managed group there was a 10% death or stroke incidence over a time interval of less than 3 years emphasizes the need to provide a low-risk cure for these patients.

Conclusion

Cerebral AVMs represent a heterogenous group of lesions. Current classification systems provide a foundation for clinical decision making in the treatment of ruptured and unruptured AVMs. Microsurgical resection is the primary recommendation for class A or Spetzler-Martin grades I and II AVMs. Class B or Spetzler-Martin grade III AVMs should be considered for multimodality therapy. Class C or Spetzler-Martin grades IV and V AVMs should be managed conservatively unless the patient suffers progressive neurologic decline and/or multiple hemorrhages. Multimodality treatment of class C AVMs is often required when therapy is indicated. Partial treatment of an AVM does not provide any significant protection from future hemorrhage, although it may alleviate symptoms related to local ischemia from steal phenomenon. Patients presenting with unruptured AVMs still warrant consideration for treatment, using the paradigm detailed above, based on a critical evaluation of the ARUBA trial.

SPINAL ARTERIOVENOUS MALFORMATIONS

Introduction

The classification systems for spinal arteriovenous malformations include a wide array of vascular lesions in and around the spinal cord. The most widely recognized system for classifying spinal AVMs was created from the efforts of several different authors.[72-80] This classification describes four types of spinal AVMs: type I, dural arteriovenous fistulae (AVFs); type II, intramedullary glomus AVMs; type III, juvenile or combined AVMs; and type IV, intradural perimedullary AVFs. The type I lesions consist of an abnormal connection between a dural branch of a radicular artery and dural veins at the nerve root sleeve, resulting in arterialization of the perimedullary venous plexus. Type II lesions are located within the tissue of the spinal cord. Type III lesions involve the intradural and extradural compartment and are frequently referred to as juvenile or metameric AVMs. Type IV spinal AVMs are intradural fistulae located ventrally, with arterial input typically from the anterior spinal artery. Recently, this classification system was modified by the senior author in order to more effectively characterize these lesions.[81,82] This system is based on specific anatomic and pathophysiologic characteristics of the varying lesions and is summarized in Table 72-3. The modified classification system is compared below to the prior system and is used to discuss therapeutic recommendations.

Extradural Arteriovenous Fistulae

Extradural AVFs are the result of an abnormal connection between an arterial branch of a radicular artery and the epidural venous plexus (Fig. 72-4). This type of fistula commonly becomes symptomatic when dilation of the epidural veins results in nerve root or spinal cord compression. Vascular steal and venous hypertension can also contribute to the symptomatic presentation. Prior classification systems do not explicitly include this type of fistulae. This is likely secondary to the observation that these are extremely uncommon lesions. Endovascular treatment is the first-line treatment for these lesions, with surgical resection limited to cases requiring decompression after embolization.

Intradural Dorsal Arteriovenous Fistulae

Intradural dorsal AVFs consist of an abnormal connection between a radicular artery and the venous drainage of the

TABLE 72-3 Classification and Treatment Recommendations for Spinal Arteriovenous Malformations

Type of Spinal AVM*	Treatment Recommendations
Extradural AVF	Endovascular or combined
Intradural dorsal AVF	Surgical
Intradural ventral AVF	
A – small	Surgical
B – intermediate	Surgical
C – giant	Combined
Extradural and intradural AVM	Combined
Intramedullary AVM	
Compact	Surgical or combined
Diffuse	Surgical or combined
Conus medullaris AVM	Combined

AVM, arteriovenous malformation; AVF, arteriovenous fistula.
*Data from Kim LJ, Spetzler RF. Classification and surgical management of spinal arteriovenous lesions: arteriovenous fistulae and arteriovenous malformations. *Neurosurgery* 2006;59(5 Suppl 3):S195–201; discussion S3–13.

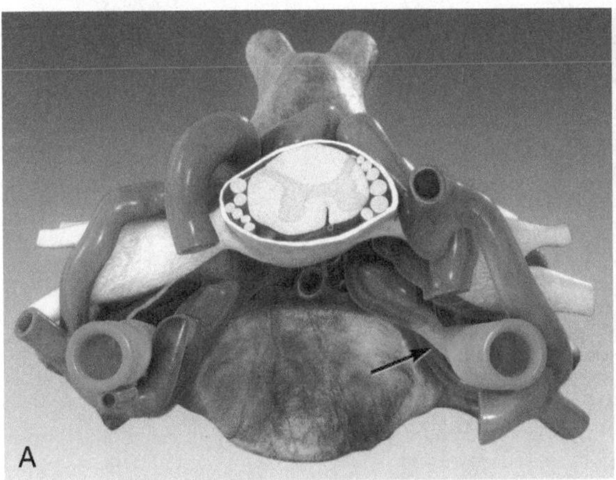

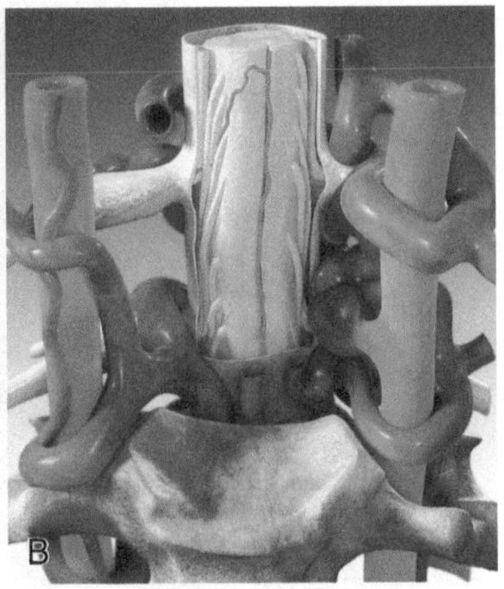

Figure 72-4. A, Axial illustration demonstrating an extradural arteriovenous malformation along a perforating branch of the left vertebral artery (arrow). B, Illustration of the anterior view demonstrating that engorgement of epidural veins can produce symptomatic mass effect on adjacent nerve roots and spinal cord. *(Used with permission from Barrow Neurological Institute, Phoenix, Arizona. Figure legend from Kim LJ, Spetzler RF. Classification and surgical management of spinal arteriovenous lesions: Arteriovenous fistulae and arteriovenous malformations. Neurosurgery 2006;59[5 Suppl 3]:S195–201, discussion S3–13, with permission from Lippincott, Williams & Wilkins.)*

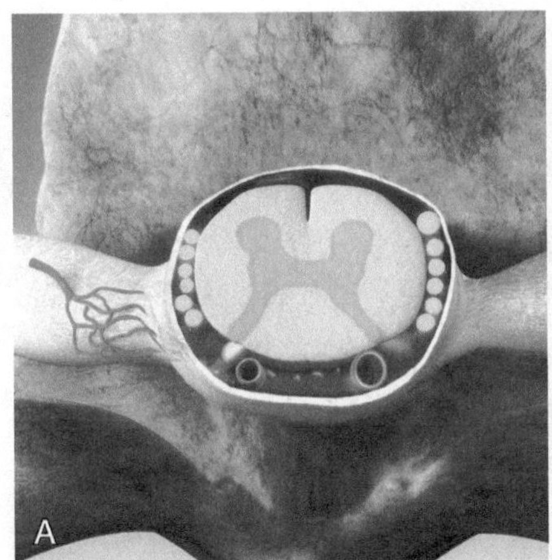

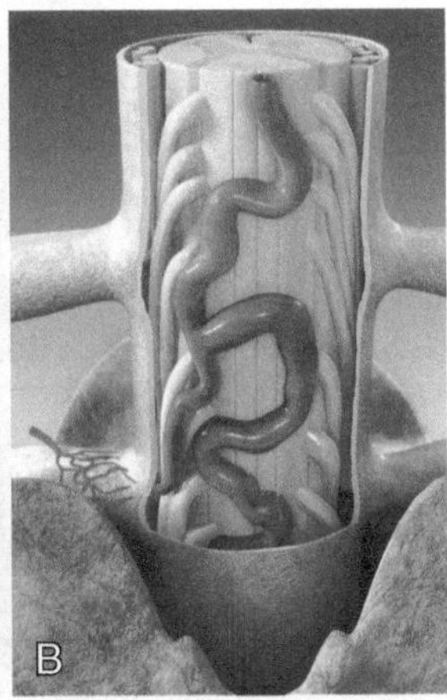

Figure 72-5. A, Axial illustration of an intradural dorsal arteriovenous malformation demonstrating an abnormal radicular feeding artery along the nerve root on the right. The glomerular network of tiny branches coalesces at the site of the fistula along the dural root sleeve. B, Illustration of the posterior view demonstrating the dilatation of the coronal venous plexus. In addition to venous outflow obstruction (not shown), arterialization of these veins produces venous hypertension. Focal disruption of the point of the fistula by endovascular or microsurgical methods will obliterate the lesion. *(Figure used with permission from Barrow Neurological Institute, Phoenix, Arizona. Figure legend from Kim LJ, Spetzler RF. Classification and surgical management of spinal arteriovenous lesions: Arteriovenous fistulae and arteriovenous malformations. Neurosurgery 2006;59[5 Suppl 3]:S195–201, discussion S3–13, with permission from Lippincott, Williams & Wilkins.)*

spinal cord at the dural sleeve of the nerve root (Fig. 72-5). The arterialization of the venous drainage of the spinal cord can cause congestive myelopathy, also known as Foix-Alajouanine syndrome. These fistulae were previously classified as type I dural AVFs.

Treatment of these fistulae can be achieved with endovascular or open surgical techniques.[83] However, the durability and safety of the treatment tend to be optimized with surgical management.[77,84–87] Both endovascular and open surgical treatment require meticulous spinal angiography to delineate the anatomy of the fistula as well as the normal irrigation of the spinal cord. These lesions are best managed with a posterior approach for exposure. With careful intraoperative planning, a minimally invasive unilateral hemilaminotomy can be used to access the lesion. The dura is opened, extending slightly above and below the exiting nerve root. The operating microscope is then used to identify the arterialized vein, which can typically be traced back to its pathologic connection at the dural root sleeve. Intraoperative indocyanine green or other angiography can be used to assist in confirmation of the fistula as well as its obliteration. Bipolar coagulation and sharp sectioning of the vein at the dural sleeve are typically all that is needed to completely eliminate the fistula. Direct measurement of venous pressure prior to and after interruption of the fistula can also be used to confirm therapeutic treatment.

INTRADURAL VENTRAL ARTERIOVENOUS FISTULAE

Intradural ventral arteriovenous fistulae are located in the subarachnoid space and consist of an abnormal communication between the anterior spinal circulation and the venous drainage of the spinal cord (Fig. 72-6). These fistulae are subclassified into types A, B, and C based on size, with type A lesions being small, B intermediate, and C giant. High flow through these fistulae can result in symptoms of vascular steal

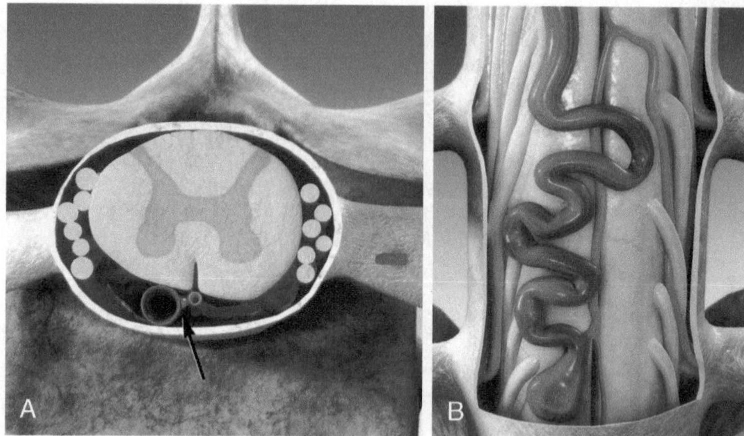

Figure 72-6. A, Axial illustration demonstrating an intradural ventral arteriovenous malformation, a midline lesion derived from a fistulous connection (arrow) between the anterior spinal artery and the coronal venous plexus. B, Illustration of the anterior view demonstrating the fistula along the anteroinferior aspect of the spinal cord. Proximal and distal to this type A lesion, the course of the anterior spinal artery is normal. *(Figure used with permission from Barrow Neurological Institute, Phoenix, Arizona. Figure legend from Kim LJ, Spetzler RF. Classification and surgical management of spinal arteriovenous lesions: Arteriovenous fistulae and arteriovenous malformations. Neurosurgery 2006;59[5 Suppl 3]:S195–201, discussion S3–13, with permission from Lippincott, Williams & Wilkins.)*

as well as venous congestive myelopathy. These fistulae were previously classified as type IV AVFs.

Type A and the majority of type B fistulae can be managed with primary surgical resection. The risks of accessing these lesions endovascularly can be high when the anterior spinal artery must be catheterized. Exposing the patient to this risk is generally not necessary when managing type A or the majority of type B lesions. However, some type B and the majority of type C lesions should be considered for endovascular therapy to reduce flow and palliate symptoms while surgical resection can be considered as an adjunct to embolization.[88–90] Surgical approaches to these lesions should maximize exposure of the anterior spinal artery. Successful surgical resection hinges on the surgeon's ability to identify and preserve the normal branches of the anterior spinal artery during obliteration of the fistula. Anterior, lateral, and posterolateral approaches are options for accessing these lesions.[91,92] In some cases destabilizing procedures provide the best exposure and spinal instrumentation and fusion must be performed.

Extradural-Intradural Arteriovenous Malformations

Extradural-intradural AVMs typically involve a discrete somite level and are commonly referred to as type III, juvenile, or metameric AVMs (Fig. 72-7). These complicated lesions can have cutaneous, muscular, bone, spinal cord, and nerve root involvement. Cobb syndrome refers to cutaneous as well as underlying vascular malformation in a pattern consistent with a single somite level.

Metameric AVMs are challenging lesions to manage, and endovascular treatment should be the primary therapeutic consideration. Surgical treatment should be reserved for symptomatic management and only in rare cases for resection. Complete resections have been reported; however, in most cases the goal of treatment is palliation of symptoms by managing vascular steal, venous hypertension, and removal of mass effect.[93,94] When indicated, individually tailored approaches, typically involving multiple surgical disciplines, are necessary for the successful operative management of these AVMs.

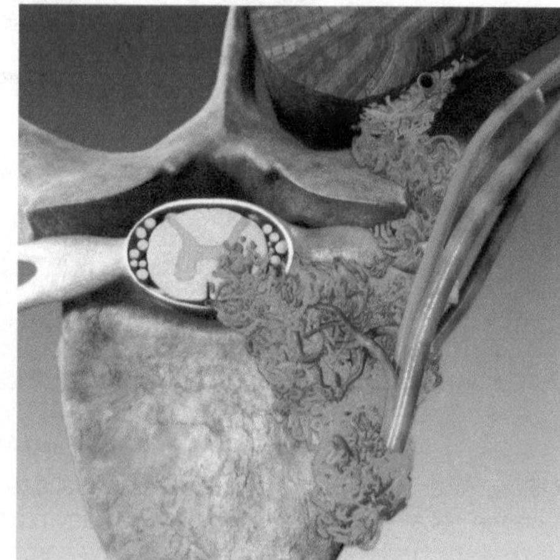

Figure 72-7. Axial illustration demonstrating an extradural–intradural arteriovenous malformation. These treacherous lesions can encompass soft tissues, bone, spinal canal, spinal cord, and spinal nerve roots along an entire spinal level. Considerable involvement of multiple structures makes these entities extremely difficult to treat. Although cures have been reported, the primary goal of treatment is usually palliative. *(Figure used with permission from Barrow Neurological Institute, Phoenix, Arizona. Figure legend from Kim LJ, Spetzler RF. Classification and surgical management of spinal arteriovenous lesions: Arteriovenous fistulae and arteriovenous malformations. Neurosurgery 2006;59[5 Suppl 3]:S195–201, discussion S3–13, with permission from Lippincott, Williams & Wilkins.)*

Intramedullary Arteriovenous Malformations

Intramedullary AVMs are located within the parenchyma of the spinal cord and can have single or multiple feeding arteries and draining veins. These AVMs are subclassified into diffuse or compact lesions based on the angioarchitecture of the lesion (Figs 72-8, 72-9). Intramedullary AVMs were previously classified as type II or glomus AVMs. The size of the AVM and the subclassification are important determinants of treatment success. Small compact intramedullary AVMs are typically

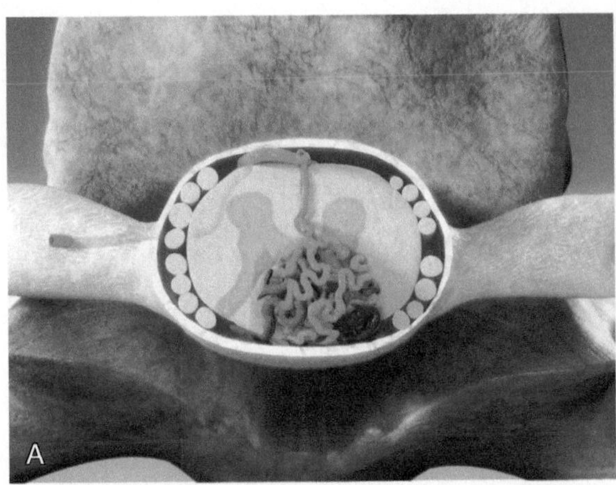

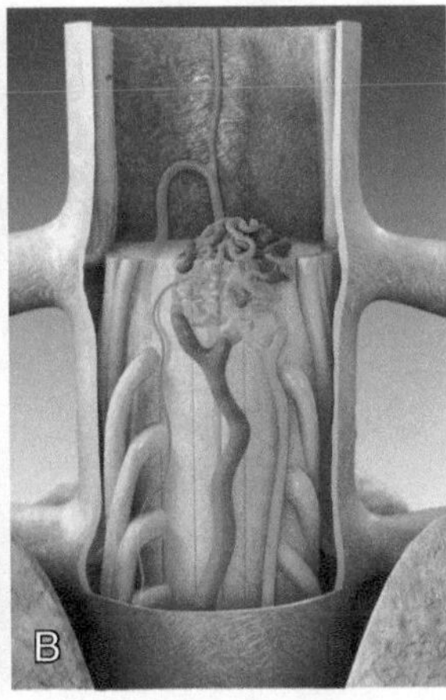

Figure 72-8. A, Axial illustration demonstrating a compact intramedullary arteriovenous malformation (AVM). In this figure, an arterial feeder from the anterior spinal artery is identified. Note the discrete, compact mass of the AVM. B, Posterior view demonstrating additional feeding branches from the posterior spinal artery and reemphasizing the compact nature of this type of spinal AVM. Portions of the AVM are evident along the surface of the spinal cord. Surgical resection is the mainstay of treatment. Preoperative embolization is reserved for select cases only. *(Figure used with permission from Barrow Neurological Institute, Phoenix, Arizona. Figure legend from Kim LJ, Spetzler RF. Classification and surgical management of spinal arteriovenous lesions: Arteriovenous fistulae and arteriovenous malformations. Neurosurgery 2006;59[5 Suppl 3]:S195–201, discussion S3–13, with permission from Lippincott, Williams & Wilkins.)*

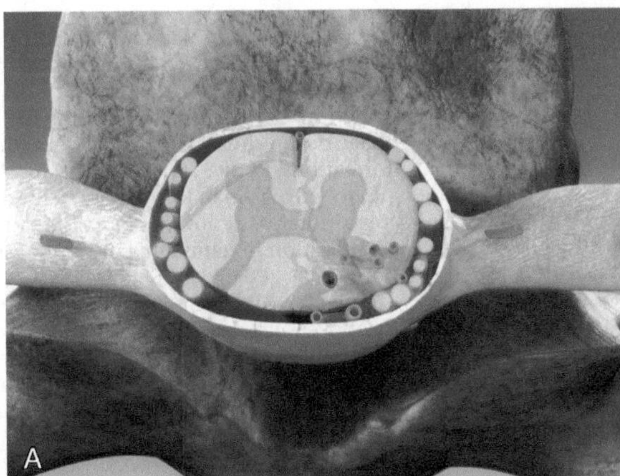

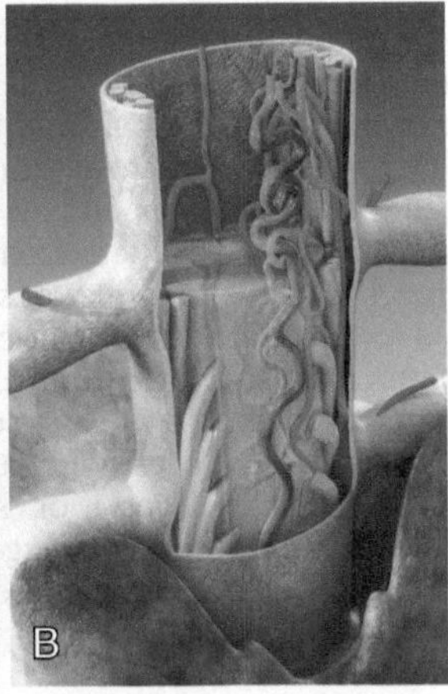

Figure 72-9. A, Axial illustration demonstrating a diffuse intramedullary arteriovenous malformation (AVM) with areas of intervening neural tissue between the intraparenchymal loops of AVM. Portions of the AVM also course along the pial surface and subarachnoid space. B, Illustration of the oblique posterior view demonstrating the loops of the AVM coursing in and out of the spinal cord. Normal neural tissue is evident between intraparenchymal portions of the AVM. This view accentuates the diffuse character of these lesions. *(Figure used with permission from Barrow Neurological Institute, Phoenix, Arizona. Figure legend from Kim LJ, Spetzler RF. Classification and surgical management of spinal arteriovenous lesions: Arteriovenous fistulae and arteriovenous malformations. Neurosurgery 2006;59[5 Suppl 3]:S195–201, discussion S3–13, with permission from Lippincott, Williams & Wilkins.)*

better candidates for both endovascular obliteration and surgical resection.

Surgical resection of intramedullary AVMs is the primary treatment for these lesions, with endovascular embolization being considered as an adjunct or salvage therapy in most cases.[82,95] Preoperative embolization can be beneficial for complex, multipedicled, or diffuse AVMs. Most commonly, these lesions are approached from a posterior or posterolateral exposure. However, the origin of the main feeding arteries must be considered and in some cases an anterior approach is preferred. Microsurgical resection of these lesions should be performed with tight adherence to the coils of the AVM. Vascular loops extending out of the AVM into the parenchyma of the cord are best truncated at the natural border of the malformation. This technique helps to avoid "chasing" vessels into normal tissue and risking neurologic injury. Intraoperative indocyanine green angiography can be used in a similar fashion as it is for cerebral AVMs, to assist in delineating anatomy. Postoperative spinal angiography is essential to demonstrate a surgical cure. Motor and sensory evoked potentials should be utilized when the patient has baseline function that can be monitored. Larger lesions can be managed with staged procedures and complete surgical resection can be achieved in approximately 90% of cases in the senior author's experience.[82]

Conus Medullaris Arteriovenous Malformations

Conus medullaris AVMs tend to be diffuse and classically have multiple feeding vessels that originate from the posterior and the anterior spinal arteries (Fig. 72-10). Venous congestion, ischemia from vascular steal, hemorrhage, and mass effect can

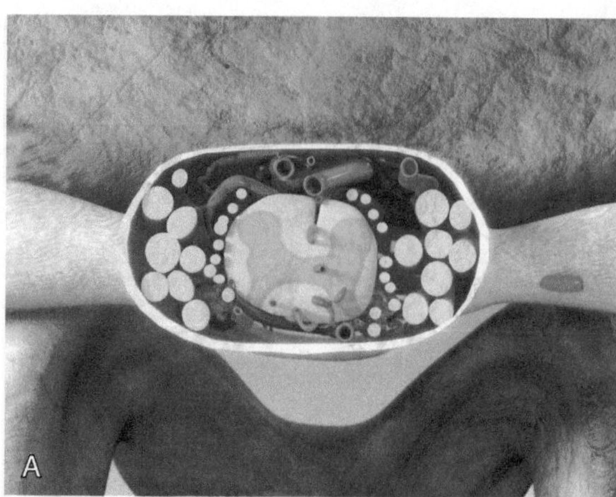

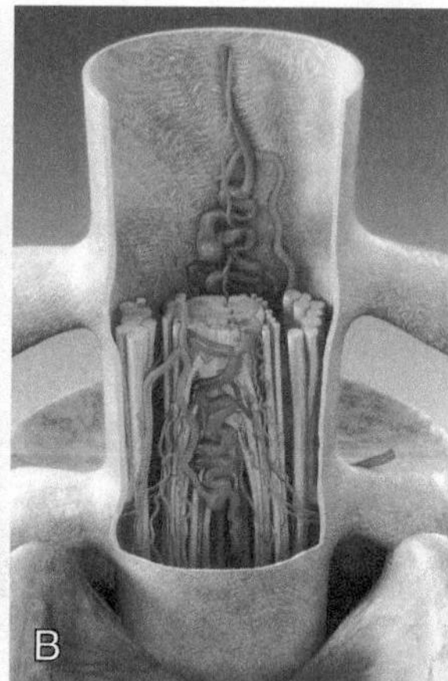

Figure 72-10. A, Axial illustration demonstrating a conus medullaris arteriovenous malformation (AVM) and the feeding arteries and draining veins from both the anterior and posterior aspects of the spinal cord. Note the proximity of the AVM to branches of the cauda equina. B, Illustration of the posterior view recapitulating the complexity of the angioarchitecture of these lesions. Anterior and posterior spinal arteries, radicular arteries, and anterior and posteriorly draining veins are involved simultaneously. Portions of the AVM can consist of direct arteriovenous shunts as well as regions of true AVM nidus. During endovascular treatment, surgical treatment, or both, it is crucial to identify the en passage branches of the anterior and posterior spinal arteries. *(Figure used with permission from Barrow Neurological Institute, Phoenix, Arizona. Figure legend from Kim LJ, Spetzler RF. Classification and surgical management of spinal arteriovenous lesions: Arteriovenous fistulae and arteriovenous malformations. Neurosurgery 2006;59[5 Suppl 3]:S195–201, discussion S3–13, with permission from Lippincott, Williams & Wilkins.)*

all contribute to the symptomatic presentation of these AVMs. Uniquely, patients with these lesions can present with both upper and lower motor neuron pathologic findings.

A combined endovascular and microsurgical therapeutic approach is recommended for conus medullaris AVMs. Exposure for these lesions is usually adequate from a posterior or posterolateral approach. Large venous dilations are common with these AVMs and when microsurgical resection is executed, it is important to also achieve adequate neural decompression from mass effect exerted by these veins. As mentioned in regard to ventral AVFs, early identification and preservation of the anterior and posterior spinal artery branches are crucial for successful surgical management. In the senior author's experience, these lesions can recur more frequently than other spinal AVMs and close follow-up is recommended.

Conclusions

Spinal vascular malformations are a heterogenous and complex conglomeration of pathologies. This chapter outlines an updated system for the classification and management of spinal AVMs and AVFs. Despite the challenging nature of these lesions, appropriate therapeutic strategies can achieve acceptable neurologic outcomes. The detailed endovascular and adjunctive radiosurgical management of these lesions is beyond the scope of this chapter, but deserve attention by those caring for these patients.

REFERENCES

1. Kim H, Hysi PG, Pawlikowska L, et al. Common variants in interleukin-1-Beta gene are associated with intracranial hemorrhage and susceptibility to brain arteriovenous malformation. Cerebrovasc Dis 2009;27:176–82.
2. Oikawa M, Kuniba H, Kondoh T, et al. Familial brain arteriovenous malformation maps to 5p13-q14, 15q11-q13 or 18p11: linkage analysis with clipped fingernail DNA on high-density SNP array. Eur J Med Genet 2010;53:244–9.
3. Hernesniemi JA, Dashti R, Juvela S, et al. Natural history of brain arteriovenous malformations: a long-term follow-up study of risk of hemorrhage in 238 patients. Neurosurgery 2008;63:823–9.
4. Al-Shahi R, Warlow C. A systematic review of the frequency and prognosis of arteriovenous malformations of the brain in adults. Brain 2001;124:1900–26.
5. Fullerton HJ, Achrol AS, Johnston SC, et al. Long-term hemorrhage risk in children versus adults with brain arteriovenous malformations. Stroke 2005;36:2099–104.
6. Achrol AS, Guzman R, Varga M, et al. Pathogenesis and radiobiology of brain arteriovenous malformations: implications for risk stratification in natural history and posttreatment course. Neurosurg Focus 2009;26(5):E9.
7. Gabriel RA, Kim H, Sidney S, et al. Ten-year detection rate of brain arteriovenous malformations in a large, multiethnic, defined population. Stroke 2010;41(1):21–6.
8. Stapf C, Mast H, Sciacca RR, et al. The New York Islands AVM Study: design, study progress, and initial results. Stroke 2003;34(5):e29–33.
9. Crawford PM, West CR, Chadwick DW, et al. Arteriovenous malformations of the brain: natural history in unoperated patients. J Neurol Neurosurg Psychiatry 1986;49:1–10.
10. Gross BA, Du R. Natural history of cerebral arteriovenous malformations: a meta-analysis. J Neurosurg 2013;118:437–43.
11. Stapf C, Mast H, Sciacca RR, et al. Predictors of hemorrhage in patients with untreated brain arteriovenous malformation. Neurology 2006;66(9):1350–5.
12. Spetzler RF, Martin NA. A proposed grading system for arteriovenous malformations. J Neurosurg 1986;65(4):476–83.
13. Spetzler RF, Ponce FA. A 3-tier classification of cerebral arteriovenous malformations. Clinical article. J Neurosurg 2011;114(3):842–9.
14. Du R, Keyoung HM, Dowd CF, et al. The effects of diffuseness and deep perforating artery supply on outcomes after microsurgical resection of brain arteriovenous malformations. Neurosurgery 2007;60(4):638–46.
15. Stapleton CJ, Armstrong DL, Zidovetzki R, et al. Thrombospondin-1 modulates the angiogenic phenotype of human cerebral arteriovenous malformation endothelial cells. Neurosurgery 2011;68(5):1342–53.
16. Hashimoto T, Lam T, Boudreau NJ, et al. Abnormal balance in the angiopoietin-tie2 system in human brain arteriovenous malformations. Circ Res 2001;89(2):111–13.
17. Hashimoto T, Lawton MT, Wen G, et al. Gene microarray analysis of human brain arteriovenous malformations. Neurosurgery 2004;54(2):410–23.
18. Mahajan A, Manchandia TC, Gould G, et al. De novo arteriovenous malformations: case report and review of the literature. Neurosurg Rev 2010;33(1):115–19.

19. Sabba C, Pasculli G, Lenato GM, et al. Hereditary hemorrhagic telangiectasia: clinical features in ENG and ALK1 mutation carriers. J Thromb Haemost 2007;5(6):1149–57.
20. Achrol AS, Pawlikowska L, McCulloch CE, et al. Tumor necrosis factor-α-238G>A promoter polymorphism is associated with increased risk of new hemorrhage in the natural course of patients with brain arteriovenous malformations. Stroke 2006;37(1): 231–4.
21. Hartmann A, Mast H, Mohr JP, et al. Morbidity of intracranial hemorrhage in patients with cerebral arteriovenous malformation. Stroke 1998;29(5):931–4.
22. Kim H, McCulloch CE, Johnston SC, et al. Comparison of 2 approaches for determining the natural history risk of brain arteriovenous malformation rupture. Am J Epidemiol 2010;171(12): 1317–22.
23. Kim H, Sidney S, McCulloch CE, et al. Racial/Ethnic differences in longitudinal risk of intracranial hemorrhage in brain arteriovenous malformation patients. Stroke 2007;38(9):2430–7.
24. Stapf C, Mohr JP, Pile-Spellman J, et al. Epidemiology and natural history of arteriovenous malformations. Neurosurg Focus 2001; 11(5):e1.
25. Brown RD Jr, Flemming KD, Meyer FB, et al. Natural history, evaluation, and management of intracranial vascular malformations. Mayo Clin Proc 2005;80(2):269–81.
26. da CL, Wallace MC, Ter Brugge KG, et al. The natural history and predictive features of hemorrhage from brain arteriovenous malformations. Stroke 2009;40(1):100–5.
27. Batjer H, Suss RA, Samson D. Intracranial arteriovenous malformations associated with aneurysms. Neurosurgery 1986;18(1): 29–35.
28. Kader A, Young WL, Pile-Spellman J, et al. The influence of hemodynamic and anatomic factors on hemorrhage from cerebral arteriovenous malformations. Neurosurgery 1994;34(5):801–7.
29. Miyasaka Y, Yada K, Ohwada T, et al. An analysis of the venous drainage system as a factor in hemorrhage from arteriovenous malformations. J Neurosurg 1992;76(2):239–43.
30. Turjman F, Massoud TF, Vinuela F, et al. Correlation of the angioarchitectural features of cerebral arteriovenous malformations with clinical presentation of hemorrhage. Neurosurgery 1995;37(5):856–60.
31. Marks MP, Lane B, Steinberg GK, et al. Hemorrhage in intracerebral arteriovenous malformations: angiographic determinants. Radiology 1990;176(3):807–13.
32. Duong DH, Young WL, Vang MC, et al. Feeding artery pressure and venous drainage pattern are primary determinants of hemorrhage from cerebral arteriovenous malformations. Stroke 1998;29(6):1167–76.
33. Waltimo O. The change in size of intracranial arteriovenous malformations. J Neurol Sci 1973;19(1):21–7.
34. Graf CJ, Perret GE, Torner JC. Bleeding from cerebral arteriovenous malformations as part of their natural history. J Neurosurg 1983;58(3):331–7.
35. Hartmann A, Stapf C, Hofmeister C, et al. Determinants of neurological outcome after surgery for brain arteriovenous malformation. Stroke 2000;31(10):2361–4.
36. Heros RC, Korosue K, Diebold PM. Surgical excision of cerebral arteriovenous malformations: late results. Neurosurgery 1990; 26(4):570–7.
37. Hamilton MG, Spetzler RF. The prospective application of a grading system for arteriovenous malformations. Neurosurgery 1994;34(1):2–6.
38. Pik JH, Morgan MK. Microsurgery for small arteriovenous malformations of the brain: results in 110 consecutive patients. Neurosurgery 2000;47(3):571–5.
39. Schaller C, Schramm J. Microsurgical results for small arteriovenous malformations accessible for radiosurgical or embolization treatment. Neurosurgery 1997;40(4):664–72.
40. de OE, Tedeschi H, Raso J. Multidisciplinary approach to arteriovenous malformations. Neurol Med Chir (Tokyo) 1998; 38(Suppl.):177–85.
41. de OE, Tedeschi H, Raso J. Comprehensive management of arteriovenous malformations. Neurol Res 1998;20(8):673–83.
42. Lawton MT. Spetzler-Martin Grade III arteriovenous malformations: surgical results and a modification of the grading scale. Neurosurgery 2003;52(4):740–8.
43. Davidson AS, Morgan MK. How safe is arteriovenous malformation surgery? A prospective, observational study of surgery as first-line treatment for brain arteriovenous malformations. Neurosurgery 2010;66(3):498–504.
44. Lawton MT, Kim H, McCulloch CE, et al. A supplementary grading scale for selecting patients with brain arteriovenous malformations for surgery. Neurosurgery 2010;66(4):702–13.
45. Vates GE, Lawton MT, Wilson CB, et al. Magnetic source imaging demonstrates altered cortical distribution of function in patients with arteriovenous malformations. Neurosurgery 2002;51(3): 614–23.
46. Mohr JP, Parides MK, Stapf C, et al., for the international ARUBA investigators. Medical management with or without interventional therapy for unruptured brain arteriovenous malformations (ARUBA): a multicentre, non-blinded, randomised trial. Lancet 2014;383:614–21.
47. Potts MB, Young WL, Lawton MT. Deep arteriovenous malformations in the Basal Ganglia, thalamus, and insula: microsurgical management, techniques, and results. Neurosurgery 2013;73(3): 417–29.
48. Kiran NA, Kale SS, Kasliwal MK, et al. Gamma knife radiosurgery for arteriovenous malformations of basal ganglia, thalamus and brainstem – a retrospective study comparing the results with that for AVMs at other intracranial locations. Acta Neurochir (Wien) 2009;151(12):1575–82.
49. Kano H, Kondziolka D, Flickinger JC, et al. Stereotactic radiosurgery for arteriovenous malformations, Part 4: management of basal ganglia and thalamus arteriovenous malformations. J Neurosurg 2012;116(1):33–43.
50. Pollock BE, Gorman DA, Brown PD. Radiosurgery for arteriovenous malformations of the basal ganglia, thalamus, and brainstem. J Neurosurg 2004;100(2):210–14.
51. Garcia MR, Alvarez H, Goulao A, et al. Posterior fossa arteriovenous malformations. Angioarchitecture in relation to their hemorrhagic episodes. Neuroradiology 1990;31(6):471–5.
52. Batjer H, Samson D. Arteriovenous malformations of the posterior fossa. Clinical presentation, diagnostic evaluation, and surgical treatment. J Neurosurg 1986;64(6):849–56.
53. Drake CG, Friedman AH, Peerless SJ. Posterior fossa arteriovenous malformations. J Neurosurg 1986;64(1):1–10.
54. Solomon RA, Stein BM. Management of arteriovenous malformations of the brain stem. J Neurosurg 1986;64(6):857–64.
55. Kelly ME, Guzman R, Sinclair J, et al. Multimodality treatment of posterior fossa arteriovenous malformations. J Neurosurg 2008;108(6):1152–61.
56. da CL, Thines L, Dehdashti AR, et al. Management and clinical outcome of posterior fossa arteriovenous malformations: report on a single-centre 15-year experience. J Neurol Neurosurg Psychiatry 2009;80(4):376–9.
57. Higashi K, Hatano M, Yamashita T, et al. Coexistence of posterior inferior cerebellar artery aneurysm and arteriovenous malformation fed by the same artery. Surg Neurol 1979;12(5): 405–8.
58. Turjman F, Massoud TF, Vinuela F, et al. Aneurysms related to cerebral arteriovenous malformations: superselective angiographic assessment in 58 patients. AJNR Am J Neuroradiol 1994; 15(9):1601–5.
59. Cunha e Sa MJ, Stein BM, Solomon RA, et al. The treatment of associated intracranial aneurysms and arteriovenous malformations. J Neurosurg 1992;77(6):853–9.
60. Brown RD Jr, Wiebers DO, Forbes GS. Unruptured intracranial aneurysms and arteriovenous malformations: frequency of intracranial hemorrhage and relationship of lesions. J Neurosurg 1990;73(6):859–63.
61. Redekop G, TerBrugge K, Montanera W, et al. Arterial aneurysms associated with cerebral arteriovenous malformations: classification, incidence, and risk of hemorrhage. J Neurosurg 1998;89(4): 539–46.
62. Pandey P, Marks MP, Harraher CD, et al. Multimodality management of Spetzler-Martin Grade III arteriovenous malformations. J Neurosurg 2012;116(6):1279–88.
63. Deruty R, Pelissou-Guyotat I, Mottolese C, et al. Prognostic value of the Spetzler's grading system in a series of cerebral AVMs treated by a combined management. Acta Neurochir (Wien) 1994;131(3–4):169–75.

64. Nataraj A, Mohamed MB, Gholkar A, et al. Multimodality treatment of cerebral arteriovenous malformations. World Neurosurg 2014;82(1-2):149–59.
65. Horton JC, Chambers WA, Lyons SL, et al. Pregnancy and the risk of hemorrhage from cerebral arteriovenous malformations. Neurosurgery 1990;27(6):867–71.
66. Robinson JL, Hall CJ, Sedzimir CB. Subarachnoid hemorrhage in pregnancy. J Neurosurg 1972;36(1):27–33.
67. Robinson JL, Hall CS, Sedzimir CB. Arteriovenous malformations, aneurysms, and pregnancy. J Neurosurg 1974;41(1):63–70.
68. Ogilvy CS, Stieg PE, Awad I, et al. Recommendations for the management of intracranial arteriovenous malformations: a statement for healthcare professionals from a special writing group of the Stroke Council, American Stroke Association. Circulation 2001;103(21):2644–57.
69. Young WL, Kader A, Pile-Spellman J, et al. Arteriovenous malformation draining vein physiology and determinants of transnidal pressure gradients. The Columbia University AVM Study Project. Neurosurgery 1994;35(3):389–95.
70. Sadasivan B, Malik GM, Lee C, et al. Vascular malformations and pregnancy. Surg Neurol 1990;33(5):305–13.
71. van BJ, van der Worp HB, Buis DR, et al. Treatment of brain arteriovenous malformations: a systematic review and meta-analysis. JAMA 2011;306(18):2011–19.
72. Di CG, Doppman J, Ommaya AK. Selective arteriography of arteriovenous aneurysms of spinal cord. Radiology 1967;88(6):1065–77.
73. Djindjian R. Embolization of angiomas of the spinal cord. Surg Neurol 1975;4(5):411–20.
74. Kendall BE, Logue V. Spinal epidural angiomatous malformations draining into intrathecal veins. Neuroradiology 1977;13(4):181–9.
75. Newton TH, Adams JE. Angiographic demonstration and nonsurgical embolization of spinal cord angioma. Radiology 1968;91(5):873–6.
76. Riche MC, Reizine D, Melki JP, et al. Classification of spinal cord vascular malformations. Radiat Med 1985;3(1):17–24.
77. Rosenblum B, Oldfield EH, Doppman JL, et al. Spinal arteriovenous malformations: a comparison of dural arteriovenous fistulas and intradural AVM's in 81 patients. J Neurosurg 1987;67(6):795–802.
78. Yaşargil MG, DeLong WB, Guarnaschelli JJ. Complete microsurgical excision of cervical extramedullary and intramedullary vascular malformations. Surg Neurol 1975;4(2):211–24.
79. Bao YH, Ling F. Classification and therapeutic modalities of spinal vascular malformations in 80 patients. Neurosurgery 1997;40(1):75–81.
80. Heros RC, Debrun GM, Ojemann RG, et al. Direct spinal arteriovenous fistula: a new type of spinal AVM. Case report. J Neurosurg 1986;64(1):134–9.
81. Kim LJ, Spetzler RF. Classification and surgical management of spinal arteriovenous lesions: arteriovenous fistulae and arteriovenous malformations. Neurosurgery 2006;59(5 Suppl. 3):S195–201.
82. Spetzler RF, Detwiler PW, Riina HA, et al. Modified classification of spinal cord vascular lesions. J Neurosurg 2002;96(2 Suppl.):145–56.
83. Narvid J, Hetts SW, Larsen D, et al. Spinal dural arteriovenous fistulae: clinical features and long-term results. Neurosurgery 2008;62(1):159–66.
84. Oldfield EH, Di CG, Quindlen EA, et al. Successful treatment of a group of spinal cord arteriovenous malformations by interruption of dural fistula. J Neurosurg 1983;59(6):1019–30.
85. Mourier KL, Gelbert F, Rey A, et al. Spinal dural arteriovenous malformations with perimedullary drainage. Indications and results of surgery in 30 cases. Acta Neurochir (Wien) 1989;100(3–4):136–41.
86. Ommaya AK, Di CG, Doppman J. Ligation of arterial supply in the treatment of spinal cord arteriovenous malformations. J Neurosurg 1969;30(6):679–92.
87. Symon L, Kuyama H, Kendall B. Dural arteriovenous malformations of the spine. Clinical features and surgical results in 55 cases. J Neurosurg 1984;60(2):238–47.
88. Glasser R, Masson R, Mickle JP, et al. Embolization of a dural arteriovenous fistula of the ventral cervical spinal canal in a nine-year-old boy. Neurosurgery 1993;33(6):1089–93.
89. Halbach VV, Higashida RT, Dowd CF, et al. Treatment of giant intradural (perimedullary) arteriovenous fistulas. Neurosurgery 1993;33(6):972–9.
90. Riche MC, Scialfa G, Gueguen B, et al. Giant extramedullary arteriovenous fistula supplied by the anterior spinal artery: treatment by detachable balloons. AJNR Am J Neuroradiol 1983;4(3):391–4.
91. Hida K, Iwasaki Y, Ushikoshi S, et al. Corpectomy: a direct approach to perimedullary arteriovenous fistulas of the anterior cervical spinal cord. J Neurosurg 2002;96(2 Suppl.):157–61.
92. Martin NA, Khanna RK, Batzdorf U. Posterolateral cervical or thoracic approach with spinal cord rotation for vascular malformations or tumors of the ventrolateral spinal cord. J Neurosurg 1995;83(2):254–61.
93. Spetzler RF, Zabramski JM, Flom RA. Management of juvenile spinal AVM's by embolization and operative excision. Case report. J Neurosurg 1989;70(4):628–32.
94. Touho H, Karasawa J, Shishido H, et al. Successful excision of a juvenile-type spinal arteriovenous malformation following intraoperative embolization. Case report. J Neurosurg 1991;75(4):647–51.
95. Connolly ES Jr, Zubay GP, McCormick PC, et al. The posterior approach to a series of glomus (Type II) intramedullary spinal cord arteriovenous malformations. Neurosurgery 1998;42(4):774–85.

73 Surgical Cavernous Malformations and Venous Anomalies

Najib E. El Tecle, Samer G. Zammar, Christopher S. Eddleman, Tarek Y. El Ahmadieh, James P. Chandler, Bernard R. Bendok, Hunt H. Batjer, Issam A. Awad

Evidence Classifications

Recommendation	Evidence Classification
1. Treatment may be considered for incidentally discovered cerebral cavernous malformations (CCMs) and CCMs that have bled once based on a case-by-case analysis.	Class IIb/Level C
2. Treatment is reasonable for CCMs that have bled more than once or for CCMs causing seizures.	Class IIa/Level C
3. Typical curative treatment of CCMs is surgical resection. Stereotactic radiosurgery may be considered for progressively symptomatic CCMs for which surgical resection is not an option.	Class IIb/Level C

For more details refer to the AHA Evidence-based Classifications on Page xvii.

KEY POINTS

- Cerebral cavernous malformations (CCMs) are typically surrounded by hemosiderin which is typically the result of either previous hemorrhage or an ongoing blood leakage into the surrounding brain.
- Three gene loci have been implicated in the pathogenesis of CCMS: Loci on chromosomal arms 7q CCM1(KRIT1), 7p CCM2(MGC4607, OSM, Malcavernin), and 3q CCM3(PDCD10, TFAR15).
- Sporadic lesions and lesions with the CCM1 genotype have a slightly more benign natural history.
- Presentation of CCMs to the pial surface determines whether safe and effective surgical extirpation is possible.
- Stereotactic radiosurgery management could be an alternative management option for progressively symptomatic CCM lesions for which surgical resection is not an option.
- Venous angiomas are venous channels with normal histologic structure traversing atypical or anomalous courses in brain parenchyma.
- Management of venous angiomas is typically observational and expectant.

The definition and classification of cerebrovascular malformations have undergone much iteration throughout history.[1–4] Before modern imaging modalities, they were once considered "angiomatous tumors." However, Bailey and Cushing[5] described these lesions as probably arising from cerebral arterial or venous structures, and Wyburn-Mason[6] described several different "phases" of potential development in the same brain suggesting a potential pathologic continuum. However, the development of advanced imaging modalities and, more particularly, magnetic resonance imaging (MRI) engendered a paradigm shift in our understanding of these lesions and for the first time allowed precise categorization of the distinct lesions during life, the detection of asymptomatic lesions, and the evolution of vascular pathology in association with clinical behavior. In the widely accepted modern classification, as refined by McCormick,[7] the cerebrovascular malformations are of four types: arteriovenous, venous, cavernous, or capillary. The cerebral arteriovenous malformations (AVMs) traditionally harbor the more dangerous natural history, and capillary malformations (or telangiectasias) are typically viewed as incidental benign lesions. The cavernous and venous malformations can manifest variable and occasionally significant clinical sequelae. It is, therefore, imperative for the clinician to characterize the lesion with sufficient specificity so as to better predict clinical behavior and more accurately select management strategy. In this chapter, we specifically address the pathologic and biologic features as well as approaches to diagnosis, natural history, and clinical management of the cerebral cavernous malformations (CCMs) and venous anomalies (VAs).

PATHOLOGIC FEATURES

Detailed pathologic description of cerebrovascular malformations in general, and of CCMS and VAs in particular, is often determined by the quality of the sample. The tendency of these lesions to bleed and the possible dynamic nature of their growth might also conceal their pathologic features. CCMs are vascular hamartomas, they have a multilobulated, mulberry-like appearance formed by clusters of thin-walled vascular sinusoid channels (dilated capillaries or caverns) lined by multilaminar endothelial cells and lacking elements of mature vessel wall (smooth muscle, elastin laminae, etc.).[1,3,8,9] The endothelial cells lie on a dense collagenous matrix lacking pericytes and smooth muscle cells. The caverns are filled with blood in a low-flow state, which allows stagnation-dependent processes to occur. Specifically, the low flow state leads to the development of thrombi at varying stages of organization and to calcium deposition in the lesion. The CCM stroma is typically formed of loose collagen without intervening neuroglial parenchyma, except in cauliflower-like projections into adjacent brain. Lesions are most often surrounded by hemosiderin deposits and gliosis, representing uniform signatures of previous hemorrhage or ongoing leakage of blood into adjacent brain. Electron microscopy analysis of the CCM–parenchyma interface often reveals a disrupted blood–brain barrier with poorly developed tight and adherens junctions, which allows for red blood cells migration into the parenchyma and the eventual deposition of hemosiderin around the malformation.[10] There is uniform angiogenic activity within CCMs, the endothelial cells lining the caverns exhibit proliferative activity,[2,11] and the lesions have been shown to exhibit a robust immune response with oligoclonal features.[11] The reddish purple lesions are variable in size, ranging from 1 mm to several centimeters and can be multiple of single. The CCMs are also known as cavernous hemangiomas, angiomas, or cavernomas.

The VAs are venous channels with normal histologic structure, but traversing atypical or anomalous courses in brain parenchyma rather than the typical superficial and deep venous patterns. They have been described with characteristic "caput medusae" branching and are best viewed as regional venous dysmorphism.[1,4] VAs do not typically manifest any arteriovenous shunting and are associated with normal intervening brain tissue, although associated capillary telangiectasias in adjacent brain have been described. They most often lack any evidence of associated hemorrhage, but a small fraction of the lesions are associated with single or multiple hemorrhagic clusters with the typical histology of CCMs. VAs do not typically exhibit angiogenic or inflammatory activity except within associated CCMs. The VAs are also known as venous developmental anomalies or venous angiomas.

EPIDEMIOLOGY

The prevalence estimates for these lesions in the general population have been made on the basis of large autopsy series and large cohorts undergoing MRI.[3,7,12] The VAs are thought to be the most common cerebrovascular malformation, found in up to 2.6% of all autopsied brains.[3,7] CCMs have been reported in 0.3–0.5% in autopsy series and of patients undergoing MRI.[2,3,7,13] VAs form, therefore, 60–70% of all vascular malformations whereas CCMs form 10–15% of all vascular malformations. Female patients with CCM may manifest a more aggressive clinical course, but the prevalence of CCMs and VAs is thought to be approximately equal in males and females.[3,7,13] From a genetics standpoint, sporadic and familial cases of CCMs have been described, the latter accounting for at least 6% of the cases.[14] Over 50% of patients with the familial form harbor more than one malformation, whereas multiple lesions are found in only 20% of the patients with the sporadic form.[15–18]

The VAs by their nature likely reflect congenital venous dysmorphism, whereas CCMs have been shown to develop after birth.[2,4,8,12,19–22] The CCMs are known to occur in two forms, namely a non-hereditary (sporadic) form and a hereditary (familial-autosomal dominant) form. Sporadic CCMs are more often associated with a VA, but this association is uncommon in familial CCMs.[23] As mentioned above, sporadic vascular lesions are typically solitary, whereas most familial cases of CCMs have multiple lesions, which are especially evident with more sensitive gradient-echo (GRE) and other magnetic-susceptibility MRI sequences. Multiple CCMs may cluster within a single VA, and are documented in the setting of previous brain irradiation.[1,3,24–29] Some CCMs can exhibit mixed or transitional features of venous, capillary, or arteriovenous histopathology, implying related pathobiologic mechanisms.[30]

Genetics

Sporadic cases of CCMs typically present with a single lesion and are not inherited. Familiar CCMs on the other hand are characterized by the presence of multiple lesions and result from an autosomal dominant, germline mutation.[31] To date, three gene loci have been implicated in the pathogenesis of CCMs.[2,32–38] Loci on chromosomal arms 7q CCM1(KRIT1), 7p CCM2(MGC4607,OSM,Malcavernin),and3qCCM3(PDCD10, TFAR15) have been identified and have been shown to have clinical penetrance of 88%, 100%, and 63%, respectively,[39–42] although respective penetrance is likely much higher when magnetic-susceptibility MRI is performed. More than 150 distinct germline mutations in CCM1, CCM2, and CCM3 are known and they all appear to cause loss of function.[43]

While this genetic pattern is typical of familial CCMs it is interesting that it is also found in cases with multifocal lesions without overt family history. Genetic analysis in a vast majority of these cases has demonstrated that they either have a *de novo* mutations or a mutation inherited from an asymptomatic parent.[44,45] For this purpose, it is useful to differentiate multiple CCMs clustered around a VA or in the field of prior irradiation (where germline mutations are rare), from other multifocal CCMs (where CCM germline mutations are common even in the absence of family history).

Knudson's two hit mechanism was proposed by Gault et al.[46] to explain why a carrier of an autosomal dominant disease would develop multiple lesions. According to this hypothesis, loss of both "normal" CCM alleles is required for individual cells to initiate the formation of a CCM. Familial CCM patients would have only one normal allele in every germline cell, which if compromised by a somatic mutation would potentially lead to the development of a CCM. Somatic mutations have been confirmed in endothelial cells microdissected from the lining of caverns.[19] The Knudsonian hypothesis was further confirmed in a larger study of resected human lesions by Ackers et al.[47] It was supported by the genesis of lesions recapitulating the human CCM phenotype in mice heterozygous for CCM genes and engineered to enhance somatic mutations.[48,49] More recently, postnatal homozygous knockout of CCM genes in endothelial cells has generated an aggressive CCM phenotype.[50,51] Yet our understanding of the two hit hypothesis in CCMs pathogenesis remains limited. It is possible that epigenetic factors might be involved in the process as well.

Cerebral Cavernous Malformation Proteins and Pathologic Implications

The loss of any of the CCM genes leads to very similar disease phenotype despite dissimilar protein products.[31] The CCM proteins can form a CCM protein complex when expressed in vitro. However, they are also expressed in different locations, different complexes and in unique patterns.[38,52–54] The loss of any of the three CCM genes in cultured endothelial cells results in the expression of stress fibers and impaired junctional integrity, mediated by RhoA kinase (ROCK). In fact, heterozygous loss of CCM proteins results in hyperpermeability of brain, lung and skin, in the absence of lesions, and this hyperpermeability is rescuable by ROCK inhibition.[55,56] This has led to the consideration of ROCK inhibition as a potential therapeutic strategy to prevent lesion genesis and maturation.[57] The CCM proteins also likely play a role in cardiovascular development, and are involved in complex signaling interactions,[58] with likely relevance to disease development.

It has been shown that the KRIT1 protein is expressed by the arterial and microvascular elements but not by the venous elements.[39–41] Interestingly, the gene product is also expressed in neuroglial cells, in particular the astrocytes forming the neurovascular unit.[12,32,35,37,59–61] Malcavernin and PDCD10 were also found to have this pattern of expression.[12,34,35,62] This has been invoked to explain lesion predominance in the central nervous system parenchyma.

NATURAL HISTORY AND CLINICAL MANIFESTATIONS

The clinical presentation of CCMs is highly variable, ranging from an asymptomatic incidental discovery through radiographic imaging for non-specific symptoms or at autopsy to associated headache, hemorrhagic stroke, epilepsy, or focal neurologic deficits. Symptomatic presentation is far more common with CCMs than VAs. Prospective risks of hemorrhage and new seizures are also more common with CCMs, in the range of 0.5–4% per year and 1–3% per year respectively, although these complications are rare in VAs except in association with CCMs. Hemorrhage in VAs has been reported in only 0.22–0.68% of lesions per year, and most verified cases have included associated CCMs. Pediatric presentation of CCMs occurs in a bimodal distribution, normally manifesting in patients either younger than 3 years or in their early teens.[4,22,43] The adult population typically presents with symptoms between the third and fifth decade of life, but the lesions can occur at any point in life.

In one of the most recent meta-analyses of the natural history of CCMs, Gross et al. analysed data from 10 natural history studies spanning 837 patients.[63] Among the 10 studies, nine provided data on CCM location, 76% of the CCMs were supratentorial, 23% infratentorial and 9% both. Also, nine series provided data on the initial presentation, 37% of the patients presented with seizures, 36% presented with hemorrhage, 23% with headaches, 22% with focal neurologic deficit and 10% were asymptomatic at presentation. The authors attempted to correct for a higher rate of hemorrhage in familial cases and reported the overall annual hemorrhage rate to be 2.4% (1.6–3.1%) per patient per year, the familial annual hemorrhage rate to be 5.1% (4.3–13%) per patient per year. The adjusted annual hemorrhage rate per lesion per year was found to be similar between familial cases and sporadic cases at 0.7% and 0.8% per lesion per year respectively. Annual rebleeding rates varied widely in the literature from 0% to 22.9%.[64–67] However, the two studies with enough power to demonstrate rebleeding rate,[63,64,67] showed values of 4.5% and 22.9% per year. This wide spectrum of values may be partially due to the lack of a standard definition of prior bleeding in CCMs as virtually all lesions exhibit some form of microhemorrhaging whereas clinically significant hemorrhage – either extending beyond the confines of the hemosiderin ring or producing neurologic symptoms – is not common.[3,68,69] A precise definition of clinically significant hemorrhage has been proposed,[70] and findings of the many conflicting clinical series and natural history studies should be interpreted in light of this strict definition.

In the gross meta-analysis, size and the presence of multiple lesions were not shown to be predictive of a higher annual rate. Age younger than 40 was predictive of higher hemorrhage rates in only one out of the ten reviewed studies[64] and female sex was predictive of higher hemorrhage rate in three out of the five studies reporting on sex relation with hemorrhage rate.[17,64,65] The major study reporting on higher risk of hemorrhage among female patients, showed an annual hemorrhage rate of 4.2% per patient per year for females and 0.9% per patient per year for males.[17] Only one prospective series showed location to be an independent predictor of hemorrhage with an annual hemorrhage rate of 4.1% per patient per year for deep lesions (hemispheric or brainstem).[66] No known host or extrinsic factor has been demonstrated to impact lesion behavior, although recent trauma and anticoagulation have been linked to symptomatic bleeds.[3,71–76] Reports have demonstrated a slightly more benign natural risk in sporadic lesions and in the setting of the CCM1 genotype, as compared with the CCM3 genotype, which apparently demonstrates the most aggressive clinical course.[19,44]

Despite the fact that CCMs do not include functional brain tissue, seizures thought to be a result of supratentorial lesions, most commonly frontal or temporal lesions, can be of any type and are believed to be related to multiple factors, including focal irritation and compression from an expanding hematoma, the presence of iron products after red blood cell breakdown secondary to multiple microhemorrhages, the formation of cortical scars, and resultant encephalomalacia.[77–84] However, in up to 6% of cases involving CCMs and epilepsy, the lesion itself is found to not be the epileptogenic trigger.[77]

As with most intracranial lesions, the type of presenting neurologic deficit is related to the location of the lesion. Most deep vascular malformations that manifest do so with hemorrhage and focal neurologic deficits, at rates ranging from 15% to 45% of cases, and with more serious neurologic compromise.[3,4,21,60] Presentation of CCMs to the pial surface determines whether safe and effective surgical extirpation is possible.[8,9,71,74–76,85] Radiosurgical strategies can be considered for inaccessible lesions, but this strategy remains controversial.[2,82,86–88]

In Figure 73-1, a 49-year-old male patient had new onset of seizures. A left temporal gyrus cavernoma was identified as the source and was surgically resected.

CEREBRAL CAVERNOUS MALFORMATIONS

Diagnostic Imaging

CCMs are angiographically occult lesions. This has earned them the name of "cryptic vascular malformations". Their low-flow status and the absence of arteriovenous shunting are thought to be responsible for this cryptic nature.

CT imaging has limited sensitivity and diagnostic specificity for CCMs. While CT scans have the ability to demonstrate calcifications, acute or chronic hemorrhage products, and cystic components, they fail to specifically demonstrate CCMs since these findings are non-specific and can be often observed with numerous other central nervous system lesions. Despite these limitations, CT has been used to follow the size of CCMs after initial hemorrhages as well as to look for new hemorrhage products. This choice, however, should be made while keeping in mind the increased radiation exposure resulting from CT scans.

MRI has proved to be the superior modality of imaging CCMs owing to the various sequences that can be employed, especially gradient echo and other magnetic-susceptibility sequences, which have been shown to be more sensitive in distinguishing CCMs.[24,71,89–92] Susceptibility weighted imaging (SWI) was investigated by De Champfleur et al. who showed that it is more sensitive than T2*GRE sequence, particularly in detecting multifocal/familial CCMS.[93] On the basis of the correlation of MRI characteristics and pathologic specimens, Zabramski et al.[20] classified CCMs into four MRI lesion types, although no relation to clinical outcome has been reported. The MRI appearance of CCM is quite specific, but the differential diagnosis may include, but is not limited to, thrombosed AVMs, hematomas, hemorrhagic tumors, and inflammatory lesions mimicking CCM features. The clinical context (including familiality), MRI associations (other lesions, such as VAs and occult CCMs), close imaging follow-up of lesions, which may rarely include catheter angiography (to exclude AVM), or surgical biopsy may be needed to establish a diagnosis.

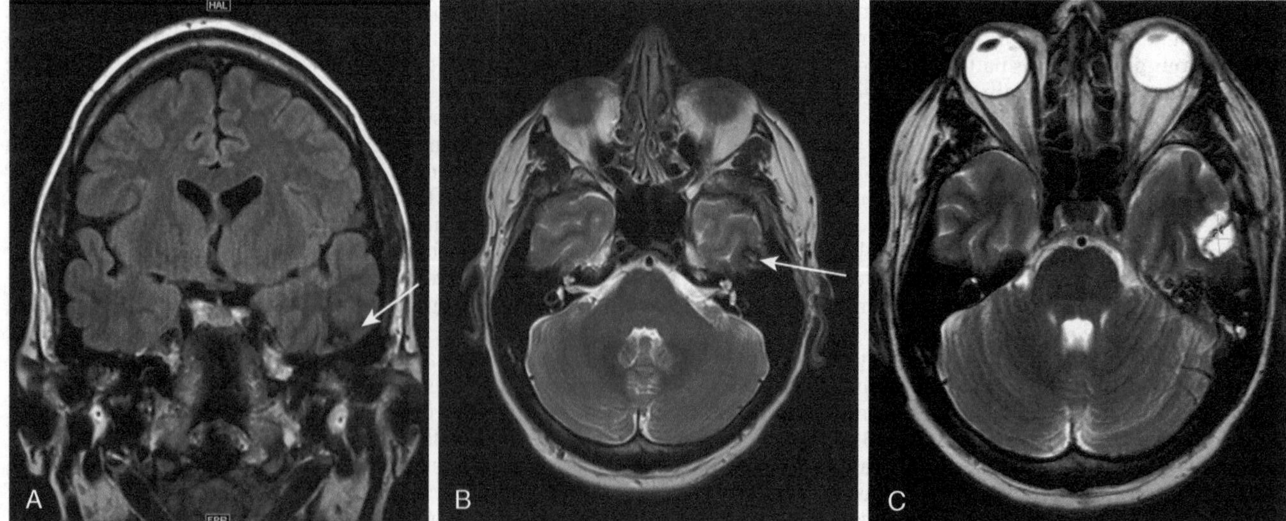

Figure 73-1. A, Coronal MRI showing a left temporal gyrus field inhomogeneity suggestive of a cavernoma. B, Axial T2 image showing the left temporal gyrus cavernoma C, Post-surgical MRI demonstrating lesion excision and the surgical cavity.

Novel MR imaging sequences have also been used to quantitatively evaluate CCMs. Hart et al. recently reported on the use of dynamic contrast enhanced MRI DCEMRI evaluation of CCMs.[94] DCEMRI is sensitive for slow transfer rate for gadolinium and though it demonstrated a large spectrum of heterogeneity in terms of transfer rate of gadolinium inside the lesions, correlation of these heterogeneities with biologic behavior are still to be determined. More recently, Tan et al. reported validations of iron concentration in CCM lesions using quantitative susceptibility mapping (QSM) technique. Mikati et al. reported increased iron content in CCM lesions with greater dynamic permeability,[95] essentially cross-validating the two techniques as potential biomarkers of CCM disease activity and potential candidate therapies.

Novel MR imaging has also been used to assess the impact of CCM on brain function in cortical locations[96] and its disruption of subcortical tracts.[97] In Figure 73-2, a 28-year-old male patient presented with numbness of the right arm and leg. MRI demonstrated a cavernoma of the cervico-medullary junction (Fig. 73-2A) as well as in the medial right thalamus, medial left high parietal lobe and the right occipital lobe (Fig. 73-2B). Diffusion tensor imaging (DTI) demonstrated poor visualization of the white matter tracts at the level of the cavernoma with the ascending and descending fibers splaying around the lesion (Fig. 73-2C). Progression of the symptoms prompted surgical excision of the cervico-medullary cavernoma (Fig. 73-2D).

Clinical Management

The most appropriate treatment for CCMs depends on a multitude of factors regarding the lesion and the patient, including, but not limited to, natural history, the age and gender of the patient, and the location and clinical manifestations of the lesion. The most common management schemes of CCMs involve expectant follow-up, management of associated seizures, microsurgical excision, and radiosurgery. The generally accepted indications for procedural therapy of CCMs are intractable seizures, worsening neurologic deficits, and symptomatic hemorrhage (acute or recurrent) in both adult and pediatric cases. Other cases may be treated in consideration of prospective natural history risk and lesion accessibility.

Expectant Follow-up and Medical Management

Although fatal events can occur from CCMs, such as intractable seizures and hemorrhages leading to death, their incidence is extremely low.[3,77,81] Therefore, emergency procedural management of CCMs after their detection is not always necessary. Advances in imaging technology have improved the ability, not only to detect CCMs, but also to follow their natural course in association with clinical symptoms. As such, observation of asymptomatic or mildly symptomatic lesions is feasible and considered first-line management in many cases. However, several situations can dictate more expeditious treatment, including lowering the prospective lifetime hemorrhage risk, decreasing the psychological burden on the patient, and reducing the costs of continued imaging and follow-up. Patient counseling is paramount in these situations and should be extremely detailed regarding the natural history of the lesion, risks of surgery, expectations of surgery, and post-procedural recovery. Patients followed-up expectantly typically undergo serial imaging of the lesion, especially in association with new or worsened symptoms.

Expectant management is also indicated in both adults and pediatric patients who have symptomatic lesions that are surgically inaccessible. However, the benefits of surgical resection in eloquent areas of the brain may yield significant benefits in younger patients and may thus be justified, as opposed to the small gain in older patients, with lower cumulative prospective risk in their remaining lifetimes.[98]

Patients presenting with seizures are initially treated with anticonvulsants, which have varying degrees of control and side effects, especially when seizures are associated with small or less accessible CCMs, or multiple lesions.[68,98] Later-generation anticonvulsant agents have a better side effect profile, but not necessarily greater effectiveness. In patients for whom anticonvulsants are not effective, careful analysis of seizure semiology and electrophysiologic localization might determine whether the CCM is the likely causative factor or merely an incidental association.[77,81,84] This determination may be particularly problematic in patients with multiple CCMs. In cases in which the CCM has been shown to be the epileptogenic factor, the more protracted the seizure history, the less likely the patient will be seizure free after resection.[68,69,99] As such, if the CCM is shown to be the

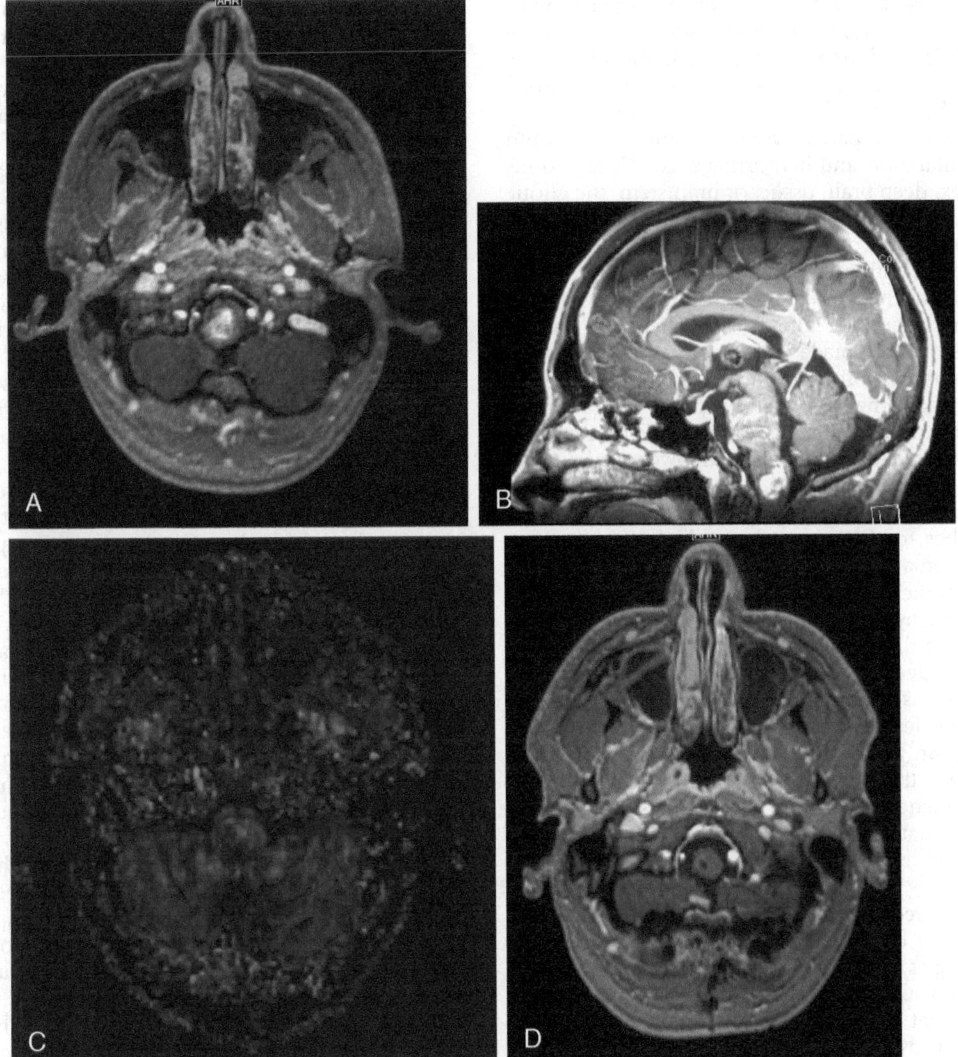

Figure 73-2. A, Axial MRI showing local field inhomogeneities at the cervico–medullary junction suggestive of a cavernoma. B, Sagittal MRI demonstrating a second cavernoma in the hypothalamic region. C, Diffusion tensor image with minimal visualization of the tracts at the level of the lesion. D, Axial MRI showing post-surgical changes with total resection of the cavernoma.

epileptogenic factor, it is recommended that surgical resection be considered earlier rather than later, so as to increase the patient's chances of being seizure free, and possibly off anticonvulsants, and to avoid lesion growth and possible extension or recalcitrant transformation of the epileptogenic region as well as future hemorrhage.[42,53,56] In cases in which other lesions are present with a first seizure in association with overt brain hemorrhage or lesion expansion, excision may be considered (see later).

Microsurgical Excision

As with any intracranial lesion being considered for surgical management, a thorough pre-operative assessment must be completed such that the benefits of surgical resection outweigh the potential risks of the procedure. Careful planning should include detailed imaging studies, such as those of the surrounding brain parenchyma and vascular structures in the cases of associated vascular anomalies, as well as functional consideration of eloquence in adjacent brain and in the proposed surgical corridor. Stereotactic guidance should always be considered so that the surgical approach can be most efficiently chosen.[100] In cases of CCMs present in eloquent areas of the brain, functional mapping by MRI activation, electrocorticography, or cortical stimulation, with the patient awake or under general anesthesia, should be carefully considered in order to avoid inadvertent or unnecessary damage to eloquent structures.[101,102]

Timing of surgery should also be carefully considered after hemorrhagic events. Sufficient time should be allowed for the reactive, post-hemorrhagic brain to stabilize and for better identification of the CCM lesion. Conversely, the hematoma cavity itself may provide a sufficient surgical conduit for resection. Significant and symptomatic mass effect from resultant hematomas or medically intractable seizures may also dictate an earlier resection.

In most cases of CCM resection, standard surgical approaches are used with the goal of minimizing injury to the surrounding normal parenchyma while maximizing exposure for an adequate lesion resection. Intraoperative stereotactic guidance has improved over the last decade with the use of frameless tracking systems calibrated to handheld wands and operative microscopes.[100] This adjunct is especially useful for optimizing the planning of the incision and bony exposure, corticectomy, and resection corridor as well as localization of deep lesions. For CCM lesions in non-eloquent brain, total resection of the CCM and the accompanying hemosiderin ring is advocated. Any associated VAs should not be disturbed because despite being an aberrant vascular structure, they likely drain normal brain parenchyma and obliteration could lead to venous infarction and hemorrhage. For CCM lesions in eloquent cortex, deep brain tissue, or brainstem, the gliotic tissue and surrounding hemosiderin ring should often be left undisturbed in order to avoid unnecessary destruction of vital structures and neural pathways. However, it is thought that, in the cases of epileptogenic CCMs, the causative agent may be the hemosiderin material or gliotic scar. Therefore, careful clinical decisions must be made in these cases so as to avoid unnecessary resection. Another adjunct to aid in the monitoring of eloquent areas of the brain is electrophysiological monitoring and mapping utilizing somatosensory evoked potentials, brainstem auditory evoked potentials, and lower cranial nerve monitoring.[88]

Multiple reports have been published regarding common surgical approaches for CCM resection, which are based on intracranial location and closest area of pial exposure.[3,8,72,74,75] Resection of superficial lesions of the supratentorial and infratentorial parenchyma often results in 95–100% complete removal, with more than 80% of cases having good or excellent outcomes.[3,8,74] Deep CCMs present in the brainstem, basal ganglia, and thalamus represent a more formidable challenge and invariably have less favorable outcomes, with 13–60% of cases worsening or being associated with serious sequelae.[3,72,74,75] However, this fact must be considered in the light of similar consequences of hemorrhage in these same locations and the fact that more than 80% of patients ultimately recover to good or better neurologic function despite the initial setback.[3,9,72,75,85] Skull base surgical approaches have been optimized in recent years for various lesion locations presenting to pial or ependymal surfaces, and intraoperative monitoring strategies have been advocated to monitor the function of various associated nuclei and pathways. Studies have also shown that improvements in patient selection and operative approach as well as close post-operative care can result in good long-term results, with about 96% of patients with brainstem, basal ganglia, or thalamic CCMs having excellent or good long-term outcomes.[75,85] In Figure 73-3, a 38-year-old female patient presented with a 1-month history of difficulty swallowing and mild hoarseness associated with right facial numbness and tingling. Brain MRI demonstrated a brainstem cavernoma (Fig. 73-3A). One month later, MRI showed an increase in the cavernoma size with increased symptoms. The patient elected to have the cavernoma removed (Fig. 73-3B, Fig. 73-3C and Video 73-1). Post-operative MRI demonstrated no residual lesion (Fig. 73-3D). The patient was discharged home on post-operative day 4 with minimal residual symptoms and kept improving on clinical follow-up.

Stereotactic Radiosurgery

The management of CCMs with stereotactic radiosurgery (SRS) remains controversial. Although microsurgical resection of non-eloquent, superficial lesions is achievable with acceptable low rates of morbidity, the management of deep-seated lesions, especially in the diencephalon or brainstem, presents a dilemma. The effect of SRS on CCMs is varied. Irradiation itself can cause de novo genesis of CCMs.[25,27] CCMs are not eliminated by SRS, and irradiated CCMs can still grow and hemorrhage.[67,82,86,87] Furthermore, the continued task of defining the natural history and relative hemorrhage rates before and after irradiation have further complicated decisions about the potential favorable impact of SRS. SRS management has typically been advocated for progressively symptomatic CCM lesions, for which surgical resection was not an option. The aim of treatment is progressive scarring and hyalinization of vascular structures in response to irradiation, ultimately resulting in decreased hemorrhage rates. Kondziolka et al.[67] reported that the hemorrhage risk after institution of SRS in patients with at least two prior hemorrhages dropped from 32% to 1.1% per year within 3 years. Lunsford et al. also studied SRS for symptomatic solitary CCMs considered high risk for resection.[103] In their study of 103 patients, the annual rate of hemorrhage was significantly reduced from 10.8% per year before SRS to 1.06% per year after SRS. As discussed in the guidelines for radiosurgical management of CCMs, which were published in 2012 by Niranjan et al. The typical delivered radiation isodose at the CCM margin should be within the range of 12–18 Gy and thought a significant decrease in annual hemorrhage rate is noted within the first 2 years after SRS; this change is more pronounced 2 years after the procedure.[104]

Huang et al.[61] reported a post-linear-acceleration (LINAC) treatment hemorrhage rate in 30 CCM patients to be 1.1% per year. Similarly, Fuetsch et al. reported their experience with 14 patients who underwent LINAC for CCM and found that the re-hemorrhage rate was also decreased to reach approximately 1% per year 10 years after treatment.[105] No significant difference has been found between gamma knife and linear accelerator radiosurgery in terms of reduction of hemorrhage risk or seizure control,[3,22,67,86] but treatment risks have been closely related to the dose and volume of lesion treated and lesion location, regardless of SRS modality. Recent studies have advocated a lower margin dose of 12–14 Gy, or hypofractionated SRS dosimetry, and a target margin within (purposely excluding) the CCM hemosiderin ring.[106,107]

Post-SRS complications include re-hemorrhage, edematous change, temporary neurologic deficit, and post-treatment seizures.[3,22,67,86] The spectrum of long-term complications is not well defined yet but might include radiation necrosis and development of new oncologic or vascular brain lesions including new cavernous malformations.[108,109] It is clear that outcome with microsurgery is better than that with SRS in terms of hemorrhage prevention or seizure control, but SRS remains an unproven option for progressively symptomatic cases in which surgical resection would be unacceptably risky. A more defined role for SRS treatment of CCMs may be determined as more centers report outcomes of various lesions and dosimetries.

VENOUS ANOMALIES

Diagnostic Imaging

A variety of imaging tools can be used to visualize VAs. Most lesions are found incidentally in association with frequent complaints of non-specific symptoms such as headache and dizziness. Non-contrast-enhanced CT scan usually fails to visualize a VA except if it is associated with a CCM or thrombosed. However, a so-called caput medusa, radial pattern of vessels with a larger central vein, can be visualized using a contrast-enhanced CT.[1,3,29,90] MRI sequences frequently demonstrate the same pattern with additional sequences to examine surrounding edema or hemorrhage, potentially suggesting associated capillary telangiectasia (punctate contrast enhancement) or frank CCM (hemosiderin signal on magnetic-susceptibility sequences). In a large retrospective series, Lee et al.[110] concluded that CT angiography and MRI with contrast could yield an excellent visualization of the VA as opposed to MRA. Cerebral angiography also demonstrates the lesion and its associated venous dysmorphism and could exclude arteriovenous shunting, but is usually not necessary because

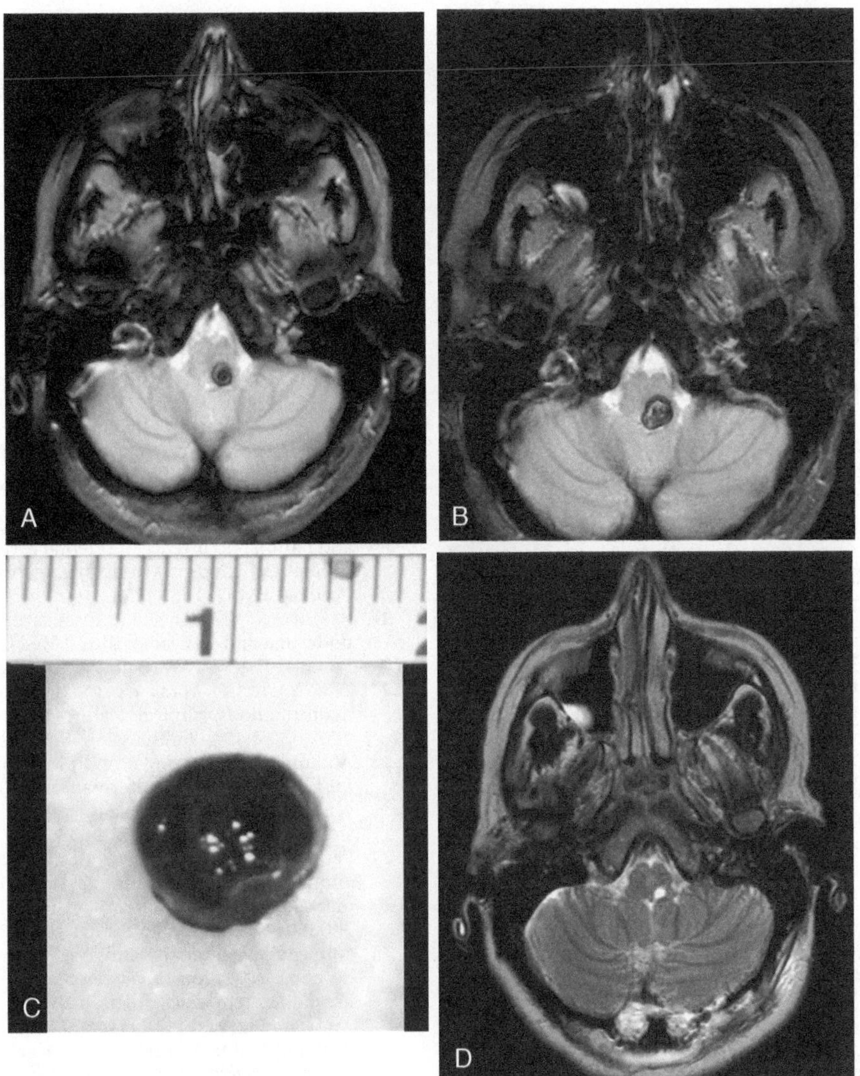

Figure 73-3. A, Axial MRI imaging demonstrating a brainstem cavernoma. B, Increase in the size of the cavernoma at 1-month follow-up. C, Cavernoma as seen after resection. D, Post-operative MRI demonstrating total resection of the cavernoma.

non-invasive imaging is sufficient to characterize the lesion.[1,3,29,90] However, Roccatagliata et al.[111] identified 11 symptomatic VAs retrospectively and showed that all these lesions were associated with a peculiar capillary stain at angiography. Thus the authors reported that conventional angiography can be useful in recognizing symptomatic VAs. Furthermore, a whole brain DSA and CT perfusion imaging can visualize the appearance of altered VA hemodynamic parameter and reveal the superior cortices of the cerebrum and cerebellum anomalies.[112] The differential diagnosis of a VA may include prominent venous drainage of an AVM and malignant neoplasm. If either is suspected, repeat imaging or catheter cerebral angiography may be necessary for final diagnostic determination.

Clinical Management

In light of their extremely low risk of hemorrhage, the management of VAs is most frequently observational and expectant. Moreover, since VAs are thought to arise from dysmorphic venous drainage of normal brain, surgical manipulation of that drainage could lead to venous infarction, hemorrhage, and even death. However, VAs can sometimes lead to hemorrhage, neurological deficits, seizures or a combination of these symptoms.[1,3,29,90,113] In these cases, an associated CCM or, less likely, an AVM is normally found on radiographic workup or surgical exploration. Therefore, when removing an associated vascular malformation with the VA, special caution should be taken to preserve the VA. Natagani et al.[113] reported a rare case of massive intracerebral hemorrhage (ICH) caused only by a developmental venous anomaly (DVA) which was treated by evacuation of the hematoma and surgical resection of the DVA. VAs presenting with seizures can be treated medically with anticonvulsants without surgical intervention.[1,3,29] However, VAs associated with intractable epilepsy may require resection of epileptogenic brain in the region of VA, which can be safe as long as the brain parenchyma drained by the VA is also resected. Clinical treatment and management of thrombosed VAs has not been established. However, anticoagulation seems to yield a favorable outcome in some reported series.[114-118] The use and risks of SRS in VAs is not justified, given these lesions' benign natural history. The association with a CCM seems to be the most important feature leading to an increase in the risk of hemorrhage in the future. As such, the use of gradient-echo or magnetic-susceptibility MRI sequences is advocated to identify such lesions, which should be followed expectantly like other CCMs. Other patients with isolated VAs are reassured and cleared to live normal lives without restrictions.

FUTURE CONSIDERATIONS

The natural course of individual CCMs and VAs remains highly variable. Other than lesion excision or irradiation, there is currently no known treatment intervention to modify lesion behavior, and there are no reliable markers predicting aggressive clinical behavior. Scientific knowledge regarding the pathobiology and pathophysiology of cerebrovascular malformations is expected to affect their clinical management. As the genetic signatures of CCMs are becoming more defined, the possibility of large prospective studies of genotype–phenotype associations can be entertained, potentially identifying other genetic modifiers of aggressive clinical course. Host and environmental factors may be identified that may also impact lesion behavior. Furthermore, elucidation of the mechanism(s) of CCM genesis with and without associated VAs should be better defined, including somatic mutations in molecular pathways involving disease genes, the involvement of antigen-driven or inflammatory mechanisms in lesion genesis or progression, and the relationships between neuroglial and vascular mechanisms and enhanced angiogenic activity in CCMs. These studies may also shed some light on why a small fraction of VAs result in associated CCMs and subsequent clinical manifestations, but the vast majority remains benign. The convergence of clinical and scientific observations will provide future clinicians with improved knowledge and tools for more specific diagnoses, individual prognostication, and novel and better-focused therapeutic interventions.

REFERENCES

1. Abla A, Wait SD, Uschold T, et al. Developmental venous anomaly, cavernous malformation, and capillary telangiectasia: spectrum of a single disease. Acta Neurochir (Wien) 2008;150: 487–9, discussion 489.
2. Awad IA. Unfolding knowledge on cerebral cavernous malformations. Surg Neurol 2005;63:317–18.
3. Brown RD Jr, Flemming KD, Meyer FB, et al. Natural history, evaluation, and management of intracranial vascular malformations. Mayo Clinic Proc 2005;80:269–81.
4. Raychaudhuri R, Batjer HH, Awad IA. Intracranial cavernous angioma: a practical review of clinical and biological aspects. Surg Neurol 2005;63:319–28, discussion 328.
5. Bailey P, Cushing H. A classification of the tumors of the glioma group on a histogenic basis with a correlated study of prognosis. Philadelphia: J.B. Lippincott Company; 1926;8:175.
6. Wyburn-Mason R. Arteriovenous aneurysm of mid-brain and retina, facial naevi and mental changes. Brain 1943;66:163–203.
7. McCormick WF, Hardman JM, Boulter TR. Vascular malformations ("angiomas") of the brain, with special reference to those occurring in the posterior fossa. J Neurosurg 1968;28:241–51.
8. D'Angelo VA, De Bonis C, Amoroso R, et al. Supratentorial cerebral cavernous malformations: clinical, surgical, and genetic involvement. Neurosurg Focus 2006;21:e9.
9. Jung YJ, Hong SC, Seo DW, et al. Surgical resection of cavernous angiomas located in eloquent areas–clinical research. Acta Neurochir Suppl 2006;99:103–8.
10. Clatterbuck R, Eberhart C, Crain B, et al. Ultrastructural and immunocytochemical evidence that an incompetent blood-brain barrier is related to the pathophysiology of cavernous malformations. J Neurol Neurosurg Psychiatry 2001;71:188–92.
11. Shenkar R, Shi C, Check IJ, et al. Concepts and hypotheses: inflammatory hypothesis in the pathogenesis of cerebral cavernous malformations. Neurosurgery 2007;61(4):693–702, discussion 702–3. PubMed PMID: 17986930.
12. Denier C, Labauge P, Bergametti F, et al. Genotype-phenotype correlations in cerebral cavernous malformations patients. Ann Neurol 2006;60(5):550–6. PubMed PMID: 17041941.
13. Del Curling O Jr, Kelly DL Jr, Elster AD, et al. An analysis of the natural history of cavernous angiomas. J Neurosurg 1991;75(5): 702–8. PubMed PMID: 1919691.
14. Kraemer DL, Awad IA. Vascular malformations and epilepsy: clinical considerations and basic mechanisms. Epilepsia 1994; 35(s6):S30–43.
15. Zabramski JM, Wascher TM, Spetzler RF, et al. The natural history of familial cavernous malformations: results of an ongoing study. J Neurosurg 1994;80(3):422–32.
16. Rigamonti D, Hadley MN, Drayer BP, et al. Cerebral cavernous malformations. New Engl J Med 1988;319(6):343–7.
17. Moriarity JL, Wetzel M, Clatterbuck RE, et al. The natural history of cavernous malformations: a prospective study of 68 patients. Neurosurgery 1999;44(6):1166–71.
18. Toldo I, Drigo P, Mammi I, et al. Vertebral and spinal cavernous angiomas associated with familial cerebral cavernous malformation. Surg Neurol 2009;71(2):167–71. PubMed PMID: 18207546.
19. Gault J, Sain S, Hu LJ, et al. Spectrum of genotype and clinical manifestations in cerebral cavernous malformations. Neurosurgery 2006;59(6):1278–84, discussion 1284–5. PubMed PMID: 17277691.
20. Maiuri F, Cappabianca P, Gangemi M, et al. Clinical progression and familial occurrence of cerebral cavernous angiomas: the role of angiogenic and growth factors. Neurosurg Focus 2006;21(1):e3. PubMed PMID: 16859256.
21. Revencu N, Vikkula M. Cerebral cavernous malformation: new molecular and clinical insights. J Med Genet 2006;43(9):716–21. PubMed PMID: 16571644. Pubmed Central PMCID: 2564569.
22. Zhao Y, Du GH, Wang YF, et al. Multiple intracranial cavernous malformations: clinical features and treatment. Surg Neurol 2007;68(5):493–9, discussion 499. PubMed PMID: 17707490.
23. Abdulrauf SI, Kaynar MY, Awad IA. A comparison of the clinical profile of cavernous malformations with and without associated venous malformations. Neurosurgery 1999;44(1):41–6, discussion 46–7. PubMed PMID: 9894962.
24. Perrini P, Lanzino G. The association of venous developmental anomalies and cavernous malformations: pathophysiological, diagnostic, and surgical considerations. Neurosurg Focus 2006;21(1):e5. PubMed PMID: 16859258.
25. Nimjee SM, Powers CJ, Bulsara KR. Review of the literature on de novo formation of cavernous malformations of the central nervous system after radiation therapy. Neurosurg Focus 2006; 21(1):e4. PubMed PMID: 16859257.
26. Beall DP, Bell JP, Webb JR, et al. Developmental venous anomalies and cavernous angiomas: a review of the concurrence, imaging, and treatment of these vascular malformations. J Okla State Med Assoc 2005;98(11):535–8. PubMed PMID: 16379482.
27. Burn S, Gunny R, Phipps K, et al. Incidence of cavernoma development in children after radiotherapy for brain tumors. J Neurosurg 2007;106(5 Suppl):379–83. PubMed PMID: 17566205.
28. Kovacs T, Osztie E, Bodrogi L, et al. Cerebellar developmental venous anomalies with associated vascular pathology. Br J Neurosurg 2007;21(2):217–23. PubMed PMID: 17453792.
29. Wurm G, Schnizer M, Fellner FA. Cerebral cavernous malformations associated with venous anomalies: surgical considerations. Neurosurgery 2005;57(1 Suppl):42–58, discussion 42–58. PubMed PMID: 15987569.
30. Awad IA, Robinson JR Jr, Mohanty S, et al. Mixed vascular malformations of the brain: clinical and pathogenetic considerations. Neurosurgery 1993;33(2):179–88, discussion 188. PubMed PMID: 8367039.
31. Fischer A, Zalvide J, Faurobert E, et al. Cerebral cavernous malformations: from CCM genes to endothelial cell homeostasis. Trends Mol Med 2013.
32. Gianfrancesco F, Cannella M, Martino T, et al. Highly variable penetrance in subjects affected with cavernous cerebral angiomas (CCM) carrying novel CCM1 and CCM2 mutations. Am J Med Genet B Neuropsychiatr Genet 2007;144(5):691–5.
33. Gianfrancesco F, Esposito T, Penco S, et al. ZPLD1 gene is disrupted in a patient with balanced translocation that exhibits cerebral cavernous malformations. Neuroscience 2008;155(2): 345–9.
34. Liquori CL, Penco S, Gault J, et al. Different spectra of genomic deletions within the CCM genes between Italian and American CCM patient cohorts. Neurogenetics 2008;9(1):25–31.

35. Stahl S, Gaetzner S, Voss K, et al. Novel CCM1, CCM2, and CCM3 mutations in patients with cerebral cavernous malformations: in-frame deletion in CCM2 prevents formation of a CCM1/CCM2/CCM3 protein complex. Hum Mutat 2008;29(5): 709–17.
36. Sürücü O, Sure U, Gaetzner S, et al. Clinical impact of CCM mutation detection in familial cavernous angioma. Childs Nerv Syst 2006;22(11):1461–4.
37. Tanriover G, Boylan AJ, DiLuna ML, et al. PDCD10, the gene mutated in cerebral cavernous malformation 3, is expressed in the neurovascular unit. Neurosurgery 2008;62(4):930–8.
38. Voss K, Stahl S, Schleider E, et al. CCM3 interacts with CCM2 indicating common pathogenesis for cerebral cavernous malformations. Neurogenetics 2007;8(4):249–56.
39. Brouillard P, Vikkula M. Genetic causes of vascular malformations. Hum Mol Genet 2007;16(R2):R140–9.
40. Dashti SR, Hoffer A, Hu YC, et al. Molecular genetics of familial cerebral cavernous malformations. Neurosurg Focus 2006;21(1): 1–5.
41. Guclu B, Ozturk AK, Pricola KL, et al. Cerebral venous malformations have distinct genetic origin from cerebral cavernous malformations. Stroke 2005;36(11):2479–80.
42. Hanjani SA. The genetics of cerebrovascular malformations. J Stroke Cerebrovasc Dis 2002;11(5):279–87.
43. Riant F, Bergametti F, Ayrignac X, et al. Recent insights into cerebral cavernous malformations: the molecular genetics of CCM. FEBS J 2010;277(5):1070–5.
44. Labauge P, Denier C, Bergametti F, et al. Genetics of cavernous angiomas. Lancet Neurol 2007;6(3):237–44.
45. Gaetzner S, Stahl S, Sürücü O, et al. CCM1 gene deletion identified by MLPA in cerebral cavernous malformation. Neurosurg Rev 2007;30(2):155–60.
46. Gault J, Shenkar R, Recksiek P, et al. Biallelic somatic and germ line CCM1 truncating mutations in a cerebral cavernous malformation lesion. Stroke 2005;36(4):872–4.
47. Akers AL, Johnson E, Steinberg GK, et al. Biallelic somatic and germline mutations in cerebral cavernous malformations (CCMs): evidence for a two-hit mechanism of CCM pathogenesis. Hum Mol Genet 2009;18(5):919–30.
48. McDonald DA, Shenkar R, Shi C, et al. A novel mouse model of cerebral cavernous malformations based on the two-hit mutation hypothesis recapitulates the human disease. Hum Mol Genet 2011;20(2):211–22. PubMed PMID: 20940147. Pubmed Central PMCID: 3005897.
49. Plummer NW, Gallione CJ, Srinivasan S, et al. Loss of p53 sensitizes mice with a mutation in Ccm1 (KRIT1) to development of cerebral vascular malformations. Am J Pathol 2004;165(5): 1509–18. PubMed PMID: 15509522. Pubmed Central PMCID: 1618670.
50. Riant F, Bergametti F, Fournier H-D, et al. CCM3 mutations are associated with early-onset cerebral hemorrhage and multiple meningiomas. Mol Syndromol 2013;4(4):165–72.
51. Fischer A, Zalvide J, Faurobert E, et al. Cerebral cavernous malformations: from CCM genes to endothelial cell homeostasis. Trends Mol Med 2013;19(5):302–8.
52. Hilder TL, Malone MH, Bencharit S, et al. Proteomic identification of the cerebral cavernous malformation signaling complex. J Proteome Res 2007;6(11):4343–55.
53. Li X, Zhang R, Zhang H, et al. Crystal structure of CCM3, a cerebral cavernous malformation protein critical for vascular integrity. J Biol Chem 2010;285(31):24099–107.
54. Zawistowski JS, Stalheim L, Uhlik MT, et al. CCM1 and CCM2 protein interactions in cell signaling: implications for cerebral cavernous malformations pathogenesis. Hum Mol Genet 2005; 14(17):2521–31.
55. Whitehead KJ, Chan AC, Navankasattusas S, et al. The cerebral cavernous malformation signaling pathway promotes vascular integrity via Rho GTPases. Nat Med 2009;15(2):177–84.
56. Stockton RA, Shenkar R, Awad IA, et al. Cerebral cavernous malformations proteins inhibit Rho kinase to stabilize vascular integrity. J Exp Med 2010;207(4):881–96.
57. McDonald DA, Shi C, Shenkar R, et al. Fasudil decreases lesion burden in a murine model of cerebral cavernous malformation disease. Stroke 2012;43(2):571–4. PubMed PMID: 22034008. Pubmed Central PMCID: 3265629.
58. Fisher OS, Boggon TJ. Signaling pathways and the cerebral cavernous malformations proteins: lessons from structural biology. Cell Mol Life Sci 2013;1–12.
59. Hogan BM, Bussmann J, Wolburg H, et al. ccm1 cell autonomously regulates endothelial cellular morphogenesis and vascular tubulogenesis in zebrafish. Hum Mol Genet 2008;17(16): 2424–32.
60. Zhao Y, Tan Y-Z, Zhou L-F, et al. Morphological observation and in vitro angiogenesis assay of endothelial cells isolated from human cerebral cavernous malformations. Stroke 2007;38(4): 1313–19.
61. Shimizu T, Sugawara K-I, Tosaka M, et al. Nestin expression in vascular malformations: a novel marker for proliferative endothelium. Neurol Med Chir (Tokyo) 2006;46(3):111–17.
62. Liquori CL, Berg MJ, Squitieri F, et al. Low frequency of PDCD10 mutations in a panel of CCM3 probands: potential for a fourth CCM locus. Hum Mutat 2006;27(1):118.
63. Gross BA, Lin N, Du R, et al. The natural history of intracranial cavernous malformations. Neurosurg Focus 2011;30(6):E24.
64. Aiba T, Tanaka R, Koike T, et al. Natural history of intracranial cavernous malformations. J Neurosurg 1995;83(1):56–9.
65. Robinson JR, Awad IA, Little JR. Natural history of the cavernous angioma. J Neurosurg 1991;75(5):709–14.
66. Porter PJ, Willinsky RA, Harper W, et al. Cerebral cavernous malformations: natural history and prognosis after clinical deterioration with or without hemorrhage. J Neurosurg 1997;87(2): 190–7.
67. Kondziolka D, Lunsford LD, Kestle JR. The natural history of cerebral cavernous malformations. J Neurosurg 1995;83(5): 820–4.
68. Awad I, Jabbour P. Cerebral cavernous malformations and epilepsy. Neurosurg Focus 2006;21(1):e7. [Epub 2006/07/25]; PubMed PMID: 16859260.
69. Ferroli P, Casazza M, Marras C, et al. Cerebral cavernomas and seizures: a retrospective study on 163 patients who underwent pure lesionectomy. Neurol Sci 2006;26(6):390–4. [Epub 2006/04/08]; PubMed PMID: 16601930.
70. Al-Shahi R, Bhattacharya JJ, Currie DG, et al. Prospective, population-based detection of intracranial vascular malformations in adults: the Scottish Intracranial Vascular Malformation Study (SIVMS). Stroke 2003;34(5):1163–9. [Epub 2003/04/19]; PubMed PMID: 12702837.
71. Cordonnier C, Salman RA-S, Bhattacharya JJ, et al. Differences between intracranial vascular malformation types in the characteristics of their presenting haemorrhages: prospective, population-based study. J Neurol Neurosurg Psychiatry 2008; 79(1):47–51.
72. Batay F, Bademci G, Deda H. Critically located cavernous malformations. Minim Invasive Neurosurg 2007;50(2):71–6.
73. Chen X, Weigel D, Ganslandt O, et al. Diffusion tensor imaging and white matter tractography in patients with brainstem lesions. Acta Neurochir (Wien) 2007;149(11):1117–31.
74. de Oliveira JG, Rassi-Neto A, Ferraz FA, et al. Neurosurgical management of cerebellar cavernous malformations. Neurosurg Focus 2006;21(1):1–8.
75. Majchrzak H, Tymowski M, Majchrzak K, et al. Surgical approaches to pathological lesions of the middle cerebellar peduncle and the lateral part of the pons - clinical observation. Neurol Neurochir Pol 2007;41(5):436–44. PubMed PMID: 18033644.
76. Sola R, Pulido P, Pastor J, et al. Surgical treatment of symptomatic cavernous malformations of the brainstem. Acta Neurochir (Wien) 2007;149(5):463–70.
77. Awad I, Jabbour P. Cerebral cavernous malformations and epilepsy. Neurosurg Focus 2006;21(1):1–9.
78. Baumann CR, Acciarri N, Bertalanffy H, et al. Seizure outcome after resection of supratentorial cavernous malformations: a study of 168 patients. Epilepsia 2007;48(3):559–63.
79. Baumann CR, Schuknecht B, Lo Russo G, et al. Seizure outcome after resection of cavernous malformations is better when surrounding hemosiderin-stained brain also is removed. Epilepsia 2006;47(3):563–6.
80. Giulioni M, Zucchelli M, Riguzzi P, et al. Co-existence of cavernoma and cortical dysplasia in temporal lobe epilepsy. J Clin Neurosci 2007;14(11):1122–4.

81. Ferroli P, Casazza M, Marras C, et al. Cerebral cavernomas and seizures: a retrospective study on 163 patients who underwent pure lesionectomy. Neurol Sci 2006;26(6):390–4.
82. Hsu P-W, Chang C-N, Tseng C-K, et al. Treatment of epileptogenic cavernomas: surgery versus radiosurgery. Cerebrovasc Dis 2007;24(1):116–20.
83. Noto S, Fujii M, Akimura T, et al. Management of patients with cavernous angiomas presenting epileptic seizures. Surg Neurol 2005;64(6):495–8.
84. Paolini S, Morace R, Di Gennaro G, et al. Drug-resistant temporal lobe epilepsy due to cavernous malformations. Neurosurg Focus 2006;21(1):1–5.
85. Recalde RJ, Figueiredo EG, de Oliveira E. Microsurgical anatomy of the safe entry zones on the anterolateral brainstem related to surgical approaches to cavernous malformations. Neurosurgery 2008;62(3):9–17.
86. Huang Y-C, Tseng C-K, Chang C-N, et al. LINAC radiosurgery for intracranial cavernous malformation: 10-year experience. Clin Neurol Neurosurg 2006;108(8):750–6.
87. Iwai Y, Yamanaka K, Yoshimura M. Intracerebral Cavernous Malformation Induced by Radiosurgery. Neurol Med Chir (Tokyo) 2007;47(4):171–3.
88. Sugano H, Shimizu H, Sunaga S. Efficacy of intraoperative electrocorticography for assessing seizure outcomes in intractable epilepsy patients with temporal-lobe-mass lesions. Seizure 2007; 16(2):120–7.
89. Jinhu Y, Jianping D, Xin L, et al. Dynamic enhancement features of cavernous sinus cavernous hemangiomas on conventional contrast-enhanced MR imaging. Am J Neuroradiol 2008;29(3): 577–81.
90. Pozzati E, Marliani AF, Zucchelli M, et al. The neurovascular triad: mixed cavernous, capillary, and venous malformations of the brainstem. 2007.
91. De Souza J, Domingues R, Cruz L, et al. Susceptibility-weighted imaging for the evaluation of patients with familial cerebral cavernous malformations: a comparison with T2-weighted fast spin-echo and gradient-echo sequences. Am J Neuroradiol 2008; 29(1):154–8.
92. Tong K, Ashwal S, Obenaus A, et al. Susceptibility-weighted MR imaging: a review of clinical applications in children. Am J Neuroradiol 2008;29(1):9–17.
93. de Champfleur NM, Langlois C, Ankenbrandt WJ, et al. Magnetic resonance imaging evaluation of cerebral cavernous malformations with susceptibility-weighted imaging. Neurosurgery 2011;68(3):641–8.
94. Hart BL, Taheri S, Rosenberg GA, et al. Dynamic contrast-enhanced MRI evaluation of cerebral cavernous malformations. Transl Stroke Res 2013;4(5):500–6.
95. Mikati AG, Tan H, Shenkar R, et al. Dynamic permeability and quantitative susceptibility related imaging biomarkers in cerebral cavernous malformations. Stroke 2014;45(2):598–601.
96. Schlosser MJ, McCarthy G, Fulbright RK, et al. Cerebral vascular malformations adjacent to sensorimotor and visual cortex. Functional magnetic resonance imaging studies before and after therapeutic intervention. Stroke 1997;28(6):1130–7. PubMed PMID: 9183338.
97. McLaughlin N, Kelly DF. Corticospinal tractography as a prognosticator for motor improvement after brainstem cavernoma resection. Br J Neurosurg 2013;27(1):108–10. PubMed PMID: 22931358.
98. Chang HS, Hongo K, Nakagawa H, et al. Surgical decision-making on cerebral cavernous malformations. J Clin Neurosci 2001; 8(5):416–20. [Epub 2001/09/06]; PubMed PMID: 11535007.
99. Noto S, Fujii M, Akimura T, et al. Management of patients with cavernous angiomas presenting epileptic seizures. Surg Neurol 2005;64(6):495–8, discussion 498–9. [Epub 2005/11/19]; PubMed PMID: 16293460.
100. Zhao J, Wang Y, Kang S, et al. The benefit of neuronavigation for the treatment of patients with intracerebral cavernous malformations. Neurosurg Rev 2007;30(4):313–18, discussion 319. [Epub 2007/07/17]; PubMed PMID: 17629759.
101. Sugano H, Shimizu H, Sunaga S. Efficacy of intraoperative electrocorticography for assessing seizure outcomes in intractable epilepsy patients with temporal-lobe-mass lesions. Seizure 2007;16(2):120–7. [Epub 2006/12/13]; PubMed PMID: 17158074.
102. Pouratian N, Bookheimer SY, Rex DE, et al. Utility of preoperative functional magnetic resonance imaging for identifying language cortices in patients with vascular malformations. J Neurosurg 2002;97(1):21–32. [Epub 2002/07/24]; PubMed PMID: 12134916.
103. Lunsford LD, Khan AA, Niranjan A, et al. Stereotactic radiosurgery for symptomatic solitary cerebral cavernous malformations considered high risk for resection: Clinical article. J Neurosurg 2010;113(1):23–9.
104. Niranjan A, Lunsford LD. Stereotactic radiosurgery guidelines for the management of patients with intracranial cavernous malformations. Prog Neurol Surg 2013;27:166–75.
105. Fuetsch M, El Majdoub F, Hoevels M, et al. Stereotactic LINAC radiosurgery for the treatment of brainstem cavernomas. Strahlenther Onkol 2012;188(4):311–18.
106. Gross BA, Batjer HH, Awad IA, et al. Cavernous malformations of the basal ganglia and thalamus. Neurosurgery 2009;65(1):7–18, discussion 18–9. PubMed PMID: 19574821.
107. Pham M, Gross BA, Bendok BR, et al. Radiosurgery for angiographically occult vascular malformations. Neurosurg Focus 2009;26(5):E16. PubMed PMID: 19408994.
108. Nanney IIIAD, El Tecle NE, El Ahmadieh TY, et al. Intracranial aneurysms in previously irradiated fields: literature review and case illustration. World Neurosurg 2014;81:511–19.
109. Viegas C, Santiago B, Tomé JB, et al. De novo cavernous malformation after radiosurgery. Open J Mod Neurosurg 2013;3:1.
110. Lee M, Kim MS. Image findings in brain developmental venous anomalies. J Cerebrovasc Endovasc Neurosurg 2012;14(1):37–43. [Epub 2012/12/05]; PubMed PMID: 23210028. Pubmed Central PMCID: 3471249.
111. Roccatagliata L, van den Berg R, Soderman M, et al. Developmental venous anomalies with capillary stain: a subgroup of symptomatic DVAs? Neuroradiology 2012;54(5):475–80. [Epub 2011/06/15]; PubMed PMID: 21667050.
112. Hanson EH, Roach CJ, Ringdahl EN. Wet al. Developmental venous anomalies: appearance on whole-brain CT digital subtraction angiography and CT perfusion. Neuroradiology 2011;53(5):331–41. [Epub 2010/07/24]; PubMed PMID: 20652805. Pubmed Central PMCID: 3077751.
113. Nagatani K, Osada H, Takeuchi S, et al. Surgical resection of developmental venous anomaly causing massive intracerebral haemorrhage: A case report. Br J Neurosurg 2013;[Epub 2013/07/12]; PubMed PMID: 23841660.
114. Griffiths D, Newey A, Faulder K, et al. Thrombosis of a developmental venous anomaly causing venous infarction and pontine hemorrhage. J Stroke Cerebrovasc Dis 2013;22(8):e653–5. [Epub 2013/06/25]; PubMed PMID: 23791470.
115. Masson C, Godefroy O, Leclerc X, et al. Cerebral venous infarction following thrombosis of the draining vein of a venous angioma (developmental abnormality). Cerebrovasc Dis 2000; 10(3):235–8. [Epub 2000/04/25]; PubMed PMID: 10773651.
116. Prasad S, Hurst RW, Kasner SE. Postpartum thrombosis of a developmental venous anomaly. Neurology 2009;72(1):92–3. [Epub 2009/01/06]; PubMed PMID: 19122037.
117. Walsh M, Parmar H, Mukherji SK, et al. Developmental venous anomaly with symptomatic thrombosis of the draining vein. J Neurosurg 2008;109(6):1119–22. [Epub 2008/11/28]; PubMed PMID: 19035729.
118. Pilato F, Calandrelli R, Gaudino S, et al. Thrombosis of a developmental venous anomaly in inflammatory bowel disease: case report and radiologic follow-up. J Stroke Cerebrovasc Dis 2013; 22(7):e250–3. [Epub 2013/01/05]; PubMed PMID: 23287422.

74 Indications for Carotid Endarterectomy in Patients with Asymptomatic and Symptomatic Carotid Stenosis

John A. Braca III, Markus J. Bookland, Daniel M. Heiferman, Christopher M. Loftus

KEY POINTS

- The risk of stroke in untreated carotid artery stenosis for symptomatic and asymptomatic patients has been estimated as 26% versus 6% over 2 years, respectively.
- Diagnostic tests include carotid duplex (technician-variable), magnetic resonance angiography (MRA) (may overestimate stenosis), computed tomography angiography (CTA) (may underestimate stenosis), and digital subtraction angiography (DSA) (gold standard).
- Medical management of carotid stenosis includes cardiovascular risk modification, glycemic control, blood pressure control, serum lipid monitoring, smoking cessation, statins, and most importantly aspirin.
- Randomized trials confirm that surgical intervention is appropriate for patients with >50% symptomatic extracranial carotid artery stenosis and >60% for asymptomatic stenosis.
- Carotid endarterectomy (CEA) is the preferable option given acceptable surgical risk and if performed by a qualified surgeon with reproducible results.
- Carotid artery stenting (CAS) with distal protective devices is an innovative new technique for the treatment of carotid stenosis with a place in disease management.

INTRODUCTION

Extracranial carotid artery stenosis has been associated with roughly 16% of all strokes and 20% of ischemic strokes alone.[1] Overall, its prevalence has been estimated to be between 0.1% and 9% among the general population, with rates rising towards 60% among those over the age of 65 years, current smokers, hypertensives, those with coronary artery disease, and individuals suffering recent strokes.[2-5] The identification and modification of extracranial carotid artery disease has become a vigorous and fruitful area of research and therapeutic endeavor over the last century, generating spirited debate and a myriad of novel treatment regimens. This chapter will review the pathophysiology of stenosis formation, basic diagnostic methods used in identifying carotid artery stenosis, current treatment modalities, and preferred surgical therapy.

PATHOPHYSIOLOGY

Plaque formation at the extracranial carotid artery bifurcation results from turbulent flow, activation of clotting factors, inflammation, and aberrant blood vessel wall endothelium. These processes may occur virtually anywhere throughout the cardiovascular tree, so patients with carotid artery stenosis should always be investigated for systemic occlusive vascular disease. When endothelial injury, inflammation and platelet aggregation do form plaque along the common carotid artery, it will most commonly be along the posterior vessel wall, within 2 cm of the bifurcation and focus within the internal carotid artery, creeping slightly into the common and external carotid arteries.

Even partial occlusion of the internal carotid artery via plaque formation can lead to ischemic sequelae.[6] Ultrasound observations of the internal carotid artery and direct visualization of retinal arteries have noted micro-emboli proceeding from internal carotid artery stenosis. These emboli can pass cephalad to retinal and cerebral vasculature leading to transient and permanent ischemic events.[7] The severity of ischemic events will vary from patient to patient and depend largely on the vessel occluded, duration of occlusion, and degree of collateral flow to the affected tissues. Often, patients with symptomatic vascular disease at the proximal internal carotid artery will have a degree of impaired vasoreactivity within the cerebral vasculature, limiting their ability to compensate for acute embolic events.[8]

Left untreated, extracranial internal carotid artery stenosis may progress to complete occlusion. If there is inadequate collateralization at the time of total occlusion, this may lead to severe stroke. Even after obliteration of a single internal carotid artery, the low flow state created near the occlusion point can continue to generate thrombus that may propagate distally. The risk of ischemic events following total internal carotid artery occlusion does decrease with time, and it becomes negligible 1 year following total occlusion.[9]

Some specific plaque characteristics appear to portend cerebral ischemia. The percentage of luminal occlusion created by a plaque has been the most clearly and thoroughly studied quality of carotid plaques. As we will review in greater detail, based on the NASCET, VASST, and ECST trials, a symptomatic patient with radiographic evidence of extracranial carotid artery stenosis >50% will risk an approximate 26% 2-year incidence of stroke. Likewise, based on ACAS and ACST, an asymptomatic patient with radiographic evidence of extracranial carotid artery stenosis >60% has roughly an 11% 5-year risk of stroke.[10] It should be carefully noted that NASCET and ECST used different methods to evaluate the internal carotid artery stenosis. In NASCET the internal carotid artery stenosis was related to the more distal normal internal carotid artery. In ECST it was related to the assumed diameter of the carotid syphon. The result is that a 50% NASCET stenosis corresponds to a 70% ECST stenosis.[11] Nevertheless, these data convincingly correlate increasing linear stenosis and vessel occlusion with cerebral ischemia and have been the foundation for current recommendations regarding surgical intervention. Plaque ulceration, rupture, and hemorrhage have also been posited as indicators of an unstable carotid artery plaque that is more likely to generate thrombus and emboli. There is, however, little data, to date, to confirm that any of these plaque qualities reliably predict cerebral ischemia; and several studies have noted comparable incidences of ulceration and hemorrhage in both symptomatic and asymptomatic patients.[12,13]

Let us examine this in greater detail. Patients with asymptomatic carotid stenosis are frequently incidentally identified by non-invasive screening tests such as carotid ultrasonography, by auscultation of a carotid bruit during routine physical examinations, or during evaluation of a contralateral symptomatic carotid stenosis. Our published knowledge base of the natural history of asymptomatic CAS has been obtained from screening and follow-up studies, studies comparing carotid endarterectomy (CEA) with medical treatment, and studies in patients undergoing CEA for ipsilateral symptomatic stenosis who have concomitant asymptomatic contralateral disease. Three specific factors have been shown to affect outcome: (1) severity of stenosis, (2) progression of stenosis, and (3) presence or absence of plaque ulceration.[14]

Effect of Stenosis Severity

The literature suggests that the risk of an ipsilateral neurologic event is directly related to the degree of asymptomatic carotid stenosis. Rijbroek et al.[15] found that the published annual risk of a neurologic event ensuing in patients with asymptomatic carotid stenosis of less than 50%, 50–80%, and greater than 80% was between 0–3.8%, 2–5%, and 1.7–18%, respectively. It should be noted, however, that the majority of these events were transient ischemic attacks or amaurosis fugax. The annual risk of a stroke was determined to be less than 1%, 0.8–2.4%, and 1–5% for asymptomatic carotid stenosis of less than 50%, 50–80%, and greater than 80%, respectively.

Effect of Stenosis Progression

Although most studies demonstrate an increased rate of ipsilateral neurologic events with stenosis progression, the annual incidence of stroke in the patients who progressed remains low (<5%). This is particularly true for stenosis greater than 80%.[16–18] The risk of progression of an asymptomatic carotid stenosis increases with time and is highly unpredictable. Estimated progression rates range anywhere from 4% to 29% per year, depending on the studied population and how stenosis progression is defined.[15]

Effect of Plaque Ulceration

The presence of plaque ulceration as well as the size and extent of the ulcer has been found to be a marker of future cerebrovascular events. Ulcer size can be measured by multiplying the length and the width in millimeters on conventional angiography. On the basis of these measurements, ulcers are classified into small type A (<10 mm^2), large type B (10–40 mm^2), and compound type C (>40 mm^2).[19] Independent of associated carotid stenosis, the presence of a type C ulcer has been shown to result in an annual stroke rate of 7.5%.[19] Type A ulcers, on the other hand, have a more benign prognosis: they are associated with an annual stroke rate of just 0.4%.[20] The natural history of type B ulcers remains unclear because of conflicting reports regarding the risk of future neurologic events.[14]

DIAGNOSIS

Many patients with carotid artery stenosis will present without any premonitory neurologic complaints. They often reach the attention of clinicians thanks to careful physical examination and the detection of a cervical bruit. A bruit can best be auscultated by placing the bell of a stethoscope over the lateral neck between the angle of the mandible and the superior margin of the thyroid cartilage. A good surgeon should always be wary of a bruit as the only evidence of stenosis, however. Venous hums, cardiac murmurs, thoracic bruits, thyromegaly, and upper extremity arteriovenous fistulas can all mimic a carotid bruit.[21–23] In many instances, the easiest way to distinguish a true carotid bruit from the many other causes of cervical bruits is to auscultate proximally along the carotid. If the sound crescendos, then the source likely originates from the arms or thoracic cavity, whereas a true carotid bruit will decrescendo as the examiner moves away from the bifurcation. The venous hum can defy this rule, but likewise may be differentiated by a simple maneuver. Venous hums obliterate with Valsalva maneuvers and lying down, while carotid bruits will remain constant.[21] Unfortunately, the absence of a cervical bruit does not rule-out carotid disease, and physicians should not shrug off the diagnosis of carotid artery stenosis for lack of a bruit if there exist other symptoms suggestive of the disease. Twenty to 35% of patients with high-grade extracranial carotid artery stenosis will have no auscultatable bruit.[24]

Once a patient with a carotid bruit or other indication of stenosis presents for surgical evaluation a careful history becomes critical. Whether or not the patient presents as asymptomatic or suffering from an ischemic neurologic event, we obtain a thorough history searching for the details of transient or permanent focal visual changes, language difficulty, facial paresis, dysarthria, numbness, or weakness. These cues can help lateralize ischemic injuries. When those ischemic events lie ipsilateral to the carotid stenosis, there is a greater indication for surgical intervention. In addition, the risk of stroke in untreated carotid artery stenosis for symptomatic and asymptomatic patients differs markedly (26% vs 6.2% over 3 years, respectively).[25,26] Computed tomography and magnetic resonance imaging can also be used to identify silent ischemic disease that would otherwise be undetectable on a history and physical.

In the end, radiographic adjuncts will always be necessary to verify the diagnosis of carotid artery stenosis. It is debatable whether carotid artery ultrasound is sufficient to establish the diagnosis of high-grade stenosis. As ultrasound evaluations tend to be very dependent on the skill of the technician, it has been suggested that carotid ultrasound only be used as a standalone diagnostic tool if its positive predictive value for >50% stenosis exceeds 90% after institutional verification.[27] Computed tomography angiography (CTA) and magnetic resonance angiography (MRA) have become increasingly useful screening modalities, as well, in the delineation of carotid artery disease. However, these methods have still not been validated to the degree of digital subtraction angiography (DSA), with some reports finding false carotid occlusions in 11% of CTAs of the neck.[28] In our experience, MRA data are not adequate to resolve the difference between high grade ICA stenosis and/or complete ICA occlusion, nor is it adequate to show us the extent of distal ICA disease, necessary information to plan a safe and effective surgery. CTA is much better at resolving these questions, but can give falsely low readings in the presence of calcium at the carotid bulb, which is often seen in carotid atheroma cases. So, at present, the authors attempt to plan surgery based on CTA if possible, or as a default DSA imaging, and both can give us anatomic cues, such as the relationship of the bifurcation to the angle of the mandible, that cannot be accurately discerned by ultrasound.

EVALUATION OF TREATMENT OPTIONS ONCE STENOSIS IS IDENTIFIED

There is an enormous literature evaluating various aspects of carotid artery treatment, and we have reviewed it extensively in three previous publications.[29-31] Most of the observational evidence has become obsolete now that level 1 cooperative trial data are available. We accept and acknowledge that clinical trials have achieved a growing role in the contemporary practice of medicine, owing in part to the advent of improved methodology for multicenter studies, increasing public awareness of clinical trials, the role of clinical trials in determining reimbursement policies, and a general consensus in the medical community that any treatment administered should be proven effective according to rigorous scientific criteria.

Medical Therapies

Initial management of carotid stenosis should attend to modifying possible concurrent disease elsewhere in the cardiovascular tree, limiting potential thromboembolic risks. Regardless of whether or not a patient with carotid artery stenosis finally requires surgical treatment, their risk of future myocardial infarctions, strokes, or peripheral vascular syndromes over 5 years exceeds 20%; and they should be counseled that future cardiovascular monitoring and care will be needed by their primary physician.[32,33]

The cornerstone underpinning such cardiovascular risk modification, aside from glycemic control, blood pressure control, serum lipid monitoring, and smoking cessation, is aspirin. All patients presenting with carotid artery stenosis should be begun on aspirin. There exists Class I evidence that perioperative low-dose aspirin (81–325 mg) reduces the risk of stroke post-operatively for up to 6 months.[34,35] Additionally, despite its known ability to precipitate gastrointestinal bleeding and hemorrhagic cerebral infarctions, a meta-analysis of >95,000 asymptomatic patients enrolled in six randomized controlled trials (RCTs) found that daily low-dose aspirin reduced critical cardiovascular events by 0.07% per year compared to placebo (P = 0.0001).[36] These results have been shown to be blunted among elderly patients and diabetics, and, as such, routine aspirin therapy remains controversial among asymptomatic patients within these populations. Overall, though, aspirin therapy should be a mainstay of initial carotid stenosis medical management in most patients.[37]

Beyond the routine implementation of aspirin therapy, current recommendations regarding medical treatments for carotid artery stenosis have evolved from a series of clinical trials over the last 40 years that progressively expanded the pharmacologic armamentarium available to internists and cardiologists. Based upon some of these early studies, many physicians have begun aggressively treating carotid artery stenosis with novel antiplatelet agents and statins. Preliminary data reviewing both symptomatic and asymptomatic patients with intra- and extracranial carotid artery stenosis have suggested that combinations of these new medications may provide stroke reduction benefits approaching that of CEA. A study evaluating symptomatic carotid artery stenosis, including intracranial disease, and combination aspirin/clopidogrel, noted a significant reduction in transcranial ultrasound demonstrated microemboli (RRR 42.4%, P = 0.025). Such radiographic reductions would, presumably but not necessarily, correlate with the likelihood of future ischemia.[38] Testing the clinical validity of clopidogrel administration for the prevention of cerebral ischemic events, several RCTs have been designed and executed to compare aspirin, clopidogrel and combination aspirin/clopidogrel treated patients. The ESPS-2 and ESPRIT studies both noted a significant relative risk reduction for stroke when patients received both aspirin and clopidogrel compared to either medication individually (aspirin/clopidogrel: 37% vs aspirin: 18%, P = 0.039).[39,40] These results have not always been durable, however, and other RCTs have noted significantly more hemorrhagic complications with combination antiplatelet agent therapy without a relative reduction in cerebral ischemia.[41,42]

The data for statin use in carotid stenosis patients are, perhaps, slightly more impressive. Subgroup analysis of 1007 patients with carotid stenosis and no attendant coronary disease in the SPARCL trial demonstrated an impressive 33% reduction in stroke risk among those patients randomized to 80 mg of atorvastatin vs placebo (P = 0.006).[43] Additionally, laboratory data evaluating endothelial injury, nitric-oxide mediated vasodilation, and platelet aggregation in hydroxyl-methyl-glutaryl-CoA reductase treated patients have shown that statins inhibit the early stages of endothelial injury associated with carotid artery atherosclerotic changes.[44]

These findings would recommend statins in comparison to surgical intervention, and they intimate that previously reported rates of stroke and death noted in the North American Symptomatic Carotid Endarterectomy Trial (NASCET)[25] and the Asymptomatic Carotid Atherosclerosis Study (ACAS)[45] trials may no longer be realistic representations of modern carotid stenosis patients (1.6% vs 3.9%). Some now argue that current rates of stroke and death among carotid stenosis patients on maximal medical therapy lie on a par with or even superior to 5-year rates post CEA or carotid artery stenting (CAS).[46] Such claims should be considered with reservation, however, as studies have likewise shown that statin usage has reduced 30-day stroke rates among CEA and CAS patients, as well (CEA: (0.0% vs 3.1%, P = 0.02; CAS: 18.4% vs 35.0%, P = 0.031).[47,48] Happily, the literature suggests that modern medical therapies may be lowering stroke rates across treatment modalities rather than driving any one method into obsolescence, though such a statement remains pure speculation. Like antiplatelet agents, no well-designed head-to-head study has yet been performed comparing statin usage alone with combined CEA or CAS and statin use, making it impossible to recommend with confidence a departure from NASCET, ACAS or similar cooperative trial data. Several groups have begun to organize a multicenter RCT hoping to ascertain whether novel, intensive medical therapy can produce reductions in stroke and death comparable or superior to surgical intervention; but no data have yet been released.[49] In the absence of such data, the NASCET, ACAS, ECST, and ACST trials remain the preeminent, if dated, studies and from these trials' data have come the endorsement of timely surgical and endovascular treatments for extracranial carotid artery stenosis.

Surgical/Endovascular Therapies

Early studies had suggested that medical management with blood pressure control and antiplatelet agents surpassed surgical intervention.[50] This thinking has changed since the 1990s. Gratifying and unimpeachable results from recent multicenter trials have advocated surgical therapy over medical management in specific cases. The data are as follows.

Asymptomatic Carotid Trials

Carotid Artery Stenosis with Asymptomatic Narrowing: Operation Versus Aspirin (CASANOVA). CASANOVA was the first study, published in 1991.[51] This was a multicenter trial consisting of 410 patients with asymptomatic CAS measuring 50–90%. Patients were randomly assigned after angiography to surgery versus medical therapy alone. All patients received daily aspirin and dipyridamole. The minimum follow-up period was 3 years. The study demonstrated no significant difference in the number of strokes and death between the surgical and medical groups. Unfortunately, the study had an unusually complicated protocol and excluded patients with greater than 90% stenosis. Furthermore, the combined complication rate of angiography and surgery was exceedingly high (6.9%).

Mayo Asymptomatic Carotid Endarterectomy Study Group Trial (MACE). In 1992, MACE was published.[52] This was a single center study comparing CEA alone with aspirin therapy. The study was terminated early, only after 71 patients had been randomly assigned, because of a significantly higher number of myocardial infarctions and transient cerebral ischemic events in the surgical group. It was presumed that these events were related to the absence of aspirin use in the patients undergoing CEA and therefore reinforced the importance of aspirin administration throughout the peri-operative period and beyond. Although there had been more ischemic events in the surgical group than in the medical group, the small number of patients and short follow-up did not allow any conclusions to be drawn.

Asymptomatic Carotid Atherosclerosis Study (ACAS). ACAS, published in 1995, was a prospective randomized multicenter trial comparing the efficacy of CEA and medical therapy to best medical therapy (BMT) alone in preventing ipsilateral stroke during a 5-year period.[53] The study comprised 1662 patients from 39 centers across the United States and Canada with asymptomatic CAS greater than 60%. The median follow-up was 2.7 years, and 9% of patients completed 5 years of follow-up. The estimated 5-year risk of ipsilateral stroke and any peri-operative stroke or death was 5.1% and 11.0% for the surgical and medical groups, respectively. CEA reduced the 5-year stroke risk by 66% in men and by 17% in women. Overall, the risk of ipsilateral stroke was reduced by 53% and remained statistically significant at 3 years' follow-up. CEA, however, did not significantly protect against major strokes or death. The surgical morbidity and mortality rate was surprisingly low: 1.5% and 0.1%, respectively. Approximately half of the total morbidity was related to angiography. A statistical benefit from CEA was seen within less than 1 year after surgery.

Veterans Affairs Cooperative Study (VAAST). In 1993, VAAST was published and demonstrated a reduction of ipsilateral neurologic events after CEA plus aspirin–antiplatelet therapy as compared with antiplatelet therapy alone (8% vs 20.6%).[54] Unfortunately, the proposed sample size was not large enough to provide statistical power, and the study failed to show a reduction of ipsilateral strokes or death. Nonetheless, after a 4-year follow-up period, the ipsilateral stroke rate in the surgical group was 4.7% in contrast to 9.4% in the medical group. However, when the peri-operative mortality (1.9%) was added to the surgical stroke rate, the difference between the two groups did not reach statistical significance. Most deaths were secondary to myocardial infarction. The trial did not include women.

Asymptomatic Carotid Surgery Trial (ACST). ACST was published in 2004 and is the largest multicenter trial to date.[55] The study consisted of 3120 patients with greater than 60% asymptomatic stenosis (diagnosed by duplex ultrasound) randomly assigned to immediate CEA or medical therapy at the discretion of the treating physician. Of the patients randomly assigned to CEA, 50% underwent surgery within 1 month and 88% underwent surgery within 1 year. Exclusion criteria included poor surgical risk, prior ipsilateral CEA, and probable cardiac emboli. Surgeons were required to have a peri-operative morbidity and mortality rate of less than 6%. The mean follow-up was 3.4 years. The peri-operative morbidity and mortality rate was 3.1%. The net 5-year risk of all strokes and death including peri-operative stroke and death was 6.4% and 11.8% in the CEA and medical groups, respectively. Fatal or disabling strokes rates were 3.5% vs 6.1%. Fatal stroke rates alone were 2.1% vs 4.2%. Both men and women benefited from CEA, although there was a greater benefit in men. CEA did not demonstrate a statistically significant benefit for patients older than 75 years. In contrast to the ACAS study, the ACST did not show statistical benefit in the immediate CEA group until nearly 2 years after surgery. This was most likely due to the lower peri-operative event rates demonstrated in the ACAS.

The Special Case of Carotid Endarterectomy and Asymptomatic Contralateral Carotid Artery Disease. The impact of contralateral carotid artery disease on asymptomatic CAS must be considered with regard to its natural history and the risk of surgical intervention. There are, however, conflicting data in the literature.

In a post hoc analysis of the ACAS that compared 163 patients with baseline contralateral occlusion with 1485 patients with patent contralateral carotid arteries, it was found that the 5-year ipsilateral stroke rate in the surgically treated patients was 5.5% vs 5%, which suggests that there is no increased surgical risk in patients with contralateral occlusion.[45] Interestingly, however, medically treated patients with contralateral occlusion had a better clinical outcome than those without contralateral disease (5-year ipsilateral stroke rate, 3.5% versus 11.7%), which suggests a relatively benign natural history. This was believed to be due to development of collateral circulation secondary to the contralateral occlusion. These findings suggest that prophylactic endarterectomy for asymptomatic CAS in the presence of contralateral occlusion provides no long-term benefit in preventing stroke and death and may actually be harmful.

In contrast, a worse natural history was reported by Irvine et al.[56] in a retrospective study consisting of 487 patients with asymptomatic CAS followed-up for a mean of 41 months. The presence of bilateral carotid artery disease was found to significantly increase the risk of overall, but not ipsilateral strokes (relative risk, 2.35). Patients with unilateral asymptomatic carotid artery disease had an overall stroke rate of less than 5% in the first year after presentation as compared with a stroke rate of 9.6% in patients with unilateral asymptomatic CAS and concomitant contralateral stenosis greater than 90%. Similar results were reported by AbuRahma et al.[57] in a prospective study consisting of 82 patients with greater than 60% asymptomatic carotid stenosis and contralateral carotid occlusion. Patients were treated with maximal medical therapy for a mean follow-up period of 59.5 months. Late strokes occurred in 33% (23% ipsilateral and 10% contralateral) and transient ischemic attacks occurred in 27% of patients (9% ipsilateral and 18% contralateral), which suggests a higher incidence of ipsilateral stroke than that reported by the ACAS study.

The risk of CEA in the presence of contralateral carotid artery occlusion is debatable. The NASCET reported a combined perioperative stroke and death rate of 14.3% in patients with contralateral carotid occlusion as compared with 4% and 5.1% in patients with patent and mild-to-moderate stenosis of the contralateral carotid artery, respectively.[58] A similarly higher risk was reported in the Acetylsalicylic Acid and Carotid Endarterectomy (ACE) trial.[59] This was a multicenter prospective randomized study evaluating the dose and role of acetylsalicylic acid in patients undergoing CEA. The study included 2804 patients, of which 54% (1512) were asymptomatic. Contralateral carotid artery occlusion (n = 236) was found to increase the perioperative risk of stroke and death by 2.3-fold. In a retrospective analysis of 1370 (54% asymptomatic) consecutive CEAs performed at a single institution, Reed et al.[60] evaluated the effect of various preoperative risk factors on the incidence of peri-operative (30-day) stroke and death. The overall stroke and death rates were 0.8% and 1.2%, respectively. Univariate analysis demonstrated that contralateral carotid occlusion (n = 75) was the only significant predictor of adverse outcome (6.7%) among the variables tested, and the relative risk was 4.3 on multivariate analysis ($P = 0.01$). Furthermore, the 5-year survival rate in patients with contralateral occlusion was found to be significantly lower than patients with patent contralateral carotid arteries (38% vs 67%). Similar findings were reported by Duncan et al.[61] in a single institutional retrospective study consisting of 1609 consecutive CEAs of which 97 had contralateral carotid artery occlusion. The same-admission stroke and mortality rate was 5.2% as compared with 1.3% ($P = 0.01$) in patients with and without contralateral occlusion, respectively. Despite these findings, several large community observational studies involving both symptomatic and asymptomatic patients demonstrate no early or long-term significant differences between patients with and without contralateral carotid occlusion.[62–65]

In conclusion, although several studies have found no statistically significant difference in the peri-operative stroke, death, and survival rates between CEAs in patients with or without contralateral carotid disease, there is a trend toward higher surgical risk in patients with contralateral carotid occlusion. Furthermore, there is a higher incidence of intraoperative electroencephalography (EEG) changes and subsequent shunt requirements in such patients. In two studies the incidence of intra-operative shunting was 46% and 52.9% in patients with contralateral carotid occlusion as compared with 13.5% and 4.8% in patients without contralateral occlusion.[62,63]

Symptomatic Carotid Trials

The major studies evaluating the use of CEA for symptomatic stenosis are the North American Symptomatic Carotid Endarterectomy Trial (NASCET),[25] the European Carotid Surgery Trial (ECST),[66] and the V.A. Symptomatic Stenosis Trial (VASST).[67] These trials, published in the early 1990s, demonstrated that in patients with symptomatic high-grade (>70%) stenosis, CEA resulted in lower stroke risk than medical therapy; the benefits of CEA, however, were realized only if the morbidity of surgery could be kept reasonably low (6%). Guidelines for CEA published by the American Heart Association in 1995[13] were updated 10 years later,[68,69] and the number of CEAs performed in this country continue to rise.

European Carotid Surgery Trial (ECST). ECST[66] entered patients with mild (defined as less than 30%), moderate (30–69%) or severe (70–99%) carotid stenosis who were then randomly assigned to either surgical or non-surgical treatment. Interim analysis of 2200 patients (mean follow-up = 2.7 years) led to premature termination of the trial for the mild and severe stenosis groups. Among the 374 patients with mild stenosis, there was no significant difference in ipsilateral stroke between the surgical and non-surgical groups. There were more treatment failures in the surgical group, which was attributed to the 2.3% risk of death or disabling stroke during the first 30 days after surgery. For severe stenosis, however, surgery was shown to be beneficial in preventing stroke. There was a 7.5% risk of ipsilateral stroke or death within 30 days of surgery. At 3 years of follow-up, there was an additional 2.8% risk of stroke in the surgical group (total = 10.3%) compared with 16.8% in the non-surgical group ($P < 0.0001$). More importantly, the risk of death or ipsilateral disabling stroke was 11% in the non-surgical group compared with 6% in the surgical group.

North American Symptomatic Carotid Endarterectomy Trial (NASCET). NASCET[25] prematurely stopped randomly assigning patients with carotid stenosis greater than 70% because of the highly significant stroke risk reduction observed in the surgical group. A total of 659 patients in this category of stenosis were assigned to surgical (n = 331) or non-surgical (n = 328) therapy. At a mean follow-up of 24 months, ipsilateral stroke was noted in 26% of patients receiving nonsurgical therapy, compared with 9% of patients who had undergone CEA, for an overall risk reduction of 17% (relative risk reduction = 71%). The benefit for surgical patients was highly significant ($P < 0.001$) for a variety of outcomes, including stroke in any territory, major stroke, and major stroke or death from any cause. A perioperative morbidity/mortality of 5.8% was rapidly surpassed in the non-surgical group, such that surgical benefit was apparent by 3 months. In addition, the protective effect of surgery was durable over time, with few strokes noted in the endarterectomy group beyond the peri-operative period. There was a direct correlation between surgical benefit and the degree of angiographic stenosis.

V.A. Symptomatic Stenosis Trial (VASST). Enrollment in VASST[68] was discontinued in early 1991 on the basis of preliminary data consistent with the NASCET findings. Subsequent analysis demonstrated a statistically significant reduction in ipsilateral stroke or crescendo TIA for patients with carotid stenosis greater than 50% who underwent surgery.[67] A total of 193 men aged 35–82 years (mean = 64.2 years) were randomly assigned to surgical (n = 91) or non-surgical (n = 98) treatment. Two-thirds of the patients demonstrated angiographic internal carotid artery stenosis greater than 70%. At a mean follow-up of 11.9 months, there was a significant reduction in stroke or crescendo TIA in patients receiving CEA (7.7%) compared with non-surgical patients (19.4%), or a risk reduction of 11.7% (relative risk reduction = 60%; $P = 0.028$). Among subgroups, the benefit of surgery was most prominent in patients with TIA in comparison with those with transient monocular blindness (TMB) or stroke, although these differences were not statistically significant. The benefit for surgery was apparent as early as 2 months after randomization and persisted over the entire period of follow-up. The efficacy of CEA was durable, with only one ipsilateral stroke beyond the 30-day peri-operative period. With one pre-operative stroke discounted, perioperative morbidity of 2.2% and mortality of 3.3% (total = 5.5%) were achieved over multiple centers among relatively high-risk patients.

The Special Case of ASA in the Setting of Carotid Surgery – The Acetylsalicylic Acid and Carotid Endarterectomy (ACE) Trial. ASA and Carotid Endarterectomy (ACE) trial[34] is a multinational, prospective, randomized trial of 2849 patients enrolled at 74 centers who were scheduled for carotid endarterectomy for arteriosclerotic disease and were randomized into four treatment groups of acetylsalicylic acid (ASA) 81 mg, 325 mg, 650 mg, or 1300 mg from 1994 to 1998. Patients also needed to tolerate 1300 mg of acetylsalicylic acid daily to be enrolled in the study. Exclusion criteria included taking acetylsalicylic acid or other antiplatelet agent that could not be stopped during the trial, recent disabling stroke, had undergone cardiac surgery in the previous 30 days or were schedule for cardiac surgery in the next 30 days. Surgeons were required to have a personal peri-operative stroke and death rate less than 6% to be eligible for participation in the study. Because patients with both symptomatic (46% of patients enrolled) and asymptomatic (54% of patients enrolled) carotid disease were enrolled in this trial and the significant evidence towards acetylsalicylic acid benefitting patients with history of TIA or stroke, it was determined to be unethical to have a purely placebo arm of the study. Follow-up was documented at 30 days and 3 months, with no patients and two patients being lost to follow-up, respectively. Treatment compliance was documented 91–93% across the four groups at 30 days and 86–89% at 3 months. The authors report there was a statistically significant decrease in strokes (3.2% vs 6.9%), myocardial infarctions (0.9% vs 3.3%), and death (1.6% and 2.2%) at 3-month follow-up for the low-dose groups (81 mg and 325 mg) as compared to the high-dose groups (650 mg and 1300 mg), respectively. As such, the relative risk increase for high-dose ASA, as compared to low-dose ASA was 25–38% across these three adverse outcome endpoints. Upon further analysis, there was no significant difference found between patients taking 81 mg and 325 mg groups, or between 650 mg and 1300 mg groups. While these data show evidence towards the use of low-dose aspirin in the peri-operative setting of carotid endarterectomy, the authors caution reads on generalizing this evidence to the use in non-operative stroke risk reduction.

Carotid Endarterectomy Symptomatic Trial Meta-analyses and Other Post Hoc Analyses

Because only three properly powered trials on symptomatic therapy CEA have been published, considerable attention has focused on the individual results from these trials. However, although the trials had similar outcomes, the inclusion and exclusion criteria and enrollment variables (degree of stenosis measurements, for example) were somewhat different. Nevertheless, because the cohorts in all three trials were relatively homogeneous, it was possible to retrospectively standardize and pool the original data. Additionally, given the volume of pertinent data on demographic and risk indices, it was possible to generate post hoc analyses examining different outcome measures and baseline variables.

In 2003, the investigators of the three symptomatic CEA trials published a meta-analysis in which raw trial data were pooled and analyzed.[70] Data (6092 patients, 35,000 patient-years of follow-up) included all patients randomly assigned to treatment in one of the three trials in the 2 decades following trial results publication, which included 95% of patients ever included in CEA trials. Original carotid angiograms were reassessed for degree of stenosis to standardize the data among trials. Outcome events were redefined when necessary for the same purpose. This analysis demonstrated that surgery was associated with a higher 5-year risk of ipsilateral ischemic stroke in patients with less than 30% carotid stenosis, no effect in patients with 30–49% risk, and marginal benefit in those with 50–69% risk; CEA was highly beneficial in preventing stroke in those with greater than 70% stenosis, provided that there was no near-occlusion. Furthermore, analysis by degree of stenosis showed the benefit proportionately increased within the 70–99% range.[70]

Another analysis of pooled data (restricted to the combined ECST and NASCET patient databases) evaluated the risk of ipsilateral stroke with medical therapy, the peri-operative risk of stroke and death, and the overall benefit from surgery in relation to seven predefined and seven post-hoc-defined subgroups.[71] Predefined variables, that is, those studied in the original trials, were as follows: sex (male, female), age (<65, 65–74, >75 years), time since last event (<2, 2–4, 4–12, >12 weeks), primary symptomatic event (ocular only, cerebral TIA, stroke), presence or absence of diabetes, plaque surface (smooth, irregular, or ulcerated), and contralateral ICA occlusion. Post hoc subgroups were: duration of cerebral TIA (<1 hour, >1 hour), previous TIA or stroke (yes/no), and presence or absence of myocardial infarction, angina, treated hypertension, treated hyperlipidemia, and smoking. Data were analyzed from 5893 patients including 33,000 patient-years of follow-up. In unoperated patients, risk of ipsilateral stroke was found to be higher in close proximity to the last ischemic event and increased with age, male gender, diabetes, in patients with prior hemispheric strokes, and in patients with ulcerated plaques. Peri-operative risk was higher in women, diabetics, and patients with hemispheric qualifying events, contralateral carotid occlusion, and ulcerated plaques. In the post-hoc subgroups, the peri-operative risk was reduced in patients with angina and increased in those with hypertension and previous TIA or stroke.

More specific subgroup correlations identified the highest benefit for surgery in men aged over 75 years operated on within 2 weeks.[71] Benefit fell sharply beyond 2 weeks, such that in order to prevent one ipsilateral stroke in a patient with greater than 50% carotid stenosis at 5 years, one would need to operate on five patients if the surgery were done within 2 weeks of random treatment assignment as opposed to 125 patients if surgery were performed beyond 12 weeks.

Several post hoc analyses restricted to the NASCET trial patients have been performed.[72–75] Among 681 patients from the NASCET trial evaluated for the correlation between collateral blood supply (anterior communicating artery, posterior communicating artery, and ophthalmic retrograde flow) and risk of ipsilateral stroke, good collateral formation was found to reduce the risk of stroke in both the medically treated group and patients undergoing CEA.[72] Patients from NASCET who had concomitant intracranial atherosclerotic disease were found to have an increased risk of ipsilateral stroke when treated medically, but not when treated surgically. Furthermore, the stroke risk was reduced for those undergoing CEA.[73] For 193 NASCET patients with leukoaraiosis, although leukoaraiosis did confer an increased risk of stroke for the medically treated group as well as a higher perioperative risk in the group undergoing surgery, CEA reduced the subsequent stroke risk in this cohort.[74] Analysis of 659 patients with more than 70% stenosis in the NASCET trial revealed an increased risk of stroke in patients found to have an angiographically demonstrated ulcerated plaque who were treated medically. CEA was very successful in this subgroup, reducing the risk of stroke by approximately half at 24 months.[75]

In executive summary, the NASCET data, released in two phases, and corroborated by ECST, indicated that CEA benefited all symptomatic patients with lesions causing more than a 70% reduction in luminal diameter and for specific subgroups of symptomatic patients with more than 50% stenosis. Likewise, the ACAS and ACST data indicated that asymptomatic patients with more than 60% stenosis had a better outcome with CEA than with medical management. Thanks largely to these well-designed, RCTs CEA has become the therapy of choice for select patients with >50% carotid artery stenosis, with the caveats that peri-operative morbidity and mortality must be limited to <3% and patient life-expectancy should be >5 years.[76]

The Carotid Endarterectomy versus Carotid Artery Stenting-A Conundrum

These multiple excellent studies elevated surgical intervention for carotid artery stenosis beyond pharmacologic therapy alone, but in the generation since their publications novel technologies in the form of endovascular CAS have presented other potential alternative treatments. As of this chapter's writing, the debate between the merits of open surgical repair and endovascular repair of carotid artery stenosis continues with vigorous input from supporters of each intervention. There are now over 11 RCTs comparing CEA and CAS.[77–86] Despite much enthusiasm, the results have, for the most part, failed to validate CAS as a non-inferior treatment for carotid artery stenosis. More to the point, several have found CAS to bear a much higher risk of subacute CVAs than carotid surgery. In 1998, the Leicester trial, though limited by a small sample size, found a 45% increase in periprocedure CVAs among CAS patients compared to CEA patients; and, in 2001, the WALLSTENT multi-center RCT demonstrated an alarming rate of ipsilateral strokes and deaths among CAS patients (CAS 12.1% vs CEA 3.6%).[82,87] These results have been cause for much concern, but supporters of CAS have often only responded by citing the nascent understanding of CAS and lack of experience with the procedure during these early studies.

As such, a number of RCTs since WALLSTENT have attempted to reverse the stigma of 30-day and 1-year infarcts from carotid stenting. Largely, they failed. The SPACE trial was mildly, but not statistically, favorable to surgery vs CAS.[79] The EVA-3S trial clearly showed that outcomes were statistically far superior with surgery than with stenting.[78] The SAPPHIRE trial, released in 2004, stands as the lone exception. It showed in a group of 334 high-risk randomized patients a 24.6% and 30.3% stroke rate between CAS and CEA.[85] The difference was not statistically significant. We note, however, that there were an enormous number of patients (415 of the original 741 patients), nearly all stented, who were treated outside of the trial, which always introduces the specter of selection bias against surgery. In addition, the SAPPHIRE results claiming equipoise have not been reproducible in subsequent, larger RCTs.[85,86]

The latest and most comprehensive RCT investigating the efficacy and safety of CAS and CEA in the treatment of carotid artery stenosis, as of this chapter's publication, is the Carotid Revascularization Endarterectomy versus Stenting Trial (CREST).[88] This multicenter RCT attempted to address the numerous failings of past RCTs comparing CEA and CAS and so provide a convincing answer to the debate between the two treatments.

A total of 2,502 patients (1,262 CEA and 1,240 CAS) were enrolled in CREST. The study included both asymptomatic and symptomatic patients with either ≥60% or ≥50% stenosis of the carotid artery by angiography (other radiographic studies were permitted for diagnosis, though with higher cutoffs). Symptomatic patients needed to present within 6 months of randomization, and all surgeons and interventionalists had to be certified for their procedure in order to participate in the trial. Within the CAS arm of the study, an embolic protection device had to be employed wherever feasible. The primary endpoint for the study was all periprocedural stroke, myocardial infarction, and death, as well as any stroke or myocardial infarction ipsilateral to the diseased artery up to 4 years following.

In the final analysis, the authors of CREST noted no difference in primary endpoints between the two treatment arms (7.2% CAS vs 6.8% CEA; 95%CI, 0.81–1.51; $P = 0.51$). Though these results are offered as evidence of equipoise between CAS and CEA, the data underpinning these conglomerate endpoint data lead to a different interpretation. Looking at stroke and myocardial infarction independently, the two largest endpoints comprising CREST's general endpoint, the study found an elevated peri-procedural stroke rate among CAS patients (4.1% CAS vs 2.3%, $P = 0.012$), on par with previous studies, and an elevated myocardial infarction rate among CEA patients (1.1 CAS vs 2.3%, $P = 0.032$). Looking at quality of life measures recorded over the study's 4-year follow-up (Medical Outcomes Study 36-Item Short-Form Health Survey (SF-36)), myocardial infarctions had no demonstrable effect on patients' quality of life, while peri-procedural strokes did. Further, the rate of major ipsilateral stokes among CAS-treated patients, despite the use of an embolic protection device, ran nearly double that of the CEA patients (15.2% CAS vs 8.0% CEA).[89]

Taken in total, these subset data from CREST beg similar conclusions as previous trials. CREST seems to have reaffirmed that CAS bears a materially higher risk of periprocedural stroke compared to CEA and that this risk is not significantly reduced by the use of modern distal embolic protection devices. The failure of distal protection devices to limit CAS-related stroke likely derives from aortic arch disease concurrent with carotid stenosis. Such plaques must be traversed by endovascular interventionalists long before these embolic protection devices can even be deployed.

Finally we should consider ICSS and the interim data from this study. The International Carotid Stenting Study (ICSS) is an ongoing multicenter, international, randomized trial of CEA versus CAS in carotid stenosis of greater than 50% that has been symptomatic in the last 12 months.[90] Patients for whom CEA posed standard risk were eligible for inclusion in the trial (with only prior CEA as the surgical high-risk exclusionary criterion) and had to be candidates for either CEA or CAS. The 120-day interim analysis of 1713 patients randomly assigned to undergo one of the procedures found no difference in rates of disabling stroke or death between CEA (3.2%) and CAS (4.0%) cohorts, but there was a significantly higher rate of any stroke, myocardial infarction and all-cause death in those patients undergoing CAS (8.5%) than in those undergoing CEA (5.2%; $P = 0.006$). Thirty day post-procedure rates of any stroke or death were also significantly higher in the CAS cohort. The investigators concluded that CEA for symptomatic carotid stenosis should remain the first-line treatment for patients deemed suitable candidates for surgery.

While CAS (with distal protective devices) has been an innovative new technique for the treatment of carotid stenosis, and no doubt has its place in the management of this disease, the evidence to date strongly favors open surgical repair. Numerous RCTs have demonstrated consistent and reproducible evidence for a lower 30-day stroke and death rate for patients randomized to CEA. In the absence of novel data to support CAS, though, current evidence-based medicine continues to confirm the superiority of CEA over CAS for the management of carotid stenosis patients.

Carotid Revascularization and Coronary Artery Bypass Graft

Currently, there are no clearly defined indications for managing asymptomatic carotid artery stenosis in patients undergoing general and vascular procedures, except in the case of coronary artery bypass grafting (CABG).[91] In 2011, Naylor et al.[92] published an update on his meta-analysis from 2002 in an attempt to further determine the role of carotid artery disease in the pathogenesis of post-CABG stroke through analysis of primarily single-center, non-randomized, retrospective studies. The perioperative risk of stroke was found to be 1.8% for patients with no significant carotid artery disease (<50% stenosis), while the 30-day stroke risk with either asymptomatic or symptomatic >50% stenosis was 7.4%, and 9.1% for 80–99% stenosis or occlusion. Asymptomatic 50–99% stenosis was associated with a 3.8% risk of stroke and 70–99% stenosis with a lower, 2.0%, risk. Additionally, bilateral, asymptomatic 50–99% stenosis or 50–99% stenosis with contralateral occlusion was associated with a 6.5% risk of perioperative stroke.

Also in 2011, the American College of Cardiology Foundation and American Heart Association published updated CABG surgery guidelines,[93] which included recommendations on carotid stenosis in this setting, although all recommendations are based on low-level evidence given the limited nature of the studies on this topic. They recommend screening carotid ultrasounds for patients with high risk factors including: age >65 years, left main coronary stenosis, peripheral artery disease, and with a history of cerebrovascular disease. The guidelines give a class IIa recommendation of carotid revascularization in conjunction with CABG in symptomatic 50–99% stenosis, noting that the severity of cerebral and myocardial dysfunction are to be weighed to determine the timing of the procedures, whether staged or simultaneous. Finally, they give a class IIb recommendation to consider carotid revascularization surgery in asymptomatic bilateral 70–99% stenosis or unilateral 70–99% with contralateral occlusion.

To further delineate the timing of carotid surgery in relation to cardiac surgery in recommended situations, in 2013, Shishehbor et al.[94] published a retrospective study of 350 patients who underwent either staged CEA before open heart surgery (CEA-OHS) (n=45), combined CEA-OSH under single anesthesia (n=145) and staged carotid artery stenting before OHS (CAS-OSH) (n=110). They found that CAS-OHS and combined CEA-OHS had similar early phase (<1 year) composite (myocardial infarction (MI), stroke and death) outcomes, whereas staged CEA-OHS was associated with the highest risk in the early phase due to 24% interstage MI rate. Finally, staged CAS-OHS patients experienced significantly fewer late phase (>1 year) composite events as compared to both staged and combined CEA-OHS.

Carotid Artery Interventions and Women

There is some evidence to indicate that female gender may negatively impact the outcome of carotid artery interventions (both CEA and CAS).[95] Perioperative risk of stroke following CEA may be higher in women as compared to men. This phenomenon may be attributed to the fact that in some studies there is a disparity between the preoperative care women receive as compared to their age-controlled male cohort (diagnostic imaging, statin use).[96,97]

Several large databases have revealed an advantage of CEA over CAS in women, and this is not demonstrated in men. However, there is no consensus on whether CEA benefits over CAS hold true in both asymptomatic and symptomatic women.[98]

The effect of hormone replacement therapy (HRT) on arterial remodeling has been postulated as a possible explanation for gender-based differences in neurologic outcomes of CEA. Lane et al. evaluated HRT on outcomes of CEA in symptomatic and asymptomatic patients. The perioperative stroke rate was higher among women receiving HRT (8.7%) than women who were not receiving HRT (1.2%), although this did not reach statistical significance. There is, therefore, no need to discontinue postmenopausal HRT in women who undergo CEA (Grade B recommendation).

The various mechanisms responsible for gender-based disparities in outcomes of carotid artery interventions (CEA or CAS) are likely multifactorial. Gender equality and stringency of standardization of the pre-operative phase of patient care will possibly shed more light on the specifics germane to the risk in women undergoing carotid artery intervention versus medical therapy.[95]

CONCLUSION

Decision Making and Patient Selection

Extracranial carotid artery stenosis affects roughly 60% of individuals over the age of 65 years and has been associated with 16% of all cerebral ischemic events.[1,2] Its formation results from chronic turbulence and injury along the endothelium of the carotid bifurcation and may be modified by the treatment or prevention of known contributing risk factors such as hypertension, diabetes, and smoking.[99-103] Based upon data from the NASCET and ACAS trials, symptomatic patients with <50% stenosis of the extracranial carotid artery, and <60% in asymptomatic patients, as determined by DSA or certified carotid ultrasonography, should be managed with aggressive medical therapy, including aspirin, statins, and modification of the risk factors noted above. Those individuals with >50% symptomatic extracranial carotid artery stenosis (again >60% for asymptomatic) should be referred for evaluation for CEA, as arteriotomy and removal of the blockage has been shown to provide reductions in 5-year morbidity and mortality superior to medical therapy alone.[25,31,66,76,103] While we embrace in theory the concept and appeal of carotid stenting, we have not been presented with data that shows that these techniques, at present, offer superior or even equivalent outcomes in the majority of carotid disease patients. In our practice, we have endovascular specialists on our neurosurgical staff, and we offer a CAS option to all patients, with the caveat that it remains at present a less preferable treatment if CEA is performed by a qualified surgeon with reproducible results.

REFERENCES

1. Fung AY, Saw J. Epidemiology and significance of carotid artery stenosis. In: Saw J, Exaire JE, Lee DS, et al., editors. Handbook Of Complex Percutaneous Carotid Intervention Contemporary Cardiology. Totowa, NJ: Humana Press Inc; 2007. p. 3–10.
2. Fine-Edelstein JS, Wolf PA, O'Leary DH, et al. Precursors of extracranial carotid atherosclerosis in the Framingham Study. Neurology 1994;44:1046–50.
3. Longstreth WT Jr, Shemanski L, Lefkowitz D, et al. Asymptomatic internal carotid artery stenosis defined by ultrasound and the risk of subsequent stroke in the elderly. The Cardiovascular Health Study. Stroke 1998;29:2371–6.
4. Meissner I, Whisnant JP, Khandheria BK, et al. Prevalence of potential risk factors for stroke assessed by transesophageal echocardiography and carotid ultrasonography: the SPARC study. Stroke Prevention: Assessment of Risk in a Community. Mayo Clin Proc 1999;74:862–9.
5. Pujia A, Rubba P, Spencer MP. Prevalence of extracranial carotid artery disease detectable by echo-Doppler in an elderly population. Stroke 1992;23:818–22.
6. Kistler JP, Ropper AH, Heros RC. Therapy of ischemic cerebral vascular disease due to atherothrombosis. N Engl J Med 1984; 311:27–34.
7. Fisher CM. Observations of the fundus oculi in transient monocular blindness. Neurology 1959;9:333–47.
8. Hedera P, Bujdakova J, Traubner P. Effect of collateral flow patterns on outcome of carotid occlusion. Eur Neurol 1995;35:212–16.
9. Kleiser B, Widder B. Course of carotid artery occlusions with impaired cerebrovascular reactivity. Stroke 1992;23:171–4.
10. Loftus CM, editor. Carotid endarterectomy: principles and technique. New York: Informa Healthcare; 2007.
11. Rothwell PM, Gibson RJ, Slattery J, et al. Equivalence of measurements of carotid stenosis. A comparison of three methods on 1001 angiograms. European Carotid Surgery Trialists' Collaborative Group. Stroke 1994;25:2435–9.
12. Hatsukami TS, Ferguson MS, Beach KW, et al. Carotid plaque morphology and clinical events. Stroke 1997;28:95–100.
13. Carr S, Farb A, Pearce WH, et al. Atherosclerotic plaque rupture in symptomatic carotid artery stenosis. J Vasc Surg 1996;23: 755–63.
14. Moore WS, Barnett HJ, Beebe HG, et al. Guidelines for carotid endarterectomy. A multidisciplinary consensus statement from the ad hoc committee, American Heart Association. Stroke 1995;26:188–201.
15. Rijbroek A, Wisselink W, Vriens EM, et al. Asymptomatic carotid artery stenosis: Past, present and future. How to improve patient selection? Eur Neurol 2006;6:139–54.
16. Roederer GO, Langlois YE, Lusiani L, et al. Natural history of carotid artery disease on the side contralateral to endarterectomy. J Vasc Surg 1984;1:62–72.
17. Johnson BF, Verlato F, Bergelin RO, et al. Clinical outcome in patients with mild and moderate carotid artery stenosis. J Vasc Surg 1995;21:120–6.
18. Mackey AE, Abrahamowicz M, Langlois Y, et al. Outcome of asymptomatic patients with carotid disease. Asymptomatic Cervical Bruit Study Group. Neurology 1997;48:896–903.

19. Dixon S, Pais SO, Raviola C, et al. Natural history of nonstenotic, asymptomatic ulcerative lesions of the carotid artery. A further analysis. Arch Surg 1982;117:1493–8.
20. Moore WS, Boren C, Malone JM, et al. Natural history of nonstenotic, asymptomatic ulcerative lesions of the carotid artery. Arch Surg 1978;113:1352–9.
21. Jones FL. Frequency, characteristics and importance of the cervical venous hum in adults. N Engl J Med 1962;267:658.
22. Sauve JS, Laupacis A, Ostbye T, et al. Does this patient have a clinically important carotid bruit? JAMA 1993;270:2843–5.
23. Caplan LR. Carotid artery disease. N Engl J Med 1963;315: 886.
24. Davies KN, Humphrey PRD. Do carotid bruits predict disease of the internal carotid arteries? Postgrad Med J 1994;70:433.
25. North American Symptomatic Carotid Endarterectomy Trial Collaborators. Beneficial effect of carotid endarterectomy in symptomatic patients with high-grade carotid stenosis. N Engl J Med 1991;325:445–53.
26. Toole JF, Baker WH, Castaldo JE, et al. Endarterectomy for asymptomatic carotid artery stenosis. JAMA 1995;273:1421–8.
27. Ballotta E, DaGiau G, Abbruzzese E, et al. Carotid endarterectomy without angiography: can clinical evaluation and duplex ultrasonographic scanning alone replace traditional arteriography for carotid surgery workup? A prospective study. Surgery 1999;126:20–7.
28. Raoult H, Gauvrit JY, Schmitt P, et al. Non-ECG-gated unenhanced MRA of the carotids: Optimization and clinical feasibility. Eur Radiol 2013;23:3020–8.
29. Loftus CM, editor. Carotid Endarterectomy: Principles and Technique. St. Louis: Quality Medical Publishing; 1995.
30. Loftus CM, Kresowik TF, editors. Carotid Artery Surgery. New York: Thieme Medical Publishers; 2000.
31. Loftus CM, editor. Carotid Artery Surgery: Principles and Technique. 2nd ed. New York: Informa Publishing; 2006.
32. Anderson KM, Odell PM, Wilson PW, et al. Cardiovascular disease risk profiles. Am Heart J 1991;121:293–8.
33. Anderson KM, Wilson PW, Odell PM, et al. An updated coronary risk profile: a statement for health professionals. Circulation 1991;83:356–62.
34. Taylor DW, Barnett HJ, Haynes RB, et al. Low-dose and high-dose acetylsalicylic acid for patients undergoing carotid endarterectomy: A randomised controlled trial. ASA and Carotid Endarterectomy (ACE) Trial Collaborators. Lancet 1999;353: 2179–84.
35. Lindblad B, Persson N, Takolander R, et al. Does low-dose acetylsalicylic acid prevent stroke after carotid surgery? A double-blind, placebo-controlled randomized trial. Stroke 1993;24: 1125–8.
36. Antithrombotic Trialist's Collaboration. Aspirin in the primary and secondary prevention of vascular disease: collaborative meta-analysis of individual participant data from randomized trials. Lancet 2009;373:1849–60.
37. Wolff T, Miller T, Ko S. Aspirin for the prevention of cardiovascular events: An Update of the Evidence for the U.S. Preventive Services Task Force. Ann Intern Med 2009;150:396–404.
38. Wong KS, Chen C, Fu J, et al. Clopidogrel plus aspirin versus aspirin alone for reducing embolisation in patients with acute symptomatic cerebral or carotid artery stenosis (CLAIR study): a randomized, open-label, blinded-endpoint trial. CLAIR Study Investigators. Lancet Neurol 2010;9:489–97.
39. Diener HC, Cunha L, Forbes C, et al. European Stroke Prevention Study 2. Dipyridamole and acetylsalicylic acid in the secondary prevention of stroke. J Neurol Sci 1996;143:1–13.
40. Halkes PH, van Gijn J, Kapelle LJ, et al. Aspirin plus dipyridamole versus aspirin alone after cerebral ischaemia of arterial origin (ESPRIT): randomized controlled trial. Lancet 2006;367: 1665–73.
41. Diener HC, Bogousslavsky J, Brass LM, et al. Aspirin and clopidogrel compared with clopidogrel alone after recent ischaemic stroke or transient ischaemic attack in high-risk patients (MATCH): randomized, double-blind, placebo-controlled trial. MATCH Investigators. Lancet 2004;364:331–7.
42. Bhatt DL, Fox KA, Hacke W, et al. Clopidogrel and aspirin versus aspirin alone for the prevention of atherothrombotic events. CHARISMA Investigators. N Engl J Med 2006;354:1706–17.
43. Sillesen H, Amarenco P, Hennerici MG, et al. Atorvastatin reduces the risk of cardiovascular events in patients with carotid atherosclerosis: a secondary analysis of the Stroke Prevention by Aggressive Reduction in Cholesterol Levels (SPARCL) trial. Stroke 2008;39:3297–302.
44. Tuñón J, Martin-Ventura JL, Blanco-Colio LM, et al. Mechanisms of action of statins in stroke. Expert Opin Ther Targets 2007;11: 273–8.
45. Baker WH, Howard VJ, Howard G, et al. Effect of contralateral occlusion on long-term efficacy of endarterectomy in the asymptomatic carotid atherosclerosis study (ACAS). ACAS Investigators. Stroke 2000;31:2330–4.
46. Chang J, Ahn J, Landsman N, et al. Efficacy of contemporary medical management for asymptomatic carotid artery stenosis. Am Surg 2013;79:987–91.
47. Patti G, Tomai F, Melfi R, et al. Strategies of clopidogrel load and atorvastatin reload to prevent ischemic cerebral events in patients undergoing protected carotid stenting. Results of the randomized ARMYDA-9 CAROTID (Clopidogrel and Atorvastatin Treatment During Carotid Artery Stenting) study. J Am Coll Cardiol 2013;61:1379–87.
48. Heyer EJ, Mergeche JL, Bruce SS, et al. Statins reduce neurologic injury in asymptomatic carotid endarterectomy patients. Stroke 2013;44:1150–2.
49. Kolos I, Loukianov M, Dupik N, et al. Optimal medical treatment versus carotid endarterectomy: the rationale and design of the Aggressive Medical Treatment Evaluation for Asymptomatic Carotid Artery Stenosis (AMTEC) study. Int J Stroke 2013;[Epub ahead of print].
50. Fields WS, Maslenikov V, Meyer JS, et al. Joint Study of Extracranial Arterial Occlusion. V. Progress report of prognosis following surgery or nonsurgical treatment for transient cerebral ischemic attacks and cervical carotid artery lesions. JAMA 1970; 211:1993–2003.
51. The CASANOVA Study Group. Carotid surgery versus medical therapy in asymptomatic carotid stenosis. Stroke 1991;22:1229–35.
52. Mayo Asymptomatic Carotid Endarterectomy Study Group. Results of a randomized controlled trial of carotid endarterectomy for asymptomatic carotid stenosis. Mayo Clin Proc 1992;67:513–18.
53. Executive Committee for the Asymptomatic Carotid Atherosclerosis Study. Endarterectomy for asymptomatic carotid artery stenosis. JAMA 1995;273:1421–8.
54. Hobson RW 2nd, Weiss DG, Fields WS, et al. Efficacy of carotid endarterectomy for asymptomatic carotid stenosis. The Veterans Affairs Cooperative Study Group. N Engl J Med 1993;328(4): 221–7.
55. Halliday A, Mansfield A, Marro J, et al. Prevention of disabling and fatal strokes by successful carotid endarterectomy in patients without recent neurological symptoms: Randomised controlled trial. MRC Asymptomatic Carotid Surgery Trial (ACST) Collaborative Group. Lancet 2004;363:1491–502.
56. Irvine CD, Cole SE, Foley PX, et al. Unilateral asymptomatic carotid disease does not require surgery. Eur J Vasc Endovasc Surg 1998;16:245–53.
57. AbuRahma AF, Metz MJ, Robinson PA. Natural history of > or =60% asymptomatic carotid stenosis in patients with contralateral carotid occlusion. Ann Surg 2003;238:551–61.
58. Gasecki AP, Eliasziw M, Ferguson GG, et al. Long-term prognosis and effect of endarterectomy in patients with symptomatic severe carotid stenosis and contralateral carotid stenosis or occlusion: Results from NASCET. North American Symptomatic Carotid Endarterectomy Trial (NASCET) Group. J Neurosurg 1995;83:778–82.
59. Taylor DW, Barnett HJM, Haynes RB, et al. Low-dose and high-dose acetylsalicylic acid for patients undergoing carotid endarterectomy: a randomised controlled trial. Lancet 1999;353:2179–84.
60. Reed AB, Gaccione P, Belkin M, et al. Preoperative risk factors for carotid endarterectomy: Defining the patient at high risk. J Vasc Surg 2003;37:1191–9.
61. Duncan JM, Reul GJ, Ott DA, et al. Outcomes and risk factors in 1,609 carotid endarterectomies. Tex Heart Inst J 2008;35:104–10.
62. Mackey WC, O'Donnell TF Jr, Callow AD. Carotid endarterectomy contralateral to an occluded carotid artery: Perioperative risk and late results. J Vasc Surg 1990;11:778–83.

63. Ballotta E, Da Giau G, Baracchini C. Carotid endarterectomy contralateral to carotid artery occlusion: Analysis from a randomized study. Langenbecks Arch Surg 2002;387:216–21.
64. Pulli R, Dorigo W, Barbanti E, et al. Carotid endarterectomy with contralateral carotid artery occlusion: Is this a higher risk subgroup? Eur J Vasc Endovasc Surg 2002;24:63–8.
65. Rockman CB, Su W, Lamparello PJ, et al. Reassessment of carotid endarterectomy in the face of contralateral carotid occlusion: Surgical results in symptomatic and asymptomatic patients. J Vasc Surg 2002;36:668–73.
66. European Carotid Surgery Trialists' Collaborative Group. MRC European Carotid Surgery Trial: Interim results for symptomatic patients with severe (70-99%) or with mild (0-29%) carotid stenosis. Lancet 1991;337:1235–43.
67. Mayberg MR, Wilson SE, Yatsu F, et al. Carotid endarterectomy and prevention of cerebral ischemia in symptomatic carotid stenosis. Veterans Affairs Cooperative Studies Program 309 Trialist Group. JAMA 1991;266:3289–94.
68. Adams RJ, Albers G, Alberts MJ, et al. Update to the AHA/ASA recommendations for the prevention of stroke in patients with stroke and transient ischemic attack. Stroke 2008;39: 1647–52.
69. Sacco RL, Adams R, Albers G, et al. Guidelines for prevention of stroke in patients with ischemic stroke or transient ischemic attack: A statement for healthcare professionals from the American Heart Association/American Stroke Association Council on Stroke: co-sponsored by the Council on Cardiovascular Radiology and Intervention: The American Academy of Neurology affirms the value of this guideline. Stroke 2006;37:577–617.
70. Rothwell PM, Eliasziw M, Gutnikov SA, et al. Analysis of pooled data from the randomised controlled trials of endarterectomy for symptomatic carotid stenosis. Lancet 2003;361(9352): 107–16.
71. Rothwell PM, Eliasziw M, Gutnikov SA, et al. Endarterectomy for symptomatic carotid stenosis in relation to clinical subgroups and timing of surgery. Lancet 2004;363(9413):915–24.
72. Henderson RD, Eliasziw M, Fox AJ, et al. Angiographically defined collateral circulation and risk of stroke in patients with severe carotid artery stenosis. North American Symptomatic Carotid Endarterectomy Trial (NASCET) Group. Stroke 2000;31: 128–32.
73. Kappelle LJ, Eliasziw M, Fox AJ, et al. Importance of intracranial atherosclerotic disease in patients with symptomatic stenosis of the internal carotid artery. The North American Symptomatic Carotid Endarterectomy Trial. Stroke 1999;30:282–6.
74. Streifler JY, Eliasziw M, Benavente OR, et al. Prognostic importance of leukoaraiosis in patients with symptomatic internal carotid artery stenosis. Stroke 2002;33:1651–5.
75. Eliasziw M, Streifler JY, Fox AJ, et al. Significance of plaque ulceration in symptomatic patients with high-grade carotid stenosis. North American Symptomatic Carotid Endarterectomy Trial. Stroke 1994;25:304–8.
76. Loftus CM. Carotid endarterectomy: The asymptomatic carotid. In: Batjer HH, editor. Cerebrovascular Disease. New York: Lippincott-Raven; 1996. p. 409–20.
77. Halliday AW, Thomas D, Mansfield A, et al. The Asymptomatic Carotid Surgery Trial (ACST). Rationale and design. Eur J Vasc Surg 1994;8:703–10.
78. Mas JL, Chatellier G, Beyssen B, et al. Endarterectomy versus stenting in patients with symptomatic severe carotid stenosis. EVA-3S Investigators. N Engl J Med 2006;355:1660–71.
79. Ringleb PA, Allenberg J, Brückmann H, et al. 30 day results from the SPACE trial of stent-protected angioplasty versus carotid endarterectomy in symptomatic patients: a randomised non-inferiority trial. Lancet 2006;368:1239–47.
80. CAVATAS Investigators. Endovascular versus surgical treatment in patients with carotid stenosis in the Carotid and Vertebral Artery Transluminal Angioplasty Study (CAVATAS): a randomised trial. Lancet 2001;357:1729–37.
81. CARESS Steering Committee. Carotid Revascularization using Endarterectomy or Stenting Systems (CARESS): phase I clinical trial. J Endovasc Ther 2003;10:1021–30.
82. Naylor AR, Bolia A, Abbott RJ, et al. Randomized study of carotid angioplasty and stenting versus carotid endarterectomy: a stopped trial. J Vasc Surg 1998;28:326–34.
83. Brooks WH, McClure RR, Jones MR. Carotid angioplasty and stenting versus carotid endarterectomy: randomized trial in a community hospital. J Am Coll Cardiol 2001;38:1589–95.
84. Alberts MJ, McCann R, Smith TP. A randomized trial of carotid stenting versus endarterectomy in patients with symptomatic carotid stenosis: study design. J Neurovasc Dis 1997;2: 228–34.
85. Yadav JS, Wholey MH, Kuntz RE, et al. Protected carotid-artery stenting versus endarterectomy in high risk patients. Stenting and Angioplasty with Protection in Patients at High Risk for Endarterectomy (SAPPHIRE) Investigators. N Engl J Med 2004; 351:1493–501.
86. Gurm HS, Yadav JS, Fayad P, et al. Long-term results of carotid stenting versus endarterectomy in high-risk patients. SAPPHIRE Investigators. New Engl J Med 2008;358:1572–9.
87. Alberts MJ. Results of a multicenter prospective randomized trial of carotid artery stenting vs carotid endarterectomy. Stroke 2001; 32:325.
88. Brott TG, Hobson RW 2nd, Howard G, et al. CREST Investigators: Stenting versus endarterectomy for treatment of carotid-artery stenosis. N Engl J Med 2010;363:80–2.
89. Silver FL, Mackey A, Clark WM, et al. Safety of stenting and endearterectomy by symptomatic status in the Carotid Revascularization Endarterectomy Versus Stenting Trial (CREST). CREST Investigators. Stroke 2011;42:675–80.
90. International Carotid Stenting Study investigators, Ederle J, Dobson J, et al. Carotid artery stenting compared with endarterectomy in patients with symptomatic carotid stenosis (International Carotid Stenting Study): An interim analysis of a randomised controlled trial. Lancet 2010;375:985–97.
91. Paciaroni M, Caso V, Acciarresi M, et al. Management of asymptomatic carotid stenosis in patients undergoing general and vascular surgical procedures. J Neurol Neurosurg Psychiatry 2005; 76:1332–6.
92. Naylor AR, Mehta Z, Rothwell PM, et al. Carotid artery disease and stroke during coronary artery bypass: A critical review of the literature. Eur J Vasc Endovasc Surg 2002;23:283–94.
93. Hillis LD, Smith PK, Anderson JL, et al. 2011 ACCF/AHA Guideline for Coronary Artery Bypass Graft Surgery: A Report of the American College of Cardiology Foundation/American Heart Association Task Force on Practice Guidelines. Circulation 2011; 124:e652–735.
94. Shishehbor MH, Venkatachalam S, Sun Z, et al. A direct comparison of early and late outcomes with three approaches to carotid revascularization and open heart surgery. J Am Coll Cardiol 2013;62:1948–56.
95. Hedayati N, Humphries MD, Zhou W. Gender and outcomes of carotid artery interventions. Vasc Endovascular Surg 2014;48: 99–105.
96. Di Carlo A, Lamassa M, Baldereschi M, et al. Sex differences in the clinical presentation, resource use, and 3-month outcome of acute stroke in Europe: data from a multicenter multinational hospital-based registry. Stroke 2003;34:1114–19.
97. Poisson SN, Johnston SC, Sidney S, et al. Gender differences in treatment of severe carotid stenosis after transient ischemic attack. Stroke 2010;41:1891–5.
98. Vouyouka AG, Egorova NN, Sosunov EA, et al. Analysis of Florida and New York state hospital discharges suggests that carotid stenting in symptomatic women is associated with significant increase in mortality and perioperative morbidity compared with carotid endarterectomy. J Vasc Surg 2012;56: 334–42.
99. ALLHAT Officers and Coordinators for the ALLHAT Collaborative Research Group. Major outcomes in high-risk hypertensive patients randomized to angiotensin-converting enzyme inhibitor or calcium channel blocker vs diuretic: The Antihypertensive and Lipid-Lowering Treatment to Prevent Heart Attack Trial (ALLHAT). JAMA 2002;288:2981–97.
100. Neal B, MacMahon S, Chapman N. Blood Pressure Lowering Treatment Trialists' Collaboration. Effects of ACE inhibitors, calcium antagonists, and other blood-pressure-lowering drugs: results of prospectively designed overviews of randomised trials. Lancet 2000;356:1955–64.
101. Collins R, Peto R, MacMahon S. Blood pressure, stroke, and coronary heart disease, part 2: short-term reductions in blood

pressure: overview of randomised drug trials in their epidemiological context. Lancet 1990;335:827–38.

102. Colhoun HM, Betteridge DJ, Durrington PN, et al. Primary prevention of cardiovascular disease with atorvastatin in type 2 diabetes in the Collaborative Atorvastatin Diabetes Study (CARDS): multicentre randomised placebo-controlled trial. CARDS investigators. Lancet 2004;364:685–96.

103. Executive Committee for the Asymptomatic Carotid Atherosclerosis Study. Endarterectomy for asymptomatic carotid stenosis. JAMA 1995;273:1421–8.

75 Extracranial to Intracranial Bypass for Cerebral Ischemia

David W. Newell, Marcelo D. Vilela, William J. Powers

KEY POINTS

- Extracranial to intracranial bypass is effective in providing additional blood flow to the middle cerebral artery from the extracranial circulation for cerebral ischemia.
- Prospective randomized trials have shown that the procedure does not reduce subsequent stroke in patients presenting with ischemic symptoms and carotid occlusion with hemodynamic impairment.
- Bypass is frequently used to treat patients with moyamoya and cerebral ischemia, although controlled trials regarding its efficacy for stroke prevention are lacking.

Bypass is used to augment blood flow to prevent cerebral ischemia with planned vessel occlusion for complex aneurysms or skull-base tumor.

Providing additional blood supply to the brain in order to treat or prevent stroke has been a goal of neurosurgeons and neurologists for many decades. The concept of an extracranial to intracranial (EC–IC) bypass to increase brain blood flow in patients with symptoms caused by complete carotid artery occlusion was first suggested by C Miller Fisher[1] in 1951. The development of the operating microscope and advances in microsurgical techniques led to the field of cerebrovascular microsurgery and the possibility for surgical creation of direct connections between the extracranial and intracranial vasculature. In 1963, Woringer and Kunlin[2] sutured a saphenous vein graft from the cervical portion of the internal carotid artery (ICA) to its intracranial portion (intracranial ICA). The graft remained patent at the time of the patient's death from coronary artery disease a few days later. A subsequent report by Pool and Potts[3] describes an intracranial bypass graft to the anterior cerebral artery for a giant aneurysm. In 1967 the first superficial temporal artery to middle cerebral artery (STA–MCA) bypass was performed in a human by M.G. Yasargil, which led to the development of a series of new procedures for cerebral revascularization. During the decades that followed, this technique and other variations were employed as surgical treatments for occlusive cerebrovascular disease of the extracranial and intracranial cerebral vessels, skull base tumors, aneurysms, cerebral vasospasm, moyamoya disease, and cerebral ischemia from other causes. This chapter reviews the development of EC–IC bypass and the current status of this procedure for the treatment of cerebral ischemia.

HISTORICAL ASPECTS

Development of the Surgical Technique

The introduction of microvascular surgery to neurosurgery was made possible by the combined efforts and ideas of surgeons between 1960 and 1970. Some of the early investigators of the applications of these techniques were surgeons at the University of Vermont in Burlington. Jacobson and Suarez[4] employed the microscope to repair vessels in small animals using the principles and techniques introduced by Alexis Carrel, and were successful in achieving a 100% patency rate after reconstructing carotid arteries in animals using 7.0 atraumatic silk. R.M.P. Donaghy, in the division of Neurosurgery at the University of Vermont, conducted early investigations in the applications of microvascular techniques to the field of neurosurgery reconstructing vessels less than 1 mm in diameter.[5,6]

M.G. Yasargil, working in the Department of Neurosurgery in Zurich under Professor Hugo Krayenbuhl, also became interested in neurosurgical applications of microvascular surgery. In 1965, Yasargil received training in Professor Donaghy's laboratory in Burlington, Vermont, in microvascular techniques utilizing the femoral and carotid arteries of small animals.[7] In 1966, the availability of a bipolar coagulator, together with the use of 9-0 sutures, allowed a major advance in the development of microsurgical revascularization, enabling the dissection of intracranial structures in a clean field and meticulous repair of intracranial vessels.[6] An approach of performing a bypass from the STA to the MCA was utilized. By the end of 1966, more than 30 such STA–MCA operations in dogs had been performed, and the technique was later published in detail.[8]

Yasargil returned to Zurich and performed the first STA–MCA bypass on October 30, 1967, on a patient with Marfan's syndrome and a complete occlusion of the MCA.[6,9] Another STA–MCA bypass procedure was performed independently 1 day later by Donaghy. Yasargil later published a manuscript describing a series of nine cases in which STA–MCA bypass had been performed, in seven for occlusion of the internal carotid or middle cerebral artery and in two as an adjuvant to the surgical treatment of complex intracranial aneurysms.[6] The feasibility of creating an EC–IC shunt was thereby demonstrated, and a major step was made into the field of reconstructive intracranial vascular microneurosurgery.

Most EC–IC bypasses in the past were STA–MCA bypasses done for atherosclerotic cerebrovascular disease, but the procedure also became useful as an adjunct in the treatment of certain intracranial aneurysms or tumors that required flow augmentation, for planned vessel sacrifice, in carotid dissections with ischemia (Figs 75.1–75.3), and for moyamoya disease.[10] Subsequently, bypass grafts using other donor arteries and the creation of interposition vein grafts between extracranial and intracranial arteries[11] (Fig. 75.1, *right*) as well as direct intracranial arterial to arterial anastomoses have been developed.[12,13] The use of non-suture techniques for STA–MCA bypass has also been described.[14]

EXTRACRANIAL TO INTRACRANIAL BYPASS IN ACUTE STROKE

In the past, the idea of performing an emergency cerebral revascularization procedure for acute ischemic stroke was reasonable, given the knowledge of ischemic thresholds for

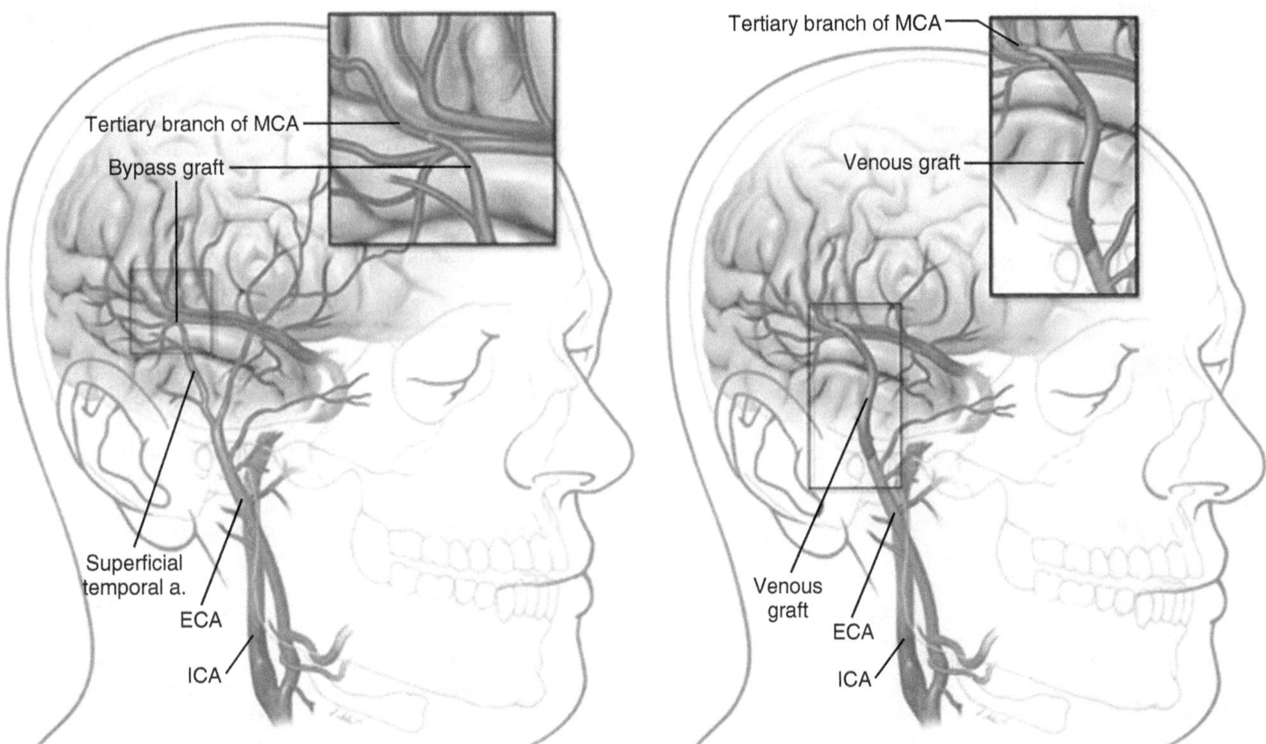

Figure 75-1. *Left,* Illustration of the completed superficial temporal artery (STA) to middle cerebral artery (MCA) (STA-MCA) bypass showing the frontoparietal branch of the STA connected to a distal surface branch of the MCA, immediately after it emerges from the distal portion of the Sylvian fissure. *Right,* Illustration of an extracranial to intracranial bypass using a saphenous vein interposition graft from the proximal STA to a distal MCA branch. ECA, external carotid artery; ICA, internal carotid artery.

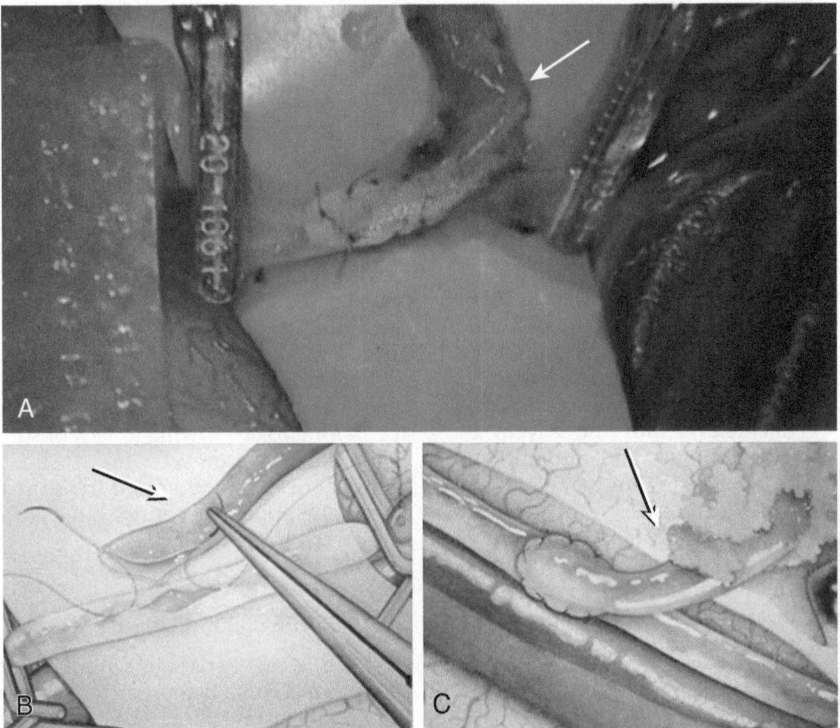

Figure 75-2. Intra-operative photographs (A and C) and drawing (B) of direct superficial temporal *(arrows)* to middle cerebral artery bypass using a microsuture technique with 10-0 suture to accomplish an end-to-side microvascular anastomosis at a cortical surface branch of the middle cerebral artery.

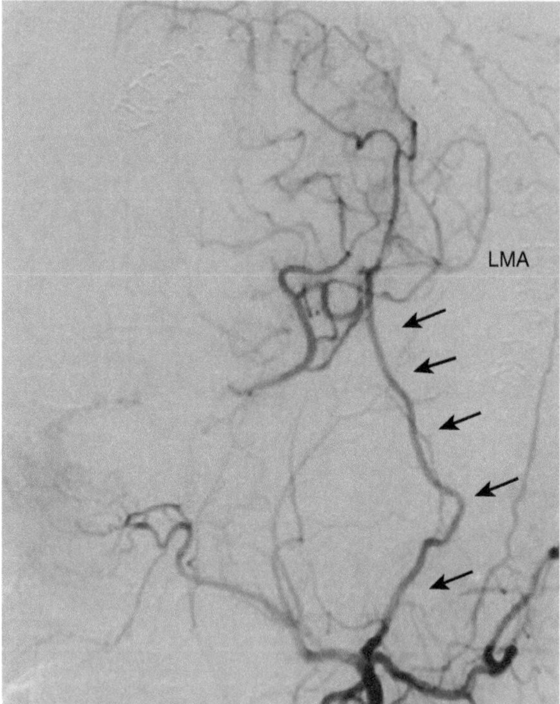

Figure 75-3. Angiogram of a selective injection of the external carotid artery leading to a superficial temporal artery *(arrows)* to middle cerebral artery bypass showing filling of the middle cerebral artery distribution from the graft. LMA, Left middle cerebral artery.

infarction and the concept of ischemic penumbra.[15] A method to provide additional blood flow to areas of the brain where the regional cerebral blood flow (rCBF) was insufficient to stop cellular function but not low enough to produce infarction was rational. Some encouraging results were initially published, but other subsequent studies reported that acute cerebral ischemia was a relative contraindication to an emergency bypass owing to poor results and a high rate of complications.[15-17]

Differentiation between regions of acute infarction and potentially salvageable regions with low flow (ischemic penumbra) is now possible with a combination of diffusion-weighted imaging (DWI) MRI, perfusion MRI, perfusion CT/CTA, and PET scans.[18-21] Within the penumbra zone, it may also be possible to differentiate those areas that will infarct without reperfusion from those regions that will most likely survive even without reperfusion.[19,20] More recently, anecdotal case reports on emergency surgical revascularization for acute stroke have demonstrated restoration of normal flow to regions of ischemic penumbra and improvement in perfusion–diffusion mismatch.[22,23] Nonetheless, with the advent of interventional neuroradiology techniques and thrombolytic therapies,[24,25] the interest in performing emergency EC–IC bypass for acute ischemic stroke decreased.[26] On the other hand, even though urgent surgical revascularization procedures for acute stroke would seem a reasonable area of interest in those patients with a contraindication to thrombolytic therapy, high rates of recanalization have been demonstrated with the use of new endovascular revascularization devices.

Experience with Bypass for Ischemia from Cerebral Vasospasm

Batjer and Samson[27] reported on 11 patients who received an STA–MCA bypass in the setting of symptomatic vasospasm. Six patients improved in the first 24 hours after surgery, and deficits were stabilized in two other patients. Benzel and Kesterson[28] also reported encouraging results and reversal of neurologic deficits in a patient with symptomatic vasospasm refractory to medical therapy who underwent STA–MCA bypass. This indication for the procedure, however, did not gain wide acceptance and the use of nimodipine, induced hypertension, endovascular techniques such as balloon angioplasty and intra-arterial injection of vasodilators are now favored in the management of cerebral vasospasm.[29,30]

Bypass for Occlusive Cerebrovascular Disease Not Amenable to Carotid Endarterectomy

Yasargil's first report of STA–MCA bypass described its use for occlusive cerebrovascular disease of the internal carotid or middle cerebral artery.[6,9] The procedure was still considered experimental at that time, however, because of a lack of proof of efficacy in stroke prevention and uncertain indications.[31,32]

The North American EC–IC Bypass Study was initiated in 1977, to compare best medical therapy with STA–MCA bypass plus medical therapy for patients with symptomatic occluded or high-grade atherosclerotic stenotic lesions of the MCA or internal carotid artery (ICA) not amenable to endarterectomy.[32] The objective of the study was to determine whether an STA–MCA anastomosis would decrease the incidence of stroke and stroke-related death in those patients. The study randomly assigned 714 patients to best medical treatment and 663 patients to an STA–MCA bypass plus best medical treatment. The 30-day surgical mortality and major stroke morbidity rates were 0.6% and 2.5%, respectively. In the surgical group, fatal and non-fatal strokes occurred earlier and more frequently. The study investigators concluded that the STA–MCA bypass was ineffective in preventing cerebral ischemia in patients with atherosclerotic disease of the MCA and ICA not amenable to endarterectomy.[32,33,34] There was no evidence that any subgroup of patients benefited from the procedure. Even though the study was considered well conducted regarding its methodology and follow-up,[34] a number of criticisms of the study included the issues regarding selection bias and generalizability.[35-38]

Subsequently, a committee appointed by the American Association of Neurological Surgeons was then encouraged to examine the study with emphasis on two aspects: *the randomized trial cohort* and *patients operated on outside the trial.*[39] Within the randomization trial cohort, none of the issues listed was judged to compromise either the design of the trial or any conclusions of the study. Regarding the number of patients operated on outside the trial, a report by Sundt indicated that at least 2500 patients underwent bypass done outside the study in participating centers.[39,40] This fact raised the concern whether the EC–IC bypass trial study conclusions could or could not be generalizable to the entire population at risk for stroke.[40] Owing to lack of sufficient data, this question could not be answered fully.[40] The study investigators also pointed out that randomized trials involve only a small fraction of the population at risk but this fact does not prevent a study from being valid.[41]

Occlusive Cerebrovascular Disease with Hemodynamic Insufficiency

After the EC–IC bypass trial results, a few centers continued to perform EC–IC bypass surgery for the treatment of symptomatic occlusion of the ICA in selected patients, with good outcomes. Indications for the procedure were based on evidence of perfusion abnormalities on imaging studies or presence of symptoms despite maximal medical management.[42-49]

This group of patients included those with demonstrated reduced cerebrovascular reserve and either recurrent ischemic symptoms or disabling transient ischemic attacks (TIAs), including limb-shaking TIAs.

The occurrence of ischemic symptoms and stroke in occlusive cerebrovascular disease can usually be attributed to thromboembolic phenomena, a decrease in cerebral perfusion pressure, or a combination of the two mechanisms.[51,52] A prospective study by Powers et al.[53] identified stroke risks of 0% at 2 years and 4.4% at 3 years in the group of never-symptomatic patients, in contrast to stroke risks of 7.7% at 1 year, 19% at 2 years, and 21% at 3 years for symptomatic patients with ICA occlusion.

Several studies have evaluated the prognostic value of measurements of cerebral hemodynamics on stroke risk in symptomatic carotid occlusion or MCA stenosis/occlusion. Data on vasomotor reactivity to acetazolamide or hypercapnia in predicting subsequent stroke have been inconsistent.[54–61] Different techniques rely on different physiologic mechanisms from which the presence of reduced perfusion pressure is inferred. Evidence that hemodynamic impairment by one method of assessment predicts subsequent stroke risk does not prove the predictive value of a similar method. For example, in a well-conducted prospective study, Ogasawara and colleagues showed that quantitative measurement of the ipsilateral CBF response to acetazolamide with xenon-133 was significantly associated with the subsequent risk of stroke, whereas the use of the change in hemisphere asymmetry index was not.[59,60] In contrast, increased oxygen extraction fraction (OEF) measured by positron emission tomography (PET) has been consistently shown to be a predictor of subsequent ipsilateral ischemic stroke. The aggregate 2-year risk for ipsilateral ischemic stroke from four studies that provide these data are 22/71 (31%) for those with increased OEF and 7/200 (3.5%) for those without.[62–65]

Several investigators have described the effects of STA–MCA bypass on improvement of rCBF, regional cerebral metabolic rate for oxygen ($rCMRO_2$), cerebral blood volume (CBV), and OEF, in patients with occlusive cerebrovascular disease. More importantly, there were a demonstrable reversal of the state of "misery perfusion" and marked improvements in regional CBF and $CMRO_2$ in the subpopulation of patients with hemodynamic impairment who underwent a revascularization procedure.[43–46,50,66–70]

The evidence that patients with carotid occlusion and increased OEF have an increased risk of stroke and the substantiation that an EC–IC bypass may reverse this stage of "misery perfusion" served as the basis for the Carotid Occlusion Surgery Study (COSS).

COSS was a prospective, randomized, blinded end-point, controlled trial conducted in 49 clinical centers and 18 PET centers in the United States and Canada beginning in 2002. COSS was designed to determine whether EC–IC bypass can reduce subsequent ipsilateral ischemic stroke at 2 years in participants with recent hemispheric symptoms from internal carotid artery occlusion and hemodynamic cerebral ischemia identified by an ipsilateral increased OEF.

In 2010, COSS was stopped by the Data, Safety and Monitoring Board based on a futility analysis of 139 patients who had already completed 2-year follow-up. The final intention-to-treat analysis based on all 195 randomized patients (98 randomized to medical therapy only and 97 randomized to additional EC–IC bypass surgery) showed no difference between the two groups. The 2-year ipsilateral stoke rates were 21.0% for the surgical group and 22.7% for the non-surgical group ($P = 0.78$). Ipsilateral ischemic strokes occurred in 14 surgical patients in the 30-day post-operative period. Only six additional surgical patients experienced an ipsilateral stroke within the subsequent 2 years. Thirty-day graft patency was 98% and patency at last follow-up was 96%. The mean OEF ratio in the surgical group improved from 1.258 at baseline to 1.109 at the 30–60-day post-operative repeat PET scan (87 with data).[70]

Although COSS failed to prove the clinical efficacy of EC–IC bypass for stroke prevention in a sample of patients with recently symptomatic carotid occlusion and increased OEF who were at high risk for recurrent stroke, it confirmed the predictive accuracy of PET OEF for identifying a high-risk subgroup (22.7 % stroke rate at 2 years) and confirmed the hypothesis that improving cerebral hemodynamics in these patients will greatly reduce the risk of subsequent stroke. However, the peri-operative stroke rate was sufficient to nullify any overall benefit of surgery.

The Japanese EC–IC Bypass Trial (JET) used the combination of reduced baseline cerebral blood flow and reduced cerebral blood flow increase to the vasodilator acetazolamide as an eligibility criterion. Two-hundred and six patients with recently symptomatic (less than or equal to 3 months) major cerebral artery occlusive disease of the internal carotid artery or middle cerebral artery were enrolled from 1998–2002. Final results of the 2-year follow-up were due in 2004. In 2006, a second interim analysis with data for 196 patients followed through January 2002 reported primary endpoints in 14/98 medically treated patients and 5/98 surgically treated patients ($P = 0.046$ by Kaplan-Meier analysis).[71] Examination of the published Kaplan–Meier curves show no endpoints within the first month in the surgical group. There is no explicit mention whether the results include 30-day post-operative morbidity and mortality, but it seems unlikely that this rate was 0 given that it was 12% in the original EC–IC bypass trial and 15% in COSS. There has been no publication of the final results.

CURRENT TRENDS IN THE USE OF EXTRACRANIAL TO INTRACRANIAL BYPASS

Basic Surgical Technique

Standard STA–MCA Bypass

The patient is placed in the supine position, with the head turned to the contralateral side and a roll under the shoulder. The hair is shaved in an appropriate distribution along the course of the STA. A selective angiogram with selective external injection of the STA is quite helpful in defining the path of the artery (see Fig. 75.1). Surface mapping with portable continuous-wave Doppler ultrasound is performed to map out the course of the donor branch of the STA. A linear incision is made directly over the artery to its distal portion approximately 4 cm from the midline with use of a needle-point (Colorado tip) cautery unit (Colorado Biomedical, Inc., Evergreen, CO). The STA is then dissected from the surrounding galeal tissue with the needle-point cautery unit. Jeweler's bipolar forceps are also used to coagulate larger branches.

A point is selected approximately 6 cm superior to the external auditory meatus for the center of the bone flap, which allows selection of the most appropriate distal branch of the MCA as a recipient artery. The ideal recipient artery is on the surface, has an adequate straight portion without significant branching, and has a diameter of approximately 1.5 mm. The arachnoid is then divided directly over the recipient artery with an arachnoid knife and microscissors. A 1.5- to 2-cm segment of the artery is isolated, and a small rubber barrier is placed under the artery, allowing the arteriotomy and the anastomosis to be performed.

Attention is then directed to the distal portion of the STA. The artery is divided with sharp scissors in an angled fashion and is then spatulated with microscissors (see Fig. 75.2). The length of the spatulation should be approximately two times the diameter of the artery. After preparation of the donor artery, it is then brought onto the rubber barrier, where the recipient artery has been isolated.

After the arteriotomy, the recipient vessel is irrigated with heparinized saline solution, which also prevents sticking from residual blood products. With a tapered needle, a 10-0 microsuture is then used to anchor the spatulated end of the donor artery to the end of the arteriotomy made on the recipient vessel. A second suture is then placed at the distal portion of the vessel, and it is anchored to the contralateral end of the arteriotomy site. Surgeon's knots are tied at both ends to prevent slippage. Interrupted sutures are then placed on each side of the arteriotomy to complete the anastomosis (see Fig. 75.2). Alternatively, a running suture technique can be used to complete the anastomosis. The temporary clips are then removed from the vessels, establishing flow through the anastomosis.

The bone flap is then rongeured around the entry site of the donor artery through the craniotomy to ensure that there is no compression. Occasionally, the inside of the bone flap can be drilled out to create a groove for the artery if this is necessary. A generous space for the artery to pass through the bone and muscle is left. The STA in some patients may be inadequate to serve as donor vessel for an STA–MCA bypass. Several conditions could be responsible for an inadequate STA donor vessel. If no suitable artery exists, using a short vein graft as described by Little et al.[11] is a viable option.

Short Saphenous Vein Graft

The incision is made in front of the tragus and is carried down to the base of the ear. The dissection is carried along the tragus down to the tragal point. This step helps locate the facial nerve, which is typically within 1 cm inferior and anterior to the tragal point. The posterosuperior portion of the parotid gland is also typically found in this location. The gland is then mobilized forward so that the trunk of the STA can be identified. Intra-operative Doppler ultrasound is also helpful in locating the artery. The artery is then dissected, and a generous portion is mobilized to allow a 1- to 2-cm working segment.

Preparation of the Saphenous Vein Graft and Anastomosis

A short segment of saphenous vein graft is harvested from the leg for use as an interpositional graft. The distal portion of the saphenous vein is often smaller and more suitable for use than the proximal portion. We prefer performing the distal anastomosis first, a step that allows superior and inferior manipulation of the vessel and an easier placement of the sutures for the end-to-side anastomosis. After completion of the distal anastomosis in a manner similar to the technique described earlier, the vein graft is brought into apposition with the trunk of the STA. The vein is cut to the appropriate length in an angled fashion, and the end is spatulated. The STA trunk is prepared in a similar fashion, with an angled cut and spatulation. A 7-0 running vascular suture is then used to complete the end-to-end anastomosis (see Fig. 75.2B).

Occlusive Cerebrovascular Disease

Based on the results of the international EC–IC Bypass Trial and COSS and with the uncertainty surrounding the outcome of the JET study, EC–IC bypass should not be performed to prevent subsequent stroke in patients with ACAO or in any subgroups selected by clinical, arteriographic, or hemodynamic criteria [Class III, A].[72]

Moyamoya Disease

The first case of moyamoya disease treated with a direct STA–MCA bypass was performed in 1972 by Yasargil on a 4-year-old child, who had remarkable improvement following the procedure.[10] Post-operative angiograms showed patency of the anastomosis and evidence of collaterals from the vertebrobasilar system and other extracranial sources. In 1980 an indirect STA–MCA bypass for bilateral occlusion of the supraclinoid ICA was performed on a patient who had recurrent symptoms of hemiparesis and aphasia.[73] A direct STA–MCA bypass was planned, but at operation no suitable recipient cortical vessel was found and the STA and surrounding tissue were laid over the cerebral hemisphere and sutured to the arachnoid. The patient had a remarkable clinical recovery, and post-operative angiograms showed extensive collateral vessel formation, establishing the effectiveness of an indirect STA–MCA bypass as a form of cerebral revascularization.

In children the benefits of EC–IC bypass for improving symptoms, reversing neurologic deficits, enabling normal intelligence development, preventing further ischemic episodes, decreasing seizure activity, and even disappearance of involuntary movements have been observed.[74–84] Several studies addressing the efficacy of the direct and the indirect bypass techniques have been done in pediatric patients, and better clinical and angiographic results are usually seen when a direct bypass can be performed.[78,83–86]

Various studies have also demonstrated the benefits of STA–MCA bypass in ischemic adult moyamoya disease, preventing further ischemic episodes and improving clinical symptoms and cerebral hemodynamics.[79,87–94]

The occurrence of cerebral hyperperfusion syndrome following a STA–MCA bypass in moyamoya patients seems to be higher than previously thought and appropriate measures should be employed to prevent and/or treat symptomatic patients so as to avoid new neurological deficits.

On the other hand, in patients who present with hemorrhage, the effectiveness of revascularization in preventing hemorrhage still remains a controversy.[87,89,92,95] A large retrospective study involving 57 neurosurgical institutions in Japan analyzed 290 patients with the hemorrhagic form of moyamoya disease. Conservative treatment was given to 138 patients, and 152 patients received surgical revascularization. In the nonsurgical group, 28.3% of the patients had a recurrent hemorrhage during follow-up, in contrast to 19.1% in the surgical group. Another retrospective study, conducted in China, included 97 patients with hemorrhagic moyamoya disease, among whom 54 received a revascularization procedure (40 patients had a STA–MCA bypass either alone or in combination with an indirect procedure) and 43 were managed conservatively. During a mean follow-up period of 7.2 years, 21 patients had a rebleeding episode, four in the bypass group and 17 in the conservative group ($P < 0.001$), suggesting that a revascularization procedure might be effective in preventing new episodes of hemorrhage.[96–98] A large prospective randomized trial is ongoing in Japan to evaluate the effectiveness of STA–MCA bypass for the prevention of cerebral hemorrhage in moyamoya disease.

Aneurysms and Tumors

The specific threshold of lowered rCBF performed in conjunction with balloon occlusion tests indicating that the collateral circulation will be inadequate to prevent ischemia after permanent parent vessel occlusion remains to be determined.[99] The use of the STA–MCA bypass remains an important resource for the management of complex aneurysms and/or skull-base low-grade meningiomas in most centers, especially in cases in which there is a high likelihood of either parent and/or branch vessel occlusion during difficult clipping, which may indicate a role for EC–IC bypass as an adjunct to clip reconstruction and/or endovascular techniques.[100] New STA–MCA bypass techniques[14] may be useful in certain circumstances when a two-limb end-to-end bypass with good blood flow and short anastomotic time are needed.

CONCLUSIONS

The EC–IC bypass is a very elegant procedure, and the STA–MCA bypass developed by M.G. Yasargil was first applied on a widespread basis for the treatment of occlusive cerebrovascular disease. The STA–MCA bypass proved to be feasible with a low complication rate, but it has been shown to be ineffective in preventing stroke in populations harboring occlusive carotid or MCA disease, even in those with increased oxygen extraction fraction who have high risk of stroke. An international multicenter trial will probably further define the role of the STA–MCA bypass in the setting of hemorrhagic moyamoya disease. This elegant surgical technique will likely remain an important tool in properly selected patients for the management of intracranial aneurysms, skull-base tumors, and moyamoya disease.

Acknowledgments and Disclosure Statement

No financial support was provided for the completion of this study. There are no conflicts of interest disclosed by the authors. We would like to thank Raquel L. Abreu for her illustrations in Figure 75.2. Portions of this manuscript appear in the following article by the same authors: Vilela MD, Newell DW: Superficial temporal artery to middle cerebral artery bypass: Past, present, and future. *Neurosurg Focus* 24:E2, 2008.

REFERENCES

1. Fisher CM. Occlusion of the internal carotid artery. Arch Psychiatry 1951;65:346.
2. Woringer E, Kunlin J. Anastomose entre la carotide primitive et la carotide intra-craniene ou la sylvienne par greffon selon la technique de la suture suspendue. Neuro-Chir 1963;9:181–8.
3. Pool JL, Potts DG. Aneurysms and arteriovenous anomalies of the brain. New York: Hoeber; 1964. p. 221–2.
4. Jacobson JH, Suarez EL. Microsurgery in anastomosis of small vessels. Surg Forum 1960;243–5.
5. Jacobson JH 2nd, Wallman LJ, Schumacher GA, et al. Microsurgery as an aid to middle cerebral artery endarterectomy. J Neurosurg 1962;19:108–15.
6. Yasargil M, editor. Microsurgery applied to neurosurgery. Stuttgart: Georg Thieme; 1969.
7. Yasargil M. A legacy of microneurosurgery: Memoirs, lessons, and axioms. Neurosurgery 1999;45:1025–92.
8. Crowell RM, Yasargil MG. End-to-side anastomosis of superficial temporal artery to middle cerebral artery branch in the dog. Neurochirurgia (Stuttg) 1973;16:73–7.
9. Yasargil MG, Krayenbuhl HA, Jacobson JH. Microneurosurgical arterial reconstruction. Surgery 1970;67:221–33.
10. Krayenbuhl H. The moyamoya syndrome and the neurosurgeon. Surg Neurol 1975;4:353–60.
11. Little JR, Furlan AJ, Bryerton B. Short vein grafts for cerebral revascularization. J Neurosurg 1983;59:384–8.
12. Newell DW, Skirboll SL. Revascularization and bypass procedures for cerebral aneurysms. Neurosurg Clin North Am 1998; 9:697–711.
13. Onesti ST, Solomon RA, Quest DO. Cerebral revascularization: A review. Neurosurgery 1989;25:618–29.
14. Newell DW, Dailey AT, Skirboll SL. Intracranial vascular anastomosis using the microanastomotic system. Technical note. J Neurosurg 1998;89:676–81.
15. Crowell RMJJ. Emergency cerebral revascularization. Clin Neurosurg 1986;33:281–305.
16. Diaz FG, Ausman JI, Mehta B. Acute cerebral revascularization. J Neurosurg 1985;63:200–9.
17. Gratzl O, Schmiedek P, Spetzler RF. Clinical experience with extra-intracranial arterial anastomosis in 65 cases. J Neurosurg 1976;44:313–24.
18. Rohl L, Ostergaard L, Simonsen CZ. Viability thresholds of ischemic penumbra of hyperacute stroke defined by perfusion-weighted MRI and apparent diffusion coefficient. Stroke 2001;32: 1140–6.
19. Schaefer PW, Ozsunar Y, He J. Assessing tissue viability with MR diffusion and perfusion imaging. AJNR Am J Neuroradiol 2003; 24:436–43.
20. Sobesky J, Zaro Weber O, Lehnhardt FG, et al. Does the mismatch match the penumbra? Magnetic resonance imaging and positron emission tomography in early ischemic stroke. Stroke 2005;36:980–5.
21. Sobesky J, Zaro Weber O, Lehnhardt FG, et al. Which time-to-peak threshold best identifies penumbral flow? A comparison of perfusion-weighted magnetic resonance imaging and positron emission tomography in acute ischemic stroke. Stroke 2004;35: 2843–7.
22. Ogasawara K, Sasaki M, Tomitsuka N. Early revascularization in a patient with perfusion computed tomography/diffusion-weighted magnetic resonance imaging mismatch secondary to acute vertebral artery occlusion. Case report. Neurol Med Chir 2005;45:306–10.
23. Krishnamurthy S, Tong D, McNamara KP. Early carotid endarterectomy after ischemic stroke improves diffusion/perfusion mismatch on magnetic resonance imaging: Report of two cases. Neurosurgery 2003;52:238–41.
24. Broderick JP, Hacke W. Treatment of acute ischemic stroke. Part I: Recanalization strategies. Circulation 2002;106: 1563–9.
25. Tissue plasminogen activator for acute ischemic stroke: The National Institute of Neurological Disorders and Stroke rt-PA Stroke Study Group. N Engl J Med 1995;333:1581–7.
26. Pikus HJ, Heros RC. Stroke: Indications for emergent surgical intervention. Clin Neurosurg 1997;45:113–27.
27. Batjer H, Samson D. Use of extracranial-intracranial bypass in the management of symptomatic vasospasm. Neurosurgery 1986;19:235–46.
28. Benzel EC, Kesterson L. Extracranial-intracranial bypass surgery for the management of vasospasm after subarachnoid hemorrhage. Surg Neurol 1988;30:231–4.
29. Elliot JP, Newell DW, Lam DJ, et al. Comparison of balloon angioplasty and papaverine infusion for the treatment of vasospasm following aneurysmal subarachnoid hemorrhage. J Neurosurg 1998;88:277–84.
30. Eskridge JM, Newell DW, Pendleton GA. Transluminal angioplasty for treatment of vasospasm. Neurosurg Clin North Am 1990;1:387–99.
31. Tew JJ. Reconstructive intracranial vascular surgery for prevention of stroke. Clin Neurosurg 1975;22:264–80.
32. The EC-IC: Bypass Study Group. Failure of extracranial-intracranial arterial bypass to reduce the risk of ischemic stroke. N Engl J Med 1985;313:1191–200.
33. Haynes B, Mukherjee J, Sackett DL. Functional status changes following medical or surgical treatment for cerebral ischemia. Results of the extracranial–intracranial bypass study. JAMA 1987;257:2043–6.
34. Peerless S. Indications for the extracranial–intracranial arterial bypass in light of the EC–IC bypass study. Clin Neurosurg 1986;33:307–26.
35. Awad IA, Spetzler RF. Extracranial–intracranial bypass surgery: A critical analysis in light of the International Cooperative study. Neurosurgery 1986;19:655–64.
36. Ausman JI, Diaz FG. Critique of the extracranial–intracranial bypass study. Surg Neurol 1986;26:218–21.
37. Day AL, Rhoton AL, Little JR. The extracranial–intracranial bypass study. Surg Neurol 1986;26:222–6.
38. Barnett HJM, Fox A, Hachinski V. Further conclusions from the extracranial–intracranial bypass trial. Surg Neurol 1986;26: 227–35.
39. Goldring S, Zervas N, Langfitt T. The extracranial–intracranial bypass study: A report of the committee appointed by the American Association of Neurological Surgeons to examine the study. N Engl J Med 1987;316:817–20.

40. Sundt TJ. Was the international randomized trial of extracranial-intracranial bypass representative of the population at risk? N Engl J Med 1987;316:814–16.
41. Barnett HJM, Sackett D, Taylor DW. Are the results of the extracranial-intracranial bypass trial generalizable? N Engl J Med 1987;316:820–4.
42. Mendelowitsch A, Taussy P, Rem JA, et al. Clinical outcome of standard extracranial-intracranial bypass surgery in patients with symptomatic atherosclerotic occlusion of the internal carotid artery. Acta Neurochir (Wien) 2004;146:95–101.
43. Schmiedek P, Piepgras A, Leisinger G. Improvement of cerebrovascular capacity by EC-IC arterial bypass surgery in patients with ICA occlusion and hemodynamic cerebral ischemia. J Neurosurg 1994;81:236–44.
44. Takagi YHN, Iwama T, Hayashida K. Improvement of oxygen metabolic reserve after extracranial-intracranial bypass surgery in patients with severe haemodynamic insufficiency. Acta Neurochir (Wien) 1997;139:52–7.
45. Iwama T, Hashimoto N, Hayashida K. Cerebral hemodynamic parameters for patients with neurological improvements after extracranial-intracranial arterial bypass surgery: Evaluation using positron emission tomography. Neurosurgery 2001;48:504–12.
46. Kobayashi H, Kitai R, Ido K. Hemodynamic and metabolic changes following cerebral revascularization in patients with cerebral occlusive diseases. Neurol Res 1999;21:153–60.
47. Nussbaum ES, Erickson DL. Extracranial-intracranial bypass for ischemic cerebrovascular disease refractory to maximal medical therapy. Neurosurgery 2000;46:37–42.
48. Neff KW, Horn P, Dinter D. Extracranial-intracranial arterial bypass surgery improves total brain blood supply in selected symptomatic patients with unilateral internal carotid artery occlusion and insufficient collateralization. Neuroradiology 2004;46:430–7.
49. Amin-Hanjani SBW, Ogilvy CS, Carter BS, et al. Extracranial-intracranial bypass in the treatment of occlusive cerebrovascular disease and intracranial aneurysms in the United States between 1992 and 2001: A population-based study. J Neurosurg 2005;103: 794–804.
50. Baron JC, Bousser MG, Rey A. Reversal of focal "misery-perfusion syndrome" by extra-intracranial bypass in hemodynamic cerebral ischemia. Stroke 1981;12:454–9.
51. Grubb RL Jr, Derdeyn CP, Fritsch SM. Importance of hemodynamic factors in the prognosis of symptomatic carotid occlusion. JAMA 1998;280:1055–60.
52. Belden JR, Caplan LR, Pessin MS, et al. Mechanisms and clinical features of posterior border-zone infarcts. Neurology 1999;53: 1312–18.
53. Powers WJ, Derdeyn CP, Fritsch SM. Benign prognosis of never symptomatic carotid occlusion. Neurology 2000;54:878–82.
54. Webster MW, Makaroun MS, Steed DL, et al. Compromised cerebral blood flow reactivity is a predictor of stroke in patients with symptomatic carotid artery occlusive disease. J Vasc Surg 1995;21:338–44.
55. Yokota C, Hasegawa Y, Minematsu K, et al. Effect of acetazolamide reactivity on long-term outcome in patients with major cerebral artery occlusive diseases. Stroke 1998;29:640–4.
56. Vernieri F, Pasqualetti P, Passarelli F, et al. Outcome of carotid artery occlusion is predicted by cerebrovascular reactivity. Stroke 1999;30:593–8.
57. Klijn CJ, Kappelle LJ, van Huffelen AC, et al. Recurrent ischemia in symptomatic carotid occlusion: prognostic value of hemodynamic factors. Neurology 2000;55:1806–12.
58. Derdeyn CP, Grubb RLJr, Powers WJ. Cerebral hemodynamic impairment: Methods of measurement and association with stroke risk. Neurology 1999;53:251–9.
59. Ogasawara K, Ogawa A, Terasaki K, et al. Use of cerebrovascular reactivity in patients with symptomatic major cerebral artery occlusion to predict 5-year outcome: comparison of xenon-133 and iodine-123-IMP single-photon emission computed tomography. J Cereb Blood Flow Metab 2002;22:1142–8.
60. Ogasawara K, Ogawa A, Yoshimoto T. Cerebrovascular reactivity to acetazolamide and outcome in patients with symptomatic internal carotid or middle cerebral artery occlusion: a xenon-133 single-photon emission computed tomography study. Stroke 2002;33:1857–62.
61. Vernieri F, Pasqualetti P, Matteis M, et al. Effect of collateral blood flow and cerebral vasomotor reactivity on the outcome of carotid artery occlusion. Stroke 2001;32:1552–8.
62. Kleiser B, Widder B. Course of carotid artery occlusion with impaired cerebrovascular reactivity. Stroke 1994;23:171–4.
63. Hokari M, Kuroda S, Shiga T, et al. Impact of oxygen extraction fraction on long-term prognosis in patients with reduced blood flow and vasoreactivity because of occlusive carotid artery disease. Surg Neurol 2009;71:532–8.
64. Yamauchi H, Fukuyama H, Nagahama Y, et al. Significance of increased oxygen extraction fraction in five-year prognosis of major cerebral arterial occlusive diseases. J Nucl Med 1999;40: 1992–8.
65. Yamauchi H, Higashi T, Kagawa S, et al. Is misery perfusion still a predictor of stroke in symptomatic major cerebral artery disease? Brain 2012;135:2515–16.
66. Gibbs JM, Wise RJ, Thomas DJ. Cerebral hemodynamic changes after extracranial-intracranial bypass surgery. J Neurol Neurosurg Psychiatry 1987;50:140–50.
67. Grubb RL, Ratcheson RA, Raichle ME. Regional cerebral blood flow and oxygen utilization in superficial temporal-middle cerebral artery anastomosis patients. An exploratory definition of clinical problems. J Neurosurg 1979;50:733–41.
68. Powers WJ, Martin WRW, Herscovitch P. Extracranial-intracranial bypass surgery: Hemodynamic and metabolic effects. Neurology 1984;34:1168–74.
69. Samson Y, Baron JC, Bousser MG, et al. Effects of extra-intracranial arterial bypass on cerebral blood flow and oxygen metabolism in humans. Stroke 1985;16:609–6315.
70. Powers WJ, Clarke WR, Grubb RL Jr, et al. Extracranial-intracranial bypass surgery for stroke prevention in hemodynamic cerebral ischemia: the Carotid Occlusion Surgery Study randomized trial. JAMA 2011b;306:1983–92.
71. Ogasawara K, Ogawa A. Jet study (Japanese EC-IC Bypass Trial). Nippon Rinsho 2006;64(Suppl. 7):524–7.
72. Garrett MC, Komotar RJ, Starke RM, et al. The efficacy of direct extracranial-intracranial bypass in the treatment of symptomatic hemodynamic failure secondary to athero-occlusive disease: A systematic review. Clin Neurol Neurosurg 2009;111: 319–26.
73. Spetzler RF, Roski RA, Kopaniky DR. Alternative superficial temporal artery to middle cerebral artery revascularization procedure. Neurosurgery 1980;7:484–7.
74. Amine ARC, Moody R, Meeks W. Bilateral temporal-middle cerebral artery anastomosis for moyamoya syndrome. Surg Neurology 1977;8:3–6.
75. Golby AJ, Marks MP, Thompson RC, et al. Direct and combined revascularization in pediatric moyamoya disease. Neurosurgery 1999;45:50–8.
76. Holbach KH, Wassman H, Wappenschmidt J. Superficial temporal-middle cerebral artery anastomosis in moyamoya disease. Acta Neurochir 1980;52:27–34.
77. Houkin K, Kuroda S, Nakayama N. Cerebral revascularization for moyamoya disease in children. Neurosurg Clin N Am 2001;12:575–84.
78. Ishikawa T, Houkin K, Kamiyama H, et al. Effects of surgical revascularization on outcome of patients with pediatric moyamoya disease. Stroke 1997;28:1170–3.
79. Karasawa J, Kiruchi H, Furuse S. Treatment of moyamoya disease with STA-MCA anastomosis. J Neurosurg 1978;49:679–88.
80. Karasawa J, Touho H, Ohnishi H. Long-term follow-up study after extracranial-intracranial bypass surgery for anterior circulation ischemia in childhood moyamoya disease. J Neurosurg 1992;77:84–9.
81. Olds MV, Griebel RW, Hoffman HJ. The surgical treatment of childhood moyamoya disease. J Neurosurg 1987;66:675–80.
82. Sakamoto K, Kitano S, Yasui T, et al. Direct extracranial-intracranial bypass for children with moyamoya disease. Clin Neurol Neurosurg 1997;99:S128–33.
83. Suzuki Y, Negoro M, Shibuya M. Surgical treatment for pediatric moyamoya disease: Use of the superficial temporal artery for both areas supplied by the anterior and middle cerebral arteries. Technique and application. Neurosurgery 1997;40:324–30.
84. Matsushima T, Inoue T, Suzuki SO. Surgical treatment of moyamoya disease in pediatric patients-comparison between the

results of indirect and direct revascularization procedures–clinical study. Neurosurgery 1992;31:401–5.
85. Goda M, Isono M, Ishii K. Long-term effects of indirect bypass surgery on collateral vessel formation in pediatric moyamoya disease. J Neurosurg 2004;100(Suppl. Pediatrics):156–62.
86. Scott RM, Smith ER. Moyamoya disease and moyamoya syndrome. N Engl J Med 2009;360:1226–37.
87. Houkin K, Kamiyama H, Abe H. Surgical therapy for adult moyamoya disease. Can surgical revascularization prevent the recurrence of intracerebral hemorrhage? Stroke 1996;27:1342–6.
88. Houkin K, Kuroda S, Ishikawa T, et al. Neovascularization (angiogenesis) after revascularization in moyamoya disease. Which technique is most useful for moyamoya disease? Acta Neurochir (Wien) 2000;142:269–76.
89. Kawagushi S, Okuno S, Sakaki T. Effect of direct arterial bypass on the prevention of future stroke in patients with the hemorrhagic variety of moyamoya disease. J Neurosurg 2000;93:397–401.
90. Kuroda S, Houkin K, Kamiyama H, et al. Effects of surgical revascularization on peripheral aneurysms in moyamoya disease: Report of three cases. Neurosurgery 2001;49:463–8.
91. Morimoto M, Iwama T, Hashimoto N. Efficacy of direct revascularization in adult moyamoya disease: Haemodynamic evaluation by positron emission tomography. Acta Neurochir (Wien) 1999;141:377–84.
92. Okada Y, Shima T, Nishida M. Effectiveness of superficial temporal artery-middle cerebral artery anastomosis in adult moyamoya disease. Cerebral hemodynamics and clinical course in ischemic and hemorrhagic varieties. Stroke 1998;29:625–30.
93. Fukui M. Guidelines for the diagnosis and treatment of spontaneous occlusion of the circle of Willis (moyamoya disease). Research Committee on Spontaneous Occlusion of the Circle of Willis (moyamoya disease) of the Ministry of Health and Welfare, Japan. Clin Neurol Neurosurg 1997;99:S238–40.
94. Han DH, Kwon OK, Byun BJ, et al. A co-operative study: Clinical characteristics of 334 Korean patients with moyamoya disease treated at neurosurgical institutes (1976–1994). Acta Neurochir (Wien) 2000;142:1263–74.
95. Ikezaki K, Fukui M, Inamura T. The current status of the treatment for hemorrhagic type moyamoya disease based on a 1995 nationwide survey in Japan. Clin Neurol Neurosurg 1997;99:S183–6.
96. Yoshida Y, Yoshimoto T, Shirane R, et al. Clinical course, surgical management and long-term outcome of moyamoya patients with rebleeding after an episode of intracerebral hemorrhage. Stroke 1999;30:2272–6.
97. Miyamoto S. Japan Adult Moyamoya Trial Group. Study design for a prospective randomized trial of extracranial-intracranial bypass surgery for adults with moyamoya disease and hemorrhagic onset—The Japan Adult Moyamoya Trial Group. Neurol Med Chir (Tokyo) 2004;44:218–19.
98. Liu X, Zhang D, Shuo W, et al. Long term outcome after conservative and surgical treatment of haemorrhagic moyamoya disease. J Neurol Neurosurg Psychiatry 2013;84:258–65.
99. Latchaw RE, Yonas H, Hunter GJ, et al. Guidelines and recommendations for perfusion imaging in cerebral ischemia. Stroke 2003;34:1084–104.
100. Bulsara KR, Patel T, Fukushima T. Cerebral bypass surgery for skull base lesions: technical notes incorporating lessons learned over two decades. Neurosurg Focus 2008;24(2):E11.

76 Decompressive Craniectomy for Infarction and Hemorrhage

Hermann Neugebauer, Eric Jüttler, Patrick Mitchell, Werner Hacke

KEY POINTS

- Patients with subtotal or complete infarction of the middle cerebral artery (MCA) territory are at high risk for space-occupying edema formation and increased ICP. Close monitoring for neurological worsening during the first days after stroke is recommended.
- The diagnosis of malignant MCA infarction is based on clinical and radiological criteria. Patients who present with a severe hemispheric syndrome, deterioration of consciousness with reduced ventilator drive, and definite infarction on neuroimaging of at least two-thirds of the MCA territory including the basal ganglia are at high risk for malignant brain edema. In addition, a lesion volume on DWI of >82 mL has a high positive predictive value for malignant MCA infarction and may guide early treatment.
- The effectiveness of medical therapies is not supported by adequate evidence from clinical trials of space-occupying edema. However, if patients deteriorate due to increased ICP, these therapies may be considered in addition to decompressive hemicraniectomy.
- Decompressive hemicraniectomy for malignant MCA infarction increases the odds of survival, but it is not without controversy. In patients older than 60 years, mortality is reduced, but survival with severe disability is more frequent.
- The decision towards surgery should be taken on an individual basis after advising patients and families about potential outcome states.
- The degree of disability that is "still acceptable" for the individual patient with malignant MCA infarction is not known, but survivors of such strokes and their caregivers indicate satisfaction with life with moderate or severe disability (mRS 4) or most severe disability (mRS 5). This contrasts with results of surveys on normal people who generally state that they would not wish to survive with severe disability.
- In large space-occupying cerebellar infarction with clinical deterioration both ventriculostomy (EVD) or additional, followed by suboccipital decompressive craniectomy (SDC) with or without stroke ectomy are options depending on the specific features of the individual patient. In older patients and patients with additional brainstem infarction the treatment decision should be made carefully on an individual basis.
- In cerebellar hemorrhage, surgical hematoma evacuation and/or EVD placement are frequently performed in patients with large (>3 cm) hematoma, basal cistern, and brainstem compression, and clinical deterioration due to hydrocephalus.
- Decompressive craniectomy is not the treatment of first choice for spontaneous cerebral hemorrhage, subarachnoid hemorrhage, and cerebral venous thrombosis. It may, however, be considered for the treatment of refractory increased ICP in these disorders. If decompressive hemicraniectomy is considered, the procedure should be performed early to prevent secondary neurologic damage and herniation. If decompressive hemicraniectomy is considered in spontaneous cerebral hemorrhage it is reasonable to consider additional hematoma evacuation.

INTRODUCTION

Life-threatening space-occupying mass effect is a common finding in various subtypes of cerebral ischemia and intracranial hemorrhages. It occurs because of acute intracranial masses such as hematomas, subacute development of severe brain edema, or both. Irrespective of the underlying cause, transtentorial or transforaminal herniation is the common endpoint and the cause of death in most of these patients who require prompt and adequate evaluation and management. This chapter deals with the surgical decompression of acute space-occupying malignant middle cerebral artery (MCA) infarction, large cerebellar infarction, intracerebral and intracerebellar hemorrhage, subarachnoid hemorrhage, and cerebral venous thrombosis.

PATHOLOGY OF BRAIN EDEMA

Regardless of the subtype of stroke or the underlying pathology, all types of intracranial masses carry the risk of severe brain tissue shifts, compression of healthy brain structures, critical increase in intracranial pressure (ICP), and subsequent complications such as compromise of cerebral blood flow (CBF) and energy supply.

In ischemic stroke, mass effect is due to local brain swelling caused by brain edema. In general, *brain edema* is defined as abnormal accumulation of fluid in the brain parenchyma. Three major subtypes of edema have traditionally been classified: cytotoxic, vasogenic, and interstitial. Cytotoxic edema results from cell swelling after decreased oxygen supply, substrate and energy failure, and the subsequent breakdown of the cell membrane ion pumps. Vasogenic edema occurs in the context of breakdown of the blood–brain barrier (BBB) due to increased vascular permeability. Interstitial edema is associated with impaired absorption of cerebrospinal fluid (CSF) and acute hydrocephalus. A combination of these subtypes is found in severe ischemic stroke, with cytotoxic brain edema playing the leading role. However, brain edema formation is a complex molecular and pathophysiologic process that is only incompletely understood.[1–4]

Malignant Middle Cerebral Artery Infarction

From 1% to 10% of patients with supratentorial ischemic infarcts suffer from subtotal or complete middle cerebral artery (MCA) territory infarctions, occasionally with additional infarction of the anterior cerebral artery (ACA) or the posterior cerebral artery (PCA) or both (Fig. 76-1).[5] These infarcts are commonly associated with serious brain swelling, which usually manifests between the 2nd and the 5th days after stroke onset and reaches a maximum at the 4th day in the majority of patients.[6–10] These massive cerebral infarctions with brain swelling are life-threatening events with a poor prognosis: up to 80% of patients with such infarcts die within the 1st week after symptom onset owing to transtentorial or transforaminal herniation.[5,11,12] For such infarcts, the term malignant MCA infarction was coined.[5]

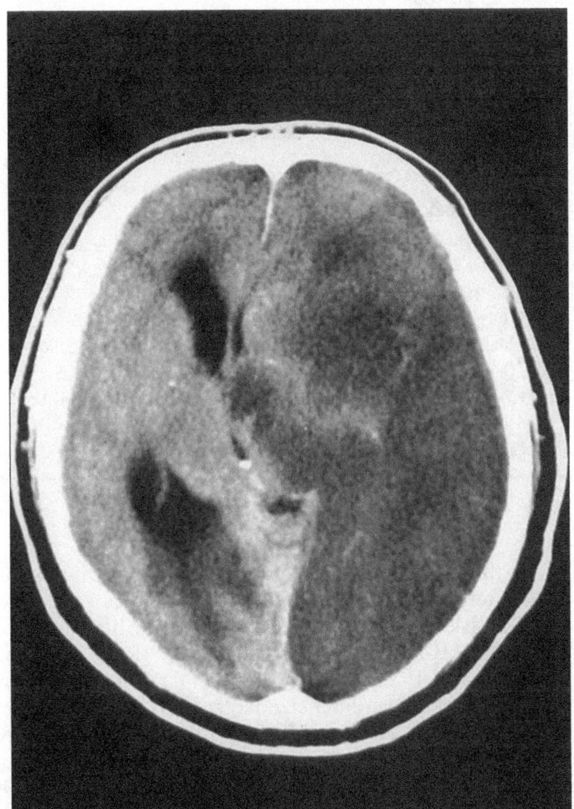

Figure 76-1. Non-contrast CT scan of a patient with malignant left middle cerebral artery (MCA) infarction plus infarction of the left posterior cerebral artery (PCA) 4 days after symptom onset under conservative treatment who died from transtentorial herniation.

The therapeutic goal is to interrupt the vicious circle of brain swelling, mass effect, increase in ICP, reduced cerebral perfusion pressure (CPP) and energy supply, and further brain tissue damage that may lead to further edema formation. Conservative therapy strategies aim to optimize CPP and oxygen delivery and to minimize cerebral metabolic demands by general measures such as adequate oxygen supply, maintenance of adequate blood pressure, optimal body and head positioning, and specific interventions, including deep sedation, barbiturates, buffers, hypothermia, osmotic therapy, steroids, and controlled hyperventilation.[13,14] However, none of these therapies is supported by adequate evidence from randomized clinical trials in space-occupying intracranial hypertension (Table 76-1).[13–15] Several reports suggest that the measures are ineffective or even detrimental.[13–20] For example, osmotic therapy is based on the presence of an intact BBB, which is largely disrupted in the infarct territory. In so far as it works at all the therapy appears to shrink normal brain tissue and so make space for swelling of infarcted tissue, potentially aggravating shifts. Mild-to-moderate hypothermia represents a promising medical treatment option, which, however, is currently not supported by evidence from larger clinical trials.[22]

ICP-lowering therapies are often used as escalating treatment options based on ICP measurement not applied until increases of ICP are evident. However, in space-occupying ischemic stroke, clinical deterioration may be due to local swelling and brain tissue shifts without, or preceeding, increases in global ICP. In patients with large MCA territory strokes and significant intracranial space, such as those with pre-existing cerebral atrophy, increases of ICP commonly occur late, after local mass effect has already led to anatomical distortion of vital brain structures.[21]

In contrast to more complex pathophysiologic theories of conservative measures, decompressive surgery is based on pure mechanical thinking: the rationale of removing a part of the neurocranium is simply to create space for the expanding brain, preventing or reducing brain tissue shifts, preventing ICP-elevation and secondary damage of unaffected brain areas.[23,24] Powerful as it sounds, this simple argument has two problems. Firstly raised pressure limits swelling so that one consequence of decompression is increased swelling. For large craniectomies, the evidence is clear that ICP is reduced despite a modest increase in swelling. The second problem with the simple mechanistic argument for decompression is that as well as reducing ICP, the operation lowers blood pressure by relaxing the reflex arterial hypertension that occurs with intracranial hypertension, and this probably leaves cerebral perfusion pressure largely unchanged.[25]

DIAGNOSIS

Although the term malignant brain infarction was introduced in 1996, there is currently no generally accepted definition of this condition.[5] The reliable early prediction of a malignant course of the ischemic lesion may justify early and more aggressive intervention. On the other hand, in the majority of cases, patients who have acute MCA infarction do not experience a malignant course and probably do not benefit from intensive care treatment or surgery and recover with conservative treatment. Currently the diagnosis of malignant brain infarction is based on (1) clinical neurologic findings, (2) a typical clinical course, and (3) neuroimaging findings (Box 76-1):

TABLE 76-1 Classification of Treatment Recommendation and Level of Evidence for Decompressive Craniectomy for Infarction and Hemorrhage[72,73]

Treatment Recommendation	Classification of Recommendation, Level of Evidence
In patients up to 60 years of age who suffer from malignant MCA infarction DHC should be performed within 48 hours from symptom onset. Decision to perform surgery depends on the willingness to survive with at least mild-to-moderate disability	I, B
In older patients with malignant MCA infarction DHC should be performed within 48 hours from symptoms onset to reduce mortality and increase the chance of survival without complete dependency. Outcome in older patients is clearly worse than in younger patients. The decision towards surgery depends on the willingness to survive with at least moderate-to-severe disability	IIb, C
External DHC with duraplasty of at least 12 cm in diameter should be performed as the procedure of choice for surgical treatment of malignant MCA infarction	I, B
Conservative therapies may be considered in addition to decompressive hemicraniectomy in patients who deteriorate due to elevated ICP	IIA, C
It is reasonable to treat patients with larger space-occupying cerebellar infarction and clinical deterioration surgical (ventriculostomy, suboccipital decompressive craniectomy, strokectomy)	I, B
It is reasonable to treat patients with cerebellar hemorrhage and clinical deterioration surgical (ventriculostomy, hematoma evacuation, decompressive craniectomy)	I, B
In patients with refractory increased ICP secondary to spontaneous cerebral hemorrhage, subarachnoid hemorrhage, and cerebral venous thrombosis, early DHC with additional hematoma evacuation in cerebral hemorrhage may be considered	IIB, C

MCA, middle cerebral artery; DHC, decompressive hemicraniectomy; ICP, intracranial pressure.
For more details refer 'AHA Evidence box index' in the FM.

1. Clinically, patients with malignant MCA infarctions present with dense hemiplegia, head and eye deviation, multimodal hemineglect, and global aphasia when the dominant hemisphere is involved. Note that the National Institutes of Health Stroke Scale (NIHSS) underestimates the severity of non-dominant infarction.[26] NIHSS score typically ranges from higher than 16–20 when the dominant hemisphere is involved, and from higher than 15–18 when the non-dominant hemisphere is involved.[26-29] Furthermore, patients with malignant MCA infarction show an impaired level of consciousness, with a score of at least 1 on item 1a of the NIHSS or less than 14 on the Glasgow Coma Scale.[5,26-28]
2. Patients with malignant MCA infarctions show a progressive deterioration of consciousness over the first 24–48 hours and frequently a reduced respiratory drive requiring mechanical ventilation.[5,27]
3. Neuroimaging shows definite infarction of at least two-thirds of the MCA territory, including the basal ganglia, with or without additional infarction of the ipsilateral ACA or the PCA territory.[27-31] Measurement of early infarct volume in stroke magnetic resonance imaging (MRI) using diffusion-weighted imaging (DWI) or apparent diffusion coefficient (ADC) mapping has a high predictive value for the development of a malignant course and may be used for early diagnosis in these patients together with computed tomography (CT).[29,32,33]

BOX 76-1 Patients with Acute Middle Cerebral Artery Infarction, with a High Risk of a Malignant Course, and Candidates for Early (<48 Hours) Hemicraniectomy

- Age 18 to 60 year
- Severe middle cerebral artery (MCA) syndrome: dense hemiplegia, head and eye deviation, multimodal neglect, global aphasia (in dominant-hemisphere infarction)
- National Institutes of Health Stroke Scale (NIHSS) score >15 (in non-dominant-hemisphere infarction) or >20 (in dominant-hemisphere infarction)
- Level of consciousness: score of ≥1 on item 1a of the NIHSS or <14 on Glasgow Coma Scale (GCS)
- Deterioration of consciousness within the first 48 hour after symptom onset and/or reduced ventilatory drive
- Neuroimaging: definite infarction of ≥2/3 of the MCA territory, at least partially including the basal ganglia; additional infarction of the anterior or posterior cerebral artery optional (CT or MRI using diffusion-weighted imaging [DWI] and perfusion imaging); *and/or* DWI lesion volume >145 mL on DWI *and/or* >82 mL on apparent diffusion coefficient [ADC] maps (MRI)

Computed Tomography

Non-contrast CT is widely available in clinical practice and detects severe ischemic changes and brain edema formation early enough to predict a malignant course in most cases. The positive predictive value (PPV) and negative predictive value (NPV) for detecting ischemic changes covering more than 50% of the MCA territory are reported to be 85% and 83% within 5 hours from symptom onset.[34] Advanced CT technologies using multimodal imaging including CT angiography (CTA) and perfusion CT (PCT) is thought to be of additional value.[35-37] In a systematic review and meta-analysis on clinical and neuroimaging findings by Hofmeijer et al.,[31] infarct size of more than 50% and perfusion deficit larger than 66% of the MCA territory within 6 hours from symptom onset were the major risk factor for the development of life-threatening edema after MCA infarction (relative risk [RR], 10.0; confidence interval [CI], 2.1–51, and RR, 7.7; CI, 2.5–24). PPV and NPV were highest in infarct size larger than 66% of the MCA territory (86% and 90%). Additional infarction of the ACA or PCA territory or both also had a high positive predictive value (86%), but a lower negative predictive value (69%) (Fig. 76-2). Intracranial carotid artery (ICA) occlusion had a comparatively low PPV (63%), although it was a significant predictor of a malignant course. Clinical variables including stroke severity did neither reach the significance nor the accuracy of CT imaging. However, overall predictive values of

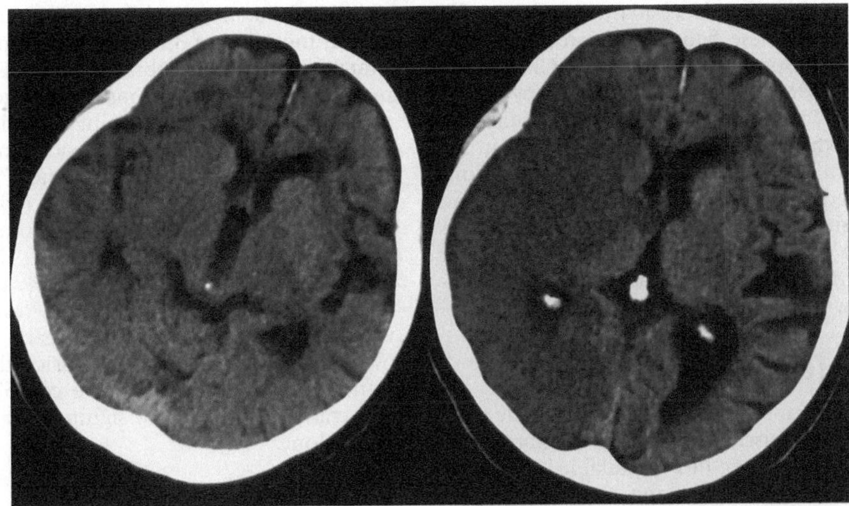

Figure 76-2. Diagnosis of malignant middle cerebral artery (MCA) infarction by non-contrast CT scans, 3 hours (*left*) and 30 hours (*right*) after symptom onset, showing infarction of the complete right MCA territory, including the basal ganglia, plus additional infarctions of the anterior cerebral artery and posterior cerebral artery territories, with incipient space-occupying effect indicated by narrowing of the frontal horn of the lateral ventricle.

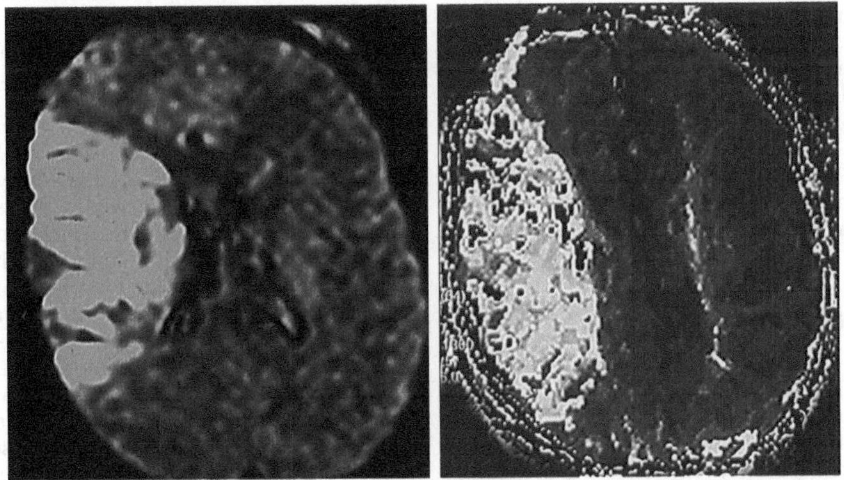

Figure 76-3. Diagnosis of malignant middle cerebral artery (MCA) infarction by MRI. *Left*, diffusion-weighted imaging (DWI); *right*, perfusion imaging 4 hours after symptom onset. A diffusion lesion of more than two-thirds of the MCA territory and a perfusion deficit of the complete MCA territory can be seen. This constellation is highly predictive for a malignant course.

routine CT imaging are too low to reliably predict a malignant course.

Magnetic Resonance Imaging

MRI allows a more accurate prediction of life-threatening brain edema in acute MCA infarction. Two retrospective studies found a lesion volume greater than 145 mL on DWI within 14 hours and greater than 82 mL on ADC maps within 6 hours from symptom onset highly predictive for the development of a malignant course with PPV of 91% and 82% and NPV of 100% and 92%, respectively.[32,33] The latter finding was reproduced in a prospective multicenter study by Thomalla et al. with high PPV, but low NPV (88% and 52%).[38] Therefore, large DWI lesions may be useful to guide early therapy by identifying patients who are at immediate risk for malignant infarct swelling. In patients with low infarct volumes despite persisting middle cerebral artery (MCA) and/or internal carotid artery (ICA) occlusion and severe stroke (NIHSS > 18) early follow-up imaging within 12 hours from stroke onset is recommended.[33,38] In contrast to DWI and ADC mapping, the value of MR perfusion imaging for the prediction of a malignant course is still controversial (Fig. 76-3).

Single-Photon Emission Computed Tomography

There are only few studies evaluating single-photon emission CT (SPECT) for the prediction of a malignant course in MCA infarction.[39-41] Berrouschot et al.[39] performed CT and technetium-99m ethylcysteinate dimer (Tc-99m ECD) SPECT, which measures perfusion and metabolic status of brain tissue, within 6 hours of symptom onset in 108 patients with acute stroke, 11 of whom died owing to MCA infarction. The sensitivity of Tc-99m ECD SPECT for predicting fatal outcome was 82% in both visual and semiquantitative analyses; specificity was 98% for visual analysis and 99% for semiquantitative analysis. These figures compared favorably with the sensitivity and specificity of baseline CT studies, which were 36% and 100%, respectively.[39] In a study by Lampl et al.[40] who performed Tc-99m diethylenetriaminepentaacetic acid (DTPA) SPECT, which measures BBB disruption, in 25 patients with MCA infarction at 36 hours after symptom onset, five patients died of herniation. Whereas stroke volume on CT was only marginally increased in these five patients in comparison with the other 20 patients, the extent of DTPA distribution, including more than one vascular territory, significantly correlated with herniation.[40]

Positron Emission Tomography

Positron emission tomography (PET) still represents the gold standard for defining the ischemic core, penumbra, and oligemia in acute stroke. However, PET is available in very few centers for patients with acute stroke and is, therefore, currently used mainly for scientific purposes and clinical studies. Only a few studies on malignant MCA infarction involve performance of PET.[42–44]

Dohmen et al.[45] investigated 34 patients with acute MCA infarction involving more than 50% of the MCA territory on non-contrast CT performed within 12 hours after symptom onset. PET was performed within 24 hours after symptom onset using flumazenil tagged with radioactive carbon (^{11}C) to assess CBF and irreversible neuronal damage. Results showed significantly larger volumes of the ischemic core and larger volumes of irreversible neuronal damage in patients with a malignant than in patients with a benign course (144.5 mL versus 62.2 mL and 157.9 mL versus 47.0 mL, respectively). In addition, mean CBF values within the ischemic core were significantly lower and the volume of the ischemic penumbra was significantly smaller in patients with malignant MCA infarction.[42]

Invasive Neuromonitoring

Multimodal invasive monitoring, including the placement of probes allowing measurement of ICP, CPP, microdialysis, and continuous electroencephalography (EEG) monitoring is an interesting instrument for close observation in patients suffering from severe strokes. Yet, except for ICP and CPP measurements, multimodal invasive monitoring is currently also restricted to a few, mostly academic centers using these tools within clinical studies and is not available for routine use. There are several studies providing data on patients with malignant MCA infarction. Dohmen et al.[45] performed invasive neuromonitoring in addition to PET. They found close correlations between a number of parameters mainly reflecting neuronal cell metabolism and the development of a malignant course after MCA infarction. These included increased ICP, decreased CPP and impaired cerebral autoregulation, increased extracellular concentrations of transmitter amino acids and decreased extracellular concentrations of non-transmitter amino acids, increased concentrations of lactate, and decreased partial tissue oxygen pressure. In particular, increased ICP to more than 26.6 mm Hg and decreased CPP to less than 56 mm Hg both showed positive and negative predictive values of 100%.[42,43,45]

Animal Studies

Several animal models of ischemic stroke provide evidence that decompressive surgery improves cerebral perfusion, reduces the volume of infarction, and significantly reduces mortality.[46–51] Using an endovascular occlusion of the MCA technique, Forsting et al.[46] demonstrated an absolute reduction in mortality of 35% after decompressive craniectomy in a rat model of focal cerebral ischemia. Furthermore, there were marked absolute reductions in average infarct volume compared with controls of 84% in animals subjected to craniectomy 1 hour after MCA occlusion and of 63% in animals subjected to craniectomy at 24 hours.[46]

Engelhorn et al.[49,50] compared reperfusion and craniectomy or both in a rat model of focal ischemia after MCA occlusion. They found significant absolute reductions in infarct volume by craniectomy at 1, 4, and 12 hours after MCA occlusion of 57%, 52%, and 33%, respectively. These results were comparable to those after early reperfusion, probably owing to improved cerebral perfusion through collaterals after craniectomy.[51] Interestingly, the combination of reperfusion and craniectomy was not significantly better than one treatment alone.[49,50]

Technical Aspects

There are a variety of techniques for decompressive surgery. External (craniectomy, removal of the cranial vault) is differentiated from internal (removal of nonviable, edematous tissue) decompression. The two can be combined.[52,53] In patients with diffuse brain edema without midline shift, bilateral craniectomy is a reasonable approach, whereas in patients with unilateral swelling of one hemisphere and midline shift, hemicraniectomy is the recommended procedure (Fig. 76-4).

For hemicraniectomy, usually a large question-mark-shaped skin incision based at the ear is made, and a bone flap containing parts of the frontal, parietal, temporal, and occipital squama is removed.[54] Alternatively, a T-shaped skin incision can be made in order to protect the occipital artery. Another approach is to make a straight incision in the midline along the superior sagittal sinus from the hairline to the vertex. A further incision is made at an angle of 120° to this and taken down behind the ear. An additional incision can be made on the other side if bilateral decompression is required at the time, or added later as required. Skull flaps are then made leaving a 30-mm-wide skull strip over the superior sagittal sinus. This gives a "tulip scalp opening" and "flower basket craniotomy" where the strip over the superior sagittal sinus is the "handle" of the basket. This operation gives the largest craniectomy. Osteoplastic craniectomy should include parts of the frontal, parietal, and temporal squamae and should be not less than 10 cm across, the larger the better. They may be extended to the skull base in the anterior and middle fossae, but this makes subsequent cranioplasty more difficult, dangerous and gives poorer cosmetics due to repeated surgery on the bulk of the temporalis muscle (Fig. 76-5). In the past, craniectomies were performed without opening of the dura, but it is now recognized that decompression is achieved mainly by dural opening. Therefore, after dura enlargement, either an autologous or artificial dural patch should be inserted (Fig. 76-6). Some centers prefer to leave the dura open,[55] but this increases the difficulty and hazard of later cranioplasty as there is then no layer to protect the brain from dissection. The need for additional tissue removal (i.e., in the case of malignant MCA infarction, temporal lobectomy) has been discussed over the years. It has been suggested that resection of the temporal lobe may reduce the risk of uncal herniation but this technique is more complicated because it is difficult to distinguish between already infarcted and potentially salvageable tissue, and a benefit has never been proven by clinical studies. Meanwhile, there is a broad consensus among neurosurgeons that external decompressive surgery by hemicraniectomy is sufficient.[55] The bone flap may be stored where facilities exist and

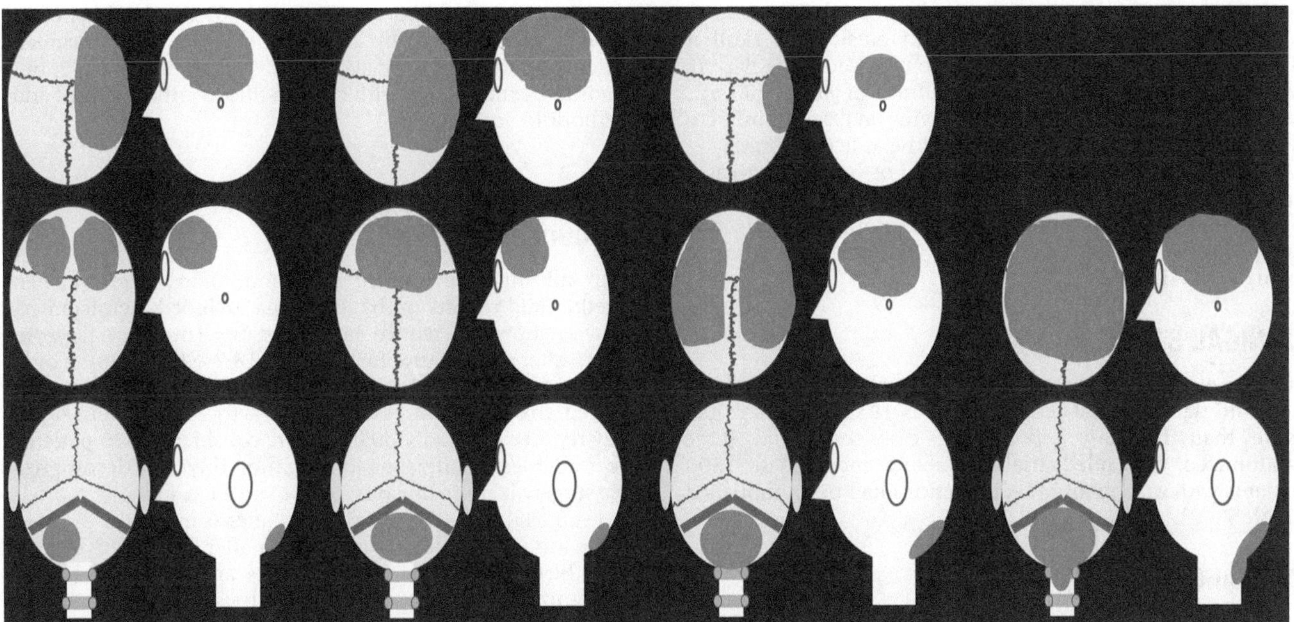

Figure 76-4. Different types of craniectomy: *Upper row, from left to right,* Unilateral frontotemporoparietal decompression (hemicraniectomy) not exceeding the sinus sagittalis superior; frontotemporoparietal decompression exceeding the sinus sagittalis superior; temporal decompression (usually with resection of the temporal lobe). *Middle row, from left to right,* Bifrontal decompression not exceeding the sinus sagittalis superior; bifrontal decompression exceeding the sinus sagittalis superior; bilateral frontotemporoparietal decompression (bilateral hemicraniectomy); total calvarectomy. *Lower row, from left to right,* Unilateral suboccipital decompression; bilateral suboccipital decompression without opening of the foramen magnum; bilateral suboccipital decompression with opening of the foramen magnum; bilateral suboccipital decompression, without opening of the foramen magnum and resection of the atlantic arch.

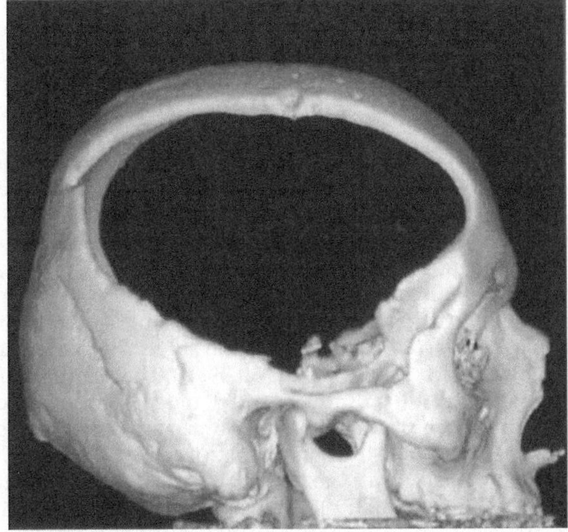

Figure 76-5. Bone defect after hemicraniectomy carried out over the entire lateral temporal lobe down to the floor of the temporal fossa.

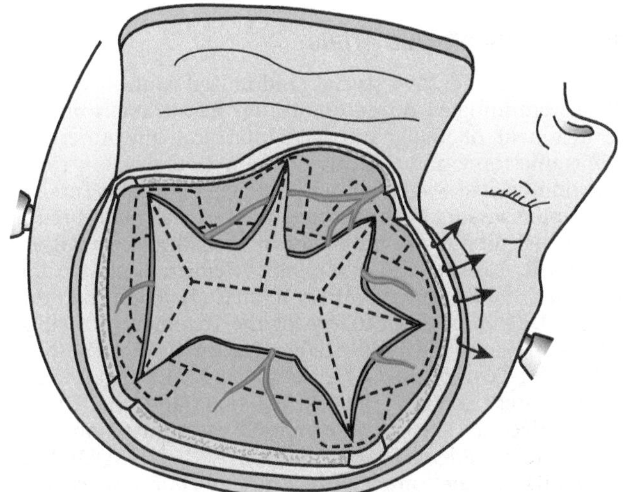

Figure 76-6. The "surgeon's eye view" of the large bone flap removal required in hemicraniectomy and surgical decompression for middle cerebral artery (MCA) territory infarction. Stellate dural incisions permit smooth brain expansion. Areas over the bulged brain are covered with either autologous or artificial dural substitute (duraplasty).

later replaced or an artificial plate can be inserted. The initial brain swelling usually subsides within 3 to 4 weeks of the stroke and repair of the cranial defect (cranioplasty) can be done at any point after this, generally the earlier the better.

Serious or life-threatening complications of craniectomy are not uncommon, including post-operative wound and bone infections, epidural or subdural hematomas, hygroma, and hydrocephalus.[52,56–58] Insufficient craniectomy can lead to local shear stress and venous congestion at the bone margins or, at worst, even to herniation through the craniectomy defect. Wagner et al.[59] analyzed post-operative CT scans of 60 patients in order to determine the occurrence of hemicraniectomy-associated infarcts and hemorrhages. Infarcts or hemorrhages of any size occurred in 70% of all patients; most lesions, however, were small (<2 mL). There was a significant association between the frequency of hemorrhage and the size of the bone defect: the smaller the bone defect, the more often lesions were encountered.[59] Therefore, the size of craniectomy is critical, not only to prevent complications, but also for craniectomy to be effective, that is, to create enough additional space outside the skull. The volume of brain tissue to be allowed to shift outside the skull is directly related to the diameter of the removed bone flap. In order to compensate additional volumes of 80 to 100 mL, which usually occur in space-occupying malignant infarcts, the diameter of the craniectomy must be at least 12 cm.

The morbidity of cranioplasty has not been investigated adequately and rates differ widely between studies. Most complications arise because of bone flap resorption, hematomas, and post-operative wound infections, with infections reported as high as 7–16%.[60-65]

CLINICAL STUDIES

Hemicraniectomy in space-occupying stroke is by no means new and dates back at least as early as 1935.[66] Up to 2009, more than 100 case reports and case series and three randomized controlled trials involving more than 1800 patients with malignant MCA infarctions had been published (Table 76-2).[27,67]

Clinical Case Series

Most of the clinical case studies and reports are retrospective, with low numbers of patients, using control groups that are often historical and not directly comparable because of higher age, more frequent lesions of the dominant hemisphere, different comorbidity, largely different conservative treatment concepts, and difference in operation techniques, cooling modes and durations of hypothermia, concomitant therapies, and patient monitoring. Most of all, however, inclusion criteria vary largely among these studies, because there is still no generally accepted definition for malignant MCA infarction.

Clinical Randomized Trials

Between 2000 and 2004 several randomized controlled trials (RCT) were initiated on decompressive hemicraniectomy in the treatment of malignant MCA infarction: the American Hemicraniectomy and Durotomy Upon Deterioration from Infarction-Related Swelling Trial (HeADDFIRST), the Turkish DEcompressive surgery for the treatment of Malignant Infarction of the middle cerebral artery in a TURkish population (DEMITUR TRIAL), the Philippian Hemicraniectomy for Malignant Middle Cerebral Artery Infarcts (HeMMI) trial, the German DEcompressive Surgery for the Treatment of malignant INfarction of the middle cerebral arterY (DESTINY) trial, the French DEcompressive Craniectomy In MALignant middle cerebral artery infarcts (DECIMAL) trial, and the Dutch Hemicraniectomy After Middle cerebral artery infarction with Life-threatening Edema Trial (HAMLET).[27-29,68-70] HeADDFIRST and DEMITUR were completed in 2003 and 2007, respectively. While HeADDFIRST was finally published in 2014, DEMITUR has not been published as a written paper yet. HeMMI is still recruiting patients. DESTINY, DECIMAL, and HAMLET have all been published as individual papers between 2007 and 2009. In addition, the results of a prospectively planned pooled analysis including all patients from DESTINY and DECIMAL and 23 patients from HAMLET which were 18 to 60 years old and treated by early hemicraniectomy within 48 hours from stroke onset were published in 2007.[71] Today, the results of the pooled analysis provide the best available evidence and the basis for the treatment recommendations on decompressive hemicraniectomy in malignant MCA infarction in current stroke guidelines.[72,73] After the final publication of HAMLET, two meta-analyses were published.[27,74] To investigate the effectiveness of decompressive hemicraniectomy in patients older than 60 years of age, the German DESTINY-II trial was conducted between 2009 and 2012 and published in 2014.[75] Another RCT by Zhao et al. which also included patients up to 80 years of age and was published in 2012, but needs to be interpreted with caution due to critical ethical and methodological aspects.

Mortality and Functional Outcome in Younger Patients

With all the results from non-randomized studies taken together and reports on hypothermia excluded, hemicraniectomy is shown to reduce early mortality (in hospital) from 66.5% after conservative treatment to 18.7% (−47.8%). If only patients for whom at least one follow-up is available are considered, this effect decreases from 50% to 24.9% (−25.1%). If only reports with individual data are considered, 370 patients are available: the effect in reducing mortality after decompressive surgery is more obvious: 81.1% vs 12.6% for early mortality (−68.5%) and 82.1% vs 17.8% after 6 months (−64.3%) (there are no individual patient data after conservative treatment beyond 1 year).[67] These results are supported by the randomized trials: In pooled met-analysis of all patients from DESTINY, DECIMAL, and HAMLET mortality at 1 year was significantly decreased by two-thirds from over 60% in the conservative group to 20% in the surgery group.[71,74] If surgery is delayed more than 48 and up to 99 hours after symptom onset, this effect is no longer seen: rates are 27.3% after decompressive surgery and 35.7% after conservative treatment (−8.4%) (see Table 76-2).[27,71]

In non-randomized studies, 31.7% of all patients undergoing decompressive surgery showed no or mild-to-moderate disability (modified Rankin Scale [mRS] score 0 to 3; Glasgow Outcome Scale [GOS] score 4 to 5; Barthel Index [BI] 60 or higher) at outcome visits, compared with 12.2% of patients undergoing conservative treatment (+19.5%). Taking into account individual patient data only, 41.5% of patients showed no or mild-to-moderate disability after decompressive surgery, compared with 0% after conservative treatment (+41.5%).[67] The meta analysis of randomized trials is complicated by the different time windows from stroke onset over which they recruited. In the five trials published to date a total of 173 patients were randomized and analyzed. When all patients are included in meta-analysis there were 92 patients in the surgical group of whom 20 died (21.7%), 55 had a mRS score of 4 or more including deaths (59.8%) and 78 had a mRS of 3 or more including deaths (84.8%). In the non-surgical group there were 81 patients of whom 49 died (60.5%), 60 had a mRS score of 4 or more including deaths (74.1%) and 78 had a mRS of 3 or more including deaths (96.3%). Three of the trials did not recruit patients beyond 48 hours from stroke onset (DESTINY,[28] DECIMAL,[29] Zhao et al.) and two recruited to 96 hours (HAMLET,[27] HeADDFIRST[69]). If the patients recruited after 48 hours are excluded then more patients in the surgery group had a mRS score of 3 or less (42.7% vs 23.4%; +19.3%). A mRS score of 4 or less was reached by 70.7% vs 26.6% (+44.1%) after decompressive surgery. If surgery is delayed more than 48 and up to 99 hours after symptom onset, 29.4% of patients after surgical treatment compared with 35.3% after conservative treatment survive with a mRS score of 3 or less (−5.9%), and 70.6% of patients after surgical treatment, compared with 64.7% after conservative treatment, survive with a mRS score of 4 or less (+5.9) (see Table 76-2).[27-29,68-70,74]

However, in the nonrandomized studies, the number of severely disabled patients (mRS score, 4 to 5; GOS score 2 to 3; BI <60) increased after hemicraniectomy from 37.8% to 43.5% (+5.7%) in all patients and from 17.9% to 40.7% (+22.8%) in reports with individual data.[67] In the pooled

TABLE 76-2 Outcome after Malignant Middle Cerebral Artery (MCA) Infarction: Comparison of Conservative Treatment and Hemicraniectomy*

	Conservative Treatment	Decompressive Surgery	Absolute Risk Reduction (%)
Non-randomized studies (all patients)	n = 471	n = 790	
In hospital mortality	66.5	18.7	−47.8
Non-randomized studies (all patients with follow-up)	n = 98	n = 543	
Independent (%)	1.0	6.1	5.1
Mild-to-moderate disability (%)	11.2	25.6	14.4
Severe disability (%)	37.8	43.5	5.7
Death (%)	50.0	24.9	−25.1
Non-randomized studies (individual data)	n = 61	n = 309	
Independent (%)	0.0	5.9	5.9
Mild-to-moderate disability (%)	0.0	35.6	35.6
Severe disability (%)	17.9	40.7	22.8
Death (%)	82.1	17.8	−64.3
Pooled analysis of randomized trials, treatment ≤48 hours, age ≤ 60 years	n = 42	n = 51	
Independent (%)	0.0	0.0	0.0
Mild-to-moderate disability (%)	21.4	43.1	21.7
Severe disability (%)	7.1	35.3	28.2
Death (%)	71.4	21.6	−49.9
Meta-analysis of randomized trials, all patients treated ≤48 hours, age ≤ 60 years	n = 56	n = 64	
Independent (%)	0.0	0.0	0.0
Mild-to-moderate disability (%)	21.4	43.8	22.4
Severe disability (%)	8.9	34.4	25.5
Death (%)	69.6	21.9	−47.7
Meta-analysis of randomized trials, treatment >48–99 hours, age ≤ 60 years	n = 29	n = 26	
Independent (%)	0.0	3.8	3.8
Mild-to-moderate disability (%)	31.0	19.2	−11.8
Severe disability (%)	24.1	50.0	26.9
Death (%)	44.8	26.9	−17.9
Meta-analysis of randomized trials, treatment ≤99 hours, age ≤ 60 years	n = 81	n = 92	
Independent (%)	0.0	0.0	0.0
Mild-to-moderate disability (%)	25.9	40.2	14.3
Severe disability (%)	13.6	38.0	24.4
Death (%)	60.5	21.7	−38.8
Meta-analysis of randomized trial, treatment ≤48 hours, age > 60 years	n = 75	n = 64	
Independent (%)	0.0	0.0	
Mild-to-moderate disability (%)	4.0	7.8	3.8
Severe disability (%)	21.3	56.3	35.0
Death (%)	74.7	35.9	−38.8

*Functional outcome classified as (1) independent outcome (modified Rankin Scale [mRS] score 0 to 1; or Glasgow Outcome Scale [GOS] score 5; or Barthel Index [BI] ≥ 90); (2) mild to moderate disability (mRS score 2 to 3; or GOS score 4; or BI 60 to 85); (3) severe disability (mRS score 4 or 5; or GOS score 2 to 3; or BI < 60); and (4) death. In cases in which more than one outcome scale is given, outcome is classified according to the following priority: mRS/GOS/BI.

analysis of the randomized trials, very severe disability (mRS score, 5) was rare, and similar with and without hemicraniectomy within 48 hours after symptom onset (4% after surgery versus 5% after conservative treatment; −1%), whereas analysis of data from all patients from DESTINY, DECIMAL, and HAMLET shows the number to increase from 3.9 to 12.1% (+8.2%). In contrast, the number of moderately to severely disabled patients (mRS score, 4) increased substantially from 2.4% after conservative treatment to 31.4% after hemicraniectomy (+29.0%) in the pooled analysis, or from 2.0% to 27.6% (+25.6%) in analysis of data from all patients from DESTINY, DECIMAL, and HAMLET. If surgery is delayed more than 48 and up to 99 hours, the number of patients with very severe disability (mRS score, 5) is not increased (+/− 0% irrespective of treatment) and the number of moderately to severely disabled patients (mRS score, 4) is increased from 35.7% after conservative treatment to 45.5% after hemicraniectomy (+9.7%) (see Table 76-2).[27,71]

In conclusion, decompressive hemicraniectomy in patients between 18 and 60 years of age is most effective in the most severely affected cases. It reduces the chance of dying by two thirds or more and this reduction in mortality is highly statistically significant. The extra survivors attain a functional level in the mRS range of 4 to 5. Surgery may increase the chance of surviving with an mRS of 3 or less but the effect is modest and not statistically significant.

Treatment of Elder Patients

Although the percentage of young patients with malignant MCA infarction is comparatively high, more than 60% of patients are older than 50 years, and more than 40% are older than 60 years.[76] Several studies indicate unfavorable outcomes and poor quality of life in elder patients, suggesting an age limit of 50, 55, or 60 years.[77–89] Interpretation of these findings is limited by the fact that in most of these studies, older patients were operated on significantly later and treated less aggressively than younger patients. The subgroup analyses of the randomized trials did not indicate poorer outcome in patients 50 years or older than in younger patients.[27,71] However, the age limit for inclusion in these trials was 60 years. To assess the effects of early decompressive hemicraniectomy within 48 hours form stroke onset in patients older than 60 years of age, the DESTINY-II trial was conducted. The trial met its primary endpoint by significantly improving the chance to survive without most severe disability 6 months after decompressive hemicraniectomy (mRS 0–4: 38% vs 18%). This difference was mainly driven by the lower mortality rate in the surgery group (33% vs 70%). At 12 months, death was less frequent after hemicraniectomy (43% vs 76%), while most severe disability was more frequent (mRS 5: 19% vs 8%). The chance to survive with moderate disability (mRS 3) was only low (6% vs 5%) and not a single patient achieved independency in both groups.[75] From these figures it is obvious, that although DESTINY-II is a positive trial and mortality is significantly reduced, functional outcome after decompressive hemicraniectomy in patients older than 60 years is considerably worse than in younger patients. Although 32% remain in a mRS of 4, which is similar to figures in younger patients, 19% remain very severely disabled, only few patients were capable of walking without assistance, and none reached functional independency. Therefore, decompressive hemicraniectomy should be considered very carefully in older patients on an individual basis (see Table 76-1).[72,73]

Assessment of Functional Outcome

Assessment of functional outcome remains a debated issue. Standard outcome measures such as the BI, GOS, and mRS, with their emphasis on motor abilities, may not account for all remaining deficits, particularly cognitive impairments and communication skills in patients with dominant-hemisphere infarctions. Moreover, the dichotomization between favorable and unfavorable outcomes is controversial.[90,91] There is strong reluctance among many physicians to regard a score on the mRS of more than 2 as a favorable outcome. On the other hand, most physicians primarily caring for patients with such a life-threatening and primarily severely disabling disease as malignant MCA infarction, a mRS score of 3 may be considered a favorable outcome. There is also agreement that a mRS score of 5 is clearly unfavorable. Therefore, the discussion is mainly related to the group of patients surviving with a mRS score of 4. In this group of patients, the terms "favorable" and "unfavorable" may mislead and should be considered in terms of "acceptable" and "unacceptable." It is the patients and their closest relatives or caregivers who should decide on which condition may be "acceptable" and which may not. Indeed, a recent systematic review, which sought to determine the outcome after surviving malignant MCA infarction from the perspective of the patients and caregivers, reported that the majority (76.6%) indicated satisfaction with their lives despite moderate severe disability (mRS 4).[92,93] The evaluation of the quality of life and the question of retrospective consent to treatment may further help in this issue, always bearing in mind that death is the most probable alternative.

Quality of Life

There are currently only scarce data on the quality of life of patients after malignant MCA infarction treated by hemicraniectomy, and available studies came to divergent results. Data of these small trials suggest that most survivors of malignant MCA infarction show an average quality of life comparable to patients with other types of stroke.[77,94–97] One trial revealed a more profound reduction in the quality of life for those surviving MCA infarction.[78] Interpretation of these findings is limited, however, because there are insufficient data on patients treated conservatively.

Treatment of Patients with Dominant-Hemisphere Infarction

The treatment of patients with malignant MCA infarction of the dominant hemisphere is another controversial issue. In many centers decompressive surgery was rarely done in these patients. The inability to communicate and severe hemiplegia, especially of the dominant upper extremity, were considered too disabling, and hemicraniectomy was often restricted to patients with a non-dominant-hemisphere infarction. From the randomized trials and larger prospective case series, there is currently no indication that patients with dominant malignant infarctions do not profit from treatment.[27,71,75] Neither mortality nor functional outcome depends on the side of the lesion in any of the larger prospective studies.[79] Indeed, the handicap caused by aphasia may be balanced by the neuropsychological deficits that are less obvious to clinical observation but may be no less disabling; that is, the severe attention deficit, apraxia, and others, in patients with infarction of the non-dominant hemisphere.[95,98] In addition, the long-term aphasia in dominant-hemisphere malignant MCA infarction is rarely complete and often shows improvement.[52,56,80,95,96] So far, there are no indications that surgery should not be considered in patients with dominant-hemisphere infarction.

Timing of Hemicraniectomy

In a review of 138 patients from retrospective and uncontrolled case series, Gupta et al.[79] found that neither time to surgery, presence of signs of herniation, nor additional lesions in other vascular territories was an independent predictor for poor outcome.[79] The randomized trials indicate that a benefit of hemicraniectomy is greatest when it is performed within 48 hours of symptom onset; however, the numbers of patients randomly assigned to treatment after 48 hours in these trials is too small to allow definite conclusions to be drawn. Furthermore, the lack of effectiveness after 48 hours in HAMLET is more due to the low mortality in the control group compared to patients treated within 48 hours (36% vs 78%). Because low mortality may be due to a selection effect in the later time window, delayed decompressive hemicraniectomy cannot be dismissed as ineffective.[27,71] Some studies suggest improved outcome if hemicraniectomy is performed within less than 24 hours after stroke onset in comparison with later surgery, especially when signs of herniation are present.[52,99] On the other hand, in other case series and non-randomized studies, time to treatment had no influence on outcome.[80,97] Currently, hemicraniectomy should be performed as soon as possible once the decision for surgical intervention has been made.

RELATED DISORDERS

Decompressive Surgery in Space-Occupying Cerebellar Infarction

Space-occupying edema is a common but frequently overlooked complication in 8–39% of large cerebellar infarctions, particularly those affecting the posterior inferior cerebellar artery territory or multiple arterial territories. The timing of edema formation is variable but in most cases reaches its maximum between the 2nd and the 4th days after stroke onset.[98–106] The tight posterior fossa provides only a small space for compensation of mass effect, and life-threatening complications may develop rapidly, including: (1) obstructive hydrocephalus due to the blockage of the fourth ventricle, (2) direct compression of the midbrain and pons, (3) upward herniation of the superior vermis cerebelli through the tentorial notch, and (4) downward herniation of the cerebellar tonsils through the foramen magnum.[101,102,108–112]

Compression of the brainstem typically manifests with ipsilateral sixth nerve palsy, facial weakness, and eventually Horner's syndrome. As compression continues, patients lose consciousness and become comatose over several hours and often demonstrate pinpoint pupils and decerebrate posturing from pontine compression. Ataxic respiration and apnea ultimately occur because of medullary compression from tonsillar herniation shortly before death.[100–108]

In the case of extensive mass effect, conservative treatment strategies are usually unsuccessful. It is widely accepted among neurosurgeons and neurologists that surgery is the treatment of choice. However, the time point at which to start surgical treatment and which factors should trigger intervention remain unclear. Furthermore, the large number of available procedures – ventriculostomy (either by extraventricular drainage [EVD] or by endoscopic third ventricle ventriculostomy [EVT]), suboccipital decompressive surgery of the posterior fossa (SDC) with or without resection of necrotic tissue (strokectomy), and a combination of both – have not been tested or compared with another in larger prospective or randomized trials. Most clinicians agree that alert and clinically stable patients should be treated conservatively and monitored closely.[110,112] Others recommend early or preventive intervention, because clinical signs of deterioration are unspecific and neuroradiologic parameters are uncertain or may be detected too late.[113–115] For patients with impaired consciousness or those whose status deteriorates, some authorities recommend ventriculostomy as the first choice, decompressive surgery being considered only when there is further clinical deterioration.[110,116] Others, however, consider this approach to be dangerous because of possible upward herniation and because it does not relieve brainstem compression. In this setting, most surgeons favor suboccipital decompression as first-choice treatment, with or without duraplasty[106,112] and with or without additional resection of infarcted tissue,[110] or a combination of ventriculostomy in addition to decompressive surgery as first choice, especially when occlusive hydrocephalus is present.[102,117,118] There is evidence showing benefit for surgery on patients who are comatose or show signs of herniation. In one prospective study, 47% of patients who were comatose had a good outcome.[115]

According to the available data, close monitoring and repeated neuroimaging, if possible using MRI to detect brainstem infarction, is the recommended procedure in patients with large cerebellar infarcts. Early surgical intervention is recommended in those patients whose status deteriorates because of mass effect rather than additional brainstem infarction, because brainstem compression, occlusive hydrocephalus, and herniation can most often be reversed or even prevented by suboccipital craniectomy (Fig. 76-7, Fig. 76-8, see Table 76-1).

If the decision for suboccipital craniectomy is made, patients should be placed in prone or semiprone (park bench) position. After vertical midline skin incision from the external occipital protruberance to the upper cervical spine (Fig. 76-9), separation of skin and subcutaneous tissue from the underlying fascia, which is cut through laterally to the spinous processes of the upper cervical spine, and disconnection of muscles from these spinous processes and the occiput, osteoplastic craniotomy should be performed beneath the transverse sinus and enlarged laterally. The foramen magnum should be opened sufficiently to decompress the cerebellar tonsils. In this context additional laminectomy and resection of the atlantic arch may be considered, particularly if the tonsils are significantly below the foramen magnum. To maximize the decompressive effect, the dura should be opened (Y-shaped) above the cerebellum and the medulla oblongata. After that step, some neurosurgeons recommend resection of necrotic tissue by suction. Duraplasty (see Fig. 76-4) may be used or the dura left open with nucial fascia closed to encourage a pseudomenigocoele. Complications include injury of the vertebral arteries, the induction of major bleeding, as well as epidural and subdural hematoma and hygroma.[119]

In general, surgical treatment is associated with much higher survival rates than conservative treatment: 81.6% in patients treated with EVD, 76.8% in patients treated with SDC, and 77.5% in patients treated with EVD and SDC compared to an overall 57.1% in patients treated conservatively and 15% in patients who progress to coma under conservative treatment. Overall functional outcome after surgery seems to be good with 40.6–54.4% of patients suffering from no or mild disability (mRS 0–1) and 20.3–41.0% suffering from moderate disability (mRS 2–3) while severe disability (mRS 4–5) is reported in only 11.4–18.8% of patients. These figures should be, however, interpreted with caution as they derive from uncontrolled retrospective case series of limited cohort size and other selection biases.[119] Little is known about the long-term outcome in survivors. In contrast to the general belief that outcome after space-occupying cerebellar infarction is generally good, two retrospective studies with long-term follow-up suggest that 4 years after stroke only 60% of patients are alive and only 38% show a favorable outcome (mRS 0–2), with age and the presence of brainstem infarction as independent negative prognostic factors.[120,121]

CEREBELLAR HEMORRHAGE

Spontaneous cerebellar hemorrhage represents approximately 10% of all cases of intracerebral hemorrhage and 15% of cerebellar strokes.[122,123] Although hypertension is the most important causative factor, amyloid angiopathy, arteriovenous malformation, distal PICA aneurysm, and cavernous malformation can cause cerebellar hemorrhage. The latter should be ruled out with CTA or angiography.[124–127] Hypertensive cerebellar hemorrhage usually occurs in the dentate nuclei and often extends into the hemispheric white matter, brainstem, and fourth ventricle. The most feared complications are, therefore, obstructive hydrocephalus with elevation of ICP – either by compression of the forth ventricle or

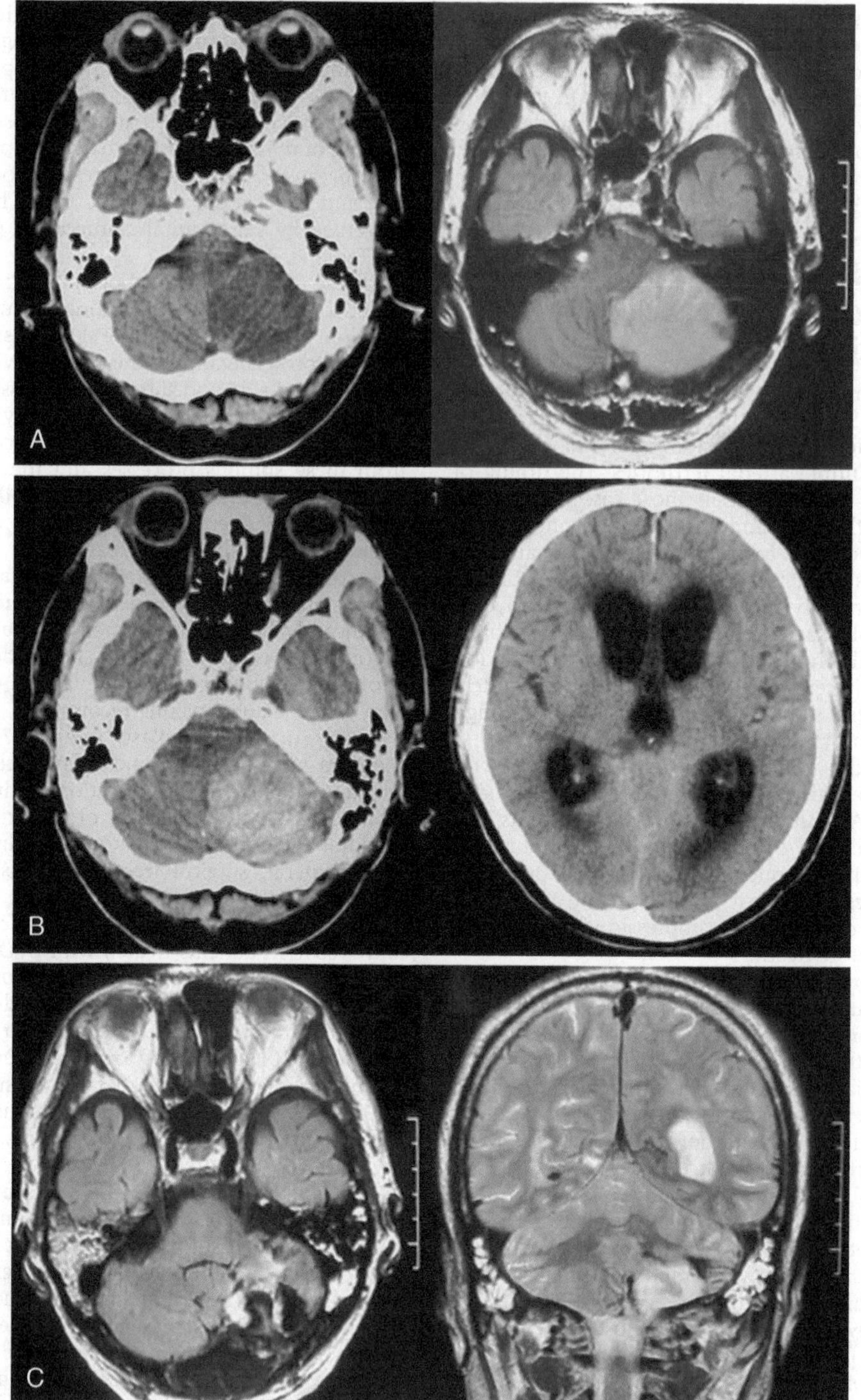

Figure 76-7. A, CT scan *(left)* and fluid-attenuated inversion recovery (FLAIR) MR image *(right)* demonstrating a cerebellar infarction in the left side. B, CT scans obtained at patient deterioration under conservative treatment disclosing a hemorrhagic transformation and hydrocephalus. C, Axial FLAIR *(left)* and coronal T2-weighted *(right)* MR images, obtained 1 month after surgery, showing the posterior fossa slack with no evidence of brainstem injury.

by intraventricular hemorrhage – compression of the brainstem, and upward or downward transtentorial herniation. In contrast to the slowly progressive increase of ICP in large cerebellar infarcts, which is due to edema formation, ICP elevation in cerebellar hemorrhage occurs rapidly due to space-occupying hematoma growth or re-bleeding. Therefore, signs of raised ICP such as headache, vomiting, and alterations in the level of consciousness are present early on in most cases.

Surgical hematoma evacuation and/or EVD placement to treat increased ICP are the treatments of choice in patients with signs of elevated ICP and/or clinical deterioration. The key surgical indicators are based on the level of consciousness, the clinical course, and the size of the hematoma. Surgery is indicated in patients with large (>3 cm) cerebellar hemorrhage, basal cistern and brainstem compression and/or hydrocephalus (Figs 76-10–76-12, see Table 76-1).[122,126,128] A suggested treatment algorithm is outlined in Figure 76-13.

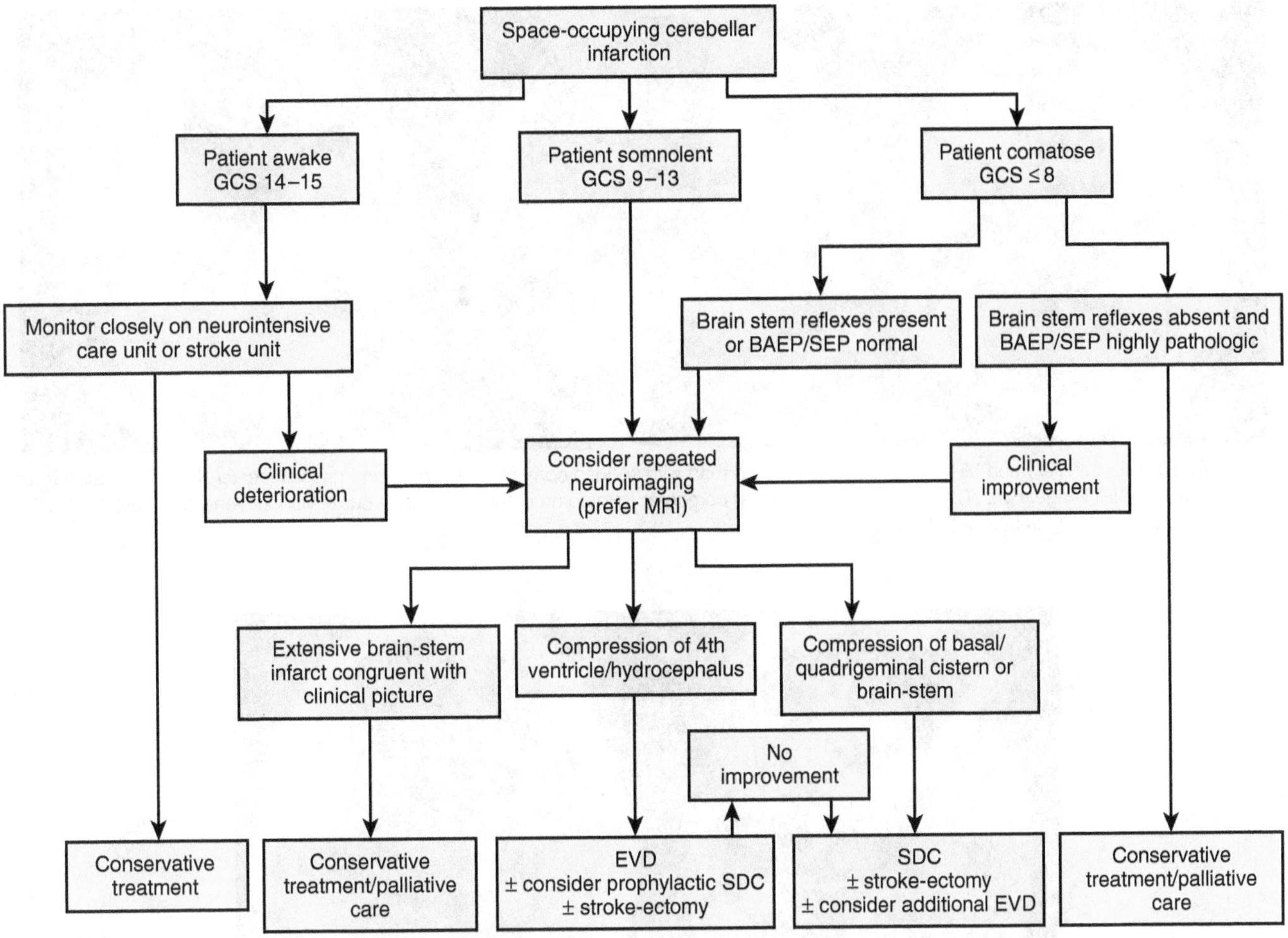

Space-occupying cerebellar infarction

Patient awake GCS 14–15

Patient somnolent GCS 9–13

Patient comatose GCS ≤8

Monitor closely on neurointensive care unit or stroke unit

Brain stem reflexes present or BAEP/SEP normal

Brain stem reflexes absent and BAEP/SEP highly pathologic

Clinical deterioration

Consider repeated neuroimaging (prefer MRI)

Clinical improvement

Extensive brain-stem infarct congruent with clinical picture

Compression of 4th ventricle/hydrocephalus

Compression of basal/ quadrigeminal cistern or brain-stem

No improvement

Conservative treatment

Conservative treatment/palliative care

EVD ± consider prophylactic SDC ± stroke-ectomy

SDC ± stroke-ectomy ± consider additional EVD

Conservative treatment/palliative care

Figure 76-8. Suggested treatment algorithm for space-occupying cerebellar infarction. GCS, Glasgow Coma Scale; EVD, extraventricular drain; SDC, suboccipital decompressive craniectomy; BAEP, brainstem auditory-evoked potentials; SEP, somatosensory-evoked potentials. *(Reprinted with kind permission of* Neurosurgical Focus *34:E8, 2013.)*

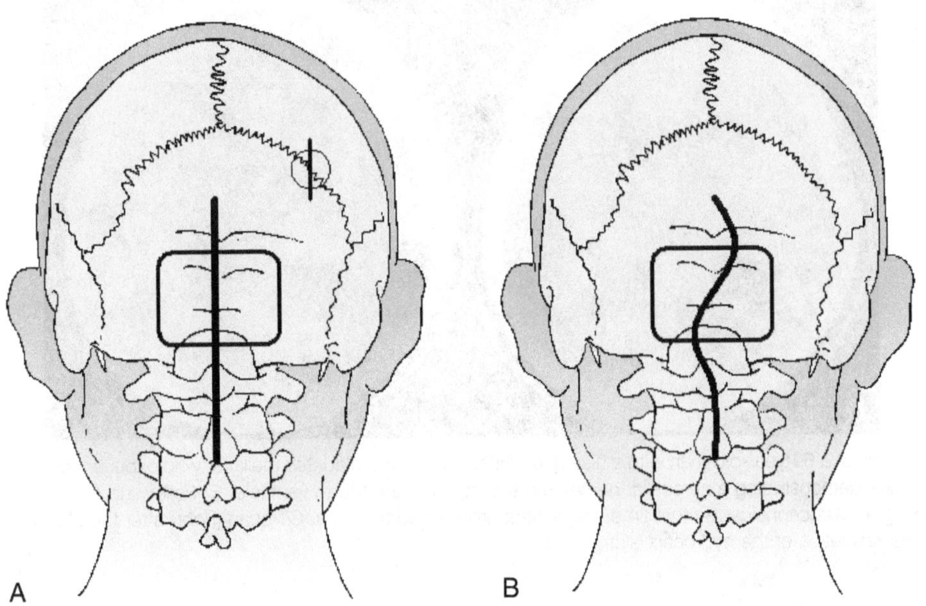

Figure 76-9. Skin incisions for suboccipital craniectomy and ventricular drainage. A, Linear incision. B, Waved skin incision. Note that the waved incision has cosmetic advantages: The post-operative scar is invisible even when the hair is wet.

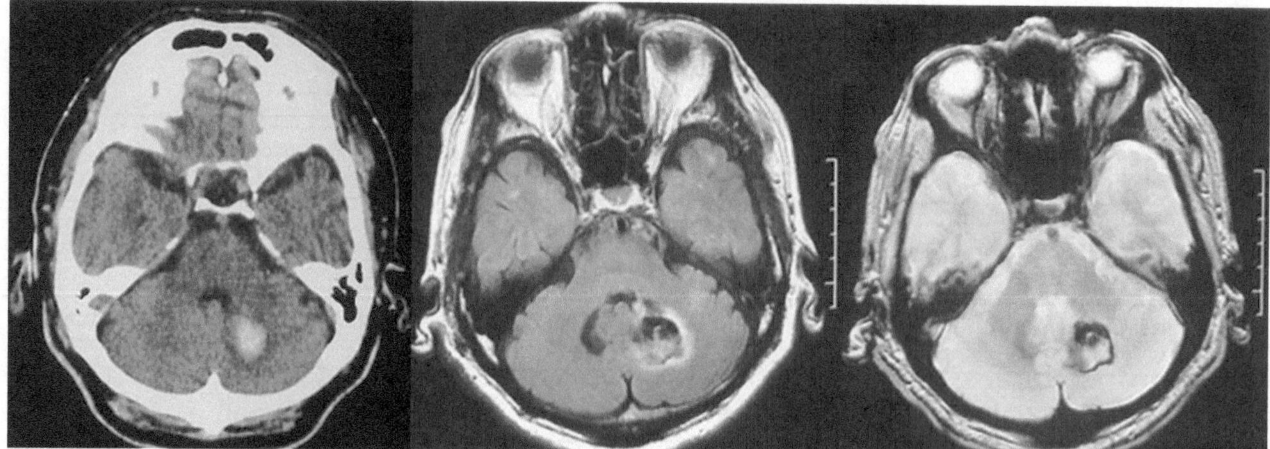

Figure 76-10. CT scan *(left)* and MR images of a 67-year-old man with sudden complaint of vertigo and nausea (*center,* fluid-attenuated inversion recovery [FLAIR] image; *right,* T2* image) showing a small cerebellar hematoma in the left dentate nuclei without ventricular perforation. The patient was conservatively treated with full recovery.

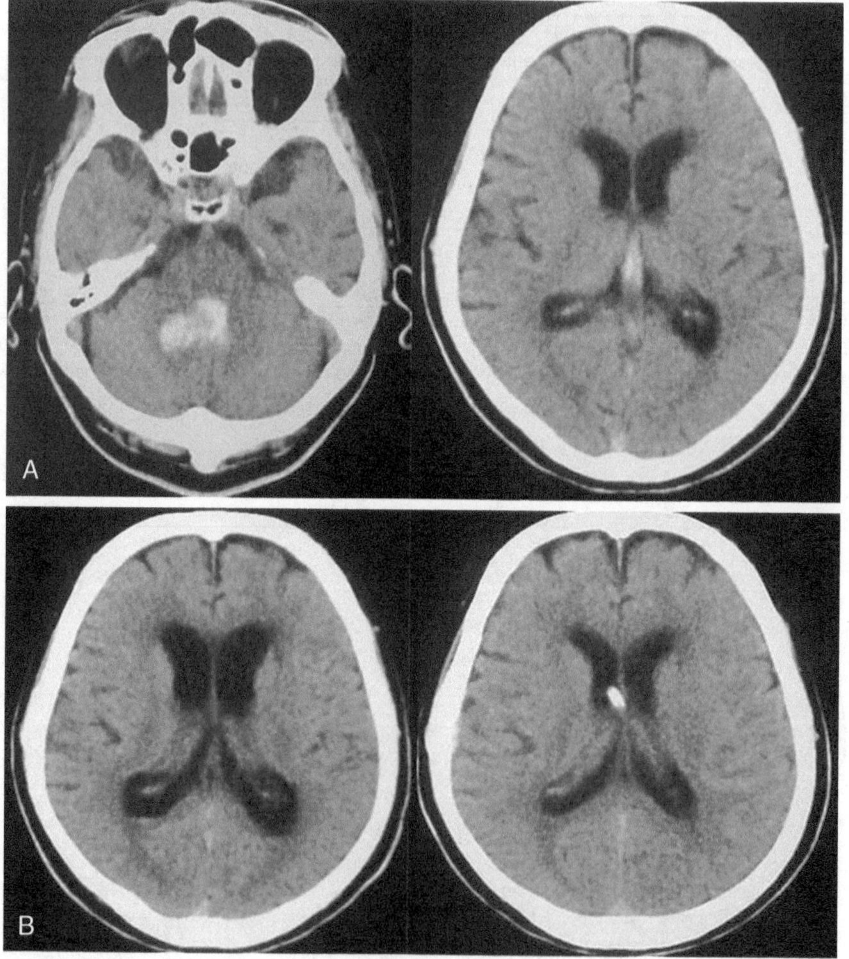

Figure 76-11. A, CT scans of a 69-year-old man with a history of hypertension and diabetes mellitus, who experienced sudden onset of vomiting and ataxia of the right side demonstrating a cerebellar hematoma extending to the fourth ventricle. B, Follow-up CT scan *(left)*, obtained 6 hours after admission, showing a hydrocephalus. By that time, the patient progressed to coma. CT scan *(right)* after the placement of ventricular drain tube revealing complete resolution of the hydrocephalus.

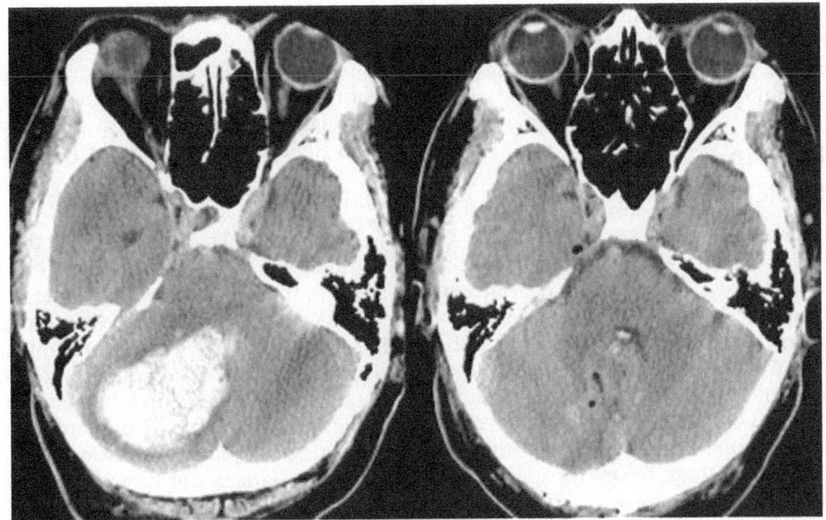

Figure 76-12. CT scan before *(left)* and after *(right)* surgery of a 46-year-old man who presented with consciousness disturbance following headache and vomiting. The initial CT scan (*left*) demonstrated a large high-density area in the right cerebellum (>3 cm). The post-operative CT (*right*) scan showed complete removal of the hematoma.

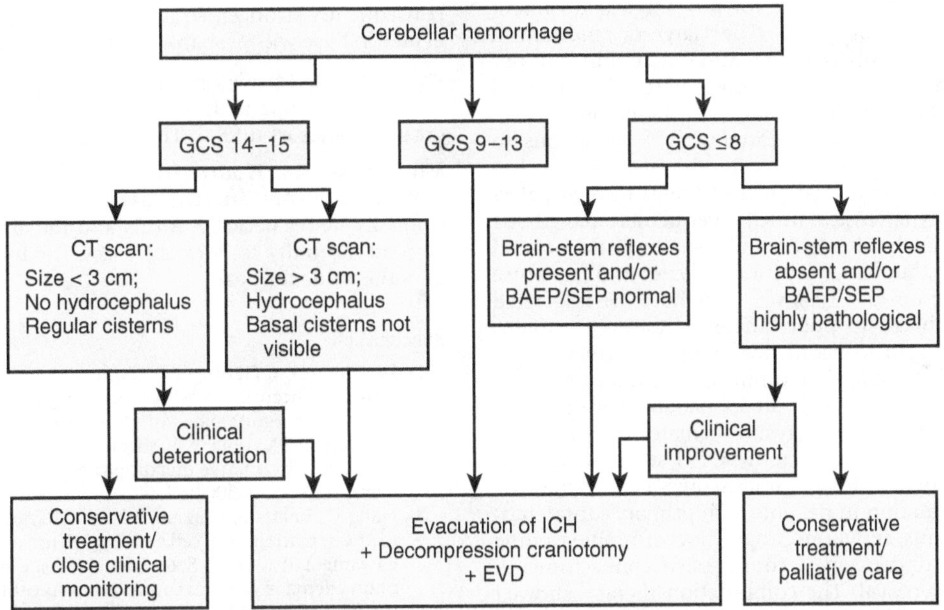

Figure 76-13. Suggested treatment algorithm for cerebellar hemorrhage. GCS, Glasgow Coma Scale; EVD, extraventricular drain; BAEP, brainstem auditory-evoked potentials; SEP, somatosensory-evoked potentials. *(Reprinted with kind permission of Witsch J, Neugebauer H, Zweckberger K, et al. Primary cerebellar haemorrhage: complications, treatment and outcome.* Clin Neurol Neurosurg *2013;115:863–9.)*

Surgical approaches range from small "key-hole" or "bore hole" craniotomies with subsequent endoscopic removal of the blood clot to large decompression craniotomies of the posterior fossa. Resection of the atlantic arch and duraplasty might be necessary to achieve a sufficient decompression in cases of additional space occupying edema. The extent of the exposure depends on the location and size of the hematoma and whether severe compression of the 4th ventricle or brainstem is present. Midline suboccipital craniectomy is recommended if the vermis or both cerebellar hemispheres should be accessed. Paramedian suboccipital craniectomy is advised if the hematoma is located to one hemisphere. Small craniotomies with (CT-guided) aspiration may be preferred in hematomas that are located to the cortical surface or in near proximity to the skull.[129,130]

Benefits of surgery on survival are not clearly supported by the literature. Pooled mortality rates were reported to be 33% in patients treated with EVD only, 29.1% with surgical treatment with or without EVD, and 33.3 in conservatively treated patients. However, these figures have to be interpreted cautiously as they derive from extremely heterogeneous studies. In contrast, single studies report mortality rates between 0% and 90% for surgical and conservative management. The same applies to functional outcome in survivors with figures ranging from 20.7% to 78.7% for no to mild disability (mRS 0–1), 6.4–39.5% for moderate disability (mRS 2–3), and 14.9–48.3% for severe disability (mRS 4–5). The few data on long-term outcome in cerebellar hemorrhage are comparable to large cerebellar infarctions with 40% of patients deceased after a period of 4 years. Factors predicting worse prognoses are large hematoma size and midline location, intraventricular hemorrhage, hydrocephalus, brainstem damage and secondary causes of hemorrhage, while GCS before surgery was not consistently found to be a reliable prognostic marker.[130]

Decompressive Surgery in Subarachnoid Hemorrhage

Only a few studies involving very small numbers of patients are available on decompressive surgery for the treatment of refractory increased intracranial pressure in subarachnoid hemorrhage (SAH), demonstrating heterogeneous results.[131-134] Early decompressive surgery seems to be more beneficial,[131] and patients without radiologic signs of ischemia seem to benefit most.[135] The use of prophylactic craniectomy was investigated in one small study of eight patients with high-grade SAH from MCA aneurysms with associated large Sylvian fissure hematomas. In seven patients, ICP was effectively decreased after decompressive surgery, with favorable outcomes in five patients (see Table 76-1).[132]

Decompressive Surgery for Spontaneous Intracerebral Hemorrhage

There is no convincing evidence for any surgical treatment option in spontaneous ICH. The largest randomized controlled trials so far, International Surgical Trial in Intracerebral Haemorrhage (STICH) and STICH II, included 1634 patients and found no benefit of early hematoma evacuation regarding outcome and mortality.[136,137] Analogous to malignant MCA infarction, not only lesion volume, but also subsequent edema formation contributes to mass effect and intracranial hypertension in ICH. Perihematomal edema develops immediately after ICH and usually peaks around the 3rd or 4th day, but has a very inhomogeneous time course and may increase up to 2 weeks.[138] Whether ICH-associated brain edema is linked to poor outcome, however, remains controversial.[139-143] In concordance with this uncertainty, there is little evidence about decompressive surgery following ICH. Murthy and colleagues report 12 patients with primary supratentorial ICH who underwent hematoma evacuation plus decompressive hemicraniectomy. Of 11 survivors, six had a favorable functional outcome (mRS score ≤3).[143] In another study on clot evacuation in patients with primary supratentorial ICH, 15 patients, in whom progression of brain swelling was anticipated, underwent decompressive craniectomy in addition to clot removal. The combination therapy showed promising results in this subgroup of severely compromised patients (see Table 76-1).[144]

Decompressive Surgery in Cerebral Venous Thrombosis

In the majority of cases, cerebral venous thrombosis (CVT) naturally takes a benign course, but in a subgroup of patients, large hemorrhagic venous infarctions and brain edema occur, eventually leading to mass effect and intracranial hypertension.[145] These patients may be candidates for more aggressive interventions. In the few reports on craniectomy in the context of CVT, favorable outcomes were reported for most cases especially if treatment was started early before signs of herniation developed.[146-148] This is in line with data from a multinational registry of patients with acute cerebral venous thrombosis and impending herniation. Decompressive surgery was lifesaving and resulted in favorable functional outcome in most cases, even in a third of patients with bilateral fixed pupils before surgery.[149] However, the registry was retrospective and thus prone to selection and recall bias while case reports are prone to a severe publication bias, and cases with unfavorable outcomes are less likely to be reported. What can be concluded from the available data is that decompressive surgery may be considered in refractory intracranial hypertension in otherwise clinically desperate situations (see Table 76-1).

Conclusions for Clinical Practice

The evidence tells us the effect of decompressive craniectomy with fair clarity and consistency, but it does not tell us what to do in individual cases. The operation substantially reduces the risk of death after strokes with raised ICP and those saved from death survive with significant disability. Effects on outcomes in the mRS 1–3 range were not significant and are at best small. The decision whether to use the treatment should be informed by this evidence, but made on a case-by-case basis respecting the patient's personal, social and religious context. This summarizes the best evidenced situation of malignant middle cerebral territory infarction. There are three areas with material differences from this.

Posterior Fossa Infarction or Hemorrhage. In this case drainage of hydrocephalus and/or posterior fossa decompression has a similar effect on mortality but with more chance of a recovery in the mRS 1–3 range. The indication for surgery is consequently stronger, equipoise is rarer and the randomized evidence base will probably always be weaker.

Age over 60. In this case decompression has a similar effect on mortality, but with worse disability in survivors with a greater chance of mRS 5. The indication is, therefore, weaker.

More than 48 Hours from Stroke Onset. Early death removes the worst-affected cases from this group. Survival is generally better because of this and the effect of decompression on mortality consequently less. The indication is weaker, as is the evidence base.

REFERENCES

1. Baethmann A, Oettinger W, Rothenfusser W, et al. Brain edema factors: Current state with particular reference to plasma constituents and glutamate. Adv Neurol 1980;28:171–95.
2. Rosenberg GA, Yang Y. Vasogenic edema due to tight junction disruption by matrix metalloproteinases in cerebral ischemia. Neurosurg Focus 2007;22:E4.
3. Liang D, Bhatta S, Gerzanich V, et al. Cytotoxic edema: Mechanisms of pathological cell swelling. Neurosurg Focus 2007;22:E2.
4. Kawamata T, Mori T, Sato S, et al. Tissue hyperosmolality and brain edema in cerebral contusion. Neurosurg Focus 2007;22:E5.
5. Hacke W, Schwab S, Horn M, et al. "Malignant" middle cerebral artery territory infarction: Clinical course and prognostic signs. Arch Neurol 1996;53:309–15.
6. Silver FL, Norris JW, Lewis AJ, et al. Early mortality following stroke: A prospective review. Stroke 1984;15:492–6.
7. Shaw CM, Alvord EC, Berry RG. Swelling of the brain following ischemic infarction with arterial occlusion. Arch Neurol 1959;1: 161–77.
8. Frank JI. Large hemispheric infarction, deterioration, and intracranial pressure. Neurology 1995;45:1286–90.
9. Ropper AH, Shafran B. Brain edema after stroke. Clinical syndrome and intracranial pressure. Arch Neurol 1984;41:26–9.
10. Bounds JV, Wiebers DO, Whisnant JP, et al. Mechanisms and timing of deaths from cerebral infarction. Stroke 1981;12: 474–7.
11. Berrouschot J, Sterker M, Bettin S, et al. Mortality of space-occupying ("malignant") middle cerebral artery infarction under conservative intensive care. Intensive Care Med 1998;24:620–3.
12. Kasner SE, Demchuk AM, Berrouschot J, et al. Predictors of fatal brain edema in massive hemispheric ischemic stroke. Stroke 2001;32:2117–23.
13. Hofmeijer J, van der Worp HB, Kappelle LJ. Treatment of space-occupying cerebral infarction. Crit Care Med 2003;31:617–25.

14. Bardutzky J, Schwab S. Antiedema therapy in ischemic stroke. Stroke 2008;38:3084–94.
15. Bereczki D, Liu M, Prado GF, et al. Cochrane report: A systematic review of mannitol therapy for acute ischemic stroke and cerebral parenchymal hemorrhage. Stroke 2000;31:2719–22.
16. Muizelaar JP, Marmarou A, Ward JD, et al. Adverse effects of prolonged hyperventilation in patients with severe head injury: A randomized clinical trial. J Neurosurg 1991;75:731–9.
17. Stringer WA, Hasso AN, Thompson JR, et al. Hyperventilation-induced cerebral ischemia in patients with acute brain lesions: Demonstration by xenon-enhanced CT. AJNR Am J Neuroradiol 1993;14:475–84.
18. Schwab S, Spranger M, Schwarz S, et al. Barbiturate coma in severe hemispheric stroke: Useful or obsolete? Neurology 1997;48:1608–13.
19. Kaufmann AM, Cardoso ER. Aggravation of vasogenic cerebral edema by multiple-dose mannitol. J Neurosurg 1992;77:584–9.
20. Juttler E, Schellinger PD, Aschoff A, et al. Clinical review: Therapy for refractory intracranial hypertension in ischaemic stroke. Crit Care 2007;11:231.
21. Poca MA, Benejam B, Sahuquillo J, et al. Monitoring intracranial pressure in patients with malignant middle cerebral artery infarction: is it useful? J Neurosurg 2010;112:648–57.
22. Schwab S, Schwarz S, Spranger M, et al. Moderate hypothermia in the treatment of patients with severe middle cerebral artery infarction. Stroke 1998;29:2461–6.
23. Yoo DS, Kim DS, Cho KS, et al. Ventricular pressure monitoring during bilateral decompression with dural expansion. J Neurosurg 1999;91:953–9.
24. Jaeger M, Soehle M, Meixensberger J. Improvement of brain tissue oxygen and intracranial pressure during and after surgical decompression for diffuse brain oedema and space occupying infarction. Acta Neurochir Suppl 2005;95:117–18.
25. Mitchell P, Gregson BA, Piper I, et al. Blood pressure in head-injured patients. J Neurol Neurosurg Psychiatry 2007;78: 399–402.
26. Krieger DW, Demchuk AM, Kasner SE, et al. Early clinical and radiological predictors of fatal brain swelling in ischemic stroke. Stroke 1999;30:287–92.
27. Hofmeijer J, Kappelle LJ, Algra A, et al. Surgical decompression for space-occupying cerebral infarction (the Hemicraniectomy After Middle Cerebral Artery infarction with Life-threatening Edema Trial [HAMLET]): A multicentre, open, randomised trial. Lancet Neurol 2009;8:326–33.
28. Juttler E, Schwab S, Schmiedek P, et al. Decompressive Surgery for the Treatment of Malignant Infarction of the Middle Cerebral Artery (DESTINY): A randomized, controlled trial. Stroke 2007;38:2518–25.
29. Vahedi K, Vicaut E, Mateo J, et al. Sequential-design, multicenter, randomized, controlled trial of early decompressive craniectomy in malignant middle cerebral artery infarction (DECIMAL Trial). Stroke 2007;38:2506–17.
30. Barber PA, Demchuk AM, Zhang J, et al. Computed tomographic parameters predicting fatal outcome in large middle cerebral artery infarction. Cerebrovasc Dis 2003;16:230–5.
31. Hofmeijer J, Algra A, Kapelle LJ, et al. Predictors of life-threatening brain edema in middle cerebral artery infarction. Cerebrovasc Dis 2008;25:176–84.
32. Oppenheim C, Samson Y, Manaï R, et al. Prediction of malignant middle cerebral artery infarction by diffusion-weighted imaging. Stroke 2000;31:2175–81.
33. Thomalla G, Kucinski T, Schoder V, et al. Prediction of malignant middle cerebral artery infarction by early perfusion- and diffusion-weighted magnetic resonance imaging. Stroke 2003;34: 1892–9.
34. Von Kummer R, Meyding-Lamade U, Forsting M, et al. Sensitivity and prognostic value of early CT in occlusion of the middle cerebral artery trunk. AJNR Am J Neuroradiol 1994;15:9–15.
35. Lee SJ, Lee KH, Na DG. Multiphasic helical computed tomography predicts subsequent development of severe brain oedema in acute ischemic stroke. Arch Neurol 2004;61:505–9.
36. Ryoo JW, Na DG, Kim SS, et al. Malignant middle cerebral artery infarction in hyperacute ischemic stroke: Evaluation with multiphasic perfusion computed tomography maps. J Comput Assist Tomogr 2004;28:55–62.
37. Dittrich R, Kloska SP, Fischer T, et al. Accuracy of perfusion-CT in predicting malignant middle cerebral artery brain infarction. J Neurol 2008;255:896–902.
38. Thomalla G, Hartmann F, Juettler E, et al. Prediction of malignant middle cerebral artery infarction by magnetic resonance imaging within 6 hours of symptom onset: A prospective multicenter observational study. Ann Neurol 2010;68:435–45.
39. Berrouschot J, Barthel H, von Kummer R. 99m technetium-ethyl-cysteinate-dimer single-photon emission CT can predict fatal ischemic brain edema. Stroke 1998;29:2556–62.
40. Lampl Y, Sadeh M, Lorberboym M. Prospective evaluation of malignant middle cerebral artery infarction with blood-brain barrier imaging using Tc-99m DTPA SPECT. Brain Res 2006;1113: 194–9.
41. Limburg M, van Royen EA, Hijdra A, et al. Single-photon emission computed tomography and early death in acute ischemic stroke. Stroke 1990;21:1150–5.
42. Dohmen C, Bosche B, Graf R, et al. Prediction of malignant course in MCA infarction by PET and microdialysis. Stroke 2003;34:2152–8.
43. Bosche B, Dohmen C, Graf R, et al. Extracellular concentrations of non-transmitter amino acids in peri-infarct tissue of patients predict malignant middle cerebral artery infarction. Stroke 2003;34:2908–13.
44. Heiss WD, Dohmen C, Sobesky J, et al. Identification of malignant brain edema after hemispheric stroke by PET-imaging and microdialysis. Acta Neurochir Suppl 2003;86:237–40.
45. Dohmen C, Bosche B, Graf R, et al. Identification and clinical impact of impaired cerebrovascular autoregulation in patients with malignant middle cerebral artery infarction. Stroke 2007;38: 56–61.
46. Forsting M, Reith W, Schabitz WR, et al. Decompressive craniectomy for cerebral infarction. An experimental study in rats. Stroke 1995;26:259–64.
47. Doerfler A, Engelhorn T, Heiland S, et al. Perfusion- and diffusion-weighted magnetic resonance imaging for monitoring decompressive craniectomy in animals with experimental hemispheric stroke. J Neurosurg 2002;96:933–40.
48. Doerfler A, Forsting M, Reith W, et al. Decompressive craniectomy in a rat model of "malignant" cerebral hemispheric stroke: Experimental support for an aggressive therapeutic approach. J Neurosurg 1996;85:853–9.
49. Engelhorn T, Doerfler A, Kastrup A, et al. Decompressive craniectomy, reperfusion, or a combination for early treatment of acute "malignant" cerebral hemispheric stroke in rats: Potential mechanisms studied by MRI. Stroke 1999;30:1456–63.
50. Engelhorn T, von Kummer R, Reith W, et al. What is effective in malignant middle cerebral artery infarction: Reperfusion, craniectomy, or both? An experimental study in rats. Stroke 2002;33:617–22.
51. Walberer M, Ritschel N, Nedelmann M, et al. Aggravation of infarct formation by brain swelling in a large territorial stroke: A target for neuroprotection? J Neurosurg 2008;109:287–93.
52. Schwab S, Steiner T, Aschoff A, et al. Early hemicraniectomy in patients with complete middle cerebral artery infarction. Stroke 1998;29:1888–93.
53. Mori K, Ishimaru S, Maeda M. Unco-parahippocampectomy for direct surgical treatment of downward transtentorial herniation. Acta Neurochir (Wien) 1998;140:1239–44.
54. Unterberg A, Juettler E. The role of surgery in ischemic stroke: Decompressive surgery. Curr Opin Crit Care 2007;13:175–9.
55. Hutchinson P, Timofeev I, Kirkpatrick P. Surgery for brain edema. Neurosurg Focus 2007;22:E14.
56. Rieke K, Schwab S, Krieger D, et al. Decompressive surgery in space-occupying hemispheric infarction: Results of an open, prospective trial. Crit Care Med 1995;23:1576–87.
57. Waziri A, Fusco D, Mayer SA, et al. Postoperative hydrocephalus in patients undergoing decompressive hemicraniectomy for ischemic or hemorrhagic stroke. Neurosurgery 2007;61: 489–93.
58. Uhl E, Kreth FW, Elias B, et al. Outcome and prognostic factors of hemicraniectomy for space occupying cerebral infarction. J Neurol Neurosurg Psychiatry 2004;75:270–4.
59. Wagner S, Schnippering H, Aschoff A, et al. Suboptimum hemicraniectomy as a cause of additional cerebral lesions in

patients with malignant infarction of the middle cerebral artery. J Neurosurg 2001;94:693–6.
60. Neugebauer H, Witsch J, Zweckberger K, et al. Space-occupying cerebellar infarction: complications, treatment, and outcome. Neurosurg Focus 2013;34:E8.
61. Broughton E, Pobereskin L, Whitfield PC. Seven years of cranioplasty in a regional neurosurgical centre. Br J Neurosurg 2014; 28:34–9.
62. Coulter IC, Pesic-Smith JD, Cato-Addison WB, et al. Routine but risky: A multi-centre analysis of the outcomes of cranioplasty in the Northeast of England. Acta Neurochir 2014;156:1361–8.
63. Gooch MR, Gin GE, Kenning TJ, et al. Complications of cranioplasty following decompressive craniectomy: analysis of 62 cases. Neurosurg Focus 2009;26:E9.
64. Lee L, Ker J, Quah BL, et al. A retrospective analysis and review of an institution's experience with the complications of cranioplasty. Br J Neurosurg 2013;27:629–35.
65. Walcott BP, Kwon CS, Sheth SA, et al. Predictors of cranioplasty complications in stroke and trauma patients Clinical article. J Neurosurg 2013;118:757–62.
66. Greco T. Le thrombosi posttraumatiche della carotide. Arch Ital Chir 1935;39:757–84.
67. Juttler E, Kohrmann M, Aschoff A, et al. Hemicraniectomy for space-occupying supratentorial ischemic stroke. Future Neurol 2008;3:251–64.
68. Frank JI, Krieger D, Chyatte D. Hemicraniectomy and durotomy upon deterioration from massive hemispheric infarction: A proposed multicenter, prospective, randomized study. Stroke 1999; 30:243.
69. Frank JI, Schumm LP, Wroblewski K, et al. Hemicraniectomy and durotomy upon deterioration from infarction-related swelling trial: randomized pilot clinical trial. Stroke 2014;45:781–7.
70. Stroke Trials Registry. <www.strokecenter.org/trials>.
71. Vahedi K, Hofmeijer J, Juettler E, et al. Early decompressive surgery in malignant infarction of the middle cerebral artery: A pooled analysis of three randomised controlled trials. Lancet Neurol 2007;6:215–22.
72. Wijdicks EF, Sheth KN, Carter BS, et al. Recommendations for the management of cerebral and cerebellar infarction with swelling: a statement for healthcare professionals from the American Heart Association/American Stroke Association. Stroke 2014;45: 1222–38.
73. Morgenstern LB, Hemphill JC 3rd, Anderson C, et al. Guidelines for the management of spontaneous intracerebral hemorrhage: a guideline for healthcare professionals from the American Heart Association/American Stroke Association. Stroke 2010;41: 2108–29.
74. Mitchell P, Gregson BA, Crossman J, et al. Reassessment of the HAMLET study. Lancet Neurol 2009;8:602–3.
75. Jüttler E, Unterberg A, Woitzik J, et al. Hemicraniectomy in older patients with extensive middle-cerebral-artery stroke. N Engl J Med 2014;370:1091–100.
76. Balzer B, Stober T, Huber G, et al. Space-occupying cerebral infarct. Nervenarzt 1987;58:689–91.
77. Erban P, Woertgen C, Luerding R. Long-term outcome after hemicraniectomy for space occupying right hemispheric MCA infarction. Clin Neurol Neurosurg 2006;108:384–7.
78. Foerch C, Lang JM, Krause J, et al. Functional impairment, disability, and quality of life outcome after decompressive hemicraniectomy in malignant middle cerebral artery infarction. J Neurosurg 2004;101:248–54.
79. Gupta R, Connolly ES, Mayer S, et al. Hemicraniectomy for massive middle cerebral artery territory infarction: A systematic review. Stroke 2004;35:539–43.
80. Kastrau F, Wolter M, Huber W, et al. Recovery from aphasia after hemicraniectomy for infarction of the speech-dominant hemisphere. Stroke 2005;36:825–9.
81. Pillai A, Menon SK, Kumar S. Decompressive hemicraniectomy in malignant middle cerebral artery infarction: An analysis of long-term outcome and factors in patient selection. J Neurosurg 2007;106:59–65.
82. Holtkamp M, Buchheim K, Unterberg A, et al. Hemicraniectomy in elderly patients with space occupying media infarction: Improved survival but poor functional outcome. J Neurol Neurosurg Psychiatry 2001;70:226–8.
83. Leonhardt G, Wilhelm H, Doerfler A, et al. Clinical outcome and neuropsychological deficits after right decompressive hemicraniectomy in MCA infarction. J Neurol 2002;249:1433–40.
84. Maramattom BV, Bahn MM, Wijdicks EMF. Which patient fares worse after early deterioration due to swelling from hemispheric stroke? Neurology 2004;63:2142–5.
85. Yao Y, Liu W, Yang X, et al. Is decompressive craniectomy for malignant middle cerebral artery territory infarction of any benefit for elderly patients? Surg Neurol 2005;64:165–9.
86. Kilincer C, Asil T, Utku U, et al. Factors affecting the outcome of decompressive craniectomy for large hemispheric infarctions: A prospective cohort study. Acta Neurochir 2005;147: 587–94.
87. Harscher S, Reichart R, Terborg C, et al. Outcome after decompressive craniectomy in patients with severe ischemic stroke. Acta Neurochir (Wien) 2006;148:31–7.
88. Rabinstein AA, Mueller-Kronast N, Maramattom BV, et al. Factors predicting prognosis after decompressive hemicraniectomy for hemispheric infarction. Neurology 2006;67:891–3.
89. Chen CC, Cho DY, Tsai SC. Outcome of and prognostic factors for decompressive hemicraniectomy in malignant middle cerebral artery infarction. J Clin Neurosci 2007;14:317–21.
90. Puetz V, Campos CR, Eliasziw M, et al. Assessing the benefits of hemicraniectomy: What is a favourable outcome? Lancet Neurol 2007;6:580.
91. Vahedi K, Hofmeijer J, Juettler E, et al. Assessing the benefits of hemicraniectomy: What is a favourable outcome? Authors' reply. Lancet Neurol 2007;6:580–1.
92. Rahme R, Zuccarello M, Kleindorfer D, et al. Decompressive hemicraniectomy for malignant middle cerebral artery territory infarction: is life worth living? J Neurosurg 2012;117:749–54.
93. Kelly AG, Holloway RG. Health state preferences and decision-making after malignant middle cerebral artery infarctions. Neurology 2010;75:682–7.
94. Vahedi K, Benoist L, Kurtz A, et al. Quality of life after decompressive craniectomy for malignant middle cerebral artery infarction. J Neurol Neurosurg Psychiatry 2005;76:1181–2.
95. Walz B, Zimmermann C, Böttger S, et al. Prognosis of patients after hemicraniectomy in malignant middle cerebral artery infarction. J Neurol 2002;249:1183–90.
96. Woertgen C, Erban P, Rothoerl RD, et al. Quality of life after decompressive craniectomy in patients suffering from supratentorial brain ischemia. Acta Neurochir (Wien) 2004;146:691–5.
97. Curry WT Jr, Sethi MK, Ogilvy CS, et al. Factors associated with outcome after hemicraniectomy for large middle cerebral artery territory infarction. Neurosurgery 2005;56:681–92.
98. De Haan RJ, Limburg M, Van der Meulen JH. Quality of life after stroke: Impact of stroke type and lesion location. Stroke 1995; 26:402–8.
99. Cho DY, Chen TC, Lee HC. Ultra-early decompressive craniectomy for malignant middle cerebral artery infarction. Surg Neurol 2005;60:227–32.
100. Hornig CR, Rust DS, Busse O, et al. Space-occupying cerebellar infarction: Clinical course and prognosis. Stroke 1994;25: 372–4.
101. Kase CS, Norrving B, Levine SR, et al. Cerebellar infarction. Clinical and anatomic observation in 66 cases. Stroke 1993;24: 76–83.
102. Tohgi H, Takahashi S, Chiba K, et al. Clinical and neuroimaging analysis in 293 patients – Tohoku Cerebellum Infarction Study Group. Stroke 1993;24:1697–701.
103. Auer LM, Auer TH, Sayama I. Indications for surgical treatment of cerebellar haemorrhage and infarction. Acta Neurochir 1986;79:74–9.
104. Baldauf J, Oertel J, Gaab MR, et al. Endoscopic third ventriculostomy for occlusive hydrocephalus caused by cerebellar infarction. Neurosurgery 2006;59:539–44.
105. Busse O, Laun A. Therapy of space-occupying cerebellar infarction. Akt Neurol 1988;15:6–8.
106. Chen HJ, Lee TC, Wei CP. Treatment of cerebellar infarction by decompressive suboccipital craniectomy. Stroke 1992;23: 957–61.
107. Koh MG, Phan TG, Atkinson JLD, et al. Neuroimaging in deteriorating patients with cerebellar infarcts and mass effect. Stroke 2000;31:2062–7.

108. Macdonell RAL, Kalnins RM, Donnan GA. Cerebellar infarction: Natural history, prognosis, and pathology. Stroke 1987;18: 849–55.
109. Heros RC. Surgical treatment of cerebellar infarction. Stroke 1992;23:937–8.
110. Raco A, Caroli E, Isidori A, et al. Management of acute cerebellar infarction: One institution's experience. Neurosurgery 2003;53: 1061–6.
111. Shenkin HA, Zavala M. Cerebellar strokes: Mortality, surgical indications and results of ventricular drainage. Lancet 1982;21: 429–32.
112. Langmayr JJ, Buchberger W, Reindl H. Cerebellar hemorrhage and cerebellar infarct: Retrospective study of 125 cases. Wien Med Wochenschr 1993;143:131–3.
113. Busse O, Laun A, Agnoli L. Obstructive hydrocephalus in cerebellar infarcts. Fortschr Neurol Psychiatr 1984;52:164–71.
114. Mathew P, Teasdale G, Bannan A, et al. Neurosurgical management of cerebellar haematoma and infarct. J Neurol Neurosurg Psychiatry 1995;59:287–92.
115. Jauss M, Krieger D, Hornig CR, et al. Surgical and medical management of patients with massive cerebellar infarctions: Results of the German-Austrian Cerebellar Infarction Study. J Neurol 1999;246:257–64.
116. Cioffi FA, Bernini FP, Punzo A. Surgical management of acute cerebellar infarction. Acta Neurochir (Wien) 1985;74: 105–12.
117. Ho SU, Kim KS, Berenberg RA, et al. Cerebellar infarction: A clinical and CT study. Surg Neurol 1981;16:350–2.
118. Jones HR, Millikan CH, Sandok BA. Temporal profile (clinical course) of acute vertebrobasilar system cerebral infarction. Stroke 1980;11:173–7.
119. Neugebauer H, Jüttler E. Hemicraniectomy for malignant middle cerebral artery infarction: current status and future directions. Int J Stroke 2013;9:460–7.
120. Jüttler E, Schweickert S, Ringleb PA, et al. Long-term outcome after surgical treatment for space-occupying cerebellar infarction: experience in 56 patients. Stroke 2009;40:3060–6.
121. Pfefferkorn T, Eppinger U, Linn J, et al. Long-term outcome after suboccipital decompressive craniectomy for malignant cerebellar infarction. Stroke 2009;40:3045–50.
122. Kobayashi S, Sato A, Kageyama Y, et al. Treatment of hypertensive cerebellar hemorrhage: Surgical or conservative management? Neurosurgery 1994;34:246–51.
123. Morioka J, Fujii M, Kato S, et al. Surgery for spontaneous intracerebral hemorrhage has greater remedial value than conservative therapy. Surg Neurol 2006;65:67–73.
124. Little JR, Tubman DE, Ethier R. Cerebellar hemorrhage in adults. Diagnosis by computerized tomography. J Neurosurg 1978;48: 575–9.
125. Luparello V, Canavero S. Treatment of hypertensive cerebellar hemorrhage: Surgical or conservative management? Neurosurgery 1995;37:552–3.
126. Mayer SA, Rincon F. Treatment of intracerebral haemorrhage. Lancet Neurol 2005;4:662–72.
127. Horiuchi T, Tanaka Y, Hongo K, et al. Characteristics of distal posterior inferior cerebellar artery aneurysm. Neurosurgery 2003;53:589–96.
128. Broderick J, Connolly S, Feldmann E, et al. Guidelines for the management of spontaneous intracerebral hemorrhage in adults: 2007 update: A guideline from the American Heart Association/American Stroke Association Stroke Council, High Blood Pressure Research Council, and the Quality of Care and Outcomes in Research Interdisciplinary Working Group. Stroke 2007;38:2001–23.
129. Yamamoto T, Nakao Y, Mori K, et al. Endoscopic hematoma evacuation for hypertensive cerebellar hemorrhage. Minim Invasive Neurosurg 2006;49:173–8.
130. Witsch J, Neugebauer H, Zweckberger K, et al. Primary cerebellar haemorrhage: complications, treatment and outcome. Clin Neurol Neurosurg 2013;115:863–9.
131. Schirmer CM, Hoyt DA, Malek AM. Decompressive hemicraniectomy for the treatment of intractable intracranial hypertension after aneurysmal subarachnoid hemorrhage. Stroke 2007;38: 987–92.
132. Smith ER, Carter BS, Ogilvy CS. Proposed use of prophylactic decompressive craniectomy in poor-grade aneurysmal subarachnoid hemorrhage patients presenting with associated large sylvian hematomas. Neurosurgery 2002;51:117–24.
133. Mitka M. Hemicraniectomy improves outcomes for patients with ruptured brain aneurysms. JAMA 2001;286:2084.
134. D'Ambrosio AL, Sughrue ME, Yorgason JG, et al. Decompressive hemicraniectomy for poor-grade aneurysmal subarachnoid hemorrhage patients with associated intracerebral hemorrhage: Clinical outcome and quality of life assessment. Neurosurgery 2005;56:12–19.
135. Buschmann U, Yonekawa Y, Fortunati M, et al. Decompressive hemicraniectomy in patients with subarachnoid hemorrhage and intractable intracranial hypertension. Acta Neurochir (Wien) 2007;149:59–65.
136. Mendelow AD, Gregson BA, Fernandes HM, et al. Early surgery versus initial conservative treatment in patients with spontaneous supratentorial intracerebral haematomas in the International Surgical Trial in Intracerebral Haemorrhage (STICH): A randomised trial. Lancet 2005;365:387–97.
137. Mendelow AD, Gregson BA, Rowan EN, et al. Early surgery versus initial conservative treatment in patients with spontaneous supratentorial lobar intracerebral haematomas (STICH II): a randomised trial. Lancet 2013;382:397–408.
138. Hoff JT, Xi G. Brain edema from intracerebral hemorrhage. Acta Neurochir Suppl 2003;86:11–15.
139. Zazulia AR, Diringer MN, Derdeyn CP, et al. Progression of mass effect after intracerebral hemorrhage. Stroke 1999;30:1167–73.
140. Ropper AH. Lateral displacement of the brain and level of consciousness in patients with an acute hemispheral mass. N Engl J Med 1986;314:953–8.
141. Strbian D, Tatlisumak T, Ramadan UA, et al. Mast cell blocking reduces brain edema and hematoma volume and improves outcome after experimental intracerebral hemorrhage. J Cereb Blood Flow Metab 2007;27:795–802.
142. Gebel JM Jr, Jauch EC, Brott TG, et al. Relative edema volume is a predictor of outcome in patients with hyperacute spontaneous intracerebral hemorrhage. Stroke 2002;33:2636–41.
143. Murthy JM, Chowdary GV, Murthy TV, et al. Decompressive craniectomy with clot evacuation in large hemispheric hypertensive intracerebral hemorrhage. Neurocrit Care 2005;2:258–62.
144. Maira G, Anile C, Colosimo C, et al. Surgical treatment of primary supratentorial intracerebral hemorrhage in stuporous and comatose patients. Neurol Res 2002;24:54–60.
145. Ferro JM, Canhao P, Stam J, et al. Prognosis of cerebral vein and dural sinus thrombosis: Results of the International Study on Cerebral Vein and Dural Sinus Thrombosis (ISCVT). Stroke 2004;35:664–70.
146. Stefini R, Latronico N, Cornali C, et al. Emergent decompressive craniectomy in patients with fixed dilated pupils due to cerebral venous and dural sinus thrombosis: Report of three cases. Neurosurgery 1999;45:626–9.
147. Coutinho JM, Majoie CB, Coert BA, et al. Decompressive hemicraniectomy in cerebral sinus thrombosis. Consecutive case series and review of the literature. Stroke 2009;40:2233–5.
148. Keller E, Pangalu A, Fandino J, et al. Decompressive craniectomy in severe cerebral venous and dural sinus thrombosis. Acta Neurochir Suppl 2005;94:177–83.
149. Ferro JM, Crassard I, Coutinho JM, et al. Decompressive surgery in cerebrovenous thrombosis: a multicenter registry and a systematic review of individual patient data. Stroke 2011;42: 2825–31.

Index

Page numbers followed by "*f*" indicate figures, "*t*" indicate tables, and "*b*" indicate boxes.

C

D

F

G

J

K

M

O

P

W

X

Y

Z